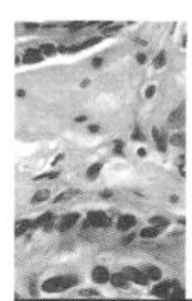

UNIT IX
Genital and Reproductive Function, 770

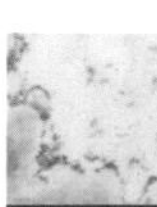

UNIT X
Gastrointestinal Function, 858

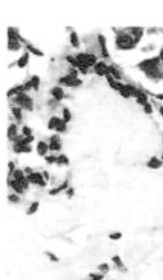

UNIT XI
Endocrine Function, Metabolism, and Nutrition, 962

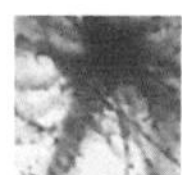

UNIT XII
Neural Function, 1044

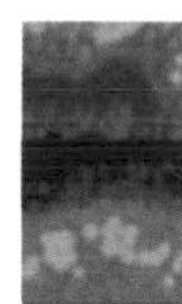

UNIT XIII
Neuropsychological Function, 1190

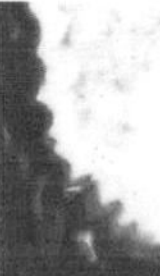

UNIT XIV
Musculoskeletal Support and Movement, 1228

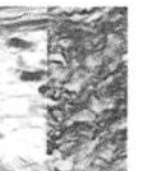

UNIT XV
Integumentary System, 1292

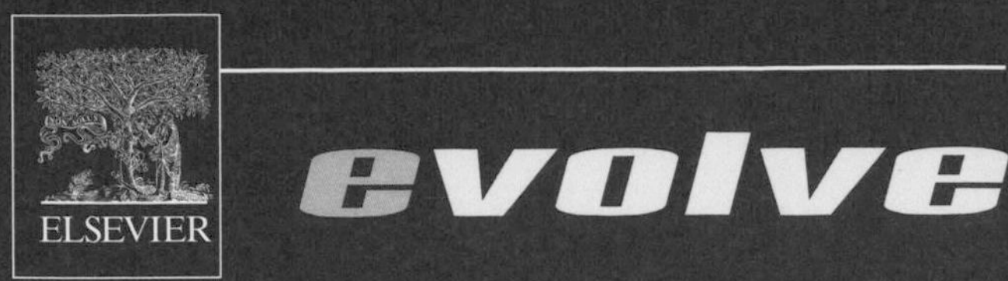

To access your Student Resources, visit the web address below:

http://evolve.elsevier.com/Copstead

- **Case Studies**
  Patient case studies that initiate the critical thinking process will assist you in the application of pathophysiologic concepts in clinical situations.
- **Disease Profiles**
  An outlined, at-a-glance review provides you with a quick study of clinically significant conditions.
- **WebLinks**
  This useful resource links you to hundreds of websites carefully chosen to supplement the content of your textbook. The WebLinks are regularly updated, with new ones added as they develop.

PATHOPHYSIOLOGY

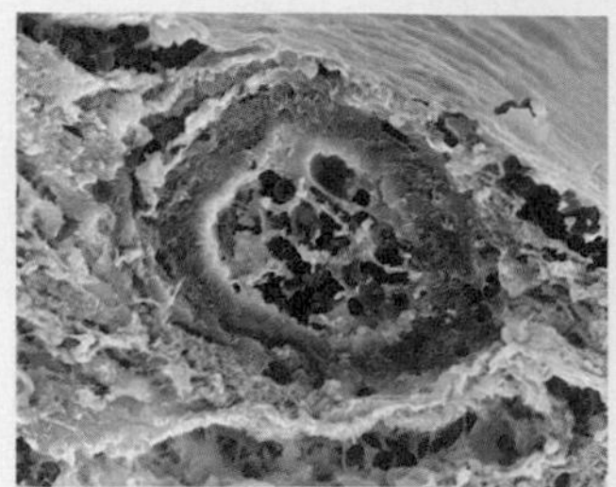

Blood Vessel by Dee Breger. Blood vessels are the conduits of the body's blood delivery system. This dynamic color-enhanced scanning electron micrograph details the interior of a blood vessel showing red blood cells (erythrocytes) moving through the vessel.

Dee Breger is the Director of Microscopy at Drexel University, Philadelphia, Pa.

PATHOPHYSIOLOGY

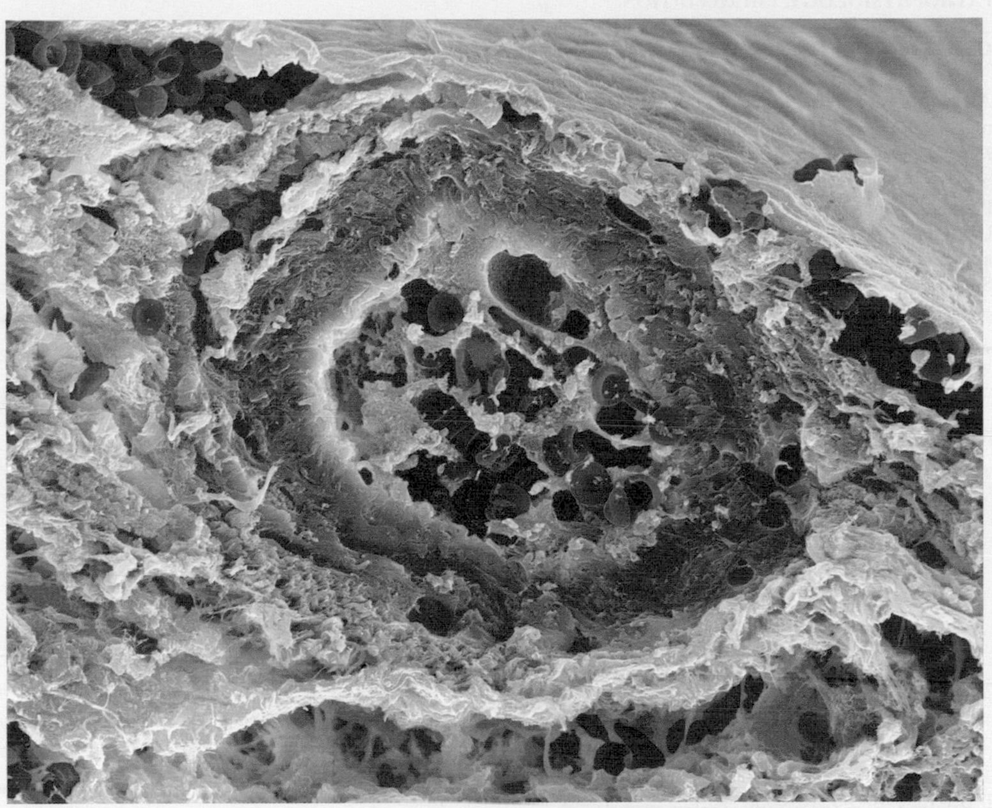

THIRD EDITION

LEE-ELLEN C. COPSTEAD, PhD, RN
Associate Dean for Education and Research
Western Campus
University of Wisconsin–Madison School of Nursing
Madison, Wisconsin
and
Administrative Director
Nursing Education and Research
Gundersen Lutheran Medical Foundation
La Crosse, Wisconsin

JACQUELYN L. BANASIK, PhD, ARNP
Associate Professor
WSU Intercollegiate College of Nursing
Washington State University
Spokane, Washington

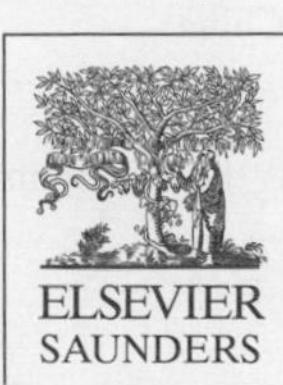

ELSEVIER
SAUNDERS

ELSEVIER
SAUNDERS

11830 Westline Industrial Drive
St. Louis, Missouri 63146

PATHOPHYSIOLOGY, THIRD EDITION

NOTICE

Pathophysiology is an ever-changing field. Standard safety precautions must be followed, but as new research and clinical experience broaden our knowledge, changes in treatment and drug therapy may become necessary or appropriate. Readers are advised to check the most current product information provided by the manufacturer of each drug to be administered to verify the recommended dose, the method and duration of administration, and contraindications. It is the responsibility of the licensed prescriber, relying on experience and knowledge of the patient, to determine dosages and the best treatment for each individual patient. Neither the publisher nor the author assumes any liability for any injury and/or damage to persons or property arising from this publication.

ISBN-13: 978–0–7216–0338–4
ISBN-10: 0–7216–0338–6

Executive Publisher: Darlene Como
Managing Editor: Brian Dennison
Developmental Editor: Barbara Watts
Editorial Assistant: Katherine V. Judge
Publishing Services Manager: Deborah L. Vogel
Project Manager: Deon Lee
Design Manager: Teresa McBryan

Printed in China

Last digit is the print number: 9 8 7 6 5 4 3

Dedicated to the memory of Michael J. Kirkhorn. He left an indelible impression on my life—as a spouse, author, teacher, and friend. Dedicated to my young daughter, Amelia Charlotte, for her spirit and creativity. Also to Dean Katharyn May, DNSc, FAAN, University of Wisconsin–Madison, School of Nursing, and Arthur J. Ross III, MD, MBA, Dean, Chicago Medical School—forces in my life who have inspired excellence as outstanding leaders and teachers.

Lee-Ellen C. Copstead

To friends and family for their interest and encouragement.

To Ray, Brent, and Brianne Banasik for their patience and love.

To researchers, teachers, and students for their knowledge and inspiration.

Jacquelyn L. Banasik

CONTRIBUTORS

Arnold A. Asp, MD
Endocrinologist
Gundersen Lutheran Medical Center
La Crosse, Wisconsin

Donna W. Bailey, MN, PhDc
School of Nursing
University of North Carolina
Chapel Hill, North Carolina

Jacquelyn L. Banasik, PhD, ARNP
Associate Professor
WSU Intercollegiate College of Nursing
Washington State University
Spokane, Washington

Carolyn Spence Cagle, PhD, RNC
Associate Professor
Harris College of Nursing
Texas Christian University
Forth Worth, Texas

Robert H. Caplan, MD
Endocrinologist
Gundersen Lutheran Medical Center
La Crosse, Wisconsin

Katherina P. Choka, RN, MSN, ARNP, FNP-C
Clinical Assistant Professor
WSU Intercollegiate College of Nursing
Washington State University
Spokane, Washington

Lee-Ellen C. Copstead, PhD, RN
Associate Dean for Education and Research
Western Campus
University of Wisconsin–Madison School of Nursing
Madison, Wisconsin
and
Administrative Director
Nursing Education and Research
Gundersen Lutheran Medical Foundation
La Crosse, Wisconsin

Cynthia Fryhling Corbett, PhD, RN
Associate Professor
WSU Intercollegiate College of Nursing
Washington State University
Spokane, Washington

Carol L. Danning, MD
Rheumatology
Gundersen Lutheran Medical Center
La Crosse, Wisconsin

Roberta J. Emerson, PhD, CCRN
Associate Professor
WSU Intercollegiate College of Nursing
Washington State University
Spokane, Washington

Marvin J. Van Every, MD
Urology
Gundersen Lutheran Medical Center
La Crosse, Wisconsin

Linda Felver, PhD, RN
Associate Professor
School of Nursing
Oregon Health & Science University
Portland, Oregon

Jane M. Georges, PhD, RN
Associate Professor
Hahn School of Nursing and Health Science
University of San Diego
San Diego, California

Fadi Ghandour, MD, FACP
Nephrology
Gundersen Lutheran Medical Center
La Crosse, Wisconsin

Ronald S. Go, MD
Section of Hematology
Department of Internal Medicine
Gundersen Lutheran Medical Center
La Crosse, Wisconsin

Timothy A. Harbst, MD
Chairman, Department of Physical Medicine and Rehabilitation
Gundersen Clinic
Gundersen Lutheran Medical Center
La Crosse, Wisconsin

K. John Hartman, MD
General Surgery Resident
Gundersen Lutheran Medical Center
La Crosse, Wisconsin

Marie L. Kotter, PhD
Professor, Clinical Laboratory Science
Chair of Health Sciences Department
Weber State University
Ogden, Utah

Naomi Lungstrom, MN, RN, CCRN
Clinical Assistant Professor
WSU Intercollegiate College of Nursing
Washington State University
Spokane, Washington

David W. Metzler, MS, MD
Behavioral Medicine
Gundersen Lutheran Medical Center
La Crosse, Wisconsin

David Mikkelsen, MD
Spokane Urology
Spokane, Washington

Kurt K. Mueller, MD
Staff Physician, Department of Dermatology
Gundersen Lutheran Medical Center
La Crosse, Wisconsin
and
Mohs Surgery Fellow
Northwestern Skin Cancer Institute
Chicago, Illinois

Joni D. Nelsen-Marsh, MN, ARNP
Family Nurse Practitioner
South Hill Family Medicine
Spokane, Washington

Linda Denise Oakley, PhD, NP
University of Wisconsin–Madison
School of Nursing
Madison, Wisconsin

Susan G. Osguthorpe, MS, RN, CNA
Clinical Associate Professor
College of Nursing
University of Utah
and
Clinical Support Manager for Specialty Care
John E. Wahlen Department of Veterans Affairs Medical Center
Salt Lake City, Utah

Nirav Patel, MD, FACS
Chief, Division of Trauma
Gundersen Lutheran Medical Center
La Crosse, Wisconsin

Faith Young Peterson, BS, MS, FNP
Family Nurse Practitioner and Clinic Manager
Terry Reilly Health Services, Marsing Clinic
Marsing, Idaho

Mark Puhlman, RN, ARNP
Clinical Research Coordinator
Mechanical Heart Coordinator
Sacred Heart Coordinator
Spokane, Washington

Jeffrey S. Sartin, MD
Infectious Diseases
Gundersen Lutheran Medical Center
La Crosse, Wisconsin

Lorna Schumann, PhD, ARNP, APRN,BC, NP-C, FAANP, CCRN
Associate Professor
WSU Intercollegiate College of Nursing
Washington State University
Spokane, Washington
and
Staff Nurse, Intensive Care Unit/Cardiac Care Unit
Valley Hospital and Medical Center
Spokane, Washington
and
Group Health Northwest
Spokane, Washington

Paul D. Silva, MD
Reproductive Endocrinologist
Gundersen Lutheran Medical Center
La Crosse, Wisconsin

Gregory P. Thompson, MD
Pulmonary and Critical Care Medicine
Gundersen Lutheran Medical Center
La Crosse, Wisconsin

Peter A. Valen, MD
Chief, Section of Rheumatology
Gundersen Lutheran Medical Center
La Crosse, Wisconsin

Marvin J. Van Every
Staff Urologist, Gundersen Clinic
Gundersen Lutheran Medical Center
La Crosse, Wisconsin

Marc S. Williams, MD
Clinical Geneticist
Gundersen Lutheran Medical Center
La Crosse, Wisconsin

REVIEWERS

Chockchai Chareandee, MD, FASN
Nephrologist
Gundersen Lutheran Medical Center
La Crosse, Wisconsin

Katherina P. Choka, RN, MSN, ARNP, FNP-C
Clinical Assistant Professor
WSU Intercollegiate College of Nursing
Washington State University
Spokane, Washington

Marye Dorsey Kellermann, RN, MSN, CRNP, PhDc
Adult and Gerontological Nurse Practitioner
Associate Professor, Coppin State University FNP Program
and
President—Necessary NP Review of Educational Entities
Baltimore, Maryland

Bernadette M. Lombardi, RN, MSN, MA, MS, PhDc
Assistant Director
Memorial and Samaritan Hospital Schools of Nursing
Albany, New York

Leila McKinney, RN, BSN
Instructor of Health Sciences
Palm Harbor University High School
Center for Wellness and Medical Professions
Palm Harbor, Florida

Douglas W. Mitchell, RN, MSN
Clinical Nurse Educator
Paradise Valley Hospital
Phoenix, Arizona

Angela Starkweather, RN, PhD, CCRN, CNRN
Assistant Professor
WSU Intercollegiate College of Nursing
Washington State University
Spokane, Washington

Debra S. Wellman, RN, MSN, CAN
Clinical Assistant Professor
Indiana University School of Nursing–Bloomington
Bloomington, Indiana

Jonathan A. Zlabek, MD
Director, Vascular Medicine
Associate Program Director
Internal Medicine Residency
Gundersen Lutheran Medical Center
La Crosse, Wisconsin

PREFACE

The scientific basis of pathophysiology is rapidly expanding and becoming increasingly well understood at the genetic and cellular levels. Accelerated progress in human genetics has virtually transformed our understanding of the living world. To be clinically relevant and useful to health care students and professionals, a text must be able to synthesize a vast amount of knowledge about a multitude of individual structures, functions, and dysfunctions into overarching concepts that can be applied to individual diseases. In the third edition of *Pathophysiology,* attention has been given to the development of practical, student-centered learning aids that support learning and mastery of content. Discussions of advanced biochemistry and basic sciences have been simplified to make them easier to understand. This third edition has been updated extensively with sensitivity to the unique needs of today's students to better prepare them as practitioners in an ever-changing health care environment.

ORGANIZATION

Pathophysiology is a comprehensive text and reference that uses a systems approach to content, beginning with a thorough treatment of normal physiology, followed by pathophysiology and application of concepts to specific disorders. The text is organized into 15 units, each of which includes a particular system or group of interrelated body systems and the pertinent pathophysiology concepts and disorders.

Unit I (Chapters 1 and 2) sets the stage for understanding major elements of the pathophysiologic processes in individuals and population groups. The purpose of these chapters is to give students an appreciation for the complex nature of disease and illness, including sociocultural influences and the significant contributions of stress, adaptation, and coping. The unifying concepts of pathophysiologic processes—etiology, pathogenesis, clinical manifestations, and implications for treatment of disease—are explained.

Unit II (Chapters 3 through 7) addresses cellular mechanisms. Chapter 3 describes normal cells to give students an insight into how cells function, with an emphasis on cellular signaling and communication. Chapter 4 discusses cellular pathology and the processes of injury, apoptosis, aging, and death. Chapters 5 and 6 describe gene structure and function, development, and genetic and congenital disorders. Chapter 7 describes the cellular biology of tumor growth, focusing on the roles of proto-oncogenes and tumor suppressor genes. Revisions reflect new knowledge about apoptosis, genetics, and cancer biology

Unit III (Chapters 8 through 12) addresses key cellular defense mechanisms and the basic processes of infectious disease, inflammation, immunity, autoimmune disease, hypersensitivity, hematologic malignancies and HIV-AIDS. Unit III was extensively revised to reflect new knowledge about immune mechanisms, classification of hematologic malignancies, and therapy for HIV disease.

Unit IV (Chapters 13 through 16) includes content pertaining to the transport of oxygen in the circulation, hemostasis, vascular regulation of flow, blood pressure regulation, and the pathologies relevant to these functions.

Unit V (Chapters 17 through 20) includes concepts related to cardiac physiology and pathophysiology. Content has been extensively updated to reflect new knowledge in the areas of coronary atherosclerosis, vulnerable plaques, acute coronary syndrome, and heart failure.

Unit VI (Chapters 21 through 23) provides a thorough description of pulmonary anatomy and physiology including concepts of ventilation, perfusion, and gas exchange. The content on obstructive disorders has been extensively rewritten.

Unit VII (Chapters 24 and 25) describes concepts basic to understanding the alterations in fluid, electrolyte, and acid-base homeostasis that accompany many disease processes.

Unit VIII (Chapters 26 through 29) provides a thorough description of renal anatomy and physiology, abnormalities of renal function, bladder dysfunction, and strategies for interpreting common laboratory values in the context of kidney or bladder diseases.

Unit IX (Chapters 30 through 34) includes extensive information on male and female genital anatomy and reproductive physiology as well as common disorders. Chapter 34 provides thorough coverage of common sexually transmitted infections.

Unit X (Chapters 35 through 38) provides a review of normal gastrointestinal anatomy, physiology, and disorders, with separate chapters dedicated to pancreatic and biliary dysfunction and liver disease.

Unit XI (Chapters 39 through 42) addresses alterations in endocrine control, metabolism, and nutrition. General concepts of endocrine control systems and pituitary mechanisms are discussed, with an emphasis on disorders of growth hormone, thyroid, and adrenal gland function. A separate chapter is dedicated to the growing problem of diabetes mellitus. Protein calorie malnutrition, chronic disease states, and age and critical illness are emphasized in Chapter 42.

Unit XII (Chapters 43 through 47) has been extensively revised to reflect new information on neural growth and more detail on synaptic mechanisms of neural function. Chapter 45 has been rewritten to provide a better understanding of common chronic diseases including Alzheimer disease and Parkinson disease. New information on migraine headache, fibromyalgia, and neuropathy has been included in Chapter 47.

Unit XIII (Chapters 48 and 49) covers current concepts in the pathophysiology of psychobiology including anxiety, mood, thought, and personality disorders.

Unit XIV (Chapters 50 through 52) includes alterations in musculoskeletal support and movement, with separate chapters dedicated to normal bone and muscle anatomy and physiology, disorders of bone and muscle, and rheumatic disorders.

Unit XV (Chapters 53 and 54) includes alterations affecting the largest system of the body—the integumentary system. Chapter 53 includes normal integumentary structure and function and a survey of common skin disorders. Chapter 54 covers burn injury, emphasizing the multiple stresses that are encountered in patients with these complex injuries.

FEATURES

An understanding of normal structure and function of the body is necessary for any detailed understanding of its abnormalities and pathophysiology. The first chapter in most units includes a fully illustrated *review of normal physiology.* Changes in structure and function as a result of normal development and aging are also addressed where appropriate. Changes due to aging are highlighted in *Aging Process* boxes. Where appropriate, pediatric and geriatric implications presented within the narrative discussion are denoted with icons:

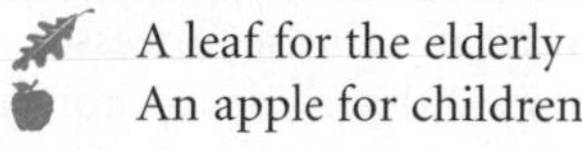

A leaf for the elderly

An apple for children

Each unit opens with *Frontiers of Research,* a short essay that engages students by encouraging them to relate the material to their own lives. Each chapter opens with *Key Questions,* which are designed to develop a strong pathophysiology knowledge base and to serve as the foundation for critical thinking. These Key Questions integrate the essential information in each chapter, emphasizing *concepts* rather than small details. *Chapter Outlines* are also included at the beginning of each chapter to help the reader locate specific content. Within every chapter, *Key Concepts* are identified at the end of every major discussion and are presented in short bulleted lists. These recurring summaries help readers to focus on the main points.

Nearly 1000 illustrations elucidate both normal physiology and pathophysiologic changes. The entire book is in *full color* for the first time, with color used generously in the illustrations to better explain pathophysiologic concepts. More than 250 of the illustrations are new to this edition, and more than 225 illustrations from the previous edition have been updated in full color. Wherever possible, we have used realistic colors in these drawings to enhance the reader's understanding and to avoid detracting from content.

To help students master the new vocabulary of pathophysiology, *key terms* appear in boldface within each chapter, and these terms are defined in a comprehensive *Glossary,* which appears at the end of the text. Throughout this text, the nonpossessive forms of eponyms (e.g., *Down* syndrome) are used consistently when referring to the person for whom a disease is named. Clinical and laboratory values are provided in the *Appendix.*

ANCILLARIES

CD Companion

This **CD-ROM,** which comes with every new copy of the book, contains a variety of useful tools for additional study, review, and exploration, including *Review Questions and Answers* for every chapter, over 650 in all; the *Key Concepts* reviews from the book, included here for convenience; the *Glossary* from the book, which is enhanced on the CD with audio pronunciations for selected terms; 24 *Disease Profiles,* which provide a snapshot of major diseases; and 18 *Animations,* to help readers visualize pathophysiologic processes.

Student Learning Resources on Evolve

The student section of the book's website hosted on Evolve evolve offers *Case Study Worksheets, Disease Profiles,* and *WebLinks* to hundreds of carefully chosen Internet sites pertaining to pathophysiology. Visit the Evolve website at **http://evolve.elsevier.com/Copstead/.**

Study Guide

Pathophysiology can be a daunting subject for students because of the large volume of factual material to be learned.

The student **Study Guide** is designed to help students focus on important pathophysiologic concepts. Activities to check recall of normal anatomy and physiology are included in each unit. A number of activities to help the student focus on similarities and differences between often confused pathologic processes are included. *Self-assessment test questions* with answers are included for each unit to help students check their understanding and build confidence for examinations. *Case studies* are used to help students begin to apply pathophysiologic concepts to clinical situations.

Instructor's Course Resources CD-ROM

The **Instructor's Course Resources CD-ROM** to accompany this text provides a number of instructional aids to instructors who require the text for their students. The materials include a *Computerized Test Bank* with more than 1200 test items, a *PowerPoint lecture guide* with more than 550 slides to facilitate classroom presentations, an *Image Collection* of more than 600 color images from the text, and *Suggested Answers to the Case Study Worksheets* found in the student section of the Evolve website.

Instructor Learning Resources on Evolve

All of the **Instructor's Course Resources** are also available on evolve Evolve, along with the Evolve Course Management System, to instructors who adopt the text. The Evolve Course Management System provides instructors and students with online communication and organization tools including discussion boards, e-mail, chat rooms, calendars, address books, and task organizers. Instructors can customize course content, build online tests, create assignments, enter grades, post announcements, and manage student groups. Instructors are encouraged to contact their Elsevier sales representative for more information about integrating Evolve into their curriculum.

ACKNOWLEDGMENTS

Many creative and unique efforts grace the pages of this work. It is exceedingly difficult to know how to best recognize every one. Writing this text has been possible only because of the tremendous dedication of authors, artists, reviewers, and editors. Our sincere gratitude goes to all who helped with this and previous editions. In particular, grateful appreciation is extended to all of the contributing authors—recognized experts—who gave exhaustively of their time to write chapters and create illustrations. We are indebted to the many thoughtful experts who gave of their time to read and critique manuscripts and help ensure excellence in chapter content throughout the text.

No project of this magnitude could be accomplished without wonderfully supportive colleagues and students who provided a source of continual motivation and encouragement. We are most keenly aware of the inspiration provided by the faculty, staff, and students of Washington State University Intercollegiate College of Nursing, Gundersen Lutheran Medical Center, and University of Wisconsin Western Campus for Nursing.

Grateful recognition is made to the staff at Elsevier. In particular, Barb Watts deserves our heartfelt thanks for helping with the illustrations and keeping track of a mountain of material. Deon Lee paid superb attention to the many details of copyediting, proofreading, and page layout. And Teresa McBryan's elegant and colorful design helped give the book its polished format. In addition, Darlene Como believed in the book and oversaw the revision from beginning to end, Brian Dennison helped with the planning and management of the project, and Katherine Judge assisted with the permissions and too many other tasks to list here.

We would like to recognize those who provided a foundation for the revised text through their contributions to the first edition: Mary Sanguinetti-Baird, Linda Belsky-Lohr, Tim Brown, Karen Carlson, Leslie Evans, Jo Annalee Irving, Debby Kaaland, Rick Madison, Maryann Pranulis, Edith Randall, Bridget Recker, Cleo Richard, Gary Smith, Pam Springer, Martha Snider, Patti Stec, Julie Symes, Lorie Wild, and Debra Winston-Heath. We also would like to thank those who contributed to the second edition of the book: Barbara Bartz, Arnold Norman Cohen, Karen Groth, Christine M. Henshaw, Carolyn Hoover, Marianne Genge Jagmin, Anne Roe Mealey, David Mikkelsen, Billie Marie Severtsen, and Jacqueline Siegel.

To the late Dr. Michael J. Kirkhorn, we give acknowledgment and thanks for writing the provocative and thoughtful essays that begin each unit.

CONTENTS

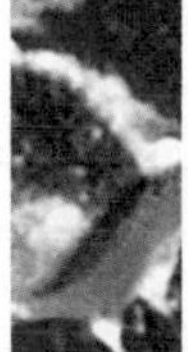

UNIT IV
Oxygen Transport, Blood Coagulation, Blood Flow, and Blood Pressure, 316

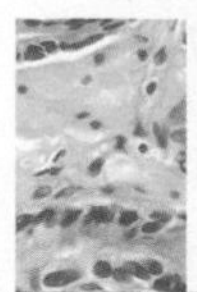

UNIT IX
Genital and Reproductive Function, 770

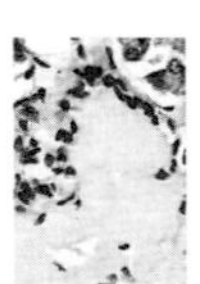

PATHOPHYSIOLOGY

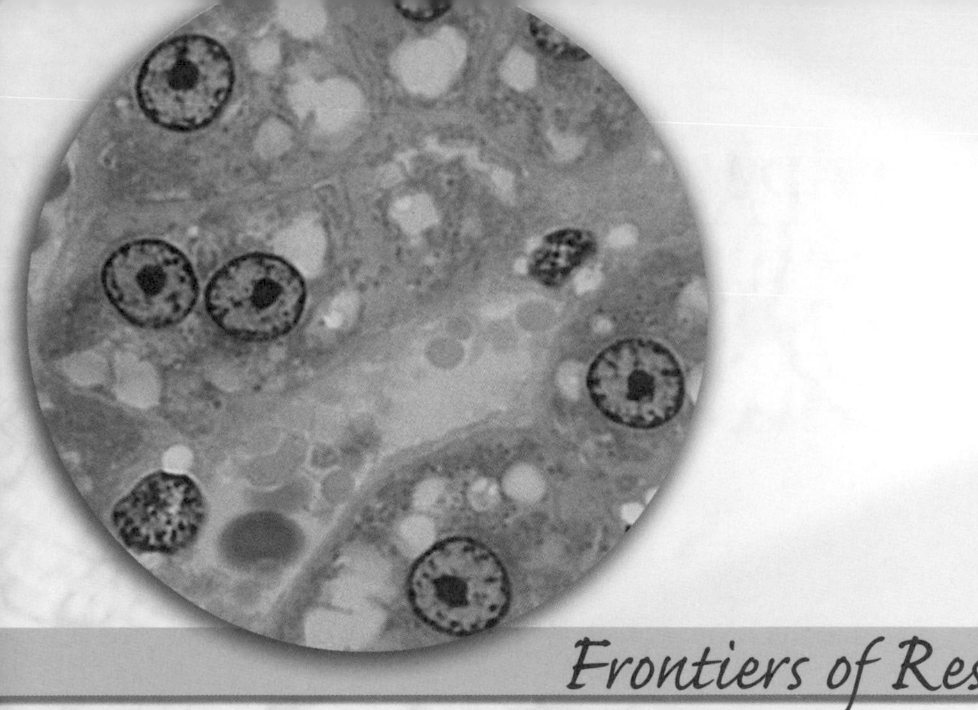

Frontiers of Research

The Complex Nature of Disease

Lee-Ellen C. Copstead and Michael J. Kirkhorn

In the not-so-distant past, people held fairly simple beliefs about disease. Health was a blessing; disease was a curse. Health was a state of wellness and an absence of bothersome or disabling symptoms. Disease was the dreaded underminer.

Deep inside, many people still believe these simple precepts. They feel lucky when they are healthy and unlucky when they are not, as if health were a natural state of goodness and disease an unexpected evil.

Scientific understanding is much more complex. The late Lewis Thomas, noted author and physician, said that disease "usually results from inconclusive negotiations for symbiosis, an overstepping of the line by one side or the other, a biological misinterpretation of borders." It is a matter of delicate balance, timing, and close calls. At the cellular level, where the relationship between health and disease is being studied most extensively, health appears to be a condition in which the body's dynamic systems of intercellular signals are translated and effected, and disease seems to be related to breakdowns in cellular communication. When a DNA error is not repaired, the cell passes on its defective gene to new cells, which may lead to many biochemical events that over time cause normal tissues to become diseased.

We are making progress. We now know—and our understanding is increasing rapidly—more about the processes of disease than ever before. The revelations produced by broad advances in genetic research signal the most dramatic of the directions in which research is carrying us. We are vastly increasing our information about age, racial and gender differences, and other factors that allow us to see disease not as an "evil visitor" but as an inherent factor in the spectrum of possibilities presented to each human being at birth. We also know more and more about the effects of outside factors, such as environmental pollution and tobacco smoking, that may turn a likelihood—a susceptibility or inherited weakness—into actual disease.

We search outside the single diseased body for patterns of disease in human communities. Epidemiologists, who study those patterns, continue to teach us more about the occurrence of disease. This science is particularly important in determining the causes of disease when environmental agents are suspected—contaminants with which the miners of radioactive materials have been brought into contact, for example, or heavy air pollution in areas with high incidences of lung disorders. Epidemiologists also remind us to keep a clear sense of balance when we think about disease. Some diseases are highly publicized, often for good reason and with beneficial effects, but a good public health epidemiologist will notice that a community may suffer as much or more when its older citizens encounter an epidemic of a mundane illness such as influenza.

In our attempts to put health and disease into perspective, the terms "normal" or "abnormal" can be easily misapplied because determining norms in health and disease often involves the as-

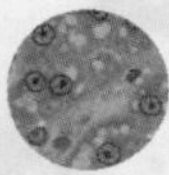

Cell nuclei. (From Gartner LP, Hiatt JL: Color textbook of histology, *ed 2, Philadelphia, 2001, Saunders, p 52.)*

UNIT I

Pathophysiologic Processes

sessment of individuals who vary greatly in their susceptibilities and in their abilities to withstand, cope, and even thrive while they are living through what is considered a diseased state.

The balance that we find in those enjoying good health or in people with disease who have settled at plateaus of stability, however impaired, is significant. That balance is as precious in those suffering from disease as it is for those who have no affliction. However, the natural human optimism that glories in good health and detests disease conveys an inadequate sense of the actual symbiosis in which agents of disease and health struggle, commingle, or quietly ignore each other in the body.

Those interested in disease will find guidance in history. The medical historian Logan Clendening found the first written descriptions of disease in Egyptian papyruses almost 3000 years old. Some of the ancient remedies, diagnoses, and treatments from early Egyptian, Greek, and Arabic medicine remain plausible today. So do some of the aphorisms of Hippocrates, if only because his observations invoke that valuable commodity common sense. "When sleep puts an end to delirium, it is a good symptom," Hippocrates said, and "In every movement of the body, whenever one begins to endure pain, it will be relieved by rest."

In our time, rest is not easy to find. We do not live restful lives. In fact, more often we find ourselves "stressed out." Stress is hard to isolate as a cause of disease, but increasingly over the past few decades health professionals have recognized the harmful consequences of living in a body that is tense and taut in a posture of fear or anxiety.

Our understanding of the nature of disease and therefore of health is proceeding with unusual speed and confidence. Researchers expect that in the near future genetic research could produce a number of astonishing cures, as well as new kinds of diagnosis, immunization, prevention, anticipation of disease, and preemptive therapy. Genetic research into the nature of disease promises to precisely locate the origin of many diseases and thus allow us to either prevent or correct them with therapies unavailable to past generations. It promises to decode our physical nature and reveal the qualities that we associate with defects of the body, mind, or spirit. So disease is being tracked to its most secret refuge, where it is naturally coded in the body. The findings of genetic research may someday cure the ills that plague us—severe acute or chronic diseases, in addition to lesser ailments. Current research also promises prevention of life-threatening diseases, including particularly tragic diseases that kill prematurely. In breast cancer, for example, current research indicates that through T-cell vaccines and T-cell therapy the cancer patient's own immune system can be strengthened in ways that fight cancer and offer possible lifelong protection against relapse.

Hippocrates would have been impressed.

chapter 1

Core Pathophysiologic Concepts

Lee-Ellen C. Copstead

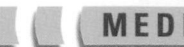

MEDIA RESOURCES

Additional Material for Study, Review, and Further Exploration

CD Companion ◆ Review Questions and Answers ◆ Key Concepts Review ◆ Glossary *(with audio pronunciations for selected terms)* ◆ Disease Profiles ◆ Animations

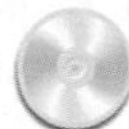

evolve Website at http://evolve.elsevier.com/Copstead/ ◆ Case Studies ◆ Disease Profiles ◆ WebLinks

KEY QUESTIONS

- What is pathophysiology, and why is it important for clinical practice?
- How might disease disrupt homeostasis?
- Why do homeostatic control mechanisms generally function as negative feedback systems?
- How are normal and abnormal physiologic parameters defined?
- What factors, other than disease, might result in "abnormal" physiologic values?
- What general factors affect the expression of disease in a particular person?
- What kinds of information about disease can be gained through application of epidemiologic methods of investigation?

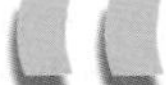

CHAPTER OUTLINE

An explosion in knowledge of DNA, especially since the late 1970s, has virtually transformed definitions of the living world and has permeated every branch of biological science. The benefits of this new biology have been awesome: a deeper understanding of evolution, greater insights into immune mechanisms, and nearly every advance against cancer and acquired immunodeficiency syndrome (AIDS). But genetic manipulation also raises sensitive and complex ethical and moral questions that did not exist half a century ago. Scientists are now able to crack and manipulate the genetic code. Mammalian cloning has become a reality. Scientists can experiment with what genes do and how they do it. These scientific breakthroughs will dramatically alter medical practice, especially the management of inherited diseases. New capabilities have led to experimental treatments such as gene therapy—molecular surgery powerful enough to cure and alter the next generation. When gene therapy is perfected as a biomedical technique, and when its attendant ethical and moral dilemmas have been resolved, the diagnosis and management of genetic defects may well be commonplace.

The study of pathophysiology takes on new importance as genetic research reveals fresh insights regarding human diseases. **Physiology** is the study of the specific characteristics and functions of a living organism and its parts; *patho* comes from the Greek *pathos,* which means suffering or disease. Together, as **pathophysiology,** these terms refer to study of the disorder or breakdown of the human body's function. Concepts of homeostasis, disease and illness, key elements of pathophysiologic processes, an agreed common terminology, and basic epidemiology are all important considerations and provide a solid foundation for this text.

CONCEPTS OF HOMEOSTASIS

Knowledge of homeostasis has contributed greatly to the fields of physiology and pathophysiology. Homeostasis has engendered a sense of order and unity to the study of biological processes. First described by the American physiologist Walter B. Cannon in his classic 1932 text, *The Wisdom of the Body,* the concept of homeostasis has elucidated the interdependence of the body's systems. For example, the circulatory, endocrine, and nervous systems are no longer regarded as isolated units, operating independently of one other. Rather, they are part of a functioning whole, working together to enable the individual to survive emergencies and everyday stresses. Bodily changes and adjustments that formerly seemed to conflict can now be better understood as adaptive or compensatory manifestations of homeostasis and as functions related to the total needs of the individual. Homeostasis has enabled us to see physiology as a dynamic process of continuous self-regulation and self-adjustment. Consequently, we can better

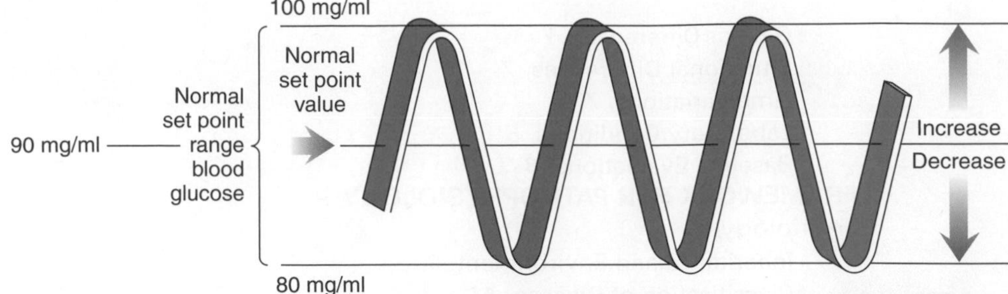

FIGURE 1-1 ■ Upper and lower limits of homeostasis. The range over which homeostasis of blood glucose, for example, is maintained. Note that the concentration of glucose fluctuates above and below a normal set point value (90 mg/ml) within a normal set point range (80 to 100 mg/ml). (Redrawn from Thibodeau GA, Patton KT: *Anatomy and physiology,* ed 5, St Louis, 2003, Mosby, p 21.)

understand the many fluctuations and oscillations that occur constantly within the body.

Although the term **homeostasis** is derived from two Greek words *homoios* ("the same") and *stasis* ("standing"), research with a variety of radioisotopes has demonstrated that homeostasis does not mean standing still or staying constant. The idea of homeostasis as a *dynamic* steady state is much more accurate. The fat or protein content of the body may not vary much from day to day, but the substances that make up the fat and protein—fatty acids and amino acids—can vary widely. The enzymes in a healthy person are constantly synthesizing and breaking down these substances. The process of synthesis and breakdown of all bodily substances is known as turnover. Hence, **homeostasis** may be defined as a dynamic steady state, representing the net effect of all turnover reactions. Maintenance of internal homeostasis is an essential feature of the normal body.

Physiologically, all cells in the body need a *balance* of oxygen and nutrients for their continuing survival and also require an environment that affords such things as narrow ranges of temperature, water content, acidity, and salt concentration. Homeostasis refers to the body's tendency to maintain balance in the presence of continual environmental variation. Parameters such as temperature, cardiac output, blood pressure, oxygen and carbon dioxide levels, acid-base balance, fluid volume, and electrolyte composition are closely regulated to maintain homeostasis.

The idea of homeostatic balance represents an ideal. Actually, in every self-regulating system some degree of deviation occurs from what is optimal or normal for that system—a range over which a given value is maintained (Figure 1-1).

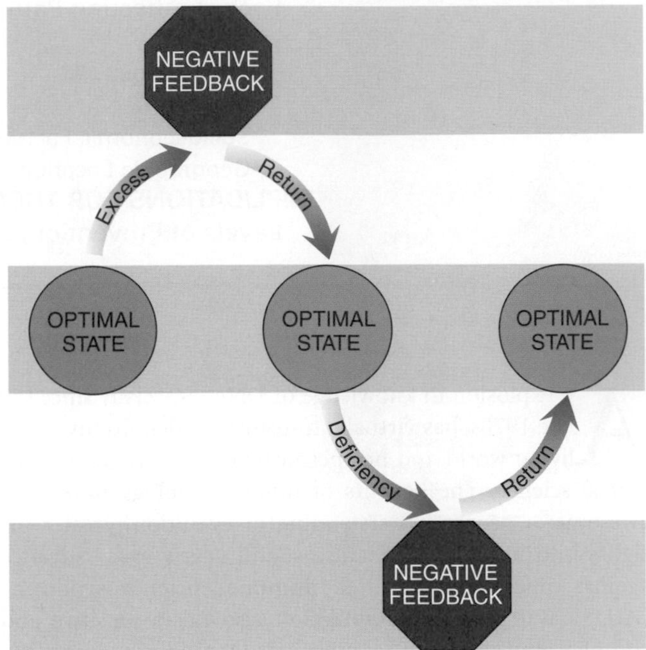

FIGURE 1-2 ■ Homeostatic systems tend to be negative feedback systems and regulate deviations from normal, leading the organism back to an optimal state and thereby negating any attempts toward radical excess or deficiency.

Homeostatic Control Mechanisms

Most homeostatic control mechanisms in the body function on the principle of **negative feedback,** which causes the controller to respond in a manner that opposes or *negates* deviation from normal (set point) level (Figure 1-2). The variable to be controlled must be "sensed" to be regulated. Thus, the controller responds by bringing the variable back to normal (set point) level. For example, when body temperature deviates from normal, negative feedback restores homeostasis. The temperature (variable) is sensed and the body responds by sweating.

Each cell of the body, each tissue, each organ, and each system plays an important role in homeostasis. These diverse regulatory systems employ feedback and feedforward mecha-

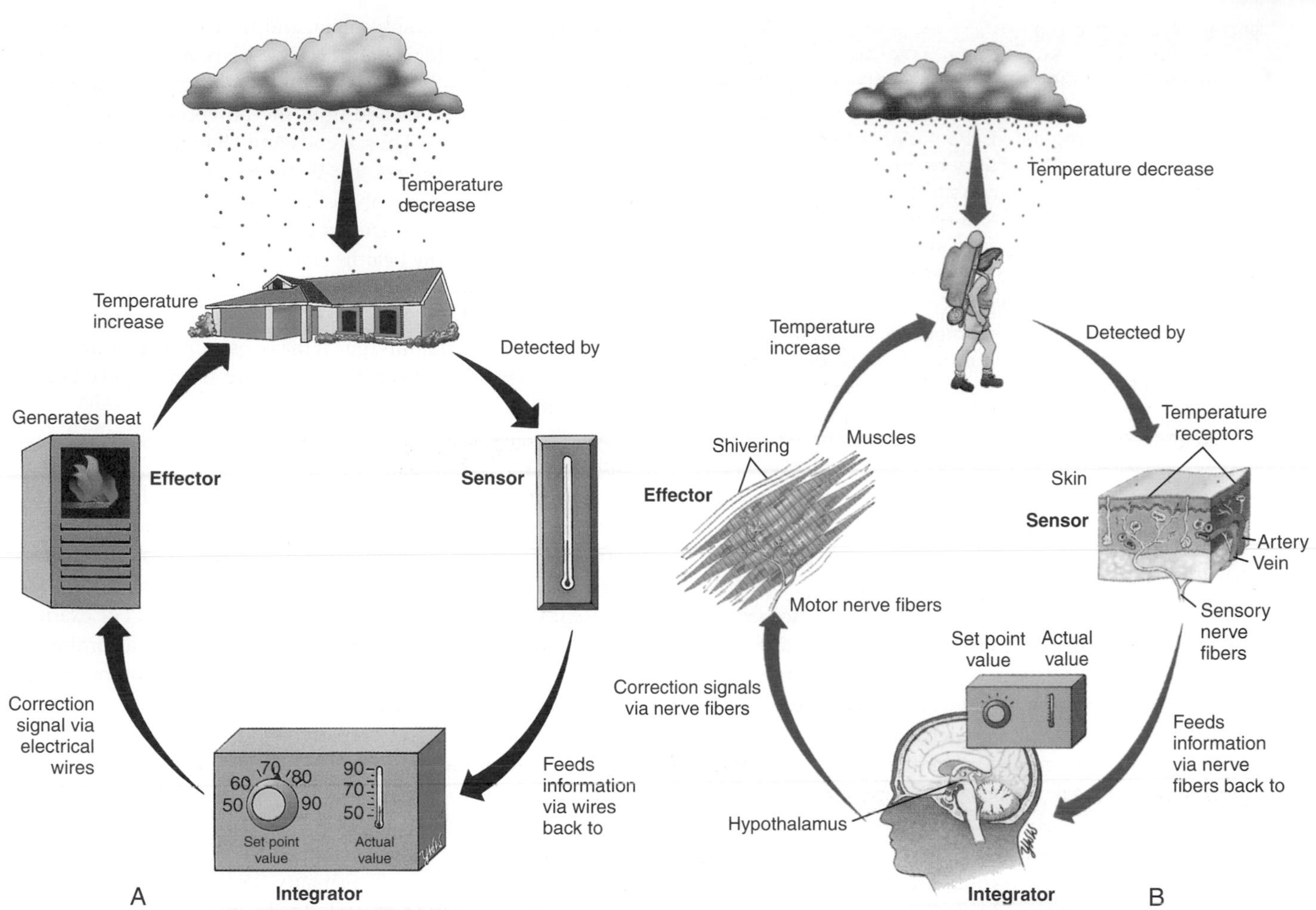

FIGURE 1-3 ■ Basic components of homeostatic control mechanisms. **A,** Heat regulation by a furnace controlled by a thermostat. **B,** Homeostasis of body temperature. In both of these examples, a stimulus (drop in temperature) activates a sensor mechanism (thermometer or body temperature receptor) that sends input to an integrating or control center (thermostat or hypothalamus), which then sends input to an effector mechanism (furnace or contracting muscle). The resulting heat that is produced maintains the temperature in a "normal range." Feedback of effector activity to the sensor mechanism completes the loop. (From Thibodeau GA, Patton KT: *Anatomy and physiology,* ed 5, St Louis, 2003, Mosby, p 24.)

nisms that far surpass our most brilliant electronic achievements. If circumstances occur that require changes or more intense regulation of the internal environment, appropriate control mechanisms must be available in the body to respond to the change and also to restore and maintain normalcy. Sensory neurons and endocrine glands are primary homeostatic sensors. Sensors then supply feedback to a regulatory center (usually the brain), which integrates all relevant input and initiates a response. The response is carried out by effectors (muscles and glands) (Figure 1-3).

Although negative feedback systems are by far the most common homeostatic systems in the body, another type of feedback exists, known as **positive feedback.** With positive feedback, an initial disturbance in a system sets off a chain of events that does not favor stability and often abruptly displaces a system away from its steady-state operating point. Only a few positive feedback examples operate in the body under normal conditions. However, events that lead to a simple sneeze, the birth of a baby, and formation of a blood clot involve several important positive-feedback relationships.

KEY CONCEPTS

- Maintenance of internal homeostasis is an essential feature of the normal body.
- In order to be regulated, the variable to be controlled must be "sensed." Sensory neurons and endocrine glands are primary homeostatic sensors. Sensors then provide feedback to a regulatory center (usually the brain), which integrates all relevant input and initiates a response. The response is carried out by effectors (muscles and glands).
- Most homeostatic control mechanisms in the body function on the principle of negative feedback, which tends to favor stability. Positive feedback, by comparison, abruptly displaces a system away from its steady-state operating point.

CONCEPTS OF DISEASE AND ILLNESS

Disease can be viewed as a disruption of homeostasis. Homeostasis can be disrupted by processes that interfere with the function of homeostatic sensors, regulatory centers, or effectors. A common notion is that disease and illness represent *abnormal* states, or at least an extension or distortion of the normal life processes going on in the individual. Disease, however, is actually the *sum* of the deviations from normal. Even in the case of an obviously infectious disease, in which the body is literally invaded, the infectious agent does not constitute the disease but only evokes the changes in the subject that ultimately manifest as disease. Attempted management with antibiotics alone may not be a sufficient cure if proper attention is not directed to the intrinsic bodily processes and the external environment of the affected individual.

Disease is *dynamic* rather than static. To the affected individual, disease means discomfort, or exactly what the word says, *dis*-ease. The complex nature of the disease process includes the interplay between injury and reaction to injury, which is a kaleidoscopic series of actions and counteractions. The signs and symptoms of disease in a given person may change daily as the biological equilibrium shifts and compensatory mechanisms are brought into play. Every disease has a range of manifestations and a natural history that varies from individual to individual.

Factors Affecting Determination of Normality

To understand and adequately manage disease, one must take into account the normal processes that have been altered, the nature of the disturbances, and the effects that such disturbances have on other vital processes.

Variations in physiologic processes may be a result of factors other than disease or illness. Age, gender, genetic and ethnic background, geographic area, and time of day may influence various physiologic parameters.[1-3] Care must be taken to interpret "abnormal" findings in the light of these possible confounding factors. In addition, the potential for spurious findings always exists. Thus, trends and changes in a particular individual are more reliable than single observations.

By means of a variety of clinical and laboratory tests, it is possible to measure characteristics of normalcy as well as deviations from it. In the healthy state, a certain value is consistently obtained for a particular factor, within specific laboratory definitions. This range of values or indices is considered to be within normal limits, given the constraints of laboratory variables. Deviations from this range are usually considered abnormal.

Genetic Variations

No absolute normal value exists for any biological parameter. There are genetic variations in many diseases; in addition, genetic responses to treatment vary and may lead to differences in clinical presentation. What is usual for one person may be different for another because of genetic variations. For example, a blood pressure reading of 120/80 mm Hg is a common value. Yet some people who consistently have a blood pressure reading of 90/70 mm Hg are in good health; this value represents their normal blood pressure. By sampling a large number of people, an "average normal" and a range of normal can be determined.

Occasionally, a person may consistently show a value outside the usual range for the factor yet function well. Although the person may have an abnormality for that characteristic in terms of the population as a whole, the unusual value may be normal for that individual.

Cultural Considerations

To place these considerations in perspective, it should be noted that the notion of what constitutes normalcy and even illness is, to a certain extent, arbitrary and influenced by culture as well as genetics. Each culture defines health and illness in a manner that reflects its experience.[4] In some cultures, women must have approval by males to receive medical attention. Dietary considerations often are culturally determined, and cultural factors determine which signs, symptoms, or behaviors are perceived as abnormal.[5] For example, a person from a literate culture with a significant reading disability would be labeled as having an abnormality, whereas the same defect would not be identified in a nonliterate culture. Furthermore, a trait such as very short stature is average and thus normal in a population of Japanese elders, yet it would be considered distinctly abnormal in a population of U.S. National Basketball Association players. An infant from an impoverished culture with "normal" chronic diarrhea and poor weight gain would be viewed as abnormal in a progressive culture such as a well-baby clinic in Sweden. Given cultural variations that affect definitions of normal and abnormal, the resulting pattern of behaviors or clinical manifestations is what the culture labels as illness.[6]

Age Differences

Many biological factors vary with age, and the normal value for a person at one age may be abnormal at another. A number of physiologic changes, such as hair color, skin turgor (tension), and organ size, vary with age. In general, most organs shrink; exceptions are the male prostate and the heart, which enlarge with age. Gray hair, wrinkled skin, and receding gums, normal in an elderly person, are abnormal in a child. Special sensory changes, such as severely diminished nearsight, high-tone hearing loss, and loss of taste discriminations for sweet and salty, are normal in an elderly adult and abnormal in a middle-aged adult or child. There are fewer sweat glands and less thirst perception in an elderly person than in a young adult or child. Elderly persons have diminished temperature sensations and can therefore sustain burn injuries—from a heating pad or bath water—because they do not perceive heat with the same intensity as do middle-aged adults. A resting heart rate of 120 beats per minute is normal for an infant but not for an adult.

Gender Differences

Some laboratory values, such as levels of sex hormones and growth hormones, show gender differences. The complete blood cell count shows differences by gender in hematocrit, hemoglobin, and red blood cell (RBC) count.[1] For example, the normal range of hemoglobin concentration for adult women is lower than that for adult men. For adult women, the normal range is 12 to 16 g/100 ml of blood; for adult men the normal range is 13 to 18 g/100 ml of blood.[1] Blood calcium ranges are slightly higher in adult women than in adult men.[2] There are also gender differences in large granular lymphocytes[2,3] and in the erythrocyte sedimentation rate (ESR). Normally, in males, the ESR is less than 13 mm/hr; it is slightly higher in females.[1] There are also differences by gender in creatinine values. For females, the normal serum creatinine level is 0.4 to 1.3 mg/dl; for males, the normal range is 0.6 to 1.5 mg/dl.[1] Research into gender differences also suggests that, on average, males snore more than females,[4-6] have longer vocal cords, have better daylight vision, have higher metabolic rates, and are more likely to be left-handed. Research also suggests that females and males have different communication styles and respond differently to similar conditions.[7]

Situational Differences

In some cases, a deviation from the usual value may occur as an adaptive mechanism, and whether the deviation is considered abnormal or not depends on the situation. For example, the RBC count increases when a person moves to a high altitude.[8] This increase is a normal adaptive response to the decreased availability of oxygen at a high altitude and is termed **acclimatization.** A similar increase in the RBC count at sea level would be abnormal.

Time Variations

Some factors vary according to the time of day; that is, they exhibit a **circadian rhythm** or **diurnal variation.** In interpreting the result of a particular test, it may be necessary to know the time at which the value was determined. For example, body temperature and plasma concentrations of certain hormones (such as growth hormone and cortisol) exhibit diurnal variation. Reflecting fluctuation in plasma levels, the peak rate in urinary excretion for a particular steroid (17-ketosteroid) occurs between 8 AM and 10 AM for persons who customarily get up early in the morning, and is about two to three times greater than the lowest rate in the same people, which occurs between midnight and 2 AM, usually during sleep.[9,10] The urinary excretion of ions (e.g., potassium) also exhibits diurnal variation. Figure 1-4 illustrates circadian rhythms of several physiologic variables for persons living on a standard day-active schedule.

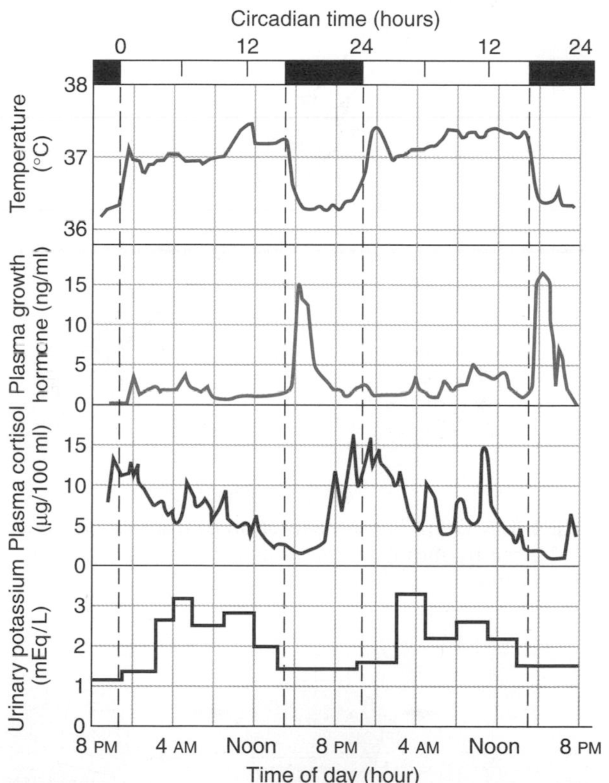

FIGURE 1-4 ■ Circadian rhythms of several physiologic variables in a human subject depict the effect of light and dark. In an experiment with lights on (*open bars* at top) for 16 hours and off (*black bars* at top) for 8 hours, temperature, plasma growth hormone, plasma cortisol, and urinary potassium levels exhibit diurnal variation. (Redrawn from Vander AJ, Sherman JH, Luciano DS: *Human physiology,* ed 7, New York, 1998, McGraw-Hill.)

Laboratory Conditions

Some clinical and laboratory measurements vary according to methods used. For example, prothrombin time is sensitive to the *reagent* used. For example, in one method of determining prothrombin time, the reagent—a substance composed of thromboplastin and calcium—is added to decalcified plasma to create a reaction—in this case, clot formation. The prothrombin time is then determined by measuring the length of time it takes for clotting to occur after this reagent is added.

In the United States alone, there are several different reagent companies and a variety of lot numbers representing each reagent. Although a given laboratory may keep the same lot number for up to a year, the reagent that is used in specific testing situations likely varies among laboratories. Industrial and possible human error may also cause variations in laboratory results.

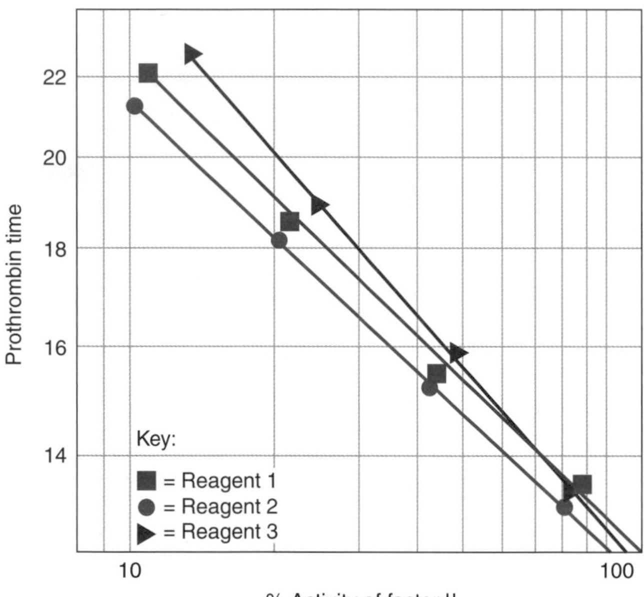

FIGURE 1-5 ■ Graphic representation of the relative sensitivity of three hypothetical reagents in determining a prothrombin time.

Whenever a new reagent is obtained, a corresponding range of normal values must be calculated. For example, to determine the range of normal for a particular reagent, a normal study using a minimum of 30 specimens—carefully controlled for age and sex and excluding all drugs, including nicotine—is conducted. The values obtained from this study determine what are called the *population mean* and the *reference range.* Figure 1-5 illustrates hypothetical examples of different reagent sensitivities in determining the prothrombin time using the procedure described above.

Baseline Evaluations

Often, when assessing a person's health status, a change in some value or factor is more significant than the actual value of the particular factor. A blood pressure of 90/70 mm Hg may not be significant if that is the usual value. However, if a person usually has a blood pressure of 120/80 mm Hg, a reading of 90/70 mm Hg would be very significant, especially if it is obtained on more than one occasion. Individuals are typically evaluated more than once—generally three times and under three different circumstances in order to establish deviation from their usual value. Deviation can be indicative of disease, especially in the presence of other signs and symptoms.

Because of these considerations, determining a normal range of variation from an average value is a complex matter. This complexity includes knowing the degree of physiologic oscillation of a particular measurement, accounting for the degree of variation among normal individuals under baseline conditions, and figuring the precision of the measurement method. Finally, the biological significance of the measurement must be estimated. Single measurements, observations, or laboratory results that seem to indicate abnormality must always be judged in the context of the entire health picture of the individual. One slightly elevated blood glucose level does not mean clinical diabetes, a single high blood pressure reading does not denote hypertension, a temporary feeling of hopelessness does not indicate clinical depression, and a single hemoglobin value lower than the average does not define anemia. The concept of physiologic oscillation may be depicted schematically as a spinning top, rotating around "ideal" conditions (Figure 1-6).

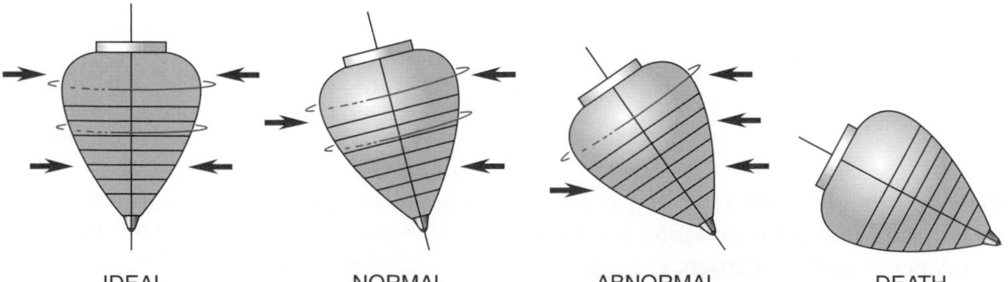

FIGURE 1-6 ■ Example of physiologic oscillation. The movement of a spinning top represents the fluctuation of a physiologic variable around ideal conditions. A disturbance in either direction could send the top whirling into danger—for our purposes, the disease state. If the disturbance is so extreme that it topples, death results.

KEY CONCEPTS

- Disease may be viewed as a disruption of homeostasis.
- Homeostasis can be disrupted by processes that interfere with the function of homeostatic sensors, regulatory centers, or effectors.
- Disease represents the *sum* of the deviations from normal.
- Variations in physiologic processes may be a result of factors *other than* disease or illness. Age, gender, genetic and ethnic background, geographic area, and time of day may influence various physiologic parameters.
- Care must be taken to interpret "abnormal" findings in the light of these possible confounding factors. In addition, the potential for spurious findings always exists.
- Trends and changes in a particular individual are more reliable than single observations.

FRAMEWORK FOR PATHOPHYSIOLOGY

Three aspects of a disease process form a framework for understanding pathophysiology. They are as follows: its cause **(etiologic process);** the mechanisms of its development **(pathogenesis),** including the structural and biochemical alterations induced in the cells and organs of the body; and the functional consequences of these changes (**clinical manifestations**) (Figure 1-7). Structure is an expression of altered chemistry, and dysfunction is an inevitable consequence. Structure, composition, and function are inseparably interrelated. Treatment for pathophysiologic disorders is "implied" by the etiologic process, pathogenesis, and clinical manifestations and is described later in this chapter.

Etiology

Etiology, in its most general definition, is the study of the causes or reasons for phenomena.[11] *Staphylococcus aureus,* a pathogen, is designated as the *etiologic agent* of an infection. Other etiologic factors in the development of the disease that influence the course of the infection include the age, health, and general nutritional status of the person. It is important to repeat that even in the case of an infectious disease such as a staphylococcal infection, the agent itself does not constitute the disease. Rather, the result of *all* of the responses to that agent, that is, *all* of the abnormalities of biological processes, constitutes the disease.

A description of etiologic process includes the identification of those causal factors that, acting in concert, provoke the particular disease or cause traumatic injury. When the cause is unknown, a condition is said to be **idiopathic.** If the cause is due to an unintended or unwanted medical treatment, the resulting condition is said to be **iatrogenic.**

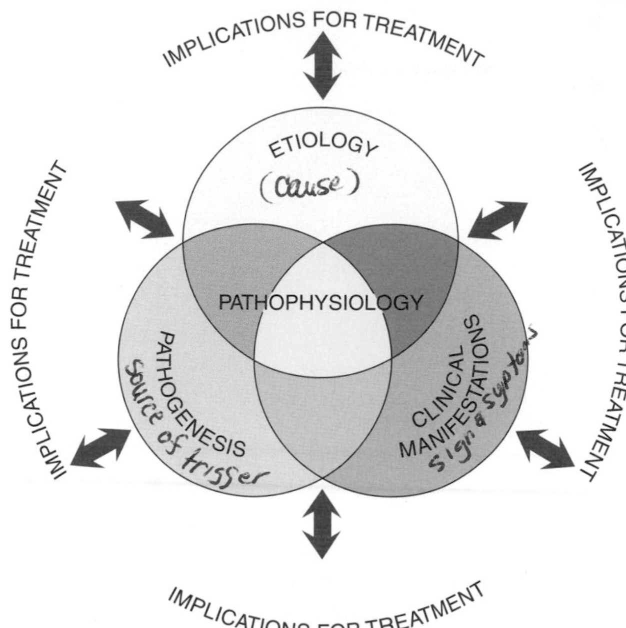

FIGURE 1-7 ■ Three interrelated aspects of a disease process form a framework for understanding pathophysiology: (1) its cause (etiologic process); (2) the mechanisms of its development (pathogenesis), including the structural and biochemical alterations induced in the cells and organs of the body; and (3) the functional consequences of these changes (clinical manifestations). Treatment for pathophysiologic disorders is "implied" by the etiologic process, pathogenesis, and clinical manifestations.

Inheritance and Environment

In the etiologic development of a particular disease, physical, chemical, infectious, or nutritional factors in the environment as well as a variety of intrinsic characteristics of the person are important considerations. For example, the influence of environmental factors in producing the barrel-shaped chests of natives of the Andes Mountains is extremely significant. Here, the altered chest shape represents not a genetic difference between the people and their lowland compatriots, but rather an irreversible acclimatization induced during the first few years of life by exposure to the low-oxygen environment of high altitude. The altered chest size—an adaptive response to the environment—remains although the individual may move to the lowlands later in life and stay there. Lowland persons who have suffered oxygen deprivation from heart or lung disease during their early years show precisely the same chest shape, further demonstrating the importance of environmental factors.

The relative impact of genes and environment varies with each disease. Some diseases, such as Down syndrome, which is an entirely genetic disorder resulting from an extra chromosome, occur in all environments. New research into the etiologic development of certain diseases, such as schizophrenia, reveals a greater relative impact of genetic control than was previously understood. By comparison, retrolental fibroplasia (vasoconstriction of the immature retinal vessels resulting

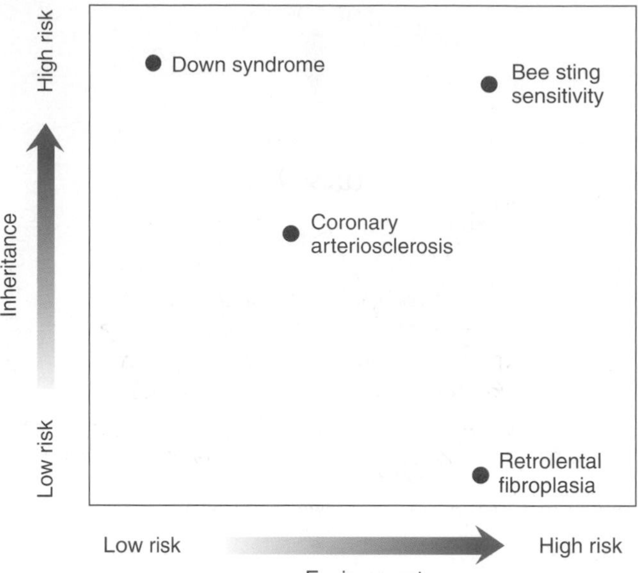

FIGURE 1-8 ■ Relative contributions of inheritance and environmental factors to the development of four disorders. Retrolental fibroplasia requires the unusual environment of premature birth and high oxygen concentration; this combination causes damage to the retina, resulting in blindness. In contrast, Down syndrome, an inherited condition, is expressed in all environments. Bee sting sensitivity requires a high-risk genotype as well as exposure to a high-risk environmental factor. Coronary arteriosclerosis is a common disease involving many genotypes and a variety of environmental agents. (Adapted from Martin G, Hoehn H: *Human pathology,* Philadelphia, 1974, Saunders.)

from exposure of a premature newborn to a high oxygen concentration) has an entirely environmental basis. Furthermore, a hypersensitivity disease can result when a bee sting occurs; both genetic predisposition and exposure to venom are required for the disease. Finally, coronary arteriosclerosis results from many predisposing genetic and environmental factors. This widely occurring disease has multiple causes. Figure 1-8 depicts one way of describing the relative contribution of inheritance (genotype) and environmental factors to the occurrence of four disorders.

Note that agents present in one environment may be hurtful to some but not all persons. Unfortunate combinations and instances of hereditary factors may combine with environmental factors. For example, the abnormal hemoglobin of sickle cell anemia—an inherited condition that causes red blood cells to form sickle shapes when the oxygen concentration is low—leads to headaches, dizziness, and pain in the abdomen when the sickled erythrocytes plug small blood vessels in the brain and liver.[12] With exposure to low oxygen concentrations, unconsciousness may be induced in affected persons, yet the unaffected are not harmed (Figure 1-9).

In short, the cause of human disease is intimately linked to two factors: genetic makeup and environmental interaction. Some regard disease as a means by which nature judges the desirability of an individual's genetic makeup in a given environment. "Survival of the fittest," the theme of darwinian evolution, or the struggle between nature (genetic makeup or inheritance) and nurture (environment), is ongoing.[13] This struggle is encompassed by the term *ecogenetics.* Identical

A
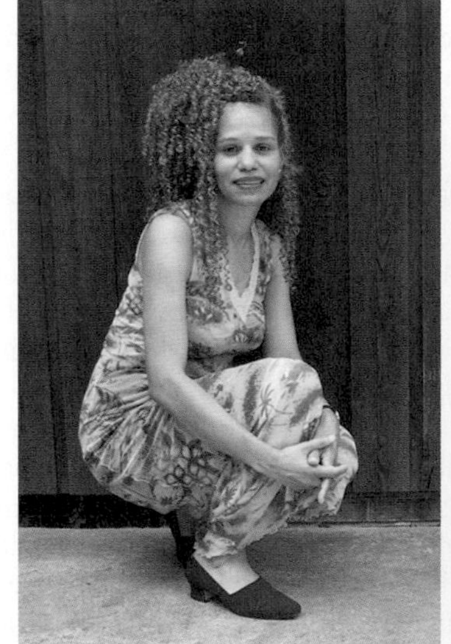
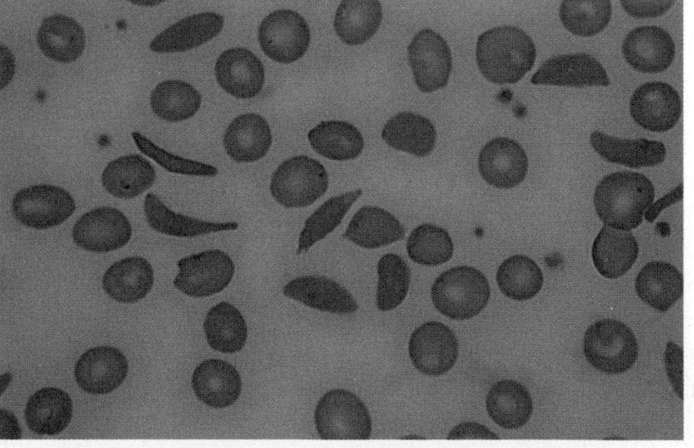
B

FIGURE 1-9 ■ Sickle cell anemia. Many African Americans **(A)** carry the same genetic protection against malaria that baffled early European Caucasian explorers in West Africa, nearly all of whom died from "the fever." However, the gene responsible for this protection can be deadly: a double dose of it produces a variant blood protein known as hemoglobin S, which induces sickle cell anemia. The abnormal hemoglobin causes red blood cells to form sickle shapes **(B)** when the oxygen concentration is low. When the sickled erythrocytes plug small blood vessels in the brain and liver, serious headache, dizziness, and abdominal pain result. (**A,** Photographed by Therese A. Capal, Rockville, Md. **B,** From Rodak BF: *Diagnostic hematology,* Philadelphia, 1995, Saunders, p 257.)

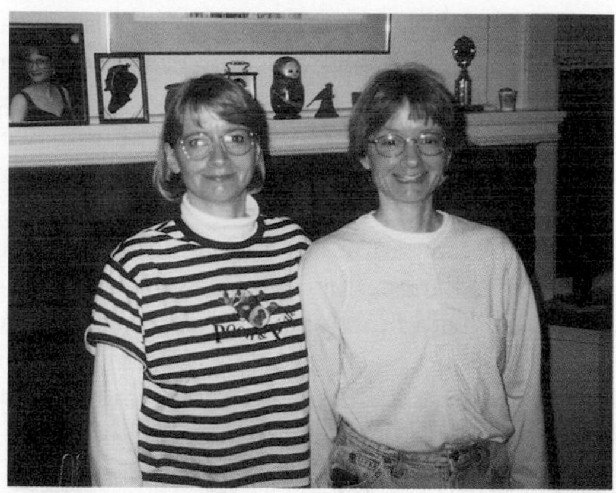

FIGURE 1-10 ■ Identical twins, produced by division of one fertilized egg, have virtually identical genetic endowments and similar appearance. Even as infants, and now as adults, characteristics visibly distinguish them. Yet their *invisible* traits, including IQ, temperament, and tendency to develop behavioral disorders, are either predetermined by genetics or subject to environmental modification. (Photographed by Robert Barnett, Richmond, Va.)

twins, for example, have the same genetic makeup; differences in them are largely due to the influence of the environment (Figure 1-10). Emphasis may be placed on the fact that inheritance provides certain conditions for diseases that are induced by environmental agents.

Classification of Disease

Myriad etiologic agents can initiate disease. Figure 1-11 depicts one way of representing these agents in broad, general terms.

No single etiologic classification is truly comprehensive. Some diseases fall into multiple categories, and many diseases have unknown causes. Some diseases may actually receive different designations in the future, as further research reveals new data. Box 1-1 summarizes the etiologic classification of diseases.

The reader will find more detailed information on each of these categories in the subsequent chapters of this book. A brief explanation of the etiologic categories presented in Box 1-1 follows.

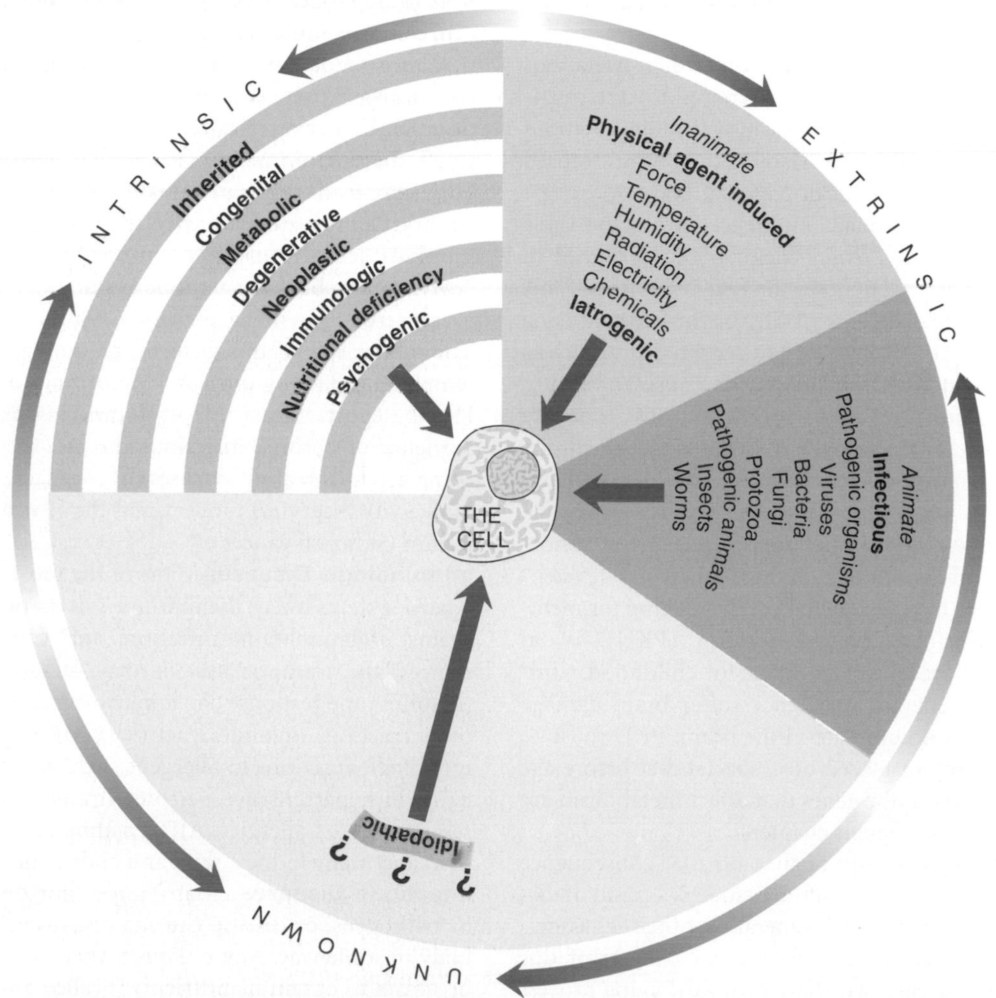

FIGURE 1-11 ■ Etiologic classification of disease. Illustrated here are the contributions of intrinsic, extrinsic, and unknown factors to disease causation.

Box 1-1

Etiologic Classification of Diseases

Inherited diseases
Congenital (inborn) diseases or birth defects
Metabolic diseases
Degenerative diseases
Neoplastic diseases
Immunologic diseases
Infectious diseases
Physical agent–induced diseases
Nutritional deficiency diseases
Iatrogenic diseases
Psychogenic diseases
Idiopathic diseases

Inherited Diseases. Altered or mutated genes can cause abnormal proteins to be made. These abnormal proteins often do not perform their intended function, resulting in the absence of an essential function. In other cases, such proteins may actually perform an abnormal, disruptive function. Either case poses a potential threat to the body's internal homeostasis.[14]

Most genetic mutations are lethal, but other mutations cause problems only when a person is exposed to certain environmental agents. Other mutations cause problems without any environmental contribution. Many abortions are caused by mutations induced by chemicals or radiation.

Congenital Diseases. Prenatal influences are responsible for most neonatal deaths. *Prenatal* denotes the period of in utero life, whereas *neonatal* denotes the first 2 months of life. During infancy, the first 2 years of life, birth defects arising from the pregnant mother's ingestion of certain drugs, such as thalidomide, or viral infection are major causes of death. These agents can deform the brain or other organs. There are also idiopathic congenital anomalies that can affect the heart, lung, or skin of the newborn—unrelated to ingestion of drugs or viral infection.

Metabolic Diseases. Metabolic diseases arise from abnormalities in the chemistry of the body. More than 100 deficiencies of vital enzymes have genetic bases.[15] Screening for metabolic disorders, such as phenylketonuria (PKU), is an important aspect of preventive medicine for childhood. Children with the PKU enzyme deficiency suffer brain damage when toxic chemicals accumulate in the brain. PKU must be diagnosed and the infant placed on a special diet before age 1 year.[16] Abnormalities in the genes that affect metabolism are further discussed in subsequent chapters.

Degenerative Diseases. Although a normal consequence of aging, degeneration of one or more tissues as a result of disease can occur at any time. The degeneration of tissues associated with aging is discussed in nearly every chapter of this book. Degenerative diseases associated with the aging process are increasing in frequency as persons are living beyond the fifth decade. Heart attacks and strokes combined account for more than half of all deaths in the United States.[17] Other degenerative diseases affect the musculoskeletal system including osteoarthritis and degenerative joint disease. Diseases affecting vital organs, including cirrhosis of the liver and emphysema of the lungs, cause chronic illness and numerous deaths.

Aging and degeneration have been linked to excessive caloric intake, radiation, the winding down of biological clocks, errors in gene function, and a loss of immunologic vigor. Most medicine practiced in the United States is conducted in hospitals and clinics that evaluate and treat individuals with degenerative diseases. The average life span in the United States of 75.4 years[17] is not likely to be extended much because degenerative and neoplastic diseases are difficult to prevent and cure.

Neoplastic Diseases. Neoplastic diseases (tumors), especially the malignant variety, are a menace. Cancers cause death when they spread from their site of origin. Generally, cancers are signaled by a lump, an increase in the size of an ulcer, loss of weight, anemia, or pain.

Of the deaths from cancer in 2003, approximately 50% were caused by a few common types involving the lung, stomach, colon-rectum, liver, and breast.[18]

Cancer probably arises from mutagenic agents such as chemicals, viruses, sunlight, irradiation, and chronic irritation. The clustering of cancer in selective geographic areas also implicates environmental factors as possible etiologic agents. For example, Burkitt's malignant lymphoma, a rare cancer, is confined almost exclusively to tropical Africa, where specific humidity, temperature, and altitude may provide an optimal environment. Burkitt's lymphoma is also associated with the presence of Epstein-Barr virus, a lymphotropic herpesvirus. The precise role of this virus in the development of Burkitt's lymphoma remains unclear.[19] According to a current World Health Report, at least 15% of all cancers worldwide are a consequence of chronic infectious disease, the most important being hepatitis B and C viruses (liver cancer), the human papilloma virus (cervical cancer), and the *Helicobacter pylori* bacterium (stomach cancer).[18]

Immunologic Diseases. One of the most extensively investigated systems today, the immune system provides protection against inflammation, infection, and cancer. In some instances, the immune system may attack one's own body (autoimmune response) or it may overreact (e.g., hypersensitivity reaction) or underreact (e.g., AIDS). Anaphylactic immunologic reactions to allergens such as bee venom could be lethal in hypersensitive persons. Immunologic reactions are responsible for allergies, AIDS, asthma, rheumatic heart disease, and many kidney, skin, and endocrine diseases.

Infectious Diseases. Many important diseases are caused by **pathogens,** or disease-causing organisms, that damage the body in some way. Any organism that lives in or on another organism to obtain its nutrients is called a *parasite.* The presence of microscopic or larger parasites may interfere with normal body functions of the host, causing disease. Besides para-

Table 1-1

Major Pathogenic Organisms

Organism	Description
Prions (proteinaceous infections particles)	Proteins that convert normal proteins of the nervous system into abnormal proteins, causing loss of nervous system function. The abnormal form of the protein may also be inherited. A newly discovered type of pathogen, not much is known about how the prion works to cause such diseases as bovine spongiform encephalopathy (BSE, "mad cow disease") or Creutzfeldt-Jakob disease (CJD).
Viruses	Intracellular parasites that consist of a DNA or RNA core surrounded by a protein coat and, sometimes, a lipoprotein envelope; they invade human cells and cause them to produce viral components
Bacteria	Tiny, primitive cells that lack nuclei; they cause infection by parasitizing tissues or otherwise disrupting normal function
Fungi	Simple organisms similar to plants but lacking the chlorophyll pigments that allow plants to make their own food; because they cannot make their own food, fungi must parasitize other tissues, including those of the human body
Protozoa	Protists, or one-celled organisms larger than bacteria whose DNA is organized into a nucleus; many types of protozoa parasitize human tissues
Pathogenic animals	Large multicellular organisms, such as insects and worms; such animals can parasitize human tissues, bite or sting, or otherwise disrupt normal body function

Data from Thibodeau GA, Patton KT: *Anatomy and physiology,* ed 5, St Louis, 2003, Mosby, p 29.

sites, organisms exist that poison or otherwise damage the human body to cause disease. Bioterrorism, food- and waterborne illness, and infection are becoming major threats to public safety. Some of the key pathogenic organisms are briefly described in Table 1-1. Figure 1-12 illustrates some of these pathogens.

Physical Agent–Induced Diseases. Agents such as toxic or destructive chemicals, extreme heat or cold, mechanical injury, and radiation can affect the body.[20] Violent injury (trauma) or death from mechanical, chemical, or physical agents are common among young people. Traffic accidents, homicide, suicide, and trauma from accidents at home, work, and war are examples. In addition, some genetically predisposed persons react adversely to certain drugs or chemicals.[21] Such persons may injure the skin, lungs, intestinal tract, liver, and kidneys from adverse drug reaction. The liver and kidneys are often damaged because these organs concentrate and excrete toxic drugs and chemicals.

Within the body, mechanical failures can occur. An intestinal loop can slip through a defect in the abdominal wall and become trapped. This is called a *hernia.* The intestine can also become twisted or telescoped within itself. Pain in the abdomen and urinary tract infection occur when a blood vessel or stricture blocks the flow of urine. Similarly, gallstones commonly form in the gallbladder; they can pass into the bile ducts and mechanically obstruct them, causing abdominal pain, nausea, and vomiting.

Nutritional Deficiency Diseases. Deficiencies in nutrients are responsible for many diseases. On a worldwide basis, deficiencies of proteins, calories, and vitamins are rampant; more than 300 million preschool-aged children are malnourished and vulnerable to infectious diseases.[18] In developing countries, tuberculosis and malnutrition are the most common causes of death. Also, deficiencies in vitamins or iodine may induce nutritional deficiency diseases.[18]

Iatrogenic Diseases. Many diseases are caused by a physician or health professional; such diseases are **iatrogenic** in origin. The first dictum of health care is to do no harm; violation of this dictum may result in iatrogenic disease. In 2000, a presidential task force labeled medical errors a "national problem of epidemic proportions." Members estimated that the "cost associated with these errors in lost income, disability, and health care costs is as much as $29 billion annually." That same year the Institute of Medicine released a historic report entitled "To err is human: building a safer health system." The report's authors concluded that 44,000 to 98,000 people die each year as a result of errors during hospitalization. They noted that "even when using the lower estimate, deaths due to medical errors exceed the number attributable to the 8th-leading cause of death." The addition of nonhospital errors may drive the numbers of errors and deaths much higher. As the authors note, the hospital data "offer only a very modest estimate of the magnitude of the problem since hospital patients represent only a small proportion of the total population at risk, and direct hospital costs are only a fraction of total costs."

Moreover, numerous drugs cause disease.[22] Historically, pregnant women threatened with spontaneous abortions were given the drug diethylstilbestrol. Approximately 20 to 25 years

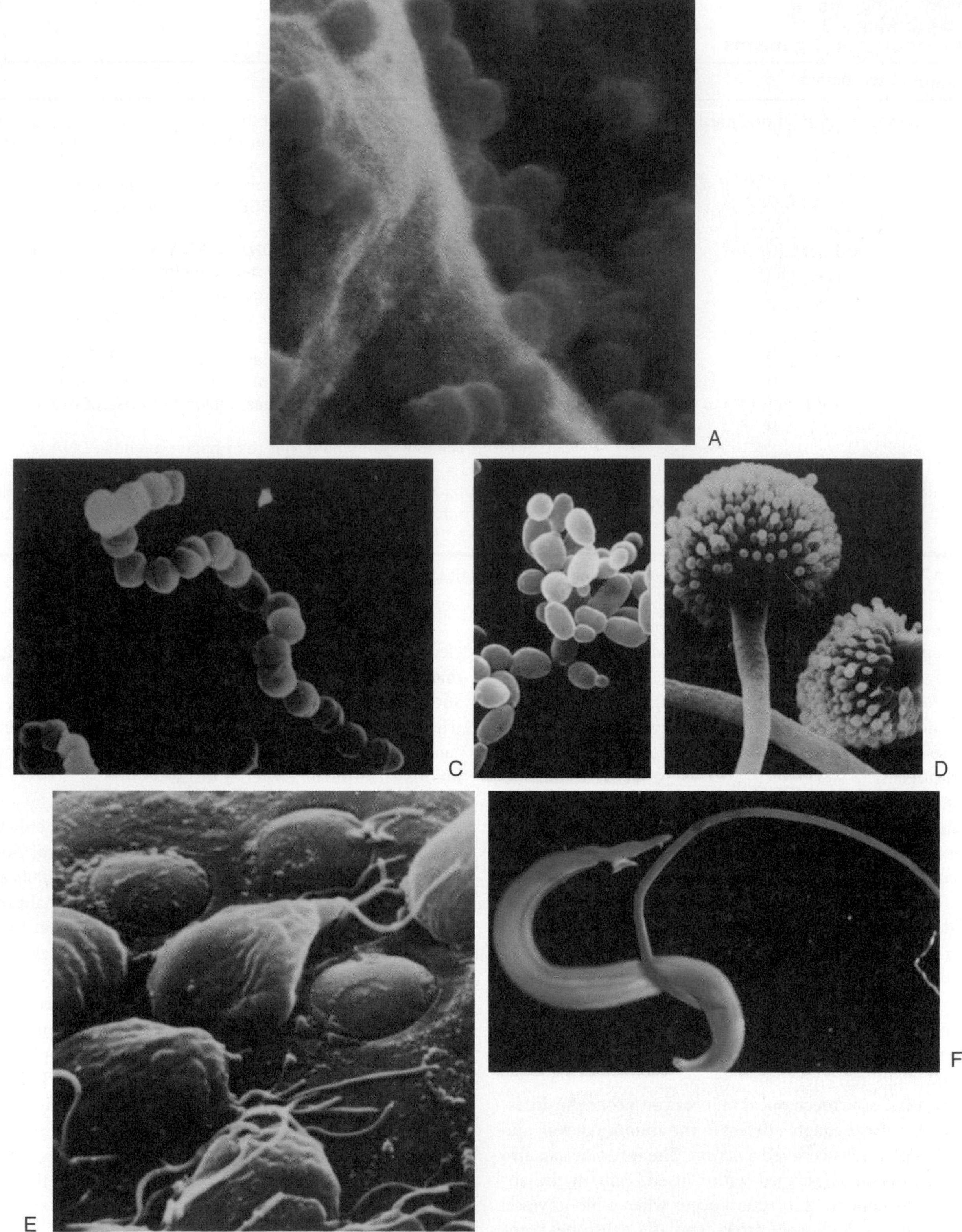

FIGURE 1-12 ■ Examples of pathogenic organisms. **A,** Viruses (the human immunodeficiency virus [HIV] that causes AIDS). **B,** Bacteria (*Streptococcus* bacteria that causes strep throat and other infections). **C,** Fungi (yeast cells that commonly infect the urinary and reproductive tracts). **D,** Fungi (the mold that causes aspergillosis). **E,** Protozoans (the flagellated cells that cause traveler's diarrhea). **F,** Pathogenic animals (the parasitic worms that cause snail fever). (**A** and **F,** From Thibodeau GA, Patton KT: *Anatomy and physiology,* ed 5, St Louis, 2003, Mosby. **B-D,** © Visuals Unlimited, Inc., Swanzey, NH. **E,** From Erlandsen SL, Magney J: *Color atlas of histology,* St Louis, 1992, Mosby.)

later, many young women born of these pregnancies developed vaginal cancer. A subcategory of drug-induced iatrogenic disease is growing in importance. Approximately 2% to 5% of hospitalized patients are ill because of a drug-induced disease.[18] Misuse of radiation by those not realizing its potential danger has resulted in the development of cancers of the liver, skin, thyroid gland, and blood.

Psychogenic Diseases. Psychogenic diseases are illnesses that appear to originate from emotional or mental causes rather than disease-causing organisms or other strictly physiologic entities. In addition, a variety of gastrointestinal disorders, such as peptic ulcer, ulcerative colitis, and spastic colon, may be aggravated by **psychogenic** or emotional factors. Some forms of asthma and dermatitis have important psychological components, explained in subsequent chapters. Psychogenic factors are extremely important in determining the course of certain diseases. Many diseases are encompassed by **psychosomatic medicine,** the discipline involving the physiologic impact of psychic stress on the emergence of disease.

According to a recent survey conducted by the Centers for Disease Control (CDC), from January through June 2003, 3.2% (95% CI = 2.8% to 3.5%) of adults aged 18 years and over experienced serious psychological distress during the past 30 days. The annual percentage of adults who experienced serious psychological distress during the past 30 days declined significantly from 3.3% in 1997 to 2.4% in 1999, and then increased from 2.4% in 1999 to 3.0% in 2002.

Idiopathic Diseases. The term *idiopathic* means "of undetermined cause." Although it is tempting to suggest that much is known about the etiologic development of disease, most diseases are idiopathic! Examples of diseases with unknown causes abound. One example is hypertension. Persistent elevation of blood pressure to greater than 140/90 mm Hg is a sign of underlying disease. Only 10% of persons with hypertension have an identifiable cause, termed **secondary hypertension.** Approximately 90% have no discernible cause for the disorder[23]; such individuals have **idiopathic hypertension.**

Pathogenesis

Pathogenesis refers to the development or evolution of a disease.[24] A description of the pathogenesis of a staphylococcal infection, for example, would include the *mechanisms* whereby invasion of the body by the pathogen ultimately led to the observed abnormalities. The study of pathogenesis—from the initial stimulus to the ultimate expression of the manifestations of the disease—remains one of the main domains of pathophysiology and is addressed for each disorder in subsequent chapters throughout the text.

It is difficult to characterize the mechanism of disease development in general terms because pathogenesis varies with the causative agent and with the type of cell, tissue, and organ affected. Nevertheless, some common manifestations of the immediate response to injury include depression and/or stimulation of cells. Stimulation of cells is expressed as increased metabolism and, frequently, an increase in the size or number of cells. Stimulation, also expressed as hyperfunction, may be shown by increased secretion (e.g., excessive mucus production) or by an increase in a mechanical function (e.g., muscle spasm). Depression, by comparison, is expressed as decreased metabolism, hypofunction, or a reduction in the size or number of cells. The type and degree of response are determined by the specific causative agent and its virulence; the quality, quantity, and duration of exposure; and the unique characteristics of the affected cells, tissues, and organs. Following the immediate action, the counteraction is almost always complex and indirect. It is the result of many combined factors acting over a period of time.

Consider, for example, a severe bacterial infection causing an abscess in a tooth. First, local invasion of cells by the bacteria and their products takes place, and an immediate direct action is expressed as cellular degeneration. Then changes occur in circulation and vascular permeability, which are important in development of the inflammatory process. Connective tissue also has a role. After this, mixed responses develop—depression and stimulation of cells, with repercussions that go far beyond the local area of infection and inflammation. These reactions include fever, an increased white blood cell count, accelerated heart rate, accelerated respiratory rate, and altered blood chemical constituents. Widespread morphologic effects occur as well: hyperplasia of the spleen, lymph nodes, and bone marrow; and cellular changes in the liver, kidneys, and heart. Refer to Unit III for an in-depth look at the processes of infection, inflammation, and immunity.

Consider high blood pressure as another example. As a result of a causative agent, mechanisms produce spasms of arterioles throughout the body, which results in increased resistance to arterial blood flow. The left ventricle of the heart responds to the stress of an increased workload, first by slight dilation, then by increased forcefulness of the heartbeat. This counteracts the increased peripheral resistance and restores circulation to normal—a homeostatic mechanism. If the stress increases, the complex pattern of counteraction will develop further, and it is likely that a failure of adaptation will occur—a gross break in the constantly shifting balance to maintain stability (hypertension)—and heart failure may result. This brings a variety of manifestations such as epigastric tenderness and abdominal discomfort (from congestion of the liver, spleen, and intestines), dyspnea (difficult, labored breathing, from pulmonary venous congestion), edematous swelling of the feet and ankles (from increased capillary filtration pressure and sodium retention), and a host of other functional, chemical, and structural changes. Units IV and V provide the background for understanding the complexities of altered cardiac function. All of this action and counteraction, a dynamic, ever-changing process, describes the pathogenesis of disease.

Factors Affecting Pathogenesis

Some of the factors that influence pathogenesis include time, quantity, location, and morphologic changes.

Time. In the case of an infectious disease, the length of *time* for which the body is invaded by a pathogen has an important effect on the reaction, qualitatively as well as quantitatively. The time at which a diseased patient is examined influences what one sees to such an extent that different stages of a disease often appear quite unrelated unless the succession of events that led from one stage to the next in time is appreciated. One must always ask the questions, "Is the disease in its early or late stages?" and "Is the process acute or chronic?"

Quantity. *Quantity* is often as important in invasion, action, and counteraction as quality. "How much?" may be the crucial question, even more important than "What?" Although it is often difficult to precisely measure bodily reactions or tissue lesions, in the case of tissue trauma, one can give at least a semiquantitative indication by using such terms as *slight, moderate,* or *marked.* Furthermore, the *virulence* or strength of the pathogen—as in the case of infectious disease—may be measured by its ability to induce serious disease.[25]

Location. The *location* of invasion and reaction is also of great importance. An invasion, such as by a tumor, that is trivial in one part of the body (e.g., a benign skin tag) may be lethal in another (e.g., an inoperable brain tumor). Furthermore, different cells have their own peculiar patterns of reaction.

Morphologic Changes. *Morphologic changes* refer to the structural and associated functional alterations in cells or tissues that are either characteristic of the disease or diagnostic of the etiologic process.[26] The cell is the structural unit of the body, and the significance of cellular abnormality in disease can hardly be overemphasized.

Clinical Manifestations

Signs and Symptoms

As certain biological processes are encroached upon, the person begins to feel subjectively that something is wrong. These subjective feelings are termed **symptoms** of disease. By definition, symptoms are subjective and can only be reported by the affected individual to an observer. However, manifestations of the disease that involve objectively identifiable aberrations are termed **signs** of disease. Nausea, malaise, and pain are symptoms, whereas fever, reddening of the skin, and a palpable mass are signs. Although signs and symptoms are distinct terms, they are often used interchangeably.

A **syndrome** is a collection of different signs and symptoms that occur together.

A demonstrable structural change produced in the course of a disease is referred to as a **lesion.** Lesions may be evident at a gross or microscopic level.

Stages

Early in the development of a disease, the etiologic agent or agents may provoke a number of changes in biological processes that can be detected by laboratory analysis, although no recognition of these changes by the patient has occurred. Thus, many diseases progress through several stages. The interval between exposure of a tissue to an injurious agent and the first appearance of signs and symptoms may be called a *latent period* or, in the case of infectious diseases, an *incubation period.* The *prodromal* period, or *prodrome,* refers to the appearance of the first signs and symptoms indicating the onset of a disease. Prodromal symptoms often are nonspecific, such as headache, malaise, anorexia, and nausea. During the *stage of manifest illness,* or the *acute phase,* the disease reaches its full intensity, and signs and symptoms attain their greatest severity. Sometimes during the course of a disease, the signs and symptoms may become mild or even disappear for a time. This interval may be called a *silent period* or *latent period.* For example, in the total-body irradiation syndrome, a latent period may occur between the prodrome and the stage of manifest illness. Another example is syphilis, which may have two latent periods: one occurring between the primary and secondary stages and another occurring between the secondary and tertiary stages.

A number of diseases have a *subclinical* stage during which the patient functions normally although the disease processes are well established. It is important to understand that the structure and function of many organs provide a large reserve or safety margin, so that functional impairment may become evident only when disease has become quite advanced anatomically. For example, chronic renal disease can completely destroy one kidney and partly destroy the other before any symptoms related to decreased renal function are perceived. Therefore, health care professionals should be especially sensitive to the fact that many of their patients do not exhibit any indication of illness despite having quite established or advanced disease.

Some diseases (e.g., some types of leukemia) follow a course of alternating exacerbations and remissions. An **exacerbation** is a relatively sudden increase in the severity of a disease or any of its signs and symptoms. A **remission** is an abatement or decline in severity of the signs and symptoms of a disease. If a remission is permanent, we say that the person is *cured.*

Convalescence is the stage of recovery after a disease, injury, or surgical operation. Occasionally a disease produces aftereffects. A condition caused by and following a disease is called a **sequela** (plural: **sequelae**). For example, the sequela of an inflammatory process in a given tissue might be scarring in that tissue. The sequelae of acute rheumatic inflammation of the heart might be scarring and deformation of cardiac valves. A **complication** of disease is a new or separate process that may arise secondarily because of some change produced by the original entity. For example, bacterial pneumonia may be a complication of viral infection of the respiratory tract.

Acute or Chronic Disease

Disease processes are often classified as acute or chronic. An **acute** condition has relatively severe manifestations but runs a short course. A **chronic** condition lasts for a long time. Sometimes chronic disease processes begin with an acute phase and become prolonged when the body's defenses are insufficient to overcome the causative agent or stressor. In other cases, chronic conditions develop insidiously and never have an acute phase. An **intercurrent** condition is one that occurs during the course of an existing disease.

KEY CONCEPTS

- Pathophysiologic processes are generally studied by examining etiologic factors, pathogenesis, and clinical manifestations.
- Etiology refers to study of the proposed cause or causes of a particular physiopathologic process. Etiology is a complex notion because most diseases are multifactorial, resulting from interplay between genetic constitution and environmental influences.
- Pathogenesis refers to the proposed mechanisms whereby a disease or disorder leads to typically observed clinical manifestations. Pathogenesis describes the direct effects of a particular disorder as well as the usual physiologic responses and compensatory mechanisms.
- Clinical manifestations describe the signs and symptoms that typically accompany a particular pathophysiologic process. Manifestations may vary depending on the stage of the disorder, individual variation, and acuity or chronicity.

CONCEPTS OF EPIDEMIOLOGY

Differences among *individuals* are, of course, very important in determining the diseases to which they are susceptible and their reactions to the diseases once contracted. But **epidemiology**, or the study of *patterns of disease* involving aggregates of people, provides yet another important dimension (Figure 1-13). Information may be gained by examining the occurrence, incidence, prevalence, transmission, and distribution of diseases in large groups of people or populations.

A disease that is native to a local region is called an endemic disease. If the disease spreads to many individuals at the same time, the situation is called an **epidemic. Pandemics** are epidemics that affect *large geographic* regions, perhaps spreading *worldwide.* Because of the speed and availability of human travel around the world, pandemics are more common than they once were. Almost every flu season, a new strain of influenza virus quickly spreads from one continent to another.

Factors Affecting Patterns of Disease

Principal factors affecting patterns of disease in human populations include the following: (1) age (i.e., time in the life cycle), (2) ethnic group, (3) gender, (4) socioeconomic factors and lifestyle considerations, and (5) geographic location.

Age

In one sense, life is entirely different during the 9 months of gestation. The structures and functions of tissues are different: they are primarily dedicated to differentiation, development, and growth. Certainly the environment is different; the individual is protected from the light of day, provided with predigested food (even preoxygenated blood), suspended in a fluid buffer, and maintained at incubator temperature. This is fortunate because the developing embryo or fetus has relatively few homeostatic mechanisms to protect it from environmental change. The factors that produce disease in utero are discussed in Unit II. Diseases that arise during the postuterine period of life and affect the neonate include immaturity, respiratory failure, birth injuries, congenital malformations, nutritional problems, metabolic errors, and infections. These conditions are discussed in separate chapters.

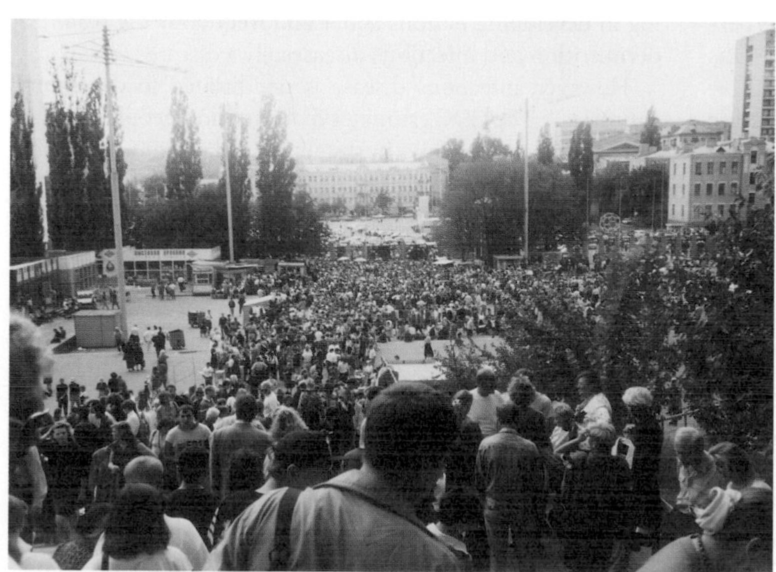

FIGURE 1-13 ■ The aggregate focus in disease: crowds at a public market in Russia.

Accidents, including poisoning, take their toll in childhood. Infections in children reflect their increased susceptibility to agents of disease. Consideration of other childhood diseases is addressed in each chapter as appropriate. The study of childhood processes and of changes that occur in this period of life is the domain of pediatrics; specific diseases that occur during maturity (age 15 to 60 years) are the primary emphasis of this text.

The term **atrophy** is used to describe the wasting effects of age. In addition to structural atrophy, the functioning of many physiologic control mechanisms also decreases and becomes less precise as age advances.

The changes in function that occur during the early years of life are termed *developmental processes.* Those that occur during maturity and postmaturity (age 60 years and beyond) are called *aging processes.* The study of aging processes and other changes that occur during this period of life is called *gerontology.* The effects of aging on selected body systems are so important physiologically that they receive separate consideration throughout the text. The immune, cardiac, respiratory, musculoskeletal, neurologic, special sensory, endocrine, gastrointestinal, and integumentary systems are all affected by the process of aging.

Ethnic Group

It is difficult to differentiate sharply between the effects of ethnicity on patterns of disease and the socioeconomic factors, religious practices, customs, and geographic considerations with which ethnicity is inseparably bound. For example, carcinoma of the penis is virtually unknown among Jews and Moslems who practice circumcision at an early age (avoiding the carcinogenic stimulus that comes from accumulation of smegma about the glans penis).

However, comparisons reveal significant differences in occurrence of certain disease states in ethnic groups that seem to be more closely related to genetic predisposition than to environmental factors. For example, sickle cell anemia has a much higher rate of occurrence in African populations, whereas pernicious anemia occurs more frequently among Scandinavians and is rare among black populations worldwide.

The study of racial and ethnic group variation in disease states is the domain of medical anthropology. Volumes have been written about disease-specific differences that relate to racial or ethnic group differences. In clinical practice, recognition of diversity in disease risk by racial or ethnic group is useful in disease diagnosis, prevention, and management. Ethnic group–specific differences, where important, are presented in individual chapters.

Gender

Particular diseases of the genital system obviously show important differences between the sexes; men do not have endometriosis nor do women have hyperplasia of the prostate, and carcinoma of the breast is more common in women than in men. Pyelonephritis is more common in young women than in men of comparable age (before they develop prostatic hyperplasia) because the external urethral orifice of women is more readily contaminated, and bacteria can more easily travel up a short urethra than a long one. Less obviously related to the reproductive system, the onset of severe atherosclerosis in women is delayed some 20 years or so over that in men, presumably because of the protective action of estrogenic hormone.

There are also gender-specific factors that defy explanation.[27] For example, systemic lupus erythematosus is much more common in women.[28] Toxic goiter and hypothyroidism are also more common in women.[29] Rheumatoid arthritis is more common in women, but osteoarthritis affects men and women with equal frequency.[30] Thromboangiitis obliterans (a chronic, recurring inflammatory peripheral vascular disease) occurs more commonly in men.[25] Gender differences in predisposition to cancer and other diseases are presented throughout the text.

Socioeconomic Factors and Lifestyle Considerations

The environment and the political climate of countries determine how people live and the health problems that are likely to ensue. The importance of poverty, malnutrition, overcrowding, and exposure to adverse environmental conditions, such as extremes of temperature, is obvious. Volumes have been written about the effects of socioeconomic status on disease. Sociologists study the influence of these factors. Social class influences education and also the type of occupation a person is likely to have.

Disease is related to occupational exposure to such agents as coal dust, noise, or extreme stress.[31] Closely related to socioeconomic factors are lifestyle considerations. People living in the United States, for example, consume too much food, alcohol, and tobacco and do not exercise enough. Childhood obesity is a problem in the United States. Arteriosclerosis; cancer; diseases of the kidney, liver, and lungs; and accidents cause most deaths in the United States. By contrast, people living in developing nations suffer and frequently die from undernutrition and infectious diseases.

However, infectious disease is not limited to developing countries.[32] The CDC estimates that 2 million people annually acquire infections while hospitalized and 90,000 people die from those infections. More than 70% of hospital-acquired infections have become resistant to at least one of the drugs commonly used to manage them, largely due to the overprescribing of antibiotics by physicians.[22] *Staphylococcus,* the leading cause of hospital infections, is now resistant to 95% of first-choice antibiotics and 30% of second-choice antibiotics. Poor staff hygiene is considered the leading source for infections acquired during hospitalizations. However, efforts to get medical workers to improve safety through means as simple as more frequent and thorough hand washing have met with only modest success.

The incidence of many parasitic diseases is closely tied to socioeconomic factors and lifestyle considerations. Worm in-

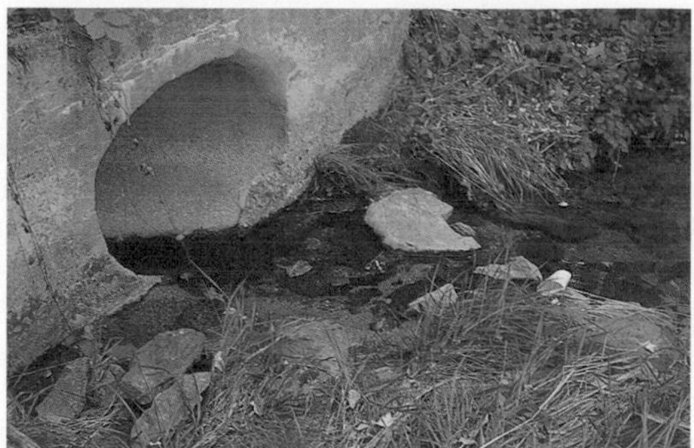

FIGURE 1-14 ■ Risk factors in the development of schistosomiasis include the widespread use of irrigation ditches that harbor the intermediate snail host. (Photographed by Therese A. Capal, Rockville, Md.)

fections, for example, are related to the use of human feces as fertilizer. In some areas, such as Africa and tropical America, the frequency of schistosomiasis (a parasitic infestation by blood flukes) is tied directly to the widespread use of irrigation ditches that harbor the intermediate snail host.[33] The fact that children play in the ditches or that clothes are washed there gives adequate opportunity for human infection (Figure 1-14).

Trichinosis (a disease caused by the ingestion of *Trichinella spiralis*) comes almost entirely from eating inadequately cooked, infected pork. People who are fond of raw meat and inadequately cooked sausage are at highest risk.

Education is often very effective in changing lifestyle patterns that contribute to disease. In Tokyo, for example, mass public education about minimizing the use of sodium—a common ingredient in most traditional Japanese cooking—has been effective in changing current dietary practices and thus affecting the control of hypertension.

Examples of educational efforts directed at lifestyle modification in the United States are numerous.[34-36] Antidrug, antismoking, and profitness messages fill the media and are prevalent on the Internet. Choosing healthy alternatives to unhealthy ones is made easier through positive peer pressure and support groups.

Geographic Location

Patterns of disease vary greatly by geographic location. Certainly there is considerable overlap with ethnicity, socioeconomic factors, and lifestyle choices, but physical environment is also an important aspect. Obviously, frostbite in Antarctica and dehydration in the Sahara are examples of disorders that are more prevalent in specific geographic settings. But important patterns of disease occur within individual countries. For example, the incidence and kind of malnutrition vary tremendously by geographic region.

Many diseases have a geographic pattern for reasons that are clear. For example, malaria, an acute and sometimes chronic infectious disease due to the presence of protozoan parasites within red blood cells, is transmitted to humans by the bite of an infected female *Anopheles* mosquito. The *Anopheles* mosquito can live only in certain regions of the world (Figure 1-15).[37]

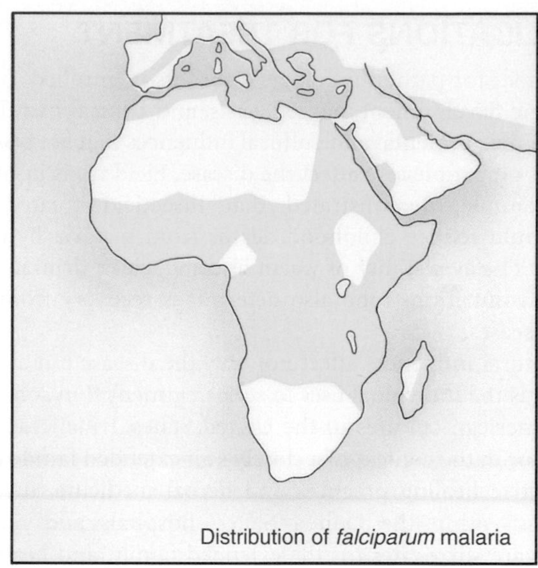

FIGURE 1-15 ■ Geographic distribution of malaria. (From Thibodeau GA, Patton KT: *Anatomy and physiology,* ed 5, St Louis, 2003, Mosby, p 973.)

Fungal diseases are more common and more serious in hot, humid regions. But some infectious diseases are highly limited geographically for reasons that are not well understood. For example, bartonellosis, which is also called Carrión disease, is found only in Peru, Ecuador, Chile, and Colombia.[25] This disease resembles malaria superficially in that the minute rickettsia-like organisms invade erythrocytes and destroy them. Humans are infected by the bite of the sand fly. Although conditions in other parts of the world should be favorable for this disease, it remains limited geographically.

Taking a world view, there is widespread recognition of the importance of geographic factors in influencing human disease.[38] The World Health Organization (WHO) and the National Institutes of Health (NIH) have been deeply concerned with geographic problems in disease. Consult WHO and NIH home pages on the World Wide Web for additional information. (Web locations are provided on the Evolve site.)

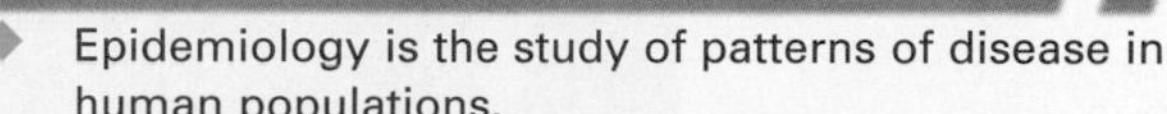

KEY CONCEPTS

- Epidemiology is the study of patterns of disease in human populations.
- Age, ethnicity, gender, lifestyle, socioeconomic status, and geographic location are epidemiologic variables that influence the occurrence and transmission of disease.
- Understanding the epidemiologic aspects of a disease is essential for effective prevention.

IMPLICATIONS FOR TREATMENT

Treatment for pathophysiologic disorders is "implied" by the etiologic development, pathogenesis, and clinical manifestations. Environmental and cultural influences that are brought to bear on people also affect the disease. Field trials in Africa, for example, demonstrated that insecticide-treated bed nets could reduce childhood deaths from malaria by up to 35%.[18] The availability of warm housing, clean drinking water, and nutritious food also determines recovery from certain diseases.

Cultural influences affect not only the disease but also the methods the individual uses to seek treatment.[39] In some Native American cultures in the United States, tribal elders are cared for in the context of a closely knit extended family using alternative healing practices and herbal medicine. In other cultures within the United States, hospitals and nursing homes are surrogates for the extended family, and healing is practiced exclusively within the context of traditional Western medicine.

Levels of Prevention

Prevention of ill health is too narrow to be the goal of health care. What is needed instead is some notion of positive health or physical "wholeness" that extends beyond the absence of ill health. WHO defines health as complete physical, mental, and social well-being, and not merely the absence of disease or infirmity.[40] For some individuals, health implies the ability to do what they regard as worthwhile and to conduct their lives as they want. Aging and ill health are not synonymous, and many elders enjoy excellent health, even in the face of chronic disease (Figure 1-16).

Epidemiologists suggest that treatment implications fall into categories called *levels of prevention*. There are three levels of prevention: primary, secondary, and tertiary. **Primary prevention** is prevention of disease by altering susceptibility or reducing exposure for susceptible individuals. **Secondary prevention** (applicable in early disease, i.e., preclinical and clinical stages) is the early detection, screening, and management of the disease. **Tertiary prevention** (appropriate in the stage of advanced disease or disability) includes rehabilitative and supportive care and attempts to alleviate disability and restore effective functioning.[41]

Primary Prevention. Prolongation of life has resulted largely from decreased mortality from infectious disease. Primary prevention in terms of improved nutrition, economy, housing, and sanitation of persons living in developed countries is also responsible for increased longevity. Certain childhood diseases—measles, poliomyelitis, pertussis (whooping cough), and neonatal tetanus—are decreasing, owing to a rapid increase in coverage by immunization programs. More than 120 million children younger than 5 years in India were immunized against poliomyelitis in a single day in 1996.[18] Globally, coverage of children immunized against six major childhood diseases increased from 5% in 1974 to 80% in 1995.[18] In 1985, Rotary International launched the PolioPlus program to protect children worldwide from the cruel and fatal consequences of polio. In 1988, the World Health Assembly challenged the world to eradicate polio. Since that time, Rotary's efforts and those of partner agencies, including the WHO, the United Nations Children's Fund, the CDC, and

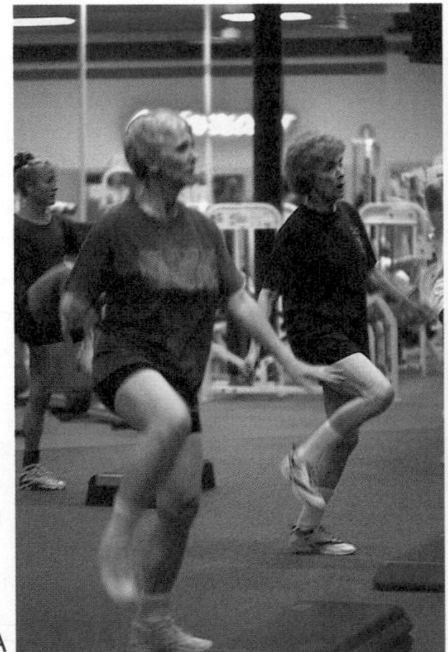

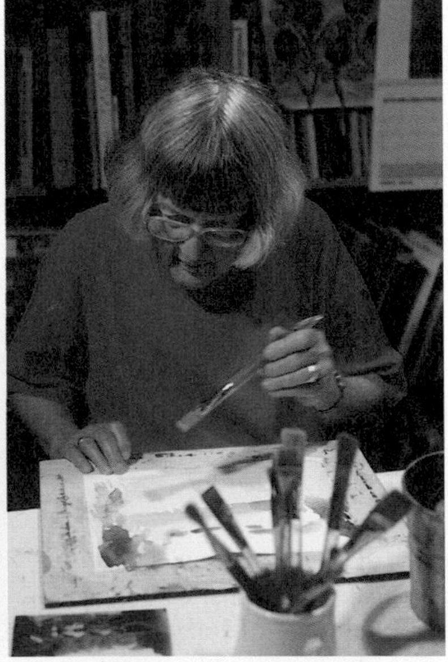

FIGURE 1-16 ■ Healthy aging: elders exercising in an aerobics class **(A)** and painting **(B)** illustrate the concept that aging and disease are not synonymous. The artist, a healthy woman in her mid-70s, is also a breast cancer survivor. (Photographed by Therese A. Capal, Rockville, Md.)

governments around the world, have achieved a 99% reduction in the number of polio cases worldwide. The PolioPlus program has been enormously successful; the goal is celebration of global eradication of polio in 2005.

Cardiovascular diseases in developed countries (except those in Eastern Europe) are on the wane, thanks to the spread of health education and promotion. Infant and child mortality rates and the overall death rate are continuing to decrease globally.

High school education programs about abstinence from sex and ways to say no to drugs, alcohol, and tobacco are other examples of primary prevention making a difference in the lives of people. Primary prevention also includes adherence to safety precautions, such as wearing seat belts, observing the posted speed limit on highways, and taking precautions in the use of chemicals and machinery. Violent crimes involving dangerous weapons must be stopped to prevent traumatic or fatal injuries.

Environmental pollutants poison the organs. Some experts fear an epidemic of cancer due to carcinogenic chemicals blighting the environment.[42] Public health measures to ensure clean food, air, and water prevent many diseases, including cancer. As air, water, and soil quality is improved, the risk of exposure to harmful carcinogens is minimized.

Secondary Prevention. Yearly physical examinations can lead to the early diagnosis of disease and, in some cases, cures. The routine use of Papanicolaou (Pap) smears has led to a decline in the incidence of invasive cancer of the uterine cervix.[43] Also, more women are examining their own breasts monthly for cancer; thus earlier diagnoses are achieved.

Prenatal diagnosis of certain genetic diseases is possible. New diagnostic laboratory techniques provide definitive information for the genetic counseling of parents. This information can aid in predicting chances of involvement or noninvolvement of offspring for a given genetic disorder (e.g., Down syndrome). One technique, *amniocentesis,* consists of removing a small amount of fluid from the amniotic sac that surrounds the fetus and analyzing the cells and chemicals in the fluid. Blood samples can also be obtained from the fetus by amniocentesis; the amniotic fluid and fetal blood are then studied for defects in enzymes, to determine sex, and to measure substances associated with defects in the spinal cord and brain.

Tertiary Prevention. Once a disease becomes established, treatment—within the context of traditional Western medicine—generally falls into one of the following two major categories: medical (including such measures as physical therapy, pharmacotherapy, psychotherapy, radiation therapy, chemotherapy, immunotherapy, and experimental gene therapy) and surgical. Numerous other subspecialties of medicine and surgery have also evolved to focus on a given organ or technique. In a clinical setting, a large array of professional caregivers provide rehabilitative and supportive services to the diseased individual. Every professional brings the perspective of his or her discipline to the caregiving situation. Each makes clinical judgments about the patient's needs and problems and decides which goals and intervention strategies are most beneficial.

KEY CONCEPTS

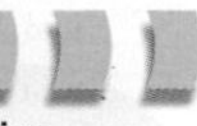

- Treatment for pathophysiologic disorders is "implied" by the etiologic development, pathogenesis, and clinical manifestations.
- Prevention is more desirable than treatment.
- Education, regular examinations and immunizations, and lifestyle management are important factors for all levels of prevention.

SUMMARY

Most people recognize what it is to be healthy and would define disease or illness as a change from or absence of that state. Under closer scrutiny, the concept of health is difficult to describe in simple, succinct terms. Correspondingly, the concepts of disease and illness are also complex. Environment, genetic constitution, socioeconomic status, lifestyle, and previous physical health all affect the timing and ultimate expression of disease.

Within the context of physical, mental, and social facets of ill health, two major concepts govern our understanding of disease and illness: disease and illness distort normal life processes and disrupt homeostasis. In the future, it is likely that more energy will be directed to the homeostatic aspects of health with the goal of preventing or at least recognizing disease and controlling its incipient forms before the body's autoregulative mechanisms are stretched to the breaking point. Until then, there is still much to learn about the pathophysiology of manifest disease, which all too often runs a fatal course because it is not fully understood.

MEDIA RESOURCES

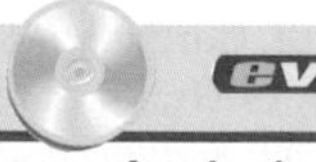

evolve

Remember to check out the ***CD Companion*** included with this book for Review Questions, Key Concepts Review, Glossary (with audio for selected terms), Disease Profiles, and Animations.

PLUS, visit the ***Evolve website*** at http://evolve.elsevier.com/Copstead/ for Case Studies, Disease Profiles, and WebLinks.

References

1. Tietz NW: *Clinical guide to laboratory tests,* ed 4, Philadelphia, 2004, Saunders.
2. Lieu PT et al: The roles of iron in health and disease, *Mol Aspects Med* 22(1-2):1-87, 2001.
3. Woods SC, Gotah K, Clegg DJ: Gender differences in the control of energy homeostasis, *Exp Biol Med* 228(10):1175-1180, 2003.

4. Weissbluth M, Davis AT, Poncher J: Night waking, sleep-wake organization, and self-soothing in the first year of life, *J Dev Behav Pediatr* 22(4):226-233, 2001.
5. Scher A: Attachment and sleep: a study of night waking in 12-month old infants, *Dev Psychobiol* 38(4):274-285, 2001.
6. Lipson JG, Dibble SL, Minarik PA, editors: *Culture and nursing care: a pocket guide,* San Francisco, 1996, UCSF Nursing Press.
7. Bendelow G et al, editors: *Gender, health, and healing: the public/private divide,* London, 2002, Routledge.
8. Schobersberger W et al: The effects of moderate altitude (1,700 m) on cardiovascular and metabolic variables in patients with metabolic syndrome, *Eur J Appl Physiol* 88(6):506-514, 2003.
9. Ticher A et al: Human circadian time structure in subjects of different gender and age, *Chronobiol Int* 11(6):349-355, 1994.
10. Redfern P, Minors D, Waterhouse J: Circadian rhythms, jet lag and chronobiotics: an overview, *Chronobiol Int* 11(4):253-265, 1994.
11. Layng TV: Causation and complexity: old lessons, new crusades, *J Behav Ther Exp Psychiatry* 26(3):179-190, 1995.
12. Feldman SD, Tauber AI: Sickle cell anemia: reexamining the first "molecular disease," *Bull Hist Med* 71(4):623-650, 1997.
13. Herlihy B, Maebius NK: *The human body in health and illness,* ed 2, Philadelphia, 2003, Saunders.
14. Scriver CR: Realities and virtual realities of inborn errors of metabolism: biochemical genetics in the molecular genetic era, *Am J Med Genet* 69(1):1-6, 1997.
15. Hommes FA: Quality control for selective screening of inborn errors of metabolism, *Eur J Pediatr* 153(7 suppl 1):S17-S22, 1994.
16. Scriver CR et al, editors: *The metabolic and molecular basis of inherited disease,* ed 8, vol 1, New York, 2001, McGraw-Hill.
17. National Center for Health Statistics: Deaths–leading causes, website: http://www.cdc.gov.nchs.fastats.lcod.htm.
18. World Health Organization, website: http://www.who.itn/en/.
19. Yarbro CH: *Cancer nursing: principles and practice,* Sudbury, Mass, 2000, Jones & Bartlett.
20. Dixit SN, Bushara DO, Brooks BR: Epidemic heatstroke in a Midwest community: risk factors, neurological complications, and sequelae, *Wis Med J* 96(5):39-41, 1997.
21. Kohn LT, Corrigan JM, Donaldson MS, editors: Committee on Quality of Health Care in America, Institute of Medicine: *To err is human: building a safer health system,* Washington, DC, 2000, National Academy Press, pp 1-48.
22. Sartin J et al: Medical management issues surrounding community-acquired pneumonia in adults, *Gundersen Lutheran Med Found J* 1(2):6-9, 2003.
23. Perry HM Jr, Miller JP: Difficulties in diagnosing hypertension: implications and alternatives, *J Hypertens* 10:88-97, 1992.
24. National Center for Biotechnology Information, website: http://www.ncbi.nlm.nih.gov/omim/.
25. *Dorland's illustrated medical dictionary,* ed 29, Philadelphia, 2000, Saunders.
26. O'Toole MT, editor: *Miller-Keane encyclopedia and dictionary of medicine, nursing, and allied health,* ed 7, Philadelphia, 2003, Saunders.
27. Young RF, Kahena E: Gender, recovery from late life heart attack, and medical care, *Women Health* 20(1):11-31, 1993.
28. Robinson DR: Systemic lupus erythematosus. In Dale DC, Federman DD, editors: *Scientific American medicine,* New York, 1996, Scientific American, pp 1-17.
29. Federman DD: Thyroid. In Dale DC, Federman DD, editors: *Scientific American medicine,* New York, 1997, Scientific American, pp 1-22.
30. Klippel JH: *Primer on the rheumatic diseases,* ed 12, Atlanta, 2001, Arthritis Foundation, pp 86-93, 184-190.
31. McGregor D: Industrial chemical and human cancer, *Biotherapy* 11(2-3):181-188, 1998.
32. Moore M, Onorato IM, McCray E, Castro KG: Trends in drug-resistant tuberculosis in the United States, 1993-1996, *JAMA* 278(10):833-837, 1997.
33. World Health Organization: Tropical diseases research, website: http://www.who.int/en/.
34. Novotny TE et al: The public health practice of tobacco control: lessons learned and directions for the states in the 1990s, *Annu Rev Public Health* 13:287-318, 1992.
35. Winslow E et al: Lifestyle modification: weight control, exercise, and smoking cessation, *Am J Med* 101(4A):25S-33S, 1996.
36. Bartfay WJ, Bartfay E: Promoting health in schools through a board game, *West J Nurs Res* 16(4):438-446, 1994.
37. World Health Organization: World malaria situation, website: http://www.who.int/en/.
38. Smith MN, Whitney GM: Caring for the environment: the ecology of health. In Chinn P, editor: *Anthology on caring,* New York, 1991, National League for Nursing Press, pp 59-69.
39. Borkan JM, Neher JO: A developmental model of ethnosensitivity in family practice training, *Fam Med* 23:212-217, 1991.
40. World Health Organization, website: http://www.who.int/en/.
41. Jekel JF: *Epidemiology, biostatistics, and preventive medicine,* Philadelphia, 2001, Saunders.
42. Dockery DW et al: An association between air pollution and mortality in six U.S. cities, *N Engl J Med* 329:1753-1759, 1993.
43. American Cancer Society: ACS cancer detection guidelines: cervical cancer, website: http://www.cancer.org/docroot/PED/content/PED_2_3X_ACS_Cancer_Detection_Guidelines_36.asp?sitearea=PED.

chapter 2

Stress, Adaptation, and Coping

Linda Denise Oakley

MEDIA RESOURCES

Additional Material for Study, Review, and Further Exploration

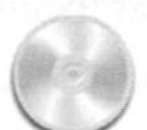

CD Companion ◆ Review Questions and Answers ◆ Key Concepts Review
◆ Glossary *(with audio pronunciations for selected terms)*
◆ Disease Profiles ◆ Animations

evolve ***Website*** at http://evolve.elsevier.com/Copstead/
◆ Case Studies ◆ Disease Profiles ◆ WebLinks

KEY QUESTIONS

- What are the links between the stress response and the development of disease?
- What are the key features of the Selye general adaptation syndrome?
- How are the neuroendocrine and immune systems and stress response related?
- How is the stress response influenced by age, gender, culture, and ethnicity?
- How is genetic background related to the stress response?

CHAPTER OUTLINE

One fundamental principle of human biology is that in order to survive humans must adapt biologically to their environment. The human organism maintains highly complex biological interactions with the environment, and these interactions can play key roles in the etiologic progression of disease. Researchers have linked a wide range of both physical and psychological health problems to the biological systems that support human adaptation.

Every day many people face potentially overwhelming environmental stressors such as isolation, overcrowding, competition, noise, dirt, pollution, and infectious organisms. Environmental stressors such as these challenge human adaptation. Through their own experiences, people become familiar with the health effects of their environments and their environmental stressors. Everyone experiences some degree of this stress most of the time. And stress is not always detrimental to health. Healthy stress is vital and necessary. For example, the physical stress of physical activity and exercise, such as walking or running, stimulates the bone osteoblastic activity and calcification needed to promote bone density, shape, and strength. Healthy stress also increases mental and physical alertness and enhances performance and productivity. Healthy stress, such as the stress of completing a demanding yet rewarding task, is likely to be perceived as pleasant, positive, or exciting. In short, stress, particularly environmental adaptation stress, is a part of life.

Stress is a dynamic state. Psychological, sociocultural, and environmental stressors produce biological responses; biological stressors produce psychological, sociocultural, and environmental responses. Although much has been learned about the dynamic biological systems and human-environment interactions involved, stress is personal. No two people respond alike, and individual stress responses change with time and changes in circumstances. This chapter provides a historical review of stress and homeostasis and a description of stress biology.

HOMEOSTASIS AND STRESS

Homeostasis is a state of equilibrium that is maintained by a dynamic process of feedback and regulation. Homeostasis represents an interaction between catabolism and anabolism; a process of constant change in both positive and negative directions. Because organisms are constantly disturbed, challenged, or threatened by internal and external forces or stressors, the dynamic steady state required for successful adaptation is produced through counteracting and/or reestablishing forces. Living organisms survive by maintaining an immensely complex, dynamic, and harmonious equilibrium called homeostasis. These forces represent biological and mental adaptation responses to stress.

Stress is defined as a state of tension that can lead to disruption or threaten homeostasis. Through photographic distortions, Figure 2-1 illustrates a person whose image literally seems to be "falling apart" due to extreme stress. The amount of stress a person can tolerate without disruption or loss of homeostasis depends on the person's adaptive capacity. Individuals differ in their adaptive capacity, and the limits of their capacity are, in part, genetically determined. When the adaptive response is successful, a dynamic steady state (homeostasis) is maintained or restored. When the adaptive response is insufficient, inappropriate, or ineffective, homeostasis will be disrupted. Persistent or prolonged disruption can result in illness.

Historical Perspectives

Contemporary homeostasis concepts have a long history. The Greek philosopher Heraclitus (ca. 500 BC) was the first to suggest that a static, unchanged state was not the natural condition and the capacity to undergo constant change was intrinsic to all things.[1] Shortly afterward, Empedocles, also a philosopher, proposed the corollary that all matter consisted of elements and qualities that were in dynamic opposition or al-

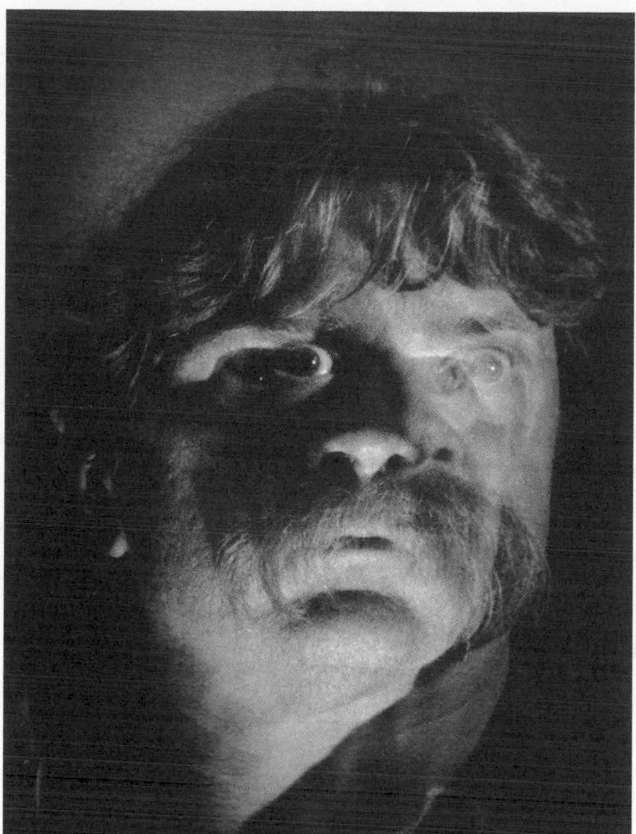

FIGURE 2-1 ■ Photographic distortions create the illusion of terror and fear. The individual literally seems to be "falling apart" due to extreme stress. (Photographed by William Kostelec, Spokane, Wash.)

liance to one another and that balance or harmony was a necessary condition for the survival of living organisms.[1] About 100 years later, Hippocrates equated health to the harmonious balance of the elements, and illness and disease to the systematic disharmony of these elements.[1] The terms dyscrasia and idiosyncrasy are derived from Hippocratic concepts of health and disease and are defined, respectively, as the defective or peculiar mixing of the elements.[1] Hippocrates also suggested that the disturbing forces that produced disharmony (disease) and counterbalancing (adaptive) forces were both derived from natural rather than supernatural sources. He introduced the idea that nature is the healer of disease. This concept was later echoed by Roman references to counterbalancing forces as *vis medicatrix naturae,* or the healing powers of nature.[1]

During the European Renaissance, Thomas Sydenham expanded the Hippocratic concept of disease as a system of disharmony brought about by disturbing forces by adding that an individual's adaptive response could itself be capable of producing pathologic changes.[1] Claude Bernard expanded the concept of harmony or steady state in the 19th century by adding *"milieu intérieur"* or the principle of dynamic internal physiologic equilibrium.[1]

In 1935, Walter B. Cannon published *Stresses and Strains of Homeostasis*[2] in which he applied basic engineering concepts of stress and strain to human physiology. Cannon also added to the concept of homeostasis by including emotional as well as physical states. He described the *"fight or flight"* reaction; the sudden increase in the physiologic ability to run or confront danger through increased alertness, focused attention, and increased levels of oxygen and glucose. Cannon connected these responses to the actions of epinephrine and norepinephrine. These findings followed Cannon's initial observations that a cat exhibiting a rage response to anesthesia had a faster rate of blood clotting than a cat that was not in a state of rage.[3] At about the time Cannon was developing these concepts, Hans Selye was developing his concepts of stress.

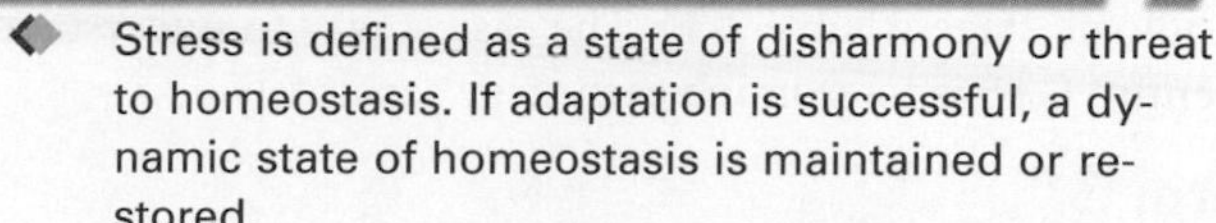

- Stress is defined as a state of disharmony or threat to homeostasis. If adaptation is successful, a dynamic state of homeostasis is maintained or restored.
- Stress evokes the fight-or-flight reaction of increased alertness, focused attention, increased energy, and a readiness to run or confront.

SELYE'S CONTRIBUTIONS TO STRESS RESEARCH

Selye was experimenting with hormonal preparations in rats when he serendipitously uncovered a biological basis for stress. He was expecting to find different changes in rats injected with different hormonal preparations but, to his amazement, the same three changes occurred each time. In every animal tested, the cortex of the adrenal gland enlarged, lymphatic organs (thymus, spleen, and lymph nodes) shrank, and stomach and duodenum bleeding ulcers developed. When Selye experimented with noxious agents, such as loud noise, toxic substances, or pituitary gland, kidney, or spleen extractions, the same three changes occurred. The changes seemed to occur simultaneously and did not appear to be related to any particular kind of injury. Any and all kinds of harmful stimuli produced the observed changes. Selye termed the harmful stimuli **stressors** and concluded that the changes observed represented a nonspecific response to any noxious stimulus. Because so many different agents caused the same changes, Selye called it a **general adaptation syndrome (GAS)** with three components: *an alarm reaction, a stage of resistance,* and *a stage of exhaustion.*[4] According to Selye's theory, individuals move through the first two stages repeatedly and consequently become adapted or habituated to the stressors they encountered during ordinary life.[5] For example, when one first gazes at a bright light, the light acts as a stressor, triggering an *alarm* reaction. As one continues to look at the light, *adaptation* in the eye occurs, marking the stage of resistance.

The stage of *exhaustion* occurs if one continues to look at the bright light allowing the eye to become permanently damaged. Further observations of the stages of alarm, resistance, and exhaustion led to efforts to differentiation between focal stressors (stimuli) and contextual stressors (stimuli) such as the descriptions developed by Roy and Roberts[6] and Roy and Andrews.[7]

Pathologic development occurs at the stage of exhaustion and is manifested as a diagnosis of one or more diseases—usually chronic—such as hypertension. If the stressor is extraordinarily severe or affects multiple body systems to produce profound pathologic processes, such as cardiac arrest, the resulting systemic exhaustion can lead to death.

General Adaptation Syndrome

Components of the GAS can be subdivided into three unique physiologic stages (Table 2-1). The easiest way to understand the entire GAS is to examine each stage separately.

Alarm

The alarm stage has been called the fight-or-flight response because it gives the body a boost of energy to either run or confront. Muscles receive increased blood supply that is enriched with both oxygen and glucose. Respiration is increased leading to increased oxygen consumption. The liver releases stored glucose into the bloodstream.

The alarm stage begins when the hypothalamus perceives a need to activate the GAS in response to a stressor (Figure 2-2). The stressor might be an argument with a friend, an upper respiratory tract infection, running a marathon, or winning the lottery. The hypothalamus perceives the experience as a stressor and mediates the activation of the sympathetic nervous system. Sympathetic nervous system activation enables the body to react very quickly to the stressor and coordinates other responses (Figure 2-3). The hypothalamus also notifies the pituitary gland, which in turn releases a variety of hormones (Figure 2-4). Once the pituitary gland is activated the alarm stage cannot be turned off or deactivated; it must run its course and progress to the stage of resistance. During the alarm stage, the hypothalamus synthesizes corticotropin-releasing hormone (CRH), which in turn triggers the anterior pituitary to release adrenocorticotropic hormone (ACTH), and the posterior pituitary gland to synthesize and release antidiuretic hormone (ADH).

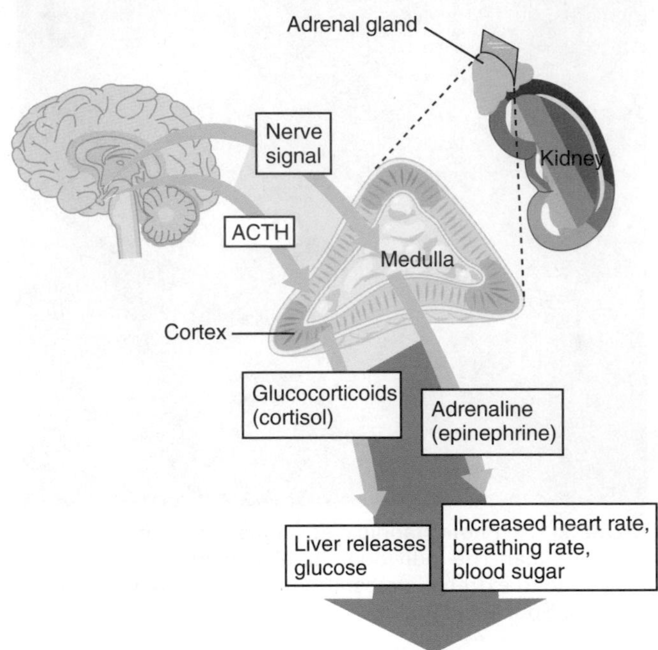

FIGURE 2-2 ■ The alarm reaction. Note the interaction of nervous and hormonal responses. *ACTH,* Adrenocorticotropic hormone. (From Thibodeau GA, Patton KT: *Anatomy and physiology,* ed 5, St Louis, 2003, Mosby, p 672.)

Table 2-1

The Three Stages of the General Adaptation Syndrome

Alarm	Resistance	Exhaustion
Increased secretion of glucocorticoids and resultant changes	Glucocorticoid secretion returns to normal	Increased glucocorticoid secretion but eventually markedly decreased secretion
Increased activity of sympathetic nervous system	Sympathetic activity returns to normal	Stress triad (hypertrophied adrenals, atrophied thymus and lymph nodes, bleeding ulcers in stomach and duodenum)
Increased norepinephrine secretion by adrenal medulla	Norepinephrine secretion returns to normal	
Fight-or-flight syndrome of changes	Fight-or-flight syndrome disappears	Loss of resistance to stressor; may lead to death
Low resistance to stressors	High resistance (adaptation) to stressor	

From Thibodeau GA, Patton KT: *Anatomy and physiology,* ed 5, St Louis, 2003, Mosby, p 673.

Resistance

If activation of the alarm stage were to continue unabated, the body would soon suffer undue wear and tear and become subject to permanent damage. The resistance stage allows adaptation and the return to a state of homeostasis. As the body moves into the stage of resistance, **cortisol** and **aldosterone** are secreted in excess. **Aldosterone** is a potent mineralocorticoid synthesized by the renin-angiotensin system that conserves sodium, producing increased water retention and consequently increased blood volume. **Cortisol** is a potent glucocorticoid (steroid hormone) released by the adrenal gland that causes an increase in blood glucose level by promoting liver gluconeogenesis. Cortisol is a key link between stress and the immune system. The resistance stage allows the body to respond to the alarm stage and, if the stressor is addressed and resolved, returns the organism to homeostasis.

Selye postulated that adaptation or the return to homeostasis requires energy. Adaptation or habituation to stress refers to either the length of time needed to reach the stage of resistance or the vigor and scope of physiologic responses to the stressor. For example, loud noise is a known stressor. Yet some people who live close to busy airports reach a point at which they barely notice the loud noises from planes flying over their homes. They become *habituated* to the stressor (loud noise).

Adaptation to a particular stressor can come about in several ways. Perception of the stressor can be altered to reduce the negative impact of the stressor. For example, perceptions of loud noises can be related to uncertainty about the meaning of the noise. People who live near an airport can develop their understanding of the loud noises and, based on their understanding, become reassured by the predictable sounds of takeoffs and landings. On a conscious level, the normal loud noises from the airport mean that everything is as it should be.

One important way to habituate to a stressor is to manipulate or "train" the hypothalamus to react less forcefully to a perceived threat or stressor. Repeatedly ignoring a specific stressor prevents the inappropriate triggering of the GAS. The result is a more acceptable level of stress response. Techniques that accomplish this **desensitization** work by changing the predominant brain waves of the individual from beta waves to alpha waves that are slower and more normal. Biofeedback, visualization, and meditation are examples of therapies that use this principle. Practicing these techniques for 20 to 30 minutes daily can enhance the ability to alter how a stressor is

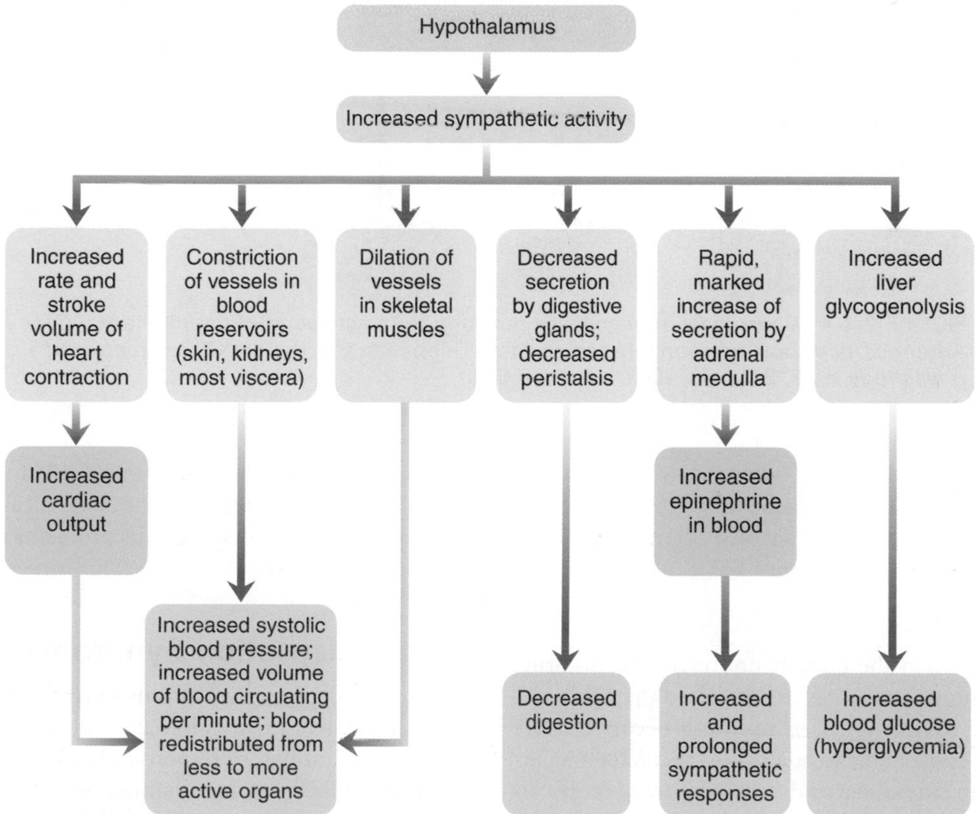

FIGURE 2-3 ■ Alarm reaction responses resulting from increased sympathetic activity. Note that these are the responses commonly referred to as the "fight-or-flight" reaction. (Modified from Thibodeau GA, Patton KT: *Anatomy and physiology,* ed 5, St Louis, 2003, Mosby, p 673.)

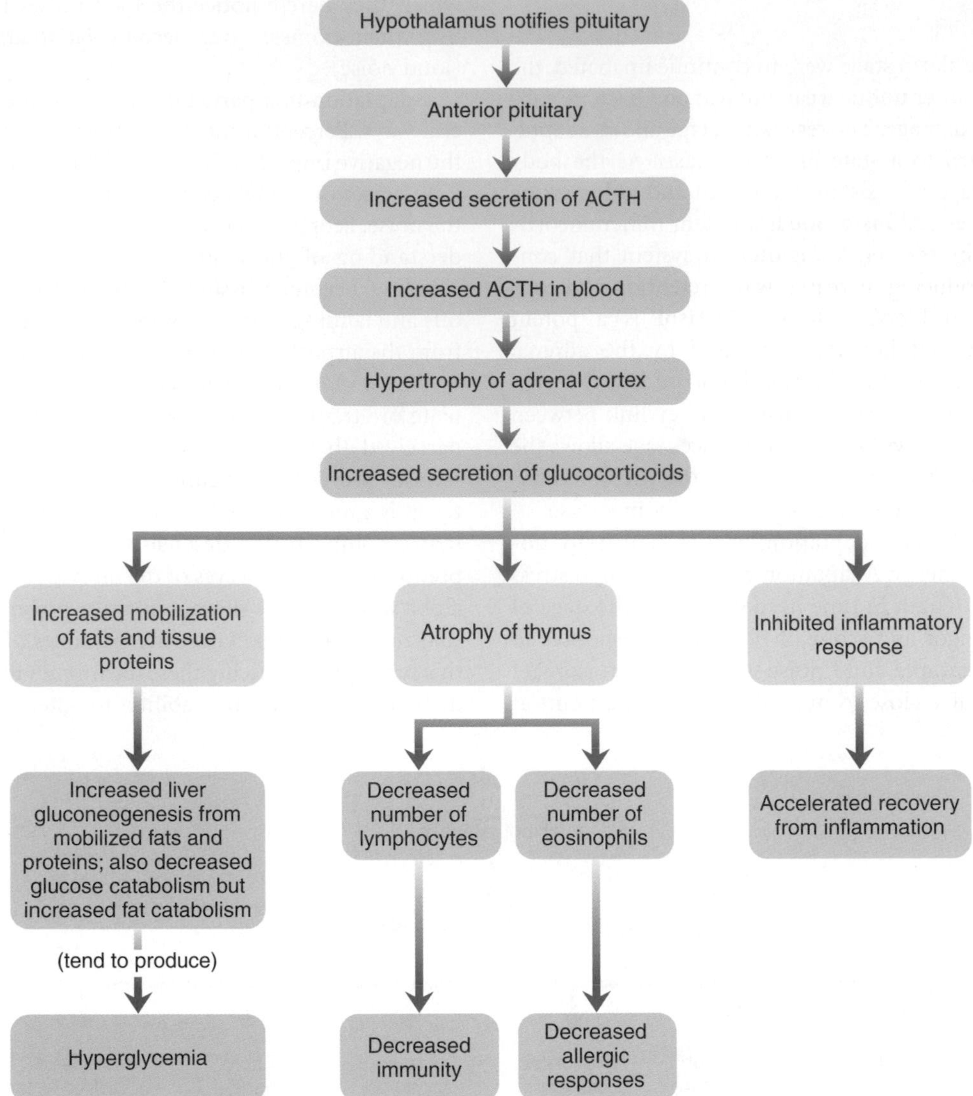

FIGURE 2-4 ■ Alarm reaction responses resulting from activation of the pituitary. *ACTH,* Adrenocorticotropic hormone. (Adapted from Thibodeau GA, Patton KT: *Anatomy and physiology,* ed 5, St Louis, 2003, Mosby, p 672.)

perceived and moderate the stress response. Migraine headache, chronic back pain, and hypertension are common stress-related conditions that have been successfully managed with desensitization methods.

Exhaustion

Exhaustion occurs when the body is no longer able to bring about a return to homeostasis. Selye postulated that when energy resources are completely used up death occurs because the organism is no longer able to adapt. He speculated that individuals have both superficial and deep adaptive energy. Superficial adaptive energy can be replaced from deeper adaptive energy stores. However, when the deep adaptive energy stores are depleted, no other resource exists to facilitate stress recovery. Often, it is at this point that the person seeks professional health care. He or she is no longer able to achieve a healthy adaptation to the stressor without medical or nursing intervention or has developed serious problems resulting from unhealthy adaptation.

Local Adaptation Syndrome

The local adaptation syndrome (LAS) is literally a localized GAS. The phenomenon, initially isolated by Selye, represents a classic inflammatory response. (See Unit III for a full explanation of infection and inflammation.) Localized signs of inflammation include redness, swelling or edema, pain, in some instances drainage, and movement limitations. Inflammation is a process whereby encapsulation separates the inflamed entity from the rest of the body, followed by attempts to destroy

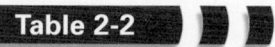

Table 2-2

Comparison of Local Adaptation Syndrome and General Adaptation Syndrome

Local Adaptation Syndrome	General Adaptation Syndrome
Physiologic response is localized; entire body not involved	Physiologic response involves entire organism
Adaptive response to a stressor	Adaptive response to a stressor
Short-term response without long-term consequences	Long-term response; depletes reservoir of adaptive energy
Restorative response: organism returns to homeostasis	Restorative response: organism returns to homeostasis (stage of resistance) or deteriorates (stage of exhaustion)

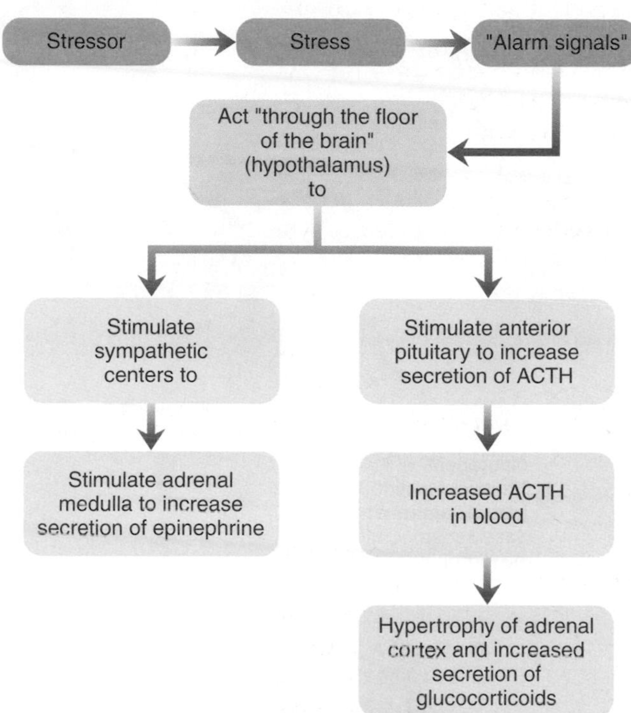

FIGURE 2-5 ■ Selye's hypothesis about activation of the stress response. *ACTH,* Adrenocorticotropic hormone. (Redrawn from Thibodeau GA, Patton KT: *Anatomy and physiology,* ed 5, St Louis, 2003, Mosby, p 674.)

the source of the inflammation using enzymes and inflammatory cell attacks. A comparison of LAS and GAS is presented in Table 2-2. Selye's concepts and hypotheses are summarized in Figure 2-5.

Although Selye's work has been widely disseminated and has provided a theoretical foundation for a considerable volume of research in nursing and other disciplines, his theory also has been widely criticized. The premise of stress as a purely physiologic response has rightly been challenged by other stress researchers. Clearly, it is almost impossible to absolutely determine whether a physical stressor alone may produce the neuroendocrine stress response or if individual thoughts and feelings about a stressor have produced the response.

Physiologists have consistently challenged Selye's GAS concept of nonspecificity. Their models present adaptive bodily responses as selective and organized to specifically counteract the bodily changes that elicit them. For example, it is not easy to explain how nonspecific physiologic and biochemical responses could help the body to adapt to both cold and heat.[8] No single stress hormone responds to all stressors in the nonspecific fashion implied in Selye's definition of the GAS. Physiologically, the body adapts to cold by using peripheral vasoconstriction to conserve heat and shivering to produce additional heat. Adaptation to heat is accomplished by using peripheral vasodilatation and sweating to increase heat loss and decrease heat production.

Selye's definitions of stress differed from the definitions proposed in physics, the field that first originated the term. This difference led to more confusion and less precision. Others criticized Selye's formulations because, as an endocrinologist, he was not viewed as being "eminently qualified" to conduct mind-body research or generate mind-body interaction theory. Nevertheless, Selye's formulations made sense to the general public and to many life science professionals. His contributions to modern stress, coping, and adaptation theory are considered important and have become the fundamental basis for today's biochemical models of stress. Other pioneering stress researchers include Holmes,[9] Rahe,[10] Mason,[11] and Lazarus.[12] Advances in basic science have allowed today's stress researchers to develop cellular models of stress that incorporate individual genetics, cell anatomy and physiology, biochemistry, psychology, behavior, gender, age, and ethnicity. Central to these advances are interactions model using the three essential systems of the stress response: nervous system, endocrine system, and immune system.

Selye's Concepts

Selye discovered that a number of noxious stimuli or stressors evoked the same type of response in experimental animals. He called this generalized response the general adaptation syndrome (GAS). Three common physiologic responses occurred in response to stress: (1) hyperplasia of the adrenal cortex, (2) atrophy of lymphoid tissues, and (3) ulceration of the stomach and duodenum.

Selye described three phases of the stress response: alarm, resistance, and exhaustion. The *alarm* reaction is the initial response to stress. The major features of the alarm reaction are attributable to activation of the sympathetic nervous system.

During the stage of *resistance,* sympathetic activity declines while secretion of adrenocortical hormones is high. If the stressor continues, habituation or adaptation may occur such that the hypothalamus fails to respond with alarm. If the stressor is too great or prolonged, energy reserves may be depleted, leading to the stage of *exhaustion.*

Selye characterized localized inflammatory processes as the LAS. Localized inflammation is characterized by redness, swelling, pain, and altered function.

CURRENT CONCEPTS

With ongoing research, Selye's original view of the stress response has been revised. Current concepts are presented in Figure 2-6.

Activation of the stress system is intended to lead to changes that improve the organism's ability to regain homeostasis, decrease the risk of exhaustion, and thereby increase the probability of survival and adaptation.

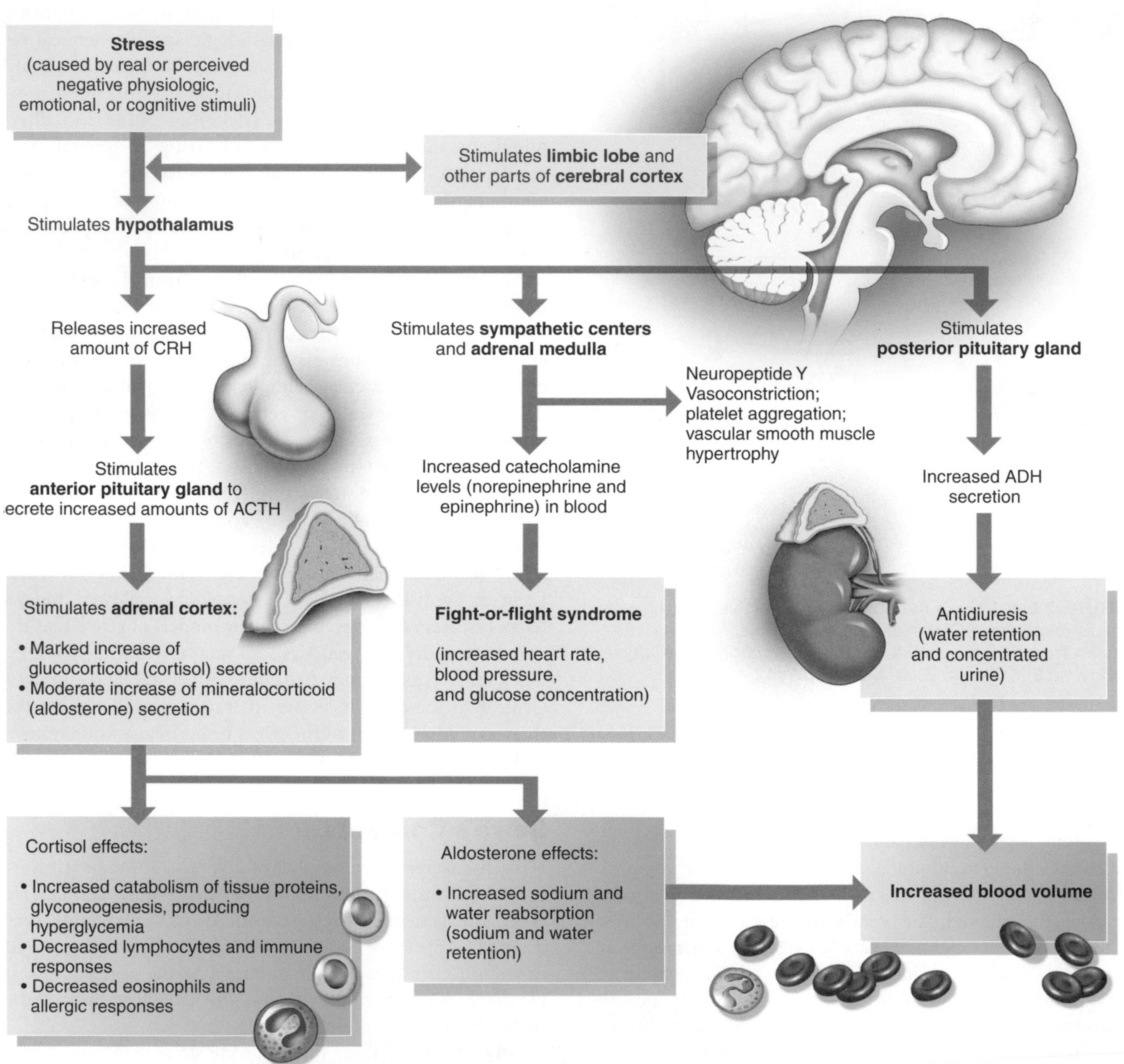

FIGURE 2-6 ■ Current concepts of the stress syndrome. *ACTH,* Adrenocorticotropic hormone; *ADH,* antidiuretic hormone; *CRH,* corticotropin-releasing hormone. (From Thibodeau GA, Patton KT: *Anatomy and physiology,* ed 5, St Louis, 2003, Mosby, p 675.)

Neuroendocrine Interactions

Catecholamine Release

The endocrine system reacts to stress by secreting hormones that can alter metabolic processes and restore homeostasis. The released hormones literally enable the body to respond to stress. Both the brain and the autonomic nervous system, primarily the sympathetic nervous system, direct the endocrine system. These neuroendocrine actions and interactions in response to stressors are summarized in Figure 2-7.

The hypothalamus prompts the release of catecholamines from the sympathetic (excitatory) nervous system. Catecholamines (epinephrine and norepinephrine) are synthesized locally by neurons in the sympathetic nervous system (norepinephrine) and by the adrenal medulla (epinephrine and norepinephrine). Catecholamines cannot cross the blood-brain barrier. Instead, they circulate in the plasma in a loose association with albumin. Circulating catecholamines have essentially the same effects as direct sympathetic stimulation. They cause increased heart rate, increased blood

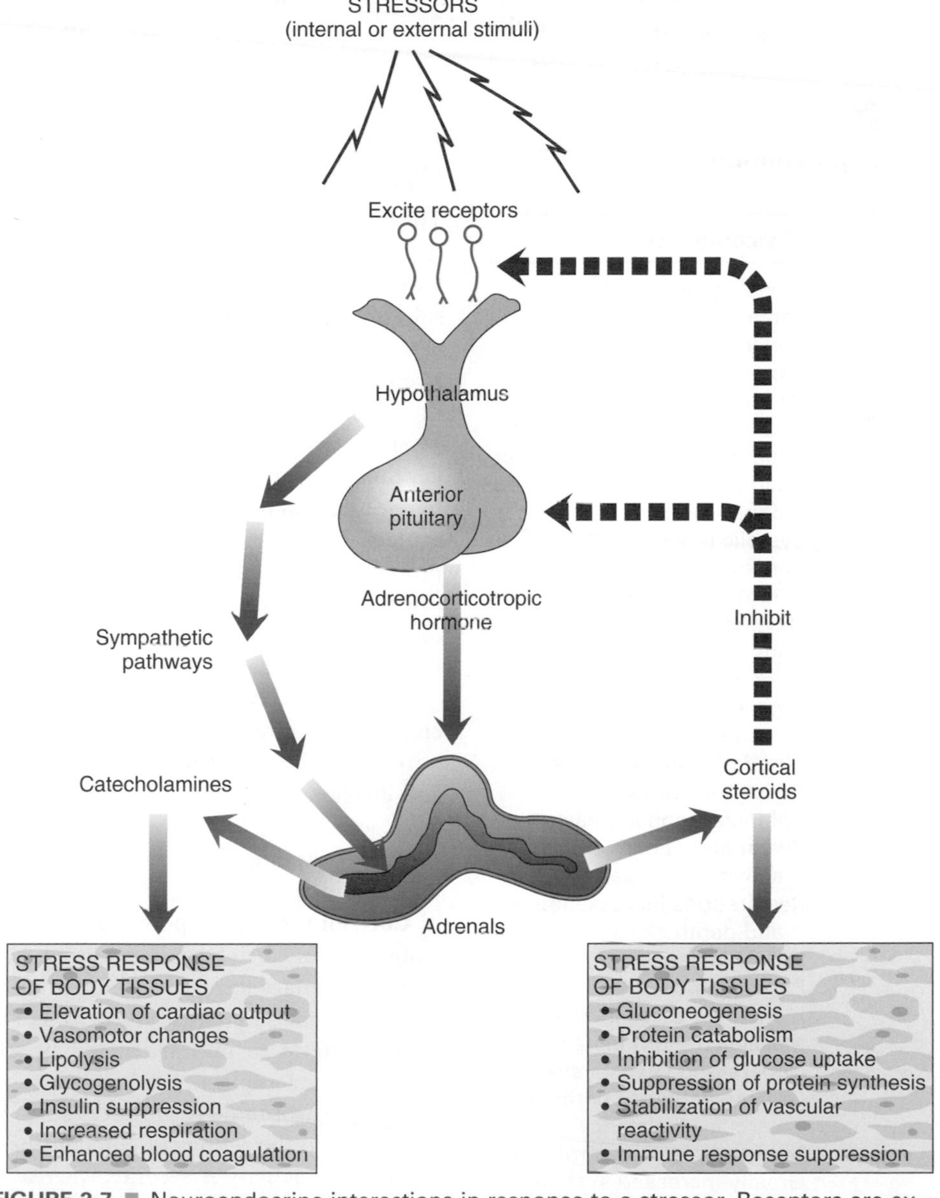

FIGURE 2-7 ■ Neuroendocrine interactions in response to a stressor. Receptors are excited by stressful stimuli and relay the information to the hypothalamus. The hypothalamus signals the adrenal cortex (by way of the pituitary) and the sympathetic pathways (by way of the autonomic nervous system). Most of the stress response is then mediated by secretions of catecholamines (epinephrine and norepinephrine) and cortical steroids (cortisol and aldosterone).

pressure, and increased blood flow to skeletal muscles. Increased circulating catecholamines contribute to the increase in strength that can be experienced in the alarm phase of the stress response.

Norepinephrine is released from the adrenal medulla and enters the liver and skeletal muscle where it is rapidly metabolized. Very little adrenal norepinephrine ever reaches distal tissue. Norepinephrine effects during the stress response are primarily derived from the sympathetic nervous system. Norepinephrine is the primary constrictor of smooth muscle in all blood vessels and therefore regulates blood pressure. During stress, the release of norepinephrine raises blood pressure by constricting peripheral vessels. At the same time, norepinephrine also reduces gastric secretion and causes dilation of the eye pupils producing the "wide-eyed" appearance of persons experiencing stress.[13]

Epinephrine produces some of the same effects as norepinephrine but has a greater influence on cardiac action. Epinephrine enhances myocardial contractility, increases heart rate, and increases venous return to the heart, thus increasing cardiac output and blood pressure. Epinephrine also has the metabolic effects of increasing glycogenolysis and increasing the release of glucose from the liver. The actions of epinephrine give persons experiencing stress sudden increases in muscular strength and aggressiveness. In the brain, the increased blood flow and increased availability of glucose lead to increases in mental attention, vigilance, and alertness. Together, these changes prepare the body for physical action, whether the action is to "fight or flee."[13] Table 2-3 summarizes the physiologic effects of epinephrine and norepinephrine.

Table 2-3 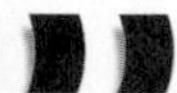

Physiologic Effects of Epinephrine and Norepinephrine

Substance	Physiologic Effect
Epinephrine	Heart rate increases
	Force of heart contractions increases
	Cardiac output increases
	Peripheral vascular bed constricts
	Renal blood vessels constrict
	Gastrointestinal vascular bed constricts
	Systolic blood pressure rises
	Metabolic rate increases to 100% above normal
	Oxygen utilization increases
	Body temperature rises
	Liver and muscle glycogenolysis increases
	Insulin secretion inhibited
	Blood glucose levels rise
	Peristalsis slows
	Sphincter tone increases
	Sweat and apocrine gland activity increases
	Respirations increase in rate and depth
	Bronchi dilate
	Pupils dilate
	Mental alertness increases
	Muscle strength increases
Norepinephrine	Generalized vasoconstriction
	Greatly increased peripheral vascular resistance
	Moderate cardiac stimulation
	Greatly increased systolic and diastolic blood pressures
	Mild metabolic effects

From Monahan FD, Neighbors M: *Medical surgical nursing, foundations for clinical practice,* Philadelphia, 1998, Saunders, p 1216.

Hypothalamic-Pituitary-Adrenal Axis

The hypothalamic-pituitary-adrenal (HPA) axis is the system that mediates the stress response by enabling the release of CRH, ACTH, ADH, glucocorticoid steroid hormones (cortisol), and mineralocorticoid steroid hormones (aldosterone) (Figure 2-8). Ordinarily, the release of cortisol, the primary stress hormone with significant health effects, continues until the released cortisol signals its own shutdown. Prolonged or persistent release of cortisol has been proposed as a possible key link between stress and disease. Activation of the HPA axis to release stress hormones is most adaptive when triggered by acute or immediate stressors. Persistent stress overwhelms the process appearing to break down the autoregulation mechanism. Instead of promoting a healthy stress response, unchecked HPA activity and stress hormone release contributes to the onset of a wide range of health problems.[13]

Aldosterone is at least 95% of the **mineralo**corticoid secreted by the adrenal cortex. The primary effect of this steroid hormone is increased renal tubular reabsorption of sodium and increase renal excretion of potassium. Through osmotic force, water tends to follow sodium; therefore, excessive reabsorption of sodium leads to increased extracellular fluid volume and increased blood pressure.[13]

Cortisol is the most potent **gluco**corticoid. The hypothalamus secretes corticotropin-releasing factor (CRF), CRF signals the pituitary to release ACTH into the blood. ACTH signals the adrenals to release glucocorticoids, primarily cortisol. Cortisol affects the immune system by affecting natural killer (NK) cells, macrophage production of cytokines, T cells, and B cells. Cortisol initially produces stress response effects that are similar to the actions of epinephrine, but the duration of epinephrine activity is seconds whereas cortisol activity can last for minutes or hours. For this reason epinephrine is more closely associated with the **alarm** stage of stress and cortisol with **resistance** and **exhaustion.** The primary effects of cortisol are stimulation of gluconeogenesis in the liver and a six- to tenfold increase in the rate of amino acid conversion to keto acids and glucose. Gluconeogenesis ensures an adequate supply of glucose for body tissues in general, but nerve cells have priority. If necessary, cortisol may act to preserve available glucose for nerve cell use by limiting the uptake and oxidation of glucose by other cells in the body.[14]

Cortisol promotes increased blood glucose through the actions of other hormones, including epinephrine, glucagon, and somatotropic growth hormone. The process of cortisol promotion of blood glucose is *permissive* in that it allows for the actions of the other hormones. Cortisol also is necessary for the maintenance of normal blood pressure and cardiac output and thus also is *permissive* for the actions of the catecholamines.

Cortisol affects protein metabolism. It has an *anabolic* effect leading to increased rates of protein synthesis and RNA in liver. Cortisol has a *catabolic* effect in muscle tissue, lymphoid tissue, adipose tissue, skin, and bone. This protein breakdown effect produces a negative nitrogen balance and increased

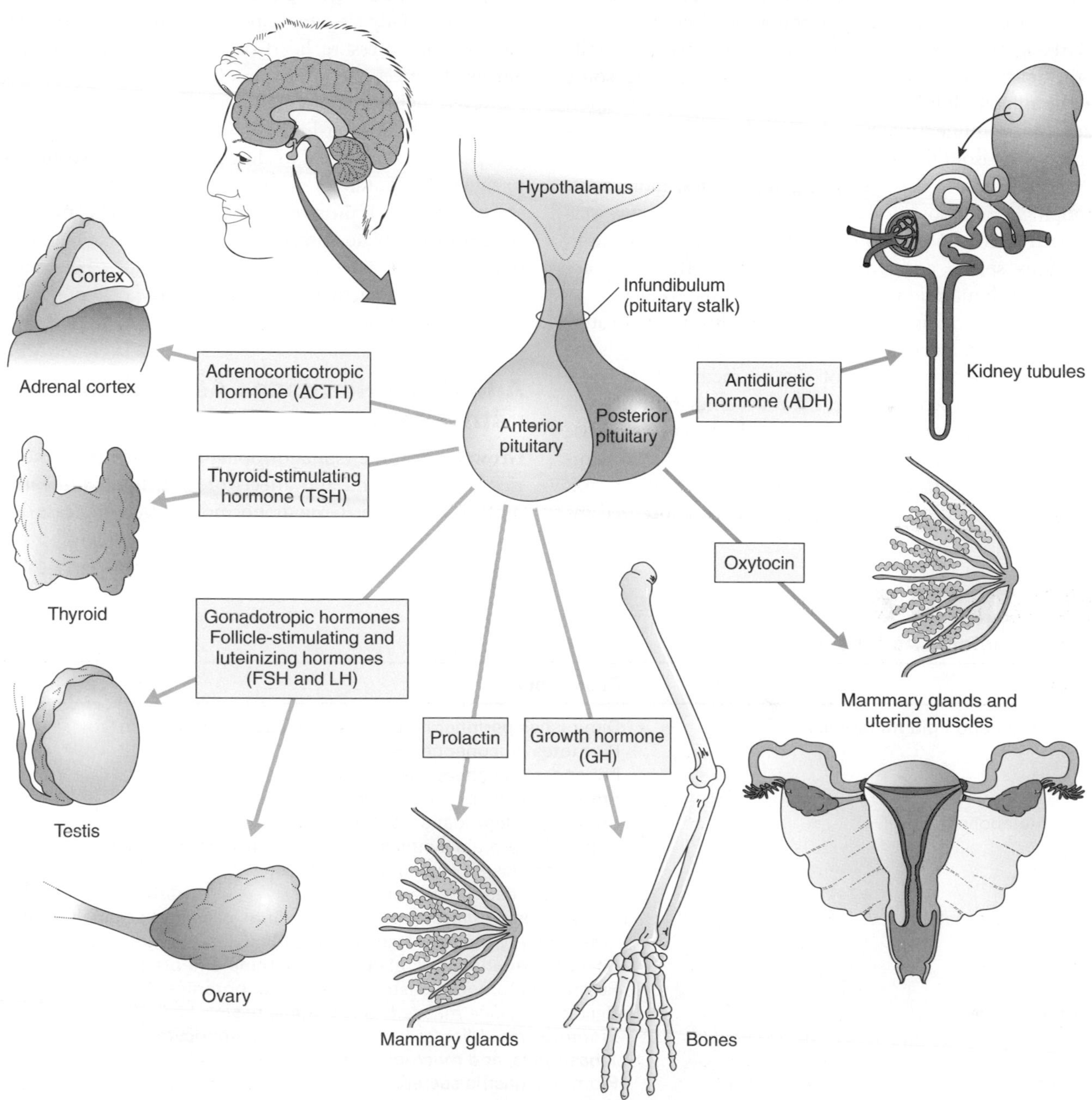

FIGURE 2-8 ■ The pituitary gland is suspended from the hypothalamus by a stalk of neural tissue. The hormones secreted by the anterior and posterior lobes of the pituitary gland and their target tissues are shown. (From Solomon EP: *Introduction to human anatomy and physiology,* ed 2, St Louis, 2003, Mosby, p 152.)

circulating amino acids. The resulting pooling of amino acids from catabolized proteins ensures amino acid availability. Preliminary research findings suggest that, in response to stress, cortisol may depress the transport of amino acids into muscle cells while enhancing their uptake into the liver, where they are converted to glucose.[14]

In the gastrointestinal tract, cortisol in response to stress promotes gastric secretion. This effect is the opposite effect of norepinephrine that reduces gastric secretion. Excessive cortisol activity and excessive gastric secretion can increase the risk for ulceration of the gastric mucosa and thus may account for Selye's early observations of gastrointestinal ulceration.

Cortisol acts as an immunosuppressant, in part, by inhibiting the macrophage production of cytokines and in some cases by directly inhibiting the proliferation and activation of specific immune system cells by inhibiting specific cytokines.[15] Cortisol literally reduces the numbers of nearly all immune response cells, including lymphocytes, monocytes, eosinophils, and basophils. Large doses of steroid medications have been shown to promote atrophy of lymphoid tissue in the thymus, spleen, and lymph nodes. These effects may account for the lymphoid tissue atrophy observed by Selye.

The ability of cortisol and other steroid hormones to suppress the inflammatory response of the immune system is the basis for the therapeutic use of steroid medications. These medications are used to inhibit the accumulation of cells at the site of inflammation and inhibit the leukocyte release of substances directly involved in producing the inflammatory process (e.g., kinins, plasminogen-activating factor, prostaglandins, and histamine). At the site of a localized inflammatory response or wound, excessive cortisol activity could inhibit fibroblast proliferation and functioning, accounting for the poor wound healing, increased susceptibility to infection, and decreased inflammatory response often seen in individuals with excess glucocorticoid levels.[15] Table 2-4 summarizes the major physiologic effects of cortisol.

Cortisol and the glucocorticoids are believed to facilitate the wide spread peripheral changes brought about by stress activation of the HPA axis. When temporary, these changes are adaptive in that energy resources are redirected as needed. Oxygen and nutrients are redirected to the central nervous system and body sites that are under stress, resulting in enhanced blood pressure, heart rate, respiratory rate, and blood glucose to meet the demands of the alarm stage of stress. However, high levels of cortisol activity in response to stress are intended to be self-limiting. Ideally, the offending stressor is coped with or adapted to allowing the high cortisol activity to signal the shutdown of the HPA axis and immune system stress responses. If the stress response, or alarm, continues, the system adapts by no longer responding to cortisol without reducing cortisol activity. Severe, prolonged, or persistent increase in cortisol activity is thought to play a major role in the stress-disease process.

Additional Hormones Associated with Stress

Growth hormone (somatotropin) is released from the anterior pituitary gland and affects protein, lipid, and carbohydrate metabolism. Growth hormone levels increase in the

Table 2-4

Major Physiologic Actions of Cortisol

Action	Description
Carbohydrate and lipid metabolism	Diminishes peripheral uptake and utilization of glucose Promotes gluconeogenesis in liver cells Enhances gluconeogenic response to other hormones Promotes lipolysis in adipose tissue
Protein metabolism	Stimulates degradation of body protein Depresses protein synthesis (including immunoglobulin) Increases plasma level of amino acids Stimulates deamination in the liver
Membrane permeability	Suppresses membrane permeability of all cells and organelles, but particularly those of lysosomes, and capillary endothelium Inhibits formation and release of histamine and bradykinin Permissive for vasoconstrictive action of norepinephrine
Immune reserve	Decreases tissue mass of all lymphatic tissues Promotes rapid decrease in circulating lymphocytes, eosinophils, basophils, and macrophages
Other effects	Promotes gastric secretion Enhances urinary excretion Decreases proliferation of fibroblasts in connective tissue

From Ramsey JM: *Basic pathophysiology: modern stress and the disease process,* Menlo Park, Calif, 1982, Addison-Wesley, p 56. Reproduced with permission.

blood following a variety of intensely stressful physical or psychological stimuli, such as strenuous exercise or extreme fear. In most circumstances, increased levels of growth hormones only occur with parallel rises in cortisol secretion.[16]

Prolactin is released from the anterior pituitary gland and is necessary for lactation and breast development. Plasma prolactin levels can become increased by a variety of stressful physical and psychological experiences. Unlike growth hormone, prolactin levels show little change after exercise. However, like growth hormone, increased prolactin levels appear to require stimuli that is much more intense than the stimuli needed to increase catecholamine or cortisol levels.[13]

Estrogen effects on the HPA stress response have been observed in humans. Estrogen appears to attenuate the HPA stress response, resulting in higher HPA stress responses in females than males. A well-designed small study of women who had undergone natural or surgical menopause showed that the application of transdermal estrogen patches significantly lessened cortisol activity in response to a low-dose injection of a bacterial endotoxin.[17] Findings such as these suggest the possibility of significant gender differences in the HPA-mediated stress response, but more research is needed before such observations can be generalized. Critics have suggested that observed gender differences in HPA stress responses more likely imply that the basic fight-or-flight model fails to characterize the female stress response.[18] Alternatively, yet another group of researchers who conducted a direct comparison of male and female stress responses associated with depressing life events observed no gender differences in stress response but significant gender differences in the type of experiences that males and females found stressful. Men were more sensitive to divorce, separation, and work problems whereas females were more sensitive to relationship problems involving people who were important to them.[19] Although many interesting differences have been observed, the effects of estrogen on HPA-mediated stress response remain largely undefined.

Testosterone regulates male secondary sex characteristics and libido. Decreased testosterone levels have been observed following exposure to physically and psychologically stressful stimuli but the mechanism that produces this effect is unknown. An interesting comparison study of the cardiovascular and endocrine stress responses and stress recovery of males and females showed that males experienced greater increases in blood pressure (alarm) and poor recovery (resistance).[20] Similarly, a direct comparison study of the urinary epinephrine, norepinephrine, and cortisol levels of male and female college students found significantly higher levels in males and students who were older.[20] Those students who were younger and females who were taking hormone replacement medications had significantly lower levels. It is not clear whether testosterone may increase male stress response or is somehow less effective than estrogen in moderating the stress response.

Stress Response and Endorphin Release

Self-analgesia involves the biological generation of natural endorphins.[21] The term *endorphin* comes from *endogenous* and *morphine.* Like the drug morphine, endorphins raise the pain threshold and produce sedation and euphoria. As endorphin levels rise, individuals experience pleasurable relief from anxiety. The stress of exercise (Figure 2-9), the excitement of dance, the anticipation of enjoying delicious food, the shock of combat, and the competition of contact sports all can produce meaningful increases in endorphin levels. During stress, specialized immune cells can secrete opioids that activate opioid receptors and produce analgesia. These immune-related opioids apparently play a key role in the modulation of inflammatory pain.[22] For example, up to a point, extreme physical exercise, such as running a marathon, will produce inflammatory pain as well as immune system opioids to reduce the pain.

Stress Response and the Immune System

The endocrine system is inextricably linked to the nervous system and to virtually every other physiologic system including the immune system. Sympathetic innervation of the blood

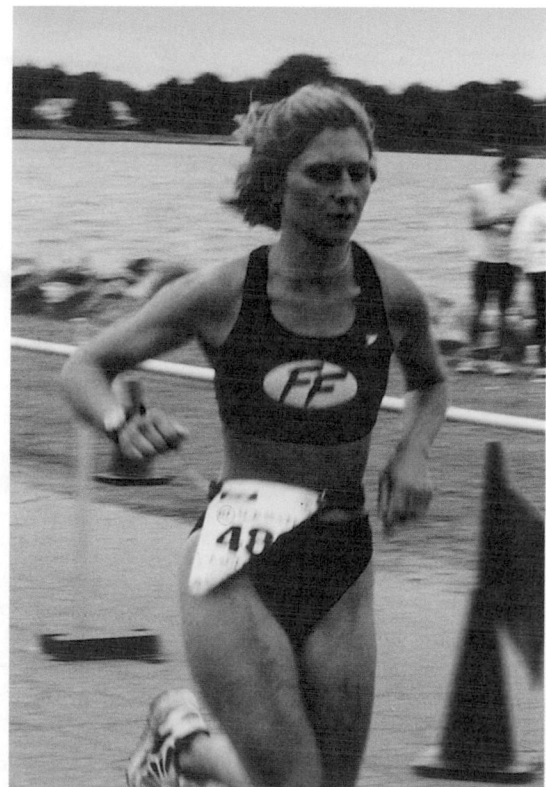

FIGURE 2-9 ■ Endorphin levels in the blood may increase in response to the stress of intense exercise. (Photographed by Therese A. Capal, Rockville, Md.)

vessels that supply the organs of the immune system create a direct mechanism for nervous system influence on immune function. Psychoneuroimmunology (PNI),[23] the study of stress-induced changes in immune functioning, has yielded invaluable scientific advances. Leaders in PNI research, such as Ronald Glaser,[24] have shown that severe and persistent psychological stress can down-regulate, or suppress, immune functioning. Immune system suppression brought about by severe or persistent stress represents a direct link between stress and disease. This link has been observed with both minor and major stressors as well as acute and chronic stress responses.[24]

For example, through immune system activation, the presence of bacteria associated with an infection would activate the HPA system resulting in acute increase in the secretion of ACTH and glucocorticoids (Figure 2-10).

Glucocorticoids, particularly cortisol, interfere with normal immune system functioning. At least three different hypotheses have been proposed to explain how this might occur. Immune cell production of soluble factors that act on the hypothalamus and thereby influence the HPA axis may raise blood glucocorticoid levels.[25] A second possibility is that activation of the immune cell production of neuroactive peptides may act on local lymphocytes. A third possibility is that thymosin peptides may stimulate T-cell differentiation and functioning.[26] Figure 2-11 illustrates a proposed role of thymosins in helping to mediate brain–immune system interactions.

The glucocorticoid resistance model[27] proposes a specific link between stress, immunity, and disease. Rather than viewing disease as a result of increased vulnerability due to stress, this model proposes that overwhelming stress reduces the sensitivity of the immune system to cortisol. Parts of the immune system respond to high cortisol levels by terminating the inflammatory response. In this way, the association of glucocorticoid resistance and disease is analogous to that of insulin resistance and diabetes. Normally, increased cortisol levels soon reach the set point that signals immune cells to terminate the immune response.

Persistently high cortisol levels are harmful to neurons, particularly in the hippocampal region of the brain, and immune system functioning. In the immune system, persistently high cortisol levels appear to cause a down-regulation or reduction of available immune cell cortisol receptors. Fewer cortisol receptors means less communication between cortisol and immune cells. Under these conditions, inflammatory disease processes are able to progress unchallenged. Researchers have tested the glucocorticoid resistance model by investigating whether persistent psychological stress could alter the ability of oral dexamethasone (synthetic cortisol) to inhibit

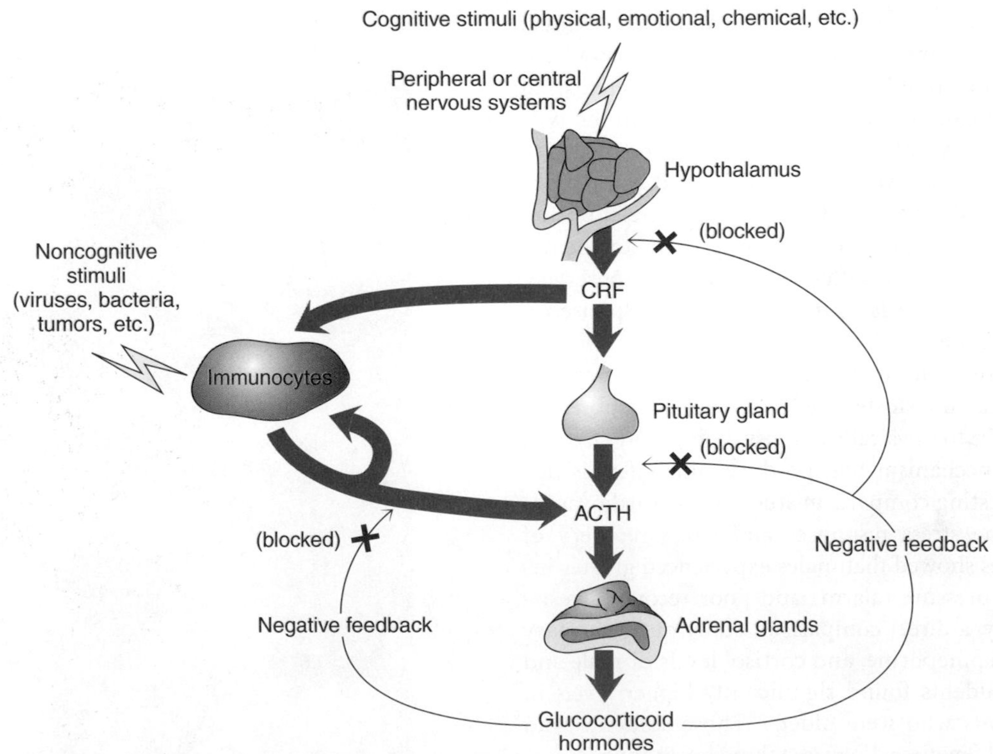

FIGURE 2-10 ■ Illustration of apparent connections between the hypothalamic-pituitary-adrenal axis and cells of the immune system. *ACTH,* Adrenocorticotropic hormone; *CRF,* corticotropin-releasing factor. (Redrawn from Blalock JE, Harbour-Menamin D, Smith EM: Peptide hormones shared by the neuroendocrine and immunologic systems, *J Immunol* 135:859s, 1985. Used with permission.)

the production of proinflammatory cytokines released by white blood cells.

The various immune functions performed by cytokines include directing white blood cells to their targets and enhancing the kill effectiveness of NK white blood cells. The researchers studied two groups: parents with and parents without a child undergoing treatment for cancer. Parents with a seriously ill child showed more depression and less immune system response to oral synthetic cortisol.[27] In other words, persistent stress caused persistently high cortisol levels that were not self-limiting. High cortisol levels have been linked with numerous immune system disorders and diseases including anorexia nervosa, obsessive-compulsive disorder, depression, alcoholism, difficult-to-manage diabetes, and hyperthyroidism.

Endorphins also have been shown to have a complex role in elevating the number of lymphocytes (both the number of active T cells and the number of cells in some T-cell subsets). It may be that endogenous opioids (endorphins) also modulate the immune system. A schematic diagram summarizing neural and neurohormonal mechanisms by which stress and morphine might affect the immune system is presented in Figure 2-12.

It is clear that stress, coping, and maintaining homeostatic balance within the human body is enormously complex. Figures 2-10 and 2-11 emphasize the variety of biological response modifiers that can influence brain–immune system interactions.

Stress Response and Disease

Adaptive stress response means the body has the capacity to respond to stressors quickly and the ability to respond to counterregulatory signals that prevent overresponse to stressors. All aspects of the stress response, including

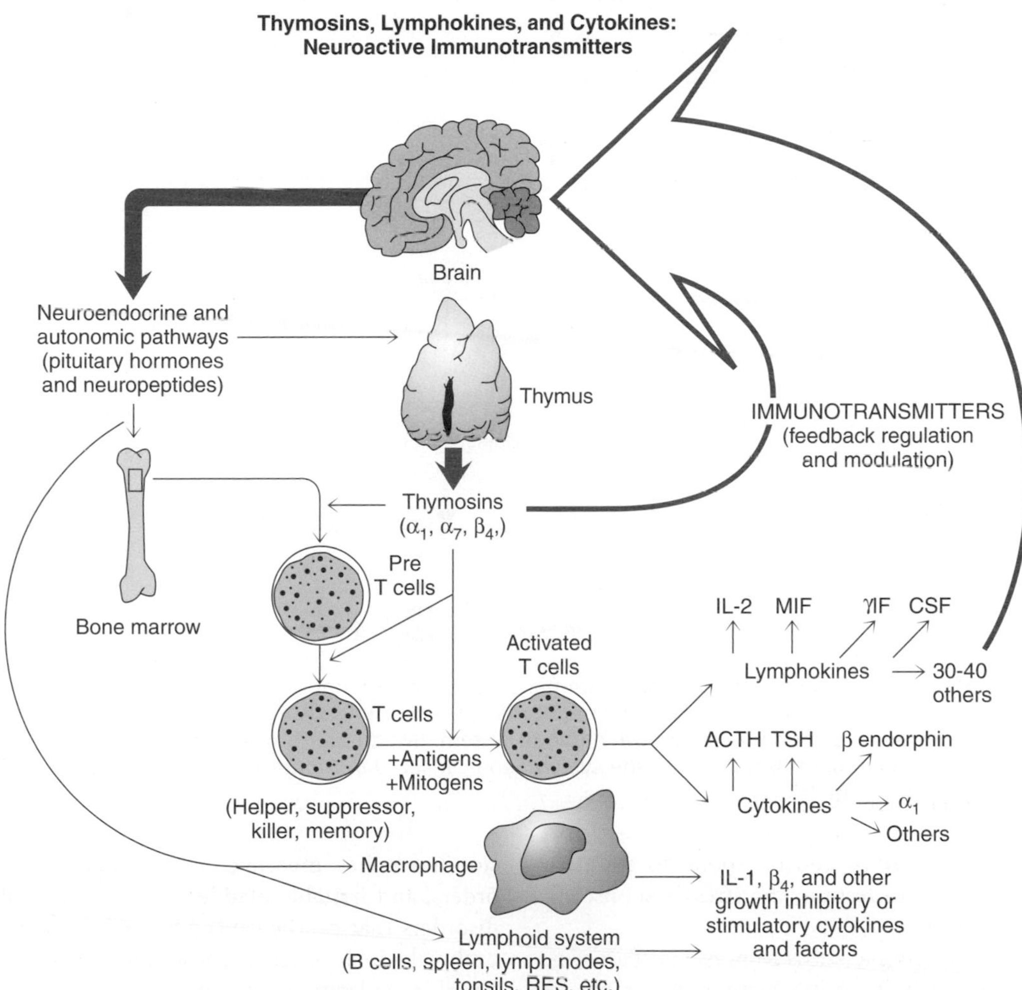

FIGURE 2-11 ■ Illustration of proposed role of thymosins in helping to mediate brain-immune interactions. *ACTH,* Adrenocorticotropic hormone; *CSF,* colony-stimulating factor; *MIF,* migration-inhibitory factor; *RES,* reticuloendothelial system; *TSH,* thyroid-stimulating hormone; *IL,* interleukin. (Redrawn from Hall NR et al: Evidence that thymosins and other biological response modifiers can function as neuroactive immunotransmitters, *J Immunol* 135:807s, 1985. Used with permission.)

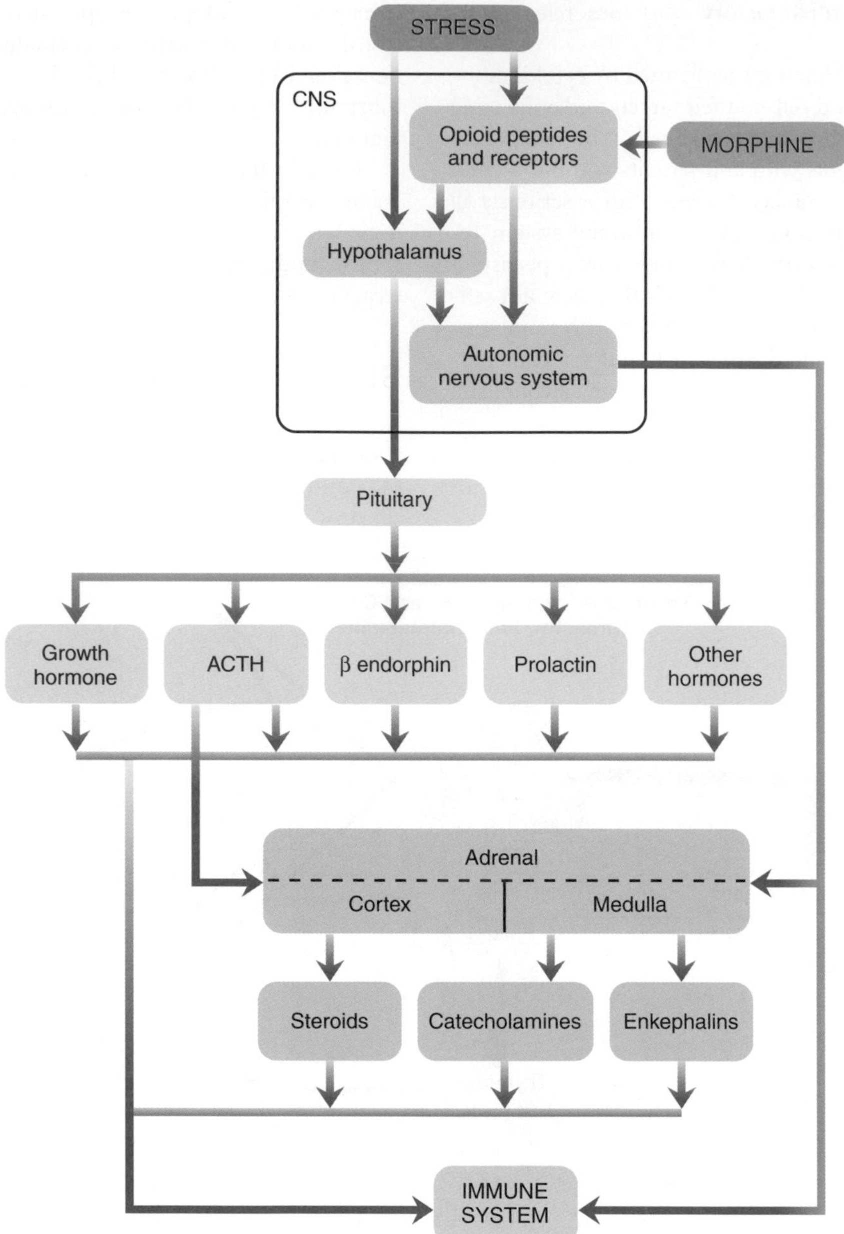

FIGURE 2-12 ■ Schematic diagram summarizing neural and neurohormonal mechanisms by which stress and morphine might affect the immune system. *ACTH,* Adrenocorticotropic hormone; *CNS,* central nervous system. (Modified from Shavit Y et al: Stress, opioid peptides, the immune system, and cancer, *J Immunol* 135:836s, 1985. Used with permission.)

inflammatory/immune reactions, must respond to counterregulatory forces designed to restrain the stress response effectively and immediately.

Maladaptive or dysfunctional stress response is characterized by persistent hyperactivity or hypoactivity in a range of pathophysiologic states that cut across the traditional boundaries of health care, from psychiatric and endocrine disorders to inflammatory disease.

Hair loss, emotional tension, mouth sores, asthma, heart palpitations, neuromuscular movement disorders (tics), tension headaches, muscle contraction backache, digestive disorders, and irritable bladder are just a few of the common disorders that can be caused by or worsened by stress. Skin outbreaks such as acne, reproductive disorders such as menstrual irregularity in women, and male impotence also have been linked with the effects of severe stress. Box 2-1 summarizes some of the physiologic and psychological effects of excessive stress. Figure 2-13 depicts the multiple organs that can be involved in the stress response by showing dysregulation.

Box 2-1

Physical and Behavioral Indicators of High Stress

Physiologic Indicators

Elevated blood pressure
Increased muscle tension
Elevated pulse
Increased respiration
Sweaty palms
Cold extremities (hands and feet)
Fatigue
Tension headache
Upset stomach: nausea, vomiting, diarrhea
Change in appetite
Change in weight
Increased blood catecholamine level
Hyperglycemia
Restlessness
Insomnia

Behavioral and Emotional Indicators

Anxiety (nonspecific fears)
Depression
Increased use of mind-altering substances (e.g., alcohol, chemical substances)
Change in eating, sleeping, or activity pattern
Mental exhaustion
Feelings of inadequacy; loss of self-esteem
Increased irritability
Loss of motivation
Decreased productivity
Inability to make good judgments
Inability to concentrate
Increased absenteeism and illness
Increased proneness to accidents

The study of potential links between immunity and stress has resulted in highly promising results. In particular, PNI studies of human immunodeficiency virus (HIV) disease progression associated with stress have greatly advanced the field. PNI studies that measured HIV viral load, antiretroviral medication effects, immune cell count, and immune cell cytotoxic over time have shown that the experience of severe life stress can significantly lower both immune system effectiveness and treatment response.[28] Increased stress levels also have been associated with increased HIV morbidity and mortality rates. Researchers caution that much still remains to be learned regarding the links between stress and HIV. However, lower NK cell counts and lower suppressor cell counts have been observed in individuals with HIV who experience stressful life events more frequently. Other experts have hypothesized that high cortisol levels associated with stress might directly affect HIV pathogenesis by increasing viral replication rates or lowering immune system defenses to other pathogens.

Stress response has been linked with more common conditions such as hypertension. A longitudinal study of high and low cardiovascular response to stressors showed that the link between stress and hypertension might be influenced by genetic and environmental factors. The study found that high cardiovascular responders who had one or more hypertensive parent and high daily stress had seven times the risk for developing systolic hypertension than their counterparts with low daily stress.[26] Similar findings have been reported for stress and atherosclerosis. Researchers showed that acute mental stress reduced radial artery vasodilatation responses by as much as half and the reduction lasted nearly an hour. According to the researchers, diminished arterial vasodilatation in response to stress could precipitate myocardial ischemia or infarction.

Stress Response and Age

The stress response of healthy infants and children is robust and timely. Specific stressors and stress-producing experiences commonly experienced by infants and young children include hospitalization, separation from parents, losses of any kind, and pain. Child growth and development is affected by a variety of conditions and circumstances including the child's perception of stressful experiences and caregiver attitudes toward the child. Duration and intensity of stressors also are important. A very brief dental visit may produce a high degree of stress in a toddler despite the fact that the toddler's exposure to the stressor is relatively brief. Acute and chronic illnesses are additional examples of moderate- to high-intensity stressors of varying duration.

Aging itself is a stressful life experience. Although age-related changes in organs and body systems occur gradually and are almost imperceptible to the affected individual, such changes have an impact on how well stress is tolerated. It has been hypothesized that stress and stress responses may augment age-related changes in the body. For example, researchers have speculated that stress may promote anatomic and biochemical neuromuscular changes that reduce the availability of chemical communication transmitters, such as acetylcholine, and thereby decrease nerve cell to muscle cell communication. These changes can result in chronic fatigue and reduced physical strength.

In addition to such physiologic changes, social changes (such as retirement, loss of income, and the death of friends or relatives) and the loss of social support such relationships offered also alter stress management and coping abilities. Elderly adults are not only at increased risk for stress-related disorders; immune system functioning also declines with age.

Some experts now speculate that the young may be as vulnerable to stress-related disease as older adults. Researchers have shown an association in animals between fetal exposure to prenatal stress and high glucocorticoid levels with low birth weight and increased risk of adult stress-related cardiovascular and metabolic disorders such as hypertension and type 2 diabetes. Increased cortisol levels have been linked with increased risk of hypertension in adolescents, particularly males, who exhibit "white coat hypertension"[29] or elevated blood pressure during health care appointments. The

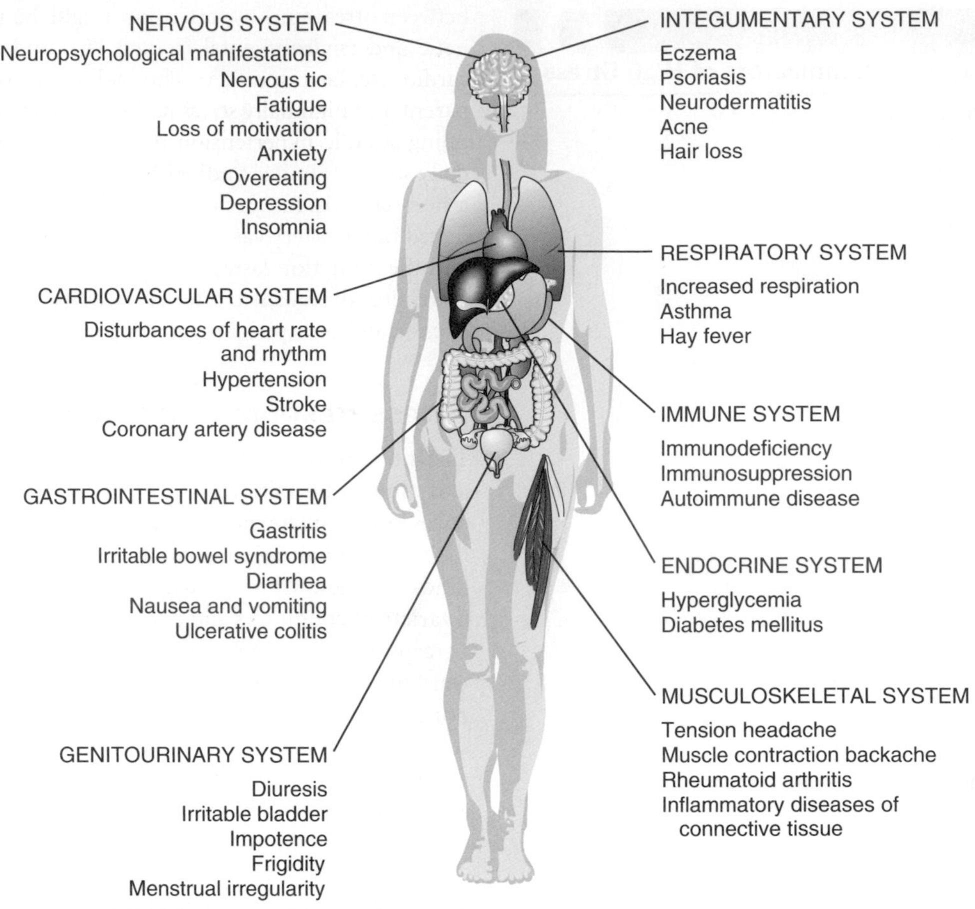

FIGURE 2-13 ■ Effects of excessive stress on target organs or systems.

researchers concluded that adolescent white coat hypertension might be an early yet recognizable sign of increased risk for developing essential hypertension. A direct comparison study of adolescent stress as either the cause of or the result of early age onset cigarette smoking showed that high stress levels preceded smoking onset.[30] Adolescents, particularly females, who had experienced more stress, stress-related depression, and anxiety might have smoked to blunt severe negative mood states. Meaningful differences in health and behavior related to cortisol level also have been reported in children aged 8 to 12 years.[31]

KEY CONCEPTS

- The stress response involves three major body systems: nervous, endocrine, and immune. These systems work together in a coordinated manner to summon the body's defenses in response to a variety of stressors including psychological, physiologic, and immunologic.
- The primary role of the nervous system is appraisal of a stimulus as stressful and activation of the sympathetic nervous system. Norepinephrine released from sympathetic nerve endings increases heart rate and contractility, constricts blood vessels, enhances blood flow to skeletal muscle, reduces gastrointestinal motility and secretion, and dilates the pupils.
- Important stress-related endocrine hormones include epinephrine from the adrenal medulla, cortisol from the adrenal cortex, and ADH from the posterior pituitary.
- Epinephrine's actions are similar to those of norepinephrine and are particularly important for increasing cardiac performance and the release of glucose from the liver.
- Cortisol has synergistic effects with catecholamines in regulating vascular smooth muscle and is antiinflammatory.
- ADH is important for blood volume regulation.
- Secretion of a number of hormones is altered with stress, but a precise role in the stress response is unknown. Growth hormone may increase or decrease, depending on the stress level. Prolactin increases and testosterone and thyroid-stimulating hormone decrease with stress.
- Endorphins increase, leading to decreased perception of pain, sedation, and euphoria.

- The role of the immune system in the stress response is less well characterized. Catecholamines and stress hormones affect the activity of immune cells, and immune-released cytokines, such as neuroactive peptides (e.g., neuroleukin), may influence the neuroendocrine system.
- A number of disorders are thought to be related to excessive stress or inappropriate stress responses. These include asthma, palpitations, headaches, menstrual irregularity, rashes, and digestive disturbances.
- Aging itself is stressful. Furthermore, stress and stress-related mechanisms augment age-related changes in the body.

STRESS AND STRESSORS

The amount of stress humans can withstand without harm varies from individual to individual and from situation to situation. The magnitude of stress response depends on the nature of the stressor, the magnitude of the stressor, and the meaning the stressor holds for the individual who is affected. Personal perceptions both conscious and unconscious significantly impact the magnitude of stress response. Genetic makeup, early stress conditioning, previous stressful experiences, and cultural expectations shape personal perceptions. A college graduate with a successful career is not likely to perceive conflict with co-workers as a major stressor. However, a person with less education and limited work opportunities is likely to appraise co-worker conflict as extremely stressful, especially if few job alternatives exist. Besides the perception of a stressor, other mediating factors, particularly internal and external resources and coping strategies, can affect the response to a major stressor. Stress is triggered in countless ways, but the most common triggers are stressful life events.

Despite many recent scientific advances, the main ingredients of the link between stress and illness continues to elude researchers. Even the link with the most accepted explanatory evidence, namely, the link between stressful life events and depression, is subject to any number of factors, one of the most important being whether the individual views the stressful life event as life in general or something that is highly specific to the individual.[32]

Stressors are agents or conditions that are capable of producing stress. Stressors may be external (e.g., air pollution) or internal (e.g., low blood glucose level or threat to self-esteem) to the individual. Common general stressors are physical (e.g., extreme hot or cold air temperature), chemical (e.g., auto exhaust), biological (e.g., bacteria), social (e.g., overcrowding), cultural (e.g., behavior norms), or psychological (e.g., feelings of hopelessness).

Stressors vary in scope, intensity, and duration, but inherent personal characteristics allow for a great deal of variation in the way humans respond to stressors. During war, individuals exposed to combat eventually become nonfunctional, although no two people are likely to experience this at the same time or in response to the same combat stressors. But no one can experience intense combat for a long time and still remain functional. Take for example a war refugee who suffers from diabetes and hypertension who is seeking safety by hiding in rugged terrain.

The combined stressors of (1) being hunted by enemy forces, (2) not having a good or secure source of food and shelter, (3) not being able to manage underlying health problems because of lack of medicine or therapy, and (4) needing to stay "on the run" are likely to adversely affect the refugee's ability to elude capture and successfully escape. The scope, intensity, and duration of these stressors likely will render the person nonfunctional.

Stressors can affect the same person in different ways at different times. Throughout life, a person goes through a number of critical developmental stages. At critical stages of development, people are likely to become more vulnerable to certain stressors than they are at less critical development stages. For example, a high level of bilirubin in the blood can cause brain damage in a newborn because the blood-brain barrier is still immature at this stage of development, permitting bilirubin to enter the brain. In an adult, however, the blood-brain barrier is impermeable to bilirubin and high plasma concentrations of bilirubin will not have a neurotoxic effect.

Stressors may be classified as low or high intensity. However, a stressor perceived as having low intensity initially may still produce negative effects if it persists for years. For example, living or working for years in a crowded, hostile social environment might produce physiologic changes that in turn can promote symptoms of hypertension. Just as a stressor initially perceived as high-intensity from the outset—such as being involved in a car accident, may prove less damaging because it is resolved more quickly.

Stressors may have a wide or narrow scope. An individual with a mildly sunburned nose has experienced a narrow-scope stressor. In this case, the stress of sunburn literally only affects a small area of skin briefly. By comparison, a newly divorced single parent with bronchitis facing a 60% reduction in household income and loss of health insurance is experiencing wide-scope stressors that affect multiple dimensions of daily life.

Less commonly noted but extremely powerful stressors are psychosocial experiences linked with individual characteristics over which a person may have little or no personal control. Acculturative stress,[32] defined as stress associated with moving from one's culture of origin to another culture, can produce many of the stress responses described in this chapter. The same can said for racial stressors[33] and socioeconomic stressors.[34] Personal psychosocial characteristics can indirectly increase or decrease the impact of most stressors. For example, novelty or sensation seeking has been identified as a personality characteristic that can indirectly buffer or reduce the impact of psychosocial stressors.[35] Based on early morning cortisol level, researchers observed that, compared with less adventurous persons, sensation seekers do not find novel situations stressful and thus have lower rise in cortisol levels and lower stress response. A study of body fat, cortisol levels, and ACTH levels considered body type as an individual characteristic that might greatly influence the perception of a stressor and the stressor's impact on the individual. Previous research findings have suggested that higher levels of body fat may be associated with chronic HPA hyperactivity and increased cortisol levels. In women, greater abdominal fat was found to counteract HPA suppression.[36] Although these findings are inconclusive, taken as a whole, they show the high potential for individual variation in HPA and cortisol response to stressors.

Stressors and Biological Synchronizing Cycles

Biological cycles act as synchronizing agents that sustain vital organism functions. For example, one of the most powerful external synchronizing agents is the cycle of daylight and darkness. To varying extents, human biological functioning is synchronized with this cycle. Biological synchronizing cycles have varying time lengths, such as the lunar (28 days) and circadian (about 1 day) cycles. The human female menstrual cycle typically follows a lunar cycle whereas human body temperature, hormone levels, and rest and activity drives tend to follow a circadian cycle. As a result of circadian and lunar cycles, individual physiologic and psychological systems are likely to differ at different hours of the day or days of the month. The effects of a stressor are influenced by the phase of biological synchronizing cycle the person is in at the time the stressor is experienced. The effects of long-lasting stressors or stress may be influenced by the extent to which the stress also interferes with innate biological synchronizing cycles. For example, persons who work overnight are persistently stressed as they essentially strive to resist their circadian cycle. Such workers tend to be more vulnerable to the onset of stress-related disorders such as depression and the common cold.

KEY CONCEPTS

- Stressors are agents or conditions capable of producing stress.
- Response to a stressor depends on its magnitude and the meaning that the stressor has for an individual. Stressors may be perceived as more or less stressful. Perception depends on genetic constitution, past experiences and conditioning, and cultural influences. Stressors may be external or internal. They may be physical, chemical, biological, sociocultural, or psychological.
- Stressors may be perceived differently at different times, and individuals may be more vulnerable to effects of stressors at certain times. The stage of development, circadian rhythms, and the effects of other previous or concurrent stressors all contribute to the stress response.

CULTURE, COPING, AND ADAPTATION

Culture refers to customs, attitudes, values, and shared beliefs that bind people together to form a society. As depicted by television programs and other popular media, Americans are fascinated by the bizarre, natural disasters, and violence. This response leads to massive outpourings of generosity and caring toward the immediate victims of such events. Paradoxically, this response also supports the avoidance of painful reality and supports attitudes that allow individuals to remain disconnected from the burdens and sufferings of those near them. This avoidance and disconnection are manifested in the American value that idealizes unemotional or highly controlled emotional response to ordinary stressful life events and stressful life circumstances. Fascination, avoidance, and disconnection are behavioral values that support the idealization of individuality as the most prized American cultural norm. Belief in going it alone and succeeding against impossible odds is an accepted reality rather than a questioned fantasy. Few cultures match the American cultural celebration of the heroic ideal in entertainment, sports, politics, religion, business, and education. Nevertheless, this cultural norm conflicts with most of what now is understood regarding stress and successful coping and adaptation.

Coping has become a commonly used expression. For example, observations such as, "He's coping so well with the death of his wife. He arranged the entire funeral and the care of his three children and returned to work the day after the funeral" and "She just fell apart after her baby died. She didn't want to see anyone and cried for days. It's a month now and she still hasn't returned to work" speak volumes.

As suggested in the above examples, coping is a biopsychosocial process of thinking and functioning that is appropriate and effective, *as culturally defined*, when an individual is faced with a stressful experience situation and that allows an individual or a group to successfully withstand the stressful experience and/or the stress response generated by the experience.[37] Popular American culture norms define coping as the ability to carry on with daily life activities with little or no display of emotional reaction during and after the stressful experience. Coping implies *standing firm* and is demonstrated in (1) the ability to communicate emotions verbally and nonverbally, (2) the ability to control emotions, (3) verbal demonstrations of the ability to accurately perceive reality, (4) verbal demonstrations of the ability to think logically and to engage in problem-solving activities, and (5) the ability to cooperate with others in the performance of desired activities.

Cultural mandates aside, the stressor that has been experienced will elicit the actual coping response that occurs. The empirically based, cognitive appraisal theory of coping described by Lazarus and Folkman[38] is perhaps the most widely accepted and tested of all the coping theories developed in the latter half of the 20th century. Unlike those who acknowledged the importance of threat appraisal but remain focused on emotion as the driving force behind coping responses,

Lazarus and Folkman focused on the lead role of cognitive appraisal in the entire stress-coping-adaptation sequence. They proposed that an event or potential stressor is viewed as a situation that is a challenge, a threat, or benign (nonchallenging, nonthreatening). In his earlier formulations, Lazarus proposed that coping responses are provoked only by events viewed as threatening.

Lazarus and Folkman[38] described two types of coping strategies: problem-focused strategies and emotion-focused strategies. The goal of problem-focused strategies was the resolution of the problem or the stressful situation, whereas the goal of emotion-focused strategies was to reduce the painful emotions associated with the stressful situation. Figure 2-14 illustrates both types of coping strategies. Initially, Lazarus gave primacy to the importance of problem-focused strategies and suggested that emotion-focused strategies were immature if not dysfunctional. However, in their more recent theorizing, Lazarus and Folkman give increased emphasis to the importance of emotions in the stress-coping-adaptation sequence and credits the insightful work of Janis as a major contribution to coping science.

A coping strategy can be considered effective or functional if it helps resolve either the situation or the feelings. A coping strategy is considered ineffective or dysfunctional if it does not achieve the desired goal. Coping that achieves unintended goals is considered dysfunctional. Because they are almost inseparable processes that both are integral to life, the terms coping and adapting often are used interchangeably. However, coping implies standing firm whereas adapting implies change.

Potential coping outcomes include (1) resolution of the stressful experience, (2) adaptation to the stressor, (3) or exacerbation of the stressful experience or the stress response. For example, a study of newlywed couples[39] measured plasma epinephrine, norepinephrine, cortisol, and ACTH levels, cardiovascular reactivity, mood, personality, and coping responses. Each couple then was reevaluated 10 years later. The researchers compared still-married couples with couples who had divorced or separated. Baseline stress hormone levels were the strongest predictors of marital status 10 years later. Divorced couples had 34% higher baseline epinephrine levels and significantly higher norepinephrine and ACTH levels than still-married couples. An elevated stress response during the newlywed period appeared to predict poor coping ability later. No other factors, including emotional moods and personality, matched the predictive value of stress hormone levels as the couples faced the many challenges of marriage. Coping

A

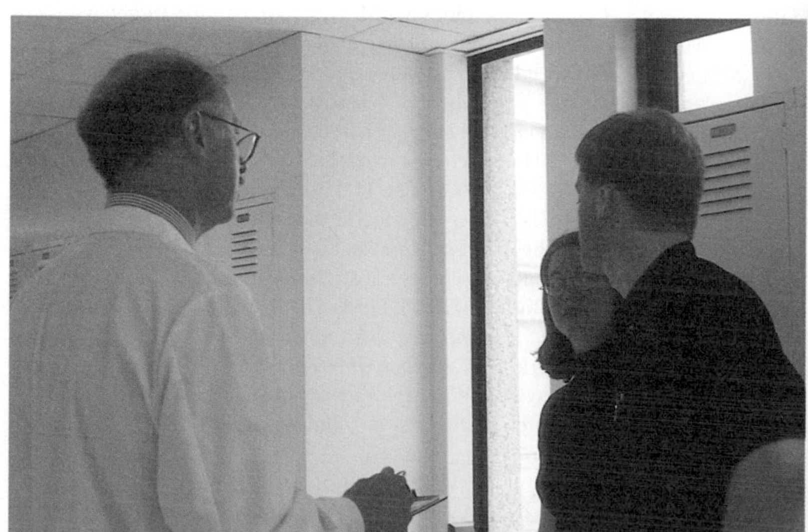

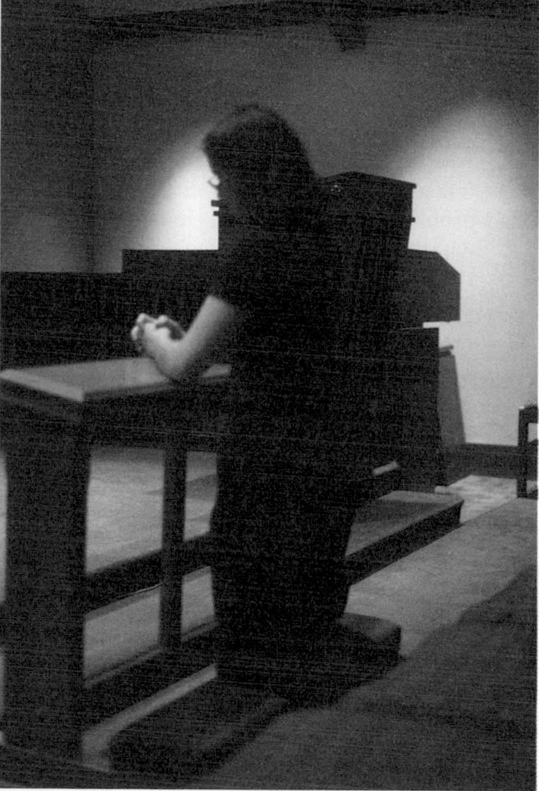

B

FIGURE 2-14 ■ Problem-focused and emotion-focused coping strategies. **A,** Problem-focused coping emphasizes the problem, in this case a medical diagnosis. **B,** Emotion-focused coping emphasizes resolution of the painful emotions associated with the diagnosis. Both coping strategies are used for different purposes. (Photographed by Therese A. Capal, Rockville, Md.)

is a highly complex process subject to a range of biopsychosocial influences, but HPA axis activity may determine actual coping effectiveness.

Adaptation refers to the biopsychosocial process of change in response to new or altered circumstances. Change in itself often is stressful and capable of provoking multiple stress responses. Proponents of life event theories assert that life events are stressful and thus provoke a stress response. Both pleasant life events, such as marriage, the anticipated birth of a child, and a job promotion, as well as unpleasant events, such as the death of a loved one or job loss, require adaptive responses. Encountering favorable or unfavorable life events require multiple levels of biological, personal, and social change or adaptation that are external as well as internal. **Maladaptation** refers to ineffective, inadequate, or inappropriate change in response to new or altered circumstances. When this occurs, the individual has little choice other than continue to expend a great deal of energy and resources attempting to cope with circumstances. Adaptation implies an improved fit between the person and the circumstances at hand, a fit that does not provoke a stress response.

KEY CONCEPTS

- Coping is the biopsychosocial process of thinking and functioning appropriately, as culturally defined, in a stressful situation. In some American cultures, coping is usually viewed as the ability to carry on normal activities without excessive emotional reactions.
- Two types of coping strategies are (1) problem-focused strategies, in which the goal is to resolve the problem, and (2) emotion-focused strategies, in which the goal is to reduce emotional pain. A coping strategy is considered functional if it helps resolve the situation or the feelings.
- Adapting is the biopsychosocial process of changing to become suited to a new or changed situation. Changing situations or life events are potential stressors that may provoke a stress response. Any event may be an actual or potential stressor.

SUMMARY

Recent technological advances have permitted improved understanding of many disease and disorder links with the human stress response. There has been an exponential increase in knowledge regarding the complex interactions of the brain via the HPA axis; the immune system via stress hormones; coping responses intended to regulate emotion, cognitive, and behavioral function; and the impact of cultural stressors.

The study of stress and related biological systems can be traced as far back as written science. As humans strive to adapt to the constant change that is modern life, the study of stress and stress-related disease has become vital to public health. Physiologic stress responses to technological, social, environmental, and biological stressors, complicated by American norms of individuality, routinely challenge ordinary daily coping efforts. Advances in the field of psychoneuroimmunology continue to contribute to the development of increasingly sophisticated models of health and illness.

MEDIA RESOURCES

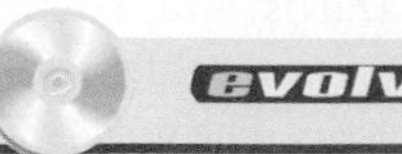

Remember to check out the ***CD Companion*** included with this book for Review Questions, Key Concepts Review, Glossary (with audio for selected terms), Disease Profiles, and Animations.

PLUS, visit the ***Evolve website*** at http://evolve.elsevier.com/Copstead/ for Case Studies, Disease Profiles, and WebLinks.

References

1. Clendening L: *Sourcebook of medical history,* New York, 1942, Dover Publications.
2. Cannon WB: Stresses and strains of homeostasis, *Am J Med Sci* 189:1-14, 1935.
3. Cannon WB: The influence of emotional states on the function of the alimentary canal, *Am J Med Sci* 137:480-487, 1909.
4. Selye H: The general adaptation syndrome and the diseases of adaptation, *J Clin Endocrinol* 6:117-230, 1946.
5. Selye H: *The stress of life,* ed 2, New York, 1976, McGraw-Hill.
6. Roy C, Roberts SL: *Theory construction in nursing: an adaptation model,* Englewood Cliffs, NJ, 1981, Prentice-Hall.
7. Roy C, Andrews HA: *The Roy adaptation model: the definitive statement,* Norwalk, Conn, 1991, Appleton & Lange.
8. Lindsay AM, Carrieri VK: Stress response. In Carrieri-Kohlman VK, Lindsay AM, West CM, editors: *Pathophysiological phenomena in nursing: human responses to illness,* ed 2, Philadelphia, 1993, Saunders.
9. Holmes TH, Rahe RH: The social readjustment rating scale, *J Psychosom Res* 11:213-218, 1967.
10. Rahe RH: Life-change measurement as a predictor of illness, *Proc R Soc Med* 61:1124-1128, 1968.
11. Mason JW: A reevaluation of the concept of non-specificity in stress theory, *J Psychiatr Res* 8:1977-1981, 1971.
12. Lazarus RS: Psychological stress and coping in adaptation and illness. In Lipowski ZJ, Lipsih DR, Whybrow PC, editors: *Psychosomatic medicine: current trends and clinical applications,* New York, 1977, Oxford University Press.
13. Sapolsky RM: *Why zebras don't get ulcers: an updated guide to stress, stress-related diseases, and coping,* New York, 1998, WH Freeman.
14. O'Connor TM, Halloran DJ, Shanahan F: The stress response and the hypothalamic-pituitary-adrenal axis: from molecule to melancholia, *QJM* 93:323-333, 2000.
15. Kelly S, Hertzman C, Daniels M: Searching for the biological pathways between stress and health, *Annu Rev Public Health* 18:437-462, 1997.
16. Kronfol Z, Remick DG: Cytokines and the brain: implications for clinical psychiatry, *Am J Psychiatry* 157(5):683-694, 2000.

17. Puder JJ et al: Estrogen modulates the hypothalamic-pituitary-adrenal and inflammatory cytokine responses to endotoxin in women, *J Clin Endocrinol Metab* 86:2404-2408, 2001.
18. Kendler KS, Thornton LM, Prescott CA: Gender differences in the rates of exposure to stressful life events and sensitivity to their depressiogenic effects, *Am J Psychiatry* 158:587-593, 2001.
19. Mathews KA, Gump BB, Owens JF: Chronic stress influences cardiovascular and neuroendocrine responses during acute stress and recovery, especially in men, *Health Psychol* 20(6):403-410, 2001.
20. Deane R, Chummun H, Prashad D: Differences in urinary stress hormones in male and female nurses at different ages, *J Adv Nurs* 37(3):304-310, 2002.
21. Shephard RJ: Exercise under hot conditions: a major threat to the immune response? *J Sports Med Phys Fitness* 42:368-378, 2002.
22. Machelsk H, Stein C: Immune mechanism in pain control, *Anesth Analg* 95:1002-1008, 2002.
23. Kiecolt-Glaser JK et al: Psychoneuroimmunology: psychological influences on immune function and health, *J Consult Clin Psychol* 70(3):537-547, 2002.
24. Glaser R et al: Stress induced immunomodulation: implications for infectious diseases? *JAMA* 281(24):2268-2270, 1999.
25. Maccari S et al: Prenatal stress and long-term consequences: implications of glucocorticoid hormones, *Neurosci Biobehav Rev* 27:119-127, 2003.
26. Light KC et al: High stress responsivity predicts later blood pressure only in combination with positive family history and high life stress, *Hypertension* 33:1458-1464, 1999.
27. Miller G, Cohen S, Ritchey AK: Chronic psychological stress and the regulation of pro-inflammatory cytokines: a glucocorticoid-resistance model, *Health Psychol* 21(6):531-541, 2002.
28. Leserman J: HIV disease progression: depression, stress, and possible mechanisms, *Biol Psychiatry* 54:295-306, 2003.
29. Vaindirlis I et al: White coat hypertension in adolescents: increased values of urinary cortisol and endothelin, *J Pediatr* 136(3):359-364, 2000.
30. Wills TA, Sandy JM, Yaeger AM: Stress and smoking in adolescence: a test of directional hypotheses, *Health Psychol* 21(2):122-130, 2002.
31. van Goozen SHM et al: Hypothalamic-pituitary-adrenal axis and autonomic nervous system activity in disruptive children and matched controls, *J Am Acad Child Adolesc Psychiatry* 39(11):1438-1445, 2000.
32. Joiner TE, Walker RL: Construct validity of a measure of acculturative stress in African Americans, *Psychol Assess* 14(4):462-466, 2002.
33. Utsey S et al: Effect of ethnic group membership on ethnic identity, race-related stress, and quality of life, *Cult Divers Ethnic Minor Psychol* 8(4):366-377, 2002.
34. Steptoe A et al: Socioeconomic status and hemodynamic recovery from mental stress, *Psychophysiology* 40:184-191, 2003.
35. Roberti JW: Biological responses to stressors and the role of personality, *Life Sci* 73:2527-2531, 2003.
36. Pasquali R et al: Cortisol and ACTH response to oral dexamethasone in obesity and effects of sex, body fat distribution, and dexamethasone concentrations: a dose-response study, *J Clin Endocrinol Metab* 87(1):166-175, 2002.
37. Kendler KS, Karkowske LM, Prescott CA: Causal relationship between stressful life events and the onset of major depression, *Am J Psychiatry* 156:837-841, 1999.
38. Lazarus RS, Folkman S: *Stress, appraisal, and coping,* New York, 1984, Springer.
39. Kiecolt-Glaser JK et al: Love, marriage, and divorce: newlyweds' stress hormones foreshadow relationship changes, *J Consult Clin Psychol* 71(1):176-188, 2003.

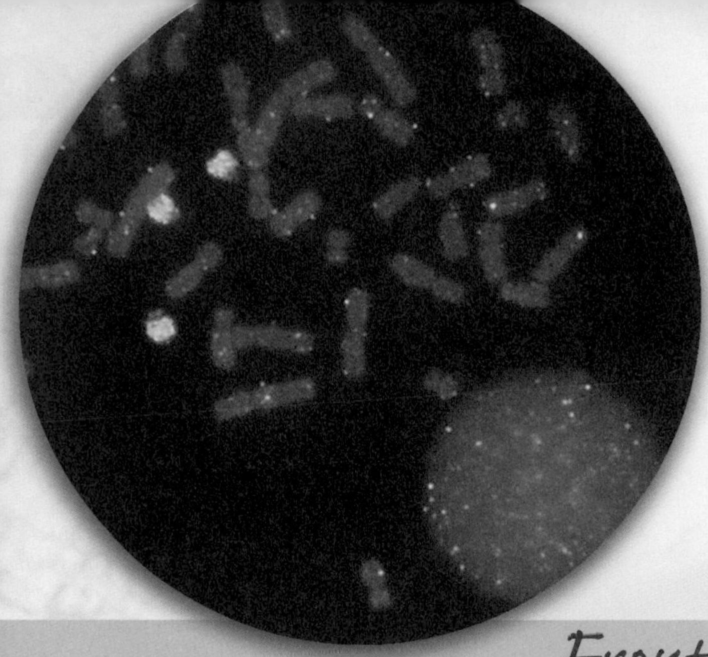

Frontiers of Research

Genes and Genetic Disorders

Marc S. Williams and Michael J. Kirkhorn

The year 2003 represented a milestone in biology and genetics. Not only was the 50th anniversary of Watson and Crick's discovery of the structure of DNA celebrated, but the final sequence of the human genome has been published. Three billion base pairs and about 30,000 genes that produce about 100,000 proteins will keep generations of biologists busy. The 20th century is recognized for a myriad of technological advances, but the 21st century is likely to be remembered as the century of the biological revolution. The completion of the human DNA sequence is the first shot in this revolution.

Genetics is the study of variation. The genome project has shown us that human beings are 99.9% similar to one another at the DNA level. Although 0.1% variation seems minimal, it represents about 3 million base pairs. Within this variation lies a wealth of information about disease susceptibility, individual drug response, so-called idiopathic reactions, as well as factors that may well influence a variety of complex traits such as intelligence, learning ability (and disability), and personality.

In October 2002, an international consortium announced a Genetic Variation Mapping Project (International HapMap Project). This project is to be completed in 3 years at a cost of $100 million. The expectation is that this will accelerate the identification of genes responsible for a variety of disorders including asthma, cancer, diabetes, and heart disease.

It is important to recognize that in most cases the changes in these genes will not represent traditional mutations that dramatically affect the function of the gene (as is seen in more traditional genetic disorders such as cystic fibrosis or Marfan syndrome). These changes mostly represent single nucleotide polymorphisms (SNPs) that have mini-

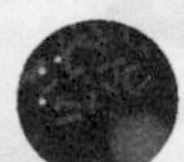

Chromosome painting with a library of chromosome 22–specific DNA probes. The presence of three fluorescent chromosomes indicates that the patient has trisomy 22. (From Kumar V, Abbas AK, Fausto N: Robbins and Cotran pathologic basis of disease, *ed 7, Philadelphia, 2005, Saunders, p 173. Courtesy Dr. Charleen M. Moore, The University of Texas Health Science Center at San Antonio, Tex.)*

Cellular Function

UNIT II

mal effect by themselves in creating susceptibility to disease. Disorders such as diabetes are likely due to the presence of many genetic variants that individually have a relatively weak contribution to the development of the disease. Only when several of these factors are present is the risk increased. Environment and other nongenetic factors also play a role in this susceptibility.

It is estimated that there are about 10 million SNPs in the genome, or 1 roughly every 300 base pairs. Identifying these SNPs and comparing specific patterns (or haplotypes) in individuals affected with a certain condition will yield a pattern of SNPs that increases an individual's risk for developing a given disorder.

At first blush, it would appear difficult to translate this information into something that is clinically useful. However, by adapting the technology developed to print circuits on silicon chips for the computer industry, researchers have been able to create "gene chips" that hold tens to hundreds of thousands of short DNA fragments. A single drop of patient blood applied to a chip of this type would yield a complete SNP susceptibility profile. Mapping an individual patient's haplotypes also may be used in the future to help customize medical treatment. Genetic variation has been shown to affect the response of patients to drugs, toxic substances, and other environmental factors. Some already envision an era in which drug treatment is customized, based on the patient's haplotypes, to maximize the effectiveness of the drug while minimizing side effects.

Francis Collins, director of the National Human Genome Research Institute, is on record as saying, "Within 50 years, we expect comprehensive genomic-based health care to be the norm in the USA." Let the revolution commence.

chapter 3

Cell Structure and Function

Jacquelyn L. Banasik

MEDIA RESOURCES

Additional Material for Study, Review, and Further Exploration

CD Companion ◆ Review Questions and Answers ◆ Key Concepts Review ◆ Glossary *(with audio pronunciations for selected terms)* ◆ Disease Profiles ◆ Animations

evolve ***Website*** at http://evolve.elsevier.com/Copstead/ ◆ Case Studies ◆ Disease Profiles ◆ WebLinks

KEY QUESTIONS

- What are the major cellular structures and their functions?
- How do cells acquire and use energy?
- How are substances transported across the cell membrane?
- Why is it that some cells can produce action potentials and others cannot?
- How do cells in a multicellular organism communicate with one another?
- What are the normal mechanisms of cellular growth control?

CHAPTER OUTLINE

A basic principle of biology states that the cell is the fundamental unit of life. As more diseases are understood on the cellular and molecular level, it appears that the cell is also the fundamental unit of disease. A knowledge explosion is currently occurring in the fields of cell and molecular biology, leading to a better understanding of human physiology and the cellular aspects of disease. Detailed knowledge of cellular dysfunction has led to the development of more specific and appropriate prevention and treatment modalities for many disease processes. Thus, an understanding of cellular mechanisms is essential for health care providers and fundamental to the discussions of pathophysiologic processes presented throughout the remainder of this text.

Cells are complex, membrane-bound units packed with a multitude of chemicals and macromolecules. They are able to replicate and thus form new cells and organisms. The very first cells on earth probably arose from the spontaneous association of organic (carbon-containing) and inorganic molecules about 3.5 billion years ago.[1] Over billions of years, the self-replicating molecules now known as deoxyribonucleic acid (DNA) and ribonucleic acid (RNA) are believed to have evolved by chance association and natural selection. Evolution of the cell membrane created a closed compartment that provided a selective advantage for the cell and accomplished the first separation of life (inside) from nonlife (outside). In this protected environment, the early cells continued to evolve and develop. Today, a number of different cell types exist, but many of the basic biochemical mechanisms of these cell types are remarkably similar. Scientists believe that all modern cells, from bacteria to human neurons, evolved from common primordial cells.[2] It is therefore possible to unlock many of the secrets of human cellular physiology by studying easily grown and rapidly proliferating cells such as yeasts and bacteria.

Much of our knowledge of cell physiology has derived from study of the class of cells known as **prokaryotic,** which includes bacteria and archaea. Prokaryotic cells are smaller and simpler than **eukaryotic** cells, having no defined nucleus or cytoplasmic organelles. Fungi, plants, and animals belong to the eukaryotic class of cells, which possess a membrane-bound nucleus and a host of cytoplasmic organelles (Figure 3-1). In this chapter, the essentials of eukaryotic cell structure, physiology, metabolism, and communication are reviewed.

PLASMA MEMBRANE

Membrane Structure

All cells are enclosed by a barrier composed primarily of lipid and protein called the **plasma membrane** (plasmalemma). This cell membrane is a highly selective filter that shields internal cell contents from the external environment. The plasma membrane performs a variety of functions, including transport of nutrients and waste products, generation of membrane potentials, and cell recognition, communication, and growth regulation. The cell membrane is a sensor of signals that enables the cell to respond and adapt to changes in its environment.

According to the fluid mosaic model, described in the 1960s by Singer and Nicolson,[3] the plasma membrane is a dynamic assembly of lipid and protein molecules. Most of the lipids and

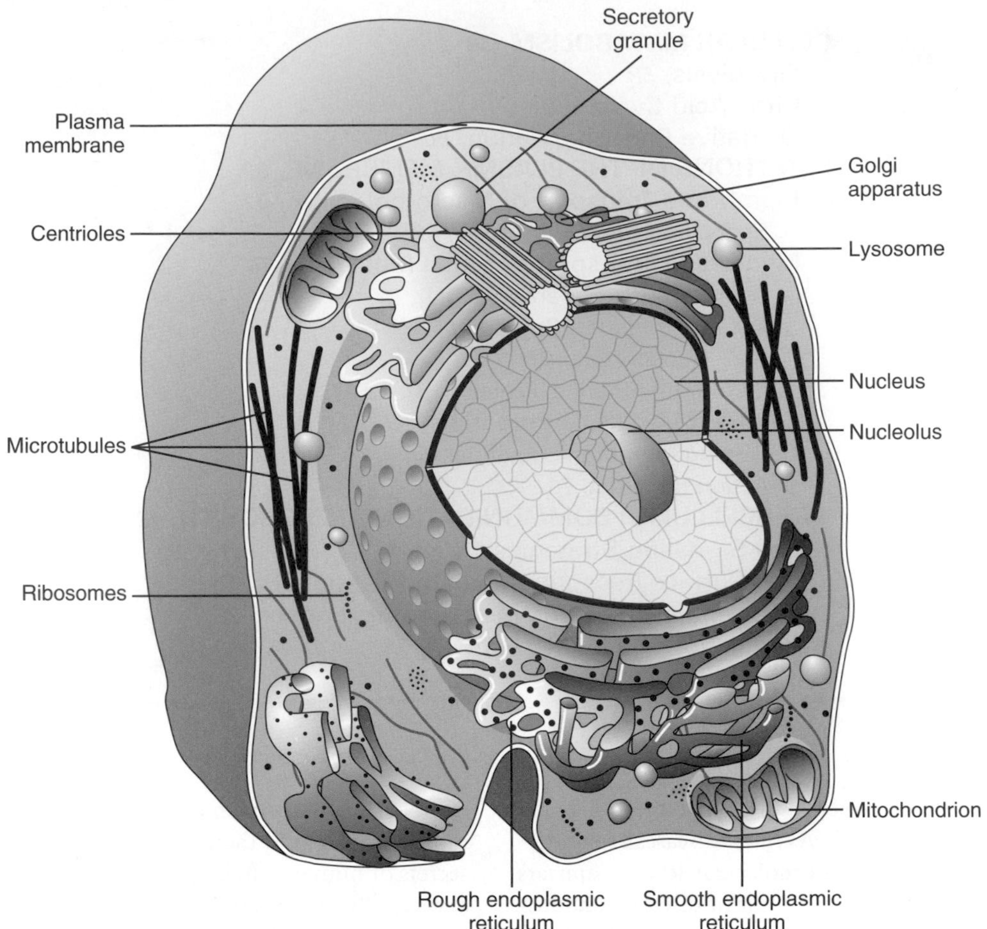

FIGURE 3-1 ■ Structure of a typical eukaryotic cell showing intracellular organelles.

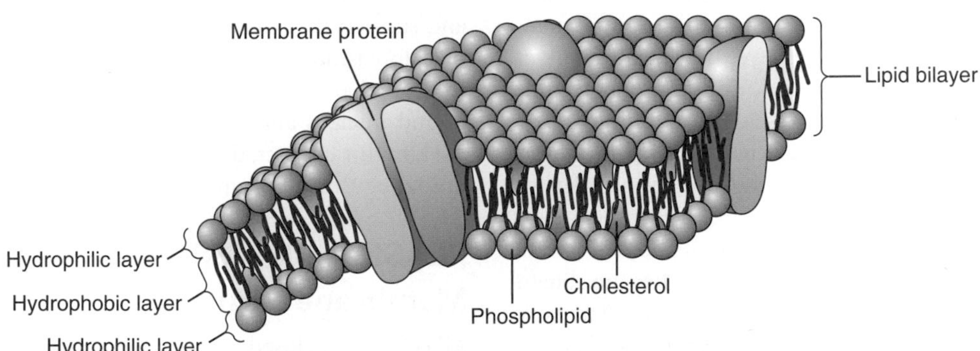

FIGURE 3-2 ■ Section of the cell membrane showing the lipid bilayer structure and integral membrane proteins.

proteins move about rapidly in the fluid structure of the membrane. As shown in Figure 3-2, the lipid molecules are arranged in a double layer, or **lipid bilayer,** which is highly impermeable to most water-soluble molecules, including ions, glucose, and proteins. A variety of proteins embedded or "dissolved" in the lipid bilayer perform most of the membrane's functions. Some membrane proteins are involved in the transport of specific molecules into and out of the cell; others function as enzymes or respond to external signals; and some serve as structural links that connect the plasma membrane to adjacent cells. The lipid structure of the plasma membrane is similar to the membrane that surrounds the cell's organelles (nucleus, mitochondria, endoplasmic reticulum, Golgi apparatus, lysosomes).

Lipid Bilayer

The bilayer structure of all biological membranes is related to the special properties of lipid molecules, which cause them to spontaneously assemble into bilayers. The three major types of membrane lipids are cholesterol, phospholipids, and glyco-

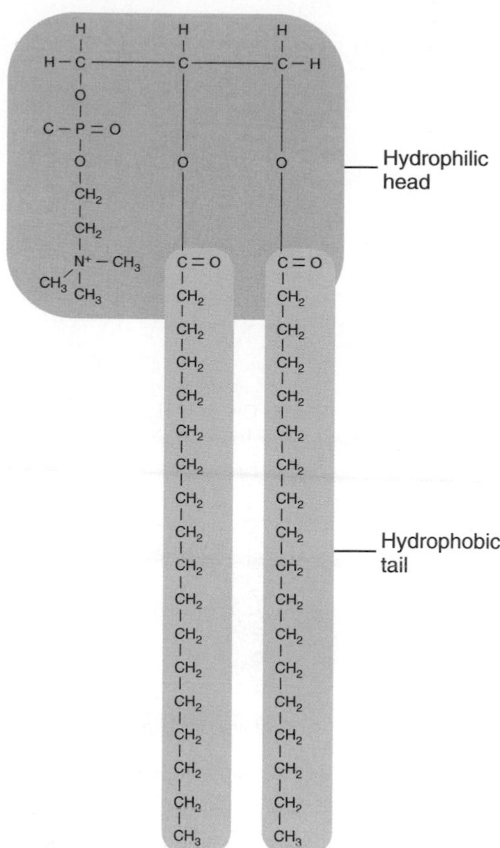

FIGURE 3-3 ■ Schematic drawing of a typical membrane phospholipid molecule showing the amphipathic nature of the structure.

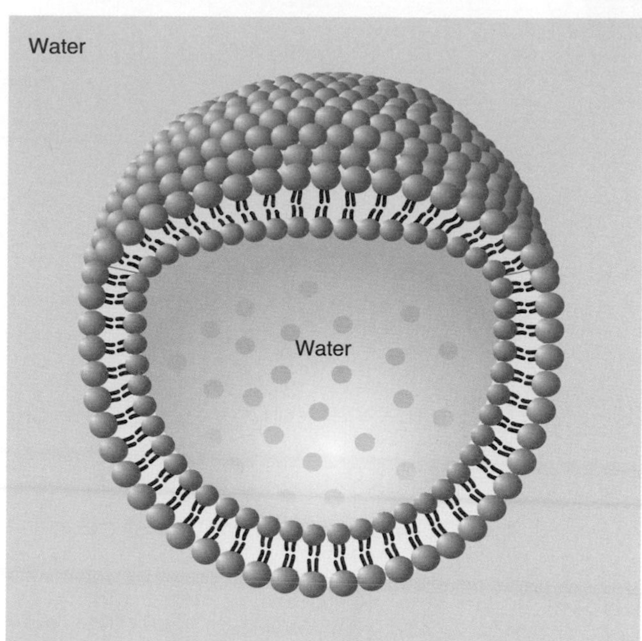

FIGURE 3-4 ■ The amphipathic nature of membrane lipids results in bilayer structures that tend to form spheres.

lipids. All three have a molecular structure that is **amphipathic**; that is, they have a hydrophilic (water-loving) charged or polar end and a hydrophobic (water-fearing) nonpolar end.[1] This amphipathic nature causes the lipids to form bilayers in aqueous solution. A typical phospholipid molecule is shown in Figure 3-3. The hydrophobic nonpolar tails tend to associate with other hydrophobic nonpolar-tail groups to avoid association with polar water molecules. The hydrophilic polar head groups preferentially interact with the surrounding aqueous environment. A bilayer, with tails sandwiched in the middle, allows both portions of the lipid molecules to be chemically "satisfied." In addition, the lipid bilayers tend to close on themselves, forming sealed, spherical compartments (Figure 3-4). If the membrane is punctured or torn it will spontaneously reseal itself to eliminate contact of the hydrophobic tails with water.

For the most part, individual lipid and protein molecules can diffuse freely and rapidly within the plane of the bilayer, but flip from one side to the other infrequently.[4] The degree of membrane fluidity depends on the lipid composition. Saturated lipids have straight tails that can pack together and tend to stiffen the membrane, whereas lipids with bent unsaturated hydrocarbon tails tend to increase fluidity. About 50% of the lipid in eukaryotic cell membranes is cholesterol, which serves to decrease membrane permeability and prevent leakage of small water-soluble molecules. In addition to affecting fluidity by the degree of saturation of tail groups, the phospholipids that inhabit the membrane also differ in the size, shape, and charge of the polar head groups. Figure 3-5 shows the structures of the four most prevalent membrane phospholipids: phosphatidylethanolamine, phosphatidylserine, phosphatidylcholine, and sphingomyelin. Some membrane-bound proteins require specific phospholipid head groups to function properly. Some lipids, sphingolipids and cholesterol in particular, may bind together transiently to form rafts in the sea of moving lipids. These rafts may surround and help organize membrane proteins into functional units. For example, a membrane receptor and its intracellular target proteins may associate together in a raft to facilitate transfer of information across the membrane.[4]

Glycolipids contain one or more sugar molecules at the polar head region. Interestingly, glycolipids and glycoproteins are found only in the outer half of the lipid bilayer, with the sugar groups exposed at the cell surface (Figure 3-6). The functional significance of membrane glycolipids remains largely a mystery, although they are thought to be involved in cell recognition and cell-to-cell interactions.[5]

Membrane Proteins

Approximately 50% of the mass of a typical cell membrane is composed of protein. The specific types of membrane proteins vary according to cell type and environmental conditions. Some membrane proteins, called *transmembrane proteins*, extend across the membrane bilayer and are in contact with both the extracellular and intracellular fluids. Transmembrane proteins serve a variety of functions, including transport of charged and polar molecules into and out of cells and transduction of extracellular signals into intracellular messages.

Phosphatidylethanolamine | Phosphatidylserine | Phosphatidylcholine | Sphingomyelin

FIGURE 3-5 ■ Chemical structures of the four most common membrane phospholipids.

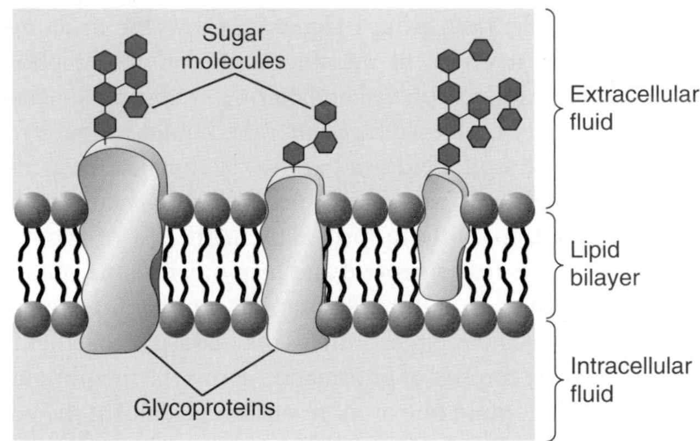

FIGURE 3-6 ■ Portion of the cell membrane showing orientation of membrane glycoproteins toward the outer surface of the cell.

Other peripheral membrane proteins are less tightly anchored to the membrane. The common structural orientations of membrane proteins are shown in Figure 3-7. The amino acid structure of membrane proteins determines the way they are arranged in the membrane. Nonpolar amino acids tend to inhabit the hydrophobic middle of the membrane, whereas charged and polar amino acids stick out into the aqueous fluid or associate with polar lipid head groups. The three-dimensional structure of many membrane proteins is complex with numerous twists and turns through the lipid bilayer.

The type of membrane proteins in a particular cell depends on the cell's primary functions. For example, a kidney tubule cell has a large proportion of transmembrane proteins, which are needed to perform the kidney's function of electrolyte and nutrient reabsorption. In contrast, the human red blood cell (RBC) contains mainly peripheral proteins attached to the inner surface of the membrane.[6] One of these proteins, spectrin, has a long, thin, flexible rod-like shape that forms a supportive meshwork or **cytoskeleton** for the cell. It is this cytoskeleton that enables the RBC to withstand the membrane stress of being forced through small capillaries.

Although proteins and lipids are generally free to move within the plane of the cell membrane, many cells are able to confine certain proteins to specific areas. Using the example of the kidney tubule cell again, it is important for the cell to keep transport proteins on its luminal side to reabsorb filtered molecules (Figure 3-8). This segregation of particular proteins is thought to be accomplished primarily by intercellular connections called **tight junctions,** which connect neighboring cells and function like a fence to confine proteins to an area of membrane. Membrane proteins also can be immobilized by tethering them to cytoskeleton or extracellular matrix structures.

KEY CONCEPTS

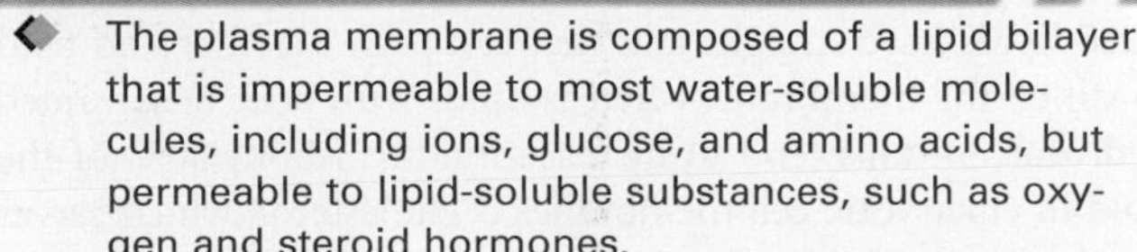

- The plasma membrane is composed of a lipid bilayer that is impermeable to most water-soluble molecules, including ions, glucose, and amino acids, but permeable to lipid-soluble substances, such as oxygen and steroid hormones.

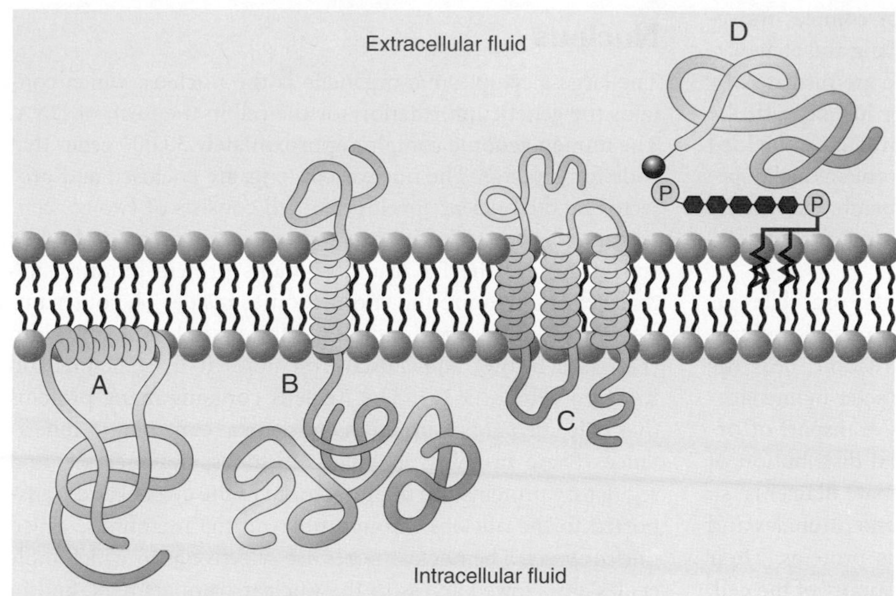

FIGURE 3-7 ■ Structural orientation of some proteins in the cell membrane. **A,** Membrane protein with noncovalent attachment to plasma lipids. **B,** Membrane protein with noncovalent attachment to another membrane protein. **C,** Transmembrane protein extending through the lipid bilayer. **D,** Covalently attached peripheral membrane protein.

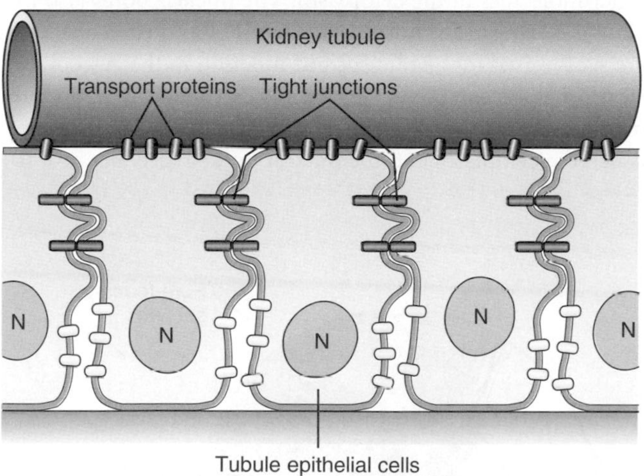

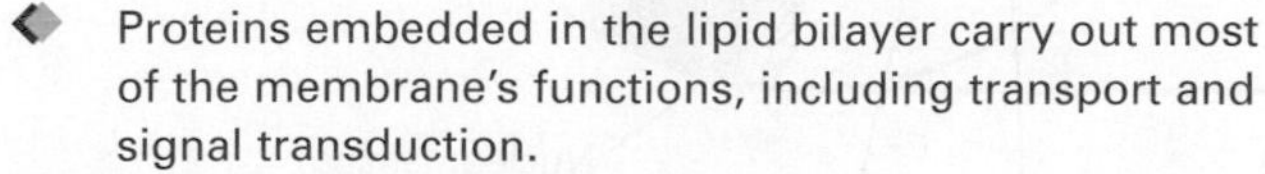

FIGURE 3-8 ■ Transport proteins may be confined to a particular portion of the cell membrane by tight junctions. Segregation of transport proteins is important for the absorptive functions of the kidney epithelial cells. *N,* Nucleus.

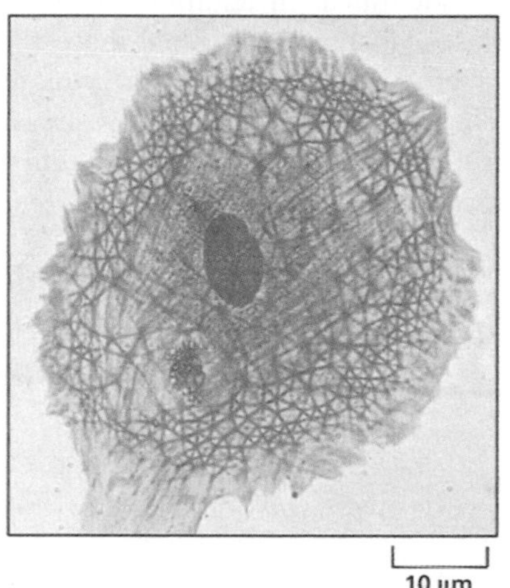

FIGURE 3-9 ■ Schematic of the cytoskeleton showing two of the major protein structures, actin and intermediate filaments. (From Alberts B et al, editors: *Molecular biology of the cell,* ed 4, New York, 2002, Garland Science, p 907.)

◆ Proteins embedded in the lipid bilayer carry out most of the membrane's functions, including transport and signal transduction.

ORGANIZATION OF CELLULAR COMPARTMENTS

Cytoskeleton

Eukaryotic cells have a variety of internal compartments, or **organelles,** which are membrane bound and carry out distinct cellular functions. The cell's organelles are not free to float around haphazardly in the cytoplasmic soup; rather, they are elaborately organized by a protein network called the *cytoskeleton* (Figure 3-9).[7] The cytoskeleton maintains the cell's shape, allows cell movement, and directs the trafficking of substances within the cell. Three principal types of protein filaments make up the cytoskeleton: actin filaments, microtubules, and intermediate filaments.

All three types of filaments are made up of small proteins that can assemble (polymerize) into filaments of varying length. The filament structures are dynamic and can be rapidly disassembled and reassembled according to the changing needs of the cell.[7] Actin filaments, also known as microfilaments, play a pivotal role in cell movement. As one might expect, muscle cells are packed with actin filaments, which allows the cell to perform its primary function of contraction. However, nonmuscle cells also possess actin filaments that are important for complex movements of the cell membrane, such as cell crawling and phagocytosis. Such movements of the cell membrane are mediated by dense networks of actin filaments that cluster just beneath the plasma membrane and interact with specific proteins embedded in it. Actin and some of the other cytoskeletal proteins make specific contacts with and through the plasma membrane and are involved in information transfer from the extracellular environment to signaling cascades within the cell.

Organization of the cytoplasm and its organelles is achieved primarily by microtubules. In animal cells, microtubules originate at the cell center, or **centrosome,** near the nucleus and radiate out toward the cell perimeter in fine lacelike threads. Microtubules guide the orderly transport of organelles in the cytoplasm as well as the equal distribution of chromosomes during cell division. Intermediate filaments, so named because their size is between that of microtubules and actin filaments, are strong, ropelike, fibrous proteins. Their primary function seems to be mechanical support of the cell. A variety of intermediate filaments that differ from tissue to tissue have been identified. In addition to the three main groups of cytoskeletal filaments described above, a large number of accessory proteins are essential for cytoskeletal function. For example, the accessory protein, myosin, is needed to bind with actin to achieve motor functions. Different accessory proteins are present in different cell types.

Nucleus

The largest cytoplasmic organelle is the **nucleus,** which contains the genetic information for the cell in the form of **DNA.** The human genome contains approximately 30,000 genes that code for proteins. The nuclear contents are enclosed and protected by the nuclear envelope, which consists of two concentric membranes. The inner membrane forms an unbroken sphere around the DNA and contains protein-binding sites that help to organize the chromosomes inside. The outer nuclear membrane is continuous with the endoplasmic reticulum (ER) (see below) and closely resembles it in structure and function (Figure 3-10). The nucleus contains many proteins that help mediate its functions of genetic control and inheritance. These proteins, including histones, polymerases, and regulatory proteins, are manufactured in the cytosol and transported to the nucleus through holes in the membrane called *nuclear pores.* The nuclear pores are selective as to which molecules are allowed access to the nuclear compartment, and in this way they protect the genetic material from enzymes and other molecules in the cytoplasm. The nuclear pores also mediate the export of products such as RNA and ribosomes that are synthesized in the nucleus but function in the cytosol. Nuclear pores are complexes of proteins that span across both the inner and outer nuclear membrane creating a pathway between the cytoplasm and the nuclear lamina (see Figure 3-10).

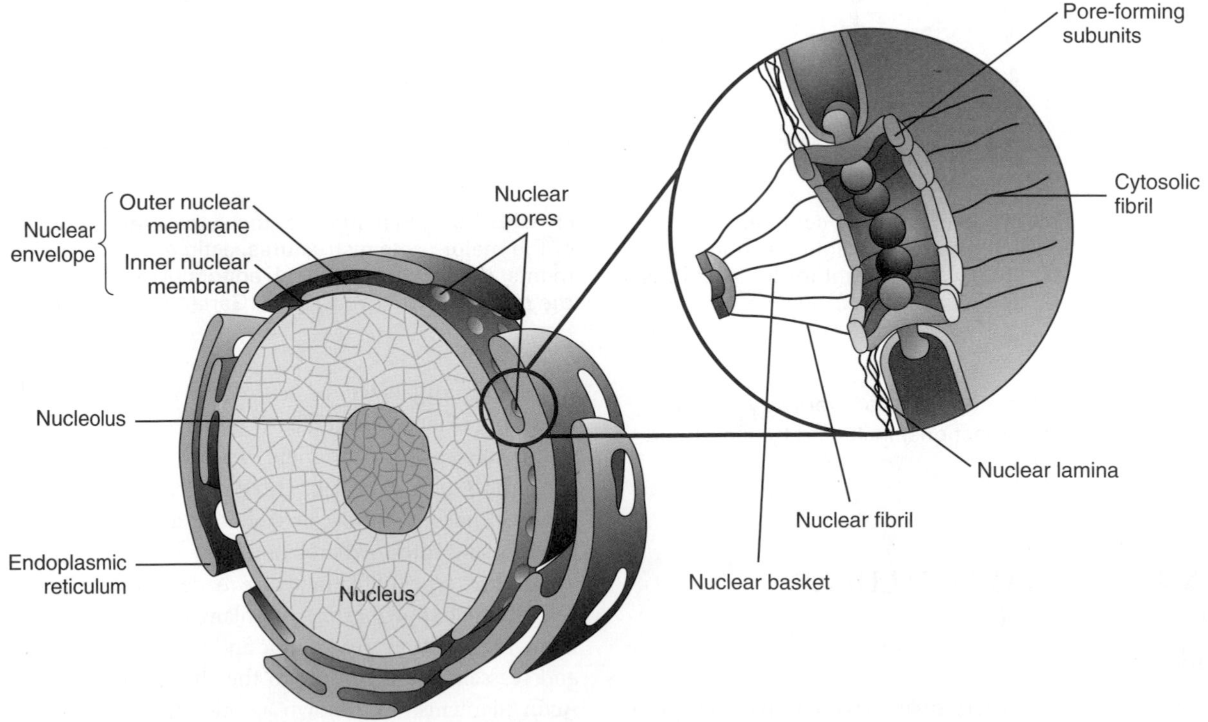

FIGURE 3-10 ■ Structure of the double-membrane envelope that surrounds the cell nucleus.

A major function of the nucleus is to protect and preserve genetic information so that it can be replicated exactly and passed on during cell division. However, the nucleus is continuously functioning even when the cell is not actively dividing. The nuclear DNA controls the production of cellular enzymes, membrane receptors, structural proteins, and other proteins that define the cell's type and behavior. (The structure and function of DNA are discussed in Chapter 5.)

During mitosis, the complex structure of the nuclear membrane and its pore-forming proteins breaks up into small bits that diffuse through the cell cytoplasm. After cell division is complete, bits of nuclear membrane surround and gather up the chromosomes and then fuse together to form a new nuclear membrane. Nuclear proteins and pore structures are then recruited back to their normal nuclear locations.[8]

Endoplasmic Reticulum

The ER is a membrane network that extends throughout the cytoplasm and is present in all eukaryotic cells (Figure 3-11). The ER is thought to have a single continuous membrane that separates the lumen of the ER from the cytosol—it could be likened to a "gastrointestinal tract" in the cell. The ER plays a central role in the synthesis of membrane components, including proteins and lipids, for the plasma membrane and cellular organelles as well as in the synthesis of products to be secreted from the cell. The ER is divided into rough and smooth types based on its appearance under the electron microscope. The **rough ER** is coated with ribosomes along its outer surface. **Ribosomes** are complexes of protein and RNA, which are formed in the nucleus and transported to the cytoplasm. Their primary function is the synthesis of proteins (see Chapter 5). Depending on the destination of the protein to be created, ribosomes may float free in the cytosol or may bind to the ER membrane. Proteins synthesized by free-floating ribosomes are released within the cytosol of the cell. Proteins to be transported into the ER have a special sequence of amino acids that binds the ribosome responsible for its synthesis to the ER membrane. The protein is then translocated through a pore in the ER membrane as it is being synthesized. After processing in the ER and Golgi apparatus, the protein is eventually transported to the appropriate organelle or secreted at the cell surface. Free-floating and rough ER ribosomes are identical and interchangeable; their location depends on the amino acid structure of the protein they are producing at the time.[9]

Regions of ER that lack ribosomes are called **smooth** ER. The smooth ER is involved in lipid metabolism. Most cells have very little smooth ER, but cells specializing in the production of steroid hormones or lipoproteins may have significant amounts of smooth ER. For example, the hepatocyte (liver cell) has abundant smooth ER containing enzymes (P450) responsible for the manufacture of lipoproteins as well as the detoxification of harmful lipid-soluble compounds, such as alcohol. The cellular smooth ER can double in surface area within a few days if large quantities of drugs or toxins enter the circulation. Cells in the adrenal cortex and gonads that produce steroid hormones also have abundant smooth ER. In addition to synthetic functions, the ER also sequesters large amounts of calcium ions by pumping them from the cytoplasm. In response to specific signals, the ER releases calcium ions as part of important second-messenger cascades. Muscle cells have extensive smooth ER (sarcoplasmic reticulum) dedicated to the sequestration of calcium. When the cell is stimulated, the sarcoplasmic reticulum releases the calcium ions needed to accomplish muscle contraction.

Golgi Apparatus

The **Golgi apparatus** or Golgi complex is composed of a stack of smooth membrane-bound compartments resembling a stack of hollow plates (see Figure 3-11). These compartments

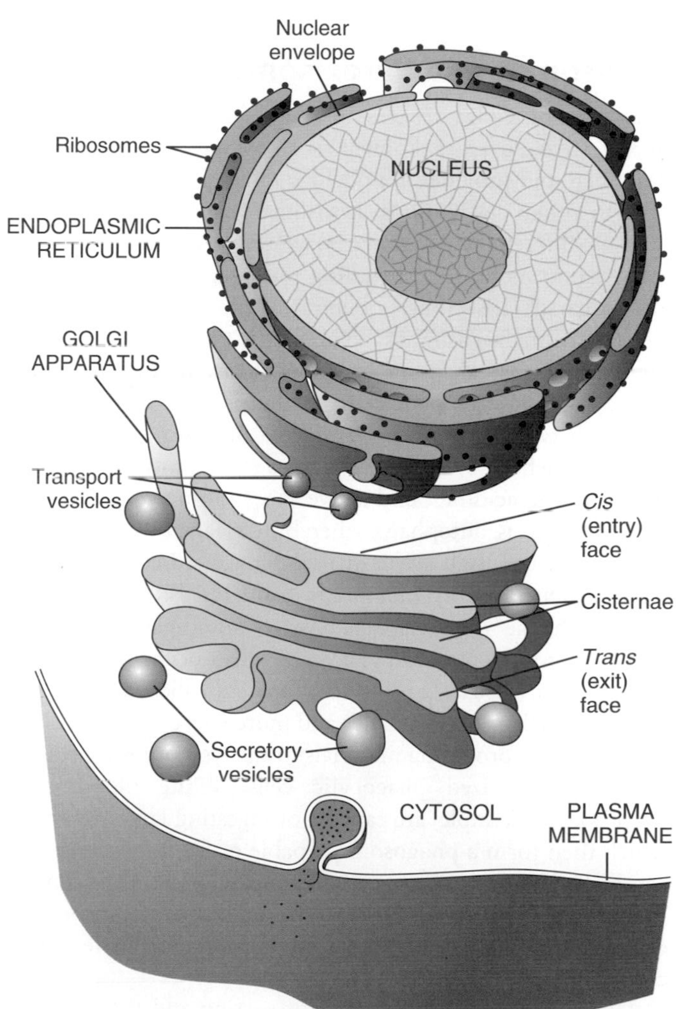

FIGURE 3-11 ■ Schematic drawing of the endoplasmic reticulum and its relationship to the Golgi apparatus and nuclear envelope.

or *cisternae* are organized in a series of at least three processing compartments. The first compartment (*cis* face) lies next to the ER and receives newly synthesized proteins and lipids by way of ER transport vesicles. These transport vesicles bud off from the ER membrane and diffuse to the Golgi where they bind and become part of the Golgi apparatus membrane. The proteins and lipids then move through the middle compartment (medial) to the final compartment (*trans* face), where they depart for their final destination. As the lipid and protein molecules pass through the sequence of Golgi compartments, they are modified by enzymes that attach or rearrange sugar molecules. After specific arrangement of these sugars has occurred, the lipids and proteins are packaged into Golgi transport vesicles (secretory vesicles). The particular configuration of sugar molecules on the lipid or protein is thought to serve as an "address label," directing them to the correct destination within the cell. Golgi vesicles transport their contents primarily to the plasma membrane and to lysosomes.

Lysosomes and Peroxisomes

Transport of Golgi vesicles to the membrane-bound bags of digestive enzymes known as **lysosomes** has been well described and provides a model for Golgi sorting and transport to other destinations. Lysosomes are filled with more than 40 different acid hydrolases, which are capable of digesting organic molecules, including proteins, nucleotides, fats, and sugars.[10] Lysosomes obtain the materials they digest from three main pathways.[10] The first is the pathway used to digest products taken up by endocytosis. In this pathway, endocytotic vesicles bud off from the plasma membrane to fuse with endosomes. Endosomes mature into lysosomes as the Golgi delivers lysosomal enzymes to them; the pH inside the lysosome acidifies, and active digestion occurs. The second pathway is autophagy whereby damaged and obsolete parts of the cell itself are destroyed. Unwanted cellular structures are enclosed by membrane from the ER, which then fuses with the lysosome, leading to autodigestion of the cellular components. Autophagy may also occur during cell starvation or disuse, leading to a process called **atrophy**, in which the cell becomes smaller and more energy efficient. The third pathway providing materials to the lysosomes is present only in specialized phagocytic cells. White blood cells (WBCs), for example, are capable of ingesting large particles, which then form a **phagosome** capable of fusing with a lysosome. The final products of lysosomal digestion are simple molecules, such as amino acids, fatty acids, and sugars, which can be utilized by the cell or secreted as cellular waste at the cell surface.

Discovery of the mechanism for sorting and transport of lysosomal enzymes was aided by studying patients suffering from the lysosomal storage diseases.[11] Patients with I-cell (inclusion cell) disease, for example, accumulate large amounts of debris in lysosomes, which appear as spots or "inclusions" in the cells. These lysosomes lack nearly all of the hydrolases normally present and thus are unable to perform lysosomal digestion. However, all the hydrolases missing from the lysosomes can be found in the patient's bloodstream. The abnormality results from "missorting" by the Golgi apparatus, which erroneously packages the enzymes for extracellular secretion rather than sending them to the lysosomes. Studies of this rare genetic disease resulted in the discovery that all lysosomal enzymes have a common marker, mannose-6-phosphate, which normally targets the enzymes to the lysosomes. Persons with I-cell disease lack the enzyme responsible for attaching this marker.

Peroxisomes (microbodies), like lysosomes, are membrane-bound bags of enzymes that perform degradative functions. They are particularly important in liver and kidney cells, where they detoxify various substances, such as alcohol. In contrast to lysosomes, which contain hydrolase enzymes, peroxisomes contain oxidative enzymes. These enzymes use molecular oxygen to break down organic substances by an oxidative reaction that produces hydrogen peroxide. The hydrogen peroxide is then used by another enzyme (catalase) to break down other organic molecules, including formaldehyde and alcohol. Catalase also prevents accumulation of excess hydrogen peroxide in the cell by converting it to water and oxygen. Peroxisomes also oxidize fatty acids (β oxidation) to produce acetyl coenzyme A (acetyl CoA) that is used in cellular metabolism. Unlike lysosomes, which acquire their enzymes from Golgi vesicles, peroxisomes import enzymes directly from the cytoplasm.

Mitochondria

The **mitochondria** have been aptly called the "powerhouses of the cell" because they convert energy to forms that can be used to drive cellular reactions. A distinct feature of mitochondria is the large amount of membrane they contain. Each mitochondrion is bounded by two specialized membranes. The inner membrane forms an enclosed space, called the *matrix,* which contains a concentrated mix of mitochondrial enzymes. The highly convoluted structure of the inner membrane with its numerous folds, called cristae (Figure 3-12), provides a large surface area for the important membrane-bound enzymes of the respiratory chain. These enzymes are essential to the process of oxidative phosphorylation, which generates most of the cell's **adenosine triphosphate (ATP)**. The outer membrane contains numerous porin transport proteins forming large aqueous channels that make the membrane porous like a sieve. Fairly large molecules, including proteins up to 5000 daltons, can pass freely through the outer membrane such that the space between the outer and inner membranes is chemically similar to the cytosol. However, the inner membrane is quite impermeable even to small molecules and ions. Specific protein transporters are required to

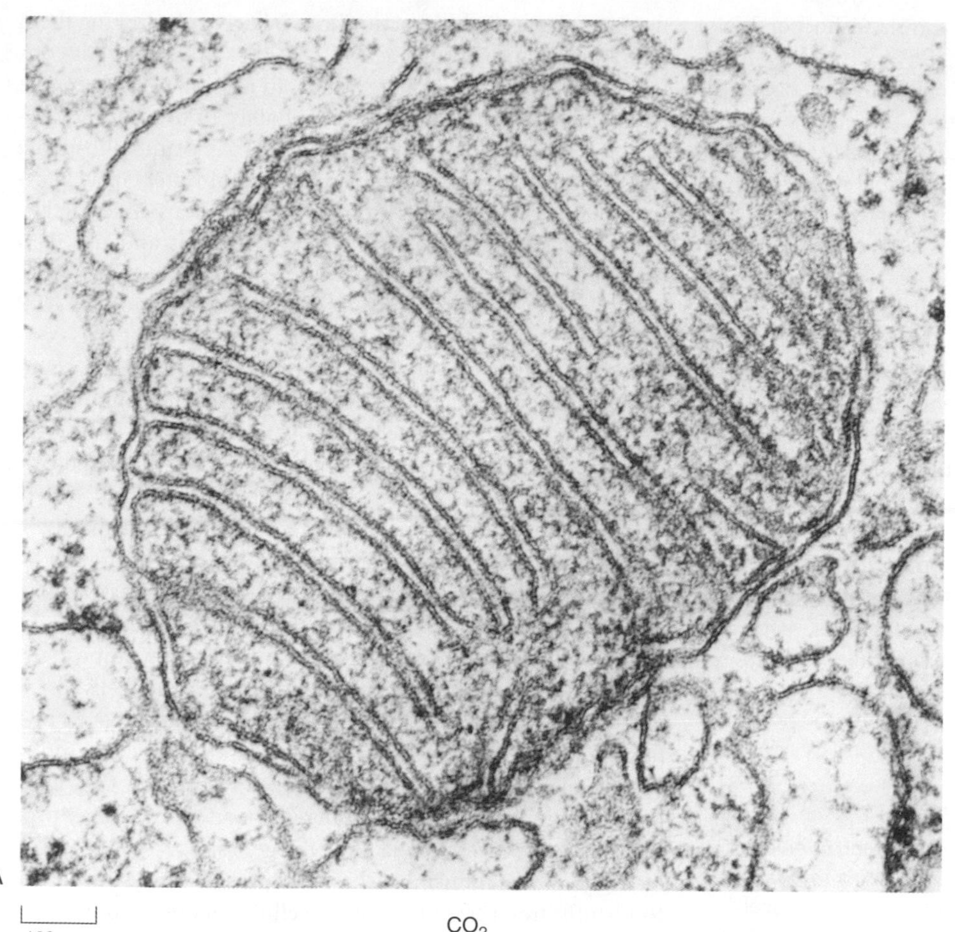

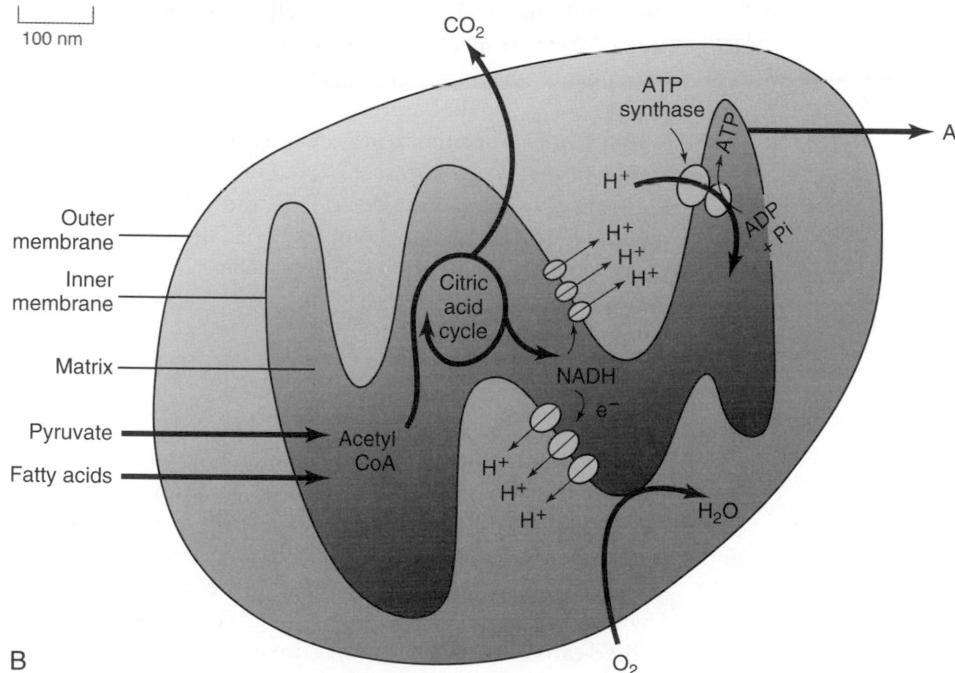

FIGURE 3-12 ■ Electron micrograph **(A)** and schematic drawing **(B)** of the mitochondrial structure. The highly convoluted inner membrane provides a large surface area for membrane-bound metabolic enzymes. (**A,** From Alberts B et al, editors: *Molecular biology of the cell*, ed 4, New York, 2002, Garland Science, p 31. Micrograph courtesy of Daniel S. Friend.)

shuttle the necessary molecules across the inner mitochondrial membrane.

Mitochondria are believed to have originated as bacteria that were engulfed by larger cells and they still retain some of their own DNA. Mitochondrial DNA codes for several transfer RNA molecules and 13 proteins.[12,13] During evolution the majority of mitochondrial genes were transferred to locations within the nuclear genome. Thus only a few of the mitochondrial enzymes are produced from DNA located in the mitochondria; the majority are transcribed from nuclear DNA. Nuclear genes are translated into protein in the cytoplasm and then transported to the mitochondria, whereas mitochondrial gene-derived proteins are made within the mitochondria. The number and location of mitochondria differ according to cell type and function. Cells with high energy needs, such as cardiac or skeletal muscle, have many mitochondria. These mitochondria may pack between adjacent muscle fibrils such that ATP is delivered directly to the areas of unusually high energy consumption. The details of mitochondrial energy conversion are discussed in the next section. Mitochondria also have an important role in programmed cell death, called *apoptosis,* which is discussed in Chapter 4.

KEY CONCEPTS

- The cytoskeleton is made up of actin, microtubules, and intermediate filaments. These proteins regulate cell shape, movement, and the trafficking of intracellular molecules.
- The nucleus contains the genomic DNA. These nuclear genes code for the synthesis of proteins. There are about 30,000 protein-coding genes in the human genome.
- The endoplasmic reticulum and the Golgi apparatus function together to synthesize proteins and lipids for transport to lysosomes or to the plasma membrane.
- Lysosomes and peroxisomes are membrane-bound bags of digestive enzymes that degrade intracellular debris.
- Mitochondria contain tricarboxylic acid and respiratory chain enzymes necessary for oxidative phosphorylation to produce ATP. Mitochondria have their own small number of genes that code for some of the mitochondrial proteins.

CELLULAR METABOLISM

All living cells must continually perform essential cellular functions such as movement, ion pumping, and synthesis of macromolecules. Many of these cellular activities are energetically unfavorable (i.e., they are unlikely to occur spontaneously). Unfavorable reactions can be driven by linking them to an energy source such as ATP. ATP is a molecule that contains high-energy phosphate bonds. In normal cells where the ATP concentration is high, approximately 11 to 13 kcal of energy per mole of ATP is liberated when one of the phosphate bonds is hydrolyzed (broken with the aid of water) in a chemical reaction.[13] Enzymes throughout the cell are able to capture the energy released from ATP hydrolysis and use it to break or make other chemical bonds. In this way, ATP serves as the "energy currency" of the cell. A specific amount of ATP is "spent" to "buy" a specific amount of work. Most cells contain only a small amount of ATP, sufficient to maintain cellular activities for just a few minutes. Because ATP cannot cross the plasma membrane, each cell must continuously synthesize its own ATP to meet its energy needs. ATP is synthesized primarily from the breakdown of glycogen and fat.

An average adult has enough glycogen stores (primarily in liver and muscle) to supply about 1 day's needs but enough fat to last for a month or more. After a meal, the excess glucose entering the cells is used to replenish glycogen stores or to synthesize fats for later use. Fat is stored primarily in adipose tissue and is released into the bloodstream for other cells to use when needed. When cellular glucose levels fall, glycogen and fats are broken down to provide glucose and fatty acyl molecules, which are ultimately metabolized to provide ATP. During starvation, body proteins can also be used for energy production by a process called gluconeogenesis.

Cellular metabolism is the biochemical process whereby foodstuffs are utilized to provide cellular energy and biomolecules. Cellular metabolism includes two separate and opposite phases: anabolism and catabolism. **Anabolism** refers to *energy-using* metabolic processes or pathways that result in the synthesis of complex molecules such as fats. **Catabolism** refers to the *energy-releasing* breakdown of nutrient sources such as glucose to provide ATP to the cell. Both of these processes require a long, complex series of enzymatic steps. The catabolic processes of cellular energy production are briefly discussed below. (See Chapter 42 for a detailed discussion of metabolism.)

Glycolysis

The catabolic process of energy production begins with the intestinal digestion of foodstuffs into small molecules: proteins into amino acids, polysaccharides into simple sugars, and fats into fatty acids and glycerol. The second stage of catabolism occurs in the cytosol of the cell, where sugar molecules are further degraded by **glycolysis** into pyruvate (three-carbon atoms). Glycolysis involves 10 enzymatic steps to break the six-carbon glucose molecule into a pair of three-carbon pyruvate molecules (Figure 3-13).[13] Glycolysis requires the use of two ATP molecules in the early stages but produces four ATP molecules in the later steps, for a net gain of two ATP molecules per glucose molecule. The pro-

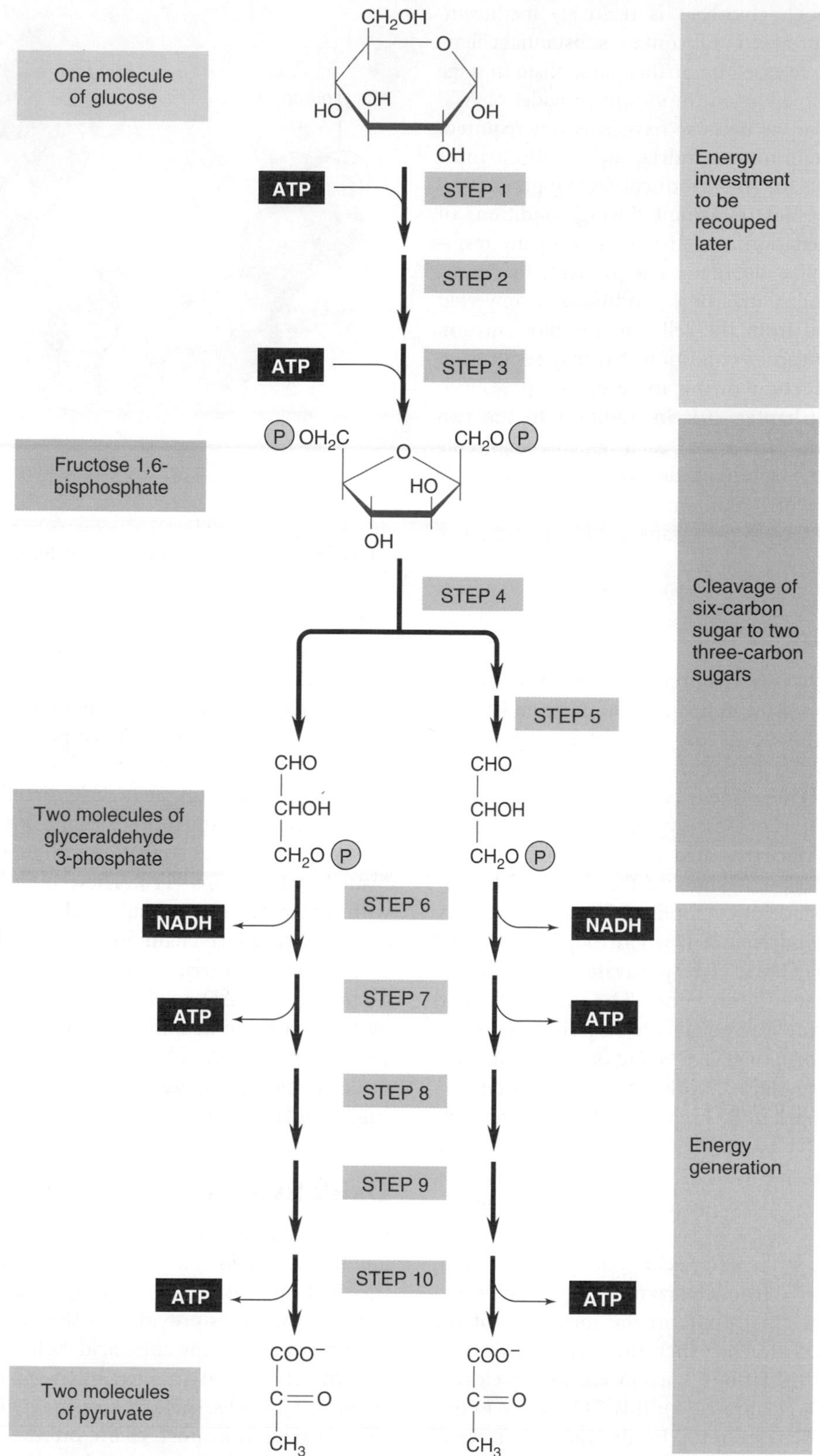

FIGURE 3-13 ■ Glycolysis involves 10 enzymatic steps to break glucose into two 3-carbon pyruvate molecules. A net gain of two ATP molecules is achieved. (From Alberts B et al, editors: *Molecular biology of the cell*, ed 4, New York, 2002, Garland Science, p 94.)

duction of ATP through glycolysis is relatively inefficient, and the pyruvate end products still contain substantial chemical energy that can be released by further catabolism in stage 3. However, glycolysis may be an important provider of ATP under *anaerobic* conditions because oxygen is not required. Cells that do not contain mitochondria, such as RBCs, must rely totally on glycolysis for ATP production. ATP production by glycolysis also becomes important during conditions of reduced cellular oxygenation, which may accompany respiratory and cardiovascular disorders. The pyruvate that accumulates during prolonged anaerobic conditions is converted to lactate and excreted from the cell into the bloodstream. Lactic acidosis is a dangerous condition that may result from excessive lactate production owing to severe or prolonged lack of oxygen (see Chapter 20). In addition to the two molecules of ATP and pyruvate, each glucose molecule produces two reduced nicotinamide adenine dinucleotide (NADH) molecules, which contain high-energy electrons that are transferred to the electron transport chain in the mitochondria.

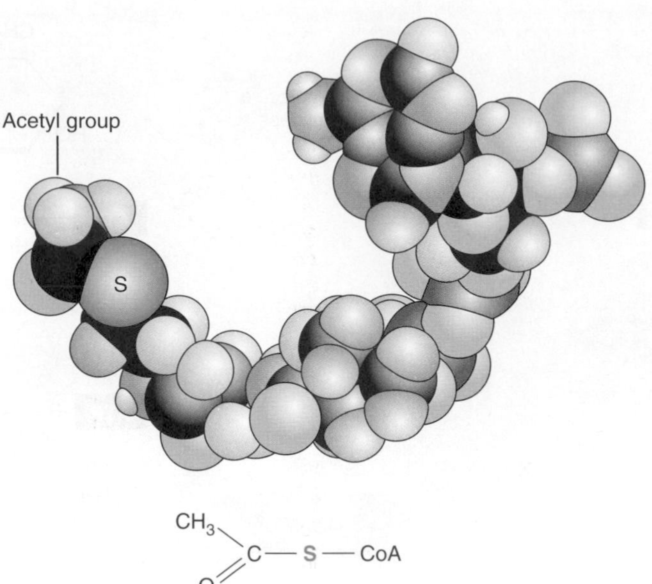

FIGURE 3-14 ■ Space-filling model of acetyl coenzyme A.

Citric Acid Cycle

For most cells, glycolysis is only a prelude to the third stage of catabolism, which takes place in the mitochondria and results in the complete oxidation of glucose to its final end products, CO_2 and H_2O. The third stage begins with the citric acid cycle (also called the Krebs cycle or the tricarboxylic acid cycle) and ends with the production of ATP by oxidative phosphorylation.[13] The purpose of the citric acid cycle is to break, by oxidation, the C—C and C—H bonds of the compounds produced in the second stage of catabolism. Pyruvate and fatty acids enter the mitochondrial matrix where they are converted to acetyl CoA (Figure 3-14). The pyruvate dehydrogenase complex cleaves pyruvate to form one CO_2, one NADH, and one acetyl CoA molecule. Fatty acids are cleaved by a process called β oxidation to form one NADH and one reduced flavin adenine dinucleotide ($FADH_2$, another type of electron carrier). No CO_2 is produced in this reaction. Patients who have difficulty excreting CO_2 because of respiratory disease are sometimes given a high-fat, low-carbohydrate diet to take advantage of the lower CO_2 production that accompanies fat metabolism.

In the first reaction of the citric acid cycle, the two-carbon acetyl group is transferred from coenzyme A to a four-carbon oxaloacetate molecule. This results in the formation of the six-carbon molecule citrate, for which the cycle is named. In a series of enzymatic oxidations, carbon atoms are cleaved off in the form of CO_2 (Figure 3-15); this CO_2 is free to diffuse from the cell and be excreted by the lungs as a waste product. Two carbon atoms are removed to form two CO_2 molecules for each complete turn of the cycle. The extra oxygen molecules needed to create CO_2 are provided by the surrounding H_2O; therefore the citric acid cycle does not require molecular oxygen from respiration. However, the cycle will shut down in the absence of oxygen because the carrier molecules, NADH and $FADH_2$, cannot unload their electrons onto the electron transport chain (which does require oxygen) and thus are unavailable to accept electrons from the citric acid cycle.

Although the citric acid cycle directly produces only one ATP molecule (in the form of guanosine triphosphate [GTP]) per cycle, it captures a great deal of energy in the form of activated hydride ions (H^-). These high-energy ions combine with larger carrier molecules, which transport them to the electron transport chain in the mitochondrial membrane. Two important carrier molecules are nicotinamide adenine dinucleotide (NAD^+), which becomes NADH when reduced by H^-, and flavin adenine nucleotide (FAD), which becomes $FADH_2$ when reduced by H^-. The energy carried by these molecules is ultimately used to produce ATP through a process called *oxidative phosphorylation.*

Oxidative Phosphorylation

Oxidative phosphorylation follows the processes of glycolysis and the citric acid cycle and results in the formation of ATP by the reaction ADP + $P_i \longrightarrow$ ATP. The energy to drive this unfavorable reaction is provided by the high-energy hydride ions (H^-) derived from the citric acid cycle. This energy is not used to form ATP directly; a series of energy transfers is required.[13] In eukaryotic cells, this series of energy transfers occurs along the **electron transport chain** on the inner mitochondrial membrane. The transport chain consists of three major enzyme complexes and two mobile electron carriers that shuttle electrons between the protein complexes (Figure 3-16). The hydrogen molecules and their associated electrons are transported to the electron transport chain by the carrier molecules

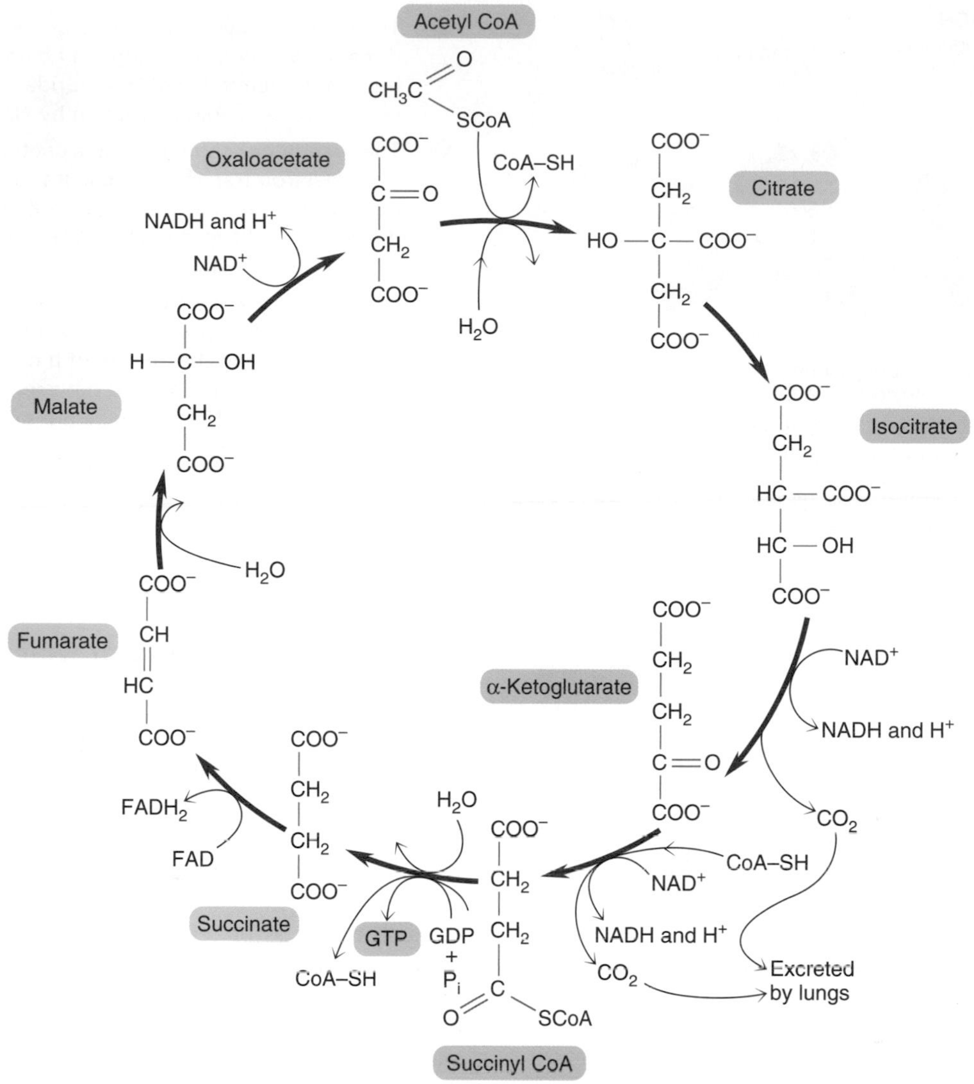

FIGURE 3-15 ■ Chemical structures of the compounds of the citric acid cycle (Krebs cycle). In a series of enzymatic reactions, carbon atoms are cleaved to form CO_2 and high-energy hydride ions, which are carried by FAD and NAD.

NADH or $FADH_2$. Each NADH carries two electrons and donates them readily to the first enzyme in the respiratory chain complex. The path of electron flow is NADH ⟶ NADH dehydrogenase complex ⟶ ubiquinone ⟶ b-c_1 complex ⟶ cytochrome c ⟶ cytochrome oxidase complex. As the electrons pass from one complex to the next they transfer energy, which is used to pump hydrogen ions (H^+) out of the mitochondrial matrix. Each transfer of one electron provides enough energy to pump one or two protons across the membrane. At the very end of the transport chain, low-energy electrons are finally transferred to O_2 to form H_2O. Oxidative phosphorylation is called *aerobic* because of this oxygen-requiring step. The last enzyme in the chain, cytochrome oxidase, collects four electrons and then transfers all four at once to a molecule of O_2 to create two water molecules. If electrons are not transferred to oxygen in the correct ratio, then oxygen free radicals may be produced and damage the cell. Free radical generation is discussed in Chapter 4.

Thus far, no ATP synthesis has been accomplished. However, the enzymes of the transport chain have harnessed energy from the transported electrons in the form of a proton (H^+) gradient. Finally, the proton gradient is used to power the synthesis of ATP. A special enzyme in the inner mitochondrial membrane (ATP synthase) allows protons to flow back into the mitochondria down their electrochemical gradient. The energy of the proton flow is used to drive ATP synthesis (Figure 3-17). A total of about 30 ATP molecules are formed from the complete oxidation of glucose into CO_2 and H_2O. Two of these are from glycolysis, two from the citric acid cycle (in the form of GTP), and the remainder from oxidative phosphorylation.[13] The ATP formed within the mitochondria is transported to the cytosol by protein transporters in the mi-

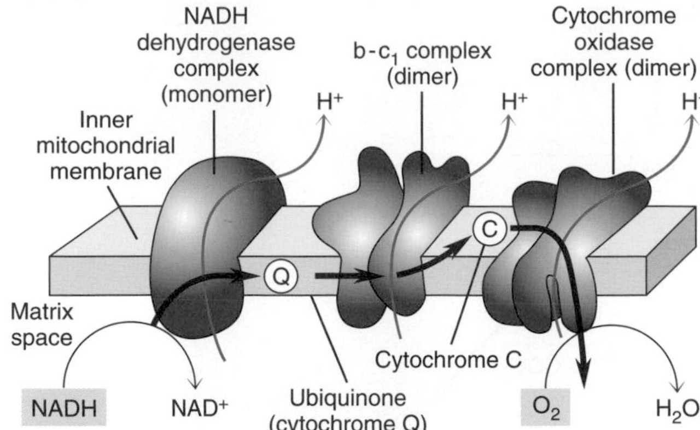

FIGURE 3-16 ■ A representation of the electron transport chain located in the inner mitochondrial membrane. High-energy electrons are passed along the chain until they combine with oxygen to form water. The energy released at each electron transfer is used to pump H^+ across the membrane.

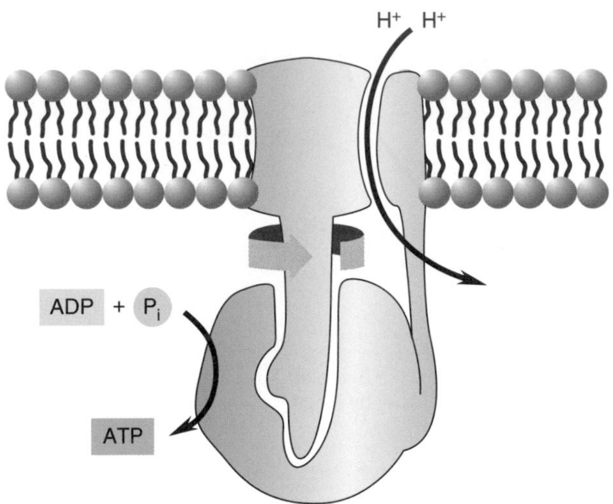

FIGURE 3-17 ■ The inner mitochondrial ATP synthetase captures the potential energy of the H^+ gradient in a manner similar to a turbine. The proton gradient drives the synthesis of ATP from adenosine diphosphate *(ADP)* and inorganic phosphate *(P_i)*.

tochondrial membrane. The ATP is then available to drive a variety of energy-requiring reactions within the cell.

KEY CONCEPTS

- Energy-requiring reactions within cells are driven by coupling to ATP hydrolysis.
- ATP is not stored and must be continuously synthesized by each cell to meet the cell's energy needs.
- Glycolysis is an anaerobic process that produces two ATP molecules, two NADH molecules, and two pyruvate molecules per glucose molecule. Pyruvate enters the mitochondria and is converted to acetyl CoA with release of a CO_2 molecule.
- The citric acid cycle in the mitochondrial matrix oxidizes the acetyl groups supplied by acetyl CoA to form large quantities of H^- (hydride ions), which are carried to the respiratory chain by NADH and $FADH_2$.
- The respiratory chain enzymes capture the energy from electron transfer and use it to produce an H^+ (proton) gradient. Molecular oxygen is required at this stage to accept the electrons from the last enzyme in the transport chain.
- ATP is produced by ATP synthase, a protein in the mitochondrial membrane. ATP synthase produces ATP by capturing the energy of the proton gradient and using it to form a bond between ADP and P_i. In total, about 30 ATP molecules are produced per glucose molecule.

FUNCTIONS OF THE PLASMA MEMBRANE

Membrane Transport of Macromolecules

Endocytosis and Exocytosis

The transport of large molecules, such as proteins and polysaccharides, across the plasma membrane cannot be accomplished by the membrane transport proteins discussed earlier. Rather, macromolecules are ingested and secreted by the sequential formation and fusion of membrane-bound vesicles. **Endocytosis** refers to cellular ingestion of extracellular molecules. The process of cellular secretion is called **exocytosis.** There are two types of endocytosis, which are differentiated by the size of the particles ingested. **Pinocytosis,** or "cellular drinking," is the method of ingesting fluids and small particles and is common to most cell types. **Phagocytosis,** or "cellular eating," involves the ingestion of large particles, such as microorganisms, and is practiced mainly by specialized phagocytic WBCs. Endocytosis begins at the cell surface by the formation of an indentation or "pit" in the plasma membrane, which is coated with special proteins, including clathrin *(coated pit).* The indentation invaginates and then pinches off a portion of the membrane to become a **vesicle** (Figure 3-18). Each vesicle thus formed is internalized, sheds its coat, and fuses with an endosome. The contents of these endocytic vesicles generally end up in lysosomes, where they are degraded.

Endocytosis of certain macromolecules is regulated by specific receptors on the cell surface. These receptors bind the molecules (ligands) to be ingested and then cluster together in coated pits. The receptor-ligand complexes are internalized by the invagination process described above. The vesicles generally fuse with endosomes where the ligand is removed from the receptor for processing by the cell. The receptor may be degraded in the lysosome or may be recycled to the cell surface to be used again. Receptor-mediated endocytosis allows the cell to be selective about the molecules ingested and to regulate the amount taken into the cell. The cell can produce

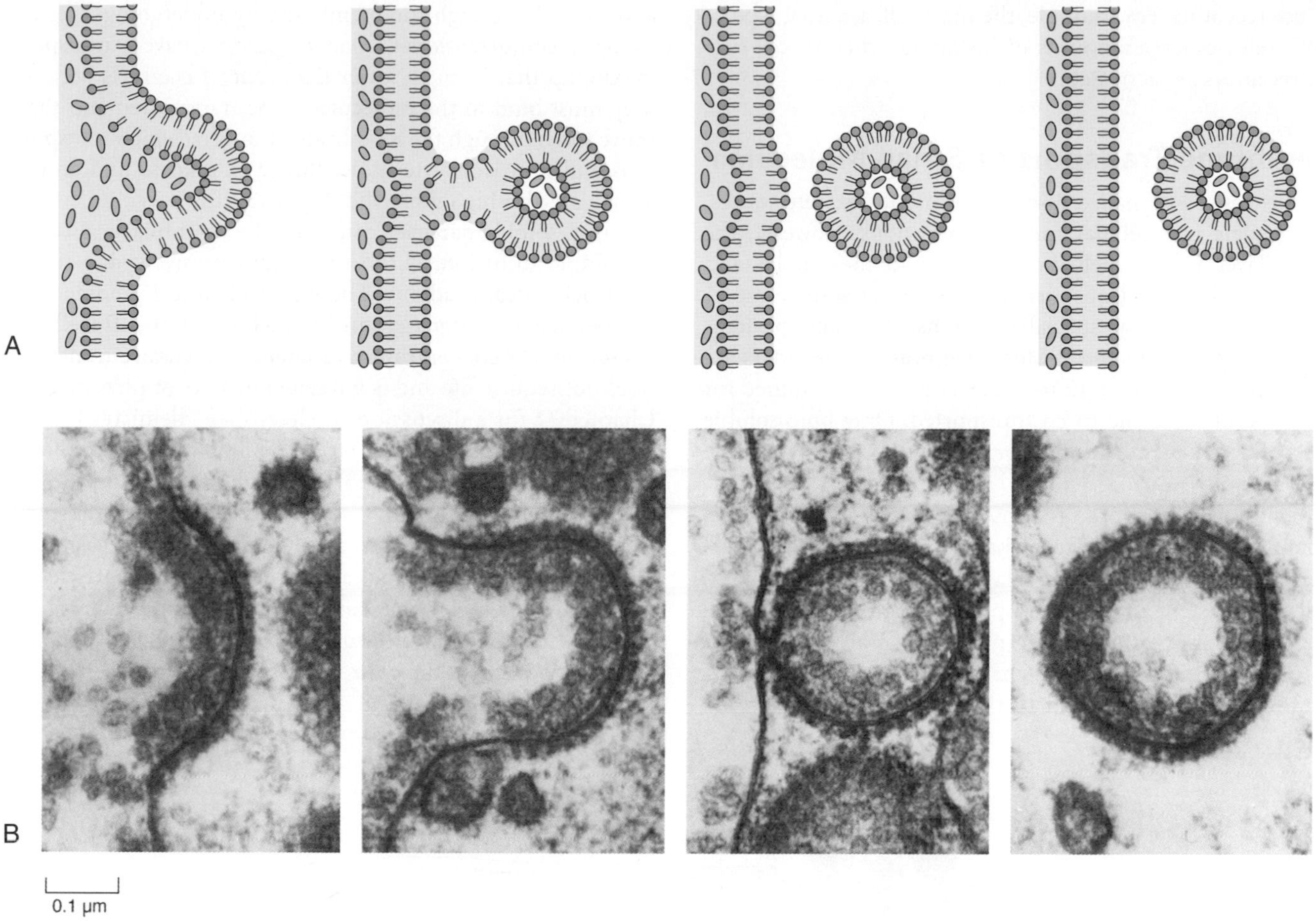

A

B

0.1 μm

FIGURE 3-18 ■ **A,** A representation of the steps of endocytosis. An invagination of the membrane occurs and pinches off to form a vesicle. Exocytosis progresses in essentially the reverse. **B,** Electron micrograph showing the steps of endocytosis. (**B,** From Perry M, Gilbert A: Yolk transport in the ovarian follicle of the hen *(Gallus domesticus):* lipoprotein-like particles at the periphery of the oocyte in the rapid growth phase, *J Cell Sci* 39:257-272, 1979.)

greater numbers of cell surface receptors to ingest more ligand.

An example of receptor-mediated endocytosis is cellular uptake of cholesterol. The process of cholesterol uptake by cells is shown in Figure 3-19. Most cholesterol in the blood is transported by protein carriers called low-density lipoproteins (LDLs). The cell can regulate the number of LDL receptors on its cell surface to increase or decrease the uptake of cholesterol. Once the LDL binds to its receptor, this complex is rapidly internalized in a coated pit. The coated vesicle thus formed sheds its coat and fuses with an endosome. In the endosome, the LDL receptor is retrieved and recycled to the cell surface to be used again. The LDL is transported to lysosomes and degraded to release free cholesterol, which the cell uses for synthesis of biomolecules such as steroid hormones.

Dangerously high blood cholesterol levels occur in some individuals who lack functional LDL receptors. These individuals inherit defective genes for making LDL receptor proteins and are incapable of taking up adequate amounts of LDL. Accumulation of LDL in the blood predisposes these individuals to development of atherosclerosis (hardened arteries) and heart disease (see Chapter 18).

Exocytosis is essentially the reverse of endocytosis. Substances to be secreted from the cell are packaged in membrane-bound vesicles and travel to the inner surface of the plasma membrane. There the vesicle membrane fuses with the plasma membrane and the contents of the vesicle arrive at the cell surface. Some secreted molecules may remain embedded in the cell membrane, others may be incorporated into the extracellular matrix, and still others may enter the extracellular fluids and travel to distant sites. Many substances synthesized by the cell, including new membrane components, are constantly being packaged and secreted. This continuously operative and unregulated pathway is termed *constitutive.* In some specialized cells, selected proteins or small molecules are packaged in secretory vesicles, which remain in the cell until the cell is triggered to release them. These special secretory vesicles are typically regulated by stimulation of cell surface receptors. For example, the mast cell, a special type of WBC, releases large amounts of histamine when its cell surface receptors are activated.

Membrane Transport of Small Molecules

All cells must internalize essential nutrients, excrete wastes, and regulate intracellular ion concentrations. However, the lipid bilayer is extremely impermeable to most polar and charged molecules. Transport of small water-soluble molecules is achieved by specialized transmembrane proteins called *transporter proteins.*[14] Most membrane transporters are highly specific—a different transporter protein is required for each type of molecule to be transported. Only lipid-soluble molecules can permeate the lipid bilayer directly by simple diffusion.

Membrane transport proteins are of two kinds: **channel proteins** and **carrier proteins.** Channel proteins form a water-filled pore through the lipid bilayer. These pores are able to open and close to allow ions to pass through the membrane. The particular structure of the protein channel ensures that only ions of a certain size and charge can move through. Carrier proteins, however, bind to the solute to be transported and move it through the membrane by undergoing a structural, or **conformational,** change. Carriers have a transport maximum that is much lower than that of channels because they must bind to the molecules to be transported and then move them through the membrane. Carriers, which transport ions and nonelectrolyte molecules (e.g., glucose and amino acids), are also highly specific (Figure 3-20).

Lipid-soluble particles can cross the lipid bilayer directly by simple diffusion. Diffusion occurs passively due to an **electrochemical gradient.** The electrochemical gradient exists because of differences in intracellular and extracellular charge and/or concentration of chemicals. Passive transport does not require life and is governed by laws of physics. (See Chapter 24 for a discussion of electrolyte chemistry.) Polar or charged molecules must cross the membrane via protein channels or carriers. Transport through membrane proteins may be a passive or an active process. Passive transport through membrane proteins is called *facilitated diffusion.* All channel proteins and some carrier proteins allow particles to move down their electrochemical gradient passively by facilitated diffusion. Passive diffusion of water is called *osmosis.* Water moves across the plasma membrane through channels called *aquaporins.*

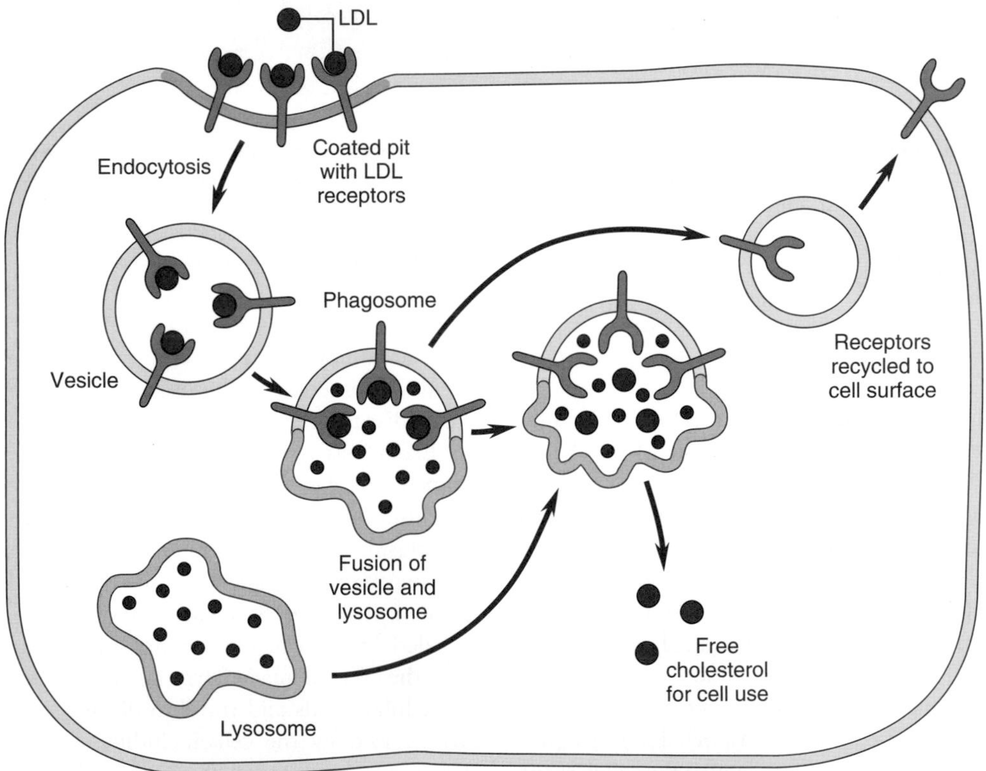

FIGURE 3-19 ■ Steps in the process of receptor-mediated endocytosis of cholesterol. Cholesterol is carried in the blood by low-density lipoproteins *(LDL).* The uptake of LDL with its associated cholesterol is mediated by a specific LDL receptor protein on the cell surface. Once internalized, the cholesterol is removed from the LDL-receptor complex and used by the cell. The LDL receptors are sent back to the cell surface to bind more LDL.

Active transport is the process whereby carrier proteins move or "pump" solutes across the membrane against an electrochemical gradient. Active transport requires metabolic energy, which may be supplied by ATP hydrolysis or by an ion gradient. Carrier proteins are thought to undergo reversible conformational (shape) changes that alternately expose the solute-binding site first on one side and then on the other side of the membrane (Figure 3-21).[14,15] A large number of membrane carrier proteins continually function to maintain the ionic and nutrient balance within the cell.

Active Transport Carriers

Sodium-Potassium Ion Pump. The sodium-potassium (Na^+-K^+) pump is present in the plasma membranes of virtually all animal cells. It serves to maintain low sodium and high potassium concentrations in the cell.[16] The Na^+-K^+ transporter must pump ions against a steep electrochemical gradient. Almost one third of the energy of a typical cell is consumed by the Na^+-K^+ pump. ATP hydrolysis provides the energy to drive the Na^+-K^+ transporter. The Na^+-K^+ pump behaves as an enzyme in its ability to split ATP to form adenosine diphosphate (ADP) and inorganic phosphate (P_i), leading to the protein being termed *Na^+-K^+ ATPase.*

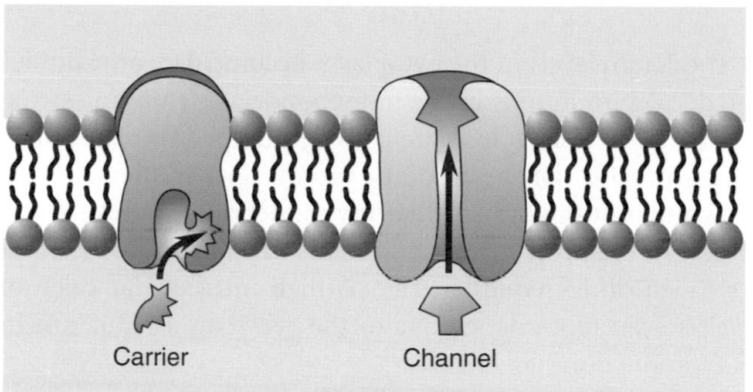

FIGURE 3-20 ■ Carrier and channel proteins in the plasma membrane are highly selective about the type of molecule allowed to pass through. Carriers bind to the substance to be transported and move it across by changing three-dimensional formation. Channels allow ions to flow through a water-filled pore in the core of the channel.

Transport of sodium and potassium ions through the Na^+-K^+ carrier protein is *coupled;* that is, the transfer of one ion must be accompanied by the simultaneous transport of the other ion. The transporter moves three sodium ions *out* of the cell for every two potassium ions moved *into* the cell (Figure 3-22). The Na^+-K^+ pump is important in maintaining cell volume. It controls the solute concentration inside the cell, which in turn affects the osmotic forces across the membrane. If Na^+ is allowed to accumulate within the cell, the cell will swell and could burst. The role of the Na^+-K^+ pump can be demonstrated by treating cells with ouabain, a drug that inhibits Na^+-K^+ ATPase. Cells thus treated will indeed swell and often burst. The Na^+-K^+ pump is responsible for maintaining a steep concentration gradient for Na^+ across the plasma membrane. This gradient can be harnessed to transport small molecules across the membrane in a process called secondary active transport. Carriers that use ATP directly are engaging in primary active transport.

Membrane Calcium Transporters. Numerous important cellular processes, such as cell contraction and growth initiation, are dependent on the intracellular calcium concentration. Intracellular calcium concentration is normally very low and tightly regulated. Two types of calcium pumps present in the plasma membrane function to remove excess calcium from the cell cytoplasm.[17] Both calcium transporters are energy-requiring carrier proteins, but each utilizes a different energy source.

One of these transporters utilizes ATP as its energy source, much as the Na^+-K^+ transporter does (Figure 3-23). The other Ca^{2+} transporter utilizes the electrochemical gradient of Na^+ to power the transport of Ca^{2+} out of the cell. The dependence

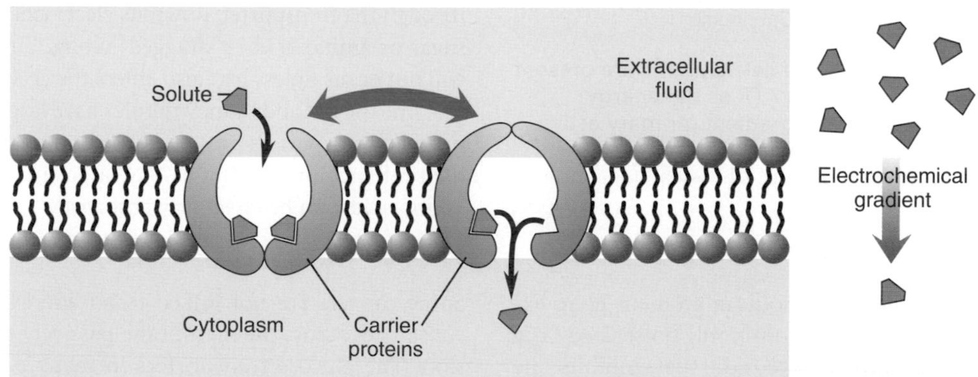

FIGURE 3-21 ■ Carrier proteins are thought to move molecules across the membrane by alternately exposing the solute-binding site first on one side and then on the other side of the membrane. Some carriers are passive and move a solute down its electrochemical gradient (shown), whereas others are linked to an energy source and can move substances against a gradient.

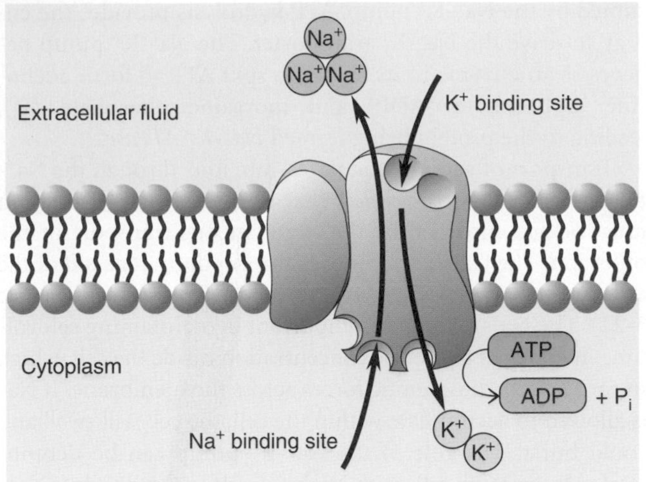

FIGURE 3-22 ■ Schematic drawing of the sodium-potassium transport protein, which uses ATP to pump Na^+ out of the cell and K^+ into the cell against steep electrochemical gradients. This transporter is responsible for maintaining a low intracellular concentration of Na^+ and a large Na^+ gradient across the membrane. The energy of this Na^+ gradient can be harvested by other transporters to actively transport substances.

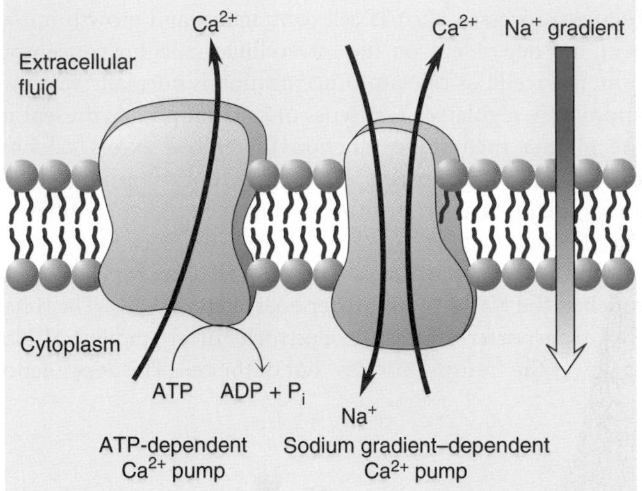

FIGURE 3-23 ■ Two transporters of calcium ions are present in some cell membranes. One uses ATP as the energy source to pump calcium against a gradient (primary active transport). The other captures the potential energy of the sodium gradient to pump calcium out of the cell (secondary active transport).

of this calcium transporter on the sodium gradient helps explain the cardiotonic effects of the commonly prescribed drug digitalis. Digitalis is a cardiac glycoside that inhibits the Na^+-K^+ pump and allows the accumulation of intracellular Na^+. The Na^+ gradient across the membrane is thus decreased, leading to less efficient calcium removal by the Na^+-dependent Ca^{2+} pump. A more forceful cardiac muscle contraction results from the increased intracellular Ca^{2+}.

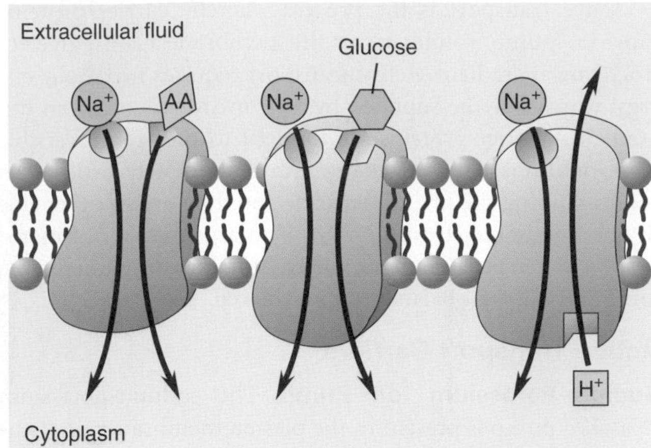

FIGURE 3-24 ■ The sodium gradient is used by some cell types to provide the energy to transport amino acids *(AA)* and glucose and to exchange sodium ions for hydrogen ions. All of these are examples of secondary active transport.

If calcium levels in the cytoplasm become dangerously elevated, calcium pumps in the mitochondrial membrane swing into action. Calcium ions are actively pumped into the mitochondria using the energy of the proton (H^+) gradient. This is the same proton gradient that the mitochondria uses to synthesize ATP, and ATP production falls when the mitochondria are called on to sequester Ca^{2+}. A high intracellular calcium level is even more dangerous to the cell than a reduction in ATP production.

Other Na^+-Driven Carriers. In animal cells, the Na^+ gradient created by the Na^+-K^+ pump is used to power a variety of transporters in addition to the calcium pump described above (Figure 3-24). The Na^+-H^+ exchange carrier uses the Na^+ gradient to pump out excess hydrogen ions to help maintain intracellular pH balance. The Na^+ gradient also can be used to bring substances into the cell. For example, glucose and amino acid transport into epithelial cells is coupled to Na^+ entry. As Na^+ moves through the transporter, down its electrochemical gradient, the sugar or amino acid is "dragged" along. Entry of the nutrient will not occur unless Na^+ also enters the cell. The epithelial cells that line the gut and kidney tubules have large numbers of these nutrient transporters present in the luminal (apical) surfaces of their cell membranes. In this way, large amounts of glucose and amino acids can be effectively absorbed.

Passive Transport Carriers

Some carriers are not linked to an energy source and move substances across the membrane passively by facilitated diffusion. The glucose transporters in many cell types belong to this class of transporters. In β cells of the pancreas, for example, the glucose transporters (Glut-2) are always present in the plasma membrane and let glucose into the cell according to its concentration in the extracellular fluid. In this way the pancreas detects blood glucose levels and releases an appropriate

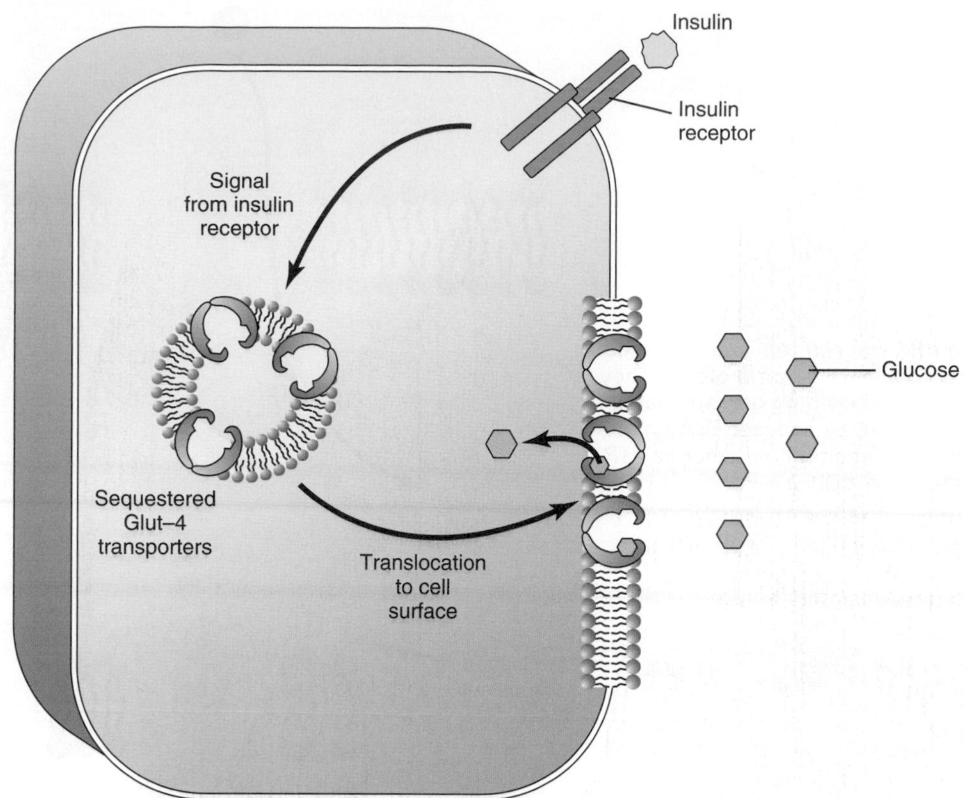

FIGURE 3-25 ■ In response to insulin binding to its receptor on the cell surface, carrier proteins that transport glucose *(Glut-4)* are moved to the cell surface where they passively transport glucose into the cell (facilitated diffusion).

amount of insulin. In insulin sensitive cells, such as muscle, liver, and adipose cells, the glucose carriers are sequestered inside the cell until insulin binds to its receptor at the cell surface. Receptor activation causes the glucose carriers (Glut-4) to move to the cell surface where they allow passive influx of glucose (Figure 3-25).

ABC Transporters

Another important class of carrier proteins is the ABC transporter family. These transporters all have a common ATP-binding domain, called the *A*TP *b*inding *c*assette (ABC), which hydrolyzes ATP to provide energy for the transport process (Figure 3-26). This family of membrane transporters is the largest of all, but the members of the family and their functions are just beginning to be described. A clinically important member of this family of carriers is a chloride channel in the plasma membrane of epithelial cells. A defect in this transporter is responsible for cystic fibrosis, a common genetic disorder that affects the lungs and pancreas (see Chapter 22). Bacteria use ABC transporters to pump out antibiotics and develop drug resistance (see Chapter 8).

Membrane Channel Proteins

In contrast to carrier proteins, which bind molecules and move them across the membrane by a conformational transformation, channel proteins form water-filled pores in the membrane. All known channel proteins are involved in transport of ions and may be referred to as ion channels. Ions can flow through the appropriate channel at very high rates (10^7 ions/sec); this is much faster than carrier-mediated transport.[14,18] However, channels are not linked to an energy source, so ions must flow passively down an electrochemical gradient. The channel proteins in the plasma membranes of animal cells are highly selective, permitting only a particular ion or class of ions to pass. More than 100 different types of ion channels have been described. Ion channels are particularly important in allowing the cell to respond rapidly to a variety of external stimuli. Most channels are not continuously open, but they open and close according to membrane signals. Ion channels may be stimulated to open or close in three principal ways: (1) *voltage-gated* channels respond to a change in membrane potential; (2) *mechanically gated* channels respond to mechanical deformation; and (3) *ligand-gated* channels respond to the binding of a signaling molecule (a hormone or neurotransmitter) to a receptor on the cell surface (Figure 3-27). In addition, some channels open without apparent stimulation and are referred to as *leak* channels. Ion channels are responsible for the development of membrane potentials and are of vital importance in nerve and muscle function, as discussed in the next section.

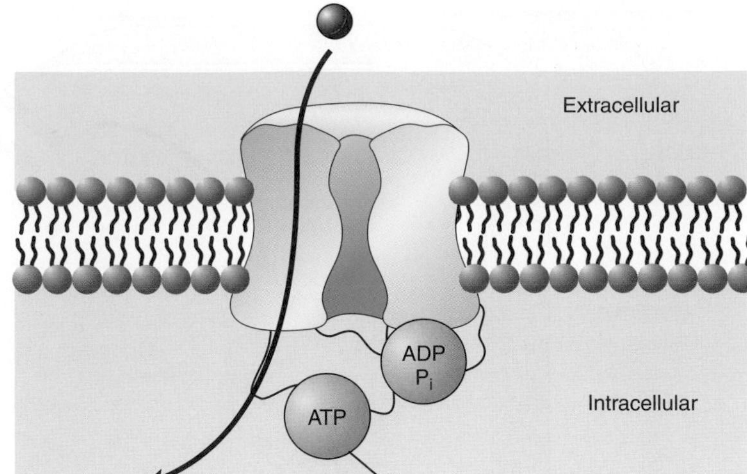

FIGURE 3-26 ■ The ABC transporters are the largest known family of membrane transport proteins. They are characterized by an ATP-binding domain that causes a substrate pocket to be exposed first on one side of the membrane and then on the other as ATP is bound and hydrolyzed to ADP and P_i.

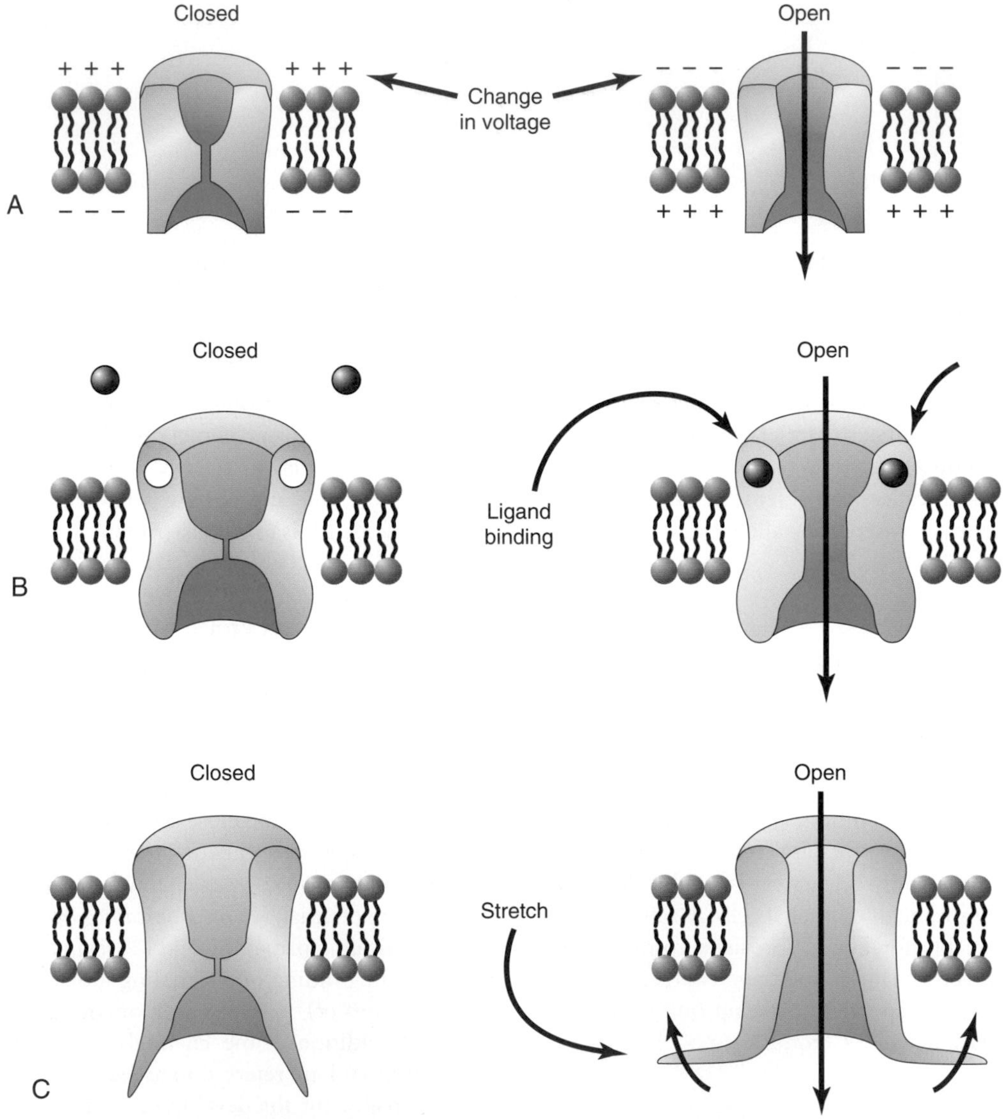

FIGURE 3-27 ■ Gating of ion channels. **A,** Voltage-gated channel. **B,** Ligand-gated channel. **C,** Mechanically gated channel.

KEY CONCEPTS

- Large, lipid-insoluble molecules are transported across the plasma membrane by endocytosis and exocytosis.
- Small, lipid-insoluble molecules are transported across the plasma membrane by two kinds of membrane proteins: carriers and channels.
- Carrier proteins may have active or passive transport functions. Examples of active transport include Na^+-K^+ pumps, Ca^{2+} pumps, ABC transporters, and those that use the Na^+ gradient for secondary active transport of glucose and amino acids. Passive carriers include those that allow glucose entry into insulin-sensitive cells.
- Channels are always passive and allow ions to move down their electrochemical gradient only. Channels open and close in response to specific signals, such as voltage changes, ligand binding, and mechanical pressure.

Cellular Membrane Potentials

Animal cells typically have a difference in the electrical charge across the plasma membranes. There is a slight excess of negative ions along the inner aspect of the membrane and extra positive ions along the outer membrane. This separation of charges creates a membrane potential that can be measured as a voltage. Positive and negative ions separated by the plasma membrane have a strong attraction to one another that can be utilized by the cell to perform work, such as the transmission of nerve impulses. A relatively large membrane potential is created by the separation of a very small number of ions along the membrane (Figure 3-28).

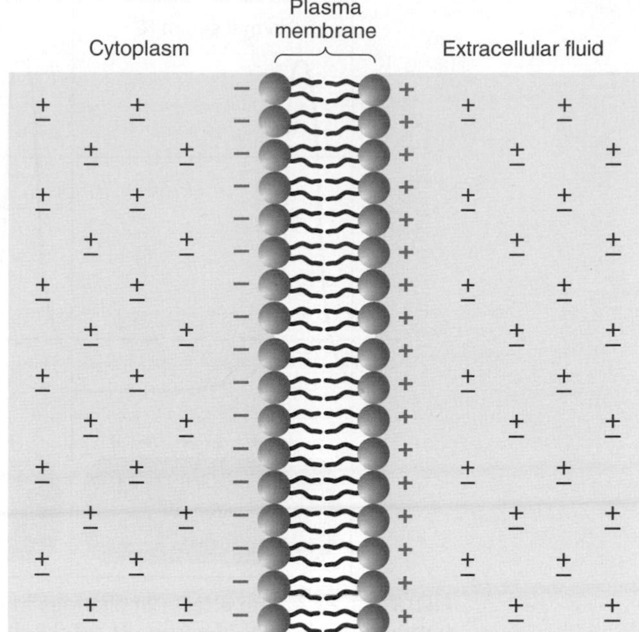

FIGURE 3-28 ■ A relatively large membrane potential results from the separation of a very small number of ions across the plasma membrane.

Resting Membrane Potential

When there is no net ion movement across the plasma membrane the electrical charge present inside the cell is called the resting membrane potential (RMP). The major determinant of the resting membrane potential is the difference in potassium ion concentration across the membrane.[14,19] The concentration of potassium inside the cell is much greater (about 30 times greater) than the extracellular potassium concentration. At rest the membrane is permeable to K^+ but not to other positively charged cations including Na^+ and Ca^{2+}. Potassium ions remain inside the cell because of the attraction of fixed intracellular anions (negatively charged organic molecules such as proteins that cannot diffuse out of the cell). Because the cell membrane is impermeable to Na^+ and Ca^{2+}, only K^+ is available to balance these negative intracellular ions. Thus, two opposing forces are acting on the potassium ion. The negative cell interior attracts K^+ into the cell, whereas the huge K^+ concentration gradient favors movement of K^+ out of the cell. When the cell is at rest and not transmitting impulses, these forces are balanced and although the membrane is permeable to K^+, there is no net movement. The voltage required to exactly balance a given potassium concentration gradient can be calculated mathematically.* The measured membrane potential is very close to that predicted mathematically and varies directly with changes in extracellular K^+ ion concentration.

For example, a typical nerve cell has a normal resting potential of about –85 mV. If the extracellular K^+ level is increased, fewer K^+ ions will leave the cell, owing to the reduced concentration gradient. These extra positive intracellular ions will neutralize more of the negative cellular anions, and the cell will *hypopolarize*, or become less negative. Conversely, if extracellular K^+ levels fall, more K^+ will exit the cell, owing to a greater concentration gradient. Fewer intracellular anions will be neutralized, and the cell interior will become more negative, or *hyperpolarized* (Figure 3-29). Changes in RMP can have profound effects on the ease of action potential generation in cardiac and nerve cells.

The RMP is described by the potassium equilibrium potential because the cell is relatively impermeable to other ions at rest. Under certain conditions, the membrane may become highly permeable to an ion other than potassium. The membrane potential will reflect the equilibrium potential of the most permeant ion.

Long-term maintenance of the potassium concentration gradient across the cell membrane is accomplished primarily

*The numerical value of the resting potential *(M)* can be calculated from the ratio of extracellular to intracellular K^+ using the Nernst equation:

$$M \text{ (in millivolts)} = 61 \log(K^+_{outside} \div K^+_{inside})$$

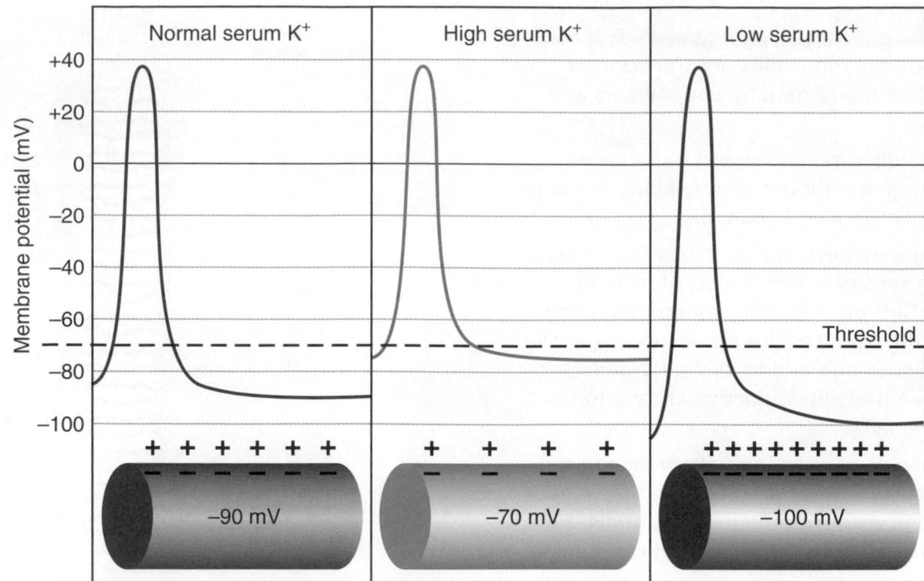

FIGURE 3-29 ■ The effects of changes in extracellular K^+ on the resting membrane potential. A high level of serum K^+ results in a hypopolarization of the membrane. A low serum K^+ level results in membrane hyperpolarization. With high serum K^+ levels, the resting membrane potential is closer to threshold, making it easier to achieve an action potential. A low serum K^+ level moves the resting membrane potential away from threshold, making it more difficult to achieve an action potential.

by the Na^+-K^+ pump. The Na^+-K^+ pump also contributes to the negative RMP in that it extrudes *three* Na^+ for every *two* K^+ brought into the cell. However, this pump can be inhibited for minutes to hours in some tissues with little immediate effect on the resting membrane potential. When the potassium ion concentration gradient finally dissipates the RMP will degrade toward zero.

Action Potential

Nearly all animal cells have negative resting membrane potentials, which may vary from –20 to –200 mV, depending on the cell type and organism. The cell membranes of some specialized cell types, mainly nerve and muscle, are capable of rapid changes in their membrane potentials. These cells are electrically "excitable" and can generate and propagate action potentials. In classic experiments, action potentials were determined to be rapid, self-propagating electrical excitations of the membrane that are mediated by ion channels that open and close in response to changes in voltage across the membrane (voltage-gated ion channels).[20-24] An action potential is triggered by membrane depolarization.

In nerve and muscle cells, the usual trigger for depolarization is binding of a neurotransmitter to cell surface receptors. Transmitter binding causes channels or pores in the membrane to open, allowing ions (primarily Na^+) to enter the cell. This influx of positive ions results in a shift in the membrane potential to a less negative value, resulting in depolarization. *Threshold* is reached when a patch of the membrane becomes sufficiently depolarized (approximately –65 mV in animal neurons) to activate voltage-gated sodium channels in the membrane. At threshold, these channels open rapidly and transiently to allow the influx of Na^+ ions. A self-propagating process follows whereby Na^+ influx in one patch of membrane causes membrane depolarization of the next patch and opens more voltage-gated Na^+ channels, allowing more Na^+ to enter the cell. This process repeats over and over again as the action potential proceeds along the length of the cell (Figure 3-30). In this way, action potentials can transmit information rapidly over relatively long distances.

A typical neuronal action potential is shown in Figure 3-31. The various changes in membrane potential during the time course of the action potential are attributable to the flow of ions through membrane ion channels. The steep upstroke of the action potential corresponds to Na^+ influx through "fast" sodium channels as described above. *Fast channels* are so termed because they open and close rapidly, with the entire process lasting less than a millisecond. This phase of rapid depolarization is terminated when the fast Na^+ channels suddenly close and the repolarization phase begins. Fast Na^+ channels are interesting in that they can assume at least three conformations (three-dimensional forms).[25] In addition to the open and closed conformations, the fast Na^+ channel has a refractory form during which the channel will not open again in response to another depolarizing stimulus (Figure 3-32). This refractory period limits the rate at which action potentials can be generated.

Two major factors contribute to cellular repolarization: sodium conductance (inflow) is stopped by closing Na^+ chan-

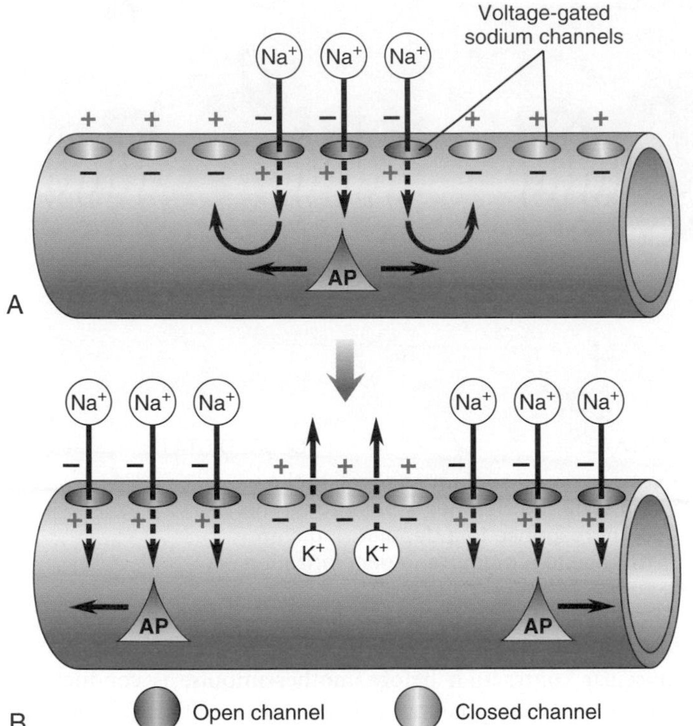

FIGURE 3-30 ■ The action potential *(AP)* in excitable cells is propagated along the membrane by the sequential opening of voltage-gated sodium channels in adjacent sections of membrane. **A,** An action potential is initiated by the opening of sodium channels in a section of membrane. **B,** The action potential is regenerated in adjacent sections of membrane as more sodium channels open. The initial segment repolarizes as sodium channels close and potassium ions move out of the cell.

nels, as described previously, and K^+ conductance (outflow) through voltage-gated K^+ channels increases. These K^+ channels respond to depolarization of the membrane in the same manner as fast Na^+ channels, but they take much longer to open and close. When K^+ channels open, K^+ flows out of the cell, owing to the concentration gradient and the loss of intracellular negativity that accompanies Na^+ influx. The loss of positive intracellular potassium ions helps to quickly return the membrane potential to its negative RMP value.

Action potentials in muscle cells are more complex than the neuronal ones just described. Recall that muscle contraction depends on the presence of intracellular calcium ions. Since Ca^{2+} carries a charge, its entry into the cell is reflected in

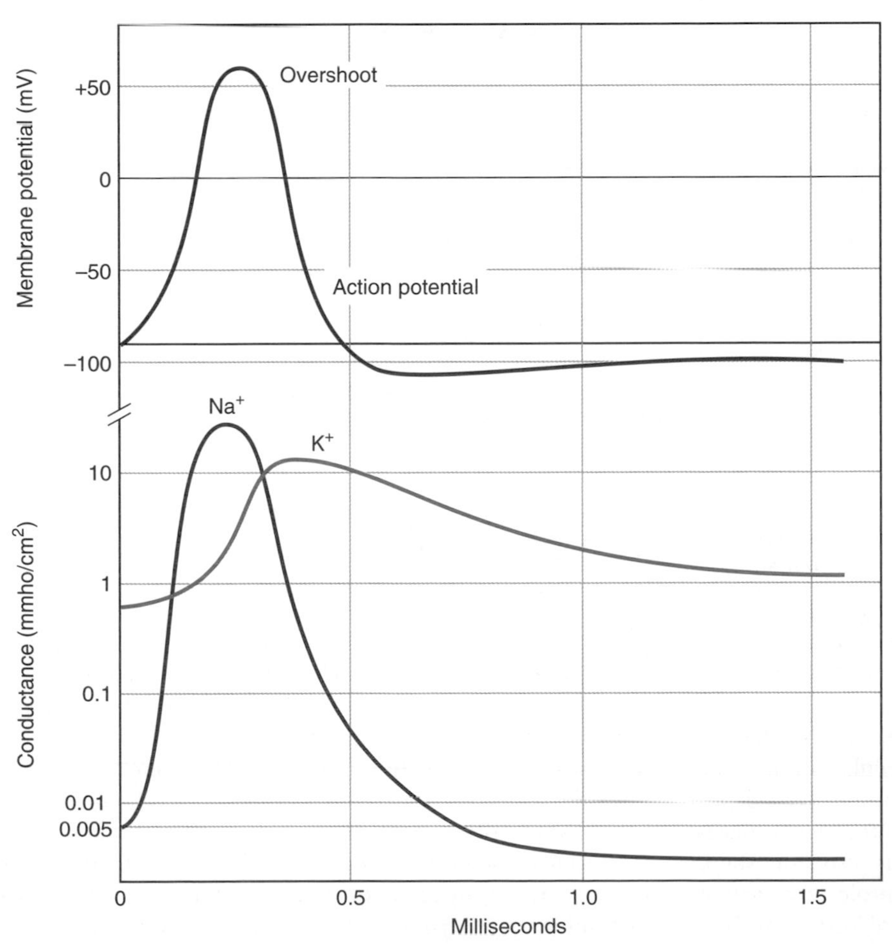

FIGURE 3-31 ■ A typical neuronal action potential showing changes in membrane potential and the associated ion conductances. Note: mmho is a measure of conductance (amperes per volt), also called millisiemens (mS). The steep upstroke of the action potential is attributed to the sudden influx of Na^+ through voltage-gated "fast" sodium ion channels. Voltage-gated K^+ channels open more slowly and stay open longer to allow K^+ efflux from the cell, which aids in repolarization.

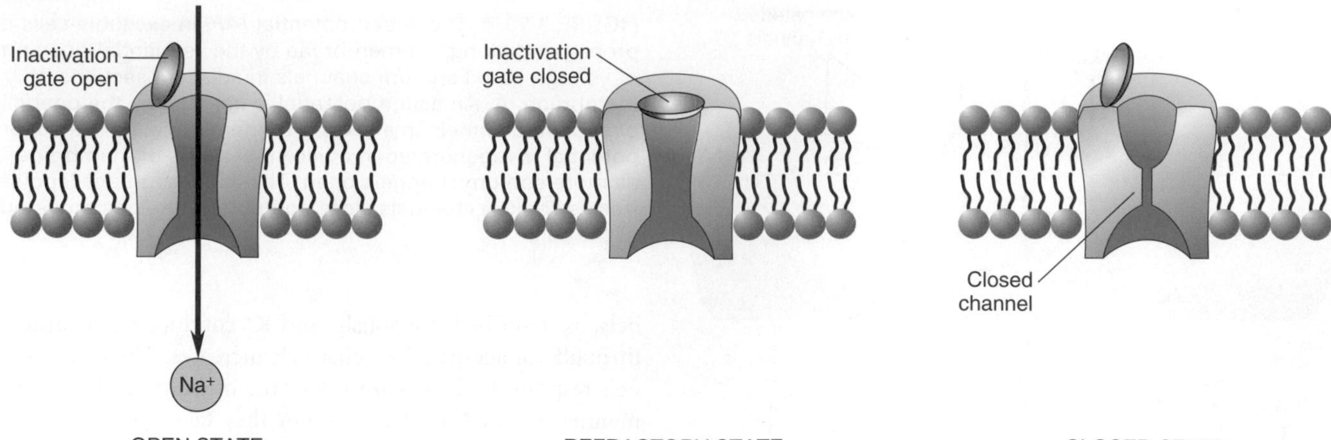

FIGURE 3-32 ■ The three possible states of the voltage-gated sodium channel. In the open state, Na^+ is allowed to pass; in the inactivated state the channel is blocked by the inactivation gate and is refractory and will not open in response to a depolarizing stimulus. In the closed state the channel will open in response to a membrane depolarization.

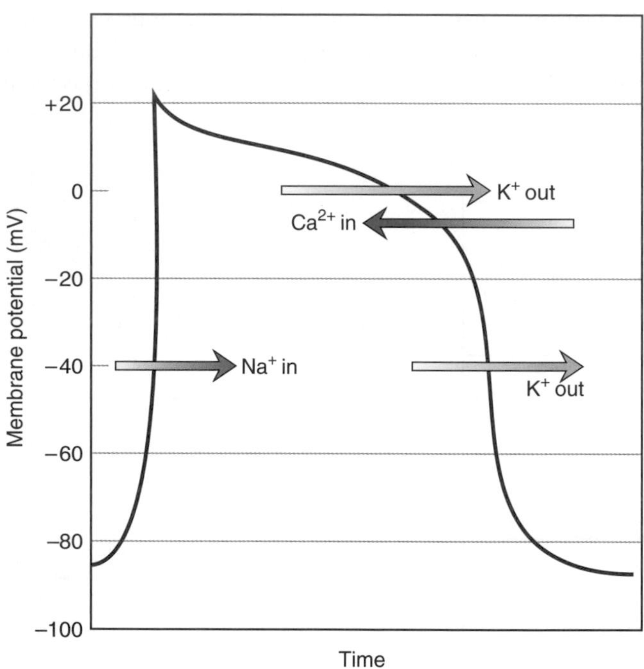

FIGURE 3-33 ■ A typical cardiac muscle cell action potential showing the ion fluxes associated with each phase. Note that the repolarization phase is prolonged in comparison to the nerve action potential in Figure 3-31. This occurs because Ca^{2+} influx offsets the repolarizing effect of K^+ efflux and a plateau in the membrane potential is seen. When the Ca^{2+} channels close, the membrane quickly repolarizes.

the membrane potential. In skeletal muscle, most of the free cytosolic calcium ions come from intracellular stores (sarcoplasmic reticulum) that are released when the cell is depolarized. In cardiac muscle cells, Ca^{2+} entry through voltage-gated channels in the plasma membrane is also important. Calcium conductance into the cell tends to prolong the action potential, resulting in a plateau phase (Figure 3-33). This is of functional importance in cardiac tissue, as it allows time for muscular contraction before another impulse is conducted and prevents the potentially disastrous condition of cardiac muscle tetany. (For a thorough discussion of cardiac electrophysiology, see Chapter 17.)

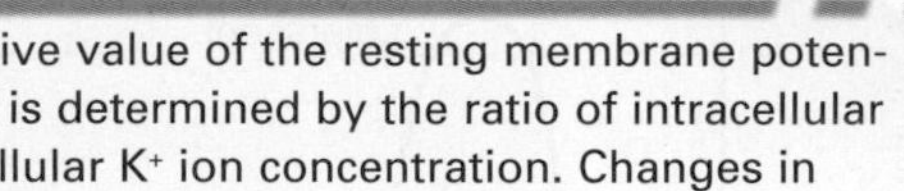

- The negative value of the resting membrane potential (RMP) is determined by the ratio of intracellular to extracellular K^+ ion concentration. Changes in serum K^+ can have profound effects on the RMP.
- Cells with voltage-gated ion channels are excitable and can produce and conduct action potentials. An action potential results from the opening of "fast" Na^+ channels, which allows Na^+ to rush into the cell.
- Repolarization is due to closure of Na^+ channels and efflux of K^+ from the cell. In cardiac muscle, repolarization is prolonged owing to Ca^{2+} influx through "slow" Ca^{2+} channels.

INTERCELLULAR COMMUNICATION AND GROWTH

Cell Signaling Strategies

Cells in multicellular organisms need to communicate with one another and respond to changes in the cellular environment. Coordination of growth, cell division, and the functions of various tissues and organ systems is accomplished by three principal means of communication: (1) through gap junctions that directly connect the cytoplasm of adjoining cells, (2) by direct cell-to-cell contact of plasma membranes or the extracellular molecules associated with the cell (extracellular matrix), and (3) by secretion of chemical mediators (ligands) that influence cells some distance away (Figure 3-34).[26]

REMOTE SIGNALING BY SECRETED MOLECULES

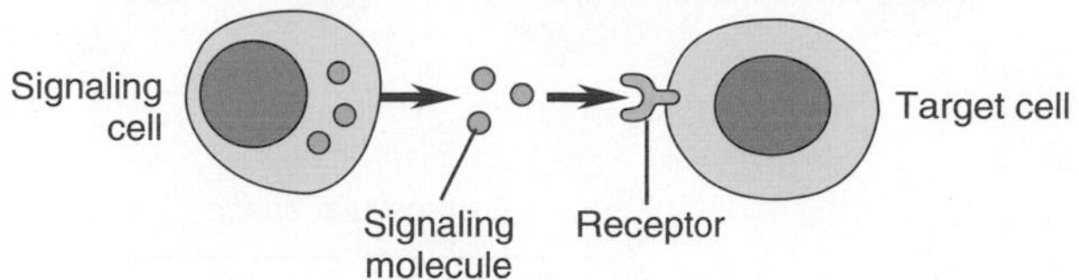

DIRECT SIGNALING BY PLASMA MEMBRANE–BOUND MOLECULES OR EXTRACELLULAR MATRIX

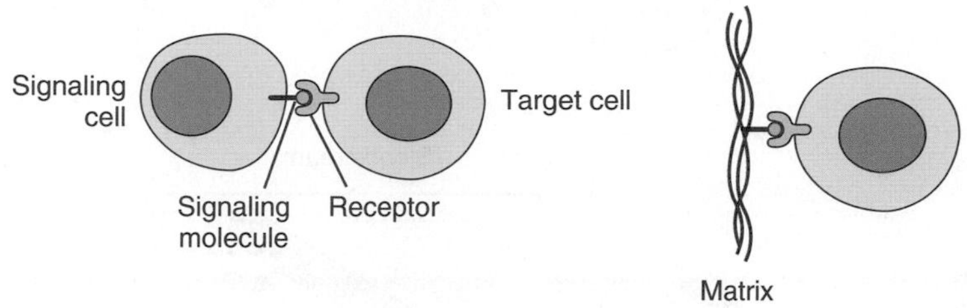

DIRECT SIGNALING VIA GAP JUNCTIONS

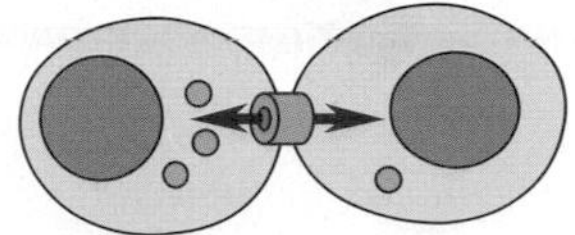

FIGURE 3-34 ■ Methods used for intercellular communication.

Gap junctions are found in large numbers in most tissues. They are connecting channels between adjacent cells that allow the passage of small molecules from one cell to the next. These junctions are formed by special transmembrane proteins that associate to form pores of about 1.5 nm in width. Small molecules, such as inorganic ions, sugars, amino acids, nucleotides, and vitamins, may pass through the pores, whereas macromolecules (proteins, polysaccharides, and nucleic acids) are too large to pass through. Gap junctions are particularly important in tissues in which synchronized functions are required, such as cardiac muscle contraction and intestinal peristaltic movements. Gap junctions appear to be important in embryogenesis as well. Cellular differentiation may be mediated in part through chemical signaling through gap junctions. (See Chapter 5 for a discussion of the development and differentiation of tissue types.)

Direct contact of cell membrane receptors with signaling molecules present on the surface of other cells or extracellular matrix is an important means of local communication among cells in tissues. Contact-dependent signaling is particularly important for the development of the immune response. Such cell-to-cell contact during fetal development is thought to allow the cells of the immune system to discriminate between foreign and self tissues and to develop self-tolerance. If cell-to-cell contact does not occur during fetal life, the immune cells may later attack the body's own cells, leading to the development of autoimmune diseases. (See Chapter 10 for a discussion of autoimmunity.) Contacts between cells and with the extracellular matrix provide signals that maintain cell survival and differentiated cell types.

The best understood form of cell communication is signaling through secreted molecules or *ligands.* Three strategies of intercellular chemical signaling have been described, relating to the distances over which they operate (Figure 3-35). *Synaptic* signaling is confined to the cells of the nervous system and occurs at specialized junctions between the nerve cell and its target cell. The neuron secretes a chemical neurotransmitter into the space between the nerve and target cell; the neurotransmitter then diffuses across and binds receptors on the postsynaptic cell. Synaptic signaling occurs over very small distances (50 nm) and involves only one or a few postsynaptic target cells. In *paracrine* signaling, chemicals are secreted into a localized area and are rapidly destroyed, so that only cells in the immediate area are affected. Growth factors (GFs), for example, act locally to promote wound healing without affecting the growth of the entire organism. *Endocrine* signaling is accomplished by specialized endocrine cells that secrete hormones that travel via the bloodstream to target cells widely distributed throughout the body. Endocrine signaling is slow in comparison to nervous signaling because it relies on diffusion and blood flow to target tissues.

Autocrine signaling occurs when cells are able to respond to signaling molecules that they secrete. Autocrine communication provides a feedback signal to the secreting cell and is commonly linked to pathways that regulate ligand secretion rates. Abnormal autocrine stimulation is thought to be a mechanism in some forms of cancer (see Chapter 7).

Target cells respond to ligand signaling through specific protein *receptors.* Cells can respond to a particular ligand only if they possess the appropriate receptor. For example, all cells

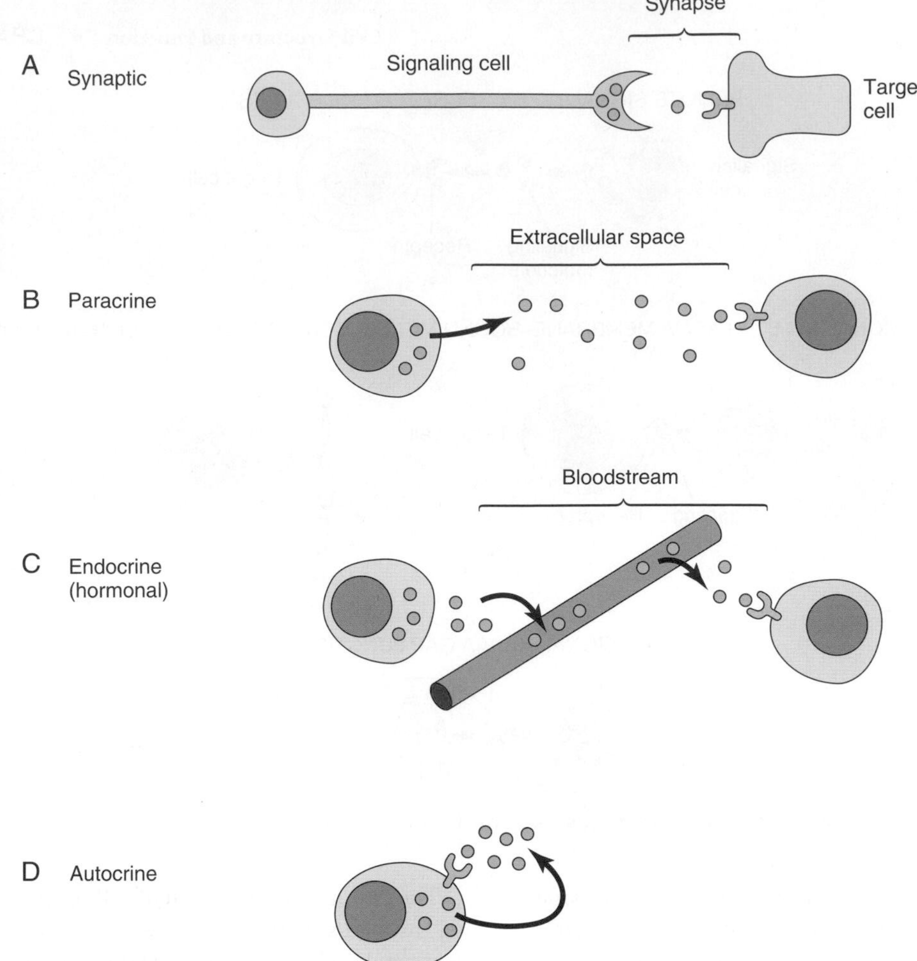

FIGURE 3-35 ■ Signaling by secreted ligands can occur over variable distances. **A,** Synaptic signaling over very small distance between neuron and target cell. **B,** Paracrine signaling through the extracellular fluid between cells in a tissue. **C,** Long-range signaling from endocrine cells through the blood stream to distant targets. **D,** Localized autocrine signaling in which the secreting cell is also the target cell.

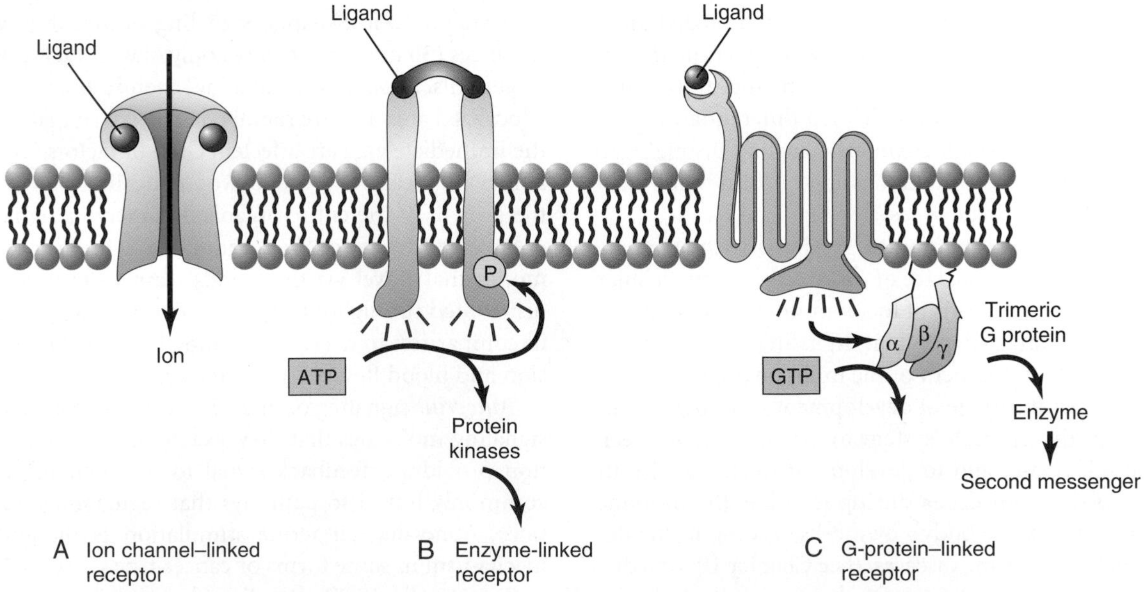

FIGURE 3-36 ■ There are three major types of cell surface receptor proteins. **A,** Ion channel–linked receptors are also called ligand-gated channels. When the ligand binds they open to allow specific ions through the membrane. **B,** Enzyme-linked receptors become activated kinases when a ligand binds to them. Kinases phosphorylate target proteins and change their activity. **C,** G-protein–linked receptors have seven membrane-spanning segments with a ligand binding pocket on the outside and a G-protein–activating portion on the inside. G-protein–linked receptors activate G proteins, which in turn activate enzymes that produce second messengers.

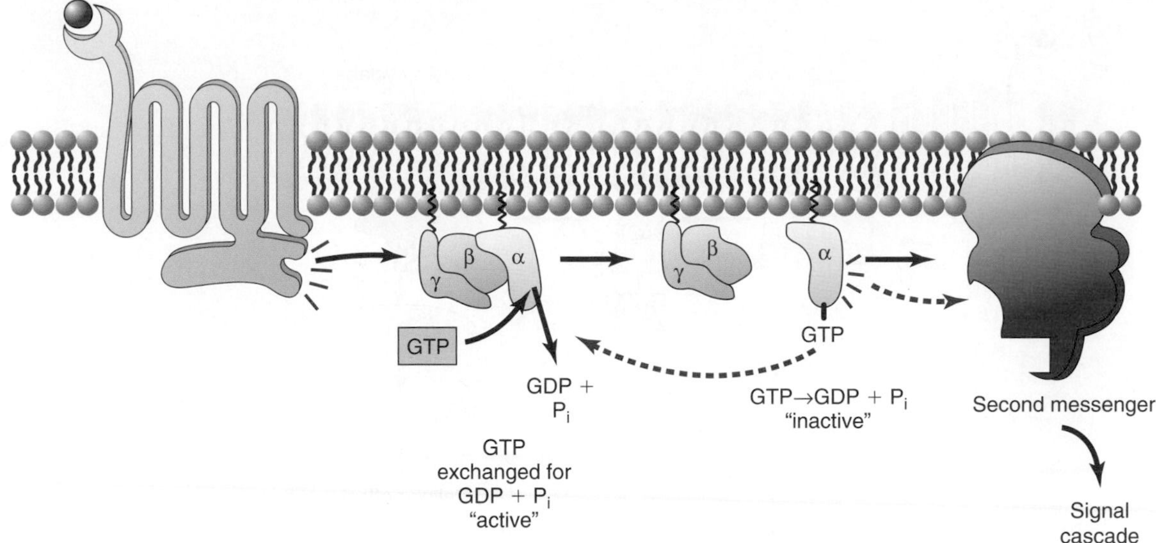

FIGURE 3-37 ■ Schematic of the proposed role of guanosine triphosphate *(GTP)*–binding proteins in the transduction of extracellular signaling messages. When the ligand binds the receptor an intracellular domain is changed into an active configuration that can interact with inactive trimeric G proteins. The receptor induces the G protein to release its bound GDP and P_i in exchange for a GTP molecule. When GTP binds to the α subunit of the G protein it is activated and diffuses away from the γβ subunits to find its target enzyme. The α GTP stimulates its target enzyme to produce a second messenger, which in turn activates a signaling cascade within the cell. After a time the α subunit hydrolyzes its GTP to GDP and P_i and becomes inactive. The α subunit is now in the correct conformation to reassociate with the γβ subunits and await another signal from the receptor.

of the body are exposed to thyroid-stimulating hormone (TSH) as it circulates in the blood, but only thyroid cells respond because they alone possess TSH receptors. However, cells that possess the same receptor may respond very differently to a particular ligand. For example, binding of acetylcholine to its receptor on a glandular cell may induce secretion, whereas binding to the same receptor on a cardiac muscle cell causes a decrease in contractile force. The cellular response to signaling molecules is regulated not only by the array of receptors the cell carries but also by the internal machinery to which the receptors are linked.

Cell Surface Receptor–Mediated Responses

Most hormones, local chemical mediators, and neurotransmitters are water-soluble molecules that are unable to pass through the lipid bilayer of the cell. These ligands exert their effects through binding with a receptor on the surface of the target cell, which then changes or transduces the external signal into an intracellular message. There are at least three major classes of cell surface receptor proteins: ion channel linked, enzyme linked, and G protein linked (Figure 3-36).[26]

Ion channel–linked receptors bind neurotransmitters, causing specific ion channels in the membrane to open or close. This type of signaling is prevalent in the nervous system, where rapid synaptic signaling between neurons is required. *Enzyme-linked* receptors catalyze enzyme reactions when they are activated by appropriate ligands. Nearly all enzyme-linked receptors function as *protein kinases;* that is, they mediate the transfer of phosphate groups from ATP (or GTP) to proteins (phosphorylate) and thus affect the activity of those proteins. The insulin receptor and most GF receptors are protein kinase receptors that phosphorylate and activate intracellular enzyme cascades. A large number of signaling ligands bind to *G-protein–linked receptors.* More than half of known drugs have their effects through G-protein–linked cascades.

G-protein–linked receptors act indirectly through a membrane-bound trimeric G protein that binds and hydrolyzes GTP. The activated G-protein then activates target enzymes or ion channels within the membrane. The target enzymes of G-protein receptors produce second messengers that trigger specific intracellular cascades and alter cell function (Figure 3-37).

There are three principal G-protein–linked signaling systems that when activated alter the intracellular concentration of one or more second messengers (Figure 3-38). Numerous G-protein–linked receptors activate trimeric G proteins whose α subunit stimulates adenylyl cyclase to produce the second messenger cyclic adenosine monophosphate (cAMP). These G proteins are called G_s. An increase in cAMP is linked to different signaling cascades in different cell types. For example, cAMP causes glycogen breakdown in liver cells, increased force of contraction in cardiac cells, and increased secretion by glandular cells. Various cell types respond

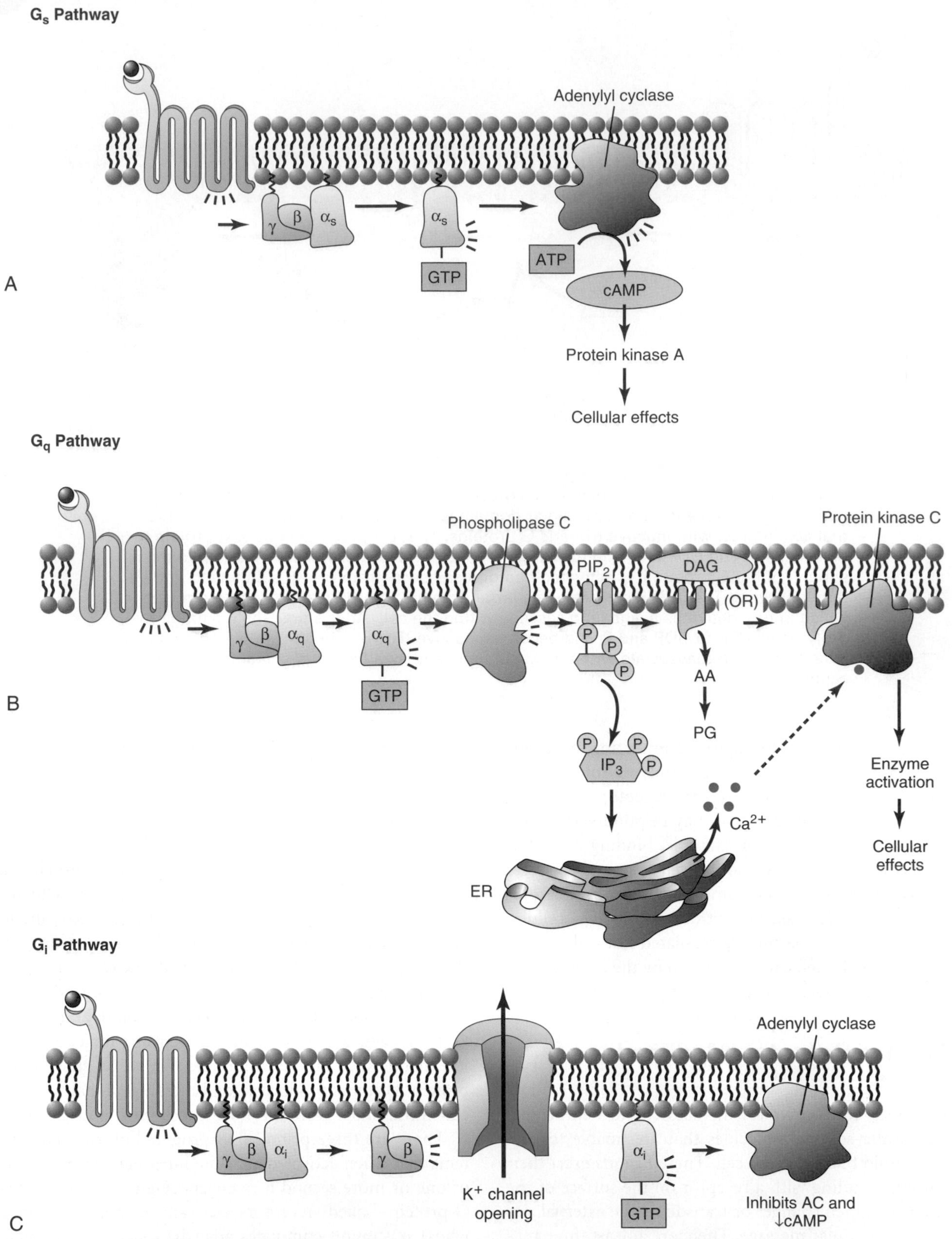

G_s Pathway

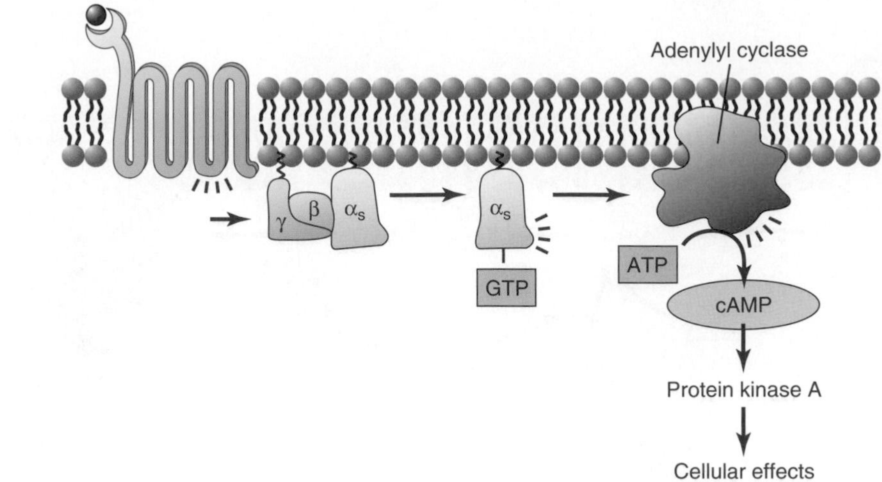

A

G_q Pathway

Phospholipase C
Protein kinase C
PIP_2
DAG
(OR)
β
α_q
γ
α_q
GTP
P
P
P
AA
PG
P
P
IP_3
P
Enzyme activation
Cellular effects
Ca^{2+}
ER

B

G_i Pathway

Adenylyl cyclase
β
α_i
γ
β
γ
α_i
K^+ channel opening
GTP
Inhibits AC and ↓cAMP

C

FIGURE 3-38 ■ Ligand binding to membrane receptors leads to activation of G proteins, which in turn regulate membrane-bound enzymes (adenylyl cyclase *[AC]* and phospholipase C). These enzymes catalyze the formation of second messengers (cyclic adenosine monophosphate *[cAMP]*, inositol 1,4,5-triphosphate *[IP_3]*, diacylglycerol *[DAG]*). Second messengers then activate enzyme cascades within the cell or affect intracellular Ca^{2+} concentration. **A,** The G_s pathway increases the production of cAMP. **B,** The G_q pathway increases the production of IP_3 and DAG, and releases intracellular Ca^{2+}. **C,** The G_i pathway is inhibitory to the production of cAMP. In some cases the γβ unit also has functional activity and may regulate ion channels. *PKC,* Protein kinase C; *ER,* endoplasmic reticulum.

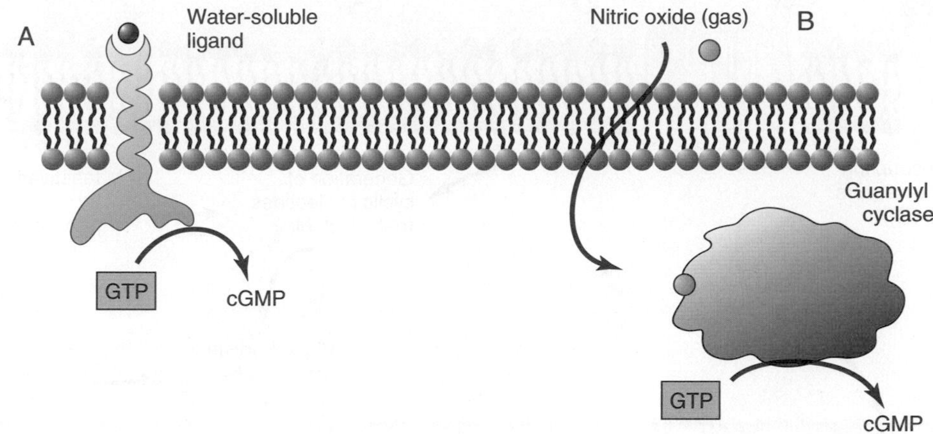

FIGURE 3-39 ■ Cyclic GMP *(cGMP)* is an important second messenger. **A,** It can be synthesized by enzyme-linked receptors that are activated by water-soluble ligands. **B,** Nitric oxide is an important signaling molecule that is lipid soluble and can diffuse across the cell membrane. Nitric oxide binds to and stimulates the enzyme guanylyl cyclase to produce cGMP.

differently to the same second messenger because of differences in enzymes and other proteins in the cell.

Another important G-protein–linked cascade is mediated by G proteins called G_q whose α subunit stimulates the enzyme phospholipase C. Phospholipase C cleaves a membrane phospholipid (PI[4,5]P_2) to form two second messengers, inositol 1,4,5-trisphosphate (IP_3) and diacylglycerol (DAG) (see Figure 3-38). The IP_3 travels to the endoplasmic reticulum where it stimulates the release of Ca^{2+} into the cytoplasm. The Ca^{2+} then triggers a change in cell function. DAG remains bound to the inner surface of the plasma membrane and can trigger several different intracellular cascades. Two important targets are the protein kinase C pathway and the eicosanoid pathway. Protein kinase C is a key enzyme in the growth response. The eicosanoid pathway results in the production of several arachidonic acid derivatives including prostaglandins. These products are often secreted by the cell as signaling molecules to other nearby cells. Prostaglandins are important mediators of inflammation and platelet function.

The third trimeric G-protein type is called G_i because it is inhibitory to the production of cAMP. G-protein–linked receptors such as the acetylcholine receptor in the heart activate G_i whose α subunit then inhibits adenylyl cyclase (see Figure 3-38). In this case, the γβ subunit of G_i is also activated and opens membrane potassium channels in the heart, which tend to slow the heart rate.

In addition to the four second messengers already mentioned (cAMP, IP_3, DAG, and Ca^{2+}) there is a fifth called cyclic guanosine monophosphate (cGMP), which is produced by the enzyme guanylyl cyclase (Figure 3-39). The primary activator of guanylyl cyclase is a small lipid-soluble gas molecule called nitric oxide. Nitric oxide is an important signaling molecule with widespread targets. It functions as a neurotransmitter in the brain and is an important smooth muscle relaxant in the vascular system. cGMP is also produced by a special class of enzyme-linked receptors (see Figure 3-39).

To be effective at communicating signals, all of the receptor systems must be quickly turned back off so that they can be responsive to the next incoming signal. A variety of strategies are used to quench the signaling cascades (Figure 3-40). For example, phosphodiesterases are enzymes that convert the cyclic nucleotides cAMP and cGMP to their inactive forms, AMP and GMP, and help to remove these second messengers soon after they are formed. Some drugs, such as caffeine and sildenafil citrate (Viagra), are phosphodiesterase inhibitors that slow the normal breakdown of cyclic nucleotides and prolong their activity. Many of the intracellular signaling cascades rely on kinases that phosphorylate their target proteins so as to change their activity. The action of kinases is countered by numerous phosphatase enzymes that quickly cleave the phosphates back off the target proteins and inhibit their activity.

The cell can also regulate the activity and number of receptors on the cell surface.[26] Generally a cell decreases the number or activity of receptors when it is exposed to excessive concentrations of signaling molecules (see Figure 3-40). Receptors can be internalized in the cell where they are inactive but are available for later use, or they can be sent to lysosomes for degradation. Destruction of receptors in lysosomes is called down-regulation. (The production of extra receptors is called up-regulation.) Receptors that remain in the membrane can also be inhibited by phosphorylation, which blocks them from interacting with their intracellular targets. Receptors that can bind ligand but do not produce a response are said to be uncoupled. The proteins that phosphorylate G-protein receptors are called G-protein receptor kinases (GRKs). The mechanisms that "turn off" signaling cascades are vitally important to maintaining a responsive communication system.

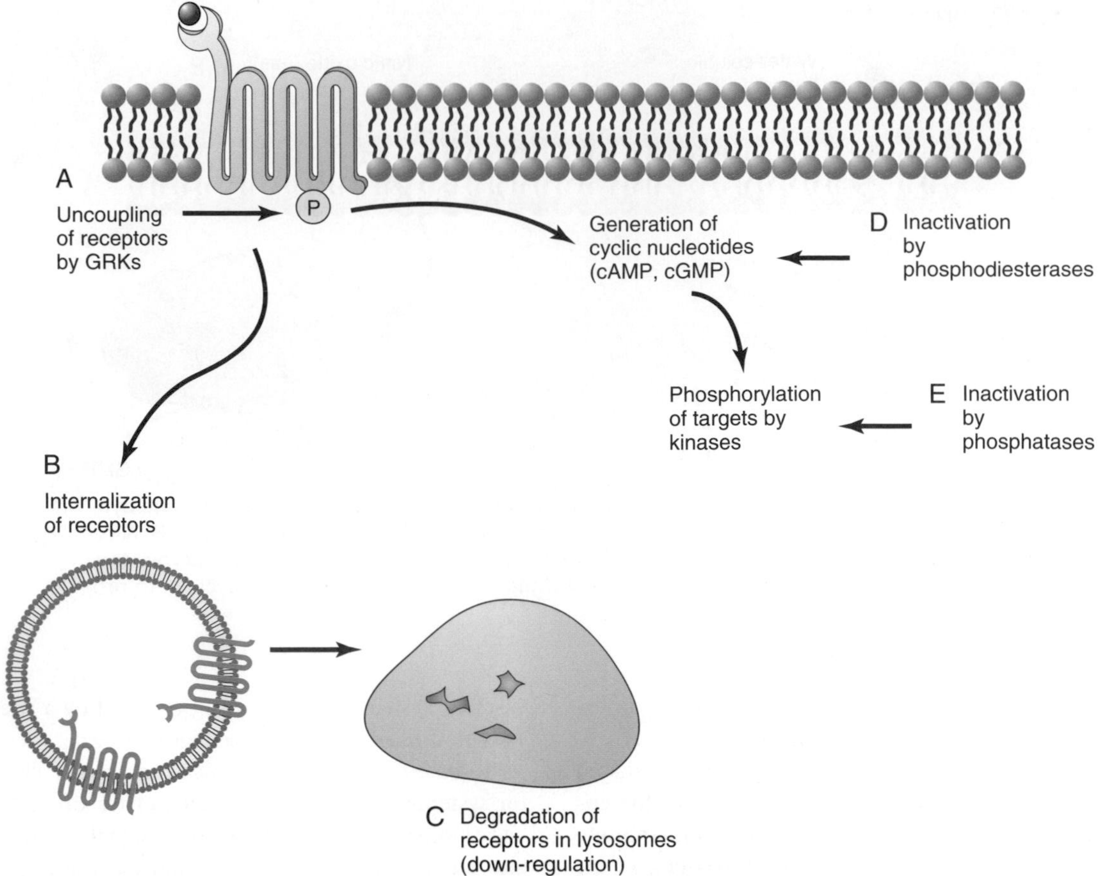

FIGURE 3-40 ■ A variety of mechanisms exist to inhibit receptor-mediated signaling cascades. **A,** Phosphorylation of the receptor by receptor kinases such as G-protein receptor kinase *(GRK)* uncouples the enzyme from its intracellular cascade. **B,** Receptor internalization temporarily reduces the number of receptors displayed at the cell surface. **C,** Receptor degradation results in a long-term reduction in receptors (down-regulation). **D,** The cyclic nucleotide second messengers can be degraded by phosphodiesterase enzymes to stop the intracellular cascade. **E,** Phosphatase enzymes counteract the phosphorylating activities of kinases and inhibit the intracellular cascade.

Intracellular Receptor–Mediated Responses

A small number of hormones are lipid soluble and can pass directly through the cell membrane to interact with receptors *inside* the cell. These receptors are located in the cell cytosol (e.g., cortisol) or may be associated with the cell nucleus (e.g., thyroid). Intracellular receptors are specific for a particular ligand, just as surface receptors are. Binding of the ligand causes the receptor to become activated. The activated cytosolic receptor then travels to the nucleus, where it binds with specific genes and regulates their activity (Figure 3-41). Since lipid-soluble ligands enter the cell directly, no second messengers are needed. Steroid hormones such as cortisol usually bind to receptors in the cytosol, whereas the thyroid receptor is already bound to DNA in the absence of its ligand. When thyroid hormone finds its nuclear receptor the complex dissociates and removes an inhibitory influence on gene transcription. Cellular responses to these gene regulatory receptor complexes are slow in comparison to the cell surface receptor responses and generally last longer.

Regulation of Cellular Growth

In multicellular organisms such as humans, the growth of cells and tissues must be strictly controlled to maintain a balance between cell birth rate and cell death rate. The system must be capable of rapidly increasing growth of a particular tissue to replace cells lost to injury and normal wear and tear while simultaneously inhibiting unwanted growth or proliferation of other cells. Special intercellular communication systems function to regulate the replication of individual cells in the body. Two important strategies of growth control have been described. First, a variety of protein GFs are required in specific combinations for growth and proliferation of particular cell types. Second, cells respond to spatial signals that indicate how much room is available. When conditions favor cell proliferation the cell proceeds through the stages of the cell cycle

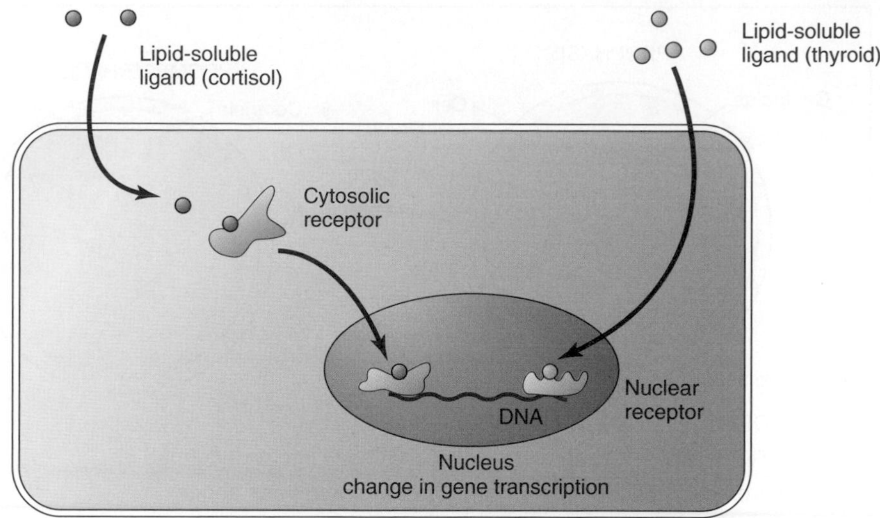

FIGURE 3-41 ■ Lipid-soluble ligands such as steroid hormones, thyroid hormones, and gases can diffuse across the cell membrane and interact with receptors located within the cell cytoplasm or nucleus. When the ligand binds to its intracellular receptor it forms a functional gene regulatory protein that affects the rate of transcription of its target genes. The response of the cell to intracellular ligands is generally slow and long lasting.

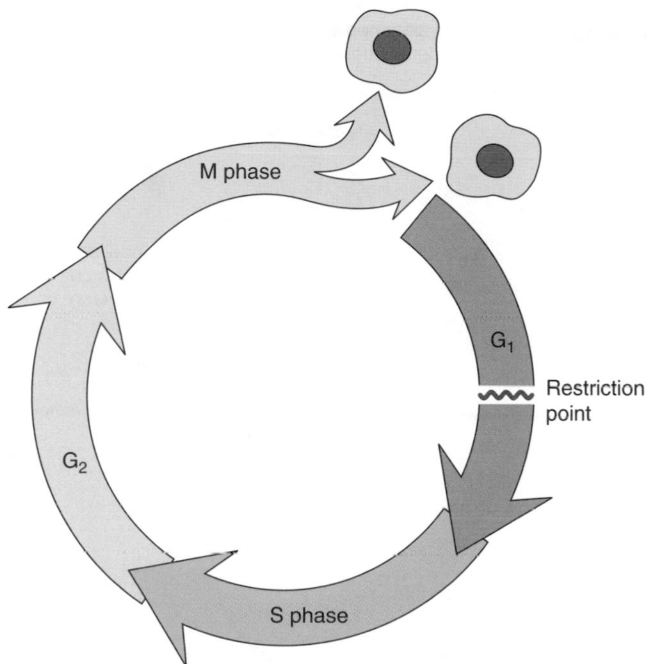

FIGURE 3-42 ■ Events of the cell cycle. The cycle begins late in G_1 when the cell passes a restriction point. The cell then proceeds systematically through the S phase (synthesis), G_2, and M phase (mitosis).

(Figure 3-42). Dormant cells remain in G_1 phase indefinitely. Cycling cells proceed through G_1, S phase (synthesis), G_2, M phase (mitosis), and cell division. S phase is characterized by duplication of DNA and synthesis of intracellular components in preparation for cell division. M phase or mitosis proceeds through six stages, beginning with prophase, in which the chromosomes condense and become visible, and ending with cytokinesis, when cell division is accomplished. The chromosomes of body cells are duplicated and distributed equally to the cell's progeny when it divides by mitosis such that each daughter cell receives an identical full set of 46 chromosomes. The stages of mitotic cell division are explained in Figure 3-43. Mitosis is responsible for the proliferation of body cells in which little genetic variation is needed or desired. A more elaborate cell division process, meiosis, occurs in the germ cells (egg and sperm) where significant chromosomal rearrangements occur (see Chapter 6).

The **cell cycle** has been the subject of intense study in recent years because of its importance in cancer biology. Cancer cells continue to grow and divide unchecked, despite the lack of appropriate signals to stimulate them. A clearer understanding of the roles of numerous genes in regulating the cell cycle is beginning to emerge. Of particular interest are the events that prod the cell from its dormant state and cause it to begin the cycle. A simplified picture of a major component of this complex process is shown in Figure 3-44. The RB protein (or pRB) is of central importance in preventing a cell from proceeding through the cell cycle.[27] The RB protein functions to bind up gene regulatory factors called E2F so that they are unable to bind to DNA promoter regions and begin the processes of cell replication. The RB protein can be induced to let go of the E2F transcription factors when appropriate growth activating signals arrive at the cell surface. These growth-promoting signals at the cell surface are transmitted to the RB protein by way of cyclin-dependent signaling pathways within the cell. Proteins called *cyclins* accumulate in the cell and then bind to and activate cyclin-dependent kinases (cdk). The cdk then phosphorylates the RB protein changing its affinity for E2F so that it lets go. The E2F then translocates to specific regions of DNA where it promotes gene transcription, allowing cell replication to begin.

To respond to a GF, a cell must have the corresponding GF receptor on its cell surface. Many cells in the body synthesize and secrete GFs, which then influence the growth of other cell types in a paracrine or endocrine fashion. Platelet-derived growth factor (PDGF) was one of the first GFs to be discovered. It is secreted by platelets when they form blood clots in response to an injury. PDGF stimulates fibroblasts and

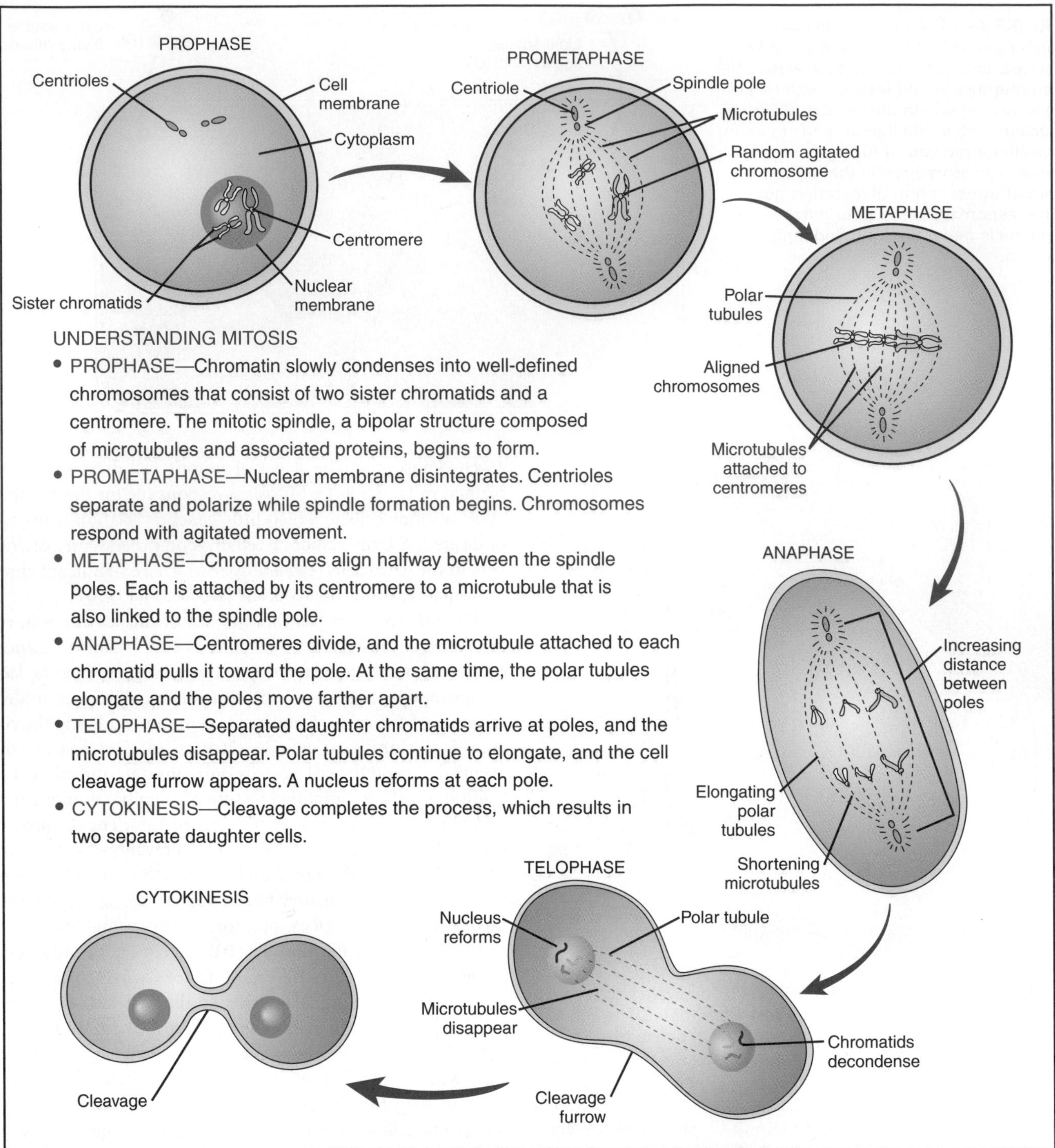
PROPHASE
Centrioles
Cell membrane
Cytoplasm
Centromere
Nuclear membrane
Sister chromatids
PROMETAPHASE
Centriole
Spindle pole
Microtubules
Random agitated chromosome
METAPHASE
Polar tubules
Aligned chromosomes
Microtubules attached to centromeres
UNDERSTANDING MITOSIS
• PROPHASE—Chromatin slowly condenses into well-defined chromosomes that consist of two sister chromatids and a centromere. The mitotic spindle, a bipolar structure composed of microtubules and associated proteins, begins to form.
• PROMETAPHASE—Nuclear membrane disintegrates. Centrioles separate and polarize while spindle formation begins. Chromosomes respond with agitated movement.
• METAPHASE—Chromosomes align halfway between the spindle poles. Each is attached by its centromere to a microtubule that is also linked to the spindle pole.
• ANAPHASE—Centromeres divide, and the microtubule attached to each chromatid pulls it toward the pole. At the same time, the polar tubules elongate and the poles move farther apart.
• TELOPHASE—Separated daughter chromatids arrive at poles, and the microtubules disappear. Polar tubules continue to elongate, and the cell cleavage furrow appears. A nucleus reforms at each pole.
• CYTOKINESIS—Cleavage completes the process, which results in two separate daughter cells.
ANAPHASE
Increasing distance between poles
Elongating polar tubules
Shortening microtubules
TELOPHASE
Nucleus reforms
Polar tubule
Microtubules disappear
Chromatids decondense
Cleavage furrow
CYTOKINESIS
Cleavage

FIGURE 3-43 ■ The six stages of mitotic cell division. (From Nichols FH, Zwelling E, editors: *Maternal-newborn nursing: theory and practice,* Philadelphia, 1997, Saunders, p 307.)

smooth muscle cells in the damaged area to divide and replace cells lost to the injury. Numerous GFs have been identified, and most cells require an appropriate combination of GF signals before they can enter the cell cycle.[28] There are many signaling steps in the pathway from GF receptor to DNA activation. Some GFs promote an increase in cell size whereas others stimulate cell division, and many GFs appear to do both. Similar signaling pathways are used to trigger cell death (apoptosis) when cells have to be reduced or removed during tissue development and remodeling. The processes of abnormal cellular proliferation and cancer are further detailed in Chapter 7. The process of apoptosis is described in Chapter 4.

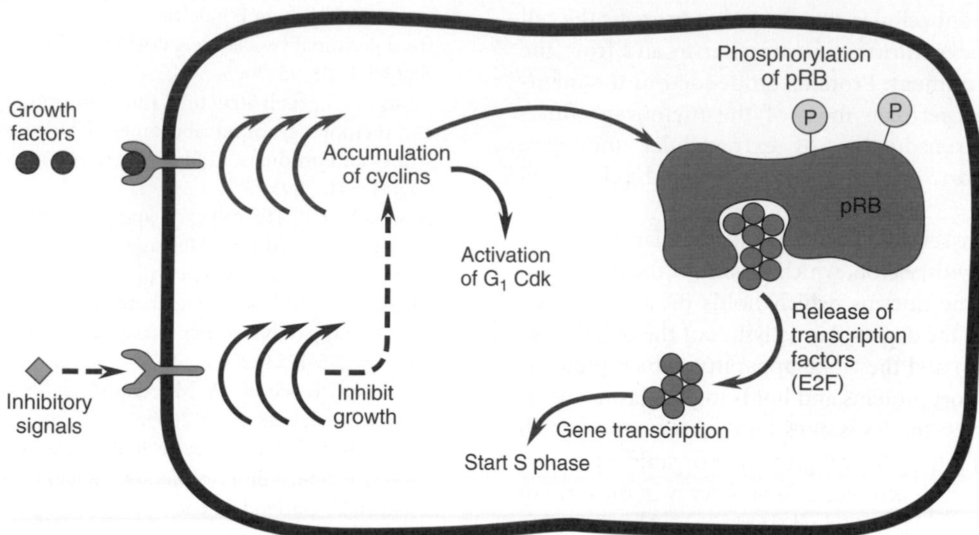

FIGURE 3-44 ■ The mechanism of initiation of cellular replication requires appropriate stimulation by extracellular growth factors that bind their complementary receptors on the cell surface. Activation of the receptor stimulates signaling pathways within the cell that increase cyclin proteins. The cyclins bind to cyclin-dependent kinases *(Cdk)* to form active enzyme complexes. The active cyclin-Cdk enzymes phosphorylate RB protein *(pRB),* inducing it to let go of E2F transcription factors that initiate replication. In the absence of appropriate growth factor signals, the RB protein functions to inhibit unwanted cell proliferation.

KEY CONCEPTS

- Intercellular communication is accomplished by three principal means: (1) gap junctions, which directly connect the cytoplasm of adjoining cells; (2) direct cell-to-cell surface contact; and (3) secretion of chemical mediators (ligands). Most ligands are water soluble molecules that interact with receptors on the cell surface. These receptors are of three general types: ion channel linked, enzyme linked, and G protein linked.
- Binding of a ligand to a G-protein receptor usually results in the production of second messengers (cAMP, IP_3, DAG, Ca^{2+}) within the target cell that alter cell function.
- Somatic cells divide by a process called mitosis in which daughter cells each receive an identical and complete set of 46 chromosomes.
- Cell replication normally requires specific extracellular GFs that activate signaling systems within the cell. Cyclin proteins and cyclin-dependent kinases alter the function of RB protein, causing it to release transcription factors that begin the process of cell replication.

SUMMARY

Detailed knowledge of cell physiology is essential to understanding disease processes. Cells are complex, membrane-bound units that perform a variety of functions necessary to the maintenance of life. The major cell components and their functions are summarized in Table 3-1. The cell mem-

Table 3-1 

Structure and Function of Major Cellular Components

Cellular Structure	Functions
Plasma membrane	Protective barrier separates life from nonlife Extracellular message transduction Transport of materials into and out of the cell Maintenance and transmission of membrane potentials Cell-to-cell recognition, interaction
Cytoskeleton	Maintenance of cell shape Cell movement Trafficking within the cell
Nucleus	Protection of genetic material Regulation of cell type and function through control of protein synthesis
Endoplasmic reticulum	Protein and lipid synthesis Lipid metabolism and detoxification
Golgi apparatus	Protein and lipid modification and sorting Transport of proteins and lipids to appropriate destinations
Lysosomes	Hydrolytic breakdown of organic waste
Peroxisomes	Oxidative breakdown of organic waste
Mitochondria	Cellular energy production (ATP)

ATP, Adenosine triphosphate.

brane is an important cellular structure that protects the cell interior and mediates information transfer to and from the extracellular environment. Proteins embedded in the membrane lipid bilayer perform most of the membrane functions, including transduction of extracellular messages, membrane transport, electrical excitation, and cell-to-cell communication.

Human cells have several important intracellular organelles. These include the cytoskeleton, which organizes the intracellular compartment; the nucleus, which holds the cell's genetic material and directs the day-to-day activities of the cell; the endoplasmic reticulum and the Golgi apparatus, which produce, package, and transport proteins and lipids to the plasma membrane and lysosomes; the lysosomes and peroxisomes, which perform the task of intracellular digestion of organic waste; and the mitochondria, which produce cellular energy in the form of ATP. The energy released by ATP hydrolysis is used by the cell to drive the many energetically unfavorable reactions needed to maintain cellular functions. Multicellular organisms have developed complex communication systems to control cell behavior, such as growth and differentiation into specialized cell types. Disruption of these cellular processes is at the root of pathophysiologic processes and disease.

MEDIA RESOURCES

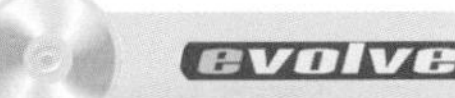

evolve

Remember to check out the ***CD Companion*** included with this book for Review Questions, Key Concepts Review, Glossary (with audio for selected terms), Disease Profiles, and Animations.

PLUS, visit the ***Evolve website*** at http://evolve.elsevier.com/Copstead/ for Case Studies, Disease Profiles, and WebLinks.

References

1. Alberts B et al: The cell cycle and programmed cell death. In Alberts B et al, editors: *Molecular biology of the cell*, ed 4, New York, 2002, Garland Science, pp 3-45.
2. Lahava N, Nira S, Elitzurb A: The emergence of life on Earth, *Progr Biophys Mol Biol* 75:75-120, 2001.
3. Singer SJ, Nicolson GL: The fluid mosaic model of the structure of cell membranes, *Science* 175:720-731, 1972.
4. Alberts B et al: The cell cycle and programmed cell death. In Alberts B et al, editors: *Molecular biology of the cell*, ed 4, New York, 2002, Garland Science, pp 583-614.
5. Hakomori S: Structure, organization, and function of glycosphingolipids in membrane, *Curr Opin Hematol* 10(1):16-24, 2003.
6. Bennett V, Baines A: Spectrin and ankyrin-based pathways: metazoan inventions for integrating cells into tissues, *Physiol Rev* 81:1353-1392, 2001.
7. Alberts B et al: The cell cycle and programmed cell death. In Alberts B et al, editors: *Molecular biology of the cell*, ed 4, New York, 2002, Garland Science, pp 907-82.
8. Lenart P, Ellenberg J: Nuclear envelope dynamics in oocytes: from germinal vesicle breakdown to mitosis, *Curr Opin Cell Biol* 15(1):88-95, 2003.
9. Johnson AE, et al: Structure, function, and regulation of free and membrane-bound ribosomes: the view from their substrates and products, *Cold Spring Harb Symp Quant Biol* 66:531-541, 2001.
10. Alberts B et al: The cell cycle and programmed cell death. In Alberts B et al, editors: *Molecular biology of the cell*, ed 4, New York, 2002, Garland Science, pp 711-766.
11. Cheng SH, Smith AE: Gene therapy progress and prospects: gene therapy of lysosomal storage disorders, *Gene Ther* 10(16):1275-1281, 2003.
12. Chinnery PF, Schon EA: Mitochondria, *J Neurol Neurosurg Psychiatry* 74(9):1188-1199, 2003.
13. Alberts B et al: The cell cycle and programmed cell death. In Alberts B et al, editors: *Molecular biology of the cell*, ed 4, New York, 2002, Garland Science, pp 767-830.
14. Alberts B et al: Membrane transport of small molecules and the electrical properties of membranes. In Alberts B et al, editors: *Molecular biology of the cell*, ed 4, New York, 2002, Garland Science, pp 615-658.
15. Daniel H, Rubio-Aliaga I: An update on renal peptide transporters, *Am J Physiol Renal Physiol* 284(5):F885-F892, 2003.
16. Clausen T: The sodium pump keeps us going, *Ann N Y Acad Sci* 986:595-602, 2003.
17. Martonosi AN, Pikula S: The network of calcium regulation in muscle, *Acta Biochim Pol* 50(1):1-30, 2003.
18. Karpen JW, Ruiz M: Ion channels: does each subunit do something on its own? *Trends Biochem Sci* 27(8):402-409, 2002.
19. Lamas JA, Reboreda A, Codesido V: Ionic basis of the resting membrane potential in cultured rat sympathetic neurons, *Neuroreport* 13(5):585-591, 2002.
20. Hodgkin AL: *The conduction of the nervous impulse*, Liverpool, England, 1971, Liverpool University Press.
21. Baker PF, Hodgkin AL, Shaw T: The effects of changes in internal ionic concentrations of the electrical properties of perfused giant axons, *J Physiol* 164:355-374, 1962.
22. Hodgkin AL, Huxley AF: Currents carried by sodium and potassium ions through the membrane of the giant axon of *Loligo*, *J Physiol* 116:449-472, 1952.
23. Hodgkin AL, Huxley AF, Katz B: Measurement of current-voltage relations in the membrane of the giant axon of *Loligo*, *J Physiol* 116:424-448, 1952.
24. Hodgkin AL, Katz B: The effect of sodium ions on the electrical activity of the giant axon of the squid, *J Physiol* 108:37-77, 1949.
25. Bezanilla F: Voltage sensor movements, *J Gen Physiol* 120(4): 465-473, 2002.
26. Alberts B et al: The cell cycle and programmed cell death. In Alberts B et al, editors: *Molecular biology of the cell*, ed 4, New York, 2002, Garland Science, pp 831-906.
27. Stiegler P, Giordano A: The family of retinoblastoma proteins, *Crit Rev Eukaryot Gene Expr* 11(1-3):59-76, 2001.
28. Alberts B et al: The cell cycle and programmed cell death. In Alberts B et al, editors: *Molecular biology of the cell*, ed 4, New York, 2002, Garland Science, pp 983-1026.

chapter 4

Cell Injury, Aging, and Death

Jacquelyn L. Banasik

MEDIA RESOURCES

Additional Material for Study, Review, and Further Exploration

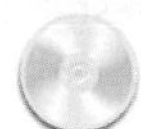

CD Companion ◆ Review Questions and Answers ◆ Key Concepts Review
◆ Glossary *(with audio pronunciations for selected terms)*
◆ Disease Profiles ◆ Animations

evolve ***Website*** at http://evolve.elsevier.com/Copstead/
◆ Case Studies ◆ Disease Profiles ◆ WebLinks

KEY QUESTIONS

- What are the usual cellular responses to reversible injury?
- How are reversible and irreversible cellular injuries differentiated?
- How do necrosis and apoptosis differ?
- To what kind of injuries are cells susceptible?
- What are the usual physiologic changes of aging and how are these differentiated from disease?

CHAPTER OUTLINE

Disease and injury are cellular phenomena. Although pathophysiologic processes are often presented in terms of systemic effects and manifestations, ultimately it is the *cells* that make up the systems that are affected. Even complex multisystem disorders such as cancer ultimately are due to alterations in cell function. Increasingly, the mysterious mechanisms of diseases are being understood on the cellular and molecular level, allowing better methods of treatment and prevention. This chapter presents the general characteristics of cellular injury, adaptation, aging, and death that underlie the discussions of systemic pathophysiologic processes in later chapters of this text.

Cells are confronted by many challenges to their integrity and survival and have efficient mechanisms for coping with an altered cellular environment. Cells respond to environmental changes or injury in three general ways: (1) If the change is mild or short lived, the cell may withstand the assault and completely return to normal. This is called a *reversible cell injury.* (2) The cell may adapt to a persistent but sublethal injury by changing its structure or function. Generally, adaptation also is reversible. (3) Cell death may occur if the injury is too severe or prolonged. Cell death is irreversible and may occur by two different processes termed *necrosis* and *apoptosis.* Necrosis is cell death caused by external injury, whereas apoptosis is triggered by intracellular signaling cascades that result in cell suicide. Necrosis is considered to be a pathologic process associated with significant tissue damage, whereas apoptosis may be a normal physiologic process in some instances and pathologic in others.

REVERSIBLE CELL INJURY

Regardless of the cause, reversible injuries and the early stages of irreversible injuries often result in cellular swelling and the accumulation of excess substances within the cell. These changes reflect the cell's inability to perform normal metabolic functions owing to insufficient cellular energy in the form of adenosine triphosphate (ATP) or dysfunction of associated metabolic enzymes. Once the acute stress or injury has been removed, by definition of a reversible injury, the cell returns to its preinjury state.

Hydropic Swelling

Cellular swelling due to accumulation of water, or hydropic swelling, is the most common manifestation of reversible cell injury.[1] Hydropic swelling results from malfunction of the sodium-potassium (Na^+-K^+) pumps that normally maintain ionic equilibrium of the cell. Failure of the Na^+-K^+ pump results in accumulation of sodium ions within the cell, creating an osmotic gradient for water entry. Because Na^+-K^+ pump function is dependent on cellular ATP, any injury that results in insufficient energy production will also result in hydropic swelling (Figure 4-1).[1] Hydropic swelling is characterized by a large, pale cytoplasm, dilated endoplasmic reticulum, and swollen mitochondria. With severe hydropic swelling, the endoplasmic reticulum may rupture and form large water-filled

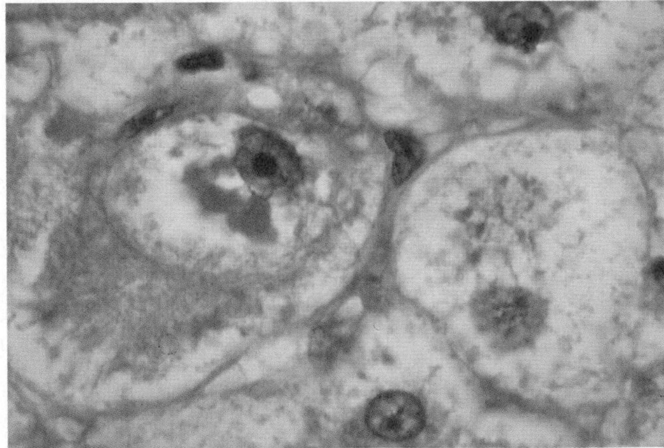

FIGURE 4-1 ■ Cellular swelling in hepatocytes in alcoholic liver disease. Cellular morphology typical of hydropic swelling. (From Kumar V, Cotran RS, Robbins SL, editors: *Basic pathology,* ed 7, Philadelphia, 2003, Saunders, p 24. Photograph courtesy Dr. James Crawford, Department of Pathology, Brigham and Women's Hospital, Boston.)

vacuoles. Generalized swelling in the cells of a particular organ will cause the organ to increase in size and weight. Organ enlargement is indicated by the suffix *-megaly* (e.g., *splenomegaly* denotes an enlarged spleen, *hepatomegaly* denotes an enlarged liver).

Intracellular Accumulations

Excess accumulations of substances in cells may result in cellular injury because the substances are toxic or provoke an immune response or merely because they occupy space needed for cellular functions. In some cases, accumulations do not in themselves appear to be injurious but rather are indicators of cell injury. Intracellular accumulations may be categorized as (1) excessive amounts of normal intracellular substances such as fat, (2) accumulation of abnormal substances produced by the cell because of faulty metabolism or synthesis, and (3) accumulation of pigments and particles that the cell is unable to degrade (Figure 4-2).

Normal intracellular substances that tend to accumulate in injured cells include lipids, carbohydrates, glycogen, and proteins. Faulty metabolism of these substances within the cell results in excessive intracellular storage. In some cases, the enzymes required for breaking down a particular substance are absent or abnormal as a result of a genetic defect. In other cases, altered metabolism may be due to excessive intake, toxins, or other disease processes.

A common site of intracellular lipid accumulation is the liver, where many fats are normally stored, metabolized, and synthesized. Fatty liver is often associated with excessive intake of alcohol.[2] Mechanisms whereby alcohol causes fatty liver remains unclear, but it is thought to result from direct toxic effects as well as the preferential metabolism of alcohol instead of lipid (see Chapter 38 for a discussion of fatty liver). Lipids may also accumulate in blood vessels, kidney, heart, and other organs. Fat-filled cells tend to compress cellular components to one side and cause the tissue to appear yellowish and greasy (Figure 4-3). In several genetic disorders, the enzymes needed to metabolize lipids are impaired; these include Tay-Sachs disease and Gaucher disease, in which lipids accumulate in neurologic tissue.

Glycosaminoglycans (mucopolysaccharides) are large carbohydrate complexes that normally make up the extracellular matrix of connective tissues. Connective tissue cells secrete most of the glycosaminoglycan into the extracellular space, but a small portion remains inside the cell and is degraded by lysosomal enzymes. The *mucopolysaccharidoses* are a group of genetic diseases in which the enzymatic degradation of these molecules is impaired and they collect within the cell. Mental retardation and connective tissue disorders are common.

Like other disorders of accumulation, *excessive glycogen storage* can be the result of inborn errors of metabolism, but the most common cause is diabetes mellitus.[1] Diabetes mellitus is associated with impaired cellular uptake of glucose, which results in high serum and urine glucose levels. Cells of

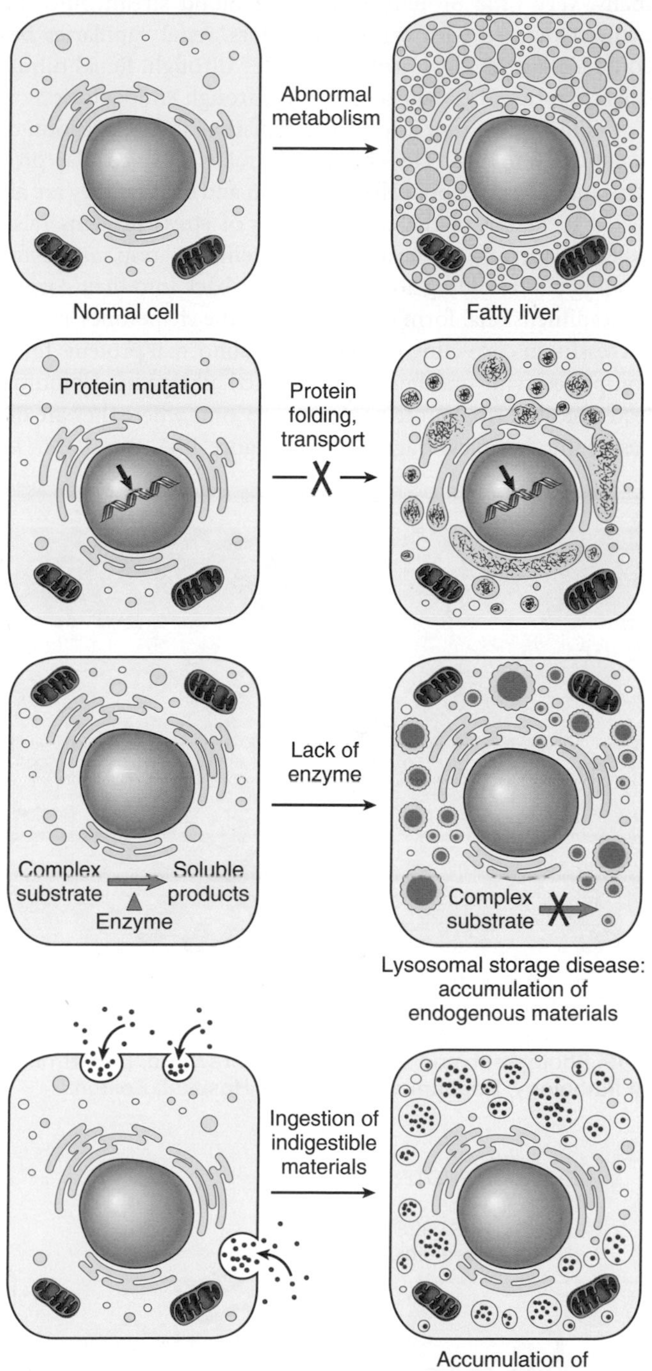

FIGURE 4-2 ■ General mechanisms of intracellular accumulation: (1) abnormal metabolism as in fatty change in the liver, (2) mutations causing alterations in protein folding and transport so that defective proteins accumulate, (3) deficiency of critical enzyme responsible for lysosomal degradation, and (4) an inability to degrade phagocytosed particles such as coal dust. (From Kumar V, Cotran RS, Robbins SL, editors: *Basic pathology,* ed 7, Philadelphia, 2003, Saunders, p 18.)

the renal tubules reabsorb the excess filtered glucose and store it intracellularly as glycogen. The renal tubule cells are also a common site for abnormal accumulations of proteins. Normally, very little protein escapes the blood stream into the urine. However, with certain disorders, renal capillaries become leaky and allow proteins to filter through. Renal tubule cells recapture the escaped proteins through endocytosis.

Cellular stress may lead to accumulation and aggregation of denatured proteins. The abnormally folded intracellular proteins may cause serious cell dysfunction and death if they are allowed to persist in the cell. A family of stress proteins (also called chaperone or heat-shock proteins) is responsible for binding and refolding aberrant proteins back into their correct three-dimensional form (Figure 4-4). If the chaperones are unsuccessful in correcting the defect, the abnormal proteins form complexes with another protein called ubiquitin. Ubiquitin leads the abnormal proteins to a proteosome where they are digested into harmless fragments (see Figure 4-4).

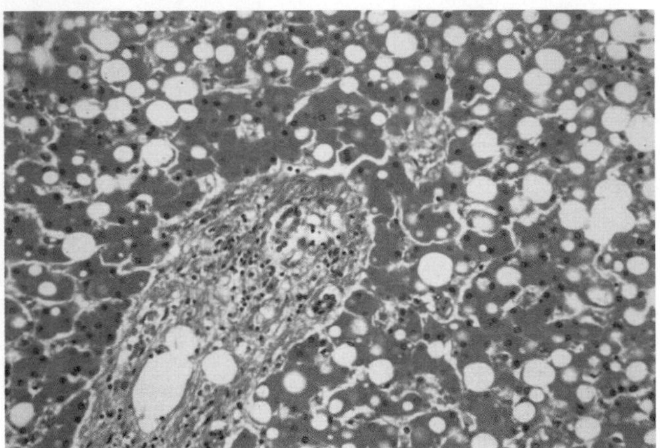

FIGURE 4-3 ■ Fatty liver showing large intracellular vacuoles of lipid. (From Kumar V, Cotran RS, Robbins SL, editors: *Basic pathology,* ed 7, Philadelphia, 2003, Saunders, p 19. Photograph courtesy Dr. James Crawford, Department of Pathology, Brigham and Women's Hospital, Boston.)

In some cases, the accumulated substances are not metabolized by normal intracellular enzymes. In diabetes, for instance, high serum glucose levels result in excessive glucose uptake by neuronal cells. Neurons possess an enzyme that converts the glucose to sorbitol.[3] The sorbitol is not metabolized by normal glycolytic enzymes and thus accumulates in the cell, where some of it is converted to fructose. Both sorbitol and fructose are osmotic particles that pull water into the cell, interfering with nerve impulse conduction and contributing to altered sensation in the person with diabetes. (Diabetes mellitus is discussed in Chapter 41.)

Finally, a variety of pigments and inorganic particles may be present in cells. Some pigment accumulations are normal, such as the accumulation of melanin in tanned skin, whereas others signify pathophysiologic processes. Pigments may be produced by the body (endogenous) or may be introduced from outside sources (exogenous). In addition to melanin, the iron-containing substances hemosiderin and bilirubin are endogenous pigments that, when present in excessive amounts, indicate disease processes. Hemosiderin and bilirubin are derived from hemoglobin. Excessive amounts may indicate abnormal breakdown of hemoglobin-containing red blood cells (RBCs), prolonged iron administration, and hepatobiliary disorders. Inorganic particles that may accumulate include calcium, tar, and mineral dusts such as coal, silica, iron, lead, and silver. Mineral dusts generally are inhaled and accumulate in lung tissue (Figure 4-5). Inhaled dusts cause chronic inflammatory reactions in the lung, which generally result in destruction of pulmonary alveoli and capillaries and the formation of scar tissue. Over many years the lung may become stiff and difficult to expand because of extensive scarring.

Deposits of calcium salts occur in conditions of altered calcium intake, excretion, and metabolism. Impaired renal excretion of phosphate may result in the formation of calcium phosphate salts that are deposited in the tissues of the eye, heart, and blood vessels. Calcification of the heart valves may cause obstruction to blood flow through the heart or interfere with valve closing. Calcification of blood vessels may result in

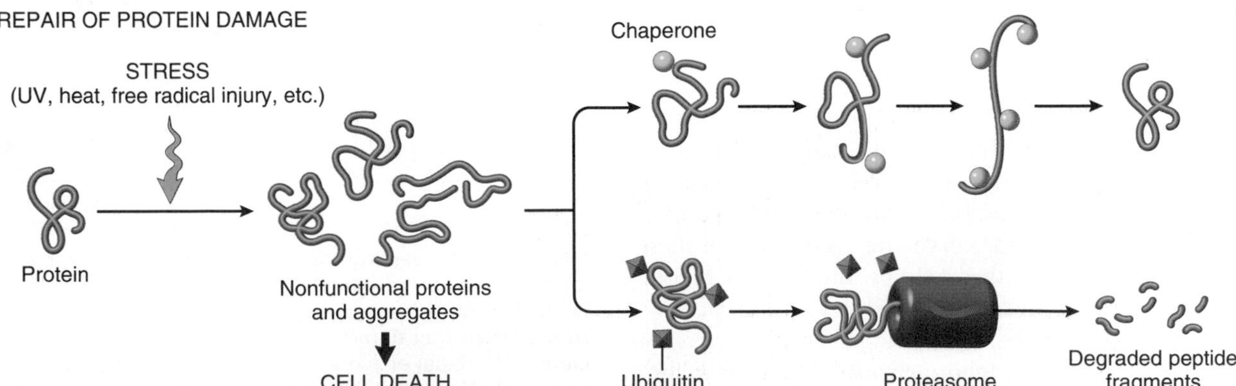

FIGURE 4-4 ■ Roles of chaperone proteins in protein refolding and ubiquitin in protein degradation after stress-induced protein damage. (From Kumar V, Cotran RS, Robbins SL, editors: *Basic pathology,* ed 7, Philadelphia, 2003, Saunders, p 17.)

narrowing of vessels and insufficient blood flow to distal tissues. Dead and dying tissues often become calcified (filled with calcium salts) and appear as dense areas on x-ray films. For example, lung damage due to tuberculosis often is apparent as calcified areas, called *tubercles.*

With the exception of inorganic particles, the intracellular accumulations generally are reversible if the causative factors are removed.

KEY CONCEPTS

- Hydropic swelling is an early indicator of cell injury. It results from Na^{+}-K^{+} pump dysfunction at the cell membrane.
- Intracellular accumulations of abnormal endogenous or exogenous particles indicate a disorder of cellular metabolism.
- Damage from accumulation of abnormal intracellular protein is limited by chaperone proteins that attempt to refold the protein into its correct shape and by the ubiquitin-proteosome system that digests targeted proteins into fragments.

CELLULAR ADAPTATION

The cellular response to persistent, sublethal stress reflects the cell's efforts to adapt. Cellular stress may be due to an increased functional demand or a reversible cellular injury. Although the term **adaptation** implies a change for the better, in some instances an adaptive change may not be beneficial. The common adaptive responses are atrophy (decreased cell size), hypertrophy (increased cell size), hyperplasia (increased cell number), metaplasia (conversion of one cell type to another), and dysplasia (disorderly growth) (Figure 4-6). Each of these changes is potentially reversible when the cellular stress is relieved.

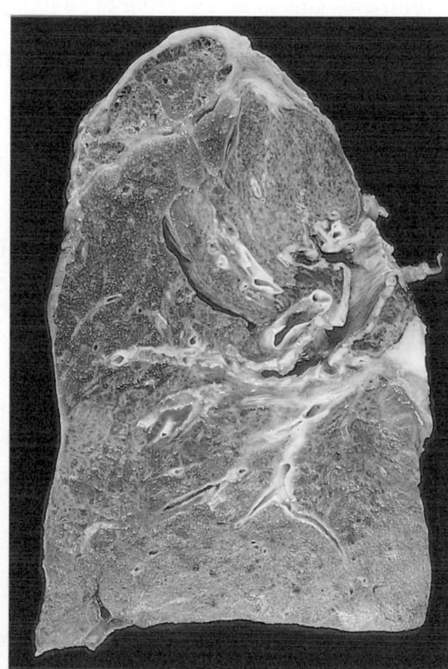

FIGURE 4-5 ■ Accumulations of silicon dust in tissues of the lung. (From Kumar V, Cotran RS, Robbins SL, editors: *Basic pathology,* ed 7, Philadelphia, 2003, Saunders, p 272. Photograph courtesy Dr. John Goldeski, Brigham and Women's Hospital, Boston.)

Atrophy

Atrophy occurs when cells shrink and reduce their differentiated functions in response to a variety of normal and injurious factors. The general causes of atrophy may be summarized as (1) disuse, (2) denervation, (3) ischemia, (4) nutrient starvation, (5) interruption of endocrine signals, (6) persistent cell injury, and (7) aging. Apparently, atrophy represents an effort by the cell to minimize its energy and nutrient consumption by decreasing intracellular organelles and other structures.

A common form of atrophy is due to a reduction in functional demand, sometimes called **disuse atrophy.** For example, immobilization by bed rest or casting of an extremity results in shrinkage of skeletal muscle cells. On resumption of activity, the tissue resumes its normal size. Denervation of skeletal muscle results in a similar decrease in muscle size due to loss of nervous stimulation. Inadequate blood supply to a tissue is known as **ischemia.** If the blood supply is totally interrupted, the cells will die, but chronic sublethal ischemia usually results in cell atrophy. The heart, brain, kidneys, and lower leg are common sites of ischemia. Atrophic changes in the lower leg due to ischemia include thin skin, muscle wasting, and loss of hair. Atrophy also is a consequence of chronic nutrient starvation, whether due to poor intake, absorption, or distribution to the tissues. Many glandular tissues throughout

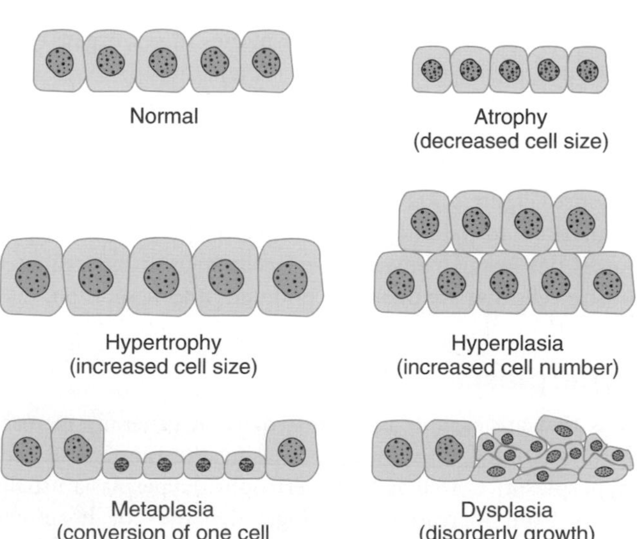

FIGURE 4-6 ■ The adaptive cellular responses of atrophy, hypertrophy, hyperplasia, metaplasia, and dysplasia.

the body depend on growth-stimulating (trophic) signals to maintain size and function. For example, the adrenal cortex, thyroid, and gonads are maintained by trophic hormones from the pituitary gland and will atrophy in their absence. Atrophy due to persistent cell injury is most commonly related to chronic inflammation and infection.

The biochemical pathways that result in cellular atrophy are imperfectly known; however, two pathways for protein degradation have been implicated. The first is the previously mentioned ubiquitin-proteosome system, which degrades targeted proteins into small fragments (see Figure 4-4). The second involves the lysosomes that may fuse with intracellular structures leading to hydrolytic degradation of the components. Certain substances apparently are resistant to degradation and remain in the lysosomal vesicles of atrophied cells. For example, lipofuscin is an age-related pigment that accumulates in residual vesicles in atrophied cells, giving them a yellow-brown appearance.

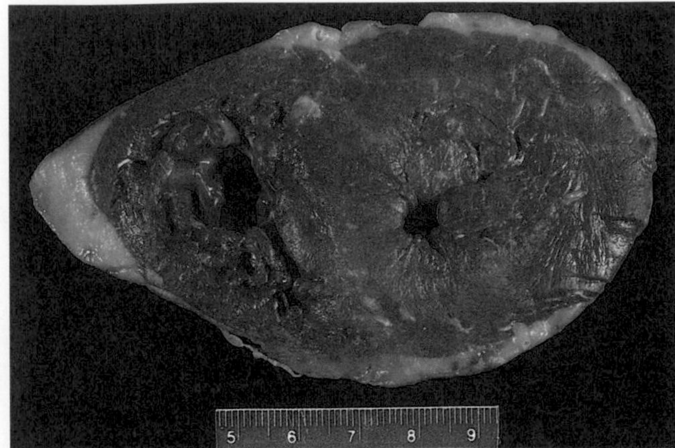

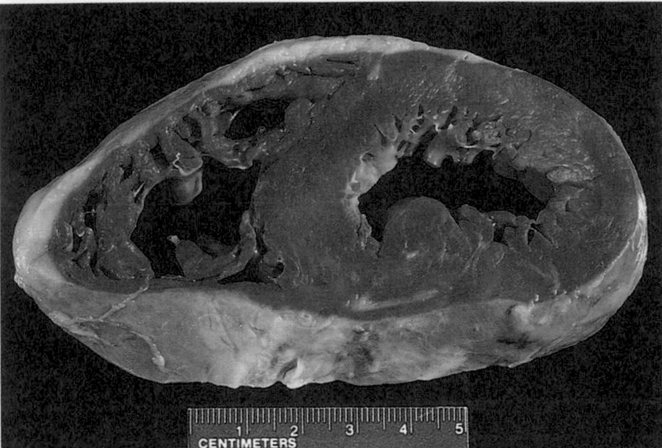

FIGURE 4-7 ■ **A,** Hypertrophy of cardiac muscle in the left ventricular chamber. **B,** Compare with the thickness of the normal left ventricle. This is an example of cellular adaptation to an increased cardiac workload. (From Kumar V, Cotran RS, Robbins SL, editors: *Basic pathology,* ed 7, Philadelphia, 2003, Saunders, p 5.)

Hypertrophy

Hypertrophy is an increase in cell mass accompanied by an augmented functional capacity. Cells hypertrophy in response to increased physiologic or pathophysiologic demands. Cellular enlargement results primarily from a net increase in cellular protein content.[4] Like the other adaptive responses, hypertrophy subsides when the increased demand is removed; however, the cell may not entirely return to normal because of persistent changes in connective tissue structures. Organ enlargement may be a result of both an increase in cell size (hypertrophy) and an increase in cell number (hyperplasia). For example, an increase in skeletal muscle mass and strength in response to repeated exercise is primarily due to hypertrophy of individual muscle cells, although some increase in cell number is also possible because muscle stem cells (satellite cells) are able to divide. Physiologic hypertrophy occurs in response to a variety of trophic hormones in sex organs—the breast and uterus, for example. Certain pathophysiologic conditions may place undue stress on some tissues, causing them to hypertrophy. Liver enlargement in response to bodily toxins and cardiac muscle enlargement in response to high blood pressure (Figure 4-7) represent hyperplastic and hypertrophic adaptations to pathologic conditions. Hypertrophic adaptation is particularly important for cells such as differentiated muscle cells that are unable to undergo mitotic division.

Hyperplasia

Cells that are capable of mitotic division generally increase their functional capacity by increasing the number of cells (**hyperplasia**) as well as by hypertrophy. Hyperplasia usually results from increased physiologic demands or hormonal stimulation. Persistent cell injury also may lead to hyperplasia. Examples of demand-induced hyperplasia include an increase in RBC number in response to high altitude and liver enlargement in response to drug detoxification. Trophic hormones induce hyperplasia in their target tissues. Estrogen, for example, leads to an increase in the number of endometrial and uterine stromal cells. Dysregulation of hormones or growth factors can result in pathologic hyperplasia such as that which occurs in thyroid or prostate enlargement.

Chronic irritation of epithelial cells often results in hyperplasia. Calluses and corns, for example, result from chronic frictional injury to the skin. The epithelium of the bladder commonly becomes hyperplastic in response to the chronic inflammation of cystitis.

Metaplasia

Metaplasia is the replacement of one differentiated cell type with another. This almost always occurs as an adaptation to persistent injury, with the replacement cell type better able to tolerate the injurious stimulation.[1] Metaplasia is fully reversible when the injurious stimulus is removed. Metaplasia often involves the replacement of glandular epithelium with squamous epithelium. Chronic irritation of the bronchial mucosa by cigarette smoke, for example, leads to the conversion of ciliated columnar epithelium to stratified squamous epithelium. Metaplastic cells generally remain well differentiated and of the same tissue type, although cancerous transformations can occur. Some cancers of the lung, cervix, stomach, and bladder appear to derive from areas of metaplastic epithelium.

Dysplasia

Dysplasia refers to the disorganized appearance of cells because of abnormal variations in size, shape, and arrangement. Dysplasia occurs most frequently in hyperplastic squamous epithelium, but it may also be seen in the mucosa of the intestine. Dysplasia probably represents an adaptive effort gone astray. Dysplastic cells have significant potential to transform into cancerous cells and are usually regarded as *pre*neoplastic lesions.[1] (See Chapter 7 for a discussion of cancer.) Dysplasia that is severe and involves the entire thickness of the epithelium is called *carcinoma in situ.* Mild forms of dysplasia may be reversible if the inciting cause is removed.[1]

KEY CONCEPTS

- Adaptive cellular responses indicate cellular stress due to altered functional demand or chronic sublethal injury.
- Hypertrophy and hyperplasia generally result from increased functional demand. Atrophy results from decreased functional demand or chronic ischemia. Metaplasia and dysplasia result from persistent injury.

IRREVERSIBLE CELL INJURY

Pathologic cellular death occurs when an injury is too severe or prolonged to allow cellular adaptation or repair. Two different processes may contribute to cell death in response to injury: necrosis and apoptosis. Necrosis usually occurs as a consequence of ischemia or toxic injury and is characterized by cell rupture, spilling of contents into the extracellular fluid, and inflammation. Apoptosis occurs in response to injury that does not directly kill the cell but triggers intracellular cascades that activate a cell suicide response. Apoptotic cells generally do not rupture and are ingested by neighboring cells with minimal disruption of the tissue and without inflammation. Apoptosis is not always a pathologic process and occurs as a necessity of development and tissue remodeling.

Necrosis

Necrotic cells demonstrate typical morphologic changes, including a shrunken (pyknotic) nucleus that is subsequently degraded (karyolysis), a swollen cell volume, dispersed ribosomes, and disrupted plasma and organelle membranes (Figure 4-8). The disruption of the permeability barrier of the plasma membrane appears to be a critical event in the death of the cell.[5] Necrotic cell death is not reversible.

Localized injury or death of tissue is generally reflected in the entire system as the body attempts to clear away dead cells and works to compensate for loss of tissue function. Several

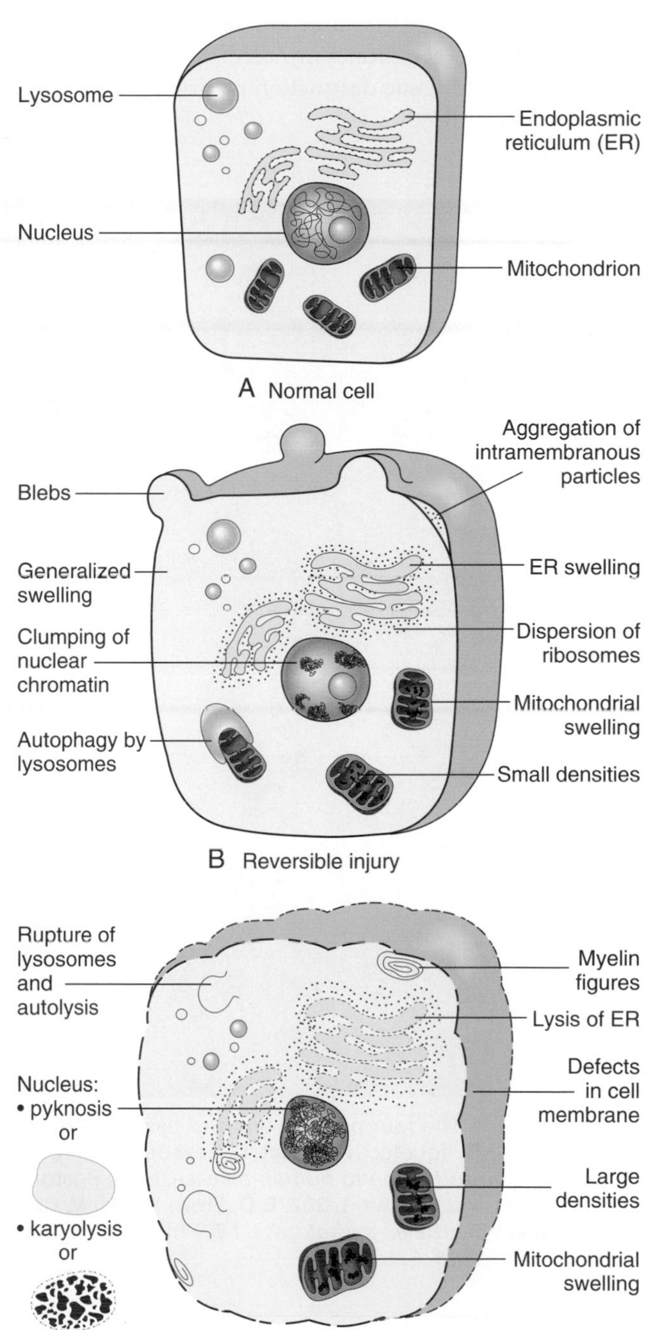

FIGURE 4-8 ■ Cellular features of cell necrosis **(C)** compared with a normal cell **(A)** and a reversibly injured cell **(B)**. (From Kumar V, Cotran RS, Robbins SL: *Basic pathology,* ed 7, Philadelphia, 2003, Saunders, p 22.)

manifestations indicate that the system is responding to cellular injury and death. A general inflammatory response is often present, with general malaise, fever, increased heart rate, increased white blood cell (WBC) count, and loss of appetite. With the death of necrotic cells, intracellular contents are released and often find their way into the blood stream. The presence of specific cellular enzymes in the blood is used as an indicator of the location and extent of cellular death. For example, an elevated serum amylase level indicates pancreatic damage, and an elevated creatine kinase (MB isoenzyme) or cardiac troponin level indicates myocardial damage. The location of pain due to tissue destruction may also aid in the diagnosis of cellular death.

Four different types of tissue necrosis have been described: coagulative, liquefactive, fat, and caseous (Figure 4-9). They differ primarily in the type of tissue affected. *Coagulative* necrosis is the most common. Manifestations of coagulative necrosis are the same, regardless of the cause of cell death. In general, the steps leading to coagulative necrosis may be summarized as follows: (1) ischemic cellular injury, leading to (2) loss of the plasma membrane's ability to maintain electrochemical gradients, which results in (3) influx of calcium ions and mitochondrial dysfunction, and (4) degradation of plasma membranes and nuclear structures (Figure 4-10). The area of coagulative necrosis is composed of denatured proteins and is relatively solid. The coagulated area is then slowly

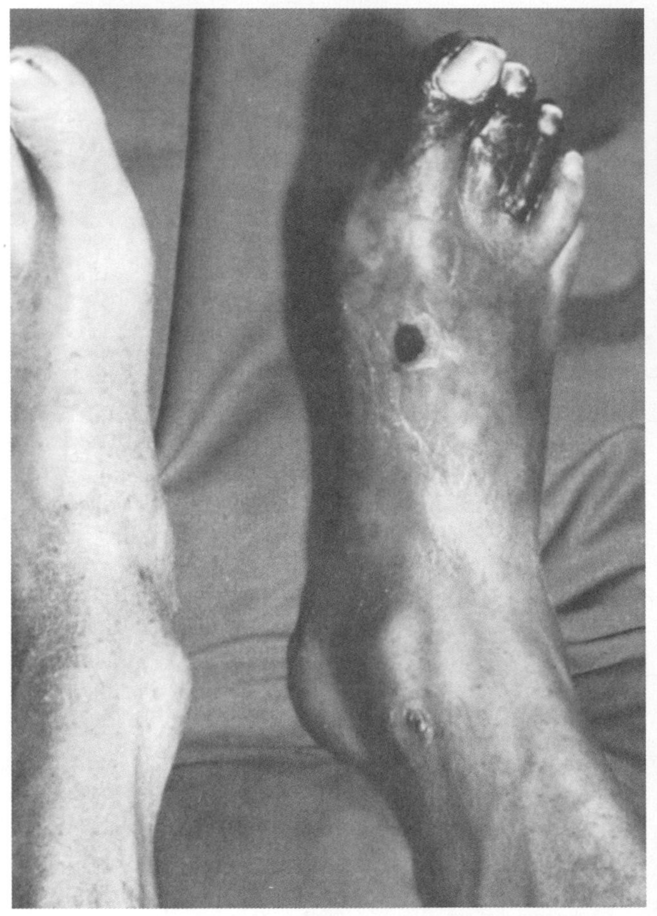
A

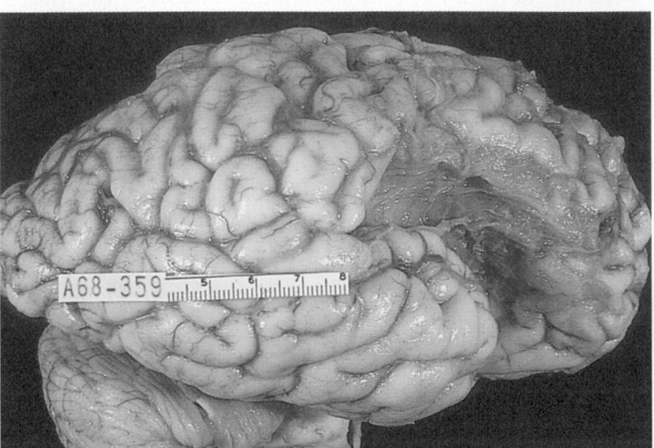

B

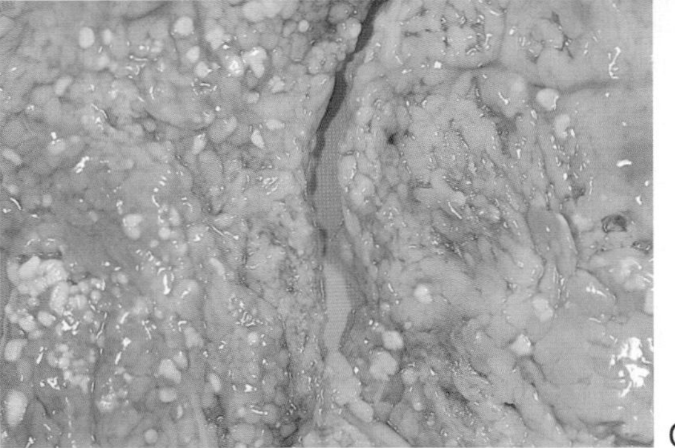
C

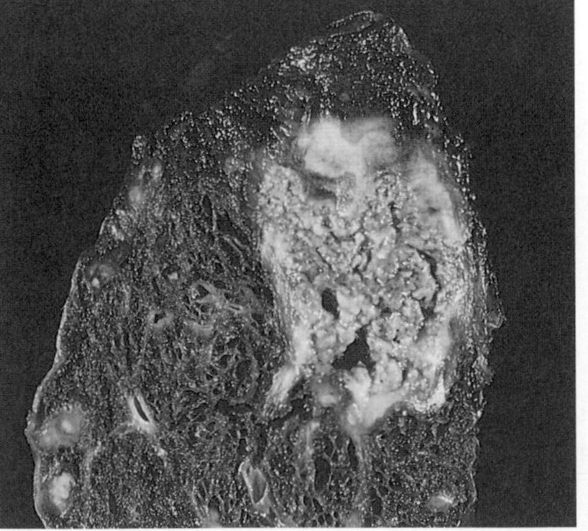
D

FIGURE 4-9 ■ The four primary types of tissue necrosis. **A,** Coagulative; **B,** liquefactive; **C,** fat; **D,** caseous. (**A,** From Crowley L: *Introduction to human disease,* ed 4, Boston, 1996, Jones and Bartlett, p 302. **B-D,** From Kumar V, Cotran RS, Robbins SL: *Basic pathology,* ed 7, Philadelphia, 2003, Saunders, pp 815, 826.)

dissolved by proteolytic enzymes and the general tissue architecture is preserved for a relatively long time (weeks). This is in contrast to liquefactive necrosis.

When the dissolution of dead cells occurs very quickly, a liquefied area of lysosomal enzymes and dissolved tissue may result and form an abscess or cyst. This type of necrosis, called *liquefactive necrosis,* may be seen in the brain, which is rich in degradative enzymes and contains little supportive connective tissue. Liquefaction may also result from a bacterial infection that triggers a localized collection of WBCs. The phagocytic WBCs contain potent degradative enzymes that may completely digest dead cells, resulting in liquid debris.

Fat necrosis refers to death of adipose tissue and usually results from trauma or pancreatitis. The process begins with the release of activated digestive enzymes from the pancreas or injured tissue. The enzymes attack the cell membranes of fat cells, causing release of their stores of triglycerides. Pancreatic lipase can then hydrolyze the triglycerides to free fatty acids, which precipitate as calcium soaps (saponification). Fat necrosis appears as a chalky white area of tissue.

Caseous necrosis is characteristic of lung tissue damaged by tuberculosis. The areas of dead lung tissue are white, soft, and fragile, resembling clumpy cheese. Dead cells are walled off from the rest of the lung tissue by inflammatory WBCs. In the center, the dead cells lose their cellular structure but are not totally degraded. Necrotic debris may persist indefinitely.

Gangrene is a term used to describe cellular death involving a large area of tissue. Gangrene usually results from interruption of the major blood supply to a particular body part, such as the toes, leg, or bowel. Depending on the appearance and subsequent infection of the necrotic tissue, it is described as dry gangrene, wet gangrene, or gas gangrene. *Dry* gangrene is a form of coagulative necrosis characterized by blackened, dry, wrinkled tissue that is separated from adjacent healthy tissue by an obvious line of demarcation (see Figure 4-9, *A*). It generally occurs only on the extremities. Liquefactive necrosis may result in *wet* gangrene, which is typically found in internal organs, appears cold and black, and may be foul smelling due to the invasion of bacteria. Rapid spread of tissue damage and the release of toxins into the blood stream make wet gangrene a life-threatening problem. *Gas* gangrene is characterized by the formation of bubbles of gas in damaged muscle tissue. Gas gangrene is due to infection of necrotic tissue by anaerobic bacteria of the genus *Clostridium.* These bacteria produce toxins and degradative enzymes that allow the infection to spread rapidly through the necrotic tissue. Gas gangrene may be fatal if not managed rapidly and aggressively.

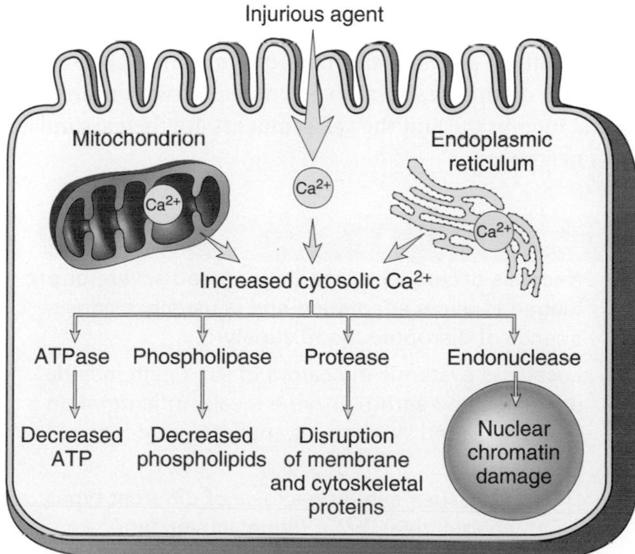

FIGURE 4-10 ■ Cellular injury as a consequence of intracellular calcium overload. (From Kumar V, Cotran RS, Robbins SL: *Basic pathology,* ed 7, Philadelphia, 2003, Saunders, p 8.)

Apoptosis

The number of cells in tissues is tightly regulated by controlling the rate of cell division and the rate of cell death. If cells are no longer needed they activate a cellular death pathway resulting in cell suicide. In contrast to necrosis, which is messy and results in inflammation and collateral tissue damage, apoptosis is tidy and doesn't elicit inflammation. Apoptosis is not a rare event; large numbers of cells are continually undergoing cell suicide as tissues remodel. During fetal development, for example, more than half of the nerve cells that form undergo apoptosis. It is estimated that more than 95% of the T lymphocytes that are generated in the bone marrow are induced to undergo apoptosis after reaching the thymus. These are normal physiologic processes that regulate normal system function. Apoptosis has also been implicated in pathologic cell death and disease. For example, it has been estimated that the area of tissue death following a myocardial infarction (heart attack) is about 20% necrotic and 80% apoptotic.[6] Death of cancer cells in response to radiation or chemotherapy is believed to be primarily caused by apoptotic mechanisms. When the rate of apoptosis is greater than the rate of cell replacement, tissue or organ function may be impaired. Apoptosis is now recognized as a primary factor in diseases such as heart failure (Chapter 19) and dementia (Chapter 45). The mechanisms regulating apoptosis are complex, and only major concepts are included here.

There are two types of environmental signals that may induce apoptosis. First, apoptosis may be triggered by withdrawal of "survival" signals that normally suppress the apoptotic pathways.[7] Normal cells require a variety of signals from neighboring cells and from the extracellular matrix in order to stay alive (Figure 4-11). If these contacts or signals are removed, the cell suicide cascade is activated. Cancer cells are notorious for their ability to survive despite the lack of appropriate survival signals from their environment (see Chapter 7). A second mechanism of triggering apoptosis involves extracellular signals that bind to the cell and actively trigger the

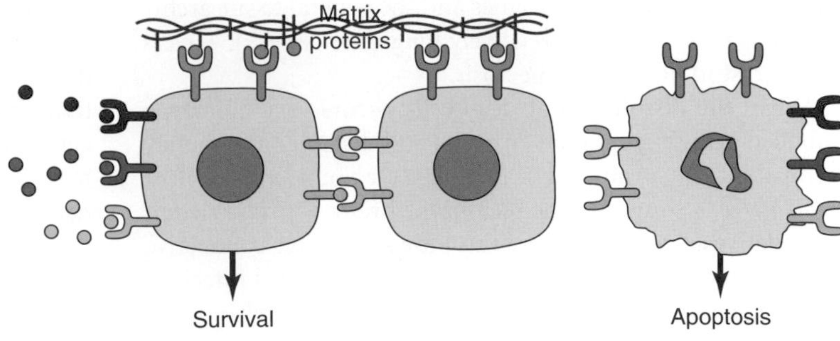

FIGURE 4-11 ■ Each cell displays a set of receptors that enable it to respond to extracellular signals that control growth, differentiation, and survival. Extracellular signals are provided by the neighboring cells, secreted signaling molecules, and the extracellular matrix. Withdrawal of these survival signals induces the cell to initiate apoptosis.

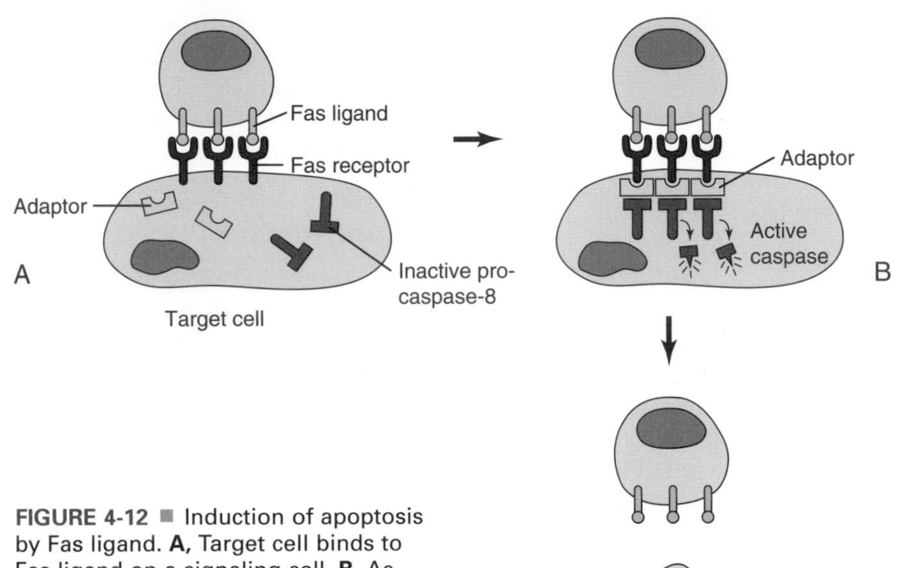

FIGURE 4-12 ■ Induction of apoptosis by Fas ligand. **A,** Target cell binds to Fas ligand on a signaling cell. **B,** Active Fas receptors organize and activate caspases. **C,** The caspases degrade the nucleus and trigger cell death.

death cascade, such as the *fas* ligand or "death receptor" (Figure 4-12). Cells also have a way to monitor their condition and usefulness internally. When excessive, irreparable damage occurs to the cell's DNA or other vital structures, growth and division stalls for a while to permit repair. If the damage is too great, the cell will trigger its own death. This apoptotic pathway is governed by a protein called p53 (TP53). The amount of p53 in a cell is normally quite low but increases in response to cellular DNA damage. If high levels of p53 are sustained, apoptosis will occur.[8] Thus p53 is important in preventing the proliferation of cells with damaged DNA. A large number of cancers are associated with a mutation in the p53 gene, which allows cancer cells to escape this monitoring system.

Regardless of the initiating event, apoptosis involves numerous intracellular signals and enzymes (Figure 4-13). A family of enzymes called caspases is the main component of the proteolytic cascade that degrades key intracellular structures leading to cell death. The caspases are proenzymes that are activated in a cascade. Activation of a few *initiator* caspases at the beginning of the cascade results in a rapid domino effect of caspase activation. Some caspases cleave key proteins such as the nuclear lamina to destroy the nuclear envelope, whereas others activate still more enzymes that chop up the DNA. All of this destruction is contained within an intact plasma membrane and the cell remnants are then assimilated by its neighbors.

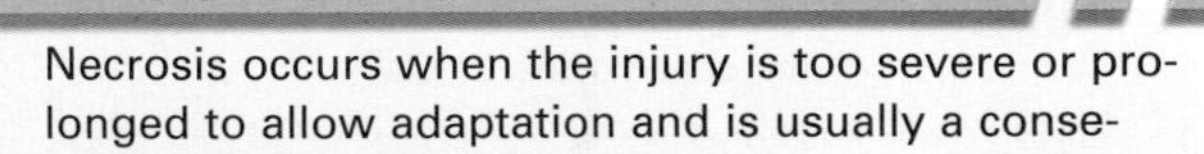

KEY CONCEPTS

- Necrosis occurs when the injury is too severe or prolonged to allow adaptation and is usually a consequence of disrupted blood supply.
- Local and systemic indicators of cell death include pain, elevated serum enzyme levels, inflammation (fever, elevated WBC count, malaise), and loss of function.
- Different tissues exhibit necrosis of different types: heart (coagulative), brain (liquefactive), lung (caseous), and pancreas (fat).
- Gangrene refers to a large area of necrosis, which may be described as dry, wet, or gas gangrene. Gas gangrene and wet gangrene may be rapidly fatal.

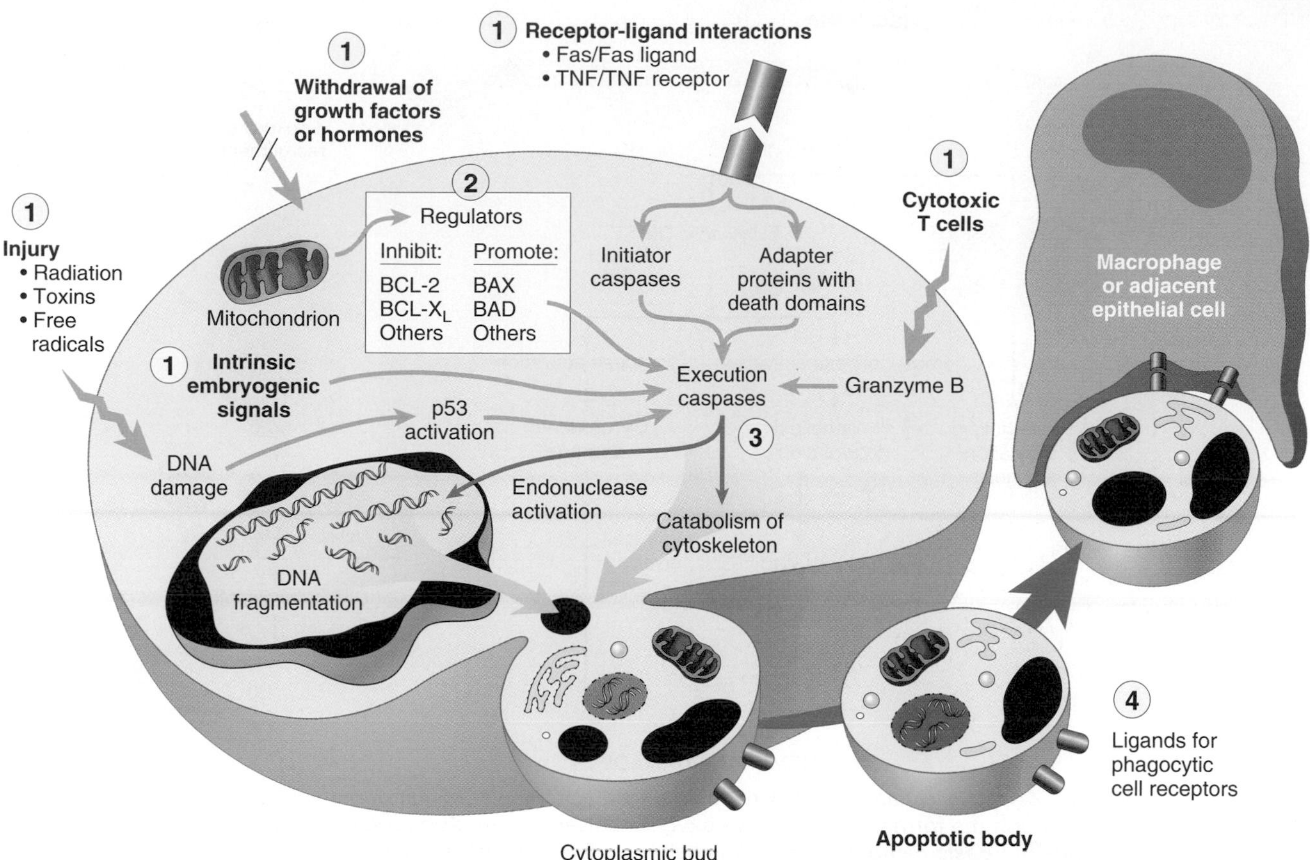

FIGURE 4-13 ■ Schematic of the events of apoptosis. *(1)* Numerous triggers can initiate apoptosis including withdrawal of survival factors, various cell injuries, binding to Fas ligand, interaction with cytotoxic cells or intrinsic signals. *(2)* Regulatory proteins may inhibit or promote the activation of caspases. *(3)* Caspase activation begins the process of cellular degradation. *(4)* Apoptotic cell fragments are internalized by phagocytic cells. (From Kumar V, Cotran RS, Robbins SL: *Basic pathology,* ed 7, Philadelphia, 2003, Saunders, p 29.)

◆ Apoptosis is cell death resulting from activation of intracellular signaling cascades that cause cell suicide. Apoptosis is tidy and not usually associated with systemic manifestations of inflammation.

ETIOLOGY OF CELLULAR INJURY

Cellular injury and death result from a variety of cellular assaults, including lack of oxygen and nutrients, infection and immune responses, chemicals, and physical and mechanical factors. The extent of cell injury and death depends in part on the duration and severity of the assault and in part on the prior condition of the cells. Well-nourished and somewhat adapted cells may withstand the injury better than cells that are poorly nourished or unadapted. Common causes of cellular injury include hypoxic injury, nutritional injury, infectious and immunologic injury, chemical injury, and physical and mechanical injury.

Ischemia and Hypoxic Injury

Living cells must receive a continuous supply of oxygen to produce ATP to power energy-requiring functions. Lack of oxygen (**hypoxia**) results in power failure within the cell. Tissue hypoxia is most often due to *ischemia,* or the interruption of blood flow to an area, but it may also result from heart disease, lung disease, and RBC disorders. Ischemia is the most common cause of cell injury in clinical medicine and injures cells faster than hypoxia alone. Faster injury occurs because ischemia not only disrupts the oxygen supply, but also allows metabolic wastes to accumulate and deprives the cell of nutrients for glycolysis. The cellular events that follow oxygen deprivation are shown in Figure 4-14. Decreased oxygen delivery to the mitochondria causes ATP production in the cell to stall and ATP-dependent pumps, including the Na^+-K^+ and Ca^{2+} pumps, to fail. Sodium accumulation within the cell creates an osmotic gradient favoring water entry, resulting in hydropic swelling. Excess intracellular calcium collects in the mitochondria,

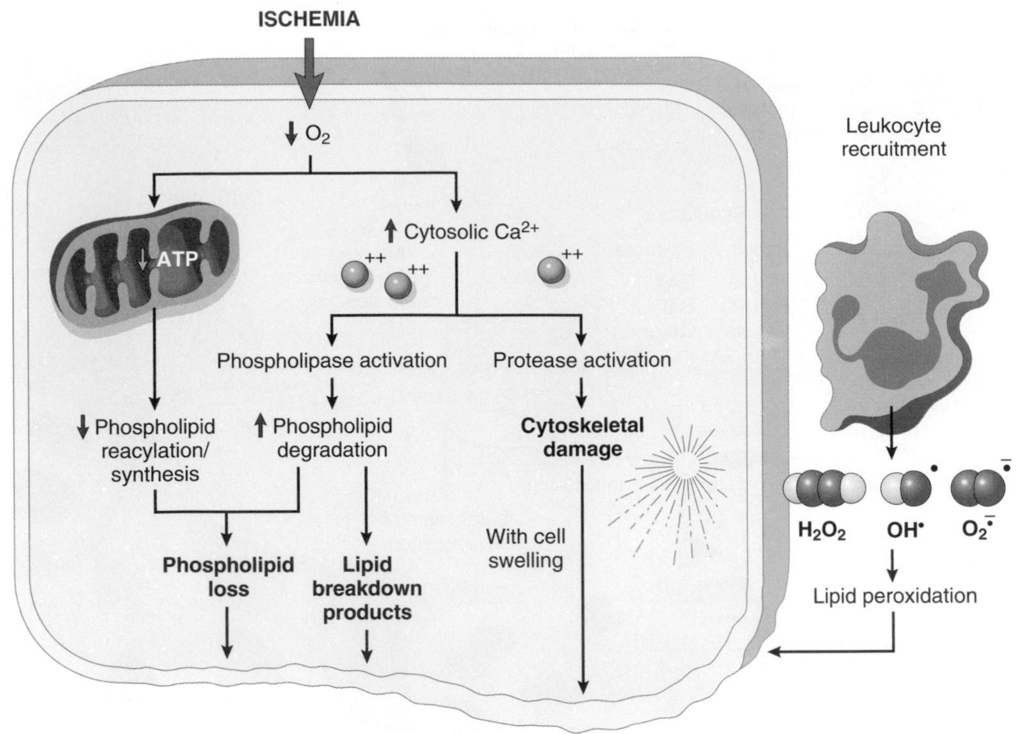

FIGURE 4-14 ■ Mechanisms of ischemia-induced cell injury. Cellular damage often occurs through the formation of reactive oxygen radicals. (From Kumar V, Cotran RS, Robbins SL: *Basic pathology,* ed 7, Philadelphia, 2003, Saunders, p 23.)

further interfering with mitochondrial function. A small amount of ATP is produced by anaerobic glycolytic pathways, which break down cellular stores of glycogen. The pyruvate end products of glycolysis accumulate and are converted to lactate, causing cellular acidification. Lactate can escape into the blood stream resulting in **lactic acidosis,** which can be detected by laboratory tests. Cellular proteins and enzymes become progressively more dysfunctional as the pH falls. Up to a point, ischemic injury is reversible, but when the plasma and mitochondrial membranes are critically damaged cell death ensues.

Cell death due to oxygen deprivation is slow to develop, generally taking many minutes to hours. In fact, most cellular damage occurs after the blood supply to the tissues has been restored—a so-called *reperfusion injury.* Ischemia-reperfusion is a complex phenomenon, but three critical components have been identified: (1) calcium overload, (2) formation of reactive oxygen molecules, and (3) subsequent inflammation.

Restoration of blood flow to ischemic cells bathes them in a fluid high in calcium ions at a time when their ATP stores are depleted and they are unable to control ion flux across the cell membrane. Accumulation of calcium ions in the cytoplasm can trigger apoptosis or activate enzymes that degrade lipids in the membrane (lipid peroxidation).

The ischemic episode also primes cells for abnormal generation of reactive oxygen molecules such as, superoxide (O_2^-), peroxide (H_2O_2), and hydroxyl radicals (OH^-).[9] These reactive oxygen species are free radicals that have an unpaired electron in an outer orbital. They steal hydrogen atoms and form abnormal molecular bonds. Molecules that react with free radicals are in turn converted to free radicals, continuing the destructive cascade. Reactive oxygen species damage cell membranes, denature proteins, and disrupt cell chromosomes. Oxygen free radicals also have been linked to initiation of the inflammatory cascade (see Figure 4-14).

Ischemia primes cells for generation of oxygen radicals by allowing the buildup of ATP precursors such as adenosine diphosphate (ADP) and pyruvate during the period of hypoxia. When oxygen supply is reestablished, there is a disorganized burst of high-energy electrons that partially reduce oxygen, forming oxygen radicals. The ischemia-reperfusion event frequently is followed by a generalized inflammatory state,[10] which may lead to ongoing cellular and organ damage for days and weeks following the initial event. White blood cells recruited to the area stick and release enzymes and other chemicals that further damage the cells in the area. (Mechanisms and causes of ischemic tissue injury are described further in Chapter 20.)

Nutritional Injury

Adequate amounts of fats, carbohydrates, proteins, vitamins, and minerals are essential for normal cellular function. Most of these essential nutrients must be obtained from external sources because the cell is unable to manufacture them. The cell is unable to synthesize many of the 20 amino acids needed to form the proteins of the body. Likewise, most vitamins and minerals must be obtained from exogenous sources. Cell injury results from deficiencies as well as excesses of essential nutrients.

Certain cell types are more susceptible to injury from particular nutritional imbalances. Iron deficiency, for example, primarily affects RBCs, whereas vitamin D deficiency affects bones. All cell types must receive glucose for energy, and fatty acid and amino acid building blocks to synthesize and repair cellular components. Nutritional deficiencies result from poor intake, altered absorption, impaired distribution by the circulatory system, or inefficient cellular uptake. Common causes of malnutrition include (1) poverty, (2) chronic alcoholism, (3) acute severe illness, (4) self-imposed dietary restrictions, and (5) malabsorption syndromes.[11] Vitamin deficiencies are common even in industrialized countries because of pervasive use of processed foods. Some examples of vitamin deficiency disorders are shown in Table 4-1. Deficiencies of minerals, especially iron, also are common (Table 4-2).

Nutritional excesses primarily result from excessive intake, although deficient cellular uptake by one cell type may contribute to excess nutrient delivery to other cell types. For example, in the condition of diabetes mellitus, some cell types have deficient receptors for insulin-dependent glucose uptake, which causes excessive amounts of glucose to remain in the blood stream. As a result, cells that do not require insulin to take in glucose, such as neurons, may have abnormally high intracellular glucose levels. An excess of caloric intake above metabolic use produces overweight and obesity syndromes. Excess body fat can be estimated by measuring the ratio of body weight (in kilograms) to height (in meters squared) to derive the body mass index (BMI). A BMI greater than 27 kg/m^2 imparts a heath risk and a BMI greater than 30 kg/m^2 is considered to be obesity.[12] Numerous health problems are associated with excess body fat including heart and blood vessel disease, musculoskeletal strain, diabetes, hypertension, and gallbladder disease.

Infectious and Immunologic Injury

Bacteria and viruses are common infectious agents that may injure cells in a variety of ways. The virulence of a particular biological agent depends on its ability to gain access to the cell and its success in altering cellular functions. (See Chapter 8 for a detailed discussion of infectious processes.) Some of the injurious effects are directly due to the biological agent, but added injury may be done indirectly by triggering the body's immune response.

Most bacteria do not gain entry into the cell and so accomplish their injurious effects from the outside. (Notable exceptions include *Mycobacterium tuberculosis, Shigella, Legionella, Salmonella,* and *Chlamydia.*) Some bacteria produce and secrete powerful destructive enzymes that digest cellular membranes and connective tissues. For example, collagenase and lecithinase are produced by *Clostridium perfringens.* Other bacteria produce **exotoxins,** which interfere with specific cellular functions when released from the bacterium. *Clostridium botulinum* and *Clostridium tetani,* for example, produce life-threatening toxins that disrupt normal neuromuscular transmission. Cholera and diphtheria are well-known examples of exotoxin-related diseases. Exotoxins are primarily proteins and are generally susceptible to destruction by extremes of heat. Certain gram-negative bacteria (e.g., *Escherichia coli, Klebsiella pneumoniae*) contain another type of toxin, **endotoxin,** in their cell wall. On lysis of the bacteria, the endotoxin is released, causing fever, malaise, and even circulatory shock.[13]

The indirect cellular injury due to the bacteria-evoked immune response may be more damaging than the direct effects of the infectious agent. White blood cells secrete many enzymes and chemicals meant to destroy the invading organism, including histamines, kinins, complement, proteases, lymphokines, and prostaglandins. Normal body cells may be exposed to these injurious chemicals because they are too close to the site of immunologic battle. Immune cells are particularly adept at producing free radicals, which can attack host cell membranes and induce significant cell injury.

Viruses are small bits of genetic material that are able to gain entry into the cell. They may be thought of as intracellular parasites that use the host cell's metabolic and synthetic machinery to survive and replicate. Viral infections tend to follow two distinct pathways. In some cases the virus remains in the cell for a considerable time without inflicting lethal injury. In other cases the virus causes rapid lysis and destruction of the host cell. The mechanisms that determine which course the virus will take are poorly understood.

The polio virus is an example of a virus that is directly cytopathic: it kills the host cell directly without immune system participation.[14] The polio virus is made up of RNA, which the cell recognizes as any other messenger RNA molecule and translates into viral proteins. Some of the virally coded proteins insert into the plasma membrane of the cell, forming pores or channels that allow ions to diffuse across. The cell dies as the vital ion gradients are dissipated.

Other viruses remain in the cell for long periods, unobtrusively making and releasing viral copies of themselves without causing lethal cell injury. The virally infected cells may not escape death, however, because they express cell surface proteins that are foreign to the host's immune system. The hepatitis B virus is an example of such an indirectly cytopathic virus that causes immune-mediated cell death. The hepatitis B virus consists of double-stranded DNA that gets incorporated into the host cell's nucleus, where it can be transcribed by the normal DNA polymerases. The mRNA transcripts of the viral genes are transported to the cytoplasm and translated into structural proteins and enzymes, which are used to make more copies of the virus. Such virally infected cells may remain functional virus factories until they are destroyed by the host's immune system.

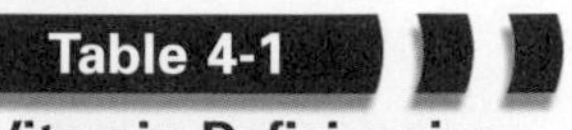

Vitamin Deficiencies

Function	Basis of Deficiency	Changes in Deficiency	Toxicity
Vitamin E (Fat Soluble)			
Encompasses eight tocopherols and tocotrienols, α-tocopherol most active Antioxidants and free radical scavengers Acts along with selenium in maintenance of cell (neuronal) membranes	Abundant in vegetables, grains, and nuts Primary deficiency rare Secondary deficiency In premature infants With a fat malabsorption With abetalipoproteinemia	Increased RBC fragility and hemolytic anemia Peripheral neuropathy Degeneration of spinal cord posterior columns and spinocerebellar tracts May favor oxidation of LDL and development of atherosclerosis and cardiovascular disease	Depresses vitamin K procoagulant levels
Vitamin K (Fat Soluble)			
Required cofactor for liver carboxylation of glutamic acid residues in many proteins (e.g., clotting factors VII, IX, and X; prothrombin; and anticoagulant proteins C and S) Required cofactor for osteocalcin (in bone matrix) and for renal epithelium	Derived from endogenous bacteria and green vegetables Deficiency uncommon except In breast-fed newborns (lacking endogenous flora) With fat malabsorption With broad-spectrum antibiotics With large doses of vitamin E or anticoagulants	Bleeding diathesis (e.g., hemorrhagic disease of newborn)	In infants: hemolytic anemia
Vitamin B_1—Thiamine (Water Soluble)			
Becomes phosphorylated to form thiamine pyrophosphate, involved in many α-ketoacid decarboxylation and transketolation reactions such as in synthesis of ATP May also have role in neuronal conduction	Widely available except in refined foods (e.g., polished rice, white flour) Deficiency syndrome With diets largely of polished rice In chronic alcoholism With renal dialysis	Classic deficiency syndrome is beriberi "Wet" beriberi with cardiac failure and edema "Dry" beriberi with peripheral neuropathy Focal hemorrhages into mammillary bodies, periventricular thalamus (Wernicke-Korsakoff syndrome) Various combinations of above	Rare Fleeting lethargy, ataxia
Vitamin B_2—Riboflavin (Water Soluble)			
Component of coenzymes flavin mononucleotide and flavin adenine dinucleotide in various redox reactions	Widely available in meat, dairy products, and vegetables Deficiency syndrome In economically deprived Frequently in conjunction with lack of other B vitamins Rare as secondary deficiency in alcoholic patients, and in debilitated (e.g., cancer) patients	Ariboflavinosis characterized by: Cheilosis—fissures at angles of mouth Glossitis—tongue atrophy Eye changes—interstitial keratosis Dermatitis—nasolabial folds Sometimes anemia	Unreported in humans

From Kumar V, Cotran RS, Robbins ST: *Robbins basic pathology,* ed 7, Philadelphia, 2003, Saunders, pp 301-302.
LDL, Low-density lipoprotein; *RBC,* red blood cell.

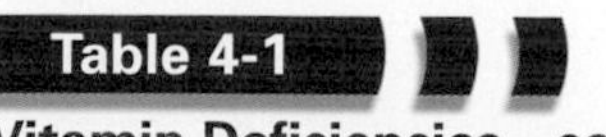

Vitamin Deficiencies—cont'd

Function	Basis of Deficiency	Changes in Deficiency	Toxicity
Niacin—Vitamin B_3 (Water Soluble)			
Generic term nicotinic acid and nicotinamide Latter component of nicotinamide adenine dinucleotide (NAD) and its phosphate (NADP) Widely involved as electron acceptors and hydrogenases	Widely available in grains, beans, and seed oils Can be endogenously synthesized from tryptophan Deficiency can occur from lack of B_3 or lack of tryptophan Deficiency seen usually: In chronic alcoholism In chronic illnesses With diets largely of corn (maize), in which niacin is tightly bound Deficiency also seen in carcinoid syndrome where tryptophan is diverted to synthesis of serotonin and other products Prolonged use of antituberculosis drug isoniazid	Deficiency state is known as *pellagra* (three D's): Diarrhea Dementia owing to loss of neurons in brain Dermatitis symmetric on exposed skin	Formerly seen with pharmacological doses as hypolipidemic agent Flushing, hyperglycemia, and possible liver damage
Vitamin B_6 (Water Soluble)			
Three substances—pyridoxine, pyridoxal, and pyridoxamine—together with phosphates are called pyridoxine Phosphate forms serve as coenzymes in metabolism of lipids and amino acids (e.g., synthesis of niacin from tryptophan)	Deficiency rare in primary form because B_6 is present in all natural foods, but destroyed in processing Bottle-fed babies at risk Deficiency usually in combination with other vitamin B deficiencies, and in chronic alcoholism because acetaldehyde enhances degradation	Usually combined with lack of other B vitamins Changes are indistinguishable from those related to other B deficiencies (e.g., angular cheilitis, stomatitis, glossitis)	Peripheral neuropathies with chronic use of large doses

Chemical Injury

Toxic chemicals or poisons are plentiful in the environment (Table 4-3 and Table 4-4). Some toxic chemicals cause cellular injury directly, whereas others become injurious only when metabolized into reactive chemicals by the body. Carbon tetrachloride (CCl_4) is an example of the latter.[15] Carbon tetrachloride, a formerly used dry-cleaning agent, is converted to a highly toxic **free radical,** $CCl_3^{\cdot}$, by liver cells. The free radical is very reactive, forming abnormal chemical bonds in the cell and ultimately destroying the cellular membranes of liver cells, causing liver failure. In high doses, acetaminophen, a commonly used analgesic, may have similar toxic effects on the liver.

Many toxins are inherently reactive and do not require metabolic activation to exert their effects. Common examples are heavy metals (e.g., lead and mercury), toxic gases, corrosives, and antimetabolites. Some toxins have an affinity for a particular cell type or tissue, whereas others exert widespread systemic effects. For example, carbon monoxide binds tightly and selectively to hemoglobin, preventing the red cell from carrying sufficient oxygen. Lead poisoning, however, has widespread effects, including effects on nervous tissue, blood cells, and the kidney. Extremely acidic or basic chemicals are directly corrosive to cellular structures. Certain chemicals interfere with normal metabolic processes of the cell. Some of these antimetabolites have been put to use in the form of cytotoxic agents for the management of cancer (see Chapter 7).

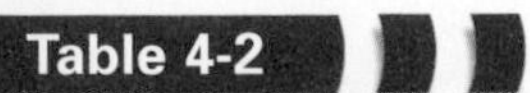

Selected Trace Elements and Deficiency Syndromes

Element	Function	Basis of Deficiency	Clinical Features
Zinc	Component of enzymes, principally oxidases	Inadequate supplementation in artificial diets Interference with absorption by other dietary constituents Inborn error of metabolism	Rash around eyes, mouth, nose, and anus called acrodermatitis enteropathica Anorexia and diarrhea Growth retardation in children Depressed mental function Depressed wound healing and immune response Impaired night vision Infertility
Iron	Essential component of hemoglobin as well as a number of iron-containing metalloenzymes	Inadequate diet Chronic blood loss	Hypochromic microcytic anemia
Iodine	Component of thyroid hormone	Inadequate supply in food and water	Goiter and hypothyroidism
Copper	Component of cytochrome *c* oxidase, dopamine β-hydroxylase, tyrosinase, lysyl oxidase, and unknown enzyme involved in cross-linking collagen	Inadequate supplementation in artificial diet Interference with absorption	Muscle weakness Neurologic defects Abnormal collagen cross-linking
Fluoride	Mechanism unknown	Inadequate supply in soil and water Inadequate supplementation	Dental caries
Selenium	Component of glutathione peroxidase Antioxidant with vitamin E	Inadequate amounts in soil and water	Myopathy Cardiomyopathy (Keshan disease)

From Kumar V, Cotran RS, Robbins ST: *Robbins basic pathology,* ed 7, Philadelphia, 2003, Saunders, p 303.

Table 4-3

Major Outdoor Air Pollutants

Pollutant	Origin(s)	Consequences
Ozone (O_3)	Interactions of oxygen with various pollutants such as oxide of nitrogen, sulfur, and hydrocarbons	Is highly reactive and oxidizes polyunsaturated lipids that become irritants and induce release of inflammatory mediators affecting all airways down to bronchoalveolar junctions
Nitrogen dioxide	Combustion of fossil fuels such as coal, gasoline, and wood	Dissolves in secretions in airways to form nitric and nitrous acids, which irritate and damage linings of airways
Sulfur dioxide	Combustion of fossil fuels such as coal, gasoline, and wood	Yields sulfuric acid, bisulfites, and sulfites, which irritate and damage linings of airways; together with nitric acid, contributes to acid rain
Carbon monoxide	Incomplete combustion of gasoline, oil, wood, and natural gas	Combines with hemoglobin to displace oxyhemoglobin and thus induce systemic asphyxia
Particulates	Great variety of finely divided (and therefore airborne) pollutants ranging from relatively innocuous plaster dust to highly dangerous asbestos dust (see discussion of pneumoconiosis in Chapter 23) May include lead, ash, hydrocarbon residues (some may be carcinogenic), and other industrial and nuclear wastes	Major contributor to smog and a major cause of respiratory disease (see discussion of pneumoconiosis in Chapter 23)

From Kumar V, Cotran RS, Robbins ST: *Robbins basic pathology,* ed 7, Philadelphia, 2003, Saunders, p 266.

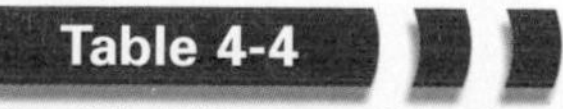

Health Effects of Indoor Air Pollutants

Pollutant	Population at Risk	Effects
Carbon monoxide	Adults and children	Acute poisoning
Nitrogen dioxide	Children	Increased respiratory infections
Wood smoke	Children	Increased respiratory infections
Formaldehyde	Adults and children	Eye and nose irritation, asthma
Radon	Adults and children	Lung cancer
Asbestos filters	Maintenance and abatement workers	Lung cancer; mesothelioma
Manufactured mineral fibers	Maintenance and construction workers	Skin and airway irritation
Bioaerosols	Adults and children	Allergic rhinitis, asthma

From Kumar V, Cotran RS, Robbins ST: *Robbins basic pathology,* ed 7, Philadelphia, 2003, Saunders, p 267.

Physical and Mechanical Injury

Injurious physical and mechanical factors include extremes of temperature, abrupt changes of atmospheric pressure, mechanical deformation, electricity, and electromagnetic radiation.[11]

Extremes of cold result in the hypothermic injury known as frostbite. Before actual cellular freezing, severe vasoconstriction and increased blood viscosity may result in ischemic injury. With continued exposure to cold, a vasodilatory response may occur, leading to intense swelling and peripheral nerve damage. The cytoplasmic solution may freeze, resulting in the formation of intracellular ice crystals and rupture of cellular components. Frostbite generally affects the extremities, ears, and nose and is often complicated by gangrenous necrosis.

Extremes of heat result in hyperthermic injury or burns. High temperatures cause microvascular coagulation and may speed up metabolic processes in the cell. Burns result from direct tissue destruction by high temperatures and are classified according to the degree of tissue destruction. Burns are discussed in Chapter 54.

Abrupt changes in atmospheric pressure may result from high-altitude flying, deep sea diving, and explosions. Pressure changes may interfere with gas exchange in the lungs, cause the formation of gas emboli in the blood stream, collapse the thorax, and rupture internal organs. A well-known example of pressure injury is the condition of "the bends," which afflicts deep-sea divers who surface too quickly. The rapid decrease in water pressure results in the formation of bubbles of nitrogen gas in the blood, which may block the circulation and cause ischemic injury.

Destruction of cells and tissues due to mechanical deformation ranges from mild abrasion to severe lacerating trauma. Cell death may result from direct trauma to cell membranes, resulting blood loss, or obstruction of blood flow and hypoxia. Nonpenetrating trauma generally results from physical impact with a blunt object such as a fist, a car steering wheel, or the pavement. Common causes of penetrating trauma are knives and guns. Trauma-induced inflammatory swelling may further compromise injured tissues.

Electrical injury may occur when the cells of the body act as conductors of electricity. The electrical current damages tissues in two ways: (1) by disrupting neural and cardiac impulses, and (2) by hyperthermic destruction of tissues. Resistance to the flow of electrons results in heat production, which damages the tissues. The current tends to follow the path of least resistance—through neurons and body fluids—causing violent muscle contractions, thermal injury, and coagulation in blood vessels. In general, greater electrical injury is suffered with high-voltage alternating current applied to a low-resistance area (wet skin).

There are many forms of electromagnetic radiation, ranging from low-energy radio waves to high-energy γ rays or photons (Figure 4-15). Radiation is capable of injuring cells by three general mechanisms: (1) direct breakage of chemical bonds, (2) ionization, and (3) heat production.[11] Cellular DNA is particularly susceptible to damage from radiation exposure.[16] A direct hit of the radiant energy on the DNA molecule may result in breakage of the chemical bonds holding the linear DNA together. This type of direct bond breakage generally results from the high-energy forms of radiation, such as x and γ rays. The molecular bonds of DNA may also be indirectly disrupted by ionizing radiation. *Ionization* refers to the ability of the radiant energy to split water molecules by knocking off orbital electrons (**radiolysis**). Radiolysis creates activated oxygen molecules that behave as free radicals, stealing electrons from other molecules and disrupting chemical bonds. Many forms of radiation are capable of ionization, but the medium-energy α and β particles that result from decay of atomic nuclei are especially destructive. Low-energy electromagnetic radiation, such as that from microwaves, ultrasound, computers, and infrared light, cannot break chemical bonds, but it can cause rotation and vibration of atoms and molecules.[17] The rotational and vibrational energy is then converted to heat. It is probable that the resulting localized hyperthermia may result in cellular injury. Some studies have documented a higher incidence of certain cancers in persons occupationally exposed to radiofrequency microwave electromagnetic radiation whereas others have found no relationship.[11]

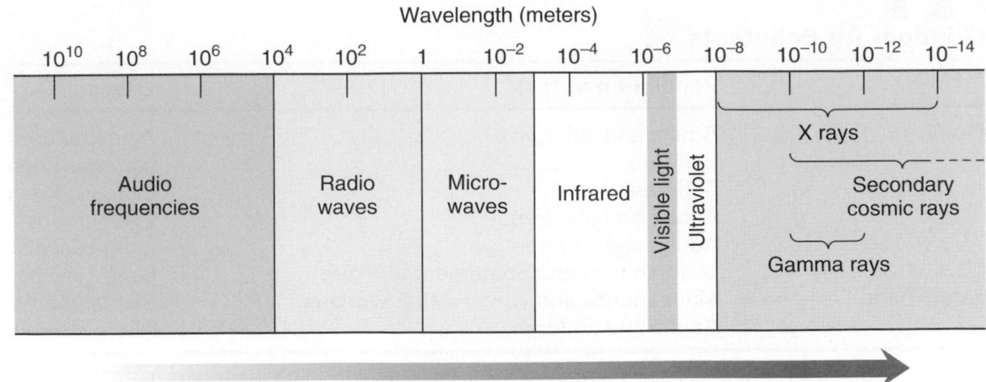

FIGURE 4-15 ■ Types of electromagnetic radiation.

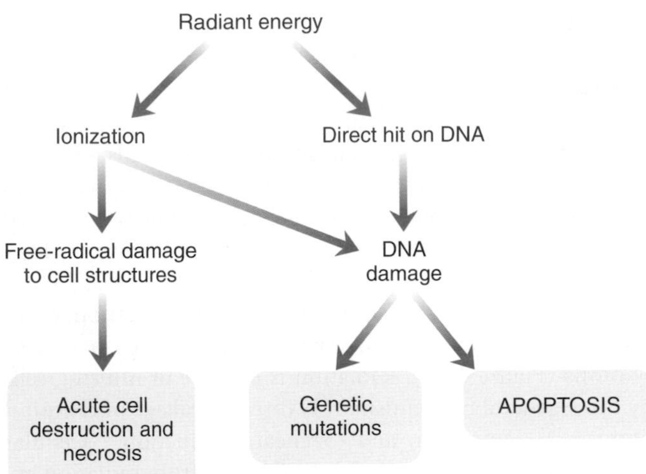

FIGURE 4-16 ■ The mechanism of radiation-induced genetic and cell injury.

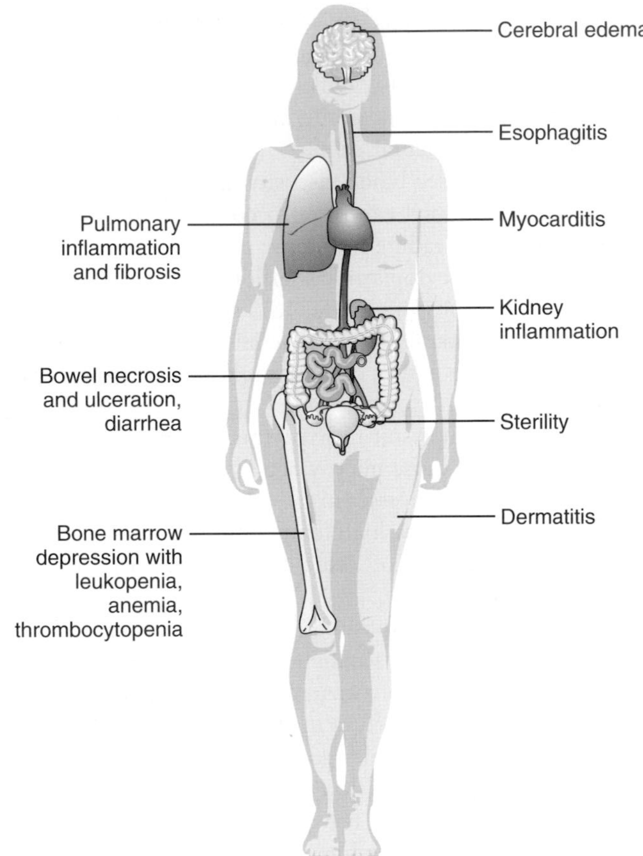

FIGURE 4-17 ■ Signs and symptoms of acute radiation sickness.

At the cellular level, radiation has two primary effects: (1) genetic damage and (2) acute cell destruction (Figure 4-16). The vulnerability of a tissue to radiation-induced genetic damage depends on its rate of proliferation. Genetic damage to the DNA of a long-lived, nonproliferating cell may be of little consequence, whereas tissues with rapid cellular division have less opportunity to repair damaged DNA before passing it on to the next generation of cells. (Genetic mutation is discussed in Chapter 6.) Hematopoietic, mucosal, gonadal, and fetal cells are particularly susceptible to genetic radiation damage.

Radiation-induced cell death is attributed primarily to the radiolysis of water, with resulting free radical damage to the plasma membrane. Whole-body exposure to sufficiently high levels of radiation (300 rad) results in acute radiation sickness with hematopoietic failure, destruction of the epithelial layer of the gastrointestinal tract, and neurologic dysfunction. The high levels of irradiation that cause acute radiation sickness are associated with events such as nuclear accidents and bombings. Radiation exposure from diagnostic x rays, cosmic rays, and natural radiant chemicals in the earth are far below the level that would result in acute radiation sickness. The signs and symptoms of acute radiation sickness are shown in Figure 4-17. The fact that radiation induces cell death in proliferating cells is used to advantage in the management of some forms of cancer. Radiation therapy may be used when a cancerous growth is confined to a particular area. Injury associated with radiation therapy is generally localized to the irradiated area. Small arteries and arterioles in the area may be damaged, leading to blood clotting and fibrous deposits that compromise tissue perfusion. Most irradiated cells are thought to die through the process of apoptosis rather than from direct killing effects of radiation.[18] Radiation induces cell damage that triggers the apoptotic pathway in cells that cannot efficiently repair the damage. Cells most susceptible to apoptotic death are those that tend to have high rates of division.

KEY CONCEPTS

- Hypoxia is an important cause of cell injury that usually results from poor oxygenation of the blood (hypoxemia) or inadequate delivery of blood to the cells (ischemia).
- Reperfusion injury to cells may occur when circulation is restored, owing to the production of partially reduced oxygen molecules that damage cell membranes and trigger immune-mediated injury.
- Nutritional injury is a common cause of dysfunction and disease. Malnutrition is rampant in many poor countries, whereas industrialized nations are facing an epidemic of obesity-related disorders, including heart disease and diabetes.
- Cellular damage due to infection and immunologic responses is common. Some bacteria and viruses damage cells directly, others stimulate the host's immune system to destroy the host's cells.
- Chemical, physical, and mechanical factors cause cell injury in various ways. Chemicals may interfere with normal metabolic processes in the cell. Injury due to physical factors, such as burns and frostbite, causes direct destruction of tissues. Radiation-induced cell death is primarily a result of radiolysis of water, with resulting free radical damage to the cell membrane.

CELLULAR AGING

The inevitable process of aging and death has been the subject of interest and investigation for centuries. Despite scientific study and the search for the fountain of youth, a satisfactory explanation for the process of cellular aging and methods for halting the aging process have not been revealed. The maximal human life span has remained constant at about 90 to 110 years, despite significant progress in the management of diseases.[19] It seems apparent that aging is distinct from disease, and that the life span is limited by the aging process itself rather than by the ravages of disease. Although the elderly are certainly more vulnerable to diseases, the aging process and disease processes are generally viewed as different phenomena. In practice, the distinction between aging and disease may be difficult to make. For example, the aging skeleton normally loses some bone mass, but too much bone loss results in osteoporosis—a disease process. Likewise, a loss of blood vessel elasticity is generally viewed as a normal aging change, but at what point does too much "hardening of the arteries" become abnormal? This confusion results from the continued inability to identify the irreversible and universal processes of cellular aging as separate from the potentially reversible effects of disease.

Cellular Basis of Aging

The two major schools of thought regarding aging hold that it is caused either by **extrinsic** events that progressively damage cells or by **intrinsic** genetic programs of the cells themselves.[1] Although many theories have been proposed to explain different aspects of aging, it is clear that cell senescence is multifactorial. Each of the following theories of aging explains certain manifestations of the aging process: the somatic mutation theory, the free radical theory, the immunologic theory, the error theory, the neuroendocrine theory, and the programmed senescence theory.

The *somatic mutation theory* is based on the idea that chronic exposure to normal background environmental radiation results in random genetic damage in cells. The cell dies when genetic damage becomes extensive enough to impair critical functions. This theory was proposed to explain the observation that long-term irradiation shortens the life span of experimental animals. This theory suggests that people living in places with increased levels of background radiation, such as at high altitudes, would age more quickly. No such difference has yet been reported.

The *free radical theory* was prompted in part by the observation that larger animals, which have slower metabolic rates, generally have longer life spans.[1] Metabolic rate, in turn, determines the production of activated oxygen free radicals. Aging is thought to result from the cumulative and progressive damage to cell structures, particularly the cell membrane, by these oxygen radicals. The accumulation of lipofuscin pigment, the brown aging pigment, in older cells is taken as evidence of the progressive destruction of membrane lipids by the free radicals. However, no evidence of increased free radical production with aging has been found.

The functional capacity of the immune system declines with age, and the ability to distinguish between self tissue and foreign tissue appears to become impaired. Autoimmune disorders, in which the immune system attacks the body's own cells, are more prevalent in the elderly. The *immunologic theory* of aging maintains that aging is due to failure of the immune system, resulting in the progressive destruction of body cells. The immune theory does not explain the process of aging in simple animals that do not have a well-developed immune system.

The *error theory* of aging is based on the idea that random errors in the translation of key cellular proteins eventually leads to cell death.[20,21] This theory holds that if errors occur in transcriptional and translational enzymes, which control their own synthesis, the errors will be multiplied with time until an "error catastrophe" results in cell death. Although this theory has drawn much interest, it has accumulated little supportive evidence.

The invariable sequence of cell death in certain tissues and organs during embryogenesis has suggested to some researchers that aging is controlled by some intrinsic genetic program or *clock genes.* The *neuroendocrine theories* suggest that the hypothalamic-pituitary system, as the master timekeeper of the body, controls the aging process.[22] Age-related changes in the structure and function of certain hormones have been reported.

The *programmed senescence theory* also holds that aging is the result of an intrinsic genetic program. Support for the theory of a genetically programmed life span comes primarily from studies of cells in culture. In classic experiments by Hayflick, fibroblastic cells in culture were shown to undergo a finite number of cell divisions.[23] Fibroblasts taken from older individuals underwent fewer cell divisions than those from younger individuals. Given an adequate environment, the information encoded in the cellular genome is thought to dictate the number of possible cell replications; after which damaged or lost cells are no longer replaced. Recently, it has been postulated that cells undergo a finite number of replications because the chromosomes shorten a bit with each cell division until some critical point is reached (Figure 4-18), at which time the cell becomes dormant or dies. The end caps of the chromosomes, called **telomeres,** are the sections that shorten with each cell division.[24] Certain cells are able to replenish their telomeres, which gives them potential immortality. The enzyme that rebuilds the telomeres has been named *telomerase.* Interestingly, a number of cancer cell types have been found to produce telomerase, whereas most normal cells do not (Chapter 7). The discovery of telomere shortening with cellular division lends support to the genetic theory of aging.

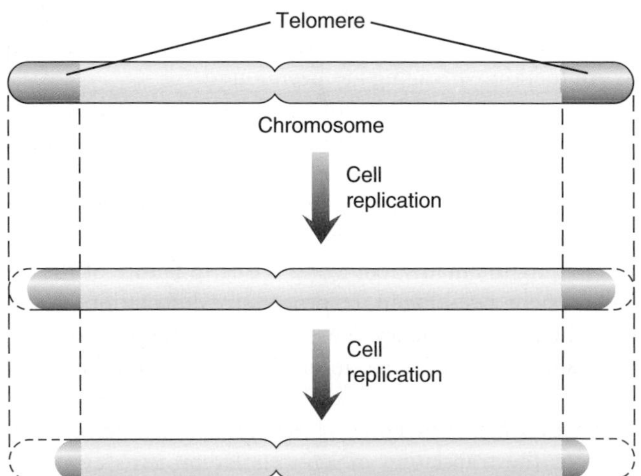

FIGURE 4-18 ■ The end caps of the chromosomes are called *telomeres.* In most body cells, the telomeres progressively shorten with each cell replication until a critical point is reached, at which time the cell becomes dormant or dies.

Physiologic Changes of Aging

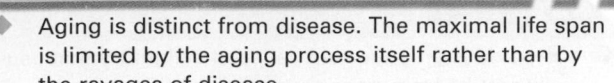

All of the body systems show age-related changes that can be generally described as a decrease in functional reserve or inability to adapt to environmental demands. An overview of the tissue and systemic changes of aging is presented in Table 4-5. The details of age-related changes in the various body systems are described in later chapters of this book.

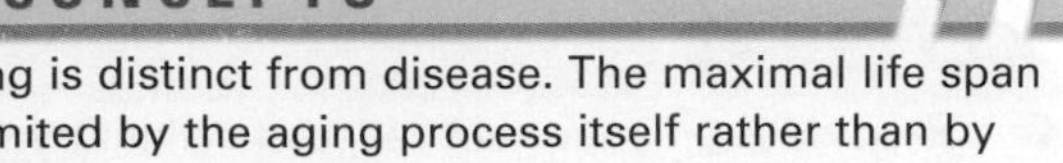

- Aging is distinct from disease. The maximal life span is limited by the aging process itself rather than by the ravages of disease.
- Aging theories are of two general schools. According to the first school, aging is caused by extrinsic events that progressively damage cells. Aligned with this school are the somatic mutation theory, the free radical theory, and the immunologic theory of aging. According to the second school, aging is caused by intrinsic genetic programs. Representatives of this school are the neuroendocrine theories and the programmed senescence theory. The discovery of telomere shortening with each cell division supports the genetic theory of aging.
- Age-related changes in body systems can generally be described as a decrease in functional reserve and a reduced ability to adapt to environmental demands.

SOMATIC DEATH

Death of the entire organism is called *somatic death.* In contrast to localized cell death, no immunologic or inflammatory response occurs in somatic death. The general features of somatic death include the absence of respiration and heartbeat. However, this definition of death is insufficient because in some cases breathing and cardiac activity may be restored by resuscitative efforts. Within several minutes of cardiopulmonary arrest, the characteristics of irreversible somatic death become apparent. Body temperature falls, the skin becomes pale, and blood and body fluids collect in dependent areas. Within 6 hours, the accumulation of calcium and the depletion of ATP result in perpetual actin-myosin cross-bridge formation in muscle cells. The presence of stiffened muscles throughout the body after death is called *rigor mortis.* Rigor mortis gives way to limpness or flaccidity as the tissues of the body begin to deteriorate. Tissue deterioration or putrefaction becomes apparent 24 to 48 hours after death.[25] Putrefaction is associated with the widespread release of lytic enzymes in tissues throughout the body, a process called *postmortem autolysis.*

The determination of "brain death" has become necessary because of technological ability to keep the heart and lungs working through artificial means even though the brain is no longer functional. Criteria for determining brain death as proof of somatic death may vary by geographic area but gen-

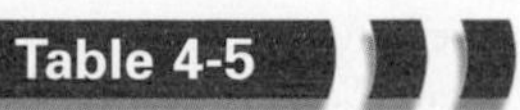

Overview of the Physiologic Changes of Aging

System	Physiologic Changes
Cardiovascular	↓ Vessel elasticity due to calcification and connective tissue (↑ pulmonary vascular resistance)
	↓ No. of heart muscle fibers with ↑ size of individual fibers (hypertrophy)
	↓ Filling capacity
	↓ Stroke volume
	↓ Sensitivity of baroreceptors
	Degeneration of vein valves
Respiratory	↓ Chest wall compliance due to calcification of costal cartilage
	↓ Alveolar ventilation
	↓ Respiratory muscle strength
	Air trapping and ↓ ventilation due to degeneration of lung tissue (↓ elasticity)
Renal/urinary	↓ Glomerular filtration rate due to nephron degeneration (↓ one third to one half by age 70 yr)
	↓ Ability to concentrate urine
	↓ Ability to regulate H^+
Gastrointestinal	Muscular contraction
	↓ Esophageal emptying
	↓ Bowel motility
	↓ Production of HCl, enzymes, and intrinsic factor
	↓ Hepatic enzyme production and metabolic capacity
	Thinning of stomach mucosa
Neurologic/sensory	Nerve cells degenerate and atrophy
	↓ Of 25%-45% of neurons
	↓ Neurotransmitters
	↓ Rate of conduction of nerve impulses
	Loss of taste buds
	Loss of auditory hair cells and sclerosis of eardrum
Musculoskeletal	↓ Muscle mass
	Bone demineralization
	Joint degeneration, erosion, and calcification
Immune	↓ Inflammatory response
	↓ In T-cell function due to involution of thymus gland
Integumentary	↓ Subcutaneous fat
	↓ Elastin
	Atrophy of sweat glands
	Atrophy of epidermal arterioles causing altered temperature regulation

erally include unresponsiveness, flaccidity, absence of brainstem reflexes (e.g., swallowing, gagging, pupil and eye movements), absence of respiratory effort when the subject is removed from the mechanical ventilator, absence of electrical brain waves, and lack of cerebral blood flow.

KEY CONCEPTS

- Somatic death is characterized by the absence of respirations and heartbeat. Definitions of brain death have been established to describe death in instances in which heartbeat and respiration are maintained mechanically.
- After death, body temperature falls, blood and body fluids collect in dependent areas, and rigor mortis ensues. Within 24 to 48 hours the tissues begin to deteriorate and rigor mortis gives way to flaccidity.

SUMMARY

Cells and tissues face many challenges to survival, including injury from lack of oxygen and nutrients, infection and immune responses, chemicals, and physical and mechanical factors. Cells respond to environmental changes or injury in three general ways: (1) If the change is mild or short lived, the cell may withstand the assault and return to its preinjury status. (2) The cell may adapt to a persistent but sublethal injury by changing its structure or function. (3) Cell death by apoptosis or necrosis may occur if the injury is too severe or prolonged. Characteristics of reversible cell injury include hydropic swelling and the accumulation of abnormal substances. Cell necrosis is characterized by irreversible loss of function, release of cellular enzymes into the blood stream, and an inflammatory response. The disruption of the permeability barrier of the plasma membrane appears to be a critical event in necrotic cellular death. Apoptosis is characterized by a tidy, noninflammatory autodigestion of the cell.

Aging is a normal physiologic process characterized by a progressive decline in functional capacity and adaptive ability. The biological basis of aging remains largely a mystery, but several theories have been proposed to explain certain aspects of the process. At present, most sources differentiate between the biological alterations of aging and the alterations consequent to disease processes. In practice, however, the distinction may be difficult to make.

MEDIA RESOURCES

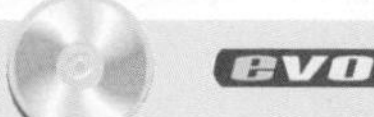

Remember to check out the ***CD Companion*** included with this book for Review Questions, Key Concepts Review, Glossary (with audio for selected terms), Disease Profiles, and Animations.

PLUS, visit the ***Evolve website*** at http://evolve.elsevier.com/Copstead/ for Case Studies, Disease Profiles, and WebLinks.

References

1. Mitchell R, Cotran R: Cell injury, adaptation, and death. In Kumar V, Cotran R, Robbins S, editors: *Robbins basic pathology,* ed 7, Philadelphia, 2003, Saunders, pp 3-32.
2. Crawford J: The liver and biliary tract. In Kumar V, Cotran R, Robbins S, editors: *Robbins basic pathology,* ed 7, Philadelphia, 2003, Saunders, pp 591-634.
3. Clare-Salzler M, Crawford J, Kumar V: The pancreas. In Kumar V, Cotran R, Robbins S, editors: *Robbins basic pathology,* ed 7, Philadelphia, 2003, Saunders, pp 635-656.
4. Yarasheski KE: Exercise, aging, and muscle protein metabolism, *J Gerontol A Biol Sci Med Sci* 58(10):M918-M922, 2003.
5. Nieminen AL: Apoptosis and necrosis in health and disease: role of mitochondria, *Int Rev Cytol* 224:29-55, 2003.
6. Nadal-Ginard B et al: Myocyte death, growth, and regeneration in cardiac hypertrophy and failure, *Circ Res* 92:139-150, 2003.
7. Alberts B et al: Cell communication. In Alberts B et al, editors: *Molecular biology of the cell,* ed 4, New York, 2002, Garland Science, pp 831-906.
8. Alberts B et al: The cell cycle and programmed cell death. In Alberts B et al, editors: *Molecular biology of the cell,* ed 4, New York, 2002, Garland Science, pp 983-1026.
9. White BC et al: Brain ischemia and reperfusion: molecular mechanisms of neuronal injury, *J Neurol Sci* 179(S1-2):1-33, 2000.
10. Chan RK et al: Ischaemia-reperfusion is an event triggered by immune complexes and complement, *Br J Surg* 90(12): 1470-1478, 2003.
11. Kumar V, Cotran R, Robbins S: Environmental disease. In Kumar V, Cotran R, Robbins S, editors: *Robbins basic pathology,* ed 7, Philadelphia, 2003, Saunders, pp 265-306.
12. *Clinical guidelines on the identification, evaluation, and treatment of overweight and obesity in adults,* NIH Publication No. 98-4083, National Institutes of Health, 1998.
13. Van Amersfoort ES, Van Berkel TJ, Kuiper J: Receptors, mediators, and mechanisms involved in bacterial sepsis and septic shock, *Clin Microbiol Rev* 16(3):379-414, 2003.
14. Samuelson J: General pathology of infectious disease. In Kumar V, Cotran R, Robbins S, editors: *Robbins basic pathology,* ed 7, Philadelphia, 2003, Saunders, pp 307-322.
15. Weber LW, Boll M, Stampfl A: Hepatotoxicity and mechanism of action of haloalkanes: carbon tetrachloride as a toxicological model, *Crit Rev Toxicol* 33(2):105-136, 2003.
16. Huang L, Snyder AR, Morgan WF: Radiation-induced genomic instability and its implications for radiation carcinogenesis, *Oncogene* 22(37):5848-5854, 2003.
17. Osepchuk JM, Petersen RC: Historical review of RF exposure standards and the International Committee on Electromagnetic Safety (ICES), *Bioelectromagnetics* 24(suppl 6):S7-S16, 2003.
18. Rupnow BA, Knox SJ: The role of radiation-induced apoptosis as a determinant of tumor responses to radiation therapy, *Apoptosis* 4(2):115-143, 1999.
19. Troen BR: The biology of aging, *Mt Sinai J Med* 70(1):3-22, 2003.
20. Orgel L: The maintenance of the accuracy of protein synthesis and its relevance to aging, *Proc Natl Acad Sci U S A* 49: 517-521, 1963.
21. Orgel L: The maintenance of the accuracy of protein synthesis and its relevance to aging: a correction, *Proc Natl Acad Sci U S A* 67:1476, 1970.
22. Dillman VM: *The neuroendocrine theory of aging and degenerative disease,* Pensacola, Fla, 1992, Center for Bio-Gerontology.
23. Hayflick L: The biology of human aging, *Adv Pathobiol* 7(2):80-99, 1980.
24. Djojosubroto MW et al: Telomeres and telomerase in aging, regeneration and cancer, *Mol Cell* 15(2):164-175, 2003.
25. Shennan T: *Postmortems and morbid anatomy,* ed 3, Baltimore, 1935, William Wood.

Molecular Genetics and Tissue Differentiation

chapter 5

Jacquelyn L. Banasik

MEDIA RESOURCES

Additional Material for Study, Review, and Further Exploration

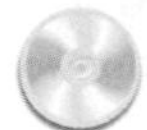

CD Companion ◆ Review Questions and Answers ◆ Key Concepts Review
◆ Glossary *(with audio pronunciations for selected terms)*
◆ Disease Profiles ◆ Animations

evolve ***Website*** at http://evolve.elsevier.com/Copstead/
◆ Case Studies ◆ Disease Profiles ◆ WebLinks

KEY QUESTIONS

- How is genetic information stored in the cell and transmitted to progeny during replication?
- How does the simple four-base structure of DNA serve as a template for synthesis of proteins that may contain 20 varieties of amino acids?
- What roles do genes play in determining cell structure and function?
- How is gene expression regulated?
- By what mechanisms can the cells of an organism, which all contain identical genes, become differentiated into divergent cell types?
- What are the general structures and functions of the four main tissue types: epithelial, connective, muscle, and nerve?

CHAPTER OUTLINE

The ability of scientists to study and manipulate genes has evolved at an incredible pace, including the recent sequencing of all the nucleotides in an entire human genome. A better understanding of the role that genetics plays in cellular function and disease has spurred efforts to develop therapies to correct genetic abnormalities. The science of genetics developed from the premise that invisible, information-containing elements called **genes** exist in cells and are passed on to daughter cells when a cell divides. The nature of these elements was at first difficult to imagine: what kind of molecule could direct the day-to-day activities of the organism and also be capable of nearly limitless replication? The answer to this question was discovered in the late 1940s and was almost unbelievable in its simplicity. It is now common knowledge that genetic information is stored in long chains of stable molecules called **deoxyribonucleic acid (DNA).** The human genome contains approximately 30,000 genes encoded by only four different molecules. These molecules are the deoxyribonucleotides containing the bases *adenine* (A), *cytosine* (C), *guanine* (G), and *thymine* (T). Genes are composed of varying sequences of these four bases, which are linked together by sugar-phosphate bonds. By serving as the templates for the production of body proteins, genes ultimately affect all aspects of an organism's structure and function. Some knowledge of the basic principles of genetics is therefore prerequisite to understanding a variety of disease processes. This chapter examines the biochemistry of genetics (molecular genetics), concepts of regulation of gene expression, and the processes of tissue differentiation. Principles of genetic inheritance precede the discussion of genetic diseases in Chapter 6.

MOLECULAR GENETICS

Structure of DNA

In humans, DNA encodes genetic information in 46 long double-stranded chains of nucleotides called chromosomes.[1] The **nucleotides** consist of a five-carbon sugar (deoxyribose), a phosphate group, and one of the four nucleotide bases (Figure 5-1). The nucleotide bases are divided into two types based on their chemical structure. The pyrimidines, cytosine and thymine, have single-ring structures. The purines, guanine and adenine, have double-ring structures (Figure 5-2). DNA polymers are formed by the chemical linkage of these nucleotides. The sugar-phosphate linkages, also called *phosphodiester bonds,* join the phosphate group on one sugar (attached to the 5-carbon) to the 3-carbon of the next sugar (see Figure 5-1). The four kinds of bases (A, C, G, T) are attached to the repeating sugar-phosphate chain. The bases of one strand of DNA form weak bonds with the bases of another strand of DNA. These noncovalent hydrogen bonds are specific and complementary (Figure 5-3). The bases G and C bond together and the bases A and T bond together. Nucleotides that are able to bond together are called *base pairs.*

In the early 1950s, Watson and Crick proposed that the structure of DNA was a double helix.[2] In this model, DNA can be envisioned as a twisted ladder, with the sugar-phosphate bonds as the sides of the ladder and the bases forming the rungs (see Figure 5-3). There is one complete turn of the helix every 10 base pairs. The two strands of DNA must be complementary to form the double helix; that is, the bases of one strand must pair exactly with their complementary bases on the other strand. The helix is wound around proteins called histones to form *nucleosomes* (Figure 5-4). DNA coupled to histones and other nuclear proteins is termed *chromatin.* When a cell is not dividing, the chromatin is loosely packed within the nucleus and not visible under the light microscope. During cell division the chromatin becomes tightly condensed into the 46 chromosomes that become visible during mitosis.

The discovery of the double-helix model was profound because it immediately suggested how information transfer could be accomplished by such simple molecules. Because each DNA strand carries a nucleotide sequence that is exactly complementary to the sequence of its partner, both strands can be used as templates to create an exact copy of the original DNA double helix. When a cell divides to form two daughter cells, each daughter cell must receive a complete copy of the parent cell's DNA. The process of DNA replication requires separation of the DNA double helix by breaking the hydrogen bonds between the base pairs. Specific replication enzymes then direct the attachment of the correct (complementary) nucleotides to each of the single-stranded DNA templates. In this way two identical copies of the original DNA double helix are formed and passed on to the two daughter cells during cell division.

FIGURE 5-1 ■ A nucleotide consists of a sugar (deoxyribose), a phosphate group, and one of the four nucleotide bases. Nucleotides are joined by repeating sugar-phosphate bonds to form long chains, called *polymers. A,* Adenine; *C,* cytosine; *G,* guanine; *T,* thymine.

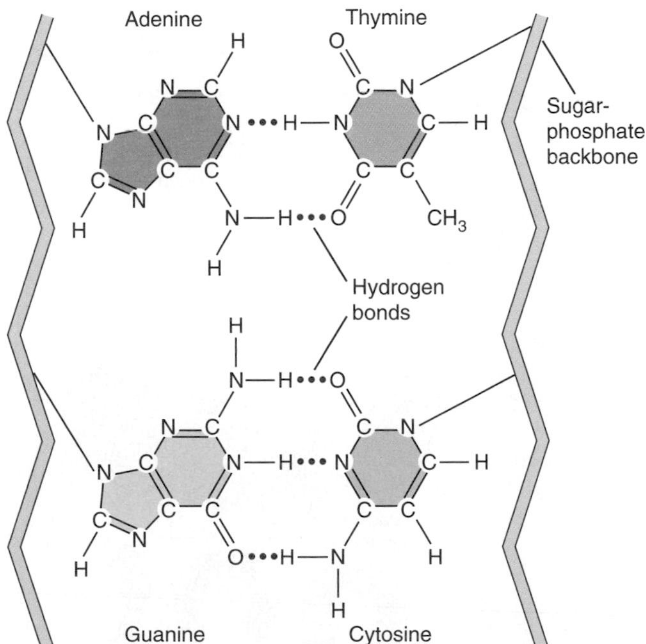

FIGURE 5-2 ■ The two types of DNA bases are the single-ring pyrimidines and the double-ring purines. Thymine (T) and cytosine (C) are pyrimidines, and adenine (A) and guanine (G) are purines. Base pairing occurs between A and T and between C and G because of hydrogen bonds *(dots).*

DNA Replication

Although the underlying principle of gene replication is simple, the cellular machinery required to carry out the replication process is complex, involving a host of enzymes and proteins.[3] These "replication machines" can duplicate DNA at a rate of 1000 nucleotides per second and complete the duplication of the entire genome in about 8 hours.[4] The DNA double helix must first separate so that new nucleotides can be paired with the old DNA template strands. The DNA double helix is normally very stable: the base pairs are locked in place so tightly that they can withstand temperatures approaching the boiling point. DNA replication is started by special proteins called "initiator proteins" that pry the DNA strands apart at specific places along the chromatin, called replication origins. Then special enzymes called DNA helicases are needed to rapidly unwind and separate the DNA strands, whereas helix-destabilizing proteins (also called single-stranded DNA-binding proteins) bind to the exposed DNA strands to keep them apart until replication can be accomplished (Figure 5-5).

Once a portion of the DNA double helix has been separated, special enzymes called **DNA polymerases** bind the single strands of DNA and begin the process of forming a new complementary strand of DNA. The polymerases match the appropriate base to the template base and catalyze the formation of the sugar-phosphate bonds that form the backbone of the DNA strand. Replication proceeds along the DNA strand in one direction only: from the 3' end toward the 5' end.[4] The

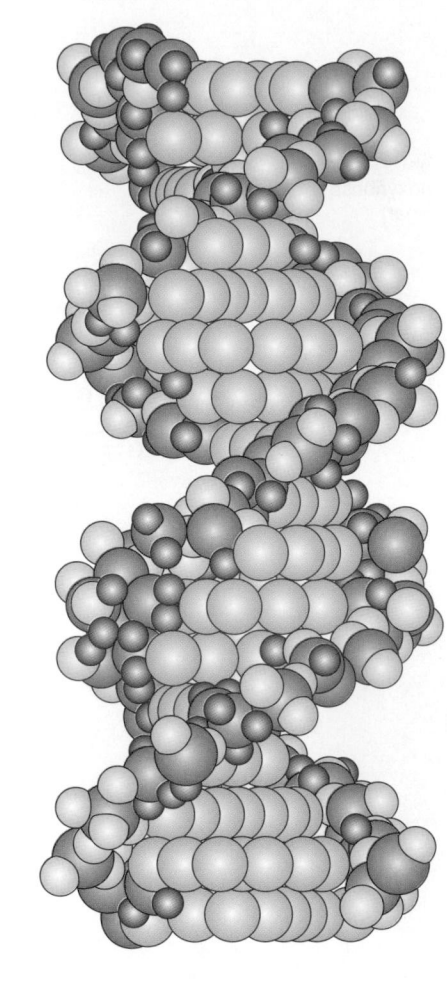

FIGURE 5-3 ■ A schematic and space-filling model of the DNA double helix as proposed by Watson and Crick. The pairing of bases is specific and complementary: Cytosine *(C)* always pairs with guanine *(G),* and adenine *(A)* always pairs with thymine *(T).*

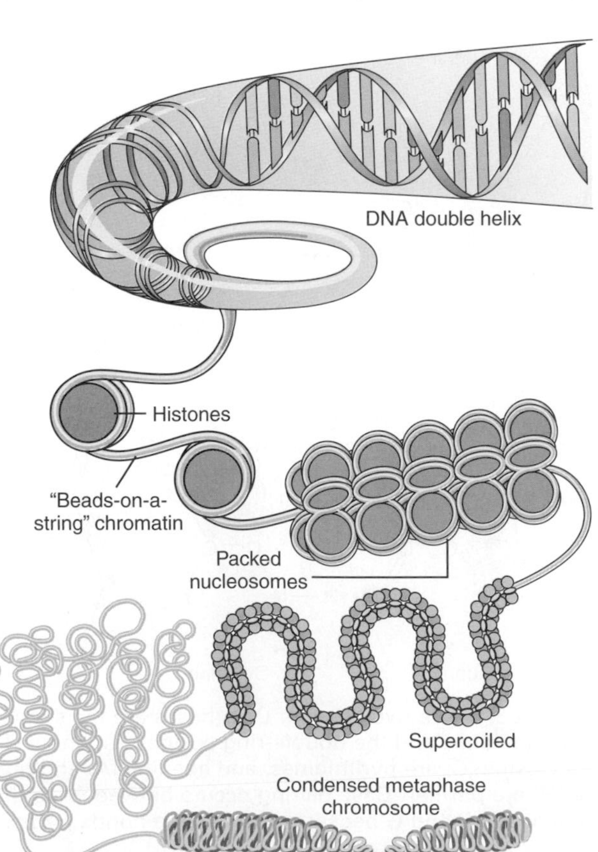

FIGURE 5-4 ■ DNA is packaged by wrapping around protein complexes called *histones* to form beadlike structures called *nucleosomes.* During cell division the coiled DNA becomes very condensed into chromosomes that are visible under the light microscope. During interphase and when genes are being transcribed, the DNA is more loosely packaged and not visible.

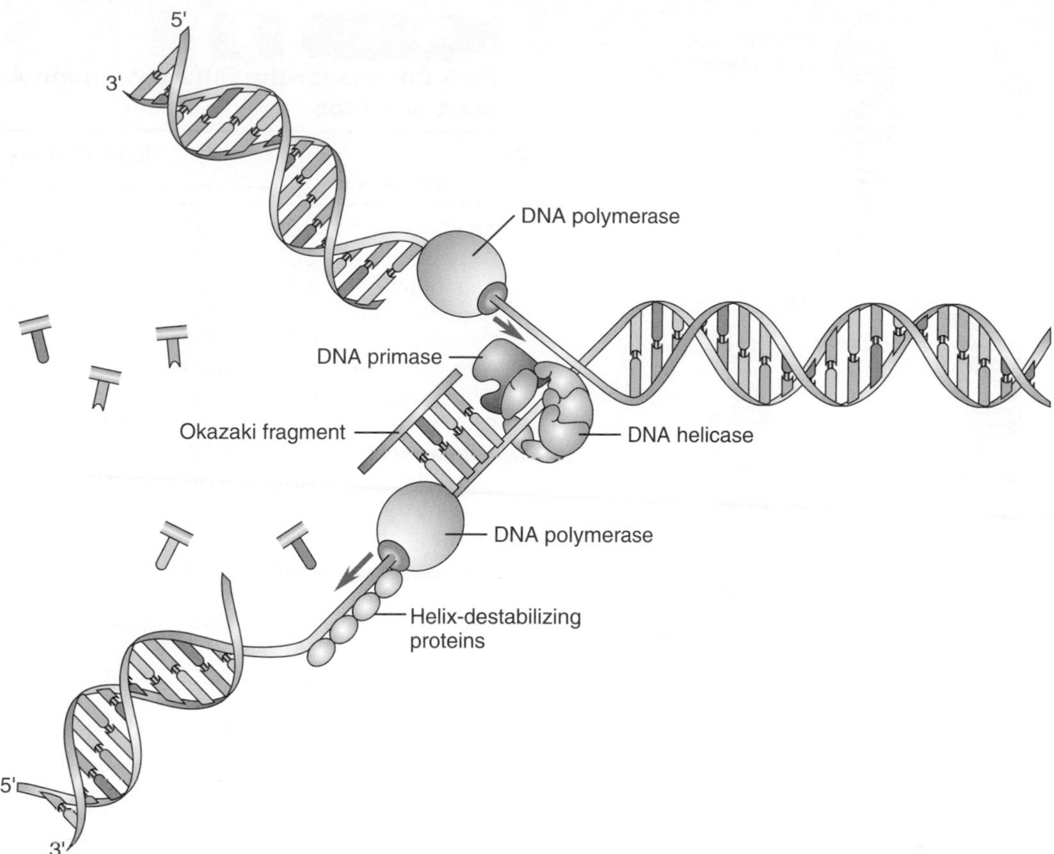

FIGURE 5-5 ■ Summary of the major proteins of the DNA replication fork. Helicase unwinds the DNA double helix, while helix-destabilizing proteins keep the strands from reuniting. Okazaki fragments are formed in a "backstitching" direction and then sealed together with DNA ligase.

ends of the DNA strands are labeled 3' and 5' according to the exposed carbon atom at that end. Because two complementary DNA strands are antiparallel, DNA replication is asymmetrical; one strand, the leading strand, is replicated as a continuous polymer, but the lagging strand must be synthesized in short sections in a "backstitching" process. The backstitched fragments of DNA, called Okazaki fragments, are then sealed together by DNA ligase to form the unbroken DNA strand. DNA polymerase is unable to replicate DNA located at the very ends of the chromosomes (the telomeres) and another special enzyme complex, called telomerase, is needed for this. In many somatic cell types, telomerase is not present and the cell's chromosomes get a bit shorter with each cell division. Chromosomal shortening has been proposed as a mechanism of "counting" the number of replications and may be important in cellular aging and prevention of cancer (see Chapter 7). DNA replication is said to be semiconservative because each of the two resulting DNA double helices contains one newly synthesized strand and one original (conserved) strand (Figure 5-6).

The DNA polymerase also has an ability to proofread the newly synthesized strands for errors in base pairing. If an error is detected, the enzyme will back up, remove the incorrect nucleotide, and replace it with the correct one. The fidelity of copying during DNA replication is such that only about one error is made for every 10^9 base pair replications.[5] The self-correcting function of the DNA polymerases is extremely important because errors in replication will be passed on to the next generation of cells.

Genetic Code

How do an organism's genes influence its structural and functional characteristics? The prevailing theory in biology holds that genes direct the synthesis of proteins in cells. It is the presence (or absence) and relative activity of various structural proteins and enzymes that produce the characteristics of the cell. Proteins are composed of one or more chains of amino acids (polypeptides) that fold into complex three-dimensional structures. Cells contain 20 different types of amino acids that join together in a specific sequence to form a particular protein (Table 5-1). Each type of protein has a unique sequence of amino acids that dictates its structure and activity.

If genes are to direct the synthesis of proteins, the information contained in just four kinds of DNA nucleotide bases must in some way code for 20 different amino acids. This

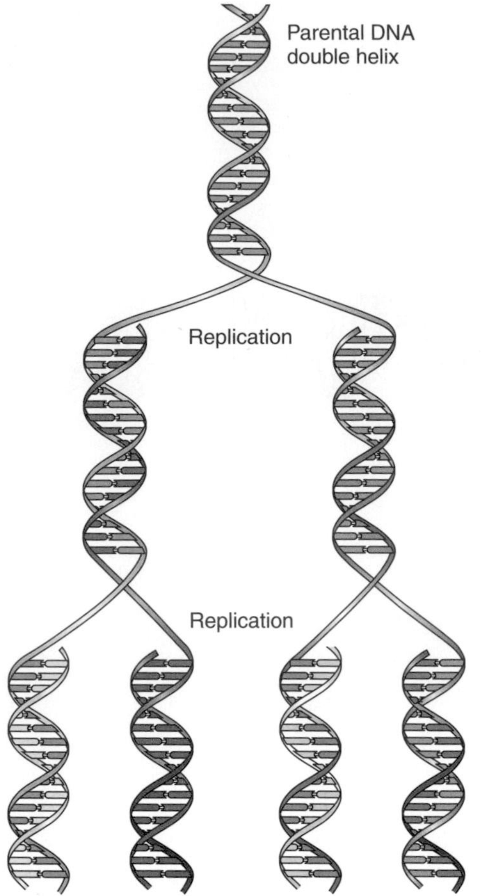

FIGURE 5-6 ■ DNA replication is semiconservative. Each of the new DNA double helices contains one newly synthesized strand and one original strand.

so-called genetic code was deciphered in the early 1960s.[6,7] It was determined that a series of three nucleotides (triplet) was needed to code for each of the 20 amino acids. Because there are four different bases, there are 4^3 or 64 different possible triplet combinations. This is far more than needed to code for the 20 known amino acids. Three of the nucleotide triplets or **codons** do not code for amino acids and are called stop codons because they signal the end of a protein code. The remaining 61 codons all code for one of the 20 amino acids (see Table 5-1). Obviously, some of the amino acids are specified by more than one codon. For example, the amino acid arginine is determined by six different codons. The code has been highly conserved during evolution and is essentially the same in organisms as diverse as humans and bacteria.

Several intermediate molecules are involved in the process of DNA-directed protein synthesis, including the complex protein-synthesizing machinery of the ribosomes and **ribonucleic acid (RNA)**. With few exceptions, the flow of information transfer is from DNA to RNA to protein. RNA is structurally similar to DNA except that the sugar molecule is ribose rather than deoxyribose, and one of the four bases is different in that uracil replaces thymine. Because of the biochemical

Table 5-1

RNA Codons for the Different Amino Acids and for Start and Stop

Amino Acids	RNA Codons					
Alanine	GCU	GCC	GCA	GCG		
Arginine	CGU	CGC	CGA	CGG	AGA	AGG
Asparagine	AAU	AAC				
Aspartic acid	GAU	GAC				
Cysteine	UGU	UGC				
Glutamic acid	GAA	GAG				
Glutamine	CAA	CAG				
Glycine	GGU	GGC	GGA	GGG		
Histidine	CAU	CAC				
Isoleucine	AUU	AUC	AUA			
Leucine	CUU	CUC	CUA	CUG	UUA	UUG
Lysine	AAA	AAG				
Methionine	AUG					
Phenylalanine	UUU	UUC				
Proline	CCU	CCC	CCA	CCG		
Serine	UCU	UCC	UCA	UCG	AGC	AGU
Threonine	ACU	ACC	ACA	ACG		
Tryptophan	UGG					
Tyrosine	UAU	UAC				
Valine	GUU	GUC	GUA	GUG		
Start (CI)	AUG					
Stop (CT)	UAA	UAG	UGA			

From Guyton AC, Hall JE: *Textbook of medical physiology,* ed 10, Philadelphia, 2000, Saunders, p 28.
CI, Chain initiation; *CT,* chain termination.

similarity of uracil and thymine, both can form base pairs with adenine. In addition, RNA forms stable single-stranded molecules, whereas DNA strands anneal together forming a double-stranded molecule.

Several functionally different types of RNA are involved in protein synthesis and cell function. Researchers estimate that only 2% of the DNA in human chromosomes codes for proteins. Some transcription units code for functional RNA molecules that have direct activities in cells and do not code for protein. The function of the vast majority of DNA is unknown. Ribosomal RNA (rRNA) is found associated with the ribosome (see Chapter 3) in the cell cytoplasm. Messenger RNA (mRNA) is synthesized from the DNA template in a process termed **transcription** and carries the protein code to the cytoplasm, where the proteins are manufactured. The amino acids that will be joined together to form proteins are carried in the cytoplasm by the third type of RNA, transfer RNA (tRNA), which interacts with mRNA and the ribosome in a process termed **translation.**

Transcription

Transcription is the process whereby mRNA is synthesized from a single-stranded DNA template. The process is similar

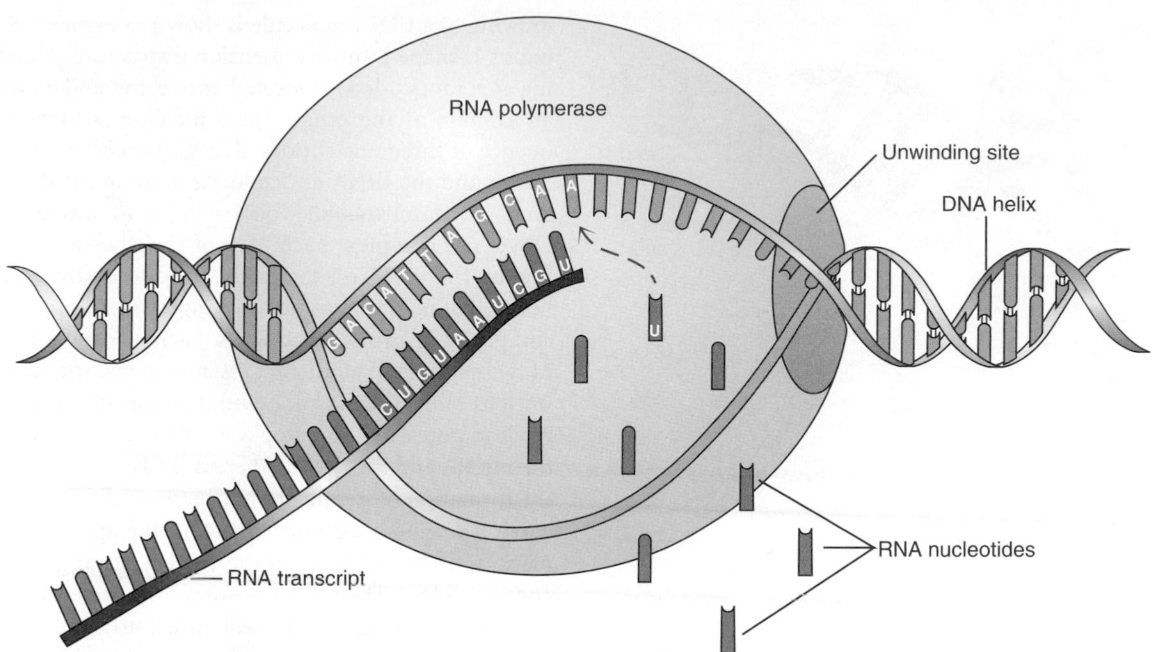

FIGURE 5-7 ■ A moving RNA polymerase complex unwinds the DNA helix ahead of it while rewinding the DNA behind. One strand of the DNA serves as the template for the formation of mRNA.

to DNA replication. Double-stranded DNA must be separated in the region of the gene to be copied, and specific enzyme complexes (DNA-dependent RNA polymerases) orchestrate the production of the mRNA polymer. Only one of the DNA strands contains the desired gene sequence and serves as the template for the synthesis of mRNA. This strand is called the *sense strand.* The other strand is termed the *nonsense* or *antisense strand* and is not transcribed into an RNA message.

Some genes are continuously active in certain cells, whereas others are carefully regulated in response to cellular needs and environmental signals. Special sequences of DNA near a desired gene may enhance or inhibit its rate of transcription. In general, a gene is transcribed when the RNA polymerase–enzyme complex binds to a promoter region just upstream of the gene's start point. The RNA polymerase directs the separation of the DNA double helix and catalyzes the synthesis of the RNA message by matching the appropriate RNA bases to the DNA template (Figure 5-7). The RNA message is directly complementary to the DNA sequence, except that uracil replaces thymine.

In higher organisms, the DNA template for a particular protein is littered with stretches of bases that must be removed from the original RNA transcript *(pre-mRNA)* before it can be translated into a protein. These unwanted areas, called **introns,** are removed in the nucleus by a complex splicing process, resulting in an mRNA sequence that contains only the wanted segments, called **exons.** Introns range from 10 to 100,000 nucleotides in length.[8] A single gene may contain dozens. The function of introns remains largely a mystery, although they are believed to be important in the evolution of new genetic information and in the regulation of gene activity during embryonic development. Many of these intron sequences are conserved across species, which implies an important function. The removal of introns and splicing of the RNA transcript is mediated by a group of small RNA-protein complexes located in specialized areas of the nucleus called the *spliceosomes.* The *snRNPs,* or small nuclear ribonucleoproteins in *spliceosomes,* attach to the pre-mRNA and prevent its escape through the nuclear envelope until all of the necessary splicing has been accomplished.[9] Most pre-mRNA transcripts can be spliced in different ways to increase the number of different protein forms produced by a single gene.[8]

The processed mRNA is finally transported to the cell cytoplasm through pores in the nuclear membrane that contain complexes which inspect the mRNA for certain structural characteristics that distinguish it from RNA debris. The mRNA then directs the synthesis of a protein in cooperation with tRNA and the ribosomes. Each mRNA may serve as a template for thousands of copies of protein before it is degraded.

Translation

Translation is the process whereby messenger RNA is used to direct the synthesis of a protein. The mRNA is read in linear fashion from one end to the other, with each set of three nucleotides serving as a codon for a particular amino acid. The codons in the mRNA do not directly recognize the amino acids. Intermediary molecules or "translators" are required. These intermediaries are the tRNA molecules. A schematic

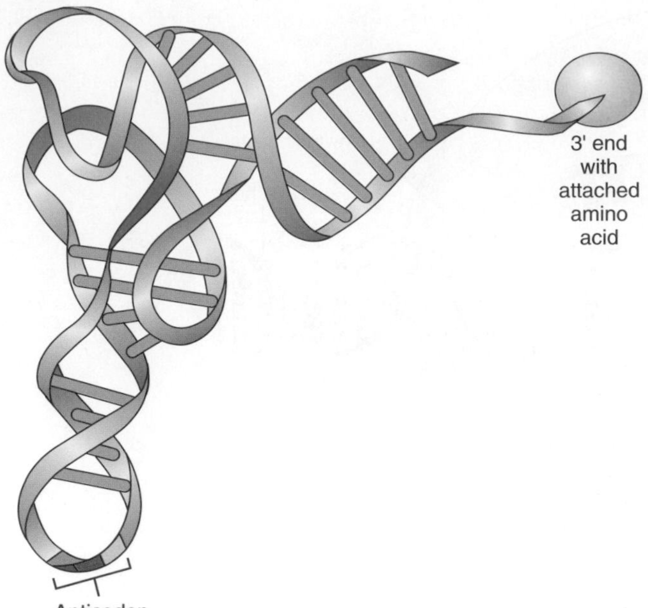

FIGURE 5-8 ■ Schematic drawing of a transfer RNA (tRNA) molecule. Each tRNA binds a specific amino acid, which corresponds with the three-base sequence at the anticodon end.

drawing of a tRNA molecule is shown in Figure 5-8, illustrating its L-shaped, three-dimensional structure. A codon reading area (anticodon) is located at one end and an amino acid attachment at the other. The anticodon is formed by a sequence of three nucleotides. Recognition between the mRNA codon and the tRNA anticodon is accomplished by the same kind of complementary base pairing as was described for DNA. The complex machinery of the ribosome is needed to line up the tRNA on the mRNA and to catalyze the peptide bonds that hold the amino acids together. **Ribosomes** are large complexes of protein and RNA. Each ribosome is composed of two subunits that are first assembled in a special part of the nucleus called the *nucleolus* and then transported through the nuclear pores to the cytoplasm. The smaller subunit binds the mRNA and the tRNA, whereas the larger subunit catalyzes the formation of peptide bonds between the incoming amino acids. The ribosome must first find the appropriate starting place on the mRNA to set the correct reading frame for the codon triplets. Then the ribosome moves along the mRNA, translating the nucleotide sequence into an amino acid sequence, one codon at a time (Figure 5-9).[10] The newly synthesized protein chain is released from the ribosome when a "stop codon" signaling the end of the message is reached.

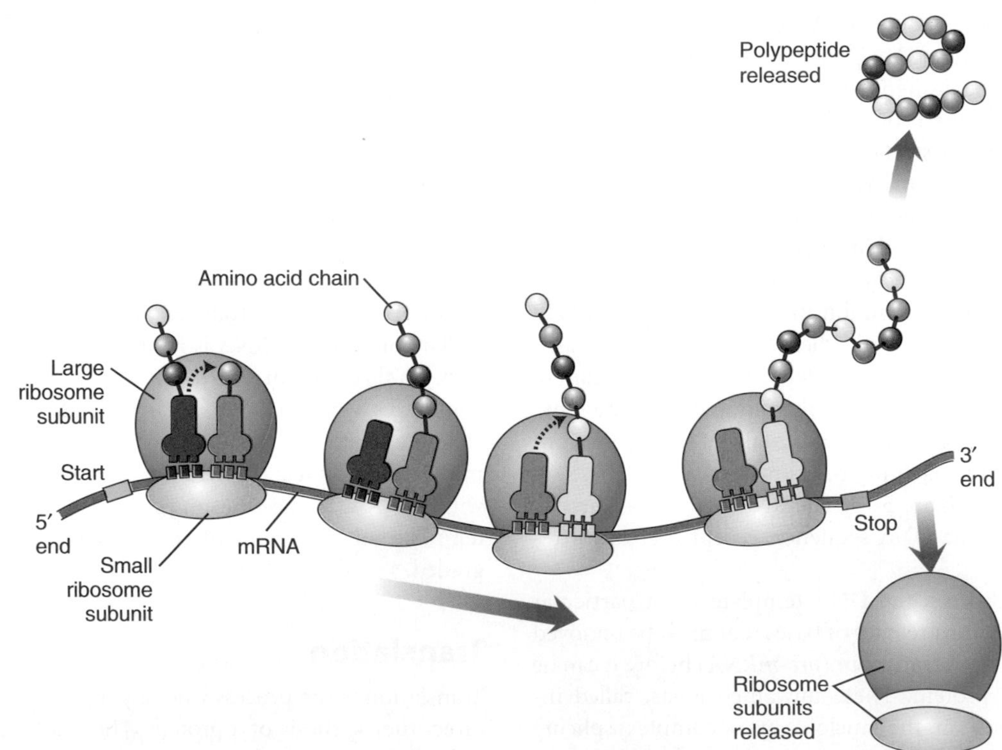

FIGURE 5-9 ■ Synthesis of a protein by the ribosomes attached to a messenger RNA *(mRNA)* molecule. Ribosomes attach near the start codon and catalyze the formation of the peptide chain. The mRNA strand is read in groups of three nucleotides (codons) until the stop codon is reached and the peptide is released. Several ribosomes may translate a single mRNA into multiple copies of the protein.

KEY CONCEPTS

- Genes are the basic units of inheritance and are composed of DNA located on chromosomes. Genes direct the day-to-day activities of the cell by controlling the production of proteins.
- The structure of DNA can be envisioned as a twisted ladder, with the sugar-phosphate bonds as the sides of the ladder and the four nucleotide bases (adenosine, cytosine, guanine, and thymine) forming the rungs. The nucleotides form complementary base pairs, C with G and A with T.
- The DNA double helix must separate into single strands to provide a template for synthesizing new, identical DNA strands that can be passed on to daughter cells during cell division. DNA replication is accomplished by the enzyme complex DNA polymerase. DNA synthesis has extremely high fidelity.
- A linear sequence of DNA that codes for a particular protein is called a gene. During transcription, genes provide a template for the synthesis of mRNA by the enzyme complex RNA polymerase.
- After appropriate cutting and splicing of the pre-mRNA transcript, the mRNA is transported to the cytoplasm and translated into a protein. Each nucleotide triplet (codon) in the mRNA codes for a particular amino acid. Protein synthesis is accomplished by ribosomes, which match the mRNA codon with the correct tRNA anticodon and then catalyze the peptide bond to link amino acids together into a linear protein.

REGULATION OF GENE EXPRESSION

The genome contains the genetic information of the cell and ultimately determines its form and function. All the various cells in a multicellular organism contain the same genome, and differences in cell type are thought to be due to differences in DNA *expression.* To maintain the cell's phenotype, some genes must be actively transcribed, whereas other genes remain quiescent. In addition, the cell must be able to change the expression of certain genes in order to respond and adapt to changes in the cellular environment. At any one time a cell expresses 10,000 to 20,000 of its approximately 30,000 genes.[11] Some basic principles about the mechanisms that control gene expression are beginning to emerge, but much remains to be determined. There is evidence that gene expression can be regulated at each of the steps in the pathway from DNA to RNA to protein synthesis. The proteins made by a cell can be controlled in the following ways: (1) regulating the rate and timing of gene transcription; (2) controlling how the mRNA is spliced; (3) selecting which mRNAs are transported to the cytoplasm; (4) selecting which mRNAs are translated by ribosomes; (5) selectively destroying certain mRNAs in the cytoplasm; or (6) selectively controlling the activity of the proteins after they have been produced.[11]

For a majority of genes, the most important regulators of expression are the transcriptional controls. Animal cells contain DNA-binding proteins that are able to enhance or inhibit gene expression. These gene regulatory proteins recognize and bind only particular DNA sequences and thus are specific to the genes they regulate.[12] A cell contains many gene regulatory proteins, each of which works in combination with others to control numerous genes. The ability to regulate gene expression allows the cell to alter its structure and function in response to signals from its environment.

Transcriptional Controls

The gene regulatory proteins described in the preceding paragraphs are thought to control gene transcription by binding near the promoter sequence of DNA, where the RNA polymerase must attach to initiate transcription of the gene.[13] Binding of the regulatory protein may either enhance or inhibit RNA polymerase binding and subsequent transcription of the gene. This is sometimes referred to as "turning on" or "turning off" a gene. The DNA-binding proteins are able to recognize their specific binding sites because of small variations in structure of the external surface of the DNA double helix and do not require separation of the strands to bind. These regulatory DNA-binding proteins can be categorized as positive controls that turn on or activate transcription *(activators)* or negative controls that inhibit transcription *(repressors).*

In humans, the strategies for gene regulation are complex. Gene regulatory proteins often bind DNA segments far from the gene being regulated, and binding of several gene regulatory proteins in combination is often necessary. A critical step in initiating gene transcription in human cells is the assembly of general transcription factors at the promoter region.[14] General transcription factors are a group of proteins necessary for RNA polymerase activity, and initiation of transcription does not occur without them. Regulatory gene activator proteins help to collect the transcription factors at the promoter of the correct gene by first recognizing and binding to a specific DNA sequence and then coordinating the assembly of the transcription factors (Figure 5-10).

Inhibition of transcription is achieved by gene repressor proteins, which also recognize and bind specific DNA sequences but inhibit the assembly of transcription factors at the site. Some repressor proteins may work simply by binding to and physically blocking the promoter region, but most appear to exert their effects through more complex mechanisms, such as compacting the DNA to make it difficult to pry open, interfering with activator proteins, and binding up or inhibiting transcription factors. Inappropriate transcription of genes in a particular cell may have dire consequences for the cell or for the organism as a whole and is a carefully regulated process.

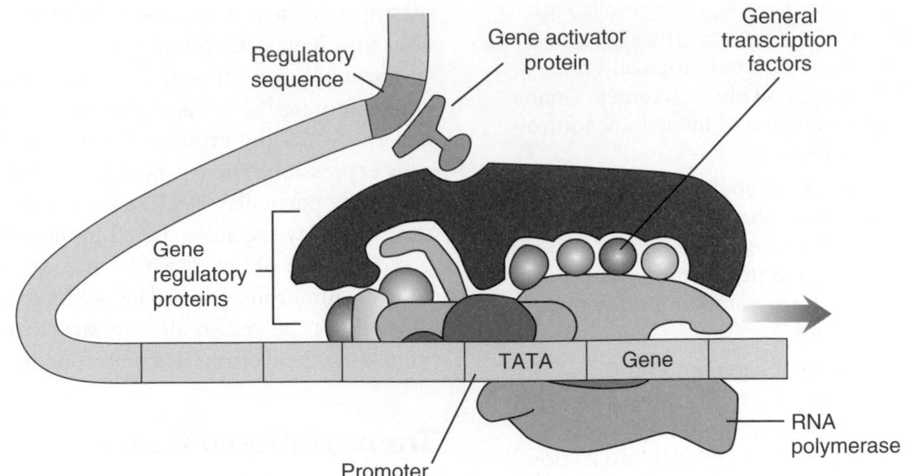

FIGURE 5-10 ■ Gene activator proteins coordinate the assembly of general transcription factors at the promoter region of the gene to be transcribed. RNA polymerase is unable to bind and begin transcription until the requisite transcription factors are in place.

KEY CONCEPTS

- All the cells in an individual have essentially the same DNA; however, cells differ greatly in structure and function. This occurs because genes are selectively expressed in particular cells.
- Gene expression can be regulated at any step in the pathway from DNA to RNA to protein synthesis. The most important regulators are transcriptional controls.
- A critical step for initiation of gene transcription is the assembly of general transcription factors at the promoter region of the gene.
- The actions of general transcription factors and RNA polymerase are controlled by a large number of regulatory proteins that specifically bind to DNA. The presence of certain DNA-binding proteins at specific sites can activate or repress the transcription of a particular gene in response to signals in the cell's environment.

DIFFERENTIATION OF TISSUES

Cell Diversification and Cell Memory

The cells of a multicellular organism tend to specialize so as to perform particular functions in coordination with other cells and tissues of the body. Cells not only must become different during development; they must also remain different in the adult, after the original cues for cell diversification have disappeared. The differences among cell types are ultimately due to the differentiating influences experienced in the embryo. Differences are maintained because the cells somehow remember the effects of those past influences and pass the memory on to their descendants. When a skin cell divides to replace lost skin cells, the daughter cells are also skin cells; when a liver cell divides, its daughter cells are liver cells; and so on. The behavior of cells of higher organisms is governed not only by their genome and their present environment, but also by their developmental history.

There is substantial evidence that the differences in tissue structure and function in a particular organism are not due to deletions or additions to the genome.[15] All of the cells of an organism contain essentially the same genes. Many genes are expressed in nearly all cell types (e.g., the so-called *housekeeping genes* that code for RNA and proteins essential for cell viability). It is the expression of a relatively few tissue-specific genes that results in differences among cell types.[11] The exact mechanisms leading to the stable expression of tissue-specific genes in particular cell types are largely unknown; however, differences in DNA packaging and the combination of gene regulatory proteins passed on during cell division are thought to be important. It is apparent that in order for a gene to be expressed, it must be accessible to the transcriptional machinery of the nucleus. The DNA in human cells is extensively packaged, so that 40 in. of linear DNA can be compacted to fit into the cell nucleus[1] (see Figure 5-4).

Some regions of DNA, called **heterochromatin,** are so condensed that they are not open to transcription. It is thought that the pattern of packaging as well as the DNA-binding proteins that regulate it are transmitted to progeny when a cell divides such that the pattern of gene expression is maintained in a sort of cell memory. An example of this mechanism is the inactivation of one of the X chromosomes in females.[16] In mammals, all female cells contain two X chromosomes (XX), whereas male cells contain an X and a Y chromosome (XY). One of the X chromosomes in females is permanently inactivated early in development by condensed packaging. This apparently occurs to prevent a double dose of the X gene products. Which of the two X chromosomes is inactivated in a particular cell is a random event. However, the same X chromosome will be inactive in all of the cell's progeny. The pattern of inactivated genes in a particular cell type is "remembered" in subsequent generations of cells and may explain how differentiated tissues remain differentiated in the adult.

Mechanisms of Development

Embryonic development is associated with selective gene expression that controls four essential processes to enable a single cell to develop into a complex organism: (1) cell proliferation, (2) cell differentiation, (3) cell-to-cell communication, and (4) cell movement and migration.[17] Very early in embryonic development, cells begin to divide asymmetrically so that daughter cells are not identical. Each time a cell divides it must retain memory of the developmental events that have preceded the division so that it can progress along a developmental pathway toward becoming a differentiated tissue. Interactions with nearby cells, chemical gradients and extracellular matrix components provide environmental clues to guide the cell to its appropriate form and location in the developing organism. Chemicals that control the patterning of fields of nearby tissue are termed **morphogens.** For example, cells in the head region may specialize to secrete a "position signal" for other cells. The morphogen is progressively degraded as it diffuses through the neighboring tissue such that it has higher concentration close to the source. A particular cell will have information regarding its proximity to the head region based on the surrounding concentration of the chemical. Morphogens are thought to be effective only over small distances. Thus the gross distinctions—between head and tail, for example—must be made very early in the embryo, and morphogens can provide only a general pattern for future development. Successive levels of detail can be filled in later by other positional signals.

The organization of molecules surrounding the cell surface also provides positional information. The extracellular matrix is composed of a large meshwork of molecules that is produced locally by cells in the area. Some common components include the proteins collagen and elastin, long polysaccharide chains called glycosaminoglycans, and a variety of peptides, growth factors, and hormones. The extracellular matrix is highly organized, with components binding to each other and to the cell membrane in specific ways. The extracellular matrix is thought to be important in cell development through its ability to screen or modulate the transport of molecules, such as growth factors, to the cell membrane and through direct contacts with the cell membrane that bring about changes in cell structure and function.[18]

The extracellular matrix surrounding the cells in different locations may provide positional information to cells that must migrate to their final destination.[18] In vertebrates, connective tissue cells appear to provide much of this positional information. As the migratory cell travels through the connective tissue, it may continually "test" the surroundings, searching for cues to guide it. Migratory cells with specific cell surface receptors may interact differentially with the extracellular matrix in different areas. In this way the migratory cell can be guided along particular paths and induced to settle in particular areas. Once the migratory cell has settled, local extracellular matrix molecules may further affect the cell's growth rate, differentiation, and likelihood of survival.

Interactions between the extracellular matrix and nearby cells are mediated primarily by binding proteins called **integrins.**[19] Integrins are transmembrane proteins that tie the cell's cytoskeleton to particular matrix structures. They enable the cytoskeleton and extracellular matrix to communicate across the plasma membrane in specific ways. In addition to inducing cells to bind in a particular location, integrins have been shown to activate intracellular signaling pathways, which may influence cell behavior in numerous ways (e.g., cell shape, polarity, metabolism, development, and differentiation).

The steps leading to the development of differentiated tissues in a multicellular organism are such that, once differentiated, a cell type generally does not revert to earlier forms. Some tissues are said to be terminally differentiated and have limited capacity to change form or replicate. Other tissues maintain less differentiated stem cells that are able to develop into a variety of cell types, depending on environmental cues.

Differentiated Tissues

The more than 200 different cell types in the adult human are generally classified into four major tissue categories: epithelium, connective tissue, muscle, and nerve.[20] The tissue types with some of their subtypes are summarized in Table 5-2. Most of the organ systems of the body are combinations of these four tissue types mixed together in a highly organized and cooperative manner.

Epithelial Tissue

Epithelial cells cover the majority of the external surfaces of the body and line the glands, blood vessels, and internal surfaces. Epithelial cells adopt a variety of shapes and functions, depending on their locations. For example, the *stratified* epithelium that makes up the epidermis of the skin is several layers thick and is primarily protective in function. New epithelial skin cells are formed from stem cells in the deepest part of the epidermis, where it contacts the basal lamina. As cells mature, they move outward toward the surface until they become keratinized and finally flake away (Figure 5-11). Keratin is a tough protective protein that is present in large quantities in the outer skin layers of flattened, dead epithelial cells. The epidermis in humans is completely replaced about once per month, but turnover can occur more rapidly after injury to the skin.[20]

In addition to stratified epithelium, the epithelium may be characterized as simple or pseudostratified according to the number and arrangement of cell layers (Figure 5-12). *Simple* epithelium consists of a single layer of cells, all of which contact the basement membrane. Simple epithelium is found in

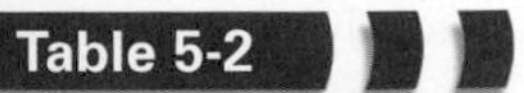

Table 5-2

Major Categories and Location of Body Tissues

Tissue Type	Locations
Epithelium	
Simple squamous	Lining of blood vessels, pulmonary alveoli, Bowman capsule
Simple cuboidal	Thyroid, sweat, and salivary glands; kidney tubules
Simple columnar	Lining of intestine, glandular ducts
Pseudostratified (mixed cell shapes)	Male urethra, respiratory passages
Stratified squamous	Skin, mucous membranes
Stratified columnar	Epiglottis, anus, parts of pharynx
Stratified transitional (layers of different cell shapes)	Bladder
Connective Tissue	
Loose	Widespread locations, dermis of skin, adipose, tissue organs
Dense/supportive	Cartilage, bone, tendons, joints, fascia surrounding muscles
Hematopoietic	Bone marrow, lymph tissue, plasma
Muscle	
Skeletal	Voluntary muscles of body
Cardiac	Heart (myocardium)
Smooth	Intestine, blood vessels, bladder, uterus, airways
Myoepithelial	Mammary, sweat, and salivary glands
Nervous	
Neurons	Central and peripheral nerves
Neuroglia	Primarily central nervous system

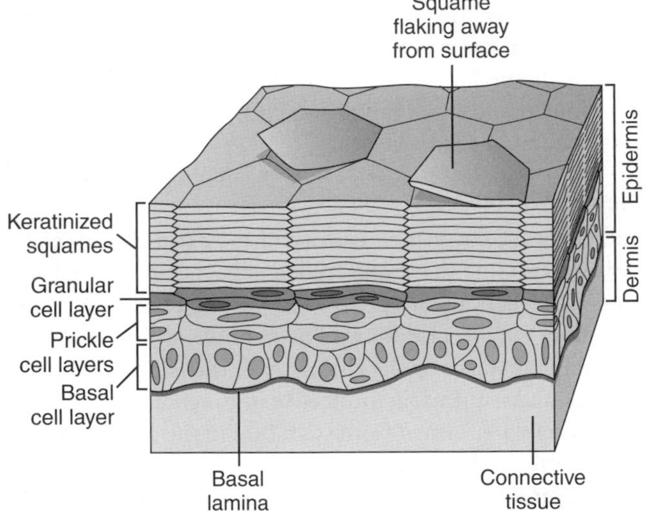

FIGURE 5-11 ■ Organization of epidermal skin layers, showing the flattened keratinized outer layer. Epithelial cells are continually produced by stem cells at the basal lamina and then migrate to the surface.

the lining of blood vessels and body cavities, in many glands, and in the alveoli of the lungs. The simple epithelium that lines the blood vessels is called endothelium. Simple epithelium also forms the kidney tubules and lines the intestine, where absorption is its primary function. *Stratified* epithelium consists of two or more layers of epithelial cells and is found in mucous membranes, such as the mouth, and in the skin, as mentioned previously. Epithelium that appears to be more than one layer thick because of a mixture of cell shapes but is actually a single layer is called *pseudostratified* epithelium. The linings of the respiratory tract and some glands contain pseudostratified epithelium.

Epithelial cells may also be classified according to cell shape. The three basic cell shapes are squamous, cuboidal, and columnar. Squamous cells are thin in comparison to their surface area and have a flattened appearance. Cuboidal cells are approximately equal in width and height, similar to a cube. Columnar cells are a bit taller than they are wide, resembling a rectangular column. Several classifications of epithelial tissue are given in Table 5-2 using both shape and layering as criteria.

Connective Tissue

Connective tissue is the most abundant and diverse tissue in the body, including cell types as different as bone cells, fat cells, and blood cells.[20] Connective tissue commonly functions as a scaffold on which other cells cluster to form organs, but it does much more than hold tissues together. Connective tissue cells often form an elaborate extracellular matrix, which is thought to be important in the maintenance of cell differentiation (Figure 5-13). Connective tissue cells play an important part in the support and repair of nearly every tissue and organ in the body. Three major classifications of connective tissue

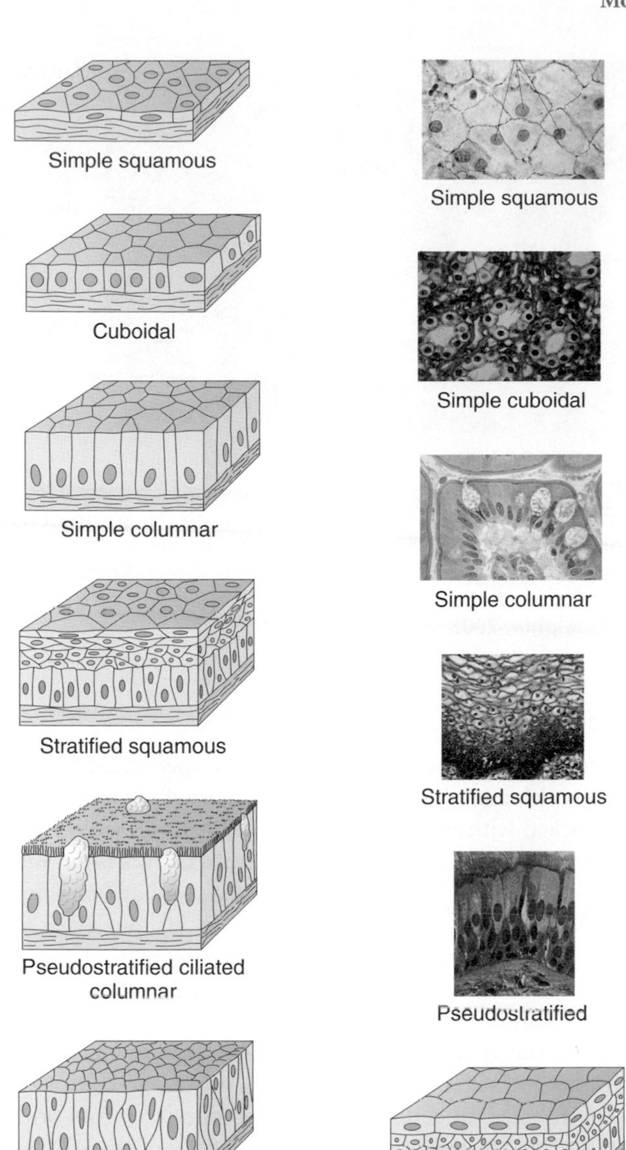

FIGURE 5-12 ■ Various epithelial tissue shapes and layering.

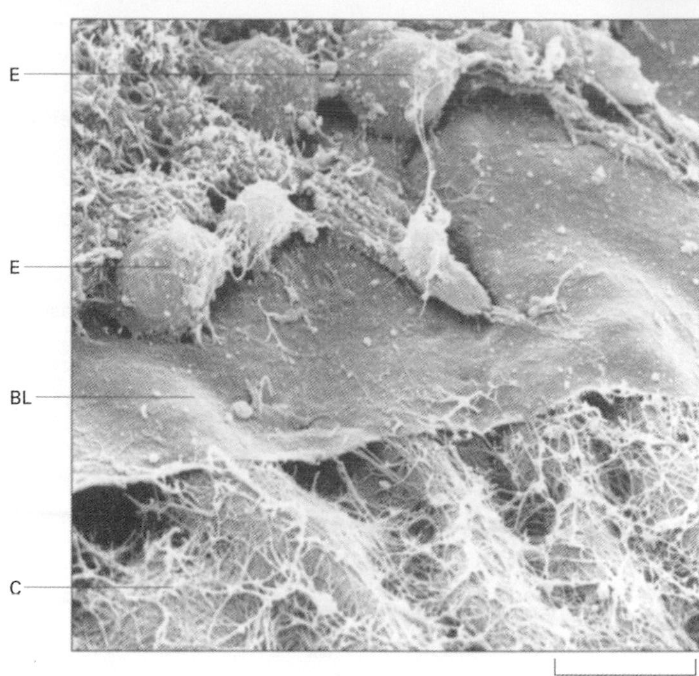

FIGURE 5-13 ■ Scanning electron micrograph of epithelial cells *(E)* attached to the basal lamina *(BL)* in the cornea of a chick embryo. Note the underlying network of loose connective tissue *(C)*. (From Alberts B et al, editors: *Molecular biology of the cell,* ed 4, New York, 2002, Garland Science, p 1297. Micrograph courtesy Robert Trelstad.)

are commonly identified: loose connective tissue, dense or supportive tissue, and hematopoietic tissue.

Loose connective tissue appears unstructured, with a fair amount of space between fibers of the extracellular matrix. The matrix contains a number of cell types and an elaborate meshwork of protein and other molecules (Figure 5-14). The primary protein constituents are collagen, elastin, and reticular fibers. Collagen is composed of tough, nonelastic bundles of protein fibers that are secreted by fibroblasts. It gives structural strength to skin, tendons, ligaments, and other tissues. The ability of a structure to withstand deforming and stretching forces is due, in large part, to elastin, which can return to its original length after being stretched, like a rubber band. Elastin is important to the function of structures such as the aorta, which must expand to accept the blood ejected from the heart during systole and bounce back to its original shape during diastole. Reticular fibers are short branching fibers that provide networks for the attachment of connective tissue to other cell types, such as epithelial cell attachments in glands, hematopoietic cells in bone marrow, and the parenchymal cells (functional cells) in organs. Cell types associated with loose connective tissue include the fibroblasts, mast cells, and adipocytes (fat cells).

Dense or supportive connective tissue is rich in collagen, which gives strength to structures such as cartilage, tendon, bone, and ligaments. The collagen fibers are more organized and densely packed than in loose connective tissue. Cartilage cells or chondrocytes may be found in the trachea, joints, nose, ears, vertebral disks, organs, and the young skeleton. Once formed, the collagenous extracellular matrix structures require little maintenance and do not receive a blood supply. Bone is a very dense form of connective tissue composed of a mixture of tough collagen fibers and solid calcium phosphate crystals in approximately equal proportions. Throughout the bone's hard extracellular matrix are channels and cavities occupied by living cells (osteocytes) (Figure 5-15). These cells incessantly model and remodel their bony environment, responding to environmental signals. These osteocytes are of two kinds: the cells that erode old bone are called *osteoclasts,* whereas the cells that form new bone are called *osteoblasts.* Osteoblasts detect when a bone is subjected to a greater load

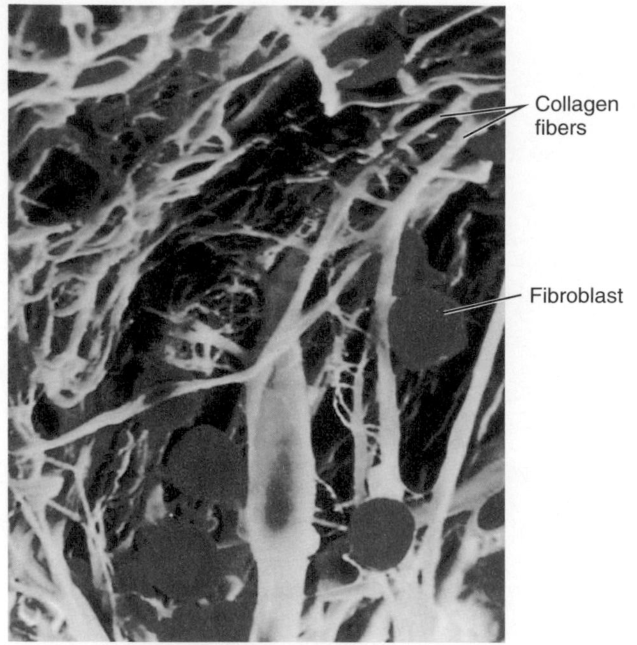

Loose connective tissue

FIGURE 5-14 ■ Scanning electron micrograph of fibroblasts in loose connective tissue of a rat cornea. The matrix is composed primarily of collagen fibers (magnification ×440). (From Solomon EP: *Introduction to human anatomy and physiology,* ed 2, Philadelphia, 2003, Saunders, p 34.)

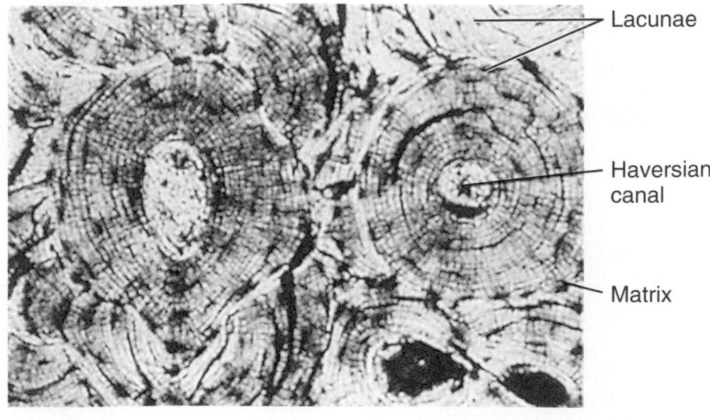

Bone

FIGURE 5-15 ■ Photomicrograph of a section of compact bone showing circular networks formed by the action of osteoclasts and osteoblasts as they remodel the bone. The osteocytes occupy the lacunae and canals. (From Solomon EP: *Introduction to human anatomy and physiology,* ed 2, Philadelphia, 2003, Saunders, p 34.)

stress and adapt by strengthening the bone mass. Conversely, when the load is removed as during bed rest, the osteoclasts busily digest the bone away, often resulting in some of the common complications of immobility. Osteoclasts, like macrophages, are derived from monocytes that are produced in the bone marrow. The monocytes travel via the blood stream and collect at sites of bone resorption, where they fuse together to become osteoclasts.[21] Osteocyte activity is essential for bone growth and the repair of bone injuries. (See Chapter 50 for a detailed description of the musculoskeletal system.)

The blood-forming organs of the body are formed by a specialized type of connective tissue called *hematopoietic* tissue. The blood cells include the red cell, or **erythrocyte,** which is specialized for the transport of oxygen; the platelet, or **thrombocyte,** which is important in blood coagulation; and a host of white cells, or **leukocytes,** which mediate immune function. Blood-forming tissue is located in the bone marrow, spleen, and lymphatic tissue. Hematopoietic cells are necessarily nomadic, traveling to distant areas of the body, sometimes settling in a particular organ, sometimes moving continuously (Figure 5-16). Blood cells have a short life span in comparison to other cells and must continually be replenished. This is accomplished by the hematopoietic stem cells. Stem cells reside primarily in the bone marrow and are pluripotent; they may differentiate into any of the blood cell types. This results in a system that can respond quickly to the changing needs of the body.

Muscle Tissue

The term *muscle* refers to tissues that are specialized for contraction. Muscle cells, or myocytes, are usually long and thin and packed with the proteins actin and myosin, which make up the contractile apparatus. In mammals, there are four main categories of muscle cells: skeletal, cardiac, smooth, and myoepithelial (Figure 5-17).[20] Contraction in all four types depends on intracellular calcium and occurs because of interactions between actin and myosin filaments. Actin and myosin filaments differ among cell types with regard to amino acid sequence, arrangement within the cell, and the mechanisms that control contraction. The mechanism of muscle contraction has been called the sliding filament hypothesis or cross-bridge theory. These terms describe the interactions of the actin and myosin filaments as they form bonds and pull past each other, causing the muscle cell to shorten. Contraction is initiated by an increase in intracellular free calcium and requires energy in the form of adenosine triphosphate (ATP). A detailed description of actin-myosin cross-bridging and the role of calcium, troponin, and tropomyosin can be found in Chapter 17.

Skeletal muscle is responsible for nearly all voluntary movements. Skeletal muscle cells fuse together to form long multinucleated fibers that can be huge, up to 0.5 m in length. Once fused and differentiated into mature skeletal muscle cells, they cannot enter the cell cycle and divide to produce new cells. Skeletal muscle stem cells (satellite cells) are retained in the muscle tissue and can proliferate in response to muscle damage. The actin and myosin proteins in skeletal muscle are aligned in orderly arrays, giving the tissue a striped appearance under the microscope, which in turn has led to the term *striated muscle.* Skeletal muscle contracts in response to stimulation from the motor neurons of the nervous system. As in other types of muscle, stimulation results in an increase in free calcium within the cell. In skeletal mus-

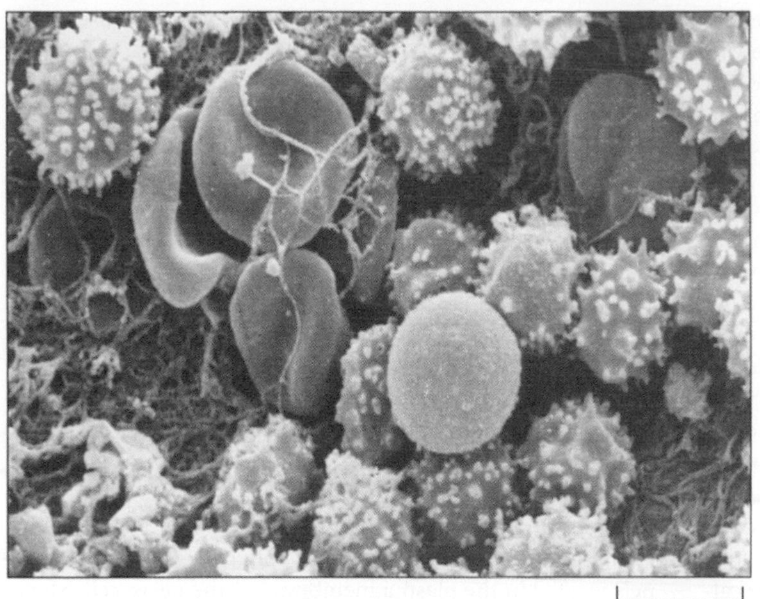

FIGURE 5-16 ■ Scanning electron micrograph of red and white blood cells in the lumen of a blood vessel. Red cells are smooth and concave, whereas white cells are rough and rounded. (From Alberts B et al, editors: *Molecular biology of the cell,* ed 4, New York, 2002, Garland Science, p 1284. Courtesy Ray Moss.)

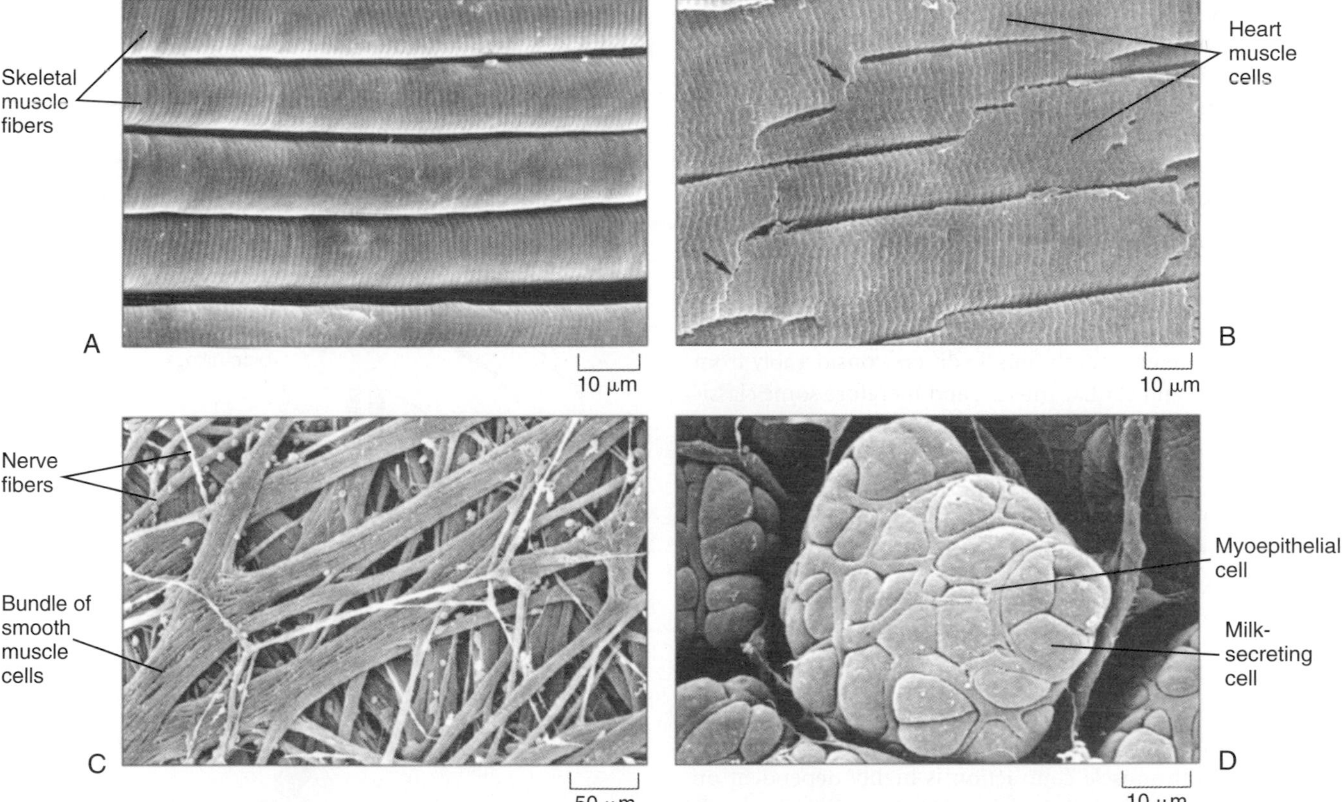

FIGURE 5-17 ■ The four classes of muscle cells. **A,** Skeletal muscle. **B,** Heart (cardiac) muscle. **C,** Smooth muscle (bladder). **D,** Myoepithelial cells in a mammary gland. (**A** and **C,** From Alberts B et al, editors: *Molecular biology of the cell,* ed 4, New York, 2002, Garland Science, p 1297. **A,** Courtesy Junzo Deskati. **B,** From Fujiwara T: Cardiac muscle. In Canal ED, editor: *Handbook of microscopic anatomy,* Berlin, 1986, Springer-Verlag. **C,** Courtesy Satoshi Nakasiro. **D,** From Nagato T et al: A scanning electron microscope study of myoepithelial cells in exocrine glands, *Cell Tissue Res* 209:1-10, 1980.)

cle, the calcium comes from internal storage sites in the sarcoplasmic reticulum. Contraction is initiated when the calcium binds troponin, a regulatory protein attached to the actin filament. Because of the high energy requirements of contracting skeletal muscle, the cells are packed with energy-producing mitochondria.

Like skeletal muscle, *cardiac muscle* also has a striated appearance due to the systematic organization of its actin and myosin filaments. Cardiac muscle cells are linked by special structures, called *intercalated disks,* that cause the tissue to behave as a **syncytium:** all of the cells contract synchronously. Cardiac muscle contracts in response to autonomic innervation and blood-borne chemicals, but it also has the special property of automaticity. Automaticity refers to the inherent ability of the cell to initiate a contraction without outside stimulation. The contractile mechanisms of cardiac muscle are similar to those of skeletal muscle, requiring free calcium to interact with troponin, resulting in the formation of actin-myosin cross-bridges. In cardiac muscle, some of the free calcium comes from the sarcoplasmic reticulum, but diffusion into the cell through channels in the cell membrane is also necessary. These membrane calcium channels represent an important difference from skeletal muscle, as they can be manipulated by drugs (calcium channel blockers) without disrupting skeletal muscle control. (Cardiac muscle is discussed in Chapter 17.)

Smooth muscle comprises a diverse group of tissues located in organs throughout the body. Smooth muscle generally is not under voluntary control and therefore is called *involuntary muscle.* Some types of smooth muscle are able to contract intrinsically, and most are influenced by the autonomic nervous system. Smooth muscle is found in blood vessels and in the walls of hollow organs such as those of the gastrointestinal tract, uterus, and large airways.

The structure of smooth muscle differs considerably from that of skeletal and cardiac muscle, and therefore some classification schemes consider it to be a member of the connective tissue family.[20] The actin and myosin filaments are less organized in smooth muscle, and the muscle does not have striations. Smooth muscle contraction tends to be slower and can be maintained indefinitely. This is critical to the function of blood vessels, which must maintain a degree of contraction or vascular tone to maintain the blood pressure. Smooth muscle differs in the way actin-myosin cross-bridges are formed and in the calcium-binding regulatory proteins. When calmodulin, the calcium-binding protein in smooth muscle, binds calcium, it stimulates the rate of cross-bridge formation by myosin. Smooth muscle contraction is highly dependent on the diffusion of extracellular calcium into the cell through calcium channels in the plasma membrane (sarcolemma). Thus, like cardiac muscle, smooth muscle can also be affected by drugs that alter the calcium channel's ability to conduct calcium. For example, calcium channel–blocking drugs are used to cause the smooth muscle in arterial blood vessels to relax as a treatment for high blood pressure.

Myoepithelial cells represent the fourth class of muscle cells. They are located in the ducts of some glands (e.g., mammary, sweat, and salivary). Unlike all other types of muscle, myoepithelial cells lie in the epithelium and are derived from embryonic ectoderm, whereas skeletal, cardiac, and smooth muscle are derived from embryonic mesoderm. Myoepithelial cells contract in response to specific stimuli (e.g., oxytocin in the mammary gland) and serve to expel the contents from the gland.

Nervous Tissue

Nervous tissue is widely distributed throughout the body, providing a rapid communication network between the central nervous system and various body parts. Nerve cells are specialized to generate and transmit electrical impulses very rapidly. Like muscle, nerves are excitable; they respond to stimulation by altering their electrical potentials. This excitability is due to the presence of voltage-sensitive ion channels located in the plasma membrane of the nerve cell. Move-

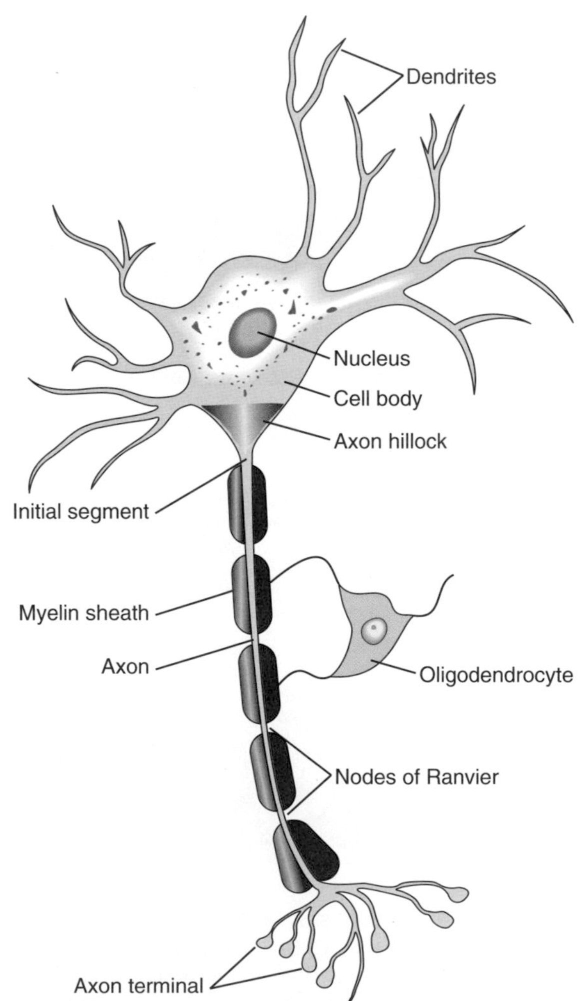

FIGURE 5-18 ■ Diagram of a typical neuron showing the cell body, axon, and dendrites. Neurons have many shapes and sizes.

ment of ions through these channels results in the production and propagation of action potentials along the length of the neuron. Neurons communicate their action potentials to other nerve and muscle cells through synapses. At the synapse, the presynaptic neuron releases a chemical neurotransmitter into the space between itself and the next neuron, where it diffuses across and interacts with the postsynaptic neuron.

A typical neuron is composed of three parts: a cell body, an axon, and one or more dendrites (Figure 5-18). The cell body contains the nucleus and other cytoplasmic organelles. The axon is generally long (as long as 1 m) and may be encased in a myelin sheath. The axons usually conduct impulses away from the cell body, whereas the dendritic processes usually receive information and conduct impulses toward the cell body. Neurons are classified on the basis of the number of projections extending from the cell body. Neurons are terminally differentiated and incapable of replicating. However, some neural stem cells are located in certain areas of the brain and may replicate to form either neurons or glial cells in response to specific signals (see Chapter 43).

In addition to neurons, nervous tissue contains a variety of supportive cells, termed **neuroglia** ("nerve glue"), that nourish, protect, insulate, and clean up debris in the central nervous system. These include the astrocytes, oligodendroglia, ependymal cells, and microglia. (See Chapter 43 for a detailed description of nervous system anatomy and physiology.)

KEY CONCEPTS

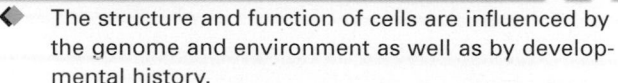

- The structure and function of cells are influenced by the genome and environment as well as by developmental history.
- Embryonic development is associated with selective gene expression that controls four essential processes to enable a single cell to develop into a complex organism: (1) cell proliferation; (2) cell differentiation; (3) cell-to-cell communication; and (4) cell movement and migration.
- Differentiated cell types have different capacities to divide. Some tissues, such as nerve and cardiac muscle, are terminally differentiated and have limited ability to divide. Other cell types, such as skin and bone marrow, maintain more stem cells, which have great capacity to proliferate.
- Different cell types in the adult human are classified into four major categories: epithelium (e.g., skin, glands, endothelium), connective tissue (e.g., bone, cartilage, fat, blood), muscle (e.g., skeletal, cardiac, smooth), and nervous tissue (e.g., neuronal, glial).

SUMMARY

The development, differentiation, and day-to-day activities of a cell are directed by its genes. Genes are sequences of nucleotides that provide the template for the production of cellular proteins. In large part, the kinds and amounts of cellular proteins determine cell structure and function. All of the cells of the body possess essentially the same DNA, but through complex processes of differentiation they become specialized to perform particular functions. It is believed that different sets of genes are active in different cell types. The four major classes of differentiated tissues are epithelial, connective, muscle, and nerve. These four tissues interdependently form the functioning systems of the body.

MEDIA RESOURCES

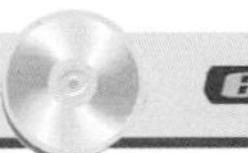

evolve

Remember to check out the ***CD Companion*** included with this book for Review Questions, Key Concepts Review, Glossary (with audio for selected terms), Disease Profiles, and Animations.

PLUS, visit the ***Evolve website*** at http://evolve.elsevier.com/Copstead/ for Case Studies, Disease Profiles, and WebLinks.

References

1. Alberts B et al: DNA and chromosomes. In Alberts B et al, editors: *Molecular biology of the cell,* ed 4, New York, 2002, Garland Science, pp 191-234.
2. Watson JD, Crick FHC: Molecular structure of nucleic acids: a structure for deoxyribose nucleic acid, *Nature* 171:737-738, 1953.
3. Hubscher U, Seo YS: Replication of the lagging strand: a concert of at least 23 polypeptides, *Mol Cell* 12(2):149-157, 2001.
4. Alberts B et al: DNA replication, repair and recombination. In Alberts B et al, editors: *Molecular biology of the cell,* ed 4, New York, 2002, Garland Science, pp 235-298.
5. Kunkel TA, Bebenek K: DNA replication fidelity, *Annu Rev Biochem* 69:497-529, 2000.
6. Crick FHC: The genetic code: III, *Sci Am* 215(4):55-62, 1966.
7. Frisch L, editor: The genetic code. In *Cold Spring Harbor symposia on quantitative biology,* Cold Spring Harbor, NY, 1966, Cold Spring Harbor Laboratory.
8. Alberts B et al: How cells read the genome from DNA to protein. In Alberts B et al, editors: *Molecular biology of the cell,* ed 4, New York, 2002, Garland Science, pp 299-374.
9. Gravely BR: Sorting out the complexity of SR functions, *RNA* 6(9):1197-1211, 2000.
10. Frank J: The ribosome: a macromolecular machine par excellence, *Chem Biol* 7:R133-R141, 2000.
11. Alberts B et al: Control of gene expression. In Alberts B et al, editors: *Molecular biology of the cell,* ed 4, New York, 2002, Garland Science, pp 375-466.
12. Emerson BM: Specificity of gene regulation, *Cell* 109(3): 267-270, 2003.
13. Hochheimer A, Tjian R: Diversified transcription initiation complexes expand promoter selectivity and tissue-specific gene expression, *Genes Dev* 17(11):1309-1320, 2003.
14. Warren AJ: Eucaryotic transcription factors, *Curr Opin Struct Biol* 12(1):107-114, 2002.
15. Gurdon JB: The developmental capacity of nuclei taken from intestinal epithelium cells of feeding tadpoles, *J Embryol Exp Morphol* 10:622-640, 1962.

16. Lyon MF: X-chromosome inactivation and human genetic disease, *Acta Paediatr Suppl* 91(439):107-112, 2002.
17. Alberts B et al: Development of multicellular organisms. In Alberts B et al, editors: *Molecular biology of the cell,* ed 4, New York, 2002, Garland Science, pp 1157-1258.
18. Holly SP, Larson MK, Parise LV: Multiple roles of integrins in cell motility, *Exp Cell Res* 261(1):69-74, 2000.
19. Bokel C, Brown NH: Integrins in development: moving on, responding to, and sticking to the extracellular matrix, *Dev Cell* 3:311-321, 2002.
20. Alberts B et al: Histology: the lives and deaths of cells in tissues. In Alberts B et al, editors: *Molecular biology of the cell,* ed 4, New York, 2002, Garland Science, pp 1259-1312.
21. Yang TT et al: Human mesenchymal tumour-associated macrophages differentiate into osteoclastic bone-resorbing cells, *J Bone Joint Surg Br* 84(3):452-456, 2002.

chapter 6

Genetic and Developmental Disorders

Jacquelyn L. Banasik

MEDIA RESOURCES

Additional Material for Study, Review, and Further Exploration

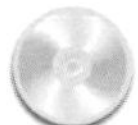

CD Companion ◆ Review Questions and Answers ◆ Key Concepts Review
◆ Glossary *(with audio pronunciations for selected terms)*
◆ Disease Profiles ◆ Animations

evolve *Website* at http://evolve.elsevier.com/Copstead/
◆ Case Studies ◆ Disease Profiles ◆ WebLinks

KEY QUESTIONS

- How are genes transmitted from parent to offspring?
- How is pedigree analysis used to determine if a trait is inherited as autosomal dominant, autosomal recessive, or X-linked?
- How might abnormal meiosis lead to alterations in chromosome number or structure?
- What are the inheritance patterns and general clinical features of some common genetic disorders?
- What is the role of the environment in development of congenital disorders?
- What methods of genetic testing are available?

CHAPTER OUTLINE

Geneticists and parents alike have marveled at the development of a recognizable human baby, with eyes and ears, toes and fingers, from its simple beginning as a single cell containing one set of genes. Considering the enormous list of potentially disastrous genetic and environmental influences, the birth of a healthy normal child does indeed seem like a miracle. Although the risk of bearing a child with mental or physical defects is small for most parents, it is real and is often a source of worry during the prenatal period. It has been estimated that most people harbor one or two defective genes that are recessive and therefore of little consequence until they are transmitted to offspring.[1] In addition, there are many known and unknown environmental hazards to which the parent and fetus may be exposed. Structural defects that are due to errors in development and are present at birth are called **congenital malformations.** It is estimated that about 3% of newborns have a major malformation of cosmetic or functional significance.[2] Based on birth statistics in 2002,[3] it is estimated that each year in the United States more than 120,000 infants are born with physical or mental damage.

Congenital disorders are generally grouped according to genetic or environmental causes. Approximately one half of all birth malformations have no identifiable cause.[4] In this chapter, the general principles of inheritance, genetic and environmental causes of congenital disorders, and the principles of diagnosis, counseling, and gene therapy are described.

PRINCIPLES OF INHERITANCE

"Whom does the baby look like?" is frequently asked of new parents. It is common knowledge that traits tend to run in families, but Gregor Mendel, a 19th century monk turned geneticist, was the first to notice that traits were transmitted in a predictable way from parent to offspring.[5] Height, weight, skin color, eye color, and hair color are some of the physical traits that characterize an individual. **Phenotype** refers to the physical and biochemical attributes of an individual that are outwardly apparent. These traits are a result of the expression of the individual's unique genetic makeup, or **genotype.** In humans, these genes are organized into 46 different chromosome units that become visible under the microscope only during cell division.

During meiosis, chromosomes look like Xs of varying sizes and shapes. The X-shaped chromosome is really made up of two identical linear chromosome units, called **chromatids,** which separate during meiosis. The point at the middle of the X at which the two sister chromatids are joined together is the **centromere** (Figure 6-1). Human chromosomes are **diploid;** they occur as pairs. One member of the pair comes from the mother and one member comes from the father. Under the microscope the members of a pair appear to be identical (**homologous**) although they are different in DNA sequence. Chromosomes are characterized on the basis of total size, length of the arms of the X, and their characteristic banding patterns when exposed to certain stains (karyotype) (Figure 6-2).

Of the 23 pairs of chromosomes, 22 are homologous and are called **autosomes.** The remaining pair, the **sex** chromosomes, differs in males and females. Females receive an X chromosome from each parent (homologous), whereas males receive an X chromosome from their mothers and a Y chromosome from their fathers (hemizygous). Thus, the genotype is a result of the union of 23 maternal and 23 paternal chromosomes at conception. Sexual reproduction allows the mixing of genomes from two different individuals to produce offspring that differ genetically from one another and from their parents. This source of genetic variability is advantageous to the species because it allows for adaptation and evolution in a changing environment.

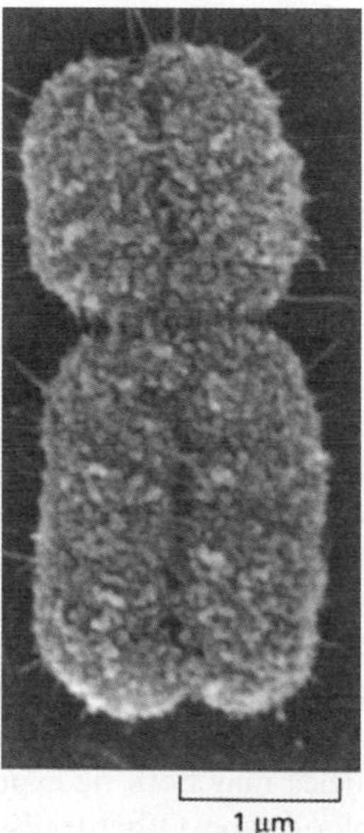

FIGURE 6-1 ■ Scanning electron micrograph of a chromosome showing the two sister chromatids attached at the centromere. Sister chromatids separate during meiosis with one chromatid being distributed to each daughter cell. (From Alberts B et al, editors: *Molecular biology of the cell,* ed 4, New York, 2002, Garland Science, p 206. Courtesy Terry D. Allen.)

For two germ cells (egg and sperm) to combine to form a cell with the normal complement of 46 chromosomes (23 pairs), each germ cell must contribute only half of the total. **Meiosis** refers to this special form of cell division, which results in germ cells that are **haploid;** they have half of the normal number of chromosomes. In contrast to mitosis (see Chapter 3), meiosis involves two divisions of the chromosomal DNA. A comparison of meiotic and mitotic cell division is shown in Figure 6-3.

During the first phase of meiosis, duplicated sister chromatids come in close contact with their homologous pairs. Portions of the homologous chromosomes are exchanged in a process called *crossing over* (Figure 6-4). This results in a mixing of the maternal and paternal genes of the cell to form a new combination of genes within the chromosomes. Genetic recombination is very precise, such that genes are exchanged intact and not interrupted in the middle. On average, each homologous pair of chromosomes has two or three crossover events occurring during the first meiotic division.[6] The first cellular division of meiosis results in two cells, each with 46 chromosomes. These two cells undergo a second division in which the sister chromatids are pulled apart (similar to normal mitosis), resulting in four cells, each having only 23 chromosomes. Each of the germ cells has a different combination of genes that, when passed on through sexual reproduction, will form a new, genetically unique individual.

The genes that code for a particular trait, such as eye color, are located at a particular position (locus) on the chromosome and come in several forms, or **alleles.** In the case of eye color, there are two common alleles, blue and brown. A person actually has two alleles for each gene, one received from each parent. If both alleles for a trait are identical, the individual is **homozygous** for that trait. If two different alleles are present, the individual is **heterozygous** for the trait. Using the eye color example again, if an individual receives a blue eye color allele from each parent, he or she is homozygous for eye color. If a blue eye color allele is received from one parent and a brown eye color allele is received from the other parent, the individual is heterozygous for that trait.

Some traits, like eye color, involve only one gene locus and are called single-gene traits. (Variations in shade may be determined by other genes.) The transmission of single-gene traits from parent to offspring follows predictable patterns that can be demonstrated using the Punnett square (Figure 6-5). In the Punnett square, the alleles for a gene are repre-

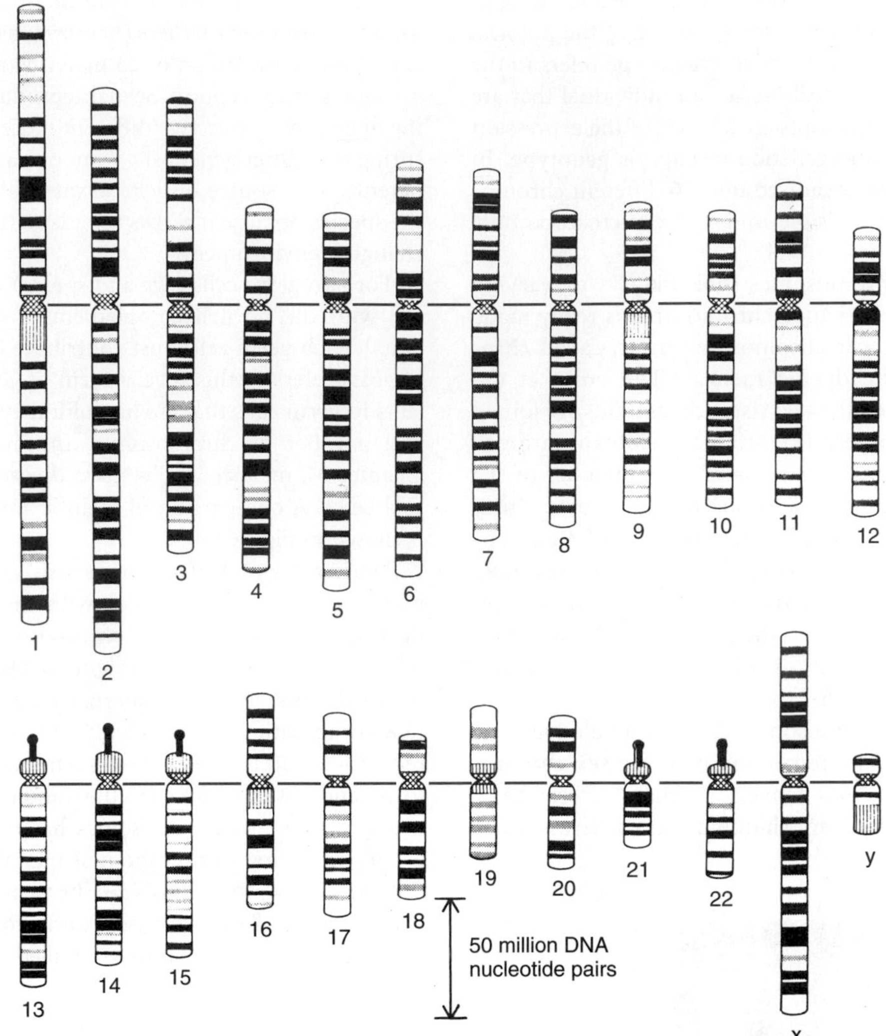

FIGURE 6-2 ■ A standard map of the banding pattern of each of the 23 chromosomes of the human. Somatic cells contain two copies of each chromosome. The centromere region is marked by the line. (From Alberts B et al, editors: *Molecular biology of the cell,* ed 4, New York, 2002, Garland Science, p 199.)

sented by capital and lowercase letters. The capital letter represents the **dominant** allele and the lowercase letter is the **recessive** allele. As the term implies, the trait of the dominant allele is apparent and will mask the recessive allele. A recessive trait is apparent only if *both* alleles for the trait are recessive (homozygous). Dominant genes often code for functional enzymes or structural proteins and recessive genes code for nonfunctional ones. The Punnett square is based on the mendelian principle that all genes are independent and will be inherited in a random manner. Thus, if both parents are heterozygous for a dominant trait (Aa), the offspring will have a 25% probability of being AA, a 50% probability of being Aa, and a 25% probability of being aa. Persons having the AA and Aa genotypes will *express* the trait in a similar manner. The trait will be absent in the aa genotype. Many genetic diseases are carried in the recessive allele and are manifested only by the homozygous (aa) genotype. Persons who are heterozygous for the disease (Aa) are said to be **carriers** because they are able to pass the defective recessive gene to their offspring even though they do not exhibit the trait.

Some alleles are not clearly dominant or recessive and result in a blending or *codominant* expression of the trait. Blood type, for example, has three distinct alleles: A, B, and O. The A and B alleles may both be expressed together, resulting in the AB blood type. Other traits result from the interaction of several gene loci and are called **polygenic** or multifactorial. Polygenic traits are heritable, but predicting their occurrence is more difficult. Polygenic traits are often affected by environmental factors. As examples, height, weight, and blood pressure are polygenic traits; however, dietary intake certainly influences the ultimate expression of these genes.

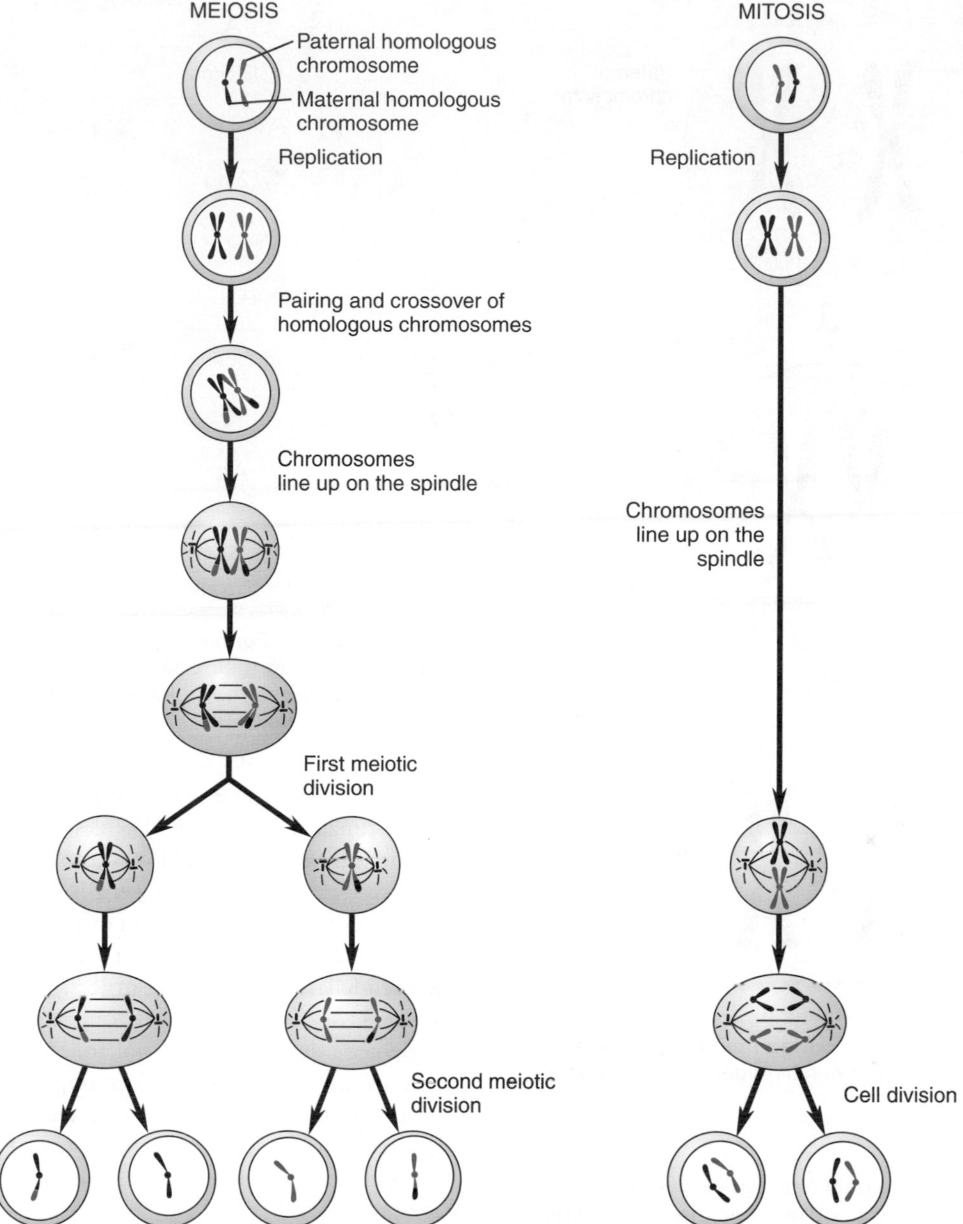

FIGURE 6-3 ■ A comparison of meiosis and normal mitotic cell division, showing only one homologous chromosome pair. In meiosis, the homologous chromosomes form a pair and exchange sections of DNA in a process called *crossing over.* Two nuclear divisions are required in meiosis to form the haploid germ cells.

KEY CONCEPTS

- Human DNA is organized into 46 chromosomes (23 pairs). Paired chromosomes look similar under the microscope but differ in DNA sequence. One member of each pair is inherited from the mother, the other from the father.
- Twenty-two pairs of chromosomes are autosomes. The remaining pair, the sex chromosomes, confers maleness (XY) or femaleness (XX).
- During meiotic cell division, the chromosomes are distributed to daughter cells. Meiosis results in four daughter cells, each having one-half the normal number of chromosomes (23).
- Genes that code for a particular trait come in several forms or alleles. Genotype refers to the particular set of alleles an individual receives. Phenotype refers to an individual's observable attributes. People with different genotypes may have similar phenotypes.

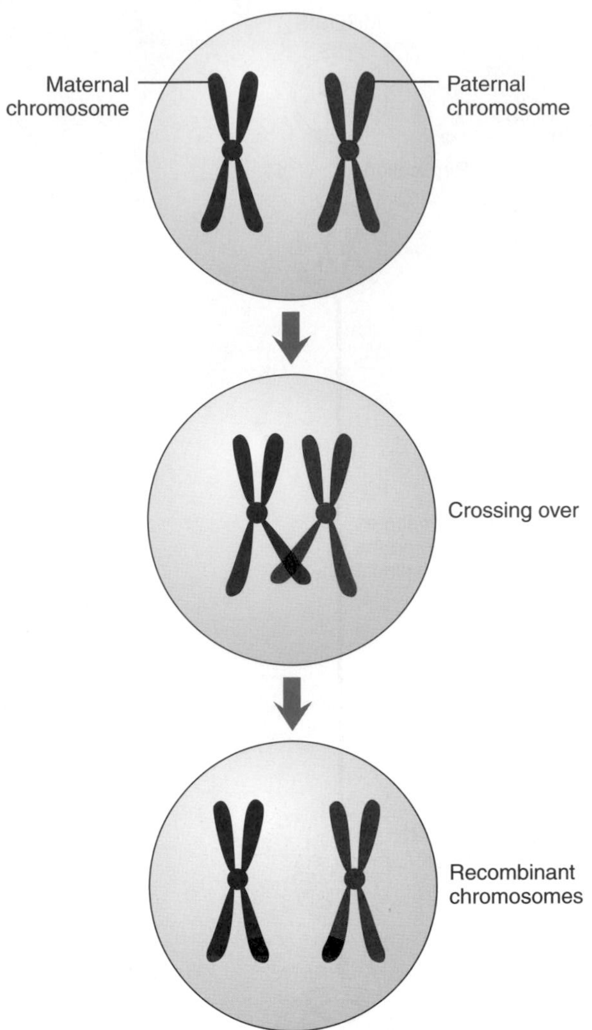

FIGURE 6-4 ■ Crossing over during meiotic prophase I results in a reassortment of genes between homologous chromosomes.

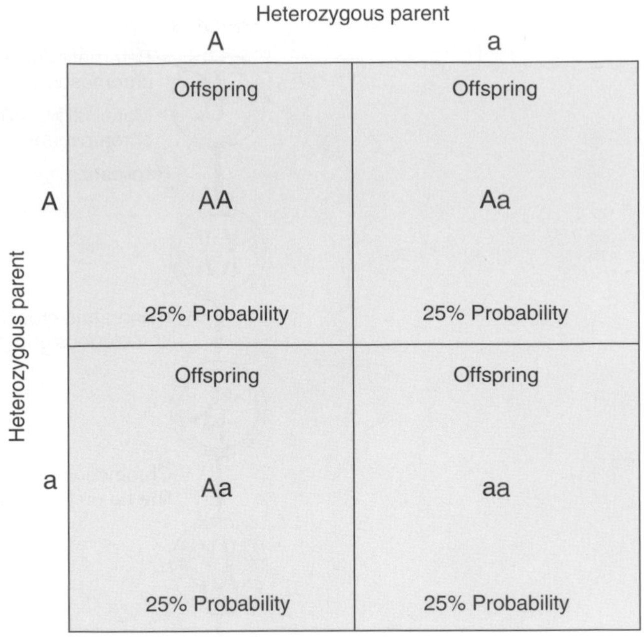

Heterozygous parent (columns) × Heterozygous parent (rows)

	A	a
A	Offspring AA 25% Probability	Offspring Aa 25% Probability
a	Offspring Aa 25% Probability	Offspring aa 25% Probability

FIGURE 6-5 ■ A Punnett square shows the distribution of parental genes to their offspring. This example shows the mating of two heterozygous individuals. *A,* Dominant genes; *a,* recessive genes.

◆ Some traits involve only one gene locus and are called single-gene traits. The transmission of these traits from parent to offspring follows predictable patterns. The expression of single-gene traits is determined by whether the gene is dominant or recessive. Dominant genes usually code for functional enzymes; recessive genes do not. Traits resulting from the interaction of several genes are polygenic and do not follow predictable patterns of inheritance.

GENETIC DISORDERS

Genetic disorders may be apparent at birth or may not be clinically evident until much later in life. The great majority of genetic disorders are inherited from the affected individual's parents. However, 15% to 20% represent new mutations that arise during fetal development.[4] The genetic disorders encountered clinically are only a small percentage of those that occur, representing the less extreme aberrations that permit live birth. It has been estimated that about 50% of spontaneous first-trimester abortions have demonstrable chromosomal abnormalities, and many more may have hidden genetic defects.[4]

Disorders that are genetic in origin traditionally have been divided into three groups: (1) chromosomal aberrations, (2) mendelian single-gene disorders, and (3) multifactorial or polygenic disorders. A fourth group encompasses a number of single-gene defects that do not follow the classic mendelian patterns of inheritance. This group includes triplet-repeat mutations, mitochondrial gene mutations, and mutations influenced by genomic imprinting. General principles of transmission and selected examples are included for each of the four groups.

CHROMOSOMAL ABNORMALITIES

Chromosomal defects are generally due to an abnormal number of chromosomes or alterations in the structure of one or more chromosomes. These defects usually result from errors in the separation or crossing over of chromosomes during meiosis or mitosis. Approximately 1 in 200 newborn infants has some form of chromosomal abnormality.[4]

Aberrant Number of Chromosomes

The union of sperm and egg results in a fertilized egg (zygote) with the full complement of 46 chromosomes: 22 pairs of autosomes and 2 sex chromosomes (euploid). **Aneuploidy** refers to an abnormal number of chromosomes—in humans, either more or less than 46. The usual causes of aneuploidy are

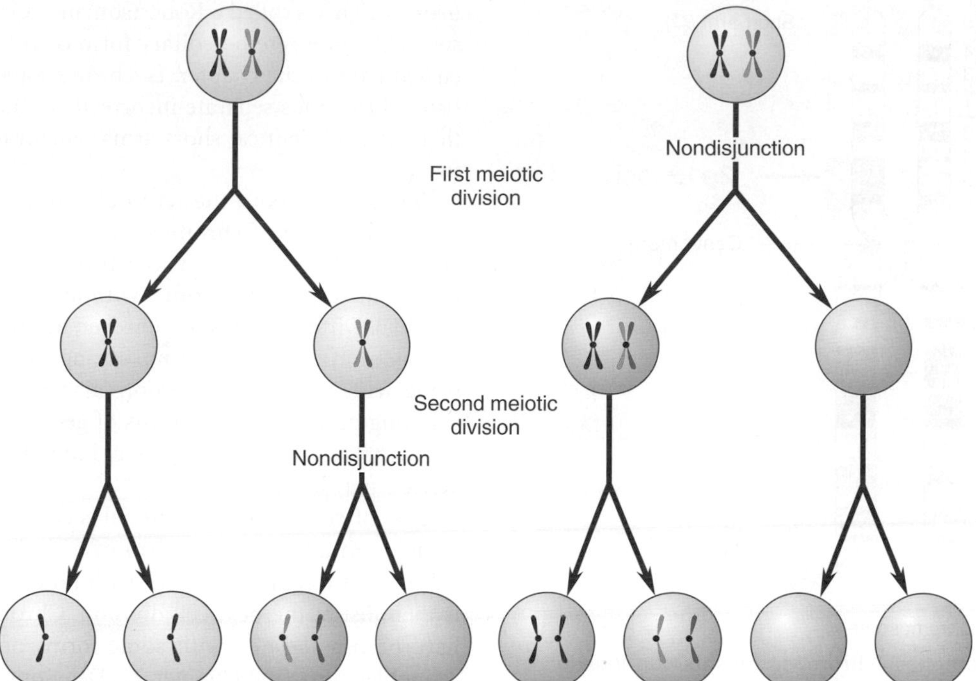

FIGURE 6-6 ■ Mechanism of nondisjunction leading to aneuploidy. For simplicity, only one pair of chromosomes is shown.

nondisjunction and anaphase lag.[7] **Nondisjunction** means that the paired homologous chromosomes fail to separate normally during either the first or second meiotic division (Figure 6-6). The resulting germ cells then have an abnormal number of chromosomes: one will have 22 chromosomes and one will have 24. When the chromosomes from the abnormal germ cell are combined with a normal germ cell containing 23 chromosomes, the fertilized cell will either be deficient by one chromosome (45) or have an extra chromosome (47). In anaphase lag, one chromosome lags behind and is therefore left out of the newly formed cell nucleus. This results in one daughter cell with the normal number of chromosomes and one with a deficiency of one chromosome, a condition called **monosomy. Polysomy** refers to the condition of having too many chromosomes.

The causes of abnormalities in chromosome number are poorly understood. Radiation, viruses, and chemicals have been implicated because they can interfere with mitosis and meiosis in experimental animals. Their role in causing aneuploidy in humans is unproved. Two conditions are known to increase the risk of abnormalities in chromosome number in humans: advanced maternal age and abnormalities in parental chromosome structure.[8] There is no precise explanation for the higher risk of nondisjunction with these conditions.

In general, monosomy involving the autosomes is not compatible with life. Autosomal polysomy may result in a viable fetus. The extra autosomal chromosomes are nearly always associated with severe disabilities. Disorders involving extra or missing sex chromosomes are more common and less debilitating.

Abnormal Chromosome Structure

Alterations in chromosome structure are usually due to breakage and loss or rearrangement of pieces of the chromosomes during meiosis or mitosis. During meiosis, the homologous chromosomes normally pair up and exchange genetic alleles in a process called crossing over. Normal crossing over involves precise gene exchange between homologues only, with no net gain or loss of DNA. When the normal process of crossing over goes awry, portions of chromosomes may be lost, attached upside down, or attached to the wrong chromosome. Mitosis also presents opportunities for chromosomal breakage and rearrangement. The severity of the chromosomal rearrangement ranges from insignificant to lethal, depending on the number and importance of the gene loci involved. Gene locations can be described by their location on the long arm (q arm) or the short arm (p arm) of the chromatid. For example, the gene locus 2p13 is located on the short arm of chromosome 2 at region 1, band 3 (Figure 6-7). The common types of chromosomal rearrangements are translocations, inversions, deletions, and duplications (Figure 6-8).

Chromosomal *translocations* result from the exchange of pieces of DNA between nonhomologous chromosomes. If no genetic material is lost, as in a reciprocal translocation, the individual may have no symptoms of the disorder. However, an individual with a reciprocal translocation is at increased risk of producing abnormal gametes. The exchange of a long chromatid arm for a short one results in the formation of one very large chromosome and one very small chromosome (see Fig-

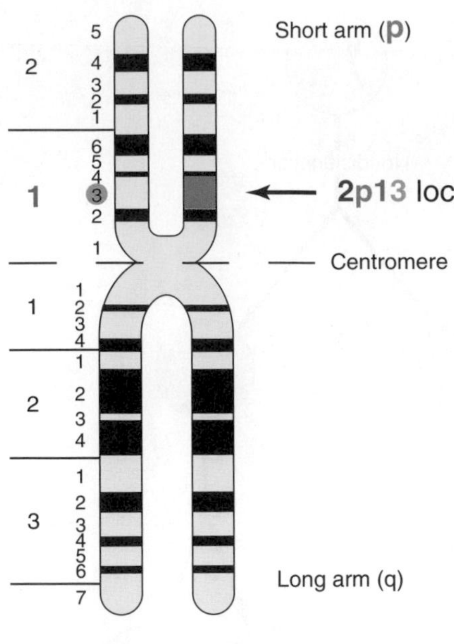

FIGURE 6-7 ■ Metaphase chromosome showing location of centromere and long and short arms of the chromatids. Gene loci are described by the chromosome number, location on short *(p)* or long *(q)* arm, region, and band.

ure 6-8). This is called a Robertsonian translocation and is responsible for a rare hereditary form of Down syndrome, discussed later in the chapter. Isochromosomes occur when the sister chromatids separate incorrectly at the centromere such that the two identical short arms remain together, as do the two long arms.

Inversion refers to the removal and upside-down reinsertion of a section of chromosome (see Figure 6-8). Like balanced translocations, inversions involve no net loss or gain of genetic material and are often without consequence to the individual. Difficulties result, however, when homologous chromosomes attempt to pair up during meiosis. The chromosome with an inverted section may not pair up properly, resulting in duplications or loss of genes at the time of crossing over. Thus, the offspring of an individual harboring an inversion may be affected.

Loss of chromosomal material is called *deletion.* Deletions result from a break in the arm of a single chromosome, resulting in a fragment of DNA with no centromere. The piece is then lost at the next cell division. Chromosomal deletions have been associated with some forms of cancer, including retinoblastoma (see Chapter 7). Deletions at both ends of a chromatid may cause the free ends to attach to one another, forming a ring chromosome.

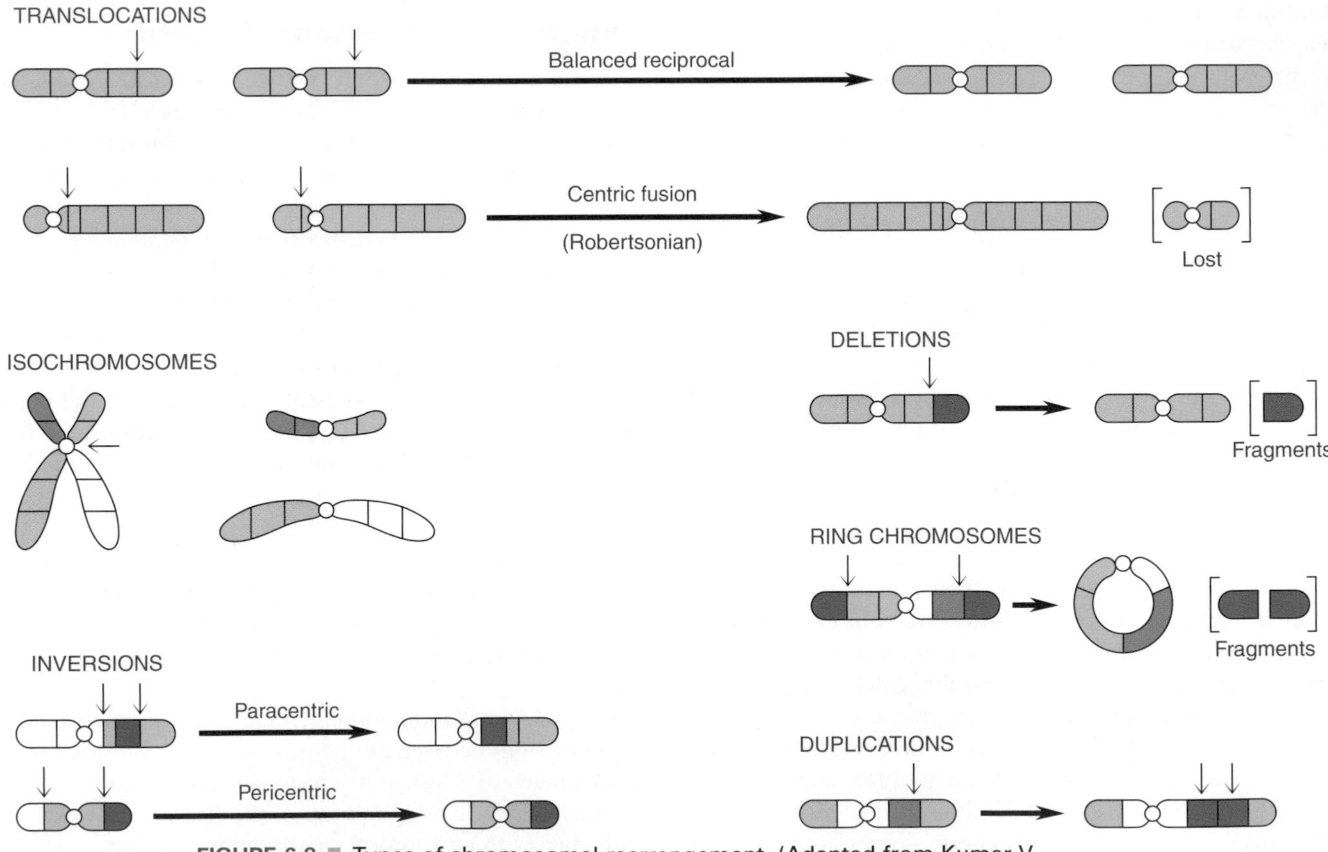

FIGURE 6-8 ■ Types of chromosomal rearrangement. (Adapted from Kumar V, Cotran RS, Robbins ST: *Robbins basic pathology,* ed 7, Philadelphia, 2003, Saunders, p 229.)

In contrast to a deletion, where genes are lost, *duplication* results in extra copies of a portion of DNA. The consequences of duplications are generally less severe than those from loss of genetic material.

Examples of Autosomal Chromosome Disorders

Trisomy 21 (Down Syndrome)

Trisomy 21 is a chromosomal disorder in which individuals have an extra 21st chromosome. It is the most common of the chromosomal disorders and a leading cause of mental retardation, occurring in about 1 in 700 live births.[9] A lower incidence of about 1 in 1000 live births has been reported in many countries because of a trend toward prenatal diagnosis and termination of pregnancies.[9] The syndrome, first described by Langdon Down in 1866,[10] includes mental retardation, protruding tongue, low-set ears, epicanthal folds, poor muscle tone, and short stature (Figure 6-9). Children with Down syndrome often are afflicted with congenital heart deformities, such as atrial septal defect, and an increased susceptibility to respiratory infections and leukemia. A majority of fetuses known to have trisomy 21 are either stillborn or aborted.[9]

A rare form of Down syndrome (occurring in about 4% of cases) is due to a chromosomal translocation of the long arm of chromosome 21 to another chromosome. It is believed that inheritance occurs by passing of the chromosome from parent to offspring. In contrast, the cause of trisomy 21 is not well understood, although it is clearly associated with advanced maternal age.[11] Table 6-1 demonstrates a rise in the incidence of Down syndrome from maternal age 20 to 45 years. The reason for increased susceptibility of the ovum to nondisjunction with age remains unknown. In 95% of cases, the extra chromosome 21 is thought to be of maternal origin[4]; however, some studies have reported a correlation with paternal age.[12,13]

Table 6-1 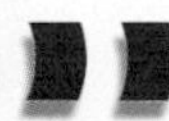

Frequency of Trisomy 21 (Down Syndrome) in Relation to Maternal Age

Age of Mother at Birth (yr)	Frequency of Trisomy 21 at Birth
20	1/1470
25	1/1333
30	1/935
35	1/353
37	1/200
39	1/112
41	1/68
43	1/46
45	1/36
50	1/26

Data from Morris JK et al: Comparison of models of maternal age-specific risk for Down syndrome live births, *Prenat Diagn* 23:252-258, 2003.

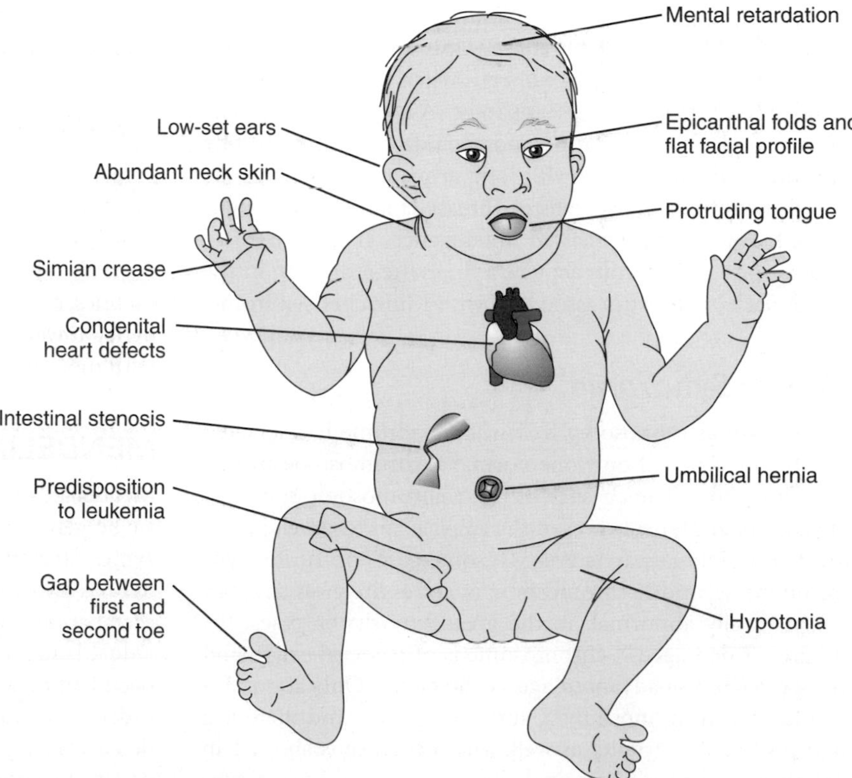

FIGURE 6-9 ■ Typical clinical manifestations of trisomy 21 (Down syndrome).

Trisomy 18 (Edwards Syndrome) and Trisomy 13 (Patau Syndrome)

Trisomy of chromosomes 18 or 13 is much less common than trisomy 21 and more severe. Mental retardation is quite severe, and average life expectancy is only a few weeks beyond birth. Trisomies involving chromosomes 8, 9, and 22 also have been described but are extremely rare.

Cri du Chat Syndrome

Deletion of the short arm of chromosome 5 results in a syndrome characterized by severe mental retardation, round face, and congenital heart anomalies. The syndrome was so named because of the characteristic cry of the affected infant, which resembles a cat crying. Some children afflicted with this syndrome survive to adulthood, and they generally thrive better than those with the trisomies.

Examples of Sex Chromosome Disorders

Klinefelter Syndrome

The incidence of Klinefelter syndrome is about 1 in 500 to 1 in 1000 live births, making it one of the most common genetic diseases of the sex chromosomes.[14,15] Individuals with Klinefelter syndrome usually have an extra X chromosome (an XXY genotype). However, individuals with more than one extra X (XXXY and XXXXY) have also been described. The presence of the Y chromosome determines the sex of these individuals to be male; however, the extra X chromosomes result in abnormal sexual development and feminization. The condition is rarely diagnosed prior to puberty, when lack of secondary sex characteristics becomes apparent. Associated symptoms reflect a lack of testosterone and include testicular atrophy and infertility, tall stature with long arms and legs, feminine hair distribution, gynecomastia (breast enlargement), high-pitched voice, and impaired intelligence (Figure 6-10).[15] Testosterone therapy can achieve a dramatic reduction in the feminine characteristics associated with Klinefelter syndrome.

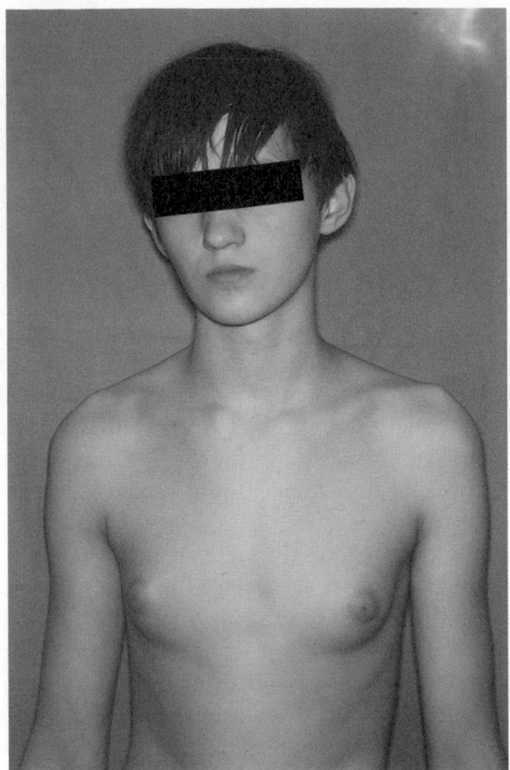

FIGURE 6-10 ■ Typical clinical manifestations of Klinefelter syndrome. (From Moore KL, Persuad TVN: *The developing human: clinically oriented embryology,* ed 7, Philadelphia, 2003, Saunders, p 165.)

Turner Syndrome

Also known as monosomy X, Turner syndrome is associated with the presence of only one normal X chromosome and no Y chromosome. The absence of the Y chromosome results in a female phenotype; however, the ovaries fail to develop, and affected individuals are sterile. In some cases of Turner syndrome the second X chromosome is not entirely missing but is structurally abnormal. In the great majority of cases, the missing or damaged X chromosome is of paternal origin and may be related to advanced age of the father. Only about 3% of infants with monosomy X survive to birth, and there is a high postnatal mortality as well. The incidence is about 1 in 3000 female births.[16] Principal characteristics of Turner syndrome include short stature, webbing of the neck, fibrous ovaries, sterility, amenorrhea, a wide chest, and congenital heart defects (Figure 6-11).

Multiple X Females and Double Y Males

A relatively common disorder of the sex chromosomes is the presence of an extra copy of the X chromosome in females (XXX) or of the Y in males (XYY). Most individuals appear normal; however, females may experience menstrual abnormalities, and males will generally be taller than average. A tendency toward mental retardation has been noted in females with more than four X chromosomes.

MENDELIAN SINGLE-GENE DISORDERS

Mendelian disorders result from alterations or mutations of single genes. The affected genes may code for abnormal enzymes, structural proteins, or regulatory proteins. An individual has two variants or alleles of each gene (one allele from each parent). A recessive gene is expressed only when the individual is homozygous for the gene, that is, the individual has two identical copies. Dominant genes require only one allele in order to be expressed. Mendelian disorders are generally classified according to the *location* of the defective gene (autosomal or sex chromosome) and the *mode of transmission* (dominant or recessive). The great majority of mendelian disorders are fa-

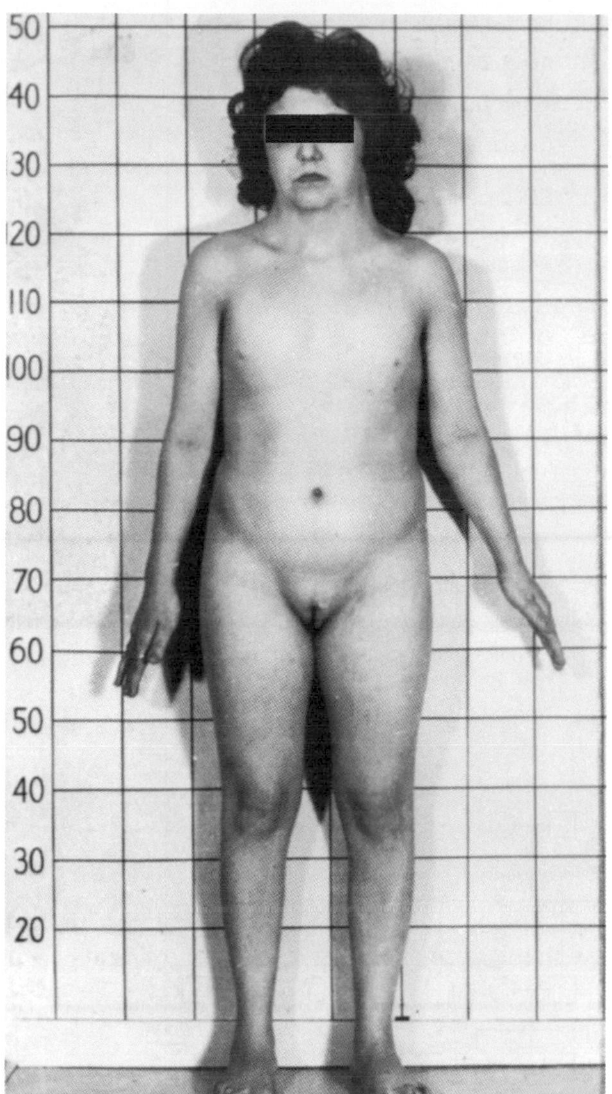

FIGURE 6-11 ■ Typical clinical manifestations of Turner syndrome. (From Connor JM, Ferguson-Smith MA: *Essential medical genetics,* ed 5, London, 1997, Blackwell Scientific, p 123.)

milial (mutant genes inherited from the parents), but 10% to 15% represent new mutations. In many cases the particular gene responsible for a mendelian disease has not been identified. A detailed **pedigree** may be used to trace the transmission of the disease through the history of a family. The pedigree chart (Figure 6-12), showing family relationships and which members have been affected by the disease, is a useful tool in determining the pattern of inheritance as recessive, dominant, or sex linked. Mendelian genetics is based on the principle that single genes are randomly and independently transmitted to offspring such that there is a 50:50 chance of receiving one or the other of a parent's alleles for a particular gene. There are many exceptions to these rules, but the rules generally are useful in predicting transmission patterns for a number of single-gene disorders. The number of known single-gene disorders is now greater than 5000.[4] A comprehensive database of the chromosomal location and sequence of single-gene disorders, called *Online Mendelian Inheritance in Man*, can be accessed at http://www.ncbi.nlm.nih.gov/omim.

DNA Mutation and Repair

The term **mutation** refers to a permanent change in DNA structure. Genetic mutation is a rare event despite the daily exposure of cells to numerous mutagenic influences. Radiation, chemicals, viruses, and even some products of normal cellular metabolism are all potential **mutagens.** In a typical cell, more than 5000 adenine and guanine DNA bases are lost and more than 100 cytosine bases are damaged each day owing to thermal disruption.[17] Many other types of DNA damage also occur, but only a few of these changes result in permanent alterations (mutations). The stability of the genes, and thus the low mutation rate, depends on efficient DNA repair mechanisms.

There are a variety of cellular DNA repair mechanisms. All require the presence of a normal complementary DNA template to correctly repair the damaged strand of DNA. Single-stranded breaks or loss of bases from only one DNA strand are readily repaired. Double-stranded breaks, involving both strands of complementary DNA, may result in permanent loss of genetic information at the break point where the broken strands are reunited. Different types of DNA damage are detected and repaired by different enzyme systems. The steps in one type of DNA repair are shown in Figure 6-13.

Genetic mutations are generally of two types: a point mutation, which involves a single base pair substitution, or a frameshift mutation, which often changes the genetic code dramatically. A sequence of three DNA bases (codon) is required to code for each amino acid. A point mutation in the gene may cause the affected codon to signify an abnormal amino acid. The inclusion of the abnormal amino acid in the sequence of the protein may or may not be of clinical significance. Sickle cell anemia and α_1-antiprotease deficiency are examples of point mutation disorders in which a single amino acid substitution causes significant dysfunction. A frameshift mutation is due to the addition or removal of one or more bases, which changes the "reading frame" of the DNA sequence. The DNA sequence is normally "read" in groups of three bases, with no spaces between. All of the codon triplets will be changed in the DNA region downstream from the mutation, resulting in a protein with a greatly altered amino acid sequence (Figure 6-14).

Autosomal Dominant Disorders

Autosomal dominant disorders are due to a mutation of a dominant gene located on one of the autosomes. Autosomal dominant disorders follow predictable patterns of inheritance (Figure 6-15), which may be summarized as follows:

- Males and females are equally affected.
- Affected individuals usually have an affected parent.
- Unaffected individuals do not transmit the disease.

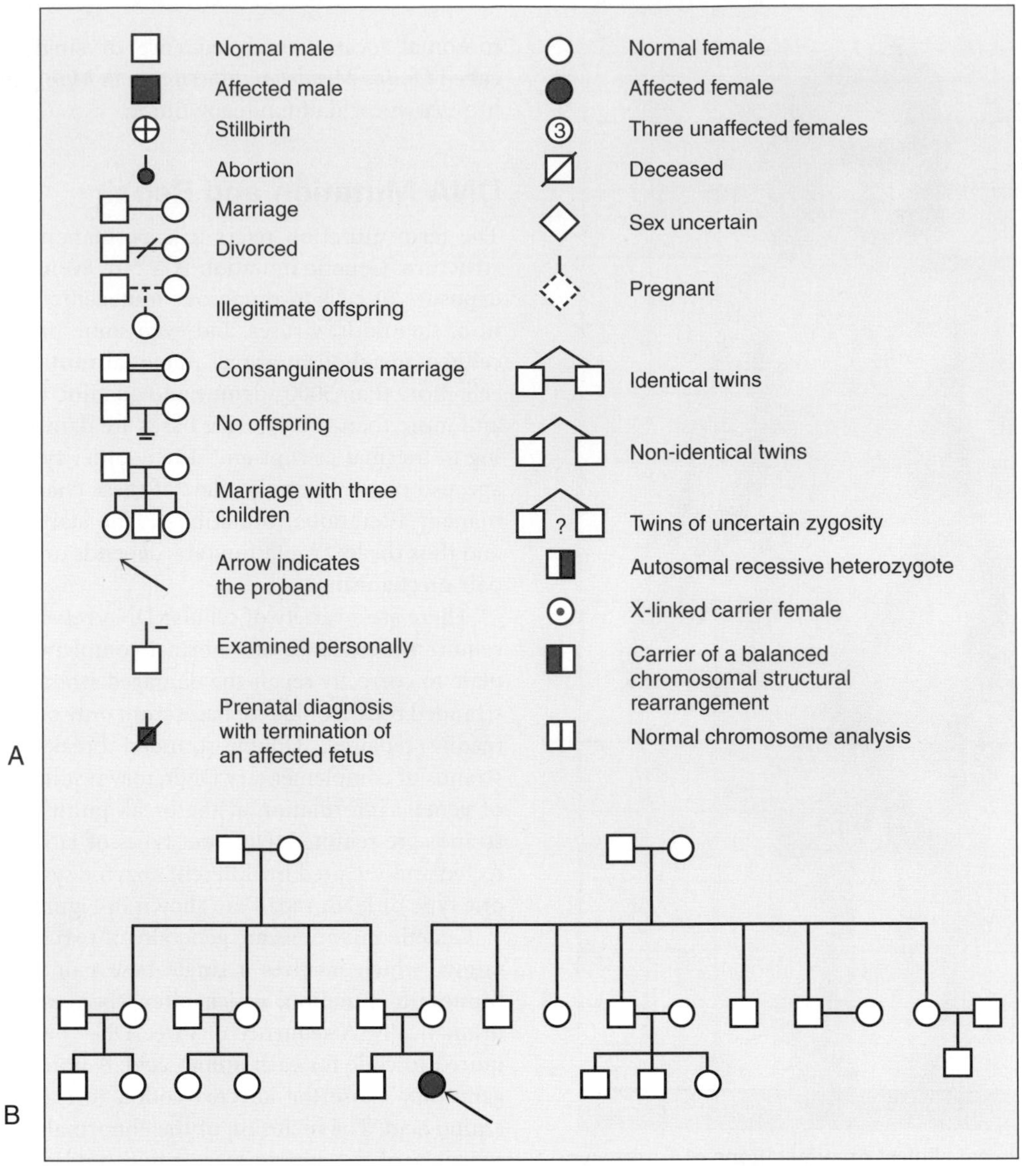

Normal male
Affected male
Stillbirth
Abortion
Marriage
Divorced
Illegitimate offspring
Consanguineous marriage
No offspring
Marriage with three children
Arrow indicates the proband
Examined personally
Prenatal diagnosis with termination of an affected fetus
Normal female
Affected female
3
Three unaffected females
Deceased
Sex uncertain
Pregnant
Identical twins
Non-identical twins
?
Twins of uncertain zygosity
Autosomal recessive heterozygote
X-linked carrier female
Carrier of a balanced chromosomal structural rearrangement
Normal chromosome analysis
A
B

FIGURE 6-12 ■ **A,** Common symbols for pedigree analysis. **B,** Typical family pedigree chart.

Normal DNA
DNA damage
Removal of damaged base pair (step 1)
DNA polymerase inserts new base pair using good strand as a template (step 2)
DNA ligase repairs nick (step 3)

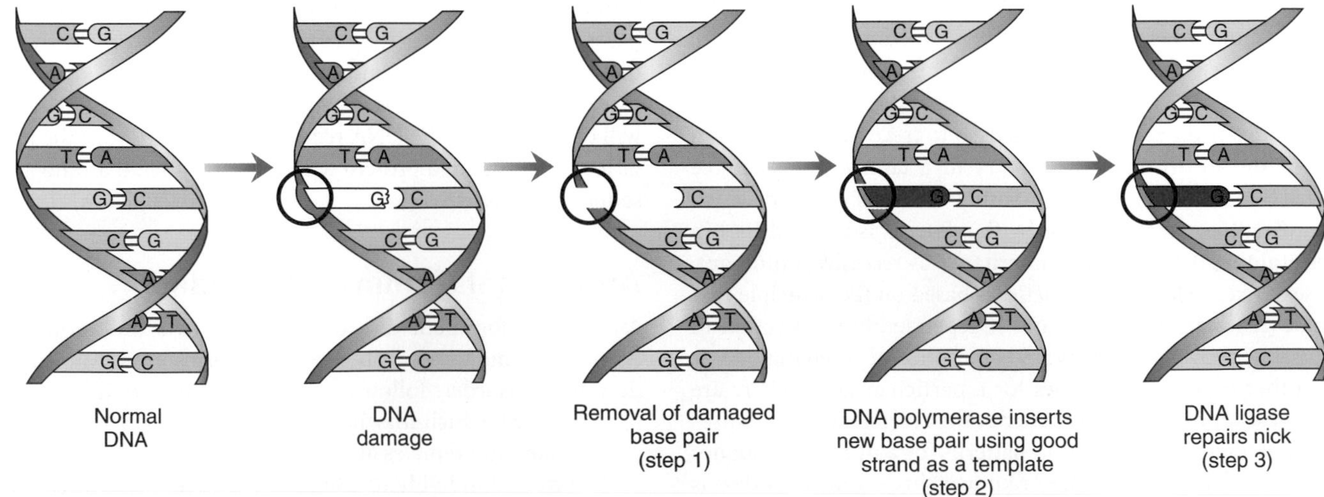

FIGURE 6-13 ■ The steps of DNA repair. In step 1 the damaged section is removed; in steps 2 and 3 the original DNA sequence is restored.

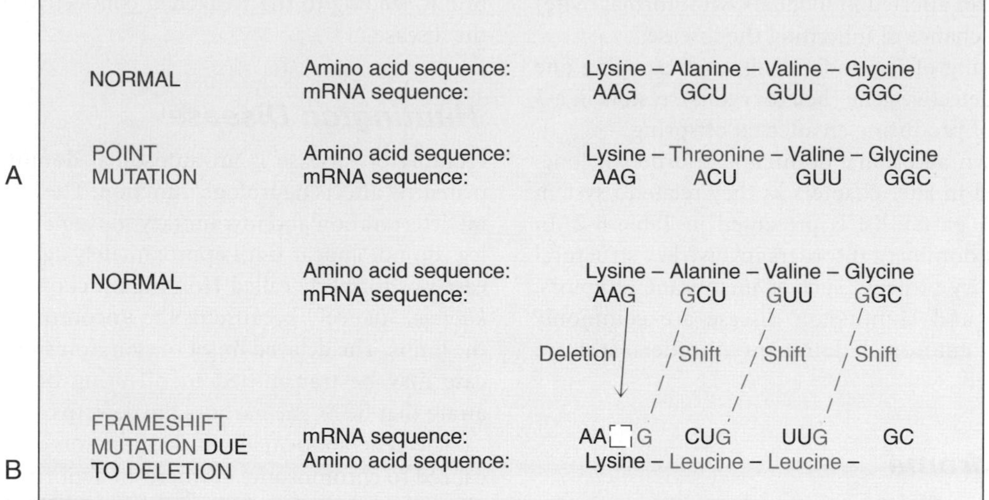

FIGURE 6-14 ■ Schematic illustration of mutations that alter the messenger RNA sequence and the resulting protein amino acid sequence. **A,** Point mutation alters one amino acid. **B,** Frameshift mutation alters all downstream amino acids.

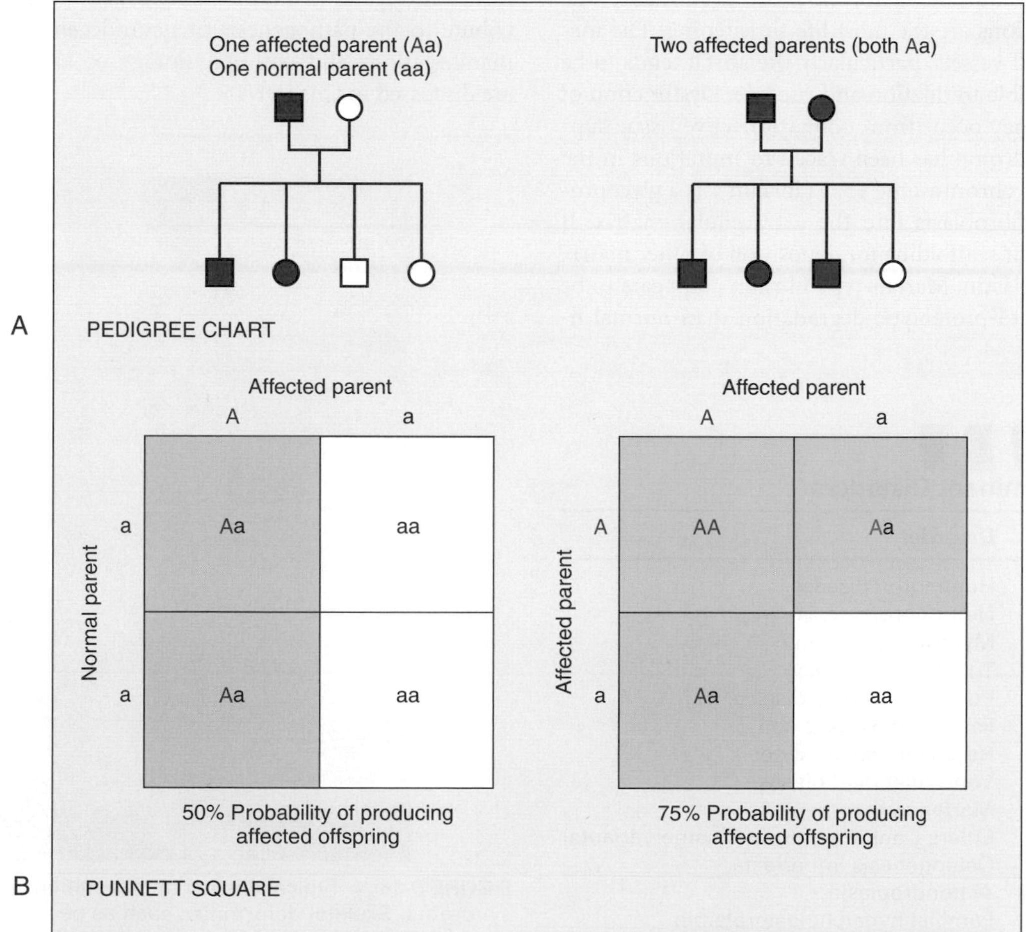

FIGURE 6-15 ■ Typical pattern of inheritance of an autosomal dominant trait (e.g., Marfan syndrome). **A,** Pedigree chart. **B,** Punnett square.

- Offspring of an affected individual (with normal mate) have a 1 in 2 chance of inheriting the disease.
- The rare mating of two individuals, each carrying one copy of the defective gene (heterozygous), results in a 3 in 4 chance of producing an affected offspring.

The list of known autosomal dominant disorders is long. Many are described in later chapters as they relate to system pathophysiology. A partial list is presented in Table 6-2. In general, autosomal dominant disorders involve key structural proteins or regulatory proteins, such as membrane receptors. Marfan syndrome and Huntington disease are commonly cited examples of autosomal dominant disorders and are briefly described here.

Marfan Syndrome

Marfan syndrome is a disorder of the connective tissues of the body. Individuals with Marfan syndrome are typically tall and slender with long, thin arms and legs (Figure 6-16). Because of the long, thin fingers, this syndrome has also been called arachnodactyly ("spider fingers"). It is commonly suggested that President Abraham Lincoln may have had this disorder. Although skeletal and joint deformities are problematic, the cardiovascular lesions are the most life threatening. The medial layer of blood vessels, particularly the aorta, tends to be weak and susceptible to dilation and rupture. Dysfunction of the heart valves may occur from poor connective tissue support. Marfan syndrome has been traced to mutations in the fibrillin 1 gene on chromosome 15.[18] Fibrillin 1 is a glycoprotein secreted by fibroblasts into the extracellular matrix. It provides important scaffolding for deposition of other matrix proteins such as elastin. Marfan-type fibrillin 1 appears to be more susceptible to proteolytic degradation than normal fibrillin, leading to the weakened connective tissues typical of the disease.

Table 6-2

Autosomal Dominant Disorders

System	Disorder
Nervous	Huntington disease
	Neurofibromatosis
	Myotonic dystrophy
	Tuberous sclerosis
Urinary	Polycystic kidney disease
Gastrointestinal	Familial polyposis coli
Hematopoietic	Hereditary spherocytosis
	Von Willebrand disease
Skeletal	Marfan syndrome
	Ehlers-Danlos syndrome (some variants)
	Osteogenesis imperfecta
	Achondroplasia
Metabolic	Familial hypercholesterolemia
	Acute intermittent porphyria

From Kumar V, Cotran RS, Robbins ST: *Robbins basic pathology,* ed 7, Philadelphia, 2003, Saunders, p 215.

Huntington Disease

Huntington disease is an autosomal dominant disease that primarily affects neurologic function. The symptoms of mental deterioration and involuntary movements of the arms and legs do not appear until approximately age 40 years. The disease was formerly called Huntington chorea (from the Greek *khoreia,* "dance") because of the uncontrolled movements of the limbs. The delayed onset of symptoms means that the disease may be transmitted to offspring before the carrier is aware that he or she harbors the defective gene.

The gene abnormality in Huntington disease has been localized to chromosome 4, where an abnormally large number of triplet repeats (CAG) has been noted.[19,20] Triplet repeats of more than 39 are reliably associated with development of the disease, and the greater the number of triplet repeats, the earlier the onset of symptoms.[20] The Huntington disease protein (huntingtin) has a long segment of glutamine amino acids that are coded for by the CAG triplet repeat. The protein forms aggregates in brain tissue, which are thought to contribute to the pathogenesis of neurodegeneration.[21] Clinical manifestations and pathophysiology of Huntington disease are discussed in Chapter 45.

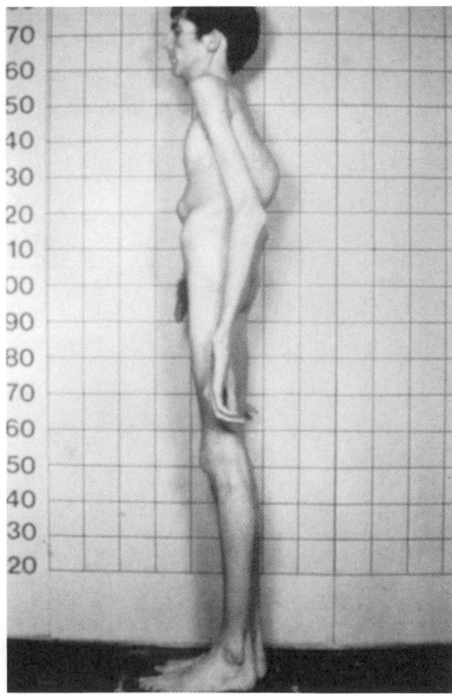

FIGURE 6-16 ■ Typical clinical manifestations of Marfan syndrome. Skeletal deformities such as pectus excavatum and abnormal curvature of the thoracic spine are common findings. (From Connor JM, Ferguson-Smith MA: *Essential medical genetics,* ed 5, London, 1997, Blackwell Scientific, p 142.)

Autosomal Recessive Disorders

Autosomal recessive disorders are due to a mutation of a recessive gene located on one of the autosomes. Autosomal recessive disorders follow predictable patterns of inheritance (Figure 6-17), which may be summarized as follows:

- Males and females are equally affected.
- In most cases the disease is not apparent in the parents or relatives of the affected individual, but both parents are carriers of the mutant recessive gene.
- Unaffected individuals may transmit the disease to offspring.
- The mating of two carriers (heterozygous) results in a 1 in 4 chance of producing an affected offspring and a 2 in 4 chance of producing an offspring who carries the disease.

It is believed that nearly everyone carries one or more mutant recessive genes. Related individuals are more likely to carry the *same* recessive genes. Because recessive diseases are only expressed when both alleles for a particular gene are mutant (homozygous), they are often associated with **consanguinity**—the mating of related individuals.[1] The closer the biological relationship, the greater the proportion of shared genes and the greater the risk of producing affected offspring.

Recessive disorders often involve abnormal enzymatic functions. The gene for a particular enzyme may be absent or present in a mutant, and therefore nonfunctional, form. The enzyme deficiency usually is not apparent in heterozygotes carrying one normal gene and one mutant gene because the normal gene produces enough of the necessary enzyme. In the homozygous state, neither gene for the enzyme is functional, resulting in an enzyme deficiency. A partial list of the large number of autosomal recessive disorders that have been identified is given in Table 6-3. Many of these diseases involve inability to metabolize nutrients (inborn errors of metabolism) or to synthesize cellular components because of enzyme deficiencies. Albinism, phenylketonuria, and cystic fibrosis are described here as representative examples. Other disorders are described in the discussions of system pathophysiology in later chapters.

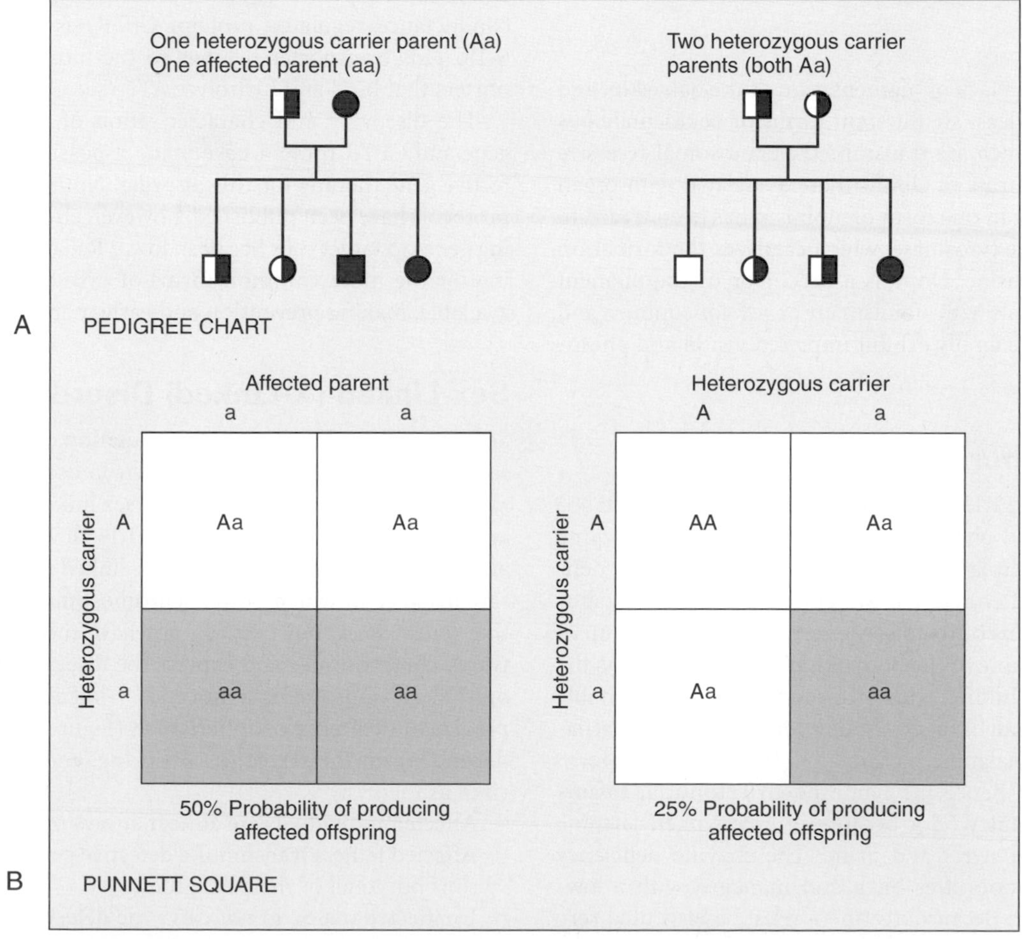

FIGURE 6-17 ■ Typical pattern of inheritance of an autosomal recessive trait (e.g., cystic fibrosis, sickle cell anemia). **A,** Pedigree chart. **B,** Punnett square.

Table 6-3

Autosomal Recessive Disorders

System	Disorder
Metabolic	Cystic fibrosis Phenylketonuria Galactosemia Homocystinuria Lysosomal storage disease α_1-Antitrypsin deficiency Wilson disease Hemochromatosis Glycogen storage diseases
Hematopoietic	Sickle cell anemia Thalassemias
Endocrine	Congenital adrenal hyperplasia
Skeletal	Ehlers-Danlos syndrome (some variants) Alkaptonuria
Nervous	Neurogenic muscular atrophies Friedreich ataxia Spinal muscular atrophy

From Kumar V, Cotran RS, Robbins ST: *Robbins basic pathology,* ed 7, Philadelphia, 2003, Saunders, p 216.

Albinism

Albinism refers to a lack of pigmentation of the hair, skin, and eyes. There are at least six different forms of oculocutaneous albinism, all of which are transmitted as autosomal recessive disorders. Some forms of albinism are associated with organ defects. The defect in one form of albinism has been traced to lack of the enzyme tyrosinase, which catalyzes the formation of dopa from tyrosine. Dopa is a precursor of the pigment melanin. Individuals with albinism are at risk for sunburn and skin cancer, and generally exhibit impaired vision and photosensitivity.[22]

Phenylketonuria

Phenylketonuria (PKU) results from an inability to metabolize the amino acid phenylalanine due to lack of the enzyme phenylalanine hydroxylase. It is one of several enzyme deficiencies that are often referred to as inborn errors of metabolism. The symptoms of the disorder are due to the buildup of dietary phenylalanine in the body, which primarily affects the nervous system. Children with PKU tend to be overly irritable and tremorous and have slowly developing mental retardation. Excess phenylalanine is excreted in the urine in the form of phenylketones; hence the name phenylketonuria. Infants typically have a musty odor because of excess phenylalanine byproducts in the sweat and urine. The enzyme deficiency can be detected soon after birth and managed with a low-phenylalanine diet. Because treatment must be instituted very early to prevent mental retardation, routine screening for PKU is performed at birth.

Cystic Fibrosis

Cystic fibrosis is one of the most common single-gene disorders, with about 5% of white Americans harboring the defective gene.[4,23] The incidence of cystic fibrosis is approximately 1 in 2500 live births. The clinical abnormalities associated with cystic fibrosis have been traced to a defect in a membrane transporter for chloride ions in epithelial cells. The alteration in chloride transport is associated with production of abnormally thick secretions in glandular tissues. The lung bronchioles and pancreatic ducts are primarily affected, often resulting in progressive destruction of these organs (see Chapter 22).

The cystic fibrosis gene was isolated in 1989 and mapped to chromosome 7. A number of different mutations of this gene have been identified, all of which cause a similar defect in chloride transport across the cell membrane. The most common mutation, accounting for about 70% of cystic fibrosis cases, is due to a deletion of three nucleotides that normally code for a phenylalanine at position 508.[23] The absence of this single amino acid apparently causes the protein to fold abnormally, preventing its release from the endoplasmic reticulum, where it is eventually degraded. A schematic of the normal chloride transporter (called cystic fibrosis transmembrane conductance regulator protein, CFTR) is shown in Figure 6-18. This transporter belongs to the family of ABC transporters that bind and hydrolyze ATP (see Chapter 3).

The discovery and characterization of the cystic fibrosis gene and CFTR protein have made it possible to envision effective gene therapy for this disorder. Numerous clinical trial protocols have been published, however, efficiency for delivering genes to target cells has been low.[24] Reliable genetic screening for the more common forms of cystic fibrosis is readily available, making prevention and early management possible.

Sex-Linked (X-Linked) Disorders

Sex-linked disorders are due to a mutation of the sex chromosomes. Disorders linked to the Y chromosome are extremely rare, and for that reason the terms "sex linked" and "X linked" are often used interchangeably. Nearly all X-linked disorders are recessive. Females express the X-linked disease only in the rare instance in which both X chromosomes carry the defective gene. Males, however, do not have the safety margin of two X chromosomes and express the disease if their one and only X chromosome is abnormal. X-linked disorders follow predictable patterns of inheritance (Figure 6-19), which are dependent on the sex of the offspring, and may be summarized as follows:

- Affected individuals are almost always male.
- Affected fathers transmit the defective gene to none of their sons but to all of their daughters.
- Unaffected males do not carry the defective gene.
- A carrier female has a 1 in 2 chance of producing an affected son and a 1 in 2 chance of producing a carrier daughter.

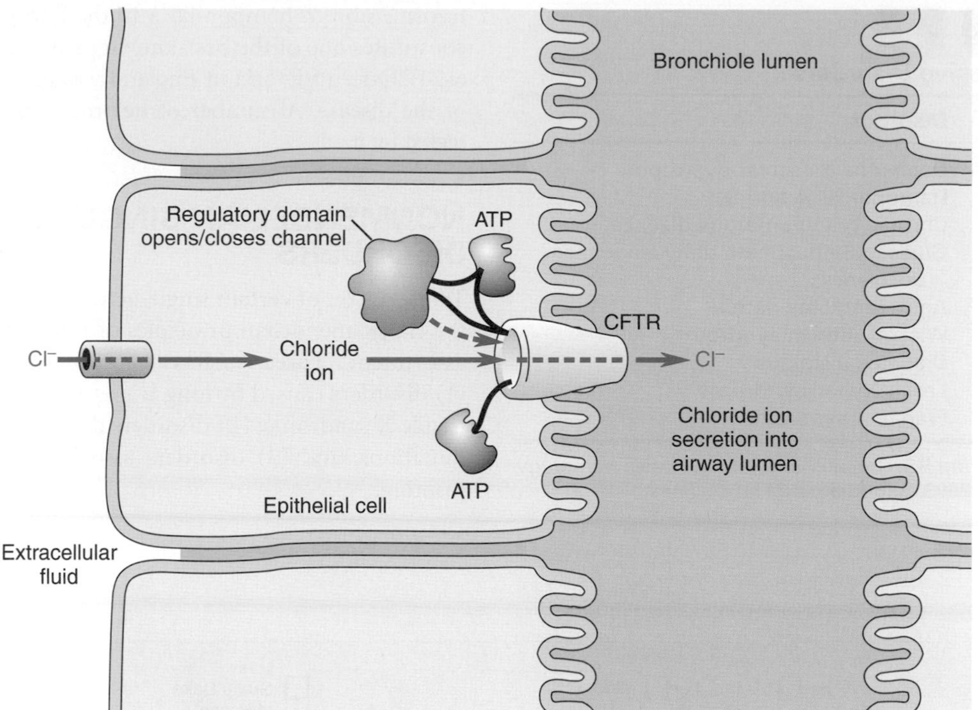

FIGURE 6-18 ■ Schematic illustration of the cystic fibrosis transmembrane conductance regulator *(CFTR)* located in an epithelial cell. CFTR is a transmembrane protein that transports chloride from the cytoplasm into the lumen of the bronchiole. Mutations in the CFTR transporter gene are believed to cause the thick secretions typical of cystic fibrosis.

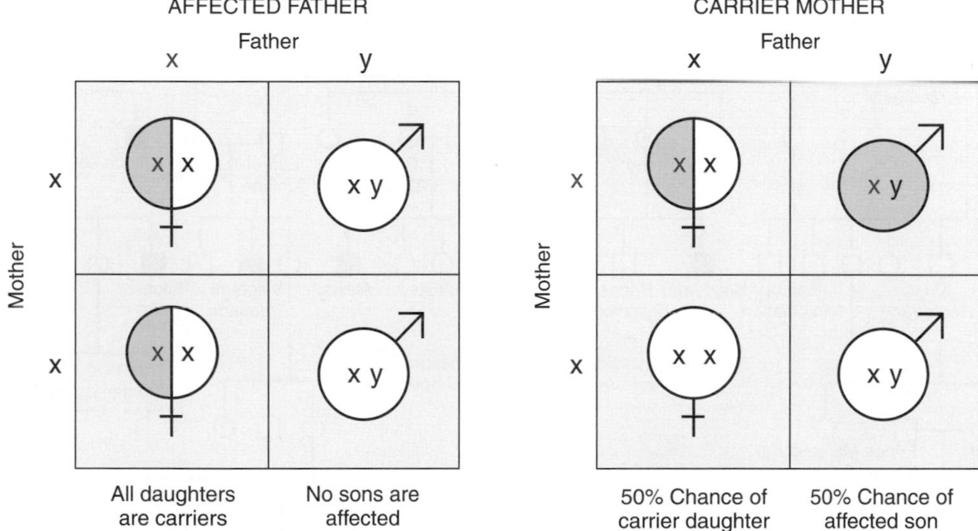

FIGURE 6-19 ■ Typical inheritance pattern for X-linked disorders. The risk of disease varies according to the gender of the offspring.

- Females are affected only in the rare homozygous state that may occur from the mating of an affected or carrier mother and an affected father.

Several X-linked recessive disorders have been identified, as presented in Table 6-4. A well-known example of an X-linked disease is hemophilia A.

Hemophilia A

Hemophilia A is a bleeding disorder associated with a deficiency of factor VIII, a protein necessary for blood clotting. Individuals afflicted with hemophilia A bleed easily and profusely from seemingly minor injuries (see Chapter 14). The

Table 6-4

X-Linked Recessive Disorders

System	Disorder
Musculoskeletal	Duchenne muscular dystrophy
Blood	Hemophilias A and B
	Chronic granulomatous disease
	Glucose-6-phosphate dehydrogenase deficiency
Immune	Agammaglobulinemia
	Wiskott-Aldrich syndrome
Metabolic	Diabetes insipidus
	Lesch-Nyhan syndrome
Nervous	Fragile X syndrome

From Kumar V, Cotran RS, Robbins ST: *Robbins basic pathology,* ed 7, Philadelphia, 2003, Saunders, p 217.

transmission of hemophilia A in the European royal families constitutes one of the best-known pedigrees available (Figure 6-20). Queen Victoria of England was the first known carrier of the disease. A number of her male descendants were affected by it.

NONMENDELIAN SINGLE-GENE DISORDERS

Transmission of certain single-gene disorders does not follow the classic mendelian principles of random and independent assortment. Three such categories have been described: (1) disorders caused by long triplet repeat mutations, such as fragile X syndrome; (2) disorders due to mitochondrial DNA mutations; and (3) disorders associated with genomic imprinting.

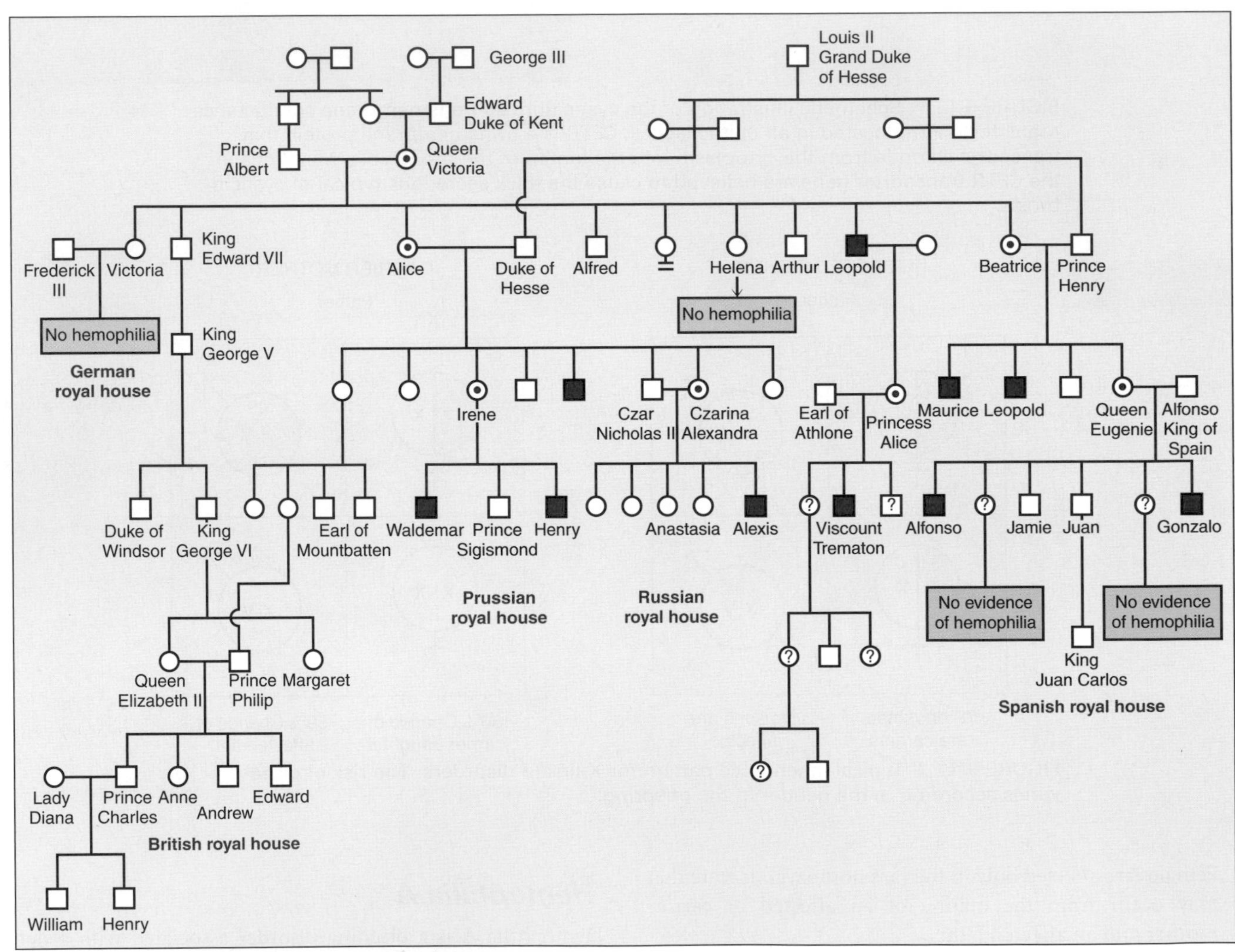

FIGURE 6-20 ■ Pedigree chart for the transmission of the X-linked disease hemophilia A in the royal families of Europe.

Triplet Repeat Mutations

Fragile X syndrome is a prototypical example of disorders characterized by long repeating sequences of three nucleotides, called *triplet repeats.* Fragile X syndrome is the most common cause of familial mental retardation, exhibiting a prevalence rate of about 1 in 4000.[25] A typical constriction on the long arm of the X chromosome can be detected on cytogenic studies. The area is composed of long repeating triplets of the sequence CGG. Normal individuals have an average of 29 CGG triplet repeats at this gene locus. Persons with fragile X syndrome have significantly more: 230 to 4000 triplet repeats. Persons who have an intermediate number of repeats (52 to 230) are said to have a *pre*mutation and are at significant risk for producing affected offspring, although they themselves are unaffected.[4] The premutation is unstable and predisposed to amplification during oogenesis, but not spermatogenesis. As the premutation is passed on through the female lineage, the number of triplet repeats tends to increase as does the risk of mental retardation in the offspring. As might be guessed, the transmission patterns of this disorder are quite unusual. Males with fragile X syndrome tend to be more severely affected, apparently because the presence of a second X chromosome in females moderates the clinical symptoms. The protein normally produced by the fragile X gene *(FMR1)* is a ribosome-associated protein.[25] It is found in the dendrite area of neurons and may be involved in synthesis of neuronal proteins.

Mitochondrial Gene Mutations

Nearly all cellular genes are located in the cell nucleus; however, several mitochondrial genes are passed on to daughter cells within the mitochondria when a cell divides. Essentially all mitochondria are contributed to a zygote by the egg and are therefore of maternal origin because sperm contain few if any mitochondria.[4] (A rare case of paternal transmission of a mitochondrial gene defect has been described.) Mothers transmit mitochondrial DNA to both sons and daughters, but only daughters can transmit the genes to their offspring. Mitochondrial DNA codes for enzymes involved in oxidative phosphorylation reactions, and mutations tend to cause dysfunction in tissues with high utilization of ATP such as nerve, muscle, kidney, and liver. Mitochondrial gene disorders exhibit tricky inheritance patterns and are very rare.

Genomic Imprinting

The concept of genomic imprinting challenges the long-held belief that the parental origin of a gene does not matter to the cells that inherit them. Genomic imprinting is a poorly understood process whereby maternal and paternal chromosomes are marked differentially within the cell. Genomic imprinting can be illustrated by considering two very different syndromes, which at first glance appeared to be a result of the same chromosomal defect. Prader-Willi syndrome and Angelman syndrome both result from a deletion at the same location on chromosome 15.[26] Prader-Willi syndrome is characterized by mental retardation, short stature, obesity, poor muscle tone, and hypogonadism. Patients with Angelman syndrome are also mentally retarded, but they have ataxia and tend to laugh inappropriately. The fact that two different syndromes resulted from the same mutation was puzzling until it was discovered that the Prader-Willi mutation is always on the paternally derived chromosome 15, whereas the Angelman syndrome mutation is always on the maternally derived chromosome 15. These findings imply that the cell is not blind to the parental origin of chromosomes and that homologous chromosomes may be marked and function differently within the cell.

MULTIFACTORIAL (POLYGENIC) DISORDERS

Multifactorial disorders are thought to involve two or more mutant genes that act together to produce the trait. Multifactorial disorders are greatly influenced by environmental factors, so they do not follow clear-cut modes of inheritance but do tend to "run in families." Characteristics that are governed by multifactorial inheritance tend to have a range of expression in the population. For example, height, weight, and intelligence are multifactorial. Most multifactorial disorders also present a range of severity, although a few disorders are either present or absent. In the latter case, it may be that a certain threshold number of defective genes must be inherited before the disease is expressed.[4]

It is extremely difficult to predict the risk of occurrence of multifactorial disorders based on family history. The risk of recurrence of a typical multifactorial disorder is in the range of 2% to 7%.[4] Thus, the parents of one affected child have a 2% to 7% chance of bearing a second affected child. The risk rises to about 9% after the birth of a second affected child. The number of genes contributing to the disorder, the degree to which the disease is expressed, and environmental influences (most of which may be undetermined) all affect the true risk of recurrence. It is apparent why multifactorial inheritance has been called "a geneticist's nightmare."

In contrast to single-gene and chromosomal abnormalities, which are rare, multifactorial disorders are very common. High blood pressure, cancer, diabetes mellitus, cleft lip, and several forms of congenital heart defects are governed by multifactorial inheritance. This list is destined to grow as knowledge of the role of genetic mechanisms in cellular function and disease expands.

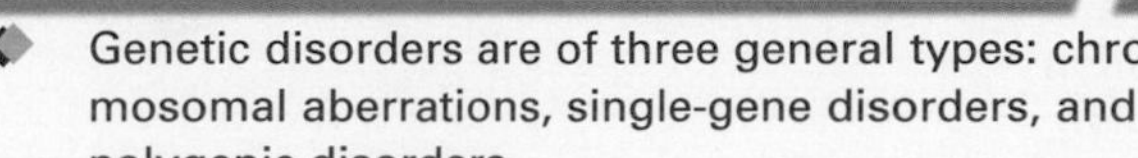

- Genetic disorders are of three general types: chromosomal aberrations, single-gene disorders, and polygenic disorders.

- Chromosome disorders result from an abnormality in number or structure. The presence of only one chromosome of a homologous pair is termed *monosomy* (e.g., Turner syndrome), and the presence of an excessive number of chromosomes is called *polysomy* (e.g., Down syndrome). Abnormal rearrangement of portions of the chromosomes (translocation, inversion, deletion, duplication) can result in loss or unusual expression of genes.
- Single-gene disorders result from mutations that alter the nucleotide sequence of one particular gene. Mendelian disorders are transmitted predictably and include autosomal dominant (e.g., Huntington disease), autosomal recessive (e.g., cystic fibrosis), and sex-linked (e.g., hemophilia) disorders.
- Some single-gene disorders have unusual transmission patterns, which violate Mendel's laws. These include triplet repeat mutations, mitochondrial DNA mutations, and genomic imprinting disorders.
- Polygenic disorders are very common and result from the interaction of multiple genes. Disorders such as high blood pressure, cancer, and diabetes are polygenic.

ENVIRONMENTALLY INDUCED CONGENITAL DISORDERS

Adverse influences during intrauterine life are a significant cause of errors in fetal development that result in congenital malformations. The study of developmental anomalies is called *teratology* (from the Greek *teras,* or "monster"). Most malformations are associated with genetic causes; however, numerous environmental influences that may adversely affect the developing fetus, such as chemicals, radiation, and viral infections, have been identified (Table 6-5). Factors that cause congenital malformation are called **teratogens.** Many substances are thought to have teratogenic potential, based on experiments in animals, but few are proved in humans. Exposure to a known teratogen may, but need not, result in a congenital malformation. Susceptibility to a teratogen depends on the amount of exposure, the developmental stage of the fetus when exposed, the prior condition of the mother, and the genetic predisposition of the fetus.[4]

Periods of Fetal Vulnerability

The timing of the exposure to a teratogen greatly influences fetal susceptibility and the resulting type of malformation. The intrauterine development of humans can be divided into two stages: (1) the embryonic period, which extends from conception to 9 weeks of development, is followed by (2) the fetal period, which continues until birth. Prior to the third week of gestation, exposure to a teratogen generally either damages so few cells that the embryo develops normally, or damages so many cells that the embryo cannot survive and spontaneous abortion occurs. Between the third and ninth week of gestation the embryo is very vulnerable to teratogenesis, with the fourth and fifth weeks being the time of peak susceptibility.[4] Organ development (organogenesis) occurs during this period and is very sensitive to injury, regardless of the cause. Each organ has a critical period during which it is most vulnerable to malformation (Figure 6-21). Unfortunately, an embryo may be exposed to teratogens during the vulnerable period because the mother does not yet realize she is pregnant. The fetal period, from 3 to 9 months, is primarily concerned with further growth and maturation of the organs, and susceptibility to errors of morphogenesis is significantly less. Fetal insults occurring after the third month are more likely to result in growth retardation or injury to normally formed organs.

Table 6-5

Causes of Congenital Malformations in Humans

Cause	Malformed Live Births (%)
Genetic	
Chromosomal aberrations	10-15
Mendelian inheritance	2-10
Multifactorial	20-25
Environmental	
Maternal/placental infections (e.g., rubella, toxoplasmosis, syphilis, cytomegalovirus infection, human immunodeficiency virus infection)	2-3
Maternal disease states (e.g., diabetes, phenylketonuria, endocrinopathies)	6-8
Drugs and chemicals (e.g., alcohol, folic acid antagonists, phenytoin, thalidomide, warfarin)	~1
Irradiation	~1
Unknown	40-60

Adapted from Stevenson RE et al, editors: *Human malformations and related anomalies,* New York, 1993, Oxford University Press, p 115. In Kumar V, Cotran RS, Robbins ST, editors: *Robbins basic pathology,* ed 7, Philadelphia, 2003, Saunders, p 240.

Teratogenic Agents

The teratogenic potential of many agents is unknown. Several chemicals, some infections, and large doses of radiation are definitely associated with a higher risk of congenital disorders. In general, teratogens cause errors in morphogenesis by interfering with cell proliferation, migration, or differentiation. The specific mechanisms of action of most teratogens are unknown.

Chemicals and Drugs

The list of proved teratogenic chemicals and drugs includes thalidomide, alcohol, anticonvulsants, warfarin, folate antagonists, androgenic hormones, angiotensin-converting enzyme inhibitors, and organic mercury. Almost no drugs or chemicals are considered to be totally safe, and the current trend is to discourage pregnant women from using *any* drugs or chemicals. Two agents, thalidomide and alcohol, illustrate the teratogenic potential of chemicals.

In the 1960s, a jump in the incidence of congenital limb deformities was traced to maternal use of thalidomide, a tranquilizer, between the 28th and 50th day of pregnancy.[2] Exposure during the vulnerable period was associated with a very high risk (50% to 80%) of fetal malformation. Typically, the arms were short and flipperlike, although deformities ranged from mild abnormalities of the digits to complete absence of the limbs. Damage to other structures, particularly the ears and heart, also occurred. Thalidomide is one of the most potent teratogens known.

The chronic ingestion of large amounts of alcohol is known to cause a group of congenital anomalies referred to as *fetal alcohol syndrome* (FAS). It is estimated that between 1 and 5 of every 1000 newborns suffer from alcohol-induced anomalies.[27] The incidence in the United States is more than 20 times that in Europe and is highly associated with low socioeconomic status. Affected infants suffer from growth retardation, neurologic disorders, malformations of the head and face, and atrial septal heart defects. Data are insufficient to determine what, if any, level of alcohol intake during pregnancy is safe. It is clear that factors other than the absolute amount of alcohol intake during pregnancy are important in determining risk of FAS. Low socioeconomic status may be a permissive factor, allowing the teratogenic effects of alcohol to affect the fetus to a greater extent.[28] The mechanisms of alcohol teratogenesis include maternal-fetal hypoxia and excessive free radical production. Alcohol

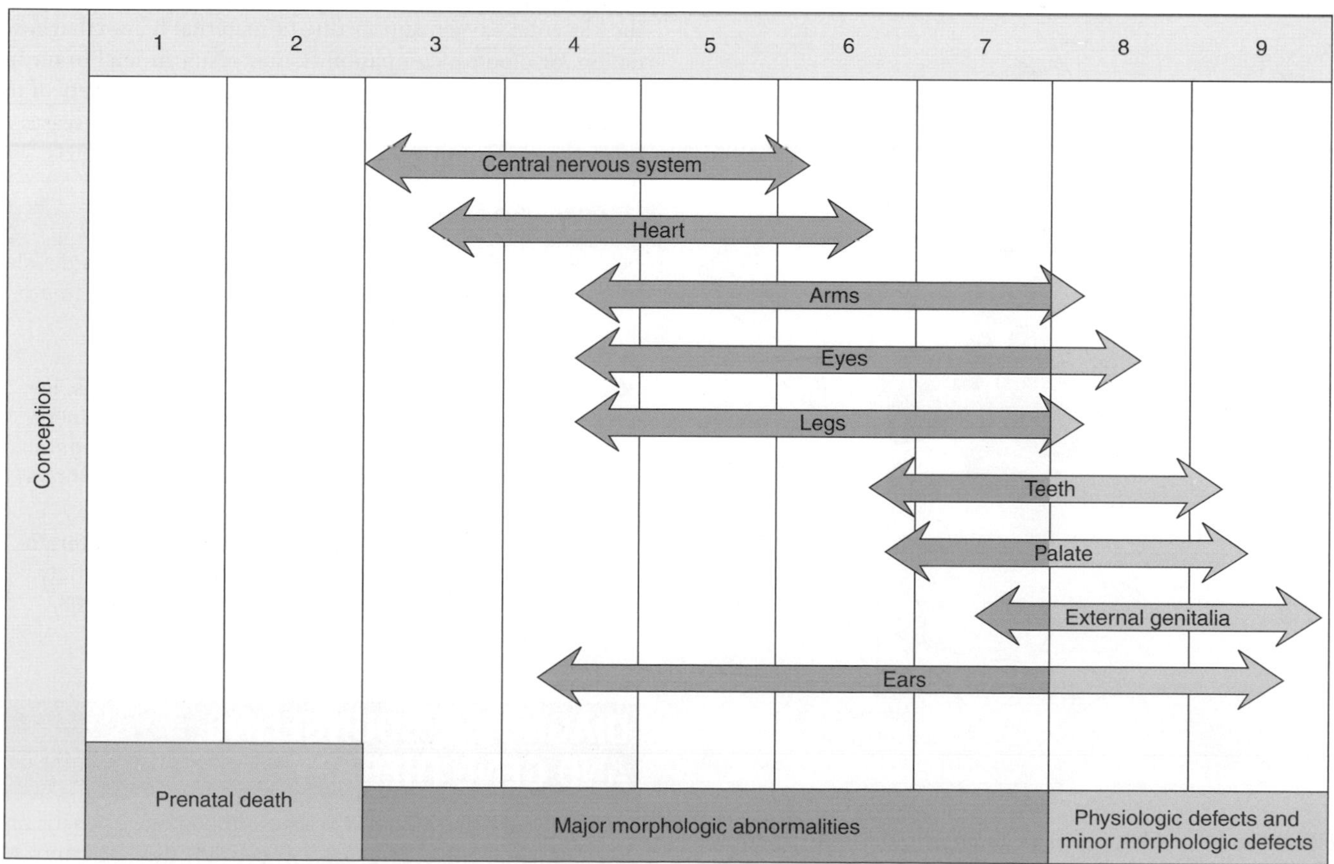

FIGURE 6-21 ■ The vulnerable periods of fetal organ development.

causes acute and transient collapse of the umbilical cord, which could damage the fetus by interrupting its oxygen supply. Complete abstinence from alcohol during pregnancy is generally recommended.

Infectious Agents

A number of perinatal infections have been implicated in the development of congenital malformations.[2] Certain viral infections appear to carry the greatest threat, although protozoa and bacteria have also been implicated. As with other teratogens, the gestational age of the fetus at the time of infection is critically important. Perhaps the best known viral teratogen is rubella. The risk period for rubella infection begins just prior to conception and extends to 20 weeks gestation, after which the virus rarely crosses the placenta. Rubella-induced defects vary but typically include cataracts, deafness, and heart defects. Several other organisms cause a similar constellation of congenital defects, so the acronym **TORCH** was developed to alert clinicians to the potential teratogenicity of these infections. TORCH stands for toxoplasmosis, others, rubella, cytomegalovirus, herpes. The major features of the TORCH complex are shown in Figure 6-22. The category of "others" includes several less frequently seen causes: hepatitis B, coxsackievirus B, mumps, poliovirus, and others. All microorganisms of the TORCH complex are able to cross the placenta and infect the fetus.

Toxoplasmosis is a protozoal infection that can be contracted from ingestion of raw or undercooked meat and from contact with cat feces. Cytomegalovirus and herpes simplex virus are generally transmitted to the fetus by chronic carrier mothers. Cytomegalovirus and herpes simplex virus often colonize the genital area of the mother. Infants who escape infection in utero may still acquire the virus as they pass through the birth canal (see Chapter 34).

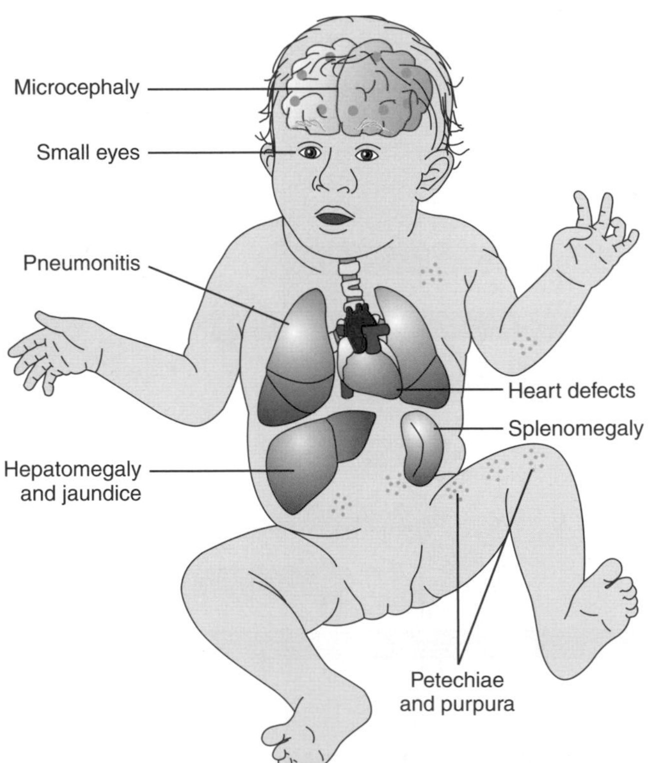

FIGURE 6-22 ■ Major clinical findings in the TORCH (toxoplasmosis, others, rubella, cytomegalovirus, herpes) complex of infective congenital disorders.

Radiation

In addition to being mutagenic, radiation is also teratogenic. The teratogenic potential of radiation became apparent from the increased incidence of congenital malformations in children born to women who underwent irradiation of the cervix for cancer and in the children of atomic bomb victims in World War II. It is not known if lower levels of radiation, such as those used in diagnostic x-rays, are teratogenic. It is generally recommended that pregnant women avoid diagnostic x-rays or use appropriate lead shielding.

Other Disorders of Infancy

An infant may be afflicted with a variety of problems at birth that do not fall into the category of genetic or developmental malformations. These problems generally arise later in uterine life and often involve mechanical factors or problems with the health of the mother and placenta. For example, babies with low birth weight or immaturity at birth may have difficulty breathing and taking in adequate nutrition. Interruption of the placental oxygen supply due to maternal hemorrhage, sedation, or blood incompatibility may result in fetal brain injury. A difficult labor and delivery may result in a variety of injuries during the birth process. The details of these diseases of infancy and childhood may be found in specialized texts.

KEY CONCEPTS 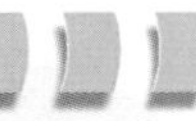

- Environmental factors that adversely affect the developing fetus are called *teratogens.* Exposure to teratogens is particularly dangerous during the third to ninth weeks of gestation.
- Known teratogens include chemicals and drugs, infections, and radiation. The teratogenic potential of many chemicals and drugs is unknown, so pregnant women are usually advised to avoid all drugs if possible.
- Of the infectious agents, viruses are the most teratogenic, particularly organisms of the TORCH variety (toxoplasmosis, others, rubella, cytomegalovirus, herpesvirus).

DIAGNOSIS, COUNSELING, AND GENE THERAPY

In recent years, the ability to diagnose and manage genetic and developmental disorders has improved dramatically. Although pedigree analysis continues to be an important method for identifying at-risk individuals, for a number of disorders it is now possible to determine if parents carry defective genes or if a particular fetus is afflicted. Currently, the ability to detect genetic mutations far exceeds the ability to offer definitive genetic treatment, giving rise to many ethical concerns.[29,30] Unfortunately, many individuals at risk for transmitting recessive genetic diseases are not identified until the birth of an afflicted child. Genetic counseling and prenatal assessment then become extremely important in assisting the family in regard to future pregnancies.

Prenatal Diagnosis and Counseling

A number of conditions are associated with a higher risk of congenital anomalies and are indications for instituting counseling and prenatal diagnostic examination. These conditions include (1) maternal age of 35 years or greater; (2) having borne a child with a chromosomal disorder (such as trisomy 21); (3) having a known family history of X-linked disorders; (4) having a family history of inborn errors of metabolism; (5) the occurrence of neural tube anomalies in a previous pregnancy; and (6) being a known carrier of a recessive genetic disorder. As diagnostic methods become more cost effective, general screening for other risk factors may be possible.

At present, ultrasound and amniocentesis are the mainstays of prenatal diagnostic examination. **Ultrasound** is a noninvasive procedure that uses sound waves to produce a reflected image of the fetus. It is commonly used to determine gestational age, fetal position, and placental location. Ultrasound is also useful in detecting visible congenital anomalies such as spina bifida (neural tube defect), heart defects, and malformations of the face, head, body, and limbs. It is useless for determining biochemical or chromosomal alterations.

Amniocentesis may be performed to determine genetic and developmental disorders not detectable by ultrasound. During amniocentesis, a needle is inserted through the abdomen or vagina and into the uterus. A sample of amniotic fluid containing skin cells shed by the fetus is removed for analysis. The amniotic fluid can be analyzed for abnormal levels of certain substances secreted by the fetus, such as α-fetoprotein, which may indicate neural tube defects. The live skin cells can be cultured and subjected to biochemical and chromosomal analysis. Only certain genetic and developmental disorders can be reliably detected by these procedures, and they may not provide the needed information until relatively late in the pregnancy. Amniocentesis cannot generally be performed prior to the 16th week of gestation, and 2 or 3 more weeks may be required to culture skin cells and subject them to analysis. **Chorionic villus sampling** involves the removal of a bit of tissue directly from the chorion (the outer membrane of the fetal sac). It can be performed at 8 weeks gestation.

Embryoscopy allows direct visualization of the embryo as early as the first trimester of pregnancy. The scope is inserted through the cervix and into the uterus. Embryoscopy can be used to identify developmental progress and to diagnose structural anomalies. An exciting application of this technique is the potential to directly manage genetic disorders with targeted gene or stem cell therapy.[31] The early diagnosis of congenital disorders allows a greater number of treatment options. Some disorders can be managed in utero; others may require early delivery, immediate surgery, or cesarean section to minimize fetal trauma. Early warning of fetal difficulties allows parents time to prepare emotionally for the birth of the child. In some instances, termination of the pregnancy may be the treatment of choice.

Genetic Analysis and Therapy

Painstaking pedigree analysis has allowed geneticists to assign a number of genetic traits and diseases to particular locations on the chromosomes. The process of determining the chromosomal location of genes is called *mapping.* Recent techniques in genetic analysis have radically improved the ability to assign genes to specific chromosomal locations. Not only are the locations of many genes being found, but the entire DNA sequence of many genes has been determined.

An exciting outcome of the human genome project is the potential for gene therapy—the treatment of genetic disease by replacing the defective gene with a normal, healthy one. This idea once sounded like science fiction, but clinical trials are already under way to manage a number of genetic disorders.[32] The first federally approved gene therapy procedure was performed in 1990 to treat a child who suffered from a rare condition called severe combined immunodeficiency (SCID) by introducing a functional gene for the enzyme adenosine deaminase. In the past, children who suffered from SCID had severely compromised immune systems and generally died from overwhelming infections unless their environment was strictly controlled. Use of gene therapy has been successful in improving immune function and allowing these children to live in the outside world.

Gene therapy has the potential for alleviating human suffering by curing genetic diseases, but it is accompanied by a number of moral and ethical dilemmas.[33] Tampering with the human gene pool could have serious implications for human evolution. There is also the potential for using the technology to create "new and improved" human beings or human clones.

Recombinant DNA Technology

Over the past 25 years, DNA has gone from being the hardest cellular molecule to study to being the easiest. The great advances in molecular genetics during this time are due to the development of recombinant DNA technologies. It is now possible to select a specific region of DNA, produce unlimited copies of it, determine its nucleotide sequence, use it to make unlimited quantities of a desired protein, or alter its DNA sequence at will (genetic engineering) and reinsert it into a living cell. These tools provide the means to uncover the nucleotide sequence of the entire human genome, to create DNA probes to explore an individual's genetic makeup for specific mutations, to mass produce therapeutic proteins and vaccines, and to cure genetic disorders by replacing mutant cellular genes with normally functioning ones.

Recombinant DNA technology comprises a number of techniques, the most important of which are briefly described here.

- The long, difficult-to-handle DNA strands are more easily studied if cut into smaller pieces. This is accomplished by restriction enzymes that cleave DNA at specific sites. The resulting pieces then can be separated by electrophoresis according to their size. A section of DNA can be collected and efficiently sequenced by automated means.
- Nucleic acid hybridization techniques take advantage of the natural tendency for DNA and RNA to find and bind to a complementary nucleotide sequence. A labeled piece of DNA or RNA can therefore be used to search for or "probe" for its complementary sequence among the many millions of sequences in a cell or cell extract. For example, in a fluorescence in situ hybridization assay, a probe for a specific site on a chromosome is attached to a fluorescent label and incubated with a cell. The fluorescence then identifies the location and number of copies of the particular chromosome sequence (Figure 6-23). Without the hybridization technique, finding a desired gene among the 10^9 base pairs in the human genome could take many years of intense effort, like finding the proverbial needle in a haystack.
- DNA cloning is the technique used to produce many identical copies of a DNA sequence containing a gene of interest. The availability of large quantities of a purified gene sequence makes study and gene manipulation possible. A number of different techniques can be used to clone DNA. The polymerase chain reaction (PCR) technique is very efficient if the DNA sequence is already partially known. Basically, the DNA sequence of interest is mixed with special DNA polymerases that use the DNA sequence as a template to produce double-stranded DNA. Each DNA thus produced can in turn act as a template for production of another DNA. Large quantities can be produced very rapidly by PCR. The DNA can also be cloned by inserting it into bacteria by use of a viral or plasmid vector. Bacteria that take up the desired gene are identified by hybridization with a labeled probe. The desired bacteria then are allowed to proliferate, making a copy of the DNA sequence along with their own genome with each cell division.
- Genetic engineering refers to a process whereby a gene of interest is altered from its original form. The changed (mutant) genes can be reintroduced into a cell to disclose the effect on cell function and thus elucidate the normal function of the original gene and its protein product. Genetic engineering has been applied to plants to increase their value as food crops. Genetically engineered cells can be turned into protein factories to produce hormones, such as insulin, in large quantity.

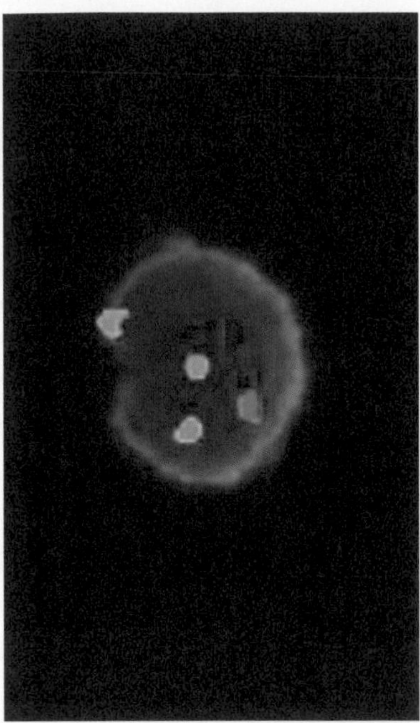

FIGURE 6-23 ■ Fluorescence in situ hybridization assay showing an interphase nucleus from a male patient with suspected trisomy 18. Three different fluorescent probes have been used: The red probe hybridized to the Y chromosome, the green probe hybridized to the X chromosome, and the blue probe hybridized to the centromere of chromosome 18. Three copies of chromosome 18 are identified, confirming the diagnosis. (From Kumar V, Cotran RS, Robbins ST, editors: *Robbins basic pathology,* ed 7, Philadelphia, 2003, Saunders, p. 258. Photograph courtesy Dr. Nancy R. Schneider and Jeff Doolittle, University of Texas Southwestern Medical Center, Dallas.)

Gene therapy relies heavily on these techniques to facilitate identification of genetic mutations, study of gene function, and development of methods to repair or replace mutant genes. Many more applications of recombinant DNA technology will become apparent as research on the genetic basis of human function and disease proceeds.

KEY CONCEPTS

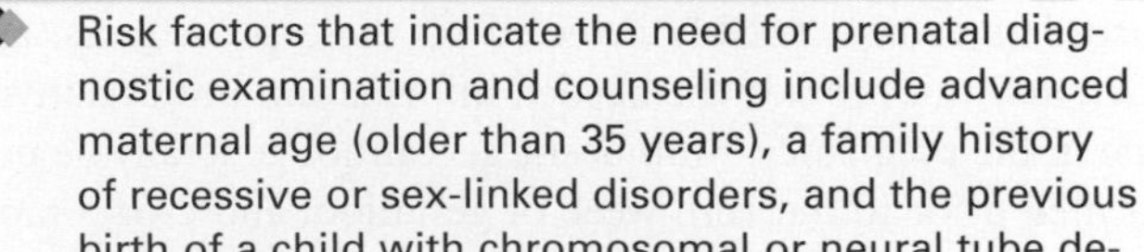

- Risk factors that indicate the need for prenatal diagnostic examination and counseling include advanced maternal age (older than 35 years), a family history of recessive or sex-linked disorders, and the previous birth of a child with chromosomal or neural tube defects.
- Ultrasound, amniocentesis, and chorionic villus sampling are the mainstays of prenatal assessment for genetic disorders.
- DNA sequences that are complementary to a gene of interest can be synthesized and used to probe the genome to determine if and where the gene is pres-

ent. These hybridization techniques make screening for genetic disorders relatively fast and simple.

- Gene therapy is the treatment of genetic disease by replacing defective genes with normal genes. Gene therapy is possible because of the advances attained in recombinant DNA technology over the past 25 years.

SUMMARY

Genetic and developmental disorders are responsible for a number of congenital malformations. Congenital disorders are caused by genetic and environmental factors that disrupt normal fetal development. Genetic disorders are classified as (1) chromosomal alterations, including structural and numeric abnormalities; (2) mendelian disorders, including autosomal dominant, autosomal recessive, and X-linked disorders; and (3) nonmendelian single-gene disorders, including triplet repeats, mitochondrial gene defects, and genetic imprinting disorders. Known environmental teratogens include radiation, infectious organisms, and various chemicals and drugs. The embryo is particularly susceptible to teratogens during the period of organogenesis, which extends from the third to the ninth week of gestation. Pedigree analysis, ultrasound, amniocentesis, and chorionic villus biopsy may provide helpful information regarding genetic risk and the prenatal condition of at-risk infants. DNA sequencing of normal and mutant genes has made it possible to efficiently screen for genetic disorders and develop gene therapies for a variety of genetic diseases.

MEDIA RESOURCES

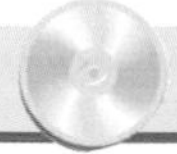

evolve

Remember to check out the ***CD Companion*** included with this book for Review Questions, Key Concepts Review, Glossary (with audio for selected terms), Disease Profiles, and Animations.

PLUS, visit the ***Evolve website*** at http://evolve.elsevier.com/Copstead/ for Case Studies, Disease Profiles, and WebLinks.

References

1. Modell B, Darr A: Science and society: genetic counselling and customary consanguineous marriage, *Nat Rev Genet* 3(3):225-229, 2002.
2. Kalter H: Teratology in the 20th century: environmental causes of congenital malformations in humans and how they were established, *Neurotoxicol Teratol* 25(2):131-282, 2003.
3. Martin J et al: Births: final data for 2002, *Natl Vital Stat Rep* 52(10):1-113, 2002.
4. Maitra A, Kumar V: Genetic and pediatric diseases. In Kumar V, Cotran RS, Robbins ST, editors: *Robbins basic pathology,* ed 7, Philadelphia, 2003, Saunders, pp 211-264.
5. Bateson W: *Mendel's principles of heredity,* London, 1902, Cambridge University Press.
6. Alberts B et al: Germ cells and fertilization. In Alberts B et al, editors: *Molecular biology of the cell,* ed 4, New York, 2002, Garland Science, pp 1127-1156.
7. Hassold T, Hunt P: To err (meiotically) is human: the genesis of human aneuploidy, *Nat Rev Genet* 2(4):280-291, 2001.
8. Petersen MB, Mikkelsen M: Nondisjunction in trisomy 21: origin and mechanisms, *Cytogenet Cell Genet* 91(1-4):199-203, 2000.
9. Roizen NJ, Patterson D: Down's syndrome, *Lancet* 361(9365):1281-1289, 2003.
10. Down JHL: Observations on an ethnic classification of idiots, *Clin Lect Rep London Hosp* 3:259-262, 1866.
11. Morris JK et al: Comparison of models of maternal age–specific risk for Down syndrome live births, *Prenat Diagn* 23(3):252-258, 2003.
12. Fisch H et al: The influence of paternal age on Down syndrome, *J Urol* 169(6):2275-2278, 2003.
13. Wyrobek AJ et al: Mechanisms and targets involved in maternal and paternal age effects on numerical aneuploidy, *Eviron Mol Mutagen* 28(3):254-264, 1996.
14. Bojesen A, Juul S, Gravholt CH: Prenatal and postnatal prevalence of Klinefelter syndrome: a national registry study, *J Clin Endocrinol Metab* 88(2):622-626, 2003.
15. Manning MA, Hoyme HE: Diagnosis and management of the adolescent boy with Klinefelter syndrome, *Adolesc Med* 13(2):367-374, viii, 2002.
16. De Vigan C et al: EUROSCAN Working Group: contribution of ultrasonographic examination to the prenatal detection of chromosomal abnormalities in 19 centres across Europe, *Ann Genet* 44(4):209-217, 2001.
17. Alberts B et al: DNA replication, repair, and recombination. In Alberts B et al, editors: *Molecular biology of the cell,* ed 4, New York, 2002, Garland Science, pp 235-298.
18. Collod-Beroud G, Boileau C: Marfan syndrome in the third millennium, *Eur J Hum Genet* 10(11):673-681, 2002.
19. The Huntington's Disease Collaborative Research Group: A novel gene containing a trinucleotide repeat that is expanded and unstable on Huntington's disease chromosomes, *Cell* 72:971, 1993.
20. Margolis R, Ross CA: Diagnosis of Huntington disease, *Clin Chem* 49(10):1726-1732, 2003.
21. Bates G: Huntingtin aggregation and toxicity in Huntington's disease, *Lancet* 361(9369):1642-1644, 2003.
22. Okulicz JF et al: Oculocutaneous albinism, *J Eur Acad Dermatol Venereol* 17(3):251-256, 2003.
23. Bobadilla JL et al: Cystic fibrosis: a worldwide analysis of CFTR mutations—correlation with incidence data and application to screening, *Hum Mutat* 19(6):575-606, 2002.
24. Griesenbach U, Geddes DM, Alton EW: Update on gene therapy for cystic fibrosis, *Curr Opin Mol Ther* 5(5):489-494, 2003.
25. Stevenson RE, Schwartz CE: Clinical and molecular contributions to the understanding of X-linked mental retardation, *Cytogenet Genome Res* 99(1-4):265-275, 2002.
26. Vogels A, Fryns JP: The Prader-Willi syndrome and the Angelman syndrome, *Genet Couns* 13(4):385-396, 2002.
27. Abel EL: An update on the incidence of FAS: FAS is not an equal opportunity birth defect, *Neurotoxicol Teratol* 17(4):437-443, 1995.
28. Abel EL, Hannigan JH: Maternal risk factors in fetal alcohol syndrome: provocative and permissive influences, *Neurotoxicol Teratol* 17(4):445-462, 1995.

29. Fleming DA: Ethical considerations of genetic testing, *J Clin Ethics* 13(4):316-323, 2002.
30. Milunsky JM, Milunsky A: Genetic counseling in perinatal medicine, *Obstet Gynecol Clin North Am* 24(1):1-17, 1997.
31. Crombleholme TM, Johnson MP: Fetoscopic surgery, *Clin Obstet Gynecol* 46(1):76-91, 2003.
32. Russell SJ, Peng KW: Primer on medical genomics. X: gene therapy, *Mayo Clin Proc* 78(11):1370-1383, 2003.
33. Ott BB: The Human Genome Project: an overview of ethical issues and public policy concerns, *Nurs Outlook* 43(5):228-231, 1995.

chapter 7

Neoplasia

Jacquelyn L. Banasik

MEDIA RESOURCES

Additional Material for Study, Review, and Further Exploration

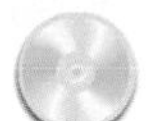

CD Companion ◆ Review Questions and Answers ◆ Key Concepts Review
◆ Glossary *(with audio pronunciations for selected terms)*
◆ Disease Profiles ◆ Animations

evolve *Website* at http://evolve.elsevier.com/Copstead/
◆ Case Studies ◆ Disease Profiles ◆ WebLinks

KEY QUESTIONS

- How do neoplastic cells differ from normal cells?
- In what ways do benign and malignant tumors differ?
- How might overexpression of proto-oncogenes lead to abnormal cellular proliferation?
- How might underexpression of tumor suppressor genes lead to abnormal cellular proliferation?
- What properties are gained during tumor progression that contribute to malignant behavior and metastasis?
- How are tumor grading and staging used to guide the selection of cancer therapies?
- How might lifestyle and carcinogen exposure contribute to cancer risk?
- How can tumor cells be eradicated from the body?

CHAPTER OUTLINE

Neoplasia means "new growth." In common use, the term implies an *abnormality* of cellular growth and may be used interchangeably with the term *tumor.* Neoplasia is associated with uncertain and sometimes life-threatening consequences. It is no surprise that the discovery of a tumor in an individual can evoke feelings of disbelief, anger, and dread. Characterization of the tumor cells is of critical importance to determine whether the tumor is benign or malignant (cancerous). The diagnosis of a **benign** growth is received with great relief inasmuch as the tumor is generally easily cured. The diagnosis of a **malignant** cancer, on the other hand, may herald months of intensive and often uncomfortable treatment with uncertain outcomes. Cancer remains the second leading cause of death in the United States for both men and women.

It is increasingly clear that cancer is associated with *altered expression of cellular genes* that normally regulate cell proliferation and differentiation. A unified theory of cancer causation has emerged, and new methods for cancer therapy continue to be developed. Cancer is a complex, multifaceted disorder with each individual cancer having some unique properties. A better understanding of the molecular characteristics of individual cancers is encouraging the development of specific therapies that target the cancer's weaknesses.

BENIGN VERSUS MALIGNANT GROWTH

Characteristics of Benign and Malignant Tumors

The terms *benign* and *malignant* refer to the overall consequences of a tumor to the host. Generally, malignant tumors have the potential to kill the host if left untreated, whereas benign tumors do not. This difference is not strict because some benign tumors may be located in critical areas. For example, a benign tumor may be life threatening if it causes pressure on the brain or blocks an airway or blood vessel. Histologic examination of a tumor is the primary mode for determining its benign or malignant nature. Certain tumor characteristics have historically been shown to indicate malignant potential. Important considerations include localization of the tumor and the differentiation of tumor cells.

Benign tumors do not invade adjacent tissue or spread to distant sites. Many benign tumors are encapsulated by connective tissue, which is an indication of strictly local growth. Any evidence that tumor cells have penetrated local tissues (invasiveness), lymphatics, or blood vessels suggests a malignant nature with potential to spread to distant sites (metastasize).

As a general rule, benign cells more closely resemble their tissue type of origin (e.g., skin, liver) than do malignant cells. The degree of tissue-specific differentiation has traditionally been used to predict malignant potential. A lack of differentiated features in a cancer cell is called **anaplasia,** and a greater degree of anaplasia is correlated with a more aggressively malignant tumor.[1] Anaplasia is indicated by variation in cell size and shape within the tumor, enlarged nuclei, abnormal mitoses, and bizarre-looking giant cells (Figure 7-1). Regardless of histologic appearance, invasion of local tissue or evidence of **metastasis** to distant sites confirms the diagnosis of malignancy.

Other differences between benign and malignant tumors have been noted (Table 7-1). Benign tumors generally grow more slowly, have little vascularity, rarely have necrotic areas, and often retain functions similar to those of the tissue of origin. Conversely, malignant tumors often grow rapidly and may initiate vessel growth in the tumor. They frequently have necrotic areas and are dysfunctional.

Tumor Terminology

General rules for the naming of tumors have been developed to indicate the tissue of origin and the benign or malignant nature of the tumor. The suffix *-oma* is used to indicate a benign tumor, whereas *carcinoma* and *sarcoma* are used to indicate malignant tumors. Carcinoma refers to malignant tumors of epithelial origin and sarcoma to malignant tumors of mesenchymal (nerve, bone, muscle) origin. Thus a benign tumor of glandular tissue would be called an adenoma, but a malignant tumor of the same tissue would be called an adenocarcinoma (Table 7-2). Some notable exceptions to the rules are lymphomas, hepatomas, and melanomas, which are all highly malignant despite their *-oma* suffix. Leukemia refers to a malignant growth of white blood cells. The great majority of

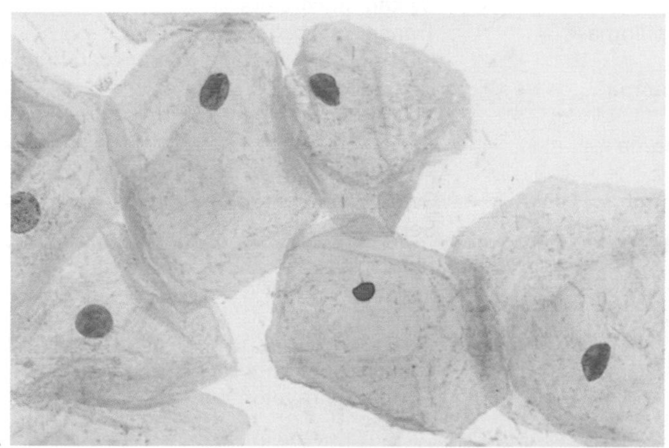

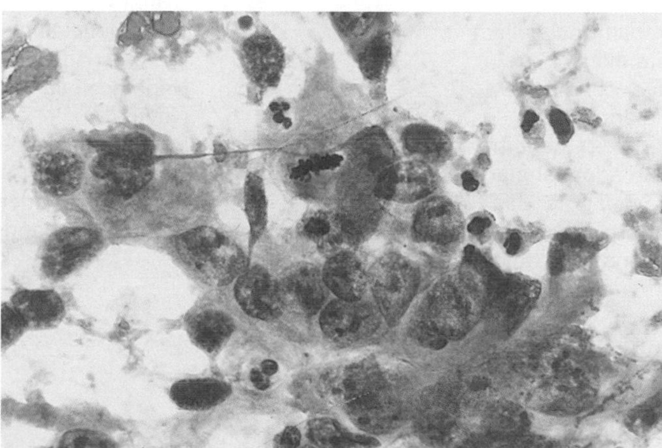

FIGURE 7-1 ■ **A,** Normal Papanicolaou smear from the uterine cervix showing large, flat epithelial cells with small nuclei. **B,** Typical histologic appearance of anaplastic tumor cells showing variation in cell size and shape, with large, hyperchromic nuclei. (From Kumar V, Cotran RS, Robbins SL: *Basic pathology,* ed 7, Philadelphia, 2003, Saunders, p 208. Courtesy Dr. Richard M. DeMay, Department of Pathology, University of Chicago.)

Table 7-1 

General Characteristics of Benign and Malignant Tumors

Characteristic	Benign	Malignant
Histology	Typical of tissue of origin Few mitoses	Anaplastic, with abnormal cell size and shape Many mitoses
Growth rate	Slow	Rapid
Localization/metastasis	Strictly local, often encapsulated/no metastasis	Infiltrative/frequent metastases
Tumor necrosis	Rare	Common
Recurrence after treatment	Rare	Common
Prognosis	Good	Poor if untreated

human cancers (90%) are carcinomas from malignant transformation of epithelial cells.[2]

The Cancerous Phenotype

Cells growing in normal tissue have predictable relationships with neighboring cells. In a particular tissue, the rate of cell growth is precisely matched to the rate of cell death. Normal cells require constant reassurance from their environment that their continued existence is desirable, and they proliferate only when space is available and appropriate growth-stimulating signals are present. Normal cells also respond to signals instructing them to commit suicide by actively killing themselves in a process called *apoptosis* (see Chapter 4). Tumor cells, however, do not obey the rules; they have escaped the normal mechanisms of growth control. A number of antisocial properties develop in tumor cells that allow them to proliferate at the expense of other cells and tissues of the body. These antisocial behaviors can be summarized as follows:

- Cancer cells proliferate despite lack of growth-initiating signals from the environment.
- Cancer cells escape signals to die and achieve a kind of immortality in that they are capable of unlimited replication.
- Cancer cells lose their differentiated features and contribute poorly or not at all to the function of their tissue.
- Cancer cells are genetically unstable and evolve by accumulating new mutations at a much faster rate than normal cells.
- Cancer cells invade their local tissue and overrun their neighbors.

Table 7-2

Nomenclature for Neoplastic Diseases

Cell or Tissue of Origin	Benign	Malignant
Tumors of Epithelial Origin		
Squamous cells	Squamous cell papilloma	Squamous cell carcinoma
Basal cells	—	Basal cell carcinoma
Glandular or ductal epithelium	Adenoma	Adenocarcinoma
	Cystadenoma	Cystadenocarcinoma
Transitional cells	Transitional cell papilloma	Transitional cell carcinoma
Bile duct	Bile duct adenoma	Bill duct carcinoma (cholangiocarcinoma)
Liver cells	Hepatocellular adenoma	Hepatocellular carcinoma
Melanocytes	Nevus	Malignant melanoma
Renal epithelium	Renal tubular adenoma	Renal cell carcinoma
Skin adnexal glands		
Sweat glands	Sweat gland adenoma	Sweat gland carcinoma
Sebaceous glands	Sebaceous glands adenoma	Sebaceous glands carcinoma
Germs cells (testis and ovary)	—	Seminoma (dysgerminoma), embryonal carcinoma, yolk sac carcinoma
Tumors of Mesenchymal Origin		
Hematopoietic/lymphoid tissue	—	Leukemia, lymphoma, Hodgkin disease, multiple myeloma
Neural and retinal tissue		
Nerve sheath	Neurilemmoma, neurofibroma	Malignant peripheral nerve sheath tumor
Nerve cells	Ganglioneuroma	Neuroblastoma
Retinal cells (cones)	—	Retinoblastoma
Connective tissue		
Fibrous tissue	Fibromatosis (desmoid)	Fibrosarcoma
Fat	Lipoma	Liposarcoma
Bone	Osteoma	Osteogenic sarcoma
Cartilage	Chondroma	Chondrosarcoma
Muscle		
Smooth muscle	Leiomyoma	Leiomyosarcoma
Striated muscle	Rhabdomyoma	Rhabdomyosarcoma
Endothelial and related tissues		
Blood vessels	Hemangioma	Angiosarcoma
		Kaposi sarcoma
Lymph vessels	Lymphangioma	Lymphangiosarcoma
Synovium	—	Synovial sarcoma
Mesothelium	—	Malignant mesothelioma
Meninges	Meningioma	Malignant meningioma

From Murphy GP, Lawrence W, Lenhard RE, editors: *American Cancer Society textbook of clinical oncology,* Atlanta, 1995, American Cancer Society, p 77. Reproduced by permission of the American Cancer Society, Inc.

- Perhaps worst of all, cancer cells gain the ability to migrate from their site of origin to colonize distant sites where they do not belong.

Cancers are thought to arise from stem cells that are present in tissues. Tissue stem cells are not terminally differentiated and are capable of entering the cell cycle, whereas the other differentiated tissue cells do not replicate. What cellular derangement converts a normally cooperative stem cell to a competitive one? The answer, it seems, is in its genes.

KEY CONCEPTS

- Malignant tumors kill the host, whereas benign tumors generally do not. The primary difference between malignant and benign tumors is the propensity of malignant tumors to invade adjacent tissue and spread to distant sites (metastasize).
- The suffix *-oma* is used to indicate a benign tumor (e.g., fibroma). *Carcinoma* and *sarcoma* are used to indicate malignancy (e.g., fibrosarcoma). Exceptions include melanomas, lymphomas, hepatomas, and leukemia, all of which are malignant.
- Cancer cells exhibit antisocial properties that allow them to ignore growth-controlling signals from the environment. Cancer cells proliferate excessively, become immortal, invade locally, and may travel to distant sites where they establish new colonies.

GENETIC MECHANISMS OF CANCER

Despite much progress in our understanding of how mechanisms of growth control and cellular differentiation may go awry, there is still no simple answer to the question, "What causes cancer?" It is increasingly evident, however, that cancer is primarily a disorder of gene expression. Early support for a genetic basis of cancer came from the observation that cancer often resulted from agents known to damage deoxyribonucleic acid (DNA). In the 1970s a number of potential cancer-causing agents (**carcinogens**) were identified by demonstrating their mutagenic potential.[3] The suggestion that mutant genes were the basis for cancer launched intense research to identify the cancer-causing gene or genes.

It is now apparent that two major categories of critical cancer genes are involved in the regulation of cellular growth and that dysfunction of these genes is a factor in most forms of cancer.[2] The first category is **proto-oncogenes,** which code for components of the cellular growth-activating pathways. *Overactivity* of proto-oncogenes enhances cell proliferation and predisposes to the development of cancer. The second category of cancer-related genes is **tumor suppressor genes,** which inhibit cell proliferation. Cancers may arise when tumor suppressor gene function is lost. To achieve malignant transformation, a cell must generally suffer mutations in a combination of these growth regulatory genes. A cell thus transformed passes on these mutations to its progeny when it divides and forms a clone of abnormally proliferating cells. Numerous studies have begun to unravel the details of how proto-oncogenes and tumor suppressor genes may dysfunction and contribute to the cancerous phenotype. In addition to the genes that regulate the cell cycle, the genes that regulate apoptosis are important in cancer development. For cancer cells to achieve immortality and avoid replicative senescence, a defect in the apoptotic pathway is necessary.

Proto-Oncogenes

Proto-oncogenes were the first of the tumor-associated genes to be discovered, and about 100 different ones have been described to date.[2] As often happens in the study of genes, a gene associated with a disease process is identified long before its normal cellular function is elucidated. Thus genes associated with cancer are traditionally named for the cancer in which they were first discovered (in mutant form) rather than their normal cellular function. Many of the first cancer-associated genes, called **oncogenes,** were initially identified in viruses and still retain the name reflecting their viral discovery. The term *proto-oncogene* was created to label the normal cellular counterpart of the oncogene. A representative list of known proto-oncogenes is shown in Table 7-3.

The majority of proto-oncogenes described to date code for components of cell-signaling systems that promote cell proliferation.[2] These components can be lumped into four

Table 7-3 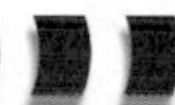

Examples of Proto-Oncogenes and Their Mechanisms of Action

Factor	Type of Cancer
Proto-Oncogenes for Growth Factors	
PDGF	Glioma (brain tumor
FGF	Melanoma
EGF	Breast
TGF-α	Breast, numerous others
Proto-Oncogenes for Receptors	
ERBB1 (EGF receptor)	Breast, brain
HER-2 (ERBB2)	Breast, ovarian
RET	Thyroid
Proto-Oncogenes for Cytoplasmic Signaling Molecules	
RAS	Lung, ovarian, colon, pancreatic
ABL	Leukemia
Proto-Oncogenes for Transcription Factors	
C-MYC	Leukemia, breast, lung
N-MYC	Neuroblastoma
L-MYC	Lung
MYB	Various
JUN	Various
FOS	Various
REL	Various

EGF, Epidermal growth factor; *FGF,* fibroblast growth factor; *PDGF,* platelet-derived growth factor; *TGF,* transforming growth factor.

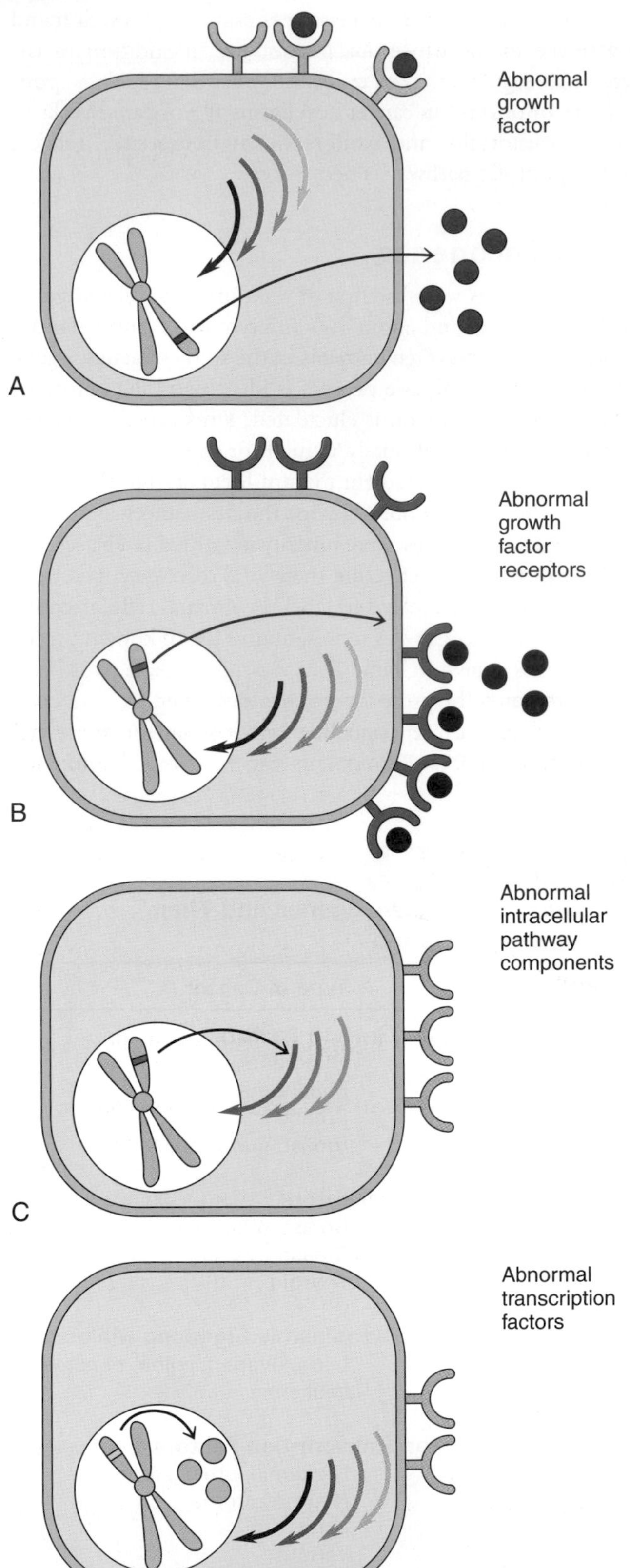

FIGURE 7-2 ■ Possible effects of proto-oncogene activation on growth signaling pathways. **A,** Production of growth factors. **B,** Production of growth factor receptors. **C,** Intracellular pathway disturbances. **D,** Activation of transcription factors for growth.

broad categories: (1) growth factors, (2) receptors, (3) cytoplasmic signaling molecules, and (4) nuclear transcription factors (Figure 7-2). Excessive activity in any of these components may release the cell from environmental feedback and allow it to proliferate abnormally.

Growth Factors

The first proto-oncogenes to be discovered coded for growth factors. A great deal of intercellular communication is accomplished through the cell-to-cell transmission of growth factors. Growth factors are small peptides that are manufactured by cells and secreted into the extracellular space. They diffuse to nearby cells and interact with receptors on the target cell surface. Binding of growth factors to cell surface receptors activates growth-promoting cascades within the cell. As a general principle, stem cells do not produce growth factors sufficient to stimulate their own proliferation. The growth-stimulating signals must be produced by the cell's environment. The cell's environment also conveys growth-inhibiting signals. Overproduction of stimulatory growth factors by a mutant proto-oncogene can shift the balance of signals and produce excessive self-stimulated growth (**autocrine signaling**). Examples of tumor-secreted growth factors include platelet-derived growth factor, transforming growth factor-α, and epidermal growth factor. Certain cancer types typically secrete particular growth factors. For example, platelet-derived growth factor is commonly oversecreted in glial cell cancers (brain tumors) and connective tissue cancers (sarcomas).

Growth Factor Receptors

Peptide growth factors cannot penetrate the cell membrane directly, so their presence at the cell surface must be transmitted intracellularly by cell surface receptors. Receptors are transmembrane proteins with the growth factor–binding area on the outside of the cell and an enzyme-activating area on the inside of the cell. These receptors are extremely specific; they will bind with only one particular growth factor. Binding activates a series of reactions within the cell that eventually leads to cell proliferation.

A mutational event may allow the expression of receptors that should not be present at all or allow excessive amounts of normally present receptors, or it may produce receptors with abnormally high affinity. All of these changes result in excessive responsiveness to the growth factors normally present in the cell's environment. Some mutant receptors may even be active in the absence of growth factors and spur the cell to divide despite the absence of environmental signals to do so. An important example of a receptor abnormality is the overexpression of human epidermal growth factor receptor type 2 (HER2) receptors in about 25% of breast cancers. The overactive receptors stimulate proliferation of tumor cells even when there is little or no growth factor bound to them.

Cytoplasmic Signaling Pathways

A third way in which oncogenes may allow growth factor independence is by the manufacture of excessive or abnormal components of the intracellular growth-signaling pathways. These pathways involve numerous enzymes and chemicals that are only partly known. They normally function to transmit growth signals from activated receptors at the cell surface to the cell nucleus. An oncogene that codes for excessive or abnormal cytoplasmic signaling components could cause activation of the pathway even though no signal was received at the cell surface. The best understood example of this mechanism is mutations of the *ras* gene family. Proteins encoded by *ras* genes are G proteins that transmit growth signals from receptors at the cell surface into the interior of the cell. The ras protein is active when it has guanosine triphosphate (GTP) bound to it, but it quickly hydrolyzes the GTP, thus automatically turning itself off after a brief period of activity. A mutation in the *ras* gene can code for a protein that is unable to hydrolyze GTP, so it remains persistently active and stimulates cell growth inappropriately. Mutations of the *ras* genes occur in about 30% of all human cancers, including leukemias and lung, ovarian, colon, and pancreatic cancer.

Transcription Factors

The entire growth factor pathway, including the growth factor, the receptor, and the second-messenger cascade, ultimately affects transcription of a set of genes in the nucleus that spur the cell to enter S phase. A number of proto-oncogenes have been identified that code for transcription factors in the nucleus. Transcription factors are proteins that must be assembled at the promotor area to begin gene transcription (see Chapters 3 and 5). Transcription factors are normally sequestered and prevented from indiscriminate activity until appropriate signals cause their release. Mutations in transcription factor genes may cause overproduction of transcription factors or interfere with the normal mechanisms for keeping them in check. *Myc, jun,* and *fos* are examples of proto-oncogenes that code for nuclear transcription factors. Abnormalities of the *myc* genes are found in numerous cancers, including lung and breast cancer, leukemia, and neuroblastoma.

From Proto-Oncogene to Oncogene

Proto-oncogenes become activated oncogenes when mutations alter their activity so that proliferation-promoting signals are generated inappropriately. At least four general ways in which proto-oncogenes can be activated are known (Figure 7-3): (1) oncogenes may be introduced into the host cell by a retrovirus; (2) a proto-oncogene within the cell may suffer a mutagenic event that changes its structure and function; (3) a DNA sequence that normally regulates proto-oncogene expression may be damaged or lost and allow the proto-oncogene to become abnormally active; and (4) an error in chromosome replication may cause extra copies of the proto-oncogene to be included in the genome (amplification).

In the early 1960s it was discovered that certain viruses were associated with cancer in various animal models. Researchers speculated that a virus could introduce a mutant, cancer-causing gene (oncogene) into the host's cells. Indeed, malignant cells containing the cancer-causing viruses were shown to have incorporated a small number of viral genes into their cellular DNA.[4] The presence of these oncogenes was required to maintain the malignant state of the cell.

Only a few types of human cancers are thought to be associated with viruses. The clearest associations involve viruses called retroviruses. At least three retroviruses are thought to be causative factors in some human cancers: human immunodeficiency virus is associated with Kaposi sarcoma, Epstein-Barr virus with Burkitt lymphoma, and human T-lymphocyte virus type I with adult T-cell leukemia-lymphoma.

Retroviruses are composed of RNA and possess a unique enzyme, reverse transcriptase, which directs the synthesis of a DNA copy of the viral RNA. The DNA copy can then be incorporated into the cellular DNA and become part of the host's genome. The degree of viral oncogene expression depends on where the oncogene is inserted in the host DNA. Insertion near a promoter sequence may result in continuous transcription of the oncogene. Viral oncogenes are not subject to normal DNA transcription controls and are thus not responsive to growth-suppressing signals. Where did the viral oncogenes originate? Apparently, the tendency of retroviruses to slip in and out of host genomes allows them to pick up some of the host's genes, namely, the growth-promoting proto-oncogenes.

Proto-oncogene expression is tightly regulated in a normal cell. A number of different mutations can affect proto-oncogene expression and activity. A point mutation in the coding region of the proto-oncogene can alter the structure of its protein product and make it hyperactive. An example of this mechanism is the abnormal ras protein described earlier. Even though the protein is made in normal quantity, its activity is enhanced. Other mutations may lead to overproduction of a protein with normal structure. Gene amplification and chromosomal rearrangement during mitosis may release the proto-oncogene from its normal regulation and allow excessive transcription (Figure 7-4).

In summary, mutational events in the cell's genome cause overexpression of normal proto-oncogene products or production of altered and hyperactive proteins. Most known oncogenes act by releasing the cell from its dependence on growth-promoting signals in the environment. This effect may be accomplished by abnormal production of growth factors, receptors, cytoplasmic signaling molecules, or nuclear transcription factors.

Tumor Suppressor Genes

To become malignant, cells must devise ways to evade the normal inhibitory mechanisms that keep the brakes applied to cell division. It is not enough to simply overstimulate growth-promoting signals. Critical elements of the proliferation-inhibiting pathways are defective in most cancers. The components of the inhibitory machinery are specified by the so-called *tumor suppressor genes.* Tumor suppressor genes are difficult to study because they are noticeable only when they are not there. The first tumor suppressor gene to be discovered was the *Rb* gene, so named because of its role in

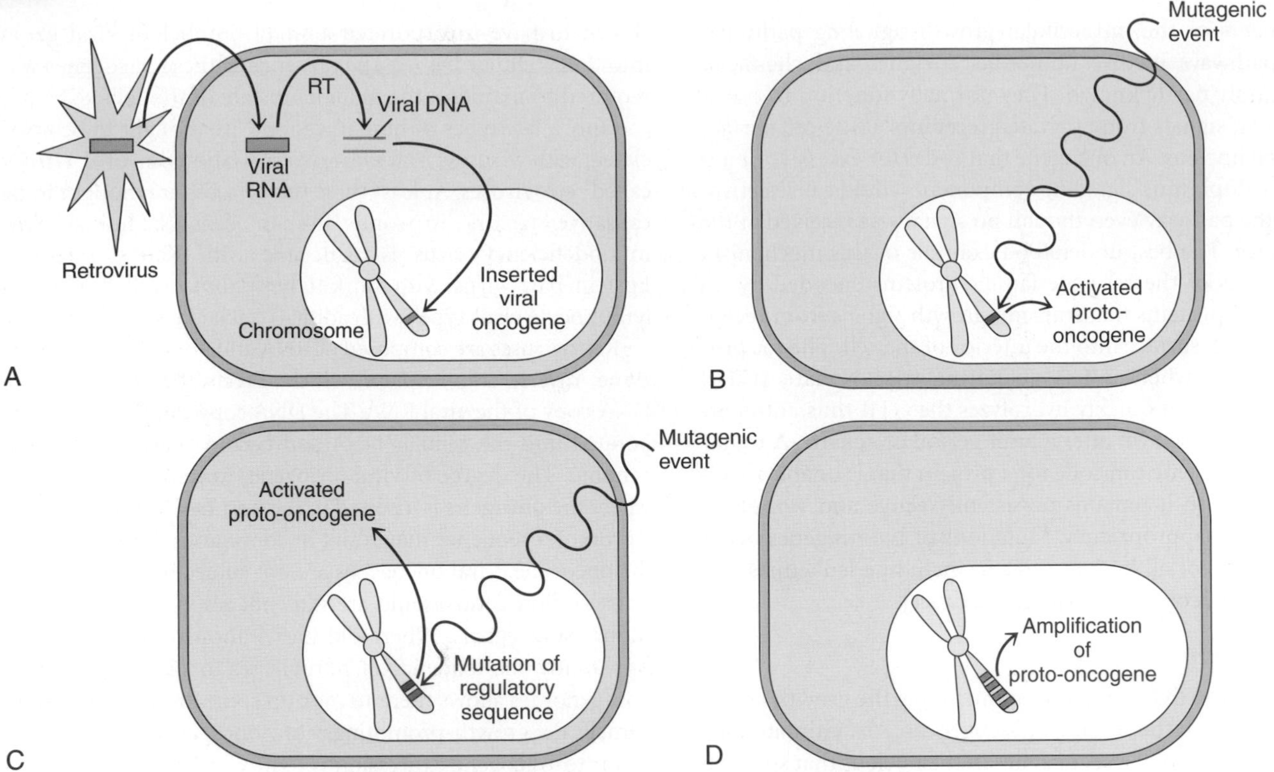

FIGURE 7-3 ■ Mechanisms of proto-oncogene activation. **A,** Retroviral insertion. **B,** Proto-oncogene mutation. **C,** Regulatory sequence mutation. **D,** Proto-oncogene amplification. *RT,* Reverse transcriptase.

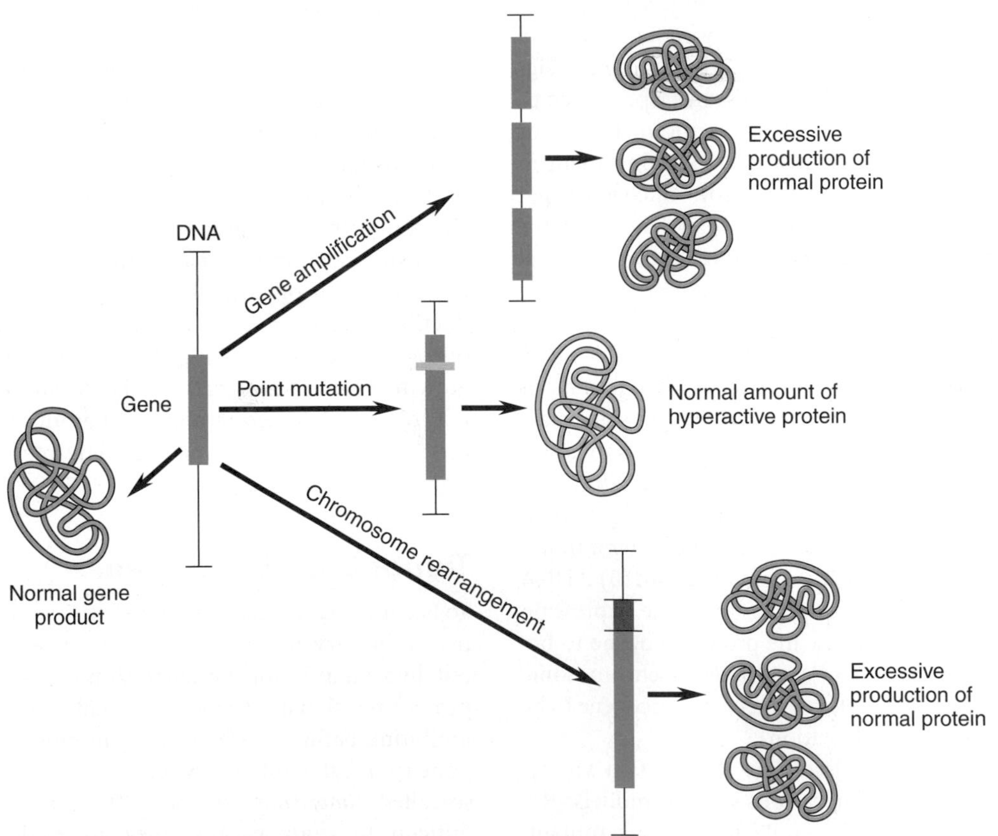

FIGURE 7-4 ■ Overactivity of proto-oncogenes may be due to normal production of an abnormal protein (mutation in coding sequence) or excessive production of a normal protein (gene amplification or chromosome rearrangement).

retinoblastoma, a cancer of the eye (also called PRB).[5] A familial form of retinoblastoma is associated with the transmission of a genetic defect; a portion of chromosome 13 is missing, which is where the *Rb* gene is normally located. An absent *Rb* gene predisposes an individual to cancer, but cancer will not develop unless the other copy of the *Rb* gene (from the other parent) is also damaged (Figure 7-5).

Since the initial discovery of the *Rb* tumor suppressor gene, researchers have compiled an impressive list of other genes that appear to function as inhibitors of cellular proliferation

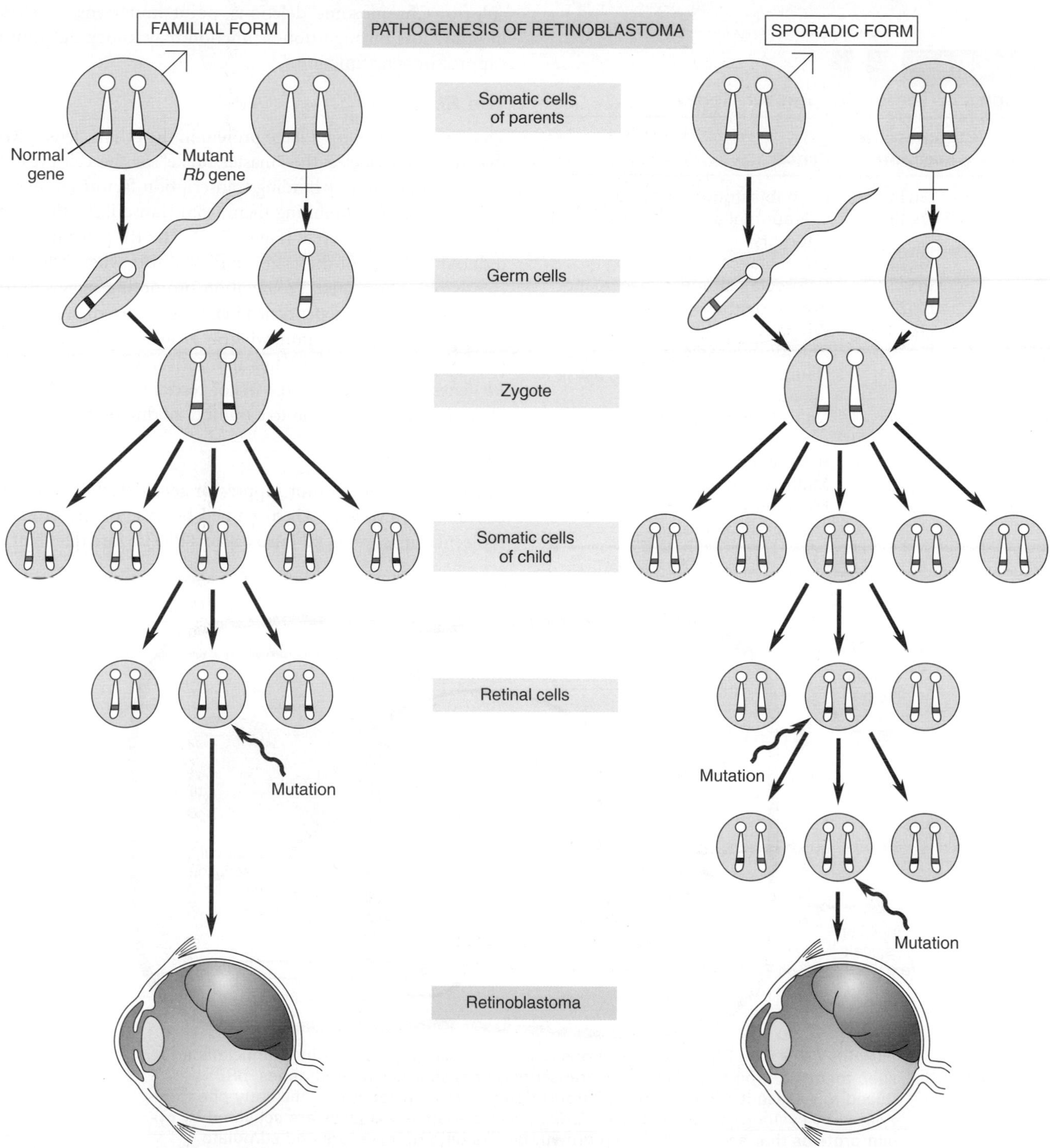

FIGURE 7-5 ■ Both DNA copies (alleles) of the *Rb* tumor suppression gene must be dysfunctional for retinoblastoma to occur. Inheriting a defective *Rb* gene predisposes an individual to the development of cancer because only a single mutational event is required to inactivate pRB function. (Redrawn from Kumar V, Cotran RS, Robbins SL: *Basic pathology,* ed 7, Philadelphia, 2003, Saunders, p 184.)

(Table 7-4). As with the *Rb* gene, both copies of the tumor suppressor genes must be inactivated for cancer to develop. A person who inherits a defective copy of a tumor suppressor gene from one parent has a much higher risk of cancer than one who inherits two healthy copies. Knowledge about the sequence of many of these genes provides the opportunity to screen individuals with familial cancers to determine whether they carry a defective gene. Detection of defective tumor suppressor genes is easier than figuring out their normal cellular functions, but steady progress is being made.

Why do tumor suppressor genes stop functioning? As with proto-oncogene activation, genetic mutations are the usual culprits. Chromosome deletions, point mutations, or chromosome loss through nondisjunction may knock out tumor suppressor gene function.

Table 7-4

Examples of Tumor Suppressor Genes

Gene	Chromosome Location	Cancer
RB	13q14	Retinoblastoma, sarcoma
P53	17p13	Li-Fraumeni syndrome, 50% of all tumors
DCC	18q21	Colorectal carcinoma
APC	5q21	Colorectal, stomach, pancreatic
BRCA1	17q21	Breast, ovarian
WT1	11p13	Wilms tumor
WT2	11p15	Rhabdomyosarcoma
NF1	17q11	Neurofibromatosis type 1, astrocytoma
NF2	22q12	Neurofibromatosis type 2, meningioma
VHL	3p25	Renal cell carcinoma
MEN1	11q23	Multiple endocrine neoplasia
MTS1	9p21	Melanoma, leukemia, sarcomas, several carcinomas

The *Rb* Gene

The *Rb* gene codes for a large protein in the cell nucleus (pRB) that has been labeled the "master brake" of the cell cycle. It blocks cell division by binding transcription factors (primarily E2F) and thereby inhibiting them from transcribing the genes that initiate the cell cycle (Figure 7-6). The RB protein can be induced to let go of the transcription factors when it is sufficiently phosphorylated. Proliferation-promoting signals in the cell increase cyclin-dependent kinase (cdk) enzymes and promote pRB phosphorylation, whereas growth-inhibiting signals prevent phosphorylation. Thus an inactivating mutation of the *Rb* genes removes one of the major restraints on cell division. Defective pRB is common to a number of different cancers.

The *P53* Gene

The most common tumor suppressor gene defect identified in cancer cells involves *P53*, so named because of the protein's molecular mass of 53 kd (also called TP53). More than half of

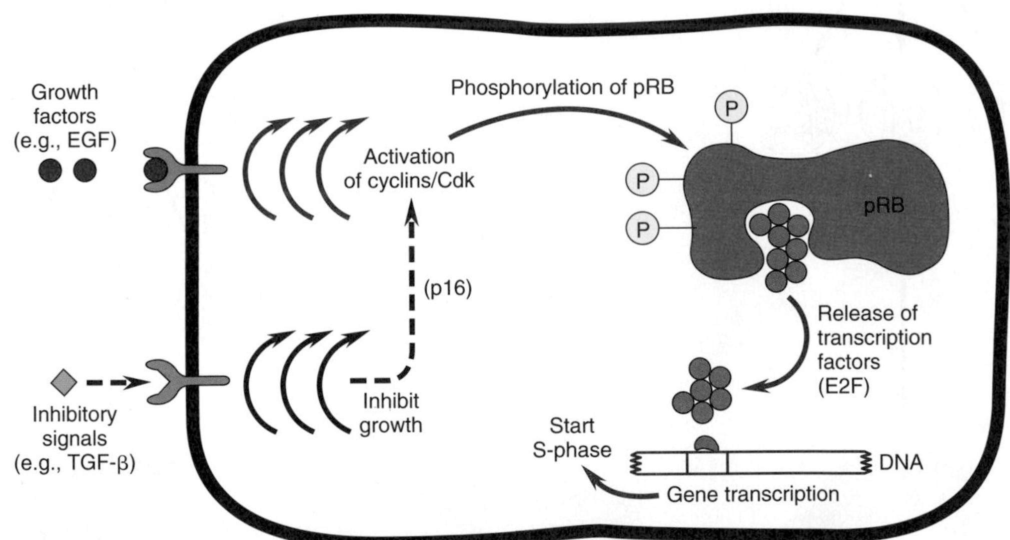

FIGURE 7-6 ■ The RB protein functions to bind transcription factors in the nucleus and keep them from participating in the transcription of cell cycle–related genes. pRB is induced to release its hold on the E2F transcription factors when it is sufficiently phosphorylated by cyclin-dependent kinases *(Cdk)*. Cyclin-dependent kinases are activated by cyclin proteins that accumulate when growth factors bind to receptors and stimulate growth pathways. Other signals, such as transforming growth factor-β *(TGF-β)*, inhibit the activity of cyclin/Cdk through activation of inhibitory proteins such as p16. A loss of pRB function removes the "major brake" on cell division. *P*, Phosphate group; *EGF*, epidermal growth factor.

all types of human tumors lack functional *P53*. The p53 protein, like pRB, inhibits cell cycling. Unlike pRB, however, normally very little p53 is found in cells, and it accumulates only after cellular, particularly DNA, damage. P53 binds to damaged DNA and stalls cell division, presumably to allow time for DNA repair before DNA replication in S phase (Figure 7-7). In the face of excessive damage (or other distress signals), p53 may direct the cell to initiate apoptosis. A defect in p53 function disrupts this important quality control system, allowing genetically damaged and unstable cells to survive and continue to replicate (see Figure 7-7). Genetically unstable cells have a propensity to accumulate more cancer-promoting mutations as they proliferate. The *P53* gene is important for therapeutic reasons as well. Chemotherapy- and radiation-induced cell death is mediated in large part by p53. These agents usually do not kill cancer cells directly; rather, they cause enough cellular damage in the target cell to trigger p53-mediated cell suicide. Cancer cells that lack functional p53 may therefore be resistant to some radiation and chemotherapeutic protocols.

BRCA1 and *BRCA2*

Many tumor suppressor genes have been identified through studies of inherited predisposition to certain types of cancer. The breast cancer genes *BRCA1* and *BRCA2* are important examples. Women with an inherited defect in the *BRCA1* gene

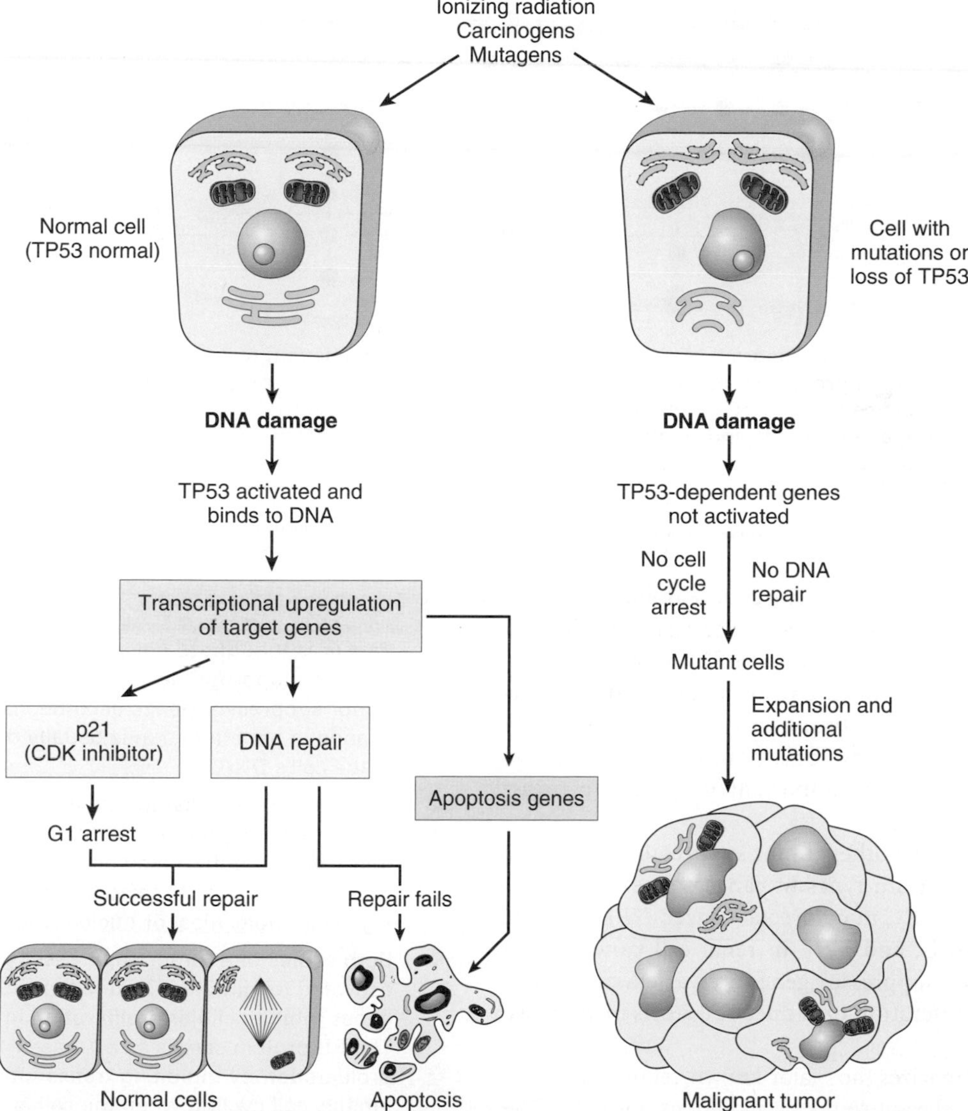

FIGURE 7-7 ■ The role of *TP53* in maintaining the integrity of the genome. Damage to DNA in cells with functional *TP53* stalls the cell cycle so that DNA can be repaired. If repair fails then the cell undergoes apoptosis to prevent the proliferation of DNA-damaged cells. If the *TP53* is not functional, genetically unstable cells may be allowed to survive and proliferate. (Redrawn from Kumar V, Cotran RS, Robbins SL: *Basic pathology,* ed 7, Philadelphia, 2003, Saunders, p 187.)

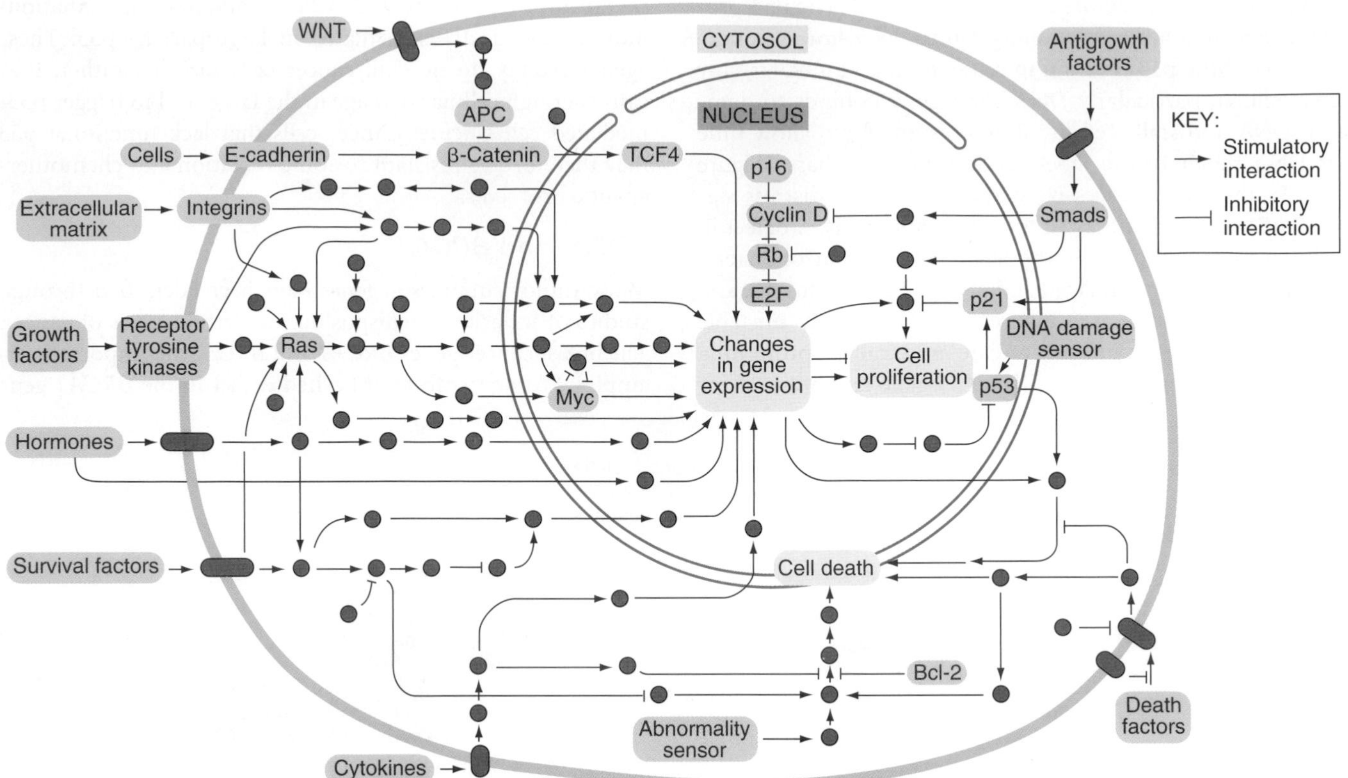

FIGURE 7-8 ■ Diagram of the major signaling pathways relevant to human cancer. Overactivity of proto-oncogenes and underactivity of tumor suppressor genes result in enhanced cell proliferation and inhibition of appropriate cell death. More than 100 proto-oncogene products and numerous tumor suppressor gene products have been identified. (From Alberts B et al, editors: *Molecular biology of the cell,* ed 4, New York, 2002, Garland Science, p 1343.)

have about an 85% risk of breast cancer developing and a 40% to 60% risk of ovarian cancer.[6] The age of onset of inherited breast cancer is earlier than the onset of noninherited (sporadic) forms, and the prevalence of bilateral breast cancer is higher. Inherited forms of breast cancer account for only about 5% to 10% of all cases of breast cancer, but study of the genes involved is providing important insights into breast cancer biology in general.

Defects in numerous other tumor suppressor genes have been identified in certain types of cancers (see Table 7-4), including *APC* and *DCC* in colorectal cancer, *NF1* and *NF2* in neurofibromatosis, and *VHL* in renal cell cancers. The functions of tumor suppressor genes are varied, but all appear to inhibit proliferation or induce apoptosis in defective cells.

Figure 7-8 summarizes the major known cellular signaling pathways that are relevant to the development of cancer. The functions of oncogenes and tumor suppressor genes are shown to interact to determine cell proliferation, cell survival, and cell death. In general, any cellular alteration that promotes proliferation or inhibits cell death can contribute to an increased risk of tumor development.

KEY CONCEPTS

- Cancer is thought to develop when proto-oncogenes become inappropriately activated in a cell or when tumor suppressor genes become inactivated. This change in gene function is usually due to mutations in the cell's DNA.
- Proto-oncogenes disrupt the intercellular communication pathway that normally regulates cell proliferation. This disruption may occur through abnormal production of growth factors, receptors, cytoplasmic signaling molecules, or nuclear transcription factors.
- Both copies of a tumor suppressor gene must be inactivated to eliminate its function. Tumor suppressor genes inhibit cellular proliferation in various ways. The RB protein serves as a "master brake" on cell proliferation by inhibiting transcription factors. p53 inhibits cell cycling when the cell is damaged to allow time for DNA repair. p53 is also important in initiating apoptosis of damaged or unwanted cells.

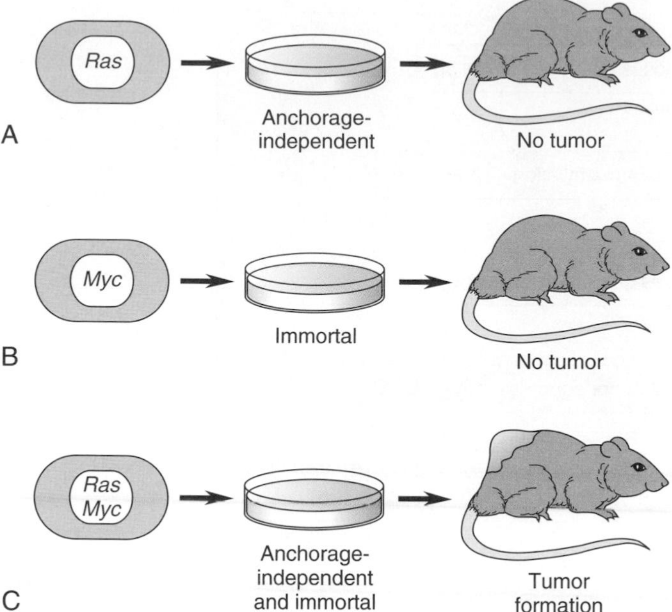

FIGURE 7-9 ■ Synergy between oncogenes may be necessary to initiate malignant growth. **A,** The *ras* gene only. **B,** The *myc* gene only. **C,** Synergy between *ras* and *myc* genes.

MULTISTEP NATURE OF CARCINOGENESIS

From the preceding discussion it might seem that simply introducing an oncogene into a normal cell or knocking out a tumor suppressor gene would be sufficient to transform it into a malignant cell. Such has not proved to be the case. Growth regulation of mammalian cells appears to be organized in such a manner that a single aberrant gene is unable to induce conversion to full malignancy. Different genes work in distinct ways and may effect only a subset of the changes necessary to achieve full malignancy. For example, introduction of the *ras* oncogene into normal cells in culture causes them to show anchorage independence, but they are unable to form tumors when inoculated into an animal. Anchorage independence is a typical feature of most transformed cells and means that they are capable of proliferating even if they are not attached to a matrix. Normal cells will not divide and will initiate apoptosis if they do not have a space on the matrix on which to anchor themselves. Similarly, the *myc* oncogene allows cells to grow indefinitely in culture, but these immortal cells are still unable to induce tumor formation. However, when both the *ras* and *myc* oncogenes are introduced into normal cells, they become fully malignant (Figure 7-9).[7]

These culture experiments support the clinical observation that carcinogenesis is a multistep phenomenon.[2] The steps of carcinogenesis have been labeled initiation, promotion, and progression (Figure 7-10).

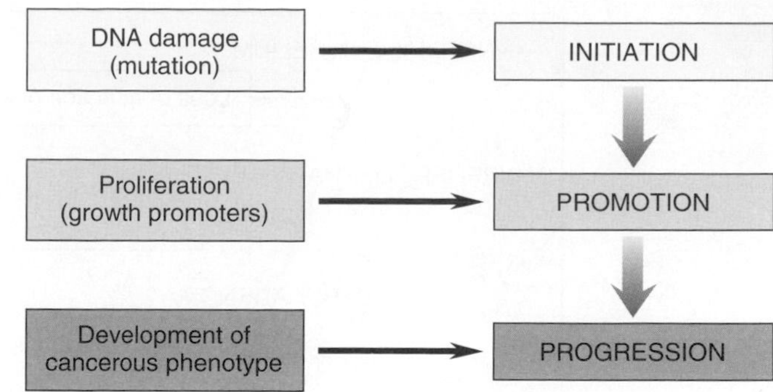

FIGURE 7-10 ■ Theoretical steps in the development of cancer include initiation, promotion, and progression.

Initiation

Initiating events are thought to be genetic mutations that activate proto-oncogenes and inactivate tumor suppressor genes. However, the genetic mutations are not evident until the mutant cell proliferates. *Proliferation* is a requirement for cancer development, and nonproliferating cells cannot cause cancer. This explains why terminally differentiated tissues that have few or no stem cells, such as cardiac or nerve, rarely become cancerous. It has been suggested that six or more mutations may be necessary to achieve full malignancy.[8] The development of colorectal cancer is a well-documented example of these sequential changes (Figure 7-11). Each individual cancer is likely to have its own unique combination of mutations that eventually lead to malignant behavior.

A number of etiologic agents are thought to be important initiators of cancer. The term *carcinogen* is applied to agents and substances capable of inducing cancer. Some carcinogens are complete carcinogens capable of the initiation of genetic damage as well as the promotion of cellular proliferation, whereas many others are only partial carcinogens. Partial carcinogens are often promoters that stimulate growth but are incapable of causing genetic mutations sufficient to initiate cancer by themselves. Examples of known carcinogens are ultraviolet and ionizing radiation, certain viruses, asbestos, and numerous chemicals. Most known chemical carcinogens are encountered through repeated occupational exposure (Table 7-5).

Promotion

Promotion is the stage during which the mutant cell proliferates. The transition from initiation to promotion may involve the activation of another oncogene or the inactivation of a tumor suppressor gene that has kept proliferation in check. Nonmutating factors may also be important in promoting cellular proliferation. For example, nutritional factors and infection may provide a stimulus for cellular proliferation. As previously described, cellular growth is regulated by numerous hormonal growth factors. It is not surprising, then, that hormones may act as promoters of certain types of cancer.

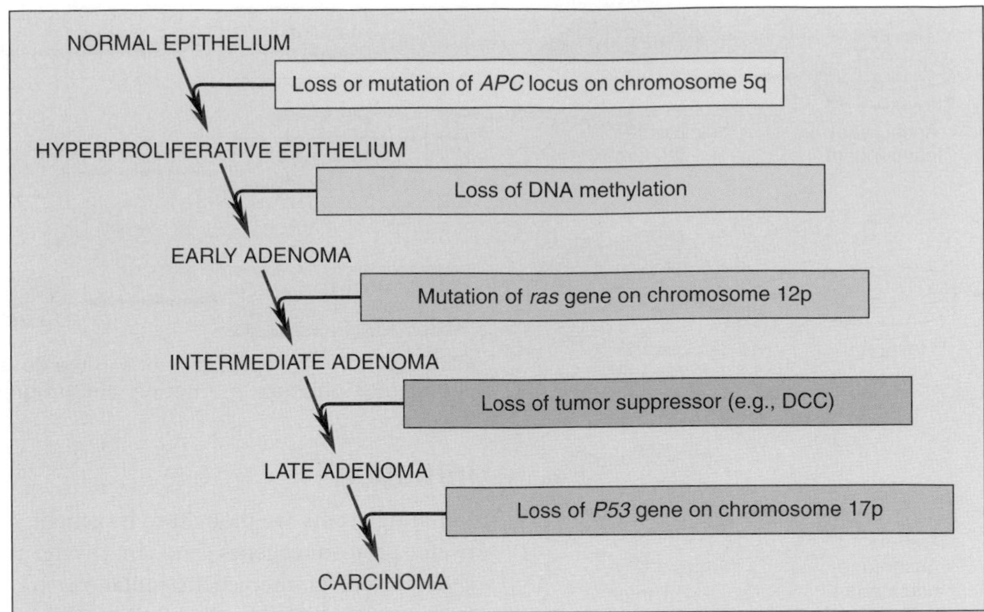

FIGURE 7-11 ■ The development of colorectal cancer illustrates the concept of multistep carcinogenesis. Derangement of several genes is likely to occur in most types of cancer. (Modified from Alberts B et al, editors: *Molecular biology of the cell,* ed 4, New York, 2002, Garland Science.)

The relationship between estrogen hormones and breast, ovarian, and uterine cancer is an important example. Epidemiologic studies indicate that the greater the number of menstrual cycles experienced, the higher the risk of these types of cancer developing. Women with early menarche, late first pregnancy, lack of breast-feeding, and late menopause have a greater risk of developing breast, uterine, and ovarian cancer. This enhanced susceptibility is thought to occur in part because of the greater lifetime estrogen exposure. Estrogen is a trophic hormone for these tissues and may therefore be viewed as having promoter effects. Treatment protocols using antiestrogen agents (tamoxifen) indicate that breast cancer risk may be reduced by blocking the effects of estrogen.[9,10] However, estrogen is not considered to be carcinogenic and does not cause genetic mutations.

A similar relationship has been identified for prostate cancer and testosterone hormones. In males, testosterone is secreted primarily from the testes under the influence of pituitary gonadotropins. Testosterone is a growth factor for the prostate gland and can act as a promoter of tumor formation in this tissue. This relationship is supported by the fact that therapeutic blocking of testosterone activity in persons with prostate cancer can help shrink the tumor.

Whereas the association between trophic hormones and reproductive cancers is well established, much less is known about the role of hormonal promoters in other tissue types. The apparent associations between cancer and dietary intake, body weight, and economic class are likely to be linked to hormonal regulation at the cellular level. For example, increased insulin exposure as a result of high carbohydrate and caloric intake may have promoting effects because of insulin's growth-enhancing properties. Further study is needed to clarify the role that hormonal factors may play in cancer promotion.

Progression

Progression is the stage during which the mutant, proliferating cells begin to exhibit malignant behavior. Generally, the mutation suffered during initiation is not sufficient to cause the biochemical changes necessary for malignant behavior. The proliferating cells are genetically unstable and may undergo chance mutations that give them a growth advantage. Clones of mutant cells exhibit a wide variation in phenotype. *Phenotype* refers to the cell's traits, such as morphology, metabolism, and biochemical makeup. Cells whose phenotype gives them a growth advantage proliferate more readily. With each cycle of proliferation an opportunity for chance variation arises. In the end, highly evolved tumor cells are generated that differ significantly from their normal ancestors. These cells have developed characteristics such as laminin receptors, lytic enzymes, and anchorage independence that enable them to behave malignantly.[11]

Cancer cells often have numerous abnormalities of chromosome structure, and the karyotype can be quite bizarre with bits and pieces of chromosomes attached in the wrong places and extra or missing chromosomes. An example of the chromosomes obtained from a breast cancer cell is shown in Figure 7-12. The color stains are specific for a particular chromosome, and each chromosome pair should be one color.

Table 7-5

Carcinogenicity to Humans for Selected Substances from the IARC Monograph Database

Chemical Family	Category*
PAHs	
TCDD (dioxin)	1
2,3,7,8-tetrachlorodibenzo-*p*-dioxin benzo[a]pyrene	2A
Benzo[a]anthracene	2A
PCBs (polychlorinated biphenyls)	2A
Benzo[b]fluoranthene	2B
AAs	
4-Aminobiphenyl	1
Benzidine	1
IQ (2-amino-3-methlimidazo[4,5-*f*]quinoline)	2A
MeIQ (2-amino-3,4-dimethylimidazo [4,4-*f*]quinoline)	2B
PhIP (2-amino-1-methy-6-phenylimidazo [4,5-*b*]pyridine)	2B
4-Nitropyrene	2B
Alkylating Agents	
Sulfur mustard	1
DMS, DES, ENU	2A
EDB (ethylene dibromide)	2A
NNK [4-(*N*-nitrosomethylamino)-1-(3-pyridyl)-1-butanone]	2B
Many nitrosamines	2B
DMN (*N*-nitrosodimethylamine)	2A
Mycotoxins	
Aflatoxins (naturally occurring)	1
Aflatoxin M1	2B
Sterigmatocystin	2B
Metals (as compounds)	
Nickel	1
Chromium	1
Cadmium	1
Arsenic	1
Beryllium	1
Cobalt	2B
Fibers	
Silica (asbestos)	1
Wood dust	1
Ceramic fibers	2B
Glasswool	2B
Acrylic fibers	3
Others	
Vinyl chloride	1
Tobacco smoke	1
Tobacco products	1
Cyclophosphamide	1
Sulfur mustard	1
Nitrogen mustard	1
Formaldehyde	2A
Cisplatin	2A
Methylene chloride	2B
Hydrazine	2B
Hydrogen peroxide	3
Ethylene	3

From Loechler E, Henry B, Seo K: Cellular responses to chemical carcinogens. In Coleman W, Tsongalis G, editors: *The molecular basis of human cancer,* Totowa, NJ, 2002, Humana Press, p 204.

*Categorization by group based on the following criteria of evaluation for agents as stated in the Preamble to the IARC Monographs. Group 1, The agent is carcinogenic to humans. This category is used when there is sufficient evidence of carcinogenicity in humans. Group 2, This category includes agents for which, at one extreme, the degree of evidence of carcinogenicity in humans is almost sufficient, as well as those for which, at the other extreme, there are no human data but for which there is evidence of carcinogenicity in experimental animals. Agents are assigned to either group 2A (probably carcinogenic to humans) or group 2B (possibly carcinogenic to humans). Group 3, The agent is not classifiable as to its carcinogenicity to humans. This category is used most commonly for agents, mixtures, and exposure circumstances for which the evidence of carcinogenicity is inadequate in humans and inadequate or limited in experimental animals. Group 4, The agent (mixture) is probably not carcinogenic to humans.

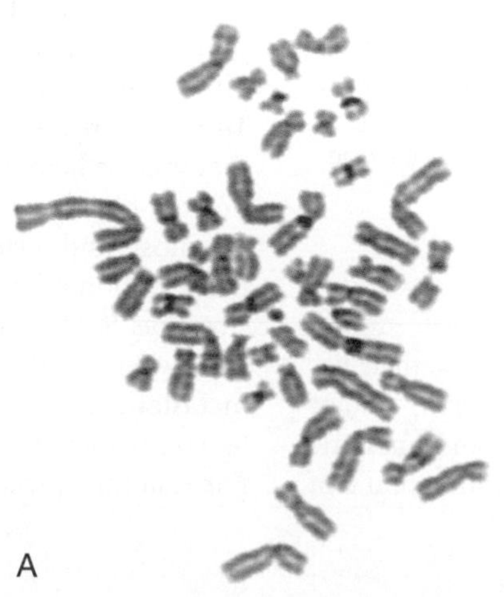

A

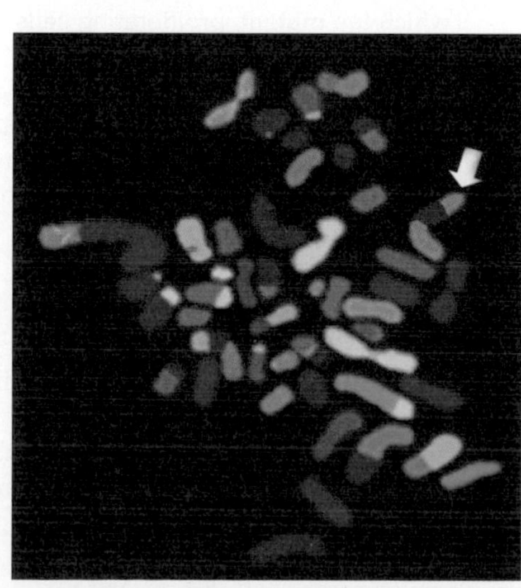

B

FIGURE 7-12 ■ Chromosomes from a breast tumor showing abnormalities in number and structure. **A,** General DNA stain. **B,** A combination of fluorescent stains that give a different color for each human chromosome. Translocations are seen where chromosomes are multicolored. There are 48 chromosomes instead of the usual 46. (From Alberts B et al, editors: *Molecular biology of the cell,* ed 4, New York, 2002, Garland Science, p 1321. Courtesy Joanne Davidson and Paul Edwards.)

Note the numerous multicolored chromosomes indicating multiple translocations of chromosome pieces.

To become malignant, cancer cells must also overcome the normal limits on the number of cell replications allowed before a cell stops dividing and dies. In the early 1970s it was discovered that normal somatic cells replicate only a finite number of times in culture: fetal cells may replicate 80 or so times, whereas cells from older individuals divide only 20 or 30 times.[12] A mechanism whereby cells can track their history of cell division, as well as the way in which cancer cells may overcome it, has been proposed.[13] Each time a cell divides, it must replicate its DNA, but DNA polymerase is unable to copy the DNA strands all the way to the very tips of the chromosomes (called *telomeres*). The telomere thus shortens a bit with each cell division until some critical length is reached and cell division stops (see Chapter 4). Unicellular organisms and germ cells produce an enzyme called telomerase that promotes resynthesis of the telomere ends and permits these cell types to replicate indefinitely. Most cancer cells synthesize telomerase as they acquire the malignant phenotype, thus rescuing themselves from critical telomere shortening and gaining a mechanism for achieving immortality. In addition, the majority of cancers are deficient in P53 activity, which allows them to escape apoptosis despite gross derangements in DNA structure.

The fact that conversion from a normal cell type to a malignant cell type requires multiple steps implies many opportunities to intervene in the process. Prevention of the initiating mutation may be difficult inasmuch as carcinogens are ubiquitous; however, therapies to prevent promotion and progression could render the initial mutation harmless. As the biochemical processes governing promotion and progression become clearer, strategies for blocking these stages continue to be developed.

KEY CONCEPTS

- Full expression of cancer in a host is a multistep process. These steps have been described as initiation, promotion, and progression. The initiating event is thought to be a genetic mutation. Promotion refers to the stage in which the mutant cell is induced to proliferate. Progression is the stage during which the mutant, proliferating cells begin to exhibit malignant behavior.
- Malignant cells commonly produce telomerase, an enzyme that repairs the telomeres and may be a key for attaining immortality. The majority also have insufficient P53, which allows the tumor cells to escape apoptosis despite DNA damage.

METASTASIS

Metastasis is the process whereby cancer cells escape their tissue of origin and initiate new colonies of cancer in distant sites. For tumor cells to gain access to the blood or lymphatic circulation, they must first escape the basement membrane of the tissue of origin, move through the extracellular space, and penetrate the basement membrane of the vessel. This process is thought to involve loss of cell-to-cell adhesion and binding to matrix components such as laminin via specific laminin receptors on the tumor cell, followed by release of enzymes such as proteases and collagenases that digest the basement membrane.[14] The cancer cell then squeezes through the rift by ameboid movement. The process is repeated at the vessel basement membrane to access the blood or lymphatic vessel. When the cell reaches the tissue to be colonized, it must again traverse the basement membranes by using similar mechanisms (Figure 7-13). Once in a new tissue setting, the cancer cell colony must acquire nutrients and a blood supply and cope with an environment that may differ considerably from its origin. In general, more poorly differentiated cancer cells are better able to adapt to foreign tissues and survive.

Patterns of Spread

The survival of tumor cells in the circulation is not guaranteed. They may be detected by immune cells and destroyed, or they may undergo apoptosis unless they quickly find a matrix on which to stick. Fewer than 1 in 10,000 of the cancer cells that enter the circulation survive to form a new tumor at a distant site.[14] Some tumor cell types appear to prefer specific target organs. Sometimes the pattern of metastasis is related to the circulatory flow. For example, metastatic tumors from the colon often seed the liver because they travel in the portal vein. The localization of most metastatic tumors is not so easily explained by blood flow patterns, and some tumor cells appear to "home" to specific targets. This homing tendency is poorly understood but may involve chemotactic signals from the organ to which the tumor cells respond. Cell surface receptors of the integrin and cell adhesion molecule families, which mediate cell-to-matrix and cell-to-cell adhesion, are likely to influence the choice of tissues that cancer cells invade. Spread via lymphatics is somewhat more predictable than spread by blood flow. Generally, the lymph nodes that immediately drain the tissue of cancer origin are colonized first, and then the tumor cells tend to spread contiguously from node to node. Hodgkin disease, a lymphoma, is particularly noted for its orderly spread via the lymphatics.

Because tumor cells exhibit various degrees of differentiation or resemblance to the parent tissue of origin, it may be difficult to determine the metastatic cancer's tissue of origin. **Tumor markers** are substances associated with tumor cells that may be helpful in identifying their tissue type. Identification of the tissue of origin has important implications for prognosis and selection of treatment. Tumor markers rely on the retention of at least some characteristics of the parent tissue type. Some tumor markers are released into the circulation, whereas others must be identified through biopsy of the metastatic tissue. Enzymes and other proteins that are specific to a particular cell type are commonly used as tumor markers. For example, production of thyroglobulin protein is specific

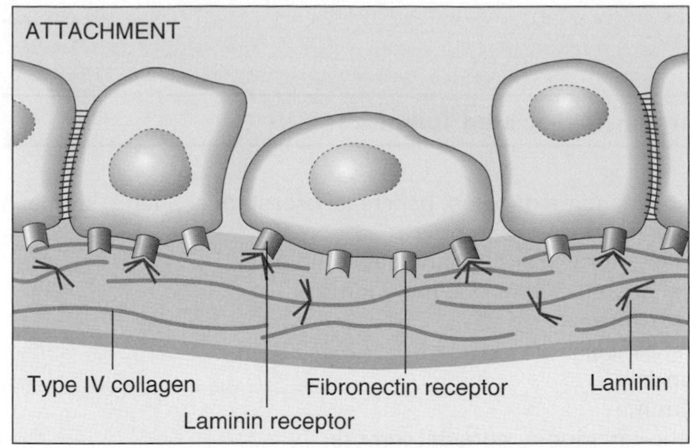

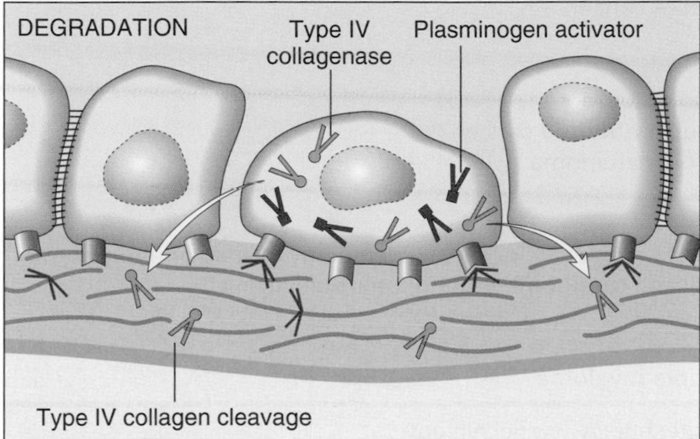

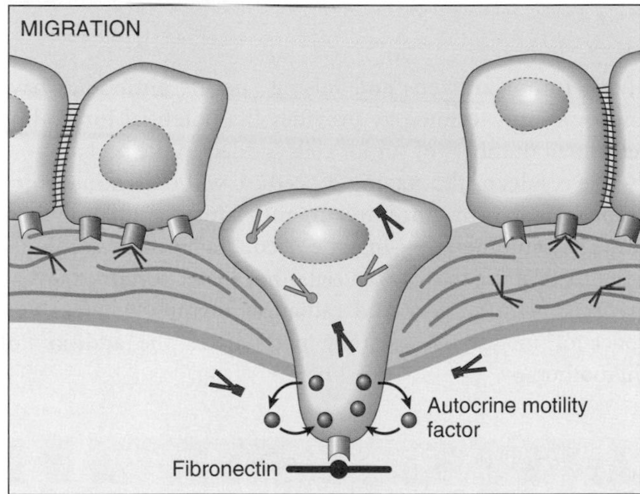

FIGURE 7-13 ■ The mechanisms of tumor invasion allow tumor cells to escape the site of origin, penetrate the basement membrane, and travel to distant sites. **A,** Tumor cells produce laminin and fibronectin receptors that allow attachment and migration toward the basement membrane. **B,** Enzymes that break down proteins are released into the area to form a rift. **C,** The tumor cell migrates away from the site of origin with the help of autocrine factors that enhance its mobility. (From Kumar V, Cotran RS, Robbins SL, editors: *Basic pathology,* ed 7, Philadelphia, 2003, Saunders, p 191.)

for thyroid tumor cells. Melanoma cells express the antigens HMB-45 and S-100, which is helpful in identification as melanocytes. Unfortunately, most tumor markers are not very specific for cancer since the normal cells in the tissue of origin also produce them. Tumor markers are most useful as indicators for further diagnostic evaluation and to track the tumor burden. An increasing blood concentration of a specific tumor marker may indicate progression and proliferation of the cancer cells (increased tumor burden). See Table 7-6 for other examples of antigen, hormone, and enzyme markers used to identify tumor cell types.

Angiogenesis

Tumors cannot enlarge more than about 2 mm in diameter unless they grow blood vessels into the tumor mass to provide oxygen and nutrients. Angiogenesis is the process of forming new blood vessels. Most tumors do not induce angiogenesis until late in the stage of cancer development and so remain small and nonvascularized for years. The triggers that spur the cancer to begin angiogenesis are not completely understood. Tumor cells may begin to produce angiogenic factors such as vascular endothelial growth factor (VEGF) in response to hypoxia or other signals. VEGF stimulates proliferation of vascular endothelial cells, which then migrate to the tumor and orchestrate blood vessel development. Metastatic tumors must also initiate angiogenesis in their new locations or they will not survive. Therefore inhibition of angiogenesis is an important therapeutic goal to limit tumor growth and metastasis and continues to be an area of active research.

Grading and Staging of Tumors

Grading and staging of tumors are done to predict the clinical behavior of a malignant tumor and to guide therapy. **Grading** refers to the histologic characterization of tumor cells and is basically a determination of the degree of anaplasia. Most grading systems classify tumors into three or four classes of increasing degrees of malignancy. A greater degree of anaplasia indicates a greater malignant potential. The correlation between the grade of the tumor and its biological behavior is not perfect. Some low-grade tumors have proved to be quite malignant.

The choice of treatment modality is usually influenced more by the stage of the tumor than by its histologic grade. **Staging** describes the location and pattern of spread of a tumor within the host. Factors such as tumor size, extent of local growth, lymph node and organ involvement, and presence of distant metastases are considered. Several staging systems exist; however, the international TNM (*t*umor, *n*ode, *m*etastasis) system is used extensively as a general framework for staging tumors.[15] Particular staging criteria vary with tumors in different organ systems. Examples of staging criteria for breast and colon cancer are shown in Tables 7-7 and 7-8.

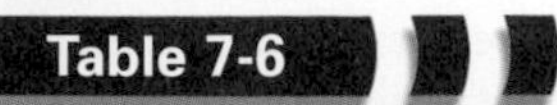

Selected Markers Useful for Tumor Identification

Marker	Commonly Associated Tumor
Antigens	
Carcinoembryonic antigen (CEA)	Adenocarcinoma of colon, pancreas, breast, ovary, lung, stomach
Desmin	Myogenic (muscle) sarcoma
CA 125	Ovarian, uterus, cervix, pancreas, others
CA 19-9	GI, pancreatic carcinoma; melanoma
CA 15-3	Breast cancer
CA 27-29	Breast cancer
HMB-45	Melanoma
S-100 protein	Melanoma
α-Fetoprotein	Hepatic carcinoma, gonadal tumors
Prostate-specific antigen (PSA)	Prostate cancer
Hormones	
Human chorionic gonadotropin	Gonadal tumors
Calcitonin	Medullary thyroid cancer
Thyroglobulin	Thyroid carcinoma
Isoenzymes	
Prostatic acid phosphatase	Prostate adenocarcinoma, leukemia, non-Hodgkin lymphoma
Neuron-specific enolase	Small cell carcinoma of lung, neuroblastoma
Immunoglobulins	
Monoclonal Ig	Multiple myeloma

Data from National Cancer Institute, National Institutes of Health, website: http://www.nci.nih.gov.

In the past, tumor staging was based primarily on results of radiography and exploratory surgery. The availability of computed tomography (CT) and magnetic resonance imaging (MRI), as well as other highly sophisticated imaging techniques, has revolutionized cancer detection.[16] These imaging modalities allow noninvasive exploration of the tissues of the entire body. The computer-generated images can then be scrutinized for any signs of abnormality that might signal the presence of hidden tumors. CT and MRI rely primarily on detection of differences in tissue density and are therefore not totally specific for tumors. They can, however, guide the selection of sites for exploration and biopsy and potentially reduce unnecessary surgery. Positron emission tomography (PET) is another promising staging technology because it facilitates cancer detection based on molecular and biochemical processes within the tumor tissues. PET may be used in certain clinical situations in which CT has known limitations, such as differentiation of benign from malignant lymph nodes or other lesions, differentiation of residual tumor from scar tissue, or detection of unsuspected distant metastases.[16]

Antibodies can also be used to track down cancer cells in the body. Antibodies can be raised against specific antigens present on the surface of tumor cells. The antibodies are also bound to a tracer (e.g., a radioactive isotope such as iodine 125), which can be detected by imaging. As methods for identifying tumor antigens and raising specific antibodies have improved, this technology provides the potential for finding very small numbers of tumor cells hidden in the body.

The results of the staging procedure will determine which of the mainstays of cancer treatment—surgery, radiation therapy, or chemotherapy—may be used, singly or in combination, to destroy the cancer cells. Localized tumors may be managed with surgery and radiation therapy, whereas evidence of metastasis generally necessitates the addition of chemotherapy.

KEY CONCEPTS

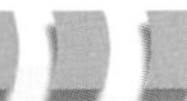

- Malignant cells produce specialized enzymes and receptors to enable them to escape their tissue of origin and metastasize.
- The spread of tumors generally occurs by way of the blood stream or lymphatics. Tumor cells often lodge in the capillary beds of the organs that drain them, such as liver and lung. Some tumors appear to "home" to certain tissues.
- Grading and staging are done to predict tumor behavior and guide therapy. Grading is the histologic characterization of tumor cells, whereas staging describes the location and pattern of tumor spread within the host.

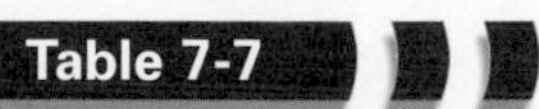

TNM Staging Criteria for Breast Cancer

Primary Tumor (T)

TX	Primary tumor cannot be assessed
T0	No evidence of primary tumor
Tis	Carcinoma in situ, intraductal carcinoma, lobular carcinoma in situ, or Paget disease of the nipple with no tumor
T1	Tumor 2 cm or less in greatest dimension
T1mic	Microinvasion 0.1 cm or less in greatest dimension
T1a	Tumor 0.5 cm or less in greatest dimension
T1b	Tumor more than 0.5 cm but not more than 1 cm in greatest dimension
T1c	Tumor more than 1 cm but not more than 2 cm in greatest dimension
T2	Tumor more than 2 cm but not more than 5 cm in greatest dimension
T3	Tumor more than 5 cm in greatest dimension
T4	Tumor of any size with direct extension to chest wall or skin
T4a	Extension to chest wall, not including pectoralis muscle
T4b	Edema (including peau d'orange) or ulceration of skin of the breast or satellite nodules confined to the same breast
T4c	Both T4a and T4b
T4d	Inflammatory carcinoma

Lymph Node (N)

NX	Regional lymph nodes cannot be assessed (e.g., previously removed)
N0	No regional lymph node metastasis
N1	Metastasis to movable ipsilateral axillary lymph node(s)
N2	Metastasis to ipsilateral axillary lymph node(s) fixed to one another or to other structures
N2a	Metastasis in ipsilateral axillary lymph nodes fixed to one another (matted) or to other structures
N2b	Metastasis only in clinically apparent* ipsilateral internal mammary nodes and in the *absence* of clinically evident axillary lymph node metastasis
N3	Metastasis in ipsilateral infraclavicular lymph node(s) with or without axillary lymph node involvement, or in clinically apparent* ipsilateral internal mammary lymph node(s) and in the *presence* of clinically evident axillary lymph node metastasis; or metastasis in ipsilateral supraclavicular lymph node(s) with or without axillary or internal mammary lymph node involvement
N3a	Metastasis in ipsilateral infraclavicular lymph node(s)
N3b	Metastasis in ipsilateral internal mammary lymph node(s) and axillary lymph node(s)
N3c	Metastasis in ipsilateral supraclavicular lymph node(s)

Distant Metastasis (M)

MX	Presence of distance metastasis cannot be assessed
M0	No distant metastasis
M1	Distant metastasis

Stage Grouping

Stage 0	Tis	N0	M0
Stage I	T1	N0	M0
Stage IIA	T0	N1	M0
	T1	N1	M0
	T2	N0	M0
Stage IIB	T2	N1	M0
	T3	N0	M0
Stage IIIA	T0	N2	M0
	T1	N2	M0
	T2	N2	M0
	T3	N1	M0
	T3	N2	M0
Stage IIIB	T4	Any N	M0
Stage IIIC	Any T	N3	M0
Stage IV	Any T	Any N	M1

Adapted from Greene F: *AJCC cancer staging handbook*, ed 6, New York, 2002, Springer-Verlag, pp 263-266.
**Clinically apparent* is defined as detected by imaging studies (excluding lymphoscintigraphy) or by clinical examination or grossly visible pathologically.

Table 7-8

TNM Staging Criteria for Colon Cancer

Primary Tumor (T)

TX	Primary tumor cannot be assessed
T0	No evidence of primary tumor
Tis	Carcinoma in situ: intraepithelial or invasion of lamina propria
T1	Tumor invades submucosa
T2	Tumor invades muscularis propria
T3	Tumor invades through the muscularis propria into the subserosa, or into nonperitonealized pericolic or perirectal tissues
T4	Tumor directly invades other organs or structures, and/or perforates visceral peritoneum

Regional Lymph Nodes (N)

NX	Regional lymph nodes cannot be assessed
N0	No regional lymph node metastasis
N1	Metastasis in 1-3 regional lymph nodes
N2	Metastasis in 4 or more regional lymph nodes

Distant Metastasis (M)

MX	Distant metastasis cannot be assessed
M0	No distant metastasis
M1	Distant metastasis

Stage Grouping

Stage 0	Tis	N0	M0
Stage I	T1	N0	M0
	T2	N0	M0
Stage IIA	T3	N0	M0
Stage IIB	T4	N0	M0
Stage IIIA	T1-T2	N1	M0
Stage IIIB	T3-T4	N1	M0
Stage IIIC	Any T	N2	M0
Stage IV	Any T	Any N	M1

Adapted from Greene F: *AJCC cancer staging handbook*, ed 6, New York, 2002, Springer-Verlag, pp 131-132.

◆ The TNM staging system is used to describe the tumor size, lymph nodes affected, and degree of metastasis.

EFFECTS OF CANCER ON THE BODY

The effects of cancer on the host vary widely, depending on the location of the tumor and the extent of metastasis. Early-stage cancer may be asymptomatic. As the tumor increases in size and spreads through the body, a number of symptoms become apparent, including pain, cachexia, immune suppression, and infection. Once treatment has begun, patients may also suffer hair loss and sloughing of mucosal membranes. The American Cancer Society has published the seven warning signs of cancer as a way of encouraging the public to seek early evaluation of potential cancers (Box 7-1). The presentation of cancer in children differs from that in adults, and special warning signs have been identified for the pediatric population (Box 7-2).

Box 7-1

Cancer's Seven Warning Signs

Change in bowel or bladder habits
A sore that does not heal
Unusual bleeding or discharge
Thickening or lump in breast or elsewhere
Indigestion or difficulty swallowing
Obvious change in wart or mole
Nagging cough or hoarseness

Pain is often the most feared complication of the disease process. Pain may be due to invasion of metastatic cells into organs or bone and subsequent activation of pain and pressure receptors in these tissues. Tissue destruction and inflammation may contribute to cancer pain. Pain is strongly influenced by fear and fatigue. Cancer treatment may contribute to overall pain because of procedures requiring biopsy and drug administration through veins. Fortunately, pain can usually be well controlled through the use of analgesics. The use of pa-

Box 7-2

Cancer's Warning Signs in Children

Continued, unexplained weight loss
Headaches with vomiting in the morning
Increased swelling or persistent pain in bones or joints
Lump or mass in abdomen, neck, or elsewhere
Development of whitish appearance in pupil of the eye
Recurrent fevers not caused by infections
Excessive bleeding or bruising
Noticeable paleness or prolonged tiredness

tient-controlled analgesia has been effective in reducing patient fears of inadequate therapy for pain (see Chapter 47).

Cachexia refers to an overall weight loss and generalized weakness (Figure 7-14). Many factors contribute to cancer cachexia, including loss of appetite (anorexia) and increased metabolic rate. Anorexia accompanies many disease processes and may result from toxins released by the cancer cells or immune cells. Cancer patients may have aversions to specific foods and may feel full after only a few bites. Nausea and vomiting are common complications of cancer therapy and contribute to decreased nutrient intake. Despite the minimal nutrient intake, body metabolism remains high. Cancer cells may compete with normal cells for available nutrients. Nutrients are mobilized from fat and protein stores in the body and consumed by the hypermetabolic cells. Some patients may require nutritional supplementation by enteral or parenteral routes.

Individuals with cancer often demonstrate deficits in immune system competence. Cancer cells secrete substances that suppress the immune system. Individuals with cancer may have reduced populations of T and B cells and may respond poorly to injected antigens. The mechanisms by which cancer cells depress immune responses are not well understood, but the prognosis for cancer recovery is poorer when the immune system is depressed. Immune cells, including cytotoxic T cells and natural killer (NK) cells, actively detect and destroy cancer cells.

In addition to the general immunodepressive effects of cancer, some cancer cells have developed ways to elude immune system detection.[17] For example, cancer cells can internalize their immunoreactive cell surface antigens when antibodies attach to them. A reduction in antigenic sites decreases the likelihood of further stimulation of antibody production. Some tumors escape detection because they are coated with normal extracellular matrix molecules such as glycoproteins. The glycoproteins physically cover up the antigenic tumor markers. Tumor cells that closely resemble normal cells may trigger the production of regulatory T cells that suppress the activity of other immune cells. Regulatory T cells are a subclass of T lymphocytes. The conditions that activate them are as yet poorly understood, but they are probably important in keeping the immune system in check so that normal tissues are not attacked. Difficulty differentiating between the tumor

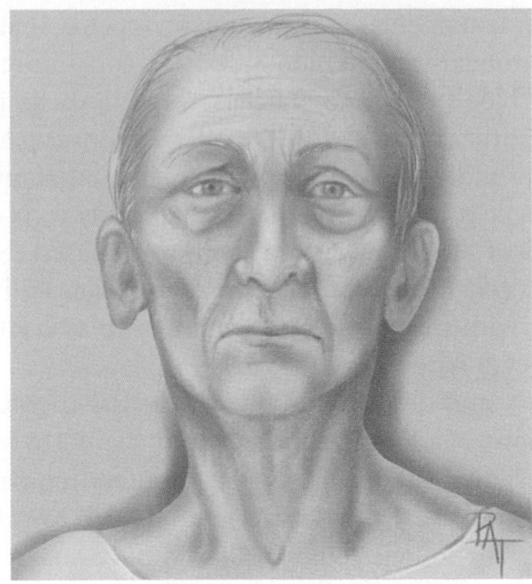

FIGURE 7-14 ■ General emaciated appearance in cancer cachexia. (From Jarvis C: *Physical examination and health assessment,* ed 2, Philadelphia, 1996, Saunders, p 297.)

cell and a normal cell may result in the production of regulatory T cells that actually aid tumor cell growth.

Bone marrow suppression contributes to the anemia, leukopenia, and thrombocytopenia that often accompany cancer. Bone marrow suppression may be due to invasion and destruction of blood-forming cells in the bone marrow, poor nutrition, and chemotherapeutic drugs. *Anemia* refers to a deficiency in circulating red cells. In addition to decreased production of blood cell precursors in the bone marrow, anemia may result from chronic or acute bleeding. The signs and symptoms of anemia, such as fatigue, increased heart rate, and increased respiratory rate, are related to a decrease in oxygen-carrying capacity.

Leukopenia refers to a decrease in circulating white blood cells (leukocytes). Malignant invasion of the bone marrow is a primary cause of leukopenia, with malnutrition and chemotherapy being contributing factors. A deficiency in white blood cells reduces the patient's ability to fight infection, which is a major cause of morbidity and mortality in cancer patients. Often the offending organism is *opportunistic;* it is unable to infect an immunocompetent host and becomes virulent only when a person is immunocompromised. Infections are very difficult to manage because the host is unable to mount an effective immune response. Infections are also difficult to prevent because the majority of the infecting organisms are from the patient's own endogenous flora (skin, gastrointestinal tract). The development of severe leukopenia or infection during treatment may necessitate changes in the chemotherapeutic regimen to allow bone marrow recovery.

Thrombocytopenia is a deficiency in circulating platelets, which are important mediators of blood clotting. Platelet deficiencies predispose to life-threatening hemorrhage. A platelet count of less than 20,000/mm^3 has been associated with spontaneous hemorrhage.

Anemia, leukopenia, and thrombocytopenia may be managed by administration of blood products containing red blood cells, white blood cells, and platelets, respectively. In fact, blood replacement therapy is used more often in cancer patients than in any other medical condition. When chemotherapy is terminated, stem cells in the bone marrow generally recover and the production of blood cells resumes. In some cases, the production of red and white blood cells can be enhanced by treating the patient with specific growth factors, such as erythropoietin or granulocyte-stimulating factors.

Hair loss and the sloughing of mucosal membranes are complications of radiation therapy and chemotherapy. Treatment is designed to kill the rapidly proliferating cancer cells, but normal cells with high growth rates such as mucosal epithelia and hair follicle cells are also damaged. Damaged mucosa is a primary source of cancer pain and anorexia, and may provide a portal for the invasion of organisms from the skin or gastrointestinal tract.

Paraneoplastic syndromes are symptom complexes that cannot be explained by obvious tumor properties and occur in 10% to 15% of patients with cancer. Many of the syndromes are associated with excessive production of hormones or cytokines by the tumor. Common paraneoplastic syndromes include (1) Cushing syndrome secondary to excess adrenocorticotropic hormone (ACTH) secretion, and (2) hyponatremia and water overload secondary to excess antidiuretic hormone (SIADH, syndrome of inappropriate ADH) secretion. Small cell carcinoma of the lung is commonly the culprit for excess ACTH and ADH syndromes. Hypercalcemia (elevated serum calcium) is another important paraneoplastic syndrome associated with abnormal production of parathyroid hormone–related protein (PTHrP) by the tumor cells. Unexplained hypercalcemia is regarded as evidence of cancer until proven otherwise. Hypercalcemia may be a consequence of metastatic bone cancer, and in this case it would be an expected finding rather than a paraneoplastic syndrome.

If left untreated, cancer has the potential to kill the host. The cause of death is multifactorial. Infection, hemorrhage, and organ failure are the primary causes of cancer death. The failure of cancer-ridden organs such as liver, kidney, brain, and lung results in the loss of life-sustaining functions. Treatment for cancer can also be detrimental to the host by contributing to immunosuppression and platelet deficiencies. The additive effects of one or more of these factors may lead to death.

KEY CONCEPTS

- Regardless of the type of malignancy, affected individuals exhibit characteristic signs and symptoms, including pain, cachexia, bone marrow suppression, and infection.
- Bone marrow suppression is manifested as anemia, leukopenia, and thrombocytopenia.
- Immunosuppression with consequent infection is a primary cause of cancer-associated death.

CANCER THERAPY

The overall 5-year survival rate for patients with cancer is approximately 60%, with some types of cancer having much higher or lower rates.[18] Early detection of cancer, while it remains localized in the tissue of origin, is associated with the best prognosis for cure. Patients with metastatic invasion of regional lymph nodes still have a good opportunity for cure with appropriate therapy. Widespread invasion of multiple tissues and organs is associated with a poor prognosis, and therapy may be aimed at palliation of symptoms rather than cure. The mainstays of cancer therapy are surgery, radiation therapy, and chemotherapy. In some hormone-sensitive tumors (breast, prostate), hormonal blocking drugs may be used. Immunotherapy and targeted molecular therapies have begun to emerge as important treatments for specific cancers. Transplantation of stem cells from the bone marrow or peripheral blood is an increasingly important aspect of cancer treatment for leukemia, lymphoma, and some solid tumors. The choice of treatment depends largely on the results of the staging procedure. A greater degree of metastasis generally requires a more aggressive therapeutic approach.

Surgery

The majority of patients with solid tumors are treated surgically, which can be curative in some localized cancers. The main benefit of surgery is removal of a tumor with minimal damage to other body cells. The surgeon generally removes a margin of normal-appearing tissue around the resected tumor to ensure complete tumor removal. Lymph nodes are subjected to biopsy and also removed if evidence of metastasis is present. Surgical resection of some tumors can be tricky if vital structures such as neurons or blood vessels are involved.

Surgery involves risks related to anesthesia, infection, and blood loss. The surgical procedure may be disfiguring or may result in loss of function. Surgical resection as the sole treatment for solid tumors is curative in a minority of patients because most patients already have undetectable metastases at the time of diagnosis.[19] There is evidence that tumor surgery can alter the behavior of the tumor and predispose the patient to recurrence.[19] Therefore, surgical resection is commonly accompanied by radiation therapy or chemotherapy. Even one remaining cancer cell could be sufficient to reinitiate tumor formation.

Radiation Therapy

Ionizing radiation is used for two principal reasons: to kill tumor cells that are not resectable because of location in a vital or inaccessible area and to kill tumor cells that may have escaped the surgeon's knife and remain undetected in the local area. Radiation kills cells by damaging their nuclear DNA. Cells that are rapidly cycling are more susceptible to radiation death because there is little time for DNA repair. Radiation may not kill cells directly; rather, it may initiate apoptosis. The *P53* tumor suppressor gene is an important mediator of this response. Many tumors have mutant *P53* and may be less susceptible to radiation-induced cell death.

It is difficult to kill all the cells of a large tumor by irradiation because they are heterogeneous; they are in different phases of mitosis and are cycling at different rates. A radiation dose large enough to kill all the tumor cells would be sufficient to kill the normal cells as well. Radiation is most effective at eradicating small groups of tumor cells.[20] It is often used in combination with surgery. Radiation is also useful for palliative reductions in tumor size. Pain from bone and brain tumors may be effectively managed with radiation therapy that shrinks the tumor. Tumors with bleeding surfaces may be coagulated with radiation to decrease blood loss.

A certain degree of destruction of normal cells in the irradiated field is expected with radiation therapy. The guiding principle behind radiation therapy is to give the maximal dose that normal tissues can tolerate and hope that it kills the tumor. Radiation is best used when tumor cells are regionally located. Total-body irradiation to kill tumor cells in disseminated locations is not recommended because of the likelihood of life-threatening tissue damage, although it may be used in preparation for bone marrow or peripheral stem cell transplantation.

Chemotherapy

Chemotherapy refers to the systemic administration of anticancer chemicals as treatment for cancers that are known or suspected to be disseminated in the body. Unlike surgery or radiation therapy, which are locally or regionally applied, chemotherapeutic drugs can find their cancer cell targets in areas throughout the entire body. Examples of standard chemotherapeutic agents are listed in Table 7-9.

Most chemotherapeutic agents are cytotoxic because they interfere with some aspect of cell division. The more rapidly dividing cells are more susceptible to the killing effects of chemotherapeutic agents. In a large tumor mass, the rates of cell division are very diverse, with many slowly dividing cells. At any one time, only a portion of the tumor cells are in a cell cycle stage that is susceptible to chemotherapy. Several courses of chemotherapy are generally necessary to ensure that all tumor cells have been killed. It is difficult to kill slowly cycling tumor cells without also killing normal cells that are cycling at approximately the same rate. Small tumors are easier to eradicate because rates of cell division are generally faster. To effect a cure, the "stem" cells that give rise to clones of malignant cells must be destroyed. Unfortunately, stem cells may not divide as rapidly as other cells. Resection or irradiation to reduce tumor size may prompt the stem cells to divide, thus making them more susceptible to chemotherapy. Tumor cells with mutations of the *P53* gene may be resistant to chemotherapeutic agents that work by damaging DNA, so other drugs may be more effective.

Chemotherapeutic agents are not selective for tumor cells, and a certain amount of normal cell death also occurs. Rapidly dividing cells, particularly those of the bone marrow, intestinal epithelia, and hair follicles, are most affected. Bone marrow depression is a most serious side effect inasmuch as it predisposes the patient to anemia, bleeding, and infection.

New approaches to cancer drug therapy have emerged that indirectly inhibit tumors rather than seeking to kill tumor cells directly. A promising approach is to interrupt the tumor's blood supply. To proliferate, solid tumors must be supplied by a progressively expanding network of capillaries. The development of new capillaries, called *angiogenesis,* is accomplished by migration and growth of endothelial cells. Drugs that block angiogenesis (antiangiogenics) are in various phases of clinical trials.

Immunotherapy

It has been suggested that the cancerous transformation of cells may be a relatively common event in life, yet few of these cells survive to give rise to cancer. The immune system may play a role in the detection and eradication of these cancerous cells.[21] The primary support for this view comes from the observation that people who are immunocompromised have a greater incidence of cancer. Support for the immune surveillance theory has waxed and waned over the years, but it has provided the basis for research on possible ways to use the immune system to fight the battle against cancer. Harnessing the power of the immune system to fight cancer is a particularly appealing idea because of the potential for *specificity.*

Traditional forms of treatment are not selective for cancer cells and result in unavoidable damage to normal tissue. The immune system, on the other hand, is noted for its ability to make subtle distinctions between normal and abnormal or foreign cells. Recognition of tumor cells as different from their normal counterparts is the basis of tumor immunology. Recognition depends on the expression of abnormal molecules or antigens on the cancer cell surface (Figure 7-15). Unfortunately, most tumor-associated antigens are also expressed to some degree on normal cells, which makes it difficult to develop strategies to target cancer cells selectively.

Despite much progress in understanding the immune system in the last several years, the hope for effective immunotherapy for cancer has not yet been fully realized. Current modes of immunomodulation primarily involve the use of interferons, interleukins, and monoclonal antibodies. These therapies are generally used as adjuncts to surgery, irradiation, and chemotherapy.

Interferons are glycoproteins produced by immune cells in response to viral infection. Interferons inhibit cell proliferation and are stimulatory to NK cells, T cells, and macrophages. Interferon-α has been used successfully to treat hairy cell leukemia (a rare B-cell malignancy), chronic myelogenous leukemia, and multiple myeloma.[22] Interferon therapy

Table 7-9
Examples of Chemotherapeutic Agents

Class	Drug	Mechanism of Action
Alkylating agents	Altretamine Carmustine Dacarbazine Procarbazine Temozolomide Mechlorethamine Melphalan Chlorambucil Cyclophosphamide Ifosfamide Thiotepa Busulfan	DNA alkylation leading to strand breaks and cross-links that disrupt DNA replication and transcription; active throughout the cell cycle
Antimetabolites	Methotrexate 5-Fluorouracil Cytarabine 6-Mercaptopurine 6-Thioguanine Fludarabine 6-Mercapturine Pentostatin 6-Thioguanine Gemcitabine	Substitute for or compete with a metabolite, thus interfering with DNA and RNA synthesis; active mainly during S phase
Antitumor antibiotics	Actinomycin D Bleomycin Mitomycin C Doxorubicin Daunorubicin Dactinomycin Idarubicin Valrubicin Mitoxantrone	Various effects on DNA such as fragmentation, binding, and cross-linking strands; interfere with transcription
Plant alkaloids	Vincristine Vinblastine Etoposide Docetaxel Irinotecan Paclitaxel Teniposide Topotecan Vinorelbine	Bind to mitotic proteins (tubulin) and prevent formation of mitotic spindle; cells arrest in mitosis
Hormones	Estrogens (diethylstilbestrol) Gonadotropin-releasing hormone	Decrease luteinizing hormone secretion and inhibit prostate tumor growth
	Tamoxifen	Estradiol antagonist; inhibits estrogen-dependent tumors (breast)
	Corticosteroids	Bind to and lyse lymphoid cancer cells
Heavy metal agents	Cisplatin Carboplatin Oxaliplatin	Activated platinum causes DNA cross-linking
Monoclonal antibodies	Alemtuzumab	Binds to CD52 on immune cells
	Bevacizumab	Binds to VEGF and inhibits angiogenesis
	Gemtuzumab	Binds to CD33 on leukemic blasts
	Rituximab	Binds to CD20 on B lymphocytes
	Trastuzumab	Binds to HER-2 receptor on breast cancer cells

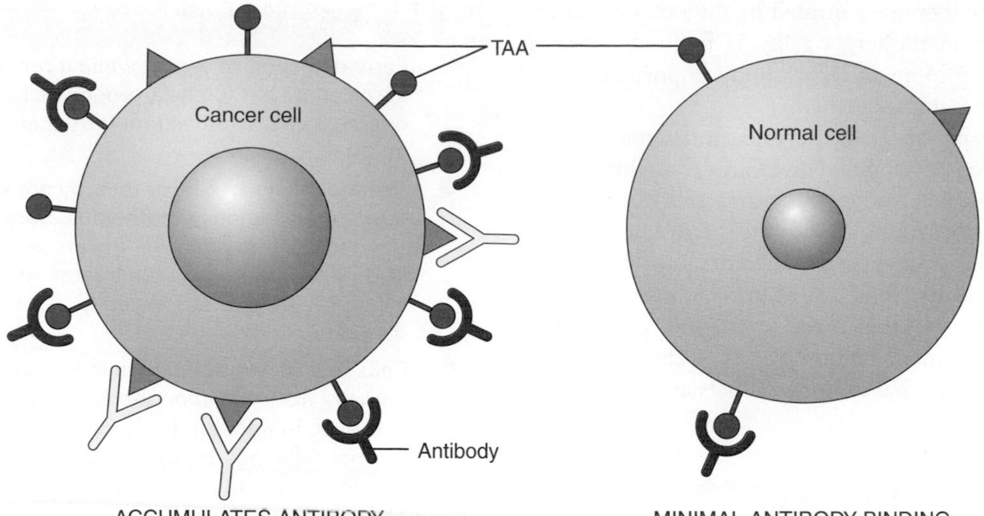

FIGURE 7-15 ■ Cancer cells express abnormal antigens (tumor-associated antigens *[TAA]*) on their cell surface that can activate immune cells or be used as targets for monoclonal antibodies.

produces symptoms similar to those of a viral infection: fever, chills, and muscle aches.

Interleukins are peptides produced and secreted by white blood cells. They are also called lymphokines or cytokines. Interleukin-2 (IL-2) is an important cytokine secreted by activated T-helper cells. It stimulates the proliferation of T cells, NK cells, and macrophages. IL-2 can be used to stimulate the growth of these immune cells in culture. Immune cells taken from a patient's blood can be grown in culture in the presence of IL-2. Then the greatly expanded number of immune cells can be given back to the patient, along with intravenous infusions of IL-2. Such treatment has been associated with regression of some tumors (melanoma, renal cell carcinoma).[23] Because IL-2 toxicity is high and many individuals have severe allergic reactions, the benefit of therapy must be weighed against the risks for each individual situation.

The use of monoclonal antibodies (antibodies having identical structure) in cancer therapy is currently the subject of intense investigation. Monoclonal antibodies specifically bind with target antigens and can therefore be used in several ways as treatment for cancer. Antibodies can be used to deliver a cytotoxic drug preferentially to the cancer cell and thus minimize drug interactions with normal cells. Similarly, antibodies can be used to direct other cytotoxic cells, such as NK and T cells, to tumor cells lurking in the body. Antibodies can be attached to a radioactive label and injected into a patient to screen for recurrence of tumor growth. Antibodies can also be directed against cells that support tumor growth.

Monoclonal antibodies have been developed for management of several cancers (see Table 7-9). For example, nearly 25% of breast cancers have overexpression of the HER2 receptor on the surface of malignant cells. The monoclonal antibody trastuzumab specifically binds to this HER2 protein and helps immune cells to find and kill the tumor cells.

Gene and Molecular Therapy

Because cancer is fundamentally a disorder of gene function, the use of gene therapy to alter the malignant behavior of cells may have high therapeutic potential. As specific gene derangements are identified for particular tumors, gene therapy may be used to suppress overactive oncogenes or replenish missing tumor suppressor function. Current uses of gene therapy for cancer include genetic alteration of tumor cells to make them more susceptible to cytotoxic agents or immune recognition and genetic alteration of immune cells to make them more efficient killers of tumor cells. A number of these approaches to therapy have shown promise in clinical trials.

For example, human brain tumors have been managed by insertion of a viral gene for thymidine kinase. Introduction of this gene makes the tumor cells susceptible to subsequent treatment with the antiviral drug ganciclovir.[24] Tumor cells can also be made more recognizable to immune cells by insertion of genes that cause the tumor cells to express "foreign" proteins on their cell surface. This type of gene therapy has shown some benefit in melanoma and renal carcinoma. Replacement of genes for P53 is an attractive therapy because tumor cells would be more susceptible to apoptosis. Gene replacement of other tumor suppressors such as PRB or APC in those tumors that are deficient could help inhibit tumor proliferation.

Gene therapy can be directed at cells other than tumor cells to enhance the body's cancer defenses. One such approach involves harvesting immune cells from the cancer patient, inserting IL-2 genes, and then returning the genetically enhanced immune cells to the patient. The enhanced immune cells attack the tumor cells more vigorously than normal immune cells do and have been shown to persist in the body for 6 months or longer.

At present, gene therapy is limited by difficulty in delivering the new genes to the target cells. As methods improve, gene therapy will become an increasingly important part of cancer prevention and management.

Molecular therapies that target cytoplasmic signaling pathways have also been developed. For example, in chronic myelogenous leukemia a chromosomal rearrangement results in the abnormal production of an enzyme, BCR/ABL. This enzyme stimulates cell proliferation and contributes to the overproduction of leukemic cells. An agent that specifically inhibits this enzyme has been approved and promises to improve the management of this disease. Other drugs that specifically target abnormal tumor products are under development.

Stem Cell Transplantation

Transplantation of hematologic stem cells is used to manage life-threatening disorders in which the patient's bone marrow is incapable of manufacturing white blood cells, red blood cells, or platelets. Most often, nonfunctional marrow is a consequence of the high-dose chemotherapy and radiation used to manage hematologic malignancies such as leukemia and lymphoma. Stem cell transplantation also has been applied to other malignancies (e.g., breast cancer) and to nonmalignant disorders (e.g., aplastic anemia, sickle cell anemia, and thalassemia).

Stem cells can be harvested from aspirates of bone marrow or from the donor's peripheral blood stream. Bone marrow is rich in stem cells, but the peripheral blood is poor. To obtain adequate stem cells from the blood, the cells are first mobilized by cytokines, chemotherapy drugs, or both, and then the immune cells are collected from the enriched blood through a process called *pheresis.* The stem cell donor can be a tissue-matched individual (allogeneic), an identical twin (syngeneic), or the patient in question (autologous). A closer match between donor and recipient is associated with a better outcome.

Before infusion of donor stem cells, the patient's own immune cells must be suppressed to prevent transplant rejection. It is also necessary to eliminate any residual malignant cells from the body to avoid relapse of the cancer. Both of these objectives are accomplished through high-dose chemotherapy and total-body irradiation regimens, which leave the patient susceptible to severe anemia, infection, and bleeding. The therapeutic goal of stem cell transplantation is to restore immune and hematopoietic function. It may take weeks to months for the infused stem cells to set up housekeeping and begin to proliferate in their new host. During this time, the transplant recipient requires intensive monitoring and management of complications.

The success of stem cell transplantation depends on a number of factors, including the patient's age, closeness of tissue matching, stage of cancer, and general health status before transplantation. Transplantation is an expensive undertaking but may significantly improve disease survival rates in some malignancies.[25]

KEY CONCEPTS

- Early detection of cancer while it remains localized is associated with the best prognosis for cure. The overall 5-year survival rate for patients with cancer is about 60%.
- The mainstays of cancer therapy are surgery, radiation therapy, and chemotherapy. Surgery and radiation therapy are effective for cancers that are localized. Chemotherapy is the treatment of choice for cancers known or suspected to be disseminated in the body.
- Cells that divide rapidly are the most susceptible to damage from radiation therapy or chemotherapy. However, in addition to cancer cells, rapidly dividing normal cells may be killed. Cells of the bone marrow, hair follicles, and gastrointestinal mucosa are particularly susceptible.
- Immunotherapy has the potential to specifically target cancer cells. At present, interferon, IL-2, and monoclonal antibodies are being used to boost the immune system's ability to locate and destroy cancer cells.
- Gene therapy may be used to alter cancer cells to suppress oncogenes, enhance tumor suppressor genes, or make tumor cells more susceptible to cytotoxic agents.
- Transplantation of hematopoietic stem cells is an important adjunct to cancer therapy that provides a method to restore bone marrow function after high-dose irradiation or chemotherapy.

EPIDEMIOLOGY AND CANCER RISK FACTORS

Cancer accounts for approximately 25% of all deaths, which makes it the second leading cause of death in the United States. Most cancer deaths (77%) occur in persons older than 55 years. The American Cancer Society estimates that men have almost a 1 in 2 lifetime risk of developing cancer and women have slightly higher than a 1 in 3 risk. The 5-year relative survival rate for all cancers combined is about 62%.[18] Fortunately, the current view of cancer causation predicts that most cancer is preventable. Indeed, one third of cancer-related deaths may be attributed to lifestyle factors. Life-style factors of particular importance are tobacco use, nutrition, and obesity. Sun exposure is a significant risk factor for skin cancer (Chapter 53), and sexual exposure to certain strains of human papillomavirus predisposes to cervical cancer (Chapter 34). The high incidence and relative ease of screening for breast, cervical, colorectal, and prostate cancers has prompted the development of guidelines for early detection of these cancers. The current recommendations for early detection of cancer in average-risk, asymptomatic persons are shown in Table 7-10. Statistics regarding some of the major forms of cancer are shown in Figure 7-16.

Further discussions of particular cancers can be found in chapters relating to corresponding body systems.

Tobacco Use

The impact of tobacco use on cancer-related death can be most vividly seen by looking at cancer death rates in the United States from 1930 to 1999 (Figure 7-17). Whereas all other cancer-related death rates declined or remained relatively stable, the death rate from lung cancer increased dramatically. The increase is attributable almost entirely to smoking. Lung cancer remains the leading cause of cancer death in both men and women, accounting for 30% of all cancer deaths. Lung cancer has one of the worst survival rates of all cancers—only 15%. In addition to lung cancer, tobacco use has been linked with cancer of the pancreas, bladder, kidney, mouth, esophagus, and cervix. Smoking prevalence among adults in the United States declined an average of 1% per year between 1993 and 2000. In

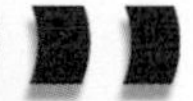

Table 7-10

Screening Guidelines of the Early Detection of Cancer in Asymptomatic People

Site	Recommendation
Breast	Women 40 and older should have an annual mammogram and an annual clinical breast examination (CBE) by a health care professional, and should perform monthly breast self-examination (BSE). Ideally the CBE should occur before the scheduled mammograms. Women ages 20 to 39 should have a CBE by a health care professional every 3 years and should perform BSE monthly.
Colon and rectum	Beginning at age 50, men and women should follow one of the examination schedules below: A fecal occult blood test (FOBT) every year A flexible sigmoidoscopy (FSIG) every 5 years Annual fecal occult blood test and flexible sigmoidoscopy every 5 years* A double-contrast barium enema every 5 years A colonoscopy every 10 years
Prostate	The PSA test and the digital rectal examination should be offered annually, beginning at age 50, to men who have life expectancy of at least 10 years. Men at high risk (African-American men and men with a strong family history of one or more first-degree relatives diagnosed with prostate cancer at an early age) should begin testing at age 45. For both men at average risk and high risk, information should be provided about what is known and what is uncertain about the benefits and limitations of early detection and management of prostate cancer so that they can make an informed decision about testing.
Uterus	Cervix: Screening should begin approximately 3 years after a woman begins having vaginal intercourse, but no later than 21 years of age. Screening should be done every year with regular Pap tests or every 2 years using liquid-based test. At or after age 30, women who have had three normal test results in a row may get screened every 2 to 3 years. However, doctors may suggest a woman get screened more often if she has certain risk factors, such as HIV infection or weak immune system. Women 70 years and older who have had three or more consecutive normal Pap tests in the last 10 years may choose to stop cervical screening. Screening after total hysterectomy (with removal of the cervix) is not necessary unless the surgery was done as a treatment for cervical cancer. Endometrium: The American Cancer Society recommends that all women should be informed about the risks and symptoms of endometrial cancer, and strongly encouraged to report any unexpected bleeding or spotting to their physicians. Annual screening for endometrial biopsy beginning at age 35 should be offered to women with or at risk for hereditary nonpolyposis colon cancer (HNPCC).
Cancer-related checkup	For individuals undergoing periodic health examinations, a cancer-related checkup should include health counseling, and depending on a person's age, might include examinations for cancers of the thyroid, oral cavity, skin, lymph nodes, testes, and ovaries, as well as for some nonmalignant diseases.

American Cancer Society guidelines for early cancer detection are assessed annually in order to identify whether there is new scientific evidence sufficient to warrant a reevaluation of current recommendations. If evidence is sufficiently compelling to consider a change or clarification in a current guideline or the development of a new guideline, a formal procedure is initiated. Guidelines are formally evaluated every 5 years regardless of whether new evidence suggests a change in the existing recommendations. There are nine steps in this procedure, and these "guidelines for guideline development" were formally established to provide a specific methodology for science and expert judgment to form the underpinnings of specific statements and recommendations from the Society. These procedures constitute a deliberate process to ensure that all Society recommendations have the same methodological and evidence-based process at their core. This process also employs a system for rating strength and consistency of evidence that is similar to that employed by the Agency for Health Care Research and Quality (AHCRQ) and the US Preventive Services Task Force (USPSTF).

*Combined testing is preferred over either annual FOBT or FSIG every 5 years alone. People who are at moderate or high risk for colorectal cancer should talk with a doctor about a different testing schedule.

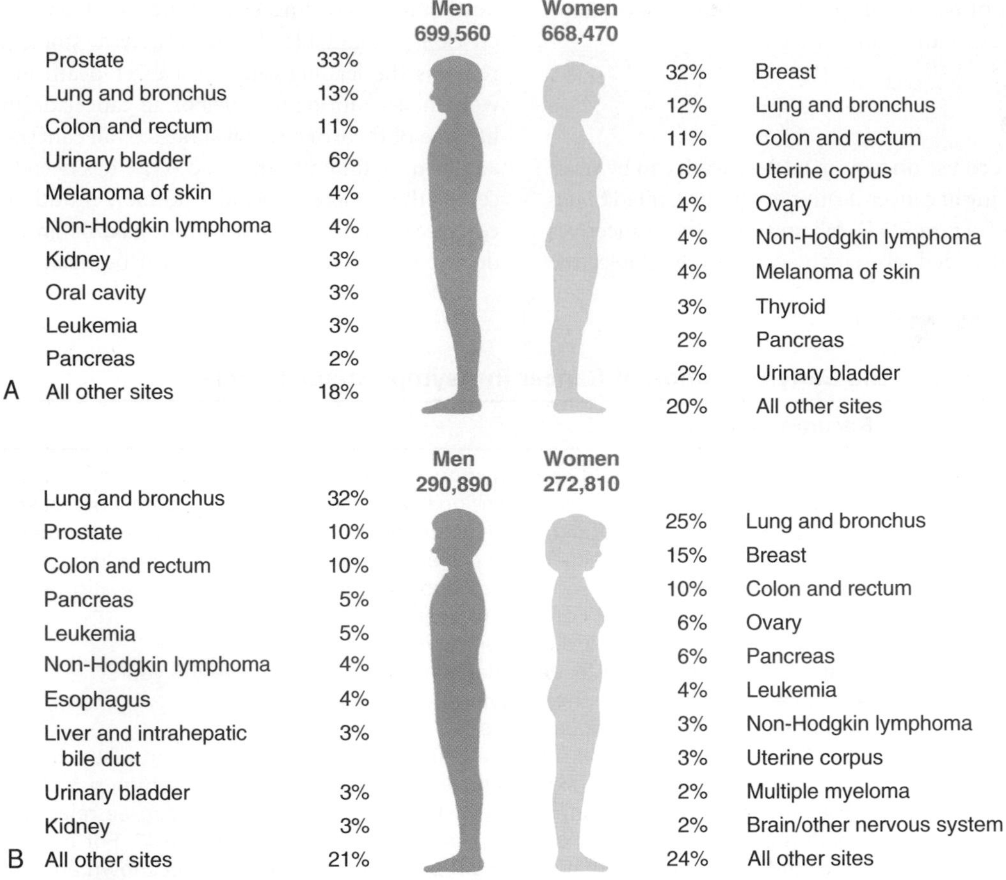

FIGURE 7-16 ■ United States 2004 estimated new cancer cases **(A)** and estimated cancer deaths **(B)** in 10 leading sites by sex. Excludes basal and squamous cell skin cancers and in situ carcinomas except urinary bladder. (From American Cancer Society: *Cancer facts and figures—2004,* Atlanta, 2004, The Society.)

the year 2000, 46.5 million U.S. adults were current smokers. Twenty-six percent of adult men and 21% of adult women smoked. Approximately 14% of high school students reported being current, frequent cigarette smokers in 2001.[18]

Carcinogens can be grouped into two major types: those that cause genetic damage (initiators) and those that promote growth of the tumor (promoters). Tobacco smoke contains hundreds of compounds, many of which have known genotoxicity (e.g., polycyclic aromatic hydrocarbons, nicotine derivatives) and probably serve as initiators. Tobacco smoke also contains promoters, which spur the mutant cells to proliferate. Promotion appears to be dose dependent, with the risk of cancer increasing sharply as use increases above 20 cigarettes per day.[26] However, the number of years of smoking is a better predictor of risk than the number of cigarettes smoked per day.[27] Cessation of smoking results in a decline in cancer risk owing to the removal of promoters.

Nutrition

The results of studies on the relationship between cancer and certain nutrients remain confusing and contradictory. The general opinion is that diet is associated with cancer risk, but there is little agreement as to what that association might be. A lack of fruits and vegetables in the diet may be a significant contributor to cancer risk, but the mechanisms are unclear. Dietary factors believed to be related to cancer risk include fat, fiber, alcohol, and antioxidants. It is not yet clear how single nutrients, nutrient combinations, overnutrition, or body fat distribution affect the risk of developing cancer, and more research is needed.[28]

Fat

Several epidemiologic studies done in the 1970s and early 1980s suggested a relationship between high-fat diets and the development of breast, colon, and prostate cancer. In some studies, however, higher fat intake was found to be protective against some cancers. A pooled analysis of seven large studies found no link between fat intake and the risk of breast cancer.[29] Further research on the specific type of fat intake and other cofactors is needed to clarify the fat-cancer relationship. One explanation for discrepant results might be that high-fat diets tend to be high-calorie diets. Several studies in animals have shown that regardless of fat intake, tumor growth may be inhibited by caloric restriction. Some investigators have pro-

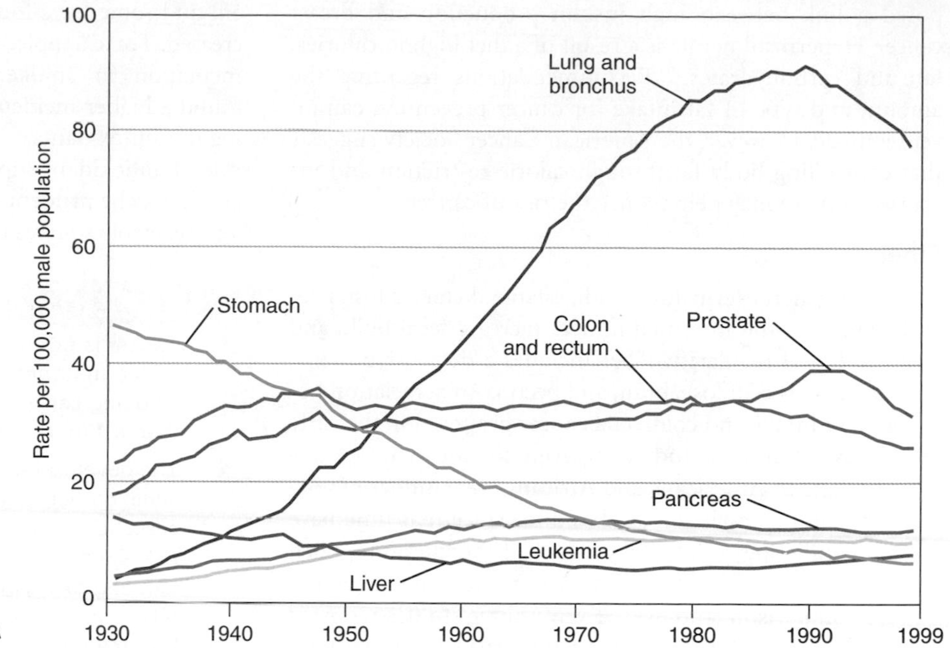

Per 100,000, age-adjusted to the 2000 US standard population.
Note: Due to changes in ICD coding, numerator information has changed over time. Rates for cancers of the liver, lung and bronchus, and colon and rectum are affected by these coding changes.
Source: US Mortality Public Use Data Tapes 1960-1999, US Mortality Volumes 1930-1959, National Center for Health Statistics, Centers for Disease Control and Prevention, 2002.
American Cancer Society, Surveillance Research, 2003

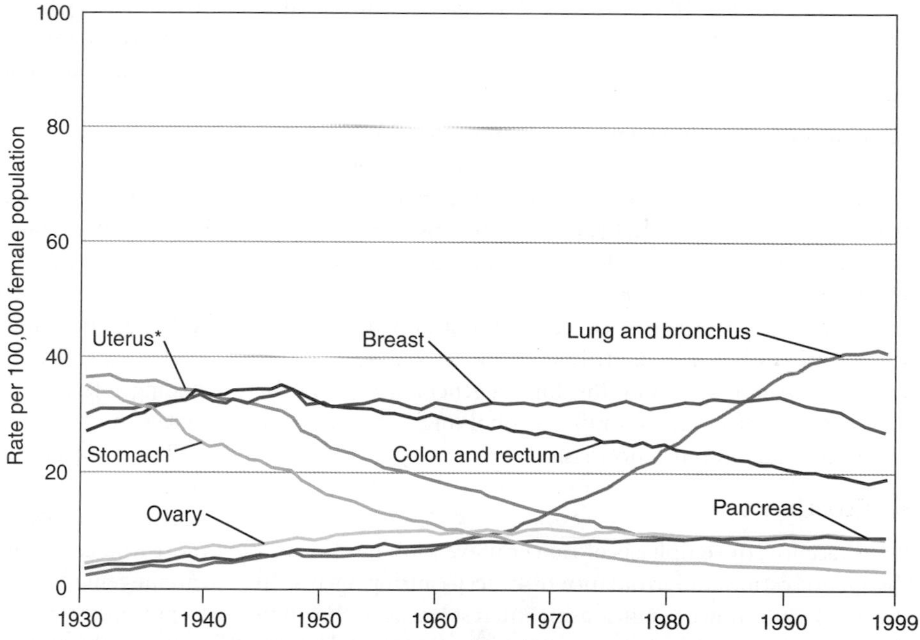

Per 100,000, age-adjusted to the 2000 US standard population.
*Uterus cancer death rates are for uterine cervix and uterine corpus combined.
Note: Due to changes in ICD coding, numerator information has changed over time. Rates for cancers of the liver, lung and bronchus, colon and rectum, and ovary are affected by these coding changes.
Source: US Mortality Public Use Data Tapes 1960-1999, US Mortality Volumes 1930-1959, National Center for Health Statistics, Centers for Disease Control and Prevention, 2002.
American Cancer Society, Surveillance Research, 2003

FIGURE 7-17 ■ U.S. age-adjusted cancer death rates for selected sites in men **(A)** and women **(B)** from 1930 to 1999. (Redrawn from American Cancer Society: *Cancer facts and figures—2003,* Atlanta, 2003, The Society.)

posed a link between high insulin production and breast cancer. Hyperinsulinemia is a result of a diet high in calories, fat, and carbohydrates.[30] Recommendations regarding the amount and type of fat intake for cancer prevention cannot yet be made. However, the American Cancer Society suggests that controlling body fat through calorie restriction and increased activity may help reduce the risk of cancer.

Fiber

Fiber is a general term for nondigestable dietary substances that remain in the intestinal lumen, increase fecal bulk, and improve bowel regularity. Fiber includes a diversity of compounds such as cellulose, bran, and pectin. An association between fiber intake and colorectal cancer proposed in the early 1970s was based on a study comparing the incidence of certain ailments in Americans and Africans.[31] A number of correlational and comparison studies done since that time have yielded conflicting results. In a review of the literature, Pilch related the findings of 44 studies (22 correlational studies and 22 case comparison studies).[32] Twenty-three studies reported a protective role for fiber in colon cancer; 14 found no relationship. Seven studies showed that fiber increased the risk of colon cancer. Two large clinical trials assessing the effects of a high-fiber diet on colon cancer failed to find a significant benefit.[33,34] Part of the difficulty may be linked to the way that different studies define dietary fiber. Because fiber is associated with beneficial effects on digestion and elimination, fiber intake in the range of 10 to 13 g per 1000 calories consumed is generally recommended.

Alcohol

Alcohol intake has been linked to a number of cancers, including breast, esophageal, laryngeal, and liver cancer. Alcohol may exert its cancer-promoting effects through impairment of the liver's ability to metabolize harmful substances and endogenous hormones. Moderate alcohol intake has been shown to increase estrogen levels, which may account for its promoting effects on breast cancer.[35] As a carbohydrate-dense substance, alcohol may contribute to cancer risk through its effects on insulin secretion. Insulin is a general growth factor for a number of tissues. Limiting alcohol intake may provide a modest reduction in cancer risk.

Antioxidants

Until recently, the emphasis of cancer prevention has been on the identification and avoidance of cancer-causing agents. In the last decade, however, increasing interest has been shown in finding substances with cancer-protective properties. The fact that DNA damage is an important step in cancer initiation, coupled with the knowledge that oxygen free radicals can impart this damage, led to the idea that antioxidants may have protective effects for cancer.

Vitamin A and the antioxidant trio of vitamin E, β-carotene, and vitamin C have been most widely studied. The use of antioxidants to prevent cancer sounds like a good idea; however, several large-scale studies have failed to reveal a benefit and some have found that the risk of cancer may be increased. For example, two studies using β-carotene supplementation in smokers and asbestos-exposed individuals found a higher incidence of lung cancer in the group receiving the antioxidants.[36,37] Further research is needed before the role of antioxidant supplementation can be defined. At present, it may be prudent to consume a diet high in natural fruit and vegetable sources of antioxidants.

KEY CONCEPTS

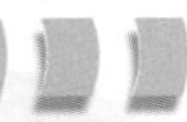

- Cancer is primarily a disease of the elderly. It is estimated that men have almost a 1 in 2 chance of developing cancer whereas women have a little more than a 1 in 3 chance.
- The development of many cancers is related to lifestyle, particularly tobacco use and nutrition. Smoking cessation is considered important in reducing cancer risk. Guidelines regarding nutrition are less clear. Limiting excessive fat, carbohydrate, and alcohol intake while increasing dietary fiber, fruit, and vegetables may be of benefit.

SUMMARY

Neoplasia is abnormal cell proliferation of a benign or malignant nature. Benign tumors resemble their parent cells and are strictly local, whereas malignant tumors are anaplastic, invade local tissues, and may spread to distant sites (metastasize). The most important consideration for cancer management is the degree of cancer spread in the body, which can be determined by staging procedures. Cancer is managed by surgical removal, radiation therapy, chemotherapy, and immunotherapy.

Cancer cells have complex relationships with the host. The host immune system is capable of but not always successful in recognizing and killing cancer cells. Cancer cells exert immunosuppressive effects on the host and eventually cause pain, cachexia, and bone marrow suppression. If untreated, cancer has the potential to kill the host by multifactorial processes, including infection, hemorrhage, and organ failure. If treated, cancer has an overall 5-year survival rate of approximately 62%.

The primary cause of cancer is thought to be a carcinogenic lifestyle, with other environmental carcinogens playing a lesser role. Tobacco use and improper nutrition are the two most studied carcinogenic lifestyle factors. Tobacco is clearly carcinogenic through its ability to cause genetic damage and to promote the growth of mutant cells. The evidence linking nutritional factors such as fat and fiber intake to cancer risk is less convincing.

Cancer is thought to develop when proto-oncogenes become inappropriately activated in the cell or tumor suppressor genes become inactivated. This change in activation is usually due to a mutational event in the cell's DNA. Oncogenes are thought to disrupt intercellular communication, which normally exerts growth-controlling effects on the cell. This disruption is accomplished primarily through the production of abnormal growth factors, growth factor receptors, cytoplasmic signaling molecules, or nuclear transcription factors that allow the cancer cell to manufacture its own growth-promoting signals. The tumor suppressor genes *Rb* and *P53* are important inhibitors of cell replication. The RB protein binds and sequesters transcription factors, whereas p53 monitors the integrity of cellular DNA and may initiate apoptosis (cell suicide) when significant cell damage occurs.

MEDIA RESOURCES

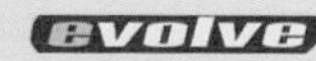

Remember to check out the ***CD Companion*** included with this book for Review Questions, Key Concepts Review, Glossary (with audio for selected terms), Disease Profiles, and Animations.

PLUS, visit the ***Evolve website*** at http://evolve.elsevier.com/Copstead/ for Case Studies, Disease Profiles, and WebLinks.

References

1. Kumar V, Cotran R, Robbins S: Neoplasia. In Kumar V, Cotran R, Robbins S, editors: *Robbins basic pathology,* ed 7, Philadelphia, 2003, Saunders, pp 165-210.
2. Alberts B et al: Cancer. In Alberts B et al, editors: *Molecular biology of the cell,* ed 4, New York, 2002, Garland Science, pp 1313-1362.
3. McCann J, Ames BN: Detection of carcinogens as mutagens in the *Salmonella*/microsome test: assay for 300 chemicals: discussion, *Proc Natl Acad Sci U S A* 73:950-955, 1976.
4. Dulbecco R: Cell transformation by viruses, *Science* 166: 962-968, 1969.
5. Weinberg RA: Tumor suppressor genes, *Science* 254:1138-1146, 1991.
6. Charpentier A, Aldaz C: The molecular basis of breast carcinogenesis. In Coleman W, Tsongalis G, editors: *The molecular basis of human cancer,* Totowa, NJ, 2002, Humana Press, pp 347-363.
7. Hunter T: Cooperation between oncogenes, *Cell* 64:249-270, 1991.
8. Vogelstein B, Kinzler KW: The multistep nature of cancer, *Trends Genet* 9(4):138-141, 1993.
9. Lindley C: Breast cancer. In Dipiro J et al, editors: *Pharmacotherapy: a pathophysiologic approach,* ed 5, New York, 2002, McGraw-Hill, pp 2223-2252.
10. Clemons M, Goss P: Estrogen and the risk of breast cancer, *N Engl J Med* 344(4):276-285, 2001.
11. Murphy PM: Chemokines and the molecular basis of metastasis, *N Engl J Med* 345(11):833-835, 2001.
12. Hayflick L: The biology of human aging, *Adv Pathobiol* 7(2): 80-99, 1980.
13. Shay JW, Wright WE: Telomerase: a target for cancer therapeutics, *Cancer Cell* 2(4):257-265, 2002.
14. Cairns RA, Khokha R, Hill RP: Molecular mechanisms of tumor invasion and metastasis: an integrated view, *Curr Mol Med* 3(7):659-671, 2003.
15. Greene F: *AJCC cancer staging manual,* ed 6, New York, 2002, Springer-Verlag.
16. Jerusalem G et al: PET scan imaging in oncology, *Eur J Cancer* 39(11):1525-1534, 2003.
17. Khong HT, Restifo NP: Natural selection of tumor variants in the generation of "tumor escape" phenotypes, *Nat Immunol* 3(11):999-1005, 2002.
18. American Cancer Society: *Cancer facts and figures—2003,* Atlanta, 2003, The Society.
19. Coffey JC et al: Excisional surgery for cancer cure: therapy at a cost, *Lancet Oncol* 4(12):760-768, 2003.
20. Fleming ID et al: Basis for major current therapies for cancer. In Murphy GP, Lawrence W, Lenhard RE, editors: *American Cancer Society textbook of clinical oncology,* Atlanta, 1995, American Cancer Society, pp 96-134.
21. Platsoucas CD et al: Immune responses to human tumors: development of tumor vaccines, *Anticancer Res* 23(3A): 1969-1996, 2003.
22. Kirkwood J: Cancer immunotherapy: the interferon-alpha experience, *Semin Oncol* 29(3 suppl 7):18-26, 2002.
23. Dutcher J: Current status of interleukin-2 therapy for metastatic renal cell carcinoma and metastatic melanoma, *Oncology (Huntingt)* 16(11 suppl 13):4-10, 2002.
24. Bolognani F, Goya RG: Gene therapy in the neuroendocrine system: its implementation in experimental models using viral vectors, *Neuroendocrinology* 73(2):75-83, 2001.
25. Serna DS et al: Trends in survival rates after allogeneic hematopoietic stem-cell transplantation for acute and chronic leukemia by ethnicity in the United States and Canada, *J Clin Oncol* 21(20):3754-3760, 2003.
26. Weisburger JH, Williams GM: Causes of cancer. In Murphy GP, Lawrence W, Lenhard RE, editors: *American Cancer Society textbook of clinical oncology,* Atlanta, 1995, American Cancer Society, pp 10-39.
27. Flanders WD et al: Lung cancer mortality in relation to age, duration of smoking and daily cigarette consumption: results for Cancer Prevention Study II, *Cancer Res* 63(19):6556-6562, 2003.
28. American Cancer Society: *Cancer prevention and early detection,* Atlanta, 2003, The Society.
29. Hunter DJ, Willett WC: Nutrition and breast cancer, *Cancer Causes Control* 7(1):56-68, 1996.
30. Giovanucci E: Insulin, insulin-like growth factors and colon cancer: a review of the evidence, *J Nutr* 131(11 suppl): 3109S-3120S, 2001.
31. Burkitt DP, Walker ARP, Painter NS: Dietary fiber and disease, *JAMA* 229:1068-1074, 1974.
32. Pilch SM, editor: *Physiological effects and health consequences of dietary fiber,* Bethesda, Md, 1987, Federation of American Societies for Experimental Biology.
33. Alberts DS et al: Lack of effect of a high-fiber cereal supplement on the recurrence of colorectal adenomas. Phoenix Colon Cancer Prevention Physicians' Network, *N Engl J Med* 342(16):1156-1162, 2000.
34. Schatzkin A et al: Lack of effect of low-fat, high-fiber diet on the recurrence of colorectal adenomas. Polyp Prevention Trial Study Group, *N Engl J Med* 342(16):1149-1155, 2000.
35. McTiernan A: Behavioral risk factors in breast cancer: can risk be modified? *Oncologist* 8:326-334, 2003.
36. Omenn GS et al: Risk factors for lung cancer and for intervention effects in CARET, the Beta-Carotene and Retinol Efficacy Trial, *J Natl Cancer Inst* 88(21):1550-1559, 1996.
37. Albanes D et al: Effects of Alpha-Tocopherol Beta-Carotene Cancer Prevention Study, *Am J Clin Nutr* 61:1427S-1430S, 1995.

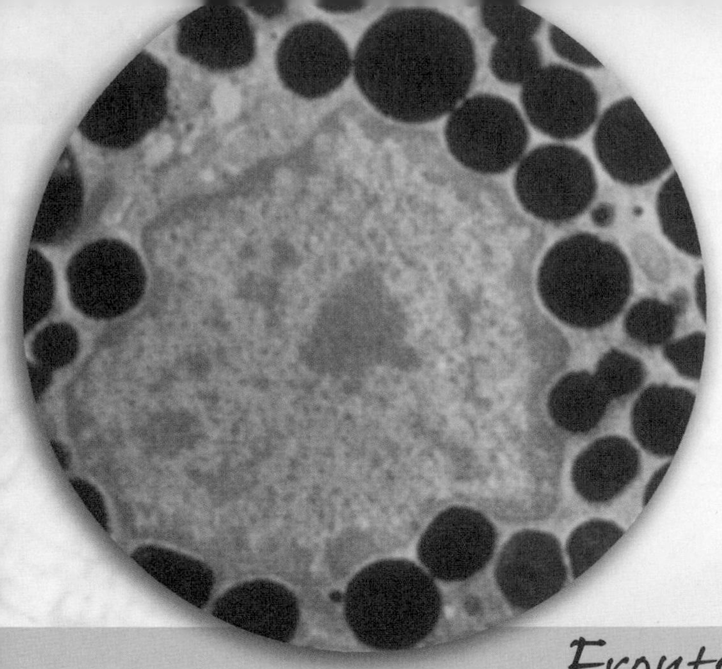

Frontiers of Research

Immune System Responses

Peter A. Valen and Michael J. Kirkhorn

The human body is under constant attack by outside and, occasionally, unrecognized inside invaders. These invaders, including microbes and cancer cells, overcome recognition and establish a foothold. The body's "homeland security" is provided by the immune system, which functions to recognize foreign invaders, mobilize defense forces, and attack. Occasionally the system fails to mount an adequate defense or mistakes our own healthy tissue as foreign, and disease results.

Today, largely through research into autoimmune disease, cancer, and the virus that causes acquired immunodeficiency syndrome (human immunodeficiency virus [HIV]), we are learning more about how the immune system works.

The immune system is an intricate network of organs, cells, and soluble proteins that functions to distinguish between "self" and "nonself." The immune system can be divided into innate immunity, with which we are born, and learned or adaptive immunity, which is acquired during life as we encounter foreign substances (antigens).

The components of the immune system involved in innate immunity—including macrophages, neutrophils, and complement—recognize a wide range of foreign antigens. Adaptive immunity, on the other hand, is specific to the particular antigen encountered. Because of adaptive immunity, the immune system can remember a previously encountered antigen and can respond in a quick and vigorous way. This memory is carried by lymphocytes, which are long-lived cells. This immune response is why people generally have infectious diseases like chickenpox and measles only once, and it is also responsible for the success of vaccinations in preventing disease.

The human immune system may be outsmarted by new forms of infection, such as viruses transmitted from another species, quickly evolving pathogens or viruses like HIV, exposure to novel pathogens as a result of rapid worldwide travel, or drug-resistant strains of organisms.

Occasionally the immune system malfunctions by misinterpreting the body's tissues as foreign, resulting in autoimmune disease. These diseases can be triggered in several ways. If tissue that is normally sequestered and therefore "hidden" from the immune system, such as fluid in the eyeball, escapes as a result of disease or injury, the immune system may react against it. Normal body tissues may be altered by viruses, drugs, sunlight,

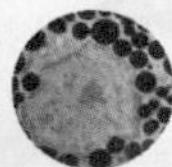

Mast cell. This colorized micrograph shows a mast cell filled with dense red granules of the inflammation mediator called histamine. *(From Wilson SF, Thompson JM:* Respiratory disorders, *St Louis, 1990, Mosby.)*

Defense

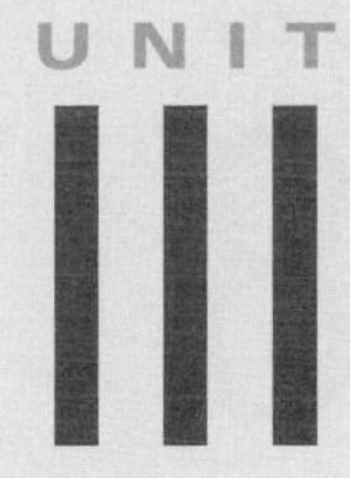

or radiation and therefore become immunogenic. The immune system, responding to a foreign antigen, may mistakenly attack normal tissues that resemble the foreign antigen, as occurs in rheumatic fever following a streptococcal infection. Finally, lymphocytes may be transformed by viruses or cancer and overproduce antibodies against normal human tissue. Examples of autoimmune diseases include multiple sclerosis, systemic lupus, Graves disease, rheumatoid arthritis, and type I diabetes mellitus. These conditions are common, affecting about 5% of adults in Europe and North America, and predominate in women.

Research on the causes and treatment of these and other autoimmune diseases is proceeding rapidly. We are learning more about the precise genetic factors involved in the pathogenesis of these conditions. The Human Genome Project has demonstrated that there are approximately 30,000 genes. Other research initiatives have led to information on gene markers and gene expression. Linkage studies can demonstrate whether a particular genetic variant is more often present in affected family members than in healthy family members. This methodology can identify areas of chromosomes associated with susceptibility to certain diseases. Ultimately, if a gene mutation responsible for a particular disease can be identified, as in severe combined immunodeficiency (SCID), for example, gene-transfer therapy may yield a cure.

Advances in genetic engineering and immunology are also leading to more effective vaccines. One such exciting development is the use of DNA vaccines. DNA coding for a foreign antigen is injected into an animal, resulting in direct production of the foreign antigen by host cells. These vaccines should result in fewer side effects because the foreign antigen is coming from the host itself. These vaccines should also be easier and less expensive to produce than conventional vaccines. Trials are under way using DNA vaccines against influenza, herpes simplex, T-cell lymphoma, and HIV. Potential risks include the possibility that the vaccine's DNA will be integrated into host chromosomes and turn on oncogenes or turn off suppressor genes or that prolonged immunostimulation by foreign antigens could lead to autoimmune disease.

Understanding the immune system and its various responses is critical to an understanding of not only the causes, but also the prevention, treatment, or even cure of human diseases.

Infectious Processes

Mark Puhlman

MEDIA RESOURCES

Additional Material for Study, Review, and Further Exploration

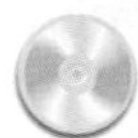

CD Companion ◆ Review Questions and Answers ◆ Key Concepts Review
◆ Glossary *(with audio pronunciations for selected terms)*
◆ Disease Profiles ◆ Animations

evolve ***Website*** at http://evolve.elsevier.com/Copstead/
◆ Case Studies ◆ Disease Profiles ◆ WebLinks

KEY QUESTIONS

- What is the role of epidemiology in the identification, definition, and prevention of infectious diseases?
- What factors influence the transmission of infectious agents?
- How do infectious microorganisms, including bacteria, viruses, fungi, and parasites, differ in structure, life cycle, and infectious processes?
- What conditions compromise host defenses against microorganisms?
- What are opportunistic infections and when do they develop?

CHAPTER OUTLINE

Infection is the cause of death for many people afflicted with a chronic or critical illness, with the very young and the very old being particularly susceptible to infection. Infections are caused by microorganisms that gain entry into the body. Once a microorganism adheres to or invades the human body, the signs and symptoms generally associated with infection are generated. The microorganisms that cause infection and disease are called pathogens, and the major types of microorganisms that can cause infections include bacteria, viruses, fungi, and parasites.

Different pathogens inhabit various environments such as hospitals, the food supply, water, and animal or human vectors. For example, many hospitalized patients are at risk for the development of sepsis, an overwhelming infection that may lead to multiple organ failure, irreversible hypotension, and death. Food-borne pathogens and the methods of preserving the food supply have an impact on transmission of infections, as do the location, density, and sanitary practices of a population. Globalization of the world's population with the associated rapidity and extent of air travel has major implications for the worldwide spread of infectious agents before the infected individual becomes symptomatic or identifiable.

Infection with pathogenic microorganisms has become a tool of war and terrorism in the world. "Weapons of mass destruction" are nuclear, chemical, and biological in nature. Whether it is anthrax spores sent through the mail or the threat of smallpox being introduced to a nonimmunized population, infection and the methods of preventing it have a key role in the defense of humanity. Health care professionals have a vital role in the prevention, early detection, and management of infections.

EPIDEMIOLOGIC CONCEPTS

Epidemiology is the study of health events and disease, their distribution, and associated causative factors in a defined population.[1] This science arose from the study of epidemics but now encompasses both infectious (e.g., human immunodeficiency virus [HIV] epidemic) and noninfectious (e.g., atherosclerosis) diseases. This chapter will confine its discussion to infectious disease, although some concepts are common to both.

The goals of epidemiology are to define the disease, identify outbreaks, assist in the development and evaluation of treatment protocols, and develop prevention strategies. This science attempts to attain these goals by conducting epidemiologic studies of disease. These studies can be broadly divided into observational studies, which describe events, exposures, and diseases occurring in a defined population, and experimental studies, which attempt to intervene in a controlled environment to study the effect of an intervention on the course of a disease.[2] Giving a randomly selected group of at-risk individuals educational programs about HIV prevention to determine the effect on risk taking behavior is an example of an experimental study. Studying the natural history of the Ebola virus outbreak in Zaire in 1976 is an example of an observational study.

The U.S. Centers for Disease Control and Prevention and the World Health Organization have pivotal roles in identifying diseases, tracking their natural history, and defining protocols for their control and prevention. An example of how these organizations can control disease is the virtual eradication of smallpox from the world. The World Health Organization, with the cooperation of other health organizations such as the Centers for Disease Control and Prevention, mandated immunizations for all those susceptible to the disease who were living in or traveling to areas where smallpox was prevalent. This immunization program, coupled with the lack of a viral host other than humans, led to the eradication of smallpox, except in the laboratory. Only the fear of the reintroduction of the virus into the population in a bioterrorism attack or biological warfare may mandate the continued immunization of susceptible populations such as health care workers, emergency personnel, and the military.

Transmission of Infection

Transmission of disease requires a chain of events that must occur unbroken to allow one human to infect another.[1,2] The pathogenic organism must live and reproduce in a reservoir (Figure 8-1). In this reservoir the organism multiplies to numbers adequate to infect another. The reservoir may be a human being, as in the influenza virus; an animal, as in bats and rabies; or soil, as in enterobiasis (pinworm infestation).

The **pathogen** must have a portal of exit with a mode of transmission from the reservoir to a susceptible victim. The portal of exit is usually closest to the breeding site of the organism. For example, *Neisseria gonorrhoeae*, the organism that

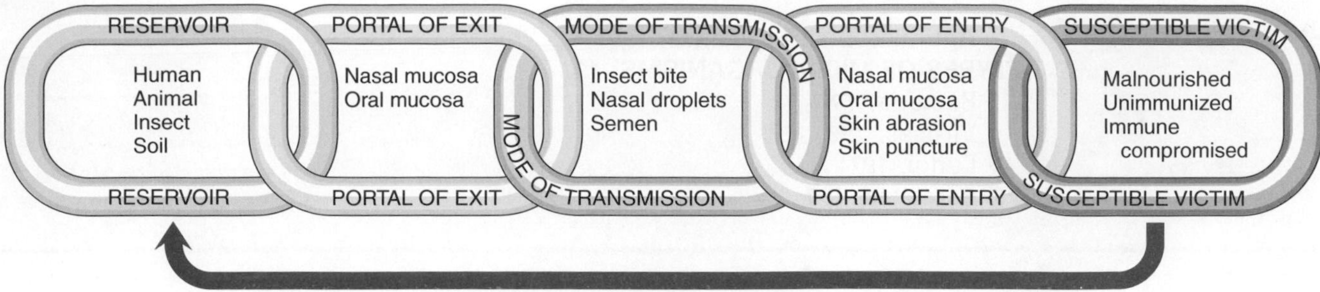

FIGURE 8-1 ■ Chain of transmission of microorganisms from host to victim.

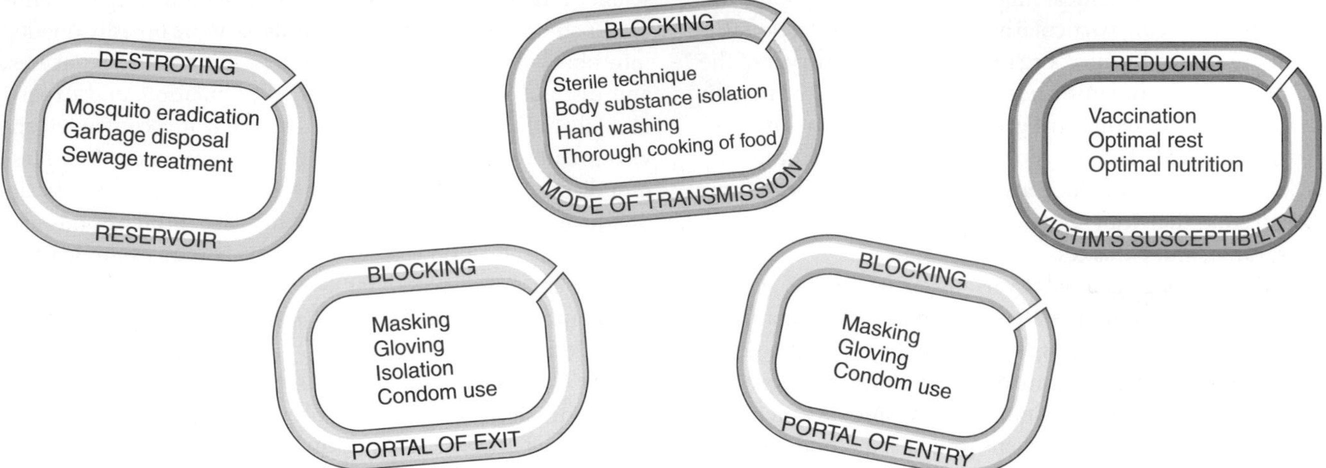

FIGURE 8-2 ■ Breaking the chain of transmission of microorganisms from host to victim.

is responsible for gonorrhea, usually resides in the urethra of the male and the vaginal canal of the female. The microorganism is transmitted by sexual contact.

Transmission of the pathogen can be either direct or indirect.[2-4] Direct transmission occurs when direct contact is made between the reservoir and the new host.[4] This contact can be physical or effected by fecal contamination or airborne droplets. Indirect contact occurs when the reservoir deposits the organism on an inanimate object (**fomite**), which then transmits the pathogen to the new host. An example of this mode of transmission is enterobiasis (pinworm) infestation, in which the eggs are deposited on soil, clothing, and bedding and ingested by hand-to-mouth contamination. The pathogen gains entry to the victim through a portal, usually close to the breeding area in the body. If the host is susceptible to the pathogen, the microorganism grows in numbers to overwhelm the host's immune system and infection occurs. Thus the entire cycle repeats itself.

If a balance is established between the "victim" and the microorganism to control the location of the pathogen and numbers of microorganisms on the victim's body, pure *colonization* occurs. The microorganism does not cause infection in that individual, but the organism continues to live and can be passed on to other victims. An example of this is *Staphylococcus aureus*, which can be found on the nasal passages of 25% to 30% of the population.[5] In these individuals, the bacteria does not cause disease but can be given to another immune-compromised individual and cause severe or life-threatening infection.

Control of disease occurrence depends on breaking this chain of transmission in one or more places[4] (Figure 8-2). A pathogen can be vulnerable in one or more links of the transmission chain. The goal of epidemiology is to identify these vulnerabilities and exploit them to stop disease transmission. Some pathogens (e.g., bacteria) are susceptible to direct attack with antibiotics. Antibiotics are designed to directly kill the pathogen or hold it in check so that the body's defenses can eradicate it. Some microorganisms have developed a resistance to antibiotics through repeated exposure to subtherapeutic doses and their indiscriminant use for nonbacterial infections. This "antibiotic resistance" is a major threat to the success of management of bacterial infections. The emergence of vancomycin-resistant *Enterococcus* (VRE) and methicillin-resistant *S. aureus* (MRSA) is a very troubling development in infectious disease management.

Destroying nonhuman reservoirs and vectors of the pathogen can also break the chain of transmission. For example, controlling the number of mosquitoes with insecticides

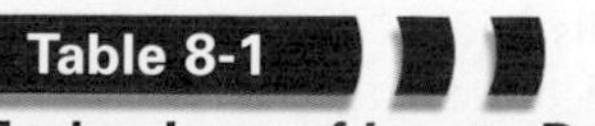

Mechanisms of Innate Defense

Mechanism	Description
Species resistance	Genetic characteristics of the human species protect the body from certain pathogens
Mechanical and chemical barriers	Physical impediments to the entry of foreign cells or substances
Skin and mucosa	Forms a continuous wall that separates the internal environment from the external environment, preventing the entry of pathogens
Secretions	Secretions such as sebum, mucus, and enzymes chemically inhibit the activity of pathogens
Inflammation	The inflammatory response isolates the pathogens and stimulates the speedy arrival of large numbers of immune cells
Phagocytosis	Ingestion and destruction of pathogens by phagocytic cells
Neutrophils	Granular leukocytes that are usually the first phagocytic cell to arrive at the scene of an inflammatory response
Macrophages	Monocytes that have enlarged to become giant phagocytic cells capable of consuming many pathogens; often called by more specific names when found in specific tissues of the body
Natural killer cells	Group of lymphocytes that kill many different types of cancer cells and virus-infected cells
Interferon	Protein produced by cells after they become infected by a virus; inhibits the spread or further development of a viral infection
Complement	Group of plasma proteins (inactive enzymes) that produce a cascade of chemical reactions that ultimately cause lysis (rupture) of a foreign cell; the complement cascade can be triggered by specific or nonspecific immune mechanisms

From Thibodeau GA, Patton KT: *Anatomy and physiology,* ed 5, St Louis, 2003, Mosby, p 645.

and other biological means is a method used to curb the spread of malaria and West Nile. Immunization of domesticated animals against rabies eliminates one reservoir of potential rabies transmission. Distribution of clean needles in the intravenous drug user community is aimed at removing a common transmission vector (contaminated needles) for HIV, the causative pathogen responsible for acquired immunodeficiency syndrome (AIDS).

Blocking the portal of exit can also block transmission of the pathogen. For example, having patients with tuberculosis wear masks as they move through the hospital and implementing respiratory isolation techniques to stop droplet transmission are interventions aimed at blocking the portal of exit.

Standard precautions are infection control guidelines designed to block the pathogen's portal of exit, route of transmission, and portal of entry.[2] Hand washing is one of the most effective ways to break the chain of transmission by blocking an important mode of transmission—contaminated hands.

Finally, host susceptibility is an important aspect of the transmission of a pathogen. Factors such as age, gender, ethnic group, and genetic makeup all affect the susceptibility of the host. Although these factors cannot be changed, improving the host's immune system by improving his or her nutritional status, decreasing stress, and limiting fatigue can decrease the host's susceptibility to infection. Immunization of the host also has a key role in blocking the transmission of infection. Immune globulin given the host can provide passive immunity to some infections.

Antibiotic use has had a tremendous impact in the susceptibility of microorganisms to common antibiotics. Limiting the use or overuse of antibiotics and instructing patients in the appropriate use of those antibiotics (take full course, etc.) can limit the increase of antibiotic resistance. Limiting the use of antibiotics in the food supply can also limit the population's exposure to antibiotics and the development of antibiotic resistance.

Role of Host

The host defense system is multifaceted and consists of a **innate immune response** (Table 8-1) composed of mechanical and biochemical barriers, phagocytes, and chemical mediators, as well as a **specific immune response.**[3,6,7] (Host immune systems are discussed in greater detail in Chapter 9.) The body's exterior is an effective mechanical and biochemical barrier to most organisms and infectious agents. The epithelium is difficult for organisms to penetrate because of its structure, pH, continual cell-sloughing process, attachment prevention, the passage of secretory IgA through the epithelium from lymphocytes, and the production of biochemical agents. These barriers may be interrupted or destroyed by medical interventions. For example, endotracheal tubes, urinary catheters, and invasive monitoring catheters interfere with protective epithelial surfaces.[3]

Host Characteristics

Epithelial Barriers

The skin and mucous membrane are important mechanical and biochemical barriers (Figure 8-3). Intact physical barriers act as a blockade to foreign material entering the body. The epithelial cells of the skin provide multilayer protection from the many microorganisms with which the body comes in contact. The dry surface of the skin does not promote the growth of organisms because moisture is preferred. Constant shedding of the epidermis and mucosal membranes aids in the removal of any microorganisms that are attached to their surfaces. For example, an intestinal epithelial cell half-life is 30 hours, which limits the number of bacteria that could attach to the cell. The high fat content of the skin inhibits the growth of bacteria and fungi.[6,8]

The mucous membrane linings of the gastrointestinal and genitourinary tracts provide a barrier separating the sterile internal body from the external environment. The lungs are protected with a layer of mucous lining. The sticky consistency of mucus traps microorganisms, and the cilia sweep the microorganisms away. The mucociliary system and alveolar macrophages are important for ridding the lungs of trapped microorganisms.[6,8] Mechanisms such as coughing, sneezing, and urinating help to remove particles trapped on mucous membranes of the body.

Chemical barriers enhance the effectiveness of the mechanical barriers.[6,8] The acidic environment of the skin, urine, and vagina inhibits bacterial growth. The secretion of hydrochloric acid with a pH of 1 to 2 by the stomach results in the killing of microorganisms. Saliva, mucus, tears, and sweat contain antimicrobial chemicals such as lysozyme, an enzyme that destroys bacterial cell walls and is thus bactericidal.[6,8] Lactoferrin is another mucosal protein that keeps bacterial replication low by reducing the availability of free iron needed for bacterial growth. Sebaceous gland secretions act as antifungals. In addition, immunoglobulins (IgA, IgG) are present in many of the body's secretions and prevent entry of bacteria and viruses through mucous membranes. (See Chapter 9 for a discussion about immunoglobulins.)

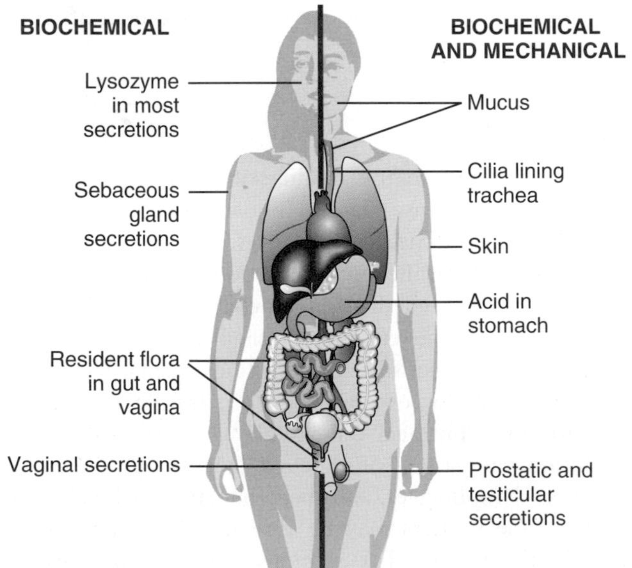

FIGURE 8-3 ■ Some of the mechanical and biochemical barriers of the human body.

Removal or degradation of the body's mechanical and biochemical barriers creates a setting in which infection is likely. For example, burn victims who have lost portions of their skin barrier are at high risk for infection. Hospitalized patients who have incisions or intravenous and urinary catheters are at risk for infection because their skin barrier has been breached. The normal action of cilia in the respiratory tract in removing foreign particles is blocked by endotracheal tubes. When a urinary catheter is in place, flushing of bacteria from the urinary tract opening (meatus) is bypassed.

Risk Factors

Nutritional Status. Adequate nutrition is necessary to maintain a healthy immune system. It has long been recognized that malnutrition is a risk factor for the development of infections. Protein energy malnutrition is associated with defects in cell-mediated immunity (specific), impaired intracellular killing by neutrophils, reduced complement activity, and decreased levels of secretory IgA.[9]

Vitamin and trace element deficiencies have been associated with specific defects in the immune system. Severe iron deficiency alters the functioning of some of the cellular components of the immune system and is believed to increase the susceptibility to infection. Excess amounts of trace elements and fatty acids may also depress the immune system, which emphasizes the need for the intake of optimal amounts of nutrients.[9-11]

A host responding to an infection will need additional protein and nutrients to fight the microbial invasion. Decreased nutrition during this period can lead to a negative nitrogen balance. Anergy in a preoperative patient has been a marker for increased postoperative morbidity and sepsis. Anergy, or the failure to mount a localized response to a known antigen when given intradermally, can result from protein energy malnutrition.

Chronic Illness. Chronic illnesses such as diabetes, cancer, heart disease, and renal failure are associated with an increased risk of infection. Deaths in patients with chronic illnesses are frequently directly related to an infectious process. Infections are cited as the leading cause of death in patients with acute renal failure and diabetes.[12,13]

Diabetes alters the host's ability to resist infection. Phagocytosis is impaired with hyperglycemia, and detection of the pain of infection may be delayed because of neuropathies. The virulence of some microorganisms is increased when exposed to hyperglycemic environments. With increased glucose levels, *Candida* has been shown to flourish because of increased resistance to phagocytosis.[12]

Circulatory problems associated with cardiac failure or peripheral vascular disease are risk factors for infection. The cellular components of the immune system are dependent on the circulatory system to deliver them to the site of infection. In addition, antimicrobial agents need to be transported to the site of infection. Many pathogens thrive in areas with poor tissue perfusion.[6,12]

Age. Age is also a variable in the ability to resist infections. Infants are at an increased risk for infection owing to an immature immune system. The lack of previous exposure to microorganisms makes the immune system naive and less efficient in mounting a defense. A newborn is susceptible to gram-negative bacterial infections and sepsis because of the lack of IgM. Detection of infection in the newborn is based on a high level of suspicion and accurate recognition of the subtle signs of lethargy, feeding difficulties, temperature control problems, and changes in vital signs.[6]

The elderly are more susceptible to infection because of declining function of the immune system. Depressed cell-mediated immunity, changes in T-lymphocyte functioning, and atrophy of the thymus gland are some of the factors that may cause decreased immunity.[14] Greater morbidity and mortality are associated with infection in the elderly. The lungs and urinary tract are the most common sites of infection in the elderly.[15] However, the increased diversity and types of infections in the elderly in comparison with other age groups leads to a higher frequency of sepsis and bacteremia.[15] Infection may also be manifested atypically, with absence of fever and the sudden onset of confusion. The subtle changes and lack of fever obscure clinical recognition of the presence of an infectious process.[15,16]

Immunosuppression. Immunosuppression may result from a systemic disease involving the immune system or from the treatment for a disease. Defects may occur in one or more of the components of the immune response: phagocytic, complement, cellular, or humoral. A person is considered immunocompromised when such a defect is known to exist. The defect may be caused by a disease such as AIDS, by complement deficiencies, or by the absence of humoral antibody production. The defect may also be drug induced. Agents that can cause immunosuppression are antimetabolites, corticosteroids, cyclosporine, and antibiotics.[17] Immunocompromised hosts are highly susceptible to life-threatening infections, so meticulous care in the prevention of infection is a high priority for such patients.

Stress has been implicated in predisposing an individual to an infectious process. An example is the outbreak of a latent herpes simplex infection in response to stress. Stress hormones such as corticosteroids are known for their effect of depressing the immune system. Complex interactions exist between the immune system and the neuroendocrine system. Hormones such as corticosteroids, endorphins, and lymphokines participate in the regulatory loop between the two systems. (For further discussion, see Chapter 2.)

Abdominal trauma may result in spleen injury and possible therapeutic splenectomy. Patients with splenectomy are at high risk for overwhelming infection by *Streptococcus pneumoniae.* The spleen normally facilitates the phagocytosis of encapsulated bacteria. Prevention of life-threatening infections is aided by vaccination of all splenectomy patients with pneumococcal vaccine[18] as well as yearly influenza immunizations.

Role of Immunization

Immunization of a population is the most cost-effective method of altering the host's susceptibility to a pathogen for which a vaccine has been developed.[1] There are two goals. The first is to confer immunity to the host by direct exposure to the altered pathogen. The second is to decrease the number of susceptible hosts in the population, thereby limiting the possibility of transmission of the disease. By this method, known as herd immunity, the disease can be controlled or eliminated without immunizing everyone, as long as a high enough percentage of the population is immunized. If the percentage of adequately immunized individuals drops, epidemics may result.

Immunization exposes the potential host to altered bacteria, viruses, or their derivatives, which stimulates the body to produce antibodies against these pathogens without causing the disease. These antibodies allow the body to destroy the pathogen before it has a chance to cause disease when the potential host is again exposed to the pathogen. The number of susceptible hosts in the population decreases as immunization rates increase. When a critical percentage of the susceptible population is immunized, the chain of transmission is broken and the disease outbreak averted. Immunization often requires repeated exposure to the altered pathogens in the form of vaccines, such as those recommended by the American Academy of Pediatrics.[19]

Role of Environment

Multiple environmental factors affect the prevalence and transmission of various infections and infestations. To illustrate, parasitic infections are facilitated by hot and humid climatic conditions, overcrowded living conditions, the presence of insect vectors in bed linen or clothing, improper sewage disposal or treatment such as the use of raw human sewage as fertilizer, the lack of clean water, and the consumption of contaminated raw or undercooked meat or vegetables.

Infections may be transmitted by inhalation of polluted dust or air. For example, the fungus *Coccidioides immitis,* which causes Valley Fever, is pandemic in the southwestern United States. Toxoplasmosis is caused by inhalation or ingestion of dirt, sand, or litter dust contaminated with cat feces that contain the causative protozoon *Toxoplasma gondii.*

Fecal contamination of meat and vegetables by improper cleaning or slaughtering techniques leads to many infections in the general population. *Salmonella* contamination of poultry during slaughter and dressing of the meat, coupled with improper preparation and incomplete cooking, leads to numerous *Salmonella* infections each year. In the early 1990s, fecal contamination of beef during the slaughter and dressing of the meat, coupled with incomplete cooking of the contaminated hamburger, led to *Escherichia coli* infection of many people in the northwestern United States. Contamination of apples used in the processing of unpasteurized fruit juices also led to an *E. coli* outbreak.

Tuberculosis and poliomyelitis are known to occur in crowded living environments under conditions of poor nutrition and hygiene. Viral hepatitis type A is transmitted by the fecal-oral route, usually following consumption of contaminated food or water or ingestion of sewage-contaminated clams.[20]

Some infections occur only in certain regions of the world. African sleeping sickness, caused by the parasite *Trypanosoma brucei rhodesiense,* occurs only in woodland and savanna areas south and east of Lake Tanganyika. This environmental limitation is related to the environmental range of its vector, the tsetse fly, *Glossina morsitans.*[4]

Many infections are known to have seasonal patterns. For example, poliomyelitis occurs during the summer and fall in temperate zones and throughout the year in the tropics. Septic meningitis also tends to occur during the summer and fall. Epidemic typhus caused by *Rickettsia prowazekii* occurs in the winter or in cool climates under conditions of poor sanitation and poor hygiene. It is under these conditions that the human host is most likely to be wearing clothes and can be bitten by the human louse, which is the vector for this disease. Lyme disease is more prevalent in the summertime in wooded areas when people are more likely to be in the forest and be bitten by the deer tick, the insect vector of the disease.[4,21]

KEY CONCEPTS

- Epidemiology is the study of health events and disease, their distribution, and associated causative factors in a defined population. Goals of epidemiology are to define a disease, identify outbreaks, assist in the development and evaluation of treatment protocols, and develop prevention strategies.
- Transmission of disease requires a chain of events that includes passing of the pathogen from the reservoir of the infection through a portal of exit to a susceptible host through a portal of entry by a circumscribed mode of transmission.
- The host has several lines of defense to prevent and fight infection. The skin and mucous membranes provide a first line of defense through mechanical and biochemical barriers. Shedding of epithelium, cilia action, acidic secretions, and enzymes help remove or destroy microorganisms before they gain access to the body.
- Malnutrition may depress immune function because many components require adequate proteins, vitamins, and minerals for synthesis. Immunoglobulins, complement factors, and clotting factors require adequate protein metabolism by the liver.
- Chronic illnesses such as diabetes and cardiovascular disease predispose to infection because circulation of immune components may be impaired and a high-glucose medium may enhance bacterial growth.
- Trauma, burns, invasive instrumentation, antibiotics, and immunosuppressive therapies, which may accompany acute illnesses, predispose an individual to infection by altering normal host defenses.
- The very young and very old are more susceptible to infection because of immature or degenerating immune function.
- Stress is associated with increased secretion of corticosteroids, which are believed to depress immune function. Exogenous steroids and other immunosuppressive therapies (radiation, antibiotics, anticancer drugs, and antirejection drugs) also increase the risk of infection.
- Immunizations alter the susceptibility of the host by stimulating the immune system to create antibodies to the pathogen.
- Environmental factors influence the likelihood of exposure and infection by microorganisms. Sanitation, air quality, living conditions, and climate are important factors.

HOST-PARASITE RELATIONSHIP

Normal Microbial Flora

The interactions between a host, such as a human, and the microorganisms that reside on or in the host are referred to as the **host-parasite relationship.** Large numbers of microorganisms reside on the skin and in the gastrointestinal tract and vagina of the human host. These microbes normally cause no harm to the host. They are parasites that depend on the host's environment—temperature, moisture, nutrients, and other parasites. They obtain nutrients from the host in order to grow and reproduce. The host and normal parasitic flora usually balance their interactions to the benefit of each in order to grow and survive—a symbiotic relationship.

Interestingly, these bacteria have a role in protecting the host from other pathogens by using nutrients and thus preventing other microbial colonization. Normal bacterial flora also participate in metabolic processes such as the synthesis of vitamin K in the colon.[13] Harmless inhabitation of the skin or mucous membranes by these microorganisms is called **colonization.**

Resident floras are usually of specific types and occupy a certain environment in or on the host. These floras recolonize quickly if disturbed. For example, normal resident floras of the skin include bacteria such as *Corynebacterium, Staphylo-*

coccus epidermidis, and *Streptococcus viridans,* as well as fungi, yeasts, and even mycobacteria.[6]

Normal floras can become pathogenic if they gain entry to the body when the immune system is compromised. These infections are referred to as **opportunistic.** An increased number of people are at risk for opportunistic infections because of diseases of the immune system, such as AIDS, and because of therapies that depress the immune system, such as the use of steroids in the management of asthma.[17]

When a microorganism is capable of consistently causing disease in all infected hosts, the organism is considered to be **virulent.** As summarized by Boutotte, "Virulence thus represents the interaction between the properties of the host and the pathogen that permits expression of the pathogenic properties of a parasite to the detriment of the host."[23]

The human body is well designed to defend itself against pathogens with its innate and specific immune systems. The first line of defense is the innate immune system, which includes the skin and mucous membranes. These structures prevent the entry of microorganisms into the body. If pathogens do enter the body and thus make it a host, components of the immune system detect their presence and attempt to destroy them. In healthy humans, potentially infectious parasites are usually defeated before the body becomes a host. Infectious disease occurs when pathogens enter a host and cause signs and symptoms of illness.[1]

The ability of the human body to resist infection requires an intact defense system. Host and environmental factors such as nutrition, age, illness, air quality, sanitation, and stress may alter the host's resistance to infection. In addition, characteristics of the pathogen such as virulence, toxins, adherence, and invasiveness may allow it to evade the human defense system and colonize.[4] This relationship between the host, the parasite, and the environment, as shown in Figure 8-4, is the framework for understanding infectious processes.[1]

Microorganism Characteristics

Microorganisms possess certain characteristics that assist in their penetration and survival in the host despite the presence of an intact defense system. Virulence, toxin production, microbial adherence, and invasiveness are microorganism factors that influence the development of infection in the host.

Microbial adherence is the ability of the microorganism to latch onto and gain entrance into the host. Without the ability to either directly penetrate a host or stick to the host's tissue surface, pathogens are removed by normal host defenses. Entry into the host can occur directly, as with a surgical wound, arthropod bite, or direct penetration. An infected female *Anopheles* mosquito can inject *Plasmodium vivax* with its bite and cause malaria. *Ancylostoma duodenale* (hookworm) directly penetrates the skin when the skin comes in contact with infected soil.

Entry can also occur through the microorganism's ability to adhere to the host's epithelial cells because of adhesion molecules on the cell surface of certain microorganisms. The type of adhesion varies. For example, the mechanism of adhesion of *E. coli* is protein K88, and that for group A streptococci is lipoteichoic acids. Some bacteria, such as *E. coli,* have pili or fimbriae (hairlike structures) that enable them to attach to glycoproteins containing mannose on their hosts. Microbes are also attracted to and able to attach to certain cell surface

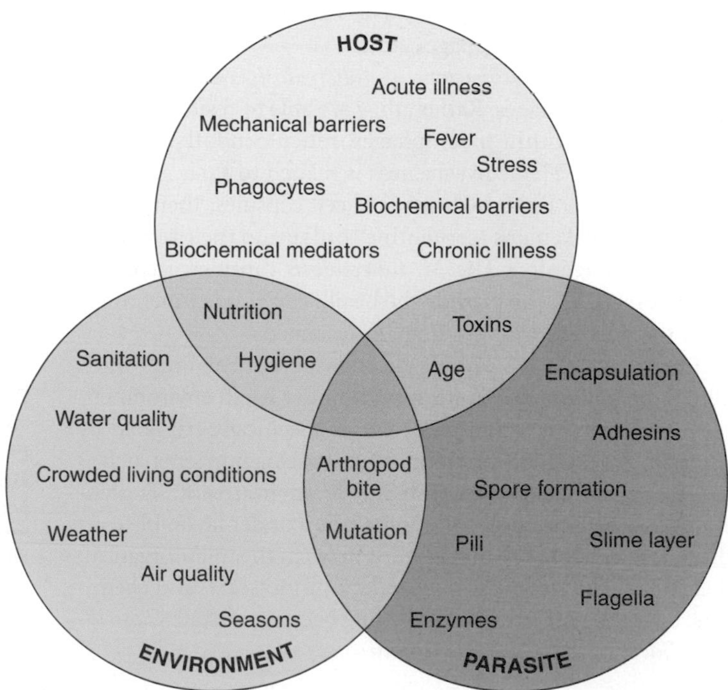

FIGURE 8-4 ■ This depiction of the interactions of host, parasite, and environment provides a framework for understanding infectious processes.

proteins such as fibronectin or to the rough surfaces of intravascular or intracavity catheters.

Microbial development of a slime layer also facilitates adherence. The slime layer is the result of extracellular synthesis of a substance, usually a mucopolysaccharide, by enzymes on the surface of the bacteria. The slime layer, called glycocalyx, acts as a glue or adhesive that sticks the bacteria to host surfaces. For example, the slime layer produced by *Streptococcus mutans* allows bacteria to adhere to tooth enamel and form plaque.[4]

Virulence and invasiveness factors include a variety of mechanisms that microorganisms have evolved to elude and block host defenses or assist in host invasion. These characteristics contribute to the pathogenicity of the microorganism by enabling it to penetrate natural barriers, resist death by phagocytosis, or survive antimicrobial therapy (e.g., methicillin-resistant *S. aureus*). Examples include bacterial enzymes, encapsulation, mutation, mobility, endospore formation, and resistance to phagocytosis and antimicrobial therapy.

Bacterial enzymes (such as fibrinolysin, coagulase, and hyaluronidase) aid in the microorganism's ability to spread or invade tissues. Most enzymes dissolve or hydrolyze blood, collagen, or connective tissue components. Fibrinolysin, produced by streptococci, dissolves coagulated plasma and allows local microbial spread into host tissues. Hyaluronidase is secreted by staphylococci, clostridia, streptococci, and other organisms.[24] This enzyme helps microbes to spread locally by dissolving a connective tissue component called hyaluronic acid.

Encapsulation prevents opsonization (recognition and binding) by antibodies and thus prevents the microorganism from being phagocytized. For example, *S. pneumoniae* (pneumococci) diplococci have a polysaccharide capsule that protects them from phagocytosis. The bacterial slime layer also protects bacteria from phagocytosis.

To illustrate, *Mycobacterium tuberculosis* bacilli are not killed by macrophages. Rather, they are able to reside engulfed in endosomes within macrophages, reticuloendothelial cells, and giant cells. Their invasiveness is related to their ability to form tiny, hard, lipid, hydrophobic cell capsules; their ability to form parallel chains (serpentine cords); and their resistance to chemical agents.[23] The *M. tuberculosis* capsules are called tubercles. Within the capsule the bacilli can reside indefinitely until the host's immune system is weakened.[25]

Other bacteria are capable of endospore formation, which allows the microorganism to survive under harsh environmental conditions. The endospore state is specifically triggered by bacterial genes under conditions of decreasing nutrients such as decreasing nitrogen or carbon in the environment. The endospore, which is capable of regeneration under favorable conditions, is a resting cell that is released when the microorganism dies. It is highly resistant to heat, lack of moisture, and chemicals. Examples of endospore-forming bacteria include *Clostridium, Bacillus,* and *Coxiella burnetii.*

Antimicrobial Resistance

Antimicrobial resistance is conferred to microorganisms that are able to mutate in response to changes in the host's environment in order to successfully infect the host.[7,26,27] For example, the development of methicillin-resistant *S. aureus* is the result of successful mutation of the organism and selection of resistant strains in response to antibiotic exposure. The ability of *S. aureus* to become antibiotic resistant was recognized with the introduction of penicillin and continues today[7,26,28] (Table 8-2).

Another contributor to antibiotic resistance is the tendency for persons treated with antibiotics to take only part of their daily dose rather than completing the full course.[23,29] This practice may allow relatively resistant microorganisms that can survive a low-dose antibiotic course to become the dominant species. The resistant form may then be transmitted to other individuals and become common in the general population.

Mobility is a characteristic of bacteria with **flagella,** motile appendages that allow the bacterium to move or swim toward nutrients in a favorable environment. This movement, called *chemotaxis,* is usually toward sugar or amino acid concentrations in the environment. Other microorganisms block aspects of the host's immune system, such as by obstructing antigen processing and encouraging the growth of suppressor cells.

Microorganisms may also produce toxins in the host that can affect the host's cells systemically or locally. The toxins are classified as exotoxins or endotoxins. **Exotoxins** are polypeptide toxins that are produced and released by the organism. They are highly antigenic, highly toxic, and unstable when exposed to heat. They cause illness and death by binding to specific receptors in target organs and by interfering with vital metabolic pathways.[30] Some exotoxin-producing bacteria in-

Table 8-2

Historical Progression of *Staphylococcus aureus* Resistance to Antibiotics

Antibiotic and Year Introduced	Year Resistance Appeared
Penicillin, 1941	1940s
Streptomycin, 1944	Mid-1940s
Tetracycline, 1948	1950s
Erythromycin, 1952	1950s
Gentamicin, 1964	Mid-1970s
Methicillin, 1959	Late 1960s

Data from Morita MM: Methicillin-resistant *Staphylococcus aureus:* past, present and future, *Nurs Clin North Am* 28:625-637, 1993; and Rosenberg J: Methicillin-resistant *Staphylococcus aureus* (MRSA) in the community: who's watching? *Lancet* 346:132-133, 1995.

clude *Clostridium botulinum, Clostridium tetani, S. aureus,* and *Shigella dysenteriae.*[4] For example *C. tetani* produces an exotoxin called tetanospasmin, which is a powerful neurotoxin. Tetanospasmin interferes with synaptic transmission of inhibitory interneurons in the spinal cord, which leads to tetany, muscle spasms, characteristic "lockjaw" (trismus), and seizures.

Endotoxins are associated with gram-negative bacteria such as enterobacteria, common causative agents of septic shock. Endotoxin is an immunogenic part of the bacterial cell wall (lipopolysaccharide) that triggers a massive immune response when the bacterium lyses.[30] The subsequent immune response leads to shock, vascular collapse, and multiple organ failure.[17] (See Chapter 20 for a further discussion of septic shock.)

KEY CONCEPTS

- A number of microorganisms are considered resident flora because they live on or in the host without causing disease. Resident flora benefits the host by synthesizing molecules and inhibiting the growth of nonresident microorganisms. If the host's immune system is compromised, resident flora may become pathogenic and cause opportunistic infection.
- Microorganisms possess characteristics that enhance their pathogenic potential. Adherence is improved by the presence of adhesion molecules, slime layers, and pili. Escape from immune detection and destruction is enhanced by encapsulation, spore formation, mutation, flagella, and toxin production. Microorganisms that possess these characteristics are more virulent and thus more likely to cause disease.

TYPES OF MICROORGANISMS

Refer to Figure 1-12 for photographic examples of pathogenic organisms.

Bacteria

Bacteria are single-celled organisms that have no internal organelles (Figure 8-5). They live in the intestines of humans and other creatures and participate in digestion. They live in the soil and are responsible for its fertility. They degrade dead tissue and break it down for other organisms to use. Among the countless types of bacteria that exist, only a small percentage are known to be harmful to humans.[6,24]

Bacteria are classified into four major groups based on their cell wall shape and mechanism of movement: gliding bacteria (e.g., myxobacteria), spirochetes (e.g., *Treponema pallidum* [Figure 8-6]), mycoplasmas (e.g., *Mycoplasma pneumoniae*), and rigid bacteria. The rigid bacteria are further broken down into actinomycetes (e.g., *Mycobacterium tuberculosis*) and unicellular forms.

The unicellular forms of rigid bacteria include **intracellular** obligate parasites and **free-living bacteria.** Intracellular obligate parasites consist of rickettsiae and chlamydiae and must live within a host cell to survive.

Free-living bacteria are classified by morphology (shape) and their response to Gram staining. They have three basic shapes. **Cocci** are round and nonmotile. They may stick together in clumps that look like bunches of grapes (e.g., staphylococci), in pairs (e.g., diplococci), or in long strands (e.g., streptococci). **Bacilli,** by comparison, are rod shaped and may be motile (e.g., *Pseudomonas aeruginosa*) (see Figure 8-5). About half of the species are motile and half are nonmotile. The third shape is the **spiral** (e.g., *Spirillum*).

Bacteria are further differentiated by their ability or inability to retain a basic dye after iodine fixation, known as the **Gram stain** reaction. Gram staining separates bacteria into gram-positive organisms, which look dark purple under the microscope; gram-negative organisms, which look pink; or acid-fast organisms, which resist staining but, once stained, resist decoloration. Further differentiation of bacteria is based on nutritional requirements (such as whether the organism is anaerobic or aerobic), on colony characteristics, and on antibiotic resistance.

Pathogenic bacteria owe the ability to infect humans to their structure and proteins. For example, pili enhance certain bacteria's capacity to adhere to the host's surface and thereby improve the bacteria's virulence. Other bacteria have mucopolysaccharide layers or enzymes that facilitate their invasiveness. Figure 8-7 classifies examples of pathogenic bacteria according to the part of the human body that they commonly infect. Bacteria are introduced to the host in a variety of ways. Once they have penetrated the initial defense mechanisms, the microorganism divides and creates a colony. In an attempt to contain and eliminate the invading microorganism an acute inflammatory reaction in the body occurs.

Phagocytic cells such as neutrophils and macrophages are recruited to the area, where they ingest and destroy the microorganisms. If these responses are insufficient to contain the infection, the microorganisms move throughout the body through the natural currents of fluids (i.e., blood stream, lymph system, or intrastitial fluids). If the microorganisms are not contained, they move through the lymph system to the lymph nodes where the infectious agent stimulates an immune response. If they are present in sufficient numbers to overwhelm the lymph nodes, circulating clumps of microorganisms can cause bacteremia and microabscesses. In severe cases, sepsis, hypotension, organ system failure, and death can occur.

Box 8-1 summarizes primary pathogens associated with specific infections in the human host.[31] Numerous antibiotics have been developed to decrease the risk (prophylaxis) or severity of infection by specific bacteria. Table 8-3 summarizes antimicrobial selection based on the infecting organism.[29]

Microscopic Morphology of Bacteria

Cocci

in clusters

in chains

in pairs

in tetrads

Bacilli

Coccobacilli

Bacilli occur in many sizes

Fusiform bacilli

Palisading

Spirochetes

A

Glycoprotein

Envelope

Capsomer

Nucleic acid

Capsid

Nucleocapsid

Core protein

B

Chlamydospore

Blastospore

C

FIGURE 8-5 ■ Types of microorganisms. **A,** Bacteria. **B,** Virus. **C,** Fungus. (**A,** From Mahon CR, Manuselis G: *Textbook of diagnostic microbiology,* ed 2, Philadelphia, 2000, Saunders. **B** and **C,** From Gould BE: *Pathophysiology for the health professions,* ed 2, Philadelphia, Saunders, 2002, p 62.)

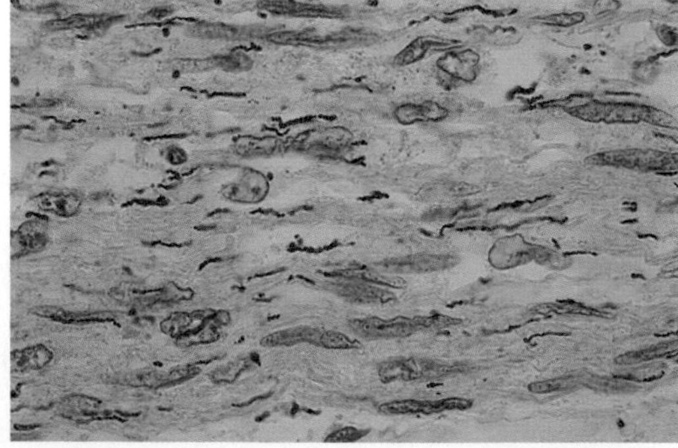

FIGURE 8-6 ■ Spirochetes (e.g., *Treponema pallidum*): immunohistochemistry of the muscular layer in the small intestine of a newborn with congenital syphilis. Multiple spirochetes are shown in red (both cross-sections and entire treponemes can be noted, (100). (Courtesy Jeannette Guarner, MD, and Sherif R. Zaki, MD, PhD, Centers for Disease Control and Prevention, Atlanta.)

Viruses

Viruses, the smallest known infective agents, range in size from 20 to 300 nm.[22] They are composed of DNA or RNA and a capsule surrounding the genetic material. Viruses have only enough genetic information to code for 2 to 60 proteins. They are totally dependent on the host cell for energy and the "machinery" to replicate. A comparison of viruses and other microorganisms is presented in Table 8-4.

Viruses were once differentiated only by size. With advances in gene sequencing and use of the electron microscope, viruses can now be classified by the genetic makeup of the organism, the mode of replication, the structure of the viral capsule (also known as the capsid), and the specific host cell that the virus invades.

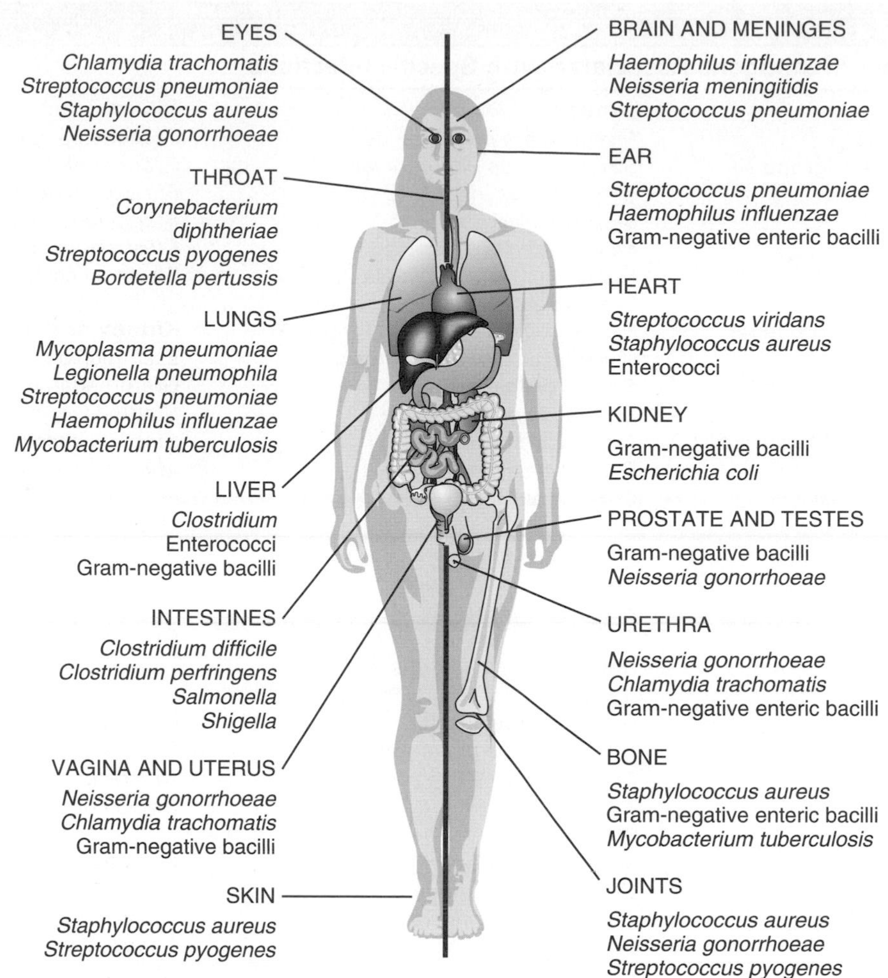

FIGURE 8-7 ■ Examples of pathogenic bacteria classified according to the part of the human body that they commonly infect.

All viruses must enter a host cell to replicate, and invasion of a host cell is accomplished by several methods. A virus can adhere to the cell membrane and cause phagocytosis. Once inside the host cell, the virus capsule is removed to expose viral genetic material to the cell's interior. Another way that a virus can invade a host cell is by sticking to the surface of the cell and injecting viral genetic material directly into the interior.

Some viruses direct the manufacture of an envelope that surrounds the viral capsid. The envelope is made of host cell membrane and viral proteins. The virus may be released from the host cells by budding from the cell's surface without destroying the host cell (Figure 8-8).

Viruses that do not manufacture an envelope are usually released by *lysing* the host cell, thus destroying it. The mechanism of lysis seems to be a progressive breakdown of the host cell's maintenance mechanisms with resultant buildup of waste products intracellularly and lack of nutrient transport into the cell. Ultimately, the cell wall is disrupted and the cell lyses.

Two major categories of viruses exist: those that contain DNA and those that contain RNA (Table 8-5). RNA viruses are characterized either as **retroviruses** or as straight replicating viruses.

The DNA viruses (e.g., herpes simplex virus) produce messenger RNA in the host cell's nucleus with the host cell's enzymes. The proteins and the DNA of the virus are thus replicated and assembled in the host cell.

By comparison, RNA viruses, such as influenza virus (Figure 8-9), replicate their genetic information in one of two ways. Retroviruses contain encoding information for the enzyme **reverse transcriptase** so that they can create both messenger RNA and DNA from their own genome. The viral DNA is incorporated into the host cell's DNA, and when the host cell replicates, the viral DNA also replicates, thus perpetuating the viral genome as long as the host cell line survives. Viral proteins and RNA are manufactured by using the virus's messenger RNA and the host cell's organelles. HIV, the retrovirus that causes AIDS, is an example of a virus that causes permanent change in the genome (mutation) and function of the host cell.

In contrast to RNA retroviruses, the straight replicating viruses reproduce in one of two ways, depending on whether the single-stranded RNA is a positive or a negative copy. Viruses

Box 8-1

Examples of Primary Pathogens Associated with Specific Infections

Burns
Staphylococcus aureus
Streptococcus pyogenes (group A)
Pseudomonas aeruginosa
Gram-negative bacilli

Skin Infections
Staphylococcus aureus
Streptococcus pyogenes (group A)
Gram-negative bacilli
Treponema pallidum

Decubitus and Surgical Wounds
Staphylococcus aureus
Gram-negative enteric bacilli
Pseudomonas aeruginosa
Streptococcus pyogenes (group A)
Anaerobic streptococci
Clostridium spp.
Enterococcus
Bacteroides spp.

Meninges
Neisseria meningitidis
Haemophilus influenzae
Streptococcus pneumoniae
Streptococcus spp.
Escherichia coli
Gram-negative bacilli
Streptococcus pyogenes (group A)
Staphylococcus aureus
Mycobacterium tuberculosis
Listeria monocytogenes
Enterococcus (neonatal period)
Treponema pallidum
Leptospira

Brain Abscess
Streptococci (aerobic and anaerobic)
Bacteroides spp.
Staphylococcus aureus

Paranasal and Middle Ear
Streptococcus pneumoniae
Streptococcus pyogenes (group A)
Haemophilus influenzae
Gram-negative enteric bacilli
Pseudomonas aeruginosa
Anaerobic streptococci
Staphylococcus aureus

Throat
Streptococcus pyogenes (group A)
Neisseria gonorrhoeae
Bacteroides spp.
Fusobacterium
Spirochetes
Corynebacterium diphtheriae
Bordetella pertussis

Lungs
Mycoplasma pneumoniae
Streptococcus pneumoniae
Haemophilus influenzae
Staphylococcus aureus
Klebsiella
Pseudomonas aeruginosa
Gram-negative bacilli
Streptococcus pyogenes (group A)
Mycobacterium tuberculosis
Chlamydia psittaci
Legionella pneumophila
Anaerobic streptococci
Bacteroides spp.
Coxiella burnetii

Lung Abscess
Anaerobic streptococci
Bacteroides spp.
Fusobacterium
Staphylococcus aureus
Klebsiella
Gram-negative bacilli
Streptococcus pneumoniae
Enterococcus

Pleura
Staphylococcus aureus
Streptococcus pneumoniae
Haemophilus influenzae
Gram-negative bacilli
Anaerobic streptococci
Bacteroides spp.
Fusobacterium
Streptococcus pyogenes (group A)
Mycobacterium tuberculosis

Endocardium
Viridans group of streptococci
Staphylococcus aureus
Enterococcus
Other streptococci
Staphylococcus epidermidis
Gram-negative enteric bacilli
Pseudomonas aeruginosa

Peritoneum
Escherichia coli
Gram-negative bacilli
Enterococcus
Bacteroides fragilis
Anaerobic streptococci
Clostridium spp.
Streptococcus pneumoniae
Streptococcus pyogenes (group A)
Neisseria gonorrhoeae
Mycobacterium tuberculosis

Biliary Tract
Escherichia coli
Gram-negative bacilli
Enterococcus spp.
Staphylococcus aureus
Clostridium spp.
Streptococci (aerobic and anaerobic)

Kidney and Bladder
Escherichia coli
Gram-negative bacilli
Staphylococcus aureus
Staphylococcus epidermidis
Mycobacterium tuberculosis

Urethra
Neisseria gonorrhoeae
Chlamydia trachomatis
Trichomonas vaginalis
Gram-negative enteric bacilli
Ureaplasma urealyticum

Prostate
Gram-negative enteric bacilli
Neisseria gonorrhoeae
Staphylococcus aureus

Epididymis and Testes
Gram-negative bacilli
Neisseria gonorrhoeae
Chlamydia trachomatis
Mycobacterium tuberculosis

Bone (Osteomyelitis)
Staphylococcus aureus
Salmonella
Gram-negative enteric bacilli
Streptococcus pyogenes (group A)
Mycobacterium tuberculosis
Anaerobic streptococci
Pseudomonas aeruginosa

Joints
Staphylococcus aureus
Neisseria gonorrhoeae
Streptococcus pyogenes (group A)
Gram-negative enteric bacilli
Pseudomonas aeruginosa
Streptococcus pneumoniae
Neisseria meningitidis
Haemophilus influenzae (in children)
Mycobacterium tuberculosis

Data from Ewald GA, McKenzie CR, editors: *Manual of medical therapeutics,* ed 28, St Louis, 1995, Washington University School of Medicine.

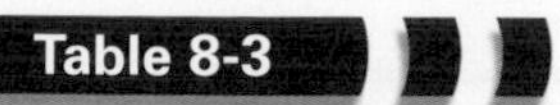

Antimicrobial Selection Based on Organisms

Organism	First Drug of Choice	Alternative Drugs
Gram-Positive Cocci		
Staphylococcus aureus		
Non–penicillinase producing	Penicillin G or V	A cephalosporin, vancomycin, clindamycin, imipenem
Penicillinase producing	A penicillinase resistance penicillin	Vancomycin, cephalosporin, clindamycin, amoxicillin-clavulanic acid, ticarcillin-clavulanic acid, ampicillin-sulbactam, piperacillin tazobactam, imipenem, TMP-SMZ
Methicillin resistant	Vancomycin ± gentamicin Vancomycin ± rifampin	TMP-SMZ, minocycline, Quinupristin/Dalfopristin, Linezolid
Streptococcus, hemolytic groups A, B, C, G	Penicillin G or V	Erythromycin, a cephalosporin, vancomycin, clindamycin, azithromycin, clarithromycin
Viridans	Penicillin G ± aminoglycoside	Cephalosporin, vancomycin
Anaerobic	Penicillin G	Clindamycin, cephalosporin
Enterococcus	Ampicillin + gentamicin	Vancomycin + gentamicin
Vancomycin resistant	Linezolid	
Pneumococcus	Penicillin G or V	Erythromycin, cephalosporin, vancomycin, TMP-SMZ, chloramphenicol, clindamycin, azithromycin, clarithromycin
Gram-Negative Cocci		
Neisseria meningitidis (meningitis or septicemia)	Penicillin G	Cefotaxime, ceftizoxime, ceftriaxone, ampicillin, chloramphenicol
Neisseria gonorrhoeae (genital)	Ceftriaxone or cefixime	Ciprofloxacin, spectinomycin, ofloxacin, cefpodoxime proxetil
Moraxella catarrhalis	TMP-SMZ	Cefuroxime, cefotaxime, ceftizoxime, ceftriaxone, cefuroxime axetil, erythromycin, tetracycline, azithromycin, amoxicillin-clavulanic acid, clarithromycin
Gram-Positive Bacilli		
Bacillus anthracis	Penicillin G	Erythromycin, tetracycline
Listeria monocytogenes	TMP-SMZ	Ampicillin ± aminoglycoside
Clostridium tetani	Penicillin G	Metronidazole, chloramphenicol, clindamycin, imipenem
Clostridium perfringens	Penicillin	Cephalosporin
Corynebacterium diphtheriae	Erythromycin	Penicillin G
Gram-Negative Bacilli		
Escherichia coli (first UTI)	Sulfonamide, TMP-SMZ	Ampicillin, cephalosporin, ciprofloxacin, ofloxacin
Escherichia coli (sepsis)	Cefotaxime, ceftizoxime, ceftriaxone, ceftazidime	Ampicillin, TMP-SMZ, ciprofloxacin, imipenem, aminoglycoside, ofloxacin
Klebsiella pneumoniae	Cefotaxime, ceftizoxime, ceftriaxone, ceftazidime	TMP-SMZ, aminoglycoside, imipenem, ciprofloxacin, ofloxacin, piperacillin, mezlocillin
Enterobacter	TMP-SMZ, imipenem	Aminoglycoside, ciprofloxacin, ofloxacin, aztreonam
Legionella pneumophila	Erythromycin + rifampin	TMP-SMZ, clarithromycin, azithromycin, ciprofloxacin
Serratia	Cefotaxime, ceftizoxime, ceftriaxone, ceftazidime	TMP-SMZ, aminoglycoside, ciprofloxacin, ofloxacin, imipenem
Proteus mirabilis	Ampicillin	Aminoglycoside, TMP-SMZ, ciprofloxacin, ofloxacin
Pseudomonas aeruginosa	Aminoglycoside + antipseudomonal penicillin	Ceftazidime ± aminoglycoside, imipenem ± aminoglycoside, aztreonam ± aminoglycoside, ciprofloxacin ± piperacillin, ciprofloxacin ± ceftazidime

Continued

Table 8-3

Antimicrobial Selection Based on Organisms—cont'd

Organism	First Drug of Choice	Alternative Drugs
Gram-Negative Bacilli—cont'd		
Pseudomonas cepacia	Ceftazidime	Chloramphenicol, tetracycline, TMP-SMZ, amoxicillin-clavulanic acid, imipenem
Helicobacter pylori	Tetracycline + metronidazole + bismuth subsalicylate	Amoxicillin + metronidazole + bismuth subsalicylate, tetracycline + clarithromycin + bismuth subsalicylate
Salmonella	Ceftriaxone, ciprofloxacin, ofloxacin	TMP-SMZ, ampicillin, chloramphenicol
Shigella	Ciprofloxacin, ofloxacin	Ampicillin, TMP-SMZ, ceftriaxone
Haemophilus influenzae		
Meningitis or epiglottiditis	Cefotaxime, ceftizoxime, ceftriaxone, ceftazidime	Chloramphenicol
Other sites	TMP-SMZ	Ampicillin, amoxicillin, doxycycline, azithromycin, clarithromycin, cefotaxime, ceftizoxime, ceftriaxone, cefuroxime, cefuroxime, axetil
Bordetella pertussis	Erythromycin	TMP-SMZ
Brucella	Tetracycline + gentamicin	TMP-SMZ ± gentamicin. Chloramphenicol ± gentamicin
Acinetobacter	Imipenem	Minocycline, TMP-SMZ, doxycycline, aminoglycosides, piperacillin, ciprofloxacin, ofloxacin, ceftazidime
Campylobacter	Erythromycin	Tetracycline, ciprofloxacin, ofloxacin
Pasteurella (plague)	Streptomycin	Chloramphenicol, tetracycline, gentamicin
Vibrio cholerae	Tetracycline	TMP-SMZ, ciprofloxacin, ofloxacin, ceftazidime
Spirochetes		
Treponema pallidum	Penicillin G	Tetracycline, ceftriaxone
Treponema pertenue	Penicillin G	Tetracycline
Leptospira	Penicillin G	Tetracycline
Borrelia burgdorferi (Lyme disease)	Tetracycline	Amoxicillin, ceftriaxone, cefuroxime axetil, azithromycin, clarithromycin, penicillin
Acid-Fast Bacilli		
Mycobacterium		
Mycobacterium tuberculosis	Isoniazid + rifampin + pyrazinamide ± ethambutol or streptomycin	
Mycobacterium leprae	Dapsone + rifampin + clofazimine	Minocycline, ofloxacin, clarithromycin
Special Considerations		
Chlamydia psittaci	Tetracycline	Chloramphenicol
Chlamydia trachomatis	Doxycycline, azithromycin	Ofloxacin, sulfisoxazole
Mycoplasma pneumoniae	Tetracycline	Erythromycin, clarithromycin
Rickettsia	Tetracycline	Chloramphenicol, ciprofloxacin, ofloxacin

Data from Tierney LM, McPhee SJ, Papadakis MA: *Current medical diagnosis and treatment,* ed 40, Stamford, Conn, 2001, Appleton & Lange.
TMP-SMZ, Trimethoprim-sulfamethoxazole; *UTI,* urinary tract infection.

Table 8-4

Comparison of Viruses and Other Microorganisms

Organism	Grows in Nonliving Media	Contains Both DNA and RNA	Contains Ribosomes	Sensitive to Antibiotics
Bacteria	Yes	Yes	Yes	Yes
Mycoplasmas	Yes	Yes	Yes	Yes
Rickettsiae	No	Yes	Yes	Yes
Chlamydiae	No	Yes	Yes	Yes
Viruses	No	No	No	No

in which the RNA is a single positive copy use the strand as a direct template to make viral proteins and a complementary RNA strand. The complementary strand then serves as a template for making more positive strands that can be packaged into new viruses. The RNA viruses that possess a negative copy replicate in a similar manner, except that the RNA must be transcribed to a positive complementary copy before it can produce proteins or viral RNA. Most viral infections are self-limited, and few antimicrobial agents have been developed to treat them. Effective vaccines are available for some viruses, including polio, measles, rubella, and hepatitis A and B.

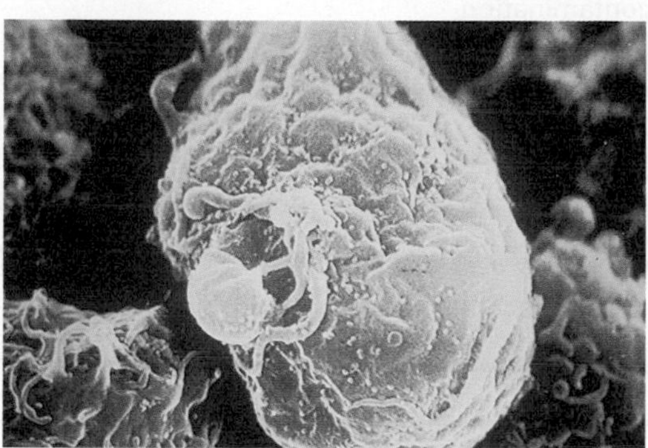

FIGURE 8-8 ■ Scanning electron micrograph of HIV-1–infected T4 lymphocyte. Large numbers of HIV virions are budding from the plasma membrane of the lymphocytes. (Courtesy Centers for Disease Control and Prevention, Atlanta.)

Fungi

Fungi are nonphotosynthetic, eukaryotic protists that are disseminated through the environment. They can reproduce by

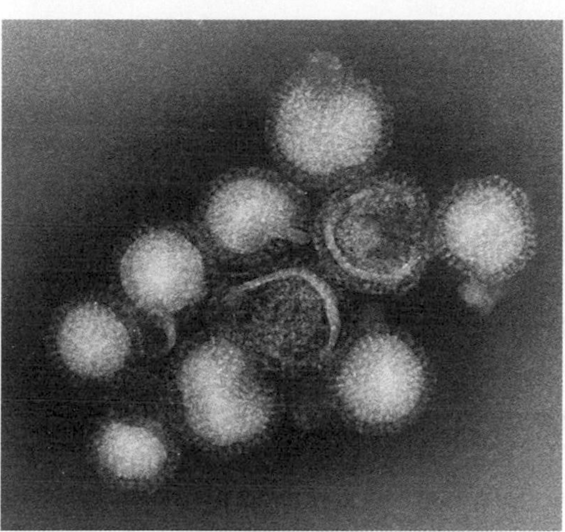

FIGURE 8-9 ■ Electron micrograph of influenza virus, an RNA virus (×150,000). (Courtesy Dr. F. A. Murphy, Centers for Disease Control and Prevention, Atlanta.)

Table 8-5 

Examples of Primary Viral Pathogens Associated with Specific Infections

Family	Viral Example	Disease	Type of Nucleic Acid
RNA Viruses			
Astroviridae	Astrovirus		SS (+) RNA
Arenaviridae	Lymphocytic choriomeningitis virus	Meningitis	2 circular SS (antisense) RNA segments
Bunyaviridae	California encephalitis virus	California encephalitis	3 circular SS (antisense) RNA segments
Caliciviridae	Norwalk virus		SS (+) RNA
Coronaviridae	Coronaviruses		SS (+) RNA
Filoviridae	Ebola virus	Ebola virus	SS (–) RNA
Orthomyxoviridae	Influenza viruses	Influenza	8 SS (–) RNA*
Paramyxoviridae	Measles virus	Measles	SS (–) RNA
Picornaviridae	Poliovirus	Polio	SS (+) RNA
Reoviridae	Rotaviruses		10-12 DS RNA segments
Retroviridae	HIV-1	AIDS	2 identical SS (+) RNA segments
Rhabdoviridae	Rabies virus	Rabies	SS (−) RNA
Togaviridae	Rubella virus	Rubella	SS (+) RNA
DNA Viruses			
Adenoviridae	Human adenoviruses		DS DNA
Hepadnaviridae	Hepatitis B	Hepatitis B	DS DNA without SS portions
Herpesviridae	Herpes simplex virus	Herpes	DS DNA
Papovaviridae	JC virus	Warts	Circular DS DNA
Parvoviridae	Human parvovirus	Parvo	SS (+) or (–) DNA
Poxviridae	Vaccinia virus		DS DNA

Data from Mandell GL, Bennett JE, Dolan R, editors: *Principles and practice of infectious disease,* ed 5, New York, 2000, Churchill Livingstone.
DS, Double stranded; *SS,* single stranded; *(+),* message sense; *(–),* antimessage sense.
*Influenza C: seven segments.

Table 8-6
Fungal Infections

Infection	Distribution	Mode of Transmission	Vector
Cryptococcosis	Everywhere	Inhalation	Pigeon feces
Candidiasis	Normal flora	Ever present	N/A
Phycomycosis (mucormycosis)	Everywhere	Inhalation, ingestion, wound contamination	Decayed matter, soil
Histoplasmosis	River valleys (e.g., California), southwestern USA (Arizona, Nevada)	Inhalation	Bird and bat feces
Coccidioidomycosis (San Joaquin Valley fever)	Semiarid USA (e.g., California), southwestern USA (Arizona, Nevada)	Inhalation	Dust, dirt
Blastomycosis	Southeastern USA south central USA midwestern USA, Great Lakes region	Inhalation	Unknown
Aspergillosis	Everywhere	Inhalation	Decaying vegetation

simply dividing (asexually) or by combining their genetic information before dividing (sexually). Infections caused by fungi are called mycotic infections, or **mycoses.** Fungi cause infection first by colonizing the area. The fungus adheres to and proliferates on the site of infection. The next phase requires invasion of the epithelium. Anything that breaks the integrity of the skin (e.g., maceration) facilitates the invasion. Polymorphonuclear leukocytes attempt to phagocytize and digest the invading fungi. Neutrophils, monocytes, and eosinophils can destroy fungi in the body, causing edema, erythema, and itching at the site of infection.[1]

Certain fungi live as normal flora (e.g., *Candida*). When the body's defense mechanisms are compromised, the fungi can overgrow and cause local or systemic infections. Patients who have been given antibiotics lose some of their normal flora along with the targeted pathogen. The fungi that are not affected by the antibiotic overgrow to fill that niche. Some patients with AIDS, being treated with chemotherapy or immunosuppressive agents, lack the immune system to prevent fungi from overgrowing, and are therefore more susceptible to fungal infections (opportunistic fungi). Examples of opportunistic fungi are *Candida,* Phycomycetes, *Aspergillus,* and *C. immitis.*

Superficial mycoses, such as that caused by the dermatophytes (e.g., tinea pedis), occur only on superficial, dead, keratinized tissue like hair, epidermis, and nails.[6]

Subcutaneous mycoses occur when fungi are introduced into subcutaneous tissue during trauma. These fungi, when present in tissue, cause chronic granulomatous disease. An example is *Sporothrix schenckii.* This fungus causes sporotrichosis, which may spread throughout the lymph system.[4]

Systemic mycoses may occur in both healthy and immunocompromised hosts. Because the fungi causing systemic infections are usually found in soil, the infections tend to be endemic to certain regions where the fungus is found.[1,4] Infection is caused by inhalation of dust containing the fungus. Because of the endemic nature of these fungi, large segments of the population in the endemic area may have been exposed and infected as children without any symptoms. If symptoms develop, they are usually self-limiting and mild. However, for those with altered immune systems, the disease becomes severe and disseminated. Examples of systemic mycoses are histoplasmosis, blastomycosis, and coccidiomycosis.

To illustrate, *Histoplasma capsulatum* is a fungus that commonly occurs in soil in the central and eastern United States. *Histoplasma* also occurs in soil rich with chicken feces or bat guano. Humans and animals exposed to dust storms in endemic areas or contaminated with these feces are most likely to be infected. They may also have positive histoplasmin skin tests and may show calcified sites of infection in their lungs.[4,17]

Conditions that predispose an individual to the potential for an opportunistic fungal infection or to a disseminated pathogenic fungal infection are AIDS, leukemia, cancer chemotherapy, organ transplantation with immune-suppressing therapy, alcoholism, drug abuse, and malnutrition. Opportunistic infections also thrive when the natural flora has been altered with antibiotics or when the environment contains more nutrients in which the fungi can grow, such as the hyperglycemic blood stream of a diabetic, or the vaginal tract of a female who has been given antibiotics.[1,17]

Generally, cultures of fungi are difficult to grow artificially in a laboratory. The most common method of identification is

Symptoms	Location of Infection: Primary Site(s)	Location of Infection: Secondary Site(s)
Fever, cough, weight loss, pleuritic pain, CNS disturbances	Pulmonary system	Meninges, skin, bone
Mucocutaneous pain and itching at site of infection	Fungemia, endocarditis	Kidneys, eyes, heart
Rhinocerebral mucormycosis: destruction of CN II, IV, V, VI; erosion of carotid artery; meningitis; brain abscess Pulmonary mucormycosis: dyspnea, chest pain, hemoptysis	Nose, brain, lung	Rare
Flulike: cough, fever, myalgias, weight loss, anemia, leukopenia, thrombocytopenia, painful oropharyngeal ulcers	Pulmonary system	Bone marrow
Cough, fever, pleuritic chest pain, weight loss, dyspnea, chest pain, CNS disturbances	Pulmonary system	Skin, bone, joints, meninges
Flulike: pleuritic chest pain, arthralgias, erythema nodosum, weight loss, fever, cough, chest pain	Pulmonary system	Skin, bone, joints, male GU tract
Dyspnea, chest pain, hemoptysis, wheezing	Pulmonary system	Brain, kidney, liver

by visualizing their characteristic shapes on a slide of infected tissue.

Drugs used to systemically manage fungal diseases include ketoconazole, amphotericin B, caspofungin, and voriconazole. Systemic treatment is used more commonly on the immune compromised patient. Topical treatment of cutaneous fungal infections can include clotrimazole, ketoconazole, or miconazole. Systemic treatment is usually reserved for disseminated disease inasmuch as the local infection is usually self-limited. Table 8-6 summarizes important aspects of the most common fungi.

Parasites

Parasites are representative of four families of the animal kingdom: protozoa, or single-celled animals (Figure 8-10); nemathelminths, or roundworms; platyhelminthes, or flatworms; and arthropoda, or invertebrate animals with jointed appendages.[4,21] These parasites live on or in the human body during some part of their life cycle. They depend on their human host for shelter and sustenance. Many parasites have very complicated life cycles that include a larval and adult stage. They rely on particular hosts and vectors to transmit the infection from host to host. Host resistance depends on macrophages, neutrophils, eosinophils, and platelets, which kill both protozoa and worms. T cells are required to develop immunity against these organisms. This explains the high incidence of *Toxoplasma* and *Pneumocystis carinii* infection in HIV patients who are low on CD4 T cells.[32]

The symptoms of parasitic infection depend on the area in which the infestation develops. Protozoan infestation of the gastrointestinal tract produces cramping, abdominal pain, and bloody diarrhea (amebiasis). Infestation of the blood produces fever, chills, rigor, and later anemia, all of which are associated with malaria (*Plasmodium* infection). Acute pruritus and rash occur after infection of the skin with *Sarcoptes scabiei* (scabies).[4]

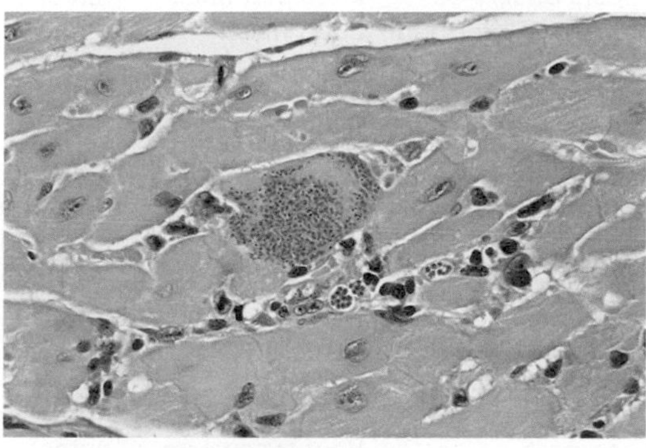

FIGURE 8-10 ■ Protozoa: mouse heart infected with *Trypanosoma cruzi.* Amastigotes are seen inside a muscle fiber (pseudocyst), as well as inside inflammatory cells (hematoxylin and eosin stain, (63). (Courtesy Jeannette Guarner, MD, Centers for Disease Control and Prevention, Atlanta.)

Identification of the infectious agent is usually accomplished by visualizing either the adult parasite or its ova by direct observation of the area (inspection of the skin or hair) or by microscopic examination of blood, feces, or tissue samples. Table 8-7 summarizes various parasitic infections of humans, including the common name, location, symptoms, and mode of transmission.

Table 8-7

Parasitic Infections

Parasitic Agent	Common Name of Disease	Location of Infection	Symptoms	Mode of Transmission
Helminths (Worms)				
Ancylostoma duodenale	Hookworm	Blood vessels of gut	Anemia	Skin penetration
Ascaris lumbricoides	Giant roundworm	Small intestine, lungs	Pneumonitis (rare), intestinal obstruction (rare)	Oral (fecal contamination), autoinfection
Enterobius vermicularis	Pinworm	Cecum	Anal pruritus	Oral
Onchocerca volvulus	River blindness	Skin, eye	Blindness	Insect inoculation
Strongyloides stercoralis	Strongyloidiasis	Small intestine, lungs	Eosinophilia, urticaria, rash, abdominal pain, pneumonitis	Skin penetration, autoinfection
Trichinella spiralis	Trichinosis	Muscles	Muscular pain, eosinophilia, fever, periorbital edema	Oral (infected meat)
Trichuris trichiura	Whipworm	Intestine	Rectal prolapse	Oral (fecal contamination)
Wuchereria bancrofti	Filariasis	Lymphatics	Elephantiasis	Insect (mosquito)
Trematodes				
Clonorchis sinensis	Liver fluke	Liver	Biliary obstruction (rare)	Oral-raw fish
Fasciola hepatica	Liver fluke	Liver	Fever, right upper quadrant abdominal pain, eosinophilia	Oral
Fasciolopsis buski	Intestinal fluke	Liver	Abdominal pain, diarrhea	Oral
Paragonimus westermani	Lung fluke	Lung, intestine	Eosinophilia, cough, chest pain, bronchitis	Oral: poorly cooked freshwater crab or crayfish
Schistosoma haematobium	Blood fluke	Urinary tract	Acute: rash, fever, cough, chest, chills	Skin inoculation
Schistosoma japonicum	Blood fluke	Mesenteric blood vessels	Hepatomegaly, splenomegaly	Skin inoculation
Schistosoma mansoni	Blood fluke	Mesenteric blood vessels	Lymphadenopathy, eosinophilia	Skin inoculation
Cestodes (Tapeworms)				
Diphyllobothrium latum	Fish tapeworm	Intestine	Megaloblastic anemia	Oral: poorly cooked fish
Taenia saginata	Beef tapeworm	Intestine	Mild abdominal pain	Oral: poorly cooked beef
Taenia solium	Pork tapeworm	Intestine	Mild abdominal pain	Oral: poorly cooked pork
Echinococcus granulosus	Hydatid cyst	Lung, liver	Cholestasis, liver congestion and atrophy, biliary obstruction	Oral: inoculation with sheep, cattle, or dog feces
Protozoa				
Entamoeba histolytica	Amebic dysentery	Intestine	Bloody, mucoid diarrhea; colicky abdominal pain	Contaminated water, raw vegetables
Plasmodium spp.	Malaria	Liver, erythrocytes	High fever, chills, rigor, anemia, headache, malaise, chest pain, abdominal pain	Female *Anopheles* mosquito
Leishmania spp.	Kala azar; cutaneous leishmaniasis	Reticuloendothelial cells of the body; disseminates to spleen, liver, bone marrow, lymph glands	Chronic: abdominal discomfort, ascites, fever, weakness, pallor, weight loss, cough Acute: sudden fever, chills	All transmission accomplished through the bite of sandflies after biting specific infected mammals
Trypanosoma spp.				
T. cruzi	Chagas disease	Blood stream	Local inflammation, lymphadenopathy, muscular necrosis including myocardium (heart failure), esophagus, and colon (dilation); fever, malaise, anorexia, edema of face	Insects—hematophagous (blood drinking) *Triatoma*

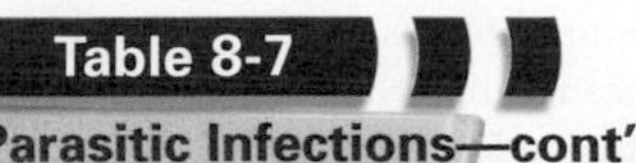

Table 8-7
Parasitic Infections—cont'd

Parasitic Agent	Common Name of Disease	Location of Infection	Symptoms	Mode of Transmission
Protozoa				
T. brucei	African sleeping sickness	Blood stream	Fever, malaise, headache, rash, CNS disturbances	Glossina flies (tsetse flies)
Toxoplasma gondii	Toxoplasmosis	Throughout body	Acute: usually asymptomatic Immunosuppressed: encephalitis, myocarditis, pneumonitis Newborn: impaired vision, neurologic disorders	Eating raw or undercooked meat, poultry, or dairy foods; oral inoculation with cat feces
Pneumocystis carinii	Pneumonitis	Lungs	Fever, cough, tachypnea, costal retractions, cyanosis	Inhalation
Giardia lamblia	Epidemic diarrhea	Intestine	Acute, self-limited diarrhea; occasionally malabsorption with weight loss	Fecal contamination of water; person to person
Trichomonas vaginalis	Trichomoniasis (vaginitis)	Vagina	Irritation, discharge	Sexually transmitted
Ectoparasites				
Pediculus humanus				
Var. *corporis*	Body louse	All hair-covered parts of body	Pruritus Nits at base of hair shaft	Person to person, by fomites
Var. *capitis*	Head louse	Head area		
Pediculus pubis	Pubic louse	Pubic area		
Sarcoptes scabiei (var. *hominis*)	Scabies	Skin	Pruritus, worse at night; linear burrows in folds of fingers, elbows, knees, axillae, pelvic girdle	Person to person
Maggots (larvae of dipterous flies)	Myiasis	Necrotic tissue	Depends on location of infestation	Dipterous flies
Chiggers (mites)		Skin	Intense pruritus, hemorrhagic papules	Inhabit dogs, rabbits, cats, rats; foul cheese, flour, house dust
Ticks		Skin	Can transmit tick paralysis, Lyme disease	Reside in wooded and grassy areas

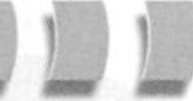

KEY CONCEPTS

- Microorganisms responsible for infections in humans include bacteria, viruses, fungi, and parasites.
- Bacteria are characterized according to shape (cocci, rods, spirals), reaction to stains (gram negative, gram positive, acid fast), and oxygen requirements (aerobic, anaerobic).
- Viruses are bits of genetic material (DNA, RNA) with associated proteins and lipids. The smallest infective agents known, viruses are intracellular pathogens that use the host's energy sources and enzymes to replicate. Viral replication may or may not destroy the host cell. DNA viruses may be incorporated directly into the host genome. RNA viruses serve as templates for the production of viral RNA and proteins.
- Retroviruses are RNA viruses that contain a special enzyme called reverse transcriptase that mediates the synthesis of a DNA copy of the RNA virus. The DNA can then be incorporated into the host genome and passed on to daughter cells when the cell divides.
- Fungal infections can be superficial (e.g., ringworm, athlete's foot), subcutaneous (e.g., sporotrichosis), or systemic (e.g., histoplasmosis). Systemic fungal infections tend to be more serious and usually do not occur unless the host's immune system is compromised.
- Parasites include protozoa, helminths (roundworms, flatworms), and arthropods. Manifestations of parasitic infections vary depending on the organism and site of infection. Common sites of parasitic infestation are the skin and gastrointestinal tract.

SUMMARY

This chapter has described the infectious process and the roles of immunization and the environment in the transmission of infection between hosts. The process of transmission of infection can be thought of as a chain with links that flow from the host or reservoir of the microorganism to the next susceptible victim. The goal of infection control is to block transmission of the microorganism to susceptible victims by severing the chain at one or more links.

Four basic types of microorganisms exist: bacteria, or single-celled organisms with cellular organelles that allow them to live independently in the environment; viruses, or tiny genetic parasites that require the host cell to replicate and spread; fungi, or nonphotosynthetic, eukaryotic single or multicellular creatures that are found throughout the environment; and parasites, which include protozoa, roundworms, flatworms, and arthropods. These organisms can be helpful or harmful to the host. When harmful, a microorganism is considered pathogenic. The study of pathogenic organisms and the way that they spread is called epidemiology.

The host-parasite relationship is determined by the characteristics of both the microorganism and the host. Microorganism factors that affect the relationship include whether the parasite must kill the host cell to propagate, the reaction of the host to the invading microorganism and its endotoxins, and the ability of the microorganism to live independently from the host in the environment. Host factors such as the integrity of barriers to transmission, nutritional status, age, and drug regimen all have an impact on this relationship.

Health care professionals have a key role in the prevention and early detection of infectious processes in hospital and community settings. The identification of high-risk individuals who are more susceptible to infection will assist in earlier detection of the manifestations of infection. Management of infections requires optimizing the client's host defense system and is supplemented by pharmacologic and nutritional interventions.

MEDIA RESOURCES

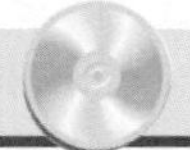

evolve

Remember to check out the ***CD Companion*** included with this book for Review Questions, Key Concepts Review, Glossary (with audio for selected terms), Disease Profiles, and Animations.

PLUS, visit the ***Evolve website*** at http://evolve.elsevier.com/Copstead/ for Case Studies, Disease Profiles, and WebLinks.

References

1. Mandell GL, Gennett JE, Dolin R: *Principles and practice of infectious diseases,* ed 5, New York, 2000, Churchill Livingstone.
2. Garner JS: Guideline for isolation precautions in hospitals, *Am J Infect Control* 24:24-52, 1996.
3. Chulay M, Guzzetta C, Dossey B: *AACN handbook of critical care nursing 1995,* Stamford, Conn, 1996, Appleton & Lange.
4. Chin J, editor: *Control of communicable diseases in man,* ed 17, Washington, DC, 2000, American Public Health Association.
5. U.S. Centers for Disease Control and Prevention: Boulder County Department of Health, 2002. Website: http://www.cdc.gov/.
6. Price SA, Wilson LM: *Pathophysiology: clinical concepts of disease processes,* ed 6, St Louis, 2002, Mosby.
7. Guyton AC: *Textbook of medical physiology,* ed 10, Philadelphia, 2000, Saunders.
8. Vander AJ, Sherman JH, Luciano DS: *The mechanisms of body function: human physiology,* ed 8, New York, 2001, McGraw-Hill.
9. Redmond HP et al: Immunosuppressive mechanisms in protein-calorie malnutrition, *Surgery* 110:311-316, 1991.
10. Moore FA et al: Early enteral feeding compared with parenteral reduces postoperative septic complications: the results of a meta analysis, *Ann Surg* 216:172-183, 1992.
11. Kudsk KA et al: Enteral versus parenteral feeding: effects on septic morbidity after blunt and penetrating abdominal trauma, *Ann Surg* 215:503-513, 1992.
12. Kehn CR, Wein GC: *Joslin's diabetes mellitus,* ed 13, Philadelphia, 1994, Lea & Febiger.
13. Hoyt MJ: Host defense mechanisms and compromises in the trauma patient, *Crit Care Nurs Clin North Am* 1:753-765, 1989.
14. Yoshikowa TT, Norman DC: Antibiotic therapy: what to consider when treating geriatric patients, *Hosp Formulary* 29(8):754-768, 1993.
15. Patrick M: *Respiratory problems: nursing management for the elderly,* ed 3, Philadelphia, 1993, Lippincott.
16. Stark JL: *The renal system: core curriculum for critical care nursing,* ed 4, Philadelphia, 1991, Saunders.
17. Deitch E, editor: Surgical infections, *Surg Clin North Am* 74(3):537-557, 1994.
18. Marshall J, Sweeny D: Microbial infection and the septic shock response in critical surgical illness, *Arch Surg* 125:17-23, 1990.
19. American Academy of Pediatrics: *Recommended childhood immunization schedule,* Elk Grove, Ill, 1997, The Academy.
20. Okoth FA: Viral hepatitis, *East Afr Med J* 73(5):308-312, 1996.
21. Cooper RB: *Everything you needed to know about diseases,* Springhouse, Pa, 1996, Springhouse.
22. Guyton AC: *Textbook of medical physiology,* ed 10, Philadelphia, 2000, Saunders.
23. Boutotte J: TB: the second time around and how you can help control it, *Nursing* 23(5):42-50, 1993.
24. Rakel RE: *Conn's current therapy 2002,* ed 2, Philadelphia, 2002, Saunders.
25. George RB et al: *Chest medicine,* ed 3, Baltimore, 1995, Williams & Wilkins.
26. Chadwick PR: Making real sense of methicillin-resistant *Staphylococcus aureus, Lancet* 348:1525-1526, 1996.
27. Schrieber JR, Goldman DA, editors: Antimicrobial resistance in pediatrics, *Pediatr Clin North Am* 42(3):519-537, 1995.
28. Rosenberg J: Methicillin-resistant *Staphylococcus aureus* (MRSA) in the community: who's watching, *Lancet* 346:132-133, 1995.
29. Tierney LM, McPhee SJ, Papadakis MA: *Current medical diagnosis and treatment,* ed 38, Stamford, Conn, 1998, Appleton & Lange.
30. Danner RL et al: Endotoxemia in human septic shock, *Chest* 99:169-175, 1991.
31. Ewald GA, McKenzie CR, editors: *Manual of medical therapeutics,* ed 28, St Louis, 1995, Washington University School of Medicine.
32. Roitt I, Brostoff J, Male D: *Immunology,* ed 4, St Louis, 1998, Mosby.

chapter 9

Inflammation and Immunity

Jacquelyn L. Banasik

MEDIA RESOURCES

Additional Material for Study, Review, and Further Exploration

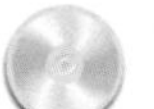

CD Companion ◆ Review Questions and Answers ◆ Key Concepts Review
◆ Glossary *(with audio pronunciations for selected terms)*
◆ Disease Profiles ◆ Animations

evolve ***Website*** at http://evolve.elsevier.com/Copstead/
◆ Case Studies ◆ Disease Profiles ◆ WebLinks

KEY QUESTIONS

- What are the major organs and cellular components of the body's defense against foreign antigens?
- How do immune cells communicate through cell-to-cell interactions and through secreted cytokines?
- How do innate and adaptive immune mechanisms differ?
- How do macrophages, granulocytes, and lymphocytes work together to locate, recognize, and eliminate pathogens?
- What is the role of MHC class I and II proteins in cell-mediated immunity?
- Why is an immune response usually more effective on subsequent exposure to an antigen than after the first exposure?
- How do noncellular immune system components, including antibodies, complement, and clotting factors, aid the immune response?

CHAPTER OUTLINE

The immune system is a complex network of cells and tissues that work together to protect the body against foreign invaders. The wide variety of potential pathogens requires a defense system that is diversified and adaptable. Several types of white blood cells (WBCs) are of primary importance in localizing, recognizing, and eliminating foreign substances. These immune cells are strategically situated in diverse locations so that pathogens may be detected quickly. The dispersed nature of these defensive cells necessitates a complex system of intercellular communication to effectively mobilize reinforcements to areas of need. A tremendous amount of information has accumulated in the last 10 years about how immune cells communicate and the processes that enable them to migrate to particular locations. The impact of this research goes far beyond the traditional immune disorders such as immunodeficiency diseases and hypersensitivity reactions. Indeed, it is now difficult to identify many pathophysiologic processes that do not involve the immune system in some way. The immune system has been implicated in the pathogenesis of disorders as diverse as atherosclerosis, myocardial infarction, shock, diabetes, and stroke. Therefore, an understanding of immune function is fundamental to the study of a wide variety of diseases. This chapter describes the organs and cells that constitute the immune system, the mechanisms of action of innate and adaptive defenses, and the communication processes whereby immune cells achieve a coordinated response. Underreactions and overreactions of the immune system, immune system malignancies, and human immunodeficiency virus disease are described in Chapters 10, 11, and 12, respectively.

COMPONENTS OF THE IMMUNE SYSTEM

The structures of the immune system include (1) skin and mucous membranes; (2) the mononuclear phagocyte system; (3) the lymphoid system, including spleen, thymus gland, and lymph nodes; and (4) bone marrow. All these structures are inhabited by different types of WBCs (leukocytes) that mediate **inflammation** and **immunity.** Leukocytes are responsible for locating and eliminating pathogens and foreign molecules. They are aided in their task of bodily defense by a number of chemical mediators, including **complement, kinins,** clotting factors, and **cytokines.**

Components of the immune system are often categorized into specific or innate defenses according to the mechanisms whereby antigens are recognized. Innate defenses require no previous exposure to mount an effective response against an **antigen,** and a wide variety of different antigens are recognized. Natural killer (NK) cells and phagocytic cells such as **neutrophils** and **macrophages** are mediators of innate defenses. In contrast, specific defenses respond more effectively on second exposure to an antigen (adaptive) and are highly restricted in the ability to recognize antigens. B lymphocytes (B cells) and T lymphocytes (T cells) are the agents of specific immunity.

Although separating immune components into specific and innate systems is helpful for studying inflammation and immunity, it is an artificial division because they function in a highly integrated manner. The approach used in this chapter is to first describe the major components of the immune system, discuss innate and specific adaptive defenses separately, and then summarize the integrated function of the entire system and its regulation.

EPITHELIAL BARRIERS

The skin and mucous membranes are sometimes called the "first line of defense" because they are frequently the initial sites of microbial invasion. Intact epithelia in skin and mucous membranes provide mechanical and chemical barriers that prevent microorganisms from gaining access to the body's tissues. The skin epithelium produces antimicrobial peptides called *defensins* that can kill a wide variety of bacteria and fungi. The intestinal epithelium produces another form of bactericidal peptide called *cryptocidins* that prevent bacteria from colonizing the intestinal wall.[1] Resident microorganisms may aid in providing this line of defense by making conditions inhospitable for pathogens (see Chapter 8). Disruption of the normal epithelial barriers increases the likelihood that pathogens will successfully establish an infection. Physical trauma (e.g., burns, lacerations, erosions) and biochemical alterations (e.g., pH changes, increased glucose concentration, decreased enzyme production) predispose to infection. Pathogens that breach the skin or mucous membranes are generally first detected by cells of the mononuclear phagocyte system. These cells are thought to derive from monocytes produced in the bone marrow. Specialized antibody-secreting cells also locate to the mucous membranes where they produce antibodies of the immunoglobulin A (IgA) class. IgA antibodies bind antigens on the mucosal surface and prevent them from entering more deeply into the tissues.

MONONUCLEAR PHAGOCYTE SYSTEM

The mononuclear phagocyte system (previously called the reticuloendothelial system) is composed of monocytes and macrophages that are widely distributed throughout the body. Monocytes from the circulating blood migrate to organs and tissues to become macrophages. Macrophages are found throughout the body and go by various names in different tissues, such as alveolar macrophages in the lungs, microglial cells in the brain, Kupffer cells in the liver, and histiocytes in connective tissue (Figure 9-1). Dendritic cells are a monocyte-derived cell type that specializes in capturing and presenting antigens to T cells. Dendritic cells are strategically located in subcutaneous and submucosal tissues.

Macrophages and dendritic cells are often the first immune system cells to encounter a pathogen or foreign antigen after

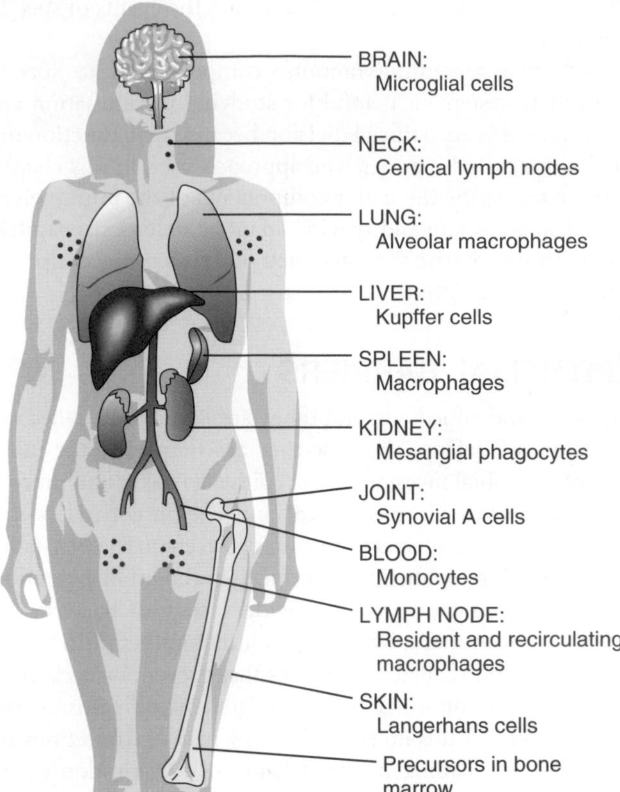

FIGURE 9-1 ■ Cells of the mononuclear phagocyte system. (Redrawn from Schindler LW: *Understanding the immune system,* NIH Pub No 92-529, Bethesda, Md, 1991, U.S. Department of Health and Human Services, p 9.)

it has entered the body, and they are instrumental in communicating news of the invasion to other immune cells. This communication is accomplished through secretion of chemical signaling molecules called cytokines and by presentation of captured antigen to the specific, adaptive immune cells. Macrophages have many other roles in the immune response in addition to their sentry function. Macrophages are powerful phagocytes, each capable of ingesting numerous microbes. Macrophages are called on to clean up the area after an inflammatory reaction in which dead neutrophils and inflammatory debris have accumulated, and they have a role in wound healing.

LYMPHOID SYSTEM

The primary lymphoid organs are the bone marrow and thymus gland, which are the structures where lymphocytes develop. All types of lymphocytes are produced from stem cells in the bone marrow (Figure 9-2). T lymphocytes then migrate to the thymus for development, whereas B lymphocytes stay in the marrow to develop. NK cells are a third population of lymphocytes that lacks both T-cell and B-cell markers. NK cells are produced and released from the bone marrow and function in innate immune responses. NK cells are found mainly in the circulation and spleen. Once mature, T and B lymphocytes migrate to the secondary lymphoid organs where they await activation by antigens. Secondary lymphoid organs include the tonsils, spleen, lymph nodes, and Peyer patches (Figure 9-3).

Primary Lymphoid Organs

Bone marrow is contained in all the bones of the body. The primary function of bone marrow is **hematopoiesis,** or the formation of blood cells. There are two kinds of bone marrow: red and yellow. Hematopoiesis is carried out by red (functioning) marrow. By adulthood, red marrow is confined to the pelvis, sternum, ribs, cranium, ends of the long bones, and vertebral spine. Yellow or fatty bone marrow is found in the remaining bones. It does not contribute to hematopoiesis.

B lymphocytes (B cells) are produced and develop in the bone marrow. B cells migrate from the outer edges toward the center of the bone marrow as they develop. Pre-B cells are subjected to a highly selective quality control process, and less than 25% of the developing B cells are allowed to survive. B cells that leave the bone marrow to colonize secondary lymphoid organs are called naive B cells because they have not yet encountered antigen.

T lymphocytes (T cells) develop in the thymus, which is located in the anterior mediastinum overlying the heart. Pre-T cells initially enter the outer aspect (cortex) of the thymus lobules, and many die as they migrate to the center (medulla) of the thymus. The selection process for T cells is even more rigorous than that for B cells; only about 5% of the cells entering the thymus survive to reenter the circulation and colonize secondary lymphoid organs. The thymus is relatively large at birth and progressively increases in size until puberty. After puberty, the thymus steadily atrophies and only a low level of new T-cell development continues into adulthood.[2] The thymus produces interleukin-7 (IL-7), a cytokine that promotes T-cell proliferation.

Secondary Lymphoid Organs

Once mature, lymphocytes leave their primary lymphoid organs and travel through the blood to localize in peripheral, or secondary, lymphoid tissues, including lymph nodes, spleen, tonsils, and Peyer patches in the intestine. These naive T cells and B cells express specific receptor proteins on their cell surfaces that allow them to "home" to specific locations in lymph tissue. Naive B cells and T cells have a short life span of a few days to weeks unless they encounter an antigen. Antigens are carried to the naive cells in the lymph nodes by the specialized antigen-presenting dendritic cells. When exposed to antigen, T cells and B cells migrate toward each other within the lymph nodes and begin to proliferate. Activated T cells may then migrate to lymph vessels and travel to the blood stream, where

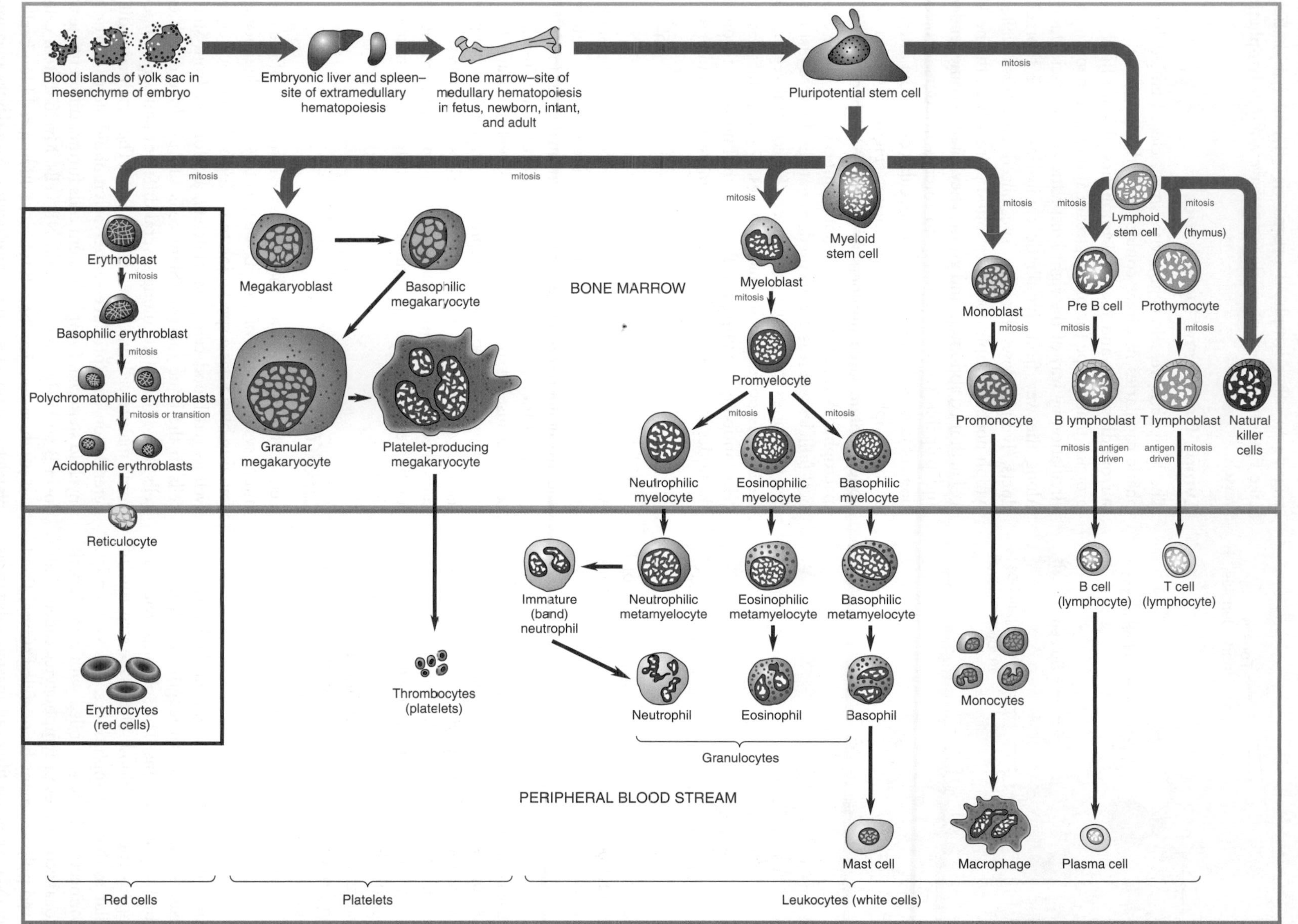

FIGURE 9-2 ■ Maturation of human blood cells showing pathways of cell differentiation from the pluripotent stem cell to mature granulocytes, monocytes, lymphocytes, thrombocytes, and erythrocytes. Production begins in embryo blood islands in the yolk sac. As the embryo matures, production shifts to the liver, spleen, and bone marrow. In an adult, nearly all hematopoiesis occurs in the bone marrow. The two major differentiation pathways are the myeloid pathway and the lymphoid pathway. The lymphoid pathway produces lymphocytes, whereas the myeloid pathway produces granulocytes, monocytes, platelets, and red cells.

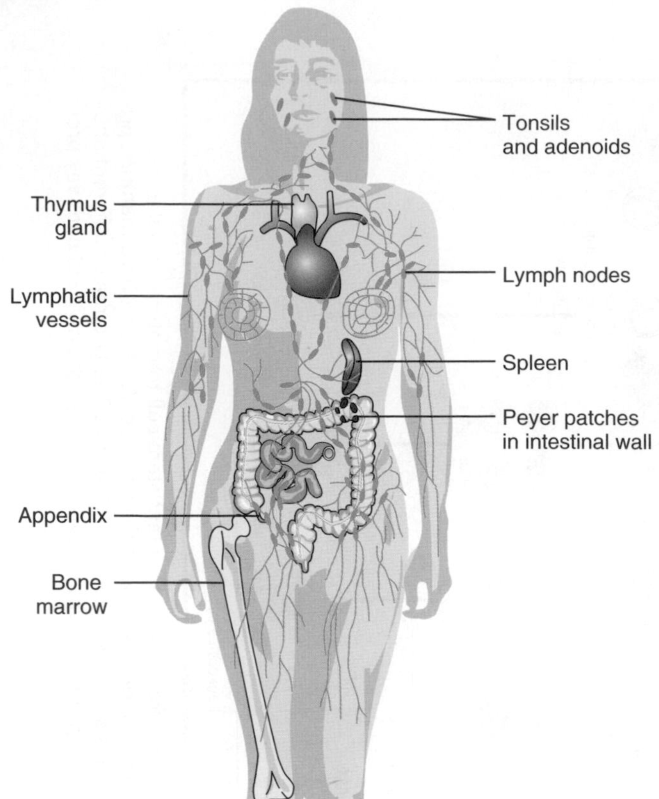

FIGURE 9-3 ■ Principal organs of the lymphoid system.

they are dispersed throughout the system. The majority of B cells stay in the lymph node where they mature into antibody-secreting plasma cells.

Tonsils

Tonsils are aggregates of lymphoid tissue located in the mouth and pharynx. The tonsils are strategically located at the entrance to the digestive and respiratory systems, where they are likely to encounter microorganisms. Unlike lymph nodes, tonsils have no afferent (incoming) lymphatic vessels. They do have efferent lymphatic drainage so that activated lymphocytes from the tonsils can migrate to other lymphoid organs. Tonsils normally make an important contribution to immune function; however, they may occasionally become chronically infected, and surgical removal (tonsillectomy) is then necessary.

Spleen

The spleen is located under the diaphragm on the left side of the body. It measures about 12 cm in length, which makes it the largest of the lymphoid organs. The spleen provides an important filtering function for blood. The tissue structure of the spleen is similar to that of lymph nodes. It is surrounded by a capsule of connective tissue and filled with a meshwork of red pulp and localized masses of lymphocytes called white pulp. Within the red pulp are many blood-filled sinuses lined with macrophages. Macrophages filter out foreign substances and old red blood cells. Lymphocytes located in the white pulp are in a strategic position to come in contact with blood-borne antigens. Lymphocytes thus activated in the spleen can migrate to other lymphoid organs via efferent lymphatics. Like the tonsils, the spleen does not have afferent lymphatic vessels.

Lymph Nodes and Lymphatics

The lymphatic vessels begin with small, closed-ended lymphatic capillaries in direct contact with the interstitial fluid surrounding cells and tissues. Lymphatics pick up fluid and proteins that escape the blood stream and return them to the circulation by way of the right lymphatic and thoracic ducts. Along the way from lymphatic capillaries to the thoracic ducts, lymph flows through specialized structures called lymph nodes. Lymph nodes are found primarily in the neck, axilla, thorax, abdomen, and groin. They often become tender and palpable when responding to foreign invaders. Projections of connective tissue called trabeculae divide the interior of the lymph node into compartments (Figure 9-4). Lymph nodes contain large numbers of B and T lymphocytes and macrophages. B cells are the predominant cell type in the cortical follicles whereas T cells predominate in the area just under the cortex called the paracortex. The central region, or medulla, is populated by macrophages, B cells, and plasma cells (antibody-secreting B cells). Lymph fluid flows through the nodes in a way that allows these immune cells to filter, detect, and react to foreign material.

Peyer Patches

Aggregates of lymphoid tissue can be found scattered throughout the body, particularly in the gastrointestinal, respiratory, and urogenital tracts. These structures are analogous to lymph nodes, but they are not encapsulated and contain primarily B cells. Because of their location these structures have been termed mucosa-associated lymphoid tissue (MALT) or gut-associated lymphoid tissue (GALT). These structures, also called Peyer patches, are of particular importance in producing antibodies to microorganisms that tend to invade mucosal tissue.

LEUKOCYTES

Leukocytes, or WBCs, are the primary effector cells of the immune system. Each of the six different types of leukocytes found in blood has a special job to perform. All leukocytes, as well as red blood cells and platelets, are formed from stem cells in the bone marrow. Stem cells can produce daughter cells that differentiate along several different pathways to become mature cell types (see Figure 9-2). The first major differentiation step produces either a lymphoid stem cell or a myeloid stem cell. Lymphoid stem cells further differentiate to form B and T lymphocytes and NK cells. Myeloid stem cells can produce a variety of cell types, including red blood cells, platelets, monocytes, and **granulocytes.** Monocytes that migrate to tissues are called macrophages. Granulocytes are fur-

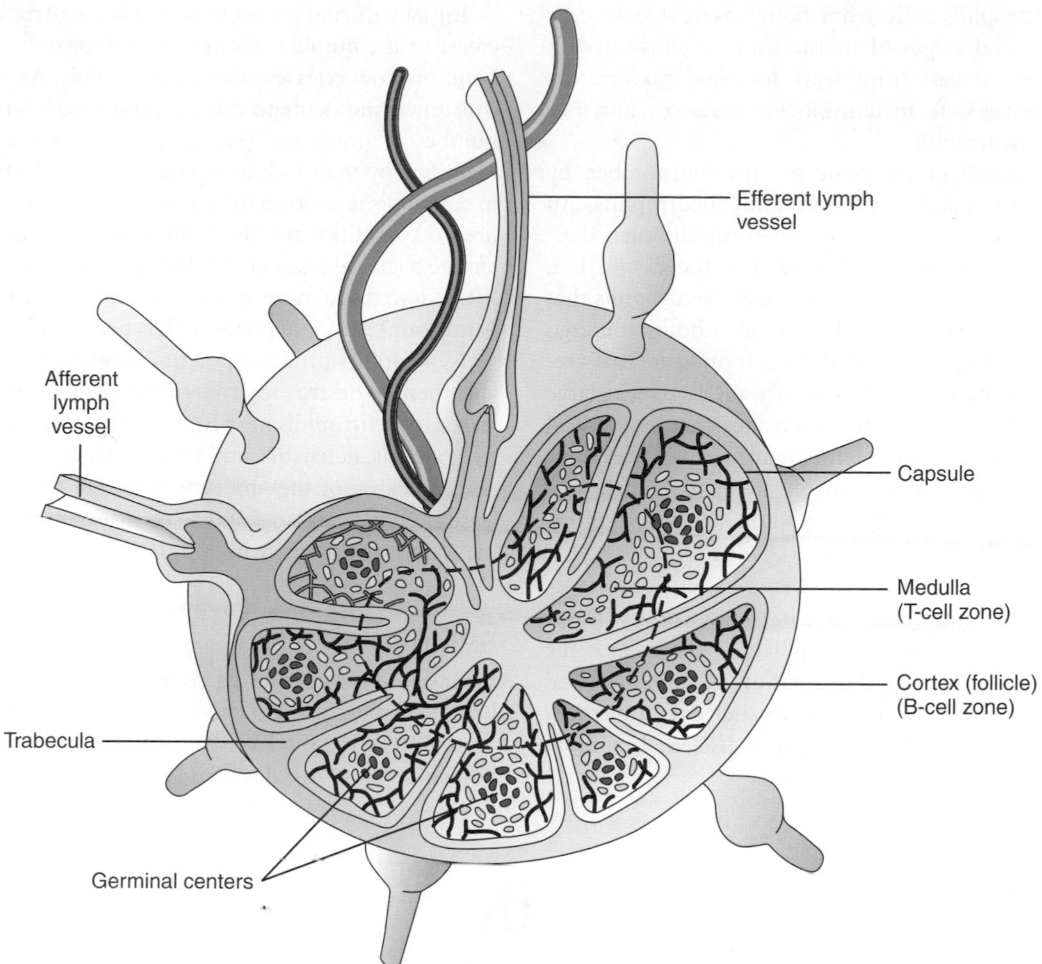

FIGURE 9-4 ■ Schematic drawing of a typical lymph node showing afferent and efferent lymph vessels, as well as B-cell and T-cell zones.

Table 9-1

Leukocyte Proportions and Functions

Type	Percentage*	Role in Inflammation
Neutrophils	60-80	First to appear after injury, phagocytosis
Lymphocytes	20-30	Immune response
Monocytes (macrophages)	3-8	Phagocytosis
Eosinophils	1-6	Allergic reactions, parasite infection
Basophils	0-2	Contain histamine, mediate type I allergic reactions, initiate inflammation

*Total white cell count, 3500 to 10,000/μl.

ther divided into neutrophils, eosinophils, and basophils. Basophils are precursors of the mast cells located in tissues.

Development of these cell types is influenced by hormonal signaling molecules called cytokines. Cytokines are produced locally in the bone marrow and by various other cells. Certain cytokines stimulate stem cell growth, proliferation, and differentiation into particular cell types. The WBC count and differential are commonly measured laboratory tests used to evaluate white cell production. A normal WBC count and differential are shown in Table 9-1. The general features of each of the six WBC types are summarized in the following sections.

Neutrophils

Neutrophils are circulating granulocytes that are also known as polymorphonuclear leukocytes (polys or PMNs). They account for 60% to 80% of the total WBC count. Neutrophils normally have two to five nuclear lobes and coarse, clumped chromatin. Neutrophils arise from bone marrow stem cells and undergo several stages of maturation. As illustrated in Figure 9-2, these stages, from least to most mature, are myeloblast, promyelocyte, metamyelocyte, band cell, and mature segmented neutrophil.

Neutrophils stored in the bone marrow outnumber, by about 10-fold, the quantity of circulating neutrophils. An adult produces more than 1×10^{11} neutrophils each day.[1] These stored neutrophils are released into the circulation, where they have a half-life of 4 to 10 hours. Neutrophils that are not recruited into tissues within about 6 hours undergo programmed cell death (apoptosis). Neutrophils are early responders to an acute bacterial infection and arrive in large numbers very quickly. They are phagocytes that engulf and degrade microorganisms. Circulating neutrophils have receptors on their cell surfaces that enable them to bind to endothelial cells in areas of inflammation. These receptors, called L-selectins, allow neutrophils to stick and roll along the capillary surface.[3] Other interactions between neutrophil integrin receptors and extracellular matrix then facilitate movement of neutrophils through the capillary wall and into the tissue. Neutrophils are attracted to areas of inflammation and bacterial products by **chemotactic** factors such as complement fragments and cytokines. This process is discussed in more depth in the acute inflammation section.

Initially during an acute infection, **neutrophilia,** or an increase in the number of circulating neutrophils, occurs as the bone marrow releases stored neutrophils. As neutrophils are consumed and demand exceeds production, an increase in the number of immature (band) neutrophils occurs. Bands are identified by their lack of nuclear segmentation. This increase in band cells is referred to as a "shift to the left of normal" (Figure 9-5). Traditionally, the band count has been used to differentiate bacterial from viral infections, and a greater shift to the left is viewed as a more severe infection. The utility of using the band count for these purposes has been called into question.[4]

Neutrophils produce potent chemical mediators that enable them to destroy microorganisms. More than 50 toxins released by neutrophils have been identified, including oxidizing free radicals, defensins, and proteolytic enzymes, such as elastase.[5] Because of the ability to generate free radicals and release enzymes, neutrophils can cause extensive damage to normal tissue during their inflammatory response.

Eosinophils

Eosinophils are circulating granulocytes that have two nuclear lobes and stain brilliant red-orange with eosin. They make up 1% to 6% of the total WBC count. Eosinophils mature in the bone marrow (3 to 6 days) and circulate in the blood for about

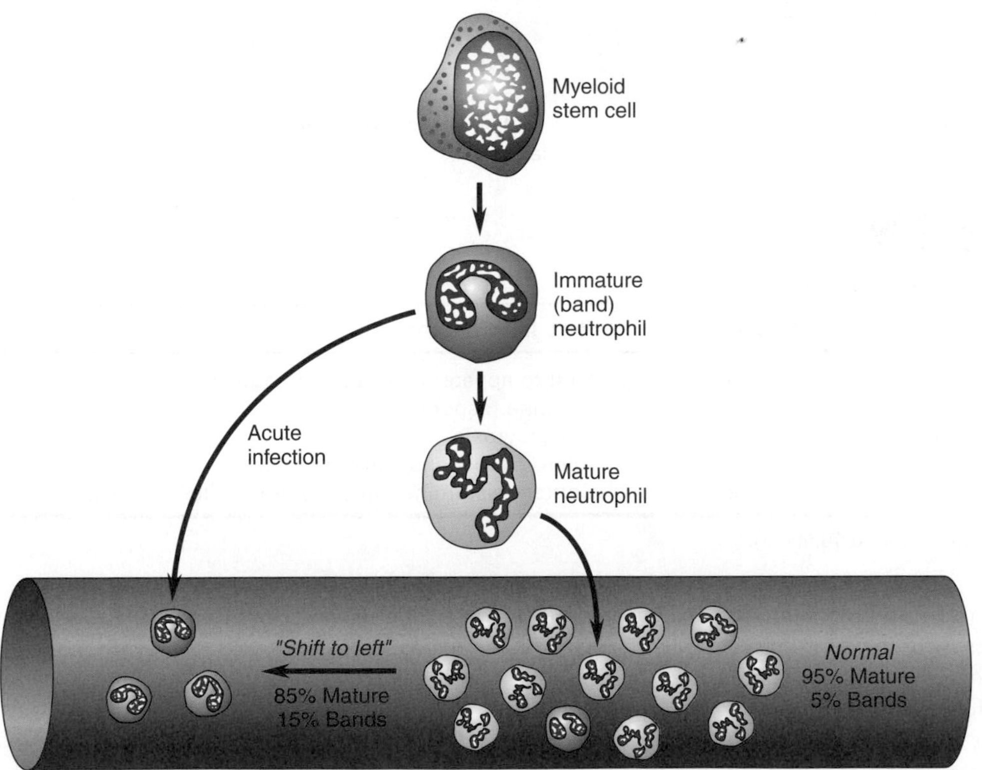

FIGURE 9-5 ■ Inflammatory cytokines stimulate the release of more immature neutrophils, called "bands," from the bone marrow. An increased ratio of bands to mature neutrophils is termed a "shift to the left." This clinical term evolved from the practice of listing bands to the left of mature cells on the laboratory report sheet. A shift to the left is commonly seen with acute bacterial infections.

30 minutes. They have a half-life of 12 days in tissue. Eosinophils arise from myeloid stem cells and undergo a maturation process similar to that of neutrophils.

Eosinophils are particularly associated with and increase in number during allergic reactions and infection by intestinal parasites. The role of eosinophils in allergic reactions is less well characterized than that of mast cells. Eosinophils are recruited into areas of inflammation where they release inflammatory chemicals, such as lysosomal enzymes, peroxidase, prostaglandins, and leukotrienes. The triggers that stimulate eosinophil degranulation and their role in inflammation are not well understood. The primary function of eosinophils is to kill parasitic helminths (worms). Helminths are too large to be phagocytosed by neutrophils or macrophages, and their exterior is resistant to attack by complement or mast cell products. Eosinophils produce specialized molecules such as major basic protein and eosinophil cationic protein, which may be more effective against helminths.[1] Eosinophils recognize helminths that have been opsonized (coated) with IgE antibody. They bind to the IgE and then release their stored chemicals onto the surface of the opsonized helminth. Parasitic infections are a significant problem in much of the world, with one third of the population being affected.

Basophils and Mast Cells

Basophils are granulocytes characterized by granules that stain blue with basophilic dyes. Basophils account for 0% to 2% of the total leukocyte count. Basophils are structurally similar to mast cells. Mature basophils circulate in the vascular system, whereas mast cells are found in connective tissue, especially around blood vessels and under mucosal surfaces. When stimulated, mature basophils can migrate to connective tissue, but once in the tissue, basophils (then called mast cells) do not reenter the circulation.

The average basophil life span is measured in days, whereas mast cells can live for weeks to months. Mast cells and basophils have IgE receptors that allow them to bind and display IgE antibodies on their cell surfaces. When an appropriate stimulus occurs, such as antigen binding to the IgE **antibodies,** mast cells and basophils release granules (**degranulate**) containing proinflammatory chemicals.

Mast cell and basophil granules contain histamine, platelet-activating factor, and other vasoactive amines that are important mediators of immediate hypersensitivity responses. Degranulation of mast cells and basophils begins the inflammatory response that is characteristically associated with allergic reactions. Mast cells and basophils are also involved in wound healing and chronic inflammatory conditions (see Chapter 10).

Monocytes and Macrophages

Monocytes and macrophages, like granulocytes, originate from bone marrow stem cells of the myeloid lineage. Monocytes are immature macrophages and account for about 5% of the total WBC count. Monocytes circulate in the blood stream for about 3 days before they enter tissue to become macrophages. As described earlier, macrophages are found in widespread locations as part of the mononuclear phagocyte system.

Phagocytosis by macrophages is similar to that by neutrophils except that neutrophils are short lived and die in the process of fighting infection. Macrophages, in contrast, may live for months to years and can migrate in and out of tissue. Macrophages are more efficient phagocytes than neutrophils are and can ingest several times as many microorganisms. Macrophages are capable of cell division and may proliferate at the site of inflammation.

Macrophages are covered with a variety of receptor proteins on their cell surface (Figure 9-6). Some of these receptors help macrophages locate antigens that have been coated by antibodies. These receptors are called Fc receptors because they bind to the part of an antibody called the constant fragment, or Fc. Macrophages also have receptors for the complement component C3b. Complement, like antibodies, can coat an antigen and make it more recognizable to macrophages. Coating of antigen by antibodies or by complement is called **opsonization.** Macrophages have receptors that help them recognize bacteria directly. These receptors bind to particular molecules prevalent in the bacterial cell wall. For example, mannose receptors and at least 10 different Toll-like receptors on macrophages allow them to recognize common microbial structures (see Figure 9-6). Other receptors, called selectins and integrins, help macrophages stick to capillary walls, enter and move through tissue. Integrin receptors bind to proteins in the extracellular matrix and help macrophages target or "home" to certain areas.

In addition to their phagocytic function, macrophages have important secretory function. Some of the substances secreted by macrophages are cytokines, which help to coordinate the activities of other immune cells (Figure 9-7). Macrophage cytokines include IL-1, IL-6, IL-12, and tumor necrosis factor α (TNF-α). These cytokines promote inflammation, as well as the activity of other WBCs, including neutrophils and lymphocytes (see the section on cytokines).

Macrophages secrete a number of proteins that are important in wound healing. Some of these proteins are enzymes that break down tissue (collagenase, elastase, plasminogen activator), whereas others stimulate the growth of new granulation tissue (fibroblast growth factor, angiogenic factors).

A third function of macrophages, in addition to phagocytosis and secretion, is antigen presentation. For T cells to recognize antigens, these antigens must first be processed and presented on the surface of an antigen-presenting cell such as dendritic cells, macrophages, or B cells. Macrophages accomplish this task by first engulfing the antigen, then processing it into smaller pieces, and finally combining the antigen fragments with special membrane proteins. The antigen complexes are then displayed on the macrophage cell surface, where T lymphocytes (T helper cells) can recognize and become activated by them. Antigen presentation is explored in more detail in the section on Specific Adaptive Immunity.

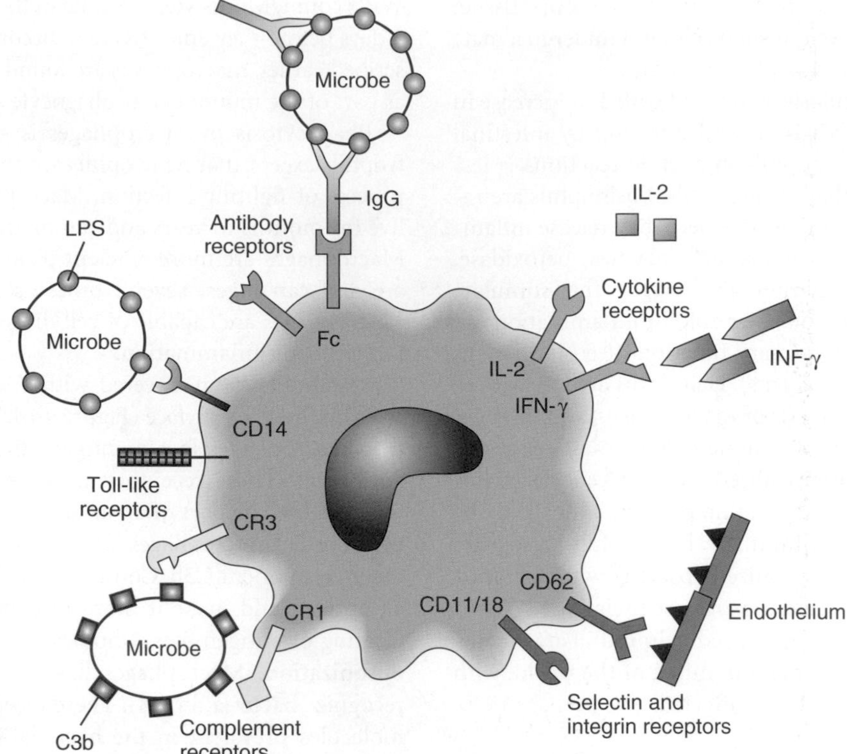

FIGURE 9-6 ■ Macrophage surface receptors. Macrophages display receptors for a number of extracellular molecules that enhance their function such as cytokines, complement, selectins, integrins, and antibody *(Fc)*. Toll-like receptors recognize patterns of microbial components and trigger intracellular signaling cascades in the macrophage. *IFN-γ*, Interferon γ; *IL*, interleukin; *LPS*, Lipopolysaccharide.

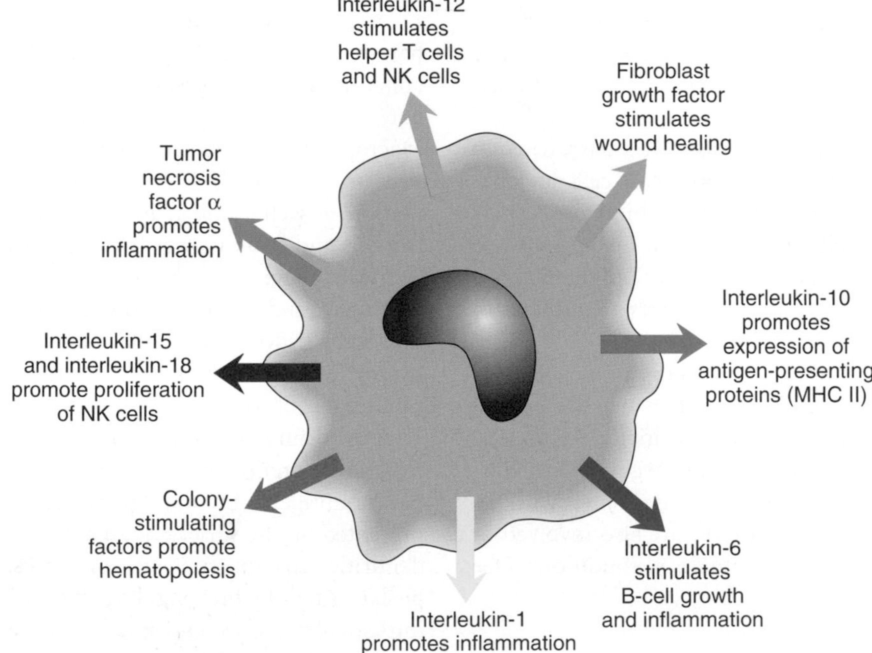

FIGURE 9-7 ■ Macrophages are of central importance in initiating inflammation and recruitment of other leukocytes to areas of need. Macrophages secrete a variety of cytokines that induce inflammation and chemotaxis. Some macrophage cytokines stimulate the growth and differentiation of other white blood cell types.

Lymphocytes

The three major types of lymphocytes are NK cells, T cells, and B cells. NK cells function in innate immunity, whereas B and T lymphocytes are the cells responsible for specific, adaptive immunity. B and T cells have the capacity to proliferate into "memory cells," which provide long-lasting immunity against specific antigens. NK, T, and B cells are derived from a common lymphoid stem cell in the bone marrow that is stimulated to proliferate by bone marrow–derived cytokines including IL-7. T cells then migrate to the thymus, where they mature. B cells remain in the bone marrow during their maturation phase. NK cells are released into the circulation. Together NK, B, and T lymphocytes compose approximately 20% of the total WBC count. Mature NK cells circulate and populate the spleen, whereas T and B cells home to secondary lymphoid organs.

Structurally, lymphocytes are small, round cells with a large, round nucleus. Despite their relatively uniform appearance, lymphocytes can be sorted into a number of subpopulations based on characteristic surface proteins called cluster of differentiation (CD) markers. More than 250 different CD markers have been identified thus far, with different immune cell types displaying different combinations on their cell surfaces. Lymphocytes have many complex and differentiated functions, and only the major lymphocyte subtypes are discussed in this chapter.

Natural Killer Cells

NK cells have no B- or T-cell markers and are not dependent on the thymus for development. NK cells are considered to be innate immune cells because they can effectively kill tumor cells and virally infected cells without previous exposure. NK cells kill their target cells by a mechanism similar to that used by cytotoxic T cells. Unlike T and B cells, NK cells can respond to a variety of antigens and are therefore not specific for a particular antigen. Like neutrophils and macrophages, NK cells recognize antibody-coated target cells with their Fc receptors. This process is called antibody-dependent cell-mediated cytotoxicity (ADCC). NK cells also target virally infected cells and tumor cells. They are thought to be able to recognize these cells because virally infected cells lack certain normal self proteins on their cell surface (major histocompatibility complex I, or MHC I, proteins). Cells that display normal MHC I are protected from NK cell cytotoxicity.

T Lymphocytes

Two major classes of T lymphocytes can be differentiated by the presence or absence of CD4 and CD8 surface proteins (Figure 9-8). T cells that possess CD4 proteins ($CD4^+$) are called

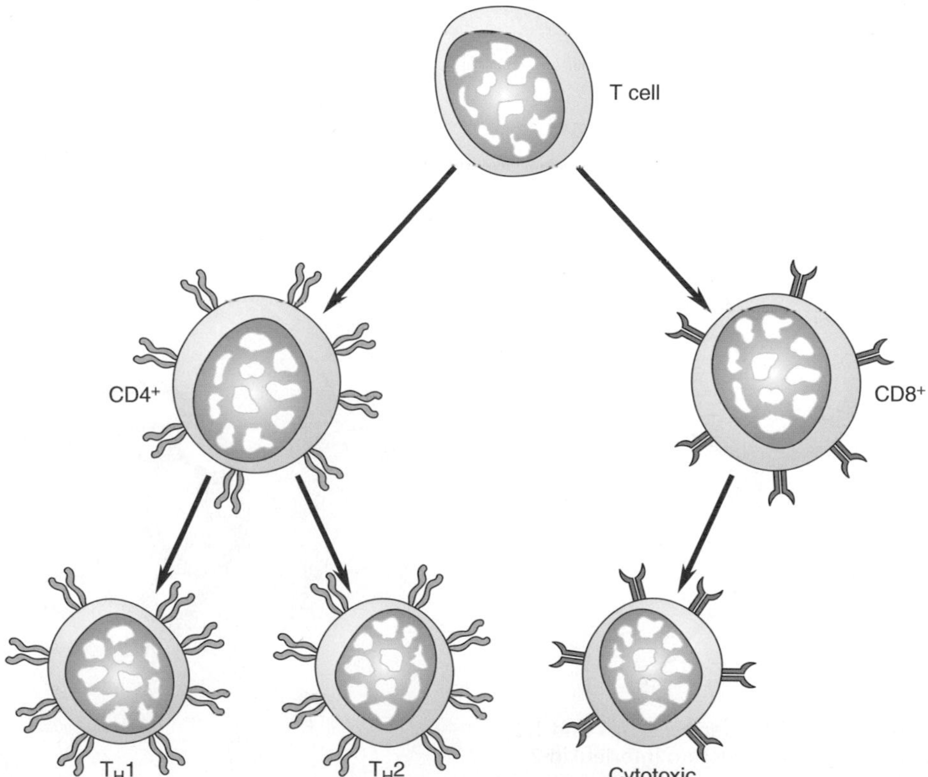

FIGURE 9-8 ■ The two major classes of T lymphocytes can be differentiated by CD markers on the cell surface. T helper cells have CD4 markers, whereas cytotoxic T cells have CD8 markers. CD4 cells can be further differentiated into T_H1 and T_H2, which secrete different cytokines. CD8 cells are cytotoxic T cells.

T helper cells. T helper cells interact with antigens presented on the surface of specialized antigen-presenting cells such as dendritic cells, macrophages, and B cells. T helper cells can be further divided into two subclasses called T_H1 and T_H2 based on the types of cytokines that they secrete (Figure 9-9). The T_H1 subset of T helper cells develops in response to IL-12 from macrophages and, when activated, secretes cytokines that activate other T cells (IL-2) and macrophages (interferon γ [IFN-γ]). T_H2 cells develop in response to IL-4 from activated T helper cells and secrete cytokines that stimulate B-cell proliferation and antibody production (e.g., IL-4, IL-5, IL-10, IL-13).[6]

The presence of CD8 protein ($CD8^+$) on a T lymphocyte characterizes it as a cytotoxic T cell. Cytotoxic T cells recognize antigen presented in association with surface proteins that can be found on all nucleated cells of the body (MHC I). When a $CD8^+$ T cell recognizes a foreign antigen on a cell, the antigen-presenting cell is killed; thus the name cytotoxic T cell. $CD8^+$ cells are particularly effective at destroying virally infected cells, foreign cells, and mutant cells. Proliferation of activated cytotoxic T cells is enhanced by T helper cell cytokines, particularly IL-2.

B Lymphocytes

B cells are distinguished from other lymphocytes by their ability to produce antibodies and by the presence of antibody-like receptors (B-cell receptors [BCRs]) on their cell surfaces. Each B cell carries many copies (100,000) of identical BCRs and is able to respond to only one antigen **epitope**[7] (Figure 9-10). B cells require "help" from T helper cells to respond efficiently to protein antigens. B cells bind and internalize the protein antigen, then process and present it to T helper cells. T cells that recognize the presented peptides bind to and are activated by the B cell. T-cell help is provided to the B cell by physical cell-to-cell contact through coreceptor binding, as well as through secreted cytokines. Some B cells can respond to nonprotein antigens such as bacterial sugar and lipid molecules. B-cell responses to nonprotein antigens are T cell independent because T cells respond only to peptide antigens. Exposure to antigens stimulates B cells to mature into antibody-secreting plasma cells and memory cells. B-cell memory cells form a reserve of cells that can quickly mount an immune response on subsequent exposure to the same antigen. Memory cells are able to survive for months to years, whereas most antibody-secreting plasma cells live for only a few days. Plasma cells are able to secrete antibodies at a rate of about 2000 per second per cell.[7] Memory B cells and plasma cells develop in germinal centers located in secondary lymphoid organs, including the lymph nodes and spleen. A few long-lived

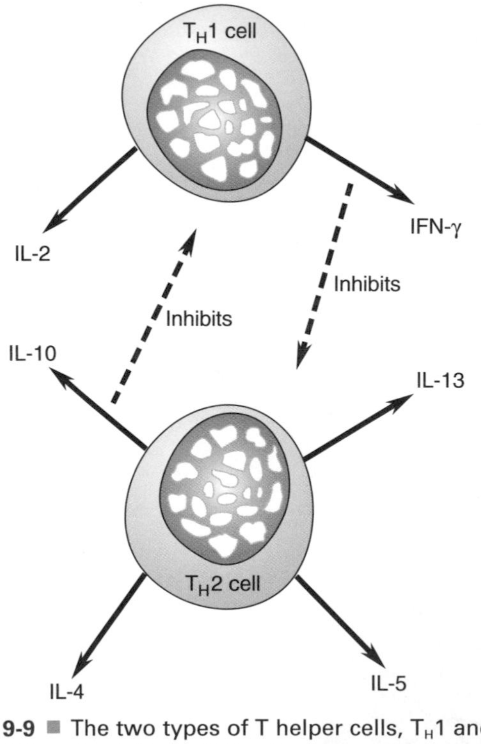

FIGURE 9-9 ■ The two types of T helper cells, T_H1 and T_H2, secrete different cytokines. T_H1 cells secrete interleukin-2 and interferon γ, which stimulate T cells and macrophages. T_H2 cells secrete a number of cytokines that affect B cells. T_H1 and T_H2 cells inhibit the release of cytokines from one another and thus help regulate the immune response. *IFN-γ,* Interferon γ; *IL,* interleukin.

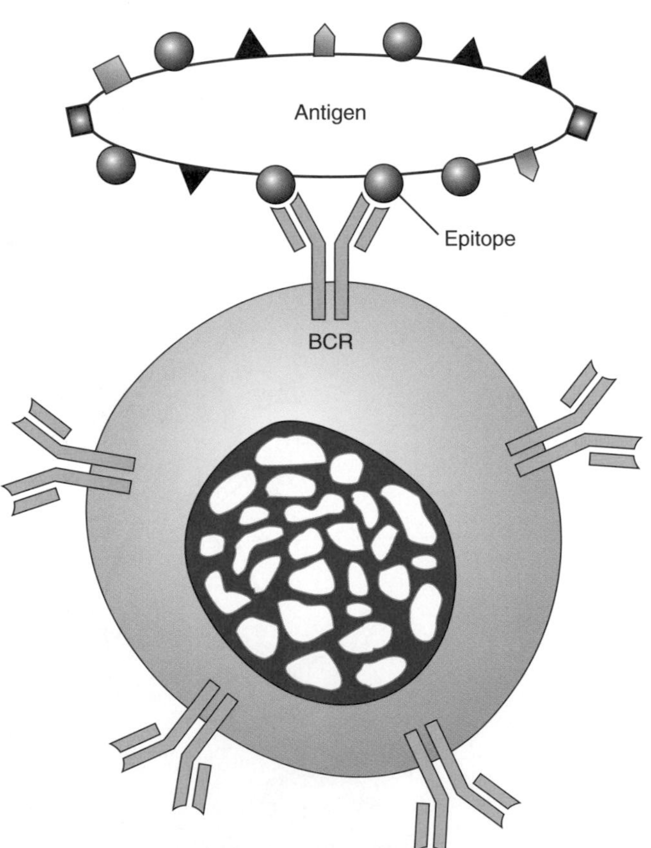

FIGURE 9-10 ■ A typical B cell showing a number of identical B-cell receptors *(BCR)* on the cell surface. Each BCR is capable of binding to two identical antigen epitopes.

plasma cells inhabit the bone marrow and continue to produce a low level of antibody, which provides immediate protection on second exposure to the same antigen. The mechanisms of specific adaptive immunity are explored later in the chapter.

CHEMICAL MEDIATORS OF IMMUNE FUNCTION

Complement

The complement system consists of about 20 plasma proteins that interact to enhance inflammation, chemotaxis, and lysis of target cells. Complement proteins are synthesized in the liver and by macrophages and neutrophils. They circulate in the blood in an inactive form. Activation of the complement cascade occurs via two different pathways: classical and alternative. In both pathways, the inactive complement proteins are converted to their active form in a sequence of reactions. Major actions of complement proteins include cell lysis, facilitation of phagocytosis by opsonization, inflammation, and chemotaxis (Figure 9-11).

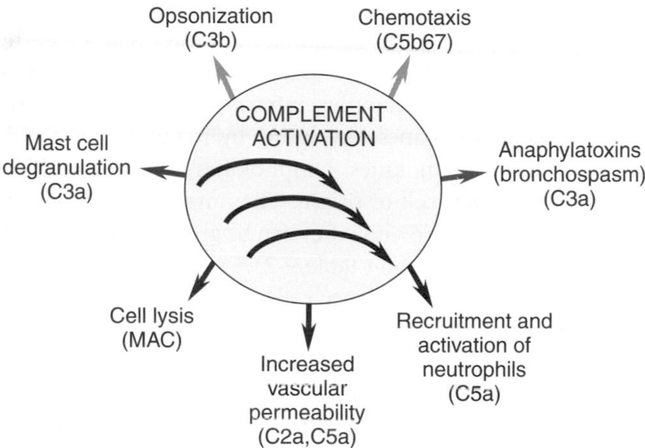

FIGURE 9-11 ■ Activation of the complement cascade results in the production of products that perform a variety of functions to augment the immune response. *MAC,* Membrane attack complex.

The classical pathway is usually triggered by IgG or IgM antibody-antigen complexes. The alternative pathway can be initiated on first exposure to an antigen. Lipopolysaccharide, in bacterial cell walls, and endotoxin are effective triggers of the alternative pathway. In the classical pathway, an antibody hooked onto an antigen combines with C1, the first of the complement proteins. This step sets in motion a domino effect called the complement cascade (Figure 9-12). The alternative pathway begins with the activation of C3. The alternative pathway can be activated on first exposure and is part of the innate immune response.[8] C3 spontaneously degrades into active C3b fragments in plasma. If microbial cell surfaces are present the C3b fragment can bind directly to the microbe. Two other complement proteins, factors B and D, combine with C3b to initiate the alternative pathway. C3 is the most important and plentiful of the complement proteins. C3 breaks down into two fragments called C3a and C3b. C3a is a proinflammatory protein that causes histamine release from mast cells, contraction of smooth muscle, and increased endothelial cell permeability. C3b initiates the next step in the cascade by cleaving C5 into its active fragments C5a and C5b. Complement protein fragment C5a is both a powerful inflammatory chemical and a potent chemotactic agent. C5a chemotaxis stimulates neutrophils and monocytes to migrate to the inflamed tissue. C5a also activates neutrophils by trig-

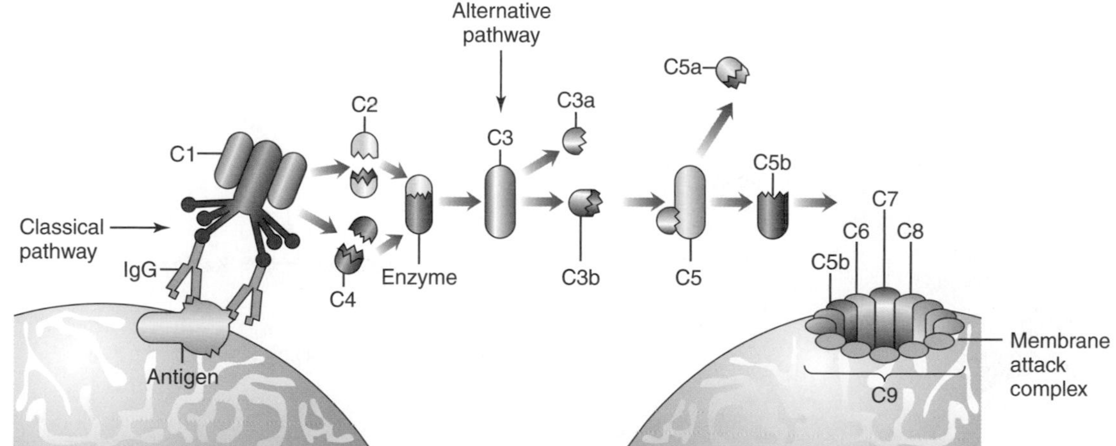

FIGURE 9-12 ■ The complement cascade is activated by the first complement molecule, C1, which binds an antigen-antibody complex. This event begins a domino effect, with each of the remaining complement proteins performing its part in the attack sequence. The end result is a hole in the membrane of the offending cell and destruction of the cell. (Redrawn from Schindler LW: *Understanding the immune system,* NIH Pub No 92-529, Bethesda, Md, 1991, U.S. Department of Health and Human Services, p 11.)

gering their oxidative activity and increasing their glucose uptake.

The C5b fragment combines with C6, C7, C8, and multiple units of C9 to form a large porelike structure (C5b6789) called the membrane attack complex. The membrane attack complex has a direct cytotoxic effect by attacking cell membranes and disrupting the lipid bilayer. This action allows free movement of sodium and water into the target cell, which causes it to rupture (Figure 9-13). The complement system is a potent inflammatory and cytotoxic system that is carefully regulated by a number of inhibitory factors. Normal host cells produce membrane and plasma proteins that prevent complement binding to their surface (e.g., C1 inhibitor, protein S).

Kinins

Bradykinin and kallidin are two of the many kinins present in the body. Kinins are small polypeptides that cause powerful vasodilation. They are especially active in the inflammatory process. The kinin system is linked to the clotting system via the Hageman factor (XII) and is activated with the activation of clotting.[1] The first step in this process is the conversion of factor XII to factor XIIa (Figure 9-14). Factor XIIa converts a substance known as prekallikrein to kallikrein. Kallikrein converts precursor substances known as kininogens to kinins. The most prevalent is kallidin, which is then converted to bradykinin. Activated kinins cause increased vascular permeability, vasodilation, and smooth muscle contraction. Kinins are also responsible for pain, which is one of the classic signs of inflammation.

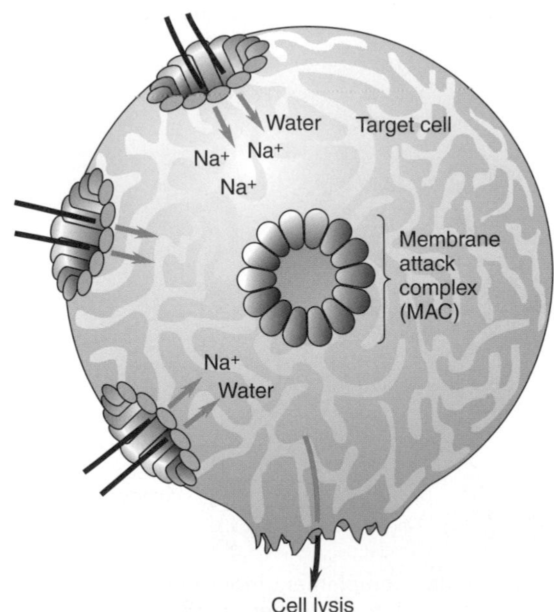

FIGURE 9-13 ■ Activation of the complement cascade results in the formation of membrane attack complexes that insert in the cell membrane. These porelike structures allow sodium and water influx, which causes the cell to swell and rupture.

Clotting Factors

The blood coagulation cascade's major purpose is to stop bleeding. It is also intimately involved in inflammation and triggering of the kinin system. The key linkage between the inflammatory response and clotting system is activated factor XII (Hageman factor) (see Figure 9-14). (The blood coagulation cascade is discussed in detail in Chapter 14.) Activation of the coagulation cascade results in the formation of insoluble fibrin strands, which provide an effective barrier to the spread of infection. Clot formation also activates the fibrinolytic cascade, which breaks down fibrin proteins. Some of the fibrin degradation products are chemotactic signals for neutrophils.

Cytokines

Cytokines are polypeptide signaling molecules that affect the function of other cells by stimulating surface receptors. Cytokines function in a complex intercellular communication network. WBC cytokines have gone by many names previously, including monokines, lymphokines, and interleukins, depending on their cell of origin. The number of known cytokines is large and growing; they can be grouped according to their source and function (Table 9-2).

Macrophages and T helper cells are the main sources of immune system cytokines. These cytokines generally function as chemotactic factors (chemokines), antiviral factors, mediators of inflammation, hematopoietic factors, or activation signals for specific types of WBCs. The major cytokines produced by macrophages are shown in Figure 9-7. T helper cells of the T_H1 subclass produce two main cytokines, IL-2 and IFN-γ, whereas T_H2 cells secrete a number of cytokines important to B-cell function (see Figure 9-9). Cytokines function to enhance and coordinate both innate and specific immune defenses. They are discussed in more detail in the sections that follow.

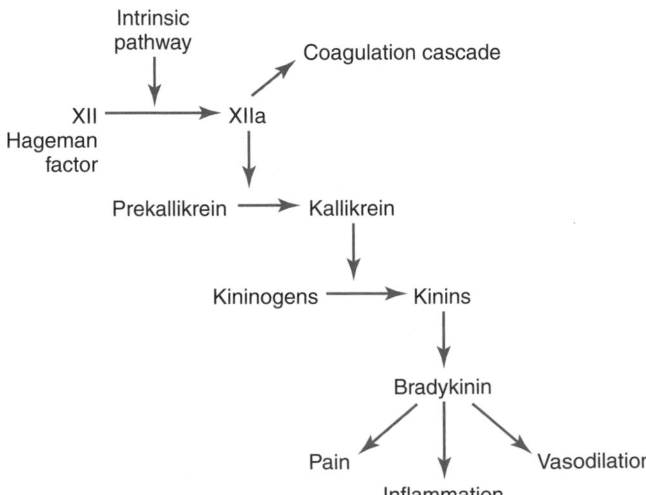

FIGURE 9-14 ■ The common linkage of the kinin and coagulation systems through the activation of factor XII (Hageman factor). *XIIa,* Active factor XII.

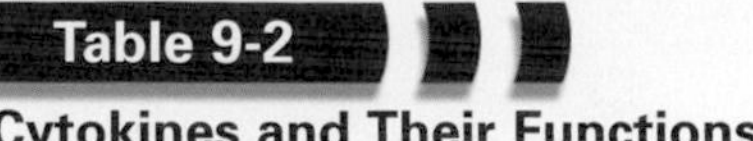

Cytokines and Their Functions

Cytokine	Origin	Function
IFN-α	Secreted by macrophages and induced by RNA or DNA viruses and by single- or double-stranded polyribonucleotide	Inhibits virus replication, toxic to cancer cells, stimulates leukocytes, facilitates NK cell activity, produces fever, increases B- and T-cell activity
IFN-β	Secreted by fibroblasts and induced by RNA or DNA viruses and by single- or double-stranded polyribonucleotide	Inhibits virus replication, toxic to cancer cells, facilitates NK cell activity, produces fever
IFN-γ	Lymphokine secreted by activated T cells, (T_H1 and $CD8^+$) and NK cells	Inhibits virus replication, promotes antigen expression, activates macrophages, inhibits cell growth, induces myeloid cell lines, promotes B-cell switch to IgG
IL-1	Monokine, mononuclear phagocyte	Stimulates T cells and macrophages; induces acute phase reaction of inflammation, IL-2 secretion, fever production; similar to TNF and endogenous pyrogen
IL-2	Lymphokine secreted mainly by T helper cells (T_H1)	Promotes growth of T cells, enhances function of NK cells, assists T-cell maturation in thymus, B-cell proliferation
IL-3	Synthesized by T cells, endothelial cells, fibroblasts, other cells	Induces proliferation and differentiation of other lymphocytes, pluripotent stem cells, mast cells, granulocytes
IL-4	T helper cells (T_H2)	Promotes T-cell/B-cell interactions, promotes synthesis of IgE by B cell and T_H2 cell growth, promotes mast cell and hematopoietic cell growth
IL-5	Lymphokine secreted by T helper cells (T_H2)	Promotes growth and differentiation of B cells to secrete IgA, induces differentiation of eosinophils
IL-6	Cytokine secreted by mononuclear phagocytes, T helper cells (T_H2), tumors, and nonlymphoid cells (e.g., endothelium)	Promotes immunoglobulin secretion by B cells, induces fever, promotes release of inflammation factors from liver cells, promotes differentiation of hematopoietic stem cells and nerve cells
IL-7	Stromal cells in bone marrow	Stimulates immature lymphocytes to divide
IL-8	Macrophages	Enhances inflammation and chemotaxis (CXCL chemokine)
IL-9	T_H2 cells	Enhances growth of T helper cells
IL-10	T_H2 cells and macrophages	Inhibits activation of T_H1 cells and macrophages, inhibits IL-12 production
IL-11	Stromal cells in bone marrow	Stimulates platelet production
IL-12	Macrophages, dendritic cells	Enhances T_H1 cell activities and release of IFN-γ by T cells and NK cells
IL-13	T_H2 cells	Stimulates B-cell growth and IgE production, suppresses macrophages
IL-14	T cells	Induces B-cell proliferation
IL-15	Macrophages (esp. viral infection)	Similar actions to IL-2, enhances proliferation of T cells (CD8) and NK cells
IL-16	$CD8^+$ T cells	$CD4^+$ cell chemotaxis, suppresses viral replication of HIV
IL-17	$CD4^+$ T cells	Stimulates production of TNF-α, IL-l, and chemokine
IL-18	Macrophages in response to microbes	Increases NK cell proliferation and secretion of IFN-γ by T_H1
IL-19	Uncertain	Similar to IL-10?
IL-20	Uncertain	Similar to IL-10?
IL-21	Uncertain	Similar to IL-15, stimulates production of NK cells
IL-22	Uncertain	Similar to IL-10?
IL-23	Uncertain	Similar to IL-12, stimulates cell-mediated immunity
IL-24	Uncertain	Similar to IL-10?
IL-25	T_H2 cells	Stimulates production of cytokines by the T_H2 cells
TNF-α	Macrophages	Induces leukocytosis, fever, weight loss, inflammation, necrosis of some tumors; stimulates lymphokine synthesis; activates macrophages; toxic to viruses and tumor cells
TNF-β	T cells	Inhibits B-cell and T-cell proliferation
G-CSF, M-CSF, GM-CSF	Macrophages, T cells, fibroblasts	Stimulates granulocyte and monocyte production in the bone marrow
TGF-β	T cells, macrophages	Inhibits T cells, B cells, and macrophages
Chemokines		
CXCL 1-13	Macrophages and various cells in tissues	Recruitment of neutrophils, macrophages, lymphocytes
CCL 1-28	Macrophages and various cells in tissues	Recruitment of neutrophils, macrophages, lymphocytes

GM-CSF, Granulocyte-macrophage colony-stimulating factor; *HIV,* human immunodeficiency virus; *IFN,* interferon; *IL,* interleukin; *NK,* natural killer; *TNF,* tumor necrosis factor; *TGF,* transforming growth factor.

KEY CONCEPTS

- The primary lymphoid organs are the thymus and bone marrow. T cells develop in the thymus, whereas B cells develop in the bone marrow. Mature lymphocytes then migrate to secondary lymphoid structures, including the spleen and lymph nodes.
- Blood cells are produced in the bone marrow in response to specific hematopoietic growth factors. Granulocytes (neutrophils, basophils, eosinophils) and monocytes (macrophages) are phagocytic cells that provide innate protection. Lymphocytes (B cells, T cells) are specific cells that react only to particular antigens. NK cells are lymphocytes that lack T and B cell markers and function in innate immune responses. Other blood components produced by bone marrow are erythrocytes and platelets.
- Neutrophils are the most numerous WBCs in blood. A large storage pool lies in the bone marrow and can be mobilized in response to antigen. Neutrophils are the predominant WBC type in early infection. They migrate to the area by following chemotactic factors and perform phagocytic functions. During acute bacterial infection, larger numbers of immature neutrophils (bands) are released into the blood, which is termed a "shift to the left."
- Monocytes located in tissue are called macrophages. Monocytes and macrophages are distributed in strategic locations throughout the body, including the skin, lungs, gastrointestinal tract, liver, spleen, and lymph. Macrophages are powerful phagocytes and are predominant in late inflammation.
- T lymphocytes, the major effectors of cell-mediated immunity, interact with specific antigens on cell surfaces. They are important in immunity against foreign, infected, or mutant cells. In addition, they secrete cytokines that boost the immune response of B cells and other cell types. T cells are composed of two main subtypes called CD4 (helper) and CD8 (cytotoxic). B lymphocytes are the major effectors of antibody-mediated immunity.
- The complement system consists of about 20 plasma proteins that interact in a cascade fashion to produce important mediators of inflammation and immunity. The cascade can be activated by microbial antigens (alternative pathway) or by antigen-antibody complexes (classical pathway).
- Cytokines are peptide factors released by immune cells. They have many functions, including as inflammatory mediators, chemotaxins, intercellular communication signals, growth factors, and growth inhibitors. Macrophages and lymphocytes are important sources of immune cytokines.

INNATE DEFENSES AND INFLAMMATION

Inflammation occurs when cells are injured, regardless of the cause of the injury. It is a protective mechanism that also begins the healing process. The inflammatory response has three purposes: (1) to neutralize and destroy invading and harmful agents, (2) to limit the spread of harmful agents to other tissue, and (3) to prepare any damaged tissue for repair. Inflammatory reactions increase capillary permeability such that phagocytic cells, complement, and antibodies can leave the blood stream and enter tissues where they are needed.

Five cardinal signs of inflammation have been described: (1) redness (rubor), (2) swelling (tumor), (3) heat (calor), (4) pain (dolor), and (5) loss of function (functio laesa). The suffix *itis* is commonly used to describe conditions associated with inflammation. For example, appendicitis, tendinitis, and nephritis refer to inflammation of the appendix, tendon, and kidney, respectively.

Inflammation can be caused by many conditions. Any injury to tissue will evoke an inflammatory response. Injury can arise from sources outside the body (exogenous) or from sources inside the body (endogenous). Surgery, trauma, burns, and skin injury from chemicals are all examples of exogenous injuries. Endogenous injuries may result from tissue ischemia such as myocardial infarction or pulmonary embolism.

Inflammation and infection are commonly confused because they often coexist. Under normal conditions, infection is always accompanied by inflammation; however, not all inflammation involves an infectious agent. For example, inflammation can occur with sprain injuries to joints, myocardial infarction, sterile surgical incisions, thrombophlebitis, and blister formation as a result of either temperature extremes or mechanical trauma.

Inflammation may be categorized as either acute or chronic. Acute inflammation is short in duration, lasting less than 2 weeks, and involves a discrete set of events. Chronic inflammation tends to be more diffuse, extends over a longer period, and may result in the formation of scar tissue and deformity.

INFLAMMATION

The inflammatory response is remarkably the same, regardless of the cause. Events in the inflammatory process include (1) increased vascular permeability, (2) recruitment and emigration of leukocytes, and (3) phagocytosis of antigens and debris. The inflammatory response is outlined in Figure 9-15.

Increased Vascular Permeability

Immediately after injury, the precapillary arterioles around the injured area contract briefly, which causes a short period of vasoconstriction. The amount of vasoconstriction depends on the degree of vascular injury and is usually of little significance.[9] Vasoconstriction is followed by a prolonged period of vasodilation. A number of vasoactive chemicals are released during the inflammatory process, including histamine, prostaglandins, and leukotrienes (Table 9-3). Mast cells are an important source of these inflammatory chemicals. Mast cells in the area of injury degranulate and release packets of histamine and other inflammatory chemicals. One of the early actions of these mediators is to vasodilate and cause endothelial cells to begin contraction and rounding up, thus increasing capillary permeability. The greater volume of blood increases the amount of pressure within the blood vessels (hydrostatic pressure). The increased pressure along with increased permeability pushes fluid out of the blood vessels and into the surrounding tissue. Because of the dilated blood vessels and open capillaries, more blood is carried to the injured area and contributes to the redness, pain, heat, and swelling of inflammation (Figure 9-16).

Histamine is an early mediator of this inflammatory response. It is such a potent vasodilator that it can cause significant reductions in blood pressure when released in excessive amounts. Histamine also causes bronchial constriction and mucus production. Histamine receptor blocking agents are widely used in allergic reactions to suppress these inflammatory actions of histamine.

Prostaglandins and leukotrienes are phospholipid compounds formed from arachidonic acid. The prostaglandins involved in inflammation contribute to vasodilation, increased

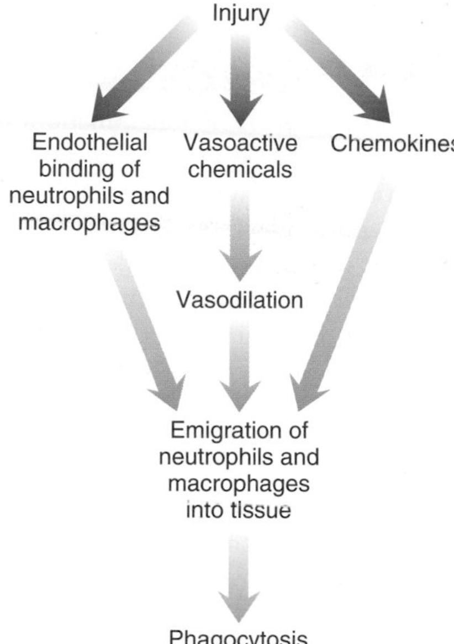

FIGURE 9-15 ■ Tissue injury stimulates the release of a number of chemical mediators that promote vasodilation, chemotaxis, and binding of neutrophils and macrophages to area capillaries. These events facilitate the emigration of neutrophils and macrophages into the tissue, where they begin phagocytosis.

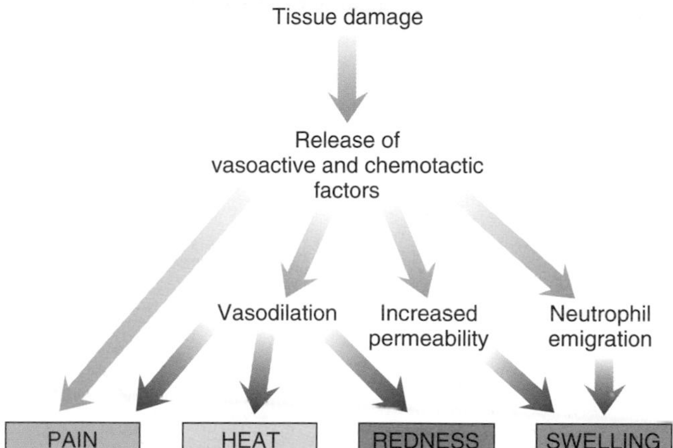

FIGURE 9-16 ■ The cardinal signs of acute inflammation result mainly from vasodilation and increased vascular permeability.

Table 9-3

Mediators of Acute Inflammation

Mediator	Vasodilation	Increased Permeability: Immediate	Increased Permeability: Sustained	Chemotaxis	Opsonin	Pain
Histamine	+	+++	–	–	–	–
Serotonin (5-HT)	+	+	–	–	–	–
Bradykinin	+	+	–	–	–	++
Complement 3a	–	+	–	–	–	–
Complement 3b	–	–	–	–	+++	–
Complement 5a	–	+	–	+++	–	–
Prostaglandin (E_2)	+++	+	+?	–	–	–
Leukotrienes (B_4, D_4)	–	+++	+?	+++	–	–
Lysosomal proteases	–	–	++*	–	–	–
Oxygen radicals	–	–	++*	–	–	–

Data From Roitt I et al: *Immunology,* ed 6, St Louis, 2001, Mosby.
*Proteases and oxygen-based free radicals derived from neutrophils are believed to mediate a sustained increase in permeability by means of their damage to endothelial cells.

permeability, and platelet aggregation (Figure 9-17). Prostaglandin D_2 also acts as a chemotactic factor and stimulates neutrophil emigration. Prostaglandins cause pain by enhancing the sensitivity of pain receptors.[9] They arise from the cyclooxygenase pathway and can be inhibited by drugs that block enzymes in this pathway, such as aspirin.

Five types of leukotrienes are generated from the lipoxygenase pathway: A_4, B_4, C_4, D_4, and E_4. Leukotriene B_4 is a potent chemotactic agent that causes aggregation of leukocytes; leukotrienes C_4, D_4, and E_4 all cause smooth muscle contraction, bronchospasm, and increased vascular permeability.[9] Leukotriene receptor blocking agents can be used to inhibit the inflammatory actions of these chemicals.

During the early phase of tissue inflammation, platelets move into the site and adhere to exposed vascular collagen. The platelets release fibronectin to form a meshwork trap and stimulate the intrinsic clotting cascade to help reduce bleeding. Platelets release a number of peptide growth factors, including platelet-derived growth factor and insulin-like growth factor.[10] Platelet-derived growth factor stimulates fibroblast cell proliferation, and insulin-like growth factor type I is a potent vascular endothelial cell chemotactic factor. Triggering of the blood coagulation cascade also occurs and leads to the formation of a fibrin clot. Usually, early clot formation occurs within several minutes. Fibrin is also deposited in the lymph system, where it causes lymphatic blockage. Lymphatic blockage "walls off" the area of inflammation from the surrounding tissue and delays the spread of toxins.

The vascular changes that occur soon after injury are beneficial to the injured tissue because irritating or toxic agents are diluted by the fluid that leaks out of the blood vessels into surrounding tissue. In addition, when the fluid leaves the blood vessels, the remaining blood becomes viscous (thick) and circulation is slowed, facilitating neutrophil emigration.

Emigration of Leukocytes

As blood flows through areas of inflammation, neutrophils move to the sides of the blood vessels and roll along the endothelium of the vessel wall. This process is referred to as margination or pavementing. Normally, neutrophils slide past the capillary endothelial cells and do not stick. Injured tissue triggers the expression of adhesion molecules on the surface of endothelial cells, and the adhesion molecules bind to receptors on neutrophils (Figure 9-18). These receptors, called se-

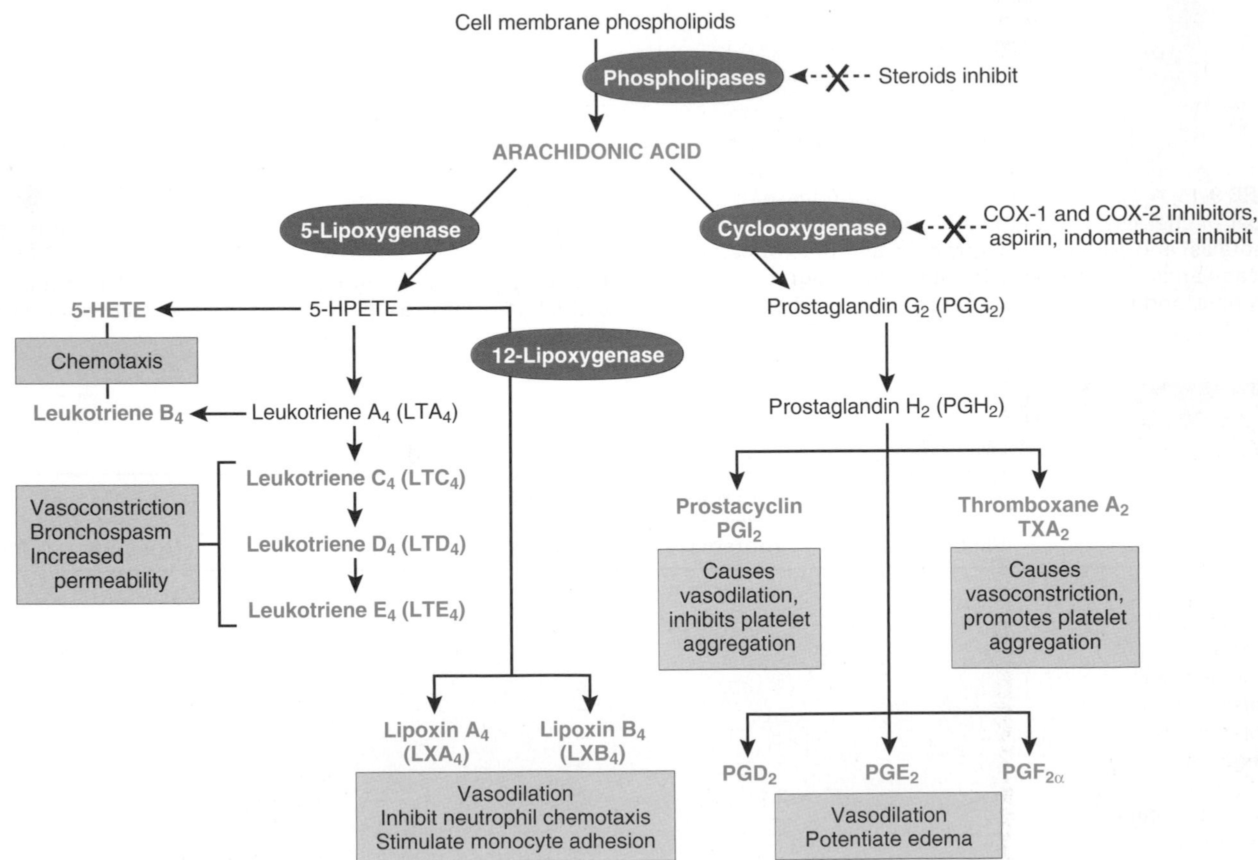

FIGURE 9-17 ■ Generation of prostaglandins, thromboxane, and leukotrienes from arachidonic acid and roles in inflammation. (From Kumar V, Cotran RS, Robbins SL: *Robbins basic pathology,* ed 7, Philadelphia, 2003, Saunders, p 281.)

lectins, help neutrophils stick and roll along the capillary endothelial surface.[3] Binding to and subsequent movement through the capillary wall are accomplished by another group of receptors called integrins. Chemokines present on the endothelium enhance the binding affinity of integrins so the neutrophil can attach firmly to the vessel wall. This process of passing through the blood vessel walls and migrating to the inflamed tissue is referred to as emigration or diapedesis. Diapedesis begins within a few minutes to hours of injury. Even though the spaces between endothelial cells lining the vessels are much smaller than the neutrophils, neutrophils are able to slide through a small portion at a time.

Neutrophils are attracted to the inflamed tissue by a process called **chemotaxis.** Biochemical mediators that attract neutrophils include bacterial toxins, degenerative products of the inflamed tissue, the C5a complement fragment, and other substances. Neutrophils are thus guided through the tissue to an area of injury by these chemicals. Because neutrophils are highly mobile, they are first on the scene to begin phagocytosis and production of collagenase to break down dead tissue. Monocytes are slightly slower to arrive at an area of inflammation but use a similar process of emigration to gain entry to the area of tissue injury.

Eosinophils and NK cells also respond to the site of inflammation. Eosinophils are rich in chemical mediators such as hydrolases and peroxidases, which may contribute to the inflammatory process. NK cells are most effective in recognizing virally infected cells and opsonized microbes.

Phagocytosis

Once neutrophils and monocytes (macrophages) enter the tissue, they begin the process of phagocytosis (Figure 9-19). These cells produce a wide variety of enzymes that digest protein structures. Some of these enzymes include lysozyme, neutral proteases, collagenase, elastase, and acid hydrolases. Neutrophils and macrophages specialize in collagen and extracellular matrix degradation. Peptide bonds are cleaved in the extracellular matrix by collagenase, elastase, proteinase, and gelatinase. If the microbe is small enough to be internalized, it will be captured by the phagocyte and endocytosed into a phagosome. The phagosome then merges with a lysosome con-

On blood test (WBC) if neutrophils are high or left sided shift something acute going on.

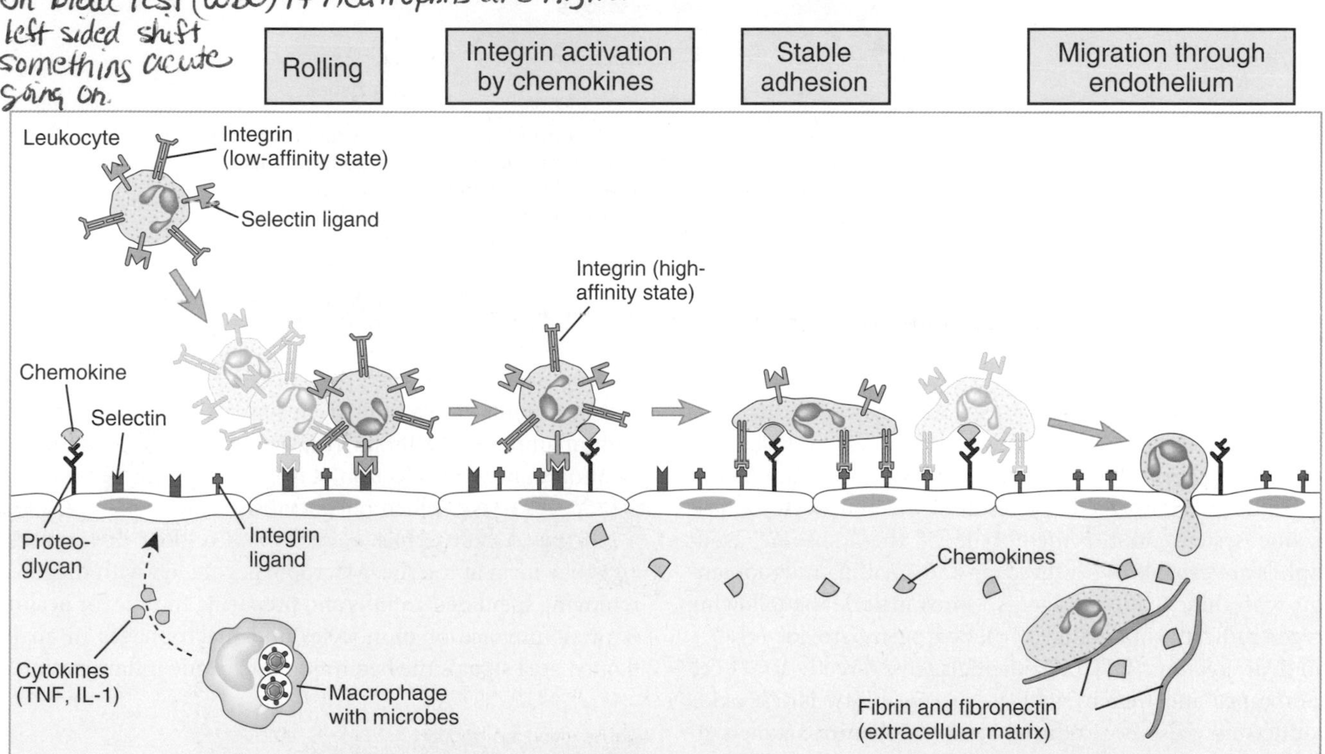

FIGURE 9-18 ■ Emigration of neutrophils from the blood stream into tissue is mediated by receptor interactions with the capillary endothelium. With inflammation and injury, endothelial cells begin to express binding molecules on their cell surfaces (selectins). Leukocytes also have selectins, which can bind to endothelial adhesion proteins. The selectin interactions cause the leukocytes to stick and roll. Chemokines on the surface of endothelial cells interact with neutrophils (and macrophages) to increase the binding affinity of integrin receptors on leukocytes. Firm attachment and diapedesis through the capillary wall is facilitated by integrins, which allow the neutrophils to bind to endothelial cells and extracellular matrix and then pull themselves into the tissue. *TNF,* Tumor necrosis factor; *IL,* interleukin. (From Abbas AK, Lichtman AH: *Cellular and molecular immunology,* ed 5, Philadelphia, 2003, Saunders, p 281.)

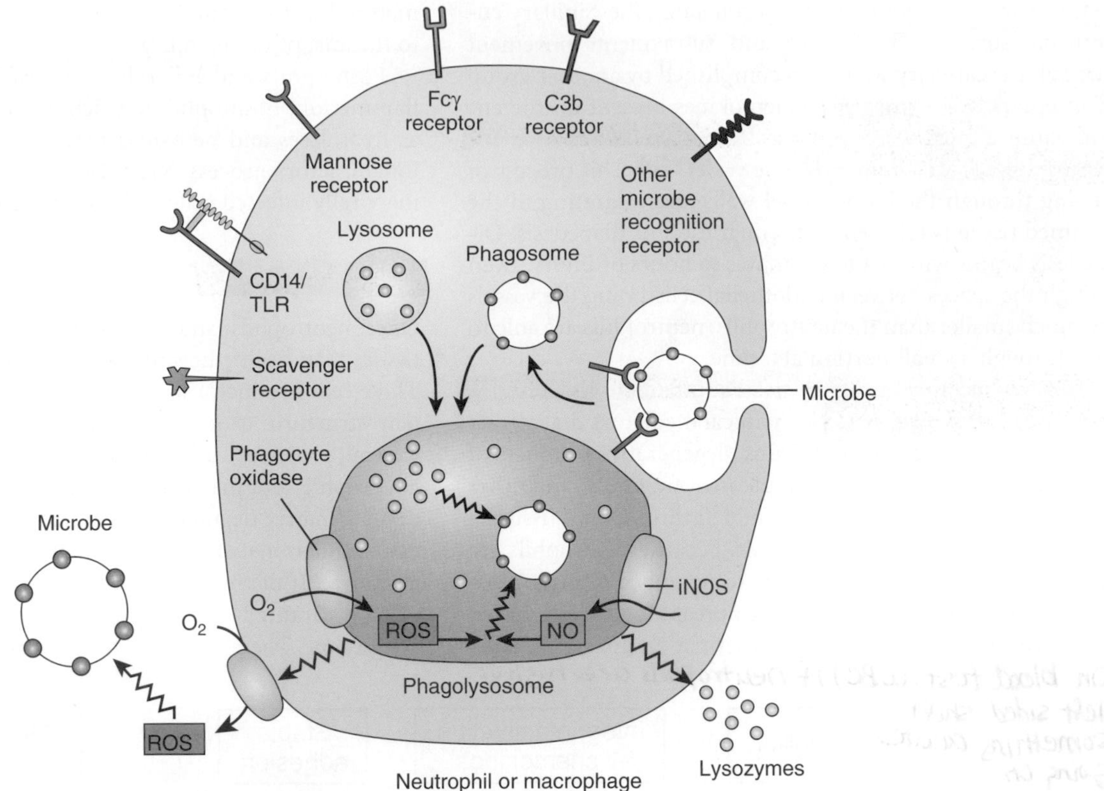

FIGURE 9-19 ■ Neutrophils and macrophages have a number of different receptors on their surface that enable them to bind to components of microbes or to opsonins like IgG and complement. Bound microbes are internalized into phagosomes that fuse with lysosomes containing numerous enzymes. Some of these enzymes degrade proteins (proteolytic) and others such as oxidase and inducible nitric oxide synthase *(iNOS)* produce free radicals that attack molecular bonds. When phagocytes are strongly stimulated or microbes are too large to internalize, the lysosomal enzymes may be activated or released at the cell surface causing tissue damage and inflammation. *ROS,* Reactive oxygen species.

taining degradative enzymes. Large antigens may trigger the neutrophil to release its degradative enzymes extracellularly.

Oxidizing agents, the most destructive of the inflammatory cell products, are formed as a result of the phagocyte oxidase enzyme system on the membrane of the lysosome. Neutrophils are capable of synthesizing and assailing microorganisms with these oxidizing agents, which include the following oxygen radicals: superoxide (O_2^-), hydrogen peroxide (H_2O_2), and hydroxyl ions (OH^-). Oxidizing agents directly attack cell membranes and thereby increase permeability. Nitric oxide products may also be produced by inducible nitric oxide synthase (iNOS) and function in concert with oxygen radicals to attack microbial molecules[1] (see Figure 9-19).

Because acute inflammation can cause severe tissue damage, it is not surprising that a system of inactivators is present. An important inhibitor of inflammatory damage is α_1-antiprotease. Antiproteases are made in the liver and circulate continuously in the blood stream. α_1-Antiprotease inhibits the destructive proteases released from activated neutrophils. A deficiency of antiproteases can predispose an individual to inflammatory tissue destruction.

Neutrophils have a limited capacity to phagocytose foreign and inflammatory debris. Once the neutrophil leaves the circulation to fight an infection, it is unable to exit the tissue and will die at the site. When phagocytosis is incomplete, a collection of dead neutrophils, bacteria, and cellular debris, called pus, may form at the site. Macrophages are left with the job of removing spent neutrophils and preparing the site for healing. A predominance of monocytes and macrophages in an inflamed area signals the beginning of chronic inflammation.

Chronic Inflammation

Macrophages are essential for wound healing because of their phagocytic and débridement functions. Macrophages produce proteases that help in removing foreign protein from the wound. Macrophages also release tissue thromboplastin to facilitate hemostasis and stimulate fibroblast activity. Macrophages secrete other peptide growth factors such as angiogenic factor, which encourages the growth of new blood vessels. Macrophages also phagocytose spent neutrophils and their degradation products so they do not interfere with healing. Prolonged inflammation may impair healing and result in an accumulation of macrophages, fibroblasts, and collagen, called a granuloma. Granulomas are usually evident on examination of tissue biopsy as clusters of macrophages surrounding particulate matter or resistance microbes such as *Mycobacterium tuberculosis.* Fibrosis and scarring are evident because normal parenchyma is replaced with fibrous tissue.

HEALING

Inflammatory responses can terminate or be resolved in several ways over time. Usually the reconstructive phase begins 3 to 4 days after injury and persists for 2 weeks. The major cells involved in this phase include fibroblasts, endothelial cells, and myofibroblasts.

Fibroblasts are found all over the body and are thought to originate in mesenchymal primitive tissue. They synthesize connective tissue and are able to migrate. Fibroblasts are stimulated to make collagen, proteoglycans, and fibronectin by a variety of growth factors.[10] Macrophages secrete lactate and release growth factors that stimulate fibroblasts. Fibroblasts respond to contact and density inhibition and thereby facilitate orderly cellular growth. Myofibroblasts develop at the wound edge and induce wound contraction.

Endothelial cells grow into the connective tissue gel stimulated by angiogenic substances. They usually develop capillary beds from existing vessels. The new capillaries can bring in nutrients for tissue repair and wound healing. However, because the new capillaries are leaky, they contribute to continuing edema.

Regeneration of damaged tissue into the preexisting tissue type requires survival of the basement membrane and tissue stem cells. Some cell types regenerate constantly; among these types are the epithelial cells of the skin and mucous membranes, bone marrow cells, and lymphoid cells. Cells of the liver, pancreas, endocrine glands, and renal tubules are also able to regenerate when necessary. However, some cell types, such as neurons and muscle cells, regenerate poorly. The maturation phase of wound healing occurs several weeks after the injury and may last for 2 years or more. It is characterized by wound remodeling by fibroblasts, macrophages, neutrophils, and eosinophils. Wound remodeling is the process of collagen deposition and lysis with débridement of the wound edges. During this phase the wound changes color from bright red to pink to whitish. As long as a wound is pink, the maturation phase is not completed.

INFLAMMATORY EXUDATES

Exudate is fluid that leaks out of blood vessels, combined with neutrophils and the debris from phagocytosis. Exudates may vary in composition, but all types have similar functions, including (1) transport of leukocytes and antibodies, (2) dilution of toxins and irritating substances, and (3) transport of the nutrients necessary for tissue repair.

Serous exudate is watery, has a low protein content, and is similar to the fluid that collects under a blister. This type of exudate generally accompanies mild inflammation. With mild inflammation, the permeability of the blood vessels is not greatly changed. As a result, only some protein molecules escape from vessels, and serous exudate, with a low protein content, develops.

With greater injury, more inflammation occurs and the blood vessels become more permeable. Because of this increased permeability, more protein can pass through the vessel walls. Fibrinogen, a large protein molecule, can pass through a highly permeable blood vessel wall. *Fibrinous exudate* is sticky and thick and may have to be removed to allow healing; otherwise, scar tissue and adhesions may develop. However, in some instances fibrinous exudate may be beneficial. In the case of acute appendicitis, fibrinous exudate may actually wall off and localize the infection and prevent its spread.

Purulent exudate is called pus. Purulent exudate generally occurs in severe inflammation accompanied by bacterial infection and is primarily composed of neutrophils, protein, and tissue debris. Large pockets of purulent exudate, called abscesses, must generally be removed or drained for healing to take place.

Hemorrhagic exudate has a large component of red blood cells. This type of exudate is usually present with the most severe inflammation. Hemorrhagic exudate occurs with severe leakage from blood vessels or after necrosis or breakdown of blood vessels.

SYSTEMIC MANIFESTATIONS OF INFLAMMATION

Inflammation is associated with both localized and systemic signs and symptoms. The localized symptoms, described previously, occur with both acute and chronic inflammation. Depending on the magnitude of injury and the resistance of the individual, localized inflammation can lead to systemic involvement. Systemic responses include fever, neutrophilia (increased blood neutrophil count), lethargy, and muscle catabolism. Three macrophage-derived cytokines—IL-1, IL-6, and TNF-α—are responsible for most of the systemic effects of inflammation.[9]

TNF-α and IL-1 act on the brain to raise body temperature, induce sleep, and suppress appetite. By raising the set point for body temperature, these cytokines induce conservation of heat through vasoconstriction, as well as increased heat production through shivering. An increase in body temperature is assumed to improve the immune response; however, the mechanism is unclear. IL-1 is responsible for stimulating the release of neutrophils from bone marrow storage sites, thus producing neutrophilia. All three cytokines act on skeletal muscle to enhance protein catabolism, which provides an available pool of amino acids for efficient antibody production by plasma cells.

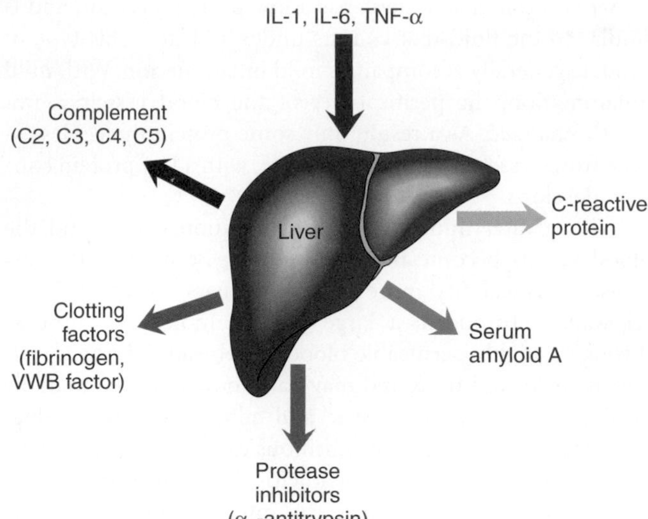

FIGURE 9-20 ■ The liver is a target for three important cytokines, interleukin-1 *(IL-1),* IL-6, and tumor necrosis factor α *(TNF-α).* In response to these cytokines, the liver releases a number of proteins, collectively called acute phase proteins.

The liver is an important target for IL-1, IL-6, and TNF-α. These cytokines induce the liver to release a number of proteins collectively called acute phase proteins, which include complement components, clotting factors, and protease inhibitors (Figure 9-20). Two of the most important acute phase proteins are C-reactive protein (CRP) and serum amyloid A. Both are thought to have important roles in controlling inflammation to prevent excessive tissue damage.[9]

When the liver releases acute phase proteins, the level of fibrinogen in the serum is increased. Fibrinogen coats the surface of red blood cells and reduces their charge so that they aggregate more readily. A blood test called the erythrocyte sedimentation rate (ESR, "sed. rate") provides a simple measure of the level of inflammation in an individual. Thus an elevated ESR indicates the presence of inflammation in the body. The greater the inflammation, the faster the red blood cells settle to the bottom of a test tube and the higher the ESR. The ESR is a nonspecific but clinically useful indicator of inflammation. Serum CRP activity is also used as a nonspecific indicator of inflammation in a manner similar to the ESR.

KEY CONCEPTS

- Previous exposure to foreign antigens is not required for the activation of innate immune defenses. Inflammation is an important aspect of innate immunity that involves localization of harmful agents and the bringing of phagocytic cells to the area. Classic manifestations of inflammation are redness, swelling, heat, pain, and loss of function.
- Inflammatory chemicals such as histamine, prostaglandins, and leukotrienes are released from injured tissues, mast cells, macrophages, and neutrophils. These chemicals increase vascular permeability, vasodilate, and attract immune cells to the area (chemotaxis).
- Phagocytes migrate to the inflamed area, collect at the side of the vessel, and squeeze through into the tissue. Emigration of neutrophils and macrophages is facilitated by selectins and integrins present on the surface of endothelial cells and leukocytes. Neutrophils arrive in large numbers in acute bacterial infection and begin active phagocytosis. Neutrophils and macrophages produce proteolytic enzymes and oxidizing agents to destroy and digest antigens. With chronic inflammation, macrophages and lymphocytes predominate.
- Healing is mediated by growth factors released from platelets and immune cells that stimulate fibroblasts to divide and manufacture extracellular matrix proteins. Endothelial cells respond to angiogenic growth factors by forming capillary networks.
- Inflammatory exudate functions to transport immune cells, antibodies, and nutrients to the tissue and dilute the offending substances. Serous exudate is watery and low in protein; fibrinous exudate is thick, sticky, and high in protein; purulent exudate contains infective organisms, leukocytes, and cellular debris; and hemorrhagic exudate contains red blood cells.
- Systemic manifestations of inflammation include fever, neutrophilia, lethargy, muscle catabolism, increased acute phase proteins (CRP), and increased ESR. These responses are attributable to the IL-1, IL-6, and TNF-α released from macrophages and inflamed tissues.

SPECIFIC ADAPTIVE IMMUNITY

The specific immune system uses remarkably effective and adaptive defense mechanisms capable of recognizing foreign invaders, destroying them, and retaining a memory of the encounter such that an even more effective defense (adaptive) will be achieved after subsequent exposure. As previously described, B and T lymphocytes are the cellular mediators of specific adaptive immunity. B cells are said to provide "humoral" immunity because the antibodies they produce are found in body fluids, or "humors." T cells provide "cell-mediated" immunity because they recognize antigen presented on the surface of cells. To achieve immunity against specific antigens, B and T lymphocytes must be capable of recognizing an enormous range of foreign antigen yet not be reactive to self tissues.

Differentiation between self and nonself requires a complex lymphocyte development process in which self-reactive lymphocytes are destroyed and potentially useful lymphocytes are preserved. The MHC proteins have a primary role in enabling lymphocytes to react to foreign antigen while remaining tolerant to self antigen. Self tolerance is not always effectively main-

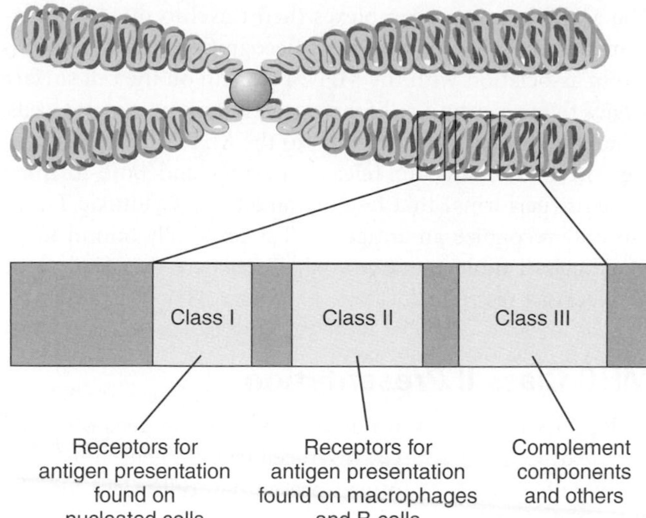

FIGURE 9-21 ■ Major histocompatibility complex genes are categorized into three main groups known as class I, II, and III. Class I and II genes code for antigen-presenting proteins, whereas class III genes code for a heterogeneous group of proteins, many of which serve immune functions.

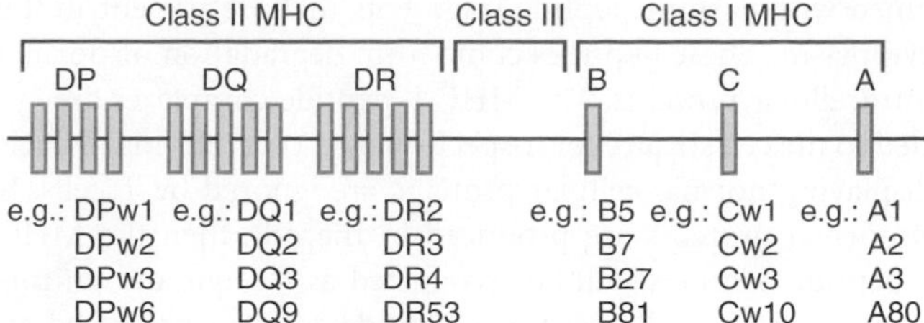

FIGURE 9-22 ■ Each individual receives six class I major histocompatibility complex *(MHC)* genes including pairs of A, B, and C genes. One member of the pair is inherited from each parent. MHC class I genes are expressed in all nucleated cells of the body. Each individual also receives six class II MHC genes, three from each parent. However, class II proteins are composed of two polypeptide chains such that an individual may have 10 to 20 different MHC class II protein molecules. Class II MHC proteins are expressed on the surface of specialized antigen-presenting cells like macrophages, dendritic cells, and B cells. The structure of an individual's MHC proteins is assessed to determine the "tissue type" when matching for tissue transplantation procedures.

tained, and impairment in self tolerance can result in the development of autoimmune disorders (see Chapter 10).

MAJOR HISTOCOMPATIBILITY COMPLEX

A cluster of genes on chromosome 6 is known as the **major histocompatibility complex.** In humans, the MHC is also known as the **human leukocyte antigen** (HLA) complex. The proteins made by these genes are displayed on the surface of body cells and mark them as "self." The MHC contains three classes of genes: I, II, and III (Figure 9-21). Class I and II genes code for proteins that display or "present" antigens on the surface of cells. Antigen presentation is a vital first step in the initiation of an immune response. T lymphocytes cannot recognize foreign antigens unless they are displayed on MHC proteins on the surface of a cell. Class III genes code for a variety of proteins, many of which are of importance to inflammatory reactions, including several complement proteins.

A great deal of **polymorphism** is found in the MHC class I and II genes, which means that it is very unlikely that an individual will have exactly the same MHC genotype as another. For example, three gene loci for MHC class I proteins (A, B, C) are located on each chromosome 6, and an individual inherits one chromosome from each parent for a total of six MHC class I genes. Each of these genes has many different forms (alleles) such that each of the six is likely to be different (Figure 9-22). Related individuals will generally be more similar but not identical (unless identical twins). The "matching" of MHC gene expression is an important consideration for tissue and organ transplantation. The closer the match is, the less likely that the host will reject the transplant. An individual also receives six MHC class II genes that are expressed on specialized antigen-presenting cells, such as dendritic cells, macrophages, and B cells. Because of the potential for mixing and matching of class II MHC gene products, an individual may express 10 to 20 different MHC class II proteins.[1] It is the MHC class I and II proteins on the surface of cells that display both self and foreign antigens for inspection by T cells. Cells displaying foreign antigens stimulate an immune response, whereas those displaying self antigens do not. Genetic diversity in MHC gene expression is believed to be important to the preservation of a species because new pathogens are likely to encounter at least some individuals with MHC genotypes that can recognize and eliminate these pathogens.

ANTIGEN PRESENTATION BY MHC

Nucleated cells in the body are capable of expressing MHC class I proteins on their cell surfaces, whereas only certain specialized cells, primarily dendritic cells, macrophages, and B cells, are able to express MHC class II proteins. Cytotoxic T cells are able to recognize antigen bound to MHC class I proteins, whereas T helper cells recognize antigen bound to MHC class II proteins. T cells are screened during development in the thymus so that they recognize and are tolerant to self MHC proteins and do not react to self peptides displayed by self MHC proteins. This concept is explored further in the section on cell-mediated immunity. The sources of antigen, mechanism of antigen processing, and T-cell response to antigen are quite different for MHC I and MHC II reactions.

MHC Class I Presentation

Nucleated cells continuously produce MHC class I proteins on the rough endoplasmic reticulum (ER) where they are combined with various peptide fragments that are present in the cytoplasm. These peptides come from degradation of normal intracellular proteins. The MHC I–peptide complexes are cycled to the cell surface for inspection by T cells. Normal MHCs displaying normal cellular proteins are ignored by T cells. If abnormal proteins are produced in the cell, then the MHC I–peptide complex will be recognized as foreign and an immune response will occur. The peptide antigens presented on MHC I are of intracellular origin. Because viruses are able to gain access to cells on their own, viral protein is a common source of foreign MHC class I antigens. Abnormal cellular proteins produced by mutant cells may also be presented on MHC I, thus targeting them for immune destruction. Before intracellular proteins can be presented at the cell surface, they must be processed and transported to the ER, where they are combined with newly synthesized MHC class I protein (Figure 9-23). Peptide fragments are generated in the cytoplasmic proteasomes and escorted through the ER by special transporters called *transporters associated with antigen processing* (TAPs). The TAP transporters are located near the MHC I complexes on the ER membrane and target the peptides to the MHC I binding cleft. The MHC I binding cleft can accommodate peptide fragments of 8 to 11 amino acids[1] (Figure 9-24). The MHC I–antigen complexes then travel to the cell membrane, where they are displayed. Recognition of foreign antigen in association with the MHC I protein on the cell surface targets the presenting cell for destruction by cytotoxic T cells. When the cytotoxic T cell binds to the MHC I–antigen complex, it is stimulated to release enzymes and pore-forming proteins (perforins) that lyse the target cell. Cytotoxic T cells can only recognize an antigen if it is physically bound to an MHC class I molecule. Cytotoxic T cells are thus said to be MHC class I restricted.

MHC Class II Presentation

MHC class II proteins are used to present antigens obtained from extracellular sources. Extracellular antigens must first be engulfed by the antigen-presenting cell. Cells of the monocyte-macrophage lineage, dendritic cells, and B cells are responsible for presenting antigen by MHC II. Macrophages and dendritic cells obtain foreign antigens by phagocytosis and are thus able to process and present a large number of different antigens. They are said to be "nonspecific" for this reason. B cells, on the other hand, are very particular about the antigens that they engulf. The antigen must specifically bind

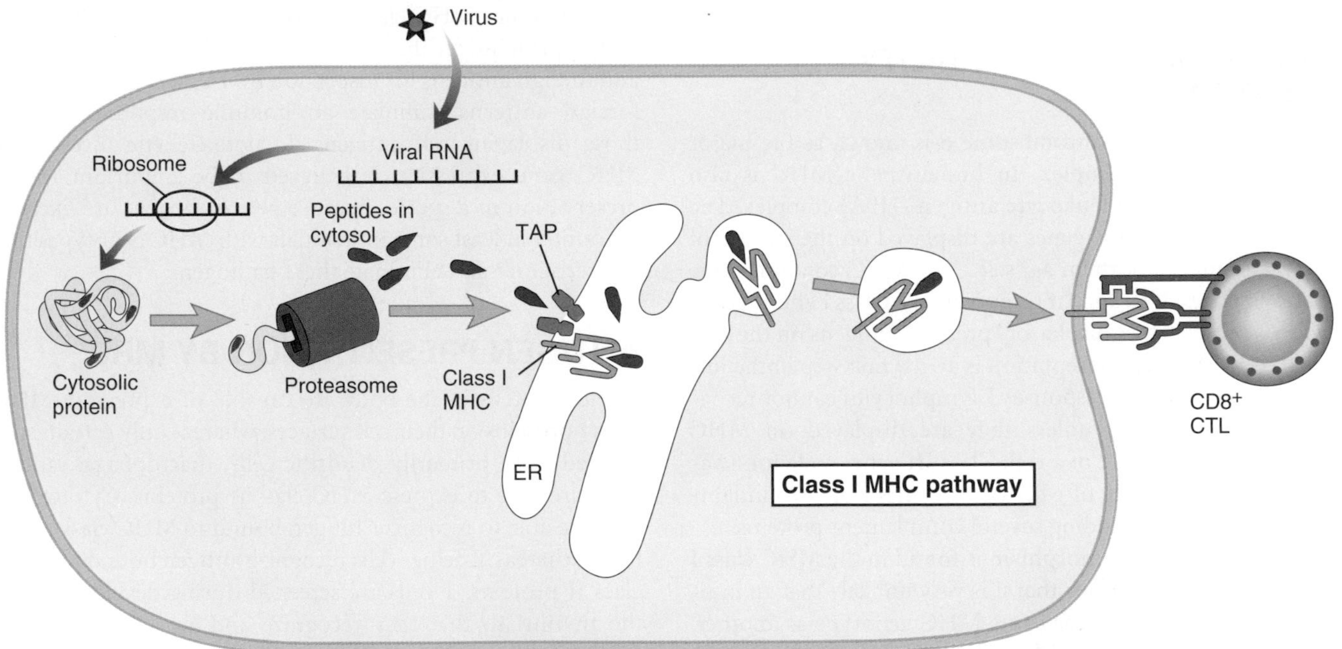

FIGURE 9-23 ■ Nearly all nucleated cells of the body are able to process and display antigen in association with major histocompatibility complex *(MHC)* class I protein. The antigens come from the intracellular compartment, and a common source of foreign antigen is viral infection. The viral proteins made within the cell's cytoplasm are processed into peptide fragments in the proteasome and then enter the endoplasmic reticulum *(ER)* through TAP transporters. There they combine with MHC class I proteins. The MHC class I–antigen complex then shuttles to the cell surface within a vesicle. When the vesicle combines with the plasma membrane, the MHC class I–antigen complex is displayed on the cell surface. *TAP,* Transporter associated with antigen processing; *CTL,* cytotoxic T lymphocyte. (From Abbas AK, Lichtman AH: *Cellular and molecular immunology,* ed 5, Philadelphia, 2003, Saunders, p 91.)

to the BCR to be ingested by a B cell. Each B cell has only one type of BCR and therefore processes and presents only one specific antigen. The specificity of the BCR corresponds to the antibody that the activated B cell will produce. The process of B-cell activation is explored in the section Mechanisms of Humoral Immunity.

After the antigen-presenting cell has ingested an antigen, it is degraded into fragments within the cellular phagosomes (endocytic vesicle). MHC II proteins are synthesized on the rough ER and pick up an antigen from the phagosome on their way to the plasma membrane (Figure 9-25). The class II MHC molecule is formed by two protein chains, and the binding cleft is more flexible than that of MHC I proteins (Figure 9-26). Peptides displayed by MHC class II proteins range in size from 10 to 30 amino acids.[1] The MHC II–antigen complexes are then displayed at the cell surface where T helper cells can detect them. T helper cells can only recognize a foreign antigen if it is physically bound to an MHC II protein. T helper cells are thus said to be MHC II restricted. Naive T cells located in lymph nodes are usually presented with antigen by dendritic cells. Dendritic cells populate the body surfaces and mucous membranes. When they engulf antigen, they break their tissue attachments and home to lymph nodes where they interact with T helper cells.

MECHANISMS OF CELL-MEDIATED IMMUNITY

T cells are able to recognize foreign antigen displayed on the surface of antigen-presenting cells through specialized receptors called T-cell receptors (TCRs). Each T cell has tens of thousands of identical TCRs on its cell surface.[7] Each T cell is thus able to recognize and respond to only a single antigenic epitope. This property is what makes T cells specific. The binding specificity of the TCR is randomly determined by recombination and rearrangement within the genes that code for the TCR-binding domain. Billions of different TCR amino acid sequences are possible, thus providing a tremendous diversity of potential antigen-binding specificities. This diversity increases the likelihood that one or more T cells will have the right TCRs to allow recognition of any of the various pathogens that may gain access to the body. The drawback to this random approach is that many TCRs will be useless or may bind self antigens. A rigorous selection process occurs in the thymus such that self-reactive T cells are eliminated. This selection process requires at least two steps. In the first, T cells must demonstrate an ability to recognize self MHC proteins displayed on the surface of specialized thymic cells. Portions of the TCR must make appropriate contact with the MHC

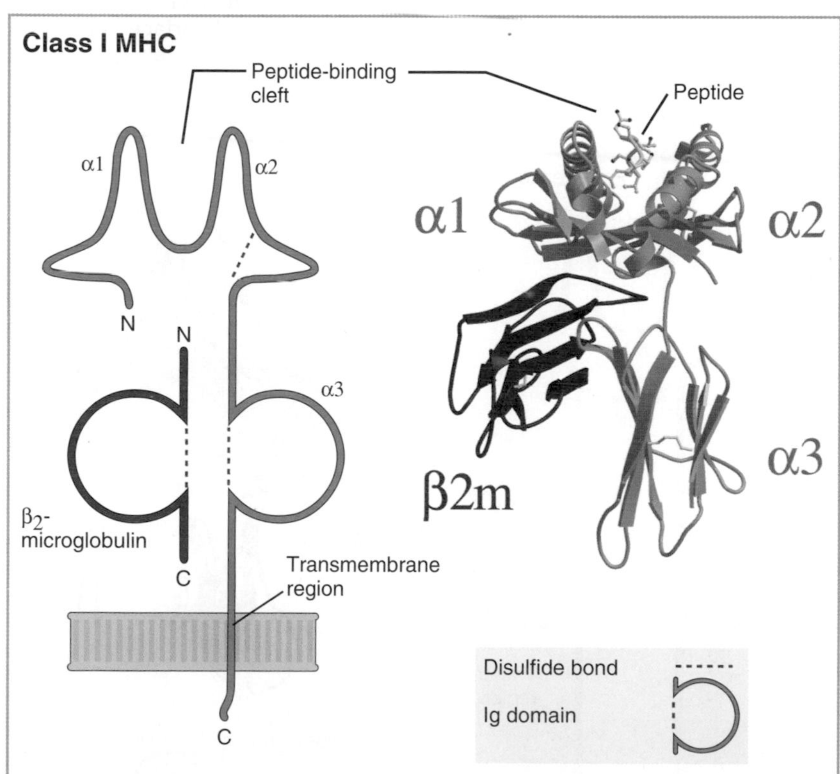

FIGURE 9-24 ■ Schematic diagram of the class I major histocompatibility complex molecule. Note that the peptide binding cleft is formed from one polypeptide chain that restricts the size of peptide in the pocket to 8 to 11 amino acids. (From Abbas AK, Lichtman AH: *Cellular and molecular immunology,* ed 5, Philadelphia, 2003, Saunders, p 91.)

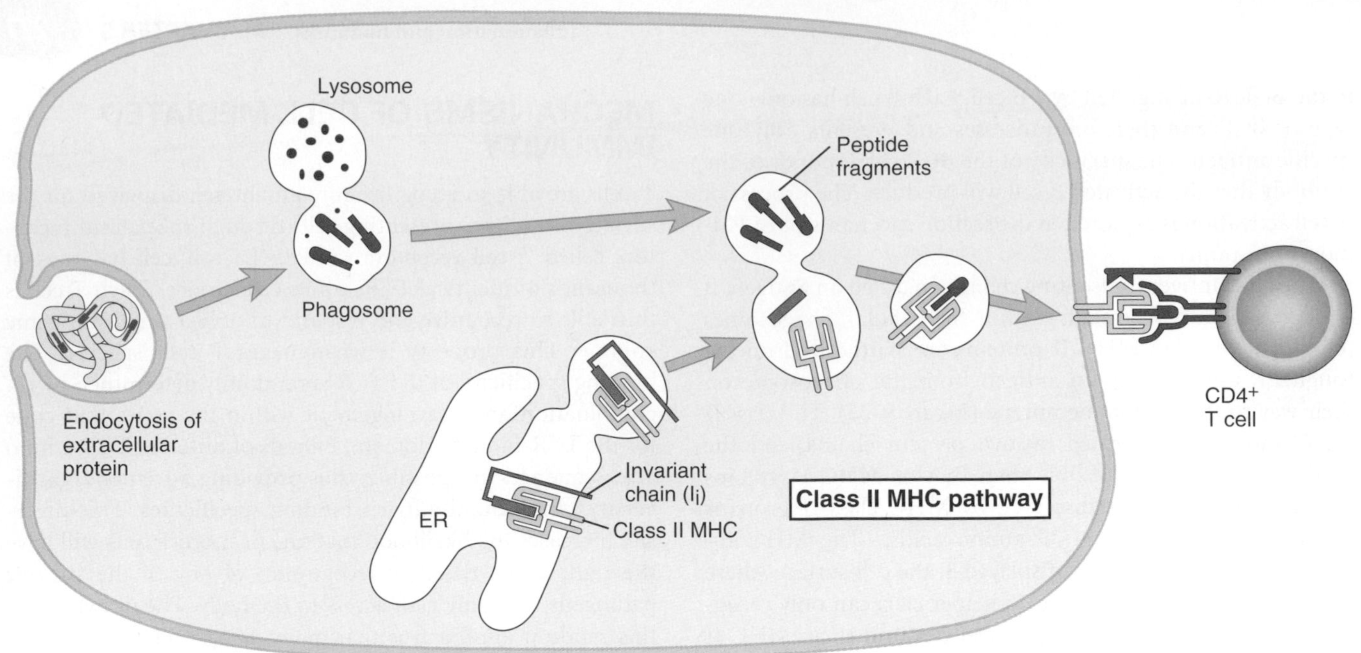

FIGURE 9-25 ■ Only specialized cells are able to obtain extracellular antigen for processing and presentation in association with major histocompatibility complex *(MHC)* class II protein. These cells are primarily dendritic cells, macrophages, and B cells. The antigen is first engulfed into a vesicle called a phagosome, which fuses with a lysosome. Enzymes within the phagosome break the protein down into pieces. MHC II molecules are synthesized on the endoplasmic reticulum *(ER)* and then transported to the phagosome in a vesicle. The binding cleft of the MHC II protein is complexed with a blocking protein to prevent it from picking up peptide before it reaches the phagosome. The phagosome and vesicle fuse, and the MHC II loses its blocking protein and picks up an antigen peptide. The complex then migrates to the cell surface and combines with the cell membrane. The MHC II–antigen complex is then displayed on the cell surface. (From Abbas AK, Lichtman AH: *Cellular and molecular immunology,* ed 5, Philadelphia, 2003, Saunders, p 91.)

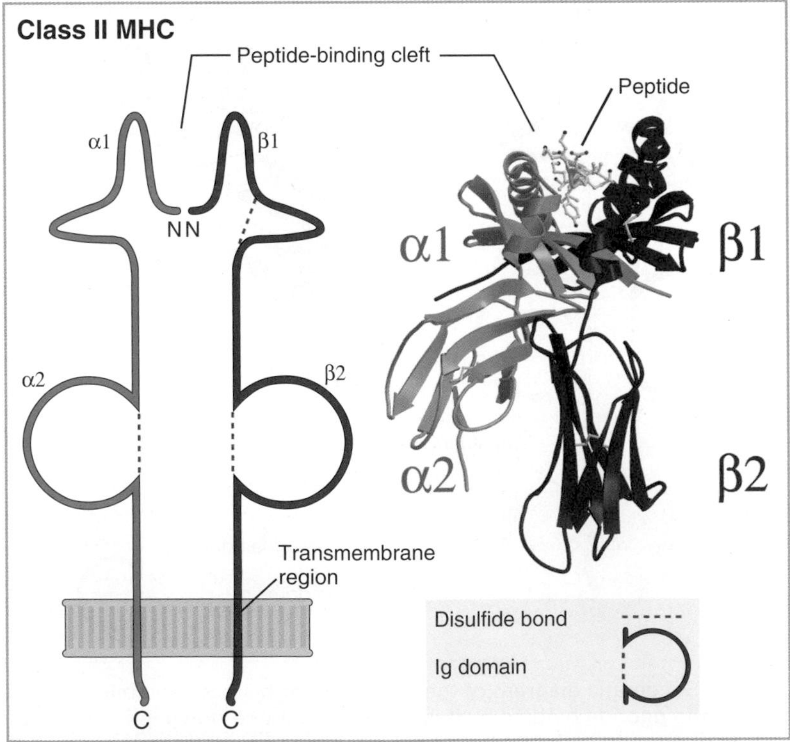

FIGURE 9-26 ■ Schematic diagram of the class II major histocompatibility complex *(MHC)* molecule. Note that the peptide-binding cleft is formed from two separate polypeptide chains, which allows the size of peptide in the pocket to be 10 to 30 amino acids. (From Abbas AK, Lichtman AH: *Cellular and molecular immunology,* ed 5, Philadelphia, 2003, Saunders, p 73.)

protein or the T cell will not be able to respond to antigens presented on the cell surface.[11] The expression of either CD4 or CD8 on the T cell helps determine which class of MHC the T cell must fit. T cells that do not have functional TCRs undergo apoptosis in the thymus. The second requirement is that the TCR does not bind tightly to MHC proteins that are displaying normal self-derived peptides. Tight binding to self peptides also triggers the cell to initiate apoptosis. T cells that pass these tests migrate to secondary lymphoid tissues to await foreign antigens. Exposure of a T cell to its corresponding antigen results in expansion of the T cell into a clone of cells that all recognize the same antigen. This process ensures that useful T cells are maintained in the body as memory cells, whereas T cells that do not encounter antigen will die out. Members of the T-cell clone migrate to lymphoid organs throughout the body, where they can respond rapidly should the same antigen reenter the system. The life span of mature T cells is long, but the numbers of memory cells in a clone will decline over time. However, intermittent exposure to the antigen is likely to occur and will stimulate proliferation and maintain immunity.

The two major types of T cells, T helper cells and cytotoxic T cells, react very differently to activation of their TCRs by antigen and are therefore described separately in the following sections.

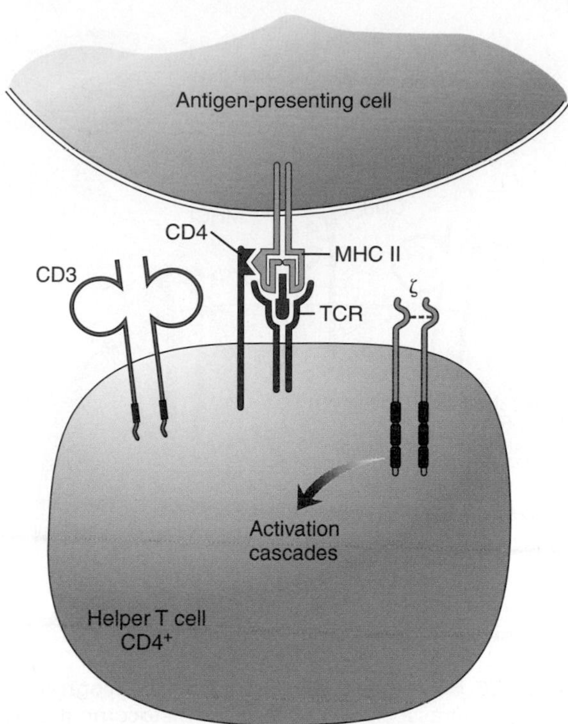

FIGURE 9-27 ■ T helper cells can recognize and bind antigen in association with major histocompatibility complex *(MHC)* class II molecules. The T-cell receptor *(TCR)* on the T helper cell binds to the antigen, and the CD4 protein recognizes the MHC class II protein. Binding is very specific because the TCR must match the antigen fragment precisely. Once binding is achieved, CD3 and ζ proteins associated with the TCR are activated to initiate intracellular enzyme cascades.

T Helper Cells (CD4$^+$)

T helper cells recognize antigen in association with MHC class II molecules. The CD4 protein is needed to enable T helper cells to bind the MHC II protein, whereas the TCR recognizes the specific antigen being presented (Figure 9-27). Binding of the TCR to its corresponding antigen generates a signaling cascade in the cytoplasm of the T helper cell. The TCR is linked to this signaling cascade through another protein called CD3. Stimulation of CD3 results in the activation of enzymes (kinases) in the cytoplasm that mediate the production of two second messengers, inositol triphosphate and diacylglycerol (see Chapter 3). Inositol triphosphate initiates a rise in the concentration of intracellular calcium ion, which also acts as a second messenger to change cell behavior. Other protein kinases turn on the genes for cytokines (e.g., IL-2, IFN-α, and others), IL-2 receptors, and other cell surface proteins. As previously mentioned, the two subtypes of T helper cells, T_H1 and T_H2, secrete somewhat different amounts and types of cytokines. These cytokines provide the "help" that T helper cells give to other cells of the immune system. For example, IL-2 activates helper and cytotoxic T cells, NK cells, and macrophages, and IFN-α is a potent activator of macrophages. IL-2 and IFN-α are the main cytokines secreted by T_H1 cells. The cytokines secreted by T_H2 cells have stimulatory effects on B cells (e.g., IL-4, IL-5, IL-6, IL-13). In addition, when a B cell is serving as the antigen-presenting cell, T helper cells provide specific B-cell help through direct cell-to-cell contact by receptor proteins.

Cytotoxic T Cells (CD8$^+$)

Cytotoxic T cells recognize antigen displayed in association with MHC class I protein. The CD8 protein is needed to facilitate binding to the MHC I, whereas the TCR specifically recognizes the presented antigen (Figure 9-28). Binding of the TCR to its corresponding antigen triggers a number of responses in the cytotoxic T cell. This process is similar to that described for T helper cells and involves signal transduction through CD3 proteins. Antigen binding by cytotoxic T cells is not sufficient to activate them. Cytotoxic T cells also require costimulation by IL-2 cytokines. IL-2 is secreted primarily by activated T helper cells (T_H1). Thus, cytotoxic T cells require T helper cell "help" before they are effective. Cytokines are generally not enough to induce significant proliferation of target cells unless other costimulators are also present. This helps ensure that the cells that specifically recognize a particular antigen are the ones that get the help. Costimulators are often present on the surfaces of the presenting and responding cells (Figure 9-29). Once activated, cytotoxic T cells proliferate into memory cells as well as effector cells. Effector cells accomplish their cytotoxic functions in two ways, through perforins and through CD95.

Perforins are proteins manufactured in the cytotoxic T cell and stored in granules (vesicles) within the cytoplasm. A

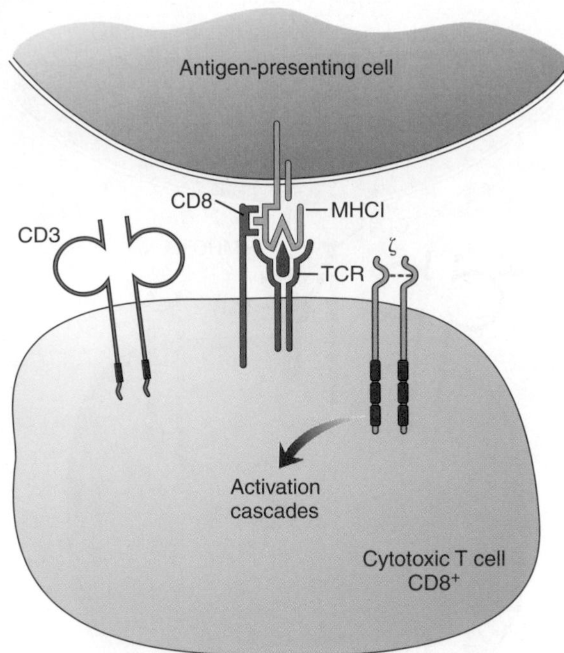

FIGURE 9-28 ■ Cytotoxic T cells are able to recognize and bind antigen in association with major histocompatibility complex (MHC) class I molecules. The T-cell receptor on the cytotoxic T cell binds to the antigen, and the CD8 protein recognizes the MHC I protein. Binding is specific. Once binding is achieved, CD3 proteins initiate intracellular enzyme cascades.

number of proteolytic enzymes (granzymes) are located in the granules along with the perforins. Binding to the target cell causes the granules to migrate to the contact site, where they are released onto the target cell membrane (Figure 9-30). The perforins assemble into pores, which then allow the granzymes to move into the target cell. Granzymes degrade DNA and trigger target cell death (apoptosis).

Perforins function in a similar manner to the complement membrane attack complex previously described. It is not entirely clear how the cytotoxic T cell manages to escape injury in this process. Presumably, the perforins and granzymes are focused on the target cell in some controlled manner.

The CD95 protein on cytotoxic T cells is called the CD95 ligand (CD95L) or the FAS ligand.[12] It can bind specifically to complementary CD95 proteins (FAS) found on the surface of target cells. Normal, healthy cells do not express CD95 and are not recognized by cytotoxic cells. Binding of the CD95L to CD95 triggers programmed cell death (apoptosis) of the target cell (see Figure 9-30). This system is thought to be particularly important in culling senescent cells and self-reactive lymphocytes.

MECHANISMS OF HUMORAL IMMUNITY

B cells are responsible for antibody-mediated (humoral) immunity. B cells have two major subpopulations: memory cells and plasma cells. Memory B cells contain antigen receptors and function in a manner similar to memory T cells. In other words, memory of exposure to an antigen is stored in a clone of memory B cells. When exposed to the same type of antigen in the future, these memory B cells are able to respond rapidly with appropriate antibodies.

Some B cells differentiate into short-lived antibody-producing factories called plasma cells. All of the plasma cells in a clone secrete antibodies with identical antigen-binding specificity (monoclonal antibody). The secreted antibodies circulate in the blood and body fluids and bind specifically to the antigen that triggered their production. Once antigen is cleared, the population of plasma cells declines and the antibody concentration (titer) falls. However, some long-lived plasma cells continue to secrete a level of antibody sufficient to provide immediate protection upon the next exposure to the same antigen.[1]

Antigen Recognition by B Cells

During their development in the bone marrow, B cells begin to express BCRs on their cell surfaces. The structure of the antigen-binding area on the BCR is randomly determined in a manner similar to that described for TCRs. Each BCR is coded for by two distinct types of genes: one for the variable region, which makes up the antigen-binding site, and one for the constant region, which is essentially the same for all antibodies of a given class (Figure 9-31). The antibody class of the BCR bound to the B-cell surface is IgM. Rearrangement, recombination, and selective splicing of variable-region genes allow for great diversity of BCR binding specificities. The potential number of different BCRs is enormous (1×10^{16}). Some of these combinations are unsuitable for BCR assembly, and it has been estimated that a typical human B-cell population can recognize approximately 10 million different antigenic epitopes.[1] As is the case with T cells, useful B cells—ones activated by antigen—will be preserved in the body, whereas B cells that encounter no antigen will die out.

The growth and activity of B cells that recognize protein antigens are carefully regulated by T cells. Binding of antigen to the B cell's BCR is a necessary but insufficient stimulus to produce an effective B-cell clone. To be effectively activated, the B cell must engulf some of the antigen, process it, and present it to T helper cells. This activity will initiate cell-to-cell contact between the B cell and its complementary T-cell helper. A number of receptor interactions bind the T and B cells together, in addition to the main MHC II–TCR interaction, and include B7-CD28 and CD40L-CD40 (Figure 9-32). These cell-to-cell binding interactions stimulate intracellular signaling pathways in the B cell (and T helper cell) that promote clonal expansion and differentiation. B cells also require certain cytokines to proliferate and begin antibody synthesis. B cells are quite dependent on T cell help during the initial exposure to antigen (primary response), but less so on subsequent exposures. Some types of B cells have BCRs that bind nonprotein antigens, such as bacterial sugars and lipids. Since T cells only recognize peptides, these types of B-cell responses

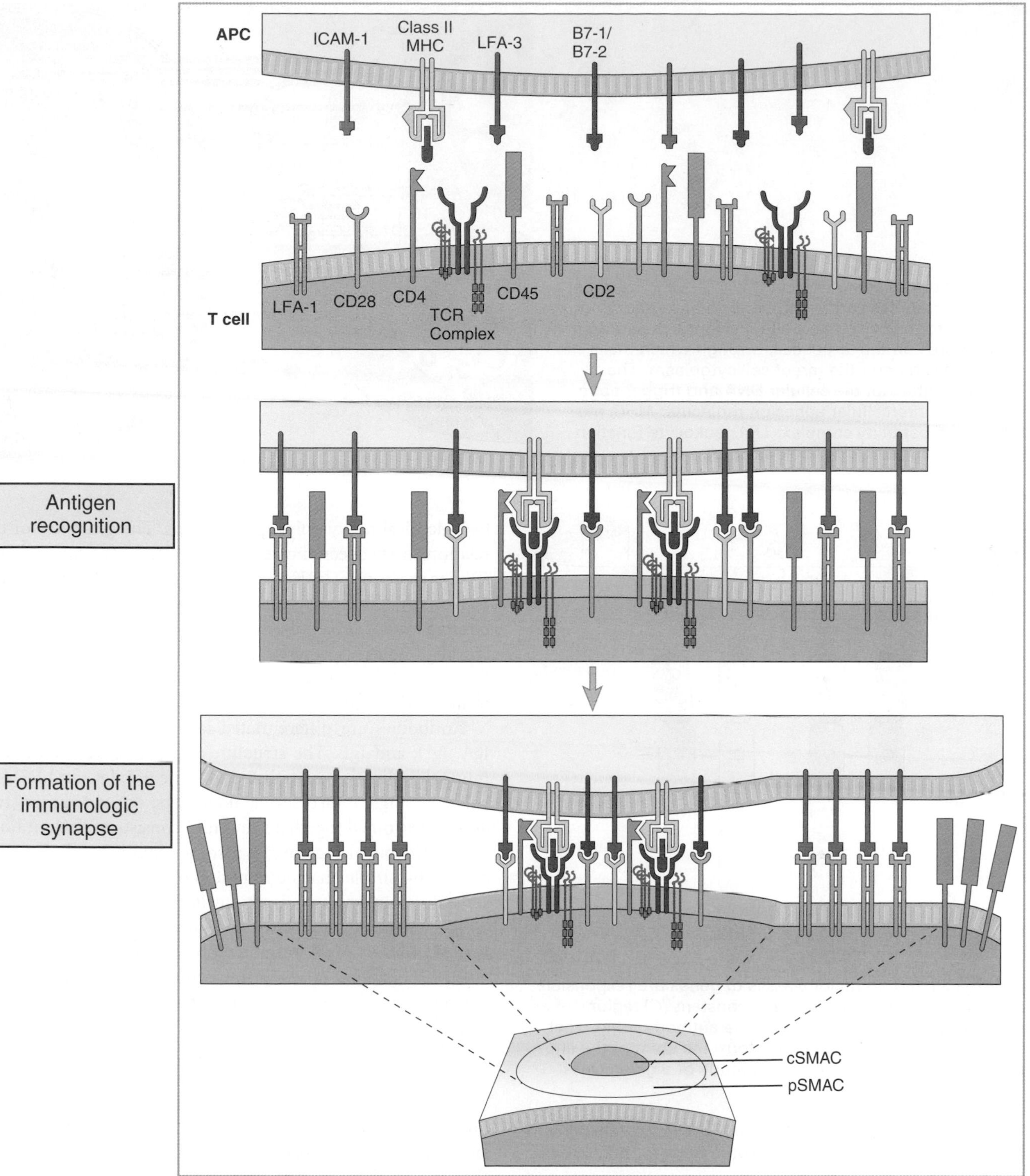

FIGURE 9-29 ■ Schematic diagram illustrating the formation of the "immunologic synapse." Numerous receptor-ligand interactions bind a T cell to an antigen-presenting cell *(APC)*. When the receptors and ligands interact in concert, the T cell and antigen-presenting cells are activated. *ICAM,* Intercellular adhesion molecule; *MHC,* major histocompatibility complex; *LFA,* leukocyte function–associated antigen; *TCR,* T-cell receptor; *cSMAC,* central supramolecular activation cluster; *pSMAC,* peripheral supramolecular activation cluster. (From Abbas AK, Lichtman AH: *Cellular and molecular immunology,* ed 5, Philadelphia, 2003, Saunders, p 176.)

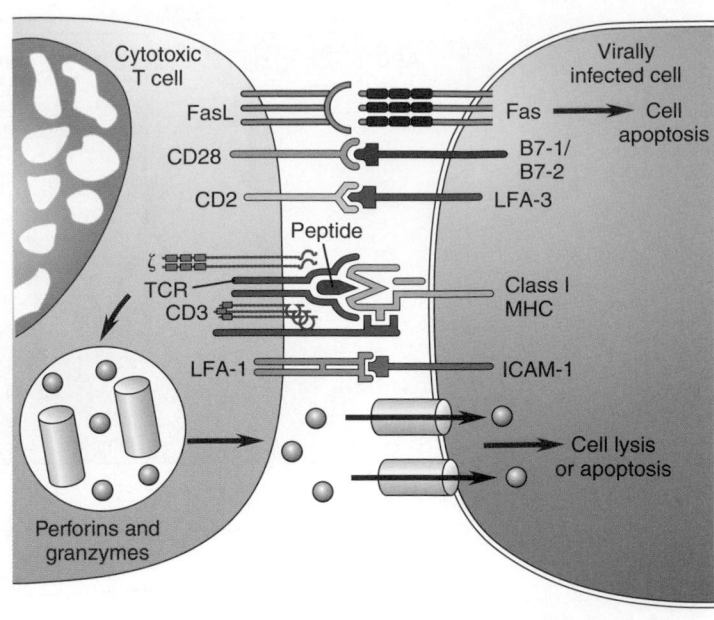

FIGURE 9-30 ■ Binding of a cytotoxic T cell to its target stimulates granules containing perforin and granzymes to migrate to the cell contact site. Perforins then assemble into pores on the target cell, through which the granzymes can enter the target cell cytoplasm. The granzymes interrupt the cellular DNA and trigger apoptosis. *ICAM,* Intercellular adhesion molecule; *MHC,* major histocompatibility complex; *LFA,* leukocyte function–associated antigen; *TCR,* T-cell receptor.

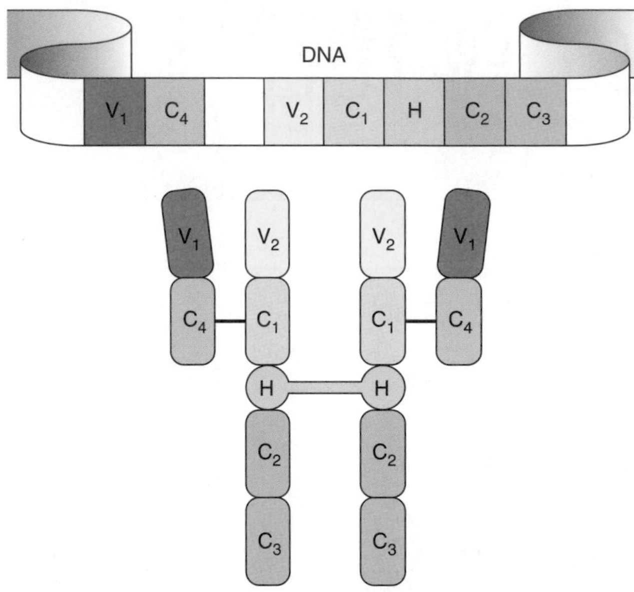

FIGURE 9-31 ■ Two major classes of genes are responsible for coding for the variable *(V)* and constant *(C)* regions of an antibody. Variable genes code for the antibody region that binds to antigen. Constant genes form the stem of the antibody and are the same for any antibody of a given class.

are T cell independent. Other costimulatory signals, such as the complement fragment C3d on the antigen, may provide the necessary costimulation to achieve a B-cell response and antibody production. It is doubtful that memory cells are formed in this process[1] (Figure 9-33).

Antibody Structure

Each antibody (immunoglobulin) molecule contains two identical light polypeptide chains joined by disulfide bonds to two identical heavy polypeptide chains. The geometry of the relationship between the heavy (H) and light (L) chains forms a Y-like structure. The H chains form the stem of the Y and the L chains are on the outside of the arms of the Y. The antigen-binding end of the antibody is often called the Fab (antigen-binding fragment), whereas the stem is called the Fc (constant fragment). It is the structure of the constant fragment that determines the antibody class.

Antibodies are differentiated into five classes: IgG, IgM, IgA, IgD, and IgE. The structure and properties of the immunoglobulin classes are listed in Table 9-4. IgG and IgE circulate as single molecules or monomers; IgA is a dimer (two antibodies joined together); and IgM consists of five antibody molecules joined together to form a pentamer. IgD is found on the B-cell plasma membrane. Different antibody classes serve different immune functions in the body.

IgG, the most common type of immunoglobulin, accounts for 75% to 80% of all immunoglobulins. It is found in nearly equal proportions in the intravascular and interstitial compartments and has a long half-life of about 3 weeks. IgG is the smallest of the immunoglobulins and can more easily escape the blood stream to enter the interstitial fluid surrounding tissues.

IgM accounts for about 10% of circulating immunoglobulins and is predominantly found in the intravascular pool.[13] Its large pentamer structure prevents it from migrating through the capillary wall. IgM has a half-life of 5 days. It is the first immunoglobulin to be produced on exposure to antigens or after immunization and is the major antibody found on B-cell surfaces. IgM is the antibody class that works best to activate complement, which is important for cytotoxic functions in the immune system. Only one molecule of IgM is needed to activate complement, whereas two molecules of IgG are needed to do the same.

Receptor-mediated endocytosis of antigen
Antigen processing and presentation
Antigen presentation to helper T cell
Activation of T cell; expression of CD40 ligand,cytokine secretion
Activation of B cell by cytokines and CD40 ligation
B cell
Microbial protein antigen
Class II MHC-peptide complex
CD40
B cell
T cell
B7-1, B7-2
CD28
CD40 ligand
Cytokines
CD40 ligand
Cytokines

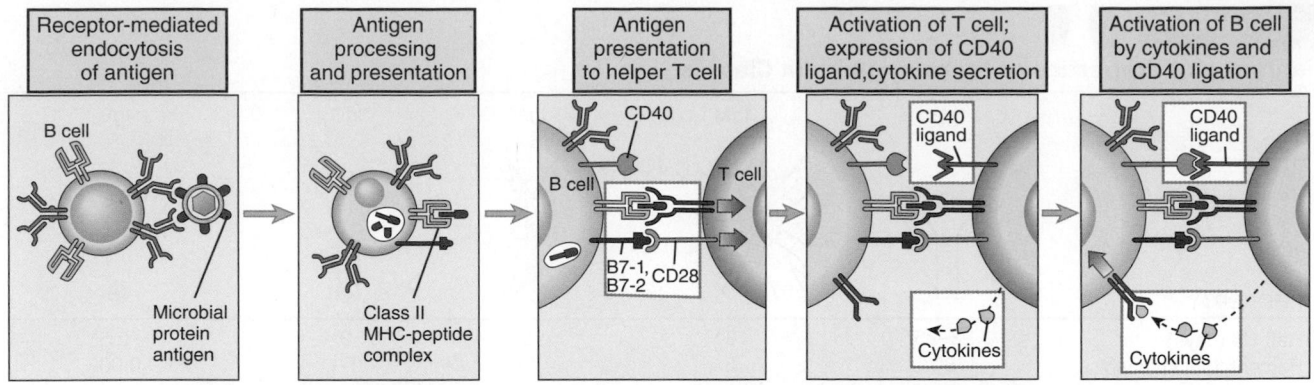

FIGURE 9-32 ■ Activation of a B cell requires T helper cell "help." This help is given through a number of cell-to-cell interactions via receptors, as well as through the secretion of cytokines that stimulate B-cell growth and differentiation. *MHC,* Major histocompatibility complex. (Redrawn from Abbas AK, Lichtman AH: *Cellular and molecular immunology,* ed 5, Philadelphia, 2003, Saunders, p 201.)

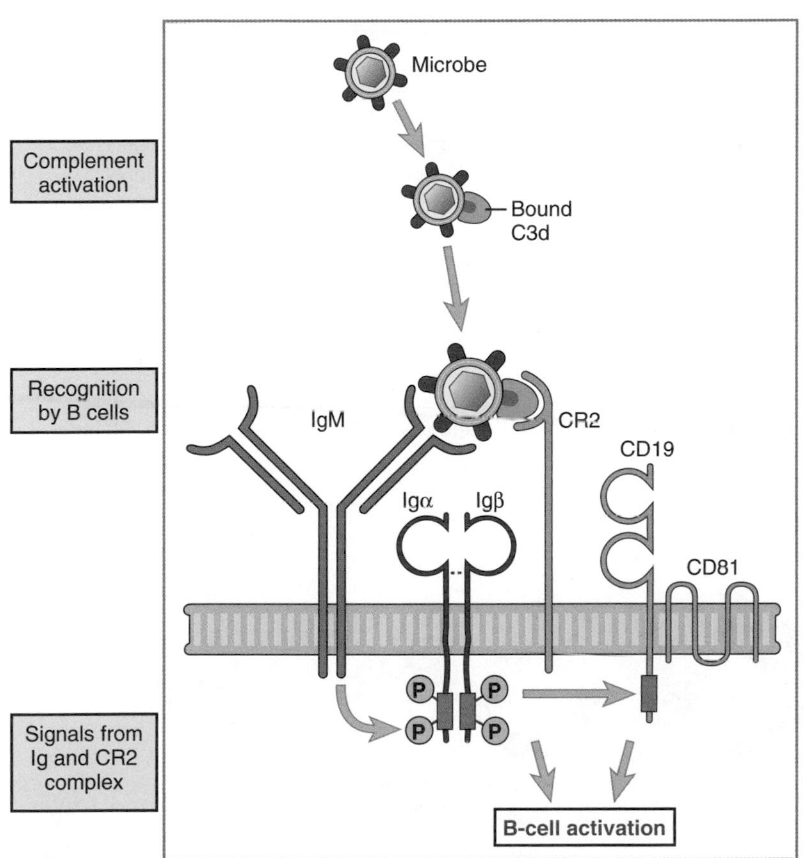

FIGURE 9-33 ■ In response to nonprotein antigens (T cell independent) B cells can be activated by complement opsonins on the microbial antigen. The complement-receptor *(CR)* interaction provides a costimulatory signal to the B-cell receptor–antigen signal. (Redrawn from Abbas AK, Lichtman AH: *Cellular and molecular immunology,* ed 5, Philadelphia, 2003, Saunders, p 195.)

IgA is produced by plasma cells located in the tissue under the skin and mucous membranes. IgA is primarily found in saliva, tears, tracheobronchial secretions, colostrum, milk, and gastrointestinal and genitourinary secretions. Transport of IgA into secretions is facilitated by binding to a secretory component produced by epithelial cells. This complex is called secretory IgA (Figure 9-34). The half-life of IgA is about 6 days.

IgD is found in trace amounts in the serum (1%) and is located primarily on the membranes of B cells along with IgM. IgD has a half-life of 3 days. Little is known about its function, but it is thought to be a cellular antigen receptor acting to stimulate the B cell to multiply, differentiate, and secrete other specific immunoglobulins.

IgE is found bound by its Fc tail to receptors on the surface of basophils and mast cells (Figure 9-35). Only trace amounts

Table 9-4

Diagram and Properties of Immunoglobulin Classes

PROPERTY	IgG	IgM	IgA	IgD	IgE
Half-life (days)	23–25	5	6	3	2.5
Percent total immunoglobulin	80	6	13	0–1	0.002
Molecular wt (daltons)	146,000	900,000	160,000	184,000	200,000
Complement fixation	++	+++	–	–	–
Placental transfer	+++	–	–	–	–
Receptor for macrophage	+++	–	–	–	–
Reaction with staph protein A	+++	–	–	–	–
Passive cutaneous anaphylaxis	+++	–	–	–	+
Transported across epithelium	–	Occasionally	+	–	–
Prominent antibody activity	Anti-Rh against infections	ABO isoagglutinins, rheumatoid factor	Against infections	Binds to B cells in presence of IgM	Mast cell sensitization, cytophilic antibody skin sensitizing antibody
Cell binding functions:					
Mononuclear cells	+	–	–	–	?/+
Neutrophils	+	–	+	–	–
Mast cells/basophils	–	–	–	–	+++
T cells/B cells	+	+	+	+	+
Platelets	+	+	–	–	?

Data from Roitt IM: *Immunology,* ed 6, St Louis, 2001, Mosby; and Abbas AK: *Cellular and molecular immunology,* ed 5, Philadelphia, 2003, Saunders.

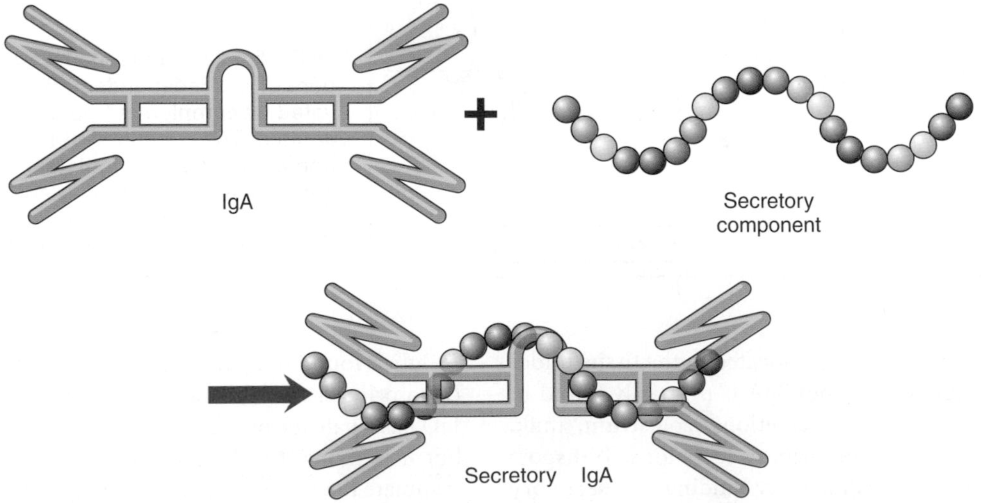

FIGURE 9-34 ■ IgA is often combined with a protein called secretory component, which helps bind two IgA molecules together at their F_c ends.

of IgE are identified in the serum. IgE has a half-life of 2.5 days. It has a role in immunity against helminthic parasites (worms) and is responsible for initiating inflammatory and allergic reactions (e.g., asthma, hay fever). IgE functions as a signaling molecule and causes mast cell degranulation when antigen is detected at the mast cell surface (see Chapter 10).

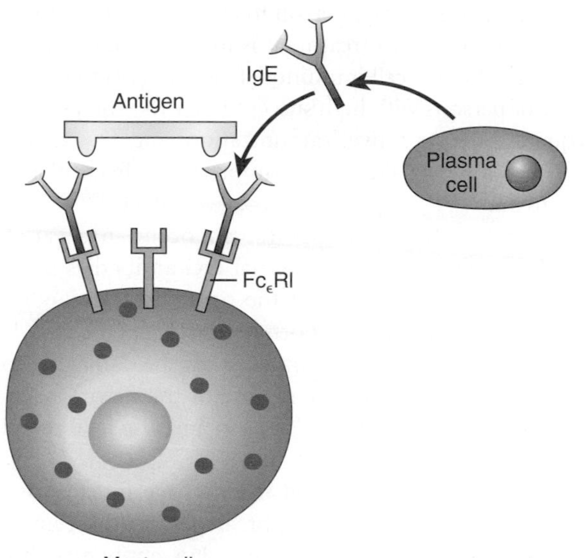

FIGURE 9-35 ■ Mast cells bind IgE antibody with their F_c receptors *($Fc_{\epsilon}RI$)* and display the IgE on the cell surface, where they are available to bind antigens.

Class Switching and Affinity Maturation

During the course of an antibody response, the class of antibody manufactured by a particular B cell usually changes. The antigen-binding site does not change and remains specific for the particular antigen that initiated the response. To switch class, the B cell selects different constant region genes to splice to the antigen-binding fragment. Thus, most B cells begin by using genes that code for IgM and IgD. Then the B cell switches to produce IgG, IgE, or IgA.[14] The triggers that determine the class of antibody a particular B cell will produce are incompletely understood. Some cytokines have a role in class switching. For example, IFN-γ promotes IgG production, IL-4 promotes IgE production, and transforming growth factor β (TGF-β) promotes IgA production[14] (Figure 9-36).

Knowledge about the normal progression of class switching may be helpful in determining whether an infectious process is acute or chronic. For example, a person newly infected with hepatitis B virus would be expected to have primarily IgM antihepatitis B, whereas in chronic or previous infection, B cells would switch class to produce mainly IgG. The relative concentrations of antihepatitis B IgM and IgG can help identify the time of onset of the infection.

Over the course of a B-cell antibody response, the affinity with which the antibodies bind to antigen often increases. This is thought to occur because of a process called affinity maturation during which B cells produce random changes in the antigen-binding pocket of the BCR.[15] Those that bind antigen most avidly are stimulated to proliferate to a greater

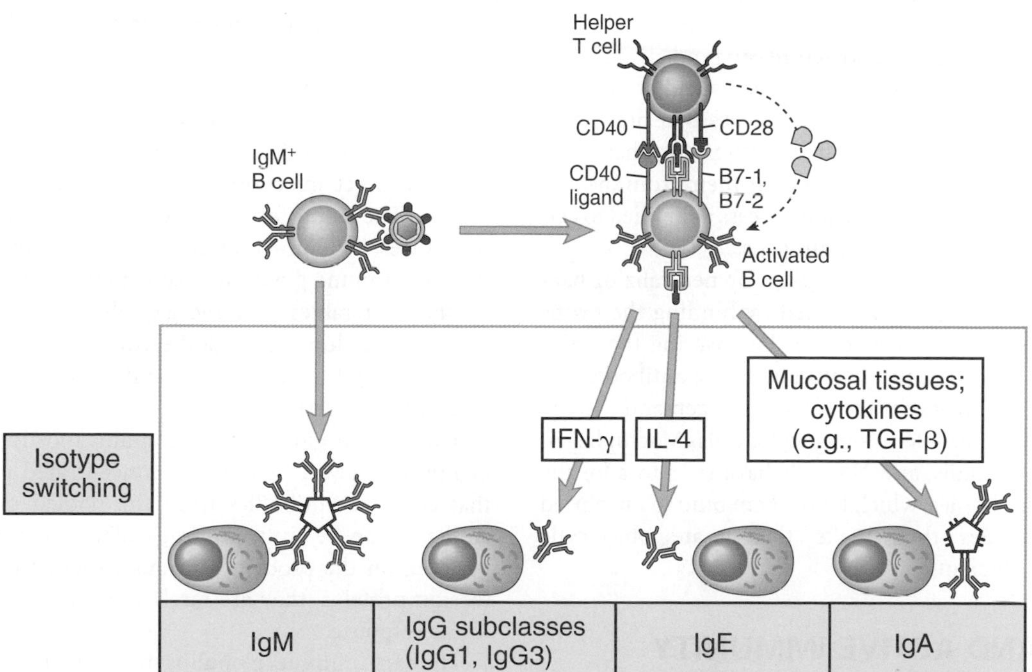

FIGURE 9-36 ■ Activated B cells undergo class switching from IgM to IgG, IgE, or IgA. Class switching is influenced by the presence of specific cytokines. *IFN,* Interferon; *IL,* interleukin; *TGF,* transforming growth factor. (Redrawn from Abbas AK, Lichtman AH: *Cellular and molecular immunology,* ed 5, Philadelphia, 2003, Saunders, p 205.)

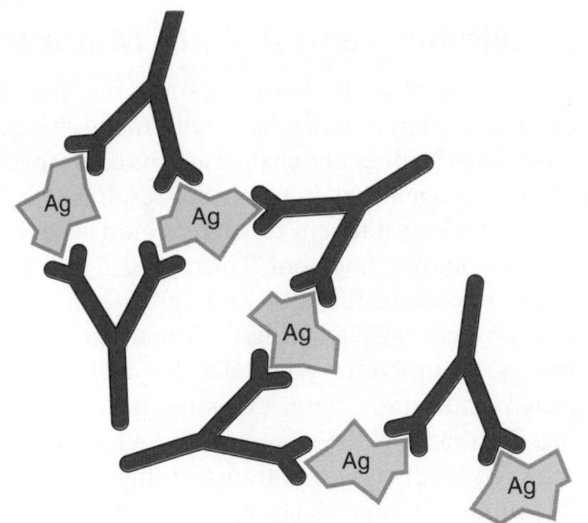

FIGURE 9-37 ■ Large antigen *(Ag)*-antibody complexes tend to precipitate out of solution, which makes it easier for phagocytic cells to find and eliminate the antigens.

extent. Thus, the antibodies formed later in an immune response are more efficient in binding antigen at lower and lower concentrations. Affinity maturation occurs in specialized germinal centers in the lymph nodes.

Antibody Functions

Antibodies function in a number of ways to enhance the localization and removal of antigens from the body. These functions can generally be summarized as precipitation, agglutination, neutralization, opsonization, and complement activation. Precipitation and agglutination occur because each arm of the immunoglobulin Y structure can bind an antigenic epitope. This structure allows the antibodies and antigens to bind together into large insoluble complexes that precipitate out of body fluids (Figure 9-37). It is efficient for phagocytic cells to find the large complexes and clear them from the system. Agglutination refers to the same process as applied to cellular antigens rather than soluble antigens.

Antibodies can function as antitoxins by neutralizing bacterial toxin. This role is accomplished by binding the toxins before they can interact with cells or by covering the active portions of the toxin and inactivating it. Some antibodies are effective opsonins. They coat the foreign antigen and thereby make it more recognizable to phagocytic cells. Macrophages, neutrophils, eosinophils, and NK cells have receptors for the Fc ends of the antibodies, which helps them bind to opsonized antigens. Antibodies thus make the innate phagocytic processes more efficient.

PASSIVE AND ACTIVE IMMUNITY

Immunity is a state of resistance against infection from a particular pathogen. Immunity is provided primarily by adequate levels of circulating antibodies. Antibody levels can be measured by a blood test called an antibody titer. A sufficiently high antibody titer confers immunity by removing pathogens from the body before they cause signs and symptoms of illness. Immunity can be achieved passively or actively.

Passive Immunity

Passive immunity involves the transfer of plasma (sera) containing preformed antibodies against a specific antigen from a protected or immunized person to an unprotected or nonimmunized person. Such treatment is indicated in the following situations: (1) in B-cell immunodeficiencies; (2) following exposure of persons with high susceptibility to a disease without adequate time for active immunization; and (3) when antibody injection may alleviate or suppress the effects of an antigenic toxin.

Passive transfer of antibodies can occur in a variety of ways. In the fetus, certain maternal IgG antibodies can cross the placental barrier. Most of the time these antibodies are beneficial and assist the newborn in resisting pathogens. However, in some cases, these antibodies can be damaging to the fetus, as occurs in hemolytic disease of the newborn. In this disorder, maternal antibodies bind to and lyse fetal red blood cells (see Chapters 10 and 13).

Antibody, complement, and macrophage function is deficient at birth. Newborns who are breast-fed may have improved immune function. Newborns receive IgA antibodies through breast milk. The infant's immature gastrointestinal tract and low proteolytic enzyme activity do not destroy all protein, which allows some of the IgA antibodies to be absorbed. These antibodies assist the infant in defending against bacterial and viral infections during infancy. It has been hypothesized by some researchers that IgA antibodies in breast milk may modify the ways that proteins cross the infant's highly permeable intestinal mucosa and help prevent food allergies in later life.[16]

Another method of passive immunity, called serotherapy, involves direct injection of antibodies into an unprotected person. The unprotected individual can receive a variety of substances, including immune globulin (human) such as IgG; specific immune globulins like hepatitis B immune globulin (human) or rabies immune globulin (human); and plasma containing all human antibodies; or animal antibodies such as diphtheria antitoxin, tetanus antitoxin, botulism antitoxin, and antirabies serum.

Human immune globulin contains mostly IgG with traces of IgA and IgM. It is a sterile, concentrated protein solution that contains antibodies from the pooled plasma of many adults. It can be given intramuscularly or intravenously, depending on the product. Although these antibodies contain foreign proteins, they are rarely the cause of an adverse immune response.

Human immune globulins may be used as prophylaxis against hepatitis B and as therapy for the following conditions: antibody deficiency disorders, pediatric acquired immunodeficiency syndrome, and hypogammaglobulinemia after bone marrow transplantation.

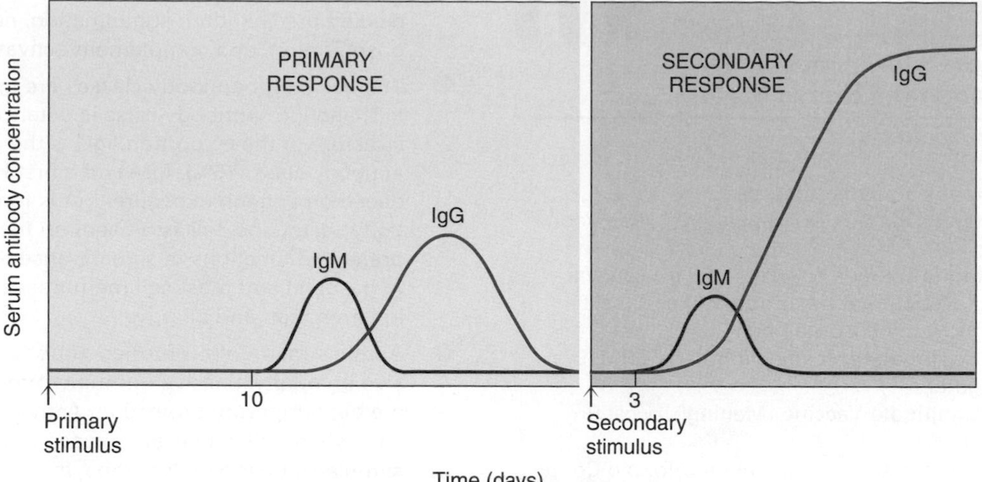

FIGURE 9-38 ■ Time phases in the immune response. The primary response takes much longer to develop and falls off rapidly. On second exposure, a much quicker and greater antibody response is achieved.

Animal antibodies are given in specific situations only when necessary because of significant allergic risks with animal sera. Patients who have specific animal allergies or a history of asthma, allergic rhinitis, or other allergies are highly susceptible to serum sickness, anaphylaxis, or acute febrile reactions. Serum sickness occurs when antibodies bind to foreign proteins in the injected sera forming immune complexes that precipitate into capillaries and joints causing inflammation. Animal antibodies may be given to ameliorate toxins or venoms, including botulism, diphtheria, rabies, tetanus, snake bite, and spider bite.

Active Immunity

Active immunity confers a protected state owing to the body's immune response as a result of active infection or immunization. The development of active immunity requires the maturation and maintenance of memory B cells. On second exposure to antigen, the antibody response is much greater and more rapid (Figure 9-38). Exposure to antigen can be achieved through active infection or through immunization. The immune system must be exposed to the antigen long enough and in sufficient dose to stimulate an immune response.

Immunization tricks the immune system into responding to a perceived infection. Vaccines contain altered microorganisms or toxins that retain their ability to stimulate the immune system (antigenic properties) but do not have pathogenic properties. Vaccines can contain live and attenuated (altered) or killed infectious agents.

Vaccines that contain live altered virus or bacteria cause active infection but little injury to the vaccinated individual. These vaccines provide good humoral and cellular immunity with longer lasting memory and often lifetime immunity. Examples of vaccines registered in the United States are listed in Box 9-1.

KEY CONCEPTS

- Specific immunity refers to functions of B and T lymphocytes. Each lymphocyte recognizes and reacts to only one particular antigen. On initial exposure to an antigen, lymphocytes undergo clonal expansion so that many lymphocytes are distributed throughout the body that can recognize and react to that particular antigen. These cells are called memory cells. Subsequent exposure results in a much faster and larger lymphocyte response.
- T lymphocytes are able to bind antigens only when they are displayed on the surface of cells. Cytotoxic T cells ($CD8^+$) react to cells that have foreign MHC class I proteins on their surface. T helper cells ($CD4^+$) bind to cells that have MHC class II proteins on their surface. MHC class II proteins are found on antigen-presenting cells (B cells, dendritic cells, and macrophages). These cells engulf foreign antigens and combine the antigens with MHC class II proteins on their cell surface.
- T cells, which mature in the thymus, have two major subgroups: T helper cells and cytotoxic T cells. T helper cells perform a central role in specific immunity. Activation of T helper cells results in secretion of the cytokines necessary for clonal expansion of T and B lymphocytes. Cytotoxic T cells locate and lyse abnormal cells through the actions of perforins.
- B- and T-cell functions are interdependent. T cells cannot respond to soluble antigens. B cells can process free antigen and present it to T cells. On first exposure, B cells are minimally activated by antigen unless they are stimulated by cytokines and coreceptors from T cells.
- B lymphocytes mature in bone marrow and lymph tissue. B cells have receptors on their surfaces that can bind antigens. Each B cell binds only one partic-

Box 9-1

Vaccines Licensed for Immunization and Distributed in the United States

Anthrax Vaccine Adsorbed
BCG Live
Diphtheria & Tetanus Toxoids Adsorbed
Diphtheria & Tetanus Toxoids & Acellular Pertussis Vaccine Adsorbed
Diphtheria & Tetanus Toxoids & Acellular Pertussis Vaccine Adsorbed, Hepatitis B (recombinant) and Inactivated Poliovirus Vaccine Combined
Haemophilus b Conjugate Vaccine (Diphtheria CRM197 Protein Conjugate)
Haemophilus b Conjugate Vaccine (Meningococcal Protein Conjugate)
Haemophilus b Conjugate Vaccine (Tetanus Toxoid Conjugate)
Haemophilus b Conjugate Vaccine (Meningococcal Protein Conjugate) & Hepatitis B Vaccine (Recombinant)
Hepatitis A Vaccine, Inactivated
Hepatitis A Inactivated and Hepatitis B (Recombinant) Vaccine
Hepatitis B Vaccine (Recombinant)
Influenza Virus Vaccine, Live, Intranasal
Influenza Virus Vaccine, Trivalent, Types A and B
Japanese Encephalitis Virus Vaccine Inactivated
Measles Virus Vaccine, Live
Measles and Mumps Virus Vaccine, Live
Measles, Mumps, and Rubella Virus Vaccine, Live
Meningococcal Polysaccharide Vaccine, Groups A, C, Y, and W-135 Combined
Mumps Virus Vaccine Live
Pneumococcal Vaccine, Polyvalent
Pneumococcal 7-Valent Conjugate Vaccine (Diphtheria CRM197 Protein)
Poliovirus Vaccine Inactivated
Rabies Vaccine
Rubella Virus Vaccine Live
Smallpox Vaccine, Dried, Calf Lymph Type
Tetanus and Diphtheria Toxoids Adsorbed for Adult Use
Tetanus Toxoid
Typhoid Vaccine Live Oral Ty21a
Varicella Virus Vaccine Live
Yellow Fever Vaccine

Updated February 2, 2004. FDA/Center for Biologics Evaluation and Research.

ular antigen. With appropriate T helper cell "help," antigen binding causes the B cell to divide (clonal expansion). Some of the daughter cells become plasma cells, which actively produce and secrete antibodies. Other daughter cells (memory cells) resemble the original cell and are distributed in lymph throughout the body. On subsequent exposure to the antigen, antibody production is rapid.

- Antibodies are proteins that specifically bind a particular antigen. Antibodies have several functions, including precipitation, agglutination, neutralization, opsonization, and complement activation.
- The five major antibody classes are IgG, IgM, IgA, IgD, and IgE. Antibody class is determined by the structure of the Fc portion. IgG is the most prevalent antibody class (75%). IgM is the first kind to be produced on antigen exposure. IgA is found primarily in body secretions. IgD is present on the B-cell membrane and functions in signal transduction. IgE binds to basophil and mast cell membranes and mediates inflammation and allergy.
- Administration of preformed antibodies confers passive immunity. Passive immunity provides immediate but temporary protection. Active immunity occurs when individuals are exposed to antigen that stimulates their own lymphocytes to produce memory cells. Active immunity confers long-term protection but may take several weeks to develop.

INTEGRATED FUNCTION AND REGULATION OF THE IMMUNE SYSTEM

The innate and adaptive cells of the immune system work interdependently to protect the host from foreign antigens. Efficient interdependent function depends on a complex communication network that allows coordination of various immune components. One of the reasons that the immune system uses such a complex communication system is to ensure that normal healthy tissue is not injured. The destructive powers of the immune system must be tightly regulated to avoid undue tissue damage. These regulatory controls can be affected by aging and disease. The effects of aging on immune function are described in The Aging Process: Changes in the Immune System. In the following sections, major events in the immune response to a new antigen are summarized and mechanisms of immune regulation are described.

INTEGRATED RESPONSE TO NEW ANTIGEN

A new antigen entering the body through the skin or mucous membranes will generally encounter tissue macrophages and dendritic cells stationed in strategic locations in the body as part of the mononuclear phagocyte system. Macrophages initiate activity of both the innate and specific immune components (Figure 9-39). First, activated macrophages release cytokines that initiate inflammation and chemotaxis. Some of these cytokines (TNF-α, IL-1) induce capillary endothelial cells to express selectins and integrin ligands that help circulating leukocytes to stick to the capillary wall (margination) and then move into the tissue locations of antigens (emigration). Neutrophils, macrophages, and NK cells are attracted to

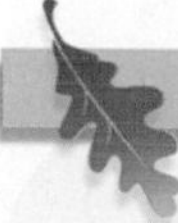

THE AGING PROCESS

Changes in the Immune System

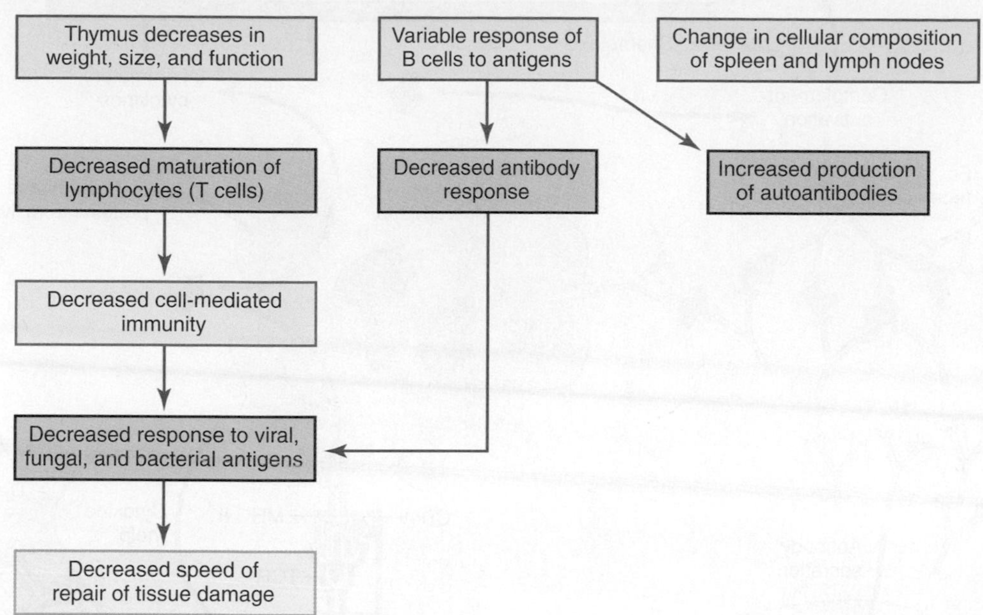

In the elderly, immune system function is altered with a decreased ability to respond to antigenic stimulation. The elderly are able to respond to infections with previously produced "remembered" antibodies. However, they are less able to respond to new antigens. As a result of these changes, there is decreased speed of repair of tissue damage and increased vulnerability to disease. The cells of the immune system in elderly persons are not able to proliferate or reproduce as effectively as those in younger persons. Although the total number of T cells remains the same, T-cell function is decreased. T cells are less able to proliferate and have decreased cytotoxicity. Antibody production also decreases, especially antibodies such as IgG. There is also a rise in autoantibody production, which may influence the increase in autoimmune disease in the elderly. Thymus size decreases after puberty, causing a decline in thymic hormone production, decreased T-cell differentiation, and reduced T-cell–related B-cell differentiation. Usually thymic hormone secretions stop after age 60 years. However, the role of thymus involution in elderly immune system changes is currently uncertain.

the infected area by chemotactic factors, some of which are released by macrophages whereas others are products of the complement cascade and tissue injury. The complement cascade is activated by the alternative pathway on primary exposure to an antigen. Complement fragments C3a and C5a are potent inflammatory agents. Complement activation also results in the formation of membrane attack complexes that directly lyse cellular antigens.

Tissue injury associated with the infectious process also activates the coagulation cascade, which forms a fibrin meshwork to help entrap and localize the agent, and the kinin system, which promotes vasodilation to increase blood flow to the area. A number of other vasodilatory chemicals may be released from mast cells in the area when they degranulate. These inflammatory chemicals lead to the classic manifestations of inflammation: warmth, swelling, redness, pain, and loss of function. Neutrophils, macrophages, and NK cells that emigrate to the tissue find their targets through innate receptors on their cell surfaces. Thus, they are as effective on first exposure to an antigen as they are on subsequent exposures. These receptors bind to complement opsonins and molecules expressed on microbes such as lipopolysaccharide and mannose. NK cells release cytotoxins onto their targets; macrophages and neutrophils phagocytose and digest their targets.

Dendritic cells and macrophages ingest protein antigens to process and present them to T helper cells in association with MHC class II proteins. Dendritic cells move from the tissue and travel to the T cell zones of lymph nodes. Activation of T helper cells results in the secretion of a variety of cytokines that boost the growth and activity of many immune cells, including macrophages, neutrophils, NK cells, cytotoxic and T helper cells, and B cells. Some of the cytokines produced by activated T cells and macrophages stimulate stem cells in the bone marrow to produce more WBCs (neutrophilia). Other

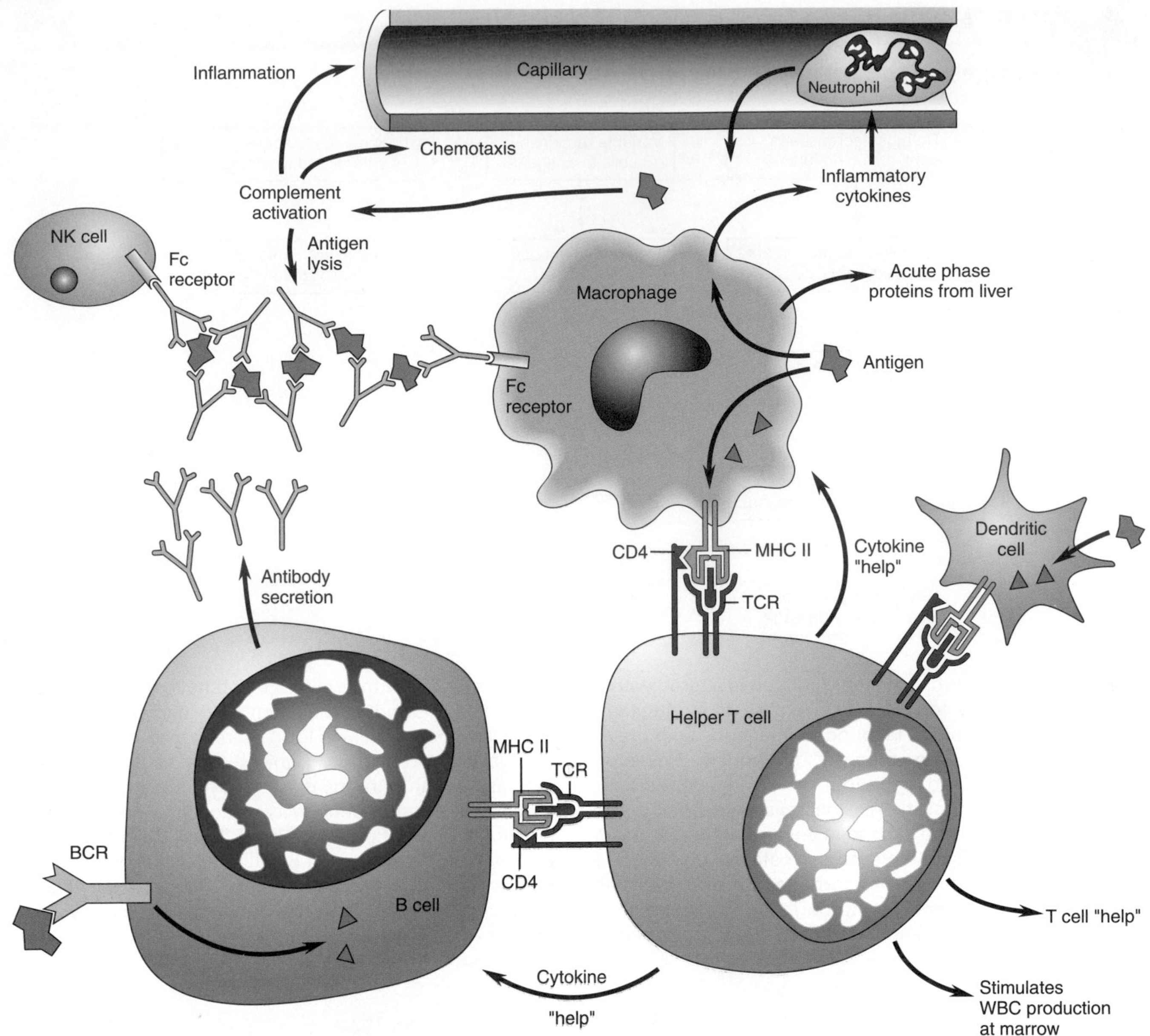

FIGURE 9-39 ■ Diagram showing the integrated function of a number of immune components. Note that the macrophage is at the center of many immune functions, including chemotaxis and inflammation, presentation of antigen to T cells, and phagocytosis of antibody-antigen complexes. *NK,* Natural killer; *MHC,* major histocompatibility complex; *BCR,* B-cell receptor; *TCR,* T-cell receptor; *WBC,* white blood cell.

cytokines affect the brain (inducing fever, lethargy, and anorexia) and the liver (producing acute phase proteins).

Meanwhile, certain B cells that encounter the antigen in the lymph nodes will have the right BCR to bind and internalize it. Internalized antigen is then processed and presented to T helper cells in association with B cell MHC II proteins. Complementary T helper cells then bind the B cell (via MHC II–TCR–CD4 interactions) and provide help to the B cell through the secretion of cytokines and through coreceptor-mediated second-messenger signals. B cells thus activated proliferate into a clone of cells, some of which become memory cells whereas others become plasma cells. Plasma cells synthesize and secrete antibodies that specifically bind the antigen. Significant antibody production takes 10 to 14 days to occur, and the infected individual may have signs and symptoms of illness during this time.

Antibodies enhance the function of innate phagocytic cells by collecting antigen into large complexes that are easier for nonspecific cells to locate and phagocytose. Activated T helper cells also secrete cytokines such as IL-2 and IFN-γ, which enhance the effectiveness of macrophages. After the antigen is cleared from the body, macrophages perform clean-up functions to remove inflammatory debris and dead neutrophils from the tissue. Macrophages also secrete enzymes and growth factors that stimulate tissue healing.

After the primary infection, B and T memory cells populate the body in much larger numbers and can mount an effective immune response very quickly on second exposure. The individual then has immunity for the particular pathogen because the antigen will usually be cleared from the system before significant illness occurs.

If the infectious agent is a virus, the story is somewhat different. Virally infected cells initiate cytotoxic T-cell activity, which serves to kill the infected cells. Natural killer cells are important for detecting and destroying virally infected cells that have down-regulated their MHC I proteins, making themselves invisible to cytotoxic T cells.[17] Helper T cell responses and B-cell production of antibody to the virus occur by the processes previously described. However, neutrophils are less important in the response to viral infection.

REGULATION OF IMMUNE FUNCTION

The mechanisms that promote inflammation and enhance immune function are much better understood than those that negatively regulate these processes. However, the mechanisms for turning off an immune response and keeping inflammation in check are just as important. The destructive powers of the immune system can cause severe tissue damage unless carefully controlled.

Inhibition of immune responses occurs in a number of different ways. The process of inducing tolerance to self antigens is of primary importance. Because both T and B lymphocytes produce antigen-binding receptors by a random process, generation of self-reactive lymphocytes cannot be prevented. As previously mentioned, B and T cells are subjected to a rigorous selection process as they mature in the bone marrow or thymus. Several theories have been proposed to explain how self-reactive cells are detected and eliminated. The clonal deletion theory suggests that cells in the thymus process and present self antigens to developing T cells. Those lymphocytes that avidly bind self antigens are triggered to initiate programmed cell death (apoptosis).[18] There appears to be a critical time in fetal development when self antigens begin to be differentiated from foreign antigens. Before that time, antigens introduced into the fetus will be viewed as "self" and tolerance to them will develop. By the same token, self antigens that do not get presented to T cells in the thymus may be viewed as foreign. This situation may occur with certain so-called sequestered antigens as would be found in the interior of the eye or testes. If these antigens are later released by trauma, an immune response may be directed against them.

Clonal deletion may not rid the body of all self-reactive lymphocytes; therefore many safeguards are in place to prevent their activation. A complex process of antigen processing and presentation is required before T and B cells can be effectively activated. A certain "dose" of antigen must be present to achieve an effective response.[1] Antigen in very high dose appears to cripple lymphocyte responsiveness and may initiate apoptosis. Self antigens may be present in such high quantity that reactive lymphocytes are killed. Because dendritic cells, macrophages, and B cells are important antigen-presenting cells, they can exert some influence on T-cell activation by controlling the dose of antigen presented. Certain cytokines are known to influence the production of MHC proteins and can therefore alter the amount of antigen to which T cells are exposed.

B-cell activation requires a number of costimulatory signals from different sources. This complexity helps ensure that B cells will be activated appropriately. These signals include antigen binding to the BCR, T helper binding to the B-cell MHC class II protein, expression of costimulatory ligands and receptors, and secretion of cytokines that promote B-cell growth and differentiation into memory cells and plasma cells. In addition, B cells are subject to negative feedback by circulating antibodies. Circulating IgG antibodies can bind to special receptors (Fc) on the B-cell membrane and inhibit B-cell activity.[19] As B cells switch from IgM to IgG and soluble IgG-antigen complexes begin to accumulate, the immune complexes can bind to the Fc receptors on B cells and block further antibody production (Figure 9-40).

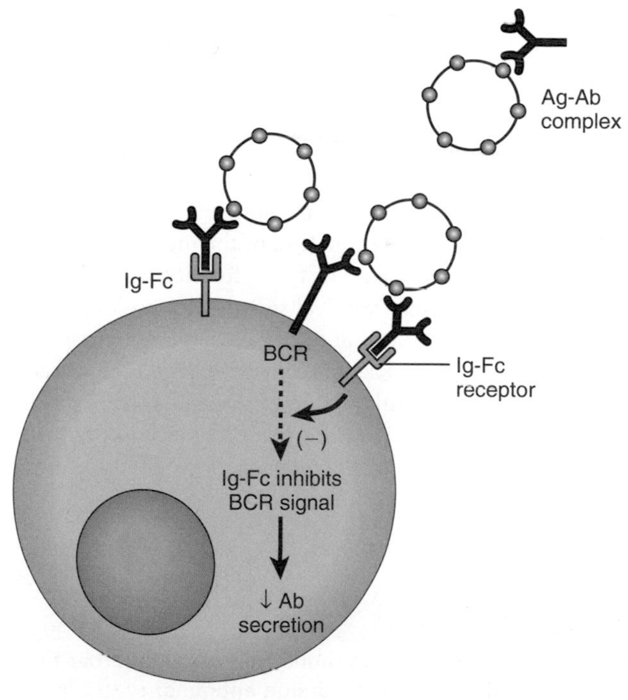

FIGURE 9-40 ■ IgG antibody can bind to antigen to form antigen-antibody *(Ag-Ab)* complexes that attach to special F_c receptors on the surface of B cells. Binding of the antigen-antibody complexes in this manner inhibits B-cell production of antibody. This process is called negative-feedback regulation. *BCR,* B-cell receptor.

Another mechanism of immune suppression is accomplished through cells that secrete inhibitory chemicals. These cell types have not been definitively identified, but some studies suggest that a subtype of CD4 T cell may perform regulatory functions. They may inhibit immune responses by secreting immunosuppressive cytokines such as IL-10 and TGF-β.

Control of the complement, kinin, and clotting systems is achieved by a number of inhibitory binding proteins. C1 inhibitor, a glycoprotein, inhibits both the Hageman factor (factor XII) and activated portions of C1. Other portions of the complement system are regulated by other binding proteins (e.g., factor I, factor H, and S protein). S protein is of particular importance. It prevents the complement membrane attack complex from attaching to and lysing cell membranes.

The production of oxygen free radicals by neutrophils can be inhibited through a number of antioxidant enzymes, including superoxide dismutase, glutathione peroxidase, and catalase. Vitamin E and β-carotene are fat-soluble vitamins that react with oxygen radicals and prevent membrane damage. Uric acid and vitamin C neutralize oxidizing agents in the cytoplasm.[20] Neutrophils also release proteolytic enzymes that injure tissues. Protease inhibitors produced by the liver, such as α_1-antitrypsin, help reduce excessive protein destruction.

The neuroendocrine system also has a role in immune regulation. Immune cells have receptors for glucocorticoid hormones and a number of neuropeptides, including enkephalins, endorphins, adrenocorticotropic hormone, oxytocin, somatostatin, and substance P.[21,22] It is a well-known phenomenon that stress and depression can lead to reduced immune function. Some of these hormones are believed to be responsible for this effect. The immune system also affects the nervous system through secreted cytokines such as IL-1 and TNF-α, which induce sleep and malaise.

One of the most important mechanisms of terminating an immune reaction is the elimination of the inciting antigen. As the antigen is cleared, many of the cytokines and costimulators are reduced so that "survival signals" are no longer given to lymphocyte populations and they undergo apoptosis.

Despite these complex and effective regulatory mechanisms, immune and inflammatory disorders are extremely common. Chapter 10 describes the pathophysiology of the common overreactions and underreactions of the immune system.

KEY CONCEPTS

- Specific and innate immune cells work together to protect the body from foreign antigens. Macrophages and dendritic cells play a central role because they are commonly the first immune cells to encounter the antigen. Macrophages secrete cytokines that stimulate WBC production and help WBCs locate the area. Tissue reactions activate the clotting cascade and kinin system, which help to localize the antigen and promote movement of fluid and immune cells into the tissue.
- Macrophages and dendritic cells are antigen-presenting cells that engulf and display antigen on their cell surface in association with MHC class II proteins. T helper cells are specifically activated by these antigen-presenting cells. T helper cells secrete cytokines that stimulate the production of WBCs in the marrow, initiate proliferation of mature B and T cells, and stimulate the phagocytic potential of macrophages and neutrophils.
- B-cell proliferation and antibody secretion usually require T-cell help. B cells internalize and present antigen to T cells, which then stimulate B-cell proliferation. B cells secrete antibodies that help phagocytic cells localize and destroy antigens.
- The immune response to primary exposure is slow and often insufficient to prevent illness. Memory cells that develop during primary exposure can mount a more effective response on subsequent exposure and usually prevent manifestations of illness.
- T and B lymphocytes must be tolerant to self. T lymphocytes capable of reacting with self tissue are thought to be destroyed or permanently inactivated during development in the thymus. One theory suggests that lymphocytes must come in contact with all self antigens during development, and those that do not specifically bind self antigens are allowed to survive.
- B cells are subject to careful regulation by T helper cells and by negative feedback from high concentrations of circulating antigen-antibody complexes.
- Mechanisms to inhibit and control the immune response include regulatory T-cell cytokines, complement inhibitors, degradation of inflammatory mediators, circulating antiproteases, and antioxidants.

SUMMARY

Cells and tissues throughout the body participate in defense against foreign antigens. Some components of the immune system are able to react to almost any foreign invader upon first exposure. These innate components are essential for protecting the body while the specific immune defenses are being activated. Innate defenses include physical and biochemical barriers of the skin and mucous membranes, cells of the mononuclear phagocyte system, neutrophils, NK cells, and a large number of chemical mediators such as complement, clotting factors, kinin, and cytokines. Immunity to specific antigens is provided by B and T lymphocytes. T helper cells are important regulators of the immune system because they secrete cytokines that enhance T-cell, B-cell, and macrophage function.

The forces of inflammation and immunity must be carefully controlled to prevent excessive tissue damage. Extensive measures are used to rid the body of self-reactive lymphocytes and to control reactions once a foreign antigen has been cleared. A well-functioning immune system effectively protects against foreign invaders, learns from the process such that it is even more effective on subsequent exposure, yet leaves healthy normal tissue unharmed.

MEDIA RESOURCES

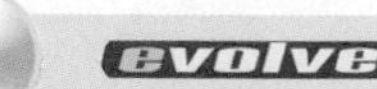

Remember to check out the ***CD Companion*** included with this book for Review Questions, Key Concepts Review, Glossary (with audio for selected terms), Disease Profiles, and Animations.

PLUS, visit the ***Evolve website*** at http://evolve.elsevier.com/Copstead/ for Case Studies, Disease Profiles, and WebLinks.

References

1. Abbas AK, Lichtman AH: *Cellular and molecular immunology,* ed 5, Philadelphia, 2003, Saunders.
2. Lydyard PM, Grossi CE: Cells, tissues and organs of the immune system. In Roitt I, Brostoff J, Male D, editors: *Immunology,* ed 6, St Louis, 2001, Mosby, pp 15-45.
3. McIntyre TM et al: Cell-cell interactions: leukocyte-endothelial interactions, *Curr Opin Hematol* 10(2):150-158, 2003.
4. Cornbleet PJ: Clinical utility of the band count, *Clin Lab Med* 22(1):101-136, 2002.
5. Aldridge AJ: Role of the neutrophil in septic shock and the adult respiratory distress syndrome, *Eur J Surg* 168(4):204-214, 2002.
6. Agnello D et al: Cytokines and transcription factors that regulate T helper cell differentiation: new players and new insights, *J Clin Immunol* 23(3):147-161, 2003.
7. Guyton AC, Hall JE: Resistance of the body to infection: II. Immunity and allergy. In Guyton AC, Hall JE, editors: *Textbook of medical physiology,* ed 10, Philadelphia, 2000, Saunders.
8. Blatteis CM et al: Signaling the brain in systemic inflammation: the role of complement, *Front Biosci* 9:915-931, 2004.
9. Mitchell RN, Cotran RS: Acute and chronic inflammation. In Kumar V, Cotran RS, Robbins SL, editors: *Robbins basic pathology,* ed 7, Philadelphia, 2003, Saunders, pp 33-60.
10. Mitchell RN, Cotran RS: Tissue repair: cell regeneration and fibrosis. In Kumar V, Cotran RS, Robbins SL, editors: *Robbins basic pathology,* ed 7, Philadelphia, 2003, Saunders, pp 61-78.
11. Faro J et al: The impact of thymic antigen diversity on the size of the selected T cell repertoire, *J Immunol* 172(4):2247-2255, 2004.
12. Kojima Y et al: Localization of Fas ligand in cytoplasmic granules of $CD8^+$ cytotoxic T lymphocytes and natural killer cells: participation of Fas ligand in granule exocytosis model of cytotoxicity, *Biochem Biophys Res Commun* 296(2):328-336, 2002.
13. Turner M: Antibodies. In Roitt I, Brostoff J, Male D, editors: *Immunology,* ed 6, St Louis, 2001, Mosby, pp 65-85.
14. Li Z et al: The generation of antibody diversity through somatic hypermutation and class switch recombination, *Genes Dev* 18(1):1-11, 2004.
15. Neuberger MS et al: Memory in the B-cell compartment: antibody affinity maturation, *Philos Trans R Soc Lond B Biol Sci* 355(1395):357-360, 2000.
16. Hanson LA, Korotkova M, Telemo E: Breast-feeding, infant formulas, and the immune system, *Ann Allergy Asthma Immunol* 90(6 suppl 3):59-63, 2003.
17. French AR, Yokoyama WM: Natural killer cells and viral infections, *Curr Opin Immunol* 15(1):45-51, 2003.
18. Palmer E: Negative selection: clearing out the bad apples from the T-cell repertoire, *Nat Rev Immunol* 3(5):383-391, 2003.
19. Heyman B: Feedback regulation by IgG antibodies, *Immunol Lett* 88(2):157-161, 2003.
20. Winklhofer-Roob BM et al: Effects of vitamin E and carotenoid status on oxidative stress in health and disease. Evidence obtained from human intervention studies, *Mol Aspects Med* 24(6):391-402, 2003.
21. Haddad JJ, Saade NE, Safieh-Garabedian B: Cytokines and neuro-immune-endocrine interactions: a role for the hypothalamic-pituitary-adrenal revolving axis, *J Neuroimmunol* 133(1-2):1-19, 2002.
22. Pert CB, Dreher HE, Ruff MR: The psychosomatic network: foundations of mind-body medicine, *Altern Ther Health Med* 4(4):30-41, 1998.

chapter 10

Alterations in Immune Function

Faith Young Peterson

MEDIA RESOURCES

Additional Material for Study, Review, and Further Exploration

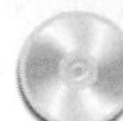

CD Companion ◆ Review Questions and Answers ◆ Key Concepts Review ◆ Glossary *(with audio pronunciations for selected terms)* ◆ Disease Profiles ◆ Animations

evolve *Website* at http://evolve.elsevier.com/Copstead/ ◆ Case Studies ◆ Disease Profiles ◆ WebLinks

KEY QUESTIONS

- What are the potential mechanisms whereby erroneous reaction of the immune system with self tissue leads to autoimmune diseases?
- How do type I, II, III, and IV hypersensitivity reactions differ according to the immune cell types involved and the mechanism of tissue injury?
- What are the common features of autoimmune disorders and certain types of hypersensitivity disorders?
- How are hypersensitivity disorders detected, prevented, and treated?
- How do the etiologic processes of primary and secondary immune deficiency disorders differ?
- What are the clinical features of the common immunodeficiency disorders?

CHAPTER OUTLINE

The purposes of the immune system are to defend the body against invasion or infection by foreign substances called **antigens,** to assist the body to maintain a steady state, and to patrol for and destroy cells that are abnormal or damaged. Normally, the immune system works efficiently to accomplish these purposes, but in some situations inappropriate immune responses lead to disease.

These disorders can be divided into two general categories: (1) excessive immune responses and (2) deficient immune responses. The category of excessive immune responses includes disorders in which the immune system is overfunctioning or hyperfunctioning. Examples are autoimmunity and hypersensitivity disorders.

The category of deficient immune responses includes disorders in which the immune response is ineffective because of congenital, genetic, or acquired dysfunction. Examples of deficient immune responses are severe combined immunodeficiency (SCID) syndrome, DiGeorge syndrome, and selective IgA deficiency. Human immunodeficiency virus/acquired immunodeficiency syndrome (HIV/AIDS) is a primary acquired immunodeficiency disorder that is discussed in Chapter 12. The secondary immunodeficiencies associated with white blood cell malignancies are included in Chapter 11.

EXCESSIVE IMMUNE RESPONSES

Excessive immune response disorders result from a functional increase in the activity of the immune system. Autoimmunity and hypersensitivity are types of excessive immune response disorders. They are often related, and both may be present in patients with excessive immune responses. It may be helpful to think of autoimmunity as a way of describing the *etiologic process,* or cause, of abnormal excessive immune responses toward self tissues. Hypersensitivity disorders describe *mechanisms* of injury, or how the injury occurs, which may or may not involve autoimmunity. Autoimmunity occurs when the body attacks its own tissues. Autoimmune reactions toward self tissues are mediated through type II and III hypersensitivity mechanisms. For this reason, many autoimmune diseases are also considered hypersensitivity reactions. For example, myasthenia gravis is both an autoimmune disease and a type II hypersensitivity reaction. Immune complex glomerulonephritis is both an autoimmune disease and a type III hypersensitivity reaction.

The cause of immune system overreactions is poorly understood. Interplay between genetic factors, particularly major histocompatibility complex (MHC) genes, and environmental factors is thought to be important in the development of autoimmune disorders. Certain hypersensitivity disorders have familial tendencies also, but the specific genes and environmental agents remain to be discovered. Some evidence suggests that excessive immune responses may be due to glucocorticoid resistance in target tissues. For example, the number of glucocorticoid receptors in circulating leukocytes is decreased 50% in patients with rheumatoid arthritis. This decrease in receptors would prevent adequate suppression of leukocyte activity and could further enhance inflammation.

AUTOIMMUNITY

Autoimmunity occurs when the immune system recognizes a person's own cells ("self") as foreign and mounts an immune response that injures self tissues. It is a breakdown of self tolerance. Identification and tolerance of self antigens occur during embryonic development. During this time, aggressive or intolerant self-reactive (autoreactive) lymphocytes are eliminated or suppressed (see Chapter 9). Autoimmune diseases result when self tolerance is lost and reactions between self antigens and the immune system occur.

Several theories have been proposed to explain how various immune system components and environmental triggers might interact to produce autoimmunity. However, no single theory can yet explain the loss of self tolerance that occurs in autoimmune diseases. A number of genetic and environmental factors interacting together most probably contribute to the development of autoimmunity.

The theory of antigenic mimicry emphasizes the similarities between certain molecular segments of foreign antigens called *epitopes* and the person's own cells.[1] For example, all cells, whether self or foreign, are made up of proteins, carbohydrates, nucleic acids, and lipids. Certain viruses and bacteria evolve to look like "self" and use "molecular mimicry" to slip past the immune system defenses. Self cells with the same or similar molecular segments as these foreign epitopes can "fit" lymphocyte receptors. Therefore, these self antigens can be attacked as foreign under certain circumstances when the normal cell has been altered, such as by a viral infection that stimulates the immune response.

Another theory proposes that release of sequestered antigens triggers the autoimmune response. This theory suggests that certain self antigens are isolated from the immune system within an organ during the neonatal period. They are not in contact with antigen-processing cells during the embryonic period when self tolerance usually occurs. These hidden self antigens occur in sites such as the cornea of the eye, the testicles, or other areas not drained by lymphatics. If and when these sites are damaged later in life, the hidden or sequestered self antigens are exposed to the immune system, which does not recognize them as self. Therefore, the damaged cells are attacked.

A number of T-cell theories of autoimmunity have been proposed, including thymus gland defects, decreased suppressor T-cell function, and altered T helper cell function. The theories attributing autoimmunity to thymus gland defects state that maturation and differentiation of T cells are affected by either decreased hormone secretion or failure of the thymus to expose T cells to all self products. In this theory, the thymus gland is responsible for exposing developing T cells to self products produced in the thymus or carried to the thymus gland. If some self products are not exposed to the developing T cells, the product will not be recognized as self and will subsequently be attacked. This lack of exposure to self products is thought to be a major factor in the development of generalized autoimmune diseases such as systemic lupus erythematosus (SLE). The theory attributing autoimmunity to decreased suppressor T-cell activity states that decreased numbers of suppressor T cells fail to repress immunoglobulin activity. However, this theory does not adequately explain tissue-specific or organ-specific autoimmune damage, but it may explain generalized autoimmunity as seen in SLE. The altered T helper cell function theory asserts that changed T helper cells lose their self tolerance through a variety of mechanisms.

A number of B-cell theories of autoimmunity have also been proposed. The theory attributing autoimmunity to escape of B-cell tolerance proposes that certain B cells lose their responsiveness to suppressor T-cell messages. The B-cell activation theories, which are well supported clinically and experimentally, suggest that extrinsic factors or intrinsic, genetic B-cell defects cause autoantibody production and an increase in the number and activity of B cells. A number of extrinsic factors, including viruses, bacteria, antibiotics, proteolytic enzymes, and lipopolysaccharides, have been found to be B-cell–activating factors that could trigger autoantibody production.

Genetic Factors

Genetic predisposition seems to be an important factor in the development of autoimmune disorders. Recent studies show that different cytokine profiles can be associated with autoimmunity. Those with genetically low levels of tumor necrosis factor α (TNF-α) and high levels of interleukin-10 (IL-10) may be more tolerant than those with normal levels.[1] The role of genetics is supported by the observation that certain MHC genes—also called human leukocyte antigen (HLA) genes—are frequently associated with certain autoimmune disorders (Table 10-1). Gender, which is genetically determined, also influences the expression of autoimmune disorders. The exact mechanisms of gender and genetic influence on autoimmune expression have not been established, but the relationship is significant.

Certain MHC genes appear to increase the risk of development of autoimmune disease. The strongest correlation of MHC molecules with autoimmune disease is the linkage between the HLA-B27 phenotype and ankylosing spondylitis. In this case, 95% of all people with ankylosing spondylitis have a positive B27 phenotype. However, not everyone with a positive B27 phenotype develops ankylosing spondylitis both be-

Table 10-1

Major Histocompatibility Genes and Autoimmune Disease

Disease	HLA (MHC) Antigen	Frequency in Patients (%)	Frequency in Controls (%)	Relative Risk
Ankylosing spondylitis				
Caucasians	B27	89	43	69
Japanese	B27	85	<1	207
Rheumatoid arthritis	DR4	68	25	3.8
Graves disease	Dw3	56	25	3.7
Type 1 diabetes mellitus	DR3/DR4 heterozygous			33
Systemic lupus erythematosus	DR4	73	33	5
Narcolepsy	DR2	100	34	358

Data from Tierney LM, McPhee SJ, Papadalkis MA: *Current medical diagnosis and treatment,* ed 37, Stamford, Conn, 1998, Appleton & Lange.

cause of differences in the way antigen is presented to the immune system and because of environmental factors. Other diseases are associated with different MHC phenotypes, but the correlation between risk for disease and presence of the disease marker is much lower. For example, Addison disease is associated with the DR3 phenotype, but it has only a 6% risk correlation. Juvenile rheumatoid arthritis is strongly associated with HLA-DR5.

An individual's mix of T_H1 and T_H2 cells may contribute to allergic reactivity. T_H2 cells release IL-4 and IL-5, which stimulates B cells to produce IgE. T_H1 cells secrete interferon-γ and IL-2, which may inhibit IgE production by B cells.

Environmental Triggers

Viral infections may also be associated with the development of autoimmunity. Viruses can activate B cells, decrease the function of T cells, contribute to the development of antigenic mimicry, or insert viral components on cell surfaces and trigger immune reactions. For example, Epstein-Barr virus has been frequently cited as a cause of autoimmune disease. Other factors that may contribute to autoimmunity include environmental triggers leading to inflammation or lymphokine release that activates antiself T cells.

Although the etiology of autoimmunity continues to be investigated, the mechanisms whereby autoantibodies injure tissues are better understood. The autoantibodies produced by autoimmune disorders affect tissue by the mechanisms described for type II and type III hypersensitivity reactions found later in this chapter.

Pharmacotherapies

Although no particular treatment for autoimmune disorders has been established, immunosuppressive therapy is the treatment most often used. Because autoimmunity is expressed in different ways, the immunosuppressive treatment for each type of autoimmune disease is individualized depending on disease expression. Immunosuppressive therapy has become increasingly important in the armamentarium of medicine. These drugs are essential for inhibiting excessive or aberrant immune responses. The ideal immunosuppressive medication would be an agent that inhibits only the abnormal immune response without limiting the positive and protective functions of the immune system or causing any organ toxicity. Unfortunately, no immunosuppressive medications like that exist.

Immunosuppressive agents include corticosteroids and cytotoxins. Corticosteroids decrease the number of lymphocytes and decrease antibody formation as well as alter the functional activities of lymphocytes. They also have many other activities as a result of their glucocorticoid function. Corticosteroids tend to be the first line of treatment for many autoimmune diseases, such as asthma and allergies, and are the oldest of the immunosuppressive drugs. They act by altering cellular metabolism, readily crossing cell membranes and binding to receptors within cells. They are often used intermittently in other autoimmune diseases such as rheumatoid arthritis. Examples include methylprednisolone (Solu-Medrol) and fluticasone (Flovent, Flonase). Cytotoxins were originally used as anticancer agents but are now increasingly used to manage autoimmune disorders. They can kill actively proliferating cells. In autoimmune treatment, they are used to kill lymphocytes after they are transformed from their resting G_0 state to actively proliferating cells. The key to the use of cytotoxins is to effectively apply their killing activity without hurting the rest of the body. These medications are widely used for the management of rheumatoid arthritis, SLE, psoriatic arthritis, Wegener granulomatosis, and rheumatoid vasculitis. An example of a cytotoxin is methotrexate.

Cyclosporine (Sandimmune) is an immunosuppressant that is more selective than corticosteroids or cytotoxins. It selectively and reversibly suppresses T helper cells in the G_0 or G_1 phase of the cell cycle without killing them. As a result, it inhibits the development of killer or cytotoxic T cells without decreasing the numbers of cells. It also impairs the ability of T cells to respond effectively to foreign antigens. It is used to suppress reactions during tissue or organ transplantation.

Antirheumatic agents are used in rheumatoid arthritis, SLE, and ankylosing spondylitis but are increasingly used in other autoimmune diseases. These agents work as disease modifiers. An example of a disease modifier is etanercept (Enbrel), a drug that binds to and blocks the activity of TNF-α and TNF-β. Etanercept also modulates TNF-mediated responses such as leukocyte migration and expression of adhesion molecules. Other examples include azathioprine (Imuran); leflunomide (Arava), and infliximab (Remicade).

Therapeutic plasmapheresis is another type of therapy occasionally used in the management of autoimmune diseases. Plasmapheresis is analogous to dialysis and involves the selective filtering or removal of plasma or a plasma cell type. The patient's whole blood is filtered and the plasma component containing the autoantibodies removed and replaced with albumin or another colloid solution. This type of therapy has been effective in the management of myasthenia gravis, thrombocytopenic purpura, multiple sclerosis, and Rh-negative hemolytic disease of the newborn.

KEY CONCEPTS

- Autoimmune disorders occur when the immune system erroneously reacts with "self" tissues. These disorders are thought to be polygenic and multifactorial; however, the exact etiologic process is unknown.
- The antigenic mimicry theory proposes that since self and foreign antigens are composed of the same basic building blocks—proteins, carbohydrates, nucleic acids, and lipids—small alterations in self tissue may lead to immunogenic attack.
- The theory involving release of sequestered antigens suggests that self antigens that do not come in direct contact with lymphocytes during fetal development may cause autoimmune reactions if they are subsequently released from sequestration.
- Abnormal production of subclasses of T lymphocytes, particularly suppressor T cells, has been proposed as a reason for the development of autoimmunity, as well as the development of abnormal B cells that do not respond to suppressor T cell signals.
- A genetic component is probable inasmuch as certain autoimmune disorders are more commonly associated with particular MHC types and female gender.
- Viruses may also be causative in the development of autoimmune disorders. Viruses may alter self cells, thus precipitating an immune attack. Formed antibodies may then cross-react with similar but uninfected cells.
- Autoantibodies injure body tissues through the mechanisms described for type II and type III hypersensitivity reactions.

HYPERSENSITIVITY

Hypersensitivity is a normal immune response that is inappropriately triggered or excessive or produces undesirable effects on the body. The basic mechanism that triggers hypersensitivity is a specific antigen-antibody reaction or a specific antigen-lymphocyte interaction. Four classes or types of hypersensitivity are differentiated. Each type is characterized by a specific cellular or antibody response. Hypersensitivity types I, II, and III are mediated by antibodies produced by B lymphocytes. Type IV hypersensitivity is mediated by T cells. Hypersensitivity reactions are specific to a particular antigen and do not usually occur on first exposure to the antigen. Although the diseases or syndromes associated with each type differ in their clinical signs and symptoms, the underlying pathophysiologic process is similar within each type. In Table 10-2 the four major types of hypersensitivity are contrasted.

Type I Hypersensitivity

Etiology. Increasing evidence indicates that genetic mechanisms influence type I hypersensitivity. There is a strong genetic or hereditary linkage regarding the IgE response to antigens (allergens). This genetic component involves both the ability to respond to an allergen and the general ability to produce an IgE antibody response. For example, children born to two allergic parents have a 50% chance of being allergic. Children born to one nonallergic and one allergic parent have a 30% chance of being allergic.

Researchers are currently exploring two genetic avenues that influence hyperresponsiveness and allergies. These directions include research on IgE levels and suppressor T-cell function. High IgE levels have been found in some hypersensitive people. It has also been found that low levels of suppressor T cells are associated with high IgE levels and the MHC genes *HLA-B8* and *HLA-Dw3*. *HLA-B8* may be linked to suppressor T-cell control of immune responses. These findings suggest that IgE production is under T-cell control. However, not all allergic people have high IgE levels.

Several other hypotheses regarding the causes of allergic, type I hypersensitivity reactions have been proposed. It is hypothesized that a suppressor T-cell deficiency or abnormal mediator feedback increases mast cell degranulation and the inflammatory response. Environmental pollutants may play a role by increasing mucosal permeability and enhancing antigen (allergen) entry into the body. This increased entry would subsequently increase IgE responsiveness.

In addition, an allergic breakthrough hypothesis has been devised to explain type I hypersensitivity reactions. This hypothesis suggests that in both high-IgE and low-IgE responders, overt expression of clinical symptoms is seen only when some allergic breakthrough level is exceeded. Exceeding this hypothesized level may depend on the presence of concomitant factors, such as viral infections of the upper respiratory tract, transient IgA deficiency, or decreased suppressor T-cell activity.

Table 10-2

The Four Types of Hypersensitivity

Characteristic	Type I: Atopic, Anaphylactic	Type II: Cytotoxic, Cytolytic	Type III: Immune Complex (Arthus Reaction)	Type IV: Delayed Hypersensitivity
Mediated by	IgE	IgM or IgG	IgG	T_{DTH} lymphocytes
Complement activation	No	Yes	Yes	No
Immune response	Ag plus IgE, leading to mast cell degranulation	Surface Ag and Ab, leading to killer cell cytotoxic action or complement-mediated lysis	Ag-Ab complex in tissues; complement activated and PMNs attracted	Ag-sensitized T cells release lymphokines, leading to inflammatory reactions, and attract macrophages, which release mediator
Peak action	15-30 min	15-30 min	6 hr	24-48 hr
Serum transferability	Yes	Yes	Yes	No
Cell transferability	No	No	No	Yes (T cells)
Genetic mechanisms	Familial High IgE level HLA-linked *Ir* genes General hyperresponsiveness	HLA linked in some cases	Familial (autoimmune) HLA specificities	Unknown
Causes of reaction	T-cell deficiency Abnormal mediator feedback Environmental factors and Ag	Exposure to Ag or foreign tissue, cells, or graft	Persistent infection—microbe Ag Extrinsic environmental Ag Autoimmunity—self Ag	Intradermal Ag Epidermal Ag Dermal Ag
Manifestation (examples)	Asthma, rhinitis, atopic eczema, bee-sting reaction	ABO transfusions, hemolytic disease of newborn, myasthenia gravis	Glomerulonephritis, SLE, farmer's lung, arthritis, vasculitis	Guillain-Barré disease, tuberculin test, contact dermatitis, multiple sclerosis

Ab, Antibody; *Ag,* antigen; *Ig,* immunoglobulin; *DTH,* delayed-type hypersensitivity; *PMN,* polymorphonuclear leukocyte; *HLA,* human leukocyte antigen; *SLE,* systemic lupus erythematosus.

Pathogenesis. Type I hypersensitivity is also known as immediate hypersensitivity, meaning that the hypersensitivity reaction is immediate. It is a sensitization reaction characterized by signs and symptoms of an allergic reaction immediately after contact with an antigen (allergen). The reaction usually occurs 15 to 30 minutes after exposure to the allergen.

At the cellular level, immunoglobulin E (IgE) is the principal antibody mediating this reaction. IgE is produced by specialized plasma B cells and circulates in very small amounts in the blood. When an individual is exposed to an allergen to which he or she is allergic, selected plasma B cells produce IgE. It usually takes repeated exposures to the allergen to cause significant levels of IgE to be present in the blood.

Mast cells are the principal effector cells, although there are many other cells with histamine and other mediators that are or can be involved in the reaction. These may include neutrophils, eosinophils, lymphocytes, macrophages, epithelial cells, endothelial cells, and particularly basophils. Mast cells are found throughout the body in all loose connective tissue. They are covered with IgE receptors—up to 500,000 on their cell surfaces—and they are filled with vesicles or granules containing potent vasoactive, proinflammatory chemical mediators (especially histamine) that produce inflammation when they are released. The IgE receptors on mast cells bind the Fc portion of an IgE antibody. The IgE antigen-binding sites are then displayed on the mast cell surface where they can bind to antigens that pass by the mast cell (Figure 10-1). This process makes the mast cells responsive to particular antigens.

The initial incident during a type I hypersensitivity response is the cross-linking of two IgE receptors to one antigen on the mast cell located at the site of the allergen's entry into the body (see Figure 10-1). Cross-linking of IgE and the antigen causes an increase in intracellular calcium (Ca^{2+}) that results in immediate, massive, local mast cell degranulation of preformed and newly formed proinflammatory mediators. The release of mediators causes an inflammatory response.

Mast cells, basophils, and other effector cells release many chemicals. Some of the mediators are preformed and stored in

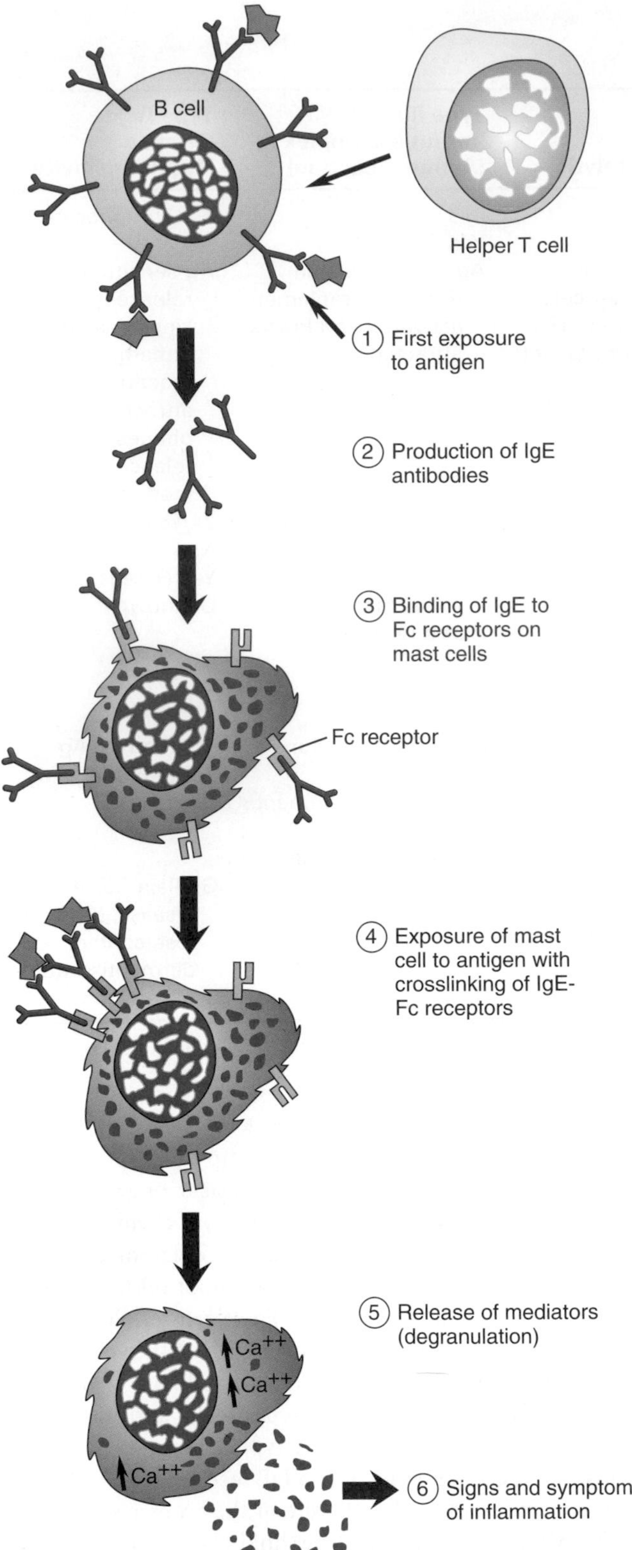

FIGURE 10-1 ■ Type I hypersensitivity reaction.

vesicles, such as histamine, heparin, proteolytic enzymes, and chemotactic factors. Other mediators are formed during the degranulation process. Examples of newly formed mediators include superoxide, prostaglandins, thromboxanes, leukotrienes, bradykinin, and interleukins (see Chapter 9).

One of the most important mediators of type I hypersensitivity is histamine. Histamine binds to H_1 (histamine 1), H_2, and H_3 receptors, which are located on many types of cells. Mast cells have receptors for H_1, H_2, and H_3 with H_1 receptors being the most active. Basophils express predominantly H_2 receptors, whereas neutrophils and eosinophils have both H_1 and H_2 receptors. Recent evidence shows that H_1 and H_2 receptors are present on monocytes and macrophages with an increase in H_1 receptors when monocytes differentiate into macrophages.[2] The histamine that binds to H_1 receptors is responsible for increased vascular permeability, vasodilatation (flushing), urticaria formation (hives), smooth muscle constriction (bronchial asthma with wheezing and coughing), increased mucus secretion and pruritus (increased itching), and increased gut permeability. The histamine that binds to H_2 receptors causes smooth muscle relaxation in the lower airways, augments gastric acid secretion from parietal cells, and in high concentrations has an inhibitory effect on inflammatory cells decreasing degranulation, and decreasing neutrophil chemotaxis. The H_3 receptors are located in postganglionic cholinergic nerves in lung bronchi.[2]

The proteolytic enzymes kininogenase and tryptase activate the kinin pathway and C3 activates the complement cascade via the alternative pathway. Heparin decreases clot formation. The chemotactic factors recruit or activate other inflammatory and immune cells. Leukotrienes cause smooth muscle contraction and increase vascular permeability.

Manifestations. Manifestations of an immediate hypersensitivity reaction vary in severity and intensity. For many people, type I hypersensitivity reactions are annoying, such as hives (urticaria), seasonal allergic rhinitis, eczema, or mild asthma symptoms. In other people, the symptoms are more problematic, including tightening of the throat, localized edema, wheezing, and tachycardia such as associated with localized angioedema reactions or more severe asthma reactions. In a very small number of highly allergic people, the type I hypersensitivity reaction can be expressed as a life-threatening allergic reaction known as anaphylaxis such as that associated with bee sting, seafood, or peanut allergic reactions. Common allergenic medications, insects, and foods that can trigger type I hypersensitivity reactions are listed in Box 10-1.

Treatment. Treatment for type I hypersensitivity primarily involves pharmacologic management with antihistamines, β-adrenergics, theophyllines, cromolyn sodium, corticosteroids, anticholinergics, or a combination. Antihistamines such as diphenhydramine (Benadryl) are used to block the effect of histamine. This action decreases vascular permeability and bronchoconstriction. β-Adrenergic sympathomimetics and theophyllines are used to decrease bronchoconstriction

Box 10-1

Possible Causes of Human Anaphylaxis

Medications
Penicillin, penicillin analogues, and other antibiotics
Radiographic contrast media
Aspirin, indomethacin, and other analgesics
Allergenic extracts

Biological Agents
Serum proteins, including γ-globulin
Insulin and other hormones
Vaccines
Enzymes such as penicillinase
Local anesthetics
Hymenoptera (stinging) insects
Polistes wasps
Honeybees
Fire ants
Hornets and yellow jackets

Foods
Nuts
Seafood, especially shellfish
Eggs
Fruit, especially citrus and strawberries
Tartrazine, yellow dye no. 5
Inorganic chemicals
Nickel
Aluminum
Zinc

and bronchospasm. Available orally, parenterally, and via inhalers, these medications have a rapid onset. **Epinephrine** is a major β-adrenergic given subcutaneously or intravenously during acute allergic reactions, especially after food or bee sting reactions. Most patients with severe allergies to food or insect bites are given prescriptions for epinephrine in the form of Epipen with an autoinjector. Other β-adrenergics that can be given include metaproterenol (Alupent), terbutaline (Brethaire), and albuterol (Ventolin). Theophyllines given include aminophylline, theophylline (Theo-Dur), and oxtriphylline. Cromolyn sodium (Intal) stabilizes mast cell membranes and thereby prevents degranulation and release of inflammatory mediators. It is not used during acute attacks but may be helpful in preventing reactions in the future. Corticosteroids are used to decrease the inflammatory response. Anticholinergics are used to block the parasympathetic system and thus allow greater sympathetic activity. This action indirectly causes bronchodilation.

Prevention. Some protective, proactive actions taken during pregnancy are thought to decrease the likelihood that type I hypersensitivity will develop in children from families with a history of allergies. These actions include avoiding foods to which the mother is allergic, limiting excesses of one type of food during the last trimester of pregnancy, avoiding whole eggs during the last month before delivery and while breast-feeding, and limiting cow's milk to two glasses per day. Other actions that may be helpful during the child's infancy include avoiding exposure to environmental pollution, breast-feeding for a minimum of 6 months, supplementation with non–cow's milk products such as soy milk, giving solid foods only after the infant is 6 months old, keeping the infant's room as free of dust and molds as possible, and keeping pets (dogs, cats, birds) out of the home.

Pharmacotherapeutic Prevention. Another avenue for prevention of type I hypersensitivity reactions involves the use of cromolyn sodium or desensitization therapy (immunotherapy). Cromolyn sodium (Intal) stabilizes mast cells and inhibits mast cell degranulation, which decreases release of the vasoactive mediators. This medication is used primarily for patients with asthma.

Desensitization, or immunotherapy, is more successful in patients with hay fever than in those with other types of allergies. It involves both environmental control of external allergens and titrated pharmacologic exposure to allergens. Environmental control involves a systematic plan to decrease exposure to house dust, molds, and animal dander. Pets are kept out of the house. The person must avoid food allergens, wool carpets, goose down or feather pillows, dried plants, and exposure to other animal and vegetable products. The person is urged to use air conditioning and electronic air filters.

Pharmacologic desensitization involves injecting a person with sufficient antigen (allergen) on a regular basis over a course of months or years, followed by periodic maintenance or booster therapy. Gradually the dose is increased until the person can tolerate the allergen without a type I hypersensitivity reaction. The goal of this therapy is a change in immunoglobulins so that there is an increase in IgG and IgA blocking antibodies, no increase in IgE during allergy season, decreased basophil reactivity, and decreased lymphocyte reactivity to allergens.

Type II Hypersensitivity

Etiology and Pathogenesis. Type II hypersensitivity, also known as tissue-specific, cytotoxic, or cytolytic hypersensitivity, is characterized by antibodies that attack antigens on the surface of specific cells or tissues. Often the reaction is immediate (15 to 30 minutes after exposure to the antigen). However, the reaction can occur over time such as in thyroiditis or myasthenia gravis. The mechanisms that encompass type II tissue-specific hypersensitivity all occur after the binding of antibody to tissue-specific antigens. The reaction is mediated by the complement system and a variety of effector cells, including tissue macrophages, platelets, killer cells, neutrophils, and eosinophils. IgG and IgM are the principal antibodies. Examples of this type of hypersensitivity reaction include ABO transfusion reactions, hemolytic disease of the newborn, myasthenia gravis, thyroiditis, hyperacute graft rejection, and autoimmune hemolytic anemia (Table 10-3). Transfusion reactions, hemolytic disease of the newborn, and

Table 10-3

Disease and Autoantibodies Associated with Type II Hypersensitivity

Disease	Antigen/Autoantibody
Type 1 diabetes	Islet cells
Insulin-resistant diabetic states	Insulin receptor
Myasthenia gravis	Acetylcholine receptor
Addison disease	Adrenal epithelial cells
Autoimmune hemolytic anemia	Red cell membrane
Immune thrombocytopenic purpura	Platelet membrane
Autoimmune neutropenia	Neutrophil antigens
Pernicious anemia	Intrinsic factor, gastric parietal cells
Lymphocytic thyroiditis	Thyroglobulin
Graves disease	Receptor for thyroid-stimulating hormone
Pemphigus vulgaris	Desmosomes
Hyperacute graft rejection	Donor antigens

graft rejection are examples of **isoimmunity**, a condition in which the immune system reacts against antigens on tissues from other members of the same species.

The initial mechanism during a type II hypersensitivity response is exposure to antigen on the surface of foreign cells. The Fab portion of IgG or IgM antibodies binds to antigens on the target foreign cell to form an antigen-antibody complex (Figure 10-2). (Refer also to Chapter 9 for a discussion of IgG and IgM antibodies.) The Fc region of the IgG or IgM antibodies sticks out away from the cell membrane surface. The Fc region then acts as a bridge between the antigen and complement or the effector cells. This antigen-antibody binding with Fc bridging is the key and leads to cytotoxic or cytolysis reactions by one of several mechanisms. One mechanism is complement-mediated lysis. Complement-mediated lysis occurs through the classical pathway for activation of complement. The classical pathway of complement generates the activated complement component C3b via splitting of C4 and C2 by C1. The activated complement component C3b is bound to the target cell by the Fc region of IgG or IgM. C3b increases opsonization, which in turn increases the capacity of the system to allow lysis by other effector cells or by complement itself. Lysis of the foreign cell is by complement via the C5-C9 membrane attack complex dissolving the plasma membrane of the cell.

Transfusion Reaction

An example of this type of mechanism is a blood transfusion reaction. It occurs when a person receives blood from someone with a different blood group type (Table 10-4). If a person with type A blood having type A antigens and anti-B antibodies incorrectly receives type B blood with B antigens and anti-A antibodies, the anti-B antibodies will attach to the surface of the infused type B red blood cells and the anti-A antibodies in the infusion will attach to the surface of the circulating type A red blood cells. This event will stimulate the destruction of large numbers of red cells. The resulting signs and symptoms of this major blood group reaction include fever, chills, flushing, tachycardia, hypotension, low back pain, pleuritic chest pain, nausea, vomiting, restlessness, anxiety, oliguria, and headache. The reaction may progress to anaphylaxis, shock, and death.

Hemolytic Disease of the Newborn

A second mechanism for antigen-antibody binding in type II hypersensitivity reactions is direct destruction by Fc-bearing effector cells such as macrophages. The macrophage can link to exposed Fc antibody regions. Once this bridging occurs, the foreign cell is phagocytized and destroyed by lysosomes within the effector cell. This can be mediated with or without complement involvement. An example of this type of mechanism is hemolytic disease of the newborn or erythroblastosis fetalis.

This condition occurs during pregnancy when an Rh-negative mother is sensitized to her fetus's Rh-positive red cell group antigens because of exposure during her current or a previous pregnancy. The mother's IgG Rh-positive antibodies cross the placental barrier and attack the fetus's red blood cells. The mother's exposure usually occurs during birth or miscarriage of a previous Rh-positive child, when mixing of fetal and maternal blood takes place. However, it can occur with bleeding at any time during the pregnancy. After this exposure, Rh-positive antibodies develop in the mother and affect her subsequent children. It takes as little as 1 cm^3 of blood for antibodies to Rh-positive red cells to develop in the mother. Usually, the first Rh-positive child is not affected unless placental tearing or leakage into the mother's circulation occurs. Antibody screens are routinely performed during pregnancy and RhoGAM administered at 28 weeks and at delivery for prevention of Rh-positive antibodies. RhoGAM contains antibodies against Rh antigens on fetal blood cells and is given to the mother to destroy fetal cells that may be present in her circulation before her immune system becomes activated and begins to produce anti-Rh antibodies. RhoGAM is not effective if the mother already has a positive antibody titer for fetal Rh antigens.

Myasthenia Gravis and Graves Disease

A third mechanism for antigen-antibody binding is seen in myasthenia gravis, an autoimmune disorder. In this case, antibodies form to the acetylcholine receptor on muscle membrane surfaces, primarily the motor end-plate (Figure 10-3). With antigen-antibody formation at the receptor site, complement attacks the receptor. Effector cells are not thought to be

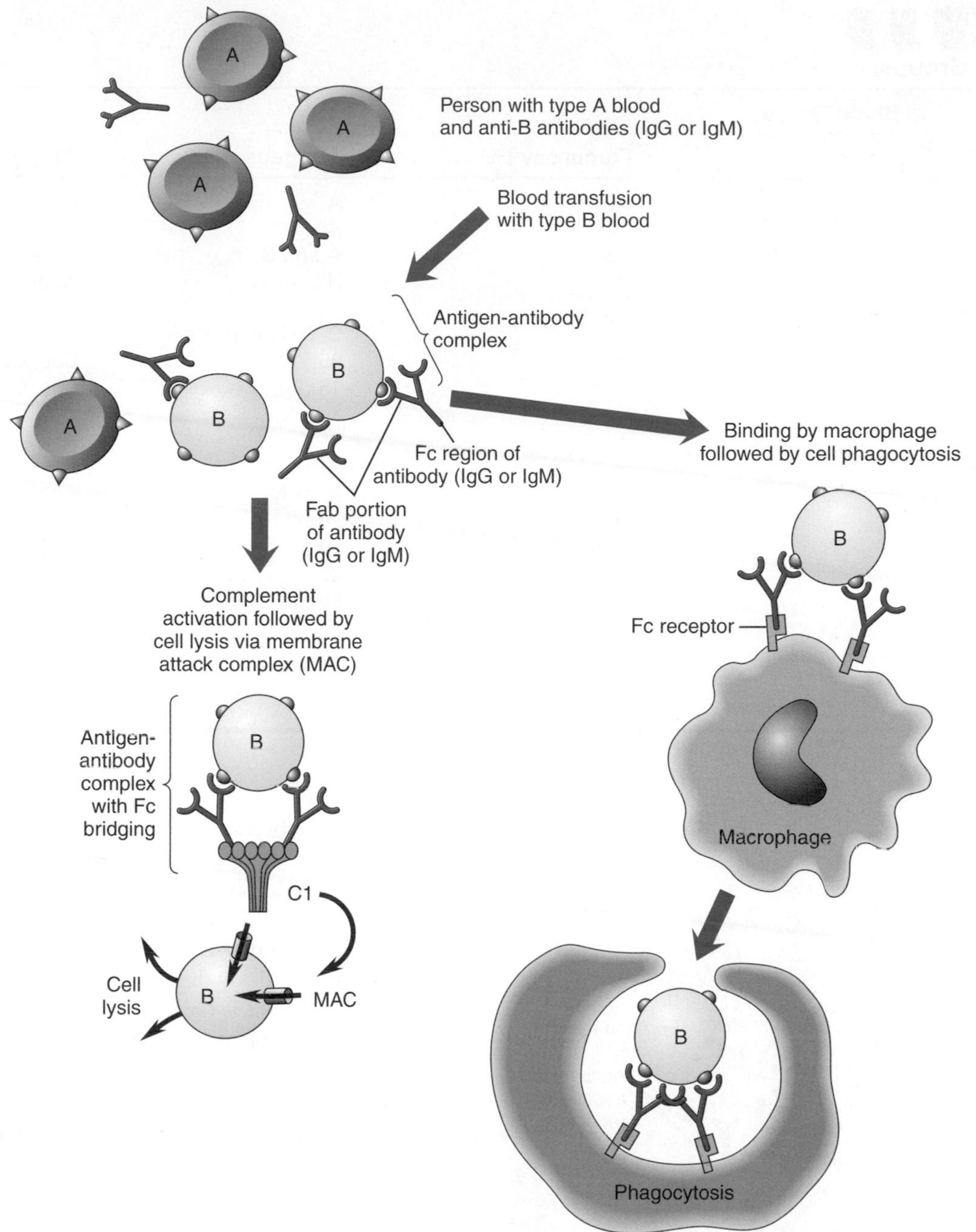

FIGURE 10-2 ■ Type II hypersensitivity reactions.

involved in this type II hypersensitivity reaction. The loss of acetylcholine stimulation at the motor end-plate causes the extreme muscular weakness associated with myasthenia gravis.

A fourth mechanism for antigen-antibody binding in type II hypersensitivity reactions is also mediated by effector cells. The effector cells in this case do not directly engulf and destroy the complex because the tissue is too large for the cells to engulf and destroy. Therefore, the effector cells, such as neutrophils, bind to the target cells and block the receptors from normal functioning causing injury to or malfunction of the involved tissue. Lymphocytic thyroiditis and Graves disease are examples of this type of disorder.

Hyperacute Graft Rejection

Another type II hypersensitivity mechanism for antigen-antibody binding involves both effector cells and complement as in hyperacute graft rejection that affects transplanted tissues. It occurs when the transplanted donor tissue has an antigen to which the recipient has preformed antibodies. For example, when tissue from a blood type A or B donor is transplanted

Table 10-4

Major Blood Groups

Blood Group			
Phenotype	**Frequency (%)**	**Antigens**	**Antibodies in Serum**
A	42	A	Anti-B
B	8	B	Anti-A
AB	3	A and B	None
O	47	H	Anti-A, anti-B
Other major blood group systems:			
Rhesus (Rh)		C, D, E, c, d, e	
	Rh^+	85	Cde, CDE
	Rh^-	15	Cde, CdE
Kell		K or k	
	K	9	K
	k	91	k
MN		M or N	
	MM	28	MM
	MN	50	MN
	NN	22	NN
Duffy		Fy^a, Fy^b, Fy	
	Fy^aFy^b	46	Fy^a, Fy^b
	Fy^a	20	Fy^a
	Fy^b	34	Fy^b
	Fy	0.1	Fy

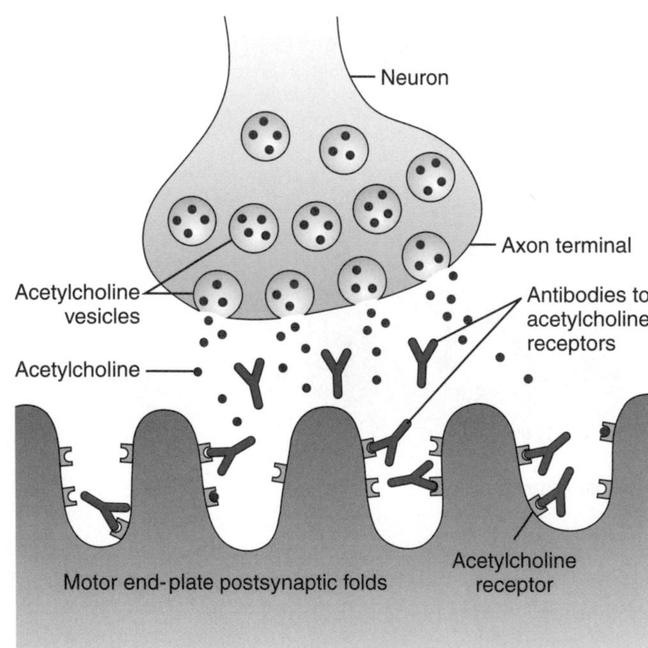

FIGURE 10-3 ■ Type II hypersensitivity reaction in a person with myasthenia gravis. Having limited receptors available for acetylcholine impairs neuromuscular transmission.

into a blood type O recipient, the recipient has anti-A and anti-B antibodies. These antibodies will immediately attack the foreign transplanted tissue.

Onset begins immediately after revascularization occurs in the transplant procedure. At this time, the blood supply from the patient is established in the newly transplanted organ. The patient's antibodies attack the foreign protein antigens and form an antigen-antibody complex. Effector cell infiltration and complement-mediated lysis of donor tissues, inflammation, vascular thrombosis, and hemorrhage occur. The reaction happens so quickly that within 48 hours after transplantation the graft tissue is ravaged and no longer functioning.

To prevent hyperacute graft rejection, tissue and blood typing of donors and recipients of transplanted tissue is extensive. Lists of potential recipients are matched to donors through organ donation laboratories both regionally and nationally. Only rarely has hyperacute graft rejection occurred because of an error in tissue or blood typing.

Type III Hypersensitivity

Etiology. Type III hypersensitivity results from failure of the immune and phagocytic systems to get rid of antigen-antibody immune complexes and is not tissue specific. It is also known as an immune complex or Arthus reaction. Type III hypersensitivity is characterized by antigen-antibody complex deposition into tissues, with consequent activation of complement and a subsequent inflammatory reaction. It is not an immediate reaction in that it occurs over a period of several hours and is often ongoing.

Three possible scenarios can precipitate type III hypersensitivity. First, persistent low-grade infection by a microbial or viral agent can stimulate a weak antibody response. The continuing nature of persistent infection and antibody response

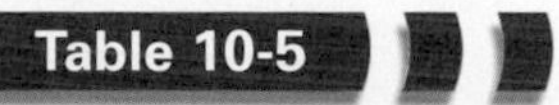

Diseases Associated with Type III Hypersensitivity

Disease	Antigen
Immune complex glomerulonephritis	GBM, exogenous antigens, drugs
Systemic lupus erythematosus (SLE)	Double-stranded DNA, DNA-histone complex, Sm, RNP, Ro:SSA, La:SSB, centromere
SLE-associated glomerulonephritis	Double-stranded DNA, DNA-histone complex, Sm, RNP, Ro:SSA, La:SSB
Acute allergic alveolitis	Various puffball spores from moldy dwellings
Farmer's lung disease	Thermophilic actinomycetes from contaminated hay or grains
Chemical worker's lung	Isocyanates
Still disease—postinfectious arthritis	RANA, or none identified
Rheumatoid arthritis	RANA
Serum sickness	Lymphocytes or thymocytes from heterologous serum
Henoch-Schönlein purpura	Upper respiratory viruses, drugs (antibiotics and thiazides), foods (milk, fish, eggs, rice, nuts, beans), and immunizations
Drug-induced vasculitis	Drugs (antibiotics and thiazides)
Polyarteritis nodosa	Antineutrophil cytoplasmic
Wegener granulomatosus	Antineutrophil cytoplasmic
Goodpasture syndrome	GBM

SLE, Systemic lupus erythematosus; *GBM,* glomerular basement membrane; *Sm,* Smith; *RNP,* ribonucleoprotein; *Ro,* Robert; *La,* Lane; *SS,* single stranded; *RANA,* rheumatoid arthritis nuclear antigen.

leads to chronic immune complex production. These immune complexes are not successfully removed from the blood and are deposited in many sites, including blood vessels, glomeruli, and joints. Second, an extrinsic environmental antigen from molds, plants, or animals can be inhaled into the lung where it is exposed to antibody in the body fluid. This inhalation of antigen causes antigen-antibody complex formation in alveoli with immune complex deposition in the alveolar walls. Third, an autoimmune process can develop in which autoantibodies attack self antigens. In this case, the body forms both parts of the immune complex. Autoantibodies to either circulating or tissue-fixed self antigens such as IgG or DNA may be produced by the target organ itself. Because the self antigens persist over time, chronic immune complex production and deposition in tissues take place.

The mechanism of injury in type III hypersensitivity reactions is from activation of complement and other proinflammatory mediators in response to the antigen-antibody complex deposition. The antibody-antigen complex deposition does not cause the injury. The tissue injury is caused by an inflammatory reaction to the antibody-antigen complex. Therefore, it is not a tissue-specific reaction. The onset of this reaction occurs up to 6+ hours after exposure to the antigen. IgG and IgM are the principal antibodies. The principal effector cells are neutrophils and mast cells. The principal mediator of the reaction is complement. Examples of type III hypersensitivity reaction include SLE, immune complex glomerulonephritis, serum sickness, and drug-induced vasculitis. Table 10-5 lists diseases associated with type III hypersensitivity.

Pathogenesis. Type III hypersensitivity reactions tend to be ongoing with variations in symptoms based on changing antibody-antigen ratios, amount of complement available to mediate the inflammation, and the dynamic nature of the antibody-antigen reaction. It is sometimes difficult to differentiate between type II and type III hypersensitivity reactions. The key differences between a type II and a type III reaction are the location of antigen and the mechanism of injury. As previously described, type II reactions occur in response to tissue-specific antigen located on cell surfaces and involve direct cell death or malfunction from the antigen-antibody reaction. Type III hypersensitivity reactions involve antigens forming antigen-antibody complexes that precipitate out of the blood or body fluid and are deposited into tissues.

Type III hypersensitivity reactions involve a sequential process that begins with interaction between a circulating soluble antigen and soluble antibody or between an insoluble antigen and a soluble antibody. Depending on the concentration of antigen and antibody, multiple cross-linking of antigen and antibody occurs and immune complexes are formed. Most immune complexes are removed effectively before they can cause injury. In type III hypersensitivity, the immune complexes are not removed and thus cause tissue injury.

When both antigen and antibody are small or intermediate in size and soluble, the immune complex precipitates out of the body fluid and is deposited into tissues. When only the antibody is soluble, the antibody reacts with fixed antigen in the tissues. Then the antibody within the complex links with the complement system by its Fc receptors (Figure 10-4).

Activation of the classic complement cascade causes release of C3a and C5a, as well as the membrane attack complex. C3a stimulates the release of histamine from mast cells, indirectly increasing vascular permeability and vasodilation. Bronchial smooth muscle contraction occurs, resulting in bronchial constriction, wheezing, and coughing. C3a also causes the rounding up of endothelial cells, thereby increasing vascular

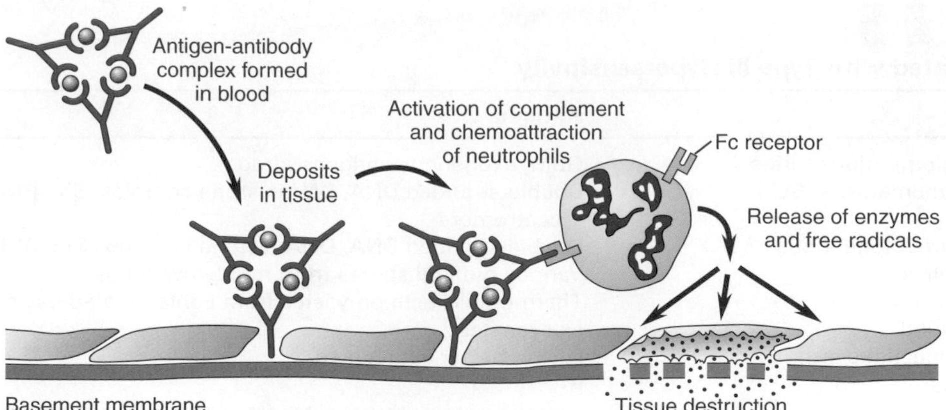

FIGURE 10-4 ■ Type III hypersensitivity reaction.

permeability. The increased vascular permeability leads to edema formation, which allows cellular inflammatory components to move around more easily. It also dilutes and limits the duration of action of mediators. C5a is an even more powerful component than C3a. It causes a powerful release of proinflammatory mediators with actions the same as those of C3a. It is also a powerful chemotactic agent for neutrophils. C5a also causes a respiratory burst within neutrophils in which oxygen consumption is increased to 50 times normal along with increased glucose uptake and procoagulant activity.

As a result of the activation of complement, neutrophils, macrophages, and mast cells are attracted to the area and are activated. These cells begin lysis and destruction of tissue via the release of cytokines and the inflammatory response. The inflammation causes tissue destruction, scarring, and further reaction of the immune system against the damaged tissue (see Figure 10-4).

Tissue Deposition. Antigen-antibody complex deposition in tissues is affected by a number of factors. Size appears to be an important factor. Smaller immune complexes are able to circulate for longer periods, which may increase the immune response. However, small complexes can also be removed more easily because they can pass through the glomerular basement membrane via urine. The very large complexes can be phagocytized more easily because they are easily marked or fixed by complement and bound to red blood cells. The large complexes can then be transported to the liver, where they are phagocytized by the reticuloendothelial system—particularly the Kupffer cells in the liver—and easily removed from the system. However, large complexes can become stuck in the kidney where they are unable to cross the glomerular basement membrane.

Increased vascular permeability as a result of histamine or other vasoactive mediator release is also hypothesized to be an important factor in tissue deposition. Researchers have found that small immune complexes can be deposited in tissues treated with vasoactive mediators. Sites of increased turbulence and blood pressure tend to have increased immune complex deposition. These sites include the glomerular capillaries, joint linings, ciliary body, pulmonary alveolar membranes, and vascular endothelial linings, especially around curves or bifurcations.

Intermediate-sized immune complexes tend to be deposited because they do not fix complement well, do not bind with red blood cells well after fixation, and are not removed by the mononuclear phagocyte system well. Large numbers of any size immune complex can be deposited if they are so numerous that the phagocytic cells are overwhelmed. Deposition of immune complexes also depends on their immunoglobulin class and the affinity between the antigen and antibody. Finally, deposition may be affected by the type of antigen or by the relationship between the immune complex and sites with increased collagen. Because DNA and collagen have strong affinity, an increased quantity of DNA–anti-DNA immune complexes may be deposited in collagen membranes such as in the kidney. The electrical charge of the immune complex may affect where it is deposited. For example, a positively charged immune complex may be attracted by a negatively charged basement membrane.

Immune Complex Glomerulonephritis

Etiology. Immune complex glomerulonephritis (an inflammatory renal disorder) is an example of a type III hypersensitivity reaction caused by persistent low-grade infection. It involves the interaction of soluble exogenous antigen with soluble antibody and is the cause of most glomerulonephritis cases. Glomerulonephritis typically occurs 10 days to 2 weeks after infection with a *Streptococcus* bacterial strain. The immune complex is deposited in the glomerular capillary wall and mesangium.

Clinical Manifestations and Treatment. This deposition causes damage to the glomerular basement membrane with resultant proteinuria, hematuria, hypertension, oliguria, and red cell casts in the urine (see Chapter 27). In some types of glomerulonephritis, the client may have edema, nephrotic syndrome, and acute renal failure that may progress to chronic renal failure.

Treatment of glomerulonephritis involves the use of corticosteroids to decrease inflammation. In certain situations, cyclophosphamide and azathioprine may be used as immunosuppressives. Antihistamines and antiserotonins have been tried in attempts to decrease vasoactive mediators and vascular permeability. Anticoagulants and antiplatelet medications such as aspirin, as well as plasmapheresis, are currently being studied. In plasmapheresis, plasma is removed from the blood and fresh frozen plasma or albumin is used to replace the withdrawn plasma.

Systemic Lupus Erythematosus

Etiology. SLE is another example of a type III hypersensitivity reaction caused by autoantibody production. It is a member of the group of diseases variably called autoimmune, connective tissue, collagen vascular, or inflammatory disorders. SLE tends to occur more frequently in women than in men, with an incidence of 7.6 per 100,000. It is primarily characterized by the development of antibodies against nuclear antigens such as DNA, deoxyribonucleohistone, and RNA. Production of autoantibodies to red blood cells, neutrophils, platelets, lymphocytes, and other organs or tissues may also occur. SLE is associated with decreased serum complement levels.

In SLE, antinuclear and anti-DNA autoantibodies attack and are deposited on collagen-rich tissues, including the glomerular basement membrane and the dermal-epidermal junction. The exact mechanism causing cell damage and the release of DNA with the subsequent development of anti-DNA is not known. However, once formed, the anti-DNA autoantibodies can react with DNA from damaged cells anywhere in the body. The resulting inflammatory response causes increased cell damage and further antigen-antibody immune complex formation, thus leading to a cyclic process. The immune complex deposition and resulting inflammatory response cause the signs and symptoms of SLE.

Clinical Manifestations. The disorder has a variety of signs and symptoms because any organ system can be involved in SLE. Kidney involvement leads to nephritis and glomerulonephritis. Skin symptoms include an erythematous rash on exposed skin, purpura, alopecia, mucosal ulcerations, subcutaneous nodules, and splinter hemorrhages. The client may have symptoms of arthritis or polyarthralgia, pleurisy, pericarditis, restrictive pulmonary disease, retinal changes, thrombocytopenia, anemia, and gastrointestinal ulceration. Central nervous system involvement includes neuritis, seizures, depression, or psychosis.

Treatment. Treatment of SLE ranges from administration of nonsteroidal antiinflammatory agents such as aspirin to systemic corticosteroids. Corticosteroids decrease inflammation and provide immunosuppression, which can decrease symptoms and add to the patient's quality of life. Antimalarials such as hydroxychloroquine or chloroquine are occasionally used in cases with skin involvement because they bind and alter DNA. If the patient does not respond to corticosteroids, immunosuppressives such as cyclophosphamide, chlorambucil, or azathioprine or cytotoxic agents can be used.

Type IV Hypersensitivity

Type IV hypersensitivity is also known as delayed hypersensitivity. Delayed hypersensitivity is characterized by tissue damage resulting from a delayed cellular reaction to an antigen. Unlike other hypersensitivity reactions, primary antibody involvement is absent. The principal mediators are lymphocytes, including lymphokine-producing T cells (Td) that mediate the reaction by releasing lymphokines (cytokines) and/or antigen-sensitized cytotoxic T cells (Tc) that can directly kill cells. The principal effector cells are lymphocytes and macrophages with mast cells involved in the early phases. Neutrophils are not involved in type IV hypersensitivity reactions. This reaction is slow in onset, beginning 24 hours after exposure and lasting up to 14 days after exposure.

Type IV hypersensitivity reactions involve a series of events evolving gradually. Mast cell degranulation occurs early in the evolution of a delayed hypersensitivity reaction, followed by lymphocyte and macrophage invasion. The mast cells are gatekeepers that regulate leukocyte migration in the microvasculature. Unlike that occurring in type I hypersensitivity reactions, the mast cell degranulation is more limited and localized. The reaction is also limited by the action of suppressor T cells, which inhibit other T-cell actions. Why and how the mast cells are limited in this type of hypersensitivity reaction is not well understood. However, the combined action of mast cell and T-cell mediators recruits other T cells and macrophages to the site.

Several types of delayed hypersensitivity reactions are recognized, including cutaneous basophil hypersensitivity (Jones-Mote sensitivity), contact hypersensitivity, tuberculin-type hypersensitivity, and granulomatous hypersensitivity.

Cutaneous Basophil Hypersensitivity

Cutaneous basophil is the most rapid type of delayed hypersensitivity reaction. It is a lymphocyte-mediated basophil reaction. Soluble antigen that has been injected intradermally or antigens introduced into the dermis trigger T-cell activation and subsequent release of cytokines and activation of basophils, which infiltrate the area. The reaction peaks with skin swelling in 24 hours and can last 7 to 10 days. An example of this type of hypersensitivity is skin graft reactions and rejection.

Contact Hypersensitivity

Contact hypersensitivity is the most familiar type IV hypersensitivity. It is an immune or inflammatory response to a wide variety of plant oils, chemicals, ointments, clothing, cosmetics, dyes, and adhesives. Contact hypersensitivity is an epidermal phenomenon. As a delayed reaction, it peaks in 48 to 72 hours.

The reaction is slow because the skin-penetrating antigen is very small and in an incomplete form. This incomplete, lipid-soluble antigen is called a **hapten.** The hapten must first penetrate the epidermis, where it links with a normal body protein in the epidermis called a carrier. Only after the hapten combines with the carrier is it a complete antigen—often called a hapten conjugate.

The complete antigen is processed by epidermal macrophages called Langerhans cells, which are located in the suprabasal epidermis. The Langerhans cells move to the local lymph channel, where they migrate to the regional lymph node. Within the lymph node, the Langerhans cells display the now processed complete antigen to CD4+ T cells in the paracortex. Then the antigen-sensitized CD4+ T cells release lymphokines, which initiate an inflammatory response and attract other effector cells. The primary lymphokines include IL-2, IL-3, interferon, TNF, and macrophage-stimulating factors (Figure 10-5).

Lymphokines (cytokines) and prostaglandins are important in contact hypersensitivity. The presentation of antigen to T cells by Langerhans cells causes the lymphokine cascade of vasoactive and cytoactive substances. These substances cause inflammation as well as activation of other cells. After about 72 hours, the reaction begins to decrease because of degradation of the antigen and production of prostaglandin E, which inhibits IL-1 and IL-2 production.

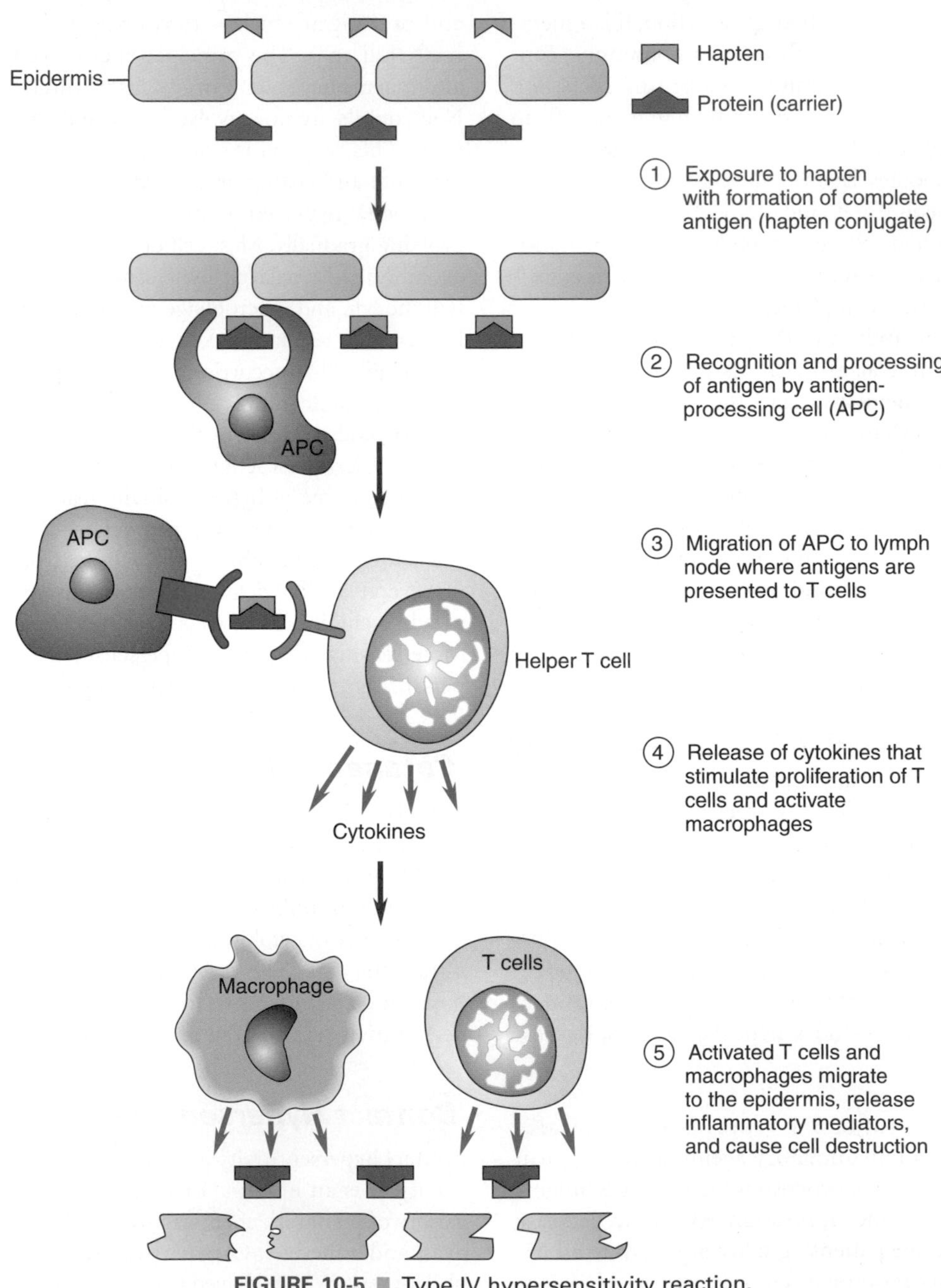
Epidermis
Hapten
Protein (carrier)
1 Exposure to hapten with formation of complete antigen (hapten conjugate)
APC
2 Recognition and processing of antigen by antigen-processing cell (APC)
APC
Helper T cell
3 Migration of APC to lymph node where antigens are presented to T cells
Cytokines
4 Release of cytokines that stimulate proliferation of T cells and activate macrophages
Macrophage
T cells
5 Activated T cells and macrophages migrate to the epidermis, release inflammatory mediators, and cause cell destruction

FIGURE 10-5 ■ Type IV hypersensitivity reaction.

After primary exposure or immunization, a cellular reaction takes place at each subsequent exposure site. Cross-reactivity with related substances also occurs in contact hypersensitivity. For example, a person with contact dermatitis to nickel will react when exposed to a variety of nickel alloys, including the metal in earrings, zippers, and belt buckles. Skin symptoms resulting from contact dermatitis include redness, edema, itching, and blisters. People with sensitivities may also experience respiratory symptoms if exposed to aerosolized hapten. This situation could occur when a person is downwind from burning poison ivy or burning tires.

Tuberculin-Type Hypersensitivity

Tuberculin-type hypersensitivity occurs when someone who has tuberculosis antibodies is exposed to tuberculin in a tuberculin test. It is a dermal phenomenon that peaks in 48 to 72 hours. The person experiences redness, induration, and inflammation at the site of the intradermal injection. Because the amount injected is so small, the reaction disappears when the antigen has degraded. However, people with severe reactions may experience tissue necrosis at the site.

Granulomatous Hypersensitivity

Granulomatous hypersensitivity reaction is a primary defense against intracellular infections and represents a chronic type IV hypersensitivity reaction. It is a protective defense reaction that eventually causes tissue destruction because of persistence of the antigen. In this type of hypersensitivity, antigen is not destroyed within the macrophages either because of failure of lysosome-phagosome fusion, as in tuberculosis and leprosy, or because of the resistance of various materials to internal lysozymes, as in retained suture material or talc. In an effort to protect the host, lymphocytes and macrophages actually cause the tissue damage by releasing cytokines and stimulating an inflammatory response.

Antigen is engulfed and ingested by macrophages attempting to destroy the antigen, but these actions are unsuccessful in type IV hypersensitivity. The macrophages form a core of inflammatory cells that include lymphocytes, tissue histiocytes, eosinophils, plasma cells, giant cells, and epithelioid cells. This collection of inflammatory cells develops into a ball-like mass called a granuloma. The predominant cell in the granuloma is the macrophage. Epithelioid cells come from macrophages and are large, flat cells with a large amount of endoplasmic reticulum. When epithelioid cells fuse, they form multinucleated giant cells. This core is surrounded by lymphocytes. Gradually, fibroblastic activity and increased collagen synthesis cause the granuloma to become fibrotic with scar formation. Often, central necrosis occurs within the granuloma and is called caseous or cheesy necrosis. Patients with granulomatous diseases have a variety of symptoms. Table 10-6 lists the granulomatous diseases and the pathogens associated with them.

Table 10-6 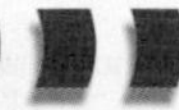

Granulomatous Disease Associated with Type IV Hypersensitivity

Disease	Bacterium
Tuberculosis	*Mycobacterium tuberculosis*
Leprosy	*Mycobacterium leprae*
Histoplasmosis	*Histoplasma capsulatum*
Coccidioidomycosis	*Coccidioides immitis*
Brucellosis	*Brucella abortus*
	Brucella suis (less common)
	Brucella melitensis (less common)
Tularemia	*Francisella (Pasteurella) tularensis*

KEY CONCEPTS 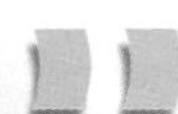

- Type I hypersensitivity is an immediate allergic or anaphylactic type of reaction mediated primarily by sensitized mast cells. The reaction is initiated when IgE antibodies located on the mast cell membrane are bound by antigen, with subsequent cross-linking of IgE receptors. Mast cell degranulation releases chemicals that mediate the signs and symptoms of anaphylaxis. Released histamine, kinin, prostaglandins, interleukins, and leukotrienes cause increased vascular permeability, vasodilation, hypotension, urticaria, and bronchoconstriction. Examples of type I reactions include drug reactions, bee sting reactions, and asthma.
- Type II hypersensitivity occurs when antibodies are formed against antigens on cell surfaces, usually resulting in lysis of target cells. Cell lysis may be mediated by activated complement fragments (membrane attack complex) or by phagocytic cells that are attracted to target cells by the attached antibodies. Examples include transfusion reactions, erythroblastosis fetalis, myasthenia gravis, and hyperacute graft rejection.
- Type III hypersensitivity reactions occur when antigen-antibody complexes are deposited in tissues and result in the activation of complement and subsequent tissue inflammation and destruction. Antigen-antibody complexes activate the complement cascade and subsequently attract phagocytic cells to the tissue. Persistent low-grade infections, inhalation of antigens into alveoli, and autoimmune production of antibodies may result in chronic production of antigen-antibody complexes. Examples include glomerulonephritis and SLE.
- Type IV hypersensitivity reactions are T cell mediated and do not require antibody production, in contrast to type I, II, and III reactions. Sensitized T cells react with altered or foreign cells and initiate inflammation. Contact dermatitis, tuberculin reactions, transplant rejection, and graft-versus-host disease are examples.

DEFICIENT IMMUNE RESPONSES

Deficient immune responses result from a functional decrease in one or more components of the immune system. These disorders can affect lymphocytes, antibodies, phagocytes, and complement proteins. Two types of immune deficiency are differentiated: primary and secondary. Primary disorders are immune deficiencies not attributable to other causes; these may be congenital or acquired. Examples of primary immunodeficiency disorders include SCID syndrome, DiGeorge syndrome, selective IgA deficiency, and AIDS. Secondary immunodeficiency disorders are a consequence of other processes or treatments in the body. Examples of secondary disorders include those associated with hyperlipidemia or malnutrition, medical treatments such as cancer chemotherapy, or biopsychosocial stress such as postsurgical immune system problems.

PRIMARY IMMUNODEFICIENCY DISORDERS

Primary immunodeficiency disorders are either acquired by infection with a virus or are congenital and result from abnormal development or maturation of immune cells. The congenital genetic disorders are often sex linked. The most common primary disorders are listed in Table 10-7. The first clinical indicators of immunodeficiency disorders are the signs and symptoms of infection, and the disorders are often first suspected when an individual has severe recurrent, un-

Table 10-7

Primary Immunodeficiency Disorders

Disorder	Functional Deficiency	Error
Bruton X-linked agammaglobulinemia	Antibody	*BTK* gene mutant
Common variable (acquired) hypogammaglobulinemia	Antibody	
Selective IgA deficiency	IgA antibody	
Secretory component deficiency—chronic mucocutaneous candidiasis	Secretory IgA	
Selective IgM deficiency	IgM antibody	
Selective deficiency of IgG subclasses	IgG antibody subclass	
Immunodeficiency with elevated IgM	IgG and IgA antibodies	
Transient hypogammaglobulinemia of infancy	Low antibodies	
Antibody deficiency with nearly normal immunoglobulins	Antibody	
Duncan X-linked lymphoproliferative disease	Anti–Epstein-Barr virus–linked antigen antibody	
DiGeorge syndrome (congenital thymic hypoplasia or aplasia)	Primarily T cells	Chromosome 22q11.2 deletion syndrome
Nezelof syndrome	T cells, antibody, neutropenia	
Autosomal recessive SCID	T cells, antibody	Defects of JAK3
Autosomal recessive SCID with ADA deficiency	T cells, antibody	
X-linked recessive SCID	T cells, antibody	Defects of *IL2RG* gene
Defective expression of MHC antigens	T cells, antibody	
SCID with leukopenia (reticular dysgenesis)	T cells, antibody, granulocytes	
Wiskott-Aldrich syndrome (immunodeficiency with eczema and thrombocytopenia)	Antibody, T cells	Defect of short arm of X chromosome at Xp11.3/mutation of *WASP* gene
Ataxia, telangiectasia	Antibody, T cells	
Cartilage-hair hypoplasia	T cells	
Immunodeficiency with thymoma	T cells, antibody	
Hyperimmunoglobulinemia E	Excessive IgE	
Lymphocyte function antigen 1 deficiency	Cytotoxic cells, phagocytic cells	
Chédiak-Higashi syndrome	Natural killer cells, phagocytic cells	
Chronic granulomatous disease of childhood	Phagocytic cells	
Acquired immunodeficiency syndrome	T cells, CD4 cells	

SCID, Severe combined immunodeficiency; *ADA,* adenosine deaminase; *MHC,* major histocompatibility complex.

usual, or unmanageable infections. HIV disease and AIDS are discussed separately in Chapter 12.

B-Cell and T-Cell Combined Disorders

Severe Combined Immunodeficiency Disorders

Etiology and Pathogenesis. Severe combined immunodeficiency (SCID) disorders are due to embryonic defects and are characterized by severe immune system dysfunction and a variety of clinical features. The most common SCID disorders are autosomal recessive (or Swiss type), autosomal recessive with deficiency of the enzyme adenosine deaminase, X-linked recessive, defective expression of MHC antigens, and SCID with leukopenia or reticular dysgenesis. Most of these disorders are due to mutations of recombination activating genes *(RAG)* 1 or 2, both of which are involved in the process of antigen receptor gene assembly.[3]

The most severe form of SCID, called reticular dysgenesis, causes failure of all white blood cell development. Complete failure of lymphoid and myeloid stem cells during fetal development is not generally compatible with life—most infants die in utero or shortly after birth. Infants with reticular dysgenesis have failure of both lymphocyte and granulocyte development. Although the fetus grows normally, the infant is severely affected, with decreased numbers of lymphocytes, decreased antibodies, and decreased phagocytic cells. For those infants who survive birth, either umbilical cord blood or HLA-haploidentical (i.e., identical HLA-type) hematopoietic stem cell transplantation has been tried with mixed results.

The X-linked recessive type is due to a defect of the *IL2RG* gene that is responsible for encoding common γ chain which is needed by several cytokine receptors.[4] It is the most common type (50% of cases), affecting boys more often than girls. Infants with SCID caused by autosomal recessive or X-linked recessive disease lack circulating T cells and usually have a normal to increased number of B cells that do not function normally. The enzymes or other essential components necessary for immune cell functioning are deficient—particularly enzymes linked with purine nucleoside phosphorylase or adenosine deaminase metabolism. As a result, the infant accumulates toxic metabolites of purine or adenosine that affect lymphocytes. Antibody titers are decreased because of lack of antibody formation after immunization. T cells are low in number (less than 1000/μl) or absent, but the ratio of $CD4^+$ to $CD8^+$ cells is not inverted as in AIDS. Some infants have increased numbers of B cells, but they are unable to function. Generally, most patients have small, hypoplastic thymus glands indicative of poor or absent T-cell development.

Clinical Manifestations and Treatment. Infants with SCID caused by defective expression of MHC antigens have poor antibody production with decreased IgG, IgM, and IgA. Lymphocyte numbers are normal to slightly decreased. T-cell function is decreased.

Infants with these syndromes are usually ill by 3 months of age and often have thrush, severe *Candida* diaper dermatitis, or infections such as otitis, pneumonia, and diarrhea. They are prone to sepsis, opportunistic infections with such pathogens as *Candida albicans* or *Pneumocystis carinii,* infections with such viruses as cytomegalovirus or herpesvirus, and common childhood diseases such as varicella and measles. Because of their severity, infections in infants with SCID are medical emergencies.

Management of SCID includes bone marrow transplantation and gene therapy. In 2000, gene therapy was used for the first time to treat these patients. They received gene-modified $CD34^+$ hematopoietic cells using ex vivo gene transfer involving retroviral vectors.[5]

Wiskott-Aldrich Syndrome

Etiology and Pathogenesis. Wiskott-Aldrich Syndrome is an X-linked immunodeficiency disorder that affects both T cells and B cells. The gene deficiency is caused by a mutation of the WAS protein (WASP) gene and has been mapped to the short arm of the X chromosome at Xpll.23. The *WASP* gene is involved in cytoplasmic signaling and in reorganization of the actin cytoskeleton. In this syndrome, IgM is decreased. Other antibody concentrations are variable, with IgE and IgA usually elevated and IgG normal to low. This antibody variability is due to increased antibody catabolism. Platelet deficiency is also associated with Wiskott-Aldrich syndrome. T cells are present but function deficiently. Affected infants have particular difficulty mounting immune responses to protein and polysaccharide antigens, including bacterial cell walls (e.g., *Pseudomonas aeruginosa, Staphylococcus pneumoniae*).

Clinical Manifestations and Treatment. Wiskott-Aldrich syndrome is clinically characterized by the presence of eczema, thrombocytopenic purpura, and infection. Affected children are prone to pneumococcal infections, including pneumonia, meningitis, otitis media, and sepsis. They are also subject to renal disease and malignancies. The average age of these infants at death is 3.5 years without treatment.

Infants with Wiskott-Aldrich syndrome are treated with antibody replacement therapy, and antibiotic therapy. Bone marrow transplantation, stem cell transplantation, and gene therapy are used to manage this disorder in affected children.

T-Cell Disorders

DiGeorge Syndrome

Etiology and Pathogenesis. DiGeorge syndrome, or thymic hypoplasia, is a developmental T-cell disorder associated with total or partial loss of thymus gland function. The development of DiGeorge syndrome is due to a chromosomal 22q 11.2 deletion (del 22q11). There may also be associated genetic modifiers that can vary the syndrome clinically. In this disorder, the aplastic or hypoplastic thymus is unable to assist in the maturation of T cells. Therefore, T cells are deficient. B cells are normal.

Clinical Manifestations and Treatment. Because this is a developmental disorder, it is often associated with other congenital problems such as cardiac and great vessel anomalies, hypoparathyroidism with hypocalcemia, esophageal atresia, genital anomalies, and unusual facial features including mandibular hypoplasia and low-set ears.

Infants with partial loss of thymus function may not have trouble with infections. However, infants with total loss of thymus function resemble children with SCID and rarely live to the age of 6 years without treatment. For these children, thymic transplantation has been helpful in reestablishing T-cell populations.

Chronic Mucocutaneous Candidiasis

Etiology and Pathogenesis. Chronic mucocutaneous candidiasis is an autosomal recessive T-cell disorder characterized by a selective deficiency of cell-mediated immunity against *Candida albicans.* In this case, T cells do not produce the correct cytokines needed for the cell-mediated immunity to *Candida.* This causes persistent or recurrent severe skin, nail, and mucous membrane infections with *Candida albicans.* B-cell and T-cell functions are usually normal, except for the inability of the T cells to respond to *Candida* infections. Occasionally IgA or other antibody levels may be affected.

Clinical Manifestations and Treatment. The goal of treatment is to reduce the severity of skin and mucous membrane infection and decrease the disfigurement from infection and scarring. This disorder is also associated with an autoimmune disorder called autoimmune polyendocrinopathy-candidiasis-ectodermal dystrophy (APECED).[6] The most common components of APECED are chronic mucocutaneous candidiasis, hypoparathyroidism, and Addison disease.

B-Cell Disorders

IgA Deficiency

Etiology and Pathogenesis. The most common B-cell primary immunodeficiency disorder is selective IgA deficiency. This disorder affects 1 in 400 persons. It is a B-cell disorder characterized by failure of IgA-bearing lymphocytes to become plasma cells, with resulting lack of serum and secretory IgA. Genetically, it can be an autosomal recessive or autosomal dominant disease.

Clinical Manifestations and Treatment. People with this disorder are prone to respiratory, gastrointestinal, and genitourinary tract infections. They tend to have many autoantibodies (including anti-IgA antibodies), with a high incidence of vascular and collagen autoimmune diseases. They often react to cow's milk, and inflammatory bowel conditions can develop. Because they have severe allergic reactions to blood or blood products containing IgA, exogenous IgA replacement is contraindicated. Treatment includes prevention of infection and management of infection with appropriate antibiotics.

Bruton X-Linked Agammaglobulinemia

Etiology and Pathogenesis. Bruton X-linked agammaglobulinemia, or congenital hypogammaglobulinemia, is a B-cell genetic disorder caused by a lack of normal bursal-equivalent tissue. In this case, the B-cell precursors are unable to complete maturation in the bone marrow. The disorder is linked to a mutation of a gene called *btk* (Bruton tyrosine kinase) located on the long arm of the X chromosome at position Xq21,1-11. In 1952 it was the first immunodeficiency disorder identified. In this case, a mutation in a cytoplasmic signal-transducing molecule encoded by the *btk* gene results in B-cell deficiency with decreased serum concentrations of IgG and no detectable IgA or IgM. The number of T cells is increased and the cells function normally. The thymus also functions normally. The disease is characterized by recurrent bacterial infection and profound hypogammaglobulinemia due to decreased numbers of circulating B cells. Male infants are affected, but this disorder is not usually diagnosed until they are 9 to 12 months old because of passive maternal IgG protection.

Clinical Manifestations and Treatment. Frequent infections, most often due to *H. influenzae* and *S. pneumoniae,* occur in these infants, causing pneumonia, otitis media, meningitis, sinusitis, and septicemia. The recurrent infections can lead to tissue destruction and injury.

Despite the infections, these infants can grow normally if treated with antibiotics and recurrent administration of human immune globulin. However, passive immunotherapy is not always effective. Many children die before the age of 6. If the child survives to adulthood, life expectancy is decreased and large joint arthritis is common.

Transient Hypogammaglobulinemia

Transient hypogammaglobulinemia of infancy is a self-limiting condition in which the infant is slow to acquire normal immunoglobulin levels. The infant experiences a lengthened period of low IgG levels after birth. Affected infants can demonstrate normal immunoglobulin levels and immune system function by approximately age 4. During the period of low antibody levels they are more susceptible to infections, particularly respiratory tract infections.

SECONDARY IMMUNODEFICIENCY DISORDERS

A number of physical, psychosocial, nutritional, environmental, and pharmacologic factors can singly or in combination lead to the development of secondary immunodeficiency disorders. Many of these linkages are discussed in Chapter 8.

The direct and indirect linkages between the brain and the endocrine and immune systems are well known. As a result, excessive or defective neuroendocrine responses can lead to disease. For example, an excessive neuroendocrine response to stress with increased corticosteroids increases one's susceptibility to infectious agents and tumors but enhances resistance to autoimmune disease. On the other hand, a defective neuroendocrine response to stress with low corticosteroid levels enhances autoimmune disease and inhibits infections and tumors.[2] Individuals experiencing physical and psychosocial stress, decreased social support, depression, and bereavement show decreased immune system functioning.

T-cell and B-cell numbers decrease after surgery. This temporary deficiency can last up to 1 month and is most likely a result of the stress of surgery. Some types of surgery, such as splenic surgery, actually reduce the effectiveness of the immune system. Removal of the spleen reduces serum IgM and the antibody response to encapsulated bacteria (e.g., *S. pneumoniae, H. influenzae, Staphylococcus aureus*). Disease states such as diabetes mellitus, drug- or alcohol-induced cirrhosis, severe burns, severe trauma, sickle cell anemia, malignancies, and severe infections are associated with secondary immune deficiencies. Pregnancy and infancy are also associated with secondary immune dysfunction.

A number of pharmaceuticals affect the functioning of the immune system. Cytotoxins and other cancer pharmacotherapeutic drugs cause a state of generalized immunosuppression. For example, methotrexate is a phase-specific cytotoxin in which cells are killed only if they are in the S or DNA-synthetic phase. Cyclophosphamide is toxic to cells in any mitotic phase, although it is better at killing active cells. Anesthetics (halothane, cyclopropane, nitrous oxide, ether), alcohol, antibiotics, antithyroids, anticonvulsants, antihistamines, and steroids decrease cellular or humoral immunity by various methods. For example, chronic nitrous oxide toxicity leads to cell-mediated immune deficits. Therapeutic radiation (x-rays) also affects the immune system by destroying rapidly proliferating cells. In states when T-cell and B-cell clones are needed, irradiation eliminates these cells, thus blunting or reducing the effectiveness of the body's response.

A number of studies have linked immune system competency and nutritional status. Malnutritional states can lead to protein depletion, as well as carbohydrate, lipid, vitamin, and mineral deficiencies. Protein and calorie depletion leads to T-cell reductions and dysfunction. Antibodies are composed of proteins, levels of which are also low in a state of depletion. Low levels of zinc, an enzyme cofactor needed for lymphocyte function, as well as low levels of folic acid and vitamins B_6, A, and E, can lead to T-cell and B-cell dysfunction. Overnutrition, especially hyperlipidemia, can lead to lymphocyte and granulocyte dysfunction. Kinsella and Lokesh[7] in 1990 stated that deficiencies, imbalances, or excess nutritional factors may impair the development of all stem cells, alter the recognition and processing of antigens, hurt immune cell proliferation, reduce phagocytic and cytolytic capacity, and harm cooperative interactions between cells in the immune system.

In the elderly, immune system function is altered. The response to antigenic stimulation is variable. The elderly are less able to respond to "new" antigenic stimuli. The cells of the immune system in the elderly are not able to proliferate or reproduce as effectively as in younger persons. Although the total number of T cells remains the same, T-cell function is decreased. T cells are less capable of proliferating and have decreased cytotoxicity. Antibody production also decreases. A rise is also seen in autoantibody production, which may influence the increase in autoimmune disease in the elderly.

KEY CONCEPTS

- Primary deficiencies in immune function may be congenital, genetic, or acquired.
- Secondary deficiencies are conditions that impair immune function as a result of other processes, such as poor nutrition, stress, or drugs.
- Impairment in T cells and B cells results in SCID. Functional B and T lymphocytes are lacking, and infants with SCID easily succumb to sepsis and opportunistic infections. Other types of primary immunodeficiency disorders affect a particular cell type: DiGeorge syndrome occurs with T-cell agenesis related to a lack of thymus function; chronic mucocutaneous candidiasis is due to abnormal T cells that cannot respond to *Candida;* and selective IgA deficiency is caused by B-cell abnormality.
- Problems in neuroendocrine and immune system interactions are a cause of secondary immunodeficiencies. Excessive neuroendocrine response to stress with increased corticosteroid production increases susceptibility to infection.
- Medications such as cytotoxins and other cancer pharmacotherapeutic drugs cause generalized secondary immunosuppression. However, other medications, such as anesthetics, alcohol, antibiotics, and steroids, also affect the immune response and can lead to secondary immunosuppression.
- Malnutrition, a major cause of immune system dysfunction, leads to lymphocyte dysfunction and altered stem cell development.

SUMMARY

Human beings live in internal and external environments teeming with antigens capable of producing immunologic responses. Contact with an antigen or antigens usually leads to induction of a normal protective immune response. However, some individuals experience disease caused by either excessive immune responses or deficient immune responses.

Both excessive and deficient immune reactions are damaging to tissue. The tissues that are affected depend on the type of antigen, the type of antigen exposure, and the degree of immune responsiveness. In children with immune system dysfunction caused by embryonic defects, the lack or dysfunction of T cells, B cells, and antibodies can lead to lethal or recurrent infections that severely limit the child's ability to interact with the environment. As a result of their immune disorder, some of these children may never reach maturity. In the elderly, malnutrition, medications, and decreased immune system function as a result of aging, surgery, stress, decreased social support, depression, and bereavement lead to increased infections and autoimmune disease. Autoimmune disease is a type of excessive immune reaction in which the immune system "attacks" the body's own cells. Many autoimmune diseases are also hypersensitivity reactions.

Excessive immune reactions are common and involve a complex interplay between antigen and components of the immune system. Hypersensitivity disorders are differentiated by the cell type involved and the time course of the reaction. For example, type I hypersensitivity is a rapid response caused by a host of lethal chemicals generated by but involving only one antibody, IgE, and one effector cell, the mast cell. It is an antigen-antibody reaction causing the release of potent chemicals that can lead to extreme, even life-threatening reactions in susceptible individuals. Type II hypersensitivity is also immediate but is tissue specific involving IgG and IgM antibodies, a host of effector cells, and the complement system. It is a linkage between antigen on target cells and the Fab portion of IgG or IgM antibodies. Examples include blood transfusion reactions, hemolytic anemia, and myasthenia gravis.

Type III hypersensitivity reactions, which involve IgG as the major antibody and neutrophils and mast cells as the effector cells, take several hours to develop. These reactions involve the deposition of antigen-antibody immune complexes into tissue and activation of the complement system. This reaction is a deposition problem that depends on the solubility of the antigen-antibody complex and the vascular system. The tissues that have the antigen-antibody complex deposited into them become inflamed. SLE is the major example of type III hypersensitivity. Type IV hypersensitivity takes days to develop and involves cytotoxic T cells but no antibodies. Examples include poison ivy, contact dermatitis, and organ transplant rejection.

MEDIA RESOURCES

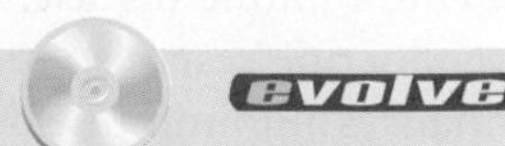

Remember to check out the ***CD Companion*** included with this book for Review Questions, Key Concepts Review, Glossary (with audio for selected terms), Disease Profiles, and Animations.

PLUS, visit the ***Evolve website*** at http://evolve.elsevier.com/Copstead/ for Case Studies, Disease Profiles, and WebLinks.

References

1. Check E: The virtue of tolerance, *Nature* 418:364-366, July 2002.
2. Bachert C: The role of histamine in allergic disease: re-appraisal of its inflammatory potential, *Allergy* 57(4):287-296, 2002.
3. Villa A, et al: V(D)J recombination defects in lymphocytes due to RAG mutations: severe immunodeficiency with a spectrum of clinical presentations, *Blood* 97(1):81-88, 2001.
4. Notarangelo LD, et al: Combined immunodeficiencies due to defects in signal transduction: defects of the gammac-JAK 3 signaling pathway as a model, *Immunobiology* 202(2):106-119, 2000.
5. Herzog RW, Hagstrom JN: Gene therapy for hereditary hematological disorders, *Am J Pharmacogenomics* 1(2):137-144, 2001.
6. Halonen M, et al: AIRE mutations and human leukocyte antigen genotypes as determinants of the autoimmune polyendocrinopathy-candidiasis-ectodermal dystrophy phenotype, *J Clin Endocrinol Metab* 87(6):2568-2574, 2002.
7. Kinsella JE, Lokesh B: Dietary lipids, eicosanoids, and the immune system, *Crit Care Med* 18(suppl):S94-S113, 1990.

chapter 11

Malignant Disorders of White Blood Cells

Jacquelyn L. Banasik

MEDIA RESOURCES

Additional Material for Study, Review, and Further Exploration

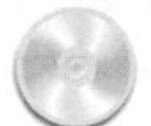

CD Companion ◆ Review Questions and Answers ◆ Key Concepts Review ◆ Glossary *(with audio pronunciations for selected terms)* ◆ Disease Profiles ◆ Animations

evolve ***Website*** at http://evolve.elsevier.com/Copstead/ ◆ Case Studies ◆ Disease Profiles ◆ WebLinks

KEY QUESTIONS

- How do the various types of leukemia, lymphoma, and plasma cell myeloma differ based on the cell type of malignant transformation?
- How do the clinical presentations, prognosis, and management of types of acute and chronic leukemia differ?
- Why are malignant disorders of white blood cells commonly associated with bone marrow depression?
- How is Hodgkin disease clinically and histologically differentiated from other types of lymphoma?
- What is the purpose and process of staging procedures for malignant lymphoma?
- What clinical and laboratory findings would suggest a diagnosis of plasma cell myeloma?
- What are the expected side effects and common complications of chemotherapy and radiation therapy?
- What is disease remission and how does it differ from cure?

CHAPTER OUTLINE

Leukemia, lymphoma, and plasma cell myeloma (multiple myeloma) are common neoplastic disorders of the bone marrow and lymphoid tissues. Depending on the location and specific types of white blood cells involved, these malignancies can be further divided into a number of specific subtypes. Leukemias can be conceptualized as circulating tumors that are disseminated from the beginning of the disease process and primarily involve the blood and bone marrow. Lymphoma tends to localize in lymph tissues but is often disseminated to other sites at the time of diagnosis. Plasma cell myeloma has a predilection to form localized tumors in bony structures.

Malignancies of the blood-forming tissues and lymphatic structures often present with nonspecific symptoms. Malaise, weakness, unexplained fever, night sweats, and recurrent infections should raise suspicion of malignancy. Enlarged, nontender lymph nodes (lymphadenopathy) are a common finding in lymphoma. Often, white blood cell malignancies are found by chance during routine assessment of the complete blood cell count (CBC). A very high total white blood cell count or the presence of abnormal cell types should precipitate an assessment for hematologic cell malignancy. In general, earlier detection of malignancy is associated with a better prognosis for cure.

CLASSIFICATION OF HEMATOLOGIC NEOPLASMS

Various classification schemes have been used to group hematologic neoplasms, with clinicians favoring schemes that use clinical findings and pathologists preferring morphologic criteria. With the advent of technologies to identify specific genetic alterations and molecular characteristics of neoplastic cells, the traditional classification systems have become less useful. However, many clinicians and organizations, such as the American Cancer Society, continue to use traditional groupings to collect statistics and to provide information to the public. The approach used in this chapter incorporates the most recent World Health Organization (WHO) classifications for hematologic neoplasms and also includes common clinical terminology. A major force behind the adoption of the WHO classification is the recognition that lymphoid leukemias and lymphomas are not separate disorders and represent different stages of the same biological disease. Thus, the major categories of the WHO system are based on the cell type of the neoplasm, rather than its location in the body.[1] Neoplasms involving cells of the myeloid lineage (Box 11-1) are separated from those of the lymphoid lineage (Box 11-2). The myeloid lineage includes red cells, platelets, monocytes, and granulocytes; the lymphoid lineage includes B cells, T cells, and natural killer (NK) cells (Figure 11-1). There are four major categories of myeloid neoplasms: myeloproliferative diseases; myelodysplastic/proliferative diseases; myelodysplastic syndromes; and acute myeloid leukemia (AML). There are three major categories of lymphoid neoplasms: B-cell neoplasm, T-cell and NK cell neoplasm, and Hodgkin disease. The term non-Hodgkin lymphoma is still in clinical usage and refers to lymphomas of B-cell, T-cell, and NK cell origin. Non-Hodgkin lymphoma includes such a large and diverse group of malignancies that it has little relevance to prognosis or treatment. The WHO classification does not use this term. Other classification systems in current use include the FAB (French-American-British) system for subtypes of myeloid leukemia (Table 11-1). There are many etiologic, pathogenic and treatment similarities among the hematologic malignancies, and these are addressed in a general way first, followed by sections on specific diseases.

ETIOLOGY OF MYELOID AND LYMPHOID NEOPLASMS

As in other malignant processes, the exact cause of hematologic neoplasms is unknown. The basic mechanism of malignant transformation involves genetic damage to cells, which

Box 11-1

Proposed WHO Classification of Myeloid Neoplasms

Myeloproliferative Diseases (MPD)

Chronic myelogenous leukemia, Philadelphia chromosome (Ph1) (t[;22][qq34;q11], bcr/abl)+
Chronic neutrophilic leukemia
Chronic eosinophilic leukemia/hypereosinophilic syndrome
Chronic idiopathic myelofibrosis
Polycythemia vera
Essential thrombocythemia
Myeloproliferative disease, unclassifiable

Myelodysplastic/Myeloproliferative Diseases

Chronic myelomonocytic leukemia (CMML)
Atypical chronic myelogenous leukemia (aCML)
Juvenile myelomonocytic leukemia (JMML)

Myelodysplastic Syndromes

Refractory anemia (RA)
With ringed sideroblasts (RARS)
Without ringed sideroblasts
Refractory cytopenia (myelodysplastic syndrome) with multilineage dysplasia (RCMD)
Refractory anemia (myelodysplastic syndrome) with excess blasts (RAEB)
5q-syndrome
Myelodysplastic syndrome, unclassifiable

Acute Myeloid Leukemias (AML)

Acute myeloid leukemias with recurrent cytogenetic translocations
- AML with t(8;21) (q22;q22), AML1(CBFα)/ETO
- Acute promyelocytic leukemia (AML with t(15;17)(q22;q11-12) and variants, PML/RARα)
- AML with abnormal bone marrow eosinophils (inv(16)(p13q22) or t(16;16)(p13;q11), CBFβ/MYHIIX)
- AML with 11q23 (MLL) abnormalities

Acute myeloid leukemia with multilineage dysplasia
- With prior myelodysplastic syndrome
- Without prior myelodysplastic syndrome

Acute myeloid leukemia and myelodysplastic syndrome, therapy related
- Alkylating agent related
- Epipodophyllotoxin related (some may be lymphoid)
- Other types

Acute myeloid leukemia (AML) not otherwise categorized
- AML minimally differentiated
- AML without maturation
- AML with maturation
- Acute myelomonocytic leukemia
- Acute monocytic leukemia
- Acute erythroid leukemia
- Acute megakaryocytic leukemia
- Acute basophilic leukemia
- Acute panmyelosis with myelofibrosis

Acute Biphenotypic Leukemias

From Jaffe ES et al, editors: *World Health Organization classification of tumours: pathology and genetics of tumors of haematopoietic and lymphoid tissues,* Lyon, France, 2001, IARC Press, p 194.

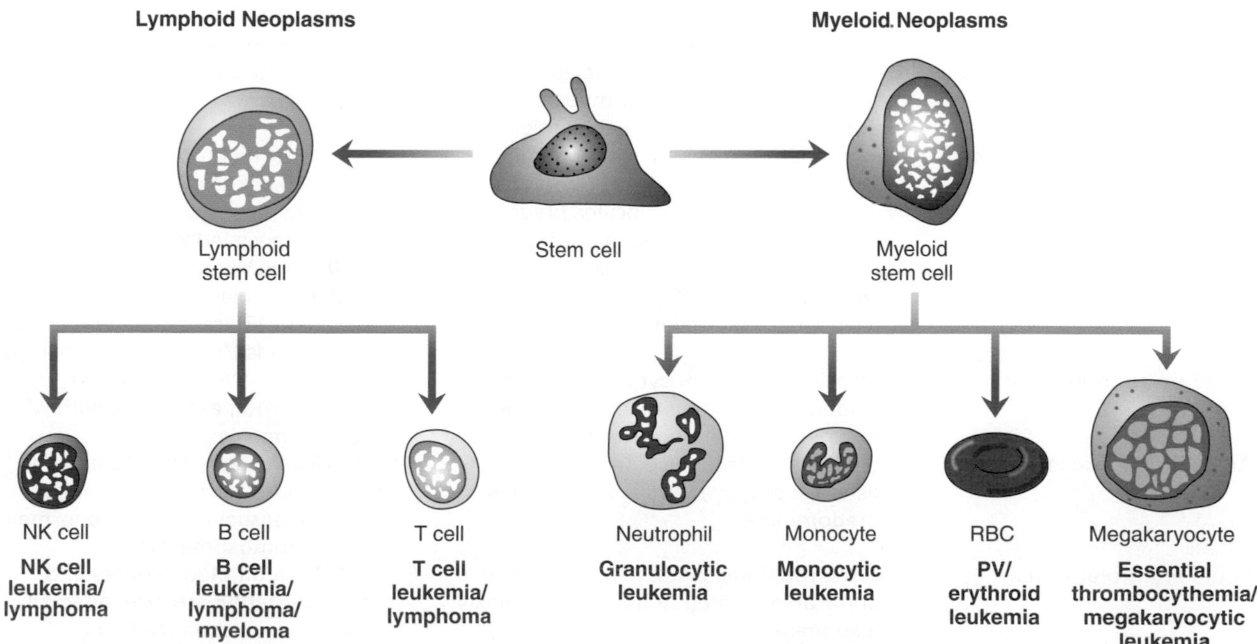

FIGURE 11-1 ■ Division of hematologic neoplasms into myeloid and lymphoid lineages. *PV,* Polycythemia vera.

Box 11-2

Proposed WHO Classification of Lymphoid Neoplasms

B-Cell Neoplasms

- Precursor B-cell neoplasm
  - Precursor B-lymphoblastic leukemia/lymphoma (precursor B-cell acute lymphoblastic leukemia)
- Mature (peripheral) B-cell neoplasms*
  - B-cell chronic lymphocytic leukemia/small lymphocytic lymphoma
  - B-cell prolymphocytic leukemia
  - Lymphoplasmacytic lymphoma
  - Splenic marginal zone B-cell lymphoma (± villous lymphocytes)
  - Hairy cell leukemia
  - Plasma cell myeloma/plasmacytoma
  - Extranodal marginal zone B-cell lymphoma of MALT type
  - Nodal marginal zone B-cell lymphoma (± monocytoid B cells)
  - Follicular lymphoma
  - Mantle cell lymphoma
  - Diffuse large B-cell lymphoma
    - Mediastinal large B-cell lymphoma
    - Primary effusion lymphoma
  - Burkitt lymphoma/Burkitt cell leukemia

T- and NK-Cell Neoplasms

- Precursor T-cell neoplasm
  - Precursor T-lymphoblastic lymphoma/leukemia (precursor T-cell acute lymphoblastic leukemia)
- Mature (peripheral) T-cell neoplasms
  - T-cell prolymphocytic leukemia
  - T-cell granular lymphocytic leukemia
  - Aggressive NK-cell leukemia
  - Adult T-cell lymphoma/leukemia (HTLV1$^+$)
  - Extranodal NK/T-cell lymphoma, nasal type
  - Enteropathy-type T-cell lymphoma
  - Hepatosplenic $\gamma\delta$ T-cell lymphoma
  - Subcutaneous panniculitis-like T-cell lymphoma
  - Mycosis fungoides/Sézary syndrome
  - Anaplastic large cell lymphoma, T/null cell, primary cutaneous type
  - Peripheral T-cell lymphoma, not otherwise characterized
  - Angioimmunoblastic T-cell lymphoma
  - Anaplastic large cell lymphoma, T/null cell, primary systemic type

Hodgkin Lymphoma (Hodgkin Disease)

- Nodular lymphocyte predominance Hodgkin lymphoma
- Classical Hodgkin lymphoma
  - Nodular sclerosis Hodgkin lymphoma (Grades 1 and 2)
  - Lymphocyte-rich classical Hodgkin lymphoma
  - Mixed cellularity Hodgkin lymphoma
  - Lymphocyte depletion Hodgkin lymphoma

From Jaffe ES et al, editors: *World Health Organization classification of tumours: pathology and genetics of tumors of haematopoietic and lymphoid tissues,* Lyon, France, 2001, IARC Press, p 195.
More common entities are underlined.
*B and T/NK cell neoplasms are grouped according to major clinical presentations (predominantly disseminated/leukemic, primary extranodal, predominantly nodal).

Table 11-1

FAB Classification of Acute Myeloblastic (Myelocytic) Leukemias

Class	Morphology	Comments
M0: Minimally differentiated AML	Blasts lack definitive cytologic and cytochemical markers of myeloblasts but express myeloid lineage antigens	2% to 3% of AML
M1: AML without differentiation	Very immature myeloblasts predominate; few granules or Auer rods	20% of AML; Ph chromosome, present in 10% to 15% of cases, worsens prognosis
M2: AML with differentiation	Myeloblasts and promyelocytes predominate; Auer rods commonly present	30% of AML; presence of t(8;21) translocation associated with good prognosis
M3: Acute promyelocytic leukemia	Hypergranular promyelocytes, often with many Auer rods per cell; may have reniform or bilobed nuclei	5% to 10% of AML; disseminated intravascular coagulation common; presence of t(15;17) translocation is characteristic; responds to retinoic acid therapy
M4: Acute myelomonocytic leukemia	Myelocytic and monocytic differentiation evident; myeloid elements resemble M2; peripheral monocytosis	20% to 30% of AML; presence of inv16 or del16q associated with better prognosis
M5: Acute monocytic leukemia	Monoblasts (peroxidase negative, esterase positive) and promonocytes predominate	10% of AML; usually in children and young adults; gum infiltration common; associated with abnormalities of chromosome 11q23
M6: Acute erythroleukemia	Bizarre, multinucleated, megaloblastoid erythroblasts predominate; myeloblasts also present	5% of AML; high blood counts and organ infiltration are rare; affected persons are of advanced age
M7: Acute megakaryocytic leukemia	Blasts of megakaryocytic lineage predominate; react with antiplatelet antibodies; myelofibrosis or increased bone marrow reticulin	

From Kumar V, Cotran RS, Robbins SL, editors: *Basic pathology,* ed 7, Philadelphia, 2003, Saunders, p 437.
AML, Acute myeloblastic (myelocytic) leukemia; *Ph,* Philadelphia.

disrupts growth control and differentiation pathways. These processes are thought to be similar to those described for solid tumors (see Chapter 7).

Viruses have long been suspected as agents in some neoplasms, particularly retroviruses and herpesviruses. In most cases, viruses are considered to be risk factors for neoplasia rather than causal agents. Close associations have been found between a small number of viruses and particular malignancies. For example, human T-cell leukemia virus (HTLV-1) is linked to the development of adult T-cell lymphoma/leukemia and human immunodeficiency virus (HIV) is linked to B-cell lymphomas. Epstein-Barr virus (EBV) has been implicated in both Hodgkin disease and Burkitt lymphoma.[2] EBV is nearly ubiquitous in the population worldwide, with 90% of adults having evidence of previous infection (seropositive). It is possible to obtain EBV-transformed B cells from nearly all EBV-seropositive individuals, but progression to malignancy is rare.[2] Effective immune surveillance is thought to keep proliferation in check and prevent progression in immunocompetent individuals.

Radiation exposure is an important etiologic factor for leukemia and lymphoma. Because of the relatively high turnover of hematologic cells, they are more susceptible to radiation-induced damage than most other cell types. An acute whole-body dose of radiation like that which occurs with nuclear explosions is known to increase the risk of leukemia. In Japanese survivors of the atomic bomb the estimated lifetime risk of leukemia is 0.85%, sixfold higher than the norm.[3] There are substantial uncertainties about the risk of low-level, long-term exposure to radiation. The average annual exposure from usual exposures including cosmic rays and medical procedures is very low and estimated to account for less than 5% of leukemia cases.

Despite intensive scrutiny only a small number of chemicals have been shown unequivocally to increase the risk of hematologic malignancies. Benzene has been implicated in numerous studies as has cigarette smoking. Other suggested carcinogens have failed to be confirmed, including exposure to hair dye, alcohol, and marijuana.[4] On the other hand, a study from the Children's Cancer Group found a link between high maternal intake of products high in bioflavonoids (beans, fresh vegetables, and fruit) and an increased incidence of infant leukemia.[5] These bioflavonoids were enzyme inhibitors (topoisomerase II inhibitors) that caused DNA cleavage and chromosome translocations. The antineoplastic drugs used to treat cancers, especially the alkylating agents, are significant factors in the development of posttreatment hematologic neoplasia. Any drugs that suppress the bone marrow or immune function are also believed to predispose to the emergence of malignancies.

A number of disease conditions have been linked to the development of leukemia, although the mechanisms are unclear. A reduction or alteration in normal hematopoiesis, as occurs in such disorders as Fanconi anemia and aplastic anemia (see Chapter 13), is associated with a higher incidence of leukemia. A higher risk also has been noted in some genetic diseases, including Down syndrome and Klinefelter syndrome (see Chapter 6).

GENERAL PRINCIPLES OF MANAGEMENT

Diagnosis of Hematologic Neoplasms

Clinical manifestations of leukemia are related to bone marrow suppression and organ dysfunction secondary to leukemic infiltration. Bone marrow suppression results in varying degrees of **leukopenia, anemia,** and **thrombocytopenia.** It is these three deficiencies that cause the most common clinical manifestations and may prompt the patient to seek care. Common manifestations of hematologic malignancies are shown in Box 11-3.

Anemia, with a hematocrit of 25% to 30% or hemoglobin of 8 to 10 g/dl, may manifest with pallor, fatigue, malaise, shortness of breath, and decreased activity tolerance. The severity of symptoms is determined by the rate of red blood cell decrease as well as the absolute deficiency. Chronically low hemoglobin and hematocrit may be tolerated better than a drastic drop. Depending on symptoms, transfusion may be indicated when the hematocrit falls below 30%.

Box 11-3

Common Manifestations of Hematologic Malignancies

History
Fever
Weight loss
Night sweats
Itching (pruritus)
Fatigue
Bone pain (sternum, tibia, femur, back)
Abdominal fullness
Bleeding episodes (epistaxis, menorrhagia)
Bruising, petechiae
Frequent infections
Headache, nausea, vomiting

Physical
Enlarged spleen
Enlarged liver
Enlarged lymph nodes
Hyperplasia of gums

Laboratory
Anemia or polycythemia
Thrombocytopenia or thrombocythemia
Leukopenia or leukocytosis
Blasts on peripheral blood smear
Elevated uric acid
Elevated alkaline phosphatase
Hypercalcemia

Thrombocytopenia, with a platelet count below 20,000 cells/μl, can manifest as petechiae, easy bruising, bleeding gums, occult hematuria, or retinal hemorrhages. Spontaneous intracranial bleeding can occur and may be fatal. In general, the risk of bleeding increases proportionately to the fall in platelet count. Platelet transfusion may be given when the risk of bleeding is high.

Insufficient numbers of functional leukocytes leaves the patient at high risk for development of infection and the complete blood count is routinely monitored. **Neutropenia** is an absolute neutrophil count less than 500 cells/μl, and an affected patient requires protective isolation (neutropenic precautions) to prevent infection. Infections may be caused by bacterial, viral, fungal, or protozoal organisms. Often, the microorganisms are of the opportunistic variety. That is, they are part of the patient's own flora, which normally do not cause disease unless the host's immune system becomes incompetent. It is very difficult to protect patients from their own flora, and infection is the most common cause of death in the immunocompromised leukemic patient. The presence of infection is suspected if fever develops. Infections are managed aggressively with antibiotic agents to prevent development of life-threatening sepsis.

Infiltrative manifestations include lymphadenopathy, joint swelling and pain, weight loss, anorexia, hepatomegaly, and splenomegaly. Sternal tenderness is frequently present in chronic myeloid leukemia (CML). Gingival hyperplasia occurs in acute myeloid leukemia (AML). Meningeal involvement is frequently encountered in children with acute lymphoid leukemia (ALL). Central nervous system (CNS) infiltration can occur with any type of leukemia and may be difficult to manage because of the poor ability of chemotherapeutic agents to cross the blood-brain barrier. CNS involvement can present with increased intracranial pressure, seizures, or changes in mental ability. Increased intracranial pressure should be suspected in the leukemia patient who complains of nausea, vomiting, headache, and visual changes.

A key aspect of diagnosis is the evaluation of a peripheral blood sample. Blood cell number and morphology is indicative; however, definitive diagnosis is usually made after bone marrow aspiration or lymph node biopsy. Malignant cells can be subtyped according to genetic and molecular characteristics to better determine prognosis and choice of treatment.

Principles of Treatment

To make informed treatment decisions, the patient and family need information about the nature and prognosis of their disease as well as about the risks and benefits of various treatment options. Many treatment protocols are experimental, and the outcomes may be uncertain. Sometimes the side effects of treatment and poor chance of effectiveness will weigh in favor of palliative care. Treatment decisions are complex and stressful for all concerned. A great deal of support must be available during the diagnostic, treatment, and monitoring phases.

The management of hematologic malignancies relies primarily on the use of combination chemotherapy to eradicate malignant cells and stem cell transplant to rescue and restore bone marrow function. In some cases radiation may be used as an adjunct to drug therapy. Unfortunately, the treatment regimen usually causes many serious side effects that must be monitored and treated.

The goal of chemotherapy is to induce long-term remission, that is, the absence of any detectable neoplastic cells in the body. A complete remission (CR) is defined as a return to normal hematopoiesis with normal red cell, neutrophil, and platelet count and no detectable neoplastic cells. For leukemia, the bone marrow must have less than 5% blasts and be maintained for at least 4 weeks.[6] CR is not synonymous with cure, and it is estimated that up to a billion neoplastic cells can still be present and undetectable when the above parameters of CR have been met. Therefore, most treatment protocols include several cycles of chemotherapy to eradicate the undetected cells. The choice of antineoplastic agents varies with the type of neoplasia and the stage of clinical disease (Box 11-4). Most chemotherapeutic agents work by disrupting some aspect of DNA synthesis or cell replication and induce **apoptosis** (cell suicide; see Chapter 4). In general, rapidly dividing cells are more susceptible to apoptosis because they have less time for repair. Neoplasms with genetic defects that impair apoptotic pathways may be more difficult to eradicate and require more intense therapy. Unfortunately, these high doses are toxic to normal stem cells as well and can produce fatal bone marrow failure. Therefore, to effect a cure, high-dose chemotherapy is often followed by bone marrow "rescue" with transplantation of functional stem cells.

Chemotherapy usually includes two or three treatment phases: (1) remission induction phase, (2) postremission or consolidation phase, and (3) remission maintenance phase. The aim of treatment during the remission induction phase is to eliminate all detectable neoplastic cells and achieve a CR. Postremission consolidation therapy begins after CR is attained in an attempt to eliminate the population of undetected cells that may have escaped initial induction phase treatment. Maintenance phase treatment is used in the management of some neoplasms to prolong the remission interval. Intermittent chemotherapy may be continued for 2 to 3 years after initial induction of remission. Drugs that target the neoplastic cells specifically, such as monoclonal antibodies or molecular therapies, are generally less toxic than other agents and may be used for long-term maintenance in patients with residual disease.

In children and adults, the CNS can act as a sanctuary for neoplastic cells, and conventional routes of chemotherapy are unsuccessful because they do not permit drug to cross the blood-brain barrier efficiently. Chemotherapeutic agents administered into the cerebrospinal fluid (CSF) via lumbar puncture (intrathecal route) can effectively eliminate leukemic cells in the CNS. This therapy carries significant risk for temporary or permanent neurologic damage. A number of

Box 11-4

Typical Roles of Specific Cytotoxic Drugs in the Treatment of the Leukemias

Acute Lymphoblastic Leukemia

Induction: Vincristine + prednisone + two or three other drugs from an anthracycline (daunorubicin or idarubicin), cyclophosphamide, L-asparaginase

Intensive consolidation: Cytarabine (Ara-C), other drugs including an anthracycline (daunorubicin or idarubicin), epipodophyllotoxins (etoposide or teniposide), antimetabolite (methotrexate or 6-thioguanine)

Maintenance (2 years): Oral methotrexate and mercaptopurine

CNS prophylaxis: Intrathecal methotrexate

Acute Myeloid Leukemia

Induction: Ara-C + an anthracycline (daunorubicin or idarubicin) + etoposide or 6-thioguanine

Intensive postremission therapy: High-dose Ara-C or bone marrow/stem cell transplantation

Acute Promyelocytic Leukemia

Induction: Retinoic acid alone or with anthracycline/Ara-C combination

Postremission therapy: Anthracycline/Ara-C if retinoic acid is used as a single agent in induction

Chronic Lymphoid Leukemia

Chlorambucil ± prednisone; cyclophosphamide, vincristine, prednisone (CVP) in relapsed or resistant patients

Chronic Myeloid Leukemia

Hydroxyurea and/or busulfan; interferon-α

From Henderson ES, Lister TA, Greaves MF: *Leukemia,* ed 7, Philadelphia, 2002, Saunders, p 404.

different chemotherapeutic agents can be administered safely by the intrathecal route, including methotrexate.[7]

Prevention and Management of Complications

Maintenance of adequate nutrition in patients with hematologic malignancy is a major challenge. Anorexia, weight loss, nausea, vomiting, and **stomatitis** are common findings, especially during the treatment phase. Children and adolescents on chemotherapy may experience significant growth delay, and measures to maintain protein and caloric intake are necessary. Newer antiemetic agents have been helpful in reducing nausea, vomiting, and anorexia associated with chemotherapy and should be considered in patients experiencing these symptoms.

Infection is the most troublesome of complications for the immunosuppressed patient. Constant vigilance in prevention, early detection, and rapid management of infections can profoundly affect the outcome of chemotherapy. When the neutrophil count falls below a critical level, attempts to isolate the patient from infectious agents are often instituted. Intramuscular injections are avoided because they damage skin integrity and may also cause excessive bleeding into the tissues. Rectal temperatures, enemas, and suppositories are avoided to prevent infections associated with mucosal damage.

An elevated temperature in the neutropenic patient is a worrisome finding. A thorough search for the site of infection is indicated, with cultures being taken from potential sites such as throat, urine, sputum, blood, and all indwelling intravenous lines and tubes. Early initiation of broad-spectrum antibiotic therapy to cover likely organisms is undertaken while awaiting culture results.

The length of time that a patient remains neutropenic can be shortened with the use of growth factors to stimulate bone marrow production of granulocytes. These growth factors are similar to the natural colony-stimulating factors produced within the body. When administered to the immunosuppressed patient, they can reduce the chances of infection by enhancing the neutrophil count. Neutrophils are responsible for rapid defense against infectious organisms. They are normally produced and mobilized in great numbers during bacterial invasions. Once the neutrophils leave the blood stream to kill and ingest bacteria, they live for only a short period. Thus, neutrophils must be continuously produced to maintain immunocompetence. Both the neoplastic process and the chemotherapeutic agents used to manage it suppress bone marrow production of neutrophils. The longer a patient remains neutropenic, the more likely is the development of life-threatening infection. Administration of granulocyte colony-stimulating factors reduces the period of neutropenia and enhances immunocompetence. Thus, granulocyte colony-stimulating factors are commonly used during high-dose chemotherapy protocols, and also after bone marrow transplantation, to enhance grafting and speed bone marrow recovery time.

Bone marrow transplantation has been an important part of the management of acute leukemia for many years. The intense chemotherapy used to induce remission often leads to bone marrow failure. Stem cells can be reintroduced into the host's bone marrow by bone marrow transplantation. The transplanted cells are given intravenously; they find their way to the host's bone marrow, where they establish residence and begin to produce functional white blood cells, red blood cells, and platelets. A close match between donor and host is necessary for a successful transplantation. Otherwise, the transplanted cells can mount an immune attack on the host's tissues—a life-threatening problem called *graft-versus-host disease* (see Chapter 10). In past years, bone marrow for transplantation was obtained by aspiration from the marrow of a suitable donor. *Peripheral stem cell transplantation* allows stem cells to be harvested from the circulating blood stream. This procedure can be used to collect stem cells from the patient's own blood to be stored and then reinfused after chemotherapy and irradiation. This type of transplant is called *autologous,* whereas a transplant from a closely matched relative is called *allogeneic* (Figure 11-2). Use of autologous transplants eliminates the problem of graft-versus-host disease and reduces transplant-related mortality, but the potential for recurrence is higher than with allogeneic transplants.

It has been noted that in AML and CML, transplantation with allogeneic cells is much more successful in curing leukemia than is autologous transplantation. Transplanted cells in the allograft are thought to detect and kill leukemic cells in a process termed *graft versus leukemia.* Autologous transplants are appropriate in some cases, especially when a matched donor is not available, because they may extend life even though cure is unlikely. Autologous transplants are well tolerated and cause fewer complications than allografts. Methods to purify a patient's collected peripheral blood by selectively removing neoplastic cells are available to reduce the risk of reintroducing malignant cells during autologous transplantation. Increased availability of stem cell transplants allows patients to undergo more intensive chemotherapy, aimed at cure rather than palliation, based on the knowledge that bone marrow rescue is possible.

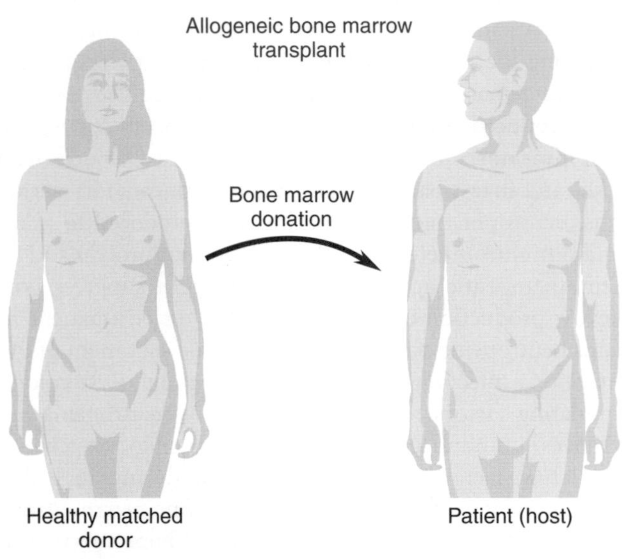

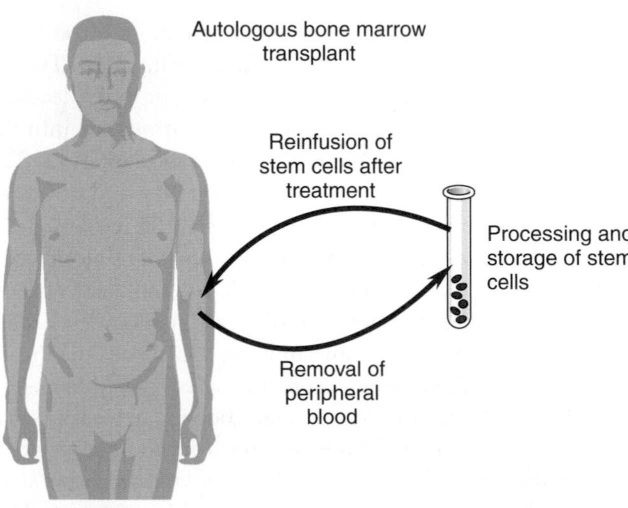

FIGURE 11-2 ■ A comparison of allogeneic bone marrow transplant and autologous stem cell transplant.

Anemia is a common complication of leukemia and chemotherapy. Red blood cell production by the bone marrow is suppressed, but the size and shape of red cells present in the blood are normal. This is called *normocytic,* normochromic anemia. Administration of erythropoietin growth factors can enhance red blood cell production and moderate anemic episodes. However, patients frequently require red blood cell transfusion therapy to maintain adequate red blood cell counts. Patients with frequent or significant bleeding episodes are also predisposed to severe anemia, and efforts to prevent bleeding will help to minimize anemia.

Platelet deficiency (thrombocytopenia) with resultant hemorrhage can be a life-threatening complication of leukemia and chemotherapy. Careful monitoring of skin, mucous membranes, urine, stool, and emesis for the presence of obvious or occult blood is necessary. Spontaneous intracranial hemorrhage is a serious complication of thrombocytopenia and may be apparent as sudden severe headache and altered level of consciousness. In patients at high risk of bleeding, fresh frozen plasma or pooled platelets may be given to inhibit bleeding. Patients must be protected from trauma and may be placed on activity restrictions.

Pain is a common complication of the diagnostic and treatment protocols used in the cancer patient as well as of the disease process itself. Pain most commonly involves the bones and joints, and is due to pressure caused by infiltration and accumulation of neoplastic cells in the bone marrow. *Hemarthrosis* (bleeding into joints) can cause acute episodes of joint pain. Chemotherapy may help reduce bone pain, as the number of neoplastic cells is reduced drastically. Patients are subjected to numerous painful procedures during diagnosis, treatment, and monitoring. Frequent blood and bone marrow sampling, placement of intravenous access lines for drug administration, and unpleasant drug side effects all contribute to the pain experience. Nausea and mouth pain (stomatitis) are frequent complaints during chemotherapy. Pain management with a variety of strategies, including narcotic and nonnarcotic drugs, distraction, and biofeedback, are generally helpful. (See Chapter 47 for a discussion of pain and pain management.)

Epithelial cells, with normally high rates of turnover, are particularly susceptible to damage by radiation and chemotherapy. Sloughing of skin and mucous membranes and hair loss are common. Loss of skin and mucous membrane integrity increases the risk of infection and can contribute significantly to the pain and discomfort of treatment. **Alopecia** leads to an altered body image and may interfere with the individual's ability to cope with the treatment protocol. It is helpful to reassure the patient that hair loss is a temporary consequence of the chemotherapeutic regimen and will grow back once therapy is completed.

Abnormalities in growth, development, and fertility are complications of particular concern in children undergoing radiation and chemotherapy. Cranial irradiation and methotrexate infusions have been associated with declines in cognitive function, memory, and reading and mathematics proficiency. Children who undergo total-body irradiation in preparation for bone marrow transplantation are likely to experience growth failure and gonadal dysfunction. Growth failure may improve with the administration of human growth hormone. Sexual development is frequently impaired in both girls and boys. Girls usually experience ovarian failure and require hormone replacement therapy. Boys generally recover testosterone production and do not require replacement, but spermatogenesis and fertility usually remain impaired.

KEY CONCEPTS

- Classification of the types of leukemia is based on cell type involved (lymphoid or myeloid) and degree of cell maturation. Common myeloid neoplasms include CML, polycythemia vera, essential thrombocythemia, and AML. Common lymphoid neoplasms include chronic lymphoid leukemia (CLL), acute lymphoblastic leukemia, plasma cell myeloma, Hodgkin disease, and various forms of non-Hodgkin lymphoma.
- Risk factors for the development of hematologic neoplasms include exposure to chemical, viral, and radiation mutagens; chemotherapy drugs; and immunodeficiency disorders.
- Common manifestations of hematologic neoplasia are due to insufficient production of normal white blood cells, red blood cells, and platelets, as evidenced by leukopenia, anemia, and thrombocytopenia. Anemia manifests as pallor, fatigue, dyspnea, and decreased activity tolerance. Thrombocytopenia causes petechiae, bleeding gums, hematuria, and prolonged bleeding time. Leukopenia manifests as frequent, recurrent infections. Other manifestations may occur with infiltration of tissues and organs. These include weight loss, anorexia, lymphadenopathy, bone pain, and CNS dysfunction.
- Chemotherapy is the mainstay of management for most hematologic neoplasms. Several courses may be needed to kill neoplastic stem cells. Most chemotherapeutic agents interfere with some aspect of DNA replication and cell division to induce apoptosis (cell suicide).
- Treatment is associated with a number of potential complications including anemia, infection, and bleeding. Rapidly dividing hair cells and mucous membranes are also affected, leading to alopecia and stomatitis. Transfusion of blood products or stimulation of endogenous production with colony-stimulating factors and erythropoietin may be necessary. Bone marrow transplantation may be undertaken in some cases to restore stem cell function.

MYELOID NEOPLASMS

Myeloid neoplasms result from transformation and proliferation of a precursor stem cell in the bone marrow (Figure 11-3). The progeny of the aberrant stem cell forms a clone of abnormal cells that accumulate in the bone marrow and are released into the circulation. In many cases, the abnormal stem cell is multipotent and causes the overproduction of more than one cell type, resulting in myeloproliferative disease. The cells produced in myeloproliferative diseases are usually functional and have a normal morphologic appearance. The common myeloproliferative diseases are chronic myeloid leukemia (CML), polycythemia vera (PV), and essential thrombocythemia (ET), referring respectively to an excess of granulocytes, red blood cells, and platelets. These insidious and indolent disorders have few clinical symptoms and are commonly discovered on routine CBC analysis. Common features of CML, PV, and ET include involvement of a multipotent hematopoietic progenitor cell; marrow hypercellularity; overproduction of one or more functional blood cells; chromosomal abnormalities involving chromosomes 1, 8, 9, 13, and 20; eventual spontaneous conversion to AML or development of marrow fibrosis.[8]

In contrast to the myeloproliferative diseases, the myelodysplastic syndromes and AML are characterized by neoplastic cells that are morphologically and functionally abnormal.

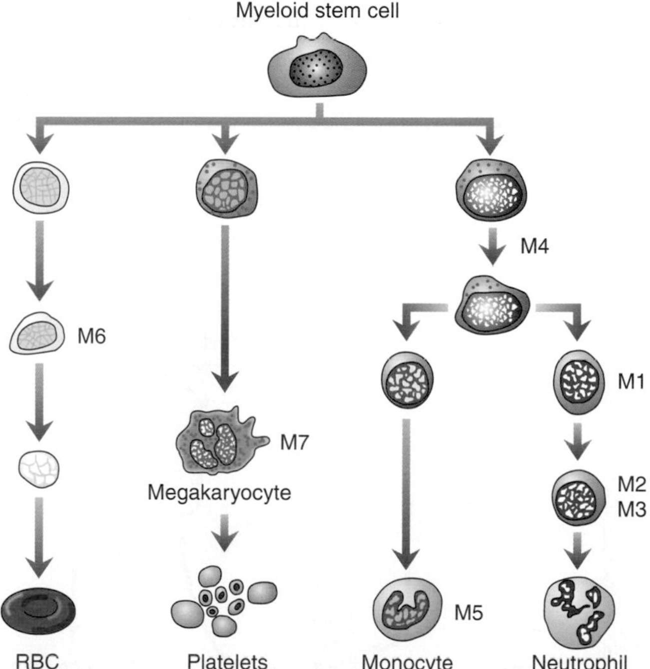

FIGURE 11-3 ■ Maturation pathways of myeloid cells showing the different types of leukemia associated with various stages of development. M1, M2, and M3 types result in granulocytic leukemia; M4 has characteristics of monocytic and granulocytic leukemia; M5 is monocytic; M6 is associated with erythroid leukemia; and M7 is associated with megakaryocytic leukemia. *RBC,* Red blood cell.

The prognosis for myelodysplastic syndromes and AML is poor, and intensive treatment is necessary to extend life. AML and the myeloproliferative disease CML are described below. A discussion of PV and ET can be found in Chapters 13 and 14, respectively.

Chronic Myeloid Leukemia

Pathogenesis and Clinical Manifestations. CML represents approximately 15% of all cases of leukemia in the United States. The average age of onset is between 40 and 50 years, and CML occurs only occasionally in childhood and adolescence.[9] The majority of CML cases are characterized by malignant granulocytes that carry a unique chromosomal abnormality, the Philadelphia chromosome (Ph^+). The Philadelphia chromosome is formed because of a balanced translocation between chromosomes 9 and 22 (Figure 11-4). The translocation causes two genes to be juxtaposed, resulting in a new fusion gene called *bcr/abl.* This mutation is thought to be critical in the development of CML. Molecular studies have revealed that the protein product of the fusion gene is a functional enzyme that spurs cell proliferation and reduces apoptotic cell death. CML is unusual among human cancers because a single oncogene, *(bcr/abl),* is capable of conferring a malignant state.[10] Numerous mutations are necessary for development of most other cancers (see Chapter 7). Following the characterization of the fusion protein, drugs targeted to inhibit its action were developed (e.g., imatinib). The goal of anti-bcr/abl therapy is to reduce the number of leukemic cells with the bcr/abl genotype to undetectable levels. It is not known whether imatinib can cure CML or what duration of treatment is necessary to permanently suppress the leukemic cell population. Some patients with CML have developed drug resistance against imatinib, and research is ongoing. The cells in CML are more mature than those found in AML, as noted by the greater degree of nuclear segmentation (Figure 11-5).

The usual clinical presentation of CML includes a high granulocyte count on the CBC and splenomegaly. Symptoms, when present, may include fatigue, weight loss, sweats, bleeding, and abdominal discomfort from the enlarged spleen.

Prognosis and Treatment. CML does not respond well to chemotherapy. Although most patients will achieve a temporary remission, the overall survival time is poor. In untreated patients the median survival is about 2 years.[11] The only known curative treatment is **allogeneic** bone marrow transplantation from a suitable donor. It is believed that the donor cells detect and kill the host's leukemic cells. Even with a human leukocyte antigen (HLA)–identical sibling donor, the probability of transplant-related mortality is about 25% and the likelihood of long-term disease-free survival is 50% to 60%.[10,11] Transplant-related mortality is about 50% if the HLA-matched donor is unrelated.[10] Bone marrow transplantation with cells harvested from the patient's own blood (autografting) during the early stages of CML may also be done, but it is less effective in curing the disease. For those not able to undergo stem cell transplantation, standard chemotherapy during the chronic phase may be instituted. Chemotherapy may include hydroxyurea, interferon α (IFN-α), cytosine arabinoside (cytarabine, Ara-C), and imatinib. A standard treatment algorithm for CML is shown in Figure 11-6. Once CML has progressed to the blast phase, the prognosis is very poor regardless of treatment, with an expected median survival of 3 to 4 months.

Acute Myeloid Leukemia

Pathogenesis and Clinical Manifestations. AML is primarily a disease of adults, comprising 80% of cases of acute leukemia in this population while accounting for only 20% of the cases of acute leukemia of childhood.[9] The median

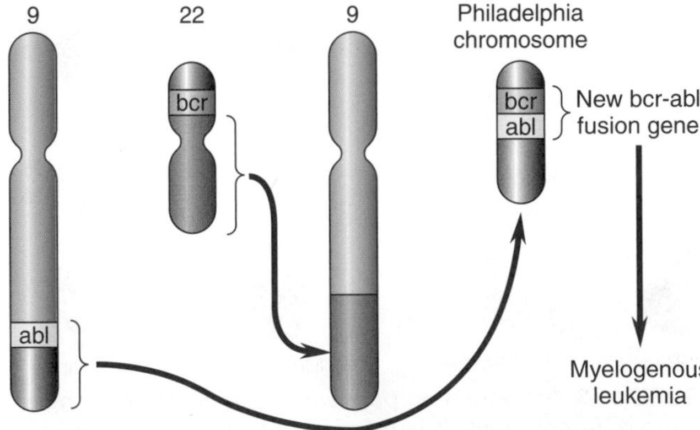

FIGURE 11-4 ■ A balanced translocation between chromosomes 9 and 22 results in the formation of a Philadelphia chromosome. The translocation causes two genes, *abl* and *bcr,* to become juxtaposed, resulting in a fusion gene. This fusion gene, *bcr-abl,* is thought to be essential for the development of chronic myeloid leukemia.

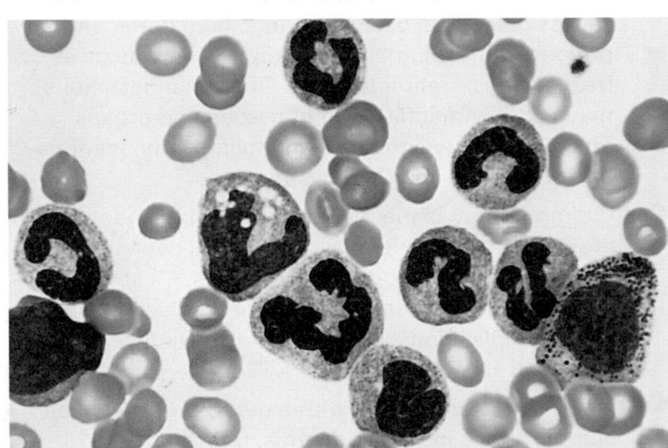

FIGURE 11-5 ■ A peripheral blood smear from a patient with chronic myeloid leukemia (CML). Note that a greater degree of neutrophil segmentation is found in CML than in acute myelogenous leukemia (see Figure 11-7), reflecting a more advanced stage of development. (From Kumar V, Cotran RS, Robbins SL, editors: *Robbins basic pathology,* ed 7, Philadelphia, 2003, Saunders, p 439. Photograph courtesy Dr. Robert W. McKenna, Department of Pathology, University of Texas Southwestern Medical School, Dallas.)

age at presentation is 64 years. Like CML, AML is a malignant disorder associated with transformation of a myeloid stem cell. The bone marrow aspirate must have more than 20% blasts to be classified as AML.[12] AML can present in a variety of ways because of the potential for myeloid stem cells to produce different cell types. Thus, AML has a number of subtypes, which are identified by the stage at which cell development stops (see Figure 11-3). The FAB system for classifying AML as M0 through M7 is in common use (see Table 11-1). Acute granulocytic leukemia is the most common type of disorder, and the term is often used interchangeably with AML. Myeloblastic cells have a large, nonsegmented nucleus and fine chromatin (Figure 11-7). AML is also subtyped according to genetic abnormalities. Worse outcomes are noted with loss of *TP53* or *RB* tumor suppressor gene function. The WHO classification of AML recognizes four common types of genetic abnormalities (see Box 11-1). Most are chromosomal translocations or inversions. If cytogenetic class is not apparent, then AML is classified by morphologic characteristics, including myeloid cell of origin and degree of differentiation or maturation. Correct classification increases the accuracy of prognosis and may influence the choice of treatment.

AML presents in a manner very similar to that of ALL, and the two are difficult to distinguish by clinical findings alone. Acute leukemia causes bone pain, anemia, thrombocytopenia, and increased susceptibility to infection. The onset of symptoms is abrupt, with most patients seeking care within a few weeks of disease onset. The prognosis is much worse for AML than for ALL, with fewer than 50% of children and only about 30% of adults achieving long-term survival.[6,13] An exception is the promyelocytic subtype of AML. Although it accounts for only 10% to 15% of AML cases, acute promyelocytic leukemia (APL) deserves special consideration because it is the most curable of all AML subtypes, with a 70% to 80% 5-year disease-free survival.[6] APL is characterized by a chromosomal translocation between 8 and 21, which forms a fusion gene called *PML/RARα*. The PML/RARα protein binds to a repressor complex in the cell nucleus and inhibits myeloid cell differentiation. RARα is a retinoic acid receptor that can be induced to release its inhibitory hold on differentiation when all-*trans* retinoic acid (ATRA) is administered. Addition of ATRA to the chemotherapy management of patients with APL significantly improves disease-free survival.[6]

Prognosis and Treatment. Treatment protocols for AML are increasingly incorporating the cytogenetic profile of the leukemic cells to individualize therapy and monitor response. Traditionally the management of AML has two phases: remission induction and consolidation/postremission. A CR is attempted in the remission induction phase, with an attempt to eliminate any undetected residual leukemic cells during the consolidation/postremission phase. Patients with AML who are able to complete only one or two cycles of their chemotherapy because of toxicity almost invariably have recurrence of leukemia even when CR was achieved. To induce remission, most protocols use two cycles of a combination of agents (e.g., idarubicin + Ara-C + etoposide, called the ICE protocol; or daunorubicin + Ara-C + 6-thioguanine, called the DAT protocol). Postremission therapy commonly includes high dose Ara-C in younger patients while the elderly require lower dose regimens. Drug treatment is constantly being evaluated and altered to obtain better outcomes. At present patients younger than 60 years have a 4-year survival of 30% to 40%, whereas elderly patients have a 2-year survival of 20%.[6] With the advent of allogeneic stem cell transplantation, the chances for cure may improve; however, procedure-related mortality is 10% to 25%. New therapies using monoclonal antibodies to detect and destroy leukemic cells have been used and show promise for improving outcomes in AML.

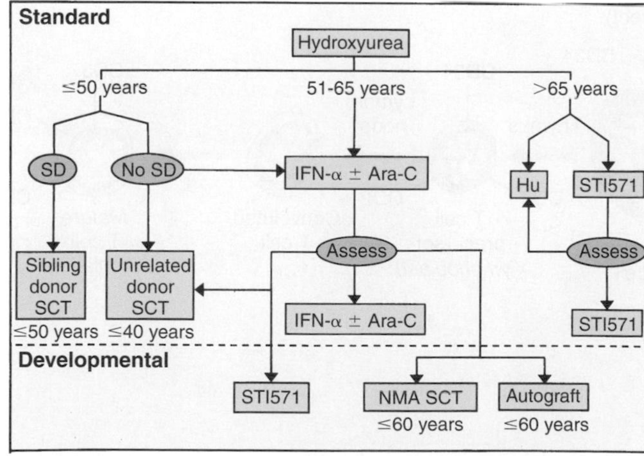

FIGURE 11-6 ■ Treatment algorithm for patients presenting with chronic myeloid leukemia in the chronic stage. *SD,* Sibling donor (HLA identical); *IFN,* interferon; *Ara-C,* cytosine arabinoside (cytarabine); *Hu,* hydroxyurea; *NMA SCT,* nonmyeloablative stem cell transplantation. (From Henderson ES et al, editors: *Leukemia,* ed 7, Philadelphia, 2003, Saunders, p 593.)

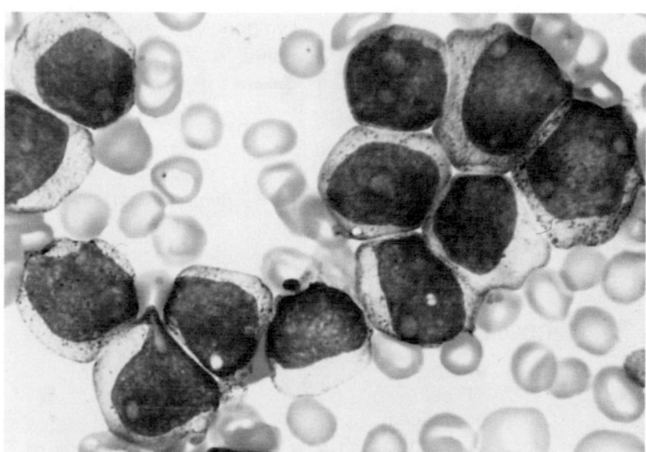

FIGURE 11-7 ■ A peripheral blood smear showing typical cells of acute myelogenous leukemia. (From Kumar V, Cotran RS, Robbins SL, editors: *Robbins basic pathology,* ed 7, Philadelphia, 2003, Saunders, p 424.)

KEY CONCEPTS

- CML is a myeloproliferative disorder that affects adults primarily, has an insidious onset, and responds poorly to chemotherapy. CML is characterized by the presence of a gene translocation (Philadelphia chromosome) that produces a fusion gene called *bcr-abl.* The product of this gene is thought to be responsible for producing the malignancy. This molecular abnormality is the target of new drug therapies to eliminate neoplastic cells. The prognosis of CML remains relatively poor but may be improved with allogeneic bone marrow transplantation in which transplanted cells destroy leukemic cells.
- AML affects adults primarily, has an acute onset, responds fairly well to treatment, and has a prognosis somewhat worse than that of ALL. AML is usually a malignancy of granulocytes, although other myeloid cell types may be affected. Several gene abnormalities have been identified in AML that may indicate better or worse prognosis. The median survival of patients younger than 60 years is 30% to 40% at 4 years.

LYMPHOID NEOPLASMS

The lymphoid neoplasms include malignant transformations of B cells, T cells, and NK cells. When present in blood and bone marrow, lymphoid neoplasms are called leukemias, and when they are localized in lymphoid tissues they are called lymphomas. The location of lymphoid neoplasms is a consequence of the stage of the disease. The WHO classification uses cell type rather than stage to classify the lymphoid neoplasms, resulting in some difficulty with the traditional conceptualization of leukemias and lymphomas. The factors that determine whether a particular neoplastic cell will present as leukemia or as lymphoma are not presently known. Subcategories of the B-cell and T-cell/NK groups are based on the maturity of the neoplastic cells (see Box 11-2). The *precursor cell* neoplasms are characterized by cells that have arrested development in the early blast stage, whereas the *mature cell* neoplasms are more differentiated and often located in peripheral sites (Figure 11-8).

Chronic Lymphoid Leukemia

Pathogenesis and Clinical Manifestations. CLL accounts for about 30% of all cases of leukemia in the United States. In 95% of cases, a malignant B-cell precursor is at fault.[14] Only 5% of cases of CLL are associated with T-cell transformation, but this type is more aggressive.[4] In general, B-cell CLL follows an indolent course, which is usually asymptomatic. Often CLL is found by accident on routine blood count examinations. When CLL becomes symptomatic, patients may experience fatigue, weight loss, and anorexia. Because the leukemic B cells do not produce antibodies normally, an increased susceptibility to certain types of infection may occur. Malignant lymphocytes invade lymphoid tissues and bone marrow, disrupting function. Lymphoid invasion often presents as enlarged, painless lymph nodes (lymphadenopathy) or enlarged spleen. Bone marrow infiltration reduces the production of normal blood components. A typical

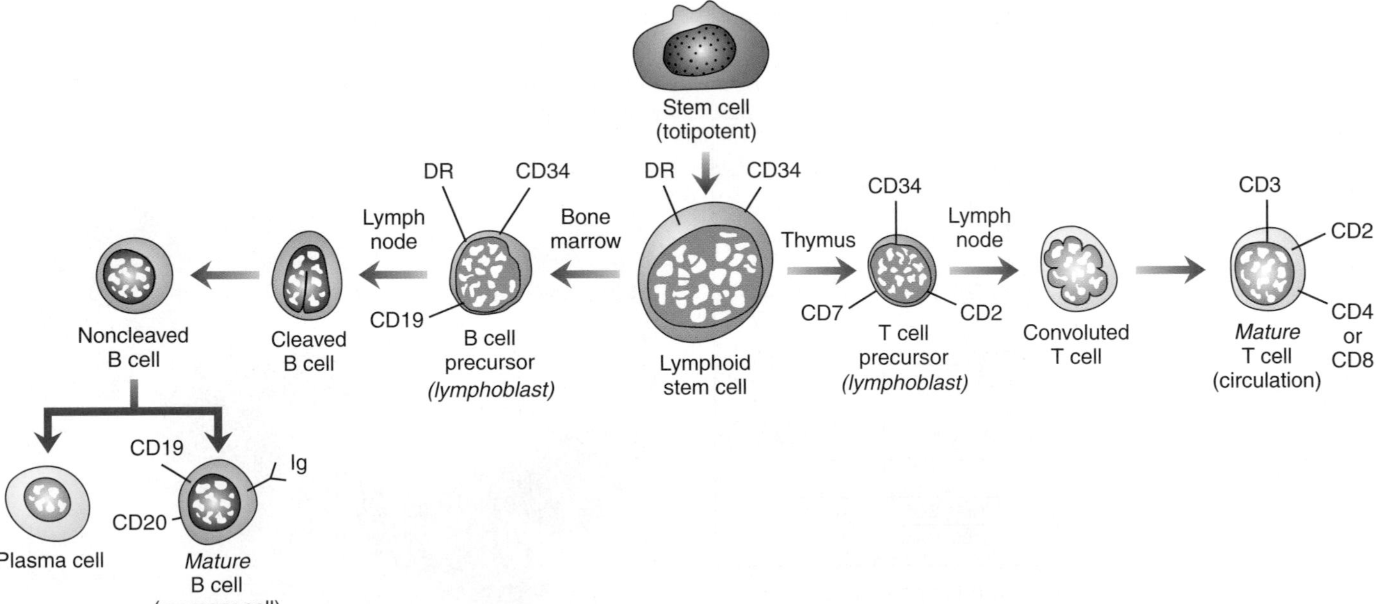

FIGURE 11-8 ■ Maturation pathways of T and B lymphocytes showing the stages at which lymphocyte development is typically arrested in leukemia. Different markers are present on the surface of B cells and T cells at progressive stages of development, which are helpful in identifying the neoplastic cell type and maturity.

slide of a bone marrow aspirate from a patient with CLL is shown in Figure 11-9. Note the preponderance of lymphoid cells. CLL cells are characterized by defective apoptosis and live longer than they should. They are derived from mature peripheral B cells.

Prognosis and Treatment. Certain genetic lesions confer better or worse prognosis. A mutation in the variable region of the immunoglobulin gene (IgV) is associated with a median survival of 24 years or more, whereas those who lack the IgV gene mutation have a median survival of less than 8 years.[15] CLL cell types demonstrating short telomere lengths and TP53 dysfunction have poor outcomes. Since the average age of patients with CLL is about 65 to 70 years, those with indolent disease may not be treated; they are more likely to die of another disorder rather than CLL. Patients with cell types likely to progress rapidly may receive therapy (e.g., rituximab) to induce remission. Those without complete response may consider stem cell transplantation to prolong the duration of remission.

Acute Lymphoblastic Leukemia/Lymphoma

Pathogenesis and Clinical Manifestations. ALL is a malignant disorder of the lymphoid cell lineage. The great majority of cases are the result of malignant transformation of B cells (80%), with the remainder involving T cells.[16] The abnormal cells resemble immature lymphocytes, called *lymphoblasts* (Figure 11-10). Most lymphoblastic neoplasms present as leukemias, but lymphoblastic lymphomas are thought to be the same disease at a different stage. B-cell leukemias are categorized into cytogenetic groups based on common chromosomal translocations. One of these transformations results in the *bcr/abl* fusion gene discussed previously in the context of CML. Three other types of translocations also form fusion genes that produce abnormal signaling components. These gene derangements have different prognoses and may respond differently to alternative treatment protocols.

Lymphoblasts do not mature and accumulate in large numbers in the blood and bone marrow. At least 20% of the bone marrow cells must be leukemic lymphoblasts to meet the diagnostic criteria for ALL.[16] Accumulation of leukemic cells in the bone marrow crowds out the production of normal red blood cells, platelets, and leukocytes. Circulating blasts are poorly functioning cells and do not provide effective immunocompetence.

ALL is primarily a disorder of children. It is the most common malignancy and the second leading cause of death in this population.[9] The peak incidence occurs between the ages of 3 and 7 years. A second rise in incidence occurs in middle age. The onset of symptoms is abrupt, with complaints of bone pain, bruising, fever, and infection being common. Children may refuse to walk and their parents may report loss of appetite, fatigue, and abdominal pain. The spleen, liver, and lymph nodes may be enlarged from leukemic infiltration. A small number of children (3%) may present with CNS signs from leukemic infiltration of brain tissues.[17]

Prognosis and Treatment. ALL is highly curable in the pediatric population, but less so in adults. The 5-year survival rate is 85% in children and 30% to 50% in adults.[17] Certain forms of ALL are more responsive to therapy. For example, children with pre–B-cell type have a 90% cure rate, whereas those with mature B-cell or immature T-cell leukemia have a poorer prognosis.

Chemotherapy for ALL remission induction includes cyclical administration of drug combinations, usually including vincristine, prednisolone, and an anthracycline (see Box 11-4).[18] Postremission chemotherapy with or without stem cell transplantation is indicated for most patients. In general,

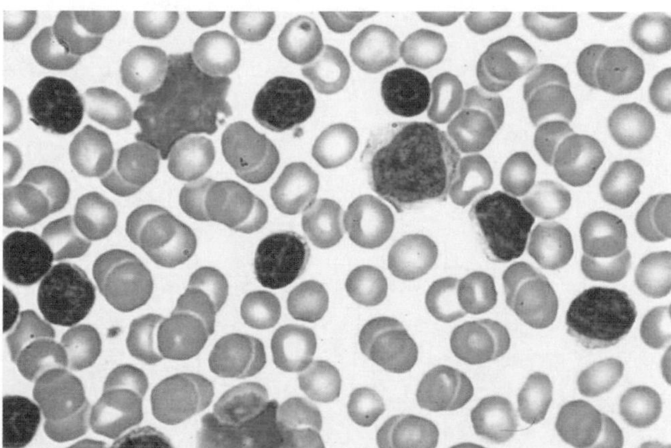

FIGURE 11-9 ■ Bone marrow aspirate showing small lymphocytes with condensed nuclear chromatin typical of chronic lymphocytic leukemia, B-cell type. (From Henderson ES et al, editors: *Leukemia,* ed 7, Philadelphia, 2003, Saunders, color plate 11-28.)

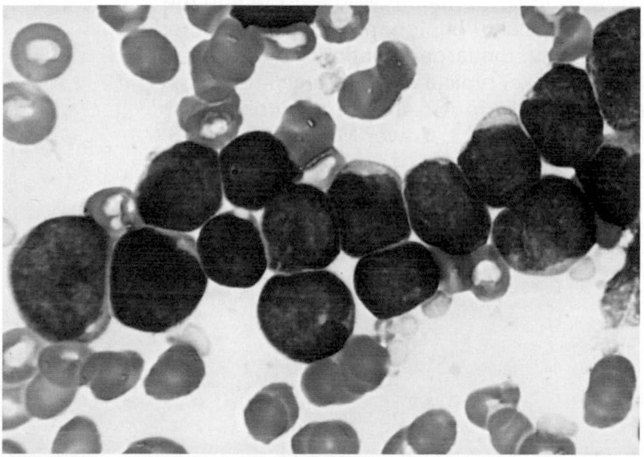

FIGURE 11-10 ■ Peripheral blood smear showing typical cells of acute lymphocytic leukemia. (From Kumar V, Cotran RS, Robbins SL, editors: *Robbins basic pathology,* ed 7, Philadelphia, 2003, Saunders, p 424.)

adults with ALL require more intense therapy than children to achieve CR. Monoclonal antibodies may be used in patients whose tumors express specific antigens (e.g., anti-CD18 and anti-CD20 antibodies).

Hairy Cell Leukemia

Pathogenesis and Clinical Manifestations. Hairy cell leukemia is a rare, chronic type of leukemia of unknown cause. The disease represents about 2% of adult leukemias, but it is of interest because of its highly treatable nature. The median age at presentation is about 55 years and there is a 5-to-1 predominance of males.[19] Hairy cell leukemia has a B-cell phenotype and is characterized by the presence of peculiar cells with hair-like projections on their surface (Figure 11-11). At diagnosis, patients have hairy cells in the peripheral blood as well as reduced numbers of granulocytes, platelets, and red blood cells. Splenomegaly is a common finding, being present in 90% of patients.

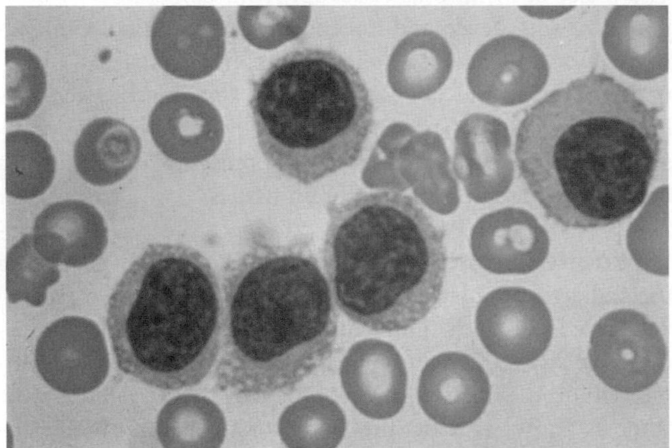

FIGURE 11-11 ■ Peripheral blood smear showing cells typical of hairy cell leukemia. (From Henderson ES et al, editors: *Leukemia,* ed 7, Philadelphia, 2003, Saunders, color plate 11-29.)

Prognosis and Treatment. Treatment may be instituted when a patient becomes symptomatic with an enlarged spleen, recurrent infection, bleeding disorder, or anemia. The treatment of choice is the purine analog 2-chlorodeoxyadenosine [2-CdA]) daily for 5 to 7 days, which produces CR rates of 80%.[20]

Plasma Cell Myeloma (Multiple Myeloma)

Pathogenesis and Clinical Manifestations. Plasma cell myeloma, also known as multiple myeloma, is a malignant disorder of mature, antibody-secreting B lymphocytes, called *plasma cells.* Malignant plasma cells have a predilection to invade bone and form multiple tumor sites. Other tissues may be targeted also, including lymph nodes, liver, spleen, and kidneys. Plasma cell myeloma occurs exclusively in the adult population, usually affecting individuals older than 40 years, with a median age at presentation of 65 years.[20] Men are affected more often than women.

As with other forms of neoplasia, the exact etiologic process of plasma cell myeloma is unknown, but abnormalities in chromosome structure and number are commonly found.[21] The malignant plasma cells all belong to a single clone, and the antibodies they produce are identical monoclonal antibodies. Excessive production of antibodies results in accumulation in the blood stream, which can be detected by serum protein electrophoresis. Normally, serum antibod-

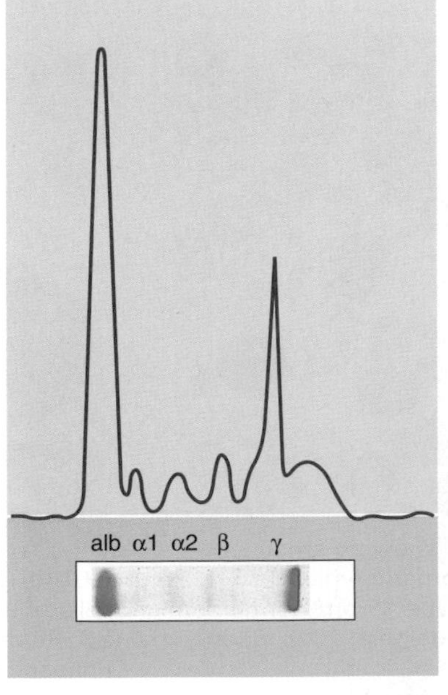

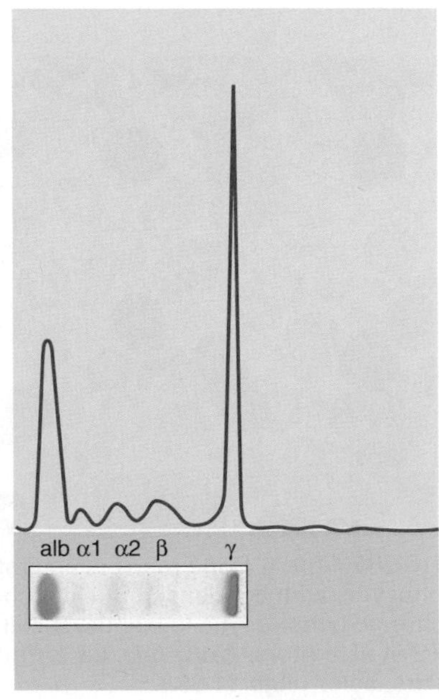

FIGURE 11-12 ■ Serum protein electrophoresis comparing abnormal myeloma protein in the γ region typical of benign monoclonal gammopathy **(A)** with the large quantity of monoclonal antibody (spike) typical of plasma cell myeloma **(B).** (From Skarin AT: *Atlas of diagnostic oncology,* London, 2003, Gower Medical, pp 536-537.)

ies are of many forms (polyclonal) and show a varied distribution of size on the electrophoresis test. In plasma cell myeloma, there is a large amount of one type of antibody, which forms a characteristic spike on the gel (Figure 11-12). Excessive production of light-chain antibody fragments by malignant plasma cells results in their accumulation in blood and urine. When found in urine, these light-chain fragments are called **Bence Jones protein.** In addition to helping to confirm the diagnosis, Bence Jones protein is important to the pathogenesis of plasma cell myeloma because it can cause kidney damage. Malignant plasma cells tend to accumulate in bone where they enhance osteoclastic activity and produce bone lesions.[21] Pathologic fractures, especially compression fractures of the vertebral column, are common. Bone destruction releases calcium into the blood stream, with resultant hypercalcemia.

Most of the clinical manifestations of multiple myeloma are due to bone and renal damage. The diagnosis of plasma cell myeloma is suspected based on the monoclonal antibody peak, the presence of Bence Jones protein, hypercalcemia, and evidence of bone lesions. The diagnosis is confirmed by bone marrow biopsy. Normally, the plasma cell component of the marrow comprises about 5%. In multiple myeloma, plasma cells may occupy 30% to 95% of the bone marrow (Figure 11-13). A minimum of at least 10% to 15% bone marrow plasma cells is necessary for the diagnosis of plasma cell myeloma.[21] The likelihood of bone marrow dysfunction increases as the plasma cell component increases. Normal production of erythrocytes, platelets, and leukocytes can be impaired to varying degrees.

The onset of plasma cell myeloma is generally slow and insidious. A premalignant stage of plasma cell myeloma is apparent in some individuals who have excess production of monoclonal antibodies but no evidence of bone lesions or Bence Jones protein in the urine. This stage is called monoclonal gammopathy of undetermined significance (MGUS). Approximately 25% of patients with MGUS progress to malignant disease.[16] In most affected individuals the disease remains asymptomatic until it is fairly advanced. The asymptomatic stage often lasts for many years after malignant transformation. During this time the only complaint may be that of frequent infections. Diagnosis during the asymptomatic phase is usually made because of the presence of protein in the urine or high serum calcium levels on routine examination. Bone pain usually heralds the onset of the symptomatic phase. Sometimes the evaluation of a fracture or back pain leads to the identification of suggestive lesions in a skeletal structure. Anemia, recurrent infections, and bleeding tendencies suggest the complication of bone marrow depression.

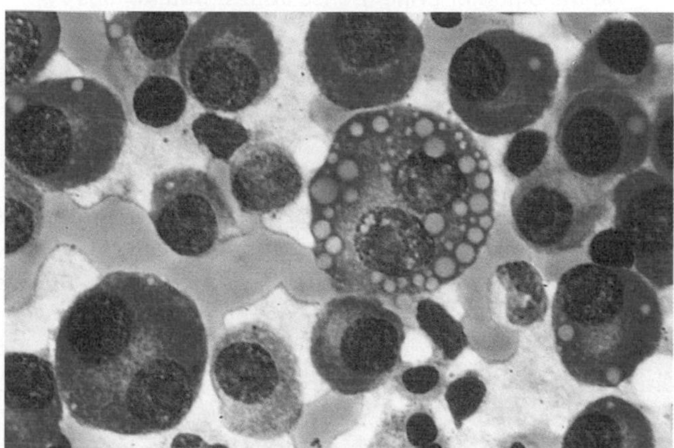

FIGURE 11-13 ■ A bone marrow aspirate from a patient with multiple myeloma showing a large number of abnormal plasma cells with multiple nuclei and cytoplasmic droplets. (From Kumar V, Cotran RS, Robbins SL, editors: *Robbins basic pathology,* ed 7, Philadelphia, 2003, Saunders, p 430.)

Renal insufficiency is a complication experienced by approximately 50% of patients with plasma cell myeloma.[21] Impairment of renal function is due to a combination of factors, including hyperproteinemia, Bence Jones protein, hypercalcemia, and hyperuricemia. Impaired function may initially present as excessive urination and frequent nocturnal urination. As the glomerular filtration rate falls, the serum creatinine and blood urea nitrogen levels may be increased, and the quantity of urine output may fall.

Bone involvement is a consistent feature of plasma cell myeloma. Radiologic studies of ribs, spine, skull, and pelvis show a characteristic "honeycomb" appearance, due to lucid areas of demineralized bone (Figure 11-14). Minimal trauma is likely to result in fractures. Sometimes fractures occur with no known trauma; these are called *pathologic* fractures.

Prognosis and Treatment. Antineoplastic agents may be used to induce and maintain a remission in plasma cell proliferation. The best chemotherapy regimen has not yet been determined. The combination of vincristine, Adriamycin (doxorubicin), and dexamethasone (VAD) is commonly used. The remission induction rate with these agents is about 60%, with a median survival of about 3 years after initiation of therapy.[21] High-dose chemotherapy followed by allogenic bone marrow transplantation is becoming more common and offers a better CR rate. However, the mortality rate associated with transplantation is high (approximately 40% to 50%).[16] Autologous stem cell transplantation is considered to be the optimal initial therapy for most patients. Thalidomide and its derivatives have shown promising results in some studies.

Pharmacologic management of renal dysfunction is often employed. Diuretics to increase renal blood and urine flow may be helpful in flushing harmful substances. Diuretics may also be employed to reduce hypercalcemia by increasing renal excretion. During chemotherapy, when rapid cell lysis is expected, drugs to enhance excretion of byproducts, such as

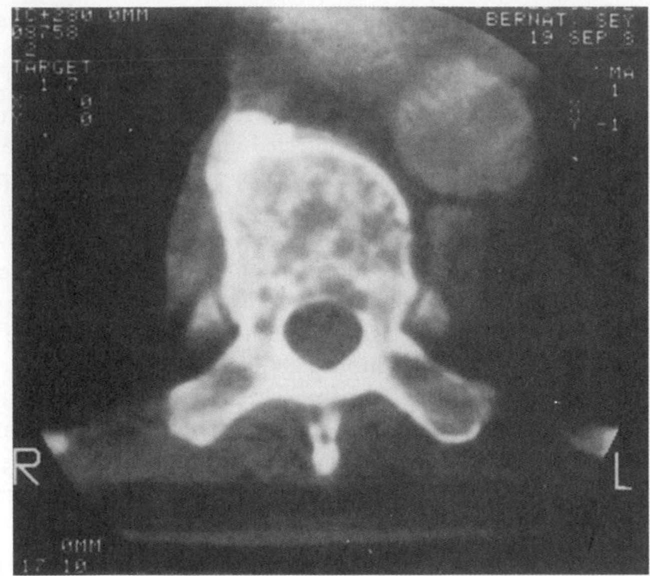
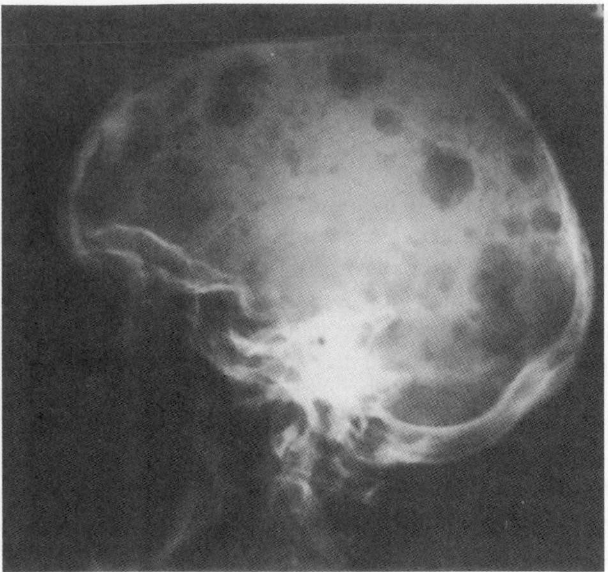

FIGURE 11-14 ■ Vertebral body **(A)** and skull **(B)** radiographs showing the characteristic "honeycomb" appearance of demineralized bone associated with multiple myeloma. (Courtesy Marvin J. Stone, MD, Sammons Cancer Center, Baylor University Medical Center, Dallas.)

uric acid, may be used. Allopurinol, a drug also used for gouty arthritis, is helpful in preventing uric acid **nephropathy** due to the high uric acid load. Acute renal failure can be precipitated in the plasma cell myeloma patient if dehydration occurs. Careful monitoring and management of fluid intake is essential, especially when patients are receiving diuretic therapy.

Chronic bone pain is a common problem in the myeloma patient that may require use of multiple remedies. Narcotic and nonnarcotic pain relievers are often necessary. Localized application of radiation to bone lesions may reduce bone pain in some cases.

KEY CONCEPTS

- CLL is a neoplastic transformation of a mature, peripheral B cell that affects adults primarily and has an insidious onset. CLL is usually asymptomatic. Disease in certain genotypes is associated with long survival times and does not require therapy; in other cases, disease is progressive and may be managed with stem cell transplantation or administration of monoclonal antibodies.
- ALL affects children primarily, has an acute onset, responds well to therapy, and has a good prognosis. ALL is associated with transformation of precursor "blasts" in the bone marrow. ALL often manifests with bone pain, infections, and a tendency to bleeding. A significant number of children with ALL have CNS involvement and intrathecal chemotherapy is necessary.
- Plasma cell myeloma is due to malignant transformation of antibody-secreting B lymphocytes. It primarily affects older adults. The onset of symptoms is insidious, with most patients experiencing a 4- to 10-year period of clinical latency. Some patients have a preneoplastic phase called monoclonal gammopathy of undetermined significance. When present, symptoms include bone pain, pathologic fractures, anemia, thrombocytopenia, leukopenia, and renal insufficiency. Malignant plasma cells all secrete the same monoclonal antibody, and detection of this antibody in the blood or urine (Bence Jones protein) aids in diagnosis.

Hodgkin Disease

Hodgkin disease represents about 30% of all cases of malignant lymphoma, accounting for approximately 7000 new cases annually in the United States.[9] It occurs across the age continuum, with half of cases occurring in persons between the ages of 20 and 40 years. The overall incidence of Hodgkin disease is higher in males, and it carries a worse prognosis in males. The overall 5-year survival rate for treated Hodgkin disease, including all stages, is about 85%.[9]

Pathogenesis and Clinical Manifestations. Hodgkin disease is a malignant disorder of the lymph nodes characterized by the presence of **Reed-Sternberg** cells on histologic examination. Reed-Sternberg cells originate from B cells in the germinal centers of lymph nodes.[22] Reed-Sternberg

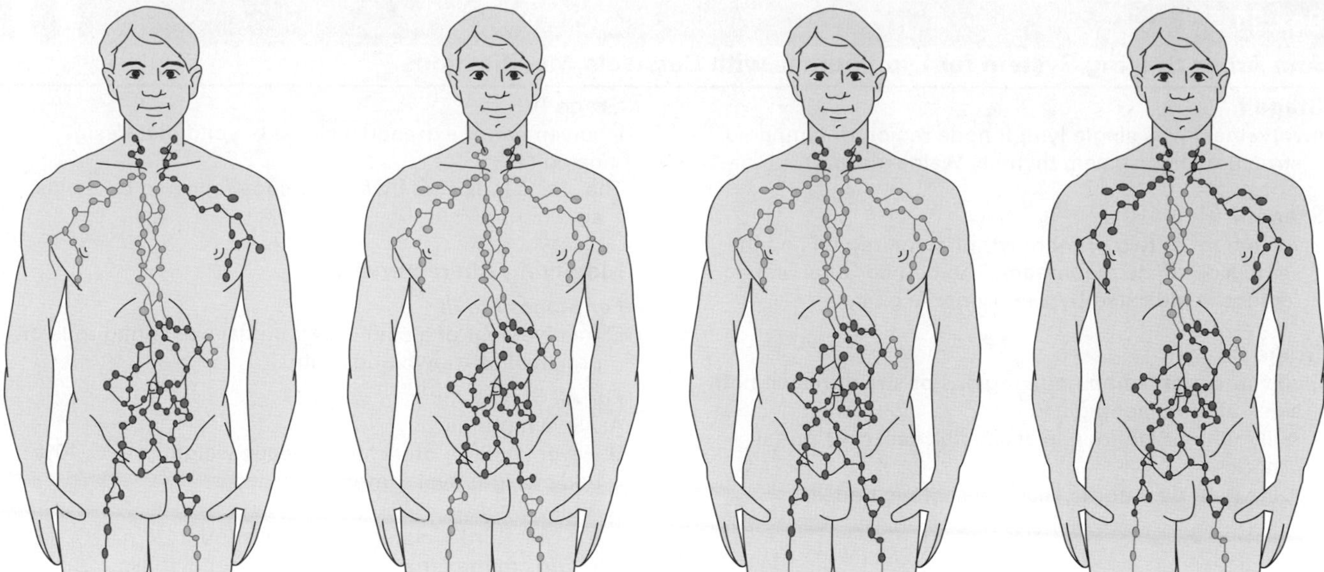

FIGURE 11-15 ■ Schematic drawing showing the orderly, contiguous, and predictable spread of Hodgkin disease. (Redrawn and modified from Rosenberg SA: Hodgkin disease: no stage beyond cure, *Hosp Pract* 21[8]:97, 1986. After original illustrations by Bunji Tagawa.)

cells are malignant, but they tend to grow and spread in a very predictable manner. This predictability sets Hodgkin disease apart from other types of lymphoma. Hodgkin disease usually metastasizes along contiguous lymphatic pathways (Figure 11-15). Epstein-Barr virus is frequently found in the genome of transformed Reed-Sternberg cells and is thought to be important in the pathogenesis of Hodgkin disease. The malignant cells are clonal, originating from a single mutant precursor cell, and usually present in a single node or localized chain of nodes. In addition to malignant Reed-Sternberg cells, inflammatory cells accumulate within the node (Figure 11-16). Neoplastic Reed-Sternberg cells constitute only a small minority (2%) of the cells in the lymph node tumor.[22]

There are two types of Hodgkin disease: (1) the rare lymphocyte predominance type, which accounts for 5% of cases, and (2) the classical type (cHD) representing the other 95%. The classical type can be divided further into four subtypes according to the relative number of reactive cells in the tumor. The histologic pattern does not seem to predict the prognosis, and the stage of Hodgkin disease is more relevant than the histologic features.[22]

Clinical manifestations of Hodgkin disease are dependent on the site of origin as well as on the stage of dissemination. Lymphomas often are asymptomatic in the early stages. The usual clinical presentation includes painless lymph node enlargement that may be accompanied by fever, night sweats, pruritus, weight loss, and malaise. Usually lymph node enlargement occurs in nodes above the diaphragm, the cervical nodes being the most common site. Other supradiaphragmatic nodes are the supraclavicular, axillary, and mediastinal nodes. Less commonly, nodes below the diaphragm are the primary site. The inguinal nodes are the most common subdiaphragmatic site. As the disease spreads from the site of origin, other lymph nodes and organs may become involved, including the spleen and bone marrow. Staging procedures are performed to determine the extent of metastasis at the time of diagnosis. Staging dictates the treatment modality best suited to provide the patient with the greatest chance for long-term survival.

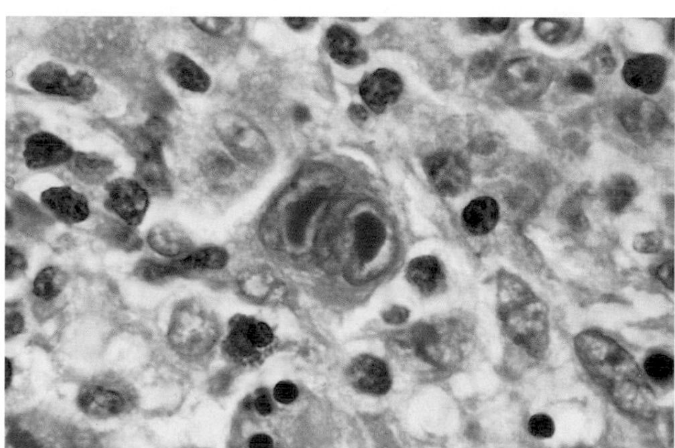

FIGURE 11-16 ■ Histologic sample showing the typical binucleate Reed-Sternberg cells found in Hodgkin disease. An eosinophil can be seen below the Reed-Sternberg cell. (From Kumar V, Cotran RS, Robbins SL, editors: *Robbins basic pathology,* ed 7, Philadelphia, 2003, Saunders, p 432. Courtesy Dr. Robert W. McKenna, Department of Pathology, University of Texas Southwestern Medical School, Dallas.)

Prognosis and Treatment. The staging protocol commonly used today was first adopted in 1971 at the Ann

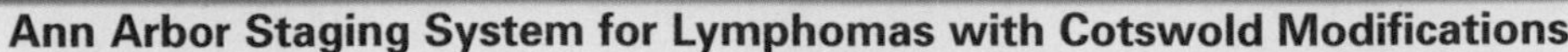

Box 11-5

Ann Arbor Staging System for Lymphomas with Cotswold Modifications

Stage I

Involvement of a single lymph node region or lymphoid structure (e.g., spleen, thymus, Waldeyer ring)

Stage II

Involvement of two or more lymph node regions on the same side of the diaphragm. The number of anatomic regions is indicated by a subscript (e.g., II_3)

Stage III

Involvement of lymph node regions or structures on both sides of the diaphragm

- III_1: with or without splenic, hilar, celiac, or portal nodes
- III_2: with para-aortic, iliac, mesenteric nodes

Stage IV

Involvement of extranodal site(s) beyond that designated "E"

The site is indicated by a letter code followed by a plus sign (+)

Modifying Characteristics

For Stages I to III

E: Involvement of a single, extranodal site contiguous or proximal to known nodal site

For All Stages

A: No symptoms

B: Fever (>38(C), drenching sweats, weight loss (>10% body weight over 6 months)

X: Bulky disease

- >One third widening of mediastinum
- >10 cm maximal dimension of nodal mass

CS: Clinical stage is based on history, physical examination, laboratory studies, CT scans.

PS: Pathologic stage is based on tissue sampling obtained through invasive procedures such as laparotomy and biopsy.

Site notations: *N,* nodes; *H,* liver; *L,* lung; *M,* bone matter; *S,* spleen; *P,* pleura; *O,* bone; *D,* skin.

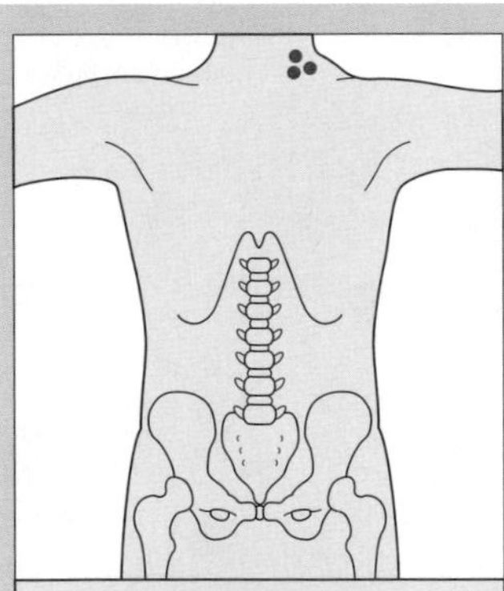

Stage I

- Involvement of single lymph node region
  or
- Involvement of single extralymphatic site (stage I_E)

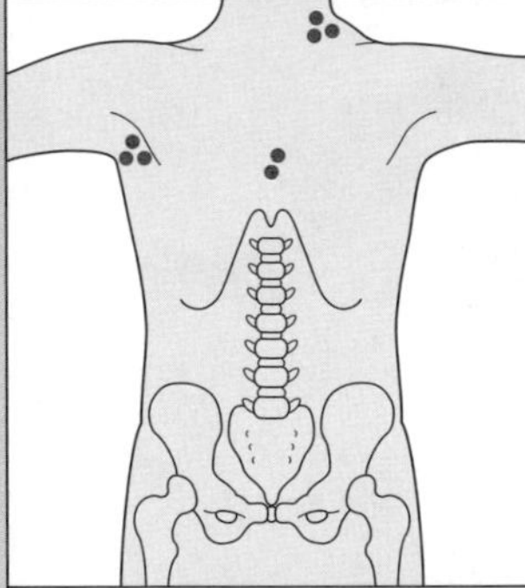

Stage II

- Involvement of ≥2 lymph node regions on same side of diaphragm
- May include localized extralymphatic involvement on same side of diaphragm (stage II_E)

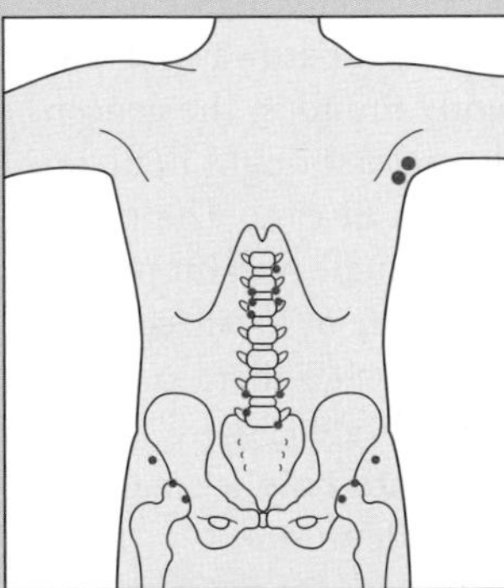

Stage III

- Involvement of lymph node regions on both sides of diaphragm
- May include involvement of spleen (stage III_S) or localized extranodal disease (stage III_E) or both (III_{E+S})

For Hodgkin disease:

III_1
- Disease limited to upper abdomen—spleen, splenic hilar, celiac, or porta hepatic nodes

III_2
- Disease limited to lower abdomen—periaortic, pelvic, or inguinal nodes

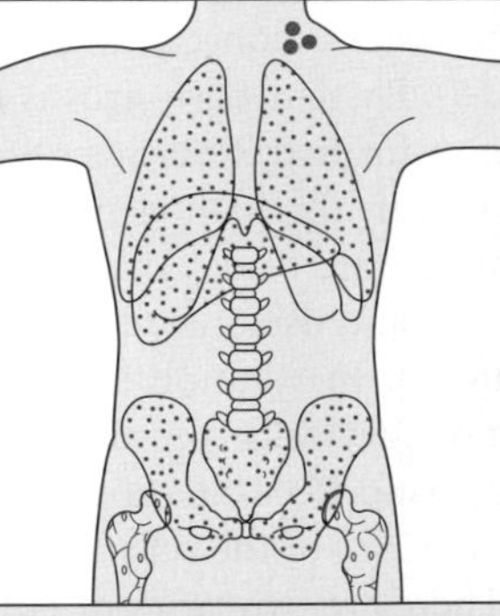

Stage IV

- Disseminated (multifocal) extralymphatic disease involving one or more organs (e.g., liver, bone marrow, lung, skin), with or without associated lymph node involvement
  or
- Isolated extralymphatic disease with distant (nonregional) lymph node involvement

NOTE: Stage designation "B" indicates unexplained weight loss >10% of body weight in preceding 6 months and/or fevers of >38°C and/or night sweats. Stage designation "A" indicates the absence of the features characterizing "B."

FIGURE 11-17 ■ Depiction of the locations of malignant cells in the various stages of lymphoma using the Ann Arbor staging system. (From Skarin AT: *Atlas of diagnostic oncology,* London, 2003, Gower Medical, p 479.)

Box 11-6

Recommended Procedures for Proper Staging

- Adequate surgical biopsy reviewed by an experienced hemopathologist; in primary extranodal lymphomas, biopsy should also include a lymph node when palpable
- Detailed history with special attention to the presence or absence of systemic symptoms
- Careful physical examination, emphasizing node chains, size of liver and spleen, Waldeyer's ring inspection, and bony tenderness
- Routine laboratory tests: complete blood count, erythrocyte sedimentation rate, liver function tests, serum uric acid, serum lactate dehydrogenase
- Chest radiograph (posteroanterior and left lateral) with measurement of mediastinal mass/thorax ratio
- Bipedal lymphangiography in selected cases if adequately trained radiologists are available
- Chest and abdominal CT (or MRI) scan, and abdominal ultrasound
- Radioisotopic evaluation with ^{67}gallium, especially if mediastinum is involved
- Core needle biopsy of bone marrow from unilateral posterior iliac crest
- Cytologic examination of any effusion
- ^{18}Fluorodeoxyglucose positron emission tomography in suspicious cases
- Any further study when suggested by clinical symptoms or sign (e.g., bone scan)

From Wiernik PH et al, editors: *Neoplastic diseases of the blood,* ed 4, New York, 2003, Cambridge University Press.

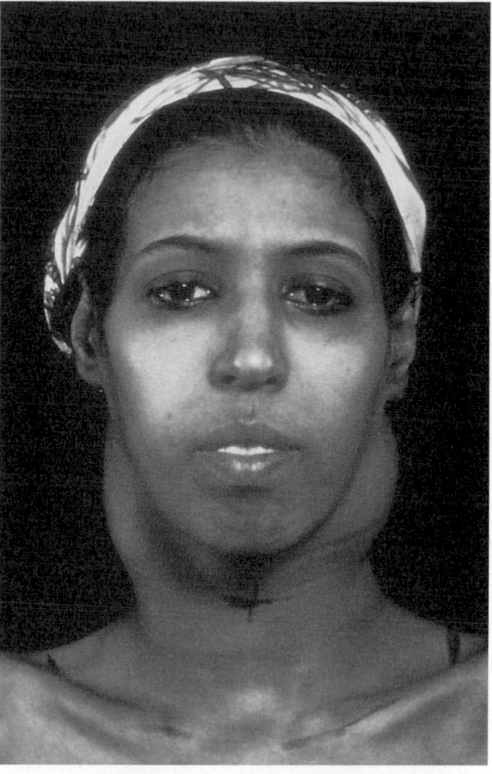

FIGURE 11-18 ■ Hodgkin disease (stage IIA). Marked enlargement of cervical lymph nodes is present in this patient. It is usually painless and may be confined to only one area or may affect two or more areas. (From Skarin AT: *Atlas of diagnostic oncology,* London, 2003, Gower Medical, p 482.)

Arbor symposium on staging in Hodgkin disease and modified in 1989 at the Cotswold meeting (Box 11-5).[23,24] The same procedure is also used for staging non-Hodgkin lymphomas. This protocol uses the presence or absence of certain clinical symptoms as well as the locations of affected nodes to determine the clinical stage of disease. The four stages are shown in Figure 11-17. The letter A denotes the absence of clinical symptoms, whereas the letter B is used when symptoms are present at the time of staging. These symptoms include loss of more than 10% of body weight, unexplained fevers, and night sweats. The clinical stage (CS) is based on history, physical examination, and noninvasive procedures such as computed tomography (CT) scanning. The pathologic stage (PS) is determined by the results of invasive procedures such as laparotomy and tissue biopsy. Clinical and pathologic staging procedures are summarized in Box 11-6. The staging workup determines the locations of tumors in the body, thereby identifying the extent of spread (Figure 11-18). The stage dictates the treatment modalities used. In general, localized tumors are more amenable to application of radiation therapy, whereas disseminated disease responds better to systemic chemotherapeutic agents. Since Hodgkin disease often is detected while localized, radiation therapy is commonly used, with good results.

Patients with nonbulky, stage IA or IIA disease may be candidates for radiation as sole therapy. However, a relatively high rate of relapse has been noted, and combined chemotherapy with limited field radiation is often used.[22] For those patients receiving radiation therapy a determination of appropriate radiation field and dosing is important to maximize tumor kill while preventing radiation damage and excessive destruction of normal cells. Careful shielding procedures are used to limit the field of radiation (Figure 11-19). Patients with bulky disease, "B" symptoms, or stage III and IV disease require chemotherapy with or without radiation. Favorable stage disease is usually treated with 2 to 4 cycles of ABVD (Adriamycin [doxorubicin], bleomycin, vinblastine, and dacarbazine) followed by radiation to the involved lymph nodes.[25] In early stage disease this protocol produces a 90% 10-year disease-free survival. The ABVD protocol is preferred over the original MOPP regimen because there is less gonadal toxicity and reduced sterility.[25] The MOPP regimen includes the drugs mechlorethamine (Mustargen), Oncovin (vincristine), procarbazine, and prednisone. The CR rate with the MOPP regimen is about 80%. Some common chemotherapeutic combinations are shown in Table 11-2. More aggressive chemotherapy is indicated for patients with advanced Hodgkin disease (Table 11-3). Radiation and chemotherapy are associated with a

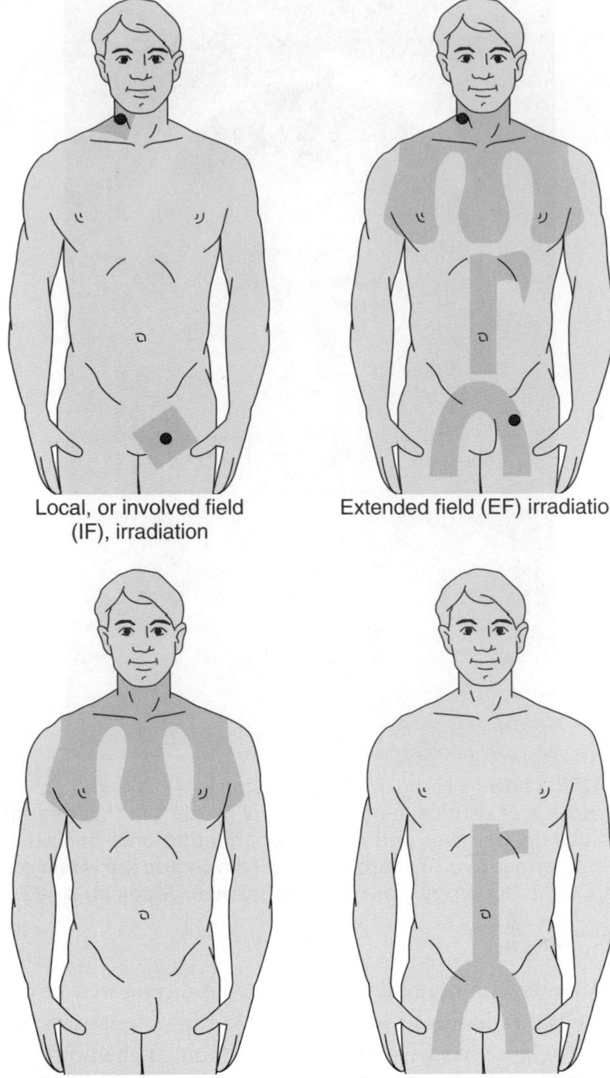

FIGURE 11-19 ■ Typical radiation fields for lymphoma. Different fields of radiation may be used depending on the location of disease.

Table 11-2

Combination Chemotherapy Regimens for Hodgkin Disease

Drug	Dose (mg/m²)	Route	Days
MOPP			
Mechlorethamine	6	IV	1, 8
Oncovin (vincristine)	1.4	IV	1, 8
Procarbazine	100	PO	1-14
Prednisone	40	PO	1-14
ABVD			
Adriamycin (doxorubicin)	25	IV	1, 15
Bleomycin	10	IV	1, 15
Vinblastine	6	IV	1, 15
Dacarbazine	375	IV	1, 15
ChlVPP			
Chlorambucil	6	PO	1-14
Vinblastine	6	IV	1, 8
Procarbazine	100	PO	1-14
Prednisone	40	PO	1-14
MOPP/ABVD			
Alternating months of MOPP and ABVD			
MOPP/ABV Hybrid			
Mechlorethamine	6	IV	1
Oncovin (vincristine)	1.4	IV	1
Procarbazine	100	PO	1-7
Prednisone	40	PO	1-14
Adriamycin (doxorubicin)	35	IV	8
Bleomycin	10	IV	8
Vinblastine	6	IV	8

Adapted from Dipiro JT et al, editors: *Pharmacotherapy: a pathophysiologic approach,* ed 5, New York, 2002, McGraw-Hill, p 2339.

number of side effects including bone marrow depression, with resultant immunosuppression, anemia, and bleeding. Heart failure may be a late consequence in patients receiving radiation to the mediastinum.

B-Cell, T-Cell, and NK-Cell Lymphoma (Non-Hodgkin)

The malignancies included in the classification of non-Hodgkin lymphoma are the malignant lymphomas that do not have the characteristic Reed-Sternberg cells of Hodgkin disease. The majority of cases of non-Hodgkin lymphoma arise from lymph nodes, but they can originate in any lymphoid tissue. With the exception of a few subtypes, most cases of non-Hodgkin lymphoma occur in older adults (95%), and males are at a slightly higher risk than females. The incidence of non-Hodgkin lymphoma is on the rise, particularly in areas with large AIDS populations. More than 50,000 new cases of non-Hodgkin lymphoma are diagnosed annually in the United States.[9] The lifetime risk of developing a non-Hodgkin lymphoma is about 1 in 50.

Most cases of Non-Hodgkin lymphoma arise from B cells, T cells, or NK cells. Some of the more common types of non-Hodgkin lymphoma are summarized in Table 11-4. The prognosis and recommended treatment protocols vary according to type. A general schema for grouping non-Hodgkin lymphoma according to indolent or aggressive types is in common usage.[26] Generally, indolent disease is associated with longer survival times whereas aggressive lymphomas tend to be disseminated at presentation and carry a generally poorer prognosis. As a group, the non-Hodgkin types of lymphoma are more likely to spread early and unpredictably in comparison with Hodgkin disease.

Table 11-3

General Treatment Recommendations for Hodgkin Disease*,†

Early stage disease	
Favorable prognosis (CS I or II with no risk factors)	Extended field radiation or 4-6 cycles of ABVD or EBVP plus involved field radiation
Unfavorable prognosis (CS I or II with risk factors)	4-6 cycles of ABVD or MOPP/ABV plus involved field radiation
Advanced stage disease (CS III or IV)	6-8 cycles of ABVD, or MOPP/ABV, or ChlVPP, or MOPP plus radiation to residual lymphoma or sites of bulky disease
Relapsed disease	
Relapse after radiation	6-8 cycles of chemotherapy with or without radiation (treat as if this were primary advanced disease)
Relapse after primary chemotherapy‡,§	Salvage chemotherapy at conventional doses or high-dose chemotherapy and autologous hematopoietic stem cell transplantation

From Dipiro JT et al: *Pharmacotherapy: a pathophysiologic approach,* ed 5, New York, 2002, McGraw-Hill, p 2339.
CS, Clinical stage.
*Patients should be considered for clinical trials when possible.
†In general, patients with large mediastinal adenopathy should be treated with chemotherapy followed by radiation to the mediastinum.
‡A standard regimen or approach does not exist.
§Highly selected patients may be treated with radiation alone.

Pathogenesis and Clinical Manifestations. The etiologic process of non-Hodgkin lymphoma is unknown, but it is thought to be similar to that of other malignant transformations. The tumor cells are all derived from a single mutant precursor cell and are clonal. Viruses are suspected in the development of some types of lymphoma. In particular, Burkitt lymphoma is strongly associated with the presence of Epstein-Barr virus.[2] Adult T-cell lymphomas are associated with infection by human T-cell leukemia virus, type 1 (HTLV-1).[2] The overall 5-year survival rate for all types of non-Hodgkin lymphomas combined is about 50%.[9]

Most patients with non-Hodgkin lymphoma present with advanced disease (stage III or IV). Clinical manifestations may include painless lymphadenopathy, fever, night sweats, weight loss, malaise, and pruritus (similar to Hodgkin disease). A comparison of the features of Hodgkin disease and non-Hodgkin lymphoma is shown in Table 11-5. Extranodal involvement occurs early in the course of non-Hodgkin lymphoma, and patients may present with infiltrative disease of the skin, gastrointestinal tract, bone, or bone marrow. Complications occur more frequently in non-Hodgkin lymphoma than in Hodgkin disease. Two of the most serious oncology emergencies are obstruction of the superior vena cava and spinal cord compression. Infection, bone metastasis, and joint effusions are also common. Staging of non-Hodgkin lymphoma is done in the same way as for Hodgkin disease, and the classification system is not different. Earlier clinical stages are associated with the best prognosis for survival.

Prognosis and Treatment. The effectiveness of therapy for non-Hodgkin lymphoma is variable. Favorable outcomes are likely in stage I and II disease. However, non-Hodgkin lymphoma is likely to present as stage III or IV disease, which has a poor prognosis. Therapeutic management is determined by the clinical stage, histologic type, age of the patient, and bone marrow integrity at the time of diagnosis.[27] Current standard treatment options for indolent and aggressive forms of non-Hodgkin lymphoma at different stages are shown in Box 11-7. Multiagent protocols similar to the ones used for late-stage Hodgkin disease are used commonly. Bone marrow transplantation may be used in the management of lymphoma complicated by bone marrow failure.

KEY CONCEPTS 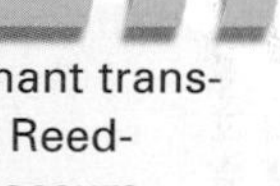

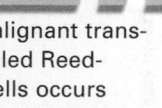

- Hodgkin disease is characterized by malignant transformation of B cells in lymph nodes called Reed-Sternberg cells. Spread of malignant cells occurs along predictable, contiguous pathways. Most commonly, a single cervical lymph node is involved initially, with slow progression to nearby nodes.
- Non-Hodgkin lymphoma constitutes a diverse group of malignant diseases of lymphoid tissue. The characteristic Reed-Sternberg cell of Hodgkin disease is not present. Non-Hodgkin lymphoma is unpredictable in its spread and is often disseminated at diagnosis.
- Manifestations of Hodgkin disease and non-Hodgkin lymphoma are similar. These include painless lymph node enlargement, fever, night sweats, and weight loss. Early stage disease is often asymptomatic.
- Staging is done to determine the degree of dissemination of disease. When affected lymph nodes are localized to one area (stage I) or one side of the diaphragm (stage II), the prognosis for cure is very

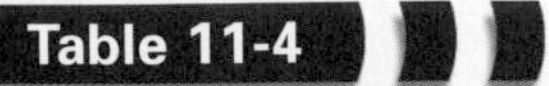

Table 11-4

Summary of the More Common Lymphoid Neoplasms (Non-Hodgkin Type)

Entity	Frequency	Salient Morphology	Immunophenotype	Comments
B-Cell Lymphoma				
Follicular lymphomas	40% of adult lymphomas	Germinal center cells arranged in a follicular pattern	$CD10^+$, $BCL2^+$ mature B cells expressing surface immunoglobulin	Occur in older patients; generalized lymphadenopathy; associated with t(14;18); leukemia less common than in small lymphocytic lymphoma; indolent course but difficult to cure
Mantle cell lymphoma	3%-4% of adult lymphomas	Diffuse or vaguely nodular pattern with small cleaved cells	$CD5^+$ mature B cells expressing surface immunoglobulin and cyclin D1	Occurs predominantly in older males; disseminated disease in nodes, spleen, marrow, and gastrointestinal tract common; t(11;14) is characteristic; aggressive and difficult to cure
Extranodal marginal zone lymphoma (MALT lymphoma)	About 5% of adult lymphomas; more common in parts of Europe (Italy)	Variable; small round to irregular lymphocytes predominate; 40% show plasmacytic differentiation; B cells invade epithelium in small nests (lympho-epithelial lesions)	Mature B cells expressing surface immunoglobulin $CD5^-$, $CD10^-$	Occurs at extranodal sites involved by chronic inflammation. Very indolent; may be cured by local excision
Diffuse large B-cell lymphomas	40%-50% of adult lymphomas	Various cell types; predominantly large germinal center-like cells; others with immunoblastic morphology	Mature B cells, ± surface immunoglobulin	Occur in older patients as well as pediatric age group; greater frequency of extranodal, visceral disease; marrow involvement and leukemia very uncommon at diagnosis and poor prognostic sign; aggressive tumors, but up to 50% are curable
Burkitt lymphoma	<1% of lymphomas in the United States	Cells intermediate in size between small lymphocytes and immunoblasts; prominent nucleoli; high mitotic rate; starry sky appearance caused by high rate of apoptosis	Mature B cells expressing CD10 and surface immunoglobulin	Endemic in Africa; sporadic elsewhere; increased frequency in the immunosuppressed; predominantly affects children; extranodal visceral involvement presenting features; rapidly progressive but responsive to therapy
T-Cell Lymphoma				
Mycosis fungoides/ Sézary syndrome	Most common type of cutaneous lymphoma	Variable; in most cases, small cells with markedly convoluted nuclei predominate; cells often infiltrate the epidermis (Pautrier abscess)	$CD4^+$ mature T cells ($CD3^+$)	Presents with local or more generalized skin involvement. Very indolent course. Sézary syndrome associated with diffuse erythroderma and peripheral blood involvement
Peripheral T-cell lymphoma, not otherwise specified	Most common type of T-cell lymphoma in adults	Variable; usually a spectrum of small to large tumor cells with irregular nuclei	Mature T-cell phenotype ($CD3^+$)	Not clearly a specific entity. Often presents as disseminated disease. Generally poor prognosis

Modified from Kumar V, Cotran RS, Robbins ST: *Robbins basic pathology,* ed 7, Philadelphia, 2003, Saunders, p 437.
MALT, Mucosa-associated lymphoid tissue.

Table 11-5

Clinical Differences in Hodgkin Disease and Non-Hodgkin Lymphoma

Characteristic	Hodgkin Disease	Non-Hodgkin Lymphoma
Pattern of spread	Contiguous spread	Noncontiguous spread
Extranodal disease	Uncommon	More common involvement of gastrointestinal tract, testes, bone marrow
Site of disease	Mediastinal involvement common	Mediastinal involvement less common
	Bone marrow involvement uncommon	Bone marrow involvement common
	Liver involvement uncommon	Liver involvement common
Extent of disease	Often localized	Rarely localized
B symptoms	Common	Uncommon

Box 11-7

Standard Treatment Options for Non-Hodgkin Lymphoma

Indolent Stage I or Contiguous Stage II

1. Involved field irradiation
2. Chemotherapy with radiation therapy
3. Extended (regional) irradiation to cover adjacent prophylactic nodes
4. Chemotherapy alone or watchful waiting if radiation therapy is not feasible
5. Subtotal or total lymphoid irradiation (rarely indicated)

Aggressive Stage I or Contiguous Stage II

1. Chemotherapy with radiation therapy
   - CHOP

Indolent (Noncontiguous) Stages II, III, and IV

1. For asymptomatic patients, deferred therapy with careful observation
2. Purine nucleoside analog:
   - Fludarabine
   - 2-Chlorodeoxyadenosine
3. Oral alkylating agents (with or without steroids):
   - Cyclophosphamide
   - Chlorambucil
4. Combination chemotherapy alone:
   - CVP: cyclophosphamide + vincristine + prednisone
   - C(M)OPP: cyclophosphamide + vincristine + procarbazine + prednisone
   - CHOP: cyclophosphamide + doxorubicin + vincristine + prednisone
   - FND: fludarabine + mitoxantrone + dexamethasone
5. Anti-CD20 monoclonal antibody (rituximab) may be considered as first-line therapy, either alone or with combination chemotherapy
6. Yttrium-90–labeled ibritumomab tiuxetan is available commercially, and iodine-131–labeled tositumomab is under clinical evaluation for patients with minimal (<25%) or no marrow involvement with lymphoma
7. Intensive therapy with chemotherapy and total-body irradiation followed by autologous or allogeneic bone marrow or peripheral stem cell transplantation is under clinical evaluation
8. Phase III trials comparing chemotherapy alone versus chemotherapy followed by anti-idiotype vaccine.

Aggressive or Noncontiguous Stages II, III, and IV

1. CHOP plus rituximab
2. Combination chemotherapy alone:
   - CHOP
3. Autologous bone marrow or peripheral stem cell or allogeneic bone marrow transplantation for patients at high risk of relapse is under clinical evaluation

From National Cancer Institute, National Institutes of Adult Health, 2003, at www.cancer.gov.adult.

good. Dissemination to lymph nodes above and below the diaphragm (stage III) or to extralymphatic organs or tissues (stage IV) carries a poorer prognosis.

- Radiation of the involved field is commonly used for malignant lymphoma in early stages. More disseminated disease may be treated with chemotherapeutic protocols (e.g., ABVD for Hodgkin disease and CHOP for non-Hodgkin lymphoma). Non-Hodgkin lymphoma is routinely treated with chemotherapy because the location of malignant cells is often uncertain. Treatment may lead to bone marrow suppression and may predispose the patient to anemia, thrombocytopenia, and leukopenia.

SUMMARY

Malignant disorders of white blood cells are classified according to cell type and fall into two major categories: myeloid neoplasms and lymphoid neoplasms. Myeloid neoplasms commonly present as leukemia and usually involve transformation of granulocytes. Lymphoid neoplasms may present as leukemia, lymphoma or plasma cell myeloma. Leukemia is a malignant neoplasm of immature stem cells that is characterized by diffuse replacement of the bone marrow by neoplastic blasts. In most cases the leukemic cells spill over into the blood, where they may be seen in large numbers. These cells may also infiltrate the liver, spleen, lymph nodes, and other tissues throughout the body. Lymphoma is characterized by malignancy of cells found in lymphoid tissues and usually arises in the lymph nodes. Hodgkin disease is a special category of malignant lymphoma that is characterized by the presence of Reed-Sternberg cells. Hodgkin disease is more predictable in its spread than the non-Hodgkin types of lymphoma, and it is generally curable in the early stages. Non-Hodgkin lymphoma types comprise a large number of different disorders that involve malignant transformation of B cells, T cells, or NK cells. As with Hodgkin disease, earlier stages are more easily cured. However, the non-Hodgkin lymphomas tend to be unpredictable in their spread, and the prognosis is less certain. Plasma cell myeloma is a malignant transformation of mature, antibody-secreting B cells. Malignant plasma cells are monoclonal and all produce identical antibodies, which accumulate in the blood. These cells have a predilection to settle in skeletal structures where they cause bone demineralization and destruction. Hypercalcemia, bone fractures, and renal damage are common complications of plasma cell myeloma. Treatment for the various types of hematologic neoplasms continues to evolve, and excellent disease-free survival is commonly achieved when the disease is caught in the early stages.

MEDIA RESOURCES

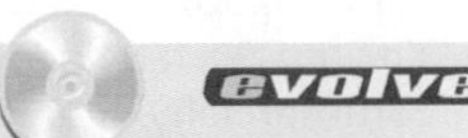

evolve

Remember to check out the ***CD Companion*** included with this book for Review Questions, Key Concepts Review, Glossary (with audio for selected terms), Disease Profiles, and Animations.

PLUS, visit the ***Evolve website*** at http://evolve.elsevier.com/Copstead/ for Case Studies, Disease Profiles, and WebLinks.

References

1. Jaffe ES et al, editors: *World Health Organization classification of tumours: pathology and genetics of tumours of haematopoietic and lymphoid tissues,* Lyon, France, 2001, IARC Press.
2. Schulz TF, Neil JC: Viruses and leukemia. In Henderson ES, Lister TA, Greaves MF, editors: *Leukemia,* ed 7, Philadelphia, 2002, Saunders, pp 200-226.
3. Boice JD: Radiation-induced leukemia. In Henderson ES, Lister TA, Greaves MF, editors: *Leukemia,* ed 7, Philadelphia, 2002, Saunders, pp 152-170.
4. Pedersen-Bjergaard: Chemicals and leukemia. In Henderson ES, Lister TA, Greaves MF, editors: *Leukemia,* ed 7, Philadelphia, 2002, Saunders, pp 171-199.
5. Ross JA et al: Maternal exposure to potential inhibitors of DNA topoisomerase II and infant leukemia (United States): a report from the children's cancer group, *Cancer Causes Control* 7(6):581-590, 1996.
6. Lowenberg B, Griffin JD, Tallman MS: Acute myeloid leukemia and acute promyelocytic leukemia, *Hematology (Am Soc Hematol Education Program)* 82-101, 2003.
7. Gaynon PS, Siegel SE: Childhood acute lymphoblastic leukemia. In Henderson ES, Lister TA, Greaves MF, editors: *Leukemia,* ed 7, Philadelphia, 2002, Saunders, pp 601-620.
8. Spivak JL et al: Chronic myeloproliferative disorders, *Hematology (Am Soc Hematol Education Program)* 200-224, 2003.
9. *Cancer Facts and Figures, 2003,* Dallas, 2003, American Cancer Society.
10. Melo JV, Hughes TP, Apperley JF: Chronic myeloid leukemia, *Hematology (Am Soc Hematol Education Program)* 132-152, 2003.
11. Barnett MJ, Eaves CJ: Chronic myeloid leukemia. In Henderson ES, Lister TA, Greaves MF, editors: *Leukemia,* ed 7, Philadelphia, 2002, Saunders, pp 583-600.
12. Vardiman JW, Harris NL, Brunning RD: The World Health Organization (WHO) classification of the myeloid neoplasms, *Blood* 100:2292-2302, 2002.
13. Robatiner A, Lister TA: Acute myelogenous leukemia. In Henderson ES, Lister TA, Greaves MF, editors: *Leukemia,* ed 7, Philadelphia, 2002, Saunders, pp 485-517.
14. Keating MJ: Chronic lymphocytic leukemia. In Henderson ES, Lister TA, Greaves MF, editors: *Leukemia,* ed 7, Philadelphia, 2002, Saunders, pp 656-691.
15. Keating MJ et al: Biology and treatment of chronic lymphocytic leukemia, *Hematology (Am Soc Hematol Education Program)* 153-175, 2003.
16. Aster J: The hematopoietic and lymphoid systems. In Kumar V, Cotran R, Robbins S, editors: *Robbins basic pathology,* ed 7, Philadelphia, 2003, Saunders, pp 395-452.
17. Gaynon PS, Siegel SI: Childhood acute lymphoblastic leukemia. In Henderson ES, Lister TA, Greaves MF, editors: *Leukemia,* ed 7, Philadelphia, 2002, Saunders, pp 601-620.
18. Joel SP, Robatiner A: Pharmacology of antileukemic drugs. In Henderson ES, Lister TA, Greaves MF, editors: *Leukemia,* ed 7, Philadelphia, 2002, Saunders, pp 394-440.
19. Hoffman M, Rai K: Hairy cell leukemia. In Henderson ES, Lister TA, Greaves MF, editors: *Leukemia,* ed 7, Philadelphia, 2002, Saunders, pp 693-703.
20. Linker CA: Blood. In Tierney LM, McPhee SJ, Papadakis MA, editors: *Current medical diagnosis and treatment,* ed 42, New York, 2003, McGraw-Hill, pp 469-521.
21. Barille-Nion S et al: Advances in biology and therapy of multiple myeloma, *Hematology (Am Soc Hematol Education Program)* 248-278, 2003.
22. Diehl V et al: Hodgkin's lymphoma: biology and treatment strategies for primary, refractory and relapsed disease, *Hematology (Am Soc Hematol Education Program)* 225-247, 2003.
23. Carbone PP et al: Report of the committee on Hodgkin's disease staging classification, *Cancer Res* 31:1860-1861, 1970.
24. Lister TA et al: Report of a committee convened to discuss the evaluation and staging of patients with Hodgkin's disease: Cotswold meeting, *J Clin Oncol* 7(11):1630-1636, 1989.
25. Adult Hodgkin's Lymphoma (PDQ): National Cancer Institute, http://www.nci.nih/gov, 2003.
26. Non-Hodgkin's Lymphoma (PDQ): National Cancer Institute, http://www.nci.nih/gov, 2003.
27. Vose JM et al: Update on epidemiology and therapeutics for non-Hodgkin's lymphoma, *Hematology (Am Soc Hematol Education Program)* 241-262, 2003.

chapter 12

HIV Disease and AIDS

Faith Young Peterson

MEDIA RESOURCES

Additional Material for Study, Review, and Further Exploration

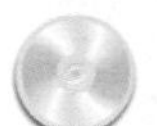

CD Companion ◆ Review Questions and Answers ◆ Key Concepts Review
◆ Glossary (with audio pronunciations for selected terms)
◆ Disease Profiles ◆ Animations

evolve ***Website*** at http://evolve.elsevier.com/Copstead/
◆ Case Studies ◆ Disease Profiles ◆ WebLinks

KEY QUESTIONS

- What are the common modes of HIV transmission and how can infection be prevented?
- What is the scope of the HIV/AIDS epidemic in the United States and the world?
- How does infection with HIV lead to progressive immunodeficiency and AIDS?
- How has knowledge of the HIV life cycle led to the development of multidrug treatment strategies?
- How are $CD4^+$ cell counts and various clinical findings used to classify the stages of HIV disease and AIDS?
- What are the common systemic manifestations of AIDS and associated opportunistic infections?
- What are the current treatment recommendations for HIV disease and AIDS?

CHAPTER OUTLINE

Human immunodeficiency virus (HIV) infection and acquired immunodeficiency syndrome (AIDS) are primary acquired immunodeficiency disorders resulting in defective immune functioning. The hallmark of HIV infection is defective cell-mediated immunity, especially the decrease in $CD4^+$ or T-helper/inducer lymphocytes. $CD4^+$ T cells are necessary for appropriate immune responsiveness because they are the cells that mediate between the antigen-presenting cells and other immune cells such as B cells and other T cells. $CD4^+$ lymphocytes are characterized by the presence of the CD4 receptor.

This chapter focuses on HIV disease and AIDS—from epidemiology to pathogenesis and management. HIV is the prototypical public health infectious disease of the late 20th century. HIV is an infectious organism. It was originally thought to be a rapid killer; however, it does not act like other infectious organisms that overwhelm the immune system. HIV infection is a chronic illness associated with widespread and diverse organ involvement with varying signs and symptoms, and it causes long-term suffering. It encompasses all of the armamentarium of a viral infection that has completed the evolutionary jump from animal to human. HIV has done more than just confuse and captivate scientists and health professionals; it has also mobilized risk groups and placed medicine and society at a crossroads of opinion. In this epidemic, the lines between privacy and public health and between morality and compassion have been argued. HIV disease is complex, but in its complexity it has opened the door to better understanding of the immune system.

EPIDEMIOLOGY

HIV infection is a primary immunodeficiency disease caused by the retroviruses, HIV type 1 and HIV type 2. The emergence of HIV worldwide has triggered major research efforts to better understand and combat its lethal effects on the immune system. Despite research and public health surveillance and prevention activities, the virus has continued mutating and spreading globally. HIV has caused a nondiscriminatory pandemic. It infects people worldwide without regard for age, race, gender, or social class. However, HIV infection is increasingly becoming a disease of poor, uneducated, or undereducated people of color.

Since its identification in the early 1980s, more than 42 million people have been infected with HIV and more than 16 million have died, and these numbers are increasing, particularly in third world countries. Currently, two thirds or more of all cases occur in sub-Saharan Africa, particularly South Africa, and in Southeast Asia and Latin America where it is spreading in epidemic proportions. In third world countries, those infected with HIV have limited access to medication for treatment, and dissemination of prevention information and education for the general public is lacking.

In the United States, it is estimated that 1.4 million people were infected with HIV from 1981 to 2001.[1] Among those individuals, there have been 816,149 cases of AIDS and 467,910 deaths due to AIDS.[1] The numbers of deaths in the United States and other industrialized countries are stable or declining where access to medication, care, and prevention is greater (Figure 12-1).

In the United States, when the epidemic was first identified in the early 1980s, most of the cases (60%) were in Caucasians, with African-Americans and Hispanic persons accounting for most of the other cases (39%).

Current statistics show a changing picture of the people diagnosed with AIDS in the United States; 41% are black, 38% white, 20% Hispanic, 1% Asians/Pacific Islanders, and less than 1% Native Americans and Alaska Natives. In males living with AIDS, 57% contracted the disease through sex with other men (MSM), 24% were intravenous drug users (IVDs), 8% were combined MSM/IVDs, and 9% were exposed via heterosexual contact.[2] In women with AIDS, 57% were exposed via heterosexual contact and 39% were IVDs.[2] Ninety percent of children younger than 13 years were infected perinatally.[2] The number of HIV-infected individuals continues to increase despite prevention education. The U.S. Centers for Disease Control and Prevention (CDC) suggests that up to 280,000 people in the United States may be unaware that they are infected with HIV because of late testing.[2] It is also disturbing that the number of men with HIV infection is again increasing.

History

Retroviruses were one of the first viruses discovered at the turn of the century as the cause of cancer in chickens.[3] Originally, retroviruses were identified only in nonhuman species, where their presence was generally harmless or occasionally associated with tumors and slowly progressive cardiovascular, pulmonary, or neurologic diseases. Retroviruses have subsequently been identified in most animal species.

HIV is very closely related to primate retroviruses, particularly the green monkey virus and macaque monkey virus, termed simian immunodeficiency virus or simian T-cell lymphotropic virus type III (STLV-III). This primate retrovirus does not cause disease in monkeys. It is hypothesized that a virus similar to STLV-III may have crossed species into humans and undergone a series of mutations that became HIV as early as 1675. It established itself in Africa as an epidemiologic disease after 1930.

In 1980 the first human retroviruses were found to affect T cells. Human T-cell lymphotropic virus type I (HTLV-I) was found to infect T cells and cause adult T-cell leukemia. HTLV-II was subsequently discovered and found to be associated with the development of hairy cell leukemias and T-cell leukemias. HTLV-IV is associated with chronic lymphomas, but this relationship is not well established. These transforming, cancer-causing viruses were originally thought to be closely linked to HIV. Such has proved not to be correct. However, their discovery enlightened Gallo, Essex, and Montagnier, who were able to narrow their search for the cause of AIDS.

In 1981 the first descriptions of immunodeficiency disease in previously healthy persons appeared in the medical literature. However, the specific retrovirus causing HIV infection and AIDS was not isolated until 1983 (Montagnier) and 1984 (Gallo).

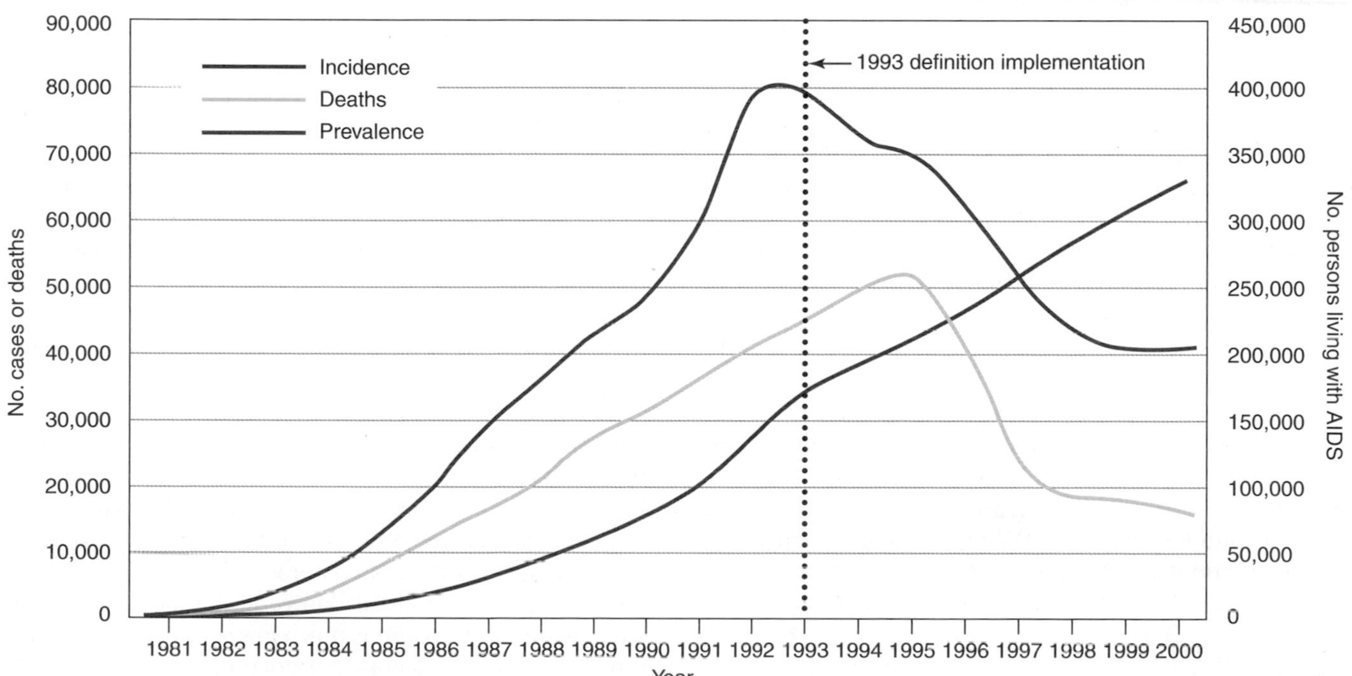

FIGURE 12-1 ■ Estimated AIDS incidence and deaths among persons with AIDS, by year of diagnosis or death and year-end prevalence, United States, 1981 to 2000. Data were adjusted for delays in reporting of cases and deaths. (From Update: AIDS—United States, 2000, *MMWR Morb Mortal Wkly Rep* 51[27]:592-595, 2002.)

HIV has been identified as a type of retrovirus from the subfamily Lentivirinae, with *Lentivirus* being its only genus. This subfamily is so named from the Latin (*lentus,* "slow") because infection develops gradually. It was originally labeled human HTLV-III but was renamed HIV. HIV-2, a related but distinct retrovirus, was later identified in 1986 and is most closely related to simian immunodeficiency virus. HIV-2 is differentiated from HIV-1 by a longer clinical latency period from the onset of infection to the development of symptoms.

Although the syndrome of AIDS was not reported until 1981, isolated cases of HIV or HIV-like infections were reported in the 1950s and 1960s. Positive tests on serum for HIV-1 antibodies were found in samples taken from a man in Leopoldville (now Kinshasa), Congo, a small region in Central Africa, in the 1950s with implications that the virus emerged sometime in the 1930s to 1940s.[4] This infection appears to have remained localized before spreading to the rest of Central Africa during the late 1960s and early 1970s. It is commonly thought that HIV reached Haiti in the late 1970s and may have reached Europe and the Americas from there.

In the United States, the first suspected case occurred in 1968. A sexually active 15-year-old African-American male who was admitted to St Louis City Hospital in 1968 had extensive lymphedema, chlamydial infection in most of his body fluids, and disseminated Kaposi sarcoma.[5] Tests on frozen autopsy tissue from 1969 confirm that he was infected with a virus closely related or identical to the AIDS virus. However, it was not until 1981 when previously healthy young homosexual men in increasing numbers contracted unusual diseases for their age group, such as *Pneumocystis carinii* pneumonia (PCP) and Kaposi sarcoma, that researchers identified HIV. These young men in San Francisco, Los Angeles, and New York provided the basis of inquiry into the HIV infection. The first evidence of alternative forms of transmission of the virus by blood and blood products appeared in 1982. All of these early patients were shown to have a type of HIV virus called HIV-1. It was at this time that the term acquired immunodeficiency syndrome (AIDS) was first used.

HIV-1 antibody testing technology was developed in 1985, at which time it was licensed by the Food and Drug Administration. In 1985, blood samples from Guinea-Bissau in West Africa revealed a new virus related to HIV-1 but distinctly different called HIV-2. In the United States, HIV-2 was not identified until December 1987 in a visitor from West Africa. It is hypothesized that the independence wars and socioeconomic upheavals in the 1960s and 1970s led to its epidemic growth.[6] The first anti-HIV drug was approved in 1987. By 1988, the World Health Organization (WHO) declared December 1 as the first World AIDS Day.

Types of HIV

Both HIV-1 and HIV-2 are found worldwide. They are similar in structure and function but are differentiated from each other by their envelope glycoproteins, point of origin, and latency periods. HIV-1 is thought to have originated in Central Africa and HIV-2 was originally isolated in West Africa. HIV-1 is the causative organism of most AIDS cases found in Central Africa, the United States, Europe, and Australia. HIV-2 is found primarily in West Africa.[6] HIV-2 has the same genetic structure as HIV-1 but has different envelope glycoproteins. HIV-2 produces a milder form of the disease and appears to be less virulent with a longer latency period than HIV-1.

Many subspecies or strains of HIV also exist because of the rapid rate of HIV virion mutation. The subspecies may exist in different hosts, as well as within an individual host. Currently, at least 10 subtypes of HIV-1 have been identified: group N (YBF30), group O, and group M with 8 subtypes (A, B, C, D, E, F, G, H). Research is currently focusing on the identification of HIV subtypes and strains in different populations and geographic areas. For example, in the United States, Europe, and Australia, most infected persons have HIV-1, subtype B, whereas in India, HIV-2 and HIV-1 strains A, B, and C are usually found.

Transmission

HIV-1 and HIV-2 can infect people through three major types of transmission: sexual transmission via semen or vaginal and cervical secretions through homosexual, bisexual, or heterosexual intercourse; parenteral transmission via blood, blood products, or blood-contaminated needles or syringes; and perinatal transmission in utero, during delivery, or in breast milk. In very low titers, HIV is known to be present but has not been shown to be transmitted via urine, saliva, tears, cerebrospinal fluid, amniotic fluid, and feces. HIV is not known to be transmitted via saliva particulates or aerosol routes.

Common modes of transmission include needle/syringe sharing between intravenous drug users, unprotected sex with infected partners, receipt of HIV-contaminated blood or blood products or infected semen during artificial insemination, unanticipated needle or scalpel injury during care or surgical treatment of infected patients, and neonatal transmission from an infected mother to her infant. Blood bank screening and testing procedures have nearly eliminated the transmission of HIV-contaminated blood in the United States. However, this route of transmission is high in third world countries, where the blood supply is highly contaminated and much of the blood and blood products are not screened before use.[1]

Health care workers who are exposed to blood or infected body fluids or needles/sharp instruments are at risk of contracting HIV. The risk of developing HIV is greatest for those health care workers who have a deep injury with visible blood from a contaminated needle or sharp instrument or who have a direct puncture into an artery or vein. They also are at risk if they have prolonged blood-skin contact, especially if extensive. The risk of infection is much lower with the use of universal precautions and postexposure prophylaxis.

Transmission from an infected mother to her infant may occur either in the intrauterine period, in the intrapartum period at the time of delivery, or postpartum via breast-feeding or primary maternal infection during pregnancy. Of these, intrapartum transmission at the time of delivery is thought to be the most common route. HIV infection does not cause any specific congenital abnormalities, but there is an increased risk of spontaneous abortion. The overall risk to the fetus of HIV transmission is estimated to be between 15% and 40% for each pregnancy, with increasing risk in subsequent pregnancies for each HIV-positive fetus born. Increased risks of antepartum transmission include increased maternal viral load; advanced maternal clinical disease as evidenced by low $CD4^+$ counts; primary infection during pregnancy with viremia, HIV, or other infection of the placenta; and breaks in the placental barrier. Increased risks of intrapartum transmission include high maternal viral load at the time of delivery, prolonged ruptured membranes (more than 4 hours), infant exposure to blood/secretions, abruptio placentae, infant prematurity, and the presence of coinfections. The rate of HIV perinatal transmission is reduced to less than 10% with the use of zidovudine (azidothymidine, AZT) during pregnancy and during the first months of the infant's life.

In the United States, those at greatest risk of HIV infection include (1) homosexual and bisexual men; (2) intravenous drug users who share needles or syringes; (3) sexual partners of those in high-risk groups, particularly heterosexual women; and (4) infants born to infected mothers. Sexual intercourse, particularly heterosexual transmission in the presence of another sexually transmitted disease, is the cause of the greatest increase in infection rate. These are the areas that require preventive education and practices.

Worldwide, HIV has infected more than 42 million people. Heterosexual intercourse with infected partners, contaminated blood, and prenatal or perinatal transmission are the major routes of transmission of HIV in Africa, South and Southeast Asia, and developing countries. In these countries an equal proportion of males and females are infected. The major risks for HIV transmission in third world countries include multiple sexual partners, sex with prostitutes, history of other sexually transmitted diseases, and genital lesions or abrasions of any kind.

Since the introduction of multiple drug therapy against HIV, the number of patients diagnosed with and dying from AIDS has declined in the United States. However, the number of HIV-infected persons continues to increase at a rate of 40,000 per year despite prevention education.[2] The CDC estimates that up to 280,000 people in the United States may be unaware that they are infected with HIV because of late testing. Greater proportions of persons becoming infected are exposed during heterosexual contact, live in the south, are female, and are black or Hispanic.[2] Approximately 10% to 11% of all HIV cases involve people over the age of 50, representing 15% of the total number of AIDS cases. The death rate is higher in the older AIDS population than in the younger AIDS population.

Most heterosexual transmission is due to sexual intercourse with IVDs or bisexual men. Consequently, women are the fastest growing risk group. Women with other sexually transmitted diseases or vaginal/cervical inflammation are at higher risk for the development of HIV/AIDS.

Routine social contact with people who are HIV positive does not increase one's risk of HIV infection. For example, using public restrooms, swimming in public swimming pools, touching or hugging someone who is HIV positive, and eating with community utensils or in restaurants are safe practices. One cannot get HIV infection from insects such as mosquitoes.

Exposure to HIV does not mean that one will contract HIV or AIDS, and it does not mean rapid progression. The interacting forces between viral and host factors influence whether an individual will contract HIV infection, particularly the amount and virulence of the virus and the host's response by T-cell–mediated cytotoxicity or by cytokines. In studies of hemophiliacs who received tainted blood products, 10% to 25% of the individuals evaded infection.

Researchers have identified an HIV resistance allele or deletion mutant of the *CCR5* gene in certain people.[7] When inherited from both parents, the mutant *CCR5* gene appears to protect individuals from infection even after multiple exposures. When only one gene is inherited, the progression to AIDS tends to be slower. The gene is not equally distributed among people. Persons of Caucasian-American and Caucasian-European descent have the highest number of mutant allele genes, and Native American, African, and East Asian people have the lowest number of mutant alleles.[7] Researchers have also found that stromal-derived factor (also known as pre–B-cell growth-stimulating factor) can down-regulate cell factors important for HIV binding to lymphocytes (CXCR4) on cells effectively blocking HIV-1 infection.[8]

Prevention of Transmission

Because effective management of HIV is expensive and cure not yet possible, prevention is essential. However, one-time exposure to information or a single message is usually less successful than programs that teach prevention skills and reinforce positive behavior. The primary way to prevent transmission is to use safe sex practices. Safe sex practices include the following: abstaining from sex, using a condom (barrier protection) during sexual intercourse, avoiding multiple sexual partners, and knowing the HIV status of all sexual partners. It is important that education regarding safe sex practices be tailored to appropriate age groups, ethnicity, culture, and sexual preference. Health care provider–patient dialogue may be helpful, but most providers do not use the visit to speak about HIV protection, leading to a missed opportunity.

Spermicides such as nonoxynol 9 or C31G do not inactivate HIV and other sexually transmitted microorganisms. No studies on the effect of using progestins such as levonorgestrel (Norplant) or medroxyprogesterone (Depo-Provera), the diaphragm, or oral contraceptives on the transmission of HIV suggest any benefit. The early use of antepartum and intrapartum antiretroviral therapy and avoidance of breast-feeding can prevent maternal-child HIV infection.

HIV infection in drug users can be prevented with the use of sterile needles via improved access to clean needles and avoidance of dirty or shared needles. Such intervention includes needle/syringe exchange programs for IVDs and cleaning of dirty needles with bleach before use. When using bleach, the user must rinse out all blood first; then fill the needle and syringe with full-strength bleach at least three times for 30 to 60 seconds.

Medical and health care personnel are at risk through occupational exposure to blood and body fluids. Self-protection through the use of standard precautions can decrease risk by reducing exposure. Health care providers should carefully wash their hands before and immediately after patient contact. It is essential to wear disposable gloves for any actual or potential contact with blood or body secretions, when handling items contaminated with blood or body fluids, when performing fingersticks or heelsticks, or when the health care provider has scratches or cuts on the hand.

Gowns or plastic aprons, masks, goggles, or face shields should be worn to protect the face and clothing when there is risk of splashes and airborne droplets of blood or body fluids. Protective gear should be changed between patients. Careful prevention of parenteral exposure when using needles or other equipment should be emphasized. Needles and sharp implements should be disposed of in rigid, puncture-proof containers. Such implements should not be bent, broken, or recapped before disposal. In combative patients who must have blood drawn or injections given, careful use of humane and limited restraint devices may be necessary to prevent injury to the involved health care workers. Resuscitation bags and masks should be readily available to minimize the need for mouth-to-mouth procedures.

Unfortunately, accidents necessitating the development of postexposure prevention protocols do occur. If a health care worker sustains an injury with significant exposure to HIV-infected blood or body fluids such as a needlestick, a postexposure prevention protocol should be initiated as soon as possible and preferably before 72 hours. Such protocols involve the administration of two reverse transcriptase inhibitors, either zidovudine (Retrovir) and lamivudine, or stavudine and didanosine. The length of administration of the agents depends on multiple factors and may be 4 weeks or longer. If the HIV-infected patient has advanced disease, the health care worker should take a protease inhibitor such as nelfinavir (Viracept) or indinavir (Crixivan) in addition to the reverse transcriptase inhibitors. This same protocol has been advocated for use as post-sexual exposure prophylaxis. However, its use is controversial.

KEY CONCEPTS

- HIV disease is a primary immunodeficiency disorder caused by viral infection of $CD4^+$ cells. It is a major health concern because it causes chronic, severe, long-term disease in the first world and very poor prognosis and death in the third world. It carries a very poor long-term prognosis.
- HIV types 1 and 2 are retroviruses that primarily infect $CD4^+$ lymphocytes and macrophages. HIV-1 is the primary causative virus infecting persons in Central Africa, the United States, Europe, and Australia.
- HIV is acquired primarily through sexual transmission via semen and vaginal and cervical secretions; through parenteral transmission via blood, blood products, and contaminated needles/syringes; and through perinatal transmission from an infected mother to her infant antepartum, intrapartum, and postpartum via breast milk.
- HIV is known to be present in but is not believed to be transmitted via urine, saliva, tears, cerebrospinal fluid, amniotic fluid, feces, or aerosols.
- Those at greatest risk of HIV infection include homosexual and bisexual men, IVDs who share needles or syringes, sexual partners of those in high-risk groups, and infants born to infected mothers.
- The use of safe sex practices such as condoms and the use of safe parenteral practices such as sterile needles/syringes decrease the risk of infection.
- Exposure to blood and body fluids of infected individuals through skin, mucous membranes, and accidental needlesticks is the primary risk factor for health care workers. The universal use of standard precautions decreases the risk of infection.
- After significant accidental exposure to HIV-infected blood or body fluids, it is recommended that health care workers take postexposure antiretroviral medication as soon as possible after exposure and as needed for 4 weeks after exposure.

ETIOLOGY

HIV Structure

HIV is an RNA retrovirus that causes a defect in cell-mediated immunity that progresses to AIDS. The viral RNA must be converted to DNA before the viral genes can be expressed to make copies of the RNA virus. Like other retroviruses, HIV differs from DNA viruses in that the RNA genome cannot replicate without undergoing conversion into DNA.

HIV consists of a core or nucleocapsid containing two strands or chains of RNA, protein, and enzymes surrounded and protected by a spherical lipid bilayer viral envelope that is 0.0001 mm across. Between the envelope and core is a protein layer called p17. The nucleocapsid or core is composed of a protein called p24. Within the nucleocapsid, the two strands of RNA compose the HIV genome (Figure 12-2). The HIV genome consists of at least nine genes. The *gag* gene encodes the core antigen proteins. The *pol* gene encodes reverse transcriptase proteins. The *env* gene encodes the viral envelope protein glycoprotein gp160, which is split into two fragments, gp120 and gp41, by cellular protease.

Several other genes have been identified, including *tat, rev, nef, vif, vpr,* and *vpu.* These genes are primarily regulatory genes. The *tat* gene encodes proteins that regulate HIV repli-

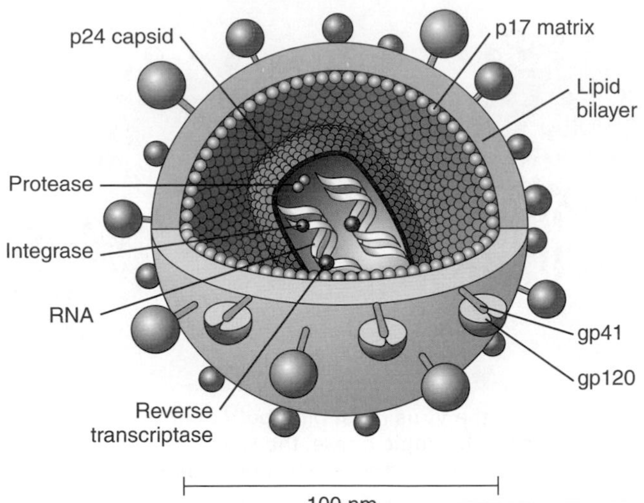

FIGURE 12-2 ■ HIV particle showing the p24 capsid protein surrounding the two strands of viral RNA.

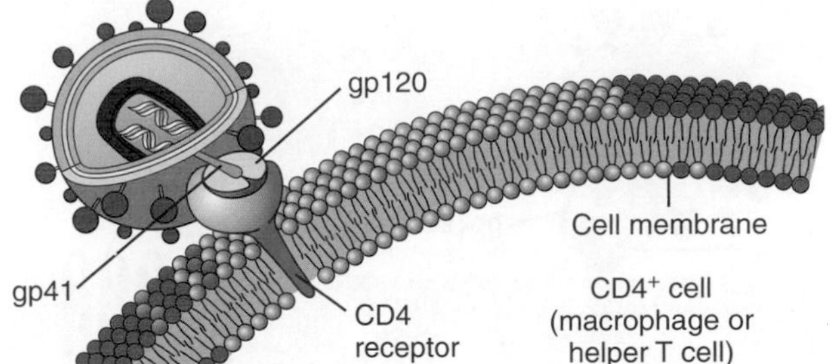

FIGURE 12-3 ■ Schematic view of a retrovirus particle. The core is surrounded by an envelope that is derived from host membranes enriched with viral glycoproteins (gp120, gp41). Interaction of the envelope glycoproteins with a host-encoded cell surface receptor (CD4) is shown.

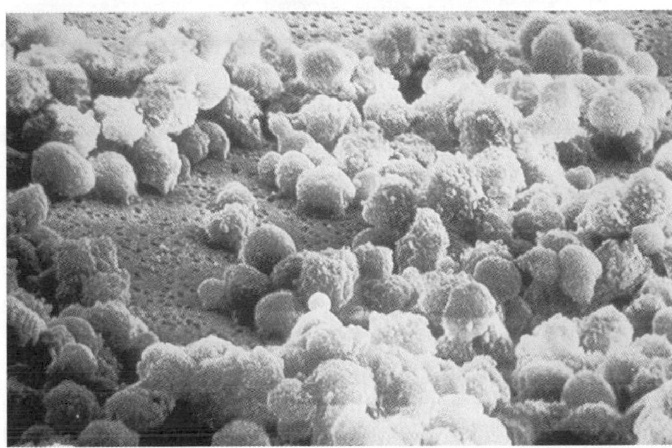

FIGURE 12-4 ■ Scanning electron micrograph (low magnification) of a population of HIV-infected lymphocytes. (Courtesy Centers for Disease Control and Prevention, Atlanta.)

cation and can accelerate HIV viral protein production. It is controlled by *tat*-binding protein. The *rev* gene encodes proteins that regulate viral messenger RNA expression. Rev proteins inhibit regulatory proteins and enhance viral structural gene production. The *vif* (virion infectivity factor) gene appears to increase the ability of the virus to infect other cells. It suppresses the human protein (CEM 15) that inhibits HIV-1.[9]

The HIV genome contains all of the information regulating the virus's structural format and growth during its life cycle. The enzymes within the core are also very important because they facilitate the conversion of RNA to DNA. This conversion is the means of information transfer with this virus. The enzymes include reverse transcriptase, integrase, and protease. Reverse transcriptase is composed of two associated enzymes called polymerase and ribonuclease. Reverse transcriptase is the unique enzyme in HIV that allows the virus to copy RNA into DNA. Protease is a complex enzyme that works as a "molecular scissors." It splits the other viral components by a process known as autocatalysis. Immature virions containing inactive gag/pol, a long precursor protein, are released in the plasma where they are cleaved by protease into smaller active units. Protease also clips p55, the core gag viral protein precursor, into smaller molecules and is needed to facilitate final mature viral assembly for HIV to be infectious.

The viral envelope consists of a membrane derived from the host cell. Viral glycoprotein studs protruding from the cell membrane make it look like a studded ball (Figure 12-3). Gp120 and gp41 are the two HIV envelope proteins that cover the viral particle surface. Gp120 is the most external and distal part of each "stud," whereas gp41 is the bridge that holds it onto the virion surface. The surface envelope also contains other cell surface proteins derived from the host cell containing adhesion molecules. Although the viral particle (virion) is roughly spherical, great diversity is found in size and shape, such as comet-shaped virions and virions with tails.

HIV Binding and Infection

Once inside the body, HIV particles are attracted to cells with receptors on their surface called CD4. The HIV envelope protein gp120 specifically binds to the CD4 receptor. Which $CD4^+$ cells are attracted to the virus changes over time. The CD4 receptor is found on many types of cells, including T cells, microglial cells, monocyte-macrophages, follicular dendritic cells, immortalized B cells, retinal cells, Langerhans cells in the skin, bone marrow stem cells, cervical cells, bone marrow–derived circulating dendritic cells, and enterochromaffin cells in the colon, duodenum, and rectum. Vaginal cells do not contain CD4 receptors. Of these cells, the $CD4^+$ T-helper/inducer cells and macrophages are most often implicated and involved in the process of infection. Figure 12-4 illustrates a group of HIV-infected $CD4^+$ cells imaged by scanning electron micrography. Initially the virus is attracted to macrophages and the virus is called "M tropic."[7] Later the virus becomes either dual tropic and affects both macrophages and T cells, or "T tropic" and affects primarily T cells.[7]

Usually T cells are infected before the onset of symptoms. $CD4^+$ T cells are composed of two subsets: T-helper-1 (T_H1) and T-helper-2 (T_H2). The T_H1 subset produces interferon-γ

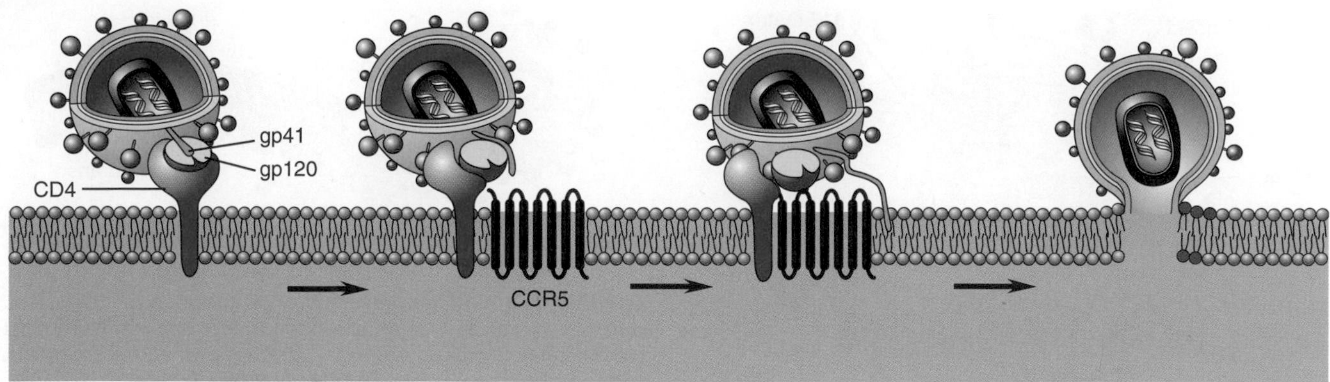

FIGURE 12-5 ■ Early HIV infection, M tropic. In HIV infection, the virus must bind both a CD4 receptor and a coreceptor to fuse with the host cell. In the M-tropic phase, the key coreceptor is CCR5.

and interleukin-2 (IL-2). The T_H2 subset produces IL-4, IL-6, and IL-10. Of these two subsets, the T_H1 subset is the one that is markedly decreased in advanced disease.

However, CD4 alone is not sufficient for fusion of the virion and host cell. A number of important coreceptors called chemokines are necessary for the virus to gain entry into cells. These important chemokine coreceptors must be present for the virion to fuse with the host cell. The chemokine called CCR5 must be present for the HIV particles to bind to the $CD4^+$ cells in early infection during the M-tropic phase, and another chemokine receptor called CXCR4 must be present in later infection during the dual or T-tropic phase.[7] These coreceptors, particularly CCR5, are essential for HIV infection. Since 1996 when the coreceptors were first discovered, a number of other coreceptors have been identified, including APJ, CCR2b, CCR3, CCR8, CCR9, CX3CR1, CXCR4, GPR1, GPR15, STRL33, US28, and V28.[10] The function of most of these coreceptors is unknown. It is hypothesized that some of the coreceptors may be needed for various strains of HIV, for HIV infection in babies and children, or for infection of the brain and nervous system.

The gp120 portion of the virion envelope must combine with the first receptor, CD4, and then change shape by refolding. In the second shape, it combines with the second receptor, either CCR5 or CXCR4, to fuse with the cell. Once the HIV particle is bound to both the CD4 receptor and the chemokine receptor on the host cell, gp41 implants itself in the cell membrane (Figure 12-5). This sequence of events causes the viral particle and the cell to fuse. The core of the virus is then injected into the cytoplasm of the host cell and infection is produced.

Once in the cytoplasm, a single-stranded DNA copy is made by reverse transcriptase from the viral RNA. Using the single-stranded DNA as a template, DNA polymerase copies it to make a second DNA strand and destroys the original RNA strands. The accuracy of DNA transcription is poor, with mutations occurring frequently. This tendency to mutate makes HIV highly resistant to antiviral medications.

Once formed, the new viral DNA migrates to the cell nucleus. Inside the nucleus, integrase splices the viral DNA, called HIV **provirus,** into the host cell's DNA. Once in the host cell's DNA, the viral DNA (provirus) will be replicated together with the host cell's DNA during every cell division. Now the viral DNA is permanently part of the host cell's DNA (Figure 12-6).

When $CD4^+$ cells decline, the diversity of $CD4^+$ cells is affected. With antiretroviral therapy, the naïve T cells that can respond to new infections persist in low numbers despite an increase in memory T cells. Therefore, persons with HIV who are receiving antiretroviral therapy can respond to old but not new infections. This phase is indicative of deterioration in immune system function despite any temporary increase in $CD4^+$ cell counts and decreased viral load from antiretroviral therapy.

Several researchers hypothesize that HIV-infected T cells can directly infect non–CD4-bearing epithelial cells.[11] From electron micrographic studies they believe that infected T cells attracted to inflamed vaginal epithelial cells attach to the cells. The HIV virions are released from the bottom of the T cells, migrate through the cellular gap between the cells, and are ingested by the epithelial cells.[11] An opposing view is that infection in the presence of inflammation is due to the presence of $CD4^+$ macrophages or Langerhans cells that lie directly under the epithelial cells.[11]

KEY CONCEPTS

- HIV is an RNA virus known as a retrovirus. It must undergo reverse transcription within infected cells to form viral DNA.
- HIV consists of a nucleocapsid containing two strands of RNA, protein, and enzymes surrounded by a spherical lipid bilayer viral envelope. At least nine genes make up the HIV genome.
- The HIV genome contains all of the information regulating the virus's structural format and growth, including the conversion of RNA to DNA.

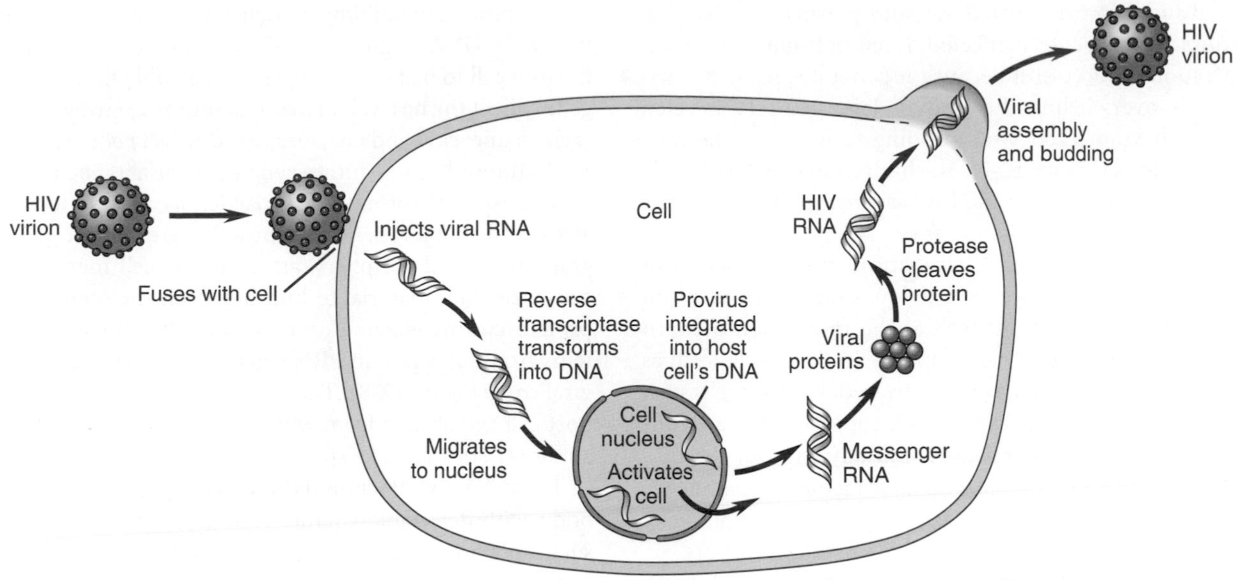

FIGURE 12-6 ■ HIV life cycle. A schematic representation from the time of initial HIV fusion with a host cell, integration into the host cell's DNA, and ending with the replication of a new virion.

- The enzymes needed to convert HIV RNA to DNA include reverse transcriptase, integrase, and protease.
- HIV gains access to $CD4^+$ cells by attaching to the CD4 receptor on the cell surface. Viral envelope protein gp120 and coreceptor chemokines such as CCR5 or CXCR4 mediate attachment.

PATHOGENESIS

Effect of HIV on Immune Cells at the Cellular Level

The hallmark of HIV infection is the decrease in $CD4^+$ T-helper/inducer lymphocytes. T-helper/inducer cells are necessary for appropriate immune responsiveness because they are the cells that mediate between the antigen-presenting cells and other immune cells such as B cells and other T cells. $CD4^+$ lymphocytes are characterized by the presence of the CD4 receptor.

Macrophages have CD4 receptors and act as both targets and reservoirs for HIV. As the infection progresses, they become more functionally impaired with defective phagocytosis and chemotaxis, abnormal antigen presentation, and abnormal cytokine production. They also contribute to the T-cell decline by increasing $CD4^+$ cell death.

In addition to these cellular immune system abnormalities, humoral immune system dysfunction is also present. B-cell numbers usually remain normal. Immunoglobulin G_1 (IgG_1) and IgG_3 levels are usually elevated from hypergammaglobulinemia. IgM levels are elevated in early infection, whereas IgA levels are elevated in late infection. Despite these elevations, the responsiveness to polysaccharide (bacterial cell wall) antigens that require $CD4^+$ cell activation of B cells is decreased. Immune complexes are increased, and B-cell differentiation and response to antigens are decreased. Autoantibodies, especially against erythrocytes, platelets, lymphocytes, neutrophils, nuclear proteins, myelin, and spermatozoa, occur either in association with disease processes (e.g., HIV-associated thrombocytopenia) or spontaneously. HIV antibodies are produced, but they are ineffective against the disease.

The envelope glycoproteins (gp120 and gp41) on the surface of virions are prime targets for antibody production. However, the success of the HIV infection is such that these viral envelope glycoproteins are not very antigenic or immunogenic. Several researchers believe that this property is due to the large amount of carbohydrate on the surface of gp120. Within the human body, high-carbohydrate substances look like "self" to the immune system. Therefore, the virus "hides" under the cover of the glycosylation. Another factor that allows HIV envelope proteins to escape the early antibodies is the way that gp120 and gp41 are bound together. Although the interface between gp120 and gp41 is an area that is highly immunogenic, the gp120 and gp41 molecules are noncovalently bonded together. Early antibodies cannot bind the assembled, functional envelope glycoprotein complex. Later neutralizing antibodies are effective against the complex, but by that time the infection is well established.

Viral Production and Cell Death

The key element in the success of HIV infection is that HIV replicates prolifically from the onset of infection. The high level of infection is characterized by a high level of virion turnover (HIV replication) and a high level of $CD4^+$ cell turnover (host cell death). At least 10 billion HIV particles are produced and destroyed each day, with a plasma virus half-life of 6 hours and an acutely infected T-cell half-life of 1.1 days. The infection is successful because it generates so many virions that it overwhelms the body's defenses. HIV-infected $CD4^+$ cells have marked viral budding to generate and produce new virions (Figure 12-7). In children infected with HIV, the virus is more aggressive and leads more rapidly to immune system dysfunction.

Despite its prolific virion generation, the production of new virus is variable between individuals and dependent on the host's cellular activity, as well as the interaction between HIV regulatory genes *(tat, nef, rev, vif)*. In some cells such as T cells, HIV can lie dormant until activated. In other cells such as macrophages and monocytes, RNA copies of HIV are consistently being made and released, initially without destruction of the host cell. Other host cellular factors that influence viral production of HIV include lack of proteins, inhibition by other proteins, or low concentrations of initiation factors.

Sheehy et al have identified a human protein CEM15 that is part of the innate antiviral defense system in the body.[12] It can repress or inhibit HIV-1 if present in the cell. However, not all cells produce CEM15. Those that do are called nonpermissive whereas those that do not are called permissive. *Vif* is needed by the HIV-1 virus to overcome the defense that CEM15 provides in nonpermissive cells. In permissive cells, the virus can reproduce freely without restriction whether *vif* is present or not.[12]

Several features associated with long-term survival of patients with HIV have been identified. Most importantly, long-term survivors have a low viral load and strong $CD8^+$ killer T-cell activity. This $CD8^+$ killer T-cell activity suppresses viral replication and thus slows progression of the disease, especially in the early stages of the disease. It is also thought that a strong immunologic defense preserves the manufacture of $CD4^+$ T cells that especially recognize and react to HIV. If this ability is lost, these cells may not regenerate even with treatment. Finally, the longer presence of a weaker strain of the M-tropic type may lead to longer survival.

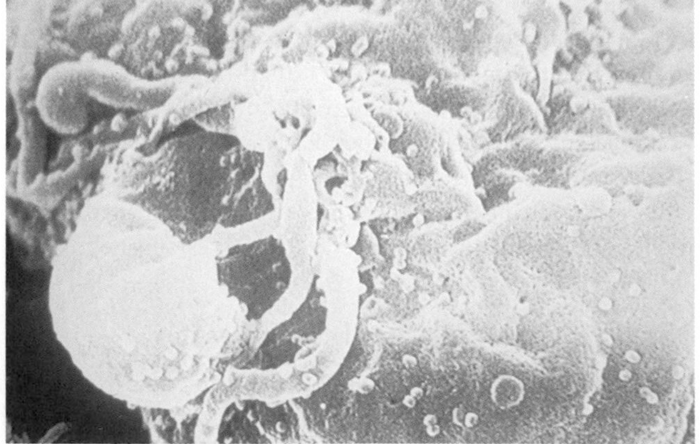

FIGURE 12-7 ■ Scanning electron micrograph of HIV-1–infected $CD4^+$ lymphocytes showing virus budding from the plasma membrane of the lymphocytes. (Courtesy Centers for Disease Control and Prevention, Atlanta.)

The process of building new virus particles begins within the host cell's DNA. Segments at the end of the viral genome tell the host cell to make RNA copies of the viral DNA. Some of the genes direct the host cell to manufacture viral envelope proteins (gene name: *env*) and enzymes (gene name: *pol*), whereas other RNA strands become future genetic material (gene name: *gag*).

The assembly of new virus particles, called **virions,** occurs at the cell membrane. Three proteins are produced and migrate to the cell periphery, attach to the cell membrane, and cause the viral material to bud out from the membrane. The protein-cutting enzyme protease separates the envelope proteins from enzymes and RNA genetic material and binds the viral core (Figure 12-8). Therefore, the completed virion has a host cell membrane from which the envelope proteins gp120 and gp41 stick out like spikes.

During early infection, HIV is widespread throughout the body, with detectable viremia and viral seeding of lymph tissues. This process progresses to an asymptomatic phase of infection with little detectable virus in the blood. During this period, seeded HIV replicates in the lymph nodes and gradually destroys lymph tissue during the infection. The infection in the lymph nodes is more intense with higher HIV RNA expression in comparison with the low to moderate plasma concentration of virus. This phase of the infection is associated with chronic lymphadenopathy and a persistent, gradual decline in $CD4^+$ T-cell numbers. The lymphadenopathy is caused by a vigorous intralymphoid immune response against HIV infection. At the end of the lymphoreticular infection after destruction of lymph tissue, viremia again occurs. It is hypothesized that the destroyed lymph nodes are no longer capable of removing or holding virus, thus allowing viral escape into the blood stream. Even with combination antiretroviral treatment, HIV-1 can persist for several years in pools of resting, memory $CD4^+$ T cells. This pool of memory $CD4^+$ cells remains lost or unavailable to immune system attack inasmuch as such cells lack HIV surface antigens because they carry only provirus DNA.

Once viral production starts or restarts in activated resting cells, death of the infected cells can occur. Cells may die from the accumulation of intracellular viral DNA or the loss of normal cellular protein synthesis because of the infection. Most methods of host cell death involve the envelope protein gp120 or immune processes. Cross-linking of CD4 and gp120 can trigger a type of automatic preprogrammed T-cell death called **apoptosis.** CD4 and gp120 cross-linking can also cause the cell to stop dividing and decreases the cell's ability to fight new infections—a condition called **anergy.** Profuse viral production with multiple CD4 receptors in close proximity can rip holes in the cell membrane and cause host cell death (Figure 12-9). Multiple virion buds with gp120 on their surfaces attach to the surrounding host cell membrane CD4 receptors. This attachment causes tearing of the host cell membrane with subsequent cellular edema and death.

Another process of cell death occurs when multiple uninfected cells become fused together with infected cells by the virus. This mass of cells, called a **syncytium,** can lead to a large number of cell deaths from a single event. The T-tropic strains tend to produce syncytia and cause even faster depletion of T cells.

New research shows that myeloid-derived dendritic cells (MDDCs) can aid in the formation of syncytium when they patrol the body, engulfing the virus and presenting the virus to T cells for processing.[13] HIV is engulfed by the MDDCs, which are highly mobile. When an MDDC interacts with a T cell, there is a concentration of virus, receptor, and coreceptor that facilitates both infection of $CD4^+$ T cells and the development of a syncytium.[12]

Cell death can occur when the immune system makes antibodies to the viral envelope protein. When gp120 is shed, it binds to uninfected CD4 receptors. Then the immune system attacks the uninfected but antibody-coated cells with the complement system or killer T cells and kills the uninfected host cells via antibody-dependent cellular cytotoxicity or natural killer cell cytotoxicity.

Cell death can be secondary to a type III hypersensitivity reaction. Gp120 and gp41 have characteristics similar to those of major histocompatibility class (MHC) antigens—carbohydrate-covered protein. In this case, the body may fail to recognize the difference between gp120 and "self MHC markers" and attack normal cells as nonself. This phenomenon causes the destruction of large numbers of T cells. Cells may also be affected by T-cell–mediated cytotoxicity or by cytokines and inflammation resulting from infection.

Progression of HIV Infection from Seroconversion to AIDS

HIV disease is an infectious state that progresses over time to AIDS with its many manifestations. AIDS is a syndrome, not a disease, which means that the virus can express itself in many ways. No one symptom typifies either HIV infection or AIDS. However, groups of signs and symptoms are useful in staging progress of the infection.

Once the HIV virion enters the body, it rapidly replicates (Figure 12-10). It is present in the blood and cerebrospinal

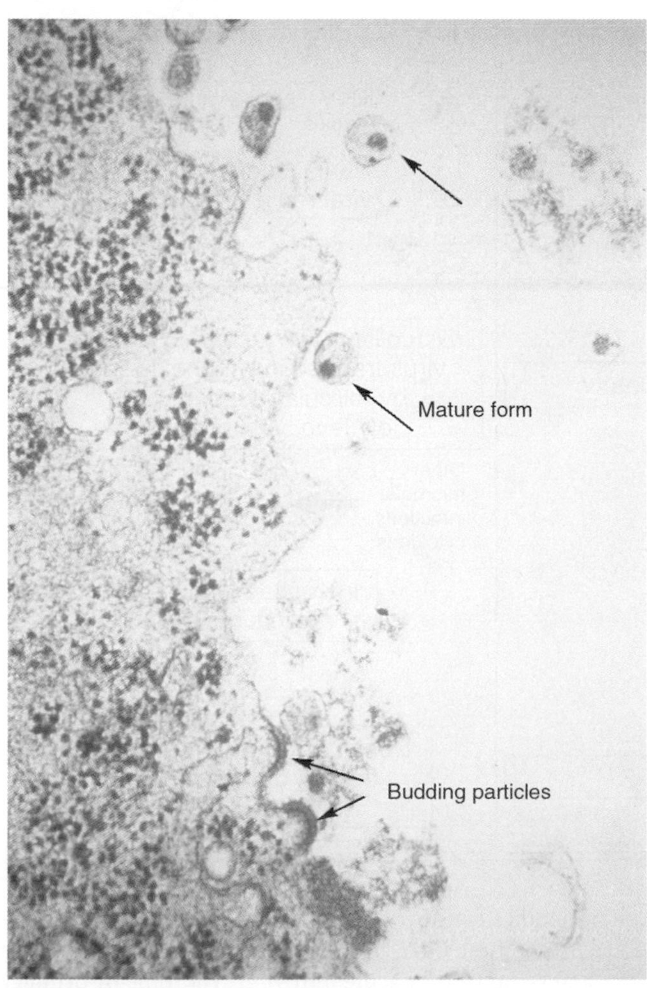

FIGURE 12-8 ■ HIV-1/lymphadenopathy virus found in a hemophiliac patient with AIDS. Virus particles range in size from 90 to 120 nm. Viral budding and the production of new virions are facilitated by protease. (Courtesy Centers for Disease Control and Prevention, Atlanta.)

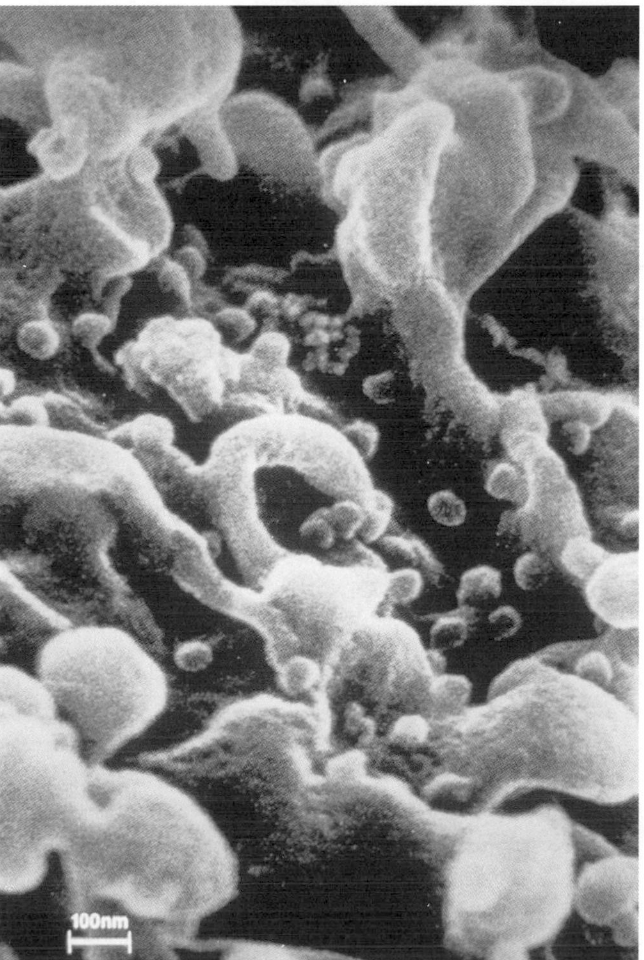

FIGURE 12-9 ■ High magnification of a $CD4^+$ lymphocyte infected with HIV-1. Note the large number of budding HIV virions, which can lead to host cell death by membrane tearing or syncytium formation. (Courtesy Centers for Disease Control and Prevention, Atlanta.)

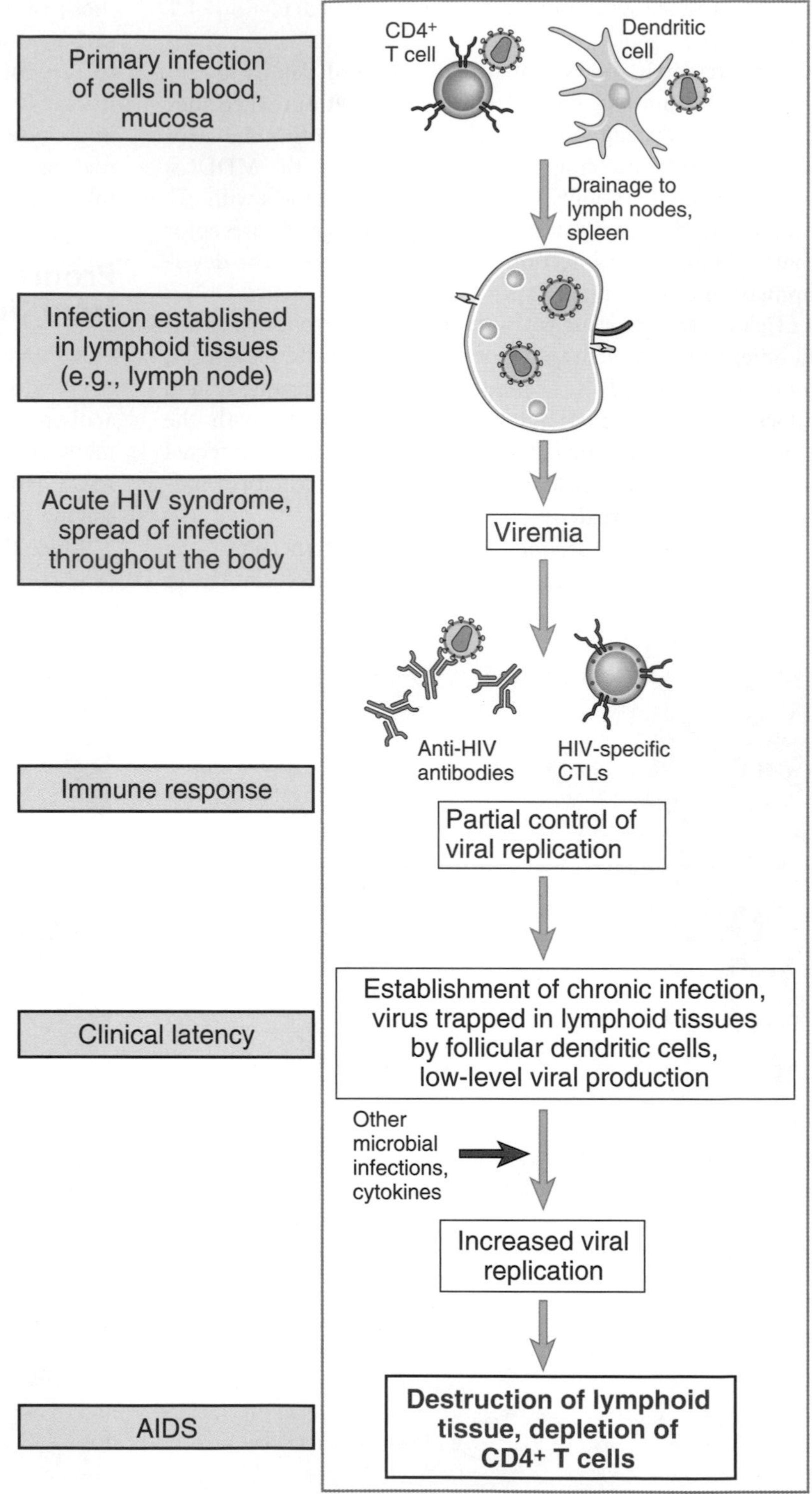

FIGURE 12-10 ■ Progression of HIV infection. The clinical stages of HIV disease correlate with a progressive spread of HIV from the initial site of infection to lymphoid tissues throughout the body. The immune response of the host temporarily controls acute infection but does not prevent the establishment of chronic infection of cells in the lymphoid tissues. Cytokine stimuli induced by other microbes serve to enhance HIV production and progression to AIDS. *CTLs,* Cytotoxic T lymphocytes. (From Abbas AK, Lichtman AH: *Cellular and molecular immunology,* ed 5, Philadelphia, 2003, Saunders, p 469.)

fluid but is not detected on laboratory test results because no antibodies have formed yet. Usually no symptoms are present. It is a time of rapid virus replication. The person is infectious but does not know it.

Seroconversion occurs between 3 weeks and 6 months after exposure but may take as long as 14 months. This means that antibodies are now present in the blood and can be detected. At the time of seroconversion, the person experiences signs and symptoms of acute retroviral syndrome or primary HIV infection. At this time, the symptoms of primary HIV infection includes flulike or mononucleosis-like symptoms, including fever, chills, headaches, nausea, vomiting, fatigue, weakness, arthralgias, sore throat, stiff neck, photophobia, irritability, and rash. The rash is not the same in everyone and may be maculopapular, vesicular, or urticarial. Encephalopathy may even develop. The CD4$^+$ T-cell count is greater than 400. The number of white blood cells, including lymphocytes, is decreased except for an increased number of CD8$^+$ T cells. Platelets are also decreased. The person has an elevated erythrocyte sedimentation rate. Then after the first few weeks, the symptoms disappear. However, HIV is still present and the person continues to be infectious throughout the rest of the course of the infection.

After this period of seroconversion, the patient experiences the latency period which can last 3 to 12 years. Antiviral immune activity is ongoing. Production of virus is maintained or stabilized at a set level. The person feels well but may experience some chronic lymphadenopathy or mild symptoms only. The CD4$^+$ T-cell count is greater than 400. Stabilization of the serum level of virus at a certain point is attributable to the antiviral response, the number of CD4$^+$ cells, and the virulence of the HIV strain. During this period of asymptomatic or mild infection, however, the provirus is producing large numbers of virions and is destroying the body's immune system. Up to 2 million viral particles can be produced daily. The key point is that although the infection is clinically asymptomatic, the virus is active and is not latent.

Immediately after the latency period of infection, there is a period of rapid virus production occurring for up to 18 months. A persistent and continuous drop in the CD4$^+$ T-cell count to less than 400 takes place. The antiviral innate immune activity is less effective as the viral load (level of virus in the blood) increases.

As the viral loads increase and the immune system declines, the patient enters the stage of symptomatic, chronic HIV infection. At this time, the patient goes from partially responding to skin testing (partial anergy) to complete anergy with no response to skin testing. Severe viral or fungal infections of the skin and mucous membranes develop. Oral and genital herpes simplex and candidiasis usually develop, as well as oral hairy leukoplakia. The person may have cytomegalovirus (CMV) infection, Epstein-Barr virus infection, or both as well as other opportunistic infections.

By the time the patient has developed AIDS, the CD4$^+$ T-cell count is usually less than 100. The person typically has one or more opportunistic infections, including PCP, *Toxoplasma gondii*–associated neural toxoplasmosis, cryptosporidiosis (gastroenteritis), and *Mycobacterium* tuberculosis. The person usually has one or more tumors or cancers, including Kaposi sarcoma (a connective tissue skin cancer), lymphomas, or cancer of the rectum or tongue.

Disease progression in infants and children is determined by when the child became infected (timing), viral load, the child's immune response, and viral virulence. In general, children with HIV progress more rapidly than adults. Most children fall into two distinct groups: those with rapidly progressive disease and those with slower disease progression. In those with rapidly progressing disease, symptoms develop within the first 6 months of life, sustained decreases in CD4$^+$ cell counts are noted, and AIDS develops within the first 2 years of life. Early aggressive treatment in perinatally infected infants may slow disease progression and prolong immune function.

CDC HIV Classification System

The CDC HIV classification system is a simple matrix classification system for adults and children and is the preferred method of staging. In this system, CD4$^+$ T-cell counts are linked with clinical symptomatology. The CDC has defined three CD4$^+$ T-cell categories and three clinical categories that are mutually exclusive. The CD4$^+$ T-cell categories define three T-cell ranges. In category 1, the CD4$^+$ T-cell count is greater than or equal to 500/μl; in category 2, the CD4$^+$ T-cell counts range from 200 to 499/μl; and in category 3, the CD4$^+$ T-cell count is less than 200/μl.[14]

In adults, the clinical categories are labeled A through C. Category A includes a variety of clinical conditions such as asymptomatic, persistent generalized lymphadenopathy and a history of or current acute HIV infection with accompanying illness. Category B includes conditions that are secondary to impaired cell-mediated immunity such as candidiasis (oral or vaginal), fever, persistent diarrhea, oral hairy leukoplakia, shingles, idiopathic thrombocytopenic purpura, pelvic inflammatory disease, listeriosis, and peripheral neuropathy. Category C includes conditions that are listed in the AIDS surveillance case definition. An individual in category C will remain in this category. The CDC classification matrix is given in Table 12-1. An HIV-positive person with a CD4$^+$ count less than 200/μl or a category C AIDS indicator condition is diagnosed with AIDS.

In children, category N is an asymptomatic phase with no signs or symptoms of disease. Category A is a mildly symptomatic phase with two or more of the following conditions: lymphadenopathy, hepatomegaly, splenomegaly, dermatitis, parotitis, or recurrent/persistent upper respiratory infection, sinusitis, or otitis media. Category B is a moderately symptomatic phase in which the child exhibits some opportunistic infections as a result of impaired cell-mediated immunity or impaired bone marrow function. These conditions include anemia, thrombocytopenia, bacterial meningitis, pneumonia or sepsis, candidiasis, thrush, CMV, diarrhea, hepatitis, herpes simplex infection, herpes zoster infection, leiomyosarcoma, nephropathy, persistent fever, toxoplasmosis, and varicella. The category C phase is severely symptomatic with AIDS. The revised pediatric HIV classification system based on age-specific CD4$^+$ T-cell counts and percentage is given in Table 12-2.

DIAGNOSTIC TESTING

To diagnose HIV infection, laboratory tests such as the enzyme-linked immunosorbent assay (ELISA) and the Western blot are used to detect the presence of HIV antibodies, which in infected

Table 12-1

CDC HIV/AIDS Classification Matrix

CD4+ T-Cell Categories	A Asymptomatic Acute HIV	B Symptomatic, Not (A) or (C)	C AIDS Indicator
	Clinical Categories		
1 ≥500/μl	A1	B1	C1
2 200-499/μl	A2	B2	C2
3 <200/μl AIDS indicator T-cell count	A3	B3	C3

From Centers for Disease Control and Prevention: 1993 Revised classification system for HIV infection and expanded surveillance case definition for AIDS among adolescents and adults, *MMWR Morb Mortal Wkly Rep* 41(RR-17):1-6, 1993.

Table 12-2

Revised Pediatric HIV Classification Matrix*

Immune Categories	CD4+ T-Cell Counts <12 mo	1-5 yr	6-12 yr
Category 1: No suppression	>1500/μl >25%	>1000/μl >25%	>500/μl >25%
Category 2: Moderate suppression	750-1499/μl 15%-24%	500-999/μl 15%-24%	200-499/μl 15%-24%
Category 3: Severe suppression	<750/μl <15%	<500/μl <15%	<200/μl <15%

From Foundation for Care Management, Dunn JM, editor: Special considerations in treating HIV positive children, *HIV Hotline* 7(5):7-12, 1997.
*Based on age-specific CD4+ count per microliter and percentage.

persons are found in measurable quantities. The ELISA test result is positive for HIV antibodies if the blood or oral mucosal transudate of an infected person reacts with the surface antigen of a killed HIV virus. The ELISA test uses purified viral proteins placed on plastic beads or in multiwell trays. When the test serum or oral mucosal transudate from a patient comes in contact with the purified viral proteins, an antigen-antibody reaction occurs. Antihuman antibody added to the reaction can be detected calorimetrically and indicates whether any antigen-antibody compounds have formed. This test is highly sensitive (more than 99%) and specific (more than 99%) in high-risk populations. For the test to be specific, however, it must be performed with both HIV-1 and HIV-2 viral antigens.

When the ELISA test result is positive, a second test, the Western blot, is used to confirm the presence of HIV antibodies. The Western blot test uses an expensive process called electrophoresis, so usually it is used only as a confirmatory test. This test identifies specific antibodies against the HIV protein antigens. The specificity of this test in combination with the ELISA is greater than 99.9%. The problem with this additional testing is that the patient must wait up to 1 to 2 weeks for confirmation.

There is a new, rapid, fingerstick-based HIV assay that is being used as well: OraQuick Rapid HIV-1 Antibody test results can be obtained in about 20 minutes. However, positive results must be confirmed by a Western blot. It is also important to remember that false negative tests can occur during the initial period of HIV infection before seroconversion.

Testing neonates for HIV is difficult because of maternal transmission of IgG antibodies against HIV. These passive maternal antibodies cross the placenta and can last as long as 15 months. Therefore, the best method to determine whether a neonate has HIV is to culture the virus from blood and peripheral tissue.

Another important test is the absolute $CD4^+$ cell count. The $CD4^+$ count is a specific indicator of disease progression of HIV to AIDS. As the $CD4^+$ cell count declines, the risk of progression to AIDS and the development of opportunistic infections and malignancies increase. Highly virulent communicable diseases can still occur when the $CD4^+$ count is high. However, when the $CD4^+$ cell count drops below 200 cells/μl the number and severity of low-virulence diseases and opportunistic infections increase. It is at this level that many patients begin taking prophylactic medications to prevent opportunistic and other infections. Also used is the $CD4^+$ lymphocyte percentage, which is more stable and has less variation over time. When the $CD4^+$ lymphocyte percentage is less than 20%, the risk of AIDS developing is higher.

Another useful test is the plasma viral load, which indicates the amount of viral replication and the effectiveness of therapy and helps predict disease progression. The level of HIV RNA in plasma is the strongest predictor of outcome over time. When the plasma HIV RNA content is low, the risk of disease progression declines. The plasma viral load helps the clinician to assess the effectiveness of various therapies and is the basis for initiating more aggressive therapies to decrease the viral load. Usually, HIV RNA levels should drop after the onset of therapy and by 6 months should be undetectable. The viral load assay counts copies of HIV RNA in 1 ml of plasma and is either a reverse transcriptase polymerase chain reaction (RT-PCR) or a branched DNA (bDNA) assay. Because each virion contains two strands of RNA, the actual virion level is half the HIV RNA counted. Tests are currently sensitive to 50 copies per milliliter. If the patient continues to have disease progression despite treatment, genotypic and phenotypic resistance tests may be ordered. These tests are expensive and have not been standardized or approved by the Food and Drug Administration. Genotypic testing identifies viral mutations whereas phenotypic testing identifies the concentration of antiretroviral drug needed to inhibit viral replication in culture medium. Ideally this testing would allow the best drugs to be given to the patient.

Another common test is an anergy test or a delayed hypersensitivity (type IV) test for such organisms as *M. tuberculosis* or mumps or measles virus. In early HIV infection, these test results are normal. However, in advanced cases, the patient will have no response to testing because of the loss of macrophage and $CD4^+$ T-cell functioning.

Two other tests may be used: β_2-microglobulin and p24 antigen. β_2-Microglobulin is a cell surface protein that indicates macrophage stimulation. Levels greater than 3.5 are associated with rapid progression of the disease. P24 antigen is indicative of active HIV replication and confirms the diagnosis of HIV infection. It is positive before seroconversion and may be used before the ELISA result would be positive. It is also elevated in later stages of the disease, a period when antibody testing may be unreliable.

Other laboratory and diagnostic tests can assist in the treatment of persons infected with HIV, including a complete blood cell count (CBC), a chemistry panel or screen, and chest radiographs. These tests are routinely used to detect infections and changes in a patient's physiologic status (Box 12-1). The CBC detects the development of anemia (as a result of infection or chronic illness or secondary to therapy) and neutropenia and thrombocytopenia, which may occur in advanced disease.

Box 12-1

Tests Used to Evaluate Progression of HIV Infection

Complete Blood Cell Count
White blood cell count normal to decreased
Lymphopenia (<30% of the normal number of WBCs)
Thrombocytopenia (decreased platelet count)

Lymphocyte Screen
Reduced $CD4^+/CD8^+$ T-cell ratio
$CD4^+$ (helper) lymphocytes decreased
$CD8^+$ lymphocytes increased

Quantitative Immunoglobulin
IgG increased
IgA frequently increased

Chemistry Panel
Lactate dehydrogenase increased (all fractions)
Serum albumin decreased
Total protein increased
Cholesterol decreased
AST and ALT elevated

Anergy Panel
Nonreactive (anergic) or poorly reactive to infectious agents or environmental materials (e.g., pokeweed, phytohemagglutinin mitogens and antigens, mumps, *Candida*)

Hepatitis B Surface Antigen
To detect the presence of hepatitis C

Blood Cultures
To detect septicemia

Chest Radiograph
To detect *Pneumocystis carinii* infection or tuberculosis

AST, Aspartate aminotransferase; *ALT,* alanine aminotransferase.

KEY CONCEPTS

- HIV virions are attracted to cells with CD4 receptors such as T cells, microglial cells, monocyte-macrophages, follicular dendritic cells, immortalized B cells, retinal cells, Langerhans cells in the skin, bone marrow stem cells, cervical cells, bone marrow–derived circulating dendritic cells, and enterochromaffin cells in the colon, duodenum, and rectum.
- The hallmark of AIDS is a decrease in $CD4^+$ cells, including T-helper lymphocytes and macrophages. B-cell responsiveness is decreased because of dependence on T-helper cell cytokines.
- The key element in HIV infection is the high level of virion production and the high level of $CD4^+$ cell death.
- $CD4^+$ cell death occurs via several mechanisms. Cross-linking of CD4 receptors by viruses may result in T-cell death, apoptosis, or anergy. Virions may cause the linkage of infected and uninfected cells, followed by cell fusion and death. B cells may form antibodies against infected T cells. Viral budding may cause excessive loss of cell membrane.
- Laboratory testing for HIV is accomplished by using either the enzyme-linked immunosorbent assay (ELISA) or the Western blot test. Usually the ELISA test is performed first. If it is positive, the Western blot test is performed to confirm the presence of specific antibodies against HIV protein antigens.
- HIV is an infectious disease that progresses to AIDS and is characterized by different clinical manifesta-

tions at each stage. Individuals move through the stages at different rates.

- Flulike symptoms and the formation of anti-HIV antibodies (seroconversion) characterize the early stage of viral seeding. Next, symptoms of early immune dysfunction are present, including lymphadenopathy, fever, and night sweats. A surge in viral production and a drop in the $CD4^+$ lymphocyte count follow this stage.
- In the later stages, $CD4^+$ counts continue to fall and the person is subject to a number of opportunistic infections and tumor formation. An HIV-positive individual is diagnosed with AIDS when the $CD4^+$ T-cell count is less than 200/μl or when a category C AIDS indicator condition is present.
- Children often have rapidly progressive disease, with onset of AIDS between ages 4 and 8 years.

CLINICAL MANIFESTATIONS

HIV affects all body systems, particularly the cutaneous, pulmonary, gastrointestinal (GI), neurologic, and ocular systems. GI manifestations develop in nearly all persons with HIV. Pulmonary and cutaneous symptoms develop in approximately 50% to 75% of all persons with HIV, and neurologic symptoms develop in 50% to 60%. Box 12-2 outlines the common agents of infection in patients with AIDS.

Systemic Manifestations

As implied in the classification systems presented earlier, the course of HIV infection parallels the functioning of the immune system. As immune function declines, the number of opportunistic infections and malignancies increases. The most significant systemic symptom is malnutrition or wasting syndrome. This is defined as unintended, involuntary loss of greater than 10% body weight due to HIV infection.[15] There is major muscle wasting, associated with the weight loss and malnutrition. The malnutrition is due to a combination of factors, including an elevated metabolic rate, chronic inflammation, malabsorption, anorexia, decreased intake of food, and the effect of multiple opportunistic insults. In addition, tumor necrosis factor, which increases the breakdown of fat and decreases the synthesis of fatty acids, is elevated in HIV/AIDS patients with secondary infections. In Africa, HIV is known as "slim disease" because of the wasting. Malnutrition is a leading cause of death among AIDS patients in the United States. Prevention is key, involving assessment of nutritional parameters as well as nutritional education and exercise. Patient's body mass index, weight, calorie and protein intake, prealbumin, serum albumin, and triglyceride levels are frequently measured.

To prevent or delay the wasting process, medications are being evaluated, including ketotifen, thalidomide, testosterone, anabolic steroids such as nandrolone (Deca-Durabolin) and oxandrolone, dehydroepiandrosterone, and a combination of medications. Ketotifen is a tumor necrosis factor inhibitor and antihistamine that is used because its side effects are appetite stimulation and weight gain. Thalidomide, which is also a tumor necrosis factor inhibitor, appears to be effective against wasting syndrome and increases fat-free mass.[15] Oxandrolone is an anabolic steroid designed specifically to promote weight gain, particularly lean body mass. Megestrol acetate (Megace), a progestational agent, and dronabinol, an antiemetic, are often used to decrease nausea and increase appetite. Use of human growth hormone (somatropin, Serostim) may also be given (6 mg/day intramuscularly) to increase lean body mass.[15]

Vitamins A, C, and E; the B vitamins; zinc; selenium; sulfur amino acids; and other antioxidants are also used. The use of these nutrients can prevent the up-regulation of inflammatory cytokines and thereby decrease inflammation. High-protein, high-calorie meals and snacks are recommended, along with

Box 12-2

Common Agents of Infection in Patients with AIDS

Viruses
Herpes simplex 1 and 2
Herpes zoster
JC virus
Epstein-Barr virus
Human papillomavirus
Varicella
Adenovirus

Bacteria
Campylobacter spp.
Shigella spp.
Neisseria spp.
Salmonella spp.
Chlamydia spp.
Staphylococcus spp.
Haemophilus influenzae spp.
Legionella spp.
Treponema spp.
Mycobacterium spp.

Fungi
Candida albicans
Cryptococcus neoformans
Histoplasma capsulatum
Coccidioides immitis
Nocardia

Protozoa
Pneumocystis carinii
Toxoplasma gondii
Isospora belli
Cryptosporidium
Giardia lamblia
Entamoeba histolytica

Data from Stites DP, Terr AI: *Basic and clinical immunology,* ed 7, Los Altos, Calif, 1991, Appleton & Lange; Ungvarski PJ, Schmidt J: AIDS patients under attack, *RN* 55(11):35-44, 1992; and Anastasi JK, Rivera JL: Identify the skin manifestations of H.I.V., *Nursing* 92(11):58-61, 1992.

nutritional supplements. High-fat foods should be avoided because they increase diarrhea, as can lactose-containing foods. Nutritional supplements, which provide both protein and calories, are full of nutrients and can be formulated either with or without lactose and with or without medium-chain triglyceride oil (a more easily digested fat). For example, Carnation Instant Breakfast or Ensure can provide 240 calories of protein, carbohydrates, fat, vitamins, and minerals; Nitrofuel, Sustacal Plus, Advera, and Lipisorb can provide even more protein (14 g) and are lactose free. Lipisorb also provides medium-chain triglyceride oil, is more easily absorbed, and leads to less diarrhea. Questran, a bile acid sequestrant, is sometimes used to decrease or bind the excess fat that causes diarrhea. Total parenteral nutrition as well as gastrostomy or jejunostomy tube feeds are reserved for those with severe malnutrition and GI manifestations.

Gastrointestinal Manifestations

GI manifestations are nearly universal in persons with HIV. In fact, the GI tract may be the major target organ in HIV infection. HIV may or may not be a significant direct pathogen in the GI tract. The major HIV GI complication is chronic diarrhea. The diarrhea, often watery or bloody, causes malabsorption and consequently severe weight loss. This complex of HIV-related malnutrition causes muscle loss leading to increased morbidity and risk of death. Use of antiemetics and antidiarrheals are often useful in controlling symptoms.

Whenever chronic diarrhea or other GI symptoms develop in a patient with HIV, it is important to determine the cause. GI symptoms can be due to multiple opportunistic infectious agents and are rarely due to tumors occurring in the GI tract. Some of the most significant infectious agents are viruses such as CMV and herpes simplex; fungi such as *Candida;* bacteria such as *Salmonella, Shigella, Clostridium difficile, Chlamydia trachomatis,* and *Campylobacter;* and parasites such as *Giardia, Isospora, Entamoeba histolytica,* and *Cryptosporidium.* GI symptoms include chronic diarrhea, oral candidiasis, anorexia, nausea, vomiting, mucous membrane ulcers, retrosternal pain on swallowing, abdominal pain, and low serum vitamin B_{12}. Ulcerations occur as a primary manifestation or secondary to the inflammation. Treatment involves the use of antibiotics such as vancomycin (Vancocin), amikacin (Amikin), ampicillin, ciprofloxacin (Cipro), erythromycin, trimethoprim-sulfamethoxazole (Bactrim), metronidazole (Flagyl), clotrimazole troches (Mycelex), ganciclovir (Cytovene), spiramycin (Rovamycine), and eflornithine (Ornidyl), depending on the offending organism.

A common cause of diarrhea is the protozoa *Cryptosporidium.* It infects the intestinal epithelium lining the microvillus border. This organism is transmitted via water, food, animals, and other humans. The onset of cryptosporidiosis is generally acute and associated with explosive diarrhea within 4 to 14 days after infection. In nonimmunocompromised persons, the symptoms last up to 2 weeks, but in immunocompromised persons, the diarrhea and symptoms can persist indefinitely. Cryptosporidiosis causes nausea, vomiting, severe watery nonbloody diarrhea, abdominal pain, cramping, electrolyte disturbances, and dehydration. It is characterized by massive amounts of highly infectious diarrhea (more than 15 to 20 L).

Diagnosis is made by stool examination for ova and parasites and by bacterial culture and sensitivity. Antibiotic treatment is not always effective, but paromomycin (Humatin), nitazoxanide (NTZ), octreotide, azithromycin (Zithromax), and clarithromycin (Biaxin) have been used. In the acute phase, some patients must be given intravenous hydration for support. Thereafter, increased oral intake, along with low-residue, high-protein, high-calorie diets, and loperamide (Imodium) tablets, up to 16 to 18 per day, are used to help control the diarrhea.

Prevention of *Cryptosporidium* infection is most important. Preventive activities include routine testing of well water, using water filters at home, avoiding ice or unfiltered tap water both at home and in restaurants, and avoiding fresh fruit or vegetables rinsed with unfiltered water. Fruit and vegetables can be washed in bottled water, filtered water, or water with 20 drops of 2% iodine per gallon.

Oropharyngeal and/or esophageal *Candida albicans* infections occur in most patients with HIV at some time during the course of their disease. Most often, oral *candidiasis* is pseudomembranous in type, with white plaques that bleed when removed and leave an erythematous surface. *Candida* oropharyngeal lesions produce pain and discomfort during eating, loss of taste, and **xerostomia.** *Candida* esophageal lesions cause pain with swallowing, dysphagia, and a feeling of "throat swelling." These lesions lead to worsening wasting syndrome. Management of oropharyngeal *candidiasis* includes the use of topical agents such as clotrimazole (Mycelex) or nystatin (Mycostatin) suspension or lozenges. Side effects include an unpleasant taste and GI side effects, with inconvenient dosing regimens (up to six times per day). In persistent cases, oral medications such as fluconazole (Diflucan), itraconazole (Sporanox), and ketoconazole (Nizoral) may be used. Management of esophageal *candidiasis* is done with oral medications, particularly fluconazole.

Pulmonary Manifestations

Pulmonary manifestations are a major source of morbidity and mortality in AIDS patients. Pulmonary diseases include opportunistic pneumonias such as those associated with *P. carinii,* CMV, *M. tuberculosis, Histoplasma,* or *Staphylococcus,* as well as parenchymal lung diseases including Kaposi sarcoma, lymphoma, nonspecific pneumonitis, and adult respiratory distress syndrome. Infection with *M. tuberculosis* occurs in 4% of patients with HIV and is particularly problematic in third world countries where the TB comorbidity rates are up to 50%. Patients who have tuberculosis have an increased risk of being infected with a multidrug-resistant type of organism.

PCP is the most common initial opportunistic infection in AIDS. However, the incidence of *P. carinii* has decreased with the use of prophylaxis. *P. carinii* is classified as a protozoa, but recent research indicates that it may be related to yeasts. This organism prefers alveolar environments and infects most people during early childhood. Children usually have *Pneumocystis* antibodies by 2 to 3 years of age, but the organism does not cause disease in immunocompetent persons. With immunodeficiency and CD4$^+$ cell counts below 200/μl, *Pneumocystis* becomes activated and causes PCP. The nonspecific symptoms of PCP resemble those of early HIV infection—flulike fever, fatigue, and weight loss. The major pulmonary feature of PCP is severe hypoxemia with a PaO_2 less than 60 mm Hg. The most severe pulmonary symptoms are similar to those of adult respiratory distress syndrome (Figure 12-11). These symptoms include decreased phospholipid (surfactant) production, early dry cough, dyspnea, tachypnea, chest discomfort, and marked pallor and cyanosis.

Diagnosis of PCP is by chest radiography, and organisms are identified in sputum with Wright-Giemsa stain. Sputum is induced by using 3% saline via nebulizer, and patients must avoid brushing their teeth, using mouthwash, or eating for 8 hours prior. Other tests that can be performed include bronchoalveolar lavage or biopsy and gallium scanning. Treatment includes the use of intravenous or oral trimethoprim-sulfamethoxazole (Bactrim, Septra) and parenteral and aerosolized pentamidine (NebuPent, Pentam 300). If these medications are not tolerated, other treatments include the use of dapsone-trimethoprim, dapsone-pyrimethamine, atovaquone (Mepron), clindamycin-primaquine, eflornithine, and trimetrexate (Neutrexin).

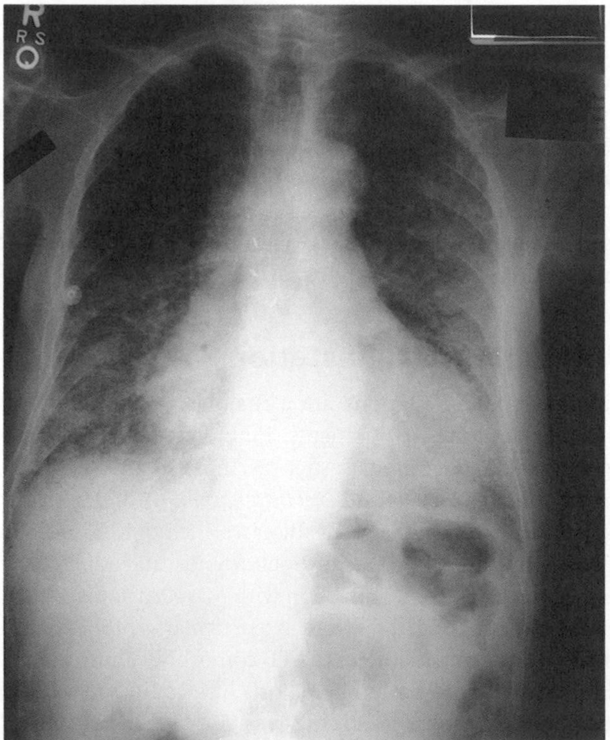

FIGURE 12-11 ■ *Pneumocystis carinii.* A chest radiograph shows bilateral lower lobe interstitial infiltrates. (Courtesy Dr. Paula Karvalho, Veterans Administration Medical Center, Boise, Idaho.)

To prevent other PCP infections by prophylaxis, patients with CD4$^+$ counts of less than 200 cells/μl are given one to two double-strength trimethoprim-sulfamethoxazole tablets either daily or three times per week to prevent the recurrence of infection. This is a very effective suppressive therapy that prevents life-threatening PCP. If patients cannot tolerate it, substitutes include aerosolized pentamidine 300 mg/month, dapsone 200 mg twice weekly, or dapsone with pyrimethamine and leucovorin.

Mucocutaneous Manifestations

Mucocutaneous manifestations occur both early and late in the course of HIV infection. The viral exanthem of HIV infection, associated with seroconversion, is an erythematous, fine maculopapular rash found on the face, trunk, and arms. HIV viral exanthem is a self-limited manifestation that occurs in 40% to 60% of all HIV-infected persons. It is generally seen within 2 to 6 weeks of exposure and lasts up to 1 to 2 weeks. It is associated with mild pruritus, fever, malaise, night sweats, fatigue, pharyngitis, weight loss, diarrhea, headache, and lymphadenopathy.

Other mucocutaneous manifestations may be allergic, infectious, or neoplastic in origin. Cutaneous symptoms depend on the cause and location. Allergic causes may be due to drug reactions or the development of seborrheic dermatitis, psoriasis, or skin-colored papular eruptions.

Viral causes include herpes simplex, varicella zoster, Epstein-Barr virus, and human papillomavirus (Figure 12-12). The development of genital warts (condylomata acuminata) from human papillomavirus is an early symptom of HIV disease in women. For mucocutaneous viral infections, acyclovir (Zovirax) or vidarabine is the recommended antiviral agent.

Oral hairy leukoplakia is an example of an oral mucous membrane viral infection thought to be due to Epstein-Barr virus or human papillomavirus. Oral hairy leukoplakia is characterized by white to gray thickened, raised lesions with vertical folds, corrugations, or "hairs" that form on the tongue

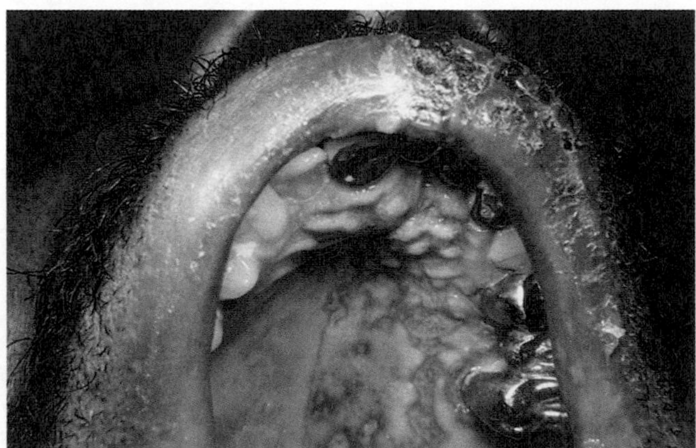

FIGURE 12-12 ■ Herpes zoster in an HIV-infected individual. (From Callen JP: *Color atlas of dermatology,* Philadelphia, 1993, Saunders, p 382.)

and buccal mucosa. Usually they form on the sides of the tongue (Figure 12-13). These lesions cannot be removed or scraped off with a tongue blade, which differentiates this infection from oral candidiasis or thrush. These lesions only occur as the $CD4^+$ count declines. They are not usually painful.

In HIV-infected persons, herpes simplex viruses 1 and 2 cause the formation of large groups of painful vesicles on an erythematous base; these vesicles rupture and crust and become large, ulcerative, and occasionally necrotic. They are chronic, painfully persistent, and usually occur on the genitalia, digits, and perianal or perioral areas. Herpes simplex virus may produce protein that enhances the replication of HIV.

Bacterial infectious causes of mucocutaneous manifestations include *M. avium* or *Staphylococcus aureus. Staphylococcus* is a common bacterial skin infection in patients with HIV associated with folliculitis, furuncles (boils), or bullous impetigo. Occasionally sepsis may occur. Treatment includes topical antibiotics such as clindamycin or mupirocin, use of an antibacterial soap such as chlorhexidine, and systemic antibiotics as needed, including dicloxacillin, cephalosporins, fluoroquinolones, or erythromycin. Abscesses may have to be drained. In patients with recurrent infections, intranasal mupirocin may be used weekly in addition to the aforementioned agents.

Fungal skin infectious agents include *Candida, Cryptococcus,* or *Histoplasma* (Figure 12-14). Vaginal candidiasis is the most common early skin symptom in HIV-positive women. Other infectious agents include parasites such as the mites that cause scabies.

Neoplasms can also occur, including Kaposi sarcoma, squamous cell carcinoma, basal cell carcinoma, or cutaneous lymphomas. Kaposi sarcoma is an AIDS-related malignancy that affects the skin and mucous membranes, lymphatics, and other internal organs. It is one of the few neoplasms indicative of immune system dysfunction.

Before 1981, Kaposi sarcoma was rarely found in the United States except in elderly men of Mediterranean or Eastern European Jewish ancestry. With the AIDS epidemic, it is now found in young, formerly healthy persons who live in the United States, are homosexual or bisexual, and in whom AIDS develops. It rarely occurs in other high-risk groups or in women in the United States. Kaposi sarcoma is the most common tumor found in HIV-infected homosexual men.

The skin lesions of Kaposi sarcoma are individual tumors that begin as flat or macular subcutaneous patches. The patches initially range from light pink to deep purple and are painless, nonblanching, and nonpruritic (Figure 12-15). The lesions evolve from patches into thickened plaques or large nodules that may change to brown over time, especially in darkly pigmented persons. They may occur anywhere on the body, although they usually begin on the head—the face, eyelids, conjunctivae, pinnae, scalp, or buccal membranes (Figure 12-16). Lesions range in size from a few millimeters to coalesced patches covering large areas of the body. The lesions are highly vascular but do not bleed excessively. The lesions may also occur internally in either the lungs or intestines in approximately 40% of patients.

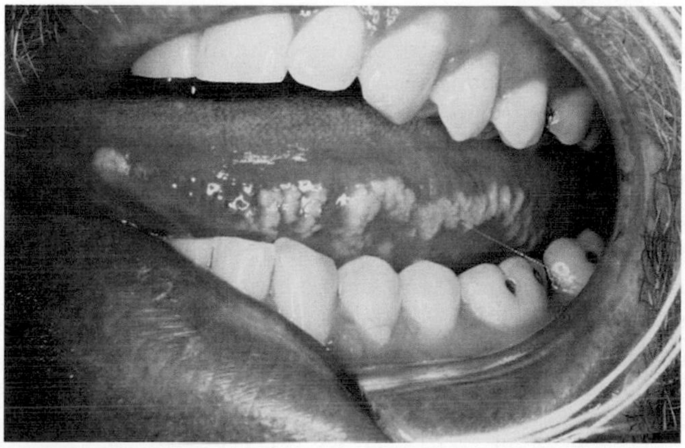

FIGURE 12-13 ■ Oral hairy leukoplakia, a manifestation of Epstein-Barr virus infection in HIV-infected individuals. (From Callen JP: *Color atlas of dermatology,* Philadelphia, 1993, Saunders, p 377.)

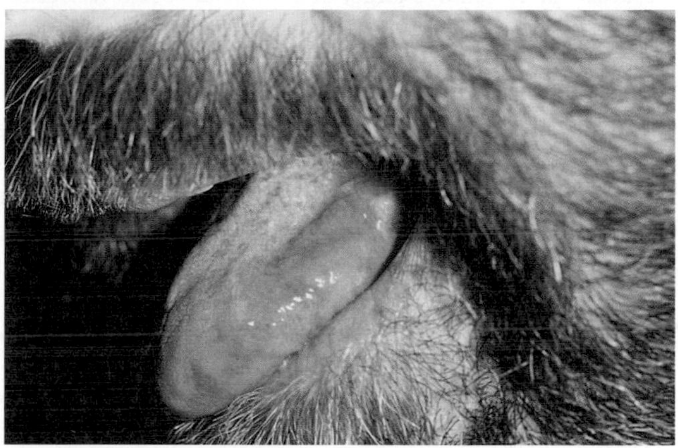

FIGURE 12-14 ■ *Candida albicans* in an HIV-infected person. (From Callen JP: *Color atlas of dermatology,* Philadelphia, 1993, Saunders, p 386.)

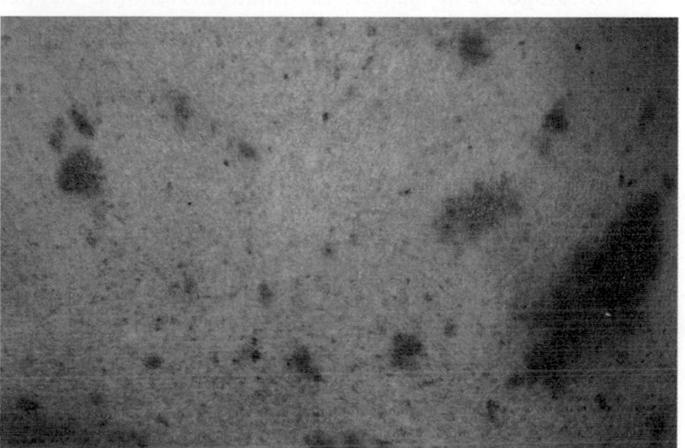

FIGURE 12-15 ■ HIV-associated Kaposi sarcoma in the macular stage. (From Callen JP: *Color atlas of dermatology,* Philadelphia, 1993, Saunders, p 55.)

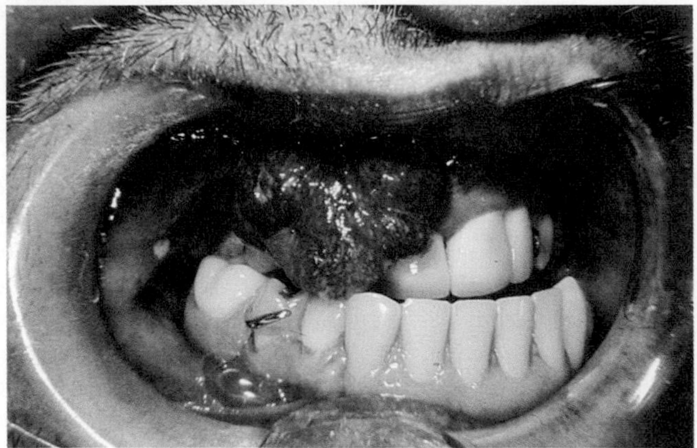

FIGURE 12-16 ■ HIV-associated Kaposi sarcoma in the nodular stage. (From Callen JP: *Color atlas of dermatology,* Philadelphia, 1993, Saunders, p 379.)

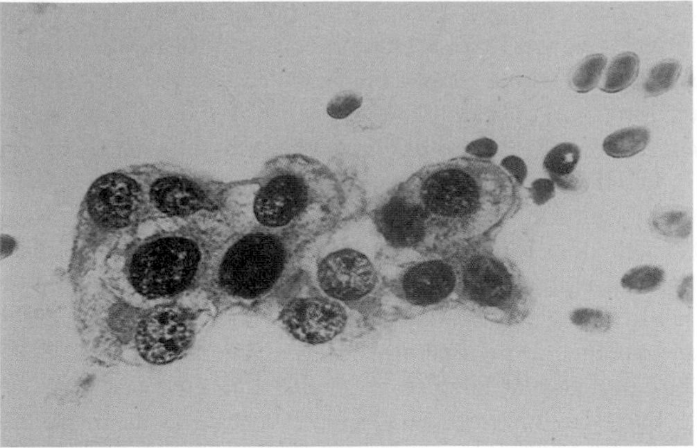

FIGURE 12-17 ■ Cervical dysplasia. Women with AIDS require more frequent monitoring because cervical dysplasia commonly occurs and progresses rapidly.

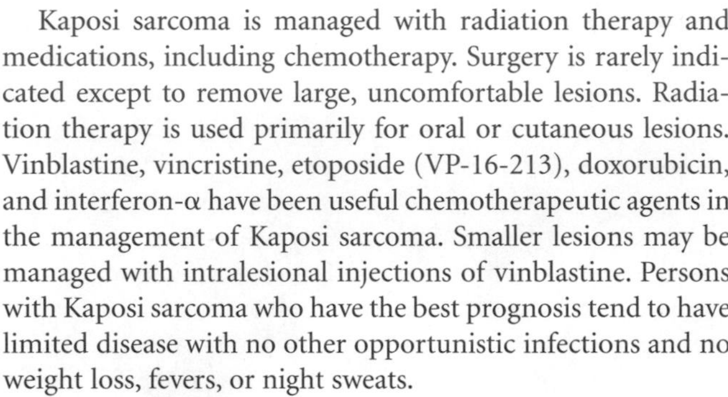

Kaposi sarcoma is managed with radiation therapy and medications, including chemotherapy. Surgery is rarely indicated except to remove large, uncomfortable lesions. Radiation therapy is used primarily for oral or cutaneous lesions. Vinblastine, vincristine, etoposide (VP-16-213), doxorubicin, and interferon-α have been useful chemotherapeutic agents in the management of Kaposi sarcoma. Smaller lesions may be managed with intralesional injections of vinblastine. Persons with Kaposi sarcoma who have the best prognosis tend to have limited disease with no other opportunistic infections and no weight loss, fevers, or night sweats.

Gynecologic Manifestations

Gynecologic manifestations of HIV disease are marked by persistent monilial vaginitis secondary to *C. albicans,* cervical dysplasia, and neoplasia, as well as pelvic inflammatory disease. Cervical dysplasia affects 40% of HIV-infected women (Figure 12-17). Cervical dysplasia has no symptoms, but the cell changes can lead to neoplasia. Therefore, either Papanicolaou smears or colposcopic examinations should be performed every 6 months to detect cervical cancer early in HIV-positive women. Cervical cancer is particularly aggressive in women with HIV. Pelvic inflammatory disease is more common in HIV-positive women. Pelvic inflammatory disease is caused by the same type of organisms, including *C. trachomatis,* and is managed with the same antibiotics as used in non–HIV-infected women.

Neurologic Manifestations

Neurologic manifestations are often the reason that people with HIV seek treatment. HIV invades the neurologic system early in the course of its infection. It infects glial cells, endothelial cells, and brain macrophages. Central and peripheral nervous system manifestations may be due to HIV infection directly or may be due to infectious agents causing meningitis or neoplasms causing space-occupying lesions. Opportunistic infectious agents affecting the neurologic system include *Toxoplasma* and *Cryptococcus.* A variety of peripheral neuropathies can result from HIV infection directly, although some may be due to herpes zoster infection.

HIV encephalopathy (AIDS dementia complex, subacute or AIDS encephalopathy) is the most common neurologic encephalopathic manifestation. HIV encephalopathy is due directly or indirectly to HIV infection or viral products, cytokine-related cellular damage, and the competition or interference between gp120 and neuroleukin, a nerve growth factor. This disorder can affect both adults and children. It occurs when other opportunistic infections begin to appear later in the disease process.

HIV encephalopathy is a syndrome characterized by progressive cognitive impairment or subcortical dementia. In other words, the patient is alert but demented and confused. Computed tomography shows diffuse atrophy in the cerebral cortex, widened sulci, ventricular enlargement, and shrinking of the basal ganglia. Cerebrospinal fluid analysis shows elevated protein and abnormal IgG levels. Symptoms may wax and wane over the course of a day, with intermittent periods of lucidity and confusion.

The cognitive neurologic symptoms associated with HIV encephalopathy include inattentiveness, confusion, forgetfulness, loss of concentration, slower verbal response, headache, apathy, and inability to complete or perform complex tasks. These symptoms can lead to global dementia associated with marked memory impairment and disorientation. Before the motor strength declines, the patient may forget time, place, person, and activities, which can lead to safety issues such as wandering, leaving appliances on, and forgetting to take medications.[16] The associated focal motor deficits include slower motor responses, clumsiness, weakness, loss of balance, handwriting changes, and slurred speech. As HIV encephalopathy progresses, motor strength declines with subsequent large muscle weakness and difficulty walking and moving. Associated generalized symptoms consist of fever and mild metabolic acidosis. Behavioral symptoms include personality changes, social withdrawal, depression, poor hygiene and grooming, lack of insight, apathy, agitation, and, less commonly, anxiety and hyperactivity. In children, head circumference does not increase with age.

As the disorder progresses, the neurologic symptoms become more severe. Ataxia, hypertonia, tremors, and incontinence appear. The person may be alert but cognitively impaired, mute, and paraplegic. Hemianopia (partial blindness), myoclonus, and seizures may also develop. The person may become comatose and lethargic with other systemic dysfunctions. Management of HIV encephalopathy includes treatment with zidovudine (Retrovir), an antiretroviral agent. Other treatment includes coordinating home and environmental safety and patient/family support. A neuroleptic such as haloperidol is occasionally used to control agitation.

Ocular Manifestations

Ocular manifestations of HIV infection may be of infectious or noninfectious origin. Noninfectious causes of ocular problems include HIV retinopathy and malignancy. Infectious causes include bacteria such as *Treponema pallidum* (syphilis) and *Staphylococcus;* fungi including *Candida, Cryptococcus,* and *Histoplasma;* protozoa such as *Pneumocystis* and *Toxoplasma;* and viruses such as herpes simplex and CMV.

The most severe type of ocular infection is CMV retinitis. After an insidious onset, ocular CMV precipitates perivascular hemorrhages, fluffy exudates, and vasculitis in the retina. The CMV retinal infection leads to destruction and necrosis of the retina, with resulting blindness. Management of CMV retinitis includes ganciclovir (Cytovene) intravenously or orally, trisodium phosphonoformate (Foscavir, foscarnet) intravenously, and cidofovir intravitreally. Oral ganciclovir, 1000 mg three times a day (4 tablets three times a day) after the use of intravenous therapy, is a potential prophylactic agent. An intraocular sustained-release ganciclovir implant is also available for the management of acute and chronic CMV retinitis.

HIV-associated retinopathy causes the development of cotton-wool spots and microvascular retinal changes. Cotton-wool spots are small, indistinct white spots with associated hemorrhage. These changes are not as severe as CMV retinitis and may remit spontaneously.

Manifestations in Other Systems

A study by Bozzette et al indicates no increased risk for cardiovascular or cerebrovascular events in patients with HIV. The increased hyperglycemia and hyperlipidemia due to medications for HIV do not seem to increase risk. Therefore, the myocardial infarction and stroke rates are not higher in HIV patients.[17]

Renal impairment can also occur with HIV infection. HIV can affect the kidneys and cause AIDS-associated nephropathy (AIDS-related glomerulopathy), drug-induced ischemia, and renal failure. Hematologically, individuals with HIV have anemia, thrombocytopenia, and granulocytopenia.

HIV-related endocrine dysfunction is usually associated with changes in hormone secretion secondary to the stress response; destruction of endocrine tissue from infection, cancer, or inflammation; or the use of pharmacologic agents. The adrenal gland is the organ most affected by HIV infection. Adrenal secretion of cortisol may be elevated at the expense of other hormones. Injury to the adrenal gland rarely leads to frank cortisol deficiencies. Most endocrine dysfunction is subtle, with few overt manifestations. Triiodothyronine, thyroxine, and thyroid-binding globulin levels may be elevated.

Rheumatologic manifestations of HIV infection are varied and include osteoporosis, osteopenia, as well as musculoskeletal infections such as infectious arthritis and osteomyelitis, which are due to a decrease in the number of T cells. In patients with musculoskeletal infections, the most common organisms involved are *S. aureus, Streptococcus pneumoniae, C. albicans, Mycobacterium kansasii,* and *Mycobacterium avium-intracellulare.* Other manifestations are due to immune-mediated arthritis, such as Reiter disease, psoriatic arthritis, and undifferentiated spondyloarthropathy syndromes, or due to disorders occurring as a direct result of the immune response to HIV, including polymyositis, vasculitis, and immune complex diseases related to the production of autoantibodies. However, the increasing incidence of osteopenia and osteoporosis in the HIV population is significant.[18] The actual cause for this increase is unclear but may be related to antiretroviral therapy. Treatment includes using biphosphonate medications and selective estrogen receptor moderators. The treatment is more difficult in men.

Manifestations in Children

Children with HIV become symptomatic much faster than adults—usually within their first year of life. Because of the invasion of virus, children's growth and development are markedly affected, including physical growth retardation with failure to thrive, impaired intellectual development, and impaired motor functioning with decreased coordination. The infant develops normally until the virus begins its nervous system invasion. After that time, neurologic impairment is characterized by development of weakness, loss of previously accomplished developmental milestones, hypotonia, or hypertonia.

More serious bacterial and viral infections also develop in children who undergo repeated bouts of communicable diseases such as chickenpox. Extensive candidiasis without any relationship to antibiotic therapy may be an early symptom. Respiratory problems, including the development of PCP, are common.

Because lactose intolerance is common in these children, soy formulas are often used. Dairy products may be introduced into the diet gradually as tolerated. Children need particular attention to their diet; increased calories and protein, as well as nutrient-rich snacks such as raisins and peanuts for growth and development, are advisable.

KEY CONCEPTS

- All body systems are affected by HIV.
- Early HIV infection is characterized by fever, chills, headaches, nausea, vomiting, diarrhea, fatigue, weakness, arthralgia, sore throat, stiff neck, photophobia, irritability, and rash.
- The most significant systemic symptom is malnutrition or wasting, which is due to a combination of various factors, including an elevated metabolic rate, chronic inflammation, malabsorption, anorexia, and the effect of multiple opportunistic insults.
- GI symptoms occur frequently in patients with HIV. Symptoms include diarrhea caused by *Cryptosporidium* or other agents, ulceration, and candidiasis, as well as multiple opportunistic infections.
- Pulmonary symptoms include opportunistic pneumonias (particularly PCP), tuberculosis, and adult respiratory distress syndrome.
- Mucocutaneous symptoms occur both early and late in the course of HIV infection. One of the first symptoms is the viral exanthem that occurs during the primary infection. Other manifestations may be allergic; infectious, such as candidiasis or herpes, human papillomavirus, and Epstein-Barr virus infections; or neoplastic, such as Kaposi sarcoma.
- Neurologic manifestations include peripheral neuropathy, encephalopathy with dementia, headache, apathy, and focal deficits.
- Gynecologic manifestations include persistent monilial vaginitis, cervical dysplasia, and pelvic inflammatory disease.
- Ocular manifestations include HIV-associated retinopathy, CMV retinitis, malignancy, and a variety of infectious causes.
- AIDS, the end stage of HIV infection, is characterized by opportunistic infections and tumor formation.
- Children with HIV have growth and development problems, including impaired physical growth, intellectual development, and motor functioning.

TREATMENT

Antiretroviral Therapy Recommendations

The goal of medication and therapeutic management of HIV/AIDS is to delay disease progression, decrease resistance, minimize clinical manifestations, and ultimately prolong survival. Drug management of HIV infection has evolved from monotherapy, or therapy with one agent, to the use of multiple medications—called highly active antiretroviral therapy (HAART). This polydrug therapy approach involves the administration of two or three antiretroviral agents; it provides better viral suppression, thereby decreasing viral load, increasing CD4 counts, and decreasing resistance for a longer period. The objective of HAART is to provide the greatest viral suppression for the longest time to prevent viral mutations. This approach makes good sense. If one drug blocks 90% of viral replication, the others may eliminate the rest of the resistant virions. However, even with HAART, complete viral eradication is not possible with current treatment strategies.

Arguments have been made both for and against early antiretroviral therapy. Those for early antiretroviral therapy wish to preserve as much of the functional immune system as possible; once destroyed, it cannot be regenerated. Those against are concerned about preventing viral resistance, particularly when infected individuals must comply with complex and undesirable dosing schedules. However, HAART is most advocated due to the optimal goal of therapy with maximal viral suppression.

HIV drug treatment failures are due to HIV resistance, which is a widespread problem and concern. Failure of HIV drug treatment is usually due to poor adherence to HAART, poor toleration of the drugs, prior exposure to single or multiple antiretroviral drug therapy, or counteracting interactions among the drugs used. It is easy to see why persons taking the multidrug regimen may fail to comply with nutritional and drug therapy because of the sheer volume of drugs to be taken in a day. A person infected with HIV must take at least 13 to 30 pills per day; he or she must also remember which ones should be taken with food or on an empty stomach and which ones cannot be taken together at the same time. In addition, some persons with HIV/AIDS may be demented because of the disease, homelessness, or addiction to intravenous drugs, any of which limits their ability to adhere to the strict treatment regimens. Finally, some of the treatments for opportunistic infection or cancer involve many other drugs: intravenous, oral, and intracavital.

Current recommendations for antiretroviral therapy for HIV include starting therapy for all HIV-infected persons with detectable HIV RNA plasma levels or for anyone with levels above 5000 to 10,000 copies per milliliter of plasma. In patients with low HIV RNA plasma levels (less than 500 copies per milliliter) and high $CD4^+$ counts, therapy may be withheld and the patient reevaluated every 3 to 6 months. Early antiretroviral treatment seems to be better tolerated by patients and helps to prolong life. However, there is increased risk of medication and metabolic complications, osteoporosis, and hyperlipidemia.[17]

Some of the current medications available to adults with HIV have not been recommended for children younger than 13 years. In the past, treatment was often delayed weeks or months before starting therapy. Now it is recommended that multidrug therapy be begun at birth; however, virion levels are usually not detectable for up to 2 weeks after birth. Therefore, some physicians recommend intensive therapy for all infants born to HIV-positive women even though the infant may not have infection. This controversial method is not universal but does take into consideration the rapid progression of infection in infants.

The three major classes of antiretroviral medications are nucleoside analogs or nucleoside reverse transcriptase inhibitors, nonnucleoside reverse transcriptase inhibitors or nonnucleoside analogs, and protease inhibitors. All of these antiretroviral medications block viral replication within cells by inhibiting either reverse transcriptase or protease. The current optimal combination of medications is multidrug therapy with two nucleoside analogs and one or two protease inhibitors or two nucleosides and a nonnucleoside reverse transcriptase inhibitor, which is called *protease sparing regimen.* Viral resistance to treatment is reduced by the complete suppression of virus (Figure 12-18). However, multidrug therapy retails at approximately $900 to $1400 per month, and compliance with complicated drug therapy that has many side effects is variable. Virus resistance increases with treatment protocol noncompliance. Total drug holidays for periods of time may actually bolster patient compliance and not affect resistance.

Nucleoside Reverse Transcriptase Inhibitors

Nucleoside reverse transcriptase inhibitors resemble the natural substances used by the virus to build HIV DNA. Nucleoside reverse transcriptase inhibitors prevent HIV replication by preventing HIV DNA synthesis and have been found to slow progression of the disease (Table 12-3).

Nucleoside analogs include zidovudine, didanosine, zalcitabine, stavudine, lamivudine, and abacavir. All of them must be converted to an active state intracellularly. Class side effects include pancreatitis, bone marrow toxicity, peripheral neuropathy, and hepatic toxicity. Of the nucleoside reverse transcriptase inhibitors, the first and most widely used is zidovudine (3-azido-3-deoxythymidine, AZT, Retrovir). Zidovudine is rapidly absorbed when taken orally and can penetrate the blood-brain barrier. Its efficacy decreases in 1 to 3 years if used alone. It may improve platelet counts in cases of immune thrombocytopenia. Usual dosages include 200 to 600 mg orally every 8 hours or 300 mg in a slow-release formulation orally every 12 hours (usually one pill twice per day). Typical side effects include headache, nausea, vomiting, insomnia, malaise, myalgia, confusion, hepatitis, neutropenia, and bone marrow suppression. Subjective side effects, such as headache and nausea, usually decrease or end within 6 weeks. A CBC with differential must be done every 3 months when stable. Zidovudine is usually given to HIV-infected women during pregnancy as early as the 14th week of gestation. It is a pregnancy category C drug. Exactly how AZT blocks transmission to the fetus is unknown, but passive transplacental drug transport does occur. The long-term consequences of AZT use in pregnancy are unknown.

Stavudine (d4T, Zerit) is most often used as a substitute for zidovudine in initial combination therapy. It is a potent antiviral that does penetrate cerebrospinal fluid well. It should not be combined with zidovudine. The usual dosage is 20 to 40 mg orally twice daily (usually one pill twice per day). Side effects include dose-related peripheral neuropathy and, rarely, pancreatitis. Liver function studies should be performed every 3 months.

Didanosine (ddI, Videx) is the second oldest nucleoside analog. It is sometimes effective in patients resistant to zidovudine. It is available as a capsule, chewable tablet, or powder for oral solution. It must be taken on an empty stomach. Usual dosages are 125 to 300 mg orally every 12 hours (usually two pills twice per day). Side effects include dry mouth, nausea, vomiting, diarrhea, abdominal pain, painful dose-related peripheral neuropathy, and pancreatitis. It can also cause severe lactic acidosis. Patients cannot use alcohol concurrently, and in the case of sodium-sensitive patients, didanosine contains sodium. The new capsule form is buffered and causes less diarrhea. Didanosine cannot be given with

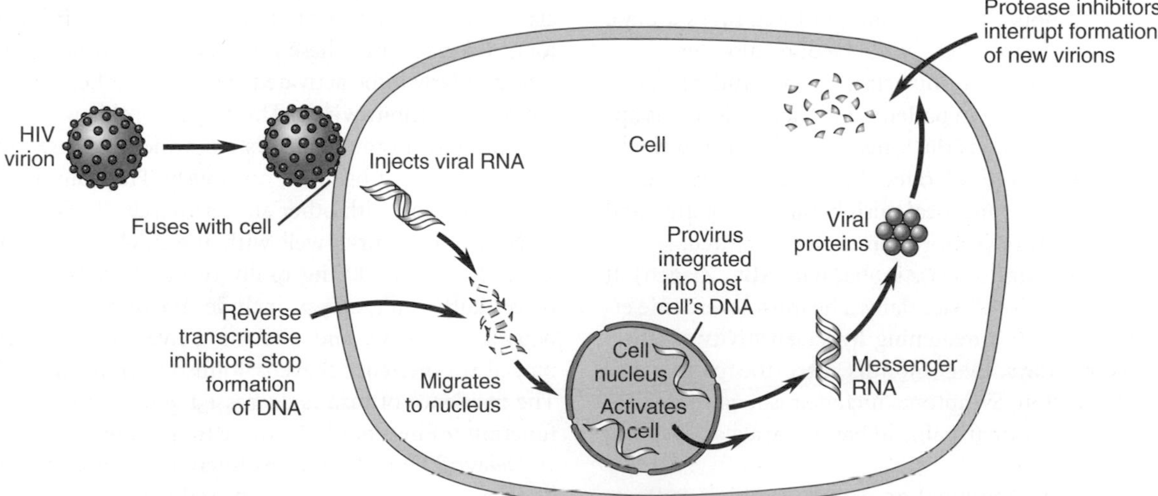

FIGURE 12-18 ■ Antiretroviral therapy. The stages in the life cycle of HIV in which antiretroviral therapy is effective are shown.

Table 12-3

Nucleoside Reverse Transcriptase Inhibitors

Class side effects: Pancreatitis, bone marrow toxicity, peripheral neuropathy, hepatic toxicity

Drug/Brand Name	Dosage	Additional Side Effects	Laboratory Work Needed	Cautions
Zidovudine (AZT, Retrovir)	200-600 mg po q8h *or* 300 mg XR q12h *Children:* 90-180 mg/m^2 up to 200 mg q8h	Headache, nausea, vomiting, insomnia, malaise, myalgia, confusion	CBC q3mo	—
Stavudine (d4T, Zerit)	20-40 mg po bid (usually 1 pill bid) *Children:* 1 mg/kg bid (for children <30 kg)	—	Liver function studies q3mo	Do not give with zidovudine
Didanosine (ddl, Videx)	125-300 mg po q12h *Children:* 120 mg/m^2 po bid	Dry mouth, nausea, vomiting, *diarrhea,* abdominal pain, severe lactic acidosis	CBC, potassium, and liver function studies q1mo	Must be taken on empty stomach
Zalcitabine (ddc, Hivid)	0.375-0.75 mg q8h	Oral and esophageal ulcers	CBC and liver function studies q1mo	Must be taken on empty stomach
Lamivudine (3TC, Epivir)	150 mg po bid *or* 300 mg po qd *Children:* 4 mg/kg up to 150 mg po bid	Nausea, malaise, fatigue, headaches	CBC and liver function studies q3mo	—
Abacavir (ABC, Ziagen)	300 mg bid *Children >3 mo:* 8 mg/kg up to 300 mg bid	Life-threatening hypersensitivity reaction	CBC and liver function studies q3mo	Never rechallenge if hypersensitivity occurs

CBC, Complete blood cell count; *XR,* extended release.

zalcitabine. CBC and potassium and liver function studies must be performed every month.

Zalcitabine (ddC, Hivid) is the least potent in this nucleoside class. It is associated with oral and esophageal ulcers, peripheral neuropathy, and pancreatitis. The usual dosage is 0.375 to 0.75 mg orally every 8 hours (usually one pill three times a day). CBC and liver function studies should be done monthly.

Another medication in this class is lamivudine (3TC, Epivir), which is also used in patients with hepatitis B. It is approved for children and has the longest half-life. It is well absorbed and generally well tolerated. Side effects include nausea, malaise, fatigue, headaches, peripheral neuropathy, and pancreatitis. Pancreatitis is more common in children.

The newest agent in this class is abacavir (ABC, Ziagen). It is very potent and is given twice daily. The most severe side effect is a potentially life-threatening hypersensitivity reaction occurring several days to 6 months after the patient has started the medication. Symptoms include rash, nausea, vomiting, diarrhea, abdominal pain, lethargy, myalgia, dyspnea, and cough.

There are two new combination drugs: Combivir containing zidovudine 300 mg and lamivudine 150 mg; and Trizivir containing abacavir 300 mg, lamivudine 150 mg, and zidovudine 300 mg.

Nonnucleoside Reverse Transcriptase Inhibitors

Nonnucleoside reverse transcriptase inhibitors also inhibit reverse transcriptase, but by a different mechanism. Drugs in this class include nevirapine (Viramune) and delavirdine (Rescriptor), and efavirenz. These medications need not be converted intracellularly to be activated. The greatest benefit is that they are potent antiretrovirals. The biggest problem is that they affect the cytochrome P-450 system, which increases drug interactions and must be given cautiously. They can only be given in combination with other antiretrovirals (Table 12-4).

Nevirapine works well with the nucleoside analogs. The usual dosage is 200 mg orally twice a day (usually one pill twice daily). Side effects include maculopapular rash, fever, nausea, headache, and abnormal liver function tests. They may also experience Stevens-Johnson syndrome or hepatitis. The incidence of rash is decreased when started slowly. Liver function testing should be done frequently.

Delavirdine is difficult to tolerate because four pills must be taken three times per day mixed with water and not given within an hour of antacids or didanosine. It can cause similar side effects as those listed with nevirapine. It does not cross the blood-brain barrier.

Table 12-4

Nonnucleoside Reverse Transcriptase Inhibitors

Class side effects: Affect cytochrome P-450 system, maculopapular rash, nausea, headache, hepatitis, or elevated liver function test results

Drug/Brand Name	Dosage	Additional Side Effects	Laboratory Work Needed	Cautions
Nevirapine (Viramune, NVP)	200 mg bid (start with 200 mg qd × 14 days) *Children <8 yr:* 7 mg/kg bid *Children ≥8 yr:* 4 mg/kg bid	Stevens-Johnson syndrome	Liver function tests q1-3mo	—
Delavirdine (Rescriptor, DLV)	400 mg tid *Children ≥16 yr:* 400 mg po tid	Stevens-Johnson syndrome	Liver function tests q1-3mo	Must not give within 1 hr of antacids or didanosine
Efavirenz (Sustiva, EFV)	*Adults/children >40 kg:* 600 mg capsules qd *Children ≥3 yr and 10-15 kg:* 200 mg po qhs *Children ≥3 yr and 15-20 kg:* 250 mg po qhs *Children 20-25 kg:* 300 mg qhs	Dizziness, drowsiness, problems concentrating, insomnia, "hangover," vivid dreams	Liver function tests q1-3mo	Do not give with a high-fat meal Best taken between 6 and 9 PM

Efavirenz (EFV, Sustiva) can be given once daily in 600-mg capsules. It can be taken with meals or on an empty stomach. It is best taken between 6 and 9 PM to allow the patient to sleep through many of the side effects. Side effects include central nervous system effects (dizziness, drowsiness, concentration problems, insomnia, vivid dreams, and "hangover" in the morning), rash, nausea, vomiting, diarrhea, and liver enzyme elevations.

Protease Inhibitors

Protease inhibitors attack at another phase in the viral life cycle. These medications inhibit the enzyme protease, whose action is to clip the viral protein precursors to the appropriate size. These precursors are essential for HIV maturation, infection, and replication. Protease inhibitor therapy is extremely expensive, with a retail price of approximately $6000 to $8000 per year. Protease inhibitors are never used as single agents because of the potential for a patient to develop resistance. They have poor CNS penetration and cause lipodystrophy, including development of "buffalo hump," increased abdominal girth, and increased breast size. They also interact with the cytochrome P-450 system. Protease inhibitors include saquinavir, ritonavir, indinavir, nelfinavir, and amprenavir (Table 12-5).

Saquinavir (Invirase [hard-gel], Fortovase [soft-gel]) is highly active against HIV, especially when used in combination with zidovudine, didanosine, or zalcitabine. It is the best tolerated of the protease inhibitors and should be taken with high-fat meals. Saquinavir is easily absorbed but quickly metabolized in the liver by cytochrome P-450 and thus has poor bioavailability. Only 4% of the drug is available in the blood stream. It should be given cautiously with other medications. The usual dosage is 1200 mg orally every 8 hours (usually six pills three times per day). Side effects include abdominal discomfort, nausea, diarrhea, rash, and hyperlipidemia.

Ritonavir (Norvir) is a potent inhibitor of HIV that is found in high concentrations in serum and lymph nodes. It is well absorbed but must be taken with food to reduce side effects. Ritonavir no longer has to be refrigerated and can be kept at room temperature. It contains alcohol. It is conveniently dosed at 600 mg orally every 12 hours (usually six pills twice a day). The side effects of ritonavir are related to its plasma level and are quite severe and poorly tolerated. Side effects include asthenia, nausea, diarrhea, vomiting, anorexia, abdominal pain, taste perversion, and circumoral and peripheral paresthesias. These side effects have caused some patients to stop taking the medication. It also interacts with many medications. Liver function tests and triglyceride levels should be monitored. The medication has an unpleasant taste, but there are many ways to disguise it by coating the mouth with peanut butter, licorice, chocolate syrup, jelly, honey, popsicles, or chewing gum.

Table 12-5

Protease Inhibitors

Class side effects: Lipodystrophy, increased abdominal girth, interaction with cytochrome P-450 system, hyperlipidemia, nausea, diarrhea

Drug/Brand Name	Dosage	Additional Side Effects	Laboratory Work Needed	Cautions
Saquinavir (Invirase, Fortovase)	1200 mg (6 tablets of 200 mg) q8h *Children:* 33 mg/kg po tid	Rash	Lipid panel, glucose, liver function tests	Take with high-fat meal Use with caution with other medications
Ritonavir (Norvir)	600 mg (6 tablets of 100 mg) q8h	Unpleasant taste, taste perversion, anorexia, circumoral and peripheral paresthesias	Lipid panel, glucose, liver function tests	Must take with food Soft gel capsules contain 43% alcohol; usually poorly tolerated
Indinavir (Crixivan)	800 mg (2 tablets of 400 mg) q8h	Insomnia, taste changes, renal calculi, hemolytic anemia	Lipid panel, glucose, liver function tests, CBC	Must take on empty stomach or light, low-fat, low-protein meal Must take only q8h
Nelfinavir (Viracept)	750 mg q8h or 1250 mg (5 tablets of 250 mg) bid *Children:* 20-45 mg/kg po tid	Flatulence, hyperglycemia	Lipid panel, glucose, liver function tests, CBC	Diarrhea (responds to Imodium)
Amprenavir (Agenerase)	1200 mg (8 tablets of 150 mg) bid *Children <50 kg:* 20 mg/kg up to 1200 mg	Rash, perioral numbness, fatigue, paresthesias	Lipid panel, glucose, liver function tests, CBC	Contains sulfonamide, so patients allergic to sulfa cannot take

CBC, Complete blood cell count.

Indinavir (Crixivan) has good antiviral properties but also moderately inhibits cytochrome P-450. The usual dosage is 800 mg orally every 8 hours (usually two pills three times daily). It should be taken on an empty stomach or with a light, low-fat, low-protein meal. Side effects include vomiting, nausea, abdominal pain, insomnia, lipodystrophy, pharyngitis, taste changes, elevated bilirubin, flank pain with the development of renal calculi. Hemolytic anemia may occur. Some believe that indinavir is the best of the class because of its modest side effects.

Nelfinavir (Viracept) is popular because of its less complicated dosing. Patients can take 750 mg three times per day or five tablets (1250 mg) twice per day. Its most bothersome side effect is diarrhea, although it does respond to loperamide (Imodium). Other side effects include flatulence, rash, headache, nausea, lipodystrophy, hyperlipidemia, and hyperglycemia.

Amprenavir (Agenerase) is the drug of choice when patients are resistant to other protease inhibitors. The pill burden is high—eight tablets (1200 mg) twice per day. It also contains a large amount of vitamin E and is a sulfonamide. Therefore, patients with sulfa allergy cannot take this medication. It should not be given during pregnancy. Side effects include rash, nausea, vomiting, diarrhea, headache, perioral numbness and tingling, fatigue, and paresthesias.

Other Treatments and Vaccines

Human granulocyte colony-stimulating factor (filgrastim [Neupogen]) is also being used to increase nonspecific immunity by increasing neutrophils in persons with neutropenia. This agent is particularly helpful in decreasing medication-induced neutropenia. It is given daily in a subcutaneous dose calculated by weight (usually 5 μg/kg). Epoetin alfa (erythropoietin) is also used to manage medication-induced anemia secondary to AZT use. The starting dosage is 8000 U subcutaneously per week and may be increased to 48,000 U/wk until the hematocrit is 35% to 40%. An associated side effect is hypertension. Intravenous immunoglobulin can sometimes be used in HIV-infected children with T-cell counts above 200/μl. It shows a decrease in the incidence of serious bacterial, minor bacterial, viral, and opportunistic infections.

Other studies are being conducted in an effort to find ways to rebuild the immune system. Researchers want to make sure that the T cells cloned after initiation of antiretroviral therapy will respond to both new and old infections. Currently, interleukin-2 (IL-2), a T-cell growth factor, is being infused intravenously or given subcutaneously intermittently for 5 days every 8 weeks. The strategy is effective in increasing populations of T cells, but it also increases the viral load transiently during treatment.

Prevention of HIV infection by active immunity conferred by vaccine is the ultimate goal of current research. This task is extremely difficult because of variability between strains of HIV and the frequency of HIV mutations. At this time, several experimental vaccines are being tested in either phase I or phase II trials. The HGP-30 vaccine contains a synthetic copy of p17, a core HIV protein, which is simple and inexpensive to prepare. The concern is whether it could become a provirus and be integrated into cellular DNA. Gp160 vaccine has been developed from a genetically engineered form of gp160, an HIV envelope protein. The results of the study by VaxGen released in 2003 were disappointing and showed no benefit of vaccine over placebo. A humanized monoclonal antibody vaccine against either the CD4-gp120 binding site or the immunodominant V_3 loop of gp120 is also being studied. This vaccine is currently in phase I and II trials. Unfortunately, to date vaccine-elicited antibodies have failed to recognize HIV in patients. A vaccine developed by Jonas Salk is made from inactivated HIV that has had its envelope removed and its immunogenic proteins enhanced. This vaccine would boost the immune response to HIV in persons already infected. Other vaccines, including HIV peptides, live vector viruses, and pseudovirions, are currently in some phase of trials. Ongoing research is being carried out in an effort to quantify the effectiveness of these vaccines in stimulating both cellular and humoral responses to HIV.

KEY CONCEPTS

- Management of HIV and AIDS includes the use of antiretroviral medications, including nucleoside reverse transcriptase inhibitors, nonnucleoside reverse transcriptase inhibitors, and protease inhibitors.
- The current optimal combination of medications is triple therapy with two reverse transcriptase inhibitors and a protease inhibitor.
- Efforts to stimulate immune function with peptide growth factors and the development of vaccines are under investigation.
- Aggressive treatment of opportunistic infections with appropriate antibiotics and antivirals is a large part of the treatment regimen.

SUMMARY

HIV is an RNA virus that primarily infects and destroys the immune system. In so doing it destroys one of the basic foundations of human regulation and protection. HIV decreases the body's ability to fight organisms, opens the door to opportunistic infections, and allows neoplasms to emerge with ease. HIV can infect anyone of any age. The ultimate parasite, it slowly destroys the host while manufacturing billions of copies of itself. Study of this virus has improved our understanding of the immune system as well as cellular function.

MEDIA RESOURCES

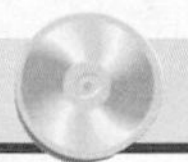

evolve

Remember to check out the ***CD Companion*** included with this book for Review Questions, Key Concepts Review, Glossary (with audio for selected terms), Disease Profiles, and Animations.

PLUS, visit the ***Evolve website*** at http://evolve.elsevier.com/Copstead/ for Case Studies, Disease Profiles, and WebLinks.

References

1. Janssen RS et al: Advancing HIV prevention: new strategies for a changing epidermic—United States, 2003, *MMWR Morb Mortal Wkly Rep* 52(15):329-332, 2003.
2. Update: AIDS—United States, 2000, *MMWR Morb Mortal Wkly Rep* 51(27):592-595, 2002.
3. Varmus H: Retroviruses, *Science* 240:1427-1435, 1988.
4. Balter M: Virus from 1959 sample marks early years of HIV, *Science* 279:801, 1998.
5. Garry RF et al: Documentation of an AIDS virus infection in the United States in 1968, *JAMA* 260(14):2085-2087, 1988.
6. Lemey P et al: Tracing the origin and history of the HIV-2 epidemic, *Proc Natl Acad Sci U S A* 10.1073/pnas.0936469100, 2003.
7. O'Brien SJ, Dean M: In search of AIDS-resistance genes, *Sci Am* 40(3):41-44, 1997.
8. Winkler C et al: Genetic restriction of AIDS pathogenesis by an SDF-1 chemokine gene variant, *Science* 279:389-393, 1998.
9. Pomerantz RJ: A tough viral nut to crack, *Nature* 48(6898):594-595, 2002.
10. Balter M: AIDS researchers negotiate tricky slopes of science, *Science* 280:825-826, 1998.
11. Cohen J: Women: absent term in the AIDS research equation, *Science* 269(5225):777-780, 1995.
12. Sheehy AM et al: Isolation of a human gene that inhibits HIV-1 infection and is suppressed by the viral vif protein, *Nature* 48(6898):646-650, 2002.
13. McDonald D et al: Recruitment of HIV and its receptors to dendritic-cell–T-cell junctions, *Science* 300(5623):1295-1297, 2003.
14. Centers for Disease Control and Prevention: 1993 Revised classification system for HIV infection and expanded surveillance case definition for AIDS among adolescents and adults, *MMWR Morb Mortal Wkly Rep* 41(RR-17):1-6, 1992.
15. Wooland S: Wasting syndrome in HIV-AIDS patients: a guide to prevention and management, *Adv Nurse Practitioners* 9(9):42-48, 2001.
16. Coyne PJ, Lyne ME, Watson AC: Symptom management in people with AIDS, *Am J Nurs* 102(9):48-55, 2002.
17. Bozzette SA et al: Cardiovascular and cerebrovascular events in patients treated for human immunodeficiency virus infection, *N Engl J Med* 348:702-710, 2003.
18. Greene MD: Older HIV patients face metabolic complications, *Nurse Practitioner* 28(66):17-28, 2003.

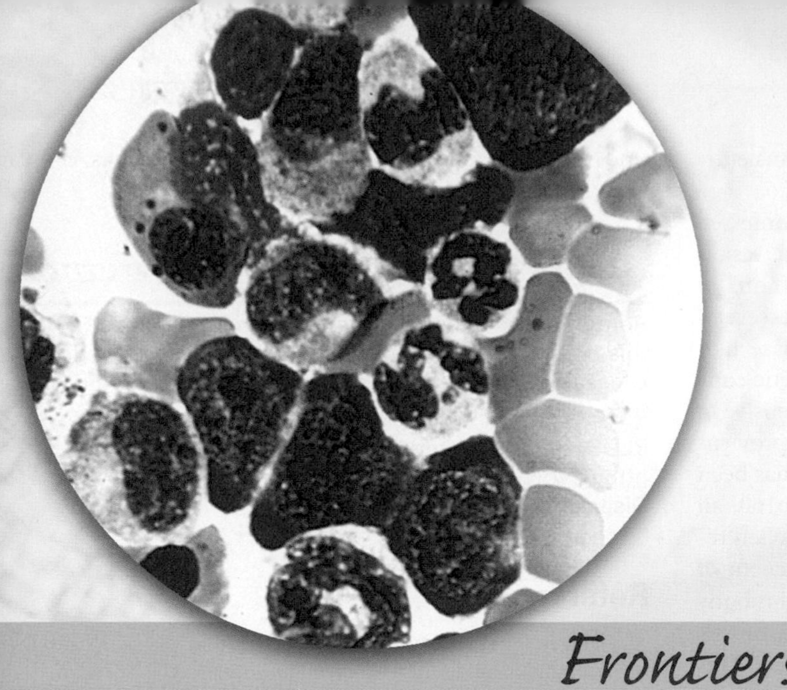

Frontiers of Research

Blood and Circulatory Disorders

Ronald S. Go and Michael J. Kirkhorn

Voluntary blood donors are among the heroines and heroes of our time. They provide the precious fluid that allows the survival of accident victims and surgical patients. However, at times voluntarism is not enough. When blood replacement supplies run low, an additional concern is added to the multitude of worries that attend therapy and healing; such shortages revive one of the dreams of medicine: to find ways to bypass the donor. Gene therapy may eventually produce the means for therapeutic production of blood cells.

Donors donate, but the producers of blood cells are hormones—specifically, hematopoietic growth factors, or hemopoietins. They provide the variety of blood cell types that the body requires.

All of the many types of blood cells develop from a single type that originates in the bone marrow, stem cells, which have been called the one of the most primitive cells known to exist in the body. Stem cells reside in the bone marrow—in adults, principally the marrow of membranous bones. The supply of red blood cells issuing from the marrow is regulated by a feedback cycle that ensures an adequate supply of cells for tissue oxygenation. When oxygen carried to the tissues decreases, the bone marrow immediately begins to produce more red blood cells, as it does in response to various forms of anemia. White blood cells, or leukocytes, which are indispensable to the immune system's ability to resist disease, are formed in the bone marrow and in lymph tissue.

In November 1998, scientists at the University of Wisconsin and Johns Hopkins University announced that they had isolated and grown embryonic stem cells. The development of therapies from this discovery will require years of laboratory work, but the culturing of these cells is crucial because it places medical science at the bedrock of cell development, the gestational stage at which cells are differentiated for the development of body organs. It could lead to therapies for previously untreatable diseases by creating new cells that could replace diseased cardiac, brain, or renal tissue; introduce nerve cells to repair tissue lost in spinal injury; or restore bone marrow to replace blood-forming organs damaged by disease or radiation.

Because the blood is contained in a dynamic system and that system is influenced by the ordinary details of daily life—what we eat and how much, whether we exercise, the state of our emotions—healthy blood flow is also a frontier of research. Nowhere is this frontier more evident than in our increasing understanding of the serious health consequences of high blood pressure and the simple daily choices that can prevent illness.

The human body is a container of carefully balanced pressures. The flow of blood is monitored by the body. When pressures exceed the limits tolerated by monitoring systems, the body's controls

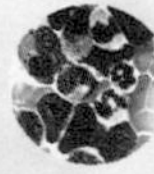

Megaloblastic anemia (bone marrow aspirate). (From Kumar V, Abbas AK, Fausto N: Robbins and Cotran pathologic basis of disease, *ed 7, Philadelphia, 2005, Saunders. Courtesy Dr. Jose Hernandez, Department of Pathology, University of Texas Southwestern Medical School, Dallas.)*

Oxygen Transport, Blood Coagulation, Blood Flow, and Blood Pressure

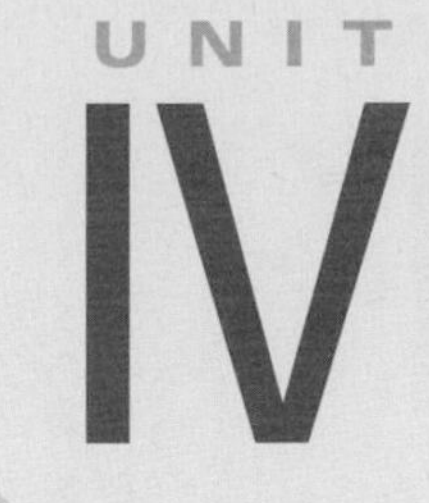

may be activated. Blood flow to each tissue is monitored by microvessels, which measure what each tissue needs, thus controlling local blood flow. Nervous control of circulation also helps control tissue blood flow.

The heart pays attention to the demands of the tissues by responding to the return of blood through the veins and to nerve signals that make it pump the required amounts of blood. The arterial pressure itself is carefully regulated; if it falls below its normal mean level, immediate circulatory changes—increased heart pumping, contraction of venous reservoirs, constriction of arterioles—provide more blood for the arteriolar tree. Kidneys play their part by secreting pressure-controlling hormones and by regulating blood volume.

Hypertension, or high blood pressure, is a concern because it influences a number of disorders, including stroke, coronary artery disease, and renal disease. Current estimates indicate that about 50 million Americans, slightly less than 20% of the population, suffer from high blood pressure.

Findings from the Treatment of Mild Hypertension Study reported in 1993 have contributed to understanding the effects of lifestyle modifications, including weight reduction, restriction of sodium consumption, aerobic exercise, and reduction of alcohol drinking, in subjects with only marginally high blood pressure.

An article in the *Journal of the American Medical Association* suggests that the results of this long-term study—a significant reduction in blood pressure and no additional treatment required for 59% of the volunteer subjects—indicate that "lifestyle modification be used as definitive or adjunctive therapy in all hypertensive patients." Citing another study by the Veterans Administration Cooperative Study Group on Antihypertensive Agents, the same article points out that the lifestyle study interventions produced results equaling those achieved with diltiazem hydrochloride, which was shown by the Veterans Administration study to be the drug most successful in lowering diastolic blood pressure.

The importance of lifestyle—our daily habits, guided or unguided by prudence—is substantiated by other recent findings. A report on the Framingham Study, in which a group of men and women with no initial signs of hypertension were monitored for 18 to 20 years to determine whether anxiety and anger influenced the onset of hypertension, showed that "feelings of anxiety or tension may increase the risk of hypertension among middle-aged men." In this study, no relationship between anxiety and hypertension was found in middle-aged women. The researchers recommended consideration of "behavioral treatment for hypertension . . . as part of a nonpharmacologic treatment program among anxious middle-aged men with mild to moderate hypertension" and as an adjunct to treatment with antihypertensive drugs.

chapter 13

Alterations in Oxygen Transport

Marie L. Kotter • Susan G. Osguthorpe

MEDIA RESOURCES

Additional Material for Study, Review, and Further Exploration

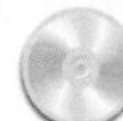

CD Companion ◆ Review Questions and Answers ◆ Key Concepts Review ◆ Glossary *(with audio pronunciations for selected terms)* ◆ Disease Profiles ◆ Animations

evolve ***Website*** at http://evolve.elsevier.com/Copstead/ ◆ Case Studies ◆ Disease Profiles ◆ WebLinks

KEY QUESTIONS

- What factors are necessary for normal red blood cell production?
- How do red blood cells transport oxygen and carbon dioxide in the circulation?
- How are laboratory tests used to detect anemia and polycythemia?
- What are the general effects of anemia on body systems?
- How are history, clinical manifestations, and laboratory studies used to differentiate the various forms of anemia?
- How are history, clinical manifestations, and laboratory studies used to differentiate the various forms of polycythemia?
- What are the appropriate treatment measures for each of the common types of anemia and polycythemia?

CHAPTER OUTLINE

Blood is a critical body fluid composed of formed elements and cells suspended in plasma that circulates through the cardiovascular system. As the primary transport system of the body, blood is involved in the physiologic and pathologic activities of all organs. The **red blood cell** (RBC), or **erythrocyte,** is essential to oxygen transport within the circulatory system. Red cells contain large numbers of hemoglobin molecules, which are designed to move oxygen efficiently from the lungs to other body tissues. Hemoglobin also aids in acid-base balance. In addition, RBCs carry carbon dioxide away from the cells and back to the lungs for expiration.

COMPOSITION OF BLOOD

The total blood volume averages 75.5 ml/kg in men and 66.5 ml/kg in women, which is 5 to 6 L or 7% to 8% of body weight. The blood cells make up approximately 45% and blood plasma 55% of the blood volume. Blood **plasma** is composed of about 92% water and 7% plasma proteins (Figure 13-1). The arterial pH of normal blood is 7.35 to 7.45.

Organic and Inorganic Components

The plasma proteins are formed mainly in the liver. They are nondiffusible and assist in regulating blood volume and the body's fluid balance. Plasma proteins contribute to blood viscosity, which is important in maintaining blood pressure. There are three general types of plasma proteins. The first is serum albumin, which is an essential factor in maintaining blood volume and pressure. The second is serum globulin, which is composed of three general fractions. The α fraction is associated with the transport of bilirubin, lipids, and steroids; the β fraction is associated with the transport of iron and copper in plasma; and the γ fraction contains the antibody molecules. Fibrinogen is the third major type of plasma protein. It is the precursor of fibrin, which forms the frame-

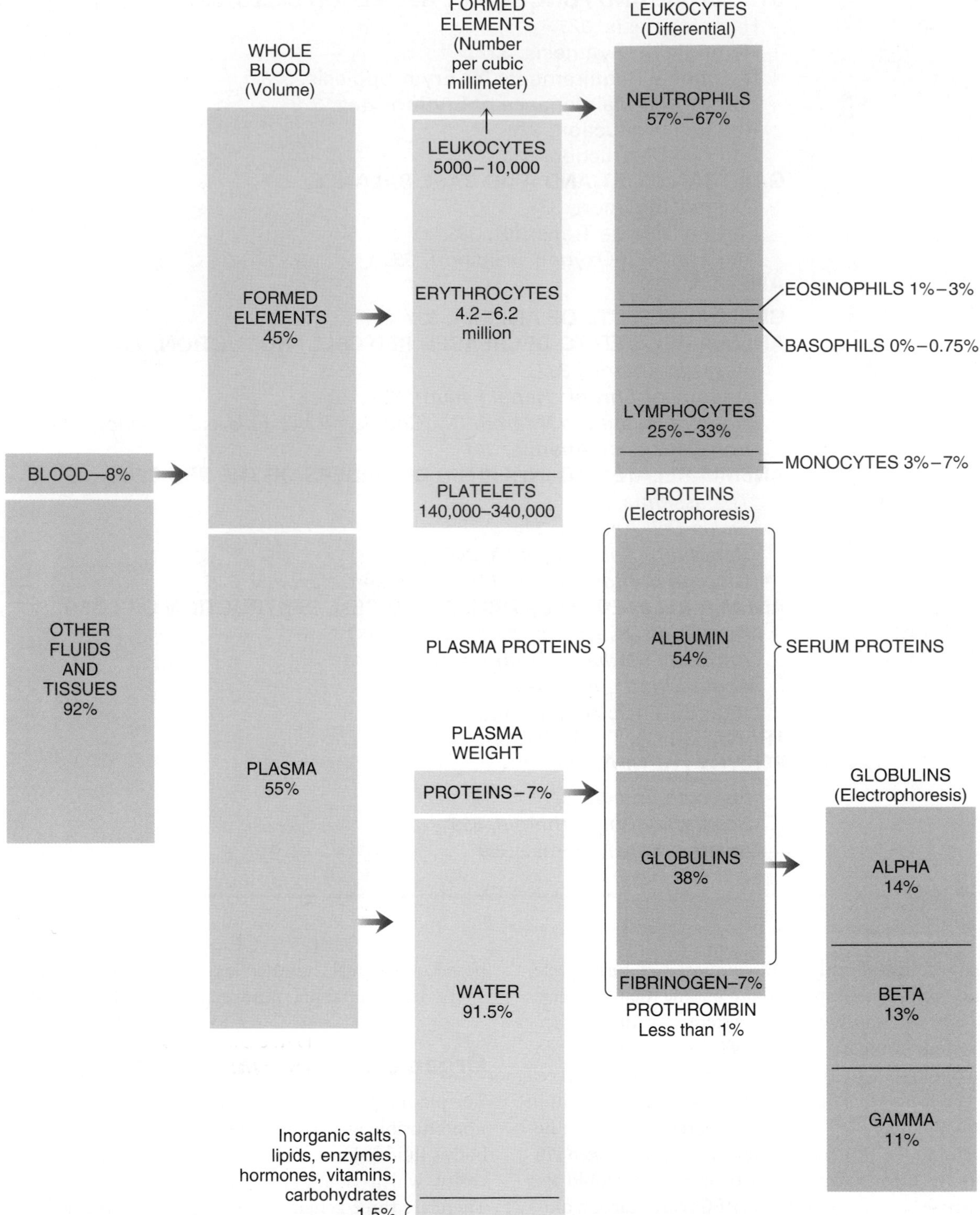

FIGURE 13-1 ■ Composition of blood in the normal adult. (Redrawn from Jacob SW, Francone CA: *Elements of anatomy and physiology,* ed 2, Philadelphia, 1989, Saunders, p 164.)

work of blood clots. Regulatory proteins, such as hormones and enzymes, are also present in the plasma. Diffusible nonorganic substances, such as sodium chloride, calcium, potassium, iodine, and iron, are used by body cells and make up 0.9% of plasma. Diffusible organic constituents, such as urea, uric acid, xanthine, creatine, creatinine, and ammonia, are products of tissue activity that are transported from the tissues to the kidneys and skin for excretion. Also included in this category are nutritive organic materials, such as amino acids, glucose, fats, and cholesterol, which are foodstuffs in solution absorbed from the gastrointestinal (GI) tract. They are transported to other body tissues for utilization and storage (Table 13-1).[1]

Cellular Components

Erythrocytes

Of the cellular elements of blood (Table 13-2), **RBCs,** or **erythrocytes,** are the most numerous, with normal concentrations ranging from 4.2 to 6.2 million cells/mm^3. RBCs are responsible for transporting oxygen to the tissues, removing carbon dioxide from the tissues, and buffering blood pH.

Table 13-1

Organic and Inorganic Components of Blood

Constituent	Amount/Concentration	Major Functions
Water	92% of plasma weight	Medium for carrying all other constituents
Electrolytes	Total <1% of plasma weight	Keep H_2O in extracellular compartment; act as buffers; function in membrane excitability
Na^+	136-145 mEq/L (142 mM)	
K^+	3.5-5 mEq/L (4 mM)	
Ca^{2+}	4.5-5.5 mEq/L (2.5 mM)	
Mg^{2+}	1.5-2.5 mEq/L (1.5 mM)	
Cl^-	100-106 mEq/L (103 mM)	
HCO_3^-	27 mEq/L (27 mM)	
Phosphate (mostly HPO_4^{2-})	3-4.5 mEq/L (1 mM)	
SO_4^{2-}	0.5-1.5 mEq/L (0.5 mM)	
Proteins	6-8 g/dl (2.5 mM)	
Albumin	3.5-5.5 g/dl	Provide colloid osmotic pressure of plasma; act as buffers; bind other plasma constituents (e.g., lipids, hormones, vitamins, metals)
Globulins	1.5-0.3 g/dl	Enzymes; enzyme precursors; antibodies (immune globulins); hormones
Fibrinogen	0.2-0.4 g/dl	Clotting factor
Gases, arterial plasma		
CO_2 content	22-30 mmol/L of plasma	Byproduct of metabolism; most CO_2 content is from HCO_3^- and acts as a buffer
O_2	Pao_2, 80 mm Hg or greater (arterial); $P\bar{v}o_2$, 30-40 mm Hg (venous)	Oxygenation
N_2	0.9 ml/dl	Byproduct of protein catabolism
Nutrients		Provide nutrition and substances for tissue repair
Glucose and other carbohydrates	70-105 mg/dl (5.6 mM)	
Total amino acids	40 mg/dl (2 mM)	
Total lipids	450 mg/dl (7.5 mM)	
Cholesterol	150-250 mg/dl (4-7 mM)	
Individual vitamins	0.0001-2.5 mg/dl	
Individual trace elements	0.001-0.3 mg/dl	
Waste products		
Urea (BUN)	10-20 mg/dl (5.7 mM)	End product of protein catabolism
Creatinine	0.7-1.5 mg/dl (0.09 mM)	End product of energy metabolism
Uric acid	2.5-8 mg/dl (0.3 mM)	End product of protein metabolism
Bilirubin	0.3-1.1 mg/dl	End product of red blood cell destruction
Direct conjugated	0.1-0.5 mg/dl	
Indirect unconjugated	0.1-0.7 mg/dl	
Individual hormones	0.000001-0.05 mg/dl	Functions specific to target tissue

Adapted with permission from Vander AJ, Sherman JH, Luciano DS: *Human physiology: the mechanisms of body function,* ed 7, New York, 1998, McGraw-Hill.

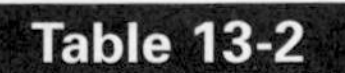

Table 13-2

Characteristics of Blood Cells

Cell	Structural Characteristics	Normal Amounts in Circulating Blood*	Function	Life Span
Erythrocyte (red blood cell)	Nonnucleated biconcave disk containing hemoglobin	Males: 4.7-6.1 $\times$ 10^{12}/L Females: 4.2-5.4 $\times$ 10^{12}/L	Gas transport to and from tissue cells and lungs	80-120 days
Leukocyte (white blood cell)	Nucleated cell	4.8-10.8 $\times$ 10^9/L	Body defense mechanisms	See below
Lymphocyte	Mononuclear immunocyte	1.2-3.4 $\times$ 10^9/L; 20%-44% leukocyte differential	Humoral and cell-mediated immunity	Days or years, depending on type
Neutrophil	Segmented polymorphonuclear granulocyte with neutrophilic granules	1.4-6.5 $\times$ 10^9/L; 50%-70% leukocyte differential	Phagocytosis, particularly during early phase of inflammation	5 days
Eosinophil	Segmented polymorphonuclear granulocyte with eosinophilic granules	0-0.7 $\times$ 10^9/L; 0%-4% leukocyte differential	Phagocytosis, antibody-mediated defense against parasites, participate in mucosal immune response	Unknown
Basophil	Segmented polymorphonuclear granulocyte with basophilic granules	0-0.2 $\times$ 10^9/L; 0%-2% leukocyte differential	Transport and release of heparin and histamine, involved in immune and inflammatory responses	Unknown
Monocyte-macrophage	Large mononuclear phagocyte	0.11-0.59 $\times$ 10^9/L; 2%-9% leukocyte differential	Phagocytosis; process and present antigens	Months to years
Platelet	Discoid cytoplasmic fragment derived from megakaryocytes	130-400 $\times$ 10^9/L	Hemostasis following vascular injury; forms hemostatic plug, provides cofactors, maintains vascular endothelium	9.5 days

Illustrations from GA Thibodeau, Patton KT: *Anatomy and physiology,* ed 5, St Louis, 2003, Mosby.
*Given in SI units.

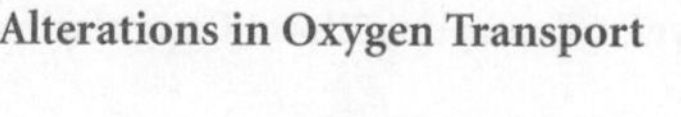

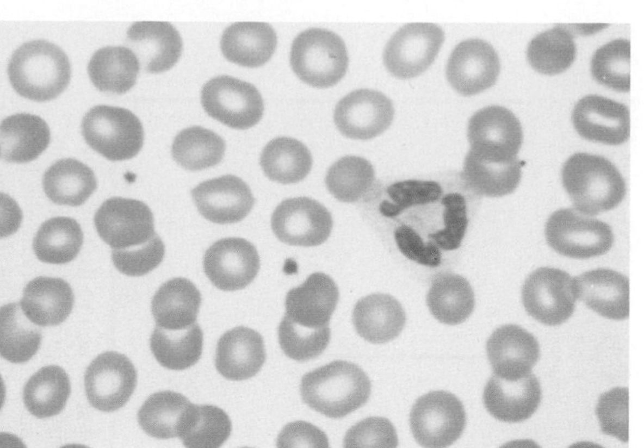

FIGURE 13-2 ■ Mature erythrocytes. A mature neutrophil is also shown. (Courtesy Beth Payne, Sacred Heart Medical Center, Spokane, Wash.)

They have no cytoplasmic organelles, nucleus, mitochondria, or ribosomes. Therefore, RBCs cannot synthesize protein or carry out oxidative reactions. Instead the erythrocyte's cytoplasm consists of a solution containing proteins, hemoglobin, and electrolytes that regulates diffusion through the cellular membrane. RBCs live for 80 to 120 days in the circulation; then they die and are replaced. Hemoglobin is the main functional constituent of the red cell. It is a protein that enables the blood to transport 100 times more oxygen than could be transported in plasma alone. An enzyme inside RBCs, carbonic anhydrase, is responsible for the buffering mechanism of red cells.[2]

The erythrocyte's size and shape also contribute to its function as a gas carrier (Figure 13-2). It is a small, biconcave disk, about 7.2 μm in diameter, that must circulate through splenic sinusoids and capillaries, which are only 2 μm in diameter. This remarkable feat is accomplished through a property called reversible deformability, which allows the RBC to assume a torpedo-like conformation and then return to a biconcave disk shape.[2]

Leukocytes

White blood cells (WBCs), or **leukocytes,** protect the body by phagocytosis of microorganisms and other debris and participate in immune antibody formation. Leukocytes act primarily in the tissues but are also transported in the circulatory and lymphatic systems. The average adult has approximately 5000 to 10,000 leukocytes per cubic millimeter of blood. Monocytes and granulocytes are WBCs that share a common lineage with RBCs and platelets. Due to the interrelationship of RBCs, WBCs, and platelets, which are all derived from the myeloid stem cell (Figure 13-3), abnormalities in these cells are seen in some red cell diseases.[3] Leukocyte structure and function are discussed in detail in Chapter 9.

Platelets

Platelets are essential in the formation of blood clots and in the control of bleeding. They are not cells but are circulating cytoplasmic fragments of megakaryocytes and are incapable of mitotic division. They contain cytoplasmic granules that release biochemical mediators involved in the hemostatic process. Normally, 150,000 to 400,000 platelets/mm^3 circulate freely in the blood. An additional third of the body's platelets are in a reserve pool in the spleen. The average life span of platelets in the peripheral blood is approximately 4 to 5 days.[4]

The amounts of the different cellular components in the blood vary with age. Table 13-3 gives normal values from birth to 21 years.[5]

KEY CONCEPTS

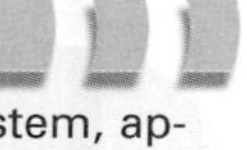

- Of the 4 to 6 L of blood in the circulatory system, approximately 45% is blood cells and 55% is plasma. The plasma fraction contains dissolved substances, including nutrients, ions, plasma proteins, metabolic wastes, hormones, and enzymes.
- Red cells function to carry oxygen and carbon dioxide in the blood. They have a limited life span of 80 to 120 days because they contain no cytoplasmic organelles and thus are incapable of replacing lost or damaged cellular components. The normal red cell concentration is 4.2 to 6.2 million cells/mm^3.
- Leukocytes, or WBCs, are the other cell type present in blood. Leukocytes circulate in much lower numbers than RBCs (5000 to 10,000/mm^3). Leukocytes are important mediators of immunity.
- Platelets are not cells but are small fragments of megakaryocytes. The normal platelet count is 150,000 to 400,000 cells/mm^3.

STRUCTURE AND FUNCTION OF RED BLOOD CELLS

The cellular components of blood originate in the yolk sac mesenchyme, move to the liver and spleen during fetal life, and finally are limited to the marrow of the body skeleton (Figure 13-4). Bone marrow provides a special environment for hematopoietic cell proliferation and maturation. Developing cells are held in a fine reticular meshwork, which provides free access to plasma nutrients but retains developing cells until their maturity allows penetration of the endothelial barrier. In times of need, immature cells (reticulocytes and nucleated red blood cells, or NRBCs) are released early into the circulation; their presence in increased numbers is a sign that the hematopoietic system is stressed or is experiencing disease.[5]

Hematopoiesis

Hematopoiesis is the developmental process leading from pluripotential stem cells to mature, differentiated red cells, neutrophils, eosinophils, basophils, monocytes, and platelets. **Lymphopoiesis** describes this process for lymphocytes. Both hematopoietic and lymphopoietic stem cells probably derive from a single totipotent stem cell pool in fetal development,

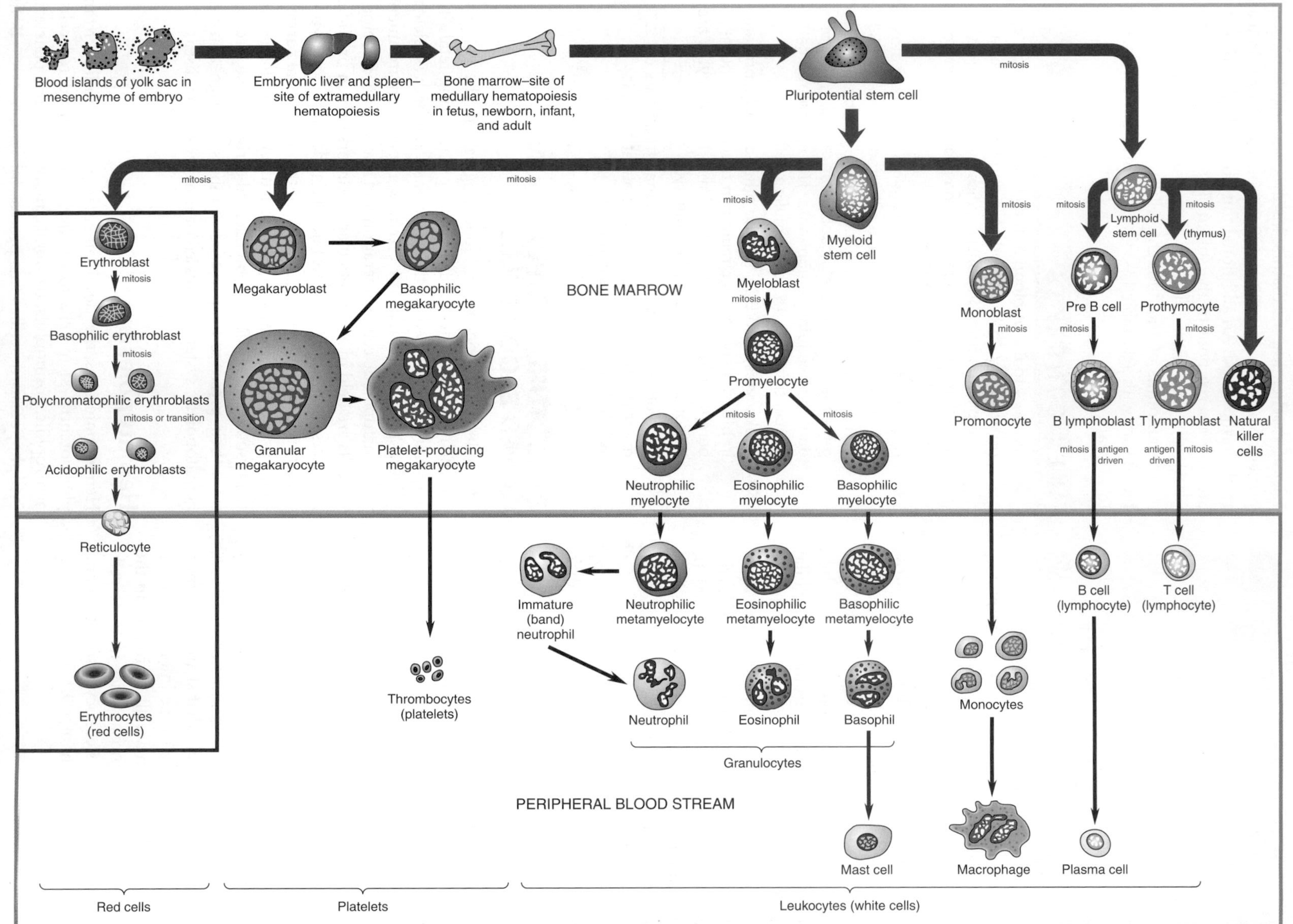

FIGURE 13-3 ■ Maturation of human blood cells. Probable pathways of blood cell differentiation from the pluripotential stem cell to mature leukocytes, erythrocytes, and platelets. Production of cells begins in embryo blood islands of the yolk sac. As the embryo matures, production shifts to the liver and spleen (extramedullary hematopoiesis) and progresses to bone marrow (medullary hematopoiesis). In an adult, all production is in the bone marrow. Current thinking is that all cell production begins with a pluripotential stem cell, which differentiates into either a myeloid stem cell or a lymphoid stem cell, which then differentiates into a specific blast cell. For example, red cell differentiation begins with the proerythroblast, which matures into a basophilic erythroblast, to a polychromatophilic erythroblast, and to an acidophilic erythroblast, all of which are found in the bone marrow. Red cell differentiation concludes with production of reticulocytes and mature red cells (erythrocytes), which normally are found only in the peripheral blood.

Table 13-3

Age-Related Changes in Hematologic Values

Age	Hemoglobin (g)	Hematocrit (%)	RBC Count (millions/mm³)	Platelets (thousands/mm³)	Reticulocytes (%)	WBC Count (/mm³)	PMN Count Adult	Band Forms (%)	Eosinophils (%)	Basophils (%)	Lymphocytes (%)	Monocytes (%)
Birth	17.6	55	5.5	350.0	5.0	9000-30,000 (avg., 18,000)	9400 (52%)	9.1	2.2	0.6	31	5.8
24 hr	18.0	56	5.3	400.0	5.2	9400-34,000 (avg., 19,045)	9800 (52%)	9.2	2.4	0.5	31	5.8
1 wk	17.0	54	5.0	300.0	1.0	5000-21,000 (avg., 12,279)	4700 (39%)	6.8	4.1	0.4	41	9.1
2 mo	12.4	30	4.3	260.0	0.5	5500-18,000 (avg., 11,000)	3300 (30%)	4.4	2.7	0.5	57	5.9
6 mo	11.5	34	4.6	250.0	0.8	6000-17,500 (avg., 11,900)	3300 (28%)	3.8	2.5	0.4	61	4.8
2 yr	12.9	40	4.8	250.0	1.0	6000-17,000 (avg., 10,680)	3200 (30%)	3.0	2.6	0.5	59	5.0
6 yr	14.1	42	4.8	250.0	1.0	5000-14,500 (avg., 8500)	4000 (48%)	3.0	2.7	0.6	42	4.7
14 yr	15.0	M: 45 F: 42	5.1	250.0	1.0	4500-13,000 (avg., 7900)	4200 (53%)	3.0	2.5	0.5	37	4.7
21 yr	15.0	M: 45 F: 42	5.1	250.0	1.0	4500-11,000 (avg., 7400)	4200 (56%)	3.0	2.7	0.5	34	4.0

From Platt W: *Color atlas and textbook of hematology,* ed 2, Philadelphia, 1979, Lippincott, p 4. Reproduced by permission of William R. Platt, MD.

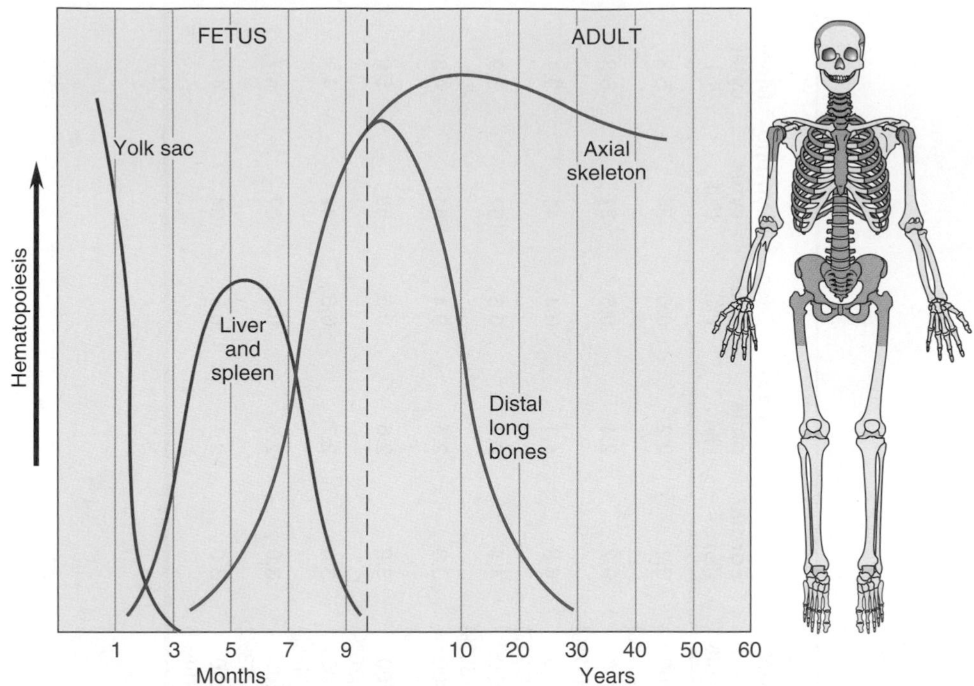

FIGURE 13-4 ■ Location of active marrow growth in the fetus and adult. During fetal development, hematopoiesis is first established in the yolk sac mesenchyme, later moves to the liver and spleen, and finally is limited to the bony skeleton. From infancy to adulthood, there is progressive restriction of productive marrow to the axial skeleton and proximal ends of the long bones, which appear as shaded areas on the drawing of the skeleton. (Redrawn from Hillman RS, Finch CA, editors: *Red cell manual,* ed 6, Philadelphia, 1992, FA Davis, p 2.)

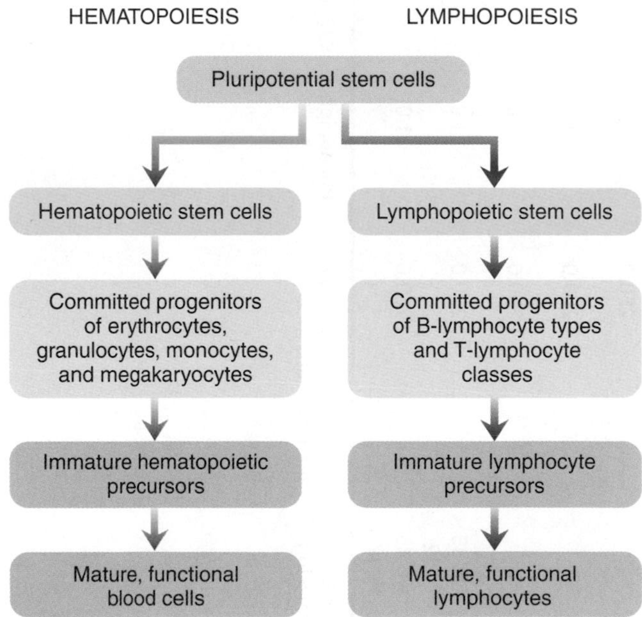

FIGURE 13-5 ■ Stem cells and normal hematopoiesis. (Data from Williams WJ et al, editors: *Hematology,* ed 4, New York, 1990, McGraw-Hill, p 152.)

but it is uncertain if this is the functioning stem cell after birth (Figure 13-5). Research suggests that a pluripotential stem cell that is stimulated by erythropoietin and other poietins to cause further differentiation into separate cell lines may be the primary stem cell in adults.[6]

Hematopoiesis is a two-stage process that involves mitotic division or proliferation and maturation or differentiation. Each type of blood cell has stem cells that undergo mitosis when stimulated by a specific biochemical signal, which indicates that the number of circulating cells has decreased. Medullary or bone marrow hematopoiesis continues throughout life and can be accelerated by several mechanisms, including (1) an increase in differentiation of daughter cells, (2) an increase in number of stem cells, and (3) conversion of yellow (fatty) bone marrow (which does not produce cells) to red marrow (which does produce cells). Marrow conversion is stimulated by erythropoietin, which is the hormone from the kidney that stimulates erythrocyte production. In adults, extramedullary hematopoiesis, or production of blood cells in tissue other than bone, is usually a disease symptom.[7]

Erythrocyte development is shown in detail in Figure 13-3. During this process, the cell changes from a large nucleated cell, rich in ribosomes, to a reticulocyte, which is a small disk that has lost its nucleus. The reticulocyte (Figure 13-6) leaves the marrow, enters the blood stream, and matures into an

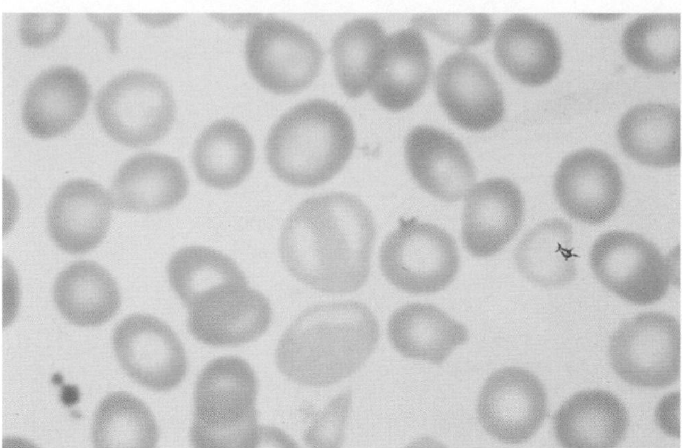
FIGURE 13-6 ■ Reticulocytes seen on peripheral blood smear. The two reticulocytes in the center still contain remnants of intracellular organelles. (Courtesy Beth Payne, Sacred Heart Medical Center, Spokane, Wash.)

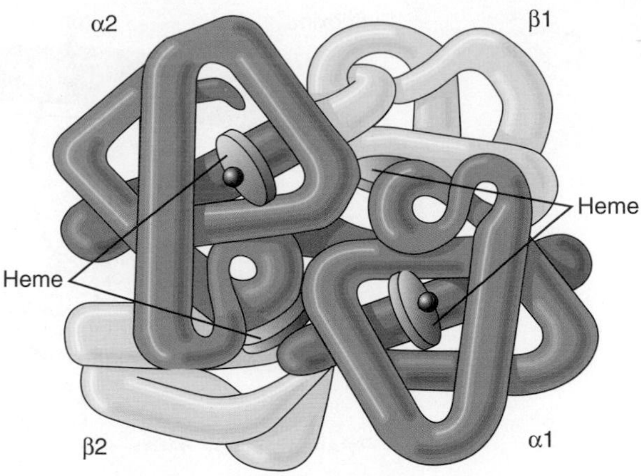

FIGURE 13-7 ■ Molecular structure of hemoglobin. The molecule is a spherical tetramer weighing approximately 64,500 daltons. It contains two α- and two β-polypeptide chains and four heme groups.

erythrocyte in 24 to 48 hours. During this period, mitochondria and ribosomes disappear, and the cell can no longer synthesize hemoglobin. The cell relies on glycolysis for adenosine triphosphate (ATP) production. The normal reticulocyte count is 1% of the total RBC count. This makes it a useful test to determine effective erythropoietic activity,[7] as erythropoietin stimulates uncommitted stem cells to differentiate into proerythroblasts.

Hemoglobin Synthesis

The immature red cell can be viewed as a factory for hemoglobin synthesis. In a mature red cell, **hemoglobin,** the oxygen-carrying protein, composes about 90% of the cell's dry weight in the form of approximately 300 hemoglobin molecules.[2] Hemoglobin that is carrying oxygen is called oxyhemoglobin. Hemoglobin is composed of two pairs of polypeptide chains, the globins. Each globin has an attached heme molecule that is composed of iron plus a protoporphyrin molecule (Figure 13-7).[8]

After dietary iron is absorbed in the duodenum and proximal jejunum, it is transported through the plasma by the protein transferrin to transferrin iron receptors on the RBC membrane. The transferrin-receptor complex is engulfed by the cell into an invagination of the cell surface. The invagination becomes sealed off and forms an intracytoplasmic vacuole. Iron is then released and either stored as ferritin or used to synthesize heme (Figure 13-8).[5] About 67% of total body iron is bound to heme in erythrocytes and muscle cells, and 30% is stored bound to ferritin or hemosiderin-containing macrophages and hepatic parenchymal cells. The remaining 3% is lost daily in urine, sweat, bile, and epithelial cells that are shed in the intestines.

The mitochondria are responsible for the synthesis of protoporphyrin. The final heme molecule consists of four por-

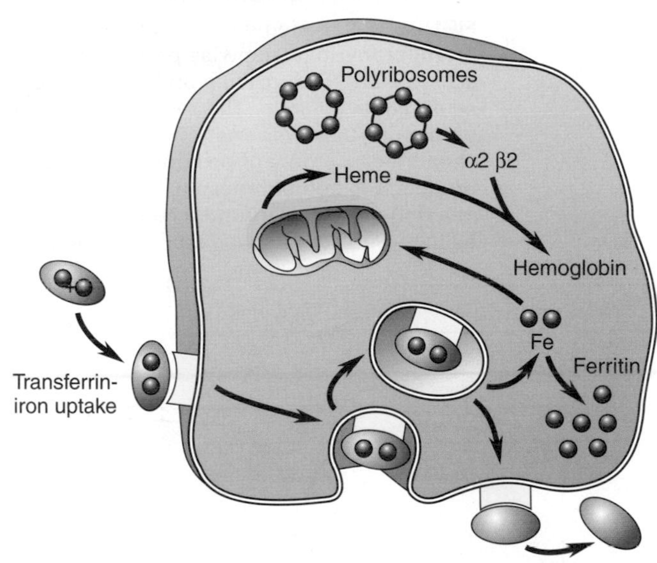

FIGURE 13-8 ■ Intracellular pathways for iron uptake and incorporation into hemoglobin. The iron-transferrin complex is picked up by a membrane-associated receptor and brought into the cell by invagination and formation of an intracytoplasmic vacuole. The iron is then released and stored as intracytoplasmic ferritin or used to synthesize heme, the precursor of hemoglobin. The transferrin-receptor complex is returned to the cell membrane, where the apotransferrin is expelled back into the circulation. (Redrawn from Hillman RS, Finch CA, editors: *Red cell manual,* ed 6, Philadelphia, 1992, FA Davis, p 8.)

phyrin moieties assembled in a ring structure around a central iron molecule (Figure 13-9).[5]

Globin is assembled from two pairs of polypeptide chains produced on specific ribosomes. The protein chain produced in fetal life is altered after birth by sequential gene suppression and activation. At birth, red cells contain mainly fetal hemoglobin (hemoglobin F), which is composed of two α chains

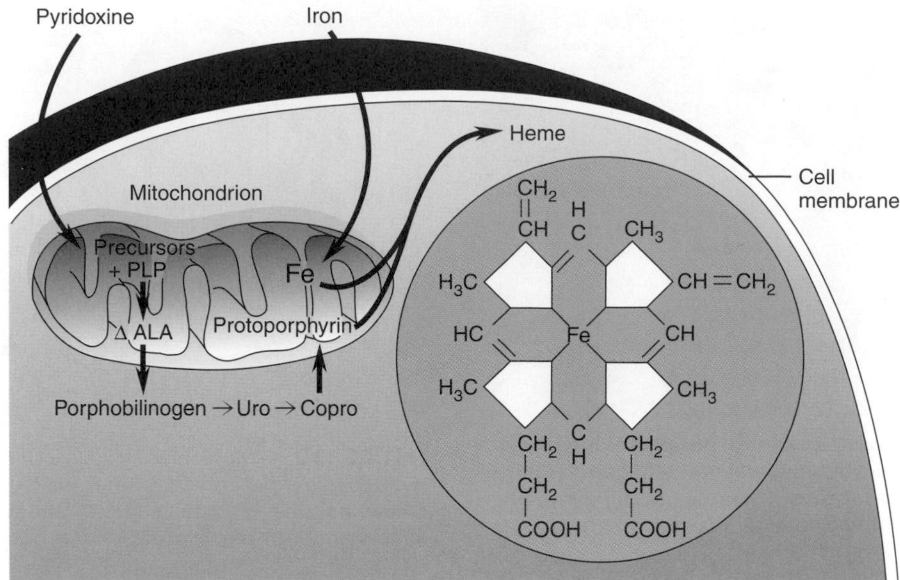

FIGURE 13-9 ■ Heme formation. The mitochondrion is responsible for the synthesis of protoporphyrin, a stepwise process beginning with the formation of Δ-aminolevulinic acid *(Δ-ALA)* from glycine and succinyl coenzyme A, with pyridoxal-5-phosphate *(PLP)* as an essential cofactor. The sequence of porphobilinogen, uroporphyrin *(Uro),* and coproporphyrin *(Copro)* formation then occurs in the cytoplasm, followed by an intramitochondrial assembly of protoporphyrin and iron to form heme. The structure of the final product, the heme molecule, is shown. It consists of four porphyrin moieties assembled in a ring structure around a central iron molecule. (Redrawn from Hillman RS, Finch CA, editors: *Red cell manual,* ed 6, Philadelphia, 1992, FA Davis, p 9.)

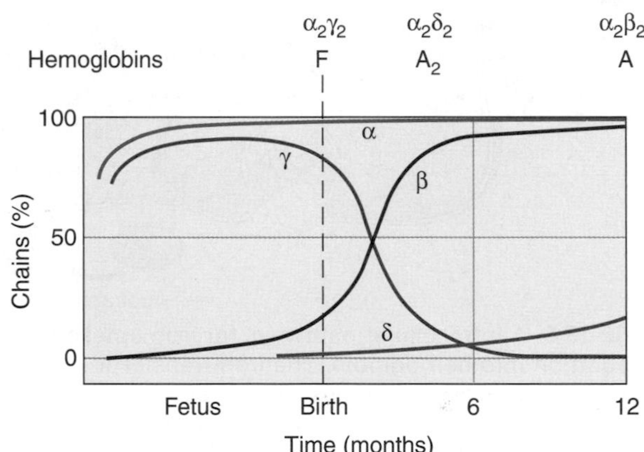

FIGURE 13-10 ■ Changes in hemoglobin with development. Sequential suppression and activation of individual globin genes in the immediate postnatal period result in a switch from fetal hemoglobin (hemoglobin F: two α chains and two γ chains) to adult hemoglobin (hemoglobin A: two α chains and two β chains). A small amount of hemoglobin A_2 (two α chains and two δ chains) is also present in the adult. (Adapted from Hillman RS, Finch CA, editors: *Red cell manual,* ed 6, Philadelphia, 1992, FA Davis, p 9.)

and two γ chains. Hemoglobin F is a more efficient gas carrier under decreased oxygen tension than hemoglobin A and releases CO_2 more readily. Within 120 days, fetal hemoglobin disappears and is replaced by adult hemoglobin (hemoglobin A) (Figure 13-10). This switch is the result of globin genes and is not well understood. Hemoglobin A is composed of two α chains and two β chains and makes up 97% of the hemoglobin found in adults. Hemoglobin A_2 makes up 2% to 3% of hemoglobin found in adults and is composed of $\alpha_2\delta_2$.[8,9]

Several hundred abnormal hemoglobinopathies have been described that have changes in the two α chains and two β chains. Most are characterized by the substitution of only one amino acid and are classified by the polypeptide chain in which the substitution occurs.[8]

Nutritional Requirements for Erythropoiesis

In addition to iron, which is required for hemoglobin synthesis, the normal development of erythrocytes requires adequate supplies of protein, vitamins, and minerals. Erythropoiesis cannot proceed in the absence of vitamins, especially B_{12}, folate, B_6, riboflavin, pantothenic acid, niacin, ascorbic acid, and vitamin E. Folates and vitamin B_{12} (cobalamin) are absorbed from food by the ileal mucosa. Folate deficiencies or vitamin B_{12} deficiencies lead to impaired DNA synthesis in erythroid cells because the vitamins are coenzymes in a large number of key reactions in cellular metabolism. Absorption of vitamin B_{12} requires intrinsic factor in the gastric juice. Intrinsic factor is secreted by the stomach parietal cells and binds to vitamin B_{12}. The complex then moves down the gastrointestinal tract to the ileum, where it attaches to specific

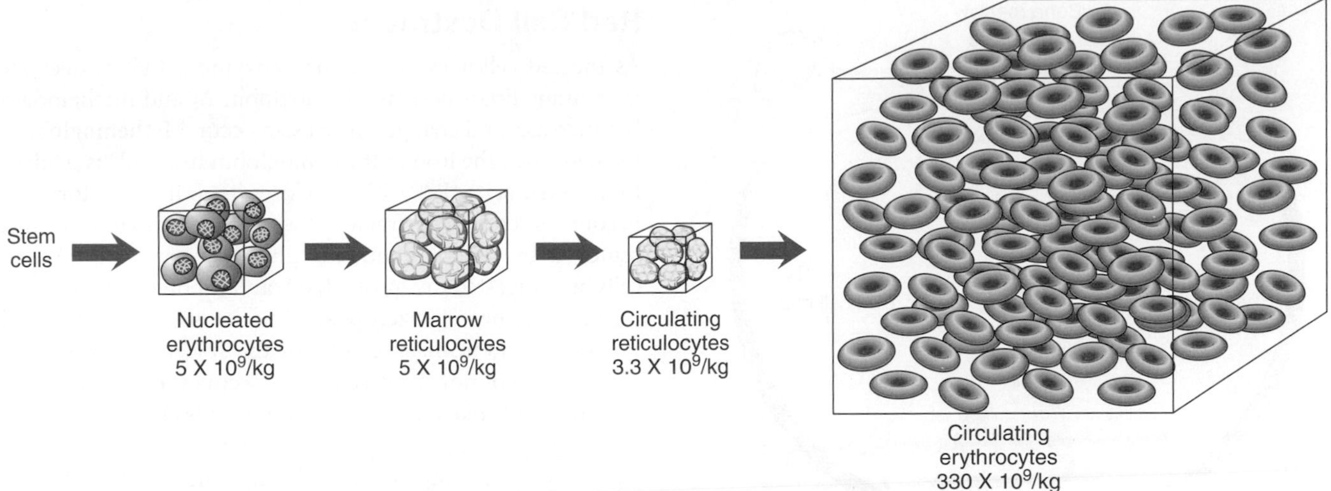

FIGURE 13-11 ■ Scale model of the erythron, showing the relative proportions of each of the components. The numbers below each box indicate the average number of cells per kilogram of body weight. (Redrawn from Wintrobe M et al, editors: *Clinical hematology,* ed 8, Philadelphia, 1981, Lea & Febiger, p 109.)

receptor sites on the ileum mucosal cell. It is absorbed into the cell, released, and transported in the blood to the tissues and liver.[10,11]

Energy and Maintenance of Erythrocytes

For the RBC to perform efficiently and survive in the circulation for the full 120-day life span, it must have a source of energy. Without an energy source, the red cell becomes sodium logged and potassium depleted. The shape changes from a biconcave disk to a sphere, and it is quickly removed from the circulation by the filtering action of the spleen and the mononuclear phagocyte system. The metabolism of the RBC is limited due to the absence of a nucleus, mitochondria, and other subcellular organelles. Although the binding, transport, and release of O_2 and CO_2 is a passive process that does not require energy, other energy-dependent metabolic processes occur that are essential to the RBC viability. The chief metabolic pathway, accounting for about 90% of the glucose used, is the anaerobic or Embden-Meyerhof pathway. The Embden-Meyerhof pathway provides ATP for regulation of intracellular Na^+, K^+, Ca^{2+}, and Mg^{2+} concentration via cation pumps. About 10% of the glucose undergoes aerobic glycolysis in the hexose monophosphate shunt. The hexose monophosphate shunt provides nicotinamide adenine dinucleotide phosphate (NADPH) and glutathione (GSH) to reduce cellular oxidants. This protects the cell from permanent oxidant injury. The methemoglobin reductase pathway protects hemoglobin from oxidation via NADH and methemoglobin reductase. Last, the Rapoport-Leubering pathway forms 2,3-diphosphoglycerate (DPG), which facilitates oxygen release to the tissues. These pathways contribute energy for maintaining (1) high intracellular K^+, low intracellular Na^+, and very low intracellular Ca^{2+} (cation pumps); (2) reduced hemoglobin; (3) high levels of reduced GSH; and (4) membrane integrity and deformability.[2] Deficiencies of enzymes that regulate these pathways can be due to natural causes, such as the normal aging process, or to an inherited deficiency of an enzyme.[2,12]

Red cell membrane structures are matrices formed from a double layer of phospholipids. In the red cell membrane, the globular proteins floating on the "sea of lipids" form a protein network on the cytoplasmic surface of the membrane. One half of the mass of the membrane is lipid, which is partially responsible for many of its physical characteristics. Both passive cation permeability and mechanical flexibility can be significantly influenced by changing the lipid composition of the membrane. Maintenance and renewal of membrane lipids in well-developed RBCs is important, and problems in these pathways result in premature cell death.[13]

Red Cell Production

When blood is described as a single body system, it is called the **erythron** (Figure 13-11). The erythron includes the blood cells and their bone marrow precursors, so that it is much larger than the liver. The size of the erythron increases or decreases based on the erythropoietic process and the pathologic changes in red cells seen in anemia.[14] **Erythropoiesis** is controlled by a system sensitive to alterations in the concentration of hemoglobin in the blood. A decrease in hemoglobin decreases the tissue oxygen tension in the kidney. In response to this hypoxia, the kidney secretes a hormone, **erythropoietin,** that stimulates primitive stem cells in the bone marrow to differentiate into proerythroblasts or pronormoblasts, thereby increasing the erythron (Figure 13-12).[2,15] Hypoxia from causes other than low hemoglobin level can also initiate this response.

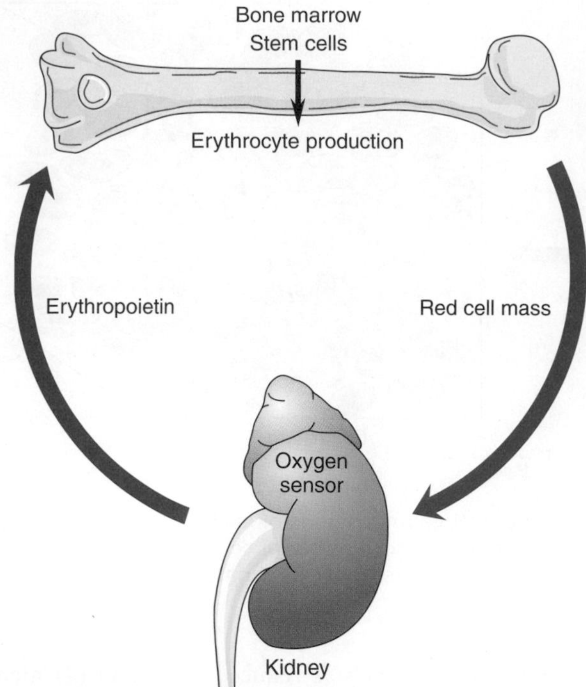

FIGURE 13-12 ■ Feedback circuit illustrating the role of erythropoietin in the regulation of red cell mass.

Red Cell Destruction

As the red cell ages, the various enzyme activities decrease, membrane lipids decrease, hemoglobin A_2 and methemoglobin increase, and changes in cell size occur. **Methemoglobin** is formed when the iron of the hemoglobin molecule is oxidized to the ferric state (Fe^{3+}). The cell loses its ability to deform and becomes increasingly fragile. These aging red cells are then removed by the mononuclear phagocytic system. The red cells are digested by proteolytic and lipolytic enzymes in phagolysosomes of macrophages. Some 80% to 90% of this process occurs in macrophages of the spleen and liver. Only 10% to 20% of normal destruction occurs intravascularly.[2,16]

Globin is broken down into amino acids and the iron is recycled. Porphyrin is reduced to **bilirubin,** which is transported to the liver and conjugated by the enzyme glucuronyl transferase. Finally, conjugated bilirubin is excreted in the bile as glucuronide. Bacteria in the intestine convert conjugated bilirubin into urobilinogen, which is excreted primarily in the stool but also in the urine. Any condition causing increased red cell destruction increases the load of bilirubin to be cleared, which leads to increased serum levels of unconjugated bilirubin and increased excretion of urobilinogen. Increased levels of circulating bilirubin give the skin a yellow tone,

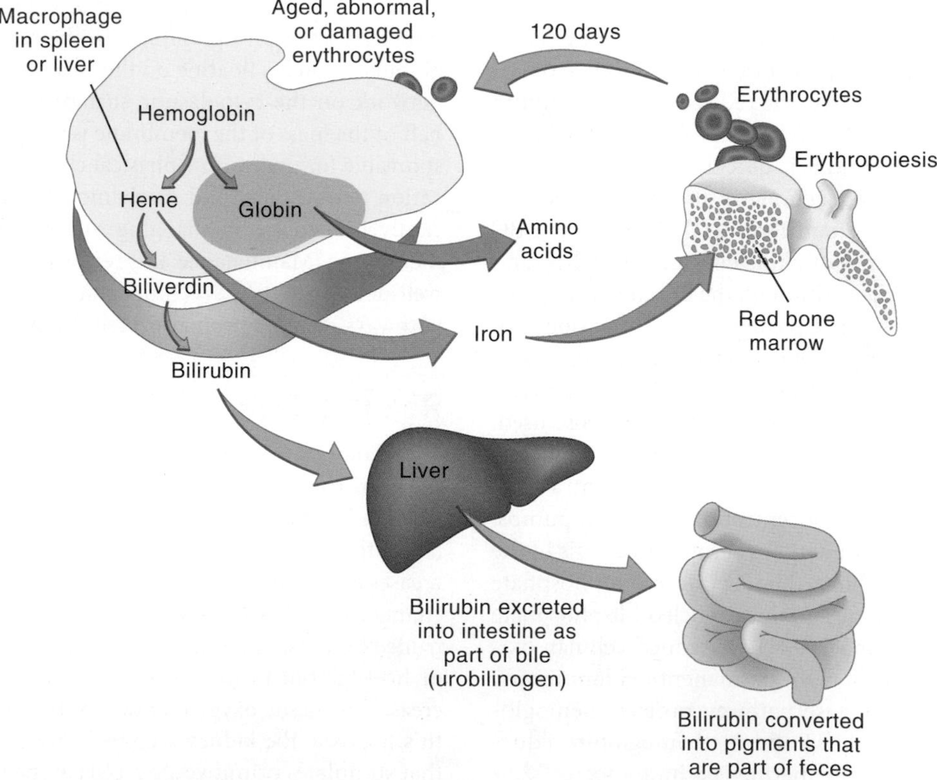

FIGURE 13-13 ■ Most hemoglobin degradation occurs in the macrophages of the spleen. The globin and iron portions are conserved and reused. Heme is reduced to bilirubin, eventually degraded to urobilinogen, and excreted in the feces. Thus, indirect indicators of erythrocyte or erythrocyte destruction include the blood bilirubin level and urobilinogen concentration in the feces. (From Thibodeau GA, Patton KT: *Anatomy and physiology,* ed 5, St Louis, 2003, Mosby, p 537.)

which is called jaundice. In newborns, the albumin levels for bilirubin transport are low and liver glucuronidase for bilirubin conjugation is low, which may cause an accumulation of toxic unconjugated bilirubin. Unconjugated bilirubin is toxic because in this form it is lipid soluble and can easily cross cell membranes. This form of bilirubin has a high affinity for basal ganglia of the central nervous system. The conjugated form of bilirubin is water soluble but lipid insoluble, and it cannot cross cell membranes (Figure 13-13).[2,16]

KEY CONCEPTS

- Red cell development from pluripotential stem cells in the bone marrow is stimulated by a hormone growth factor called erythropoietin. Erythropoietin is secreted into the blood stream by kidney cells in response to low oxygen tension in the blood.
- During development, red cells lose their nuclei and other cytoplasmic organelles. A reticulocyte is an immature red cell that still retains some cellular organelles. An increased blood reticulocyte count is a useful indicator of increased red cell production.
- Hemoglobin is the major component of red cells. It is composed of two pairs of polypeptide chains, each of which has a heme molecule attached. Oxygen can bind reversibly to an iron molecule at the center of each heme. When fully saturated, a hemoglobin molecule carries four oxygen molecules, or 1.34 ml of oxygen per gram of hemoglobin, and is referred to as oxyhemoglobin.
- Red cell production requires adequate amounts of several nutrients, particularly iron, vitamin B_{12}, and folate. Lack of intrinsic factor inhibits absorption of B_{12} from the small intestine and is a risk factor for anemia.
- Red cells rely on glycolysis for energy production because they do not contain mitochondria. As energy production declines due to red cell aging and loss of essential glycolytic enzymes, the cell swells, gets trapped in the spleen, and is removed from the circulation. Red cell degradation releases bilirubin, a toxic substance that is conjugated in the liver and excreted in urine and bile.

GAS TRANSPORT AND ACID-BASE BALANCE

RBCs have many important functions in the body related to gas transport and acid-base balance.[2,16,17] RBCs contain hemoglobin, which is responsible for oxygen transport to the body tissues.[2,16] Oxygen combines with the heme portion of hemoglobin to form oxyhemoglobin in a loose and reversible bond in the pulmonary capillary with a high partial pressure of oxygen (Po_2) and is carried to the tissues with a low Po_2, where it is released.[17] Large quantities of carbonic anhydrase in RBCs catalyze the reaction between CO_2 and water produced by cellular metabolism in the tissues to form carbonic acid and subsequently hydrogen and bicarbonate ions for elimination by the lungs and kidneys. Finally, the hemoglobin protein directly binds with CO_2 to form carbaminohemoglobin for CO_2 transport, which is an acid-base buffer responsible for as much as 50% of the whole blood–buffering power.[2,16]

Oxygen Transport

Transport of oxygen to the body tissues and removal of carbon dioxide is a complex process involving interdependent function of the lungs, heart, and blood (Figure 13-14). Approximately 97% of oxygen in the blood is transported on red cells loosely and reversibly combined with hemoglobin (oxyhemoglobin), and 3% is dissolved in plasma. Each hemoglobin molecule can bind four atoms of oxygen. Despite a combining potential of 1.39 ml of oxygen per gram of hemoglobin in pure hemoglobin, a maximum of about 1.34 ml of oxygen per gram of hemoglobin is available, owing to a reduction of about 4% by impurities such as methemoglobin. The blood of a normal person contains approximately 15 g of hemoglobin per 100 ml of blood. Therefore, in the average person, the hemoglobin in 100 ml of blood can combine with approximately 20 ml of oxygen if the hemoglobin is 100% saturated. This value is expressed as 20 vol%.[17,18]

$$\text{Oxygen } (O_2) \text{ capacity of hemoglobin (Hb)} = \text{Hb (g/100 ml)} \times 1.34 \text{ ml } O_2/\text{g Hb} = 15 \text{ g/100 ml} \times 1.34 \text{ ml } O_2/\text{g Hb} = 20.1 \text{ ml } O_2/100 \text{ ml (or vol\%)}$$

The partial pressure of oxygen (Po_2) reflects the pressure or tension that oxygen exerts when it is dissolved in blood. Partial pressure is measured in millimeters of mercury (mm Hg). In the pulmonary capillaries, where Po_2 is high, oxygen binds efficiently with hemoglobin, but in the tissue capillaries, where Po_2 is low, oxygen is released from hemoglobin. The partial pressure affects the tendency of oxygen to bind with hemoglobin.[19] The partial pressure of oxygen in arterial blood (Pao_2) is usually 80 to 100 mm Hg, whereas the partial pressure of oxygen in venous blood ($P\bar{v}O_2$) is usually 35 to 40 mm Hg. The amount of hemoglobin bound to oxygen relative to the total amount of hemoglobin is expressed as the oxygen saturation, in a percentage.[19,20] Saturation of arterial blood with oxygen (Sao_2) is normally 95% to 100%, whereas that of venous blood ($S\bar{v}O_2$) is 60% to 80%.[17-20]

The oxygen-hemoglobin dissociation curve (Figure 13-15) describes the relationship between Po_2 and So_2. The upper part of the curve represents oxygen uptake in the lungs and demonstrates that significant changes in Po_2 result in only small changes in So_2 to help ensure adequate oxygen delivery to the tissues.[18,19] On the steep lower portion of the curve, reflecting the venous blood, small changes in venous Po_2 result in large changes in $S\bar{v}o_2$.[19] Therefore, the tissues are protected with an available oxygen reserve as large quantities of oxygen are released from the blood for relatively small decreases in Po_2. Normally, tissue Po_2 does not rise above 40 mm Hg to en-

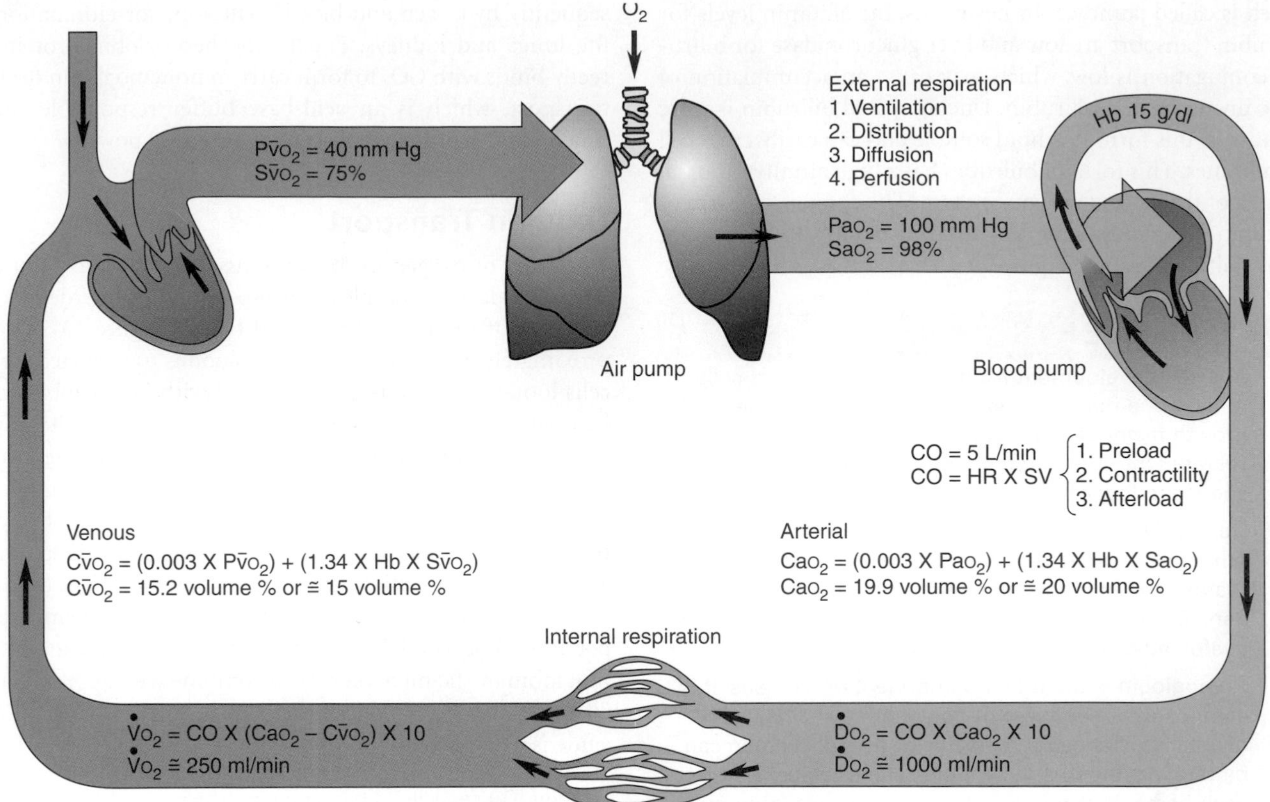

FIGURE 13-14 ■ Oxygen transport. Diffusion of oxygen into the pulmonary capillaries occurs when alveolar Po_2 exceeds capillary Po_2. Maintenance of this gradient is dependent on adequate alveolar ventilation and perfusion. Delivery of oxygenated blood to the tissues *($\dot{D}o_2$)* is determined by the content of oxygen in the blood *(Cao_2)* and the cardiac output *(CO)*. The difference between arterial and venous oxygen is a reflection of oxygen consumption by tissues *($\dot{V}o_2$)*. *Hb,* Hemoglobin; *HR,* heart rate; *SV,* stroke volume.

hance diffusion of oxygen from the blood to the tissues. The strength of the bond between hemoglobin and oxygen is called the oxygen-hemoglobin affinity. For any given Po_2, hemoglobin saturation will be higher when affinity is increased and saturation will be lower when affinity is decreased. Changes in hemoglobin affinity are represented by shifts in the oxyhemoglobin dissociation curve (see Figure 13-15). Shifts in the oxyhemoglobin curve affect the ability of hemoglobin to pick up O_2 in the lungs and release it in the tissues. The ability of hemoglobin to release oxygen to the tissues is commonly assessed at point P_{50} on the oxygen-hemoglobin dissociation curve. The P_{50} is the Po_2 at which 50% of the hemoglobin is saturated. A decrease in oxygen affinity (shift to the right on the oxyhemoglobin dissociation curve) or an increase in oxygen affinity (shift to the left) can be caused by the conditions listed in Figure 13-15.[18]

A shift of the oxyhemoglobin dissociation curve due to changes in the blood levels of Pco_2 and the H^+ concentration is important to enhance oxygen uptake by the blood in the lungs and the release of oxygen from the hemoglobin to the body tissues. This is called the Bohr effect.[17]

A shift of the oxyhemoglobin dissociation curve to the right enhances oxygen release to the cell. The shift provides the increase in oxygen delivery that is needed during exercise and other types of stress, as well as in chronic disease states. A shift of the oxyhemoglobin dissociation curve to the left is seen with a decrease in H^+ ion concentration, with a decrease in Pco_2, with an increase in pH, with a decrease in temperature, with a decrease in 2,3-DPG, in some congenital hemoglobinopathies, and with carboxyhemoglobin.

Another important factor affecting O_2 delivery to tissues is the arterial oxygen content (Cao_2).[17,18,20] Arterial blood oxygen content (Cao_2) and venous blood oxygen content ($C\bar{v}o_2$) can be calculated by adding the amount of oxygen combined with hemoglobin, and the amount of oxygen dissolved in plasma (Table 13-4).

Oxygen delivery, or $\dot{D}o_2$, is the amount of oxygen (in milliliters) delivered per minute to the tissues.[18] It is calculated by multiplying the arterial oxygen content (Cao_2) by the cardiac output (CO). Cardiac output is usually between 4 and 8 L/min. Therefore, oxygen delivery is approximately 1000 ml/min.

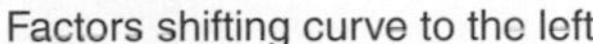

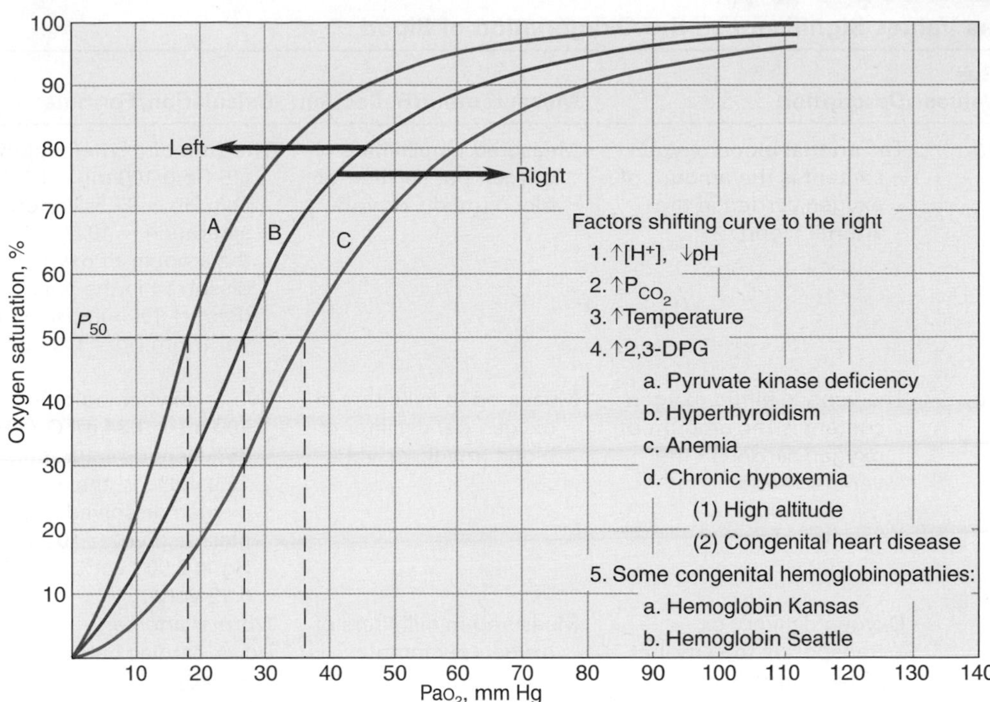

FIGURE 13-15 ■ Oxygen-hemoglobin dissociation curve: factors affecting hemoglobin's affinity for oxygen. Curve *B* is the standard oxyhemoglobin dissociation curve. Factors that shift the curve to the left are represented in curve *A;* factors that shift the curve to the right are represented in curve *C.* (Redrawn from Gottlieb JE: Breathing and gas exchange. *2,3-DPG,* 2,3-diphosphoglycerate. In Kinney MR, Packa DR, Dunbar SB, editors: *AACN's clinical reference for critical care nursing,* ed 3, New York, 1993, McGraw-Hill, p 672.)

Oxygen consumption (VO_2) is the amount of oxygen consumed by the tissues and is measured in milliliters of oxygen per minute. Once the oxygen reaches the tissues, oxygen consumption is controlled by the rate of energy expenditure within the cells or the rate at which adenosine diphosphate (ADP) is formed from ATP to provide energy. The increasing concentration of ADP enhances the metabolic utilization of oxygen.[17] Oxygen consumption can be determined by subtracting the oxygen remaining in the venous blood (CvO_2) from the oxygen delivered to the tissues by the arteries (CaO_2), and is known as the Fick equation.[20]

Gas values (pressure and content) relative to the oxygenation of blood are summarized in Table 13-4.

Carbon Dioxide Transport

RBCs are important in the transport of carbon dioxide in the blood. Carbon dioxide, a byproduct of cellular metabolism, is transported in three forms in the blood: (1) as dissolved gas, (2) as bicarbonate ion (HCO_3^-), and (3) in association with hemoglobin (Figure 13-16).[17] The partial pressure of carbon dioxide (PCO_2) reflects the pressure or tension that carbon dioxide exerts when it is dissolved in the blood. Partial pressure is measured in millimeters of mercury (mm Hg). In the pulmonary capillaries, carbon dioxide easily dissociates from hemoglobin and then diffuses across the alveolar membrane into the alveolar sacs. In the body tissues, the carbon dioxide inside the cells diffuses into the blood and attaches to the hemoglobin as oxygen is released to the tissues. The partial pressure of carbon dioxide in the arterial blood (PaCO_2) is usually 40 mm Hg and in the venous blood (PvCO_2) is usually 45 mm Hg.[17] Dissolved carbon dioxide combines slowly with water in the plasma to form carbonic acid (H_2CO_3), but in the red cell the presence of carbonic anhydrase acting as a catalyst significantly accelerates this reaction.[17,20] Carbonic acid rapidly dissociates into hydrogen ions (H^+) and bicarbonate ions (HCO_3^-).[17,20] As the concentration of HCO_3^- in the red cell increases, it diffuses into the plasma, whereas the H^+ remains, causing chloride to diffuse from the plasma into the red cell to maintain electrical neutrality. This is referred to as the **chloride shift.**[18]

Hemoglobin provides an excellent acid-base buffer by reacting with the free hydrogen ions and directly with carbon dioxide to form carbaminohemoglobin (Hb-CO_2), which is easily dissociated in the lungs as carbon dioxide for exhalation.[17] Unloading of oxygen in the tissue facilitates the loading of carbon dioxide and is referred to as the Haldane effect.[17,18]

Table 13-4

Gas Values Significant to the Oxygenation of Blood

Gas Values	Description	Measurement/Reflection	Calculation/Formula	Normal Value/Formula
Cao_2	The arterial blood oxygen content is the amount of oxygen carried in the arterial blood	Measured in milliliters of oxygen per deciliter of blood (ml/dl), or vol%	The sum of oxyhemoglobin (15 Hb g/100 ml × 1.34 ml O_2/g Hb × 97.5% arterial saturation = 19.6 vol%) + the amount of oxygen dissolved in the plasma (Pao_2 = 100 mm Hg × 0.003 vol%/mm Hg = 0.3 vol%)	~20 vol% Formula: 19.6 vol% oxyhemoglobin + 0.3 vol% dissolved in plasma = 19.9 vol%
$C\bar{v}o_2$	The venous blood oxygen content is the amount of oxygen carried in the venous blood	Measured in milliliters of oxygen per deciliter of blood (ml/dl), or vol%	$C\bar{v}o_2$ = oxyhemoglobin (15 Hb/100 ml × 1.34 ml O_2/g Hb × 75% venous saturation = 15.0 vol%) + the amount of oxygen dissolved in the plasma ($P\bar{v}o_2$ = 40 mm Hg × 0.003 vol%/mm Hg = 0.12 vol%)	~15 vol% Formula: 15 vol% oxyhemoglobin + 0.12 vol% dissolved in plasma = approximately 15 vol%
$\dot{D}o_2$	Oxygen delivery or transport is the amount of oxygen delivered to the tissues	Measured in milliliters of oxygen per minute (ml/min)	*Normal arterial:* $\dot{D}o_2$ = cardiac output (L/min) × Cao_2 × 10 *Normal venous:* $\dot{D}o_2$ = cardiac output (L/min) × $C\bar{v}o_2$ × 10	*Normal arterial:* ~1000 ml of O_2/min *Normal venous:* ~750 ml of O_2/min
Pao_2	The partial pressure of oxygen in arterial blood	Measured in millimeters of mercury (mm Hg) Reflects the tension or pressure that is exerted by oxygen when it is dissolved in plasma		Normal Pao_2 is 80-100 mm Hg
$Paco_2$	The partial pressure of carbon dioxide in arterial blood	Measured in millimeters of mercury (mm Hg) Reflects the tension or pressure that is exerted by carbon dioxide when it is dissolved in plasma		Normal $Paco_2$ is 35-45 mm Hg
$P\bar{v}o_2$	The partial pressure of oxygen in venous blood	Measured in millimeters of mercury (mm Hg) Reflects the tension or pressure that is exerted by oxygen when it is dissolved in plasma		Normal Pvo_2 is 35-40 mm Hg
$P\bar{v}co_2$	The partial pressure of carbon dioxide in venous blood	Measured in millimeters of mercury (mm Hg) Reflects the tension or pressure that is exerted by carbon dioxide when it is dissolved in plasma		Normal Pvo_2 is 41-51 mm Hg
Sao_2	The amount of hemoglobin bound to oxygen relative to the total amount of hemoglobin, both reduced and bound, in arterial blood	Expressed as a percentage		Normal Sao_2 is 95%-100%

Table 13-4

Gas Values Significant to the Oxygenation of Blood—cont'd

Gas Values	Description	Measurement/Reflection	Calculation/Formula	Normal Value/Formula
$S\bar{v}O_2$	The amount of hemoglobin bound to oxygen relative to the total amount of hemoglobin, both reduced and bound, in venous blood	Expressed as a percentage		Normal $S\bar{v}O_2$ is 60%-80%
$\dot{V}O_2$	Oxygen consumption is the amount of oxygen consumed by the tissues	Measured in milliliters of oxygen per minute (ml/min)		
		Oxygen consumption is derived from the difference between arterial oxygen transport and venous oxygen transport	$\dot{V}O_2$ = cardiac output × ($CaO_2 - C\bar{v}O_2$) × 10	Normal $\dot{V}O_2$ is 200-250 ml of O_2/min

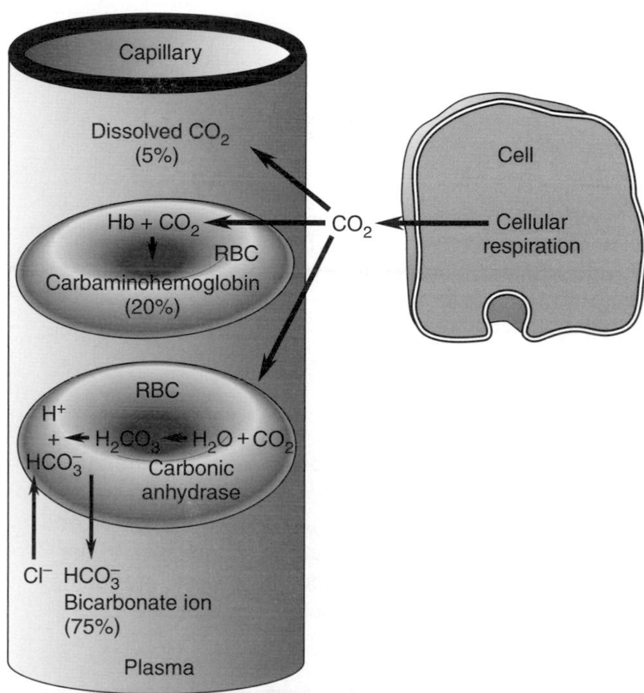

FIGURE 13-16 ■ Carbon dioxide is transported in three forms in the blood: (1) as dissolved gas, (2) as bicarbonate ion (HCO_3^-), and (3) in association with hemoglobin *(Hb)*.

Alterations in Oxygen Transport

There must be sufficient circulating hemoglobin mass to meet the metabolic needs of the body. A feedback mechanism ensures that when the oxygen reaching the tissues decreases, a compensatory increase occurs in the production of red cells.[2] The feedback mechanism regulating RBC production is under the control of erythropoietin. As stem cells differentiate into the erythroid committed line, the most primitive stem cell is referred to as the erythroid burst-forming unit (BFU-E), which is controlled by growth factors derived from T lymphocytes and macrophages and, to a lesser degree, by erythropoietin.[3,5] The BFU-E further differentiates into erythroid colony-forming units (CFU-E) more responsive to erythropoietin, and subsequently into normoblasts and mature RBCs.[2,3,5] The majority of erythropoietin is actively secreted by the kidney. Another 10% of erythropoietin is formed elsewhere in the body.[2,5]

Factors that decrease hemoglobin mass (such as anemia) or decrease arterial saturation (such as hypoxia from either cardiac or pulmonary conditions) impair oxygen delivery to the body tissues. This stimulates an increased release of erythropoietin and the production of RBCs.[2] Figure 13-17 illustrates the compensatory regulation of erythropoiesis that is seen in hypoxia, anemia, and polycythemia vera.

KEY CONCEPTS

- Nearly all (97%) of the oxygen transported in blood is bound to hemoglobin within the red cells. Only 3% is dissolved in plasma. It is this 3% which is measured as PaO_2. At a normal PaO_2, hemoglobin is 95% to 100% saturated with oxygen. About 25% of the bound oxygen is unloaded to the tissues, resulting in a venous hemoglobin saturation of about 75%.
- The oxyhemoglobin dissociation curve describes the relationship between the partial pressure of oxygen and hemoglobin saturation. In the lung, where PO_2 is high (100 mm Hg), oxygen is loaded onto hemoglobin. In the tissues, where PO_2 is low (40 mm Hg), oxygen is unloaded from hemoglobin to tissues.

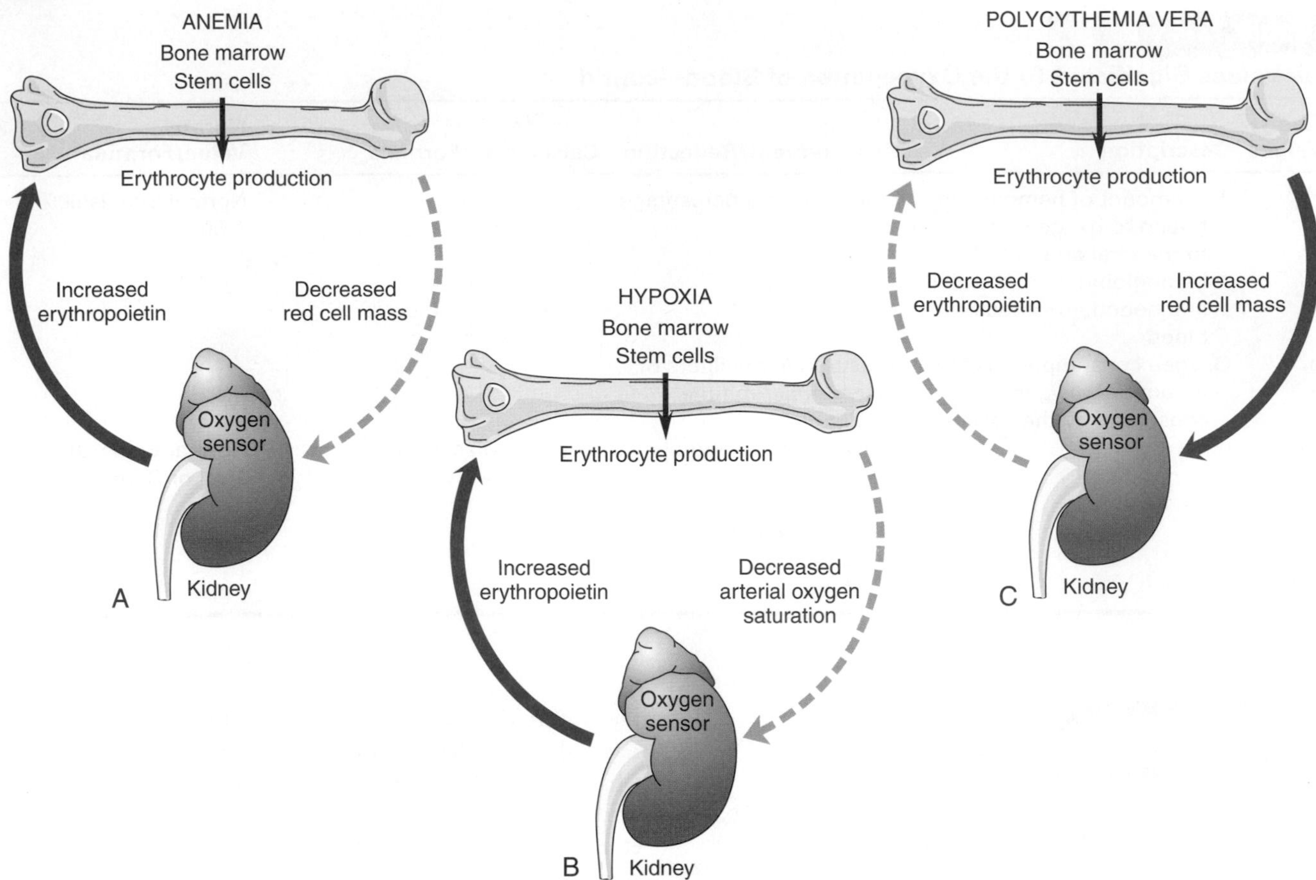

FIGURE 13-17 ■ Alterations in the erythropoietin feedback circuit. Any factor decreasing oxygen delivery to the oxygen sensor cells results in increased secretion of erythropoietin and a compensatory increase in erythrocyte production as illustrated in **A** for anemia, with a decrease in erythrocyte mass, and in **B** for hypoxia, with a decrease in arterial oxygen saturation. An increase in erythrocyte mass, as occurs with polycythemia vera **(C)**, decreases erythropoietin production.

- The affinity of hemoglobin for oxygen is affected by temperature, acid-base status, 2,3-DPG levels, and carbon dioxide. Affinity decreases at the tissue level due to increased levels of acid, 2,3-DPG, and carbon dioxide. This shift to the right of the oxyhemoglobin dissociation curve enhances unloading of oxygen to the tissue. A shift to the left occurs in the lungs, where blood is more alkalotic and carbon dioxide levels are lower. The increased affinity of hemoglobin for oxygen at the lung facilitates oxygen binding.
- The oxygen content of arterial blood is calculated by adding the amount bound to hemoglobin (Hb) plus the amount dissolved in plasma: $Cao_2 = (Hb \times 1.34 \times Sao_2) + (Pao_2 \times 0.003)$. Oxygen delivery to the body tissues is calculated by multiplying Cao_2 by cardiac output (CO): $\dot{D}o_2 = Cao_2 \times CO \times 10$.
- The consumption of oxygen by tissues can be estimated using the Fick equation: $\dot{V}o_2 = CO \times (Cao_2 - C\bar{v}o_2) \times 10$. Oxygen consumption increases with increased tissue metabolism.
- Hemoglobin is an important factor in carbon dioxide transport in the blood. In the tissues, hemoglobin binds carbon dioxide to form carbaminohemoglobin, which then releases carbon dioxide in the lungs. RBCs contain the enzyme carbonic anhydrase, which greatly increases conversion of carbon dioxide and water into HCO_3^- and H^+ at the tissue level. In the lungs, the reaction proceeds in reverse, producing carbon dioxide, which is eliminated by the lungs.

ANEMIA

Erythrocyte disorders are divided into two groups: (1) **anemia,** defined as a deficit of red cells, and (2) **polycythemia,** defined as an excess of red cells.[21,22] In discussing the various erythrocyte disorders in terms of the classification system given in Box 13-1, it is possible to review the more common types of anemia without the comprehensive review detailed in hematology reference books. An anemic patient has tissue hypoxia due to the low oxygen-carrying capacity of the blood. In contrast, a patient with polycythemia has increased whole-blood viscosity and blood volume due to the increase in number of RBCs.[22] (Polycythemia is discussed in greater detail later in this chapter.)

Box 13-1

Classification of Anemia and Polycythemia

Anemia

A. Relative
   1. Macroglobulinemia
   2. Pregnancy
   3. Athletes
   4. Postflight astronauts

B. Absolute
   1. Decreased red cell production
      a. Stem cell failure
         (1) Aplastic anemia
         (2) Anemia of leukemia and of myelodysplastic syndromes
      b. Progenitor cell failure
         (1) Pure red cell aplasia
         (2) Renal failure
         (3) Chronic disorders
         (4) Endocrine disorders
      c. Precursor cell failure
         (1) Megaloblastic anemias
         (2) Iron deficiency anemia
         (3) Thalassemia
         (4) Hemoglobinopathies
         (5) Congenital enzyme deficiencies
   2. Increased red cell destruction or loss
      a. Hereditary
         (1) Membrane defects
         (2) Globin defects
         (3) Enzyme defects
      b. Acquired
         (1) Macroangiopathic (traumatic)
         (2) Microangiopathic
         (3) Antibody mediated
         (4) Hypersplenism
         (5) Acute blood loss

Polycythemia (Erythrocytosis)

A. Relative (decreased plasma volume)
   1. Dehydration
   2. Apparent (normal plasma and red cell volume)
   3. Stress or smoker's erythrocytosis

B. Absolute (increased red cell volume)
   1. Primary
      a. Polycythemia vera
      b. Erythrocytosis (erythremia)
   2. Secondary
      a. Appropriate
         (1) Altitude
         (2) Cardiopulmonary disorder
         (3) Increased hemoglobin affinity for oxygen
      b. Inappropriate
         (1) Renal cysts and tumors
         (2) Hepatoma
         (3) Cerebellar hemangioblastoma
         (4) Essential

From Williams WJ et al, editors: *Hematology,* ed 3, New York, 2001, McGraw-Hill, pp 372, 374.

Relative anemia is characterized by normal total red cell mass with disturbances in the regulation of plasma volume. For example, in pregnant women the average plasma volume is 43% greater than in nonpregnant women, which causes a "dilutional anemia."[21]

Absolute anemia includes those types of anemia with an actual decrease in numbers of red cells. This can be caused by decreased production of red cells or increased destruction of red cells.[21]

GENERAL EFFECTS OF ANEMIA

The clinical manifestations of anemia include a reduction in oxygen-carrying capacity, tissue hypoxia, and compensatory mechanisms to restore tissue oxygenation.[21,22] Increased pulmonary and cardiac function increases the oxygen supply, and an increase in oxygen extraction occurs to protect tissues. Specific adaptations to anemia to increase oxygenated blood flow include an increase in the heart rate, cardiac output, circulatory rate, and preferential increase in blood flow to vital organs. Specific adaptations to anemia to increase oxygen utilization by tissues include an increase in 2,3-DPG in erythrocytes and a decreased oxygen affinity of hemoglobin in tissues. Selective tissue perfusion provides shunting to vital organs in short-term compensation, and increased erythropoietic activity is stimulated to provide long-term compensation.[6] The extent of the physiologic adaptations is influenced by (1) the severity of the anemia; (2) the competency of the pulmonary and cardiac systems; (3) the oxygen requirements of the individual, which are dependent on physical and metabolic activity; (4) the duration of the anemia; (5) the underlying disease or condition; and (6) the presence and severity of coexisting disease.[21] Specific symptoms related to anemia are vasoconstriction, pallor, tachypnea, dyspnea, tachycardia, transient murmurs, angina pectoris, heart failure, intermittent claudication, night cramps in muscles, headache, light-headedness, tinnitus, roaring in the ears, and faintness.[6]

ANEMIA RELATED TO DECREASED RED CELL PRODUCTION

Aplastic Anemia

Etiology and Pathogenesis. Aplastic anemia is an example of a stem cell disorder that is characterized by a reduction of hematopoietic tissue in the bone marrow, fatty marrow replacement, and pancytopenia. The decrease in functional bone marrow mass is usually caused by toxic, radiant, or immunologic injury to the bone marrow stem cells, which causes a decrease in red cells, white cells, and platelets, or **pancytopenia.**[23]

Aplastic anemia can be classified as acquired or familial. Acquired aplastic anemia can be caused by chemical and physical agents listed in Table 13-5. Other causes include certain viral infections (e.g., hepatitis, Epstein-Barr virus, human immunodeficiency virus [HIV], dengue), some mycobacterial infections, diffuse eosinophilic fasciitis, pregnancy, Simmonds disease, and sclerosis of the thyroid. Familial aplastic anemia is associated with Fanconi constitutional pancytopenia, pancreatic deficiency in children, and putative hereditary defect in cellular uptake of folate.[24]

Laboratory Features. Pancytopenia in aplastic anemia is characterized by low red cell, white cell, and platelet counts. The magnitude of the **granulocytopenia** is very important for

Table 13-5

Drugs Associated with Aplastic Anemia*

Category	High Risk	Moderate Risk	Low Risk
Analgesic			Phenacetin, aspirin, salicylamide
Antiarrhythmic			Quinidine, tocainide
Antiarthritic		Gold salts	Colchicine
Anticonvulsant		Carbamazepine, hydantoin, felbamate	Ethosuximide, phenacemide, primidone, trimethadione
Antihistamine			Chlorpheniramine, pyrilamine, tripelennamine
Antihypertensive			Captopril, methyldopa
Antiinflammatory		Penicillamine, phenylbutazone, oxyphenbutazone	Diclofenac, ibuprofen, indomethacin, naproxen, sulindac
Antimicrobial			
Antibacterial		Chloramphenicol	Dapsone, methicillin, penicillin, streptomycin, β-lactam antibiotics
Antifungal			Amphotericin, flucytosine
Antiprotozoal		Quinacrine	Chloroquine, mepacrine, pyrimethamine
Antineoplastic			
Alkylating agents	Busulfan, cyclophosphamide, melphalan, nitrogen mustard		
Antimetabolites	Fluorouracil, mercaptopurine, methotrexate		
Cytotoxic antibiotics	Daunorubicin, doxorubicin, mitoxantrone		
Antiplatelet			Ticlopidine
Antithyroid			Carbimazole, methimazole, methylthiouracil, potassium perchlorate, propylthiouracil, sodium thiocyanate
Sedative and tranquilizer			Chlordiazepoxide, chlorpromazine (and other phenothiazines), lithium, meprobamate, methyprylon
Sulfonamides and derivatives			
Antibacterial			Numerous sulfonamides
Diuretic		Acetazolamide	Chlorothiazide, furosemide
Hypoglycemic			Chlorpropamide, tolbutamide
Miscellaneous			Allopurinol, interferon, pentoxifylline

From Shadduck RK: Aplastic anemia. In Beutler E et al, editors: *Williams hematology,* ed 6, New York, 2001, McGraw-Hill, pp 375-389. This list was compiled from the AMA Registry, Publications of the International Agranulocytosis and Aplastic Anemia Study, other reviews and studies, previous compilations of offending agents, and selected reports.

*Drugs that invariably cause marrow aplasia with high doses are termed high risk; drugs with 30 or more reported cases are listed as moderate risk; other are less often associated with aplastic anemia (low risk).

the immediate prognosis. An absolute granulocyte count of less than 200/mm^3 results in immediate susceptibility to infectious complications. Coagulation tests are generally normal except for the bleeding time, which reflects the low platelet count.[24]

Clinical Manifestations. The onset is usually insidious, and patients often present only after the late manifestations of **pancytopenia** are evident. The symptoms due to the gradual fall of RBCs include weakness, fatigue, lethargy, pallor, dyspnea, palpitations, onset of transient murmurs and the tachycardia of anemia. Fever, chills, and bacterial infections (particularly in the mouth or perirectal area) are seen secondary to **neutropenia.** Petechiae, bruising, nosebleeds, retinal hemorrhage, and increased menstrual flow are seen due to **thrombocytopenia.**[23]

Treatment. Treatment for aplastic anemia is multifaceted and dependent on the severity of the disease. Treatment includes (1) identification and avoidance of further toxin exposure; (2) human leukocyte antigen (HLA) and ABO typing of family members to identify serologically defined loci and potential bone transplant donors; (3) maintenance of minimally essential levels of hemoglobin and platelets; (4) prevention and management of infection; (5) determination of efficacy of bone marrow transplantation; and (6) other forms of therapy, such as immunosuppressive therapy or stimulation of hematopoiesis and bone marrow regeneration in patients not suited to receive a transplant.[23-26] In patients with severe disease, the major curative approach is allogenic bone marrow transplantation; however, only one third of all patients have compatible donors.[23-26] Preparative regimens using cyclophosphamide and antithymocyte globulin have resulted in a 90% disease-free survival rate for patients with hematopoietic cell transplantation with bone marrow derived from an HLA-matched sibling donor.[27]

Course and Prognosis. Bone marrow transplantation is highly successful and curative for 75% to 85% of untransfused patients and 55% to 60% of patients with multiple previous transfusions. Twenty to thirty percent of transplantation survivors experience severe graft versus host disease, which can be significantly improved by immunosuppressive therapy in 50% to 70% of patients.[22] Prognosis is related to the absolute neutrophil count and the platelet count. Children respond better than adults with both bone marrow transplantation and immunosuppression therapy, especially in patients with mild to moderate disease. Aplastic anemia is usually fatal unless managed with bone marrow transplantation.[23-27]

Anemia of Chronic Renal Failure

Etiology and Pathogenesis. The anemia of chronic renal failure occurs primarily from (1) failure of the renal endocrine function, which causes impaired erythropoietin production and bone marrow compensation, and secondarily from (2) failure of the renal excretory function, leading to hemolysis, bone marrow cell depression, and blood loss.[28]

Laboratory Features. This anemia is characterized by a decreased red cell count and low hemoglobin and hematocrit values. Some red cells appear grossly deformed with a few large spicules (Figure 13-18). The total leukocyte differential cell count, leukocyte counts, and platelet count are usually normal. The red cell indices—mean corpuscular volume (MCV), mean corpuscular hemoglobin (MCH), and mean corpuscular hemoglobin concentration (MCHC)—are also normal.[28,29]

Clinical Manifestations. Any of the clinical manifestations described earlier (see General Effects of Anemia) may be evident in chronic renal failure. In addition, pericardial effusions may occur. The hematocrit falls in proportion to the degree of renal insufficiency, and uremia occurs as the glomerular filtration rate falls below 40 ml/min. Signs and symptoms usually manifest when the hematocrit falls to 20% or below.[29]

Treatment. Therapy consists of administration of erythropoietin to achieve the target hematocrit of 33% to 36% and target hemoglobin of 11 to 12 g/dl. In adults the initial dose should be 80 to 120 units per kilogram per week divided into two or three subcutaneous injections or 120 to 180 units per kilogram per week given as three intravenous injections. The hematocrit and hemoglobin are monitored at least every 2 weeks. When the target hematocrit is achieved, adult patients can be maintained by administering 50 to 100 units per kilogram per week in divided doses. Pediatric patients younger than 5 years usually require higher initial and maintenance doses.[28-33] It is important to maintain adequate iron stores. The National Kidney Foundation prefers intravenous iron, but an oral iron preparation providing at least 100 mg of elemental iron per day is often used. Vitamin B_{12} and folic acid are also administered. Hypertension, especially in patients

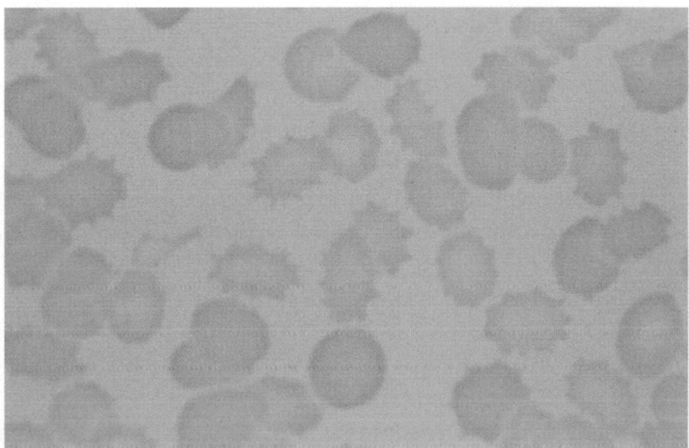

FIGURE 13-18 ■ Burr cells found in acute kidney disease. (Courtesy Beth Payne, Sacred Heart Medical Center, Spokane, Wash.)

with this previously existing condition, is often seen and should be managed with medication.[28-33]

Course and Prognosis. More than 95% of patients respond to erythropoietin therapy. Patients who do not respond or first respond when larger doses are given should be evaluated for an adequate iron supply, infection, or excessive splenic hemolysis. Occasionally aluminum toxicity is responsible for resistance to treatment.[28-33]

Anemia Related to Vitamin B_{12} (Cobalamin) or Folate Deficiency

Etiology and Pathogenesis. The anemia resulting from a deficiency of either vitamin B_{12} (cobalamin) or folate is caused by a disruption in DNA synthesis of the blast cells in the bone marrow. This disruption produces very large abnormal bone marrow cells called **megaloblasts.** In the peripheral blood the red cells are larger than normal (**macrocytic**), the granulocytes are hypersegmented, and the numbers of red cells, white cells, and platelets are decreased.[34,35] All of these signs can be seen on the peripheral blood smear.

The classic anemia in this classification is pernicious anemia. The fundamental defect causing pernicious anemia is the lack of intrinsic factor. Without it, vitamin B_{12} cannot be absorbed, thus leading to vitamin B_{12} deficiency. This deficiency results in disordered nucleic acid metabolism, which causes **megaloblastic dysplasia,** a condition involving abnormal production and maturation of red cell, white cell, and platelet systems. There is strong evidence that pernicious anemia develops as a result of genetically determined autoimmune disease, which is manifested by serum and gastric juice antibodies against intrinsic factor and parietal cells.[34] The biochemical basis of the neurologic lesions in pernicious anemia is not known. There can be peripheral nerve degeneration, degeneration of the posterior columns of the spinal cord, or both. There is some evidence of abnormal fatty acid metabolism in the peripheral nerves and degeneration of the white matter in the spinal cord in animals.[34,35]

Laboratory Features. The peripheral blood shows low RBC counts of 500,000 to 750,000 cells/mm^3, low WBC counts of 4000 to 5000 cells/mm^3, and low platelet counts of 50,000 cells/mm^3. These counts are usually not as low as those seen in aplastic anemia. The bone marrow shows megaloblastic dysplasia, which results in a peripheral blood picture of macrocytosis and hypersegmented neutrophils. The red cell indices show normal MCH and MCHC and increased MCV. The Schilling test, which measures excretion of radioactive vitamin B_{12}, indicates low levels, and the serum level of vitamin B_{12} is low. Gastric analysis reveals a lack of free hydrochloric acid in the gastric juice (achlorhydria).[34,35]

Folate deficiencies resemble vitamin B_{12} deficiencies except for the neurologic disease, which is more characteristic of vitamin B_{12} deficiency. Folate deficiencies are usually the result of dietary deficiencies, alcoholism and cirrhosis, pregnancy, or infancy.

Clinical Manifestations. The clinical features of vitamin B_{12} deficiency include paranoid ideation, dementia, cognitive dysfunction, delusions, and hallucinations, often referred to as "megaloblastic madness."[34] The neurologic abnormalities include symmetric paresthesias of the feet and hands with vibratory sense and proprioception disturbances. The paresthesias progress to spastic ataxia owing to degenerative changes of the dorsal and lateral columns of the spinal cord. Cerebral signs include irritability, somnolence, memory impairment, and perversion of taste, smell, and vision.[34,35] Manifestations of pure folate deficiency include a blunted affect in general demeanor with evidence of depression, sleep deprivation, and irritability. History of circumstances likely to result in folic acid deficiency includes poor or fad diet, frank malabsorption, or alcoholism. In folate deficiency, cerebral symptoms, such as irritability, memory loss, and personality changes, are seen.[34,35] Clinical manifestations that are seen in both vitamin B_{12} and folate deficiencies include pedal edema, nocturia, tachypnea, dyspnea, and tachycardia associated with heart congestion; glossitis, weight loss, malabsorption, and episodic or chronic diarrhea with steatorrhea are gastrointestinal manifestations. Musculoskeletal symptoms of arthralgia and frank arthritis are seen in autoimmune diseases; nocturnal pain and upper and/or lower extremity cramps often indicate spinothalamic tract involvement. Dermatologic symptoms include blotchy brown skin pigmentation, especially in nail beds and skin creases. When this is associated with vitiligo, autoimmune processes should be suspected.[34,35]

Recent research has reported an association between low folate levels and the risk of neural tube defects and abnormalities of the heart, urinary tract, and limbs in neonates. These data support the routine supplementation before pregnancy of all women who might become pregnant with 1.0 mg/day of folic acid.[34,35] This is the largest dose that will not mask vitamin B_{12} deficiency.

Treatment. Routine treatment with full doses of parenteral vitamin B_{12} (1 mg/day) and oral folate (1 to 5 mg/day) before the cause of the deficiency is identified should only be used in critically ill patients. In managing the anemia related to vitamin B_{12} or folate deficiency, it is important to (1) recognize that megaloblastic anemia is present, (2) ascertain if vitamin B_{12}, folate, or a combined deficiency is the cause, and (3) diagnose the underlying disease and mechanism responsible for the deficiency. Replacement of vitamin B_{12} and folic acid is indicated in vitamin B_{12} and folic acid deficiency anemia, respectively (Table 13-6). Transfusion therapy may be indicated in elderly or critically ill patients. Serum hypokalemia should be managed with potassium supplements to prevent sudden death, reportedly associated with a sharp drop in serum potassium level seen in vitamin B_{12} therapy.[34,35]

Table 13-6

Replacement Therapy for Vitamin B_{12} and Folic Acid Deficiency Anemia

	Vitamin B_{12} Deficiency	Folate Deficiency
Vitamin form	Cyanocobalamin (B_{12})	Folic acid
Route	Intramuscular	Oral
Dose		
Initial	Cyanocobalamin IM: Week 1: 1 mg/day Week 2: 1 mg twice weekly Week 4: 1 mg/wk for 4 weeks followed by maintenance or Cyanocobalamin IM: Weeks 1 and 2: 1 mg/day Week 3: 1 mg/day weekly until hematocrit is normal	1 mg/day
Maintenance	Cyanocobalamin IM: 1 mg/mo for life Note: For patients who prefer oral therapy, 1 mg/day	1 mg/day
Neurologic treatment	Cyanocobalamin IM: 1 mg every 2 wk for 6 mo	
Prophylaxis	Total gastrectomy Infants of mothers with pernicious anemia Infants on specialized diets Lactoovovegetarians/vegans	All women contemplating pregnancy Pregnancy/lactation Prematurity Hemolytic anemias Hyperproliferative hemolytic states Rheumatoid arthritis or psoriasis patients on methotrexate therapy

From Antony AC: Megaloblastic anemias. In Hoffman R et al, editors: *Hematology, basic principles and practice,* ed 3, New York, 2000, Churchill Livingstone, p 475.

Course and Prognosis. The majority of patients respond well to replacement therapy; however, continued assessment and monitoring of these patients is essential to prevent hematologic or neurologic relapse secondary to inadequate therapy.[34,35] In patients with neurologic signs and symptoms, the reversibility of the neurologic damage is slow, with a maximal response requiring up to 6 months. Further substantial increases in recovery are unlikely after 12 months. In 90% of patients with subacute combined degeneration, major improvement is seen.[34] The degree of functional recovery is inversely related to the extent of the disease and duration of the signs and symptoms. Patients with signs and symptoms of less than 3 months duration may have complete reversal.[34,35]

Iron Deficiency Anemia

Etiology and Pathogenesis. Iron deficiency, the most common nutritional deficiency in the world, is the most common cause of anemia. Iron deficiency results in the unavailability of iron for hemoglobin synthesis. This may be due to low intake, diminished absorption, physiologic increase in requirements (such as pregnancy), excessive iron loss (such as acute or chronic hemorrhage), or chronic renal failure, hemodialysis, and idiopathic iron loss. Iron is one of the most carefully conserved body substances, and under normal conditions very little is lost except as a result of bleeding. Normal dietary requirements, if 10% is absorbed, are as follows: adult men, 12 mg/day; adult women aged 14 to 30 years, 15 mg/day; and adult women aged 60 years or more, 10 mg/day. Pregnant women require up to 30 mg/day, and children require 10 mg/day. A normal diet supplies the adult with about 10 to 15 mg/day.[36-40]

Laboratory Features. In latent iron deficiency there may be no anemia, but after receiving iron patients respond with a significant increase in blood hemoglobin level. In a typical case caused by chronic bleeding, the reduction in hemoglobin concentration is proportionately greater than the reduction in the red cell count. The red cells are smaller and paler than normal cells due to the decreased amount of hemoglobin and are described as **hypochromic, microcytic red cells.** Therefore, the red cell indices MCV, MCH, and MCHC are decreased. The white cell counts are usually normal. The platelet count varies, depending on the cause of the deficiency. In severely anemic children and infants, thrombocytopenia may be present. In patients who are bleeding, thrombocytosis may be present. The serum ferritin level is decreased, the serum iron level is decreased, total iron binding capacity (TIBC) is increased, and tissue iron stores are decreased.[36-40]

Clinical Manifestations. In the majority of patients anemia is asymptomatic; however, patients may experience general symptoms of anemia such as pallor, weakness, fatigue, dyspnea, palpitations, new and transient heart murmurs, irritability, headaches, light-headedness, and pica (craving for nonfood substances such as dirt, clay, ice, laundry starch, cardboard, or hair). Restless legs are seen at night, especially in the elderly. In severe cases, gastrointestinal symptoms are seen, such as glossitis, dysphagia, erosions at the corners of the mouth, esophageal webbing, and atrophic gastritis, as well as changes in the fingernails, conjunctival pallor, and splenomegaly.[36-40]

Treatment. Iron deficiency anemia is managed with oral administration of ferrous sulfate (150 to 200 mg daily in three or four doses between meals) until hematologic normality is reached. Infants may be given 50 to 100 mg daily in divided doses. Thereafter it is important to continue the treatment for 4 to 6 months to build iron stores. Urgent treatment may be accomplished with iron-dextran infusions. Although iron therapy remediates the iron deficiency anemia, the underlying cause must be sought and corrected.[36-40]

Course and Prognosis. The symptoms may be alleviated in the first few days of treatment. The reticulocyte count is an index of erythropoiesis. The reticulocyte count increases as the RBC production increases and usually reaches maximal levels in 7 to 12 days, and the hemoglobin is usually normal by 2 months. The prognosis is excellent if the underlying cause is benign; however, even in patients with incurable disease states, management of iron deficiency anemia with iron therapy can increase the comfort level.[36-40]

ANEMIA RELATED TO INHERITED DISORDERS OF THE RED CELL

Thalassemia

Anemia can also be caused by increased destruction, or **hemolysis,** of red cells. Hemolytic anemias are characterized by decreased red cell survival rates. The thalassemias are examples of a type of anemia caused by decreased red cell survival rates. The red cells produced are abnormal and prone to destruction. This destruction is based on an intrinsic defect in the red cells.[41-44]

Etiology and Pathogenesis. The thalassemias are a group of diseases associated with the presence of mutant genes that suppress the rate of synthesis of globin chains. Thalassemias are classified according to the polypeptide chain or chains with deficient synthesis, such as α-thalassemia or β-thalassemia.[41-44]

A deficiency in one or more polypeptide chains causes decreased hemoglobin synthesis and an imbalance between α- and non–α-chain production. Because of the lack of hemoglobin, the anemia is severe, and the peripheral cells are microcytic and hypochromic. The disruption of the globin balance causes the normal chains to build up and precipitate within the cytoplasm. This damages the cell membranes, which leads to premature cell destruction. The most clinically severe form of the thalassemias is thalassemia major, which occurs in homozygous patients. Thalassemia minor is the term used to describe the heterozygous carrier state. For example, in homozygous β-thalassemia, the deficiency of β-chain synthesis results in the accumulation of α chains, which aggregate to form insoluble inclusions in bone marrow erythroid precursors (Figure 13-19). These inclusions cause early destruction of 70% to 85% of marrow erythroblasts. In response to this massive destruction, erythroid cell proliferation in homozygous β-thalassemia is significant.[41-44]

Patients who are significantly anemic have an increased intestinal iron absorption that is related to the degree of expansion of the RBC precursor population. This can be decreased with blood transfusions. The iron accumulates in the Kupffer cells of the liver, the macrophages in the spleen, and the parenchymal cells of the liver.[41]

Laboratory Features. Laboratory values vary, depending on the severity of the imbalance, which is determined by the genetic pattern. Due to the decrease in hemoglobin, the red cells are hypochromic and microcytic, and red cell indices—MCV, MCH, and MCHC—are decreased. Many target cells are present. In homozygous or major syndromes the hemoglobin is often less than 7 g/dl, and there are nucleated red cells in the peripheral blood. The leukocyte number is usually increased but the platelet number is normal. The bone marrow is hypercellular, with profound erythroblastic hyperplasia. There is evidence of hemolysis with increased unconjugated bilirubin levels and increased excretion of urobilin and urobilinogen. Hemoglobin electrophoresis is performed to determine the type of abnormal hemoglobin. An increased level of fetal hemoglobin ranging from 10% to 90% is characteristic of homozygous α-thalassemia. No hemoglobin α is produced. Excess γ chains form γ4 homotetramers or Bart's hemoglobin. Excess β chains form β4 homotetramers or hemoglobin H.[41-44]

Clinical Manifestations. Patients may have any of the clinical manifestations described earlier (see "General Effects of Anemia"). The clinical findings are the result of deficient α-globin production in α-thalassemia or α-globin chain excess and persistent hemoglobin F production in β-thalassemia.[41-44]

α-Thalassemia is found primarily in Asian individuals; however, it has also been documented in increasing numbers in individuals of Mediterranean or African descent. Usually patients with α-thalassemia minor are silent carriers or present with mild to moderate anemia. They are identified during familial studies following the identification of a family

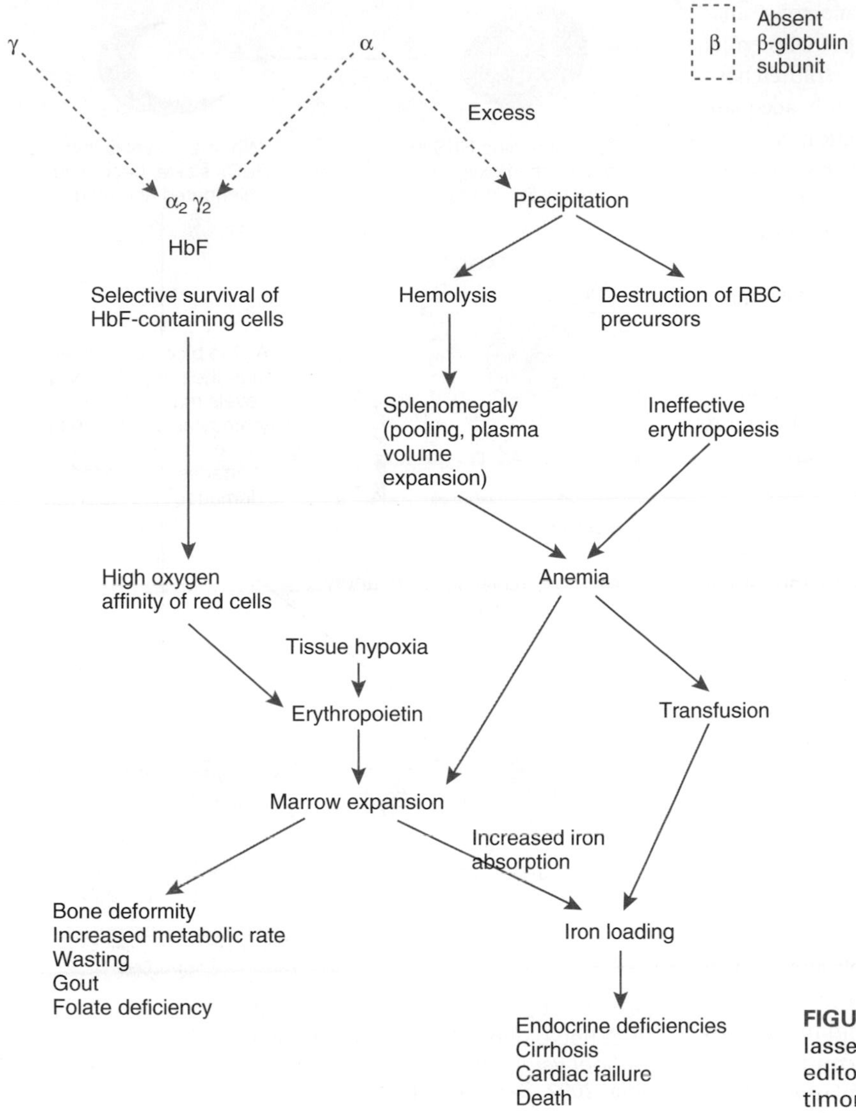

FIGURE 13-19 ■ The pathophysiology of β-thalassemia. *HbF,* Hemoglobin F. (From Lee GR et al, editors: *Wintrobe's clinical hematology,* ed 10, Baltimore, 1998, Williams & Wilkins, p 560.)

member with Bart's hemoglobin hydrops fetalis or hemoglobin H disease (α-thalassemia major). Infants with Bart's hemoglobin hydrops fetalis are pale and edematous and have hepatomegaly, splenomegaly, and ascites. Individuals with hemoglobin H disease have typical facies and bone changes seen in β-thalassemia, splenomegaly, and hepatomegaly.[41-43]

β-Thalassemia occurs mainly in individuals of Mediterranean descent and presents as thalassemia major, intermedia, or minor. It is also seen in the Middle East, parts of India and Pakistan, and throughout Southeast Asia. Untreated patients with thalassemia major have skull bone deformities from intramedullary and extramedullary bone marrow expansion, mongoloid facies, bowing and **rarefaction** of long bones, extension of bone marrow into paraspinal or intraabdominal tumors, **icterus,** hepatomegaly, splenomegaly, and cardiac failure or endocrinopathies, such as diabetes mellitus and hypogonadism from excessive intestinal iron absorption. Patients with thalassemia intermedia show fewer effects of iron overload, growth retardation, marrow expansion, and splenomegaly; however, deforming bone and joint disease, chronic leg ulceration, and infection are common in this form of thalassemia. Thalassemia minor is usually relatively asymptomatic.[41-44]

Treatment. Children with thalassemia are treated with blood transfusion therapy to maintain a hemoglobin level of 9.5 to 14 g/dl to ensure normal growth and development and to avoid skeletal deformities. Recent studies support maintaining the lower hemoglobin level of 9.5 g/dl to reduce iron loading while maintaining normal growth and development. Iron supplements are avoided, and chelation therapy is started when the serum ferritin levels reach 1000 μg/dl. Subcutaneous infusion with deferoxamine, an iron-chelating agent, is given 8 to 12 hours daily 5 days a week at doses of 20 mg/kg. Vitamin C (100 to 200 mg/day taken orally increases iron excretion) is required for management of iron overload. Splenectomy is indicated in cases with hypersplenism, but it requires aggressive management of infection following the procedure. Bone marrow transplantation has been used with success in severe β-thalassemia. The best candidates are younger children, as older children have a high rejection and mortality rate. Children with adequate treatment with iron chelation prior to transplantation have disease-free survival rates of 90% to 93% with a 4% risk of mortality related to the procedure. Venesection is another treatment to remove excess body iron prior to transplantation. Folic acid administration is used. As this is a genetically transmitted disease, it is important for patients and parents to receive appropriate genetic counseling.[41-44]

Course and Prognosis. Infants with Bart's hemoglobin hydrops fetalis inherit an α-thalassemia gene from both parents who only have the α-thalassemia trait. These infants are usually stillborn or die within hours to days of birth. Some patients with hemoglobin H disease live a full life. Patients with β-thalassemia intermedia can expect to live until middle age; however, iron loading and crippling bone disease occur in the third and fourth decades. In one study individuals with β-thalassemia major who were adequately treated with transfusions and chelation therapy and who maintained a reduction of body iron at less than 2500 μg/L over 12 years had a cardiac disease–free survival of 91% compared to others with higher levels and a survival rate of less than 20%.[41] Two promising future treatments include gene therapy and manipulation of the hemoglobin F to A switch. Both therapies could significantly prolong life.[41,43]

Sickle Cell Anemia

Etiology and Pathogenesis. Sickle cell anemia is a genetically determined defect of hemoglobin synthesis. In hemoglobin S, valine is substituted for glutamic acid in the sixth position of the β chain, rather than the normal configuration. This apparently minor change in the molecular structure causes profound changes in hemoglobin stability and solubility. Under decreased oxygen tension, hemoglobin S undergoes polymerization, which causes the red cell to assume a sickled shape (Figure 13-20). Patients who are homozygous produce only hemoglobin S. No hemoglobin A is synthesized because all the β chains are S chains, which combine with normal α chains to form hemoglobin S. In heterozygous patients with sickle cell trait, both normal and S chains are formed. Because fewer abnormal chains are produced than normal ones, the amount of hemoglobin A usually exceeds that of hemoglobin S. It has been suggested that preferential sickling of cells with malarial parasites reduces the number of parasites and allows children with sickle cell trait who are infected with these parasites to reach reproductive age. This may have provided a selective advantage to the hemoglobin S trait, thereby preventing S from being genetically eliminated.[45-48]

The pathogenetic signs and symptoms of sickle cell disease all relate to the red cell sickling. Sickled red cells have a decreased survival time, which causes anemia. Sickled cells cause vascular occlusion, which results in capillary stasis, venous thrombosis, and arterial emboli. The most dangerous feature of sickle cell anemia is the occurrence of acute episodes of "crisis," which can be hemolytic or vascular (Box 13-2).[45-48]

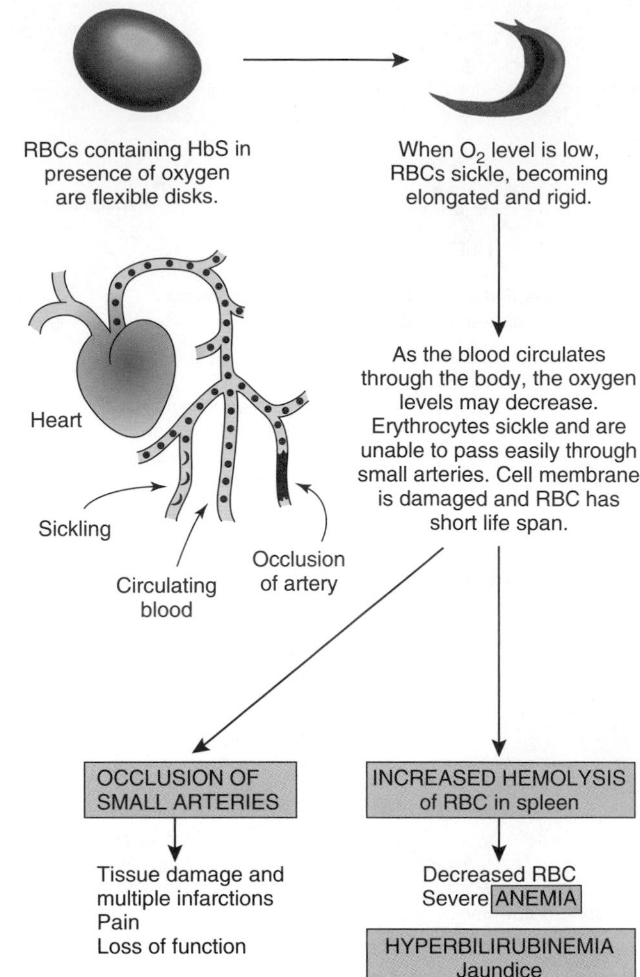
RBCs containing HbS in presence of oxygen are flexible disks.
When O_2 level is low, RBCs sickle, becoming elongated and rigid.
Heart
Sickling
Circulating blood
Occlusion of artery
As the blood circulates through the body, the oxygen levels may decrease. Erythrocytes sickle and are unable to pass easily through small arteries. Cell membrane is damaged and RBC has short life span.
OCCLUSION OF SMALL ARTERIES
Tissue damage and multiple infarctions
Pain
Loss of function
INCREASED HEMOLYSIS of RBC in spleen
Decreased RBC
Severe ANEMIA
HYPERBILIRUBINEMIA
Jaundice

FIGURE 13-20 ■ Sickle cell anemia: the effects of sickling. *RBC,* Red blood cell; *HbS,* hemoglobin S. (From Gould BE: *Pathophysiology for the health professions,* ed 2, Philadelphia, 2002, Saunders, p 247.)

Laboratory Features. The laboratory features in sickle cell anemia are distinctive. The anemia is usually severe, with red cells of different shapes and sizes. Target red cells are present, and occasionally sickled cells can be seen on smears (Figure 13-21). Red cell breakdown products are increased, which increases serum bilirubin, urobilinogen, and urobilin levels. Acute hemolytic crisis is characterized by hemoglobinuria, leukocytosis, and normoblastosis; diffuse intravascular coagulation may develop.[45-48]

Clinical Manifestations. Sickle cell anemia and sickle cell trait are found almost entirely in the black race.[45-48] Hemolysis of the sickle cells occurs in the spleen or vascular space, and vasoocclusive events occur in the small capillaries and venules caused by sickle cells.[45] The red cell life span is already shortened by the sickling and may precipitate a hemolytic crisis with jaundice. Sudden massive pooling of red

Box 13-2

Complications of Sickle Cell Anemia

Decreased RBC Survival
Anemia
Reticulocytosis
Hyperbilirubinemia
Increased pigment excretion
Cholelithiasis
Hyperplastic bone marrow
Osteoporosis
Osteosclerosis
Siderosis

Acute Hemolytic Crisis
Leukocytosis
Reticulocytosis
Hyperbilirubinemia
Hemoglobinuria
Normoblastosis
Diffuse intravascular coagulation (consumption coagulopathy)

Vascular Occlusion (Capillary Stasis, Venous Thrombosis, Arterial Emboli)
Splenomegaly
Splenic infarction
Splenic atrophy
Hepatomegaly
Cirrhosis
Hematuria
Sickle cell dactylitis
Aseptic necrosis of bones
Infarction of bone marrow
Infarction of various organs
Priapism
Skin ulcers
Pulmonary embolism

Painful Crisis (Occlusive Vascular Crisis)
Fever
Pain
Sudden death

Data from Miale J, editor: *Laboratory medicine hematology,* ed 6, St Louis, 1982, Mosby, p 637.

cells, particularly in the spleen, can create a sequestration crisis, which is thought to result in the deaths that occur in the first years of life.[45-48] Infarctive crises or painful episodes are a result of obstruction of blood vessels, tissue hypoxia, and tissue death, and may occur throughout the body. Vasoocclusive events are described in Table 13-7. Children with sickle cell anemia are shorter and experience delayed puberty, but they attain normal height with late adolescent growth. Bony abnormalities, "hand-foot" syndrome with periostitis of the metacarpal and metatarsal bones, splenomegaly, inability to concentrate urine, priapism with subsequent impotence, underdeveloped genitalia and hypogonadism, hepatomegaly, jaundice, gallstones, tachycardia, acute chest syndrome (fever, chest pain, increasing WBC count, and pulmonary infiltrates), retinal vessel obstruction, cerebrovascular accidents, leg ulcers, and infections are all seen in sickle cell disease patients. Pregnant women may exhibit signs of pyelonephritis, pulmonary infarction, pneumonia, antepartum hemorrhage, premature fetal delivery, and fetal death.[45-48]

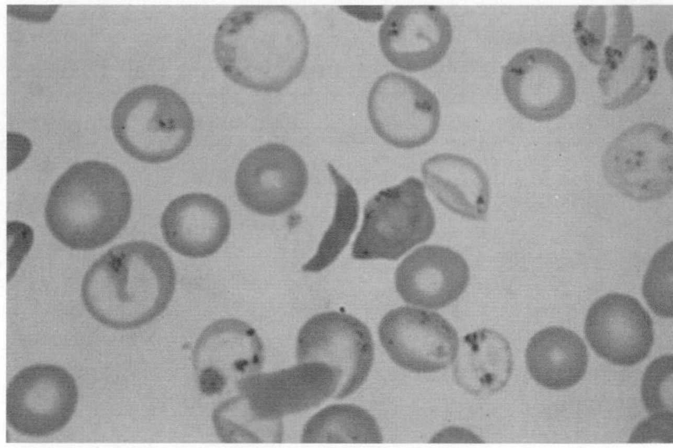

FIGURE 13-21 ■ Blood smear showing sickle cells in sickle cell anemia. (Courtesy Beth Payne, Sacred Heart Medical Center, Spokane, Wash.)

Treatment. Stem cell transplantation is curative and the treatment of choice. Currently there are no safe, effective antisickling agents, and treatment is primarily supportive. To avoid precipitation of a vasoocclusive crisis, it is important to prevent dehydration, infection, fever, acidosis, hypoxemia, and cold exposure.[45-48] As salicylates impose an acid load, acetaminophen is the preferred antipyretic.[46] Vaccination for pneumococcal pneumonia should be done before 2 years of age in patients with sickle cell anemia and booster vaccinations given 3 to 5 years later. Penicillin prophylaxis is important to prevent streptococcal pneumonia and pneumococcal septicemia. Other vaccinations include *Haemophilus influenzae* type B and hepatitis B. Transfusions are used to restore normal hematocrit levels, and splenectomy is performed in children with sequestration syndrome. Treatment with hydroxyurea increases fetal hemoglobin levels and can ameliorate crisis. During pregnancy, folic acid should be given to prevent neural tube defects. If iron deficiency is present, iron supplements should also be given. Transfusion should be used only when clinical and hematologic indicators are present.[45-48]

Course and Prognosis. Successful stem cell transplantation cures sickle cell anemia; however, mortality in young children with a good family donor match is 10%. Sickle cell anemia is a serious disorder, and without stem cell transplantation many patients die in childhood, especially in sequestration crisis. In young children with sickle cell anemia, there is a 30% incidence of splenic sequestration crisis with a 15% mortality. Functional hyposplenia predisposes individuals to infections, such as pneumonia and chronic pyelonephritis with renal failure. Heart failure, bone marrow and fat emboli, shock, and organ failure are common causes of death. In developed countries, patients who have not undergone stem cell transplantation may survive into

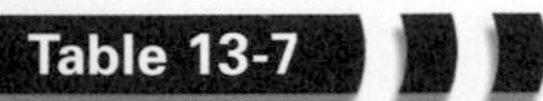

Vasoocclusive Consequences of Sickle Cell Disease

Event	Incidence	Features
Acute		
Painful episodes	>50% of patients with HbSS and HbSβ-thalassemia	Mild to severe pain; one or several areas
Chest syndrome	10%-20% of adults	Difficult to distinguish from pneumonia; may involve entire lung
Priapism	10%-40% of males	Can have a more chronic form; causes impotence
Cerebrovascular accidents	1%-10% of children	Usually subarachnoid bleeding in adults
Hepatopathy	<2% of adults	Bilirubin may reach >80 mg/dl
Chronic		
Aseptic bone necrosis	10%-25% of adults	Hips and shoulders, common in HbSC
Proliferative retinopathy	50% of adults with HbSC; <5% HbSS	Can lead to retinal detachment
Leg ulcers	10%	Can be severe and disabling
Functional asplenia and autosplenectomy	Starts in infancy; >90% of adults with HbSS	Predispose to sepsis
Nephropathy	Renal failure in older patients	Nephritic syndrome, renal failure

From Sternberg MH: Hemoglobinopathies and thalassemias. In Stein JH et al, editors: *Internal medicine,* ed 5, St. Louis, 1998, Mosby, p 658.
HbS, Hemoglobin S (sickle hemoglobin); *HbSC,* hemoglobin SC disease; *HbSS,* hemoglobin SS (sickle cell anemia).

the third and fourth decades, whereas survival past childhood in underdeveloped countries is unusual.[45-48] The survival rates have increased dramatically due to stem cell transplantation, newborn screening, early diagnosis, preventive measures to avoid sequestration crisis, and patient education.[45-48]

Hereditary Spherocytosis

Etiology and Pathogenesis. In hereditary spherocytosis, the red cells have defective red cell membrane skeletons, altered membrane properties, and altered cell metabolism. This causes them to have a decreased survival time in patients with an intact spleen. The disease is inherited as an autosomal dominant trait and is characterized by red cells that are fragile microspherocytes. In addition, there is increased destruction of **spherocytes** (abnormal spherical erythrocytes) in the spleen. Patients have anemia, intermittent jaundice, splenomegaly, and uniform responsiveness to splenectomy. The principal cellular defect is a loss of membrane surface area due to defects of several membrane proteins, including ankyrin, band 3, α-spectrin, and β-spectrin.[49-52]

Laboratory Features. The concentration of hemoglobin within the red cells is increased. Reticulocytosis is present, and microspherocytes are seen on the blood smear. Osmotic fragility is increased, and serum unconjugated bilirubin is increased. Following splenectomy, the hemoglobin is in the high-normal range.[49-52]

Clinical Manifestations. Hereditary spherocytosis is the most common hereditary hemolytic anemia and is most common in people with a northern European background. The major clinical manifestations are anemia, jaundice, splenomegaly, bile pigment gallstones, and chronic leg ulcers. The anemia is usually mild due to compensation by the erythropoietic bone marrow cells. Aplastic crisis precipitated by an infection may be seen with associated fever, abdominal discomfort, nausea, vomiting, rapidly increasing weakness, pallor, tachycardia, low blood pressure, and shock.[49-52]

Treatment. Treatment usually consists of splenectomy, which may be performed in infancy in severe cases but more commonly is done in late childhood. Folic acid therapy to prevent folate deficiency is necessary as well. Transfusion is usually indicated only in aplastic crisis.[49-52]

Course and Prognosis. Most patients have no or mild anemia, fluctuating degrees of jaundice, and episodes of aplastic or hemolytic anemia. Splenectomy is usually curative; however, the subsequent risk of acquiring a serious infection is significant.[49-52]

Glucose-6-Phosphate Dehydrogenase Deficiency

Etiology and Pathogenesis. An example of an intracellular defect caused by an enzyme deficiency is glucose-6-phosphate dehydrogenase (G6PD) deficiency. The energy required for RBC membrane function and cellular integrity is derived from the anaerobic metabolism of glucose. Traditionally, hemolytic anemias caused by enzyme deficiencies have been called nonspherocytic to distinguish them from classic

Table 13-8

Drugs and Chemicals to Be Avoided by Individuals with Glucose-6-Phosphate Dehydrogenase Deficiency

Category	Drug/Chemical
Analgesics/antipyretics	Acetanilide, acetophenetidin (phenacetin), aminopyrine, antipyrine, aspirin, probenecid, pyramidone
Miscellaneous	α-Methyldopa, ascorbic acid, dimercaprol (BAL), hydralazine, mestranol, methylene blue, nalidixic acid, naphthalene, niridazole, phenylhydrazine, toluidine blue, trinitrotoluene, urate oxidase, vitamin K (water soluble), phenazopyridine, quinine
Antimalarials	Chloroquine, hydroxychloroquine, mepacrine (quinacrine), pamaquine, pentaquine, primaquine, quinine, quinocide
Cytotoxics/antibacterials	Chloramphenicol, co-trimoxazole, furazolidone, furmethonol, nalidixic acid, neoarsphenamine, nitrofurantoin, nitrofurazone, para-aminosalicylic acid
Cardiovascular drugs	Procainamide, quinidine
Sulfonamides/sulfones	Dapsone, sulfacetamide, sulfa-5-methoxypyrimidine, sulfanilamide, sulfapyridine, sulfasalazine, sulfisoxazole
Miscellaneous (dietary)	Fava beans. Some individuals also avoid red wine, all legumes, blueberries (including yogurts containing these), soy products, tonic water, camphor

Ethnasios R: G6PD deficiency reference guide, Associazione Italiana Favismo—Deficit di G6PD (ONLUS). http://www.favism.org.

hereditary spherocytosis. When black soldiers receiving the antimalarial drug primaquine began suffering hemolytic episodes, a type of hemolytic anemia caused by a deficiency of G6PD (an enzyme in the red cell glycolytic pathway) was discovered. When G6PD-deficient RBCs are challenged by one of several drugs, glutathione is depleted and glucose utilization is inhibited. These events cause RBC membrane damage, which results in removal of the damaged cells by mononuclear phagocytes. Except in rare instances, G6PD-deficient persons do not have hemolytic anemia unless challenged by drugs.[53-58] G6PD deficiency is the most common metabolic disease of the RBC, and 130 million people are affected worldwide. This gene is found in 11% of African-American males and in Sephardic Jews. As the responsible gene is an X-linked recessive gene, close relatives of affected individuals should be screened. Because G6PD deficiency is found in areas where malaria was once endemic, G6PD deficiency is thought to have conferred selective advantage against *Plasmodium falciparum* malaria infection.[58]

Laboratory Features. Usually this anemia is first recognized during or after an infectious illness or following exposure to a suspect drug or chemical. The hematologic tests reflect the severity of the hemolytic episode. The diagnosis is made using a specific test that measures G6PD activity.[53-58]

Clinical Manifestations. Most individuals have no clinical manifestations of this disease. When such manifestations occur, hemolytic anemia is triggered by drug administration, infection, diabetic acidosis, the newborn period, and, in one subset, exposure to fava beans.[53-58] Drugs and chemicals that should be avoided by persons with G6PD deficiency are listed in Table 13-8.[55]

Treatment. Treatment is usually preventive and consists of avoidance of drugs that trigger hemolytic episodes and aggressive infection management. Some patients may require transfusion therapy or exchange transfusion in the case of life-threatening hemolysis.[53-58]

Course and Prognosis. The prognosis is generally good as the episodes of hemolytic crisis are usually self-limiting, except in fava bean–susceptible individuals, in whom shock may develop in a short time.[55]

ANEMIA RELATED TO EXTRINSIC RED CELL DESTRUCTION OR LOSS

The final category of types of absolute anemia includes those caused by extrinsic abnormalities. The most important of these category types is immune hemolytic anemia caused by antibodies to red cells. Immune hemolytic anemias are further subdivided into those caused by isoantibodies, which may be the result of accidental immunization of individuals (e.g., hemolytic disease of the newborn), and those caused by autoantibodies (in individuals whose bodies create antibodies against their own red cells).[59-64]

Hemolytic Disease of the Newborn

Etiology and Pathogenesis. When fetal red cells cross the placenta, they may stimulate the production of maternal antibodies against antigens on the fetal red cell not inherited from the mother. These maternal antibodies cross into the fetal circulation and cause destruction of fetal cells. In severe cases, hydrops fetalis may result. Fetal-maternal ABO incompatibility is the most common cause of hemolytic disease of the newborn (HDNB), but Rh incompatibility is clinically more important because of the severity of the hemolytic disease in the fetus. With the introduction of Rh treatment, the total incidence of HDNB in Rh-negative women has been greatly reduced.[60,63]

Laboratory Features. Anemia, **reticulocytosis** (an increased number of circulating reticulocytes), and nucleated red cells are seen in the peripheral blood of the infant. There is a rough correlation between the hemoglobin levels and the severity of the disease. Untreated infants may experience a rapid fall in hemoglobin levels after birth. Leukocytosis is present, but platelet counts are usually normal. Infants with severe disease may have thrombocytopenia. Serum bilirubin, a hemolytic breakdown product, is readily transferred across the placenta. At birth, the baby's bilirubin level reflects both the severity of the hemolytic process and the ability of the baby's liver enzyme system to conjugate and excrete bilirubin. The total bilirubin value equals the sum of the direct (conjugated water-soluble) bilirubin plus the indirect (unconjugated fat-soluble) bilirubin. Cord blood red cells show a characteristic positive direct antiglobulin test (**Coombs test**), reflecting the maternal antibodies attached to the infant's red cells.[60,63]

During pregnancy, laboratory tests of amniotic fluid for bilirubin and antibodies and tests of the mother's peripheral blood for maternal sensitization are useful in predicting whether infants will be affected by HDNB.[60,63]

Clinical Manifestations. The clinical manifestations of HDNB are hemolytic anemia, extramedullary erythropoiesis, and hyperbilirubinemia. Jaundice, petechial hemorrhages, hepatomegaly, splenomegaly, heart failure (with pulmonary edema, pleural effusions, ascites, and edema), kernicterus (a condition in the newborn marked by severe neural symptoms, associated with high levels of bilirubin in the blood), and diffuse intravascular coagulation are seen in these infants. Many infants die in utero.[60,63]

Treatment. A standard 300-μg dose of anti-Rh immunoglobulin (RhoGAM) is given to the mother before or after delivery. This immunoglobulin destroys the baby's RBCs before they can sensitize the mother. This dose protects the mother against 30 ml of Rh-positive blood. Amniocentesis and fetal blood sampling are used to evaluate the severity of the disease. In severe cases, in utero transfusion and early delivery have been performed on fetuses with severe **erythroblastosis.** Exchange transfusion lowers the serum bilirubin and the antibody content of the neonatal blood and removes cells susceptible to hemolysis. Phototherapy and phenobarbital are used to lower the bilirubin level. Albumin has been used to increase the albumin-binding capacity and to reduce the risk of kernicterus and the need for exchange transfusion.[60,63]

Course and Prognosis. The consequences of HDNB range from death, to possible retardation, to a barely perceptible hemolytic process. Severe anemia correlates with equally severe hyperbilirubinemia and high risk of central nervous system complications.[60,63] Many infants appear normal at birth, only to develop jaundice within 2 to 3 hours. Petechial hemorrhages develop soon after birth, and kernicterus is usually seen late in the second day of significant jaundice. Successful RhoGAM administration prevention programs have reduced the perinatal mortality to about 1% to 2%.[60,63]

Antibody-Mediated Drug Reactions

Etiology and Pathogenesis. Drug-induced immune hemolytic anemia is an example of a disease in which exposure to a drug causes destruction and lysis of the allergic or sensitized person's own red cells. Drugs can lead to red cell hemolysis by four different immune mechanisms (Table 13-9).[53,59,61,62,64]

Hapten Mechanisms. In the hapten mechanism, which is seen with penicillin, cephalosporins, and tetracycline, the drug combines with a component of the RBC membrane. An antibody is developed against the drug. When the drug is given again, it coats the red cells, and the antibody attaches to the drug–red cell complex. The antigen-antibody complex then causes hemolysis.[53,59,61,62,64]

Neoantigen Formation. The old terminology for neoantigen formation is immune complex formation. In this situation, the drug combines with the RBC membrane and the antibody reacts with the new antigenic sites created by the

Table 13-9

Mechanisms of Drug-Induced Hemolysis or Positive Direct Antiglobulin Test

	Drug Absorption	Neoantigen	Autoimmune	Nonimmune Adsorption
Prototype drug	Penicillin	Quinidine/stibophen	α-Methyldopa	First-generation cephalosporins
Role of drug	Cell-bound hapten	Antibody binds drug + RBC	Induces drug-independent RBC antibody	Modifies RBC membrane; adsorbs proteins nonspecifically
Typical DAT	IgG	C3	IgG	Nonimmunoglobulin
Antibody reactions	Reacts only with drug-coated cells	Reacts only with drug present	Drug independent; panagglutinin	No antibody present
Typical clinical presentation	Subacute onset; mild to severe hemolysis	Acute onset; severe hemolysis	Insidious onset; chronic mild hemolysis	No hemolysis

From Lee GR et al, editors: *Wintrobe's clinical hematology,* ed 10, Philadelphia, 1998, Lea & Febiger, p 1254.
RBC, Red blood cell; *DAT,* direct antiglobulin test; *C3,* complement third component.

combination of the drug and membrane. The RBC is hemolyzed. The immune complex can also bind to platelet and leukocyte membranes, causing anemia, leukopenia, and thrombocytopenia. Quinidine, hydrochlorothiazide, sulfonamides, isoniazid, tetracycline, and cephalosporin are common drugs that causes this type of reaction.[53,59,61,62,64]

Membrane Modification. In membrane modification, seen in cephalosporin sensitivity, the drug alters the RBC membrane protein. Plasma proteins attach to the altered RBC protein and cause a positive serologic test but no cell hemolysis.[61]

Autoantibody Induction. This mechanism was first studied in cases of hemolytic anemia with patients who were taking the antihypertensive agent methyldopa (Aldomet). The drug appears to induce antibody formation to red cell membrane Rh antigens. About 29% of the patients receiving this drug develop a positive antiglobulin test response.[53,59,61,62,64]

Laboratory Features. The laboratory features for all mechanisms show increased red cell turnover and anemia if hemolysis exceeds the rate of RBC production. Serologic tests, such as the direct antiglobulin test, will be positive. In hapten antibody–mediated drug reactions and in immune complex formation, the antiglobulin reaction is positive for immunoglobulins. In autoantibody induction, the antiglobulin reaction is positive for complement. Fragmented RBCs may be seen on the peripheral blood smear. These fragments are called schistocytes (Figure 13-22). Leukopenia and thrombocytopenia are sometimes seen with drug-induced platelet or leukocyte destruction.[53,59,61,62,64]

Clinical Manifestations. Types of immune drug-induced hemolytic anemia vary in symptoms and severity, depending on the mechanism involved. Hapten (e.g., penicillin) and autoimmune (e.g., methyldopa) drug-induced hemolytic anemias have an insidious onset of symptoms over a period of weeks. The neoantigen formation (e.g., quinine or quinidine) may present with sudden, severe hemolysis with hemoglobinuria and result in acute renal failure. Other clinical manifestations include acute respiratory distress syndrome and respiratory arrest.[53,59,61,62,64]

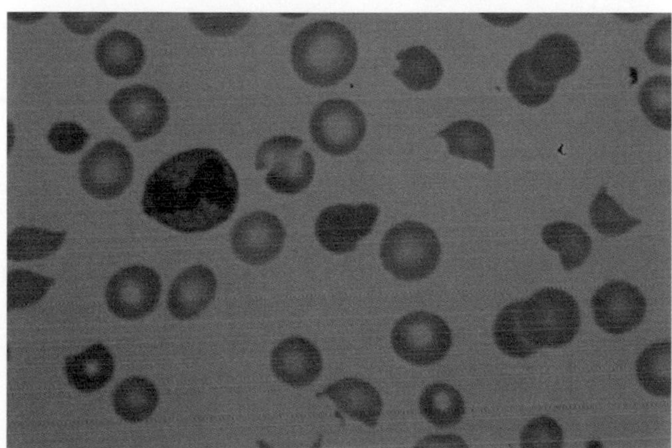

FIGURE 13-22 ■ Schistocytes are fragments of red blood cells produced by hemolytic pathologies. (Courtesy Beth Payne, Sacred Heart Medical Center, Spokane, Wash.)

Treatment. Recognition and discontinuation of the responsible drug are usually the only treatment necessary. Steroid therapy and transfusions may be required in cases of severe hemolysis.[53,59,61,62,64]

Course and Prognosis. Immune hemolytic anemia due to drugs is usually mild and the prognosis is good; however, with severe hemolysis, death can occur.[53,59,61,62,64] Laboratory findings for erythrocyte disorders are summarized in Table 13-10.

Acute Blood Loss

Etiology and Pathogenesis. Acute blood loss anemia may present after trauma or secondary to a disease process. Acute blood loss anemia decreases the overall blood volume and impairs oxygen delivery.[65,66]

Laboratory Features. A decrease occurs in both hematocrit and hemoglobin level due to blood loss. The hematocrit is less than 40% in men and 37% in women. The hemoglobin concentration is less than 14 g/dl in men and 12 g/dl in women.[65] Anemia may not be apparent in the early stages because the cells and plasma are diminishing simultaneously. As replacement fluids move into intravascular space, the anemia becomes apparent in later laboratory tests. The cells have normal MCV, MCH, and MCHC values, and they are normocytic and normochromic.

Clinical Manifestations. In a normal 70-kg person with a 5000-ml total blood volume, 10% loss of blood (500 ml) rarely causes any clinical signs except occasional vasovagal syncope. A 20% loss (1000 ml) usually causes no clinical symptoms at rest, but tachycardia is seen with exercise, and a slight postural drop in blood pressure occurs.[65,66] A person with a 30% loss (1500 ml) usually presents with flat neck veins when supine, postural hypotension, and exercise tachycardia. A 40% loss (2000 ml) causes the central venous pressure, cardiac output, and arterial blood pressure to fall below normal while the patient is supine and at rest, with associated air hunger, tachycardia, and cold, clammy skin. A 50% loss of total blood volume (2500 ml) often causes shock and death.[65,66]

Treatment. Blood volume replacement therapy with crystalloid solutions, colloid solutions (plasma protein, albumin, or dextran), and fresh whole blood is essential in the early management of acute hemorrhage to restore blood volume and to prevent shock. Complete reliance on fresh whole blood for managing acute blood loss is contraindicated and should be reserved for patients with a low red cell mass, in whom tissue hypoxia is a threat. Replacement of red cell mass by increased red cell production is a gradual process, which occurs over 2 to 5 days as the marrow stem cells proliferate

Table 13-10

Laboratory Findings for Erythrocyte Disorders

Disease	Hct	Hb	MCV	MCH	MCHC	RETIC	RBC	WBC	PLT
Relative anemia	Low	Low	Normal	Low	Low	Normal	Low	Low	Low
Absolute Anemia Caused by Decreased Production									
Aplastic anemia	Low	Low	Normal	Low	Low	Low	Low	Low	Low
Chronic renal failure	Low	Low	Normal	Normal	Normal	Low	Low	Normal	Normal
Pernicious anemia	Low	Low	High	High	Normal	Low	Low	Low	Low
Folate deficiency	Low	Low	High	High	Normal	Low	Low	Low	Low
Iron deficiency	Low	Low	Low	Low	Low	Normal or high	Low	Normal	Normal
Thalassemia	Low	Low	Low	Low	Low	High	Low	Normal	Normal
Absolute Anemia Caused by Increased Destruction									
Intrinsic Abnormality									
Sickle cell	Low	Low	Normal	Normal	Normal	High	Low	Normal	Normal
Hereditary spherocytosis	Low	Low	Normal	Normal	Normal to high	High	Low	Normal	Normal
G6PD deficiency	Low	Low	Normal	Normal	Normal	High	Low	High	Normal
Extrinsic Abnormality									
HDNB	Low	Low	Normal	Normal	Normal	High	Low	High	Normal
Antibody-mediated drug reactions	Low	Low	Normal	Normal	Normal	High	Low	Normal	Normal
Acute blood loss	Normal to low	Normal to low	Normal	Normal	Normal	High	Normal to low	Normal to low	Normal to low
Polycythemias									
Relative polycythemia	High	High	Normal	Normal	Normal	Normal	High	High	High
Absolute polycythemia vera	High	High	Normal	Normal	Normal	High	High	High	High
Secondary polycythemia	High	High	Normal	Normal	Normal	High	High	Normal	Normal

Hct, Hematocrit; *Hb,* hemoglobin; *MV,* mean corpuscular volume; *MCH,* mean corpuscular hemoglobin; *MCHC,* mean corpuscular hemoglobin concentration; *RETIC,* reticulocytosis; *RBC,* red blood cell; *WBC,* white blood cell; *PLT,* platelets; *G6PD,* glucose-6-phosphate dehydrogenase; *Segs,* segmented neutrophils; *HDNB,* hemolytic disease of the newborn; *NRBCs,* nucleated red blood cells.

and mature. Maximal red cell production is seen by the 10th day after hemorrhage.[65,66]

Course and Prognosis. With adequate replacement therapy, the prognosis is excellent; however, the underlying cause must be identified and managed. Chronic blood loss anemia usually presents as iron deficiency anemia. It is associated with gastric ulcers and other diseases of the gastrointestinal system in men. In women it is also seen in conjunction with heavy and/or prolonged menstrual bleeding or hormonal imbalances related to the menstrual cycle.

Other Extrinsic Abnormalities

Other *mechanisms,* such as mechanical heart valves or cardiopulmonary bypass machines, may cause physical damage

Blood Smear	Other Laboratory Tests	Other Diagnostic Characteristics
Normal	Plasma volume increased, causing relative decrease in number of cells	Increased volume can be caused by pregnancy, splenomegaly, IV infusions
Normocytic, hypochromic RBCs; lack of neutrophils; increased lymphocytes	HbF may be increased; erythropoietin increased; bone marrow aplastic	Specific cause should be identified and removed from environment
Normocytic, normochromic RBCs; RBCs often have spicules	Erythropoietin decreased; bone marrow production suppressed	Kidney tests abnormal
Oval macrocytes; hypersegmented segs	Decreased B_{12} level; positive Schilling test	Neurologic symptoms; increased bilirubin
Oval macrocytes; hypersegmented segs	Decreased folic acid level; negative Schilling test	No neurologic symptoms
Microcytic, hypochromic RBCs	Serum iron decreased; iron-binding increased; ferritin decreased	Bone marrow iron decreased
Microcytic, hypochromic RBC target cells, basophilic stippling	Decreased osmotic fragility; hemoglobin electrophoresis diagnostic; serum iron, TIBC, and ferritin normal	Hereditary disease
Normocytic, normochromic RBC target cells; sickle cells; NRBCs	HbS present on electrophoresis	Hereditary disease
Spherocytes present	Bilirubin elevated; haptoglobins reduced; abnormal RBC fragility	Hereditary disease
Heinz body smear positive	Tests only abnormal in hemolytic episodes	Hereditary disease
Spherocytes, NRBCs	Bilirubin elevated; Coombs test positive; urinary urobilinogen increased	Jaundice; edema; hepatosplenomegaly
Polychromatic RBCs due to increased reticulocytes	Bilirubin elevated; Coombs test positive; urinary urobilinogen increased	Jaundice
Appears normal until reticulocytes increase	Values depend on severity of hemorrhage and when blood is drawn	
Normal	Plasma volume decreased, causing relative increase in number of blood cells	Decrease in volume
Teardrops, macrocytes, and NRBCs may be present; shift to left on differential	O_2 saturation normal; bone marrow hypercellular; all three cell lines increased	
Normal	Hypoxemia may be evident; serum erythropoietin elevated	Lung disease may be present

to the red cells, resulting in hemolysis. Drugs and chemicals, physical agents (e.g., burns), or infectious diseases (e.g., malaria) may result in anemia. Venom from bee and wasp stings, spider and scorpion bites, and snake bites has been associated with hemolytic anemia. Finally, hypersplenism and splenomegaly can cause anemia, leukopenia, or **thrombocytopenia** severe enough to require splenectomy.[67]

TRANSFUSION THERAPY

Medical indications for transfusion therapy are restorations or maintenance of oxygen carrying capacity, blood volume, hemostasis, and leukocyte function. A summary of blood components, indications, actions, contraindications, precautions, and hazards is presented in Table 13-11.[66,68] Types of transfu-

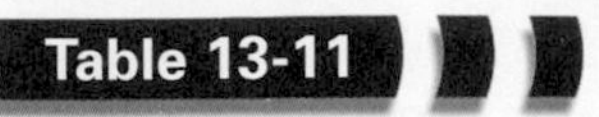

Summary of Blood Components

Component*	Major Indications	Action	Not Indicated for These Conditions
Whole blood	Symptomatic anemia with large volume deficit	Restoration of oxygen-carrying capacity, restoration of blood volume	Condition responsive to specific component
Whole blood irradiated	See *Whole blood;* risk for GVHD	See *Whole blood;* GVHD is reduced	See *Whole blood*
RBCs; RBCs (adenine-saline added)†	Symptomatic anemia	Restoration of oxygen-carrying capacity	Pharmacologically treatable anemia; coagulation deficiency
RBCs (deglycerolized)	See *RBCs;* IgA deficiency with anaphylactoid reactions	See *RBCs;* deglycerolization removes plasma protein; risk of allergic and febrile reactions reduced	See *RBCs*
RBCs irradiated	See *RBCs;* risk for GVHD	See *RBCs;* γ irradiation inactivates donor lymphocytes; GVHD is reduced	See *RBCs*
RBCs (leukocyte-poor)	Symptomatic anemia, febrile reactions from leukocyte antibodies	Restoration of oxygen-carrying capacity	Pharmacologically treatable anemia; coagulation deficiency
RBC washed	See *RBCs;* IgA deficiency with anaphylactoid reactions; recurrent severe allergic reactions to unwashed red cell products	See *RBCs*; washing reduces plasma proteins; risk of allergic reactions may be reduced	See *RBCs*
Fresh-frozen plasma (FFP)	Deficit of labile and stable plasma coagulation factors and TTP	Source of labile and nonlabile plasma factors	Condition responsive to volume replacement
Liquid plasma, plasma, and thawed plasma	Deficit of stable coagulation factors	Source of nonlabile factors	Deficit of labile coagulation factors or volume replacement
Plasma, cryoprecipitate reduced	TTP	See *FFP;* deficient in Factors I, VIII, vWF, and XIII; deficient in high molecular weight; vWF multimers as compared to FFP	See *FFP;* deficiency of coagulation factors known to be depleted in this product, Factors I, VIII, vWF, XIII; volume replacement
Cryoprecipitated AHF; cryoprecipitated AHF, pooled	Hemophilia A,‡ von Willebrand disease,‡ hypofibrinogenemia, factor XIII deficiency	Provides factor VIII, fibrinogen, vWF, factor XIII	Deficit of any plasma protein other than those enriched in cryoprecipitated AHF
Platelets; platelets pooled	Bleeding from thrombocytopenia or platelet function abnormality	Improves hemostasis	Plasma coagulation deficits; some conditions with rapid platelet destruction (e.g., ITP, TTP) unless life-threatening hemorrhage
Platelets, pheresis†	Bleeding from thrombocytopenia or platelet function abnormality	Improves hemostasis	Plasma coagulation deficits and some conditions with rapid platelet destruction (e.g., ITP)
Platelets irradiated; platelets pooled irradiated; platelets pheresis irradiated	See *Platelets*; risk of GVHD	See *Platelets*; γ irradiation inactivates donor lymphocytes; reduced risk of GVHD	See *Platelets*
Platelets (leukocytes reduced); platelets pheresis (leukocytes reduced)	See *Platelets*; febrile reactions; prevention of HLA alloimmunization	See *Platelets*; reduction of leukocytes reduces risk of febrile reactions, HLA alloimmunization, and CMV	See *Platelets;* leukocytes reduction; should not be used to prevent GVHD
Granulocytes, pheresis	Neutropenia with infection	Provides granulocytes	Infection responsive to antibiotics
Granulocytes pheresis irradiated; granulocytes platelets irradiated	See *Granulocytes;* see *Platelets*	Provides granulocytes with or without platelets	See *Granulocytes;* see *Platelets*

AHF, Antihemophilic factor; *TTP,* thrombotic thrombocytopenic purpura; *GVHD,* graft-versus-host disease; *ITP,* idiopathic thrombocytopenic purpura; *vWF,* von Willebrand factor.
*For all cellular components there is a risk that the recipient may become alloimmunized.
†RBCs and platelets may be processed in a manner that yields leukocyte-reduced components for which the main indications are prevention of febrile, nonhemolytic transfusion reactions and prevention of leukocyte alloimmunization. Risks are the same as for standard components, except for reduced risk of febrile reactions.
‡When virus-inactivated concentrates are not available.

Special Precautions	Hazards	Rate of Infusion
Must be ABO identical; labile coagulation factors deteriorate within 24 hr after collection	Infectious diseases; septic/toxic, allergic, febrile reactions; circulatory overload; GVHD	For massive loss, as fast as patient can tolerate
See *Whole blood*	See *Whole blood*	See *Whole blood*
Must be ABO compatible	Infectious diseases; septic/toxic, allergic, febrile reactions, GVHD	As patient can tolerate, but <4 hr
See *RBCs*		See *RBCs*
See *RBCs*	See *RBCs*	See *RBCs*
Must be ABO compatible	Infectious diseases; septic/toxic, allergic reactions (unless plasma also removed [e.g., by washing]); GVHD	As patient can tolerate, but <4 hr
See *RBCs*	See *RBCs*	See *RBCs*
Should be ABO compatible	Infectious diseases, allergic reactions, circulatory overload	<4 hr
Should be ABO compatible	Infectious diseases, allergic reactions	<4 hr
Must be ABO compatible	See *FFP*	<4 hr
Frequent repeat doses may be necessary	Infectious diseases, allergic reactions	<4 hr
Should not use some filters (check manufacturer's instructions); should be ABO compatible with plasma	Infectious diseases; septic/toxic, allergic, febrile reaction; GVHD	<4 hr
Should not use some microaggregate filters (check manufacturer's instructions)	Infectious diseases; septic/toxic, allergic, febrile reactions; GVHD	<4 hr
See *Platelets*	See *Platelets*	See *Platelets*
See *Platelets*	See *Platelets*	See *Platelets*
Must be ABO-compatible; do not use depth-type microaggregate filters	Infectious diseases; allergic, febrile reactions; GVHD	One unit over 2-4 hr period; observe closely for reactions
See *Granulocytes;* see *Platelets*	See *Granulocytes;* see *Platelets*	See *Granulocytes;* see *Platelets*

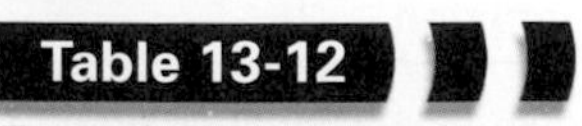

Transfusion Reactions

Type	Signs and Symptoms	Usual Cause
Acute intravascular hemolytic (immune)	Hemoglobinemia and hemoglobinuria, fever, chills, anxiety, shock, disseminated intravascular coagulation (DIC), dyspnea, chest pain, flank pain, nausea/vomiting, headache, pain at needle site and along venous tract	Incompatibility due to clerical errors; involves ABO (primarily) or other erythrocyte antigen-antibody incompatibility
Delayed extravascular hemolytic (immune)	Fever, malaise, indirect hyperbilirubinemia, increased urine urobilinogen, falling hematocrit	Destruction of RBCs; usually involves non-ABO antigen-antibody incompatibility occurring 3-10 days post-transfusion
Graft versus host disease (GVHD)		Viable T lymphocytes react against tissue antigens in recipient Immunocompromised recipients most at risk
Febrile	Fever, chills, rarely hypotension	Antibodies to leukocytes or plasma proteins
Allergic	Urticaria (hives), flushing, wheezing, laryngeal edema, rarely hypotension or anaphylaxis	Antibodies to plasma proteins
Hypervolemic	Dyspnea, rales, hypertension, pulmonary edema, cardiac arrhythmias, precordial pain, cyanosis, dry cough, distended neck veins	Too rapid or excessive blood transfusion
Noncardiogenic pulmonary edema	Dyspnea, pulmonary edema, normal cardiac pressures	Anti-HLA or antileukocyte antibodies
Hypothermia	Chills, low temperature, irregular heart rate, possible cardiac arrest	Rapid infusion of cold blood products
Electrolyte disturbances, hyperkalemia	Nausea, diarrhea, muscular weakness, flaccid paralysis, paresthesia of extremities, bradycardia, apprehension, cardiac arrest	Massive transfusions or in patients with renal problems
Citrate intoxication (hypocalcemia)	Tingling in fingers, tetany, muscular cramps, carpopedal spasm, hyperactive reflexes, convulsions, laryngeal spasm, respiratory arrest	Massive transfusion of blood
Air emboli	Sudden difficulty in breathing, sharp pain in chest, apprehension, respiratory or cardiac arrest	Air emboli from blood administered under pressure
Bacterial sepsis	Shock, chills, fever	Contaminated blood component
Delayed reactions, transmission of infection	Signs of infection after transfusion (e.g., jaundice from hepatitis; bacterial or toxin contamination—high fever, severe headache or substernal pain, hypotension, intense flushing, vomiting/diarrhea)	Hepatitis, AIDS, malaria, syphilis, bacteria, viruses, other

Adapted with permission from Whaley LR, Wong L, editors: *Nursing care of infants and children,* ed 4, St Louis, 1991, Mosby; and Pisciotto PT, Civarel Roberts SC, editors: *Blood transfusion therapy: a physician's handbook,* ed 3, Arlington, Va, 2000, American Association of Blood Banks.

sion reactions, signs and symptoms, usual causes, treatment, and precautions are summarized in Table 13-12.

Before transfusion therapy can occur, various donor tests are run on the blood unit sample. These include ABO and Rh(D); syphilis; HIV antigen and antibodies; hepatitis B and C antigens; and human T-cell lymphotropic virus. Blood centers, which are producing plasma for fractionation, also run a test for alanine aminotransferase.[68]

Specific pretransfusion testing using blood samples from the recipient and the donor unit must be done to ensure that

Treatment	Precautions
Stop transfusion; hydrate; support blood pressure and respiration; induce diuresis; treat shock and DIC	Positively identify donor and recipient blood types and groups before transfusion is begun; verify with one other nurse or physician. Transfuse blood slowly for first 15-20 min and/or initial one-fifth volume of blood; remain with patient. In event of signs or symptoms, stop transfusion immediately, maintain patent IV line, and notify physician. Save donor blood to recrossmatch with patient's blood. Monitor blood pressure for shock. Insert urinary catheter and monitor hourly outputs. Send sample of patient's blood and urine to laboratory for presence of hemoglobin (indicates intravascular hemolysis). Observe for signs of hemorrhage resulting from DIC. Support medical therapies to reverse shock.
Monitor hematocrit, renal function, coagulation profile; no acute treatment generally required	Observe for post-transfusion anemia and decreasing benefit from successive transfusion
	Use γ-irradiated components to prevent GVHD
Stop transfusion; give antipyretics, acetaminophen (or aspirin if patient not thrombocytopenic)	Use of leukocyte-poor RBCs is less likely to cause reaction
Stop transfusion; give antihistamine; if severe, give epinephrine and/or steroids	Pretransfusion antihistamine; use of washed RBC components
Induce diuresis; phlebotomy; support cardiorespiratory system as needed	Transfuse blood slowly. Prevent overload by using packed RBCs or administering divided amounts of blood. Use infusion pump to regulate and maintain flow rate. If signs of overload, stop transfusion immediately. Place patient in semi-Fowler position to increase venous resistance
Support blood pressure and respiration (may require intubation)	Use washed RBCs; avoid unnecessary transfusion
Monitor temperature; if markedly subnormal, stop transfusion	Allow blood to warm at room temperature ($<$1 hr). Use an electric warming coil to rapidly warm blood
Kayexalate enemas if potassium $>$5.0 mEq/L	Use washed RBCs or fresh blood if patient at risk
Stop transfusion; administer IV calcium if severe	Infuse blood slowly (citrate reaction less likely to occur). If signs of tetany occur, clamp tubing immediately, maintain patent intravenous line, and notify physician
Stop transfusion; turn patient on left side; aspirate right atrial/ventricular air emboli	When infusing blood under pressure before container is empty, if air is observed in tubing, clamping tubing immediately below air bubble, clear tubing of air by aspirating air with syringe or disconnecting tubing and allowing blood to flow until air has escaped
Stop transfusion; support blood pressure; give antibiotics	Care in blood collection and storage
Stop transfusion; do culture and sensitivity tests; treat specific infection	Blood is tested for HBsAg (hepatitis B), syphilis, and, in most centers, HIV (AIDS); positive units are destroyed. Individuals at risk for carrying certain viruses are deferred from donation. Observe for signs of infection.

the blood component will not harm the recipient and the blood component will have an acceptable survival when transfused. ABO and Rh typing and RBC antibody detection tests are run, and then a crossmatch between the donor unit and the recipient is performed.[68]

ABO compatibility is crucial as the recipient's plasma may contain ABO naturally occurring antibodies depending on blood type. Table 13-13 illustrates the antigens and antibodies occurring in various ABO types. Table 13-13 lists the percentage of each blood type by various populations. If a type O per-

Table 13-13

ABO Blood Groups

Blood Type	Antigen (RBC membrane)	Antibody (plasma)	Can receive blood from	Can donate blood to
A (40%)	A antigen	Anti–B antibodies	A, O	A, AB
B (10%)	B antigen	Anti–A antibodies	B, O	B, AB
AB* (4%)	A antigen, B antigen	No antibodies	A, B, AB, O	AB
O† (46%)	No antigen	Both Anti–A & Anti–B antibodies	O	O, A, B, AB

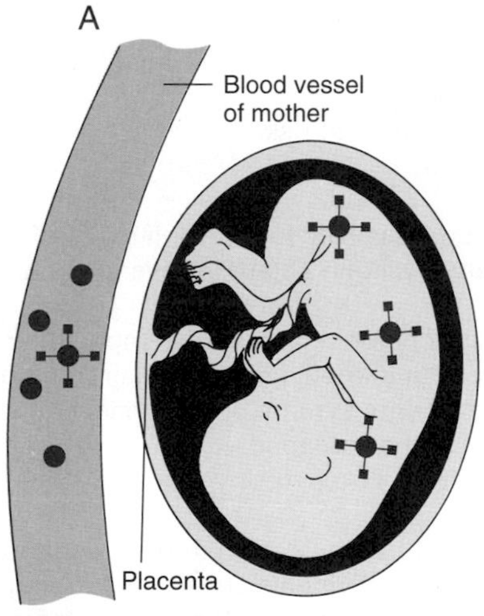

A few Rh+ RBCs leak across the placenta from the fetus into the mother's blood.

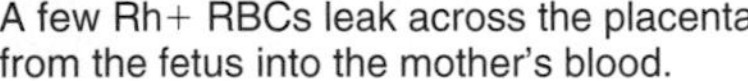

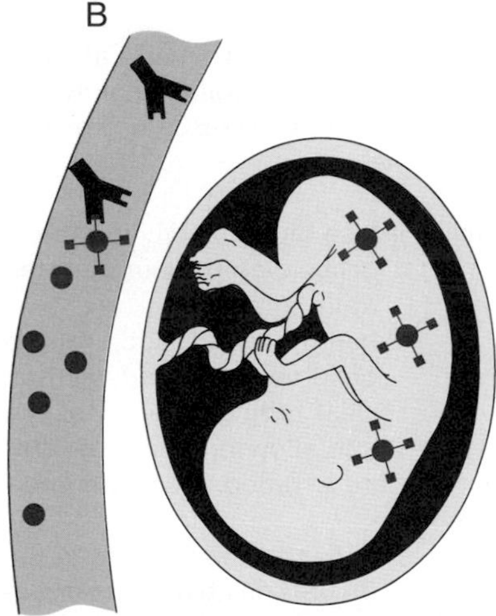

The mother produces anti-Rh antibodies in response to Rh antigen on Rh+ RBCs.

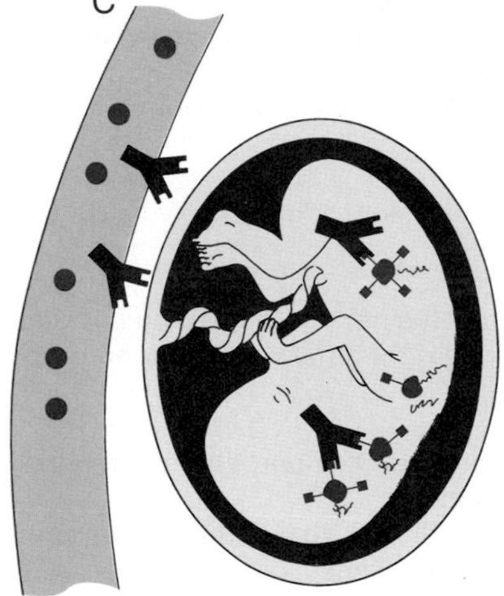

During subsequent pregnancies anti-Rh antibodies cross the placenta and enter the blood of the fetus. Hemolysis of Rh+ blood occurs. The fetus may develop erythroblastosis fetalis.

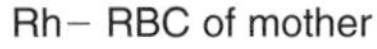

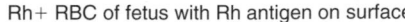

Rh− RBC of mother

Rh+ RBC of fetus with Rh antigen on surface

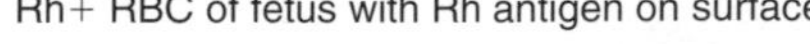

Anti-Rh antibody made against Rh+ RBC

Hemolysis of Rh+ RBC

FIGURE 13-23 ■ Rh incompatibility can cause serious problems when an Rh-negative woman and an Rh-positive man produce an Rh-positive offspring. **A,** During the first pregnancy, some Rh^+ red blood cells leak across the placenta from the fetus into the mother's blood. **B,** The mother produces antibodies in response to the antigens on the Rh^+ red blood cells. **C,** During subsequent pregnancies, some of the mother's anti-Rh antibodies cross the placenta and attack the Rh antigen of the fetus, causing agglutination and hemolysis of red blood cells *(RBCs)* (erythroblastosis fetalis). (From Solomon EP: *Introduction to human anatomy and physiology,* ed 2, St Louis, 2003, Mosby, p 172.)

son, who has both anti-A and anti-B antibodies in his or her plasma, receives a transfusion of type A, B, or AB blood, the donor cells will be agglutinated and hemolysed immediately (Figure 13-23).

Rh(D) compatibility is also tested to ensure that the recipient does not become sensitized and begin making anti-Rh(D) antibodies. This is particularly important in females of childbearing age as anti-Rh(D) antibodies can cross the placenta and cause hemolytic disease of the newborn. In Figure 13-23 the maternal sensitization has occurred with the first baby. With the advent of RhoGAM prevention programs (see "Hemolytic Disease of the Newborn"), this cause has been reduced and transfusions remain as one of the methods that can cause the production of maternal anti-Rh(D) antibodies.

KEY CONCEPTS

- The general effects of anemia are due to tissue hypoxia and efforts to compensate for low oxygen carrying capacity. Vasoconstriction, pallor, tachypnea, dyspnea, tachycardia, ischemic pain, lethargy, and light-headedness may be present. In addition, signs and symptoms relating to the specific cause of the anemia may be present. These accompanying manifestations are helpful in determining the cause of the anemia.
- Anemia may be due to abnormally low production of red cells and/or excessive loss or destruction. Decreased production of red cells may be due to stem cell failure (aplastic anemia), lack of erythropoietin (renal disease), or nutritional deficiencies of iron, vitamin B_{12}, or folate. Excessive red cell loss may be due to hemolysis (e.g., ABO and Rh incompatibility, drugs) or bleeding (e.g., surgery, trauma). Inherited disorders of red cells often impair production and increase destruction of red cells.
- Determination of the cause of anemia is based on the history, differential signs and symptoms, and results of laboratory studies. The important differentiating features of the major types of anemia are as follows:
  Aplastic anemia: History of toxic or radiation injury to bone marrow. Accompanying leukopenia and thrombocytopenia. Red cells are normocytic and normochromic.
  Chronic renal failure: History of renal disease. Decreased erythropoietin level and erythropoietin responsiveness. Red cells are normocytic and normochromic.
  Vitamin B_{12} and folate deficiency: History of poor intake or gastrointestinal disease. Accompanying neurologic dysfunction. Red cells are megaloblastic (macrocytic).
  Iron deficiency: History of poor intake or chronic blood loss. Decreased serum ferritin and iron levels. Red cells are microcytic and hypochromic.
  Hemolytic: History of ABO or Rh incompatibility or drug exposure. Increased bilirubin, jaundice, positive direct antiglobulin. Red cells are normocytic and normochromic.
  Acute blood loss: History of trauma, surgery, or known bleeding. Accompanying manifestations of volume depletion. Red cells are normal. Anemia may not be apparent until fluid loss is replaced.
- Inherited disorders of the red cell (thalassemia, sickle cell anemia, spherocytosis, G6PD deficiency) predispose red cells to early destruction because of abnormalities in hemoglobin structure, cell shape, membrane structure, or energy production. Manifestations of hemolysis (e.g., bilirubin, jaundice) are often present.
- The general management of anemia is aimed at removing the cause, if possible; restoring oxygen carrying capacity with blood transfusion when necessary; and preventing the complications of ischemia (e.g., with rest, oxygen therapy) and hemolysis (e.g., increased fluid intake, management of high bilirubin levels).

POLYCYTHEMIA

In polycythemia, red cells are present in excess, which increases the whole-blood viscosity, which in turn causes clinical manifestations such as hypertension. The three types of polycythemia are classified according to cause. *Polycythemia vera* is associated with neoplastic transformation of bone marrow stem cells. *Secondary polycythemia* is due to chronic hypoxemia, with a resultant increase in erythropoietin production. *Relative polycythemia* is due to dehydration, which causes a spurious increase in the RBC count.

Polycythemia Vera

Etiology and Pathogenesis. Polycythemia vera or primary polycythemia is a type of chronic **panmyelosis** and is part of the spectrum of myeloproliferative disorders. Polycythemia vera arises from transformation of a single stem cell into a cell with a selective growth advantage that gradually becomes the predominant source of marrow precursors. There is overproduction of normal red cells, white cells, and platelets. The cause is unknown. Possible mechanisms for the proliferation include (1) unregulated neoplastic proliferation of stem cells, (2) presence of abnormal myeloproliferative factor acting on normal stem cells, and (3) increase of stem cell sensitivity to erythropoietin and other hematopoietins.[69-73] Some researchers have postulated that it is damage to the undifferentiated stem cell by a virus, radiation, drugs, or other agents that causes mutation and neoplastic transformation.[69-73]

Laboratory Features. The diagnosis depends primarily on results of laboratory studies, which show an absolute increase in red cell mass and leukocytosis and thrombocytosis. The bone marrow shows **hyperplasia** of red cells, white cells, and platelets and extension of active hematopoietic marrow into bones of the extremities. Uric acid is increased due to excessive cell proliferation, which results in the destruction of an increased number of cells. Arterial oxygen saturation is normal, which differentiates polycythemia vera from secondary (hypoxemic) erythrocytosis. Secondary findings include elevated serum vitamin B_{12} and elevated leukocyte alkaline phosphatase levels (Table 13-14).[69-73]

Clinical Manifestations. Symptoms include headache, backache, weakness, fatigue on exertion, pruritus, dizziness, sweating, visual disturbances, weight loss, paresthesias, dyspnea, joint complaints, and epigastric distress and pressure.[69-73] Common clinical manifestations include hypertension, occlusive vascular lesions, and mucosal hemorrhage due to engorgement of retinal and sublingual veins, but each phase of the disease presents somewhat differently. Most of the clinical symptoms of polycythemia vera are related to the increased red cell mass, which gives rise to an increased blood viscosity. The liver and spleen become congested, which increases the risk of clots, acidosis, and organ infarction. The onset is insidious, with variable manifestations in virtually any organ system. Clinical symptoms appear between 60 and 80 years of age, and they appear more often in men and whites. The disorder is rarely seen in children. In the preerythrocytic or developmental phase, hepatosplenomegaly, night sweats, and postbathing pruritus are common. Other patients experience mild thrombohemorrhagic symptoms or **erythromelalgia** (painful erythematous palms and soles from an increased number of circulating platelets).[69-73]

The evolution of polycythemia vera is shown in Table 13-15. The phases include an asymptomatic phase, a plethoric or erythrocytic phase, an inactive phase, and a spent phase when anemia develops. The final evolutionary phase of polycythemia vera is that of acute myeloid leukemia.[69-73]

In the erythrocytic phase, occlusive vascular lesions, such as transient ischemic attacks, cerebrovascular accidents (strokes), myocardial ischemia or infarctions, portal venous obstruction, or superficial venous thrombosis, occur and may be the first indication of the presence of the disease. The hyperviscosity produces symptoms of reduced cerebral blood flow, such as headaches, dizziness, and visual disturbances. Walking may induce leg pain and spasm, called intermittent claudication.[69-73]

Mucosal hemorrhagic manifestations include epistaxis, ecchymosis, and gastrointestinal and genitourinary bleeding. Progressive splenomegaly, intermittent claudication, peptic ulcer, hyperuricemia, and gout are often seen. The most striking feature is a ruddy or florid face, telangiectasis (chronic dilation of capillaries and small arterial branches producing small, reddish tumors of the skin) of the cheeks and nose, and purplish cyanosis of the lips and ears. Hypertension is seen in about half of patients. Distention of the retinal veins with a dark purple coloration is another important clinical finding. As the disease develops into the spent or postpolycythemia myeloid metaplasia phase, many patients complain only of **asthenia;** however, progressive hepatosplenomegaly, severe anemia, hemorrhage (particularly cutaneous), weight loss, and wasting often occur. The final phase is the development of acute myeloid leukemia.[69-73]

Treatment. There is no cure. Treatment is directed at reducing the increased blood volume, blood viscosity, red cell mass, and platelet counts by phlebotomy, radioactive phosphorus, and chemotherapeutic agents. Phlebotomy of 450 to 500 ml every 2 to 4 days until a normal hematocrit is reached alleviates many symptoms for most patients. Phlebotomy of

Table 13-14

Typical Laboratory Findings in Patients with Polycythemia Vera, Secondary Polycythemia, and Relative Polycythemia

Findings*	Polycythemia Vera	Secondary Polycythemia	Relative Polycythemia
Splenomegaly	Present	Absent	Absent
Leukocytosis	Present	Absent	Absent
Thrombocytosis	Present	Absent	Absent
Abnormal primary wave of epinephrine-induced platelet aggregation	Present	Absent	Absent
Red blood cell mass	Increased	Increased	Normal
Arterial oxygen saturation	Normal	Decreased or normal	Normal
Serum vitamin B_{12}	Increased	Normal	Normal
Leukocyte alkaline phosphatase	Increased	Normal	Normal
Marrow	Panhyperplasia	Erythroid hyperplasia	Normal
EPO level	Decreased	Increased	Normal
Endogenous CFU-E growth	Present	Absent	Absent

From Beutler E et al, editors: *Williams hematology,* ed 6, New York, 2001, McGraw-Hill, p 695.
EPO, Erythropoietin; *CFU-E,* erythroid colony-forming unit.
*The differences listed are not present in all patients.

only 200 to 300 ml should be considered for elderly patients or those with cardiovascular disease. In the past, a hematocrit of 50% was used as the upper limit of hematocrit tolerated before phlebotomy was used. Studies have found that increased vascular complications, decreased cerebral blood flow, and decreased mental alertness occurred when hematocrit levels exceeded 45%. Phlebotomy is effective in controlling red cell mass, but myelosuppressive therapy is needed when the platelet count increases to more than 800,000 to 1,000,000/μl to control hepatosplenomegaly and thrombocytosis. The agent of choice for myelosuppressive therapy is hydroxyurea 500 mg either once or twice daily. Another agent is radioactive phosphorus (2 to 4 mCi) given intravenously following an initial series of phlebotomies, and may require a follow-up dose based on the initial dose response in 6 to 8 weeks to bring the disease under control. It is effective in 75% to 85% of cases, and remissions lasting 6 to 24 months often occur. Chemotherapy with the alkylating agents such as busulfan and chlorambucil were widely used; however, they are no longer routinely used due to the associated risk of leukemia.[69-73] A combination of platelet pheresis and cytotoxic chemotherapy (hydroxyurea or busulfan) has been successfully used for symptomatic patients with thrombocytosis. The efficacy of interferon remains to be determined.[69-73]

Course and Prognosis. Unmanaged polycythemia vera has a poor prognosis, with a survival of less than 2 years. The prognosis depends on the nature and severity of the complications, the duration of the erythrocytotic phase before commencing the postpolycythemic myeloid metaplasia phase, and the duration of the acute myeloid leukemia phase. Treatment in the erythrocytotic phase is essential or the patients are at extremely high risk for thromboses. The development of thrombosis, hemorrhage, and myeloproliferative syndromes is common. Treated patients have a median survival of 10 to 15 years, with the most common causes of death being thrombosis, hemorrhage, leukemia, and other myeloproliferative conditions.[69-73]

Table 13-15

Evolution of Polycythemia Vera

Stage	Clinical Findings
Asymptomatic phase	Splenomegaly Isolated erythrocytosis Isolated thrombocytosis
Erythrocytotic phase	Erythrocytosis Thrombocytosis Leukocytosis Splenomegaly Thrombosis Hemorrhage Pruritus
Inactive phase	No longer requires phlebotomy or chemotherapy Iron deficient
Postpolycythemic myeloid metaplasia	Anemia Leukoerythroblastosis Thrombocytopenia or thrombocytosis Enlarging splenomegaly Systemic symptoms (fever, weight loss) Acute myeloid leukemia

From Hoffman R et al, editors: *Hematology: basic principles and practice,* ed 3, New York, 2000, Churchill Livingstone, p 1130.

Secondary Polycythemia

Etiology and Pathogenesis. Secondary polycythemia is absolute erythrocytosis caused by increased stimulation of RBC production, usually in response to tissue hypoxia caused by, for example, high altitude or lung disease. There are other types of secondary polycythemia that are caused by renal or other organ tumors, which cause an increase in erythropoietin production.[70,74]

As this type of polycythemia demonstrates an increase in red cell mass with no involvement of other marrow elements, it is most commonly seen in association with a known hypoxic stimulus, increased erythropoietin, or excess adrenocortical steroids or androgens.[70,74]

Laboratory Features. The laboratory findings confirm increased red cell production with no increase in white cells or platelets. Erythropoietin levels are increased.[70,74]

Clinical Manifestations. The symptoms are those of the underlying disease state, such as cardiovascular disease with right-to-left shunt, chronic lung disease or alveolar hypoventilation, low barometric pressure, living at high altitudes, or abnormal hemoglobin concentration.[70,74]

Treatment. As this condition is a physiologic compensation, the clinical treatment is directed at identifying and managing the underlying cause. Phlebotomy has been used to reduce cardiovascular work and appears to be helpful in both cardiovascular and chronic obstructive pulmonary disease. Oxygen administration is helpful in chronic lung diseases.

Course and Prognosis. The course and prognosis are influenced by the underlying disease process.

Relative Polycythemia

Etiology and Pathogenesis. **Relative** (spurious) **polycythemia** is characterized by an increased hematocrit in the presence of normal or decreased total RBC mass. Two types of patients manifest this characteristic. In the first group, the laboratory finding is secondary to an obvious disturbance in fluid balance such as is seen in severe dehydration or endocrinologic disorders. Patients in the other group, often described as having stress polycythemia, have hypertension, increased hematocrit levels, and no increase in total RBC mass or obvious fluid loss. Research is continuing on the etiologic process and pathogenesis.[69,74,75]

Laboratory Features. All hematologic tests are normal except for elevated hematocrit, hemoglobin level, and RBC count. The size of the red cell is normal. Increased levels of cholesterol and uric acid are common.[70,74,75]

Clinical Manifestations. The manifestations are contingent on the underlying cause. In dehydration, the patient will have flat neck veins, decreased skin turgor, thirst, tachycardia, and, in severe cases, low cardiac output and blood pressure. If the underlying condition is stress related, the symptoms are those of a catecholamine stress response. Patients are usually white middle-aged men. In patients with spurious polycythemia due to smoking, the problem is usually chronic, and the symptoms that are due to the hyperviscosity described for polycythemia vera are often found.[70,74,75]

Treatment. As this is a spurious form of polycythemia, it is important to recognize and manage the underlying cause. Fluid administration and management will resolve dehydration; however, spurious polycythemia is likely to be associated with a long-term condition that will require concurrent medical management. When the condition is a result of stress, identification of the stressors and stress management are indicated, with long-term follow-up. In spurious polycythemia due to smoking, the patient must stop smoking in order for the condition to resolve.[70,74,75]

Course and Prognosis. The long-term prognosis is excellent if the underlying condition is identified and resolved, but patients with chronic anxiety or an inability to quit smoking may experience the same complications related to erythrocytosis as are seen in polycythemia vera.[70,74,75]

KEY CONCEPTS

- Three types of polycythemia have been identified, according to cause. Polycythemia vera is associated with neoplastic transformation of bone marrow stem cells. Secondary polycythemia is due to chronic hypoxemia, with a resultant increase in erythropoietin production. Relative polycythemia is due to dehydration, which causes a spurious increase in RBC count.
- Differential diagnosis of the type of polycythemia is based on the history and accompanying manifestations.
- *Polycythemia vera:* Absence of hypoxemia and dehydration, accompanied by leukocytosis and thrombocytosis.
- *Secondary polycythemia:* History of lung disease or living at high altitude. Hypoxemia evident on blood gas evaluation. Erythropoietin level is elevated.
- *Relative polycythemia:* History of fluid loss or poor intake. Accompanying manifestations of dehydration.
- Treatment of polycythemia is aimed at removing the cause, if possible. Phlebotomy and bone marrow–suppressing agents may be used for polycythemia vera. Major complications of polycythemia are increased blood viscosity and the risk of thrombi.

SUMMARY

The purpose of the erythron is to ensure adequate oxygen delivery with respect to oxygen demand. This is enhanced by the unique ability of hemoglobin in RBCs to carry and release oxygen at a suitable tension to support energy-generating systems in the body tissues. Anemia, a deficit in RBCs, poses a serious threat to oxygen transport and to the ability of the body to receive adequate oxygenation. Intense research in RBC physiology and pathophysiology continually yields new information for a better understanding of erythrocyte disorders, improved treatment modalities, and improved prognoses.

MEDIA RESOURCES

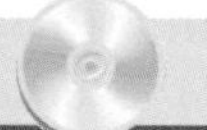

evolve

Remember to check out the ***CD Companion*** included with this book for Review Questions, Key Concepts Review, Glossary (with audio for selected terms), Disease Profiles, and Animations.

PLUS, visit the ***Evolve website*** at http://evolve.elsevier.com/Copstead/ for Case Studies, Disease Profiles, and WebLinks.

References

1. Platt W: Introduction to hematology. In Platt W, editor: *Color atlas and textbook of hematology,* Philadelphia, 1979, Lippincott, pp 1-6.
2. McKenzie SB: The erythrocyte. *Textbook of hematology,* ed 2, Baltimore, 1996, Williams & Wilkins, pp 33-53.
3. McKenzie SB: The leukocyte. *Textbook of hematology,* ed 2, Baltimore, 1996, Williams & Wilkins, pp 55-89.
4. McKenzie SB: Primary hemostasis. *Textbook of hematology,* ed 2, Baltimore, 1996, Williams & Wilkins, pp 477-500.
5. Hillman RS, Finch CA: General characteristics of the erythron. In Hillman RS, Finch CA, editors: *Red cell manual,* ed 7, Philadelphia, 1996, FA Davis, p 8.
6. Beutler E: Production and destruction of erythrocytes. In Beutler E et al, editors: *Williams hematology,* ed 6, New York, 2001, McGraw-Hill, pp 355-368.
7. Diggs L, Sturm D, Bell A: *The morphology of human blood cells,* Abbott Park, Ill, 1985, Abbott Laboratories, pp 1-86.
8. Nagel RL: Disorders of hemoglobin function and stability. In Handin RL, Lux SE, Stossel TP, editors: *Blood: principles and*

practice of hematology, ed 2, Philadelphia, 2002, Lippincott, pp 1597-1654.
9. Telen MJ, Kaufman RE: The mature erythrocyte. In Lee GR et al, editors: *Wintrobe's clinical hematology,* ed 10, Baltimore, 1998, Williams & Wilkins, pp 193-227.
10. McKenzie SB: Megaloblastic and nonmegaloblastic macrocytic anemias. *Textbook of hematology,* ed 2, Baltimore, 1996, Williams & Wilkins, pp 177-199.
11. Carmel R, Rosenblatt DS: Disorders of cobalamin and folate metabolism. In Handin RL, Lux SE, Stossel TP, editors: *Blood: principles and practice of hematology,* ed 2, Philadelphia, 2002, Lippincott, pp 1361-1398.
12. Beutler E: Energy metabolism and maintenance of erythrocytes. In Beutler E et al, editors: *Williams hematology,* ed 6, New York, 2001, McGraw-Hill, pp 319-332.
13. Gallagher PG, Forget BG: The red cell membrane. In Beutler E et al, editors: *Williams hematology,* ed 6, New York, 2001, McGraw-Hill, pp 333-344.
14. Dessypris EN et al: Erythropoiesis. In Lee GR et al, editors: *Wintrobe's clinical hematology,* ed 10, Baltimore, 1998, Williams & Wilkins, pp 169-192.
15. Papayannopoulou T, Abkowitz J, D'Andrea A: Biology of erythropoiesis erythroid differentiation, and maturation. In Hoffman RL et al, editors: *Hematology: basic principles and practice,* ed 3, New York, 2000, Churchill Livingstone, pp 202-219.
16. Guyton AC: Red blood cells, anemia, polycythemia. In Guyton AC, Hall JE, editors: *Textbook of medical physiology,* ed 10, Philadelphia, 2000, Saunders, pp 382-391.
17. Guyton AC: Transport of oxygen and carbon dioxide in the blood and body fluids. In Guyton AC, Hall JE, editors: *Textbook of medical physiology,* ed 10, Philadelphia, 2000, Saunders, pp 463-473.
18. St. John RE: The pulmonary system. In Alspach JG, editor: *Core curriculum for critical care nursing,* ed 5, Philadelphia, 1998, Saunders, pp 1-136.
19. American Edwards Laboratories: *Continuous* Svo_2 *monitoring: theory and applications,* Irvine, Calif, n.d., The Laboratories.
20. Ahrens TS, Powers KC: Pulmonary clinical physiology. In Kinney MR, Packa DR, Dunbar SB, editors: *AACN's clinical reference for critical care nursing,* ed 4, St Louis, 1998, Mosby, pp 491-516.
21. McKenzie SB: General aspects and classifications of anemia. In *Textbook of hematology,* ed 2, Baltimore, 1996, Williams & Wilkins, pp 91-120.
22. Erslev AJ: Clinical manifestations and classification of erythrocyte disorders. In Beutler E et al, editors: *Williams hematology,* ed 6, New York, 2001, McGraw-Hill, pp 369-374.
23. Shadduck RK: Aplastic anemia. In Beutler E et al, editors: *Williams hematology,* ed 6, New York, 2001, McGraw-Hill, pp 375-390.
24. Williams DM: Pancytopenia, aplastic anemia and pure red cell aplasia. In Lee GR et al, editors: *Wintrobe's clinical hematology,* ed 10, Baltimore, 1998, Williams & Wilkins, pp 1449-1484.
25. Young NS, Maciejewski JP: Aplastic anemia. In Hoffman R et al, editors: *Hematology: basic principles and practice,* ed 3, New York, 2000, Churchill Livingstone, pp 297-331.
26. Young N: Aplastic anemia and related bone marrow failure syndromes. In Goldman L, Bennett JC, editors: *Cecil textbook of medicine,* ed 21, Philadelphia, 2000, Saunders, pp 848-853.
27. Negrin RS, Blume KG: Allogenic and autologous hematopoietic cell transplantation. In Beutler E et al, editors: *Williams hematology,* ed 6, New York, 2001, McGraw-Hill, pp 209-247.
28. Caro J, Erslev AJ: Anemia of chronic renal failure. In Beutler E et al, editors: *Williams hematology,* ed 6, New York, 2001, McGraw-Hill, pp 399-406.
29. Luke RG, Sanders CE, Curtis JJ: Chronic renal failure. In Stein JH et al, editors: *Internal medicine,* ed 5, St Louis, 1998, Mosby, pp 776-795.
30. Daniak N: Hematologic complications of renal disease. In Hoffman R et al, editors: *Hematology: basic principles and practice,* ed 3, New York, 2000, Churchill Livingstone, pp 2357-2373.
31. Curtis JJ: Treatment of irreversible renal failure. In Goldman L, Bennett JC, editors: *Cecil textbook of medicine,* ed 21, Philadelphia, 2000, Saunders, pp 578-586.
32. Means RT: Anemia of chronic disorders. In Lee GR et al, editors: *Wintrobe's clinical hematology,* ed 10, Baltimore, Williams & Wilkins, 1998, pp 1011-1021.
33. Luke RG: Chronic renal failure. In Goldman L, Bennett JC, editors: *Cecil textbook of medicine,* ed 21, Philadelphia, 2000, Saunders, pp 571-578.
34. Antony AC: Megaloblastic anemias. In Hoffman R et al, editors: *Hematology: basic principles and practice,* ed 3, New York, 2000, Churchill Livingstone, pp 446-485.
35. Babior BM: The megaloblastic anemias. In Beutler E et al, editors: *Williams hematology,* ed 6, New York, 2001, McGraw-Hill, pp 425-445.
36. Lee GR: Iron deficiency and iron-deficiency anemia. In Lee GR et al, editors: *Wintrobe's clinical hematology,* ed 10, Baltimore, 1998, Williams & Wilkins, pp 979-1010.
37. Means RT: Iron deficiency anemia, the anemia of chronic disease, sideroblastic anemia, and iron overload. In Stein JH et al, editors: *Internal medicine,* ed 5, St Louis, 1998, Mosby, pp 641-645.
38. Fairbanks VF, Beutler E et al: Iron deficiency. In Beutler E et al, editors: *Williams hematology,* ed 6, New York, 2001, McGraw-Hill, pp 447-470.
39. Brittenham GM: Disorders of iron metabolism: iron deficiency and overload. In Hoffman R et al, editors: *Hematology: basic principles and practice,* ed 3, New York, 2000, Churchill Livingstone, pp 397-427.
40. Duffy TP: Microcytic and hypochromic anemias. In Goldman L, Bennett JC, editors: *Cecil textbook of medicine,* ed 21, Philadelphia, 2000, Saunders, pp 854-859.
41. Weatherall DJ: The thalassemias. In Beutler E et al, editors: *Williams hematology,* ed 6, New York, 2001, McGraw-Hill, pp 547-580.
42. Lukens JN: The thalassemias and related disorders: quantitative disorders of hemoglobin synthesis. In Lee GR et al, editors: *Wintrobe's clinical hematology,* ed 10, Baltimore, 1998, Williams & Wilkins, pp 1405-1448.
43. Rodgers GP et al: Hemoglobinopathies: the thalassemias. In Goldman L, Bennett JC, editors: *Cecil textbook of medicine,* ed 21, Philadelphia, 2000, Saunders, pp 884-889.
44. Steinberg MH: Hemoglobinopathies and thalassemias. In Stein JH et al, editors: *Internal medicine,* ed 5, St Louis, 1998, Mosby, pp 650-660.
45. Beutler E: The sickle cell diseases and related disorders. In Beutler E et al, editors: *Williams hematology,* ed 6, New York, 2001, McGraw-Hill, pp 581-606.
46. Lukens JN: The abnormal hemoglobins: general principles. In Lee GR et al, editors: *Wintrobe's clinical hematology,* ed 10, Baltimore, 1998, Williams & Wilkins, pp 1329-1345.

47. Embury SH, Vichinsky EP: Sickle cell disease. In Hoffman R et al, editors: *Hematology: basic principles and practice,* ed 3, New York, 2000, Churchill Livingstone, pp 510-553.
48. Embury SH: Sickle cell anemias and associated hemoglobinopathies. In Goldman L, Bennett JC, editors: *Cecil textbook of medicine,* ed 21, Philadelphia, 2000, Saunders, pp 893-905.
49. Gallagher PG, Forget BG: Hereditary spherocytosis, elliptocytosis, and related disorders. In Beutler E et al, editors: *Williams hematology,* ed 6, New York, 2001, McGraw-Hill, pp 503-518.
50. Golan DE: Hemolytic anemias: red cell membrane and metabolic defects. In Goldman L, Bennett JC, editors: *Cecil textbook of medicine,* ed 21, Philadelphia, 2000, Saunders, pp 867-876.
51. Glader BE, Lukens JN: Hereditary spherocytosis and other anemias due to abnormalities of the red cell membrane. In Lee GR et al, editors: *Wintrobe's clinical hematology,* ed 10, Baltimore, 1998, Williams & Wilkins, pp 1132-1159.
52. Gallagher PG et al: Red cell membrane disorders. In Hoffman R et al, editors: *Hematology: basic principles and practice,* ed 3, New York, 2000, Churchill Livingstone, pp 576-610.
53. Winkelman JC: Hemolytic anemia. In Stein JH et al, editors: *Internal medicine,* ed 5, St Louis, 1998, Mosby, pp 661-670.
54. Vulliamy TJ, Luzzatto L: Glucose-6-phosphate dehydrogenase deficiency and related disorders. In Handin RL, Lux SE, Stossel TP, editors: *Blood: principles and practice of hematology,* ed 2, Philadelphia, 1995, Lippincott, pp 1921-1950.
55. Beutler E: Glucose-6-phosphate dehydrogenase deficiency and other red cell enzyme abnormalities. In Beutler E et al, editors: *Williams hematology,* ed 6, New York, 2001, McGraw-Hill, pp 527-546.
56. Prchal JT, Gregg XT: Red cell enzymopathies. In Hoffman R et al, editors: *Hematology: basic principles and practice,* ed 3, New York, 2000, Churchill Livingstone, pp 561-575.
57. Greene HL: Glycogen storage diseases. In Goldman L, Bennett JC, editors: *Cecil textbook of medicine,* ed 21, Philadelphia, 2000, Saunders, pp 1087-1088.
58. Glader BE, Lukens JN: Glucose-6-phosphate dehydrogenase deficiency and related disorders of hexose monophosphate shunt and glutathione metabolism. In Lee GR et al, editors: *Wintrobe's clinical hematology,* ed 10, Baltimore, 1998, Williams & Wilkins, pp 1176-1190.
59. Thomas AT: Autoimmune hemolytic anemias. In Lee GR et al, editors: *Wintrobe's clinical hematology,* ed 10, Baltimore, 1998, Williams & Wilkins, pp 1233-1263.
60. Ramasethu J, Luban NLC: Alloimmune hemolytic disease of the newborn. In Beutler E et al, editors: *Williams hematology,* ed 6, New York, 2001, McGraw-Hill, pp 665-676.
61. Packman CH: Drug-related immune hemolytic anemia. In Beutler E et al, editors: *Williams hematology,* ed 6, New York, 2001, McGraw-Hill, pp 657-664.
62. Parr D, Doukas M: Drug-induced hematologic disorders. In Dipiro JT et al, editors: *Pharmacotherapy: a pathophysiologic approach,* ed 3, Stamford, Conn, 1997, Appleton & Lange, pp 1915-1917.
63. Bowman MJ: Alloimmune hemolytic disease of the fetus and newborn. In Lee GR et al, editors: *Wintrobe's clinical hematology,* ed 10, Baltimore, 1998, Williams & Wilkins, pp 1210-1232.
64. Schwartz RS et al: Autoimmune hemolytic anemias. In Hoffman R et al, editors: *Hematology: basic principles and practice,* ed 3, New York, 2000, Churchill Livingstone, pp 611-629.
65. Hillman RS, Hershko C: Acute blood loss anemia. In Beutler E et al, editors: *Williams hematology,* ed 6, New York, 2001, McGraw-Hill, pp 677-682.
66. Schroeder ML et al: Principles and practice of transfusion medicine. In Lee GR et al, editors: *Wintrobe's clinical hematology,* ed 10, Baltimore, 1998, Williams & Wilkins, pp 817-874.
67. Beutler E: Hemolytic anemia due to chemical and physical agents. In Beutler E et al, editors: *Williams hematology,* ed 6, New York, 2001, McGraw-Hill, pp 629-632.
68. American Association of Blood Banks, America's Blood Centers: *Circular of information for the use of human blood and blood components (ARC 1751),* Arlington, Va, August 2000, American Red Cross.
69. Beutler E: Polycythemia. In Beutler E et al, editors: *Williams hematology,* ed 6, New York, 2001, McGraw-Hill, pp 689-702.
70. Means RT: Polycythemia vera. In Lee GR et al, editors: *Wintrobe's clinical hematology,* ed 10, Baltimore, 1998, Williams & Wilkins, pp 2374-2389.
71. Hoffman R: Polycythemia vera. In Hoffman R et al, editors: *Hematology: basic principles and practice,* ed 3, New York, 2000, Churchill Livingstone, pp 1130-1154.
72. Spivak JL: Myelodysplastic syndromes. In Handin RL, Lux SE, Stossel TP, editors: *Blood: principles and practice of hematology,* ed 2, Philadelphia, 2002, Lippincott, pp 379-432.
73. Hutton JJ: The leukemias and polycythemia vera. In Stein JH et al, editors: *Internal medicine,* ed 5, St Louis, 1998, Mosby, pp 682-690.
74. Means RT: Polycythemia: erythrocytosis. In Lee GR et al, editors: *Wintrobe's clinical hematology,* ed 10, Baltimore, 1998, Williams & Wilkins, pp 1538-1554.
75. Beutler E: Preservation and clinical use of erythrocytes and whole blood. In Beutler E et al, editors: *Williams hematology,* ed 6, New York, 2001, McGraw-Hill, pp 1879-1892.

Alterations in Hemostasis and Blood Coagulation

chapter 14

Naomi Lungstrom • Roberta J. Emerson

MEDIA RESOURCES

Additional Material for Study, Review, and Further Exploration

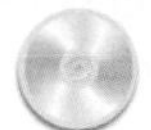

CD Companion ◆ Review Questions and Answers ◆ Key Concepts Review
◆ Glossary *(with audio pronunciations for selected terms)*
◆ Disease Profiles ◆ Animations

evolve ***Website*** at http://evolve.elsevier.com/Copstead/
◆ Case Studies ◆ Disease Profiles ◆ WebLinks

KEY QUESTIONS

- How do platelets and factors of the clotting cascade contribute to hemostasis?
- What findings from the patient history, physical, or laboratory studies would indicate a potential bleeding disorder?
- How are laboratory tests used to differentiate the various coagulation disorders?
- What vascular alterations result in abnormalities of hemostasis?
- What are the common causes of platelet deficiencies, excesses, and dysfunction?
- What are the common causes of inherited and acquired disorders of coagulation?

CHAPTER OUTLINE

The term **hemostasis** means arrest of bleeding or prevention of blood loss after a blood vessel is injured. Hemostasis is accomplished via a complex interaction involving the vessel wall, circulating platelets, and plasma coagulation proteins. If hemostasis is inadequate, bleeding results; if hemostasis is excessive, inappropriate clotting or thrombosis results.

This chapter reviews the process of hemostasis and how that process is evaluated by means of clinical assessment and laboratory tests. The focus of the chapter is on disorders of hemostasis and coagulation that result in bleeding. Disorders that result in thrombosis are discussed in Chapter 15.

THE PROCESS OF HEMOSTASIS

Stages of Hemostasis

Primary hemostasis, the initial response to vascular injury, involves the interaction between platelets and the injured blood vessel. The immediate response of the vessel to trauma is vasoconstriction to reduce blood loss. Although nervous reflex may play a part, this vasoconstriction results primarily from local myogenic spasm that may last from minutes to hours. The more trauma to the vessel, the greater the degree of vascular spasm. More vasoconstriction occurs with a blunt or crushing injury (resulting in less bleeding) than with a sharp cut to a vessel.[1]

The second component of primary hemostasis is formation of a platelet plug. Platelets not only adhere to endothelial collagen exposed by injury, they also aggregate (clump together) at the site of vessel injury. The formation of this platelet plug is usually completed within 3 to 7 minutes.

Secondary hemostasis involves the formation of a fibrin clot, or **coagulation,** at the site of injury to maintain the hemostasis already initiated. Clotting factors are activated via the **intrinsic pathway** or **extrinsic pathway,** and participate in a series of events that catalyze or facilitate the conversion of fibrinogen to fibrin. This process takes an average of 3 to 10 minutes.

Clot retraction, the final stage of clot formation, occurs when the components of the fibrin clot—the platelet plug, fibrin strands, and trapped red blood cells—are compressed or contracted to form a firm clot. This stage takes approximately 1 hour.

Platelets

Platelets have an integral role in hemostasis; thus, it is important to review their nature and function (Figure 14-1). A normal platelet count is between 150,000/mm^3 and 350,000/mm^3. Platelets, also known as *thrombocytes,* are the smallest of the formed elements in the blood. They are produced in the bone marrow from megakaryocytes, which are derived from the pluripotent stem cell. Approximately 70% of platelets are found in the circulation and 30% are sequestered in the spleen.[2] Factors such as the stress response, epinephrine, and exercise may stimulate platelet production. The average life span of a platelet is 10 days. On completion of its life span, a platelet is eliminated from the circulation by the tissue macrophage system.[1]

Platelets play a complex role in the process of hemostasis. Initially, platelets adhere to subendothelial collagen exposed by trauma (Figure 14-2). After adhesion, the platelets become activated and initiate degranulation, the release of alpha granules and dense bodies. Alpha granules release platelet thrombospondin, fibrinogen, fibronectin, von Willebrand factor, and coagulation factors V and VIII. The dense granules release

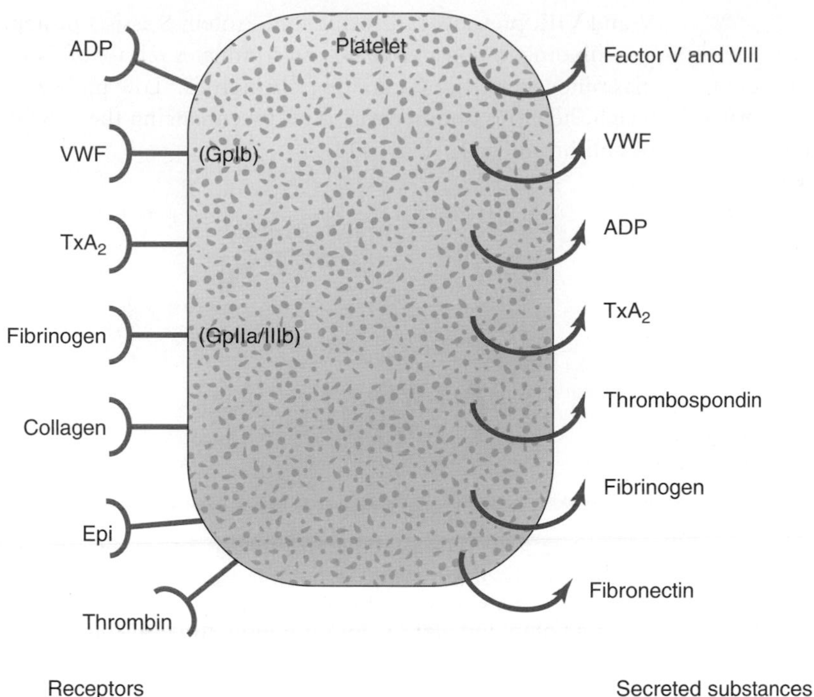

FIGURE 14-1 ■ Platelets are complex cell fragments containing numerous chemical mediators that are released when platelets are activated. Platelets display a variety of cell surface receptors that mediate both adhesion to exposed subendothelium and aggregation with other platelets. *ADP,* Adenosine diphosphate; *VWF,* von Willebrand factor; *TxA_2,* thromboxane A_2; *Epi,* epinephrine.

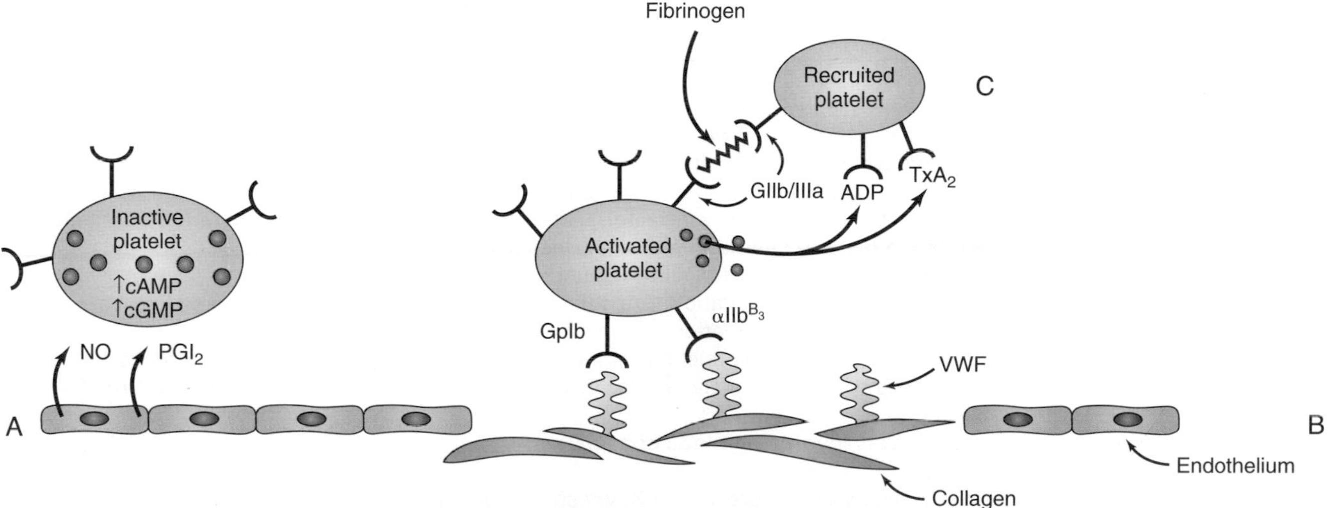

FIGURE 14-2 ■ **A,** Endothelial cells normally prevent platelet adhesion by releasing nitric oxide *(NO)* and prostaglandin I_2 *(PGI_2),* which increases platelet cGMP and cAMP levels reducing the likelihood of their being activated. **B,** Injury to the vessel wall exposes collagen and von Willebrand factor *(VWF),* which are bound by specific receptors on platelets causing them to adhere and become activated. **C,** Activated platelets release numerous chemical mediators that bind to and stimulate other nearby platelets. Groups of platelets aggregate together by binding to fibrinogen molecules through their GpIIb/IIIa receptors. *ADP,* Adenosine diphosphate; *TxA_2,* thromboxane A_2.

adenosine diphosphate (ADP), adenosine triphosphate (ATP), and serotonin. The presence of ADP and collagen encourages arachidonic acid formation, which leads to formation of thromboxane A_2 (a potent platelet aggregation agonist). Aspirin and other cyclooxygenase enzyme inhibitors can be used to block this cascade. Thromboxane A_2 stimulates the glycoprotein IIb/IIIa receptors to be expressed and further promote platelet adhesion. The glycoprotein IIb/IIIa blockers (e.g., eptifibatide) are useful antiplatelet agents.[2-5]

In addition to the major role of platelets in primary hemostasis, they are also involved in secondary hemostasis. Platelets catalyze interactions between activated coagulation factors, accelerating the conversion of prothrombin to thrombin. Platelets also have a role in clot retraction.

Blood Coagulation Factors

With the exception of tissue factor (factor III, tissue thromboplastin) and calcium, blood coagulation factors are plasma proteins that circulate in the blood stream in an inactive state. These factors are listed in Table 14-1 according to the internationally standardized nomenclature. The factors are numbered in the order of their discovery, not the order in which they participate in the clotting cascade. Some factors have both active and inactive forms; the letter "a" after the Roman numeral designates the active form.

The liver is responsible for the synthesis of coagulation factors, with the exception of part of factor VIII. Factors II, VII, IX, X, protein C, and protein S are dependent on vitamin K for synthesis and normal activity. Some of the coagulation proteins can also be synthesized by other cells such as megakaryocytes and endothelial cells.[5] Antithrombin III and protein C are protein complexes that promote anticoagulation. Antithrombin is a potent anticoagulant that binds to and inactivates free thrombin, preventing its binding and cleaving of fibrinogen. Protein C, a plasma protein that inactivates factors V and VIII, prevents clot formation. Protein S assists protein C in binding to phospholipase and stimulates release of tissue plasminogen activator, initiating fibrinolysis.[5] Low molecular weight heparins and heparin work by enhancing the activity of antithrombin III (Figure 14-3).

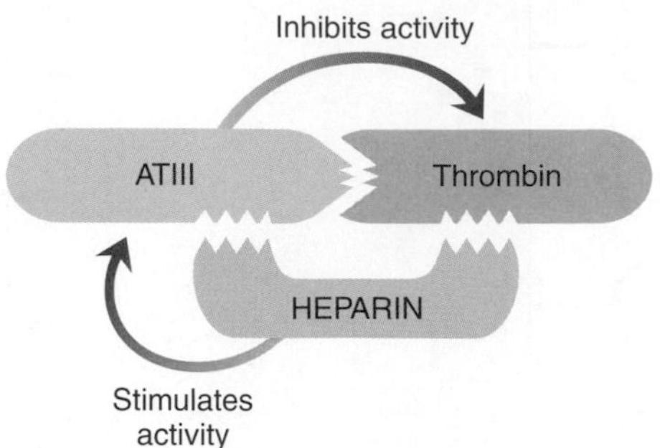

FIGURE 14-3 ■ Antithrombin III *(ATIII)* can bind and neutralize the activity of thrombin. Heparin is a catalyst that increases the activity of ATIII making it more effective. Thrombin is a potent inducer of clot formation; thus, ATIII and heparin have significant anticoagulant properties.

Table 14-1

The Clotting Factors

Factor	Action
I: Fibrinogen	Factor I is converted to fibrin by the enzyme thrombin. Individual fibrin molecules form fibrin threads, which are the scaffold for clot formation and wound healing.
II: Prothrombin	Factor II is the inactive precursor of thrombin. Prothrombin is activated to thrombin by coagulation factor X (Stuart-Prower factor). After it is activated, thrombin converts fibrinogen (coagulation factor I) into fibrin and activates factors V and VIII.
III: Tissue thromboplastin	Factor III interacts with factor VII to initiate the extrinsic clotting cascade.
IV: Calcium	Calcium (Ca^{2+}), a divalent cation, is a cofactor for most of the enzyme-activated processes required in blood coagulation. Calcium also enhances platelet aggregation and makes red blood cells clump together.
V: Proaccelerin	Factor V is a cofactor for activated factor X, which is essential for converting prothrombin to thrombin.
VI: Discovered to be an artifact	No factor VI is involved in blood coagulation.
VII: Proconvertin	Factor VII activates factors IX and X, which are essential in converting prothrombin to thrombin. Synthesis is vitamin K dependent.
VIII: Antihemophilic factor	Factor VIII together with activated factor IX enzymatically activates factor X. In addition, factor VIII combines with another protein (von Willebrand factor) to help platelets adhere to capillary walls in areas of tissue injury. A lack of factor VIII is the basis for classic hemophilia (hemophilia A).
IX: Plasma thromboplastin component (Christmas factor)	Factor IX, when activated, activates factor X to convert prothrombin to thrombin. This factor is essential in the common pathway of the intrinsic and extrinsic clotting cascades. A lack of factor IX is the basis for hemophilia B. Synthesis is vitamin K dependent.
X: Stuart-Prower factor	Factor X, when activated, converts prothrombin into thrombin. Synthesis is vitamin K dependent.
XI: Plasma thromboplastin antecedent	Factor XI, when activated, assists in the activation of factor IX. However, a similar factor must exist in tissues. People who are deficient in factor XI have mild bleeding problems after surgery but do not bleed excessively as a result of trauma.
XII: Hageman factor	Factor XII is critically important in the intrinsic pathway for the activation of factor XI.
XIII: Fibrin-stabilizing factor	Factor XIII assists in forming crosslinks among the fibrin threads to form a strong fibrin clot.

From Ignatavicus DD, Workman ML: *Medical surgical nursing: critical thinking for collaborative care,* ed 4, Philadelphia, 2002, Saunders, p 824.

Fibrin Clot

In normal hemostasis, the fibrin clot is produced through activation of the intrinsic or extrinsic pathway and, in turn, the common final pathway. Effective hemostasis is the result of interactions between all of these pathways and is commonly referred to as the *coagulation cascade.*

Figure 14-4 illustrates the coagulation cascade. The intrinsic pathway of coagulation begins when blood comes into contact with altered vascular endothelium or another negatively

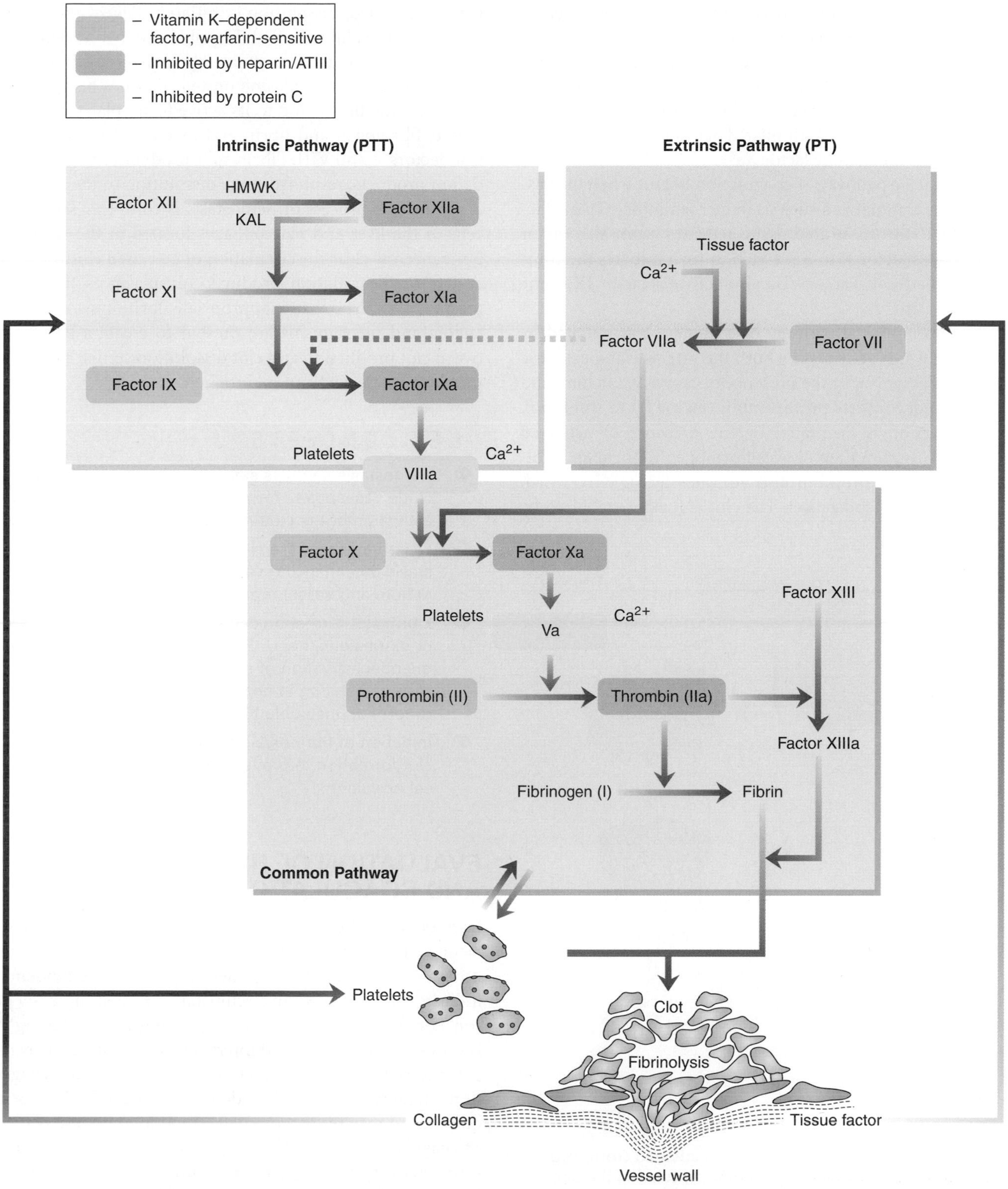

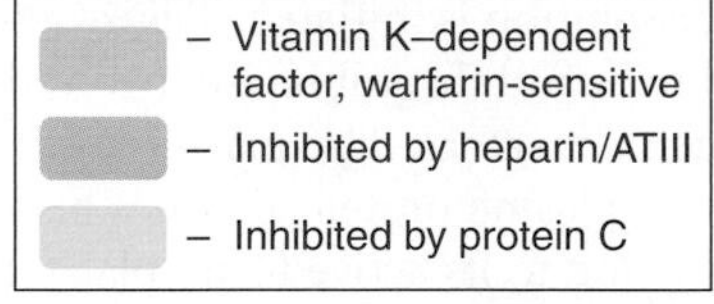

FIGURE 14-4 ■ Coagulation cascade. *PTT,* Partial thromboplastin time; *PT,* prothrombin time.

charged surface, such as glass. This contact phase of coagulation involves four factors: (1) factor XII, (2) high molecular weight kininogen (HMWK), (3) prekallikrein, and (4) factor XI. Factor XII is activated to factor XIIa, which in turn activates XI to XIa and prekallikrein to its active form, kallikrein. Kallikrein liberates bradykinin from HMWK. The release of bradykinin produces an initial vasodilation followed by release of angiotensin II and vasoconstriction. The major role of factor XIa is activation of factor IX to factor IXa in the presence of calcium. Factor IXa then activates factor X to factor Xa in the presence of factor VIII, calcium, and phospholipid. This activation usually takes place on the membrane of stimulated platelets. The common final pathway is initiated by factor Xa.

The extrinsic pathway of coagulation begins when the vascular wall is traumatized such as in a crush injury. Tissue factor (factor III) from injured tissue activates factor VII. Factor VIIa activates factor X to Xa, which in turn initiates the common final pathway. Factor VIIa also activates factor IX in the intrinsic system.

The common final pathway of coagulation is initiated by factor X, which is activated by both the intrinsic and extrinsic pathways. Factor Xa, in the presence of factor V, calcium, and phospholipid, converts prothrombin (factor II) to thrombin. This conversion is facilitated by the presence of activated platelets. Thrombin then cleaves fibrinogen to form an insoluble fibrin clot. Thrombin also activates factor XIII, which promotes fibrin stabilization. The clot is further stabilized by clot retraction. Thrombin also helps to perpetuate the clotting cascade by continuing to activate factors V and VIII.

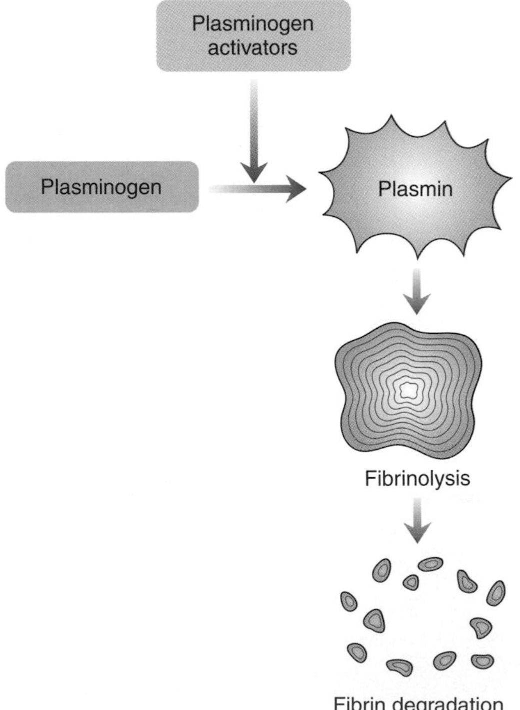

FIGURE 14-5 ■ Fibrinolysis. Plasmin, activated from plasminogen, enzymatically cleaves fibrin proteins in the clot. This results in fibrin split products, which can be measured.

Fibrinolysis

At the same time the fibrin clot is forming, the process of **fibrinolysis** or clot dissolution is initiated (Figure 14-5). Factor XII, HMWK, kallikrein, and thrombin are involved in the release of plasminogen activators. The plasminogen activators cleave plasminogen, a plasma protein that has been incorporated into the fibrin clot, to its active form, plasmin. Plasmin digests fibrinogen and fibrin and inactivates blood coagulation factors V and VIII. Fibrin split products, or fibrin degradation products, result from the dissolution of the fibrin clot.

The entire process of hemostasis is complex. The Kupffer cells of the liver and macrophages located in the spleen and bone marrow clear the circulation of activated clotting factors and fibrin degradation products. Antiplasmins that inhibit plasmin exist to prevent inappropriate fibrinolysis. All of these factors and mechanisms are present to create a balance between clot production and clot dissolution so that normal hemostasis is achieved and maintained.

KEY CONCEPTS

- Hemostasis involves several critical steps. These include vasospasm, formation of a platelet plug, and activation of the clotting cascade to form a fibrin clot.
- Factors released from platelets contribute to hemostasis by enhancing vasoconstriction, platelet aggregation, and vessel repair.
- Fibrin clot formation can be initiated by the intrinsic or extrinsic pathway. Each pathway requires the sequential activation of specific clotting factors, ultimately resulting in enzymatic cleavage of fibrinogen to form an insoluble fibrin clot.
- Initiation of fibrinolysis occurs simultaneously with clot formation to prevent excessive clotting and vessel occlusion.

EVALUATION OF HEMOSTASIS AND COAGULATION

Data obtained from clinical assessment and laboratory tests facilitate the identification and evaluation of a hemostatic abnormality. Evaluation of a patient for a bleeding tendency is indicated in the following circumstances: when there is a personal or family history of bleeding; during active bleeding that is unresponsive to standard interventions; as part of screening prior to surgery; and for ongoing evaluation of anticoagulation therapy. A bleeding tendency may be inherited or acquired, and may result from defects in blood vessels, platelets, or coagulation factors. The purpose of the evaluation process is to determine if a problem exists and to ascertain the underlying cause so that appropriate management can be initiated.

Clinical Assessment

Both the family history and the personal history are important in the evaluation of a bleeding problem (Table 14-2). A family history of bleeding in males is often linked to one of the types of hemophilia, which accounts for the majority of serious inherited coagulation problems.[4,6] The location, severity, duration, and setting in which bleeding occurs are also important clues to the type of defect that is present. Bleeding associated with vascular and platelet defects usually occurs immediately after trauma (e.g., dental extraction), involves skin or mucous membranes, and is brief. Delayed bleeding or bleeding into muscles or joints is more typical of a coagulation defect.[4]

Systemic diseases such as uremia, liver disease, systemic lupus erythematosus, and malignancies may be associated with a bleeding problem. Medication history, including use of over-the-counter medications, is another important aspect in the evaluation of a hemostatic defect. A common cause of acquired bleeding problems is drug ingestion. Specific drugs that alter hemostasis include aspirin and aspirin-containing preparations, nonsteroidal antiinflammatory agents, some antibiotics, anticoagulants, alcohol, and chemotherapeutic and thrombolytic agents.

Many of the physical findings of bleeding are manifested in the skin and mucous membranes. The individual may appear pale or jaundiced. Pallor is associated with a marked decrease in hemoglobin; jaundice is associated with liver or gallbladder disease and possible coagulation disorders and with excessive red blood cell destruction.

Petechiae are flat, pinpoint, nonblanching red or purple spots caused by capillary hemorrhages in the skin and mucous membranes (Figure 14-6). Petechiae are commonly seen with vascular and platelet disorders. They are usually present on dependent areas of the body, such as the legs, or on areas constricted by tight clothing. Not all petechiae indicate a bleeding problem. Petechiae found on other body areas not constricted by tight clothing, such as the abdomen or thorax, may be associated with infectious disease or other pathophysiologic sources. Petechiae may be seen in the newborn as a result of the trauma of delivery, not as a result of a bleeding problem.

When petechiae occur in groups or patches, the term **purpura** is used (Figure 14-7). Purpuric lesions are often pruritic (itchy). Fever and malaise may be present, as may effusions into joints or viscera, manifested by joint or abdominal pain.

Ecchymosis occurs when blood escapes into the tissues, producing a bruise (Figure 14-8). If the area is raised, it is called a **hematoma. Hemarthrosis,** manifested by swelling and pain, is bleeding into a joint. Large ecchymoses, hematomas, and hemarthroses are seen in coagulation disorders.

Telangiectasia is a lesion created by dilation of capillaries and small arteries, typically on the lips, tongue, tips of the fingers and toes, and sometimes in visceral vessels (Figure 14-9). These thin, dilated, tortuous vessels are red to violet, blanch with pressure, and tend to bleed with minimal

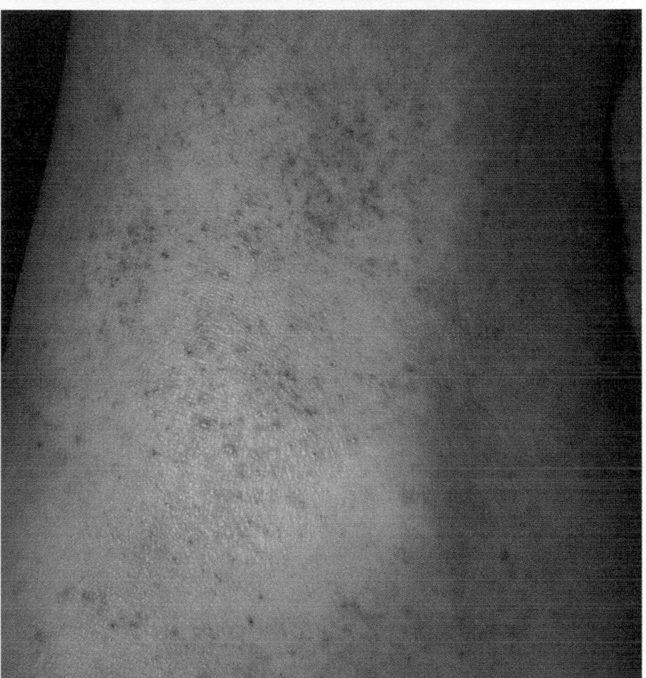

FIGURE 14-6 ■ Petechiae. (From Dockery GL: *Cutaneous disorders of the lower extremity,* Philadelphia, 1997, Saunders.)

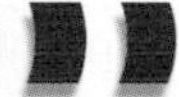

Table 14-2

Clues from Patient History Regarding Bleeding Disorders

Clue from Patient History	Possible Cause
Family history of bleeding in both males and females	Von Willebrand disease
Family history of bleeding in males	Hemophilia A or B
Newly acquired bruising	Drugs (especially aspirin and NSAIDs, anticoagulant therapy), thrombocytopenia
Excessive bleeding/bruising during/after surgery	Mild-severe deficiency of coagulation factors, von Willebrand disease; thrombocytopenia, drug ingestion
Bleeding following initial hemostasis	Factor XIII deficiency

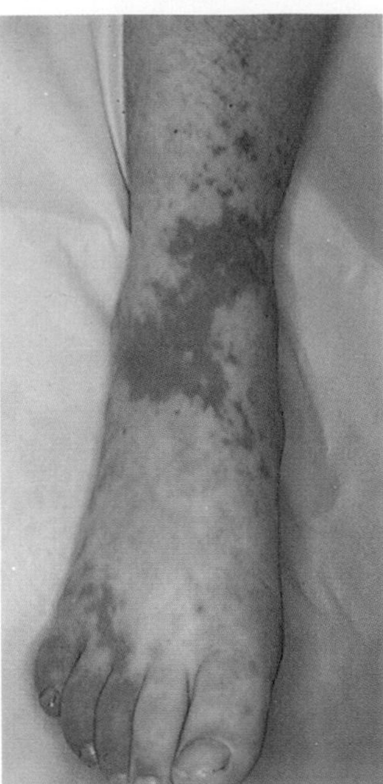

FIGURE 14-7 ■ Purpura. (From Hurwitz S: *Clinical pediatric dermatology: a textbook of skin disorders of childhood and adolescence,* ed 2, Philadelphia, 1993, Saunders, p 269.)

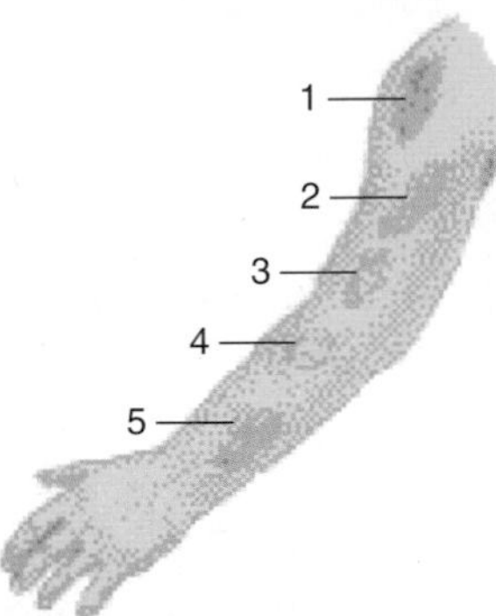

FIGURE 14-8 ■ Ecchymosis. A large patch of capillary bleeding into tissues. Color in a light-skinned person is first red-blue or purple *(1)* immediately after or within 24 hours of trauma and generally progresses to blue to purple *(2)*, blue-green *(3)*, yellow *(4)*, and brown to disappearing *(5)*. (From Jarvis C: *Physical examination and health assessment,* ed 2, Philadelphia, 2004, Saunders, p 258.)

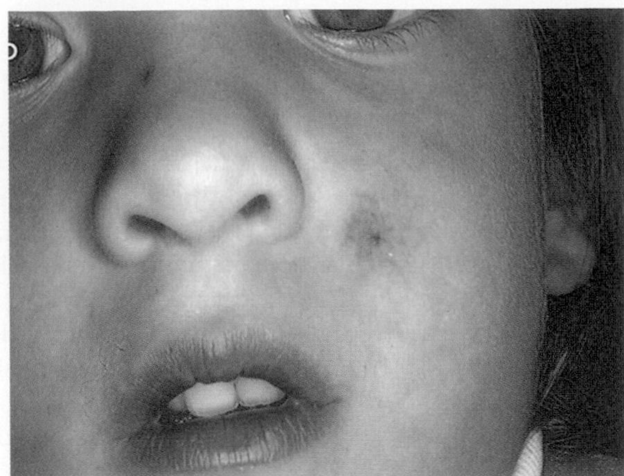

FIGURE 14-9 ■ Telangiectasia (spider or star angioma). A fiery red, star-shaped marking with a solid circular center. Capillary radiations extend from the central arterial body. With pressure, note a central pulsating body and blanching of extended legs. Develops on face, neck, or chest; may be associated with pregnancy, chronic liver disease, or estrogen therapy, or may be normal. (From Hurwitz S: *Clinical pediatric dermatology: a textbook of skin disorders in childhood and adolescence,* ed 2, Philadelphia, 1993, Saunders, p 266.)

trauma. Spider telangiectasia branch into the subcutaneous and dermal layers of the skin and are often associated with liver disease.

Other significant findings of a bleeding disorder on physical examination include blood (bright red, rusty, or black) in drainage or excreta, such as feces (**hematochezia** or **melena**), urine (**hematuria**), vomitus (**hematemesis**), gastric drainage, or sputum (**hemoptysis**). Excessive menstrual bleeding may occur (**menorrhagia**). Acute abdominal or flank pain may indicate internal bleeding. Hypovolemia from bleeding may produce a shock state and present as hypotension, tachycardia, pallor, altered mentation, and decreased urine output. The two sites at which bleeding is most life threatening are the oropharynx (resulting in airway compromise) and within the brain tissue. One of the leading causes of death in patients experiencing severe disorders of coagulation is intracerebral hemorrhage.[3]

Laboratory Tests

Many laboratory tests are available to aid in the diagnosis of hemostasis problems (Table 14-3). Basic screening includes a complete blood cell count (CBC), including a platelet count and peripheral blood smear, bleeding time, prothrombin time (PT), activated partial thromboplastin time (aPTT), and thrombin time. These screening tests evaluate both primary and secondary hemostasis. The CBC determines if anemia is present, the platelet count determines the number of platelets, and the peripheral smear indicates the number and gross morphologic characteristics of platelets. The bleeding time evaluates vascular status and platelet function. The PT and international normalized ratio (INR) assess the extrinsic pathway of coagulation, and the aPTT assesses the intrinsic pathway. Reporting prothrombin activity as a percentage of PT in seconds can pose difficulty in the adjustment of anticoagulation therapy because the PT varies with each laboratory and the reagent used there. Laboratories have tried to compensate for this variation by using the ratio of the patient's value to the laboratory's control value, which again varied with the reagent. The INR is a standardized value used worldwide that controls for this reagent variability. Thrombin time measures the time needed to convert fibrinogen to fibrin; this reflects the quantity and quality of fibrinogen as

Table 14-3

Select Laboratory Tests Used to Assess Bleeding

Test	Normal Value*	Purpose or Significance
Platelet count	150,000-350,000/mm³	Determines number of platelets; decreased in ITP, anemias, DIC, infection, chemotherapy; increased in leukemia, cancer, splenectomy
Bleeding time	3-10 min	Assesses platelet and vascular response; increased in thrombocytopenia, vascular defects, severe liver disease, DIC, von Willebrand disease, aspirin ingestion
Prothrombin time	10-14 sec; 100%	Evaluates the extrinsic pathway of coagulation; increased in vitamin K deficiency, hemorrhagic disease of the newborn, liver disease, DIC, anti-coagulant therapy. Evaluates all coagulation factors except VIII and XII
International normalized ratio	1.5 (low-level anticoagulation for atrial fibrillation) 2.0-3.0 (medium level anticoagulation for DVT, pulmonary embolism, MI, stroke prophylaxis) 2.5-3.5 (high level anticoagulation for mechanical heart valve)	Evaluates extrinsic pathway of coagulation (as prothrombin time); provides uniformity worldwide, independent of reagents
Activated partial thromboplastin time	33-45 sec	Evaluates the intrinsic pathway of coagulation; increased in hemophilia, vitamin K deficiency, liver disease, DIC, circulating anticoagulants, heparin therapy
Thrombin time	15 sec, or control + 5 sec	Measures conversion of fibrinogen to fibrin; increased in DIC, liver disease, low fibrinogen <100 mg/dl, multiple myeloma
Fibrinogen†	200-400 mg/dl	Measures fibrinogen level; decreased in liver disease, DIC
Fibrin split products or fibrin degradation products†	<3 μg/ml	Measures byproducts from breakdown of fibrin clot; increased in DIC, hypoxia, leukemia, thromboembolic disorders
Clot retraction†	1 hr: evidence of shrinking and increased firmness 24 hr: 50% of volume is clot, 50% is serum	Rough measure of platelet function; decreased in thrombocytopenia, von Willebrand disease
Platelet aggregation†	Visible aggregates form in <5 min	Measures rate and percentage of aggregation; decreased in mononucleosis, ITP, von Willebrand disease, leukemia, aspirin ingestion, thrombasthenia, Bernard-Soulier syndrome
Tourniquet test (Rumpel-Leede test, capillary fragility test)†	No petechiae or occasional petechiae	Evaluates vascular fragility and platelet function; positive test in thrombocytopenia, vascular purpuras, thrombasthenia
Euglobin lysis time†	No lysis of fibrin clot at 37° for 3 hr; clot is observed for 24 hr	Assesses fibrinolysis; increased lysis in DIC, incompatible blood transfusion, cirrhosis, cancer, obstetric complications
Plasma D-dimer assay	<200 ng/ml	Assesses fibrinolysis, increased in deep vein thrombosis, pulmonary embolism (highly non-specific), DIC (high negative predictive value)

DIC, Disseminated intravascular coagulation; *DVT,* deep vein thrombosis; *ITP,* idiopathic thrombocytopenic purpura; *MI,* myocardial infarction.
*Value may vary, depending on source.
†Tests not included in a routine coagulation screen.

well as the influence of any inhibitors. The D-dimer assay reflects fibrinolysis.

Further laboratory investigation is necessary if abnormalities are identified on the screening tests or if despite normal screening test results a bleeding problem obviously exists. Specific tests are available to assess abnormal platelet function, the presence of circulating anticoagulants, fibrin split products, and levels of individual coagulation factors. Table 14-4 reflects the alterations in laboratory values seen with the major disorders of hemostasis.

Table 14-4

Alterations in Laboratory Values Seen with Major Disorders of Hemostasis

	Laboratory Alterations							
Disorder	**Platelet Count**	**Bleeding Time**	**PT**	**aPTT**	**TT**	**FSP**	**FVIII**	**FIX**
Idiopathic thrombocytopenic purpura	↓	Prolonged	N	N	N	N	N	N
Hemophilia A	N	N/Prolonged	N	↑	↑	N	↓	N
Hemophilia B	N	N/Prolonged	N	↑	↑	N	N	↓
Von Willebrand disease	N	Prolonged	N	↑	↑	N	↓	N
Vitamin K deficiency	N	Prolonged	↑	N/↑	↑	N	N	N/↓
Disseminated intravascular coagulation	↓	Prolonged	↑	↑	↑	↑	↓	↓
ASA/NSAIDs	N	Prolonged	N	N	N	N	N	N
Heparin	N/↓	Prolonged	N	↑	↑	N	N	N
Coumadin	N	Prolonged	↑	N/↑	↑	N	N	N
Vascular purpura	N	N/Prolonged	N	N	N	N	N	N
Liver disease	N/↓	Prolonged	↑	N/↑	N	N	N	N/↓

ASA, Acetylsalicylic acid; *NSAIDs,* nonsteroidal antiinflammatory drugs; *PT,* prothrombin time; *aPTT,* activated partial thromboplastin time; *TT,* thrombin time; *FSP,* fibrin split products; *FVIII,* factor VIII; *FIX,* factor IX; *N,* normal.

KEY CONCEPTS

- Bleeding tendencies may be inherited or acquired. A history of abnormal bleeding, liver disease, and anticoagulant drug use may be important risk factors. Physical findings of petechiae, purpura, ecchymoses, telangiectasia, and occult or frank bleeding are indicative.
- Usual laboratory tests include platelet count, bleeding time, PT (extrinsic pathway), activated thromboplastin time (intrinsic pathway), and thrombin time.

VASCULAR AND PLATELET DISORDERS

Vascular Disorders

Vascular disorders of hemostasis and coagulation are those in which the primary cause of bleeding is a problem with the vascular component of primary hemostasis. The vascular defect may be acquired (e.g., related to ingestion of a specific drug) or inherited.

Vascular Purpura

Etiology. Vascular purpura is a disorder in which purpura—patches of petechiae, or pinpoint hemorrhages, on the skin—are present; the primary cause of the purpura, or more extensive bleeding in some cases, is an abnormality of the vessels or the tissues that support them (see Figure 14-7).

Allergic purpura (anaphylactoid purpura, Henoch-Schönlein purpura) is most often seen in children between the ages of 4 and 7.[7,8] Drug-induced purpura may result from many drugs, including atropine, chloral hydrate, and other sedatives; sulfa drugs; procaine penicillin; and warfarin (Coumadin). Purpuric lesions and perhaps severe hemorrhage are components of the Ehlers-Danlos syndrome and osteogenesis imperfecta, which are both inherited disorders of connective tissue.[9,10] Acquired disorders of connective tissue such as scurvy (vitamin C deficiency), senile purpura (seen in the elderly), and corticosteroid purpura (associated with steroid drug therapy) may also result in purpuric lesions.

Pathogenesis. The allergic purpuras are thought to result from an autoimmune process that produces inflammation or vasculitis of small vessels. As a result, perivascular infiltration and serosanguineous effusion occur into surrounding tissues to produce the characteristic purpuric lesion.

The pathophysiologic process of drug-induced purpura is not well understood. An autoimmune process such as that described in the preceding paragraph has been proposed.

Structural abnormalities of vessels and perivascular supportive tissue provide the mechanism for bleeding in many of the vascular purpura. These abnormalities may be inherited or acquired. In Ehlers-Danlos syndrome and osteogenesis imperfecta, the vascular abnormality is thought to result from decreased amounts or poor quality of collagen and elastin; both are necessary for perivascular support. Vitamin C deficiency, which causes scurvy, results in defective collagen synthesis. The lack of proper collagen support for the vessels leads to bleeding. In the elderly (senile purpura), loss of subcutaneous fat and changes in connective tissue allow for more mobility of the skin. Shearing force then causes rupture of small vessels. Steroids induce catabolism of proteins in supportive tissues, decreasing the mechanical strength of the microvasculature.

Clinical Manifestations. The purpuric lesions characteristically appear and fade or disappear in groups. The lesions are not elevated and do not blanch with pressure.

With allergic purpura, the lesions tend to be palpable and are found on the proximal extremities, especially on the legs and buttocks; they may be accompanied by fever, itching, arthralgia, and paresthesia. Bleeding from the lesions themselves and generalized bleeding are uncommon. Usually, allergic purpura is self-limited, and the prognosis is good.

Generalized purpura is characteristic of drug-induced vascular purpura. The lesions quickly subside when the drug is discontinued. Other bleeding manifestations are uncommon.

The purpuric lesions associated with inherited connective tissue disorders, such as Ehlers-Danlos syndrome, often are accompanied by large ecchymoses and hematomas. Although not common, bleeding into the brain tissue may result in cerebrovascular accident (stroke).[10]

The purpuric lesions seen with scurvy typically occur around hair follicles and on the medial surfaces of the thighs and buttocks. Ecchymoses and large hematomas may also occur.

Senile purpura and corticosteroid purpura generally occur on the dorsum of the hands and forearms and are aggravated by trauma. Other bleeding is uncommon.

Diagnosis and Treatment. The diagnosis of vascular purpura is one of exclusion after platelet disorders and coagulation disorders have been ruled out. An abnormal tourniquet test (positive Rumpel-Leede test) in the setting of a normal or increased bleeding time, normal platelet count, and normal coagulation study results suggests a problem with the vascular component of hemostasis.

Treatment for vascular purpura includes removal or avoidance of the causative agent if one is identified (e.g., penicillin) and interventions to relieve symptoms such as itching. If more extensive bleeding accompanies the purpura, identification of the cause and intervention to control the bleeding are necessary.

Hereditary Hemorrhagic Telangiectasia

Etiology. A telangiectasia is a dilated and/or tortuous small blood vessel, found in the skin or mucous membranes, that has a tendency to bleed spontaneously and/or following minor trauma (see Figure 14-9). Hereditary hemorrhagic telangiectasia (Osler-Weber-Rendu disease) is transmitted as an autosomal dominant trait; the vascular abnormalities can be seen in children but become more prominent after puberty, peaking between the fourth and fifth decades. As the telangiectases—the skin spots resulting from the vascular lesion—become more prominent, the frequency and severity of the bleeding increase.[11,12]

Pathogenesis. The telangiectases result from an abnormality in vascular development. The vessel wall is composed of a single layer of endothelium; thus, support and contractile properties are deficient, leading to spontaneous bleeding or bleeding as a result of minor trauma.[12] Any mucosal surface (e.g., respiratory, gastrointestinal, and genitourinary tracts) may be involved. Arteriovenous malformations in the lung, liver, and brain are the most serious complications.[13]

Clinical Manifestations. Bright red or purple lesions, ranging from pinpoint to 3 mm in diameter, can be found on the nasal mucous membranes, lips, palate, tongue, face, trunk, palms of the hands, and the soles of the feet. Recurrent epistaxis is a hallmark with increasing frequency as the patient ages. Severity of the disorder is linked to age of onset.[12] Typically the lesions are flat and blanch with pressure.

The most common clinical problem is mucous membrane bleeding, especially **epistaxis** (nosebleed). However, bleeding may occur from telangiectases in any area. Frequent bleeding episodes may result in anemia.[13]

Diagnosis and Treatment. The diagnosis is confirmed from the presence of multiple telangiectases, repeated episodes of bleeding, or a family history of bleeding in both sexes. If telangiectases are not easily visible, the diagnosis is more difficult to make.

Treatment is primarily supportive and includes use of topical hemostatic agents or cauterization if the bleeding site is accessible; nasal tamponade; and iron replacement; laser treatment for cutaneous lesions; embolization and estrogen or estrogen with progesterone for epistaxis. ε-Aminocaproic acid is used for controlling severe hemorrhage.[13] Blood transfusions or surgical intervention for uncontrolled bleeding or removal of an arteriovenous fistula may be considered in selected cases.[13]

Platelet Disorders

Platelet disorders of hemostasis and coagulation are those in which the primary cause of bleeding is an abnormality in the quantity or the quality of platelets.

Thrombocytopenia

Etiology. **Thrombocytopenia** is a common cause of generalized bleeding. Some of the many causes of thrombocytopenia are listed in Box 14-1.

Idiopathic thrombocytopenic purpura (ITP) is an immune-mediated thrombocytopenia that occurs in the absence of toxin or drug exposure or a disease known to be associated with decreased platelets. Acute ITP occurs at any age and in both sexes following an acute viral infection.[4,14-16] Resolution is usually spontaneous, and the prognosis is good. Chronic ITP is more common in adults 20 to 50 years of age. The onset is insidious, and women are affected most often. A pregnant woman with

Box 14-1

Some Causes of Thrombocytopenia

Decreased Platelet Production
Folate/B_{12} deficiency
Radiation therapy
Chemotherapy
Drugs (e.g., alcohol, thiazides, phenytoin)
Aplastic anemia
Cancer in bone marrow

Decreased Platelet Survival
Drugs (e.g., thiazides, digoxin, heparin, furosemide, certain antibiotics)
Mechanical prosthetic heart valves
Viral and bacterial infections
Circulating immune complexes
Increased destruction in the spleen
Disseminated intravascular coagulation

Splenic Sequestration (Pooling)
Splenomegaly
Hypothermia

Platelet Dilution
Massive transfusions with blood stored for more than 24 hours

ITP can deliver a thrombocytopenic infant because the antiplatelet antibody crosses the placenta. Adult ITP may precede or occur in association with diseases of altered immunity, such as systemic lupus erythematosus (see Chapter 10), lymphoproliferative disease (see Chapter 11), or acquired immunodeficiency syndrome (AIDS) (see Chapter 12).

Pathogenesis. Four general mechanisms are responsible for thrombocytopenia: decreased platelet production, decreased platelet survival, splenic sequestration (pooling), and intravascular dilution of circulating platelets (see Box 14-1). Regardless of the mechanism responsible for thrombocytopenia, there are fewer platelets available, and inadequate hemostasis is the potential result.

Platelets are produced by bone marrow megakaryocytes. Platelet production falls when the number of megakaryocytes is reduced or when the process of platelet production (thrombocytopoiesis) is ineffective. Although numerous causes of decreased platelet production are listed in Box 14-1, drugs are often responsible. Bone marrow suppression from chemotherapy and alcohol ingestion are common causes of platelet reduction.[6,16] In the elderly, thiazide diuretics are the most likely drugs to cause thrombocytopenia, affecting both platelet survival and megakaryocyte production. In chemotherapy the mechanism of platelet destruction is the result of myelotoxicity and not immune platelet destruction.[16]

The average life span of a platelet is 10 days. Decreased platelet survival may be the result of an antibody-mediated immune mechanism that destroys platelets (e.g., ITP, heparin) or the result of increased consumption of platelets, as seen in disseminated intravascular coagulation (DIC). Direct trauma to platelets from vascular or valvular prostheses may also be responsible for decreased platelet survival.

Normally, 30% of the total number of platelets can be found in the spleen and the remaining 70% are circulating. When the spleen is enlarged (splenomegaly), as much as 90% of the platelets may be pooled or sequestered in the spleen; thus, the circulating number of platelets is markedly decreased.[3,16] If the spleen cannot be felt on physical examination, platelet sequestration can be ruled out as the primary mechanism of the thrombocytopenia.

The final mechanism responsible for thrombocytopenia is dilution of circulating platelets by administration of massive transfusions. Platelets degenerate in stored blood after 24 hours; thus, when a large amount of blood deficient in platelets is transfused, thrombocytopenia results.

Clinical Manifestations. Clinical manifestations of thrombocytopenia are generally absent until the platelet count falls below 100,000/mm^3.[16] Increased bruising and prolonged bleeding following minor trauma may be seen with a platelet count of 50,000/mm^3.[16] Petechiae and purpura are prominent with platelet counts below 50,000/mm^3.[16] Spontaneous mucosal, deep tissue, and intracranial bleeding may be seen with platelet counts below 20,000/mm^3.[16]

Diagnosis. Thrombocytopenia is diagnosed by the presence of a low platelet count. The bleeding time is prolonged and clot retraction is poor or absent. PT, partial thromboplastin time, and other coagulation studies are normal. The CBC will indicate if the thrombocytopenia is isolated or if an associated problem, such as anemia or leukopenia, is present. Gross morphology of platelets, evaluated from the peripheral blood smear, and bone marrow examination provide additional information regarding the mechanism for the thrombocytopenia. Because many drugs are associated with thrombocytopenia, careful review of all medications the patient is taking is also necessary in the search for the cause of the thrombocytopenia.

Treatment. The treatment for thrombocytopenia is based on the identified cause or mechanism and may include any of the following: discontinuation of any suspected drug; avoidance of aspirin and pharmacodynamically similar drugs that alter normal platelet function; administration of corticosteroids to increase platelet production and to decrease splenic sequestration of platelets; platelet transfusions; plasma exchange (plasmapheresis); or splenectomy. Plasmapheresis is the mechanical separation of plasma from the cellular components of blood. The technique can also separate single blood components such as platelets. When large volumes of plasma are removed, a colloid solution must be administered to maintain the oncotic pressure; this is termed *plasma exchange*.[17,18] Splenectomy results in removal of a major site of platelet destruction and also eliminates a source for production of antiplatelet antibodies.

Thrombocytosis

Etiology. Thrombocytosis is generally defined as a platelet count above 400,000/mm^3. Transitory thrombocytosis is seen following stress or physical exercise. Secondary or reactive thrombocytosis occurs as a response to hemorrhage, inflammatory diseases, malignancy, infection, hemolysis, or splenectomy. Primary thrombocytosis or thrombocythemia is seen with polycythemia vera and chronic granulocytic leukemia.[4,6,16]

Pathogenesis. In all types of thrombocytosis, the number of platelets is increased, but the mechanism of the increase varies. Transitory thrombocytosis results from release of preformed platelets, not increased production. As the name implies, the elevation in platelet count is transient. Secondary thrombocytosis results from an actual increase in platelet production via an unknown mechanism. With primary thrombocytosis, there is abnormal proliferation of megakaryocytes in the bone marrow, resulting in as much as a 15-fold increase in platelet production. The pathophysiologic basis for the excessive bleeding or thrombosis that may result is not well understood.

Clinical Manifestations. In general, transitory and secondary thrombocytosis do not result in hemorrhage or thrombotic complications. Hemorrhage into the skin and mucous membranes and gastrointestinal bleeding may be seen with primary thrombocytosis. Thrombosis resulting in peripheral vascular ischemia or pulmonary embolism may further complicate the clinical picture. Thromboembolic events are the most common cause of death. However, the course of thrombocytosis is benign in most patients.

Diagnosis and Treatment. The diagnosis is made on the basis of a high platelet count. Bleeding time may be normal or prolonged, and platelet aggregation is normal or impaired. The history and clinical presentation, as well as additional laboratory tests such as bone marrow examination, aid in determining the type of thrombocytosis.

No treatment is necessary with transitory and secondary thrombocytosis. Reducing platelet production with the use of cytotoxic agents such as hydroxyurea is one approach to managing primary thrombocytosis, and anagrelide is a new drug that is being used to decrease the platelet count by up to 50% in 11 days.[17] Antiplatelet therapy (e.g., aspirin or dipyridamole) may also be employed. In the presence of acute bleeding or thrombosis, plasma exchange may be used to temporarily control the platelet count.

Qualitative Platelet Disorders

Etiology. Although the number of platelets may be normal, the ability of the platelets to function in the hemostatic process may be abnormal; thus, a qualitative platelet disorder is present. Inherited defects in platelet function such as Bernard-Soulier syndrome (giant platelet syndrome), von Willebrand disease, and thrombasthenia (Glanzmann disease) are rare. In contrast, acquired disorders of platelet function are common; they are often associated with drugs, especially aspirin; with uremia; or with a coexisting hematologic disease, such as leukemia.

Pathogenesis. Whether the qualitative platelet disorder is inherited or acquired, at least one aspect of platelet function (adhesion, aggregation, or release reaction) is abnormal; a bleeding tendency results. In both Bernard-Soulier syndrome and von Willebrand disease, platelet adhesion is abnormal. Platelet aggregation is the problem in thrombasthenia, due to the absence of the fibrinogen receptor necessary for normal platelet aggregation. Aspirin and other nonsteroidal antiinflammatory agents inhibit production of thromboxane A_2 and thus impair both platelet aggregation and the platelet release reaction.

Clinical Manifestations. The clinical presentation of a qualitative platelet disorder is some form of bleeding tendency, such as petechiae or purpura on skin and mucous membranes, epistaxis, gastrointestinal bleeding, or menorrhagia. Acquired platelet function defects may also result in excessive bleeding during and following surgical procedures.

Diagnosis and Treatment. With qualitative platelet defects, the bleeding time is prolonged but the platelet count and other routine coagulation screening test results are normal. Although a bleeding time greater than 10 minutes is associated with a slight increase in bleeding tendency, the risk is not significantly increased until the bleeding time exceeds 15 or 20 minutes.[4,14]

Special laboratory tests that more specifically evaluate platelet function, such as platelet aggregation studies, are necessary to determine the exact cause of bleeding.[4] Coexisting hematologic defects may make diagnosis of a platelet defect difficult.

If the platelet disorder is drug induced, the offending drug is discontinued. Transfusion with normal platelets is the usual intervention if treatment is necessary because of bleeding. Administration of desmopressin or cryoprecipitate is the treatment of choice when von Willebrand disease is the underlying cause of bleeding, as well as for patients with aspirin overdose and cirrhotic patients.[4] The treatment for von Willebrand disease is described in greater detail in the following section.

KEY CONCEPTS

- Disorders of the vasculature that result in altered hemostasis include inflammation (allergic purpura), structural abnormalities (collagen diseases), and weakened vessel walls (telangiectasia).
- An insufficient quantity of platelets (fewer than 50,000/mm^3) results from decreased production, sequestration, increased destruction, or dilution. Impor-

tant causes of thrombocytopenia include autoimmune destruction (ITP), DIC, and mechanical destruction (artificial valves).

- Excessive quantity of platelets (more than 400,000/mm^3) results from excessive production (proliferation of bone marrow cells). Thrombocythemia may result in excessive coagulation with thrombosis or excessive bleeding.
- A normal platelet count does not ensure adequate platelet function. Platelet adhesion, aggregation, and degranulation may be abnormal, resulting in a prolonged bleeding time. The usual cause is drug related (e.g., aspirin), but, rarely, the platelet defect is inherited (e.g., von Willebrand disease).

COAGULATION DISORDERS

Coagulation disorders or **coagulopathies** are defects of the normal clotting mechanism. They may result in bleeding due to a problem with the formation, stabilization, or lysis of the fibrin clot. Or, the result may be inappropriate activation of the coagulation cascade, producing excessive clot formation.

Hemophilia

Etiology. Hemophilia is rare in the general population, but it is the most common severe inherited coagulation disorder. Excessive bleeding following circumcision or the formation of a hematoma after vitamin K injection leads to the diagnosis in the neonate. Some children will not develop bleeding problems until they begin crawling or walking.

Hemophilia A, the classic form of the disease, accounts for approximately 85% of cases of clinical hemophilia. Hemophilia A is due to factor VIII deficiency.[1,19] The majority of patients inherit this X-linked recessive disorder; hemophilia is transmitted by an asymptomatic carrier female to an affected son. Approximately 20% of patients with hemophilia A have a negative family history because of a spontaneous mutation of the hemophilic gene.

Less common than hemophilia A is hemophilia B, also known as Christmas disease. Factor IX is deficient in this form of hemophilia.[18,19]

Hemophilia is often classified according to the extent to which the specific coagulation factor (factor VIII or IX) is deficient. Patients with severe hemophilia have less than 1% normal coagulation factor activity; patients with moderate hemophilia, 1% to 5% normal coagulation factor activity; and patients with mild hemophilia, 5% to 25% normal coagulation factor activity.[19-21]

Of critical concern in the hemophilic patient is intracranial hemorrhage and other serious bleeding episodes. Because of advances in treatment, however, a normal life span is possible for many.

Pathogenesis. Hemophilia A results from the lack of or the abnormal function of factor VIII. Hemophilia B results from the lack of or the abnormal function of factor IX. A deficiency or malfunction in either factor interferes with the normal sequence of events in the intrinsic pathway of coagulation and, in turn, the eventual production of fibrin clot. Inability to form a fibrin clot results in bleeding.

Clinical Manifestations. Once clinical evidence of bleeding is present, hemophilia A and B are indistinguishable. Patients with mild hemophilia may not experience symptoms until stressed by surgery or trauma. Prolonged bleeding from relatively minor trauma and occasional spontaneous bleeding episodes are characteristic of moderate hemophilia. With severe hemophilia, frequent episodes of spontaneous bleeding are likely.

Any of the following clinical manifestations may occur: easy bruising, prolonged bleeding from the nasal or oral mucosa, deep tissue hematomas, hemarthrosis, bleeding into muscles in the extremities, spontaneous hematuria, gastrointestinal bleeding, and intracranial bleeding. The hallmark of hemophilia is hemarthrosis. Knees, ankles, and elbows are the most often affected. Repeated episodes of hemarthrosis may result in joint deformity.[4,18,19]

Major long-term complications of hemophilia include progressive joint deformity due to repeated hemarthroses; and hepatitis, cirrhosis, and AIDS related to repeated transfusions and/or administration of virus-contaminated factor concentrates.

Diagnosis and Treatment. Hemophilia is considered as the cause of bleeding when the family history is positive for bleeding in males, there is a history of joint bleeding and hematomas, and joint deformity is present on the physical examination. Laboratory tests consistent with hemophilia include a normal or slightly prolonged bleeding time, a normal PT, and a prolonged aPTT. Factor assay verifies a deficiency in factor VIII or IX. Early in pregnancy, chorionic villus biopsy or amniocentesis may be done to identify factor deficiency; thus, prenatal diagnosis of hemophilia is possible.[3]

The patient and family must learn about hemophilia, including how to recognize and appropriately respond to bleeding episodes, what lifestyle changes will be necessary, and how the disease is transmitted. Prevention of injury and avoidance of aspirin and aspirin-like drugs, which alter platelet function in achieving and maintaining hemostasis, are important parts of treatment. Joint bleeding is managed by immobilization of the limb and application of ice.

With dental procedures requiring local anesthesia, prophylactic administration of factor VIII should be considered in the patient with hemophilia A. Bleeding episodes due to hemophilia A are managed primarily by the administration of cryoprecipitate or other preparations of factor VIII concentrate. Recombinant DNA–derived factor concentrates contain no viruses and are now available.[18,19] The goal of therapy is to obtain a factor VIII level at least 30% of normal.[19,21] Up to 20% of patients with severe hemophilia develop factor VIII inhibitor, an antibody that rapidly inactivates transfused factor VIII.[19,21] Plasmapheresis and immunosuppressive therapy are sometimes necessary to maintain adequate factor VIII levels in these patients.

Mild to moderate bleeding due to hemophilia B is managed with the administration of fresh or fresh frozen plasma or cryoprecipitate. Use of Konyne 80 or Proplex T, both of which are concentrates containing factors II, VII, IX, and X, is another therapeutic option. These concentrates are now treated in a variety of fashions (heat, pasteurization, solvent detergents, immunoaffinity purification) to prevent transmission of viruses. Their use was previously associated with the transmission of human immunodeficiency virus (HIV) and hepatitis viruses.[19,21] Mononine is a newer, highly purified factor IX concentrate that appears to be safe in terms of both adverse effects and viral transmission.[19,21]

Von Willebrand Disease

Etiology. Von Willebrand disease is inherited as an autosomal dominant disorder of factor VIII carrier protein and platelet dysfunction. In rare cases, von Willebrand disease is an autosomal recessive disorder.[4,22,23] Several less common subtypes of the disease have been identified, but all have some defect in von Willebrand factor, a plasma protein. Von Willebrand disease occurs in both females and males. Bleeding manifestations of the disease tend to become more severe with age.

Pathogenesis. Von Willebrand factor and factor VIII normally circulate in plasma as a complex. Von Willebrand factor is necessary for stabilization of factor VIII in the circulation and for normal adherence of platelets to damaged vascular endothelium.[4,23] In von Willebrand disease, the level of von Willebrand factor is decreased or absent; factor VIII may be mildly to severely depressed. Absence of platelet adhesion at the site of vascular injury and deficient factor VIII activity in the intrinsic coagulation pathway contribute to the bleeding seen in von Willebrand disease.

Clinical Manifestations. Epistaxis, mucosal bleeding, ecchymoses, gastrointestinal bleeding, and menorrhagia are common clinical manifestations of von Willebrand disease. Once hemostasis is achieved, it can usually be maintained. Hemarthrosis is rare. Although not common, von Willebrand disease should be considered as a possible cause of excessive surgical bleeding. Bleeding manifestations may decrease during pregnancy because levels of von Willebrand factor and factor VIII rise during this time.

Diagnosis and Treatment. The history and clinical presentation initially suggest the possibility of von Willebrand disease as the cause of bleeding. Laboratory tests consistent with the disease include a prolonged bleeding time, prolonged aPTT, normal platelet count, and normal PT. More specialized testing will verify that plasma von Willebrand factor is decreased and factor VIII activity is reduced.

Mild forms of classic von Willebrand disease can be managed with desmopressin, which causes release of von Willebrand factor and factor VIII from vascular endothelial cells.[4,23] Excessive menstrual bleeding can be managed with hormonal suppression. Severe bleeding is managed with cryoprecipitate that contains both factor VIII and von Willebrand factor. Humate-P, a recombinant replacement therapy, is now available. Aspirin and aspirin-containing drugs, which inhibit normal platelet function in hemostasis, should be avoided in patients with von Willebrand disease.[4,7,23]

Complications of therapy for severe von Willebrand disease include hepatitis and AIDS, related to transfusions with blood products. Antibodies that inhibit the activity of von Willebrand factor may develop, but this is rare.

Vitamin K Deficiency Bleeding in Infancy

Etiology. As the name implies, this coagulation disorder is seen in the newborn, typically 48 to 72 hours after birth, through 6 months of age.[24] Hemorrhagic disease of the newborn is more common in breast-fed babies (who do not receive vitamin K supplement) than in formula-fed babies. It is rare in Western countries because of routine administration of vitamin K to newborns.

Pathogenesis. This bleeding disorder results from a deficiency of the vitamin K–dependent coagulation factors II, VII, IX, and X. The levels of these factors are approximately 50% of normal in umbilical cord blood; the levels decline rapidly after birth, hitting their lowest at 48 to 72 hours. In a small number of infants, the decline is so significant that severe bleeding results. After 72 hours, the levels of these coagulation factors gradually increase over the course of several weeks. This increase is primarily due to absorption of vitamin K from the diet. The vitamin K content of human milk is very low compared with standard infant formulas, therefore, breast-fed babies need vitamin K supplementation.[24,25]

Hepatic immaturity may also contribute to hemorrhagic disease of the newborn. The liver may be unable to initially produce adequate levels of the vitamin K–dependent coagulation factors.[26]

Clinical Manifestations. Evidence of bleeding, such as melena (tarry, black feces composed of partially digested blood), bleeding from the umbilicus, and hematuria, appears on the second or third day of life. Life-threatening complications include intracranial hemorrhage and hypovolemic shock.

Diagnosis and Treatment. The diagnosis is primarily based on the clinical presentation, particularly the timing of the onset of bleeding. The PT is prolonged; vitamin K–dependent clotting factors are decreased.

Administration of vitamin K prophylactically to the newborn prevents the severe decline of the vitamin K–dependent coagulation factors and largely eliminates this coagulation disorder.

If evidence of hemorrhage is present, vitamin K should be administered. For severe hemorrhage, fresh plasma will replenish the deficient coagulation factors and stop the bleeding. Fresh whole blood will correct severe anemia and shock.

Premature infants may experience bleeding due to platelet abnormalities and a deficiency in several coagulation factors. Because of hepatic immaturity, vitamin K is ineffective therapy in these infants. Fresh plasma is the treatment of choice for the premature infant with bleeding complications.

Acquired Vitamin K Deficiency

Etiology. Acquired vitamin K deficiency may result in bleeding due to a coagulation defect. Vitamin K, a fat-soluble vitamin, is obtained via the diet and intestinal flora. Vitamin K is then absorbed by the intestine and stored in the liver. Normal absorption is dependent on bile acids and adequate mucosal function in the intestine. Vitamin K is necessary for normal synthesis and function of coagulation proteins (factors II, VII, IX, and X) as well as coagulation inhibitors (proteins C and S).

Vitamin K deficiency, with its associated risk for bleeding, may occur with the following: malnutrition, malabsorption (including biliary disease), chronic hepatic disease, antibiotic therapy, and oral anticoagulation therapy.

Pathogenesis. One of the many functions of the liver is the synthesis and transport of bile, which is necessary for fat digestion and normal absorption in the small intestine. Vitamin K is a fat-soluble vitamin; if fat malabsorption occurs due to a lack of bile, vitamin K is not absorbed, resulting in a vitamin K deficiency. In the newborn, especially the premature infant, vitamin K deficiency may be related to liver immaturity and the lack of vitamin K synthesis by the intestine until the gut is colonized with the flora that produce vitamin K. Coumadin-type drugs are vitamin K antagonists that inhibit the normal activity of vitamin K in the synthesis of clotting factors. The net effect is decreased clotting factor activity.

Although vitamin K is deficient, the liver continues to synthesize the vitamin K–dependent coagulation factors. However, the coagulation activity of these factors is impaired, resulting in bleeding.

Clinical Manifestations. Evidence of bleeding may present in a variety of ways, including mucosal and gastrointestinal bleeding, ecchymoses, menorrhagia, and hematuria. Surgical bleeding may be a significant problem in the patient with a vitamin K deficiency.

Diagnosis and Treatment. Vitamin K deficiency should be considered as the cause for bleeding when the PT is increased but other coagulation studies are normal. Of the vitamin K–dependent clotting factors, factor VII (extrinsic pathway) has the shortest half-life; thus, the PT is prolonged first. Ultimately, the aPTT will also be prolonged as clotting factors in the intrinsic pathway become deficient.

Parenteral administration of vitamin K rapidly restores levels in the liver with normal production of coagulation factors in 8 to 16 hours.[26] Fresh frozen plasma, with an immediate supply of clotting factors, is the treatment of choice for severe hemorrhage. Correction or removal of the cause of vitamin K deficiency is also an important part of therapy.

Disseminated Intravascular Coagulation

Etiology. Disseminated intravascular coagulation (DIC) is an acquired hemorrhagic syndrome in which both clotting and bleeding occur simultaneously (Figure 14-10). This syndrome is also known as "disseminated intravascular coagulopathy" or "disseminated intravascular consumption" in some references. Widespread clotting in small vessels leads to consumption of the clotting factors and platelets, which in turn leads to bleeding. DIC is either chronic or acute. The chronic form is seen mainly in the cancer patient with malignancy and presents in a less severe form with bleeding tendencies that are mild to moderate and thrombotic episodes.[26-28] The liver and bone marrow have sufficient time to replenish consumed factors and platelets, which leads to a more thrombotic problem.[6] Acute DIC occurs secondary to a variety of factors, including malignancy, sepsis, snake bite, abruptio placentae, trauma and crushing injuries, transfusions of incompatible blood, burns, shock, and severe liver disease.[2,3,27] DIC is estimated to occur in 1 of every 900 to 2400 adult admissions in large, urban hospitals. Mortality rates are reported to range from 50% to 80%.

Pathogenesis. DIC represents a paradox of both thrombosis and hemorrhage. Accelerated intravascular clotting in small vessels is initiated by contact of the blood with damaged vascular endothelium (sepsis, burns), release of procoagulant substances into the blood (snake venom, malignancy), generation of procoagulants in the blood (incompatible blood transfusion), or stagnant blood flow (shock). Coagulation factors, especially prothrombin, platelets, factor V, and factor VIII, are rapidly consumed. At the same time, the fibrinolytic system is activated to break down the clots. The fibrin degradation products or fibrin split products that result act as circulating anticoagulants. The combination of coagulation, anticoagulation, and fibrinolysis ultimately leads to hemorrhage.[6,27]

Clinical Manifestations. Although both bleeding and clotting are part of the syndrome, initially bleeding is more apparent clinically. Petechiae and ecchymoses on skin and

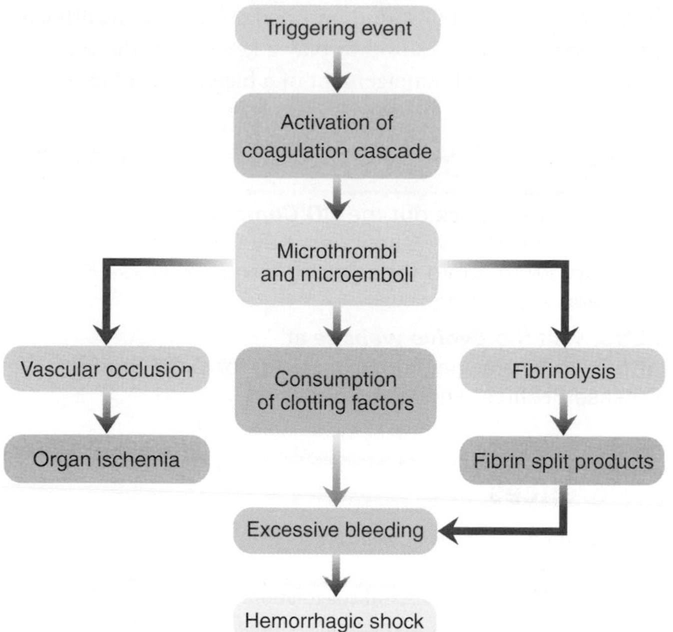

FIGURE 14-10 ■ Pathophysiology of disseminated intravascular coagulation. Clotting and bleeding occur simultaneously, resulting in organ ischemia and hemorrhagic shock.

mucous membranes, as well as bleeding from orifices and any site of injury, such as venipuncture and injection sites, may be present. Acrocyanosis (cold, mottled fingers and toes) may be apparent due to thrombi formation in the microvasculature of the extremities. Thrombi in the pulmonary microcirculation (small vessels) may result in dyspnea, hemoptysis, and crackles or rales, as blood fills alveoli. Patients with DIC are also predisposed to acute renal failure due to the presence of microthrombi in the renal microvasculature.

Diagnosis and Treatment. The diagnosis of DIC is based on a high index of suspicion drawn from the history and presenting signs and symptoms. The typical clinical picture described above, plus the presence of a predisposing cause, should make DIC a consideration. Abnormal coagulation studies that help confirm the diagnosis include increases in the bleeding time, PT, aPTT, fibrin split products, and thrombin time; the fibrinogen level and platelet count are decreased. D-Dimer is one of the most useful tests to measure fibrinolysis; this in conjunction with an elevated antithrombin complex is indicative of DIC.[26-28]

The cornerstone of treatment for DIC is removal or correction of the underlying cause and support of major organ systems. Replacement of depleted clotting factors with fresh frozen plasma, packed red blood cells, platelets, or cryoprecipitate may be necessary. Antifibrinolytics (ϵ-aminocaproic acid) may be used if there is life-threatening hemorrhage.[26] Although controversial, heparin may be utilized to minimize further consumption of clotting factors. The purpose of heparin therapy is to stop thrombin formation, thus preventing microemboli. Low-dose subcutaneous heparin appears to be as effective as high-dose heparin with fewer complications. Heparin has been found useful in chronic DIC.[27,28]

Hepatic Disease

Etiology. A common complication of many hepatic disorders is abnormal hemostasis. With the exception of part of the antihemophilic factor, all plasma protein clotting factors, fibrinolytic factors, and their inhibitors are synthesized totally or predominantly by the liver.[2,3,26] If liver function is altered by disease, bleeding is one manifestation.

Pathogenesis. Several factors may contribute to the abnormal hemostasis seen in liver disease. Liver disease alters the synthesis and transport of bile, which is necessary for normal fat digestion and absorption. Impaired absorption and metabolism of vitamin K, which is fat soluble, result in decreased hepatic synthesis of coagulation factors II, VII, IX, and X. Altered liver function also results in decreased synthesis of fibrinogen and factors V and XI.[26] A deficiency in any of the coagulation factors can interrupt the normal process of fibrin clot formation. In addition to synthesis of coagulation factors, the liver also has a role in removing activated coagulation proteins and activated fibrinolytic proteins from the circulation. Failure to adequately filter these proteins may result in an imbalance between clot formation and clot dissolution (fibrinolysis), manifesting clinically as DIC.[26,27] Liver disease may also alter normal production of inhibitors of coagulation (antithrombin III, proteins C and S), which contributes to the hypercoagulable component of DIC.[26]

Another factor contributing to the bleeding associated with liver disease is thrombocytopenia. A low platelet count is common in liver disease. The exact mechanism is unknown but may relate to splenomegaly associated with portal hypertension.[26] Sequestration of platelets in the enlarged spleen depletes the number circulating and available for normal hemostasis. The portal hypertension that develops as blood flow through the liver is retarded adds to the bleeding problem. As pressure in collateral circulatory beds increases, bleeding is manifested as esophageal varices and hemorrhoids (see Chapter 38).

Clinical Manifestations. Patients with chronic, rather than acute, liver disease are more likely to have clinical evidence of a bleeding problem. Typical clinical features may include any of the following: petechiae, ecchymoses, spider telangiectasia, bleeding from venipuncture sites or esophageal varices, and gastrointestinal bleeding. DIC may complicate the clinical presentation. Bleeding may not be a problem until the patient has surgery or a biopsy.

Diagnosis and Treatment. The patient with liver disease and associated bleeding will commonly have a decreased platelet count, normal or decreased fibrinogen levels, and prolonged PT and aPTT. More specific coagulation studies may be indicated in some situations.

Treatment may be instituted prophylactically prior to surgery or biopsy or it may be mandated by a bleeding episode. The degree of abnormality on coagulation tests or the severity of the bleeding will influence the aggressiveness of therapy. Because of the high likelihood of vitamin K deficiency, administration of vitamin K may be the initial intervention. Platelet infusions are appropriate if significant thrombocytopenia is present. Fresh frozen plasma is the primary replacement product utilized to supply coagulation factors. Administration of large quantities of plasma carries the risk of precipitating hepatic encephalopathy and fluid overload. Transfusions of whole blood or, more commonly, packed red blood cells may be necessary to manage bleeding of significant proportions.

KEY CONCEPTS

- Coagulation disorders result from defects in the clotting cascade or fibrinolytic process. These disorders may be inherited or acquired.
- Hemophilia is an inherited bleeding disorder that results from deficient clotting factor production. The most common types are hemophilia A (factor VIII) and hemophilia B (factor IX).
- Von Willebrand disease is an inherited bleeding disorder caused by abnormal factor VIII carrier protein production. The disease results in a deficiency of factor VIII in the circulation and decreased platelet function.
- Vitamin K deficiency is associated with several coagulation disorders, including hemorrhagic disease of the newborn and bleeding related to malnutrition and liver disease. Vitamin K is a necessary cofactor for liver production of factors II, VII, IX, and X.
- Disseminated intravascular coagulation (DIC) is an acquired bleeding syndrome associated with a number of etiologic factors, including trauma, malignancy, burns, shock, and abruptio placentae. DIC is characterized by widespread clot formation in small vessels. Clotting factors and platelets are consumed, leaving the patient with deficient resources for appropriate clot formation. The platelet count and fibrinogen levels are typically decreased, and PT, aPTT, thrombin time, bleeding time, and fibrin split products are elevated.

SUMMARY

The presence of unexpected overt or covert bleeding may signal an acquired or inherited problem with hemostasis. A review of normal hemostasis, as well as information on selected disorders of hemostasis and coagulation, has been presented in this chapter. With a sound knowledge base, the health care professional is in a position to play a key role in the recognition, diagnosis, and management of a bleeding problem.

MEDIA RESOURCES

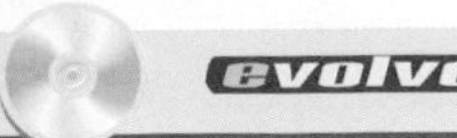

Remember to check out the ***CD Companion*** included with this book for Review Questions, Key Concepts Review, Glossary (with audio for selected terms), Disease Profiles, and Animations.

PLUS, visit the ***Evolve website*** at http://evolve.elsevier.com/Copstead/ for Case Studies, Disease Profiles, and WebLinks.

References

1. Guyton A: *Textbook of medical physiology,* ed 10, Philadelphia, 2000, Saunders.
2. Lea H: Hematopoiesis and coagulation. In Woods S et al, editors: *Cardiac nursing,* ed 4, Philadelphia, 2000, Lippincott Williams & Wilkins.
3. Handin R: Bleeding and thrombosis: disorders of coagulation and thrombosis. In Wilson J et al, editors: *Harrison's principles of internal medicine,* ed 15, New York, 2001, McGraw-Hill.
4. Triplett D: Coagulation and bleeding disorders: review and update, *Clin Chem B* 46(8):1260-1269, 2000.
5. Fuster V et al, editors: *Hurst's the heart,* ed 10, New York, 2001, McGraw-Hill.
6. George J: Platelets, *Lancet* 355:1531-1539, 2000.
7. Tizard E: Henoch-Schönlein purpura, *Arch Dis Child* 80:380-388, 1999.
8. Nunnelee J: Henoch-Schönlein purpura: a review of the literature, *Clin Exc Nurse Pract* 4(2),72-75, 2000.
9. Whilelaw S: Ehlers-Danlos syndrome, classical type case management, *Pediatr Nurs* 29(6):423-426, 2003.
10. Mao J: The Ehlers-Danlos syndrome: on beyond collagens, *J Clin Invest* 107(9):1063-1069, 2001.
11. Schneiderman P: Vascular purpuras. In Beutler E et al, editors: *Williams hematology,* ed 6, New York, 2001, McGraw-Hill.
12. Azuma H: Genetic and molecular pathogenesis of hereditary hemorrhagic telangiectasis, *J Med Invest* 47(3-4): 81-90, 2000.
13. George J: Thrombocytopenia. In Beutler E et al, editors: *Williams hematology,* ed 6, New York, 2001, McGraw-Hill.
14. Stasi R: Management of immune thrombocytopenic purpura in adults, *Mayo Clin Proc* 79(4):504-522, 2004.
15. Doyle B: Thrombocytopenia, *AACN Clin Issues* 8(3):469-480, 1997.
16. Drews R: Thrombocytopenic disorders in critically ill patients, *Am J Respir Crit Care Med* 162:347-351, 2000.
17. Rock G: Therapeutic plasmapheresis, *Curr Opin Hematol* 3(6):504-510, 1996.
18. Sherry K: Plasmapheresis in the intensive care unit. I. Technical considerations, *Care Crit Ill* 14(5):176-179, 1998.
19. Bolton-Maggs P: Haemophilias A and B, *Lancet* 361(9371):1801-1809, 2003.
20. Britton B: About hemophilia, *Nursing* 33(12):78, 2003.
21. Greer F: Vitamin K deficiency and hemorrhage in infancy, *Clin Perinatol* 22(3):759-777, 1995.

22. DiPaola J: Current therapy for rare factor deficiencies, *Haemophilia* 7(1):16-22, 2001.
23. Paper R: Can you recognize and respond to von Willebrand disease? *Nursing* 33:54-56, 2003.
24. Kumor D: Vitamin K status of premature infants: implications for current recommendations, *Pediatrics* 108(5):1117-1124, 2001.
25. Puckett R: Prophylactic vitamin K for vitamin K deficiency bleeding in neonates, *Cochrane Database Sys Rev* 4:CD002776, 2000.
26. Gralink H: Acquired disorders of coagulation. In Kelley W, editor: *Textbook of internal medicine,* ed 3, Philadelphia, 2001, Lippincott-Raven Publishers.
27. Geiter H: Disseminated intravascular coagulopathy, *Dimens Crit Care Nurs* 22(3):108-116, 2003.
28. Dressler D: DIC: coping with a coagulation crisis, *Nursing* 34(5):58-62, 2004.

chapter 15

Alterations in Blood Flow

Naomi Lungstrom • Roberta J. Emerson

MEDIA RESOURCES

Additional Material for Study, Review, and Further Exploration

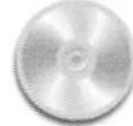

CD Companion ◆ Review Questions and Answers ◆ Key Concepts Review ◆ Glossary *(with audio pronunciations for selected terms)* ◆ Disease Profiles ◆ Animations

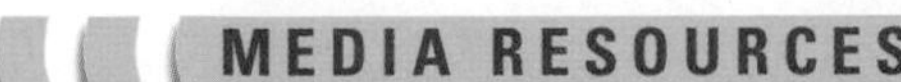

Website at http://evolve.elsevier.com/Copstead/ ◆ Case Studies ◆ Disease Profiles ◆ WebLinks

KEY QUESTIONS

- How do the structures of arteries, veins, capillaries, and lymphatics differ, reflecting the functions of each?
- What is the relationship among vessel resistance, blood pressure, and blood flow?
- How is resistance regulated centrally by the autonomic nervous system and locally by tissue?
- What are the determinants of transcapillary exchange of fluids, electrolytes, and nutrients?
- How do arterial and venous obstructions develop?
- What are the clinical consequences of acute and chronic arterial obstruction?
- What are the clinical consequences of superficial and deep venous obstructions?

CHAPTER OUTLINE

The primary functions of the circulatory system are the transportation of oxygen and nutrients and the removal of metabolic waste products within the body. To perform these functions, a complex circuitry of vessels traverses the body (Figure 15-1), powered by the pumping action of the heart. Movement of blood through the lungs is provided by the right side of the heart. Systemic blood flow is supplied by the left side of the heart.

Nutrients are absorbed into the blood as it moves through the gastrointestinal tract via the splanchnic circulation. Oxygen uptake and the release of carbon dioxide occur in the specialized vascular bed of the pulmonary circulation. The liver, with its extensive blood supply, has a major role in metabolism and generation of metabolic waste products. These, and other metabolic byproducts, are carried by the blood to the kidneys for elimination. Inadequate circulation in the lungs, liver, or kidneys may interfere with the removal of metabolic wastes from the body. Effective transportation of oxygen and nutrients and the removal of waste materials depend on proper functioning of the circulatory system.

Aging produces significant changes in the circulatory system, altering the ability of the system to carry out its functions and increasing susceptibility to certain disease processes. The effects of the aging process on the circulatory system are summarized in The Aging Process: Changes in the Circulatory System.

ORGANIZATION OF THE CIRCULATORY AND LYMPHATIC SYSTEMS

After passing through the pulmonary circulatory system and leaving the left side of the heart, blood flows through a graduated series of tubes to all cells of the body before returning to the right side of the heart. The powerful left ventricle propels the blood to the aorta, arteries, arterioles, and, finally, to the capillary beds. Here the proximity of capillary endothelium to

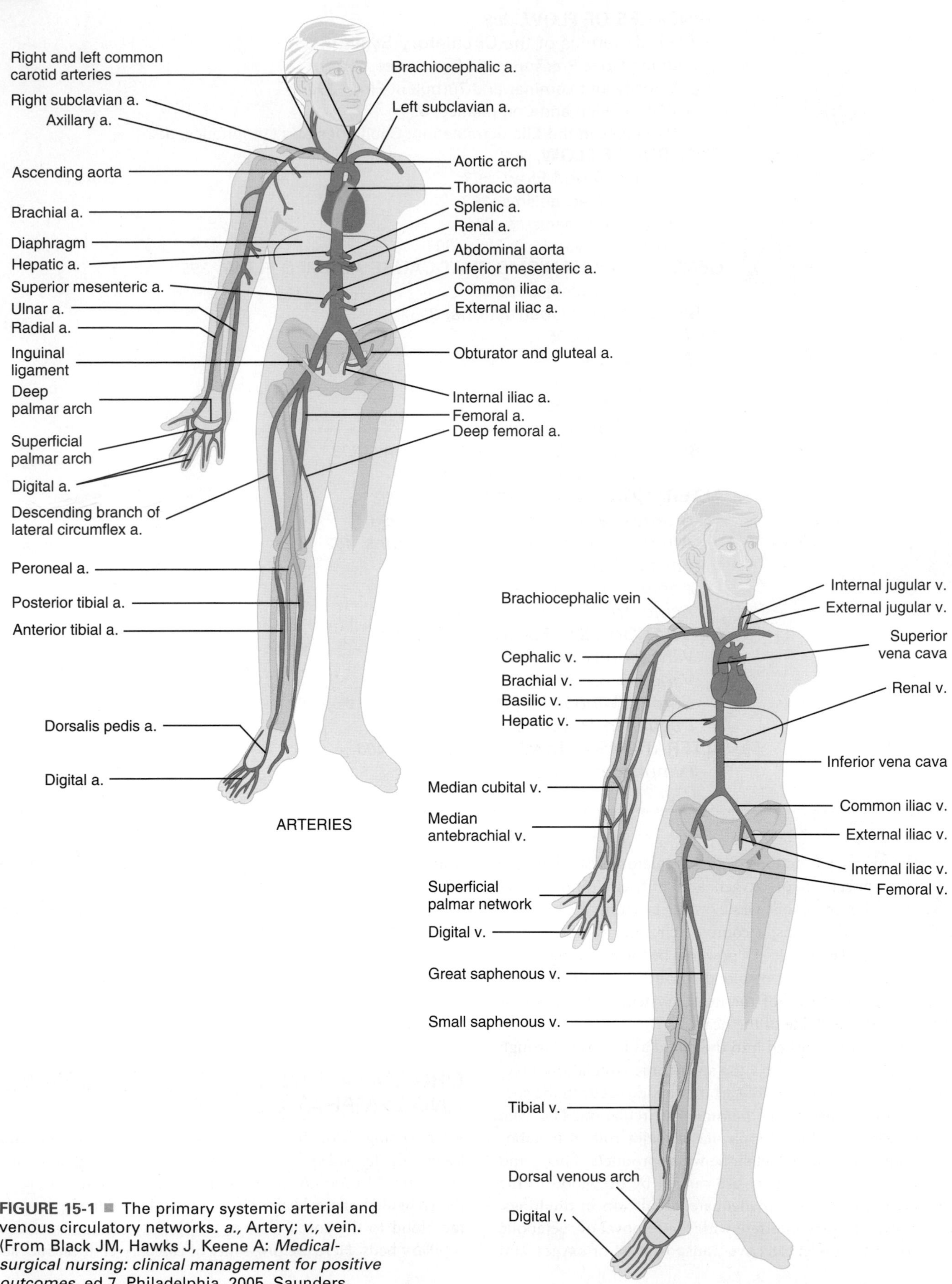

FIGURE 15-1 ■ The primary systemic arterial and venous circulatory networks. *a.,* Artery; *v.,* vein. (From Black JM, Hawks J, Keene A: *Medical-surgical nursing: clinical management for positive outcomes,* ed 7, Philadelphia, 2005, Saunders, p 1469.)

THE AGING PROCESS

Changes in the Circulatory System

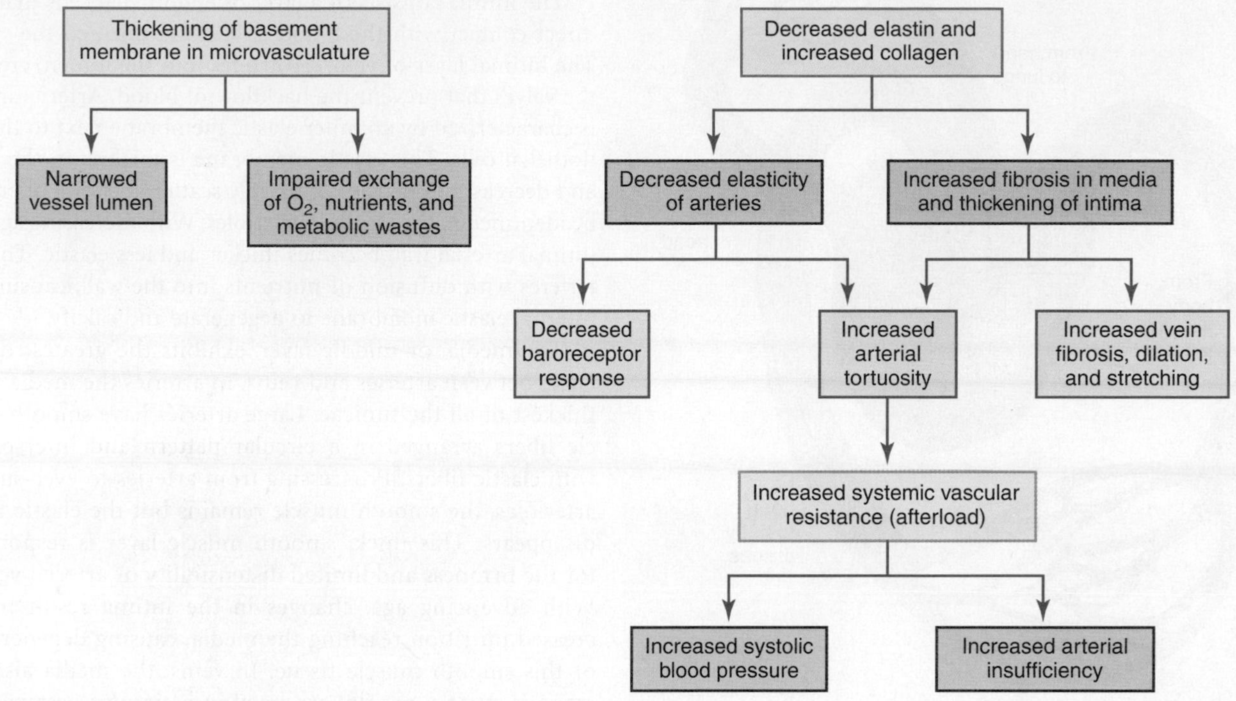

In the aging individual, changes occur throughout the vascular bed. The microvascular bed demonstrates thickening of the basement membrane. This change narrows the vessel lumen and impairs the free exchange of oxygen, nutrients, and metabolic wastes at the cellular level.

In both arteries and veins, the vascular changes occur first in the proximal portions. The intima becomes fibrotic and the endothelial cell variation increases. In the media, the amount of elastin and smooth muscle is reduced, whereas the amount of fibrotic and collagen tissue increases. With collagen cross-linking, the vessel walls lose elastic flexibility and recoil, becoming more stiff and less compliant. They become inflexible tubes with an increase in systemic vascular resistance (SVR). The increased SVR causes a reduction in tissue and organ blood flow and decreased perfusion.

Baroreceptor function is reduced because of decreased sensitivity of the receptors and diminished responsiveness of the vessels due to their rigidity. These factors decrease the body's ability to respond to hypotensive and hypertensive stimuli. The decreased compliance of the systemic vascular system increases afterload, forcing the left ventricle of the heart to work harder to meet the metabolic demands of the body.

the other cells of the body facilitates movement of nutrients and oxygen into the cells and removal of cellular metabolic wastes. Capillary blood is then collected by venules, which flow into veins, returning blood to the vena cava and the right side of the heart (Figure 15-2). The complete process, moving 5 L of blood through the entire circuit, takes only about a minute.

The lymphatic system is a specialized scheme of channels and tissues (nodes). It is not arranged in a circuit, as is the circulatory system. Instead, the lymphatic vessels begin blindly, deep in the connective tissue. One of the functions of the lymphatic system is to reabsorb fluid that leaks out of the vascular network into the interstitium and return it to the general circulation. During the process of exchange that occurs at a cellular level within the capillary bed, some fluid moves into the interstitium and fails to return to the vascular bed. This lost fluid can amount to as much as 2 to 4 L/day. At this circulatory level, lymphatic vessels lie in close proximity to the capillary vasculature. The fluid, called *lymph* at this point, is absorbed by the lymphatics and returned to the venous circulation by way of the thoracic duct and the right lymphatic duct (Figure 15-3).

Vessel Structure

To carry out their specialized functions, the circulatory vessels and lymphatic vessels are markedly different structurally. Knowledge of the morphology of these vessels enhances an

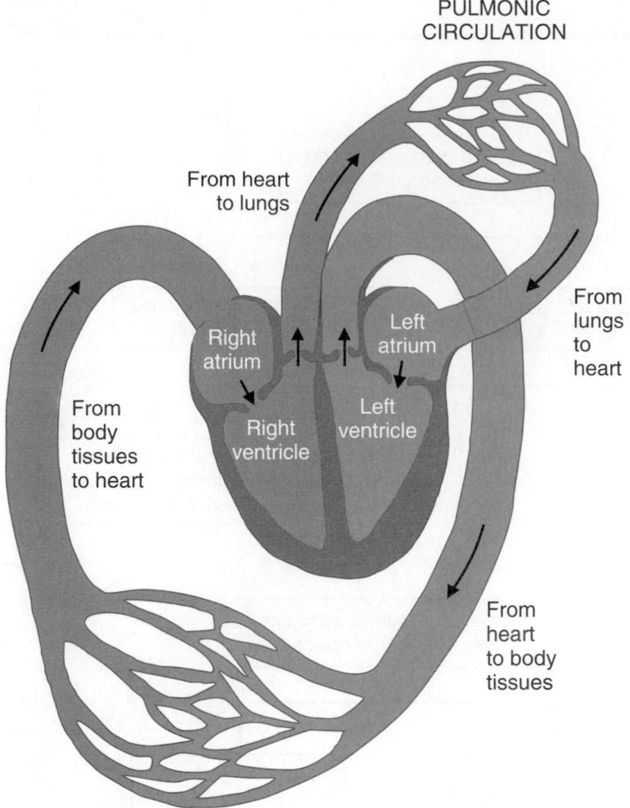

FIGURE 15-2 ■ The circulatory system. Beginning from the body tissues, blood returns to the right side of the heart, through the right atria to the right ventricle, which propels it into the lungs. In the lungs, the metabolic waste carbon dioxide is removed and oxygen is replenished. Oxygenated blood leaves the pulmonic circulation and returns to the heart via the left atrium to the left ventricle. From the left side of the heart, the oxygenated blood enters the systemic circulation, where oxygen is delivered to the tissues in exchange for metabolic wastes. (From Black JM, Hawks J, Keene A: *Medical-surgical nursing: clinical management for positive outcomes,* ed 7, Philadelphia, 2005, Saunders, p 1549.)

understanding of the alterations in function produced by disease.

Structurally, arteries, capillaries, and veins have significant variation. The primary differences between the smaller arterial and venous vessels occur in the quantities of muscle and connective tissue present. In arterioles, the principal tissue is muscle, whereas in venules, muscle is scarce and connective tissue predominates. The composition of the walls and the size and shape of the vessels vary in larger arteries and veins. Capillary walls are composed of a single layer of endothelial cells. These extremely simple structures carry out extraordinarily complex functions.

Anatomy of Arteries and Veins

The walls of both arteries and veins are composed of three microscopically distinct layers, or tunicae: the intima, the media, and the adventitia. The histologic components of these coats are similar in arteries and veins (Figure 15-4). Generally, the walls of veins are not as thick as the walls of arteries, but the lumina are larger.

The intima consists of a layer of endothelial cells that is in direct contact with the blood as it flows through the vessel. The intimal layer of veins protrudes into the lumen, creating the valves that prevent the backflow of blood. Arterial intima is characterized by an inner elastic membrane next to the endothelial cells. This elastic membrane is thickest in the aorta and decreases in density until only scattered elastic fibers can be identified in the smallest arterioles. With increasing age, the intimal arterial wall becomes thicker and less elastic. This interferes with diffusion of nutrients into the wall, causing the internal elastic membrane to degenerate and calcify.

The media, or middle layer, exhibits the greatest differences between arteries and veins. In arteries the media is the thickest of all the tunicae. Large arteries have smooth muscle fibers arranged in a circular pattern and interspersed with elastic fibers. Progressing from arteries to ever-smaller arterioles, the smooth muscle remains but the elastic tissue disappears. This thick, smooth muscle layer is responsible for the firmness and limited distensibility of arterial vessels. With advancing age, changes in the intima result in decreased nutrition reaching the media, causing degeneration of this smooth muscle tissue. In veins, the media also has smooth muscle, usually arranged in a circular pattern with some longitudinal strands. The quantity of smooth muscle decreases as the veins become larger. Venous media also contains collagenous connective tissue, but elastic tissue is rare except in the largest veins.

In veins, the adventitia is the thickest of the tunicae. It is composed of collagenous connective tissue and longitudinal smooth muscle. In larger arteries there is a discernible external elastic membrane in the adventitia. This membrane is eliminated as the arteries become smaller. Arterial adventitia consists predominantly of collagenous connective tissue. Some larger vessels also contain isolated, longitudinally arranged fibers of smooth muscle.

Anatomy of Capillaries

Capillaries are composed of a single thickness of endothelium. Moving from the end of an arteriole to the beginning of a venule, capillaries narrow to a diameter barely sufficient for a single red blood cell (RBC) to pass through. In some tissues, one or two smooth muscle cells form a precapillary sphincter that controls flow through the vessel (Figure 15-5).

There are spaces between the endothelial cells that vary in size from organ system to organ system. These spaces, or pores, permit certain constituents to pass in and out of the capillaries. For example, capillary beds in the brain have very small spaces and permit only certain very small molecules to pass through. The space between endothelial cells of the brain is so small that it is referred to as the *blood-brain barrier.* In parts of the kidneys, however, capillaries are more porous, al-

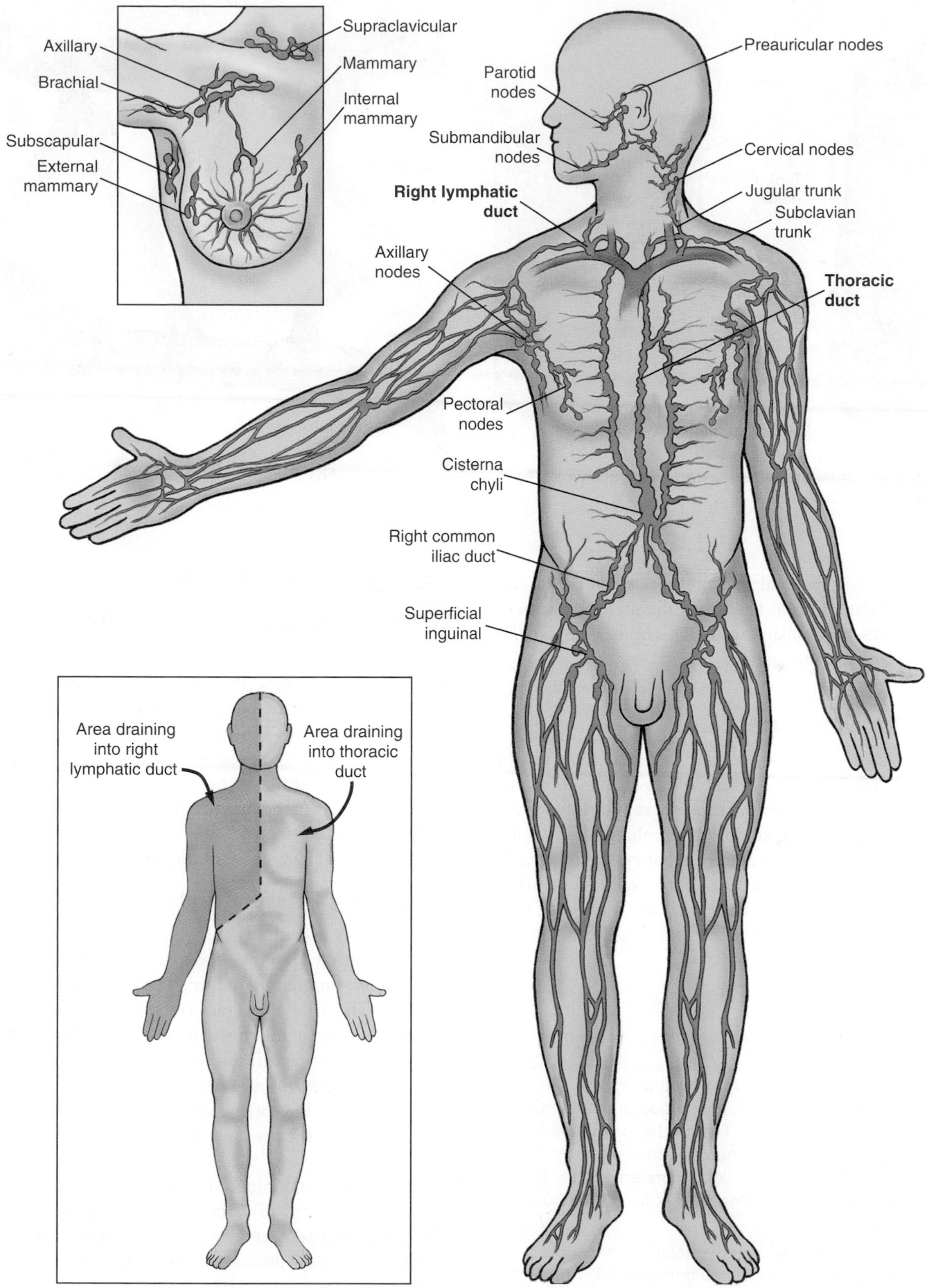

FIGURE 15-3 ■ Simplified scheme of lymphatic anatomy. The lymphatic capillaries collect vascular capillary excess fluid and return it to the venous circulation. (From Monahan FD, Neighbors M: *Medical surgical nursing: foundations for clinical practice,* ed 2, Philadelphia, 1998, Saunders, p 330.)

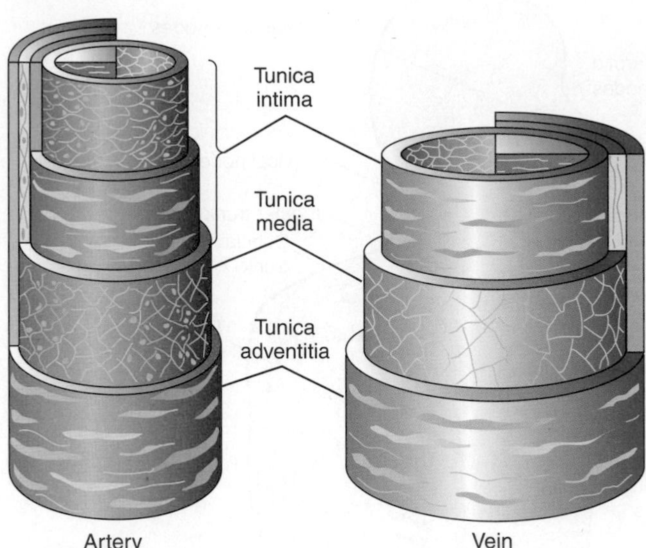

FIGURE 15-4 ■ Tunicae of arteries and veins showing the thicker walls of the arteries.

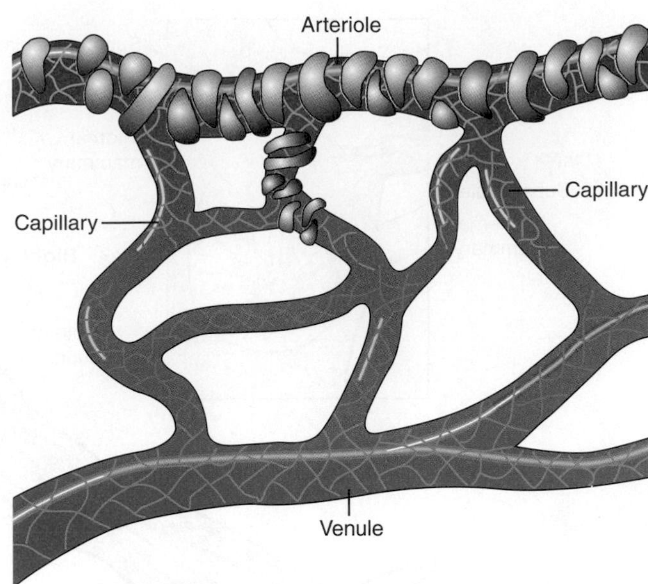

FIGURE 15-5 ■ Capillary network.

lowing much larger molecules to move between the circulation and the filtrate (urine). The size of the spaces between the endothelial cells of capillary walls determines the *capillary permeability* of a specific capillary bed.

Lymphatic Structure

Lymphatic vessels are thin walled and resemble most veins in their appearance. Like their counterparts in the circulatory system, they range in size from lymphatic capillaries to vessels of increasing diameter. Like veins, lymphatics have valves composed of folds of their inner layer that extend into the lumen of the channels (Figure 15-6). The walls of lymphatic capillaries contain contractile fibers that are stimulated when stretched, causing the vessels to contract and propel lymph along the vessel.

KEY CONCEPTS

- Arteries and veins have three distinct layers. The intima, the innermost layer, is composed of a single layer of endothelial cells. The media, or middle layer, is composed of smooth muscle and elastin. Media is thicker in arteries than in veins. The adventitia, the outermost layer, is composed of supporting connective tissue.
- Capillaries have only a single layer of endothelial cells. The permeability of capillaries is determined by how tightly the endothelial cells join together.
- Lymphatic vessels resemble veins, having thin walls and valves.

PRINCIPLES OF FLOW

Hemodynamics of the Circulatory System

The principles of blood flow are known as circulatory **hemodynamics.** These principles govern the quantity of blood passing by a given point in a specific period of time. Therefore, blood flow may be recorded as a given number of liters, milliliters, or cubic centimeters per second, minute, or hour. A discussion of the hemodynamics of the circulatory system includes the concepts of pressure, resistance, velocity, laminar and turbulent flows, wall tension, and compliance.

Blood Flow, Pressure, and Resistance

Blood flow is accomplished by movement along a pressure gradient within the vascular bed. This means that blood moves from an area of higher pressure to an area of lower pressure. The arterial and arteriolar walls with their muscular media coat provide the high-pressure end of the gradient. Seeking a lower pressure, blood moves toward the venous system. The thinner, more pliable walls of the venous vascular bed furnish the low-pressure portion of the pressure gradient. The greater the pressure difference, the greater the blood flow.

The movement of blood through the vascular system is opposed by the force of *resistance.* The relationship between blood flow and resistance is an inverse one: as resistance increases, blood flow decreases. This force has several determinants, each of which can change resistance considerably; these determinants are represented in physiology by *Poiseuille law:*

$$\text{Resistance} = \frac{8nl}{\pi r^4}$$

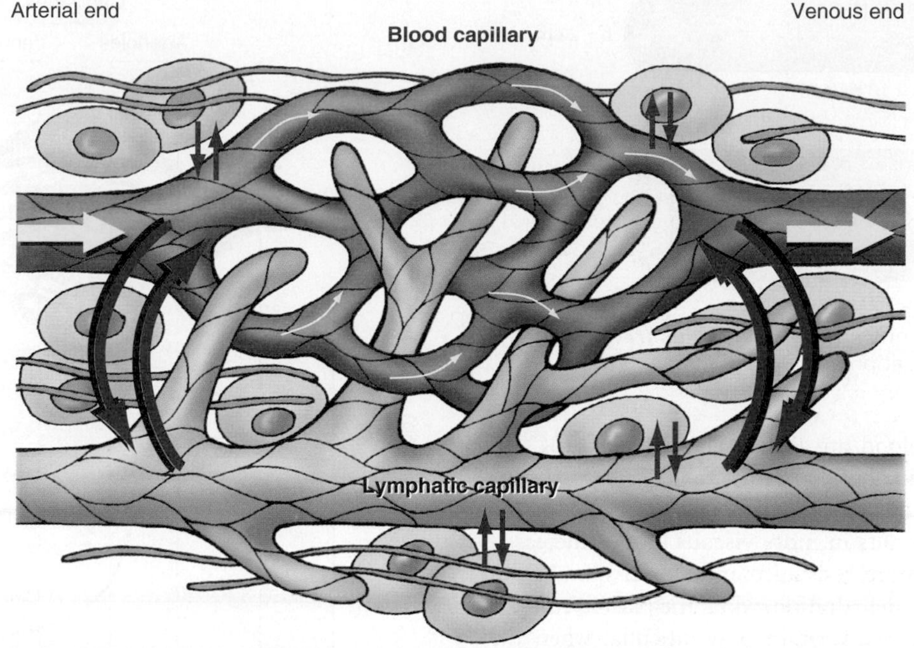

FIGURE 15-6 ■ Lymphatic network. The lymphatic system is integrally related to the systemic vascular system. Excess fluid and plasma diffuse between the capillaries, interstitial spaces, and lymphatic vessels. Because lymphatic capillaries have larger spaces between endothelial cells, they can remove excess interstitial fluid or plasma that venous capillaries cannot reabsorb.

The number 8 is a mathematical constant, as is the value of π; n represents blood viscosity; l represents the length of a given vessel; and r is the radius of the vessel. Using this formula, effects of changes on the components of resistance are very predictable.

Two of the determinants of resistance are *vessel length* and *vessel radius.* As predicted by Poiseuille law, resistance changes directly with the length of the vessel, and these changes in resistance significantly affect flow. As illustrated in Figure 15-7, given three vessels of the same radius, doubling the length increases the resistance and reduces the flow *(Q)* by 50%. Reducing the vessel length by half decreases resistance and increases the flow by 100%. These changes in flow occur when the pressure gradient remains constant and are due solely to variations in vessel length. Resistance decreases as the radius of a vessel increases. Resistance is inversely related to the fourth power of the vessel's radius, or r^4. Therefore, increasing the radius of the vessel markedly reduces resistance and produces an exponential increase in blood flow. Figure 15-8 demonstrates the effect of doubling the radius of a vessel on the flow of blood if all other factors related to flow are held constant. The resulting flow of blood is 16 times greater in the greater-diameter vessel.

Although there is variability in the length of vessels throughout the circulatory system, vessels are incapable of altering their own length. There is, however, considerable ability to change the diameter of vessel walls in normal physiology, and many disease processes (e.g., arteriosclerosis) and drug therapies (e.g., vasopressors) are associated with changes in the size of the vessel lumen. Even minor changes will produce major alterations in resistance and, hence, blood flow. This makes changes in diameter the most important determinant of resistance.

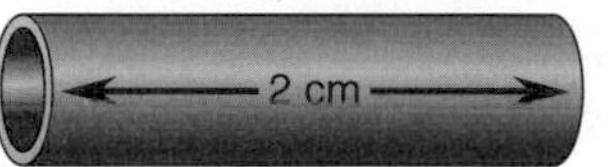

Q = 10 ml/sec

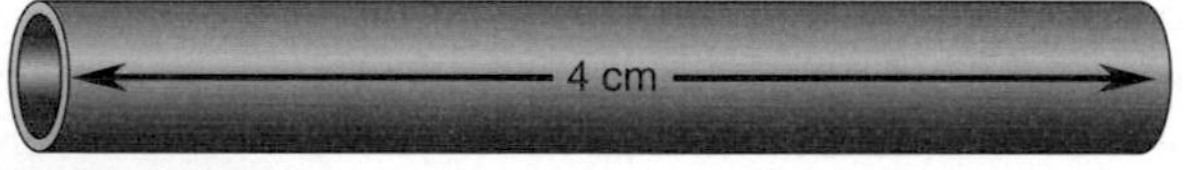

Q = 5 ml/sec

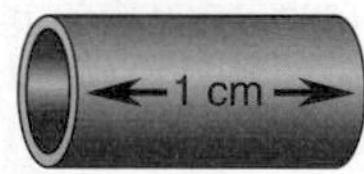

Q = 20 ml/sec

FIGURE 15-7 ■ Relationship of vessel length to blood flow *(Q)* with a constant pressure gradient.

The third determinant of resistance is the *viscosity* of the blood itself, represented in Poiseuille law as n. Viscosity denotes the thickness of a fluid. When the blood is more viscous, the friction between the cells and the liquid increases, and resistance to flow increases. Blood is composed of a suspension of cellular material and plasma. Roughly 99% of the cellular

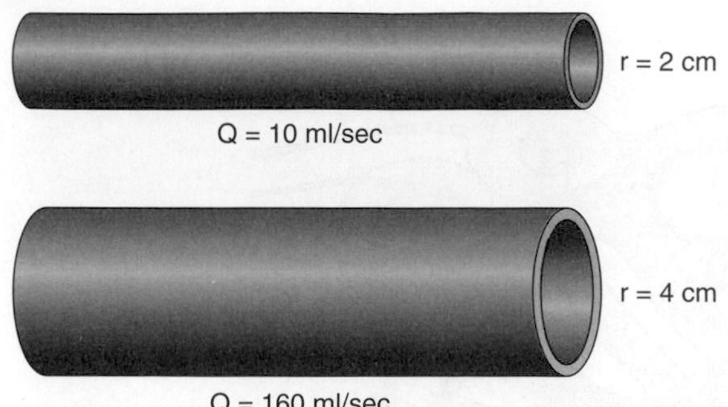

FIGURE 15-8 ■ Relationship of vessel radius *(r)* to blood flow *(Q)* with a constant pressure gradient.

constituents of the blood are RBCs. The ratio of RBCs to plasma is presented in the laboratory value *hematocrit.* Increasing the relative concentration of RBCs or decreasing the plasma component results in more viscous blood (increased hematocrit); hence, more resistance and slower blood flow. This is what occurs in dehydration, when the plasma component is relatively decreased, or in polycythemia, when the number of RBCs increases.

The relationship between the variables of driving pressure and resistance and their effect on blood flow is expressed by *Ohm's law,* as follows:

$$Q = P/R$$

where Q is the blood flow, P is the pressure difference between two points, and R is resistance. Altering any one of the determinants of resistance (vessel length, vessel radius, blood viscosity) produces a change in flow. Likewise, a change in the pressure difference within the circulatory system results in a change in the flow of blood. The arterioles are the major site of resistance in the vascular system and require a greater pressure to maintain blood flow. As the resistance decreases across the systemic vasculature, less pressure is necessary to maintain blood flow (Figure 15-9).

Total peripheral resistance refers to the resistance throughout the entire vascular system. It can be calculated on the basis of the pressure difference between the arteries and the veins. Clinically, *systemic vascular resistance* (SVR) is used to denote resistance peripheral to the heart and lungs. Because the primary determinant of SVR is the resistance vessels, or the arterioles, diseases and drug therapies that affect these vessels have the most profound impact on the SVR. Any condition that produces an increase in SVR, such as hypertension, requires more work for the heart to overcome the elevated resistance and eject its volume of blood (see Chapter 16). This increased workload means that the heart needs more oxygen and nutrients. When SVR is pathologically decreased, the blood is spread over a larger surface area and blood flow slows dramatically. Individual organs, such as the kidney and brain, may not obtain sufficient blood flow to meet metabolic needs. This is what occurs in distributive shock states (see Chapter 20).

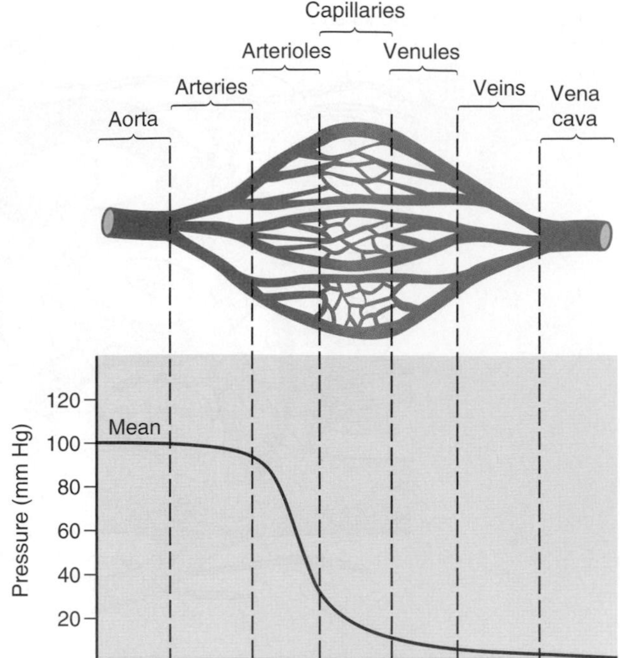

FIGURE 15-9 ■ Mean pressure changes within the systemic vasculature. A significant decrease in pressure occurs as blood flows through the arterioles into the capillaries. The figure illustrates the role of the arterioles in the determination of vascular resistance. Because of the large number of capillaries, total resistance is not increased with the decreased radius of the capillaries.

Velocity and Laminar and Turbulent Flow

As previously discussed, blood flow is defined as the volume of blood that passes a given point in a given unit of time. *Velocity* is a measure of the distance traveled in a given interval of time and is usually expressed in centimeters per second. Velocity is governed by the total cross-sectional area and varies inversely with it. An increase in the total cross-sectional area produces a decrease in velocity, whereas a decrease in the total cross-sectional area produces an increase in velocity. The total cross-sectional area of the aorta and vena cava is small, and they have the most rapid rate of flow, whereas the capillary beds combine to produce the greatest total cross-sectional area and have the slowest flow rate. The dividing and subdividing of vessels within the circulatory system results in greater velocity in the arterial and venous beds than in the capillary bed (Figure 15-10). An understanding of the concept of velocity enhances discussion of laminar and turbulent flow.

When blood flows through a long, smooth-walled vessel, it does so in layers. The velocity of the layers varies, with blood in the center moving much faster than blood in the outer layers. The blood in the center layer moves the most quickly because it is in contact with blood only. The outermost layer is in contact with the vessel wall, which exerts friction against the cellular components of the blood. Many cells stick to the intima. This layer may flow only minimally if at all. Layers of

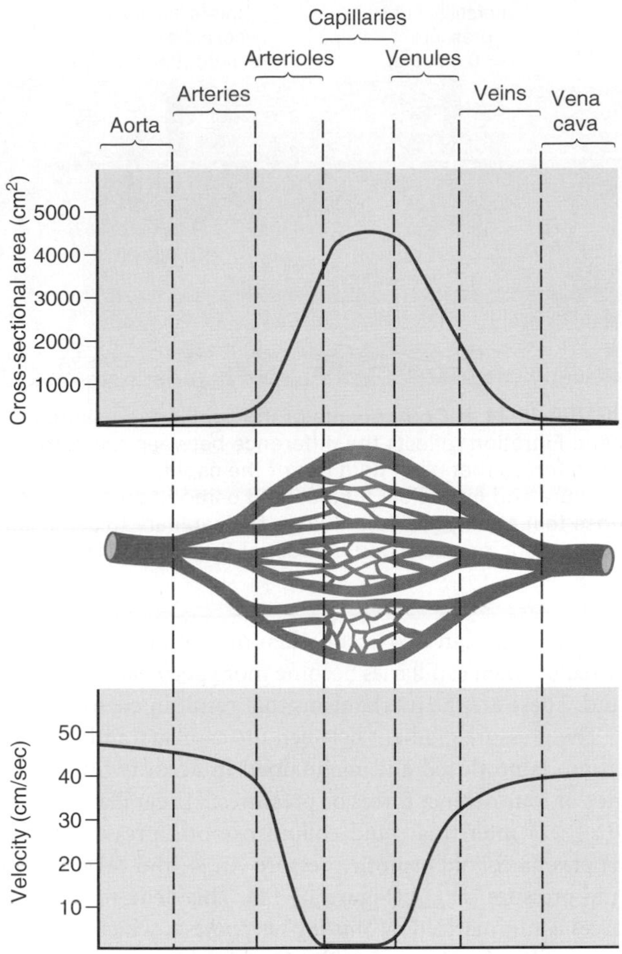

FIGURE 15-10 ■ The effect of increasing cross-sectional area on the velocity of blood flow. Increased cross-sectional area in the capillary bed results in a significant decrease in velocity when compared to the arterial and venous networks.

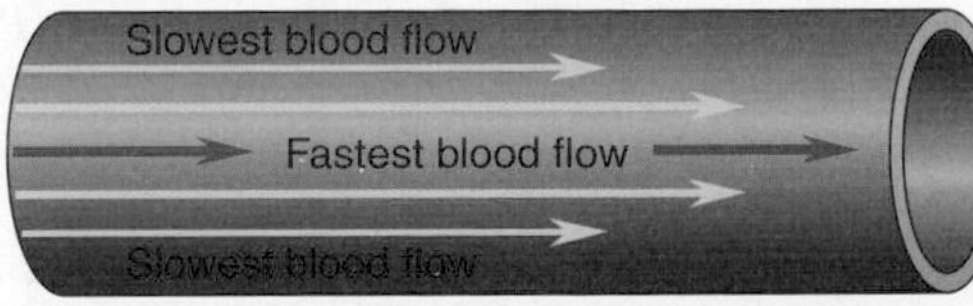

FIGURE 15-11 ■ Parabolic profile of laminar blood flow.

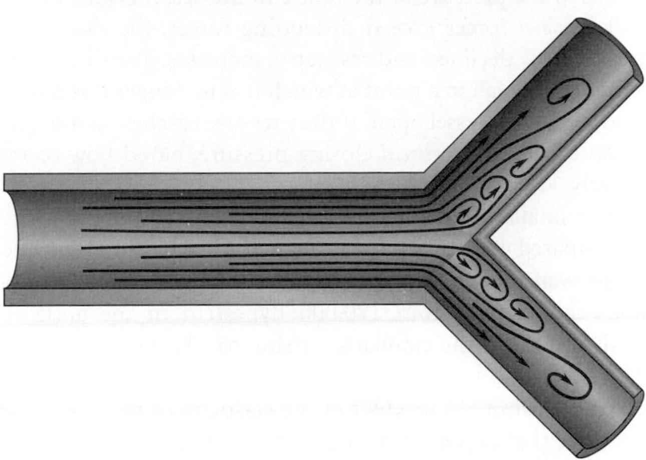

FIGURE 15-12 ■ Turbulent flow generated at a blood vessel bifurcation.

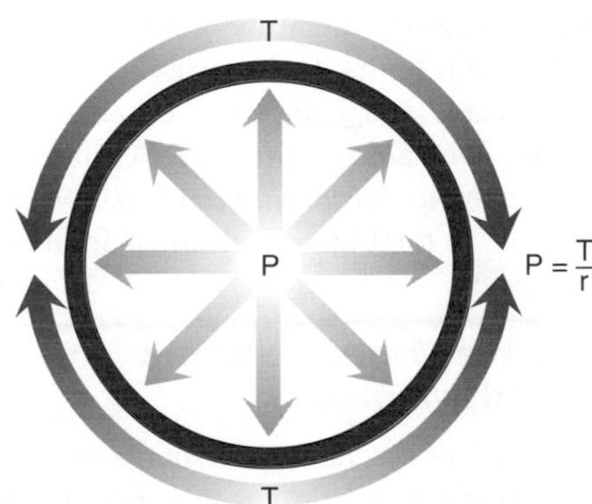

FIGURE 15-13 ■ Law of Laplace as applied to a blood vessel. Distending pressure *(P)* is the difference between the pressures on either side of the vessel and is equal to the wall tension *(T)* divided by the radius of the blood vessel *(r)*.

blood between this outer layer and the central core of blood slide over one another with increasing velocity. This is referred to as the *parabolic profile of laminar flow* and is illustrated in Figure 15-11.

The streamlined nature of laminar flow is disrupted by normal anatomy and by pathologic processes creating turbulent flow. Turbulent flow is an interruption in the forward current of blood flow by crosswise flow (Figure 15-12). The propensity for turbulent flow increases with increasing velocity and increased vessel radius, so that some turbulence can be predicted at the aortic root and in the branches of major arteries. The same process can be seen in a river, where boulders interrupting the flow produce whirlpools and the characteristic roar of rapids. In the human body, turbulent flow through blood vessels can be auscultated as a **bruit.** Sometimes it can be palpated as well, and then it is called a **thrill.** This turbulence may be due to increased velocity, blood moving through branching vessels at a sharp angle, blood flowing around an obstruction in the vessel, or blood flowing over a roughened intimal surface. Turbulent flow alters the parabolic profile seen with laminar flow, slowing velocity around the source of the turbulence. This slowing can cause cellular components of the blood to adhere to one another, to the turbulent focus, and to the intimal wall, promoting the formation of a blood clot (**thrombus**).

Wall Tension and Compliance

The relationship between distending pressure and wall tension is expressed by the *law of Laplace* and is illustrated in Figure 15-13. This physical principle has broad applications in physiology; however, the present discussion focuses on its implications for blood vessels. The distending pressure *(P)* is the transmural pressure, or pressure on one side of the vessel wall minus the pressure on the other side of the blood vessel. It is equal to the wall tension *(T)* divided by the radius of the blood vessel *(r)*. In summary, an increase in radius or distending pressure results in increased wall tension.

When the pressure of the blood in the vessel begins to fall, wall tension forces exceed distending forces, the radius decreases, flow declines, and resistance increases. The distending pressure may fall to a point at which it is no longer possible to hold the blood vessel open. If the pressure reaches 20 mm Hg, a point called the *critical* closing pressure, blood flow ceases entirely.

The smaller the radius of the blood vessel, as in a capillary as compared with an artery or a vein, the less tension is needed in the wall to balance out the distending pressure. Wall tensions fall rapidly from 170,000 dynes/cm in the aorta to 16 dynes/cm in the capillaries, rising to 21,000 dynes/cm in the vena cava.

Wall tension is a product of the elasticity of the vessel and is a force that opposes the distending pressure. How wall tension in a given vessel responds to changes in distending pressures is based on its compliance. Compliance reflects the distensibility of a blood vessel—its ability to accept an increased volume of blood. The large quantity of muscle tissue in much of the arterial system limits its distensibility. Veins, however, are highly distensible and compliant, capable of holding a large quantity of blood at a low pressure. Because of this quality, veins are referred to as *capacitance vessels.* When the body is at rest, 75% of the total blood volume is found in the systemic venous system.

Dynamics in the Microcirculation: Capillaries and Lymphatics

The smallest vessels of the vascular system and the lymphatic vessels are commonly referred to as the *microcirculation.* The primary function of the capillary bed is the essence of the circulatory system as a whole: the exchange of gases and nutrients. Blood flow in the capillary bed is largely laminar, with minimal turbulence at bifurcations. Within each organ or tissue in the body, capillary blood flow is related to the driving force, which is the difference between arterial and venous pressures, and inversely related to resistance.

The exchange of materials across the capillary endothelium through the interstitial space, to or from the cells, occurs as a continuous process. Substances pass between cells and capillaries by moving along a concentration gradient (diffusion), whereas fluid moves according to a pressure gradient (filtration).

As fluid moves through the interstitial space, most of it returns to the capillary bed. Normally, approximately 10% of the fluid remains in the interstitium and is picked up by the adjacent lymphatic system to be returned to the general circulation. Alteration in the pressure gradient responsible for filtration can allow an excessive amount of fluid to escape into the interstitial space. Increased fluid accumulation in the interstitial space can also occur when the lymphatic flow is impaired or when capillaries become more permeable and "leak" fluid. These are the mechanisms that result in **edema.**

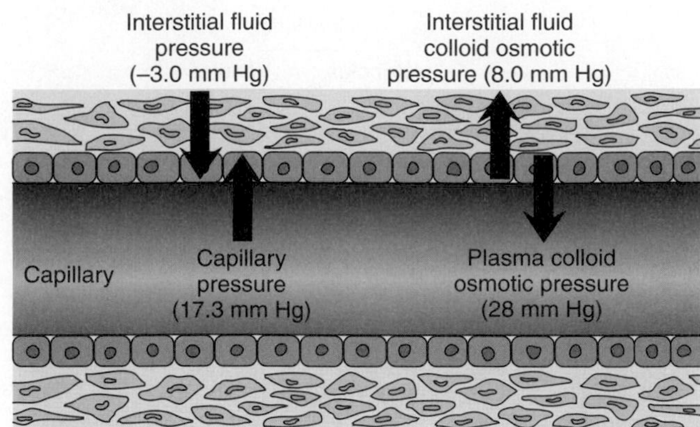

FIGURE 15-14 ■ Components of the capillary pressure gradient. Filtration reflects the difference between the combined forces that push fluid out of the capillary (capillary pressure and interstitial fluid colloid osmotic pressure) and those that attempt to hold fluid in the capillary (plasma colloid osmotic pressure and interstitial fluid pressure).

The pressure gradient between the capillary and the interstitium is produced and maintained in accord with the balance of four distinct forces or pressures: (1) capillary pressure (P_{cap}), (2) interstitial fluid colloid osmotic pressure (π_{tissue}), (3) plasma colloid osmotic pressure (π_{cap}), and (4) interstitial fluid pressure (P_{tissue}) (Figure 15-14). This delicate balance of forces is summarized by *Starling's hypothesis,* which states that the net filtration is equal to the combined forces fostering filtration minus the combined forces opposing filtration:

$$\text{Pressures favoring filtration} = P_{cap} + \pi_{tissue}$$

For example:

$$(+17.3 \text{ mm Hg}) + (+8.0 \text{ mm Hg}) = 25.3 \text{ mm Hg}$$

$$\text{Pressures opposing filtration} = P_{tissue} + \pi_{cap}$$

For example:

$$(-3.0 \text{ mm Hg}) + (+28 \text{ mm Hg}) = 25.0 \text{ mm Hg}$$

$$\text{Net filtration pressure} = (P_{cap} + \pi_{tissue}) - (P_{tissue} + \pi_{cap})$$

For example:

$$(+25.3 \text{ mm Hg}) - (+25.0 \text{ mm Hg}) = (+0.3 \text{ mm Hg})$$

Clinically, capillary fluid pressure and plasma colloid osmotic pressure are most important to a discussion of pathophysiology. Capillary fluid pressure is the blood pressure in the capillary. It is the force pushing fluid from the capillary into the interstitium and is often called the *hydrostatic pressure.* The strength of this force depends on the blood pressure and resistance within the arterial and venous systems. Pathologic conditions resulting in a change in either the blood pressure or the resistance to flow can alter this force, most frequently increasing it and propelling more fluid into the interstitial space.

Plasma proteins are responsible for the primary force resulting in fluids remaining in the capillary: plasma colloid osmotic pressure. Most plasma proteins remain in the capillaries because they are such large molecules that they cannot move through the capillary walls easily. The vast majority of plasma protein, by weight, is albumin. Although globulins and fibrinogen have greater molecular weight, albumin is present in plasma in greater quantity. The number of dissolved molecules in the plasma determines the plasma colloid osmotic pressure. In the interstitial space, the number of dissolved molecules in the interstitial space establishes the interstitial fluid colloid osmotic pressure. Albumin, as the smallest of the plasma proteins, moves with some difficulty through the capillary walls and into the interstitium. But plasma has nearly four times the concentration of proteins as the interstitium. For that reason, plasma colloid osmotic pressure normally exceeds that in the interstitium, favoring fluids remaining in the capillaries.

Applying the Starling hypothesis to the net filtration pressure in a typical capillary results in a total pressure favoring filtration of 0.3 mm Hg. This pressure difference is responsible for producing a fluid excess in the interstitial space, which is then normally picked up by the lymphatic system for eventual return to the circulation. If the pressures alter, resulting in an even greater pressure gradient, more fluid moves from the capillaries into the interstitial space. Likewise, a change in the permeability *(K)* of the capillary wall allowing plasma protein leakage or a reduction in lymphatic flow will allow fluid to collect in the interstitium. In each case, the result is **edema,** which can occur with many pathologic conditions. When lymphatic flow is impaired, allowing fluid to collect in the interstitium, it is more specifically termed **lymphedema.**

Once absorbed into the lymphatic system, interstitial fluid is referred to as *lymph.* It is similar in composition to interstitial fluid but has a lower concentration of protein. Molecules of fat and bacteria are also found in lymph. Lymph circulates throughout the body at a rate of approximately 3 L/day. Lymphatic flow can be increased by increasing the capillary pressure, decreasing the plasma colloid osmotic pressure, increasing the interstitial fluid colloid osmotic pressure, or increasing the permeability of the capillaries. The interstitial fluid hydrostatic pressure increases (becomes less negative) when any of these factors changes, producing an increase in lymphatic flow.[1]

KEY CONCEPTS

- Physical laws govern the flow of blood through the circulatory system. Predictions regarding blood flow, blood pressure, and resistance to flow can be made using these laws. The important relationships may be summarized as follows:
  1. Flow = pressure/resistance
  2. Blood pressure = flow (cardiac output) × resistance
  3. Resistance = pressure/flow
- The main factors affecting resistance to flow are radius and length of the vessels, and blood viscosity and turbulence. Usually, radius of the vessel is the most important determinant of resistance. Radius affects resistance inversely and to the fourth power. A small decrease in radius results in a large increase in resistance.
- The velocity of blood flow varies inversely with the total cross-sectional area of the vascular bed. The capillaries have the greatest total cross-sectional area and therefore the slowest flow.
- Laplace's law describes the relationships among wall tension, distending pressure, and vessel radius *($P = T/r$; $T = Pr$).* An increase in radius or distending pressure results in increased wall tension. At critical closing pressure, wall tension overwhelms distending pressure and blood flow halts.
- The transcapillary exchange of fluid and nutrients is accomplished by the processes of diffusion and filtration. Diffusion refers to movement of solute and is determined by capillary permeability and the size of the concentration gradient. Filtration refers to movement of fluid and is affected in the following way:
  1. Increased capillary fluid pressure and interstitial fluid colloid osmotic pressure enhance filtration.
  2. Increased interstitial fluid pressure and plasma colloid osmotic pressure oppose filtration.
  3. Increased permeability *(K)* enhances filtration.

CONTROL OF FLOW

Blood flow throughout the periphery is controlled by extrinsic mechanisms mediated by the autonomic nervous system, the venous and thoracic pumps, and intrinsic autoregulatory mechanisms. Lymphatic flow is controlled by increasing interstitial fluid colloid osmotic pressure and by the lymphatic pumps. In healthy people, these mechanisms of control respond to changes in the internal and external environment and compensate rapidly and efficiently; however, during states of illness these mechanisms may be inadequate to compensate for alterations in flow.

Control of Blood Flow

Extrinsic Mechanisms

The autonomic nervous system provides the primary extrinsic control of blood flow through the sympathetic nervous system (SNS). Although parasympathetic nervous system (PSNS) innervation is important to the regulation of the heart, it is not important to the regulation of peripheral resistance. Within the medulla, groups of neurons form the *vasomotor center.* This area plays a major role in the maintenance of blood pressure (see Chapter 16). The vasomotor center responds to direct stimulation and afferent stimuli of both an excitatory and inhibitory nature. A basal rate of discharge from the vasomotor center results in a continuous minimal level of contraction of vascular smooth muscle, referred to as *vasomotor tone.*

All blood vessels except the small venules and capillaries contain smooth muscle that is innervated by adrenergic fibers from the SNS. Because arteries have the most smooth muscle, they are most affected by SNS stimulation. Veins, by contrast, have little neural innervation, and venoconstriction has a minor role in controlling blood flow except in the skin and the splanchnic circulation of the gut. In general, the release of norepinephrine, the SNS postganglionic neurotransmitter, results in arterial vasoconstriction via the α_1 receptors located on the vascular smooth muscle walls. Likewise, drugs that mimic the α_1-receptor response (α_1 agonists such as phenylephrine) produce vasoconstriction, increasing vasomotor tone and diastolic blood pressure. An α_1 antagonist such as prazosin causes the blockade of receptors and vasodilation of the arterial bed.

Although β_2-adrenergic receptors located on blood vessels found in skeletal muscle produce vasodilation when stimulated, they are only minimally affected by endogenous norepinephrine from the SNS. Epinephrine, the endogenous catecholamine released by the adrenal medulla, or its exogenous pharmacologic equivalent (Adrenalin), stimulates these receptors, producing vasodilation. Therefore, their major role is not so much to maintain vasomotor tone but to increase nutrient and oxygen supplies to skeletal muscles during periods of stress.

Blood flow through the venous system is maintained by the pressure gradient from the veins into the right side of the heart and by the venous and thoracic pumps. Blood is propelled through the circuit, pushed by the force of left ventricular contraction, and moves forward toward the low-pressure side of the pump on the right side of the heart. In the peripheral veins, the venous pump is activated by skeletal muscle activity. Folds in the intimal wall of the veins create valves. Contraction of the skeletal muscles bordering the veins compresses them, forcing the valves open and propelling venous blood back toward the heart. This "venous pump" significantly facilitates venous return. Patients who are immobilized by bed rest lose this valuable mechanism, which results in a decrease in cardiac preload and increased work of the heart to maintain the cardiac output. The thoracic pump acts to increase venous return to the heart as intrathoracic pressure changes with breathing. This process, like the venous pump, enhances venous return to the heart (preload) (see Chapter 17).

Intrinsic Mechanisms

Autoregulation refers to the ability of organs themselves to maintain a relatively constant blood flow, regardless of changes in arterial pressure. This flow is *relatively* constant because it has limits; there is a range within which it is maintained, and the range varies slightly from organ to organ. A number of theories have been offered to explain how autoregulation works to meet the needs of individual organs within the body. The *myogenic hypothesis* is based on the observation that as vascular smooth muscle is stretched, it contracts. Therefore, as arterial pressure rises and arterial walls stretch, contraction is stimulated, producing vasoconstriction. The myogenic hypothesis also suggests that resistance to flow is increased with stretch by early closing of precapillary sphincters. The *metabolic hypothesis* proposes that metabolic byproducts (metabolites) or substrates exert a direct effect, altering blood flow to the area. Metabolites might include carbon dioxide or lactic acid. Histamine and prostaglandins are examples of metabolic substrates. The vascular endothelium itself can influence contraction of vascular smooth muscle, directly regulating vascular tone through the release of relaxing and contracting factors. Relaxing factors include nitric oxide, prostacyclin, and endothelium-derived hyperpolarizing factor. Angiotensin II, oxygen-derived free radicals, prostacyclin H_2, and thromboxane A_2 are among the constricting factors.[2-4] In addition, several substances that are not produced by the vascular endothelium, such as acetylcholine, bradykinin, histamine, and substance P, exert their effect by increasing the formation of nitric oxide.[5] The substances create a balance of forces in health but may be disrupted by aging, disease, or pharmacologic interventions.[6-10] Deficits of nitric oxide, or a decreased responsiveness, have been the focus of considerable recent research into the pathogenesis of hypertension (see Chapter 16).

A local increase in blood flow is referred to as **hyperemia.** The increase in local blood flow in response to increased metabolic demand is called *active* or *functional* hyperemia. *Reactive* hyperemia occurs when a temporary reduction in blood flow is reversed. The body responds by briefly increasing circulation to the area, resulting in the characteristic flushing seen, for instance, when a tourniquet is removed. The *tissue pressure hypothesis* of autoregulation postulates that an acute increase in the pressure within the arterial system causes an increase in interstitial volume and pressure. This increased tissue pressure, external to the vasculature, results in compression of small vessels, which increases resistance and reduces flow.

Control of Lymphatic Flow

The movement of lymph is expedited by lymphatic pumps. This is a general concept that encompasses the pumping action of the lymphatics themselves and the pumping effect on the lymphatic vessels produced by activity external to them. Like veins, lymphatic vessels have valves on their intimal surface that allow forward movement of fluid toward the heart and systemic circulation. Compression of lymphatic channels by adjacent skeletal muscles, the smooth muscle of organs, and the pulsatile movement of arteries force lymph toward the heart. Intrathoracic pressure changes related to breathing increase lymphatic return as well as venous return. Lymphatic flow is therefore enhanced by increased physical activity, increased blood pressure, or increased respiratory rate. Lymphatic contractions are thought to be the primary factor in lymphatic flow. Lymphatic capillaries contract when stretched, propelling lymph forward. The rate of contractions increases as the volume of lymph increases.

KEY CONCEPTS

- The blood flow through a particular vascular bed is regulated centrally by the autonomic nervous system and locally by the organ or tissue.
- In most vascular beds, the SNS causes constriction, which increases resistance and reduces flow. Smooth muscle cells in these vascular beds have α_1 receptors that bind the SNS neurotransmitter norepinephrine, causing contraction. There is no significant parasympathetic innervation of systemic vessels.
- Autoregulation refers to a tissue's ability to regulate its own flow. Autoregulation allows a tissue to maintain optimal flow despite changes in blood pressure or metabolic demands. In instances of high blood pressure or decreased metabolic demand, the arterioles and precapillary sphincters that control flow to the tissue constrict, reducing flow. In instances of low blood pressure or high demand, vessels dilate, increasing flow.
- Lymphatic vessels maintain flow by contracting when stretched with lymph. Intraluminal valves prevent backflow. External compression by contracting muscles enhances lymph flow.

GENERAL MECHANISMS THAT CAUSE ALTERED FLOW

A reduction in flow through the systemic vasculature results in impaired ability to transport gases and nutrients to and from body tissues. Cells of the body vary in their oxygen demands. *Hypoxia,* an insufficient supply of oxygen, can occur for many reasons, such as a decrease in hemoglobin formation (see Chapter 13) or diminished oxygen transport in the lungs (see Chapter 21). When flow through the arterial system is altered, the cause of hypoxia is *ischemia.* Impairment in flow through the venous system interferes with the removal of metabolic waste products and causes fluid pressure to build up in the system, a condition known as *venous engorgement* or *venous obstruction.* When the lymphatic circulation is altered, the resulting fluid and pressure changes may be visible locally or systemically.

Lymphatic Vessels

The lymphatic circulatory system may be overwhelmed when changes in capillary or interstitial oncotic pressures increase filtration or when the movement of fluid at the capillary bed is impaired. The result is **edema,** an excessive amount of fluid in the interstitial spaces. A wide variety of conditions can result in edema.

When lymphatic flow is altered due to impairment in the circulation of lymph itself, the condition is called **lymphedema.** The result is also an excessive quantity of fluid in the interstitium, but the underlying cause is an obstruction to flow.

Blood Vessels: Obstructions

Pathologic processes affecting blood flow may involve impedance of the arterial or venous system. Some obstructions to flow are specific to either the arterial or venous portion of the system, but most can occur in some form on both sides. Obstructions to flow that may interfere with arterial or venous flow are presented in detail in the following discussion. Those that are specifically arterial or venous in nature are detailed more fully later in the chapter.

Thrombosis

A **thrombus** is a stationary blood clot formed within a vessel or a chamber of the heart. Thrombosis is initiated by a change in the blood vessel resulting in localized reduction in flow. Inflammation of blood vessels may be the stimulus for thrombosis in either arteries or veins.

Etiology. Thrombosis refers to the formation of clots at these sites, to differentiate it from the clotting process that takes place as a homeostatic mechanism. Thrombi may form in the chambers of the heart in association with certain abnormal heart rhythms (see Chapter 19), following a myocardial infarction, damage to heart valves, or replacement of heart valves with artificial ones (see Chapter 18). More commonly, thrombi develop in either the arterial or the venous circulatory system. Activation of the clotting or coagulation cascade within the vessel produces a hypercoagulable state and results in thrombosis (see Chapter 14, Figure 14-4). Certain drugs, such as oral contraceptives, increase the tendency to form thrombi as well. Thrombosis is also more likely to occur when blood flow slows dramatically, becomes more turbulent, or if there is damage to intimal walls, creating a roughened surface.

Pathogenesis

Arterial. The significance of thrombosis rests in the ability of a clot within a blood vessel to reduce flow and increase turbulence, which enhances formation of more thrombi. The results of reduced blood flow vary depending on whether the arterial or venous system is involved. If the thrombus forms in the arterial system, decreased distal flow can result in **ischemia.** This is significant in several pathologic conditions, such as acute arterial occlusion (discussed in this chapter). Other examples of arterial thrombosis are explored elsewhere in this text (e.g., myocardial infarction, Chapter 18; cerebrovascular accident/stroke, Chapter 44).

Venous. In the venous system, thrombosis alters venous return, impairing removal of metabolic wastes and producing swelling (edema). When inflammation occurs in a vein (**phlebitis**) and is accompanied by the formation of a thrombus, it is called **thrombophlebitis.** The most common cause of thrombophlebitis is the inflammation produced by the placement of a needle or catheter for intravenous therapy. Thrombosis may also be initiated by a generalized reduction in flow and the release of vasoactive substances that occur in shock states (see Chapter 20). Systemic derangement in coagulation takes place in disseminated intravascular coagulation, resulting in thrombosis in the microcirculation throughout the body (see Chapter 14). Risk factors associated with thrombosis are listed in Box 15-1.

Clinical Manifestations and Treatment. Arterial thrombosis is usually manifested by intermittent claudication and pain with activity in the affected limb that improves with rest. The limb might also be cool to touch and cyanotic. A late sign is a painful arterial ulcer found usually around one toe.[11]

Symptoms for venous thrombosis may be absent or may be life-threatening secondary to pulmonary embolism. Other signs include calf or groin tenderness and swelling of the affected limb with associated increased skin temperature. Pain in the calf with dorsiflexion of the foot (Homan sign) appears in 10% of those with thrombophlebitis.[12]

Interventions in the management of thrombus formation may be medical or surgical. Ideally, thrombosis is prevented in high-risk individuals through pharmacologic or other medical approaches. The prophylactic (preventive) injection of low doses of heparin (5000 units subcutaneously every 8 to 12 hours), which inhibits activation of factor X, the rate-limiting step in the clotting cascade, is effective and commonly used for hospitalized patients. Low molecular weight heparins have become an alternative to heparin and have their effect on antithrombin III. Warfarin sodium (Coumadin) may also be given prophylactically. It is an oral anticoagulant that depresses synthesis by the liver of vitamin K–dependent clotting factors (II, VII, IX, and X). Aspirin in low doses (325 mg every 2 days) ameliorates certain thrombotic conditions such as cerebrovascular accidents (CVAs) and myocardial infarction. Ticlopidine, a platelet aggregation inhibitor, has also proved useful in the prevention of thrombotic disease. Once a thrombus has formed, anticoagulant therapy is given to prevent the formation of further thrombi, but it is not effective in dissolving an existing clot. Therapeutic doses of subcutaneous or intravenous heparin may be instituted. At these higher dosages, heparin inhibits the synthesis of thrombin and prevents the formation of a stable fibrin clot by blocking the conversion of fibrinogen to fibrin and impairing the activation of fibrin-stabilizing factor (factor XIII). Thrombolytic agents such as streptokinase, urokinase, alteplase, and reteplase are intravenous drugs that are capable of dissolving clots. They are currently used for patients with thrombi in coronary and pulmonary arteries, peripheral arteries in the legs, and cerebral arteries. Their use must be closely supervised; patients receiving thrombolytic therapy are usually in critical care settings.[13] Additional medical prophylactic interventions include the use of antiembolic stockings or sequential compression devices for immobilized patients and initiation of ambulation as soon as possible.

Because thrombi partially or completely occlude flow through the involved vessel, they can produce ischemia distal to that point in an artery or congestion behind the obstruction in a vein. A thrombus that only partially occludes a vessel continues to be affected by the force of blood flow. Eventually, it may break free from the vessel wall and become an embolus.

Box 15-1

Risk Factors Commonly Associated with Thrombosis

General (Arterial and Venous)

Hypercoagulable conditions
- Polycythemia
- Dehydration
- Platelet aggregation

Pump failure
- Congestive heart failure
- Shock

Dysrhythmias

Aging

Trauma, including surgery

Drugs
- Anesthetic agents
- Oral contraceptives
- Tobacco

Arterial

Arteriosclerosis/atherosclerosis

Venous

Immobilization

Embolus

An **embolus** is a collection of material that forms a clot within the blood stream. This traveling clot is propelled by blood flow to a distant point, where it lodges to produce a new site of obstruction.

Etiology and Pathogenesis. An embolus may be a **thromboembolus,** having begun as a thrombus that was subsequently dislodged from the vessel intima, valvular leaflets in the heart, or having formed within a chamber of the heart. Thromboemboli from the left side of the heart exit the aorta and most commonly lodge in a cerebral artery, resulting in a *cerebrovascular accident,* or *stroke* (see Chapter 44). Most thromboemboli in the venous system originate in the deep veins of the pelvis and lower extremities. They traverse the venous circulation and return to the right side of the heart, eventually lodging in the arterial side of the pulmonary vasculature and resulting in a pulmonary embolism (see Chapter 21). A thromboembolus from the right side of the heart will also result in a pulmonary embolism. Thromboemboli from the venous circulation are the most common cause of pulmonary emboli, but the cause may be nonthrombotic, as is the case for tumor, fat, air, amniotic fluid, or bacterial emboli.

Clinical Manifestations. A left-sided embolism leads to a cerebrovascular accident. Manifestations differ depending on the area of the brain affected. Symptoms include loss of cognitive function, motor changes, and different levels of sensory loss[11] (see Chapter 44). A right-sided pulmonary embolism presents with increased heart rate, increased respiratory rate, and a sense of doom in the patient. Sharp, stabbing chest pain on inspiration is also noted. Increased pulmonary pressure precipitates cardiovascular symptoms such as hypotension, syncope, and neck vein distention.[11]

Treatment. *Embolectomy* is the surgical removal of an embolus and is usually confined to thromboemboli. The use of this surgical technique is contingent on the location of the embolus. In patients who experience repeated emboli, usually originating from the peripheral venous system, a filter may be surgically implanted in the inferior vena cava. As the blood passes through the filter, emboli are trapped and cannot progress into the pulmonary circulation. The body's own thrombolytic enzyme, plasmin, destroys the trapped emboli.

Emboli Produced by Other Causes. Various other materials, some totally foreign to the blood stream, can also form emboli if present in sufficient quantity. Fat emboli are aggregates of fat molecules released into the blood after trauma or surgery involving bone. Most frequently the long bones of the legs are the source of these emboli. Increased pressure generated within the traumatized bone by the inflammatory response forces molecules of fat from the interior of the bone into the blood stream. Malignancy produces metastasis by various means, one of which is via the blood as tumor emboli. Collections of bacteria and exudate may break free from a source within the circulation, such as the leaflets of the valves of the heart in bacterial endocarditis. Once in the blood stream, the bacterial emboli travel on, eventually occluding circulation and becoming a new site of infection. Air from the external environment is a foreign material when found in the blood stream as air emboli. Bubbles of air, having most likely entered the blood through an intravenous catheter, come to rest in small blood vessels. It is difficult to identify the specific volume of air that can sufficiently obstruct flow to result in deleterious effects. In animal research, the quantity of air needed to produce death varies, partially affected by the speed with which it is injected. Under some circumstances, a 5-ml injection of air will result in death of animal models. At other times, a 100-ml bolus of air will not produce adverse effects.[14]

Increased pressure in the abdomen generated during labor and delivery may force amniotic fluid into the blood stream as emboli. Here the emboli cause a different set of problems. Amniotic fluid cannot perform the functions of the blood in carrying gases and nutrients, but as a fluid it does not produce obstruction to flow. Instead, the proteins and cells in amniotic fluid act as antigens, initiating an immune response.

Vasospasm

Vasospasm is a sudden, involuntary constriction of arterial smooth muscle that results in an obstruction to flow. In some cases, vasospasm is sufficient to produce hypoxia distally, as in variant (Prinzmetal) angina (see Chapter 18). Frequently, the cause of vasospasm is unknown. Certain individuals may be unusually sensitive to hormonal changes or food additives, which may result in vasospasm of cerebral arteries. The vasodilation following cerebral vasospasm is thought to contribute to migraine headaches. Vasospasm may be mediated by environmental factors, such as exposure to cold or emotional stress, producing a localized response.

Inflammation

Vasculitis is inflammation of the intima of an artery. Inflammation of the lining of a vein is called **phlebitis.** If superficial, these inflammations may be visible as reddened, tender streaks on the skin. Of more significance is their potential to serve as foci for the thrombotic process.

Arteritis (angiitis) is a specific term that identifies an inflammatory process of autoimmune origin in arteries. The initiating stimulus for this autoimmune disease is frequently an infectious process, whether viral or bacterial (especially streptococcal), or an adverse response to drugs such as sulfonamides or phenothiazines.

Mechanical Compression

A variety of forces external to the vascular system may result in partial or complete obstruction of blood flow. Trauma may produce direct pressure on a blood vessel, resulting in occlusion. This same effect may result from constriction due to casts or tight dressings. Swelling secondary to bleeding or edema within a fascial compartment created by fascial tissue surrounding groups of muscle, or external compression of the compartment by a tight cast, eventually compromises the circulation in vessels that pass through the compartment, producing *compartment syndrome* (see Chapter 51). Prolonged occlusion produces neurovascular alterations that can be assessed before the ischemia is irreversible. These alterations are identical to those of acute arterial occlusion, discussed later in this chapter. In an untreated patient, compartment syndrome can result in prolonged hypoxia, ischemia, and necrosis of tissues.

Blood Vessels: Structural Alterations

An assortment of pathologic conditions in blood vessel structure will produce alterations in blood flow. The structure of arteries or veins may be changed secondary to congenital anomalies or pathologic processes triggered later in life.

Types of Structural Alterations

Valvular Incompetence. The intimal folds of veins that form the valves can be damaged, interfering with the effective flow of blood through a portion of the venous system (valvular incompetence). The subsequent pathologic processes may affect superficial veins (**varicose veins**) or deep veins (**chronic venous insufficiency**), resulting in severe tissue hypoxia and venous stasis ulcers.

Arteriosclerosis/Atherosclerosis. Arteriosclerosis is a complex condition that produces structural changes in arteries. **Atherosclerosis,** a specific type of arteriosclerosis, produces an increase in the number of smooth muscle cells and a collection of lipids within the intima of medium- and large-sized arteries. This process eventually narrows the lumina and decreases their ability to dilate. Atherosclerotic changes are responsible for or contribute to many diseases throughout the body such as hypertension, renal failure, coronary artery disease (CAD), and cerebrovascular disease.

Aneurysms. An **aneurysm** is a localized dilation of an arterial wall. Aneurysms vary in the severity of their consequences, depending on their size, type, and location. All aneurysms produce an alteration in flow due to the changes in vessel diameter. But more significant is the fact that the aneurysm represents a weakened area in the artery that may eventually rupture (see the section on alterations in arterial flow in this chapter).

Arteriovenous Fistulas. An **arteriovenous fistula (AVF)** is an abnormal communication between arteries and veins. It is usually congenital in origin but may result from traumatic injury. Symptoms depend on the size and location of the fistula. Because AVFs provide a shortcut between the two vascular systems, they can result in alterations in oxygenation to the involved tissues and systemic hemodynamic changes. One of the most common and serious types of AVFs is **arteriovenous malformation (AVM).** An AVM is a tangled knot of arteries and veins found most commonly within the brain vasculature. AVMs may be the underlying cause of such conditions as headaches, CVA, dementia, or seizures (see Chapters 44 and 45). If the AVF is sufficient to cause hemodynamic changes, surgery is performed to ligate all of the branches of the fistula and isolate it from the general circulation.

KEY CONCEPTS

- Altered blood flow results from obstructive processes. Obstruction results in reduced flow beyond the obstruction (downstream) and increased pressure before the obstruction (upstream).
- In the arterial system, obstruction manifests primarily as distal ischemia. In the venous system, obstruction manifests as edema.
- The causes of vessel obstructions include thrombi, emboli, vasospasm, external compression (e.g., compartment syndrome), and structural alterations (e.g., atherosclerotic plaques, aneurysms).

ALTERATIONS IN ARTERIAL FLOW

Alterations in arterial flow result from obstruction (arteriosclerosis, atherosclerosis, arteritis, vasospasm, thrombi, emboli, and acute occlusion) or mechanical alterations (AVFs and aneurysms).

Arteriosclerosis/Atherosclerosis

Etiology and Pathogenesis. **Arteriosclerosis** is a generic term meaning "hardening of the arteries" and broadly includes three pathologic processes: Mönckeberg sclerosis (medial calcific sclerosis), arteriolar sclerosis, and atherosclerosis. Mönckeberg sclerosis is characterized by calcium deposition in the tunica media of intermediate-sized arteries. The result is thickening and increased rigidity of the vessel wall, but no reduction in flow. Arteriolar sclerosis is characterized by thickening and luminal narrowing of the small arteries that occurs in association with hypertension. Atherosclerosis, the most common arteriosclerotic process, affects intermediate-sized and large arteries. Smooth muscle cells and lipids collect along the intimal surface, producing a narrowing of the luminal diameter and a reduction in flow (Figure 15-15).

Atherosclerosis is the pathologic origin for the vast majority of arterial disease and is ultimately the cause of nearly half of the deaths in the United States and western Europe. Atherosclerosis tends to develop in large- and medium-sized arteries, most frequently the coronary, cerebral, carotid, and femoral arteries and the aorta. More than 60% of the mortality associated with atherosclerosis is due to occlusion of coronary arteries (CAD), producing myocardial ischemia and infarction. The remainder of deaths due to atherosclerosis are secondary to thrombotic or hemorrhagic processes in such organ systems as the brain, kidneys, liver, and gastrointestinal tract and the extremities. When the peripheral vascular system is affected, it is most often the lower extremities, and the disease process is called **arteriosclerosis** or *atherosclerosis obliterans.* Research results from the classic Framingham Study identified the development of lower extremity arterial disease in 5% of the subjects over the course of the 24-year data collection interval.[15] The precise pathologic mechanism of atherosclerosis is unknown; it is most likely a combination of factors. The insidiousness of the disease process has affected the speed and specificity of research. The three primary pathologic processes currently appear to be (1) a response to serum lipid levels, (2) reaction to injury of the vessel wall, and (3) cellular

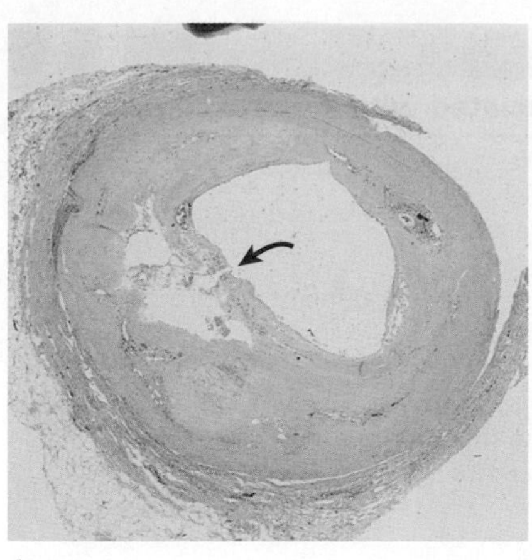
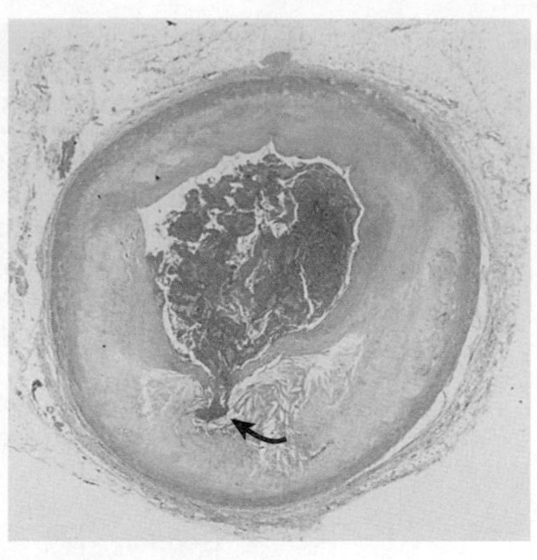
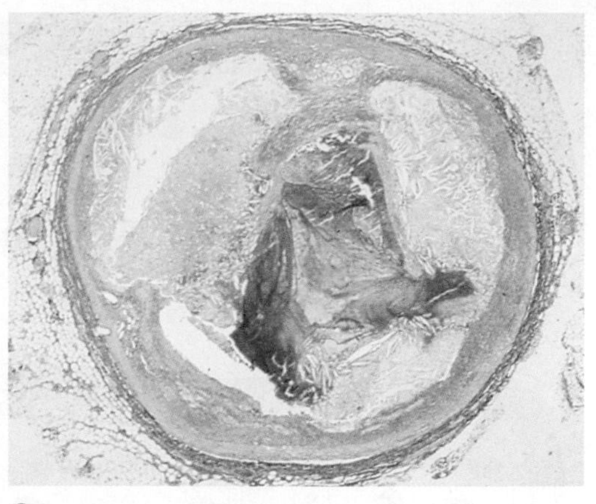

A B C

FIGURE 15-15 ■ Atherosclerotic plaque rupture. **A,** Plaque rupture without superimposed thrombus, in a patient who died suddenly. **B,** Acute coronary thrombosis superimposed on an atherosclerotic plaque with focal disruption of the fibrous cap, triggering a fatal myocardial infarction. **C,** Massive plaque rupture with superimposed thrombus, also triggering a fatal myocardial infarction (special stain highlighting fibrin in *red*). In both **A** and **B,** an *arrow* points to the site of plaque rupture. (**A** and **C,** From Kumar V, Cotran RS, Robbins ST: *Robbins basic pathology,* ed 7, Philadelphia, 2003, Saunders, p 333. **B,** Reproduced from Schoen FJ: *Interventional and surgical cardiovascular pathology: clinical correlations and basic principles,* Philadelphia, 1989, Saunders, p 61.)

transformation. Each hypothesis has spawned considerable research attention.

Lipid insudation is currently held to be the most important factor in the pathogenesis of atherosclerosis. According to the theory, high concentrations of cholesterol in the serum in the form of low-density lipoproteins (LDLs) are transported into the muscle tissues of the artery, where they produce irritation and proliferation of muscle cells (Figure 15-16).

Lipoproteins. Cholesterol is a necessary component of cellular membranes and is used in the manufacture of steroids within the body. Cholesterol itself is highly insoluble and is transported throughout the body in the form of lipoproteins, which are cholesterol cores with protein shells. Although there are several forms of lipoproteins, LDLs and high-density lipoproteins (HDLs) are most important in the discussion of atherosclerosis. Receptors on the surface of the LDL molecule bind with receptors on cell membranes, allowing the molecule to be absorbed into the cell. These receptors abound in the muscle cells of arteries. The protein coat is dissolved and the cholesterol is used to meet the cellular needs. The excess cholesterol that is not removed is stored and acts as a cellular irritant; the precise mechanism is unclear. But the correlation between high levels of serum LDLs and cholesterol is clearly significant in the development of atherosclerosis. HDL seems to serve as a protective mechanism in the formation of atherosclerosis. It is postulated that HDL can remove cholesterol from formations in the arterial walls and transport it back to the liver.[1] Consequently, cholesterol levels and lipoprotein profiles are closely supervised. An acceptable total cholesterol level for an adult who has no coronary disease is less than 200 mg/dl. Levels of LDL are felt to be detrimental if greater than 160 mg/dl. Protective levels of HDL are those greater than 40 mg/dl.[16] A major preventive intervention related to atherosclerosis is encouraging the consumption of a low-fat diet, with those fats being primarily polyunsaturated (from vegetable sources as opposed to animal).

An additional lipoprotein, Lp(a), is similar to LDL but acts as an independent risk factor for premature CAD. Premature CAD results in myocardial infarction, coronary insufficiency, angina pectoris, or sudden cardiac death before age 55. Concentrations of Lp(a) seem to be primarily genetically determined. However, current research suggests that aggressive management of LDL imbalance may result in lower Lp(a) levels.[10,17-19]

The *reaction to injury* hypothesis is grounded in nonspecific damage to the endothelial surface of the arterial intima, producing an alteration in wall permeability. The normal barrier is lost, and serum constituents such as platelets and large quantities of lipoproteins enter the intimal lining. Platelets aggregate and some are damaged, releasing platelet-derived growth factor (PDGF), which stimulates growth of smooth muscle cells. Media smooth muscle cells, normally protected by an intact intima, are drawn to the intima and proliferate. The essence of this hypothesis is the chronicity of irritation, in contrast to mild intermittent irritation, which is reversible. Chronic irritation may be due to smoking, hypercholesterolemia, and such hemodynamic stressors as hypertension, diabetes mellitus, and high levels of circulating catecholamines, angiotensin, or hormones. See Chapter 17 for further discussion of progression of atherosclerosis.

Risk Factors. Historically, health care has focused on preventing atherosclerosis by manipulation of predisposing factors. These risk factors are categorized as modifiable or non-

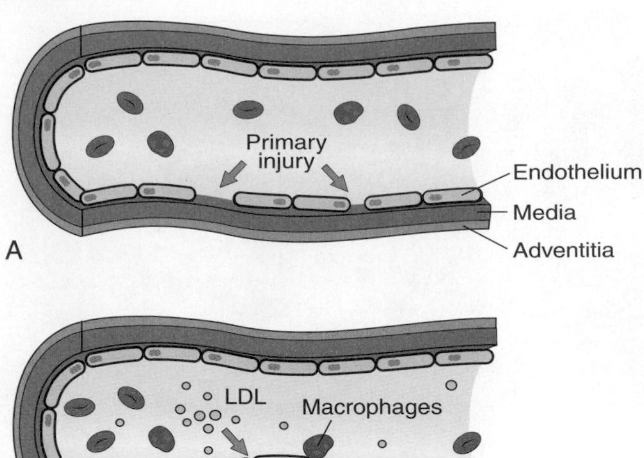

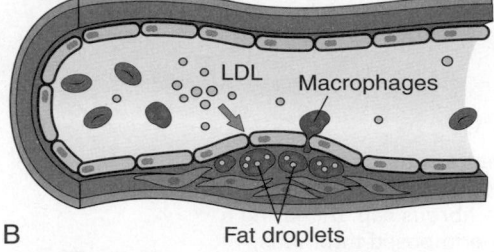

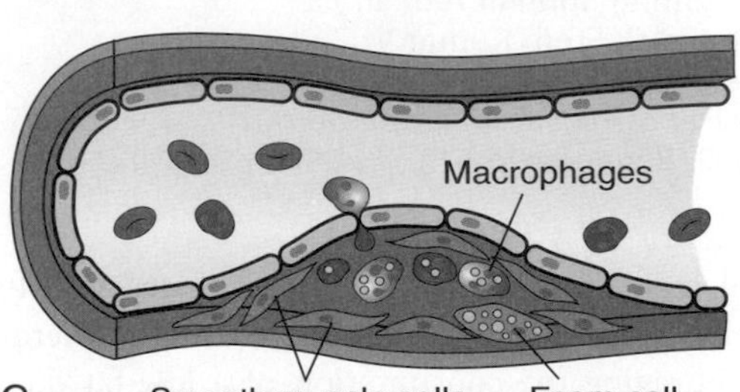

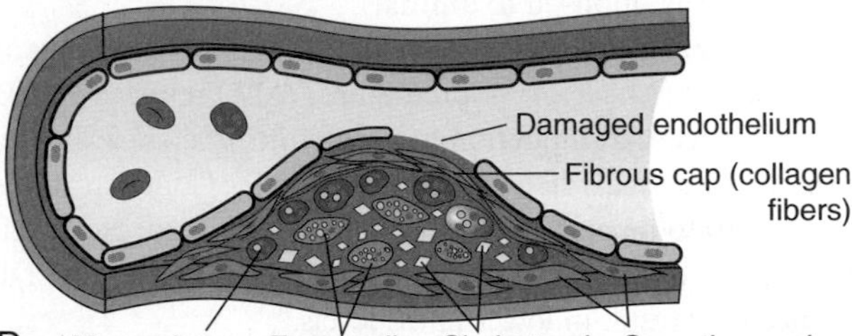

FIGURE 15-16 ■ Pathogenesis of atherosclerosis. **A,** Endothelial injury. **B,** Influx of lipids. **C,** Accumulation of lipids in vessel wall, proliferation of smooth muscle cells, and accumulation of macrophages. **D,** Atheromas consist of a lipid-rich soft part and a firm fibrous cap. *LDL,* Low-density lipoprotein. (From Damjanov I: *Pathology for the health-related professions,* ed 2, Philadelphia, 2000, Saunders, p 149.)

modifiable, according to the individual's degree of control over them (Box 15-2). It is often difficult to isolate the effect of a single risk factor because they most frequently occur in combination with one another.

The most frequently cited prospective research into atherosclerotic risk factors began in 1948 in Framingham, Massachusetts.[15] Initially, 5209 men and women between the ages of 30 and 59 volunteered to be subjects in the study. The purpose of the study was to identify factors associated with the development of atherosclerosis over a long period. The Framingham Study is ongoing, with researchers now studying the children of the original participants. Much of the available information regarding atherosclerotic risk factors is based on the results of this research.

Box 15-2

Risk Factors Associated with Atherosclerosis

Modifiable risk factors

- Smoking
- Elevated blood pressure
- Glucose intolerance
- Elevated cholesterol and low-density lipoproteins
- Decreased physical activity
- Obesity
- Weight fluctuations
- Ineffective stress management

Nonmodifiable risk factors

- Age
- Gender
- Ethnicity
- Heredity

Modifiable Risk Factors. Both the nicotine and carbon monoxide found in tobacco products have been found to cause endothelial injury, facilitating the development of atherosclerotic plaques. They appear to adversely affect serum lipid levels as well. Nicotine produces vasospasm and increased platelet aggregation, which can decrease myocardial oxygen supply. Endogenous catecholamines are released with smoking, increasing blood pressure and heart rate, which result in an increase in myocardial oxygen demand. Smoking increases the risk of coronary heart disease to two to four times normal. This risk is even greater if the individual has hypertension, hypercholesterolemia, glucose intolerance, or diabetes because these conditions have a synergistic effect with smoking.[20] Death rates after a myocardial infarction are higher among smokers.[21] Cessation of smoking results in a 50% risk reduction from coronary heart disease within the first year, and a risk equal to that in nonsmokers after 10 years.[17]

Increases in both systolic and diastolic blood pressure are associated with an increased incidence of atherosclerosis. Diastolic blood pressure elevations are probably more significant because they represent the status of the cardiovascular system when it is at rest. The risk diminishes with interventions directed to lowering the blood pressure.[11] Hypertension is often found in the presence of other risk factors. (See Chapter 16 for a discussion of hypertension.)

Elevated serum cholesterol and LDL levels were discussed in the previous section as significant contributors to the development of atherosclerosis. In addition to dietary fat intake, smoking and diabetes mellitus have been found to be associated with elevations in LDL and reduced levels of HDL.[11,16,21] Glucose intolerance is affiliated with diabetes mellitus, a disease in which an absolute lack of or a decreased response to insulin produces a derangement in metabolism (see Chapter

41). Atherosclerosis is highly correlated with glucose intolerance, probably because of the alterations in carbohydrate and fat metabolism and the direct damage to vessel basement membrane with elevated blood glucose levels. The incidence of atherosclerotic diseases is much higher among those with diabetes mellitus than in the general population, but it does not appear to be related to the degree of hyperglycemia.[21] Individuals with diabetes mellitus are also more likely to have other risk factors, such as obesity, hypertension, and elevated serum lipid levels.

Obesity, defined as a body weight 30% or greater than ideal, is thought to be a contributing risk factor for atherosclerosis in that it may accelerate the process. Abdominally distributed obesity seems to be most highly correlated with atherosclerosis.[21] Weight gain is associated with increasing serum cholesterol and LDL levels, increasing systolic blood pressure, glucose intolerance, and a sedentary lifestyle.

Physical activity has been found to increase HDL levels, the collateral circulation, and vessel size, and to decrease total cholesterol levels, glucose intolerance, body weight, and blood pressure. Clearly, all of these events can retard the development and mitigate the severity of atherosclerosis. Research likewise substantiates physical inactivity as a risk factor for cardiovascular disease.[21]

Stress and personality factors have received considerable attention as risk factors for atherosclerosis over the past 10 to 20 years. It is extremely difficult to isolate these facets and examine them quantitatively and qualitatively. Objectively, stress results in the release of endogenous catecholamines that contribute to the increased work of the cardiovascular system. Subjectively, the rushed, stressed person is less inclined to exercise and eat wisely and more inclined to smoke and be hypertensive.

Nonmodifiable Risk Factors. Certain risk factors are not modifiable and hence cannot be manipulated for prevention purposes. As an individual ages, changes occur in the proliferation of smooth muscle of blood vessels. Stem cells in the media—which yield differentiated cells—decline in their speed of replication. Thus, clonal senescence is hypothesized to be a risk factor for the eventual morphologic changes found with atherosclerosis.

Gender is another nonmodifiable risk factor. Men have a higher incidence of atherosclerosis earlier in life than women, apparently owing to the protective effects of estrogen. After menopause, this advantage is lost. It may be lost earlier if women smoke, have hypertension, have increased serum cholesterol levels, or take oral contraceptives.[22,23] Until recently, postmenopausal hormone replacement was believed to be protective against CAD, however the Woman's Health Initiative (WHI) study found a higher incidence of myocardial infarction in the group receiving HRT. Over 16,600 women were followed for 5.2 years. Women on a combination of estrogen and progesterone had a 29% increase in CHD events over those who took a placebo. No significant difference in death to CHD event was noted.[24]

A strong family history of CAD is an important predictor of its occurrence and subsequent prognosis. The specific mechanism is uncertain, but most likely it is a combination of genetic and environmental factors. Certain of the modifiable risk factors are also known to have a genetic component.

Studies of ethnicity as a nonmodifiable risk factor associated with atherosclerosis have predominantly focused on the increased incidence of CAD and hypertension among black Americans compared with white Americans.[25] Research among Hispanic Americans indicates a lower incidence of CAD and subsequent mortality than in non-Hispanic Americans.[23,25] In both cases, the overlap of genetic and environmental factors makes ethnicity, as an isolated independent variable, difficult to evaluate.

Clinical Manifestations and Diagnosis. Disease manifestations vary with the tissues involved and the severity of altered flow. Atherosclerosis is an underlying pathologic condition for much of the hypertension, renal disease, cardiac disease, peripheral arterial disease, and stroke seen in health care practice. Approaches to diagnosis and treatment of decreased organ or tissue function vary. Patient history and physical assessment provide significant information. Noninvasive tests such as Doppler flow studies may identify areas of occlusion or diminished flow. *Plethysmography* may be used to measure changes in the relative size of extremities associated with blood flow. Ankle pressures are obtained with a blood pressure cuff and Doppler ultrasonography and compared with brachial blood pressures in the ankle-brachial (A/B) index. A normal A/B index is 1.0; an index less than 1.0 is indicative of diminished arterial flow. Exercise or stress testing may be performed to evaluate the pain of arterial occlusive disease (intermittent claudication). Angiography—the radiologic study of blood flow—is the most frequently employed diagnostic examination. (See Chapter 18 for a discussion of coronary artery disease, Chapter 16 for a discussion of hypertension, Chapter 28 for a discussion of renal failure, and Chapter 44 for a discussion of cerebrovascular accidents.)

Treatment. Identification of and interventions directed toward modifiable risk factors are the major thrusts of treatment, regardless of the organs or tissues affected. Nonpharmacologic interventions, such as weight reduction, smoking cessation, exercise, and low-fat diet, are the first-line actions. Drug therapy to decrease hypercholesterolemia is considered when the nonpharmacologic approaches are found to be ineffective or inadequate or the presence of additional risk factors indicates that the patient would benefit from such interventions. Fibric acid, nicotinic acid, bile acids, and statins and their derivatives are the drugs of choice.[26-29] Balloon angioplasty, the surgical radiologic fragmentation of atherosclerotic plaques by inflation of a specially equipped catheter, is commonly performed on both coronary and peripheral arteries. Laser angioplasty is being combined with balloon angioplasty to create an opening in significantly obstructed peripheral vessels before the balloon is inflated. Balloon angioplasty with stent placement is being used. Stent placement has proven to have a good procedure success rate with fewer return visits for revascularization. Currently, when balloon angioplasty of the coronary arteries is unacceptable or fails to result in satisfactory improvement, coronary artery bypass graft (CABG) surgery is performed. Autologous donor grafts, most commonly from either the saphenous veins or the internal mammary arteries, or less commonly from a radial artery, are used. Peripheral arterial bypass grafts are named for their sites of origin and termination (e.g., aortofemoral, femoropopliteal). Synthetic graft material, such as Gore-Tex, is more commonly used for peripheral vascular bypass surgery.

Arteritis: Thromboangiitis Obliterans

Thromboangiitis obliterans (Buerger disease) is a somewhat rare inflammatory condition affecting small- and medium-sized arteries of the upper and lower extremities and producing varying degrees of obstruction.

The inflammation is accompanied by thrombosis, fibrosis, and scarring that may extend to neighboring nerves. It is associated with cigarette smoking and found most frequently in Asian rather than Western countries and in men younger than 40 years.[30,31]

Veins may also be affected, but the signs and symptoms relate to obstruction of arterial flow (Box 15-3 and Figure 15-17). With arterial occlusion, patients may complain of pain with activity (*intermittent claudication;* Figure 15-18) and also have pain at rest and be sensitive to cold. Peripheral pulses are diminished. Ulceration may occur. Patients are encouraged to cease smoking. Bypass surgery is rarely an option because the involved vessels are too distal. If the disease is not detected early and managed appropriately, amputation may be necessary.[30]

Box 15-3

Defining Characteristics of Thromboangiitis Obliterans

Skin assessment
- Cool or cold to touch
- Decreased or absent hair growth
- Dry, thin, glossy appearance
- Thickened nails
- Pallor when elevated, rubor when dependent
- Diminished or absent pulses

Pain assessment
- Sharp and stabbing
- Intensified with activity
- Relieved by rest or dependency

Ulcer assessment
- Severely painful
- Pale, gray base
- Well-defined edges
- Located on heels, lateral malleolus, between distal portions of phalanges, pretibial area

Raynaud Syndrome

An extreme vasoconstrictive response of the arteries in the hands and fingers produces the characteristic signs and symptoms of Raynaud syndrome.

Affected persons, primarily women, have numb, cold hands after exposure to stress or cold temperatures. As the ischemia progresses, the hands become cyanotic and the pain diminishes. As the vasoconstriction diminishes and reactive hyperemia occurs, the subject complains of throbbing, burning pain, and the hands become erythematous.

Various treatment modalities have been used with differing degrees of success. Because the precise cause of Raynaud syndrome is unknown, interventions have been directed to enhancing the circulation. Biofeedback and relaxation techniques may be beneficial.[32] The most widely used drugs are calcium channel blockers, which produce vasodilation by in-

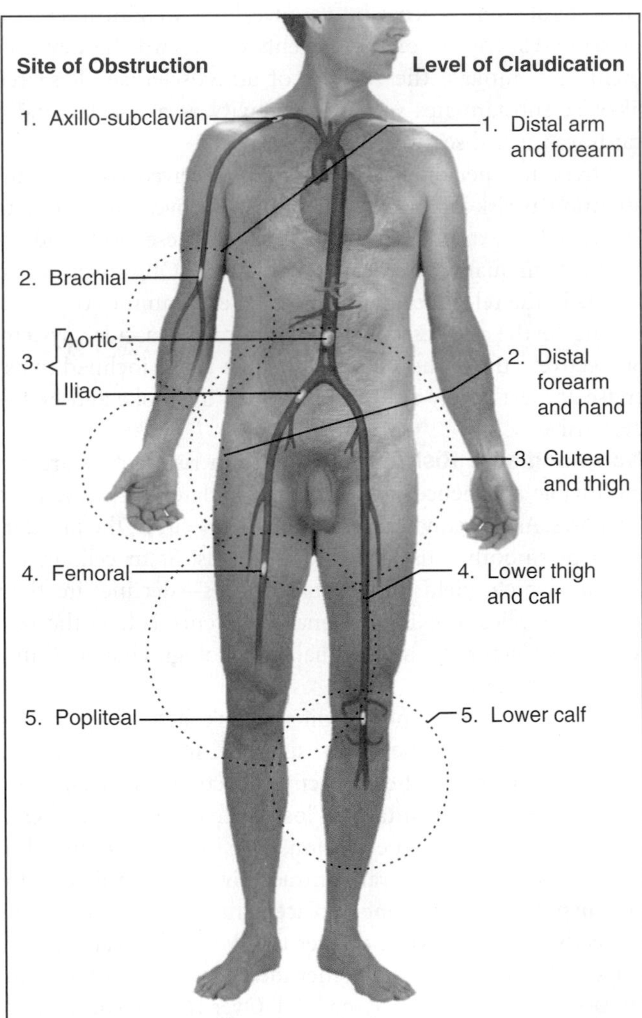

FIGURE 15-17 ■ Arterial obstructions and their corresponding areas of claudication. (From Monahan FD, Neighbors M: *Medical surgical nursing: foundations for clinical practice,* ed 2, Philadelphia, 1998, Saunders, p 332.)

terfering with calcium influx into vascular smooth muscle cells.[32,33] Sympatholytic drugs such as prazosin have been studied and found to be more effective than placebos. Prostaglandin therapy has proved helpful but is not approved at this time.[33] Persons with the syndrome are urged to protect themselves from cold temperatures, vibration, and nicotine and to use stress reduction interventions.[32,33]

Aneurysms

As described previously, aneurysms are localized arterial dilations. The arterial wall deteriorates until it is weakened sufficiently to bulge outward. The underlying cause may be atherosclerotic changes in the vessel, a congenital weakness, or a weakening induced by infection, inflammation, or a traumatic injury. Aneurysms are most frequently found in the cerebral circulation (berry aneurysm in the circle of Willis) and in the thoracic and abdominal aorta.[20]

Classifications. Aneurysms are classified as true or false, depending on the layers of the arterial wall involved (Figure 15-19). In *true aneurysms,* all three tunicae are involved (intima, media, and adventitia), whereas in *false aneurysms,* at least one tunica is left unaffected. In a false aneurysm, the muscle tissue and fascia often confine the leaking blood, which enhances thrombus formation. False aneurysms are most often due to trauma rather than vessel disease. True aneurysms are further divided. *Saccular aneurysms,* like false aneurysms, are usually secondary to trauma. Infection also produces saccular aneurysms. The weakening is confined to one side of the vessel, producing a ballooning. *Fusiform aneurysms* represent weakening on both sides of the vessel wall.

All aneurysms can affect blood flow, but of greatest clinical concern is the *dissecting aneurysm* (see Figure 15-19). Here the tear in the arterial wall creates a channel for blood flow. The tear may be between the intima and media or between the media and adventitia. As more blood escapes into the space, the layers are separated from one another in both directions from the leak, and the vessel becomes progressively weaker; it may rupture. Rupture can be explained by the law of Laplace. As the radius of the vessel increases, the tension in the wall increases. Rupture of a major vessel such as the aorta carries a high mortality.

Clinical Manifestations. Signs and symptoms of a cerebral aneurysm are associated with increasing intracranial pressure (see Chapter 44). Nondissecting aneurysms may pro-

Activity
Obstruction
Increased tissue demand for O_2
Decreased tissue supply of O_2
Anaerobic metabolism
Build up of metabolic wastes
Irritation of peripheral nerve endings
Pain
(Relief)
Decreased metabolic wastes
Rest
Decreased tissue demand for O_2
Aerobic metabolism

FIGURE 15-18 ■ Pathophysiologic process of intermittent claudication and its relief.

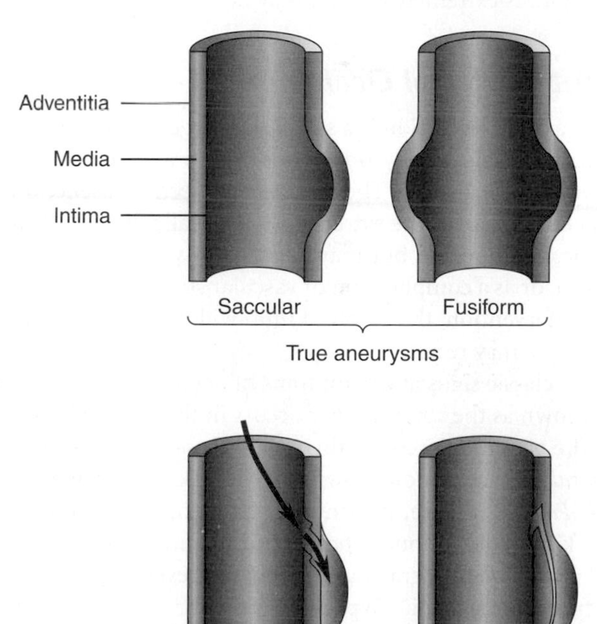

FIGURE 15-19 ■ Classification of aneurysms. All three tunicae are involved in true aneurysms (fusiform and saccular). In false aneurysms, blood escapes between tunica layers and they separate. The muscle and fascia confine the leak; a thrombus forms and seals the leak. In a dissecting aneurysm, a tear in the intima creates a channel into which blood leaks, creating a hematoma. Continued expansion of the hematoma further separates the intima from the other layers, weakening the vessel.

duce no symptoms. Dissecting aortic aneurysms often present as sudden, severe, tearing pain that radiates into the back or abdomen. The patient may show signs and symptoms of shock. Renal blood flow may be compromised, producing renal failure. If the ascending aorta is affected, arterial blood flow to the head and upper extremities may be affected. In the descending aorta, blood supply to the spinal nerves may be compromised, resulting in paraplegia. Computed tomography and transesophageal echocardiography (TEE) are the most common diagnostic modalities.[34,35] TEE has proven to be reliable and is immediately available in an emergency setting.[34,35]

Treatment. Dissecting aneurysms are emergency situations and may be managed medically and/or surgically. Medical intervention is directed at lowering the blood pressure to decrease the speed and severity of the dissection. Vasodilators such as nitroprusside (Nipride) or diazoxide (Hyperstat) are often administered parenterally. Calcium channel blockers and adrenergic blockers are also used, both for their vasodilating antihypertensive effects and for their negative inotropic effect, which decrease the force of the myocardial contraction.[11] Surgical intervention involves resection (removal) of the aneurysm and insertion of a prosthetic graft. If the aneurysm is extremely large, it may be inoperable.

Acute Arterial Occlusion

Acute arterial occlusion is a surgical emergency. An embolism lodges in a major artery, one that is usually already affected by atherosclerotic disease. The result is an effective absence of arterial circulation to the extremity. It is usually due to a thrombus or an embolism but may occur with vasospastic disease, trauma, or as a complication of vascular surgery. Without surgical intervention, the involved limb will become gangrenous and sepsis may result.

The classic signs and symptoms of acute arterial occlusion are known as the *six P's. Pallor* occurs in the involved extremity. The patient may complain of *paresthesia,* and some degree of *paralysis* may be noted, owing to the lack of oxygen to nerve cells. *Pain* is intense, continuous, and unrelated to activity. The skin is cold to touch *(polar)* and essentially *pulseless.*

Anticoagulant therapy is initiated to prevent the formation of further thrombi. Bypass surgery or revascularization through thrombolytic therapy is usually attempted.[36] Surgical removal of an embolism, as previously discussed, is referred to as *embolectomy.* If these approaches are not successful, amputation is necessary.[36]

KEY CONCEPTS

- Common causes of arterial obstruction are atherosclerosis, arteritis, Raynaud syndrome, and aneurysms. Emboli are the usual cause of acute arterial occlusion.
- Atherosclerosis is the most common cause of chronic progressive arterial obstruction. Several risk factors for the development of atherosclerosis have been proposed, among them smoking, hyperlipidemia, male gender, advancing age, sedentary lifestyle, obesity, glucose intolerance, and a relevant family history. Several theories have been advanced to explain the pathogenesis of atherosclerosis, but none has been proved.
- Acute arterial obstruction is accompanied by the classic manifestations known as the six P's: pallor, paresthesia, paralysis, pain, pulselessness, and polar (cold to touch).

ALTERATIONS IN VENOUS FLOW

Pathologic venous conditions are the result of obstruction to flow (deep vein thrombosis) or structural alterations (valvular incompetence).

Valvular Incompetence

Etiology and Pathogenesis. The intimal surface of veins folds into valves periodically (Figure 15-20). When the valves are open, blood is propelled forward by the pressure changes exerted by the skeletal muscles and the intraabdominal and intrathoracic pumps. When this pressure decreases, backward flow of blood is prevented by proper closure of the valves (valvular competency). Valvular incompetence results in *venous insufficiency.* When the superficial veins are involved, the disease process is called **varicose veins. Chronic venous insufficiency** occurs as a progression of the varicosities, when deep veins are affected.

The cause of valvular incompetence is valvular overstretching due to excessive venous pressures. Veins are designed as low-pressure systems. After the blood leaves the high-pressure arterial bed, it passes into the fine capillary network, which slows

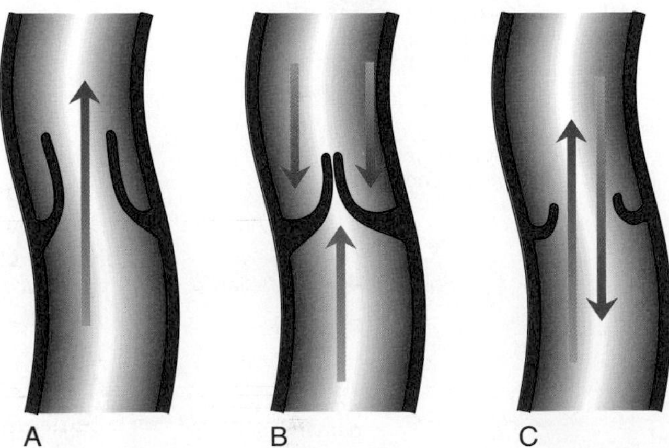

FIGURE 15-20 ■ The venous valves. **A,** Open valves permit forward blood flow. **B,** Closed valves prevent backflow of blood. **C,** Incompetent valves, unable to close fully, allow blood to flow backward, producing venous insufficiency.

flow and reduces the pressure. Blood flow through the veins is essentially pumped by forces outside the veins. The highly distensible vein walls are capable of expanding to create a reservoir of blood. When the pressure against which the pumps must push is elevated for a prolonged period, the veins stretch and the valve cusps can no longer meet. Backflow results in further engorgement of the involved veins. The process is most frequently seen in people whose occupations require them to stand for long periods. Obesity and pregnancy also elevate venous pressure and may contribute to varicosity formation.

Clinical Manifestations and Treatment. Symptoms may include a feeling of heaviness or tension and itchiness. Thrombi can promote valve obstruction and further thrombus formation. In prolonged insufficiency, edema and stasis dermatitis (discoloration along the lower calf to ankle) may develop. Long-term insufficiency can lead to ulcer formation.[11,37,38]

Prevention interventions include smoking cessation and beginning a walking program. Regular exercise has been shown to decrease future cardiovascular events.[37] Antiplatelet therapy may be started using ASA, ticlopidine, or clopedigrol.[13,37] Revascularization may be attempted by either balloon angioplasty or surgical bypass.[37]

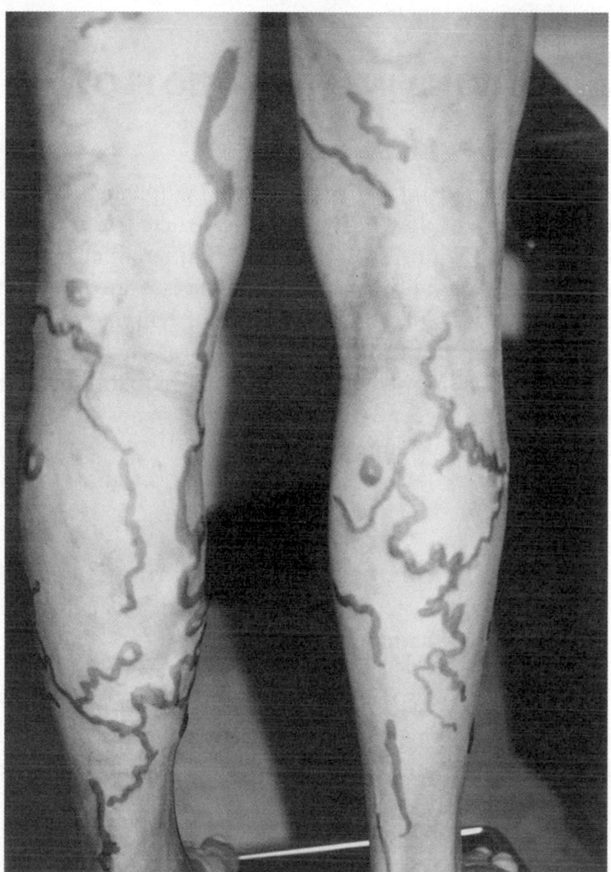

FIGURE 15-21 ■ Varicose veins. Varicosities are best observed when the patient is standing because standing increases the pressure and causes the tortuous veins to become more visible. They are outlined, as in the illustration, prior to surgical intervention. Note the tortuous pattern. (From Black JM, Hawks J, Keene A: *Medical-surgical nursing: clinical management for positive outcomes,* ed 7, Philadelphia, 2005, Saunders, p 1539.)

Varicose Veins

Etiology and Pathogenesis. Varicosities are superficial, darkened, raised, and tortuous veins (Figure 15-21). The greater saphenous vein is primarily affected, although varicosities may also develop in the lesser saphenous veins. Impaired venous return causes increased capillary pressure, and the involved limb may become edematous.

Clinical Manifestations and Treatment. Patients may complain of an aching, heavy discomfort, but they are primarily disturbed by the appearance of the varicosities.

Many of the diagnostic tests used for the arterial system are used for the identification of venous disease. The patient history and physical assessment provide important baseline information. Doppler ultrasound and impedance plethysmography are among the most frequently used assessment tools.[38]

Conservative medical interventions are designed to reduce venous pressure and enhance the venous pump, especially the skeletal muscle pump. Patients are encouraged to elevate their legs whenever they can and to avoid standing for long periods of time. Elastic stockings can facilitate venous return by enhancing the skeletal muscle pump. When sitting, patients are urged to not cross their knees or ankles. Exercise, particularly walking or swimming, is suggested. If appropriate, weight reduction is recommended. *Sclerotherapy* involves the injection of a sclerosing agent (3% sodium tetradecyl sulfate [Sotradecol]) into the involved vein. Compression of the vein following the injection prevents the formation of a thrombus. Sclerosis initiates an inflammatory process and compression forces the lumen to collapse. The intima adheres to itself and heals, and the vein is obliterated. Collateral venous circulation meets the need for venous return from the extremity. This procedure is usually limited to isolated superficial veins rather than to more generalized disease of deep veins.[38,39]

If necessary, surgical interventions for varicose veins may be selected. *Vein stripping* and *vein ligation* commonly are performed as outpatient procedures and are often combined with sclerotherapy. Vein ligation involves tying off communicating veins (e.g., those that drain into the saphenous vein). The vein, now isolated, is excised, or removed, and stripped from the extremity. Both of these treatment modalities depend on the presence of adequate deep venous structures to provide alternate routes for venous drainage.

Chronic Venous Insufficiency

Etiology and Pathogenesis. **Chronic venous insufficiency** results when valvular incompetence advances to involve the deep veins (superficial femoral, anterior and posterior tibial, peroneal) of the legs. Communicating or perforating veins

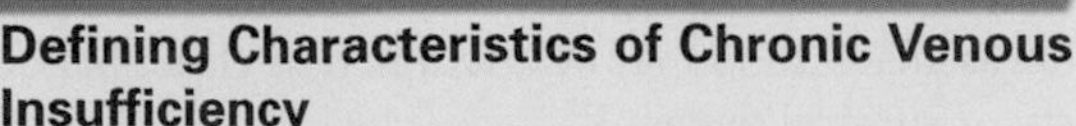

Box 15-4

Defining Characteristics of Chronic Venous Insufficiency

Skin assessment
- Warm, tough, and thickened to touch
- Pigmented areas, reddish brown
- Edema, especially at end of day
- Visible healed ulcers
- Evidence of varicose veins may be present

Pain assessment
- Aching, cramping
- Sometimes decreases with ambulation
- Relieved by elevation

Ulcer assessment
- Moderately painful
- Pink-red base
- Irregular, uneven edges
- Located on medial malleolus

provide direct access between the superficial and deep veins. As the pressure in the superficial veins remains elevated for a prolonged period, the deep veins are eventually affected.

Clinical Manifestations and Treatment. Venous stasis ulcers also develop as superficial veins rupture with the increased pressures associated with activity.[39] The skin pigmentation becomes brown as small veins rupture, leaking red blood cells, which are eventually broken down. Defining characteristics of chronic venous insufficiency are listed in Box 15-4.

The diagnostic and medical interventions described for varicose veins may prove helpful in the management of chronic venous insufficiency. Antibiotics may be necessary for secondary infections of venous stasis ulcers. Sclerotherapy and vein stripping are rarely done, for the entire venous circulation of the limb is usually affected at this point. Pentoxifylline (Trental) is also used; it increases leukocyte deformability and inhibits neutrophil adhesion and activation.[39]

Deep Vein Thrombosis

Etiology and Pathogenesis. The pathophysiologic process of thrombus formation has been previously described. Acute venous obstruction is most frequently secondary to a thrombus in a deep vein of the lower extremities. Upper extremities are less frequently affected by deep vein thrombosis.

Clinical Manifestations and Treatment. Deep vein thrombosis of the legs may be asymptomatic. Signs and symptoms, if present, typically include edema and dilated superficial veins secondary to the increased venous pressure. Pain may be present due to pressure on adjacent nerves and the inflammatory process initiated by the alteration in coagulation.

Deep vein thrombosis is treated aggressively; deep vein thrombosis of the lower extremities and pelvic veins is the most frequent source of pulmonary emboli. Most often, patients are hospitalized, and intravenous therapeutic anticoagulation therapy (heparin) is initiated. Occasionally, patients are treated on an outpatient basis with oral anticoagulants (warfarin sodium; Coumadin). Patients who have previously developed deep vein thromboses are at risk for further hypercoagulation and may undergo prophylactic anticoagulation with antiplatelet therapy (low-dose aspirin). With subsequent hospitalization, these patients frequently are given low molecular weight heparin therapy prophylactically.[13]

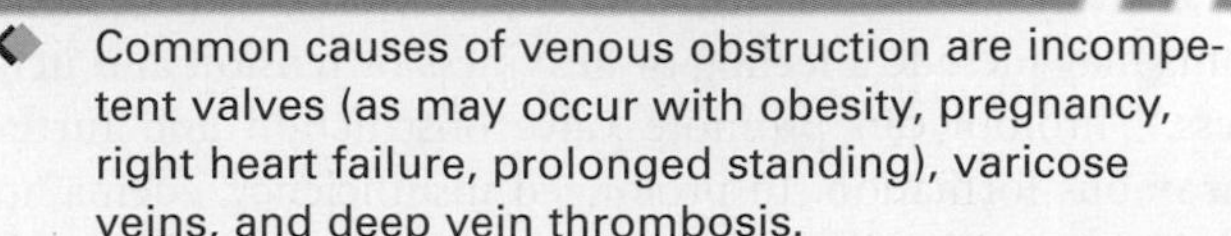

KEY CONCEPTS

- Common causes of venous obstruction are incompetent valves (as may occur with obesity, pregnancy, right heart failure, prolonged standing), varicose veins, and deep vein thrombosis.
- Edema, stasis ulcers, and pain usually accompany chronic venous obstruction.
- Deep vein thrombosis is potentially life threatening because of the likelihood of embolization to the pulmonary circulation. It is treated aggressively with immobilization of the extremity and the administration of anticoagulants.

ALTERATIONS IN LYMPHATIC FLOW

Lymphedema

Etiology and Pathogenesis. Lymphedema occurs when the normal flow of lymph is obstructed or altered in some fashion (Figure 15-22). It is often differentiated as primary or secondary. Primary lymphedema is related to a congenital absence or decreased numbers of lymphatics or obstruction of the thoracic duct or the cisterna chyli, where the upper and lower body lymphatic systems join to drain into the vascular system. Secondary lymphedema is most frequently due to the surgical removal of lymph nodes, as with breast cancer, or destruction of the lymphatics by radiation therapy in the management of various malignancies.

Clinical Manifestations and Treatment. Patients may present with bilateral or unilateral edema, usually beginning in the feet or hands and progressing centrally. This form of edema is not associated with the skin changes (pigmentation, ulceration) seen with edema originating from the systemic venous system. Chronic congestion produces subcutaneous fibrosis, resulting in thick, rough skin, often called *brawny edema*.[11,40,41]

Medical treatment includes use of external pneumatic compression devices, elastic stockings, exercise, and diuretics.[11,41] Complex decongestive physiotherapy, developed in Australia and Europe, is a 2- to 4-week treatment plan that involves diet, skin care, and massage therapy, is now being introduced into the United States.[40] Antibiotics and benzopyrones are two drug classifications with proven efficacy. Benzopyrones increase lymphatic flow (by enhancing collect-

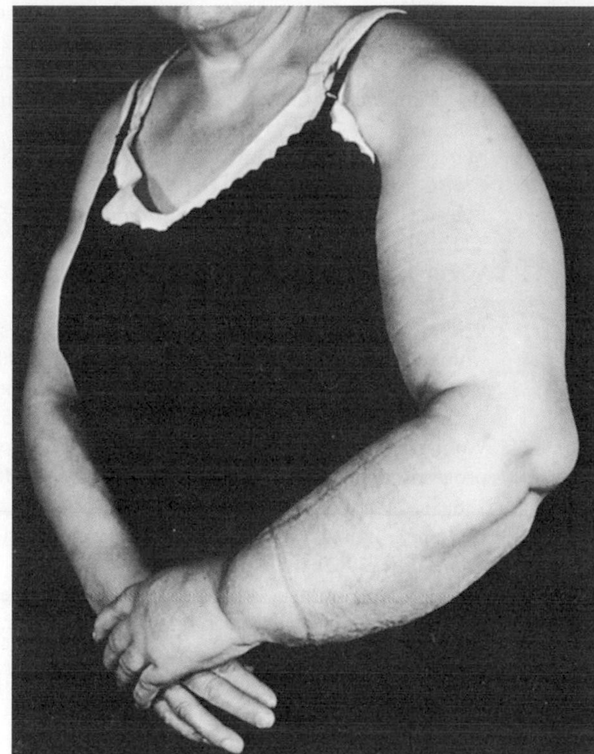
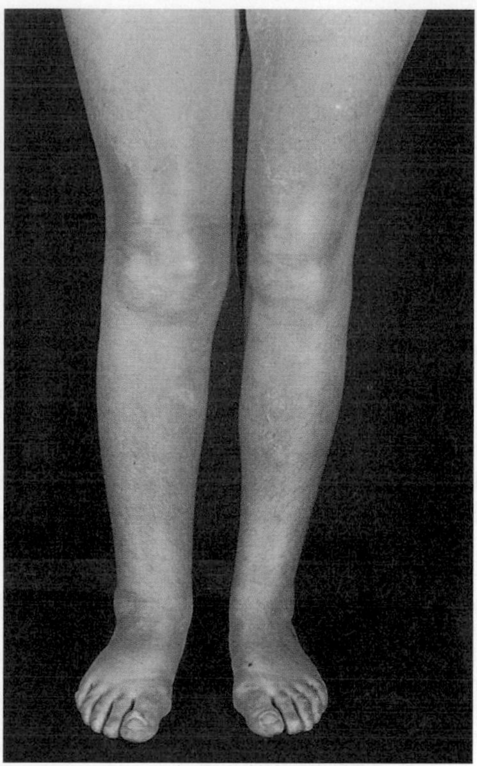

FIGURE 15-22 ■ Types of lymphedema. **A,** Lymphedema of an arm secondary to surgical alterations in the lymphatic system associated with mastectomy. **B,** Lymphedema of a leg. (From Black JM, Hawks J, Keene A: *Medical-surgical nursing: clinical management for positive outcomes,* ed 7, Philadelphia, 2005, Saunders, p 1543.)

ing lymphatic pumping capacities), increase capillary resistance and decrease their permeability, and increase macrophage proteolytic activity. Coumarin and flavonoids are the two major groups of benzopyrones used. Antibiotics are prescribed for the cellulitis that accompanies lymphedema.[41] Surgical removal of skin and subcutaneous tissue followed by split-thickness skin grafting over the muscle may be helpful, but the results are physically unattractive. Reconstructive surgery may be done to create lymphovenous bypasses, but these often result in thrombosis. Other surgical interventions have been attempted, depending on the location of the problem, with varying degrees of success.

KEY CONCEPTS

- Obstruction to lymph flow is most commonly due to surgical removal of or radiation damage to lymphatic vessels during treatment of cancer.
- Manifestations of lymphatic obstruction include regional edema and thickened subcutaneous tissue.

SUMMARY

The circulatory system is organized to facilitate its dual functions of oxygen and nutrient transport and metabolic waste product removal. The arrangement and unique structure of the circulatory vessels permit the system to carry out these functions.

An understanding of the principles and control of flow aids in the comprehension of the pathologic conditions resulting in alterations in flow. Principles of flow, or the hemodynamics of the circulation, include concepts and physical laws relating to relationships of flow, pressure and resistance, velocity, laminar and turbulent flow, and wall tension and compliance. Control of blood flow occurs through both extrinsic and intrinsic mechanisms. Lymphatic flow is controlled through the lymphatic pump system, governed by skeletal muscle, and the smooth muscle of organs and arteries.

Pathophysiologic changes that result in alterations in blood flow can be classified as due to either obstruction (thrombosis, emboli, vasospasm, inflammation, mechanical compression) or structural alterations (valvular incompetence, arteriosclerosis/atherosclerosis, aneurysms, AVFs). Conditions that produce alterations in arterial or venous flow are due to one of these primary processes. Pathologic conditions of the lymphatic system are essentially due to disruption of the normal pressure relationships or an obstruction within the circulatory system; proper functioning of the lymphatic system depends on the appropriate functioning of the vascular system.

MEDIA RESOURCES

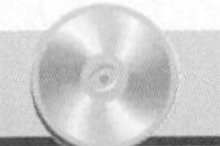

evolve

Remember to check out the ***CD Companion*** included with this book for Review Questions, Key Concepts Review, Glossary (with audio for selected terms), Disease Profiles, and Animations.

PLUS, visit the ***Evolve website*** at http://evolve.elsevier.com/Copstead/ for Case Studies, Disease Profiles, and WebLinks.

References

1. Guyton A: *Textbook of medical physiology,* ed 10, Philadelphia, 2000, Saunders.
2. Fuster V et al, editors: *Hurst's the heart,* ed 10, New York, 2001, McGraw-Hill.
3. Halcox J: Effect of sildenafil on human vascular function, platelet activation and myocardial ischemia, *J Am Coll Cardiol* 40(7):1232-1239, 2002.
4. Britten A: Clinical importance of coronary endothelial vasodilator dysfunction and therapeutic options, *J Intern Med* 245:315-327, 1999.
5. Raitakari O: Testing for endothelial dysfunction, *Ann Med* 32(5):293-304, 2000.
6. Perticone F: Prognostic significance of endothelial dysfunction in hypertensive patients, *Circulation* 104:191-196, 2001.
7. Paniagua O: Transient hypertension directly impairs endothelium-dependent vasodilation of the human microvasculature, *Hypertension* 36:941-944, 2000.
8. Taddei S: Restoration of nitric oxide availability after calcium antagonist treatment in essential hypertension, *Hypertension* 37:943-948, 2001.
9. Jensen-Urstad K: Gender difference in age-related changes in vascular function, *J Intern Med* 250:29-36, 2001.
10. Felmeden D: Low-density lipoprotein subfractions and cardiovascular risk in hypertension: relationship to endothelial dysfunction and effects of treatment, *Hypertension* 41(3):528-533, 2003.
11. Ignatavicius D et al, editors: *Medical-surgical nursing: critical thinking for collaborative care,* ed 4, Philadelphia, 2002, Saunders.
12. Tovey C, Wyatt S: Diagnosis, investigation, and management of deep vein thrombosis, *BMJ* 326:1180-1184, 2003.
13. Lehne R: *Pharmacology for nursing care,* ed 4, Philadelphia, 2001, Saunders.
14. Ganong WF: *Review of medical physiology,* ed 20, Norwalk, 2001, Appleton & Lange.
15. Dawber TR: *The Framingham Study: the epidemiology of atherosclerotic disease,* Cambridge, Mass., 1980, Harvard University Press.
16. Expert Panel on Detection, Evaluation, and Treatment of High Blood Cholesterol in Adults: Executive summary of the third report of the National Cholesterol Education Program (NCEP) expert panel on detection, evaluation and treatment of high blood cholesterol in adults, *JAMA* 285(19):2486-2497, 2001.
17. Luc G: Lipoprotein(a) as a predictor of coronary heart disease: the PRIME study, *Atherosclerosis* 163:377-384, 2002.
18. von Eckardstein A et al: Lipoprotein(a) further increases the risk of coronary events in men with high global cardiovascular risk, *J Am Coll Cardiol* 37(2)434-439, 2001.
19. Marcovina S: Lipoprotein(a) and coronary heart disease risk, *Curr Cardiol Rep* 1(2):105-111, 1999.
20. Bolego C: Smoking and gender, *Cardiovasc Res* 53:568-576, 2002.
21. Wilson J et al, editors: *Harrison's principles of internal medicine,* ed 15, New York, 2001, McGraw-Hill.
22. Redberg R: The epidemiology of cardiovascular disease in women, *Manag Care Interface* suppl A:6-9, 17, 2000.
23. Hughs S: Improving cardiovascular health in women: an opportunity for nursing, *J Cardiovasc Nurs,* 19(2):145-147, 2004.
24. Woman's Health Group: Risks and benefits of estrogen plus progestin in healthy postmenopausal women, *JAMA* 288(3):321-333, 2002.
25. Budoff M: Ethnic differences in coronary atherosclerosis, *J Am Coll Cardiol* 39(3):408-412, 2002.
26. Ansell B: Developing a clinical strategy for cholesterol management in an era of unanswered questions, *Am J Cardiol* 88(suppl):25f-30f, 2001.
27. McCormick J: Pharmacologic treatment of dyslipidemia, *Am J Nurs* 100(2):55-60, 2000.
28. Ginsberg H: Hypertriglyceridemia: new insights and new approaches to pharmacologic therapy, *Am J Cardiol* 87:1174-1180, 2001.
29. Walsh J: Drug treatment of hyperlipidemia in women, *JAMA* 291(181):2243-2252, 2004.
30. Olin JW: Thromboangiitis obliterans (Buerger's disease), *N Engl J Med* 343(12):864-869, 2000.
31. Kurata A: Thromboangiitis obliterans: classic and new morphological features, *Virchows Arch* 463:59-67, 2000.
32. Bowling J: Raynaud's disease, *Lancet* 361(9374):2078-2080, 2003.
33. Wigley F: Raynaud's phenomenon, *N Engl J Med* 347(13):1001-1008, 2002.
34. Terramani T: New approaches to abdominal aortic aneurysm, *Emerg Med* 12:22-28, 2002.
35. Beese-Biurstrom S: Aortic aneurysm and dissections, *Nursing* 34(2):36-42, 2004.
36. Nordt T: Thrombolysis: newer fibrinolytic agents and their role in clinical medicine, *Heart* 59(11):1358-1362, 2003.
37. Dorgan S: Management options for patients with intermittent claudication, *Br J Nurs* 13(8):448-451, 2004.
38. Phillips T: Current approaches to venous ulcers and compression, *Dermatol Surg* 27:611-621, 2001.
39. Cavorsi J: Venous ulcers of the lower extremities: current and newer management techniques, *Top Geriatr Rehabil* 16(2):24-34, 2000.
40. Hull M: Lymphedema in women treated for breast cancer, *Semin Oncol Nurs* 16(3):226-237, 2000.
41. Sieggreen MY, Kline RA: Current concepts in lymphedema management, *Adv Skin Wound Care* 17(4):174-178, 2004.

chapter 16

Alterations in Blood Pressure

Katherina P. Choka

MEDIA RESOURCES

Additional Material for Study, Review, and Further Exploration

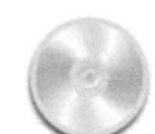

CD Companion ◆ Review Questions and Answers ◆ Key Concepts Review ◆ Glossary *(with audio pronunciations for selected terms)* ◆ Disease Profiles ◆ Animations

evolve ***Website*** at http://evolve.elsevier.com/Copstead/ ◆ Case Studies ◆ Disease Profiles ◆ WebLinks

KEY QUESTIONS

- How do changes in cardiac output and systemic vascular resistance affect blood pressure?
- How is blood pressure detected and regulated by the autonomic nervous system?
- What are the risk factors for development of primary and secondary high blood pressure?
- How is high blood pressure detected, classified, and managed?
- What are the pathologic consequences of uncontrolled high blood pressure?
- How is orthostatic hypotension defined, detected, and managed?

CHAPTER OUTLINE

A complex array of cardiovascular mechanisms work together with the actions of other systems to perfuse body tissues. Chapter 15 presented mechanisms that control blood flow. For the human body to function effectively, an adequate perfusion pressure must accompany blood flow.

Arterial blood pressure is the driving force that propels blood throughout the body. Blood pressure is closely regulated to maintain adequate perfusion pressure to vital organs. This chapter describes factors affecting blood pressure, measurement of blood pressure, and alterations in blood pressure.

FUNCTION OF THE ARTERIAL AND PULMONARY SYSTEMS

Arterial blood pressure is generated by the heart as it contracts and ejects blood into the systemic arterial vascular system. As blood travels through the vascular system, the pressure decreases: rapidly as the blood passes through the arterioles and then more slowly as it passes through the capillaries and the venous system (Figure 16-1). By the time that the blood has returned to the right atrium, the pressure is almost entirely dissipated. This decrease in pressure is due to the resistance to flow offered by the vascular system; the arterioles provide the most resistance. Because fluid moves from an area of high pressure to an area of low pressure, the pressure difference between the aorta and the right atrium is the force that propels blood through the vasculature.

Arterial blood pressure is recorded as a systolic and a diastolic value. During ventricular contraction, the pressure in the aorta and brachial artery rises to an average peak value of 120 mm Hg. This is termed the *systolic blood pressure.* Systolic blood pressure is a function of the volume ejected and the compliance of the aorta. During the diastolic phase of the cardiac cycle, the pressure within the aorta and brachial arteries falls to an average minimum value of 70 mm Hg. This is termed the *diastolic blood pressure.* Passive elastic recoil of the aorta ejects blood into peripheral arteries during this phase, and the pressure never falls to zero.[1-3] Pulmonary and systemic arteries contribute to the overall peripheral resistance. However, due to the thin-walled, highly distensible pulmonary artery systems that lacks smooth muscle, the pulmonary vascular resistance is lower (see Figure 16-1).[4]

Systemic vascular resistance (SVR) is the major determinant of diastolic blood pressure. SVR reflects arteriolar radius, the degree of constriction, and is the main variable in determining afterload. Narrowing of vessel diameter increases SVR and diastolic pressure; vasodilation reduces SVR. Many factors can increase or decrease SVR, and these will be discussed later in this chapter. Most patients that have hypertension have increased SVR with a normal cardiac output (CO). However, it has been postulated that early hypertension may be due to a raised CO and sympathetic overactivity.[3,5] Furthermore, isolated systolic hypertension is often seen in the elderly and is not always accompanied by an increase in SVR. The rise

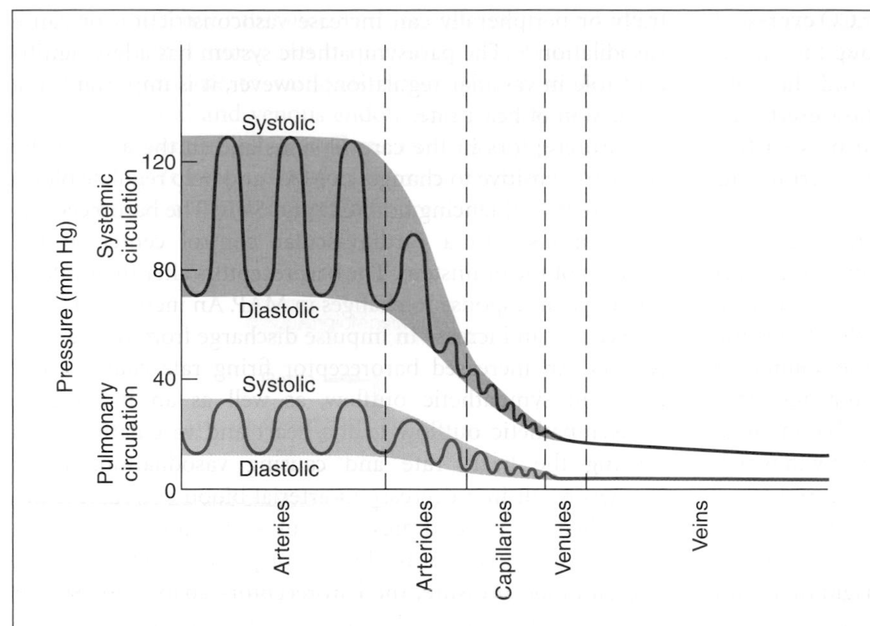

FIGURE 16-1 ■ Changes in pressure through the vascular system. (Redrawn from Vander AJ, Sherman JH, Luciano DS: *Human physiology: the mechanisms of body function,* ed 7, New York, 1998, McGraw-Hill, p 408. Reproduced by permission of McGraw-Hill.)

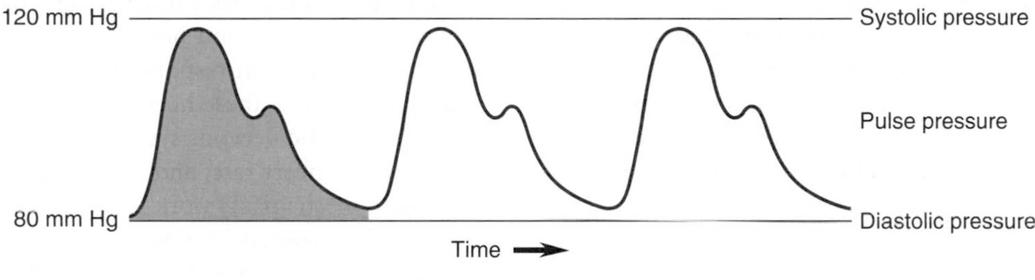

FIGURE 16-2 ■ Arterial pressure pulse showing systolic, diastolic, and pulse pressures and graphic calculation of mean arterial pressure.

in systolic blood pressure is due to the lack of elasticity of the large arteries.[6]

Arterial Pressure Pulses

The difference between systolic and diastolic blood pressure is termed the **arterial pulse pressure** (Figure 16-2). **Pulse pressure** is determined by stroke volume (the amount of blood ejected with each heart beat), the speed at which the stroke volume is ejected, and arterial distensibility.[2] A narrowed pulse pressure can be a reflection of reduced stroke volume.[4]

Mean arterial pressure (MAP) is the average pressure in the circulatory system throughout the cardiac cycle. Because more time is spent in diastole than in systole at normal heart rates, MAP is not the arithmetic average of diastolic and systolic pressure but rather reflects the relative time spent in each portion of the cardiac cycle. MAP is used to assess circulatory status and to titrate vasoactive medication. MAP is derived most accurately by using intraarterial blood pressure measurement and dividing the area under the arterial pressure curve by the time needed for one cardiac cycle (see Figure 16-2). In the absence of an intraarterial catheter, MAP may be estimated by the formula "diastolic pressure plus one third of the pulse pressure."[4] For example, when the blood pressure is 110/80 mm Hg, MAP is estimated to be 90 mm Hg in the following way:

$$\text{Pulse pressure} = 110 - 80 = 30 \text{ mm Hg}$$
$$\text{MAP} = \text{diastolic pressure} + (\text{pulse pressure}/3)$$
$$\text{MAP} = 80 \text{ mm Hg} + (30 \text{ mm Hg}/3) = 90 \text{ mm Hg}$$

This formula is based on the assumption that the heart rate is approximately 60 beats/min. With chronically ill patients who are often tachycardic, the diastolic pressure may be less than one half, making this calculation inaccurate.[4]

Determinants of Blood Pressure

The relation between pressure, flow, and resistance in a system is defined by the following formula: flow is equal to the change in pressure along the tube divided by resistance (see Chapter

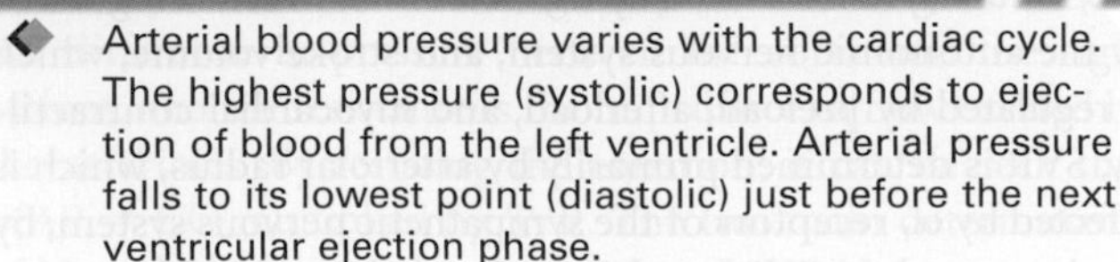

- Arterial blood pressure varies with the cardiac cycle. The highest pressure (systolic) corresponds to ejection of blood from the left ventricle. Arterial pressure falls to its lowest point (diastolic) just before the next ventricular ejection phase.
- The pulse pressure is the difference between systolic and diastolic pressure. MAP is the average pressure throughout the cardiac cycle (estimated as diastolic plus one third of the pulse pressure). MAP is the product of CO and SVR.
- Arterioles create most of the resistance in the circulation. Arteriolar diameter profoundly affects arterial resistance and therefore blood pressure.
- The aortic and carotid baroreceptors are important regulators of arterial blood pressure. A reduction in arterial pressure results in activation of sympathetic nerves to the heart and vessels and inhibition of parasympathetic influence on the heart. Blood pressure returns to normal as the heart rate, CO, and SVR increase.
- A number of chemical mediators influence arteriolar diameter and therefore blood pressure. Mediators that generally cause vasoconstriction and elevate blood pressure include angiotensin II, vasopressin, endothelin, and thromboxane A_2. Blood pressure–reducing mediators include histamine, some prostaglandins, prostacyclin, and nitric oxide.

MEASUREMENT OF ARTERIAL BLOOD PRESSURE

Methods of Measuring Arterial Blood Pressure

Indirect Methods

Blood pressure is most commonly measured indirectly with a sphygmomanometer and a stethoscope. A hollow bladder within a cuff, the sphygmomanometer is wrapped around a limb, usually the upper part of the arm. If possible, the patient's arm should be at the level of the heart and supported.[13] As the brachial or radial artery is palpated, the cuff is inflated while the observer notes at what level the pulse disappears. Cuff inflation is continued for another 30 mm Hg; the cuff is then gradually deflated until the pulse reappears. This number reflects the systolic blood pressure and may be recorded as a palpated value, such as 120/P. When the palpatory method is used, no diastolic value is obtained.[14] Assessment of the lower extremity blood pressure may be necessary in certain situations. The technique used is identical to brachial except the popliteal artery is used. Systolic pressure in the legs is 10 to 40 mm Hg higher than in the brachial artery.[14]

The technique for obtaining an auscultated blood pressure is similar to that for palpating the pulse to determine blood pressure. After the cuff is applied and inflated to 30 mm Hg above the patient's palpated systolic blood pressure, the cuff is gradually deflated while the observer listens through the stethoscope placed over the brachial artery. The return of blood flow through the artery is signaled by **Korotkoff sounds,** named after the Russian physician who first described them. The sounds are due to turbulent flow through the partially occluded artery (Table 16-1).[14]

Phase I is associated with the onset of tapping sounds heard through the stethoscope and is recorded as the systolic blood pressure. In the past, phase IV was used as the diastolic blood pressure in children. Recent studies have determined that phase V, the disappearance of Korotkoff sounds, should be used for diastolic blood pressure in both children and adults.[9-12]

Palpation of the radial artery during cuff inflation ensures that an auscultatory gap will not be missed. The **auscultatory gap** is the time during cuff deflation after systolic blood pressure measurement when the Korotkoff sounds disappear (Figure 16-5). Although the sounds disappear, the ability to palpate the pulse does not. This generally occurs between the first and second Korotkoff sounds. If the cuff was not inflated high enough initially, the resumption of Korotkoff sounds during phase III may be mistaken for the onset of sounds in phase I.

An auscultatory gap happens most frequently in persons with hypertension; if the auscultatory gap is missed, the systolic blood pressure recorded will be too low or the diastolic recorded as abnormally high. Once the blood pressure is known and an auscultatory gap is ruled out, it is not necessary to estimate blood pressure by palpating the pulse before auscultation. The palpatory method is also useful when auscultatory blood pressure is difficult to obtain, such as in persons with low blood pressure, as in shock.[14]

Another indirect method combines the Doppler technique with the use of a sphygmomanometer. Ultrasonic impulses are transmitted from a transducer placed over an artery to the blood cells flowing through the artery. The impulses are reflected back to the transducer, which translates the impulses into audible sound. As the blood pressure cuff is deflated, the transducer is placed over an artery. The onset of sounds from the Doppler instrument is equivalent to phase I Korotkoff

Table 16-1

Korotkoff Sounds

Phase	Description
I	Initiation of clear tapping sounds—systolic blood pressure
II	Murmuring or swishing sounds
III	Increase in intensity and crispness of sounds
IV	Muffling of sounds
V	Disappearance of sounds—diastolic blood pressure

sounds and signals systolic blood pressure. It is recorded as a Doppler pressure, such as 120/D. As with palpated pressures, no diastolic measurement is obtained. This technique, as with palpated measurement, is useful in persons in whom blood pressure is difficult to measure by auscultation (e.g., persons with low blood pressure).[4]

Direct Methods

Direct measurement of arterial blood pressure is also possible. A catheter is introduced into a peripheral artery such as the radial, brachial, or femoral artery and connected to a pressure transducer. Pressure from the artery is transmitted to and exerts pressure on the diaphragm at the air-fluid interface in a dome attached to the transducer. The transducer converts the pressure on the diaphragm to electrical signals. The electrical signals are amplified, filtered, and displayed on a monitor in waveforms. Digital readings of systolic pressure, diastolic pressure, and MAP are often displayed.[4]

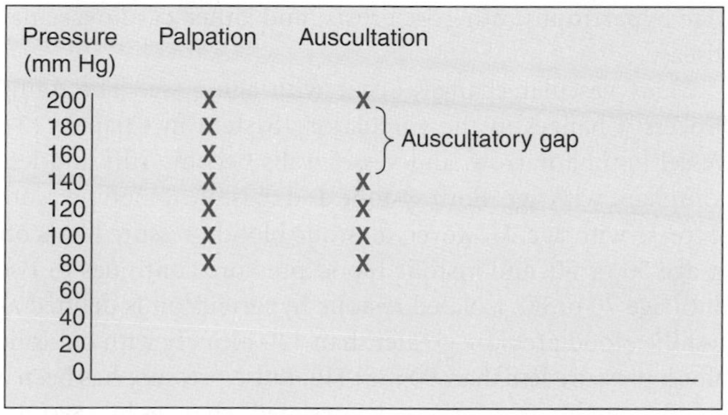

Pressure (mm Hg)	Palpation	Auscultation
200	X	X
180	X	Auscultatory gap
160	X	
140	X	X
120	X	X
100	X	X
80	X	X
60		
40		
20		
0		

FIGURE 16-5 ■ Auscultatory gap. Palpating the blood pressure (BP) before auscultation allows one to assess the true systolic BP. Palpated BP equals 200/P. Auscultated BP when the cuff is inflated to only 180 mm Hg results in a falsely low value of 140/80 mm Hg.

Factors That Affect Blood Pressure Measurement

A number of factors can affect blood pressure measurements. These factors are of two major types: technical factors and factors involving the subjective influence of the observer (Table 16-2). Technical aspects include such things as body positioning and size of the cuff used. If the arm used for blood pressure measurement is positioned above the level of the heart, the blood pressure may be artificially lowered; if the arm is positioned below the heart, blood pressure may be artificially raised. If the arm is unsupported, isometric activity by the patient in an effort to keep the arm elevated may result in falsely high readings. The American Heart Association recommends the use of a cuff with a bladder width that is 40% of the circumference of the midpoint of the limb. Use of cuffs with bladders that are too narrow results in falsely elevated blood pressure readings; use of bladders that are too wide results in erroneously low readings.[14]

Table 16-2

Technical, Subjective, and Other Factors That Influence Blood Pressure Readings

Factor	Effect on Blood Pressure
Technical Factors	
Cuff	
Too wide, too long	BP falsely low
Too narrow, too short	BP falsely high
Arm position	
Above heart	BP falsely low
Below heart	BP falsely high
Unsupported	BP falsely high
Excessive pressure on head of stethoscope	Diastolic progressively decreased with increased pressure
<1 min between readings	BP falsely high
Respiration	BP increased during inspiration
Subjective Factors	
Terminal digit preference	Tendency to end BP in zero
Observer bias	Record BP higher or lower, depending on recorder's biases
Poor hearing	Altered reading
Other Factors	
"White coat" phenomenon	Higher BP reading when measured by a physician
Eating, smoking, taking caffeine, exercising within 30 min of BP	Increased BP
Speaking while BP measured	Increased BP

BP, Blood pressure.

KEY CONCEPTS

- Arterial blood pressure is recorded as the onset of Kortkoff sounds (systolic) and the disappearance of sounds (diastolic).
- Erroneous blood pressure measurements may be due to a missed auscultatory gap, hydrostatic pressure changes with changes in arm position, inappropriate cuff size, or observer bias.

HYPERTENSION

High blood pressure is defined in adults as systemic blood pressure persistently elevated above 140 mm Hg systolic, 90 mm Hg diastolic, or both. Those with diabetes mellitus or kidney disease with greater than 1 g/day proteinuria should aim for a blood pressure of less than or equal to 130/80 mm Hg. In the United States, more than 50 million people have or are being treated for high blood pressure.[15] A classification scheme for blood pressure has been developed by the Joint National Committee on Prevention, Detection, Evaluation, and Treatment of High Blood Pressure (JNC7). Categories for classifying high blood pressure now include prehypertension with hopes that treatment can be started before complications have taken place. Table 16-3 lists the new classification of blood pressure. If the systolic and diastolic values fall in different stages, the higher stage is used to indicate appropriate treatment.[16] Primary and secondary causes of hypertension are discussed later in this chapter (see the Classification of High Blood Pressure section).

Risk Factors

Age

Blood pressure rises consistently with age, beginning at levels as low as 50/40 mm Hg in newborns and increasing to over 200 mm Hg in some elderly subjects.[8] High blood pressure in children is classified as "significant" when it is greater than or equal to the 95th percentile for age and as "severe" when it is greater than or equal to the 99th percentile for age. In addition, evaluation of the child's height is necessary to accurately interpret blood pressure (Box 16-1 and Table 16-4). Taller children have higher blood pressure and should be evaluated in terms of norms corresponding to children of equal height.[17,18] For example, a tall 16-year-old boy with a blood pressure of 130/84 would not be considered to have hypertension, but a 16-year-old boy at the 5th percentile for height with the same blood pressure would be considered to have hypertension. High blood pressure in childhood is a predictor of hypertension in adult life, especially in association with obesity. Furthermore, blood pressure elevation in children is a risk factor for early development of left ventricular hypertrophy, atherosclerosis, and other cardiovascular disease.[19,20]

Many vascular changes occur with aging (see The Aging Process: Changes in the Circulatory System in Chapter 15). Vessel lumina narrow, and vessel walls become stiff and less compliant with age. Both systolic and diastolic blood pressure increase with age. However, diastolic blood pressure levels off at age 50 or 60, and systolic blood pressure continues to rise until age 70 or 80. Isolated systolic hypertension is defined as systolic blood pressure greater than 140 mm Hg with diastolic blood pressure less than 90 mm Hg. Pulse pressure has been a helpful predictor of these age-related changes.[6,21] Systolic blood pressure has been found to be a more accurate predictor of mortality and cardiovascular events than diastolic blood pressure in the elderly.[22]

Race

Hypertension in African-Americans is among the highest in the world.[23] They have higher rates of stage 2 hypertension than whites with respectively higher cardiovascular mortality rates than the general population.[16,24] Furthermore, there is earlier evidence of target organ damage such as increased left ventricular mass than whites with similar blood pressure levels. Although the exact cause for these differences is unclear, salt sensitivity, elevated endothelin levels, and decreased renin levels have been proposed as possible factors.[5,24-26]

Table 16-3

Classification of Blood Pressure in Adults

Category	SBP (mm Hg)		DBP (mm Hg)
Normal	<120	and	<80
Prehypertension	120-139	or	80-89
Hypertension, stage 1	140-159	or	90-99
Hypertension, stage 2	≥160	or	≥100

From U.S. Department of Health and Human Services (National Institutes of Health, National Heart, Lung, and Blood Institute): *The seventh report of the Joint National Committee on Prevention, Detection, Evaluation, and Treatment of High Blood Pressure (JNC7),* NIH Publication No 03-5231, May 2003.
SBP, Systolic blood pressure; *DBP,* diastolic blood pressure.

Box 16-1

Classification of Blood Pressure in Children and Adolescents*

SBP and DBP <90th percentile	Normal
SBP or DBP ≥90th percentile and <95th percentile	High-normal†
SBP or DBP ≥95th percentile	Hypertension†

Selected data from the *Update on the task force report (1987) on high blood pressure in children and adolescents: a working group report from the National High Blood Pressure Education Program,* NIH Pub No 96-3790, Bethesda, Md, September 1996, National Heart, Lung, and Blood Institute.
SBP, Systolic blood pressure; *DBP,* diastolic blood pressure.
*For age and sex.
†For age and sex measured on at least three separate occasions.

Obesity

Excess weight is associated with elevated levels of blood pressure.[19] Obesity in childhood is a predictor of high blood pressure in adulthood. Obese persons are three times more likely to develop hypertension, with young adults having a 5.5-fold increased likelihood of developing hypertension. There is a strong relationship between hyperinsulinemia, obesity, and hypertension. Weight reduction in overweight individuals is known to reduce blood pressure.[27,28]

Table 16-4

Blood Pressure Levels for the 90th and 95th Percentiles of Blood Pressure for Boys and Girls Aged 1 to 17 Years by Percentiles of Height*

	Systolic BP (mm Hg)†							Diastolic BP (mm Hg)†						
Age (yr)‡	**5th**	**10th**	**25th**	**50th**	**75th**	**90th**	**95th**	**5th**	**10th**	**25th**	**50th**	**75th**	**90th**	**95th**
Boys														
1														
90th	94	95	97	98	100	102	102	50	51	52	53	54	54	55
95th	98	99	102	102	104	106	106	55	55	56	57	58	59	59
3														
90th	100	101	103	105	107	108	109	59	59	60	61	62	63	63
95th	104	105	107	109	111	112	113	63	63	64	65	66	67	67
6														
90th	105	106	108	110	111	113	114	67	68	69	70	70	71	72
95th	109	110	112	114	115	117	117	72	72	73	74	75	76	76
10														
90th	110	112	113	115	117	118	119	73	74	74	75	76	77	78
95th	114	115	117	119	121	122	123	77	78	79	80	80	81	82
13														
90th	117	118	120	122	124	125	126	75	76	76	77	78	79	80
95th	121	122	124	126	128	129	130	79	80	81	82	83	83	84
17														
90th	128	129	131	133	134	136	136	81	81	82	83	84	85	85
95th	132	133	135	136	138	140	140	83	85	86	87	88	89	89
Girls														
1														
90th	97	98	99	100	102	103	104	53	53	53	54	55	56	56
95th	101	102	103	104	105	107	107	57	57	57	58	59	60	60
3														
90th	100	100	102	103	104	105	106	61	61	61	62	63	63	64
95th	104	104	105	107	108	109	110	65	65	65	66	67	67	68
6														
90th	104	105	106	107	109	110	111	67	67	68	69	69	70	71
95th	108	109	110	111	112	114	114	71	71	72	73	73	74	75
10														
90th	112	112	114	115	116	117	118	73	73	73	74	75	76	76
95th	116	116	117	119	120	121	122	77	77	77	78	79	80	80
13														
90th	118	118	119	121	122	123	124	80	80	81	82	82	83	84
95th	121	122	123	125	126	127	128	80	80	81	82	82	83	84
17														
90th	122	123	124	125	126	128	128	79	79	79	80	81	82	82
95th	126	126	127	129	130	131	132	83	83	83	84	85	86	86

Selected data from the *Update on the task force report (1987) on high blood pressure in children and adolescents: a working group report from the National High Blood Pressure Education Program,* NIH Pub No 96-3790, Bethesda, Md, September 1996, National Heart, Lung, and Blood Institute.

*Compare the child's systolic and diastolic BPs with the numbers provided in the table, using the age and the height percentile. The child is normotensive if BP is below the 90th percentile. If the child's BP (systolic or diastolic) is at or above the 95th percentile, the child may be hypertensive and needs further evaluation.

†The column headings *5th, 10th, 25th, 50th, 75th, 90th,* and *95th* are height percentiles, which are determined by standard growth curves.

‡In this column, *90th* and *95th* are BP percentiles, which are determined by a single measurement.

Nutritional Factors

Evidence-based research supports sodium as the nutrient most often associated with hypertension.[29] The mechanism of sodium-related hypertension is multifactorial including elements of the renin-angiotensin-aldosterone system, nitric oxide, catecholamines, endothelin, and atrial natriuretic peptide. Salt restriction decreases the development of left ventricular hypertrophy and reduces aortic stiffness.[30,31]

Potassium, magnesium, and calcium may also have a role in hypertension. Increasing the intake of potassium to a serum level of 4.0 has an antihypertensive effect by increasing natriuresis, increasing vasodilation, and lowering cardiovascular reactivity to catecholamines and angiotensin II.[32] A low serum potassium level in itself can cause sodium retention, possibly contributing to hypertension.[30] Calcium supplementation improves vasorelaxation by enhancing hyperpolarization and improving nitric oxide sensitivity.[33] Ongoing research suggests that magnesium has a mild antihypertensive effect.[29]

Classification of High Blood Pressure

Primary High Blood Pressure

Primary (essential or idiopathic) hypertension accounts for approximately 95% of all cases of hypertension. These cases of hypertension are defined as such when secondary causes including renovascular disease, aldosteronism, pheochromocytoma, renal failure, and others are not present.[34] Genetics also plays a part in the development of high blood pressure.[35] In addition, environmental factors such as stress, moderate alcohol intake, smoking, and a sedentary lifestyle contribute to high blood pressure.[16]

As mentioned earlier, other areas of inquiry into the causes of primary hypertension include increased sensitivity to angiotensin II and the associated effects on nitric oxide in the development of hypertension. Blockage of the endogenous substance nitric oxide results in increased sympathetic firing and elevated blood pressure. Animal studies suggest that hypertensive rats are deficient in the production of nitric oxide.[7] Also, angiotensin II elevation may negate the vasodilatory properties of nitric oxide. Stress can have a role in chronically high levels of angiotensin II.[12]

Physiologic Mechanisms. Alterations in a variety of physiologic mechanisms are currently being investigated for their role in high blood pressure. The renin-angiotensin-aldosterone system and the mechanisms controlling sodium excretion are of interest. The renin-angiotensin-aldosterone system is usually activated in response to low renal perfusion, decreased sodium delivery, and sympathetic stimulation. Activation of this system results in renal retention of sodium and water and excretion of potassium, which increases vascular volume, renal perfusion, and blood pressure. In situations of low circulating fluid volume and sodium deficiency, renin activity is stimulated and sodium and water retention and vasoconstriction are produced.[9] African-Americans have been found to have low renin activity.[36] This low renin activity is linked to sodium sensitivity and excess. However, the effect is the same as in persons with high renin activity: increased vascular volume and elevated blood pressure. Most people with high blood pressure have normal renin activity levels.[25]

The vascular endothelium is now recognized to be a hormone-producing endocrine gland in its own right. There are various categories of endothelins, with endothelin-1 being most significant in relation to hypertension. Circulatory endothelin-1 has potent vasoconstrictor effects and contributes to abnormal vascular reactivity.[25]

Diabetes mellitus has been identified as a risk factor for primary hypertension. In type II diabetes, hypertension is often associated with obesity, dyslipidemia, and insulin resistance.[37] Furthermore, hyperinsulinemia and insulin resistance without a diagnosis of type II diabetes account for approximately 50% of individuals with essential hypertension.[37] Ongoing research may support earlier screening for hyperinsulinemia in preventing hypertension. The hypertensive mechanisms of insulin are not yet known; hypotheses include increased norepinephrine release, sodium retention, and increased vascular tone by affecting the sodium transport mechanisms in blood vessels. Insulin resistance is associated with enhanced sympathetic nervous system activity, as indicated by an elevated heart rate.[26] Insulin is also associated with an accelerated rate of atherosclerosis development.[27] Hyperinsulinism and insulin resistance have been noted in nonobese normotensive individuals with a family history of hypertension.[38,39]

Secondary High Blood Pressure

Hypertension that can be explained by a specific disease is termed secondary. In children with high blood pressure, most cases are attributable to an identifiable cause. Essential hypertension in children, although less common, has a strong family component.[40] However, researchers are finding more children to have no identifiable cause for their hypertension than in previous years. Early hyperinsulinemia, hyperlipidemia, and obesity require further research to determine their roles in hypertension. Hypertension in children is associated with left ventricular hypertrophy.[19,20]

Renal Disorders. Renal disease is the most common cause of secondary high blood pressure in children and adults. Conditions that produce excess secretion of renin may result in high blood pressure. For example, renal artery stenosis may cause a reduction in renal perfusion, stimulate activation of the renin-angiotensin-aldosterone system, and result in increased renin. Subsequent retention of sodium and water, along with vasoconstriction, results in elevated blood pressure. Wilms tumor, a renin-secreting tumor that causes an increase in blood pressure, activates the renin-angiotensin-aldosterone system, with resultant sodium and water retention and vasoconstriction. Any form of renal failure that results in retention of sodium and water may produce hypertension. Hypertension may also cause renal failure by damaging the arterioles that supply the kidneys.

A reduction in blood flow to the kidneys stimulates the renin-angiotensin-aldosterone system to promote sodium and water retention and vasoconstriction, which further reduces blood flow. This vicious cycle continues and aggravates the renal failure and hypertension.[40,41]

Endocrine Disorders. Elevated levels of adrenocortical hormones can result in high blood pressure. Both the glucocorticoids (e.g., cortisol) and mineralocorticoids (e.g., aldosterone) promote sodium and water retention by the kidneys and thereby result in elevated blood pressure. Examples of conditions that produce excesses of these hormones are primary aldosteronism, Cushing syndrome, and exogenous administration of glucocorticoids.[40]

Pheochromocytomas, tumors of chromaffin tissue seen most commonly in the adrenal medullae, secrete catecholamines, which produce sympathetic nervous system stimulation resulting in vasoconstriction, increased heart rate, and increased CO. This excess secretion of catecholamines dramatically elevates blood pressure and may result in death within 6 months if not treated.[8]

Other endocrine disorders that may result in high blood pressure include acromegaly, which is associated with increased aldosterone levels (producing sodium and water retention), and hypothyroidism or hyperthyroidism. Hypothyroidism causes a reduction in CO; this reduction is balanced by an increase in SVR, which produces elevated diastolic blood pressure readings. Thyroid hormone enhances the effects of the sympathetic nervous system (faster heart rate, strengthened contractility, and vasoconstriction); hyperthyroidism may therefore also cause high blood pressure.[40]

Vascular Disorders. Arteriosclerosis causes an increase in SVR and therefore an increase in blood pressure, particularly diastolic blood pressure. In addition, arteriosclerosis may cause narrowing of renal arteries resulting in stimulation of the renin-angiotensin-aldosterone system. Paradoxically, high blood pressure accelerates atherosclerosis, and a self-perpetuating cycle is produced.[8]

Coarctation of the aorta may produce high blood pressure in children and adults. Ejection of blood into the narrowed aorta results in an elevated systolic blood pressure in the arms. An identifying feature of high blood pressure caused by coarctation of the aorta is the presence of normal or lower blood pressure in the legs than in the arms. Normally, blood pressure is higher in the legs than in the arms.[40]

Neurologic Disorders. Problems that cause elevated intracranial pressure, such as intracerebral hemorrhage and subdural hematoma, may result in elevated blood pressure. Pressure on the posterior hypothalamus, the medulla, or nerve pathways (such as from tumors) may produce excessive catecholamine secretion and increased blood pressure. Benign or malignant tumors of the sympathetic nervous system may produce hypertension.[2]

Spinal cord injuries may produce hypertension in response to stimuli such as a full bladder, a phenomenon called autonomic hyperreflexia or dysreflexia (see Chapter 45).[2]

Exogenous Compounds. Many prescription and over-the-counter medications can cause elevations in blood pressure. Sympathomimetics (drugs that evoke the effects of impulses conveyed by postganglionic fibers of the sympathetic nervous system), amphetamines, tricyclic antidepressants, corticosteroids, and oral contraceptives are some of the drugs known to produce high blood pressure.[8] Caffeine and nicotine, by producing vasoconstriction, can also increase blood pressure (Box 16-2). So-called recreational drugs, particularly cocaine, may also have significant cardiovascular effects, including hypertension. Special concerns in adolescents include all of the aforementioned, plus anabolic steroid use, ethanol use, tobacco chewing, and cigarette smoking.[15,16]

Isolated Systolic Hypertension in Elderly Persons

After the age of 65 to 69, the prevalence of hypertension increases to 50%. Isolated systolic hypertension is defined as systolic blood pressure greater than or equal to 140 mm Hg with

Box 16-2 

Substances that Increase Blood Pressure

Over-the-Counter and Prescription Medications
Sympathomimetic substances
- Amphetamines
- Epinephrine
- Dopamine

Tricyclic antidepressants
Anabolic steroids
Corticosteroids
Monoamine oxidase inhibitors
Oral contraceptives

Trace Metals, Minerals, and Electrolytes
Cadmium
Lead
Mercury
Sodium
Zinc
Selenium

Dietary Substances
Foods containing tryptophan and tyramine
- Chicken liver
- Pickled herring
- Yeast extract
- Broad beans
- Matured cheeses
- Beer
- Wines
- Caffeine
- Licorice

Other
Nicotine, including chewing tobacco

a diastolic pressure of less than 90 mm Hg. Isolated systolic hypertension is more common in women than men.[21] Widened pulse pressure is characteristic of isolated systolic hypertension.[42] Furthermore, systolic blood pressure elevation is a stronger predictor of mortality than diastolic blood pressure.[6]

Decreased distensibility of the aorta and large arteries in the elderly occurs as arteriosclerosis progresses with age. This reduced distensibility produces an elevation in systolic blood pressure without an increase in diastolic blood pressure.[21] Isolated systolic hypertension is associated with a higher risk of stroke, ischemic heart disease, and death.[42]

Treatment is geared to lowering systolic blood pressure slowly. Low-dose thiazide diuretics and slow-acting/long-acting calcium antagonists may be drugs of choice.[42] However, others classes of drugs have also been effective.

Hypertension During Pregnancy

Blood pressure normally decreases during the first two trimesters of pregnancy and gradually returns to normal levels during the third trimester. The initial decrease in blood pressure is apparently due to a decrease in SVR inasmuch as CO is increased by 40% to 60% during pregnancy. As SVR returns to normal levels, blood pressure rises. During pregnancy, levels of angiotensin II and aldosterone are also increased and promote vasoconstriction and sodium and water retention.[11,43]

Approximately 12% to 22% of pregnancies are complicated by high blood pressure.[43] The Joint National Committee on Detection, Evaluation and Treatment of High Blood Pressure classifies high blood pressure during pregnancy as follows: (1) preeclampsia-eclampsia, (2) chronic hypertension, and (3) chronic hypertension with superimposed preeclampsia.[22] About one fourth of pregnant women with high blood pressure have preeclampsia and eclampsia.[16]

Because of the cardiovascular changes that occur with pregnancy, the usual criteria for adult high blood pressure do not apply. The current classification of gestational hypertension is a blood pressure of at least 140/90 mm Hg after 20 weeks of pregnancy.

Preeclampsia-Eclampsia. Preeclampsia is characterized by elevated blood pressure, proteinuria, and edema. Maternal blood supply to the fetus is interrupted by maladaptation of maternal vessels, exaggerated inflammatory response, and failure of normal invasion of trophoblast cells. The end result is poor villus formation and placental insufficiency.[43] Associated maternal complications include decreased vascular volume, edema, hypoproteinemia, thrombocytopenia, liver involvement, and increased risk of intrauterine growth retardation. The syndrome of hemolysis, elevated liver enzymes, and low platelets is called HELLP. If not rectified, preeclampsia may progress to eclampsia, involving seizures and possibly coma.[43] Usually developing after the 20th week of gestation, preeclampsia occasionally may occur earlier in the pregnancy. Onset during the second trimester is associated with increased maternal and fetal risk.[15] The condition may occur during first and subsequent pregnancies, and blood pressure returns to normal between pregnancies. Treatment with aspirin, a prostaglandin synthesis inhibitor, may prevent preeclampsia in women at high risk, but aspirin is not recommended for healthy women without risk factors. Also, adequate calcium intake is associated with a decreased risk of preeclampsia[43,44]

Chronic hypertension in pregnancy is generally defined as hypertension before pregnancy or before 20 weeks gestation.[45,46] Blood pressure fluctuations resemble those in normal pregnant women; that is, blood pressure decreases early in the pregnancy and increases during the last 3 months. These changes in blood pressure may be mistaken for preeclampsia in women with previously undiagnosed chronic hypertension. Unlike women with preeclampsia, however, women with chronic high blood pressure will remain hypertensive after delivery. Chronic high blood pressure increases the risk of preeclampsia.[46]

Transient or late high blood pressure may occur during the last trimester of pregnancy or in the early postdelivery period. Blood pressure returns to normal levels within 10 days after delivery.[45]

Accelerated High Blood Pressure

Accelerated (malignant) high blood pressure is a rapidly progressing, potentially fatal form of hypertension in which diastolic blood pressure exceeds 120 mm Hg. Although accelerated hypertension develops in only about 1% of all hypertensive persons, the 1-year mortality rate if untreated approaches 90%. This form of high blood pressure is most likely to develop in African-Americans, males, and middle-aged people. Severe emotional stress, excessive salt intake, and abrupt discontinuation of antihypertensive medication without tapering are examples of situations that may trigger a hypertensive crisis; any disease that produces high blood pressure can result in the accelerated form. The most common mechanism of malignant hypertension is bilateral renal artery stenosis. The patient is usually symptomatic with headache, blurred vision, and dyspnea.[40]

In addition to extremely high blood pressure, evidence of target organ damage is present (Figure 16-6). Any organ may be damaged, but the kidneys are most commonly involved. Damage to the afferent arterioles produces stiff, thickened arterioles that are less responsive to changes in perfusion. Renal failure may ensue because of the hypertension or due to hypoperfusion when blood pressure is lowered. Urine output and renal function must be monitored. Other potential problems resulting from arterial damage include encephalopathy, cardiac failure, dissecting aortic aneurysm, and severe retinopathy in the form of papilledema. Hypertensive

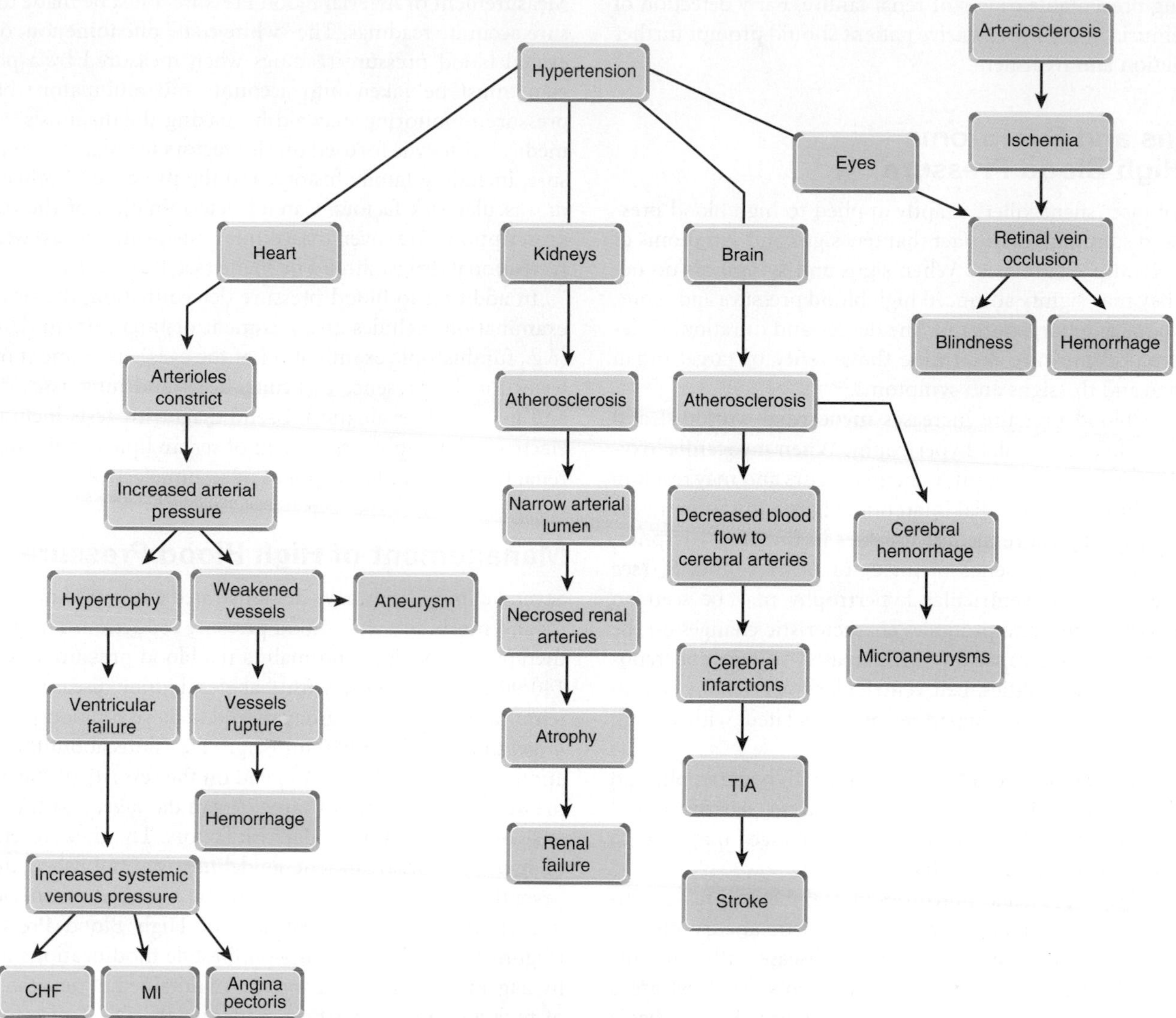

FIGURE16-6 ■ The potential effects of chronic hypertension on major target organs. *CHF,* Congestive heart failure; *MI,* myocardial infarction; *TIA,* transient ischemic attack. (From Monahan FD, Neighbors M: *Medical surgical nursing: foundations for clinical practice*, ed 2, Philadelphia, 1998, Saunders.)

retinopathy may also produce visual changes ranging from blurred vision to blindness.[40]

Effects of High Blood Pressure

Cardiac

Elevated systemic blood pressure requires that the left ventricle work harder to overcome the resistance to ejection of blood. In response, the left ventricular muscle hypertrophies, which increases myocardial oxygen demand. The workload of the left ventricle increases as blood pressure increases. When the myocardial oxygen demand exceeds the supply, ischemia develops and heart failure may ensue (see Chapter 18).[8,21]

Vascular

Sustained high blood pressure causes changes in the walls of arteries and arterioles. High blood pressure accelerates the development of atherosclerosis in the aorta and in medium-sized to large arteries; the resultant decrease in caliber of these arteries results in isolated systolic high blood pressure in the elderly. Atherosclerosis also contributes to cerebral infarction.[21,47]

Arteriosclerosis in the smaller arteries and arterioles contributes to cerebrovascular disease and peripheral vascular disease. Fibrinoid necrosis occurs in the small arterioles and produces lesions in the kidneys and in the retina. The effects of ongoing hypertension on the renal vasculature can occur rapidly and can be profound. Hypertension is one of the leading preventable causes of renal failure. Early detection of proteinuria in the hypertensive patient should prompt further evaluation and treatment.[7]

Signs and Symptoms of High Blood Pressure

The phrase "silent killer" is aptly applied to high blood pressure and summarizes the fact that few signs and symptoms of high blood pressure exist. When signs and symptoms do occur, they may signify advanced high blood pressure and represent damage to target organs. The degree and duration of elevated blood pressure determine the severity of target organ damage and the signs and symptoms.[22]

High blood pressure increases myocardial workload and produces left ventricular hypertrophy. When myocardial oxygen demand exceeds supply, ischemia occurs and may result in heart failure or myocardial infarction. Signs and symptoms of left ventricular failure include crackles in the lungs, dyspnea, fatigue, and the presence of an extra heart sound, S_3 (see Chapter 19). Left ventricular hypertrophy may be seen on chest radiographs and produces characteristic changes on the electrocardiogram consisting of increased voltage and repolarization abnormalities. Left ventricular hypertrophy is a serious consequence of hypertension associated with a high mortality rate.[6]

Acceleration of atherosclerosis along with hypertrophy and edema of vessel walls produces coronary artery narrowing and additional myocardial ischemia. These changes may lead to angina pectoris and myocardial infarction.

Other cardiovascular outcomes of high blood pressure include the development and rupture of aortic aneurysms and the development of peripheral arterial disease with intermittent claudication. Cerebrovascular accidents (strokes) are a major complication of high blood pressure. Hemorrhagic stroke is commonly associated with high blood pressure and has a high mortality rate. Signs and symptoms depend on the location of the infarct or hemorrhage, and range from weakness to aphasia and hemiplegia. Nonspecific signs and symptoms of cerebrovascular diseases caused by high blood pressure may include headache, irritability, fatigue, seizures, and coma.[47]

Arteriolar changes associated with high blood pressure cause serious problems in the kidneys. Renal artery obstruction, decreased renal perfusion, and altered nephron function result in renal failure. Consequently, proteinuria, nocturia, and azotemia may occur.[9]

Diagnosis of High Blood Pressure

A diagnosis of high blood pressure is made after a minimum of two blood pressure measurements on separate occasions reveal elevated readings. At least 2 minutes should be allowed between repeated blood pressure measurements.[19] Careful measurement of blood pressure, as described in the section on Measurement of Arterial Blood Pressure, must be made to ensure accurate readings. The **"white coat" phenomenon,** or elevated blood pressure readings when measured by a physician, must be taken into account, and ambulatory blood pressure monitoring may aid in making the diagnosis.[48] The medical history is focused on risk factors for high blood pressure, including family history, and the presence of other cardiovascular risk factors. Careful determination of the use of prescription and over-the-counter medications, as well as recreational drugs, should be made (see Box 16-2).

In addition to blood pressure determination, the physical examination includes an assessment of target organ damage (e.g., funduscopic examination of the eyes), assessment of arteries for the presence of bruits, heart and lung assessment, and neurologic evaluation. Useful diagnostic tests include an electrocardiography, assessment of serum lipids, evaluation of renal function, and assessment of serum electrolytes.[40,42]

Management of High Blood Pressure

Several clinical trials have demonstrated a decrease in mortality and morbidity with blood pressure reduction. The goal of therapy is to achieve and maintain a blood pressure less than 140/90 mm Hg. Those with diabetes, kidney disease, or proteinuria in excess of 1 g/day should achieve a blood pressure target of less than 130/80 mm Hg.[22] Decisions about the initiation and type of therapy depend on the severity of the blood pressure, the presence of target organ damage, and the presence of other cardiovascular risk factors. The most recent set of hypertension treatment guidelines was published in the Seventh Report of the Joint National Committee on Detection, Evaluation, and Treatment of High Blood Pressure[49] (Figure 16-7). The emphasis on lifestyle modifications in the management of hypertension was maintained. A new category of prehypertension has been added to the JNC7 recommendations. Prehypertension is identified in persons with systolic blood pressures between 120 and 139 mm Hg and diastolic pressures between 80 and 89 mm Hg. Prehypertensive persons are at risk for progression to classified hypertension.[49]

Lifestyle Modifications

In persons with prehypertension lifestyle modifications may be instituted initially without concomitant pharmacologic therapy both to lower blood pressure and to reduce the effects of other cardiovascular risk factors. In stage 1 and 2 hypertension, lifestyle modification will be adjunct to drug therapy. Depending on the individual patient indications and comorbid conditions, drug therapy may be started early. Patients with compelling indications such as heart failure, history of myocardial infarction, coronary artery disease, diabetes, chronic kidney disease, and recurrent stroke will require certain classes of antihypertensive drug therapy.[49] Weight reduction in overweight persons may lower blood pressure, often enough to achieve normal blood pressure levels. The blood

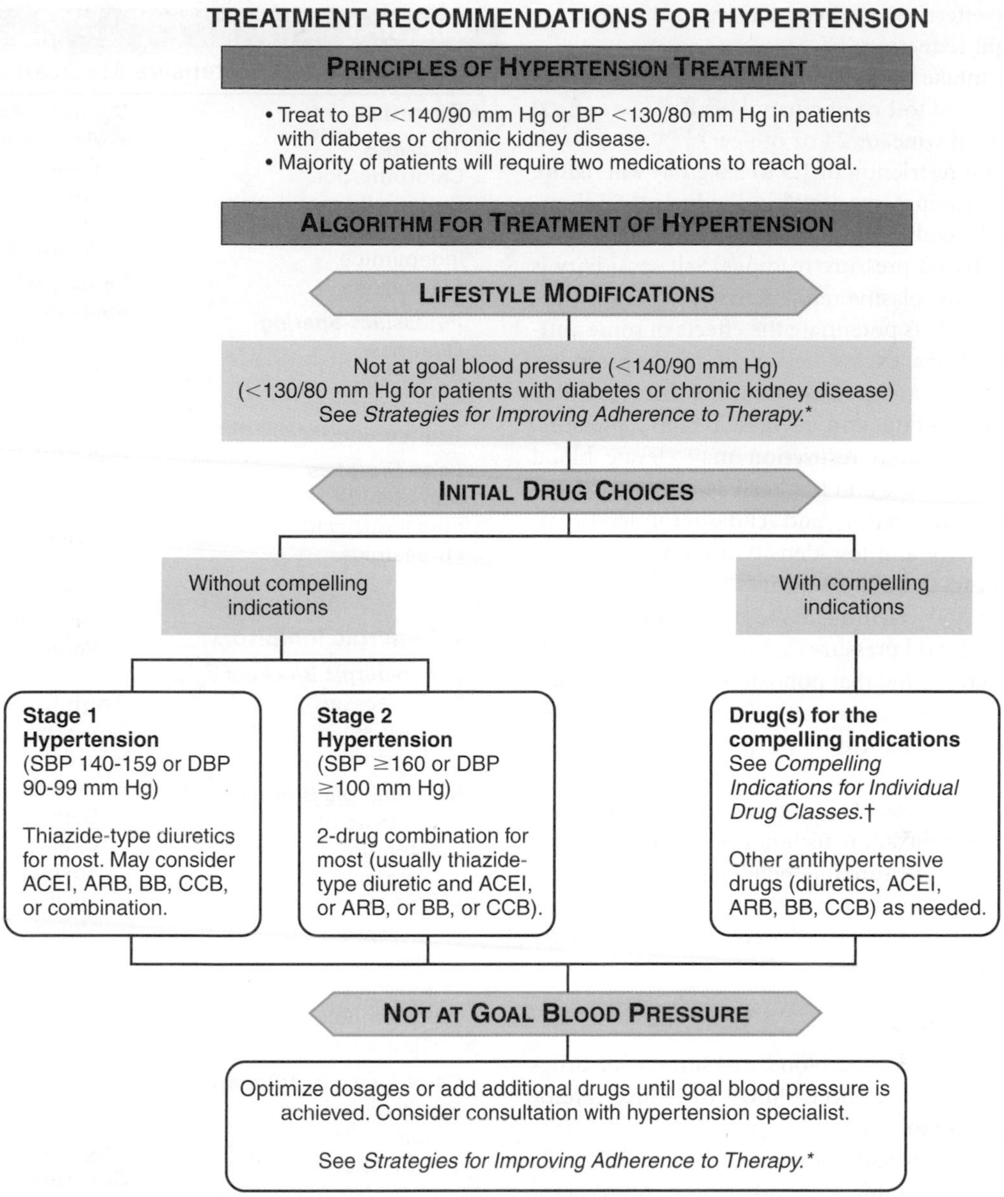

TREATMENT RECOMMENDATIONS FOR HYPERTENSION

PRINCIPLES OF HYPERTENSION TREATMENT

- Treat to BP <140/90 mm Hg or BP <130/80 mm Hg in patients with diabetes or chronic kidney disease.
- Majority of patients will require two medications to reach goal.

ALGORITHM FOR TREATMENT OF HYPERTENSION

LIFESTYLE MODIFICATIONS

Not at goal blood pressure (<140/90 mm Hg)
(<130/80 mm Hg for patients with diabetes or chronic kidney disease)
See *Strategies for Improving Adherence to Therapy.**

INITIAL DRUG CHOICES

Without compelling indications

Stage 1 Hypertension
(SBP 140-159 or DBP 90-99 mm Hg)

Thiazide-type diuretics for most. May consider ACEI, ARB, BB, CCB, or combination.

Stage 2 Hypertension
(SBP ≥160 or DBP ≥100 mm Hg)

2-drug combination for most (usually thiazide-type diuretic and ACEI, or ARB, or BB, or CCB).

With compelling indications

Drug(s) for the compelling indications
See *Compelling Indications for Individual Drug Classes.*†

Other antihypertensive drugs (diuretics, ACEI, ARB, BB, CCB) as needed.

NOT AT GOAL BLOOD PRESSURE

Optimize dosages or add additional drugs until goal blood pressure is achieved. Consider consultation with hypertension specialist.

See *Strategies for Improving Adherence to Therapy.**

***Strategies for Improving Adherence to Therapy:** Clinician empathy increases patient trust, motivation, and adherence to therapy. Physicians should consider their patients' cultural beliefs and individual attitudes in formulating therapy.

†Compelling Indications for Individual Drug Classes:

	Recommended Drugs					
Compelling Indication	Diuretic	BB	ACEI	ARB	CCB	Aldo ANT
Heart failure	●	●	●	●		●
Post–myocardial infarction		●	●			●
High coronary disease risk	●	●	●		●	
Diabetes	●	●	●	●	●	
Chronic kidney disease			●	●		
Recurrent stroke prevention	●		●			

FIGURE 16-7 ■ Lifestyle modifications for the management of high blood pressure. *BP,* Blood pressure; *SBP,* systolic blood pressure; *DBP,* diastolic blood pressure; *ACEI,* angiotensin-converting enzyme inhibitor; *Aldo ANT,* aldosterone antagonist; *ARB,* angiotensin receptor blocker; *BB,* β-blocker; *CCB,* calcium channel blocker. (From U.S. Department of Health and Human Services [National Institutes of Health, National Heart, Lung, and Blood Institute]: The seventh report of the Joint National Committee on Prevention, Detection, Evaluation, and Treatment of High Blood Pressure [JNC7], NIH Publication No 03-5231, May 2003.)

Know what's good for who?

pressure–lowering effects of antihypertensive medications are enhanced by weight reduction.[22,27]

Excess alcohol intake contributes to high blood pressure and should be restricted to 1 oz of ethanol per day (2 oz of 100 proof whiskey, 8 oz of wine, or 24 oz of beer).[22,36]

Moderate sodium restriction of 1.5 to 2.5 g/day will reduce blood pressure in "sodium-sensitive" individuals.[16] Sodium-sensitive individuals tend to be older, obese, and black and to have higher initial blood pressure readings. Salt sensitivity is also associated with low plasma renin activity.[25,30]

Sodium-restricted diets potentiate the effects of some antihypertensive medications. Excess dietary salt intake promotes the excretion of calcium and potassium in the urine, possibly promoting vasoconstriction and increased blood pressure. Conversely, extreme sodium restriction may elevate blood pressure in some individuals and has been associated with increased norepinephrine, renin, and cholesterol levels, although total cholesterol and low-density lipoprotein cholesterol elevation appears to be short term.[50,51]

High potassium and calcium intake may reduce or suppress the increase in blood pressure that occurs after salt loading. Some studies have found that potassium supplementation effects a reduction in blood pressure.[32,51] Increased calcium intake has been shown to reduce blood pressure in pregnant women.[52]

Some individuals successfully lower blood pressure by using biofeedback and relaxation techniques. Regular aerobic exercise reduces blood pressure independent of weight loss.[53] Reduction of dietary fat intake reduces serum cholesterol levels, facilitates weight loss, and possibly reduces blood pressure directly.[36]

Pharmacologic Therapy

Managing systolic and diastolic blood pressures with drugs and lifestyle modification has been shown to reduce cardiovascular morbidity and mortality.[49]

Initial drug therapy usually begins with diuretics or β-blockers (Box 16-3). ACE inhibitors and angiotensin receptor blockers are useful in hypertension, congestive heart failure, and diabetes. Drugs from other classifications, such as calcium antagonists, though effective in reducing blood pressure, have not been demonstrated to be effective in reducing morbidity and mortality. However, recent research supports using long-acting dihydropyridines for management of isolated systolic hypertension in the elderly.[16,49,54]

Other considerations in the choice of initial therapy include demographic considerations, concomitant diseases, and quality-of-life issues. Although age and gender have not been found to determine drug responsiveness, African-Americans are generally more responsive to diuretics and calcium antagonists than to β-blockers or ACE inhibitors.[16,49] However, ongoing studies may support the use of ACE inhibitors in African-Americans due to the high rate of associated renal insufficiency secondary to hypertension in this population.

Box 16-3

Selected Antihypertensive Medications

Diuretics

Thiazides
- Chlorothiazide
- Chlorthalidone
- Hydrochlorothiazide
- Indapamide
- Metolazone

Potassium-Sparing Diuretics
- Amiloride
- Spironolactone
- Triamterene

Loop Diuretics
- Bumetanide
- Ethacrynic acid
- Furosemide
- Torsemide

Adrenergic Inhibitors

α-Adrenergic Blockers
- Doxazosin
- Prazosin
- Terazosin

β-Adrenergic Blockers
- Acebutolol
- Atenolol
- Betaxolol
- Carteolol
- Metoprolol
- Nadolol
- Pindolol
- Propranolol
- Timolol

Combined α,β-Adrenergic Blockers
- Carvedilol
- Labetalol

Centrally Acting α_2-Adrenergic Agonist
- Clonidine
- Guanabenz
- Guanfacine
- Methyldopa

Peripheral Adrenergic Blockers
- Guanadrel
- Guanethidine
- Reserpine

Calcium Antagonists
- Amlodipine
- Diltiazem
- Felodipine
- Isradipine
- Nicardipine
- Nifedipine
- Verapamil

Angiotensin-Converting Enzyme Inhibitors
- Benazepril
- Captopril
- Enalapril
- Fosinopril
- Lisinopril
- Quinapril
- Ramipril
- Trandolapril

Direct Vasodilators
- Hydralazine
- Minoxidil

Angiotensin II Receptor Blockers
- Losartan
- Valsartan
- Irbesartan

Although some antihypertensive drugs worsen some diseases, other diseases may be ameliorated. For example, β-blockers may worsen asthma but may improve angina pectoris and reduce myocardial oxygen demand in patients following myocardial infarction. Use of an antihypertensive drug that is also effective in the management of a concomitant disease may simplify the medication regimen and reduce costs.[49] Many antihypertensive agents have undesirable side effects. Compliance with the medication plan may be significantly influenced by drugs that impair sexual function, impair mental acuity, or reduce exercise tolerance. The cost of therapy must be considered when selecting antihypertensive therapy. Inability to pay for the medication may be a hidden reason for failure of drug therapy.[16]

If adequate blood pressure control is not achieved with single-drug therapy, the dose is increased, a drug of a different class is substituted, or a drug of a different class is added. Addition of a drug with a different mode of action from the first will often allow smaller doses of drugs to be used, thereby reducing the incidence of side effects.[16,49]

Hypertensive Crisis

In some instances, urgent lowering of blood pressure may be necessary to avoid serious organ damage or death. Severe perioperative hypertension, accelerated hypertension, intracranial hemorrhage, and dissecting aortic aneurysms are examples of situations requiring rapid reduction of blood pressure. Intravenous agents are used in these situations and require monitoring in an intensive care unit. Examples of intravenous agents include sodium nitroprusside, nitroglycerin, hydralazine, labetalol, and methyldopa.[4]

KEY CONCEPTS

- High blood pressure is arbitrarily defined as a blood pressure above 140 mm Hg systolic, 90 mm Hg diastolic, or both. Chronic high blood pressure is associated with an increased risk of left ventricular hypertrophy, left-sided heart failure, and atherosclerosis.
- Several risk factors for the development of hypertension have been proposed: age, ethnicity and family history, obesity, and high sodium intake.
- Persons in whom primary hypertension develops have a genetic predisposition (polygenic) that can be influenced by environmental factors such as lifestyle and diet. An imbalance of endothelium-derived mediators may be important in the development of hypertension. The endothelium secretes and processes a number of vascular constricting and relaxing factors.
- Secondary hypertension refers to high blood pressure of known cause such as renal artery stenosis, renal failure, hypersecretion of aldosterone or catecholamines, hyperthyroidism, increased intracranial pressure, and drugs. It is less common in adults but is the cause of most high blood pressure in children.
- Hypertension is associated with headache, retinopathy, seizures, renal disease, cardiovascular disease, and coma; however, symptoms may be absent. The diagnosis is made after at least two elevated blood pressure readings on separate occasions.
- Treatment centers on measures to decrease vascular resistance, blood volume, or both. Weight reduction, moderation of alcohol intake, sodium and fat restriction, and relaxation may be recommended. Drugs may be used to decrease vascular resistance (ACE inhibitors, angiotensin receptor blockers, adrenergic inhibitors, calcium antagonists, direct vasodilators) and reduce blood volume (diuretics).

LOW BLOOD PRESSURE

Hypovolemia and Shock

Loss of blood volume, such as through hemorrhage or excessive diarrhea, may result in low blood pressure. Systolic blood pressure reflects the pressure exerted in the aorta and large arteries by the blood; a reduction in volume results in a reduction in the amount of pressure exerted. This reduction in pressure is sensed by the baroreceptors and triggers activation of the renin-angiotensin-aldosterone system to produce sodium and water retention and vasoconstriction in an attempt to restore blood volume and therefore pressure (see Figure 16-3).

Excessive hypovolemia results in shock.[8,9] In addition, shock may occur in response to exposure to an allergen (anaphylactic shock) or to bacterial endotoxins (septic shock). Shock is discussed in detail in Chapter 20.[8]

Orthostatic Hypotension

Successful change of position from supine to upright requires an intact cardiovascular system and adequate fluid volume. When the upright position is assumed, blood volume transiently shifts to the lower extremities. The baroreceptors in the carotid arteries and in the arch of the aorta sense a decrease in circulating volume and trigger mechanisms that cause peripheral vasoconstriction and an increased heart rate in an attempt to restore MAP. During change from a supine to an upright position, the normal postural vital sign response includes a slight decrease in systolic blood pressure (less than 10 mm Hg).[55] A drop in systolic blood pressure of more than 20 mm Hg and/or a pulse increase of 20 beats/min or more that occurs with a change to standing position is called orthostatic or postural hypotension.[14,55] Orthostatic changes can occur in patients with hypovolemia, clinical dehydration, prolonged bed rest, or blood loss, especially in the elderly. Some drugs, including diuretics, antihypertensive medications, and pain medications, can cause orthostatic hypotension. Thus a blood pressure measurement prior to administering these drugs is advised.[14,54] Symptoms of orthostatic hypotension include dizziness, light-headedness, or syncope as cerebral blood flow is reduced.

Impaired cardiovascular response constitutes the second type of problem that produces an altered vital sign response to postural change. One of two mechanisms is involved: inadequate peripheral vasoconstriction or inadequate heart rate increase that can occur with patients on β-blockers and patients with spinal cord injury. Primary dysfunction of the cardiovascular reflex may also be a problem. The vital sign response to inadequate peripheral vasoconstriction mimics that of hypovolemia, and differentiation between the two is based on client history. Peripheral neuropathy, as occurs in diabetics, may limit peripheral vasoconstriction.[56] Management of orthostatic hypotension depends on the cause. Orthostatic hypotension caused by fluid volume deficit is treated by restoring fluid volume. Unless secondary to pharmacologic therapy, persons with orthostatic hypotension caused by impaired cardiovascular responses must be taught to minimize the blood pressure changes that result from position change. Such training is accomplished by teaching the person to make position changes slowly so as to allow gradual compensation to the upright position. The same instructions should be given to persons with orthostatic hypotension resulting from pharmacologic therapy if a change in or discontinuation of the medication is not possible.

KEY CONCEPTS

- Orthostatic hypotension is due to a reduction in CO when the upright position is assumed. Activation of the baroreceptors usually minimizes the decrease in blood pressure by increasing the heart rate and vascular resistance. A drop in systolic blood pressure greater than 20 mm Hg and/or a pulse increase of 20 beats/min or more signifies orthostatic hypotension.
- The usual cause of orthostatic hypotension is intravascular volume depletion.
- An impaired baroreceptor reflex may also result in orthostatic hypotension. Adrenergic blocking drugs, peripheral neuropathy, and spinal cord injury can interrupt the normal baroreceptor reflex pathway.

SUMMARY

Arterial blood pressure, specifically MAP, is a closely regulated physiologic parameter. A variety of mechanisms interact to maintain the blood pressure needed to perfuse body tissues.

Mechanisms that elevate blood pressure may be stimulated in response to such situations as hemorrhage or low renal perfusion, as occurs in heart failure or shock, or those mechanisms may be activated in the absence of identifiable stimuli, as in primary hypertension. Primary hypertension is a significant public health problem affecting millions of Americans. Primary prevention and early detection remain key in reducing the associated mortality associated with hypertension. Reduction of elevated blood pressure is vital in preventing damage to body organs and may be achieved by lifestyle modification or pharmacologic methods.

Intact cardiovascular reflexes and sufficient fluid volume are both necessary for the maintenance of adequate blood pressure with positional change. Alterations in volume status, peripheral vasoconstriction, or the heart rate response can interfere with the ability to successfully assume an upright posture.

MEDIA RESOURCES

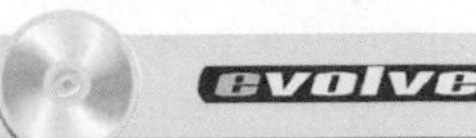

evolve

Remember to check out the ***CD Companion*** included with this book for Review Questions, Key Concepts Review, Glossary (with audio for selected terms), Disease Profiles, and Animations.

PLUS, visit the ***Evolve website*** at http://evolve.elsevier.com/Copstead/ for Case Studies, Disease Profiles, and WebLinks.

References

1. Vander AJ, Sherman JH, Luciano DS: *Human physiology: the mechanisms of body function,* ed 9, New York, 2001, McGraw-Hill.
2. Clochesy JM et al: *Critical care nursing,* ed 2, Philadelphia, 1996, Saunders.
3. Ganong WF: *Review of medical physiology,* ed 19, Norwalk, 1999, Appleton & Lange.
4. Darovic GO: *Hemodynamic monitoring: invasive and noninvasive clinical application,* ed 3, Philadelphia, 2002, Saunders.
5. Beevers G, Lip GYH, O'Brien E: *Pathophysiol Hypertens* 322:912-916, 2001.
6. Staessen JA et al: Risks of untreated and treated isolated systolic hypertension in the elderly: meta-analysis of outcome trials, *Lancet* 355:865-872, 2000.
7. Lehne RA: *Pharmacology for nursing care,* ed 4, Philadelphia, 2001, Saunders.
8. Guyton AC, Hall JE: *Textbook of medical physiology,* ed 10, Philadelphia, 2000, Saunders.
9. Givertz MM: Manipulation of the renin-angiotensin system, *Circulation* 104:e14-e18, 2001.
10. Kato N et al: Genetic analysis of the atrial natriuretic peptide gene in essential hypertension, *Clin Sci* 98(3):251-258, 2000.
11. Sander M, Chavoshan B, Ronald GV: A large blood pressure–raising effect of nitric oxide synthase inhibition in humans, *Hypertension* 33:937-942, 1999.
12. O'Keefe JH et al: Should an angiotensin-converting enzyme inhibitor be standard therapy for patients with atherosclerotic disease? *J Am Coll Cardiol* 37(1):1-7, 2001.
13. Beevers G, Lip GYH, O'Brien E: Blood pressure measurement. I. Sphygmomanometry: factors common to all techniques, *BMJ* 322:981-985, 2001.
14. Potter PA, Perry GA: *Fundamentals of nursing,* ed 5, St Louis, 2001, Mosby.
15. Sellers KW et al: Gene therapy to control hypertension: current studies and future perspectives, *Am J Med Sci* 322(1):1-6, 2001.
16. Sixth Report of the Joint Committee on Detection, Evaluation, and Treatment of High Blood Pressure, *Arch Intern Med* 157:2413-2446, 1997.
17. Nehal SU, Ingelfinger JR: Pediatric hypertension: recent literature, *Nephrology* 14:189-196, 2002.
18. Morgenstern B: Blood pressure, hypertension, and ambulatory blood pressure monitoring in children and adolescents, *Am J Hypertens* 15:64S-66S, 2001.
19. Sorof JM: Prevalence and consequence of systolic hypertension in children, *Am J Hypertens* 15:57S-60S, 2002.
20. Daniels SR: Cardiovascular sequelae of childhood hypertension, *Am J Hypertens* 15:61S-63S, 2002.
21. Rigaud AS, Forette B: Hypertension in older adults, *J Gerontol* 56A(4):M217-M225, 2001.
22. Garg J, Messerli AW, Bakris GL: Evaluation and treatment of patients with systemic hypertension, *Circulation* 105: 2458-2461, 2002.

23. Stein MC et al: Hypertension in black people: study of specific genotypes and phenotypes will provide a greater understanding of interindividual and interethnic variability in blood pressure regulation than studies based on race, *Pharmacogenetics* 11:95-110, 2001.
24. Peters RM, Flack JM: Salt sensitivity and hypertension in African American: implications for cardiovascular nurses, *Prog Cardiovasc Nurs* 15(4):138-144, 2000.
25. Adviye E: Hypertension in black patients: an emerging role of the endothelin system in salt-sensitive hypertension, *Hypertension* 36(1):62-67, 2000.
26. Weinberger MH: Salt and blood pressure, *Cardiology* 15(4):254-257, 2000.
27. Thakur V, Richards R, Reisin E: Obesity, hypertension and the heart, *Am J Med Sci* 321(4):242-248, 2001.
28. Abbasi F et al: Relationship between obesity, insulin resistance and coronary heart disease risk, *J Am Coll Cardiol* 40(5): 937-943, 2002.
29. Suter PM, Sierro C, Vetter V: Nutritional factors in the control of blood pressure and hypertension, *Nutr Clin Care* 5(1):9-19, 2002.
30. Aviv A: Salt and hypertension: the debate that begs the bigger question, *Arch Intern Med* 161:507-510, 2001.
31. Kaplan NM: The dietary guideline for sodium: should we shake it up? Nos. 1 and 2. *Am J Clin Nutr* 71:1020-1026, 2000.
32. Cohn JN et al: New guidelines for potassium replacement in clinical practice, *Arch Intern Med* 160:2429-2436, 2000.
33. Jolma P et al: High-calcium diet enhances vasorelaxation in nitric oxide–deficient hypertension, *Am J Physiol Heart Circ Physiol* 279:H1036-H1043, 2000.
34. Carretero OA, Oparil S: Essential hypertension. Part I: definition and etiology, *Circulation* 100(3):320-343, 2000.
35. Timberlake SS, O'Conner DT, Parmer R: Molecular genetics of essential hypertension: recent results and emerging strategies, *Opin Nephrol Hypertens* 10:71-79, 2001.
36. Carretero OA, Oparil S: Essential hypertension. Part II: treatment, *Circulation* 101(4):446-458, 2000.
37. American Diabetes Association: Position statement: treatment of hypertension in adults with diabetes, *Diabetic Care* 25: S71-S73, 2002.
38. McLaughlin T, Reaven G: Insulin resistance and hypertension, *Geriatrics* 55(6):28-35, 2000.
39. McFarlane S, Banerji M, Sower J: Insulin resistance and cardiovascular disease, *J Clin Endocrinol Metab* 86(2):713-718, 2000.
40. Noble J: *Textbook of primary care medicine,* ed 3, St Louis, 2001, Mosby.
41. Behrman RE, Kliegman RM, Arvin AM: *Nelson textbook of pediatrics,* ed 16, Philadelphia, 2000, Saunders.
42. Zwieten PA: Drug treatment of systolic hypertension, *Nephrol Dial Transplant* 16:1095-1097, 2001.
43. Walker JJ: Pre-eclampsia, *Lancet* 356:1260-1265, 2000.
44. Dekker G, Sibai B: Primary, secondary, and tertiary prevention of pre-eclampsia, *Lancet* 357:209-215, 2001.
45. American College of Obstetrics and Gynecology Committee on Practice: *Chronic hypertension in pregnancy*, Bulletin 98, Washington, DC, 2001, The College, pp 179-185.
46. Sibai BM: Chronic hypertension in pregnancy, *Obstet Gynecol* 199:369-377, 2002.
47. Prisant ML, Moser M: Hypertension in the elderly; can we improve results of therapy? *Arch Intern Med* 160:283-289, 2000.
48. McAlister FA, Straus SE: Measurement of blood pressure: an evidence based review, *BMJ* 322:908-911, 2001.
49. The Seventh Report of the Joint National Committee on Prevention, Detection, Evaluation, and Treatment of High Blood Pressure, *JAMA* 289:2560-2571, 2003.
50. Egan BM, Lackland DT: Biochemical and metabolic effects of very-low-salt diets, *Am J Med Sci* 320:233-239, 2000.
51. Coruzzi P et al: Potassium depletion and salt sensitivity in essential hypertension, *J Clin Endocrinol Metab* 86:2857-2862, 2001.
52. Ritchie LD, King JC: Dietary calcium and pregnancy-induced hypertension: is there a relation? *Am J Clin Nutr* 71: 1371S-1374S, 2000.
53. Lesniak KT, Dubbert PM: Exercise and hypertension, *Curr Opin Cardiol* 16:356-359, 2001.
54. Commentary: Is it time for a new approach to the initial treatment of hypertension? *Arch Intern Med* 161:1140-1144, 2001.
55. Jarvis C: Physical examination and health assessment, Philadelphia, 2000, Saunders.
56. Swartz MH: *Textbook of physical diagnosis,* ed 3, Philadelphia, 1998, Saunders.

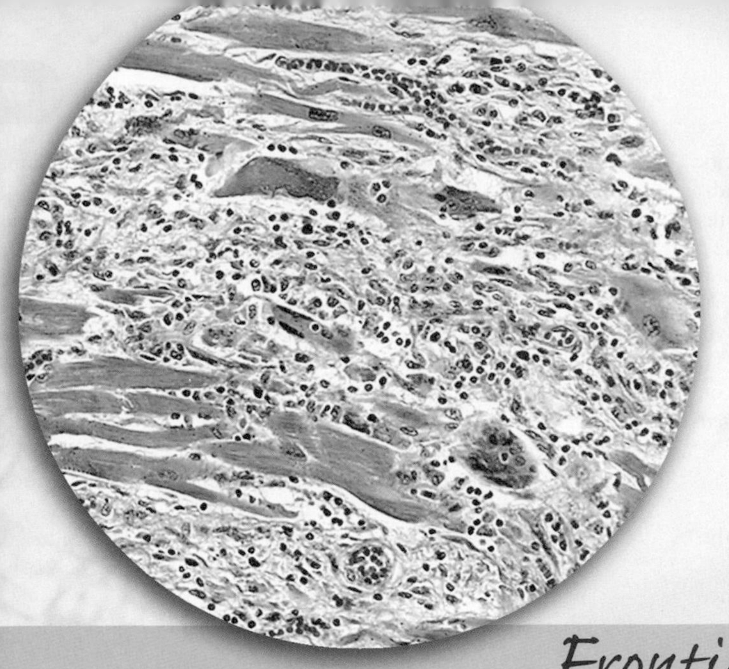

Frontiers of Research

Heart Disease and Health Habits

Jacquelyn L. Banasik and Michael J. Kirkhorn

We carry with us a primitive understanding of the body that tells us about the connection between our emotions and our hearts. Romance, surprise, fear, and excitement manifest in the quickening of the heart—our hearts go *pitter pat.* Stress and anger make us worry about *blowing our top,* a reference to the responsiveness of blood pressure to our emotions. We may even *faint with fear or joy.* Health care professionals cannot ignore the influence of psychological factors and lifestyle choices in the development of diseases of the heart.

Measures to reduce the risks of cardiovascular and other lifestyle diseases are incredibly simple yet exceedingly difficult to implement. *Don't smoke. Eat well. Engage in regular physical activity.* These are the simple instructions for a healthy body, known for generations. However, in an environment where enticements to smoke, to eat super sizes of processed food, to drive instead of walk, to work at a desk, and to entertain ourselves in front of television or computer screens, these simple instructions are difficult to implement.

In addition to the environmental pressures to eat more and be sedentary, there are a host of parties concerned not with improving the health of Americans, but in making money from the American obsession with "health" improvement. Confusing messages emanate from all corners:

Weight loss is good for your health. Weight loss is bad for you because you will gain more back. Eat a low-carbohydrate, high-protein diet. Eat a low-fat, high-carbohydrate diet. Just eat less. Moderate activity every day is enough for health. Exercise isn't effective unless it is vigorous and aerobic. No pain, no gain. Health benefits accrue from short bouts of low to moderate intensity. A healthy body must be lean and have a certain BMI. You can be fat AND fit. Obesity is a major risk factor for disease. Obesity is not a major risk factor for disease and only a marker for sedentary behavior. Lifestyle changes aren't enough; drugs must be used for maximum effect. Buy this pill, this equipment, this videotape, this magazine, this diet book, this membership, this surgery, and you will lose weight, look better, feel better, and (of course) be happier and healthier.

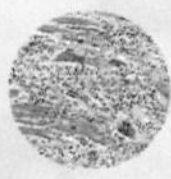

Giant cell myocarditis, with mononuclear inflammatory infiltrate containing lymphocytes and macrophages, extensive loss of muscle, and multinucleated giant cells. (From Kumar V, Abbas AK, Fausto N: Robbins and Cotran pathologic basis of disease, *ed 7, Philadelphia, 2005, Saunders.)*

UNIT V

Cardiac Function

It is no wonder that Americans throw up their hands. Health professionals are confused and unable to give sound advice about which lifestyle changes to implement and how to maintain them over time. If stress and anger are bad for the heart, the current situation in which people are made to feel guilty about their risk profiles but are unable to effectively improve upon them may increase their risk!

There is a great deal of research support for the notion that chronic cigarette smoking is a significant risk factor for heart and lung disease, and clinicians can have confidence that efforts toward smoking cessation will result in significant risk reduction. Efforts to help patients reduce stress, improve coping, and ameliorate depression are also useful. Studies have found that emotionally depressed survivors of heart attacks have five times the mortality rate of survivors not having depression. Other recommendations are less clear.

An interesting controversy about the role of obesity is brewing. Some researchers suggest that fat mass has little to do with health and that subcutaneous fat may actually improve overall mortality and protect against several diseases. These researchers suggest that weight has few health consequences as long as an individual engages in regular, moderate-intensity activity and eats a nutritious diet. Some have even concluded that efforts to lose weight are detrimental because the nearly inevitable weight regain is harmful to blood pressure control and metabolism. Other obesity researchers believe that weight loss is necessary to improve obesity-related risks for cardiovascular disease and diabetes.

It seems prudent to encourage regular, moderate-intensity activity and nutritious eating for all, with less emphasis on the difficult-to-achieve goal of weight loss. A great deal of rigorous research must be done to improve our understanding and provide a foundation for lifestyle recommendations. However, a skeptic's eye must be used to evaluate research done by those who stand to gain from the sale of products or services related to the research outcomes. Practitioners must be careful not to confuse weight loss goals for esthetic reasons with the goal of improving health. Body weight is not the only or the best indicator of health, and we must strive to avoid prejudice against fat until the health-related issues are clear.

Cardiac Function

Jacquelyn L. Banasik

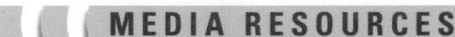

MEDIA RESOURCES

Additional Material for Study, Review, and Further Exploration

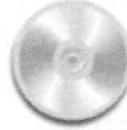

CD Companion ◆ Review Questions and Answers ◆ Key Concepts Review
◆ Glossary *(with audio pronunciations for selected terms)*
◆ Disease Profiles ◆ Animations

evolve ***Website*** at http://evolve.elsevier.com/Copstead/
◆ Case Studies ◆ Disease Profiles ◆ WebLinks

KEY QUESTIONS

- How are events of the cardiac cycle reflected in pressure and volume changes within the cardiac chambers?
- What factors affect the blood supply to myocardial tissue?
- How does sarcomere cross-bridge formation lead to muscle cell contraction?
- What is the process of excitation-contraction coupling in heart muscle cells?
- How are action potentials generated and conducted in myocardial and pacemaker cells?
- How does the electrocardiogram relate to impulse conduction through the heart?
- How do heart rate, preload, afterload, and contractility affect cardiac output and cardiac workload?
- What diagnostic tests are used to evaluate cardiac structure and function?

CHAPTER OUTLINE

The primary function of the heart is to produce the driving force that propels blood through the vessels of the circulatory system. Along with the lungs, the heart works to distribute oxygenated blood and nutrients to tissues and organs of the body. Complex regulatory mechanisms function to match the cardiac output with the metabolic needs of the tissues. Cardiac dysfunction can lead to abnormal function or death of cells in tissues throughout the body. Cardiovascular disease is the leading cause of mortality in the United States, and a significant proportion of the population suffers from physical limitations associated with impaired cardiac function. Familiarity with cardiac anatomy and physiology is requisite to understanding cardiac diseases and therapy.

CARDIOVASCULAR ANATOMY

Heart

The heart is located in the **mediastinum,** suspended between the lungs, behind the sternum, and in front of the vertebral column, thoracic aorta, and esophagus (Figure 17-1).[1] When viewed from the front, the heart appears to be rotated to the left, so that the right atrium and right ventricle are most ante-

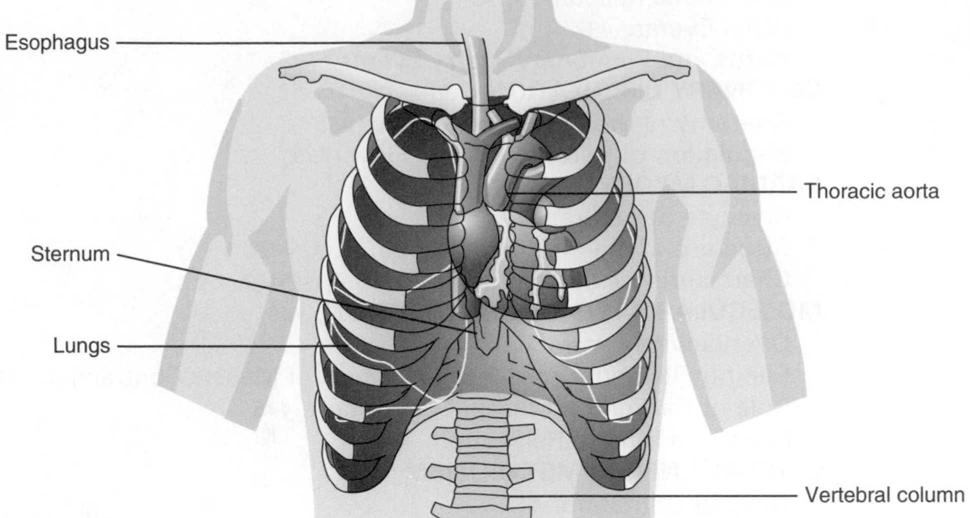

FIGURE 17-1 ■ Position of the heart in the mediastinum. The base of the heart protrudes into the right side of the chest, whereas the apex lies in the lower left side of the chest.

rior. The base of the heart protrudes somewhat into the right side of the chest and is relatively fixed in place by its attachments to the great vessels. The apex of the heart lies primarily in the left side of the chest and is directed forward toward the anterior chest wall. With each heartbeat, a characteristic thrust, or point of maximal impulse (PMI), is generated and can be palpated where the apex strikes against the chest. The PMI is normally located on the left side of the chest where the fifth intercostal space and midclavicular line intersect. Variations in heart size and position within the chest may be related to age, body size, shape, weight, or pathologic conditions of the heart and other nearby structures.

Functionally important cardiac tissues include connective tissues, which form the fibrous skeleton and valves; cardiac muscle, which produces the contractile force; and epithelial tissue, which lines the cardiac chambers and covers the outer surfaces of the heart. The fibrous skeleton consists of four rings that provide a firm scaffold for attachment of cardiac muscle and the cardiac valves. Four cardiac valves control the direction of blood flow through the heart (Figure 17-2). The **mitral valve** (bicuspid) directs blood flow from the left atrium to the left ventricle, whereas the **tricuspid valve** directs blood from the right atrium to the right ventricle. The edges of these atrioventricular (AV) valves are attached to rings formed by the fibrous skeleton. Valve leaflets are tethered to papillary muscles of the ventricular chambers by connective tissues called **chordae tendineae. Papillary muscles** attach to ventricular walls and help prevent the valve leaflets from bending backward into the atria during ventricular contraction (Figure 17-3). The AV valves open passively during diastole when the pressure of blood in the atria exceeds that in the ventricles. Ventricular contraction reverses the pressure gradient and causes AV valves to snap shut, preventing blood from flowing backward into the atria.

Two semilunar valves are located in the ventricular outflow tracts. The **pulmonic valve** lies between the right ventricle and pulmonary artery, and the **aortic valve** lies between the left ventricle and aortic artery. Compared to the AV valves, the semilunar valves are thicker and are not supported by fibrous cords. They open and close passively according to pressure gradients, just as the AV valves do. When intraventricular pressures exceed pulmonary and aortic artery pressures, the semilunar valves remain open and then close when ventricular pressures fall below aortic and pulmonary artery pressures.

The cardiac muscle layer (**myocardium**) produces the contractile force that pushes blood through the circulatory system. Heart muscle is organized into four separate chambers of varying muscular wall thickness, reflecting the degree of pressure each chamber must generate to pump blood. Atria serve primarily as conduits and have a thinner layer of muscle than the ventricles. The left ventricular muscle is two to three times thicker than that of the right ventricle because higher pressures are required to eject blood into the systemic circulation than into the pulmonic system. Normal chamber pressures are shown in Table 17-1. Alterations in chamber pressures may reflect pathologic cardiovascular changes such as valvular disorders, blood volume abnormalities, and heart failure (see Chapters 18 and 19).

Cardiac chambers and valves are lined by a layer of squamous epithelial cells called **endocardium.** The endocardial layer provides a smooth surface on which blood can slide, which prevents clotting and minimizes trauma to red cells. The endocardium is continuous with endothelium of the vascular system. Outer surfaces of the heart are also covered by a layer of epithelial cells, called **epicardium,** which is part of a protective covering called the pericardium. The **pericardium** is composed of two layers that envelop the heart like a sac (Figure 17-4). The inner layer (visceral pericardium or epi-

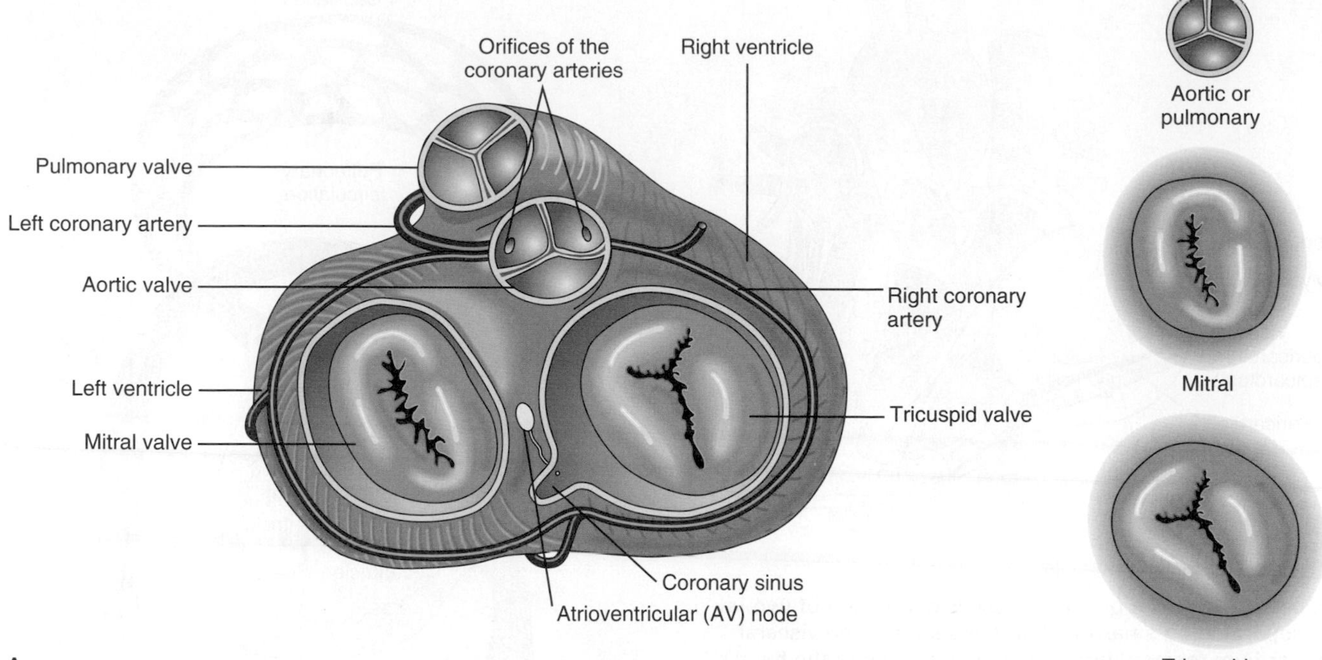

FIGURE 17-2 ■ **A,** Position of the heart valves as viewed from above. **B,** Configuration of the heart valves showing the two cusps of the mitral valve and the three cusps of the tricuspid valve. The pulmonary and aortic valves have three leaflets.

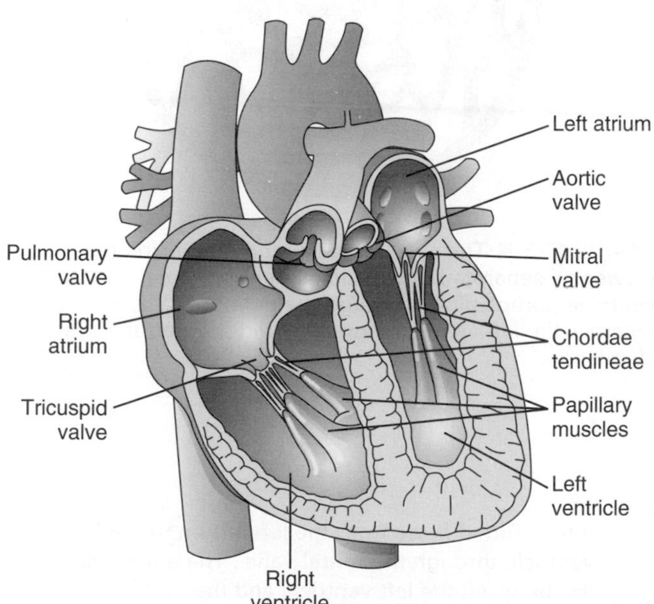

FIGURE 17-3 ■ The chordae tendineae and papillary muscles attach the mitral and tricuspid valve leaflets to the ventricular myocardium.

cardium) is attached directly to the heart's outer surface, whereas an outer layer (parietal pericardium) forms a sac around the heart. The parietal pericardium is composed of an epithelial layer and a tough fibrous layer.

Visceral and parietal pericardial layers are separated by a thin, fluid-filled space (pericardial space) that usually contains 10 to 30 ml of serous fluid. This fluid lubricates pericardial surfaces and reduces friction as the layers slide against one another during cardiac contraction. Accumulations of fluid in the pericardial space or inflammation of the pericardial sac can restrict cardiac filling and impair cardiac output.

Table 17-1

Normal Pressures in the Heart

Location	Pressure (mm Hg)*
Right atrium	0-8
Right ventricle	15-28/0-8
Pulmonary artery	15-28/4-12
Left atrium	4-12
Left ventricle	100-120/4-12
Aorta	100-120/60-80

*Right and left atrial pressures listed as means; other pressures written as systolic/diastolic.

Circulatory System

The circulatory systems of the lungs and body can be viewed as two separate but dependent systems (Figure 17-5). The left-sided heart chambers produce the force to propel blood through the vessels of the systemic (body) circulation. The left atrium receives oxygenated blood from the lungs by way of the pulmonary veins and delivers it to the left ventricle. This oxygenated blood is pumped by the left ventricle into the

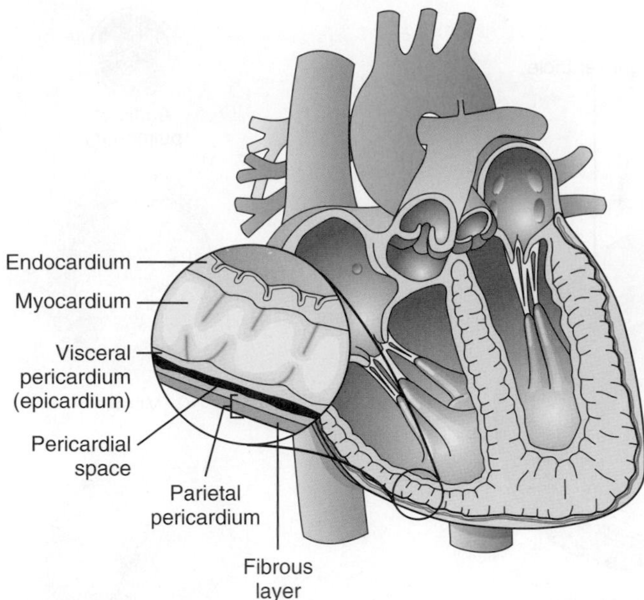

FIGURE 17-4 ■ The pericardial sac is composed of two layers separated by a narrow fluid-filled space. The visceral pericardium (epicardium) is attached directly to the heart's surface, whereas the parietal pericardium forms the outer layer of the sac.

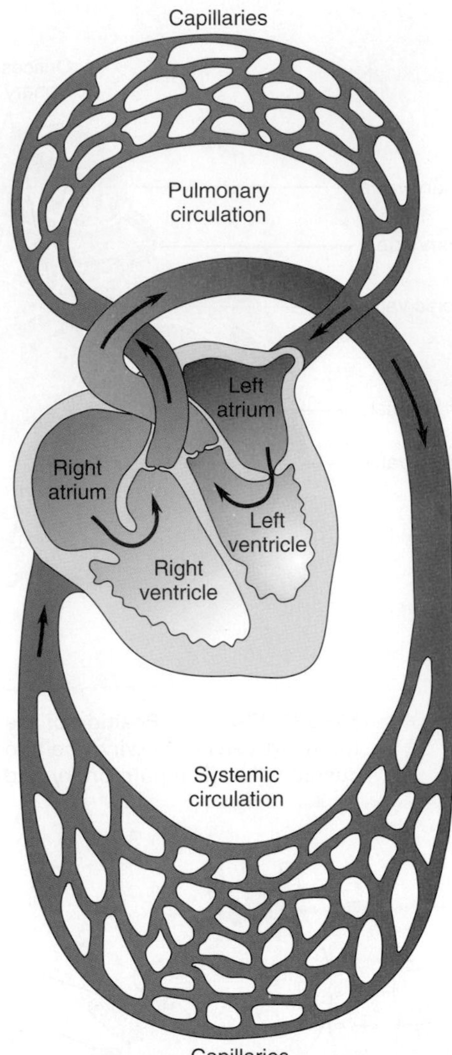

FIGURE 17-5 ■ The systemic and pulmonary circulations viewed as separate but interdependent systems. The right ventricle pumps blood through the pulmonary vasculature, whereas the left ventricle pumps blood through the systemic circulation.

aorta, which supplies the arteries of the systemic circulation. Venous blood is collected from capillary networks of the body and returned to the right atrium by way of the venae cavae. Blood from the head returns to the right atrium through the superior vena cava, and blood from the body returns via the inferior vena cava.

The right side of the heart receives deoxygenated blood from the systemic circulation and pumps it through the lungs by way of the pulmonary artery. The pulmonary artery divides into left and right branches, which subdivide to supply blood to pulmonary capillary beds. Exchange of respiratory gases occurs at the pulmonary capillaries so that blood delivered to the left atrium by the pulmonary veins is well oxygenated.

Left and right heart circulations are connected in series such that the output of one becomes the input of the other. Thus, the functions of the right and left sides of the heart are interdependent. Failure of one side of the heart to pump efficiently soon leads to dysfunction of the other side.

Characteristic changes in the anatomy and physiologic functioning of the heart and circulatory systems occur with aging (The Aging Process: Changes in the Heart). In general, these changes result in a decreased cardiac reserve and a greater predisposition to cardiac muscle ischemia.

KEY CONCEPTS

- Blood flows from the right atrium to the right ventricle through the tricuspid valve. The pulmonic valve lies between the right ventricle and the pulmonary artery. Blood flows from the left atrium to the left ventricle through the mitral valve. The aortic valve lies between the left ventricle and the aorta.
- Heart muscle (myocardium) is lined with endothelium on the inner surface and covered with epicardium on the outer surface.
- The pericardial sac envelops and protects the heart from friction.
- The right-sided heart chambers pump deoxygenated (venous) blood through the lungs. The left-sided heart chambers pump oxygenated blood through the systemic circulation.

THE AGING PROCESS

Changes in the Heart

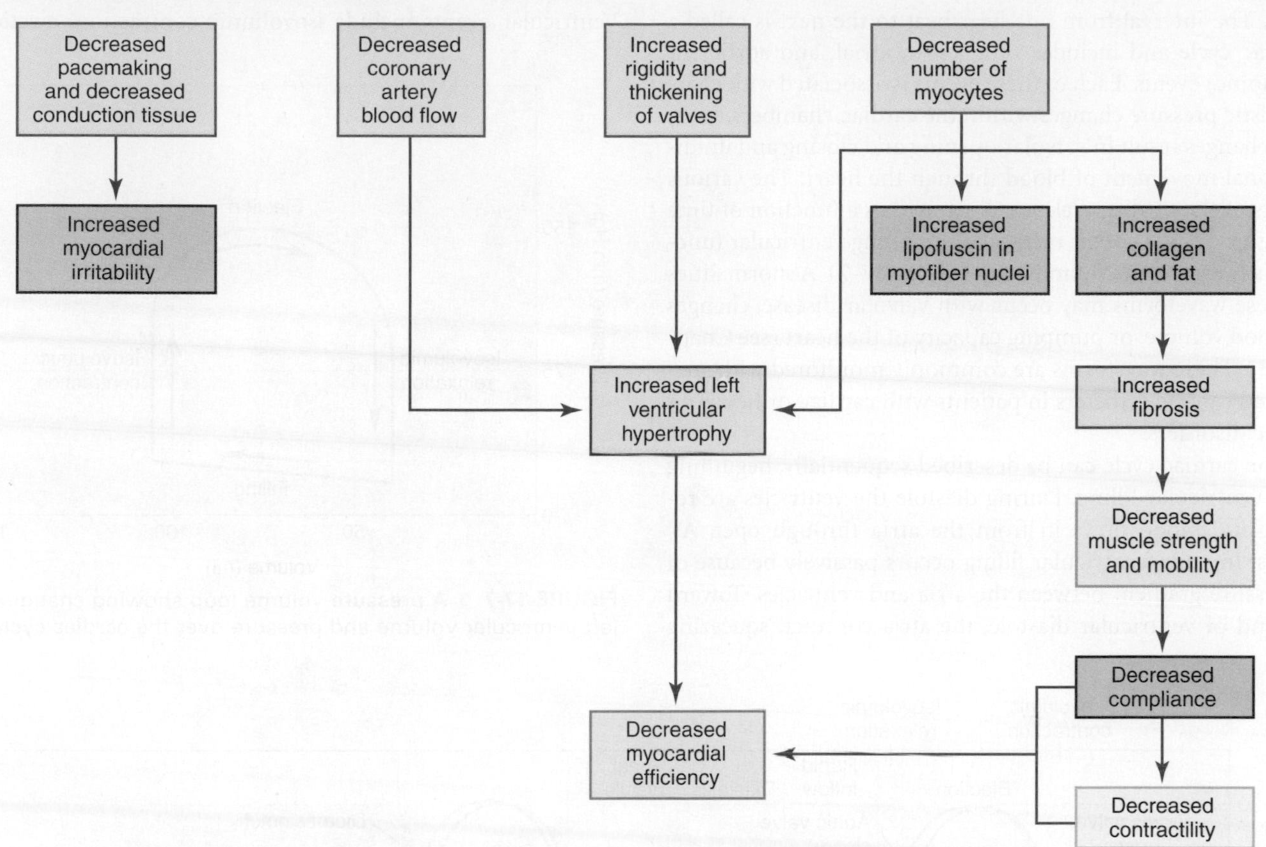

With aging, there is a decrease in the number of myocytes, but the heart size does not change appreciably. With the loss of overall cardiac muscle tissue, a corresponding expansion occurs in myocardial collagen and fat. The left ventricular muscle wall becomes thicker, with a resulting increase in oxygen demand. The endocardium becomes fibrotic and sclerosed. Cross-linking of the collagen tissue within the heart muscle increases myocardial stiffening, which causes decreased compliance. The decrease in compliance produces a decline in cardiac contractility, which reduces the heart's pumping ability. The rate of ventricular relaxation decreases.

Fibrotic changes in cardiac valves result from a combination of hemodynamic stress and generalized thickening. There is also a decrease in coronary artery blood flow to the myocardium, which affects myocardial oxygen and nutrient supply. The myocardial cells increase in size, with increased lipofuscin pigment and lipid deposition.

Within the specialized electrical conduction tissue, there is loss of myocytes in and fibrosis of conduction pathways, especially in the sinoatrial (SA) node, AV node, and bundle of His. There is a decreased number of pacemaker cells in the SA node resulting in less responsiveness of that node to adrenergic stimulation. Myocardial cell irritability increases. On the ECG, the P wave may be notched or slurred. The PR interval is longer, and the QRS amplitude decreases. The axis may shift left due to left ventricular muscle thickening (hypertrophy). The T wave may be notched, and the amplitude may decrease.

The changes previously noted affect cardiac function. The resting heart rate in the elderly is unchanged. During stress or exercise, the aging heart is unable to respond quickly with an elevated rate, and the maximal heart rate elevation is reduced. Once the heart rate is elevated, it takes a much longer time for the heart rate to return to the resting level. The cardiac stroke volume and cardiac output generally decrease with age. Oxygen consumption in the myocardium is reduced, resulting in less efficient function when stressed and an overall decreased cardiac reserve.

CARDIAC CYCLE

Each heartbeat is composed of a period of ventricular contraction (**systole**) followed by a period of relaxation (**diastole**). The interval from one heartbeat to the next is called a **cardiac cycle** and includes ventricular, atrial, and aortic (or pulmonic) events. Each of these events is associated with characteristic pressure changes within the cardiac chambers. Pressure changes result in valvular opening and closing and unidirectional movement of blood through the heart. The various events of the cardiac cycle are illustrated as a function of time in Figure 17-6. Another method of graphing ventricular function is the pressure-volume loop (Figure 17-7). Abnormalities in these waveforms may occur with valvular disease, changes in blood volume, or pumping capacity of the heart (see Chapter 18). These waveforms are commonly monitored with specialized cardiac catheters in patients with cardiac or hemodynamic disorders.

The cardiac cycle can be described sequentially, beginning with ventricular filling. During diastole the ventricles are relaxed and blood flows in from the atria through open AV valves. Initially, ventricular filling occurs passively because of a pressure gradient between the atria and ventricles. Toward the end of ventricular diastole, the atria contract, squeezing more blood through the AV valves into the ventricles. Atrial contraction increases the ventricular blood volume by 15% to 20%.[2] This "atrial kick" is particularly important during fast heart rates, when the time for ventricular filling is shortened. Ventricular events include isovolumic contraction, ejection,

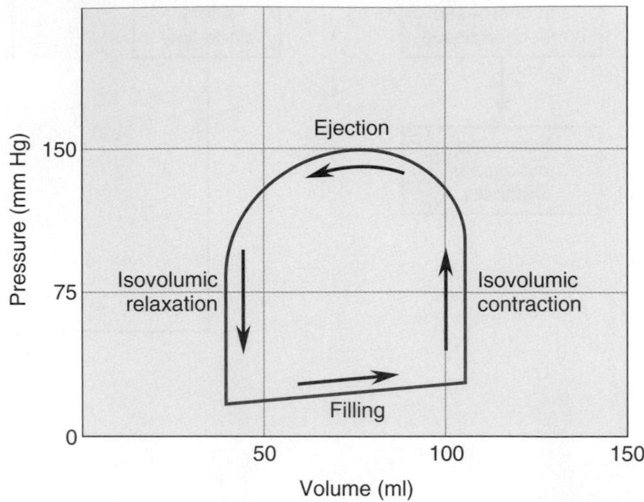

FIGURE 17-7 ■ A pressure-volume loop showing changes in left ventricular volume and pressure over the cardiac cycle.

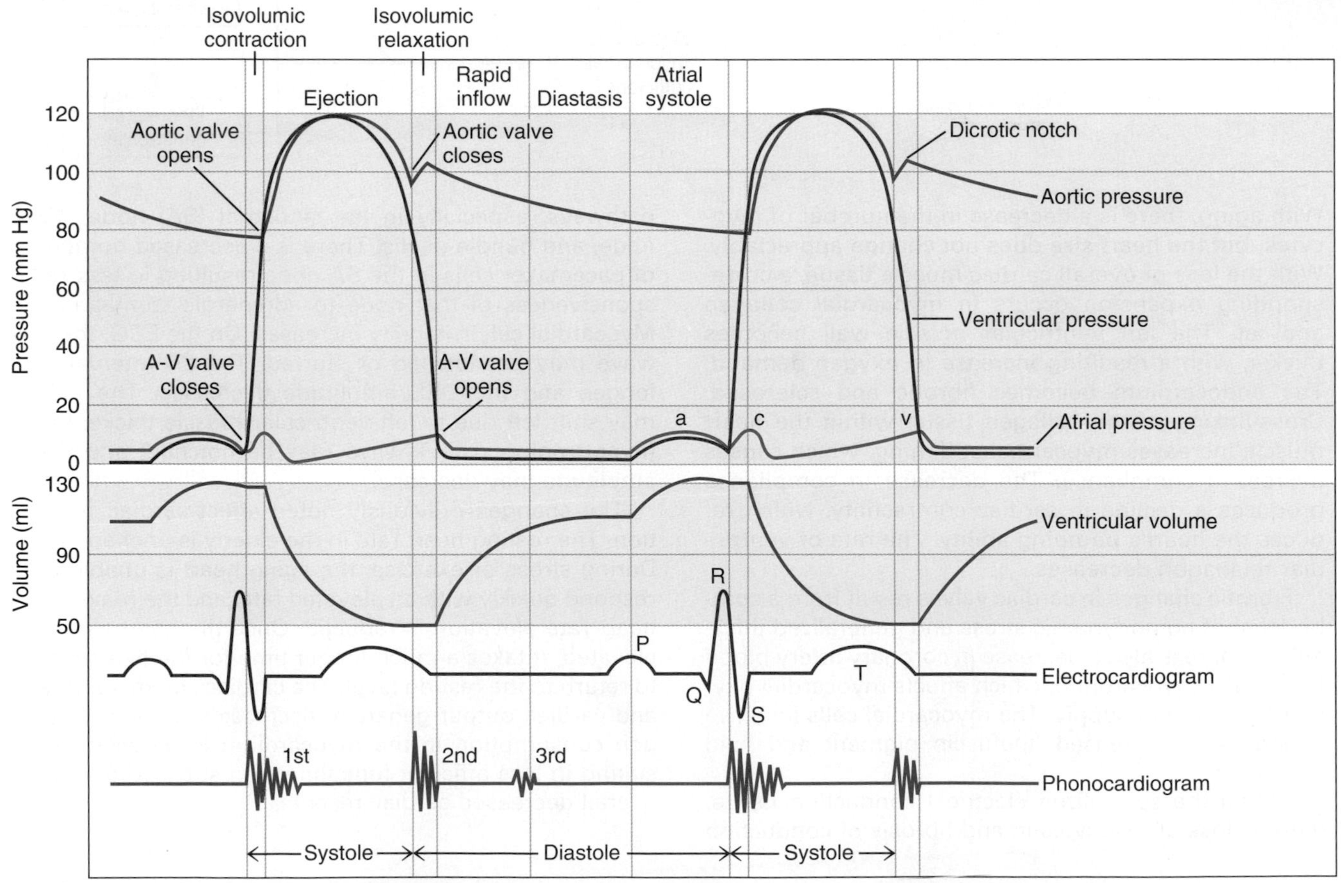

FIGURE 17-6 ■ The events of the cardiac cycle showing relationships among left atrial and ventricular pressures, ventricular volume, and aortic pressure. An identical set of events occurs on the right side of the heart although pressures are lower.

and isovolumic relaxation. Each of these cycle events is further described in the following sections.

Isovolumic Contraction

Immediately following atrial systole the ventricles begin to contract, causing intraventricular pressure to rise and the AV valves to close. AV valve closure produces a sound that can be heard at the chest wall and is termed S_1. Ventricular pressure rises rapidly during isovolumic contraction because all four cardiac valves are closed, and the volume of blood within the ventricular chamber is forcefully compressed by the powerful ventricular myocardium (see Figure 17-6, *red tracing*). Volume remains constant during this phase. The rate of rise in pressure is an indication of the contractile state of the heart. The greater a change in pressure per unit time *(dP/dT)*, the higher the contractile state. Sympathetic nervous system activation increases d*P*/d*T* whereas conditions such as heart failure are characterized by a slower rate of pressure development.

Ventricular Ejection

Ventricular contraction results in a rapid rise in ventricular pressure. As ventricular pressure exceeds aortic pressure (or pulmonic), the valve is forced open and a period of rapid ejection of blood from the ventricle follows. The rapid ejection phase is followed by a period of reduced ejection as aortic (or pulmonic) pressure rises and ventricular pressures and volumes fall. The amount of blood ejected with each contraction of the ventricle is called the stroke volume (SV). The volume of blood in the ventricle prior to ejection is the end-diastolic volume (EDV) and the amount of blood that remains in the ventricle after ejection is the end-systolic volume (ESV). Thus, stroke volume equals EDV minus ESV. An important and commonly used index of pumping effectiveness is the ejection fraction (EF), which is calculated by dividing SV by EDV. A normal EF is 60% to 80%; patients with systolic heart failure often have EF less than 40%.

Isovolumic Relaxation

The isovolumic relaxation phase begins with semilunar valve closure in response to falling ventricular pressures and ends when the AV valves open to allow ventricular filling. Ventricular blood volume remains constant during this period because all four cardiac valves remain closed. Closure of the semilunar valves causes the second heart sound, S_2. Opening of the AV valves signals the beginning of rapid ventricular filling and the start of another cardiac cycle. The rate of ventricular relaxation is indicated by the drop in ventricular pressure per unit time and is called the –d*P*/d*T*. Rapid relaxation is necessary to allow the ventricle to fill quickly and at a low pressure prior to the next systole. Impaired relaxation is a common finding in patients with heart failure and contributes to the symptoms of congestion (see Chapter 19). Relaxation of the ventricle is an energy-requiring process that becomes impaired when blood flow and oxygen delivery to the heart are inadequate.

Atrial Events

Atrial pressure waves have three characteristic curves: *a, c,* and *v* (see Figure 17-6, *green tracing*). The *a* wave corresponds to atrial contraction, which immediately precedes AV valve closure. The *c* wave occurs early in ventricular systole and is thought to represent bulging of AV valves into the atrial chambers. The *v* waves have a gradual incline, which represents filling of the atrium as blood returns from the circulation. The *v* wave drops rapidly as atrial pressure is relieved by AV valve opening. A large *v* wave is often associated with inadequate closure of the AV valve, resulting in regurgitation of ventricular blood back into the atrium during ventricular systole. The mean right atrial pressure, also called the central venous pressure (CVP), is commonly measured as an indicator of the blood volume in the heart.

Aortic and Pulmonary Artery Events

Aortic and pulmonary artery pressures rise and fall in relation to the cardiac cycle. Arterial pressures fall to their lowest value just prior to semilunar valve opening. This lowest pressure is called *diastolic blood pressure.* Arterial pressure reaches its maximum during ventricular ejection and is called *systolic blood pressure.* A characteristic notch *(dicrotic notch)* in the arterial pressure curve may be seen as the semilunar valves close (see Figure 17-6, *blue tracing*).

The difference in aortic pressure between systole and diastole is partly dependent on the aorta's elastic characteristics. During systole, the aorta stretches to accommodate blood ejected by the ventricle. The stretched aorta has "stored" or potential energy that is released during diastole to maintain driving pressure and to keep blood flowing continuously through the circulation. Aortic stiffening, as occurs with aging or arteriosclerosis, may result in higher systolic and lower diastolic blood pressures due to loss of aortic elastic properties.[3] When aortic or pulmonic pressures are chronically elevated, the ventricles must generate more pressure to open the semilunar valves and eject the stroke volume. Over time this increase in pressure work can damage the heart muscle and lead to hypertrophy or failure.

KEY CONCEPTS

- Characteristic pressure wave changes that occur during the cardiac cycle may be useful in diagnosing cardiac disease and volume status.
- The atria have three characteristic waves: *a, c,* and *v*. The *a* wave corresponds to atrial contraction, the *c* wave corresponds to AV valve bulging during ventricular contraction, and the *v* wave corresponds to atrial filling.

- The ventricles have four important phases: isovolumic contraction, ejection, isovolumic relaxation, and diastolic filling. The rate and amplitude of these pressures reflect chamber volume, contractility, and valvular function. Left ventricular pressure/volume relationships are frequently used to diagnose heart failure.
- Pressure changes in the aorta during a cardiac cycle are partly dependent on the elasticity of the aorta. Differences between systolic and diastolic pressures are less with a compliant aorta. Aortic stiffness results in higher systolic and lower diastolic pressures.

CORONARY CIRCULATION

Anatomy of the Coronary Vessels

The blood supply to heart muscle is provided by the coronary arteries (Figure 17-8). Right and left coronary artery openings are located in the sinuses of Valsalva, in the aortic root, just beyond the aortic valve.[2] The right coronary artery originates near the aortic valve's anterior cusp and passes diagonally toward the right ventricle in the AV groove. In approximately 50% of the population, the right coronary artery gives rise to a posterior descending vessel that supplies blood to the heart's posterior aspect. In 20% of the population, the left coronary artery is dominant in supplying blood to the ventricles, and in 30% of the population the right and left coronary arteries deliver about the same amount of blood and neither is dominant.[4] The *left main coronary artery* arises near the aortic posterior cusp and travels a short distance anteriorly before dividing into the *left anterior descending* and *circumflex* branches. The anterior descending branch supplies septal, anterior, and apical areas of the left ventricle, whereas the circumflex artery supplies the lateral and posterior left ventricle. The three major coronary arteries give rise to a number of smaller branches that penetrate the myocardium and branch into small arterioles and capillaries. Regular exercise and stable atherosclerotic plaques in the coronary arteries are thought to stimulate the development of more extensive collateral circulation in the heart. Collateral vessels may help limit infarct size in patients suffering acute coronary occlusions (see Chapter 18). Areas supplied by divisions of the coronary arteries are listed in Table 17-2. Most of the heart's capillary beds drain into the coronary veins, which then empty into the right atrium through the coronary sinus (Figure 17-9).

Regulation of Coronary Blood Flow

Blood flow through coronary vessels is determined by the same physical principles that govern flow through other vessels of the body, namely, driving pressure and vascular resistance to flow.[5] According to Ohm's law, an increase in driving pressure *(P)* increases blood flow *(Q)*, whereas an increase in resistance *(R)* reduces blood flow: $Q = P/R$ (see Chapter 15). Driving pressure through the coronary arteries is determined by aortic blood pressure and right atrial pressure. This relationship can be expressed in the following equation:

Coronary driving pressure ***(P)*** = ABP − RAP, where ABP is aortic blood pressure and RAP is right atrial pressure. Thus, an increase in aortic pressure enhances coronary blood flow, whereas an increase in right atrial pressure opposes coronary flow.

Coronary vascular resistance *(R)* has two major determinants: (1) coronary artery diameter and (2) the varying degree of external compression due to myocardial contraction and relaxation. Coronary artery diameter is continuously adjusted to maintain blood flow at a level adequate for myocardial demands. **Autoregulation** is the term used to describe the intrinsic ability of the arteries to adjust blood flow according to tis-

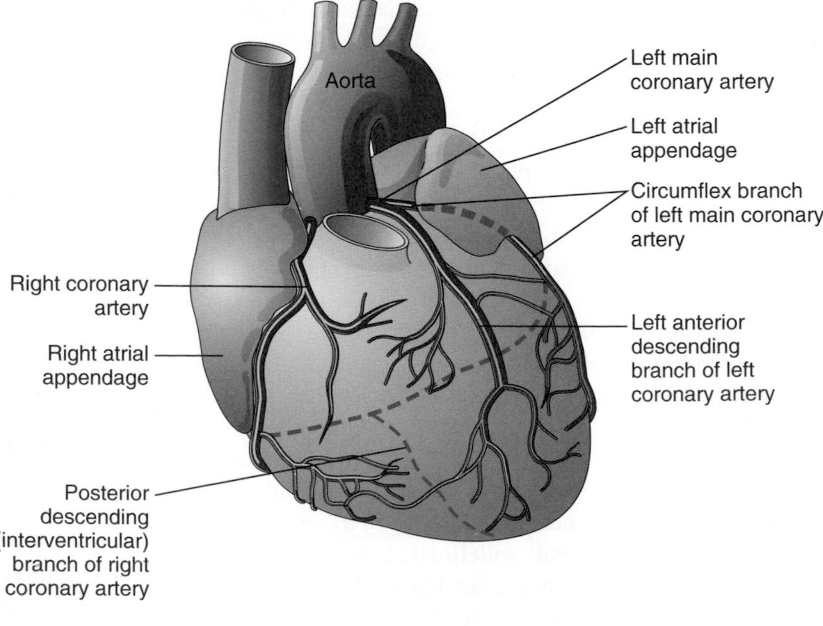

FIGURE 17-8 ■ Coronary arteries supplying the heart. The right coronary artery supplies the right atrium, ventricle, and posterior aspect of the left ventricle in most individuals. The left coronary artery divides into the left anterior descending and circumflex arteries, which perfuse the left ventricle.

sue needs. Vessel dilation *(vasodilation)* occurs in response to increased tissue metabolism or reduced driving pressure, whereas decreased metabolic activity or increased driving pressure results in a decreased vessel diameter *(vasoconstriction)*.

The mechanism of autoregulation can be explained by the metabolic hypothesis, which proposes that increased metabolism or decreased blood flow results in a buildup of vasodilatory chemicals in the vessel. Smooth muscle encircling the vessel relaxes in response to the presence of the chemicals, increasing vessel diameter. Several vasodilating substances have been proposed, including potassium ions, hydrogen ions, carbon dioxide, nitric oxide, prostaglandins, and adenosine. The endothelial cells that line vessels are known to secrete a variety of relaxing and constricting factors, which may contribute to autoregulation. An increase in the level of adenosine, a product of adenosine triphosphate (ATP) metabolism, is currently believed to be the chief vasodilatory chemical produced by the myocardium.[4] A low level of oxygen in the blood *(hypoxemia)* also may cause vasodilation of the coronary arteries. Vasodilatory substances are washed away as blood flow increases in response to increased vessel diameter. A declining level of vasodilatory chemicals results in vasoconstriction. Thus, vessel diameter is continuously adjusted according to concentrations of vasodilatory chemicals, which are directly related to the tissue's metabolic activity.

An ATP-sensitive potassium channel has been implicated in the regulation of coronary blood flow.[6] The concentration of ATP in vascular smooth muscle regulates a specific K^+ channel. As ATP levels rise in response to increased coronary flow, the channel closes, making it easier to depolarize the cell and contract vascular smooth muscle. Contraction of vascular smooth muscle reduces the diameter of the coronary arteries and reduces blood flow. The opposite also occurs: a reduction in ATP, due to low flow or increased metabolism, opens the K^+ channels. Potassium then leaks out of the vascular smooth muscle and short circuits the depolarizing influences. This inhibits vascular contraction, leading to vasodilation and increased coronary blood flow. Substances other than ATP are believed to open and close these channels and may contribute to coronary regulation during periods of ischemia or increased metabolic demand.

Nitric oxide (NO) produced by endothelial cells lining the coronary arteries is an important regulator of coronary blood flow. NO is a diffusible gas produced by the enzyme, inducible nitric oxide synthase, in response to numerous stimuli including hypoxemia and platelet factors. NO is a potent vasodilator, and inhibition of its production is associated with reduced coronary blood flow. The majority of known risk factors for coronary heart disease have been shown to impair nitric oxide–dependent vasodilation of coronary arteries.[6]

Vessel diameter also is regulated by the autonomic nervous system. The coronary arteries are primarily innervated by sympathetic nerves, but they also receive a small amount of parasympathetic innervation. The sympathetic neurotransmitter norepinephrine (NE) is a vasoconstrictor; however, autoregulatory mechanisms predominate in the heart such that an increase in sympathetic nervous system activation usually does not constrict coronary arteries. The increased metabolic activity associated with sympathetic nervous system stimulation overrides the direct effect of norepinephrine on the vessels. Parasympathetic activity contributes to vasodilation by promoting the production of nitric oxide by coronary endothelial cells.

In addition to vessel diameter, coronary resistance is affected by myocardial contraction. During systole, cardiac muscle compression creates a marked rise in coronary resistance that reduces coronary blood flow (perfusion). Blood flow to the left ventricle is greatly decreased during systole

Table 17-2

Areas Supplied by the Coronary Arteries

Artery	Area Supplied
Right coronary	Right atrium (55% of persons)
	Right ventricle
	Intraventricular septum
	Sinus node (55% of persons)
	Atrioventricular node
	Bundle of His
Left anterior descending	Right atrium (45% of persons)
	Right ventricle (minor)
	Left ventricle (anterior, apex)
	Anterior papillary muscles
	Right and left bundle branches
	Intraventricular septum
Left circumflex	Left atrium
	Left ventricle (posterior, anterior)
	Sinus node (45% of persons)

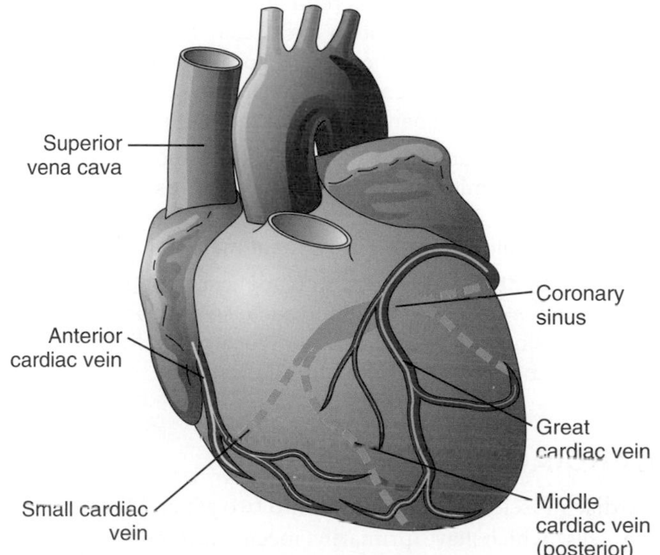

FIGURE 17-9 ■ Venous drainage of the heart. Coronary veins drain blood from the myocardial capillary bed and deliver it into the right atrium.

because of the pressures generated by the thick muscular layer. Blood vessels that penetrate the myocardium to supply the innermost endocardial areas are more compressed during contraction than are outer epicardial vessels. Even though coronary artery driving pressure is greatest during ventricular systole, little blood flow reaches the ventricles because of the high external pressure applied to the coronary vessels as the myocardium contracts. Therefore, most myocardial blood flow occurs during the diastolic interval between ventricular contractions. The time the heart spends in diastole is directly related to heart rate. Faster heart rates reduce diastolic time and decrease coronary artery blood flow.

Cardiac muscle needs a continuous supply of oxygen and nutrients to perform its pumping functions. A disruption in cardiac blood flow *(ischemia)* generally results in some degree of pump failure and damage to cardiac tissues. Myocardial ischemia may be caused by conditions that reduce coronary blood flow or increase myocardial demands for oxygen. These include (1) reduced driving pressure (e.g., low aortic blood pressure or high right atrial pressure), (2) reduced vessel diameter (e.g., hypertrophy, arteriosclerosis, thrombosis, vasoconstricting chemicals), (3) reduced perfusion time (e.g., high heart rates, some dysrhythmias), and (4) increased metabolic demands (e.g., fever, sepsis, anemia).

KEY CONCEPTS

- The right and left coronary arteries originate from the aortic root, within the sinuses of Valsalva. In most people the right coronary artery perfuses the right ventricle, AV node, sinoatrial (SA) node, and right atrium.
- The left coronary artery divides into the left circumflex artery and left anterior descending artery, which perfuse the left atrium and ventricle.
- Coronary blood flow is regulated centrally by the autonomic nervous system and locally by autoregulation. The amount of coronary flow depends on driving pressure and coronary resistance. Coronary resistance is dependent on vessel diameter.
- Adenosine and nitric oxide are two important vasodilating chemicals that are produced in response to inadequate oxygen delivery to the heart and help to increase blood flow so as to meet metabolic demands.
- Although driving pressure is highest during systole, there is little coronary flow because of vessel compression by the contracting myocardium. Most coronary blood flow occurs during diastole.

CARDIAC MYOCYTES

Cardiac muscle cells are divided into two general types: working cells, which have primarily mechanical pumping functions, and electrical cells, which primarily transmit electrical impulses. Both types are *excitable:* they are able to produce and transmit action potentials. Working myocardial cells are packed with contractile filaments and make up the bulk of the atrial and ventricular muscle. Electrical cells function to initiate and coordinate contraction of the working cells. Differentiated cardiac myocytes are unable to enter the cell cycle to proliferate; however, they can increase in size and synthesize more contractile proteins (hypertrophy). New myocardial cells can be formed from stem cells that have the potential to divide. Stem cells may be recruited from the circulation and stimulated to divide and mature into myocytes within the myocardium.[7] Conditions that increase myocardial cell death are thought to stimulate recruitment of stem cells into the myocardium. When the rate of myocardial cell loss exceeds replacement by stem cells, the condition of heart failure may ensue (see Chapter 19).

Myocyte Structure

Typical myocardial cells (myocytes) are illustrated in Figure 17-10. Cardiac myocytes are described as muscle "fibers" because of their long narrow shape. The plasma membrane (sarcolemma) of one cardiac cell is joined end to end with its neighbors by intercalated disks, which contain gap junctions that allow the rapid passage of electrical impulses from one cell to the next. The intercalated disks permit the many separate cells of the myocardium to function together in a coordinated manner. This arrangement is called a *functional syncytium.* The sarcolemma also forms membrane-lined channels that penetrate the cell and become the transverse tubules (T tubules) (Figure 17-11). The T tubules permit ex-

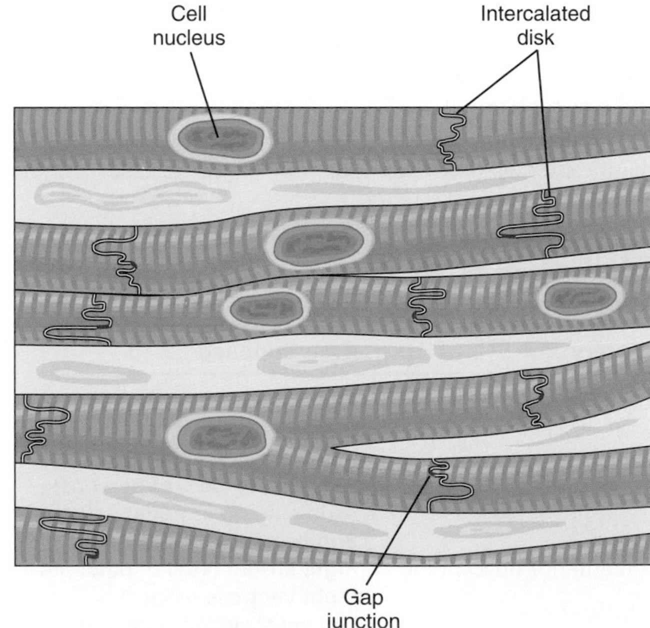

FIGURE 17-10 ■ Myocardial cells, showing long narrow shape and interconnecting junctions, forming a functional syncytium. The end of one muscle cell is fused to the next by intercalated disks. Within these connections are specialized proteins that form a fluid-filled pore (gap junction) between the fused cells. Ions can travel through the gap junctions to transport changes in membrane potential from one cell to the next.

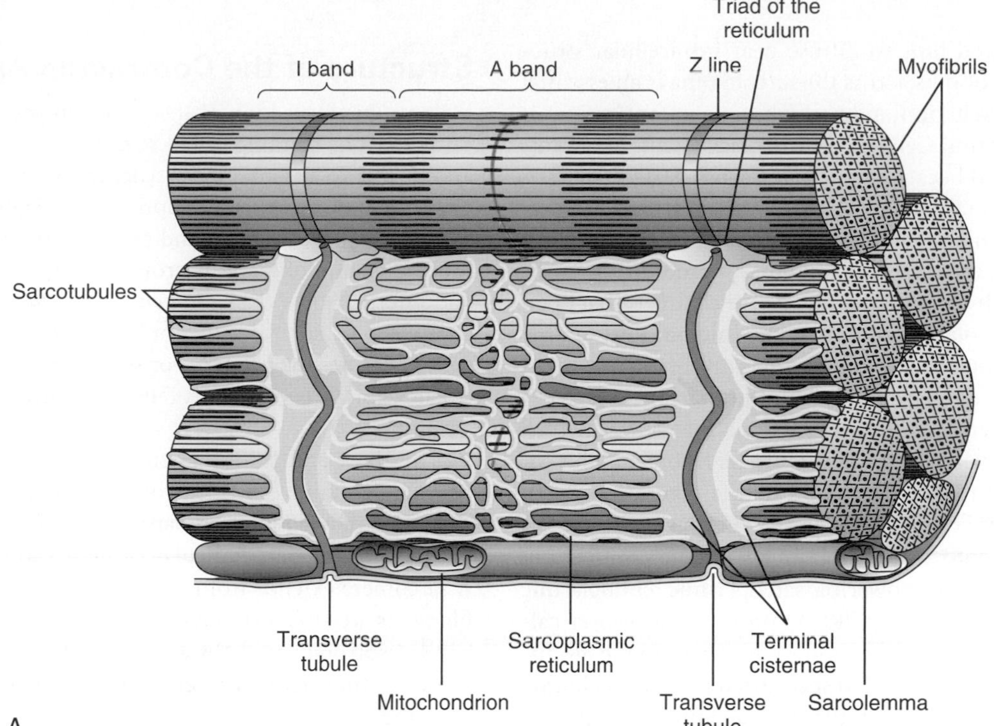

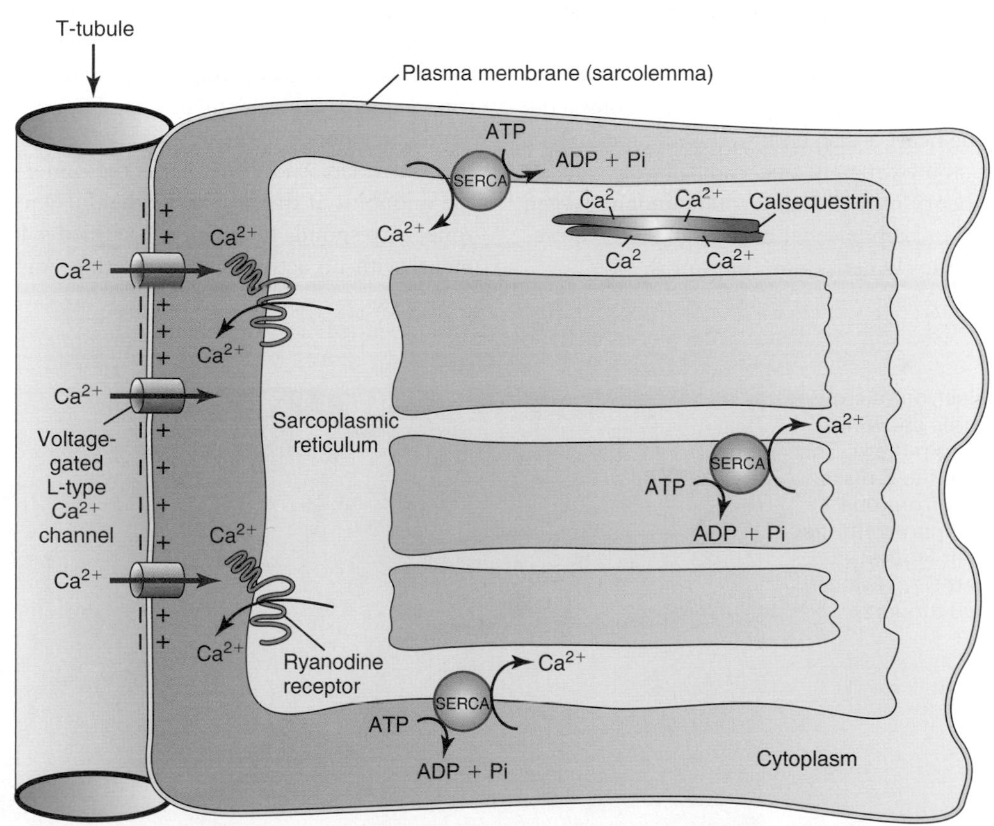

FIGURE 17-11 ■ **A,** Schematic diagram of a portion of a cardiac myocyte showing the transverse tubules (T tubules), which extend horizontally from the plasma membrane into the cell interior. The T tubules are extensions of the plasma membrane that bring the extracellular fluid into juxtaposition with the terminal ends of the sarcoplasmic reticulum (SR). The T tubule with the SR on either side of it is called the triad of the reticulum. **B,** Calcium ions that enter the cytoplasm through voltage-gated L-type channels on the T-tubule membrane interact with the ryanodine receptors on the sarcoplasmic reticulum. The activated ryanodine receptors allow calcium ions to flow into the cell cytoplasm where they initiate contraction. As soon as they are released, calcium ions are rapidly captured by the sarcoplasmic endoplasmic reticulum calcium ATPase *(SERCA)* pumps on the SR membrane.

tracellular fluid and ions to diffuse near intracellular structures. Movement of ions across the sarcolemma is an essential part of cellular excitation and the subsequent contraction of intracellular elements. Cellular contractile elements are simultaneously activated because signals at the cell surface are rapidly transmitted internally by the T tubules.[8]

The sarcoplasmic reticulum (SR) is an extensive labyrinth of hollow membrane that stores significant amounts of intracellular calcium. It contains Ca^{2+}-sensitive channels that open briefly during depolarization and allow calcium ions to flow into the cytoplasm. An action potential traveling along the T tubule opens voltage-sensitive calcium ion channels (L type) in the plasma membrane. The Ca^{2+} ions that enter the cell through these channels interact with receptors on the SR membrane called ryanodine receptors (see Figure 17-11, *B*). Activation of these receptors opens calcium gates on the SR and Ca^{2+} rushes into the cytoplasm to initiate contraction. The SR also contains powerful sarcoplasmic endoplasmic reticulum calcium ATPase (SERCA) pumps that recover calcium ions from the cytoplasm and return them to the SR. Inside the SR, calcium is bound to specialized proteins including calsequestrin. This helps keep the free calcium concentration in the SR lower such that the calcium transporters have a lower gradient to pump against.

Cardiac muscle cells are packed with numerous mitochondria that are strategically positioned along the contractile fibers of the cell. The heart is also endowed with an extensive capillary network, approximately one capillary per muscle cell. The large number of mitochondria and abundant oxygen supply are necessary to keep pace with the high ATP requirements of the contractile elements and ion pumps.

Structure of the Contractile Apparatus

Microscopic inspection of the cardiac myocyte reveals a typical pattern of banding called *striation.*[9] This striated appearance is due to an organized structure of the proteins (myofibrils) of the contractile apparatus (Figure 17-12). The contractile proteins, actin and myosin, are called *filaments* because they are long and narrow. **Myosin** filaments are larger and referred to as *thick filaments. Thin filaments* are actually composed of several different types of protein bundled together. **Actin** is the primary constituent of thin filaments, with smaller amounts of the proteins **tropomyosin** and **troponin** bound to it.

The thick and thin filaments are specifically arranged in contractile units called **sarcomeres** (Figure 17-13). Sarcomeres are defined by dark bands called *Z disks* (also called Z lines), which lie perpendicular to actin and myosin filaments. A sarcomere extends from one Z disk to the next. Thin actin filaments are attached to Z disks and extend from them. The I bands (isotropic) are light in color and correspond to the position of thin actin filaments extending in both directions from the Z disk. Thick myosin filaments lie parallel to and between the thin filaments. They are held in place by a very large and elastic protein called *titin* that extends from the Z disk to the center of the sarcomere. Each myosin filament is surrounded by six thin filaments (see Figure 17-13). The dark A band corresponds to an area where the actin and myosin filaments overlap. An M line marks the center of the A band and the midpoint of the myosin filaments. One other zone, the H zone, corresponds to a region occupied solely by myosin filaments with no actin filament overlap. An efficient, synchro-

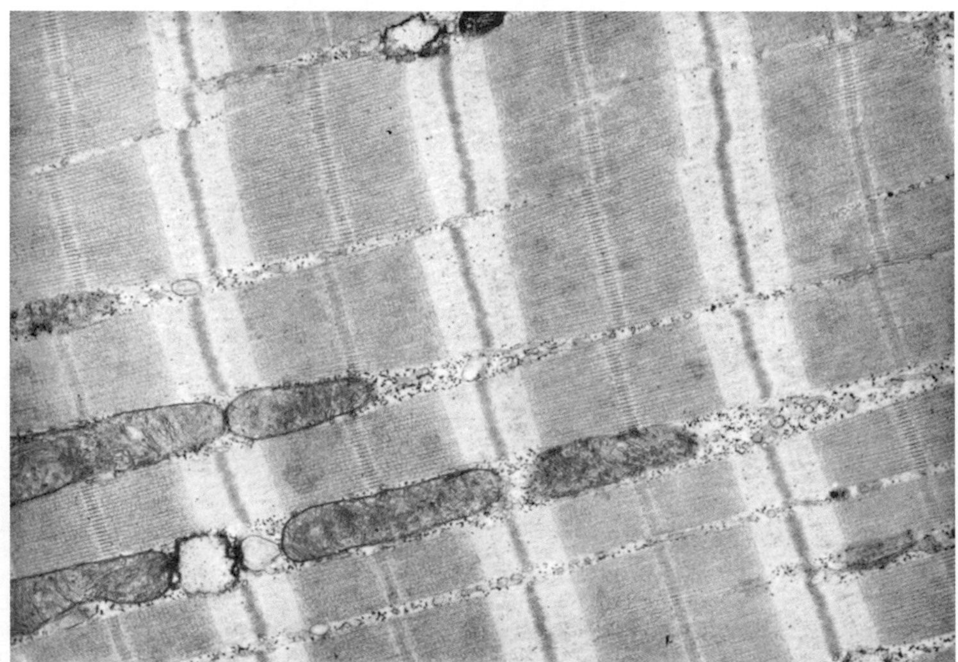

FIGURE 17-12 ■ Electron micrograph of muscle fibrils showing characteristic banding pattern. The dark vertical lines are the Z disks. A sarcomere extends from one Z disk to the next. Compare with the schematic drawing in Figure 17-13. (From Fawcett DW: *The cell,* Philadelphia, 1981, Saunders.)

nized contraction is enhanced by this precise arrangement of contractile elements.

Characteristics of Contractile Filaments

Myosin molecules are composed of six polypeptide chains, two heavy (H) chains and four light (L) chains. These light and heavy chains are organized into a tail region and two globular "head" areas (Figure 17-14). The myosin heads interact with actin filaments to produce muscle contraction. Thick filaments are made up of many myosin molecules with tail regions bundled together and heads sticking out at intervals along the bundle. The head regions are flexible and can bend and pull on actin filaments to accomplish muscle contraction. Myosin heads are oriented in opposite directions on either side of the center tail region (see Figure 17-14). Myosin heads have enzymatic properties and can cleave ATP to release energy necessary for muscle contraction. Different forms of myosin have varying rates of ATP hydrolysis which affects how quickly the muscle contracts. The level of thyroid hormone is known to affect the type of myosin produced in heart cells. Hyperthyroidism is associated with a fast cycling type and hypothyroidism with a slow type of myosin. The rate of myosin cycling can also be regulated at the light chain of the myosin protein. Cellular enzymes that attach a phosphate to the light chain speed up the rate of cycling. Phosphorylation is increased by activation of myocardial β_1 receptors and enhances contractility.[9]

As previously mentioned, thin filaments are composed of several different proteins, including actin, nebulin, tropomyosin, and troponin. Actin filaments are actually polymers of many globular actin proteins that are attached end-to-end, like two strings of beads, and then twisted together to form a helix (Figure 17-15). Each of the actin beads has a site that

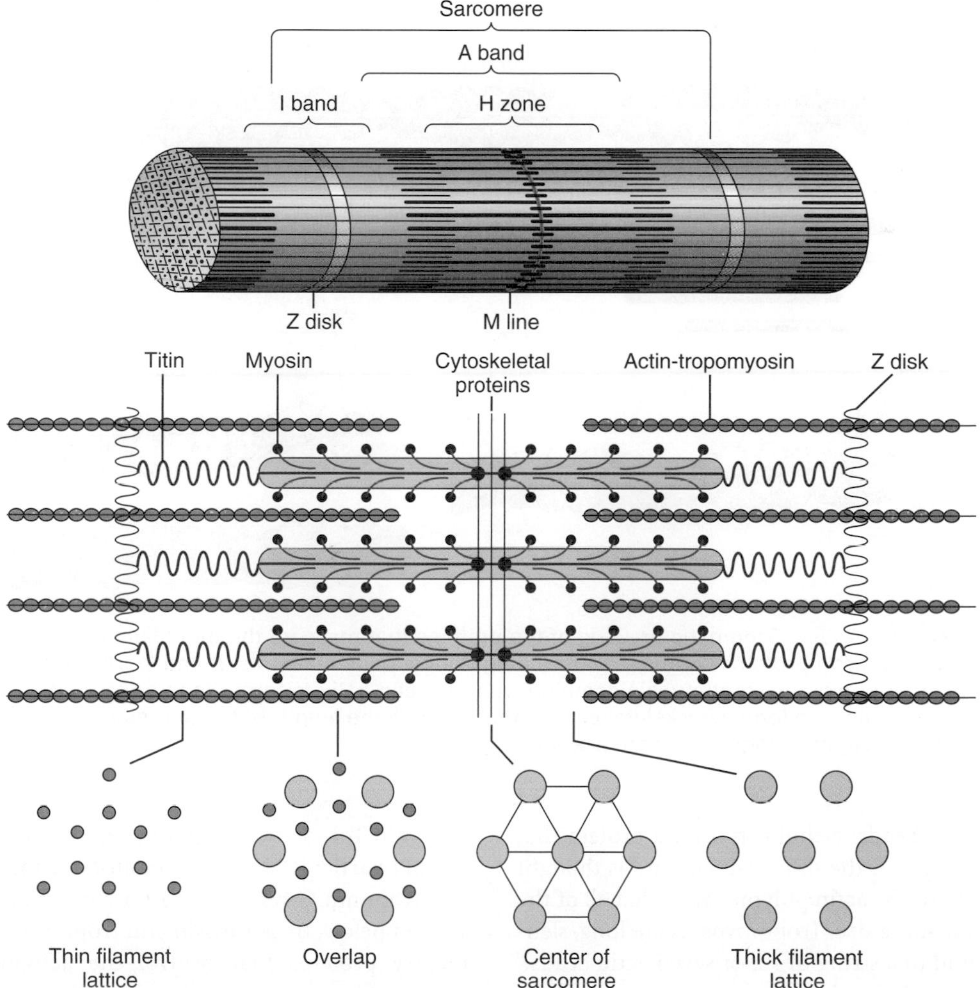

FIGURE 17-13 ■ Thick and thin filaments are organized into contractile units called *sarcomeres.* A sarcomere extends from one Z disk to the next and represents the fundamental unit of muscle contraction. See text for description of bands, zones, and lines. Overlap of thick and thin filaments in each area is shown in cross-section at the bottom. Each thick filament interacts with six thin filaments that surround it.

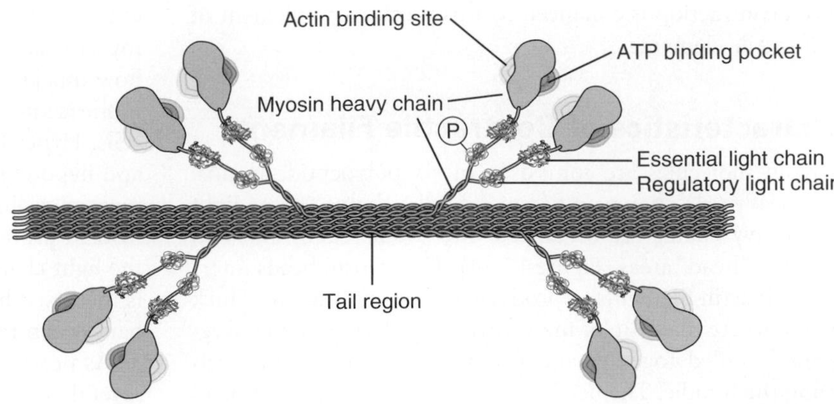

FIGURE 17-14 ■ The thick filament of the sarcomere is composed of myosin proteins. Myosin head groups are oriented in opposite directions on either side of the center tail region. Phosphorylation *(P)* of the regulatory light chain increases myosin activity and rate of cross-bridge cycling.

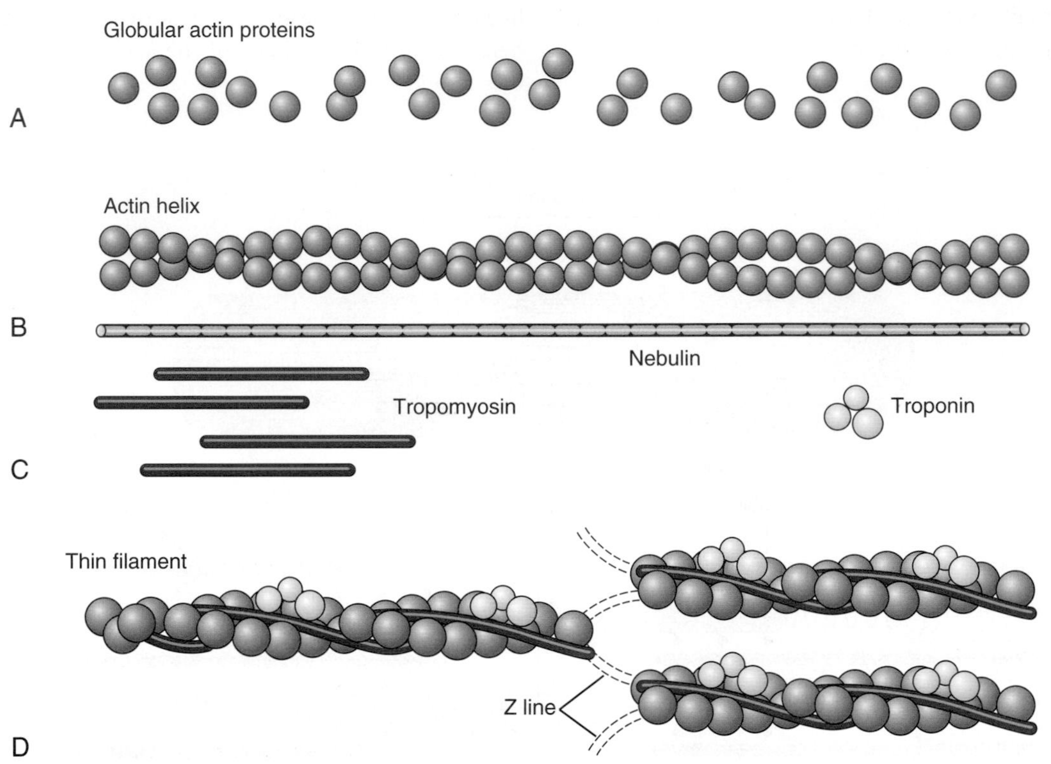

FIGURE 17-15 ■ Schematic drawing of the proteins that make up the thin filament. **A,** Globular actin proteins combine to form long double-helix filaments. **B** and **C,** The proteins troponin and tropomyosin combine with the actin helix to form the thin filament **(D).** Nebulin is a long cytoskeletal protein that extends the length of the thin filament and is thought to regulate filament length.

can bind with myosin heads. Nebulin is a long protein that extends the entire length of the thin filament and is thought to regulate the length of the actin polymer such that all of the thin filaments are the same size. Tropomyosins are long, slender proteins that bind to a string of six or seven actin beads.[9] When myocardial muscle is relaxed, tropomyosin molecules cover the myosin-binding sites on the actin beads. A third protein complex, troponin, is attached to the thin filament and regulates the availability of binding sites on the actin filament. Each troponin is composed of three subunits, called troponin T, I, and C. Troponin T binds to tropomyosin, troponin I participates in the inhibitory actions of tropomyosin, and troponin C binds up to four molecules of Ca^{2+}. As described below, tropomyosin and troponin are important regulatory proteins that control the activities of actin and myosin filaments. The specific isoforms (amino acid sequences) of troponin T and I present in heart tissue differ from those in other types of cells, and their presence in the serum can be used to detect myocardial infarction (see Chapter 18).

KEY CONCEPTS

- The myocardial cells of the heart behave as a syncytium because they are joined by gap junctions within the intercalated disks that permit the flow of ions from one cell to the next.
- Myocytes are packed with actin and myosin proteins that form the contractile apparatus. The thick filaments are composed of myosin proteins. Myosin has enzymatic activity and splits ATP, releasing energy needed for movement of the filaments.
- The thin filament is composed of actin and two regulatory proteins, troponin and tropomyosin. At rest, tropomyosin inhibits myosin-binding sites on actin. The position of tropomyosin is regulated by the calcium-binding protein troponin. Nebulin is another actin-associated protein that helps regulate thin filament length.

MOLECULAR BASIS OF CONTRACTION

Overview of Contraction

The heart's pumping action is accomplished by the additive contractions of the many myocytes that form the cardiac chambers. Because each myocyte contributes only a small amount to overall muscle shortening, all cells of the chamber must shorten simultaneously to produce a forceful contraction. The specialized cells of the conduction system function to stimulate myocardial contraction in a coordinated way. An action potential traveling down the conduction system is the usual trigger for contraction. Cardiac myocyte depolarization causes ion channels in the plasma membrane and T tubules to open, permitting sodium and calcium entry and release of calcium from the SR. The presence of free calcium in the sarcoplasm (muscle cytoplasm) results in contraction. These events describe the process of excitation-contraction coupling.

Sliding Filament/Cross-Bridge Theory of Muscle Contraction

The sliding filament, or cross-bridge, theory of muscle contraction is suggested by the anatomic configuration of the sarcomere described earlier. Muscle shortening is accomplished by increasing the amount of overlap of actin and myosin filaments. The Z disks at the ends of the sarcomere move closer together as overlapping actin and myosin filaments slide past one another. Myosin heads grip binding sites on the actin beads and pull the thin filaments toward the sarcomere's center. Each time a myosin head binds an actin bead it forms a so-called **cross-bridge.** Flexible myosin heads move in a ratchet-like manner to tug on the actin filaments (Figure 17-16). Each ratcheting motion moves actin filaments only minutely, and many sequential cross-bridge formations are required to shorten the sarcomere. Thus, myosin heads bend back and forth, binding and pulling on the actin filaments in a steplike fashion. Actin filaments are prevented from slipping back to their original position because some myosin-actin bonds are forming while others are releasing. The making and the subsequent breaking of each actin-myosin cross-bridge requires one molecule of ATP. Consequently, tremendous quantities of ATP are hydrolyzed with each cardiac contraction.

ATP hydrolysis, which occurs at the myosin head region, provides the energy for contraction and also affects the capability of myosin to bind actin.[9] Myosin has two functional states or conformations: (1) a low-affinity state in which it binds weakly and (2) a high-affinity state in which it avidly binds actin. The affinity of the myosin head for actin depends on whether ATP is bound (low affinity) or ADP and inorganic phosphate (P_i) are bound (high affinity). A proposed sequence of cross-bridge cycling is as follows (see Figure 17-16):

1. Free myosin heads bind ATP and hydrolyze it to ADP and P_i, which remain on the myosin. Myosin heads now have a high affinity for actin and are in an extended conformation.
2. If binding sites on actin are accessible, myosin binds to the actin.
3. Binding results in release of ADP and P_i and a ratchet movement of the myosin, which shortens the sarcomere (power stroke).
4. With loss of ADP and P_i, myosin can bind another molecule of ATP. The myosin heads with ATP bound now have a low affinity for actin and release from the binding site. ATP is again hydrolyzed to ADP and P_i, and another cross-bridge cycle is initiated.

Continued cross-bridge cycling is dependent on the availability of ATP and calcium ions. A lack of ATP results in fewer cross-bridge cycles and inability of the muscle to shorten normally.

Role of Calcium in Muscle Contraction

Muscle contraction is dependent on the presence of an adequate amount of calcium ion in the cytoplasm. In the absence of free intracellular calcium, muscle contraction will not take place, even though myosin head groups have high affinity for actin-binding sites. This phenomenon can be explained in the following way. At rest, myosin heads are prevented from binding to actin by tropomyosin proteins, which inhibit actin-binding sites. The position of tropomyosin protein is controlled by troponin. When calcium is absent, troponin induces tropomyosin to inhibit the actin binding sites. When calcium binds to troponin C, the troponin complex induces tropomyosin to move and expose the binding sites (see Figure 17-16, *A* and *B*). Cross-bridge formation immediately ensues because myosin heads have high affinity for these sites in the relaxed state. The concentration of free calcium ions in the myocardial cell determines how many actin sites are exposed and, therefore, the number of cross-bridges and extent of contraction. The release of Ca^{2+} into the cytoplasm is regulated by numerous neurotransmitters and hormones that affect contractility as described in later sections of this chapter.

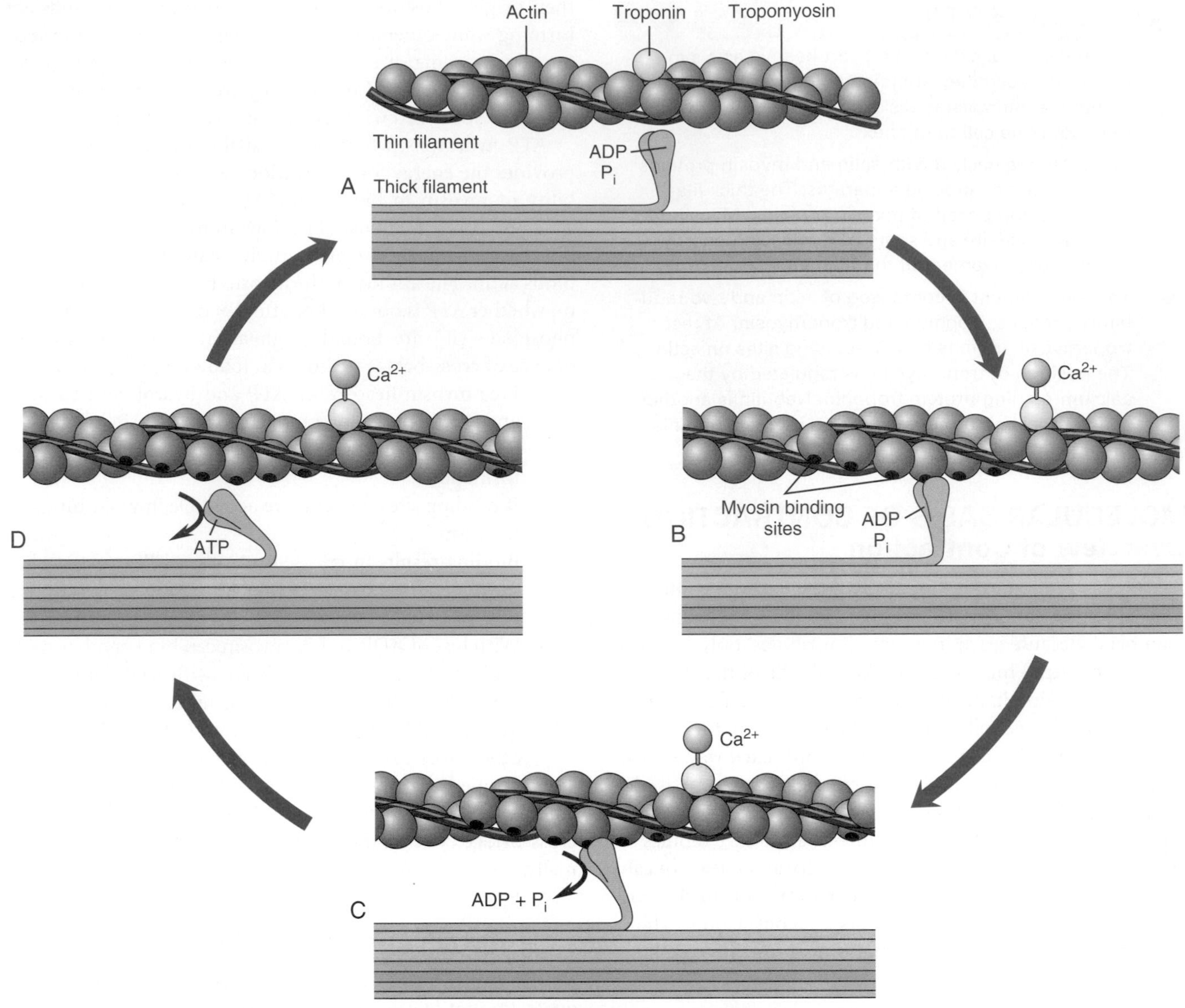

FIGURE 17-16 ■ The cross-bridge cycle of muscle contraction. **A,** The myosin head has hydrolyzed its bound adenosine triphosphate *(ATP)* to adenosine diphosphate *(ADP)* and inorganic phosphate *(P_i)*, which remain on the myosin. In this state the myosin has high affinity for actin but cannot bind because the actin-binding sites are not accessible. **B,** When calcium ion enters the cell and binds to troponin, the tropomyosin-blocking protein moves to allow myosin to bind actin, forming a cross-bridge. **C,** The act of binding changes the shape of myosin so that ADP and P_i are released. The "power stroke" is accomplished by movement of the myosin neck region. **D,** When a new molecule of ATP binds to the myosin, it changes to a low-affinity state and releases from the actin. ATP is again hydrolyzed to ADP and P_i to start the cycle again. Each cross-bridge cycle uses one ATP molecule.

Energy of Muscle Relaxation

Although muscle relaxation is generally viewed as a passive phenomenon, it actually requires significant energy to pump calcium ions out of the cytoplasm. As calcium levels fall, calcium diffuses away from the troponin molecules and tropomyosin is induced to cover the actin binding sites. With actin binding sites covered, myosin heads are unable to initiate cross-bridge formation, and thick and thin filaments slide back to their resting position. Removal of calcium ions is an energy-requiring process. Membrane pumps located in the sarcolemma and SR actively move calcium out of the sarcoplasm against a concentration gradient (Figure 17-17). The sarcolemma contains two different calcium pumps: one that requires ATP and one that uses the potential energy of the sodium gradient to remove calcium from the cell. Calcium

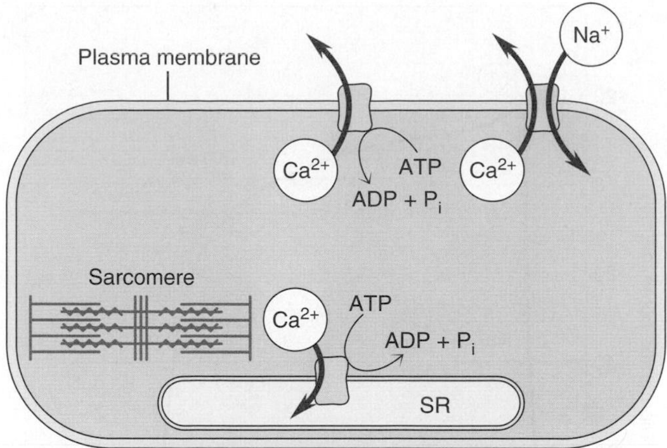

FIGURE 17-17 ■ Calcium ions *(Ca^{2+})* are removed from the cardiac muscle cell cytoplasm by energy-dependent protein transporters in the plasma membrane and sarcoplasmic reticulum *(SR)* membrane. Thus cardiac relaxation is an energy-requiring process. *ADP,* Adenosine diphosphate; *ATP,* adenosine triphosphate; P_i, inorganic phosphate.

pumps on the SR (SERCAs) require ATP. Thus energy deficiency due to myocardial ischemia can impair diastolic relaxation as well as systolic contraction of the heart muscle.

KEY CONCEPTS

- Cardiac myocytes are terminally differentiated cells, incapable of proliferation. New myocytes are formed from stem cells that are recruited from the circulation.
- Contraction of cardiac muscle is accomplished by shortening of individual sarcomeres. This is due to increased overlap of actin and myosin filaments. Myosin heads bind to specific sites on actin and pull the thin filaments toward the center of the sarcomere.
- ATP hydrolysis provides the energy for cross-bridging and also affects the affinity of myosin for actin. Myosin has high affinity for actin when ADP and P_i are bound, and low affinity when ATP is bound. Myosin cycles between high- and low-affinity states, making and breaking cross-bridges with the actin filament.
- The presence of intracellular free calcium ion (Ca^{2+}) is necessary for muscle contraction to occur. When Ca^{2+} is absent, actin-binding sites are inhibited and not accessible for cross-bridging. Binding of Ca^{2+} to troponin induces the movement of tropomyosin to expose actin-binding sites and allow cross-bridge formation.
- Muscle relaxation is due to removal of Ca^{2+} from the cytoplasm. This is an energy-requiring process.

CARDIAC ENERGY METABOLISM

The heart, like other tissues in the body, utilizes energy from ATP hydrolysis to drive its energy-requiring functions. Synthesis of ATP in cardiac muscle cells is accomplished by the same glycolytic and oxidative reactions described in detail in Chapter 3.

Oxygen Utilization

Because the heart is continuously active, its energy requirements are considerable. Very little ATP is stored in myocardial cells, so that a continuous supply of oxygen and nutrients is necessary to support ongoing ATP synthesis. Even under normal resting conditions, the heart extracts a large portion of oxygen from the blood perfusing it. Conditions of increased oxygen demand, therefore, must be met by increasing the rate of coronary blood flow. When oxygen delivery is insufficient to meet requirements for oxidative phosphorylation, the cell must rely on ATP produced by glycolysis. Unfortunately, glycolysis results in production of only enough ATP to maintain the cell for seconds to minutes. In addition, anaerobic glycolysis results in local buildup of lactic acid, which may further impair cardiac performance.

Under conditions of relative ATP excess, myocardial cells are able to transfer energy to a storage form called *creatine phosphate* (CP). This transfer is accomplished by the enzyme **creatine kinase** (CK or CPK), in the following reaction:

$$\text{ATP} + \text{creatine} \longleftrightarrow \text{ADP} + \text{CP}$$

Although amounts of cellular CP are limited, they provide an immediate source of energy when cellular ATP levels are low. Under conditions of ischemia, the enzymatic reaction would proceed in reverse, utilizing CP and adenosine diphosphate (ADP) to produce ATP.

The enzyme CK is also useful in the diagnosis of myocardial cell damage. Damaged cells leak their enzymes into extracellular fluid and eventually into the blood stream. Elevated levels of blood CK are indicative of cell membrane damage. Different types of tissue contain different forms of CK (isoenzymes). The MB form of CK is found in cardiac muscle, and elevated serum levels of this enzyme are indicative of myocardial infarction.[10] Other intracellular proteins, including troponin and myoglobin, are released during myocardial cell death and also can be used as markers of myocardial infarction (see Chapter 18).

Substrate Utilization

The primary foodstuffs that provide fuel for energy-producing enzymatic processes in cardiac muscle are glucose and fatty acids.[11] Amino acids are less important metabolic substrates for cardiac muscle except during states of starvation. The amount of fatty acids and glucose utilized by heart muscle cells depends on their relative concentrations in the blood. Fatty acids are the preferred fuel, particularly in a fasting state, when glucose levels are lower. Under fasting conditions, fatty acids account for approximately 85% of myocardial fuel and glucose contributes only 15%. After eating, when blood glucose levels rise, glucose utilization may increase to about 50%. Fatty acid metabolism requires oxygen and is therefore not useful under conditions of ischemia. The heart is also able to use lactate and ketones as sources of energy when they accumulate in the circulation.

KEY CONCEPTS

- CP is an immediately available storage form of energy. Under conditions of low ATP availability, CP is converted to ATP by the enzyme CK.
- The primary energy substrates for the heart are fatty acids and glucose.

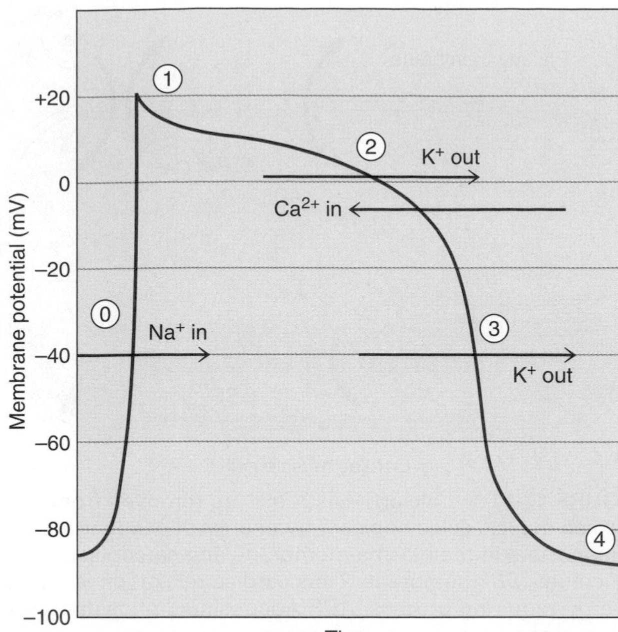

FIGURE 17-18 ■ The ventricular myocardial action potential has five characteristic phases, representing changes in ion movement through the plasma membrane. *Phase 0:* Rapid upstroke due to sodium influx. *Phase 1:* Slight repolarization due to closure of sodium channels and beginning potassium efflux. *Phase 2:* Plateau due to offsetting influx of calcium and efflux of potassium. *Phase 3:* Rapid repolarization due to closure of calcium channels and increased potassium efflux. *Phase 4:* Resting membrane potential reestablished due to closure of all voltage-sensitive channels.

CARDIAC ELECTROPHYSIOLOGY

The plasma membranes of cardiac cells are endowed with special ion channels that make the cells excitable. Excitable tissues are capable of generating and conducting action potentials. The heart is rhythmically activated by action potentials, which are generated and transmitted by a specialized conduction system. Spread of an action potential over cardiac muscle cell surfaces results in myocardial contraction. An understanding of the electrophysiologic properties of the heart is important because many cardiac disorders result in disturbances in electrical function.

Cardiac Resting Potential

Like other cells, resting cardiac cells are negatively charged on the inside with respect to the outside (see Chapter 3). Differences in potassium ion concentration across the cell membrane determine the resting membrane potential. Atrial and ventricular muscle cells generally have a resting membrane potential of –85 to –95 mV. Pacemaker cells are less polarized having a resting membrane potential of about –60 mV. An increase in extracellular potassium ion tends to depolarize the cell (make it less negative), and a lower-than-normal extracellular potassium tends to hyperpolarize the cell (make it more negative). The degree of polarization is an important determinant of the ease with which an action potential can be initiated. Abnormalities in serum potassium level are a common source of cardiac dysrhythmias.

Cardiac Action Potentials

Depolarization of cardiac cells to a threshold point results in activation of voltage-sensitive ion channels in the membrane. A myocardial action potential (Figure 17-18) results from movement of ions through these open voltage-gated channels. The action potential in atrial and ventricular cells has five characteristic phases.[12] Atrial action potentials are shorter in duration because they have a reduced Phase 2 compared with ventricular cells.

Phase 0. Phase 0 begins when the membrane potential approaches threshold and voltage-gated "fast" sodium channels open momentarily. Due to a steep electrochemical gradient for sodium entry, rapid influx of sodium ions occurs. Sodium entry depolarizes the cell by neutralizing the difference in charge (polarity) across the membrane. A steep depolarizing deflection is recorded. Class I antiarrhythmic agents such as quinidine and lidocaine block voltage-gated sodium channels and interfere with phase 0 depolarization (see Chapter 19).[13]

Phase 1. Phase 1 is identified on the monitor as a small repolarizing deflection that corresponds to closure of the fast sodium channels and beginning efflux of potassium from the cell. The interior of the cell is now more positively charged, which induces potassium ions to leave the cell.

Phase 2. Phase 2 is also called the *plateau phase* because little change in membrane potential occurs during this time, even though ions continue to move across the membrane. Phase 2 is primarily associated with an influx of calcium ions, which is offset by an efflux of potassium ions. These calcium channels open and close slowly in comparison to fast sodium channels and are thus referred to as slow channels or L-type channels (long-lasting).

The calcium that enters the cell during phase 2 is linked to muscle contraction as previously described. The L-type calcium channels can be modified by agonists that prolong the open phase, such as catecholamines, and by antagonists that shorten the open phase, such as acetylcholine. Calcium channel–blocking agents (class IV antiarrhythmic agents) are used commonly in patients with cardiovascular diseases to inhibit calcium influx.[13] β-Blockers (class II antiarrhythmics) also reduce calcium ion influx during phase 2 by indirectly inhibiting calcium channels.

Phase 3. Phase 3 is characterized by a rapid return to the resting membrane potential. This is accomplished by closure of the slow calcium channels and continued and even more rapid efflux of potassium ions from the cell. Sodium channels remain absolutely refractory during phases 1, 2, and early 3. The latter part of phase 3 represents a *relative refractory period,* when sodium channels may be induced to open, but a larger than normal depolarizing stimulus is required. If an abnormally early (premature) depolarization occurs during the relative refractory period, it will be conducted more slowly than usual because few fast Na^+ channels are ready to be activated. Slow conduction through the myocardium predisposes to cardiac dysrhythmias, such as ventricular fibrillation (see Chapter 19). Class III antiarrhythmic agents, like amiodarone, increase the refractory period by inhibiting opening of potassium channels during phase 3.[13]

Phase 4. Phase 4 corresponds to the period of time between action potentials when no changes in membrane voltage are evident and the resting membrane potential is present. The resting membrane potential in myocardial cells is flat and they do not spontaneously depolarize. In contrast, cells in the pacemaker and conduction system automatically depolarize and have a sloping phase 4. The Na^+-K^+ pump and Ca^{2+} pumps work continuously throughout all phases to maintain the internal and external concentrations of sodium, potassium, and calcium ions.

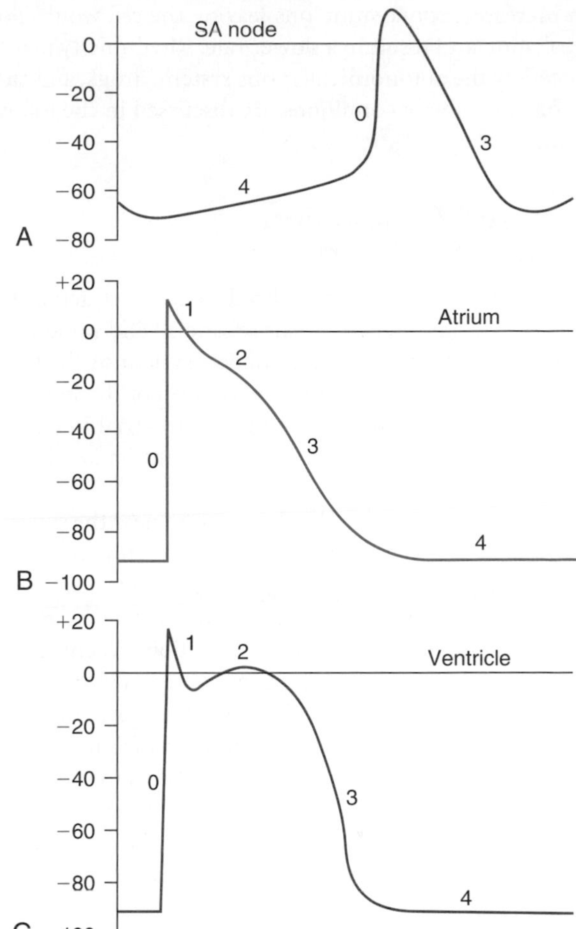

FIGURE 17-19 ■ Rhythmic cells **(A)** have a sloping phase 4, in contrast to the flat phase 4 of the atrial **(B)** and ventricular **(C)** muscle cell. Spontaneous depolarization during phase 4 allows pacemaker cells to develop action potentials automatically. *SA,* Sinoatrial. (Adapted from Hoffman BF, Cranefield PF: *Electrophysiology of the heart,* New York, 1960, McGraw-Hill.)

Rhythmicity of Myocardial Cells

Rhythmicity (automaticity) refers to intermittent, spontaneous generation of action potentials. A requirement for rhythmicity is that the cell membrane has channels that automatically open during phase 4. These channels open when the membrane potential becomes more negative during repolarization phase.[12] Progressive channel opening makes the pacemaker cells leaky to Na^+, Ca^{2+}, and K^+. Gradually the flow of positive ions into a cell depolarizes the membrane and results in generation of an action potential. Toward the end of repolarization sodium ions begin to flow into the pacemaker cell through ion channels called I_f. The I_f channels originally were named for a "funny" current and later discovered to be sodium channels that are activated by membrane repolarization. Late in phase 4, an increase in calcium ion influx occurs through voltage-gated calcium channels called T type for "transient." These channels open and close more quickly than the L-type calcium channels that open during the action potential. An action potential is initiated when phase 4 depolarization reaches the threshold for opening of voltage-gated, L-type, slow calcium channels. Repolarization is achieved in large part by an exodus of potassium ions from the cell. Rhythmic cells have a recognizable action potential that is characterized by a sloping phase 4 (Figure 17-19), in contrast to the flat phase 4 of ventricular muscle cells.

The rate of rhythmic discharge is determined by the relative influx of Na^+ and Ca^{2+} versus the efflux of K^+. In a normal heart, a cell with the fastest rate of spontaneous depolarization becomes the pacemaker for the rest of the heart. Cells in the SA node, located in the right atrium, generally function as the heart's pacemaker because they have the fastest rate of spontaneous depolarization. However, other cells in the conduction system are also capable of spontaneous depolarization and may initiate an action potential in certain circumstances.

The steepness of the slope of phase 4 depolarization determines the rate of action potential generation. Several factors determine the steepness of the slope, including membrane permeability to sodium, calcium, and potassium. For example, an increase in potassium ions leaving the cell would slow depolarization and result in a slower rate. Rhythmicity may be influenced by the autonomic nervous system, drugs, and electrolyte balance. These conditions are discussed in the following sections.

Specialized Conduction System of the Heart

Some myocardial cells are specialized to conduct action potentials throughout the heart in an organized and rapid manner. These cells make up the conduction system of the heart, as shown in Figure 17-20. Normal excitation of the heart follows a pathway beginning with the SA node, atrial internodal pathways, AV node, bundle of His, ventricular bundle branches, and, finally, Purkinje fibers.

The SA node is located in the right atrium near the superior vena cava inlet. It receives innervation from sympathetic and parasympathetic branches of the autonomic nervous system. The SA node generally serves as a pacemaker for the heart, generating about 75 (range, 60 to 100) action potentials per minute in a resting adult. SA action potentials are spread contiguously to adjacent atrial cells at a rate of about 1.0 m/sec.[12] A fibrous skeleton separates atria from ventricles and prevents spread of impulses from atrial cells to ventricular cells. There are several small bundles of atrial muscle cells that conduct impulses slightly faster than the usual atrial cell. One such bundle, the anterior interatrial band (Bachmann bundle), conducts impulses from the SA node to the left atrium. The existence of three other bundles that conduct impulses from the SA node to the AV node has been suggested. Atrial depolarization results in atrial contraction, which increases the volume delivered to the still relaxed ventricular chambers.

After traversing the atria, the impulse initiated at the SA node arrives at the AV node (AV junction) located in the posterior septal wall of the right atrium just behind the tricuspid valve. There is a characteristic slowing of impulse conduction through the AV node, which allows for completion of atrial contraction prior to beginning ventricular systole. The AV node is actually composed of several different types of fibers that have somewhat different action potential conduction times. Overall, it normally takes about 0.13 second for an impulse to pass through the AV node. The slowness of conduction through AV fibers is related to two factors: (1) cells in the AV region have less negative resting membrane potentials and therefore a slower phase O, and (2) there are few gap junctions between AV nodal cells so that cell-to-cell conduction of action potentials is more difficult due to high resistance.[12,14] The AV node is richly innervated by the autonomic nervous system. The AV node spontaneously depolarizes at a rate of 40 to 60 times per minute and usually becomes the heart's pacemaker if the SA node fails.

Purkinje cells (fibers), which lead from the AV node to ventricular myocardium, are vastly different from AV nodal cells. They are large and well structured to conduct impulses very rapidly. After penetrating the AV fibrous barrier, the bundle of

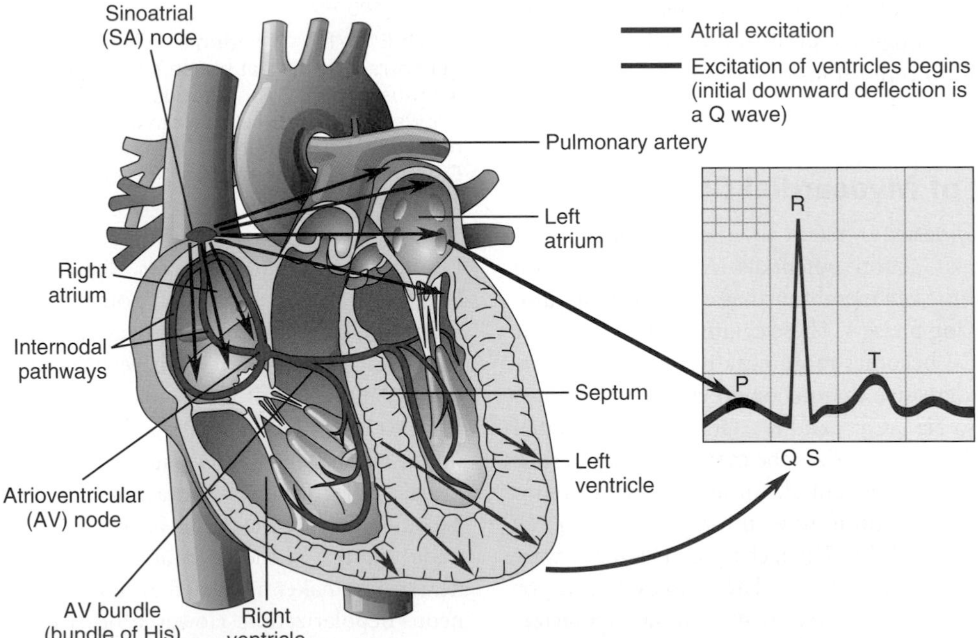

FIGURE 17-20 ■ Schematic drawing of the conducting system of the heart. An impulse normally is generated in the sinus node and travels through the atria to the AV node, down the bundle of His and Purkinje fibers, and to the ventricular myocardium. Recording of the depolarizing and repolarizing currents in the heart with electrodes on the surface of the body produces characteristic waveforms.

Purkinje fibers travels 5 to 15 mm down the intraventricular septum toward the apex. The main bundle then divides into left and right bundle branches, which travel down the left and right sides of the intraventricular septum. Successive branches of Purkinje fibers penetrate the ventricular muscle mass from the endocardial side. Intraventricular septal areas are depolarized first, followed by apical muscle and finally the lateral walls (Figure 17-21). Early septal depolarization allows the septum to contract first and provide a stable wall for the left and right ventricles to contract against.[12] The total time elapsed between main bundle branch and terminal Purkinje fiber depolarization is only 0.03 second.[14] Therefore, the entire ventricular endocardium is activated almost simultaneously. Purkinje fibers are capable of spontaneous depolarization at a rate of 15 to 40 times per minute and may become pacemakers for the heart if impulses from the SA and AV nodes are interrupted.

Action potentials are rapidly transmitted from the terminal Purkinje fibers to cardiac muscle fibers and then spread contiguously from cell to cell through the ventricular muscle. Approximately 0.03 second is required for the impulse to be transmitted through the ventricular myocardium.[14] Impulses normally travel from the terminations of Purkinje fibers at endocardial surfaces toward the epicardial surfaces. Depolarization of the right ventricle is accomplished slightly sooner than the left because of differences in muscle mass. Depolarization of the ventricular myocardium is followed by contraction and ejection of blood from the ventricles.

The capability of faster pacemakers to suppress the automatic discharge of slower pacemakers is called overdrive suppression. A slower pacemaker may be revealed if the normal pacemaker is suddenly interrupted. Sometimes it takes time for the slower pacemaker to "kick in" and begin pacing at its intrinsic rate. A previously rapid rate of depolarizations apparently enhances the activity of membrane Na^+-K^+ pumps, resulting in a period of hyperpolarization (more negative resting potential) when the faster pacemaker suddenly stops. Thus, it takes a bit longer to reach threshold and initiate the first action potential.

Autonomic Regulation of Rhythmicity

Both sympathetic and parasympathetic nerves supply the heart. Sympathetic innervation is widespread to all areas, including the ventricular myocardium. Parasympathetic innervation, by way of the vagus nerves, is localized primarily in SA and AV nodal areas. The right vagus nerve supplies the SA node, whereas the left vagus nerve supplies the AV node.[15] The autonomic nervous system exerts control over heart rate and velocity of impulse conduction. In general, sympathetic activation increases heart rate *(chronotropic effect)* and increases speed of conduction *(dromotropic effect)* as well as inducing heart muscle to contract more forcefully *(inotropic effect)*. These effects are achieved by release of NE from sympathetic nerve endings. Binding of NE to β receptors on heart muscle cell membranes opens membrane channels, which allows more rapid sodium and calcium ion entry.

Parasympathetic activation primarily results in a reduction in heart rate and speed of action potential conduction. Acetylcholine is the neurotransmitter released by parasympathetic nerve endings. Acetylcholine binding by muscarinic receptors on heart cells increases membrane permeability to potassium ions, allowing them to leak from the cell. The resulting hyperpolarization makes it more difficult to reach threshold and initiate an action potential. The resting heart is normally under a predominant parasympathetic influence, which results in an SA discharge rate of about 75 beats/min. If parasympathetic activity is blocked, the spontaneous discharge rate of SA nodal cells increases to about 100 beats/min. An increase in vagal activity can reduce heart rate significantly. Breath holding, bearing down during defecation, and pressing on the carotid arteries may increase vagal tone and reduce heart rate.

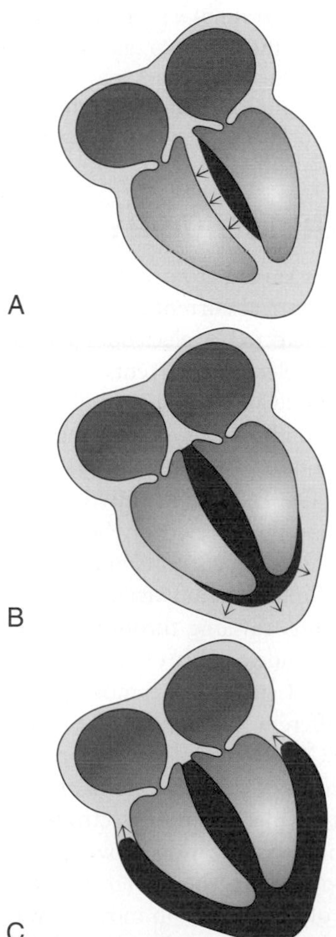

FIGURE 17-21 ■ Sequence of ventricular depolarization showing septal depolarization in a left-to-right direction **(A)**, followed by apical depolarization in an endocardial to epicardial direction **(B)**, and finally, depolarization of the lateral walls **(C)**. Repolarization proceeds in the opposite direction.

KEY CONCEPTS

- The cardiac resting membrane potential is about −90 mV. The resting membrane potential is determined by the ratio of intracellular to extracellular K^+ concentration.
- The five phases of the cardiac action potential are due to changes in ion conductance through the plasma membrane. The main changes in ion conductance result from opening of the fast Na^+ channels (phase 0), slow Ca^{2+} channels (plateau), and K^+ channels (repolarization) in the plasma membrane.
- Spontaneous generation of action potentials in automatic cells is due to progressive leak of Na^+ and Ca^{2+} into the cell via channels that automatically open after repolarization. The rate of cation leak determines the rate of pacemaker discharge. Parasympathetic influence increases K^+ efflux and slows the rate. Sympathetic influence increases influx of Na^+ and Ca^{2+} and increases the rate.
- The usual conduction pathway for depolarization of the heart begins at the SA node, progresses through the atria, enters the AV node, and activates the His Purkinje fibers. Purkinje fibers leave the AV node and divide into left and right branches that innervate the endocardial surface of the ventricular myocardium.

ELECTROCARDIOGRAPHY

As action potentials spread from cell to cell throughout the myocardium, an electrical current is transmitted to the body surface and can be detected by electrodes placed on the skin.[16] A recording of these electrical currents is called an *electrocardiogram* (ECG). The ECG is a useful indicator of abnormalities of the heart's conduction system. Irregularities in initiation of impulses, conduction rates, and conduction pathways can be identified. The ECG looks different from the cardiac action potential described previously because it registers depolarizing and repolarizing currents in the whole heart rather than the activity of individual myocytes (Figure 17-22).

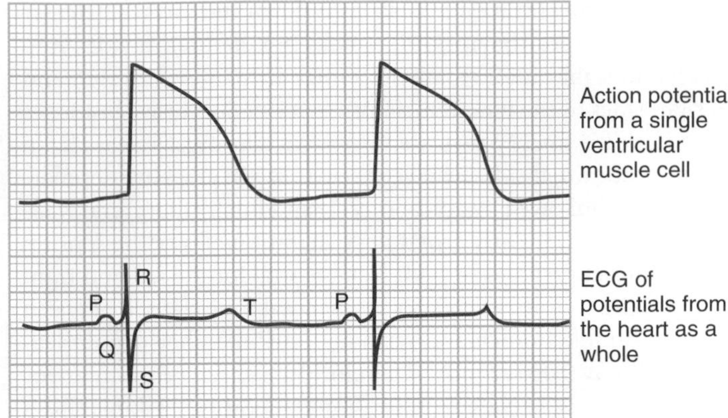

FIGURE 17-22 ■ Comparison of the action potential from a single ventricular muscle cell, showing rapid depolarization and prolonged repolarization phases, against an electrocardiogram of potentials from the heart as a whole. Ventricular myocytes remain depolarized and refractory through the entire QT interval. (Redrawn from Guyton AC, Hall JE: *Textbook of medical physiology,* ed 9, Philadelphia, 1996, Saunders.)

Electrical currents traveling through the heart have both direction and magnitude and are often described as *vectors.* At any instant, electrical currents are moving in various directions through different regions of the heart. Waveforms recorded at the ECG electrodes are algebraic sums of all of these vectors. Patterns of electrical activity shown on the ECG vary according to the placement of electrodes on the body. In general, a wave of depolarization moving toward a positive recording electrode will register as an upward deflection on the ECG. A wave of repolarization moving away from a positive electrode also will register as an upward deflection on the ECG. A downward deflection results from a wave of depolarization moving away from a positive electrode (Figure 17-23). Placement of a recording electrode on the lower left extremity (lead II) results in the typical ECG pattern shown in Figure 17-24. A description of the usual electrode placements is included in the section on diagnostic tests at the end of this chapter.

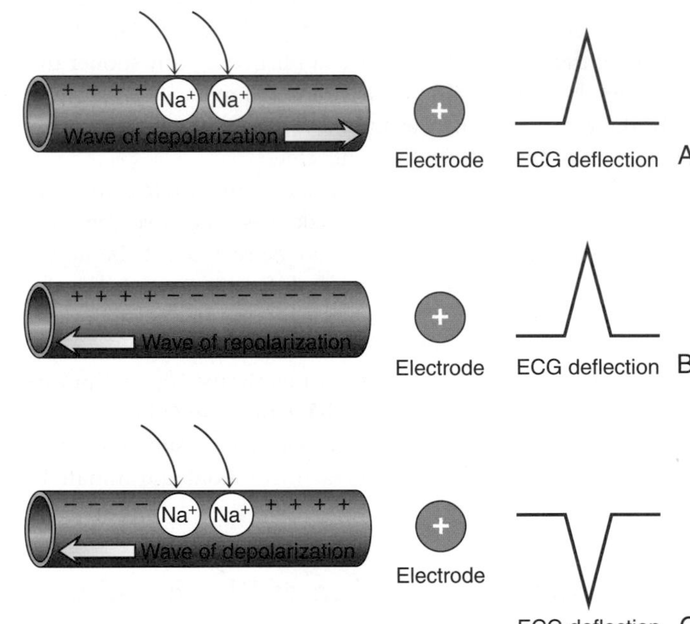

FIGURE 17-23 ■ Electrocardiographic *(ECG)* waveforms may be positive (upward) or negative (downward), depending on the location of electrodes on the chest. **A,** A wave of depolarization moving toward a positive electrode results in a positive deflection. **B,** A wave of repolarization moving away from a positive electrode results in a positive deflection. **C,** A wave of depolarization moving away from a positive electrode results in a negative deflection.

Each deflection on the ECG has a normal characteristic shape and time interval (see Figure 17-24). The three major wave complexes are the *P wave,* which corresponds to atrial de-

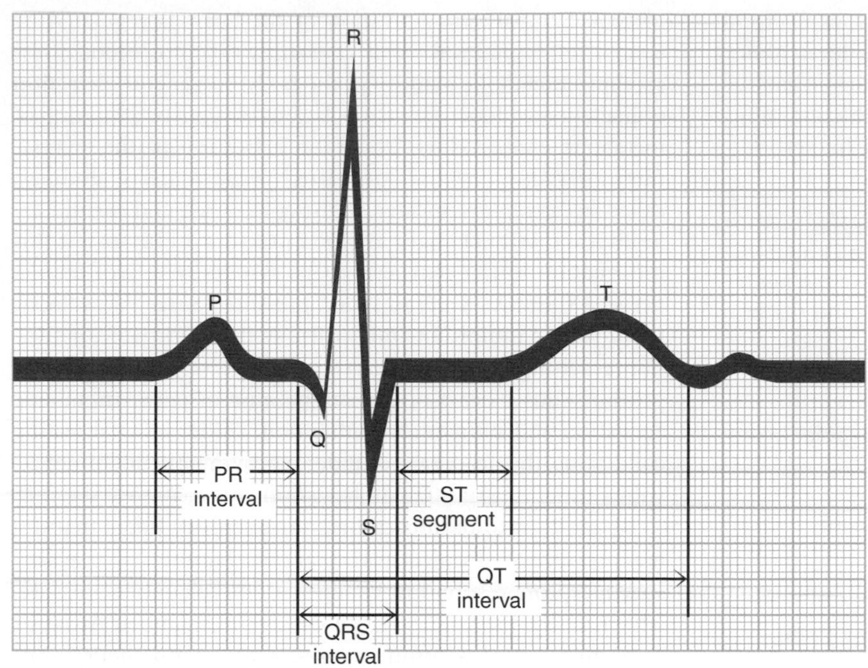

FIGURE 17-24 ■ Usual electrocardiographic pattern recorded from lead II, showing characteristic waves and intervals.

polarization, the *QRS complex,* which represents ventricular depolarization, and the *T wave,* which reflects ventricular repolarization. The PR interval, between the beginning of the P wave and the beginning of the QRS complex, includes atrial, AV node, and His Purkinje fiber depolarization. The normal sequence of ventricular depolarization begins with the septum, followed by the apex, and, finally, the base of the ventricular walls. Septal depolarization begins on the left septal surface and then travels toward the right, resulting in a negative deflection, the *Q wave* in lead II (Figure 17-25). A large upright *R wave* corresponds to a wave of depolarization traveling down the ventricles toward the apex. Depolarization of the ventricular base, because it moves in a direction away from the lower limb electrode, is recorded as a negative *S wave.* The ST interval, between the S wave and the beginning of the T wave, is isoelectric (flat), as the entire ventricle is depolarized and no detectable current is flowing. The QT interval, from the beginning of the QRS complex to the end of the T wave, is commonly measured as an indicator of ventricular systole. The T wave is normally upright in lead II, representing a wave of repolarization moving away from a positive electrode. In some patients, particularly those with slow heart rates, the T wave is

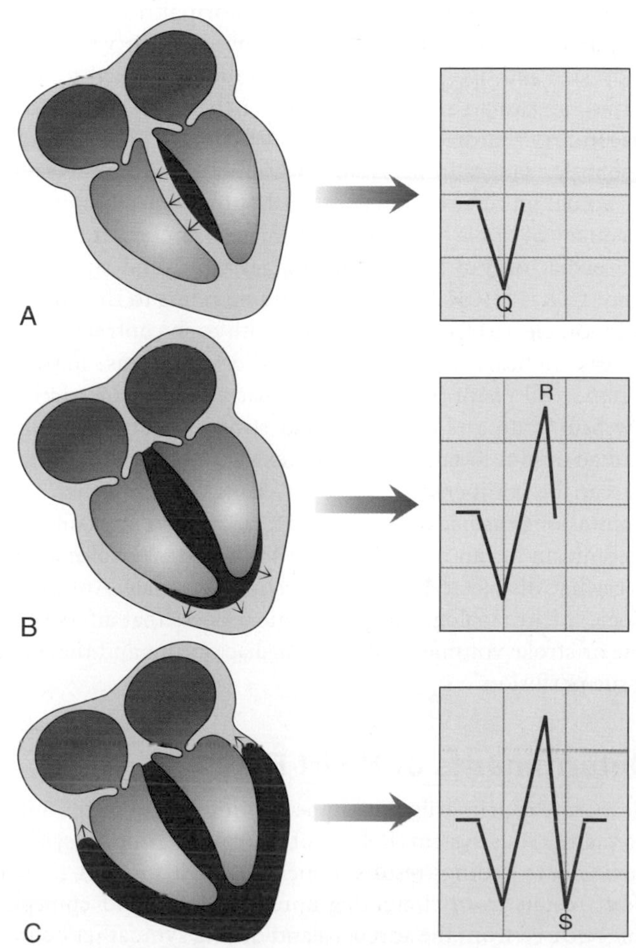

FIGURE 17-25 ■ The QRS complex results from the sequence of ventricular depolarization. **A,** In lead II, septal depolarization is in a direction away from the positive electrode, resulting in a negative Q wave. **B,** Depolarization of the apex of the heart is in a direction toward the positive electrode, resulting in a large positive R wave. **C,** Depolarization of the lateral walls and base of the ventricles is in a direction away from the positive electrode, resulting in a negative S wave.

followed by a small positive deflection, called a *U wave.* Prominent U waves also are a sign of a low potassium level. Abnormalities in any time intervals may indicate abnormal conduction pathways and enhanced or slowed conduction times. Rhythm disturbances are discussed in detail in Chapter 19.

KEY CONCEPTS

- The ECG represents an algebraic sum of all depolarizing and repolarizing currents occurring in the heart. ECGs are useful for detecting conduction and rhythm disturbances.
- The major deflections of the ECG are:
  P wave: atrial depolarization
  PR interval: atrial, AV node, and Purkinje depolarization
  Q wave: septal depolarization
  R wave: apical depolarization
  S wave: depolarization of lateral walls (base)
  T wave: ventricular repolarization

DETERMINANTS OF CARDIAC OUTPUT

Cardiac output is a measure of the amount of blood pumped out of the heart each minute. Because the heart's primary function is to pump enough blood to circulate oxygen and nutrients to tissues, cardiac output is an extremely important indicator of cardiovascular health. The normal resting cardiac output is approximately 5 to 6 L/minute, but it varies with body size and age. Cardiac output is often indexed to body surface area in an attempt to adjust for these differences (cardiac index = cardiac output/body surface area). A normal cardiac index ranges from 2.8 to 3.3 L/minute/m^2. Regardless of the actual number of liters of blood pumped per minute, the adequacy of tissue perfusion is ultimately important.

Cardiac output is a product of heart rate and stroke volume (CO = HR × SV). **Stroke volume** refers to the amount of blood ejected from the ventricle with each contraction. An increase in heart rate (to a point) and/or an increase in stroke volume will result in a greater cardiac output. Conversely, a low heart rate and/or a decreased stroke volume will cause cardiac output to fall. To a certain extent, a change in one factor can be compensated for by a change in the other, thus maintaining cardiac output at a constant level. For example, it is common for an individual with limited stroke volume due to cardiac disease to have a high resting heart rate. Any physiologic, pharmacologic, or pathologic process that alters heart rate or stroke volume may affect cardiac output and therefore tissue perfusion.

Determinants of Heart Rate

Heart rate is primarily determined by influences of the autonomic nervous system. Release of norepinephrine by sympathetic nerve endings results in increased heart rate. A similar effect results from circulating norepinephrine and epinephrine released from the adrenal gland during sympathetic stimulation. Sympathetic activation of the heart is regulated by several reflex pathways that constantly monitor blood pressure and metabolic activity in the body. In general, detection of inadequate blood pressure, a lack of oxygen, or a buildup of metabolic end products results in activation of the sympathetic nervous system. Specialized sensory nerve endings, called *baroreceptors,* located in the aortic arch and carotid arteries respond to changes in blood pressure and transmit this information to the central nervous system by way of cranial nerves IX and X. A fall in blood pressure causes parasympathetic system inhibition and cardiac sympathetic nerve activation, resulting in a rise in heart rate. Conversely, a rise in blood pressure causes heart rate to fall because of parasympathetic activation and sympathetic inhibition. Under normal resting conditions, the heart rate is under parasympathetic influence, with a usual rate of 60 to 80 beats/min.

In addition to baroreceptors, other sensory fibers that detect pressure are located in the cardiac chambers. These sensory receptors respond to changes in intrachamber pressure, which reflect the volume of blood in the chamber. Atrial or ventricular overdistention suppresses parasympathetic influence and increases heart rate (Bainbridge reflex).[15] Heart rate may also be influenced by higher CNS activities that do not involve reflex pathways. Anxiety, fear, and excitement may activate the sympathetic system, for example. A variety of drugs can mimic or block the effects of both sympathetic and parasympathetic systems and therefore influence heart rate (see Chapter 18).

In general, an increase in heart rate results in an increase in cardiac output; however, at very high heart rates, cardiac output may actually fall. At high heart rates (e.g., more than 200 beats/min), the time for diastolic ventricular filling can be significantly reduced, resulting in a low stroke volume. The benefit of increased heart rate is therefore undermined by impaired pumping efficiency.

Determinants of Stroke Volume

Three major factors influence stroke volume: (1) the volume of blood in the heart (**preload**), (2) the contractile capabilities of heart muscle (**contractility**), and (3) impedance opposing ejection of blood from the ventricle (**afterload**). Each of these factors is in turn influenced by many other physiologic, pharmacologic, and sometimes pathologic variables.

Volume of Blood in the Heart (Preload)

The heart can only pump as much blood as is delivered to it by the circulatory system. Blood returning to the heart from the circulation is often called venous return. Normally, venous return is equal to cardiac output because the circulatory system is just that—a circuit. However, there may be inequalities over several heartbeats when changes in blood volume or blood distribution occur. The heart is well suited to adjust to these beat-to-beat changes in venous return such that the healthy heart pumps essentially whatever amount is delivered to it.

The amount of blood present in the ventricles just prior to contraction (end-diastolic volume) is an important determinant of stroke volume. The relationship between diastolic volume and the force of myocardial contraction is known as the **Frank-Starling law of the heart.**[2,17] In essence, this law states that an increase in resting muscle fiber length results in a greater development of muscle tension. Ventricular muscle fiber length is determined by the volume of blood it contains, commonly called the *preload.* An increase in preload results in a greater force of contraction and a larger stroke volume. In this way, the ventricle is able to adjust its stroke volume, beat by beat, according to the amount of blood to be pumped.

The Frank-Starling law of the heart may be understood by recalling the molecular structure of contractile units of heart muscle. For contraction to occur, the actin and myosin filaments that make up the sarcomere must form cross-bridges and slide together. Stretching the muscle prior to contraction could optimize actin-myosin filament overlap and allow greater numbers of cross-bridges to form, resulting in a more forceful contraction (Figure 17-26). If sarcomere length is too short prior to contraction, further shortening is limited because actin filaments begin to abut the opposite Z disk. Stretching the muscle prior to contraction appears to make the contractile apparatus more sensitive to calcium ions such that a greater contractile force occurs for a given calcium concentration.[2]

The cardiac function curve describes the effects of preload on ventricular stroke volume (Figure 17-27). In practice, stroke volume and ventricular end-diastolic volume are difficult to measure, and other indicators, such as ventricular pressure and cardiac output, may be used. Cardiac function curves can be measured in persons with poorly functioning hearts to determine the best filling volume (preload) for optimizing cardiac output. Often, the failing heart requires a higher than normal preload to maintain a normal cardiac output.

Contractile Capabilities of the Heart (Contractility)

Heart muscle contractility depends on several factors, including (1) the amount of contractile proteins in the muscle cells, (2) the availability of ATP, and (3) the availability of free calcium ions in the cytoplasm. Contractility is, by definition, independent of fiber end-diastolic length and is therefore not affected by preload. Given an adequate ATP supply, the contractile state of the normal myocardium is primarily determined by factors that increase the availability of free calcium ions within the myocardial cell. In general, an increased intracellular free calcium level can be accomplished by enhanced release from internal stores, enhanced entry from extracellular fluid, reduced rates of sequestration in the SR, and reduced rates of extrusion across the plasma membrane.

A variety of agents, called *positive inotropes,* are associated with increased intracellular calcium levels in the heart. These include the sympathetic neurotransmitters norepinephrine and epinephrine, thyroid hormone, caffeine, digitalis, and

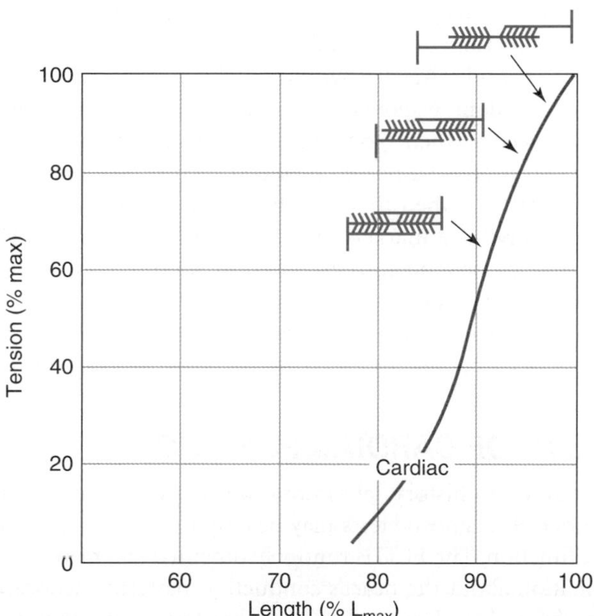

FIGURE 17-26 ■ The force of muscle contraction depends in part on its resting length before activation. At short lengths, filaments may overlap and interfere with cross-bridge formation. At optimal length, the greatest tension is developed, and cross-bridge formation is enhanced.

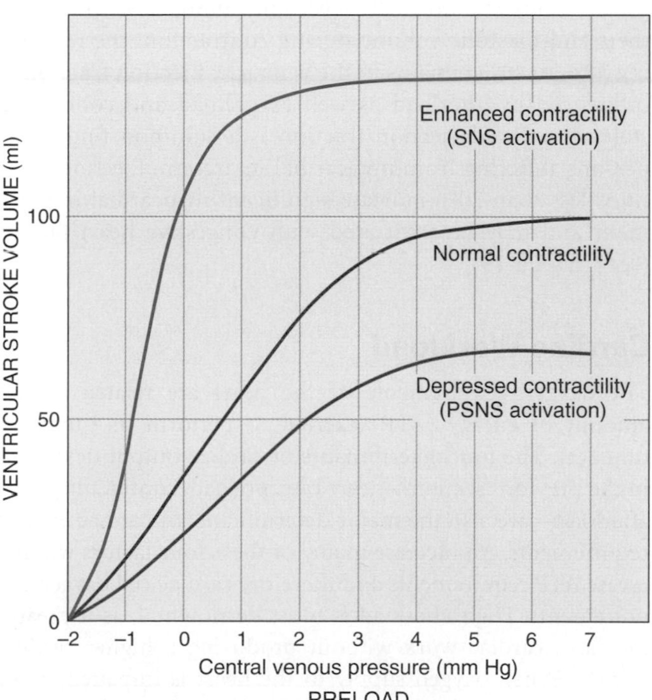

FIGURE 17-27 ■ Cardiac function curves showing the dependence of ventricular stroke volume on preload. Different hearts have different cardiac function curves and may respond differently to the same degree of preload. *PSNS,* Parasympathetic nervous system.

many others. Agents that depress contractility, called *negative inotropes*, achieve their effects by reducing intracellular calcium levels. These agents include L-type calcium channel blockers, parasympathomimetics, and sympathetic blocking drugs. The baroreceptor reflex, described previously in relation to heart rate, is also an important regulator of stroke volume through its effects on contractility.

Cardiac disease may adversely affect contractility because of an inadequate oxygen supply or because of loss of myocardial pumping cells. These disorders are discussed in Chapter 18.

Impedance to Ejection from the Ventricle (Afterload)

The third major determinant of stroke volume is afterload, which refers to the impedance or resistance that must be overcome to eject blood from the chamber. Left ventricular afterload is determined primarily by aortic blood pressure. Because high blood pressure increases left ventricular afterload, vasodilating agents that reduce blood pressure can significantly decrease afterload. Normally the aortic valve offers little impedance to flow; however, aortic valve narrowing may significantly increase afterload. An increase in afterload will result in a decrease in stroke volume unless contractility or preload (or both) is adjusted to compensate. Conversely, a decrease in afterload will allow a larger than normal volume of blood to be ejected from the heart, requiring less myocardial work.

The ventricles normally eject only about 60% to 70% of their end-diastolic volume during contraction; the remaining 30% to 40% remains in the ventricle. **Ejection fraction** is influenced by afterload as well as preload and contractile state. A reduced ejection fraction is a common finding in persons suffering from myocardial infarction. Ejection fractions less than 20% indicate significant myocardial impairment and may be associated with congestive heart failure (see Chapter 19).

Cardiac Workload

The oxygen requirements of the heart are related to the amount of energy (ATP) exerted to perform its pumping function. The four determinants of cardiac output described in the previous section—heart rate, preload, contractility, and afterload—are also the major determinants of cardiac energy requirements. An increase in any of these four factors will increase ATP requirements and therefore cardiac cell oxygen requirements. High afterload is most detrimental, as it greatly increases cardiac work without producing a higher cardiac output. When oxygen supply to the heart is impaired, as in coronary atherosclerosis, it may be beneficial to reduce myocardial oxygen demand by reducing cardiac workload. This may be accomplished by reductions in heart rate, preload, afterload, and contractility.

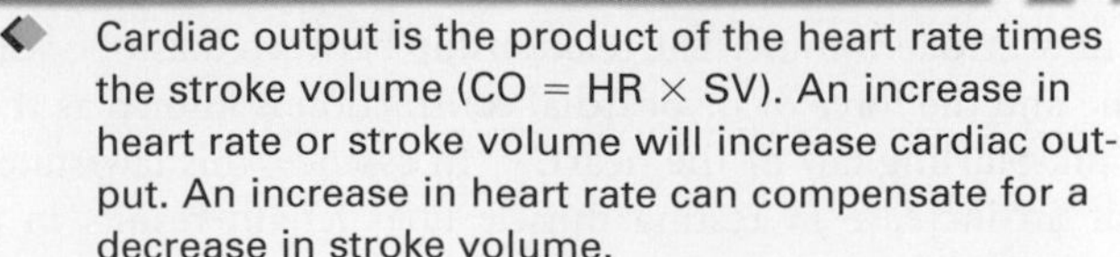

- Cardiac output is the product of the heart rate times the stroke volume (CO = HR × SV). An increase in heart rate or stroke volume will increase cardiac output. An increase in heart rate can compensate for a decrease in stroke volume.
- Heart rate is controlled primarily by the autonomic nervous system. Factors that increase heart rate include low blood pressure (baroreceptors), acidemia (chemoreceptors), atrial and ventricular overdistention (Bainbridge reflex), and emotions. Activation of the vagus nerve will decrease heart rate.
- Stroke volume is influenced by preload. According to the Frank-Starling law, increased preload stretches the sarcomere, resulting in more forceful contraction.
- Increased contractility increases stroke volume by causing a greater percentage of the ventricular volume to be ejected. Any factor that enhances availability of cytoplasmic free Ca^{2+} will increase contractility.
- Increased afterload will decrease stroke volume. Afterload is determined primarily by the resistance of the arterial system. Vasoconstriction and high aortic pressure increase afterload.
- Any factor that increases heart rate, preload, contractility, or afterload will increase the workload of the heart.

ENDOCRINE FUNCTION OF THE HEART

In addition to its pumping function, the heart also has an endocrine function: secretion of natriuretic peptides.[18] Atrial natriuretic peptide (ANP) is synthesized by myocytes in the atria and released in response to atrial stretch. Increased atrial stretch occurs when blood volume becomes excessive. The ventricles produce a related peptide called B-type natriuretic peptide (BNP) when they are chronically overdistended. An elevated BNP is a marker for congestive heart failure.[18] ANP and BNP cause enhanced excretion of sodium and water by the kidney. In general, the effects of the natriuretic peptides are antagonistic to those of the renin-angiotensin-aldosterone system (see Chapter 26).

TESTS OF CARDIAC FUNCTION

In addition to history, laboratory, and physical assessment, a number of diagnostic tests may be employed to evaluate cardiac function. The ECG is routinely obtained and provides information about the heart's conduction patterns. Echocardiography and nuclear cardiography are tests that use various modes to image the heart. A more direct assessment of cardiac function can be obtained by cardiac catheterization. In addition, a number of methods have been developed to quantify myocardial blood flow. Each of these studies is briefly described in this section.

Electrocardiography

The ECG graphically indicates electrical currents generated by cardiac cells. The current is registered by skin electrodes placed in particular positions on the body.[16] The standard ECG has 12 different leads that are obtained through 10 skin electrodes: 3 standard bipolar limb leads, 3 augmented unipolar limb leads, and 6 unipolar chest leads. Bipolar leads represent a difference in electrical potential between two electrodes, one positive and one negative. Augmented unipolar limb leads represent a difference in potential between one electrode and the average of the other two limb electrodes. Unipolar chest leads represent a difference in potential between the chest electrode and a location at the center of the heart. Each lead provides a different ECG because of its particular "view" of current flow through the heart.

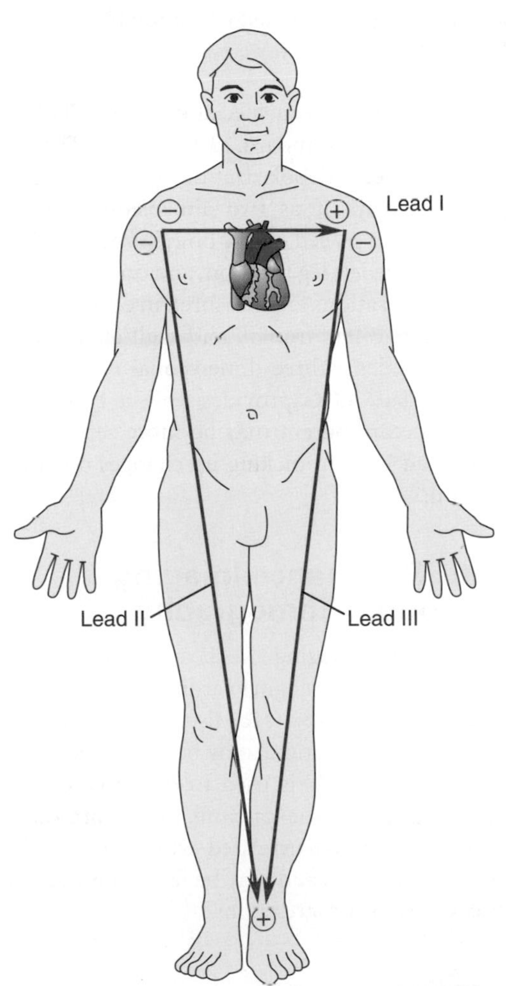

FIGURE 17-28 ■ Positions of standard bipolar limb leads I, II, and III.

The three standard bipolar limb leads are lead I, lead II, and lead III (Figure 17-28): lead I measures the current between the right arm and left arm, lead II measures the current between the right arm and left leg, and lead III measures the current between the left arm and left leg. A normal ECG from leads I, II, and III is illustrated in Figure 17-29.

Electrode placement for the augmented unipolar limb leads is illustrated in Figure 17-30. Unipolar limb lead electrodes provide the positive pole: lead aV_R is recorded from the right arm, lead aV_L is recorded from the left arm, and lead aV_F is recorded from the left leg. In these leads, *a* stands for augmented; *V* stands for voltage; and *R, L,* and *F* indicate the location of the unipolar lead (*r*ight arm, *l*eft arm, and *f*oot [left]). A normal ECG from these leads is illustrated in Figure 17-31.

Precordial unipolar chest leads are recorded from electrodes placed in six positions over the heart on the anterior chest (Figure 17-32). Chest leads are designated as V_1, V_2, V_3, V_4, V_5, and V_6. The normal ECG from the chest leads is shown in Figure 17-33. The chest leads provide a horizontal view of the heart, whereas the limb leads provide a view of the frontal plane.

Twelve-lead ECGs are usually recorded for a short period of time when the patient is resting. Sequential ECGs are useful for determining changes over time. In some cases it is necessary to monitor the ECG recording for an extended period to capture rhythm problems that occur infrequently or with particular activities. This is accomplished by continuous ambulatory monitoring (e.g., Holter monitoring) over a 24- to 48-hour period. An ECG can also be recorded during exercise

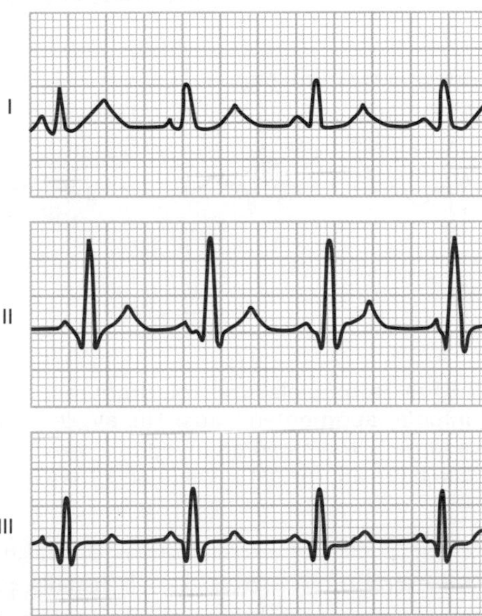

FIGURE 17-29 ■ Normal electrocardiogram recorded from the three standard bipolar limb leads. The R wave is normally upright in leads I, II, and III. (Redrawn from Guyton AC, Hall JE: *Textbook of medical physiology,* ed 10, Philadelphia, 2000, Saunders.)

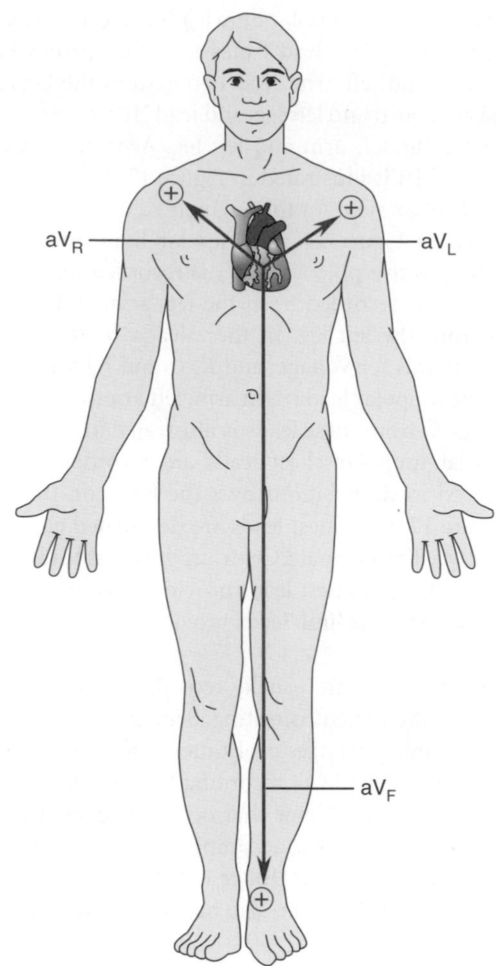

FIGURE 17-30 ■ Unipolar augmented leads aV_R, aV_L, and aV_F.

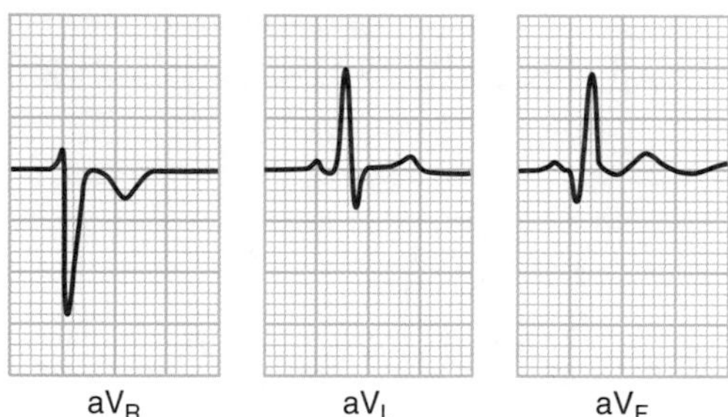

FIGURE 17-31 ■ Normal electrocardiogram recorded from the three unipolar augmented leads. The aV_R lead is characterized by a large S wave and an inverted T wave. The aV_L and aV_F leads have an upright R wave and T wave.

to monitor the effects of exercise stress on cardiovascular function. An exercise test (stress test) is usually performed while the subject progressively increases his or her effort on a treadmill or stationary bicycle. The exercise ECG is particularly useful for assessing the adequacy of coronary circulation when the myocardial workload is increased. Impaired myocardial oxygen delivery may be evident on the ECG as ST segment elevation or depression and abnormal T waves.

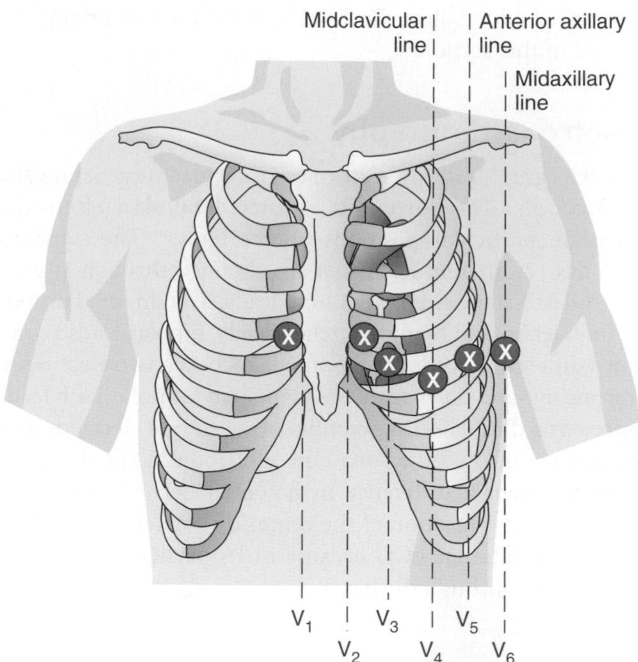

FIGURE 17-32 ■ Unipolar chest (precordial) leads V_1 through V_6.

The *vectorcardiogram* is a special kind of ECG that differs substantially from the standard 12-lead ECG. The vectorcardiogram detects heart depolarization in two planes simultaneously and displays it as two-dimensional vector loops. Seven electrodes are placed on the body surface, including five chest positions, one left leg position, and one forehead or neck position. Depolarizations are measured in each of three planes of the body: horizontal, frontal, and sagittal. Thus, a vectorcardiogram provides a three-dimensional view of the heart, whereas a standard ECG provides only a two-dimensional view. The vectorcardiogram may be more sensitive than the standard 12-lead ECG in picking up changes due to myocardial infarction.

Magnetic Resonance Imaging and Computed Tomography

Magnetic resonance imaging (MRI) and computed tomography (CT) are useful for imaging cardiac structures.[19] Myocardial thickening, pericardial sac disease, valvular structures, and congenital malformations may be visualized by MRI. Ultrafast electron beam CT is used to detect coronary plaque burden by quantifying the calcium in the arterial walls. A higher calcium score is correlated with a greater degree of coronary atherosclerosis and may be used to predict coronary artery disease risk or progression.

Echocardiography

Echocardiography uses reflected sound waves (ultrasound) to provide an image of cardiac structure and motion within the

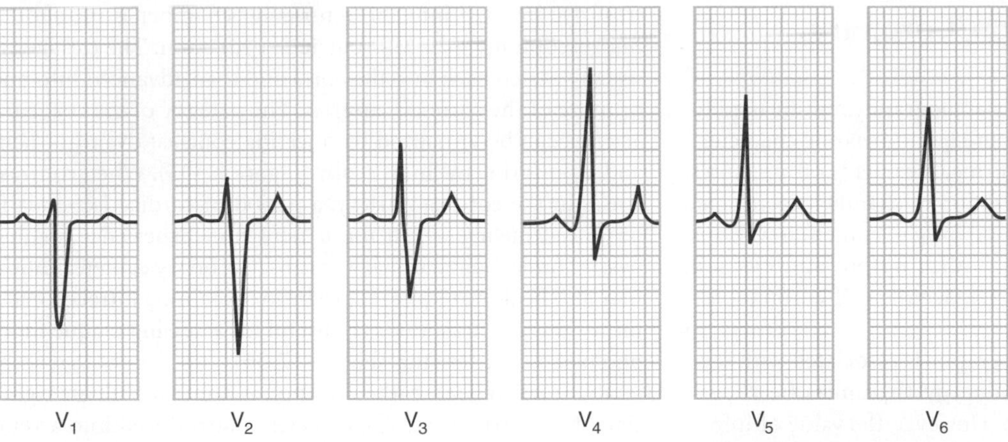

FIGURE 17-33 ■ Normal electrocardiogram recorded from the six unipolar chest leads, V_1 through V_6. Note the R-wave progression across the precordial leads as the R waves become increasingly positive. (Redrawn from Guyton AC, Hall JE: *Textbook of medical physiology,* ed 10, Philadelphia, 2000, Saunders.)

chest.[19] The cardiac echo is obtained by placing a blunt probe on the chest surface that transmits and receives high-frequency sound waves. Sound waves traveling through chest and heart structures are reflected back to the receiving probe. The time between sound wave emission and detection of reflected waves is used to calculate distances between the probe and reflecting tissue. The sound waves are not heard or felt by the subject and have no known detrimental effects on tissues. The probe is moved across the chest to assess cardiac structures of interest, and recordings are videotaped for later viewing.

Echocardiograms are particularly useful for diagnosis of heart enlargement, valvular disorders, collections of fluid in the pericardial space, cardiac tumors, and abnormalities in left ventricular motion. An echocardiogram is shown in Figure 17-34.

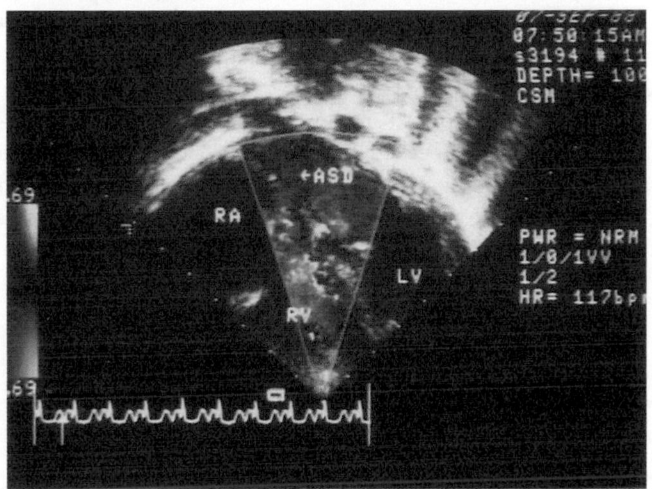

FIGURE 17-34 ■ Color echocardiogram of a child with a large atrial septal defect *(ASD).* The *red* indicates low-velocity blood flow through the defect toward the ultrasound transducer. The *yellow* indicates areas of turbulent blood flow. *RA,* Right atrium; *RV,* right ventricle; *LV,* left ventricle. (From Skorton DJ et al, editors: *Marcus cardiac imaging: a companion to Braunwald's heart disease,* ed 2, vol 1, Philadelphia, 1996, Saunders.)

Nuclear Cardiography

Radioactive substances injected into the blood stream can be used to trace the patterns of blood flow in the heart.[19] Radiation exposure is minimal, as very small amounts of radioactive substances are used. Radioactive tracers can be linked to substances that accumulate in normal myocardial cells as the tracer is delivered by coronary blood flow. Areas with impaired perfusion will take up less radioactivity and appear as "cold spots" on the scan. Alternatively, a radioactive tracer can be linked to a substance that accumulates in recently infarcted tissue and is excluded from healthy cells. The infarct appears as a "hot spot" on the scan. Scanning usually is done using single-photon emission computed tomography (SPECT), which images numerous slices through the heart or by planar imaging, which gives an overall picture in one plane only.

Thallium (^{201}Tl) and technetium-99 labeled compounds (^{99m}Tc sestamibi) are used to assess the adequacy of blood flow to cardiac tissues. After injection of the radioactive compound the heart is scanned to visualize the amount of radioactivity taken up by cardiac tissues. Healthy cardiac tissues that receive adequate blood supply actively accumulate these isotopes. Areas of inadequate blood flow or infarcted tissue do not accumulate isotope and appear as cold spots on the scan. Resting and exercise scanning are done to assess for exercise-induced perfusion defects. In recent years, scanning for the purpose of identifying infarcted tissue is less commonly done. ^{99m}Tc-labeled Sn-pyrophosphate is traditionally used because it accumulates in recently infarcted tissue creating a hot spot of radioactivity.

Gated pool scanning is used primarily to assess left ventricular motion and ejection fraction. Before it is injected intravenously, radioactive technetium is attached to albumin or red cells, and therefore it remains in the blood stream and is not taken up by cells. Computer imaging is used to analyze blood flow through the chambers of the heart over many cardiac cycles. The dynamics of ventricular motion, such as hypercontractility or hypocontractility, may be visualized.

Cardiac Catheterization/Coronary Angiography

Cardiac catheterization/coronary angiography may be used to determine important structural and hemodynamic characteristics because it affords direct measurement of pressures within cardiac chambers; visualization of chamber size, shape, and movement; sampling for blood oxygen content in various heart regions; measurement of cardiac output and ejection fraction; and visualization and management of coronary artery obstructions.[19]

Cardiac catheterization angiography is associated with several serious risks, including bleeding, dysrhythmias, heart perforation, and coronary ischemia. However, the value of information supplied is generally believed to far outweigh the risks. Catheterization is frequently used to evaluate suspected or confirmed coronary artery disease, valvular dysfunction, congenital defects, left ventricular dysfunction, and coronary bypass graft patency.

Assessment of the left side of the heart, including the coronary arteries, is achieved by passing a catheter through a femoral or brachial artery into the aorta. The catheter is then manipulated into the left ventricle or left atrium to assess chamber pressures, and a ventriculogram is obtained. Contrast dye injected into the ventricular chamber is monitored fluoroscopically to assess ventricular function. The catheter is usually pulled back into the aorta and then advanced into one or more of the coronary arteries. The patency of the coronary arteries can be visualized by injecting contrast dye into them and monitoring by fluoroscopy (Figure 17-35). When contrast dye is in the coronary artery, a period of cardiac ischemia is produced during which the patient may experience angina, dysrhythmias, and coronary spasms. Coronary catheterization may also be done to insert a probe for obtaining intracoronary ultrasounds. Ultrasounds are useful for assessing plaque morphologic characteristics (Figure 17-36).

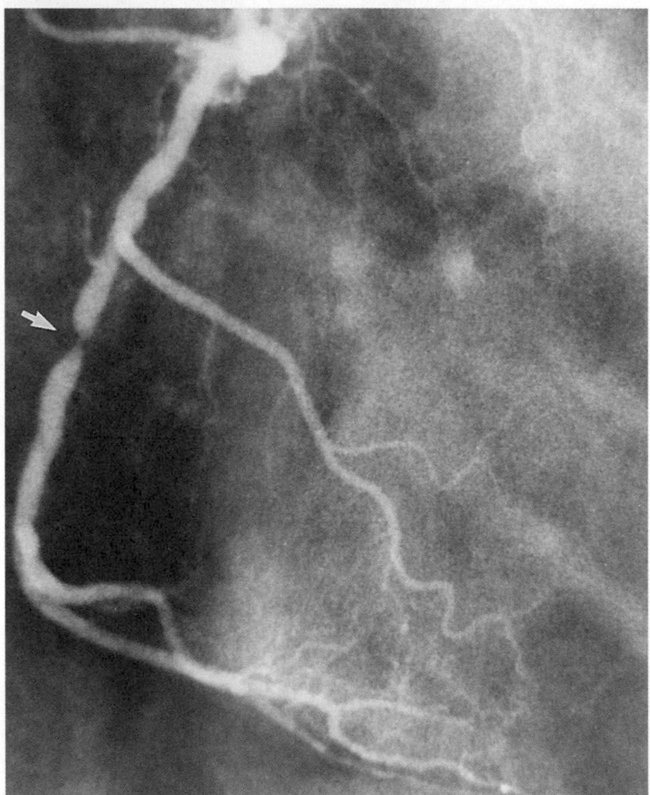

FIGURE 17-35 ■ Coronary artery angiography. The *arrow* shows an area of obstruction of the right coronary artery. (From Johnson MR: Principles and practice of coronary angiography. In Skorton DJ et al, editors: *Marcus cardiac imaging: a companion to Braunwald's heart disease,* ed 2, vol 1, Philadelphia, 1996, Saunders.)

Right-sided heart catheterization is done to evaluate right-sided heart structures. The catheter is introduced into a vein, usually femoral or antecubital, then threaded through the inferior vena cava and into the heart. Pressures and blood samples are obtained as the catheter is advanced into the right atrium, ventricle, and pulmonary artery. Right heart catheterization is useful in assessing tricuspid and pulmonary valve disorders, pulmonary hypertension, septal defects, and right ventricular function.

Coronary angiography is commonly followed by interventions to treat detected abnormalities. The coronary catheter can be used to direct thrombolytic agents to the site of coronary thrombosis and rapidly restore blood flow to ischemic areas. Laser therapy, coronary balloon angioplasty, and stent placement can also be performed during coronary angiography. These methods clear the coronary obstruction through thermal and mechanical means. The success of these approaches to management of coronary obstruction depends largely on how soon after an ischemic event they are done.

Myocardial Blood Flow Quantitation

A number of new techniques are being used to measure myocardial blood flow by invasive and noninvasive methods.[19] These procedures may help identify patients with abnormalities of the microcirculation that impair the ability to increase myocardial blood flow when needed. Coronary angiography, discussed in the previous section, is helpful only in assessing the large epicardial vessels and not the microcirculation.[18] New procedures including positron emission tomography (PET) scan, fast MRI, myocardial contrast echocardiography, and Doppler catheter studies enhance the ability to discover more subtle impairment of myocardial blood flow. These tests are especially useful in detecting a change in blood flow and can be used to evaluate blood flow responsiveness to increased myocardial oxygen demand. Patients who fail to increase myocardial blood flow appropriately despite normal coronary artery patency may have disorders of the cardiac microcirculation.

SUMMARY

The heart's primary function is to pump sufficient blood to deliver oxygen and nutrients to the body. The heart may be viewed as two separate pumps: a right-sided pump that per-

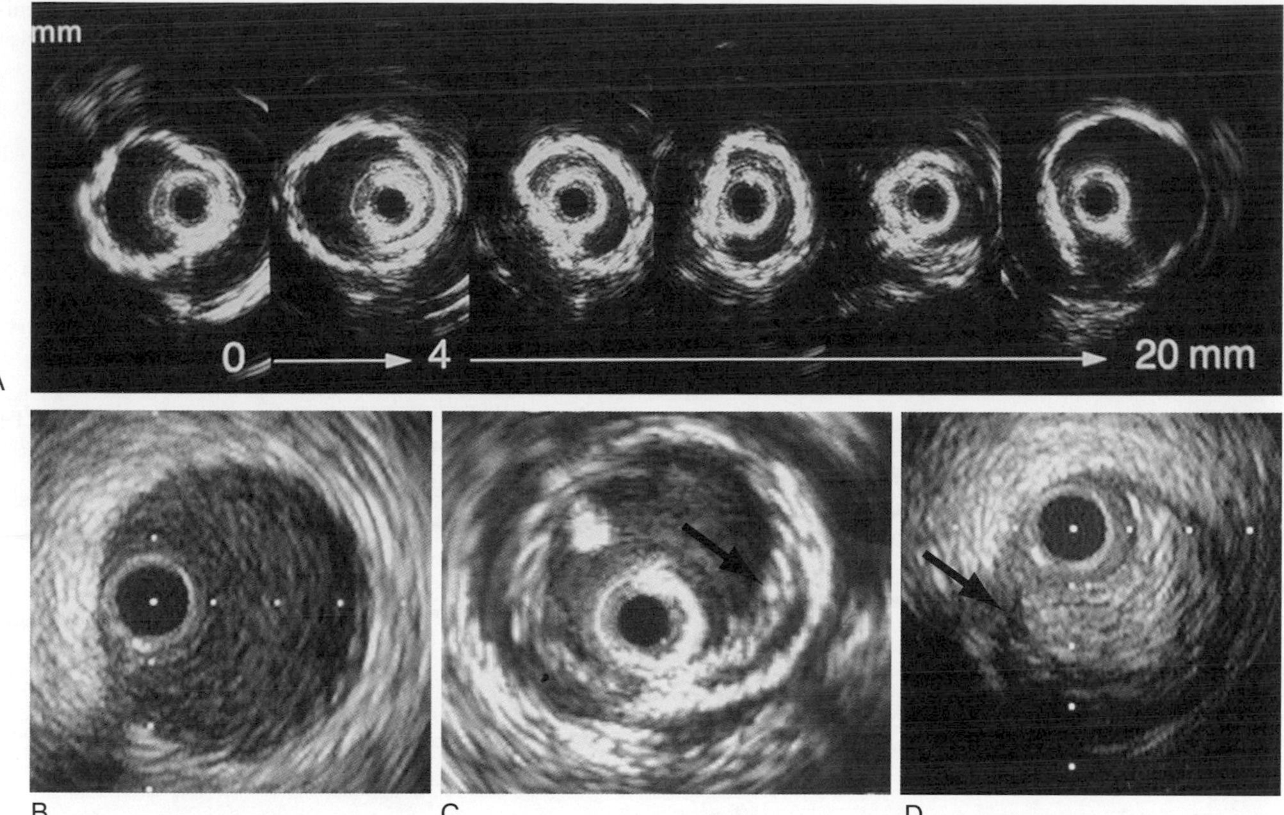

FIGURE 17-36 ■ Intracoronary ultrasonographic examples of plaque morphology. **A,** Concentric calcification of the left anterior descending artery. **B,** A normal vessel wall. **C,** Fibrous cap on coronary plaque. **D,** A soft plaque with rupture of the fibrous cap. (From Braunwald E, Zipes D, Libby P: *Heart disease: a textbook of cardiovascular medicine,* ed 6, Philadelphia, 2001, Saunders, p 416.)

fuses the lungs and a left-sided pump that perfuses the systemic circulation. The left ventricle must generate higher pressures and therefore has a thicker myocardial mass and higher energy requirements. Because little ATP storage in cardiac cells is possible, the coronary arteries must deliver a steady supply of oxygen and nutrients. Cardiac contraction can be described by the sliding filament/cross-bridge theory and occurs only in the presence of ATP and free calcium ions. Any factor that enhances intracellular calcium ion concentration will result in generation of a greater contractile force.

A coordinated cardiac contraction is possible because the heart's conduction system activates the chambers in a sequential manner. The sinoatrial node is the usual pacemaker because it has the highest intrinsic rate of diastolic depolarization. The diastolic depolarization rate is strongly influenced by the autonomic nervous system. The ECG shows the electrical activity of the heart and is a useful indicator of cardiac conduction abnormalities.

The ultimate indicator of cardiac function is the cardiac output, which is the product of heart rate and stroke volume. The autonomic nervous system is the main regulator of heart rate, whereas stroke volume is influenced by preload, afterload, and contractility. These factors are also the primary determinants of myocardial work and energy expenditure.

MEDIA RESOURCES

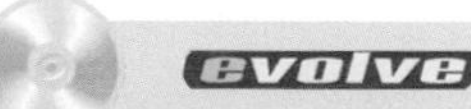

Remember to check out the ***CD Companion*** included with this book for Review Questions, Key Concepts Review, Glossary (with audio for selected terms), Disease Profiles, and Animations.

PLUS, visit the ***Evolve website*** at http://evolve.elsevier.com/Copstead/ for Case Studies, Disease Profiles, and WebLinks.

References

1. *Gray's anatomy,* ed 38, London, 1995, Churchill Livingstone.
2. Opie LH: Mechanisms of cardiac contraction and relaxation. In Braunwald E, Zipes D, Libby P, editors. *Heart disease: a textbook of cardiovascular medicine,* ed 6, Philadelphia, 2001, Saunders, pp 443-478.
3. Levy MN: The arterial system. In Berne RM et al, editors. *Physiology,* ed 5, St Louis, 2004, Mosby, pp 355-367.
4. Ganong WF: Circulation through special regions. In Ganong WF, editor: *Review of medical physiology,* New York, 2003, McGraw-Hill, pp 614-632.
5. Levy MN: Hemodynamics. In Berne RM et al, editors: *Physiology,* ed 5, St Louis, 2004, Mosby, pp 341-354.

6. Ganz P, Ganz W: Coronary blood flow and myocardial ischemia. In Braunwald E, Zipes D, Libby P, editors: *Heart disease: a textbook of cardiovascular medicine,* ed 6, Philadelphia, 2001, Saunders, pp 1087-1113.
7. Nadal-Ginard B et al: Myocyte death, growth, and regeneration in cardiac hypertrophy and failure, *Circ Res* 92:139-150, 2003.
8. Levy MN: The cardiac pump. In Berne RM et al, editors: *Physiology,* ed 5, St Louis, 2004, Mosby, pp 305-321.
9. Pollard TD, Earnshaw WC: Muscles. In Pollard TD, Earnshaw WC, editors: *Cell biology,* Philadelphia, 2004, Saunders, pp 651-670.
10. Panteghini M et al: Use of biochemical biomarkers in acute coronary syndromes. IFCC Scientific Division, Committee on standardization of markers of cardiac damage. International Federation of Clinical Chemistry, *Clin Chem Lab Med* 37:683-693, 1999.
11. Ganong WF: Excitable tissue: muscle. In Ganong WF, editor: *Review of medical physiology,* New York, 2003, McGraw-Hill, p 82.
12. Levy MN: Electrical activity of the heart. In Berne RM et al, editors: *Physiology,* ed 5, St Louis, 2004, Mosby, pp 274-304.
13. Bauman JL, Schoen MD: Arrhythmias. In Dipiro JT et al, editors: *Pharmacotherapy: a pathophysiologic approach,* ed 5, New York, 2002, McGraw-Hill, pp 273-304.
14. Guyton AC, Hall JE: *Textbook of medical physiology,* ed 10, Philadelphia, 2000, Saunders, p 109.
15. Levy MN: Regulation of the heart beat. In Berne RM et al, editors: *Physiology,* ed 5, St Louis, 2003, Mosby, pp 322-340.
16. Conover MB: *Understanding electrocardiography,* ed 8, St Louis, 2003, Mosby.
17. Starling EH: *The Linacre lecture on the law of the heart,* London, 1918, Longmans Green.
18. Stoupakis G, Klapholz M: Natriuretic peptides: biochemistry, physiology, and therapeutic role in heart failure, *Heart Dis* 5(3):215-223, 2003.
19. Braunwald E, Zipes D, Libby P: Part 2: Examination of the patient. In Braunwald E, Zipes D, Libby P, editors: *Heart disease: a textbook of cardiovascular medicine,* ed 6, Philadelphia, 2001, Saunders, pp 160-421.

Alterations in Cardiac Function

chapter 18

Jacquelyn L. Banasik

MEDIA RESOURCES

Additional Material for Study, Review, and Further Exploration

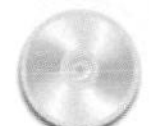

CD Companion ◆ Review Questions and Answers ◆ Key Concepts Review ◆ Glossary *(with audio pronunciations for selected terms)* ◆ Disease Profiles ◆ Animations

evolve ***Website*** at http://evolve.elsevier.com/Copstead/ ◆ Case Studies ◆ Disease Profiles ◆ WebLinks

KEY QUESTIONS

- What is the role of injury, inflammation, and lipid oxidation in coronary plaque initiation and progression?
- What factors alter the balance between myocardial oxygen supply and demand?
- How do the clinical features of the coronary heart disease syndromes differ?
- How do valvular disorders alter cardiac pressure dynamics and workload?
- What are the similarities and differences among the cardiomyopathies and myocarditis?
- How do pericarditis and pericardial effusions differ in regard to cause and significance?
- What factors determine whether a congenital heart defect will produce cyanosis?

CHAPTER OUTLINE

The incidence of cardiovascular disease increased rapidly in the United States during the last century and it now claims the lives of nearly 1 million people annually.[1] Approximately half of these deaths are due to coronary heart disease (CHD), whereas stroke, high blood pressure, congenital heart disease, and others claim the remainder. Nearly twice as many people die of cardiac disorders as all types of cancers combined. Since the late 1960s, however, a decline in cardiac mortality has been achieved in the United States because of improvements in treatment and prevention. More than 13 million people living today have a history of angina pectoris or myocardial infarction (MI).[1] Men and women are equally represented, although women tend to be older when their heart disease becomes apparent. In 2004, the economic cost of cardiovascular diseases, including stroke, was estimated at $368.4 billion annually.[1] CHD is the most important cardiovascular disorder in terms of numbers affected and economic impact.

CORONARY HEART DISEASE

CHD is characterized by insufficient delivery of oxygenated blood to the myocardium because of atherosclerotic coronary arteries. When metabolic demand for oxygen exceeds supply, the myocardium becomes ischemic, which leads to a dysfunction in cardiac pumping and predisposes to abnormal heart rhythms. If the ischemic episode is severe or prolonged, irreversible damage to myocardial cells may result in MI.

Etiology of Coronary Heart Disease

The most common cause of CHD is coronary artery atherosclerosis—sometimes called coronary artery disease (CAD) or ischemic heart disease. Atherosclerosis causes progressive narrowing of the arterial lumen and predisposes to a number of processes that can precipitate myocardial ischemia, including thrombus formation, coronary vasospasm, and endothelial cell dysfunction. Less common causes of ischemic heart disease include abnormalities of blood oxygen content (e.g., respiratory failure) and poor perfusion pressure through the coronary arteries (e.g., hypotension, hypovolemia). Sometimes patients experience the signs and symptoms of cardiac ischemia but show no evidence of coronary artery atherosclerosis when evaluated by angiography. These patients are thought to have abnormalities of the microcirculation. Abnormal vascular regulation by endothelial cells in small vessels of the heart has been suggested as a probable mechanism. Endothelial cells secrete variable quantities of vascular relaxing and contracting factors and play a key role in controlling myocardial blood flow. Abnormalities of the microcirculation are more difficult to detect than coronary artery plaque, which is evident on coronary angiography. As evaluation methods improve, disorders of the microcirculation are likely to be more frequently recognized as factors contributing to CHD.

Box 18-1

Risk Factors for Coronary Heart Disease

Nonmodifiable Risks

Age: ≥45 years for men; ≥55 years for women
Gender: male
Family history of premature coronary heart disease
- Myocardial infarction or sudden cardiac death in male first-degree relative at age less than 55 years or female first-degree relative at age less than 65 years

Lipid Risk Factors

Total cholesterol >200 mg/dl
LDL cholesterol >130 mg/dl
Triglycerides >150 mg/dl
HDL cholesterol <40 mg/dl

Nonlipid Risk Factors

Hypertension >140/90
Cigarette smoking
Thrombogenic state
Diabetes
Obesity
Physical inactivity
Poor diet (atherogenic)

Probable Risk Factors (Emerging)

Lipoprotein(a)
Small LDL particles (pattern B)
HDL subtypes
Apolipoprotein B
Homocysteine
Fibrinogen
High-sensitivity C-reactive protein
Impaired fasting glucose (100-125 mg/dl)

Data from NCEP III guidelines, 2002, NIH Publication No 02-5215.
LDL, Low-density lipoprotein; *HDL,* high-density lipoprotein.

Mechanisms of Coronary Atherosclerosis

Knowledge about mechanisms of plaque formation in the coronary arteries has rapidly accumulated in recent years. Epidemiologic studies reported in the 1960s suggested associations among certain traits and habits and the development of CHD. More recent studies have confirmed and expanded on these *risk factors,* which include several major risks (age, family history, abnormal lipids, cigarette smoking, hypertension, diabetes, and obesity) and numerous probable risks (Box 18-1).[2] Although males and females succumb to heart disease in equal numbers, male gender is a risk factor for earlier development of heart disease (on average about 10 years earlier). The risk factors for CHD are the same as those for atherosclerosis in other arteries and are discussed in Chapter 15.

The observation that atherosclerotic plaque is composed primarily of lipid prompted the idea that abnormal lipid metabolism was a probable culprit in the development of CHD, and a great deal of attention has been focused on therapies to reduce serum cholesterol in individuals with hyperlipidemia. Lipids are transported through the blood stream in combination with specific proteins (**apoproteins**). Certain lipid-protein molecules (**lipoproteins**) are associated with a greater risk of atherosclerosis. The five major kinds of lipoproteins are shown in Figure 18-1. High levels of low-density lipoproteins (LDLs), which are high in cholesterol, have been associated with the highest risk. Very-low-density lipoproteins, which have large amounts of triglycerides, also appear to increase the risk. High-density lipoproteins, on the other hand, have been correlated with a decreased risk of atherosclerosis.[2]

High-density lipoproteins are thought to transport cholesterol from the vessel back to the liver for excretion, thus clearing away atheromatous plaque. The role of low-density and, indirectly, very-low-density lipoproteins is to bring cholesterol to the peripheral tissues (Figure 18-2). Cholesterol uptake by peripheral cells is mediated by receptors (LDL receptors) on cell surfaces that bind and promote endocytosis of

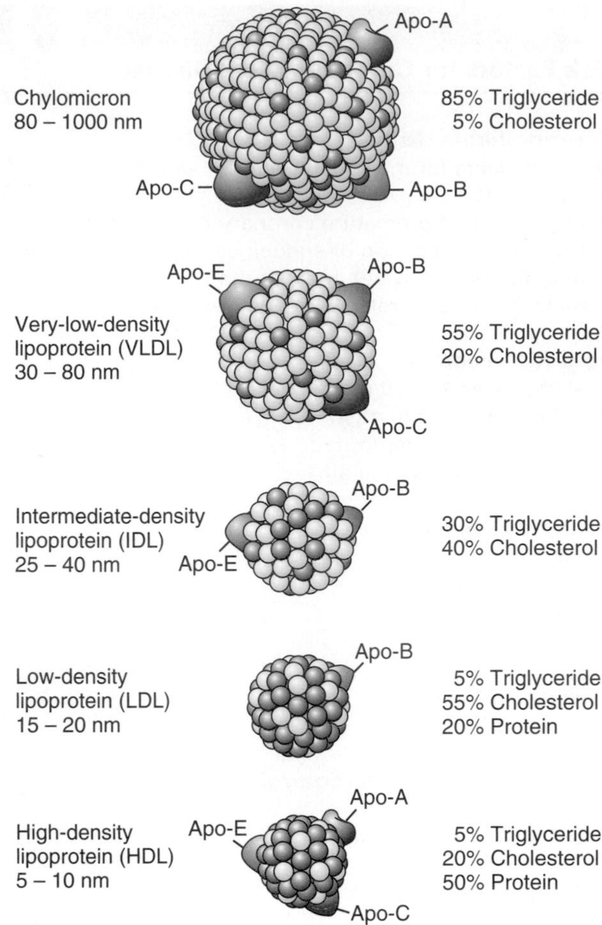

FIGURE 18-1 ■ Serum lipoprotein fractions showing lipid composition and apoprotein components. Binding of lipoproteins to receptors is mediated through apoproteins.

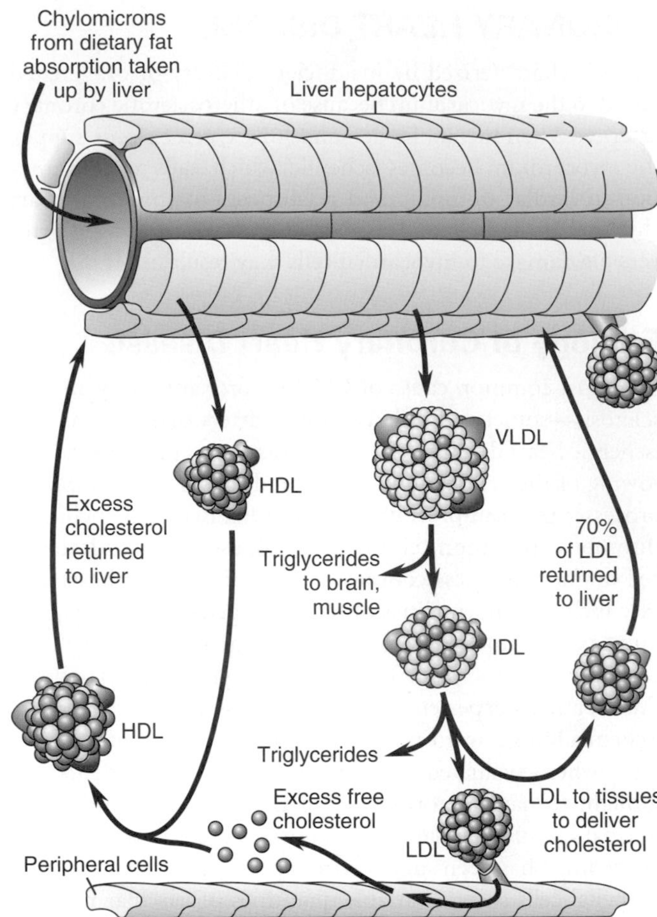

FIGURE 18-2 ■ Schematic of lipoprotein metabolism in the body. Chylomicrons from dietary fat absorption are taken up by the liver and resynthesized into high-density lipoprotein *(HDL)* and very-low-density lipoprotein *(VLDL)*. HDL circulates to the peripheral tissues and takes up excess cholesterol for transport back to the liver. Triglycerides are removed for tissue use from VLDL, which becomes intermediate-density lipoprotein *(IDL)*. More triglyceride removal leads to the formation of low-density lipoprotein *(LDL)*. LDL is taken up by peripheral tissues to obtain cholesterol. About 70% of the circulating LDL returns to the liver.

cholesterol. The liver normally binds and internalizes about 75% of the circulating LDL cholesterol.

Extreme cases of hyperlipidemia occur in individuals who have genetic derangements in lipid metabolism. These disorders run in families, and some are associated with the development of severe coronary atherosclerosis at a young age unless aggressively managed. The most common form of genetic hyperlipidemia (familial hypercholesterolemia) is associated with a defect in the LDL receptor on liver cells.[3] Inability of the liver to efficiently remove cholesterol from the blood stream results in hyperlipidemia. Genetic disorders of lipid metabolism are described in Table 18-1. Even when lipid metabolism is normal, a high-fat diet can overwhelm the liver's ability to clear LDL cholesterol from the circulation and result in hyperlipidemia. Dietary fat restriction may be beneficial in reducing cholesterol in this case.

Atherosclerotic plaques are initiated by injury to the coronary artery endothelium. The specific cause of endothelial dysfunction in the early stage of atherosclerosis is uncertain; however, several potential mechanisms have been described. These include chronic hemodynamic sheer stress, which may explain the typical localization of plaques at arterial branch points; toxins from cigarette smoke; infections and inflammatory agents; and hyperlipidemia. Once the injury occurs the endothelium may become more permeable and recruit leukocytes (Figure 18-3). LDLs leak through the endothelium and into the vessel wall (insudation) where they are oxidized by endothelial cells and macrophages.[4] Oxidized lipids are damaging to the endothelial and smooth muscle cells, and stimulate the recruitment of macrophages into the vessel wall where they engulf the lipids. Lipid-filled macrophages are called foam cells. The macrophages and foam cells release inflammatory mediators and growth factors that attract more leukocytes and stimulate smooth muscle proliferation. Excess lipid and debris begins to accumulate within the vessel wall and coalesce into a pool called the lipid core (see Figure 18-3). Ath-

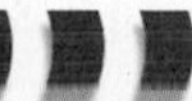

Table 18-1

Genetic Lipoprotein Disorders

Disorder	Gene
LDL Particles	
Familial hypercholesterolemia	LDL-R
Familial defective apo B-100	ApoB
Abetalipoproteinemia	MTP
Hypobetalipoproteinemia	ApoB
Familial phytosterolemia	?
Lp(a)	
Familial Lp(a) hyperlipoproteinemia	Apo(a)
Remnant Lipoproteins	
Dysbetalipoproteinemia type III	ApoE
Hepatic lipase deficiency	HL
Triglyceride-Rich Lipoproteins	
Lipoprotein lipase deficiency	LPL
ApoCII deficiency	ApoCII
Familial hypertriglyceridemia	Polygenic
Chylomicron retention disease	?
Familial combined hyperlipidemia	Polygenic
HDL Particles	
ApoAI deficiency	ApoAI
Familial HDL deficiency/Tangier disease	ABC1/CERP
Familial LCAT deficiency syndromes	LCAT
CETP deficiency	CETP

From Ridker PM, Genest J, Libby P: Risk factors for atherosclerotic disease. In Braunwald E, Zipes D, Libby P, editors: *Heart disease: a textbook of cardiovascular medicine,* ed 6, Philadelphia, 2001, Saunders, p 1016.
LDL, Low-density lipoprotein; *Lp(a),* lipoprotein a; *HDL,* high-density lipoprotein; *LCAT,* lecithin cholesterol acyltransferase; *CETP,* cholesteryl ester transfer protein.

erosclerotic plaques with large lipid cores are fragile and prone to rupture. Rupture of a plaque exposes subendothelial proteins and initiates platelet aggregation and thrombus formation. Thrombi may be asymptomatic if they are small and do not occlude the artery. Components of the thrombus may be incorporated into the plaque causing it to enlarge. Older plaques have significant collagen and fibrin, which form a cap and tend to make the plaque more stable. Numerous therapies aimed at stabilizing vulnerable plaques and preventing thrombus formation have been studied in clinical trials. Lipid-lowering therapy is a mainstay of treatment and prevention

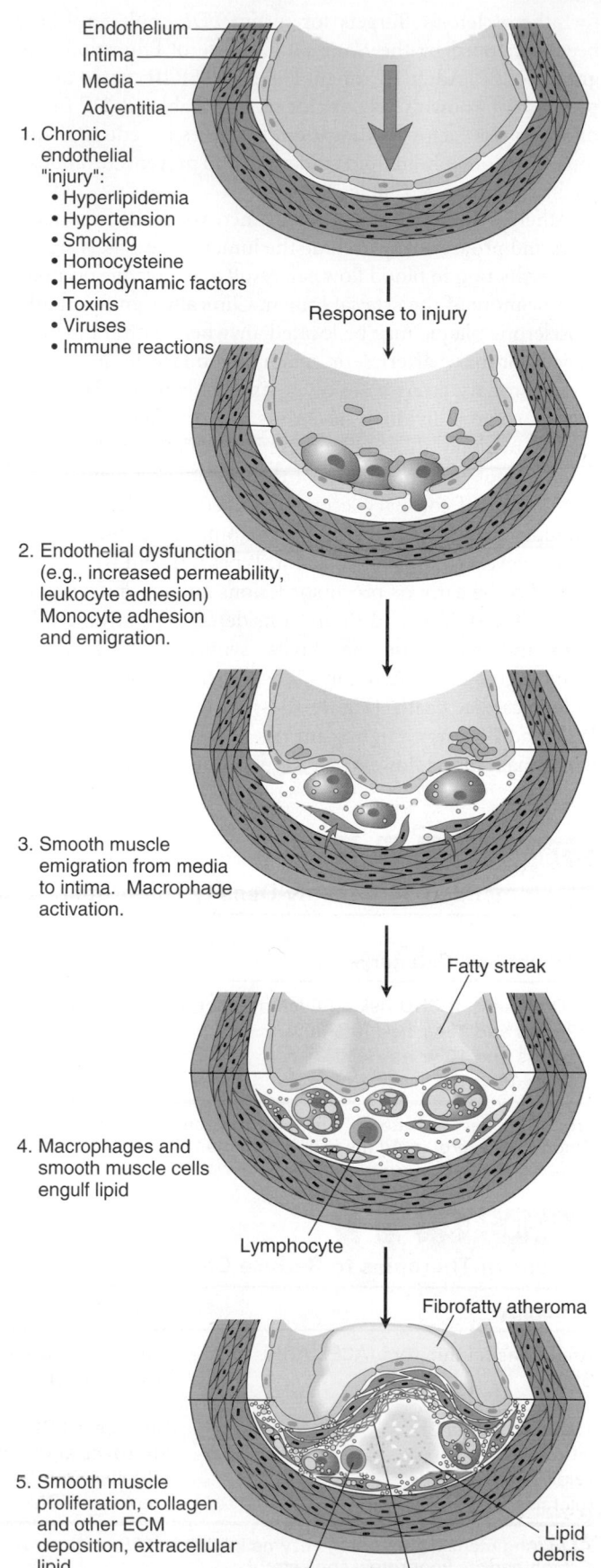

Endothelium
Intima
Media
Adventitia
1. Chronic endothelial "injury":
• Hyperlipidemia
• Hypertension
• Smoking
• Homocysteine
• Hemodynamic factors
• Toxins
• Viruses
• Immune reactions
Response to injury
2. Endothelial dysfunction (e.g., increased permeability, leukocyte adhesion) Monocyte adhesion and emigration.
3. Smooth muscle emigration from media to intima. Macrophage activation.
Fatty streak
4. Macrophages and smooth muscle cells engulf lipid
Lymphocyte
Fibrofatty atheroma
5. Smooth muscle proliferation, collagen and other ECM deposition, extracellular lipid
Lipid debris
Lymphocyte
Collagen

FIGURE 18-3 ■ Pathogenesis of atherosclerosis. *1,* Chronic endothelial injury leads to *2. 2,* Endothelial dysfunction, permeability, and inflammation. *3,* Activated monocytes infiltrate the arterial wall and smooth muscle proliferates. *4,* Macrophages engulf lipid to become foam cells. *5,* A lipid core forms in the arterial wall and fibrous cap evolves. (From Kumar V, Cotran R, Robbins S: *Robbins basic pathology,* ed 7, Philadelphia, 2003, Saunders, p 335.)

for atherosclerosis. Targets for serum LDL cholesterol have been developed by the National Cholesterol Education Program (NCEP) Adult Treatment Panel (NCEP III) based on the presence of known CHD or risk factors (Table 18-2).[2] In addition to risk factor modification, therapies to reduce plaque inflammation, inhibit lipid oxidation, and prevent thrombosis are in common use (Table 18-3).

Atherosclerotic lesions generally increase in size over many years and progressively occlude the lumen of vessels. A significant reduction in blood flow can result when plaque occupies 75% or more of the arterial lumen. Clinically significant atherosclerotic plaque may be located anywhere within the three major coronary arteries or major secondary branches. All three coronary arteries are often simultaneously affected, although some individuals have only one or two diseased vessels. Surprisingly, the extent and severity of atherosclerotic lesions are not good predictors of the severity of ischemia.

Six types of coronary lesions have been characterized and attempts made to correlate the anatomic descriptions with plaque development and behavior. Types I, II, and III are considered to be early or precursor lesions and are not symptomatic.[5] Types IV, V, and VI are considered to be advanced lesions and may cause the clinical syndromes of ischemia, including angina, infarction, ischemic cardiomyopathy, and sudden cardiac death[6] (Figure 18-4). Advanced lesions (types IV, V, and VI) carry a significant risk of producing disruptions in coronary blood flow. When a type IV or V lesion is complicated by plaque disruption and thrombus formation, it is then classified as a type VI lesion.

Stable plaques usually are asymptomatic or may be associated with exercise-induced angina pain (stable angina pectoris). However, some plaques are vulnerable to rupture or erosion, which can initiate thrombosis formation and acute coronary occlusion. A variety of factors have been identified as markers of increased plaque vulnerability (Box 18-2). These factors include (1) active inflammation within the plaque; (2) a large lipid core with a thin cap; (3) endothelial denudation (erosion) with superficial platelet adherence; (4) fissured or ruptured cap; and (5) severe stenosis predisposing to high sheer stress.[7] Acute coronary syndrome (ACS, i.e., unstable angina, MI) and sudden cardiac death are nearly always associated with acute disruption of a vulnerable plaque. Because the types of plaques that are most vulnerable often do not significantly obstruct the lumen before they rupture, ACS frequently occurs in individuals whose disease had been asymptomatic. Patients with a high risk for or known presence of vulnerable plaques benefit from therapies to improve plaque behavior and prevent thrombosis.[8]

Pathophysiology of Ischemia

Ischemia of cardiac cells occurs when the oxygen supply is insufficient to meet metabolic demands. Myocardial cells are unable to store much energy in the form of adenosine triphos-

Table 18-2

Recommended Serum Low-Density Lipoprotein Targets to Reduce the Risk of Coronary Heart Disease

Patient Risk Category	LDL-C Cut Point for Initiating Drug Therapy	LDL-C Goal
CHD present or CHD risk equivalent (≥2 risks plus 10-yr risk >20%)	>100	<100
≥2 risks and 10-yr risk 10%-20%	≥130	<130
≥2 risks and 10-yr risk <10%	≥160	<130
≤1 risk 10-yr risk <10%	≥190	<160

From National Cholesterol Education Program: Third Report of the Expert Panel on Detection, Evaluation, and Treatment of High Blood Cholesterol in Adults (Adult Treatment Panel III), *Circulation* 106:3143-3421, 2002 and modifications in 2004.
CHD, Coronary heart disease; *LDL-C,* low-density lipoprotein cholesterol.

Table 18-3

Actions of Therapies to Reduce Coronary Heart Disease

Therapy	Major Actions	Other Actions
Angiotensin inhibitors (ACEI, ARB)	Improves endothelial function	Antioxidant (LDL), antiinflammatory
Statins	Decreased LDL-C, increases HDL-C	Improve endothelial function, antiinflammatory, antioxidant (LDL)
Fish oil (omega-3)	Decreases LDL-C, increases HDL-C	Inhibits thrombosis
Fibrates	Improves endothelial function	Increases HDL
Aspirin	Inhibits thrombosis, antiinflammatory	
Exercise	Increases HDL	Improves endothelial function

ACEI, Angiotensin-converting enzyme inhibitor; *ARB,* angiotensin II receptor blocker; *LDL-C,* low-density lipoprotein cholesterol; *HDL-C,* high-density lipoprotein cholesterol.

phate (ATP) and must therefore continuously receive a supply of oxygen for aerobic synthesis of ATP. ATP is essential for powering myocardial contraction as well as for cell maintenance. Because the heart is unable to stop and rest when ATP supplies dwindle, it is essential that a steady flow of oxygen be provided.

Factors that decrease myocardial oxygen supply or increase myocardial oxygen demand can upset the balance and result in cellular ischemia. Thus, the critical factors in meeting cellular demands for oxygen are (1) the rate of coronary perfusion and (2) myocardial workload. Coronary perfusion can be impaired in several ways, including (1) large, stable atherosclerotic plaque, (2) acute platelet aggregation and thrombosis, (3) vasospasm, (4) failure of autoregulation by the microcirculation, and (5) poor perfusion pressure.

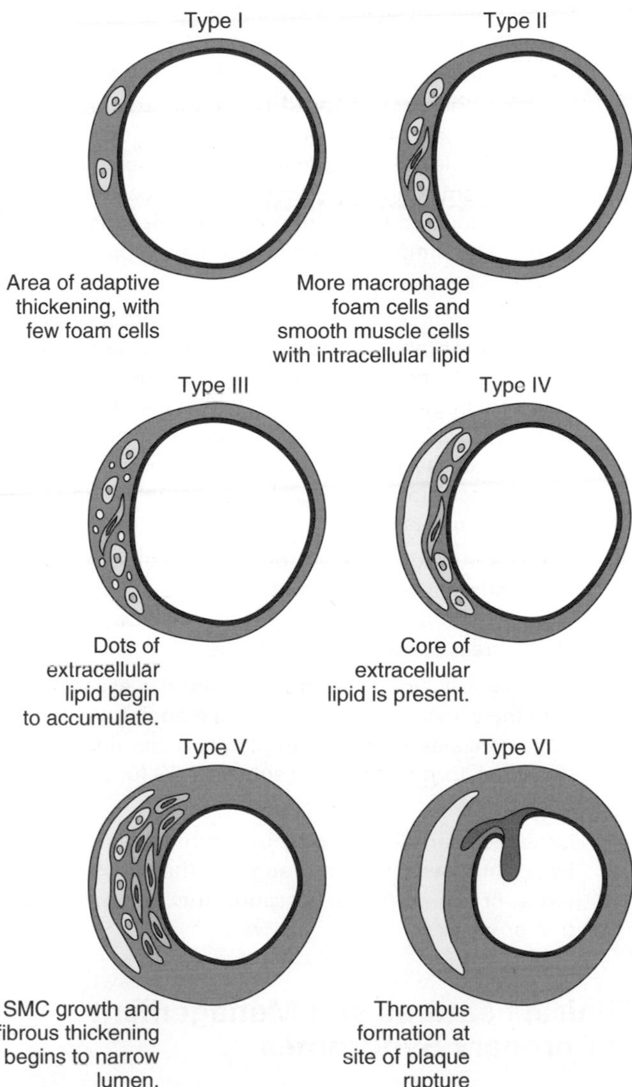
Type I
Type II
Area of adaptive thickening, with few foam cells
More macrophage foam cells and smooth muscle cells with intracellular lipid
Type III
Type IV
Dots of extracellular lipid begin to accumulate.
Core of extracellular lipid is present.
Type V
Type VI
SMC growth and fibrous thickening begins to narrow lumen.
Thrombus formation at site of plaque rupture

FIGURE 18-4 ■ Schematic drawing of plaque formation and progression in a coronary artery. Type I, II, and III lesions are asymptomatic but indicate accumulation of lipids in the arterial wall. Type IV, V, and VI lesions predispose to the ischemic syndromes. *SMC,* Smooth muscle cell.

Myocardial workload depends on heart rate, preload, afterload, and contractility (see Chapter 17). An increase in any of these variables increases myocardial oxygen requirements and may precipitate ischemia. However, even conditions resulting in very high myocardial oxygen consumption will seldom lead to ischemia unless some underlying impairment in coronary perfusion is present.

One or more of the aforementioned mechanisms are operative in producing clinically significant myocardial ischemia resulting in the acute or chronic coronary syndromes. Advanced fibrous plaque (type V) is thought to produce intermittent ischemia when 75% or more of the arterial lumen is occluded.[9] Because fibrous plaque progresses slowly over

Box 18-2

Markers of Vulnerability at the Plaque/Artery Level

Plaque

Morphologic Features/Structure

- Plaque cap thickness
- Plaque lipid core size
- Plaque stenosis (luminal narrowing)
- Remodeling (expansive versus constrictive remodeling)
- Color (e.g., yellow, glistening yellow, red)
- Collagen content versus lipid content, mechanical stability (stiffness and elasticity)
- Calcification burden and pattern (nodule versus scattered, superficial versus deep, etc.)
- Shear stress (flow pattern throughout the coronary artery)

Activity/Function

- Plaque inflammation (macrophage density, rate of monocyte infiltration, and density of activated T cell)
- Endothelial denudation or dysfunction (local nitric oxide production, anticoagulation/procoagulation properties of the endothelium)
- Plaque oxidative stress
- Superficial platelet aggregation and fibrin deposition (residual mural thrombus)
- Rate of apoptosis (e.g., apoptosis protein markers, coronary microsatellite)
- Angiogenesis, leaking vasa vasorum, and intraplaque hemorrhage
- Matrix-digesting enzyme activity in the cap (e.g., matrix metalloproteinase 2, 3, 9)
- Certain microbial antigens (e.g., heat-shock protein 60, *Chlamydia pneumoniae*)

Panarterial

- Transcoronary gradient of serum markers of vulnerability
- Total coronary calcium burden
- Total coronary vasoreactivity (endothelial function)
- Total arterial burden of plaque including peripheral (e.g., carotid intima medial thickness)

From Naghavi M et al: From vulnerable plaque to vulnerable patient: a call for new definitions and risk assessment strategies: part 1, *Circulation* 108:1664-1672, 2003.

many years, the heart has time to develop alternative pathways for myocardial blood flow. This collateral circulation can preserve blood flow despite almost total occlusion of the coronary artery. Thus stable fibrous plaque may produce no symptoms of ischemia unless the demand of the heart for oxygen is suddenly elevated, as occurs in exercise or stress. When the onset of ischemia is predictable with certain activities and subsides with rest, the patient is said to have a chronic coronary syndrome called classic or stable angina pectoris.

ACS occurs when sudden obstruction of coronary blood flow results in acute myocardial ischemia. Acute obstruction is usually associated with the formation of a clot in the coronary artery at the site of a vulnerable plaque. Rupture of the plaque exposes a rough area composed of collagen and other molecules that are thrombogenic. A high fibrinogen level, as occurs in smokers, and enhanced platelet adhesiveness, as occurs in hyperlipidemia, may enhance the risk of thrombus formation. Clot formation begins with adherence of platelets to the ruptured plaque. The platelets that initially attach release chemicals that attract more platelets, which aggregate and form a plug. The coagulation cascade may also be initiated and result in the formation of a platelet-fibrin clot that may occlude the vessel or break loose and travel farther along the vessel. Chemicals released by activated platelets include several vasoactive products (serotonin, thromboxane) that may contribute to spasm of the coronary vessel, further reducing blood flow.

Thrombosis occurs suddenly and may partially or completely obstruct the artery and cause acute ischemia. The ACS may present as unstable angina, MI, or sudden cardiac death. Appreciation of the role thrombus plays in coronary obstruction has resulted in the prophylactic use of antithrombotics, such as aspirin. Research indicates that the long-term use of small doses of aspirin reduces mortality from ischemic heart disease.[10]

Vasospasm has been proposed as a mechanism of ischemia in patients who have anginal signs and symptoms but no significant amount of fibrous plaque in the coronary arteries. Vasospasm may be the causative factor in variant, or Prinzmetal, angina. Intense vasospasm can occur in response to certain drugs, such as cocaine.

As previously mentioned, endothelial cells are important regulators of vascular tone. They secrete variable amounts of constricting and relaxing factors to control tissue perfusion. This autoregulation of blood flow allows the microvasculature to dilate when the need for oxygen in a particular area is increased. Failure of endothelial cells to appropriately regulate flow is a potential mechanism of myocardial ischemia.[11] Endothelial cells can be damaged by circulating toxins from cigarette smoke, immune cells, and infectious agents. Inflammatory disorders that may alter endothelial cell function include lupus erythematosus, Kawasaki syndrome, and polyarteritis nodosa. The importance of inflammatory processes in the pathogenesis of CHD is receiving greater recognition resulting in efforts to find markers (e.g., serum high-sensitivity C-reactive protein) and methods to reduce inflammation in those at risk.

Even if the coronary arteries and microcirculation are functioning properly, coronary perfusion may still be inadequate if perfusion pressure is low. Recall from Chapter 17 that coronary blood flow occurs primarily during diastole and depends on the driving pressure in the aorta. A fall in aortic blood pressure can significantly reduce coronary perfusion, particularly in vessels with high resistance to flow. Conditions such as shock, hemorrhage, and anesthesia may be associated with a fall in blood pressure, which decreases driving pressure and coronary perfusion and results in myocardial ischemia. However, the most common cause of cardiac ischemia is atherosclerotic coronary arteries.

KEY CONCEPTS

- Cardiac ischemia occurs when the heart's demand for oxygenated blood exceeds its supply. In most cases, ischemia is a result of impaired blood flow through the coronary arteries.
- CHD is most often associated with coronary atherosclerosis. Risk factors for CHD are the same as for atherosclerosis of other arteries and include advancing age, male gender, family history, hyperlipidemia, diabetes, smoking, hypertension, and obesity. Endothelial injury and inflammation and lipid accumulation in the intima are thought to be the primary initiators of coronary atherosclerosis.
- Atherosclerotic lesions can be divided into six types based on morphologic features. Type I, II, and III lesions are asymptomatic precursor lesions in which lipids are beginning to accumulate in the arterial wall. Type IV, V, and VI lesions are advanced lesions that may cause symptoms because of progressive arterial occlusion or acute plaque disruption and thrombus formation.
- Vulnerable plaques may rupture or become eroded, which stimulates clot formation on the plaque. Plaques with a large lipid core, thin cap, or high sheer stress are vulnerable plaques.
- Chronic occlusion of a coronary vessel is associated with the clinical syndrome of stable angina. Acute occlusion is associated with plaque disruption and thrombus formation and results in ACS (unstable angina or MI).
- Ischemic heart disease may uncommonly be caused by coronary vasospasm, trauma to the coronary arteries, or low perfusion pressure from volume depletion or shock.

Clinical Features and Management of Coronary Syndromes

Five syndromes can be differentiated according to the severity and onset of cardiac symptoms. Stable *angina pectoris* and *ischemic cardiomyopathy* are chronic syndromes that usually progress slowly and are a consequence of chronic obstruction from stable atherosclerotic plaques. The ACSs have an abrupt onset, life-threatening consequences, and are associated with acute changes in plaque morphology and thrombosis. The ACSs include *unstable angina* and *MI.* Unstable angina and MI are considered together because they are difficult to differentiate in the acute stage when therapeutic decisions must be made. Any of the coronary heart syndromes may precipitate *sudden cardiac death* and associated dysrhythmias.

Angina Pectoris

Angina pectoris is characterized by chest pain associated with intermittent myocardial ischemia. The length and the severity of the myocardial ischemia are insufficient to result in the death of cells. Bouts of chest pain and associated symptoms are generally recurrent and may be precipitated by conditions that increase myocardial oxygen demand, such as exercise, stress, sympathetic nervous system activation, and increased preload, afterload, heart rate, or muscle mass. Ischemic pain receptors from the myocardium travel to the central nervous system with the eighth cervical and first through fourth thoracic dorsal root ganglia. Sensory neurons from the jaw, neck, and arm also travel in these nerve trunks, so heart pain may be perceived as emanating from these body parts. This phenomenon is called *referred pain.* Anginal pain may be described as burning, crushing, squeezing, or choking. Pain is sometimes represented by expressions such as "an elephant is sitting on my chest" or by the patient placing a tight fist on the chest. Anginal pain may be mistakenly attributed to indigestion or dental pain.

Anginal ischemia, although temporary, may result in inefficient cardiac pumping with resultant pulmonary congestion and shortness of breath. Three patterns of angina pectoris have been described: stable or typical angina, Prinzmetal or variant angina, and unstable or crescendo angina. All these patterns are associated with underlying coronary vessel disease and may be exhibited in a particular individual at different times and under different conditions. Unstable angina may progress to acute ischemia and is discussed in the ACS section along with MI.

Stable Angina. *Stable angina* is the most common form and is therefore called classic or typical angina. Stable angina is characterized by stenotic atherosclerotic coronary vessels that reduce coronary blood flow to a critical level. The stenosed arteries dilate poorly in response to increased myocardial oxygen requirements. Under conditions of increased myocardial workload, such as during physical exertion or emotional strain, coronary perfusion is inadequate and ischemia results (Figure 18-5). The onset of anginal pain is generally predictable and elicited by similar stimuli each time. Stable angina is generally relieved by rest and nitroglycerin, a drug that causes coronary and peripheral vasodilation and reduces myocardial workload.

Prinzmetal Variant Angina. *Prinzmetal variant angina* is characterized by unpredictable attacks of anginal pain. Although most individuals with Prinzmetal angina have significant coronary atherosclerosis, the onset of ischemic symptoms is unrelated to physical or emotional exertion, heart rate, or other obvious causes of increased myocardial oxygen demand. Vasospasm has been identified as the probable mechanism leading to variant angina, although the cause of the vasospasm is unknown. Proposed mechanisms include atherosclerosis-induced hypercontractility, abnormal secretion of vasospastic chemicals by local mast cells, and abnormal calcium flux across vascular smooth muscle. Variant angina responds well to treatment with calcium channel–blocking drugs, which inhibit vascular smooth muscle contraction.

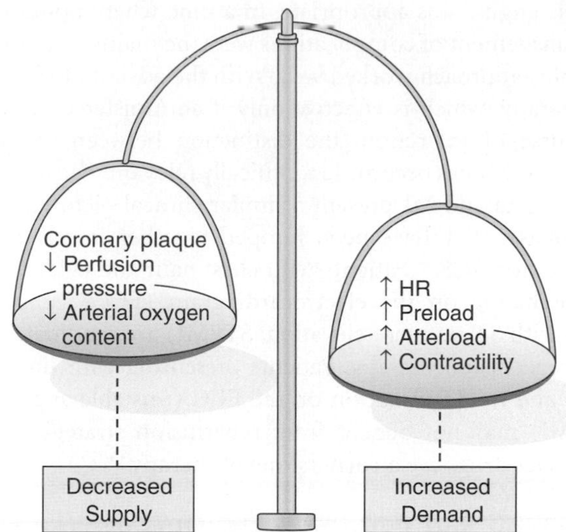

FIGURE 18-5 ■ Factors that decrease coronary blood supply or increase myocardial oxygen demand can upset the balance and lead to ischemia and anginal pain.

Patients with stable angina are at risk for developing ACS and need aggressive treatment for risk factor reduction and therapies to reduce the risk of plaque rupture, thrombosis, and dysrhythmia.

Acute Coronary Syndrome

Unstable angina and MI are difficult to distinguish on the basis of clinical manifestations and are lumped together by the term acute coronary syndrome. Both are characterized by chest pain that may be more severe and lasts longer than the patient's typical angina or may occur in individuals whose disease was previously asymptomatic. In both cases, plaque rupture with subsequent acute thrombus development is thought to occur. In unstable angina, the occlusion is partial or the clot is broken down before the death of myocardial tissue. In MI, the occlusion is complete and the thrombus persists long enough for development of irreversible damage to myocardial cells. In the past, differentiation of unstable angina and MI was based on laboratory evaluation of serum enzyme levels (e.g., MB band of creatine kinase [CK-MB], troponins I and T). If cardiac enzymes were elevated, which is indicative of necrosis, a diagnosis of MI was made; if not, a diagnosis of unstable angina was appropriate. In a time when monitoring and management of complications were the mainstay of treatment, this approach worked well. With the advent of reperfusion therapy, which is effective only if administered early in the course of infarction, the distinction between unstable angina and MI has become less clinically relevant. Because unstable angina and MI present a similar clinical picture in the acute phase, they have been lumped together in treatment protocols for ACS.[12] Patients with chest pain and evidence of acute ischemia on the electrocardiogram (ECG) (unstable angina with ST-segment elevation; STEMI) are candidates for acute reperfusion therapy. Patients presenting with unstable angina and no ST elevation on the ECG (unstable angina or NSTEMI) may not benefit from reperfusion strategies, and antiplatelet drugs are a cornerstone of therapy.[13]

Etiology and Pathogenesis. MI results when prolonged or total disruption of blood flow to the myocardium causes irreversible cellular death. Acute MI is the most important form of CHD and results in more than 500,000 deaths annually in the United States.[1] It is estimated that an American male has greater than a one in five chance of sustaining an MI or fatal ischemic event before the age of 65. An MI may occur at any age, but the frequency rises with advancing age. Females younger than 45 years have a sixfold lesser risk of MI than men of the same age. After menopause, the rate of MI in women approaches that of their male counterparts and becomes essentially equal by age 80.[9]

Two morphologic types of MI have been described, each having different clinical significance. A **transmural infarct** involves the entire thickness of the ventricular wall and is the more serious of the two types. It is also the more common. A **non–Q-wave** (subendocardial) infarct affects only the inner third to half of the ventricular wall (Figure 18-6) and is generally associated with less severe symptoms. These lesions are not exclusive: a non–Q-wave MI can extend across the ventricular wall to become a transmural MI under certain circumstances. It is believed by some investigators that the pathophysiologic process of these two types of MI is somewhat different.

As previously described, the initiating event in most MIs is believed to be development of a thrombus on top of an ulcerated or cracked atherosclerotic plaque. The initiating event is a sudden change in structure of the plaque. Platelets passing by the surface of the ruptured plaque adhere to it, initiate formation of a platelet plug, and activate the clotting cascade. The resultant thrombus grows until it occludes the vessel and triggers the transmural MI.

The thrombus theory of acute transmural MI was controversial for many years because only 50% of persons dying of transmural MI had a demonstrable thrombus at autopsy. Then DeWood and co-workers[14] demonstrated that about 90% of persons with acute MI had an intracoronary thrombus within 4 hours of the onset of symptoms but only 60% had thrombi 12 to 24 hours later. This observation suggested that

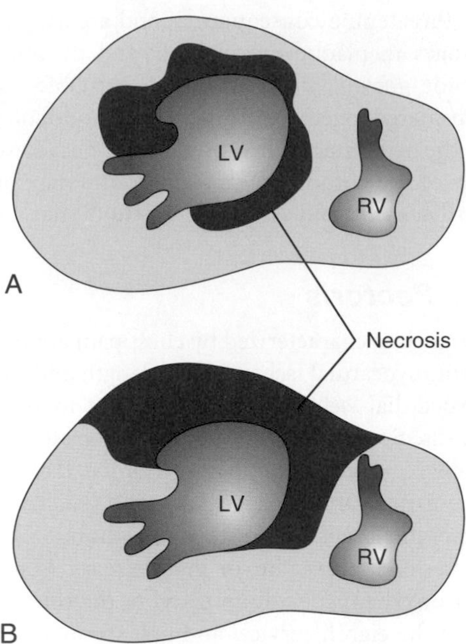

FIGURE 18-6 ■ Comparison of non–Q-wave (subendocardial) infarct **(A)** and transmural infarct **(B)**. Note that the zone of necrosis affects only the inner aspect of the left ventricle in **A** but extends completely through the wall in **B**. *LV,* Left ventricle; *RV,* right ventricle.

the thrombus was quickly dissolved by natural mechanisms after the occlusive event. Further support for the thrombus theory comes from the effectiveness of thrombolytic therapy; agents such as streptokinase and tissue plasminogen activator successfully restore flow through obstructed coronary vessels and significantly reduce mortality.[15]

The pathophysiologic progression of the subendocardial type of MI is less well established. The **subendocardium** is most vulnerable to a reduction in blood flow. The coronary arteries enter the myocardium at the outer epicardial surface and traverse thick ventricular walls before finally delivering blood to the endocardial areas. Factors such as an increased demand for oxygen in the setting of generalized atherosclerosis may be involved, although a role for thrombus has also been proposed. Underlying atherosclerotic coronary disease is almost always present, but often no critical stenosis resulting in greater than 75% occlusion.

The cellular consequences of an acute interruption in blood flow to the myocardium do not occur instantaneously or uniformly. Acute occlusion causes a range of cellular events, depending on the availability and adequacy of collateral blood flow, the relative workload, and the length of time that flow is interrupted. A typical transmural infarct has several zones composed of cells in various stages of ischemia and death.

Experiments in animal models indicate that complete occlusion of a coronary vessel results in a predictable pattern of cellular dysfunction and death.[9] Depletion of ATP in acutely ischemic cells begins immediately, followed within 1 to 2

Table 18-4

Cellular Events After Myocardial Infarction

Time	Gross	Light Microscope	Electron Microscope	Other
0-30 min	No change	No change	Reversible changes (mitochondrial swelling, relaxation of myofibrils)	Loss of enzyme activity; glycogen loss
1-2 hr	No change	Few "wavy" fibers at margin of infarct	Irreversible changes (sarcolemmal disruption, electron-dense mitochondrial deposits)	
4-12 hr	No change	Early coagulation necrosis; edema; occasional neutrophils; minimal hemorrhage		
18-24 hr	Slight pallor or mottling	Continuing coagulation necrosis (nuclear pyknosis and disintegration; cytoplasmic eosinophilia); "contraction band" necrosis at periphery of infarct; neutrophilic infiltrate		
24-72 hr	Pallor	Complete coagulation necrosis of myofibers; heavy neutrophilic infiltrate with early fragmentation of neutrophil nuclei		
4-7 days	Central pallor with hyperemic border	Macrophages appear; early disintegration and phagocytosis of necrotic fibers; granulation tissue visible at edge of infarct		
10 days	Maximally yellow, soft, shrunken; purple border	Well-developed phagocytosis; prominent granulation tissue in peripheral areas of infarct		
7-8 wk	Firm, gray	Fibrosis		

From Kumar V, Cotran RS, Robbins ST: *Robbins basic pathology,* ed 7, Philadelphia, 2003, Saunders, p 368.

minutes by an impaired ability to contract. Within 10 minutes, cellular concentrations of ATP fall to half normal, and irreversible cell injury occurs after 30 to 40 minutes of complete occlusion (Table 18-4). Ischemic necrosis begins in the subendocardial zone and spreads across the ventricular wall toward epicardial surfaces. Epicardial areas are spared for longer periods because they have the greatest collateral network of arterial vessels. The ultimate size of the infarcted tissue depends on the extent, duration, and severity of ischemia. Areas of necrosis may be intermixed with or surrounded by zones of reversibly injured cells that are marginally perfused by collaterals. In the typical infarction about 20% of the cells die from necrosis and the remaining 80% from apoptosis of injured cells that initiate programmed cell death.[16] "Rescue" of these potentially salvageable cells is an important focus of treatment. (See Chapter 4 for a discussion of apoptosis.)

Nearly all transmural infarcts are located in the left ventricular walls. Isolated right ventricular infarction occurs in only 1% to 3% of MIs. Occlusion of the left anterior descending artery causes 40% to 50% of acute MIs, the right coronary artery contributes another 30% to 40%, and the left circumflex contributes 15% to 20%.[9] The locations of the resulting infarcts are shown in Table 18-5. It is common for individuals with coronary heart disease to suffer from more than one MI during their lifetime.

The area of necrosis resulting from MI undergoes a series of morphologic changes as the infarct ages.[9] These morphologic changes generally cannot be detected on gross examination until 6 to 12 hours after infarct. After 18 to 24 hours the area of infarction becomes paler than surrounding tissues. Thereafter the area of infarction becomes obvious as it turns yellowish and soft with a rim of red vascular connective tissue (Figure 18-7). At 1 to 2 weeks the necrotic tissue is progressively degraded and cleared away. Infarcted myocardium is particularly weakened and susceptible to rupture at this time. By 6 weeks the necrotic tissue has been replaced by tough fibrous scar tissue.

Table 18-5

Location of Myocardial Infarction According to Coronary Artery Affected

Arterial Obstruction	Location of Infarct
Left anterior descending (40%-50% of infarcts)	Anterior wall of LV near apex Anterior two thirds of interventricular septum
Right coronary (30%-40% of infarcts)	Posterior wall of LV Posterior one third of interventricular septum
Left circumflex (15%-20% of infarcts)	Lateral wall of LV

Data from Kumar V, Cotran RS, Robbins ST: *Robbins basic pathology,* ed 7, Philadelphia, 2003, Saunders, p 366.
LV, Left ventricle.

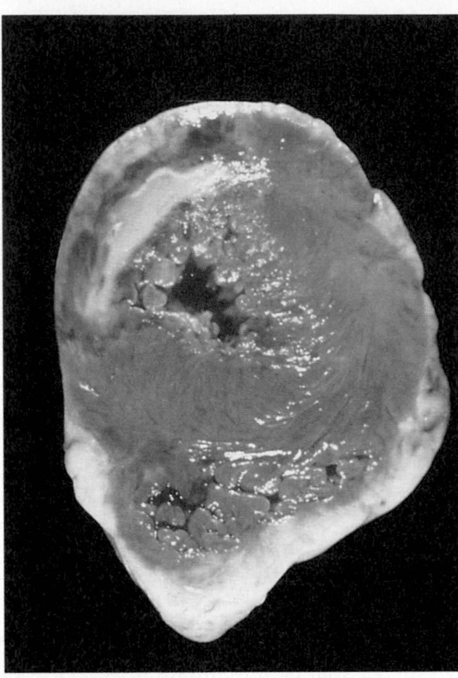

FIGURE 18-7 ■ This photograph of a 5- to 7-day-old posterolateral infarction clearly shows a large, pale yellow lesion surrounded by a dark red zone of inflammation. (From Kumar V, Cotran R, Robbins S: *Robbins basic pathology,* ed 7, Philadelphia, 2003, Saunders, p 369.)

Diagnosis of ACS. The diagnosis of ACS is based on three primary indicators: symptoms, electrocardiographic changes, and elevations of specific marker proteins in the blood. Other diagnostic examinations such as cardiac catheterization, echocardiography, and radionuclide scintigraphy may also be done to provide additional information (see Chapter 17).

Severe crushing, excruciating chest pain that may radiate to the arm, shoulder, jaw, or back is the harbinger of ACS. Pain is commonly accompanied by nausea, vomiting, diaphoresis (sweating), and shortness of breath. In contrast to anginal pain, infarction pain generally lasts more than 15 minutes and is not relieved by rest or nitroglycerin. In some instances, however, the MI is entirely asymptomatic and may elude detection. Asymptomatic MI has been called "silent MI" and may be detected only serendipitously at a later date. Pain may be difficult to assess in individuals with a tendency to ignore or deny their symptoms. Thus, although pain is an important indicator of acute ischemia, other clinical information is often needed to correctly distinguish between angina, infarction, and noncardiac sources of pain. Women, in particular, more commonly complain of atypical symptoms with MI, including, fatigue, nausea, back pain, and abdominal discomfort. Atypical complaints in patients with CHD risk factors should prompt a high suspicion of ACS.

Electrocardiographic Changes. Myocardial ischemia and infarction often result in characteristic changes on ECG waveforms. Injury and ischemia are indicated on the ECG by ST-segment changes. ST-segment elevation is thought to represent acute cell injury and ischemia. The presence of ST-segment elevation on the ECG indicates that the ischemic injury is ongoing and that efforts to improve perfusion or reduce oxygen demand may be effective in preserving myocardial muscle mass. These patients are regarded as having unstable angina with STEMI in treatment protocols for ACS. Infarcted muscle that is necrotic and no longer electrically active is indicated by the appearance of abnormally deep or wide Q waves and inverted T waves (Figure 18-8). These changes are very specific for MI and, when present, are diagnostic. Q waves are usually persistent findings, whereas ST-segment and T-wave changes may resolve over time. Q waves take time to develop and may not be present in the acute phase of an MI.

Dysrhythmias and the characteristic ST-segment changes that accompany ACS are attributed to injured and ischemic cells that have not yet become necrotic. Reversibly injured cells have limited ATP supplies to power membrane pumps and are predisposed to leakage of ions across their cell membranes. Abnormal ion flux may result in continuous current flow even when the heart is at rest. This current leak may be seen on the ECG as ST-segment elevation.

The 12-lead ECG is used to localize the injured region of the left ventricle. Various leads of the 12-lead ECG "look at" different regions of the heart. Abnormalities such as Q waves and ST-segment elevation in a particular lead or leads indicate that the damage is localized to the part of the left ventricle "seen" by that lead. MIs may thus be described as anterior, lateral, posterior, septal, inferior, or a combination of these. Spe-

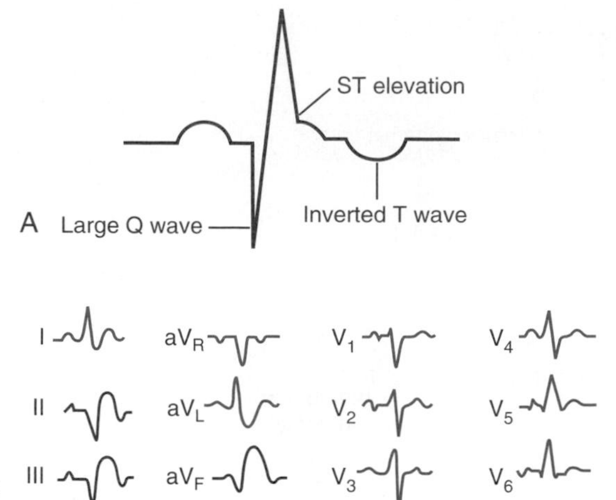

FIGURE 18-8 ■ **A,** Typical ECG infarction pattern showing abnormally large Q wave, ST elevation, and inverted T wave. **B,** Typical ECG in acute inferior myocardial infarction. Note the Q waves and ST-segment elevation in leads II, III, and aV_F.

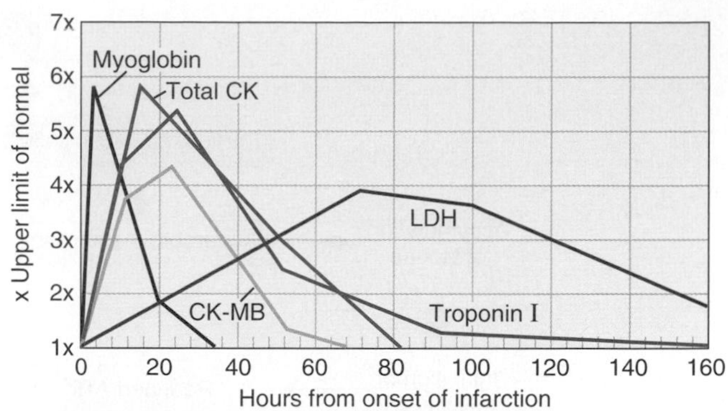

FIGURE 18-9 ■ Time course of serum marker protein elevations after acute myocardial infarction. The MB band of creatine kinase *(CK-MB)* and troponin I are the most specific of the protein markers. Myoglobin is an early marker but is not very specific. (Redrawn from Antman EM: General hospital management. In Julian DG, Braunwald E, editors: *Management of acute myocardial infarction,* London, 1994, Saunders, p 631.)

cial leads placed on the right side of the chest can be helpful in detecting right ventricular infarcts. (The 12-lead ECG is described in Chapter 17.) In some cases patients presenting with ACS do not have ST elevation on the ECG. They may have ST depression or T-wave changes. Some of these patients will develop elevated serum markers indicating MI. These patients have NSTEMI. The infarct size is generally smaller and the outcomes are better than those in patients with STEMI.[13]

Serum Markers. The appearance of certain proteins in the blood after myocardial cell death is a very sensitive and reliable indicator of MI. Myocardial cell death leads to elevated serum levels of myoglobin, troponin, lactate dehydrogenase, and creatine kinase.[9] An increase in these proteins suggests leakage from fatally damaged cells that have lost plasma membrane integrity. Cardiac cells contain particular forms of these proteins called isoenzymes. Cardiac isoenzymes have a slightly different amino acid sequence than other cell types. In particular, myocytes contain the isoenzymes CK-MB, troponin I, and troponin T. An elevated level of serum CK-MB is a highly specific indicator of MI and considered to be diagnostic. However, CK-MB remains elevated for only 48 to 72 hours after MI. Two proteins that make up part of the cardiac cell contractile apparatus, troponins I and T, have become the markers of choice for detecting MI. Cardiac troponin levels become elevated in serum at about the same time as CK-MB, but they remain elevated for a longer period. Cardiac troponins I and T are highly sensitive and specific for cardiac cell death but less helpful in detecting new infarction (reinfarction) because levels remain elevated for a prolonged period (Figure 18-9). Cardiac myoglobin levels are elevated in serum very quickly after MI and may be helpful in early detection; however, cardiac myoglobin is less specific than the other markers. All serum markers are useful diagnostically only during the acute period of MI. Patients with ACS who do not develop elevations of these serum markers are diagnosed with unstable angina.

In addition to chest pain, electrocardiographic abnormalities, and serum protein marker elevations, a person experiencing an MI may exhibit signs of cardiac inflammation, including fever, leukocytosis, and an elevated sedimentation rate. Symptoms of circulatory inadequacy, including fatigue, restlessness, anxiety, and weakness, may be present.

The events associated with ACS are summarized in Figure 18-10. Note that totally ischemic cells, which die and become electrically silent, are the source of the clinical findings of Q waves and also release the indicative serum marker proteins (CK-MB, troponins). Partially ischemic cells are potentially salvageable but are unable to maintain normal ion flux across the cell membrane. Abnormal ion flux is responsible for the ST-segment changes in acute ischemia and also predisposes to a variety of cardiac dysrhythmias, including ventricular ectopy and conduction blocks (see Chapter 19).

Neither partially ischemic nor totally ischemic cells are able to contract effectively, and poor stroke volume leads to a drop in cardiac output. Decreased stroke volume triggers a number of compensatory actions designed to improve cardiac output. In particular, activation of the sympathetic nervous system increases the heart rate, contractility, blood pressure, and fluid retention by the kidney. Unfortunately, these compensatory efforts impose a greater workload on the heart and may contribute to further ischemic damage. Compensatory mechanisms are shown in Figure 18-11 and include sympathetic nervous system activation, enhanced preload, and hypertrophy of cardiac myocytes.

Prognosis and Treatment. It is difficult to determine an overall prognosis for acute MI because many variables affect the outcome, including the extent and location of the infarct, previous cardiovascular health, age, and the presence of

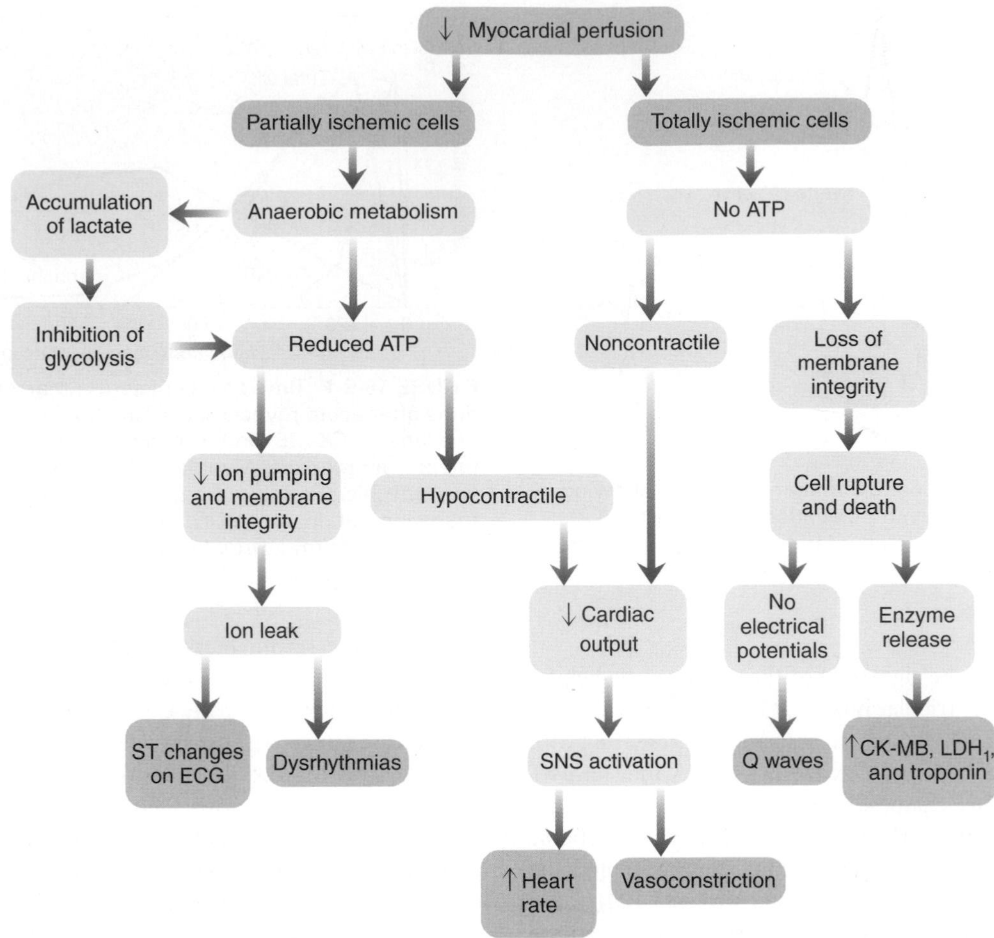

FIGURE 18-10 ■ Summary of events after myocardial infarction. *ATP,* Adenosine triphosphate; *SNS,* sympathetic nervous system; *CK-MB,* MB band of creatine kinase; *LDH,* lactate dehydrogenase; *ECG,* electrocardiography.

other disease processes. Of particular importance is the rapidity with which treatment is sought. Most deaths from MI occur before the victim reaches the hospital. Overall mortality within 1 year of MI is about 25% for men and 38% for women.[1] In approximately 10% to 20% of cases an MI is not accompanied by any complications (uncomplicated MI) and the patient recovers rapidly. However, the remaining 80% to 90% of MIs are followed by one or more complications.[9] Potential complications include cardiac dysrhythmias, congestive heart failure, cardiogenic shock, ventricular rupture, and thromboembolism.

Treatment for MI is directed at decreasing myocardial oxygen demand and increasing myocardial oxygen supply while monitoring and managing complications as they arise. Measures to reduce myocardial workload frequently include preload and afterload reduction, heart rate control, pain relief, and activity restriction. Sympathetic antagonists, nitrates, and morphine sulfate are the mainstays of drug therapy. Measures to increase oxygen delivery to ischemic areas include oxygen administration, antiplatelet therapy with aspirin and other antiplatelet agents, thrombolytic (fibrinolytic) drugs, anticoagulants, angioplasty, and coronary artery bypass grafting (CABG) (Figure 18-12). Therapies aimed at opening the blocked coronary artery are called reperfusion therapies.

Thrombolytic (fibrinolytic) therapy, when given within 2 hours of the onset of ischemia, can significantly improve outcome and limit infarct size in patients presenting with STEMI.[15] Thrombolytic agents can be administered systemically or directly into the blocked coronary artery. Common thrombolytics include streptokinase and several types of tissue plasminogen activators (e.g., alteplase, reteplase, lanoteplase, tenecteplase). These agents all predispose to hemorrhage and may be contraindicated in some individuals with bleeding disorders or trauma.

Another approach to opening an acutely occluded coronary artery is by angioplasty. In this procedure, called percutaneous transluminal coronary angioplasty (PTCA), a balloon-tipped catheter is inserted into an artery (usually femoral, brachial, or radial) and advanced up the aorta and into the coronary artery. When the balloon is correctly positioned at the site of stenosis, it is inflated to crush the stenotic area and increase vessel diameter. Unfortunately, the crushed plaque often serves as a point of thrombosis and restenosis unless fol-

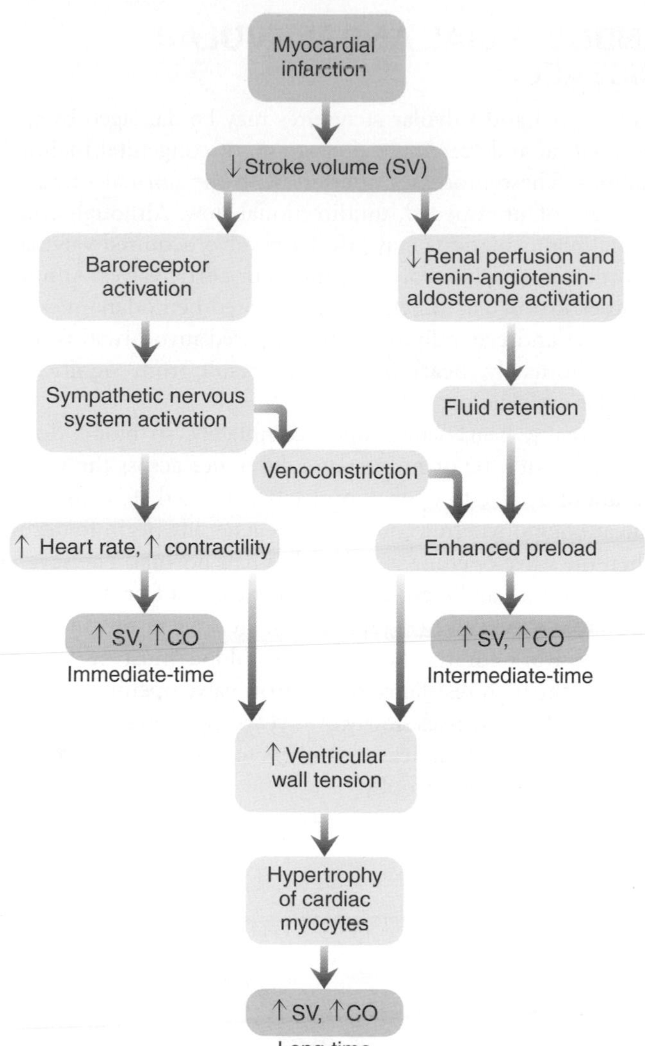

FIGURE 18-11 ■ Compensatory responses to increase stroke volume *(SV)* and maintain cardiac output *(CO)* after myocardial infarction.

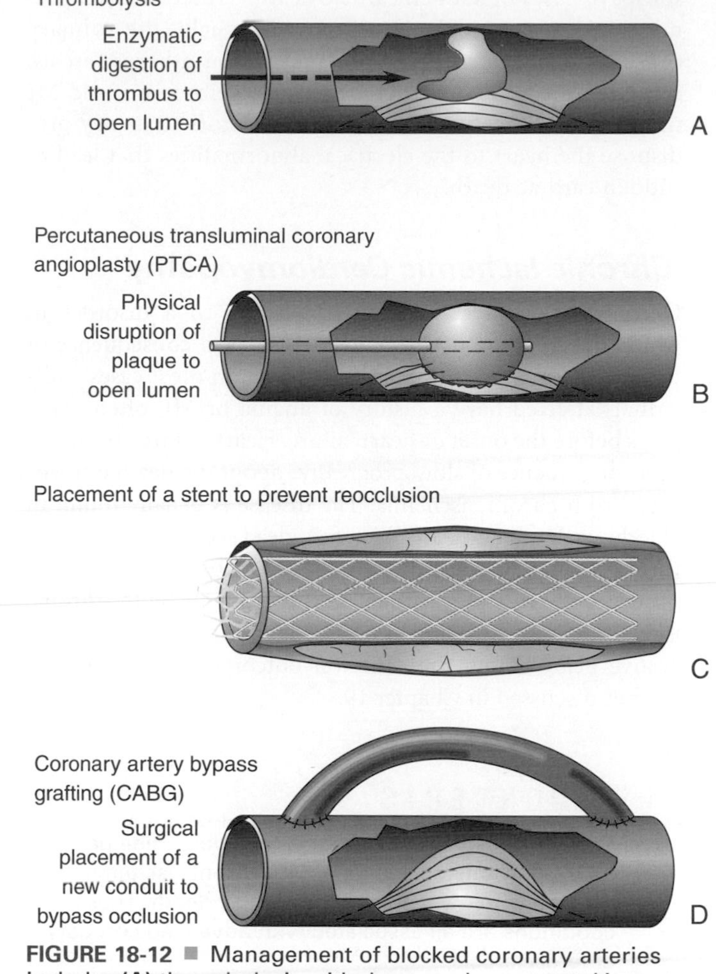

FIGURE 18-12 ■ Management of blocked coronary arteries includes **(A)** thrombolysis with drugs such as streptokinase and tissue plasminogen activator; **(B)** plaque disruption with percutaneous transluminal coronary angioplasty, followed by anticoagulation or stent placement; **(C)** placement of a stent to prevent reocclusion; and **(D)** coronary artery bypass grafting—surgical placement of a new conduit to bypass the occluded area of the artery.

lowed by anticoagulation. Insertion of a small intracoronary brace or stent is advocated by many cardiologists to prevent restenosis after PTCA (see Figure 18-12). Stents may be coated with drugs such as heparin to prevent thrombosis and reocclusion at the stent. If PTCA can be performed rapidly at the onset of STEMI the mortality rate is improved in comparison with fibrinolytic therapy.[17]

CABG may be performed as treatment for acute MI if thrombolytic therapy or PTCA is contraindicated or ineffective. More commonly, CABG is performed to alleviate angina in patients with advanced atherosclerotic plaque. This procedure uses an alternative vessel (e.g., mammary artery, radial artery, or saphenous leg vein) to circumvent the blocked portion of the coronary artery and reestablish flow downstream from an occlusion.

Early detection and management of dysrhythmias and conduction disorders are an important part of the immediate care of a patient with MI. Many dysrhythmias are life threatening and, at the very least, lead to decreased cardiac output or increased myocardial workload. Continuous electrocardiographic monitoring is generally the standard of care because of the high incidence of electrical disturbances after MI. Common dysrhythmias and conduction disorders are described in Chapter 19.

Sudden Cardiac Death

Sudden cardiac death is usually defined as unexpected death from cardiac causes within 1 hour of the onset of symptoms.[18] Coronary heart disease is at the root of the vast majority of cases of sudden cardiac death. Rarely, sudden cardiac death may be a complication of hereditary or acquired structural or electrical abnormalities. It is estimated that 300,000 to 400,000 individuals die each year in the United States of sudden cardiac death.[1] It is most often associated with coronary atherosclerosis and may be the initial manifestation of the disease. Acute MI occurs in only a small subset of cases of sudden cardiac death.[18] A lethal dysrhythmia such as ventricular fibrillation is usually the primary cause of death. Ischemia from multivessel atherosclerosis, diffuse myocardial atrophy, scarring and fibrosis of old MI tissue, and electrolyte imbalances are factors that may predispose the heart to the electrical abnormalities that lead to sudden cardiac death.

Chronic Ischemic Cardiomyopathy

Chronic ischemic cardiomyopathy refers to a disorder in which heart failure develops insidiously as a consequence of progressive ischemic myocardial damage. In most cases, individuals affected have a history of angina or MI, often many years before the onset of heart failure. Heart failure appears to be a consequence of slow, progressive apoptotic death of myocytes from chronic ischemia. The disease is usually found in elderly individuals. Atrophic and dead cells are scattered throughout the myocardium rather than being localized, as occurs with MI. The prognosis for patients with chronic ischemic cardiomyopathy is quite poor, with death from congestive heart failure the common outcome. Heart failure is further discussed in Chapter 19.

KEY CONCEPTS

- The clinical syndromes of CHD include angina pectoris, ACS (unstable angina, MI), chronic ischemic cardiomyopathy, and sudden cardiac death. These conditions are all associated with advanced coronary atherosclerosis.
- Angina is characterized by intermittent bouts of chest pain brought on by exertion and generally relieved by rest. No permanent myocardial damage occurs.
- Prolonged or severe ischemia results in MI that is characterized by severe, unrelieved chest pain, nausea and vomiting, diaphoresis, shortness of breath, and inflammation (fever, increased white blood cell count, increased sedimentation rate).
- Serum protein marker elevations and electrocardiographic changes are diagnostic of MI. The most specific and sensitive serum markers are increased CK-MB and troponin I and T. ECG changes include ST-segment elevation, large Q waves, and inverted T waves.
- A drop in cardiac output as a result of MI triggers a number of compensatory responses, including sympathetic activation. The sympathetic nervous system increases the heart rate, contractility, and blood pressure, all of which increase myocardial workload.
- Treatment of acute ischemia usually includes efforts to decrease myocardial oxygen demand (sympathetic antagonists, rest, heart rate control, pain relief, afterload reduction) and increase oxygen delivery (thrombolysis, angioplasty, coronary bypass grafting).

ENDOCARDIAL AND VALVULAR DISEASES

Endocardial and valvular structures may be damaged by inflammation and scarring, calcification, or congenital malformations. These processes interfere with the normal valvular property of unimpeded, unidirectional flow. Although congenital malformations may affect any valve, acquired valvular disorders generally involve the mitral or aortic valves. Abnormalities in valvular function cause altered hemodynamics in the heart and generally result in increased myocardial workload. Ultimately, heart failure may result from significant valvular dysfunction.

Normally, heart valves open completely, so blood flows through with little or no pressure difference across the valve. Failure of a valve to open completely is termed **stenosis.** Significant hemodynamic consequences generally begin to occur when the valve opening is reduced to half normal. The severity of stenosis can be estimated by the degree of pressure gradient across the valve (Figure 18-13). Stenosis results in extra pressure work for the heart because blood must be forced through the high resistance of a narrow valve opening. Stenosis generally progresses slowly over years to decades, which allows time for affected heart chambers to compensate through myocardial cell hypertrophy.

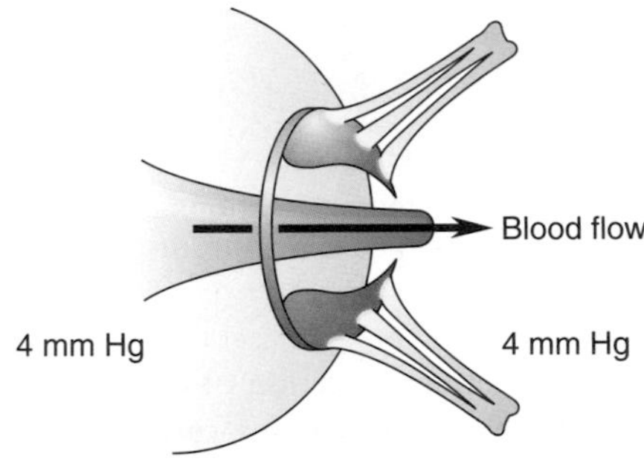

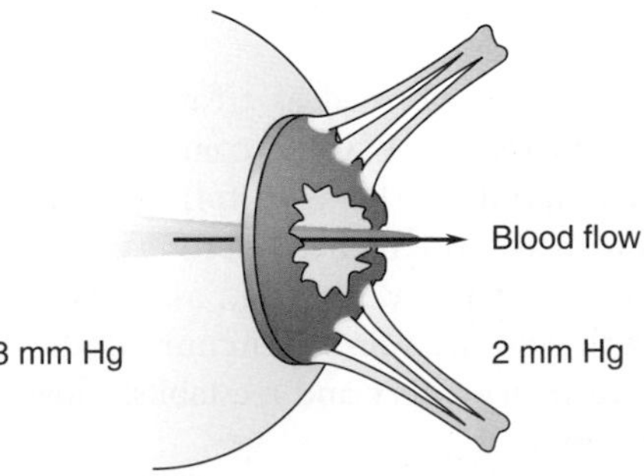

FIGURE 18-13 ■ Development of a pressure gradient across a stenosed valve. The chamber behind the narrowed valve opening must work harder to force blood through.

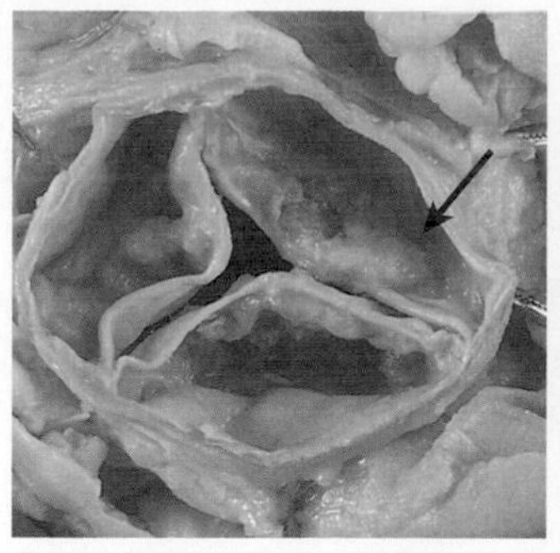

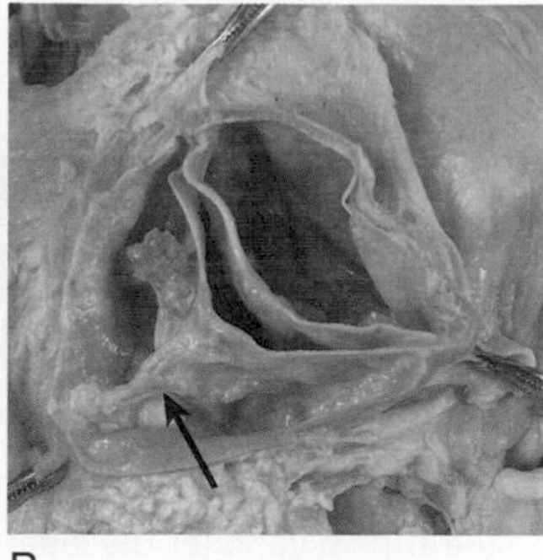

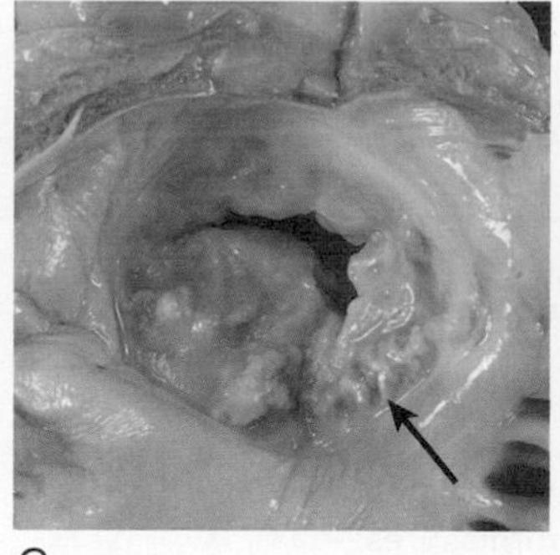

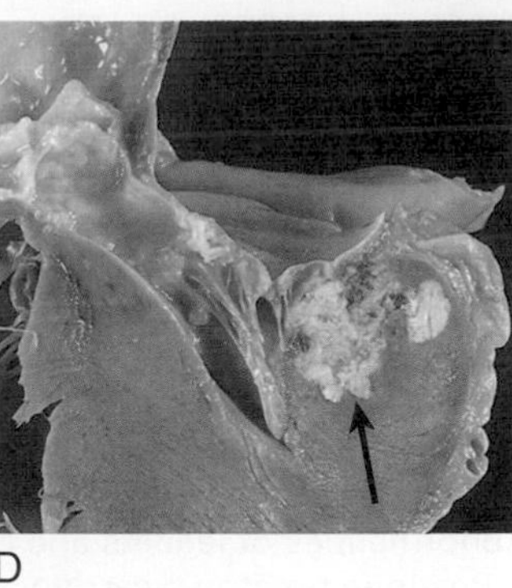

FIGURE 18-14 ■ Valvular degeneration and calcification. **A,** Calcific aortic stenosis of previously normal (three-cusp) valve. **B,** Calcific aortic stenosis of congenitally bicuspid valve. **C,** Mitral valve calcification. **D,** Cut section of valve from **C.** (From Kumar V, Cotran R, Robbins S: *Robbins basic pathology,* ed 7, Philadelphia, 2003, Saunders, p 567.)

Regurgitation or insufficiency refers to the inability of a valve to close completely, thereby allowing blood to flow in a reverse direction. Regurgitation may develop suddenly from valvular infection or rupture of a supporting papillary muscle. Sudden regurgitation is poorly tolerated inasmuch as little compensation is possible. Regurgitation results in extra volume work for the heart because more blood must be pumped to maintain adequate forward flow.

Diseased valves may exhibit elements of both stenosis and regurgitation, although one problem usually predominates. Postinflammatory scarring from rheumatic heart disease and valvular calcification with aging are the primary causes of stenosis (Figure 18-14). A wide variety of diseases of the endocardium may lead to valvular regurgitation, including rheumatic heart disease and infective endocarditis, which are discussed later in this chapter. Damaged valves are susceptible to infection, and antibiotic prophylaxis is therefore indicated for dental, surgical, and diagnostic procedures. The major causes of acquired mitral and aortic valvular diseases are listed in Table 18-6. Valvular disorders are often associated with abnormal heart sounds called murmurs. Careful assessment of the location and character of a murmur can help identify the underlying valvular abnormality. Defining characteristics of common valve disorders are described in Table 18-7.

Disorders of the Mitral Valve

Three important disorders of the mitral valve are stenosis, regurgitation, and mitral valve prolapse.

Mitral Stenosis

In *mitral stenosis* the flow of blood from the left atrium into the left ventricle is impaired. Mitral stenosis is therefore characterized by an abnormal left atrial–left ventricular pressure gradient during ventricular diastole (Figure 18-15). Normally the pressures in the atrium and ventricle are nearly equal during ventricular diastole when the mitral valve is open. Figure 18-15 shows that with mitral valve stenosis, atrial pressure remains higher than ventricular pressure throughout diastole. As the stenosis worsens, the pressure gradient often increases. In normal adults the area of the mitral valve orifice is 4 to 6 cm^2 and symptoms of stenosis do not appear until the orifice is narrowed to 2 cm^2. When the mitral valve orifice narrows to 1 cm^2, a critical stenosis is present and a pressure gradient of 20 mm Hg or more usually develops across the valve.[19] Increased pressure work of the left atrium leads to atrial chamber enlargement and hypertrophy. Progressive narrowing of the mitral valve may lead to markedly elevated left atrial pressures and subsequent increased pulmonary vascular pressure. If uncorrected, mitral stenosis may result in chronic pulmonary hypertension, right ventricular hypertrophy, and right-sided heart failure.

The signs and symptoms of mitral stenosis are due to congestion of blood volume and increased pressure in the left atrium and pulmonary circulation, as well as decreased stroke volume of the left ventricle because of deficient filling. Symptoms are exacerbated by conditions that further decrease left ventricular filling such as an increased heart rate. Atrial dysrhythmias such as atrial fibrillation are common because of excessive atrial volume. Atrial enlargement and fibrillation also predispose to the development of atrial clots, which may dislodge and result in systemic embolization. Signs and symptoms of mitral stenosis secondary to pulmonary congestion may include orthopnea, cough, dyspnea on exertion, paroxysmal nocturnal dyspnea, abnormal breath sounds, and poor arterial oxygenation. Reduced left ventricular stroke volume may be apparent as fatigue, poor activity tolerance, and weakness. Exertional dyspnea is the most common complaint. Blood rushing through the narrowed mitral valve during ventricular diastole can sometimes be heard as a low-pitched, rumbling diastolic murmur at the heart's apex. In many cases, an opening snap may also be heard.

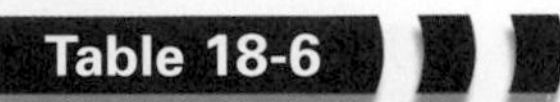

Table 18-6

Major Causes of Acquired Valvular Heart Disease

Mitral Valve Disease	Aortic Valve Disease
Stenosis	
Postinflammatory scarring (rheumatic heart disease)	Postinflammatory scarring (rheumatic heart disease) Senile calcific aortic stenosis Calcification of a congenitally deformed valve
Regurgitation	
Abnormalities of leaflets and commissures: Postinflammatory scarring Infective endocarditis Floppy mitral valve (prolapse) Scleroderma Systemic lupus erythematosus	Intrinsic valvular disease: Postinflammatory scarring (rheumatic heart disease) Infective endocarditis
Abnormalities of the tensor apparatus: Rupture of papillary muscle Papillary muscle dysfunction (fibrosis) Rupture of chordae tendineae Sarcoidosis	Aortic disease: Degenerative aortic dilation Syphilitic aortitis Ankylosing spondylitis Rheumatoid arthritis Marfan syndrome
Abnormalities of the LV cavity and/or annulus: LV enlargement (myocarditis, congestive cardiomyopathy) Calcification of the mitral ring	

Modified from Schoen FJ: Surgical pathology of removed natural and prosthetic heart valves, *Hum Pathol* 18(6):558-567, 1987; and Braunwald E, Zipes D, Libby P, editors: *Heart disease: a textbook of cardiovascular medicine,* ed 6, Philadelphia, 2001, Saunders, p 1654.
LV, Left ventricle.

Table 18-7

Defining Characteristics of Murmurs

Valve Disorder	Quality	Location, Radiation
Mitral stenosis	Low-pitched rumble, midsystolic	At apex
Mitral regurgitation	Loud, pan-systolic, high pitched, blowing	Loudest at apex, transmitted to left axilla
Aortic stenosis	Harsh, midsystolic, crescendo-decrescendo	Right second intercostal space, transmitted to neck
Aortic regurgitation	Faint, blowing, diastolic	Left sternal border, aortic area, apex

Mitral Regurgitation

Mitral regurgitation is characterized by backflow of blood from the left ventricle to the left atrium during ventricular systole. Elevation of left atrial volume and pressure by regurgitant flow leads to characteristic giant *v* waves on the atrial pressure monitor (Figure 18-16). The severity of mitral insufficiency is related to the amount of left ventricular stroke volume that is regurgitant and depends, in part, on the aortic resistance to flow (afterload). A high afterload increases the amount of regurgitant flow. The left ventricle must pump a greater volume to compensate for the regurgitant flow and maintain an effective stroke volume. Both the left atrium and ventricle generally dilate and hypertrophy to compensate for the extra volume that they are required to pump. In most patients with severe mitral regurgitation, compensation is maintained for many years.[19] If severe and uncorrected, mitral regurgitation may lead to left-sided heart failure. The signs and symptoms of mitral regurgitation are similar to those described for mitral stenosis and result from pulmonary congestion and poor cardiac output. Chronic weakness and fatigue are common complaints. The murmur of mitral regurgitation

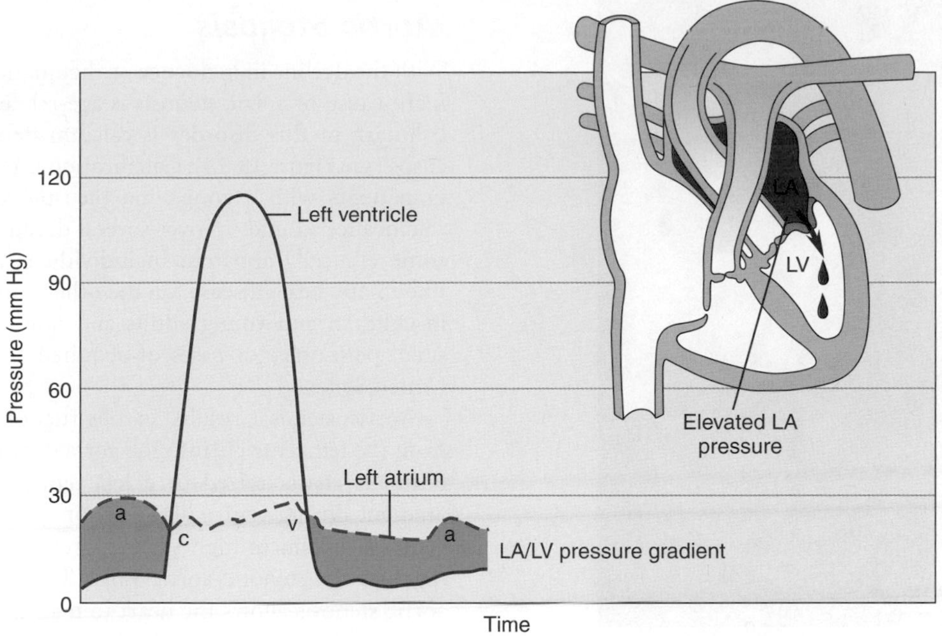

FIGURE 18-15 ■ Mitral stenosis is characterized by an abnormal left atrial *(LA)*–to–left ventricular *(LV)* pressure gradient during ventricular diastole *(shaded area).*

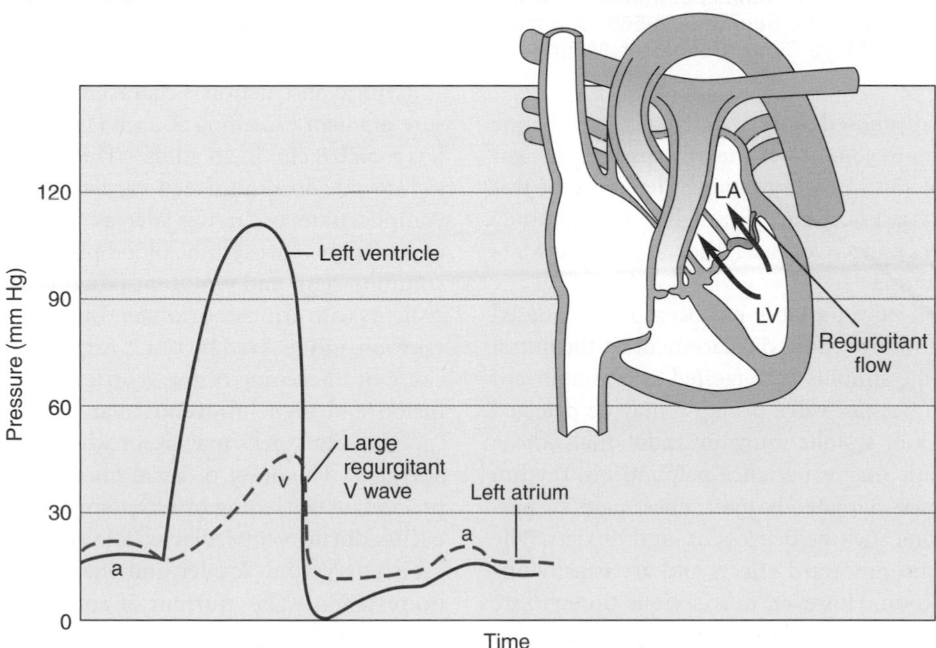

FIGURE 18-16 ■ Mitral regurgitation causes characteristic giant v waves on the left atrial *(LA)* pressure monitor. *LV,* Left ventricular.

usually occurs throughout ventricular systole (pansystolic), radiates toward the left axilla, and has a high-pitched blowing character. The arterial pulse may be helpful in distinguishing the systolic murmur of mitral regurgitation from that of aortic stenosis. The upstroke of the pulse is sharp and full in mitral regurgitation, whereas it is weaker and delayed in aortic stenosis.

Mitral Valve Prolapse

Approximately 2% to 3% of the population have mitral valves that balloon up into the left atrium during ventricular systole.[19] This condition is called *mitral valve prolapse* (Figure 18-17). Women between the ages of 20 and 40 years are most often affected. In a great majority of cases the disorder is

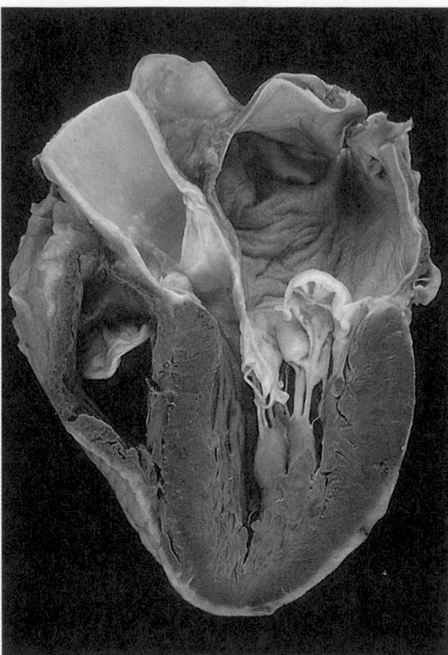

FIGURE 18-17 ■ Appearance of mitral valve prolapse. Note how the valve balloons up into the left atrium. (From Cotran RS, Kumar V, Collins T, editors: *Robbins pathologic basis of disease,* ed 6, Philadelphia, 1999, Saunders, p 569. Courtesy William D. Edwards, MD, Mayo Clinic, Rochester, Minn.)

asymptomatic and diagnosed only incidentally on routine physical examination. In some cases the prolapse is sufficient to cause a degree of mitral regurgitation. The cause of this valvular abnormality is uncertain, although it is commonly associated with other connective tissue disorders such as Marfan syndrome or scoliosis.

Historically, mitral valve prolapse has been overdiagnosed and the finding of 2 mm or more displacement of the mitral valve leaflets above the annulus is suggested as an important diagnostic criterion.[19] Mitral valve prolapse may be detected by a midsystolic click or systolic murmur. Individuals whose disease is symptomatic may experience palpitations, rhythm abnormalities, dizziness, fatigue, dyspnea, chest pain, or psychiatric manifestations such as depression and anxiety. The large majority have no untoward effects and are usually unaware of their condition. However, four serious though rare complications of mitral valve prolapse are recognized: (1) Infective endocarditis is more common and may warrant prophylactic antibiotics for invasive procedures. (2) A slow, insidious onset of mitral regurgitation may necessitate treatment. (3) Dysrhythmias may develop. (4) Sudden death may occur in association with fatal ventricular dysrhythmias, although it is considered a remote risk unless other cardiac pathologic process is also present. Surgical repair of mitral prolapse is rarely indicated.

Disorders of the Aortic Valve

The primary disorders of the aortic valve are stenosis and regurgitation.

Aortic Stenosis

With the decline in incidence of rheumatic fever, the predominant cause of aortic stenosis is age-related calcification. The hallmark of this disorder is calcium deposits on the aortic cusps (see Figure 18-14). Calcification is particularly common in patients with a congenital bicuspid aortic valve. Aortic calcifications build up over several decades and generally become clinically apparent in individuals 70 to 90 years old. Rheumatic heart disease, on the other hand, occurs primarily in children and young adults and now accounts for only a small percentage of cases of acquired aortic stenosis in the United States.

Aortic stenosis results in obstruction to aortic outflow from the left ventricle into the aorta during systole. This condition is characterized by a left ventricular–aortic pressure gradient during ventricular ejection (Figure 18-18). The left ventricle produces high systolic pressure to overcome resistance of the stenotic aortic valve. The slow development of aortic stenosis allows the heart to maintain stroke volume by compensatory left ventricular hypertrophy. The combination of high left ventricular pressure and hypertrophy predisposes the heart to ischemia and attacks of anginal pain. Continued high left ventricular afterload from a stenotic aortic valve may lead to left-sided heart failure.

Critical obstruction is characterized by a peak systolic pressure gradient exceeding 50 mm Hg and an aortic valve orifice less than 0.8 cm^2 in an adult.[19] The symptoms of aortic stenosis are due to diminished cardiac output, with pulmonary complications occurring later as the left ventricle fails. Syncope, fatigue, low systolic blood pressure, and faint pulses are common signs and symptoms. Angina occurs in two thirds of patients with critical aortic stenosis and is often brought on by exertion and relieved by rest.[19] Angina is thought to occur because of thickening of the ventricular wall with reduced perfusion and high intraventricular wall tension. Syncope and "graying out" spells may occur when cerebral perfusion is inadequate. The onset of atrial fibrillation or heart block may precipitate worsening of symptoms. A characteristic murmur occurs during ventricular systole and varies in intensity, progressively getting louder and then diminishing (crescendo-decrescendo). The murmur of aortic stenosis generally radiates to the neck. The heart rate is usually slow to allow for a necessarily long ejection phase and a prominent S_4 is usually present. Surgical correction is indicated for symptomatic aortic stenosis because medical therapy is not effective.

Aortic Regurgitation

Aortic regurgitation results from an incompetent aortic valve that allows blood to leak back from the aorta into the left ventricle during diastole. Causes of aortic regurgitation are similar to those of mitral regurgitation (see Table 18-6). Valvular incompetence may be secondary to an abnormal aortic valve or to aortic root dilation with widening of the aorta such that the valve leaflets no longer appose. The aorta may dilate be-

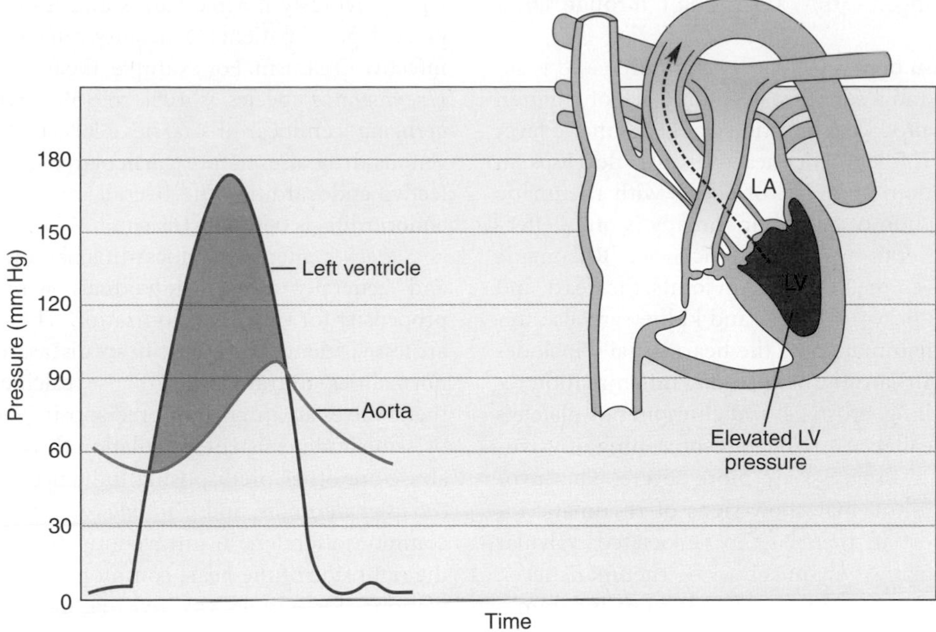

FIGURE 18-18 ■ Aortic stenosis is characterized by an abnormal left ventricular *(LV)*-to-aortic pressure gradient *(shaded area). LA,* Left atrial.

cause of degenerative changes with aging or as a consequence of connective tissue disease. The left ventricle becomes volume overloaded because it contains its usual preload, received from the atrium, plus regurgitant blood from the aorta. The left ventricle compensates for this extra volume work with hypertrophy and dilation. A larger than normal stroke volume is thus achieved to produce a high systolic blood pressure. Diastolic blood pressure is generally lower than normal because of rapid runoff of blood into the ventricle. The large stroke volume and rapid decline in diastolic blood pressure result in a bounding peripheral pulsation, and the head may bob with each systole (Figure 18-19).

Aortic insufficiency is characterized by a high-pitched blowing murmur during ventricular diastole. Patients may complain of palpitations and a throbbing or pounding heart because of the large ventricular stroke volume. The major complication of aortic regurgitation is left-sided heart failure as a result of the high ventricular workload. However, chronic aortic regurgitation is well tolerated for years, and asymptomatic individuals can delay valve replacement surgery. Acute aortic regurgitation is poorly tolerated and necessitates immediate correction.

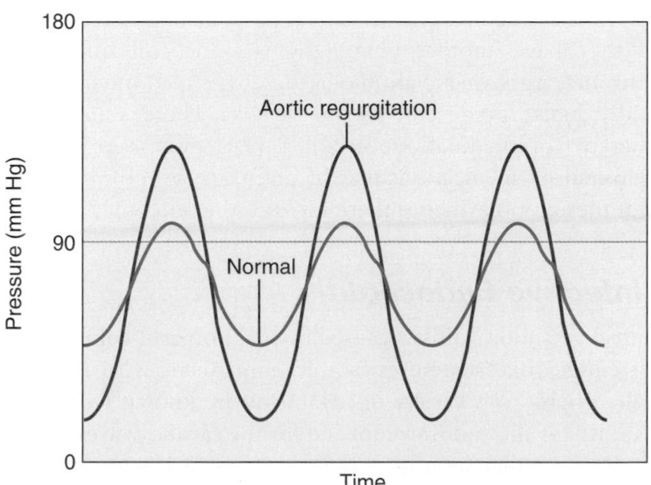

FIGURE 18-19 ■ Typical arterial pressure fluctuation in aortic regurgitation showing a high systolic pressure and a low diastolic pressure.

Diseases of the Endocardium

Rheumatic Heart Disease

Rheumatic heart disease is an uncommon but serious consequence of rheumatic fever. The incidence of rheumatic fever has steadily declined in the United States, but the disease still affects an estimated 12 million people a year worldwide.[20] Rheumatic fever is an acute inflammatory disease that follows infection with group A β-hemolytic streptococci.

Damage is due to immune attack on the individual's own tissues. For poorly understood reasons, antibodies against the streptococcal antigens are also directed against self tissues, possibly because of an autoimmune phenomenon or cross-reactivity between streptococcal antigens and certain tissue molecules. It is unknown why some individuals experience progressive tissue damage and others suffer no lasting consequences. A genetic predisposition to heightened immune responsiveness has been suggested and an association with human leukocyte antigen (HLA) types DR 1 through DR 4 has been noted.[21]

The acute infection occurs primarily in children and is accompanied by fever and a sore throat. In only 3% of children with pharyngeal streptococcal infection does rheumatic fever eventually develop.[21] Rheumatic heart disease develops in 50% to 75% of children and 35% of adults with rheumatic fever.[21] Prompt initiation of antibiotic therapy is often effective in primary prevention of rheumatic fever. Rheumatic fever diffusely affects connective tissue in joints, the heart, and the skin. The central nervous system and kidney are also frequently involved. Inflammation of the heart usually includes all layers and results in carditis. Endocardial inflammation results in valvular swelling, erosions, and clumping of platelets and fibrin on valve leaflets. Scarring and shortening of valvular structures become progressively more severe. The myocardium and pericardium may show signs of rheumatic inflammation; however, if there is no associated valvular inflammation the diagnosis is unlikely to be rheumatic fever. Other hallmarks of rheumatic fever include joint inflammation, involuntary movements (Sydenham chorea), and a distinctive truncal rash. An elevated antibody titer against streptococcal products (antistreptolysin O, anti-DNase B) may help confirm the diagnosis. Unfortunately, individuals who experience rheumatic fever have a 50% chance of recurrence if they have another pharyngeal streptococcal infection.[21] Chronic prophylactic antibiotic therapy is recommended for individuals who develop rheumatic fever. There is no specific therapy for rheumatic fever and care is supportive. Antiinflammatory medications may be given for symptom control, but there is no evidence that they alter the outcome.[21]

Infective Endocarditis

Infective endocarditis is caused by invasion and colonization of endocardial structures by microorganisms with resulting inflammation. A variety of organisms are known to have an affinity for the endocardium and for the cardiac valves in particular. Valvular lesions include growths of microorganisms enmeshed in fibrin deposits. These growths are called vegetations. They may become quite large, interfering with valvular function and predisposing to embolus formation. The most common bacterial culprits are several strains of *Streptococcus* and *Staphylococcus aureus.* A requisite for infective endocarditis is invasion of the blood stream by infective organisms. The portal of entry may be obvious, as with an overt infection, intravenous drug addiction, or invasive surgical or dental procedures. Sometimes the source may be less obvious, such as the gastrointestinal tract or the oral cavity. Once the organism enters the circulation, several factors influence its ability to attack endocardial structures and cause disease.

Acute infective endocarditis may theoretically develop in any individual if host resistance is low, if the organism is highly virulent, and if the bacterial invasion is sufficiently large. Acute infective endocarditis usually affects individuals with previously normal valves and leads to death in a large percentage of patients. Mortality rates vary with the type of infective organism. For example, the mortality associated with *Haemophilus* species is 10% to 15%, whereas *Pseudomonas aeruginosa* endocarditis carries a 50% to 89% mortality. Intravenous drug abusers are particularly susceptible to acute infective endocarditis. The overall mortality rate for infective endocarditis is between 16% and 27%.[22]

Subacute infective endocarditis has a more insidious onset and generally affects individuals with some preexisting propensity for valvular colonization. The offending organisms are less virulent. Rheumatic heart disease, congenital heart abnormalities, mitral valve prolapse, calcified valves, and prosthetic valves are important predisposing factors. Immunosuppression and persistent inoculation through intravenous drug abuse are other predisposing influences. *S. aureus, Staphylococcus epidermidis,* and *Candida,* which colonize the skin, are common offenders in intravenous drug users. The valves on the right side of the heart commonly are infected in this population.

Organisms associated with subacute infective endocarditis usually are not virulent enough to attack normal healthy endocardium but are able to gain a foothold in hearts with some underlying predisposition. Preexisting cardiac disease may allow the formation of platelet-fibrin deposits on the valves because of abnormal or stagnant blood flow patterns. These deposits become the site of organism attachment. Antibodies against the invader may further assist attachment by causing organisms to clump together.

The diagnostic findings in both acute and subacute infective endocarditis are much the same. Large, bulky, bacteria-laden vegetations hang from the heart valves and adjacent endocardial surfaces. In addition to the risk of embolization, vegetations may cause erosion or perforation of the underlying valve leaflet. In acute forms, adjacent myocardium may be eroded and abscessed. With time, valvular vegetations become fibrotic and calcified.

Unfortunately, the clinical features of subacute infective endocarditis are quite nonspecific, with low-grade fever the most consistent sign. Nonspecific fatigue, weight loss, and flu-like symptoms may be the only clues. Positive blood cultures may help confirm the diagnosis. In contrast, acute infective endocarditis has a more obvious onset with fever, chills, malaise, and, frequently, a heart murmur. Complications such as valvular insufficiency, myocardial abscess (Figure 18-20), embolization, and renal disease generally occur early in the course of the disease. The interval between initiation of bacteremia and the onset of symptoms is less than 2 weeks in the majority of cases.[22] Management of the acute and subacute types centers on antibiotic therapy, with surgical replacement of valves when indicated. Prevention through prophylactic antibiotic therapy in individuals at risk is an important consideration.

The endocardium is prey to many other disorders, such as systemic lupus erythematosus (an immunologic disease), cal-

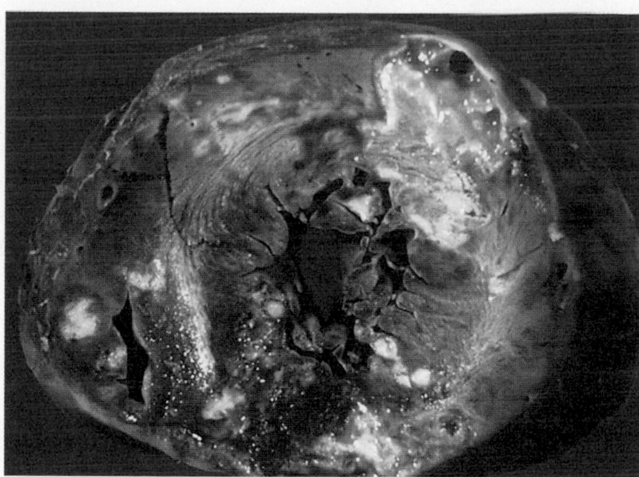

FIGURE 18-20 ■ Heart of a patient who died from acute bacterial endocarditis caused by *Staphylococcus aureus.* The left ventricle contains numerous abscesses formed by seeding from vegetations traveling in the coronary arteries. (From Kumar V, Cotran R, Robbins S, editors: *Robbins basic pathology,* ed 7, Philadelphia, 2003, Saunders, p 382.)

cium deposition secondary to renal disease, and nonbacterial thrombotic endocarditis secondary to hypercoagulable states associated with cancer.

KEY CONCEPTS

- Valvular disorders are of two primary types. Failure of stenotic valves to open properly causes an abnormal pressure gradient across the valve and increases the pressure work of the heart. Regurgitant valves allow blood to flow backward across the valve and result in extra volume work for the heart.
- Mitral stenosis is characterized by a large left atrial–to–left ventricular pressure gradient during ventricular diastole. Mitral stenosis leads to left atrial and pulmonary congestion.
- Mitral regurgitation is characterized by large *v* waves in the left atrial pressure tracing and a loud systolic murmur that radiates to the left axilla. Mitral regurgitation increases the work of the left atrium and ventricle and can lead to left-sided heart failure.
- Aortic stenosis results in obstruction to the outflow of blood from the left ventricle. It is characterized by a large left ventricular–to–aortic pressure gradient and a crescendo-decrescendo murmur during systole that radiates to the neck. The extra pressure work can lead to left ventricular hypertrophy and failure.
- Aortic regurgitation is characterized by a high systolic and low diastolic blood pressure and a bounding pulse. The murmur of aortic regurgitation occurs during diastole. Left ventricular failure may result because of the high-volume work.
- Rheumatic heart disease results from immune-mediated damage to the endocardium after group A β-hemolytic streptococcal infection.
- Acute and subacute infective endocarditis results in the growth of bacteria-laden vegetations on heart valves. In addition to valvular erosion and scarring, embolization may occur.

MYOCARDIAL DISEASES

In addition to the diseases already discussed, which secondarily affect the myocardium as a consequence of inadequate blood supply or endocardial infection, two additional categories of diseases of heart muscle are myocarditis and cardiomyopathy. Myocarditis is an inflammatory disorder of the heart muscle characterized by necrosis and degeneration of heart muscle cells. Cardiomyopathy includes several disorders of the heart muscle that may be genetic or acquired but are noninflammatory. The division of these categories is somewhat arbitrary; however, the clinical course of myocarditis is generally acute and stormy, with recovery or death from cardiac failure occurring weeks to months after the onset of symptoms. In contrast, the cardiomyopathies generally evolve more insidiously over years, with few symptoms until the heart slips into failure.

Myocarditis

Myocarditis is characterized by inflammation, leukocyte infiltration, and necrosis of cardiac muscle cells. Causes of myocarditis are many and include microbial agents, several forms of immune-mediated disease, and several physical agents. The more common causes of myocarditis are listed in Box 18-3. The true incidence of myocarditis is unknown because the diagnosis relies largely on circumstantial evidence.

Most cases of myocarditis in North America are associated with viral infection, whereas Chagas disease *(Trypanosoma cruzi)* is common in South America. Cardiac involvement generally appears days or weeks after a viral infection elsewhere in the body. Documenting a viral cause is often impossible, but a rising antibody titer supports the diagnosis. The mechanism of viral myocarditis is uncertain. Direct viral cytotoxicity may occur, or the virus may evoke an immune response directed against the heart. Most investigators currently believe the second mechanism to be most likely. In countries other than the United States, nonviral organisms are more commonly associated with myocarditis. For example, the protozoan *T. cruzi,* which is endemic in areas of Central and South America, infects about 20 million persons worldwide.[23] A myocarditis called Chagas disease eventually develops in a large number of infected individuals. Chagas disease is the leading cause of cardiovascular death in endemic countries.[23]

In some cases of myocarditis the individual's immune system appears to be the causative agent. Antibodies or activated

Box 18-3

Major Causes of Myocarditis

Infectious Agents
Viruses (e.g., coxsackievirus, echovirus, influenza virus, human immunodeficiency virus, cytomegalovirus)
Chlamydia (e.g., *C. psittaci*)
Rickettsia (e.g., *R. typhi* [typhus fever])
Bacteria (e.g., *Corynebacterium* [diphtheria], *Neisseria* [meningococcemia], *Borrelia* [Lyme disease])
Fungi (e.g., *Candida*)
Protozoa (e.g., *Trypanosoma* [Chagas disease], *Toxoplasma*)
Helminths (e.g., *Trichinella*)

Immune-Mediated Reactions
Postviral
Poststreptococcal (rheumatic fever)
Systemic lupus erythematosus
Drug hypersensitivity (e.g., methyldopa, sulfonamides)
Transplant rejection

Unknown
Sarcoidosis
Giant cell myocarditis

Modified from Kumar V, Cotran RS, Robbins SL: *Basic pathology*, ed 7, Philadelphia, 2003, Saunders, p 383.

lymphocytes are formed against heart tissue. Several drugs, including penicillin, tend to evoke a hyperactive immune response in some individuals and may cause an allergic-type reaction that affects the myocardium. Toxins and chemical causes of myocarditis include cocaine, chemotherapeutic agents, snake bite and insect venoms, lead, and numerous others. Regardless of the specific cause, inflammation of cardiac muscle is characteristic.

Acute myocarditis is most often characterized by general dilation of all four heart chambers. The ventricular myocardium is "flabby" with patchy or diffuse necrotic lesions. The heart muscle appears inflamed and edematous with white blood cell infiltrates. Endocardial structures are usually normal. The clinical course of acute myocarditis varies in severity from asymptomatic to rapidly evolving heart failure. Generalized symptoms related to the inflammatory process may be present, as well as electrocardiographic changes caused by myocardial cell death. Many persons recover completely, whereas others have progressive disease that is manifested years later as dilated cardiomyopathy. Thus myocarditis and the cardiomyopathic forms of myocardial disease overlap and are difficult to separate. Therapy is supportive and no specific treatments are available for most forms. The use of corticosteroids to suppress the immune response is controversial.

Cardiomyopathy

Cardiomyopathies can be classified by cause or by functional impairments. Those with known causes have been classified as specific cardiomyopathy by the World Health Organization (Table 18-8).[24] Those cardiomyopathies with uncertain cause are classified based on their predominant pathophysiologic features. The major functional classes are the dilated, hypertrophic, and restrictive forms (Figure 18-21). The terms primary cardiomyopathy for dysfunction of unknown cause and secondary cardiomyopathy for myocardial dysfunction of known cause are also in clinical use. Most definitions of primary cardiomyopathy exclude hypertensive, ischemic, congenital, valvular, pericardial, and inflammatory myocardial disorders.

Dilated Cardiomyopathy

Dilated or congestive cardiomyopathy (DCM) is characterized by cardiac failure associated with dilation of all four heart chambers. Four factors are suspected in the initiation of dilated cardiomyopathy: alcohol toxicity, genetic abnormality, pregnancy, and postviral myocarditis. Alcohol and its metabolites are toxic to heart muscle cells and are associated with thiamine and other nutritional deficiencies. However, the exact mechanism of alcohol-associated cardiomyopathy remains unclear, which justifies its continued inclusion in the category of primary cardiomyopathy. Peripartum cardiomyopathy is the term applied to cases of dilated cardiomyopathy discovered just before or just after delivery. A nutritional deficiency is suspected because in most instances peripartum cardiomyopathy occurs in poor women having frequent pregnancies.

In some cases, dilated cardiomyopathy runs in families and has a presumed genetic basis. At least 20% of patients with DCM have a first-degree relative with signs of DCM.[25] Genetic defects in the protein structure of myocardial cytoskeleton appear to be contributory in most genetic forms of DCM. Postviral myocarditis is an attractive pathogenetic mechanism for dilated cardiomyopathy, as previously discussed. Myocardial biopsy specimens often reveal signs of inflammatory injury; however, progression from acute myocarditis to dilated cardiomyopathy has rarely been documented. A variety of other causes have been proposed as well. In fact, dilated cardiomyopathy is a bit of a catch-all term invoked to cover cases of dilated congestive failure having no well-defined origin.

Histologic examination of hearts with dilated cardiomyopathy reveals nonspecific changes in the majority of cases.[20] An occasional hypertrophied or atrophied myocyte may be apparent, along with mild fibrosis. The clinical picture is one of slowly progressing biventricular heart failure. The diagnosis is based on exclusion of other causes. Cardiac transplantation is the only definitive treatment.

Hypertrophic Cardiomyopathy

In contrast to dilated cardiomyopathy, hypertrophic cardiomyopathy (HCM) is characterized by a thickened, hyperkinetic ventricular muscle mass. The hypertrophy is often not uniform throughout the heart, and in about 25% of patients the septum is most affected leading to the term *idiopathic hy-*

Table 18-8

Classification of the Cardiomyopathies

Disorder	Description
Dilated cardiomyopathy	Dilatation and impaired contraction of the left or both ventricles. Caused by familial/genetic, viral and/or immune, alcoholic/toxic, or unknown factors, or is associated with recognized cardiovascular disease.
Hypertrophic cardiomyopathy	Left and/or right ventricular hypertrophy, often asymmetrical, which usually involves the interventricular septum. Mutations in sarcoplasmic proteins cause the disease in many patients.
Restrictive cardiomyopathy	Restricted filling and reduced diastolic size of either or both ventricles with normal or near-normal systolic function. Is idiopathic or associated with other disease (e.g., amyloidosis, endomyocardial disease).
Arrhythmogenic right ventricular cardiomyopathy	Progressive fibrofatty replacement of the right, and to some degree left, ventricular myocardium. Familial disease is common.
Unclassified cardiomyopathy	Diseases that do not fit readily into any category. Examples include systolic dysfunction with minimal dilatation, mitochondrial disease, and fibroelastosis.
Specific Cardiomyopathies	
Ischemic cardiomyopathy	Presents as dilated cardiomyopathy with depressed ventricular function not explained by the extent of coronary artery obstructions or ischemic damage.
Valvular cardiomyopathy	Presents as ventricular dysfunction that is out of proportion to the abnormal loading conditions produced by the valvular stenosis and/or regurgitation.
Hypertensive cardiomyopathy	Presents with left ventricular hypertrophy with features of cardiac failure due to systolic or diastolic dysfunction.
Inflammatory cardiomyopathy	Cardiac dysfunction as a consequence of myocarditis.
Metabolic cardiomyopathy	Includes a wide variety of causes, including endocrine abnormalities, glycogen storage disease, deficiencies (such as hypokalemia), and nutritional disorders.
General systemic disease	Includes connective tissue disorders and infiltrative diseases such as sarcoidosis and leukemia.
Muscular dystrophies	Includes Duchenne, Becker-type, and myotonic dystrophies.
Neuromuscular disorders	Includes Friedreich ataxia, Noonan syndrome, and lentiginosis.
Sensitivity and toxic reactions	Includes reactions to alcohol, catecholamines, anthracyclines, irradiation, and others.
Peripartal cardiomyopathy	First becomes manifest in the peripartum period, but it is likely a heterogeneous group.

Derived from Richardson P et al: Report of the 1995 World Health Organization/International Society and Federation of Cardiology Task Force on the Definition and Classification of Cardiomyopathies, *Circulation* 93:841, 1996. Copyright 1996, American Heart Association. In Wynne J, Braunwald E: The cardiomyopathies and myocarditides. In Braunwald E, Zipes D, Libby P, editors: *Heart disease: a textbook of cardiovascular medicine,* ed 6, Philadelphia, 2001, Saunders, p 1751.

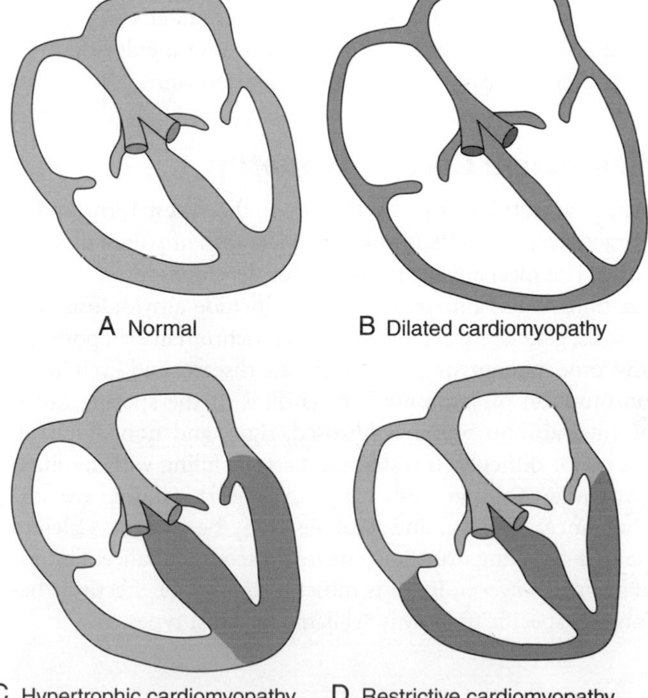

FIGURE 18-21 ■ The three types of cardiomyopathy. **A,** Normal heart. **B,** Dilated cardiomyopathy demonstrating enlargement of all four chambers. **C,** Hypertrophic cardiomyopathy showing a thickened left ventricle. **D,** Restrictive cardiomyopathy characterized by a small left ventricular volume.

pertrophic subaortic stenosis. The left ventricle is usually more involved than the right.

Substantial evidence suggests that this form of cardiomyopathy is transmitted genetically. Abnormalities of cardiac sarcomere proteins have been identified in several familial forms of the disease. Abnormalities in genes coding for myosin, tropomyosin, and troponin T have been linked to the development of HCM. It is estimated that about 30% of familial HCM cases are due to mutations of the myosin heavy chain gene, 15% due to troponin T mutation, and less than 3% to tropomyosin mutations.[25] The remaining half of cases are thought to have mutations in other cytoskeletal elements.

There is wide variation in the expression of HCM. It may be asymptomatic or may be associated with symptoms of ventricular outflow obstruction or impaired diastolic filling. Outflow obstruction is particularly problematic when the myocardial hypertrophy is localized in the subaortic septal region. Strenuous activity may precipitate profound outflow obstruction, negligible stroke volume, and sudden death. Other factors contributing to reduced stroke volume are the smaller intraventricular chamber size and a noncompliant ventricle characteristic of diastolic dysfunction. The most common symptoms of HCM are dyspnea (90%) and angina (75%). Microscopically, the hypertrophied muscle cells appear disorganized and haphazardly oriented into whorls rather than the usual linear arrangement.

The clinical course of HCM is variable, with most patients experiencing little change in cardiac function over many years. Surgery to thin the septal thickening (myectomy) is rarely performed any longer because this technique has been superseded by drug therapy. In general, drugs that increase myocardial contractility or heart rate are avoided because they further impair diastolic filling and worsen aortic outflow obstruction. β-Adrenergic antagonists and calcium channel–blocking drugs may be used to dampen the hypercontractility. Long-term survival is possible. Myocardial ischemia is common, and the risk of sudden cardiac death is high because of fatal dysrhythmias. Patients who die from HCM usually do so suddenly and most often after or during vigorous physical exertion.[25]

Restrictive Cardiomyopathy

Restrictive cardiomyopathy (RCM) is the rarest form and is characterized by a stiff, fibrotic ventricle with impaired diastolic filling. The mechanisms proposed for development of ventricular fibrosis remain speculative and include amyloidosis, sarcoidosis, genetic inheritance (e.g., hemochromatosis), postviral syndrome, malnutrition, autoimmune disease, and even heavy consumption of serotonin.[21] Regardless of the specific cause, the myocardium becomes fibrosed, rigid, and noncompliant. The major difficulty is restricted diastolic filling with resultant low stroke volume and congestive heart failure. Exercise intolerance, dyspnea, and weakness may be present. Calcium channel–blocking drugs may be instituted to enhance diastolic relaxation; however, RCM is difficult to manage effectively because no specific therapy is available for most types.

Specific Cardiomyopathy

Cardiomyopathies of presumed known origin constitute the category of specific cardiomyopathy. Box 18-4 lists causative agents associated with specific cardiomyopathy. The specific

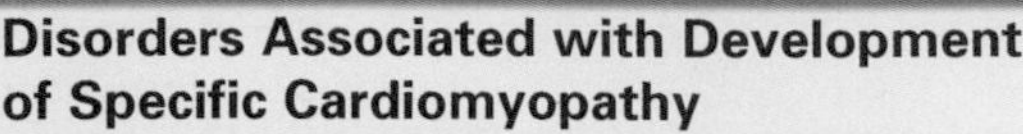
Box 18-4

Disorders Associated with Development of Specific Cardiomyopathy

Cardiac Infections
Viruses
Chlamydia
Rickettsia
Bacteria
Fungi
Protozoa

Toxic
Alcohol
Cobalt
Catecholamines
Carbon monoxide
Lithium
Hydrocarbons
Arsenic
Cyclophosphamide
Doxorubicin (Adriamycin) and daunorubicin

Metabolic
Hyperthyroidism
Hypothyroidism
Hypokalemia
Hyperkalemia
Nutritional deficiency—protein, thiamine, other avitaminoses
Hemochromatosis

Neuromuscular Disease
Friedreich ataxia
Muscular dystrophy
Congenital atrophies

Storage Disorders and Other Depositions
Hunter-Hurler syndrome
Glycogen storage disease
Fabry disease
Amyloidosis

Infiltrative
Leukemia
Carcinomatosis
Sarcoidosis
Radiation-induced fibrosis

Immunologic
Myocarditis (several forms)
Transplant rejection

From Schoen FJ: The heart. In Cotran RS, Kumar V, Collins T: *Robbins pathologic basic of disease,* ed 6, Philadelphia, 1999, Saunders, p 580.

cardiomyopathies present functionally as dilated, hypertrophic, or restrictive disorders, and the symptoms are similar.

KEY CONCEPTS

- Myocarditis is an inflammatory disorder characterized by scattered necrotic and dead heart muscle cells. Most cases are associated with viral infection. The major complication of myocarditis is dilation of the four heart chambers, with reduced contractility.
- Cardiomyopathies encompass a number of disorders of heart muscle that may be genetic or acquired but are not inflammatory. In most cases the exact cause is unknown.
- Dilated cardiomyopathy is characterized by enlargement of all four chambers and reduced contractility.
- Hypertrophic cardiomyopathy primarily affects the left ventricle and ventricular septum. Genetic mutations in myosin proteins are suspected in most cases. Conditions that increase contractility of the heart (exercise, drugs) can result in obstruction of ventricular outflow and reduced cardiac output.
- Restrictive cardiomyopathy is characterized by a stiff, fibrotic left ventricle that resists diastolic filling. Decreased cardiac output and left-sided congestive failure can result.

PERICARDIAL DISEASES

Pericardial disorders are rarely isolated processes of primary cause; rather, they are sequelae of other disorders such as systemic infection, trauma, metabolic derangement, or neoplasia. Despite the diversity of causative factors, pericardial involvement is generally manifested as an accumulation of fluid in the pericardial sac or inflammation of pericardial structures.

Pericardial Effusion

An accumulation of noninflammatory fluid in the pericardial sac is called *pericardial effusion.* Normally, the pericardial space contains only 30 to 50 ml of thin, clear fluid. Under pathologic conditions, as much as 500 ml may accumulate. The composition of the usual types of effusions are as follows:

Serous—a transudate secondary to congestive failure or hypoproteinemia

Serosanguineous—a mixture of serous fluid and blood that may follow blunt chest trauma or cardiopulmonary resuscitation

Chylous—a collection of lymph from obstruction of lymphatic drainage

Blood—hemopericardium usually resulting from penetrating trauma to the heart

Cardiac Tamponade

The accumulation of pericardial fluid is generally without clinical significance except as an indicator of underlying disease processes. However, if the fluid accumulation is large or occurs suddenly, the life-threatening condition of cardiac tamponade may ensue. Tamponade refers to external compression of the heart chambers such that filling is impaired.

Signs and symptoms of cardiac tamponade include reduced stroke volume and compensatory increases in heart rate. Systemic venous congestion occurs because blood is prevented from entering the compressed heart by way of the superior and inferior venae cavae. Venous congestion may be apparent as distended neck veins. Changes in intrathoracic pressure during respiration may have exaggerated effects on cardiac filling. The presence of waxing and waning of blood pressure in synchrony with respiration is called *pulsus paradoxus.* Significant pulsus paradoxus is usually defined as a difference of 10 mm Hg or more in systolic blood pressure between inspiration and expiration. Other manifestations of tamponade include rising filling pressures in the heart chambers, muffled heart sounds, dull chest pain, diminished electrocardiographic amplitude, and a compressed cardiac silhouette on radiographs.

Treatment is aimed at relieving the pericardial pressure by aspirating the offending fluid *(pericardiocentesis).* Failure to manage tamponade may result in drastically reduced diastolic filling, cardiovascular collapse, and death. Nonsymptomatic pericardial effusions may be aspirated or merely monitored and allowed to resolve spontaneously. Treatment is directed at the underlying cause of the effusion.

Pericarditis

Inflammation of the pericardium originates from a variety of causes (Table 18-9). Rarely is the pericardium the primary site of disease. Pericarditis is often categorized as acute or chronic; however, these forms are morphologically and etiologically

Table 18-9

Causes of Pericarditis

Infectious Agents	Miscellaneous
Viruses	Myocardial infarction
Pyogenic bacteria	Uremia
Mycobacterium tuberculosis	Post–cardiac surgery status
Fungi	Neoplasia
Other parasites	Trauma
	Radiation
Presumably Immunologically Mediated	
Rheumatic fever	
Systemic lupus erythematosus	
Scleroderma	
Postcardiotomy	
Post–myocardial infarction (Dressler) syndrome	
Drug hypersensitivity reaction	

Modified from Cotran RS, Kumar V, Collins T: *Robbins pathologic basis of disease,* ed 6, Philadelphia, 1999, Saunders, p 587.

similar.[9] Chronic pericarditis refers to a healed stage of the acute form that results in chronic pericardial dysfunction.

Acute Pericarditis

Acute pericarditis can be categorized according to the character of the inflammatory exudate: serous, fibrinous, purulent, hemorrhagic, or caseous.

MI is a common cause of acute pericarditis. The symptoms of acute pericarditis are due to the systemic effects of inflammation and pericardial damage and include fever, leukocytosis, malaise, and tachycardia. Sticking and rubbing of the visceral and parietal pericardial layers cause pain that may radiate to the back and be associated with esophageal discomfort and dysphagia (difficulty swallowing).

Acute pericarditis may be confused with anginal pain. Rubbing of the pericardial layers may be heard as a friction rub. The rub can be transient and intermittent and may sound squeaky or like scratchy sandpaper. Epicardial injury from pericarditis may be apparent on the ECG as ST-segment elevation. Treatment is generally symptom oriented and includes medications to relieve pain and minimize inflammation.

Chronic Pericarditis

Healing of an acute form of pericardial inflammation may result in chronic (healed) pericardial dysfunction of two principal kinds: adhesive mediastinopericarditis and constrictive pericarditis. Adhesive mediastinopericarditis is usually a consequence of suppurative or caseous pericarditis or a complication of previous cardiac surgery. It may also follow significant irradiation of the chest. The pericardial sac is destroyed and the external aspect of the heart adheres to surrounding mediastinal structures. The workload of the heart increases significantly because contraction is opposed by the attached surrounding structures.

Constrictive pericarditis may be a result of previous suppurative or caseous pericarditis, commonly secondary to tuberculosis. However, in many cases the cause of pericardial dysfunction is unknown. The pericardial sac becomes dense, nonelastic, fibrous, and scarred. It encases the heart like a stiff cage and impairs diastolic filling. The constrictive process generally occurs slowly and may be quite advanced by the time symptoms occur.

Symptoms may include exercise intolerance, weakness, fatigue, and systemic venous congestion. Treatment is aimed at relieving the constriction by removal of pericardium (pericardectomy) and administration of inotropic agents to improve cardiac contractility.

KEY CONCEPTS

- Large accumulations of pericardial fluid can result in cardiac tamponade. External compression of the heart chambers impairs diastolic filling and results in decreased stroke volume. Distended neck veins, pulsus paradoxus, elevated and equalized intrachamber pressures, and muffled heart sounds are indicative.
- Acute pericarditis causes sticking and rubbing of the visceral and parietal pericardial layers. A friction rub, pain radiating to the back, esophageal discomfort, and generalized signs of inflammation are usually present.
- Chronic pericarditis can lead to destruction of the pericardial sac with adhesion of the heart to surrounding mediastinal structures. Cardiac contraction may be impaired.
- Constrictive pericarditis results in a fibrous, scarred pericardium that restricts cardiac filling.

CONGENITAL HEART DISEASES

Congenital heart disease is an abnormality of the heart that is present from birth. A wide variety of defects have been described, and only the pathophysiology of the most common defects will be included. A brief description of fetal cardiac development is a necessary prelude to a discussion of congenital heart diseases.

Embryologic Development

Development of the heart involves a complex orchestration of formation and resorption of structures. Abnormalities in the development of four important heart structures are at the root of most of the common heart defects: (1) development of the atrial septum, (2) development of the ventricular septum, (3) division of the main outflow tract (truncus arteriosus) into the pulmonary and aortic arteries, and (4) development of the valves. Each of these processes is briefly reviewed.

The primitive heart begins as an enlarged tube much like a blood vessel. The tube has three layers. The inner luminal layer is thin and composed of endothelial cells. This layer will eventually line the inner chambers of the heart and valves. The outermost layer is also thin and is called the myoepicardial mantle. The outer mantle will form the epicardial and muscular structures of the heart. In between these two thin layers of cells is a thick layer of gelatinous substance called cardiac jelly. Cardiac jelly is the precursor to endocardial cushion tissue, which is important in the formation of membranes in the heart, including the septa that separate the four chambers of the heart.

By day 23, the heart tube begins to beat. The tube folds on itself to form an asymmetric loop structure (Figure 18-22). One bulge of the loop forms a primitive single atrium, another forms the future left ventricle, and a third forms the future right ventricle and common ventricular outflow tract (truncus arteriosus). The common atrium is divided into right and left atria by growth of the interatrial septum. Atrial

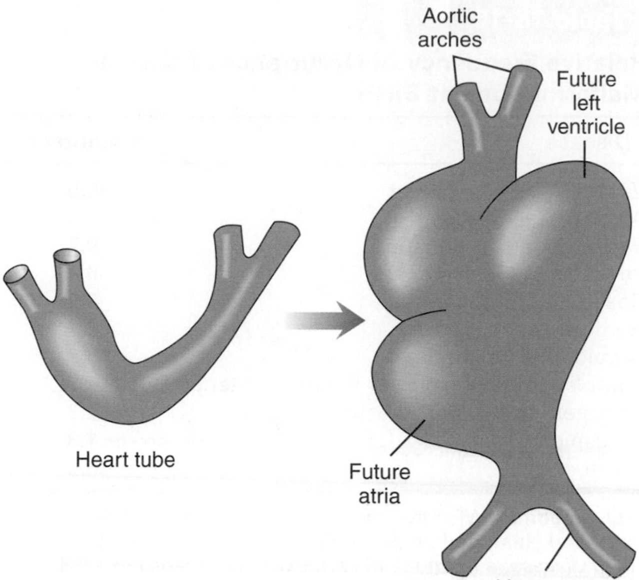

FIGURE 18-22 ■ Asymmetric loop structure in early embryonic development of the heart.

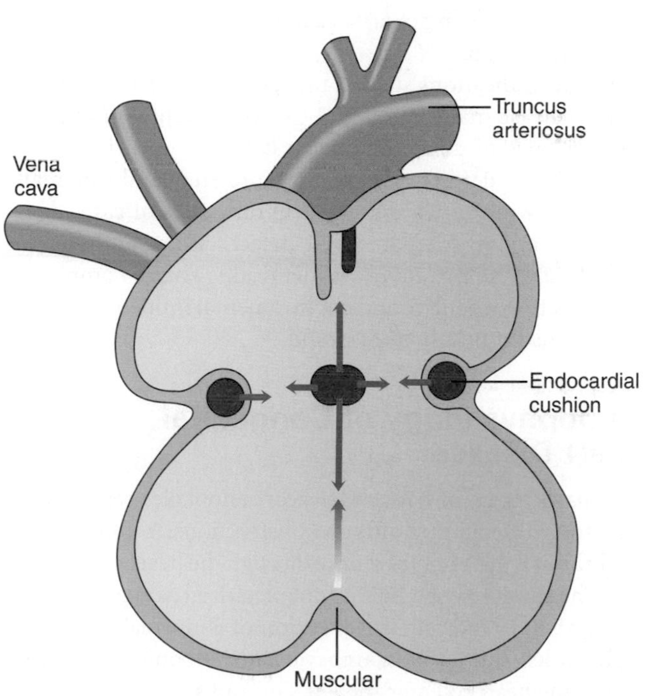

FIGURE 18-23 ■ Formation of the intracardiac septa.

septation occurs in several steps. First, the *septum primum* is formed passively in the superior surface by an indentation caused by the overlying truncus arteriosus (Figure 18-23). Next, the superior and inferior endocardial cushions grow and extend toward each other. These flaps of tissue overlap but do not fuse so that blood can pass through from the right atrium to the left atrium. A reverse in the direction of flow, as occurs at birth, would push the flap shut and close the hole. This flap-

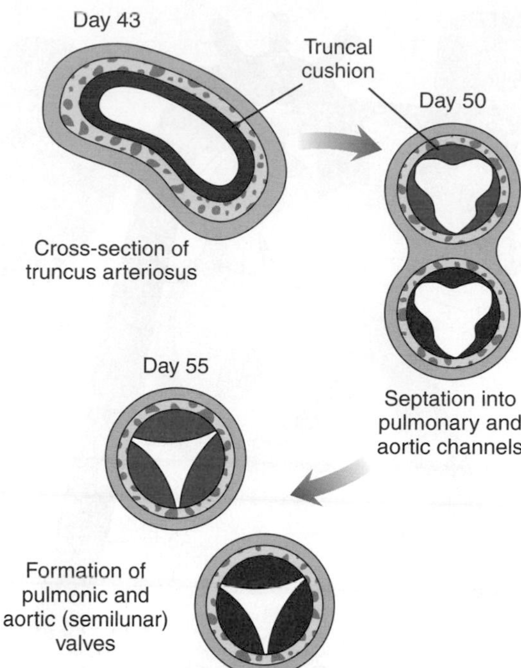

FIGURE 18-24 ■ Septation of the truncus arteriosus and formation of the semilunar valves.

like opening, called the *ostium secundum,* remains open throughout fetal life and is later called the *foramen ovale.*

Septal formation between the ventricles follows a similar pattern. The lower portion of the interventricular septum is formed by circular growth and fusing of the muscular ventricular walls. Then the muscular septum proliferates upward toward the atria. The inferior endocardial cushion tissue also grows downward to meet the uplifting muscular septum (see Figure 18-23).

At about the same time that the atrial and ventricular septal structures are being elaborated, the common ventricular outflow tract, the truncus arteriosus, is divided into the pulmonary and aortic channels. This process is accomplished by growth and eventual fusion of mounds of endocardial cushions located in the wall of the truncus arteriosus. The truncal endocardial cushions go on to form the semilunar valves as well (Figure 18-24).

The atrioventricular septum and valves are similarly formed by growth and fusion of the right and left lateral cushions. Superior and inferior cushions also contribute to formation of the septum between the atria and ventricles. Leaflets of the valves are initially formed by lumps of cushion material, which are replaced by muscle tissue from the ventricular wall. The muscle tissue also forms the chordae tendineae and papillary muscle structures. Eventually, the muscle cells of the leaflets and chordae tendineae are replaced by tough fibrous connective tissue.

When the embryonic heart is fully developed, two important passageways still permit blood flow to bypass the lungs (Figure 18-25). The foramen ovale lies between the left and

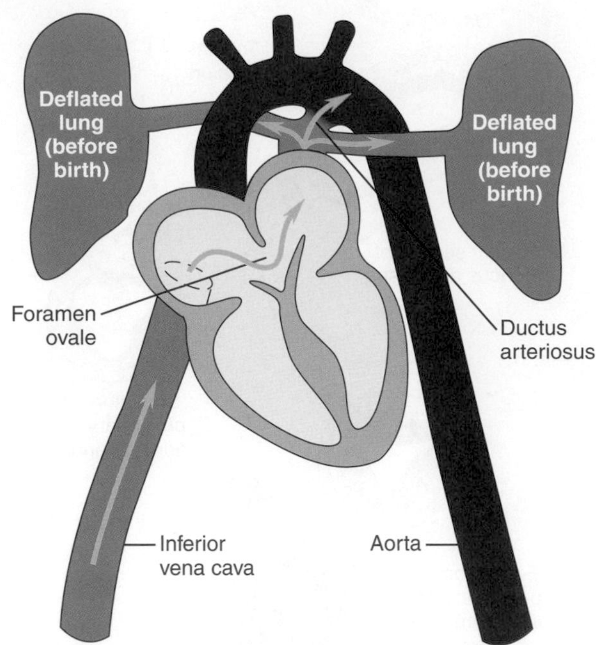

FIGURE 18-25 ■ Fully developed embryonic heart showing the foramen ovale and ductus arteriosus. These structures allow blood to bypass the pulmonary circulation during fetal life.

Table 18-10

Relative Frequency of Occurrence of Cardiac Malformations at Birth

Disease	Percentage
Ventricular septal defect	30.5
Atrial septal defect	9.8
Patent ductus arteriosus	9.7
Pulmonic stenosis	6.9
Coarctation of the aorta	6.8
Aortic stenosis	6.1
Tetralogy of Fallot	5.8
Complete transposition of the great arteries	4.2
Persistent truncus arteriosus	2.2
Tricuspid atresia	1.3
All others	16.5

From Friedman WF, Silverman N: Congenital heart disease in infancy and childhood. In Braunwald E, Zipes D, Libby P, editors: *Heart disease: a textbook of cardiovascular medicine,* ed 6, Philadelphia, 2001, Saunders, p 1506.
Data based on 2310 cases.

right atria and allows blood to bypass the right ventricle. Blood flows right to left through the atrial opening because the pressure in the left atrium is low. High resistance of the deflated lungs also causes right ventricular pressure to be high, which impedes right ventricular filling. The other important structure is the ductus arteriosus, a channel that connects the pulmonary artery and the aorta. Blood flows from the pulmonary artery into the aorta during fetal life because of high vascular resistance in the collapsed lungs. Both these communications generally close after birth when the lungs inflate and the resistance on the right side of the heart falls. Clamping the umbilical cord also serves to increase systemic vascular resistance, which further augments the reverse in pressure gradient, with left heart pressures now exceeding those on the right.

Etiology and Incidence of Congenital Heart Disease

Congenital heart disease is the most common heart disorder in children, with an overall incidence of about 0.8% of all live births.[9] The most common heart defects are listed in Table 18-10, with approximate frequencies of occurrence. In more than 90% of cases the cause of the heart defect is unknown.[9] Multifactorial inheritance with both genetic and environmental influences is probable. Very few cases of congenital malformation can be clearly attributed to environmental factors. Maternal rubella during the first trimester of pregnancy is the best documented environmental cause of heart defects. A large number of cardiac teratogens are suspected from animal studies, including hypoxia, ionizing radiation, and heavy alcohol consumption.

Several indications suggest that genetic influence is important in cardiac malformation. A twofold to tenfold increase in the incidence of congenital heart defects is seen in siblings. Several heart defects also occur more frequently in males. However, twin studies show that in only 10% of cases does a heart defect (ventricular septal defect) afflict both infants, even though their genotype is identical.[26] Thus a complex interplay between genetic and environmental influences is probable and as yet poorly understood.

Pathophysiology of Congenital Heart Disease

The many forms of congenital heart anomalies result in two primary pathologies: **shunts** and obstructions. A shunt denotes an abnormal path of blood flow through the heart or great vessels. The shunt may be further characterized as right-to-left or left-to-right to indicate the direction of abnormal blood flow. Right-to-left shunts allow unoxygenated blood from the right side of the heart to enter the left side and systemic circulation without first passing through the lungs. Infants with right-to-left shunting of blood generally have some degree of cyanosis because of the decreased oxygen content of the arterial blood (cyanotic defect). Conversely, a left-to-right shunt occurs when oxygenated blood from the left side of the heart or aorta flows back into the right side to be recirculated through the lungs. The blood reaching the systemic circulation is oxygenated and the infant is not cyanotic (acyanotic defect). However, the right side of the heart has an increased workload because of the extra shunt blood. In time, the overload of the right side of the heart can result in right ventricular hypertrophy and high right-sided heart pressures. A left-to-right shunt may then progress to a more dangerous right-to-left shunt when right heart pressures exceed left heart pressures. Congenital disorders causing abnormal blood flow through the heart include atrial septal defect, ventricular septal defect, patent ductus arteriosus, tetralogy of Fallot, transposition of the great arteries, truncus arteriosus, and tricuspid atresia.

Some heart anomalies produce obstructions to blood flow because of abnormal narrowings. Stenosis or atresia (failure to develop) of valves and coarctation of the aorta are the most common obstructive defects. Obstructions do not result in cyanosis but generally increase the workload of the affected chamber. Heart failure is a potential consequence of congenital heart defects and presents differently in infants and children than in adults (Box 18-5).

In addition to being classified according to pathologic features as obstructions or shunts, heart defects are also classified according to the clinical manifestation of cyanosis. Acyanotic disorders include the obstructive disorders and left-to-right shunts. The cyanotic category includes abnormalities causing right-to-left shunts. Specific heart defects are described further and follow this categorization.

Acyanotic Congenital Defects

Atrial Septal Defect

During the third to fifth week of fetal development, the left and right atria are separated by flaps of tissue that become the atrial septum. The foramen ovale remains patent during intrauterine life such that blood may pass from the right to the left atrium and bypass the uninflated and nonfunctional lungs (Figure 18-26). The foramen ovale normally remains open in utero because pressure on the right side of the heart is higher than that on the left. With birth, however, the pressure gradient reverses as the lungs inflate and greatly reduce pulmonary vascular resistance. The higher left-sided pressure forces the flap shut, and fusion of the foramen ovale membrane normally occurs. The majority of atrial septal defects occur at the location of the foramen ovale. The abnormal septal opening may be of variable size. Small defects (1 cm) are well tolerated. Even larger atrial septal defects may be asymptomatic for many years as long as the shunt flow is left to right and therefore acyanotic.

The long-term increase in pulmonary blood flow may eventually lead to pulmonary hypertension, right ventricular hypertrophy, and a reversal of the shunt to a right-to-left pattern. Cyanosis, respiratory difficulty, and right-sided heart failure may ensue. Large or symptomatic atrial septal defects are commonly repaired surgically early in life, before pulmonary complications occur.

Ventricular Septal Defect

A ventricular septal defect is the most common congenital cardiac anomaly. It is frequently associated with other cardiac defects such as tetralogy of Fallot, transposition of the great arteries, and atrial septal defects. The ventricular septum develops between the fifth and sixth weeks of fetal life as the membrane derived from the endocardial cushion fuses with the muscular septum (Figure 18-27).

The majority of ventricular septal defects are located in the membranous septum, very close to the bundle of His. As with atrial septal defects, the functional significance depends largely on the size of the defect. The shunt is initially left to right because left-sided heart pressures are higher. With the increase in pulmonary blood flow, pulmonary hypertension and right ventricular hypertrophy may result and cause a reversal of the shunt.

Box 18-5

Features of Heart Failure in Infants

Poor feeding and failure to thrive
Respiratory distress (mainly tachypnea)
Rapid heart rate (160 to 180 beats/min)
Pulmonary rales or wheezing
Cardiomegaly and pulmonary edema on radiogram
Hepatomegaly (peripheral edema unusual)
Gallop sounds
Color (ashen pale or faintly cyanotic)
Excessive perspiration
Diminished urine output

From Friedman WF, Silverman N: Congenital heart disease in infancy and childhood. In Braunwald E, Zipes D, Libby P, editors: *Heart disease: a textbook of cardiovascular medicine,* ed 6, Philadelphia, 2001, Saunders, p 1512.

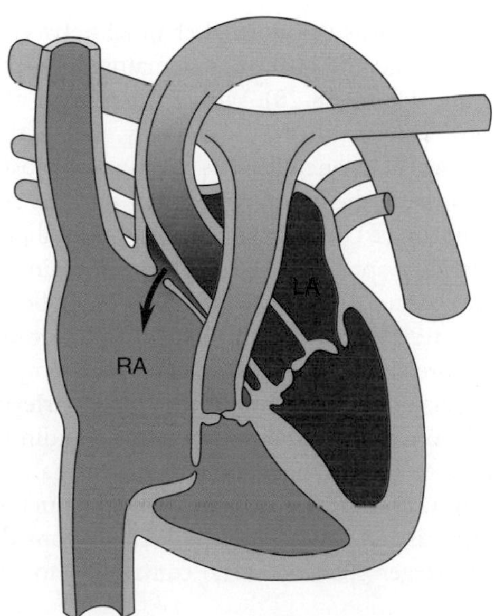

FIGURE 18-26 ■ Atrial septal defect. Blood flow through the defect is usually left to right and produces an acyanotic shunt.

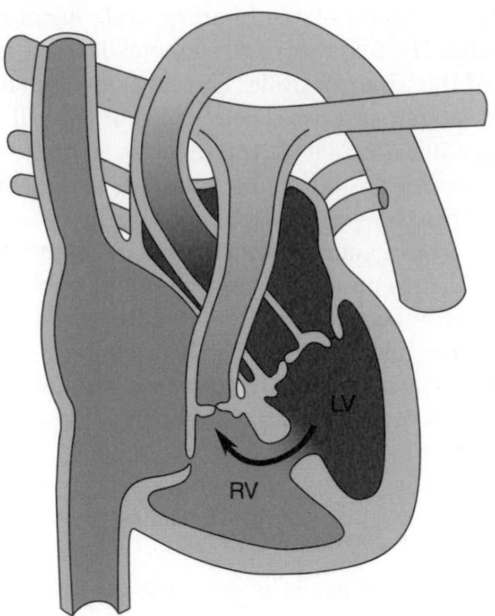

FIGURE 18-27 ■ Ventricular septal defect. Blood flow through the defect is usually left to right and produces an acyanotic shunt.

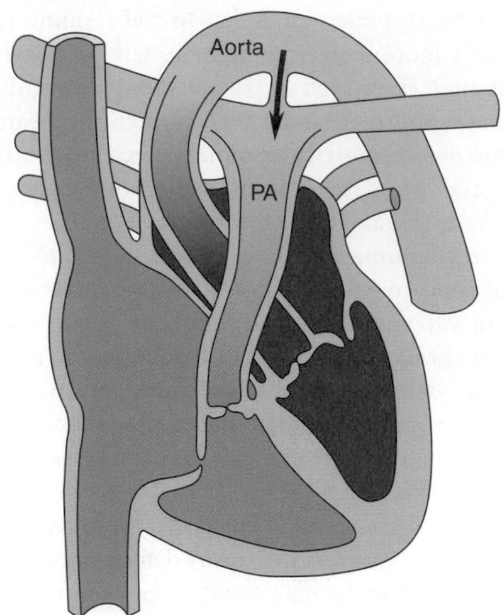

FIGURE 18-28 ■ Patent ductus arteriosus. Blood flow through the ductus is usually from the aorta to the pulmonary artery and produces an acyanotic shunt.

Large ventricular septal defects may be apparent at birth because of rapidly developing right-sided heart failure and a loud systolic murmur. Large, symptomatic defects in infants or moderate defects in older children are repaired surgically to avoid progression to pulmonary vascular disease. Small ventricular septal defects in infants are generally not immediately repaired because of the tendency of such defects to close spontaneously.

Patent Ductus Arteriosus

The ductus arteriosus is a normal channel between the pulmonary artery and the aorta that remains open during intrauterine life (Figure 18-28). Within 1 to 2 days after birth, the ductus arteriosus closes functionally, and within a few weeks it closes permanently. The ductus arteriosus allows blood to flow from the pulmonary artery into the aorta, thus bypassing the lungs. Low oxygen tension and local production of prostaglandins appear to be important in maintaining patency of the channel during fetal life. After birth, flow through the ductus arteriosus switches to left to right because of the higher pressure in the aorta. This change in flow direction brings oxygenated blood through the ductus arteriosus and stimulates it to close. A reduction in prostaglandin E appears to contribute to constriction and closure. In many cases the reason for abnormal continued patency of the ductus arteriosus after birth is not well understood. Conditions that cause low blood oxygen tension may contribute to continued patency.

Most often a patent ductus arteriosus has no clinical significance early in life because the shunt is left to right and no cyanosis is evident. Surgical management is not usually immediately undertaken because these defects tend to close spontaneously. Prostaglandin inhibitors may be given to induce closure of the defect. Continued patency of the ductus arteriosus is usually obvious because of a harsh, grinding systolic murmur and often a systolic thrill (vibration). Surgical closure of the patent ductus arteriosus is done as soon as it becomes evident that spontaneous closure is unlikely. As with other left-to-right shunt disorders, uncorrected patent ductus arteriosus results in pulmonary hypertension complicated by respiratory and right-sided heart failure. Eventual reversal of

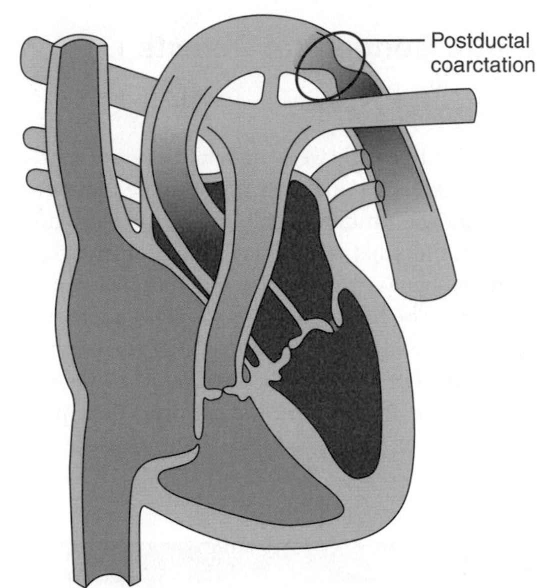

FIGURE 18-29 ■ Coarctation of the aorta. The arterial narrowing can produce a weaker pulse in the lower extremities.

the shunt to a right-to-left pattern results in cyanosis. Because the ductus is usually located distal to the origin of the subclavian artery, the lower extremities may show cyanosis whereas the upper extremities remain pink.

Coarctation of the Aorta

Coarctation refers to a narrowing or stricture that may impede blood flow. Coarctation of the aorta is a common heart defect that affects males three to four times more frequently than females. Narrowing of the aorta may occur anywhere along its length; however, in most cases the coarctation is located just before or just after the ductus arteriosus (Figure 18-29). Preductal coarctation (proximal to the ductus arteriosus) is usually more severe and often associated with other anomalies. In some instances the aortic stricture is so severe that blood flow to the lower part of the body must be maintained solely through flow through the ductus arteriosus. This situation results in a very high workload for the right side of the heart and may lead to congestive failure in the early neonatal period. Blood supply to the arms and head is unaffected because these arteries arise proximal to the stricture. Postductal coarctation is generally less severe and may go unrecognized until adulthood.

The upper extremities typically have an elevated blood pressure, with weak pulses and low blood pressure in the lower extremities. An important part of assessment of the newborn is comparison of pulses in the upper and lower extremities to assess for symmetry. All types of coarctation are usually accompanied by systolic murmurs and ventricular hypertrophy. The stricture can be repaired surgically by resection of the narrowed region. If left untreated, significant coarctation may lead to congestive heart failure, intracranial hemorrhage, or aortic rupture.

Pulmonary Stenosis or Atresia

Isolated pulmonary stenosis and atresia are included in the category of acyanotic defects because they do not themselves result in cyanosis. However, they often occur in conjunction with other anomalies that allow survival into the neonatal period. The other defects may allow shunting of blood and result in cyanosis. In pulmonary atresia, no communication is found between the right ventricle and the lungs, so that blood must enter the lungs by first traveling through a septal opening and then through a patent ductus arteriosus. The right ventricle is typically underdeveloped (hypoplasia), and the atrial septal defect is large. Pulmonary stenosis can be mild to severe, depending on the extent of narrowing of the pulmonic valve. Pulmonary stenosis is usually due to abnormal fusion of the valvular cusps. Right ventricular hypertrophy occurs secondary to the high ventricular afterload caused by the narrowed outflow opening. Isolated pulmonary stenosis is easily corrected by surgery; however, the prognosis depends in large part on the health of the right ventricle.

Aortic Stenosis or Atresia

Congenital aortic atresia is rare and not compatible with survival. Depending on its severity, aortic stenosis is correctable and associated with a good prognosis. Aortic stenosis may involve the valvular cusps or the subvalvular fibrous ring just below the cusps. The narrowed aortic outflow tract results in a high left ventricular afterload, which causes the left ventricle to enlarge. A prominent systolic murmur is usually apparent. Surgical replacement is the definitive treatment if the stenosis is severe, progresses, or becomes symptomatic.

Cyanotic Congenital Defects

Tetralogy of Fallot

The four defining features of tetralogy of Fallot are (1) a ventricular septal defect; (2) an aorta positioned above the ventricular septal opening (overriding aorta); (3) pulmonary stenosis that obstructs right ventricular outflow; and (4) right ventricular hypertrophy (Figure 18-30).

The severity of the symptoms is related primarily to the degree of pulmonary stenosis. The heart is generally enlarged because of the extensive right ventricular hypertrophy. Even if the condition is untreated, individuals with tetralogy of Fallot may live into adulthood. The defect often results in cyanosis because the overriding aorta receives unoxygenated blood from the right side of the heart as well as oxygenated blood from the left side. The degree of cyanosis depends on the amount of blood received from the right side, which in turn depends on the degree of pulmonic obstruction. Surgical

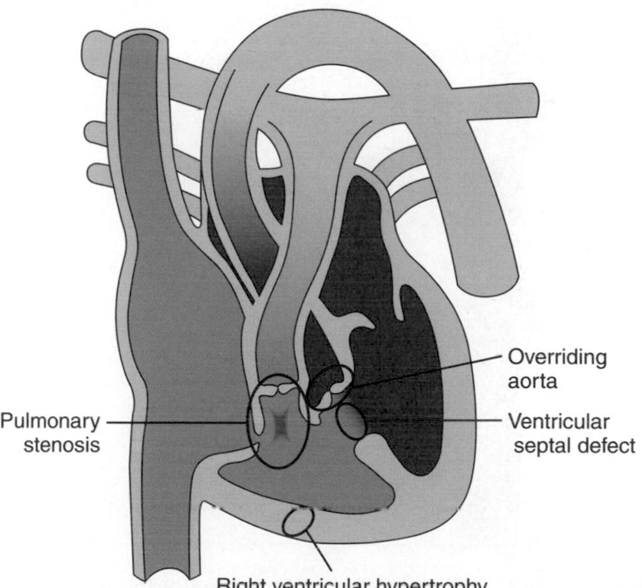

FIGURE 18-30 ■ Tetralogy of Fallot showing the four characteristic abnormalities: pulmonary stenosis, ventricular septal defect, overriding aorta, and right ventricular hypertrophy. Tetralogy of Fallot is a cyanotic defect.

correction is usually recommended because prolonged palliation carries the risk of infective endocarditis and secondary polycythemia.

Transposition of the Great Arteries

In the most common form of transposition of the great arteries, the aorta arises from the right ventricle and the pulmonary artery arises from the left ventricle (Figure 18-31). This anomaly results in the formation of two separate, noncommunicating circulations. The right side of the heart receives blood from the systemic circulation and recirculates it through the body by way of the aorta. Blood reaching the body has not passed through the lungs and is therefore not oxygenated. The left side of the heart receives oxygenated blood from the lungs and then recirculates it through the lungs by way of the pulmonary artery. Unless some mixing of these separate circulations takes place through other heart defects, such as septal defects, transposition is not compatible with life.

Nearly all infants who survive the neonatal period have an interatrial opening, and most also have a patent ductus arteriosus. A good deal of mixing must be maintained after birth for the infant to survive. Surgery may be directed at improving the mixing of systemic and pulmonary blood by enlarging or creating openings in the heart. Corrective surgery in which the aorta and pulmonary arteries are cut from the heart and sewn to the opposite ventricular outflow tract is the treatment of choice. The coronary arteries must also be reimplanted into the new left ventricular outflow tract in this procedure.

Truncus Arteriosus

Truncus arteriosus is a congenital malformation in which failure of the pulmonary artery and aorta to separate results in formation of one large vessel that receives blood from both the right and left ventricles (Figure 18-32). A large ventricular septal defect and a single valvular structure are present and lead to the single large artery. Mixing of blood from the right and left sides of the heart results in systemic cyanosis. The amount of blood entering the systemic versus the pulmonary circulation depends on the degree of vascular resistance in the two systems. Abnormally high pulmonary blood flow may progress to pulmonary hypertension and right ventricular hypertrophy. Increased pulmonary resistance causes the cyanosis to become more severe as more blood enters the systemic circulation. Surgical correction is required for survival.

Tricuspid Atresia

Absence of the tricuspid valve is almost always associated with underdevelopment of the right ventricle and an atrial septal defect. Circulation is maintained by the defect, which allows blood to bypass the right ventricle. A patent ductus arteriosus is required to perfuse the lungs. In some cases a concomitant ventricular septal defect is present and may allow some blood to pass into the right ventricle and enter the pulmonary circulation. Cyanosis is present from birth, and the mortality rate is high. Surgical correction is required for survival.

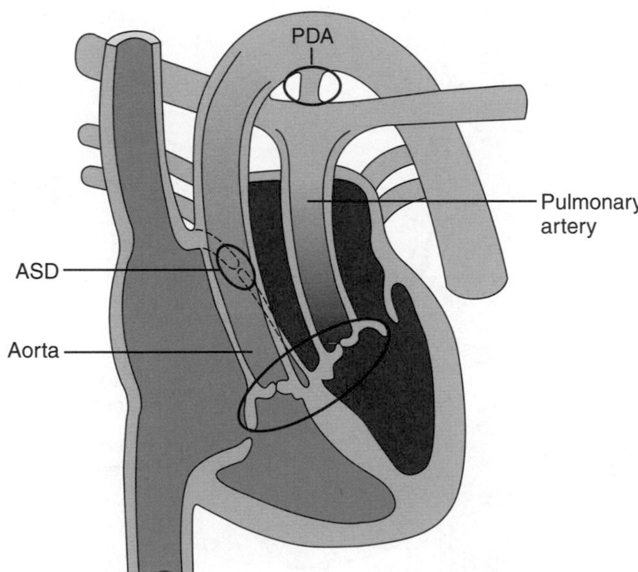

FIGURE 18-31 ■ Transposition of the great arteries. Two separate circulations are formed, which is incompatible with life unless mixing of blood occurs through other defects. *ASD,* Atrial septal defect; *PDA,* patent ductus arteriosus.

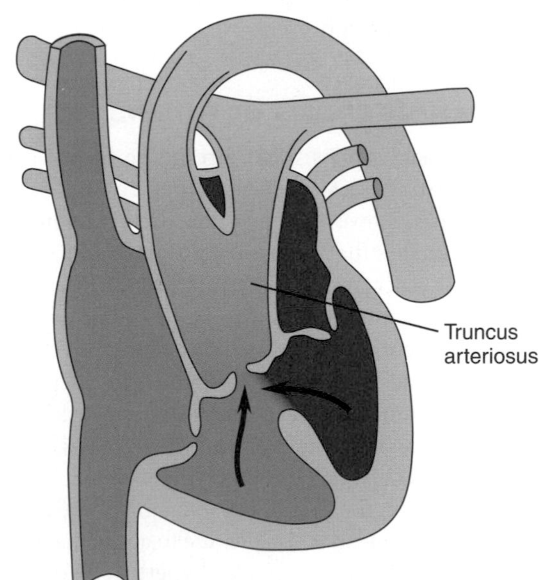

FIGURE 18-32 ■ Truncus arteriosus is a cyanotic defect. Failure of septation results in a common outflow tract from the ventricles. A ventricular septal defect is also present.

KEY CONCEPTS

- Different congenital heart anomalies result in two primary pathologic processes: (1) shunting of blood through abnormal pathways in the heart or great vessels and (2) obstruction to blood flow because of abnormal narrowing.
- Disorders that result in left-to-right shunting of blood or obstruction to flow are generally acyanotic. These disorders include atrial septal defect, ventricular septal defect, patent ductus arteriosus, coarctation of the aorta, and pulmonary and aortic stenosis and atresia.
- Disorders that result in right-to-left shunting of blood result in cyanosis. These disorders include tetralogy of Fallot, transposition of the great arteries, truncus arteriosus, and tricuspid atresia.

SUMMARY

A variety of disease processes may interfere with the heart's ability to provide the body with oxygenated blood. Among these processes are coronary heart disease, valvular and endocardial diseases, myocardial diseases, pericardial diseases, and congenital heart defects. The most important forms of coronary heart disease are angina pectoris and acute coronary syndrome, both of which usually result from coronary atherosclerosis. Stenotic coronary lesions obstruct blood flow to the myocardium and result in ischemia. Distinction between angina and MI relies primarily on the presence of myocardial enzymes in the blood. Angina is ischemia without cellular death and therefore does not result in enzyme elevation. MI, on the other hand, is associated with the death of myocardial cells and subsequent release of intracellular enzymes. MI may be complicated by dysrhythmias and failure of the heart to pump efficiently.

Valvular disorders are of two types: those that impede flow because of stenosis and those that allow regurgitation because of failure to close completely. The general consequence of valvular disorders is increased myocardial workload secondary to high afterload (stenosis) or high preload (regurgitation). The heart may eventually decompensate and proceed to congestive heart failure. The endocardial diseases rheumatic heart disease and infective endocarditis also primarily affect the heart valves and create stenosis and regurgitation.

Disorders of the myocardium include myocarditis, which is an inflammatory process, and cardiomyopathy, which is a noninflammatory process, usually of unknown cause. Most cases of myocarditis are viral; however, it is the immune system's response to the virus that appears to cause myocardial damage. Myocarditis results in a dilated, flabby heart with decreased pumping efficiency. The cardiomyopathies are a diverse group of disorders that may be classified as primary (having unknown cause) and specific (caused by a known disease process). Primary cardiomyopathies include a dilated form, a hypertrophic form, and a restrictive form. The primary problem in the dilated form is poor contractility of all heart chambers. The hypertrophic form may cause left ventricular outflow obstruction that interferes with cardiac output and increases left ventricular strain. Dysfunction in the restrictive form is caused by poor diastolic filling as a result of a stiff, fibrosed ventricular chamber.

Pericardial disorders include accumulations of fluid in the pericardial sac and acute and chronic forms of pericarditis. Pericardial fluid may be serous, serosanguineous, chylous, or frank blood. Pericardial accumulations are usually of little consequence except as indicators of underlying pathophysiologic processes. However, if the accumulation is large or rapid, it may compress the heart and interfere with diastolic filling—a process called cardiac tamponade. Pericarditis refers to inflammation of the pericardium. It is usually secondary to other disease processes. Pericardial inflammation generally causes pain and may be associated with a friction rub. Chronic pericarditis can cause erosion of the pericardial sac such that the epicardial layer of the heart may become fused to other mediastinal structures. Alternatively, chronic pericarditis may cause the pericardial sac to become fibrotic and noncompliant such that it restricts expansion of the heart during diastolic filling.

A number of heart disorders may be present at birth and can be categorized as obstructions or shunts and as cyanotic or acyanotic. In general, disorders that allow unoxygenated blood from the right heart to enter the systemic circulation (right-to-left shunt) cause cyanosis. Examples of cyanotic defects include tetralogy of Fallot, transposition of the great arteries, truncus arteriosus, and tricuspid atresia. Examples of acyanotic defects are coarctation of the aorta, atrial and ventricular septal defects, and patent ductus arteriosus.

All heart diseases discussed in this chapter may be complicated by heart failure. Heart failure occurs when the pumping efficiency of the heart is decreased such that cardiac output is subnormal. It is often accompanied by congestion of the lungs or the systemic venous system. Heart failure is discussed in Chapter 19.

MEDIA RESOURCES

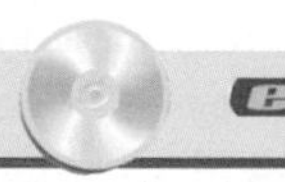

Remember to check out the ***CD Companion*** included with this book for Review Questions, Key Concepts Review, Glossary (with audio for selected terms), Disease Profiles, and Animations.

PLUS, visit the ***Evolve website*** at http://evolve.elsevier.com/Copstead/ for Case Studies, Disease Profiles, and WebLinks.

References

1. American Heart Association: *Heart disease and stroke statistics—2004 update,* Dallas, 2003, The Association.
2. Third Report of the National Cholesterol Education Program (NCEP) Expert Panel on Detection, Evaluation, and Treatment of High Blood Cholesterol in Adults (Adult Treatment Panel III), Bethesda, 2002, National Heart, Lung, and Blood Institute, National Institutes of Health.

3. Libby P: The vascular biology of atherosclerosis. In Braunwald E, Zipes D, Libby P, editors: *Heart disease: a textbook of cardiovascular medicine,* ed 6, Philadelphia, 2001, Saunders, pp 995-1009.
4. Schoen FJ, Cotran RS: Blood vessels. In Kumar V, Cotran R, Robbins S, editors: *Robbins basic pathology,* ed 7, Philadelphia, 2003, Saunders, pp 325-360.
5. Stary HC et al: A definition of initial, fatty streak, and intermediate lesions of atherosclerosis. A report from the Committee on Vascular Lesions of the Council on Arteriosclerosis, American Heart Association, *Circulation* 89(5):2462-2478, 1994.
6. Stary HC et al: A definition of advanced types of atherosclerotic lesions and a histological classification of atherosclerosis. A report from the Committee on Vascular Lesions of the Council on Arteriosclerosis, American Heart Association, *Arterioscler Thromb Vasc Biol* 15(9):1512-1531, 1995.
7. Naghavi M et al: From vulnerable plaque to vulnerable patient: a call for new definitions and risk assessment strategies: part 1, *Circulation* 108:1664-1672, 2003.
8. Forrester JS: Prevention of plaque rupture: a new paradigm of therapy, *Ann Intern Med* 137:823-833, 2002.
9. Schoen FJ: The heart. In Kumar V, Cotran R, Robbins S, editors: *Robbins basic pathology,* ed 7, Philadelphia, 2003, Saunders, pp 543-599.
10. Hennekens CH, Dyken ML, Fuster V: Aspirin as a therapeutic agent in cardiovascular disease: a statement for healthcare professionals from the American Heart Association, *Circulation* 96(8):2751-2753, 1997.
11. Triggle CR et al: The endothelium in health and disease: a target for therapeutic intervention, *J Smooth Muscle Res* 39(6):249-267, 2003.
12. Ryan TJ et al: 1999 update: ACC/AHA guidelines for the management of patients with acute myocardial infarction. A report of the American College of Cardiology/American Heart Association Task Force on Practice Guidelines (Committee on Management of Acute Myocardial Infarction), *J Am Coll Cardiol* 34(3):890-911, 1999.
13. Braunwald E et al: ACC/AHA 2002 guideline update for the management of patients with unstable angina and non-ST-segment elevation myocardial infarction—summary article: a report of the American College of Cardiology/American Heart Association Task Force on Practice Guidelines (Committee on the Management of Patients With Unstable Angina), *J Am Coll Cardiol* 40(7):1366-1374, 2002.
14. DeWood MA et al: Prevalence of total coronary occlusion during the early hours of transmural myocardial infarction, *N Engl J Med* 303(16):897-902, 1980.
15. Young JJ, Kereiakes DJ: Pharmacologic reperfusion strategies for the treatment of ST-segment elevation myocardial infarction, *Rev Cardiovasc Med* 4(4):216-227, 2003.
16. Nadal-Ginard B et al: Myocyte death, growth, and regeneration in cardiac hypertrophy and failure, *Circ Res* 92(2):139-150, 2003.
17. Waters RE II et al: Current perspectives on reperfusion therapy for acute ST-segment elevation myocardial infarction: integrating pharmacologic and mechanical reperfusion strategies, *Am Heart J* 146(6):958-968, 2003.
18. Antezano ES, Hong M: Sudden cardiac death, *J Intensive Care Med* 18(6):313-329, 2003.
19. Braunwald E: Valvular heart disease. In Braunwald E, Zipes D, Libby P, editors: *Heart disease: a textbook of cardiovascular medicine,* ed 6, Philadelphia, 2001, Saunders, pp1643-1713.
20. World Health Organization and International Society and Federation of Cardiology. Strategy for controlling rheumatic fever/rheumatic heart disease, with emphasis on primary prevention: memorandum from a joint WHO/ISFC meeting, *Bull WHO* 75:583-587, 1995.
21. Dajani AS: Rheumatic fever. In Braunwald E, Zipes D, Libby P, editors: *Heart disease: a textbook of cardiovascular medicine,* ed 6, Philadelphia, 2001, Saunders, pp 2192-2198.
22. Karchmer AW: Infective endocarditis. In Braunwald E, Zipes D, Libby P, editors: *Heart disease: a textbook of cardiovascular medicine,* ed 6, Philadelphia, 2001, Saunders, pp 1723-1747.
23. Higuchi Mde L et al: Pathophysiology of the heart in Chagas' disease: current status and new developments, *Cardiovasc Res* 60(1):96-107, 2003.
24. Richardson P et al: Report of the 1995 World Health Organization/International Society and Federation of Cardiology Task Force on the Definition and Classification of Cardiomyopathies, *Circulation* 93(5):841-842, 1996.
25. Wynne JA, Braunwald E: The cardiomyopathies and myocarditides. In Braunwald E, Zipes D, Libby P, editors: *Heart disease: a textbook of cardiovascular medicine,* ed 6, Philadelphia, 2001, Saunders, pp 1751-1806.
26. Newman TB: Etiology of ventricular septal defects: an epidemiologic approach, *Pediatrics* 76(5):741-749, 1985.

Heart Failure and Dysrhythmias: Common Sequelae of Cardiac Diseases

chapter 19

Jacquelyn L. Banasik

MEDIA RESOURCES

Additional Material for Study, Review, and Further Exploration

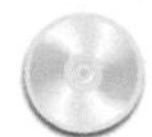

CD Companion ◆ Review Questions and Answers ◆ Key Concepts Review
◆ Glossary *(with audio pronunciations for selected terms)*
◆ Disease Profiles ◆ Animations

evolve ***Website*** at http://evolve.elsevier.com/Copstead/
◆ Case Studies ◆ Disease Profiles ◆ WebLinks

KEY QUESTIONS

- What are the common predisposing factors for development of congestive heart failure (CHF)?
- How does CHF with primarily systolic dysfunction differ from CHF with primarily diastolic dysfunction?
- How do the compensatory responses triggered in CHF work to restore cardiac output?
- How can clinical manifestations be used to differentiate left-sided heart failure from right-sided heart failure?
- How are preload, afterload, and contractility managed therapeutically in the patient with CHF?
- What are the characteristic electrocardiographic features of the common cardiac dysrhythmias?
- What is the clinical significance and usual treatment of each of the common cardiac dysrhythmias?

CHAPTER OUTLINE

Congestive heart failure (CHF) and cardiac dysrhythmias may occur in association with cardiac diseases from a number of different causes. *Heart failure* refers to inability of the heart to maintain sufficient cardiac output to optimally meet metabolic demands of tissues and organs. Heart failure is the potential end point of all serious forms of heart disease. The majority of patients with heart failure exhibit symptoms of fluid overload and are said to have CHF. Disturbances in electrical activity of the heart may signify underlying pathophysiologic processes and may also lead to insufficient cardiac output. Neither heart failure nor dysrhythmia is a primary medical disease, and underlying pathophysiologic processes must also be investigated.

Heart failure is defined as insufficient cardiac output due to cardiac dysfunction. Ineffectiveness of the cardiac pump results in congestion of blood flow in the systemic or pulmonary circulation, leading to *CHF*. CHF is an increasingly common disorder, affecting about 5 million Americans, with more than 550,000 new cases diagnosed in the United States each year.[1] Heart failure is the most common reason for hospitalization in patients older than 65 years.[2] The increasing incidence of CHF reflects an improved survival rate after myocardial infarction (MI) as well as greater longevity of the population in general. The incidence of CHF approaches 10 per 1000 population after age 65.[1]

CONGESTIVE HEART FAILURE

Etiology and Pathogenesis

A large number of disorders, including most of those discussed in Chapter 18, can lead to the development of CHF. These disorders are often grouped into ischemic cardiomyopathies and nonischemic cardiomyopathies for comparison and research purposes. The majority of cases of CHF are associated with ischemic cardiomyopathy due to coronary artery disease and hypertension.[2] Less common causes of CHF include dilated cardiomyopathy, congenital heart defects, valvular disorders, respiratory diseases, anemia, and hyperthyroidism.

Regardless of specific cause, the pathophysiologic state of heart failure results from impaired ability of myocardial fibers to contract (systolic failure), relax (diastolic failure), or both. Until the late 1980s, systolic dysfunction was thought to be the primary problem in all forms of CHF. Now it is evident that approximately half of patients with CHF have preserved systolic function but impaired diastolic function.[3] Diastolic dysfunction is more common in women, the elderly, and those with no history of MI.

Differentiation of heart failure patients into these two groups is based on the left ventricular ejection fraction (EF). Ejection fraction is calculated by dividing stroke volume by end-diastolic volume. A normal EF is 60% to 80%. Patients with systolic failure have characteristically low ejection fractions. Patients with EF greater than 50% do not have significant systolic dysfunction. Patients exhibiting congestive signs and symptoms and low cardiac output, but who have an EF greater than 50%, have a diastolic dysfunction. The overall mortality for heart failure is high, with about 50% of patients dying within 5 years of diagnosis.[2] Survival rates vary significantly between sexes, with men having a 35% survival rate at 5 years and women having a 53% survival rate.[4] The median survival time after diagnosis is 1.7 years in men and 3.2 years in women.[4] Patients with low EF but no congestive symptoms have a survival rate about the same as those with preserved EF who have congestive symptoms. The highest mortality occurs in patients with both low EF and congestive symptoms.

Systolic Failure

Patients with systolic failure have reduced myocardial contractility evidenced by a low EF and a reduced dP/dT during ventricular systole. The dP/dT is a measure of how quickly the ventricle can develop a forceful contraction. The nature of the impaired contractility is only partially understood; however, myocyte loss and dysregulation of neurohormones are believed to be critical elements.[5]

Impaired contractility due to MI is a common cause of heart failure. MI, with cell death and loss of contractile elements, reduces the heart's contractile force (**inotropy**). The degree of pump failure is related to the amount of heart muscle lost. Myocardial cells are also subject to high rates of apoptosis (programmed cell death) in patients with heart failure. Apoptosis can be triggered by excessive stimulation by certain neurohormones and by ischemia. Over time, the loss of pumping cells contributes to reduced contractility.

Inadequate supplies of oxygen to the contracting cells may impair contractility because each myosin cross-bridge cycle requires a molecule of adenosine triphosphate (ATP). When ATP production is low, fewer cross-bridge cycles may be accomplished with each contraction, resulting in a reduced EF.

β-Receptor down-regulation is thought to be an important mechanism of impaired systolic function. Chronic overexcitation of cardiac β receptors by sympathetic neurotransmitters leads to a reduction in the number of β receptors and results in a myocardium that is less responsive to sympathetic stimulation and adrenergic drug therapy. β-Receptor–blocking agents have been shown to improve EF and also to reduce mortality, lending support to the view that chronic excessive sympathetic nervous system (SNS) activation is detrimental to cardiac function.[5]

The severity of systolic failure can be estimated by measuring the amount of blood that the ventricle is able to eject into the arterial system. A reduced stroke volume, reduced cardiac output, and lowered EF are associated with heart failure. In severe systolic failure, the EF may fall below 15% or 20%. In general, the prognosis worsens as EF falls.

Diastolic Failure

Ischemic heart disease and hypertension are the two main causes of diastolic failure, just as they are the primary causes of systolic failure. It is not clear why the same disease processes result in different cardiac dynamics in different individuals. Diastolic failure is a disorder of myocardial relaxation such that the ventricle is excessively noncompliant and does not fill effectively. Two separate functional processes occur during the diastolic relaxation phase: The first is an energy-requiring process (**lusitropy**) that removes free calcium ions from the cytoplasm by pumping them back into the sarcoplasmic reticulum and across the cell membrane into the extracellular fluid. Removal of calcium ions inhibits cross-bridge formation and allows the thick and thin filaments of the sarcomere to passively slide apart. Ischemia, with subsequent ATP deficiency, interferes with the efficiency of calcium ion removal and can impair the active phase of diastolic relaxation.

The second process is passive stretch of the ventricular myocardium to accommodate filling. Passive compliance of the ventricle can be decreased by deposition of fibrin and collagen during scar formation or by hypertrophic thickening of the ventricular wall. Impairment of both active and passive processes may occur together and are difficult to distinguish clinically.

The hallmark of diastolic failure is that the patient exhibits clinical manifestations of CHF, including low cardiac output, congestion, and edema formation, but has a normal EF (usually defined as greater than 50%), indicating absence of significant systolic impairment.[3] Because treatment recommendations differ, an echocardiogram to measure EF is recommended in all pa-

Table 19-1

Features of Systolic and Diastolic Dysfunction in Congestive Heart Failure

	Systolic Dysfunction	Diastolic Dysfunction
Presentation	<65 yr Progressive dyspnea	≥65 yr Acute dyspnea
Physical examination findings	S_3 heart sound Pulmonary congestion	S_4 heart sound Pulmonary congestion Left ventricular hypertrophy
Chest x-ray findings	Cardiomegaly	Normal or small heart
Ejection fraction	<50%	≥50%

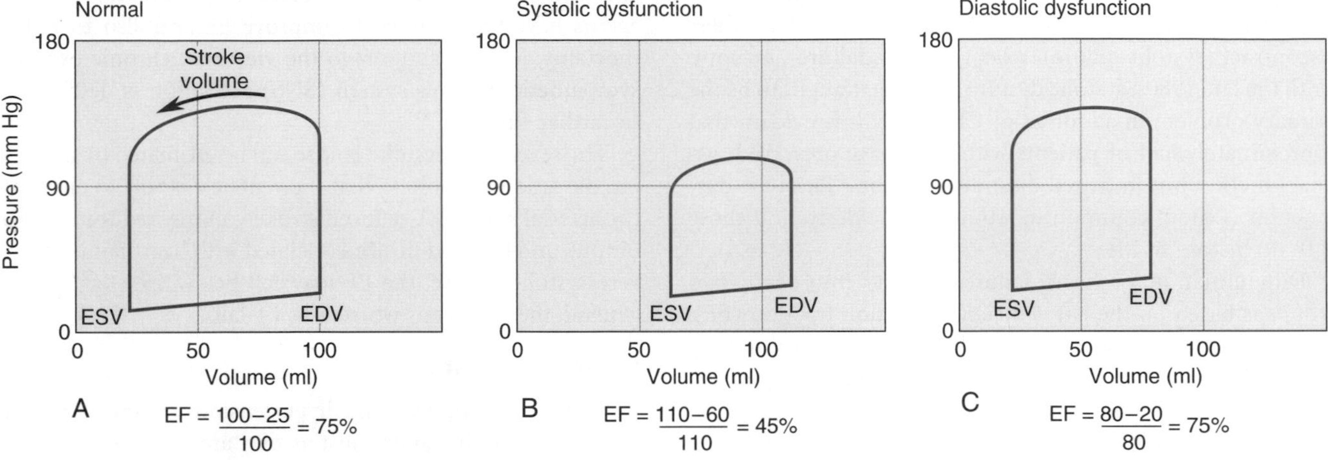

FIGURE 19-1 ■ A comparison of the left ventricular pressure-volume loop in normal heart **(A)**, systolic dysfunction **(B)**, and diastolic dysfunction **(C)**. Note that end-diastolic *pressure* is higher than normal in both systolic and diastolic failure, but end-diastolic *volume* is lower in diastolic dysfunction. *EDV*, End-diastolic volume; *ESV*, end-systolic volume; *EF*, ejection fraction.

tients with CHF to distinguish diastolic from systolic dysfunction.[3] A comparison of the features of systolic and diastolic failure is shown in Table 19-1. A comparison of the left ventricular pressure-volume loop in systolic and diastolic dysfunction is shown in Figure 19-1. Systolic failure is characterized by higher than normal diastolic volume and low EF, whereas the pressure-volume loop in diastolic failure indicates poor compliance with a low diastolic volume at a higher than normal pressure.

KEY CONCEPTS

- CHF is a potential consequence of most cardiac disorders. Heart failure occurs when the heart is unable to provide sufficient cardiac output to maintain function of the body.
- The most common cause of CHF is myocardial ischemia from coronary artery disease, followed by hypertension and dilated cardiomyopathy.
- Impaired contractility resulting in systolic failure is frequently associated with CHF. The biochemical basis of impaired contractility involves loss of cardiac muscle cells, β-receptor down-regulation, and reduced ATP production.
- In about half of CHF patients, systolic function is preserved and diastolic dysfunction predominates. Diastolic failure is particularly likely to develop in the elderly, in women, and in those without history of MI.
- Left ventricular pressure-volume loops characterize the differences in systolic and diastolic dysfunction. High diastolic volume and reduced EF indicate systolic failure, whereas diastolic failure is characterized by higher diastolic pressure and low volume.

Compensatory Mechanisms and Remodeling

When the heart fails to provide adequate cardiac output to meet tissue demands, a number of compensatory mechanisms are triggered. These mechanisms are helpful in restoring cardiac output toward normal, but in the long term they are detrimental to the heart. Much of the current management of

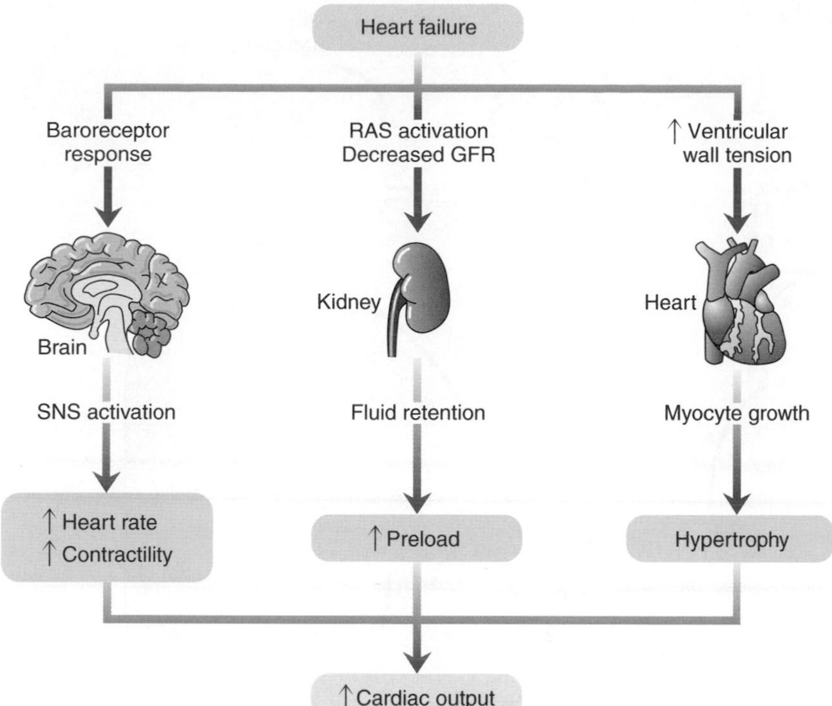

FIGURE 19-2 ■ The major compensatory mechanisms in heart failure that act to restore cardiac output. *RAS,* Renin-angiotensin-aldosterone system; *GFR,* glomerular filtration rate; *SNS,* sympathetic nervous system.

CHF is aimed at attenuating the harmful consequences of these compensatory responses.[5] Three main compensatory mechanisms are activated in heart failure: SNS activation, increased preload, and myocardial hypertrophy (Figure 19-2).

Sympathetic Nervous System Activation

Sympathetic activation of the heart is primarily a result of baroreceptor reflex stimulation. The baroreceptors (pressoreceptors) located in the aorta and carotid arteries detect a fall in pressure due to diminished stroke volume and transmit this information to the central nervous system (CNS). The CNS increases activity in the sympathetic nerves to the heart, resulting in increased heart rate and contractility. However, because of impaired contractile ability, the failing heart may have reduced responsiveness to sympathetic activation. Sympathetic activation also causes venoconstriction, which redistributes blood and increases cardiac preload. Sympathetic constriction of arterioles helps to maintain blood pressure when cardiac output is reduced. Specialized cells in the kidney called juxtaglomerular cells also receive SNS stimulation when cardiac output falls. The juxtaglomerular cells release renin and initiate the renin-angiotensin-aldosterone cascade, leading to salt and water retention by the kidney. Sympathetic activation is an early and immediate compensatory response to insufficient cardiac output.

Sympathetic activation is a very effective means for increasing cardiac output in an acute process, such as volume depletion. However, in heart failure, sympathetic activation becomes a chronic process that is ultimately deleterious. A major problem with excessive sympathetic activation is that afterload on the left ventricle can be increased significantly. A high afterload increases cardiac workload and may decrease stroke volume. In a number of studies, afterload-reducing agents, which dilate the systemic arterioles, have been shown to improve cardiac function in patients with CHF.[6]

β-Blocking agents also have been advocated in the management of CHF to block the cardiac effects of sympathetic activation. Many clinicians had been reluctant to utilize β-blockers in patients with CHF because they are negative inotropes and have the potential to reduce cardiac output. In CHF, where cardiac output is already low, the use of a negative inotrope would seem to be contraindicated. However, several randomized clinical trials have reported an improved mortality rate and better EF in patients receiving certain β-blockers.[7] Long-term SNS stimulation of the heart may also contribute to heart failure progression and remodeling of the cardiac tissue. Remodeling is a process of myocyte loss, hypertrophy of remaining cells, and interstitial fibrosis (Figure 19-3). The remodeled tissue is less functional and may predispose to worsening failure and cardiac dysrhythmias.

Increased Preload

Increased **preload** in the cardiac chambers is initially a consequence of reduced EF with a resultant increase in residual end-systolic volume. Subsequently, decreased cardiac output to the kidney reduces glomerular filtration, resulting in fluid conservation. In addition, the renin-angiotensin-aldosterone cascade is activated because of reduced blood flow to the kidney and SNS activation of the juxtaglomerular cells. Angiotensin II and aldosterone enhance sodium and water reab-

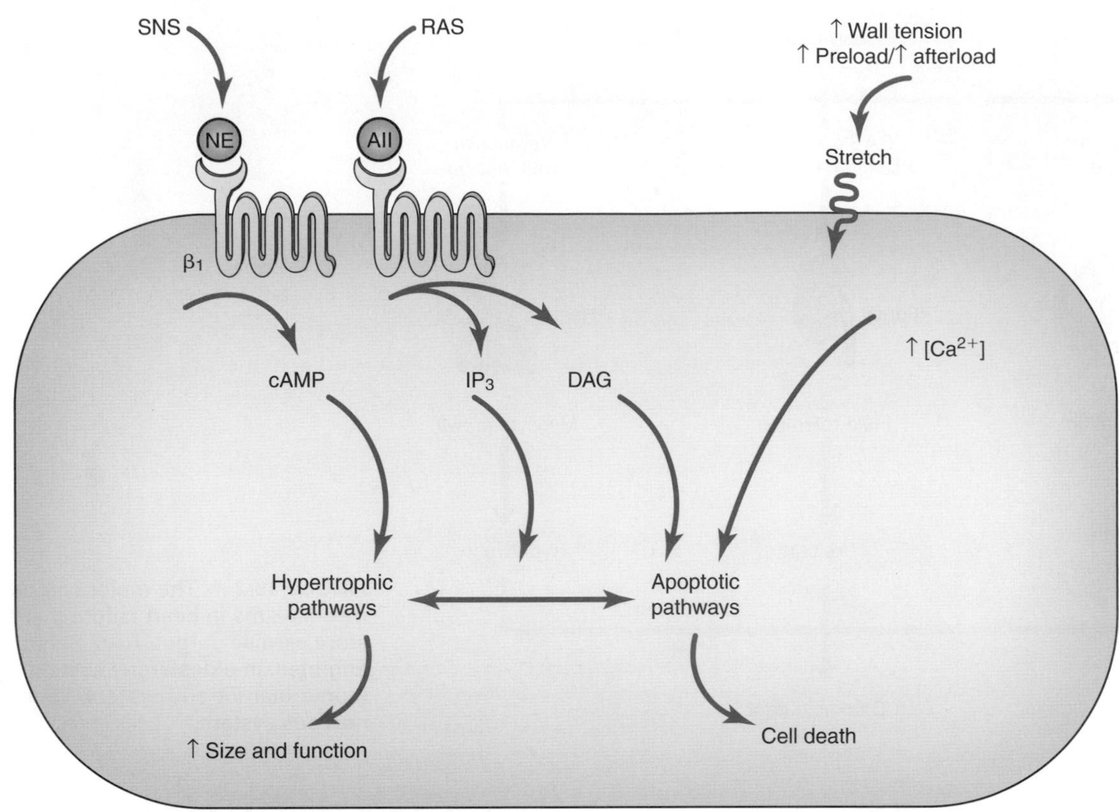

FIGURE 19-3 ■ Mechanisms of ventricular remodeling in heart failure. Activation of β_1 receptors and AII receptors along with stretch of the cell membrane trigger signaling cascades. Under some conditions these triggers lead to effective hypertrophy and an increase in size and function, and in others they trigger apoptotic cell death. *SNS,* Sympathetic nervous system; *NE,* norepinephrine; *RAS,* renin-angiotensin-aldosterone system; *AII,* angiotensin II; *cAMP,* cyclic adenosine monophosphate; *IP_3,* 1,4,5-inositol triphosphate; *DAG,* diacylglycerol.

sorption by the kidney, contributing to an elevated blood volume. Increased preload is a compensatory mechanism that enhances the ability of the myocardium to contract forcefully. An enlarged chamber volume causes the myocardial fibers to lengthen during diastole, which results in greater fiber shortening during contraction (Frank-Starling mechanism).[8] The diastolic length of the muscle fibers is thought to determine the number of effective cross-bridge cycles that can be accomplished during systole.[8] Thus, up to a point, an increase in the volume or preload of the heart will result in a greater force of contraction (Figure 19-4). The cardiac function curve flattens out at a certain point, and little further benefit is obtained despite increasing preload. Patients with systolic failure have a cardiac function curve that is flat and shifted to the right of normal. Thus, they require a higher preload to achieve a given stroke volume. However, patients with CHF often retain so much volume that their hearts are functioning on the flat part of the curve. These patients benefit from preload reduction, which will decrease congestive symptoms and cardiac workload with little or no reduction in cardiac output. Diuretics are commonly used to achieve moderate preload reduction.

Myocardial Hypertrophy and Remodeling

Hypertrophy of cardiac muscle cells is the third mechanism of compensation and generally takes much longer to occur than preload enhancement or sympathetic activation. Hypertrophy appears to result, in part, from a chronic elevation of myocardial wall tension.[9] Wall tension may be high as a result of increased diastolic blood volume (high preload) or as a consequence of high systolic pressures generated in the chamber (high afterload). The relationship between myocardial wall tension and intrachamber pressure and diameter is described by the law of Laplace: tension = transmural pressure × radius/wall thickness. When the ventricular chamber enlarges and pressures increase, more tension is created in the ventricular muscle wall (Figure 19-5). The development of high systolic pressures in the ventricle may be necessary to overcome a high afterload, such as occurs with arterial hypertension and aortic valve stenosis. The hypertrophy of contractile elements in the

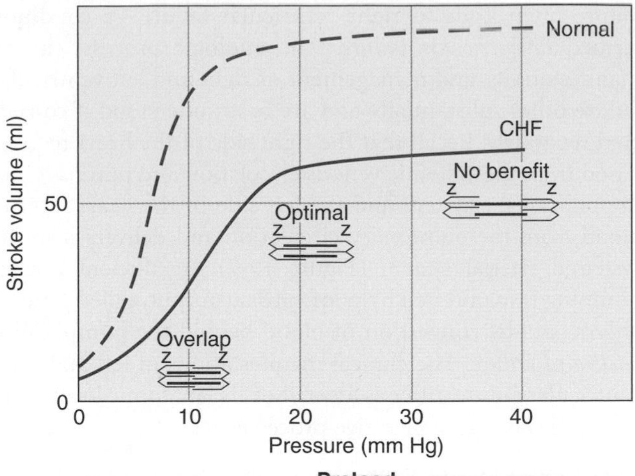

FIGURE 19-4 ■ Effect of increased preload on sarcomere length and stroke volume. Systolic failure results in a shift of the curve to the right and a dampening of maximal stroke volume. A greater preload is required to achieve a given stroke volume compared with the normal ventricle.

myocardium boosts the heart's pumping force and helps to reduce the wall tension back toward normal. In general, an increase in chamber diameter because of excessive preload is thought to contribute to eccentric hypertrophy in which the muscle fibers elongate. High afterload results in concentric hypertrophy in which the muscle fibers grow in diameter and thicken the ventricular wall (Figure 19-6).

Neurohormonal factors including norepinephrine and AII also have hypertrophic effects on the heart (see Figure 19-3). Circulating angiotensin II levels are higher than normal in CHF because of poor kidney perfusion, which triggers production of angiotensin II through the renin-angiotensin-aldosterone cascade. In heart failure, angiotensin II is also produced locally in the heart. Angiotensin II binding to its receptor on cardiac myocytes activates genes in the growth pathways. An important enzyme in the pathway of angiotensin II production is angiotensin-converting enzyme (ACE). Drugs called ACE inhibitors have been developed to block the activity of this enzyme. Numerous clinical trials have shown a significant reduction in mortality with the administration of ACE inhibitors.[10]

In summary, enhanced preload and cardiac hypertrophy may allow a heart to compensate for systolic dysfunction for an extended period. Unfortunately, these compensatory mechanisms, which serve to restore cardiac output to the tissues, also result in an increase in myocardial work and oxygen requirements and appear to cause detrimental remodeling. Progression and decompensation may occur when the primary disease plus the superimposed burdens of compensation overwhelm the heart's ability to generate adequate contractile force. The focus of therapy for CHF is to maintain a state of compensation by minimizing cardiac work while optimizing cardiac output and preventing or delaying ventricular remodeling.

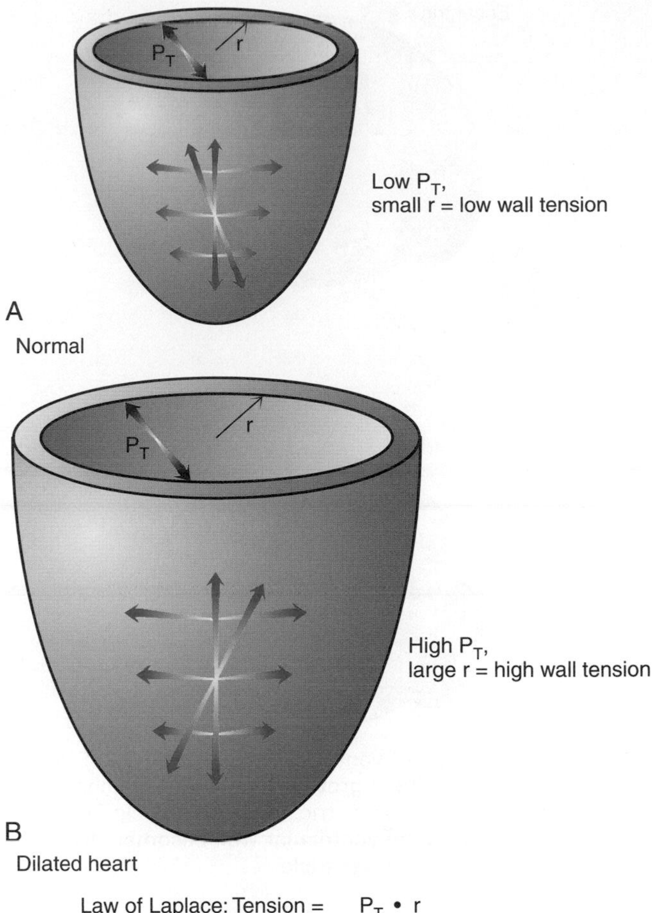

FIGURE 19-5 ■ Mechanism of myocardial hypertrophy due to increased ventricular wall tension. According to the law of Laplace, an increase in chamber radius or pressure will increase wall tension. The hypertrophic response increases wall thickness and helps to relieve wall tension. **A,** Heart with normal radius *(r)* and intraventricular pressure. **B,** Heart with enlarged chamber and high intraventricular pressure. P_T, Transmural pressure.

KEY CONCEPTS

- Compensatory mechanisms are activated in heart failure in an attempt to improve cardiac output. Unfortunately, these responses also increase myocardial workload and may perpetuate the heart failure. Treatment for CHF is aimed at attenuating the harmful effects of the compensatory responses.
- Sympathetic activation is an early response to reduced cardiac output. Sympathetic nervous system activation increases heart rate, contractility, arterial vasoconstriction, and renin release. The failing heart generally has reduced responsiveness to SNS neurotransmitters due to β-receptor down-regulation.
- Decreased cardiac output reduces kidney perfusion and leads to activation of the renin-angiotensin-

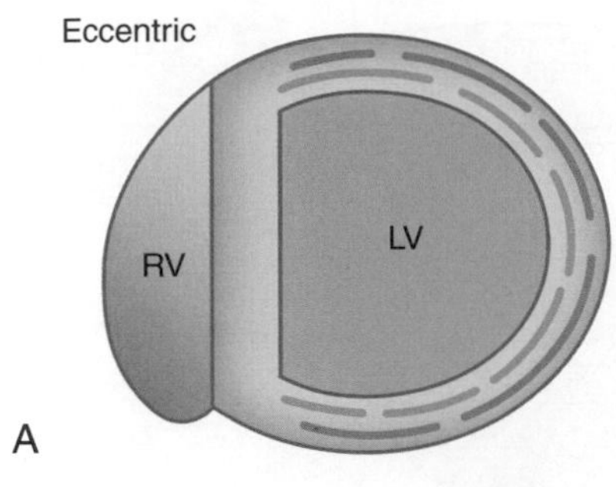

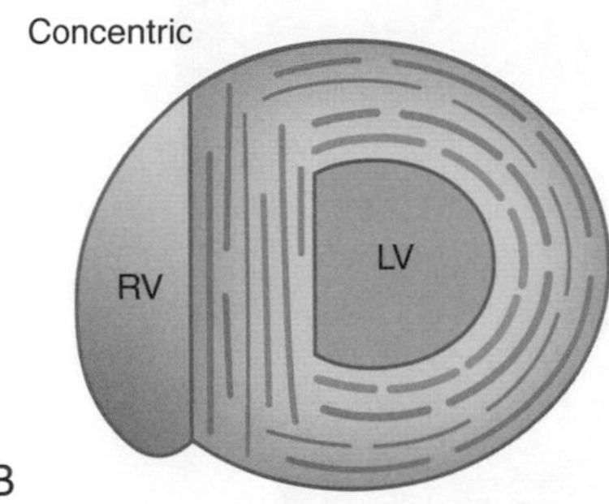

FIGURE 19-6 ■ Forms of ventricular hypertrophy. **A,** Eccentric, in which muscle fibers grow in length and the chamber diameter increases. **B,** Concentric, in which muscle fibers grow in diameter and the ventricular wall becomes thicker. *RV,* Right ventricle; *LV,* left ventricle.

aldosterone cascade and volume retention. Extra blood volume increases cardiac preload. Higher preload results in more forceful ejection of blood from the heart (Frank-Starling law) and improves cardiac output.

- Cardiac hypertrophy is stimulated by elevated myocardial wall tension and the growth-promoting actions of neurohormones, such as norepinephrine and angiotensin II. Hypertrophy adds contractile filaments and improves contractile force.
- The mechanisms that enable the heart to compensate for reduced stroke volume are detrimental in the long term. Excessive neurohormones, volume overload, and high wall tension contribute to ventricular remodeling. Gradually, the ventricle loses myocytes and accumulates fibrotic tissue. The remaining myocytes are usually hypertrophied.

Clinical Manifestations

The clinical presentation of CHF differs depending on which ventricle (left, right, or both) is failing to pump blood adequately. Left ventricular failure is the most common presentation of CHF. Because of circulatory dynamics, left ventricular failure often leads to right ventricular failure—a condition termed *biventricular failure.* The etiologic process, clinical manifestations, and management of right and left ventricular failure differ substantially and are best understood if considered separately. Recall that the right side of the heart receives blood from the systemic venous circulation and pumps it into the pulmonary system and the left side of the heart receives blood from the pulmonary circulation and delivers it to the systemic arterial system (Figure 19-7). Insufficient cardiac pumping is manifested by poor cardiac output, called *forward failure,* and by congestion of blood behind the pump, called *backward failure.* The clinical manifestations of left and right ventricular failure differ as a result of the anatomic location of the "backward" or congestive processes.

Left-Sided Heart Failure

Left-sided heart failure is most often associated with left ventricular infarction, cardiomyopathy, aortic and mitral valvular disease, and systemic hypertension.[5] The *forward* effects of left-sided heart failure are due to insufficient cardiac output with diminished delivery of oxygen and nutrients to peripheral tissues and organs (Figure 19-8). Inadequate perfusion of the brain may lead to restlessness, mental fatigue, confusion, anxiety, and impaired memory. Generalized fatigue, activity intolerance, and lethargy may be present (Figure 19-9).

Reduced perfusion of the kidney results in a decline in urine output (oliguria) with subsequent fluid retention. Activation of the renin-angiotensin-aldosterone cascade contributes to conservation of sodium and water by the kidney and may also cause vascular constriction. Vascular constriction serves to maintain blood pressure and redistribute reduced cardiac output to vital organs; however, it also increases the afterload against which the damaged left ventricle must pump. If renal blood flow becomes severely limited, the patient with left ventricular failure may develop kidney failure.

Forward failure also results in activation of the SNS because of the baroreceptor reflex. Sympathetic activation contributes to vascular constriction and helps maintain blood pressure in the face of reduced cardiac output; however, as with angiotensin II, it increases left ventricular afterload. Sympathetic activation results in a compensatory increase in heart rate that may augment cardiac output to some extent but, again, raises myocardial ATP consumption.

The *backward effects* of left-sided heart failure produce dramatic clinical symptoms due to pulmonary dysfunction (see Figure 19-8). Ineffective pumping of the left ventricle results in an accumulation of blood within the pulmonary circulation. As blood pressure (hydrostatic) builds within the pulmonary veins and capillaries, fluid is forced from the capillaries into interstitial and alveolar spaces, causing edema. Pulmonary congestion and edema are associated with a number of clinical findings (see Figure 19-9). **Dyspnea,** or breathlessness, occurs early in the progression of left-sided heart failure and may be considered the cardinal symptom. Difficulty breathing may be exacerbated by activity (dyspnea on exer-

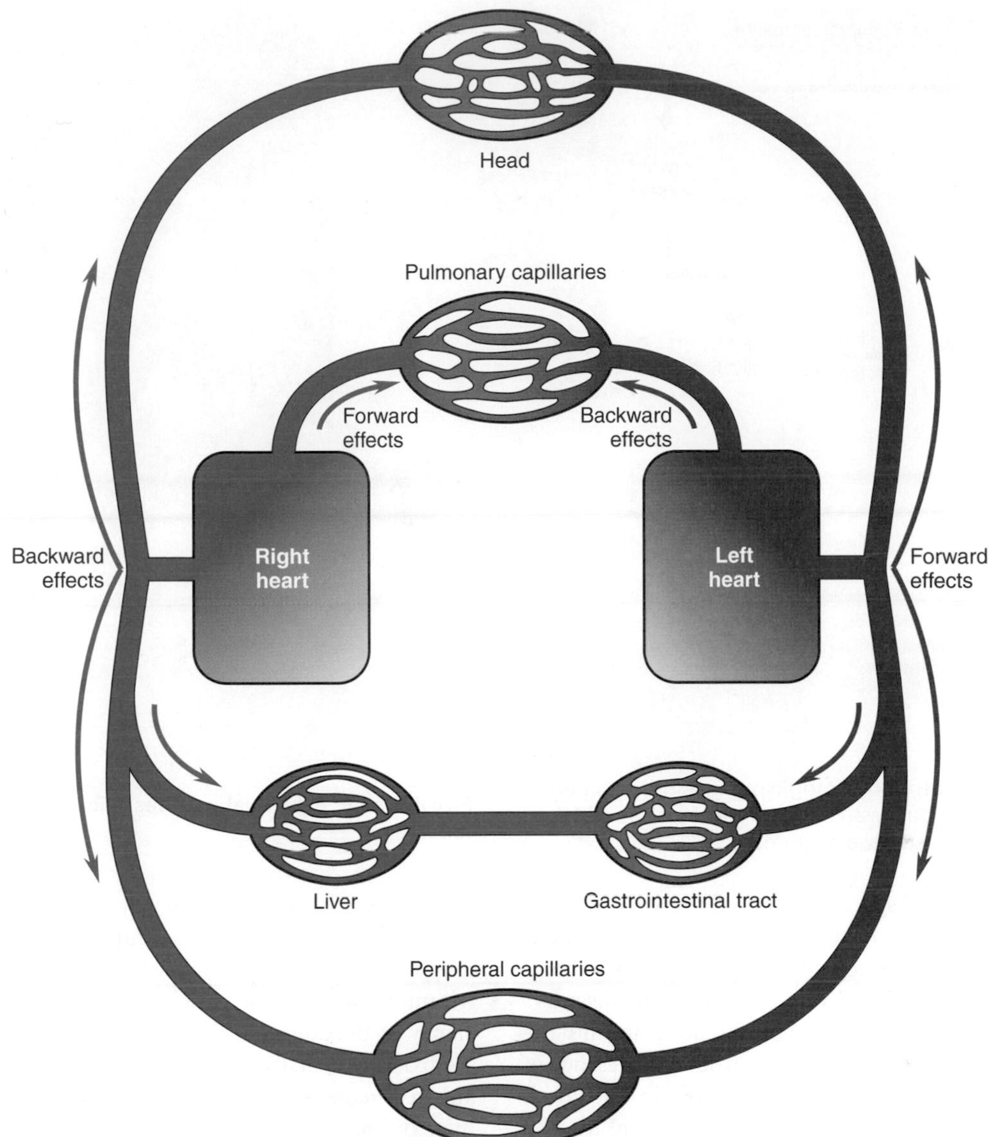

FIGURE 19-7 ■ Systemic and pulmonary circulations viewed as separate but interdependent systems.

tion), lying down (**orthopnea** and **paroxysmal nocturnal dyspnea**), and blood volume expansion. Orthopnea and paroxysmal nocturnal dyspnea are due in part to a redistribution of blood volume from the periphery to the heart when the individual lies down. The failing left ventricle is unable to effectively pump extra volume, and pulmonary congestion is worsened. The severity of orthopnea may be quantified by the degree of head elevation (e.g., number of pillows) used to relieve dyspnea. Paroxysmal nocturnal dyspnea refers to intermittent attacks of severe dyspnea during the night and is a most distressing form of orthopnea. The individual experiences a feeling of suffocation and panic at not being able to overcome the dyspnea. Sitting or standing helps to relieve the dyspnea because blood pools in the extremities, reducing pulmonary hydrostatic pressure and congestion.

Clinical signs of pulmonary congestion include cough, respiratory crackles (rales), hypoxemia, high left atrial pressure (LAP), and typical findings on x-ray film. Cough results from bronchial irritation associated with congestion. In severe cases, sputum may be blood tinged, from breakage of fragile capillaries, and frothy, due to fluid buildup in the alveoli. The severity of pulmonary edema can be estimated from the location of crackles within the lung fields. Crackles are abnormal sounds caused by the movement of air through partially fluid-filled alveoli. Edema fluid collects in dependent lung fields because of gravity and progressively moves up the lung as more edema fluid accumulates. For example, in mild pulmonary edema, crackles might be heard with a stethoscope only at the base of the upright lung, but with increasing severity they become apparent in the lower third to half of the lung. Fluid in

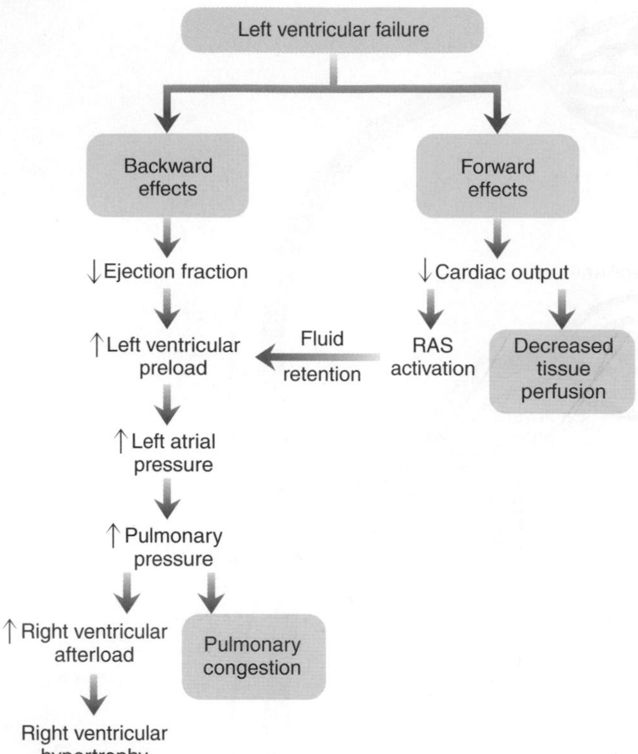

FIGURE 19-8 ■ The pathophysiologic process of left-sided heart failure, showing backward and forward effects. *RAS,* Renin-angiotensin-aldosterone system.

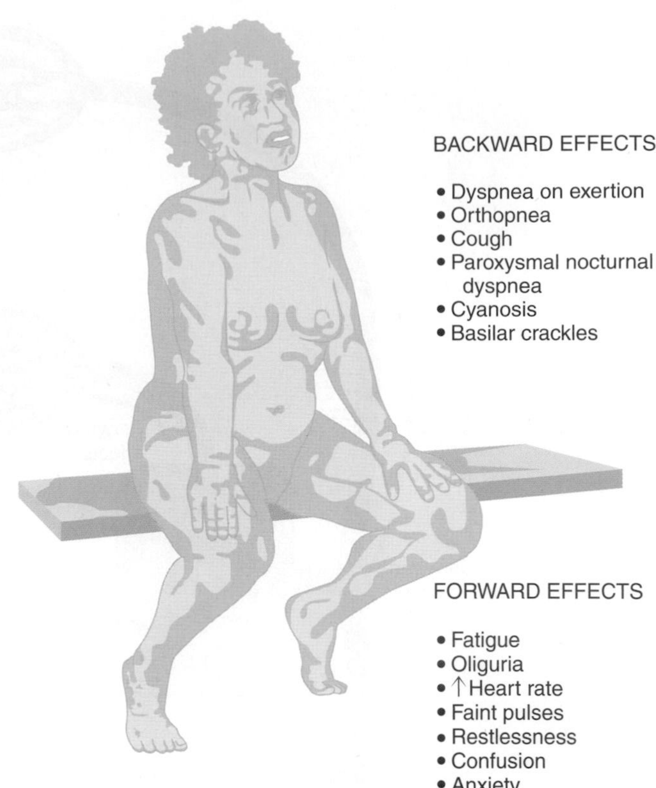

FIGURE 19-9 ■ Clinical manifestations of left-sided heart failure.

the alveoli and interstitial spaces also interferes with alveolar-capillary gas exchange and results in some degree of hypoxemia. Hypoxemia may be detected by arterial blood gas analysis and may be apparent clinically as cyanosis. **Cyanosis** refers to a blue coloration of the skin typically seen around the mouth (circumoral cyanosis) and results from the presence of significant amounts of desaturated hemoglobin in the blood. Cyanosis is a late sign and is clinically evident only when a large amount (about 5 g/dl) of hemoglobin is deoxygenated (≤75% saturated).

Elevated LAP is a common finding in left-sided heart failure due to excessive blood volume and the compensatory responses of atrial dilation and hypertrophy. Atrial pressure can be estimated by inserting a balloon-tipped catheter (Swan-Ganz) into the pulmonary artery. If LAP acutely increases to 25 mm Hg (normal, 4 to 12 mm Hg), increased capillary filtration leads to pulmonary edema. Patients with chronic elevations in LAP are more resistant to developing acute pulmonary edema and may not experience symptoms until pressures approach 40 mm Hg.[11] Typical x-ray findings include an enlarged heart and engorged pulmonary capillaries and lymphatic vessels.

Acute cardiogenic pulmonary edema is a life-threatening condition that severely impairs gas exchange, producing dramatic signs and symptoms. The patient exhibits severe dyspnea and anxiety, and a bolt-upright posture is usually assumed in order to maximize respiratory effort. Bubbly crackles may be heard all the way up the lung from the bases to the apices, and pink frothy sputum may be expectorated or may well up from the trachea. Anxiety and hypoxemia contribute to tachycardia, which may worsen the pumping efficiency of the failing heart. Cyanosis and symptoms of tissue hypoxia are usually apparent. The immediate treatment is aimed at reducing the fluid volume in the lungs and supporting oxygenation.

Right-Sided Heart Failure

Because the right and left ventricles function in series, left ventricular failure eventually increases the burden on the right ventricle and may cause it to fail as well. The causes of right ventricular failure must therefore include all the causes of left ventricular failure. Pure right ventricular failure is rare and is usually a consequence of right ventricular infarction or pulmonary disease. Only 3% of MIs occur in the right ventricle; however, right ventricular infarctions are often poorly tolerated and difficult to manage.[5] Pulmonary disorders that result in increased pulmonary vascular resistance impose a high afterload against which the right ventricle must pump. The resultant right ventricular hypertrophy, called **cor pulmonale,** may progress to right ventricular failure as the lung disease worsens.

Any lung disorder that decreases the total cross-sectional area of the lung vasculature can increase pulmonary vascular resistance and produce right ventricular strain. Hypoxemia,

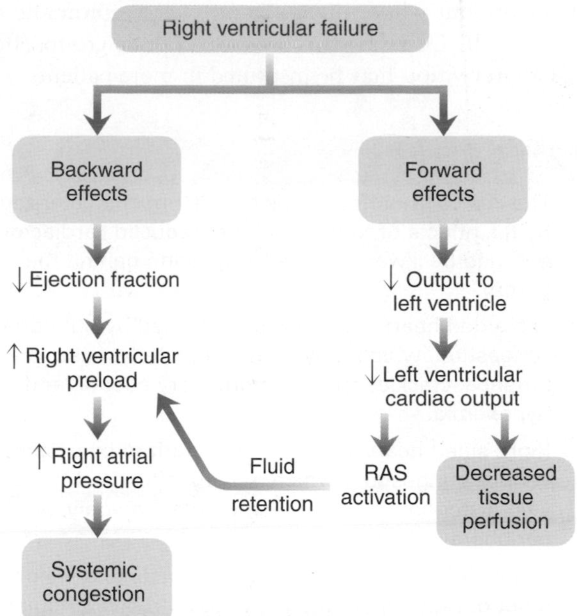

FIGURE 19-10 ■ The pathophysiologic process of right-sided heart failure, showing backward and forward effects. *RAS,* Renin-angiotensin-aldosterone system.

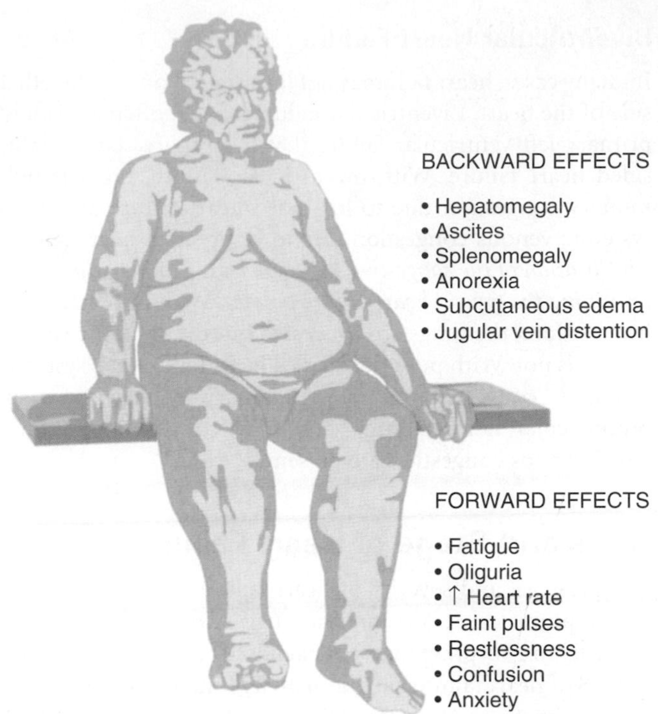

FIGURE 19-11 ■ Clinical manifestations of right-sided heart failure.

for example, causes the pulmonary arterioles to constrict, which increases pulmonary resistance. Destruction or blockage of the vascular bed, such as occurs with emphysema or pulmonary embolus, similarly reduces the cross-sectional area of the pulmonary vasculature and leads to increased pulmonary resistance. If the increase in pulmonary resistance and right ventricular workload occurs gradually, the right ventricle can compensate by increasing preload and hypertrophy. However, the thin musculature of the right ventricle has limited ability to adjust to acute changes in workload as would occur with a right ventricular infarction or large pulmonary embolus.

The *forward effects* of right-sided heart failure are very similar to those described for the left side of the heart (Figure 19-10). If the right side of the heart fails to deliver an adequate amount of blood to the left side, then systemic cardiac output will be reduced despite the fact that the left ventricle is functioning properly. The forward effects of failure include SNS activation, stimulation of renin release from the kidney with resultant volume expansion, and activity intolerance. There is no direct impairment of arterial oxygenation due to right-sided heart failure; however, peripheral tissues may suffer from hypoxia due to reduced cardiac output.

As with left-sided heart failure, congestion of blood occurs behind the failing ventricle due to inefficiency of the pump. The *backward effects* of right-sided heart failure are due to congestion in the systemic venous system (see Figure 19-10). Systemic venous congestion results in impaired function of the liver, portal system, spleen, kidneys, peripheral subcutaneous tissues, and brain (Figure 19-11).

The liver is usually somewhat increased in size and weight, but individual hepatocytes may show signs of atrophy and necrosis due to chronic passive congestion.[9] Impedance to blood flow through the liver may cause hydrostatic pressure to build in the portal system, leading to edema formation in the peritoneal cavity (ascites). Increased pressure in the portal system is reflected back to the spleen and gastrointestinal tract. The spleen is generally enlarged (congestive splenomegaly), and gastrointestinal symptoms such as anorexia and abdominal discomfort may be present.

Increased systemic venous pressure causes congestion of the kidneys, which contributes to the decreased glomerular filtration and fluid retention. Fluid retention may be perpetuated by the congested liver, which is unable to metabolize plasma aldosterone normally.[9] Excess fluid volume and venous congestion caused by right-sided heart failure result in subcutaneous edema. Edema is usually particularly apparent in the lower extremities.

Drainage of venous blood from the head and neck by way of the superior vena cava is also impeded by right-sided heart failure. The jugular veins may be abnormally distended, and mental functioning may be impaired. The hepatojugular reflux test can be done to assess the severity of right-sided heart failure. The liver is manually compressed, causing a sudden increase in venous blood returning to the right heart, while jugular neck veins are observed for sudden distention. In the absence of right-sided heart failure, the sudden increase in venous return would enter the heart unimpeded and no neck vein distention would be apparent.

Biventricular Heart Failure

In many cases, heart failure is not localized to one or the other side of the heart. Biventricular failure is most often a result of primary left ventricular failure that has progressed to right-sided heart failure. With biventricular failure, there is pulmonary congestion due to left-sided heart failure as well as systemic venous congestion due to right-sided heart failure. *The location of the congestive symptoms is a primary clue in determining the type of heart failure present.* With pure left-sided heart failure, the lungs are congested but the systemic venous system is not. With pure right-sided heart failure, the systemic system is congested but the pulmonary system is not. In biventricular failure, both pulmonary congestion and systemic venous congestion are present.

Class and Stage of Heart Failure

The presence and severity of heart failure is usually assessed by symptom scales. A commonly suggested tool for detecting heart failure in previously undiagnosed individuals is called FACES of heart failure: *f*atigue, *a*ctivity limitation, *c*ongestion, *e*dema, *s*hortness of breath. These are classic findings in CHF and, if present, indicate a need for further diagnostic assessment. Traditionally, a patient with suspected CHF would be diagnosed by x-ray and echocardiography. Recently, a blood test for B-type natriuretic peptide (BNP) has been introduced to help identify patients with CHF. BNP is similar to atrial natriuretic peptide (ANP) except that it is manufactured by the ventricular myocytes under conditions of volume overload. A significant correlation between the amount of BNP in the blood stream and the severity of CHF has been documented and a high BNP is quite specific for CHF.[12]

The severity of symptoms is used to assign a heart failure class (New York Heart Association classes [NYHA] I to IV)[13] (Table 19-2). The NYHA class is used to determine prognosis, therapy, and monitoring. Another classification scheme has been proposed to allow inclusion of patients at high risk for heart failure but whose disease is not yet symptomatic (see Table 19-2). By including this pre–heart failure group, efforts aimed at prevention may be instituted in more patients.

KEY CONCEPTS

- The clinical manifestations of CHF are characterized by the effects of forward failure (reduced cardiac output) and backward failure (congestion behind the pump).
- Left-sided heart failure is characterized by pulmonary congestion, which may manifest with dyspnea, orthopnea, crackles, cough, pulmonary edema, and hypoxemia.
- Right-sided heart failure is characterized by systemic venous congestion, which may manifest with jugular vein distention, hepatomegaly, splenomegaly, and peripheral edema.
- Left-sided heart failure frequently leads to development of right-sided heart failure. With biventricular failure, congestive signs and symptoms are found in both the pulmonary and systemic venous circulation.
- Heart failure is diagnosed by signs and symptoms, x-ray findings, and echocardiographic findings. A plasma BNP level may be used to diagnose CHF in patients with shortness of breath.
- The severity of symptoms is used to assign a heart failure class and stage.

Treatment

Therapy for CHF is aimed at improving cardiac output while minimizing congestive symptoms and cardiac workload. These objectives are obtained by manipulating preload, afterload, and contractility. When possible, specific treatment is undertaken to correct the underlying cause of the heart failure. Some pharmacologic agents commonly used in the management of heart failure are listed in Table 19-3.

Table 19-2

Stages of Heart Failure

Stage	Description	NYHA	Clinical Clues
A	Patients at high risk of developing HF	Not applicable	Coronary artery disease, hypertension, diabetes, dyslipidemia, family history of cardiomyopathy
B	Patients who have structural heart disease but have never manifested signs or symptoms of HF	I	Left ventricular hypertrophy (by ECG or echo), valvular disease, past myocardial infarction
C	Patients who have current or previous symptoms of HF	II-III	Dyspnea, fatigue, exercise intolerance, prior HF hospitalization
D	Patients with advanced structural heart disease and marked symptoms of HF at rest	IV	End-stage, awaiting transplant, receiving palliative care

Adapted from Hunt SA et al: AHA/ACC guidelines, *Circulation* 104(24):2996-3007, 2001. ©2001, American Heart Association, Inc.
HF, Heart failure.

Table 19-3

Drugs Used in the Management of Heart Failure

Category of Action	Examples
Preload-Reducing Drugs	
Diuretics	
B-type natriuretic peptide	Nesiritide
Loop diuretics	Furosemide (Lasix) Ethacrynic acid (Edecrin) Bumetanide (Bumex)
Thiazide and thiazide-like	Chlorothiazide (Diuril) Hydrochlorothiazide (Hydro-Diuril) Chlorthalidone (Hygroton) Indapamide (Lozol)
Osmotic diuretic	Mannitol (Osmitrol)
Venodilators	
Narcotic	Morphine
Nitrates	Isosorbide dinitrate (Isordil) Nitroglycerin (Nitro-Bid)
Afterload-Reducing Drugs	
Calcium-channel blockers	Nicardipine (Cardene) Nifedipine (Procardia)
Centrally acting anti-adrenergics	Clonidine (Catapres) Guanabenz (Wytensin) Methyldopa (Aldomet)
Peripherally acting anti-adrenergics	Guanethidine (Ismelin) Reserpine (Serpasil)
Direct vasodilators	Hydralazine (Apresoline) Nitroprusside (Nipride) Prazosin (Minipress) Minoxidil (Rogaine)
Inotropic Drugs (Increase Contractility)	
Cardiac glycosides	Digitoxin (Crystodigin) Digoxin (Lanoxin) Deslanoside (Cedilanid)
β-Adrenergics	Dobutamine (Dobutrex) Dopamine (Intropin) Isoproterenol (Isuprel)
Phosphodiesterase inhibitors	Amrinone (Inocor)
Neurohormonal Modulators	
β-Blocking agents	Metoprolol (Lopressor) Bisoprolol (Zebeta) Carvedilol (Coreg)
Angiotensin-converting enzyme inhibitors	Captopril (Capoten) Enalapril (Vasotec) Lisinopril (Zestril) Quinapril (Accupril) Ramipril (Altace)
Angiotensin receptor blockers	Losartan (Cozaar) Candesartan (Atacand)

Despite the large number of agents being used in the management of CHF, only a few have been associated with significant improvement in mortality risk, particularly ACE inhibitors and certain β-blockers.[10] A clearer understanding of the underlying molecular mechanisms of CHF is needed to improve pharmacologic management. Little research has been conducted to determine the best treatment for patients with primarily diastolic failure, and treatment recommendations are similar.[3]

Management of Preload

CHF is generally associated with an elevated preload due to an expanded intravascular volume and a reduced EF. According to the Frank-Starling law, an elevated preload is desirable because it will enhance systolic shortening and improve cardiac output. Unfortunately, high preload exacerbates congestive symptoms and adds to the work of an already damaged heart. The aim of therapy, then, is to optimize preload such that congestive symptoms are minimized but cardiac output is not compromised. The right ventricle is particularly sensitive to reductions in preload, and care must be taken to avoid a significant drop in right ventricular output when intravascular volume is decreased.

Several drugs may be administered to reduce intravascular volume, including diuretics and ACE inhibitors. Patients may be instructed to modify salt and fluid intake as well. Diuretics promote the excretion of fluid by increasing renal blood flow, blocking sodium and chloride reabsorption, or both. Drugs that inhibit enzymes that convert angiotensin I (inactive) to angiotensin II (active) are called ACE inhibitors. The fact that the kidney may continue to produce renin has little effect because angiotensin II and aldosterone production is blocked. Preload may also be reduced by redistribution of blood volume within the vascular system. Drugs that cause venous dilation and peripheral pooling of blood can effectively reduce preload. The BNP normally synthesized by the heart in response to volume overload has been manufactured into a drug called nesiritide. Nesiritide is administered intravenously and is a potent diuretic and antagonist of the renin-angiotensin-aldosterone system.[12] It may be used in the hospitalized patient to reduce preload and afterload. In acute congestive syndromes, such as pulmonary edema, phlebotomy (blood removal) may also be performed.

When patients are in a state of severe cardiac compromise, it may be necessary to plot a cardiac function curve to determine the optimal preload. This is accomplished by measuring cardiac output while manipulating preload with preload reducers (diuretics, venodilators) or preload enhancers (volume loading). The lowest preload that achieves an adequate cardiac output is the desired point of function.

Management of Afterload

Afterload represents the resistance against which the ventricle must pump and is an important determinant of myocardial energy consumption. Afterload may be inappropriately high in heart failure because of primary hypertension, elevated angiotensin II, or SNS activation. As mentioned previously, diminished stroke volume is detected by the aortic and carotid baroreceptors, which results in sympathetic activation. Sympathetic stimulation of the arterioles causes them to constrict, thus increasing vascular resistance, arterial blood pressure, and ventricular afterload.

Drugs that cause arteriolar dilation may be used to decrease left ventricular afterload (see Table 19-3). Arteriolar dilation is accomplished by inducing relaxation of vascular smooth muscle cells by decreasing calcium ions in the cytosol. Calcium entry into vascular smooth muscle cells can be blocked by calcium channel–blocking drugs (e.g., nifedipine) or by inhibition of vasoconstrictive neurotransmitters and peptides. Nitrates increase the production of the vasodilator substance nitric oxide. Afterload reduction improves cardiac output but may precipitate hypotension in some patients. Some of these agents have additional effects on venous smooth muscle and cardiac muscle and may reduce preload and myocardial contractility. Careful assessment is required to optimally reduce afterload while avoiding excessive reductions in preload or contractility.

In addition to drug therapy, afterload can be reduced mechanically with the intraaortic balloon pump (Figure 19-12).[14] This treatment is invasive, associated with several potential complications, and generally reserved for severe cases of left ventricular failure. A catheter with a balloon at the end is inserted, usually through the femoral artery, into the descending aorta. A machine outside the body intermittently inflates and deflates the balloon in time with cardiac contractions. During ventricular systole, the balloon is quickly deflated, which creates a vacuum effect in the aorta, reduces ventricular afterload, and promotes ventricular emptying. In addition to improving cardiac output by reducing afterload, the intraaortic balloon pump also reduces myocardial strain and improves perfusion of the coronary arteries. Coronary blood flow is enhanced during diastole when the balloon is quickly inflated, raising the driving pressure for flow through the coronary arteries. In some cases, increased coronary blood flow may improve the availability of myocardial ATP and increase contractility.

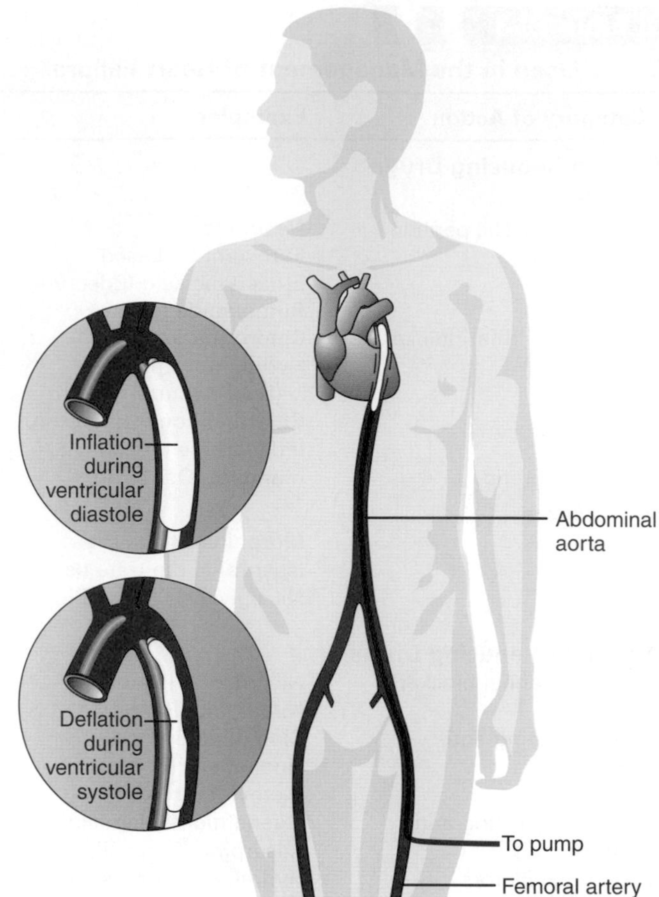

FIGURE 19-12 ■ Schematic diagram of an intraaortic balloon pump positioned in the aorta. The balloon deflates during ventricular systole to aid left ventricular emptying by reducing afterload. The balloon inflates during ventricular diastole to increase aortic diastolic pressure and improve coronary artery perfusion.

Management of Contractility

Improvements in contractility are achieved primarily through drug therapy and efforts to optimize oxygen and nutrient delivery to compromised myocardial cells. Contractility refers to the rate and extent of force generated by the ventricle during systole and is not dependent on preload.[8] Contractility is enhanced by measures that increase the availability of ATP and intracellular calcium during systole. The synthesis of sufficient ATP depends primarily on the adequacy of myocardial perfusion and oxygenation. Oxygen administration and evaluation of the hemoglobin level may be employed to support oxygen delivery. If ischemia is thought to be surgically correctable, coronary artery bypass may be considered.

When improving cardiac output is necessary to avoid shock, positive inotropic agents may be used. However, long-term use of positive inotropic agents may be associated with increased mortality. Positive inotropes work by increasing the availability of intracellular calcium ions during systole. These drugs include sympathomimetic agents, digitalis, and phosphodiesterase inhibitors. Drugs that mimic SNS effects, such as norepinephrine, isoproterenol, and dopamine, may be used to improve cardiac output but have a high potential for imposing excessive afterload and dramatically increasing myocardial oxygen consumption. Dobutamine is a drug that enhances contractility but does not increase afterload and may be better tolerated.

Digitalis or a related cardiac glycoside is the usual treatment of choice for the long-term management of severe heart failure. Cardiac glycosides directly inhibit the sodium-potassium pump present in the cell membrane of all cells. This results in an increase in intracellular sodium accumulation and a decrease in the gradient for sodium entry into the

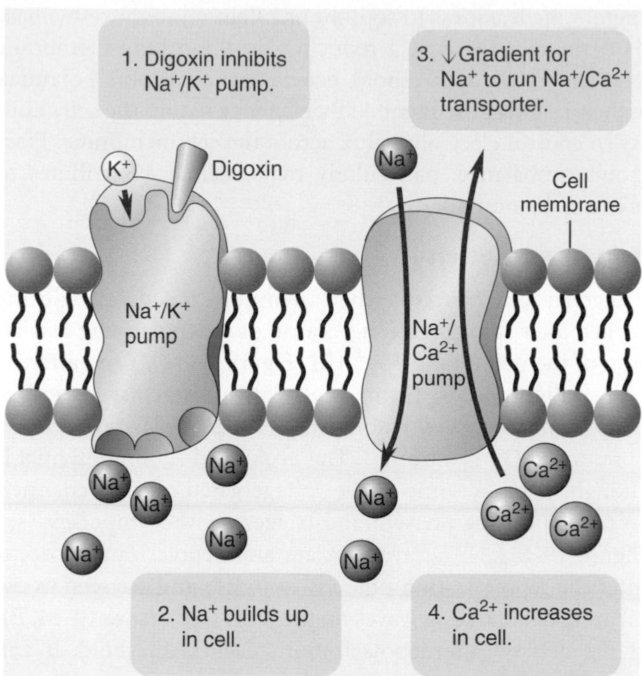

FIGURE 19-13 ■ A section of cardiac muscle cell membrane showing the effects of digoxin on the Na^+-K^+ pump, resulting in accumulation of intracellular sodium and less efficient Ca^{2+} extrusion. Digitalis competes with K^+ for the K^+ binding site on the Na^+-K^+ pump. Thus, a low serum K^+ can increase the effect of the drug.

cell (Figure 19-13). A diminished sodium gradient slows the sodium-dependent calcium pump that normally removes intracellular calcium. This allows more calcium to remain in the cell, thus strengthening myocardial contraction. Digitalis also slows the heart rate through parasympathetic system activation and promotes sodium and water excretion through improved cardiac output to the kidney. Dangerous side effects from digitalis toxicity may occur because inhibition of sodium-potassium pumps in cells throughout the body can disrupt ion balance, cellular volume control, and nerve and muscle transmission. Depletion of serum potassium (hypokalemia) may potentiate digitalis toxicity (see Figure 19-13). Unlike the other positive inotropic agents, digitalis does not appear to increase mortality.[15]

Neurohormonal Modulators

Numerous clinical trials have documented a reduced mortality risk of about 30% in heart failure patients treated with ACE inhibitors. The ACE inhibitors are indicated in all heart failure patients as standard therapy. Those who do not tolerate ACE inhibitors because of cough may benefit from angiotensin receptor blockers (ARBs). In addition, some studies have shown additional benefit with drugs that block aldosterone activity.[6] The β-blocking agents have been studied in large clinical trials of heart failure patients and found to decrease mortality by about 30%.[6,7] The patients in these studies were already on ACE inhibitors or ARBs. Because of their potential negative inotropic effects, beginning doses are small and are increased incrementally up to recommended cardioprotective doses. Patients who are unstable, volume overloaded, or experiencing heart block should be stabilized prior to β blockade.

Cardiac Resynchronization

Patients with enlarged hearts and conduction delays may benefit from pacemakers, which help to synchronize ventricular contraction. A wide QRS complex is the usual indication for resynchronization therapy in the CHF patient. Pacing electrodes are placed in the atrium and both ventricles to allow coordinated depolarization of the heart muscle. Many patients experience significant improvement in congestive symptoms and activity tolerance with resynchronization.

Future Therapies

The current view of heart failure progression implicates a high rate of myocardial cell apoptosis as a significant factor. Although recent evidence suggests that new myocardial cells are produced by stem cells in the heart, the rate of cell death outstrips the rate of production. New therapies may target stem cells to improve their replicative capacity or find ways to block apoptotic mechanisms. More research into heart failure pathophysiologic processes and treatment is needed to address the current dismal outlook for heart failure outcomes.

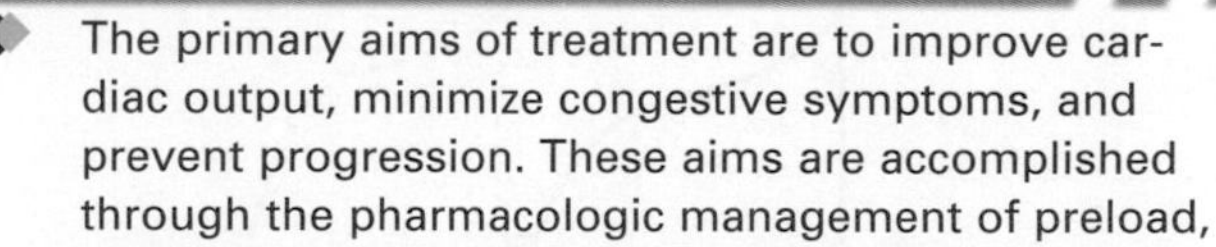

- The primary aims of treatment are to improve cardiac output, minimize congestive symptoms, and prevent progression. These aims are accomplished through the pharmacologic management of preload, afterload, contractility, and neurohormones.
- Diuretics and venodilators are used to alleviate congestion by reducing preload. Preload reduction must be approached cautiously to avoid a reduction in cardiac output.
- Sympathetic antagonists, ACE inhibitors, nitrates, and direct vasodilators are used to decrease cardiac workload by reducing afterload. Excessive reductions in blood pressure must be avoided.
- Myocardial contractility may be improved by measures that increase oxygen delivery to the heart. In addition, positive inotropic drugs such as digitalis and β agonists may be used to improve contractility.
- ACE inhibitors and some β-blocking agents have been shown to improve mortality risk in patients with CHF and should be considered for all patients.
- Resynchronization of ventricular depolarization with pacemakers may improve contraction in patients with wide QRS complexes.

CARDIAC DYSRHYTHMIAS

Dysrhythmia or arrhythmia refers to an abnormality of the cardiac rhythm of impulse generation and conduction. A normal heartbeat is initiated in the sinoatrial (SA) node and follows a consistent pathway of depolarization through the atria, atrioventricular (AV) node, His-Purkinje system, and, finally, the ventricular myocardium (see Chapter 17). Electrical depolarization of the heart is normally followed by atrial and then ventricular muscular contraction. A number of factors may lead to disturbances in heartbeat, including hypoxia, electrolyte imbalance, trauma, inflammation, and drugs. Dysrhythmias are significant for two reasons: (1) they indicate an underlying pathophysiologic disorder and (2) they can disrupt normal cardiac output. Dysrhythmias can be categorized into three major types: abnormal rates of sinus rhythm, abnormal sites (ectopic) of impulse initiation, or disturbances in conduction pathways.

Dysrhythmia Mechanisms

Atrial and ventricular dysrhythmias are believed to arise from three mechanisms: inappropriate automaticity, triggered activity, or reentrant mechanisms.

Automaticity

Inappropriate automaticity implies that an atrial or ventricular cell that is normally incapable of spontaneous depolarization acquires the ability to initiate action potentials. Plasma membrane leakiness to sodium or calcium ions at rest (phase 4) is thought to cause a reduction in the resting membrane potential toward threshold generating an action potential. Ischemia and subsequent ATP deficiency reduce the cell's ability to control electrolyte flux across the cell membrane. Electrolyte imbalance, particularly hypokalemia, contributes to abnormal automaticity.

Triggered Activity

Triggered activity occurs when an impulse is generated during or just after repolarization because of a depolarizing oscillation of the membrane potential (Figure 19-14). Early afterdepolarizations occur during the relative refractory period of phase 3 in patients with abnormally long repolarization times (prolonged QT syndrome). The prolonged action potential is thought to allow some of the voltage-gated calcium channels to reopen during phase 3 and trigger another impulse[16] (see Figure 19-14, *A*). Delayed or late afterdepolarizations occur after the repolarization phase is complete and are seen as oscillating depolarizing waves on the ECG (see Figure 19-14, *B*). If the delayed afterdepolarization reaches threshold, it will trigger an action potential. Digitalis toxicity and excessive catecholamine stimulation may contribute to this disorder. Delayed afterdepolarizations are thought to occur because calcium ions are ineffectively removed from the cytoplasm during muscle relaxation. An increase in Ca^{2+} during phase 4 can trigger release of more Ca^{2+} from the sarcoplasmic reticulum and trigger an action potential.[16]

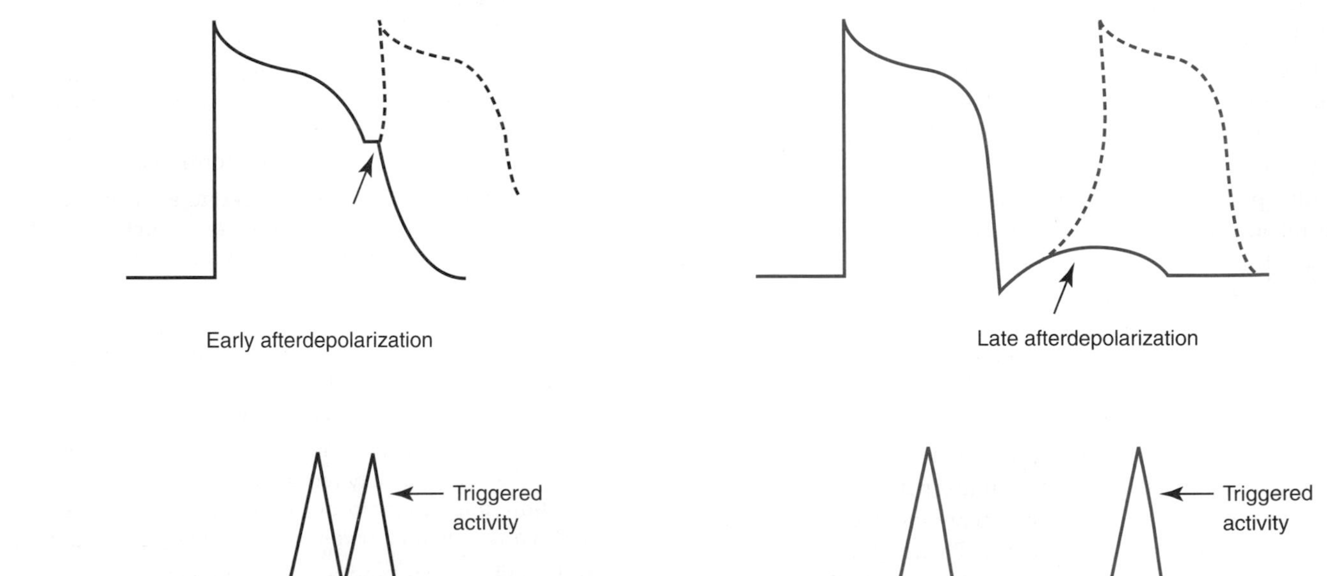

FIGURE 19-14 ■ Mechanisms of triggered activity. **A,** Early afterdepolarization in ventricular cell showing triggered action potential during the repolarization phase. The electrocardiogram *(ECG)* shows an R wave occurring on top of the T wave (R-on-T phenomenon). **B,** Late or delayed afterdepolarization occurs after the repolarization phase has been completed and results in an early beat after the T wave. If the late afterdepolarization does not reach threshold, no triggered beat will occur.

Reentry

Reentry is thought to be the culprit in most dysrhythmias. Reentry is a complex process in which a cardiac impulse continues to depolarize in a part of the heart after the main impulse has finished its path and the majority of the fibers have repolarized. If the errant impulse proceeds slowly enough, it may eventually meet with nonrefractory cells and initiate an extra, ectopic cardiac depolarization. Reentry processes are produced when electrical conduction in a portion of the heart is abnormally slowed (functional) or has an unusually long pathway (anatomic). Reentry depolarizations usually occur as complex spiral waves in which the activating wavefront follows or "chases" its repolarizing tail (Figure 19-15). If the wavefront encounters only refractory tissue, the reentrant process suddenly terminates.[17] Myocardial ischemia and electrolyte abnormalities predispose to reentry mechanisms.

Dysrhythmia Analysis

ECG recording paper is specifically designed to allow easy measurement of waveform amplitude and duration (Figure 19-16). Each small box on the ECG paper represents an amplitude of 0.1 mV and a duration of 0.04 second (paper speed at 25 mm/sec).[18] Larger boxes are also marked on the paper and correspond to 0.5 mV in amplitude (five small boxes) and 0.2 second in duration (five small boxes). These markings allow measurement of waveform amplitude, duration, and heart rate. Rhythm strips presented in this chapter are from a single lead only (usually lead II), but it should be emphasized

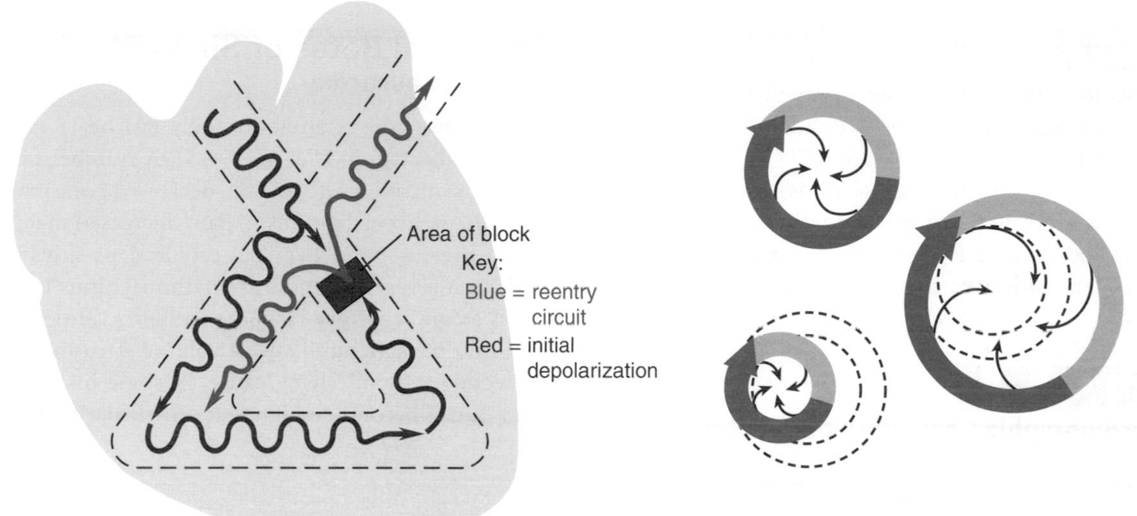

FIGURE 19-15 ■ Mechanism of reentry. **A,** A wave of depolarization that travels slowly or by an abnormal pathway may encounter myocardium that has had time to recover and can restimulate it. **B,** This may result in an extra beat, or the depolarization may continuously "chase its tail" in a circuit, causing defibrillation. The circuit can be relatively fixed or can wander into various "wavelets."

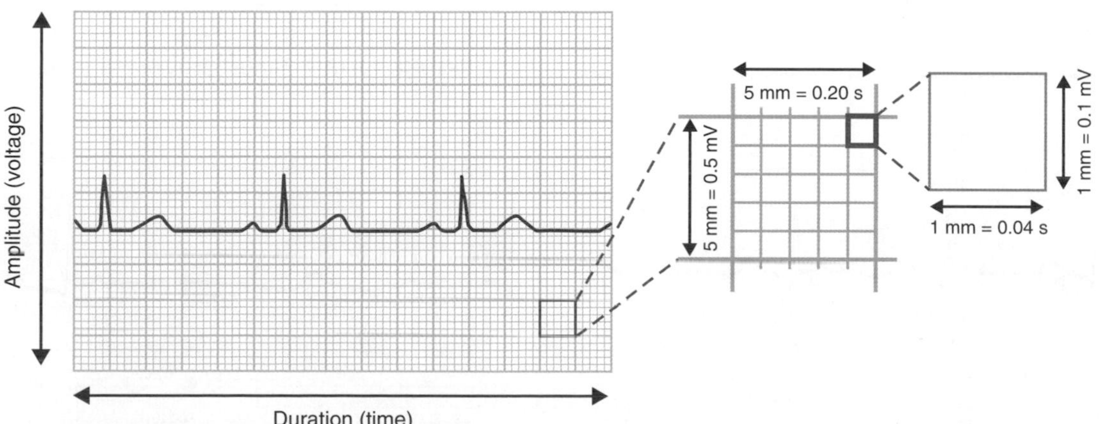

FIGURE 19-16 ■ Electrocardiographic strip showing the markings for measuring amplitude and duration of waveforms, using a standard recording speed of 25 mm/sec.

that thorough ECG interpretation often requires several leads to provide different views of electrical conduction through the heart. (Lead placement is discussed in Chapter 17.)

Normal Sinus Rhythm

Before one proceeds to the interpretation of dysrhythmias, the features of normal sinus rhythm must be understood. Normal sinus rhythm is generally defined as an impulse rate between 60 and 100 per minute that begins in the sinus node and follows the normal conduction pathway. Characteristics of normal sinus rhythm are listed in Table 19-4. The rhythm shown in Figure 19-17 is regular; there is a P wave for every QRS complex; the PR, QRS, and QT intervals are of normal duration; and there are no "funny-looking" beats.

There are several methods for figuring heart rate using the rhythm strip. The easiest but least accurate method is to count the number of QRS complexes within 6 seconds and multiply by 10. Electrocardiogram (ECG) paper has 3-second marks along the top that can be used to determine a 6-second interval. A more accurate method for determining heart rate is to count the number of small boxes between complexes. The number of boxes is divided by 1500 to determine heart rate because there are 1500 small boxes per minute (1500 × 0.04 second = 60 seconds). Neither of these methods is accurate with irregular rhythms, so heart rate must be calculated for a longer interval, usually 1 minute. With this understanding of rate calculation and methods to measure the duration and amplitude of waveforms, one can analyze dysrhythmias.

Table 19-4

Electrocardiographic Characteristics of Normal Sinus Rhythm

Characteristic	Findings
Rhythm	Regular, PP intervals and R-R intervals may vary as much as 3 mm and still be considered regular
Rate	60-100 beats/min
P waves	One P wave preceding each QRS
PR interval	0.12-0.20 second, constant
QRS duration	0.04-0.10 second, constant
QT interval	0.40 second (varies with rate)

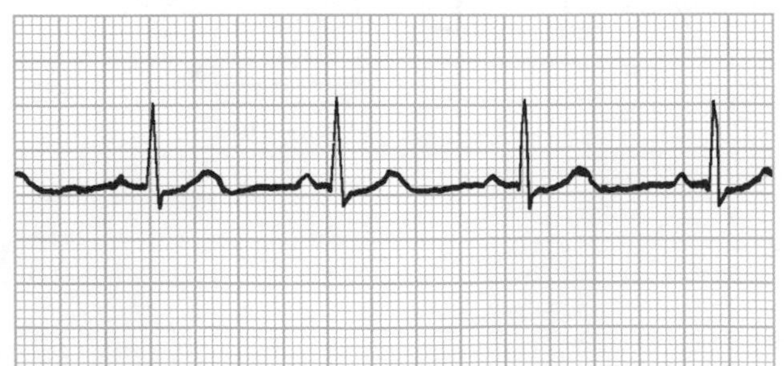

FIGURE 19-17 ■ Normal sinus rhythm (rate, 64/min).

KEY CONCEPTS

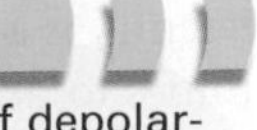

- Dysrhythmias are initiated by three types of depolarizing mechanisms: abnormal automaticity, triggered activity from afterdepolarizations, and reentrant circuits.
- Measurement of ECG waveform amplitude, duration, and frequency is necessary to analyze cardiac rhythms. ECG paper is marked in small boxes representing 0.1 mV of amplitude and 0.04 second of duration.
- Normal sinus rhythm is characterized by regular PP and RR intervals, a rate of 60 to 100 beats/min, and normal PR (0.12 to 0.20 second) and QRS (0.04 to 0.10 second) intervals.

Abnormal Rates of Sinus Rhythm

Sinus Tachycardia

Sinus tachycardia is an abnormally fast heart rate of greater than 100 beats/min (Figure 19-18). A number of factors, including sympathetic activation, decreased parasympathetic activity, fever, hyperthyroidism, pain, increased metabolism, low blood pressure, and hypoxia, can lead to sinus tachycardia, making it a very common dysrhythmia. Sinus tachycardia often is a compensatory response to increased demand for cardiac output or reduced stroke volume. Treatment is aimed at correcting the underlying cause. In some instances, however, the rate can become so high that ventricular filling is impaired

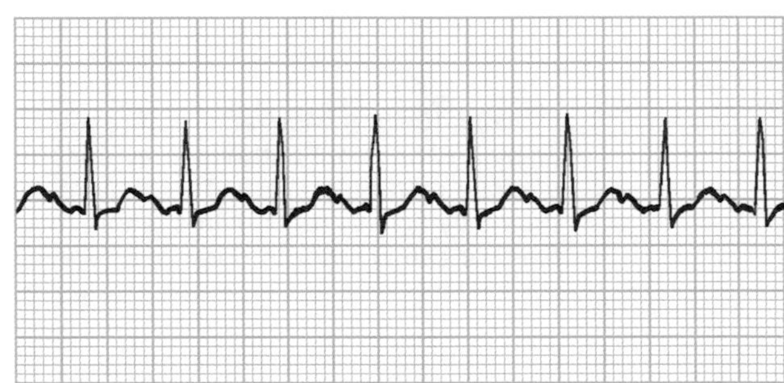

FIGURE 19-18 ■ Sinus tachycardia (rate, 150/min).

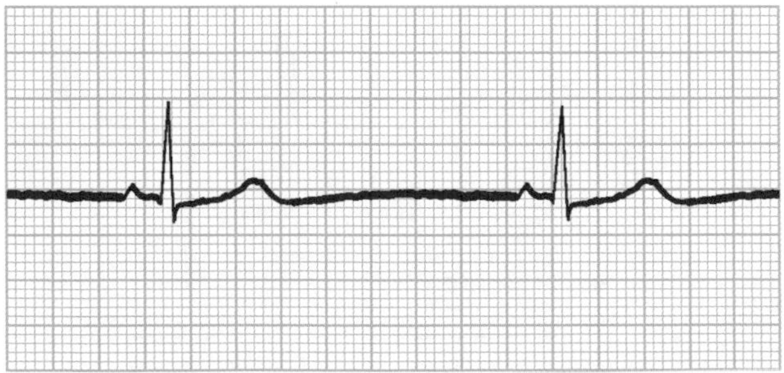

FIGURE 19-19 ■ Sinus bradycardia (rate, 35/min).

and cardiac output is compromised. Sympatholytic agents or calcium channel–blocking agents may then be indicated.

Sinus Bradycardia

Traditionally a heart rate of less than 60 beats/min is called *bradycardia;* however, lower rates are commonly encountered in physically trained individuals. Sinus bradycardia results from slowed impulse generation by the sinus node in response to parasympathetic activity, sleep, drugs, increased stroke volume, or acute hypertension (baroreceptor reflex). Important features of sinus bradycardia are shown in Figure 19-19. Sinus bradycardia may be a normal finding in well-conditioned individuals who have large resting stroke volumes. Abnormal parasympathetic activation can result from pain (vasovagal), carotid sinus massage, endotracheal suctioning, and the Valsalva maneuver (bearing down). Slow heart rates may be well tolerated by some individuals and not require treatment. If the slow heart rate precipitates low cardiac output, it is usually treated with sympathomimetic or parasympatholytic drugs.

Sinus Arrhythmia

A degree of variability in the heart rate, or sinus arrhythmia, is a normal finding associated with fluctuations in autonomic influences and respiratory dynamics. Sinus arrhythmia can be particularly pronounced in children. Sinus arrhythmia must be differentiated from a sinus node irregularity called *sick sinus syndrome,* in which alternating periods of sinus bradycardia and tachycardia occur (Figure 19-20). Sick sinus syndrome may necessitate implantation of a permanent pacemaker. Sinus arrhythmia is a normal finding and thus requires no treatment.

Sinus Arrest

The absence of impulse initiation in the heart results in electrical *asystole.* It is characterized by a flat ECG lacking recognizable waveforms (Figure 19-21). Electrical asystole results in mechanical asystole and zero cardiac output. An escape rhythm from a slower pacemaker will generally begin to fire after several seconds of sinus arrest. Sinus arrest may result from MI, electrical shock, electrolyte disturbances, acidosis, and extreme parasympathetic activity. Prolonged complete electrical asystole is unlikely, and fine ventricular fibrillation may be the underlying rhythm. Sinus arrest may be treatable with a cardiac pacemaker.

KEY CONCEPTS 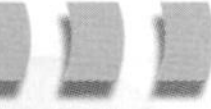

- Sinus tachycardia (more than 100 beats/min) usually occurs from sympathetic activation of the heart. SNS activation may be compensatory (e.g., occurring in

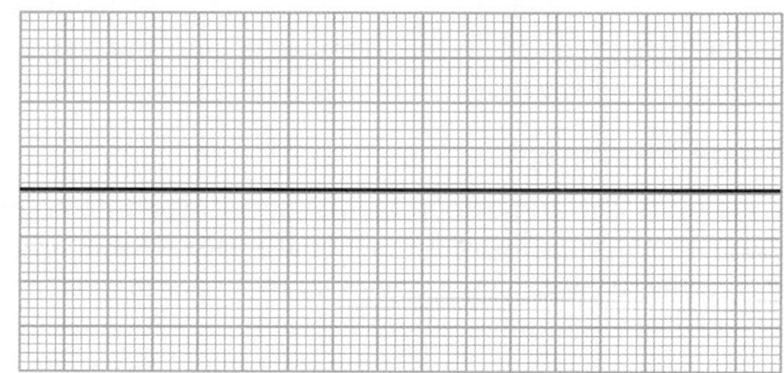

FIGURE 19-21 ■ Electrical asystole.

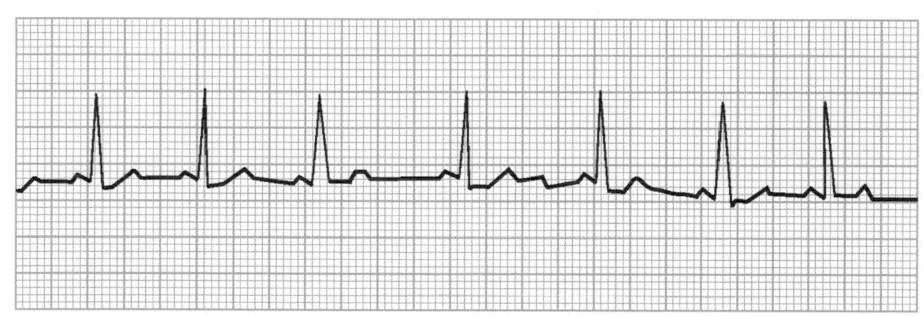

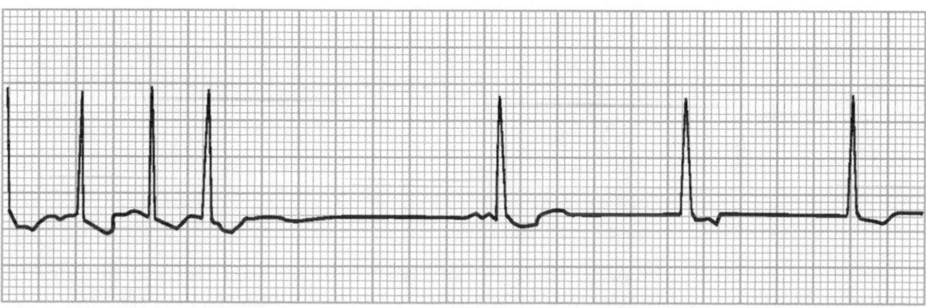

FIGURE 19-20 ■ **A,** Sinus arrhythmia is a normal finding that may be particularly pronounced in children. **B,** Sick sinus syndrome. Strips show alternating periods of tachycardia and bradycardia.

the setting of low blood pressure, low cardiac output, or hypoxemia) or may be due to pain and anxiety.

- Sinus bradycardia (less than 60 beats/min) usually occurs in response to parasympathetic activity. Bradycardia is treated if the slow heart rate precipitates inadequate cardiac output.
- Sinus arrhythmia is usually normal and more pronounced in young persons than in older adults.
- Sinus arrest may lead to prolonged intervals of electrical asystole and zero stroke volume until another pacemaker begins to fire. An artificial pacemaker may be required.

Abnormal Site of Impulse Initiation

Initiation of a cardiac impulse at a site other than the SA node occurs primarily for two reasons. First, SA node failure may allow a slower pacemaker to take over. Takeover by a slower pacemaker is called an *escape rhythm.* Second, enhanced excitability, triggered activity, or reentrant circuits may cause a premature depolarization and override the SA node.

Escape Rhythms

Escape beats can originate in the AV nodal region or in the ventricular Purkinje fibers. A junctional escape rhythm originates in the AV node, has a rate of 40 to 60 per minute, and has a normal QRS configuration (Figure 19-22). A ventricular escape rhythm originates in the Purkinje fibers, has a rate of 15 to 40, and is characterized by an abnormally wide QRS complex on the ECG (Figure 19-23). An important clue to identifying escape rhythms is the absence of normal P waves and PR intervals. After the impulse is generated in the Purkinje or nodal cell, it can be conducted backward to the atria. Thus, a P wave, if present, may be inverted and located before, during, or after the QRS complex. Escape rhythms are usually poorly tolerated because they are slow and associated with decreased cardiac output. Failure of the sinus node can be managed with a pacemaker.

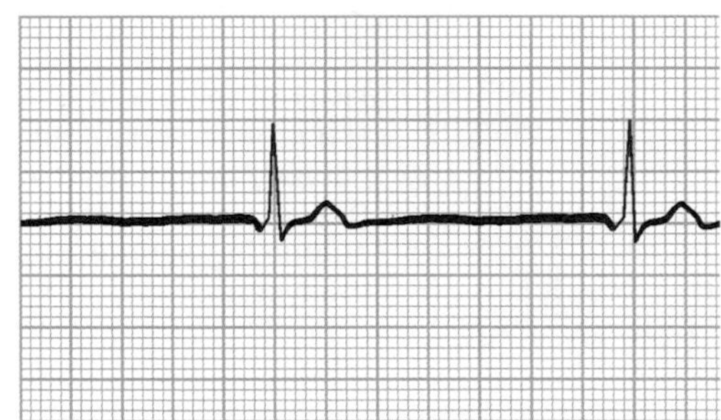

FIGURE 19-22 ■ Junctional escape rhythm (rate, 59/min).

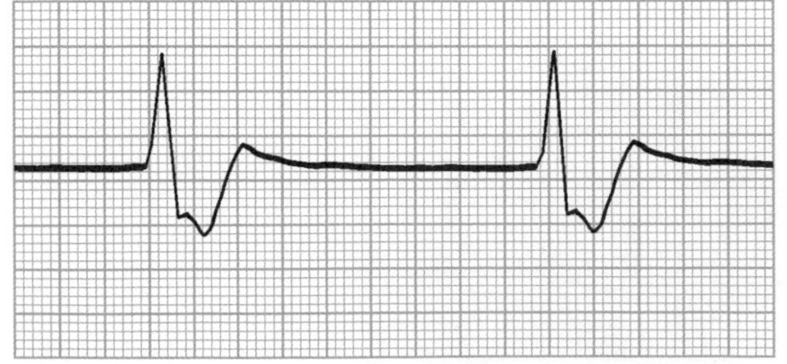

FIGURE 19-23 ■ Ventricular escape rhythm (rate, 33/min).

Atrial Dysrhythmias

Premature Atrial Complexes and Tachycardia. Premature atrial complexes (PACs) originate in the atria but not at the SA node. The PAC occurs earlier than normal, is preceded by a P wave, and has a normal QRS configuration (Figure 19-24). P waves preceding the PAC usually have a different shape (morphology) than the sinus beats. Sometimes the PAC is not conducted through the AV node to the ventricle and is not followed by a QRS complex (nonconducted P wave). Isolated or rare PACs are not clinically significant. However, frequent PACs may indicate an underlying pathophysiologic process and may be precursors to more serious dysrhythmias. Paroxysmal focal atrial tachycardia is a burst of atrial complexes resembling several PACs in a row (Figure 19-25). The rhythm is regular at a usual rate of 130 to 240 beats/min. It may be difficult to distinguish this rhythm from sinus tachycardia; however, differences in P-wave configuration are usually apparent. The period of atrial tachycardia may last for minutes, hours, or days and can result in ischemia. Focal atrial tachycar-

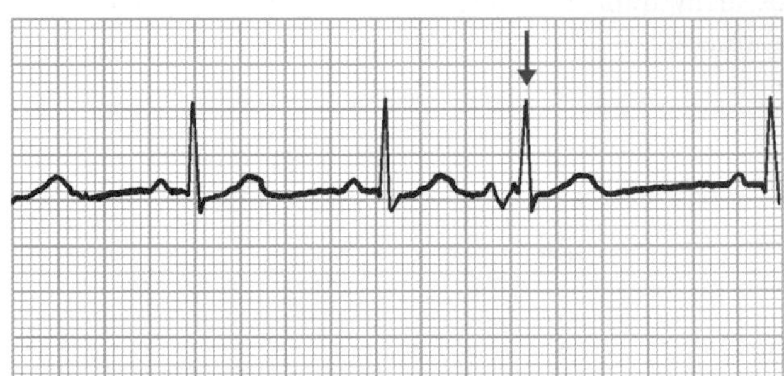

FIGURE 19-24 ■ Premature atrial complex *(arrow).* Note early P wave and different P-wave morphology.

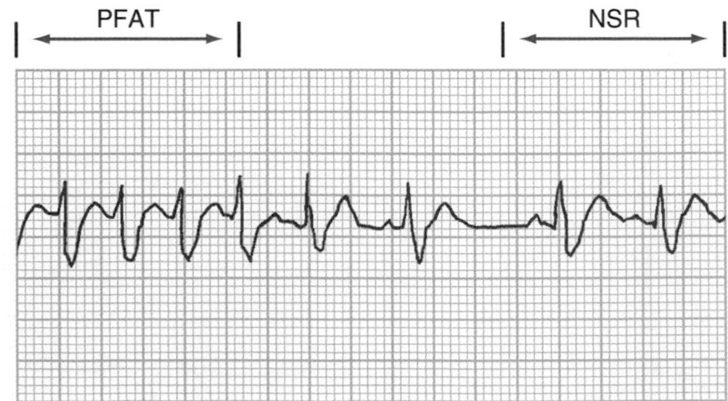

FIGURE 19-25 ■ Paroxysmal focal atrial tachycardia *(PFAT)* followed by transition to normal sinus rhythm *(NSR).*

dia can occur in persons with no underlying heart disease in response to emotional stress or drugs. An episode may start as a PAC that has an abnormally slow conduction time through the atria and AV node. This is thought to allow the wave of depolarization to reexcite previously depolarized cells, resulting in reentry and perpetuation of the abnormal rhythm.

Atrial Flutter and Fibrillation. **Atrial flutter** is typically manifested by a rapid atrial rate of 240 to 350 beats/min and a characteristic sawtooth pattern of atrial depolarizations (Figure 19-26). There is overlap in the mechanism of atrial tachycardia and atrial flutter and several types of flutter have been described. These are commonly categorized according to atrial rate; type I (typical) has rates of 240 to 350 per minute and type II has rates in excess of 350 per minute. The QRS configuration is normal; however, some of the atrial depolarizations may not conduct through the AV node, resulting in a slower ventricular rate. The ventricular rate may be irregular if there is a variable block or may be regular if there is a uniform block, such as 2:1 or 3:1. Reentry is the probable mechanism for typical atrial flutter. Persons exhibiting atrial flutter usually have underlying heart disease, fluid overload, or atrial ischemia.

Atrial fibrillation is a completely disorganized and irregular atrial rhythm accompanied by an irregular ventricular rhythm of variable rate (Figure 19-27). The atrial impulses appear as small, squiggly waves of various sizes and shapes. Atrial fibrillation is sustained by multiple reentrant "wavelets" that continually change in size and direction. The majority of atrial depolarizations are blocked at the AV node, with few reaching the ventricles and initiating ventricular contraction. Atrial fibrillation causes the atria to quiver rather than to contract forcefully. This allows blood to become stagnant in the atria and may lead to formation of thrombi. Atrial fibrillation may occur intermittently or be sustained in the long term. Patients with chronic atrial fibrillation often are treated with anticoagulant medications to prevent atrial clot formation. Atrial fibrillation is a significant risk factor for cerebrovascular stroke. Patients with heart failure may experience more symptoms when they are in atrial fibrillation because the usual "atrial kick" that normally adds 15% to 20% more blood to the ventricle prior to systole is lost and therefore cardiac output may be reduced. Cardioversion with an electrical shock to the chest is commonly used to manage atrial fibrillation. Numerous antiarrhythmic agents can be used to convert atrial fibrillation to sinus rhythm or control the ventricular response rate, including calcium channel blockers, β-blockers, digitalis, and amiodarone.

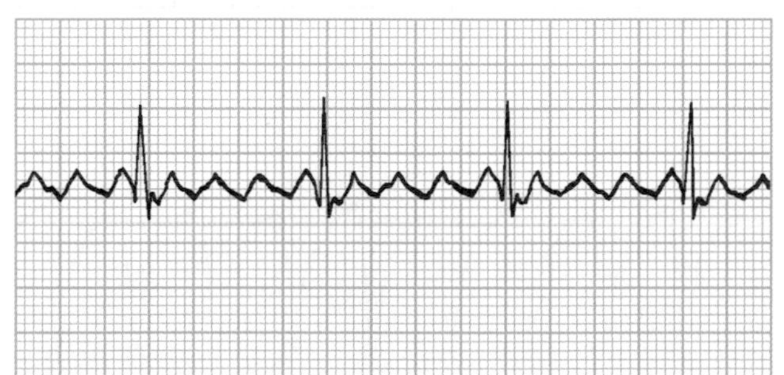

FIGURE 19-26 ■ Atrial flutter with four atrial depolarizations to one ventricular depolarization.

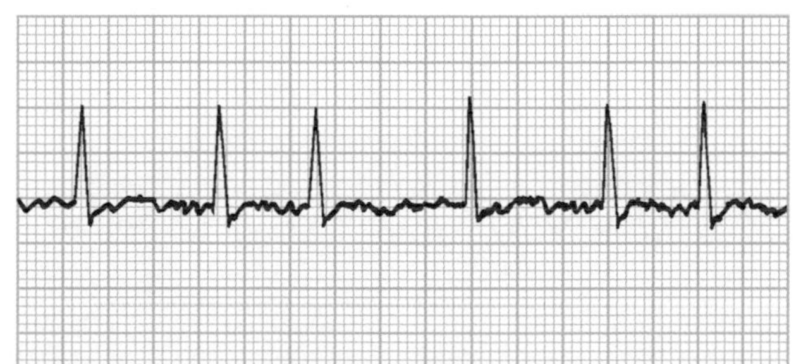

FIGURE 19-27 ■ Atrial fibrillation showing an irregularly irregular ventricular response.

Junctional Dysrhythmias

Premature junctional complexes can be initiated in two junctional zones: in the area just proximal to the AV node, where atrial fibers enter, or in the area just distal to the AV node, where nodal fibers enter the bundle of His. The impulse spreads upward into the atrium, causing a P wave, and downward into the ventricle, causing a normally configured QRS complex. The P wave may precede, follow, or be buried in the QRS complex. Premature junctional beats have the same clinical significance as PACs and are generally well tolerated.

Junctional tachycardia is a rapid junctional discharge in the range of 70 to 140 beats/min (Figure 19-28). The rhythm resembles a series of junctional premature beats, with P waves preceding, following, or buried in the QRS complexes. Differentiation of the electrocardiographic pattern produced by junctional tachycardia from that produced by atrial tachycardia is often difficult, and the term "supraventricular tachycardia" may be used for both.

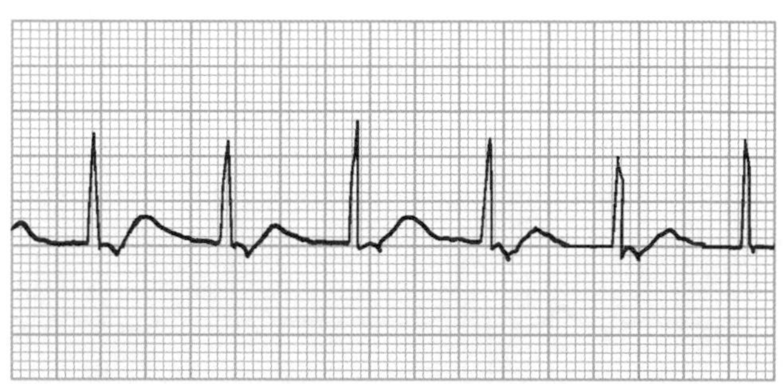

FIGURE 19-28 ■ Junctional tachycardia (rate, 108/min). Note that P waves follow the QRS waves because of retrograde depolarization spreading from the atrioventricular node to the atria. This rhythm may also be called *supraventricular tachycardia.*

Ventricular Dysrhythmias

Premature Ventricular Complexes. Premature ventricular complexes (PVCs) arise from the ventricular myocardium. The impulse depolarizes the ventricles but does not activate the atria or depolarize the sinus node. Thus, the normal rhythm of sinus discharge is not disturbed. The normal sinus impulse is generally buried in the bizarre-looking QRS from the premature ventricular beat. The sinus impulse does not result in a QRS complex because the ventricles are refractory from the premature depolarization. The next sinus beat occurs just when it would have occurred normally if there had been no premature beat. Thus, the interval between the sinus beat preceding and the sinus beat following the premature beat is twice the regular interval (Figure 19-29). This is known as a "compensatory pause" and helps confirm the diagnosis of PVCs. The QRS of the premature complex is prolonged (more than 0.10 second) and bizarre in appearance. The T wave is usually in a direction opposite to the main QRS deflection. Premature ventricular beats are commonly associated with coronary artery disease, drug overdose, and electrolyte disturbances—particularly hypokalemia and hypomagnesemia. The clinical significance depends in part on the frequency of the premature beats. With high frequency, cardiac output may be compromised. Frequent PVCs may be managed with antiarrhythmic drugs, such as amiodarone. However, prophylactic use of antiarrhythmic drugs in patients with asymptomatic disease is not recommended. In some groups (e.g., after MI), certain antiarrhythmics have been linked to higher mortality.[17]

Ventricular Tachycardia. Ventricular tachycardia consists of three or more consecutive ventricular complexes at a rate greater than 100/min (Figure 19-30). The rhythm is fairly regular and the complexes generally have the same configuration (monomorphic). With rapid rates, it may be difficult to distinguish the QRS complexes from the ST segments and T waves, and the ECG depicts a series of large, wide, undulating waves. The sinus node usually continues to discharge independently of the ventricular rhythm, and P waves, if seen, are not associated with the QRS complexes.

Reentry is the probable mechanism of ventricular tachycardia in most cases, although automaticity and triggered activity have also been implicated. Ventricular tachycardia is often associated with myocardial ischemia and infarction. Damage to the myocardium alters conduction times and conduction pathways, which sets the stage for reentry loops. High catecholamine levels and an abnormal electrolyte balance may contribute to the dysrhythmogenesis.

Ventricular tachycardia is a serious dysrhythmia that is nearly always indicative of significant heart disease. It may be fatal unless it is successfully and rapidly managed. Ventricular tachycardia may compromise cardiac output, resulting in loss of consciousness. Treatment consists of administration of antiarrhythmic drugs and, if necessary, cardiopulmonary resuscitation and administration of 10 to 100 joules (J) of electrical current to the chest (cardioversion).

Ventricular Fibrillation. Ventricular fibrillation is a rapid, uncoordinated cardiac rhythm that results in ventricular quivering and lack of effective contraction. The rhythm is generally easily identified, particularly when assessment of the patient indicates absence of pulse and loss of consciousness. The ECG is rapid and erratic, with no identifiable QRS complexes (Figure 19-31). Ventricular fibrillation results in death if not reversed within minutes.

The same conditions that result in ventricular tachycardia may cause ventricular fibrillation. A critically timed premature beat or accelerating ventricular tachycardia may be the precursor to ventricular fibrillation. The ventricular depolarization is thought to be fractionated into a number of localized reentrant currents within the myocardial mass. The uncoordinated depolarizations are sustained because of variability in conduction velocities and refractory periods.

Ventricular fibrillation must be rapidly identified and managed with cardiopulmonary resuscitation and defibrillation with electrical current. Defibrillation differs from car-

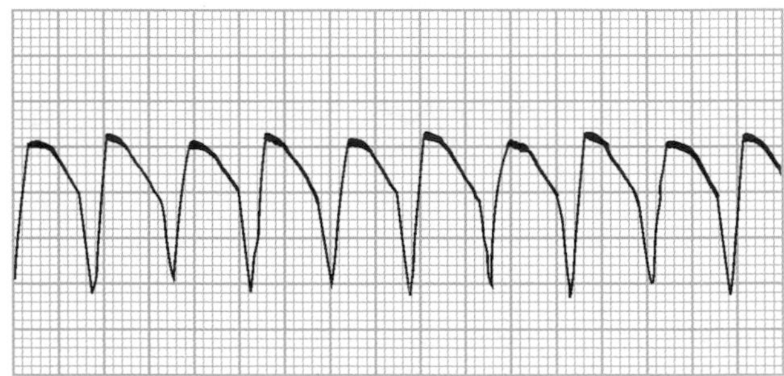

FIGURE 19-30 ■ Ventricular tachycardia (rate, 178/min).

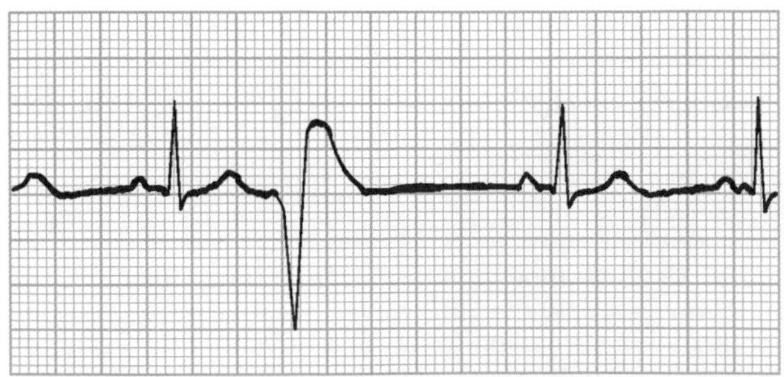

FIGURE 19-29 ■ Premature ventricular complex.

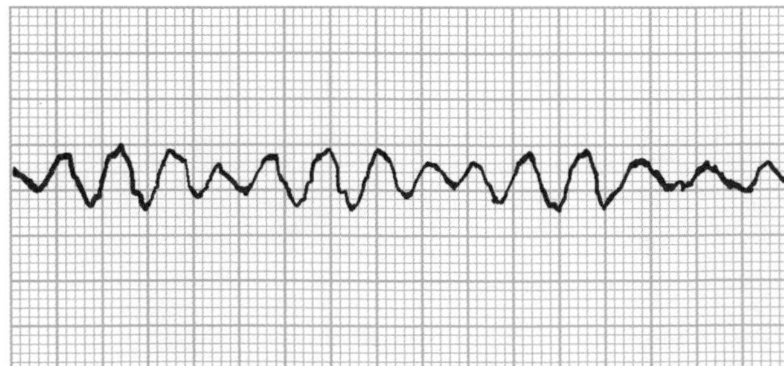

FIGURE 19-31 ■ Ventricular fibrillation.

dioversion in that the administration of current is not synchronized with the R wave and the amount of energy delivered is greater (200 to 350 J). The earlier the defibrillation is performed, the better is the chance for successful resuscitation. In some instances, the ventricular fibrillation pattern is very fine and is similar to the tracing seen in atrial arrest. Defibrillation is still indicated. Defibrillation and cardiopulmonary resuscitation are usually followed by administration of antiarrhythmic drugs.

KEY CONCEPTS

- Failure of the SA node to generate impulses may result in a junctional or ventricular escape rhythm. These rhythms are slow and may be poorly tolerated. Absence of P waves is important in determination of escape rhythms.
- In most cases, premature beats and ectopic rhythms are attributed to reentry mechanisms. Reentry circuits may be established when portions of the heart have abnormal conduction rates or pathways. Enhanced automaticity and triggered activity are alternative mechanisms for generation of ectopic complexes.
- Atrial dysrhythmias include premature atrial complexes, tachycardia, flutter, and fibrillation. Atrial dysrhythmias are usually well tolerated unless the ventricular response rate is significantly altered.
- Junctional tachycardias are difficult to distinguish from atrial tachycardias and they are often regarded together as supraventricular tachycardias.
- Frequent PVCs, tachycardia, and ventricular fibrillation are associated with a significant fall in cardiac output and must be rapidly diagnosed and managed.

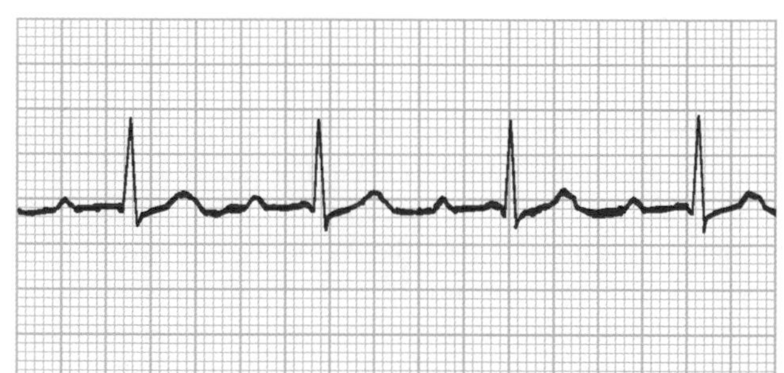

FIGURE 19-32 ■ First-degree atrioventricular block; PR interval, 0.32 second.

Conduction Pathway Disturbances

Disorders of cardiac impulse conduction include delays, blocks, and abnormal pathways. Cardiac ischemia and infarction commonly are associated with conduction blocks and delays, whereas abnormal pathways are usually congenital.

Disturbances of Atrioventricular Conduction

A disturbance in conduction between the sinus impulse and its associated ventricular response has been called *atrioventricular block.* The conduction may be abnormally slowed or completely blocked. The AV block results from a functional or pathologic defect in the AV node, bundle of His, or bundle branches. Three categories of AV block have traditionally been described: first-degree block, second-degree block (which includes types I and II), and third-degree (complete) block. These AV conduction disorders are associated with different pathologic processes and clinical implications.

First-degree block is generally identified by a prolonged PR interval (more than 0.20 second) on the ECG (Figure 19-32). The rhythm remains regular, and each P wave is associated with a QRS complex. First-degree block is a common finding and may occur in the absence of organic heart disease. Drugs and organic heart disorders, such as myocardial ischemia and congenital heart defects, may cause first-degree block. First-degree block is generally monitored but is not actively managed except to alleviate the underlying cause if possible.

Second-degree block is diagnosed when some of the atrial impulses are not conducted to the ventricles. Two types of second-degree block are identified by the pattern of nonconducted impulses. Type I (Mobitz type I, Wenckebach) is associated with progressively lengthening PR intervals until one P wave is not conducted (dropped beat). The pattern repeats, causing the QRS complexes to occur in groups. The PP intervals are constant, whereas the RR intervals vary (Figure 19-33). Type I second-degree block is usually due to reversible ischemia of the AV node, often associated with acute MI. The ischemic node is slow to recover after each depolarization, resulting in a longer and longer nodal delay until one impulse is not conducted. This gives the AV node time to recover, and the next atrial impulse is conducted more quickly, with a nearly normal PR interval, beginning the cycle again. Treatment is rarely required. If the block progresses to a type II block, a pacemaker may be required.

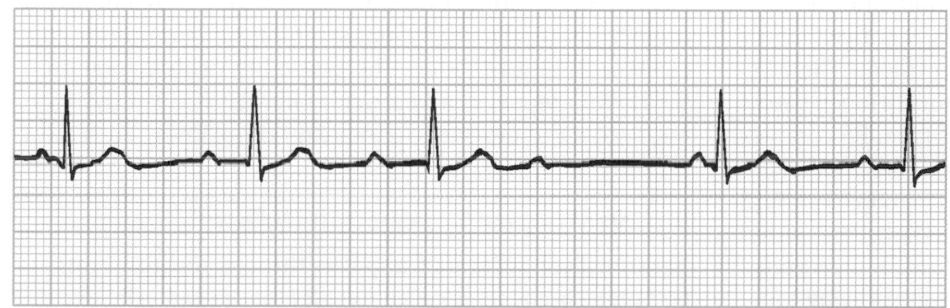

FIGURE 19-33 ■ Second-degree atrioventricular block, type I (Wenckebach, Mobitz type I). Note the progressive lengthening of the PR interval until one P wave is not conducted (dropped).

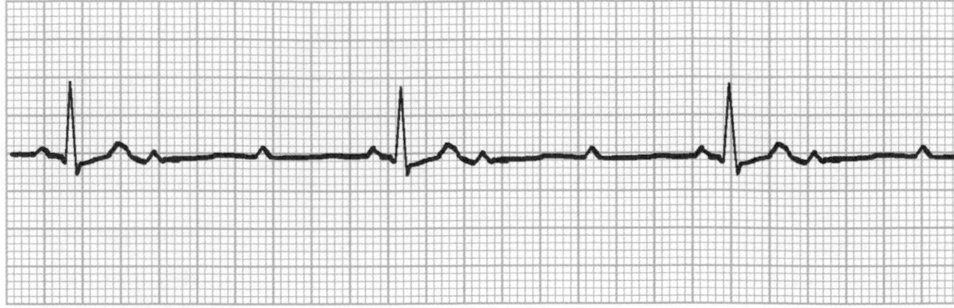

FIGURE 19-34 ■ Second-degree atrioventricular (AV) block, type II (Mobitz type II). Every third P wave is followed by a QRS complex. The other P waves are not conducted through the AV node. The PR interval on conducted impulses is constant.

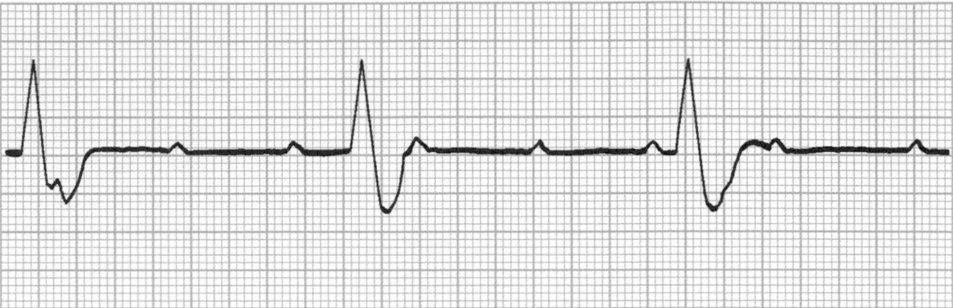

FIGURE 19-35 ■ Complete third-degree atrioventricular block. Note that there is no relationship between P waves and QRS complexes because the atria and ventricles are depolarizing independently.

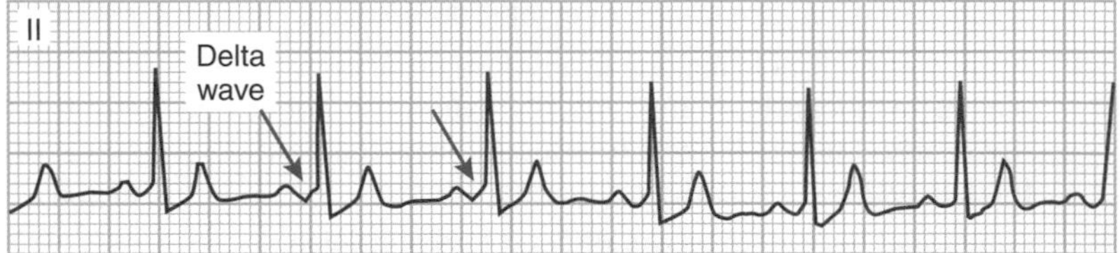

FIGURE 19-36 ■ Electrocardiogram in lead II from a patient with Wolf-Parkinson-White syndrome. Note the slurred upstroke of the R wave (delta wave). (From Conover MB: *Understanding electrocardiography,* ed 8, St Louis, 2003, Mosby, p 288.)

Type II second-degree block is identified by the presence of nonconducted P waves (dropped beats) with a consistent PR interval (Figure 19-34). The QRS complex is usually, but not always, wide (0.12 second or greater). Type II block is generally associated with pathologic lesion of the bundle of His, the right bundle branch, or both. It is the bundle branch block that causes the QRS complexes to be abnormally wide. Type II second-degree block is less common than type I but is more serious. It is usually associated with anterior septal MI or fibrosis of the conduction system. Type II block may progress to complete heart block with slow ventricular escape rhythm and poor cardiac output. Type II block may also result in severe bradycardia due to the number of dropped beats. Symptomatic type II block may require implantation of a pacemaker.

Third-degree block may occur as a result of pathologic lesion of the AV node, bundle of His, or bundle branches. No impulses are conducted from the atria to the ventricles, and a junctional or ventricular escape rhythm is evident. The ECG shows regularly occurring P waves that are totally independent of the ventricular rhythm (Figure 19-35). If the QRS complex is narrow, the block is most likely in the AV node, proximal to the bundle of His. A prolonged QRS interval (more than 0.12 second) indicates pathology distal to the bundle of His, within the bundle branches. The severity of symptoms is determined primarily by the heart rate, with slower rhythms being more serious. A pacemaker is generally required.

Abnormal Conduction Pathways

Some individuals have congenital abnormalities of the cardiac conduction system called *accessory pathways.* These extra conduction tracts provide alternative pathways for depolarization of the heart, resulting in abnormally early ventricular depolarizations following atrial depolarizations. The best known of these preexcitation syndromes is Wolff-Parkinson-White syndrome. This syndrome is caused by accessory pathways that originate in the atria, bypass the AV node, and enter a site in the ventricular myocardium. This results in more rapid activation of the ventricle, a short PR interval, initial slurring of the QRS (δ wave), and a wide QRS complex (Figure 19-36). The accessory pathway may provide a mechanism for reentry and the development of supraventricular tachycardia. Identification and treatment of individuals with preexcitation syndromes is desirable to prevent symptoms of supraventricular tachycardia and to reduce the possibility of deterioration of the rhythm to atrial or ventricular fibrillation. Antidysrhythmic agents and measures to interrupt the pathway, such as vagal stimulation, may be used.

Intraventricular Conduction Defects

Abnormal conduction of impulses through the intraventricular bundle branches is called *bundle branch block.* The two primary bundles are the right bundle branch, which supplies the

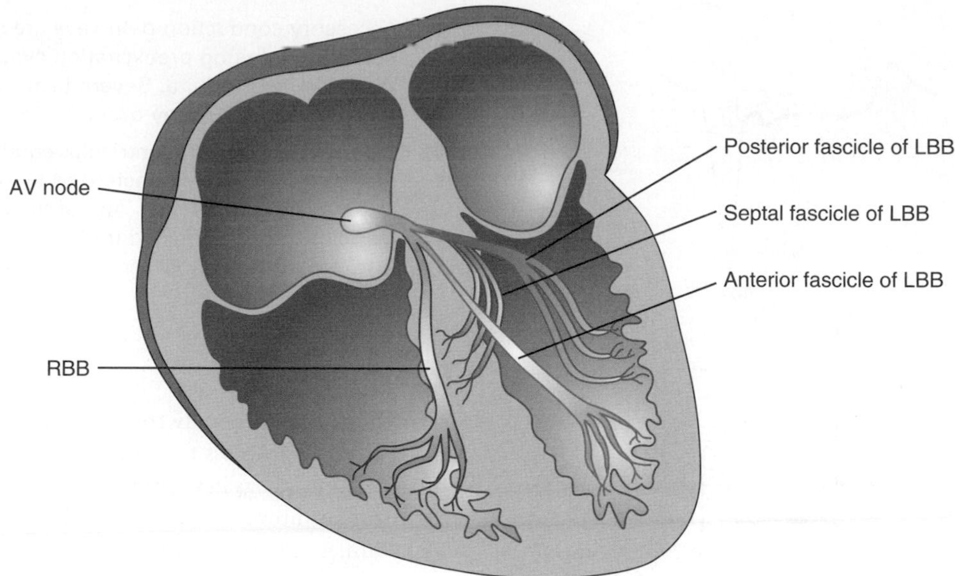

FIGURE 19-37 ■ The right bundle branch *(RBB)* innervates the right ventricle. The left bundle branch *(LBB)* has three divisions: the posterior, septal, and anterior fascicles. *AV,* Atrioventricular.

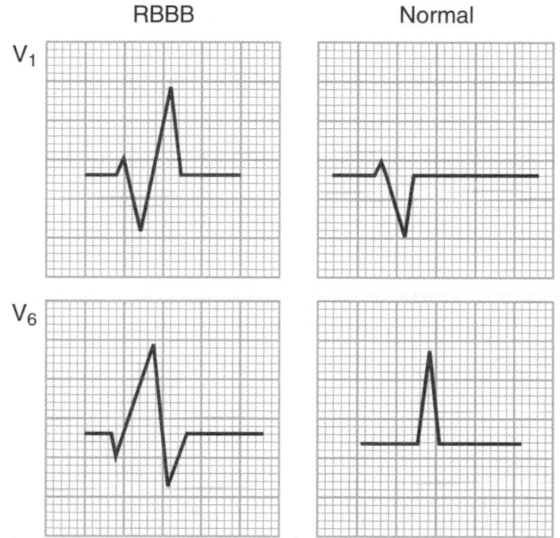

FIGURE 19-38 ■ Right bundle branch block pattern. Note late R wave in V_1 and abnormal S wave in V_6.

right ventricle, and the left bundle branch, which supplies the left ventricle. The left bundle branch is further divided into three fascicles: anterior, posterior, and septal (Figure 19-37). These supply the anterior, posterior, and septal portions of the left ventricle, respectively. Slowed or obstructed conduction occurring in one or more of these bundles results in abnormal ventricular depolarization and wide, bizarre-appearing QRS complexes. Bundle branch blocks are best detected with ECG leads V_1 and V_6.

Right bundle branch block may be present in almost any form of heart disease. It is occasionally found in individuals having no clinical evidence of heart disease. Right bundle branch block can progress to complete heart block in some cases. The electrocardiographic pattern is indicative of blocked conduction to the right ventricle such that the left ventricle depolarizes first, then spreads to the right ventricle. Right bundle branch block is classically associated with a late R wave in lead V_1 and an S wave in V_6. These changes are compared with the normal V_1 and V_6 in Figure 19-38.

Left bundle branch block causes a delay in left ventricular depolarization. The right ventricle is activated first through the right bundle branch, followed by right-to-left activation of the septum and, finally, left ventricular activation. The QRS complex is abnormally wide (more than 0.12 second) but has a nearly normal deflection pattern in V_1 and V_6. In V_1, the small R wave normally associated with septal depolarization is absent, and V_6 consists of a wide R wave (Figure 19-39).

Left anterior fascicular block is also called anterior hemiblock. Impaired conduction in the anterior fascicle causes the posterior aspect of the left ventricle to be activated first, followed by spread through the left ventricular myocardium in an upward and leftward direction. The electrocardiographic pattern shows small initial R waves followed by large S waves in leads II and III. The duration of the QRS complex is within normal limits.

Left posterior fascicular block (hemiblock) is due to a block in the posterior fascicle of the left bundle, which causes the anterior left ventricle to be activated first, followed by spread in a downward and rightward direction. The electrocardiographic findings include Q wave in leads II, III, and aV_F and R wave in leads I and aV_L. These electrocardiographic findings may mimic ventricular hypertrophy or inferolateral MI, making recognition difficult.

Slowed or obstructed conduction may occur simultaneously in more than one bundle or fascicle, leading to the terms

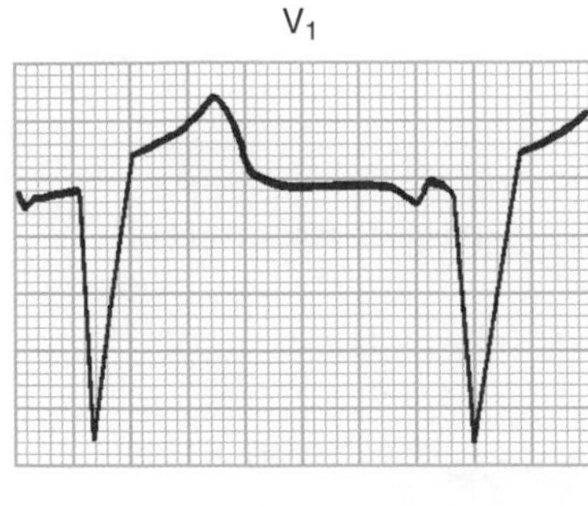

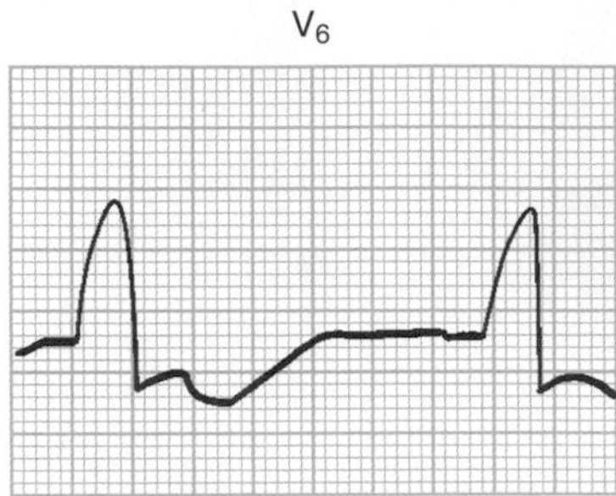

FIGURE 19-39 ■ Left bundle branch block pattern. Note wide S wave in V_1 and wide R wave in V_6.

bifascicular block and *trifascicular block*. For example, a right bundle branch block occurring in conjunction with a left posterior hemiblock is called a bilateral or bifascicular block. Trifascicular block refers to a bifascicular bundle block (most commonly right bundle branch block with left anterior hemiblock) in addition to a first-degree block (prolonged PR interval). The prolonged PR interval is usually due to incomplete block in the left posterior fascicle. Complete trifascicular block would make it impossible for a supraventricular depolarization to activate the ventricles and would be a third-degree or complete heart block.

KEY CONCEPTS

- Disturbances of AV conduction are generally referred to as AV blocks. First-degree block is characterized by a prolonged PR interval and usually requires no treatment.
- Two types of second-degree block have been identified. Type I (Wenckebach) is characterized by progressive prolongation of the PR interval until one P wave is not conducted. Type I block is associated with AV nodal ischemia. Type II second-degree block is identified by a rhythm showing a consistent PR interval with some nonconducted P waves. This block is more serious because it has a tendency to progress to complete AV (third-degree) block.
- Third-degree or complete heart block is diagnosed when there is no apparent association between atrial and ventricular conduction. This rhythm is serious, as it is typically associated with slow ventricular rhythm and poor cardiac output.
- Accessory conduction pathways are suspected in persons exhibiting preexcitation syndromes such as Wolf-Parkinson-White. Severe tachycardias and other reentrant rhythms may occur.
- Disturbances of intraventricular conduction (bundle branch blocks) are characterized by wide, bizarre-looking QRS complexes. Any of the three ventricular fascicles may be affected (right bundle, left anterior fascicle, left posterior fascicle).

Treatment

Dysrhythmias are generally treated if they are symptomatic or are expected to progress to a more serious level. A number of antiarrhythmic drugs have proved effective in managing many dysrhythmias; however, most have also been shown to cause dysrhythmias (proarrhythmic).[17] These drugs alter the properties of ion movement across cardiac membranes and affect automaticity as well as the rate and duration of depolarization and repolarization. The major electrophysiologic classes of antiarrhythmic compounds are summarized in Table 19-5. Treatment may also include measures to improve cardiac output, including pacemakers and drugs to improve contractility and blood pressure. Dysrhythmias causing severely reduced cardiac output, such as severe bradycardia, asystole, ventricular tachycardia, and ventricular fibrillation, require cardiopulmonary resuscitation until an effective cardiac rhythm is established.

Ablation procedures may be effective in eliminating a focus of dysrhythmia generation if one can be identified. An electrophysiologic study is done to evoke and analyze the dysrhythmia, followed by interruption (ablation) of the area generating it. Ablation is accomplished with high-frequency radio waves (radioablation) or by surgical excision. The electrophysiologic study requires insertion of electrodes directly into the heart by way of a venous or arterial catheter. The electrodes are used to record activity in specific locations and to deliver electric shocks to initiate or terminate an abnormal rhythm.[19] This test is useful in assessing responses to drug therapy and in identifying risk for sudden cardiac death. Those at high risk may benefit from insertion of implantable defibrillators that detect lethal rhythms and apply an electric shock to convert the rhythm.

SUMMARY

Heart failure may result from a number of cardiac and noncardiac disorders that diminish myocardial contractility or impose an excessive workload on the heart. The consequences of heart failure can be categorized as "forward" effects and "backward" effects. Forward effects are due to decreased cardiac output to the tissues and include decreased renal blood flow, fluid retention, activity intolerance, and mental fatigue. Backward effects are due to congestion of blood behind the

Table 19-5

Major Electrophysiologic Classes of Antidysrhythmic Compounds

Type	Drug	Conduction Velocity*	Refractory Period	Automaticity	Ion Block
Ia	Quinidine Procainamide Disopyramide	↓	↑	↓	Sodium (intermediate)
Ib	Lidocaine Mexiletine Tocainide	0/↓	↓	↓	Sodium (fast on-off)
Ic	Flecainide Propafenone† Moricizine‡	↓↓	0	↓	Sodium (slow on-off)
II§	β-Blockers Acebutolol Atenolol Esmolol Metoprolol Nadolol Pindolol Propranolol Timolol	↓	↑	↓	Calcium (indirect)
III	Amiodarone†, ¶ Bretylium† Dofetilide† Sotalol Ibutilide	0	↑↑	0	Potassium
IV§	Verapamil Diltiazem	↓	↑	↓	Calcium
Other	Digitalis	—	—	—	Enhances vagal tone, slows heart rate and AV node conduction
	Adenosine	0	↑	↓	Binds A_1 receptors and ↑ K^+ efflux, slows heart rate and AV conduction

*Variables for normal tissue models in ventricular tissue.
†Also has type II, β-blocking actions.
‡Classification controversial.
§Variables for sinoatrial and atrioventricular nodal tissue only.
¶Amiodarone also blocks calcium and sodium channels (fast on-off).

ineffectively pumping ventricle. With left-sided heart failure, the congestion is located in the lungs and produces a number of signs and symptoms, including dyspnea, orthopnea, hypoxemia, crackles, and frank pulmonary edema. Right-sided heart failure causes congestion in the systemic venous system leading to congestion and dysfunction of the liver, spleen, and kidney, as well as peripheral subcutaneous edema and distended neck veins. The location of congestive signs and symptoms is the primary clue in differentiating right- and left-sided heart failure.

Three major compensatory mechanisms operate to maintain cardiac output in the failing heart: (1) sympathetic activation, (2) increased preload, and (3) cardiac muscle cell hypertrophy. Unfortunately, these mechanisms also increase myocardial workload and oxygen requirements and may overwhelm the heart, causing decompensation. Heart failure is a progressive disorder that usually leads to death within about 5 years of diagnosis. Progression is related to myocardial remodeling characterized by myocyte loss and myocardial fibrosis. Therapies that slow the remodeling process may slow the progression of heart failure. The primary aims of therapy are to improve cardiac output and to minimize congestive symptoms and cardiac workload. These aims are achieved through management of preload, afterload, and contractility.

Dysrhythmia refers to an abnormality of electrical impulse generation or conduction. Dysrhythmias may occur in association with a number of cardiac and noncardiac disorders. Disturbances in electrical activity of the heart can indicate underlying pathophysiologic processes but are not themselves primary medical diseases. Dysrhythmias are significant because they can signal underlying pathophysiologic disorders and can disrupt normal cardiac output. Dysrhythmias can be categorized into three major types: (1) abnormal rates of sinus rhythm, (2) abnormal sites of impulse initiation, and (3) disturbances in conduction pathways. Treatment for dysrhythmias centers on maintaining adequate cardiac output, providing antiarrhythmic drugs as needed, and diagnosing and managing the underlying pathologic process.

MEDIA RESOURCES

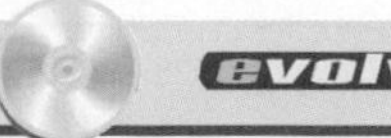

Remember to check out the ***CD Companion*** included with this book for Review Questions, Key Concepts Review, Glossary (with audio for selected terms), Disease Profiles, and Animations.

PLUS, visit the ***Evolve website*** at http://evolve.elsevier.com/Copstead/ for Case Studies, Disease Profiles, and WebLinks.

References

1. American Heart Association: *Heart disease and stroke statistics—2004 update,* Dallas, 2004, The Association.
2. National Heart Lung and Blood Institute: *Congestive heart failure data fact sheet,* Bethesda, National Institutes of Health, 1996, The Institute.
3. Angeja BG, Grossman W: Evaluation and management of diastolic heart failure, *Circulation* 107:659-663, 2003.
4. Ho KKK et al: The epidemiology of heart failure: the Framingham Study, *J Am Coll Cardiol* 22(suppl A):6A-13A, 1993.
5. Colucci WS, Braunwald E: Pathophysiology of heart failure. In Braunwald E, Zipes D, Libby P, editors: *Heart disease: a textbook of cardiovascular medicine,* ed 6, Philadelphia, 2001, Saunders, pp 600-614.
6. Johnson JA, Parker RB, Patterson JH: Heart failure. In Dipiro JT et al, editors: *Pharmacotherapy: a pathophysiologic approach,* ed 5, New York, 2002, McGraw-Hill, pp 185-218.
7. Hermann DD: Beta-adrenergic blockade 2002: a pharmacologic odyssey in chronic heart failure, *Congest Heart Fail* 8(5):262-269, 2002.
8. Levy MN: The cardiac pump. In Berne RM et al, editors: *Physiology,* ed 5, St Louis, 2004, Mosby, pp 305-321.
9. Schoen FJ: The heart. In Kumar V, Cotran R, Robbins S, editors: *Robbins basic pathology,* ed 7, Philadelphia, 2003, Saunders, pp 543-599.
10. Sackner-Bernstein JD, Hart D: Neurohormonal antagonism in heart failure: what is the optimal strategy? *Mt Sinai J Med* 71(2):115-126, 2004.
11. Gehlbach BK, Geppert E: The pulmonary manifestations of left heart failure, *Chest* 125(2):669-682, 2004.
12. Stoupakis G, Klapholz M: Natriuretic peptides: biochemistry, physiology, and therapeutic role in heart failure, *Heart Dis* 5(3):215-223, 2003.
13. Hunt SA et al: American College of Cardiology; American Heart Association: ACC/AHA guidelines for the evaluation and management of chronic heart failure in the adult: executive summary, *J Heart Lung Transplant* 21(2):189-203, 2002.
14. Richenbacher WE, Pierce WS: Treatment of heart failure: assisted circulation. In Braunwald E, Zipes D, Libby P, editors: *Heart disease: a textbook of cardiovascular medicine,* ed 6, Philadelphia, 2001, Saunders, pp 600-614.
15. The effect of digoxin on mortality and morbidity in patients with heart failure. The Digitalis Investigation Group, *N Engl J Med* 336(8):525-533, 1997.
16. Levy MN: Electrical activity of the heart. In Berne RM et al, editors: *Physiology,* ed 5, St Louis, 2004, Mosby, pp 274-304.
17. Bauman JL, Schoen MD: Arrhythmias. In Dipiro JT et al, editors: *Pharmacotherapy: a pathophysiologic approach,* ed 5, New York, 2002, McGraw-Hill, pp 273-304.
18. Conover MB: *Understanding electrocardiography,* ed 8, St Louis, 2003, Mosby.
19. Miller JM, Zipes DP: Management of the patient with cardiac arrhythmias. In Braunwald E, Zipes D, Libby P, editors: *Heart disease: a textbook of cardiovascular medicine,* ed 6, Philadelphia, 2001, Saunders, pp 700-766.

chapter 20

Shock

Jacquelyn L. Banasik

MEDIA RESOURCES

Additional Material for Study, Review, and Further Exploration

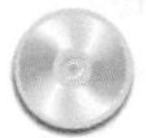

CD Companion ◆ Review Questions and Answers ◆ Key Concepts Review ◆ Glossary *(with audio pronunciations for selected terms)* ◆ Disease Profiles ◆ Animations

evolve ***Website*** at http://evolve.elsevier.com/Copstead/ ◆ Case Studies ◆ Disease Profiles ◆ WebLinks

KEY QUESTIONS

- What are the common causes of cardiogenic, hypovolemic, obstructive, and distributive shock?
- What are the common cellular and tissue responses to shock of any cause?
- How does the body try to compensate for insufficient cardiac output during shock states?
- How do clinical and hemodynamic findings differ among types of shock?
- What is the role of the immune system in septic shock and the progressive stage of other types of shock?
- How is shock managed and why does it have such a high mortality?

CHAPTER OUTLINE

Shock is a life-threatening condition characterized by hypotension and insufficient delivery of oxygenated blood to cells and tissues. In 1895, John Collins Warren described shock as a momentary pause in the act of death.[1] Despite advances in the understanding and management of this clinical syndrome, shock still has a high rate of mortality. Circulatory shock is not a primary disorder; rather, it occurs as a consequence of a previous physiologic insult. Initiating events include infections, heart disease, trauma, blood loss, and anaphylactic reactions. Early recognition and appropriate management of the primary event may prevent the development of shock syndrome. Once circulatory shock develops, a similar cascade of events follows regardless of the primary insult. This chapter presents an overview of circulatory shock, including the major causes, cellular and systemic pathogenesis, clinical manifestations, and therapeutic management. The reader is referred to other chapters in the text for a discussion of the primary disorders that may lead to shock states.

PATHOGENESIS OF CIRCULATORY SHOCK

Circulatory shock is characterized by an imbalance between oxygen supply and oxygen requirements at the cellular level.[2] When the cell does not have adequate amounts of oxygen and nutrients, it is unable to meet its metabolic demands. Cellular hypoxia results in impaired cellular function and may progress to irreversible organ damage and death. The causes of circulatory shock can be divided into four general types: cardiogenic, hypovolemic, obstructive, and distributive. Each of these types is associated with a number of primary causes (Box 20-1). Cardiogenic shock results from heart diseases that have progressed to decompensated heart failure. Hypovolemic shock is associated with loss of blood volume as a result of hemorrhage or excessive loss of extracellular fluids, such as through vomiting, diarrhea, or excessive diuresis. Obstructive shock develops when circulatory blockage disrupts cardiac output, such as a large pulmonary embolus or cardiac tamponade. Distributive shock is characterized by a greatly expanded vascular space because of inappropriate vasodilation. Vasodilation leads to hypotension and altered perfusion of tissues. Anaphylactic, neurogenic, and septic are forms of distributive shock. Each type of shock has certain unique features, but all are associated with impaired tissue oxygenation that can progress to refractory shock and organ failure.

Box 20-1

Etiology of Circulatory Shock

Cardiogenic Shock
Myocardial infarction
Cardiomyopathy
Valvular heart disease
Ventricular rupture
Congenital heart defects
Papillary muscle rupture

Hypovolemic Shock
Acute hemorrhage
Dehydration from vomiting, diarrhea
Overuse of diuretics
Burns
Pancreatitis

Obstructive Shock
Pulmonary embolism
Cardiac tamponade
Tension pneumothorax
Dissecting aortic aneurysm

Distributive Shock
Anaphylaxis
Neurotrauma
Spinal cord compression
Spinal anesthesia
Sepsis

Impaired Tissue Oxygenation

The common denominator of all forms of shock is impaired oxygen utilization by cells, which disrupts function and, if ongoing or severe, may lead to cell death, organ dysfunction, and stimulation of inflammatory reactions. Recent discoveries about the contribution of inflammatory reactions in the pathogenesis of shock have provided new insight into this complicated syndrome.

The reason for impaired oxygen utilization by cells differs in the various types of shock, but the outcomes are similar. A continuous supply of oxygen is needed by cells to allow sufficient production of energy in the form of adenosine triphosphate (ATP). Inadequate oxygen availability at the cellular level quickly impairs aerobic metabolism of glucose, fatty acids, and amino acids and causes the cells to rely on the relatively inefficient processes of glycolysis to produce cellular ATP. (A review of ATP synthesis can be found in Chapter 3.) Glycolysis is the enzymatic process of converting glucose to pyruvate, with the net production of two ATP molecules per glucose molecule. If oxygen were available, pyruvate would normally enter the mitochondria and proceed through the citric acid cycle. In the absence of cellular oxygen, the citric acid cycle is inhibited and pyruvate accumulates in the cytoplasm. Pyruvate accumulation would quickly inhibit further glycolysis and shut down ATP production entirely except that it can be converted to a substance called lactate, which diffuses from the cell and into the extracellular fluid. Accumulation of lactate in the blood stream (more than 5 mmol/L) is considered a sign of significant tissue hypoxia.[3]

An inadequate supply of cellular ATP inhibits energy-requiring cellular functions, including maintenance of ion concentrations across the plasma membrane. Because of their steep electrochemical gradients, extracellular sodium and calcium ions tend to leak into the cell. ATP-dependent pumps in the cell membrane are needed to continuously pump these ions back out. Failure of ion pumps leads to sodium and water accumulation in the cell (hydropic swelling) and an excess of intracellular free calcium. Intracellular calcium ions trigger a cascade of cellular events that further impair energy production and plasma membrane integrity. Cell death from oxygen deprivation takes from minutes to several hours, depending on the rate of metabolic activity. However, even a short period of oxygen deprivation often sets in motion a complex cascade of events that lead to further cell damage (Figure 20-1). Two important aspects of this cascade are (1) formation of oxygen radicals and (2) induction of inflammatory cytokines.

Ischemic cells may produce oxygen free radicals when oxygen supplies are restored. This process has been called reperfusion injury. Reactive oxygen molecules include superoxide (O_2^-), peroxide (H_2O_2), hydroxyl radicals (OH^-), and singlet oxygen (O). These molecules are unstable and will attack membrane structures, denature proteins, and break apart cell DNA. Another source of oxygen radicals is immune cells, particularly neutrophils, which are recruited to the area of tissue injury. Thus cellular injury may continue and progress long after the initial hypoxic insult has been resolved.

The role that immune cytokines play in shock has been studied extensively in septic shock but is thought to be similar in the late stages of other types of shock as well. Macrophages and tissue cells are stimulated to release inflammatory cytokines in response to hypoxic tissue injury and, in the case of septic shock, in response to endotoxin or other microorganism antigens.[4] The tumor necrosis factor-α (TNF-α) and interleukin-1 (IL-1) cytokines in particular have been shown to increase in the blood stream of patients with septic shock and are thought to be important mediators of vascular failure and progressive organ damage.[4] Numerous other immune cytokines and neurohormonal mediators have been implicated in the pathogenesis of shock (Table 20-1). These mediators represent potential therapeutic targets for a disorder that is notoriously difficult to manage effectively.

A hallmark of septic shock and the late stages of other types of shock is failure of the microcirculation to appropriately autoregulate blood flow. Normal tissues are able to match blood flow with metabolic needs across a wide range of blood pressures. This property ensures that blood flow is evenly distributed to tissues according to metabolic needs. In shock, autoregulation fails and excessive vascular dilation in some tissues leads to an abnormal distribution of blood flow.[5] Some capillary beds receive inadequate flow and become progressively more hypoxic, whereas other vascular routes are excessively dilated and receive too much flow.

Overall, this imbalance leads to a drop in oxygen consumption by the tissues, as well as severe hypotension, which further impairs tissue perfusion. Immune cytokines are believed to be at the root of this problem. TNF-α and IL-1 induce vascular cells to produce excessive amounts of the vasodilator nitric oxide.[4] Nitric oxide in normal quantity is thought to be protective for tissues during shock, whereas excessive production is detrimental. Nitric oxide is produced in endothelial cells and vascular smooth muscle by two enzymes, nitric oxide synthase (NOS) and inducible nitric oxide synthase (iNOS). TNF-α and IL-1 increase the activity of iNOS and thereby cause widespread, excessive production of nitric oxide (Figure 20-2).

In research studies, drugs given to nonspecifically inhibit nitric oxide synthesis were associated with improved blood pressure but higher mortality rates.[5] Specific inhibitors of iNOS that block excessive synthesis but do not inhibit baseline synthesis have been found to improve mortality in some studies.[5] In addition to the vascular dilation problem, excessive nitric oxide is also thought to contribute to free radical damage through production of the reactive metabolite peroxynitrite.[6]

Efforts to block TNF-α and IL-1 in patients with septic shock have not been effective in reducing mortality, which suggests that additional mediators are involved in the inflammatory response to shock. The inflammatory response to

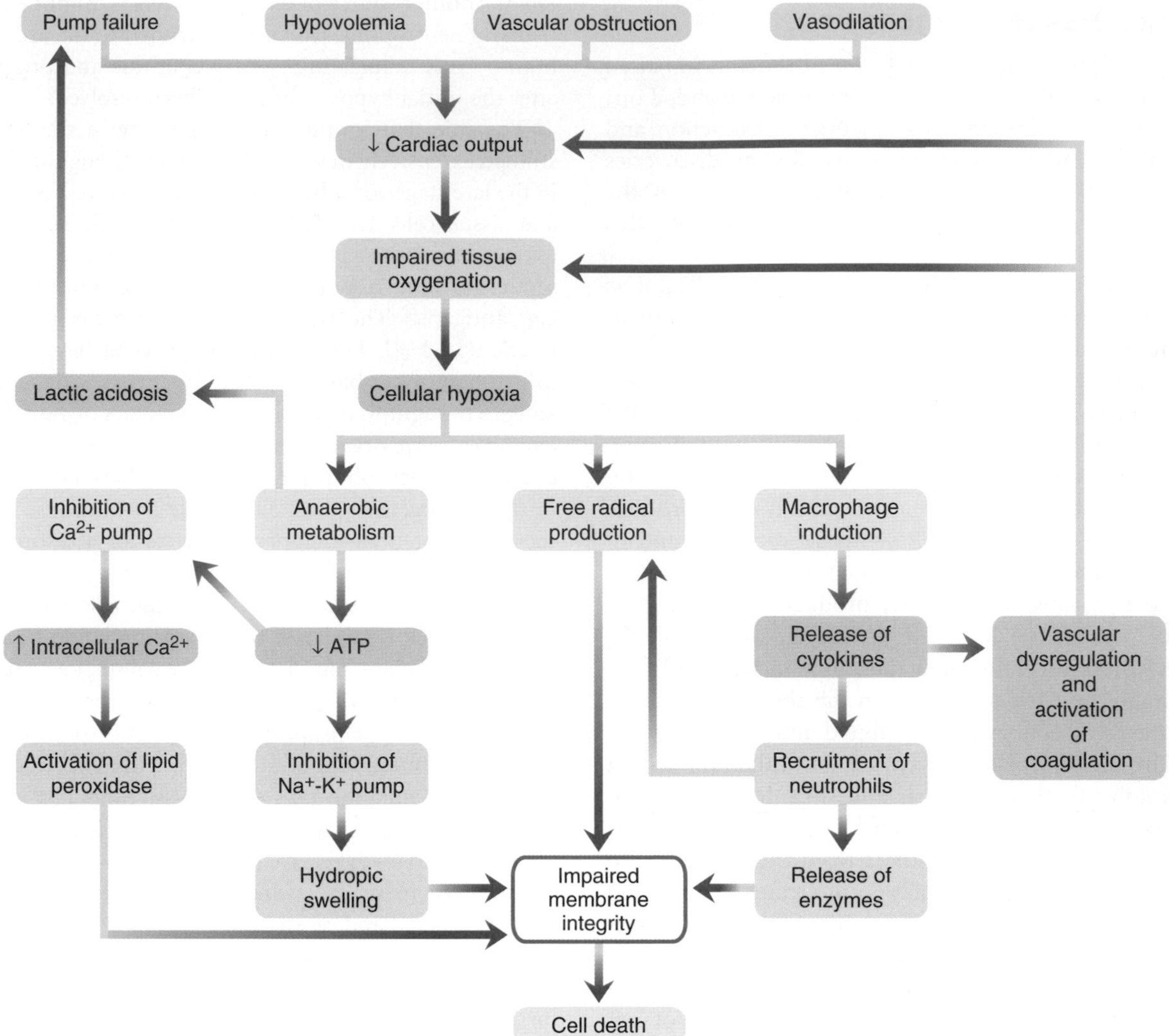

FIGURE 20-1 ■ Shock is a complex process involving cellular hypoxia, free radical formation, and systemic inflammation. All forms of shock are associated with impaired tissue oxygenation, which triggers a cascade of events leading to tissue injury and death. *ATP,* Adenosine triphosphate.

shock is responsible for most of the complications associated with organ damage discussed at the end of this chapter.

Compensatory Mechanisms in Shock

A number of compensatory responses are set in motion to restore tissue perfusion and oxygenation in the early stages of shock. Historically, these responses to shock have been divided into three clinical stages: compensated shock, progressive shock, and refractory shock. Although these stages may be useful for determining prognosis and the likelihood of the patient's recovering, the development of shock is better viewed as a continuum in which compensatory mechanisms become progressively less effective.

Insufficient cardiac output and decreased arterial blood pressure are early defects in all types of shock. Insufficient cardiac output may be a consequence of an ineffective cardiac pump or insufficient blood volume. A number of compensatory mechanisms are triggered in response to decreased cardiac output in an attempt to restore adequate perfusion pressure (Figure 20-3). Baroreceptors located in the aorta and carotid arteries quickly sense the decrease in pressure and transmit signals to the vasomotor center in the brainstem medulla. Stimulation of the sympathetic nervous system (SNS) results in increased cardiac output and vascular resistance. Because blood pressure is determined by the product of cardiac output and vascular resistance, an increase in one or both of these factors will help restore blood pressure. The SNS increases cardiac output through several mechanisms. The adrenal medulla is stimulated to release increased amounts of the catecholamines epinephrine and norepinephrine (NE), which circulate to the heart and stimulate β_1 receptors. The β_1

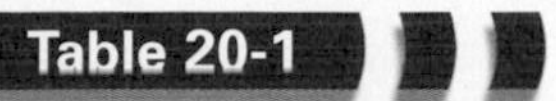

Table 20-1 Immune Cytokines and Neurohormones Associated with Circulatory Shock

Mediator	Associated Dysfunction
IL-1α	Inflammation, vasodilation, vascular leakiness
IL-1β	Inflammation, vasodilation, vascular leakiness
IL-6	Fever, increased acute phase protein
TNF-α	Inflammation, neutrophil activation
IL-10	Antiinflammatory, may suppress shock
TGF-β	Fibrosis, pulmonary edema
PAF	Platelet activation, chemotaxis
PAI-1	Increased clotting, thrombosis
Substance P	Proinflammatory
Chemokines	Neutrophil recruitment and binding to vessel endothelium
Nitric oxide	Vasodilator
C5a	Chemotactic
Protein C	Inhibits thrombus formation
Vasopressin	Improves vascular tone and responsiveness to NE/E
Cortisol	Antiinflammatory, improves vascular response to NE/E
Endothelin	Vasoconstriction
Adrenomedullin	Vasodilation
Norepinephrine	Vasoconstriction
Epinephrine	Inotropic, bronchodilation
Leukotrienes	Inflammation, bronchospasm
Histamine	Increased vascular permeability, edema
Heparin	Inhibits action of histamine
Angiotensin II	Vasoconstriction
Heat-shock proteins	Protect protein structure and function, inhibits apoptosis

IL, Interleukin; *TNF,* tumor necrosis factor; *TGF,* transforming growth factor; *PAF,* platelet-activating factor; *PAI,* plasminogen activator inhibitor; *NE,* norepinephrine; *E,* epinephrine.

receptors respond by increasing the heart rate and force of contraction in an attempt to increase cardiac output. The SNS also enhances venous return to the heart by constricting systemic arterioles and venules. Arterial vasoconstriction reduces flow through the capillary bed, which causes hydrostatic pressure in the capillaries to fall. Fluid reabsorption from interstitial spaces helps increase blood volume and improve preload. Blood vessels in the skin, kidneys, and gastrointestinal tract constrict and shunt blood to the heart and brain.

The SNS stimulates cells in the kidney to release renin, which triggers the renin-angiotensin-aldosterone cascade. Renin is also secreted from the kidneys in response to decreased blood flow and pressure in the afferent arterioles. Renin triggers the formation of angiotensin II, which is a potent vasoconstrictor and also stimulates kidney nephrons to conserve sodium and water. Conservation of volume by the kidney is further enhanced by aldosterone, which is secreted from the adrenal cortex in response to angiotensin II. Reabsorption of fluid from the kidney helps increase blood volume and enhances venous return to the heart. Another hormone, antidiuretic hormone (vasopressin), is secreted from the posterior pituitary in response to reduced blood volume. Antidiuretic hormone stimulates the kidney tubules to reabsorb water and improves the vascular response to catecholamines. In shock, urine output may fall to zero as the kidneys attempt to

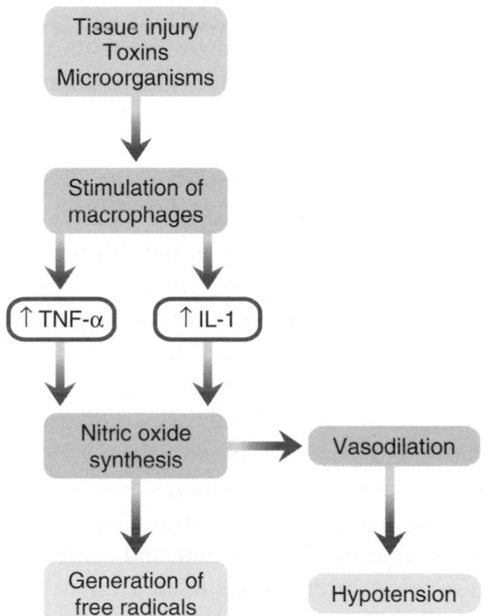

FIGURE 20-2 ■ Excess production of nitric oxide is an important mechanism of vascular failure in shock. The tumor necrosis factor-α *(TNF-α)* and interleukin-1 *(IL-1)* cytokines are promoters of inducible nitric oxide synthase. These cytokines are released from macrophages that have been activated by tissue injury or toxins.

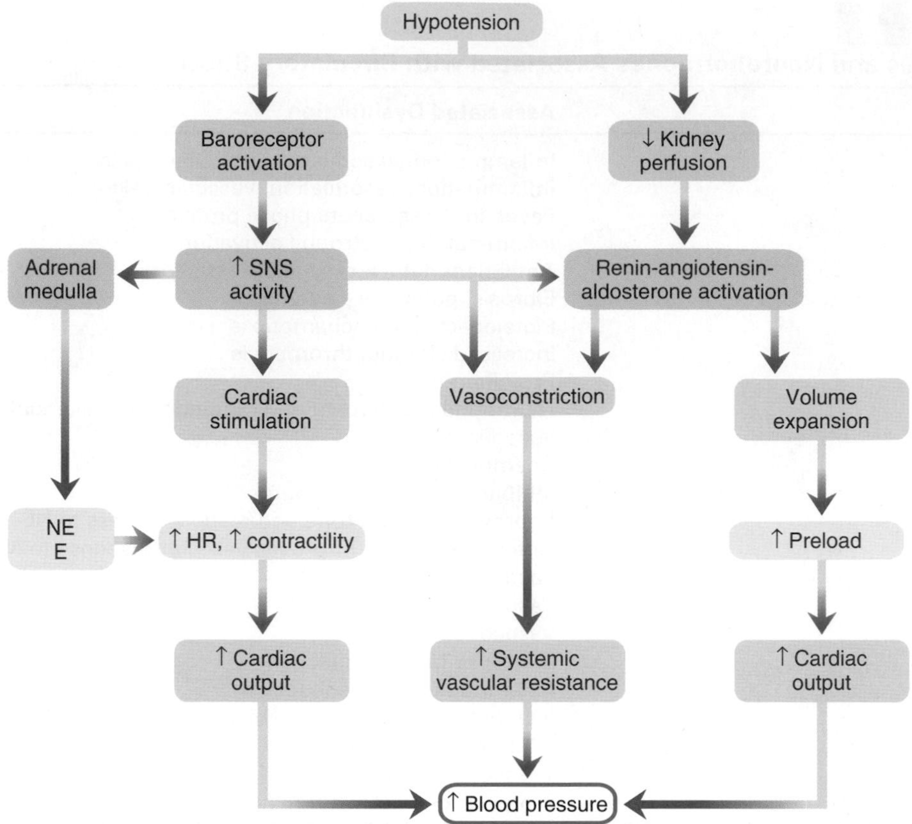

FIGURE 20-3 ■ Compensatory mechanisms are triggered in shock to help maintain arterial blood pressure despite a fall in cardiac output. *NE,* Norepinephrine; *E,* epinephrine; *SNS,* sympathetic nervous system; *HR,* heart rate.

conserve fluid to maintain blood volume and cardiac output. Unfortunately, the kidney tubules often sustain damage because of the low-flow state, which may progress to acute renal failure.

These compensatory mechanisms work well in the early stages of hypovolemic shock and may maintain blood pressure within the normal range until the volume of blood loss becomes too great (Figure 20-4). In other forms of shock, compensatory mechanisms are less effective in restoring cardiac output. In cardiogenic shock, the compensatory responses may worsen the already high preload and impose a greater workload on the failing heart. In distributive shock, the vasculature is not responsive to SNS signals to constrict. Blood pools in the peripheral tissues, which makes it difficult for the heart to maintain cardiac output despite sympathetic stimulation to increase the heart rate and contractility.

The early, compensated stages of shock may be difficult to detect clinically (Figure 20-5). A high index of suspicion is needed in patients with heart failure, trauma, blood loss, and severe infection. In addition, the following clinical findings may be present:

- A narrow pulse pressure with or without hypotension
- Tachycardia greater than 100 beats/min
- Fast and deep respirations
- Decreased urinary output
- Increased urine specific gravity
- Cool, clammy skin
- Altered mentation
- Dilated pupils

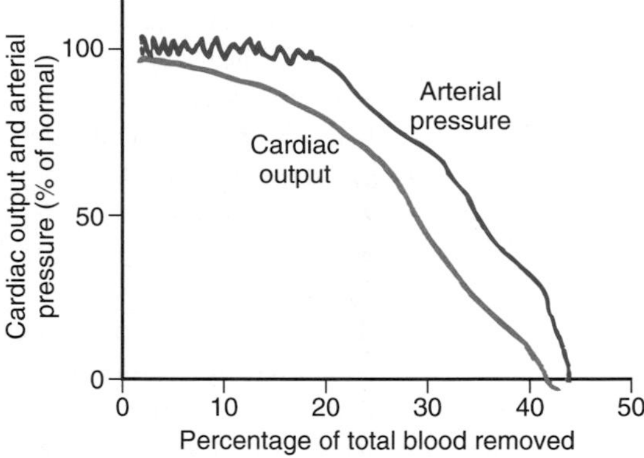

FIGURE 20-4 ■ In the early stages of hypovolemia, blood pressure is stable even though cardiac output is falling. When volume losses equal about 25% of the blood volume, blood pressure falls precipitously. (Redrawn from Guyton AC, Hall JE: *Textbook of medical physiology,* ed 10, Philadelphia, 2000, Saunders, p 254.)

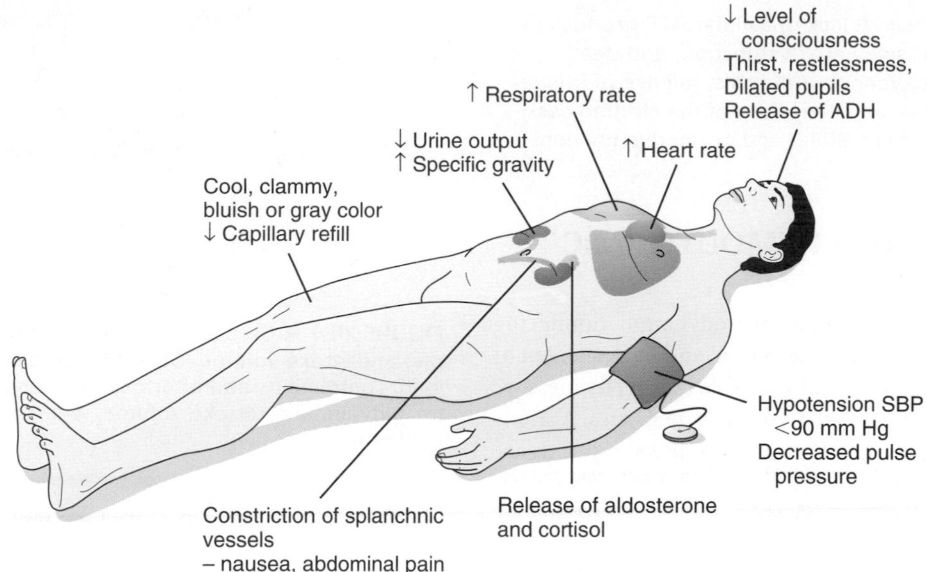

FIGURE 20-5 ■ Classical manifestations of shock. *ADH,* Antidiuretic hormone; *SBP,* systolic blood pressure.

At some point, which is variable and differs among individuals, the compensatory mechanisms can no longer sustain adequate perfusion to tissues and cells begin to suffer significant hypoxic injury. This condition is sometimes called the progressive stage of shock. Active intervention is required at this stage or the patient will probably not survive. As previously described, reduced delivery of oxygen to tissues results in hypoxic injury, free radical damage, and stimulation of the inflammatory response. Lactic acidosis may occur during the progressive stage of shock. In addition to being a marker of anaerobic metabolism, lactate can alter the acid-base balance of the blood and create a metabolic acidosis. Metabolic acidosis places a greater burden on the respiratory and renal systems and may contribute to dysfunction. Metabolic acidosis can affect electrolyte balance and contribute to cardiac dysrhythmias and conduction disturbances. In addition, myocardial depressant factors are released that impair myocardial contractility.[7] These factors contribute to reduced cardiac output and a progressive cycle of worsening tissue hypoxia.

During the later stages of shock, the vascular system begins to fail. Arterioles become unresponsive to catecholamines and previously constricted vascular beds begin to dilate. Widespread dilation and low cardiac output combine to produce severe hypotension. The low blood pressure is not sufficient for organ perfusion. At this stage the effects of shock produce more shock processes (progressive stage). Tissue damage often activates the clotting cascade, which contributes to sluggish blood flow, vascular thrombosis, and more severe tissue ischemia. Release of inflammatory mediators, along with vascular occlusion, may precipitate organ failure. The kidney, liver, and lung are particularly susceptible. The stage of refractory shock occurs when the patient becomes unresponsive to therapeutic interventions.

The progressive stage of shock is characterized by the following:

- Low blood pressure, usually lower than 90 mm Hg
- Narrow pulse pressure
- Tachycardia
- Acute renal failure (oliguria, increased blood urea nitrogen and serum creatinine)
- Decreased level of consciousness
- Increased respiratory rates
- Metabolic and respiratory acidosis with hypoxemia

KEY CONCEPTS

- Shock represents a diverse group of life-threatening circulatory conditions. The common factor among all types of shock is hypoperfusion and impaired cellular oxygen utilization. Inadequate cellular oxygenation may result from decreased cardiac output, maldistribution of blood flow, or reduced blood oxygen content.
- During the compensatory stage of shock, homeostatic mechanisms are sufficient to maintain adequate tissue perfusion despite a reduction in cardiac output. Manifestations of SNS activation are an elevated heart rate, increased myocardial stimulation, bronchodilation, vasoconstriction, cool clammy skin, dilated pupils, and decreased urine output. Blood pressure is maintained even though cardiac output has fallen.
- During the progressive stage of shock, compensatory mechanisms begin to fail and hypotension and progressive tissue hypoxia result. Shift of cells to anaerobic metabolism results in lactate production and

metabolic acidosis. A lack of cellular ATP production leads to cellular swelling, dysfunction, and death. Generation of oxygen free radicals, release of inflammatory cytokines, and activation of the clotting cascade lead to further cellular and organ dysfunction.

ASSESSMENT AND HEMODYNAMIC MONITORING

Astute assessment and appropriate hemodynamic monitoring are essential for the prevention, detection, and management of shock. Currently, it is not clinically feasible to directly measure the adequacy of cellular oxygenation in body tissues. A number of indirect measures and clinical signs and symptoms are used to help indicate when tissue hypoxia is probably occurring. These same parameters are used to tailor therapy and assess outcomes of that therapy.

Most hospitalized patients experiencing shock will have a number of monitoring devices in place to facilitate assessment of cardiac output, blood pressure, preload, vascular resistance, arterial oxygen content, and venous oxygen content. In addition, frequent measurement of serum lactate, acid-base status, and urine output can be used to indirectly assess the severity of tissue hypoperfusion and hypoxemia.

An understanding of hemodynamic principles and monitoring techniques is helpful to the discussion of shock states. A thorough discussion can be found in Chapters 15 and 17, and only the main points are reviewed here. The most important factors in determining adequate tissue oxygenation are cardiac output, arterial oxygen content, and distribution of blood flow.

Cardiac Output

The normal value for cardiac output is 4 to 8 L/min. Cardiac output is the product of heart rate and stroke volume. Stroke volume is the amount of blood ejected by the ventricle with each heartbeat. The normal value is about 70 ml per beat. Stroke volume is influenced by three major factors: preload, contractility, and afterload (Figure 20-6). **Preload,** or the amount of blood in the ventricle at the end of diastole, determines the length of the muscle fibers in the ventricular walls before the next contraction. According to the Frank-Starling law, increased muscle fiber length increases the force of contraction owing to optimal actin-myosin cross-bridging.[8] Thus an increase in preload increases stroke volume and cardiac output. In patients with low preload, a significant improvement in cardiac output can be achieved by administering blood or intravenous fluids.

Afterload is the aortic impedance that the left ventricle must overcome to eject blood during systole. The major factors determining aortic impedance are the patency of the aortic valve and the resistance in the systemic vascular system. As resistance to left ventricular ejection increases, stroke volume

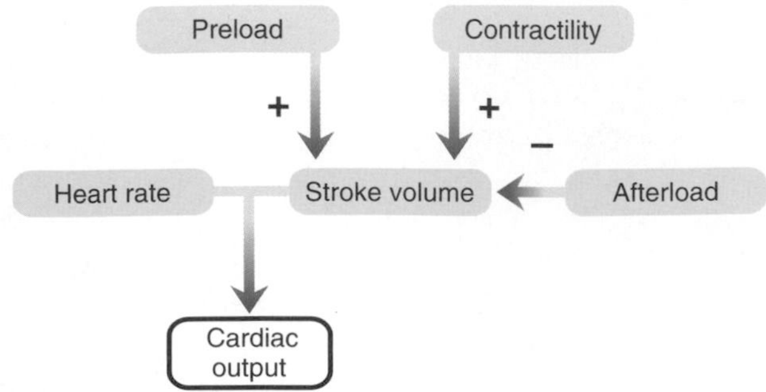

FIGURE 20-6 ■ Cardiac output is determined by the heart rate and stroke volume. Stroke volume is influenced by preload, contractility, and afterload. Increased preload and contractility enhance stroke volume, whereas increased afterload reduces it.

decreases. Conversely, as resistance falls, stroke volume increases.

Contractility is the inherent state of activation of cardiac muscle fibers. Contractility depends on the amount of free calcium ions available in the cardiac muscle cells after each electrical impulse. Contractility is influenced by sympathetic and parasympathetic nervous system neurotransmitters and other hormones and drugs. Contractility also depends on the amount of muscle mass and is influenced by myocardial ischemia and necrosis.

All of the determinants of cardiac output—heart rate, preload, afterload, and contractility—are subject to therapeutic management to optimize delivery of oxygenated blood to the tissues.

Arterial Oxygen Content

Oxygen delivery (DO_2) can be determined by multiplying cardiac output and arterial oxygen content (CaO_2). CaO_2 is the sum of dissolved oxygen and oxygen bound to hemoglobin. Adequate gas exchange in the pulmonary capillaries is necessary to fully saturate hemoglobin with oxygen. Impaired ventilation may result in reduced CaO_2 and impair DO_2. Mechanical ventilation and supplemental oxygen administration may be used to improve arterial oxygen saturation. For patients with low hemoglobin, blood transfusion may significantly improve DO_2.

A concept closely related to DO_2 is **oxygen consumption** (VO_2). Whereas DO_2 is a measure of the oxygen delivered to the tissues each minute, VO_2 is the amount of oxygen actually used by the tissues per minute. In a normal physiologic state, only about 25% of the oxygen delivered is taken up by tissues, which leaves about 75% of the oxygen to return to the heart in venous blood. When DO_2 falls because of low cardiac output, tissues extract a greater percentage of the oxygen delivered such that the amount returning in venous blood is lower. When distribution of blood flow and tissue extraction of oxygen is impaired, as in septic shock, oxygen consumption falls and the amount of oxygen returning in venous blood will be higher than it should be. The amount of oxygen returning to the heart in venous blood can be measured by a special catheter in the pulmonary artery that detects venous oxygen saturation (Svo_2). Outcomes of therapy to improve Do_2 can be assessed by monitoring Svo_2. In cardiogenic shock, for example, one would expect to see Svo_2 increase from a low value back toward 75% as cardiac output improves. In septic shock, one would expect to see Svo_2 decrease from a high value back toward 75% as distribution of blood flow to metabolically active tissues improves.

Hemodynamic Monitoring

Sophisticated monitoring equipment is available to assess the hemodynamic status of patients in shock. A flow-directed, pulmonary artery catheter can be inserted through the jugular or subclavian vein to allow measurement of intracardiac pressures, cardiac output, and Svo_2. The typical balloon-tipped flow-directed catheter used for hemodynamic monitoring has at least three lumina. When the catheter is properly positioned in the pulmonary artery, the proximal lumen lies in the right atrium and the distal lumen lies in the pulmonary artery (Figure 20-7). A third lumen is connected to a balloon at the end of the catheter, which can be blown up with air to measure left atrial pressure. Some catheters also have the potential for continuous monitoring of Svo_2.

The proximal lumen in the right atrium allows measurement of right atrial pressure. Right atrial pressure is used to indicate right ventricular end-diastolic volume or preload. The primary value of monitoring right atrial pressure is in the management of blood volume. A low right atrial pressure is associated with a low preload and may indicate a need for extracellular volume replacement to enhance cardiac output. Conversely, a high right atrial pressure may indicate a need for extracellular volume reduction to decrease cardiac workload and congestive symptoms.

The distal lumen located in the pulmonary artery allows measurement of pulmonary artery pressure. Measurement of pulmonary artery pressure is helpful in assessing pulmonary complications of shock. An increase in pulmonary artery pressure may occur in progressive shock as the lungs react to inflammatory mediators and become edematous. In the absence of lung disease, pulmonary artery diastolic pressure reflects left atrial pressure. Assessment of left atrial pressure is

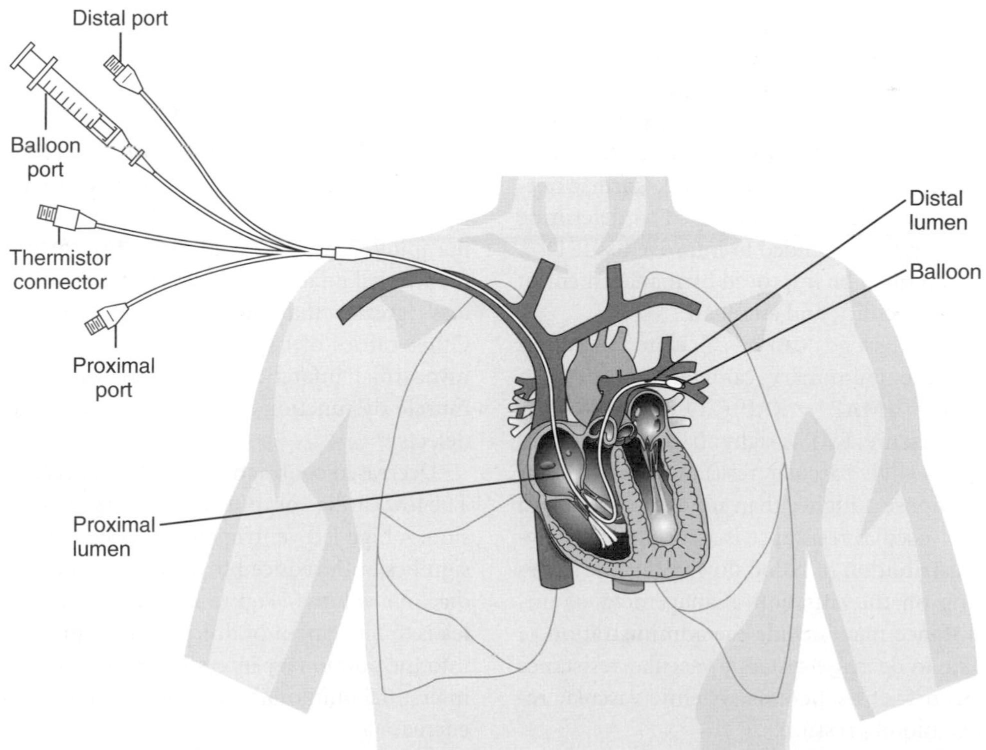

FIGURE 20-7 ■ A properly positioned pulmonary artery catheter showing the proximal port in the right atrium and the distal port in the pulmonary artery. Cardiac output determinations can be made by injecting hypothermic solution into the proximal port and measuring the degree of warm-up near the distal port. A balloon at the end of the catheter can be intermittently inflated to measure pulmonary capillary occlusion pressure. When the balloon is inflated, it will float into a small artery and wedge there. Then the distal port measures the pressure in the capillary, which is a direct reflection of left atrial pressure.

important because it indicates left ventricular preload—an important determinant of cardiac output. A more accurate assessment of left atrial pressure can be obtained by using the catheter balloon to obtain a pulmonary capillary occlusion pressure. When the balloon is inflated, the catheter tip floats into a small pulmonary artery and wedges itself there. The balloon blocks the arterial pressure events behind it and allows measurement of pressure in the capillary. Pulmonary capillary occlusion pressure is a direct reflection of left atrial pressure. Low left atrial pressure indicates reduced left ventricular preload and may indicate the need for extracellular volume replacement. Preload is also affected by the left ventricular **ejection fraction.** A poorly contracting ventricle with a low ejection fraction will tend toward a higher than normal preload because of the residual blood left in the ventricle at the end of systole. Measures to improve contractility would be expected to result in a reduction in left ventricular preload.

Cardiac output can also be measured with a pulmonary artery catheter by use of a thermodilution technique. A thermistor located at the distal end of the catheter measures a change in blood temperature between the right atrium and pulmonary artery. The change in temperature reflects the amount of blood flow through the right heart and can be used to calculate cardiac output. Some catheters work by warming blood in the right atrium and then measuring the degree of cooling at the distal thermistor. Others work by injection of a known amount of hypothermic solution into the right atrium, with measurement of the degree of warming at the distal thermistor. In either case, the greater the cardiac output, the more quickly blood temperature will return to normal. Cardiac output is an important parameter to be measured to determine the effect of various therapies intended to improve tissue Do_2. Low cardiac output can often be improved by management of heart rate, preload, contractility, and afterload.

Vascular resistance (afterload) can be calculated based on data obtained from the pulmonary catheter according to Ohm's law: resistance = (MAP − RAP)/CO, where MAP is mean arterial blood pressure, RAP is right atrial pressure, and CO is cardiac output. High vascular resistance may impair stroke volume and impose a higher than necessary workload on the ventricle. Low vascular resistance is associated with hypotension and maldistribution of blood flow in the late stages of shock. Depending on the situation, management of impaired vascular resistance may include the administration of agents that vasodilate to decrease systemic vascular resistance or agents that vasoconstrict to increase systemic vascular resistance and improve blood pressure.

To assess the adequacy of the cardiac output more accurately, the **cardiac index** can be calculated. Cardiac output does not take into account the size of the person. For example, a large person may have a cardiac output of 4 L/min, which is within the range of normal, but that value may be insufficient for a person with a large body mass. Cardiac index takes body surface area into account and gives a more accurate measurement of the heart's pumping adequacy. Cardiac index is calculated by dividing cardiac output by body surface area. Body surface area is dependent on an individual's height and weight and can be obtained from standardized charts. A cardiac index of less than 2.0 L/min/cm^2 is associated with inadequate perfusion of tissues.

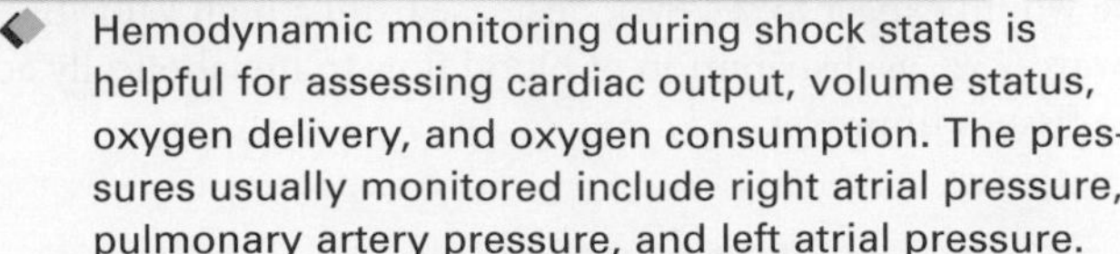

- Hemodynamic monitoring during shock states is helpful for assessing cardiac output, volume status, oxygen delivery, and oxygen consumption. The pressures usually monitored include right atrial pressure, pulmonary artery pressure, and left atrial pressure.
- Normally, about 25% of the oxygen in arterial blood is extracted by the tissues, so the mixed venous oxygen saturation (Svo_2) is approximately 75%. Low cardiac output may result in greater oxygen extraction and lower Svo_2; maldistribution of flow, as occurs in septic shock, may result in less oxygen extraction and higher Svo_2.
- Cardiac output can be measured by using a thermodilution technique. The cardiac index, derived by dividing cardiac output by body surface area, may better reflect the adequacy of cardiac performance.

TYPES OF SHOCK

Cardiogenic Shock

Etiology and Pathogenesis. Cardiogenic shock occurs primarily as a result of severe dysfunction of the left, right, or both ventricles that results in inadequate cardiac pumping. The most common cause of cardiogenic shock is myocardial infarction resulting in a significant dysfunction or loss (greater than 40%) of left ventricular myocardium.[9] Other causes of cardiogenic shock include right ventricular myocardial infarction, end-stage cardiomyopathy, papillary muscle dysfunction, free wall rupture, and congenital heart defects.[10]

Decreased contractility results in decreased cardiac output. The low cardiac output state results in decreased tissue perfusion. A high left ventricular diastolic filling pressure (preload) signifies both reduced myocardial contractility and increased diastolic volume (Figure 20-8). High left ventricular preload leads to movement of fluid from the pulmonary vascular beds into the pulmonary interstitial space, which initially results in interstitial pulmonary edema and later in alveolar pulmonary edema.

The SNS is stimulated as a compensatory mechanism to increase cardiac output. The result is an increase in heart rate and systemic vascular resistance. The increase in systemic vascular resistance makes it even more difficult for the heart to pump. Activation of the renin-angiotensin-aldosterone system results in further increases in resistance and preload. The net result of the activation of compensatory mechanisms is to increase myocardial workload and

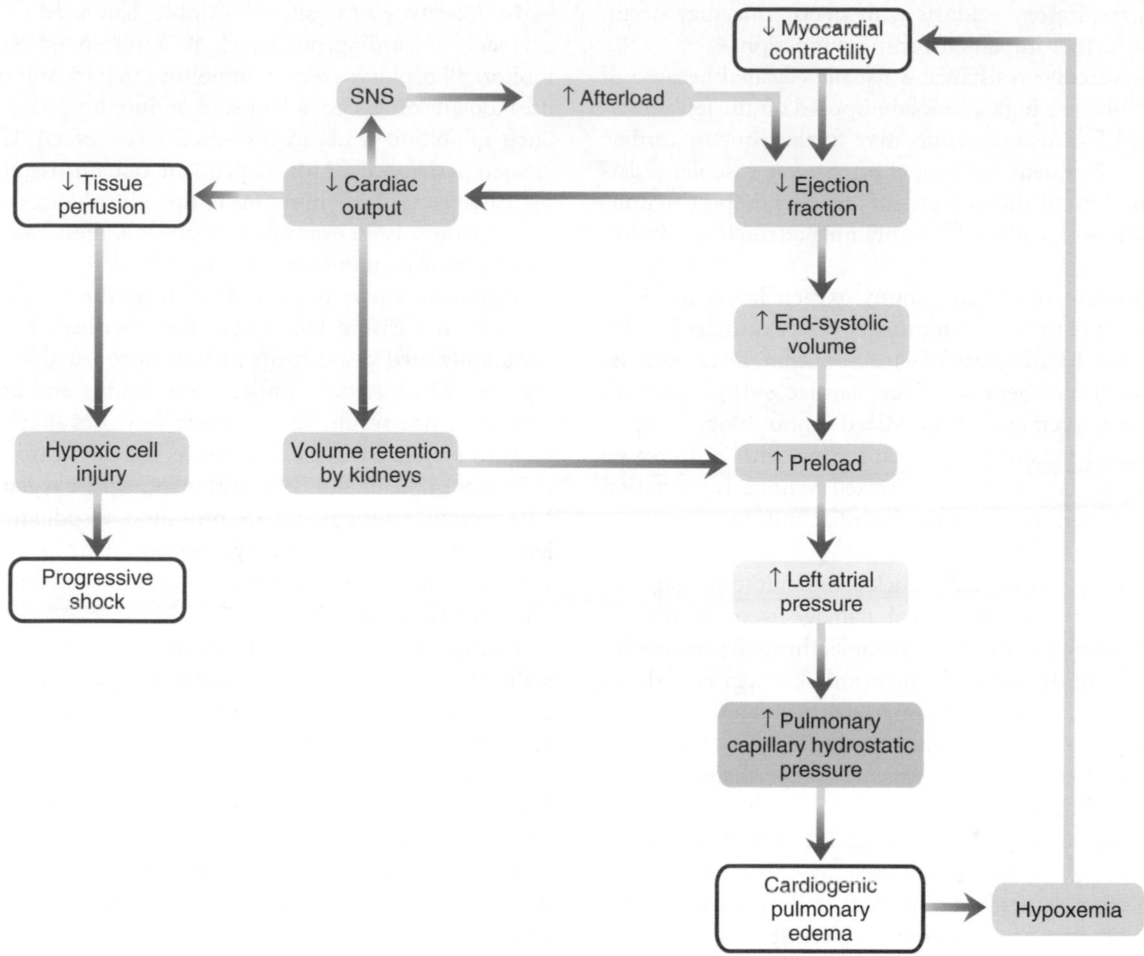

FIGURE 20-8 ■ Cardiogenic shock results in decreased tissue perfusion and cardiogenic pulmonary edema because of reduced myocardial contractility. *SNS,* Sympathetic nervous system.

oxygen demand. Thus the compensatory responses can precipitate further myocardial damage and cause a progressive decline in cardiac output.

Clinical Manifestations. Sympathetic nervous stimulation increases the heart rate and vascular resistance, which maintain blood pressure even though cardiac output has decreased. As compensatory mechanisms fail, systolic blood pressure falls and diastolic pressure increases (as a result of the sympathetic stimulation), thus narrowing the pulse pressure. Heart rates exceed 100 beats/min. Peripheral vasoconstriction occurs and produces cool, clammy skin.

Respirations become rapid and deep in the effort to increase arterial oxygenation. Auscultation of the lungs reveals coarse crackles resulting from pulmonary edema. An S_3 summation gallop may be audible over the left apex as a result of increased preload in the left ventricle.

Urine output decreases and becomes concentrated because of reabsorption of sodium and water as the kidneys work to increase blood volume. As the shock state progresses, renal ischemia may occur and renal function deteriorates. Urine output falls below 20 ml/hr, blood urea nitrogen and serum creatinine levels rise, and creatinine clearance decreases.

The patient's level of consciousness may be impaired because of low oxygen delivery to the brain. Initially the patient may be restless and confused. If cerebral hypoperfusion increases, the patient may become lethargic and unresponsive.

Frequent assessments of cardiac output and cardiac index are helpful in the clinical treatment of a patient in cardiogenic shock. Decreased myocardial contractility is responsible for decreased cardiac output and cardiac index. Pulmonary artery pressures are increased, with the pulmonary capillary occlusion pressure typically being greater than 18 mm Hg (normal, less than 12 mm Hg). When pulmonary capillary occlusion pressure acutely increases above 18 mm Hg, pulmonary congestion may develop because fluid shifts from the capillary into the interstitial and alveolar spaces.[9] Patients with chronic congestive heart failure may not develop pulmonary edema until pulmonary occlusion pressures exceed 20 to 40 mm Hg. Arterial blood gas values initially demonstrate a respiratory alkalosis secondary to hyperventilation. As pulmonary edema progresses, respiratory acidosis with hypoxemia may occur. Hypoxemia further impairs myocardial function.

Systemic vascular resistance is usually elevated because of SNS activation. The high afterload imposed on the left ventricle because of vasoconstriction may further impair cardiac performance. Frequent assessment of systemic vascular resistance is helpful in the difficult task of tailoring therapy to minimize cardiac workload while maintaining adequate perfusion pressure.

Determination of mixed venous oxygen levels in blood samples obtained from the pulmonary artery catheter is helpful in assessing the adequacy of cardiac output. Decreased tissue oxygen delivery because of low cardiac output increases the degree of oxygen extraction. Mixed venous blood samples show decreased venous oxygen saturation with a decreased cardiac output. An increase in mixed venous oxygenation would be expected with improved cardiac output.

Treatment. Cardiogenic shock is difficult to manage because the underlying myocardial damage is often not reversible. Prevention of cardiogenic shock through measures to limit infarct size during acute myocardial ischemia is desirable. Early efforts to restore coronary perfusion are associated with a decrease in the incidence of cardiogenic shock after myocardial infarction.[11] (A discussion of reperfusion therapy can be found in Chapter 18.)

The goal of treatment for cardiogenic shock is to decrease myocardial oxygen demands, increase myocardial oxygen delivery, and increase cardiac output. It is difficult to achieve these goals because interventions to increase cardiac output tend to increase myocardial oxygen demands.

Pharmacotherapy. Positive inotropic drugs are frequently used in the management of cardiogenic shock to increase contractility. Positive inotropes include β-adrenergic agonists such as NE, dobutamine, and dopamine. These drugs have the ability to increase contractility, increase cardiac output, and increase tissue perfusion; however, they all increase myocardial oxygen demand. NE is the natural neurotransmitter of the sympathetic nerves and its administration mimics SNS activation by increasing heart rate, contractility, and vascular resistance. Dobutamine increases contractility by stimulating β receptors but, unlike NE or dopamine, has minimal α-receptor activity. The major effect of dobutamine is on contractility rather than heart rate. Dobutamine may contribute to a decrease in vascular resistance and must be used with caution in hypotensive patients.[12]

Dopamine stimulates dopaminergic-, β-, and α-receptor sites. Dopaminergic activation results in increased mesenteric and renal blood flow. β-Adrenergic stimulation results in increased contractility and heart rate. α-Adrenergic stimulation results in increased systemic vascular resistance. All of the effects are dose dependent. Dopamine is often used when significant hypotension is present. Dopamine increases myocardial oxygen demands more than dobutamine does; therefore, if blood pressure is greater than 90 mm Hg, dobutamine is a better choice.[12]

Another type of positive inotropic drug used in the management of cardiogenic shock is a phosphodiesterase inhibitor. Phosphodiesterase inhibitors act by inhibiting the breakdown of cyclic adenosine monophosphate (cAMP). Such inhibition leads to increased levels of cAMP and increased activity of cAMP-dependent calcium regulation. An increased level of calcium ions in the cell enhances contractility. Milrinone is an example of a phosphodiesterase inhibitor used to increase myocardial contractility.[13]

Vasodilators may be used to decrease the workload of the heart by decreasing left ventricular afterload. Examples of commonly used vasodilators include nitroprusside and nitroglycerin. Nitroprusside causes both venous and arterial vasodilation. As a result, nitroprusside decreases afterload by decreasing systemic vascular resistance, increases cardiac output, decreases preload, and decreases myocardial oxygen demand. Nitroprusside, because of its profound vasodilating effects, has a tendency to produce hypotension. Nitroprusside has a very short duration of action and is administered by continuous intravenous infusion.[13]

Nitroglycerin is a venodilator and a coronary artery vasodilator. It is used to increase coronary artery blood flow and decrease pulmonary congestion by decreasing preload. Nitroglycerin also has a tendency to lower blood pressure, so that frequent monitoring is necessary.

Mechanical Assist Devices. Cardiogenic shock is sometimes managed by mechanical assist devices. For temporary management, **intraaortic** balloon counterpulsation may be indicated.[14] A catheter with a balloon at the distal segment is inserted through the femoral artery and positioned in the aorta just distal to the left subclavian artery (see Figure 19-12). The balloon is connected to a console that triggers the balloon to inflate in diastole and deflate in systole. The effect of balloon inflation during diastole is to increase perfusion pressure of the coronary arteries. Sudden deflation of the balloon just before ventricular systole creates a vacuum effect in the aorta that reduces left ventricular afterload. A reduction in afterload decreases left ventricular workload and increases stroke volume. Balloon counterpulsation restricts mobility and is associated with a number of vascular complications. Long-term management of patients with low cardiac output can be achieved with mechanical pumps that take over the function of the ventricle or ventricles (ventricular assist devices).[14] Ventricular assist devices are commonly used in patients awaiting heart transplantation. In some cases the temporary decrease in cardiac workload afforded by the ventricular assist device is associated with significant improvement in cardiac structure and function and the device can be removed.

Surgery. Heart transplantation is a procedure frequently performed for the treatment of refractory heart failure. Approximately 3000 transplants are done annually in the United States, with a survival rate of about 80%.[15] However, the number of persons needing heart transplantation exceeds donor availability, and other methods of surgical intervention have been developed. For example, a patient's own skeletal muscle (latissimus dorsi) can be dissected and wrapped around the heart (cardiomyoplasty) to provide ventricular assistance. A pacemaker is used to stimulate the muscle to contract at the appropriate time.[16] Despite these advanced treatment modalities, the mortality associated with cardiogenic shock remains high, and little improvement has been achieved over the past decade despite intensive supportive therapy.

KEY CONCEPTS

- Cardiogenic shock is usually a result of severe ventricular dysfunction associated with myocardial infarction. Other causes include cardiomyopathy, ventricular rupture, and congenital heart defects.
- Diagnostic features of cardiogenic shock include decreased cardiac output as a result of left ventricular dysfunction, along with elevated left ventricular end-diastolic pressure, S_3 heart sounds, and pulmonary edema. Sympathetic activation leads to an increased heart rate, vasoconstriction, and a narrow pulse pressure.
- Low cardiac output leads to reduced oxygen delivery to tissues. Tissues extract a greater percentage of oxygen from the delivered blood, which leads to reduced SvO_2.
- Therapy is aimed at improving cardiac output and myocardial oxygen delivery while reducing cardiac workload. Pharmacologic treatment often includes the use of inotropic agents (dopamine, dobutamine, amrinone), afterload-reducing agents (vasodilators), and preload-reducing agents (venodilators, diuretics). Intraaortic balloon counterpulsation may be used to reduce afterload and improve coronary artery perfusion. Ventricular assist devices may be used for longer term circulatory support, whereas heart transplantation provides definitive treatment.

Hypovolemic Shock

Etiology and Classification. Hypovolemic shock results when circulating blood volume is inadequate to perfuse tissues and decreased by at least 1000 ml.[17] The pathogenesis of early stage hypovolemic shock is straightforward: decreased intravascular volume leads to a decrease in venous return, which causes a decrease in cardiac output (Figure 20-9). The decrease in cardiac output results in decreased tissue perfusion and decreased oxygen delivery.

Circulatory volume deficits may be the result of internal or external losses. Internal losses can result from internal hemorrhage, fracture of long bones, or leakage of fluid into the interstitial spaces. External losses can result from external hemorrhage, burns, severe vomiting and diarrhea, or diuresis. External hemorrhage is the most common cause of hypovolemic shock.

The American College of Surgeons stratifies hemorrhagic shock into four classes according to the degree of blood volume lost (Table 20-2).[18] Compensated hemorrhage occurs with blood loss up to 1000 ml. Compensatory mechanisms

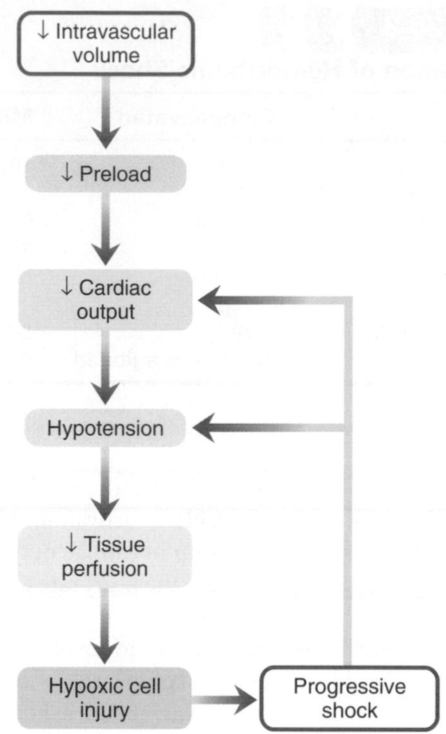

FIGURE 20-9 ■ Pathogenesis of hypovolemic shock.

maintain cardiac output, and the patient's vital signs remain within the normal range.

Mild hemorrhage is categorized as blood loss between 1000 and 1500 ml. The patient becomes anxious and restless. Blood pressure remains normal when the patient is supine but decreases when he or she is standing (orthostatic hypotension). The heart rate is between 100 and 120 beats/min. The respiratory rate is normal to mildly increased. Urine output is between 20 and 30 ml/hr. The capillary refill time may be prolonged. The capillary blanch test is performed by depressing a patient's fingernail and observing how long after release the skin color takes to return to normal. Normal capillary refill times are less than 2 seconds.

Moderate hemorrhage is a major blood loss, from 30% to 40% of total blood volume (1500 to 2000 mL). The patient is anxious and confused. Blood pressure is decreased with a narrow pulse pressure. The heart rate is greater than 120 beats/min. Respiratory rates are between 30 and 40 respirations per minute. Urine output is 5 to 20 ml/hr. The capillary refill test is prolonged.

Severe hemorrhage occurs when more than 40% of total blood volume is lost (2000 ml or more). The patient is lethargic and has severe hypotension with a narrow pulse pressure. The heart rate exceeds 140 beats/min, and the respiratory rate is markedly increased. Urine output is negligible. The capillary refill test is prolonged.

The clinical features of other forms of hypovolemic shock are similar to those of hemorrhagic shock, although the volume loss has usually occurred more gradually.

Table 20-2

Classification of Hemorrhagic Shock

Factor	Compensated	Mild	Moderate	Severe
Blood loss (ml)	≤1000	1000-1500	1500-2000	>2000
Heart rate (beats/min)	<100	>100	>120	>2000
Blood pressure	Normal	Orthostatic change	Marked fall	Profound fall
Capillary refill	Normal	May be delayed	Usually delayed	Always delayed
Respiration	Normal	Mild increase	Moderate tachypnea	Marked tachypnea: respiratory collapse
Urinary output (ml/hr)	>30	20-30	5-20	Anuria
Mental status	Normal or agitated	Agitated	Confused	Lethargic, obtunded

Clinical Manifestations. The early manifestations of hypovolemic shock are attributable to activation of the SNS. Baroreceptors quickly detect a drop in cardiac output and respond through the SNS to increase the heart rate and produce vasoconstriction. These mechanisms are effective in maintaining blood pressure in the early stages of hypovolemic shock. As the degree of blood loss increases, compensatory mechanisms begin to fail and tissue ischemia can result. If hemodynamic monitoring is instituted, the cardiac output and cardiac index are found to be decreased. Pulmonary artery pressures and pulmonary capillary wedge pressures are decreased because of the decreased preload. The finding of a low preload distinguishes hypovolemic shock from cardiogenic shock. In cardiogenic shock, preload is high and cardiac output is low. In hypovolemic shock, preload and cardiac output are both low.

Systemic vascular resistance is increased as a result of sympathetic activation. This increase is a compensatory mechanism in hypovolemia to maintain perfusion pressure. SvO_2 may be decreased because of decreased oxygen delivery and increased oxygen extraction.

Treatment. The first intervention for hemorrhagic shock is to control the source of blood loss. Second, volume losses are replaced with appropriate fluids to normalize blood pressure and cardiac output. In severe, uncontrolled hemorrhage, efforts to increase blood pressure should be postponed until the hemorrhage is under control.[17] Otherwise the increased blood pressure may worsen the hemorrhage. In all types of hypovolemic shock, fluid replacement is the primary therapy. The three main types of fluid therapy agents are colloids, crystalloids, and blood products.

Colloids are solutions that increase the serum colloid osmotic pressure within the vascular compartment. Increased colloid pressure pulls fluid from the interstitium into the vascular space. The advantage to administering colloid solutions is that only small amounts are needed to restore vascular volume. A potential disadvantage to their administration is leakage of colloid from the vascular compartment into the interstitial space if capillary permeability is increased. Examples of colloid solutions are normal human serum albumin, dextran, and hetastarch. Colloids generally are not used for hypovolemic shock unless the patient has significant interstitial edema.

Crystalloids are solutions that contain electrolytes. Isotonic solutions such as lactated Ringer solution or normal saline solution are commonly used crystalloid solutions. A disadvantage to volume replacement with crystalloid solutions is the potential for pulmonary edema to develop because of the large volumes of fluid required to restore intravascular volume. Isotonic fluids are preferred over glucose or hypotonic electrolyte solutions because isotonic solutions remain in the extracellular space and are more effective in increasing blood volume. Isotonic crystalloid fluids are preferred for volume resuscitation in hypovolemic shock that is not associated with severe anemia.[19]

When significant anemia accompanies hypovolemia, *blood products* may be the treatment of choice. Whole blood contains all of the blood components, including red cells, plasma, clotting factors, and platelets. Packed red blood cells have most of the plasma volume removed and as a result have no clotting factors. Plasma contains clotting factors but no platelets or red cells. In hemorrhagic shock, whole blood or packed red blood cells with saline may be given to replace blood loss.

In general, pharmacologic agents are not indicated for hypovolemia. Restoration of blood volume is essential. However, in some cases of shock, blood pressure remains low despite large amounts of fluid replacement, so vasoconstrictor agents must be used to support blood pressure.

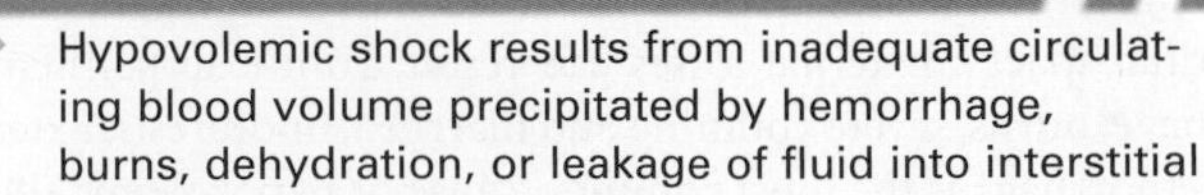

KEY CONCEPTS

- Hypovolemic shock results from inadequate circulating blood volume precipitated by hemorrhage, burns, dehydration, or leakage of fluid into interstitial spaces.
- The classic features of hypovolemic shock are the result of low cardiac output and low intracardiac pressures. Manifestations are due primarily to SNS acti-

vation: elevated heart rate, vasoconstriction, and increased myocardial contractility.

- The severity of symptoms of hemorrhagic shock correlates with the amount of blood loss: Compensated, 1000 ml blood loss, mild symptoms, and cardiac output near normal; mild, 1000 to 1500 ml blood loss, blood pressure normal, but elevated heart rate and orthostatic hypotension; moderate, 1500 to 2000 ml blood loss, decreased blood pressure, heart rate over 120 beats/min, and decreased urine output; and severe, more than 2000 ml blood loss, severe hypotension and tachycardia (140 beats/min), and oliguria.
- Therapy for hypovolemic shock is aimed at fluid replacement and control of the source of volume loss. Colloids, crystalloids, and blood products may be used as replacement fluids.

Obstructive Shock

Etiology. Obstructive shock develops when the heart is prevented from pumping because of a mechanical obstruction to blood flow. Impaired ventricular filling leads to reduced cardiac output and signs and symptoms of circulatory shock. Causes of mechanical obstruction include pulmonary embolism, cardiac tamponade, and tension pneumothorax. The presence of an obstructive mechanism may be difficult to differentiate from cardiogenic shock, and a high index of suspicion is required to rapidly diagnose the problem. Prompt relief of the obstruction is necessary to restore cardiac output and prevent cardiovascular collapse.

Clinical Manifestations. Obstructive shock is usually characterized by manifestations of right-sided heart failure. Depending on the location of the obstruction, elevated pressures in the cardiac chambers may be evident.

Pulmonary embolism results in elevated right-sided heart pressures, but left-sided pressures remain normal to low. Pulmonary emboli are usually generated in the veins of the lower extremities in patients with immobility, trauma, or hypercoagulable states. Pulmonary embolism is manifested as sudden, severe dyspnea and deteriorating arterial blood gas values. A perfusion scan of the lung may demonstrate an area of reduced blood flow. Pulmonary emboli are not generally detectable by chest radiographs.

Cardiac tamponade, which results from an accumulation of fluid in the pericardial sac, causes elevation of pressures on both the right and left side of the heart. Despite the elevated pressure, preload in the heart chambers is low, as is stroke volume. The elevated pressure is due to external compression of the heart chambers. Risks for the development of cardiac tamponade include pericarditis, blunt trauma to the chest, and cardiac surgical procedures. In pericarditis a pericardial friction rub can sometimes be heard and may help with the diagnosis.

Tension pneumothorax results in shifting and compression of mediastinal structures, including the heart, which compromises left ventricular filling. Accumulation of air in the pleural space may occur because of trauma or spontaneous rupture of lung parenchyma. A tension pneumothorax develops when the air in the pleural space begins to exert a positive pressure on lung and mediastinal structures. A deviated trachea and decreased or absent breath sounds may occur. Arterial blood gas values can deteriorate rapidly. Tension pneumothorax is detectable by chest radiography.

Treatment. Management of obstructive shock is aimed at identifying and removing the offending obstruction. Compensatory mechanisms are generally ineffective in obstructive shock, and the patient's condition may deteriorate rapidly.

If a pulmonary embolus is suspected, surgical embolectomy or thrombolytic therapy may be indicated. Administration of supplemental oxygen is indicated, and some patients may require mechanical ventilation. Pulmonary embolism is a preventable condition. Recognition of patients at risk and early treatment to avoid deep vein thrombosis are helpful in preventing pulmonary embolism. Immobile patients may need anticoagulant therapy to prevent clot formation.

Cardiac tamponade and tension pneumothorax are often associated with trauma and may be difficult to anticipate or prevent. Prompt removal of the offending fluid from the pericardial space or air from the pleural space will usually prevent circulatory shock. Pericardial fluid can be removed by needle aspiration or surgery. Tension pneumothorax is treated with chest tube insertion to relieve pressure and reestablish a negative intrapleural pressure. Measures to support blood pressure and ventilation may be required while definitive therapy is being initiated.

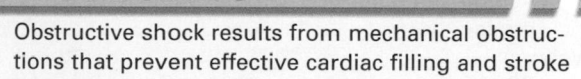

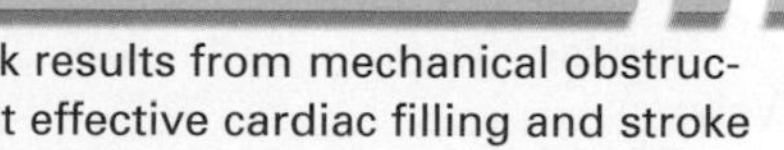

- Obstructive shock results from mechanical obstructions that prevent effective cardiac filling and stroke volume.
- Pulmonary embolism, cardiac tamponade, and tension pneumothorax are common causes of obstructive shock.
- Prompt management of the underlying obstruction is necessary to prevent cardiovascular collapse.

Distributive Shock

Distributive shock is characterized by an abnormally expanded vascular space caused by excessive vasodilation. Vasodilation results in peripheral pooling of blood and creates a relative hypovolemia. Preload and stroke volume are insufficient to maintain perfusion of the brain and tissues. Anaphylactic, neurogenic, and septic are types of distributive shock. All are characterized by vasodilation and profound hypotension, but the cause and pathogenesis of each type differ significantly.

Anaphylactic Shock

Etiology and Pathogenesis. Type I anaphylactic reactions involve an antigen/IgE antibody reaction on the surface of mast cells and basophils. IgE antibodies attach to receptor sites on these cells, where they await activation by specific antigens. Exposure to that antigen causes receptors on mast cells and basophils to cross-link and become activated. A host of vasoactive chemicals are released, including histamines, leukotrienes, bradykinins, and prostaglandins.[20] These substances result in bronchoconstriction, peripheral vasodilation, and increased capillary permeability. (A detailed discussion of type I anaphylaxis can be found in Chapter 10.) In some cases mast cell degranulation is triggered by a mechanism that does not involve IgE. These reactions may be called *anaphylactoid* (Box 20-2).

Most type I anaphylactic reactions are mild and do not result in shock. Even in more severe anaphylaxis, prompt treatment can prevent the shock syndrome. Shock occurs when peripheral dilation is massive, and a type of hypovolemic shock is precipitated. In this case blood volume is normal but the sudden enlargement of the vascular space causes blood to pool in the periphery. This condition causes cardiac preload to drop, followed by a decrease in cardiac output.

Box 20-2

Common Triggers of Anaphylaxis

Anaphylactic (IgE Dependent)

Foods
- Peanuts
- Tree nuts
- Crustaceans (crab, shrimp)

Medications
- β-Lactam antibiotics
- Other antibiotics
- Aspirin and other nonsteroidal antiinflammatory drugs

Venoms
- Bee sting
- Snake bite

Animal proteins
- Cat
- Dog
- Horse

Anaphylactoid (IgE Independent)

Radiocontrast media

Opioids

Muscle relaxants

Temperature
- Cold
- Heat

Transfusion reactions
- IgG
- IgM

Unidentified Triggers

Idiopathic

Clinical Manifestations. The onset of symptoms is usually within 2 to 30 minutes of exposure to the antigen; however, symptoms may not develop for several hours.[20] Initially the patient appears very anxious, with an increased heart rate and respiratory rate. Hypotension, urticaria, pruritus, and angioedema then develop. Often the patient has a sense of impending doom. Bronchoconstriction causes wheezing and cyanosis, and laryngeal edema results in hoarseness and stridor.

Prevention and Treatment. Prevention of anaphylactic shock is achieved by avoidance of precipitating allergens. Anaphylactic shock is most frequently associated with antibiotic therapy, in particular β-lactams.[20] Other common causes include other types of drugs, peanuts and tree nuts, insect stings, and snake bites (see Box 20-2). More than one third of cases are of unknown cause. Anaphylaxis is not a reportable disease, and the incidence is unknown; however, the estimated risk of occurrence is 1% to 3% per person in the United States.[20]

Initial therapy for anaphylactic shock is directed to removing the inciting antigen if possible. Airway management and circulatory support are critical. Tracheal intubation and assisted ventilation may be needed. Bronchodilators such as epinephrine and aminophylline can be used to manage bronchospasm. Epinephrine is also helpful in stabilizing mast cells to prevent further release of inflammatory mediators and increasing blood pressure.[20] Intravenous fluid therapy is used to increase intravascular volume and fill the enlarged vascular space. Increased preload will enhance cardiac output. A vasopressor such as dopamine or epinephrine may be given in an attempt to constrict the arterioles and raise blood pressure. Steroids may be given for their antiinflammatory effects, but the onset of action tends to be slow. Antihistamines may be administered to block histamine receptors, although their effectiveness is reduced once symptoms are present and the inflammatory mediators have been released.[20] Response to therapy for anaphylactic shock is usually rapid with a good outcome if instituted early; however, approximately 1% of anaphylactic episodes are fatal, and the majority of these are associated with antibiotics and nut allergies.[20]

Neurogenic Shock

Neurogenic shock is often transitory. It may result from depression of the vasomotor center in the medulla or from interruption of sympathetic nerve fibers in the spinal cord. Causes of neurogenic shock include brain trauma that results in depression of the vasomotor center, spinal cord injury, high spinal anesthesia, and drug overdose.

Interruption of the neural pathway for the baroreceptor reflex results in loss of sympathetic tone in the vasculature. Profound peripheral vasodilation of both arterioles and veins occurs and leads to hypotension. Peripheral pooling of blood decreases venous return to the heart; preload and cardiac output fall accordingly. Body position greatly influences the development of neurogenic shock. When the body is horizontal, venous return may be adequate and cardiac output and blood pressure are sufficient. However, when an upright position is assumed, peripheral pooling from gravitational effects causes a severe drop in cardiac output and blood pressure. Syncope and fainting will follow unless measures are taken to redistribute the blood. Elevation of the legs, slow position changes, and the use of pressure stockings on the legs may help prevent peripheral pooling. Vasoconstricting drugs and fluid expansion may sometimes be used to increase blood pressure if mechanical measures are ineffective.

Septic Shock

Septic shock is a common cause of death in intensive care units in the United States, and the incidence continues to increase. Large numbers of immunocompromised individuals in the population and extensive use of invasive technology contribute to the high rates of septic shock. The mortality associated with septic shock averages about 45%.[21]

Etiology. Sepsis results from the presence of microorganisms in the blood stream (bacteremia). However, most cases of bacteremia do not result in shock. Normally, the body's defense systems effectively destroy the bacteria and prevent widespread dissemination of the infection. Immunocompromised individuals are prone to disseminated infections called bacteremia. When the body's response to infection or other insults results in systemic signs and symptoms of widespread inflammation, the term *systemic inflammatory response syndrome* (SIRS) is applied. Septic shock is a severe systemic inflammatory reaction to infection that results in abnormal vasodilation, hypotension, and tissue hypoxia owing to the maldistribution of blood flow. Confusion about the meaning of the terms bacteremia, sepsis, septic shock, and SIRS prompted a consensus conference to provide definitions for clinical and research purposes (Table 20-3).[22]

Patients at risk for septic shock include the very young and the elderly. Patients in these age groups are less likely to be able to destroy invading microorganisms. Patients who are debilitated, malnourished, or immunocompromised by acquired immunodeficiency syndrome or chemotherapy or have chronic health problems are also at increased risk. Medical interventions that predispose a patient to septic shock include the use of invasive lines, catheters, and procedures; surgery; and immunosuppressive therapy.

Pathogenesis. Septic shock is most often associated with gram-negative septicemia. Gram-negative bacteria include *Escherichia coli, Klebsiella pneumoniae, Enterobacter aerogenes, Serratia marcescens, Pseudomonas aeruginosa,* and *Proteus* species.[23] Gram-positive organisms *(Staphylococcus aureus, Staphylococcus epidermidis, Streptococcus pneumoniae)* and fungi *(Candida*

Table 20-3

Definitions Related to Sepsis

Condition	Definition
Bacteremia (fungemia)	Presence of viable bacteria (fungi) in the blood stream.
Infection	Inflammatory response to invasion of normally sterile host tissue by the microorganisms.
Systemic inflammatory response syndrome	Systemic inflammatory response to a variety of clinical insults that can be infectious or noninfectious. The response is manifested by two or more of the following conditions: $T > 38°C$ (100.4° F) or $< 36°$ C (96.8° F); HR > 90 beats/min; RR > 20 breaths/min or $Pa_{CO_2} < 32$ Torr; WBC $> 12{,}000$ cells/mm^3, < 4000 cells/mm^3, or $> 10\%$ immature (band) forms.
Sepsis	The systemic inflammatory response syndrome secondary to infection.
Severe sepsis	Sepsis associated with organ dysfunction, hypoperfusion, or hypotension. Hypoperfusion and perfusion abnormalities may include, but are not limited to, lactic acidosis, oliguria, or acute alteration in mental status.
Septic shock	Sepsis with hypotension, despite fluid resuscitation, along with the presence of perfusion abnormalities. Patients who are on inotropic or vasopressor agents may not be hypotensive at the time perfusion abnormalities are measured
Multiple organ dysfunction syndrome	Presence of altered organ function requiring intervention to maintain homeostasis.
Compensatory antiinflammatory response syndrome	Compensatory physiologic response to systemic inflammatory response syndrome that is considered secondary to the actions of antiinflammatory cytokine mediators.

From Dipiro JT et al, editors: *Pharmacotherapy: a pathophysiologic approach,* ed 5, New York, 2002, McGraw-Hill, p 2030.
HR, Heart rate; *RR,* respiratory rate; *T,* temperature; *WBC,* white blood cell count; *Torr,* mm Hg.

species) are also important causes of septic shock. A frequent portal of entry is the genitourinary tract. Other entry sites include the gastrointestinal tract, the respiratory tract, and the skin.

Gram-negative bacteria have within their cell walls a lipopolysaccharide or **endotoxin.** It is composed of an O antigen side chain, an R core, and an inner lipid A, which is the toxic component of the endotoxin.[23] Endotoxins are released into the blood during bacterial cell lysis and initiate a chain of pathophysiologic events. Macrophages are stimulated by endotoxin to release inflammatory cytokines, including TNF-α and IL-1.[4] As previously described, TNF-α and IL-1 are thought to be major factors in the pathogenesis of septic shock because they stimulate release of more immune cytokines and the overproduction of nitric oxide.

Macrophage cytokines activate neutrophils and platelets, which release many toxic mediators such as platelet-activating factor, oxygen free radicals, and proteolytic enzymes.[4] Activation of the arachidonic acid cascade in neutrophils and platelets results in prostaglandin, leukotriene, thromboxane, and prostacyclin release, all of which have profound effects on vascular smooth muscle. Increased levels of thromboxane A_2 and B_2 produce pulmonary vasoconstriction, mediate bronchoconstriction, and act as potent platelet aggregators. Prostacyclin is a potent vasodilator and may contribute to the development of hypotension.

A number of other inflammatory cascades are activated in septic shock. The complement system is activated with release of C5a and C3a, which can produce microemboli and endothelial cell destruction. Histamine, a potent vasodilator, is released by mast cells. Histamine also increases capillary permeability, which enhances edema formation. The coagulation system is activated and may enhance the development of thrombi. The kinin system is activated and bradykinin is released, which results in vasodilation and increased capillary permeability. All these immune responses are normal reactions to microbial invasion and are necessary for eradicating infections. In overabundance, however, these mechanisms constitute a systemic inflammatory response that can result in shock. The major components of the complex pathophysiologic processes of septic shock are illustrated in Figure 20-10.

Septic shock is associated with profound peripheral vasodilation. Systemic vascular resistance is decreased, and despite the increased cardiac output, blood pressure falls. The veins also dilate, and intravascular pooling occurs in the venous capacitance system. Because of maldistribution of blood flow, some tissues are underperfused and some are overperfused. Excessive flow to areas of low metabolic demand limits oxygen extraction, which contributes to low oxygen consumption. In the initial stages of septic shock, a relative hypovolemia is present because of the increased size of the vascular compartment. Fluid administration to increase preload to a central venous pressure between 8 and 12 mm Hg is advocated at this stage even though cardiac output may already be quite high.[24] Cardiac output between 8 and 12 L/min is common in early septic shock. Even this level of cardiac output may be inadequate to perfuse the expanded vascular bed.

The generalized inflammatory response triggered in septic shock affects capillary permeability. Increased capillary permeability results in fluid movement out of the vascular beds into the interstitial space. Generalized soft tissue edema occurs and can interfere with tissue oxygenation and organ function.

Clinical Manifestations. In contrast to other forms of shock, the clinical manifestation of early septic shock is a hyperdynamic state characterized by high cardiac output and warm extremities. A comparison of the clinical findings in cardiogenic, hypovolemic, and septic shock is shown in Table 20-4.

In the hyperdynamic stage of septic shock blood pressure falls because of the decreased systemic vascular resistance and decreased venous return. Diastolic pressure falls because of a lack of sympathetic tone, and a widened pulse pressure results. The heart rate and stroke volume increase and cardiac output is higher than normal, but the patient remains hypotensive. The patient is usually febrile and may have associated chills. The skin is pink and warm to the touch as a result of peripheral vasodilation. The patient's level of consciousness may be altered as a result of cerebral ischemia. In septic shock $S\bar{v}O_2$ levels may be higher than normal because of the maldistribution of blood flow. Abnormal vasodilation causes greater flow through areas with low metabolic activity. Oxygen consumption by tissues is decreased because metabolically active tissues do not receive enough flow. Lactic acidosis may be present because of tissue hypoxemia.

In the late stages of septic shock, some patients progress to a hypodynamic phase. The hypodynamic phase is characterized by decreased cardiac output and the development of organ ischemia. The pulse pressure narrows and the skin becomes cool and clammy. Profound hypotension unresponsive to catecholamines generally occurs. Arterial blood gas analysis reveals a metabolic and respiratory acidosis with hypoxemia. Myocardial depression either from ischemia or toxins acting as myocardial depressants contributes to a falling cardiac output, deteriorating tissue perfusion, and refractory shock.

Treatment. The primary treatment in early septic shock is isotonic fluid administration to restore adequate ventricular preload.[24] If fluid administration does not restore hemodynamic stability, inotropic treatment (e.g., dopamine, dobutamine, epinephrine) may be indicated to increase cardiac output and oxygen delivery to tissues.[24] Vascular unresponsiveness to these agents may improve with administration of vasopressin. Studies have shown that the posterior pituitary is quickly depleted of vasopressin during septic shock resulting in a deficiency syndrome.[25] Vasopressin may reduce the dose of catecholamines needed to maintain blood pressure.[21]

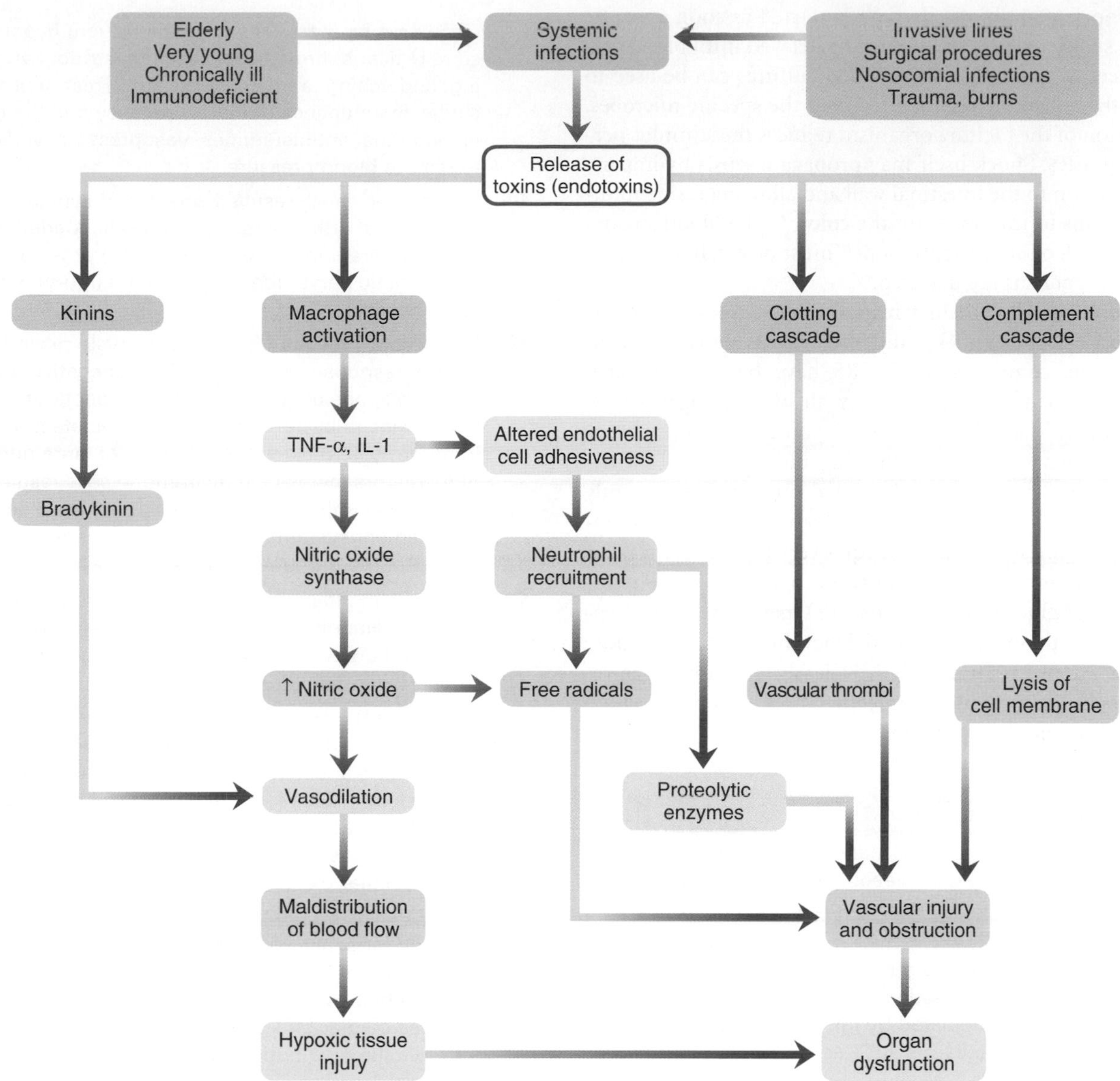

FIGURE 20-10 ■ Pathophysiologic process of septic shock. Septic shock is characterized by immune-mediated mechanisms of cellular injury and organ dysfunction. *TNF-α,* Tumor necrosis factor-α; *IL-1,* interleukin-1.

Table 20-4

Comparison of the Clinical Findings in Different Types of Shock

Parameter	Cardiogenic	Hypovolemic	Septic
Hypotension	Yes	Yes	Yes
Systemic vascular resistance	High	High	Low
Cardiac output	Low	Low	High
Cardiac preload	High	Low	Low
Venous oxygen saturation	Low	Low	High
Urine output	Low	Low	Low
Skin temperature	Cool	Cool	Warm

Appropriate antibiotic therapy is started as soon as septic shock is suspected and should not be delayed until blood cultures become positive. Positive blood cultures can be used to narrow the antibiotic regimen to cover the specific microbes. Eradication of the inciting organism reduces the stimulus perpetuating SIRS. Shock itself may propagate sepsis by impairing circulation to the intestinal wall and allowing resident microorganisms to traverse from the colon to the blood stream. Antibiotic selection for septic shock must be modified as new infective organisms are detected.

Because the inflammatory response is believed to be a critical aspect of septic shock, numerous agents designed to inhibit various components of SIRS have been investigated (Table 20-5). Unfortunately, nearly all of these agents have failed to provide significant benefit.[23] Some subgroups of septic patients may be helped by these agents, but overall the trials have been disappointing. Activated protein C is currently recommended for those with severe sepsis but does not appear helpful unless the risk of death is very high. Protein C has both antiinflammatory and antithrombotic actions. Physiologic doses of glucocorticoids (steroids) may be helpful in septic patients with documented deficiency; however, higher dose regimens are not recommended.[24] Clearly, much research remains to be done to determine the most effective ways to manage this complex syndrome.

KEY CONCEPTS

- Anaphylactic, neurogenic, and septic shock are characterized by excessive vasodilation and peripheral pooling of blood. Cardiac output is inadequate because of reduced preload.
- Anaphylactic shock is a result of excessive mast cell degranulation in response to antigen. Mast cell degranulation is mediated by IgE antibodies. Release of vasodilatory mediators such as histamine into the circulation by mast cells results in severe hypotension. Urticaria, bronchoconstriction, stridor, wheezing, and itching are usually present. Treatment includes maintenance of airway patency and the use of epinephrine, antihistamines, vasopressors, and fluids to restore blood pressure.
- Neurogenic shock results from loss of sympathetic activation of arteriolar smooth muscle. Medullary depression (brain injury, drug overdose) or lesions of sympathetic nerve fibers (spinal cord injury) are the usual causes.
- Septic shock results from a severe systemic inflammatory response to infection. Gram-negative bacteria are responsible for most cases of septic shock. Endotoxins in bacterial cell walls stimulate massive immune system activation. Release of large numbers of mediators (cytokines) by immune cells results in widespread inflammation. The clotting cascade, complement system, and kinin system are activated as part of the immune response.
- Widespread inflammation leads to profound peripheral vasodilation with hypotension, maldistribution of blood flow with cellular hypoxia, and increased capillary permeability with edema formation.
- Initially, septic shock is characterized by abnormally high cardiac output resulting from immune-mediated vasodilation and sympathetic activation of the heart. The patient is usually febrile, pink, and warm. Even though cardiac output is high, cellular hypoxia is present because of maldistribution of blood flow. Reduced cellular oxygen utilization is manifested as a high SvO_2.
- Therapy for septic shock is aimed at improving the distribution of blood flow and managing infection with antibiotics. Administration of fluid and drugs to increase cardiac and vascular performance is done to improve the distribution of blood flow.

Table 20-5 

Anti–Systemic Inflammatory Response Syndrome Agents Studied in Sepsis

Agent	Results
Monoclonal antibody against endotoxin (antilipid A)	No overall benefit
Interleukin-1 receptor antagonist	No overall benefit
Platelet-activating factor inhibitor	No overall benefit
Bradykinin antagonists	No overall benefit
Monoclonal antibody against tumor necrosis factor	No overall benefit
Tumor necrosis factor receptor components (soluble receptor)	Worsened outcome or no benefit
Suppression of nitric oxide synthases (L-NAME)	Worsened outcomes
Selective inhibition of inducible nitric oxide synthase (L-canavanine)	Remains to be seen (encouraging studies in animals)
Endothelin receptor blockers	Remains to be seen (encouraging studies in animals)
Activated protein C	No overall benefit but significant reduction in mortality in severe sepsis subgroup

Data from Dipiro JT et al, editors: *Pharmacotherapy: a pathophysiologic approach,* ed 5, New York, 2002, McGraw-Hill; and Iskit AB, GUC O: Effects of endothelin and nitric oxide on organ injury, mesenteric ischemia, and survival in experimental models of septic shock, *Acta Pharmacol Singapore* 24(10):953-957, 2003; and Bhatia M, Moochhala S: Role of inflammatory mediators in the pathophysiology of acute respiratory distress syndrome, *J Pathol* 202:145-156, 2004.

COMPLICATIONS OF SHOCK

The pathologic process of the shock state and the effects on other organs may precipitate life-threatening complications. The patient may survive the shock state only to succumb to a resulting complication. In severe shock of any cause, particularly in septic shock, a generalized inflammatory reaction may occur and is thought to contribute to the organ damage associated with shock states. Complications associated with shock include acute respiratory distress syndrome (ARDS), disseminated intravascular coagulation (DIC), acute renal failure, and multiple organ dysfunction syndrome (MODS). Damage to organ systems may be ongoing even after the initial precipitating event has been addressed. Inflammatory cytokines are thought to mediate this organ damage by altering metabolism, recruiting neutrophils, initiating the coagulation cascade, and altering capillary permeability. The complexities of this syndrome are being unraveled as the mechanisms of immune signaling are better understood.

Acute Respiratory Distress Syndrome

ARDS, a form of respiratory failure, is most commonly associated with septic shock. ARDS is characterized by the development of refractory hypoxemia, decreased pulmonary compliance, and radiologic evidence of pulmonary edema associated with normal cardiac preload (noncardiogenic pulmonary edema). The mortality in patients with shock that is complicated by ARDS ranges from 60% to 90%.[23]

The lungs are a common target of immune-mediated damage in all types of shock. Tissue ischemia, even in areas distant from the lungs, leads to neutrophil migration to pulmonary capillaries.[4] Neutrophils release destructive proteolytic enzymes, produce oxygen free radicals, and secrete inflammatory chemicals that make pulmonary capillaries leaky. A protein-rich inflammatory exudate leaks into the interstitial spaces and alveoli of the lung, where it interferes with pulmonary gas exchange. Inflammation may also damage type II pneumocytes, which normally produce surfactant. Surfactant deficiency alters alveolar surface tension and causes smaller alveoli to collapse. The effort to breathe is very great in patients with ARDS because of pulmonary edema and alveolar collapse (atelectasis).

Mechanical ventilation with positive end-expiratory pressure may be used to decrease the work of breathing, keep alveoli open, and reduce alveolar edema. Surfactant replacement therapy has been used but has little benefit. Further discussion of ARDS and its clinical manifestations can be found in Chapter 23.

Disseminated Intravascular Coagulation

DIC is a serious complication of septic shock characterized by abnormal clot formation in the microvasculature throughout the body. DIC is thought to result from endotoxin and immune activation of the clotting cascade. Obstruction of blood flow by small clots in the microcirculation leads to ischemic tissue damage. In addition, widespread clot formation consumes platelets and clotting factors, which leaves the patient at risk for serious bleeding. Laboratory assessment of the platelet count and clotting function is helpful in detecting and monitoring DIC. The platelet count and fibrinogen levels are typically low, whereas levels of fibrin degradation products (e.g., D-dimer) are elevated. Measures of the intrinsic and extrinsic clotting cascades demonstrate an elevated partial thromboplastin time and prothrombin time.

The clinical features of DIC are variable, depending on the location and severity of vascular thrombi. Vascular obstruction may be manifested as acute ischemia of the fingers and toes, with pain, pallor, and poor capillary refill. Obstruction of the kidney, liver, spleen, and lung by clots may result in signs and symptoms of organ failure. Patients may demonstrate various degrees of bleeding. Intravenous lines and catheters may begin to ooze around insertion sites. Previously stable incision lines may begin to bleed, and hematuria and hemoptysis may be present. Spontaneous intracranial hemorrhage is a particularly disastrous complication of DIC.

Treatment for DIC is complex and generally unsatisfactory. Various anticoagulant agents have been used to inhibit clot formation and prevent the consumption of clotting factors and platelets. Trials of two natural anticoagulants, antithrombin and protein C, demonstrated no overall benefit for either agent, although a subgroup with severe sepsis may have benefited in the protein C trial.[26] Heparin is an anticoagulant commonly used in DIC patients to prevent thrombosis and clotting factor consumption. There are no adequate trials to evaluate the outcomes of heparin use in DIC with sepsis. Replacement of platelets and clotting factors may be helpful in an actively bleeding patient. Further discussion of DIC can be found in Chapter 14.

Acute Renal Failure

In shock, the kidneys undergo prolonged periods of hypoperfusion. Vasoconstriction of the afferent arterioles causes decreased glomerular blood flow, decreased glomerular hydrostatic pressure, and decreased glomerular filtration rates. Hypoxic cellular damage occurs after 15 to 20 minutes of acute ischemia and results in necrosis of tubular epithelial cells. Acute tubular necrosis (ATN) is associated with decreased urinary excretion of waste products such as creatinine and urea. Rapidly increasing blood urea nitrogen and serum creatinine concentrations are indicative of ATN.

Urine output quickly falls toward zero, and the kidneys do not respond to fluids or diuretics. Epithelial cell casts in the urine indicate sloughing of tubular cells. ATN is potentially reversible, although renal function must generally be supported for a time with dialysis. Recovery of tubular function begins 1 to 2 weeks after the initial injury and may take up to a year to be completed. Further discussion of ATN can be found in Chapter 28.

Multiple Organ Dysfunction Syndrome

When organ dysfunction develops in two or more systems, the term MODS may be applied. When the patient sustains multiple organ injury from a primary insult such as trauma, the term primary MODS is used. Secondary MODS is associated with SIRS and usually develops days to weeks after the primary insult. Sepsis and septic shock are the most common causes of secondary MODS. Mortality from MODS differs depending on the number of organs affected; involvement of two organ systems carries a 54% mortality and involvement of five organs carries a 100% mortality.[27] In MODS, the body is unable to maintain homeostasis, and intensive intervention is necessary to maintain life.

As with other manifestations of septic shock, MODS is thought to be initiated by immune mechanisms that are overactive and destructive. Release of TNF-α and IL-1 from macrophages is an early event in SIRS. These cytokines and others affect endothelium throughout the body and cause recruitment of neutrophils and activation of inflammation in capillary beds. Ongoing inflammation leads to tissue destruction and organ dysfunction. Inflammatory cytokines and stress hormones stimulate an increased body metabolism, which places a greater demand on already dysfunctional organs.

At present, no specific treatment is available for MODS. Therapy is supportive, consisting of monitoring and supplementation of function until the inflammatory reactions resolve and managing complications as they arise. Depending on the organ system involved, mechanical ventilation, hemodialysis, or surgical removal of infarcted tissue may be necessary.

KEY CONCEPTS

- Shock states result in reduced or inadequate cellular oxygen consumption and may affect all organs and systems in the body. Complications of shock can be viewed as inflammatory in nature. Inflammation is triggered by hypoxic injury to cells, by antigen, or by endotoxin. Excessive or inappropriate inflammation leads to leaking capillaries, damage from proteolytic enzymes, and systemic activation of the clotting, complement, and kinin systems.
- Respiratory and kidney failure are commonly associated with shock. Inappropriate activation of the clotting cascade may result in DIC. MODS may occur with widespread cellular hypoxia and necrosis.

SUMMARY

Shock is a life-threatening syndrome associated with high mortality. Early identification of patients at risk and initiation of therapeutic measures may decrease the development of shock syndrome. Four major categories of circulatory shock have been described: cardiogenic, hypovolemic, obstructive, and distributive. Although each type of shock has specific characteristics, all are associated with a deficiency of cellular oxygen consumption. Tissue ischemia leads to hypoxic cellular dysfunction and death, generation of oxygen free radicals, and stimulation of a systemic inflammatory response. In late-stage shock and in septic shock, ongoing systemic inflammation leads to progressive organ dysfunction and can precipitate a number of shock complications, including ARDS, DIC, ATN, and MODS. New research into effective ways to intervene in the inflammatory cascade is needed to improve the management of circulatory shock.

MEDIA RESOURCES

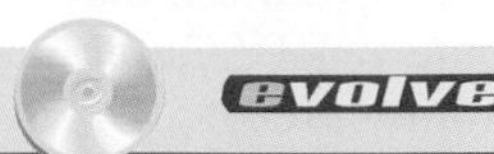

Remember to check out the ***CD Companion*** included with this book for Review Questions, Key Concepts Review, Glossary (with audio for selected terms), Disease Profiles, and Animations.

PLUS, visit the ***Evolve website*** at http://evolve.elsevier.com/Copstead/ for Case Studies, Disease Profiles, and WebLinks.

References

1. Warren JC: *Surgical pathology and therapeutics,* Philadelphia, 1895, Saunders.
2. Wilson M, Davis DP, Coimbra R: Diagnosis and monitoring of hemorrhagic shock during the initial resuscitation of multiple trauma patients: a review, *J Emerg Med* 24(4):413-422, 2003.
3. Palevsky PM, Matzke GR: Acid-base disorders. In Dipiro JT et al, editors: *A pathophysiologic approach,* ed 5, New York, 2002, McGraw-Hill, pp 995-1014.
4. Bhatia M, Moochhala S: Role of inflammatory mediators in the pathophysiology of acute respiratory distress syndrome, *J Pathol* 202:145-156, 2004.
5. Iskit AB, GUC O: Effects of endothelin and nitric oxide on organ injury, mesenteric ischemia, and survival in experimental models of septic shock, *Acta Pharmacol Sin* 24(10):953-957, 2003.
6. Dedon PC, Tannenbaum SR: Reactive nitrogen species in the chemical biology of inflammation, *Arch Biochem Biophys* 423(1):12-22, 2004.
7. Pathan N et al: Role of interleukin 6 in myocardial dysfunction of meningococcal septic shock, *Lancet* 363(9404):203-209, 2004.
8. Levy MN: The cardiac pump. In Berne RM et al, editors: *Physiology,* ed 5, St Louis, 2004, Mosby, pp 305-321.
9. Hochman JS: Cardiogenic shock complicating acute myocardial infarction: expanding the paradigm, *Circulation* 107(24):2998-3002, 2003.
10. Antman EM, Braunwald E: Acute myocardial infarction. In Braunwald E, Zipes D, Libby P, editors: *Heart disease: a textbook of cardiovascular medicine,* ed 6, Philadelphia, 2001, Saunders, pp 1114-1218.
11. Hochman JS et al: Early revascularization in acute myocardial infarction complicated by cardiogenic shock. SHOCK Investigators. Should we emergently revascularize occluded coronaries for cardiogenic shock? *N Engl J Med* 341(9):625-634, 1999.

12. Rudis MI, Dasta JF: Vasopressors and inotropes in shock. In Dipiro JT et al, editors: *Pharmacotherapy: a pathophysiologic approach,* ed 5, New York, 2002, McGraw-Hill, pp 435-452.
13. Johnson JA, Parker RB, Patterson JH: Heart failure. In Dipiro JT et al, editors: *Pharmacotherapy: a pathophysiologic approach,* ed 5, New York, 2002, McGraw-Hill, pp 185-218.
14. Richenbacher WE, Pierce WS: Treatment of heart failure: assisted circulation. In Braunwald E, Zipes D, Libby P, editors: *Heart disease: a textbook of cardiovascular medicine,* ed 6, Philadelphia, 2001, Saunders, pp 600-614.
15. Miniati DN, Robbins RC, Reitz BA: Heart and heart-lung transplantation. In Braunwald E, Zipes D, Libby P, editors: *Heart disease: a textbook of cardiovascular medicine,* ed 6, Philadelphia, 2001, Saunders, pp 615-634.
16. Rigatelli G et al: "Demand" stimulation of latissimus dorsi heart wrap: experience in humans and comparison with adynamic girdling, *Ann Thorac Surg* 76(5):1587-1592, 2003.
17. Shoemaker WC et al: Resuscitation from severe hemorrhage, *Crit Care Med* 24(suppl):S12-S23, 1996.
18. American College of Surgeons, Committee on Trauma: *Advanced trauma life support course for physicians,* Chicago, 1997, The College.
19. Erstad BL: Hypovolemic shock. In Dipiro JT et al, editors: *Pharmacotherapy: a pathophysiologic approach,* ed 5, New York, 2002, McGraw-Hill, pp 453-466.
20. Kemp SF, Lockey RF: Anaphylaxis: a review of causes and mechanisms, *J Allergy Clin Immunol* 110:341-348, 2002.
21. Dellinger RP: Cardiovascular management of septic shock, *Crit Care Med* 31(3):946-955, 2003.
22. Levy MM et al: 2001 SCCM/ESICM/ACCP/ATS/SIS International Sepsis Definitions Conference, *Crit Care Med* 31:1250-1256, 2003.
23. Kang-Birken SL, DiPiro JT: Sepsis and septic shock. In Dipiro JT et al, editors: *Pharmacotherapy: a pathophysiologic approach,* ed 5, New York, 2002, McGraw-Hill, pp 2029-2042.
24. Patel GP, Gurka DP, Balk RA: New treatment strategies for severe sepsis and septic shock, *Curr Opin Crit Care* 9:390-396, 2003.
25. Sharshar T et al: Depletion of neurohypophyseal content of vasopressin in septic shock, *Crit Care Med* 30(3):497-500, 2002.
26. Eichacker PQ, Natanson C: Recombinant human activated protein C in sepsis: inconsistent trial results, an unclear mechanism of action, and safety concerns resulted in labeling restrictions and the need for phase IV trials, *Crit Care Med* 31(1 suppl):S94-S96, 2003.
27. Awad SS: State-of-the-art therapy for severe sepsis and multisystem organ dysfunction, *Am J Surg* 186(5A):S23-S30, 2003.

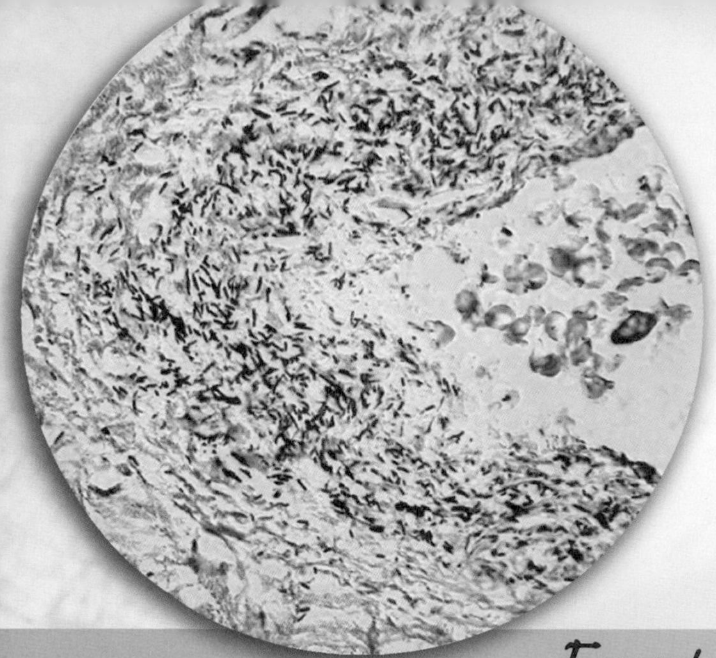

Frontiers of Research

Advances in Treatment of Respiratory Disorders

Gregory P. Thompson and Michael J. Kirkhorn

Inhale • Exhale • Hold your breath • Gasp in surprise or fright • Catch your breath • Sigh in relief • Breathe easier

Our breathing reveals us. We may conceal a moment of strong emotion by taking deep breaths. The need for conscious control only proves how meaningful breathing is. Breathing even reveals the content of our collaboration with others: to conspire is to breathe together. Anyone who inspires you is infusing or enkindling you, as though responsive breathing could fill or fire a spirit.

Our lives are sustained by respiration. Alternative medicine experts might argue that many of our common illnesses are brought on by the simple fact that most of us are shallow inhalers. Whether or not this statement is true, without doubt we jeopardize our respiration in ways that are either careless or deliberate. An estimated 46.2 million adults in the United States smoke cigarettes. Cigarette smoking is responsible for more than 440,000 deaths annually and costs more than $75 billion per year in medical expenditures. Others suffer lifelong illness from exposure to uranium dust, coal dust, asbestos, and other contaminants encountered either at work or at large in the environment.

We are slowly learning the value of prevention. In 1950, cigarette manufacturers were conspicuous advertisers in the *Journal of the American Medical Association.* One ad presented the testimonial of a "throat expert," who reported "not one single case of throat irritation due to smoking Camels." Another recommended that for "utmost enjoyment" physicians and patients alike should try Parliament cigarettes, with the "built-in filter mouthpiece."

The cost of cigarette smoking is, of course, disease—lung cancer, heart disease, and emphysema. A quick scan of the diseases and combinations of diseases of the respiratory system shows that tobacco smoking is a constant threat. Smoking causes disease or worsens any existing respiratory condition, a fact confirmed by many studies. The value of quitting permanently is clear from findings of the Lung Health Study of the National Heart, Lung, and Blood Institute of the National Institutes of Health, which concluded that quitting smoking can help up to 22% of those in whom chronic obstructive pulmonary disease might develop.

Often we inflict respiratory diseases on one another or allow our habits to aggravate allergies or illnesses in otherwise healthy people. The body has no adequate means to filter out the disease-causing ingredients of tobacco smoke or other contaminants. The nose does its complicated work of warming, humidifying, and filtering the air we breathe, but this efficient appendage cannot save those who subject themselves or are subjected to lethal contamination. Particles too small to be filtered by the nose settle into small bronchioles,

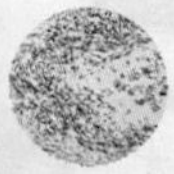

Lung section from a patient who had nosocomial Pseudomonas *pneumonia. High-powered photomicrograph demonstrates abundant bacteria* (deep blue) *invading the wall of the blood vessel. (From Kumar V, Cotran RS, Robbins SL:* Robbins basic pathology, *ed 7, Philadelphia, 2003, Saunders.)*

UNIT

VI

Respiratory Function

which is a cause of lung disease among miners. Tiny particles of cigarette smoke also escape the body's filters and cause lung disease or lung cancer.

Diseases caused or aggravated by outside contaminants are only some of the diseases found in the respiratory system. Researchers say that asthma now afflicts 1 in 15 people in the United States and Europe, and although it can be effectively controlled with inhaled corticosteroids or bronchodilators, this seeming epidemic is still of great concern. In the United States, asthma-related mortality is rising among African-Americans and Hispanics. Some advocate immunization against the contaminants that set off asthma attacks, such as dust mites, cat dander, molds, and cockroaches; partly because asthma sufferers are usually allergic to multiple aeroallergens, immunization—with a purified extract of ragweed, for example—is recommended by the National Institutes of Health only when drugs fail or when it is impossible to avoid allergens, and the British Thoracic Society recommends it not at all.

Other respiratory disorders are becoming less ominous through improvements in monitoring, treatment, and care, although they remain dangerous and troubling for the health professionals who diagnose and treat them.

Health professionals have learned to watch alertly for signs of acute respiratory distress syndrome (ARDS), which can develop slowly or suddenly, often with devastating results.

Researchers report that acute lung injury and ARDS "play pivotal roles" in most occurrences of systemic inflammatory response syndrome and multiple organ dysfunction syndrome. Understanding the pathophysiology of the lung disorders has guided researchers in their approach to often fatal system failures.

When the endothelial lining of the alveolar capillary membrane is damaged in ARDS, fluid molecules that would normally remain inside the capillaries leak into surrounding tissues. The result is edema, which disrupts normal gas exchange. Blood passes through saturated and collapsed alveoli without receiving oxygen. Supplemental oxygen cannot reach the damaged alveoli, and the heart rate and blood pressure are affected.

ARDS presents a combination of exacting responsibilities for the health care professional. Patients with ARDS require careful detection of changes in respiratory status, gas exchange, and oxygen absorption, as well as adequate nourishment. Twenty years ago, 9 in 10 ARDS patients died. The mortality is still above 50%, but a clinical response can offer the patient a good possibility for recovery.

chapter 21

Respiratory Function and Alterations in Gas Exchange

Lorna Schumann

MEDIA RESOURCES

Additional Material for Study, Review, and Further Exploration

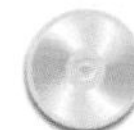

CD Companion ◆ Review Questions and Answers ◆ Key Concepts Review ◆ Glossary *(with audio pronunciations for selected terms)* ◆ Disease Profiles ◆ Animations

evolve ***Website*** at http://evolve.elsevier.com/Copstead/ ◆ Case Studies ◆ Disease Profiles ◆ WebLinks

KEY QUESTIONS

- How do the structures involved in gas exchange in the lungs differ from conducting structures?
- What factors determine the work of breathing?
- How are alveolar ventilation and oxygenation estimated and assessed?
- What factors affect the distribution of ventilation and perfusion in the lungs?
- How are oxygen and carbon dioxide transported in the circulation?
- What pathophysiologic factors might alter ventilation-perfusion matching in the lungs?
- What are the risk factors and complications of pulmonary vascular occlusion and hypertension?

CHAPTER OUTLINE

The primary function of the lungs is gas exchange. Oxygen is transported to the body tissues, and carbon dioxide, a waste product, is transported out of the body. The exchange of these gases takes place at the alveolar-capillary membrane. For effective gas exchange to occur, the processes of ventilation, perfusion, and diffusion must occur simultaneously at the alveolar-capillary interface. Problems with any of these three processes can result in hypoxemia (low arterial oxygen) or hypercarbia (high arterial carbon dioxide). An understanding of the anatomy and physiology of pulmonary gas exchange is necessary for learning about the pathophysiologic processes that follow.

FUNCTIONAL ANATOMY

Development of the Pulmonary System

On or about day 26 of embryonic development, formation of the lower respiratory system begins. This early formation consists of a laryngotracheal groove that arises from the wall of the pharynx and gives rise to the epithelium and glands of the larynx, trachea, bronchi, and pulmonary lining. The groove continues to deepen and forms a diverticulum (pouch) that develops into the laryngotracheal tube and bronchial buds.

Initially, the laryngotracheal diverticulum includes the esophagus and the trachea as a single tube. Then longitudinal ridges begin to develop along the tubular wall and form a septum (wall), which separates the esophagus from the trachea. Failure of this septum to develop leads to a **tracheoesophageal fistula** (abnormal opening), leaving a communication between the esophagus and the trachea. This abnormality occurs about once in every 2500 births. Approximately 90% of the cases of esophageal **atresia** (blind pouch) are of the type seen in Figure 21-1, *A*. Figures 21-1, *B* through *D*, show variations of tracheoesophageal fistulas.[1]

As the laryngotracheal tube continues to elongate, the lung bud divides into two bronchial buds, which become the bronchi and the right and left lung. The right bronchus becomes larger than the left. The right mainstem bronchus is normally more vertical than the left because it is the main continuation of the laryngotracheal tube and branches off the trachea at a 20-degree angle. The left bronchus branches off the trachea at an angle of 40 to 60 degrees. This normal anatomic development increases the chances that an inhaled foreign body will lodge in the right mainstem bronchus rather than the left.

Fetal lung development can be divided into four periods:

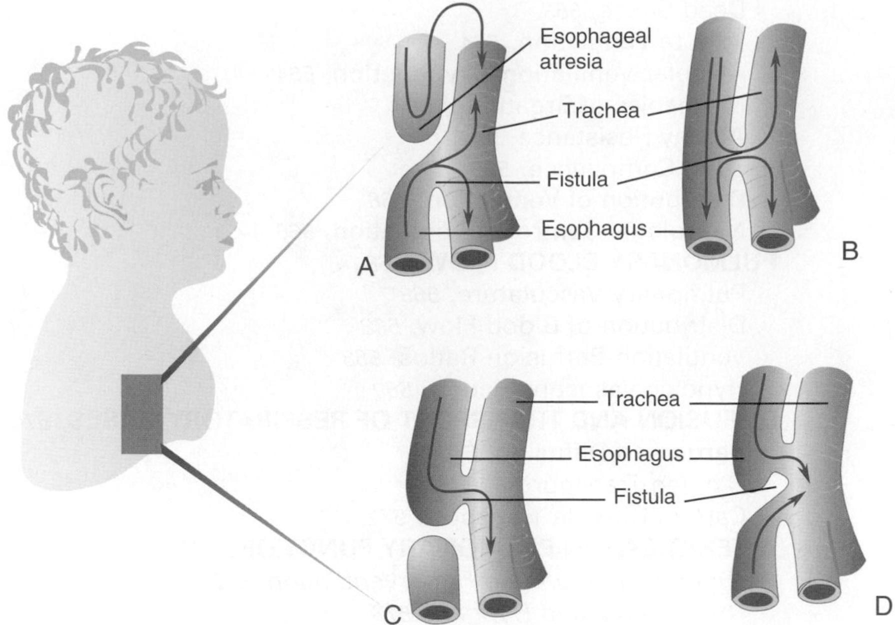

FIGURE 21-1 ■ The four primary types of tracheoesophageal fistulas. **A,** The most common type, with complete atresia (blind pouch) of the esophagus. **B,** A common opening between the trachea and esophagus. **C,** An opening from an esophageal pouch into the trachea. **D,** A double opening from two unconnected ends of the esophagus. *Arrows* indicate flow of fluid from the esophagus to the trachea.

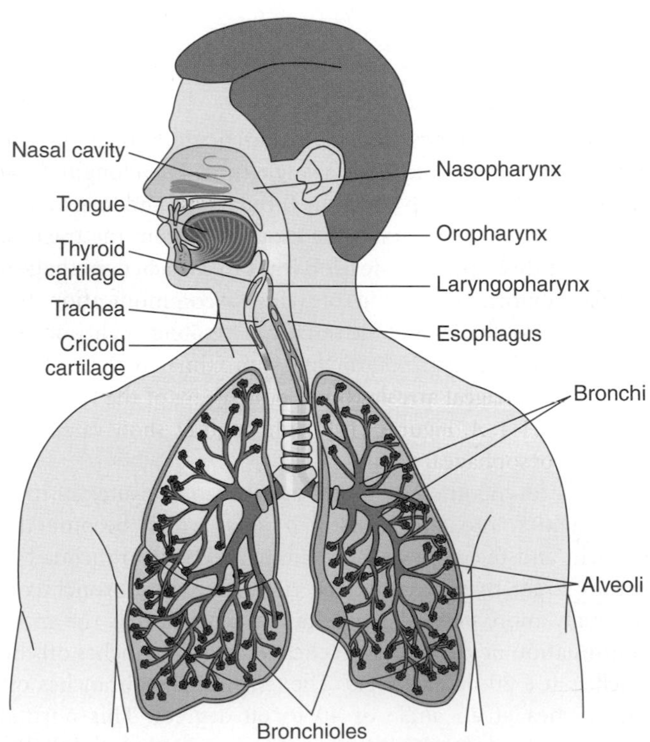

FIGURE 21-2 ■ Sagittal view diagram of the oronasal cavity (nasal cavity, nasopharynx, oropharynx, and laryngopharynx) and the respiratory passages beginning at the trachea and ending at the alveoli.

The **pseudoglandular period** (5 to 17 weeks) is the period when the bronchial divisions are differentiated, and the major elements of lung tissue are present except for those involved in gas exchange: the respiratory bronchioles and alveoli.

The **canalicular period** (16 to 25 weeks) occurs when the bronchi and bronchioles enlarge and vascularization of lung tissue takes place. At the end of this period, respiration is possible because of the development of respiratory bronchioles and primitive alveoli. Alveoli are grapelike sacs in which gas exchange occurs. Type II pneumocytes (epithelial cells that are on the internal surface of alveoli) begin to secrete surfactant at the end of this period. Surfactant is a phospholipid essential for maintaining alveolar patency.

During the **terminal sac period** (24 weeks to birth) terminal sacs become thinner, preparing the lung tissue for gas exchange. Proliferation of pulmonary capillaries is also prominent during this period. Infants born prematurely in the early weeks of this period (25 to 28 weeks) are susceptible to the development of respiratory distress syndrome (RDS) due to the immaturity of the pulmonary structures.

The **alveolar period** (late fetal life to 8 years) is the final period of lung development when alveolar ducts form from terminal sacs and alveoli mature by increasing in size and in number. Approximately one eighth to one sixth of the adult number of alveoli are present at birth.[1] During this growth period, there is a lack of structural collateral pathways necessary for maintaining open airways. This may make the individual more susceptible to

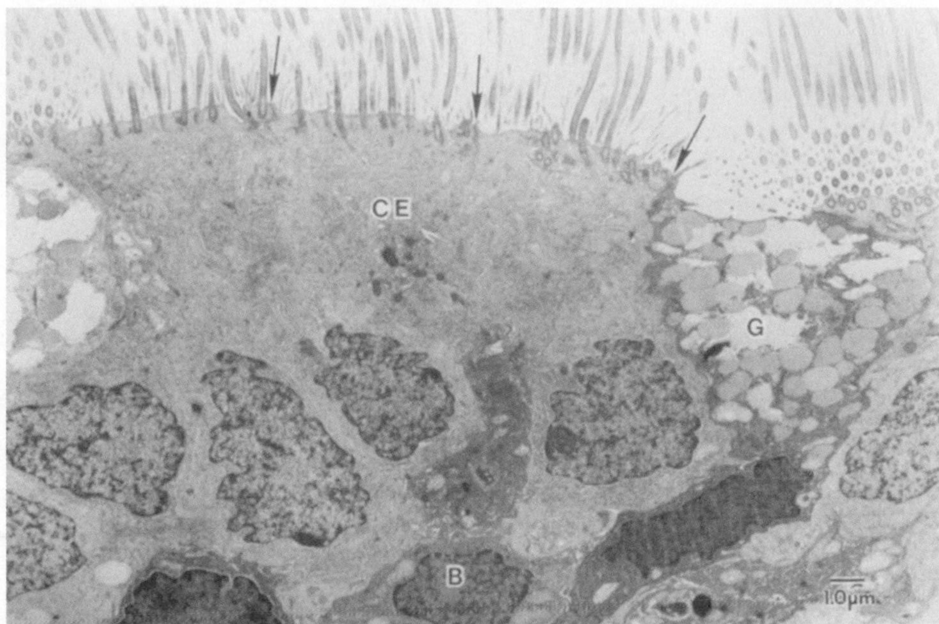

FIGURE 21-3 ■ Cells composing the bronchial epithelium are ciliated epithelial cells *(CE)*, goblet cells *(G)*, and basal cells *(B)*. Goblet cells have abundant mucus granules in the cytoplasm and their apical surface is devoid of cilia. Basal cells, as their name indicates, are located along the abluminal portion of the lining epithelium, adjacent to the basal lamina. The *arrows* at the apical surface of the airway cells indicate the location of junctional complexes between contiguous epithelial cells. (Human lung surgical specimen, transmission electron microscopy.) (From Murray JF, Nadel JA: *Textbook of respiratory medicine,* ed 3, Philadelphia, 2000, Saunders, p 9.)

atelectasis (incomplete expansion) and obstruction. Lung damage during this period may cause permanent defects in lung development.[1]

Upper Airway Structures

The respiratory system can be divided into two major anatomic areas: the upper airway and the lower airway. The upper airway consists of the nasopharyngeal cavity (nasopharynx, oropharynx, laryngopharynx) (Figure 21-2). The lower airway contains the larynx, trachea, bronchi, bronchopulmonary segments, terminal bronchioles, and the acinus (the alveolar region supplied by one terminal bronchiole, which includes numerous alveoli) (see Figure 21-2).

The nasal cavity conducts gases to and from the lungs, and filters, warms, and humidifies the air. It is a rigid box composed of two thirds cartilage and one third bone, which prevents collapse during movement of air. The convoluted turbinates (cone-shaped bones) of the nasal cavity are highly vascular, and their blood flow forms an efficient heat exchanger. Evaporation of water from the turbinate surface and from the mucus secreted by mucosal glands raises the water vapor of the inspired air to normal saturation. Therefore, air is warmed to body temperature and humidified to approximately 80% saturation.

Air is filtered by the large hairs (**vibrissae**) of the nasal cavity and cilia that line the nasal cavity. The cilia sweep foreign particles trapped by mucus into the nasopharynx, where they are swallowed or expectorated. An electron micrograph of the tracheobronchial lining is shown in Figure 21-3. Pseudostratified ciliated columnar epithelium lines the trachea and bronchi. Goblet cells and mucus-producing glands are contained in this area and are responsible for producing approximately 100 ml/day in the adult. The composition of mucus is 95% water plus mucopolysaccharides, mucoproteins, and lipids. Maintenance of water content and fluid balance is important to the mobilization of secretions. A child has more mucus-producing glands and therefore produces more mucus than an adult. In the disease state of a child, an overproduction of mucus in combination with small airway size may precipitate tracheobronchial obstruction.[2,3]

Cilia (Figure 21-4) beat in a sweeping motion like oars rowing a boat at approximately 1000 to 1500 strokes per minute.[2,3] Mucociliary transport (movement of mucus upward) is a primary defense mechanism of the tracheobronchial tree. Inhaled particles, bacteria, and macrophages are removed from the respiratory tract by ciliary clearance and cough reflex. Ciliary function is impaired by smoking, alcohol ingestion, hypothermia, hyperthermia, cold air, low humidity, starvation, anesthetics, corticosteroids, noxious gases, the common cold, and increased mucus production.[2,3]

The four paranasal sinuses are air-containing spaces adjacent to the nasal passages that provide speech resonance and

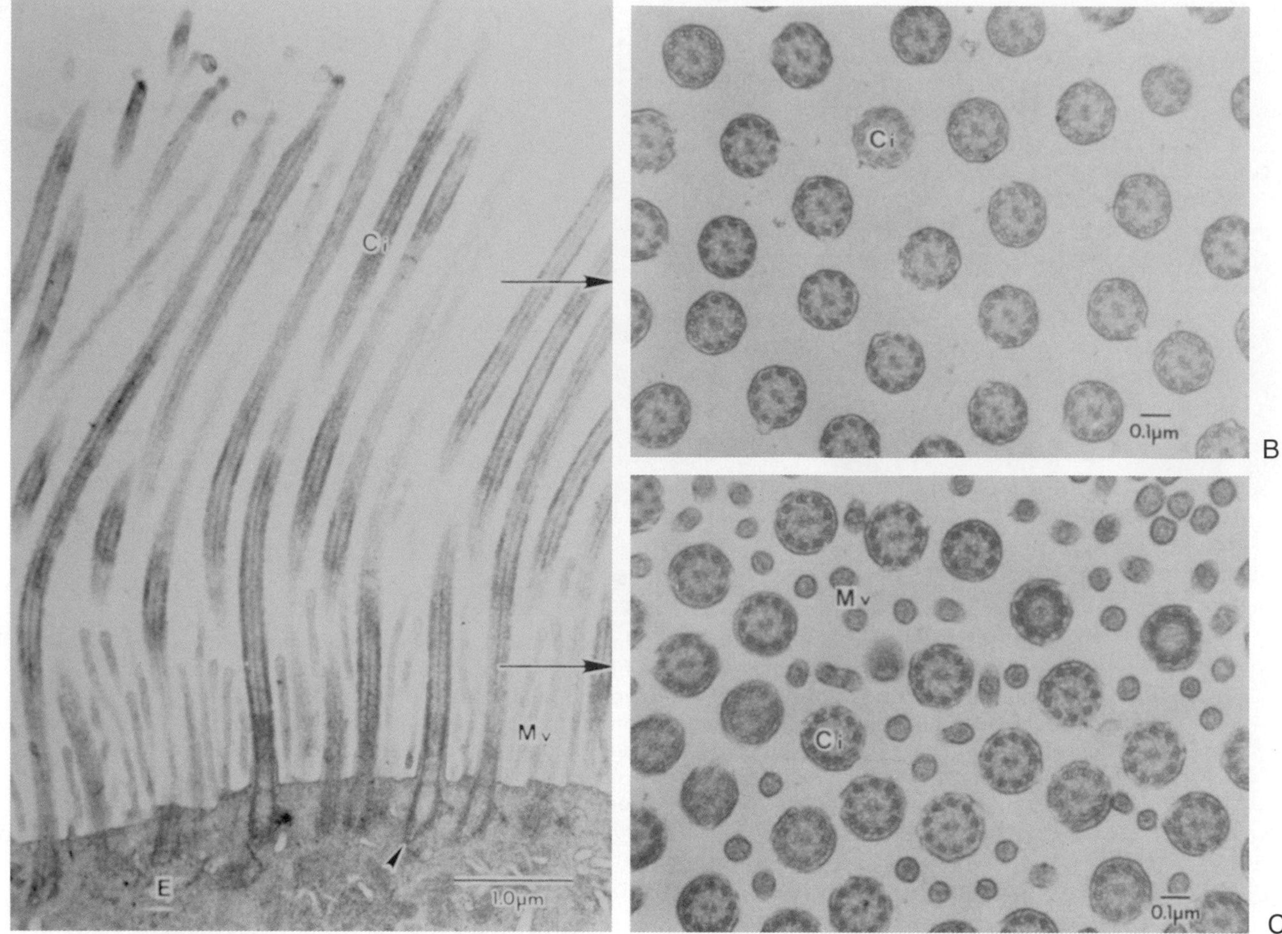

FIGURE 21-4 ■ **A,** Electron micrograph shows the ultrastructural characteristics of cilia *(Ci)* on airway epithelial cells *(E).* Each cilium has a long slender shaft that ends with a conical tip. The base of the cilium is anchored in the cell's apical cytoplasm by a curved and tapered basal foot (modified centriole; *arrowhead*). Also extending from the apical surface of ciliated airway epithelial cells are microvilli *(Mv).* The two horizontal *arrows* in **A** represent the cross-sectional planes illustrated in **B** and **C. B** and **C,** Airway cilia have the classic microtubular arrangement of motile cilia, namely, nine peripheral doublets and two central singlets. Microvilli are randomly distributed among the cilia. (Human lung surgical specimen, transmission electron microscopy.) (From Murray JF, Nadel JA: *Textbook of respiratory medicine,* ed 2, Philadelphia, 1994, Saunders, p 12.)

increase the heat and water vapor exchange surfaces. The sinuses are swept clean by mucociliary action when the communicating passages that connect them with the nasal passages remain open.

The eustachian tube between the middle ear and the posterior nasopharynx maintains the air in the middle ear at atmospheric pressure. To prevent secretions or food from entering the middle ear during swallowing, the pharyngeal muscles close the eustachian tube briefly. The nasal end of the eustachian tube is surrounded by flexible cartilage arranged in a spiral configuration. The muscles surrounding the eustachian cartilage close the opening by pulling the cartilage tighter. Because the tube is shorter in children, the potential for otitis media is increased.[2,3]

Lower Airway Structures

After air passes through the nasal cavity or oral cavity into the pharynx it passes to the larynx and finally into the tracheobronchial tree. The acinus (Figure 21-5) is located at the end of the tracheobronchial tree and is composed of bronchioles, alveolar ducts, and alveoli.

The larynx is the transition area between the upper and lower airways. Anatomically it is considered part of the lower airway, but functionally it is similar to the upper airway. The larynx contains the epiglottis, vocal cords, and cartilages. The anatomic arrangement of the larynx functions to prevent aspiration during swallowing and to assist in phonation and coughing. Each vocal cord is attached anteriorly to the thyroid

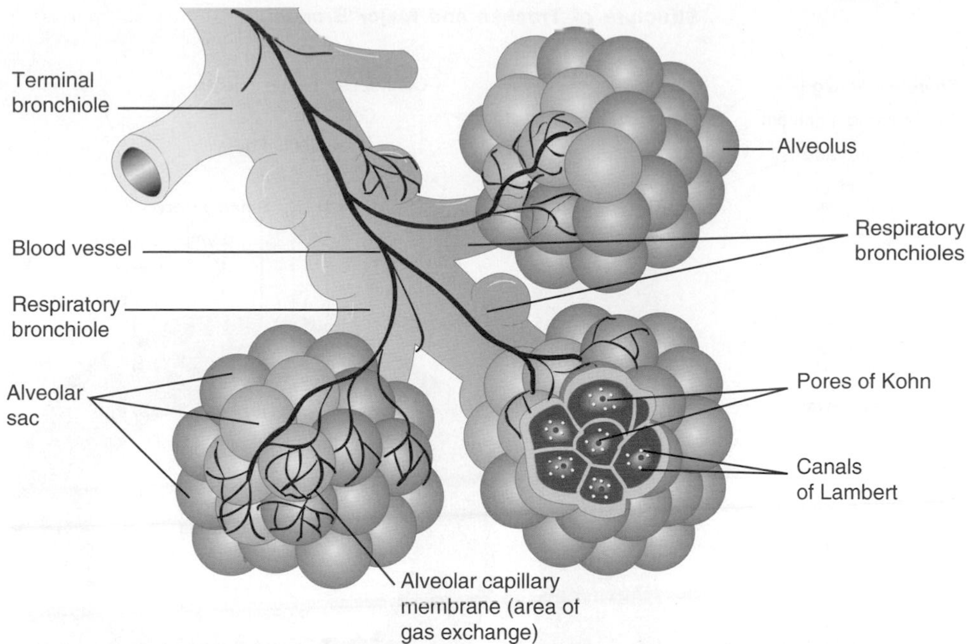

FIGURE 21-5 ■ A portion of the lower respiratory tract, including a terminal bronchiole, respiratory bronchioles, and alveoli, where interchange of O_2 and CO_2 occurs between the thin walls of the alveoli and the capillary membrane.

cartilage and posteriorly to the arytenoid cartilage. Vibration of the cords leads to phonation. Food is prevented from entering the trachea during swallowing by closure of the epiglottis. If food or fluid should bypass the epiglottis and enter the tracheobronchial tree, the cough reflex is initiated. A cough reflex is produced when the epiglottis and vocal cords close tightly against air entrapped in the lungs. When the expiratory muscles contract forcefully against the closed epiglottis and vocal cords, a pressure of approximately 100 mm Hg is created. When the cords and epiglottis suddenly open, the high-pressure buildup is allowed to escape. This reflex rapidly removes foreign matter from the tracheobronchial tree.[2,3]

The major cartilages of the larynx are the thyroid, cricoid, and arytenoid. The thyroid cartilage is a large shield-shaped cartilage often referred to as the Adam's apple. Immediately below the thyroid cartilage is the site for emergency opening (**cricothyroidotomy**) of the tracheal passageway. The cricoid cartilage lies below the thyroid cartilage and is the narrowest point in the airway of a child. It is the only complete tracheal ring, and because of its narrowness in the small child's airway, an endotracheal tube cuff is not necessary for required intubation of the airway.

The trachea, bronchi, and bronchioles make up the conducting airways that allow passage of gases to and from the gas exchange units (alveoli). These conducting airways make up a proportionately larger amount of the total airway system in the infant and child than in the adult. The trachea (Figure 21-6) contains incomplete cartilaginous rings; it is approximately 11 to 13 cm long and lies between the cricoid cartilage and the carina (ridge located at the lower end of the trachea). Individual variations in tracheal shape include U, circular, D, C, triangular, and elliptical (Figure 21-7). Of 111 adult tracheas studied, the incidence of shapes in order of frequency was 48.6%, C; 27%, U; 12.6%, D; 8.2%, elliptical; 1.8%, circular; and 1.8%, triangular.[4] These tracheal variations may affect ventilation of patients who have endotracheal tubes in their airways and require mechanical ventilation.

The majority of cough receptors lie at the carina. There the trachea divides into two mainstem (primary) bronchi, which contain cartilage and smooth muscle. Viewing the body anteriorly, the carina is located at the angle of Louis, between the sternum and manubrium at the second intercostal space.

The small size of the conducting airway in the infant and child makes even a small decrease in the size of the lumen from an obstruction critical to airway conduction.[5] Primary bronchi further divide into five (secondary) lobar branches, three to the right lung and two to the left lung. Each lobar branch enters a lobe of the lung and further divides into bronchopulmonary segments (ten segments in the right lung, nine segments in the left lung) (Figure 21-8).[2,3] Each bronchopulmonary segment is composed of 50 or more terminal bronchioles (conducting airways), which branch into respiratory bronchioles where gas exchange begins.

Nervous system control of the bronchi and bronchioles is mediated by the autonomic nervous system. Stimulation of the parasympathetic nervous system via the vagus nerve leads to constriction (by means of acetylcholine receptors) of bronchial smooth muscle. Stimulation of the sympathetic nervous system

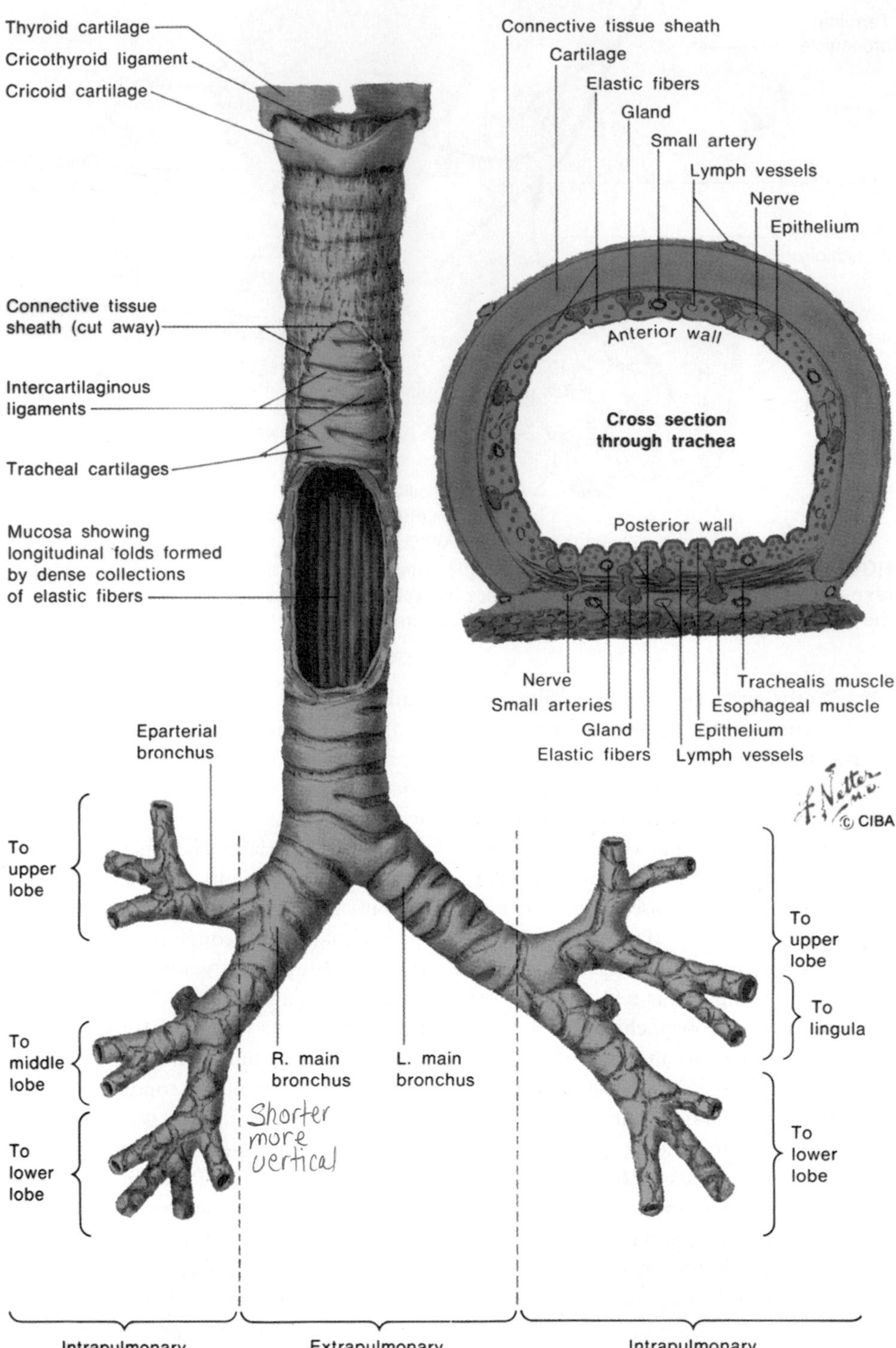

FIGURE 21-6 ■ Anterior diagram of the trachea and major bronchi. *R.,* Right; *L.,* left. (From Netter FH: *Respiratory system,* vol 7, Summit, NJ, 1979, CIBA Pharmaceutical, p 23.)

leads to relaxation of bronchial smooth muscle. Sympathetic stimulation is mediated by β_2-adrenergic receptors, which are under the control of circulating catecholamines.[5] (See the discussion in the section on neurologic control of ventilation, later in this chapter, for additional information.)

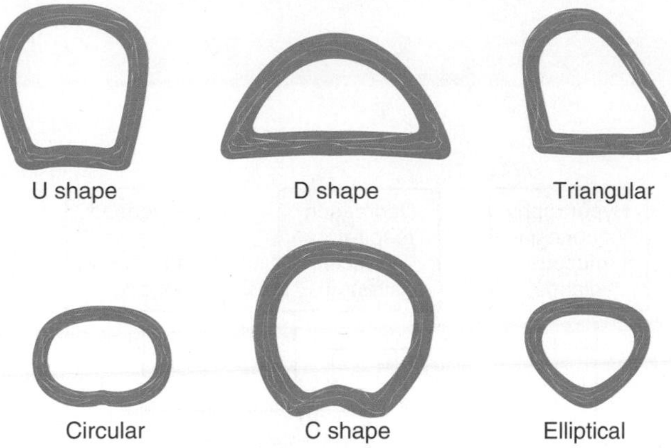

FIGURE 21-7 ■ Examples of variation in tracheal shape.

Terminal bronchioles, which include the conducting airways, further subdivide into two or more respiratory bronchioles in which gas exchange begins. The respiratory bronchioles divide into two or more alveolar ducts, which in turn supply several alveoli.

The lung is fully developed by the eighth year of life.[1,2] The large alveolar surface area in conjunction with pulmonary surfactant, a phospholipid produced by type II alveolar cells, lowers surface tension and facilitates gas exchange. Two other types of cells are found: type I alveolar cells (type I pneumocytes), which are the epithelial structural cells of the alveoli, and alveolar macrophages, which act as a defense mechanism by phagocytizing particles in the alveoli. Alveolar macrophages can be damaged by smoking and by inhalation of silica (SiO_2).

Adult lungs contain approximately 300 million alveoli, and the newborn lung contains one eighth to one sixth the adult number.[1-3] An elderly person may also have a reduction in the number of alveoli as part of the normal aging process, but many elderly people retain the same number of alveoli they had as a younger adult.

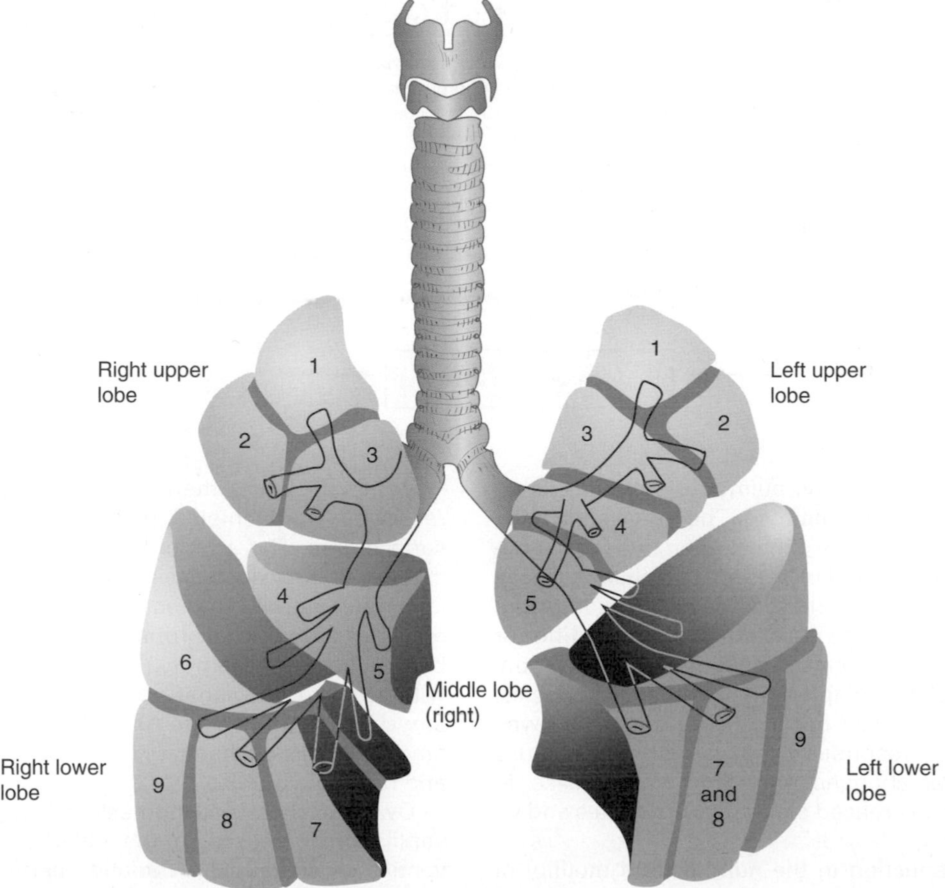

FIGURE 21-8 ■ Bronchopulmonary segments of the human lung. **Right and left upper lobes:** *1,* apical segment; *2,* posterior segment; *3,* anterior segment; **left upper lobe:** *4,* superior segment; *5,* inferior segment; **middle lobe (right):** *4,* lateral segment; *5,* medial segment; **right and left lower lobes:** *6,* superior (apical) segment; *7,* medial basal segment; *8,* anterior basal segment (on left, *7* and *8* combine to form the anteromedial basal segment); *9,* lateral basal segment; *10,* posterior basal segment.

Gas exchange occurs in the alveolar units (see Figure 21-5) where oxygen (O_2) and carbon dioxide (CO_2) transfer across the alveolar-capillary membrane. The partial pressures of gases in the alveoli are termed P_{AO_2} for oxygen and P_{ACO_2} for carbon dioxide. The partial pressures of gases in the blood are termed Pa_{O_2} for oxygen and Pa_{CO_2} for carbon dioxide. Collateral alveolar ventilation can also occur through holes in the alveolar walls, called the pores of Kohn or canals of Lambert. In addition, a small child has less collateral ventilation because of fewer pores of Kohn.[6] The alveolar membrane is thicker in the neonate and reaches the adult thinness of 0.5 mm by the age of 8 years. This thinner membrane may allow increased

THE AGING PROCESS

Changes in the Respiratory System

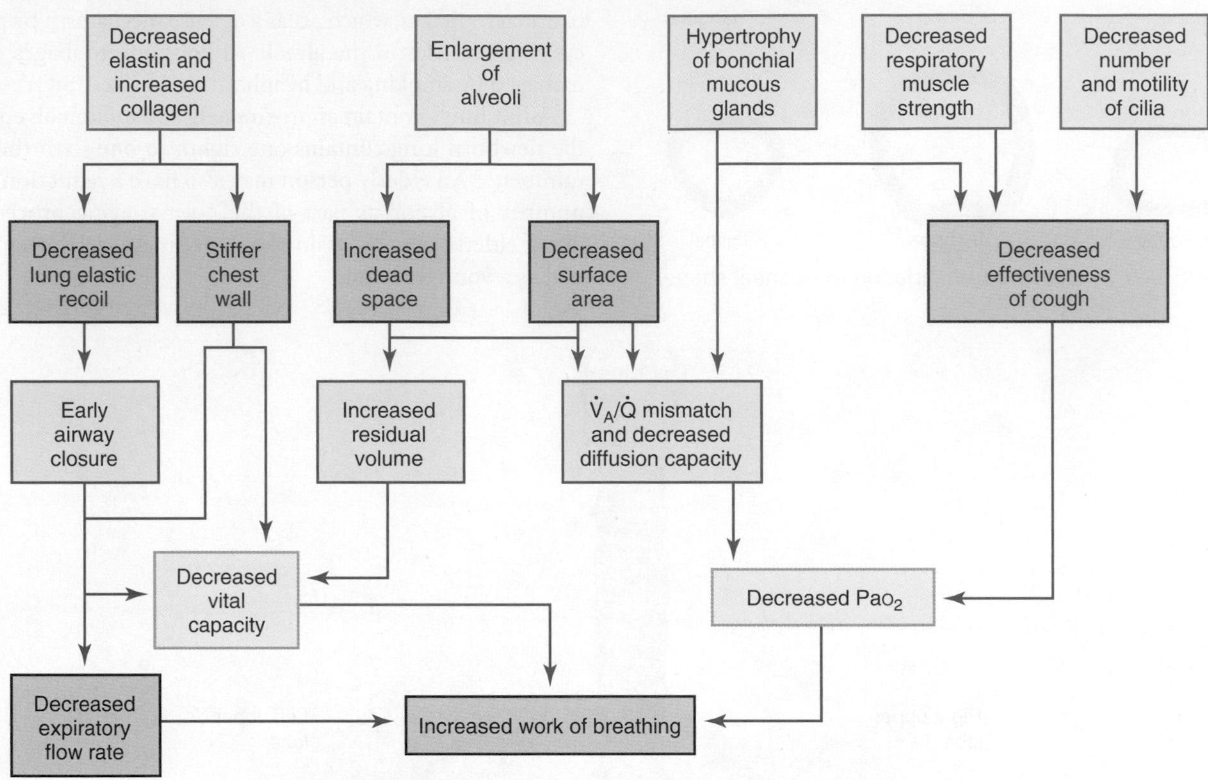

With aging, the result of all pulmonary changes is an increase in the work of breathing. The lungs show a reduction in elastin and a rise in collagen, leading to decreased elastic recoil and increased compliance. These changes give rise to increased residual volume and early airway closure. The chest wall becomes stiffer or more rigid due to rib and cartilaginous calcification. The strength of the diaphragm, intercostal muscles, and accessory muscles declines. The stiff chest wall and diminished respiratory muscle strength cause other functional changes, including an increase in dead space and decreased expiratory flow rates and vital capacity.

There is a reduction in the number and motility of cilia resulting in a decrease in respiratory clearance. There is an increase in and hypertrophy of bronchial mucous glands. The decreased respiratory muscle strength, increased mucus, chest wall stiffness, and cilia loss together reduce cough effectiveness.

Within the lungs, there is enlargement of alveoli and respiratory bronchioles with subsequent decreased surface area. The arterial blood flow through the pulmonary vessels decreases proportionally with changes in cardiac output. The loss of elastic recoil causes the enlarged respiratory bronchioles to collapse or close before the alveoli empty. Alveoli enlargement, along with reduced pulmonary artery blood flow and early airway closure, lowers diffusion capacity and the amount of gas exchange. It also increases air trapping and residual volume.

Owing to chest wall stiffness and lung rigidity, apical ventilation increases in the elderly, whereas basilar ventilation decreases. Ventilation-perfusion ($\dot{V}A/\dot{Q}$) mismatch occurs as a result of increasing apical ventilation with poor apical capillary blood flow. The result of these changes leads to reduced arterial oxygen pressure (Pa_{O_2}). Because of increased $\dot{V}A/\dot{Q}$ mismatch, the Pa_{O_2} may decrease when the elderly individual reclines.

transfer of O_2. The healthy older adult has very thin-walled, enlarged air sacs and fewer capillaries than a younger adult.[2,7] Respiratory system changes associated with normal aging are described in The Aging Process: Changes in the Respiratory System.

Pulmonary Circulation

Blood supply to the lungs comes from two sources: the bronchial artery system, which supplies a small amount of oxygenated blood to the pleura and lung tissues, and the pulmonary artery system, which provides a vast capillary network for O_2 and CO_2 exchange. The capillary networks of the neonate, young child, and elderly person are less than those in the average healthy adult. Oxygen-depleted blood leaves the right ventricle by way of the pulmonary artery trunk, which branches into the right and left pulmonary arteries. The pulmonary arteries further divide into smaller arteries and arterioles that feed into the capillary network where gas exchange occurs from the alveolar-capillary membrane.

The capillary network is a low-pressure system that can expand two to three times normal size before a significant increase in pulmonary capillary pressures is detectable. The normal pulmonary arterial pressure in a healthy adult is about 22/8 to 25/8 mm Hg. The mean pulmonary arterial pressure is approximately 15 mm Hg. This compares with the high pressure of the systemic circulation, which is normally considered to be 120/80 mm Hg, with a mean arterial pressure of 96 mm Hg.

Under normal resting conditions, only about 25% of pulmonary capillaries are perfused (filled with blood). The pulmonary circulation has two mechanisms for lowering pulmonary vascular resistance when vascular pressures are increased because of increased blood flow (Figure 21-9).[2,3,5] The first mechanism is recruitment, which allows opening of previously closed capillary vessels. The second mechanism is distention, which allows for widening of capillary vessels.

Another factor influencing pulmonary circulation is the fluid balance of the lung tissues. Fluid balance is regulated by the hydrostatic pressure, colloid osmotic pressure, and capillary permeability. When capillary hydrostatic pressure exceeds colloid osmotic pressure, fluid moves from the capillary to the interstitium. If the fluid shift is not controlled, the fluid volume will continue to increase until fluid is moved into the alveoli. Alveolar edema is more serious than interstitial edema (fluid in the interstitial space) because of its negative effects on gas exchange. Pulmonary interstitial and alveolar edema is common in disease processes such as congestive heart failure and infectious diseases of the lung. Other disease processes that also increase capillary permeability are adult respiratory distress syndrome (ARDS) and infant respiratory distress syndrome. (See Chapter 23 for further discussion.)

Age-Related Variations

Structural and physiologic variations occur at each end of the age continuum. A summary of anatomic and physiologic respiratory variations by age group is presented in Table 21-1.[8]

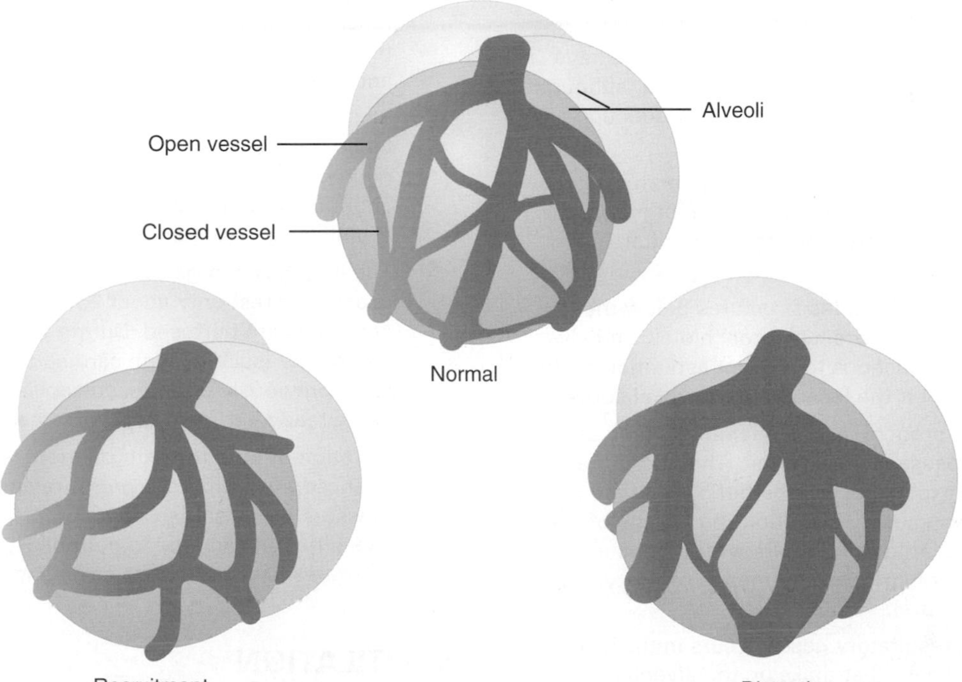

FIGURE 21-9 ■ Two mechanisms for lowering pulmonary vascular resistance in capillary vessels. Recruitment allows for opening of previously closed capillaries. Distention allows for widening of capillary vessels.

Table 21-1

Variations in Anatomy and Physiology of the Respiratory System by Age Group

	Young Newborns	Children	Adult	Elderly (>60 yr old)
Pa_{O_2} (mm Hg)	60-70	90-100	90-100	70-80
Pa_{CO_2} (mm Hg)	45-50	35-45	35-45	35-45
pH	7.3-7.4 (depends on Apgar score)	7.35-7.45	7.35-7.45	7.30-7.45
Bicarbonate (mEq/L)	20-26	22-28	24-30	24-30
Anatomic dead space	Proportional to size	Proportional to size	~150 ml	~150-200 ml
No. of alveoli	12.5%-16.5% of adult number	Adult number by 8 yr old	300,000/lung	≤300,000/lung
Thickness of alveolar membrane	Thicker than adult	Adult by 8 yr old	<0.5 μm	Thinner than adult
No. of capillaries	Less than adult	Adult by 8 yr old	Adult	Less than adult
Vital capacity	Proportionately less than adult	Proportional to size	4.7 L	Less than adult
Tidal volume	Proportional to size	Proportional to size	500 ml	Less than adult (30% less by age 80 yr)
Compliance	More compliant than adult	Similar to adult	Static compliance (90-100 ml/cm H_2O)	Less compliant
Airway resistance	Greater than adult	Greater than adult	1.0-1.5 cm H_2O/L/sec	Adult level or less

Data from Fretwell ME: Aging changes in structure and function. In Carnevali DL, Patrick M, editors: *Nursing management for the elderly,* ed 3, Philadelphia, 1993, Lippincott.

KEY CONCEPTS

- Respiratory system development begins at about day 26 of gestation. Abnormal development of the septum during this time can lead to tracheoesophageal fistula. At 25 weeks gestation, the fetal lungs have developed sufficiently to allow respiration, although alveolar development and surfactant production are just beginning.
- The upper airway includes the nasopharynx, oropharynx, and laryngopharynx. The primary functions of the upper airway are to warm, filter, and humidify inspired air.
- The lower airway includes structures below the larynx—the trachea, bronchi, bronchioles, and alveoli. The larynx functions to prevent aspiration during swallowing and is the location of the vocal cords.
- The trachea, bronchi, and bronchioles serve as conducting passageways for air. They do not engage in gas exchange. Sympathetic influence on these airways causes relaxation (by means of β_2-adrenergic receptors) and parasympathetic influence causes constriction (by means of acetylcholine receptors).
- Exchange of respiratory gases occurs in the alveoli. The epithelial cells that make up the alveoli are called type I cells (type I pneumocytes). Type II pneumocytes produce surfactant in the alveoli. The grapelike structure of the alveoli provides a huge surface area for gas exchange.
- The upper and lower airways are lined with cilia, which move rhythmically to transport mucus and trapped debris out of the respiratory tree. Ciliary function is impaired by a number of factors, among them smoking, alcohol consumption, low humidity, and anesthesia.
- The lungs are perfused by two sources: bronchial arteries bring a small amount of oxygenated blood to nourish lung tissues; pulmonary arteries bring the entire cardiac output of the right ventricle to the alveoli for gas exchange.
- The lung has a large reserve capacity for gas exchange. At rest only about 25% of the pulmonary capillaries are perfused. During periods of high lung blood flow (such as high cardiac output during exercise), previously unperfused capillaries are recruited, and already perfused capillaries become distended.
- Filtration of fluid through pulmonary capillaries is influenced by hydrostatic pressure and colloid osmotic pressure in the same way as other capillaries. Excessive filtration can lead to pulmonary edema, which interferes with normal gas exchange.

VENTILATION

Lung Volumes and Capacities

Ventilation is the process of moving air into the lungs and distributing air within the lungs to gas exchange units (alveoli) for maintenance of oxygenation and removal of CO_2.[5] Mea-

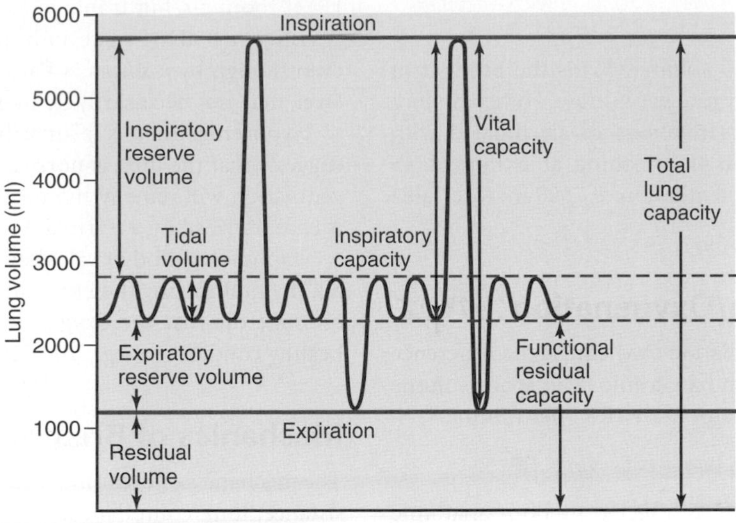

FIGURE 21-10 ■ Schematic representation of the various lung volumes and capacities for a healthy adult (see also Table 21-2).

Table 21-2

Lung Volumes and Capacities Impt

Term	Definition (Typical Volume)
Lung Volumes	
Tidal volume	A normal breath (~500 ml) or the amount of gas entering or leaving the lung during normal breathing
Inspiratory reserve volume	The amount of gas a person is able to inspire above a normal breath (e.g., maximal deep breath, ~3 L)
Expiratory reserve volume	The amount of gas expired beyond tidal volume (~1.2 L)
Residual volume	The volume of gas left in the lungs at the end of a maximal expiration (~1.2 L)
Lung Capacities	
Vital capacity	The total volume of gas that can be exhaled during maximal expiration (~4.8 L)
Inspiratory capacity	The amount of gas that can be inspired from a resting expiration (~3.5 L)
Functional residual capacity	The amount of gas left in the lungs at the end of a normal expiration (~2.4 L)
Total lung capacity	The amount of gas contained in the lungs at maximal inspiration (~6.0 L)

sures of ventilation (amount of air moved) include four lung volumes and four lung capacities. Figure 21-10 schematically presents the various lung volumes and capacities; Table 21-2 defines each term and provides further details.

Lung volumes and capacities vary with individual body size, age (decreased in the neonate, young child, and the elderly),[7-9] and the individual's body position (supine versus upright). Testing of pulmonary function to measure these volumes and capacities is covered under "Obstructive Pulmonary Disorders" in Chapter 22. Other measures important to ventilation are dead space, minute ventilation, and alveolar ventilation.

Dead Space

Dead space includes three dimensions: anatomic dead space, alveolar dead space, and physiologic dead space. Anatomic dead space includes the volume of nonusable gas (not used in gas exchange) in the conducting airways from the nose down to the respiratory bronchioles.[5,10,11] Generally in adults this area is equal to 1 ml per pound of *ideal* body weight, or approximately 150 ml. In newborns and young children, the anatomic dead space is proportionately larger for their size.[6] The anatomic dead space of elderly persons may increase slightly over that of healthy young adults because of the loss of alveolar sacs. Alveolar dead space is composed of ventilated but unperfused or underperfused areas of the lung and is often referred to as wasted ventilation.[5] Alveolar dead space increases with the development of pulmonary emboli owing to (bloodclot) decreased perfusion. Physiologic dead space (functional dead space) is the sum of the anatomic dead space and alveolar dead space.[7,11] Approximately one third of each breath occupies dead space.

Minute Ventilation

Minute ventilation or expired volume ($\dot{V}_E$) is the product of tidal volume times respiratory rate per minute. For example, a person with a tidal volume (milliliters of air inhaled with each breath) of 500 ml who is breathing at a rate of 15 breaths/minute has a minute ventilation of 7500 ml (see Table 21-2 for typical volumes).

Alveolar Ventilation/Oxygenation

By comparison, alveolar ventilation ($\dot{V}A$) equals the difference between tidal volume (VT) and anatomic dead space volume (VD) multiplied by the respiratory rate (RR) per minute.[10]

$$\text{Alveolar ventilation } (\dot{V}A) = (VT - VD) \times RR$$

Because alveolar ventilation is affected by both anatomic dead space and the respiratory rate, slow deep breathing yields a greater alveolar ventilation than rapid shallow respiration. The patient breathing 25 times/minute at a VT of 200 ml would have an alveolar ventilation as follows:

$$(200 \text{ ml} - 150 \text{ ml}) \times 25 \text{ breaths/minute} = 1250 \text{ ml}$$

A patient breathing 10 times/minute at a VT of 600 ml would have an alveolar ventilation of:

$$(600 \text{ ml} - 150 \text{ ml}) \times 10 = 4500 \text{ ml}$$

The partial pressure of oxygen in the alveoli (PAO_2) is the driving force to move O_2 into the blood and is estimated with the following equation:

$$PAO_2 = FIO_2 (PB - 47) - (PaCO_2 \div 0.8)$$

where FIO_2 is the fraction of inspired oxygen; PB, barometric pressure; 47, constant for water vapor pressure (mm Hg); 0.8, respiratory quotient; and $PaCO_2$, laboratory measurement of arterial CO_2 (mm Hg).

The value for PAO_2 is normally very close to that for PaO_2. The difference between alveolar and arterial oxygen tensions is called $A - aDO_2$. A large $A - aDO_2$ indicates poor matching of alveolar ventilation with alveolar blood flow ($\dot{V}A/\dot{Q}$ matching).

For example, to calculate $A - aDO_2$ for a person at sea level (PB = 760 mm Hg) breathing room air ($FIO_2 = 0.21$) with $PaO_2 = 75$ mm Hg and $PaCO_2 = 40$ mm Hg:

$$PAO_2 = 0.21\ (760 - 47) - (40/0.8) = 150 - 50 = 100$$

Therefore, using the arterial blood gas value obtained for the PaO_2 and the calculated PAO_2 of 100, a difference of 25 mm Hg is determined:

$$A - aDO_2 = 100 - 75 = 25 \text{ mm Hg}$$

This large of a difference indicates a significant problem with gas exchange.

In critical care settings, it is often useful to calculate the $A - aDO_2$ value to monitor the efficacy of oxygen exchange across the lung. The normal A − a gradient is less than 10 mm Hg at room air, but it increases with age and increasing FIO_2. A rising $A - aDO_2$ value indicates worsening lung function, even though hypoxemia, a PaO_2 lower than 80 mm Hg at sea level, may not necessarily be present.

Hypoxemia that is primarily caused by hypoventilation suggests that the lung is normal, and treatment that increases ventilation will remedy the problem. This type of hypoxemia is characterized by a normal $A - aDO_2$ value.

A simple method of calculating expected PAO_2 is the "law of 5's." By multiplying the FIO_2 (%) by 5, the care provider has an estimate of what the oxygen level should be under normal, healthy conditions (e.g., 5 × 21% room air = 105).

Mechanics of Breathing

The mechanics of breathing include the concepts of airway resistance, lung compliance, and opposing lung forces (elastic recoil versus chest wall expansion) of the lung. These factors affect the overall performance of gas exchange and the work of breathing.

The lungs have a natural recoil tendency, whereas the chest wall favors the expanded state. During inspiration the chest wall muscles (external intercostals) contract, elevating the ribs as the diaphragm moves downward. These two actions create a negative intrapleural pressure that causes the lung to expand. During expiration the lung deflates passively because of the elastic recoil (elastic fibers in the lung tissue), relaxation of the diaphragm, and the surface tension of the alveoli. Figure 21-11 provides a depiction of the interaction of lung forces during inspiration and expiration. In the normal resting individual, expiration is accomplished almost entirely by relaxation of the diaphragm.[5] At the end of a normal expiration, the alveoli still contain some air volume, known as the functional residual capacity. If the alveoli were allowed to empty completely, the high surface tension in the alveoli would make it more difficult to reinflate them and add significantly to the work of breathing. In the absence of surfactant, which reduces alveolar surface tension, the alveoli tend to collapse—a condition called *atelectasis.* Excessive surface tension can increase the work of breathing so much that mechanical ventilation may be required. This is often the case in ARDS and in infant respiratory distress syndrome (see Chapter 23).

Airway Resistance

Airway resistance is determined by the relationship between pressure and flow. It is influenced by airway radius and the pattern of gas flow. Resistance increases as the radius of the airway tube decreases. Resistance is calculated by the following formula:

$$\text{Resistance} = \text{pressure difference} \div \text{rate of airflow}$$

The radius of the airway decreases from the trachea to the terminal bronchioles. As mucus builds up in the airway, the passage is narrowed, and resistance to airflow increases. Other

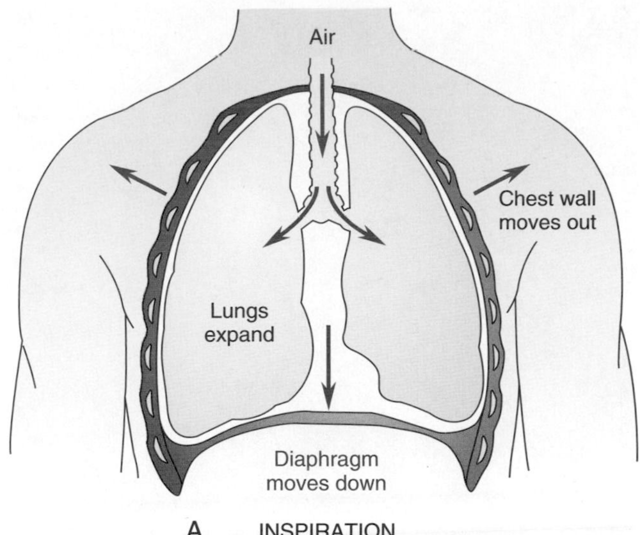

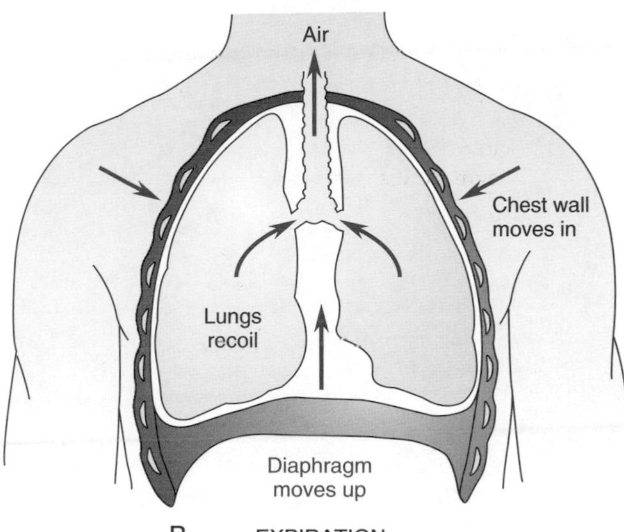

FIGURE 21-11 ■ Lung forces during inspiration and expiration. **A,** During inspiration, the respiratory muscles contract, the chest wall expands, and air flows into the lungs. **B,** During expiration, the respiratory muscles relax, the lungs recoil, and air flows passively out of the lungs.

factors affecting airway resistance include stress, pulmonary conditioning, and age.

The trachea and bronchi contain cartilage and small amounts of muscle. The cartilage assists in maintaining airway passage stability, thus preventing airway collapse. The bronchioles and terminal bronchioles do not contain cartilage but have increased amounts of smooth muscle that are innervated by the autonomic nervous system. Stimulation of cholinergic fibers leads to bronchoconstriction. Stimulation of the β_2-adrenergic receptors leads to bronchodilation. The bronchial muscles function to maintain an even distribution of ventilation. A circadian rhythm is associated with bronchial tone, with maximal bronchodilation occurring at about 6 PM and maximal bronchoconstriction occurring at 6 AM.[2]

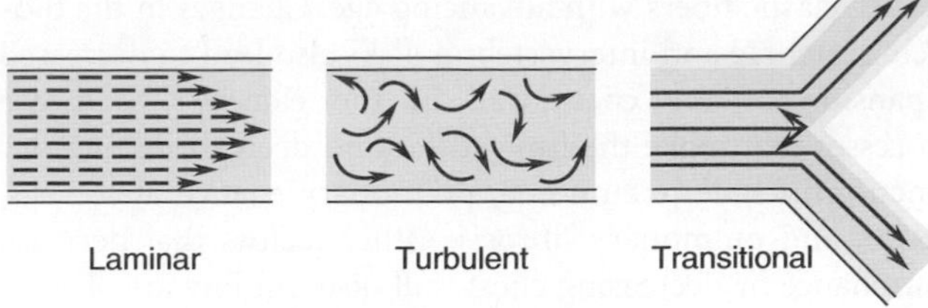

FIGURE 21-12 ■ Patterns of gas flow.

Airway resistance is also affected by the pattern of gas flow (Figure 21-12). Air movement from the nasal cavity through the large bronchi occurs by **turbulent flow,** which creates friction and increases resistance. Bronchospasm in the smaller airways and high gas flow also create turbulent flow. **Laminar flow** occurs in the small airways of the lung and creates minimal resistance to airflow. **Transitional flow** (mixed pattern of flow) occurs in the larger airways, especially at bifurcations. The highest airway resistance is at the nose because of turbulent flow with high velocities of airflow. The lowest airway resistance is in the small bronchioles where turbulent flow is low. Airway resistance is even higher in the newborn than the adult and continues to be greater than that of the adult up to the age of 5 years. Resistance changes very little in the elderly lung.[6,12,13]

Lung Compliance

Lung compliance is another factor that influences the work of breathing. Compliance represents lung expandability and the ease of lung inflation. It is best illustrated by the effort required to blow up a new balloon as compared to blowing up a balloon that has been inflated many times before. It is a measure of the relationship between pressure and volume. It is represented by the following formula:

$$\text{Compliance} = \text{change in volume} \div \text{change in pressure}$$

Two factors associated with compliance are chest wall expandability (not usually measured) and lung expandability. Lung compliance can be measured in the static (motionless) or dynamic state. Effective static compliance is determined by dividing the pressure required to deliver a volume of gas by the tidal volume as delivered by a ventilator. A more accurate measurement of compliance requires the insertion of an esophageal balloon. Normal static compliance in a healthy young adult would be 90 to 100 ml/cm H_2O.

Compliance provides an estimate of airway resistance and elasticity. Lung compliance is increased in neonates and children younger than 3.5 years because of their chest wall flexibility.[6] Lung compliance may decrease in the elderly because of increasing chest wall rigidity from calcification of costal cartilages, reduced mobility of ribs, and partial contraction of inspiratory muscles.[12,13] Compliance may be further compromised by loss in the elastic fibers of the lung that occurs with age.[12,13] There appears to be a reduction in number and thickness of elastic fibers with advancing age. Changes in the thoracic vertebrae and intervertebral disks also lead to decreased expansion of the chest wall in the elderly.[7,8,13] Disease processes that make the lung stiffer and decrease respiratory function include pneumonia, pulmonary edema, atelectasis, ARDS, and pulmonary fibrosis. Other factors that decrease compliance by decreasing chest wall distensibility are obesity, abdominal distention, kyphoscoliosis, and abdominal surgery (due to decreased respiratory effort from surgical pain). Lung compliance is increased in patients with emphysema owing to loss of alveoli and elastic tissue (see Chapter 22).

Distribution of Ventilation

Distribution of ventilation is affected by body position. In the upright individual, the alveoli at the apices of the lung are much larger than those at the base. Figure 21-13 shows the variation in structural size of alveoli at the apex compared with that at the base. In the normal upright individual, ventilation is greatest near the bottom of the lung and decreases toward the apices.[5] These regional differences are less in a supine person. The greater lung expansion at the bases results from a greater compliance of the alveoli at the bases and the downward displacement of the diaphragm, which expands the lower lobes more than the upper lobes. When an individual is in the supine lateral position, ventilation is best in the dependent lung, but the difference is not as great as that seen in the upright lung.

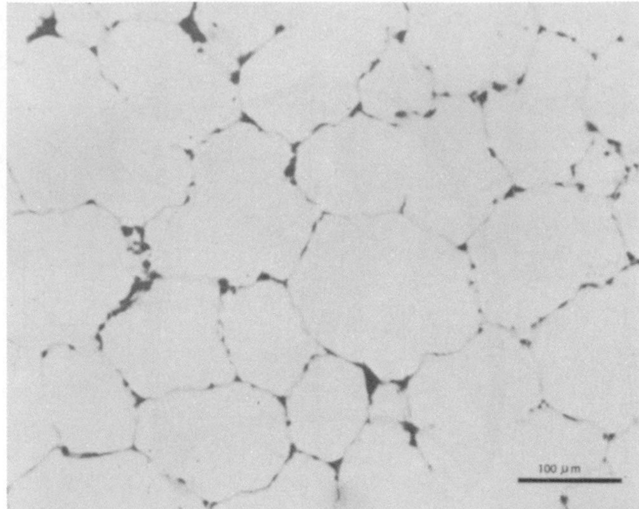

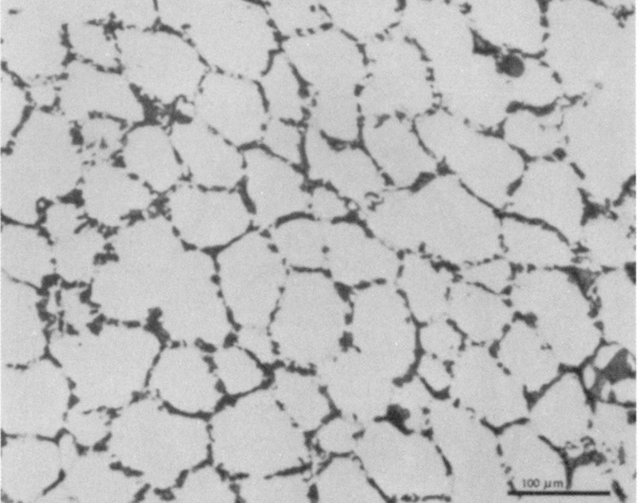

FIGURE 21-13 ■ Sections of lung from the apex *(upper panel)* and 20 cm below the apex *(lower panel)* obtained from a greyhound dog lung; specimens frozen in a vertical position. The *upper panel* shows what alveoli in the apex *(zone 1)* of the lung look like in the upright position: the air sacs are large and blood flow is diminished. The *lower panel* represents the base of the lung zone with optimal ventilation and perfusion ($\times$188). (From Murray JF: *The normal lung,* ed 2, Philadelphia, 1986, Saunders, p 110. Courtesy Jon B. Glazier, MD.)

Neurologic Control of Ventilation

Respiration is influenced by a number of factors. These include neural control centers, chemoreceptors, lung receptors, proprioceptors, and pressure receptors. The factors that regulate respiration are reviewed in this section.

Neural control of the respiratory system is located in the medulla oblongata and the pons, which is commonly referred to as the *respiratory center.* Nerve impulses travel from the brainstem by way of the phrenic nerve to the diaphragm to stimulate muscular contractions for inspiration.

The medullary respiratory center within the brainstem consists of two groups of widely dispersed neurons that function as a unit to regulate breathing. The dorsal respiratory group of neurons sends out impulses that stimulate inspiratory muscles (in the intercostals and diaphragm). The impulses are generated in increasing fashion, termed a "ramp" signal. Impulses begin slowly and increase steadily for about 2 seconds. Abrupt cessation of signals for 3 seconds allows for expiration, and then the cycle begins again.[2,3,5] This system establishes the basic respiratory rhythm. Figure 21-14 provides a schematic diagram of these interactive mechanisms on respiratory control.

The pneumotaxic center of the upper pons (see Figure 21-14) appears to influence the rate of respiration and ends inspiration by inhibition of an inspiratory ramp. In addition, input from the spinal cord, cortex, and midbrain contributes to the normal smooth pattern of respiration. The apneustic center of the lower pons (demonstrated to exist in dogs) influences the pattern of respiration and probably prevents the "switching off" of the inspiratory ramp. It may function to provide an extra driving force for the inspiratory neurons, thus prolonging inspiration.

Sensory inputs to the respiratory control center include central chemoreceptors, peripheral chemoreceptors, Hering-Breuer stretch receptors, proprioceptors, pressoreceptors, and environmental sensations.

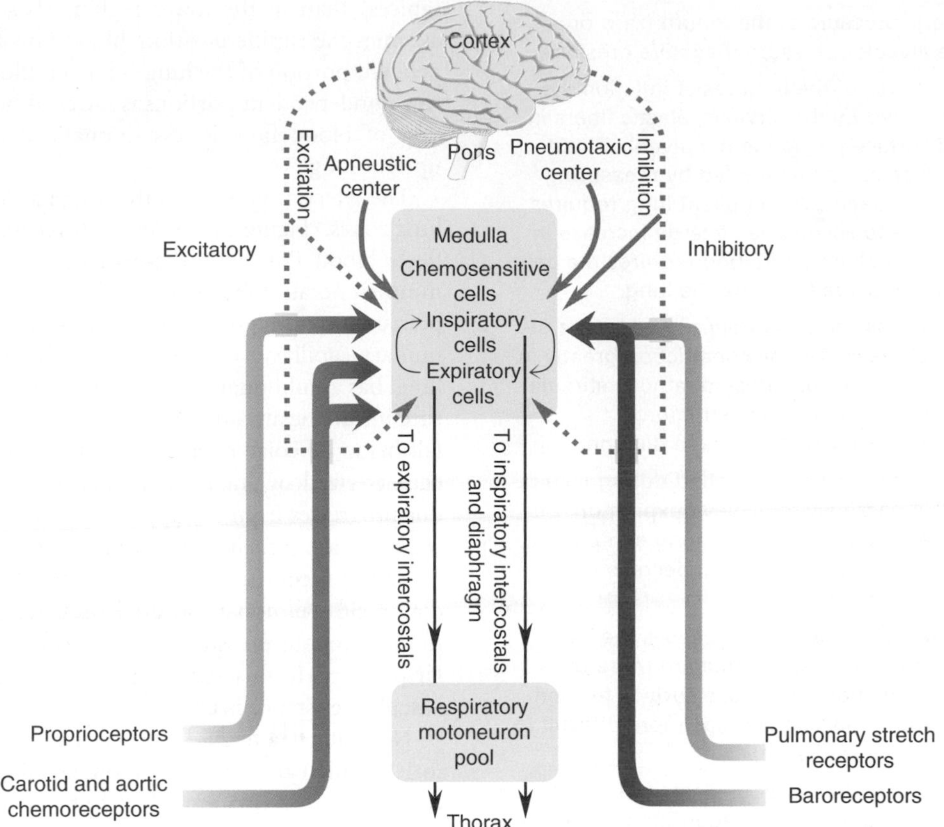

FIGURE 21-14 ■ Interactive mechanisms influencing control of respiration.

The central chemoreceptors within the medullary center respond to changes in CO_2 and pH. A person's normal stimulus to breathe occurs when a small increase in arterial carbon dioxide tension ($Paco_2$) leads to stimulation of respiration. Alveolar ventilation can increase 10-fold with an acute rise in $Paco_2$. Acidosis (decrease in pH) can also increase alveolar ventilation.

The peripheral chemoreceptors located in the aortic arch and carotid bodies respond to decreases in arterial O_2 and pH and increases in $Paco_2$. Increases in the hydrogen ion concentration (decreased pH) or the $Paco_2$ stimulate peripheral chemoreceptors, but these effects are less important than the response of central chemoreceptors.

The Hering-Breuer reflex involves stretch receptors located in the alveolar septa, bronchi, and bronchioles. Inflation of the lung initiates the response that sends neuronal impulses up the vagus nerve to the medulla to cause inhibition of inspiration. Therefore, the rate and duration of inspiration are affected. This reflex, seen primarily in neonates and at high tidal volumes (greater than 1500 ml), prevents overdistention of the lung.[2,3,5]

Proprioceptors located in the muscles and tendons of movable joints respond to body movement (exercise). The stimulus of body movement leads to stimulation of respiration (rate and depth) to maintain oxygen levels during exercise.[3]

Pressoreceptors (baroreceptors) located in the aortic arch and carotid arteries respond to changes in blood pressure. The aortic arch transmits impulses through the vagus nerve, and the carotid bodies transmit impulses through the glossopharyngeal nerve. An increase in arterial blood pressure leads to inhibition of respiration. A decrease in arterial blood pressure below a mean arterial pressure of 80 mm Hg leads to stimulation of respiration.

Environmental factors also influence respiration. Individuals demonstrate changes in respiration related to such factors as a cold shower, pin prick, and stress, as well as to airway irritation from air pollution and smoking. Infection and fever also increase the respiratory rate.

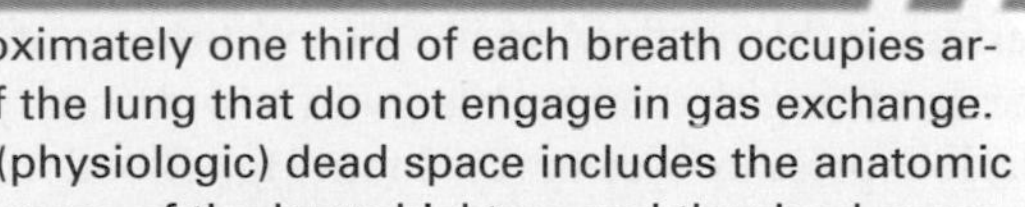

- Approximately one third of each breath occupies areas of the lung that do not engage in gas exchange. Total (physiologic) dead space includes the anatomic dead space of the bronchial tree and the dead space of unperfused alveoli.
- Alveolar ventilation may be severely compromised in persons with small tidal volumes or increased dead space. When tidal volume is not significantly greater than dead space, increased respiratory rate is not effective in restoring alveolar minute ventilation.
- To move air into the lungs, the respiratory muscles generate a negative intrapleural pressure that causes air inflow, owing to the pressure gradient between

the atmospheric pressure at the mouth (zero pressure) and the alveolar pressure (negative pressure).

- Airways and tissues of the lung resist inflation. Resistance is provided by the airways, elastic fibers in the lung, and surface tension in the alveoli. The degree of resistance can be estimated by measuring overall lung compliance. A compliant lung requires minimal pressure to accomplish a large increase in volume; a noncompliant (stiff) lung requires the generation of high pressure to inflate the lung.
- Airway resistance is primarily determined by the diameter of the airways. Airway constriction greatly increases airway resistance. Parasympathetic stimulation of the airways results in constriction; sympathetic (β_2) stimulation results in dilation.
- Elastic fibers in the lung are stretched during inspiration, then recoil passively to achieve expiration. Destruction of elastic fibers increases lung compliance; excessive fiber production (fibrosis) decreases lung compliance.
- High surface tension in an alveoli causes the surfaces to stick together, making inflation more difficult. Surfactant functions to reduce surface tension. A lack of surfactant makes the lungs more difficult to inflate (decreased compliance).
- The medulla oblongata and pons contain the neurons that integrate information regarding the ventilatory status of the body from chemoreceptors, proprioceptors, and stretch receptors. Respiratory neurons in the medulla initiate inspiration and establish the basic inspiratory-expiratory pattern. Pneumotactic center neurons in the pons primarily influence the rate and depth of respiration.
- Central chemoreceptors located within the medulla detect changes in pH and Pco_2. Peripheral chemoreceptors are located in the aorta and carotids and detect changes in arterial pH, Pco_2, and Po_2. An increase in Pco_2 or a decrease in pH or Po_2 stimulates ventilation.

PULMONARY BLOOD FLOW

Pulmonary Vasculature

Perfusion (blood flow) is the second process of respiration, the first being alveolar ventilation. The pulmonary circulation is a low-pressure system (25/8 mm Hg). Blood from the right ventricle is pumped into the main pulmonary artery and then into its branches, which divide into capillary beds throughout lung tissue. The capillary beds surround the alveoli and allow for easy exchange of O_2 and CO_2.

Distribution of Blood Flow

Distribution of blood flow (perfusion) is uneven and is affected by body position and exercise. When a person is upright, blood flow is much less in the upper regions of the lungs (apices) than in the lower regions (bases). When a person assumes the supine position, blood flow to the posterior dependent portion of the lung is higher. Blood flow to the anterior nondependent portions is lower, although the redistribution of blood flow is less dramatic than that seen in the upright lung.

The effect of gravity on the lung has led to the concept of lung zones.[5] Figure 21-15 depicts three lung zones. Zone 1 reflects blood flow in the apices of the lung. Blood flow is minimal because the enlarged alveolar sacs create an alveolar pressure that is higher than capillary pressure, leading to pulmonary capillary collapse. Zone 2, the middle region of the lung, has a pulmonary arterial pressure greater than the pressure inside the alveoli during ventricular systole, but this may fall below alveolar pressure during diastole. Thus, zone 2 is characterized by intermittent perfusion, which increases as one progresses from the upper region of the zone to the lower region of the zone in the upright position.

Zone 3 is continuously perfused throughout the entire cardiac cycle. Pulmonary arterial pressure is greater than pulmonary venous pressure, which in turn is greater than alveolar pressure. In this zone, capillary vessels are distended and vascular resistance is low.[5,6]

Normally, 1% to 2% of the cardiac output bypasses (right-to-left shunt) alveolar ventilation, creating a decrease in arterial oxygen by 3 to 5 mm Hg.[10] In bronchial anastomotic diseases, the amount of shunting may rise to 10% to 20%.[10]

Ventilation-Perfusion Ratios

The discussion about distribution of ventilation and perfusion indicates that the best overall ventilation and perfusion occurs in the dependent lung fields. A factor important to the concepts of ventilation and perfusion is the matching of an adequate volume of air in the alveoli to adequate pulmonary blood flow. In the ideal state, 4 L/min of alveolar ventilation is matched to 5 L/min of capillary blood flow in the lungs, creating a normal alveolar ventilation-to-perfusion ratio ($\dot{V}_A/\dot{Q}$) of 0.8 (Box 21-1). Two major factors that have an impact on this normal $\dot{V}_A/\dot{Q}$ ratio are right-to-left shunt and regional ventilation and perfusion changes. Other factors influencing the ratio are position changes, exercise, bed rest, and lung disease.

In a normal person in the upright position, ventilation and perfusion are lower in the upper lung (apex) than the lower lung (base). In the apex, alveoli are large and receive limited blood flow, whereas in the base, alveoli are smaller and allow for greater expansion of capillaries and thus more blood flow. In the apex, $\dot{V}_A/\dot{Q}$ is as much as 2.5 times the ideal value, causing a moderate degree of physiologic dead space. In the base, $\dot{V}_A/\dot{Q}$ is as low as 0.6 times the ideal value, representing low $\dot{V}_A/\dot{Q}$, where the blood flow exceeds ventilation. During exercise, blood flow to the upper lung region increases dramatically, thus decreasing physiologic dead space. With bed rest, the dependent area of the lungs becomes the back region in

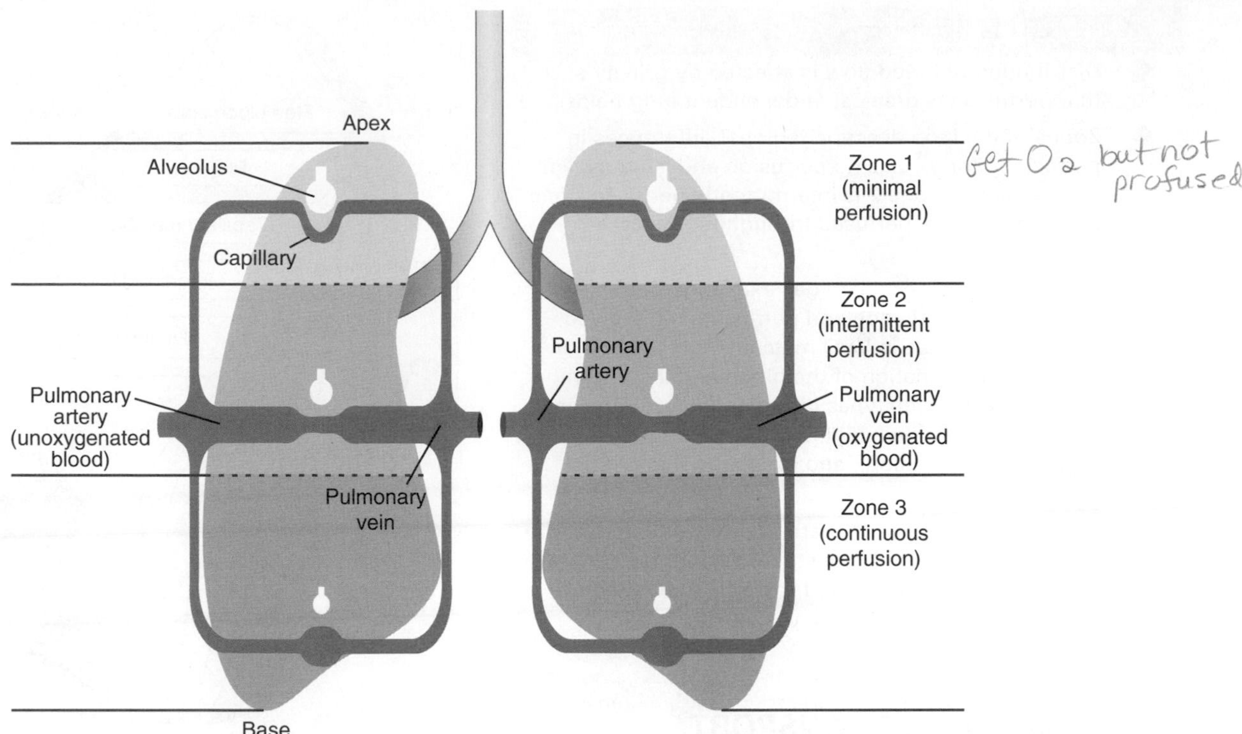

FIGURE 21-15 ■ Schematic representation of the three lung zones in which different hemodynamic conditions govern blood flow (see text for discussion).

Box 21-1

Ventilation-Perfusion ($\dot{V}A/\dot{Q}$)* Equations

Low $\dot{V}A/\dot{Q}$ (underventilated):

$$\frac{\text{2 L/min alveolar ventilation}}{\text{5 L/min blood flow}}$$

Normal $\dot{V}A/\dot{Q}$:

$$\frac{\text{4 L/min alveolar ventilation}}{\text{5 L/min blood flow}}$$

High $\dot{V}A/\dot{Q}$ (underperfused):

$$\frac{\text{4 L/min alveolar ventilation}}{\text{2 L/min blood flow}}$$

*$\dot{V}A/\dot{Q}$, where $\dot{V}A$ = alveolar ventilation and $\dot{Q}$ = blood flow.

the supine position, so that blood flow is increased to that region and alveoli are smaller.

The three types of $\dot{V}A/\dot{Q}$ imbalances are (1) high $\dot{V}A/\dot{Q}$, (2) low $\dot{V}A/\dot{Q}$, and (3) shunt. High $\dot{V}A/\dot{Q}$ is conceptually related to physiologic dead space, in which the alveolar unit is ventilated but not perfused. High $\dot{V}A/\dot{Q}$ units have a low P_{CO_2} and normal P_{AO_2} and can be viewed as a respiratory reserve, which can be used if perfusion is restored.

Low $\dot{V}A/\dot{Q}$ is conceptually related to lower Pa_{O_2} (hypoxemia). Low $\dot{V}A/\dot{Q}$ occurs regionally in areas where the airways are partially obstructed and airflow rates are low. Although an increase in total ventilation results in a decrease in alveolar CO_2, the increment in P_{AO_2} and O_2 content in end-capillary blood is minimal.[5,14,15] Low $\dot{V}A/\dot{Q}$ is responsive to treatment with oxygen because the airways are only partially obstructed, so it is possible for oxygen to enter the alveoli by diffusion.

Physiologic shunt, which is functionally equivalent to right-to-left shunt, contributes to lowering of Pa_{O_2}. Normally, in a healthy person, physiologic shunt is less than 5% of cardiac output. In patients with acute respiratory failure (ARF), physiologic shunt may rise to more than 50%.[15] Although physiologic shunt is similar to low $\dot{V}A/\dot{Q}$ in affecting low oxygen levels, shunt is not responsive to oxygen therapy because the alveoli are collapsed or consolidated and oxygen cannot gain entry into them. See the section on acute respiratory failure for details.

Hypoxic Vasoconstriction

Alveolar hypoxia leads to compensatory hypoxic vasoconstriction of the pulmonary vessels passing through poorly ventilated portions of the lungs. Blood is diverted from areas of low alveolar oxygen to areas of higher oxygen as a means of compensatory adaptation. By diverting blood flow to areas of higher oxygen concentration, the negative effects on gas exchange are reduced. Low alveolar oxygen leads to contraction of smooth muscle in the walls of the small pulmonary arterioles. One hypothesis for this reaction is that cells in the perivascular tissue release an unknown vasoconstrictor substance in response to hypoxia.[5]

KEY CONCEPTS

- Distribution of blood flow is affected by gravity such that perfusion is greatest in dependent lung fields.
- Zones of the lung describe regional differences in perfusion. Zone 1 has no perfusion and is equivalent to dead space; zone 2 is intermittently perfused; zone 3 is continuously perfused throughout the cardiac cycle.
- Optimal alveolar-capillary gas exchange depends on matching of ventilation and perfusion at the alveolus. Abnormalities in $\dot{V}A/\dot{Q}$ matching can result in inadequate oxygenation of the blood and insufficient CO_2 removal. Three types of regional $\dot{V}A/\dot{Q}$ imbalance have been described: high $\dot{V}A/\dot{Q}$ (dead space), low $\dot{V}A/\dot{Q}$ (poor ventilation), and intrapulmonary shunt (no ventilation).
- Vessels in lung areas that are poorly ventilated, and therefore hypoxic, will constrict to minimize $\dot{V}A/\dot{Q}$ imbalances by diverting blood to better ventilated areas. This is termed hypoxic vasoconstriction.

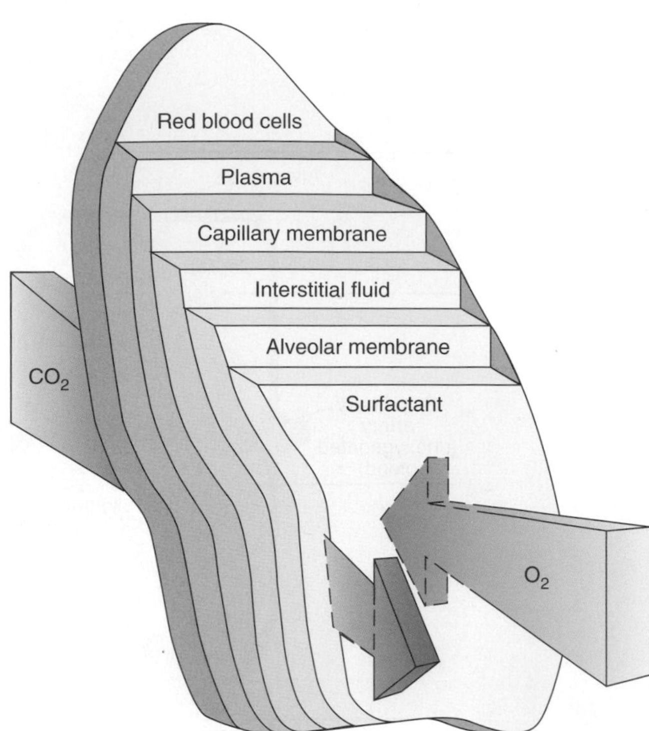

FIGURE 21-16 ■ Schematic representing the six barriers through which O_2 and CO_2 must diffuse for gas exchange to occur.

DIFFUSION AND TRANSPORT OF RESPIRATORY GASES

Barriers to Diffusion

Diffusion is the movement of gas from a high-concentration area to a low-concentration area. The alveolar-capillary membrane through which O_2 and CO_2 must diffuse consists of six barriers (Figure 21-16). For O_2 to reach the hemoglobin molecule, it must pass through surfactant, the alveolar membrane, interstitial fluid, the capillary membrane, plasma, and the red blood cell (RBC) membrane. The rate of diffusion of a gas is proportional to the tissue area and the difference in gas partial pressure between the two sides of alveoli, and inversely proportional to the tissue thickness through which the gas must move. Oxygen diffuses into the blood from the alveoli, and CO_2 diffuses out of the blood into the alveoli. Under normal conditions, O_2 and CO_2 move across the alveolar-capillary membrane in only 0.25 second. The RBC spends about 0.75 second within the pulmonary capillary system surrounding the alveoli, thus allowing an extra 0.50 second of exchange time. Even with mild disease processes, O_2 and CO_2 have adequate time for transfer.

Under abnormal conditions, such as thickening of the alveolar-capillary membrane (pneumonia, pulmonary edema, and interstitial lung disease) and decreased available surface area (emphysema), the diffusion capacity of the lung tissue is impaired. Diffusion capacity may be further impaired by increased physical activity because of the decreased time spent by the RBCs in the pulmonary capillary system. Thickening of the alveolar-capillary membrane also occurs with aging.

CO_2 is 20 times more diffusible than O_2 because of its greater solubility.[5] Factors that determine the ability and the speed of a gas to diffuse include the available surface area of alveoli and capillaries, the integrity of the capillary and alveolar membranes, the availability of hemoglobin to transport oxygen, the solubility of the gas, the **diffusion coefficient** of the gas, and the differences in partial pressure of the gases on each side of the alveolar membrane. For example, because CO_2 is 24 times more soluble than O_2, it diffuses more rapidly and requires a lower partial pressure.

Conditions that cause $\dot{V}A/\dot{Q}$ mismatch impair diffusion of gases. The decreased diffusing capacity seen in the aged person is further compromised by a decrease in the number of pulmonary capillaries and decreased lung volume and capacities. The end result is decreased PaO_2 and increased $\dot{V}A/\dot{Q}$ mismatch. The PaO_2 drops about 3 to 5 mm Hg for each decade after age 30 years.[5] Therefore, an 80-year-old individual could be expected to have a PaO_2 of 75 mm Hg. Diffusion is also decreased in the newborn because of the thickness of the alveolar membrane.[6] In a healthy adult, the PaO_2 value would be 90 to 100 mm Hg (see Table 21-1 for variations in respiratory anatomy and physiology by age grouping).

The difference between PAO_2 and PaO_2 is a good indicator of diffusion and $\dot{V}A/\dot{Q}$ matching.

Oxygen Transport

Oxygen is transported to the tissues by two mechanisms: (1) in the dissolved form in plasma and (2) in the bound state attached to the hemoglobin molecule. Only about 0.3 ml of O_2 per 100 ml is carried dissolved in the plasma.[5] The remaining

O_2 is transported on the hemoglobin molecule. A high concentration (partial pressure) of O_2 in the pulmonary capillaries causes O_2 to bind to the hemoglobin molecule. Heme is an iron-porphyrin compound that joins with the four polypeptide chains of the protein globin. Oxygen binds to each of the four heme sites to form oxyhemoglobin. At the tissue level where the partial pressure of O_2 is low, O_2 is released from the hemoglobin molecule. Depending on tissue needs, one fourth is normally unloaded at the tissues in a resting individual, which results in venous blood being 75% saturated with oxygen.

Fully bound O_2 is considered to be 100% saturated and yields a PaO_2 of 95 to 100 mm Hg. Increasing alveolar O_2 above this level will have no further effect on increasing the amount of O_2 carried on the hemoglobin molecule. Oxygen binds to the hemoglobin molecule in the lungs and is delivered to tissues. Oxygen binds when there is a high affinity of hemoglobin for oxygen (at the lungs) and releases when the affinity is decreased at the tissue level to maintain adequate metabolic processes. When PaO_2 is less than 60 mm Hg, saturation of hemoglobin for oxygen (SaO_2) falls steeply (Figure 21-17). The oxyhemoglobin dissociation curve schematic diagram shows the effects of increases and decreases in O_2 affinity at any PaO_2. Decreased O_2 affinity, also termed a "shift to the right," aids in the release of O_2 from the hemoglobin molecule, thus facilitating movement of O_2 from the blood to the tissues.

Increased O_2 affinity, termed a "shift to the left," represents a tighter binding of O_2 to the hemoglobin molecule, thus decreasing its delivery to the tissues. Although an increased affinity for O_2 reflects a higher percentage of saturated hemoglobin, its ineffective release in the tissues may be profound. Factors that affect hemoglobin affinity and shift the curve to the left (increased affinity) include alkalosis, hypothermia, decreased $PaCO_2$, and decreased 2,3-diphosphoglycerate (2,3-DPG), an end product of RBC metabolism. Factors that shift the curve to the right (decreased affinity) include acidosis, hyperthermia, increased $PaCO_2$, and increased 2,3-DPG. The availability of O_2 is also decreased by decreased cardiac output and anemia.

CaO_2 is the sum of dissolved oxygen in the plasma plus the oxygen carried on the hemoglobin (Hb) molecule. (See Chapter 13 for a more detailed discussion of oxygen carriage and transport.) Normal arterial blood oxygen content (CaO_2) is

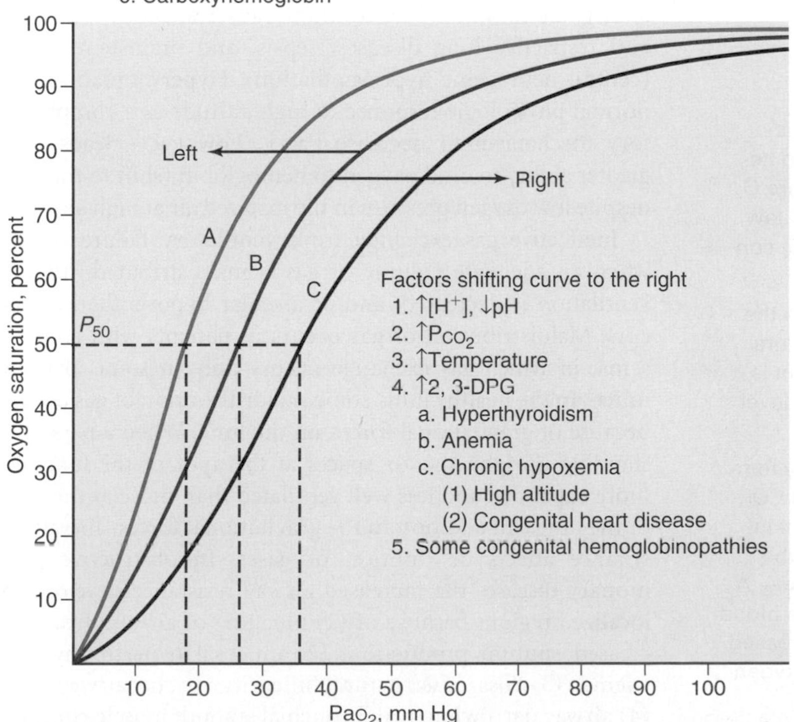

FIGURE 21-17 ■ Oxyhemoglobin dissociation curve showing factors affecting hemoglobin's affinity for oxygen. Curve *B* is the standard curve under normal conditions. Curve *A* shows a shift to the left, which represents an increased affinity of hemoglobin for oxygen. Curve *C* demonstrates a shift to the right, which represents a decreased affinity. (From Gottlieb JE: Breathing and gas exchange. In Kinney MR, Packa DR, Dunbar SB, editors: *AACN's clinical reference for critical care nursing,* ed 3, New York, 1993, McGraw-Hill, p 672.)

20 ml of O_2 per 100 ml of blood (vol%) and can be calculated by the following formula:

$$Cao_2 \text{ (vol\%)} = [\text{Hb (g/dl)} \times 1.34 \text{ (ml of } O_2\text{/g of Hb)} \times (Sao_2)] + (Pao_2 \times 0.003)$$

Carbon Dioxide Transport

Carbon dioxide, a byproduct of cell metabolism, is transported in the blood in four ways: dissolved in plasma (5% to 10% of the total CO_2 transport); as carbonic acid in the plasma (insignificant amount); as bicarbonate (60% to 70%); and as carbamino compounds on the hemoglobin molecule (20% to 30%). The greatest bulk of CO_2 transport is in the bicarbonate form. In the presence of the RBC enzyme carbonic anhydrase, CO_2 combines with water to form carbonic acid, which in turn almost instantaneously breaks down into bicarbonate ions and hydrogen ions. The released hydrogen ions attach to the hemoglobin molecule, while the bicarbonate ion diffuses into the plasma and combines with sodium. Chloride ions in the surrounding plasma shift into the RBC (chloride shift). This chemical process is reversed when the venous blood reaches the lungs, so that CO_2 can diffuse across the alveolar membrane to be exhaled.

KEY CONCEPTS

- Oxygen and CO_2 diffuse quickly across alveolar-capillary membranes. Complete equilibration of gases occurs in the first third of the capillary under normal conditions. Diffusion may be incomplete when the alveolar-capillary membrane is abnormally thickened or capillary blood flow is extremely rapid.
- Carbon dioxide is more soluble and diffuses more quickly than O_2. Disorders of diffusion often affect O_2 transfer earlier and more significantly than CO_2 transfer.
- Oxygen is carried in the blood in two forms: dissolved in solution ($Pao_2 \times 0.003$); and bound to hemoglobin (Hb × Sao_2 × 1.34). Significantly more O_2 is bound than dissolved. Low hemoglobin and low hemoglobin saturation profoundly affect the O_2 content in the blood.
- The oxyhemoglobin saturation curve describes the relationship between Pao_2 and hemoglobin saturation. At a Pao_2 of 90 to 100 mm Hg, hemoglobin is fully saturated. An increase in Pao_2 above this level does not significantly improve O_2 content.
- The affinity of hemoglobin for O_2 is affected by temperature, acid-base status, 2,3-DPG levels, and CO_2. Affinity decreases at the tissue level because of increased acid, 2,3-DPG, and CO_2. This "shift to the right" enhances the unloading of O_2 at the tissue. A "shift to the left" occurs at the lung, where the blood is more alkalotic and CO_2 levels are lower. Increased affinity of hemoglobin in the lung enhances oxygen binding.
- Carbon dioxide is transported in the blood in three major forms: dissolved, as carbaminohemoglobin, and as the bicarbonate ion. The most important of these is bicarbonate ion, which is formed from the combination of CO_2 and H_2O, forming carbonic acid (H_2CO_3). Carbonic acid breaks into HCO_3^- and H^+. At the lung, the reaction proceeds in the reverse to form CO_2, which diffuses into the alveoli.

ALTERATIONS IN PULMONARY FUNCTION

Hypoventilation and Hyperventilation

Hypoventilation occurs when delivery of air to the alveoli is insufficient to meet the need to provide oxygen and remove carbon dioxide. It is influenced by decreased rate and depth of respiration. Hypoventilation results in increased $Paco_2$ (>45 mm Hg) and resultant hypoxemia due to increased alveolar carbon dioxide, which displaces oxygen.[13] Causes may be drugs such as morphine or barbiturates, which depress the central respiratory drive, or disorders such as obesity (pickwickian syndrome), myasthenia gravis, obstructive sleep apnea, chest wall damage, or paralysis of respiratory muscles (especially the diaphragm).[5] Pain related to surgery of the thorax or abdomen often results in hypoventilation secondary to pain on inspiration.

Hyperventilation is an increase in the amount of air entering the alveoli, leading to hypocapnia ($Paco_2$ <35 mm Hg).[5,14] A physiologic cause of hyperventilation is hypoxic stimulation of peripheral chemoreceptors. Causes such as pain, fever, and anxiety are common. Less common causes include obstructive and restrictive lung diseases, sepsis, and brainstem injury (central neurogenic hyperventilation). Hyperventilation is a normal physiologic response to high altitude as a compensatory mechanism to decrease $Paco_2$. Low $Paco_2$ leads to a greater ability to bind oxygen to hemoglobin (shift to the left) despite low oxygen pressure in the inspired air at high altitude.

Ineffective gas exchange from ventilatory failure occurs when an adequate volume of gas is maldistributed, minute ventilation is decreased, and/or alveolar hypoventilation occurs. Maldistribution of gas occurs in patients with emphysema, in which gas exchange occurs only in some alveolar units.[5] In the healthy lung, some maldistribution of gas occurs because of gravitational forces on the lung. When a person is standing upright, the air spaces at the apex of the lung are more expanded and less well ventilated than those at the base of the lung.[5] In addition to the gravitational forces, airway resistance affects distribution of gases. In obstructive pulmonary diseases the increased airway resistance develops in localized regions because of (1) plugging of airways from increased sputum production, (2) mucosal hypertrophy and edema, (3) loss of structural integrity of the airway, and (4) airway narrowing from bronchial smooth muscle contraction when there is hyperactivity of the airways.[5] During expiration, air leaves the areas of least resistance first, thus creating areas of maldistribution of gas.

Hypoxemia and Hypoxia

Two terms frequently used in discussing decreased PaO_2 are **hypoxemia** and **hypoxia.** Hypoxemia refers to deficient blood oxygen as measured by low arterial O_2 and low hemoglobin saturation as measured by arterial blood gases. Hypoxia refers to a decrease in tissue oxygenation. Tissue hypoxia is difficult to measure but may be assumed when either blood flow or PaO_2 is abnormally low.

Resultant types of hypoxia can be classified into four categories: hypoxic hypoxia, anemic hypoxia, circulatory hypoxia, and histotoxic hypoxia. Hypoxic hypoxia occurs when the PaO_2 is decreased despite normal O_2 carrying capacity.[6] Causes include high altitude, hypoventilation, and airway obstruction. Oxygen therapy usually provides adequate treatment.

Anemic hypoxia results from a decrease in O_2 carrying capacity. Any disorder resulting in low hemoglobin can cause anemic hypoxia, including sickle cell anemia, carbon monoxide poisoning, and other anemias.

Circulatory hypoxia results from a low cardiac output state in which the O_2 carrying capacity is normal but blood flow is reduced. Examples of circulatory hypoxia include shock, cardiac arrest, severe blood loss, thyrotoxicosis, and congestive heart failure.

The final classification is histotoxic hypoxia, which occurs when interference of a toxic substance leads to inability of tissues to utilize available oxygen. Cyanide poisoning is an example of this hypoxic classification.

Ineffective gas exchange related to oxygen failure occurs when ventilation and perfusion are mismatched, when diffusion abnormalities exist, and when right-to-left shunt exists. During periods of normal perfusion not all capillaries are open, but the capillary system has the ability to recruit (open up) more capillaries and to distend (expand) capillaries already in use (see Figure 21-9) to increase alveolar blood flow, when it is needed as a compensatory mechanism. In addition, 1% to 3% of the total blood flow in the lung is not oxygenated because the thebesian, pleural, and bronchial veins drain unoxygenated blood into the left side of the heart and into the pulmonary veins.

Areas of low $\dot{V}A/\dot{Q}$ (see Box 21-1) may have normal perfusion but receive inadequate alveolar ventilation (Figure 21-18, *A*). This effect is similar to shunting of pulmonary arterial blood through totally unventilated units. Areas of high $\dot{V}A/\dot{Q}$ (see Figure 21-18, *B*) may have adequate ventilation but have areas of decreased perfusion. This effect is similar to having increased dead space, clinically represented by areas of ventilation without blood flow, as seen in the patient with a pulmonary embolus (PE). Although it is difficult clinically to differentiate diffusion defects from shunt effect, abnormalities occur in patients who have thickening of the alveolar-capillary membrane. Examples of diseases with thickened membranes include Goodpasture syndrome, systemic lupus erythematosus, sarcoidosis, diffuse interstitial fibrosis, and alveolar cell carcinoma.[3]

Ineffective gas exchange is also seen in patients with pulmonary shunt (see Figure 21-18, *C*). A shunt effect results from blood passing from the right side to the left side of the heart without passing through ventilated areas of the lung. Anatomic shunts may occur in patients with ventricular septal defects, atrial septal defects, and patent ductus arteriosus. Localized pneumonia and ARDS result in intrapulmonary shunts because of $\dot{V}A/\dot{Q}$ mismatch, in which alveoli are perfused but not ventilated.

Partial pressures of arterial O_2 in the newborn (60 to 70 mm Hg) and elderly (70 to 80 mm Hg) are less than those in the adult. The lower O_2 pressure is well tolerated in the newborn because of the presence of fetal hemoglobin, which has a decreased binding of 2,3-DPG, thus facilitating oxygen transfer by shifting the oxygen dissociation curve to the left.

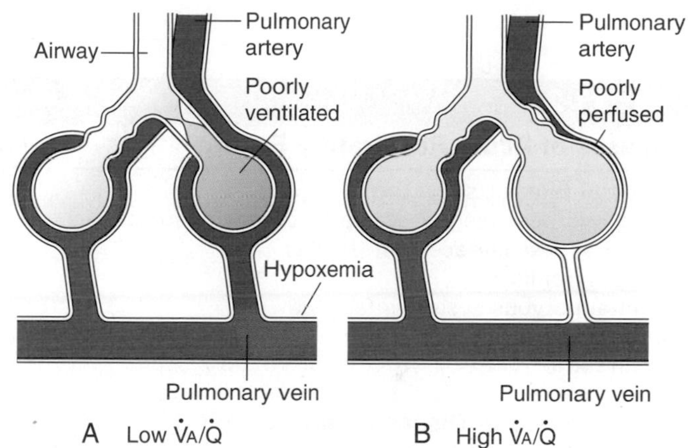

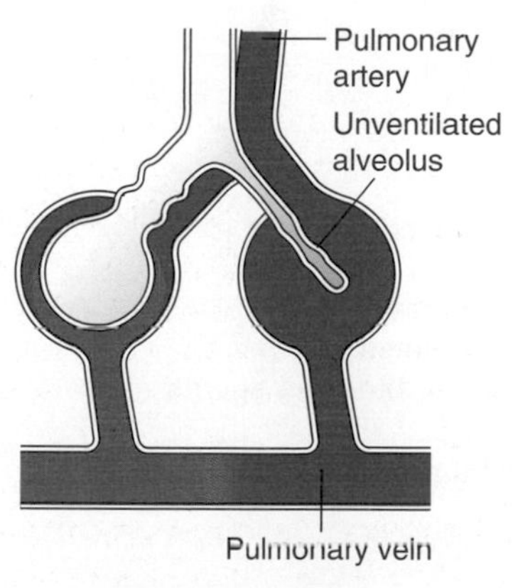

FIGURE 21-18 ■ Ventilation-perfusion abnormalities. **A,** Low $\dot{V}A/\dot{Q}$ areas that are well perfused but underventilated. **B,** High $\dot{V}A/\dot{Q}$ areas that are well ventilated but underperfused. **C,** Shunt areas that have no ventilation but are perfused (blood flow passes unventilated alveoli).

The newborn also has a higher hemoglobin concentration (20 to 21 g/dl) for the first few weeks after birth. Therefore, oxygenation is not normally a problem. The lower Pao_2 of the newborn is also associated with an increased $Paco_2$. Other blood gas values (see Table 21-1) show little difference from those of adults unless an oxygenation problem is present, such as infant respiratory distress syndrome or congenital heart disease.

Acute Respiratory Failure

Acute respiratory failure is defined as a state of disturbed gas exchange resulting in abnormal arterial blood gas values, a Pao_2 value less than 60 mm Hg (hypoxemia), and a $Paco_2$ value greater than 50 mm Hg (hypercapnia) with a pH less than 7.30 when the patient is breathing room air.[1,14] Patients with respiratory failure can be divided into three categories: (1) those with failure of respiration or oxygenation leading to hypoxemia and normal or low carbon dioxide levels; (2) those with failure of ventilation leading to hypercapnia; and (3) those with a combination of respiratory and ventilatory failure.

Etiology. The precise pathophysiologic mechanism of ARF depends on the cause or causes of the disease process. A number of conditions may cause respiratory failure (Box 21-2), including disorders of the neuromuscular chest apparatus (e.g., poliomyelitis, Guillain-Barré syndrome, quadriplegia, hemiplegia), disorders affecting the chest skeletal system (e.g., kyphoscoliosis), and chest trauma (e.g., rib and sternal fractures). Shock (septic, hypovolemic, etc.), PE, and pulmonary edema may also lead to respiratory failure. Extreme obesity may lead to alveolar hypoventilation, resulting in respiratory failure. The most common primary lung diseases causing ARF are advanced emphysema, pneumonia, asthma, and ARDS.

In general, the development of hypoxemia is related to poor matching of ventilation and perfusion. The development of hypercapnia is related to inadequate alveolar ventilation in relation to production of carbon dioxide.

Clinical Manifestations. Clinical features of ARF vary with the cause. General features include hypoxia and hypercapnia, which lead to headache, dyspnea, confusion, decreased level of consciousness, restlessness, agitation, dizziness, tremors, and initial hypertension followed by hypotension and

Box 21-2

Causes of Acute Respiratory Failure

Central Nervous System
Drug overdose (sedative, hypnotic, opioid, anesthetic)
Cerebral vascular accident (stroke)
Hypothyroidism
Central nervous system infections
Brain trauma
Brain tumor

Neuromuscular Diseases and Related Disorders
Guillain-Barré syndrome
Myasthenia gravis
Multiple sclerosis
Muscular dystrophy
Myxedema
Poliomyelitis
Polymyositis
Drug or toxin induced
- Botulism
- Aminoglycosides
- Organophosphates
- Neuromuscular blocking agents

Tetanus
Amyotrophic lateral sclerosis
Quadriplegia
Hemiplegia

Chest Wall and Diaphragm
Trauma (thoracic/abdominal)
Kyphoscoliosis
Upper abdominal or thoracic surgery
Pleural effusion
Hemo-/pneumo-/chylothorax
Massive ascites

Airways
Laryngospasm
Foreign body aspiration
Asthma
Acute exacerbation of chronic bronchitis or emphysema

Pulmonary Parenchyma Diseases
Lung contusion
Aspiration
Pneumonia
Interstitial lung diseases
Emphysema
Pulmonary fibrosis
Acute respiratory distress syndrome
Infant respiratory distress syndrome

Pulmonary Parenchyma Diseases
Pulmonary emboli (blood, fat, air, amniotic fluid)
Cardiac and noncardiac pulmonary edema
Shock
Increased CO_2 production
- Fever
- Infection
- Hyperthyroidism
- Drugs

tachycardia.[14] Early signs include rapid, shallow breathing with increased inspiratory muscle movement. Late findings include cyanosis, nasal flaring, and sternal and intercostal retractions.[1,5,7,13] The increased work of breathing may lead to cool, clammy skin, dysrhythmias, and decreased capillary refill. However, when consciousness is depressed, the latter signs may not be evident. The patient is then nearing respiratory arrest.

Diagnosis. Diagnostic tests include measurement of arterial blood gases and chest radiography. A PaO_2 of less than 60 mm Hg and a $PaCO_2$ of greater than 45 to 55 mm Hg on room air are common findings.[13] Chest radiographic findings depend on the disease process. Other supporting tests include an electrolyte panel with evidence of electrolyte imbalance and a complete blood cell count with evidence of infection or anemia.

Treatment. Maintaining ventilatory support by maintaining airway patency and ensuring adequate alveolar ventilation is the primary goal of therapy. Mechanical ventilation may be the initial treatment, followed by management of the underlying cause. If a neuromuscular problem or skeletal weakness is present, assisted ventilation with a positive-pressure volume ventilator is indicated to maintain airway patency and ensure adequate alveolar ventilation.

The primary goal of therapy is to provide adequate oxygenation at the cellular level by maintaining a PaO_2 greater than 60 mm Hg (oxygen saturation, 90%). If acute respiratory failure is caused by chronic obstructive pulmonary disease, then vigorous management of bronchospasm, infection, and heart failure is required using a combination of methylxanthines, β_2 agonists, corticosteroids (controversial), and antibiotics. Diuretics may be given for volume reduction depending on the fluid volume status of the patient. Hypotension should be managed promptly with volume replacement and/or vasopressors. The use of corticosteroids in high doses (e.g., methylprednisolone, 25 to 30 mg/kg of body weight) for the first 24 to 48 hours of the disease process is controversial because no conclusive evidence of efficacy is available.[13,14]

General supportive care consists of providing adequate nutrition to maintain fluid and electrolyte balance, providing pain management and emotional support, and preventing complications of gastrointestinal stress and bed rest. Developing a method of communication with ventilated patients is also very important. High-calorie, high-protein, low-carbohydrate nutritional support is recommended. A diet high in carbohydrates should be avoided because of its tendency to increase carbon dioxide production.[14] See Chapter 23 for specific treatments for ARDS and infant respiratory distress syndrome.

KEY CONCEPTS

- Ventilatory failure occurs when alveolar ventilation is insufficient to accomplish adequate gas exchange. Ventilatory failure may result from decreased respiratory rate, decreased tidal volume, or increased dead space. Arterial blood gas analyses demonstrate hypercarbia and hypoxemia.
- A general deficiency of O_2 in the blood (hypoxemia) results from poor diffusion at the alveoli (hypoxic hypoxia) or anemia (anemic hypoxia). Tissue hypoxia may be due to general hypoxemia or poor perfusion (circulatory hypoxia) or poor uptake of O_2 by the tissue (histotoxic hypoxia).
- Oxygenation failure occurs when diffusion of gases across the alveolar-capillary interface is impaired. Oxygenation failure may be due to $\dot{V}A/\dot{Q}$ mismatching, right-to-left shunt, or excessive barriers to diffusion. Arterial blood gas values demonstrate hypoxemia but not necessarily hypercarbia.
- Acute respiratory failure is generally diagnosed from arterial blood gas disturbances. The usual defining values are a PaO_2 less than 60 mm Hg and a $PaCO_2$ greater than 50 mm Hg when the subject is breathing room air.
- Conditions that predispose an individual to hypoventilation, ventilation-perfusion mismatch, or right-to-left shunt may lead to respiratory failure (e.g., drugs, neuromuscular weakness, chest wall deformities or trauma, and parenchymal lung diseases).
- Manifestations of respiratory failure are due to tissue hypoxia and compensatory responses and include confusion, tremors, hypotension, depressed consciousness, tachypnea, and tachycardia.
- The goal of therapy is to reduce tissue hypoxia by maintaining PaO_2 above 60 mm Hg. Depending on the underlying disease process, this may require mechanical ventilation, supplemental oxygen, nutritional supplementation, bronchodilators, and antibiotics.

ALTERATIONS IN PULMONARY VASCULATURE

Pulmonary Hypertension

Etiology. Normally the pulmonary circulation is a high-flow, low-pressure system with pressure of 25/8 mm Hg. Pulmonary hypertension is defined as a sustained increase in pulmonary arterial pressure above 30 mm Hg systolic. In some cases of pulmonary hypertension, systolic pressures may be as high as 60 to 110 mm Hg. Two broad types of pulmonary hypertension exist: primary (idiopathic) and secondary. Primary pulmonary hypertension (PPH) is rapidly progressive and is more common in women than men (1.7:1 ratio). PPH usually presents in the third to fourth decade of life.[16] The cause is unknown but can be associated with portal hypertension and cirrhosis, appetite-suppressant drugs, and human immunodeficiency virus infection. It may be familial.[14] The long-term prognosis is poor, and medical management is usually ineffective.

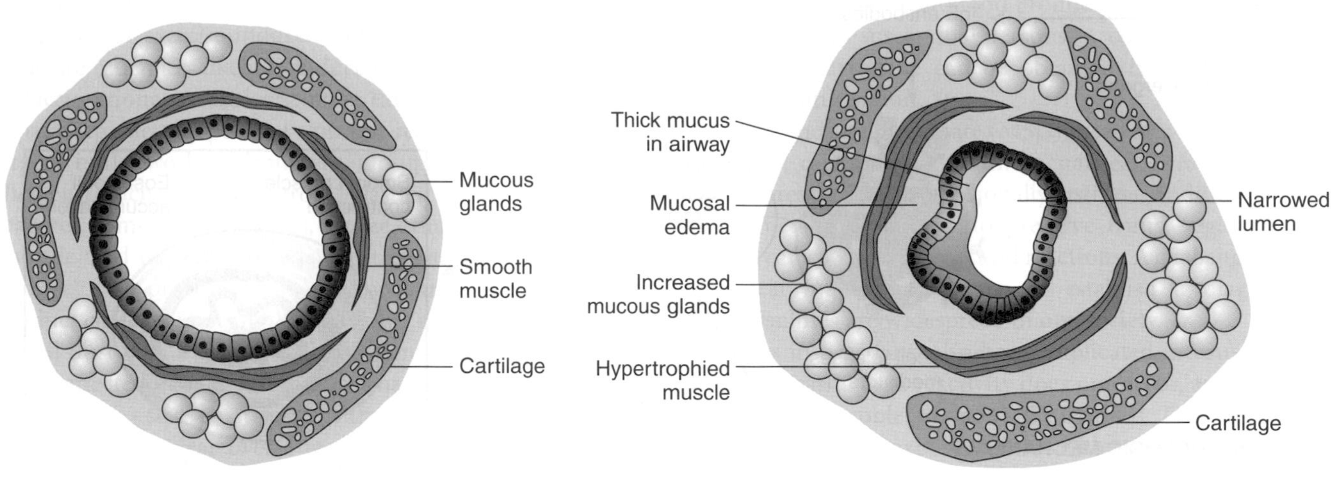

FIGURE 22-2 ■ Common bronchial wall remodeling changes in asthma are hypertrophied smooth muscle, edema, mucous gland hypertrophy, and mucus in the lumen.

that are released by the mast cell and the physiologic effect of these chemicals. With the release of chemical mediators, the normal respiratory epithelium is denuded and replaced by goblet cells, resulting in mucosal edema, inflammatory exudates, and hyperresponsiveness of the airway (bronchoconstriction and leakage).[2,11,12] Alterations in epithelial integrity lead to increased microvascular permeability. A secondary mediator response occurs 6 to 12 hours after the primary asthma attack and is more refractory to treatment. Neutrophil chemotactic factor may be the cause of this secondary response.[9] Histologic changes in the epithelial basement membrane occur over time. The basement membrane is a complex structure that separates endothelial cells from underlying stroma. The membrane provides tensile strength and physical support to surrounding structures.[7] It also functions as a filter and as a site for cell attachment. In a classic study by Hogg in 1982, the width of the basement membrane was shown to thicken in asthmatics over time.[11] The width seen in asthmatics is 17.5 μm, whereas that seen in healthy subjects is 7 μm. Airway remodeling has been detected pathologically. Patients show declines in pulmonary function over time that can progress to chronic obstructive pulmonary disease (COPD).[9] Figure 22-1 depicts the pathogenesis of asthma in relation to mast cell release and parasympathetic stimulation by way of the vagus nerve. Vagal stimulation leads to edema, mucus hypersecretion, and bronchoconstriction. The nerve endings of asthmatic patients have been found to be devoid of the bronchodilator neuropeptide vasoactive intestinal peptide.[9]

Clinical Manifestations. Common symptoms are wheezing, feelings of tightness of the chest, dyspnea, cough, and increased sputum production.[9] Some patients may have only a chronic dry cough and others have a productive cough.[8] Wheezing is caused by vibration in narrowed airways, which act like the vibrating reed of a wind instrument, yielding a musical sound.[13] Sputum is often thick, tenacious, scant, and viscid (sticky). Physical findings vary with the severity of the attack. A mild attack may be associated with a random monophonic expiratory wheezing associated with airway narrowing, tachycardia, and tachypnea. Random monophonic wheezes are located throughout the chest and come and go on examination. The area in which they are heard best is indicative of the area of obstruction (e.g., if they are heard best at the mouth, this is indicative of large airway obstruction).[13,14] Tachycardia is an early sign of hypoxemia. A more severe attack requiring medical assistance may be accompanied by the use of accessory muscles of respiration, intercostal retractions, distant breath sounds with inspiratory wheezing, orthopnea, agitation, tachypnea, and tachycardia. In the severe state, the patient may appear cyanotic, agitated, restless, and confused. The intensity of wheezing is *not* a reliable indicator of blockage of airflow. The measurement of peak expiratory flow rate (PEFR) is the best indicator of reduction in airflow (see discussion under Diagnosis). A PEFR of less than 80 L/min indicates severe obstruction.[8,15] When obstruction is the tightest, the patient cannot move enough air with enough velocity to make wheezing sounds. Isolated inspiratory wheezing may be an indicator of upper airway obstruction caused by mucus or laryngeal obstruction.[3] A patient with severe respiratory distress, prolonged expiration (indicating that the person is having difficulty moving air out of the lungs), neck and intercostal retractions, and minimal air sounds is critically ill and requires emergency intervention.

Diagnosis. The diagnosis of asthma is based on physical findings, sputum examination, pulmonary function tests, blood gas analysis, and chest radiography. Radiographic findings may be normal or may show evidence of hyperinflation with flattening of the diaphragm in progressive disease.[7] Ab-

Table 22-1

Classification of Asthma Severity

Clinical Features Before Treatment*	Symptoms†	Nighttime Symptoms	Lung Function
Step 4 Severe, persistent	Continual symptoms Limited physical activity Frequent exacerbations	Frequent	FEV_1 or PEFR ≤60% predicted PEFR variability >30%
Step 3 Moderate, persistent	Daily symptoms Daily use of inhaled short-acting β_2 agonist Exacerbation affects activity Exacerbations ≥2 times a week; may last days	>1 time a week	FEV_1 or PEFR >60% <80% predicted PEFR variability >30%
Step 2 Mild, persistent	Symptoms >2 times a week but <1 time a day Exacerbations may affect activity	>2 times a month	FEV_1 or PEFR ≥80% predicted PEFR variability 20%-30%
Step 1 Mild, intermittent	Symptoms ≤2 times a week Asymptomatic and normal PEFR between exacerbations Exacerbations brief (from a few hours to a few days); intensity may vary	≤2 times a month	FEV_1 or PEFR ≥80% predicted PEFR variability <20%

Modified from National Asthma Education and Prevention Program, National Heart, Lung, and Blood Institute, Expert Panel Report 2: Guidelines for the diagnosis and management of asthma, Washington, DC, NIH Pub No. 97-4051, July 1997.
FEV, Forced expiratory volume; *PEFR,* peak expiratory flow rate.
*The presence of one of the features of severity is sufficient to place a patient in that category. An individual should be assigned to the most severe grade in which any feature occurs. The characteristics noted in this figure are general and may overlap because asthma is highly variable. Furthermore, an individual's classification may change over time.
†Patients at any level of severity can have mild, moderate, or severe exacerbations. Some patients with intermittent asthma experience severe and life-threatening exacerbations separated by long periods of normal lung function and no symptoms.

normal physical findings include cough, wheezing, a hyperinflated chest, and decreased breath sounds. Asthmatic sputum samples reveal Charcot-Leyden crystals (formed from crystallized enzymes from eosinophilic membranes), eosinophils, and Curschmann spirals (mucous casts of bronchioles).

Forced expiratory volumes decrease during asthma attacks. PEFR is measured to determine the index of airway function. The PEFR is the maximal flow of expired air attained during a forced vital capacity (FVC) procedure.[14] The evaluation of asthma should include the measurement of forced expiratory volume over 1 second (FEV_1), FVC, and the ratio FEV_1/FVC before and after administration of a short-acting bronchodilator.[8] Airflow obstruction is indicated by a FEV_1/FVC ratio of less than 75%.[8] Classification of asthma severity (Table 22-1) is based on presenting symptoms, frequency of nighttime symptoms, and lung function.[2] Table 22-2 shows classifications of severity of acute asthma exacerbations.

Arterial blood gas values may be normal during a mild attack, but as the bronchospasm increases in intensity, respiratory alkalosis and hypoxemia become prominent findings. Elevation of arterial partial pressure of carbon dioxide (Pa_{CO_2}) is a poor prognostic sign, indicating that the patient's ability to continue breathing at a rapid rate has diminished and that exhaustion is imminent.

Respiratory failure may be evidenced by severe respiratory distress in a patient who shows no radiographic evidence of pneumothorax. As the patient improves, the wheezing becomes louder. When wheezing is no longer heard after an asthma attack, pulmonary function tests may continue to show obstructive changes for several weeks. Some patients have a slight monophonic wheeze continuously between asthma bouts and still are comfortable and functional.[13]

Determination of allergens is done by skin testing or inhalation of suspected allergens. Skin testing is usually more helpful in young patients who have extrinsic asthma. Bronchial provocation testing with histamine or methacholine[8] may be useful in confirming the diagnosis of asthma in certain cases (see Diagnostic Testing at end of chapter).

Table 22-2

Classification of Severity of Acute Asthma Exacerbations

	Mild	Moderate	Severe	Respiratory Arrest Imminent
Symptoms				
Breathlessness	While walking	While talking (infant: softer, shorter cry; difficulty feeding)	While at rest (infant: stops feeding)	
	Can lie down	Prefers sitting	Sits upright	
Talks in	Sentences	Phrases	Words	
Alertness	May be agitated	Usually agitated	Usually agitated	Drowsy or confused
Signs				
Respiratory rate	Increased	Increased	Often >30/min	
		Guide on rates of breathing in awake children:		
		Age	**Normal Rate**	
		<2 mo	<60/min	
		2-12 mo	<50/min	
		1-5 yr	<40/min	
		6-8 yr	<30/min	
Use of accessory muscles; suprasternal retractions	Usually not	Commonly	Usually	Paradoxical thoraco-abdominal movement
Wheeze	Moderate, often only end expiratory	Loud; throughout exhalation	Usually loud; throughout inhalation and exhalation	Absence of wheeze
Pulse/min	<100	100-120	>120	Bradycardia
		Guide to normal pulse rates in children:		
		Age	**Normal Rate**	
		2-12 mo	<160/min	
		1-2 yr	<120/min	
		2-8 yr	<110/min	
Pulsus paradoxus	Absent <10 mm Hg	May be present 10-25 mm Hg	Often present >25 mm Hg (adult) 20-40 mm Hg (child)	Absence suggests respiratory muscle fatigue
Functional Assessment				
PEF (% predicted or % personal best)	80%	~50%-80%	<50% predicted or personal best or response lasts <2 h	
Pa_{O_2} (on air)	Normal (test not usually necessary)	>60 mm Hg (test not usually necessary)	<60 mm Hg: possible cyanosis	
and/or				
P_{CO_2}	<42 mm Hg (test not usually necessary)	<42 mm Hg (test not usually necessary)	≥42 mm Hg: possible respiratory failure	
Sa_{O_2} % (on air) at sea level	>95% (test not usually necessary)	91%-95%	<91%	
	Hypercapnia (hypoventilation) develops more readily in young children than in adults and adolescents.			

From National Asthma Education and Prevention Program, National Heart, Lung, and Blood Institute, Expert Panel Report 2: *Guidelines for the diagnosis and management of asthma,* NIH Pub No. 97, July 1997.

Note: The presence of several parameters, but not necessarily all, indicates the general classification of the exacerbation. Many of these parameters have not been systematically studied, so they serve only as general guides.

A complete blood cell count can show an elevated number of white blood cells (WBCs) with increased eosinophils. Eosinophils are prominent in the cellular infiltrate of the bronchioles, the sputum, and the peripheral blood. A fall in the total eosinophil count is a valuable measure of effectiveness of corticosteroid treatment. With effective treatment, the total eosinophil count is depressed below 10/μl.[1,8]

Treatment. Patients should be taught to avoid those things in the environment that trigger asthma attacks. Environmental control includes dust control; removal of allergens such as feathers, molds, and animal danders; and, in some cases, removal of rugs and carpets. Other environmental control factors that help some patients with extrinsic asthma include the use of air purifiers and air conditioners. The patient should also be taught preventive therapy in regard to smoking cessation, avoidance of passive smoke, and avoidance of aerosols and odors. Patients should seek early treatment for respiratory infections.[16]

Pharmacologic therapy for all three major obstructive disorders is similar. Refer to Table 22-5 for a list of common respiratory drugs used in the management of various types of obstructive disorders. The stepwise care approach to managing asthma was developed by the National Asthma Education and Prevention Program (Table 22-3).

Figure 22-3 shows the site of action of drugs used in the management of asthma. For the ambulatory patient with infrequent attacks, inhaled short-acting bronchodilators such as albuterol, metaproterenol, and others may provide adequate control[2,8,9,16] For persons with exercise-induced asthma or children with extrinsic asthma, cromolyn sodium or nedocromil sodium (mast cell stabilizers) and inhaled short-acting bronchodilators prior to exercise are helpful. Cromolyn sodium or nedocromil sodium may be equally effective in intrinsic asthma when used continuously on a prophylactic basis. Patients with more frequent attacks require maintenance bronchodilators and inhaled corticosteroids.[2,8,9,16] Theophylline, previously used as first-line therapy for the management of asthma, has fallen into disfavor because of its numerous side effects and the availability of inhaled sympathomimetic and corticosteroid agents. In addition, many clinicians favor inhaled corticosteroids as first-line therapy.[8,9,16]

β_2-Adrenergic bronchodilator drugs, such as metaproterenol (Alupent), albuterol (Ventolin, Proventil), and terbutaline (Brethine), are effective in promoting bronchodilation. Proper administration of inhaled agents is essential for optimal therapy. The recommended method for using metered-dose nebulizers is described in Box 22-1.

Inhaled corticosteroid therapy, using beclomethasone (Vanceril, Beclovent), flunisolide (AeroBid), fluticasone (Flovent), budesonide (Pulmicort), or triamcinolone (Azmacort), is effective in most patients, and these agents are available in low, medium, and high doses. Because suppression of airway inflammation is a key component of asthma treatment, these drugs are effective. Inhaled steroids do not have the major side effects of oral steroids but are effective in decreasing the bronchial inflammatory response seen in asthmatics. Oral candidiasis can be a side effect of aerosol steroid therapy; it can be avoided by rinsing the mouth after each use. Inhaled sympathomimetics may be given 15 to 20 minutes prior to inhalation of corticosteroids to enhance delivery of the medication in the airways.[8,9,16] Inhaled corticosteroids are useful as prophylaxis but are not effective during an acute asthma episode.

Corticosteroids are used for their antiinflammatory and immunosuppressant action. Oral doses are useful for short-term use. Long-term use should be avoided if possible because of the side effects of adrenal suppression and multiple adverse effects. If long-term use is necessary, an alternate-day morning dosing schedule is effective in minimizing side effects. When oral steroid therapy must be discontinued, it is important to taper the dosage over a 7- to 10-day period. Methotrexate has been tried in patients with refractory asthma who are corticosteroid dependent. Results have not been consistently positive.[8,9] Other therapies used in more severe asthmatics include home oxygen therapy and home administration of small-volume nebulizer treatments via intermittent positive-pressure ventilation.

At home, peak flow monitoring is helpful to parents or patients in determining a treatment plan and when to seek medical assistance. Peak flow meters are also helpful in monitoring progress of the patient with around-the-clock therapy.[9]

Allergen-specific immunotherapy (hyposensitization) may be used as an adjunct to other therapies. The allergen is first identified by testing with purified allergens using the scratch, prick, or intradermal method. A positive reaction is shown by a flare or wheal occurring at the site in 15 to 20 minutes. Desensitization therapy has been shown in controlled study to reduce the frequency and severity of asthmatic episodes when a single offending allergen can be identified.[9]

Status asthmaticus (severe attack unresponsive to routine therapy) requires more rapid and intense therapy, which includes epinephrine (in young patients), subcutaneous terbutaline, and/or aminophylline. Once airflow has improved, aerosol bronchodilating inhalers may be used. Intravenous corticosteroids are the mainstay of therapy. Oxygen therapy with or without mechanical ventilation may be necessary in severe cases.

Epinephrine has been the standard emergency therapy for many years. However, many emergency rooms are now initiating therapy with nebulized β-adrenergic in combination with ipratropium bromide (Atrovent) because aerosolized drugs are associated with fewer side effects, a longer duration of action, and fewer recurrences of asthma than with epinephrine treatment. Aerosolized treatments are less traumatic to children than injections. Nebulized β-adrenergic drugs have a wide margin of safety, and dosages can be individualized to the patient.

The more patients understand about their asthma, the better they are at self-managing their symptoms. Educational

Table 22-3

Stepwise Approach for Managing Asthma in Children

Step	Long-Term Control	Quick Relief	Education
1: Mild intermittent	No daily medication needed	Short-acting bronchodilator: **inhaled β_2 agonist*** or oral β_2 agonist as needed for symptoms. Use of short-acting inhaled β_2 agonist more than twice a week may indicate the need to initiate long-term control therapy. With viral respiratory infection: bronchodilator every 4-6 hr up to 24 hr (longer with physician consult) but, in general, repeat no more than once every 6 weeks. Consider systemic corticosteroid if current exacerbation is severe or patient has a history of previous severe exacerbations.	Teach basic facts about asthma. Teach inhaler and spacer technique. Develop self-management plan. Develop an action plan for when and how to take rescue actions. Discuss appropriate environmental control measures to avoid exposure to known allergens and irritants.
2: Mild persistent	*Daily medication:* **Antiinflammatory**: either **inhaled corticosteroid** (low-dose) or **cromolyn** or **nedocromil** (infants and young children usually begin with a trial of cromolyn or nedocromil). Sustained-release theophylline (serum concentration of 5-15 μg/ml) is an alternative, but not preferred therapy. Zafirlukast or zileuton may also be considered for patients age 12 or older, though their position in therapy is not fully established.	Short-acting bronchodilator: **inhaled β_2 agonist** as needed for symptoms. Use of short-acting inhaled β_2 agonist on a daily basis or increasing use indicates the need for additional long-term control therapy.	Step 1 actions as above. Teach self-monitoring. Refer for group education if available. Review and update self-management plan.
3: Moderate persistent	*Daily medication:* **Antiinflammatory**: either **inhaled corticosteroid** (medium dose) or inhaled corticosteroid (low-medium dose) and add nedocromil or a long-acting bronchodilator, especially for nighttime symptoms: **long-acting inhaled β_2 agonist** (age 12 or older), sustained-release theophylline, or long-acting β_2 agonist tablets. *If needed:* **Antiinflammatory: inhaled corticosteroid** (medium-high dose) and long-acting **bronchodilator,** especially for nighttime symptoms; **long-acting inhaled β_2 agonist,** sustained-release theophylline, or long-acting β_2 agonist tablets.	Short-acting bronchodilator: **Inhaled β_2 agonist** as needed for symptoms. Use of short-acting inhaled β_2 agonist on a daily basis or increasing use indicates the need for additional long-term control therapy.	Step 1 and 2 actions as above.

Table 22-3

Stepwise Approach for Managing Asthma in Children—cont'd

Step	Long-Term Control	Quick Relief	Education
4: Severe persistent	*Daily medication:* **Antiinflammatory:** **Inhaled corticosteroid** (high-dose) and long-acting bronchodilator: **long-acting inhaled β_2 agonist,** sustained-release theophylline, or long-acting β_2 agonist tablets. *and* Corticosteroid tablets or syrup (2 mg/kg/day, generally not to exceed 60 mg/day) and reduce to lowest daily or alternate-day dose that stabilizes symptoms.	Short-acting bronchodilator: **Inhaled β_2 agonist** as needed for symptoms. Use of short-acting inhaled β_2 agonist on a daily basis or increasing use indicates the need for additional long-term control therapy.	Step 1 and 2 actions. Refer for individual education/counseling.
Step down Review therapy every 1-6 mo; a gradual stepwise reduction in treatment may be possible.		Step up If control is not maintained, consider stepping up. First, review patient's medication technique, compliance and environmental control (avoidance of allergens or other factors that contribute to asthma severity).	

Adapted from Expert Panel Report 2: Guidelines for the Diagnosis and Management of Asthma. NIH Publication No. 97-4051, 1997.
*Preferred treatment is indicated by bold type.

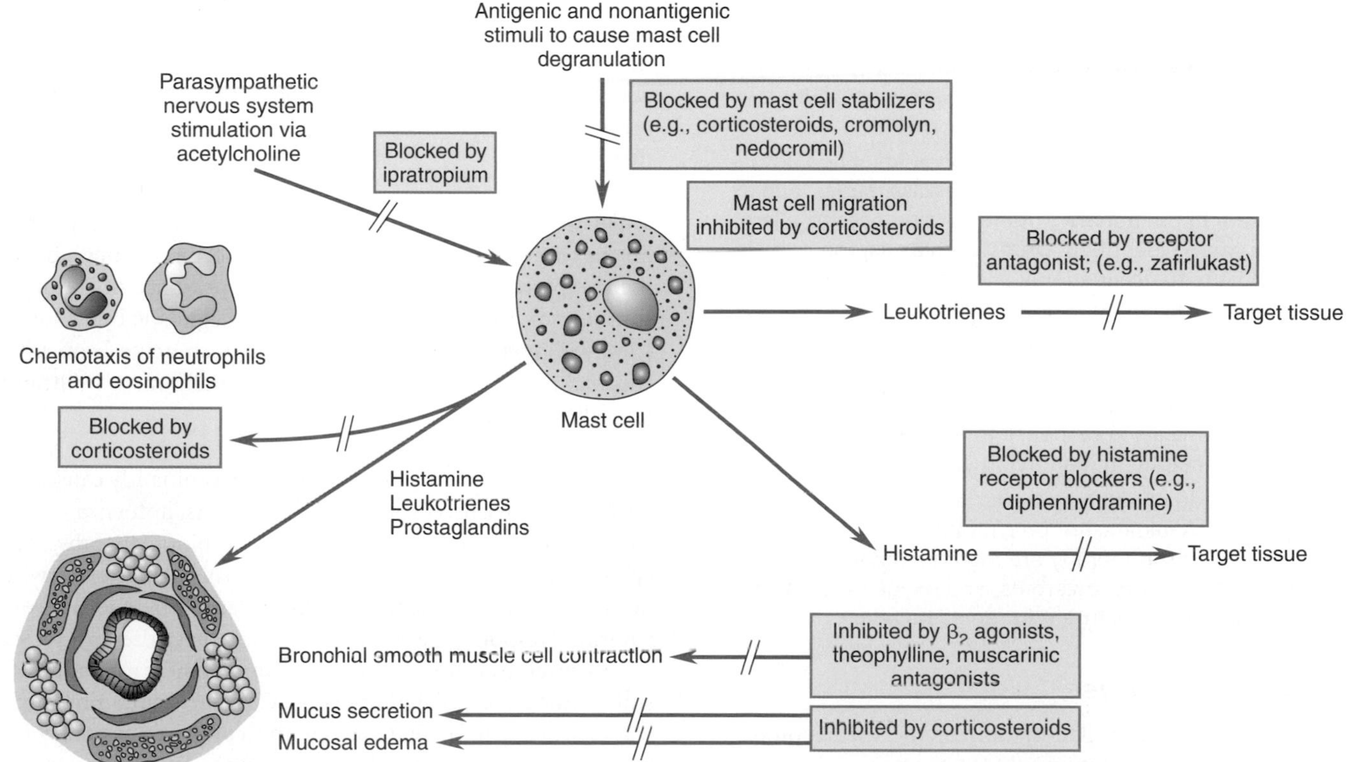

FIGURE 22-3 ■ Postulated trigger stimuli for bronchospasm and site of action of drugs used in management of asthma.

Box 22-1

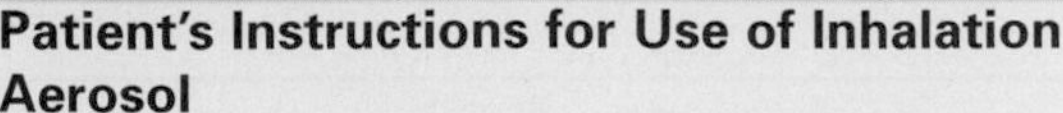

Patient's Instructions for Use of Inhalation Aerosol

1. **Shake the inhaler well** immediately before each use. Remove the cap from the mouthpiece. Inspect the mouthpiece for the presence of foreign objects before each use.
2. **Breathe out fully through the mouth.** Place the mouthpiece slightly away from the mouth, holding the inhaler in its upright position.
3. Take in a slow, deep breath while depressing the top of the canister.
4. **Hold your breath** for 10 seconds.
5. Wait 1 minute and repeat the procedure.
6. Rinse mouth with water and spit out.
7. **Clean the inhaler thoroughly and frequently.**

materials are available from the American Lung Association, the Asthma and Allergy Foundation of America, and the National Institute of Allergy and Infectious Diseases.

KEY CONCEPTS

- Asthma is characterized by acute, reversible episodes of airway obstruction. Bronchoconstriction, excessive mucus production, and swelling of the bronchial mucosa lead to the obstructive episode. Wheezing, dyspnea, hyperinflation, and cough are common features.
- An asthma episode may range in severity from mild to life threatening, depending on the degree of airway obstruction. With intense narrowing of the bronchi, severe hypoxemia may result.
- Several types of asthma have been identified. Intrinsic asthma is precipitated by exercise, stress, and exposure to pulmonary irritants, but no specific allergen can be identified. Drugs such as aspirin and exposure to occupational allergens have also been identified as etiologic agents.
- Extrinsic asthma is mediated by IgE, which is produced in response to specific antigens. The IgE binds to mast cells and causes them to release inflammatory chemicals in response to antigen. Skin testing may be helpful in identifying suspected allergens.
- Prevention of asthma attacks is an important part of therapy. Avoidance of precipitating factors and prophylactic drug therapy are recommended. Bronchodilators, corticosteroids, and oxygen therapy are mainstays of treatment for an acute attack.

Acute Bronchitis

Etiology. Acute inflammation of the tracheobronchial tree is produced most commonly (80% of cases) by a variety of viruses such as influenza virus A or B, parainfluenza virus, respiratory syncytial virus, coronavirus, rhinovirus, Coxsackie virus, and adenovirus. Nonviral causes include *Streptococcus pneumoniae, Haemophilus influenzae, Mycoplasma,* and *Chlamydia pneumoniae.* Numerous other pathogens, as well as heat, smoke inhalation, inhalation of irritant chemicals (e.g., sulfur dioxide or chlorine, bromine, or fluorine gases), and allergic reactions have also been identified.[17] Highest incidences are noted in smokers, young children, the elderly, and in winter.[7,18] The swelling of bronchial mucosa in children associated with obstruction, respiratory distress, and wheezing is known as *asthmatic bronchitis.* Acute bronchitis differs from bronchiolitis in the size of the airways affected (i.e., trachea and bronchi as opposed to the small bronchioli).[19]

Pathogenesis. The airways become inflamed and narrowed from capillary dilation, swelling from exudation of fluid, infiltration with inflammatory cells, increased mucus production, loss of ciliary function, and loss of portions of the ciliated epithelium. Many viruses and mycoplasmal bacteria inhibit macrophages and lymphocytes, temporarily promoting secondary bacterial invasion. Microorganisms may also induce long-lasting hyperirritability of the respiratory tract with associated episodes of bronchospasm.

Clinical Manifestations. The presentation of acute bronchitis is usually mild and self-limited, requiring only supportive treatment. Cough may be productive or nonproductive. Associated symptoms include low-grade fever, chest discomfort, sore throat, and fatigue. In children, the smaller airways are easily obstructed by inflammation, so that severe obstruction may occur. The smallness of airways in proportion to body size is due to a smaller lumen in relation to the vessel wall. Associated inflammation of the larynx and trachea produces croup (see section on croup in this chapter for further details).

Diagnosis. Diagnosis of acute bronchitis is usually based on the clinical presentation, with recent onset of cough being the distinctive hallmark. Neither the appearance of purulent sputum nor a WBC count is a reliable diagnostic indicator. A chest radiograph is required to distinguish acute bronchitis (normal radiograph) from pneumonia (pulmonary infiltrates on radiograph).

Treatment. Acute bronchitis is predominantly caused by viruses (rhinovirus, coronavirus, adenovirus, influenza virus). Viral infections do not respond to antibiotic therapy, and symptoms resolve spontaneously in most normal, otherwise healthy individuals. Acute bronchitis caused by bacterial organisms responds well to antimicrobial therapy (e.g., azithromycin, erythromycin, clarithromycin, trimethoprim-sulfamethoxazole, cephalosporins). Codeine-containing medications are helpful in relieving the cough associated with bronchitis. Nonpharmacologic recommendations are to increase fluid intake, avoid smoke, and use a vaporizer in the bedroom.[7,18]

The dangers of acute bronchitis include the potential for bacterial invasion, which can worsen symptoms in patients with COPD and precipitate serious infections in the aged or those with debilitating disease.

Chronic Bronchitis

Etiology. The next two sections of this chapter present chronic bronchitis and emphysema. Characteristic pathologic and clinical findings are described for each of these classifications. Clinically, pure forms of emphysema and bronchitis are rare, and most patients present a combination of several or all of these obstructive processes. Patients with emphysema and chronic bronchitis make up most cases of COPD.

The major causes of chronic bronchitis are cigarette smoking (90% cases),[20] repeated airway infections, genetic predisposition, and inhalation of physical or chemical irritants.[7,8,20,21]

Chronic bronchitis (also referred to as type B COPD or the "blue bloater"[7,8,20]) is defined *symptomatically* by hypersecretion of bronchial mucus and a chronic or recurrent productive cough of more than 3 months duration and occurring each year for two successive years in patients in whom other causes have been excluded.[8] For patients with chronic bronchitis and emphysema, airway obstruction is persistent and irreversible. The National Center for Health Statistics reports a 3:1 ratio of annual cases of chronic bronchitis to emphysema.[22]

Pathogenesis. Pathologic changes in the airway include chronic inflammation and swelling of the bronchial mucosa resulting in scarring, increased fibrosis of the mucous membrane, increased numbers (hyperplasia) of bronchial mucous glands and goblet cells, hypertrophy of bronchial glands and goblet cells, and increased bronchial wall thickness, which potentiates obstruction to airflow. Inflammation appears to predominantly be the result of neutrophil activity.[20] Interleukin-8 levels are elevated indicating sustained attraction of neutrophils to the site of inflammation. CD8 T-lymphocyte levels are also elevated. During acute exacerbations, bronchial biopsy specimens have a 30-fold increase in eosinophils.[20] Figures 22-4 and 22-5 show the histologic changes seen in chronic bronchitis. Hypertrophy of mucosal glands and goblet cells leads to increased mucus production; the mucus then combines with purulent exudate to form bronchial plugs. Chronic bronchitis patients often display bacterial colonization with *H. influenzae* and *S. pneumoniae.*[20] The mucociliary clearance action is impaired or lost, and some areas of ciliated epithelium are replaced by squamous cells (metaplasia).[20] Ciliary dysfunction occurs due to a decrease in numbers of cilia and decreased action of available cilia.

Often the inflammatory and fibrotic changes extend into the surrounding alveoli. The narrowed airways and the mucous plugs prevent proper oxygenation and potentiate airway obstruction. High airflow resistance increases the work of breathing, leading to increased oxygen demands. In areas of greater obstruction to airflow, alveoli empty and fill more slowly, leading to ventilation-perfusion ($\dot{V}A/\dot{Q}$) mismatch, thus lowering arterial oxygenation. The chronic bronchitis patient may appear as the blue bloater (Figure 22-6), reflecting the pathophysiologic process of oxygen desaturation (cyanosis) and edema associated with right-sided heart failure; hence, patients appear "blue and bloated."

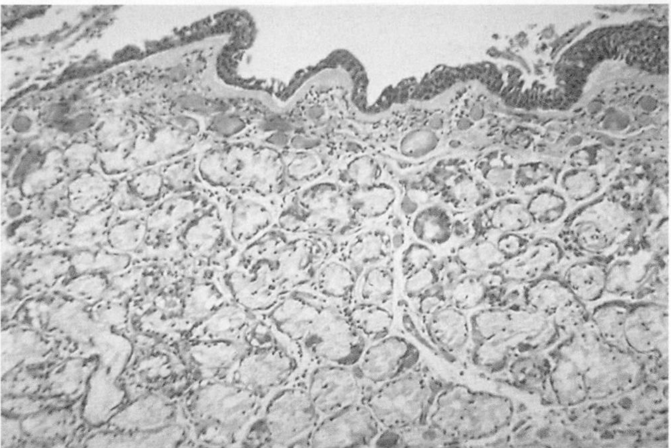

FIGURE 22-4 ■ Histologic features of chronic bronchitis. (Lumen of bronchus is above.) Note slight desquamation of mucosal epithelial cells and marked thickening (approximately twice normal thickness) of mucous gland layer. Vascular congestion is evident. (From Cotran RS, Kumar V, Robbins SL: *Robbins pathologic basis of disease,* ed 7, Philadelphia, 2003, Saunders, p 464.)

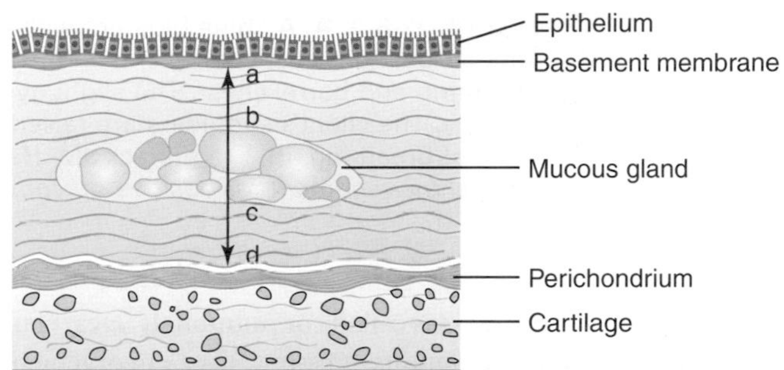

FIGURE 22-5 ■ Structure of a normal bronchial wall. In chronic bronchitis the thickness of the mucous glands increases and can be expressed as the Reid index, given by the following formula: *(b − c)/(a − d).* The ratio is normally less than 0.4. A ratio of 0.7 indicates severe bronchitis.

Involvement of small pulmonary arteries related to inflammation in the bronchial walls and the compensatory spasm of pulmonary blood vessels from hypoxia produce pulmonary hypertension. In addition, widespread bronchial narrowing and mucous plugging produce ventilation perfusion mismatch with hypoxemia and hypercarbia from impeded ventilation. The combination of hypoxia and hypercarbia increases pulmonary artery resistance and pulmonary hypertension.[20] As the process of pulmonary hypertension continues, right ventricular end-diastolic pressures increase, leading to right ventricular dilation and right-sided heart failure. Heart failure

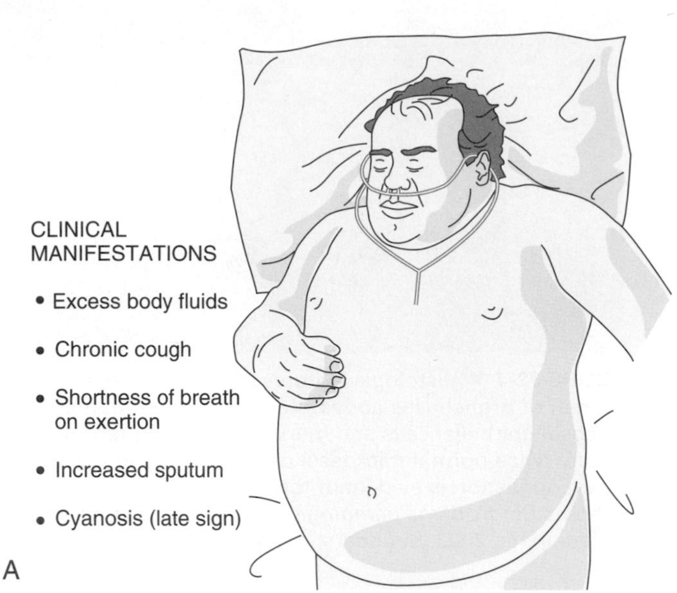

CLINICAL
MANIFESTATIONS
• Excess body fluids
• Chronic cough
• Shortness of breath on exertion
• Increased sputum
• Cyanosis (late sign)
A

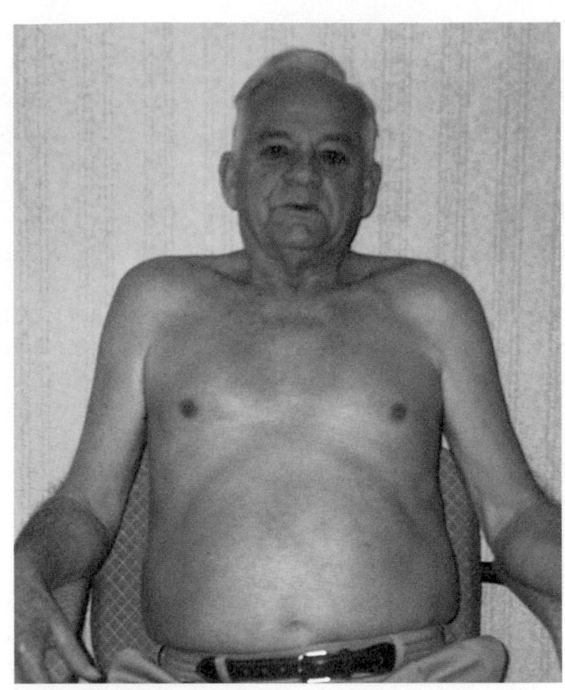

FIGURE 22-6 ■ **A,** A "blue bloater" with edema from right-sided heart failure. **B,** A client with chronic obstructive bronchitis. Note the stocky build and the presence of pursed-lip breathing and barrel chest. The slight gynecomastia is a side effect of corticosteroid therapy. The client's shoulders are raised because of shortness of breath and increased work of breathing. (**B,** From Black JM, Hawks JH, Keene AM: *Medical-surgical nursing: clinical management for positive outcomes,* ed 7, Philadelphia, 2005, Saunders, p 1819.)

resulting from lung disease is called **cor pulmonale.** Heart failure results in increased venous pressure, liver engorgement, and dependent edema. Manifestations of heart failure may occur during exacerbations of bronchitis and subside with appropriate treatment.[8,20]

Destruction of bronchial walls results in dilation of airway sacs. This is termed *bronchiectasis.* Causes of bronchial wall destruction include severe streptococcal or staphylococcal pneumonia, repeated bouts of bronchitis, infection with the mold *Aspergillus fumigatus,* mucous plugs, foreign bodies, or immunologic deficiencies. (Refer to the bronchiectasis section later in this chapter for a more detailed description of this disease process.) The dilated sacs contain pools of infected secretion that do not clear themselves and serve as sources of further infection that can spread to adjacent lung fields or can spread by the lymphatics or venous drainage to other areas of the body, commonly the brain. If bronchiectatic lesions are localized, surgical resection of the affected portions of lung may be helpful. Narrowing of the airways and turbulent airflow from mucous obstruction produce wheezing resembling asthma.

Clinical Manifestations. The typical patient is an overweight man or woman (1:2 ratio) in his or her 30s-40s[8,20,21,23] or older with shortness of breath on exertion, excessive amounts of sputum, chronic cough, evidence of excess body fluids (edema, hypervolemia), and a history of smoking. In addition, the patient often complains of chills, malaise, muscle aches, fatigue, loss of libido, and insomnia.

Sputum production may be variable and worsens with respiratory infection. Cough and sputum production are most severe in the mornings. Gradually, patients develop progressive shortness of breath on exertion. Most patients do not seek help until dyspnea becomes troublesome. By the time dyspnea on exertion is present, the disease is well advanced.[20,21]

In the end-stage disease process, the patient presents with signs of cor pulmonale (distended neck veins, a right ventricular heave, a right ventricular gallop, and peripheral edema).[20] Hypoxia leads to pulmonary hypertension. Cyanosis is a late sign.

Diagnosis. Measures used to confirm the diagnosis include chest radiography, which may show increased bronchial vascular markings, congested lung fields, an enlarged horizontal cardiac silhouette, and evidence of previous pulmonary infection. Pulmonary function tests show normal total lung capacity (TLC), increased residual volume (RV), and decreased FEV_1. Early pulmonary function testing prior to the onset of symptoms shows increased closing volume and a decrease in the maximal midexpiratory flow rate.[20] Arterial blood gas evaluation may show elevated Pa_{CO_2} and decreased Pa_{O_2} (often below 65 mm Hg). The electrocardiogram may reveal

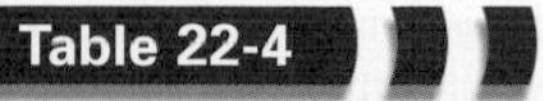

Common Distinguishing Features of Emphysema and Chronic Bronchitis*

Patient Data	Emphysema (Type A: Pink Puffer)	Bronchitis (Type B: Blue Bloater)
History		
Lifestyle	Smoker	Smoker
Weight	Weight loss	Overweight
Onset of symptoms	Usually after age 50 yr	Usually after age 40 yr
Sputum	Mild, mucoid	Excessive, purulent
Cough	Minimal or absent	Chronic; more severe in mornings
Dyspnea	Progressive exertional dyspnea	Mild to moderate, but may gradually progress to severe exertional dyspnea
Patient Complaints	Dyspnea on exertion, fatigue, insomnia	Chronic cough with mucopurulent sputum, chills, malaise, muscle aches, fatigue, insomnia, loss of libido
Physical Signs		
Edema	Absent	Present
Central cyanosis	Absent	Present in advanced disease
Use of accessory muscles to breathe	Present	Absent until end stage
Body build	Thin, wasted	Stocky, overweight
Anteroposterior chest diameter	"Barrel chest," 1:1 ratio anteroposterior chest diameter	Normal
Auscultation of chest	Decreased breath sounds, decreased heart sounds, prolonged expiration	Wheezes, crackles, rhonchi, depending on the severity of disease
Percussion	Hyperresonance	Normal
Jugular vein distention	Absent	Present
Other	Pursed-lip breathing	Evidence of right-sided heart failure (cor pulmonale)
General Diagnostic Tests		
Chest radiography	Narrowed mediastinum; normal or small vertical heart; hyperinflation; low, flat diaphragm; presence of blebs or bullae	Congested lung fields, increased bronchial vascular markings, enlarged horizontal heart
Arterial blood gas analysis	Decreased Pa_{O_2} (60-80 mm Hg); normal or increased Pa_{CO_2} (increases with advancing disease)	Decreased Pa_{O_2} (<65 mm Hg); increased Pa_{CO_2}
Electrocardiography	Normal or tall symmetrical P waves; tachycardia, if hypoxic	Right axis deviation, right ventricular hypertrophy, atrial arrhythmias
Hematocrit	Normal	Polycythemia
Pulmonary Function Tests		
Functional residual capacity	Increased	Normal or slight increase
Residual volume	Increased	Increased
Total lung capacity	Increased	Normal
Forced expiratory volume	Decreased	Decreased
Vital capacity	Decreased	Normal or slight decrease
Static lung compliance	Increased	Normal

*Clinically, features of bronchitis and emphysema are not always clear-cut because many patients have a combined disease process.[7,8,20,21]

atrial arrhythmias and evidence of right ventricular hypertrophy. Secondary polycythemia (increased numbers of red blood cells) related to continuous or nocturnal hypoxemia is common.[8,20] Nocturnal hypoxemia leads to a compensatory production of red blood cells in an attempt to carry more oxygen to the body tissues.

Depending on the severity of the disease, the physical examination may reveal scattered crackles, rhonchi, and wheezes; use of accessory muscles to breathe; jugular vein distention; and pedal and ankle edema. Table 22-4 lists the distinguishing features of both chronic bronchitis and emphysema.

Treatment. Because bronchitis and emphysema are most frequently seen in combination, the therapies covered in this section are for the combined disorder. The overall goals are to (1) block the progression of the disease, (2) return the patient to optimal respiratory function, and (3) return the patient to usual activities of daily living.

Pharmacologic treatment involves the use of inhaled short acting β agonists and inhaled anticholinergic bronchodilators (e.g., albuterol, metaproterenol, ipratropium bromide), cough suppressants (guaifenesin), and antiinfective agents for infections. Inhaled or oral corticosteroids may also be used in the treatment of some patients for acute exacerbations. Theophylline products are used less frequently due to their narrow therapeutic range and toxicity. However, many patients derive significant benefits from theophylline.[20,21]

Low-dose oxygen therapy is recommended for patients with PaO_2 levels less than 55 mm Hg.[20,21] Oxygen can be delivered through a nasal cannula (0.5 to 3 L/min) or Venturi mask (28% to 40%) at flow rates sufficient to keep the oxygen saturation above 90%. Mechanical ventilation may become necessary to get the patient over a crisis period of acute exacerbation.

Oxygen saturation can be measured by routine testing for blood gas values or by the use of noninvasive oxygen saturation monitors. Patients with hypercapnia (high levels of carbon dioxide in the blood) are sensitive to increased levels of oxygen, such as levels above 3 L/min; with oxygen therapy, carbon dioxide levels tend to be even higher. Maximal benefit of oxygen administration requires continuous administration for at least 18 hr/day.[20]

Although traditionally the mechanism of carbon dioxide retention with oxygen therapy was thought to be related to a diminished ventilatory drive, current research suggests that oxygen therapy may instead cause increased $\dot{V}A/\dot{Q}$ imbalance, precipitating a rise in carbon dioxide. It is important to remember that not all patients with a history of COPD are carbon dioxide retainers.

Patients with end-stage emphysema or oxygen levels less than 55 mm Hg[8,20,21] are frequently placed on low-level oxygen therapy at home. Home oxygen therapy has been demonstrated to retard the development of pulmonary hypertension and cor pulmonale.[8,20] Portable oxygen saturation monitors for evaluating the effectiveness of oxygen administration at home may also be used.

Smoking cessation is essential to decreasing the progression of the disease. A reduction in exposure to inhaled pulmonary irritants is also advised.[21] Supportive therapies include adequate rest, proper hydration (8 to 12 glasses of water per day unless the patient has congestive heart failure), and physical reconditioning programs using a treadmill or stationary bicycle. Low-tension, high-repetition muscle contractions provide endurance conditioning. High-tension, low-repetition muscle contractions provide strength conditioning. Alternating rest and exercise improves results on pulmonary function tests. Walking has proved to be the best form of exercise for increasing duration and intensity of activity. The patient may need to start with 5 minutes per day and then train to higher levels of activity.[20] Some authorities recommend increasing oxygen delivery by 1 L/min during exercise.[20] Some patients have benefited from the use of inspiratory muscle trainers. These devices cause the user to increase respiratory muscle strength and endurance by increasing the resistance to airflow on inspiration.[21] COPD patients also benefit from yearly influenza vaccine and pneumococcal vaccine.

KEY CONCEPTS

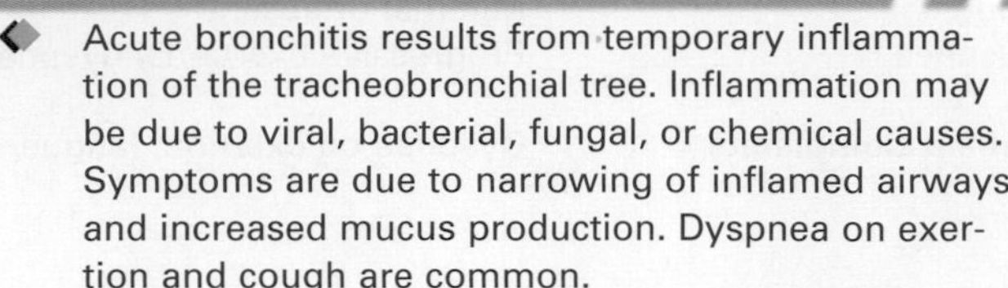

- Acute bronchitis results from temporary inflammation of the tracheobronchial tree. Inflammation may be due to viral, bacterial, fungal, or chemical causes. Symptoms are due to narrowing of inflamed airways and increased mucus production. Dyspnea on exertion and cough are common.
- Chronic bronchitis is an inflammatory disorder of the airways that most commonly results from long-term cigarette smoking. It is defined as a productive cough lasting more than 3 months per year for 2 or more consecutive years. Resultant airway damage is not reversible.
- Chronic bronchitis is associated with persistent narrowing of the airways due to chronic inflammation, scarring, and excessive mucus production. Airway obstruction leads to poor ventilation of alveoli and impaired exchange of oxygen and carbon dioxide. Blood gases are characterized by low PaO_2 and high $PaCO_2$. Persistent hypoxemia causes a compensatory increase in red blood cell production (polycythemia). Cyanosis may be evident.
- Alveolar hypoxia leads to generalized pulmonary vasoconstriction, pulmonary hypertension, and right ventricular hypertrophy (cor pulmonale) in the person with chronic bronchitis. Right-sided heart failure may occur because of the high pulmonary resistance.
- The management of chronic bronchitis centers on removing the etiologic factors (e.g., cigarette smoke), providing bronchodilator therapy, removing secretions, preventing respiratory muscle fatigue, and providing low-dose supplemental oxygen. High-dose oxygen must be used cautiously because it increases $PaCO_2$ levels.

OBSTRUCTION RELATED TO LOSS OF LUNG PARENCHYMA

Emphysema

Etiology. Emphysema (also referred to as type A COPD or the "pink puffer") is defined *pathologically* by destructive changes of the alveolar walls without fibrosis and abnormal enlargement of the distal air sacs.[7,8,20,21] Emphysema is frequently associated with chronic bronchitis. According to the National Center for Health Statistics (1997 data), of the 12.8

million Americans with COPD, 9.6 million primarily have bronchitis and 3.2 million primarily have emphysema.[23] The causes of emphysema are not fully understood, but emphysema is associated with cigarette smoking, air pollution, and certain occupations (e.g., welding, mining, and working with or near asbestos). Emphysema tends to develop over a long period and thus is seen more frequently in persons older than 50. Cigarette smoking in excess of 70 pack-years is highly predictive of COPD.[20] The normal aging process, starting at about age 30, reflects changes similar to those seen in emphysema. These changes include a loss of alveoli, an increase in the size of alveolar ducts, a loss of gas-exchanging surface area (4% per decade), and a decrease in bronchiolar musculature.[20]

When emphysema occurs in young to middle-aged adults or before the age of 50 in a smoker, it may be associated with a deficiency of α_1-antitrypsin activity in the lung. α_1-Antitrypsin deficiency is a hereditary disorder characterized by low serum levels (25 to 50 mg/dl) of α_1-antitrypsin[20,21] This subset of patients makes up less than 2% of all emphysema patients.[20] α_1-Antitrypsin is a protective enzyme that inhibits proteolytic breakdown of alveolar tissue. The protease enzymes (neutrophil derived elastase) that break down lung protein are released from neutrophils that migrate to the lung during inflammation causing alveolar wall destruction.[20]

Emphysema may follow bacterial lung infections (e.g., staphylococcal), which involves secretion of proteases that destroy the elastin proteins responsible for the normal elasticity of the lung tissue. Bacterial infections block mechanisms that normally inhibit the release of proteolytic enzymes from degenerating neutrophilic granulocytes.

Pathogenesis. The pathologic changes leading to alveolar destruction are associated with the release of proteolytic enzymes from inflammatory cells such as neutrophils and macrophages. Smoking is commonly associated with emphysema. Smoking causes alveolar damage in two ways: (1) it leads to inflammation in the lung tissue (parenchyma), thus initiating a chain of events leading to the release of proteolytic enzymes that directly damages alveolar tissue; and (2) it inactivates α_1-antitrypsin, which normally acts to protect the lung parenchyma.[20,21] Figure 22-7 illustrates the pathogenesis of emphysema.

With the loss of alveolar walls, there is also a marked reduction in the pulmonary capillary bed, which is essential for exchange of oxygen and carbon dioxide between the alveolar air and capillary blood. There is also a loss of elastic tissue in the lung, which leads to a decrease in the size of the smaller bronchioles. The loss of lung tissue leads to a loss of *radial traction*, which normally holds the airway open, and to increasing pressure around the outside of the airway lumen, which in turn increases airway resistance and decreases airflow. Figure 22-8 shows the effect of decreased radial traction on the size of small bronchioles. Air then becomes trapped in distal alveoli, leading to distended air sacs, which adds to the collapsing pressure on more proximal bronchi and increases airway obstruction. Loss of alveolar walls and air trapping lead to the formation of **bullae** (large, thin-walled cysts in the lung) that further rob the lung of its gas transport function. The appearance of the lung and lung tissue from typical emphysematous patients is shown in Figures 22-9 and 22-10.

Three major classifications of emphysema exist: (1) centriacinar (also called *centrilobular*), which is associated with both smoking and chronic bronchitis and destroys the respiratory bronchioles; (2) panacinar (also called *panlobular*), which destroys the alveoli; and (3) paraseptal, which affects the peripheral lobules. Some of the classifications of emphysema and the topographic distribution of emphysema in lung tissue are shown in Figure 22-11.

Clinical Manifestations. Patients with emphysema commonly seek help because of progressive exertional dyspnea. The typical patient with advanced disease is a thin man or woman in his or her middle 50s who has had increasing shortness of breath for the past 3 to 4 years. The difficulty in breathing is evidenced by the use of accessory muscles to breathe, progressive dyspnea, and the use of pursed-lip breathing in an effort to get more air out over a longer period of time before the small airways collapse. Cough may be minimal or absent. Decreased arterial oxygen saturation remains minor until late in the course of the disease. Late in the disease process the major symptom is dyspnea on exertion. These patients may be referred to as "pink puffers" (Figure 22-12), a term related to the physiologic matching of ventilation and perfusion. They tend to have more areas of high ventilation in relation to perfusion, thus maintaining near-normal arterial oxygen levels until end-stage disease. Ventilation-perfusion matching and a sustained high respiratory rate produce a relatively normal arterial oxygen level until late stages of the disease.[8,20,21] As with bronchitis, the incidence of emphysema is increasing in women who smoke.

Diagnosis. The diagnosis of emphysema is based on the patient's history and physical findings, pulmonary function tests, chest radiographs, arterial blood gases, and electrocardiogram. Changes seen on pulmonary function tests include an increased functional residual capacity, increased RV, increased TLC, decreased FEV_1, and decreased FVC.[8,20] Chest radiographs show hyperinflation; a low, flat diaphragm; the presence of blebs or bullae; a narrow mediastinum; and a normal or small "vertical" heart. Electrocardiographic findings may be normal or show tall P waves. Sinus tachycardia may be the first sign of decreased oxygenation. Supraventricular arrhythmias (atrial tachycardia, atrial flutter, and atrial fibrillation) and ventricular irregularities may also occur.[8] Arterial blood gas values typically reveal a mild decrease in PaO_2 (65 to 75 mm Hg) and a normal (or, in late stages, elevated) $PaCO_2$.[24]

Physical examination reveals a thin, wasted individual who is using accessory muscles to breathe and sits slightly hunched forward in an effort to breathe better. Auscultation and percussion of the lung fields reveal decreased breath sounds,

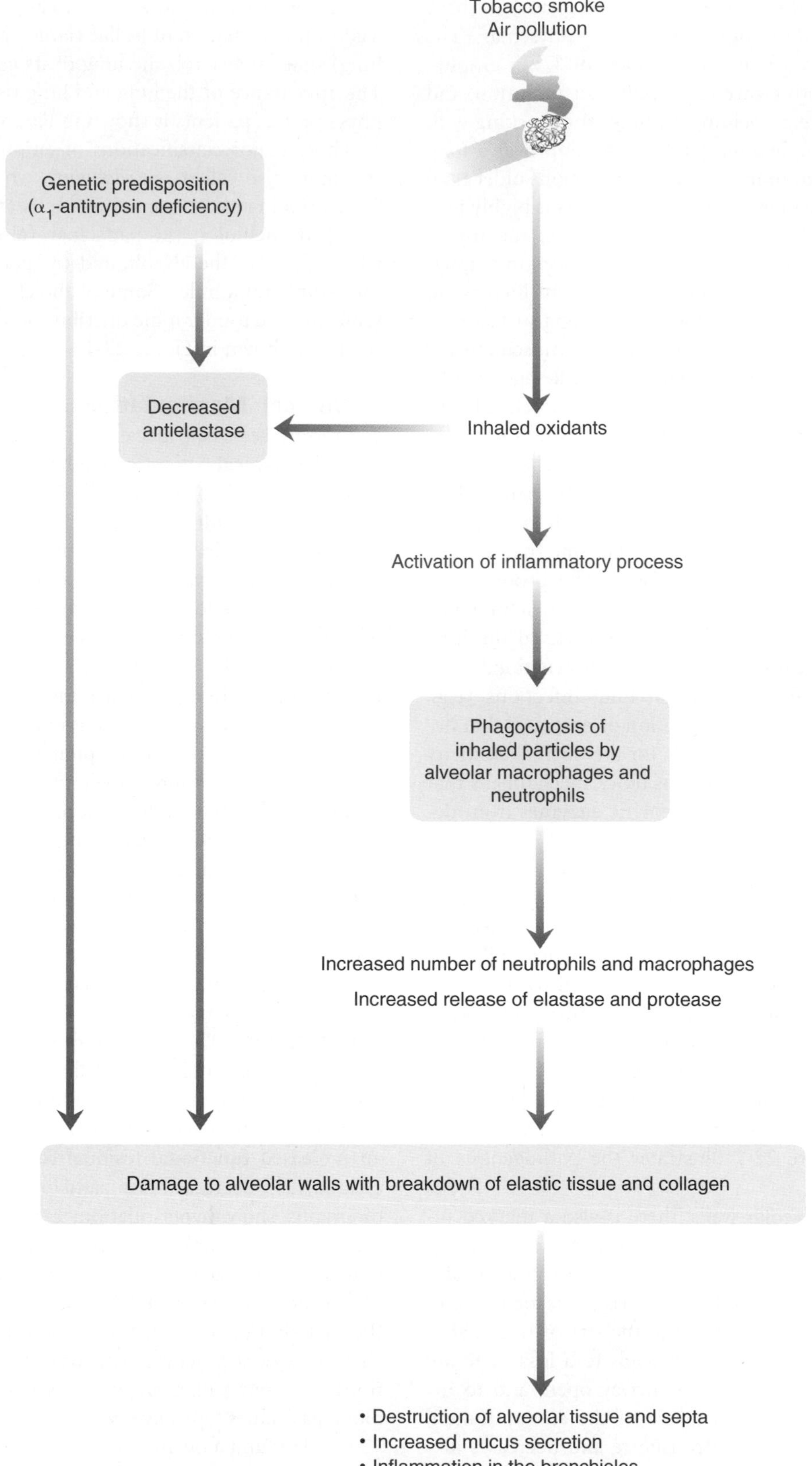

FIGURE 22-7 ■ Pathogenesis of smoke-induced emphysema.

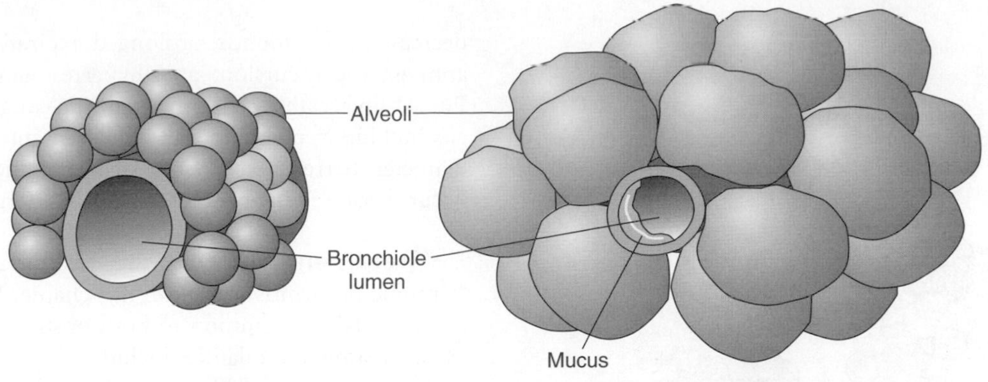

FIGURE 22-8 ■ Loss of radial traction in emphysema leads to airway collapse. **A**, Terminal bronchiole in cross-section. **B**, Terminal bronchiole with narrowed lumen resulting from loss of surrounding alveoli, leading to decreased radial traction and airway collapse.

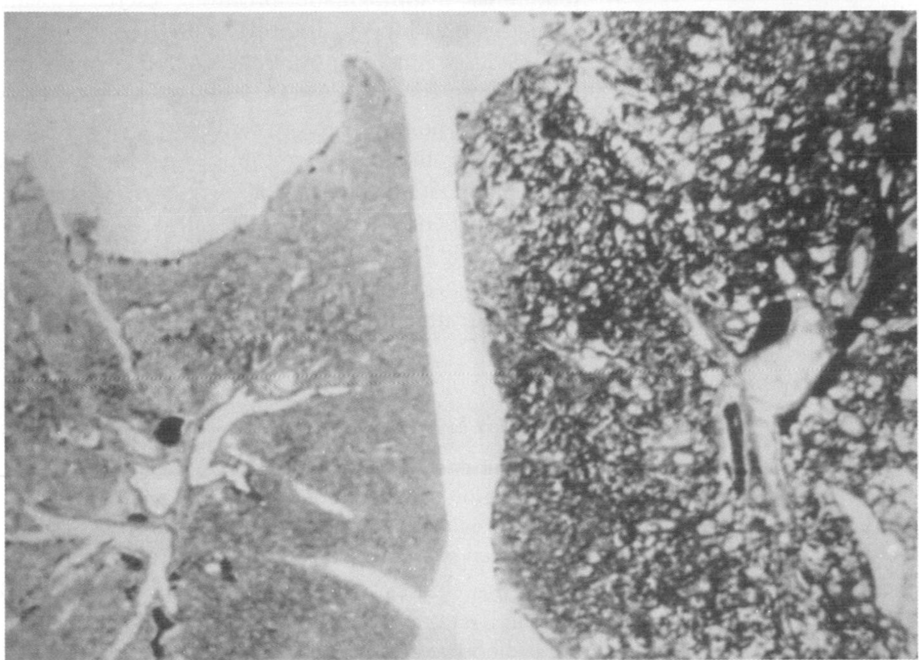

FIGURE 22-9 ■ Gross appearance of emphysematous lung. *Left,* Normal lung tissue from a nonsmoker. *Right,* Lung tissue from a smoker who has developed emphysema.

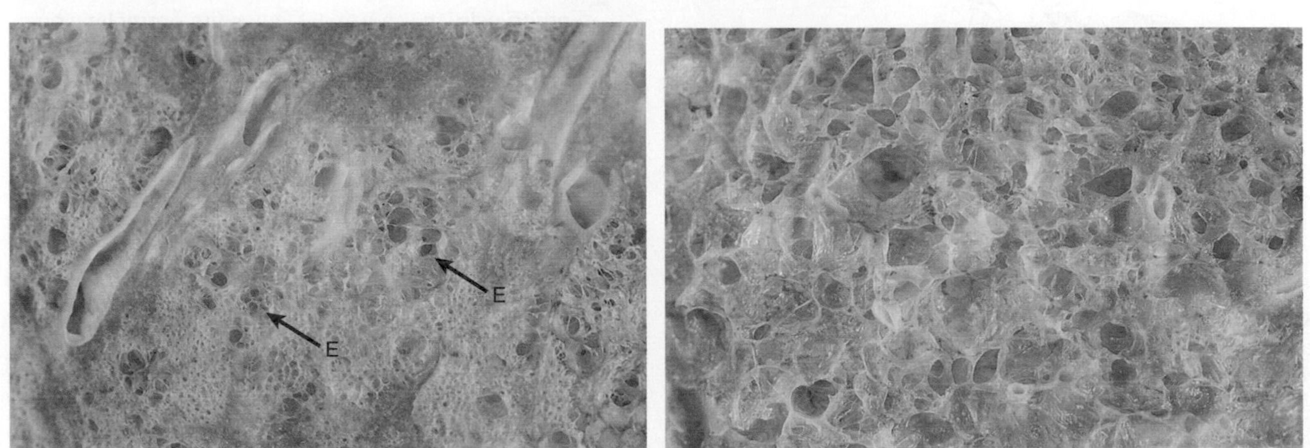

FIGURE 22-10 ■ **A,** Centriacinar (centrilobular) emphysema. Central areas show marked emphysematous damage *(E),* surrounded by relatively spared alveolar spaces. **B,** Panacinar (panlobular) emphysema involving the entire pulmonary architecture. (From Kumar V, Cotran RS, Robbins ST: *Robbins basic pathology,* ed 6, Philadelphia, 1999, Saunders, p 708.)

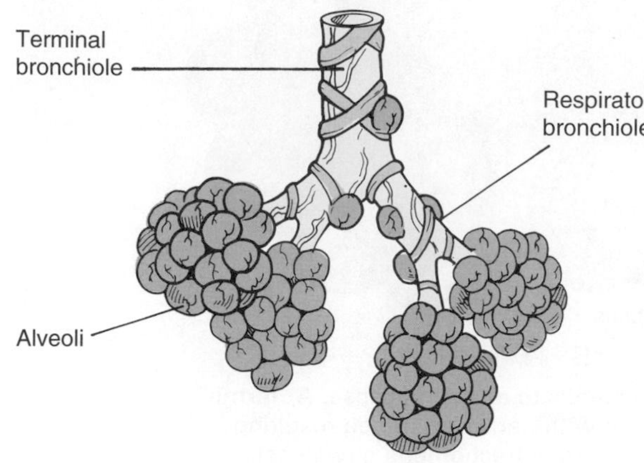

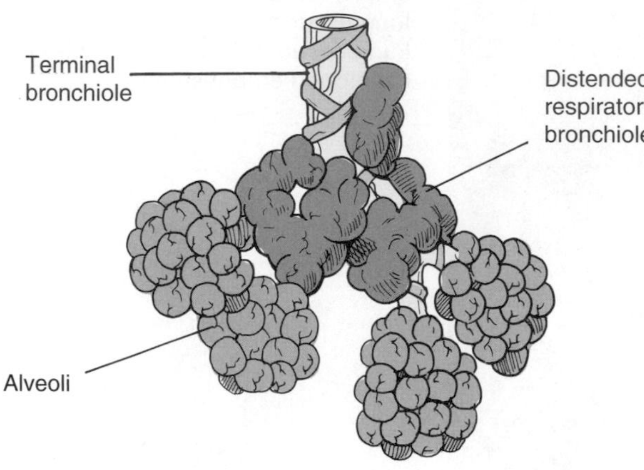

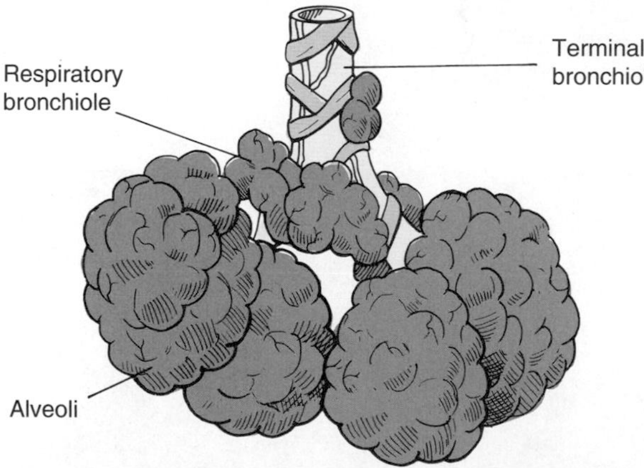

FIGURE 22-11 ■ Types of emphysema. (From Black JM, Hawks JH: *Medical-surgical nursing: clinical management for positive outcomes,* ed 7, Philadelphia, 2005, Saunders, p 1819.)

decreased heart sounds, prolonged expiration, decreased diaphragmatic excursion, and hyperresonance of the chest. Pursed-lip breathing, chronic morning cough because of mucus buildup at night, and an increased anteroposterior chest diameter (barrel chest) are also common findings. Weight loss occurs because of anorexia and lack of energy to eat.

Treatment. Refer to the treatment section under "Chronic Bronchitis" earlier in this chapter for detailed treatment modalities common to both obstructive lung diseases. Major treatment modalities include:

- Use of bronchodilators, with inhaled sympathomimetics and ipratropium bromide being preferred
- Bronchial hygiene to mobilize secretions
- Cessation of smoking
- Graded aerobic exercise
- Abdominal diaphragmatic breathing exercises with pursed-lip breathing to improve muscle conditioning for breathing and to promote exhalation of more air from the lungs
- Avoidance of pollution and irritants
- Home oxygen therapy for continuous use or only during the night and during exercise[17]

An excellent patient teaching manual called *Better Breathing: A Self-Teaching Manual* is available from PAL Medical, Inc., Maitland, Florida. Poor prognosis is associated with weight loss, so treatment is focused on maintaining proper nutrition.

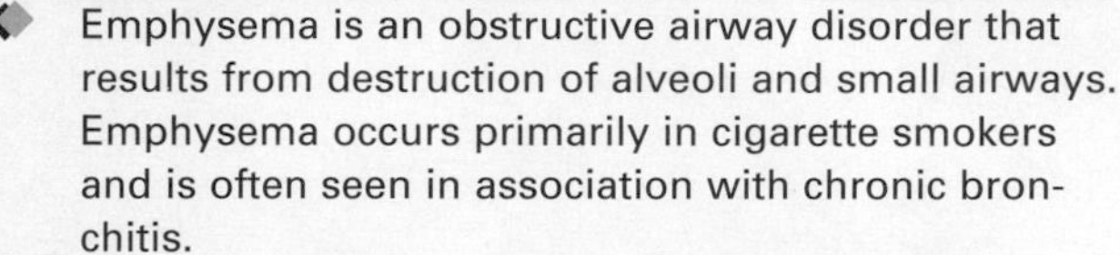

KEY CONCEPTS

- Emphysema is an obstructive airway disorder that results from destruction of alveoli and small airways. Emphysema occurs primarily in cigarette smokers and is often seen in association with chronic bronchitis.
- Alveolar destruction is due to release of inflammatory proteolytic enzymes that degrade lung proteins. Smoking also inhibits a protective enzyme, α_1-antitrypsin, that normally keeps the proteolytic enzymes in check. Genetic deficiency of α_1-antitrypsin is an uncommon cause of emphysema.
- Emphysema causes two major problems with respiration: (1) a decrease in surface area for gas exchange and (2) airway collapse due to loss of radial traction. Airway collapse is greater on expiration, resulting in air trapping and hyperinflation.
- Emphysema is characterized by dyspnea, weight loss, use of accessory muscles to breathe, a low, flat diaphragm, and a barrel chest. Cyanosis is not present until late stages of the disease. By sustaining high ventilatory effort, a patient can have blood oxygen levels that are generally maintained near normal. Carbon dioxide levels may be low due to hyperventilation.

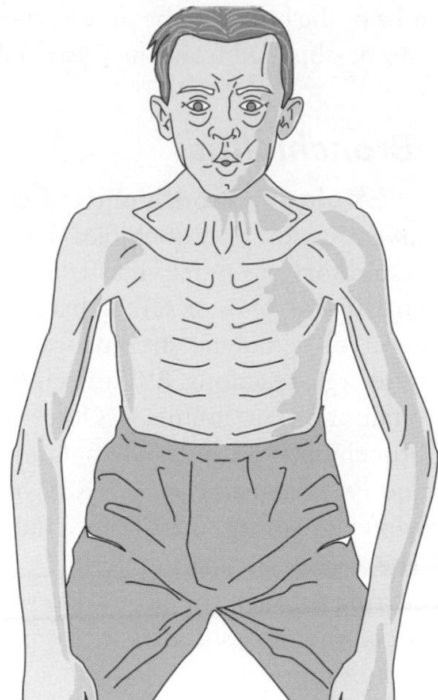

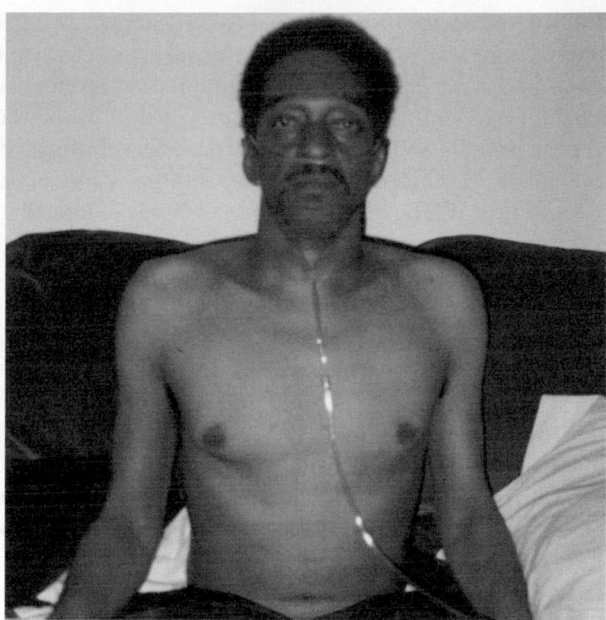

FIGURE 22-12 ■ **A,** The "pink puffer." Note the use of accessory muscles and pursed-lip breathing in an effort to get more air out of the lungs. **B,** A client with emphysema. Note the thin appearance and the presence of continuous oxygen therapy. The use of accessory muscles of respiration (neck and shoulder muscles) reflects the client's shortness of breath and increased work of breathing necessary to increase minute ventilation and to maintain adequate arterial blood gas values. (**B,** From Black JM, Hawks JH, Keene AM: *Medical-surgical nursing: clinical management for positive outcomes,* ed 7, Philadelphia, 2005, Saunders, p 1820.)

◆ Therapy for emphysema is similar to that for chronic bronchitis. Cessation of smoking is necessary to prevent progression of the disease. Present damage is irreversible. Oxygen therapy improves activity tolerance and quality of life.

OBSTRUCTION OF THE AIRWAY LUMEN

Bronchiectasis

Etiology. **Bronchiectasis** means dilation of bronchi. It is either acquired or congenital, and is classified as both an obstructive and a **suppurative** (pus-forming) disorder. Acquired bronchiectasis is now rare in the United States because of rapid diagnosis and management of bronchopulmonary infections. Cystic fibrosis is associated with 50% of the cases of bronchiectasis.[7] Children are at higher risk for development of bronchiectasis because of anatomic factors such as small, soft, elastic bronchi. Bronchi in children are easily damaged by overinflation and distention from inflammation and infection.

Bronchiectasis can be classified according to bronchial shape: saccular, with cavity-like dilatations or cylindrical, and with widening of the bronchial walls. A fusiform shape is a combination of saccular and cylindrical changes. These anatomic changes are shown in Figure 22-13. Little clinical or pathophysiologic difference in the three types has been demonstrated.

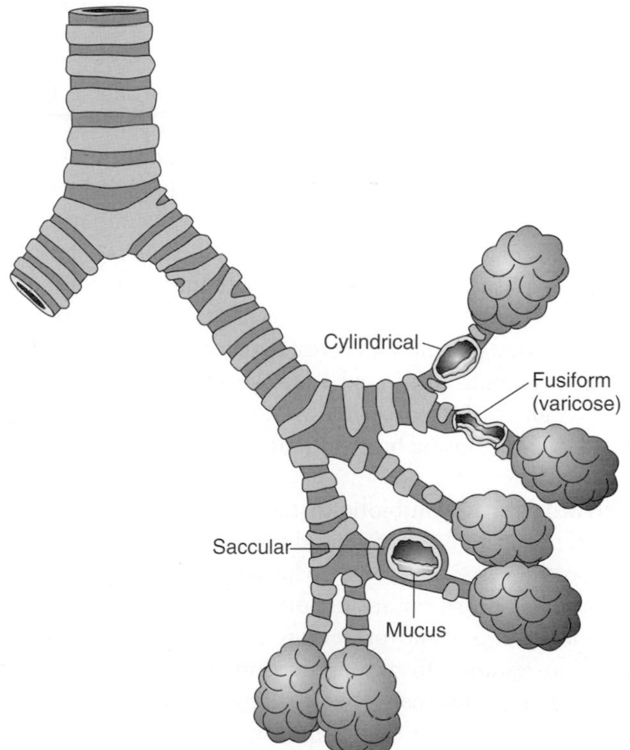

FIGURE 22-13 ■ Bronchial dilatations due to bronchiectasis. The saccular form occurs in the segmental bronchi, which are severely dilated and end blindly. The varicose form resembles varicose veins with irregular dilatations and constriction. The cylindrical form shows uniform slight dilatation.

Pathogenesis. Bronchiectasis is characterized by recurrent infection and inflammation of bronchial walls, which leads to persistent dilation of the medium-sized bronchi and bronchioles. Inflammation results in destruction of the walls of central bronchi and obliteration of peripheral bronchi and bronchioles.[22] *H. influenzae* is the most common cause of bacterial infections.[22] The destructive process leads to loss of ciliated epithelium, squamous cell **metaplasia** (abnormal transformation of normal tissue to abnormal tissue), and pus formation, which in turn leads to obstruction of airflow. Lung tissue of a patient with cystic fibrosis complicated by varicose bronchiectasis is shown in Figure 22-14.

Clinical Manifestations. The child usually presents with a chronic productive cough with copious amounts of purulent, foul-smelling, green or yellow sputum. The sputum has the characteristic of separating into three distinct layers in a sputum cup.[22] Other clinical features are **hemoptysis, crackles, rhonchi**, halitosis (bad breath), skin pallor, and, infrequently, digital clubbing. Clubbing is caused by decreased oxygenation, which leads to fibrous tissue hyperplasia in the area between the nail and distal portion of each digit. Clubbing is associated with lymphocytic extravasation, increased vascularity, and edema. The severity of clubbing parallels the severity of pulmonary disease.[19] Digital clubbing can be identified by two methods, as seen in Figure 22-15. **Hypoxemia** is seen in severe cases. Complications of bronchiectasis are malnutrition, recurrent pneumonia, right ventricular failure, and secondary visceral abscesses.[8]

Diagnosis. Generally, the diagnosis of bronchiectasis is based on a history of chronic productive cough. The patient complains about producing copious amounts of foul-smelling, purulent sputum. Radiographic abnormalities may reveal small cysts, thickening of bronchial walls, and increased bronchial markings (areas of intensity showing bronchi, which are usually not distinct). Pulmonary function tests show decreased airflow and vital capacity in advanced cases. Arterial blood gas analyses reveal hypoxemia (decreased PaO_2) and hypercapnia (increased $PaCO_2$) from obstruction to airflow. High-resolution computed tomography is the test of choice for diagnosing bronchiectasis.[8]

Treatment. Antibiotic therapy accompanied by inhalation of bronchodilators followed by vigorous chest percussion and postural drainage is the mainstay of therapy. Proper hydration and nutrition are important in promoting liquefaction of secretions and preventing increased susceptibility to infection resulting from malnutrition. Maintaining adequate nutrition is problematic due to fatigue and the energy required to eat. (Refer to the following section on cystic fibrosis for further discussion on treatment.) In severe cases, when other measures fail, bronchoscopy with bronchial lavage may be necessary to remove thick, purulent secretions. In the child with severe saccular bronchiectasis, removal of the affected area of the lung may be necessary. Patient education materials can be obtained from the Cystic Fibrosis Foundation.[25]

Bronchiolitis

Etiology. **Bronchiolitis** is characterized by widespread inflammation of bronchioles due to infectious agents such as **respiratory syncytial virus** (RSV) (50% of cases),[26] influenza virus (type A, B, or C), or bacteria (*H. influenzae,* pneumococci, or hemolytic streptococci), and occasionally produced by allergic reactions. RSV infection is a common cause of hospitalization in infants.[22] Other organisms that may cause bronchiolitis include *Mycoplasma, Chlamydia, Ureaplasma,* and *Pneumocystis carinii.*[27] RSV occurs in yearly epidemics in winter to spring, usually in children younger than 2 years.[28] The average incubation period is 5 days, with inoculation occurring through the nose and eyes.[8,27] In adults, bronchiolitis is commonly associated with smoking, toxic fumes, and immunosuppression.[8]

Pathogenesis. Once initiated by the causal agent, proliferation and necrosis of bronchiolar epithelium occur, producing obstruction and increased mucus production.[8] Production of thick, tenacious mucus leads to airway obstruction, atelectasis, and hyperinflation. Three possible mechanisms of airway obstruction may follow the inflammatory process. They include (1) development of inflammatory exudate, which may displace surfactant, leading to airway obstruction; (2) release of chemical mediators, which may produce bronchiolar constriction; and (3) development of inflammation, which may induce fibrosis and narrowing of the airway.[1,22] Goblet cell metaplasia and increased bronchial muscle mass may also occur, resulting in further airway narrowing.

Clinical Manifestations. The severity and course of the disease are variable, ranging from mild to fatal. Common clinical features include wheezing due to bronchospasm, crackles, decreased breath sounds, retractions, increased sputum, dyspnea, tachypnea (rapid, shallow respirations), and low-grade fever. Otitis media is a common complication often associated with *S. pneumoniae.*[27]

Diagnosis. Patients commonly have an elevated WBC count. The chest radiograph may show enlarged air sacs, interstitial infiltrates, atelectasis, or severe hyperinflation. Pulmonary function tests reveal severe obstruction to airflow. Rapid diagnosis of RSV may be made by identifying the viral antigen from nasal washings or nasal swab culture of secretions, using an enzyme-linked immunosorbent assay or immunofluorescent assay.

Treatment. Adequate oxygenation is maintained by providing humidified oxygen, monitoring blood gases or oxygen saturation, and providing oral, inhaled, or intravenous bronchodilator agents and, in selected cases, corticosteroids.[22]

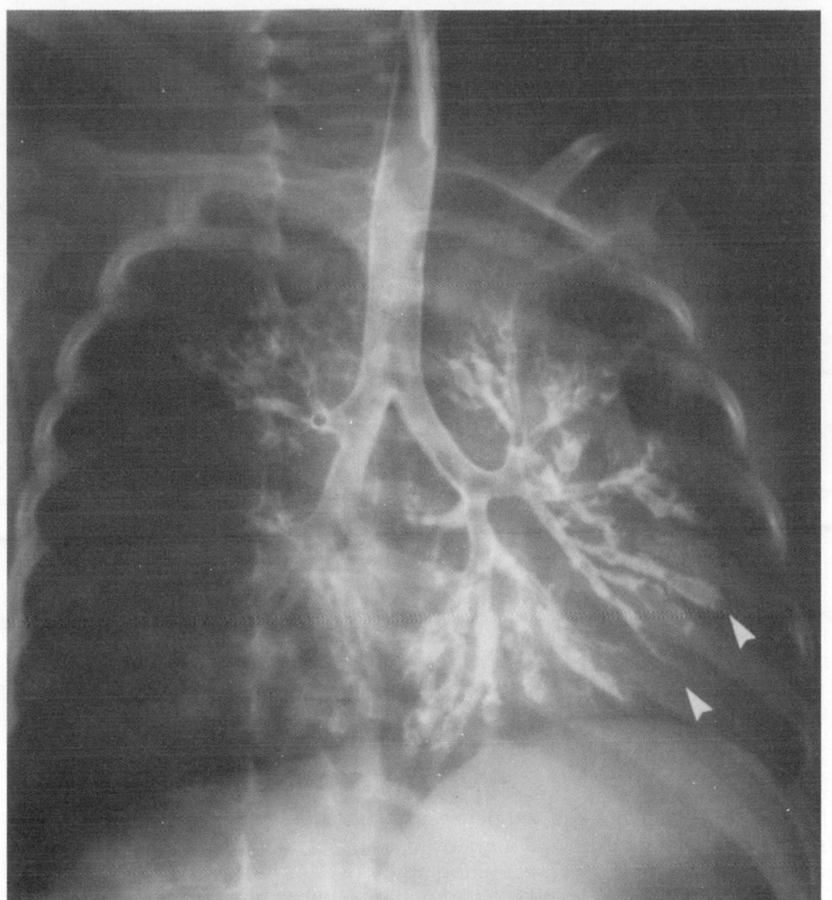

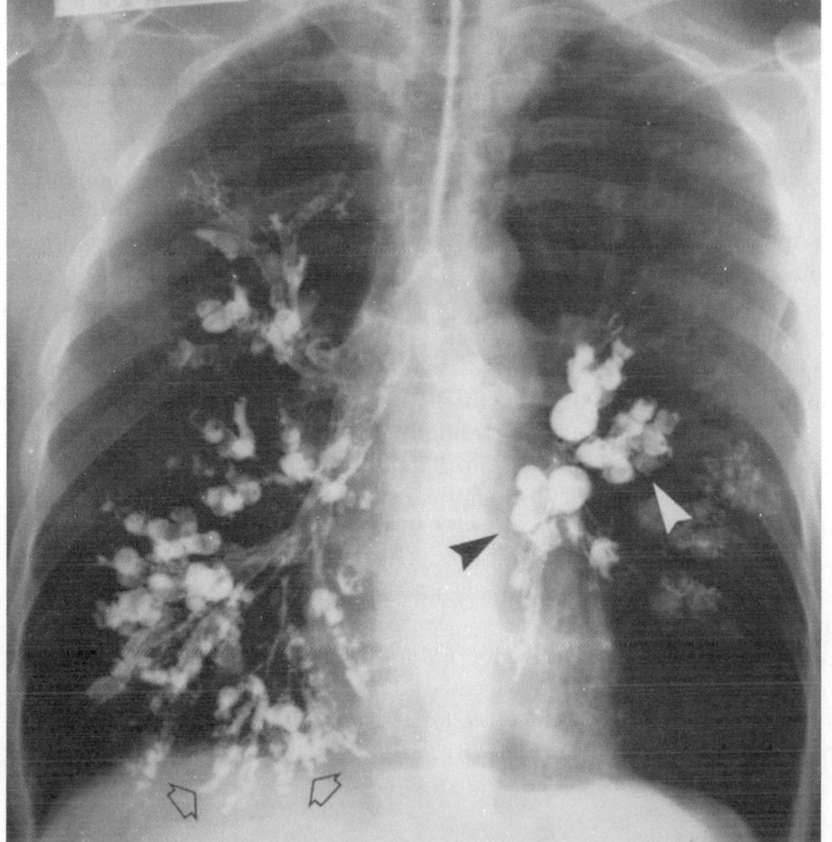

FIGURE 22-14 ■ Bronchographic features of varicose and cystic bronchiectasis. **A,** A left tracheobronchogram in a shallow posterior oblique projection reveals mildly dilated and slightly irregular bronchi that terminate after four to six generations of branchings from the trachea in a squared or bulbous appearance *(arrowheads)*. The findings are those of varicose bronchiectasis. **B,** A bilateral tracheobronchogram in the anteroposterior projection demonstrates a multitude of contrast material–filled cystic spaces resembling a cluster of grapes *(arrowheads)*, a characteristic feature of cystic bronchiectasis. Note that the cystic spaces appear after only two to three bronchial generations. Less severe bronchiectasis of the varicose type is present in the right lower lobe *(open arrows)*. (From Fraser RG et al: *Diagnosis of diseases of the chest,* ed 3, vol 3, Philadelphia, 1990, Saunders, p 2199.)

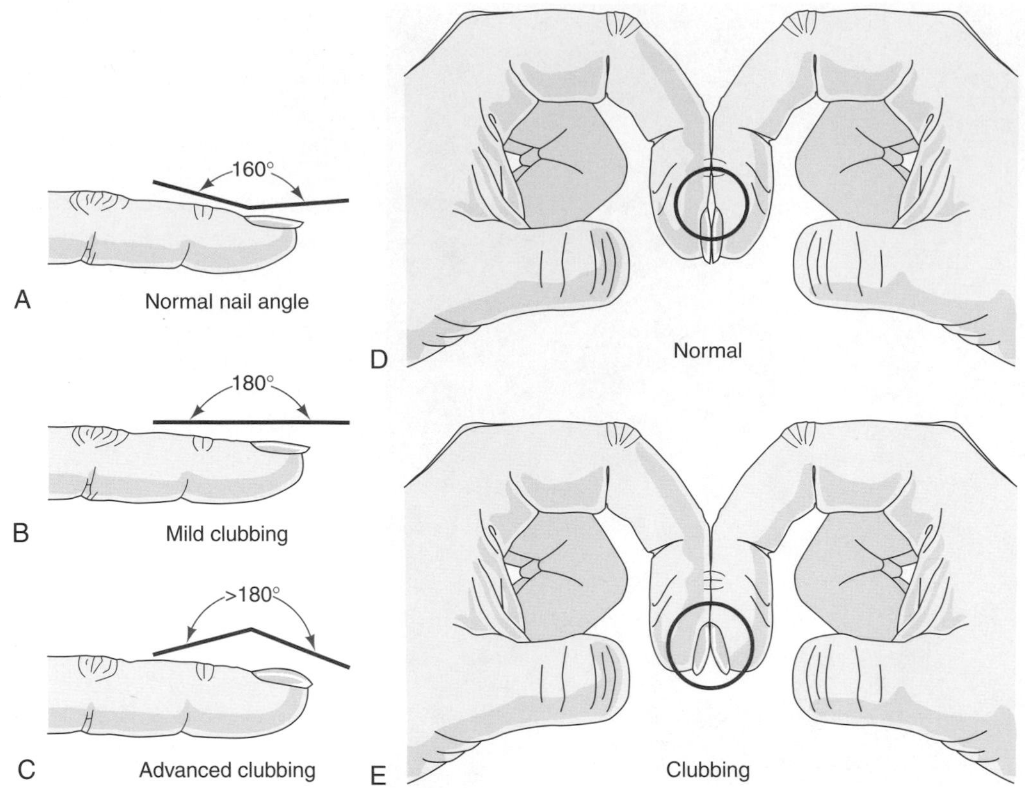

FIGURE 22-15 ■ Clubbing. **A**, Normal fingernail angle is 160 degrees. **B**, Early mild clubbing appears as flattened angle between nail and skin (180 degrees). **C**, Advanced clubbing shows a rounded (clubbed) fingertip and nail. To assess clubbing by Schamroth's diagnostic method **(D** and **E)**, place the nails of the second digits together. Obliteration of the normal diamond-shaped space between the nails is an abnormal finding, signifying clubbing.

Table 22-5 provides general information about pharmacologic agents commonly used in the management of various respiratory disorders. Use of these agents depends on the severity of the diagnosis and prescriber preference.

Aerosolized ribavirin inhibits RNA polymerase activity and inhibits the initiation and elongation of RNA fragments, resulting in inhibition of viral protein synthesis. It has been effective in treating patients with RSV but should be avoided in pregnant women. Hyperimmune RSV IgG (1500 mg/kg) is effective in combination with ribavirin in immunocompromised adults. Palivizumab, a monoclonal RSV antibody, is FDA approved for use in high-risk infants with bronchopulmonary dysplasia and congenital heart disease.[27] Other therapies include sedation for anxiety, hydration, and the administration of appropriate broad-spectrum antibiotics based on culture and sensitivity results for concomitant bacterial infections. Patients are encouraged to stop smoking and to avoid passive smoke exposure. The use of eye-nose goggles by health care workers is recommended to control the spread of RSV. The virus is spread through the air or by contact with secretions from the eye, nose, or mouth, and transmission may not be prevented by the use of masks and gowns.

Cystic Fibrosis

Etiology. Cystic fibrosis (mucoviscidosis) is an autosomal recessive disorder of the exocrine glands. It is the most common genetic lung disease in the United States, with an incidence of 1 in 2000 to 3300 Caucasian births.[8,22,29] One in 25 Caucasians are heterozygous carriers of the cystic fibrosis gene.[8] The incidence in African-Americans is rare (1 in 17,000 live births), and in Native Americans the incidence is 1 in 80,000 births.[29,30] It is almost never seen in the Asian population.[15,30] About 35% of the 30,000 cases of cystic fibrosis in the United States involve individuals older than 18 years.[8,15] Cystic fibrosis can be classified either as an airflow obstructive disorder or as a suppurative (pus-forming) disorder. Hypersecretion of abnormal, thick mucus that obstructs exocrine glands and ducts is a characteristic finding in the disease.[7]

With advances in antibiotic therapy and early recognition and management of complications, patients with cystic fibrosis are living longer into adulthood. The median survival age is now 31 years.[8,22] Some patients are now having families.

Table 22-5

Common Therapeutic Agents Used in the Treatment of Respiratory Diseases

Classification/Agent	Dosage Forms	Action
Methylxanthines		
Theophylline	Oral, IV	Bronchodilation
Aminophylline		
Oxtriphylline (Theo-Dur, Uniphyl)		
β_2 Agonists		
Catecholamines		Bronchodilation
Epinephrine (Adrenalin)	IV, inhaled	
Isoproterenol (Isuprel)	IV, inhaled	
Isoetharine	Inhaled	
Bitolterol (Tornalate)	Inhaled (nebulized)	
Resorcinols		Bronchodilation
Metaproterenol (Alupent)	Oral, inhaled	
Terbutaline (Brethine, Brethaire)	Oral, IV	
Salagen		Bronchodilation
Albuterol (Proventil, Ventolin)	Oral, inhaled	
Sustained-release albuterol (Proventil Repetabs)	Oral	
Newer agents		
Pirbuterol (Maxair)	Inhaled	
Salmeterol xinafoate (Serevent)	Inhaled	
Serevent Diskus	Inhaled	Dry powder system
Anticholinergics		
Atropine sulfate	Oral, inhaled	Blocks action of acetylcholine and increases intracellular cAMP, which lead to bronchodilation
Ipratropium bromide (Atrovent)	Inhaled	
Glucocorticoids		
Beclomethasone (Vanceril, Beclovent, QVAR)	Inhaled	Suppresses inflammation and may potentiate β_2-adrenergic agents
Budesonide (Pulmicort)	Inhaled	Dosage: 400-800 μg
Dexamethasone (Decadron)	PO/IV	
Triamcinolone acetonide (Azmacort)	IM, inhaled	
Flunisolide (AeroBid)	Inhaled	
Fluticasone (Flovent)	Inhaled	Dosage: 44, 110, 220 μg/puff
Flovent Rotadisk	Inhaled	Dry powder delivery system
Methylprednisolone	IV	
Prednisone	Oral	
Combination Inhalers		
Fluticasone and salmeterol (Advair Diskus)	Inhaled	Corticosteroid and long-acting β_2 agonist Dosage: 100/50 μg, 250/50 μg, 500/50 μg
Albuterol and ipratropium (Combivent, DuoNeb)		β_2 agonist and anticholinergic
Mast Cell Stabilizers		
Cromolyn sodium (Intal)	Inhaled	Stabilizes mast cell membranes
Nedocromil sodium (Tilade)		
Leukotriene Inhibitors		
Montelukast (Singulair)	Oral	Blocks inflammatory and bronchospastic actions of leukotrienes
Zafirlukast (Accolate)	Oral	
Zileuton (Zyflo)	Oral	

IV, Intravenous; *IM*, intramuscular; *cAMP*, cyclic adenosine monophosphate.

Pathogenesis. Cystic fibrosis is classified as an autosomal recessive disorder. More than 800 mutations in the gene that encodes for the cystic fibrosis transmembrane conductance regulator (CFTR) have been described.[8,22] One genetic defect associated with cystic fibrosis involves deletion of three base pairs in codon 508 (ΔF508) that code for phenylalanine on chromosome 7 (band q31).[15] With the loss of these three base pairs, the *CFTR* gene is dysfunctional.[8,22] This is the most common genetic mutation causing cystic fibrosis and occurs in 60% to 75% of cystic fibrosis patients tested.[8,22] *CFTR* encodes a membrane chloride channel and is expressed in the sweat glands, the lungs, and the pancreas. Mutations in the *CFTR* gene result in alteration in chloride transport and water transport across the apical surface of epithelial cells.[8,15] Cystic fibrosis primarily affects the pancreas, intestinal tract, sweat glands, and lungs, and in males causes infertility.[26] The mucus-producing glands in the gastrointestinal tract enlarge and produce excessive secretions that are thick mucoproteins. The thick eosinophilic mucous secretions plug the glands and ducts of the pancreatic acini, intestinal glands, intrahepatic bile ducts, and the gallbladder, causing dilation and fibrosis.[29,30] These changes result in decreased production of pancreatic enzymes necessary for digestion of fats, carbohydrates, and proteins, thus leading to increased fat and protein in the stool.[29,30]

The bronchopulmonary system is also affected by the thick, tenacious mucus that results from failure of chloride channels to function in the apical membranes of mucosal cells. Decreased flow of ions and water results in viscid mucus.[8,30] High concentrations of DNA in airway secretions (due to inflammation and lysis of neutrophils) increase sputum viscosity.[8,29,30] The thick mucus causes airway obstruction, atelectasis, and hyperinflation. The thick mucus also decreases ciliary action, thus contributing to mucus stasis, which provides a medium for pulmonary infection. Sweat glands, salivary glands, and lacrimal glands are also affected, leading to high concentrations of sodium and chloride in these secretions.[8,29,30]

Clinical Manifestations. Typical findings include a history of cough in a young adult or child; thick, tenacious sputum; recurrent pulmonary infections (commonly *Pseudomonas aeruginosa*); and recurrent episodes of bronchitis. These processes ultimately progress to pneumonia and bronchiectasis, cor pulmonale, and exercise intolerance.

Physical examination may reveal digital clubbing (late sign), dyspnea, tachypnea, sternal retractions, unequal breath sounds, moist basilar crackles and rhonchi, and a barrel chest that is hyperresonant to percussion.[8] Other findings that may be present are pancreatic insufficiency (85% to 90%), cirrhosis of the liver (15% to 20%), diabetes mellitus (8% to 15%), gallstones (30% to 35%), nasal polyps (15%), and failure of development of the vas deferens in males.[1,8,15,22,29-31] Infants frequently present with a history of multiple respiratory infections, meconium ileus, failure to thrive, jaundice, salt depletion, and edema.[8,15,22]

Nutritional assessment reveals depleted fat stores, steatorrhea (fatty stools), anorexia, decreased growth rate in children (weight, height, head circumference), and decreased midarm indices.[15,22]

Diagnosis. The diagnosis of cystic fibrosis is based on clinical and laboratory findings. Diagnostic studies that are routinely done include arterial blood gas measurement, pulmonary function tests, sputum culture and sensitivity with Gram stain, and chest radiography. Specific diagnostic tests for cystic fibrosis include stool examination for fat, pilocarpine iontophoresis (sweat test), and genetic testing. A 72-hour stool collection combined with the dietary history during that time is used to determine fat absorption and fecal fat excretion. A coefficient of fat absorption of less than 95% (85% in infants) can be used to define **steatorrhea** (fatty stools).[32] Arterial blood gas analyses commonly show hypoxemia and hypercapnia because of airway obstruction. Pulmonary function tests reveal decreased vital capacity, decreased airflow rates, increased airway resistance, increased functional residual capacity and decreased tidal volume. Chest radiographs show evidence of patchy atelectasis, bronchiectasis, obstructive emphysema, cystic lung fields, and peribronchial thickening.[1,15,22,29-31]

The quantitative pilocarpine iontophoresis sweat test reveals elevated sodium and chloride levels, with more than 98% of patients having levels greater than 60 mEq/L in children and greater than 80 mEq/L in adults.[7,31] A diagnostic blood test for the genetic marker ΔF-508 may be useful for confirming the diagnosis and providing genetic information to the family.[7]

Treatment. Management of cystic fibrosis involves an interdisciplinary approach. A comprehensive program that focuses on multiorgan derangements is recommended. Because pulmonary disease accounts for the majority of morbidity and mortality associated with cystic fibrosis, treatment is aimed at aggressive pharmacologic management of pulmonary infection. Treatment includes the use of bronchodilators such as albuterol or metaproterenol. Mobilization of the thick mucus by postural drainage and **chest physiotherapy** (percussion and vibration) is a priority. Alternative methods for mucus removal include the forced expiratory technique, which involves coughing (huffing) with an open glottis.[31] Recombinant human deoxyribonuclease I (Dornase alfa) acts by digesting extracellular DNA (released from lysed neutrophils) present in the viscid sputum of cystic fibrosis patients. Dornase alfa decreases the viscoelasticity of sputum, thus improving pulmonary function and decreasing the risk of infection.[7,8,31,33]

High-dose antibiotic therapy is used for acute exacerbations of respiratory infections to decrease bacterial growth in the lungs. Antibiotic therapy is primarily directed at *Staphylococcus aureus, P. aeruginosa, H. influenzae,* and Enterobacteriaceae.[7,8] Other organisms that have demonstrated antibiotic resistance are *Stenotrophomonas maltophilia* and *Burkholderia cepacia*.[8,29] This period of intense high-dose antibiotic therapy is often termed the "clean-out" regimen. Clean-out requires initial hospitalization for intravenous infusion of an aminoglycoside, such as gentamicin or tobramycin, selected on the basis of susceptibility testing and an antipseudomonal antibiotic, such as ticarcillin (Timentin), ceftazidime (Fortaz), or cefoperazone (Cefobid).[3,4,10,11,15] Long-term intermittent nebulizer treatments with tobramycin for inhalation (TOBI) improves FEV_1 and decreases the risk of symptomatic pulmonary exacerbation in *P. aeruginosa*–infected patients.[29] An annual influenza vaccine is recommended for cystic fibrosis patients because of the increased risk of complications associated with infection.[8,29]

Nutritional therapy includes unrestricted fat consumption (approximately 30% of caloric intake), a high-protein diet, and vitamin supplements (especially the fat-soluble vitamins A, D, E, and K). Other pharmacologic therapy related to nutrition is aimed at replacement of pancreatic enzymes (pancreatin or pancrelipase). Maintenance of weight in children with cystic fibrosis often requires an intake of 150% of the normal calories recommended for healthy children.[29] In some cases, enteral feedings or intravenous nutrition may be necessary on a short-term basis. Salt supplementation may be necessary in hot weather.

Heart-lung or lung transplantation is currently the only definitive treatment. Results show improved quality of life.[8] More than 200 cystic fibrosis patients worldwide have undergone transplantation, with a 3-year survival of 55%.[8] Patients receiving transplants showed marked improvement in mobility, energy, and quality of life.

Identification of the disease-related gene, the cystic fibrosis transmembrane conductance regulator *(CFTR)*,[34] has advanced prospects for corrective gene therapy (Figure 22-16).[35] Gene therapy targets the lung epithelial cell through tracheal instillation of a virus containing the recombinant gene encoding human CFTR. One limiting factor is that the gene has a short-term expression. In the experiments conducted on rats, expression persisted for only 42 days.[35]

Acute Tracheobronchial Obstruction

Etiology. Acute tracheobronchial obstruction requires immediate treatment. Causes frequently include aspiration of a foreign body (e.g., a piece of meat, peanut, coin), malpositioned endotracheal tube, laryngospasm, epiglottitis, trauma, swelling from smoke inhalation, postsurgical blood clot, and compression of the bronchus or trachea by tumors or enlarged lymph nodes. With inhaled foreign bodies the right side of the lung is affected more often than the left because of the anatomic extension of the right main bronchus from the trachea.

Pathogenesis. Obstruction by one of the etiologic agents listed earlier can be partial or complete. The health care worker must be prepared to assess the situation rapidly and act immediately to relieve the obstruction.

Clinical Manifestations. With complete obstruction, no air movement will be heard on auscultation, but the patient may still be making inspiratory chest movements. Other clinical features of complete obstruction include inability to talk, tachycardia, cyanosis, and rapid progression to unconsciousness unless the problem is quickly reversed.

With partial obstruction of the airway, the patient usually presents with stridor, sternal and intercostal retractions, wheezing, nasal flaring, tachypnea, dyspnea, tachycardia, and use of accessory muscles to breathe. Cyanosis is a late sign that usually indicates exhaustion or complete obstruction.

Diagnosis. The diagnosis of airway obstruction is based on clinical features and arterial blood gas analyses. Arterial blood gas values frequently show hypoxemia and hypercarbia. Chest radiographs may reveal the location of the obstruction.

Treatment. Treatment involves opening the obstructed airway as quickly as possible. Blows to the patient's back or use of the **Heimlich maneuver** may be necessary for the foreign body to be expelled. Aspirated contents occluding the airway are suctioned to relieve obstruction. If these methods are unsuccessful, an emergency tracheostomy should be performed in the case of a suspected upper airway obstruction in the subglottic region or above. If emergency treatment has not removed the cause of the obstruction, further intervention must be done.

Epiglottitis

Etiology. Acute epiglottitis is suspected when odynophagia (pain with swallowing) seems out of proportion to pharyngeal findings. Inability to swallow saliva with evidence of drooling is common. Epiglottitis is classified as a subtype of croup. The causative organism is primarily *H. influenzae* type B (Hib). It is most often seen in children 2 to 4 years old. Pneumococci, streptococci, and staphylococci are also causal agents.[22,36] The role of viruses in epiglottitis is unclear.[36]

Pathogenesis. The infecting agent localizes in the supraglottic area in the epiglottis and pharyngeal structures, causing rapid and potentially fatal inflammation with swelling and airway obstruction.

Clinical Manifestations. The patient frequently presents with acute respiratory difficulty that has progressed rapidly over several hours. Common signs and symptoms include drooling, dysphagia, rapid onset of fever, dysphonia, inspiratory stridor, and inspiratory retractions. The child often sits in a "sniffing dog" position, which provides the best airway patency. The oropharynx is edematous and cherry red.[26,36]

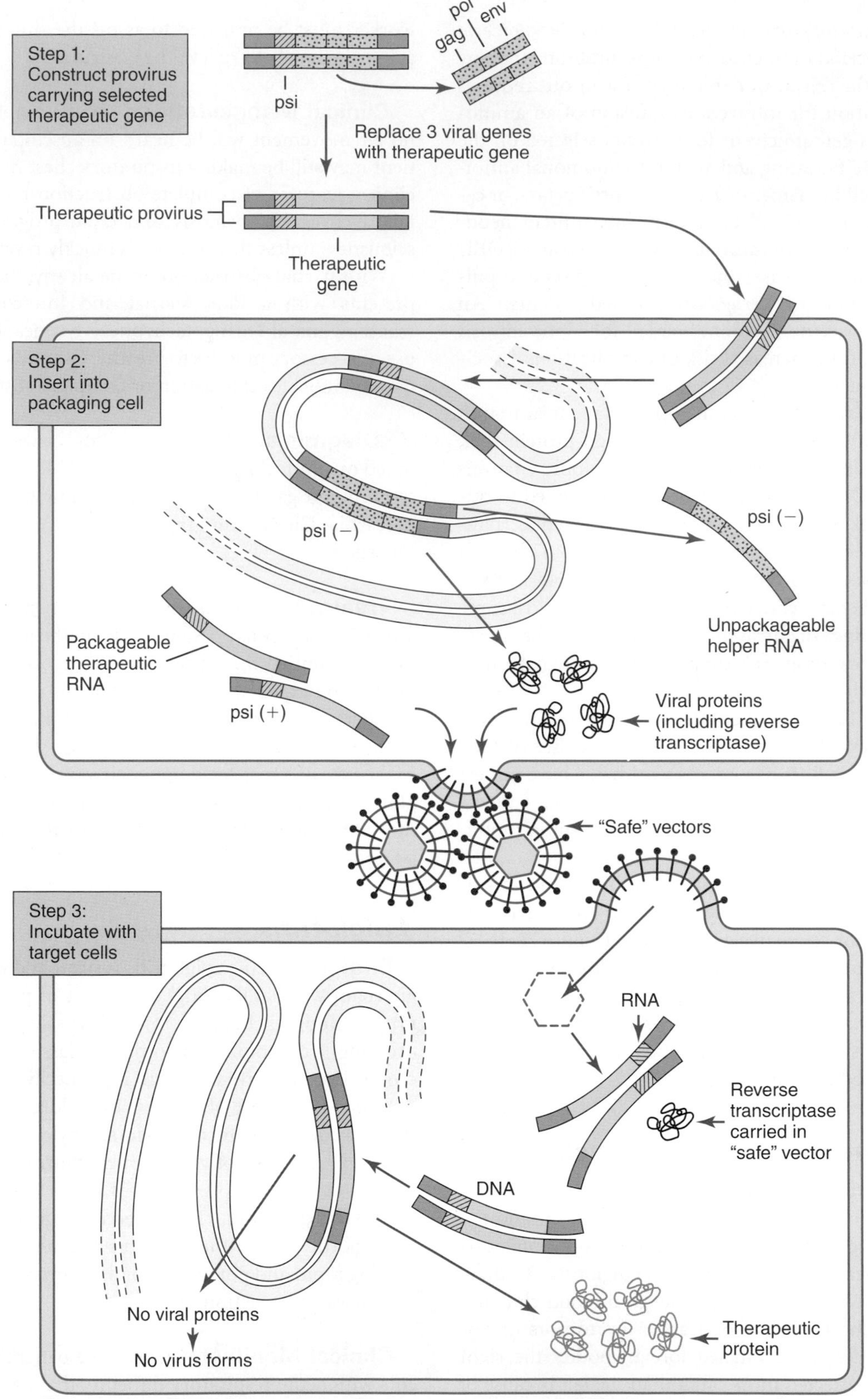

FIGURE 22-16 ■ Gene therapy may use retroviral vectors to deliver therapeutic genes. Viruses are made in which viral genes *(gag, pol,* and *env)* are removed and a therapeutic gene is substituted. The virus is then inserted into a packaging cell. Here the "therapeutic virus" is helped to replicate and repackage with the aid of a "helper" virus, which supplies the missing viral protein products to the therapeutic virus. The particles that escape the cell then carry therapeutic RNA and no viral genes. They can enter other cells and splice the therapeutic gene in the cellular DNA, but they cannot reproduce.

Diagnosis. Definitive diagnosis is obtained by direct or fiberoptic visualization of the epiglottis. Lateral neck radio graphs assist in making a definitive diagnosis and reveal a classic "thumbprint sign" (swollen epiglottis that looks like a thumbprint). A complete blood count may reveal leukocytosis with a shift to the left.[36]

Treatment. This condition is a true medical emergency and may necessitate intubation. Antibiotic therapy with ampicillin/sulbactam (Unasyn) or ceftriaxone (Rocephin) should be started immediately. Preventive treatment with the Hib vaccine is the key to decreasing the incidence of this disease.

Croup Syndrome

Etiology. Croup syndrome describes a number of acute viral inflammatory diseases of the larynx. Croup diseases include laryngotracheobronchitis (viral croup), epiglottitis (discussed previously), and bacterial tracheitis. Viral croup affects the larynx, trachea, and bronchi. It is often caused by parainfluenza virus type 1. Other potential infecting organisms include parainfluenza types 2 and 3, RSV, influenza virus, adenovirus, and *Mycoplasma pneumoniae.*[22] Croup usually occurs in the fall and early winter, affecting children aged 6 months to 3 years.[37]

Pathogenesis. The infectious agent causes inflammation along the entire airway, leading to edema formation in the subglottic area.[1]

Clinical Manifestations. The child presents with a history of upper respiratory infection or cold that has developed into a barking cough with stridor. Fever is low grade or absent. In severe cases the child may present with stridor at rest, retractions, and cyanosis.

Diagnosis. Diagnosis is based on clinical manifestations and lateral neck films to rule out epiglottitis. Direct laryngoscopy is also used to confirm the presence of epiglottitis because the clinical presentation is similar to that of croup. Lateral neck radiographs show subglottic narrowing and a normal epiglottis. The classic steeple sign associated with viral croup shows narrowing below the vocal cords.[22,37]

Treatment. Supportive treatment is used for viral croup. Mist therapy, oral hydration, and avoidance of stimulation are used in outpatient therapy. Hospitalized children are managed with oxygen therapy and pulse oximetry. Nebulized epinephrine is effective in relieving airway obstruction. Endotracheal intubation may be required for children with respiratory failure.

KEY CONCEPTS

- Obstructive disorders are associated with increased resistance to airflow.
- Bronchiectasis is associated with recurrent inflammation of the bronchial walls, chronic cough, and aneurysm-like dilatations of the bronchioles. These bronchiolar dilatations serve as pockets of infection, producing purulent, foul-smelling sputum. Treatment centers on antibiotic therapy and removal of secretions.
- Bronchiolitis refers to widespread bronchiolar inflammation, often associated with smoking and a number of infectious agents. Inflammation results in mucosal swelling, excessive mucus production, and bronchial muscle constriction—all of which narrow the airway lumen and may lead to wheezing and dyspnea. Treatment centers on bronchodilating agents and management of the underlying cause.
- Cystic fibrosis is an autosomal recessive disorder of exocrine glands and mucus cells. Secretions are excessively thick because of insufficient chloride and water transport. Thick secretions cause airway obstruction, atelectasis, and air trapping. Associated symptoms resulting from dysfunction of the exocrine pancreas are apparent. Treatment centers on removal of secretions and providing antibiotic therapy for complicating respiratory infections.
- Obstruction of the trachea or large bronchi may occur acutely, requiring immediate treatment. Usual causes include foreign body aspiration, trauma, and inflammation. With complete obstruction, no movement of air occurs, even though inspiratory efforts may be observed. Partial airway obstruction is associated with wheezing, retractions, and stridor. Treatment centers on removing the obstruction, if possible, or creating a patent airway by a tracheostomy.
- Epiglottitis is a medical emergency. *Haemophilus influenzae* type B, the primary organism associated with epiglottitis, invades the supraglottic structures (epiglottis and arytenoids), causing inflammation and edema, leading to obstruction. Key points in the clinical diagnosis are rapid onset of fever, pain and difficulty swallowing, and drooling. Lateral neck x-ray films reveal a classic thumbprint sign, which is indicative of epiglottal swelling. Airway maintenance via endotracheal intubation or tracheostomy with antibiotic therapy is the primary mode of treatment. The Hib vaccine has greatly decreased the number of cases seen in the pediatric population.
- Croup is a viral infection of the subglottic area. Children aged 6 months to 3 years present with cough and stridor following an upper respiratory infection. Humidification, oxygenation, and inhaled epinephrine are the primary treatment modalities.

DIAGNOSTIC TESTS
Pulmonary Function Testing

The primary criterion in diagnosing COPD is the demonstration of obstruction to airflow in the lungs. This may be

Table 22-6

Common Ventilatory Parameters Measured by Spirometry

Parameter	Definition
Tidal volume	Volume of air inspired and expired with a normal breath (400-500 ml or 5 ml/kg of body weight
Residual volume	Volume of gas left in lung after maximal expiration; stabilizes alveoli
Vital capacity or forced vital capacity	Maximal air that can be expired after a maximal inspiratory effort; includes inspiratory reserve volume, tidal volume, and expiratory reserve volume
Functional residual capacity	Volume of air left in lungs after a normal expiration; includes expiratory reserve volume and residual volume
Forced expiratory flow rate (FEF_{25}, FEF_{50}, FEF_{75})	Volume of air forcibly exhaled per unit time (liters per second or liters per minute) at 25%, 50%, and 75% of the FVC
Peak expiratory flow rate	Highest rate of flow sustained for 10 msec or more at which air can be expelled from the lungs

See Figure 21-10 for normal values.

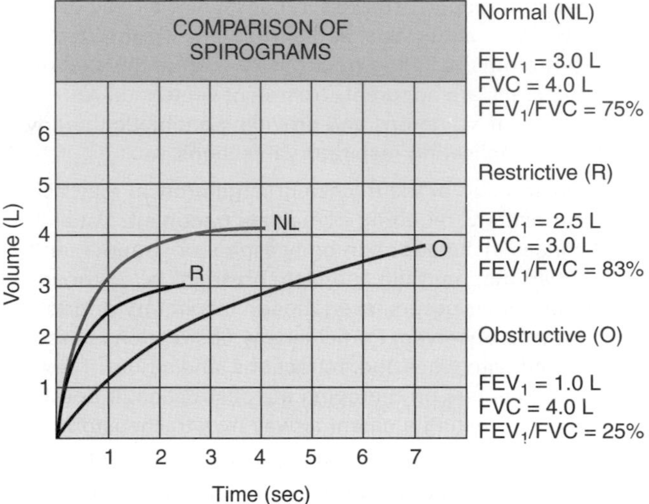

FIGURE 22-17 ■ Comparison of spirograms for normal lungs, restrictive lung disease, and obstructive lung disease. *FEV_1*, Forced expiratory volume in 1 second; *FVC*, forced vital capacity.

determined in a number of ways, but the most commonly used approach is spirometry. Table 22-6 lists common ventilatory parameters referred to in spirometry.

Spirometry is performed by asking the patient to inhale deeply and then to exhale as quickly as possible until maximal air is exhaled. The total volume of air exhaled is known as the forced vital capacity. To determine flow, the time required for exhaling the air is also measured. The volume exhaled in the first second is a reliable and reproducible index of obstructive airway disease. This value is the *forced expiratory volume in 1 second*. Figure 22-17 presents spirogram examples of normal, obstructive, and restrictive graphs for FEV_1 and FVC. For all spirometric studies, normal values are based on large population studies of healthy volunteers and are adjusted for height, weight, age, and gender data that are available for comparison.

A simple formula has been developed to define and quantify airflow obstruction. If the FEV_1/FVC ratio is 75% or greater, no significant obstruction of airflow is present. If the value obtained is between 60% and 70%, then mild obstruction of airflow is present. Moderate obstruction is defined as a value of 50% to 60%; and severe obstruction is present when the FEV_1/FVC ratio is less than 50%. Therefore, using a spirometer and measuring both volume and time, the diagnosis of chronic obstructive pulmonary disease can be made and the severity quantified.

From the spirometric ventilatory measurements (see Table 22-6), other determinations of airflow can be made from the middle to later parts of a FVC maneuver. These measures are helpful in determining the presence of small airway disease. Some investigators believe that small airway disease may be a precursor to the development of chronic bronchitis and emphysema.[1,20]

Frequently, an inhaled bronchodilator, such as albuterol or metaproterenol, may be given, with testing repeated in 15 to 20 minutes. If the FEV_1 improves by 15% or more, the patient is considered to have a positive bronchodilator response, indicative of partially reversible bronchospasm of the smooth muscles of the airways. This is most often the case with asthma or asthmatic bronchitis.

A second pulmonary function test known as the *diffusion capacity* measures the ability of the alveolar gases to diffuse into the capillary blood. The technical details of this test are beyond the scope of this book, but it is a valuable test for determining either thickening (fibrosis) of the alveolocapillary membrane or destruction (emphysema) of the membrane.

By breathing mixtures of an inert gas, such as helium, the TLC can be determined. This volume is composed of the FVC and the RV. The RV is the volume of air that remains in the lung after a person has voluntarily exhaled all of the air from the lungs (see Figure 21-10). RV/TLC is normally 30% to 35%. In some patients with airflow obstruction, air tends to

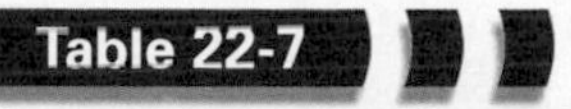

Table 22-7

Normal Arterial Blood Gas Values

Parameter	Adult*	Pregnancy	Newborn	COPD (Late Findings)
PaO_2 (mm Hg)	80-100	75-100	60-70	Decreased
$PaCO_2$ (mm Hg)	34-45	30-37	35-45	Increased
pH	7.35-7.45	7.35-7.45	7.30-7.40	Decreased
HCO_3^- (mEq/L)	24-30	20-26	20-26	Increased
Base excess (mEq/L)	±2	—	—	—
O_2 saturation (%)	96-100	95-100	90-100	Decreased

COPD, Chronic obstructive pulmonary disease.
*For elderly, PaO_2 can be estimated by the following formulas[24]: 104 − (patient's age × 0.42) for patients lying supine; and 104 − (patient's age × 0.27) for patients sitting.

get trapped in the lungs, thereby increasing the RV and resulting in overinflation of lung tissue.

Arterial blood gases are also useful as a pulmonary function measurement. Using these values, a careful assessment of both the oxygenation and the acid-base status can be determined. The normal pH is 7.40, the normal $PaCO_2$ is 40 mm Hg, and the normal PaO_2, at sea level, is 80 to 100 mm Hg. In COPD, especially in severe stage, PaO_2 falls and $PaCO_2$ rises. Table 22-7 lists normal arterial blood gas values for various groups. A thorough discussion of arterial blood gas analysis can be found in Chapter 25.

Bronchial Provocation Tests

The controlled induction of bronchospasm by inhalation of various agents is occasionally used to identify patients with hyperreactive airways and to prove whether certain inhaled substances can produce bronchospasm. Usually a series of inhalations is administered, followed by a series of ventilation measurements. Generally the test is stopped when the FEV_1 falls at least 20% more than the control measurement. This should only be done where emergency support services are available. Bronchoprovocation is contraindicated if the patient is already exhibiting symptoms or requires continual asthma medication. Allergens can be administered as solutions, dusts, or fumes. The amount administered should be no more than the patient would normally encounter in the environment. If symptoms occur, they can be readily reversed by two to four inhalations of albuterol or metaproterenol.

General hyperreactivity of the bronchi can be detected by having the patient inhale histamine phosphate solutions or methacholine (related to acetylcholine) or nebulized distilled water. A fall of more than 20% in the FEV_1 is indicative of hyperreactivity.

KEY CONCEPTS

Obstructive disorders are associated with characteristic abnormalities on pulmonary function testing. These include

- Decreased FEV_1
- Low FEV_1/FVC ratio (<70%)
- Improvement in FEV_1 after use of a bronchodilator
- Increased residual volume
- Increased functional residual capacity

SUMMARY

Health care professionals have a key role in the management of respiratory disorders in the hospital and in the community. Obstructive pulmonary diseases presented in this chapter include airway obstruction, obstruction from conditions affecting the tracheobronchial walls, and loss of lung parenchyma (emphysema). Obstructive pulmonary disorders are characterized by increased resistance to airflow. With bronchiectasis, obstruction is due to inflammation, infection, and dilation of the bronchioles. Similarly, bronchiolitis is associated with inflammation; however, in this situation, inflammation leads to mucosal edema and excessive mucus production. Airway obstruction from cystic fibrosis is related to production of excessive, thick secretions. Obstruction of the airway in croup is the result of edema and increased secretions caused by viral infection. Similarly, epiglottitis is an infectious process requiring emergency treatment. The primary organism causing epiglottitis is *H. influenzae.* The incidence of epiglottitis has been greatly reduced with the advent of the Hib vaccine.

An inflammatory process is also seen in asthma and bronchitis. The inflammation is associated with increased mucus production and edema of the tracheal bronchial mucosa in asthma and bronchitis. Bronchospasm of the tracheobronchial tree due to exposure to allergens, pulmonary irritants, stress, and exercise may result in hypoxemia. Obstruction to airflow in emphysema is due to loss of alveoli and small airways. The most common cause is cigarette smoking.

MEDIA RESOURCES

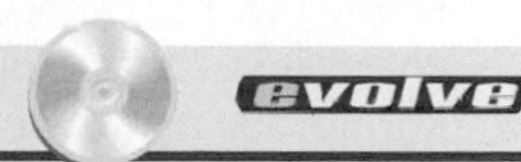

Remember to check out the ***CD Companion*** included with this book for Review Questions, Key Concepts Review, Glossary (with audio for selected terms), Disease Profiles, and Animations.

PLUS, visit the ***Evolve website*** at http://evolve.elsevier.com/Copstead/ for Case Studies, Disease Profiles, and WebLinks.

References

1. West JB: *Pulmonary pathophysiology: the essentials,* ed 5, Philadelphia, 1998, Lippincott Williams & Wilkins.
2. *National Asthma Education and Prevention Program Expert Panel Report II Guidelines for Diagnosis and Management of Asthma,* Washington, DC, 1997, US Department of Health and Human Services.
3. Vura-Weis DE: Allergies and asthma. In Sloane PD, Slatt LM et al, editors: *Essentials of family medicine,* ed 4, Philadelphia, 2002, Lippincott Williams & Wilkins, pp 301-325.
4. Brooks AM: Asthma. In Garfunkel LC, Kaczorowski J, Christy C, editors: *Mosby's pediatric clinical advisor: instant diagnosis and treatment,* St Louis, 2002, Mosby, pp 171-173.
5. Kowai K, Dubuske L: Asthma in adolescents and adults. In Rakel RE, Bope ET, editors: *Conn's current therapy, 2003,* Philadelphia, 2003, Saunders, pp 814-820.
6. Lester MR: Asthma in children. In Rakel RE, Bope ET, editors: *Conn's current therapy 2003,* Philadelphia, 2003, Saunders, pp 821-828.
7. Ferri FF: In Ferri FF, editor: *Ferri's clinical advisor: instant diagnosis and treatment,* St Louis, 2003, Mosby, pp 155, 156, 256.
8. Chesnutt MS, Prendergast TJ: Lung. In Tierney LM, McPhee SJ, Papdakis MA, editors: *Current medical diagnosis and treatment,* ed 42, New York, 2003, Lange/McGraw-Hill, pp 216-311.
9. Goroll AH, Mulley AG: Management of asthma. In Goroll AH, Mulley AG, editors: *Primary care medicine: office evaluation and management of the adult patient,* ed 3, Philadelphia, 2000, Lippincott Williams & Wilkins, pp 304-316.
10. Schneider DT: Allergic disorders and immunodeficiency. In Graef JW, editor: *Manual of pediatric therapeutics,* ed 6, Philadelphia, 1997, Lippincott-Raven.
11. Hogg JC: The pathophysiology of asthma, *Chest* 82:8s-11s, 1982.
12. Guyton AC, Hall JE: *Textbook of medical physiology,* ed 10, Philadelphia, 2000, Saunders, p 489.
13. Corwin RW: Wheezing. In Green HL, Glassock RJ, Kelley MA, editors. *Introduction to clinical medicine,* Philadelphia, 1991, BC Decker, pp 488-490.
14. Williams PV: Management of asthma, *Clin Symp* 49(3):2-32, 1997.
15. Jaskiewicz J: Cystic Fibrosis. In Garfunkel LC, Kaczorowski J, Christy C, editors: *Mosby's pediatric clinical advisor: instant diagnosis and treatment,* St Louis, 2002, Mosby, 2002, pp 263-264.
16. Boguniewicz M, Leung DYM: Allergic disorders. In Hay WW et al, editors: *Current pediatric diagnosis and treatment*, ed 15, New York, 2001, Lange/McGraw-Hill, pp 939-964.
17. Mainous AG, Hueston WJ: Acute respiratory infections. In Sloane PD et al, editors: *Essentials of family medicine*, ed 4, Philadelphia, 2002, Lippincott Williams & Wilkins, pp 259-276.
18. Kormis WA: Approach to the patient with acute bronchitis or pneumonia in the ambulatory setting. In Goroll AH, Mulley AG, editors: *Primary care medicine: office evaluation and management of the adult patient*, ed 4, Philadelphia, 2000, Lippincott Williams & Wilkins, pp 333-342.
19. Weiss EF: Clubbing. In Greene HL et al, editors: *Clinical medicine,* ed 2, St Louis, 1996, Mosby, pp 563-566.
20. Goroll AJ, Mulley AG: Management of chronic obstructive pulmonary disease. In Goroll AH, May LA, Mulley AG, editors: *Primary care medicine: office evaluation and management of the adult patient,* ed 4, Philadelphia, 2000, Lippincott Williams & Wilkins, pp 243-303.
21. Bonditt JO: Management of chronic obstructive pulmonary disease. In Rakel RE, Bope ET, editors: *Conn's current therapy, 2003,* Philadelphia, 2003, Saunders, pp 223-226.
22. Larson GL et al: Respiratory tract and mediastinum. In Hay WW et al, editors: *Current pediatric diagnosis and treatment,* New York, 2001, Lange/McGraw-Hill, pp 428-475.
23. National Center for Health Statistics: Chronic obstructive pulmonary disease (COPD), website, www.cdc.gov/nchs/fastats/copd.htm, January 2003.
24. Resnick NM: Geriatric medicine. In Tierney LM, McPhee SJ, Papadalos MA, editors: *Current medical diagnosis and treatment,* ed 37, Norwalk, Conn, 1997, Appleton & Lange, pp 48-68.
25. Cystic Fibrosis Foundation, 6931 Arlington Rd, Suite 2000, Bethesda, MD 20814; 800-344-4823, www.cff.org.
26. Behrman RE, Kliegman RM, Jenson HB: *Pocket companion to accompany Nelson textbook of pediatrics,* ed 16, Philadelphia, 2001, Saunders, pp 505-506.
27. Shandera WX, Shelburne S: Infectious diseases: viral and rickettsial. In Tierney LM, McPhee SJ, Papadakis MA, editors: *Current medical diagnosis and treatment,* ed 42, New York, 2003, Lange/McGraw-Hill, pp 1303-1395.
28. Chen S: Respiratory syncytial virus/bronchiolitis. In Garfunkel LC, Kaczorowski J, Christy C, editors: *Mosby's pediatric clinical advisor: instant diagnosis and treatment,* St Louis, 2002, Mosby, pp 635-636.
29. Froh DK: Cystic fibrosis. In Rakel RE, Bope ET, editors: *Conn's current therapy, 2003,* Philadelphia, 2003, Saunders, pp 227-229.
30. Snyder JD: Gastroenterology. In Graef JW, editor: *Manual of pediatric therapeutics,* ed 6, Philadelphia, 1997, Lippincott-Raven, pp 253-284.
31. Paranjothi S, Schuller D: Pulmonary diseases. In Ahya SN, Flood K, Paranjothi S, editors: *Washington manual of medical therapeutics,* ed 30, Philadelphia, 2001, Lippincott Williams & Wilkins, pp 216-240.
32. Heisig DG, Threatte GA, Henry JB: Laboratory diagnosis of gastrointestinal and pancreatic disorders. In Henry JB, editor: *Clinical diagnosis and management by laboratory methods,* ed 20, Philadelphia, 2001, Saunders, pp 462-478.
33. Yusen RD, Lefrak SS: Pulmonary II: Diseases. In Lin TL, Rypkema SW, editors: *The Washington manual of ambulatory therapeutics,* ed 31, Philadelphia, 2002, Lippincott Williams & Wilkins, pp 202-226.
34. Wilmott RW, Fiedler MA: Recent advances in the treatment of cystic fibrosis, *Pediatr Clin North Am* 4(3):431-451, 1994.
35. Rosenfeld MA et al: In vivo gene transfer of the human cystic fibrosis transmembrane conductance regulator gene to the airway epithelium, *Cell* 68:143-155, 1992.
36. Lieber JJ: Epiglottitis. In Ferri FF, editor: *Ferri's clinical advisor: instant diagnosis and treatment,* St Louis, 2003, Mosby, pp 310-311.
37. Jackson MA, Vahle H: Croup. In Garfunkel LC, Kaczorowski J, Christy C, editors: *Mosby's pediatric clinical advisor: instant diagnosis and treatment,* St Louis, 2002, Mosby, pp 259-260.

Restrictive Pulmonary Disorders

chapter 23

Lorna Schumann

MEDIA RESOURCES

Additional Material for Study, Review, and Further Exploration

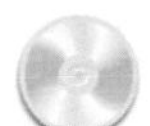

CD Companion ◆ Review Questions and Answers ◆ Key Concepts Review
◆ Glossary *(with audio pronunciations for selected terms)*
◆ Disease Profiles ◆ Animations

evolve ***Website*** at http://evolve.elsevier.com/Copstead/
◆ Case Studies ◆ Disease Profiles ◆ WebLinks

KEY QUESTIONS

- How do fibrotic lung disorders develop?
- How is the pathogenesis of acute (adult) respiratory distress syndrome similar to that of infant respiratory distress syndrome?
- How do abnormal accumulations in the pleural space affect lung function?
- What neuromuscular disorders are associated with reduced lung compliance?
- How is pulmonary tuberculosis detected and managed?
- What pulmonary function test abnormalities are characteristic of restrictive pulmonary disorders?

CHAPTER OUTLINE

Restrictive pulmonary diseases are the result of decreased expansion of the lungs due to alterations in the lung parenchyma, pleura, chest wall, or neuromuscular apparatus. These disorders may be classified as pulmonary or extrapulmonary and represent acute or chronic patterns of lung dysfunction rather than a single clinical disease. Table 23-1 lists the various disease processes that can be classified as restrictive. These diseases are characterized by a decrease in total lung capacity (TLC), vital capacity (VC), functional residual capacity (FRC), and residual volume (RV). The greater the decrease in lung volume, the greater the severity of the disease.[1] Blood gas analysis often shows decreased arterial partial pressure of oxygen (PaO_2) and normal or decreased arterial partial pressure of carbon dioxide ($PaCO_2$).

Table 23-1

Restrictive Pulmonary Disorders

Disorder Type	Representative Examples
Diseases of the Lung Parenchyma	
Neoplastic disease	—
Pneumonia	Pneumonia (viral, bacterial, fungal), hypersensitivity pneumonitis
Granulomatous disease	Sarcoidosis, tuberculosis, coccidioidomycosis, blastomycosis
Pneumoconioses	Occupational lung disease
Acute interstitial pneumonitis	—
Collagen disease	Rheumatoid arthritis, scleroderma, systemic lupus erythematosus
Atelectasis	—
Pulmonary resection	—
Vascular diseases	Pulmonary edema, pulmonary embolism
Acute respiratory distress syndrome	—
Diseases of Extrapulmonary Restriction	
Chest wall disease	Kyphoscoliosis, ankylosing spondylitis, obesity
Neuromuscular disease	Quadriplegia, hemiplegia, Guillain-Barré syndrome, myasthenia gravis, amyotrophic lateral sclerosis, muscular dystrophy
Pleural diseases	Pleural effusion, hemothorax, pneumothorax, chylothorax
Other	Abdominal distention, surgery, pregnancy

This chapter presents information related to restrictive pulmonary diseases, including lung parenchyma disorders, pleural space disorders, neuromuscular and chest wall disorders, pneumonia, and tuberculosis. Lung parenchyma disorders including interstitial fibrosis, sarcoidosis, hypersensitivity pneumonitis, and pneumoconiosis, as well as atelectatic disorders, including acute (adult) respiratory distress syndrome (ARDS) and infant respiratory disease syndrome (IRDS), are presented. Pleural space disorders, divided into pneumothorax and pleural effusions, are discussed. The section on neuromuscular and chest wall disorders is divided into neuromuscular weakness, chest wall deformities, and obesity. The final section presents the etiologic factors, pathogenesis, clinical manifestations, diagnosis, and management of pneumonia, tuberculosis, and severe acute respiratory syndrome (SARS). Table 23-2 describes variations in respiratory parameters that affect restrictive lung disease in infant and elderly populations.

LUNG PARENCHYMA DISORDERS

FIBROTIC INTERSTITIAL LUNG DISEASES

The term *interstitial lung disease* describes a group of disorders (more than 180 disease entities) that are characterized by acute, subacute, or chronic infiltration of alveolar walls by cells, fluid, and connective tissue.[1-4] If left untreated, the inflammatory process may progress to irreversible fibrosis.[4] The

Table 23-2

Age-Related Features Contributing to Restrictive Lung Disease

Anatomic Site	Impact on Restrictive Disease
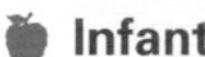 **Infant**	
Sternum and ribs are cartilaginous with soft chest wall	Diminishes effect of restrictive disease in infants
Ribs are horizontally oriented so that ribs move in and out easily	Diminishes effect of restrictive disease in infants
Accessory muscles of respiration are poorly developed	Majority of respiratory movement relies on diaphragm; restrictive diseases that compromise diaphragmatic excursion affect respiratory status; e.g., thoracic or abdominal surgery, paralysis, and abdominal masses all affect diaphragmatic excursion
Diaphragm rests horizontally and draws lower ribs inward in supine position so that diaphragmatic excursion is decreased	Leads to compromised effort of breathing
Cartilage of infant larynx is soft, so airway is compressed when neck is flexed or hyperextended	Increases airway resistance
During first month of life neonate is obligate nose breather	Nasal obstruction may lead to respiratory distress from decreased airflow
Small diameter of airway leads to increased resistance to airflow	Mucus or edema in the airway may lead to significant increase in resistance and a decrease in airway diameter
Fewer alveoli than in adults, leading to decreased radial traction applied to the airways	Increased tendency of airways to collapse
Pores of Kohn and channels of Lambert are underdeveloped, leading to fewer collateral ventilation pathways	May lead to respiratory compromise, reducing ventilatory support with restrictive diseases
Elderly	
Decreased ciliary activity	Increased incidence of infection; decreased mucus clearance in all types of respiratory disorders
Decreased chest wall compliance and decreased lung elasticity in some areas of the lung	Leads to a reduction in lung volume; leads to decreased expansion of the lungs and to decreased matching of ventilation and perfusion
Decreased stress tolerance	Increased incidence of disease and trauma with age
Decreased muscle tone	Decreased physical conditioning
Impaired immunity as evidenced by decreased T-cell function; increased autoantibodies	Decreased resistance to infection
Decreased oxygen uptake	Decreased oxygen level in the blood
Decreased vital capacity	Decreased alveolar expansion
Decreased cough reflex	Impaired ability to clear secretions and inhaled particulate matter

incidence of interstitial lung disease is 5 cases per 100,000 persons.[3]

Diffuse Interstitial Lung Disease

Etiology. Diffuse interstitial lung disease (also known as diffuse interstitial pulmonary fibrosis) is the name typically used for restrictive diseases characterized by thickening of the alveolar interstitium.[2] Synonyms frequently presented in the literature include interstitial pneumonia, diffuse parenchymal lung disease, Hamman-Rich syndrome, intrinsic fibrosing alveolitis, cryptogenic fibrosing alveolitis, and idiopathic pulmonary fibrosis. Pathogenesis of the disease is not well understood but is probably related to an immune reaction that usually begins with injury to the alveolar epithelial or capillary endothelial cells.[1,2]

Pathogenesis. Pathophysiologic changes include interstitial and alveolar wall thickening and increased collagen bundles in the interstitium (Figure 23-1). Lung tissue becomes infiltrated by lymphocytes, macrophages, and plasma cells. Persistent alveolitis may lead to obliteration of alveolar capillaries, reorganization of the lung parenchyma and irreversible fibrosis.[2] These changes in turn lead to large air-filled sacs (cysts) accompanied by dilated terminal and respiratory bronchioles.

The immune response noted in interstitial lung disease is characterized by three pathologic patterns in the alveoli: inflammation, fibrosis, and destruction.

The inflammatory pattern occurs early and is potentially reversible.[4,5] The triggering event (e.g., occupational exposure, drug ingestion, connective tissue disease) causes an inflammatory response leading to increased numbers of inflammatory cells (i.e., neutrophils, lymphocytes, macrophages).[1,2,4] An associated injury to the alveolar capillary basement membrane from the triggering event leads to increased membrane permeability and movement of fluid and debris into the alveoli. The initial injury, in association with the inflammatory pattern, leads to fibroblastic proliferation and deposition of large amounts of collagen. The fibrotic pattern is manifested

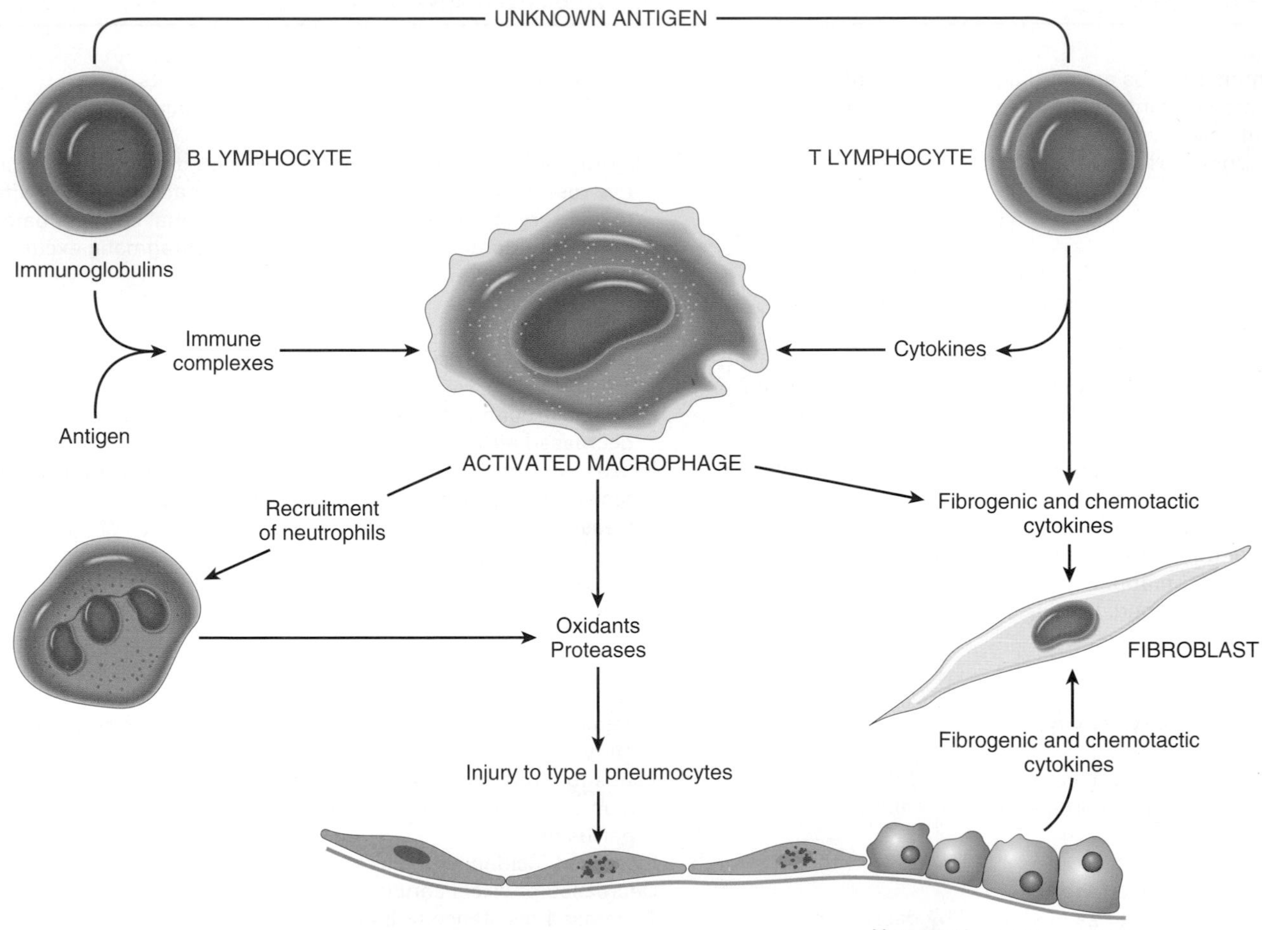

FIGURE 23-1 ■ Possible schema of the pathogenesis of idiopathic pulmonary fibrosis. (From Kumar V, Cotran RS, Robbins SL: *Basic pathology,* ed 7, Philadelphia, 2003, Saunders, p 469.)

by increases in mesenchymal cells and fibroblasts in the interstitium, and alveolar walls become thickened with increased amounts of fibrous tissue.[5-7]

The lung destruction pattern is manifested by loss of alveolar walls. Radiographically, this appears as a "honeycomb lung" and indicates end-stage disease.[2] Ground-glass appearance on chest radiograph is often an early finding.[3] The fibrotic and honeycomb patterns respond poorly to treatment.[5]

Clinical Manifestations. The most common patient complaint is progressive dyspnea with nonproductive cough.[3,5] Clinical features include rapid, shallow breathing; dyspnea; irritating, nonproductive cough; clubbing of the nail beds (40% to 80% cases)[4]; bibasilar end-expiratory[3,4] crackles (Velcro rales); and marked dyspnea with exercise. Cyanosis is a late finding. Anorexia and weight loss are noted on physical assessment. As the disease progresses, patients exhibit inability to increase cardiac output with exercise as evidenced by low maximal heart rate and high peripheral vascular resistance. Arterial oxygen desaturation occurs with exercise.[4]

Diagnosis. The chest radiograph shows a honeycomb appearance and a coarse reticular pattern indicating late stage of disease.[2,3,5-7] Ground-glass haziness is indicative of the presence of infiltrates. Open lung biopsy or transbronchial biopsy, gallium 67 scanning, and bronchoalveolar lavage may be used for diagnostic evaluation.[3] Pulmonary function testing findings are usually consistent with restrictive lung disease (decreased vital capacity, total lung capacity, and diffusing capacity).[3]

Treatment. The patient should be encouraged to avoid tobacco use and environmental exposure to the offending cause.[2-4] Primary therapy consists of administration of corticosteroids. Cyclophosphamide (Cytoxan, Neosar) and azathioprine (Imuran) are of questionable benefit, with only 20% of the sample population showing improvement.[1,2] However, these drugs have been useful in reducing the dosage of corticosteroids. Lung transplantation has been used successfully in selected patients.[3,5-7]

Sarcoidosis

Etiology. Sarcoidosis is categorized as an acute or chronic systemic disease of unknown cause, although an immunologic basis appears likely.[1] Activation of the alveolar macrophage due to an unknown antigen trigger is a possible cause.[1] The acute process occurs more commonly in women in the second or third decade of life.[1,2] The chronic form is seen more commonly in the third to fourth decades of life, with the highest incidence seen in North American blacks and northern European whites.[2]

Pathogenesis. The disease is characterized by the development of multiple, uniform, noncaseating epithelioid **granulomas** that affect multiple organ systems, most commonly the lymph nodes and lung tissue. The noncaseating granulomas are fibrotic and are surrounded by large histiocytes.[1,2,8] Sarcoid granulomas may also occur in the bronchial airways. Abnormal T-cell function is noted with this disease.[7] Other systems and/or organs frequently involved are the skin, eyes, spleen, liver, kidney, and bone marrow.[1,8]

Clinical Manifestations. Sarcoidosis is characterized by malaise, fatigue, weight loss, fever, dyspnea of insidious onset, and a dry, nonproductive cough.[2,8] Other features include erythema nodosum (lesions marked by the formation of painful nodes on the lower extremities); macules, papules, and subcutaneous nodules; hepatosplenomegaly; and lymphadenopathy. Patients with the acute disease usually present with enlarged lymph nodes and arthritis, although some patients experience no symptoms.[7] Skin lesions and lacrimal and parotid gland involvement are also noted in the acute process.[1] Iritis, uveitis, blurred vision, conjunctivitis, and ocular discomfort may develop.[8]

Diagnosis. Common laboratory findings in patients with sarcoidosis include leukopenia, anemia, increased eosinophil count, elevated sedimentation rate, and increased calcium levels (seen in 5% of patients).[2,8] Serum levels of liver enzymes may also be elevated. Approximately 70% of patients exhibit anergy (decreased sensitivity to specific antigens such as *Trichophyton*, *Candida*, mumps virus, and tuberculin).[2] Patients with active disease also demonstrate elevated levels of angiotensin-converting enzyme (40% to 80% of cases).[2]

Chest radiographs can be used to differentiate stages of the disease process: stage 0, normal; stage I, hilar adenopathy alone; stage II, hilar adenopathy and bilateral pulmonary infiltrates; and stage III, pulmonary infiltrates without adenopathy. Stage IV is characterized by advanced fibrosis with evidence of honeycombing, hilar retraction, bullae, cysts, and emphysema.[8] Pleural effusion is noted in 10% of cases of sarcoidosis.[1,2,8] Pulmonary function test results may be normal or may show evidence of restrictive disease and/or obstructive disease.[8]

Transbronchial lung biopsy demonstrates noncaseating granulomas, thus providing a definitive diagnosis (75% to 90% cases). Bronchoalveolar lavage may be used to monitor cell content in patients with sarcoidosis.[1,8] The lavage fluid is characterized by increased lymphocytes and a high CD4/CD8 cell ratio.[2]

Treatment. Administration of corticosteroids and management of symptoms is the mainstay of treatment for patients whose disease process does not resolve spontaneously and in whom progressive lung disease or evidence of extrapulmonary sarcoidosis develops. For patients with progressive disease that does not respond to corticosteroids, methotrexate or azathioprine may be used.[8] The prognosis is best for stage I disease. Death due to pulmonary insufficiency occurs in about 5% to 7% of patients.[2,8]

Table 23-3
Causes of Hypersensitivity Pneumonitis

Disease	Antigen	Allergen Source
Farmer's lung	*Thermophilia, Actinomyces*	Moldy hay, silage
Bird fancier's lung	Parakeet, pigeon, chicken	Bird excreta, feathers, and animal protein
Bagassosis	Thermophilic bacteria	Moldy sugarcane pulp
Mushroom, cork, maple bark, or malt hypersensitivity, cheese maker's lung, redwood lung	Various fungi	Handling moldy products
Grain handler's lung	Wheat weevil	Insect-infected grain
Pituitary extract hypersensitivity	Heterologous pituitary and serum proteins	—
Fish-meat worker's lung	Protein, fungi	Animal food
Humidifier lung (fever)	Thermophilic bacteria, amoebae, and fungi	Humidifiers and evaporative air coolers

Hypersensitivity Pneumonitis

Etiology. Hypersensitivity pneumonitis, also called *extrinsic allergic alveolitis,* is classified as both a restrictive disease and an occupational disease. Numerous inhaled organic dusts are responsible for the inflammatory process.[9] Table 23-3 lists various allergens related to the disease. Unlike other pulmonary diseases, hypersensitivity pneumonitis has a predominance in nonsmokers (80% to 95% of cases).[9]

Pathogenesis. The causative dust is suggested by the patient's history and confirmed by demonstration of precipitating antibodies in the serum directed to the causative antigen. The causative antigen combines with the serum antibody in the alveolar walls, leading to a type III hypersensitivity reaction. Type III hypersensitivity diseases are caused by the formation of antigen-antibody complexes[1,7] (see Chapter 10). These antigen-antibody complexes then elicit the granulomatous inflammation that leads to lung tissue injury, as evidenced by thickened alveolar walls, formation of exudate in the bronchiolar lumen, and infiltration by lymphocytes, plasma cells, and eosinophils.[1,7,10] Fibrotic lung changes occur in advanced cases.

Many individuals develop precipitating antibodies (precipitin) from organic dust exposure, but only a few develop pneumonitis.[10] Experiments in animals show that a delayed hypersensitivity (type IV) reaction to the antigen is also required before pneumonitis can occur.[10]

Clinical Manifestations. In the acute disease, symptoms start 2 to 9 hours after exposure and resolve in 12 to 72 hours.[9] General symptoms may include chills, sweating, shivering, myalgias, nausea, lethargy, headache, and malaise.[1,10,11] The patient may or may not have a fever. Respiratory symptoms may include dyspnea at rest, dry cough, tachypnea, and chest discomfort. Physical findings may include cyanosis (a late sign) and crackles (rales) in the lung bases.[1,3]

In the chronic form, progressive diffuse pulmonary fibrosis develops in the upper lobes—the hallmark of the disease.[1] In the intermediate form, the disease may manifest with acute febrile episodes and progressive fibrosis with cough, dyspnea, fatigue, and, eventually, cor pulmonale (right-sided heart failure due to lung disorders).[9]

Diagnosis. During the acute/subacute phase, transient bilateral pulmonary **infiltrates** or increased bronchial markings with alveolar nodular infiltrates may be found on chest radiographs. In the chronic phase, diffuse reticulonodular infiltrates and fibrosis are present.[10]

Skin testing with the causative antigen may produce a red, indurated, hemorrhagic reaction 4 to 12 hours after injection that lasts several days.[1] This reaction suggests precipitin-mediated sensitivity. Skin testing for most precipitating antigens is impractical because most produce irritating reactions before the precipitin reaction occurs, and many individuals without the disease have precipitating antibodies.

Common laboratory findings include an increased white blood cell count and a decreased PaO_2. Hypoxemia worsens with exercise. Pulmonary function tests show decreased lung volumes, diffusing capacity and compliance.[1,9]

Treatment. The goal of therapy is to identify the offending agent and prevent further exposure. This may require a change in environment or occupation. Oral corticosteroids may be used to decrease the inflammatory process.[9,11]

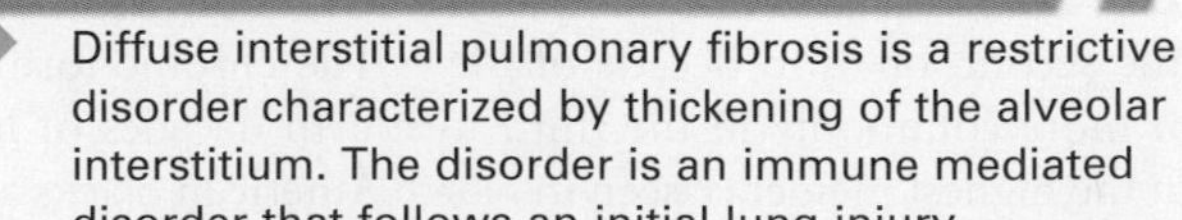
KEY CONCEPTS

- Diffuse interstitial pulmonary fibrosis is a restrictive disorder characterized by thickening of the alveolar interstitium. The disorder is an immune mediated disorder that follows an initial lung injury.
- Lung tissues are characteristically infiltrated by immune cells (macrophages and lymphocytes). Excess fibrin deposition results in stiff, noncompliant lungs. Vital capacity, tidal volume, FRC, and diffusion capac-

Table 23-4

Common Atmospheric Pollutants Contributing to Lung Disease

Pollutant	Source	Clinical Manifestations	Potential Disease Processes
Carbon monoxide	Automobile exhaust (incomplete fossil fuel combustion)	Lethargy, impairs mental skills, cherry-red mucous membranes, headache	Hypoxemia, respiratory failure
Sulfur oxides	Factories (corrosive, poisonous byproducts of combustion of sulfur-containing fuels)	Inflamed mucous membranes, eyes, upper respiratory tract, bronchial mucosa; cough	Pulmonary edema, bronchitis
Photochemical oxidants (ozone, hydrocarbons, or nitrogen oxides)	Byproduct of exposure of hydrocarbons and/or nitrogen oxides (from fossil fuel combustion with high temperatures) to sunlight	Inflammation of eyes and upper respiratory tract; cough	Tracheitis, bronchitis, pulmonary edema
Cigarette smoke	Cigarettes (carbon monoxide, nicotine, "tars")	Impaired exercise tolerance, decreased mental activity, tachycardia, hypertension, sweating	Bronchial carcinoma, chronic bronchitis, emphysema, coronary heart disease
Particulate matter	Factories/power stations; small particles, visible smoke and soot	Cough; dyspnea; itchy, watery eyes; irritated mucous membranes	Bronchitis, tracheitis, asthma

ity are generally reduced. Respiratory rate increases to compensate for the small tidal volume.

- Treatment centers on administration of drugs to depress immune system activity, such as corticosteroids.
- Sarcoidosis is a restrictive disorder associated with abnormal protein deposits (granulomas) in the lung. Granulomas are fibrotic and are associated with immune cells (histiocytes). The cause is unknown.
- Symptoms include progressive dyspnea, fever, enlarged lymph nodes, and generalized symptoms of inflammation. Pulmonary lymph nodes may be primarily affected, with progression to parenchymal involvement. Pulmonary function test results are consistent with a restrictive disorder, demonstrating reduced lung volumes and increased respiratory rate.
- Treatment centers on alleviation or relief of the symptoms. Corticosteroids may be used to reduce inflammation.
- Hypersensitivity pneumonitis includes a group of inflammatory lung disorders associated with inhalation of organic particles. Antibodies are produced in response to the inhaled particles; then antigen-antibody complexes deposit in the lung, initiating inflammation and granuloma production.
- Hypersensitivity pneumonitis is characterized by general symptoms of inflammation (e.g., fever, chills, malaise), dyspnea, dry cough, and tachypnea. Chronic exposure leads to progressive fibrosis and pulmonary dysfunction characteristic of restrictive parenchymal disease.

Occupational Lung Diseases

Etiology. Occupational lung diseases result from the inhalation of toxic gases or foreign particles. Traditionally, occupational lung diseases included pathologic conditions that were associated with the effects of exposure to inhaled dusts. However, a holistic approach to these disease entities requires consideration of atmospheric pollutants as well as natural genetic resistance and compliance with health maintenance behaviors. The distinction between occupational and environmental respiratory diseases is becoming increasingly difficult. The integration of multiple environmental areas (home, work, and leisure) further compounds the complexity of defining occupational respiratory diseases.

Although atmospheric pollutants (toxic gases) are not discussed in detail here, their impact on occupational respiratory diseases must not be minimized. The sources, potential clinical manifestations, and potential pathologic processes associated with common atmospheric pollutants are presented in Table 23-4.

Pneumoconiosis is defined as parenchymal lung disease caused by the inhalation of inorganic dust particles. Commonly, the greater the exposure to the dust, the worse the pathologic consequences. Anthracosis (coal miner's lung or black lung), silicosis (silica inhalation), and asbestosis (asbestos inhalation) are common examples of occupational lung diseases. However, exposure to several other dusts may also impair respiratory function. Included in this list are antimony ore, barium, iron, tin, fuller's earth (clay), kaolin (china clay), and talc.

Many workers are exposed to "pathogenic dust" through their jobs and the processing, packaging, or manufacturing of a specific product.[7,12] Predisposing factors such as preexisting lung disease, exposure to atmospheric pollutants, duration of dust exposure, amount of dust concentration, and particle size affect the onset and severity of the respiratory impairment.

Pathogenesis. The respiratory tract is protected by two interrelated systems: the mucociliary system and alveolar macrophages. The inhalation of inorganic particles has little effect on the mucociliary system. However, atmospheric pollutants (sulfur oxides, nitrogen oxides, and tobacco smoke) interfere with and can paralyze ciliary action.[1] As a result, the clearance effect is impaired, and inorganic particles cannot be removed.

Alveolar macrophages attempt to engulf and remove inorganic dust by one of the following methods: (1) migrating to small airways to use the mucociliary escalator; (2) engulfing dust and exiting through the lymph and/or blood system; (3) migrating through bronchial walls, depositing dust particles in extraalveolar tissue; or (4) destroying the particle (silica).[1,12]

Macrophage impairment is the primary mechanism through which inorganic particles initiate lung diseases. In an attempt to maintain a sterile alveolar environment, macrophages secrete **lysozymes** to control foreign particle activity. These enzymes, released in response to the particulate stimuli, eventually damage the alveolar walls, which may cause deposition of fibrous materials.

Although the type of inorganic particle inhaled individualizes the pathophysiologic response, the general response is similar in the context of occupational lung diseases. Silica is one of the most toxic particles to alveolar macrophages. Dense deposits of collagen material are formed around the silica particles, resulting in marked fibrotic tissue deposition and restrictive lung disease. Coal dust and asbestos initiate a similar, although less severe, response. The pathologic processes and clinical features for each of the major occupational lung diseases are summarized in Table 23-5.

Clinical Manifestations. Pneumoconioses (anthracosis, asbestosis, silicosis) generally produce no symptoms in the early stages. No physical evidence is present until the pulmonary circulation is impaired or a pulmonary infection develops. Workers may remain symptom free for up to 10 to 20 years with chronic exposure.[1,2,12] Once again, symptom manifestation is dependent on the predisposing factors.

As pneumoconioses progress, patients present with a progressive, productive cough and dyspnea, especially with exercise. In addition, patients may complain of progressive weakness and fatigue. Clubbing of fingers may also be present. Late clinical features include chronic hypoxemia, cor pulmonale, and respiratory failure.

Diagnosis. The reliability of pulmonary changes noted on chest radiographs varies with the severity of the disease. When the patient is symptom free, no changes may be noted. However, as the pneumoconioses progress, micronodular mottling and haziness become apparent.[1] In addition, nodules, fibroses, and calcifications resulting from dust particle deposition are noted. Pneumoconioses usually produce one of three radiographic findings: nodular, reticular, or linear. However, because of the insidious progression of occupational lung diseases, radiographs negative for lung disease do not exclude the presence of the disease process.

Changes in pulmonary function tests demonstrate predominantly restrictive impairment (see Figure 22-17) with a component of obstructive functional impairment, depending on the severity and type of dust inhalation.[1]

Finally, hypoxemia is evident from arterial blood gas measurements in the late disease stages. Falling PaO_2 levels are accompanied by decreased $PaCO_2$ levels as the body initially compensates for the hypoxemia with an increased respiratory drive. However, as the disease progresses, both hypoxemia and hypercapnia are evident.

Treatment. Preventive measures are the key to limiting the onset and severity of occupational lung diseases. Adherence to federal standards for dust and particulate matter, as well as continuing education of workers and employers, will have a dramatic impact on the incidence of respiratory dis-

Table 23-5

Major Occupational Lung Pneumoconioses

Pneumoconioses	Pathologic Findings	Clinical Features
Anthracosis (coal miner's lung)	*Early:* Collection of coal particles with small amount of dilation of airway *Late:* Progressive, massive fibrosis, with condensed areas of black fibrous tissue	*Early:* Minimal to no symptoms; may be seen with dyspnea with cough but often due to unrelated bronchitis or emphysema *Late:* Worsening dyspnea on exertion, productive cough, respiratory failure
Silicosis	Dense collagen deposits in respiratory bronchioles and alveoli and along lymphatics	*Early:* No symptoms noted *Late:* Productive cough, dyspnea, especially with exercise; increased risk for tuberculosis
Asbestosis	Fibrous deposits secondary to long, thin fibers, allowing deep lung penetration	Progressive dyspnea on exertion, weakness, clubbing of fingers; pleural thickening with plaque development

eases. The use of respirators for miners and the use of water sprays to decrease airborne particles in mines are two common examples of prevention techniques. Early evaluation of a work environment predisposed to occupational lung diseases is where "treatment" must begin.[12]

Two primary goals in the management of active occupational lung diseases are to prevent further parenchymal damage and to relieve signs and symptoms, when possible. Ideally, if the problematic dust can be identified, the individual should be removed from the environment. However, if a job change is unrealistic, every possible measure must be implemented to prevent further inhalation of dust particles. Included in this treatment is the evaluation of current health maintenance behaviors.

Primary treatment consists of corticosteroids, inhaled bronchodilators, oxygen therapy, and respiratory treatments (intermittent positive-pressure ventilation, postural drainage, and deep breathing exercises). The effectiveness and utilization of these therapies depend on the patient's condition and the stage of disease. Rarely are those pathologic conditions reversed with medical treatment. The primary goal is to halt symptom progression.

KEY CONCEPTS

- Occupational lung diseases result from chronic inhalation of gases and inert particles. Commonly identified particles include coal, silica, and asbestos. Smoking and environmental pollutants may be contributing factors because they depress the ciliary function necessary to remove inhaled particles.
- The presence of inert particles in the alveoli initiates macrophage activity and inflammation. Inert particles cannot be digested by phagocytes, so they are walled off by deposition of fibrous proteins.
- Manifestations of pneumoconioses are related to the restrictive nature of the pulmonary dysfunction. Progressive dyspnea, decreased vital capacity and FRC, and increased respiratory rate are common. Blood gas analyses show progressive hypoxemia; carbon dioxide levels may remain normal or low until late in the disease.
- Treatment includes prevention of further exposure and administration of corticosteroids, bronchodilators, and oxygen therapy.

ATELECTATIC DISORDERS

Acute (Adult) Respiratory Distress Syndrome

Etiology. Acute (adult) respiratory distress syndrome is characterized by damage to the alveolar-capillary membrane. Clinically, ARDS is associated with a decline in the PaO_2 that is refractory (does not respond) to supplemental oxygen therapy. Damage to the alveolar-capillary membrane causes widespread alveolar infiltrates (visible on chest radiographs) and severe dyspnea. Mortality statistics range from 30% to 63%.[1,2,13-15] Patients who recover from the acute injury can expect to return to relatively normal lung function.[1,13,14] Follow-up studies (9 months to 4 years) in ARDS survivors show a mild restrictive pulmonary function accompanied by cough, dyspnea, and sputum production.[2,13] Some individuals continue to have abnormalities in diffusing capacity, oxygenation, and lung mechanics.[2,13] This syndrome has been reported as having many causes, including severe trauma, sepsis, aspiration of gastric acid, fat emboli syndrome, and shock from any cause. Box 23-1 lists the major disorders associated with ARDS.

Box 23-1 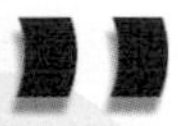

Major Disorders Associated with ARDS

Shock (any process leading to a low blood flow state)
Infectious causes
- Sepsis syndrome (primarily from gram-negative bacteria) with/without sustained hypotension (>40% cases)
- Pneumonia (viral, bacterial, fungal, mycobacterial)
- Miliary tuberculosis
- Bronchiolitis obliterans–organizing pneumonia

Trauma: pulmonary contusion
Embolism
- Fat emboli
- Air emboli
- Thrombus formation
- Amniotic fluid embolism

Head injury (increased intracranial pressure)
Aspiration (>30% cases)
- Gastric contents
- Drowning (fresh/salt water)

Drug overdose
- Heroin
- Methadone
- Propoxyphene
- Barbiturates, salicylates, thiazides, colchicine

Inhaled toxins
- Smoke inhalation
- High concentrations of oxygen (iatrogenic)
- Corrosive chemicals (ammonia, sulfur dioxide, chlorine, nitrogen dioxide)
- Free-base cocaine smoking

Radiation
Hematologic disorders
- Disseminated intravascular coagulation
- Massive blood transfusion
- Post–cardiopulmonary bypass
- Thrombotic thrombocytopenic purpura

Metabolic disorders
- Pancreatitis
- Uremia
- Paraquat ingestion

Burns
Cancer
Anaphylaxis
Eclampsia
Radiation pneumonitis
High-altitude exposure

The precise mechanism of lung injury is not known, but the common denominator appears to be increased permeability of the pulmonary vasculature and flooding of the alveoli with proteinaceous fluid, leading to the development of protein-rich pulmonary edema (noncardiogenic pulmonary edema). The acute lung injury triggers the immune system to activate the complement system and to initiate neutrophil sequestration in the lung (Figure 23-2).

Pathogenesis. The pathogenetic sequence of events in ARDS is shown in Figure 23-2. The initial injury to the alveolar-capillary membrane may be caused by direct damage,

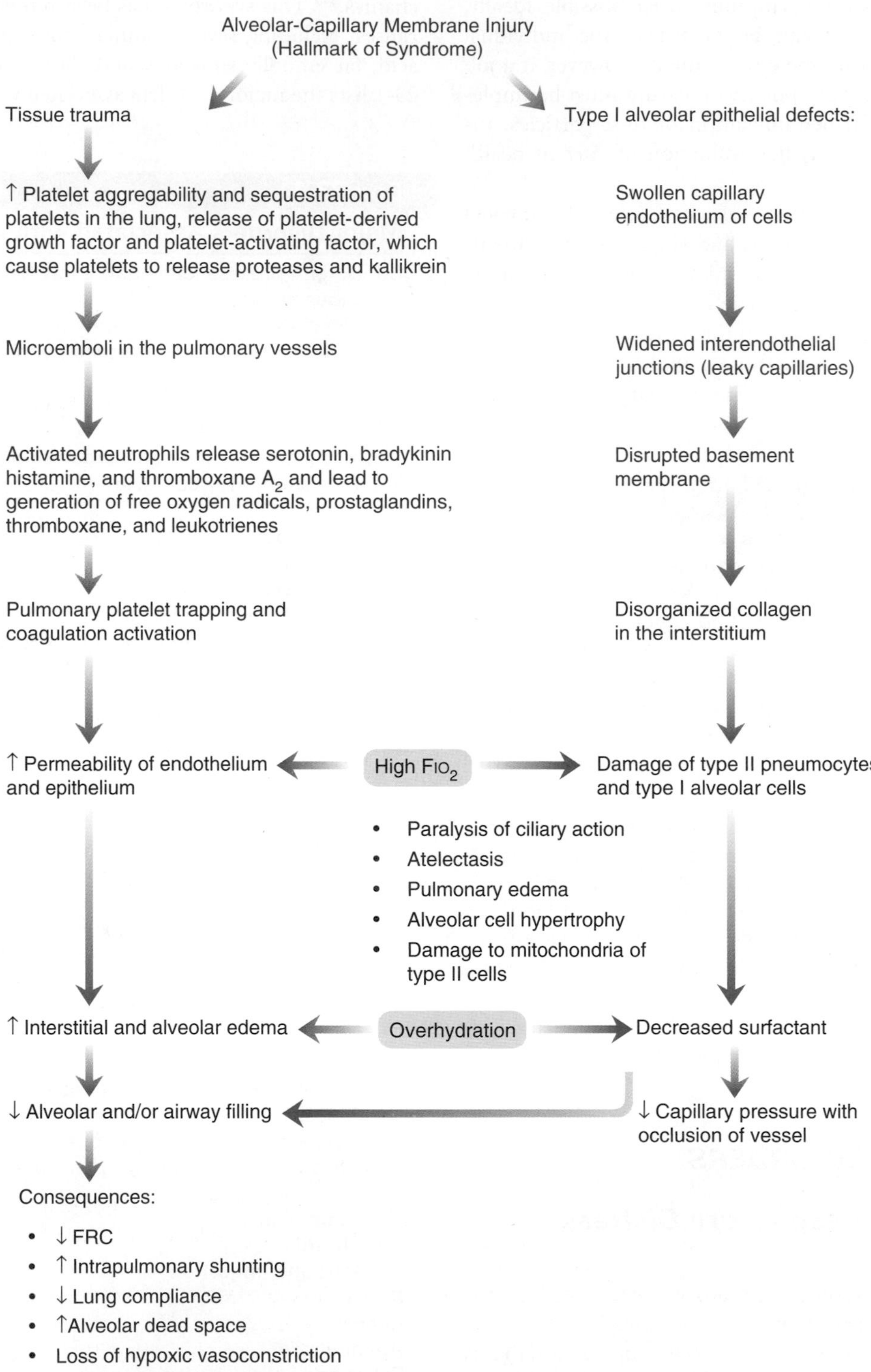

FIGURE 23-2 ■ Pathogenesis of acute respiratory distress syndrome. *FRC,* Functional residual capacity.

as seen in aspiration of acidic gastric contents, or by indirect damage, as occurs in shock from any cause. Therapeutic interventions (shown in the center boxes of Figure 23-2) may act to compound the effects of the initial lung injury. The resulting injury leads to an increase in alveolar-capillary permeability, which results in interstitial and alveolar edema.

The four characteristic pathophysiologic abnormalities of ARDS involve (1) injury to the alveoli from a wide variety of disorders, (2) changes in alveolar diameter, (3) injury to the pulmonary circulation, and (4) disruptions in oxygen transport and utilization.[13,14] Common findings in this type of injury include (1) severe hypoxemia caused by intrapulmonary shunting of blood; (2) a decrease in lung compliance; (3) a decrease in FRC; (4) diffuse, fluffy alveolar infiltrates on the chest radiograph; and (5) absence of evidence of cardiogenic pulmonary edema.[1,10,13,14]

The mechanism by which the FRC is decreased appears to be the result of very stiff, noncompliant lungs associated with alveolar edema and exudate, which exaggerate surface tension forces.[1,13,14] Early closure and continued closure lead to atelectasis and loss of lung volume.[1] The decrease in lung compliance, often severe in ARDS, is reflected in the high ventilatory pressures required to deliver an adequate volume of gas. It is thought that this decrease in lung compliance is due to loss or inactivation of surfactant with subsequent increased recoil pressure of the lungs.[1,13,14] In addition, proteinaceous fluid fills the alveoli and impairs ventilation. Figure 23-3 shows alveolar damage due to ARDS. Alveoli contain dense proteinaceous debris, desquamated cells, and hyaline membranes.

The decrease in Pa_{O_2} is a result of perfusion of large numbers of alveoli that are poorly ventilated (areas of low ventilation-perfusion) or not ventilated (areas of shunt).

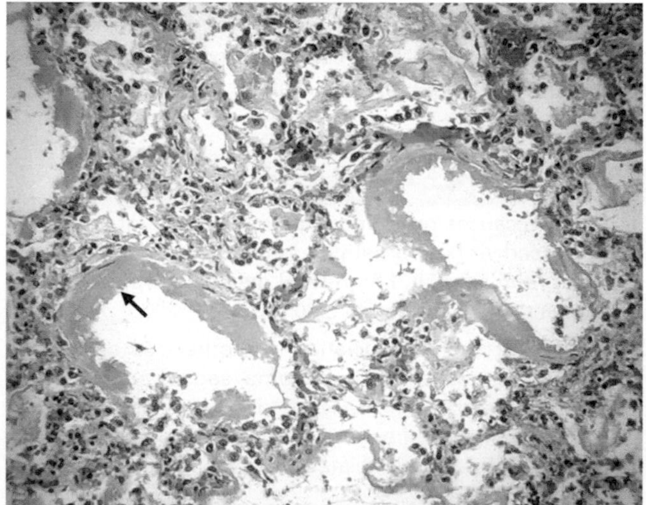

FIGURE 23-3 ■ Diffuse alveolar damage (adult respiratory distress syndrome), shown in photomicrograph. Some of the alveoli are collapsed, others are distended. Many contain dense proteinaceous debris, desquamated cells, and hyaline membranes *(arrow)*. (From Kumar V, Cotran RS, Robbins SL: *Basic pathology*, ed 7, Philadelphia, 2003, Saunders, p 468.)

Clinical Manifestations. The clinical features of ARDS usually include a history of a precipitating event that has led to a low blood volume state ("shock" state) 1 or 2 days prior to the onset of respiratory failure. The patient may complain of sudden marked respiratory distress.[1,2] Early signs and symptoms include a slight increase in pulse rate, dyspnea, and a low Pa_{O_2}. The initial presenting sign may be shallow, rapid breathing.

With progression of the disease, the patient demonstrates tachycardia, tachypnea, hypotension, marked restlessness, decreased mental status, and frothy secretions. On auscultation of lung fields, crackles and rhonchi are heard. The patient may be using accessory muscles to breathe and demonstrating intercostal and sternal retractions. A late sign is cyanosis.

Diagnosis. The hallmark of ARDS is **hypoxemia** that is refractory to increasing levels of supplemental oxygen. Uncorrected hypoxemia is associated with hypotension, decreased urine output, respiratory acidosis, metabolic acidosis, and eventual cardiopulmonary arrest. Arterial blood gas determinations reveal **hypoxia,** acidosis, and **hypercapnia.**[15] The chest radiograph may initially be normal but progresses to a diffuse "white-out" (Figure 23-4) indicative of diffuse alveolar infiltrates. The infiltrates characteristically spare the costophrenic angles.[2]

Pulmonary function tests show a marked decreased in FRC, decreased lung volumes, decreased lung compliance, and a ventilation-perfusion ($\dot{V}_A/\dot{Q}$) mismatch with a large right-to-left shunt.[1] Histologic changes found on open lung biopsy reveal atelectasis, hyaline membranes, cellular debris, and interstitial and alveolar edema[1,13] (see Figure 23-3).

Treatment. The management of ARDS entails identifying the underlying cause, addressing the cause (e.g., sepsis), maintaining fluid and electrolyte balance, and providing adequate oxygenation with the use of a volume ventilator, pressure support, and positive end-expiratory pressure (PEEP). Patients may require fraction of inspired oxygen (F_{IO_2}) levels of 1.0. The goal is to keep the PaO_2 above 60 mm Hg. Because of increased permeability of the alveolar-capillary membrane, excessive fluid administration can produce or intensify pulmonary edema.

The benefits of routine mechanical ventilation with small tidal volumes of 6 ml/kg of body weight[2,16] and PEEP have been well documented. The use of small tidal volume ventilation resulted in a 10% decrease in absolute mortality over standard large tidal volumes.[16] Use of PEEP produces a positive distending pressure across the alveoli and the airways, which maintains patency and increases FRC.

The positive effects of PEEP include (1) increasing FRC, which leads to improvement in the Pa_{O_2} by keeping alveoli open so that gas exchange is facilitated, (2) decreasing diffuse atelectasis, and (3) reducing shunting during the expiratory phase.[1,2,13,15] Another possible effect of PEEP is that it may act to conserve surfactant.

The optimal ventilatory pattern and level of PEEP are widely debated and vary from patient to patient.[15] However, it

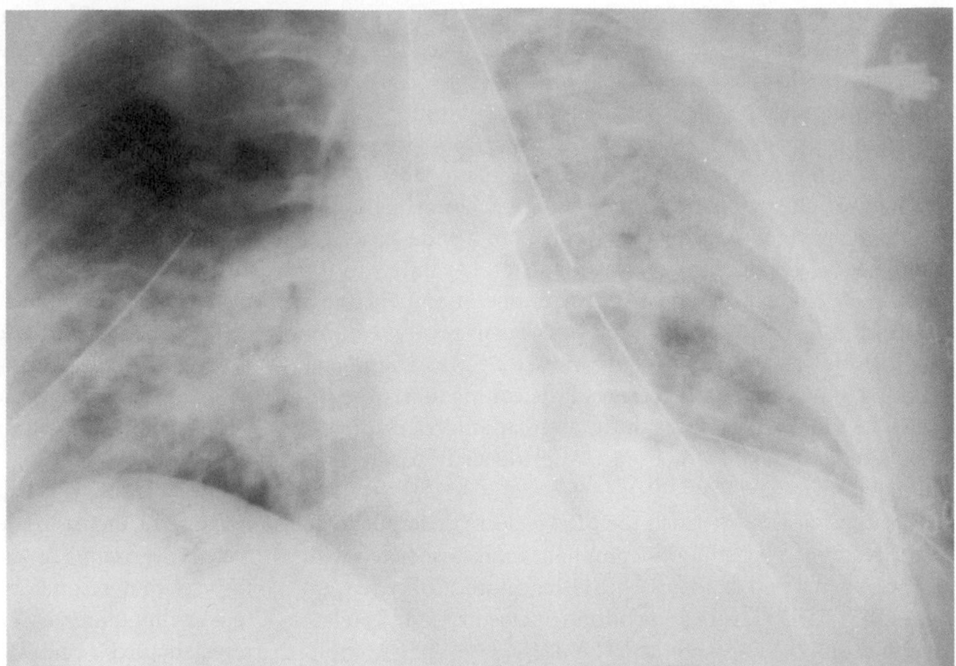

FIGURE 23-4 ■ Chest radiograph of a 28-year-old man who was involved in an automobile accident. The patient presented with multiple bilateral rib fractures and bilateral pneumothorax. Within 24 hours severe acute respiratory distress syndrome developed (note diffuse "whiteout").

is agreed that PEEP should be high enough to maintain alveolar distention throughout the entire respiratory cycle.[13] Most experts believe that PEEP should be regulated to preserve optimal cardiac output, maintain an FIO_2 at 0.6 or below, and maintain mixed venous oxygen tension (PvO_2) above 30 mm Hg.[1,2,4,13]

Complications associated with the use of PEEP are due to high pulmonary pressures and include (1) decreased cardiac output, (2) subcutaneous emphysema, (3) decreased tissue oxygenation because of a low cardiac output, which leads to lactic acidosis, (4) increased intracranial pressure, (5) increased intraocular pressure, (6) decreased urine output associated with increased antidiuretic hormone production, and (7) pneumothorax.[13]

High-frequency jet ventilation (HFJV) has been used as a treatment for respiratory distress syndrome (RDS) in both the adult and the neonate. HFJV uses rates substantially faster (60 to 3000 breaths/min) than conventional ventilation and small tidal volumes (2 to 4 ml/kg).[4,13] High-frequency jet ventilation improves carbon dioxide elimination and oxygenation. It also lowers mean airway pressures.[4] Inverse ratio ventilation (IRV) is useful in decreasing peak airway pressure, maintaining adequate alveolar ventilation, and improving oxygenation in ARDS patients. IRV uses an inspiratory-to-expiratory ratio that is greater than the standard 1:2 or 1:3. A 1:1 ratio stabilizes terminal respiratory units.[4,13] Mechanical ventilation with inhaled nitric oxide may improve gas exchange in adults and children with RDS. Inhaled nitric oxide acts as a selective pulmonary artery vasodilator leading to decreased pulmonary artery pressures and decreased intrapulmonary shunt.[2,4,13]

The goal of fluid management is to maintain the pulmonary capillary wedge pressure at the lowest level compatible with adequate cardiac output. Crystalloids should be used if needed to expand intravascular volume, and diuretics should be used to decrease intravascular volume.[2,15] Pressors such as dopamine are used to maintain blood pressure and renal perfusion.[15]

ARDS can be prevented experimentally by blocking systemic inflammatory cells. Indomethacin (Indocin), acetylcysteine, α_1-proteinase inhibitor, antitumor necrosis factor, human recombinant interleukin-1 receptor antagonist, and platelet-activating factor antagonists are being investigated.[13] Other investigational therapeutic agents include neutrophil inhibitors, such as pentoxifylline derivatives, and ketoconazole. Neutrophil inhibitors block the release of superoxide radical, which is both bactericidal and cytotoxic to host cells.[13]

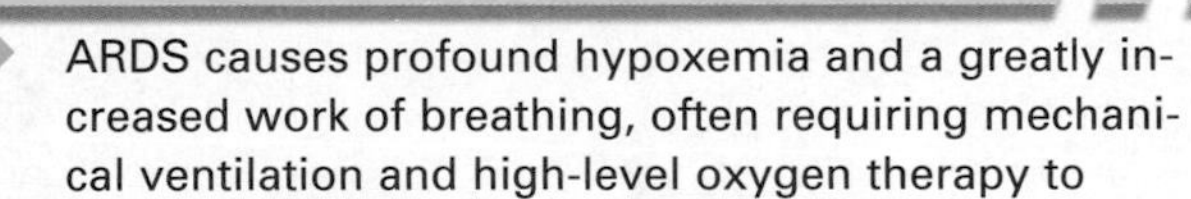

KEY CONCEPTS

- ARDS causes profound hypoxemia and a greatly increased work of breathing, often requiring mechanical ventilation and high-level oxygen therapy to maintain the PaO_2 above 60 mm Hg.
- ARDS occurs in association with other pathophysiologic processes, such as trauma, sepsis, or shock. These disorders increase the risk of development of disseminated pulmonary inflammation leading to ARDS. ARDS is associated with a mortality rate of about 50%.
- ARDS is a consequence of widespread pulmonary inflammation leading to three major pathophysiologic processes:
  1. Noncardiogenic pulmonary edema associated with "leaky" pulmonary capillaries.

2. Atelectasis associated with lack of surfactant (surfactant normally decreases surface tension in small alveoli and prevents them from collapsing).
3. Fibrosis (hyaline membranes) associated with inflammatory deposition of proteins.

- ARDS is associated with profound alterations in pulmonary function, including decreased vital capacity, decreased FRC, decreased compliance, and decreased tidal volume. Respiratory rate is increased and symptoms of tissue hypoxia may be apparent.
- Noncardiogenic pulmonary edema is evident as "whiteout" on chest radiograph. Crackles and wheezing may be heard throughout the chest. Profound dyspnea and the use of accessory muscles are common. Atelectasis and pulmonary edema result in right-to-left pulmonary shunting. Blood gas determinations show hypercarbia and hypoxemia, which do not improve much with oxygen therapy.
- Therapy is mostly supportive, i.e., to enhance tissue oxygenation until the inflammatory process resolves. Mechanical ventilation with PEEP and supplemental oxygen is the mainstay of therapy. PEEP is used to increase FRC and prevent alveolar collapse at end-expiration. PEEP may also force edema fluid out of the alveoli. High levels of oxygen (>60%) may contribute to ARDS because of absorption atelectasis. FIO_2 should be reduced as soon as possible.

Infant Respiratory Distress Syndrome

Etiology. Infant respiratory distress syndrome, also known as hyaline membrane disease, has features similar to those of ARDS. It is a syndrome of premature neonates, characterized by hemorrhagic pulmonary edema, patchy atelectasis, and hyaline (glassy) membranes.[1] Hypoxemia that is refractory to increasing levels of oxygen supplementation is the hallmark of the syndrome. The incidence is 60% in infants born at less than 30 weeks who are not treated with corticosteroids and decreases to 35% for infants receiving antenatal steroids.[17] The incidence in infants older than 34 weeks is 5%.[17,18] High-risk factors include birth prior to 25 weeks gestation, birth at advanced gestational age, poorly controlled diabetes in the mother, deliveries after antepartum hemorrhage, cesarean section without antecedent labor, perinatal asphyxia, second twin, previous infant with RDS, and Rh factor incompatibility.[17]

Pathogenesis. The primary cause of IRDS is lack of pulmonary surfactant, leading to increased alveolar surface tension and decreased lung compliance.[17] **Surfactant,** a phospholipid, is produced by type II alveolar cells in increasing quantities after 32 weeks gestation. With IRDS, lung compliance is decreased to one fifth to one tenth of normal.[1,17,18]

The neonate with IRDS must generate high intrathoracic pressures (25 to 30 mm Hg) to maintain patent alveoli. The premature neonate has a soft, compliant chest that is drawn inward with each inspiratory contraction of the diaphragm, making it difficult to maintain the high pressures needed to maintain adequate oxygenation. The end result from increased work of breathing and decreased ventilation is progressive atelectasis, increased pulmonary vascular resistance, profound hypoxemia, and acidosis.[1]

Surfactant also functions to maintain pulmonary fluid balance. Alteration of surface tension forces, normally maintained by surfactant, causes further leakage of proteinaceous fluid into the alveoli. This fluid contains fibrin and cellular debris, which causes hyaline membrane formation. Surfactant decreases surface tension in the alveolus during expiration, allowing the alveolus to remain partially open, thus maintaining FRC.[18]

A secondary cause of IRDS is immaturity of the capillary blood supply, which leads to $\dot{V}A/\dot{Q}$ mismatch, thus adding to the problems of hypoxemia and metabolic acidosis. In addition, a right-to-left shunt from an open foramen ovale or patent ductus arteriosus may increase the hypoxemia.[2]

Histologically, there is progressive damage to the basement membrane and respiratory epithelial cells. With increasing edema and loss of epithelial cells, patchy areas of atelectasis develop. Cellular damage from the disease process, excess fluid administration, and high levels of FIO_2 leads to increased capillary permeability and leakage of high-protein fluid into the alveoli.

Clinical Manifestations. The typical neonate presents with tachypnea; rapid, shallow respirations; intercostal, subcostal, or sternal retractions; diminished breath sounds; flaring of nares; hypotension; peripheral edema; low body temperature; oliguria; tachypnea (60 to 120 breaths/min); and bradycardia.[17,18] Late findings include frothy sputum, central cyanosis, and an expiratory grunting sound. Nasal flaring is a physiologic response mechanism used to increase airway diameter in an attempt to overcome airway resistance. An expiratory grunt is a physiologic response mechanism reflecting an attempt to create a physiologic PEEP by exhaling against a partially closed glottis. Paradoxical respirations ("seesaw" movement of the chest wall) may also be noted, indicating increased work of breathing.

During the first 48 to 72 hours of life, neonates with IRDS need progressively higher levels of FIO_2 to maintain adequate (60 to 80 mm Hg) oxygen levels.[17-19] As the work of breathing increases and oxygen levels decrease, metabolic acidosis occurs.[20]

Diagnosis. Initial arterial blood gas determinations reveal hypoxemia and metabolic acidosis due to lactic acid formation by hypoxic tissues. As the disease progresses, hypercapnia and respiratory acidosis develop.

The chest radiographic appearance progresses from normal, shortly after birth, to a diffuse whiteout or ground glass indicative of diffuse bilateral atelectasis and alveolar edema.

Generalized hypoinflation of the lungs is also seen on the chest study.

Measurement of the lecithin-sphingomyelin (L/S) ratio and desaturated phosphatidylcholine concentration in amniotic fluid may be done to determine the ability of the fetus to secrete surfactant. If the L/S ratio is greater than or equal to 2:1 (3:1 in mothers with diabetes), the incidence of RDS is less than 5%.[21] The presence of phosphatidylglycerol in the amniotic fluid is indicative of pulmonary maturity.[21] Administration of glucocorticoids prior to delivery may stimulate lung maturation and improve the L/S ratio.

Treatment. The mainstay of therapy is mechanical ventilation with PEEP or continuous positive-airway pressure. Prevention is a primary goal. The primary goal, as in the adult with ARDS, is to maintain adequate oxygen levels between 50 and 90 mm Hg.[1,2,19,22] The lowest FIO_2 settings should be used to maintain adequate arterial oxygen levels. High FIO_2 (100%) delivered for extended periods of time may result in further alveolar damage, primary persistent pulmonary hypertension, and retrolental fibroplasia (failure of the peripheral retina to vascularize, leading to blindness).[22] Normally, the retinal vessels vascularize at approximately 36 weeks gestation nasally and approximately 40 weeks temporally. Continuous monitoring of oxygen saturation by transcutaneous oxygen monitors has assisted the health care team in management of oxygen levels in the unstable neonate. The desired range for infants less than 34 weeks gestation is 88% to 95%.[19]

Exogenous surfactant (bovine, porcine, or synthetic) administration to premature infants has decreased the mortality rate in IRDS by 50%.[20,22] Surfactant decreases surface tension, thereby reducing the amount of pressure required to open the alveoli. In the immediate neonatal period, surfactant is necessary to maintain expansion of the lung after the first few breaths. In surfactant deficiency, the alveoli collapse after initial expansion, causing failure of oxygenation, hypoxemia, and alveolar damage. Surfactant replacement should be initiated during the first 2 hours of life.[20,22] Some surfactant products recommend repeated dosing every 6 to 12 hours up to four doses.[20,22]

High-frequency ventilation has proved to be effective in infants with severe IRDS by providing more uniform lung inflation, improving lung mechanics and improving gas exchange. Infants ventilated with high-frequency ventilation require lower mean airway pressures and have better gas exchange than those ventilated conventionally.[20,22]

General supportive therapy of adequate intravenous nutrition, fluid and electrolyte balance, minimal handling, and a neutral thermal environment should be maintained. Broad-spectrum antibiotics are prescribed for infections after cultures have been done or prophylactically until blood cultures prove negative.[19]

Complications of IRDS related to therapy include bronchopulmonary dysplasia due to anoxic damage and toxicity to high concentrations of oxygen used in treatment, pneumothorax due to mechanical ventilation, and retrolental fibroplasia. Retrolental fibroplasia is caused by high arterial oxygen levels, which cause vasoconstriction of immature retinal vessels leading to occlusion. Once the retina becomes fully vascularized, oxygen does not affect retinal vessels. In addition, the neonate is at high risk for the development of intracranial or intraventricular hemorrhage during the first few days of life.[20] The neonate is also at high risk for infections due to multiple invasive monitoring lines, catheters, and endotracheal intubation.

KEY CONCEPTS

- The symptoms of IRDS are very similar to those of ARDS. IRDS occurs most commonly in premature infants born prior to adequate development of their surfactant-producing pneumocytes (25 weeks gestation). Maturity of surfactant-producing cells can be estimated from the L/S ratio in amnionic fluid. An L/S ratio of less than 2:1 is associated with a higher risk of IRDS.
- Lack of surfactant causes atelectasis and increased work of breathing due to high alveolar surface tension. Leakage of inflammatory exudate into the alveoli results in formation of hyaline membranes.
- Symptoms of IRDS include nasal flaring, expiratory grunt, thoracic retractions, rapid shallow respirations, and bradycardia. Chest radiographs demonstrate a "whiteout." As in ARDS, blood gas values are poor, indicating severe hypoxemia and acidosis.
- Therapy for IRDS includes supportive measures, such as mechanical ventilation with PEEP or continuous positive airway pressure, and supplemental oxygen as well as specific measures to increase alveolar surfactant levels.

PLEURAL SPACE DISORDERS

Pneumothorax

Etiology. Pneumothorax is characterized by the accumulation of air in the pleural space. A primary **pneumothorax** is classified as spontaneous, occurring mainly in tall, thin men between ages 20 and 40 years without underlying disease factors.[1,2,23] A secondary pneumothorax occurs as a result of complications from preexisting pulmonary disease (such as asthma, emphysema, cystic fibrosis, infectious disease [pneumonia], interstitial lung disease, or tuberculosis). A specific category of secondary pneumothorax associated with menstruation is called *catamenial pneumothorax* (pathogenesis unknown). A catamenial pneumothorax is rare, occurs primarily in the right hemothorax, and is associated with pelvic endometriosis.[24] A third classification (tension pneumothorax) is traumatic, resulting from penetrating or nonpenetrating trauma. Other examples of traumatic pneumothorax have iatrogenic causes, such as placement of central lines, percutaneous lung biopsy, and mechanical ventilation.[2] Cigarette smoking increases the risk of spontaneous pneumothorax.[23]

Pathogenesis. Primary spontaneous pneumothorax (Figure 23-5) results from rupture of small subpleural blebs in the apices.[1] When air enters the pleural space, the lung collapses and the rib cage springs out.[1] The subpleural blebs are believed to occur in the apices as a result of negative mechanical pressures in the upper third of the upright lung field. Secondary pneumothorax occurs as a result of complications from an underlying lung problem and may be due to rupture of a cyst or bleb.[1,2] Tension pneumothorax (see Figure 23-5) results from the buildup of air under pressure in the pleural space. Air enters the pleural space during inspiration but cannot escape during expiration.[1] The lung on the ipsilateral (same) side collapses and forces the mediastinum toward the contralateral (opposite) side, thus decreasing venous return and cardiac output (see Figure 23-5). With an open, "sucking" chest wall wound, air enters during inspiration but cannot escape during expiration, leading to shift of the mediastinum (contents of the septum between the two lungs) and trachea.

Clinical Manifestations. The clinical features of pneumothorax include tachycardia, decreased or absent breath sounds on the affected side, hyperresonance, sudden chest pain on the affected side (90%), and dyspnea (80%).[23] Small pneumothoraces (less than 20%) are usually not detectable on physical examination.[24] Tension pneumothorax and a large spontaneous pneumothorax are emergency situations, with patients presenting with severe tachycardia, hypotension, a tracheal shift to the contralateral side, neck vein distention, hyperresonance, and subcutaneous emphysema. Figure 23-6 shows severe subcutaneous emphysema (air in the tissues due to tracheobronchial rupture).

Diagnosis. Arterial blood gas analysis (not commonly done) shows a decreased Pa_{O_2} and acute respiratory alkalosis. The chest radiograph shows depression of the hemidiaphragm

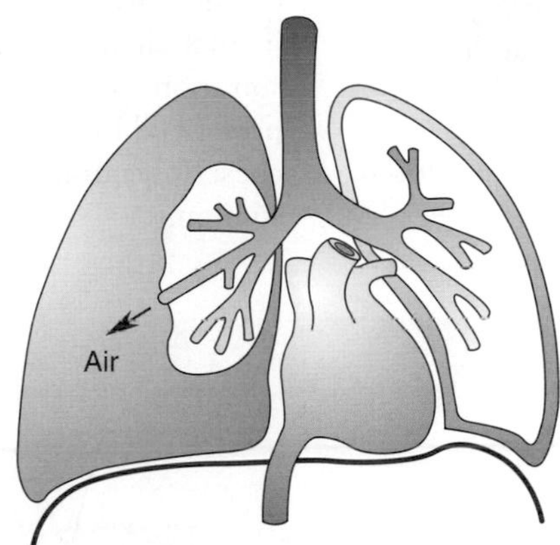

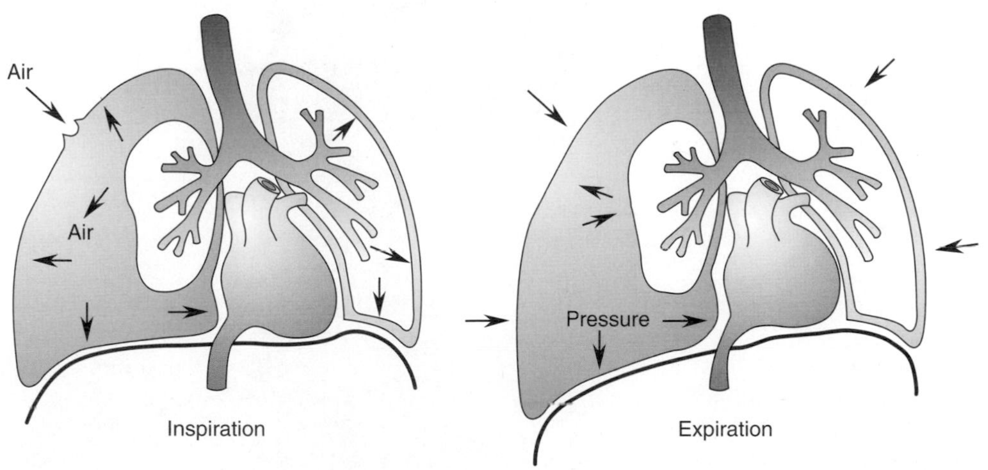

FIGURE 23-5 ■ *Top,* Spontaneous pneumothorax. *Bottom,* Tension pneumothorax: air builds up under pressure, leading to collapse of the ipsilateral lung and shift of the mediastinum to the contralateral side.

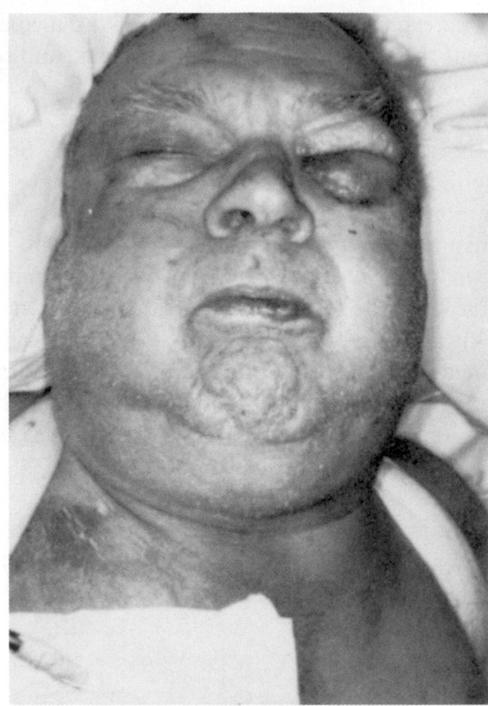

FIGURE 23-6 ■ Subcutaneous emphysema (air in the tissues) from tracheobronchial disruption and injuries of the esophagus. (From Kirsh MM, Sloan H: *Blunt chest trauma: general principles and management,* Boston, 1977, Little, Brown, p 109.)

on the side of the pneumothorax and a pleural line with absence of vessel markings peripheral to this line.[2,23,24] Chest radiography should be done with the patient standing. Expiratory films show a better demarcation of the pleural line than inspiratory films. The diagnosis may be based on clinical features without radiographic confirmation. However, a chest radiograph is usually obtained. A chest radiograph in tension pneumothorax shows a mediastinal shift (Figure 23-7). The electrocardiogram may show axis deviations, nonspecific ST-segment changes, and T-wave inversion.[25,26]

Treatment. The management of pneumothorax depends on the severity of the problem and the cause of the air leak. If the lung collapse is less than 15% to 25%, the patient may or may not be hospitalized. Typically, the patient is treated symptomatically.[2,24] A nonhospitalized patient should be monitored closely.[25,26] The expectation is for complete resolution within several weeks. If the collapse is greater than 15% to 25%, chest tube placement with water seal and suction is recommended.[1,2,23-26] Sealing the drainage chamber with a water-filled compartment prevents environmental air from being sucked into the pleural space on inspiration. The amount of suction for the chest tube is prescribed by the physician. Frequently used parameters for chest tube drainage are 2 cm H_2O seal and 20 cm H_2O suction.

FIGURE 23-7 ■ Upright posteroanterior chest radiograph showing a right-sided tension pneumothorax. Note marked deviation of trachea and cardiac silhouette into the left side of the chest. There is also depression of the right hemidiaphragm. (From Kirsh MM, Sloan H: *Blunt chest trauma: general principles and management,* Boston, 1977, Little, Brown, p 62.)

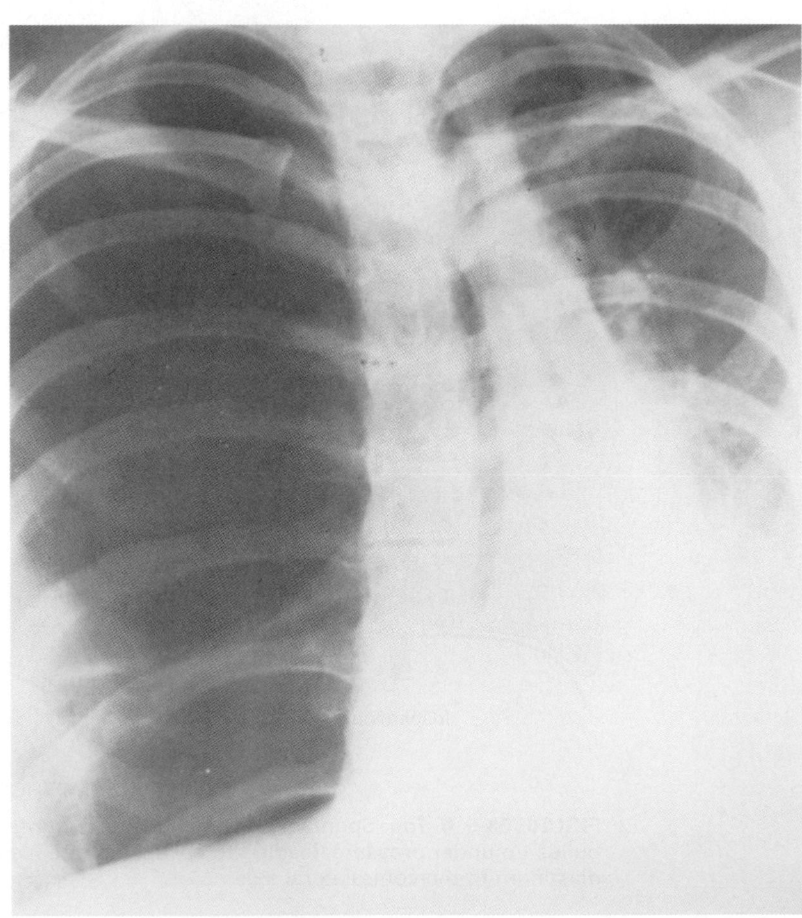

Chemical **pleurodesis** may be indicated for patients with spontaneous pneumothorax. Instillation of sterile talc, minocycline, or doxycycline into the chest wall cavity promotes adhesion of the visceral pleura to the parietal pleura to prevent further ruptures.[1,2,25,26] Lidocaine may be used in combination with these agents to provide pain control. Patients with a previous pneumothorax should be warned about exposure to high altitude, scuba diving, and smoking. A **thoracotomy** may be performed in patients in whom further spontaneous pneumothorax and blebs develop. Surgery permits stapling or laser pleurodesis of ruptured blebs.[1,2,26]

Pleural Effusion

Etiology. **Pleural effusion** is not a disease but rather a pathologic collection of fluid or pus in the pleural cavity as a result of a disease process. Normally, 5 to 15 ml of serous fluid is contained in the pleural space.[2] There is a constant movement of pleural fluid moving from parietal pleural capillaries to the pleural space, which is then reabsorbed into the parietal pleural lymphatics. The pleural membrane is a porous mesenchymal serous membrane that allows for movement of interstitial fluid. The fluid has a mucoid characteristic allowing for easy movement of the lungs.[27] The five major types of pleural effusion are (1) transudates, (2) exudates, (3) empyema due to infection in the pleural space, (4) hemothorax or hemorrhagic pleural effusions, and (5) chylothorax or lymphatic pleural effusions.[2] **Transudates** are low in protein (ratio of pleural fluid protein to serum protein is less than 0.5), low in lactate dehydrogenase (LDH; pleural fluid LDH/serum ratio less than 0.6), and have a specific gravity below 1.016.[28,29] Transudates are frequently associated with severe heart failure or other edematous states, such as cirrhosis with ascites, nephrotic syndrome, and myxedema.[2] **Exudates** are high in protein (greater than 0.5 mg/dl) and high in LDH (pleural fluid LDH/serum ratio greater than 0.6).[26,28-30] Common causes of exudates are malignancies, infections (especially pneumonia), pulmonary embolism, sarcoidosis, post–myocardial infarction syndrome, and pancreatic disease. **Empyema** is a high-protein exudative effusion resulting from infection in the pleural space. **Hemothorax** (the presence of blood in the pleural space) is often the result of chest trauma. Hemorrhagic pleural effusion contains a mixture of blood and pleural fluid. If the hematocrit of the fluid is greater than 50% of the hematocrit of peripheral blood, the fluid collection is called a **hemothorax.**[1,2] **Chylothorax** or chylous pleural effusion is an exudative process that develops from trauma as a result of leakage of chyle (lymph fluid) from the thoracic duct or from rheumatoid pleural effusion or tuberculous pleuritis.[1,2]

Pathogenesis. Pathophysiologic changes associated with the various types of effusions relate to changes in pleural capillary hydrostatic pressure, colloid oncotic pressure, or intrapleural pressure. Transudates can be caused by increased hydrostatic or decreased oncotic pressure. Exudates are associated with increased production of fluid due to increased permeability of the pleural membrane (inflammation) or impaired lymphatic drainage.[2,28,29] The imbalance in these pressures is associated with fluid formation exceeding fluid removal.

Clinical Manifestations. Clinical features vary depending on the cause of the effusion. Small effusions may be asymptomatic (which is common) in patients with less than 300 ml of fluid in the pleural cavity.[26,28] General features include dyspnea, pleuritic pain that is sharp and worsens with inspiration, dry cough, decreased chest wall movement, absence of breath sounds, dullness to percussion, and decreased tactile fremitus over the affected area.[26-30] A massive pleural effusion may lead to a contralateral tracheal shift.[26]

Diagnosis. **Thoracentesis** should be done to analyze the fluid and to reduce the amount of fluid in the pleural cavity. Evaluation of the pleural fluid is done to determine whether the cause is exudative or transudative. Pleural fluid should be analyzed for chemistry (pH, LDH, and glucose) and presence of pathogenic bacteria. Chest radiography should be done to detect pleural-based densities, infiltrates, signs of CHF, hilar adenopathy, and loculation of fluid. Computed tomography and ultrasonographic tests assist in complicated effusions and distinguish a mass from a large effusion.[26,28-30] Ultrasonography is also useful for thoracentesis guidance.

Treatment. Treatment is directed at the underlying cause of the effusion and relief of symptoms. Closed chest tube drainage in adults or thoracentesis is indicated if the effusion is large. Closed chest drainage in pediatric cases is controversial.[29] A thoracotomy to control bleeding may be required in patients with excessive bleeding (greater than 200 ml/hr).[31]

KEY CONCEPTS

- The pleural space is usually a potential space, containing only a small amount of fluid for lubrication. Accumulations of air (pneumothorax), pus (empyema), blood (hemothorax), lymph (chylothorax), or transudate in the pleural space can restrict lung expansion.
- Tension pneumothorax occurs when pleural air progressively accumulates and develops a positive pressure in the pleura. The ipsilateral (same side) lung collapses, and mediastinal structures (trachea, heart) are shifted to the opposite side. Breath sounds are diminished or absent on the affected side.
- Tension pneumothorax and a large, simple (spontaneous) pneumothorax are medical emergencies requiring treatment to remove pleural air and reexpand the lung. This usually requires insertion of a

chest tube. Chemical pleurodesis may be done in persons prone to spontaneous pneumothorax.

- A number of disease processes may result in accumulation of fluid in the pleural space. Analysis of the type of fluid (e.g., transudate, exudates, blood, pus) indicates the underlying disease process. General manifestations include dyspnea, cough, pleuritic pain, and, over the effusion, diminished breath sounds and dullness to percussion.

NEUROMUSCULAR, CHEST WALL, AND OBESITY DISORDERS

NEUROMUSCULAR DISORDERS

Diseases affecting the muscles of respiration or their nerve supply can lead to dyspnea and respiratory failure. Table 23-6 summarizes the features of these disorders.

Poliomyelitis

Poliomyelitis is a viral disease in which the poliovirus attacks motor nerve cells of the spinal cord and brainstem. The incidence of poliomyelitis in the United States is approximately 8 cases per year. All cases have been related to oral polio vaccine.[32] The diaphragm and intercostal muscles can be affected, with resulting weakness or paralysis and respiratory failure. At least 95% of infections are asymptomatic.[33] Of the patients who develop symptoms, patients with minor symptoms present with fever, headache, vomiting, diarrhea, constipation, and sore throat.[33] Patients generally recover respiratory muscle function, although occasionally patients have chronic respiratory insufficiency from previous disease. Fortunately, as the result of mass vaccination of the population, new cases are quite rare and usually occur in immigrants.[32]

Amyotrophic Lateral Sclerosis

Amyotrophic lateral sclerosis (ALS) is a degenerative disease of the nervous system that involves both upper and lower motor neurons. Commonly, muscles innervated by both spinal nerves and cranial nerves are affected. Clinically, progressive muscle weakness and wasting develop, eventually leading to profound weakness of respiratory muscles and death. Although the course of the disease is variable from patient to patient, the natural history is one of irreversibility and progressive deterioration.[2] Riluzole (Rilutek), the only medication approved for treatment, prolongs survival by 3 to 6 months (see Chapter 45).[34]

Muscular Dystrophies

Duchenne muscular dystrophy is a hereditary disease, passed from mothers to sons (X-linked recessive). The disease is characterized by progressive muscular weakness, initially in the lower extremities, and wasting. In later years (20s to 30s), respiratory muscles become involved, leading to hypoxia, hypercapnia, and frequent respiratory infections (see Chapter 51).[2]

Guillain-Barré Syndrome

Guillain-Barré syndrome, also called *acute polyneuritis,* is a disorder that is presumed to have an immunologic basis. Infection involving *Campylobacter* often precedes the diagnosis. Guillain-Barré syndrome is characterized by demyelination of peripheral nerves. Frequently, patients have a history of recent viral illness followed by development of ascending paralysis. Clinically, weakness and paralysis begin symmetrically in the lower extremities and progress or ascend proximally to the upper extremities and trunk. In severe cases, respiratory muscle weakness accompanies limb and trunk symptoms. Generally, the natural history of the disease leads to recovery, with minor residual motor deficits occurring in 15% to 20% of patients. Mortality is about 3% (see Chapter 45).[35]

Myasthenia Gravis

Patients with myasthenia gravis experience weakness and fatigue of voluntary muscles, most frequently those innervated by cranial nerves, but peripheral and respiratory muscles can also be affected. The hallmark of the disorder is weakness made worse by exercise and improved by rest. The primary abnormality is found at the neuromuscular junction, where transmission of impulses from nerve to muscle is impaired by a decreased number of receptors on the muscle. Although myasthenia gravis is a chronic illness, the manifestations can often be managed by appropriate therapy, and individual episodes of respiratory failure are potentially reversible.[2] Respiratory failure in this disorder can be due to increasing severity of illness or overmedication (see Chapter 51).

CHEST WALL DEFORMITIES

Kyphoscoliosis

Etiology. Kyphoscoliosis may develop from an unknown cause (idiopathic) or may be related to congenital disease (Pott disease) or neuromuscular disease (muscular dystrophy, Marfan syndrome, neurofibromatosis, Friedreich ataxia, or poliomyelitis).[36] Most idiopathic cases of scoliosis are found in adolescents (11 years or older). The female-to-male ratio is 7:1.[37]

Pathogenesis. Commonly, a bony deformity of the chest wall occurs as a result of kyphosis (hunchback appearance; posterior curvature deformity) and scoliosis (lateral curvature deformity) (Figure 23-8). The higher the deformity in the vertebral column, the greater the compromise of respiratory status. Lung volumes are compressed, leading to atelectasis, $\dot{V}_A/\dot{Q}$ mismatch, and hypoxemia.[2]

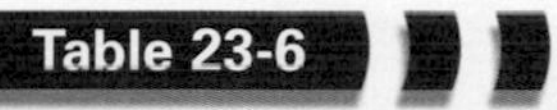

Neuromuscular Disorders Affecting the Respiratory System

Disease	Etiology	Pathophysiology	Clinical Features
Poliomyelitis (myelitis is inflammation of the spinal cord)	Develops from an enteral virus acquired by ingestion or respiratory droplet	After a 1- to 3-wk incubation period, the virus invades the intestinal blood supply; once in the circulation the virus invades all areas of the body; invasion of the central nervous system leads to neural damage and initiation of an inflammatory reaction	General symptoms are tremors, muscle weakness; bulbar poliomyelitis affects the respiratory muscle nerves, leading to respiratory paralysis; patients usually exhibit shoulder girdle paralysis first, followed by intercostal and diaphragm muscle paralysis; paralysis may be rapid or slowly progressive; also seen are diplopia, facial weakness, dysphagia, difficulty chewing, nasal voice, and loss of gag reflex
Amyotrophic lateral sclerosis	Cause unknown; current theories include autoimmune disease and a slow virus	Affects the anterior horn cells of both upper and lower motor neurons	Progressive weakness affecting distal more than proximal muscles; atrophy, fasciculations, and spasticity are noted; involvement of the respiratory muscles leads to respiratory dysfunction requiring mechanical ventilation
Muscular dystrophies (most common is Duchenne type)	Hereditary disease (X-linked recessive) passed from mothers to sons	Progressive muscular weakness noted initially in lower extremity muscles; in later years (20s-30s) respiratory muscles become involved; patients are at risk for respiratory infections	Progressive muscular weakness and wasting; skeletal deformities are also common; involvement of the respiratory muscles (diaphragm, intercostals, and accessory muscles) leads to hypoxia and hypercapnia
Guillain-Barré syndrome (acute idiopathic polyneuropathy)	Exact cause unknown, but thought to be an autoimmune disease triggered by a viral infection	The disease usually follows an infection or vaccination, peripheral nerves are affected, leading to neural inflammation, demyelination, and axon destruction	Progressive weakness and loss of motor function beginning in the feet and legs and ascending upward; sensory loss may also be noted but is not as dramatic as motor loss; loss of respiratory muscle control leads to respiratory failure, which frequently requires mechanical ventilation; autonomic nervous system symptoms may also be noted (tachycardia, arrhythmias, hypotension or hypertension, loss of ability to sweat)
Myasthenia gravis	Considered an autoimmune disease with both humoral (B cell) and cell-mediated (T cell) components	Autoantibodies and T cells bind to and damage acetylcholine receptors, leading to decreased functioning of receptors	Common symptoms are diplopia, ptosis, difficulty swallowing, increased weakness with activity, nasal voice, slurred speech, and weakness of proximal extremities; as the disease progresses, respiratory muscles become involved, leading to respiratory failure; pneumonia may result from respiratory failure and immobility

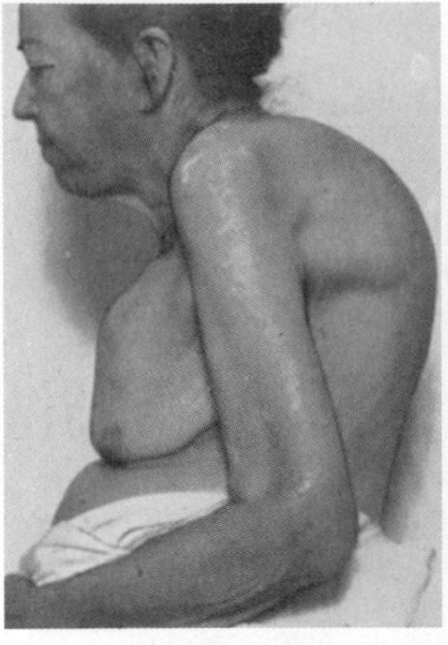
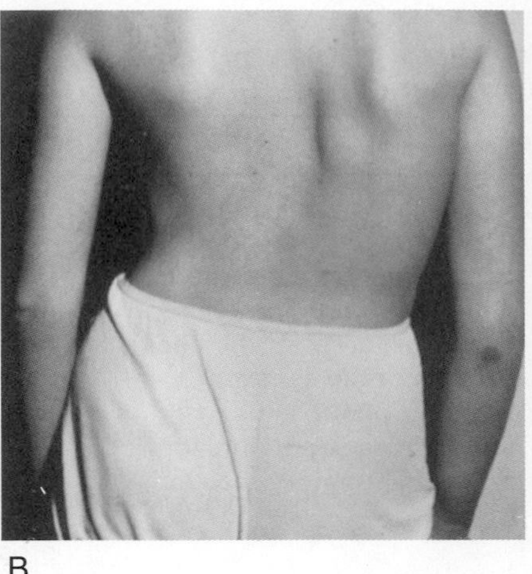
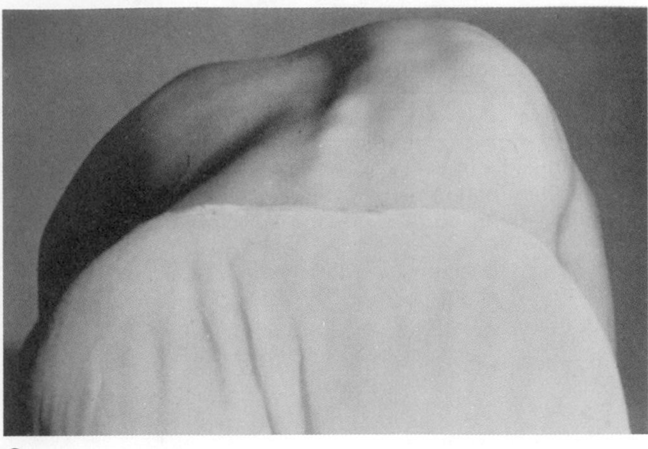

A B C

FIGURE 23-8 ■ Kyphosis **(A)** and scoliosis **(B** and **C)** are structural deformities that can interfere with ventilation. (From Delp MH, Manning RT, editors: *Major's physical diagnosis,* ed 9, Philadelphia, 1981, Saunders.)

Clinical Manifestations. Common clinical features include dyspnea on exertion; rapid, shallow breathing; and chest wall deformity as evidenced by ribs protruding backward, flaring on the convex side, and being crowded on the concave side. Hypoxemia develops later and eventually carbon dioxide retention occurs.[1]

Diagnosis. Diagnostic findings include hypercapnia, hypoxemia (due to $\dot{V}_A/\dot{Q}$ mismatch), and decreased lung volumes and lung capacities as evidenced by decreased values on pulmonary function tests. Also noted are increased pulmonary arterial pressures because of the associated pulmonary hypoxemia. Radiographs show accentuated bony curves.[1,36,37]

Treatment. Treatment depends on the severity of the deformity and the age of the patient. Kyphosis in elderly persons, especially women, is commonly due to osteoporosis. Screening for scoliosis and kyphoscoliosis in schoolchildren has proved to be an excellent method of early diagnosis of these conditions. Curvatures of less than 20 degrees should be monitored on a regular basis.[37] A postural exercise program for mild scoliosis and external braces for moderate scoliosis are recommended. For more advanced cases with curvatures greater than 40 degrees, electrical stimulation of the paraspinal muscles, spinal fusion, and spinal instrumentation (Harrington rod) placement for surgical stabilization are recommended treatments. Curvatures of greater than 60 degrees correlate with poor pulmonary function in later life.[37]

Ankylosing Spondylitis

Etiology. Ankylosing spondylitis occurs equally in both sexes and is commonly seen in the second or third decade of life.[1,38] It is characterized by chronic inflammation at the site of ligamentous insertion into the spine or sacroiliac joints. The precise cause is unknown. Ninety percent of patients with the disease have a positive HLA-B27 antigen.[38] The respiratory system is affected by limited chest expansion and by the formation of pulmonary fibrosis in the upper lobes, which later develops into bronchiectasis and cavitation.[38] Transient acute arthritis of the peripheral joints occurs in about 50% of cases.[38]

Pathogenesis. Ankylosing spondylitis is a progressive inflammatory disease leading to immobility of the vertebral joints and fixation of the ribs.[1] The inflammatory process affects the articular processes, costovertebral joints, and sacroiliac joints by inducing a fibrotic response leading to joint calcification, ligament ossification, and skeletal immobility.

Clinical Manifestations. Initial symptoms include low- to midback pain and stiffness that is more severe after prolonged rest. With exercise, the pain and stiffness decrease. As the disease process advances, rib cage movement is greatly reduced, leading to restrictive lung dysfunction.

Chest wall muscular atrophy is common and leads to further restriction of rib cage expansion. Breathing is largely accomplished by excursion of the diaphragm as the rib cage becomes immobilized. Associated problems seen with the disease include arthritis, uveitis, spondylitic heart disease, pulmonary fibrosis, and polyarteritis.[38]

Diagnosis. Pulmonary function tests show decreased vital capacity, decreased total lung capacity, and decreased compliance of the respiratory system, mainly the chest wall. Radiographs show destruction of cartilage, erosion of bone, calcification, and bony bridging of joint margins. The earliest radiologic changes are usually seen in the sacroiliac joints.[38]

Laboratory findings, although not diagnostic of the disease, include an elevated sedimentation rate in 85% of cases as well as a decreased red blood cell count and an increased white blood cell count. HLA-B27 antigen is seen in 90% of cases.[38]

Treatment. General therapy includes development of an exercise program that includes breathing exercises and mobility exercises. Pharmacologic management with nonsteroidal antiinflammatory agents provides symptomatic relief of pain and stiffness and promotes function. Indomethacin appears to be the most effective therapeutic agent.[38] Pain medications may also be used in these patients. Tumor necrosis factor inhibitors are effective in the spinal and peripheral arthritis of ankylosing spondylitis.[39]

Flail Chest

Etiology. Flail chest results from multiple rib fractures as a result of trauma to the chest wall. The ribs are fractured at two distant sites, resulting in an unstable, free floating chest wall segment that moves paradoxically inward on inspiration and outward on expiration. Bilateral costochondral separation and sternal fractures can also cause a flail segment.[40] Flail chest frequently occurs when the chest hits the steering wheel during an automobile accident.

Pathogenesis. Chest wall instability due to fracture at two distant sites on the same rib leads to an impairment of negative intrapleural pressure generation, causing decreased lung expansion on inspiration. In addition, lung parenchymal injury is common and may result in pulmonary contusion, decreased lung compliance, and respiratory failure.[40] Interstitial and alveolar hemorrhage leads to $\dot{V}A/\dot{Q}$ abnormalities.

Clinical Manifestations. Patients present after a trauma with paradoxical motion of the chest wall, either unilateral or bilateral. The injury to the chest wall is identified by careful inspection and palpation. Common features are marked shortness of breath, pain on inspiration, hypotension, cyanosis, and hypoxemia. Arterial Po_2 is often low before clinical symptoms appear.[40] Pneumothorax, hemothorax, and subcutaneous emphysema are common (see Figure 23-5).

Diagnosis and Treatment. Serial blood gas results help determine the treatment regimen. Flail chest, with large flail segments, resulting in acute respiratory failure is managed with mechanical ventilation.[40] Mechanical ventilation is achieved by positive pressure, which causes the entire chest, including the flail section, to move as a unit rather than paradoxically. Pain management may best be managed by continuous epidural anesthesia.[40]

Disorders of Obesity

Etiology. Obesity is defined as excessive body fat, with a body mass index (BMI) greater than 30 kg/m^2 based on body weight and height. Overweight is defined as BMI of 25 to 29.9 kg/m^2.[41] In most cases, obesity results from excessive caloric intake or reduced caloric expenditure. The National Health and Nutrition Exam survey reported that 59.4% of men and 49.9% of women are overweight. The findings for obesity were 19.9% of men and 25.1% of women.[42,43] A higher prevalence of obesity was found in blacks than in whites and in persons with lower incomes than in those with higher incomes.[41-43] Obese patients are at risk for a variety of disorders, the most common of which are diabetes mellitus, coronary artery disease, degenerative joint disease, gallstones, certain cancers (colon, rectum, prostate in men; uterus, biliary tract, breast, and ovary in women), and pulmonary impairment. Persons with a BMI of 30 kg/m^2 or more have an all-cause increase of mortality of 50% to 100% of those with a BMI between 20 and 25 kg/m^2.[41]

Pathogenesis. Endocrine causes of obesity are rare.[7,8] Hypothyroidism, the use of corticosteroids, and hypothalamic lesions all can lead to weight gain; however, the major cause of obesity is excess caloric intake. Several hormones act on brain receptors to regulate appetite and metabolism. Leptin binds to brain receptors, causing the release of neuropeptides that promote satiety and increase metabolic rate. Chrelin stimulates appetite. Genetic diseases such as familial partial lipodystrophy, Prader-Willi syndrome, Laurence-Moon syndrome, Bardet-Biedl syndrome, and Cohen syndrome are associated with obesity.[41-44]

Obesity may be associated with **hypoventilation.** The mechanisms of obesity hypoventilation are reduced ventilatory drive and increased work of breathing. Some patients are thought to have an abnormality in the central nervous system.[1] In addition, the increased abdominal size can force the thoracic contents upward into the chest cavity, thus decreasing lung expansion and diaphragmatic shortening. Obesity hypoventilation is also called pickwickian syndrome, after the obese boy in Charles Dickens's *Pickwick Papers.* Pickwickian syndrome is associated with hypoventilation and airway obstruction.[1]

An additional factor that contributes to the overall clinical picture in many obese patients is upper airway obstruction during sleep, that is the obstructive form of sleep apnea syndrome. Soft tissue deposits in the neck and tissues surrounding the upper airway predispose the person to episodes of complete upper airway obstruction during sleep. In a large percentage of cases, the somnolence that occurs in patients who have the obesity hypoventilation syndrome is related to obstructive sleep apnea.[42]

Clinical Manifestations. Obesity hypoventilation is characterized by decreased alveolar ventilation, somnolence, severe hypoxemia, **polycythemia,** and **cor pulmonale.** Patients complain of daytime somnolence, impotence, shortness of breath, headache, and **enuresis.**

Diagnosis. The diagnosis of obesity is self-evident on examination. There are no tests directly related to obesity;

however, tests for hypothyroidism, diabetes, and hyperlipidemia may be done to identify comorbid factors.[41] For persons with hypoventilation, arterial blood gas analyses may reveal hypoxemia and hypercapnia. Chest wall compliance, vital capacity, total lung capacity, and expiratory reserve volume are all decreased. Patients may also have an increased red blood cell count and show signs and symptoms of cor pulmonale and pulmonary hypertension.

Treatment. Primary treatment for obesity consists of weight loss. A weight loss program that includes the family members should be developed. Caloric intake that promotes an energy deficit of 500 to 1000 kcal/day is recommended. Aerobic exercise preserves lean body mass and increases energy expenditure.[41,42] Two medications are FDA approved for weight loss: sibutramine, which blocks uptake of serotonin and norepinephrine in the central nervous system, and orlistat, which reduces fat absorption in the gastrointestinal tract.[41,42] Oxygen delivery through a nasal cannula or mechanical ventilation may be necessary for patients with morbid obesity. Surgical intervention with gastric stapling or gastric bypass to decrease the gastric volume and size has proved successful in some patients.[1] These operations are intended to permanently curtail food intake.

KEY CONCEPTS

- Kyphoscoliosis is a deformity of the bony structure of the chest wall characterized by hunchback and lateral curvature of the spine. The abnormal shape of the chest interferes with the normal mechanics of breathing, resulting in small lung volumes, compression atelectasis, and hypoxemia. Compensatory tachypnea is usually present.
- Ankylosing spondylitis is a progressive inflammatory disease affecting vertebrae and ribs. Chronic inflammation leads to chest wall fibrosis and immobility. Chest wall muscle atrophy and rib cage stiffening result in pulmonary dysfunction characteristic of restrictive disorders.
- Obesity may interfere with the normal mechanics of breathing because of excessive chest weight and abdominal impingement on the chest cavity. Pickwickian syndrome is a disorder of obesity associated with hypoventilation and airway obstruction.

INFECTION OR INFLAMMATION OF THE LUNG

Pneumonia

Etiology. The term **pneumonia** (from the Greek *pneuma,* "breath") refers to an inflammatory reaction in the alveoli and interstitium of the lung, usually caused by an infectious agent. Pneumonia can result from three different sources: (1) aspiration of oropharyngeal secretions composed of normal bacterial flora and/or gastric contents; (2) inhalation of contaminants (virus, *Mycoplasma*); or (3) contamination from the systemic circulation.[2,45]

There are several ways to classify pneumonia. Pneumonias are typically classified as community acquired or hospital acquired. They are further classified as bacterial, atypical, and viral. The bacterial pneumonias may be grouped as either gram positive or gram negative, based on the staining characteristics of the organism. Staining involves applying a pigment or dye to the tissue to assist in demonstrating and classifying the organism. *Staphylococcus* and *Streptococcus* (including pneumococci) are the predominant gram-positive organisms. Gram-negative bacteria that may cause pneumonia include *Haemophilus influenzae, Klebsiella* species, *Pseudomonas aeruginosa, Serratia marcescens, Escherichia coli,* and *Proteus* species.

To assist the reader in differentiating among the various types of pneumonia, Table 23-7 presents the etiologic factors, common clinical features with age-related characteristics, radiologic findings, and antibiotic therapies for 11 forms of the disease.[2] There are many other types that are not listed.

Pathogenesis. Normally, pulmonary defense mechanisms (immune responses, cough reflex, sneezing, mucociliary clearance) protect individuals from pneumonia. Community-acquired pneumonia occurs when defense mechanisms are compromised.[2,45] A highly virulent organism may also overwhelm a person's defense mechanisms. Community-acquired pneumonias are commonly bacterial in origin.[45] After microbial agents enter the lung, they multiply and trigger pulmonary inflammation. Alveolar air spaces fill with an exudative fluid, and inflammatory cells invade the alveolar septa. Bacterial pneumonia may be associated with significant $\dot{V}A/\dot{Q}$ mismatching and hypoxemia because inflammatory exudate collects in the alveolar spaces. Chapter 21 describes $\dot{V}A/\dot{Q}$ mismatching in greater detail. Alveolar exudate tends to consolidate and becomes difficult to expectorate. Viral pneumonia does not produce exudative fluids.[13] Figure 23-9 shows the histologic progression of acute pneumonia. Patients with chronic illnesses and those who are immobile or immunosuppressed are at highest risk for developing pneumonia.[25] Disruption of the body's normal defense mechanisms leads to increased risk of pneumonia. Other patients at risk are those who have undergone thoracic or abdominal surgery or anesthesia.

Clinical Manifestations. Clinically, the pathogenic cause, severity of the disease, and age of the patient may cause variations in the presentation of pneumonia. Some patients present with fever only.[25] Rales (crackles) and bronchial breath sounds may be heard over the affected lung tissue. Patients may present with chills, cough, purulent sputum, and an abnormal chest radiograph. Patients with viral pneumonia may present with an upper respiratory prodrome (fever,

Table 23-7

Differentiating Features of Types of Pneumonia

Etiologic Organism	Common Clinical Features	Chest Radiograph	Antibiotic Treatment
Staphylococcus aureus; gram-positive cocci in clumps	Follows upper respiratory infection; fever, chills, pleuritic chest pain, cough, yellow purulent sputum; seen in patients in chronic care facilities	Consolidation, may have cavitation	Methicillin-susceptible strains: nafcillin or oxacillin with or without rifampin; methicillin-resistant strains: vancomycin with or without rifampin; alternative choice: cephalosporins, clindamycin, vancomycin
Streptococcus pneumoniae (pneumococcus); gram-positive diplococci	More common in alcoholics, also seen with chronic cardiopulmonary disease; fever, chills, pleuritic chest pain, cough, rust-colored sputum	Patchy infiltrates	Procaine penicillin G or aqueous penicillin G, amoxicillin; alternative choice: macrolides, cephalosporins, doxycycline, quinolones; prophylactic vaccine available
Haemophilus influenzae; pleomorphic gram-negative coccobacilli	Upper respiratory symptoms, fever, vomiting, irritability, cough, purulent sputum, dyspnea; affects children and older adults, affects people with chronic cardiorespiratory problems	Consolidation	Cefotaxime, ceftriaxone, doxycycline, azithromycin, TMP-SMX; alternative choice: quinolones or clarithromycin
Klebsiella pneumoniae; gram-negative encapsulated rods	Seen frequently in middle-aged men and associated with alcoholism and diabetes mellitus; rust-colored sputum	Consolidation	Aminoglycoside plus third-generation cephalosporin; alternative: aztreonam, imipenem, quinolone
Pseudomonas aeruginosa; gram-negative rods	Chronic obstructive pulmonary disease, cystic fibrosis, and mechanical ventilation; fever, chills, and copious greenish, foul-smelling sputum	Infiltrates, small pleural effusion	Aminoglycoside plus ticarcillin/ clavulanate or piperacillin/ tazobactam or aztreonam or imipenem
Escherichia coli; gram-negative rods	Complication of gastrointestinal surgery	Infiltrates, may have pleural effusion	Aminoglycoside plus third-generation cephalosporin; alternative: aztreonam, imipenem, quinolone
Virus	Fever, malaise, headache, nonproductive cough	Patchy infiltrates	Amantadine, rimantadine
Legionella species; no bacteria	Acute onset with fever, diarrhea, myalgia, and abdominal pain	Consolidation	Macrolides with or without rifampin; alternative: TMP-SMX, quinolone
Mycoplasma pneumoniae (atypical pneumonia) monocytes and neutrophils; no bacteria	Age 5-25 yr, most common in young adults; associated with otitis media and myringitis; sore throat, headache, myalgia, dry cough, fatigue, low-grade fever	Infiltrates	Erythromycin, doxycycline; alternative: quinolone or other macrolide
Pneumocystis carinii (fungus)	Immunosuppressed patients (infants, children, and adults); 60% of patients have AIDS	Diffuse infiltrates, or chest x-ray may appear normal	TMP-SMX or pentamidine; isethionate plus prednisone; alternative: dapsone plus TMP-SMX, clindamycin plus primaquine
Anaerobic pneumonia (aspiration pneumonia), mixed flora	Predisposition to aspiration, fever, weight loss, malaise, risk increases with decreased level of consciousness, artificial airway, and sedation, seen in individuals with poor dental hygiene	Infiltrates in dependent lung fields	Penicillin G; alternative choices: clindamycin, metronidazole, cefoxitin

TMP-SMX, Trimethoprim-sulfamethoxazole; *AIDS,* acquired immunodeficiency syndrome.

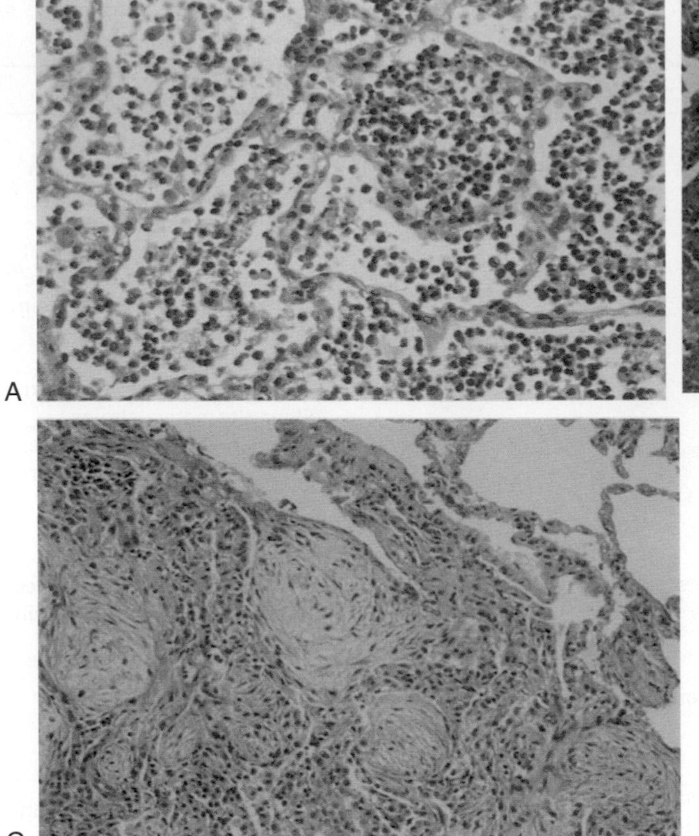

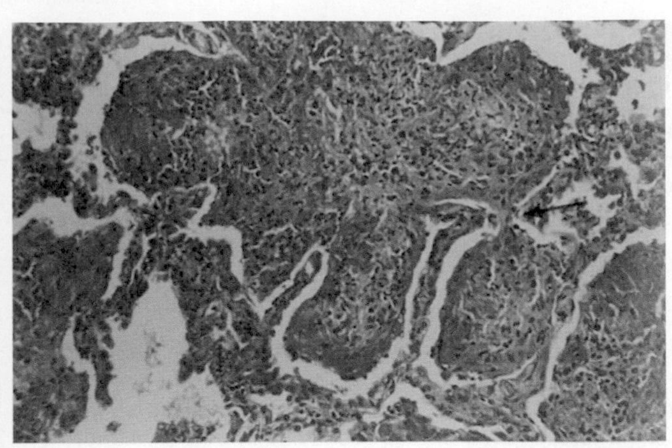

FIGURE 23-9 ■ **A,** Acute pneumonia. The congested septal capillaries and extensive neutrophil exudation into the alveoli correspond to early red hepatization. Fibrin nets have not yet formed. **B,** Early organization of intraalveolar exudate, seen in areas to be streaming through pores of Kohn. **C,** Advanced organizing pneumonia corresponding to gray hepatization and featuring transformation of exudates to fibromyxoid masses richly infiltrated by macrophages and fibroblasts. (From Cotran RS, Kumar V, Robbins SL, editors: *Robbins pathologic basis of disease,* ed 6, Philadelphia, 1999, Saunders, p 720.)

coryza, cough, hoarseness) accompanied by wheezing and/or rales.[25] Typical features of *Chlamydia* pneumonia are cough, tachypnea, rales, wheezes, and no fever. *Mycoplasma* pneumonia is a common cause of pneumonia in older children and adults.[25] Signs and symptoms include fever, cough, headache, and malaise.

Diagnosis. The chest radiograph demonstrates parenchymal infiltrates (white shadows) in the involved area, indicative of inflammatory alveolar processes.[2,25,45,46] In a patient with symptoms and clinical findings of pneumonia, a Gram stain of expectorated sputum may be obtained to distinguish bacterial from viral pneumonia and gram-negative from gram-positive organisms. Sputum Gram stains and cultures have poor positive and negative predictive values. Sputum samples that result from deep cough and are persistent give the best results.[2] If the patient had been previously healthy, the cause of the majority of these infections would either be viral, mycoplasmal, or the gram-positive pneumococcal bacterium. However, if the patient had been hospitalized or has other illnesses such as emphysema, diabetes, or alcoholism, then gram-negative organisms should be suspected. Because 24 to 48 hours may be required for culture of the etiologic agent, antibiotic therapy should be started empirically.[2] Once culture and sensitivity results are obtained, antibiotic therapy may be changed in accordance with the results of the Gram stain and culture and the patient's clinical history. Diagnosis is based on the chest radiograph, white blood cell count (greater than 15,000/μl for bacterial pneumonia[25]), and sputum culture, coupled with clinical features of fever with recurrent chills, cough, dyspnea, and rales.

Treatment. For pneumococcal pneumonia, penicillin is the drug of choice. If the patient is allergic to penicillin, macrolides, cephalosporins, or quinolones may be given.[2] If *Staphylococcus* is suspected as the etiologic agent, an alternative drug should be chosen because of the high number of penicillin-resistant strains. For staphylococcal pneumonia, intravenous nafcillin or oxacillin may be used. Cephalosporins may also be chosen as a therapeutic alternative for management of staphylococcal pneumonia. See Table 23-7 for more information.

For gram-negative pneumonia, broad-spectrum antibiotic coverage is indicated until results of laboratory cultures are known. This may be accomplished either with an aminoglycoside or a third-generation cephalosporin. The incidence of side effects increases with the use of these drugs. Nephrotoxicity and ototoxicity are known complications of aminoglycoside therapy. Blood levels of the drugs must be monitored. These levels and the rate of infusion are usually determined from peak and trough blood samples. *Peak* refers to measurement of the drug at its highest level, and *trough* is a measurement obtained when the drug level is at its lowest point. The side effects of cephalosporins include phlebitis, hypersensitivity, and bleeding disorders. Once the organism has been cultured, specific antibiotic selection is based on sensitivity of the organism to different antibiotics.

Anaerobic bacteria may present clinically as a lung abscess, necrotizing pneumonia, or empyema. These diseases are usually caused by aspiration of normal oral bacteria (such as *Bacteroides* and *Fusobacterium*) into the lung.[2] Many clinicians use high doses of penicillin G as the drug of choice for such infections, but other antibiotics such as metronidazole (Flagyl), clindamycin, and cefoxitin are acceptable alternatives.[2,25,45,46]

The most common cause of viral pneumonia is the influenza virus, but unfortunately no antibiotics are currently available for its treatment. Amantadine, an antiviral agent, may be effective in reducing symptoms; however, there have been no controlled studies testing the effectiveness of amantadine in influenza pneumonia.[2]

Mycoplasmal pneumonia is best managed with either a macrolide (first choice) or doxycycline for 3 weeks.[46,47] Mycoplasmal pneumonia is more commonly seen in the summer and fall in young adults.

Other causes of pneumonia occur less frequently in the general population. Legionnaires disease, for example, is a severe systemic illness characterized by fever, diarrhea, abdominal pain, liver and kidney failure, and pulmonary infiltrates. The organism lives in water and is transmitted by means of potable water, condensers, and cooling towers.[2] The current treatment of choice is a macrolide.

Fungal and Protozoal Pneumonia

Patients whose immune systems have been compromised by disease or by drug therapy may be susceptible to the development of opportunistic pneumonia. For example, *Pneumocystis carinii* pneumonia, an **opportunistic** infection, is commonly found in patients with cancer or with human immunodeficiency virus (HIV). Primary treatment is trimethoprim-sulfamethoxazole or pentamidine. (See Chapter 12 for further discussion of acquired immunodeficiency syndrome [AIDS].)

Aspergillus, an opportunistic fungus that is widespread in nature, may cause progressive pneumonia. *Aspergillus* is released from walls of old buildings under reconstruction. Attention should be given to the renovation of old hospitals and the placement of susceptible patients in a reconstruction area. *Aspergillus* pneumonia should be managed with amphotericin B in slowly increasing doses. Liposomal amphotericin is the drug of choice in renal insufficiency or when high dosing is necessary.[47]

KEY CONCEPTS

- Pneumonia is an inflammation of the lung that is usually associated with an infectious agent. The most common types of pneumonia are bacterial and viral. A productive cough is the primary differentiating feature between bacterial pneumonia and viral pneumonia, in which coughing is nonproductive.
- Bacterial pneumonia may be associated with significant $\dot{V}A/\dot{Q}$ mismatching and poor blood gas values because inflammatory exudate collects in the alveolar spaces. Alveolar exudate tends to consolidate and becomes difficult to expectorate. Viral pneumonia does not produce exudative fluids.
- Manifestations of bacterial pneumonia may include fever, chills, cough with purulent sputum, crackles, and areas of consolidation on chest radiograph. Dyspnea may be significant.
- The treatment of bacterial pneumonia centers on antibiotic therapy to eliminate the organism and supportive therapy to enhance ventilation and oxygenation. Most cases of viral pneumonia (influenza) are managed symptomatically, as no effective antibiotic therapy is available.
- Fungal and protozoal pneumonias are uncommon and tend to occur in immunocompromised individuals.

Pulmonary Tuberculosis

Etiology. Worldwide, 3 million people die of tuberculosis each year. There are an estimated 10 million to 15 million people in the United States with tuberculosis.[2,48] Ninety percent of cases involve reactivation of prior infection; the remainder are new infections.[48] Miliary tuberculosis is an infection of disseminated hematogenous disease. The majority of new cases occur in malnourished individuals, those living in overcrowded conditions, immunosuppressed individuals, incarcerated persons, immigrants, and elderly persons. During the past 30 years, there has been a shift in the care of such patients from specialized tuberculosis hospitals to outpatient therapy. Hospitalization of such patients may be necessary with isolation for a period of 2 to 4 weeks (longer for multidrug resistant tuberculosis). Specialized tuberculosis hospitals have reopened owing to increasing resistance of the organism to treatment and an increasing number of cases. Tuberculosis cases should be reported to local and state health departments.

Tuberculosis is caused by the bacterium *Mycobacterium tuberculosis,* an acid-fast aerobic bacillus. Any organ system can be affected by the disease, but the most common sites are the lungs and the lymph nodes. Tuberculosis is subdivided into two major classifications: primary (usually clinically and radiographically silent[2]) and reactivating. Primary disease (initial infection) may lie dormant for many years or decades.[2] When the person's immune system becomes impaired reactivation may occur. HIV, corticosteroid use, silicosis, and diabetes mellitus are associated with reactivation.[2] Reactivation may occur many years after the primary infection. Distant organ systems may be involved as a result of hematogenous spread during the primary or reactivation phase of infection. In addition, there may be disseminated disease, known as miliary tuberculosis, again resulting from hematogenous dissemination of the organisms. Strains of *M. tuberculosis* are becoming resistant to one or more first-line antituberculosis drugs.[48] Multidrug-resistant tuberculosis accounts for 15% of the tuberculosis cases in the United States. Mortality rates range from 70% to 90% in hospitals or correctional facilities in Florida and New York, with a median survival of 4 to 16 weeks.[2] Entry into the body is by inhalation of small (2 to 10 (m) droplets containing the bacteria. These droplets are produced when an infected person coughs, sneezes, or talks.

Pathogenesis. After entrance of *Mycobacterium* into the lung tissue of the susceptible person, alveolar macrophages ingest and process the microorganisms. The organisms either are destroyed or persist and multiply. Once infection becomes established, lymphatic and hematogenous dissemination occurs. T cells and macrophages surround the organisms in **granulomas** that limit multiplication and spread.[49] Dormant organisms persist for years. Reactivation may occur if the patient's immune system becomes impaired.[2,49]

The pathologic manifestation of tuberculosis is the **Ghon tubercle** or complex, which has parenchymal and lymph components. The parenchymal component is composed of a well-circumscribed necrotic nodule that later becomes fibrotic and calcified. The lymph component is found in the lymph nodes. Primary pulmonary tuberculosis is shown in Figure 23-10.

Clinical Manifestations. Clinical features include a history of contact with an infected person, low-grade fever, cough, night sweats, fatigue, weight loss, malaise, and anorexia. Chronic cough is the most common symptom.[2,49] As the disease progresses, the patient develops a productive cough with purulent sputum. Physical examination of the lung fields reveals apical crackles (rales) (*M. tuberculosis* organisms prefer lung apices due to the higher concentration of oxygen in the apices) or bronchial breath sounds over the region of lung consolidation. The patient appears malnourished and chronically ill.[2] Common sites of extrapulmonary tuberculosis are peritoneum, gastrointestinal tract, liver, spleen, bone, joints, lymph nodes, central nervous system, and genitourinary system.[49] (Please refer to Chapter 12 for a discussion of tuberculosis in HIV-infected patients.)

Diagnosis. Definitive diagnosis is made by results of sputum culture or identification of the organism by DNA or RNA amplification techniques (not routinely used).[49] Three consecutive morning sputum specimens are obtained to identify the slow-growing acid-fast bacillus. Expectoration of sputum in the early morning is ideal because the sputum is more concentrated and more plentiful. Cultures require 1 to 3 weeks for determination.[49] Gastric washings or bronchial washings may also be used for diagnostic culturing.

Chest radiographs usually show nodules with infiltrates in the lung apex and posterior segments of the upper lobes. Elderly patients may present with lower lobe infiltrates with or without pleural effusion. Figure 23-11 shows the radiographic appearance of cavitary tuberculosis in a 23-year-old man. A miliary pattern (diffuse small nodular densities) is seen with dissemination of the organism in miliary tuberculosis.[2]

Another primary diagnostic test is the tuberculin (Mantoux test) skin test (5 tuberculin units/0.1 ml of purified protein derivative injected intradermally). This test does not distinguish between current disease and past infection. If the induration in a person with HIV infection is 5 mm or greater, if the patient has close contact with individuals with tuberculosis, and if the patient has a chest radiograph consistent with tuberculosis, the likelihood of active disease is high.[1] An induration of 10 mm or greater is the reaction size for other high-risk individuals, such as intravenous drug abusers, individuals who are debilitated, children younger than 4 years or with immunosuppression, and individuals living in countries with a high incidence of the disease (Asia, Africa, Latin America). An induration of 15 mm or greater is considered positive for tuberculosis in all other persons.[2,49]

False-positive results may occur in persons with other mycobacterial infections or if they have received bacille Calmette-Guérin, a live attenuated strain of *Mycobacterium bovis* that provides active immunity against tuberculosis. False-negative results may also occur in patients who are malnourished, elderly, or immunocompromised.[2] Immunocompromised patients may not be able to mount a response (wheal) to injection of the organism. Pulmonary function tests are characteristic of restrictive diseases, with decreased lung volumes and decreased compliance.

Treatment. Primary therapy for active tuberculosis consists of (1) administering multiple drugs to which the organism is susceptible; (2) adding at least two new agents to the drug regimen when treatment failure is suspected; (3) providing the safest, most effective therapy for the shortest period of time; and (4) ensuring adherence to therapy by utilizing directly observed therapy.[2] Nonadherence to therapy due to adverse drug reactions is a major cause of treatment failure. HIV-negative individuals are typically treated for 6 to 9 months with isoniazid, rifampin, and pyrazinamide. In areas of drug resistance to isoniazid, ethambutol or streptomycin should be added. For a detailed explanation of drug therapy for tuberculosis, refer to a specialized textbook.

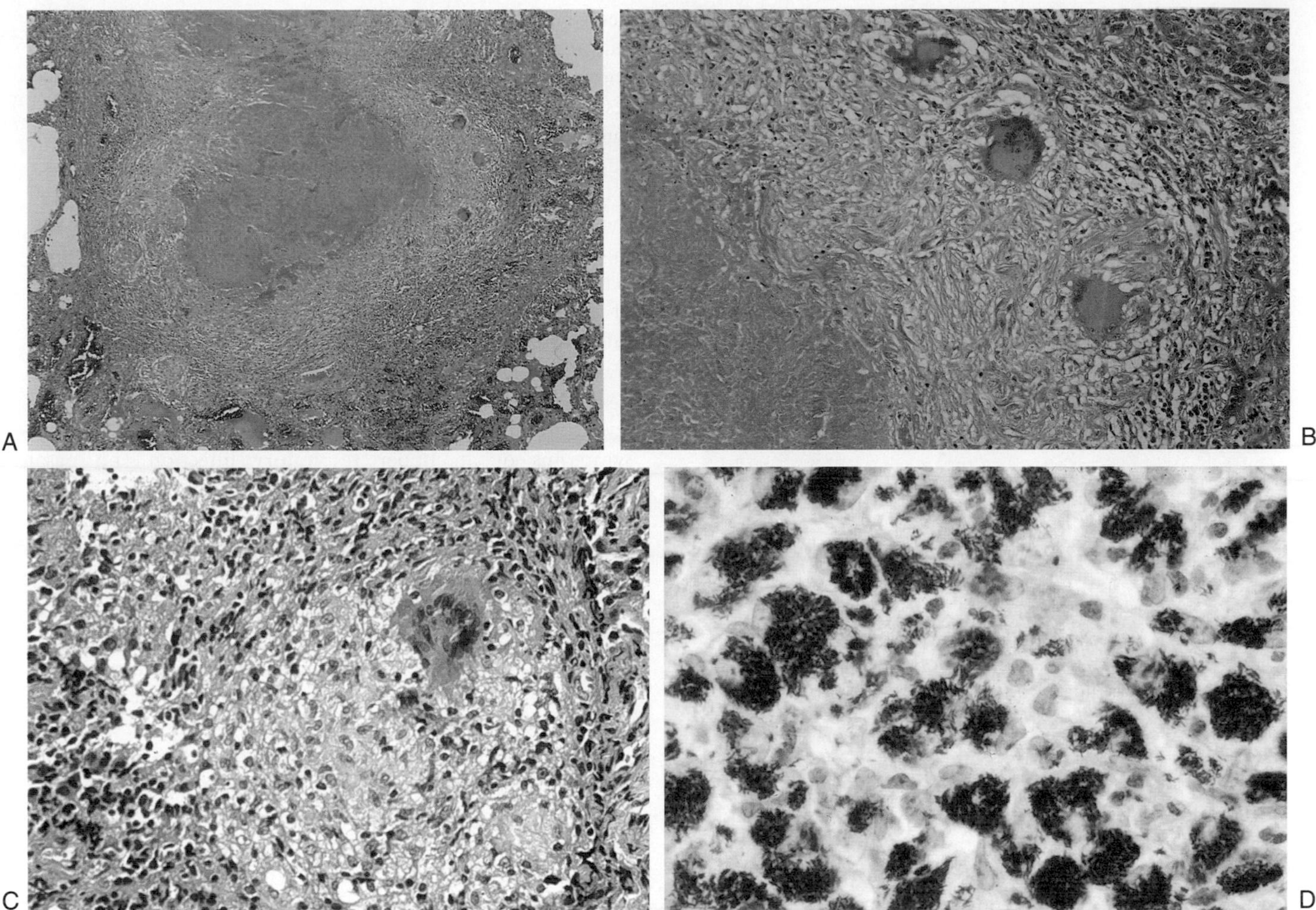

FIGURE 23-10 ■ The morphologic spectrum of tuberculosis. A characteristic tubercle at low magnification **(A)** and in detail **(B)** illustrates central granular *caseation* surrounded by epithelioid and multinucleated giant cells. This is the usual response seen in patients who have developed cell-mediated immunity to the organism. Occasionally, even in immunocompetent individuals, tubercular granulomas may not show central caseation **(C)**; hence, irrespective of the presence or absence of caseous necrosis, special stains for acid-fast organisms need to be performed when granulomas are present in histologic sections. In *immunosuppressed* individuals, tuberculosis may not elicit a granulomatous response ("nonreactive tuberculosis"); instead, sheets of foamy histiocytes are seen, packed with mycobacteria that are demonstrable with acid-fast stains **(D)**. (From Cotran RS, Kumar V, Robbins SL: *Robbins basic pathology,* ed 7, Philadelphia, 2003, Saunders, p 488. **D,** Courtesy Dr. Dominick Cavuoti, Department of Pathology, University of Texas Southwestern Medical School, Dallas.)

KEY CONCEPTS

- Tuberculosis is caused by inhalation or ingestion of the bacterium *Mycobacterium tuberculosis.* The organism spreads through the lymph and blood. Bacteria are ingested by macrophages and walled off by inflammatory proteins (granulomas). The organisms may not be killed and can persist in a dormant state for years. These walled-off areas of inflammatory cells and bacteria become fibrotic and calcified, forming Ghon tubercles—the hallmark of tuberculosis.
- Symptoms are somewhat nonspecific: low-grade fever, cough, night sweats, fatigue, and weight loss. With progression of the disease, the cough is productive of purulent sputum.
- The diagnosis is based on a positive purified protein derivative skin test for tuberculosis, positive sputum cultures, and characteristic nodules on chest radiographs.
- Isoniazid and rifampin are the agents of choice for managing tuberculosis. Drug therapy continues for 9 to 12 months for active disease and may be used for shorter periods in persons exposed to tuberculosis but having no active disease.

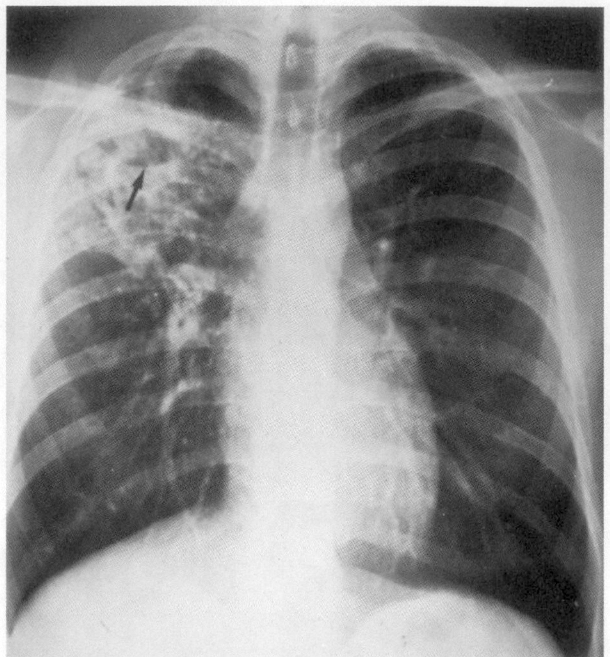

FIGURE 23-11 ■ Cavitary pulmonary tuberculosis in a 23-year-old man. (From Kersten LD: *Comprehensive respiratory nursing,* Philadelphia, 1989, Saunders, p 146.)

Severe Acute Respiratory Syndrome

Severe acute respiratory syndrome (SARS) was first reported in February 2003 as a severe form of pneumonia occurring in Asia. In that year the disease spread to more than two dozen countries in North America, South America, Europe, and Asia before the global outbreak was contained.[50] According to the World Health Organization, a total of 8089 people became sick with SARS worldwide and 774 died. Extensive efforts at identification and containment prevented further spread of the disease, and the epidemic abated in mid-2003. Only eight confirmed SARS cases occurred in the United States during the epidemic.[50] Active global surveillance for SARS in human beings had detected no further confirmed person-to-person transmission of the disease between July 2003 and August 2004. However, two cases of SARS occurred in persons working in laboratories in Southern China.

Etiology. SARS is caused by a coronavirus called SARS-associated coronavirus (SARS-CoV).[50] The primary mode of transmission appears to be through close person-to-person contact, most likely through respiratory droplets that are produced when a person coughs or sneezes. The virus also can spread through contact with contaminated objects or surfaces followed by touching the mouth, nose, or eyes.

Pathogenesis. The SARS virus epidemic was associated with milder disease in infants and children, and most of those with severe respiratory forms of the disease were adults. The median incubation period is about 4 to 6 days, and most patients become ill within 10 days after exposure.[50] Early clinical features of SARS are similar to those of other viral illnesses and include systemic signs and symptoms of an inflammatory response including fever, headache, and muscle aches. Respiratory complaints are also nonspecific and include nonproductive cough and shortness of breath. Nearly all patients develop radiographic evidence of pneumonia by day 7 to 10 of the illness, and the majority also develop lymphopenia (reduced lymphocytes in the blood).[50] The pneumonia can be severe with significant hypoxemia and an overall mortality rate of about 10%. In persons older than 60 years, the mortality rate may be close to 50%.[50]

Clinical Manifestations. Most patients present with fever, nonproductive cough, and dyspnea, often without symptoms of an upper respiratory infection (no nasal drainage). Evidence of pneumonia on chest x-ray is usually evident within 1 week of symptom onset. Lymphopenia may be evident on the complete blood count differential. There are no specific clinical manifestations for SARS, and it is unlikely as a cause of pneumonia unless there is a known history of exposure or travel to high-risk areas (mainland China, Hong Kong, or Taiwan). In the severe form of the disease, arterial blood gases reflect poor ventilation with low PaO_2.

Diagnosis. No specific laboratory or clinical clues differentiate SARS-associated pneumonia from other forms of pneumonia at presentation of the patient. Early recognition and containment rely on a high index of suspicion based on clinical and epidemiologic factors. The vast majority of SARS cases during the epidemic had a clear history of exposure to a SARS patient or to a setting in which SARS-CoV transmission was known to be occurring. Patients presenting with manifestations of viral pneumonia severe enough to cause hospitalization and a history of possible exposure should be tested for SARS. If known cases of SARS are occurring in the world, a lower threshold for testing may be instituted. Although not diagnostic, the following laboratory abnormalities have been seen in some patients with SARS: lymphopenia with a normal or low white blood cell count, elevated liver enzymes, elevated creatine kinase, elevated lactate dehydrogenase, and prolonged activated partial thromboplastin time. Definitive diagnosis requires laboratory confirmation of the SARS-CoV.[50] Respiratory specimens (e.g., from the nasopharynx, oropharynx, and sputum), blood, and stool can be tested for the presence of SARS virus.

Treatment. Currently, there are no definitive treatment recommendations for SARS. Patients with symptoms of pneumonia requiring hospitalization need supportive care, which may include administration of supplemental oxygen and mechanical ventilation. Evaluation for and treatment of other possible sources of pneumonia that may be responsive to antibiotic therapy are recommended. Isolation precautions should be instituted in cases suspicious for SARS and discontinued only after consultation with local public health authorities.

SUMMARY

Restrictive pulmonary disorders are those in which lung expansion is restricted. Restrictions are commonly caused by diseases that affect the lung parenchyma (e.g., diffuse interstitial pulmonary fibrosis), chest wall disorders, neuromuscular disorders, pleural space disorders, pneumonia, and tuberculosis. These diseases are characterized by a reduced vital capacity and a small residual lung volume. They differ from obstructive diseases, covered in Chapter 22, in that airway resistance is not increased.

MEDIA RESOURCES

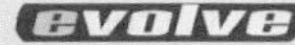

evolve

Remember to check out the ***CD Companion*** included with this book for Review Questions, Key Concepts Review, Glossary (with audio for selected terms), Disease Profiles, and Animations.

PLUS, visit the ***Evolve website*** at http://evolve.elsevier.com/Copstead/ for Case Studies, Disease Profiles, and WebLinks.

References

1. West JB: *Pulmonary pathophysiology: the essentials,* ed 5, Philadelphia, 1998, Lippincott Williams & Wilkins.
2. Chesnutt MS, Prendergart TJ: Lung. In Tierney LM, McPhee SI, Papadakis MA, editors: *Current medical diagnosis and treatment,* ed 42, New York, 2003, Lange/McGraw-Hill, pp 216-311.
3. Ferri FF: Diffuse interstitial lung disease. In Ferri FF, editor: *Ferri's clinical advisor: instant diagnosis and treatment,* St Louis, 2003, Mosby, p 270.
4. Paranjothi S, Schuller D: Pulmonary diseases. In Ahya SN, Flood K, Paranjothi S, editors, *The Washington manual of medical therapeutics,* ed 30, Philadelphia, 2001, Lippincott Williams & Wilkins, pp 216-240.
5. Moller DR, Johns CJ: Interstitial lung disease. In Stobo JD et al, editors: *The principles and practice of medicine,* ed 23, Stamford, Conn, 1996, Appleton & Lange, pp 147-154.
6. Schwartz MJ, King TE, Cherniack RM: Infiltrative and interstitial lung diseases: general principles and diagnostic approach to the interstitial lung diseases. In Murray JF, Nadel JA: *Textbook of respiratory medicine,* ed 3, Philadelphia, 2000, Saunders, pp 1803-1826.
7. Schlereter DP: Interstitial lung diseases. In Noble J et al, editors: *Textbook of primary care medicine,* ed 3, St Louis, 2001, Mosby, pp 688-697, 1560-1571.
8. Ferri FF: Sarcoidosis. In Ferri FF, editor: *Ferri's clinical advisor: instant diagnosis and treatment,* St Louis, 2003, Mosby, pp 729-730.
9. Schuyler M: Hypersensitivity pneumonitis. In Rakel RE, Bope ET, editor: *Conn's current therapy,* Philadelphia, 2003, Saunders, pp 274-275.
10. Thurlbeck WM, Miller RR: The respiratory system. In Rubin E, Farber JL, editors: *Essential pathology,* ed 3, Philadelphia, 2001, Lippincott Williams & Wilkins, pp 542-627.
11. Oliva JM: Hypersensitivity pneumonitis. In Ferri FF, editor: *Ferri's clinical advisor: instant diagnosis and treatment,* St Louis, 2003, Mosby, pp 437-438.
12. Oliver LC, Stoeckle JD: Evaluation and prevention of occupational and environmental respiratory disease. In Goroll AH, Mulley AG, editors: *Primary care medicine: office evaluation and management of the adult patient,* ed 4, Philadelphia, 2000, Lippincott Williams & Wilkins, pp 262-267.
13. Vollman KM, Aulbach RK: Acute respiratory distress syndrome. In Kinney MR et al, editors: *AACN's clinical reference for critical care nursing,* ed 4, St Louis, 1998, Mosby, pp 529-564.
14. West JB: *Pulmonary physiology and pathophysiology: an integrated, case-based approach,* Philadelphia, 2001, Lippincott Williams & Wilkins.
15. Ferri FF: Respiratory distress syndrome, acute. In Ferri FF, editor: *Ferri's clinical advisor: instant diagnosis and treatment,* St Louis, 2003, Mosby, pp 705-707.
16. The Acute Respiratory Distress Syndrome Network: Ventilation with lower tidal volumes as compared with traditional tidal volumes for acute lung injury and the acute respiratory distress syndrome, *N Engl J Med* 342(18):1301-1308, 2000.
17. Irvine LA: Neonatology. In Gunn VL, Nochyba C, editor: *The Harriet Lane handbook,* ed 16, Philadelphia, 2002, Mosby, pp 379-396.
18. Thilo EH, Rosenberg AA: The newborn infant. In Hay WW et al, editors. *Current pediatrics: diagnosis and treatment,* ed 15, New York, 2001, Lange/McGraw-Hill, pp 1059.
19. Neonatal handbook: respiratory distress syndrome. www.netsvic.org.au/nets/handbook/index.cfm, June 2002.
20. Pramanik A: Respiratory distress syndrome. www.emedicine.com/ped/topic1993.htm, July 2002.
21. Pagana KD, Pagana TJ: *Mosby's diagnostic and laboratory test reference,* ed 5, St Louis, 2001, Mosby.
22. Thompson TR: Respiratory distress in the newborn infant: evaluation and etiology, www.peds.umn.edu/divisions/neonatology/rd.htm.
23. Petropoulos P: Spontaneous pneumothorax. In Ferri FF, editor: *Ferri's clinical advisor: instant diagnosis and treatment,* St Louis, 2003, Mosby, pp 646-647.
24. Brooks AM: Spontaneous pneumothorax. In Garfunkel LC, Kaczorowski J, Christy C: *Mosby's pediatric clinical advisor,* St Louis, 2002, Mosby, pp 592-593.
25. Larsen GL et al, editors: *Current pediatrics: diagnosis and treatment,* ed 15, New York, 2001, Lange/McGraw-Hill, pp 469-470.
26. Jablons D, Cameron RB, Turley K: Thoracic wall, pleura, mediastinum and lung. In Way KW, Doherty GM, editors: *Current surgical diagnosis and treatment,* ed 11, New York, 2003, Lange/McGraw-Hill, pp 394-407.
27. Guyton AC, Hall JE: *Textbook of medical physiology,* ed 10, Philadelphia, 2000, Saunders, pp 432-443.
28. Goroll AH, Mulley AG: Evaluation of pleural effusions. In Goroll AH, Mulley AG, editors: *Primary care medicine: office evaluation and management of the adult patient,* ed 4, Philadelphia, 2000, Lippincott Williams & Wilkins, pp 279-284.

29. Toder D: Pleural effusion. In Garfunkel LC, Kaczorowski J, Christy C, editors: *Mosby's pediatric clinical advisor: instant diagnosis and treatment,* St Louis, 2002, Mosby, pp 588-589.
30. Rieger KM, Kesler KA: Pleural effusion and empyema thoracic. In Rakel RE, Bope ET, editors: *Conn's current therapy,* Philadelphia, 2003, Saunders, pp 242-244.
31. Light RW: Disorders of the pleura, mediastinum, and diaphragm. In Braunwald E et al, editors: *Harrison's principles of internal medicine,* ed 15, New York, 2001, McGraw-Hill, pp 1513-1516.
32. Policer M: Poliomyelitis. In Ferri FF, editor: *Ferri's clinical advisor: instant diagnosis and treatment,* St Louis, 2003, Mosby, pp 648.
33. Shandera WX, Shelburne S: Infectious diseases: viral and rickettsial. In Tierney LM, McPhee SI, Papadakis MA, editors: *Current medical diagnosis and treatment,* ed 42, New York, 2003, Lange/McGraw-Hill, pp 1303-1348.
34. Ferri FF: Amyotrophic lateral sclerosis. In Ferri FF, editor: *Ferri's clinical advisor: instant diagnosis and treatment,* St Louis, 2003, Mosby, p 50.
35. Ferri FF: Guillain-Barré syndrome. In Ferri FF, editor: *Ferri's clinical advisor: instant diagnosis and treatment,* St Louis, 2003, Mosby, p 362.
36. Eilert RE: Orthopedics. In Hay WW et al, editors. *Current pediatrics: diagnosis and treatment,* ed 15, New York, 2001, Lange/McGraw-Hill, pp 699-718.
37. Mercier LR: Scoliosis. In Ferri FF, editor: *Ferri's clinical advisor: instant diagnosis and treatment,* St Louis, 2003, Mosby, p 739.
38. Hellmann DB, Stone JH: Arthritis and musculoskeletal disorders. In Tierney LM, McPhee SI, Papadakis MA, editors: *Current medical diagnosis and treatment,* New York, 2003, Lange/McGraw-Hill, pp 783-838.
39. Braun J et al: New treatment options in spondyloarthropathies: increasing evidence for significant efficacy of anti-tumor necrosis factor therapy, *Curr Opin Rheumatol* 13(4):245-249, 2001.

40. Macho JR, Krupski WC, Lewis FR: Management of injured patients. In Way LW, Doherty GM, editors: *Current surgical diagnosis and treatment,* ed 11, New York, 2003, Lange/McGraw-Hill, pp 230-266.
41. Petropoulos P: Obesity. In Ferri FF, editor: *Ferri's clinical advisor: instant diagnosis and treatment,* St Louis, 2003, Mosby, pp 575-576.
42. Baron RB: Nutrition. In Tierney LM, McPhee SI, Papadakis MA, editors: *Current medical diagnosis and treatment,* ed 42, New York, Lange/McGraw-Hill, 2003, pp 1212-1244.
43. National Institute of Health, National Heart, Lung, and Blood Institute: Clinical guidelines on the identification, evaluation and treatment of overweight and obesity in adults. The evidence report. www.nhlbi.nih.gov/guidelines/obesity/ob-gdlns.pdf.
44. Fitzgerald PA: Endocrinology. In Tierney LM, McPhee SI, Papadakis MA, editors: *Current medical diagnosis and treatment,* ed 42, New York, 2003, Lange/McGraw-Hill, pp 1067-1151.
45. Levison ME: Pneumonia, including necrotizing pulmonary infections. In Braunwald E et al, editors: *Harrison's principles of internal medicine,* ed 15, New York, 2001, McGraw-Hill, pp 1475-1485.
46. Niederman MS: Bacterial pneumonia. In Rakel RE, Bope ET, editors: *Conn's current therapy,* Philadelphia, 2003, Saunders, pp 247-254.
47. McCarthy C: Pneumonia. In Garfunkel LC, Kaczorowski J, Christy C, editors: *Mosby's pediatric clinical advisor: instant diagnosis and treatment,* St Louis, 2002, Mosby, pp 590-591.
48. Alonso GO: Pulmonary tuberculosis. In Ferri FF, editor: *Ferri's clinical advisor: instant diagnosis and treatment,* St Louis, 2003, Mosby, pp 834-838.
49. Kissner D: Tuberculosis and other mycobacterial diseases. In Rakel RE, Bope ET, editors: *Conn's current therapy,* Philadelphia, 2003, Saunders, pp 275-282.
50. Centers for Disease Control and Prevention: Severe acute respiratory syndrome. www.cdc.gov/SARS, 2004.

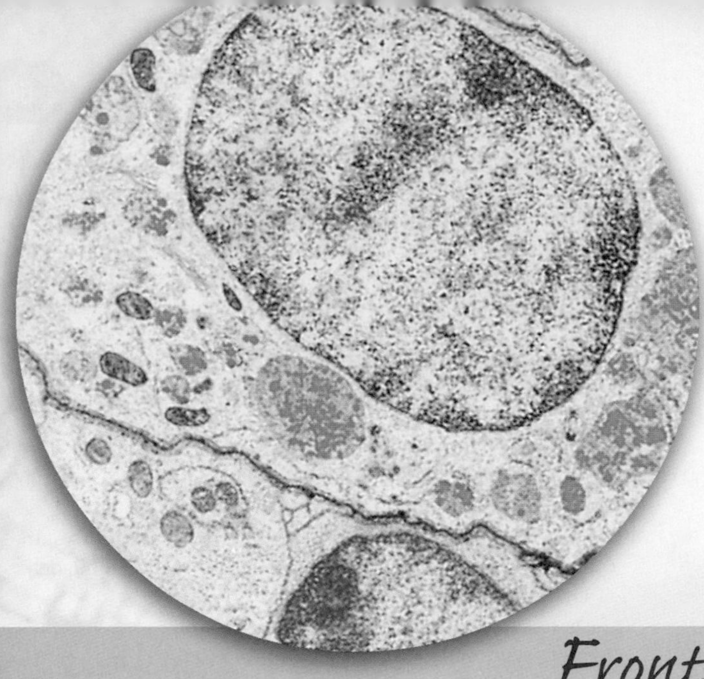

Frontiers of Research

The Sea Within Us

Linda Felver and Michael J. Kirkhorn

Humans are awash in fluids. This "sea within us" flows through our blood and lymph vessels, surrounds our cells, and even resides within them. Like the sea, our body fluids are salt water. In this salt water are sodium, chloride, potassium, calcium, magnesium, phosphate, and other electrolytes. The fluid outside cells (extracellular fluid) normally has different concentrations of these electrolytes than does the fluid inside cells (intracellular fluid). Many physiologic mechanisms combine to keep the volume, concentration, electrolyte composition, and degree of acidity (pH) of body fluids within their normal homeostatic ranges.

Persons who have chronic diseases often have risk factors for imbalances that make managing fluid and electrolytes a necessary part of their lives. Persons who have type 1 diabetes have increased risk for low plasma magnesium, extracellular fluid volume (ECV) deficit, diabetic ketoacidosis, low plasma phosphate, and either high or low plasma potassium, depending on their medications. Persons who have chronic renal failure have high risk of ECV excess; high plasma potassium, magnesium, and phosphate; and metabolic acidosis. Nurses teach individuals who have chronic diseases how to prevent imbalances and how to recognize them if they occur. Acute pathophysiologic processes bring additional needs for nursing care.

Many medications alter electrolyte homeostasis. For example, persons who take most kinds of diuretics on a long-term basis should learn to increase their intake of potassium and magnesium. They need to know which foods are rich in these electrolytes and how to recognize the muscle weakness of low plasma potassium.

Current research indicates that many persons use herbal preparations and other supplements that can cause fluid, electrolyte, or acid-base imbalances. For example, licorice root (licorice extract; *Glycyrrhiza*) causes the kidneys to excrete more potassium. In the presence of other risk factors or with excessive use, this increased potassium excretion causes symptomatic low plasma potassium. Licorice root also causes the kidneys to retain sodium and water, leading to ECV excess.

Chronic alcohol abuse frequently causes low plasma magnesium due to poor magnesium intake and absorption, diarrhea, vomiting, and alcohol-induced increased renal excretion of magnesium. Low plasma magnesium decreases plasma potassium by increasing potassium excretion in the urine. Low magnesium suppresses parathyroid

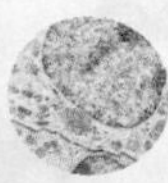

Transmission electron micrograph of glycogen granules (green) *in a liver cell. Glycogen (a polysaccharide) is the form in which human cells store glucose (a monosaccharide). (From Thibodeau GA, Patton KT:* Anatomy & physiology, *ed 5, St Louis, 2003, Mosby. Courtesy Brenda Russell, PhD, University of Illinois at Chicago.)*

Fluid, Electrolyte, and Acid-Base Homeostasis

UNIT VII

hormone, causing low plasma calcium. Chronic alcohol abuse also carries high risk for alcoholic ketoacidosis, low plasma phosphate, and ECV deficit. Alcohol-related diseases such as pancreatitis bring risk of additional imbalances. Clinicians who encounter persons who abuse alcohol need considerable knowledge of prevention, assessment, and management of these imbalances.

Assessment for fluid and electrolyte imbalances occurs in many settings. Home health nurses assess for ECV deficit in adults by measuring postural blood pressures and pulse and examining other physical signs. Telephone advice nurses can assess for the same imbalance by asking whether the person feels lightheaded when rising from a sitting or lying position. Hospital clinicians look for low serum potassium on a laboratory report. Practitioners in community settings can assess for low potassium by asking patients whether their legs feel heavy when they climb stairs.

Assessments can be adapted for persons of different ages. In adults, assessment of postural blood pressure and filling of neck veins gives useful information about ECV. These assessments are not reliable in infants and small children. Recent research on assessment of ECV deficit in children indicates that testing skin turgor and capillary refill is important. However, in older adults, poor skin turgor is not a reliable indicator.

Safe therapy for specific imbalances depends on thorough knowledge of fluid, electrolyte, and acid-base homeostasis. Nurses teach parents whose children have vomiting and diarrhea how to replace body fluids with salty liquids containing a small amount of sugar, based on research into the best composition of oral rehydration solutions. Other research has taught nurses who add potassium to flexible intravenous bags to mix them carefully end-to-end before hanging them. The medication injection port is located near the infusion outlet port on these containers. Without mixing, the potassium is delivered in a bolus, which has caused severe cardiac dysrhythmias.

Fluid, electrolyte, and acid-base imbalances may cause death. Clinicians can do much to prevent, assess, and manage these imbalances. Keeping the volume, concentration, electrolyte composition, and pH of the "sea within us," within homeostatic ranges provides the optimal environment for our cells and enables us to function as human beings.

chapter 24

Fluid and Electrolyte Homeostasis and Imbalances

Linda Felver

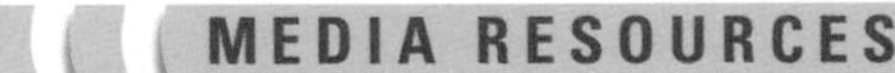

MEDIA RESOURCES

Additional Material for Study, Review, and Further Exploration

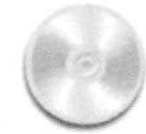

CD Companion ◆ Review Questions and Answers ◆ Key Concepts Review ◆ Glossary *(with audio pronunciations for selected terms)* ◆ Disease Profiles ◆ Animations

evolve ***Website*** at http://evolve.elsevier.com/Copstead/
◆ Case Studies ◆ Disease Profiles ◆ WebLinks

KEY QUESTIONS

- What physiologic and pathophysiologic conditions predispose an individual to disturbances in fluid intake?
- How do the compositions of plasma and interstitial fluids differ? How are they similar?
- How is water and electrolyte movement across cell membranes regulated?
- What are the usual and pathologic routes of fluid exit from the body?
- Under what conditions are saline deficit and excess likely to occur, and what are the characteristic clinical findings?
- Under what conditions are water excess (hyponatremia) and water deficit (hypernatremia) likely to occur?
- What physiologic and pathophysiologic conditions can lead to alterations in electrolyte intake, absorption, distribution, or excretion?

CHAPTER OUTLINE

The fluid of the body flows in arteries, veins, and lymph vessels; it is secreted into specialized compartments as diverse as joints, cerebral ventricles, and the intestinal lumen; it both surrounds and permeates the cells. Body fluid serves as a lubricant and as a solvent for the chemical reactions that we call metabolism; it transports oxygen, nutrients, chemical messengers, and waste products to their destinations; it plays an important role in the regulation of body temperature. Because the fluid within the body is so widespread and serves so many functions, it is not surprising that abnormalities in the volume or composition of body fluid cause clinical problems.

Disorders of fluid or electrolyte homeostasis occur as a result of many different pathophysiologic conditions. In severe cases, these disorders cause death. Although these disorders arise from many specific causes in different patient populations, these specific causes fall into general categories that arise from the principles of normal fluid and electrolyte homeostasis. This chapter first presents the principles of normal fluid homeostasis and then, building on that foundation, continues with a discussion of fluid imbalances. Similarly, the principles of electrolyte homeostasis are explained before plasma electrolyte imbalances are presented.

BODY FLUID HOMEOSTASIS

The term **body fluid,** as used in this chapter, pertains to water within the body and the particles dissolved in it. The body fluid is contained in two major compartments: **extracellular** (outside the cells) and **intracellular** (inside the cells). In all age groups except infants, approximately two thirds of body fluid is intracellular.[1] The other one third of body fluid is extracellular. Infants have more extracellular fluid than intracellular fluid; this proportion reverses within a few months as the infant grows. The extracellular fluid lies between the cells (**interstitial** compartment), in the blood vessels (**vascular** compartment), in dense connective tissue and bone, and in several minor compartments that are collectively termed the **transcellular** fluids (for example, synovial, cerebrospinal, and gastrointestinal fluids). The major body fluid compartments are depicted in Figure 24-1.

The fluids in the various body compartments have different compositions, although their total particle concentration is equal. The intracellular fluid is relatively rich in potassium, magnesium, inorganic and organic phosphates, and proteins. It is relatively low in sodium and chloride. In contrast, the ex-

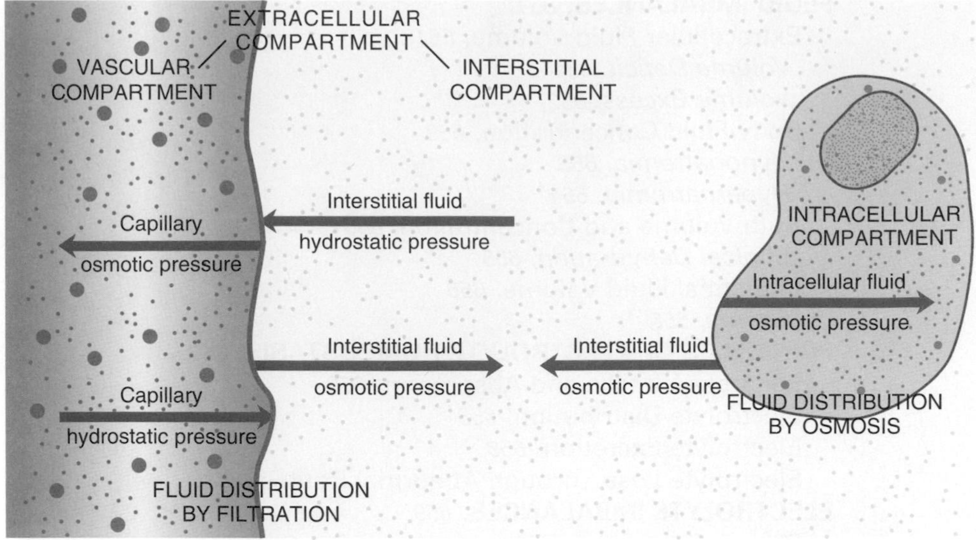

FIGURE 24-1 ■ Factors that influence body fluid distribution. Fluid distribution between the vascular and interstitial compartments is the net result of filtration across permeable capillaries. The distribution of fluid between the interstitial and intracellular compartments occurs by osmosis rather than by filtration.

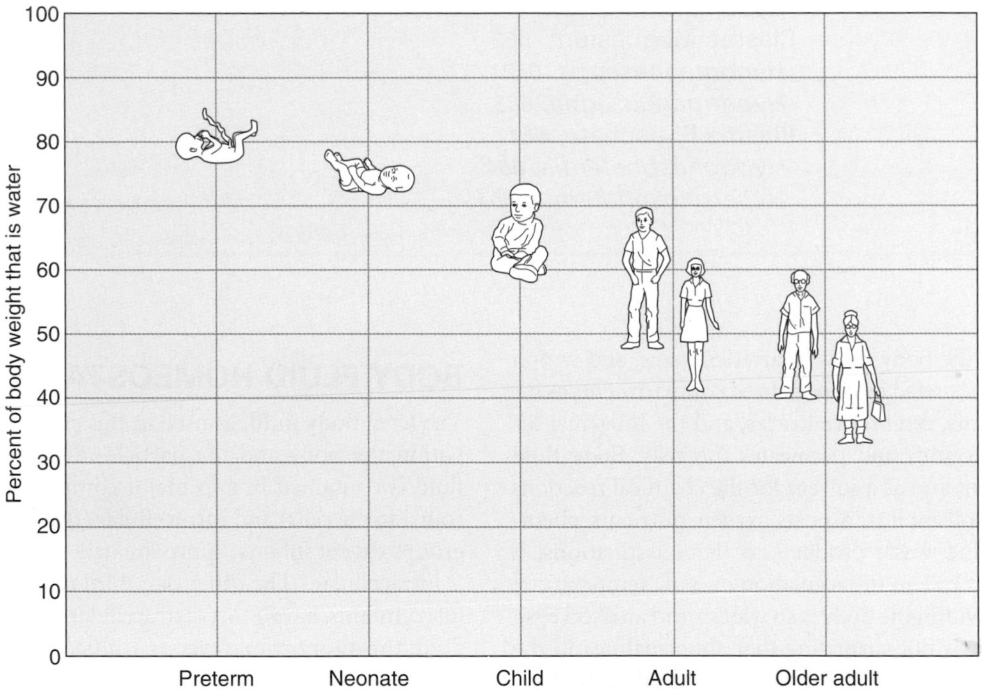

FIGURE 24-2 ■ Percentage of total body water by age. The percentage of body weight that is water is high in infancy and decreases with increasing age.

tracellular fluid in the vascular and interstitial compartments is relatively rich in sodium, chloride, and bicarbonate and relatively low in potassium, magnesium, and phosphates. The vascular portion of the extracellular fluid contains many proteins, whereas the interstitial and transcellular portions of the extracellular fluid contain very few proteins. Most transcellular fluids are secreted by epithelial cells; their composition varies according to their function.

Total body water is the total of the water in all fluid compartments. The percentage of body weight that is water varies according to a person's age and proportion of body fat (Figure 24-2). A full-term newborn infant is about 75% water by weight. (Preterm infants have an even higher percentage of water.) This percentage decreases with age. In a standard adult man, body water is about 60% of body weight. The percentage is less (about 50%) in women because they have a greater pro-

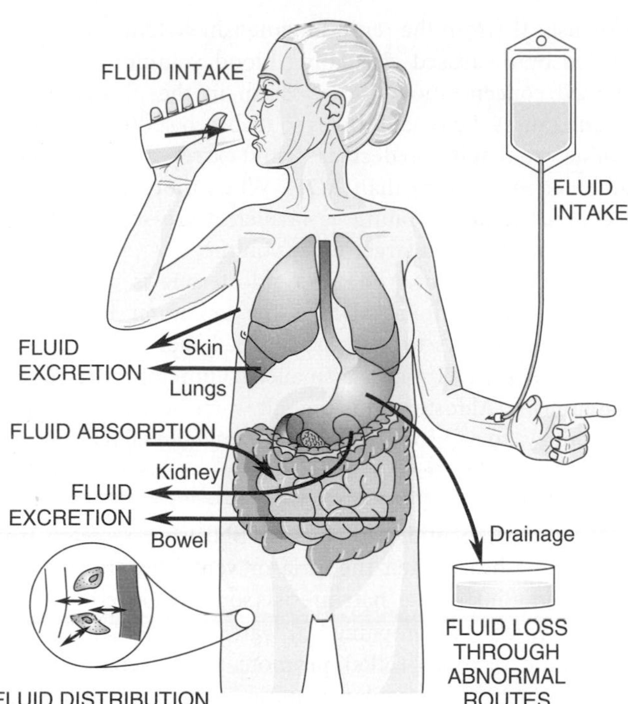

FIGURE 24-3 ■ Fluid homeostasis. Fluid homeostasis is the interplay of fluid intake and absorption, fluid distribution, fluid excretion, and fluid loss through abnormal routes.

portion of body fat than men of the same weight. In obese adults, with a much larger proportion of body fat, less of the body weight is water. In older men, 50% of the body weight is typically composed of water; in older women, it is even less. The decrease in this percentage with increased age is due primarily to the relative increase in body fat that occurs with normal aging.

One liter of water weighs 1 kg (2.2 lb). Thus, a lean, middle-aged, healthy adult man who weighs 70 kg (154 lb) has approximately 42 L of body water. Of this amount, approximately 25 L is intracellular water. The approximately 17 L of extracellular water is distributed as 3 L of plasma water, 8 L of interstitial and lymph water, 5 L of water trapped in dense connective tissue and bone, and 1 L of transcellular water.

Fluid homeostasis is a dynamic process. This process may be viewed as the net result of four subprocesses: *fluid intake, fluid absorption, fluid distribution,* and *fluid excretion.* In some persons who have pathophysiologic conditions, loss of fluid through abnormal routes also occurs. The interplay of these subprocesses is fluid homeostasis (Figure 24-3).

Fluid Intake and Absorption

Fluid intake is entry of fluid into the body by any route. Healthy persons ingest fluids orally, both by drinking and by eating (water contained in food). They also synthesize a small amount of water through cellular metabolism of the foods they eat. Fluid intake by drinking is influenced by habit, social factors, and thirst. Physiologic triggers of thirst include increased osmolality (concentratedness) of extracellular fluid (cerebral osmoreceptor–mediated thirst); decreased circulating blood volume (baroreceptor-mediated and angiotensin II and III–mediated thirst); and dryness of the mucous membranes of the mouth.[2] In older adults, cerebral osmoreceptor–mediated thirst diminishes; thus, older adults who do not have a habit of drinking fluids throughout the day may not have sufficient fluid intake to meet their needs.[3]

Additional routes of fluid intake that may occur in patients who have various pathophysiologic conditions include intravenous intake; intake tubes into the gastrointestinal tract, other body cavities, subcutaneous tissue or bone marrow; rectal intake (such as tap water enema); and, occasionally, intake through the lungs (such as near-drowning). Fluid intake by these routes is often controlled by health care professionals.

Unless fluid intake occurs intravenously, the fluid must be absorbed before it reaches the vascular compartment. Fluid absorption from the gastrointestinal tract is partially dependent on osmotic forces generated by the absorption of electrolytes and other particles.[4]

Fluid Distribution

Much of the fluid that reaches the vascular compartment is then distributed into other fluid compartments. *Fluid distribution between the vascular and interstitial compartments is the net result of filtration across permeable capillaries.* At the capillary level, two forces tend to move fluid from the capillaries into the interstitial compartment: *capillary hydrostatic pressure* (the outward push of the vascular fluid against the capillary walls) and *interstitial fluid osmotic pressure* (the inward-pulling force of particles in the interstitial fluid). Concurrently, two forces tend to move fluid from the interstitial compartment into the capillaries: *capillary osmotic pressure* (the inward-pulling force of particles in the vascular fluid) and *interstitial fluid hydrostatic pressure* (the outward push of the interstitial fluid against the outside of the capillary walls).[3]

The distribution of fluid between the vascular and interstitial compartments is analogous to two groups of people pushing on opposite sides of a swinging door—the strongest "push" will determine in which direction the door will swing. Thus, at any one point along a capillary, the direction and amount of fluid flow between the vascular and interstitial compartments are determined by the net result of opposing forces. These forces are illustrated in Figure 24-1.

In contrast, *the distribution of fluid between the interstitial and intracellular compartments occurs by* ***osmosis,*** *rather than by filtration.* Cell membranes are semipermeable membranes. This means that they are permeable to water but not to electrolytes, many of which require specialized transport mechanisms to cross a cell membrane. Thus, water can move freely through a cell membrane, but electrolytes and other particles cannot. When there is a difference in particle concentration (osmolality) inside and outside cells because the particles cannot move freely, the *water* crosses the membrane to equalize the osmolality.

The direction of movement of water by osmosis is determined by the particle concentrations on the two sides of the semipermeable cell membrane. If, on the one hand, the particle concentration (osmolality) of the interstitial fluid becomes higher than the particle concentration inside cells, water will move by osmosis from the cells to the interstitial fluid to equalize the osmolality in the two compartments. If, on the other hand, the osmolality of the interstitial fluid becomes lower than the osmolality of the intracellular fluid, then water will move from the interstitial compartment to the intracellular compartment to equalize the osmolality. In this way, the osmolality of the interstitial and intracellular compartments controls the distribution of water between them.[5]

The distribution of fluid between the intracellular and transcellular compartments is controlled by processes within the epithelial cells that secrete these fluids.

Fluid Excretion

The fourth component of fluid homeostasis is fluid excretion. Fluid excretion normally occurs through the urinary tract, bowels, lungs, and skin. Fluid is excreted through the skin as visible sweat (which may or may not occur) and as insensible perspiration (which always occurs). Another obligatory route of excretion of water is through the lungs as a person exhales. Fecal excretion of fluid occurs with normal bowel function and increases dramatically in a person who has diarrhea. In a healthy person, the largest volume of fluid is excreted in the urine.

The amount of fluid excreted in the urine is controlled primarily by the hormones antidiuretic hormone (ADH), aldosterone, and natriuretic peptides (atrial natriuretic peptide [ANP] or atrial natriuretic factor [ANF] and brain natriuretic peptide [BNP]), and to a lesser degree by minor hormones such as renal prostaglandins, and by the renal sympathetic nerves. ADH is synthesized by cells in the supraoptic and paraventricular nuclei of the hypothalamus. The axons of these cells extend down the median eminence of the pituitary stalk. The release of ADH thus occurs from the posterior pituitary gland. Factors that increase release of ADH into the blood include increased osmolality (concentratedness) of the extracellular fluid, decreased circulating fluid volume, pain, nausea, and physiologic and psychological stressors. The hormone circulates to the distal tubules and collecting ducts in the kidneys where, consistent with its name, ADH causes reabsorption of water. Reabsorption of water decreases the urine volume and makes the urine concentrated, thus decreasing fluid excretion. Factors that decrease ADH release (such as decreased osmolality of the extracellular fluid and ethanol intake) allow a large dilute urine volume.

Aldosterone is another hormone that influences urine volume. Aldosterone is synthesized and secreted by cells in the adrenal cortex. The major stimuli for its release are angiotensin II (from the renin-angiotensin system, which is activated by decreased circulating blood volume) and an increased concentration of potassium in the plasma. Aldosterone causes the renal tubules to reabsorb sodium and water (saline), so that it also decreases fluid excretion, although by a different mechanism than ADH. When more aldosterone is secreted, the urine volume is smaller; decreased secretion of aldosterone causes a larger urine volume.

A comparison of ADH and aldosterone is useful to remember their actions. ADH is the tap water hormone. It causes the kidneys to reabsorb water. Renal reabsorption of water due to ADH makes a smaller volume of more concentrated urine. Aldosterone is the salt water hormone. It causes the kidneys to reabsorb sodium and water. Renal reabsorption of sodium and water due to aldosterone makes a smaller volume of urine.

Natriuretic peptides (ANP and BNP) are secreted from cells in the heart when the atria or ventricles are stretched. ANP and BNP cause natriuresis (sodium excretion in the urine), which is accompanied by water excretion. Thus, these natriuretic peptides (NPs) promote fluid excretion in the urine. When the vascular volume increases, the heart is stretched, and more NPs are released to cause renal excretion of the excess.[6] When the vascular volume is decreased, the heart is less stretched; therefore, fewer NPs are released and the kidneys excrete less fluid. NPs oppose the action of aldosterone, but they are not as strong as aldosterone.

The urine volume that an individual produces is also highly dependent on having adequate blood pressure to perfuse the kidneys and on the glomerular filtration rate. Renal excretion of fluid is thus the end result of several factors, including hormones that respond to different stimuli and have different actions on the renal tubules.

Fluid Loss Through Abnormal Routes

Persons who have pathophysiologic conditions often experience loss of fluid through abnormal routes. Examples of these routes are emesis; tubes in the gastrointestinal tract or other body cavities; hemorrhage; drainage from fistulas, wounds, or open areas of skin; and paracentesis. The fluid lost through abnormal routes may be a significant factor in disturbing fluid homeostasis.

If the body's physiologic mechanisms are functioning well, the processes of fluid homeostasis maintain normal body fluid status. If fluid intake is large, fluid excretion is increased by the mechanisms described previously that increase urine volume (large volume of dilute urine). If fluid intake is diminished or if fluid is lost through abnormal routes, fluid excretion is decreased (small volume of concentrated urine), and thirst may cause an increase in fluid intake.

If pathophysiologic processes interfere with normal fluid homeostasis or if the normal processes become overwhelmed, then fluid imbalances result. For example, a person who has a pathophysiologic process that prevents the kidneys from excreting much fluid may accumulate too much fluid unless the fluid intake is reduced. The opposite problem will occur in a person whose fluid intake is too small to replace a large amount of fluid excreted or lost through abnormal routes.

KEY CONCEPTS

- Fluid homeostasis is a dynamic process that includes fluid intake and absorption, fluid distribution across body fluid compartments, fluid excretion, and, in some persons, fluid loss through abnormal routes.
- Habit and thirst are important regulators of fluid intake. Individuals who are unable to control their own fluid intake (such as those receiving fluids intravenously, immobile patients, and unconscious patients) are at high risk for fluid imbalance.
- Fluid (water and small particles) moves back and forth between the vascular and interstitial areas by filtration at the capillaries. Capillary hydrostatic pressure is the primary force promoting fluid movement from the capillaries to the interstitial fluid. Plasma colloid osmotic pressure is the primary force that causes interstitial fluid to move back into the capillaries.
- Water moves in and out of cells by osmosis. Electrolytes do not move freely across cell membranes but are transported by membrane channels and carriers.
- Fluid excretion may be visible (urine, feces, sweat) or invisible (respiration and insensible perspiration). Fluid loss may occur through abnormal routes such as emesis and wound drainage. To maintain fluid balance, fluid intake must counterbalance fluid excretion and loss through abnormal routes.
- Healthy kidneys adjust fluid excretion in response to blood pressure and several hormones. Aldosterone induces the kidneys to conserve saline (salt and water); natriuretic peptides (ANP and BNP) promote saline excretion. ADH causes the kidneys to retain water, thus concentrating the urine. Urine volume and concentration are important indicators of body fluid balance.

FLUID IMBALANCES

If fluid homeostasis is disturbed by pathophysiologic processes or other factors (such as medications), fluid imbalances may result. Fluid imbalances fall into two major categories: imbalances of extracellular fluid volume (**saline imbalances**) and imbalances of body fluid concentration (**water imbalances**).

Extracellular Fluid Volume

In some circumstances, individuals have too much or too little extracellular fluid. These disorders are called **extracellular fluid volume (ECV) imbalances** because they involve a change in the *amount* (volume) of the extracellular fluid. These disorders are also termed *saline imbalances* because they are disorders of **isotonic** salt water. (Isotonic saline is salt water in the same concentration as the plasma concentration.) In an ECV imbalance, the *concentration* of the extracellular fluid may be normal; there is simply too much or too little of it. Some persons have an ECV imbalance and an imbalance of body fluid concentration at the same time. In this case, both the volume and concentration (serum sodium) of the extracellular fluid are abnormal. In this section, only the volume imbalances are discussed; the concentration imbalances are discussed separately because they may occur separately.

Volume Deficit

ECV deficit is caused by removal of a sodium-containing fluid from the body. It is a decrease in saline (salt water) in the same concentration as the normal extracellular fluid, which is why the condition is sometimes termed **saline deficit.** In an uncomplicated ECV deficit, the serum sodium concentration is normal. The *concentration* of the extracellular fluid is normal; the *amount* of the extracellular fluid is abnormally decreased (Figure 24-4).

Etiology. Specific causes of ECV deficit are listed in Box 24-1. All causes of ECV deficit involve removal of a sodium-containing fluid from the extracellular compartment. The sodium-containing fluid is usually removed from the body; however, it may be sequestered in a "third space" in the body that is outside the extracellular compartment. For example, ascites (fluid in the peritoneal cavity) that develops rapidly may deplete the ECV. Another example is fluid that accumu-

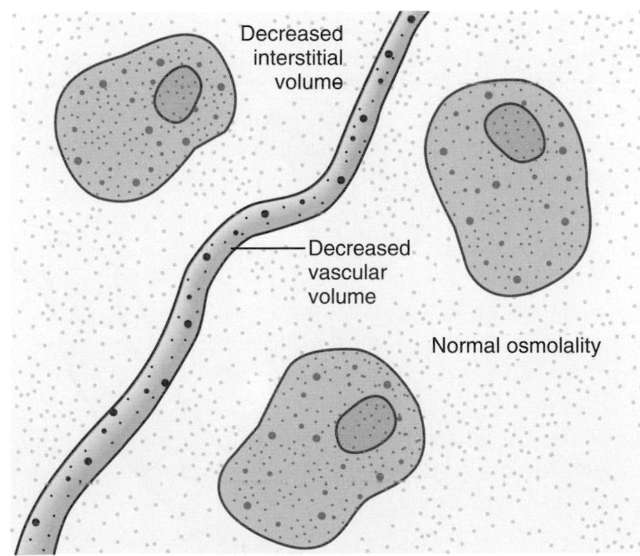

FIGURE 24-4 ■ Extracellular fluid volume deficit. Decreased volume of extracellular fluid in vascular and interstitial compartments is characteristic of extracellular fluid volume deficit.

lates rapidly in the bowel during an acute intestinal obstruction. Although the fluid in these examples remains in the body, it is no longer part of the extracellular fluid, and signs and symptoms of ECV deficit occur.

Clinical Manifestations. The signs and symptoms of ECV deficit are the result of decreased fluid volume in the vascular and interstitial areas. These clinical manifestations include sudden weight loss, postural blood pressure drop,[7] flat neck veins (or veins collapsing with inspiration) when a patient is supine, increased small-vein filling time, dizziness, and oliguria. If the kidneys are responding normally, the small volume of urine will be concentrated (and thus quite yellow). An ECV deficit that develops slowly may also be manifested by skin tenting when it is pinched up over the sternum, dryness of oral mucous membranes between cheek and gum, hard stools, soft sunken eyeballs, longitudinal furrows in the tongue, and absence of tears and sweat. An infant who develops ECV deficit has a sunken fontanel; neck veins are not reliably assessed in infants.

Sudden weight loss is a sensitive measure of ECV deficit. One liter of saline weighs 1 kg; therefore, a person who loses 1 kg in 24 hours has excreted 1 L of fluid or lost it through an abnormal route. It is not possible to lose a kilogram of fat overnight; a sudden weight loss of this magnitude results only from fluid loss, if the body weight is measured accurately. An ECV deficit may occur without a weight loss if fluid is sequestered in a third space somewhere in the body, as with ascites or intestinal obstruction.

A postural blood pressure drop denotes an inadequate circulating blood volume, which is the result of fluid depletion in the vascular compartment. If the systolic blood pressure decreases more than 15 mm Hg when a supine person stands or sits with legs dependent (hanging down), and the diastolic blood pressure decreases 10 mm Hg or more while the pulse rate increases, a postural blood pressure drop is present.[7] A severe ECV deficit may lead to hypovolemic shock.

Box 24-1

Causes of Extracellular Fluid Volume Deficit

Gastrointestinal Excretion or Loss of Sodium-Containing Fluid
Emesis
Diarrhea (includes laxative abuse)
Gastric suction or intestinal decompression
Fistula drainage

Renal Excretion of Sodium-Containing Fluid
Adrenal insufficiency
Salt-wasting renal disorders
Extensive diuretic use
Bed rest

Other Loss of a Sodium-Containing Fluid
Hemorrhage
Massive diaphoresis
Third-space fluid accumulation
Paracentesis and similar procedures
Burns

Volume Excess

ECV excess is essentially the opposite of an ECV deficit. It is the condition in which the amount of extracellular fluid is abnormally increased. Both the vascular and the interstitial areas have too much fluid (Figure 24-5). In an uncomplicated ECV

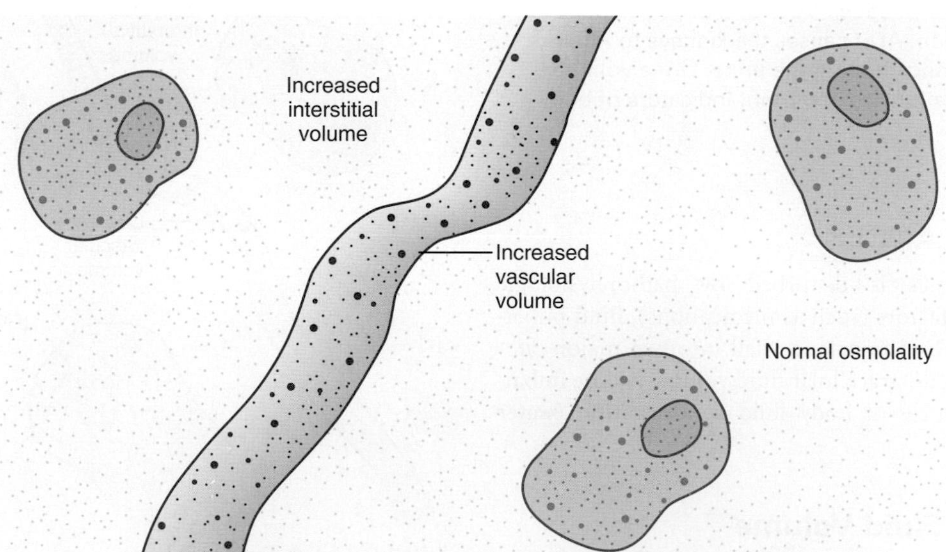

FIGURE 24-5 ■ Extracellular fluid volume excess. Increased volume of extracellular fluid in vascular and interstitial compartments is characteristic of extracellular fluid volume excess.

excess, the *concentration* of the extracellular fluid is normal, but an excessive *amount* of that fluid is present.

Etiology. ECV excess is caused by addition or retention of saline (salt water in the same concentration as the blood). For this reason, it is sometimes termed **saline excess.** As mentioned previously, the hormone aldosterone causes the kidneys to retain saline. ECV excess, therefore, may be caused by conditions that involve excessive aldosterone secretion. For example, increased aldosterone secretion is a compensatory mechanism that commonly accompanies congestive heart failure and eventually leads to ECV excess.[8] Additional causes of ECV excess are presented in Box 24-2.

Clinical Manifestations. The signs and symptoms of ECV excess are sudden weight gain, edema, and manifestations of circulatory overload: bounding pulse, neck vein distention in a person in the upright position, crackles in the dependent portions of the lungs, dyspnea, orthopnea, and even the frothy sputum of pulmonary edema. Infants who develop ECV excess have a bulging fontanel; assessment of neck veins is not effective in infants.

Sudden weight gain is a sensitive measure of ECV excess. It is impossible to gain a kilogram of fat overnight; such a sudden weight gain is accumulation of saline. People who eat salty food in a restaurant weigh more the next day because the water they drank combined with the salt in the food to make isotonic saline. The isotonic saline expands the extracellular fluid, causing a mild saline excess, until it is excreted by the kidneys. This is the reason that low-sodium diets are prescribed for persons who have pathophysiologic processes that cause saline excess (e.g., compensated congestive heart failure).

Body Fluid Concentration

In contrast to the ECV disorders just discussed, imbalances of body fluid concentration are disorders of the *concentration* rather than of the *amount* of the extracellular fluid. Body fluid concentration disorders are also called water imbalances. The serum sodium concentration reflects the osmolality (concentratedness) of the blood. Imbalances of body fluid concentration are recognized by abnormal serum sodium concentration. The normal serum sodium concentration is 135 to 145 mEq/L (may vary slightly with different laboratories). Many persons develop imbalances of both ECV and serum sodium concentration at the same time. Isolated imbalances of serum sodium concentration may also occur. In this section, the concentration imbalances are discussed separately.

Box 24-2

Causes of Extracellular Fluid Volume Excess

Excessive Intravenous Infusion of Sodium-Containing Isotonic Solutions
Normal saline (0.9% sodium chloride)
Ringer injection
Lactated Ringer injection

Renal Retention of Sodium and Water
Primary hyperaldosteronism
Congestive heart failure
Cirrhosis
Acute glomerulonephritis
Chronic renal failure
Cushing disease
Corticosteroid therapy

Hyponatremia

Natrium is the Latin word for sodium. A serum sodium concentration below the lower limit of normal indicates hyponatremia. When hyponatremia is present, the extracellular fluid contains relatively too much water for the amount of sodium present; it is more dilute than normal.

Etiology. Hyponatremia is caused by factors that produce a relative excess of water in proportion to salt in the extracellular fluid. Because the serum sodium concentration reflects the osmolality of the blood, the reduced serum sodium of hyponatremia indicates that the extracellular fluid has a reduced osmolality; it is too dilute. Hyponatremia is also called *hypotonic syndrome, hypoosmolality,* and *water intoxication.* All of these terms reflect the abnormal composition of the extracellular fluid that results when the normal proportion of salt to water in the extracellular fluid is disrupted.

A *gain of relatively more water than salt* will cause hyponatremia. As mentioned previously, the hormone ADH causes the kidneys to retain water (not sodium and water) in the body. This hormone is part of the system that normally regulates the osmolality of the extracellular fluid. However, circumstances that cause prolonged or excessive release of ADH cause the kidneys to retain too much water, which effectively dilutes the blood; hyponatremia is the result. ADH is elevated in the syndrome of inappropriate secretion of ADH (SIADH). It may also be produced **ectopically.** Small cell (oat cell) carcinoma is a type of lung tumor that frequently synthesizes and releases ADH. This ectopic production of ADH from a tumor is not subject to the feedback inhibition of normal ADH release, so inappropriate amounts of ADH are released. With continually high levels of ADH being produced by the tumor, the kidneys retain excessive amounts of water—a gain of water relative to salt. Factors that cause hyponatremia by gain of water relative to salt are presented in Box 24-3.

Hyponatremia may also be caused by a *loss of relatively more salt than water.* If salt is removed from the body while water remains, then the extracellular fluid once again will become too dilute; hyponatremia results. Factors that cause hyponatremia by loss of salt relative to water are also presented in Box 24-3. Although Box 24-3 separates causes of hyponatremia into two categories, some types of hyponatremia are

Box 24-3

Causes of Hyponatremia

Gain of Relatively More Water Than Salt
Excessive antidiuretic hormone
Barbiturate overdose
Hypotonic irrigating solutions
Excessive intravenous infusion of 5% dextrose in water
Tap water enemas
Psychogenic polydipsia (compulsive water drinking)
Forced excessive water ingestion (child abuse or club initiation)
Excessive beer ingestion (beer potomania)
Near-drowning in fresh water

Loss of Relatively More Salt Than Water
Diuretics
Salt-wasting renal disease
Replacement of water but not salt lost through emesis, diarrhea, gastric suction, diaphoresis, or burns

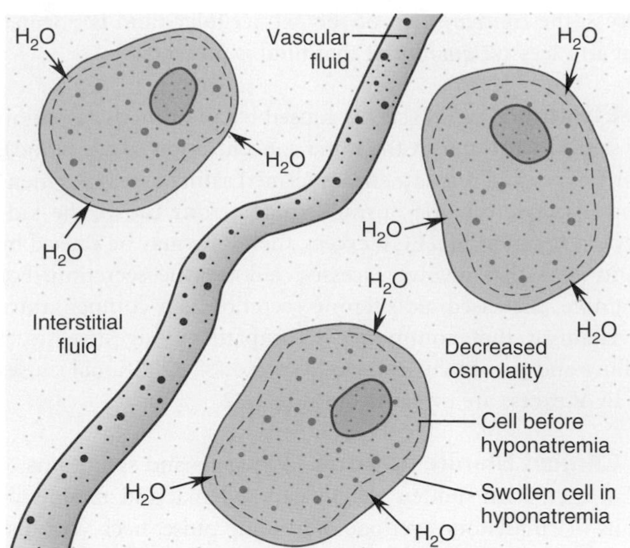

FIGURE 24-6 ■ Cell swelling in hyponatremia. Decreased osmolality (concentration) of extracellular fluid in hyponatremia causes water to move into cells by osmosis.

due to simultaneous gain of water and loss of salt. For example, compulsive water drinking in psychiatric patients (psychogenic polydipsia) and excessive beer drinking both cause hyponatremia from the combination of excessive water gain and renal sodium excretion.[9]

Clinical Manifestations. The clinical manifestations of hyponatremia are nonspecific manifestations of central nervous system dysfunction.[3] They vary from malaise, anorexia, nausea, vomiting, and headache to confusion, lethargy, seizures, and coma. Profound hyponatremia may be fatal. The signs and symptoms are caused by swelling of neurons as a result of the decreased osmolality of the extracellular fluid. As the extracellular fluid becomes too dilute, the intracellular fluid is more concentrated. Therefore, water moves into cells by osmosis (Figure 24-6). The severity of the signs and symptoms depends on the rapidity of the development of hyponatremia as well as on the absolute value of the serum sodium concentration. A rapid decrease in osmolality produces more severe manifestations than a slow decline, other factors being equal.

Hypernatremia

Hypernatremia is a serum sodium concentration above the upper limit of normal (145 mEq/L). When hypernatremia is present, the extracellular fluid contains relatively too little water for the amount of sodium present; it is too concentrated. Hypernatremia is also called *water deficit, hypertonic syndrome,* and *hyperosmolality.* These terms all reflect the relative deficit of water to salt in the extracellular fluid that occurs in hypernatremia.

Etiology. Hypernatremia is caused by a *gain of relatively more salt* than water or by a *loss of relatively more water than salt.* Both of these processes cause the body fluids to become too concentrated. Patients who receive concentrated tube feedings without enough water, especially older adults, are at high risk for hypernatremia because they gain relatively more solute than water, which causes an obligatory loss of relatively more water than salt in the urine. Hypernatremia can be prevented in these patients by administering water between feedings. Other specific factors that cause hypernatremia are presented in Box 24-4 under the two major categories.

Box 24-4

Causes of Hypernatremia

Gain of Relatively More Salt Than Water
Tube feeding
Intravenous infusion of hypertonic solution
Near-drowning in salt water
Overuse of salt tablets
Food intake with reduced fluid intake
Difficulty swallowing fluids
No access to water
Inability to respond to thirst

Loss of Relatively More Water Than Salt
Diabetes insipidus (deficient antidiuretic hormone)
Tube feeding (causes obligate water loss in urine)
Osmotic diuresis
Prolonged diarrhea or diaphoresis without water replacement

Clinical Manifestations. The signs and symptoms of hypernatremia are similar to those of hyponatremia in that they are nonspecific manifestations of central nervous system dysfunction.[3] In hypernatremia, the increased osmolality of

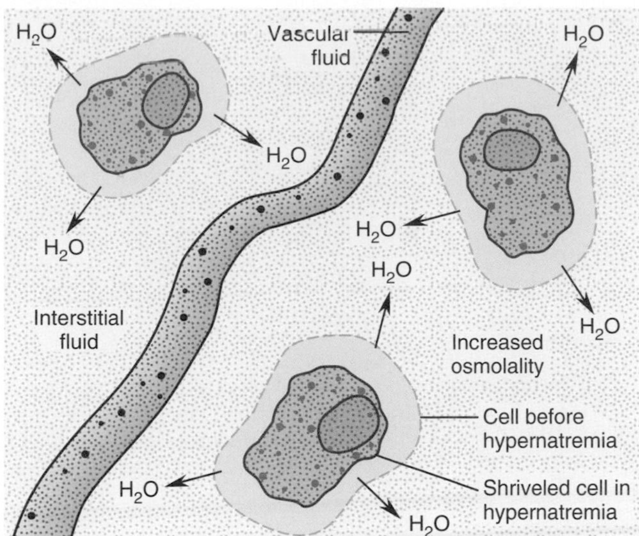

FIGURE 24-7 ■ Cell shriveling in hypernatremia. Increased osmolality (concentration) of extracellular fluid in hypernatremia causes water to move from cells by osmosis.

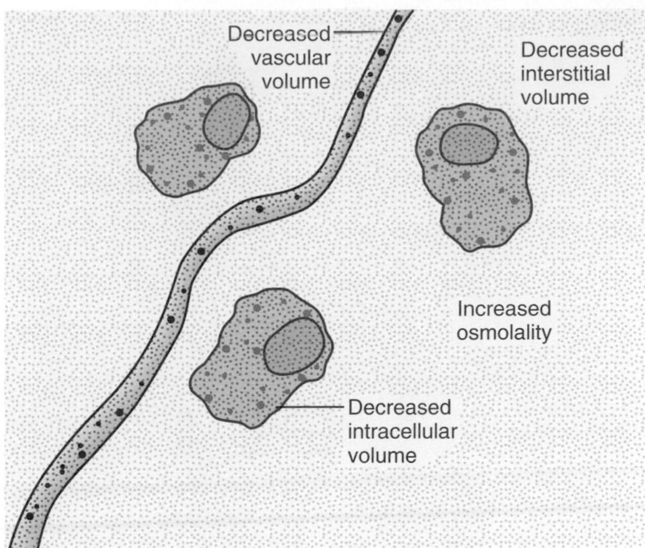

FIGURE 24-8 ■ Clinical dehydration. Decreased volume of extracellular fluid in vascular and interstitial compartments plus cell shriveling from increased osmolality of extracellular fluid are combined in clinical dehydration.

the extracellular fluid causes neurons to shrivel because water moves from the cells to the interstitial fluid by osmosis (Figure 24-7). The dysfunction ranges from confusion and lethargy to seizures and coma. Thirst and oliguria (except for hypernatremia of renal origin) are common. Severe hypernatremia may cause death.

Both Volume and Concentration

Clinical Dehydration

Clinical dehydration is usually a combination of two fluid disorders: ECV deficit and hypernatremia. A person who has clinical dehydration has too small a volume of fluid in the extracellular compartment (vascular and interstitial) and the body fluids are too concentrated (Figure 24-8).

Etiology. Clinical dehydration occurs commonly in persons who have vomiting and diarrhea and do not know how (or are unable) to replace the salt and the water that is exiting the body. Fluid excreted in diarrhea and lost by vomiting, plus the normal daily respiratory, skin, and urine excretion, is the equivalent of hypotonic saline (isotonic saline with extra water added). Removal of the saline portion of this fluid from the body causes ECV deficit. Removal of the extra water from the body causes hypernatremia.

Clinical Manifestations. The signs and symptoms of clinical dehydration are the combination of the signs and symptoms of the two separate disorders. Therefore, a person who is clinically dehydrated will have clinical manifestations as listed in Box 24-5.

Box 24-5

Signs and Symptoms of Clinical Dehydration

Sudden weight loss
Postural blood pressure drop
Dizziness on standing
Flat neck veins when supine or neck veins that collapse during inspiration (older children and adults)
Sunken fontanel (infants)
Rapid, thready pulse
Increased small-vein filling time
Oliguria
Decreased skin turgor
Dryness of oral mucous membranes
Absence of sweat and tears
Hard stools
Soft, sunken eyeballs
Longitudinal furrows in the tongue
Thirst
Confusion, lethargy
Coma
Hypovolemic shock

Interstitial Fluid Volume

Edema

Edema is an excess of fluid in the interstitial compartment. It may be a manifestation of ECV excess or it may arise from other mechanisms. The distribution of fluid between the vascular and interstitial compartments was explained previously in this chapter (see "Fluid Distribution"). An increase in the forces that tend to move fluid from the capillaries into the interstitial compartment or a decrease in forces that tend to

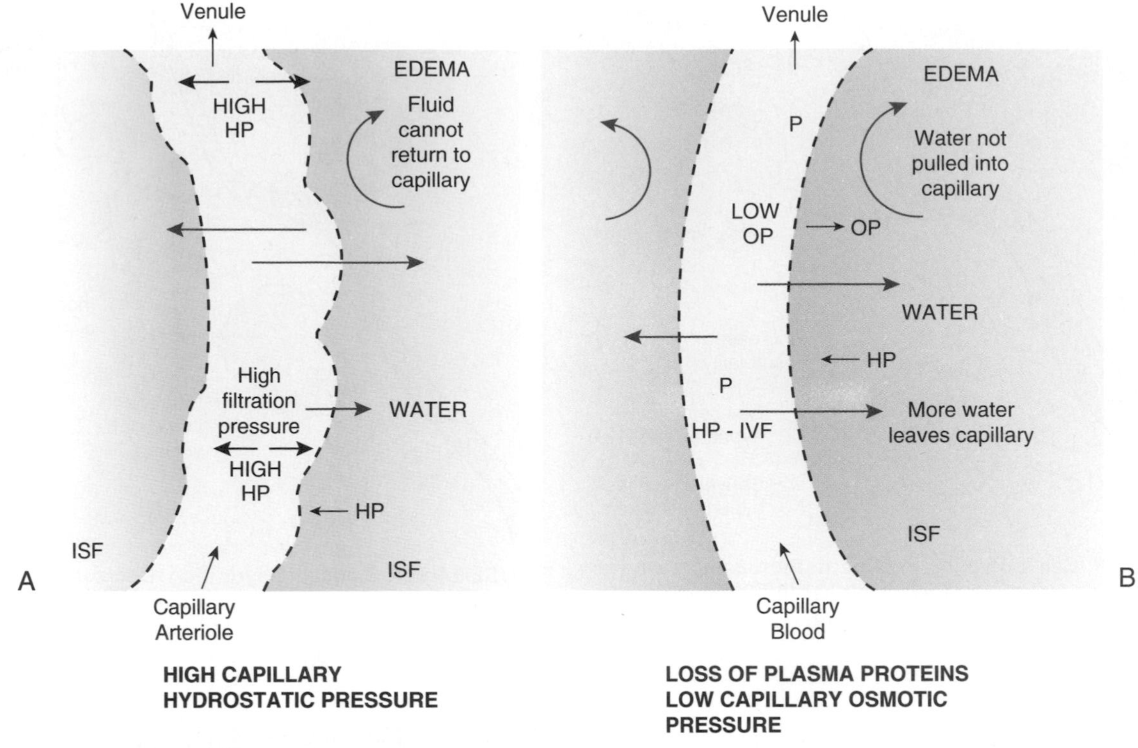

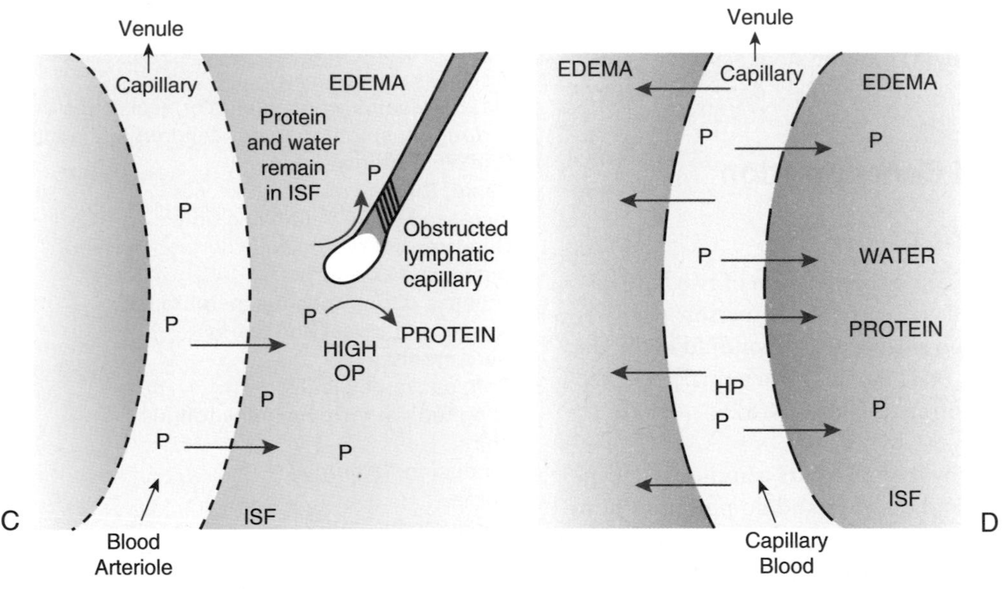

FIGURE 24-9 ■ Causes of edema. **A,** High capillary hydrostatic pressure *(HP)*. **B,** Loss of plasma proteins and low capillary osmotic pressure *(OP)*. **C,** Lymphatic obstruction. **D,** Increased capillary permeability. *P,* Protein; *ISF,* interstitial fluid; *IVF,* intravascular fluid. (From Gould BE: *Pathophysiology for the health professions,* ed 2, Philadelphia, 2002, Saunders, p 109.)

move fluid from the interstitial compartment into the capillaries will cause edema by altering normal fluid distribution between the vascular and interstitial compartments. Thus, edema may arise from increased capillary hydrostatic pressure, increased interstitial fluid osmotic pressure, blockage of lymphatic drainage, or decreased capillary osmotic pressure (Figure 24-9).

Increased capillary hydrostatic pressure is caused by increased ECV, by the increased local capillary flow that accompanies inflammation, and by venous congestion. *Increased interstitial fluid osmotic pressure* occurs when inflammation increases capillary permeability and proteins leak into the interstitial fluid. Lymphatic drainage normally removes minute amounts of protein that enter the interstitial fluid. *Blockage of lymphatic drainage* (e.g., by a tumor, parasites, fibrosis from radiation therapy, or surgical removal of lymph nodes) also causes edema when the interstitial accumulation of protein increases interstitial fluid osmotic pressure.[10] Edema resulting from increased interstitial fluid osmotic pressure or blockage of lymphatic drainage is frequently localized. *Decreased capillary osmotic pressure* occurs when the plasma proteins are decreased, as in malnutrition or liver disease (decreased protein synthesis). Edema from this cause may be extensive.

In summary, edema represents increased interstitial fluid volume, a condition that may be localized or more general. Edema may be a sign of ECV excess (which causes increased capillary hydrostatic pressure) or it may be caused by other factors that alter the distribution of fluid between the vascular and interstitial compartments.

KEY CONCEPTS

- ECV deficit (saline deficit) occurs when sodium-containing fluids are lost from the body (e.g., hemorrhage). It is an abnormally reduced volume of the vascular and interstitial fluids. Saline deficit is characterized by normal serum sodium and manifestations of volume deficit (weight loss, poor skin turgor, postural hypotension, oliguria).
- ECV excess (saline excess) is commonly due to processes that cause the kidneys to retain sodium and water. It is an abnormally increased volume of the vascular and interstitial fluids. Saline excess is characterized by a normal serum sodium level and manifestations of volume excess (weight gain, peripheral edema, distended neck veins, dyspnea).
- Hyponatremia (water excess) is associated with excessive ADH secretion or hypotonic fluid intake. It is characterized by a low serum sodium concentration, which indicates that body fluids are abnormally dilute. Clinical manifestations (confusion, lethargy, seizure, coma) occur because of cell swelling.
- Hypernatremia (water deficit) is associated with inadequate water intake or excessive water excretion or loss. It is characterized by a high serum sodium level, which indicates that body fluids are too concentrated. Clinical manifestations (confusion, lethargy, seizure, coma) occur because of cell shriveling.
- Clinical dehydration occurs commonly in persons who have gastroenteritis or other conditions that remove hypotonic sodium-containing fluids from the body. It is the combination of ECV deficit and hypernatremia. The clinical manifestations are those of both fluid disorders.
- Edema occurs when there is too much fluid in the interstitial compartment. It may be localized or generalized. The causes of edema at the capillary level are increased capillary hydrostatic pressure, increased interstitial fluid osmotic pressure, blockage of lymphatic drainage, and decreased capillary osmotic pressure.

PRINCIPLES OF ELECTROLYTE HOMEOSTASIS

The concentration of an **electrolyte** in the plasma is different from its concentration inside cells. For normal body function, the electrolyte concentration must be normal in both areas. In clinical situations, the plasma (or serum) concentration of an electrolyte is measured. Normal serum electrolyte concentrations are listed in Table 24-1. The concentration of an electrolyte in the plasma is the net result of four processes: *electrolyte intake, electrolyte absorption, electrolyte distribution,* and *electrolyte excretion.* These processes work together in a dynamic fashion to maintain electrolyte concentrations within their normal limits (Figure 24-10). Thus, if electrolyte intake increases, electrolyte excretion also may increase to normalize plasma levels. Similarly, if electrolyte intake decreases dramatically, electrolytes may be redistributed into the plasma to maintain the normal plasma concentration. This chapter discusses homeostasis and imbalances of potassium, calcium, magnesium, and phosphate. Bicarbonate is discussed in Chapter 25.

Table 24-1 

Normal Serum Electrolyte Concentrations

Electrolyte	Normal Concentration Range
Calcium (total)	9-11 mg/dl (4.5-5.5 mEq/L)
Magnesium	1.5-2.5 mEq/L
Phosphate	2.5-4.5 mg/dl (adults and older children)
	4.5-6.5 mg/dl (children)
	4.3-9.3 mg/dl (neonates)
Potassium	3.5-5.0 mEq/L
	3.9-5.9 mEq/L (neonates)
Sodium	135-145 mEq/L
	135-162 mEq/L (neonates)

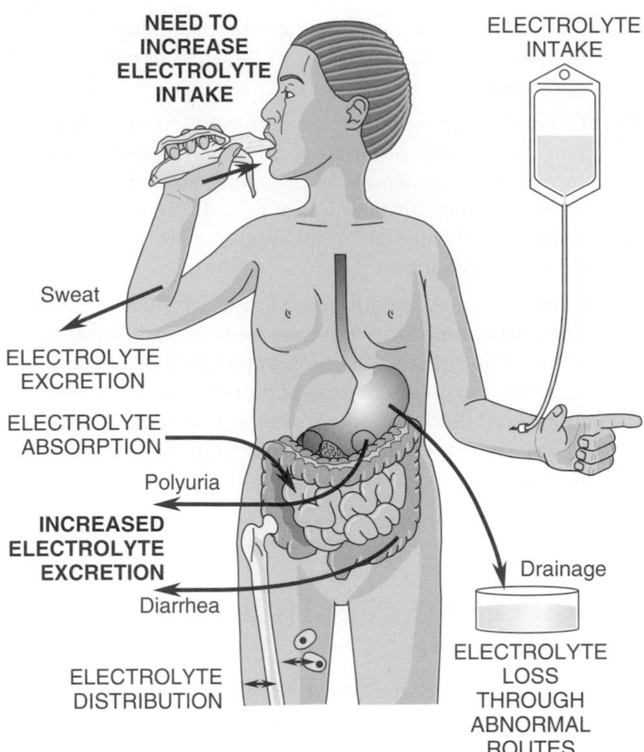

FIGURE 24-10 ■ Electrolyte homeostasis. Electrolyte homeostasis is the interplay of electrolyte intake and absorption, electrolyte distribution, electrolyte excretion, and electrolyte loss through abnormal routes. If electrolyte excretion or loss through abnormal routes increases, electrolyte intake must also increase to prevent electrolyte imbalance.

Electrolyte Intake and Absorption

Electrolyte intake normally occurs orally, through food and drink. It is important to remember that oral medications (e.g., magnesium antacids) may also be an important source of electrolyte intake. Intravenous fluids and hyperalimentation solutions are common sources of parenteral intake of electrolytes. Blood transfusions may provide significant amounts of electrolytes. Less common, but important if it occurs, is intramuscular injection of the electrolyte magnesium.

Some patients have electrolyte intake through tubes into body cavities. The most obvious examples are nasogastric and gastrointestinal feeding tubes, but more unusual situations may cause significant electrolyte intake in specific individuals (such as irrigation of the renal pelvis with magnesium-rich solutions). Rarely, electrolyte intake may occur through such unusual routes as the lungs (e.g., near-drowning in salt water, which is rich in magnesium) or the skin (e.g., through application of ointments to large areas of broken or burned skin). Electrolyte intake is controlled by the individual and by health care providers.

If electrolyte intake occurs orally, the electrolyte must be absorbed before it is physiologically useful. The absorption of some electrolytes, such as potassium, depends on concentration gradients. The absorption of other electrolytes, such as calcium, depends on the availability of binding proteins, which is influenced by the activity of vitamin D.[1] The contents of the gastrointestinal tract may influence electrolyte absorption. Many agents bind electrolytes and prevent them from being absorbed. For example, undigested fat in the intestines binds calcium and magnesium contained in food and prevents them from being absorbed. The pH of the intestinal fluid also influences the absorption of certain electrolytes, especially calcium. Medications often alter the absorption of electrolytes. Surgical removal of portions of the gastrointestinal tract can decrease electrolyte absorption.[11]

Electrolyte Distribution

Every fluid compartment contains electrolytes. However, the electrolyte concentrations of these various compartments differ. The concentration of potassium, calcium, magnesium, and phosphate inside the cells is higher than in the fluid outside the cells. The bones serve as an important reservoir of calcium, phosphate, and magnesium. The cells and the bones are often called the *electrolyte pools.*

The distribution of electrolytes between the extracellular fluid and the electrolyte pools is primarily influenced by hormones such as epinephrine (potassium), insulin (potassium and phosphate), and parathyroid hormone (calcium). Certain medications also influence electrolyte distribution. Significant movement of electrolytes between the cells and the extracellular fluid may occur within minutes.[1] In the absence of changes in electrolyte intake and excretion, a shift of electrolytes from the extracellular fluid into the electrolyte pools will decrease the plasma electrolyte concentration. Conversely, a shift of electrolyte from an electrolyte pool into the extracellular fluid will increase the plasma electrolyte concentration.

Electrolyte Excretion

Electrolyte excretion occurs through urine, feces, and sweat. The urinary excretion of some electrolytes is influenced by hormones (e.g., aldosterone increases potassium excretion), although factors such as the flow rate of renal tubular fluid are also influential. Many medications alter the rate of urinary excretion of electrolytes.[12]

Fecal excretion of electrolytes is influenced by the type of feces produced. Diarrhea increases the excretion of potassium and magnesium in particular. The composition of the feces also influences the amount of electrolyte excretion. Undigested fat in the intestines binds calcium and magnesium ions that are secreted into the gastrointestinal tract and prevents them from being reabsorbed. Thus, these electrolytes are excreted in the feces.

Electrolyte Loss Through Abnormal Routes

When electrolytes exit the body through routes other than the normal urine, feces, and sweat, this may be termed *abnormal electrolyte loss.* This factor alters electrolyte homeostasis in patients who have diverse pathophysiologic conditions. Examples of abnormal electrolyte loss are vomiting,[13] nasogastric suction, paracentesis, hemodialysis, wound drainage, and fistula drainage. Abnormal loss of electrolytes may be uncontrollable or may result from therapeutic procedures.

Electrolyte homeostasis is a dynamic interplay between the processes of electrolyte intake, electrolyte absorption, electrolyte distribution, and electrolyte excretion. In some persons, electrolyte loss through abnormal routes becomes an important factor that requires adjustment of electrolyte intake and/or electrolyte excretion to prevent development of electrolyte imbalances. Individuals who have acute or chronic illnesses have many factors that tend to cause electrolyte imbalances by disrupting or interfering with electrolyte intake, absorption, distribution, or excretion.

KEY CONCEPTS

- The electrolyte composition of the body is maintained by a careful balance of electrolyte intake, absorption, distribution, and excretion. Electrolyte imbalances result from disruption of one or more of these processes or from electrolyte loss through abnormal routes.
- The plasma concentration of an electrolyte may not reflect the intracellular concentration. Cells contain higher concentrations of potassium, calcium, magnesium, and phosphate ions, whereas the extracellular fluid contains higher concentrations of sodium, chloride, and bicarbonate ions.

ELECTROLYTE IMBALANCES

Electrolyte imbalances are widespread in many pathophysiologic conditions. An imbalance of an electrolyte may be a total body imbalance or it may be an imbalance in distribution of electrolytes within compartments, with the total body amount remaining normal. Based on the principles of electrolyte homeostasis explained in the previous section of this chapter, an excess of electrolytes in the extracellular fluid may be caused by increased electrolyte intake or absorption, shift of electrolytes from an electrolyte pool into the extracellular fluid, and decreased electrolyte excretion, either singly or in combination. Conversely, a deficit of electrolyte in the extracellular fluid may be caused by decreased electrolyte intake or absorption, shift of electrolytes from the extracellular fluid to an electrolyte pool, increased electrolyte excretion, abnormal loss of electrolytes, or some combination of these factors.

Plasma Potassium

The normal concentration of potassium ions in serum is 3.5 to 5.0 mEq/L (may vary slightly with different laboratories), except in neonates, in whom it may be higher. Most of the potassium in the body is inside the cells; the standard serum potassium measurement gives only the concentration of the small portion of potassium that is in extracellular fluid. Because a number of factors cause potassium ions to move into or out of body cells, concentration of potassium in the plasma and total body potassium content are not necessarily correlated. Whether or not they are accompanied by total body potassium imbalances, plasma potassium imbalances may cause clinically significant signs and symptoms.

Hypokalemia

Hypokalemia denotes a decreased potassium concentration in the extracellular fluid. A decrease in the plasma potassium concentration does not necessarily denote a decrease in total body potassium. Thus, hypokalemia may coexist with a total body potassium deficit, a total body potassium excess, or a normal total body potassium concentration.

Etiology. Hypokalemia is caused by factors that decrease potassium intake, shift potassium from the extracellular fluid into the cells, increase potassium excretion through the normal routes, and cause potassium loss from the body by some abnormal route. In many cases, a combination of factors leads to hypokalemia. For example, some people follow a fad diet (decreased potassium intake) and abuse diuretics (increased potassium excretion) in an attempt to lose weight. The specific causes of hypokalemia are listed in Box 24-6.

Clinical Manifestations. The ratio of intracellular to extracellular potassium ion concentration is a major determinant of the resting membrane potential of muscle cells. For this reason, potassium imbalances cause altered function of muscles (skeletal, smooth, and cardiac). In hypokalemia, both smooth and skeletal muscles are hyperpolarized (more electrical charge than usual across the cell membrane). Therefore, these muscles are less reactive to stimuli. The resulting clinical manifestations include abdominal distention, diminished bowel sounds, paralytic ileus, postural hypotension, skeletal muscle weakness, and flaccid paralysis.[14] The skeletal muscle weakness of hypokalemia is bilateral weakness that typically begins in the lower extremities and ascends. It may involve the respiratory muscles, causing respiratory paralysis more commonly than does hyperkalemia.

Many types of cardiac dysrhythmias arise from hypokalemia. Cardiac muscle cells usually become hyperpolarized with hypokalemia. However, with very low plasma potassium concentrations, hypopolarization of cardiac muscle occurs, most likely because of decreased potassium conductance. Hypokalemia also increases the rate of diastolic depolarization, which may give rise to ectopic beats, decreases conduction velocity in the atrioventricular node, prolongs cardiac action potentials by decreasing the rate of repolarization, shortens the absolute refractory period, and prolongs the relative refractory period.[7]

Hypokalemia may also cause polyuria by interfering with the action of ADH at the renal tubules. The plasma potassium concentration at which the various clinical manifestations of

Box 24-6

Causes of Hypokalemia

Decreased Potassium Intake
Anorexia
NPO (nothing by mouth) orders and intravenous solutions without potassium
Fasting
Unbalanced diet

Shift of Potassium from Extracellular Fluid to Cells
Alkalosis
Rapid correction of acidosis
Excess insulin (e.g., during total parenteral nutrition)
Excess β-adrenergic stimulation
Hypokalemic familial periodic paralysis

Increased Potassium Excretion Through Normal Routes

Renal Route
Corticosteroid therapy
Potassium-wasting diuretics
Parenteral carbenicillin or similar agents
Hypomagnesemia
Cushing disease
Hyperaldosteronism
Excessive ingestion of black licorice (contains aldosterone-like chemicals)
Amphotericin B, cisplatin, and many other drugs

Fecal Route
Diarrhea (includes laxative abuse)

Skin Route
Excessive diaphoresis

Loss of Potassium Through Abnormal Routes
Emesis
Gastric suction
Fistula drainage

hypokalemia appear depends on individual responsiveness and the presence of other concurrent electrolyte and acid-base disorders.

Hyperkalemia

If the serum potassium concentration rises above 5.0 mEq/L (the upper limit of normal), hyperkalemia is present. Hyperkalemia denotes an elevation of potassium concentration in the extracellular fluid. As mentioned previously, most of the potassium in the body is in the cells, and many factors cause potassium ions to move into or out of the cells. Thus, total body potassium may be increased, normal, or decreased in hyperkalemia, depending on its cause.

Etiology. Hyperkalemia is caused by factors that increase potassium intake, shift potassium from the cells into the extracellular fluid, and decrease potassium excretion.

Box 24-7

Causes of Hyperkalemia

Increased Potassium Intake
Excessive or too-rapid intravenous potassium infusion
Insufficiently mixed intravenous potassium
Large transfusion of stored blood
Massive doses of potassium penicillin G

Shift of Potassium from Cells to Extracellular Fluid
Acidosis caused by mineral acids
Insufficient insulin
Crushing injury
Cytotoxic drugs (tumor lysis syndrome)
Hyperkalemic periodic paralysis
β-Adrenergic blockade

Decreased Potassium Excretion
Oliguria (such as in hypovolemia or renal failure)
Potassium-sparing diuretics
Adrenal insufficiency
Angiotensin-converting enzyme (ACE) inhibitors
Angiotensin II receptor antagonists
Nephrotoxic drugs
Renin-deficient states

Large amounts of potassium released from cells after a crushing injury or massive cell death from chemotherapy will elevate the potassium concentration of the extracellular fluid.[15] Specific causes of hyperkalemia are summarized by category in Box 24-7.

Clinical Manifestations. As might be expected from the role of potassium ions in the establishment of the resting membrane potential of muscle cells, hyperkalemia causes muscle dysfunction. As hyperkalemia develops, the smooth muscle and skeletal muscle become hypopolarized. The main clinical manifestation at this stage is mild intestinal cramping and diarrhea, which occurs only in some persons. As hyperkalemia worsens, the skeletal muscle cells become hypopolarized to the extent that their resting membrane potentials lie above their threshold potential; once they have discharged, they are unable to contract again. This situation results in the skeletal muscle weakness and flaccid paralysis that is typical in hyperkalemia. This skeletal muscle weakness is an ascending weakness that appears first in the lower extremities. Both hypokalemia and hyperkalemia cause skeletal muscle weakness and/or paralysis, but the underlying alterations in the resting membrane potentials are different.

Cardiac muscle undergoes the same changes in resting membrane potential as skeletal muscle in hyperkalemia. In addition, hyperkalemia decreases the duration and rate of rise of cardiac action potentials and decreases conduction velocity in the heart. These pathophysiologic mechanisms underlie the cardiac dysrhythmias of hyperkalemia.[7] Severe hyperkalemia causes cardiac arrest.

The plasma potassium concentration at which each of these clinical manifestations occurs varies, depending on the rapidity of rise of the potassium concentration, the causes of the hyperkalemia, and other concurrent electrolyte or acid-base imbalances. Patients who have chronic renal failure often undergo potassium adaptation and have relatively mild symptoms at high plasma potassium concentrations that would be disabling in other persons. Although the mechanisms of potassium adaptation are not completely understood, increased aldosterone levels in the presence of kidney dysfunction are believed to be an important part of the mechanism. This increased aldosterone increases potassium excretion by the colon and may alter potassium distribution between the extracellular fluid and the cells to normalize the resting membrane potentials.

Plasma Calcium

Calcium in the plasma is present in three forms: some calcium ions are bound to plasma proteins (such as albumin); some are bound to small organic ions (such as citrate); and the remainder are ionized (unbound). Only the ionized calcium is physiologically active. Two laboratory measurements are available for calcium: total serum calcium and ionized calcium. The *total serum calcium* measures all of the calcium (bound plus ionized). The normal range of total serum calcium in adults is 9 to 11 mg/dl or 4.5 to 5.5 mEq/L (may vary slightly with different laboratories). Unless a calcium value specifies ionized calcium, it is total calcium. The *ionized calcium,* as the name indicates, measures only the ionized form. The normal range of ionized calcium in adults is 4.0 to 5.0 mg/dl, about half of the total calcium (varies with different laboratories). Clinically significant calcium imbalances are caused by alterations in the plasma concentration of ionized calcium.

Hypocalcemia

Hypocalcemia occurs if the serum calcium concentration drops below the lower limit of normal. If the fraction of ionized calcium in the blood is decreased by an increase in calcium binding to plasma proteins or other organic ions, the total serum calcium (the usual laboratory measurement) may be normal, but *ionized* hypocalcemia is present and may cause signs and symptoms. Clinicians frequently use formulas to adjust the total calcium if the albumin is low. These formulas are not accurate in critically ill patients. Direct measurement of ionized calcium is necessary to monitor calcium levels reliably in critically ill patients.[16]

Etiology. Hypocalcemia is caused by factors that decrease calcium intake or absorption, decrease the physiologic availability of calcium, and increase calcium excretion. The hypocalcemia of pancreatitis arises from impaired fat digestion caused by lack of pancreatic lipase. Both dietary calcium and calcium secreted into the intestine from the extracellular fluid bind to undigested fat in the intestine and are excreted from the body. Thus, both decreased calcium absorption and increased calcium excretion play a part in hypocalcemia associated with pancreatitis. Box 24-8 lists the specific causes of hypocalcemia organized according to these general etiologic factors.

Box 24-8

Causes of Hypocalcemia

Decreased Calcium Intake or Absorption
Diet with insufficient calcium and vitamin D
Excessive dietary phytates or oxalates
Pancreatitis
Steatorrhea
Chronic diarrhea (includes laxative abuse)
Malabsorption syndromes

Decreased Physiologic Availability of Calcium
Hypoparathyroidism
Excessive phosphate intake
Tumor lysis syndrome (high phosphate)
Hypomagnesemia
Alkalosis
Large transfusion of citrated blood
Rapid infusion of plasma expanders that bind calcium
Elevated plasma free fatty acids

Increased Calcium Excretion Through Normal Routes
Renal Route
Chronic renal insufficiency
Fecal Route
Steatorrhea
Pancreatitis

Clinical Manifestations. Calcium plays an important role in determining the speed of ion fluxes through nerve and muscle membranes. Thus, calcium imbalances alter normal neuromuscular irritability. The clinical manifestations of hypocalcemia are those of increased neuromuscular irritability: positive Trousseau sign; positive Chvostek sign; paresthesias; muscle twitching and cramping; hyperactive reflexes; carpal spasm; pedal spasm; tetany; laryngospasm; seizures; and cardiac dysrhythmias. The increased neuromuscular irritability of hypocalcemia is caused by a decrease in the threshold potential of excitable cells, so that action potentials are generated more easily. The cardiac effects of hypocalcemia are the result of prolongation of the plateau phase of the cardiac action potential, impairment of atrioventricular and intraventricular conduction, and impairment of myocardial contractility.[7]

A positive Trousseau sign is occurrence of a carpal spasm after occlusion of arterial blood flow to the hand for approximately 3 minutes. A positive Chvostek sign is spasm of muscles in the cheek and corner of the mouth produced by tapping the facial nerve in front of the ear. Positive Trousseau and Chvostek signs are general indicators of increased neuromuscular irritability from any cause, so they must be interpreted in the context of other clinical manifestations and specific risk factors for hypocalcemia. Chvostek sign may be positive in neonates without electrolyte imbalances.

Hypercalcemia

Hypercalcemia occurs when the serum calcium concentration rises above the upper limit of normal (11 mg/dl or 5.5 mEq/L). It indicates an elevation of the calcium concentration of the extracellular fluid.

Etiology. Hypercalcemia is caused by factors that increase calcium intake or absorption, cause a shift of calcium from bone to the extracellular fluid, and decrease calcium excretion. Many malignant tumors produce chemicals that are carried in the blood to cause release of calcium from the bones.[17] These bone-resorbing factors include osteoclast-activating factor, parathyroid hormone–related peptide, prostaglandins, and other substances not yet fully characterized. In addition, humoral factors in malignancy may decrease the renal excretion of calcium, which also contributes to hypercalcemia. Specific causes of hypercalcemia are listed by category in Box 24-9.

Clinical Manifestations.
Hypercalcemia causes decreased neuromuscular irritability. Clinical manifestations of hypercalcemia include anorexia, nausea, emesis, constipation, fatigue, polyuria, muscle weakness, diminished reflexes, headache, confusion, lethargy, personality change, and cardiac dysrhythmias. The decreased neuromuscular irritability is caused by elevation of the threshold potential of excitable cells. The cardiac effects of hypercalcemia include shortened plateau phase of the action potential, increased rate of diastolic depolarization of sinus node cells, and delayed atrioventricular conduction.[7] Renal calculi may occur in hypercalcemia due to the high calcium concentration of the urine. Pathologic fractures may appear if hypercalcemia is caused by bone resorption.

Box 24-9

Causes of Hypercalcemia

Increased Calcium Intake or Absorption
Milk-alkali syndrome
Vitamin D overdose (includes shark cartilage supplements)

Shift of Calcium from Bone to Extracellular Fluid
Hyperparathyroidism
Immobilization
Paget disease
Bone tumors
Multiple myeloma
Leukemia
Nonosseous malignancies that produce bone-resorbing factors

Decreased Calcium Excretion
Thiazide diuretics
Familial hypocalciuric hypercalcemia

Plasma Magnesium

The normal serum magnesium concentration is 1.5 to 2.5 mEq/L (may vary slightly with different laboratories). Similarly to calcium, magnesium is also present in the blood as bound (physiologically inactive) and ionized (physiologically active) forms. Ionized magnesium levels are available in some research settings. Plasma magnesium imbalances may occur concurrent with or in the absence of total body magnesium imbalances.

Hypomagnesemia

If the serum magnesium concentration decreases below the lower limit of normal (1.5 mEq/L), hypomagnesemia is present. Hypomagnesemia indicates a decreased magnesium concentration of the extracellular fluid and does not necessarily indicate a total body magnesium deficit (although the two may occur concurrently).

Etiology. The major causes of hypomagnesemia are decreased magnesium intake or absorption, increased magnesium excretion, and loss of magnesium by an abnormal route. Chronic alcoholism is a major risk factor for hypomagnesemia because it is associated with decreased magnesium intake, altered physiologic availability of magnesium, increased urinary magnesium excretion, and magnesium loss through emesis. Persons who present to health care providers with alcohol-related diseases frequently have hypomagnesemia.[18] Hypomagnesemia often causes hypokalemia by increasing urinary excretion of potassium.[19] In such cases, correction of hypomagnesemia is necessary before the hypokalemia can be corrected. Specific causes of hypomagnesemia are listed in Box 24-10.

Clinical Manifestations. Magnesium ions in the extracellular fluid depress the release of acetylcholine at neuromuscular junctions. If too little magnesium is present, excessive amounts of acetylcholine are released (Figure 24-11). Therefore, the clinical manifestations of hypomagnesemia are those of increased neuromuscular excitability. Such manifestations may include insomnia, hyperactive reflexes, muscle cramps, muscle twitching, grimacing, positive Chvostek sign,

Box 24-10

Causes of Hypomagnesemia

Decreased Magnesium Intake or Absorption
Chronic alcoholism
Malnutrition
Prolonged intravenous therapy without magnesium
Ileal resection
Chronic diarrhea (includes laxative abuse)
Malabsorption syndromes
Pancreatitis
Steatorrhea

Decreased Physiologic Availability of Magnesium
Elevated plasma free fatty acids

Increased Magnesium Excretion Through Normal Routes

Renal Route
Diabetic ketoacidosis
Chronic alcoholism
Diuretic therapy
Aminoglycoside (e.g., gentamicin) toxicity
Amphotericin B, cisplatin, or other drugs
Hyperaldosteronism

Fecal Route
Pancreatitis
Steatorrhea

Magnesium Loss Through Abnormal Routes
Emesis
Gastric suction
Fistula drainage

positive Trousseau sign, nystagmus, dysphagia, ataxia, tetany, and seizures. Cardiac dysrhythmias also occur.

Hypomagnesemia causes decreased activity of the enzyme that drives the Na^+-K^+ pump in cell membranes, so that intracellular potassium decreases in the myocardium. Increased spontaneous firing in the sinus node, shortening of the absolute refractory period, and lengthening of the relative refractory period contribute to the cardiac dysrhythmias in hypomagnesemia.[7]

Hypermagnesemia

If the serum magnesium level rises above the upper limit of normal (2.5 mEq/L), hypermagnesemia is present. Hypermagnesemia indicates an excess of magnesium in the extracellular fluid.

Etiology. The major causes of hypermagnesemia are increased magnesium intake and decreased magnesium excretion. Shift of magnesium from the bones to the extracellular fluid is seen transiently in some stages of hyperparathyroidism. Hypermagnesemia from excessive intake of magnesium in laxatives and antacids may occur in persons of any age who have unrecognized renal impairment.[20] Older adults are at highest risk from these magnesium-containing medications. Individuals who have oliguria, as in chronic renal failure, are another high-risk group for development of hypermagnesemia. Specific causes of hypermagnesemia are summarized in Box 24-11.

Clinical Manifestations. Too much magnesium in the extracellular fluid depresses neuromuscular function by decreasing the release of acetylcholine at neuromuscular junc-

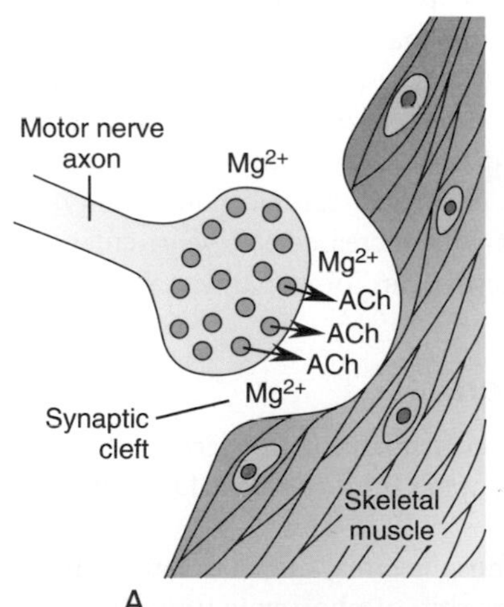

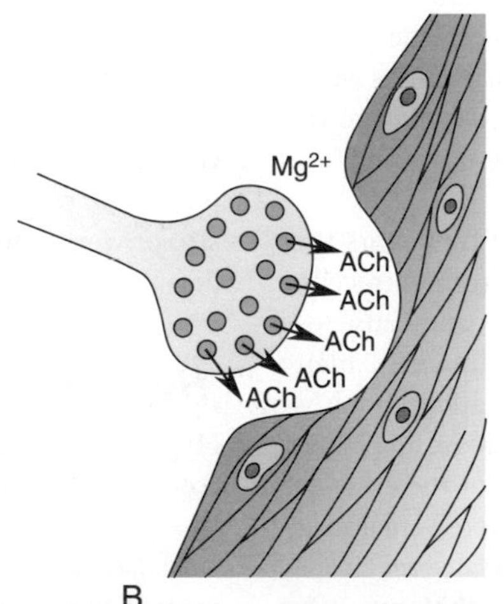

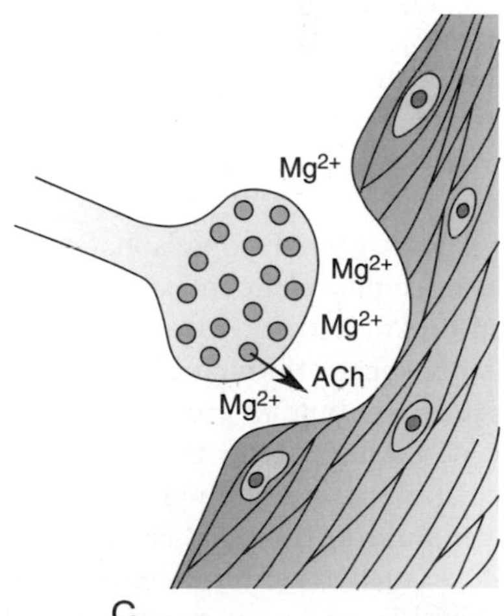

FIGURE 24-11 ■ Acetylcholine *(ACh)* release at neuromuscular junctions is altered in magnesium imbalances. **A,** Normal magnesium concentration suppresses the release of acetylcholine at neuromuscular junctions to normal levels. **B,** In hypomagnesemia, more acetylcholine is released at neuromuscular junctions, causing increased neuromuscular excitability. **C,** In hypermagnesemia, less acetylcholine is released at neuromuscular junctions, causing decreased neuromuscular excitability.

Box 24-11

Causes of Hypermagnesemia

Increased Magnesium Intake or Absorption
Ingestion or aspiration of seawater
Excessive ingestion of magnesium-containing medications (e.g., laxatives, antacids)
Excessive intravenous infusion of magnesium

Decreased Magnesium Excretion
Oliguric renal failure
Adrenal insufficiency

tions (see Figure 24-11). Thus manifestations of hypermagnesemia include decreased deep tendon reflexes, lethargy, hypotension, flushing, diaphoresis, drowsiness, flaccid paralysis, respiratory depression, bradycardia, cardiac dysrhythmias, and even cardiac arrest. The mechanisms that cause the cardiac effects of hypermagnesemia include decreased cardiac conduction and depression of membrane excitability.[7]

Plasma Phosphate

The normal range of phosphate concentration in adult plasma is 2.5 to 4.5 mg/dl (may vary slightly with different laboratories). Symptomatic phosphate imbalances are less common than other electrolyte imbalances, but, like other electrolyte imbalances, they may be fatal if untreated.

Hypophosphatemia

Hypophosphatemia is present when the phosphate concentration in the plasma decreases below the lower limit of normal (2.5 mg/dl). However, the clinical manifestations of hypophosphatemia are often not observed unless the plasma phosphate concentration is less than 1.0 mg/dl. Persons whose plasma phosphate concentration is less than 1.0 mg/dl are said to have *severe symptomatic hypophosphatemia.*

Etiology. Hypophosphatemia is caused by factors that decrease phosphate intake, shift phosphate from extracellular fluid to cells, increase phosphate excretion, and cause loss of phosphate through abnormal routes. Frequently, many factors combine to produce severe symptomatic hypophosphatemia. Any factor that causes a rapid increase in cellular metabolism will cause phosphate to shift from the extracellular fluid to the cells. Patients who are severely malnourished (such as cancer patients with advanced disease) are at high risk for severe symptomatic hypophosphatemia after nutritional replacement is started because of the increased cellular metabolism and previously depleted phosphate stores.[21] Specific factors that cause hypophosphatemia are summarized in Box 24-12.

Box 24-12

Causes of Hypophosphatemia

Decreased Phosphate Intake or Absorption
Chronic alcoholism
Chronic diarrhea
Malabsorption syndromes
Excessive or long-term use of antacids that bind phosphate

Shift of Phosphate from Extracellular Fluid to Cells
Refeeding after starvation (includes anorexia nervosa)
Total parenteral nutrition
Hyperventilation (respiratory alkalosis)
Insulin
Epinephrine
Intravenous glucose, fructose, bicarbonate, or lactate

Increased Phosphate Excretion Through the Normal Renal Route
Alcohol withdrawal
Diuretic phase after extensive burns
Diabetic ketoacidosis
Diuretic therapy

Phosphate Loss Through Abnormal Routes
Emesis
Hemodialysis

Clinical Manifestations. Phosphate is an important component of adenosine triphosphate (ATP), the major source of energy for many cellular processes. The signs and symptoms of severe symptomatic hypophosphatemia are due, in part, to decreased ATP within the cells. Another contributing mechanism is tissue hypoxia caused by decreased 2,3-diphosphoglycerate in the red blood cells. The signs and symptoms include anorexia, malaise, paresthesias, hemolysis, diminished reflexes, muscle aches, muscle weakness, respiratory failure, confusion, stupor, seizures, coma, and impaired cardiac function. The impaired cardiac function of hypophosphatemia results from decreased cardiac contractility and stroke work concurrent with increased left ventricular end-diastolic pressure. Congestive cardiomyopathy may result.[7]

Hyperphosphatemia

Hyperphosphatemia is an increase of the serum phosphate concentration above the upper limit of normal (4.5 mg/dl).

Etiology. Hyperphosphatemia may be caused by increased phosphate intake, shift of phosphate from the cells or bones to the extracellular fluid, and decreased phosphate excretion. Examples of specific causes in these categories are listed in Box 24-13. Hyperphosphatemia is common in people who have oliguric renal failure. In end-stage renal disease, re-

Box 24-13

Causes of Hyperphosphatemia

Increased Phosphate Intake or Absorption
Overzealous phosphate therapy
Excessive use of phosphate-containing enemas or laxatives

Shift of Phosphate from Cells to Extracellular Fluid
Tumor lysis syndrome
Crushing injury
Rhabdomyolysis

Decreased Phosphate Excretion
Oliguric renal failure
Adrenal insufficiency

nal phosphate excretion is severely decreased but intestinal absorption of dietary phosphate continues. In addition, elevated parathyroid hormone in end-stage renal disease releases phosphate from bones.[22]

Clinical Manifestations. The clinical manifestations of hyperphosphatemia depend on the effect of the elevated phosphate concentration on calcium ions. Typically, hyperphosphatemia causes hypocalcemia. The signs and symptoms are thus the manifestations of increased neuromuscular excitability that were presented earlier in this section in the discussion of hypocalcemia. However, in some patients, especially those who have chronic renal failure, hyperphosphatemia causes deposition of calcium phosphate salts in the soft tissues of the body.[23] These patients develop signs and symptoms such as aching and stiffness of joints, itching, and conjunctivitis, depending on the areas in which these salts precipitate.

KEY CONCEPTS

- Plasma electrolyte deficits are caused by factors that decrease electrolyte intake or absorption, shift electrolytes from the extracellular fluid to an electrolyte pool, increase electrolyte excretion, and cause abnormal loss of electrolytes.
- Plasma electrolyte excesses are caused by factors that increase electrolyte intake or absorption, shift electrolytes from an electrolyte pool to the extracellular fluid, and decrease electrolyte excretion.
- Abnormalities in plasma electrolyte concentrations may profoundly affect cellular function. Excitable cells, such as nerve and muscle, are particularly sensitive to electrolyte imbalances.
- Manifestations of potassium imbalances are due to changes in resting membrane potentials. Hypokalemia causes hyperpolarization; hyperkalemia causes hypopolarization. Both hyperkalemia and hypokalemia cause skeletal muscle weakness, flaccid paralysis, and cardiac dysrhythmias.
- Manifestations of calcium imbalances are a result of changes in threshold potential of nerve and muscle cells. Hypocalcemia decreases the threshold, resulting in hyperexcitability (twitching, tetany); hypercalcemia increases the threshold, resulting in neuromuscular depression (hyporeflexia).
- Manifestations of magnesium imbalances are similar to those of calcium imbalances. Magnesium normally inhibits release of acetylcholine at neuromuscular junctions. Hypomagnesemia increases neuromuscular excitability (hyperreflexia and twitching), and hypermagnesemia depresses excitability (hyporeflexia and flaccid paralysis).
- Severe symptomatic hypophosphatemia is characterized by manifestations of generalized cellular ATP deficiency. Hyperphosphatemia may cause hypocalcemia, with resulting increased neuromuscular excitability, or it may be associated with precipitation of calcium phosphate into soft tissues of the body.

SUMMARY

This chapter has presented the principles of fluid and electrolyte homeostasis and imbalances. Pediatric and geriatric variations are summarized in Boxes 24-14 and 24-15, respectively. Fluid and electrolyte homeostasis involves the continuous interplay of intake, absorption, distribution, and excretion of fluid and electrolytes. Loss of fluid and electrolytes through abnormal routes may also occur. When the normal mechanisms are impaired or overwhelmed, fluid and electrolyte imbalances occur. Fluid imbalances may involve the volume or the concentration of body fluid. Plasma electrolyte imbalances may be deficits or excesses and may not reflect total body electrolyte deficits or excesses. The signs and symptoms of fluid and electrolyte imbalances are summarized in Table 24-2. The pathophysiology of specific fluid and electrolyte imbalances can be derived from a working knowledge of normal fluid and electrolyte homeostasis.

MEDIA RESOURCES

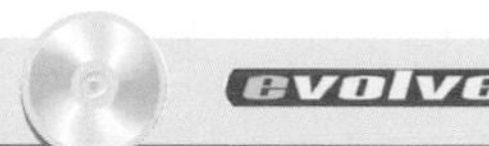

Remember to check out the ***CD Companion*** included with this book for Review Questions, Key Concepts Review, Glossary (with audio for selected terms), Disease Profiles, and Animations.

PLUS, visit the ***Evolve website*** at http://evolve.elsevier.com/Copstead/ for Case Studies, Disease Profiles, and WebLinks.

Table 24-2

Summary of Signs and Symptoms of Fluid and Electrolyte Imbalances

Imbalance	Heart	Blood Vessels	Interstitial Area	CNS	Lungs
↓ Extracellular volume	Tachycardia	Postural blood pressure drop, flat neck veins, ↑ small-vein filling time, thready pulse	↓ Skin turgor; soft, sunken eyeballs; longitudinal furrows in tongue	Dizziness	
↑ Extracellular volume		Distended neck veins, bounding pulse	Edema		Crackles, dyspnea, orthopnea, frothy sputum
↓ Na^+				Confusion, lethargy, coma, seizures	
↑ Na^+				Confusion, lethargy, coma, seizures	
↓ K^+	Dysrhythmias	Postural hypotension			
↑ K^+	Dysrhythmias, cardiac arrest				
↓ Ca^{2+}	Dysrhythmias, impaired myocardial contractility			Seizures	
↑ Ca^{2+}	Dysrhythmias			Confusion, lethargy, personality change	
↓ Mg^{2+}	Dysrhythmias			Insomnia, seizures	
↑ Mg^{2+}	Bradycardia, dysrhythmias, cardiac arrest	Hypotension, flushing		Drowsiness, lethargy	Respiratory depression
↓ P_i	Impaired cardiac function, decreased cardiac output			Confusion, stupor, coma, seizures	Respiratory failure
↑ P_i (may cause ↓ Ca^{2+})					

ECV, Extracellular fluid volume; P_i, inorganic phosphate.

Skeletal Muscle	Neuromuscular Excitability	Gastrointestinal Tract	Kidneys	Other
		Dry oral mucous membranes, hard stools	Oliguria	Sudden weight loss, sunken fontanel (infants), no tears or sweat, thirst with severe ↓ECV
		Hepatomegaly		Sudden weight gain, bulging fontanel (infants)
		Anorexia, nausea, emesis		Malaise, headache
			Oliguria	Thirst
Ascending weakness		Abdominal distention, bloating, ↓ bowel sounds, constipation, paralytic ileus	Polyuria	
Ascending weakness, flaccid paralysis		Cramping, diarrhea		
Twitching, cramping, carpal spasm, pedal spasm	Increased excitability, Trousseau sign, Chvostek sign, paresthesias, hyperactive reflexes, tetany			Laryngospasm
Weakness	Decreased excitability, depressed reflexes	Anorexia, nausea, emesis, constipation	Polyuria	Fatigue, headache
Twitching, cramping, grimacing, tremors	Increased excitability, Trousseau sign, Chvostek sign, hyperactive reflexes, tetany	Dysphagia		Nystagmus, ataxia
Flaccid paralysis	Depressed reflexes			Diaphoresis
Aching, weakness	Paresthesias, depressed reflexes	Anorexia		Malaise, hemolysis
			If Ca^{2+} remains high, damage from deposition of crystals	If Ca^{2+} remains high, pruritus, conjunctivitis, arthritis

Box 24-14

Pediatric Variations

- Infants have more extracellular fluid than intracellular fluid; this proportion reverses by a few months of age.
- About 75% of the body weight of a term infant is water; this percentage is even higher in preterm infants. The percent of body weight that is water decreases as the child grows older.
- In the first few days after birth, an infant loses fluid equal to 5% to 10% of its body weight; this is a normal process during adjustment to extrauterine life.
- Neonates have a high metabolic rate and thus a high turnover rate of water.
- Infants have increased insensible water excretion due to proportionately large body surface area, proportionately large respiratory mucosa surface area, vasomotor immaturity, and increased skin permeability. Preterm infants have even greater insensible water excretion through the skin due to flaccid extended posture (and thus greater exposed body surface area) and greater vasomotor immaturity.
- Use of phototherapy and radiant heat warmers increases insensible water excretion.
- Glomerular filtration rate is lower in infants than adults.
- The kidneys of infants have limited ability to concentrate urine or to dilute it; thus, infants are unable to excrete a large load of water effectively or to conserve fluid when needed.
- Infants communicate thirst by crying, which may not be understood by their caregivers.
- Infants and toddlers are a high-risk group for clinical dehydration.
- Assessment of extracellular volume imbalances in infants should focus on tension of fontanel rather than degree of filling of neck veins.
- Infants whose caregivers use powdered formula are at high risk for hypernatremia if the formula is reconstituted with extra powder to "strengthen" the baby.
- Laboratory normal ranges of electrolytes are generally wider for infants than older children and adults.
- Neonatal hypocalcemia may occur in infants who needed resuscitation at birth or have high-risk conditions.
- Preterm infants may have reduced body calcium stores because fetal calcium stores are built during the last trimester of pregnancy; these infants have increased incidence of neonatal hypocalcemia.
- Assessment of increased neuromuscular excitability (hypocalcemia and hypomagnesemia) in infants should not include the Chvostek sign; this sign is often positive in normal neonates. Increased neuromuscular excitability in infants includes jitteriness, hyperactive reflexes, and a high-pitched cry.
- Neonates whose mothers were given magnesium sulfate for eclampsia in the 24 hours before birth may be born with hypermagnesemia. Hypermagnesemic infants lie in a flaccid, extended posture.

Box 24-15

Geriatric Variations

- Older adults have less body water than middle-aged adults because body composition changes with increasing age (decreased muscle mass, increased fat in internal organs). About 50% of the body weight of a lean older man is water and about 45% of the body weight of a lean older woman is water; the percentage is lower in obese older adults.
- Glomerular filtration rate is lower in older adults than in middle-aged adults.
- The kidneys of older adults are less able to concentrate urine and thus less able to conserve fluid when needed. This decreased ability to concentrate urine is also responsible for nocturia, since a larger than normal volume of urine is produced at night.
- Older adults have a reduced thirst response when the osmolality of body fluids increases; thus, they may not be aware that they are becoming dehydrated.
- Older adults are a high-risk group for clinical dehydration.
- Decreased skin turgor is not reliable as a sign of extracellular fluid volume depletion in older adults, due to age-related changes in collagen and elastin. Decreased skin turgor (tenting of skin) may occur in older adults who have normal fluid volume.
- Older adults who receive tube feedings are at higher risk for hypernatremia than middle-aged adults.
- Older adults probably absorb more magnesium from antacids and cathartics than do middle-aged adults. With age-related changes in renal excretion, older adults who use oral magnesium laxatives or antacids regularly are at high risk for hypermagnesemia.

References

1. Guyton AC, Hall AE: *Textbook of medical physiology,* ed 10, Philadelphia, 2000, Saunders.
2. Stricker EM, Sved AF: Thirst, *Nutrition* 16:821-826, 2000.
3. Rose BD, Post TW: *Clinical physiology of acid-base and electrolyte disorders,* ed 5, New York, 2001, McGraw-Hill.
4. Shachar-Hill B, Hill AE: Paracellular fluid transport by epithelia, *Int Rev Cytol* 215:319-350, 2002.
5. Stein WD: Cell volume homeostasis: ionic and nonionic mechanisms. The sodium pump in the emergence of animal cells, *Int Rev Cytol* 215:231-258, 2002.
6. de Bold AJ et al: The physiological and pathophysiological modulation of the endocrine function of the heart, *Can J Physiol Pharmacol* 79:705-714, 2001.
7. Felver L: Fluid and electrolyte balance and imbalances. In Woods SL et al, editors: *Cardiac nursing,* ed 5, Philadelphia, 2005, Lippincott, pp 173-188.
8. Schrier RW, Ecder T: Unifying hypothesis of body fluid volume regulation: implications for cardiac failure and cirrhosis, *Mt Sinai J Med* 68:350-361, 2001.
9. Musch W, Xhaet O, Decaux G: Solute loss plays a major role in polydipsia-related hyponatraemia of both water drinkers and beer drinkers, *Q J Med* 96:421-426, 2003.
10. Johansson S, Svensson H, Denekamp J: Dose response and latency for radiation-induced fibrosis, edema, and neuropathy in breast cancer patients, *Int J Radiat Oncol Biol Phys* 52:1207-1219, 2002.
11. Atreja A, Abacan C, Licata A: A 51-year-old woman with debilitating cramps 12 years after bariatric surgery, *Cleveland Clin J Med* 70:417-418, 420, 423-426, 2003.
12. Greenberg A: Diuretic complications, *Am J Med Sci* 319:10-24, 2000.
13. Sugimoto T et al: Central pontine myelinolysis associated with hypokalaemia in anorexia nervosa, *J Neurol Neurosurg Psychiatry* 74:353-355, 2003.
14. Lin SH, Davids MR, Halperin ML: Hypokalaemia and paralysis, *Q J Med* 96:161-169, 2003.
15. Yang SS et al: Steroid-induced tumor lysis syndrome in a patient with preleukemia, *Clin Nephrol* 59:201-205, 2003.
16. Slomp J et al: Albumin-adjusted calcium is not suitable for diagnosis of hyper- and hypocalcemia in the critically ill, *Crit Care Med* 31:1389-1393, 2003.
17. Truong NU et al: Parathyroid hormone-related peptide and survival of patients with cancer and hypercalcemia, *Am J Med* 115:115-121, 2003.
18. Liamis G, Gianoutsos C, Elisaf M: Acute pancreatitis-induced hypomagnesemia, *Pancreatology* 1:74-76, 2001.
19. Elisaf M et al: Hypokalaemia in alcoholic patients, *Drug Alcohol Rev* 21:73-76, 2002.
20. Schelling JR: Fatal hypermagnesemia, *Clin Nephrol* 53:61-65, 2000.
21. Ladage E: Refeeding syndrome, *ORL Head Neck Nurs* 21(3):18-20, 2003.
22. Indridason OS, Quarles LD: Hyperphosphatemia in end-stage renal disease, *Adv Renal Repl Ther* 9:184-192, 2002.
23. Locatelli F et al: Management of disturbances of calcium and phosphate metabolism in chronic renal insufficiency, with emphasis on the control of hyperphosphataemia, *Nephrol Dial Transplant* 17:723-731, 2002.

chapter 25

Acid-Base Homeostasis and Imbalances

Linda Felver

MEDIA RESOURCES

Additional Material for Study, Review, and Further Exploration

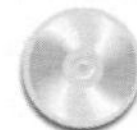

CD Companion ◆ Review Questions and Answers ◆ Key Concepts Review
◆ Glossary *(with audio pronunciations for selected terms)*
◆ Disease Profiles ◆ Animations

evolve ***Website*** at http://evolve.elsevier.com/Copstead/
◆ Case Studies ◆ Disease Profiles ◆ WebLinks

KEY QUESTIONS

- What is the chemistry and functional importance of the bicarbonate buffer system?
- What is the role of the respiratory system in regulating carbonic acid (carbon dioxide)?
- What is the role of the kidneys in regulating bicarbonate ion and acids other than carbonic acid?
- How do the lungs compensate for acid-base disturbances resulting from altered levels of metabolic acids?
- How do the kidneys compensate for acid-base disturbances resulting from altered levels of carbonic acid?
- How are arterial blood gas values used to categorize an acid-base disorder as acidosis or alkalosis, respiratory or metabolic, compensated or not?
- What pathophysiologic conditions predispose an individual to an acid-base imbalance?

CHAPTER OUTLINE

When the pH of body fluids becomes abnormal, cellular function is impaired. The pH of a fluid reflects its degree of acidity or alkalinity. Technically, pH is the negative logarithm of the hydrogen ion (H^+) concentration. The normal hydrogen ion concentration of the blood is about 40 nmol/L (40×10^{-9} mol/L), a very small number.[1] The pH (negative logarithm) of this number is 7.40, which is easier to use in clinical settings.

An alteration in pH is a change in the hydrogen ion concentration. An **acid** releases hydrogen ions. The more hydrogen ions present, the more acidic the solution. The normal pH of adult blood ranges from 7.35 to 7.45 (may vary slightly with different laboratories). The range is somewhat wider in infants and children. Table 25-1 lists normal laboratory values for pH and other acid-base parameters. If the blood and other body fluids become too acidic (reflected by a decreased pH), dysfunction occurs; if the pH of the blood falls below 6.9, death is likely to result. Similarly, if the body fluids become too alkaline, as reflected by an increased pH, dysfunction also occurs. If the pH of the blood rises above 7.8, death is again likely.

Cellular metabolism continually releases acids (carbonic and metabolic) that must be excreted from the body to prevent body fluids from becoming too acidic. This chapter presents a discussion of the normal mechanisms of acid-base homeostasis and the acid-base imbalances that arise when these homeostatic mechanisms become dysfunctional or overwhelmed.

ACID-BASE HOMEOSTASIS

The acid-base status of the body is regulated by three major mechanisms: buffers, the respiratory system, and the renal system. Laboratory measurements such as arterial blood gas values are useful indicators of the acid-base status of extracellular fluids. The partial pressure of carbon dioxide in arterial blood (Pa_{CO_2}) is an indicator of the respiratory component of acid-base balance. The plasma bicarbonate ion (HCO_3^-) concentration is an indicator of the renal (metabolic) component of acid-base balance.[1] The pH of the blood indicates the net result of normal acid-base regulation, any acid-base imbalance, and the body's compensatory responses. It is important to remember that the pH measured clinically is that of the blood and may not reflect the pH inside cells or in cerebrospinal fluid.

Table 25-1

Normal Laboratory Values for Acid-Base Parameters

Characteristic	Normal Range
Pa_{CO_2} (arterial blood)	36-44 mm Hg (adults) 30-34 mm Hg (infants)
HCO_3^- (serum)	22-26 mEq/L (adults) 19-23 mEq/L (infants)
pH (arterial blood)	7.35-7.45 (adults) 7.11-7.36 (neonates) 7.36-7.41 (infants)

Buffers

Buffers are chemicals that help control the pH of body fluids. Each buffer system consists of a weak acid, which releases hydrogen ions when the fluid is too alkaline, and a **base,** which takes up hydrogen ions when the fluid is too acidic. In this way, potential changes in pH are neutralized immediately by the action of buffers. All body fluids contain buffers. Chief among them are bicarbonate buffers (in the extracellular fluid), phosphate buffers (in intracellular fluid and urine), hemoglobin buffers (inside erythrocytes), and protein buffers (in intracellular fluid and the vascular compartment). These buffers are the first line of defense against pH disorders.

The bicarbonate buffer system is the most important buffer in the extracellular fluid. Bicarbonate ions (HCO_3^-) and carbonic acid (H_2CO_3), the two components of the bicarbonate buffer system, are in chemical equilibrium in the extracellular fluid.[2] If too much acid (e.g., lactic acid) is present, the bicarbonate ions take up the hydrogen ions (H^+) released by the acid and become carbonic acid. Through the action of the enzyme **carbonic anhydrase,** the carbonic acid is then excreted through the respiratory system in the form of carbon dioxide and water. Thus the excess acid is neutralized as bicarbonate ions are used in the buffering process.

$$HCO_3^- + H^+ \rightleftharpoons H_2CO_3 \xrightarrow[\text{carbonic anhydrase}]{} CO_2 + H_2O$$

Conversely, if too little acid is present in the extracellular fluid, the carbonic acid portion of the bicarbonate buffer system releases hydrogen ions.

$$H_2CO_3 \rightleftharpoons HCO_3^- + H^+$$

The pH of any fluid is determined by the relative amounts of acids and bases contained in it. For the pH of the blood to be within the normal range, the ratio of bicarbonate ions to carbonic acid must be 20:1, which means that 20 bicarbonate ions must be present for every carbonic acid molecule. This relationship is explained formally by the Henderson-Hasselbalch equation, which is the mathematical description of the pH of a buffered solution, here written specifically for the bicarbonate buffer system.

$$pH = pK_a + \log \frac{[HCO_3^-]}{[H_2CO_3]}$$

Square brackets, used throughout this chapter, are a standard notation for concentration. pK_a is the dissociation constant for any particular acid; it equals 6.1 for carbonic acid.[2] If the normal 20:1 ratio of bicarbonate ions to carbonic acid is present, the pH will be 7.4.

$$pH = 6.1 + \log 20$$
$$pH = 6.1 + 1.3$$
$$pH = 7.4$$

The 20:1 ratio of bicarbonate ions to carbonic acid necessary for a normal pH is an important concept in understanding the compensatory mechanisms for acid-base imbalances that will be discussed later in this chapter.

Respiratory Contribution

The respiratory system is the second defense against acid-base disorders. Body cells are continuously producing carbon dioxide (CO_2). Together, CO_2 and water (H_2O) make carbonic acid (H_2CO_3). The lungs excrete carbon dioxide and water from the body. Therefore, during the process of exhalation the lungs are effectively excreting carbonic acid. Thus, the respiratory system adjusts the amount of carbonic acid that remains in the body.

The rate and depth of respiration are strongly influenced by chemoreceptors that sense the $Paco_2$ and pH of the blood. In a healthy person, if too much carbonic acid begins to accumulate in the blood, the rate and depth of respiration increase and excess carbonic acid is removed. This response corrects the imbalance and restores blood chemistry to normal. If, on the other hand, too little carbonic acid is present in the blood, the rate and depth of respiration decrease to retain carbonic acid until it is once more present in normal amounts. Again, the imbalance is corrected and the blood chemistry returns to normal. Thus the body's **correction** of a carbonic acid excess or deficit is dependent on normal function of all components of the respiratory system, including the chemoreceptors. In older adults, the chemoreceptor response to increased $Paco_2$ may occur more slowly.

The $Paco_2$ indicates how effectively the respiratory system is excreting carbonic acid. If the $Paco_2$ is elevated, carbonic acid has accumulated in the blood. In other words, the respiratory rate and depth have been too small or lung disease has prevented sufficient carbonic acid (carbon dioxide and water) excretion.[3] Similarly, if the $Paco_2$ is decreased below normal, the lungs have excreted more carbonic acid than usual. In other words, the respiratory rate and depth have been excessive.[4]

Carbonic acid is known as a volatile acid because it can be excreted as gases (CO_2 and H_2O). It is the only volatile acid in the body. Other acids that accumulate in the body, such as lactic acid and acetoacetic acid, are nonvolatile. They are organic acids that have no gaseous form. The lungs can excrete only carbonic acid; they cannot excrete nonvolatile acids that may accumulate in the body. If a nonvolatile acid (such as lactic acid) accumulates in the blood, the rate and depth of respiration will increase because the excess hydrogen ions stimulate the chemoreceptors. This hyperventilation does not excrete lactic acid (which would correct the problem), but it does remove carbonic acid from the blood. Removing carbonic acid from the blood when another acid is present in excess helps keep the pH from dropping too low.[5] However, this response makes other values abnormal. The respiratory response to an imbalance of any acid except carbonic acid is called **compensation.** A compensatory response does not **correct** a pH disorder but it does **compensate** for it by adjusting the pH back toward normal, even though other blood chemistry values are made abnormal in the process.

The compensatory response to a deficit of any acid except carbonic acid is hypoventilation.[1] By decreasing the rate and depth of respiration, the body retains carbonic acid. This carbonic acid accumulation helps keep the pH of the blood from rising to a fatal level when another acid is deficient in the body. Respiratory compensation for an imbalance of metabolic acid requires at least several hours. Respiratory responses to changes in carbonic and metabolic acids are summarized in Table 25-2.

Table 25-2

Respiratory Responses to Changes in Carbonic and Metabolic Acids

Stimulus	Respiratory Response	Result
Increased $Paco_2$, decreased pH	Hyperventilation	Correction of imbalance
Decreased $Paco_2$, increased pH	Hypoventilation	Correction of imbalance
Decreased pH from excess of metabolic acids	Hyperventilation	Compensation for imbalance
Increased pH from deficit of metabolic acids	Hypoventilation	Compensation for imbalance

Renal Contribution

The third defense against acid-base disorders is the kidneys. The kidneys can excrete any acid from the body except carbonic acid (which is excreted by the lungs). Cells continuously produce metabolic acids during metabolism. The kidneys excrete these metabolic acids. If a metabolic acid begins to accumulate in the blood, the kidneys increase their acid excretion mechanisms to correct the problem. If a metabolic acid is deficient in the blood, the kidneys slow their acid excretion mechanisms to allow acid to accumulate to normal levels. The body's ability to correct an excess or deficit of a metabolic acid depends on normal function of the renal system. Infants excrete more bicarbonate in their urine than older children or adults do; their kidneys are less effective in excreting acid. The renal response to a large acid load is also less efficient in older adults.

The kidneys have several mechanisms that accomplish acid excretion.[2] Understanding these mechanisms requires a knowledge of basic renal physiology. At the glomerulus, fluid filtered from the blood enters the Bowman capsule, which is the beginning of the nephron. The fluid inside the nephron (renal tubular fluid) is modified by the cells that line the lumen. Renal tubular fluid that passes through the entire nephron becomes the urine.

With regard to acid excretion, bicarbonate ions (HCO_3^-) are contained in the fluid filtered from the blood at the glomerulus. They become part of the renal tubular fluid. As this fluid moves through the renal tubules, hydrogen ions are secreted into the fluid. Secretion of hydrogen ions from the blood into the renal tubular fluid occurs in the proximal tubules by the process of Na^+-H^+ exchange and in the collecting tubules by means of H^+-ATPase. The processes in the renal tubular cells that generate H^+ for secretion into the renal tubular fluid simultaneously cause the generation of HCO_3^-, which is then returned to the blood. Thus for every H^+ secreted into the renal tubular fluid, one HCO_3^- is reabsorbed (returned to the blood).

Once the H^+ are in the renal tubular fluid, most of them combine with other chemicals: urine buffers, such as phosphate and creatinine, which were filtered at the glomerulus; ammonia (NH_3), which is produced by renal tubular cells; or bicarbonate ions that were filtered at the glomerulus. Net H^+ excretion occurs after HCO_3^- has been reabsorbed in the amount that was filtered at the glomerulus. Thus net H^+ excretion is accomplished in the form of buffered H^+ (called titratable acidity) and H^+ attached to ammonia (ammonium ions, NH_4^+). Figure 25-1 illustrates these processes.

When the kidneys need to excrete more hydrogen ions, the renal tubular cells increase the production of urinary ammonium ions. Ammonium ions (NH_4^+) are not lipid soluble, so they do not easily cross from the renal tubular fluid back to the blood. Consequently, increased production of urinary ammonium ions is an effective way of trapping hydrogen ions in the renal tubular fluid so that they are excreted.

The concentration of HCO_3^- in plasma is a reflection of the effectiveness of renal regulation of metabolic acids. If metabolic acids are accumulating in the blood, they will be buffered by HCO_3^- and the HCO_3^- concentration will drop below normal. Thus a decreased concentration of HCO_3^- in plasma indicates a relative excess of metabolic acids. An increased HCO_3^- concentration in plasma indicates a relative deficit of metabolic acids (in other words, a relative excess of base).

Although the kidneys are unable to excrete carbonic acid, they can compensate for carbonic acid imbalances by adjusting the excretion of metabolic acids. Thus if carbonic acid accumulates in the blood, the kidneys can increase the excretion of metabolic acids. This compensatory action helps keep the pH of the blood from becoming too abnormal. Similarly, if a deficit of carbonic acid in the blood is prolonged, the kidneys will decrease the excretion of metabolic acids. As these metabolic acids accumulate in the blood, they will compensate for the lack of carbonic acid and return the pH of the blood toward normal. The body's compensatory response to an imbalance of one kind of acid thus returns the pH of the blood toward normal by creating an imbalance of another kind of acid. The renal compensatory response to an imbalance of carbonic acid requires several days to be fully effective.[6] Renal responses to changes in metabolic and carbonic acids are summarized in Table 25-3.

KEY CONCEPTS

- During cellular metabolism, both carbon dioxide and metabolic acids are produced. Carbon dioxide (CO_2) combines with water (H_2O) to form carbonic acid (H_2CO_3). Both carbonic and metabolic acids must be excreted to maintain acid-base homeostasis.
- Buffers are chemicals (a weak acid plus its base) that prevent large changes in pH by releasing or taking up hydrogen ions (H^+). The bicarbonate buffer system is the most important buffer in the extracellular fluid. The normal ratio of bicarbonate to carbonic acid is 20:1. Any deviation from this ratio alters the pH of the blood.
- The lungs excrete carbon dioxide. The rate and depth of respiration are normally adjusted by chemoreceptors in response to the acid-base and oxygen status. An increase in ventilation (hyperventilation) decreases the amount of carbon dioxide in blood and thus reduces the amount of carbonic acid. A decrease in ventilation (hypoventilation) allows carbon dioxide to accumulate and thus increases the amount of carbonic acid in the blood.
- The kidneys excrete metabolic acids. They can secrete H^+ into the renal tubular fluid and retain HCO_3^- in the body or may allow some HCO_3^- to be excreted, depending on the homeostatic demands. Most H^+ in the urine is buffered (titratable acidity) or in the form of ammonium ions. The concentration of

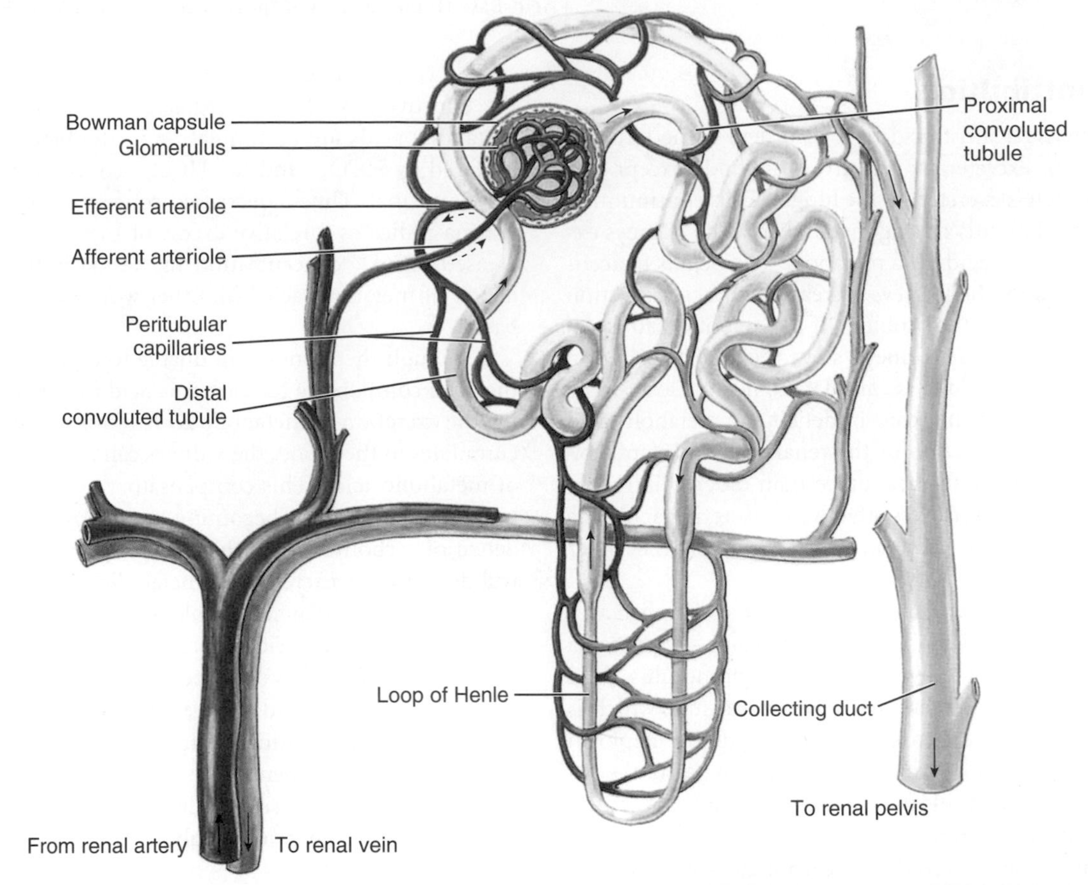

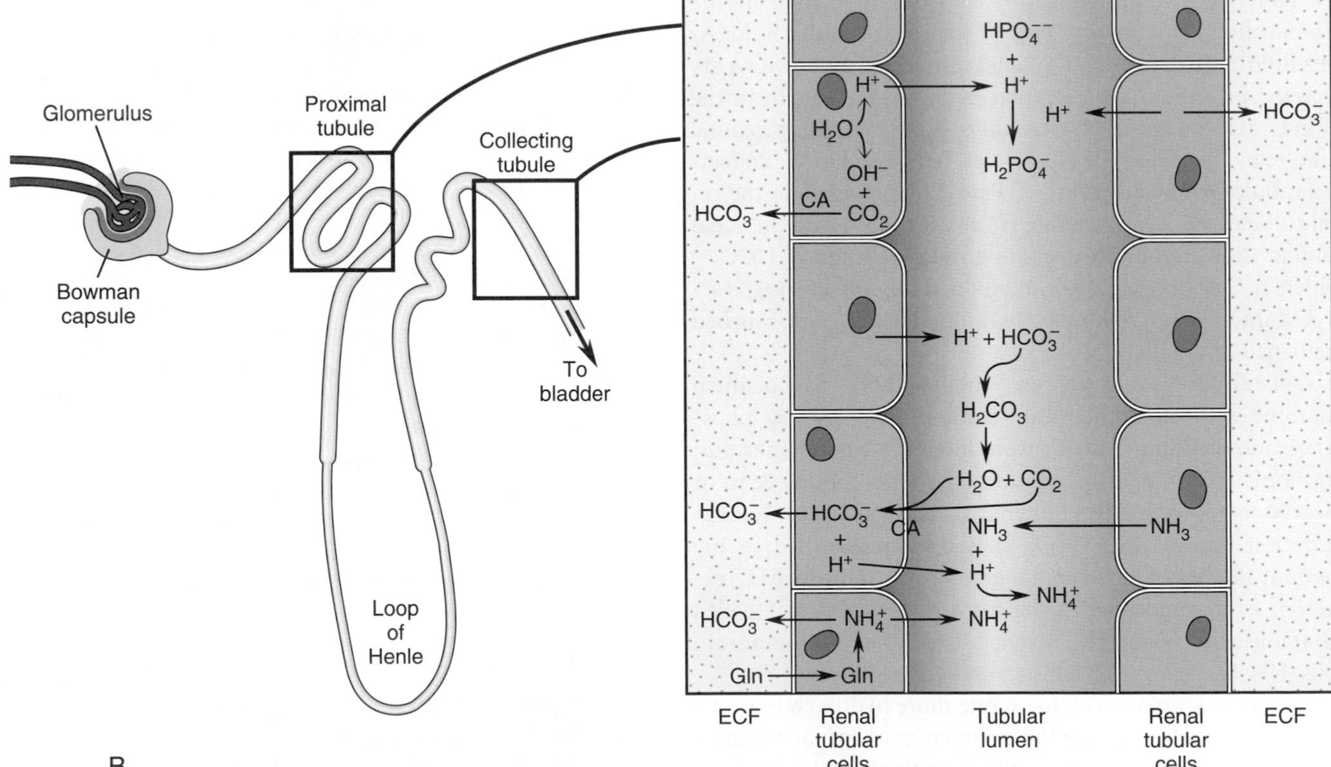

FIGURE 25-1 ■ **A,** Diagram of a nephron. **B,** Renal mechanisms for excretion of metabolic acids. Hydrogen ions secreted into the renal tubular lumen combine with buffers (phosphate buffer illustrated here), filtered bicarbonate (which is then reabsorbed), or ammonia (forming ammonium ions). These mechanisms function in both the proximal tubules and the collecting tubules. The ammonia mechanism differs slightly in the two locations. *CA,* Carbonic anhydrase, an enzyme; *ECF,* extracellular fluid; *Gln,* glutamine, an amino acid. (**A,** From Solomon EP: *Introduction to human anatomy and physiology,* ed 2, St Louis, 2003, Mosby, p 255.)

Table 25-3

Renal Responses to Changes in Metabolic and Carbonic Acids

Stimulus	Renal Response	Result
Decreased pH from excess of metabolic acids	Secrete more H^+ Make more ammonia	Correction of imbalance
Increased pH from deficit of metabolic acids	Secrete fewer H^+ Make less ammonia Excrete HCO_3^-	Correction of imbalance
Decreased pH from excess of carbonic acid	Secrete more H^+ Make more ammonia	Compensation for imbalance
Increased pH from deficit of carbonic acid	Secrete fewer H^+ Make less ammonia Excrete HCO_3^-	Compensation for imbalance

HCO_3^- in plasma is a reflection of the relative amount of metabolic acid in the blood.

- The lungs compensate for acid-base imbalances resulting from altered levels of metabolic acids; the kidneys compensate for acid-base imbalances resulting from altered levels of carbonic acid. With compensation, the pH returns toward normal but $Paco_2$ and HCO_3^- levels are abnormal.

ACID-BASE IMBALANCES

The four primary acid-base disorders are metabolic acidosis, respiratory acidosis, metabolic alkalosis, and respiratory alkalosis. **Acidosis** is the presence of a condition that tends to decrease the pH of the blood below normal (make the blood relatively more acidic). If blood pH is actually decreased, **acidemia** is also present. **Alkalosis** is the presence of any factor that tends to increase the pH of the blood above normal (make the blood relatively more alkaline). The term **alkalemia** denotes an increased blood pH. The pathophysiology of the four primary acid-base disorders is based on an understanding of the principles of acid-base homeostasis.

Metabolic Acidosis

Etiology. Metabolic acidosis is a condition that tends to cause a relative excess of any acid except carbonic acid.[7] Metabolic acidosis may be caused by an increase in acid (not carbonic), by a decrease in base, or by a combination of the two. These mechanisms decrease the normal 20:1 ratio of HCO_3^- to H_2CO_3.

An increase of any acid except carbonic acid will decrease the normal ratio of bicarbonate to carbonic acid because the bicarbonate ions are used up in buffering the excess acid. For example, when caloric intake is insufficient, as with prolonged fasting, the body begins to use its fat stores for energy. If no glucose is ingested, the fat is only incompletely metabolized and ketoacids accumulate in the blood. This condition is termed starvation ketoacidosis.[8]

Box 25-1

Common Causes of Metabolic Acidosis

Increase in Acid
Ketoacidosis (diabetes mellitus, starvation, alcoholism)
Hyperthyroidism
Severe infection
Burns
Shock
Tissue anoxia
Oliguric renal failure
Intake of acids or acid precursors

Decrease in Base
Diarrhea
Gastrointestinal fistula
Intestinal decompression
Renal tubular acidosis

Bicarbonate ions are a type of base. Any condition that causes excessive removal of bicarbonate ions from the body may cause metabolic acidosis. For example, the intestinal fluid is rich in bicarbonate ions, which are contained in pancreatic secretions. Diarrhea causes removal of this base from the body and thus contributes to the development of metabolic acidosis.[9]

Other causes of metabolic acidosis are listed in Box 25-1 under the two general mechanisms discussed: increase in acid (except carbonic acid) and decrease in base. Either mechanism tends to make the blood overly acidic. The pathophysiology of disorders that may cause metabolic acidosis is discussed in the pertinent chapters of this text.

Clinical Manifestations. The signs and symptoms of metabolic acidosis are headache, abdominal pain, and central nervous system depression (confusion, lethargy, stupor, coma).

The central nervous system depression that occurs in patients with metabolic acidosis results primarily from the decreased pH of the cerebrospinal and interstitial fluid in the brain. When the pH of the interstitial fluid falls, intracellular pH decreases, the protein structure and enzyme activity in cells are altered, and dysfunction results. Other factors specific to the cause of the acidosis may also induce central nervous system depression, such as hyperosmolality with diabetic ketoacidosis. Severe metabolic acidosis predisposes to ventricular arrhythmias (from myocardial intracellular acidity) and decreased cardiac contractility, which may be fatal.[7] Death from brainstem dysfunction usually occurs when the pH falls below 6.9.

The arterial blood gases in metabolic acidosis will show a bicarbonate concentration below normal. If the metabolic acidosis is uncompensated, the pH will also be below normal because the usual 20:1 ratio is decreased.

Uncompensated metabolic acidosis:

$$\frac{\text{Decreased } [HCO_3^-]}{\text{Unchanged } [H_2CO_3]} = \text{pH low}$$

Compensatory Response. The respiratory compensation for metabolic acidosis is hyperventilation. A decrease in pH of the blood stimulates the peripheral chemoreceptors, which then cause reflex stimulation of ventilatory neurons in the brainstem.[2] The end response is an increased rate and depth of respiration. As the rate and depth of respiration increase, more carbonic acid (carbon dioxide and water) is excreted. Although hyperventilation does not remove metabolic acid from the body, it does change the ratio of bicarbonate ion to carbonic acid in a favorable direction. Because the bicarbonate ion concentration is already decreased by the metabolic acidosis, the compensatory decrease in carbonic acid brings the ratio (and thus the pH) back toward normal.

The arterial blood gases of a person who has compensated metabolic acidosis will show decreased bicarbonate concentration (the primary imbalance), decreased $Paco_2$ (compensation), and slightly decreased or even normal pH, depending on the degree of compensation. A flow chart for interpreting laboratory measures specific to acid-base imbalances is presented in Figure 25-2. Sample laboratory val-

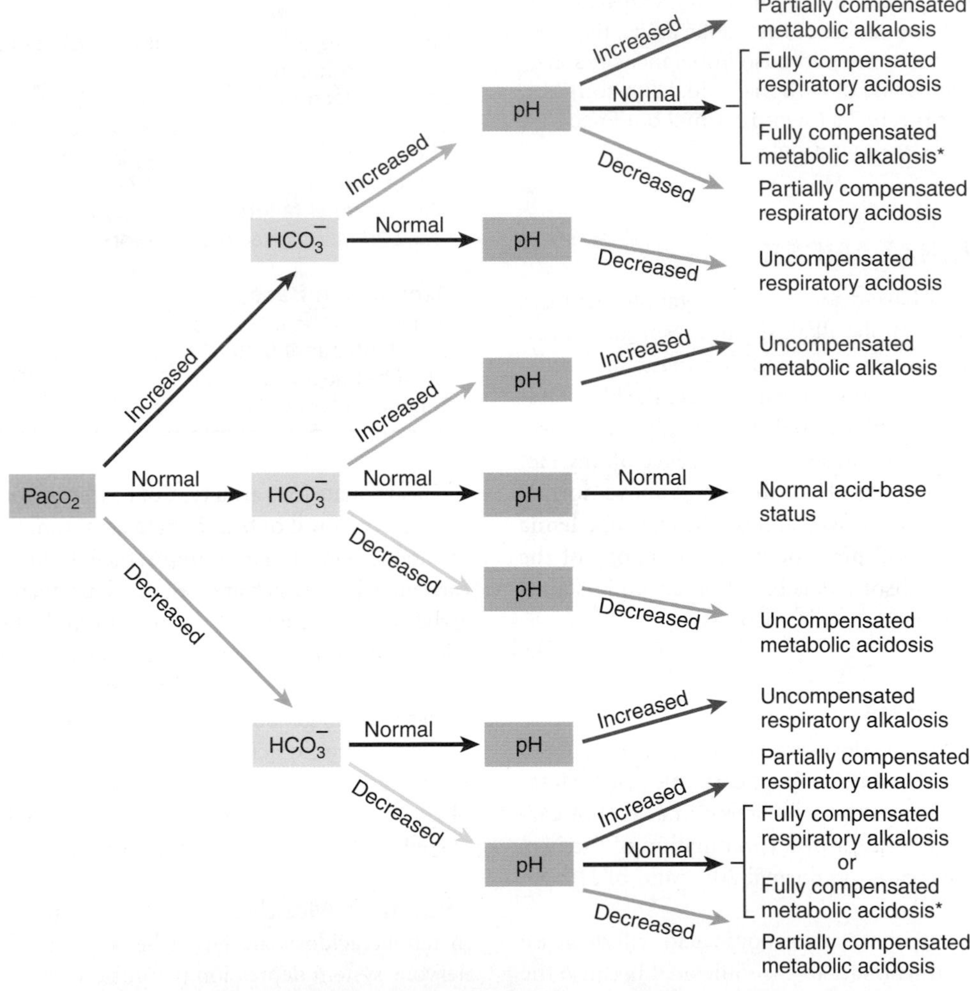

FIGURE 25-2 ■ Flow chart for interpretation of laboratory measurements specific for acid-base imbalances. Use this flow chart to determine the primary acid-base imbalance from a set of laboratory values. Begin on the left with the $Paco_2$ and follow the *arrows.* This flow chart does not include mixed acid-base imbalances.

ues for patients with metabolic acidosis are presented in Table 25-4.

Compensated metabolic acidosis:

$$\frac{\text{Decreased } [HCO_3^-] \text{ (primary)}}{\text{Decreased } [H_2CO_3] \text{ (compensatory)}} = \text{pH slightly low (partially compensated) } \textit{or} \text{ pH in the normal range (fully compensated)}$$

Respiratory Acidosis

Etiology. Respiratory acidosis is a condition that tends to cause an excess of carbonic acid.[7] This condition is aptly named because carbonic acid is excreted by the lungs in the form of carbon dioxide and water during the process of expiration.

Respiratory acidosis is caused by factors that impair the respiratory excretion of carbonic acid. Such factors include impaired gas exchange, inadequate neuromuscular function, and impairment of respiratory control in the brainstem. Box 25-2 provides examples of factors that may cause respiratory acidosis. These factors all decrease the normal 20:1 ratio of bicarbonate ion to carbonic acid (and thus decrease the pH of the blood) by increasing the carbonic acid portion of the ratio. Chronic respiratory acidosis often develops in persons who have chronic obstructive pulmonary disease. If an acute respiratory infection also develops, their acidosis may become worse.[3] Such a condition may be termed acute-on-chronic respiratory acidosis.

Clinical Manifestations. The signs and symptoms of respiratory acidosis are headache, tachycardia, cardiac ar-

Box 25-2

Common Causes of Respiratory Acidosis

Impaired Gas Exchange
- Chronic obstructive pulmonary disease
- Pneumonia
- Severe asthma
- Pulmonary edema
- Acute (adult) respiratory distress syndrome
- Obstructive sleep apnea

Impaired Neuromuscular Function
- Guillain-Barré syndrome
- Chest injury or surgery
- Hypokalemia
- Kyphoscoliosis
- Respiratory muscle fatigue

Impaired Respiratory Control (Brainstem)
- Respiratory depressant drugs (barbiturates, narcotics)
- Central sleep apnea

Table 25-4 

Sample Laboratory Values for Persons with Acid-Base Imbalances

Laboratory Value for Imbalance	Rationale
Partially Compensated Metabolic Acidosis (Diabetic Ketoacidosis)	
Pa_{CO_2} 30 mm Hg	Decreased because of compensatory hyperventilation
HCO_3^- 12 mEq/L	Decreased because of buffering of ketoacids
pH 7.22	Decreased because of excess metabolic acids; would be even lower without respiratory compensation
Uncompensated Respiratory Acidosis (Acute Asthma Episode)	
Pa_{CO_2} 55 mm Hg	Increased because of impaired gas exchange
HCO_3^- 24 mEq/L	Normal; renal compensation has not yet occurred in this acute condition
pH 7.26	Decreased because of excess carbonic acid
Fully Compensated Respiratory Acidosis (Emphysema)	
Pa_{CO_2} 60 mm Hg	Increased because of impaired gas exchange
HCO_3^- 36 mEq/L	Increased because of renal compensation in this chronic condition
pH 7.35	Normal because of renal compensation, but below 7.4
Uncompensated Metabolic Alkalosis (Repeated Emesis and ECV Depletion)	
Pa_{CO_2} 42 mm Hg	Normal, but increasing because of compensatory hypoventilation
HCO_3^- 36 mEq/L	Increased because of loss of H^+ from emesis and renal retention of HCO_3^- from ECV depletion
pH 7.52	Increased because of metabolic acid deficit
Uncompensated Respiratory Alkalosis (Hypoxemia from Pulmonary Embolism)	
Pa_{CO_2} 28 mm Hg	Decreased because of hyperventilation caused by chemoreceptor response to decreased Pa_{O_2}
HCO_3^- 24 mEq/L	Normal; renal compensation has not yet occurred in this acute condition
pH 7.52	Increased because of carbonic acid deficit

ECV, Extracellular volume.

rhythmias, and neurologic abnormalities such as blurred vision, tremors, vertigo, disorientation, lethargy, or somnolence.

Headache occurs because of dilation of blood vessels in the brain.[10,11] This cerebral vasodilation increases cerebrospinal fluid pressure; papilledema may result. Neurologic manifestations may be more prominent in patients with respiratory acidosis than in those with metabolic acidosis because carbonic acid (in the form of carbon dioxide and water) crosses the blood-brain barrier relatively easily. The neurologic manifestations result from the decreased pH of the cerebrospinal and interstitial fluid in the brain. This decreased interstitial fluid pH causes decreased intracellular pH, with resulting cellular dysfunction. Cardiac arrhythmias in patients with respiratory acidosis are also a result of decreased intracellular (myocardial cell) pH.[7] In severe respiratory acidosis, peripheral vasodilation may occur. Hypotension may result, especially if cardiac arrhythmias are also present.

Arterial blood gases in patients with respiratory acidosis will show a Pa_{CO_2} value above normal. If the respiratory acidosis is uncompensated, the pH will be below normal because the usual 20:1 ratio is decreased.[1]

Uncompensated respiratory acidosis:

$$\frac{\text{Unchanged } [HCO_3^-]}{\text{Increased } [H_2CO_3]} = \text{pH low}$$

Compensatory Response. The compensatory mechanism for respiratory acidosis is increased renal excretion of metabolic acid. This mechanism requires several days to be effective. Although the kidneys cannot excrete carbonic acid, their ability to excrete more metabolic acid changes the ratio of bicarbonate ions to carbonic acid in a favorable direction so that the pH moves toward normal. As the kidneys excrete more metabolic acid, the bicarbonate concentration increases because fewer bicarbonate ions are used for buffering. Because carbonic acid concentration is already increased, the increase in bicarbonate concentration will tend to normalize the ratio of HCO_3^- to H_2CO_3. The arterial blood gases of a person who has compensated respiratory acidosis will show increased Pa_{CO_2} (the primary imbalance), increased bicarbonate concentration (compensation), and slightly decreased or even normal pH, depending on the degree of compensation. Table 25-4 presents sample laboratory values for persons with respiratory acidosis.

Compensated respiratory acidosis:

$$\frac{\text{Decreased } [HCO_3^-] \text{ (compensatory)}}{\text{Decreased } [H_2CO_3] \text{ (primary)}} = \begin{array}{c}\text{pH slightly low} \\ \text{(partially compensated)} \\ \textit{or} \text{ pH in the normal range} \\ \text{(fully compensated)}\end{array}$$

Metabolic Alkalosis

Etiology. Metabolic alkalosis is a condition that tends to cause a relative deficit of any acid except carbonic acid.[7] Metabolic alkalosis may be caused by an increase in base (bicarbonate), by a decrease in acid, or by a combination of the two. Bicarbonate may be ingested in antacids such as baking soda and over-the-counter bicarbonate products (e.g., Alka-Seltzer). With overuse of these agents, enough bicarbonate is absorbed from the gastrointestinal tract to increase the blood bicarbonate concentration, thus increasing the pH.[12]

In addition to a gain in bicarbonate, metabolic alkalosis may also be caused by a decrease in acid. The stomach is a major reservoir of acid. Emesis and gastric suction remove acid from the body and create a relative excess of base; this situation is, by definition, metabolic alkalosis. Increased renal excretion of acid with retention of bicarbonate occurs in extracellular fluid volume depletion.[13] Metabolic alkalosis due to extracellular fluid volume depletion is often called contraction alkalosis. Hypokalemia causes hydrogen ions to shift into cells and also increases renal excretion of acid.[14]

Causes of metabolic alkalosis are summarized in Box 25-3. The pathophysiology of disorders that may cause metabolic alkalosis is discussed in the pertinent chapters of this text.

Clinical Manifestations. The signs and symptoms in patients who have metabolic alkalosis may result from the extracellular fluid volume depletion that caused the alkalosis. Thus postural hypotension may be present. Hypokalemia frequently coexists with metabolic alkalosis.[15] As described previously, hypokalemia may cause metabolic alkalosis. In addition, metabolic alkalosis that arises from another cause frequently induces hypokalemia by shifting potassium ions into cells. Thus the bilateral muscle weakness and polyuria of hypokalemia may be evident in patients who have metabolic alkalosis.

In patients who experience symptoms from the metabolic alkalosis itself, the initial manifestations are those of increased neuromuscular irritability.[16] The increased interstitial pH causes increased irritability of nerve cell membranes. The fingers and toes may tingle; signs of tetany may progress to seizures. Persons in whom metabolic alkalosis develops may become quite belligerent. With severe metabolic alkalosis, initial excitation may change to central nervous system depres-

Box 25-3

Common Causes of Metabolic Alkalosis

Increase in Base

Intake of bicarbonate or bicarbonate precursors (acetate, citrate, lactate)
Massive transfusion with citrated blood
Extracellular fluid volume depletion

Decrease in Acid

Emesis
Gastric suction
Extracellular fluid volume depletion
Hyperaldosteronism
Hypokalemia

sion. Confusion, lethargy, and coma may ensue from dysfunction of brain cells. Death occurs when the pH is around 7.8. The plasma bicarbonate concentration is elevated in patients with metabolic alkalosis.

Uncompensated metabolic alkalosis:

$$\frac{\text{Increased } [HCO_3^-]}{\text{Unchanged } [H_2CO_3]} = \text{pH high}$$

Compensatory Response. The compensatory mechanism for metabolic alkalosis is hypoventilation.[6] This shallow breathing retains carbonic acid within the body, thus increasing the lower portion of the bicarbonate ion–to–carbonic acid ratio. Because the upper portion of the ratio has been increased by the elevated bicarbonate concentration of metabolic alkalosis, the respiratory compensation tends to move the pH toward normal. Respiratory compensation for metabolic alkalosis is usually incomplete. The need for oxygen drives ventilation, even though the increased pH tends to depress it. Thus the arterial blood gases of a person who has compensated metabolic alkalosis usually show an increased bicarbonate concentration (the primary imbalance), increased Pa_{CO_2} (compensation), and a slightly increased pH. Table 25-4 presents sample laboratory values for persons with metabolic alkalosis.

Compensated metabolic alkalosis:

$$\frac{\text{Increased } [HCO_3^-] \text{ (primary)}}{\text{Increased } [H_2CO_3] \text{ (compensatory)}} = \text{pH slightly high (partially compensated)}$$

Respiratory Alkalosis

Etiology. Respiratory alkalosis is a condition that tends to cause a carbonic acid deficit.[7] With a deficit of carbonic acid, the blood is relatively too alkaline.

Respiratory alkalosis is caused by hyperventilation.[4] Carbonic acid is excreted during expiration; when the respirations are excessively rapid and deep (hyperventilation), too much carbonic acid is excreted. The resulting deficit of carbonic acid is respiratory alkalosis. In gram-negative sepsis, the respiratory center in the brainstem is often stimulated abnormally and hyperventilation results. Other causes of hyperventilation (and thus of respiratory alkalosis) are listed in Box 25-4.

Clinical Manifestations. The clinical manifestations of respiratory alkalosis are diaphoresis and increased neuromuscular irritability. Paresthesias (numbness and tingling) may occur in the fingers and around the mouth. Increased pH of the cerebrospinal fluid and cerebral interstitial fluid alters the function of brain cells. In addition, the increased pH has a direct effect of increasing membrane excitability in both central and peripheral neurons. Respiratory alkalosis also causes cerebral vasoconstriction, which reduces blood flow in the brain.[6]

The increased excretion of carbonic acid in persons with respiratory alkalosis causes the Pa_{CO_2} to be abnormally low. If the disorder is uncompensated, the pH will be abnormally high.

Uncompensated respiratory alkalosis:

$$\frac{\text{Unchanged } [HCO_3^-]}{\text{Decreased } [H_2CO_3]} = \text{pH high}$$

Compensatory Response. The compensatory mechanism for respiratory alkalosis is decreased renal excretion of metabolic acid. As metabolic acids accumulate in the blood, the bicarbonate ion concentration decreases because bicarbonate ions are used for buffering. Because the carbonic acid concentration is already decreased, renal compensation for respiratory alkalosis tends to return the ratio of bicarbonate ion to carbonic acid, and thus the pH, toward normal. Renal compensatory mechanisms take several days to be fully effective. Many of the causes of respiratory alkalosis are short lived and, for that reason, may not be compensated renally. The arterial blood gases of a person who has compensated respiratory alkalosis will show a decreased Pa_{CO_2} (the primary imbalance), decreased bicarbonate concentration (compensation), and a slightly increased or perhaps normal pH, depending on the degree of compensation. Table 25-4 presents sample laboratory values for persons with respiratory alkalosis.

Compensated respiratory alkalosis:

$$\frac{\text{Decreased } [HCO_3^-] \text{ (compensatory)}}{\text{Decreased } [H_2CO_3] \text{ (primary)}} = \text{pH slightly low (partially compensated) } \textit{or} \text{ pH in the normal range (fully compensated)}$$

Mixed Acid-Base Imbalances

In most patients, only one of the four primary imbalances discussed in this chapter arises at a time. If the imbalance persists, a compensatory imbalance arises as well. This situation has been discussed previously in this chapter. Occasionally, however, two primary imbalances arise in the same person. This latter situation is termed a **mixed acid-base imbalance.**[1] For example, a patient who has bacterial pneumonia may develop respiratory acidosis. If severe diarrhea from antibiotics devel-

Box 25-4

Common Causes of Respiratory Alkalosis (Hyperventilation)

- Anxiety, psychological distress
- Prolonged sobbing
- Hypoxemia
- Alcohol withdrawal
- Stimulation of the brainstem (salicylate overdose, meningitis, head injury)

ops at the same time, a concurrent metabolic acidosis may arise. In this mixed imbalance, the pH is likely to be very low because the two types of primary acidosis impair the effectiveness of the usual compensatory mechanisms. Specifically, the usual compensatory mechanism for metabolic acidosis is hyperventilation, which causes increased excretion of carbonic acid from the body. With bacterial pneumonia, however, the effectiveness of alveolar ventilation is already impaired and carbonic acid is being retained in the blood. Analogously, patients who have both types of primary alkalosis often have a very high pH because their usual compensatory mechanisms are impeded by the concurrent acid-base disorders.

Mixed acid-base disorders may also occur with a nearly normal pH if a primary acidosis and a primary alkalosis are involved. An example of this type of mixed disorder is a head-injured patient whose treatment includes hyperventilation by mechanical ventilation to reduce intracranial pressure (respiratory alkalosis) but who at the same time has a metabolic acidosis from acute renal failure. In this situation, the $Paco_2$ will be decreased (respiratory alkalosis), the plasma bicarbonate concentration will be decreased (metabolic acidosis), and the pH will depend on the relative severity of the two imbalances.

Box 25-5

Pediatric Variations

- Neonates often have mild metabolic acidosis. Infants younger than 1 month have a reduced ability to excrete a large acid load; their kidneys are less able to reabsorb bicarbonate, they produce less ammonia, and urinary buffers are limited in quantity. These factors increase the risk of metabolic acidosis from acid accumulation.
- Adolescents with eating disorders may have metabolic alkalosis from repeated emesis or metabolic acidosis from starvation and laxative-induced chronic diarrhea.

◆ Mixed acid-base disorders occur when two primary acid-base disorders are present independently. They may be the result of simultaneous dysfunction of the lungs and kidneys. Depending on the combination of disorders, the pH may be nearly normal or grossly abnormal.

KEY CONCEPTS

- Acidosis is a condition that tends to cause a relative excess of acid. Alkalosis is a condition that tends to cause a relative excess of base.
- Metabolic acidosis is characterized by a pH below 7.40 and an abnormally low HCO_3^-. It is caused by processes that lead to metabolic acid accumulation (e.g., lactic acidosis) or loss of HCO_3^- (e.g., diarrhea). Compensatory hyperventilation will decrease the $Paco_2$.
- Metabolic alkalosis is characterized by a pH above 7.40 and an abnormally high level of HCO_3^-. It is caused by processes that lead to metabolic acid loss (e.g., vomiting) or gain of HCO_3^- (e.g., bicarbonate antacids). Compensatory hypoventilation will increase the $Paco_2$.
- Respiratory acidosis is characterized by a pH below 7.40 and an abnormally high $Paco_2$. It is caused by processes that lead to hypoventilation by impairing gas exchange (e.g., lung diseases), neuromuscular function of the chest (e.g., hypokalemic muscle paralysis), or respiratory control mechanisms in the brainstem (e.g., barbiturate overdose). Compensatory excretion of H^+ and retention of HCO_3^- by the kidneys cause an increased HCO_3^- concentration.
- Respiratory alkalosis is characterized by a pH above 7.40 and an abnormally low $Paco_2$. It is caused by processes that lead to hyperventilation (e.g., hypoxemia, anxiety). Compensatory retention of H^+ and excretion of HCO_3^- by the kidneys cause a decreased HCO_3^- concentration.

SUMMARY

Acid-base homeostasis involves the interplay of buffers, the respiratory system, and renal mechanisms. Metabolic acids are continually produced by cellular metabolism. These metabolic acids enter the blood and are buffered and excreted by the kidneys. In healthy persons, the kidneys adjust the rate of excretion of metabolic acids to meet the demands of the acid load being produced. The concentration of bicarbonate ions in the blood indicates the effectiveness of renal excretion of metabolic acids. The carbon dioxide and water (carbonic acid) that are also produced by cellular metabolism are excreted by the lungs. In healthy persons, changes in the respiratory rate and depth adjust the rate of excretion of carbonic acid. The $Paco_2$ indicates the effectiveness of respiratory excretion of carbonic acid.

If one of the acid-base regulatory mechanisms becomes dysfunctional or overwhelmed, another mechanism can produce a compensatory response that will help normalize the pH of the extracellular fluid, even though it will not correct the acid-base imbalance. Thus the kidneys adjust their excretion of metabolic acids when the respiratory excretion of carbonic acid is abnormally altered. Similarly, the respiratory system adjusts the rate of excretion of carbonic acid if the renal regulation of metabolic acids is impaired or overwhelmed. The pH of the blood at any time is the net result of the operation of these regulatory and compensatory mechanisms.

Primary acid-base imbalances arise when the normal regulatory mechanisms for acid-base homeostasis become impaired or are overwhelmed by a large acid or alkaline load. Pediatric and geriatric variations are summarized in Boxes 25-5

Box 25-6

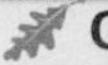

Geriatric Variations

- The chemoreceptor response to increased Pa_{CO_2} (hyperventilation) is delayed in older adults, which may delay their ability to correct respiratory acidosis
- Older adults are at increased risk of respiratory depression (and thus respiratory acidosis) from barbiturates because of increased drug half-life
- Older adults' kidneys are less able to excrete a large acid load, which increases the risk for metabolic acidosis from acid accumulation/ingestion
- Diarrhea from chronic laxative overuse may contribute to metabolic acidosis

and 25-6. Primary metabolic acidosis arises when the kidneys are unable to excrete enough metabolic acid or bicarbonate is lost from the body. The compensatory response to metabolic acidosis is hyperventilation. Primary respiratory acidosis arises when the lungs are unable to excrete enough carbonic acid. The compensatory response to respiratory acidosis is increased renal excretion of metabolic acid.

Primary metabolic alkalosis arises when the kidneys excrete too much metabolic acid or there is a gain of bicarbonate. The compensatory response to metabolic alkalosis is hypoventilation. Primary respiratory alkalosis arises when the lungs excrete too much carbonic acid. The compensatory response to respiratory alkalosis is decreased renal excretion of metabolic acid. The Pa_{CO_2} reflects the respiratory component of an acid-base imbalance, and the plasma bicarbonate concentration reflects the metabolic (renal) component of an acid-base imbalance.

A mixed acid-base imbalance occurs when two primary imbalances exist at the same time. The two primary imbalances may drive the pH to an extremely abnormal value or may nearly cancel each other's effect on the pH, although the Pa_{CO_2} and plasma bicarbonate concentration may still be very abnormal.

MEDIA RESOURCES

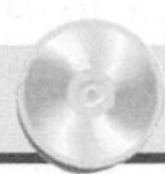

evolve

Remember to check out the ***CD Companion*** included with this book for Review Questions, Key Concepts Review, Glossary (with audio for selected terms), Disease Profiles, and Animations.

PLUS, visit the ***Evolve website*** at http://evolve.elsevier.com/Copstead/ for Case Studies, Disease Profiles, and WebLinks.

References

1. Rose BD, Post TW: *Clinical physiology of acid-base and electrolyte disorders,* ed 5, New York, 2001, McGraw-Hill.
2. Guyton AC, Hall AE: *Textbook of medical physiology,* ed 10, Philadelphia, 2000, Saunders.
3. Cham GW et al: Clinical predictors of acute respiratory acidosis during exacerbation of asthma and chronic obstructive pulmonary disease, *Eur J Emerg Med* 9:225-232, 2002.
4. Malmberg LP, Tamminen K, Sovijarvi AR: Hyperventilation syndrome, *Thorax* 56:85-86, 2001.
5. De Backer D: Lactic acidosis, *Intensive Care Med* 29:699-702, 2003.
6. Laffey JG, Kavanagh BP: Hypocapnia, *N Engl J Med* 347:43-53, 2002.
7. Felver L: Acid-base balance and imbalances. In Woods SL et al, editors: *Cardiac nursing,* ed 5, Philadelphia, 2005, Lippincott, pp 189-196.
8. Ensminger SA, Regner KR, Froehling DA: 35-year-old woman with cough, fever, and anorexia, *Mayo Clin Proc* 78:753-756, 2003.
9. Abdelgabar A et al: A case of voluminous diarrhoea with hypokalaemic acidosis, *Int J Clin Pract* 55:64-65, 2001.
10. Horiuchi T et al: Role of endothelial nitric oxide and smooth muscle potassium channels in cerebral arteriolar dilation in response to acidosis, *Stroke* 33:844-849, 2002.
11. Lindauer U et al: Cerebrovascular vasodilation to extraluminal acidosis occurs via combined activation of ATP-sensitive and Ca^{2+}-activated potassium channels, *J Cerebral Blood Flow Metab* 23:1227-1238, 2003.
12. Sahani MM et al: Metabolic alkalosis in a hemodialysis patient after ingestion of a large amount of an antacid medication, *Artif Organs* 25:313-315, 2001.
13. Greenberg A: Diuretic complications, *Am J Med Sci* 319:10-24, 2000.
14. Devendra D, Rowe PA: Unexplained hypokalaemia and metabolic alkalosis, *Postgrad Med J* 77:E4, 2001.
15. Nair S, Shoeneman MJ: Index of suspicion. Case 1. Diagnosis: hypokalemia in association with metabolic alkalosis, *Pediatr Rev* 22:67-71, 2001.
16. Simons P, Nadra I, McNally PG: Metabolic alkalosis and myoclonus, *Postgrad Med J* 79(933):414-415, 2003.

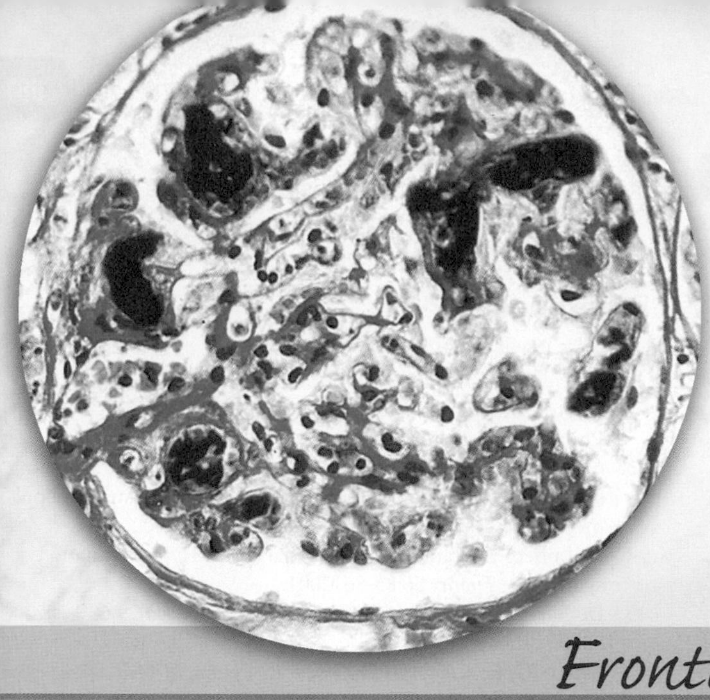

Frontiers of Research

Renal Failure and Dialysis

Fadi Ghandour and Michael J. Kirkhorn

The kidney has multiple functions. Kidneys excrete urine through the activity of about 2 million nephrons, each of which is able to filter the urine from the blood. After the urine is filtered in the glomerulus, part is reabsorbed and another passes to the renal pelvis. In this way, kidneys clean unwanted substances—metabolic end products or excess ions of sodium, potassium, chloride, or hydrogen—from the blood plasma.

The kidneys are important blood pressure regulators. The rate at which they dispose of extra cellular fluid helps keep the arterial pressure at normal levels. Kidneys are endocrine organs as well; they secrete erythropoietin, the hormone that regulates red blood cell production and converts vitamin D to its active form.

Elevated blood pressure, if not well controlled, can lead to congestive heart failure, cardiovascular accidents, and kidney failure. When diseased, the kidney can cause hypertension, and if hypertension is not controlled, it can cause kidney damage.

Chronic kidney disease is a worldwide public health problem. In the United States, the incidence and prevalence of chronic kidney disease are increasing. End-stage kidney (renal) disease (ESRD) is a drastic end point of kidney failure. The total cost of the ESRD program in the United States was $23 billion in 1999. The projected number of ESRD patients by the year 2010 has been estimated at 661,330, and the total Medicare cost has been estimated at more than $28 billion. The incidence of the disease has been increasing almost 8% to 10% each year. The severity of the disease is suggested by the fact that more than 60% of ESRD patients die within 5 years.

Diabetes is the most common cause of ESRD, followed by hypertension. There are striking racial

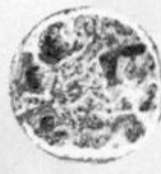

Fibrin stain showing platelet-fibrin thrombi (red) *in the glomerular capillaries, characteristic of microangiopathic disorders. (From Kumar V, Abbas AK, Fausto N:* Robbins and Cotran pathologic basis of disease, *ed 7, Philadelphia, 2005, Saunders.)*

Renal and Bladder Function

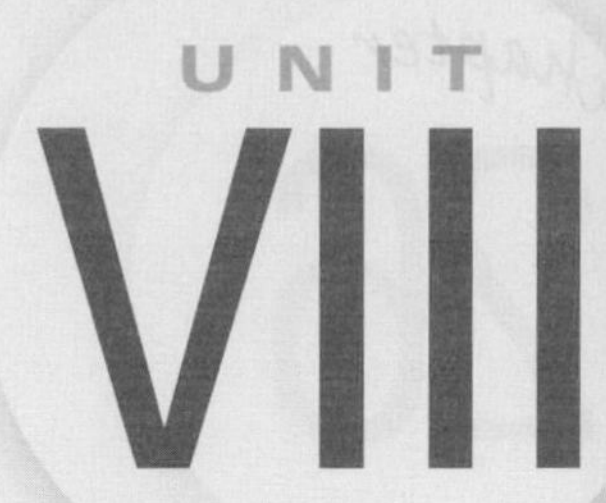

and ethnic differences in the incidence and prevalence of ESRD. African-Americans, American Indians, Alaskan Natives, Native Hawaiians, and Hispanic persons have a disproportionately high incidence and prevalence of ESRD. It is possible that differential access to health care and attention to the adequate management of chronic kidney disease for minority groups may be a cause of concern. Few studies have shown a correlation between environmental factors and the development and progression of chronic renal disease.

Transplantation is the best treatment for patients with ESRD. It prolongs and improves the quality of life. Patients need life-long medications to prevent rejection of the transplant kidney; these medications have major side effects and can cause different complications. Hemodialysis is used in patients with severely impaired kidney function. It can be inconvenient because patients have to undergo dialysis at a dialysis center three times a week for 3 to 4 hours. Peritoneal dialysis, on the other hand, offers a better lifestyle in which patients undergo dialysis at home through a peritoneal dialysis catheter in their abdomen. Both methods of dialysis carry their own complication rate and offer similar renal replacement support.

Chronic kidney disease of different etiologies is managed with blood pressure reductions, using at times several antihypertensive medications; those patients are followed up closely by their kidney doctors to help them avoid dialysis as much as possible. A few of the issues that chronic kidney dialysis patients face are fluid overload, elevated potassium level, bone disease, acid management, and special diet control.

respectively. A discussion of fluid and electrolyte imbalances and acid-base disturbances can be found in Chapters 24 and 25. The essentials of kidney structure and nephron function are presented in this chapter.

RENAL ANATOMY

The urinary system consists of the kidneys, ureters, urinary bladder, and urethra (Figure 26-1). The kidneys are located in the **retroperitoneal** space in the posterior abdomen. One kidney is on each side of the vertebral column between the level of the twelfth thoracic and third lumbar vertebrae. The costovertebral angle (CVA), the point at which the bottom of the rib cage meets the spine, is commonly used as an external landmark for finding kidney position during physical examination.[3] The right kidney is located beneath the liver and is placed slightly lower than the left kidney.

The kidneys are protected and surrounded by strong back and flank muscles, fascia, and fat. The kidneys are somewhat mobile and can be injured by high-impact activities, such as bouncing along on horseback or on a mountain bike, or by direct trauma, as might occur from falls or blunt trauma. Kidney hemorrhage results in bleeding into the retroperitoneal space but not into the peritoneal cavity.

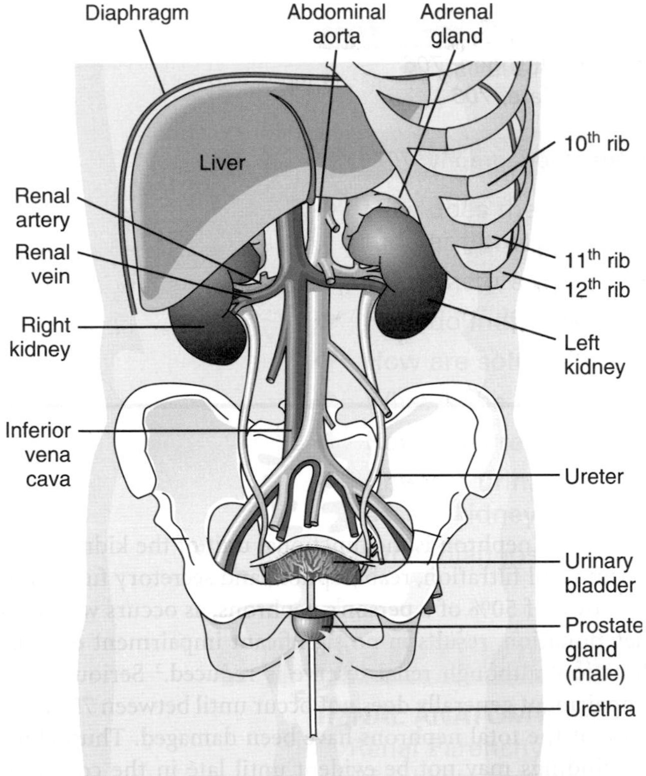

FIGURE 26-1 ■ Structure of the urinary tract. The kidneys are located in the retroperitoneal space in the posterior abdominal cavity, in contact with the diaphragm and covered on the upper portions by ribs.

The kidneys drain urine into the ureters by gravity flow. The ureters provide peristaltic action to move urine along to the bladder where it is stored. The urinary bladder collects 300 to 500 ml before stretch receptors signal a need for bladder emptying. Urine is drained from the bladder by the urethra when the internal and external sphincters are relaxed. Innervation and control of bladder function are discussed in detail in Chapter 29.

An adult kidney weighs approximately 115 to 170 g; is 11 cm long, 6 cm wide, and 3 cm thick; and is shaped like a red kidney bean, with the concave portion, termed the **hilum,** facing the vertebral column.[1] A thin, fibrous capsule covers each kidney and encloses blood vessels, lymphatic vessels, and nerve fibers, including pain receptors. Lymphatic vessels, blood vessels, and nerves enter and exit the kidney through the hilum.

Renal Parenchyma

On cross-section, the kidney is seen to contain three principal areas: the pelvis, the medulla, and the cortex (Figure 26-2). The renal pelvis is a large collecting area for the urine that drains from the many collecting ducts of the nephrons. The minor (smaller) calices collect urine as it drains from the papilla of the renal pyramids. The normal kidney has 8 to 18 minor calices and 2 to 3 major calices.[1] The major calices are large collecting spaces located between the minor calices and the upper part of the ureter.

The medulla contains 8 to 18 renal pyramids, the bases of which are adjacent to the outer cortex, whereas the apices open into the minor calices. The pyramids consist of collecting tubules, collecting ducts, long loops of Henle, and vasa recta. The papillae are the openings at the tips of the renal pyramids through which urine exits the collecting ducts.

The renal cortex, which is the outer rim of the kidney, is about 1 cm thick. The cortex contains all of the glomeruli as well as 85% of the nephron tubules. Fifteen percent of nephrons send their loops of Henle deep into the medulla and are called **juxtamedullary nephrons.** Columns of cortical tissue are found between the medullary pyramids and provide the passageway for the interlobar arteries.

Renal Lymphatics and Innervation

There are two lymphatic systems in the kidney. One system is composed of vessels that are located both in the renal capsule and immediately under the capsule in the outer cortex. The other lymphatic system is composed of vessels that accompany and wrap around the arterial blood vessels. All the lymphatic vessels, as well as blood vessels and nerves, exit the kidney through the hilum, and lymph drains into the paraaortic lymph nodes.

The kidneys are innervated by the sympathetic division of the autonomic nervous system. The lesser splanchnic nerves come from the renal plexuses, which are located next to the renal arteries. These nerve fibers travel with the renal arterial blood vessels and terminate in smooth muscle of the afferent and efferent arterioles, proximal and distal tubules, and the renin-secreting juxtaglomerular cells.[4] Stimulation of the sympathetic nervous system results in renal vasoconstriction and renin release. The renal capsule and all structures between the renal pelvis and urinary meatus are innervated with pain receptors (see Chapter 27).

Renal Blood Supply

Approximately 25% of the cardiac output is delivered to the kidneys, over 90% of which circulates through the cortex, while only 1% to 2% perfuses the medulla.[5] Total renal blood flow in both kidneys is approximately 1200 ml/min. Blood flows to the kidneys from the abdominal aorta through the renal arteries, which then divide into several interlobar arteries.[5] The interlobar arteries travel in the renal columns adjacent to the pyramids (see Figure 26-2). When the interlobar arteries reach the border of the medulla and the cortex, they branch into the arcuate arteries. The arcuate arteries then travel along the cortical medullary border parallel to the renal capsule. The arcuate arteries branch further to form small interlobular arteries, which penetrate the cortex and branch extensively to form the afferent arterioles. The afferent arterioles divide to form glomerular capillaries, which coalesce to form the efferent arterioles (Figure 26-3). The efferent arterioles branch again to form a second capillary bed. The peritubular capillaries wrap around the proximal and distal convoluted tubules. Some capillaries, called vasa recta, dip down into the medulla to surround the loops of Henle and collecting ducts. The vasa recta have a specialized loop structure that enables them to pick up interstitial fluid without excess removal of interstitial solutes. Solutes and water move into and out of the vasa recta passively such that the descending limb gains solute as it dips into the highly concentrated medulla, but then most of the solute is lost as the ascending loop makes its way back up to the cortex (Figure 26-4).

The capillaries of the peritubular system and the vasa recta join together and drain into interlobular venules. The veins that drain blood from the kidney run parallel to the arteries and are similarly named (Figure 26-5).

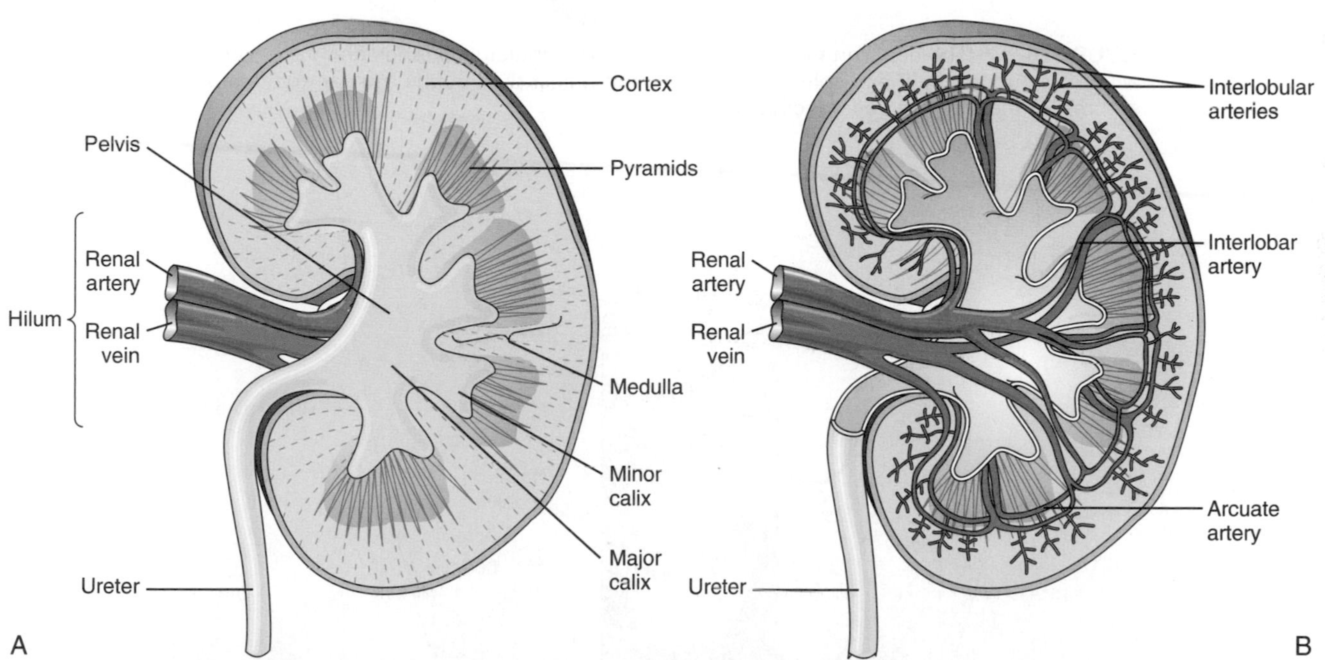

FIGURE 26-2 ■ **A,** Cross-section of the kidney showing the renal pelvis, medullary pyramids, and cortex. Normal kidneys have 8 to 18 renal pyramids and a corresponding number of minor calices. The major calices drain urine into the ureter. Blood vessels, lymphatic vessels, and nerves enter and exit through the hilum. **B,** The arterial blood supply to the kidney is derived from the renal arteries, which branch from the abdominal aorta and enter the kidney through the hilus. The renal artery branches to form several interlobar arteries, which travel toward the cortex in the renal columns. The interlobar arteries branch to form the arcuate arteries, which divide further to form the interlobular arteries. Interlobular arteries branch multiple times to provide the afferent arterioles for each of the kidney's million nephrons.

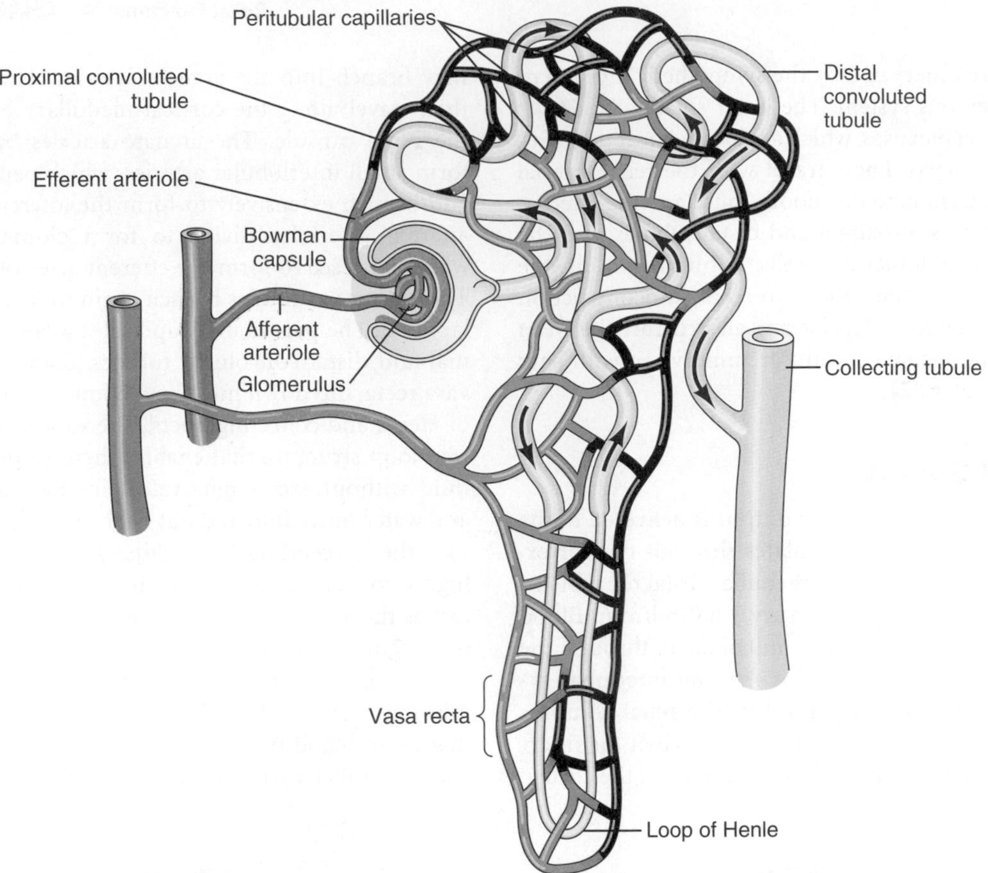

FIGURE 26-3 ■ The nephron tubule is covered by peritubular capillaries and vasa recta, which pick up the fluid and solutes that have been reabsorbed by the tubular epithelium and return them to the general circulation.

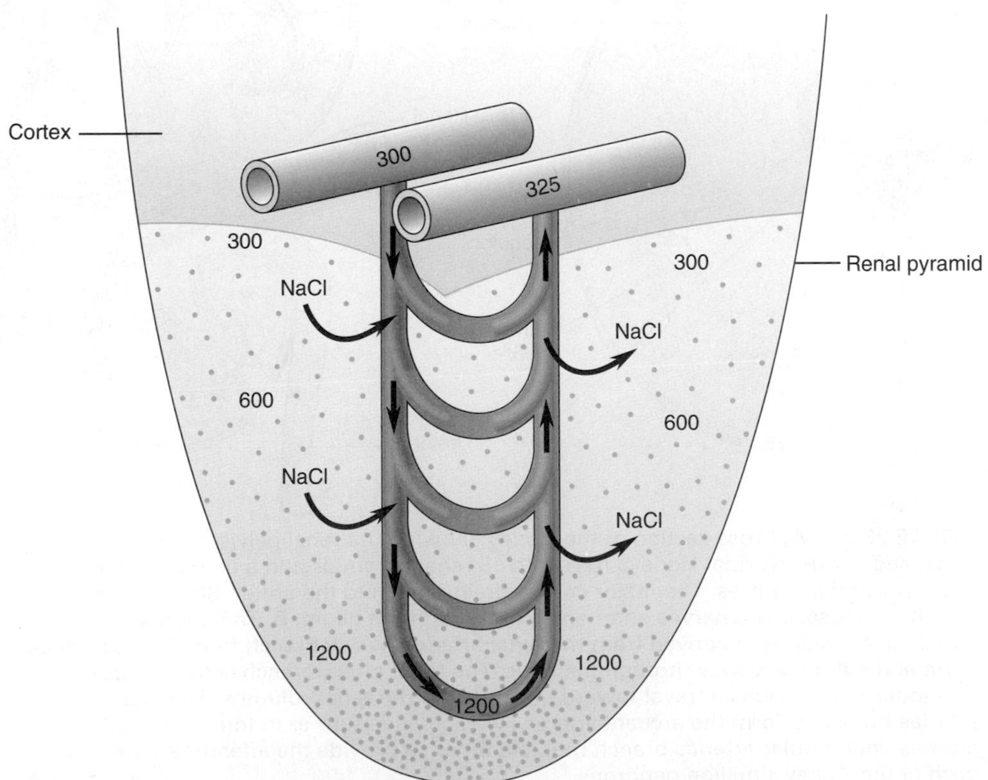

FIGURE 26-4 ■ The specialized loop structure of the vasa recta allows it to pick up interstitial water without significant solute removal. Although solutes are acquired in the descending segment, they passively diffuse back out as the ascending segment reaches the cortex.

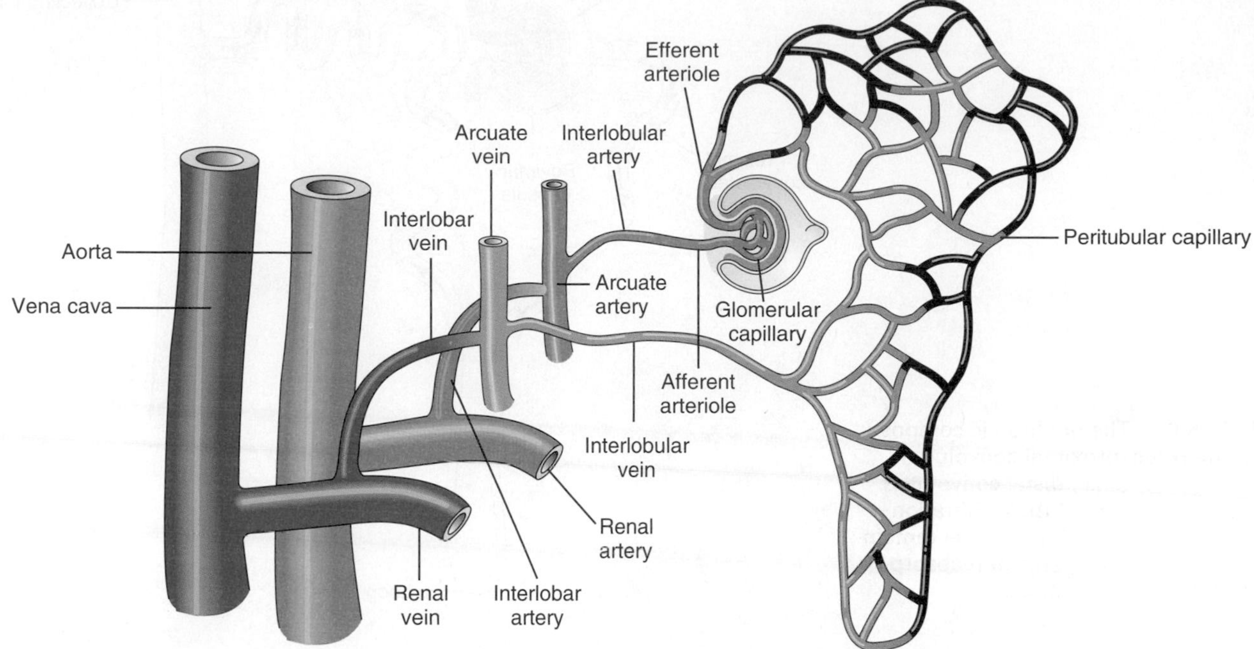

FIGURE 26-5 ■ The venous vessels of the kidney parallel the arterial vessels and are similarly named.

KEY CONCEPTS

- The kidneys are located in the retroperitoneal space, just under the diaphragm. The right kidney is slightly lower than the left. The costovertebral angle is an external landmark useful for locating the kidneys.
- The kidney can be divided into three principal anatomic sections: the pelvis, the medulla, and the cortex. The pelvis is composed of urinary collecting structures, called calices. The medulla is the middle portion and contains the renal pyramids. The cortex is the outer portion and contains glomeruli and nephron tubules.
- The kidneys are supplied with lymphatics to drain excess interstitial fluid and proteins and with sympathetic neurons to regulate blood supply and renin release.
- Blood is supplied to the kidneys by the renal artery, which divides several times to form the interlobar, arcuate, and interlobular arteries. The interlobular arteries branch multiple times to form afferent arterioles for each of the millions of kidney glomeruli.
- Each nephron has its own afferent arteriole, capillary tuft, and efferent arteriole. Efferent arterioles continue on to form peritubular capillaries, or vasa recta, which wrap around nephron structures and eventually drain into the renal veins. The loop structure of the vasa recta enables them to pick up interstitial fluid without removing excessive solute.

OVERVIEW OF NEPHRON STRUCTURE AND FUNCTION

Most of the physiologic functioning of the kidney can be understood by examining the function of an individual nephron. Thus, the nephron is said to be the functional unit of the kidney. Nephrons are organized in parallel such that each must accomplish all the necessary processing before releasing urine into the collecting ducts. Complex autoregulatory mechanisms ensure that the workload is evenly distributed among the kidneys' many nephrons.

As the unit of kidney function, a nephron must accomplish three major functions: (1) filtration of water-soluble substances from the blood; (2) reabsorption of filtered nutrients, water, and electrolytes; and (3) secretion of wastes or excess substances into the filtrate. Different segments of the nephron are specialized to accomplish each of these processes. Each nephron is composed of a glomerulus, which includes the capillary tuft and Bowman capsule, and a tubule, which includes the proximal convoluted tubule, loop of Henle, distal tubule, and collecting tubule (Figure 26-6). The nephron tubule is composed of a single layer of epithelial cells with an apical side facing the lumen and a basolateral side facing the interstitial space and capillaries (Figure 26-7). The epithelial cells in each segment of the tubule are specialized for certain functions (Table 26-1).

Glomerulus

The glomerulus is the site of fluid filtration from the blood to the nephron tubule. It is formed by a capillary tuft, which lies

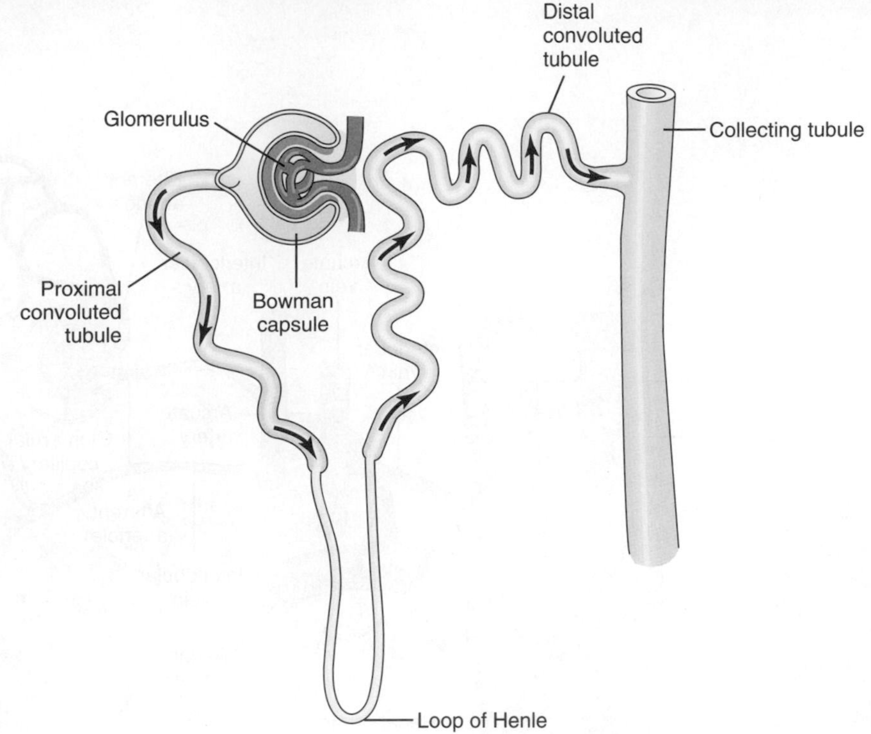

FIGURE 26-6 ■ The nephron is composed of a glomerulus, proximal convoluted tubule, loop of Henle, distal convoluted tubule, and collecting tubule. Filtration occurs at the glomerulus, and the remaining tubule segments perform reabsorption and secretion functions.

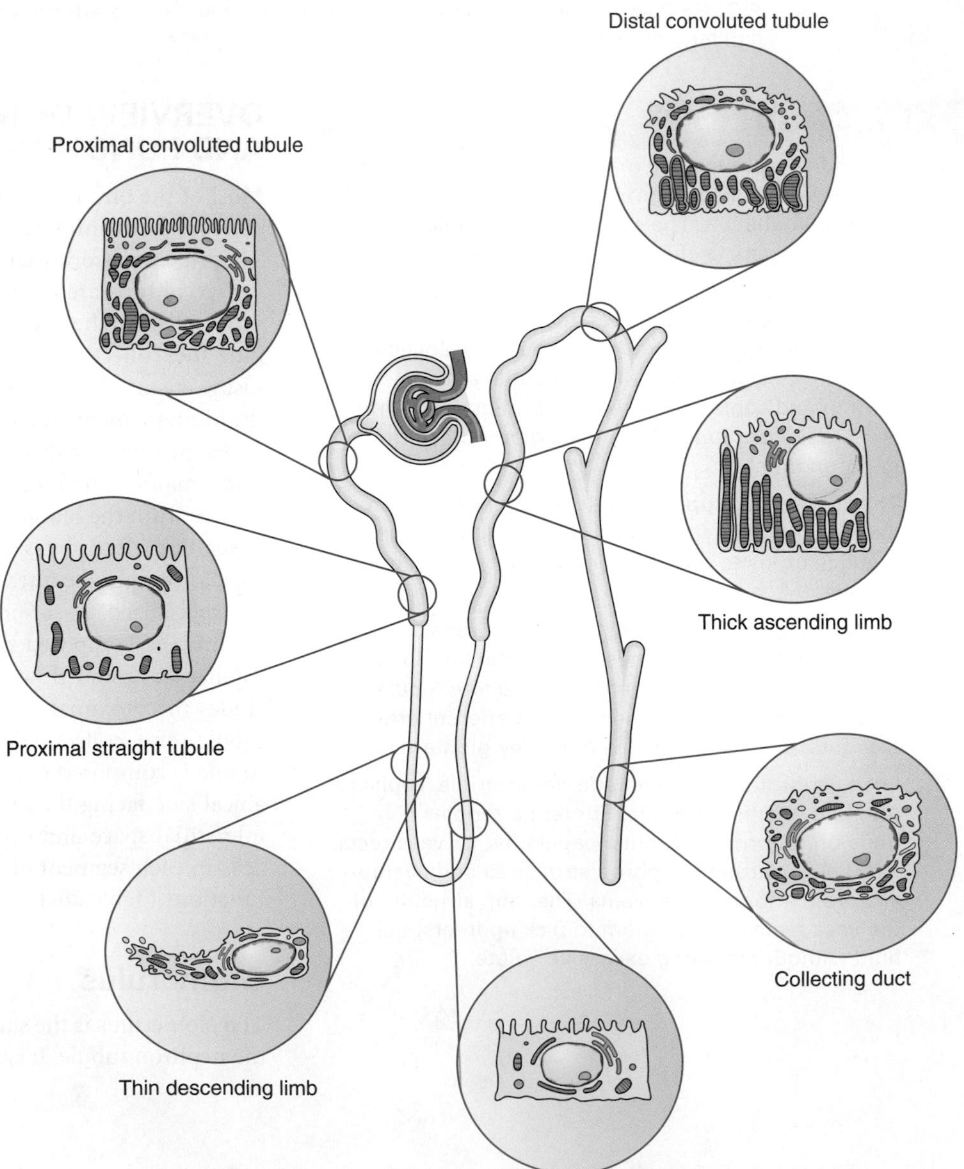

FIGURE 26-7 ■ Each segment of the nephron is specialized for certain functions, which is reflected in the type of epithelial cells that make up the tubules.

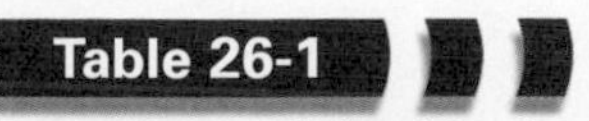

Functions of the Nephron Segments

Nephron Segment	Functions
Glomerulus	Filters fluid from the blood into Bowman capsule; prevents the passage of blood cells and proteins
Proximal convoluted tubule	Reabsorbs two thirds of the filtered water and electrolytes and all of the filtered bicarbonate, glucose, amino acids, and vitamins
Descending loop of Henle	Reabsorbs water, delivers a concentrated filtrate to the ascending loop of Henle
Ascending loop of Henle	Actively reabsorbs Na^+, K^+, Cl^- to produce a hypoosmotic filtrate and a high interstitial osmolality
Distal convoluted tubule	Reabsorbs Na^+, Cl^-, water, and urea; responsive to aldosterone; site of macula densa regulation of GFR; secretes H^+ and K^+
Collecting tubule	Reabsorption of water under the influence of ADH; secretes H^+ and K^+

GFR, Glomerular filtration rate; *ADH,* antidiuretic hormone.

between the afferent and efferent arterioles, and by the surrounding epithelial cells of Bowman capsule. The outer layer of the glomerular capsule is called the *parietal layer* and consists of a single thickness of epithelial cells resting on a layer of basement membrane (Figure 26-8). The inner (visceral) layer of the capsule is composed of specialized epithelial cells called *podocytes.* Podocytes have foot processes that surround the glomerular capillary walls (Figure 26-9). Between the podocyte and the capillary endothelium is a layer of extracellular matrix called *basement membrane* (see Figure 26-8).

Spaces between the endothelial cells are called *fenestra* and spaces between the podocyte foot processes are called *slit pores.* These intercellular spaces provide the surface area for glomerular filtration and make the glomeruli considerably more permeable than other capillaries in the body (Figure 26-10). The basement membrane is the principal selectivity barrier of the glomerulus, preventing plasma proteins, erythrocytes, leukocytes, and platelets from passing through. Cells are too large to pass through pores, and plasma proteins are negatively charged and repelled by the basement membrane.[6] Slit pores have a thin diaphragm of protein that restricts the filtration of some plasma proteins that make it through the basement membrane. *Nephrin* is an important protein in the slit pores as demonstrated by the massive proteinuria (protein in urine) that occurs when it is genetically mutated.[1] Proteins and blood cells are not usually present in the urine. If the glomerulus is injured, blood cells and proteins may filter through and be found in urine. Proteinuria is an important sign of basement membrane dysfunction.

Except for the lack of proteins and cells, the glomerular filtrate is very similar in composition to plasma. The **glomerular filtration rate** (GFR) averages about 125 ml/min.

Proximal Convoluted Tubule

Bowman capsule drains the glomerular filtrate directly into the proximal tubule segment, where two thirds of the water and electrolytes are rapidly reabsorbed[7] (Figure 26-11). Nutrients, vitamins, and small proteins normally are reabsorbed completely in the early proximal tubule. The early proximal tubule is the site of most bicarbonate ion reabsorption whereas chloride ion is reabsorbed in the late proximal tubule. The proximal tubule is made up of cuboidal epithelium and convoluted to provide a greater surface area for reabsorption. The epithelial cells in this segment have microvilli that form a brush border next to the filtrate and substantially increase the apical surface area. Proximal tubule cells have high adenosine triphosphate (ATP) requirements because most reabsorption utilizes active transport mechanisms that are dependent on Na^+-K^+ ion pumps in the basolateral membrane. The specifics of some of these transport mechanisms are discussed in subsequent sections. Water is reabsorbed passively through water channels made of proteins called aquaporin 1. Reabsorption of solutes creates the osmotic force for passive water reabsorption.

Loop of Henle

The loop of Henle is divided into the descending and ascending limbs, which differ in structure and function. The descending limb receives filtrate from the proximal convoluted tubule and delivers it to the ascending limb. The thin descending limb and initial part of the ascending segment are composed of simple epithelium. The thin part of the loop of Henle is permeable to water, but the thick ascending part is not.[4] The thick ascending segment contains powerful membrane pumps that cotransport ions (Na^+, K^+, $2Cl^-$) from the filtrate and deposit them in the interstitial fluid surrounding the loops of Henle and collecting ducts (Figure 26-12). About 15% of nephrons have extra long loops of Henle that dip down into the medulla (juxtamedullary nephrons). These nephrons are vital for creating concentrated urine.

The loop formation of the loop of Henle creates a countercurrent mechanism, which allows the ascending loop of Henle to create a high interstitial gradient in the medulla of the kidney (Figure 26-13). Because the ascending loop is

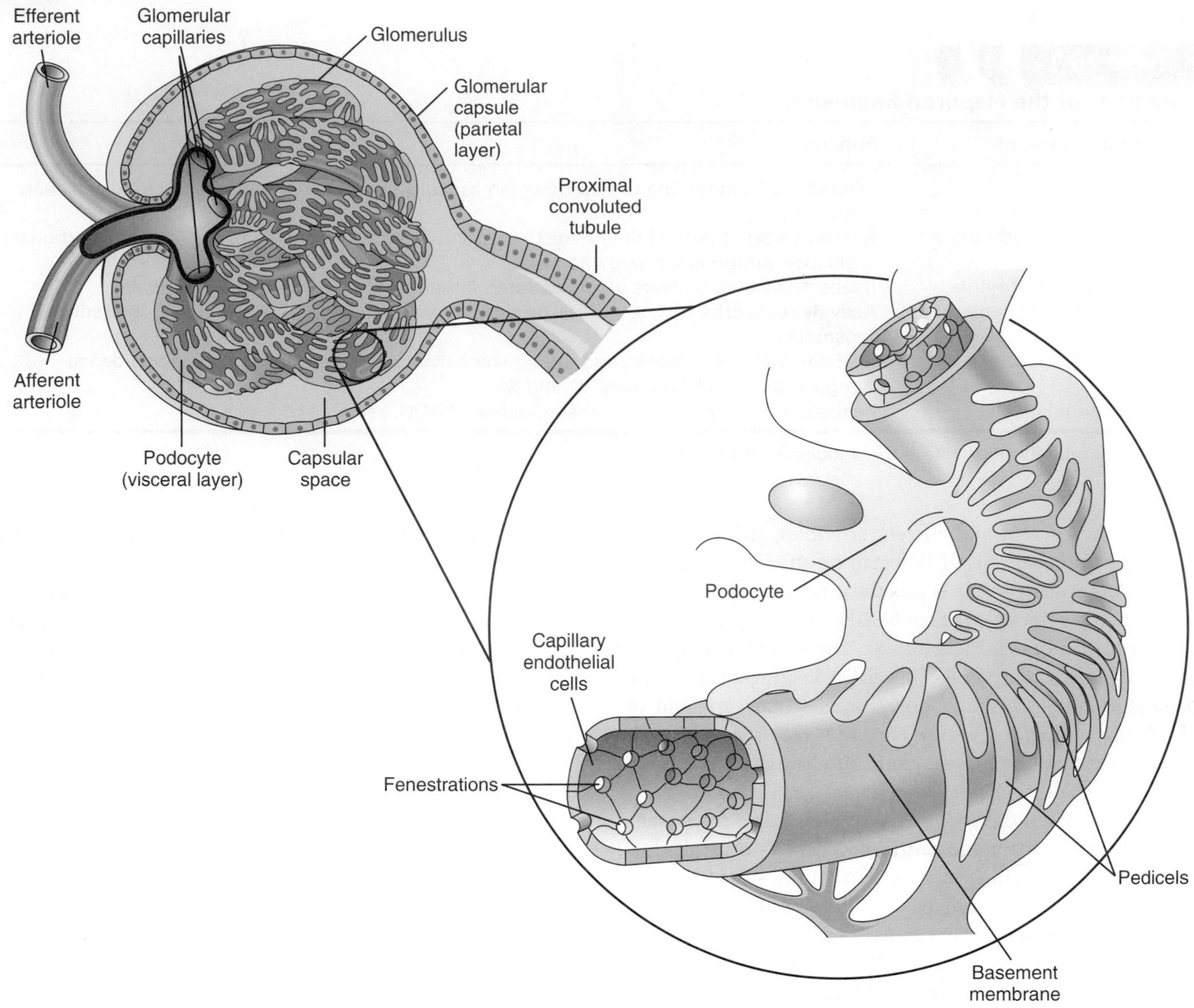

Efferent arteriole
Glomerular capillaries
Glomerulus
Glomerular capsule (parietal layer)
Proximal convoluted tubule
Afferent arteriole
Podocyte (visceral layer)
Capsular space
Podocyte
Capillary endothelial cells
Fenestrations
Pedicels
Basement membrane

FIGURE 26-8 ■ The structure of the glomerulus, including the afferent and efferent arterioles, capillary tuft, and surrounding epithelial membrane of Bowman capsule, is shown. The enlargement shows the glomerular membrane to be composed of the endothelial cells of the capillary, the podocytes of Bowman capsule, and the basement membrane between them.

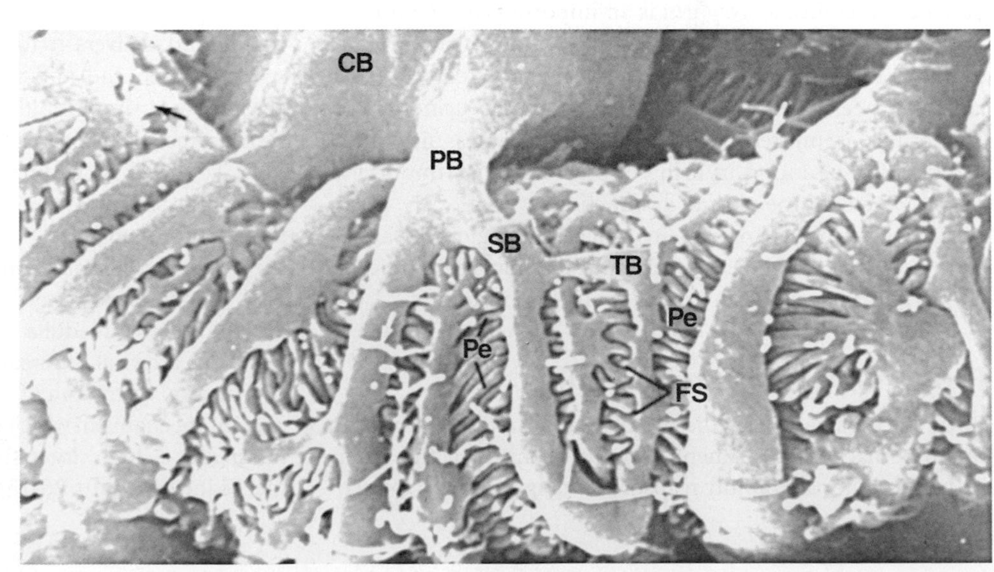

FIGURE 26-9 ■ An electron micrograph showing a close-up view of podocyte foot processes of the glomerular capillary. Note the spaces between the podocyte foot processes that contribute to a highly permeable glomerular membrane. *CB,* Podocyte cell body; *PB,* primary branch; *SB,* secondary branch; *TB,* tertiary branch; *Pe,* pedicles; *FS,* filtration slits. (From Kessel RG, Kardon RH: *Tissues and organs: a text-atlas of scanning electron microscopy,* San Francisco, 1979, WH Freeman.)

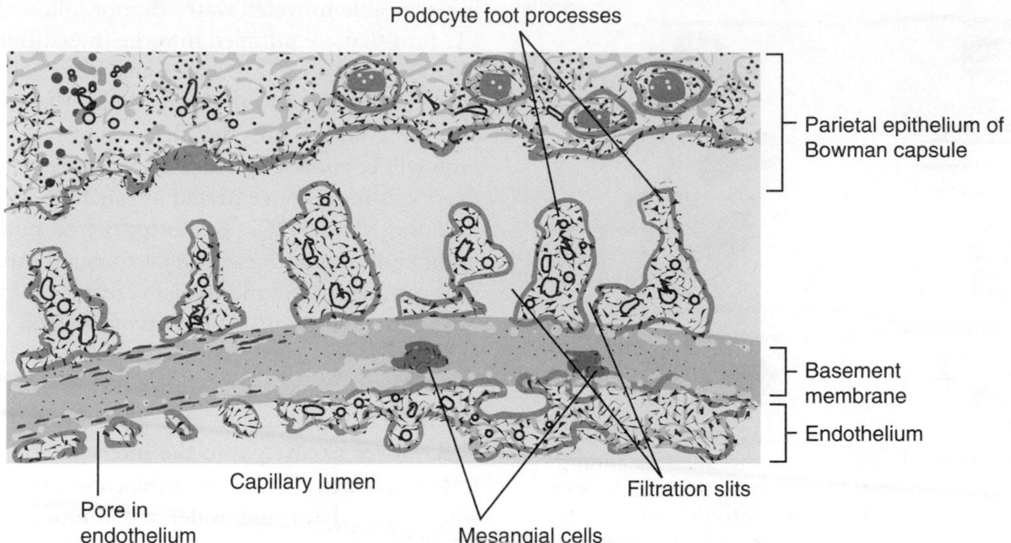

FIGURE 26-10 ■ A section of the glomerular membrane showing the large spaces between the endothelial cells and podocyte foot processes. Filtration occurs through these fenestra and slit pores. The basement membrane provides the principal selectivity barrier of the glomerulus.

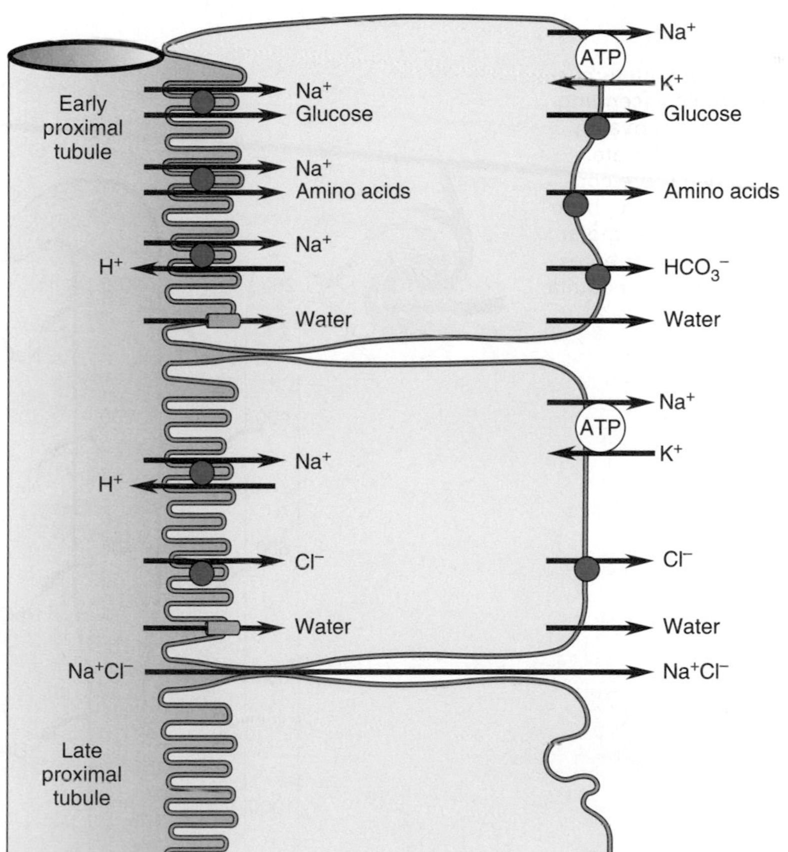

FIGURE 26-11 ■ The proximal convoluted tubule has numerous membrane transporters that function to reabsorb filtered glucose, amino acids, water, and electrolytes. The early proximal tubule reabsorbs nearly all of the filtered bicarbonate ion, whereas the late proximal tubule reabsorbs chloride ion.

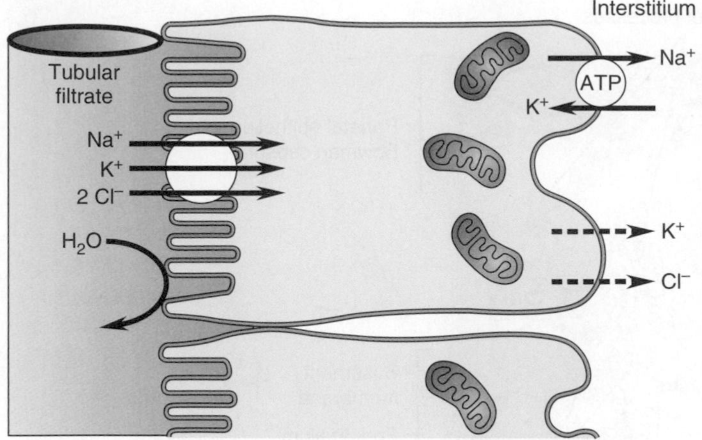

FIGURE 26-12 ■ The epithelial cells of the thick ascending loop of Henle possess powerful ion pumps that cotransport Na^+, K^+, and $2Cl^-$ ions from the filtrate into the cell. The Na^+ is then pumped out of the basolateral membrane and into the interstitium. The loop of Henle ion cotransporter is responsible for creating a highly concentrated medullary interstitium.

impermeable to water, water cannot follow the Na^+, K^+, and Cl^- ions that are pumped into the interstitium. The descending loop is permeable to water, and water will be drawn out by the extra ions that were pumped into the interstitium by the ascending limb. Thus, the filtrate that reaches the ascending limb will be more concentrated than the original filtrate. Delivery of a more concentrated filtrate to the ascending limb allows the Na^+-K^+-$2Cl^-$ cotransporter to pump out a greater number of ions and reach an even higher interstitial gradient. This countercurrent mechanism creates a maximal osmolarity of about 600 mOsm/L at the tip of the loop of Henle as compared with the usual extracellular osmolarity of 280 to 300 mOsm/L at the cortex. Another 600 mOsm/L is contributed by the accumulation of urea particles in the interstitium.[8] Urea moves passively into the interstitium down its concentration gradient. Urea becomes concentrated in the tubule when electrolytes and water are removed in the proximal tubule and loop of Henle. An overall interstitial osmolarity is generated that begins in the cortex at about 300 mOsm/L and increases progressively to about 1200 mOsm/L at a point deep in the medulla. This high interstitial osmolarity provides a gradient for water reabsorption from the collecting ducts as they pass through the medulla on their way to the renal pelvis.

FIGURE 26-13 ■ The mechanism of countercurrent multiplication. Ion pumps in the ascending loop of Henle create a gradient for removal of water from the descending loop. The filtrate reaching the ascending loop is then more concentrated, allowing the ascending loop to pump even more ions to further increase the osmolarity of the interstitial fluid. Urea also contributes to the interstitial gradient formed in the medulla.

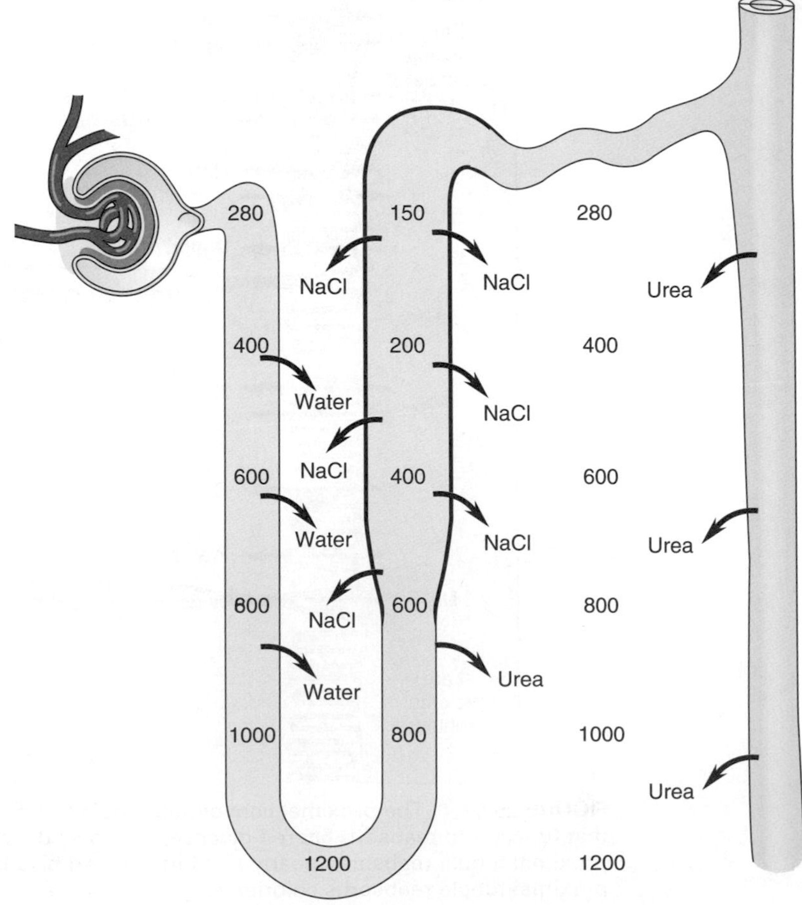

The maximal interstitial gradient attained is dependent on the length of the loops of Henle. In some animals, such as desert rats and camels, very long loops of Henle create a much higher interstitial osmolarity, which allows formation of extremely concentrated urine.

Distal Convoluted Tubule

The filtrate that reaches the distal tubule is normally hypoosmotic (150 mOsm/L) in comparison with plasma (280 mOsm/L) because electrolytes have been removed by the pumps in the ascending loop of Henle.[8] At this point in the nephron, only 10% of the original glomerular filtrate remains, and further reabsorption in the distal tubule is largely under hormonal control. Aldosterone and angiotensin II (AII) stimulate the tubule cells to reabsorb sodium and water, whereas atrial natriuretic peptide (ANP) and urodilatin inhibit reabsorption.

Collecting Duct

The distal tubules of several nephrons empty into a single collecting tubule, which then merges into progressively larger and fewer collecting ducts that run parallel to the loops of Henle. Eventually the collecting ducts form the medullary pyramids, which empty into the minor calices through the papilla. The collecting ducts travel through the high interstitial gradient of the medulla on their way to the renal pelvis. The collecting ducts have two cell types called principle cells (P cells) and intercalated cells (I cells). The majority of cells are the P type that respond to antidiuretic hormone. In the presence of antidiuretic hormone (ADH), more than 99% of the original filtrate is reabsorbed by the time it reaches the renal pelvis, creating 30 to 60 ml of concentrated urine per hour. The I cells participate in acid-base balance by regulating the secretion of acid.

KEY CONCEPTS

- The nephron is the structural and functional unit of the kidney that performs all filtration, secretion, and reabsorption functions.
- Filtration occurs at the glomerulus, a structure formed by the glomerular capillary tuft, the podocytes of Bowman capsule, and the basement membrane.
- The principal selectivity barrier for glomerular filtration is the basement membrane, which prevents the passage of cells and large proteins. The filtrate in Bowman capsule is otherwise very similar in composition to plasma.
- The proximal tubule reabsorbs about two thirds of the filtered water and electrolytes and all of the glucose, amino acids, proteins, and vitamins.
- The loop of Henle contains powerful Na^+-K^+-$2Cl^-$ cotransporters, which pump ions into the interstitium to create a high interstitial osmolarity in the renal medulla. The loop formation of the loop of Henle is essential for the countercurrent mechanism, which creates the high interstitial osmolarity.
- The distal and collecting tubules "fine-tune" sodium and water reabsorption under the influence of endocrine hormones, including aldosterone, AII, ANP, ADH, and urodilatin to create dilute or concentrated urine as needed to maintain fluid balance.

REGULATION OF GLOMERULAR FILTRATION

The GFR is determined by the filtration pressure in the glomeruli and by the permeable surface area of the glomerular membrane (K_f). Filtration pressure varies considerably from the afferent end of the glomerulus to the efferent end and is difficult to measure directly. The average net filtration pressure for the capillary as a whole is about 10 mm Hg and the permeability constant K_f is about 12.5 ml/min per mm Hg. GFR is the product of filtration pressure and K_f (10 mm Hg × 12.5 ml/min per mm Hg = 125 ml/min).[5] The GFR is determined by the physical principles of filtration across a capillary membrane (Figure 26-14).

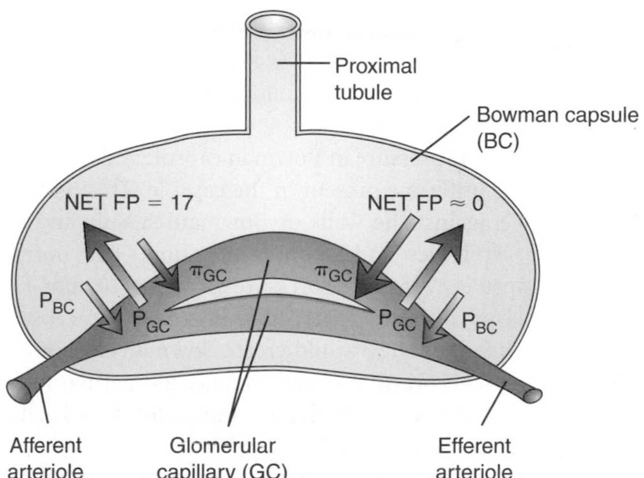

FIGURE 26-14 ■ Net filtration is higher at the afferent end of the glomerular capillary because the hydrostatic blood pressure in the capillary exceeds the pressure in Bowman capsule and the oncotic pressure in the capillary. Toward the efferent end of the capillary, the filtration pressure is low because the oncotic pressure of the blood is high and offsets the hydrostatic blood pressure. Capillary oncotic pressure gets progressively higher along the capillary because fluid is filtering out of the blood into Bowman capsule and leaving the proteins behind so they become more concentrated and exert a greater oncotic pressure. *FP,* Filtration pressure; *π,* oncotic pressure; *P,* hydrostatic pressure.

Physics of Filtration

Filtration rate is affected by factors that alter hydrostatic and oncotic pressure on either side of the glomerular membrane as shown by the following filtration equation:

$$GFR = K_f\,[(P_{gc} + \pi_{bc}) - (P_{bc} + \pi_{gc})]$$

where P_{gc} is glomerular capillary hydrostatic pressure (mm Hg); π_{bc} is oncotic pressure in Bowman capsule (mm Hg); P_{bc} is Bowman capsule hydrostatic pressure (mm Hg); and π_{gc} is oncotic pressure in the glomerular capillary (mm Hg). The following is an illustrative example resulting in a normal GFR of 125 m/min:

$$GFR = 12.5\,[(50 + 0) - (10 + 30)]$$
$$GFR = 125\text{ ml/min}$$

The main driving force for filtration is hydrostatic pressure in the glomerular capillaries. The glomerular capillary hydrostatic pressure exerts a force against the glomerular capillary walls. As blood circulates through the capillaries the hydrostatic pressure pushes blood against the walls, and fluid is filtered out. The hydrostatic pressure remains fairly constant along the length of the capillary and exerts an average force of approximately 50 mm Hg.

The glomerular capillary oncotic (colloid osmotic) pressure exists because proteins are present in the blood. Plasma proteins are negatively charged and attract positive ions, which subsequently attract water. Because ions and water are attracted to the proteins and are not pushed against the capillary wall, the glomerular capillary colloidal osmotic pressure opposes filtration by holding water and ions in the capillaries. The glomerular oncotic pressure is lower at the afferent end and becomes progressively higher along the length of the capillary (see Figure 26-14).

The hydrostatic pressure in Bowman capsule is determined by the volume of filtrate present in the capsule. This pressure exerts a force against the walls of Bowman capsule and the glomerular capillaries and opposes filtration. The normal Bowman capsule hydrostatic pressure is about 10 mm Hg. Normally plasma proteins do not filter into Bowman capsule. If they did filter, then they would create Bowman capsule oncotic pressure. This pressure would enhance glomerular filtration because proteins attract cations and water. In a healthy kidney, this pressure is negligible.

In summary, the net filtration pressure across the glomerular membrane is approximately 10 mm Hg. The filtration pressure is higher at the afferent arteriole side of the capillary and diminishes as the blood reaches the efferent end. This occurs because the capillary oncotic pressure is lower at the afferent end. As blood passes through the capillaries, continued filtration leaves a greater concentration of proteins in the capillaries, which raises the oncotic pressure. As blood reaches the efferent arterioles, filtration may cease.

Factors Affecting Filtration Pressure

One of the most important physiologic regulators of GFR is blood volume.[5] When blood volume increases because of fluid intake, the blood pressure rises slightly and causes glomerular hydrostatic pressure to increase. GFR increases, and the extra fluid is pushed into the filtrate to be excreted from the body. The opposite also occurs: when blood volume is decreased, capillary hydrostatic pressure falls, resulting in a lower GFR, and fluid is conserved. The glomerular capillary is protected from large swings in blood pressure by autoregulation. Autoregulation adjusts the arteriolar resistance to maintain a relatively steady rate of blood flow despite changes in perfusion pressure. Autoregulation is effective when mean arterial blood pressure varies between 75 and 160 mm Hg.[5] Autoregulation of renal blood flow is achieved in part by a stretch response in the vascular smooth muscle of the afferent arterioles. When blood pressure increases, the vascular smooth muscle cells reflexively constrict to keep blood flow at about the same rate. This mechanism is called *myogenic autoregulation.*

Other factors can affect GFR by altering the pressure within Bowman capsule or affecting plasma oncotic pressure. Obstruction in the tubules or collecting ducts can significantly elevate the pressure in Bowman capsule. According to the filtration equation, GFR would fall because filtration pressure would be reduced. Because plasma oncotic pressure is determined primarily by the concentration of plasma proteins, a low serum albumin would increase GFR.

Although K_f is called a constant, it is subject to change for physiologic and pathologic reasons. Specialized mesangial cells located in the glomerulus are thought to be important regulators of K_f. These cells contract and relax in response to various stimuli and alter the surface area for filtration.[9] Contraction squeezes the capillary cells together and reduces GFR, whereas relaxation allows the permeable surface area to expand. Disease processes that damage the glomerular membrane also can affect permeability. Sclerotic processes reduce K_f, whereas some inflammatory injuries may increase it.

Tubuloglomerular Feedback

Each nephron is able to regulate its own individual GFR through a process termed *tubuloglomerular feedback.* A specialized group of cells form the regulatory structure, called the **juxtaglomerular apparatus.**[10] The juxtaglomerular apparatus is composed of the glomerulus, the macula densa, and specialized juxtaglomerular cells, which are located around the glomerular arterioles (Figure 26-15). The macula densa cells are located in the distal convoluted tubule, which loops up to come in contact with the glomerulus and juxtaglomerular cells.

Macula densa cells sense changes in the volume delivered to the distal tubule. When glomerular filtration is too high an excessive volume is delivered to the distal tubule. The mecha-

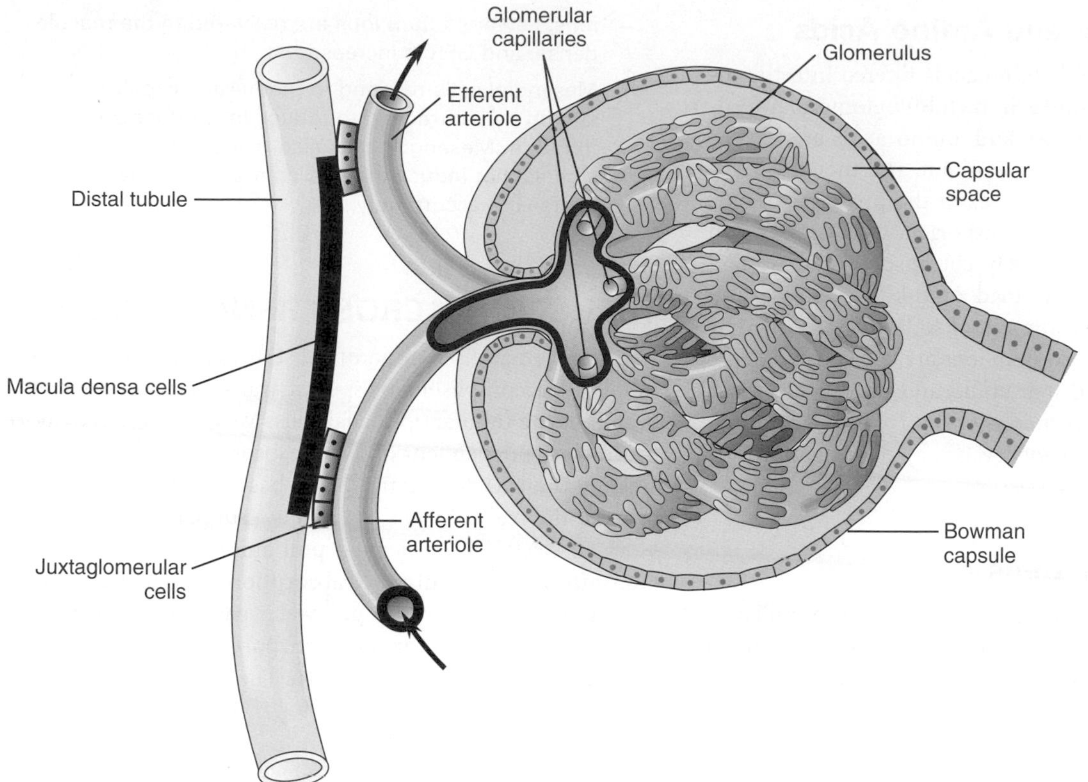

FIGURE 26-15 ■ The juxtaglomerular apparatus is composed of the macula densa cells of the distal tubule, the afferent and efferent arterioles, and the renin-secreting juxtaglomerular cells. Macula densa cells sample the distal filtrate for NaCl content and send signals to the glomerulus to adjust glomerular filtration rate.

nism whereby macula densa cells sense volume delivery is not completely understood. Some researchers suggest that it is the NaCl delivery to the macula densa cells that is sensed. A high distal tubule NaCl level means that transport processes in the previous nephron segments have been overwhelmed because GFR is too high; the macula densa sends signals to the glomerulus to reduce GFR. Conversely, a low NaCl level at the macula densa indicates that the nephron transporters are being underutilized, and GFR can be increased. Tubuloglomerular feedback helps to distribute GFR evenly among the kidneys' 2 million nephrons.

The mechanisms whereby macula densa cells are able to alter GFR are only partially understood. Glomerular filtration can be regulated by altering filtration pressure or by altering the filtration constant, K_f. The macula densa could alter GFR by regulating the resistance of the afferent and efferent arterioles and by stimulating mesangial cells to contract or relax.

Afferent dilation and efferent constriction would increase the hydrostatic pressure within the glomerulus and increase GFR. Conversely, afferent constriction and efferent dilation would reduce filtration pressure and decrease GFR. The juxtaglomerular cells that surround the afferent arteriole are thought to be mediators of this process. The juxtaglomerular cells produce and release **renin,** an enzyme that converts angiotensinogen to angiotensin I (AI). Angiotensin I is then converted to AII by endothelial cells in the glomerular capillary, which possesses angiotensin-converting enzyme (ACE) activity. AII is a potent vasoconstrictor that constricts the efferent arteriole, thus increasing GFR.[11] The signals that pass from the macula densa to the juxtaglomerular cells to regulate tubuloglomerular feedback are not completely known; however, roles for adenosine and nitric oxide have been demonstrated.[11]

Other chemical mediators are thought to be released in response to macula densa signals, including vasoactive prostaglandins. Some prostaglandins have vasodilating activities, whereas others are vasoconstrictors. The importance of prostaglandins and AII in regulating GFR is supported by the observation that drugs that inhibit their activity interfere with tubuloglomerular feedback. For example, ACE inhibitors block AII production and interfere with constriction of the efferent arteriole. This can be particularly detrimental to renal function in patients who require high filtration pressures, such as those with polycystic kidney disease or collecting system obstructions. Drugs that inhibit cyclooxygenase, such as aspirin and nonsteroidal antiinflammatory drugs, interfere with prostaglandin production and may precipitate excessive renovascular constriction in some patients.[12]

Effects of Glucose and Amino Acids

The amount of glucose and amino acids filtered into the tubular fluid can alter GFR through the tubuloglomerular feedback mechanism. Both glucose and amino acids are filtered freely through the glomerular membrane and then are reabsorbed by active transport processes in the proximal tubule. Reabsorption occurs through transporters that use sodium ion entry into the cell to actively cotransport glucose and amino acids. The greater the load of tubular glucose and amino acids, the greater the amount of sodium reabsorbed by the proximal tubule. Fewer sodium ions are transported to the macula densa cells in the distal tubule, and the macula densa perceives this as a need to increase GFR.[5] Chronically high serum glucose and amino acids levels may disrupt appropriate regulation of GFR.

Role of Mesangial Cells

Mesangial cells are located around the glomerular capillaries and are thought to participate in immune functions and to regulate the surface area available for glomerular filtration.[9] Contraction of the mesangial cells reduces surface area and relaxation increases it. Mesangial cells are responsive to glomerular stretch and are stimulated to contract when more blood enters the glomerulus. This response provides a negative feedback that decreases surface area when filtration pressure is increased. In addition, mesangial cells respond to a number of chemical mediators, including AII and endothelin (peptides that favor mesangial contraction) and ANP and nitric oxide (substances that favor relaxation). Mesangial cells thus may regulate GFR by altering the filtration constant K_f.

KEY CONCEPTS

- GFR is determined by the permeable surface area (K_f) and by capillary hydrostatic pressure and Bowman capsule oncotic pressure, which favor filtration, and by plasma oncotic pressure and Bowman capsule hydrostatic pressure, which oppose filtration. Normal GFR is about 125 ml/min.
- The filtration rate in an individual nephron is regulated by tubuloglomerular feedback in which macula densa cells sample the NaCl content (or other constituents) in the distal tubule and signal the juxtaglomerular apparatus to make appropriate adjustments in GFR.
- Afferent constriction and efferent dilation decrease GFR, whereas afferent dilation and efferent constriction increase GFR. AII and prostaglandins are important chemical mediators of arteriolar resistance.
- Excessive filtration of glucose and amino acids can result in increased GFR because their reabsorption in the proximal tubule requires cotransport of sodium ions. Fewer sodium ions are delivered to the macula densa, and GFR is increased.
- Mesangial cells respond to glomerular capillary stretch by contracting to reduce the surface area for filtration. Mesangial cells also respond to chemical signals that induce them to contract and relax, which alters GFR accordingly.

TRANSPORT ACROSS RENAL TUBULES

Reabsorption and secretion of substances across the nephron tubule are accomplished by specific transporters in the membranes of the tubular epithelial cells. Most of these transport processes are dependent on Na^+ reabsorption and made possible by the Na^+-K^+ pump in the basolateral membrane. In general, the reabsorption of cations, especially sodium, provides an electrical gradient to pull anions across the tubule and into the interstitium. Reabsorption of ions and solutes creates an osmotic force to pull water passively across the renal epithelium. A summary of transport in the various tubule segments is shown in Figure 26-16. The details of glucose, bi-

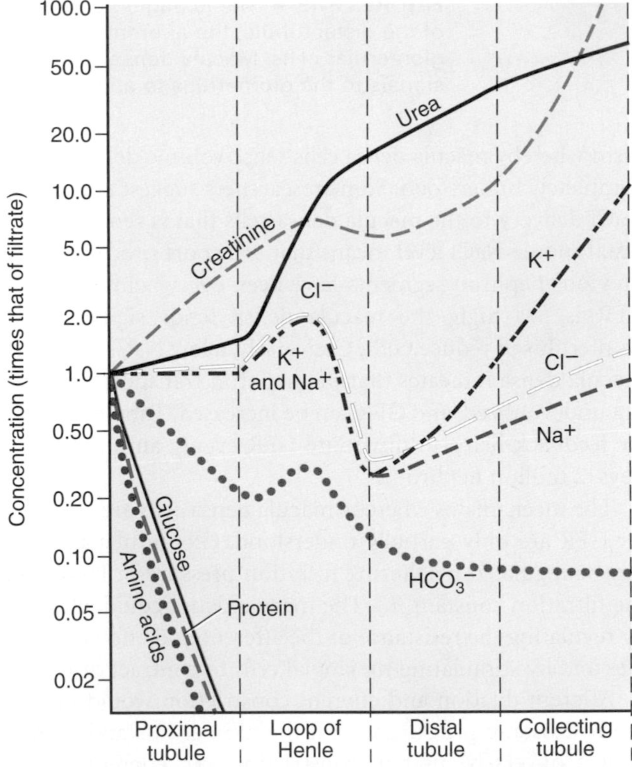

FIGURE 26-16 ■ Summary of nutrient and electrolyte composition of the filtrate in each segment of the nephron. Two thirds of the filtrate is reabsorbed in the proximal tubule. (Adapted from Guyton AC, Hall JE, editors: *Textbook of medical physiology,* ed 10, Philadelphia, 2000, Saunders, p 305.)

carbonate, H^+, and K^+ transport are described as important representative examples.

Reabsorption of Glucose

Glucose is filtered freely across the glomerular membrane such that the tubular load (in milligrams per minute) is determined by the product of serum glucose (in milligrams per milliliter) and GFR (in milliliters per minute). Normally, all of the filtered glucose is reabsorbed in the proximal tubule by a sodium-dependent cotransporter called SGLT 2 (Figure 26-17). The transport proteins have a maximal rate of transport that can be exceeded if the tubular load of glucose is too great. The transport maximum for normal kidneys is about 375 mg/min in men and 300 mg/min in women.[4] A tubular load of glucose in excess of this amount results in glycosuria. In fact, some spillage of glucose begins at a much lower tubular load because of uneven distribution of GFR to individual nephrons. Some nephrons with higher GFR may exceed their transport maximums while other nephrons are working below capacity. The point at which glucose begins to spill into the urine is called the *renal threshold.* In normal kidneys with a GFR of 125 ml/min, the renal threshold will be reached when serum glucose approaches 180 mg/dl, but significant glycosuria will not occur until the transport maximum is reached at a serum glucose level of about 300 mg/dl. Persons with low GFR associated with renal disease may not experience spillage of glucose until the serum glucose level is much higher, and glycosuria is not a reliable indicator of serum glucose level in these individuals. For example, a patient with a GFR of 50 ml/min and a serum glucose of 300 mg/dl will have a tubular glucose load of only 150 mg/min, which is well below the normal renal threshold. No glycosuria would occur despite the high serum glucose level.

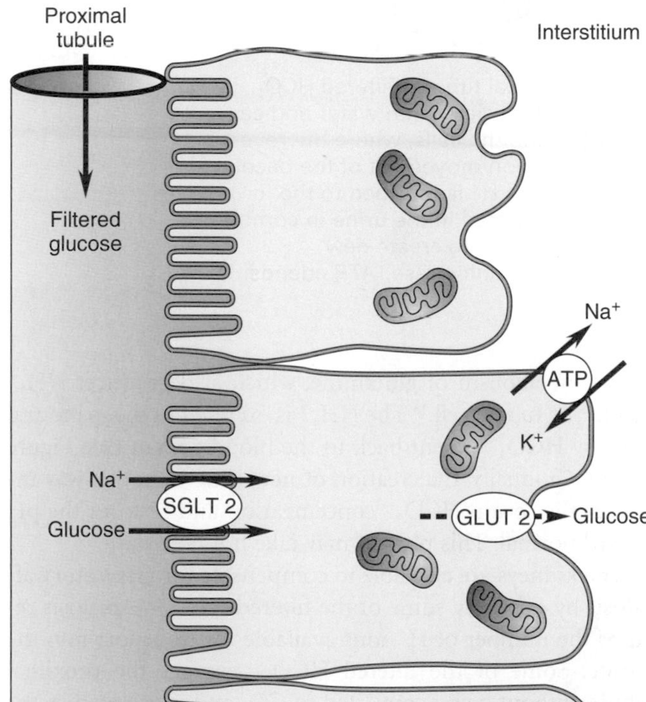

FIGURE 26-17 ■ The glucose transporter in the proximal tubule *(SGLT 2)* is dependent on sodium reabsorption from the filtrate. The Na^+-K^+ pump in the basolateral membrane keeps the intracellular sodium level low and maintains a gradient for sodium and glucose reabsorption. Glucose diffuses out of the tubule cell and back into the interstitial fluid through passive carrier proteins *(GLUT 2)*. *ATP,* Adenosine triphosphate.

Regulation of Acid-Base Balance

The kidney tubules have an important role in maintaining the pH of the blood. In addition to excreting excess H^+, the kidneys also regulate the concentration of bicarbonate (HCO_3^-) in the blood. The pH of the blood normally ranges between 7.35 and 7.45 and is determined by the ratio of acid (H_2CO_3) to base (HCO_3^-). The lungs and kidneys work together to maintain this balance. Metabolic processes create an excess of acid, which is excreted by the lungs in the form of CO_2 and by the kidneys in the form of H^+. In addition, HCO_3^- is filtered freely through the glomerulus and must be efficiently reabsorbed to maintain acid-base balance. Most HCO_3^- is reabsorbed in the proximal tubule; however, the distal segment also participates in regulating HCO_3^- and H^+ transport.

Reabsorption of HCO_3^- is complex because it is not directly transported across the apical membrane; rather, it is combined with H^+ in the tubule to form H_2CO_3, which dissociates into CO_2 and water (Figure 26-18). The H^+ for this reaction is secreted into the filtrate in exchange for Na^+. Carbonic anhydrase present in the brush border of the proximal tubule cell catalyzes the reaction. Carbon dioxide is lipid soluble and diffuses passively into the tubular cell. Once inside, intracellular carbonic anhydrase catalyzes the reverse reaction to once again form HCO_3^- and H^+. The HCO_3^- is transported out through the basolateral membrane, whereas the H^+ is recycled to the tubular fluid to bind with another HCO_3^-. The energy to power this reabsorptive process is provided by the Na^+-K^+ pump, which keeps intracellular Na^+ low so that the sodium gradient can continue to move H^+ into the tubule lumen through the Na^+-H^+ exchanger.

Normally, all of the filtered HCO_3^- is reabsorbed by this mechanism to help maintain acid-base balance.[13] Excess H^+ ions that find no HCO_3^- in the filtrate with which to bind are excreted in the urine, and urine is normally acidic. The number of H^+ ions that can be excreted in urine is limited to a pH of about 4.0. However, urine buffers, including HPO_4^{2-} and NH_3, are secreted into the filtrate and bind with excess H^+, greatly increasing the ability of the kidney to excrete an acid load (see Figure 26-18). Ammonia (NH_3) is produced by the renal epithelium via metabolism of the amino acid glutamine. Ammonia binds to H^+ to form ammonium ion (NH_4^+), whereas HPO_4^{2-} binds to H^+ to form $H_2PO_4^-$.

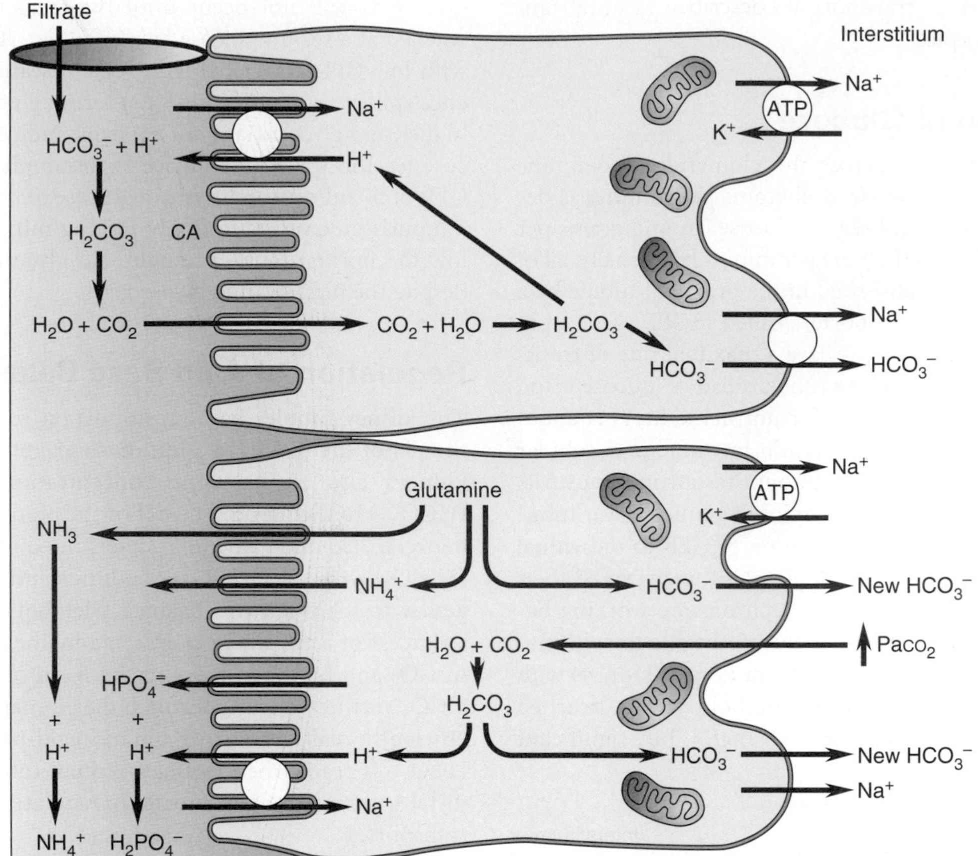

FIGURE 26-18 ■ Bicarbonate ion reabsorption across the renal tubule. Filtered HCO_3^- is combined with secreted H^+ to form carbonic acid, which dissociates into water and carbon dioxide. Carbon dioxide is lipid soluble and diffuses into the cells, where the reverse reaction converts it back to HCO_3^- and H^+. The bicarbonate ion moves out of the basolateral membrane and returns to the blood stream, whereas the H^+ is returned to the lumen to bind with another HCO_3^- ion. Excess H^+ ions are excreted in the urine in combination with phosphate and ammonia buffers. The kidney is able to create new bicarbonate as needed to maintain pH balance. *CA,* Carbonic anhydrase; *ATP,* adenosine triphosphate.

Renal Compensation Process

In some cases, the kidneys are called on to compensate for an abnormality in lung function. The lungs normally regulate the amount of carbon dioxide in the blood ($Paco_2$). When $Paco_2$ is high, more carbonic acid is formed, and the blood pH becomes acidic. The kidneys compensate by excreting more H^+ and by creating new HCO_3^- to enhance the buffering capacity of the blood. These HCO_3^- ions are additional to those already being reabsorbed from the filtrate and are, thus, new.

New HCO_3^- is created within the renal tubule cell by two processes. First, excess circulating CO_2 from respiratory acidosis diffuses into the renal cell and is converted to HCO_3^- and H^+ by the enzyme carbonic anhydrase. The new HCO_3^- is sent back to the blood stream, and the new H^+ is secreted into the urine filtrate, where it binds with a renal buffer and is excreted. The second process involves the production of ammonium ions within the tubule cell. New HCO_3^- can be formed by the metabolism of glutamine, which also produces NH_4^+ within the tubule cell.[13] The NH_4^+ is excreted in the urine and the new HCO_3^- is sent back to the blood stream (see Figure 26-18). Gradually, the creation of new HCO_3^- in this way increases the serum HCO_3^- concentration and restores the pH toward normal. This process may take hours to days.

The kidneys are also able to compensate for respiratory alkalosis by excreting some of the filtered HCO_3^-. Alkalosis reduces the number of H^+ ions available for transport into the filtrate. Some of the filtered HCO_3^- escapes the proximal tubule without being converted to CO_2 and is excreted in the urine.

Secretion of Potassium

There is normally a net excess of potassium from dietary sources that must be excreted by the kidneys. The primary transporter responsible for this process is the Na^+-K^+ pump

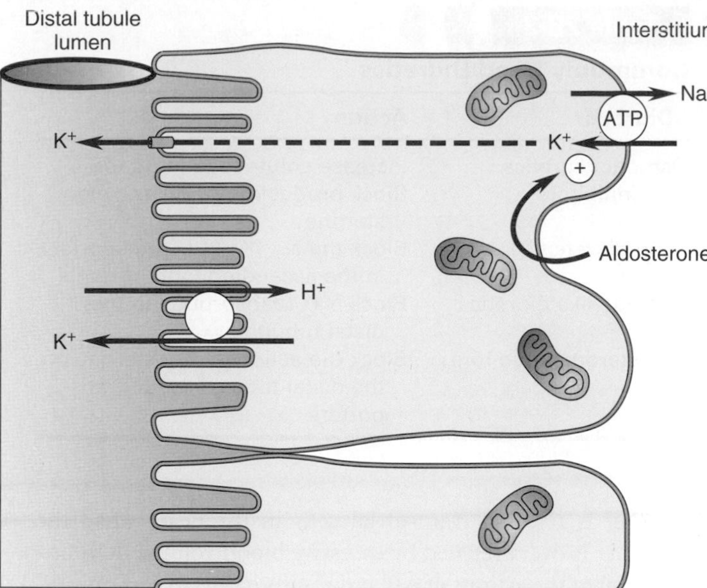

FIGURE 26-19 ■ Tubular secretion of potassium ion. Increased serum potassium and aldosterone increase the activity of the Na^+-K^+ pump and enhance K^+ secretion into the filtrate. The H^+-K^+ exchanger also regulates the secretion of K^+ ions.

in the basolateral cell membrane. The Na^+-K^+ pump moves K^+ into the tubular cell and increases the gradient for diffusion of K^+ through the apical membrane and into the filtrate (Figure 26-19). Principle cells in the distal tubule and collecting duct are the site of potassium excretion. The activity of Na^+-K^+ pumps in these segments is sensitive to aldosterone, a steroid hormone secreted by the adrenal cortex. Aldosterone increases reabsorption of Na^+ and water and excretion of K^+. Potassium excretion also is affected by the activity of the K^+-H^+ exchanger.

KEY CONCEPTS

- Reabsorption of glucose is accomplished by proximal tubule cell sodium-dependent transporters. These transporters have transport maximums that can be overwhelmed by excessive tubular loads of glucose, in which case glycosuria results.
- The kidneys participate in acid-base regulation through secretion of excess H^+ and by reabsorption and creation of HCO_3^-. Urine buffers HPO_4^{2-} and NH_3 bind excess H^+ and increase the ability of the kidney to excrete an acid load.
- HCO_3^- is not directly reabsorbed across the renal epithelium; it is first converted to CO_2 by the enzyme carbonic anhydrase. The H^+ ions needed for this reaction are provided by Na^+-H^+ pumps on the apical cell membrane.
- Secretion of potassium ions is promoted by activity of the Na^+-K^+ pump on the basolateral cell membrane. In the distal tubule, these pumps are regulated by aldosterone, which increases potassium excretion.

REGULATION OF BLOOD VOLUME AND OSMOLALITY

The kidneys play a vital role in maintaining normal blood volume and osmolality. As previously discussed, changes in blood volume alter the pressure in the glomerulus and affect GFR. An increase in blood volume results in a pressure diuresis, whereas a fall in blood volume reduces urine output. The kidney tubules are responsive to a number of hormonal signals that fine-tune tubular reabsorption. These hormones include ADH, aldosterone, AII, ANP, and urodilatin. Antidiuretic hormone is the principal regulator of osmolality, and aldosterone, AII, ANP, and urodilatin regulate extracellular volume.

Antidiuretic Hormone

ADH (also called vasopressin) is secreted from the posterior pituitary when osmoreceptors located in the hypothalamus detect a high osmolality of the extracellular fluid. Principle cells in the collecting tubules respond to ADH by translocating water pores called *aquaporin 2* to the apical membrane (Figure 26-20). These pores make the tubule permeable to water and allow water to be reabsorbed from the urinary filtrate. The high interstitial gradient of the medulla provides the osmotic force for water reabsorption. Recall that this gradient was formed by the action of powerful ion pumps in the thick ascending limb of the loop of Henle.

As water is reabsorbed into the medullary interstitium, it creates a high tissue pressure that pushes fluid into the vasa recta. The vasa recta return the reabsorbed water to the general circulation. The reabsorbed water dilutes the blood and reduces osmolality. Osmoreceptors in the brain detect the reduced osmolality and inhibit further production of ADH. When blood osmolality is too low, ADH secretion is completely inhibited, and the collecting tubules become impermeable to water. Water is not reabsorbed from the filtrate, and a large quantity of dilute urine is produced. Loss of water in excess of solute returns the blood osmolality toward normal.

An insufficiency of ADH secondary to pituitary damage results in the condition of *diabetes insipidus* in which large volumes of dilute urine are excreted leading to severe fluid imbalances. A similar problem occurs when the collecting tubules are unresponsive to ADH. This condition is called *nephrogenic* diabetes insipidus and usually results from genetic defects in either the ADH receptor (V_2) or the aquaporin 2 genes.[4]

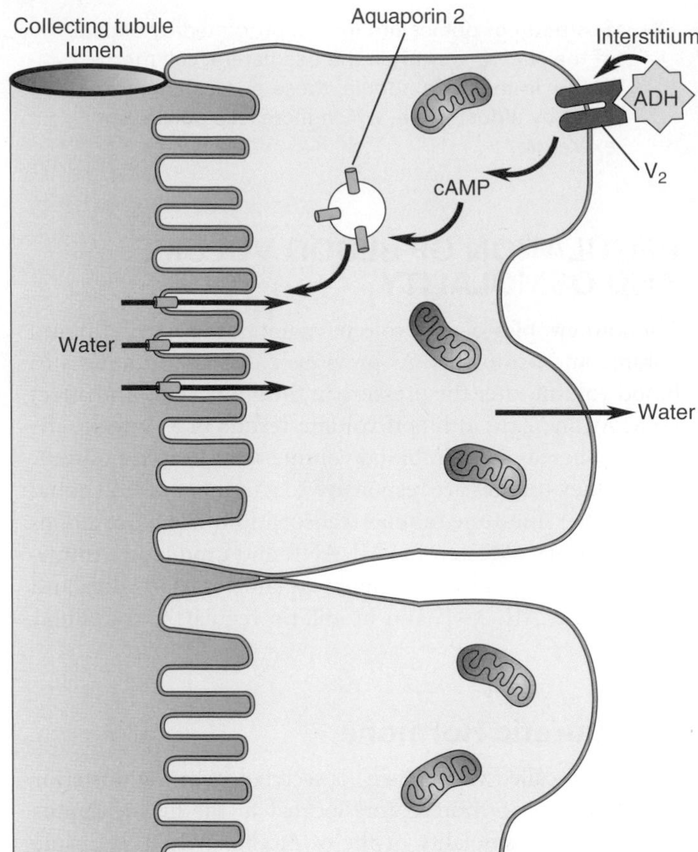

FIGURE 26-20 ■ Antidiuretic hormone *(ADH)* action on the collecting tubule epithelium. ADH binds to receptors on the basolateral cell membrane, resulting in translocation of water pores (aquaporin 2) to the apical surface. Increased water permeability results in reabsorption of water from the filtrate and into the interstitium. *cAMP,* Cyclic adenosine monophosphate; *V_2,* vasopressin-2 receptor.

Aldosterone, Angiotensin II, Atrial Natriuretic Peptide, and Urodilatin

Aldosterone, AII, ANP, and urodilatin alter blood volume without affecting its concentration. Aldosterone and AII increase reabsorption of Na^+, which provides a gradient for water reabsorption. Because salt and water are reabsorbed together, the osmolality of the reabsorbed fluid is isosmotic with plasma.

AII and aldosterone are produced when the juxtaglomerular cells in the kidney are stimulated to release renin. Renin is released in response to (1) decreased blood flow to the kidney, (2) reduced serum sodium levels, and (3) activation of sympathetic nerves to the juxtaglomerular cells.[4] Renin begins a cascade of reactions that result in the production of AII and aldosterone. When AII and aldosterone restore blood volume and blood pressure to normal, the stimuli for renin release are removed and the concentrations of AII and aldosterone fall.

Table 26-2
Commonly Used Diuretics

Diuretic	Action
Osmotic diuretics	Increase solute load in tubule
ACE inhibitors	Block production of AII and aldosterone
Loop diuretics	Block the $Na^+/K^+/2Cl^-$ transporter in the ascending loop of Henle
Thiazide-like diuretics	Block Na^+ reabsorption in the distal tubule
Aldosterone inhibitors	Block the action of aldosterone on the distal tubule Na^+/K^+ transporters

ANP is released from atrial cells in the heart when the chamber is overstretched by excessive blood volume. ANP inhibits all of the actions of AII and results in loss of sodium and water in the urine. Thus, ANP reduces extracellular volume, but the fluid losses are isosmotic with plasma, and blood osmolality remains unchanged. Urodilatin is a peptide that is secreted by distal and collecting tubule cells in response to increased circulating volume.[7] It is very similar in structure and function to ANP and inhibits Na^+ and water reabsorption by the collecting duct.

Diuretic Agents

The ability of the kidneys to reabsorb fluid can be inhibited by drugs that block sodium and water reabsorption. These agents are called *diuretics* and include osmotic diuretics, ACE inhibitors, loop diuretics, thiazide-like diuretics, and inhibitors of aldosterone activity (Table 26-2).[14] Diuretics work by altering osmotic gradients in the kidney tubules so that reabsorption of water is inhibited. Recall that water always moves passively according to an osmotic gradient. When the solute content of the filtrate is elevated, reabsorption of water is inhibited, resulting in a larger output of urine.

Osmotic diuretics (e.g., mannitol) are filtered through the glomerulus and are not reabsorbed by the tubules. The osmolality of the filtrate is increased by the presence of the solute, and more water remains in the tubule and is excreted in the urine. ACE inhibitors (e.g., captopril) inhibit the formation of AII and aldosterone, which normally stimulate the kidney tubules to reabsorb Na^+. In the absence of these hormones, more Na^+ stays in the urinary filtrate, resulting in less reabsorption of water.

Loop diuretics (e.g., furosemide) block the Na^+-K^+-$2Cl^-$ pumps in the ascending loop of Henle. The ions that would normally have been pumped into the interstitium stay in the filtrate and hold water with them. In addition, the maintenance of the high interstitial gradient in the medulla may be impaired. Washout of the gradient reduces the force for water reabsorption from the collecting ducts.

Thiazide-like diuretics (e.g., hydrochlorothiazide) block Na^+ reabsorption in the distal tubule. Sodium ions remain in the filtrate and oppose the action of the interstitial osmotic gradient.

All of these agents also increase the excretion of K^+ and are called *potassium-wasting diuretics.* Patients receiving chronic diuretic therapy with these agents usually require potassium replacement therapy.

In contrast, the aldosterone-blocking agents (e.g., spironolactone) are potassium sparing. Recall that aldosterone increases activity of the Na^+-K^+ pumps on the basolateral membrane of the distal tubule cells. These pumps promote Na^+ and water reabsorption and potassium secretion. Blockage of aldosterone reduces the activity of these pumps and results in less sodium and water reabsorption as well as less potassium excretion. Significant elevations in serum K^+ can occur with these agents.

Diuretics are used primarily in the management of high blood pressure (see Chapter 16) and congestive heart failure (see Chapter 19), but they also may be used in the diagnostic phase of acute renal failure or to manage potassium overload.

KEY CONCEPTS

- The kidneys regulate blood volume and osmolality by altering GFR and reabsorption from the urinary filtrate.
- Changes in blood volume alter the filtration pressure in the glomerulus, resulting in a pressure diuresis when blood volume is high and in reduced filtration and fluid conservation when blood volume is low.
- The kidney tubules are responsive to hormones that alter their reabsorptive properties. ADH increases the permeability of the collecting tubule to water, resulting in increased reabsorption and reduced blood osmolality.
- Aldosterone, AII, ANP, and urodilatin alter blood volume without affecting blood osmolality. Aldosterone and AII increase sodium and water reabsorption, whereas ANP and urodilatin inhibit their reabsorption.
- Diuretics alter the osmolality of the urinary filtrate and oppose the reabsorption of water, resulting in an increase in urine volume.

ENDOCRINE FUNCTIONS

The kidney is the source of two important endocrine hormones: erythropoietin and active vitamin D. Secretion of these hormones is impaired in chronic renal failure and contributes to the anemia and osteodystrophy found in this disorder (see Chapter 28).

Erythropoietin

Erythropoietin is a peptide growth factor that stimulates erythrocyte development in the bone marrow. The regulation of erythropoietin secretion is not completely understood; however, hypoxemia and decreased red cell mass are known to increase its release. Hypoxia stimulates a transcription factor (hypoxia-inducible factor, HIF) that activates erythropoietin gene transcription.[15] Presumably, an increase in red cell production increases delivery of oxygen to the kidney and inhibits further production of erythropoietin. Erythropoietin is commercially available in a recombinant form that can be given parenterally. The anemia of chronic renal failure usually responds well to erythropoietin replacement therapy.

Vitamin D

Synthesis of active vitamin D is an interdependent function of the skin, liver, and kidney. The precursors to active vitamin D can be formed in the skin in response to the ultraviolet rays in sunlight, or they can be ingested in fortified food products. These precursors (cholecalciferol) then must undergo a series of two hydroxylations to become active. The first occurs in the liver, resulting in the formation of 25-hydroxycholecalciferol. The kidney performs the second hydroxylation to form 1,25-hydroxycholecalciferol, which is the active form of vitamin D.[16] Vitamin D is a necessary cofactor for calcium absorption from the intestine. It may also facilitate calcium reabsorption in the kidney tubules.

In chronic renal failure, the production of active vitamin D is impaired, resulting in poor calcium absorption from the intestine and low serum calcium levels. A low serum calcium level is the stimulus for parathyroid hormone release, resulting in removal of calcium and phosphate from the bones. Eventually excessive parathyroid hormone activity leads to the condition of osteodystrophy and predisposes to skeletal fractures (see Chapter 28).

KEY CONCEPTS

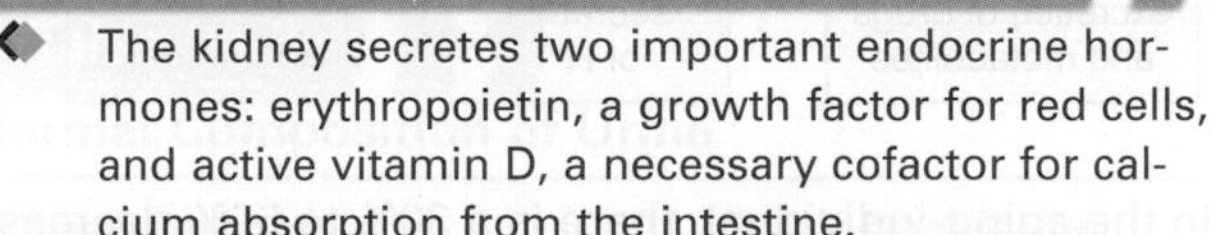

- The kidney secretes two important endocrine hormones: erythropoietin, a growth factor for red cells, and active vitamin D, a necessary cofactor for calcium absorption from the intestine.
- In chronic renal failure, impaired production of these hormones results in anemia and osteodystrophy.

AGE-RELATED CHANGES IN RENAL FUNCTION

Fetus

The fetal kidney begins to excrete urine between the 11th and 12th weeks of development.[17] Fetal urine is hypotonic to plasma because despite the fact that ADH is present and the volume receptors and osmoreceptors are functional, the renal

and drugs can change urine color. For instance, if beets have been eaten, the urine may be burgundy, and if the individual has taken phenazopyridine (Pyridium), the urine may be orange.

Normally, urine is clear and slightly acidic, although the pH range is 4.5 to 8.0. Urine allowed to stand undisturbed will become cloudy and alkaline because of the breakdown of urea to ammonia, which increases the pH. Cloudiness can result from the presence of cells, bacteria, crystals, casts, or fat substances.

Urine specific gravity and urine osmolality are measures of the concentration of solute in the urine. Urine specific gravity varies with the amount of solids in the urine, such as cells, casts, and microorganisms, but urine osmolality is not affected by these substances. Urine osmolality is a more accurate measure of the kidneys' ability to concentrate and dilute the urine. The range for specific gravity is 1.003 to 1.030, with the higher number indicating a more concentrated urine. Usually urine osmolality and specific gravity vary throughout the day and from day to day. Results that remain fixed over consecutive voidings and days could be an indicator of renal disease.

Normal urine contains no protein. A small amount of protein in the urine is insignificant, but excretion of more than 150 mg per 24 hours should be investigated, as it could indicate glomerular capillary disease. Proteinuria can cause urine to be foamy.

Glycosuria, or glucose in the urine, is abnormal and usually indicates hyperglycemia (elevated blood glucose), which can occur with diabetes mellitus or following an excessive ingestion of sugar. Rarely does glycosuria indicate renal disease.

A few epithelial cells, erythrocytes, leukocytes, and bacteria are normally found in urine. Fewer than 5 RBCs or WBCs per high-powered field is considered to be within normal limits. An excess of any of these cells may indicate a pathologic process; however, collection technique and presence of menstrual blood may be confounding factors.

Crystals and stones are not usually found in the urine. Either can originate anywhere along the urinary tract. If found in the urine, their composition should be identified and the urinary tract assessed for more crystals and stones (see Chapter 27).

When urinary casts are present, they provide important clues for differentiating renal diseases. Casts are formed in the nephron tubule and are composed of a protein meshwork with entrapped cells or cell fragments. There are many types of casts, each associated with certain renal pathologic conditions. For example, WBC casts are associated with renal infections (pyelonephritis); RBC casts indicate inflammation of the glomerulus (glomerulonephritis); and epithelial cell casts indicate sloughing of tubular cells (acute tubular necrosis).

Serum Creatinine and Blood Urea Nitrogen

Creatinine is an end product of muscle metabolism that is excreted exclusively by the kidney. The serum creatinine level averages approximately 0.7 to 1.5 mg/dl and is relatively constant throughout the day and from day to day. Creatinine levels are slightly higher in men than in women because of men's larger muscle mass.

Serum creatinine is a fairly reliable indicator of renal function because it is affected by only two factors: (1) the rate of creatinine produced from muscle, which is relatively constant in the absence of muscle breakdown; and (2) the rate of creatinine excreted by the kidney, which is determined primarily by the GFR. Therefore, the GFR is reflected in the serum creatinine level. For instance, when GFR decreases by half, the concentration of creatinine in the serum doubles. A rise in serum creatinine indicates a decrease in renal function.

Urea is an end product of protein metabolism. It is excreted primarily by the kidney and measured in the blood as **blood urea nitrogen** (BUN). The BUN averages approximately 10 to 20 mg/dl and rises with a decrease in renal function, a decrease in fluid volume, and an increase in catabolism and dietary protein intake. When a change in renal function occurs, the BUN tends to change more rapidly than creatinine does; however, BUN is less specific. Often BUN and creatinine are measured together, and the ratio is determined. Acute changes in GFR are reflected in a higher BUN-to-creatinine ratio, usually greater than 20:1.

Measures of Glomerular Filtration Rate

GFR is an important parameter in the assessment of renal function. GFR is commonly measured by evaluating the clearance of a filterable substance from the plasma. Creatinine clearance is frequently used to assess GFR, but it is not completely accurate because some secretion and reabsorption occurs in the nephron tubules. At low GFR, creatinine clearance is quite unreliable. The accuracy of creatinine clearance tests can be improved by administration of cimetidine, a drug that blocks the tubular secretion of creatinine.[19]

More accurate measurement of GFR is obtained by using inulin, an inert substance that is filtered freely at the glomerulus and is completely unaffected by tubular secretion and reabsorption. The use of inulin is more expensive and cumbersome than creatinine clearance because it must be injected. The formula for measuring clearance is the same regardless of the marker substance used. Creatinine clearance is used in the following example, but the corresponding values for inulin can be substituted in the equation.

Creatinine clearance estimates the GFR by measuring the amount of blood that is cleared of creatinine each minute. Usually a 24-hour urine specimen and a blood specimen at the midpoint of the urine collection are used to determine creatinine clearance; however, shorter intervals can be used. The measured values are calculated in the following formula:

$$\text{Clearance} = \frac{\text{urine volume (ml/min)} \times \text{urinary creatinine (mg/dl)}}{\text{Plasma creatinine (mg/dl)}}$$

Diagnostic Tests

Although studies of urine and blood are good indicators of renal function, they often are not adequate to determine the underlying pathologic process. Diagnostic tests are helpful in assessing structural abnormalities, such as tumors, obstructions, congenital anomalies, perfusion defects, and histologic abnormalities. Sometimes a combination of diagnostic tests is necessary.

Kidney, Ureter, and Bladder Roentgenography

A KUB is a plain radiograph (x-ray) taken of the abdomen to visualize the kidneys, ureters, and bladder. A KUB study shows the position, shape, size, and number of macroscopic or gross renal, ureteral, and bladder structures and surrounding bones. In addition, foreign bodies, radiopaque objects, stones, and neoplasms can be seen on KUB. The KUB may serve as a screening examination to inform further diagnostic testing.

Intravenous Urography

During intravenous urography, also called intravenous pyelography (IVP), an iodine-containing radiopaque dye is injected into a vein; it circulates through the kidney and is excreted in the urine. A rapid series of radiographs is made as the dye is being excreted. This test shows the size, shape, and location of urinary tract structures and can be used to evaluate renal excretory function. The dye is **nephrotoxic,** meaning poisonous to the kidney, and allergenic to some people. A state of hydration helps the dye to pass through the kidney and prevents renal damage. Because fecal matter and gas in the intestinal tract will interfere with visualization of the kidneys and ureters on the radiographs, a laxative or enema may be indicated before IVP.

Retrograde pyelography, also called *retrograde urography,* is an invasive procedure during which a catheter or cystoscope is passed into the bladder and ureters. A radiopaque dye is injected into the urinary tract, and x-ray films are made. Additional films are obtained as the catheters are removed, and more should be obtained approximately 15 to 30 minutes after the initial set to make sure all the dye has been excreted. This test provides anatomic information about the urinary tract from the renal pelvis through the urinary meatus and is often done when an obstruction is suspected. If desired, separate urine specimens may be obtained from each kidney before the dye is injected. Retrograde urography is often done in conjunction with cystoscopy (visualization of the bladder).

Complications associated with retrograde pyelography are urinary tract infection from retrograde movement of organisms with catheter insertion and dye injection. Hematuria can be associated with urinary tract infection or can result from injury to the urinary tract mucosa from the catheter or cystoscope. Ureteral edema can result from manipulation of the catheters and obstruct urine flow. Signs and symptoms of ureteral edema include decreased urine output and possibly pain.

Radionuclide Studies

Renograms and renal scans are diagnostic studies that use radioactive isotopes to assess kidney structure and function. In general, the renogram is more useful for assessing function, whereas the renal scan is better at detecting structural anomalies. During a renogram procedure, a small amount of filterable radioactive material is administered intravenously. It circulates through the kidney and is excreted in the urine. As the radionuclide circulates through the renal vessels and nephrons, a radiation detection probe counts the activity of the radioactive substance and simultaneously creates a graphic record of the activity. This test assesses renal function by measuring renal blood flow, glomerular filtration, and tubular secretion.

The renal scan uses a radionuclide that tends to accumulate in areas that are well perfused by blood. The renal scan images depict concentration of the radionuclide in the kidney and provide anatomic and some physiologic information. In the presence of tumors or nonfunctioning areas, the radioactive material will not be detected by the scan.

A more dynamic assessment of renal physiology can be obtained using positron emission tomography (PET) or single-photon emission computed tomography (SPECT). These modalities use scintigraphic imaging to view the kidney and can pick up subtle, dynamic changes. Regional differences in GFR, for example, can be detected by PET scan.

Radionuclide studies are safe to use with young children and when a client is allergic to radiopaque dye. There is a low incidence of allergic reactions to radiopharmaceuticals. In addition, because these substances are low-dose radiation, radionuclide studies can be repeated without deleterious effects.

Ultrasonography

Ultrasonography is a noninvasive, painless procedure that uses high-frequency sound waves to image renal structures. The sound waves are at a frequency above the limit of human hearing. Ultrasound is used because its short wavelength produces a more detailed picture or image than other types of sound waves. A probe with a transducer inside is held against the back and emits ultrasound waves that travel through tissue to the kidney and reflect off the kidney, back to the probe. The reflective waves are echoes. The returning echoes are converted by the transducer to electrical signals that a computer plots as points of light on a screen. Eventually the points build into lines, which form a picture or image.

Ultrasonography demonstrates gross renal anatomy, true kidney depth, structural abnormalities, and perirenal masses, and it can be used to distinguish between a fluid-filled cyst and a solid tumor.

Computed Tomography

Computed tomography (CT) combines roentgenograms with computer technology and is a noninvasive, painless procedure. Instead of using broad x-ray beams, CT uses thin x-ray beams, each about 10 degrees apart. The information obtained during scanning is transmitted to a computer, which constructs a tomograph and calculates its density. Because the kidneys are located deep within the abdominal cavity, they opacify better after an IV injection of a contrast agent. CT shows more detail than ultrasonography. CT can demonstrate perirenal and renal masses, renal vascular disorders, and filling defects of the collecting system.

Magnetic Resonance Imaging

Magnetic resonance imaging (MRI) is a painless, noninvasive procedure that does not use x-rays or radioactive markers. The imager applies a strong magnetic field that causes protons to align themselves with the magnetic field. Pulses of radio waves are emitted that cause the magnetic fields to rotate or resonate. The rotating fields induce electrical signals that the computer analyzes and uses to create images or pictures on a screen. The renal images are available in all planes and show more detail than the images achievable with CT. Newer methods of MRI have been developed to obtain dynamic images using the movement of contrast dye through the kidney. Sequential fast-pulse imaging (functional MRI) allows assessment of obstructions, vascular disorders, and renal insufficiency.

Renal Biopsy

The purpose of a kidney biopsy is to obtain renal tissue that may be studied to determine the nature and extent of renal disease for diagnosis, management, and prognosis. Tissue obtained during a renal biopsy is taken from the outer or cortical region of the kidney. The renal tissue is studied histologically by light and electron microscopy and immunofluorescence. Some indications for a kidney biopsy are persistent proteinuria, hematuria originating from the kidney, unexplained acute renal failure, glomerular disease, renal mass, rejection of a transplanted kidney, and renal involvement in systemic disease.[20]

Biopsy of the kidney may be accomplished by the open or closed method. Both are invasive procedures that require sterile technique. An *open renal biopsy* is rarely performed any longer and requires an operation with the subject under general anesthesia. An incision is made, the kidney is exposed, the biopsy needle is inserted into the kidney, a piece of tissue is extracted, and the area is closed and sutured. A closed renal biopsy, also called a **percutaneous** renal biopsy (percutaneous means "through the skin"), is usually done in a radiology suite, although it can be done at the bedside. A local anesthetic is given and the client is placed in a prone position with a pillow under the abdomen. Clients who have undergone kidney transplantation are positioned to maximize access to the transplanted kidney, which is usually in the groin area. The client is instructed to hold his or her breath as the biopsy needle is inserted through the skin and into the kidney. The movement of the needle as the client breathes is proof that it is in the kidney because the kidneys are in contact with the diaphragm and move with ventilation. Needle position in the kidney can also be confirmed with imaging techniques such as ultrasonography or fluoroscopy. In addition, the client usually complains of intense pressure or dull pain as the needle enters the kidney because the renal capsule is innervated by pain receptors. A small fragment of tissue is obtained, and the needle is withdrawn.

With either method of renal biopsy, hemorrhage is the most common complication. Hemorrhage may occur in the kidney, around the kidney, or into the urine. Other complications are infection, pain, clot formation in the kidney that could obstruct urine flow, aneurysm, intrarenal arteriovenous fistula, and laceration of adjacent organs or blood vessels.

Some contraindications to renal biopsy are hypertension, bleeding tendencies, documented renal neoplasm, gross sepsis, and frequent coughing or sneezing.

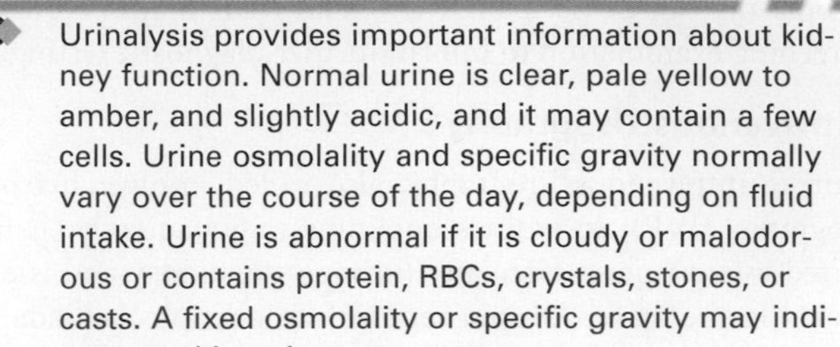

KEY CONCEPTS

- Urinalysis provides important information about kidney function. Normal urine is clear, pale yellow to amber, and slightly acidic, and it may contain a few cells. Urine osmolality and specific gravity normally vary over the course of the day, depending on fluid intake. Urine is abnormal if it is cloudy or malodorous or contains protein, RBCs, crystals, stones, or casts. A fixed osmolality or specific gravity may indicate renal impairment.
- Serum creatinine and BUN are useful indicators of renal function. Serum creatinine is a more reliable indicator of renal function than BUN. In conditions of reduced GFR, serum creatinine and BUN levels increase.
- GFR can be estimated by measuring the clearance of a filterable substance from the urine. Creatinine clearance is frequently used for this purpose, but it is not completely accurate because of some tubular processing. Inulin clearance provides a more accurate measurement of GFR.
- Diagnostic studies used to evaluate kidney structure and function include plain radiography, pyelography, radionuclide studies, ultrasound, CT, and MRI. Renal biopsy may be performed to obtain tissue for histologic examination.

SUMMARY

The kidneys have a vital role in excreting water-soluble waste products and maintaining fluid, electrolyte, and acid-base homeostasis. To perform these functions, the kidneys must have a sufficient GFR. Most waste products are removed by filtration rather than by secretion; thus, a reduced GFR results in accumulation of wastes in the blood. The kidney has a large renal reserve and accomplishes its functions well until more than 75% of the nephron mass is dysfunctional.

The nephron is the structural and functional unit of the kidney. It performs three essential functions: filtration, secretion, and reabsorption. Filtration occurs at the glomerulus at a rate of about 125 ml/min. The composition of filtrate is similar to that of blood except that proteins and blood cells are absent. Normally 99% of the filtrate is reabsorbed along the nephron tubules, resulting in the elimination of 30 to 60 ml/hr of concentrated urine. Each nephron regulates its own

GFR through tubuloglomerular feedback to prevent overloading its reabsorptive capacities.

The kidneys are responsive to a number of endocrine hormones, including ADH, aldosterone, AII, ANP, and urodilatin, which regulate blood osmolality and volume. In addition, the kidneys produce two important endocrine hormones: erythropoietin and vitamin D. Urinalysis, serum creatinine and BUN levels, and tests of GFR are important indicators of renal function. Structural abnormalities can be assessed by a variety of imaging techniques.

MEDIA RESOURCES

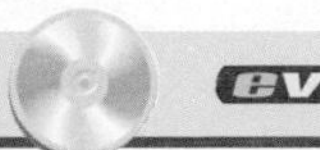

evolve

Remember to check out the ***CD Companion*** included with this book for Review Questions, Key Concepts Review, Glossary (with audio for selected terms), Disease Profiles, and Animations.

PLUS, visit the ***Evolve website*** at http://evolve.elsevier.com/Copstead/ for Case Studies, Disease Profiles, and WebLinks.

References

1. Stanton BA, Koeppen BM: Elements of renal function. In Berne RM et al, editors: *Physiology,* ed 5, St Louis, 2004, Mosby, pp 623-642.
2. Ramcharan T, Matas AJ: Long-term (20-37 years) follow-up of living kidney donors, *Am J Transplant* 2(10):959-964, 2002.
3. Jarvis C: *Physical examination and health assessment,* ed 4, Philadelphia, 2004, Saunders, p 564.
4. Ganong WF: Renal function and micturition. In Ganong WF, editor: *Review of medical physiology,* ed 21, New York, 2003, Lange/McGraw-Hill, pp 702-732.
5. Guyton AC, Hall JE: Urine formation by the kidneys: I. Glomerular filtration, renal blood flow, and their control. In Guyton AC, Hall JE, editors: *Textbook of medical physiology,* ed 10, Philadelphia, 2000, Saunders, pp 279-295.
6. Miner JH: A molecular look at the glomerular barrier, *Nephron Exp Nephrol* 94(4):e119-e122, 2003.
7. Stanton BA, Koeppen BM: Solute and water transport along the nephron: tubular function. In Berne RM et al, editors: *Physiology,* ed 5, St Louis, 2004, Mosby, pp 643-658.
8. Stanton BA, Koeppen BM: Control of body fluid osmolality and volume. In Berne RM et al, editors: *Physiology,* ed 5, St Louis, 2004, Mosby, pp 659-684.
9. Stockand JD, Sansom SC: Glomerular mesangial cells: electrophysiology and regulation of contraction, *Physiol Rev* 78:723-744, 1998.
10. Bell PD, Lapointe JY, Peti-Peterdi J: Macula densa cell signaling, *Annu Rev Physiol* 65:481-500, 2003.
11. Schnermann J, Levine DZ: Paracrine factors in tubuloglomerular feedback: adenosine, ATP, and nitric oxide, *Annu Rev Physiol* 65:501-529, 2003.
12. Gambaro G, Perazella MA: Adverse renal effects of anti-inflammatory agents: evaluation of selective and nonselective cyclooxygenase inhibitors, *J Intern Med* 253(6):643-652, 2003.
13. Stanton BA, Koeppen BM: Role of the kidneys in the regulation of acid-base balance. In Berne RM et al, editors: *Physiology,* ed 5, St Louis, 2004, Mosby, pp 703-716.
14. Carter BL, Saseen JJ: Hypertension. In Dipiro JT et al, editors: *Pharmacotherapy: a pathophysiologic approach,* ed 5, New York, 2002, McGraw-Hill, pp 157-184.
15. Fisher JW: Erythropoietin: physiology and pharmacology update, *Exp Biol Med* 228(1):1-14, 2003.
16. Silver J, Drueke TB: Master genes for bone growth, 1,25-dihydroxyvitamin D_3 synthesis, and renal conservation of phosphate and calcium, *Curr Opin Nephrol Hypertens* 7:359-361, 1998.
17. Davis ID, Avner ED: Glomerular disease. In Behrman RE, Kliegman RM, Jenson HB, editors: *Textbook of pediatrics,* ed 17, Philadelphia, 2004, Saunders, pp 1731-1735.
18. Choudhury D et al: Effect of aging on renal function and disease. In Brenner BM, editor: *Brenner and Rector's the kidney,* ed. 6, Philadelphia, 2000, Saunders, pp 2187-2216.
19. Serdar MA et al: A practical approach to glomerular filtration rate measurements: creatinine clearance estimation using cimetidine, *Ann Clin Lab Sci* 31(3):265-273, 2001.
20. Watnick S, Morrison G: Kidney. In Tierney LM, McPhee SJ, Papadakis M, editors: *Current medical diagnosis and treatment,* ed. 42, New York, 2003, Lange/McGraw-Hill, 2003, pp 867-902.

chapter 27

Intrarenal Disorders

Katherina P. Choka

MEDIA RESOURCES

Additional Material for Study, Review, and Further Exploration

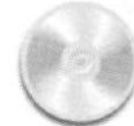

CD Companion ◆ Review Questions and Answers ◆ Key Concepts Review ◆ Glossary *(with audio pronunciations for selected terms)* ◆ Disease Profiles ◆ Animations

evolve ***Website*** at http://evolve.elsevier.com/Copstead/ ◆ Case Studies ◆ Disease Profiles ◆ WebLinks

KEY QUESTIONS

- How are the locations of renal pain and findings on urinalysis used to differentiate the causes of kidney disease?
- How do autosomal dominant and recessive forms of polycystic kidney disease differ?
- What findings help differentiate an upper urinary tract pyelonephritis from a lower urinary tract infection?
- What physiologic and pathophysiologic disorders predispose to the formation of renal calculi of differing composition?
- What effect does urinary obstruction have on glomerular filtration, urinary stasis, and infection risk?
- How are renal tumors detected and managed?
- How do the various forms of glomerulonephritis affect the permeability of the basement membrane?
- What laboratory and clinical findings suggest a diagnosis of nephrotic syndrome?

CHAPTER OUTLINE

Functional kidneys are necessary for the removal of waste products from the blood and the maintenance of fluid, electrolyte, and acid-base balance despite wide variations in intake and nonurinary losses. Systemic disorders that alter the delivery of blood flow to the kidney may adversely affect the kidney's ability to perform its filtering and homeostatic functions. In addition, many disorders occur primarily within the kidney and have the potential to result in renal insufficiency or failure.[1] In general, these disorders can be categorized as (1) congenital, (2) infectious, (3) obstructive, and (4) glomerular.

Congenital diseases discussed in this chapter are renal agenesis, which includes failure of one or both kidneys to develop, as well as autosomal dominant (ADPKD) and autosomal recessive polycystic kidney disease (ARPKD). Pyelonephritis, or kidney infection, is a fairly prevalent illness and the second leading cause of renal failure.[1] Kidney infections are the most common serious infections in pregnant women[2] and account for approximately 5% of all febrile episodes in infants.[3] Renal calculus, the most prevalent obstructive process, affects up to 10% of people in the United States.[4] Although not as common, renal tumors are often difficult to successfully manage and therefore represent a much more sinister obstructive pathologic process than calculus. At least 85% of renal tumors are diagnosed as adenocarcinoma or renal cell carcinoma, which is the cause of more than 30,000 new cases of renal cancer each year in the United States.[5,6] Glomerulopathies encompass a broad spectrum of diseases and syndromes that affect the ability of the glomeruli to filter. As a group, glomerulopathies are the leading precursors to renal failure.[7]

Whether congenital, infectious, obstructive, or glomerular, kidney pathologic processes are characterized by insufficient filtering of wastes or excessive filtering of normally retained substances and by urinary tract pain. Careful assessment of the patient's history and pain symptoms aids in the localization and diagnosis of different intrarenal and postrenal disorders. Urinalysis provides basic laboratory clues for the differential diagnosis. General descriptions of urinary tract pain and urinalysis indicators of kidney dysfunction preface the discussion of specific disorders.

MANIFESTATIONS OF KIDNEY DISEASE

Urinary Tract Pain

Assessment of the location, onset, quality, quantity, and pattern of pain, as well as interventions that relieve pain, aids in localizing the cause of the urinary tract pain. Pain associated with the urinary tract may be perceived as coming from an area slightly below the ribs to the upper part of the thighs and may be bilateral or unilateral. Typically, bladder pain is felt in the suprapubic to upper thigh area, ureteral pain in the groin or genital area, and renal pain at the **costovertebral angle** in the back. Neither renal nor ureteral pain is altered by a change in body position. Renal pain is also referred to as **nephralgia** (*-algia* is from the Greek *algos,* meaning pain).

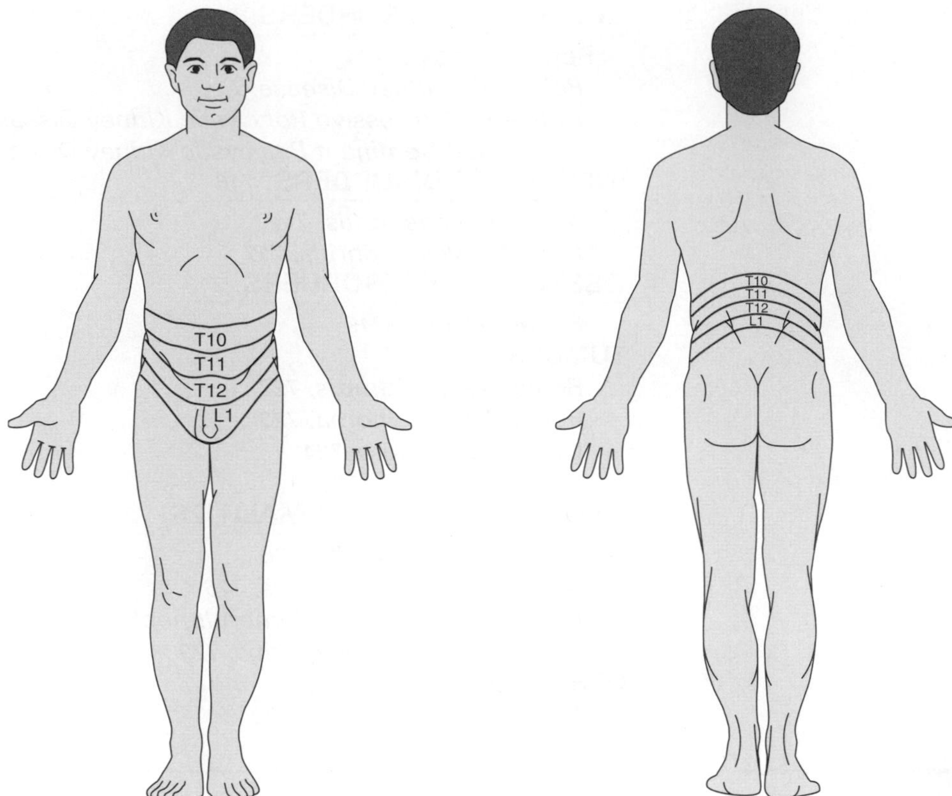

FIGURE 27-1 ■ Dermatomes T10 (thoracic) to L1 (lumbar) correspond to areas that innervate the renal structures.

Sympathetic nerves transmit information from renal and ureteral pain receptors or **nociceptors** (*noci-* is derived from the Latin *nocere,* meaning to hurt or injure) to the spinal cord between T10 and L1. Because these sympathetic nerves enter the spinal cord at this level, the pain can be felt throughout the corresponding T10-L1 dermatomes. A **dermatome** is an area of skin innervated by a specific spinal cord segment (Figure 27-1). Visceral and cutaneous afferent fibers enter the spinal cord in close proximity and converge on some of the same neurons at the spinal, thalamic, and cortical levels. When visceral pain fibers are stimulated, concurrent stimulation of cutaneous fibers occurs and the visceral pain is felt as though it had originated in the skin. Nerve fibers from the renal plexus communicate with the spermatic plexus, and because of this association, scrotal pain in males and labial pain in females may accompany renal pain.[8]

Extensive damage and even complete loss of a kidney can occur without nephralgia because most of the kidney is without pain receptors. However, the renal capsule is innervated by nociceptors, and if it is distended, inflamed, or punctured, a dull to sharp pain is felt. Distention or inflammation of the renal capsule causes a dull, constant pain. Capsular stretching can result from intrarenal fluid accumulation such as occurs with inflammation (pyelonephritis), infected or bleeding cysts, hemorrhage from blunt trauma, and neoplastic growth. In addition, whenever the renal capsule is penetrated (e.g., during biopsy or trauma), a dull pain or intense pressure is felt. Intraperitoneal and renal pain may have similar features. However, patients with renal pain characteristically move around while holding or splinting the flank area, whereas patients with intraperitoneal pain tend to lay motionless.[8]

The lower portions of the collecting system, beginning with the renal pelvis and continuing throughout the rest of the urinary tract, are innervated by many pain receptors. Obstruction of the intrarenal collecting system causes pain if the obstruction leads to distention of the renal pelvis or capsule. Large calculi, however, can develop insidiously in the renal pelvis or calices and may be painless until they start to move into the ureteral junction. Ischemia caused by the occlusion of renal blood vessels (e.g., from an embolus, arteriosclerotic disease, or tumor) results in a constant dull or sharp pain.[8]

Obstruction of the lower urinary system results in distention and intermittent sharp pain. The pain can be particularly intense if the obstruction develops rapidly. Movement of a stone down a ureter is associated with **renal colic** and excruciating pain that can radiate from the flank into the genital area. Renal colic usually increases in intensity, plateaus, and then diminishes. *Colic* refers to spasm in a tubular or hollow organ accompanied by pain.[9]

Urinalysis Indicators of Kidney Disease

Urinalysis is an essential laboratory test for all suspected problems of the genitourinary system. After history taking and a physical examination, urinalysis generally serves as a starting point for the differential diagnosis. The color, odor, and tur-

Table 27-1

Urine Dipstick Findings Associated with Kidney Disorders

Urine Dipstick Finding	Associated Renal Disorders
Specific gravity	
Decreased	Renal insufficiency
	Insufficient secretion of antidiuretic hormone
	Diabetes mellitus
pH	
Increased (6.5-8.0)	Calcium or struvite calculi
	Renal tubular acidosis
	Urinary tract infection by a urea-splitting organism
Decreased (4.5-5.5)	Uric acid or cystine calculi
Hematuria	Cystitis, nephritis
	Trauma
	Glomerulonephritis
	Calculi, malignancies, other obstructive processes
Protein	Renal hypertension
	Glomerulopathies
	Nephrotic syndromes
	Tubulopathies
	Renal artery or vein thrombosis
	Pyelonephritis
Glucose and ketones	Diabetes mellitus
	Malnutrition
Bilirubin and urobilirubin	Liver dysfunction
Leukocytes	Cystitis, nephritis
	Renal calculi and other obstructive processes
Nitrites	Cystitis, especially of gram-negative cause

Data from Brendler CB: Evaluation of the urologic patient: history, physical examination, and urinalysis. In Walsh PC et al, editors: *Campbell's urology*, ed 7, Philadelphia, 1998, Saunders, pp 131-157; Brady HR, Brenner BM: Acute renal failure. In Fauci AS et al, editors: *Harrison's principles of internal medicine*, ed 14, New York, 1998, McGraw-Hill, pp 1495-1505; Hassay KA: Effective management of urinary discomfort, *Nurse Pract* 20(2):39-46, 1995.

Table 27-2

Microscopic Urinalysis and Associated Kidney Disorders

Microscopic Urinalysis Finding	Associated Kidney Disorders
Cells	
RBCs: circular appearing	Cystitis, nephritis
	Trauma
	Calculi, malignancy, and other obstructive processes
RBCs: irregularly shaped	Glomerulopathies
WBCs	Cystitis, nephritis
	Renal calculi, malignancy, and other obstructive processes
Epithelial (irregular transitional cells)	Malignancy
Casts	
Hyaline	Chronic renal disease
	Sometimes no pathologic significance
RBCs	Glomerulonephritis
WBCs	Glomerulonephritis
	Acute or chronic pyelonephritis
	Acute tubulointerstitial nephritis
Fatty	Nephritic syndrome
Other cellular constituents	Nonspecific kidney damage
Crystals	
Cystine	Cystinuria
	Acidic urine
Uric acid	Uric acid calculi
	Acidic urine
Calcium oxalate	Calcium calculi
	Alkaline urine
Triple phosphate (struvite)	Struvite calculi
	Alkaline urine
Bacteria $>10^3$	Cystitis, nephritis
Yeast	Cystitis, yeast etiology
	Diabetes mellitus
Parasites	Vaginitis in women
	Prostatitis in men

Data from Gerber GS, Brendler CB: Evaluation of the urologic patient: history, physical examination, and urinalysis. In Walsh PC et al, editors: *Campbell's urology*, ed 8, Philadelphia, 2002, Saunders, pp 83-110.

bidity of the urine offer the first clues. Dark, strong-smelling urine may be an indicator of decreased renal function. Cloudy pungent urine generally indicates an infectious process, the turbidity being a result of leukocytes in the urine.[8] Dipstick tests and microscopic analysis provide a great deal of additional information.

Dipstick tests afford quick and inexpensive methods of gathering a variety of clinical data useful in understanding kidney diseases. Urine specific gravity, pH, and chemistry profiles, including blood, protein, glucose, ketones, and bilirubin, can be assessed. Table 27-1 lists major kidney disorders that are associated with abnormalities identified by urine dipstick testing. Microscopic urinalysis assists in further pinpointing pathologic processes by identifying cells, casts, crystals, bacteria, yeast, and parasites that are present in the urine (Table 27-2).

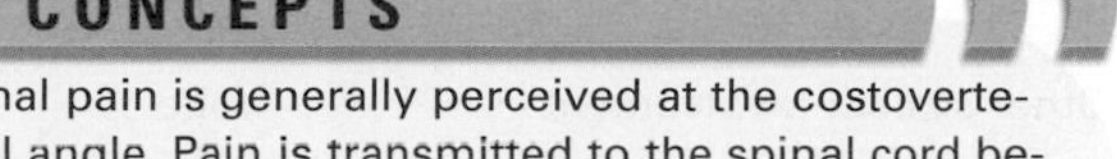

KEY CONCEPTS

- Renal pain is generally perceived at the costovertebral angle. Pain is transmitted to the spinal cord between T10 and L1 by sympathetic afferent neurons. Pain may be felt throughout the dermatomes corresponding to T10-L1.

- Renal pain is usually due to distention and inflammation of the renal capsule and has a dull, constant character. Urinary tract pain involving the ureters is usually of an intermittent, sharp, and colicky character.
- Urinalysis provides a foundation for the differential diagnosis of renal dysfunction. The presence of hematuria, crystals, casts, protein, or leukocytes is particularly indicative of urinary tract abnormalities.

CONGENITAL DISORDERS

Renal Agenesis

Renal agenesis, or failure of one or both kidneys to develop, can be found as a single entity or in combination with other congenital malformations.

Bilateral renal agenesis is found in approximately 1 in 3000 to 4000 live births. Males are affected more often than females. Bilateral agenesis results from failure of the metanephros (renal buds) to develop in the fetus.[1] Bilateral renal agenesis is incompatible with extrauterine life. Infants with bilateral renal agenesis are stillborn or die in the first few months after birth.[10] Bilateral renal agenesis is often associated with **Potter syndrome,** a collection of associated anomalies that includes (1) wide-spaced eyes with epicanthal folds, (2) low-set ears, (3) broad and flat nose, (4) hypoplastic lungs, and (5) limb anomalies.[10]

Unilateral renal agenesis is more common than bilateral renal agenesis, with the reported incidence of unilateral renal agenesis being approximately 1 in 500 live births.[11] Males are more often affected than females, and the left kidney is usually the one that fails to develop. The remaining kidney usually enlarges as a compensatory mechanism, occasionally to twice the normal size. Unilateral agenesis is often associated with concurrent anomalies, the most common being congenital cardiac problems.[10] Other concurrent abnormalities include genitourinary abnormalities (40% of cases), (2) skeletal abnormalities (30%), (3) cardiovascular and gastrointestinal abnormalities (15%), and (4) central nervous system and respiratory system abnormalities (10%). If the single kidney is normal, life expectancy is normal; however, such individuals may have an increased risk for hypertension and proteinuria.

Polycystic Kidney Disease

Polycystic kidney disease is a result of multiple dilations of the collecting ducts, which appear as if they are fluid-filled cysts. Both adults and children are affected. Autosomal recessive polycystic kidney disease (ARPKD) is usually diagnosed in infants and young children, whereas autosomal dominant polycystic kidney disease (ADPKD) is generally diagnosed in adulthood. Although the pathogenesis is similar, the ARPKD and ADPKD forms of the disease are genetically different, with distinct clinical courses (Table 27-3).

Autosomal Recessive Polycystic Kidney Disease

Etiology and Pathogenesis. **Autosomal recessive polycystic kidney disease** is a recessive disease that begins in utero, and its origins have been traced to a defect on chromosome 6. The incidence of ARPKD is reported as between 1 in 5000 and 1 in 40,000 live births.[12] One half of infants with ARPKD die within the first few days of life, and only 25% survive to the age of 10 years. The proportion of dilated collecting ducts varies from less than 10% to greater than 90%.[12] In

Table 27-3

Comparison of Autosomal Recessive and Autosomal Dominant Polycystic Kidney Disease

Feature	Autosomal Recessive Polycystic Kidney Disease	Autosomal Dominant Polycystic Kidney Disease
Gene defect	Chromosome 6	Chromosomes 4, 16
Incidence	1:5000 to 1:40,000	1:500 to 1:1000
Usual age of clinical disease onset	Perinatal	Third to fifth decades
Typical sonographic appearance	Symmetrically enlarged, homogeneous, hyperechogenic kidneys	Large cystic kidneys, sometimes asymmetric
Histology	Collecting duct ectasia, cysts derived principally from the collecting duct	Microcysts and macrocysts derived from the entire nephron
Liver	Always congenital hepatic fibrosis but of varying severity	Cysts, mostly in adults (very rarely a newborn may have congenital hepatic fibrosis)
Other system involvement	None	Intracranial aneurysms, colonic diverticula, mitral valve regurgitation, cysts of other organs

From Glassberg KI. Renal dysgenesis and cystic disease of the kidney. In Walsh PC et al, editors: *Campbell's urology,* ed 8, Philadelphia, 2002, Saunders, p 1944.

addition to the renal changes, all children will have some degree of hepatic fibrosis. In general, the less cystic involvement of the kidney, the greater the fibrotic involvement of the liver.[12] Younger mortality age is associated with more kidney involvement. Conversely, children with greater liver involvement may die of hepatic complications such as liver cirrhosis, portal hypertension, or ruptured esophageal varices.[13]

Clinical Manifestations. Fetal and newborn sonograms will show extremely enlarged hyperechogenic (increased sound vibrations) kidneys as a result of the multiple surfaces created by the cystic collecting ducts (Figure 27-2).[12] Oligohydramnios (decreased amniotic fluid) is often present because of the small amounts of fetal urine.[2,12,13] Large flank masses are a characteristic sign. Renal function varies according to the degree of cystic involvement. Urinary problems, especially chronic urinary tract infections and gross or microscopic hematuria, are often present.[12-14] Hypertension is a common finding, and Potter syndrome is sometimes associated.

Autosomal Dominant Polycystic Kidney Disease

Autosomal dominant polycystic kidney disease has an incidence rate of between 1 in 500 and 1 in 1000 and accounts for 9% to 10% of dialysis-requiring kidney failure in the United States and Europe.[12] Although sometimes called adult polycystic kidney disease, this terminology is a misnomer. The diagnosis of ADPKD can sometimes be made prenatally, and the age at diagnosis is becoming progressively lower because the prevalence of screening is increasing in families with a history of ADPKD.

Etiology and Pathogenesis. ADPKD has been linked to two chromosomes. The majority (95%) of cases are believed to be related to a defect on the short arm of chromosome 16, and the remaining 5% are due to a gene on chromosome 4.[12] The pathologic process is not clearly understood, but tubular epithelial cell hyperplasia is thought to be the primary cause of cyst development.[12] In contrast to recessive polycystic disease, cysts involve the entire nephron. Cerebral aneurysms, cardiac valve abnormalities, colonic diverticula, and cysts on other organs are the most common associated pathologic processes.[14] When present, hepatic cysts are rarely symptomatic as opposed to the morbidity and mortality associated with the hepatic fibrosis found in ARPKD.[12]

Clinical Manifestations. Symptoms associated with ADPKD most often occur between the ages of 30 and 50 years. Early manifestations include urinary tract infections, back or flank pain, hematuria, and hypertension. Scans show bilaterally enlarged kidneys. Renal function may or may not be significantly impaired at the time of diagnosis. Men generally have more renal involvement than women, and renal function deteriorates more quickly in men.[12] The age at which renal failure ensues is extremely variable, but many patients are in their 70s or 80s.[13]

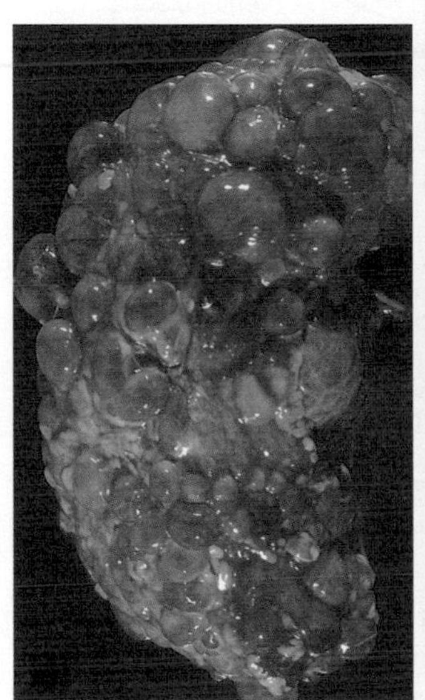
A

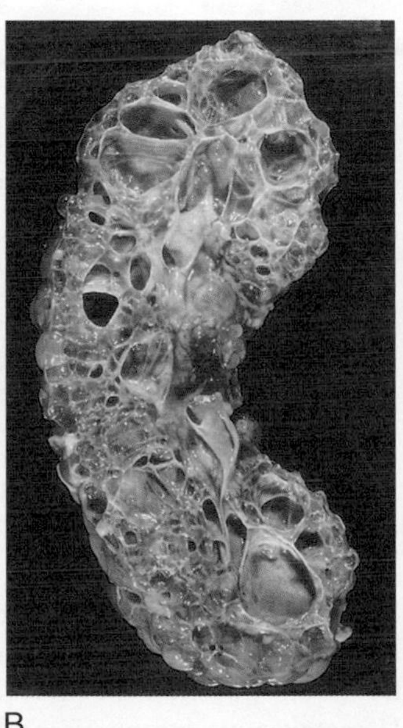
B

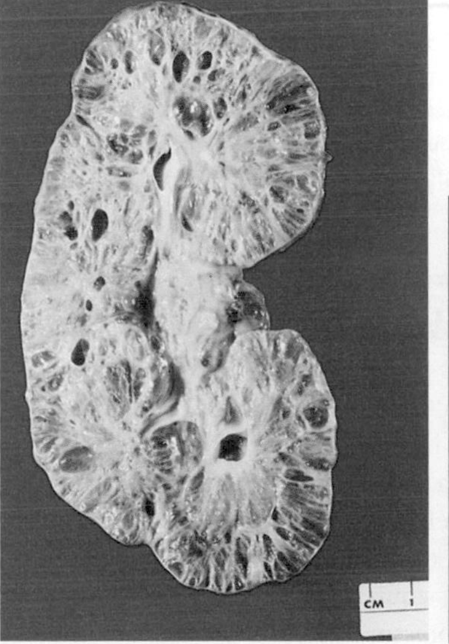

C

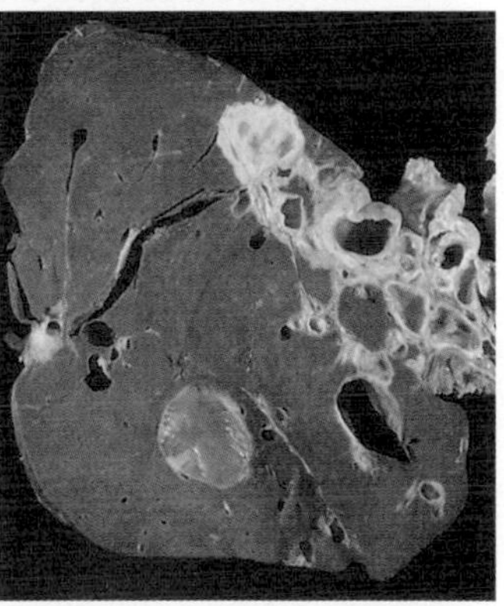
D

FIGURE 27-2 ■ **A** and **B,** Autosomal dominant polycystic kidney disease. Note the fluid-filled cysts on the external surface of the enlarged kidney **(A)** and the loss of parenchymal tissue with extensive cyst formation in the cut kidney **(B)**. **C,** A kidney from a child with autosomal recessive polycystic kidney disease. The cysts occur at right angles to the cortical surface. **D,** The liver can also become cystic in autosomal dominant polycystic kidney disease. (From Cotran RS, Kumar V, Collins T: *Robbins pathologic basis of disease,* ed 6, Philadelphia, 1999, Saunders, p 939.)

Diagnosis and Treatment. Diagnosis and treatment for both forms of polycystic disease are similar despite etiologic and pathologic differences. Diagnostic procedures include renal ultrasonography, **intravenous pyelography (IVP)**, and, occasionally, open surgical biopsy of the kidney and liver to distinguish between the recessive and dominant forms of the disease and multiple simple cysts or medullary sponge kidney.

Treatment is supportive for hypertension, urinary tract infections, cirrhosis, and renal failure. Colonic diverticula may also be present in patients with ADPKD. Renal dialysis and transplantation are appropriate treatment modalities for both types of polycystic disease. In patients in whom cirrhosis and portal hypertension develop as a result of hepatic fibrosis, the prognosis is generally poor. A familial history extending back three generations and genetic counseling are essential for either form of polycystic disease. Because ARPKD is a recessive trait, neither parent should be affected, but siblings have a 1 in 4 chance of having recessive polycystic disease. In contrast, ADPKD is a dominant trait, so half the children of patients with this disease are likely to also be affected.

KEY CONCEPTS

- Renal agenesis is relatively rare, and its presence is often associated with other congenital malformations. Bilateral renal agenesis is not compatible with life. Unilateral renal agenesis results in compensatory hypertrophy of the functional kidney. A single normal kidney is sufficient for renal function.
- Polycystic kidney disease is a genetically transmitted renal disorder. Autosomal recessive forms are evident at birth. In the autosomal dominant type, symptoms generally occur later in life. The collecting ducts have multiple dilations that progress to disrupt urine formation and flow. The inevitability of renal failure necessitates dialysis or transplantation.

INFECTIOUS DISORDERS

Normally, several mechanisms protect the renal system from infection. Chemically, the acidic pH and the presence of urea in the urine produce a relatively hostile environment for bacterial growth. Mechanically, bacteria that may exist in small numbers are washed out from the system during micturition. **Reflux** of urine from the bladder to the kidney via the ureter is prevented by the contraction of the vesicoureteral junction that occurs when the bladder fills, and pressure against the bladder wall constricts the junction into a closed position (see discussion of vesicoureteral reflux in Chapter 29). Bacteriostatic prostatic secretions in men also act as a protective mechanism.

The most common causative agents of renal system infection are gram-negative bacteria such as *Escherichia coli, Enterobacter,* and *Proteus,* which are introduced into the kidney by retrograde flow of urine from the bladder and ureter. Other causative organisms include gram-positive bacteria such as *Staphylococcus,* tuberculous bacilli, and fungi.[15] **Pyelonephritis** is an infection of the renal pelvis and interstitium. Hematogenous, lymphatic, and urinary pathways provide entry routes for infecting organisms, but admission from the lower urinary tract is by far the most common. Predisposing factors include vesicoureteral reflux (Figure 27-3), pregnancy, neurogenic bladder, instrumentation (catheterization, cystoscopy), urinary obstruction, and female sexual trauma.[2,16] Infection of the lower urinary tract is discussed in Chapter 29.

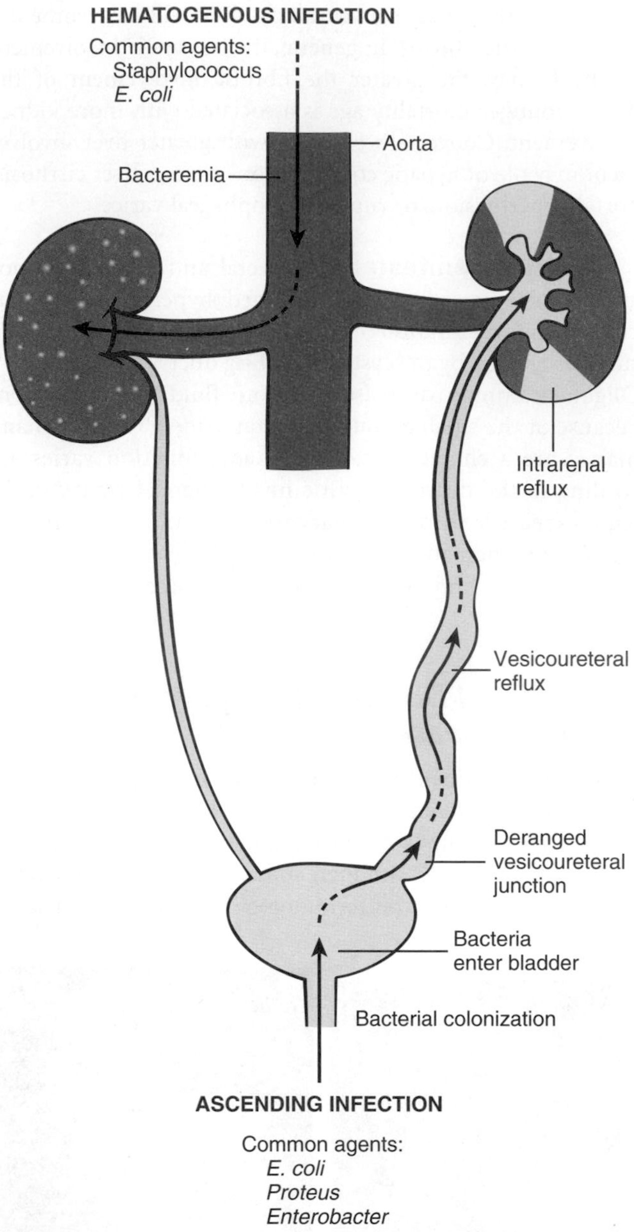

FIGURE 27-3 ■ Pathways of renal infection. Hematogenous infection results from bacteremic spread. More common is ascending infection, which results from a combination of urinary bladder infection, vesicoureteral reflux, and intrarenal reflux. (From Cotran RS, Kumar V, Collins T: *Robbins pathologic basis of disease,* ed 7, Philadelphia, 2003, Saunders, p 527.)

Acute Pyelonephritis

Pathogenesis. Bacterial colonization commonly occurs in the renal papilla as a result of the increased osmolarity. Increased osmolarity interferes with white blood cell (WBC) and complement function, thus allowing bacteria to multiply. Bacteria ascending from the lower urinary tract seed in the renal calices and papillae first, whereas infection from a hematogenous source starts in the medulla of the kidney. Regardless of the cause, within 2 to 3 days the infection spreads to the parenchyma and creates a widespread inflammatory response that results in arterial constriction and edema in the affected portions of the kidneys. Renal scarring resulting in compromised kidney function is rare in otherwise healthy adults if the infection is promptly managed. However, scarring is a more common sequela of pyelonephritis in infants, children, pregnant women, and adults with other comorbidities that inhibit either diagnosis, management, or response to antibiotic therapy.[3,15] Prevention of renal scarring is dependent on prompt and effective treatment of the infection in all age groups.

Clinical Manifestations. Symptoms of acute pyelonephritis vary among age groups and from person to person. Classic symptoms in adults are fever and chills of sudden onset, flank pain, and symptoms of urinary tract infection such as dysuria and urinary frequency or urgency. The hallmark symptom is tenderness or pain at the costovertebral angle on palpation. However, pyelonephritis may be present without these usual symptoms. Urinary tract infections, including pyelonephritis, should be suspected in infants, children, and elderly patients with more generalized symptoms such as irritability, fever and malaise, and decreased oral intake.[15] Occasionally, kidney infections are manifested by abdominal pain, nausea, and vomiting.

Diagnosis and Treatment. The diagnosis of acute pyelonephritis is based on the patient's history, symptoms, physical examination findings, and laboratory values. Urinalysis usually shows WBCs, occasional red blood cells, and WBC casts.[17] If the causative organism is fungal, commonly *Candida,* yeast will be found on urinalysis. Urine culture and sensitivity testing are required to identify the causative organism and indicate which antiinfective agent may be suitable. A complete blood cell count may reveal an elevated total WBC count and an increased percentage of neutrophils, indicative of a bacterial infection.

Upper urinary tract infections generally resolve with treatment in 10 to 14 days in the absence of obstruction or diabetes. If antibiotic therapy (Table 27-4) is successful, the bacteriuria should disappear in 24 hours, although symptoms may remain up to 72 hours. Symptoms beyond 72 hours after initiation of appropriate antibiotic therapy warrant further diagnostic evaluation for complications such as abscesses and obstructions.[17] Hydration adequate to maintain normal or nearly normal glomerular filtration is essential for recovery of the kidney. An attempt should be made to eliminate any medications that tax renal function. Prompt management of existing pyelonephritis and the prevention of future infections via education about predisposing factors are important to avert renal scarring. Children in whom pyelonephritis is diagnosed require additional diagnostic tests once the infection resolves to rule out urologic problems such as vesicoureteral reflux (see Chapter 29).

Table 27-4

Antiinfective Therapy for Pyelonephritis

Infection	Drug Formulation: Oral	Drug Formulation: Parenteral*
Acute pyelonephritis	Sulfonamides Quinolones Tetracycline Ampicillin Amoxicillin (preferred in pregnancy) Cephalosporins Co-trimoxazole-trimethoprim	Quinolones Ampicillin Cephalosporins Aminoglycosides
Recurrent or chronic pyelonephritis	Co-trimoxazole-trimethoprim Nitrofurantoin Quinolones	Aminoglycosides Quinolones

*Used if oral therapy is not tolerated or effective. Children are always initially treated parenterally.

Chronic Pyelonephritis

Chronic pyelonephritis is characterized by unilateral or bilateral pathologic changes in the kidney as a consequence of infection. Small atrophic kidneys with diffuse scarring and blunting of the calices are classic manifestations of chronic pyelonephritis[17] (Figure 27-4). Individuals at risk for chronic pyelonephritis have bacteriuria associated with obstructive uropathy such as renal calculi, neurologic deficits, vesicoureteral reflux, or intrinsic renal disease.

Pathogenesis. As a result of recurrent infections, chronic interstitial inflammation develops, with lymphocyte and plasma cell infiltration of the renal tissue. The interstitium has degrees of dilated or atrophic renal tubules with casts. Fibrosis of the interstitium, including the renal tubules, decreases the number of functional nephrons. Chronic or recurrent pyelonephritis is the second leading cause of renal failure.

Clinical Manifestations. The symptoms of chronic pyelonephritis may be minimal or similar to those of acute

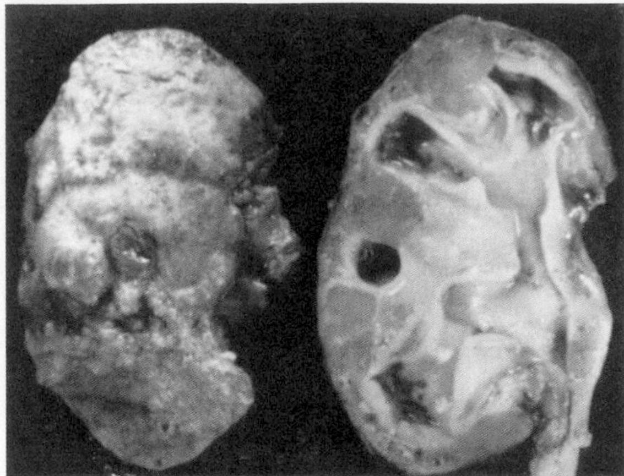

FIGURE 27-4 ■ Chronic pyelonephritis. The surface *(left)* is irregularly scarred. A cut section *(right)* reveals characteristic dilation and blunting of calices. The ureter is dilated and thickened, consistent with chronic vesicoureteral reflux. (From Cotran RS, Kumar V, Collins T: *Robbins pathologic basis of disease,* ed 6, Philadelphia, 1999, Saunders, p 976.)

pyelonephritis. Chronic pyelonephritis is often diagnosed incidentally during the diagnostic evaluation and management of such conditions as hypertension, urinary tract infection, or even **azotemia.**[17] When present, symptoms include frequency and urgency of voiding, dysuria (pain on urination), and flank pain that is vague and less intense than that associated with acute pyelonephritis.

Diagnosis and Treatment. Diagnostic testing consists of urinalysis, IVP, renal ultrasound, and, particularly in children, a voiding cystourethrogram.[17] On urinalysis, bacteriuria may or may not be present, and WBC casts may be seen. On IVP, the architecture of the kidney is distorted, with multiple wedge-shaped scars involving the cortex and papillae.[17] Ultrasonographic scans show a kidney smaller than normal, with clubbing of the affected calices. Voiding cystourethrograms are used to detect vesicoureteral reflux.

Treatment is based on the underlying cause of the disease. Obstructive pathologic processes must be resolved if present. Appropriate antibiotic treatment (see Table 27-4) is implemented according to sensitivity information. Chronic or recurrent disease may necessitate antibiotic therapy for 3 to 6 months.[18]

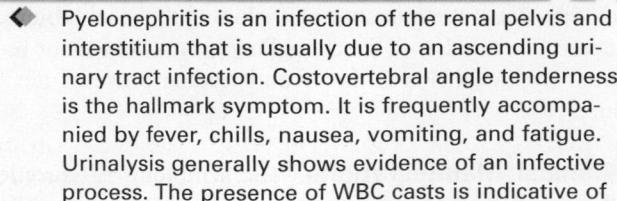

KEY CONCEPTS

- Pyelonephritis is an infection of the renal pelvis and interstitium that is usually due to an ascending urinary tract infection. Costovertebral angle tenderness is the hallmark symptom. It is frequently accompanied by fever, chills, nausea, vomiting, and fatigue. Urinalysis generally shows evidence of an infective process. The presence of WBC casts is indicative of an upper urinary tract infection as opposed to a lower urinary tract infection. When managed promptly and effectively, acute pyelonephritis does not generally result in renal scarring.
- Chronic pyelonephritis is the second leading cause of chronic renal failure. Ascending urinary tract infections are usually associated with obstructive processes leading to persistent urine stasis. Ongoing inflammation causes fibrosis and scarring with loss of functional nephrons. The diagnosis is confirmed with ultrasonography and IVP. Urinalysis may or may not show evidence of an active infection. Treatment includes correction of the underlying obstructive processes and antibiotic therapy.

OBSTRUCTIVE DISORDERS

Obstructive disorders of the renal system or urinary tract interfere with the flow of urine. Obstruction can occur at any point in the system from the renal pelvis to the urethral meatus (Figure 27-5). In general, an obstruction causes dilation of the tract proximal to the obstruction. Stasis of urine occurs and predisposes to infection and structural damage.

Disorders that are obstructive can be congenital or acquired. In children, urinary tract obstruction is usually due to anatomic abnormalities such as ureteral valves, strictures of the urethral meatus, and stenosis at the ureterovesical or ureteral pelvic junction. Obstruction in adults predominantly occurs as a result of acquired disorders and may be either intraluminal or secondary to extrinsic compression (e.g., by renal calculi or tumors) (Table 27-5).[9,10]

Changes that occur within the urinary tract as a result of obstruction are dependent on (1) the degree of obstruction (i.e., partial or complete, unilateral or bilateral) and (2) the duration and timing (acute onset or chronic) of the obstruction. Initially, hydrostatic pressure increases proximal to the obstruction as a consequence of the continued glomerular filtration and obstruction to the flow of urine. Other structures proximal to the obstruction then begin to dilate. The lower or more distal (to the kidney) the obstruction, the less dilation is seen because of the increased surface area over which the pressure is diffused.[9]

Complete obstruction of a ureter causes an accumulation of urine known as **hydroureter.** Pressure in the renal pelvis and tubules increases, with subsequent dilation of both and a flattening of the renal papillae. The glomerular filtration rate (GFR) falls, and the junctional complexes between tubular cells are disrupted. This disruption permits solutes to leak from the tubule into the capillary. Initially, renal perfusion increases because of the effects of prostaglandins on vasodilatation in the renal cortex.[19] After 24 hours, renal blood flow is approximately 55% of normal. Eventually, portions of the kidney become ischemic, and many of the nephrons have decreased filtration rates and are impaired in their ability to conserve sodium, secrete potassium,

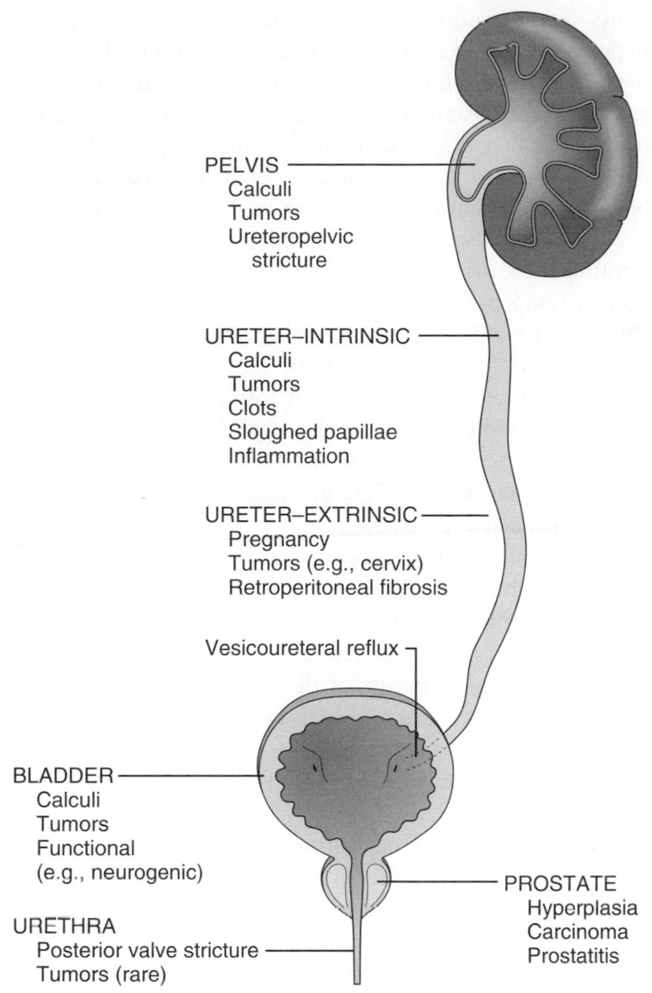

FIGURE 27-5 ■ Obstructive lesions of the urinary tract. (From Cotran RS, Kumar V, Collins T: *Robbins pathologic basis of disease,* ed 6, Philadelphia, 1999, Saunders, p 988.)

and acidify or concentrate urine. In 4 to 6 weeks, tubular atrophy and destruction of the medulla result in scar tissue and nonfunctioning or poorly functioning glomeruli. At this point the renal damage is irreversible.

In partial obstruction, the renal pelvis may become very dilated but the structural or functional disruption of the kidney may be minimal. If the obstruction is bilateral, however, clinical manifestations of fluid retention will be present. Patients often complain of symptoms such as weight gain, nausea, anorexia, malaise, headaches, increased abdominal girth, and ankle edema.[19] Functionally, partial obstruction can produce a slight to moderate decrease in blood flow and GFR and an inability to concentrate urine or secrete potassium and hydrogen ions. Normal or excessive volumes of urine may be excreted despite a reduction in GFR. The risk of dehydration and metabolic acidosis increases as a result of sodium and bicarbonate wasting.

Postobstructive diuresis usually occurs after the obstruction has been corrected, particularly in lower tract and bilateral obstruction. This diuresis is temporary and results from excretion of the sodium, urea, and water that were retained during the obstructive period. The diuresis lasts only until the composition and volume of the body's extracellular fluid return to normal, and therefore symptoms of volume depletion (postural hypotension and tachycardia) do not appear. In some cases a true salt and water wasting occurs and depletes the extracellular volume. In these cases, treatment is instituted to replace two thirds of the urine volume loss per day until the urine output returns to normal. If sodium and water excretion are severe enough to result in significant dehydration and decreased vascular volume, a defect in tubular reabsorptive function is suspected.[19]

Table 27-5

Causes of Renal System Obstruction

Type of Obstruction	Cause
Intraluminal	Calculi, clot Tumor: bladder, urethra, kidney Papillary necrosis
Extrinsic	Prostatic hypertrophy Retroperitoneal fibrosis Tumor: pelvic, retroperitoneal
Acquired	Neurogenic bladder Ureteral stricture Urethral stricture

Complications of urinary obstruction include infection, sepsis, progressive loss of renal function, and renal failure. The combination of infection and obstruction warrants emergency diagnostic testing and immediate relief of the obstruction with percutaneous nephrostomy tubes or ureteral stents to prevent renal failure and possibly death.[19] Prolonged bilateral obstruction or severe partial obstruction leads to acute and chronic renal failure. However, in many cases no clinical data can accurately predict the degree of renal function that can be attained once the unilateral or bilateral obstruction is resolved. Hence relief of the obstruction followed by close observation of renal function is the recommended treatment. Renal function may continue to improve up to 3 months after the obstruction is resolved.

Renal Calculus

Renal calculi consist of crystals of combined organic material that initially form in the calices or pelvis of the kidney.[9,20] These calculi may then migrate down the urinary tract and cause pain, obstruction, and infection. The presence of a stone or **calculus** anywhere in the urinary tract is termed **nephrolithiasis.**

Etiology and Pathogenesis. Renal calculus or nephrolithiasis occurs in 15% of Caucasian men and 6% of all women or 2% to 3% of the general population in industrial countries.[9,21] The rate of recurrence once an individual has had calculus is 50% to 60% within 10 years.[21] Calculus is four times more common in men than women, with the peak incidence occurring in 20- to 40-year-olds.[20,21] Factors influencing calculus formation are supersaturation (increased concentration of the offending solute), an abnormal urine pH, or low urine volume. The pathophysiologic process of stone formation is not completely understood. A complex interrelationship between conditions conducive to crystallization, cellular responses to crystals, the presence of matrix material to enhance mineralization, and substandard activity of the usual processes that inhibit calcium formation is involved in the etiologic progression of calculi.[9,21] Hypercalciuria is the most common physiologic abnormality found in patients with nephrolithiasis. Calcium oxalate or calcium phosphate stones make up 70% to 85% of all renal calculi.[4,9,22] Uric acid, cystine, and struvite make up the remaining portion of calculi. Table 27-6 summarizes the composition and factors contributing to the etiologic progression of different types of stones.

Because the substances that compose renal calculi are normally present in urine and do not cause calculi in everyone, mechanisms must be present that usually inhibit crystallization and supersaturation. These inhibitors are thought to include pyrophosphate, citrate, magnesium, and certain macromolecules such as glycoproteins.[9,20] Citrate seems to inhibit nephrolithiasis by forming a soluble complex with calcium and decreasing calcium activity.[9]

When citrates and magnesium, substances in the urine that inhibit stone formation, are deficient, calcium-type calculi can form. The condition of hypocitraturia can be found in patients with acidosis, chronic diarrhea, thiazide-induced hypocalcemia, and a diet high in animal protein. Hypomagnesuria is usually found in conjunction with hypocitraturia and low urine volume.[9,23] The cause of hypomagnesuria is probably a diet deficient in magnesium. Hyperoxaluria can occur in the setting of pyridoxine deficiency, excessive ascorbic acid, and enhanced absorption of dietary oxalate (enteric hyperoxaluria). Because many stones contain calcium oxalate, limiting oxalate rich foods may be recommended for the management and prevention of stones. Along with spinach and rhubarb, almonds, peanuts, chocolate, and tea may be considered high- to moderate-risk foods.[24]

Uric acid calculi are commonly found in primary gout, in conditions of low urinary pH (less than 5.5), and in hyperuricosuria. Uric acid calculi may also be found in myeloproliferative states, glycogen storage diseases, and malignancies that cause purine overproduction. Chronic diarrhea (ulcerative colitis, regional enteritis) may produce a net alkali deficit and decreased urine volume and thereby precipitate uric acid calculus formation.[22]

Cystinuria that causes cystine calculus results from an inborn error of metabolism of dicarboxylic acids. The urine may become supersaturated with cystine, particularly with a concurrently low urine pH. Struvite calculi form as a result of infection with urea-splitting organisms, usually *Proteus*.[25] *E. coli* does not produce urease and is therefore not linked to struvite calculus. Obstructed urinary drainage, instrumentation, surgery, and chronic antibiotic therapy predispose the patient to *Proteus* infection and struvite calculus.[25]

Table 27-6

Prevalence of Various Types of Renal Stones

Stone	Percentage of All Stones
Calcium oxalate (phosphate)	75
Idiopathic hypercalciuria (50%)	
Hypercalcemia and hypercalciuria (10%)	
Hyperoxaluria (5%)	
Enteric (4.5%)	
Primary (0.5%)	
Hyperuricosuria (20%)	
No known metabolic abnormality (15%-20%)	
Struvite (Mg, NH_3, Ca, PO_4)	10-15
Renal infection	
Uric acid	6
Associated with hyperuricemia	
Associated with hyperuricosuria	
Idiopathic (50% of uric acid stones)	
Cystine	1-2
Others or unknown	±10

From Kumar V, Cotran RS, Robbins ST: *Robbins basic pathology*, ed 7, Philadelphia, Saunders, 2003, p 537.

Clinical Manifestations. While the calculus is in the renal pelvis, usually no symptoms appear unless an infection or obstruction of the kidney is present. As the calculus migrates from the renal pelvis to the ureter, pain known as **ureteral colic** occurs and is the hallmark symptom of this disorder. Ureteral colic usually has an abrupt onset. It is mild at first and then becomes more severe and sharp with time. The pain is unilateral, frequently starting in the flank area and radiating to the ipsilateral (same side) portion of the groin. It results from a calculus obstructing the flow of urine in the ureter. Colicky-type pain, or pain that is rhythmic, occurs as the ureter contracts and attempts to move the stone toward the bladder. Behind the stone the ureter becomes distended with urine and inflamed from the trauma of stone passage.[21]

Diagnosis. Evaluation of a patient for renal calculus includes a thorough history of the current pain episode, as well as a medical history (including prior episodes), dietary history, and medication history. Urinalysis is performed to evaluate for hematuria, urine pH, and the presence of WBCs. Serum blood urea nitrogen (BUN) and creatinine levels are determined to assess renal function. Plain film radiography to view the kidneys, ureter, and bladder (KUB) may help in locating the size and shape of calculi. Ultrasound may be used to detect hydronephrosis, which is commonly seen with obstruction.[21] Computed tomography (CT) is often performed to determine the exact size and location of the stone. Calcium and cystine calculi are radiopaque and may be seen on a plain film. Uric acid stones are radiolucent and not usually seen. IVP may be needed to identify the site of obstruction. Recent concerns with patients using metformin (Glucophage) have led to careful use of dye-related procedures. Current recommendations of the U.S. Food and Drug Administration include discontinuing metformin before these types of procedures and retaining the patient for 48 hours after the procedure.[21]

The pain of ureteral colic is severe and sometimes accompanied by nausea and vomiting. Acute treatment involves the administration of narcotic analgesics and antiemetics and promoting a dilute urine with brisk diuresis. Dilution of the urine helps decrease supersaturation of the involved mineral. Diuresis may facilitate spontaneous movement of the calculi into the bladder. Generally, calculi less than 5 mm in diameter should pass spontaneously. Calculi greater than 5 mm size may pass, if they are located in the distal ureter. All other ureteral stones 5 mm or greater require referral to a urologist and need urologic intervention. Stones left untreated beyond 4 weeks can lead to serious complications.[21] A stone that is too large to pass spontaneously, completely obstructs the ureter or kidney pelvis, or is accompanied by infection should be removed.

Treatment. Shock wave **lithotripsy** is now widely used in the United States to fragment the calculus when it lies in the kidney, renal pelvis, or proximal end of the ureter. The smaller fragments are moved down the ureter to the bladder by urine flow. Larger fragments may be extracted surgically. Lithotripsy can be performed extracorporeally or percutaneously. In extracorporeal shock wave lithotripsy, the patient is submerged in a water tank or water-filled cushions are placed between the patient and the generator, and shock waves are administered from outside the body to precisely target and shatter the stones.[4] In the percutaneous method, a small incision is made in the patient's flank, a cystoscope or some other narrow tube is inserted, and the stone fragments are retrieved through the tube. Lithotripsy is the standard surgical treatment. Removal of stones by open procedures such as pyelolithotomy and ureterolithotomy is now a rare event.

After the acute episode has resolved, treatment is directed at preventing the formation of new calculi. Treatment entails (1) diluting the urine to 2 L or more per day so as to reduce the concentration of calculus-forming substances and (2) decreasing the amount of calculus-forming material in the urine by dietary modification or, when necessary, pharmacologic intervention. Table 27-7 delineates drugs commonly used in the treatment of nephrolithiasis. Many forms of calcium oxalate crystallization protein inhibitors are currently being investigated and may prove useful in preventing recurrent calcium-based kidney stones.[4,9]

Nutritional Considerations. Depending on the type of kidney stone, there are dietary modifications to prevent the formation and recurrence. Foods considered to be high to moderately high in oxalate include peanuts, rhubarb, tea, coffee, spinach, nuts, and chocolate. Limiting these foods has proved helpful.[9,24] Furthermore, consumption of adequate amounts of calcium and vitamin D prevents unnecessary bone reabsorption, parathyroid activation, and hypercalciuria.[26] Uric acid stone formation can be reduced by limiting the

Table 27-7

Medications Commonly Used for Nephrolithiasis Treatment

Medication	Therapeutic Effect	Indications	Potential Adverse Effects
Thiazide diuretics	Decrease urinary calcium	Hypercalciuria	Side effects, limited long-term effect
Potassium citrate	Increase urinary citrate, treat hypokalemia, correct metabolic acidosis	Hypocitraturia, hyperuricosuria, cystinuria, enteric hyperoxaluria	
Cellulose sodium phosphate (Calcibind)	Bind calcium in gut, decrease calcium absorption	Hypercalciuria	Hypomagnesemia, hypomagnesuria, hyperoxaluria
Allopurinol (Zyloprim)	Decrease uric acid secretion	Hyperuricemia, hyperuricosuria	Dermatitis liver necrosis
Penicillamine (Cuprimine, Depen) or α-mercapto-propionylglycine	Decrease urinary cystine	Cystinuria	Pancytopenia, dysgeusia, nephrotic syndrome
Captopril (Capoten)	Bind cystine	Cystinuria	
Orthophosphates	Reduce serum vitamin D and urinary calcium	Renal phosphate leak, hypercalcemia	Contraindicated with urinary tract infections
Acetohydroxamic acid (Lithostat) with antibiotics	Inhibit urease and prevent breakdown of urea into ammonia	Struvite stones	Hemolytic anemia in about 3% of patients

Adapted from Trivedi BK: Nephrolithiasis: how it happens and what to do about it, *Postgrad Med* 100(6):72, 1996.

consumption of animal protein, especially organ meats, fish, and purine-rich foods. High fluid intake, reduced sodium intake, adequate potassium, and a diet with plenty of fruit and vegetables are important factors in preventing the formation of stones of various compositions.[4,23,24]

KEY CONCEPTS

- Obstructive processes result in urine stasis, which predisposes to infection and structural damage. Common causes of obstruction include stones, tumors, prostatic hypertrophy, and strictures of the ureters or urethra.
- Complete obstruction results in hydronephrosis, decreased GFR, and ischemic kidney damage because of increased intraluminal pressure. A period of diuresis may follow relief of the obstruction.
- Stones tend to form in the urinary tract under conditions of high solute concentration, low urine volume, and abnormal urine pH. Certain substances in the urine (e.g., magnesium, citrate) are thought to inhibit stone formation. Deficiencies may predispose to stone formation.
- Most stones are composed of calcium crystals. Other forms include uric acid, cystine, and struvite. Calcium and cystine stones are radiopaque and detectable on plain radiographs. Uric acid stones are usually undetectable on radiographs.
- Stationary stones in the renal pelvis are generally asymptomatic. When the stone migrates to the ureter, intense renal colic pain ensues. Pain is usually abrupt in onset and unilateral.
- Stones may pass spontaneously or require dissolution by shock waves (lithotripsy) or surgical excision. Stones tend to recur, and attention to prevention is indicated. High fluid intake to dilute the urine and dietary changes are standard prophylactic therapy.

TUMORS

Renal tumors are divided into three groups: (1) benign, (2) primary neoplasms, and (3) secondary neoplasms (Box 27-1). All tumors distort the architecture of the kidney and renal system and thus hinder renal function. Malignant tumors also carry the threat of metastasis to distant sites.

Benign Renal Tumors

Benign renal tumors account for a small percentage of renal system tumors.

Types of Benign Renal Tumors. Renal **oncocytomas** may develop due to familial linage and are often slow growing.[27] These tumors tend to be asymptomatic and are discovered incidentally. Oncocytomas have a characteristic mahogany brown color and are well circumscribed. Histologically, oncocytomas contain large eosinophilic cells that have granular cytoplasm and round uniform nuclei.[28] **Mesoblastic nephroma** is a benign congenital tumor of infancy. Unlike Wilms tumor (nephroblastoma), this tumor is diagnosed at birth or in the child's first few months. **Renal angiomyolipoma (hamartoma)** type tumors are found in adults, including approximately 80% of patients with tuberous sclerosis (an autosomal dominant disease manifested as mental retardation, epilepsy, and fat gland adenomas).[29] These lesions are composed of abdominal blood vessels, clusters of adipocytes, and sheets of smooth muscle.[29] Discovery of the tumor may be incidental to evaluation for another condition. Larger tumors may cause abdominal discomfort, or patients may complain of flank pain with or without light-headedness and syncope from hemorrhage within the tumor.[28] Renal angiomyolipomas are often found in multiple areas in both kidneys.

Other benign renal tumors include fibromas, lipomas, leiomyomas, and hemangiomas. Fibromas are fibrous masses of the renal medulla; they are usually found in females. Lipomas consist of adipose tissue within or around the kidney. Leiomyomas are retroperitoneal tumors that form from the renal capsule or vessels. Hemangiomas are manifested by hematuria for which no other explanation can be found. A more common renal tumor is a **renal adenoma,** which is histologically similar to adenocarcinoma but is less than 3 cm in diameter. Thus controversy exists about whether these are benign tumors or very early stage malignant adenocarcinoma. Hence the term "renal neoplasm of low malignant potential" is sometimes used to describe adenomas.[28]

Treatment. Treatment for benign tumors is nephrectomy when symptoms of caliceal destruction are present.

Box 27-1

Renal Tumors

Benign Tumors
Adenoma
Oncocytoma
Mesoblastic tumor
Nephroma
Hamartoma
Leiomyoma
Hemangioma

Primary Neoplasms
Renal cell carcinoma (adenocarcinoma)
Nephroblastoma
Urothelial carcinoma
Sarcoma

Secondary Neoplasms (Listed by Primary Sites)
Adrenal carcinoma
Retroperitoneal sarcoma
Pancreatic, colon, lung, stomach, or breast cancer
Lymphoma, Hodgkin disease, multiple myeloma

Asymptomatic tumors may be observed. Treatment for renal adenomas is radical nephrectomy because of the risk of progression to renal adenocarcinoma.[6]

Renal Cell Carcinoma

Renal cell carcinoma (RCC), also known as renal adenocarcinoma, accounts for approximately 1.9% of all malignancies and 85% of newly diagnosed renal malignancies.[5] It results in more than 78,000 renal cancer related deaths per year. Interestingly, developed countries have a higher incidence of RCC than underdeveloped countries.[30]

Etiology and Pathogenesis. RCC may be diagnosed at any age but is most common in adults between 50 and 70 years old. Males are affected two to three times as often as females. Associated risk factors include occupational exposure to petroleum products, heavy metals, and asbestos; a high-protein diet; cigarette smoking; obesity; hypertension; the use of antihypertensive medications and diuretics; disease in a family member; horseshoe kidney; ADPKD; and acquired renal cystic disease from long-term (3 years or more) hemodialysis.[6,30] RCC arises from the epithelium of the proximal convoluted tubule and has been linked to a defect in chromosome 3 (Figure 27-6).[30]

Clinical Manifestations. The classic triad of symptoms in RCC consists of hematuria, flank pain, and a flank or abdominal mass that is sometimes palpable (Table 27-8) Elevated erythrocyte sedimentation rate is often an associated finding. RCC comes with poor prognosis, and approximately 40% of all patients will die within a few years.[31] However, of tumors discovered incidentally (usually when CT or ultrasound is being performed for some other reason), 75% are confined to the renal capsule (stage I), and 75% of these patients survive at least 5 years.[32]

Systemic symptoms or **paraneoplastic syndromes** are present in many patients with RCC. Fatigability, weight loss, and cachexia are common. Fever, anemia, hypertension, hepatic dysfunction, erythrocytosis, hypercalcemia, and an increased erythrocyte sedimentation rate also occur.[31] Hormone substances may be produced by RCC. Hypercalcemia can be caused by an excess of a substance generated from the tumor that mimics parathyroid hormone and prostaglandins, or it may be a sign of skeletal metastasis.[33] Hypertension occurs in 20% to 40% of patients as a result of excess renin production. Increased glucocorticoids can be manifested as Cushing syndrome. Tumor invasion into the renal vein or inferior vena cava can cause lower extremity edema. Hepatosplenomegaly and ascites can develop if the tumor extends into the hepatic vein or the inferior vena cava. Metastasis occurs in the lymph nodes, ipsilateral adrenal gland, lung, and long bones (Figure 27-7).

Diagnosis. Urinalysis is the initial study done to evaluate hematuria, but IVP is the examination performed most often to detect a tumor. Renal ultrasonography may be used to differentiate a cystic lesion from a tumor. Needle aspiration may be performed to obtain cyst fluid for cytologic analysis. CT and magnetic resonance imaging (MRI) are used in the diagnosis and staging of RCC. The TNM staging system is most widely accepted system for pathologic evaluation of RCC.[32]

Treatment. Management of adenocarcinoma generally involves radical nephrectomy (removal of the affected kidney, the ipsilateral adrenal gland, the fascia, and the local hilar lymph nodes). Partial nephrectomy is necessary for patients with bilateral RCC or carcinoma in the patient's only anatomic or functional kidney.[5] Surprisingly, 5-year survival rates after partial nephrectomy have ranged from 73% to 92% for patients with stage I disease.[34] Unfortunately, 20% to 30%

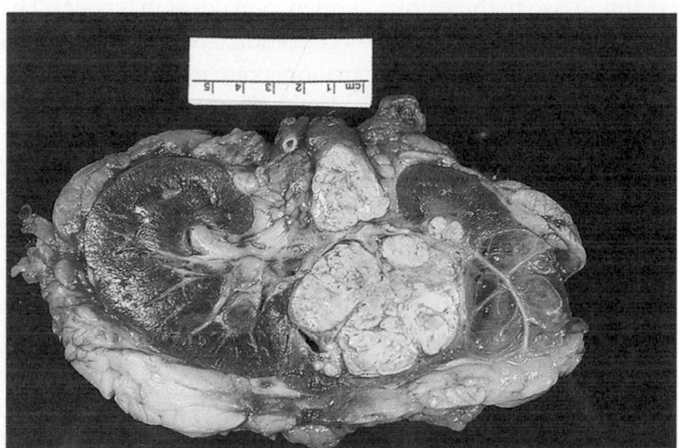

FIGURE 27-6 ■ Renal cell carcinoma with extension into the renal vein. (From Walsh PC et al, editors: *Campbell's urology,* ed 8, Philadelphia, 2002, Saunders, p 2693.)

Table 27-8

Initial Characteristics of Patients with Renal Cell Carcinoma

Characteristics	Incidence (%)
Hematuria	40-60
Flank or abdominal pain	40
Palpable mass	30
Weight loss	20-30
Anemia	20
Triad of hematuria, palpable mass, and pain	10
Fever	2-12

From Gold PJ, Fefer A, Thompson JA: Paraneoplastic manifestations of renal cell carcinoma, *Semin Urol Oncol* 14(4):216-222, 1996.

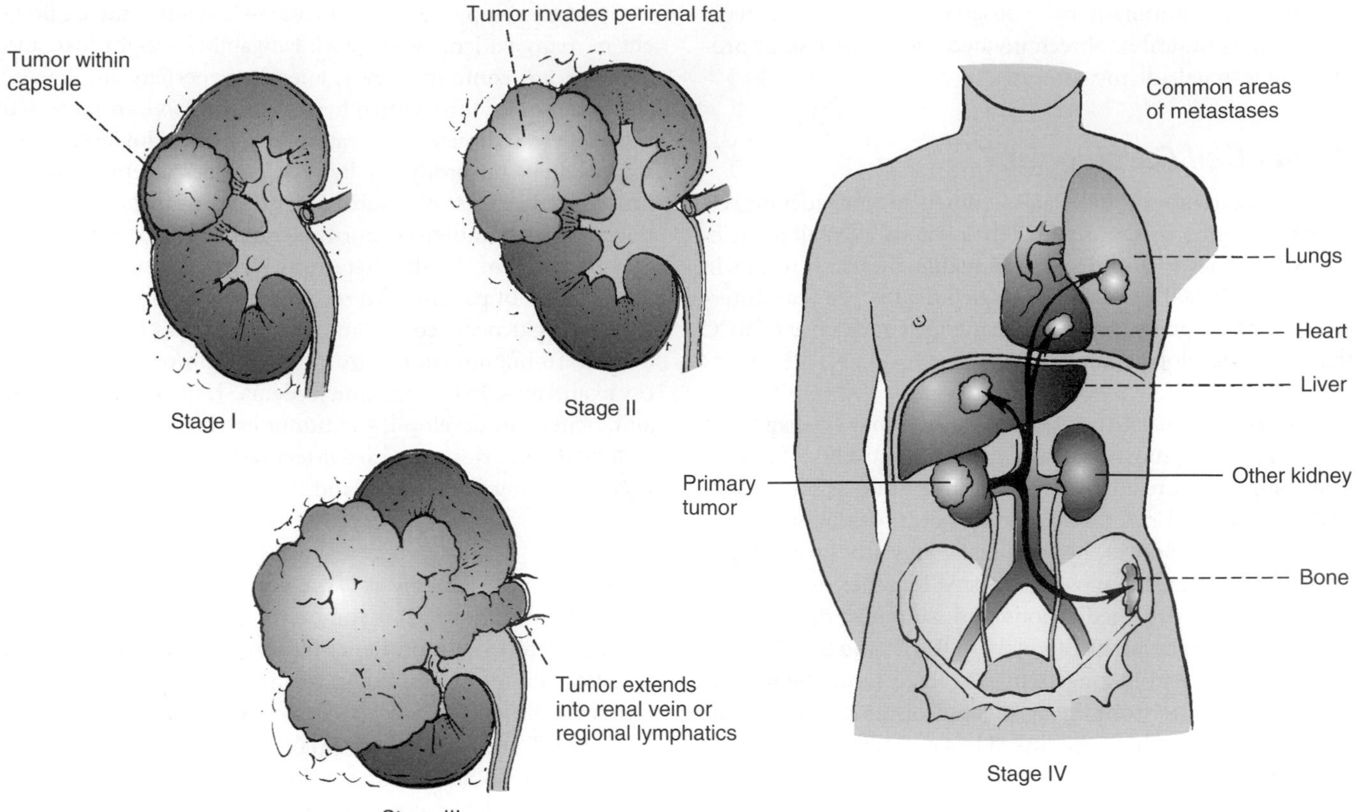

FIGURE 27-7 ■ A staging system of renal carcinoma shows the tumor confined within the renal capsule in stage I, the tumor extending beyond the renal capsule in stage II, the tumor extending into the renal vein or lymphatics in stage III, and tumor metastasis to other parts of the body in stage IV. (From Black JM, Matassarin-Jacobs E: *Medical-surgical nursing: clinical management for continuity of care,* ed 7, Philadelphia, 2005, Saunders, p 923.)

of patients with localized tumors eventually have a relapse of the disease, with lung metastasis the most common site of recurrence.[34] RCC is resistant to radiation and chemotherapy.[1] Metastatic RCC has a very poor prognosis with survival rates of 6 to 12 months from time of diagnosis. However, immunotherapy with interleukin-2 (IL-2) and interferon-α have produced antitumor responses in some patients. Ongoing research is focused at further developments in immunotherapy to improve survival rates. IL-2 activates natural killer cells, whereas interferon-α affects tumor cell growth and other mechanisms that are not yet clear.[35-37]

Urothelial Tumors

Urothelial tumors are malignant tumors of the lining of the renal pelvis, calices, ureter, and bladder. Urothelial tumors in the renal pelvis account for about 10% of all renal cancers. The majority (90%) of bladder tumors are transitional cell carcinomas. The remaining 10% are squamous cell carcinomas and adenocarcinomas.[38,39]

Etiology and Pathogenesis. Risk factors for transitional cell carcinoma include cigarette smoking; excessive coffee intake; occupational exposure to aromatics and amines; chronic abuse of analgesics containing aspirin and phenacetin; a history of urinary tract infections, calculus, or obstruction; a history of cyclophosphamide use; several familial cancer syndromes; and Balkan endemic nephropathy.[38,39] Transitional cell carcinomas are found two to three times as often in males as in females. The peak age range of occurrence of transitional cell carcinoma is 50 to 60 years. Transitional cell carcinomas are multifocal and may occur simultaneously in more than one site. Although most of the transitional cell carcinomas are located in the bladder, 5% of patients have upper tract tumors at diagnosis.[38] Furthermore, patients who have a site of disease in the renal pelvis may also have tumors in the ureter and bladder or anywhere along the urothelium. Transitional cell carcinoma grows slowly and is generally noninvasive; however, when metastasis occurs, it is usually to the lung and bone.

Clinical Manifestations and Diagnosis. Hematuria, either gross or microscopic, is an initial finding in more than 90% of patients.[38] Other manifestations include dull flank pain and acute pain with the passing of blood clots or, when tumors are more advanced, an abdominal or flank mass, bone pain, weight loss, and anorexia.[40] IVP shows a filling defect in the system. Renal ultrasonography, cystoscopy, retrograde pyelography, ureteroscopy, and nephroscopy may also be used in the diagnosis. Urine cytology studies are useful to isolate tumor cells but do not pinpoint the site of the tumor because urothelial transitional cell carcinomas are morphologically alike, regardless of where in the system they occur. CT and radionuclide scintigraphy are performed to evaluate the presence or extent of metastasis. Examination of the entire urinary tract, including the side opposite the initial tumor, is done before surgery because of the multifocal nature of transitional cell carcinoma. Evaluation of a patient with hematuria would also include complete history, physical examination, and pelvic examination and rectal examinations.[38]

Treatment. The usual treatment for renal urothelial cancer is radical nephroureterectomy, which involves a radical nephrectomy and removal of the entire ureter. The 5-year survival rate after surgery is approximately 90% because the tumors are generally low grade and noninvasive.[40] Management of transitional cell carcinoma of the bladder begins with a transurethral resection.[41] In patients with invasive or high-grade lesions, the 5-year survival rate ranges from zero to approximately 40% depending on the exact stage of the disease. Radiation therapy after surgery has led to slight improvement in local recurrence and long-term survival rates. Chemotherapy is used to manage metastatic transitional cell carcinomas.

Nephroblastoma

Nephroblastoma, or Wilms tumor, is the most common abdominal tumor in children. It can be found in adults but is rare in patients older than 15 years. In most cases, the onset is between 3 and 5 years of age.[1] Males and females are equally affected.

Etiology and Pathogenesis. A defect on chromosome 11p13 is the primary etiologic basis of Wilms tumors.[42] This defect results in abnormal growth of metanephric blastema without normal differentiation into tubules and glomeruli. Approximately 15% of children with Wilms tumors have other abnormalities, including Wilms aniridia–genital anomaly–retardation syndrome, Beckwith-Wiedemann syndrome, hemihypertrophy, musculoskeletal anomalies, and other genitourinary anomalies.[42,43]

Clinical Manifestations. Nephroblastoma is initially identified by a parent or physician on routine physical examination. A tumor or mass of the flank or abdomen is palpable in about 80% of cases. Abdominal pain, hypertension, and microscopic hematuria are other common manifestations.[44] Sudden onset of pain and fever and findings of an abdominal mass, anemia, and hypertension indicate subcapsular hemorrhage of the Wilms tumor.[44]

Diagnosis. The diagnosis of nephroblastoma is established with IVP, which usually shows caliceal distortion and occasionally calcification within the tumor mass. Renal ultrasound, CT (with contrast), and MRI are used to evaluate tumor extension and the possibility of bilateral tumors. Widespread availability will favor renal ultrasound and CT as first choices for diagnostic tests.[43] Nephroblastoma may produce a tumor thrombus in the inferior vena cava, which can lead to decreased venous return and lower extremity edema. Metastasis occurs most often to the lungs, so chest radiographs are also indicated. Other areas of metastasis are the liver, opposite kidney, central nervous system, and bone.[42,43]

Treatment. Treatment entails complete removal of the primary tumor and kidney. Survival depends on both the histologic type of the tumor and the presence of metastases. The 4-year survival rate for patients with favorable histology is 90%. Histologically, anaplasia, in which cells have extreme nuclear atypia, yields an unfavorable prognosis. Radiation and chemotherapy are administered postoperatively and may also be administered preoperatively to shrink the size of bilateral or very large or invasive tumors before resection.[43]

KEY CONCEPTS

- The kidney can be host to a number of benign and malignant primary tumors. Symptoms depend on the location of the growth. Obstruction, hematuria, and flank pain may occur. Tumor stage is usually advanced when symptoms occur.
- Tumors are usually detected with IVP. Imaging and histologic studies may be used to diagnose and stage the tumor. Nephrectomy remains the treatment of choice for renal tumors. Adjacent structures may also be removed if the tumor is malignant.
- RCC is particularly resistant to hormone therapy, radiation therapy, immunotherapy, and chemotherapy. Thus the prognosis for late-stage disease and recurrent cancer is poor.
- Nephroblastoma, or Wilms tumor, is the most common kidney cancer in children. Nephrectomy, radiation therapy, and chemotherapy are used in the management of nephroblastomas. Associated mortality rates are highly dependent on tumor stage and histopathologic state.

GLOMERULAR ABNORMALITIES

Glomerular abnormalities result from alterations in the structure and function of the glomerular capillary circulation. **Primary glomerulopathies** are disease states in which the kidney is the only or the predominant organ involved, and **secondary glomerulopathies** result from drug exposure or infection and glomerular injury in the setting of multisystem or vascular abnormalities. Alterations in glomerular capillary circulation may result in any of the following: hematuria, proteinuria, decreased GFR, and hypertension.

GLOMERULONEPHRITIS

Glomerulonephritis, or inflammation of the glomeruli, may result from immunologic abnormalities, drug exposure, toxins, or vascular and systemic disease.

Acute Glomerulonephritis

Acute glomerulonephritis is a syndrome of disorders characterized by an abrupt onset of hematuria and proteinuria in conjunction with azotemia and renal sodium and water retention.[1] RBC casts indicate glomerular bleeding and may be found microscopically.[7] Common triggers of acute glomerulonephritis are listed in Box 27-2.

Pathogenesis. The infectious processes and diseases listed in Box 27-2 indirectly cause or trigger acute glomerulonephritis by activating inflammatory cells (Figure 27-8). Circulating inflammatory cells infiltrate the glomerular capillary walls and establish antibody-antigen complexes within the glomeruli. Once the antibody-antigen complex has been established in the glomerular capillary wall, complement is deposited and attracts neutrophils and monocytes. Lysosomal enzymes are then released and damage glomerular walls. This change in the structure of the glomerular wall results in a more permeable membrane. In essence, larger gaps in the glomerular wall decrease the surface area for filtering and allow previously restricted molecules to enter the glomerular space. Two other processes are also thought to take place. Local vasoactive compounds such as angiotensin and leukotrienes contract mesangial cells and reduce perfusion to glomerular capillaries, and the Bowman space may also be damaged as a result of fibrin deposition and crescent formation (accumulation of proliferating cells within the Bowman space in the form of a crescent).[44] Fluid retention is due to a decrease in GFR and distal tubule water and sodium reabsorption.[44] Water and sodium reabsorption increases the vascular and extracellular fluid volume of the patient. Hematuria and evidence of RBC casts result because erythrocytes are now able to cross the more permeable glomerular or peritubular walls into proximal tubule fluid (which is eventually urine).

Clinical Manifestations. Urinary abnormalities may vary in severity. Gross hematuria manifested as smoky or coffee-colored urine is the most common finding. Red cell casts are classic indicators of glomerulonephritis and represent erythrocytes that have crossed from the glomerular capillary into the tubule and then assumed the shape of the tubule. White cell casts may also be present, particularly when inflammation is present in the glomerulus and interstitium.[44] Proteinuria, or the loss of more than 3 g of protein per day, is generally present. If the protein loss is extreme or continues for an extended period, the nephrotic syndrome may appear.[1]

Systemically, disruptions related to fluid volume changes are the major manifestations. Periorbital edema is the most common area for fluid retention, although edema may progress to dependent body areas and create lower extremity edema, ascites, and pleural effusion.[44] Edema occurs not only as a result of fluid volume excess but also as a result of protein loss causing a decrease in plasma oncotic pressure, which allows fluid to leave the vascular space to enter the interstitial spaces. Arterial diastolic hypertension results from increased extracellular fluid volume, increased cardiac output, and increased peripheral vascular resistance.[44]

Diagnosis. Evaluation is based on the patient's history, with particular attention to risk factors or previous symptoms

Box 27-2

Triggers of Acute Glomerulonephritis

Infectious
Poststreptococcal glomerulonephritis
Nonstreptococcal/postinfectious glomerulonephritis

Bacterial
Infective endocarditis
Meningococcemia
Pneumococcal pneumonia
Sepsis

Viral
Hepatitis B
Hepatitis C (associated cryoglobinemia)
Mononucleosis
Mumps/measles
Varicella

Parasitic
Malaria
Toxoplasmosis

Primary Disease
Berger disease (IgA nephropathy)
Mesangial proliferative
Mesangiocapillary glomerulonephritis

Multisystem Disease
Goodpasture syndrome
Henoch-Schönlein purpura
Polyarteritis nodosa
Systemic lupus erythematosus
Vasculitis

Miscellaneous
Guillain-Barré syndrome
Serum sickness
Irradiation for Wilms tumor

such as a sore throat, myalgias, arthralgias, or rash that may indicate an illness or disease that could have initiated an immune response. Progression of the symptoms is also used to determine the diagnosis. Urinalysis to detect hematuria, proteinuria, and red or white cell casts is the initial diagnostic test. If the glomerulonephritis is thought to be poststreptococcal, antibodies such as antistreptolysin O and antistreptokinase are evaluated. Serum renal indicators such as BUN and creatinine levels are evaluated to estimate the extent of renal damage. Obtaining serum complement levels such as C3 and C4 are helpful in determining hypocomplementemic states. Examples of low serum complement associated with acute glomerulonephritis include systemic lupus erythematosus, cryoglobulinemia, and subacute bacterial endocarditis.[7] A renal biopsy may be necessary for definitive diagnosis because clinical manifestations vary from person to person and different glomerular diseases have similar clinical features. Figure 27-9 presents a diagrammatic cross-section of a normal glomerular lobe, and Figure 27-10 illustrates a lobe with membranous glomerulonephritis.

Treatment. Treatment is based on the underlying causative mechanism. Commonly, azotemia is transient, with only a short period of oliguria; however, longer periods of impaired renal function are occasionally observed in which case the patient requires dialysis.[41] A diuresis then occurs in days to weeks, and the GFR returns to normal or near-normal. In otherwise healthy individuals, infectious diseases tend to respond quickly to the appropriate antiinfective agent. Medical management may also include antihypertensives, steroids, diuretics, and dietary sodium restriction.[7] It is always possible that the current episode will evolve into rapidly progressing or chronic glomerulonephritis. Many patients with poor health status before the onset of acute glomerulonephritis, especially those who are immunocompromised, may have persistent renal disease.[1]

Rapidly Progressing Glomerulonephritis

The combination of abrupt hematuria, proteinuria, and red cell casts followed by a swift decline in renal function is a syndrome known as **rapidly progressing glomerulonephritis** (RPGN).[45,46]

Etiology and Pathogenesis. RPGN is found primarily in adults and makes up 2% to 4% of all cases of glomeru-

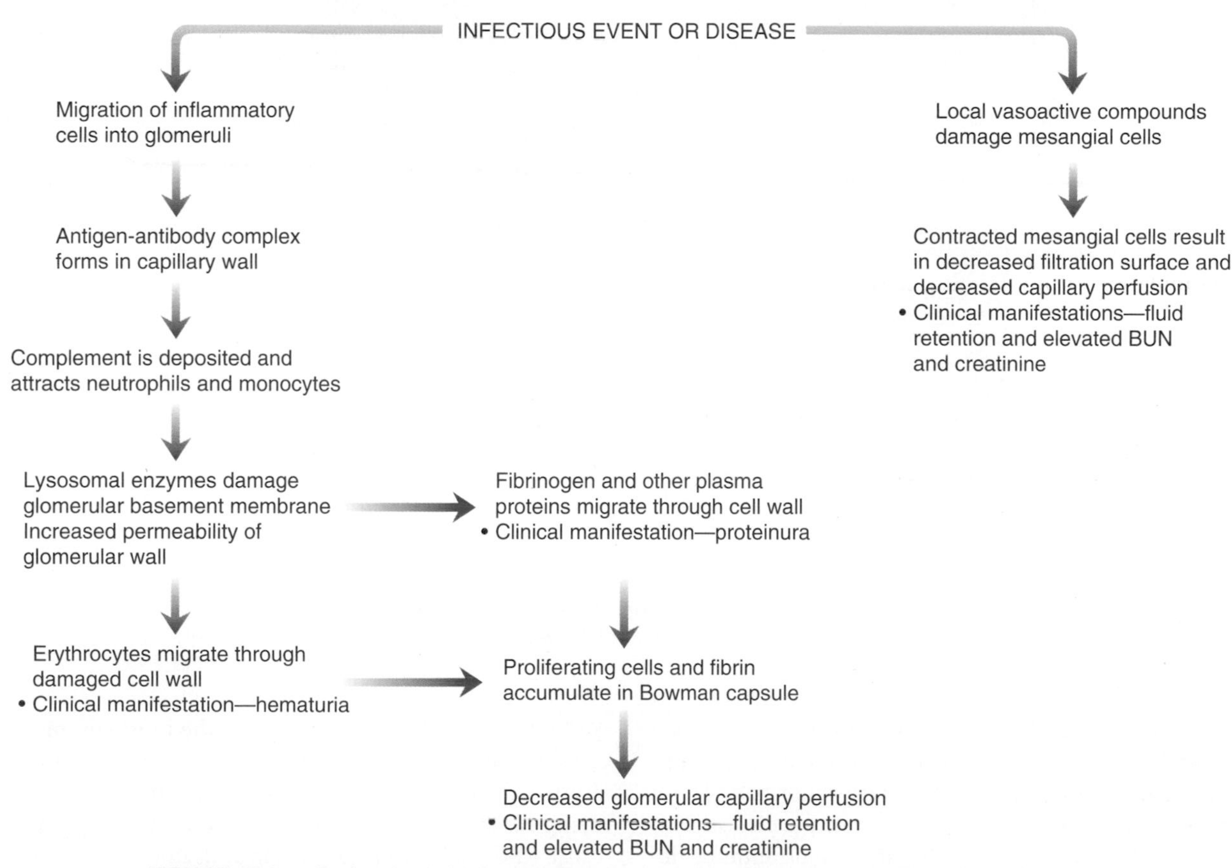

FIGURE 27-8 ■ Pathophysiologic process of acute glomerulonephritis. (Data from Brady HR, Brenner BM: Acute renal failure. In Fauci AS et al, editors: *Harrison's principles of internal medicine,* ed 14, New York, 1998, McGraw-Hill, pp 1504-1513; Glasscock RJ, Cohen AH: The primary glomerulopathies, *Dis Mon* 42:332-383, 1996; and Jennette JC, Falk RJ: Diagnosis and management of glomerular diseases, *Med Clin North Am* 81:653-677, 1997.)

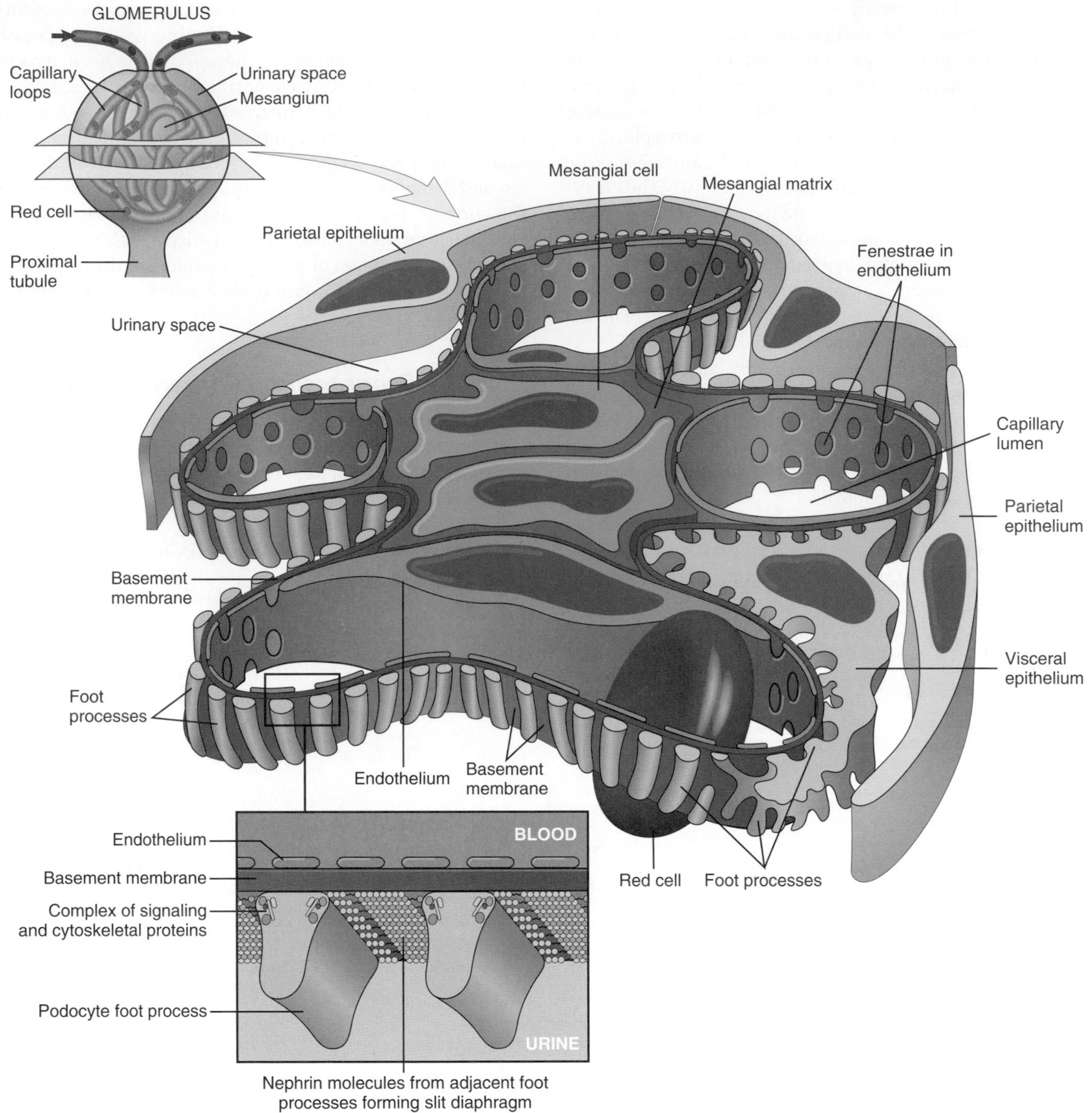

FIGURE 27-9 ■ Diagrammatic representation of a glomerular lobe. (From Cotran RS, Kumar V, Collins T: *Robbins pathologic basis of disease,* ed 7, Philadelphia, 2003, Saunders, p 511.)

lonephritis.[45] Causes of RPGN fall into four general categories: (1) complication of an acute or subacute infection; (2) complication of a multisystem disease; (3) drug exposure; and (4) as a primary disorder in the absence of other systemic disease. This type is classified based on presence or absence of immune deposits along the glomerular basement membrane.[46]

The infections most commonly associated with RPGN are poststreptococcal glomerulonephritis, infective endocarditis, visceral sepsis, and hepatitis B. The post-streptococcal state and infective endocarditis are by far the most common. Multisystem diseases associated with RPGN are systemic lupus erythematosus, Henoch-Schönlein purpura, systemic necrotizing vasculitis, and Goodpasture syndrome. Drugs that may cause RPGN are penicillamine, hydralazine, allopurinol in the presence of vasculitis, and rifampin.

Histopathologically, RPGN is characterized by crescent formation in the glomeruli.[45] The extent of the renal involvement varies. The cellular matrix of the crescents changes as the syn-

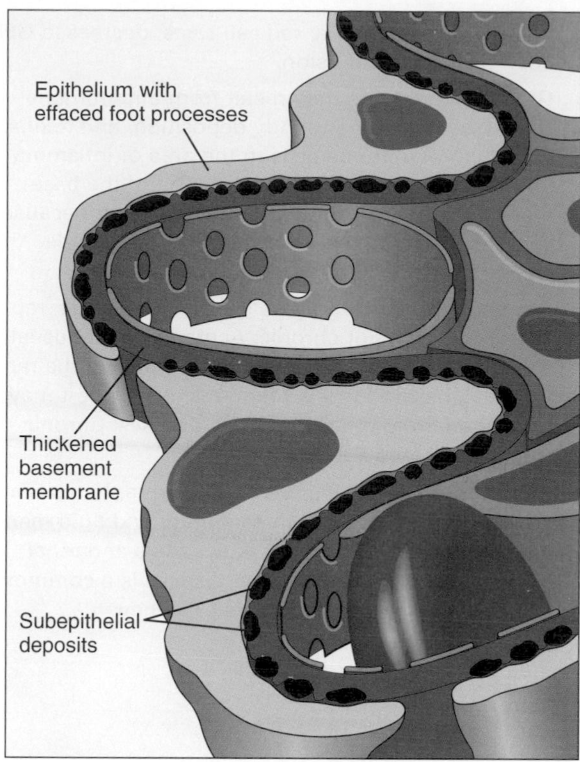

FIGURE 27-10 ■ Diagrammatic representation of membranous glomerulonephritis. (From Cotran RS, Kumar V, Collins T: *Robbins pathologic basis of disease,* ed 6, Philadelphia, 1999, Saunders, p 955.)

drome worsens. Early-stage (also called fresh or cellular) crescents consist of proliferating and invading cells and fibrin, intermediate-stage (fibrocellular) crescents contain cells and collagen, and late-stage (fibrotic) crescents are nearly entirely composed of collagen. In general, the greater the number of damaged glomeruli (those with crescents), the more severe the clinical symptoms and the poorer the renal outcome.[45]

Clinical Manifestations. Patients with RPGN may experience viral-type symptoms in the prodromal period (arthralgias, myalgias, back and abdominal pain, fever, malaise). Hypertension and edema are occasionally present. Hematuria and proteinuria in conjunction with rapidly decreasing renal function manifested by rising serum creatinine are the cardinal signs. Nausea and vomiting as a result of azotemia also occur.[45,46]

Diagnosis. Urinalysis is done to screen for hematuria, proteinuria, and casts. Serum BUN and creatinine levels and a creatinine clearance rate are determined to evaluate renal function. A streptococcal enzyme assay may also be performed to screen for the underlying mechanism. If infective endocarditis is suspected, a workup that includes blood cultures, echocardiography, and cardiac catheterization may be done. A renal biopsy is sometimes needed to differentiate the mechanism of RPGN.

Treatment. At the time of initial evaluation, up to 50% of patients are already significantly uremic and require immediate dialysis. The remaining patients need dialysis within weeks to months. If the disease is acute at this time, it is considered potentially reversible. Treatment is somewhat dependent on the underlying cause but nearly always involves sodium and fluid restriction and diuretic therapy. Immunosuppressive therapy is frequently indicated. Methylprednisolone pulse therapy has been shown to be appropriate for patients with RPGN. Large doses of the drug are given intravenously on a once-daily or alternate-day basis three times and then followed by oral prednisone. Approximately 75% of patients have shown good improvement and have attained near-normal to normal renal function. A response to drug therapy is usually evident in 5 to 10 days. Nevertheless, in some patients the condition eventually progresses to renal failure. Plasmapheresis (filtering of plasma to remove antibodies) used in conjunction with prednisone and cyclophosphamide has yielded improvement similar to that of methylprednisolone pulse therapy. Anticoagulants may be used to reduce fibrin deposition and crescent formation.[45,46]

Chronic Glomerulonephritis

Chronic glomerulonephritis is defined as continuing or persistent hematuria and proteinuria resulting in slowly progressive deterioration in renal function.[44] The end result of chronic glomerulonephritis is hypertension, small (contracted) scarred kidneys, and renal failure.

Pathogenesis. The underlying structural lesions are classified into four groups: (1) proliferative (including mesangial, or cells in the connective tissue that support the glomerular capillaries; end-capillary and extracapillary; and focal/segmental), (2) sclerosing (focal and diffuse), (3) membranous, and (4) nonspecific. Tubular atrophy and dilation may also be seen.

Within the capillary basement membranes appear to be deposits of soluble antigen-antibody complexes or formations of anti–glomerular basement membrane antibodies. Biochemical mediators of inflammation (complement, leukocytes, and fibrin) then start to damage the glomerular wall. This series of events results in changes in the renal system that were previously described in conjunction with acute glomerulonephritis.

Clinical Manifestations. The clinical manifestations of chronic glomerulonephritis are similar to those of acute glomerulonephritis. Hematuria and proteinuria are present for the duration of the disease. Tubulointerstitial inflammation and scarring are associated with decreased renal function and poorer renal prognosis.[44] Systemically, edema, fluid volume excess, and hypertension develop more insidiously than in the acute form of the disease. The disease may persist for 10 to 20 years or more from onset to end-stage renal failure.

Diagnosis and Treatment. Evaluation includes urinalysis to detect hematuria, proteinuria, and casts. Serum BUN, creatinine levels, and creatinine clearance are quantitated to estimate the degree of renal damage. Renal biopsy may be needed to differentiate the underlying pathologic abnormality. Autoimmune disorders are more likely to progress to chronic glomerulonephritis than are glomerulopathies resulting from infectious processes.

Treatment to stop or slow glomerular damage differs with the underlying mechanism. Antibiotics appropriate for the identified organism are used in infections. Corticosteroids and cytotoxic agents (e.g., cyclophosphamide) and anticoagulant and antiplatelet drugs are often used for immune-based pathologic processes.[44-46] Avoidance of nephrotoxic drug therapy or discontinuation of identified toxins is advised. Decreasing systemic and renal hypertension and controlling extracellular fluid volume, anemia, metabolic abnormalities, and uremic symptoms with dietary modification, antihypertensives (generally angiotensin-converting enzyme inhibitors), diuretics, and erythropoietin are the primary therapeutic approaches to compensate for irreversible renal damage.[44] End-stage renal disease eventually develops in many patients and necessitates long-term dialysis or renal transplantation.

KEY CONCEPTS

- Glomerular disorders are inflammatory in nature. Damage is mediated by immune processes but is not directly due to infection. Often the glomerular basement membrane is damaged, with consequent hematuria, proteinuria, red cell casts, decreased GFR, edema, and hypertension.
- Glomerulonephritis may result from autoimmune processes, antigen-antibody deposition, and toxins. Attraction of immune cells to the area of inflammation results in lysosomal degradation of the basement membrane. The GFR may fall, in part because of contraction of mesangial cells resulting in decreased surface area for filtration.
- Glomerulonephritis may be classified as acute, rapidly progressing, or chronic. Acute forms are usually due to postinfectious damage. The cause of the rapidly progressing form is often unknown, but it may be secondary to other disease processes. Chronic forms tend to be autoimmune.
- Treatment may include steroids, plasmapheresis, and supportive measures such as dietary and fluid management and management of systemic and renal hypertension. End-stage renal disease is a common outcome necessitating dialysis or kidney transplantation.

OTHER

Nephrotic Syndrome

The **nephrotic syndrome** is a collection of symptoms caused by glomerular disease. It is characterized by an increase in glomerular capillary wall permeability to serum proteins. The predominant abnormality in nephrotic syndrome is the loss of large amounts (more than 3.5 g/day) of protein in the

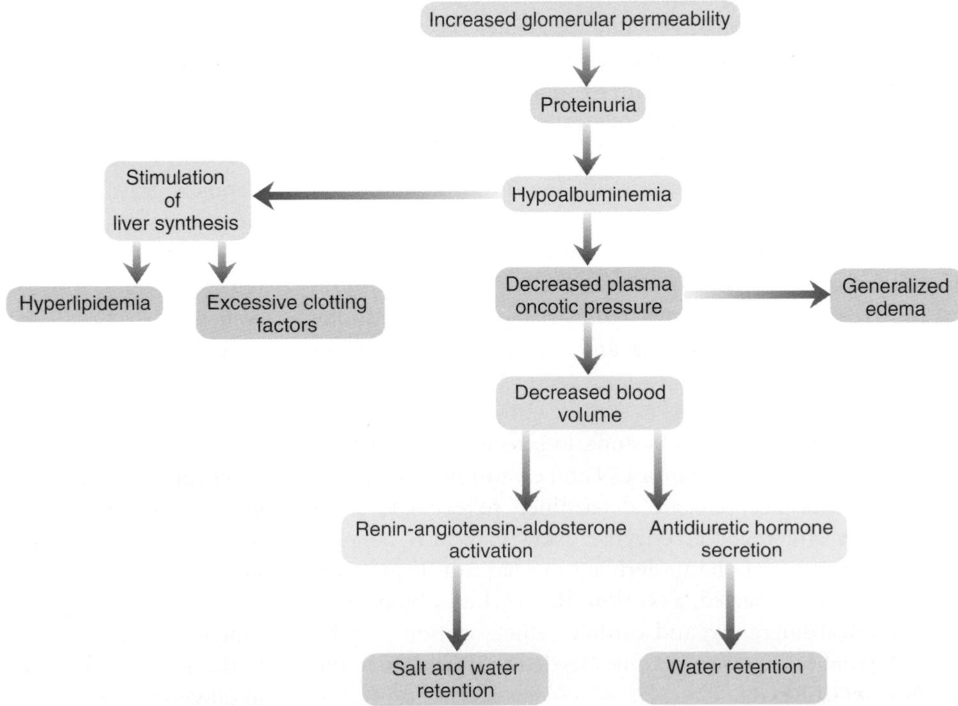

FIGURE 27-11 ■ Pathophysiologic process of nephrotic syndrome.

urine. Hypoalbuminemia, hyperlipidemia, edema, hypercoagulability, altered immunity, and lipiduria are present secondary to urine protein loss (Figure 27-11).[1,7]

Pathogenesis. More than 90% of cases of nephrotic syndrome are related to six disorders: minimal change disease (20% of adult cases and 80% of pediatric cases), focal segmental glomerulosclerosis, membranous glomerulopathy, membranoproliferative glomerulonephritis, diabetic nephropathy, and amyloidosis.[1] Diabetic nephropathy is the most common cause of nephrotic syndrome in the United States.[7] Each of these disorders increases the permeability of the glomerular wall so that it is no longer an efficient semipermeable filter. Changes in the glomerular basement membrane and foot processes (podocytes) allow proteins through the glomeruli into the collecting tubules, where they are excreted with urine (see Figure 27-10).[1,7]

Clinical Manifestations. *Hypoproteinemia* results from proteinuria. *Hypoalbuminemia* is the main protein disorder, although other proteins, such as globulins, are also lost in the urine and thus have decreased serum levels. Urinary protein loss may exceed 10 g/day and is greater than the rate at which the liver can synthesize new albumin (usually 12 to 14 g/day).

Edema results when hydrostatic and colloid oncotic pressures are not in balance. Hydrostatic pressure on the arteriole side of the vascular tree is elevated and pushes fluid into the interstitial space. Colloid oncotic pressure on the venule side exerts a pressure that pulls fluid back into the vascular space. When serum protein levels are decreased, fluid remains in the interstitial space. Edema then forms in areas where hydrostatic pressure is high (dependent areas) and where interstitial pressure is low (periorbital areas). Although fluid movement favors the interstitial space, about half of patients with the nephrotic syndrome have normal or increased plasma volume. Renal retention of sodium and fluid may account for some of this increased volume, but other factors may also contribute. Factors contributing to normal or increased plasma volume include (1) a relatively noncompliant interstitium, which resists excess fluid at a threshold; (2) a washout of interstitial oncotic pressure to less than vascular oncotic pressure as a result of increased lymph flow, which favors fluid remaining in the vascular space; and (3) decreased capillary permeability to albumin in hypoalbuminemia.

Hyperlipidemia is inversely proportional to the serum albumin concentration. It appears that increased hepatic synthesis of cholesterol, triglycerides, and lipoproteins, which may be stimulated by decreased plasma albumin levels or decreased plasma oncotic pressure, accounts for the hyperlipidemia. However, decreased catabolism of these substances may also be present. Lipiduria results from hyperlipidemia, but the level of lipiduria more closely parallels that of urine protein excretion.[44]

Hypercoagulability may be due to altered levels of clotting factors. Antithrombin III is excreted in excess via the urine. Changes in proteins C and S, hyperfibrinogenemia as a result of increased hepatic production, impaired fibrinolysis, and increased ability of platelets to aggregate are probable contributors to an increased incidence of thromboembolic events in patients with nephrotic syndrome.[44] Renal vein thrombosis, once thought to be the cause of nephrotic syndrome, is actually secondary to hypercoagulability.

Decreased immune system competence has been described in nephrotic patients. Cell-mediated immunity appears to be depressed, possibly because of hypoalbuminemia, hyperlipidemia, or a zinc deficiency. In general, nephrotic patients are predisposed to and at risk for infection.

In nephrosis, triiodothyronine and thyroid-binding globulin are decreased as a consequence of urinary loss. Trace metals, iron, copper, and zinc are deficient. Loss of cholecalciferol (vitamin D precursor) leads to a vitamin D deficiency and secondary hyperparathyroidism, hypocalcemia, and renal osteodystrophy. Drug metabolism may be altered as a result of hypoproteinemia because many medications are protein bound.

Diagnosis and Treatment. Evaluation is based on identifying the underlying pathologic mechanism, as described in previous sections. Continued assessment of symptoms and alterations is necessary to provide optimal treatment.

In children, minimal change disease (minimal pathologic change in the glomeruli) is the most common underlying disease. Standard treatment is a 12- to 16-week regimen of tapered steroids, which results in a 93% response rate.[47] Approximately 70% of patients thus treated have a relapse, and 40% to 45% have multiple relapses necessitating renal biopsy and immunosuppressive therapy (e.g., cyclophosphamide).[47]

Management of edema is conservative. Treatment is not initiated unless the condition is symptomatic. Dietary sodium restriction, rest, and the judicious use of diuretics are the most common treatment options. Intravenous albumin may be used when aggressive diuresis is needed because of severe ascites or pulmonary effusion. However, the additional albumin is lost in the urine within a short time, so this measure is only temporary.

Dietary management varies from high-protein to normal-protein diets. Some clinicians believe that an increased protein load only exaggerates protein loss. Diets low in sodium and low in saturated fats are commonly instituted. Adequate calorie and protein intake is essential for patients receiving steroid therapy.

Supplemental vitamin D, calcium, and iron are used to replace losses. Prophylactic anticoagulation is not generally used; however, anticoagulation for pulmonary embolism is appropriate. The management of renal vein thrombosis is controversial.

Nephrotic syndrome usually resolves spontaneously; however, diseases that cause nephrotic syndrome may progress to end-stage renal failure. Dialysis and renal transplantation are available as treatment options.

KEY CONCEPTS

- Nephrotic syndrome occurs because of increased glomerular permeability to proteins, which results in a urinary loss of 3.5 g of protein or more per day. Proteinuria leads to hypoalbuminemia and generalized edema as a result of decreased blood colloid osmotic pressure. Hyperlipidemia and hypercoagulability are thought to occur because of a generalized increase in liver activity stimulated by hypoalbuminemia.
- Treatment is conservative, consisting of management of symptoms and the underlying process that initiated the syndrome, when indicated (e.g., minimal change disease). Most cases resolve spontaneously. Dietary and fluid management is essential to compensate for fluid, electrolyte, and metabolic alterations.

SUMMARY

Many diseases can cause renal damage or failure. Any process that disrupts the normal architecture of the kidney will cause altered function, whether in the glomeruli, the vascular tree, or the collecting/draining system. Despite the kidney's capacity to respond to treatment and reverse the damage, ultimately any abnormality in the system has the potential to precipitate end-stage renal failure.

Glomerulonephritis and pyelonephritis are the first and second leading causes of chronic renal failure. Although glomerulonephritis is difficult to manage or prevent, pyelonephritis is a potentially preventable cause of renal failure. Obstructive processes, including stones, tumors, and congenital malformations, may precipitate acute renal failure; however, they are often amenable to treatment if detected early.

MEDIA RESOURCES

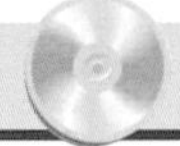

evolve

Remember to check out the ***CD Companion*** included with this book for Review Questions, Key Concepts Review, Glossary (with audio for selected terms), Disease Profiles, and Animations.

PLUS, visit the ***Evolve website*** at http://evolve.elsevier.com/Copstead/ for Case Studies, Disease Profiles, and WebLinks.

References

1. Lancaster LE: *ANNA core curriculum for nephrology nursing,* ed 4, Pitman, NJ, 2001, American Nephrology Nurses' Association.
2. Foxman B: Epidemiology of urinary tract infections: incidence, morbidity, and economic costs, *Am J Med* 113(1A):5S-13S, 2002.
3. Roberts KB: The AAP practice parameter on urinary tract infections in febrile infants and young children, *Am Fam Physician* 62:1815-1822, 2000.
4. Morton RA, Iliescu EA, Wilson JWL: Nephrology: 1. Investigation and treatment of recurrent kidney stones, *CMAJ* 166:214-218, 2002.
5. Novick AC: Nephron-sparing surgery for renal cell carcinoma, *Annu Rev Med* 53:393-407, 2002.
6. Kirkali Z, Tuzel E, Mungan MU: Recent advances in kidney cancer and metastatic disease, *BJU Int* 88:818-824, 2001.
7. Madaio MP, Harrington JT: The diagnosis of glomerular diseases, *Arch Intern Med* 161:25-34, 2001.
8. Brendler CB: Evaluation of the urologic patient: history, physical examination, and urinalysis. In Walsh PC et al, editors: *Campbell's urology,* ed 7, Philadelphia, 1998, Saunders, pp 131-157.
9. Biho G, Meyers A: Recurrent renal stone disease: advances in pathogenesis and clinical management, *Lancet* 358:651-656, 2001.
10. Gonzalez R: Urologic disorders in infants and children. In Behrman RE, Kliegman RM, Arvin AM, editors: *Nelson textbook of pediatrics,* ed 15, Philadelphia, 1995, Saunders, pp 1527-1528.
11. Pohl M et al: Toward an etiological classification of developmental disorders of the kidney and upper urinary tract, *Kidney Int* 61:10-19, 2002.
12. Glassberg KL: Renal dysplasia and cystic disease of the kidney. In Walsh PC et al, editors: *Campbell's urology,* ed 7, Philadelphia, 1998, Saunders, pp 1757-1813.
13. Bergstein JM: Anatomic abnormalities associated with hematuria. In Nelson WE et al, editors: *Nelson textbook of pediatrics,* ed 15, Philadelphia, 1996, Saunders, pp 1495-1496.
14. Gabow PA: Cystic disease of the kidney. In Bennett CJ, Plum F, editors: *Cecil textbook of medicine,* ed 21, Philadelphia, 2000, Saunders.
15. Chon CH et al: Pediatric urinary tract infections, *Pediatr Urol* 48:1441-1458, 2001.
16. Ovalle A, Levancini M: Urinary tract infections in pregnancy, *Curr Opin Urol* 11:55-59, 2001.
17. Schaeffer AJ: Infection of the urinary tract. In Walsh PC et al, editors: *Urology,* ed 8, Philadelphia, 2002, Saunders, pp 533-614.
18. Tierney Lm, McPhee SJ, Papadakis MA: *Current medical diagnosis and treatment,* ed 37, Stamford, Conn, 2002, Appleton & Lange.
19. Gulmi FA et al, editors: *Campbell's urology,* ed 7, Philadelphia, 1998, Saunders.
20. Asselman M, Verkoelen CF: Crystal-cell interaction in the pathogenesis of kidney stone disease, *Curr Opin Urol* 12:271-276, 2002.
21. Portis AJ, Sundaram CP: Diagnosis and initial management of kidney stones, *Am Fam Physician* 63:1329-1338, 2001.
22. Shekarriz B, Stoller ML: Uric acid nephrolithiasis: current concepts and controversies, *J Urol* 168:1307-1314, 2002.
23. Pearle MS: Prevention of nephrolithiasis, *Curr Opin Nephrol Hypertens* 10:203-209, 2001.
24. Heilberg IP: Update on dietary recommendations and medical treatment of renal stone disease, *Nephrol Dial Transplant* 15:117-123, 2000.
25. Kramer G, Klingler HC, Steiner GE: Role of bacteria in the development of kidney stones, *Curr Opin Urol* 10:35-38, 2000.
26. Borghi L et al: Comparison of two diets for the prevention of recurrent stones in idiopathic hypercalciuria, *N Engl J Med* 346:77-83, 2002.
27. Phillips JL et al: The genetic basis of renal epithelial tumors: advances in research and its impact on prognosis and therapy, *Curr Opin Urol* 11:463-469, 2001.

28. Belldegrun A et al, editors: *Campbell's urology,* ed 7, Philadelphia, 1998, Saunders, pp 2283-2326.
29. Dickinson M et al: Renal angiomyolipoma: optimal treatment based on size and symptoms, *Clin Nephrol* 49:281-286, 1998.
30. Godley P, Kim SW: Renal cell carcinoma, *Curr Opin Oncol* 14:280-285, 2002.
31. Mickisch GHJ: Principles of nephrectomy for malignant disease, *BJU Int* 89:488-495, 2002.
32. Gettman MT, Blute ML: Update on pathologic staging of renal cell carcinoma, *Urology* 60:209-217, 2002.
33. Gold PJ, Fefer A, Thompson JA: Paraneoplastic manifestations of renal cell carcinoma, *Semin Urol Oncol* 14:216-222, 1996.
34. Yonover MP, Flanigan RC: Should radical nephrectomy be performed in the face of surgically incurable disease? *Curr Opin Urol* 10:429-434, 2000.
35. Pantuck AJ, Zisman A, Belldegrun A: Gene and immune therapy for renal cell carcinoma, *Int J Urol* 8:S1-S4, 2001.
36. Dutcher JP: Immunotherapy: are we making a difference? *Cur Opin Urol* 10:435-439, 2000.
37. Vasey PA: Immunotherapy for renal carcinoma: theoretical basis and current standard of care, *J Clin Pharmacol* 50:521-529, 2000.
38. Metts MC et al: Bladder cancer: a review of diagnosis and management, *J Natl Med Assoc* 92:285-294, 2000.
39. Bostwick DG, Mikuz G: Urothelial papillary (exophytic) neoplasms, *Virchows Arch* 441:109-116, 2002.
40. Messing EM, Catalona W: Urothelial tumors of the urinary tract. In Walsh PC et al, editors: *Campbell's urology,* ed 7, Philadelphia, 1998, Saunders, pp 2329-2410.
41. Jung I, Messing E: Molecular mechanisms and pathways in bladder cancer development and progression, *Cancer Control* 7:325-334, 2000.
42. Pritchard-Jones K: Controversies and advances in the management of Wilms' tumour, *Arch Dis Child* 87:241-244, 2002.
43. McLorie GA: Wilms' tumor (nephroblastoma), *Curr Opin Urol* 11:567-570, 2001.
44. Brady HR, Brenner BM: Acute renal failure. In Fauci AS et al, editors: *Harrison's principles of internal medicine,* ed 14, New York, 1998, McGraw-Hill, pp 1504-1513.
45. Hricik DE, Chung-Park M, Sedor JR: Glomerulonephritis, *N Engl J Med* 339:888-899, 1998.
46. Couser WG: Glomerulonephritis. *Lancet* 353:1509-1515, 1999.
47. Roy S, Noe HM: Renal disease in childhood. In Walsh PC et al, editors: *Campbell's urology,* ed.7, Philadelphia, 1998, Saunders, pp 1664-1680.

chapter 28

Renal Failure

Katherina P. Choka

MEDIA RESOURCES

Additional Material for Study, Review, and Further Exploration

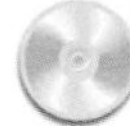

CD Companion ◆ Review Questions and Answers ◆ Key Concepts Review
◆ Glossary *(with audio pronunciations for selected terms)*
◆ Disease Profiles ◆ Animations

evolve ***Website*** at http://evolve.elsevier.com/Copstead/
◆ Case Studies ◆ Disease Profiles ◆ WebLinks

KEY QUESTIONS

- How do prerenal, intrarenal, and postrenal types of acute renal failure differ in etiology, prognosis, clinical manifestations, and management?
- What are the characteristic clinical and laboratory findings in each of the three stages of acute renal failure?
- What is the relationship between the degree of nephron loss, reduced glomerular filtration rate, and the phases of chronic renal failure?
- What are the similarities and differences between acute and chronic renal failure?
- What are the characteristic findings of uremia?
- What treatment options are available to patients with end-stage renal disease?

CHAPTER OUTLINE

The principal role of the kidneys is maintenance of homeostasis of the extracellular fluid compartment. They accomplish this task by maintaining balance between extracellular fluid and electrolytes, thereby contributing to acid-base balance, and by eliminating certain metabolic waste products such as urea from the blood stream. When these functions fail, either abruptly or insidiously, the effects are seen throughout the entire body.

ACUTE RENAL FAILURE

Acute renal failure (ARF) is a sudden, severe decrease in renal function that is potentially reversible. It is usually associated with a decrease in glomerular filtration rate (GFR), a marked decrease in urine output over several hours to several days (**oliguria** or, rarely, **anuria**), and usually **azotemia** (retention of nitrogenous wastes). Table 28-1 reviews terminology related to renal failure. ARF may be classified as oliguric (<500 ml/day) or nonoliguric (≥7800 ml/day). Approximately half of ARF patients are nonoliguric, with fewer signs and symptoms.[1] Most define the condition of ARF as an acute increase in serum creatinine (of at least 0.5 mg/dl [≥44.0 μmol/L]).[2] Despite significant advances in prevention and treatment, the mortality rate associated with ARF ranges from 40% to 60% and varies with the patient's concurrent conditions.[1,3]

Certain preexisting conditions are known to increase the risk for ARF. These chronic risk factors include preexisting renal impairment, atherosclerosis, hypertension, diabetes mellitus, heart failure, chronic liver impairment/failure, and advanced age.[4,5]

Alterations in renal function in the elderly (>65 years of age) reduce functional reserve, and aging itself can have a negative impact on the outcome of ARF because it is often an additive factor to other health problems. Aging contributes to impaired autoregulation (see Chapter 26 for a discussion of autoregulation). Autoregulation can also be negatively affected by the following medications: angiotensin-converting enzyme (ACE) inhibitors, thiazide diuretics, loop diuretics, and drugs such as aspirin and other nonsteroidal antiinflam-

Table 28-1

Terminology Related to Renal Failure

Term	Definition
Acute renal failure	Loss of kidney function that is rapid in onset and usually reversible. It may be prerenal, intrarenal, or postrenal.
Acute tubular necrosis	Acute renal failure that is intrarenal in nature. The cause is ischemic or toxic injury.
Anuria	Urinary output of less than 50 ml/day
Azotemia	Buildup of nitrogenous waste products in the blood, specifically blood urea nitrogen.
Chronic renal failure	Chronic, progressive loss of renal function that is irreversible. Causes of chronic renal failure are numerous.
Metabolic waste products	Byproducts of protein metabolism that are excreted in the urine.
Oliguria	Urinary output of less than 500 ml/day
Uremia	Clinical manifestation associated with an accumulation of nitrogenous waste products and toxins in the blood, typically associated with renal failure.

matory drugs that inhibit prostaglandin synthesis.[3] The elderly kidney has a decreased urine-concentrating ability and a reduced ability to conserve sodium, which in combination with a diminished thirst sensitivity predispose the elderly to hypovolemia and prerenal failure. The aged kidney has fewer nephrons to call on to assist renal function in the face of an intrarenal insult. There can be 50% less nephron mass by age 70.[3] Older tubular cells may also be more susceptible to damage because cellular antioxidant defenses dwindle with age. In the elderly, each case must be evaluated individually and determinations of therapeutic interventions thoughtfully considered.

Pediatric ARF is not a common occurrence and is rarely seen outside the hospitalized population. However, morbidity and mortality remain high. There are many causes of ARF in children, including prerenal processes, hypoxic/ischemic injury, and obstructive uropathies.[6] Hemolytic-uremic syndrome, nephrotoxic drugs, and glomerulonephritis are the most common causes of intrarenal failure. Hemolytic-uremic syndrome is a disease process associated with the concurrent development of hemolytic anemia, thrombocytopenia, and renal failure. Although it is most common in children and associated with a specific strain of *Escherichia coli* (0157:H7) that is ingested, it can occur in adults and may have a multifactorial etiologic development.[6] Intrarenal failure is the most common type of ARF among children. The incidence of ARF in neonates is increasing, with renal vein thrombosis and cortical necrosis among the causes. Immaturity of the kidneys predisposes neonates, whether term or preterm, to ARF. Other conditions seen in the neonatal population that may contribute to ARF include cardiac defects, lung immaturity requiring mechanical ventilation, nephrotoxic drugs, sepsis, and urinary obstruction.[6]

Box 28-1

Causes of Acute Renal Failure

Prerenal (Decreased Renal Perfusion)

Hypovolemia
- Hemorrhage
- Shock
- Third spacing (edema, ascites)
- Burns
- Dehydration (GI losses, overuse of diuretics)

Decreased cardiac output
- Cardiogenic shock
- Dysrhythmias
- Cardiac tamponade
- Congestive heart failure
- Myocardial infarction

Thromboembolic obstruction of the renal vasculature

Postrenal (Obstruction)

Benign prostatic hyperplasia
Calculi (stones)
Urinary tract infection
Tumors
Strictures
Altered bladder contraction (neurogenic bladder from medication or injury/disease)

Intrarenal (Damage to the Nephron)

Ischemic acute tubular necrosis
- Prolonged prerenal acute renal failure
- Transfusion reaction
- Rhabdomyolysis

Nephrotoxic acute tubular necrosis
- Prolonged postrenal acute renal failure
- Antibiotics (aminoglycosides, carbenicillin, amphotericin B)
- Contrast media
- Heavy metals (lead, mercury)
- Carbon tetrachloride
- Insecticides, fungicides
- Cytotoxic drugs (certain chemotherapeutic agents)
- Hemolytic-uremic syndrome

Inflammatory
- Acute glomerulonephritis
- Acute pyelonephritis

Etiology and Pathophysiology

ARF is a broad term used to organize a wide variety of potential etiologic factors. These etiologic factors are divided into three groups based on location (Box 28-1). Determination of the cause is important because it reflects differing pathologic processes, and some of the treatment interventions vary with the specific origin of the ARF.

Prerenal Failure

Prerenal ARF accounts for 60% or more of all cases of community-acquired ARF.[2] In prerenal ARF, the underlying factor is diminished perfusion of the kidney. The functional components of the kidney are intact, but decreased blood flow to the kidney ultimately results in a reduction in GFR (Figure 28-1). Normally, the kidney can maintain a stable GFR in the face of hypotension, reduced blood volume, or reduced cardiac output through autoregulation, primarily by alteration in the afferent and efferent arterioles. When mean systemic arterial pressure drops below 70 mm Hg, GFR is sharply reduced.[7,8] As noted in Box 28-1, all of the causes of prerenal failure share the commonality of reduced renal perfusion; therefore, they are often referred to as ischemic in origin. Generally, prerenal oliguria is easily reversed if identification of the specific cause and restoration of renal perfusion can be accomplished quickly. For this reason, identification of the specific event leading to prerenal renal failure is essential.[3]

Reduced GFR affects the production of filtrate and thus reduces the volume of urine eventually eliminated. Because filtrate moves more slowly through the renal tubules, more sodium (Na^+) and water are reabsorbed into the blood stream. Glomerular hypoperfusion increases the production of renin, angiotensin II, and aldosterone, which results in sodium and water retention.[6] Urine output falls to less than 500 ml/24 hr

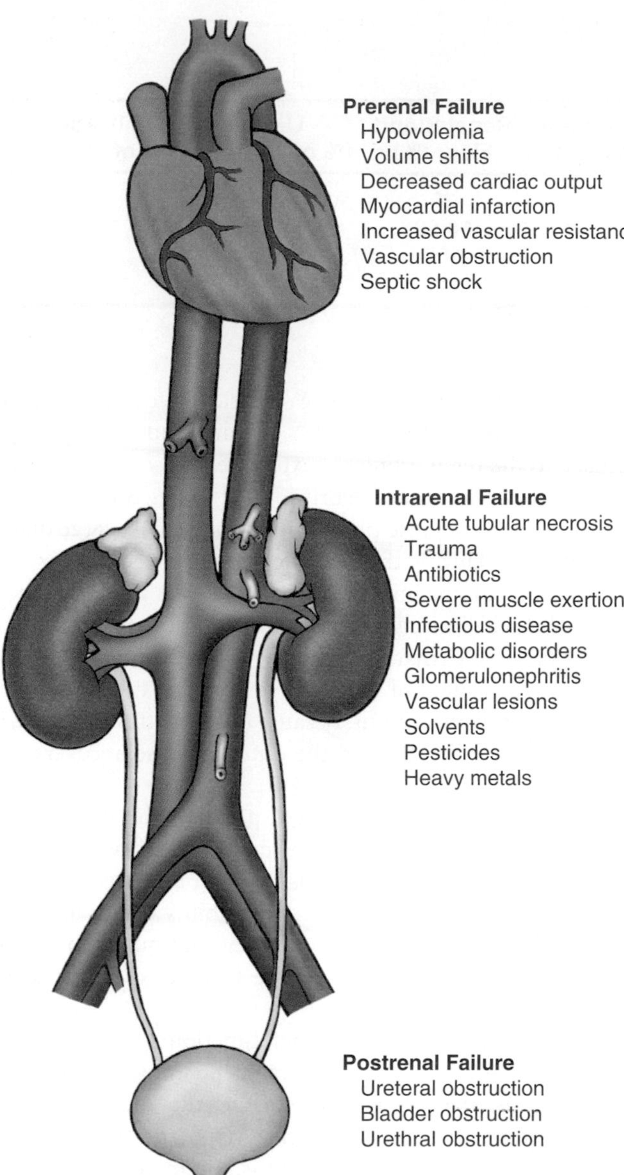

FIGURE 28-1 ■ Causes of the three types of renal failure: prerenal, intrarenal, and postrenal. (From Monahan FD, Neighbors M: *Medical-surgical nursing: foundations for clinical practice,* ed 2, Philadelphia, 1998, Saunders, p 1389.)

(oliguria) but only rarely to less than 50 ml/24 hr (anuria). Azotemia develops, indicating retention of nitrogenous waste products reflected by an elevated blood urea nitrogen (BUN) level.[9]

The hemodynamic alterations that occur in ARF if allowed to progress will lead to renal endothelial ischemia. Tissue ischemia leads to an increase in endothelin-1, a potent vasoconstrictor, and a disruption in the release of the vasodilator nitric oxide, which further reduces renal blood flow. Accumulation of inflammatory cytokines, leukocytes, and fibrin leads to obstruction in the renal microcirculation. Research suggests that the proximal tubule is highly susceptible to ischemic injury and loss of electrolyte polarity that is necessary for maintaining renal function.[6,9]

It is important to mention that many medications can contribute to a prerenal state. Nonsteroidal antiinflammatory drugs (NSAIDs) inhibit the essential vasodilatory effects of renal prostaglandins. In some individuals ACE inhibitors can cause ARF by inhibiting efferent arteriole constriction, a part of renal autoregulation of blood flow. Contrast-induced ARF is caused by acute vasoconstriction and subsequent reduction of blood flow.[3]

Postrenal Failure

The common etiologic factor in the postrenal type of ARF is obstruction of urine flow at some point distal to the kidney itself. Obstruction must be bilateral to produce renal failure. As illustrated in Box 28-1, a wide variety of conditions are capable of producing an obstruction to urine flow manifested as oliguria or anuria. This obstruction of urine flow initially produces an increase in retrograde pressure within the kidney and subsequently increases pressure in the Bowman capsule of the glomerulus. The elevated tubular pressure opposes glomerular capillary filtration pressure; production of urine is impaired because the GFR is reduced. As with prerenal ARF, azotemia develops as the kidneys' ability to carry out the function of removal of nitrogenous metabolic wastes is impaired. This accounts for 15% or less of acquired ARF and is reversed in part by removal of the obstruction.[1,3]

Intrarenal Failure

Intrarenal failure produces the most derangement in renal function. In intrarenal ARF, the functional unit of the kidney, the nephron itself, is damaged. The glomerulus may be the site of injury, as in acute glomerulonephritis, or most commonly, the renal tubules may be injured with the injury leading to acute tubular necrosis (ATN). Intrarenal ARF often has a longer course than prerenal or postrenal ARF because the nephron itself has been affected; recovery can take weeks to months.[1] In the case of severe injury, recovery may not occur in which case the patient progresses to chronic renal failure (CRF).

ATN is the most common cause of intrarenal ARF. It is important to note in Box 28-1 that prolonged ARF of either prerenal or postrenal origin can ultimately produce ATN. ATN is a result of either ischemic or nephrotoxic injury to the tubules. Generally, nephrotoxic insult without ischemia results in less severe damage to the tubules. Only the epithelial layer is affected, and it is highly capable of regeneration.[1] In ATN secondary to ischemia, however, the injury can be much more profound. "Acute tubular injury" would probably be a more appropriate term because the damage that occurs at a structural level varies considerably.[9] Tubular cells may be uninjured and functional, ischemic but capable of recovery, or frankly infarcted and necrotic.[1] As mentioned earlier with prolonged prerenal ischemia, cells located in the straight portion of the proximal tubule are the most profoundly affected.[6]

Table 28-2
Phases of Acute Renal Failure

Phase	Definition	Approximate Time Span	Renal Blood Flow (%)	Urine (% of Normal)	Filtration (% of Normal)
Oliguric	<500 ml/day	1-2 wk	25	5	10
Diuretic	≥500 ml/day to stable laboratory values	2-10 days	30-50	150-200	10-50
Convalescent	Stable laboratory values to normal function	3-12 mo	100	100	100

Cells in the tubules that are ischemic are markedly changed in terms of their surface, cytoskeleton, and the concentrations and gradients of intracellular ions, as well as their shape and borders with other cells. These changes have an impact on the progression of ARF, as well as the potential for recovery.[6]

The condition known as ATN is characterized by a distinct series of pathophysiologic events. Injured tubular epithelial cells release intracellular debris into the tubular lumen, which in combination with proteins in the tubules results in the formation of epithelial casts. These casts, along with sloughed ischemic and necrotic cells, cause luminal obstruction.[2,3] Obstructed lumina increase the pressure in the tubules, which eventually backs up to increase pressure in the Bowman capsule. Glomerular filtration is slowed profoundly. As the pressure continues to rise, further damage to glomeruli and tubules causes the filtrate to be pushed backward into the interstitium. This back leak of filtrate is an important part of the pathology of ATN.[2] As much as 50% of the already diminished glomerular filtrate may leak back into the surrounding interstitial tissue. The renal vasculature, normally able to maintain perfusion, now fails to do so and the kidney becomes increasingly hypoxic. Cytokines released by the injury to the kidney result in congestion of the vascular bed by white blood cells and platelets. Ischemic endothelial cells also release a variety of mediators such as endothelin that constrict the intrarenal blood vessels, further contributing to the vascular congestion and impaired perfusion.[6,9]

As with prerenal and postrenal failure, intrarenal failure produces the characteristic changes in urine output (oliguria or anuria) and retention of nitrogenous metabolic waste products (azotemia). The alterations in normal renal function are responsible for the clinical findings of patients in ARF.[1]

Clinical Findings

Phases of Acute Renal Failure

Acute renal failure proceeds through a series of characteristic phases (Table 28-2). Normal perfusion to the kidney is sharply diminished, which reduces the production of urine and the ability of the kidney to properly filter material delivered to it by the blood.

In the oliguric phase, urine output drops to less than 500 ml/24 hr. Occasionally the patient has anuria, or a urine output of less than 50 ml/24 hr. The oliguric phase has a duration of approximately 1 to 2 weeks. Oliguria indicates that the damage to the renal tubules is extensive and severe.[1] Oliguria is due to the collection of debris in the tubules. Some patients have little or no oliguric phase and begin to make large quantities of urine. During this diuretic phase the urine is very dilute because of the inability of the kidney to concentrate urine. This self-limiting diuresis phase signifies restoration of tubular patency. Urinary filtrate moves freely through the system, but impairment of the kidney's concentrating ability results in a large urine output. Because the patient is not oliguric and has moved directly into the diuretic phase, recovery occurs more quickly.[1]

As the kidney begins to recover, patients who initially had oliguria will progress to the diuretic phase. This period lasts a minimum of 2 days but may last as long as 2 weeks.[1] Renal blood flow increases and the filtration ability begins to slowly improve. However, the damaged kidney continues to have difficulty concentrating urine, so large volumes of dilute urine are formed.[1]

Full recovery of normal renal function may require as much as a year or as little as 8 days,[1] depending on many factors, including the specific cause of the ARF, other concomitant conditions that the patient may have, and the appropriateness of therapeutic interventions. In many cases, some degree of renal insufficiency persists. The overall mortality of ARF can be up to 50%.[1]

Laboratory Alterations

Disruption in normal functioning of the kidneys produces a wide variety of abnormal laboratory test results. Laboratory tests of the urine and blood may assist in differentiating the etiologic location of ARF (Table 28-3). Table 28-4 shows typical abnormalities in blood and urine laboratory tests associated with renal failure. Although the presence of protein in urine may not be a consistent finding in ARF, proteinuria is a strong indication that glomerular damage has occurred.[4] Protein loss contributes to an overall reduced intravascular colloidal pressure with resulting tissue edema.[4,8] The ability to manage electrolyte and acid-base balance is lost in renal failure (see Chapters 24 and 25). Most serum electrolyte levels rise in the blood and decrease in the urine. For example, a low fractional excretion of sodium (<1%) can be an indication of decreased renal

Table 28-3

Differential Diagnosis of Acute Renal Failure

Category	Urine Volume	Specific Gravity and Osmolality	Urine Sodium	Urine Microscopy	Blood Urea Nitrogen/ Creatinine Ratio
Prerenal	Oliguria or anuria	Increased	Decreased	Normal	>20:1
Intrarenal	Oliguria or non oliguria	Decreased	Increased	Casts	10:1
Postrenal	Oliguria or anuria	Variable	Variable	Increased white blood cells; bacteria possible	10:1

perfusion and compensation by the body in an attempt to improve plasma volume and perfusion.[3] Serum calcium is the one exception because of the kidney's role in maintaining calcium balance and the alterations in serum phosphorus levels. As creatinine clearance falls to less than 25 ml/min (normal is 125 ml/min), phosphorus levels in the blood begin to rise. The cycle of elevated phosphorus and reduced plasma calcium levels is the characteristic finding in renal failure. Normally, phosphorus and free ionized calcium bind to form a calcium phosphate product, which is maintained in a fairly tight range (40 mg/dl). If the calcium phosphate product is allowed to exceed 70 mg/dl (often occurring in advanced renal failure), crystals form and precipitate in various parts of the body.[4] These crystals can form in soft tissue, lungs, joints, brain, and heart.[1] This pathophysiologic process can be classified under osteodystrophies and metastatic calcifications. Parathyroid hormone (PTH) secretion has a role in the maintenance of serum calcium and phosphate levels. PTH is regulated by plasma ionized calcium concentration. Even small decreases in plasma ionized calcium levels can lead to PTH stimulation, osteoclast stimulation, bone resorption, and enhanced renal secretion of phosphate. However, the excretion of phosphate is impaired in renal failure. The kidney is also responsible for the final hydroxylation of inactive vitamin D_3 to the more active form (1,25-dihydroxycholecalciferol). This process is impaired in renal failure and contributes to reduced calcium absorption and reduced serum levels.[1,8]

Hyperkalemia is the most serious electrolyte abnormality in renal failure (Table 28-5). Dysrhythmias and even cardiac arrest may result when the serum potassium level is elevated. Serum pH falls with the retention of acidic metabolic wastes and loss of the kidney's ability to buffer hydrogen ions, resulting in metabolic acidosis.

When the kidney fails, it is unable to produce erythropoietin, a hormone growth factor that is essential for erythropoiesis in the bone marrow.[10] Without sufficient quantities of this substance, the bone marrow is inadequately stimulated, red blood cell production falls, and the hematocrit (and hemoglobin) is decreased. Hyperparathyroidism can also contribute to decreased bone marrow functioning in patients with renal failure.[10]

The reduction in GFR impairs the clearance of metabolic waste materials from the blood stream. The decrease in GFR is best reflected by decreased urine creatinine clearance.[4] Creatinine clearance is specific in its measure of GFR.[1] As nitrogenous waste products are retained in the blood, the BUN level also rises (azotemia). Characteristic of prerenal oliguria is a ratio of BUN to serum creatinine greater than 20:1. Serum creatinine and BUN rise simultaneously.[1] BUN can be elevated by other conditions, such as bleeding into the gastrointestinal tract, profound catabolic states (infection, burns, major surgery), high-protein diets, or drugs such as corticosteroids or tetracyclines.[5] Creatinine can also rise in situations involving severe muscle breakdown.[1] Laboratory tests, including BUN, serum electrolyte, creatine, calcium, phosphorus, albumin, and complete blood cell count with differential, are helpful in diagnosing and monitoring ARF.[2]

Azotemia and Uremia

An abnormally elevated BUN secondary to renal failure is termed azotemia and is due to the retention of nitrogenous waste materials. Nitrogenous wastes are produced by metabolism of amino acids. As the BUN rises, signs and symptoms related to the effects of these toxins on other body systems may develop.[11] Azotemia is a major component of what is called the uremic syndrome. Uremia includes numerous clinical symptoms, and numerous uremic toxins can contribute to the syndrome.[12,13] Table 28-6 lists some of the clinical manifestations of uremia.

KEY CONCEPTS

- ARF is an abrupt reduction in renal function accompanied by the accumulation of waste compounds in blood. Oliguria is usually present. ARF is classified into three types according to the site of disruption: prerenal, intrarenal, and postrenal. Distinction among the types of ARF is necessary to determine appropriate therapy.
- Prerenal failure is due to conditions that impair renal blood flow, such as hypovolemia, hypotension, cardiac failure, and renal artery obstruction. Prerenal failure is characterized by manifestations of a low GFR, including oliguria, high urine specific gravity and osmolality, and low urine sodium.
- Postrenal failure is due to obstruction within the urinary collecting system distal to the kidney. Obstruc-

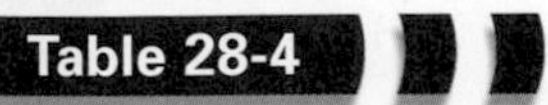

Laboratory Profile: Renal Failure

Test	Normal Range for Adults	Values in Renal Failure	Comments
Tests to Evaluate Removal of Nitrogenous Wastes			
Serum creatinine	0.6-1.1 mg/dl (women) 0.9-1.3 mg/dl (men) *Older adults:* Decreased	***In Chronic Renal Failure*** May increase by 0.5-1.0 mg/dl every 1-2 yr May be as high as 15-30 mg/dl *before* symptoms of CRF are present ***In Acute Renal Failure*** Gradual increase of 1-2 mg/dl every 24-48 hr May increase 1-6 mg/dl in 1 wk or less	Consistently elevated levels indicate decreased renal function. Serum creatinine levels are used to evaluate the effectiveness of dialysis treatments.
Blood urea nitrogen	6-20 mg/dl *Older adults:* May be slightly increased	***In Chronic Renal Failure*** May reach 180-200 mg/dl before symptoms develop ***In Acute Renal Failure*** Often increases by 10-20 mg/dl at same pace as serum creatinine level May reach 80-100 mg/dl within 1 wk	Increases depend on protein intake and other factors (see text). Rate of increase is controlled by limiting protein intake. This intervention is believed to decrease the rate of onset of systemic symptoms, such as anorexia, nausea, and vomiting. Elevations have multiple causes, including diminished renal function, excessive protein intake, sepsis, GI bleeding, dehydration, and tissue catabolism.
Electrolyte Studies			
Serum sodium	136-145 mEq/L; 136-145 mmol/L (SI units)	Normal or decreased	Clients with renal failure retain sodium. With associated water retention, serum sodium levels seem normal. With excessive water retention, serum sodium levels seem decreased owing to hemodilution. Assess the client for evidence of fluid volume excess: edema, weight increase, or elevation of diastolic blood pressure. Limit fluid intake as directed. Avoid excessive sodium intake. Monitor for signs of hypernatremia: dry skin, excessive thirst, dry mucous membranes, elevated body temperature, and flushed skin. Client may need diuretics or dialysis.
Serum potassium	*Male:* 3.5-5.0 mmol/L (SI units) *Female:* 3.4-4.4 mmol/L (SI units)	Increased	Advise the client to avoid salt substitutes and to limit potassium-containing foods. Monitor for rapidly increasing serum potassium levels in ARF. ECG changes occur with serum potassium levels $\geq$6.5. Monitor for signs of hyperkalemia: dizziness, weakness, cardiac irregularities, muscle cramps, diarrhea, and nausea. May require administration of sodium polystyrene sulfonate (Kayexalate) or other treatment.
Serum phosphorus (phosphate)	3.0-4.5 mg/dl; 0.97-1.45 mmol/L (SI units) *Older adults:* May be slightly decreased	Increased	Short-term increases have potential to cause rapid decrease in serum calcium level and cardiac rhythm disturbances. Long-term increases demineralize bones of calcium and enhance fracture potential. Phosphate-binding medications help control hyperphosphatemia and prevent calcium depletion from the bones.

From Ignatavicius DD, Workman ML: *Medical-surgical nursing: critical thinking for collaborative care,* ed 4, Philadelphia, 2002, Saunders, p 1669.
GI, Gastrointestinal; *ARF,* acute renal failure; *ECG,* electrocardiogram; *CRF,* chronic renal failure; *RBCs,* red blood cells; *WBCs,* white blood cells; *GFR,* glomerular filtration rate.

Table 28-4

Laboratory Profile: Renal Failure—cont'd

Test	Normal Range for Adults	Values in Renal Failure	Comments
Electrolyte Studies—cont'd			
Serum calcium	Total calcium: 9.0-10.5 mg/dl; 2.25-2.75 mmol/L (SI units) Ionized calcium; 4.60-5.08 mg/dl; 1.15-1.27 mmol/L (SI units) *Older adults:* slightly decreased	Decreased	Decreases in ARF may necessitate replacement. Decreases in CRF may be only slight and may or may not necessitate replacement. As the serum phosphate level increases, the serum calcium level decreases. Chronic calcium deficiency leads to renal osteodystrophy. Control of phosphate excess is usually essential before calcium replacement is initiated. Monitor for signs and symptoms of hypocalcemia: abdominal cramps, hyperactive reflexes, tingling in fingertips, and spasms in feet and wrists.
Serum magnesium	1.2-2.0 mEq/L; 0.66-1.07 mmol/L (SI units)	Increased	Advise the client to avoid compounds containing magnesium (e.g., laxatives)
Serum carbon dioxide combining power (bicarbonate)	23-29 mEq/L (venous); 23-29 mmol/L (SI units)	Decreased	Replace bicarbonate. Monitor respiratory rate and depth. Monitor for decreased orientation.
Arterial blood pH	7.38-7.42	Decreased (in metabolic acidosis) or normal	The respiratory system attempts to compensate by hyperventilation (increased rate and depth of respiration). Values are within the normal range if blood buffers and lungs can compensate. Monitor breathing rate and depth. Monitor level of consciousness.
Arterial blood bicarbonate (HCO_3^-)	21-28 mEq/L	Decreased	Provide replacement PO, IV, or by hemodialysis or peritoneal dialysis.
Arterial blood $Paco_2$	Male: 35-48 mm Hg Female: 32-45 mm Hg	Decreased	Monitor for respiratory fatigue (the client breathes more rapidly and deeply to "blow off" carbon dioxide).
Other Blood Studies			
Hemoglobin	11.7-15.5 g/dl (women); 7.4-9.9 mmol/L (SI units) 13.2-17.3 g/dl (men); 8.7-11.2 mmol/L (SI units) *Older adults:* Slightly decreased	Decreased	Decreased levels indicate anemia. Monitor for pallor, weakness, lethargy, dizziness, possible shortness of breath, and activity intolerance.
Hematocrit	*Female:* 35%-45% *Male:* 39%-49% *Older adults:* May be slightly decreased	Decreased to 20%	Same as for hemoglobin. With erythropoietin therapy, may be able to obtain levels as high as 36%.
Urinalysis*			
Specific gravity	Usually 1.016-1.022; possible range: 1.001-1.035	Usually decreased and fixed	Reflects inability of the tubules to produce a concentrated or diluted urine in response to changes in plasma osmolality. Monitor for fluid volume deficit or excess.

*Urine may become cloudy with heavy sediment. Urine output and appearance vary, depending on remaining renal function.

Continued

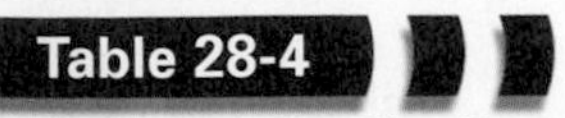

Table 28-4

Laboratory Profile: Renal Failure—cont'd

Test	Normal Range for Adults	Values in Renal Failure	Comments
Urinalysis—cont'd			
pH	Average: 5.5-6.0; possible range: 4.5-8.0	May be fixed; pH does not change with dietary changes	Collect a freshly voided specimen for testing.
Glucose	None or <15 mg/dl Usually detectable in urine of nondiabetic clients when blood level is 160-180 mg/dl	Increased	The renal threshold is often increased; therefore the blood glucose level may be >160-180 mg/dl before glucose is detectable in the urine. Monitor *blood* glucose levels.
Protein	2-8 mg/dl	Increased when there is glomerular damage or disease	Increases may be an incidental and benign finding. Transient increases occur with extreme exercise, fever, stress, or infection. Persistent proteinuria requires 24-hr collection for determination of total quantity excreted. Persistent proteinuria may indicate a serious renal problem. Instruct the client about the need for follow-up. Instruct the client in the correct procedure for collection of 24-hr specimen.
Occult blood	No RBCs or occasionally 2 or 3 RBCs per high-power field	More than 2 or 3 RBCs per high-power field Detectable hemoglobin No hemoglobin	Hemoglobin is detectable when hemolysis of RBCs has occurred. Intact RBCs are only detectable with microscopic examination. Collect a freshly voided specimen for testing.
WBCs	0-5 per high-power field	Increased in urinary tract infection	Often indicates need for urine culture.
Bacteria	Less than 1000 colonies/ml	Increased in the presence of infection, with or without an increase in WBCs	Obtain urine culture.
Casts	None or a few; composed of RBCs, WBCs, protein, or tubular cell casts such as hyaline	Casts present	Casts may be a benign occurrence or may signify that some renal injury or disease is present. Collect a freshly voided specimen for direct microscopic examination.
Creatinine clearance	97-137 ml/min (men) 88-128 ml/min (women) *Older adults:* Progressively decreased with age	Decreased	Change reflects decreases in GFR. Creatinine clearance is determined from a 24-hr urine collection and a serum creatinine value.

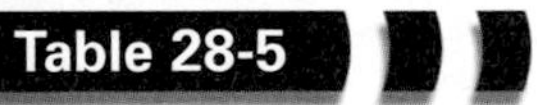

Table 28-5

Manifestations of Electrolyte Imbalances in Renal Failure

Electrolyte Imbalance	Manifestations
Hyponatremia (decreased sodium)	Headache, muscle weakness, fatigue, apathy, confusion, coma, anorexia, nausea, vomiting, abdominal cramping
Hypernatremia (increased sodium)	Dry mucous membranes, decreased urinary output, rubbery skin turgor, excitement, tachycardia
Hypokalemia (decreased potassium)	Anorexia, nausea, vomiting, abdominal distention, lethargy, confusion, mental depression, weakness, decreased standing blood pressure, arrhythmias, electrocardiographic changes
Hyperkalemia (increased potassium)	Nausea, vomiting, diarrhea, irritability, weakness, oliguria, arrhythmias, electrocardiographic changes, sudden death, numbness, tingling
Hypocalcemia (decreased calcium)	Osteoporosis, fractures, tingling, convulsions, muscle spasms, tetany, calcium deposits in tissue, nausea, vomiting, diarrhea, arrhythmias
Hypercalcemia (increased calcium)	Renal calculi, coma, decreased reflexes, lethargy, arrhythmias, muscle fatigue, bone pain, osteoporosis, fractures
Acidosis (decreased bicarbonate)	Headache, malaise, rapid deep respirations, disorientation, stupor, coma, hyperkalemia

From Monahan FD, Neighbors M: *Medical-surgical nursing: foundations for clinical practice,* ed 2, Philadelphia, 1998, Saunders, p 1390.

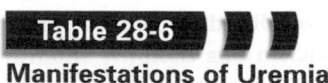

Manifestations of Uremia

System	Alteration with Uremia	Cause
Central nervous system	Uremic encephalopathy	Brain cells shrink because of osmotic gradient
Peripheral nervous system	Peripheral neuropathies	Waste interferes with nerve transmission
	Muscle weakness	
Cardiovascular	Decreased cardiac output	Increased waste has negative inotropic effect
	Pericarditis	Uremic crystals deposited in pericardium
Hematologic	Bleeding tendencies	Decreased platelet aggregation, decreased coagulation factors
	Anemia	Decreased red blood cell life span
	Infection	Decreased immune cell function
Gastrointestinal	Anorexia	Appetite suppression, vomiting
Skin	Pruritus, uremic dermatitis	Waste crystals
	Uremic frost	
	Delayed healing	Impaired collagen synthesis

tion results in elevated Bowman capsule pressure, which impedes filtration. Specific gravity, osmolality, and urine sodium are variable.

- Intrarenal failure is due to primary dysfunction of renal tubular cells and usually results in ATN. Intrarenal failure may occur with nephrotoxic, ischemic, or inflammatory insults. Intrarenal failure is characterized by manifestations of renal cell damage, including low urine specific gravity and osmolality, high urine sodium, casts, and possible proteinuria. Inadequate management or an insufficient response to management of either prerenal or postrenal failure may result in progression to intrarenal failure and ATN.
- ARF has three characteristic phases. The first phase, characterized by oliguria and progressive azotemia, may last 1 to 2 weeks. Oliguria is followed by a diuretic phase that lasts about 2 to 10 days. During the diuretic phase, urine volume increases, but tubular function is impaired and azotemia continues. The recovery phase, usually lasting from 3 to 12 months, is characterized by gradual normalization of serum creatinine and BUN. Often a degree of renal insufficiency persists.
- ARF results in characteristic alterations in laboratory tests of the blood and urine. The retention of metabolic wastes (azotemia), which is monitored by the BUN, produces widespread systemic effects (uremia).

CHRONIC RENAL FAILURE

Chronic renal failure is the progressive loss of renal function over months to years. It can be defined by a glomerular filtration rate of less than 60 ml/min/1.73 m^2 for 3 months or more.[14] Advancement of the disease can sometimes be slowed, but it is ultimately irreversible and terminates in end-stage renal disease (ESRD), the final stage of CRF. Without dialysis or kidney transplantation, the mortality associated with ESRD is 100%.[12]

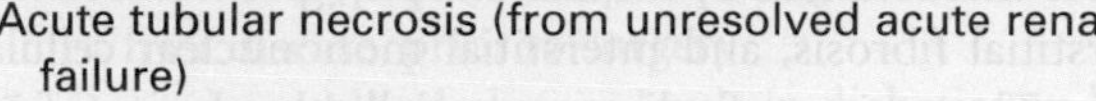

Causes of Chronic Renal Failure

Acute tubular necrosis (from unresolved acute renal failure)

Developmental/congenital conditions
- Renal agenesis
- Aplastic kidneys
- Renal hypoplasia
- Ectopic/displaced kidneys
- Fused kidneys

Cystic disorders
- Polycystic kidney disease
- Medullary cystic disease

Neoplasms
- Benign tumors of the kidney
- Malignant tumors of the kidney
- Wilms tumor

Infections
- Recurrent pyelonephritis
- Renal tuberculosis
- Poststreptococcal glomerulonephritis

Systemic conditions
- Diabetes mellitus (diabetic nephropathy)
- Diabetes insipidus
- Hypertension
- Hyperparathyroidism
- Hepatorenal syndrome
- Gout
- Amyloidosis
- Scleroderma
- Goodpasture syndrome
- Systemic lupus erythematosus

Etiology and Pathophysiology

The causes of CRF are diverse (Box 28-2) and include conditions that directly affect the kidney, as well as systemic disorders. The specific etiologic process is important because some of the treatment decisions are based on the underlying cause.[15]

research may support the recommendation for clinical use of ANP.[19]

ACE inhibitors and ARB reduce proteinuria[20] and enhance glomerular hemodynamics.[20] However, ACE inhibitors must be monitored carefully to avoid the possibility of ACE-induced ARF, which can occur in some patients. This can be defined as a progressive rise in serum creatinine ($\geq$0.5 mg/dl if serum creatinine was initially $<$2.0 and $\geq$ 1.0).[21]

Finally, management of ATN and the other conditions that may progress to CRF retards the progression to ESRD (see Chapter 27). In some cases, such as glomerulonephritis and pyelonephritis, such aggressive therapy can prevent the development of CRF altogether.

Diagnostic Tests

In addition to the renal function tests of blood and urine (see Table 28-4), which are used to diagnose and monitor renal failure, a wide variety of other diagnostic tests are used to identify renal abnormalities (Table 28-8). These tests may locate specific areas of dysfunction and thus allow interventions appropriate to the given pathologic process.

Management of Renal Failure

The objectives of management are presented in Box 28-3. Treatment of clinical problems requires an understanding of the pathology and progression of renal failure.

Pharmacology

Pharmacologic management of renal failure varies with whether the failure is acute or chronic. In ARF, after direct interventions for the specific type of cause, pharmacologic interventions are used to enhance the recovery of renal function and manage fluid and electrolyte abnormalities. Some drugs have been found to retard the progression of CRF. When ESRD has developed, drug therapy is used to manage the systemic effects of renal failure such as anemia.

In ARF pharmacologic interventions include use of the loop diuretic furosemide, which is the drug of choice in patients with ARF because it continues to be effective when the creatinine clearance is markedly decreased, it enhances renal blood flow and promotes the passage of tubular debris, and it can convert oliguric to nonoliguric ATN.[19] A decrease of 1 kg in the patient's weight corresponds to a fluid loss of 1 L. Low-dose dopamine continues to be useful for its efficacy in increasing renal perfusion. Improved perfusion of the kidney results in an increase in GFR and an increase in urine output. Therefore, in addition to monitoring patient weight, the nurse needs to closely monitor intake and output records.

The volume overload that results during the oliguric phase of ATN may prove responsive to diuretic therapy. If such treatment is ineffective, dialysis may be necessary to support this function of the kidneys until the diuretic phase is entered. Albumin may be used in hypoalbuminemic states to reverse some of the fluid that has shifted into the interstitium.[1]

Electrolyte abnormalities, especially hyperkalemia, may also be responsive to diuretic therapy in ARF. Again, dialysis remains an option, but drug therapy is usually attempted initially when the patient has ARF.[22] Elevated potassium levels may be managed pharmacologically to either remove potassium ions from the body or shift them to the cells. Sodium polystyrene sulfonate (Kayexalate) is a cation-exchange resin that exchanges potassium for sodium in the gastrointestinal tract so that excess potassium can be excreted in the stool. It is administered orally or rectally and is recommended for mild to moderate hyperkalemia.[1] Insulin carries potassium ions into the cells and decreases serum but not total-body potassium levels. It is administered with a glucose solution to prevent hypoglycemia.[1] Intravenous calcium may be administered to counteract the myocardial depressant effect of the elevated potassium levels.[1]

Clinical research into pharmacologic interventions for ARF has identified some exciting new potential therapies. Current studies are exploring the use of growth factors and adenine nucleotides to limit acute renal damage and increase the rapidity of the repair process. The future may bring a reduction in morbidity and mortality as some of these innovative approaches are initiated.[23] Future testing for renal disease will include C-reactive protein levels, which are commonly elevated in patients with renal disease.[24]

The progression of CRF to ESRD is the subject of a great deal of research. Because the incidence of ESRD doubled in the decade from 1991 to 2000 and the trend is expected to continue, any interventions that retard the process will have profound effects on quality of life and the health care budget.[12] Experts in the field suggest that the most important intervention to accomplish this goal is to control blood pressure in order to protect the kidney from the damage that hypertension produces. The use of ACE inhibitors appears to slow the progression of CRF by protecting the kidney from hemodynamically mediated glomerular damage. Calcium channel blockade has likewise been demonstrated to decelerate the progression of CRF.[21] Target blood pressure for individuals with renal disease is less than 130/80 mm Hg.[17]

The systemic effects of ESRD related to fluid and electrolyte imbalances are primarily managed by dialysis and nutritional support. Hypocalcemia and hyperphosphatemia may be additionally treated with calcium and vitamin D supplementation and phosphate binders such as aluminum hydroxide, respectively. The anemia that results from depression of erythropoietin production and uremia is managed with injections of a synthetic form of erythropoietin (Epogen). Use of this therapy has markedly reduced the need for blood transfusions.[10]

All patients in renal failure, whether acute or chronic, must have their medications carefully scrutinized. Because most medications are excreted by the kidney, dosages and frequencies must be modified. The phase of ARF or the degree of im-

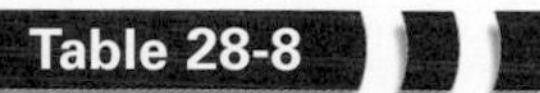

Common Radiologic and Special Diagnostic Tests for Clients with Disorders of the Renal/Urinary System

Test	Purpose	Comments
Radiography of kidneys, ureters, and bladder (KUB) (plain film of abdomen)	To screen for the presence of two kidneys To measure the kidney's size To detect gross obstruction	
Excretory urography	To measure the kidney's size To detect obstruction To assess parenchymal mass	Radiopaque contrast media may cause an allergic (hypersensitivity) reaction in iodine-sensitive clients. Contrast agent is also hypertonic and increases the risk of acute renal failure in adults with serum creatinine levels greater than 1.5 mg/dl, diabetes mellitus, multiple myeloma, or dehydration. Nephrotoxic complications can be prevented by parenteral fluid administration, the use of mannitol, and daily monitoring of serum creatinine levels.
Nephrotomography	To assess various planes of kidney tissue for cysts, tumors, or calculi	Same as for excretory urogram.
Computed tomography	To measure the size of the kidneys To evaluate contour to assess for masses or obstruction	Contrast medium may provoke acute renal failure. See comments with excretory urography for high-risk clients and preventive measures related to contrast. May be performed without contrast medium and still obtain adequate visualization.
Cystography and cystoscopy	To identify abnormalities of the bladder wall and urethral and ureteral occlusions To manage small obstructions or lesions via fulguration, lithotripsy, or removal with a stone basket	Instrumentation of the urinary tract increases the risk of infection. Monitor for infection for 48-72 hr after the procedure.
Voiding cystourethrography	To outline the bladder's contour and to detect urinary reflux from vesicourethral junctions	The risk of infection is similar to that in cystography because urinary catheterization is necessary. Monitor for postprocedure infection.
Renal arteriography	To identify vascular abnormalities within each kidney and adjacent aorta	Contrast medium may provoke acute renal failure. See comments with excretory urography for high-risk clients and preventive measures related to contrast. Essential for diagnosis and management of some vascular abnormalities, such as renal artery stenosis. Monitor for bleeding after the procedure.
Ultrasonography	To identify the size of the kidneys or obstruction in the kidneys or the lower urinary tract May detect tumors or cysts	Ultrasonography entails minimal risk to the client. Ultrasonography is a good alternative to excretory urography.
Renography (renal scanning)	To assess renal blood flow	Radioactive material is used for this test. Captopril or another angiotensin-converting enzyme (ACE) inhibitor may be used, placing the client at risk for severe hypotensive reactions during and following this procedure.

From Ignatavicius DD, Workman ML: *Medical-surgical nursing: critical thinking for collaborative care,* ed 4, Philadelphia, 2002, Saunders, p 1607.

portal vein. Dialysate fluid is placed in the peritoneal space through a surgically placed, permanent catheter (Figure 28-5).

No pressure gradient is used in this method of dialysis, so fluid moves by osmosis, drawn by hypertonic dialysate fluid from the blood vessels in the parietal and visceral membranes. The higher the concentration of glucose in the dialysate fluid, the more water is pulled out of the blood stream. Diffusion is the sole method of waste and excess electrolyte removal. The amount and type removed are determined by the length of time that the fluid remains in the peritoneum.[26] At the end of the treatment time, the patient allows the dialysate fluid to drain out of the peritoneum by gravity.

Because no vascular access is needed and no blood is outside the body, no anticoagulation is necessary with peritoneal dialysis. This method of fluid and waste removal is slow but efficient, and so is not advisable if volume overload, uremia, or electrolyte abnormalities are severe. The peritoneal membrane is a biological membrane with pores that are larger than those used in other types of dialysis. Therefore, some larger molecules such as proteins may pass through, which is usually managed by decreasing the time that the dialysate fluid remains in the body; however, albumin and total protein levels are routinely monitored. Another potential complication of this type of dialysis is peritonitis. If infection of the peritoneum occurs, this form of dialysis must be terminated and another method used until the infection is resolved.[26] Also, the dietary restrictions for patients on peritoneal dialysis are more stringent than for those on hemodialysis.

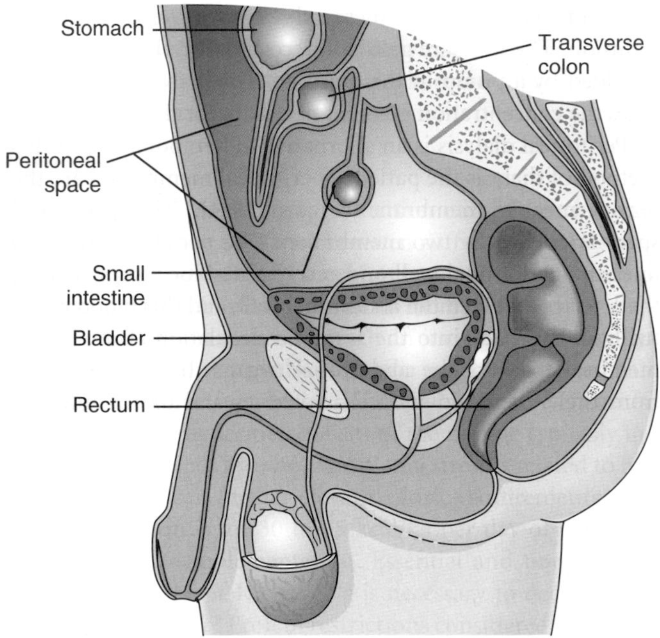

FIGURE 28-4 ■ The peritoneal space between the parietal and visceral membranes is highlighted in blue.

A major advantage of this type of dialysis is that the patient is not connected to a machine. Patients usually manage this type of dialysis themselves and go about their activities on a daily basis. The process of instilling or removing dialysate requires about 30 minutes. Between treatments, the peritoneal dialysis catheter can be tucked under clothing.

The newest method of dialysis is continuous renal replacement therapy (Figure 28-6). Its use is limited to critically ill patients whose condition is too unstable for any other form of dialysis. As with hemodialysis, vascular access is required and a special filter is used. The patient's vascular access is attached to tubing leading to the filter, and a small pump is used to propel blood through the filter. Filtered, clean blood is then returned to the patient. Waste materials and fluid, called effluent, are retained in a collection container. Although anticoagulation is required, a smaller amount of blood (80 to 100 ml) is outside the body, so that any hypotension induced by the therapy is mild.[1,22] A small pump is used to generate the pressure gradient to allow ultrafiltration and diffusion to move fluid and solutes through the filter.[1]

The several subtypes of continuous renal replacement therapy vary in their complexity in terms of whether arterial access, venous access, or both are used and whether dialysate fluid is used. This type of dialysis requires the most technically

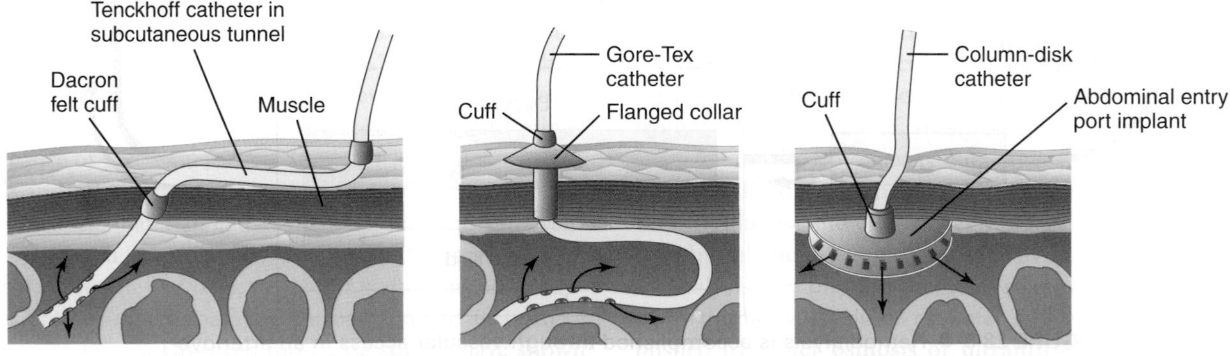

FIGURE 28-5 ■ Peritoneal dialysis catheters are surgically implanted into the abdominal cavity and may be straight, equipped with a flanged collar, or disk shaped. In all cases, they terminate within the peritoneal space. The catheters are stabilized when muscle cells attach to a Dacron cuff that is part of the catheter design. In peritoneal dialysis, fluid movement is achieved by osmosis, and toxin and electrolytes move by diffusion.

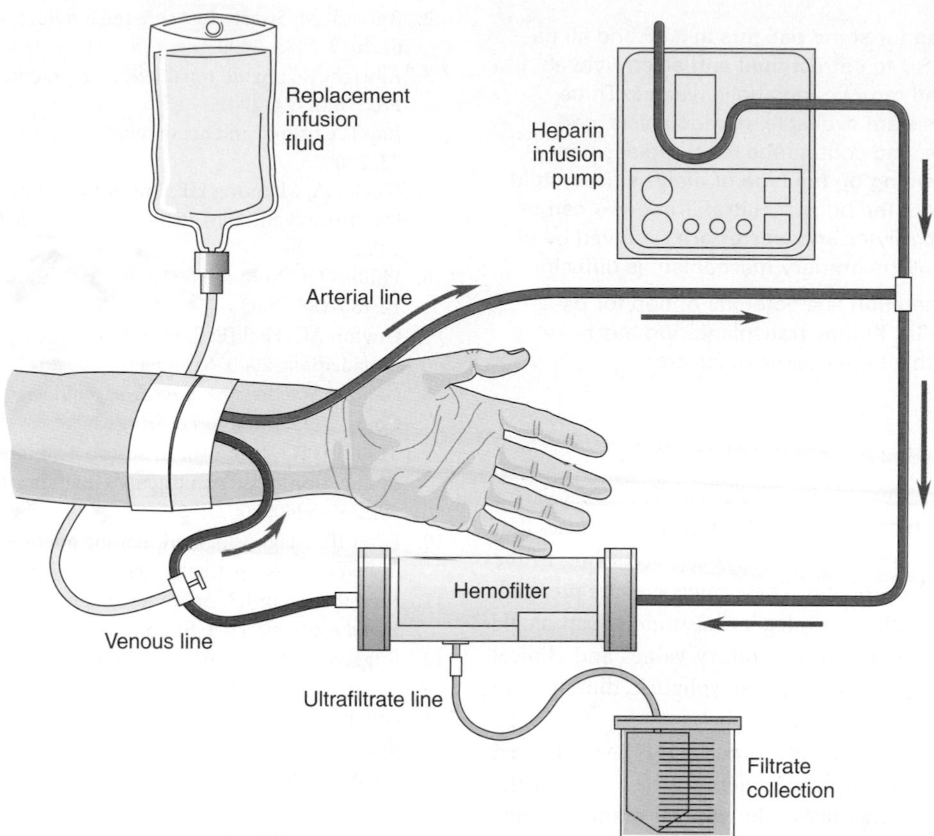

FIGURE 28-6 ■ Vascular access for continuous renal replacement therapy (CRRT) is accomplished via catheters placed in the patient's blood vessels. Toxin- and fluid-overloaded blood passes through a filter propelled by the patient's own blood pressure or a small pump. Dialysate fluid may be added to increase the removal of metabolic wastes and elevated electrolytes by diffusion. In CRRT, as with hemodialysis, fluid and some toxins move by ultrafiltration.

skilled personnel and is used for the most critically ill patients. These limitations currently restrict the use and access to continuous renal replacement therapy.[1]

Transplantation

Kidney transplantation is an alternative to dialysis for patients with ESRD. As with other conditions in which transplantation is indicated, the primary limiting factor is the availability of organs. The first successful transplantation of a human kidney occurred in 1950, but it was not until refinements in immunotherapy and surgical techniques were developed in the 1960s and 1970s that kidney transplantation became a viable option.[27]

Kidneys can be removed from brain-dead donors, or living individuals may donate a single kidney. The success of renal transplantation is greater than that of any other organ transplantation. As living unrelated donors increase and organ donation increases overall, renal transplantation will continue to be a valuable alternative treatment for patients with ESRD.[27]

KEY CONCEPTS

- Preventive interventions for intrarenal ARF include maintenance of hydration, adequate nutrition, early removal of Foley catheters, rapid intervention for hypotension, and monitoring of nephrotoxic drugs. Drug therapy with loop diuretics and dopamine may reverse ARF. Calcium channel blockers and atrial natriuretic peptides are under research for their potential use as prophylactic agents.
- Appropriate management of ATN and conditions such as diabetes that may progress to CRF may slow the progression to ESRD.
- Many diagnostic tests may be used to identify the specific area of renal dysfunction.
- Drug therapy is used in ARF to control volume overload and electrolyte abnormalities. If these therapies are insufficient, dialysis may be undertaken.
- Drug therapy in CRF is used to control hypertension, anemia, and some of the electrolyte abnormalities.
- Nutritional needs for patients in renal failure include increased calories and amino acids, as well as calcium and vitamin supplementation. Fluid, phosphorus, and potassium intake is restricted. Sodium and protein levels are determined by the underlying pathologic process.

- Dialysis is used for some patients in ARF and all patients with ESRD to correct fluid and electrolyte abnormalities and remove metabolic wastes. Three types of dialysis are available: hemodialysis, peritoneal dialysis, and continuous renal replacement therapy. Depending on the type of dialysis used, fluid is removed from the body by ultrafiltration or osmosis. Some electrolytes and wastes are removed by ultrafiltration, but the primary mechanism is diffusion.
- Renal transplantation is a potential option for patients with ESRD. Kidney transplantation has been associated with a high degree of success.

SUMMARY

Renal failure can occur at any age. ARF has multiple causes that can be classified into one of three categories according to the physical location of the problem. These categories are prerenal, intrarenal, and postrenal. Each category has unique pathologic features and some variation in laboratory values and clinical findings. ARF is divided into three phases: oliguric, diuretic, and recovery. Interventions differ for each phase.

CRF is a progressive, irreversible process. It is characterized by three stages of advancing impairment in the ability of the kidney to maintain homeostasis. The clinical manifestations of CRF are determined by the rapidity and severity of its development.

Many diagnostic tests are available to provide the nurse with information about the patient's renal function. Key aspects of care include pharmacologic management of fluid overload, electrolyte abnormalities, and metabolic wastes; nutritional management; dialysis; and renal transplantation.

Patients in renal failure are often treated with dialysis. Three forms of dialysis are available: hemodialysis, peritoneal dialysis, and continuous renal replacement therapy. Selection of the appropriate modality is determined for each individual patient.

A clear understanding of the pathophysiology related to renal dysfunction is essential for nurses caring for patients in renal failure. The impact that renal failure has on all other body systems presents many nursing challenges.

MEDIA RESOURCES

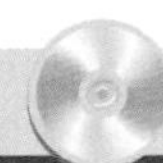

evolve

Remember to check out the ***CD Companion*** included with this book for Review Questions, Key Concepts Review, Glossary (with audio for selected terms), Disease Profiles, and Animations.

PLUS, visit the ***Evolve website*** at http://evolve.elsevier.com/Copstead/ for Case Studies, Disease Profiles, and WebLinks.

References

1. Lancaster LE: *ANNA core curriculum for nephrology nursing,* ed 4, Pitman, NJ, 2001, American Nephrology Nurses' Association.
2. Agrawal M, Swartz R: Acute renal failure, *Am Fam Physician* 61:2077-2088, 2000.
3. Albright RC: Acute renal failure: a practical update, *Mayo Clin Proc* 76:67-74, 2001.
4. Ray T: Chronic and acute renal failure, *Adv Nurse Pract* 8:69-73, 2000.
5. Block CA, Manning HL: Prevention of acute renal failure in the critically ill, *Am J Respir Crit Care Med* 165:320-324, 2002.
6. Phillips CL, Andreoli S: Acute renal failure, *Curr Opin Pediatr* 14:183-188, 2002.
7. Guyton AC, Hall JE: *Textbook of medical physiology,* ed 10, Philadelphia, 2000, Saunders.
8. Ganong WF: *Review of medical physiology,* ed 19, Stamford, Conn, 1999, Appleton & Lange.
9. Molitoris BA, Sandoval R, Sutton A: Endothelial injury and dysfunction in ischemic acute renal failure, *Crit Care Med* 30:S235-S240, 2002.
10. Foret JP: Diagnosing and treating anemia and iron deficiency in hemodialysis patients, *Nephrol Nurs J* 29:292-296, 2002.
11. Kumar S, Stein JH: Acute renal failure. In Stein JH, editor: *Internal medicine,* ed 5, St Louis, 1998, Mosby, pp 768-776.
12. Ruggenenti P, Schieppati A, Remuzzi G: Progression, remission of chronic renal diseases, *Lancet* 357:1601-1608, 2001.
13. Gutch CF, Stoner MH, Corea AL: *Hemodialysis for nurses and dialysis personnel,* ed 6, St Louis, 1999, Mosby.
14. Levey AS: Nondiabetic kidney disease, *N Engl J Med* 347:1505-1511, 2002.
15. Luke RG, Sanders CE, Curtis JJ: Chronic renal failure. In Stein JH, editor: *Internal medicine,* ed 5, St Louis, 1998, Mosby, pp 776-796.
16. Pagana KD, Pagana TJ: *Mosby's manual of diagnostic and laboratory tests,* ed 2, St Louis, 2002, Mosby.
17. Parmar MS: Chronic renal disease, *BMJ* 325:85-90, 2002.
18. Toigo G et al: Expert working group report on nutrition in adult patients with renal insufficiency (part 1 of 2), *Clin Nutr* 19:197-207, 2000.
19. Pruchnicki MC, Dasta JF: Acute renal failure in hospitalized patients: part II, *Ann Pharmacother* 36:1430-1442, 2002.
20. Herlitz H et al: The effects of an ACE inhibitor and a calcium antagonist on the progression of renal disease: the Nephros Study, *Nephrol Dial Transplant* 16:2158-2165, 2001.
21. Schoolwerth AC et al: Renal considerations in angiotensin converting enzyme inhibitor therapy, *Circulation* 104:1985-1991, 2001.
22. Ozdemir FN, Akcay A, Haberal M: Dialysis modalities in patients with acute renal failure, *Nephrol Dial Transplant* 16:18-20, 2001.
23. Nigan SK, Lieberthal W: Acute renal failure. III. The role of growth factors in the process of renal regeneration and repair, *Am J Physiol Renal Physiol* 279:F3-F11, 2000.
24. Eikelboom JW, Hankey GJ: Associations of homocysteine, C-reactive protein and cardiovascular disease in patients with renal disease, *Curr Opin Nephrol Hypertens* 10:377-383, 2001.
25. Stark J: Acute renal failure: focus on acute tubular necrosis, *Crit Care Nurs Clin* 10:159-170, 1998.
26. Gokal R, Hutchison A: Dialysis therapies for end-stage renal disease, *Semin Dial* 15:220-226, 2002.
27. Health Resources and Services Administration: *UNOS donation and transplantation nursing curriculum,* Rockville, Md, 1996, U.S. Department of Health and Human Services.

chapter 29

Disorders of the Bladder

Cynthia Fryhling Corbett

MEDIA RESOURCES

Additional Material for Study, Review, and Further Exploration

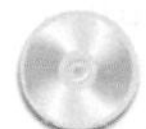

CD Companion ◆ Review Questions and Answers ◆ Key Concepts Review
◆ Glossary *(with audio pronunciations for selected terms)*
◆ Disease Profiles ◆ Animations

evolve ***Website*** at http://evolve.elsevier.com/Copstead/
◆ Case Studies ◆ Disease Profiles ◆ WebLinks

KEY QUESTIONS

- How do the pathophysiologic characteristics and management of stress, urge, overflow, and mixed incontinence differ?
- What clinical findings differentiate bladder stones from bladder tumors?
- What clinical and urinalysis findings would be indicative of a bladder infection?
- What surgical strategies are available for urine collection after management of bladder cancer with cystectomy?
- How are congenital abnormalities of the urinary collecting system detected and treated?

CHAPTER OUTLINE

The bladder is an expandable reservoir for urine, which is constantly produced by the kidney(s). A functional bladder enables one-way flow of urine from the kidney to the urethra. Bladder disorders can generally be classified as obstructive, infective, or congenital. These disorders are often overlapping. For instance, stasis of urine, which occurs with obstructive and congenital disorders, often leads to urinary tract infection (UTI). Pyelonephritis (see Chapter 27) and acute postrenal renal failure (see Chapter 28) are serious potential consequences of disorders of the lower urinary tract.

Normal bladder structure and function and selected bladder disorders affecting adults and children are presented in this chapter. Bladder disorders result in significant health problems that have tremendous physical, psychosocial, and economic ramifications for affected patients and families.[1,2] Voiding dysfunction that is manifested as **incontinence** affects more than 13 million adult Americans and 2% to 20% of children younger than 15 years.[1,3] UTIs affect millions of persons each year; without proper identification and management, such infections can lead to renal failure, sepsis, or both. Bladder cancer is steadily increasing and is the cause of approximately 12,000 deaths per year in the United States.[4] Although relatively rare, congenital disorders of the lower urinary tract have profound implications for affected children and their families. Early diagnosis and management of these bladder disorders may lessen the consequences and reduce related morbidity.

STRUCTURE AND FUNCTION OF THE BLADDER

The function of the urinary bladder is to store urine until it is released during micturition. The bladder is primarily muscle, which allows bladder distention to hold urine and bladder contraction to facilitate passage of urine through the urethra. The two principal parts of the bladder are the body and the neck (Figure 29-1). The body of the bladder, where urine collects, is made up of smooth muscle known as **detrusor muscle.** This muscle extends in all directions throughout the bladder. After the initiation of an action potential, the entire muscle contracts to allow the bladder to empty in one contraction. Ureters enter the bladder obliquely through the detrusor muscle and then travel under the bladder mucosa for 1 to 2 cm before emptying into the bladder. The mucosal lining of the body of the bladder has folds known as **rugae.** Rugae allow the bladder muscle to distend to accommodate urine without friction.

The neck of the bladder also includes the posterior urethra. The wall of the bladder neck is composed of detrusor muscle with elastic tissue. The muscle of the bladder neck is also called the internal sphincter. When the bladder neck has normal tone, the bladder is prevented from emptying until the pressure in the body of the bladder rises above a threshold.

Innervation to the bladder is supplied by the pelvic nerves, which exit the spinal cord at S2 and S3 (see Figure 29-1). Both sensory and motor nerve fibers are needed for bladder function. The sensory fibers detect stretch in the bladder wall. Signals from the posterior urethra are primarily responsible for initiating bladder emptying. The motor fibers are parasympathetic in nature.

Somatic nerve fibers control the voluntary skeletal muscle of the external bladder sphincter via the pudendal nerve. Sympathetic innervation through the hypogastric nerves at L2 is thought to stimulate blood vessels within the bladder. Sensations of fullness and pain may also be transmitted by the sympathetic fibers.

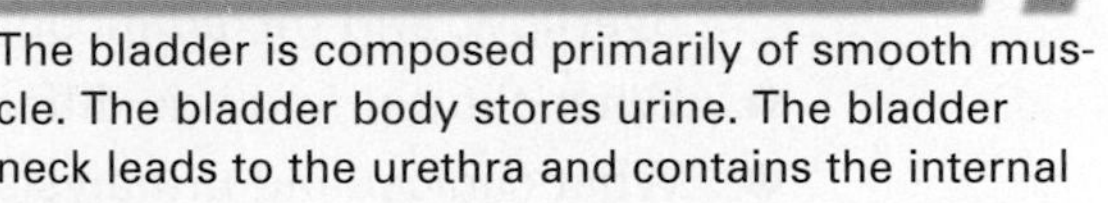

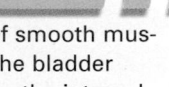

- The bladder is composed primarily of smooth muscle. The bladder body stores urine. The bladder neck leads to the urethra and contains the internal sphincter.
- Innervation of the bladder is supplied by pelvic nerves that exit the spinal cord at S2 and S3. Motor fibers to the bladder are supplied by the parasympathetic system. The somatic pudendal nerve innervates the external bladder sphincter. The sympathetic system innervates blood vessels via the hypogastric plexus.

VOIDING DYSFUNCTION

Incontinence

Voiding dysfunction and resultant urinary incontinence affect more than 13 million adult Americans. Incontinence affects approximately 29% of 30- to 60-year-old women and 1% of similar-aged men.[3] In adults older than 60, an estimated 11% to 34% of men and 17% to 55% of women in the United States have urinary incontinence.[3] More than $26 billion is spent caring for people with incontinence each year.[3]

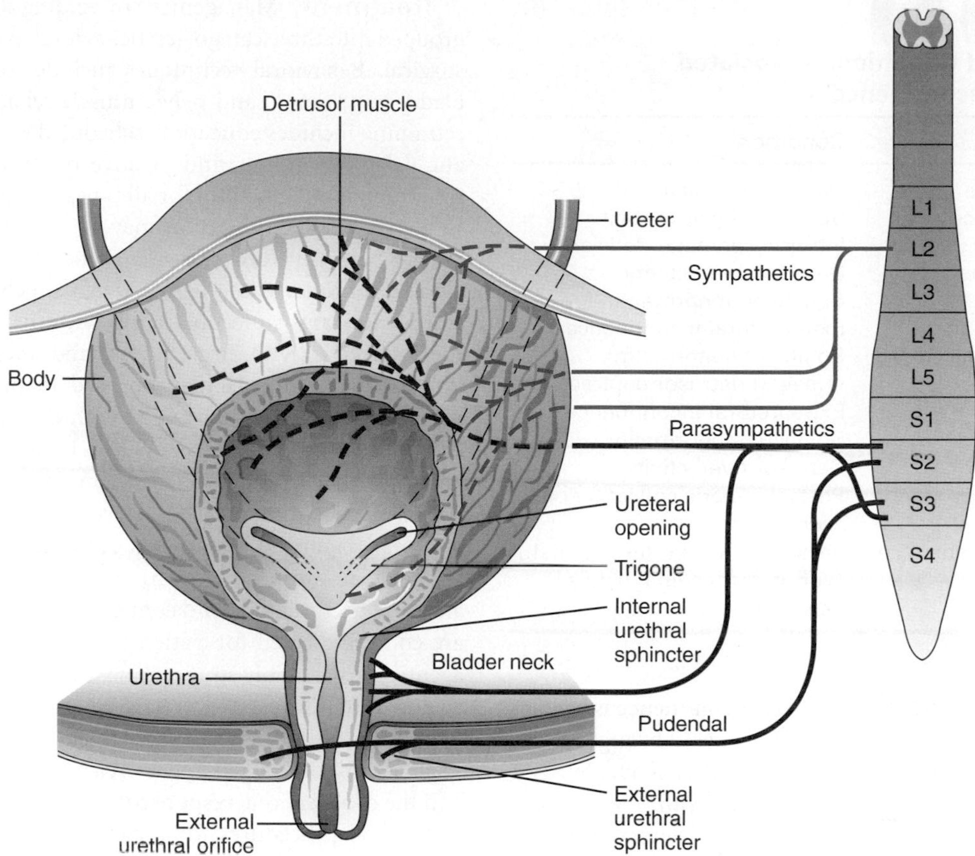

FIGURE 29-1 ■ Bladder structure and innervation.

Pathogenesis. The process of micturition is primarily a result of parasympathetic stimulation of the detrusor muscle to create contraction of the bladder. However, concomitant sympathetic stimulation of the bladder sphincters causes relaxation to allow easy passage of urine from the bladder and urethra.[3-5] Any anatomic, physiologic, or pathologic factor that disrupts this process can result in voiding dysfunction. Alternatively, voiding dysfunction may be a result of external factors such as immobility combined with age-related physiologic changes or medications that induce urinary changes (e.g., diuretics). Voiding dysfunction is usually manifested by urinary incontinence. Risk factors associated with adult urinary incontinence are listed in Box 29-1. The American Urologic Society and the Urodynamics Society have recommended that urinary incontinence be classified in the following seven symptom-based categories: urge, stress, overflow, continuous leakage, nocturnal enuresis, postvoid dribble, and extraurethral incontinence.[6] Urinary incontinence can be attributed to bladder or sphincter abnormalities. Bladder abnormalities include detrusor overactivity (instability or hyperreflexia) and poor compliance.[6] Sphincter abnormalities include urethral hypermobility and intrinsic sphincter deficiency. Table 29-1 shows abnormalities associated with each category of urinary incontinence. The term *neurogenic bladder* is frequently used to describe voiding dysfunction that has a clear neurologic basis. However, the neurologic basis results in symptoms that can be classified into one of the seven symptom categories. Table 29-1 lists the symptoms and conditions associated with urinary incontinence. *Functional incontinence* is a term commonly used to describe incontinence that is secondary to cognitive or motor deficits but not related to urinary pathologic processes.

Box 29-1

Factors Associated with Incontinence

- Immobility/chronic degenerative disease
- Impaired cognition
- Medications (e.g., diuretics)
- Morbid obesity
- Smoking
- Fecal impaction
- Delirium
- Environmental barriers
- High-impact physical activities
- Diabetes
- Stroke
- Estrogen depletion
- Low fluid intake
- Pelvic muscle weakness
- Childhood nocturnal enuresis
- Race
- Pregnancy, vaginal delivery, or episiotomy

Table 29-1

Symptoms and Conditions Associated with Urinary Incontinence

Symptom	Condition
Urge incontinence	Detrusor overactivity
Stress incontinence	Sphincter hypermobility Intrinsic sphincter deficiency
Unaware incontinence	Detrusor overactivity Sphincter abnormality Extraurethral incontinence
Continuous leakage	Sphincter abnormality Impaired detrusor contractility Extraurethral incontinence
Nocturnal enuresis	Sphincter abnormality Detrusor overactivity
Postvoid dribble	Postsphincteric collection of urine
Extraurethral incontinence	Vesicovaginal, ureterovaginal, or urethrovaginal fistula Ectopic ureter

Clinical Manifestations. **Urge incontinence** is characterized by a strong and immediate urge to void brought about by involuntary detrusor contractions (overactivity). Detrusor overactivity may or may not be associated with obvious neurologic problems such as stroke or multiple sclerosis, with obstruction, infection, or surgical trauma, or it may be idiopathic.[6] **Stress incontinence** is primarily caused by increased intraabdominal pressure combined with pelvic muscle laxity.[1,2] As such, stress incontinence is much more predominant in women than in men. Laughing, sneezing, or physical exertion may result in involuntary loss of urine. Vaginal deliveries, episiotomies, and high maternal weight gain are risk factors for stress incontinence, with the percentage of women affected increasing with greater parity.[7] Men occasionally experience stress incontinence after prostatectomy, with the probable cause being intrinsic sphincter deficiency. **Mixed incontinence** is the term used when patients have symptoms of both stress and urge incontinence. **Overflow incontinence** results from urinary retention and an overdistended bladder secondary to obstruction or detrusor underactivity or inactivity or from sphincteric malfunction. The cardinal manifestation is constant or intermittent dribbling, but symptoms similar to urge or stress incontinence may also be present. In men, prostatic hyperplasia is the most common cause of overflow incontinence. However, neurologic dysfunction and other types of outlet obstruction may also cause overflow incontinence. Unconscious or unaware incontinence is urinary leakage that is involuntary and without the individual's awareness of stress or urge. Continuous leakage is loss of urine that is constant throughout the day and night whereas nocturnal enuresis is involuntary urination at night only. Enuresis is often intermittent and may not occur every night. Leakage of urine that occurs after voiding is called postvoid dribble.[6]

Treatment. Management of voiding dysfunction can be grouped into three categories: behavioral, pharmacologic, and surgical. Behavioral techniques include toileting assistance, bladder retraining, and pelvic muscle rehabilitation. Bladder retraining includes education, scheduled voiding with systematic delay of voiding, and positive reinforcement.[1,5] Bladder retraining may be helpful for all types of bladder dysfunction. Pelvic muscle rehabilitation may be as simple as having the patient perform Kegel exercises or be more complex and include techniques with vaginal weights, pelvic floor electrical stimulation, and biofeedback.[1,5] Pelvic muscle rehabilitation is most effective with urge, stress, and mixed incontinence. Pharmacologic agents may be used to promote or inhibit physiologic activities associated with micturition, depending on the cause of voiding dysfunction (Table 29-2). Anticholinergic agents (e.g., tolterodine, oxybutynin) are used when detrusor overactivity has been determined by urodynamic testing (see Diagnostic Tests).[5,8,9] α-Adrenergic antagonists (e.g., phenoxybenzamine, prazosin) can improve bladder compliance and urethral tone and contraction.[10] α-Adrenergic agents are contraindicated for patients with hypertension. Tricyclic agents, most notably imipramine, can also be used for management of detrusor overactivity. Tricyclic antidepressants have an inhibitory effect on the bladder smooth muscle.[1,7,10] Vaginal or oral estrogen may increase vascularity, muscle tone, and the α-adrenergic response in the urethra.[1]

Surgical procedures for incontinence vary depending on the underlying anatomic or physiologic problems causing the voiding dysfunction. Voiding dysfunction that results in stress incontinence is the most amenable to surgical intervention. Surgical procedures to correct urge incontinence caused by detrusor overactivity are rare and are used as a last resort. Overflow incontinence as a result of obstruction is often surgically managed by removing the cause of the obstruction. Table 29-2 includes the surgical procedure options for each type of incontinence.

Incontinence that is not resolved by behavioral, pharmacologic, or surgical intervention must be managed by supportive devices such as intermittent catheterization, indwelling catheterization, or external collecting systems. Each of these devices creates the potential for further complications. UTIs are more likely with stasis of urine in the bladder and, in the case of catheterization, with continuous or intermittent introduction of a foreign object into the normally sterile bladder. Stasis of urine also increases the risk for bladder and renal calculi. Management of incontinence with external collecting systems predisposes patients to skin breakdown.

Enuresis

Enuresis is inappropriate wetting of clothes or beds, and the term is generally used to refer to incontinence in children. Diurnal enuresis refers to daytime wetting and nocturnal enuresis to nighttime wetting. Primary enuresis describes a child who has never achieved continence, whereas secondary enure-

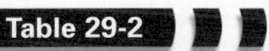

Table 29-2

Treatment Guidelines: Voiding Dysfunction

Condition	Treatment
Detrusor overactivity	Manage underlying condition (e.g., urethral obstruction, infection, bladder stones, bladder cancer, spinal cord tumors, spinal disk disease) Behavior modification Anticholinergics and/or musculotropic relaxants and/or tricyclic antidepressants (± intermittent catheterization) Electrical stimulation Biofeedback Neuromodulation Detrusor myectomy Augmentation enterocystoplasty (± intermittent catheterization) Continent urinary diversion
Low bladder compliance	Anticholinergics and/or musculotropic relaxants and/or tricyclic antidepressants (± intermittent catheterization) Neuromodulation Detrusor myectomy Augmentation enterocystoplasty (± intermittent catheterization) Continent urinary diversion
Sphincteric incontinence	Periurethral injections
Intrinsic sphincter deficiency	Pubovaginal sling Artificial urinary sphincter
Urethral hypermobility	Pelvic floor exercises (± biofeedback) Electrical stimulation Urethropexy or pubovaginal sling

sis refers to enuresis that starts after a period of at least 6 months of dryness.[11] Up to 20% of 5-year-old children, 5% of 10-year-olds, 2% of 12- to 14-year-olds, and 1% of adults have nocturnal enuresis.[12] Only about 20% of children with nocturnal enuresis also have daytime enuresis.[12] Diurnal enuresis in the absence of nocturnal enuresis is uncommon, and the cause is often related to a UTI or to the introduction of stress or change in the child's life.[13]

Etiology. The most common cause of enuresis is maturational delay.[12] Other etiologic factors include UTIs, poor toileting habits, altered or absent nocturnal arginine vasopressin (antidiuretic hormone) secretion by the pituitary gland, and anatomic abnormalities.[11,14] In female children who are wet all the time, an ectopic ureter that empties outside the bladder must be ruled out.[13]

Diagnosis. Clinical workup for enuresis includes a thorough history of elimination patterns (which may necessitate having the parents keep a diary), urinalysis, and a physical examination to identify gross anatomic abnormalities such as lesions of the spine, flank or abdominal masses, gluteal clefts, or gait problems.[12] If a UTI is detected, renal and bladder sonograms and a voiding cystourethrogram should be obtained to rule out vesicoureteral reflux (flow of urine from the bladder into the ureters toward the kidneys).[15-17] In children who remain enuretic after many months of standard treatment, urodynamic testing to eliminate the possibility of neurologic causes may be warranted.[11]

Treatment. Primary treatment for enuresis is behavioral management. If both daytime and nighttime wetting are present, daytime wetting should be addressed first to follow the normal maturational process of gaining continence. Scheduled voiding is the initial approach to daytime enuresis. More complex multidimensional approaches involve urine retention and sphincter control exercises, counseling, visualization, and hypnosis.[11,16] Research has shown that biofeedback therapy may be useful in children when other approaches have failed.[13] Nocturnal enuresis is successfully managed with bed wetting alarms in 70% of children.[11] Pharmacotherapy to manage enuresis consists primarily of synthetic arginine vasopressin and tricyclic antidepressants (e.g., imipramine).[12] Anticholinergic therapy (e.g., oxybutynin) sometimes is used but is effective in less than 40% of cases.[12] However, pharmacologic treatment is not a cure and weaning is eventually necessary.

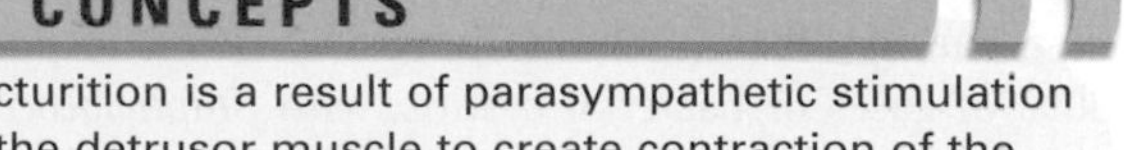

KEY CONCEPTS

- Micturition is a result of parasympathetic stimulation of the detrusor muscle to create contraction of the bladder and sympathetic stimulation to relax the bladder sphincters.

- Voiding dysfunction affects up to 25% of men and 65% of women between the ages of 20 and 60 years. It results in a health care expenditure of more than $26 billion annually in the United States.
- Detrusor overactivity results in urge incontinence.
- Weakening of pelvic muscles or intrinsic urethral sphincter deficiency results in stress incontinence.
- Obstruction or an underactive or inactive detrusor muscle causes overflow incontinence.
- Spinal cord trauma or neurologic conditions, such as multiple sclerosis, may cause reflex incontinence whereby the patient has no warning or sensory awareness of the need to void.
- Neurogenic bladder refers to loss of voluntary bladder control because of central nervous system impairment.
- Treatment options for voiding dysfunction include behavioral, pharmaceutical, and surgical interventions.
- Enuresis is inappropriate wetting, with the term usually reserved for incontinence in children.
- The primary cause of enuresis is maturational delay. Poor toileting habits and UTIs are also fairly common causes. Enuresis as a result of UTI warrants further diagnostic workup.
- Behavioral modification is the initial treatment choice for enuresis. Other methods include bed wetting alarms, pharmacotherapy, counseling, and hypnosis.

INFECTIVE OR INFLAMMATORY UROPATHIES

Cystitis

Cystitis, or inflammation of the bladder urothelium, may result from bacterial, fungal, or parasitic infections, chemical irritants, foreign bodies (e.g., stones), or trauma. By far the most common cause of cystitis—and the focus of this discussion—is bacterial infection.

Pathogenesis. Normally, bacteria are cleared from the bladder by flushing and the dilutional effects of voiding. The high urea concentration and osmolarity and low pH in urine act to kill invading bacteria in a normal bladder environment.[18] Cystitis is more common in females than males (with the exception of neonates). A shorter urethra, as well as a colonization route from the rectum and vagina to the urethra, is thought to potentiate infections in women.[18] In addition, prostatic secretions, which are antibacterial, inhibit cystitis in men younger than 50 years. *Escherichia coli* is responsible for 80% of cases of bacterial cystitis, with *Staphylococcus saprophyticus* accounting for 5% to 10% and the remaining 10% to 15% caused by either *Klebsiella* species, *Proteus mirabilis,* enterococci, or β-hemolytic streptococci.[19] Research has demonstrated that women who have recurrent bacterial cystitis have uroepithelial, vaginal, and buccal epithelial cells that enhance the binding properties of *E. coli.*[18] In addition, lower vaginal pH, lower levels of estrogen, and Lewis blood group LE(a−b−) and LE(a+b−) phenotypes are associated with an increased incidence of cystitis.[18] Other risk factors include sexual activity, use of spermicides, catheterization, diabetes mellitus, poor hygiene, and any type of bladder dysfunction causing urine stasis.

Clinical Manifestations. In about 10% of individuals with bacteriuria the infection is asymptomatic. The majority of patients with cystitis experience frequency, urgency, dysuria (painful urination), and pain in the suprapubic area, lower part of the back, or both. Flank pain is usually more serious and can indicate an infection proximal to the bladder. Visually, hematuria or cloudy urine may be evident. Urinalysis will generally show the presence (more than 10^2 colony-forming units per milliliter) of a known bacterial pathogen, as well as white blood cells, red blood cells, and nitrites.[20]

Diagnostic Test. Screening for UTI is often performed using a nitrite and leukocyte esterase dipstick. Leukocyte esterase is indicative of pyuria (white blood cells), and most urinary pathogens reduce nitrates to nitrites. The sensitivity of dipstick urinalysis combined with visual appearance has been reported at 95% for adults and 79% in children.[21,22] Consequently microscopic analysis and culture remain the gold standard for diagnosis, but in women with symptomatic disease with no complicating factors, a urinalysis that is positive for white or red blood cells or bacteriuria or a combination can provide sufficient evidence of UTI and a culture may be omitted.[20] In patients with symptomatic infection, including women with negative dipstick results, microscopic analysis and culture should be performed.

Diagnosis and Treatment. Four classifications of UTIs are differentiated in adults, and treatment is largely dependent on the classification (Figure 29-2). **Isolated infections** are first infections or those that occur more than 6 months after a previous infection. A 3-day course of a broad-spectrum antibiotic is the treatment of choice for women with isolated cystitis. Cystitis in younger men is managed with a 7- to 10-day course of antibiotics.[20] Women older than 65 should be treated with a 10-day dose of trimethoprim-sulfamethoxazole or a fluoroquinolone.[23] In older men, a minimum of 14 and up to 28 days of antibiotic therapy is recommended, with fluoroquinolones being the choice of therapy.[24,25] **Unresolved infections** are those in which bacteriuria remains after the initial treatment. The treatment of choice for unresolved infections is nitrofurantoin quinolones for 7 to 10 days.[26] Urine culture and sensitivity are also necessary to ensure antibiotic effectiveness. **Recurrent UTIs** are repeated infections within a short period after verified resolution of the earlier infection. Recurrent UTIs are fairly common in women but are rare in healthy adult men.

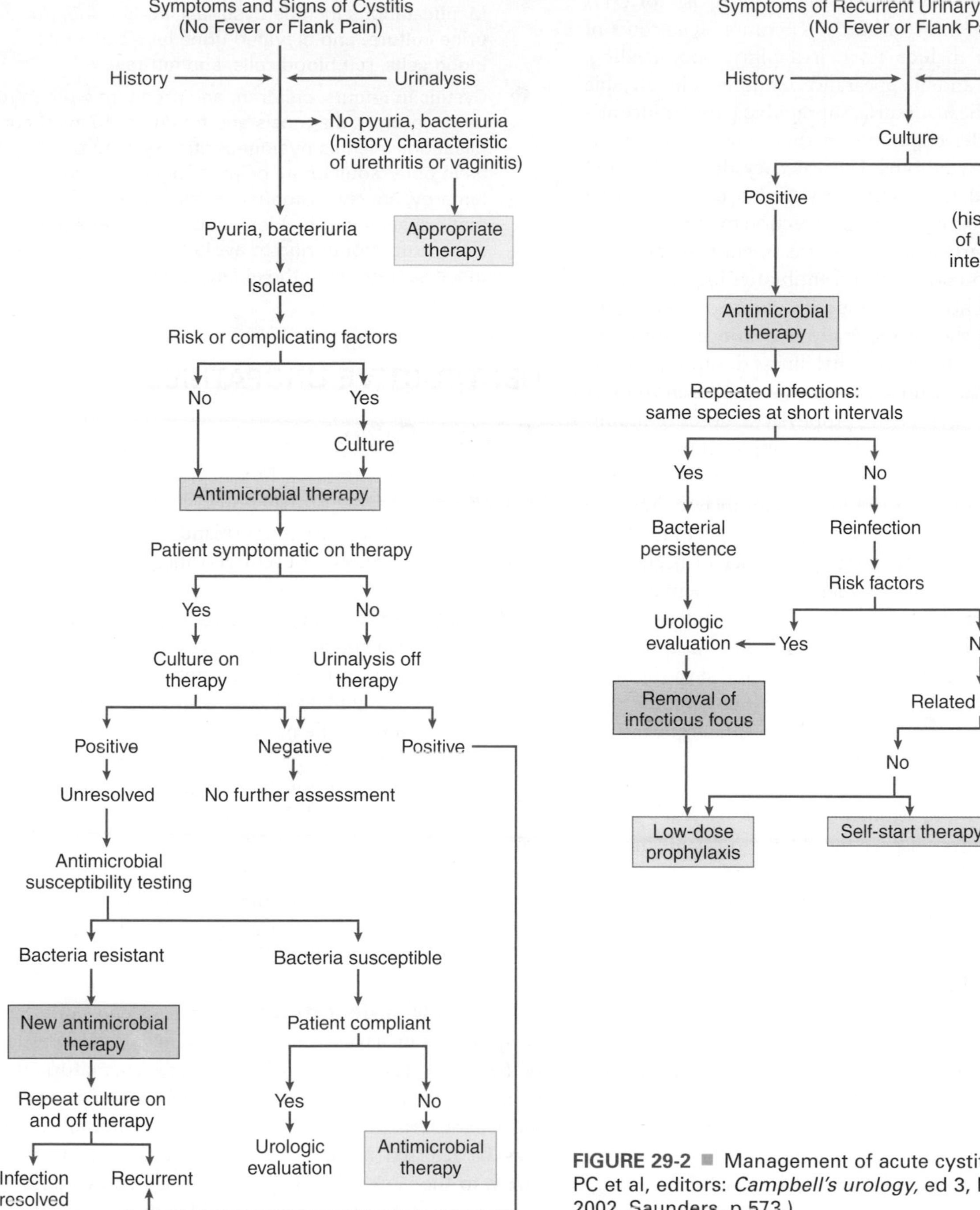

FIGURE 29-2 ■ Management of acute cystitis. (From Walsh PC et al, editors: *Campbell's urology,* ed 3, Philadelphia, 2002, Saunders, p 573.)

Recurrent infections in men should trigger a urologic examination that includes endoscopy.[20] In women, treatment includes antibiotic therapy to resolve the present infection. In addition, some female patients are optimally treated with low-dose prophylactic antibiotics or an intermittent self-start antibiotic regimen in which the woman initiates antibiotic therapy after obtaining a midstream voided specimen. In some women, recurrent infections are related to sexual intercourse, and a postcoital prophylactic antibiotic program is an effective treatment option.[19] Recurring UTIs resulting from bacterial persistence are generally indicative of the need for surgical intervention. Persistent bacterial infections are nearly always caused by an anatomic or pathologic abnormality in the urinary tract.[20] Such abnormalities include calculi, prostatitis, foreign bodies, and duplicated and ectopic ureters.[27]

Age-Related Considerations. UTIs are fairly common in children and account for 4% to 7.5% of all febrile illnesses.[28] Uncircumcised boys are particularly at risk for UTIs during the first 3 months of life.[29,30] Common symptoms of cystitis in children include fever, irritability, poor feeding, vomiting, diarrhea, and ill appearance. Children who are able to talk may also indicate dysuria, suprapubic pain, or incontinence, but even older children sometimes have difficulty localizing signs and symptoms. Untreated cystitis in children may lead to renal damage secondary to dehydration during the illness and to progression of the infection to the upper urinary tract. Hence early and effective treatment is paramount. Administration of broad-spectrum antibiotics for 7 to 14 days is the treatment of choice.[30] The specific choice of therapy, including whether to start parenterally, is contingent on many factors including age, illness severity, illness duration, and the ability to drink adequate fluids.[30,31] However, children younger than 5 years should keep taking prophylactic doses of antibiotics until radiographic evaluation is completed.[30,32] UTIs in children are often indicative of an underlying pathologic process (e.g., vesicoureteral reflux, ureteropelvic junction [UPJ] obstruction) and warrant prompt urologic evaluation.

Pregnant women have the same prevalence of bacteriuria as nonpregnant women, but diagnosis and treatment are critical in pregnant women because of the much greater propensity for pyelonephritis.[33,34] The increased likelihood of pyelonephritis is related to hydronephrosis and stasis of urine during pregnancy.[33] Antibiotic therapy must be carefully chosen to avoid fetal harm. Penicillins and cephalosporins are considered safe throughout pregnancy.

Bacteriuria significantly increases with age, so that 10% of men and at least 20% of women older than 65 years are affected.[25] Factors that predispose the elderly to cystitis include urinary tract abnormalities (e.g., calculi, benign prostatic hyperplasia, prostatitis), chronic illnesses (particularly diabetes mellitus and neurologic diseases), changes in urinary pH, decreased estrogen production in women, bowel incontinence, and greater prevalence of catheterization. A 7- to 10-day course of antibiotic treatment and close monitoring for adverse effects are recommended for symptomatic UTIs. Asymptomatic bacteriuria should not be treated in the elderly.[25] Symptoms associated with bacteriuria in the elderly may include anxiety, confusion, lethargy, and anorexia as opposed to dysuria and fever. The diagnosis is often one of exclusion, and urinalysis and culture are included in the diagnostic evaluation.[23]

KEY CONCEPTS

- Cystitis is an inflammation of the bladder lining that may be due to infection, chemical irritants, stones, or trauma. Most cases are infectious and result from bacterial invasion from the urethra.
- Factors predisposing to cystitis include female sex, age older than 65 years, catheterization, diabetes mellitus, and any disorder causing urinary stasis. Manifestations include dysuria, cloudy urine, positive urine culture, and elevated urine levels of white blood cells, red blood cells, and nitrites.
- Cystitis in infants, children, and pregnant women requires prompt diagnosis and treatment to avert complications such as pyelonephritis. Symptoms of cystitis in older adults may be atypical and include lethargy, anorexia, confusion, and anxiety. Symptomatic cystitis in the elderly should be managed with close drug monitoring to avoid toxicity. Asymptomatic bacteriuria in the elderly should not be treated.

OBSTRUCTIVE UROPATHIES

Bladder Calculi

Bladder stones are unusual but, if present, can cause symptoms of a urinary tract obstruction or infection. A stone in the bladder irritates the urothelium (bladder lining) and may obstruct the bladder neck or urethral orifice.

Pathogenesis. Bladder stones are nearly always composed of uric acid and are usually indicative of urinary retention. When the cause of retention is not evident, the finding of bladder stones should be followed with a comprehensive urologic examination to rule out common etiologic factors such as stricture of the urethra, prostatic hyperplasia, and diverticulum (small abnormal pouches in the bladder lining) of the bladder.[27] Bladder calculi are more common in men than women, with men older than 50 years at greatest risk for bladder stones. Calculi that are composed of calcium oxalate or cystine are indicative of concomitant renal stones (see Chapter 27).[26] Calculi in children are generally due to infections and/or vesicoureteral reflux.[26]

Clinical Manifestations. Bladder calculi cause general symptoms of urinary tract obstruction or infection. Irritation of the urothelial lining of the bladder causes hematuria (blood in urine), pyuria (pus in urine), and intermittent painful voiding. Characteristics of pain vary from sharp to dull, and pain may be referred to the penis, scrotum, or perineum and, rarely, to the back, hip, or foot.[35] Pain generally increases as voiding ceases. Exercise or other sudden movements that create contact between the stone and the bladder wall may also trigger pain. Bladder calculi can obstruct the bladder neck or urethral orifice and cause a sudden interruption of the urinary stream.

Treatment. Symptomatic pain management with nonsteroidal antiinflammatory agents or opioids is often required.[35] Relief of urinary obstruction and treatment of infection are the primary goals of treatment. If the urethral obstruction can be eliminated or converted to a partial obstruction with a Foley catheter, conservative treatment (consisting of acetic acid irrigation to dissolve the stone) and determination of the underlying cause can proceed. Management of infections that precipitate or result from bladder stones is based on urine culture and sensitivity. If relief of the obstruction cannot be accomplished with manipulation or catheterization, lithotripsy (sonic dissolution) or, when lithotripsy is contraindicated, surgical intervention to remove the stone may be necessary to avoid renal failure and sepsis.

Tumors

In 2002, approximately 56,500 cases of bladder cancer were diagnosed in the United States.[36] Men are three times more likely to develop bladder cancer than women.[36,37] Bladder cancer is the fourth most common cancer in the United States, and nearly 13,000 people died from bladder cancer in 2002.[36,37] Caucasians are more likely than African-Americans to have bladder cancer, but the mortality rate is higher among African-Americans.[37] Approximately 90% of all tumors are transitional cell carcinoma originating in the transitional epithelium, or urothelium, which is the lining found throughout the urinary tract.[38] The other 10% of bladder tumor types include squamous cell carcinoma, adenocarcinoma, undifferentiated carcinoma, and rhabdomyosarcoma. These tumor types are generally more resistant to treatment than transitional cell carcinoma and have a poorer prognosis.[39]

Etiology and Pathogenesis. Cigarette smoking is the greatest risk factor for bladder cancer, with up to 66% of bladder tumors in men and 25% in women attributable to cigarette smoke.[37] Approximately 20% to 30% of bladder tumors may be work related (Box 29-2). Occupations involving chemicals and rubber are associated with bladder cancer. Sewage workers and laboratory technicians are also at increased risk for bladder cancer. Specific chemicals implicated in the development of bladder cancer include α- and β-naphthylamine, benzidine, and 4-aminodiphenyl. Cigarette smoke, phenacetin analgesics, and some antineoplastic drugs have been found to act as bladder carcinogens. Cyclophosphamide treatment may create up to a ninefold increase in bladder cancer risk. Consumption of coffee, tea, or artificial sweeteners is not thought to be associated with bladder cancer.[37] Likewise, evidence suggests that heredity has a limited role in bladder cancer. However, cell-mediated or humoral immune deficiency may be a factor because urothelial tumors occur primarily in patients older than 50 years or in those receiving immunosuppressive therapy.

In children, the congenital anomaly of exstrophy of the bladder (bladder outside the abdominal cavity) may predispose to the development of bladder tumors, particularly adenocarcinomas. Recurrent UTIs are associated with squamous cell carcinomas, which are more invasive and generally have a poor prognosis in comparison with transitional cell carcinomas.[39] Parasitic infections from schistosomiasis, particularly prevalent in Egyptian males and in Africa, have been associated with squamous cell carcinoma as a result of urine-borne carcinogens formed during the infectious process and irritation by the parasitic ova.[37] Patients who have undergone urinary diversion for any reason also experience squamous metaplasia and are at risk for tumor development.

Box 29-2

Environmental Factors Associated with Bladder Cancer

Cigarette smoking
Occupational exposure to:
- Cyclic chemicals such as benzene derivatives, arylamines
- Dyes
- Rubbers
- Textiles
- Paints
- Leathers
- Many types of chemicals

Use of hair dyes
Arsenic-contaminated water
Diesel exhaust
Antineoplastic agents cyclophosphamide and chlornaphazine
Pelvic radiation
Analgesic phenacetin
Pesticides in drinking water

From: Pashos CL et al: Bladder cancer: epidemiology, diagnosis, and management, *Cancer Pract* 10:311-321, 2002.

Bladder tumors occur most often at the trigone, the ureteral orifices, and the posterior and lateral walls of the bladder (see Figure 29-1). The tumor usually spreads by a direct route through the bladder wall to adjacent organs or through lymph nodes in the pelvis and abdomen. Once treated, tumors can recur at the original site, or an entirely new tumor may develop at another site. The most common sites of metastasis are the liver, lungs, bone, and adrenals; tumor cells are carried to these sites by the blood. Other sites of metastasis are the heart, brain, and kidney.

Four features are evaluated in bladder tumors: (1) pattern of growth, (2) cell type, (3) tumor differentiation, and (4) depth of invasion. Tumor patterns include papillary, solid infiltrating, papillary and solid, and noninvasive. Cell types include transitional, squamous, and glandular. Noninvasive tumor, or carcinoma in situ, may progress to a papillary or invasive tumor in a short period or may remain inactive for years. In children, the most common bladder tumor is embryonal sarcoma, usually found at the base of the bladder. The distal ends of the ureters, the prostate, and the seminal vesicles may be involved by tumor in boys. In girls, masses at the introitus may be seen.

Clinical Manifestations. Hematuria is the initial symptom of bladder cancer in approximately 80% of cases.[37,40] However, in the early stages of bladder cancer, the hematuria

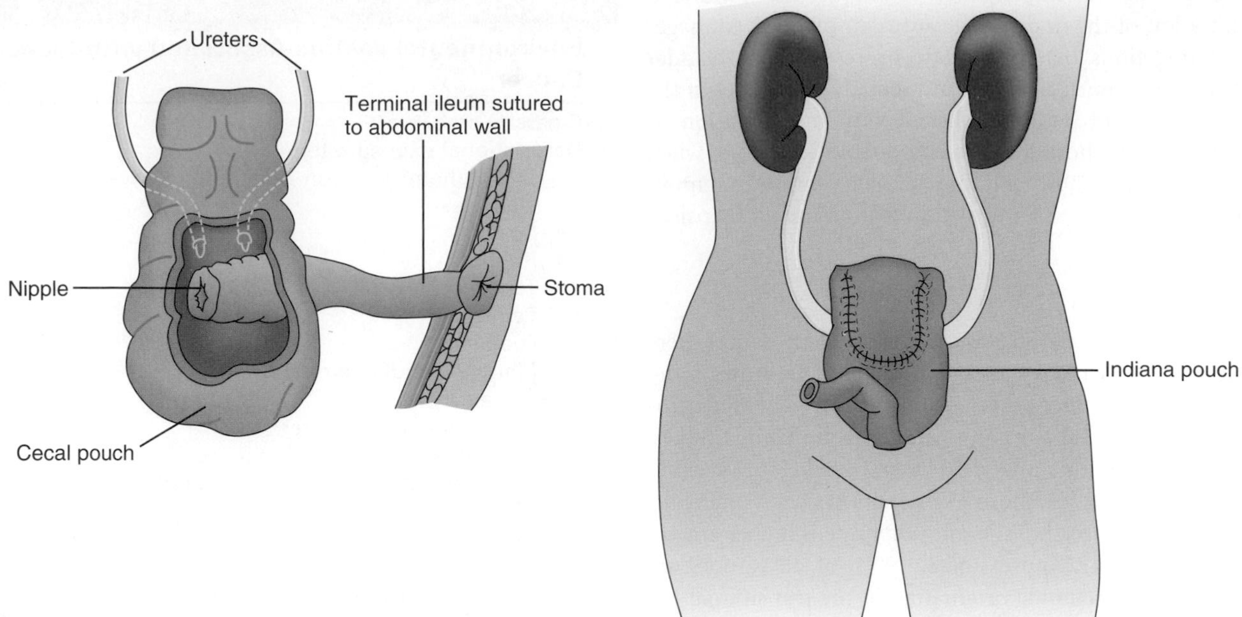

FIGURE 29-3 ■ Indiana pouch urinary diversion procedure. (From Black JM, Matassarin-Jacobs E, editors: *Medical-surgical nursing: clinical management for continuity of care,* ed 6, Philadelphia, 2005, Saunders, p 873.)

(gross and microscopic) is often intermittent. Therefore, bladder cancer should be definitively ruled out by cystoscopic examination in persons with etiologically unknown hematuria who are middle aged or older, even if hematuria is not consistently detected on repeat urinalysis.[37] Other common complaints related to bladder cancer include dysuria, frequency, and urgency, but these symptoms are nearly always accompanied by either gross or microscopic hematuria.[40]

Treatment. Treatment protocols are based on the tumor's features. For noninvasive carcinoma in situ, endoscopic resection is usually performed. Transurethral resection (TUR) with appropriate cystoscopic and cytologic follow-up is the only treatment recommended for most superficial bladder cancer.[37,40] The 30% of patients who have stage I disease and are at high risk for progression are also treated with intravesical therapy.[37,40] Immediate (within 6 hours) instillation of a chemotherapeutic agent (e.g., mitomycin C) following TUR appears to decrease the recurrence rate and prolong the recurrence-free interval of superficial bladder cancer.[41] Bacille Calmette-Guérin (BCG) immunotherapy is the treatment of choice for in situ transitional cell carcinoma of the bladder.[37] Intravesical BCG triggers a nonspecific immune response and significantly decreases tumor recurrence.[37] However, recent studies indicate that noninvasive tumors with positive p53 tumor markers are more likely to progress or recur than are non–p53-expressing tumors.[42] Hence even early-stage noninvasive p53-positive tumors may be best managed by cystectomy (see Chapter 7 for a discussion of tumor markers).[42]

Muscle-invasive tumors are usually managed with radical or simple cystectomy (removal of the bladder) and radiation therapy. Clinical trials evaluating the use of chemotherapy in conjunction with surgery and radiation are underway, but there is currently no conclusive evidence that the addition of chemotherapy decreases recurrence or mortality in persons with the disease confined to the bladder.[43] For patients with regional metastases, cisplatin may improve survival.[43] Overall survival rates for persons with metastatic bladder cancer are poor.[37] When cystectomy is necessary, urinary drainage may be accomplished via a variety of urinary diversions. When possible, continent urinary diversions that do not require external collection devices are used. The most common approach is use of the Indiana pouch (Figure 29-3).

Regardless of the specific technique, continent urinary diversions require surgical construction of a urine reservoir (usually formed by a portion of the bowel) that has a valve to prevent reflux to the upper urinary tract and a sphincter to prevent urine leakage. Orthotopic bladder replacement in which a portion of the ureter is connected to a reconstructed urinary reservoir (neoileal bladder) has also been successful in appropriate candidates (see Figure 29-3). Research suggests that orthotopic bladder substitutes have clear advantages (e.g., cosmetic, more natural voiding), with morbidity and mortality comparable to that of the standard ileal conduit.[44]

The survival rate for patients with muscle-invasive tumors is 20% to 40% at 5 years.[37] For patients with distant metastases, life expectancy averages 2 years. Chemotherapy, which may include some combination of cisplatin, methotrexate, doxorubicin, and vinblastine, is used to induce remission.

Ongoing research is being conducted on the efficacy of alternative chemotherapeutic agents. However, to date these drugs have not proved more efficacious than the more standard treatments.

KEY CONCEPTS

- Bladder stones are rare but, when present, may cause symptoms of obstruction or irritation of the bladder lining.
- Pain, especially with voiding, and hematuria may occur.
- Bladder calculi are generally the result of stasis of urine, but they may also contribute to urine stasis and infections.
- Treatment includes relief of urinary obstruction, resolution of infection, and dissolution or removal of calculi.
- Most bladder tumors originate from the transitional epithelium lining the urinary tract. Occupational exposure to carcinogenic chemicals, cigarette smoking, and chronic UTIs are thought to be the main predisposing factors.
- Bladder cancer is primarily manifested as hematuria. Dysuria, frequency, and urgency may also be present.
- Benign tumors and superficial, noninvasive tumors may be surgically removed. Tumors at high risk for progression are managed with intravesical immunotherapy.
- The treatment of choice for muscle-invasive bladder cancer is cystectomy and radiation therapy.
- Urinary diversions, in which the patient may be continent (generally requiring intermittent catheterization) or incontinent (requiring the use of an external appliance to collect urine), are created in conjunction with cystectomy.
- Some patients may be candidates for bladder reconstruction and reattachment of the ureters.

CONGENITAL DISORDERS

Vesicoureteral Reflux

Reflux of urine from the bladder to the ureter and renal pelvis, known as **vesicoureteral reflux,** is usually due to incompetence of the valvular mechanism at the ureter-bladder junction. This condition is found in childhood, usually during evaluation for recurrent UTIs. The incidence of vesicoureteral reflux in children without a UTI has been cited at 1% to 2%.[45] However, the incidence in infants and children with UTIs is much greater, with up to 50% of children with urinary infections found to have reflux.[45,46] A genetic component is also present in that siblings of children in whom reflux had been diagnosed and children of parents who have had reflux are much more likely to have reflux than are children born to families with no history of this problem. Infants who have a family history of reflux should be routinely evaluated for reflux at as early an age as possible so that appropriate medical management may be initiated.

Pathogenesis. Normally, the ureters enter the bladder at an oblique angle and then continue for 1 to 2 cm under the bladder mucosa before exiting inside the bladder cavity. As the bladder fills, pressure within it increases against the muscle wall and closes the ureteral passageway. In vesicoureteral reflux, closure of the ureteral passage is not successful, and the urine flows backward into the ureters and sometimes the kidney.

The two classifications of vesicoureteral reflux are primary and secondary. Congenital abnormalities at the ureterovesical junction are the cause of primary reflux. The mucosal ureteral tunnel is short, which decreases the efficiency of the valvular mechanism; the orifice is more lateral; and the trigone is not well developed. Primary reflux is also associated with other abnormalities of the urinary system, among them ureteral duplication, ureterocele with duplication, ureteral ectopia, and paraurethral diverticula (Figure 29-4). Secondary reflux can occur from increased pressure within the bladder (neurogenic bladder, bladder outlet obstruction), inflammatory processes, and surgical procedures at or near the ureterovesical junction. The extent of reflux is graded from I to V (Figure 29-5).

Increased renal pelvis pressure and migration of bacteria from the bladder to the kidneys may result from reflux. Dilation of the ureters, caused by grade II and higher reflux, also prevents the bladder from emptying completely and predisposes the patient to pyelonephropathy. Reflux independent of infection seems to be benign.[47,48] Hence the goal of medical management is to prevent bacteriuria, which causes renal damage.[47,48]

Clinical Manifestations and Diagnosis. Reflux is usually discovered during evaluation for recurrent UTI in children. However, the child may have voiding dysfunction, renal insufficiency, or hypertension. Diagnostic tests such as voiding cystourethrography, intravenous pyelography, radionuclide renal scintigraphy, and computed tomography are performed to evaluate the status of the kidney and bladder system.

Treatment. In nearly 80% of cases, reflux resolves spontaneously as the child grows.[47] The two main factors predictive of spontaneous resolution are younger age at diagnosis and grade I or II reflux. Renal scarring related to pyelonephritis as a result of reflux may result in decreased renal function, hypertension, and, most seriously, renal failure, which occurs in a small minority of children with vesicoureteral reflux.[17] Treatment depends on the grade of reflux. Grades I and II frequently resolve spontaneously, and observation and medical management constitute the initial approach. During the pe-

initial symptoms include a palpable flank mass in a newborn infant; abdominal, flank, or back pain; a UTI with fever; or hematuria as a result of negligible trauma. UPJ obstruction may also be asymptomatic and discovered incidentally on renal ultrasonography. If unilateral hydronephrosis is present on neonatal ultrasonography and the other kidney appears normal, no intervention is indicated. Management consists of frequent renal ultrasound to assess for hydronephrosis.

Treatment. The timing of surgical intervention to correct UPJ obstruction is controversial. Ultimately, it is a clinical decision based on the degree of obstruction, careful analysis of kidney function, and the overall health of the infant or child.[49] Early surgical repair is warranted if function of the affected kidney or kidney function in general decreases, in cases of bilateral obstruction, and in cases of congenital single kidney with obstruction. Surgical repair of UPJ obstruction usually involves removal of the stenosed area of the junction and anastomosis of the ureter and renal pelvis.

Ureteral Ectopy

An **ectopic ureter** is a single ureter implanted in a site other than normal or a duplicate ureter (see Figure 29-4). Alternative or duplicate sites of ureter implantation predispose the patient to infection and the potential for reduced renal function.

Pathogenesis. Ureters may implant anywhere along the route of migration of the mesonephric duct during fetal development. Ectopic ureters are approximately three times more common in females than males. Eighty percent of ectopic ureters are duplicated collecting systems.[51] Bilateral ectopic ureters occur in 5% to 17% of cases.[51] In males, the ureter is usually single and is most frequently found implanted in the urethra, but the bladder neck, the seminal vesicle, and the vas deferens are also common sites. In females, the ureter is generally implanted in the urethra or the vestibule; however, implantation may also occur in the vagina, cervix, or uterus.[51]

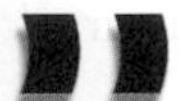

Table 29-4

Treatment Recommendations: Boys and Girls with Primary Vesicoureteral Reflux and No Renal Scarring

Clinical Presentation		Treatment: Initial (Antibiotic Prophylaxis or Open Surgical Repair)			Treatment: Follow-Up (Continued Antibiotic Prophylaxis, Cystography, or Open Surgical Repair)	
Reflux Grade/ Laterality	**Patient Age (yr)**	**Guideline**	**Preferred Option**	**Reasonable Alternative**	**Guideline**	**Preferred Option**
I-II/unilateral or bilateral	<1	Antibiotic prophylaxis				
	1-5	Antibiotic prophylaxis				
	6-10	Antibiotic prophylaxis				
III-IV/unilateral or bilateral	<1	Antibiotic prophylaxis			Bilateral: surgery if persistent	Unilateral: surgery if persistent
	1-5	Unilateral: antibiotic prophylaxis	Bilateral: antibiotic prophylaxis			Surgery if persistent
	6-10		Unilateral: antibiotic prophylaxis Bilateral: surgery	Bilateral: antibiotic prophylaxis		Surgery if persistent
V/unilateral or bilateral	<1		Antibiotic prophylaxis		Surgery if persistent	
	1-5		Unilateral: antibiotic prophylaxis Bilateral: surgery	Unilateral: surgery Bilateral: antibiotic prophylaxis	Surgery if persistent	
	6-10	Surgery				

From Greenfield SP: Management of vesicoureteral reflux in children, *Curr Urol Rep* 2:119, 2001.

Clinical Manifestations, Diagnosis, and Treatment. The diagnosis of ureteral ectopy is frequently made during maternal ultrasonography. Hydronephrosis secondary to obstruction is the typical sonographic finding.[51] Postnatally, clinical manifestations of ureteral ectopy vary depending on the site of implantation. In females the most common symptom is incontinence; other symptoms experienced by male and female patients are UTIs, obstruction, and failure to thrive. Epididymitis may be the initial problem in males. The condition is diagnosed with intravenous urography, renal ultrasonography, and endoscopy.

Surgical alternatives vary according to the site of ureteral ectopy and the function of the affected kidney(s). In the case of a single ectopic ureter, when the opposing kidney is normal, nephroureterectomy is the recommended course of treatment. If the involved kidney has adequate function, the ureter may be reimplanted in a more physiologically acceptable site. Heminephrectomy and ureteropyelostomy are not uncommon. Antenatal sonography may lead to earlier diagnosis and an increase in kidney-sparing surgery. Laparoscopic nephrectomy and heminephrectomy are increasingly used because of the reduced mortality and better visualization of the surgical field with laparoscopic procedures.[51]

Ureterocele

A **ureterocele** is a congenital cystic dilatation of the distal end of the ureter (see Figure 29-4). When the cystic structure is located entirely in the bladder, it is known as an intravesical ureterocele. The majority (75%) of ureteroceles are ectopic and are located at the bladder neck or in the urethra.

Etiology and Pathogenesis. Ureteroceles occur more often in females than males (4:1 ratio) and almost exclusively in Caucasians.[52] The embryonic development of the cystic structure is not well understood. Ureteroceles may be classified as simple structures (not associated with duplicate collecting systems), although 80% to 90% are duplicate systems with ectopic implantation. Either type of ureterocele may be unilateral or bilateral, but only about 10% are bilateral. The small orifice of the ureter acts as an obstruction in the collecting system and causes ureteral and renal calyx dilatation and often facilitates reflux and infection. If the ureterocele is large, obstruction of the bladder outlet may occur.

Clinical Manifestations, Diagnosis, and Treatment. Prenatal diagnosis of ureterocele is suspected when the maternal sonogram shows hydronephrosis and intravesical cystic dilatation. Postnatally, the most common manifestation is UTI. If the bladder outlet is obstructed, urinary retention may also be present. Patients with suspected ureterocele are treated with prophylactic antibiotics until definitive diagnosis and management are accomplished.

Anatomic deviations and pathophysiologic processes associated with ureteroceles are unique to each patient. Hence a thorough urologic workup that includes ultrasonography, voiding cystourethrography, intravenous pyelography, and nuclear scanning is done to determine the most appropriate surgical intervention. Surgical manipulation of the defect includes transurethral incision of the defect, excision of the defect with reimplantation of the ureter, or partial nephrectomy and ureterectomy.[52] Endoscopic surgery is used more and more frequently to accomplish the required procedures with less morbidity. In an acutely septic patient, percutaneous nephrostomy to drain the upper collecting system may be needed.

DIAGNOSTIC TESTS

Several common procedures are used to diagnose congenital disorders as well as the other problems discussed in this chapter. Renal ultrasound, which is painless, does not involve radiation, and provides excellent visualization of the urinary system, is the most common initial screening study for infants and children with urinary problems.[15,52]

Fluoroscopic voiding cystourethrography or radionuclide voiding cystography is generally done to yield more specific information than can be obtained by ultrasound. Fluoroscopic voiding cystourethrography involves catheterization; filling of the bladder with sterile, iodinated, dilute contrast material; and voiding.[53] Images of the bladder are taken prior to voiding to detect a ureterocele or tumor, and images taken during voiding can identify reflux or urethral abnormalities.[53] Radionuclide voiding cystography also requires catheterization and voiding to obtain images. A technetium 99m–labeled radiopharmaceutical is instilled in the bladder through the catheter followed by sterile normal saline to fill the bladder. Images are then taken with the bladder full and during voiding, but radionuclide voiding cystography does not allow visualization of the urethra.[53] The term urodynamic testing is used for procedures associated with diagnosing voiding dysfunction. There are multiple urodynamic tests and procedures and the choice of tests is based on clinical presentation and begins with the least invasive of the desired tests.[54] The most common tests are cystometry (measurement of intravesical pressure during bladder filling); urethral pressure profilometry (measurement of intraluminal pressure along the length of the urethra); uroflowmetry (noninvasive method of measuring characteristics of urine flow); and pressure-flow micturition studies (invasive method of measuring characteristics of urine flow).[54] Electrophysiologic testing may also be done to determine pathologic processes underlying voiding dysfunction. Kinesiologic studies are usually performed in a urodynamic laboratory with the purpose of examining sphincter activity during bladder filling and emptying.[54] Neurophysiologic tests allow information about the coordination between the bladder and the external sphincter.[54] Neurophysiologic tests are much more involved and are completed only in very specialized laboratories.

KEY CONCEPTS

- Congenital abnormalities of the bladder include misimplantation of ureters, strictures, an extra ureter, and ureterocele. These disorders cause problems by obstructing normal urine flow and predisposing to the retrograde flow of urine, urine stasis, and secondary infection.

SUMMARY

The bladder is a muscular reservoir that stores and eliminates urine. Unfortunately, disorders involving the bladder and lower urinary tract are quite common. In adults the most prevalent pathologic conditions are infections, malignancies, and voiding dysfunction. *E. coli* is the offending pathogen in 80% of lower UTIs. When diagnosed and managed promptly, bladder infections nearly always resolve without serious morbidity. Bladder cancer is the fourth most common type of cancer.[37] The primary clinical manifestation of bladder cancer is hematuria. Early-stage bladder cancer may be managed with partial resection and intravesical immunotherapy. Muscle-invasive bladder cancer generally requires cystectomy and radiation therapy. The ability of surgeons to reconstruct continent urinary diversion systems, including orthotopic bladders, for many patients after cystectomy is a recent milestone in bladder cancer treatment. Incontinence as a result of bladder dysfunction affects millions of adults. The prevalence of incontinence increases with age and is more common in women than men. However, incontinence is not a result of the normal aging process, and patients should be urged to seek evaluation and treatment. Behavioral, pharmacologic, and surgical approaches may be used to manage voiding dysfunction.

Lower UTIs account for 4% to 8% of all febrile illnesses in children.[30] Incontinence, generally termed enuresis, affects up to 20% of 5-year-olds, with the incidence gradually decreasing with age so that only 2% of 12- to 14-year-old children are enuretic.[13] Both UTIs and enuresis should trigger more detailed urologic evaluation to rule out congenital disorders such as UPJ obstruction, ectopic ureters, ureterocele, and vesicoureteral reflux. Vesicoureteral reflux is the most prevalent congenital lower urinary tract disorder. It predisposes children to UTIs, which can result in kidney scarring and permanent renal impairment. Most cases of vesicoureteral reflux resolve spontaneously as the child ages. Before resolution, close medical management is necessary to prevent upper UTI and kidney damage.

MEDIA RESOURCES

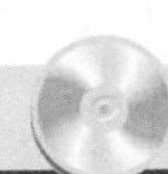

evolve

Remember to check out the ***CD Companion*** included with this book for Review Questions, Key Concepts Review, Glossary (with audio for selected terms), Disease Profiles, and Animations.

PLUS, visit the ***Evolve website*** at http://evolve.elsevier.com/Copstead/ for Case Studies, Disease Profiles, and WebLinks.

References

1. Vapneck JM: Urinary incontinence: screening and treatment of urinary dysfunction, *Geriatrics* 56(10):25-29, 2001.
2. Brown JS: Epidemiology and changing demographics of overactive bladder: a focus on the postmenopausal woman, *Geriatrics* 57(suppl 1):6-12, 2002.
3. Wood RL, Hood EH: Management of urinary incontinence, *Drug Top* 146(2):53-57, 2002.
4. de Groat WC, Yoshimura N: Pharmacology of the lower urinary tract, *Annu Rev Pharmacol Toxicol* 41:691-721, 2001.
5. Payne CK: Urinary incontinence: nonsurgical management. In Walsh PC et al, editors: *Campbell's urology,* ed 8, Philadelphia, 2002, Saunders, pp 1069-1091.
6. Blaivas JG, Groutz A: Urinary incontinence: pathophysiology, evaluation, and management overview. In Walsh PC et al, editors: *Campbell's urology,* ed 8, Philadelphia, 2002, Saunders, pp 1027-1052.
7. Criner JA: Urinary incontinence in a vulnerable population: older women, *Semin Perioperative Nurs* 10(1):33-37, 2001.
8. Smith DA, Ouslander JG: Pharmacologic management of urinary incontinence in older adults, *Top Geriatr Rehabil* 16(1):54-60, 2000.
9. Crandall C: Tolterodine: a clinical review, *J Women's Health Gender-Based Med* 10:735-743, 2001.
10. Wein AJ: Neuromuscular dysfunction of the lower urinary tract and its management. In Walsh PC et al, editors: *Campbell's urology,* ed 8, Philadelphia, 2002, Saunders, pp 931-1026.
11. Robson WLM, Leung AKC: Secondary nocturnal enuresis, *Clin Pediatr* 39:379-385, 2000.
12. Koff SA, Jayanthi VR: Non-neurogenic lower urinary tract dysfunction. In Walsh PC et al, editors: *Campbell's urology,* ed 8, Philadelphia, 2002, Saunders, pp 2261-2283.
13. Rogers J: Managing daytime and night-time enuresis in children, *Nurs Stand* 16(32):45-52, 2002.
14. Bankhead RW, Kropp BP, Cheng EY: Evaluation and treatment of children with neurogenic bladders, *J Child Neurol* 15: 141-149, 2000.
15. Berrocal T et al: Anomalies of the distal ureter, bladder and urethra in children: embryologic, radiologic, and pathologic features, *Radiographics* 22:1139-1164, 2002.
16. Muensterer OJ: Comprehensive ultrasound versus voiding cysturethrography in the diagnosis of vesicoureteral reflux, *Eur J Pediatr* 161:435-437, 2002.
17. Stenberg A, Hensle TW, Lackgren G: Vesicoureteral reflux: a new treatment algorithm, *Curr Urol Rep* 3:107-114, 2002.
18. Harrington RD, Hooton TM: Urinary tract infection risk factors and gender, *J Gender-Specific Med* 3(8):27-34, 2000.
19. Nicolle LE: Urinary tract infection: traditional pharmacologic therapies, *Am J Med* 113(1A):35S-44S, 2002.
20. Schaeffer AJ: Infections of the urinary tract. In Walsh PC et al, editors: *Campbell's urology,* ed 8, Philadelphia, 2002, Saunders, pp 515-602.

21. Gerber GS, Brendler CB: Evaluation of the urologic patient: history, physical examination, and urinalysis. In Walsh PC et al, editors: *Campbell's urology,* ed 8, Philadelphia, 2002, Saunders, pp 83-110.
22. Bachur R, Harper MB: Reliability of the urinalysis in predicting urinary tract infections in young febrile children, *Arch Pediatr Adolesc Med* 155:60-65, 2001.
23. Shortliffe LM, McCue JD: Urinary tract infection at the age extremes: pediatrics and geriatrics, *Am J Med* 113(suppl 1A):55S-66S, 2002.
24. Nicolle LE: Urinary tract infections in long-term-care facilities, *Infect Control Hosp Epidemiol* 22:167-175, 2001.
25. Matsumoto T: Urinary tract infections in the elderly, *Curr Urol Rep* 2:330-333, 2001.
26. Schwartz BF, Stoller ML: The vesical calculus, *Urol Clin North Am* 27:333-346, 2000.
27. Lingeman JE, Lifshitz DA, Evan AP: Surgical management of urinary lithiasis. In Walsh PC et al, editors: *Campbell's urology,* ed 8, Philadelphia, 2002, Saunders, pp 3361-3451.
28. Santen SA, Altieri MF: Pediatric urinary tract infection, *Emerg Med Clin North Am* 19:675-690, 2001.
29. Steele RW: The epidemiology and clinical presentation of urinary tract infections in children 2 years of age through adolescence, *Pediatr Ann* 10:653-658, 1999.
30. Roberts KB: The AAP practice parameter on urinary tract infections in febrile infants and young children, *Am Fam Physician* 62:1815-1822, 2000.
31. Shortliffe LMD: Urinary tract infections in infants and children. In Walsh PC et al, editors: *Campbell's urology,* ed 8, Philadelphia, 2002, Saunders, pp 1846-1884.
32. White CT, Matsell DG: Children's UTIs in the new millennium: diagnosis, investigation, and treatment of childhood urinary tract infections in the year 2001, *Can Fam Physician* 47: 1603-1608, 2001.
33. Smaill F: Antibiotics for asymptomatic bacteriuria in pregnancy (Cochrane review), *Cochrane Library* 3:1-23, 2002.
34. Christensen B: Which antibiotics are appropriate for treating bacteriuria in pregnancy? *J Antimicrob Chemother* 46(suppl S1):29-34, 2000.
35. Westenberg A et al: Bladder and renal stones: management and treatment, *Hosp Med* 63(1):34-41, 2002.
36. American Cancer Society: Cancer reference information. Available at http://www.nci.nih.gov/cancer_information/doc.aspx?viewid=6A5E97AF-72B-4C26-821E-AOC4F99DC22A. Accessed August 30, 2002.
37. Pashos CL et al: Bladder cancer: epidemiology, diagnosis, and management, *Cancer Pract* 10:311-322, 2002.
38. Al-Sukhun S, Hussain M: Current understanding of the biology of advanced bladder cancer, *Cancer* 97(8 suppl):2064-2075, 2003.
39. Raghaven D. Progress in the chemotherapy of metastatic cancer of the urinary tract, *Cancer* 97(8 suppl):2050-2055, 2003.
40. Randall S. Valrubicin: an alternative to radical cystectomy for carcinoma in situ of the bladder, *Urol Nurs* 21(1):30-36, 2001.
41. Malkowicz SB: Management of superficial bladder cancer. In Walsh PC et al, editors: *Campbell's urology,* ed 8, Philadelphia, 2002, Saunders, pp 2785-2817.
42. Smith ND et al: The p53 tumor suppressor gene and nuclear protein: basic science review and relevance in the management of bladder cancer, *J Urol* 169:1219-1228, 2003.
43. Schoenberg M: Management of invasive and metastatic bladder cancer. In Walsh PC et al, editors: *Campbell's urology,* ed 8, Philadelphia, 2002, Saunders, pp 2803-2817.
44. Stein JP, Skinner DG: Orthotopic urinary diversion. In Walsh PC et al, editors: *Campbell's urology,* ed 8, Philadelphia, 2002, Saunders, pp 3835-3867.
45. Smellie JM et al: Medical versus surgical treatment in children with severe bilateral vesicoureteric reflux and bilateral nephropathy: a randomized trial, *Lancet* 357:1329-1333, 2001.
46. Chertin B, Puri P: Familial vesicoureteral reflux, *J Urol* 169:1804-1808, 2003.
47. Greenfield SP: Management of vesicoureteral reflux in children, *Curr Urol Rep* 2:113-121, 2001.
48. Cataldi L, Montoro C, Benni D, Fanos V: Vesicoureteral reflux in children: old and new approaches, *Rays* 27:93-98, 2002.
49. Gonzalez R, Schimke CM: Ureteropelvic junction obstruction in infants and children, *Pediatr Clin North Am* 48:1505-1518, 2001.
50. Groshar D et al: Quantitative SPECT of ^{99m}Tc-DMSA uptake in kidneys of infants with unilateral ureteropelvic junction obstruction: assessment of structural and functional abnormalities, *J Nucl Med* 40:1111-1115, 1999.
51. Schlussel RN, Retik AB: Ectopic ureter, ureterocele, and other anomalies of the ureter. In Walsh PC et al, editors: *Campbell's urology,* ed 8, Philadelphia, 2002, Saunders, pp 2007-2052.
52. Shokeir AA, Nijman RJM: Ureterocele: an ongoing challenge in infancy and childhood, *Br J Urol Int* 90:777-783, 2002.
53. Pennington DJ, Zerin JM: Imaging of the urinary tract in children, *Pediatr Ann* 28:678-686, 1999.
54. Webster GD, Guralnick ML: The neurologic evaluation. In Walsh PC et al, editors: *Campbell's urology,* ed 8, Philadelphia, 2002, Saunders, pp 900-930.

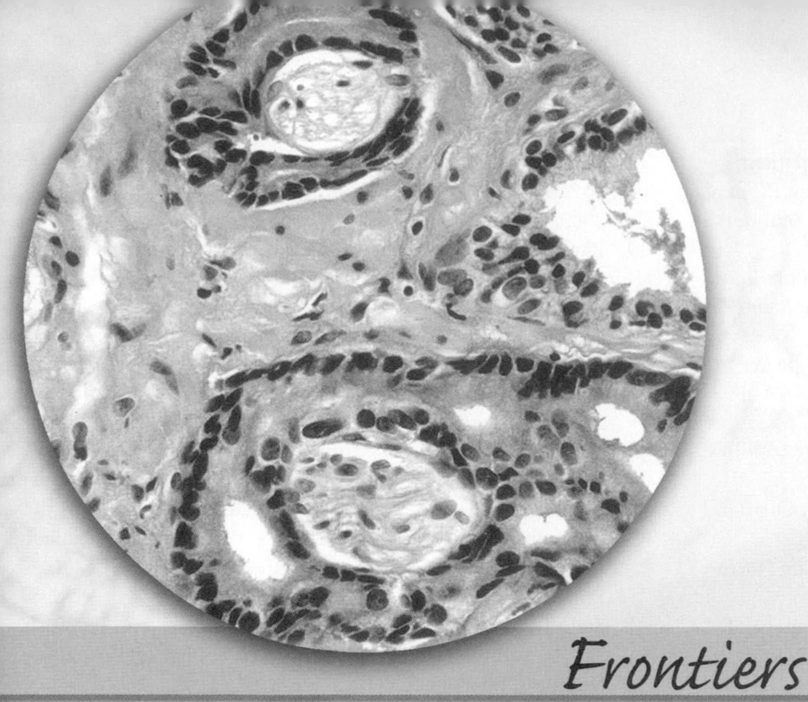

Frontiers of Research

Prostate and Breast Cancer

Ronald S. Go and Michael J. Kirkhorn

Sometimes common fears produce mutual sympathy. People do not want to find that they have one of the dread diseases, but a special dread and a sort of common concern are associated with prostate cancer and breast cancer, both of which may dwell silently in the body and spread malignant cells to other organs before they are detected.

In 2004 about 230,000 cases of prostate cancer were diagnosed, and 29,900 men died of the disease—with the mortality rate for African-American men twice as high as that for Caucasian men. Prostate cancer still ranks as the most prevalent cancer among men and the second leading cause of cancer death.

The prostate gland is a small organ near the bottom of the male bladder. It is thought to be a "sentinel" protecting the bladder from ascending bacteria, and it provides the transporting fluid for spermatozoa during ejaculation.

About 70 years ago Dr. H. H. Young found that digital rectal examination, in which the surgeon palpates the two posterior lobes of the prostate through the rectal wall and Denonvilliers fascia, was a reliable way to examine the gland for abnormalities. The posterior lobes, which contain most of the organ's glandular tissue, are the likely place for a malignancy to develop. The American Cancer Society recommends that beginning at the age of 50 years, all men who have a life expectancy of at least 10 years (5 years for African-Americans) should have a digital rectal examination and measurement of prostate-specific antigen as part of their annual checkup. One study shows that all malignant lesions will be detected if both forms of examination are used, but by itself, prostate-specific antigen is not an entirely reliable screening test.

Once a malignancy is found, physicians decide treatment by considering the man's general health, age, and life expectancy. Some physicians believe that when prostate cancer is found in an otherwise healthy and active 75-year-old man, his disease should simply be tracked because surgery and irradiation could be more deadly than the growth of tumors in elderly men. Definitive treatment is probably appropriate for a much younger man with aggressively spreading disease.

Breast cancer is the leading cause of death for women between the ages of 40 and 55 years. The disease occurs infrequently in women younger than 39 years. Breast cancer will develop in 1 woman in

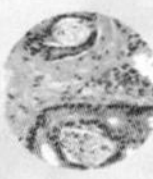

Carcinoma of the prostate showing perineural invasion by malignant glands. (From Kumar V, Abbas AK, Fausto N: Robins and Cotran pathologic basis of disease, *ed 7, Philadelphia, 2005, Saunders.)*

Genital and Reproductive Function

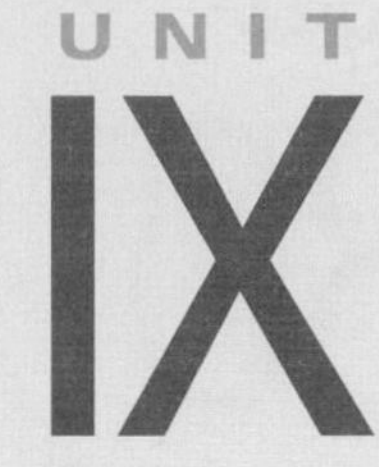

14 between 60 and 79 years of age. About 77% of all breast cancers occur in women older than 50 years. More than 30% of women in whom breast cancer is diagnosed learn that they have the disease only when it is already well advanced. This fact underscores the importance of early detection, but not until the biology of breast cancer is better understood will prevention be effective. Because breast cancer occurs more often in women who have had the disease before or whose close relatives have had the disease, health care experts recommend close surveillance of women in whom the disease is most likely to develop.

Research has revealed a number of factors that may contribute to the incidence of breast cancer. Women who smoke cigarettes, for example, are considered to be at higher risk because cigarette smoke is carcinogenic. Women exposed to ionizing radiation before the age of 40 are more likely to get breast cancer, and researchers have found evidence that women who have not given birth or who first give birth when older than 30 years are at greater risk. Alcohol intake has also been implicated as a risk factor for breast cancer. Researchers suspect that high fat intake contributes to the likelihood of breast cancer, and epidemiologic studies show that obesity increases the risk in women after menopause. Further epidemiologic investigation is needed into the effects of estrogen on breast cancer inasmuch as current studies have yielded inconclusive results. To further complicate the picture, three in four women in whom breast cancer is newly diagnosed have no known risk factors.

The American Cancer Society recommends annual mammograms for women older than 40 years. Annual clinical breast examinations are recommended for women older than 40 years, and younger women should have clinical examinations every 3 years. The American College of Obstetricians and Gynecologists takes an even stronger position and suggests that women 19 years and older consider annual clinical breast examinations.

The message to women and men is roughly the same: early detection is the best protection. Nobody can advise us with any degree of conviction that ways can be found to avoid these diseases. Nobody knows exactly what causes breast and prostate cancer. Some of the circumstances—family history, for example—are beyond control. A healthy and active lifestyle may help.

Male Genital and Reproductive Function

Marvin Van Every • David Mikkelsen • Carolyn Spence Cagle

MEDIA RESOURCES

Additional Material for Study, Review, and Further Exploration

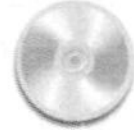

CD Companion ◆ Review Questions and Answers ◆ Key Concepts Review
◆ Glossary *(with audio pronunciations for selected terms)*
◆ Disease Profiles ◆ Animations

evolve ***Website*** at http://evolve.elsevier.com/Copstead/
◆ Case Studies ◆ Disease Profiles ◆ WebLinks

KEY QUESTIONS

- What is the role of the Sertoli cells in spermatogenesis?
- What is the function of Leydig cells?
- Which branch of the autonomic nervous system is responsible for penile erection? Ejaculation?
- Which genitourinary structures develop embryologically from the wolffian ductal system in males?
- How do the hypothalamic-pituitary gonadotropic hormones influence male reproductive function?
- How do the processes of capacitation and acrosome reaction affect the fertilization process?

CHAPTER OUTLINE

This chapter provides a foundation for comprehending male genital and reproductive disorders, which are presented in Chapter 31. The anatomy and embryology of the male genitourinary tract—those organs involved in the processes of sexual reproduction and elimination of nitrogenous wastes—will be presented first. Because these organs are derived from common embryologic structures, the anatomy and embryology of the male genitalia and urinary system will be emphasized, and the differences in embryologic development between males and females will be considered when pertinent. The remainder of this chapter will deal with the physiologic processes of male reproduction.

ANATOMY

Upper Genitourinary Tract

The upper genitourinary tract consists of the kidneys and ureters. The ureteral blood supply is derived from multiple sources. The renal pelvis and upper part of the ureter receive blood from branches of the renal artery. The arterial blood supply of the middle ureter segment comes from the internal spermatic artery, and the lowermost ureter sections receive blood from the branches of the common iliac, internal iliac, and vesical arteries (Figure 30-1). The veins of the renal pelvis and ureter are usually paired with the arteries.

Lower Genitourinary Tract

Bladder

The bladder is a hollow muscular organ that serves as a reservoir for urine. The adult bladder normally has a capacity of 450 to 500 ml. When empty, the bladder lies behind the pubic symphysis and is mainly a pelvic organ. With overdistention or chronic urine retention, the abdomen may bulge, allowing easy palpation of the bladder in the suprapubic region.

The ureters enter the bladder posteroinferiorly. The ureteral orifices are situated on a crescent-shaped ridge and are approx-

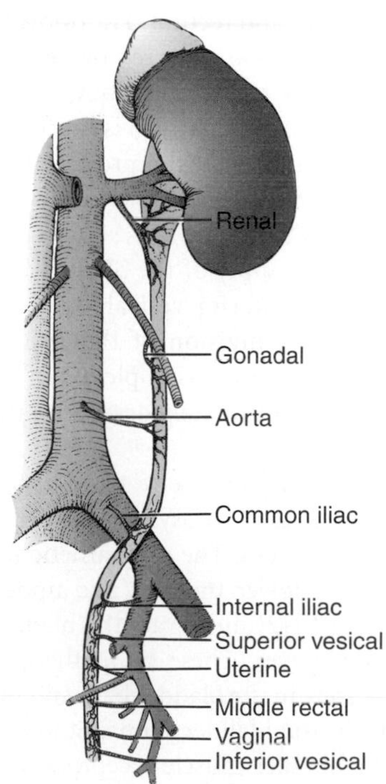

FIGURE 30-1 ■ Sources of ureteral blood supply. (From Walsh PC et al, editors: *Campbell's urology,* ed 7, Philadelphia, 1998, Saunders, p 38.)

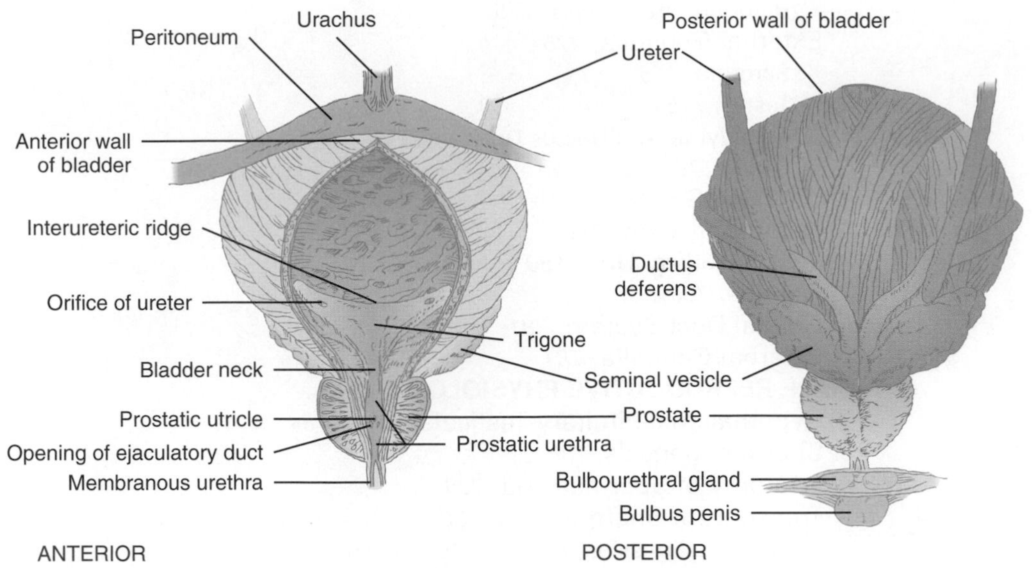

FIGURE 30-2 ■ Anterior and posterior views of the prostate gland and related structures. The triangular area demarcated by the interureteric ridge and the bladder neck is the trigone. (From Black JM, Hawks JH, Keene AM: *Medical-surgical nursing: clinical management for positive outcomes,* ed 6, Philadelphia, 2001, Saunders, p 940.)

imately 2.5 cm apart. The triangular area demarcated by this interureteric ridge and bladder neck has been labeled the **trigone** (Figure 30-2). As will be discussed later in the chapter, the trigone has a different embryologic origin from the rest of the bladder body, or fundus. The trigone is composed of mesoderm, and the fundus is composed of endoderm.

In males, the bladder lies anterior to the seminal vesicles, vasa deferentia, ureters, and rectum. The dome and part of the posterior bladder surfaces are covered by peritoneum and are thus in close proximity to the small bowel and the sigmoid colon. The neck of the bladder, which is the most inferior part, leads to the urethra. In males, the prostate lies between the bladder and the muscle layers of the pelvic floor that composes the urogenital diaphragm.

The arterial blood supply of the bladder comes from the superior, middle, and inferior vesical arteries, which originate from the anterior division of the hypogastric artery. Venous drainage occurs by a rich plexus of veins that surround the bladder and ultimately drain into the hypogastric vein.

The bladder and urethra receive their nerve supply from both the sympathetic and parasympathetic divisions of the autonomic nervous system. The sympathetic fibers, originating mainly from the lower thoracic and upper lumbar segments (T11-12 and L1-2), innervate the bladder and urethra as the hypogastric nerves. These sympathetic fibers are distributed more densely in the bladder base and proximal end of the urethra than in the bladder dome. Studies have revealed differences in the bladder muscle receptors, with cholinergic receptors concentrated in the fundus and adrenergic receptors present in the trigone and proximal end of the urethra (Figure 30-3).

The parasympathetic nerve supply originates from the sacral segments (S2-4), which proceed to form a plexus surrounding the bladder. In the male, a separate segment will reach the prostate and form the prostatic plexus. From this plexus, nerves emerge to innervate the erectile tissue of the male penis and the clitoris of the female (see Figure 30-3).

Branches of the bladder plexus penetrate the muscular coat of the bladder and become distributed throughout the detrusor. Parasympathetic muscle receptors are cholinergic in nature, and parasympathetic stimulation induces a detrusor contraction.

Urethra

The male urethra, which extends from the bladder to the external opening (urethral meatus) at the tip of the penis, functions as a conduit for both the urinary and genital systems. It is commonly divided into three segments: the *prostatic,* the *membranous,* and the *penile* or *spongy urethra* (Figure 30-4).

Auxiliary Genital Glands

The auxiliary genital glands of the male consist of the *prostate,* the *seminal vesicles,* and the *bulbourethral glands.* These glands secrete products that contribute to the seminal fluid.

Prostate

The **prostate** lies below the bladder and has both a muscular and a glandular component. The normal prostate weighs about 20 g and measures about 3.5 cm transversely and about 2.5 cm in its vertical and anteroposterior dimensions. The prostate is conical. Its base is continuous with the bladder

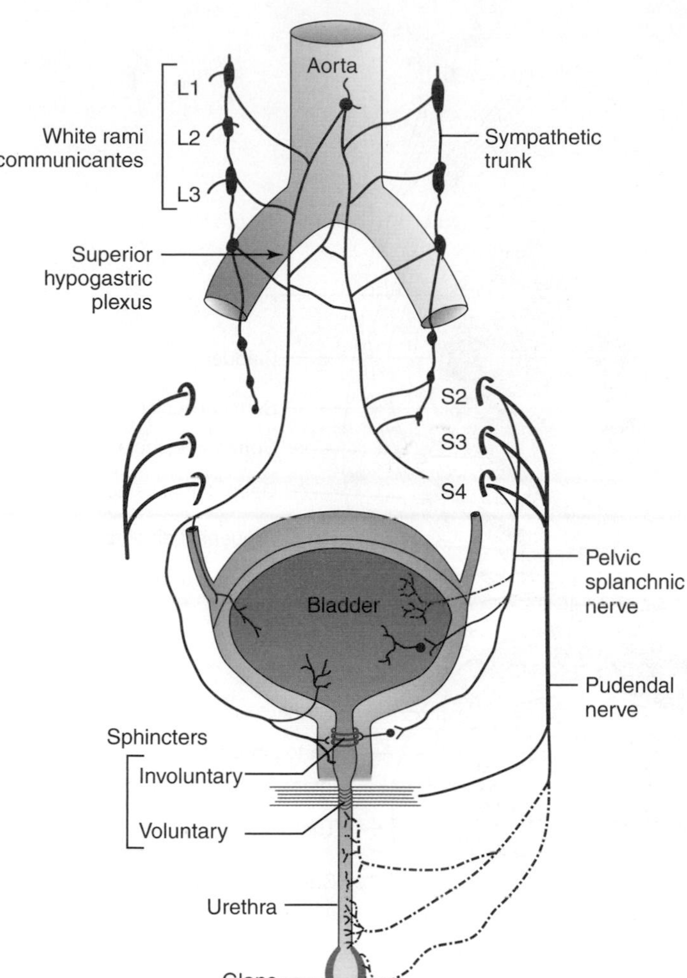

FIGURE 30-3 ■ Diagram of nerve supply to bladder and urethra. (From Sauerland EK: *Grants dissector,* ed 10, Baltimore, 1991, Williams & Wilkins, p 66.)

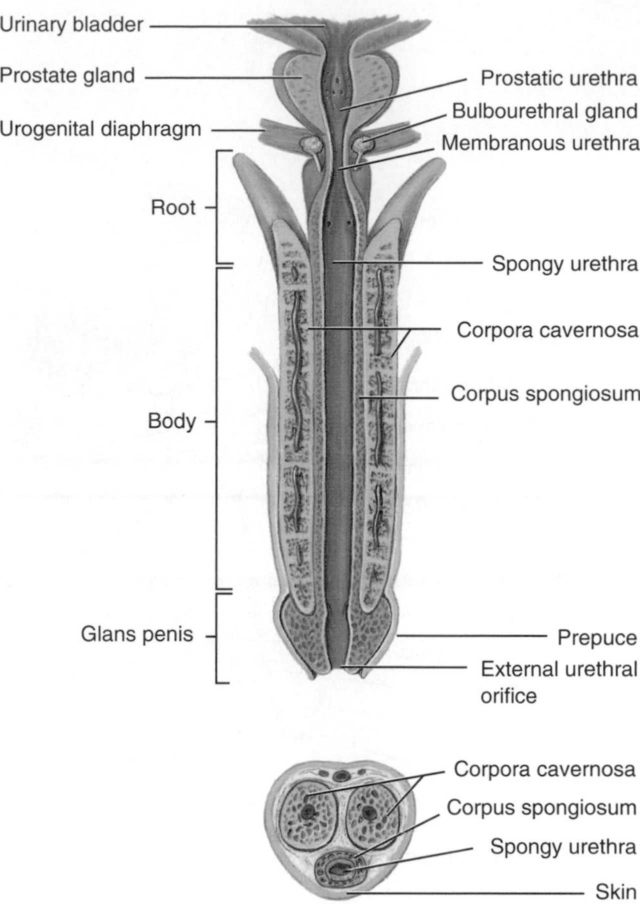

FIGURE 30-4 ■ Cross-sectional view of the penis emphasizing the membranous urethra, the urogenital diaphragm, the bulbourethral or Cowper gland, and the orifices of the bulbourethral glands. (From Applegate EJ: *The anatomy and physiology learning system: textbook,* ed 2, Philadelphia, 2000, Saunders, p 401.)

neck, and the inferior aspect of the prostate gland, or apex, lies adjacent to the urogenital diaphragm (Figure 30-5). Situated in front of the rectum, the prostate receives an excellent blood supply from a rich plexus of arteries and veins from the hypogastric vessels.

The prostate consists of a thin fibrous capsule with internally circular smooth muscle fibers and collagenous tissue that surround the urethra. Deep in this layer of connective and elastic tissue lies the prostatic stroma, which contains the prostatic epithelial glands. These glands drain into excretory ducts, which open chiefly on the floor of the urethra between the verumontanum and the vesical neck.

The main blood supply of the prostate is derived from the inferior vesical artery, a branch of the hypogastric artery. Besides the prostate, this artery also supplies the distal portion of the ureter, the seminal vesicles, and part of the bladder. A complex plexus situated between the prostate and overlying tissue freely communicates with the inferior hypogastric veins and provides venous drainage to the prostate.

Seminal Vesicles

The **seminal vesicles** are paired organs that lie next to the prostate under the base of the bladder (see Figure 30-5). Their coiled pouches secrete a fluid important to the survival of spermatozoa.

Bulbourethral Glands

The **bulbourethral** or **Cowper glands** are located on each side of the membranous urethra within the urogenital diaphragm. They add a mucoid secretion to the semen.

External Genitalia

Scrotum

The **scrotum** (see Figure 30-5) is a pouchlike sac that lies below the penis and pubic symphysis. A septum of connective tissue divides the sac into two compartments. Each compartment contains a male gonad, or testis, with its associated epididymis

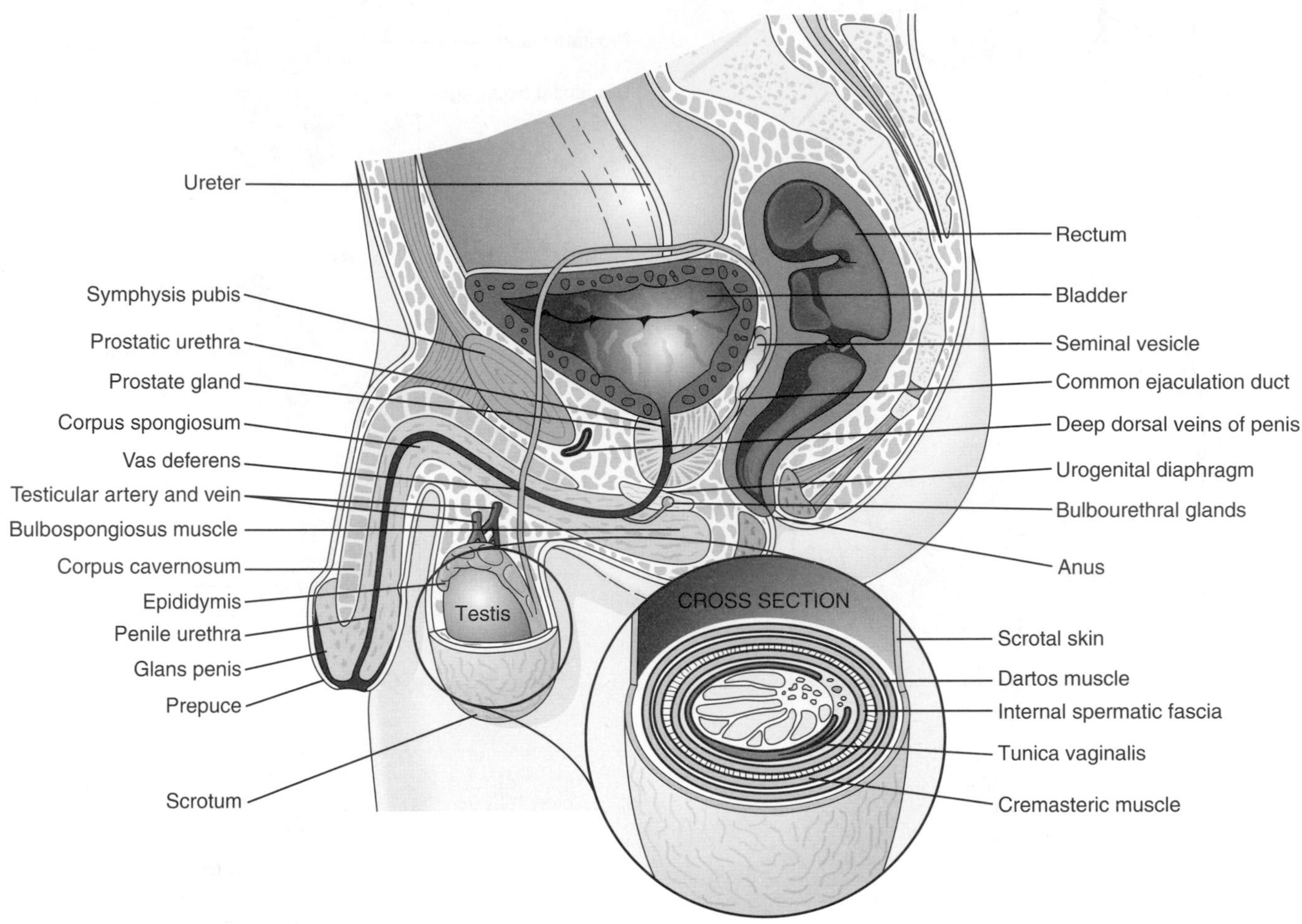

FIGURE 30-5 ■ Male genitourinary anatomy, including a cross-section of the scrotum and its layers.

and the lower portion of the vas deferens protected by the spermatic cord and its coverings. The scrotum not only supports the testes but also, by relaxation and contraction of its muscular layer, helps regulate temperature of the testes.

The scrotal sac consists of several tissue layers. The scrotal skin overlies the dartos muscle layer, whose smooth muscle fibers are embedded in loose connective tissue. The dartos muscle functions to contract the scrotal pouch with cold and expand it with heat. Under the dartos layer are several fascial layers (see Figure 30-5) that are continuous with the muscular layers of the abdominal wall and make up the covering of the spermatic cord. The external spermatic fascia is continuous with the external oblique aponeurosis of the abdominal wall. A few slips of skeletal muscle derived from the internal oblique muscle layer make up the cremasteric muscle, which adds to the upper part of the cord. The internal spermatic fascia is a continuation of the transverse fascia of the abdominal wall, with the transversus abdominis muscle not contributing to the cord layers. Finally, the peritoneum provides the tunica vaginalis layer, which is actually cut off from the abdominal cavity by obliteration of the processus vaginalis.

The scrotum receives its blood supply from the external pudendal artery, a branch of the femoral artery. In addition, the scrotum receives blood from portions of the internal pudendal artery (a branch of the hypogastric artery), the cremasteric, and testicular arteries that transverse the spermatic cord.

Testes

The **testes** are the male reproductive organs responsible for sperm production. They average about 4 to 5 cm in length and 2 to 3 cm in thickness. The testes lie within the scrotum and are suspended by the spermatic cord. The testes are covered by a thick fascial layer called the tunica albuginea. This layer invaginates posteriorly to form the mediastinum testis. This fibrous mediastinum sends fibrous septa into each testis that separate it into many different lobules. Each lobule contains one to four seminiferous tubules that if stretched to full length

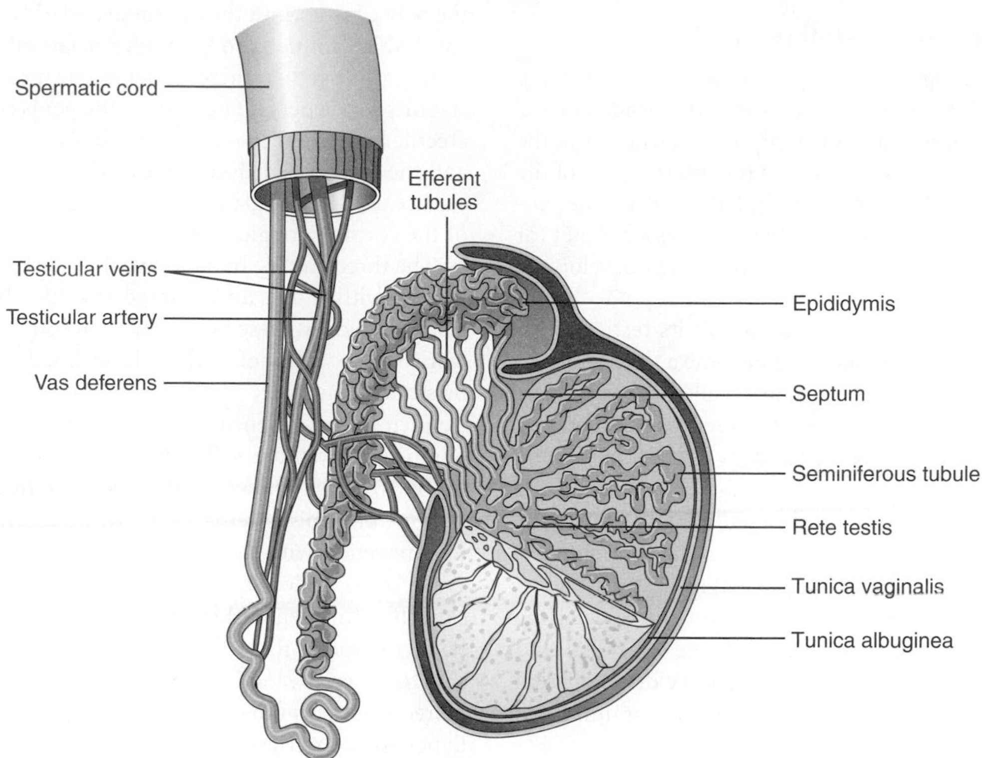

FIGURE 30-6 ■ The anatomy of the testis and epididymis. Note the numerous compartments of the testis that are filled with seminiferous tubules gathering into the rete testis; they join to form a markedly convoluted tubule that becomes the epididymis, which is continuous with the vas deferens. The epididymis attaches to the dorsomedial aspect of the testis, and the vas deferens joins the other structures of the spermatic cord.

would measure approximately 60 cm. Spermatozoa production occurs within the epithelial lining of the seminiferous tubules (Figure 30-6).

The seminiferous tubules have a basement membrane consisting of elastic and connective tissue that supports the seminiferous cells. The seminiferous cells are either **Sertoli cells** (supporting cells) or spermatogenic cells. Found between the seminiferous tubules and embedded in connective tissue, the interstitial **Leydig cells** produce and secrete testosterone, a hormone involved in the development of male sexual characteristics (Figure 30-7). The seminiferous tubules converge on the mediastinum testis. The tubules, which are connected by the straight efferent ducts, drain into the head of the epididymis.

The testicular blood supply is derived from the internal spermatics, which arise directly from the aorta below the renal arteries. They course inferiorly through the spermatic cord and anastomose with the cremasteric arteries and the arteries of the vas; these vessels also contribute to the blood supply. The blood from the testis returns through a plexus of veins in the spermatic cord (the pampiniform plexus) that forms the spermatic veins. The left spermatic vein enters the renal vein, which subsequently enters the vena cava. The right renal vein enters the vena cava directly.

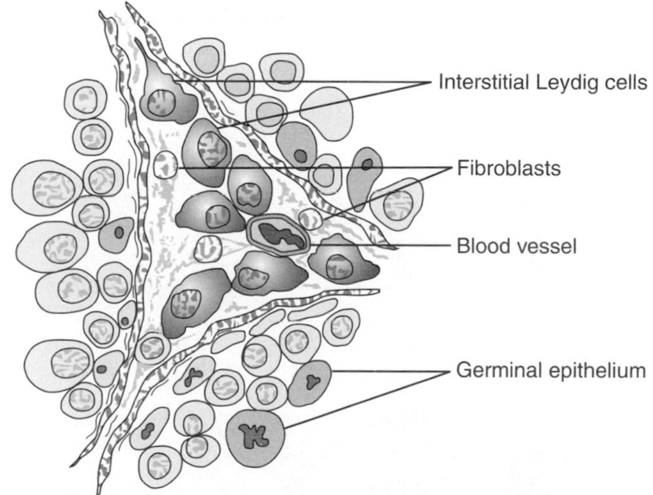

FIGURE 30-7 ■ The interstitial Leydig cells, the cells that secrete testosterone, are located in the interstices between the seminiferous tubules. (From Guyton AC, Hall JE, editors: *Textbook of medical physiology,* ed 10, Philadelphia, 2000, Saunders, p 917.)

Epididymis and Ductus Deferens

The **epididymis** is a tightly coiled tube that lies along the top of and behind each testis. It is divided into the head, situated at the upper pole of the testes; the body, lying posterior to the testes; and the tail, which is attached to the inferior pole of the testes (see Figure 30-6). The body and the tail of the epididymis form one continuous tube that serves as a conduit for maturing spermatozoa. In the epididymis, sperm develop the ability to swim.

As the convoluted tube of the tail leaves its testicular attachments, it increases in diameter to become a thick, muscular tube called the **ductus deferens,** also called the **vas deferens.** Leaving the spermatic cord, the vas follows an extraperitoneal course and passes caudally and laterally along the pelvic wall. As it passes medial to the distal end of the ureter, it bends caudally to reach the midline and lies on the posterior wall of the bladder just medial to the seminal vesicles. It terminates in a dilated ampulla that courses underneath the base of the prostate. At this point the duct of the seminal vesicle joins with the duct of the ampulla, and the ejaculatory duct is formed. The ejaculatory ducts open in the prostatic urethra at the level of the verumontanum.

Penis

The **penis** is the male organ of copulation and urinary excretion. It is composed of three erectile bodies—two paired **corpora cavernosa,** which lie dorsally, and the *corpus spongiosum,* which contains the urethra (Figure 30-8). Grossly, the penis is divided into three segments. The root of the penis consists of the proximal ends of the corpora cavernosa, which attach to the pelvic bones, and the proximal end of the corpus spongiosum, which connects to the undersurface of the urogenital diaphragm. Together these attachments provide fixation and stability to the penis. The shaft of the penis consists of all three erectile bodies: the two cavernous bodies lying on the dorsum and the corpus, which occupies a depression on their ventral surface. Finally, the glans of the penis forms the distal segment of the corpus spongiosum.

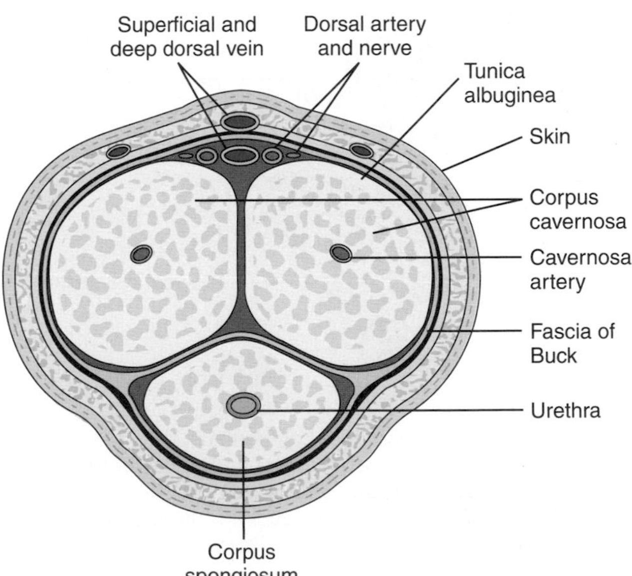

FIGURE 30-8 ■ Transverse section through the penis. The paired upper structures are the corpora cavernosa. The single lower body surrounding the urethra is the corpus spongiosum.

The three erectile bodies have the capability to become engorged with blood and enlarge considerably with erection. Microscopically, these bodies have an internal spongelike network that consists of endothelium-lined spaces surrounded by smooth muscle.

Each corpus is enclosed in a fascia sheath, the tunica albuginea, and all are subsequently surrounded by a thick fibrous envelope known as the **fascia of Buck.** The overlying skin of the penis is remarkable for its thinness and looseness of connection with the fascial sheath of the penis. The skin of the penis is folded upon itself to form the **prepuce,** or **foreskin.** It is this penile skin overlying the glans that is removed with circumcision.

The arterial blood supply is primarily derived from the paired internal pudendal arteries, which are branches of the hypogastric arteries. Each internal pudendal artery branches several times in the penis. The deep or cavernous artery supplies the entire corpus cavernosum. The urethral artery supplies the corpus spongiosum, and the bulbar artery supplies the bulb of the corpus spongiosum. The dorsal artery continues along the dorsum of the penis and lies below the fascia of Buck and between two dorsal veins. It provides additional supply to the glans (Figure 30-9).

Venous drainage of the penis is through several channels. The cavernous veins drain the corpora cavernosa, and the circumflex veins join the deep dorsal vein of the penis to also drain the corpora. The superficial dorsal vein drains the glans and part of the distal portion of the corpora. Finally, a bulbar branch drains the bulbous urethra and proximal portion of the corpus spongiosum. Together these branches coalesce and pass through the urogenital diaphragm into the retropubic venous plexus of Santorini (see Figure 30-9).

The nerve supply of the penis is formed from both parasympathetic and sympathetic components. The parasympathetic fibers arise from S2-S4, and the sympathetic component is derived from the hypogastric plexus. Although the final neurotransmitters have not been completely defined, parasympathetic stimulation from the pudendal nerve results in relaxation of vascular resistance, which increases blood flow to the penis and creates an erection. The pudendal nerve also carries sensory fibers from the penis and enters the sacral spinal cord to contribute to penile erection.

Sympathetic nerve fibers may contribute to erectile capacity, but their role has not been proved conclusively. They do innervate the proximal involuntary sphincter of the bladder neck, where contraction prevents retrograde ejaculation of semen from the prostatic urethra into the bladder. They also innervate the muscles of the seminal vesicles and prostate, which when stimulated cause ejaculation of seminal fluid into the urethra.

KEY CONCEPTS

- The upper genitourinary tract is composed of the kidneys and ureters. The lower genitourinary tract includes the bladder and urethra and the accessory male sexual organs.
- Ureters transport urine from the renal pelvis to the bladder. Ureters have several points of narrowing that predispose to obstruction: ureteropelvic junction, pelvic brim, and ureterovesical junction.
- The adult bladder has a normal capacity of 450 to 500 ml. With overdistention, the bladder may be palpable in the suprapubic region. The bladder is a muscular organ composed of several layers of muscle fibers. An important muscular landmark in the bladder is the trigone. Parasympathetic stimulation of the bladder results in bladder muscle contraction.
- The urethra extends from the bladder to the meatus at the end of the penis. In addition to transporting urine, the urethra has ducts that receive fluid from the prostate, seminal vesicles, and bulbourethral glands.
- The scrotal sac supports the testes and regulates their temperature. Testes contain several cell types important in sperm production and the development of secondary sex characteristics. Spermatogenic cells produce sperm in the testes. Sertoli cells serve to support and nurture spermatogenesis. Leydig cells produce and secrete testosterone.
- Situated in the testes, the epididymis serves as a collecting conduit for sperm. The epididymis is continuous with the ductus (vas) deferens. The vas travels along the pelvic wall and joins with the seminal vesicle duct at the prostate to form the ejaculatory duct. The ejaculatory ducts open into the urethra.
- Skin overlying the penis is very loose, which facilitates significant enlargement when the penis is engorged with blood during erection. Parasympathetic fibers forming the pudendal nerve are responsible for erection. Ejaculation is a function of the sympathetic nerve fibers.

EMBRYOLOGY

Developmental processes in the genital and urinary systems are intimately related. To facilitate understanding of this development, the two systems will be discussed in several subdivisions. The urinary system, which is composed of the nephric system and the vesicourethral unit, will be discussed first. The genital system, which is composed of the gonads, the genital ducts, and the external genitalia, will be discussed second.

Nephric System

The nephric system develops progressively through three distinct phases: the *pronephros, mesonephros,* and *metanephros.* The **pronephros** is the earliest state in humans but corresponds to the mature structure in primitive vertebrates. The pronephros consists of six to ten pairs of tubules connected by a pronephric duct. It grows caudally to join the cloaca, a blind end of the hindgut. The pronephros is a temporary structure and, except for its duct, disappears by the fourth week of intrauterine life (Figure 30-10).

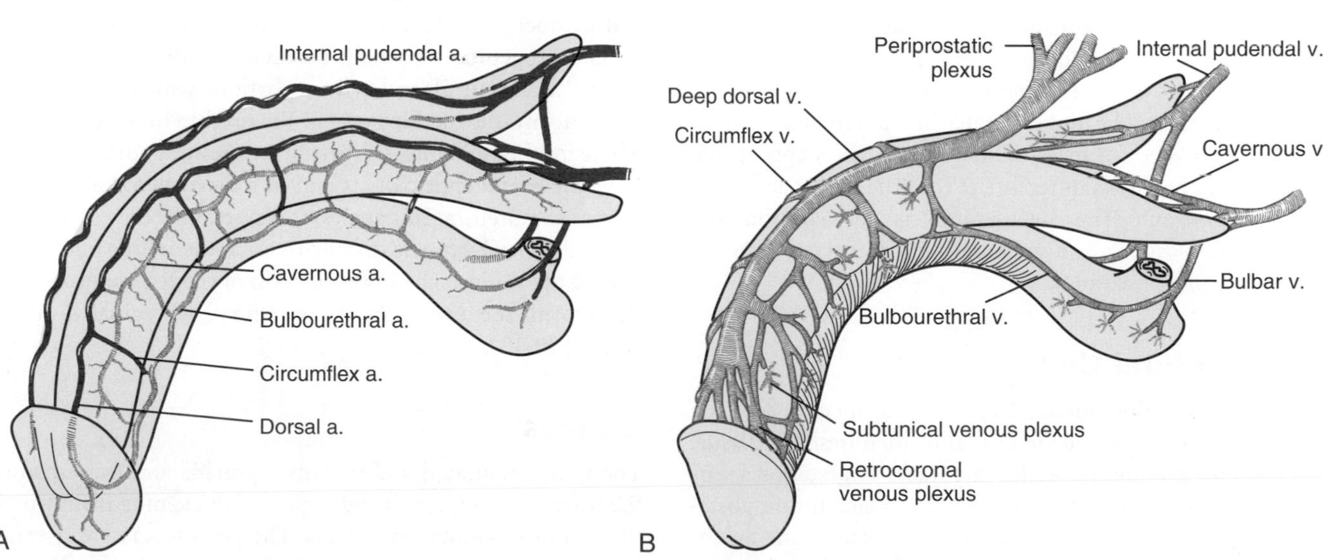

FIGURE 30-9 ■ Penile arterial supply **(A)** and venous drainage **(B)**, longitudinal views. *a.,* Artery; *v.,* vein. (From Walsh PC et al, editors: *Campbell's urology,* ed 7, Philadelphia, 1998, Saunders, p 1160.)

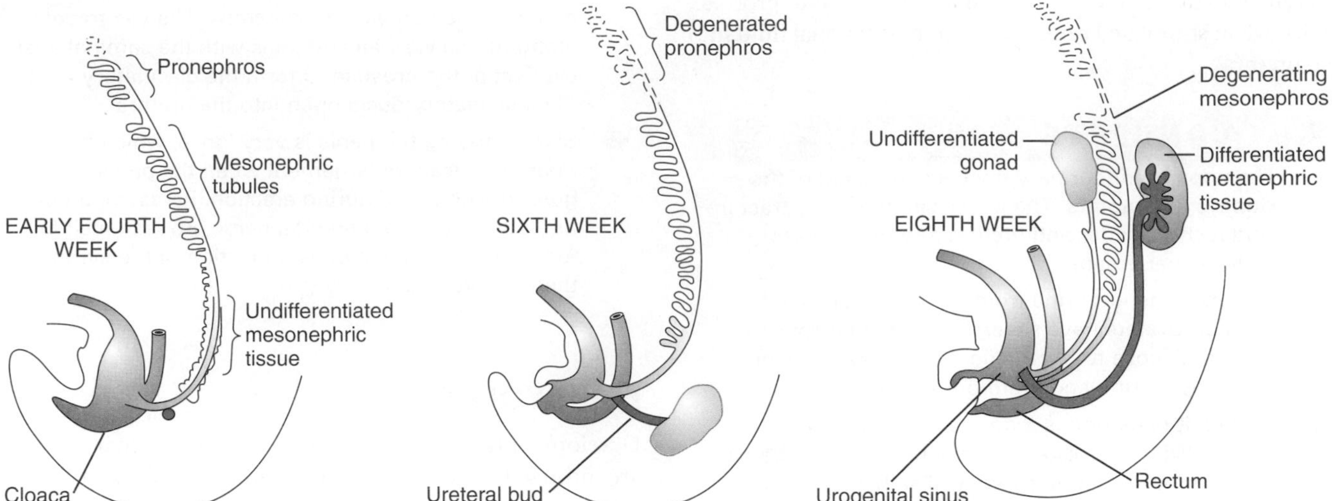

FIGURE 30-10 ■ Schematic representation of the development of the nephric system. Only a few of the tubules of the pronephros are seen early in the fourth week, whereas the mesonephric tissue differentiates into mesonephric tubules that progressively join the mesonephric duct. The first sign of the ureteral bud from the mesonephric duct is seen. At 6 weeks the pronephros has completely degenerated and the mesonephric tubules start to do so. The ureteral bud grows dorsocranially and has met the metanephrogenic cap. By the eighth week, cranial migration of the differentiating metanephros can be seen. The cranial end of the ureteric bud expands and starts to show multiple successive outgrowths. (From Tanagho EA, McAninch JW, editors: *Smith's general urology,* ed 13, East Norwalk, Conn, 1992, Appleton & Lange, p 18.)

The **mesonephros** corresponds to the mature excretory organ of some amphibians. In humans it begins developing at about the fourth to fifth week of gestation.[1-4] The tubules of the mesonephros are more numerous and form a cuplike outgrowth into which capillaries push to form a primitive glomerulus. The tubules communicate with the mesonephric duct, which is derived from the preceding pronephric duct. The number of mesonephros tubules reaches a maximum by about 8 weeks of gestation and then degenerate.

The final stage of development, the **metanephros,** begins in the fourth week when the ureteral bud grows out of the mesonephric duct. The bud elongates in a dorsocranial direction, where it meets a mass of mesoderm, the nephrogenic blastema, and begins to differentiate into the ureter and renal collecting system.[1,4] The metanephros is derived from the nephrogenic blastema and eventually differentiates into the mature mammalian kidney.

Vesicourethral Unit

The blind end of the caudal hindgut forms the cloaca, which is separated from the outside by a thin membrane of tissue, the urogenital membrane. At about 4 weeks of gestation a septum grows downward and separates the cloaca into a posterior compartment, which will become the rectum, and an anterior compartment, which will form the urogenital sinus.

The urogenital sinus receives the mesonephric duct, which is progressively absorbed into this structure. The mesonephric duct distal to the ureteral bud is absorbed into the sinus, and its mesenchyme subsequently forms the bladder trigone. The ureter, which is derived from the ureteral bud, and the mesonephric duct, which differentiates into the vas deferens, merges into the sinus as well. In a complex pattern of development, the opening of the ureteral bud, which will eventually become the ureteral orifice, migrates upward and laterally. The opening of the mesonephric duct, which will become the ejaculatory duct, migrates downward and medially (Figure 30-11).

The urogenital sinus can be divided into two main segments. The ventral and pelvic portion, which receives the ureter, forms the bladder, part of the urethra in males, and the whole urethra in females. A phallic or urethral portion will receive the mesonephric ducts and in males will form a second part of the urethra. In females, this portion receives the müllerian ducts, which fuse distally to form the uterus and upper part of the vagina. The lower portion of the female urogenital sinus forms the lower part of the vagina and vaginal vestibule (Figure 30-12).

Gonads

The undifferentiated and primitive **gonads** are derived from the urogenital ridge, a dorsal region of thickening from which the primitive kidney also forms. The gonads serve as precursors to the testes in males and the ovaries in females. During the seventh week an individual gonad begins to assume the characteristics of either a testis or an ovary.

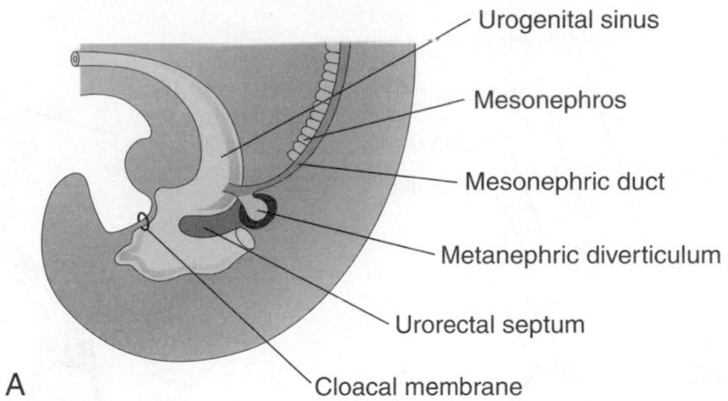

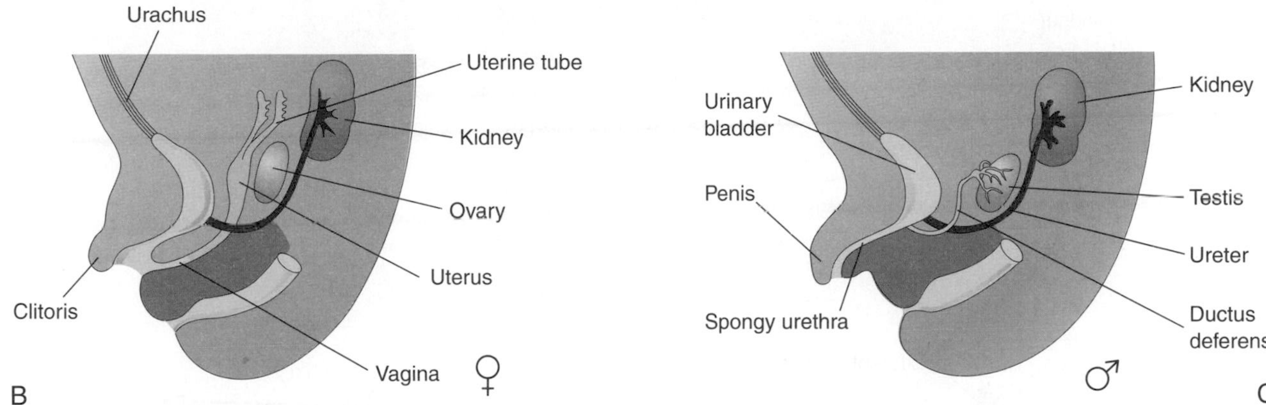

FIGURE 30-11 ■ Diagrams showing division of the cloaca into the urogenital sinus and rectum; absorption of the mesonephric ducts; development of the urinary bladder, urethra, and urachus; and changes in location of the ureters. **A,** Lateral view of the caudal half of a 5-week embryo. The stages shown in **B** and **C** are reached by the 12th week. (From Moore KL, Persaud TVN, editors: *The developing human: clinically oriented embryology,* ed 7, Philadelphia, 2003, Saunders, p 302.)

In the presence of testis-determining factor, which is located on the Y chromosome, a gonad develops into a testis. The gland increases in size, and the cells of the epithelium grow centrally into the organ's mesenchyme. These ingrowths become radially arranged, form cords, and begin to converge on the posterior aspect of the testis. The cords eventually differentiate into the seminiferous tubules, which produce spermatozoa. The testes descend behind the abdominal cavity in the retroperitoneal space and into the scrotum, usually by the eighth month of gestation.

In the absence of testis-determining factor, a gonad differentiates into an ovary, and a cortex forms from the germinal epithelium and ultimately gives rise to ovarian follicles containing ova. It descends only partially through the abdominal cavity and eventually lies adjacent to the fallopian tubes.

Genital Duct System

As the embryo develops, two different but related kinds of ducts form beside the undifferentiated gonads. The mesonephric, or **wolffian, ducts,** as previously explained, develop as nephric ducts but will go on to form the male genital ducts. The **müllerian ducts** develop alongside the mesonephric ducts (paramesonephric) and are genital structures from the start.

Early in development, each of the two müllerian ducts arises lateral to the mesonephric ducts, either directly from the mesonephric ducts themselves or possibly from the adjacent epithelium of the primitive abdominal cavity. Both ducts grow caudally to enter the urogenital sinus.

If a gonad differentiates into a testis, the wolffian ducts subsequently develop into the male duct system consisting of the epididymis, vas deferens, seminal vesicles, and ejaculatory ducts. The müllerian ducts, except for a few rudimentary fragments, rapidly atrophy.

If, on the other hand, a gonad develops into an ovary, the müllerian ducts proceed to form the uterus, fallopian tubes, and upper part of the vagina. The mesonephric, or wolffian, ducts fail to develop further and remain rudimentary (see Figure 30-12).

External Genitalia

Development of the external genitalia begins at about 12 intrauterine weeks. Prior to this point, three small protuberances appear on the external aspect of the cloacal membrane.

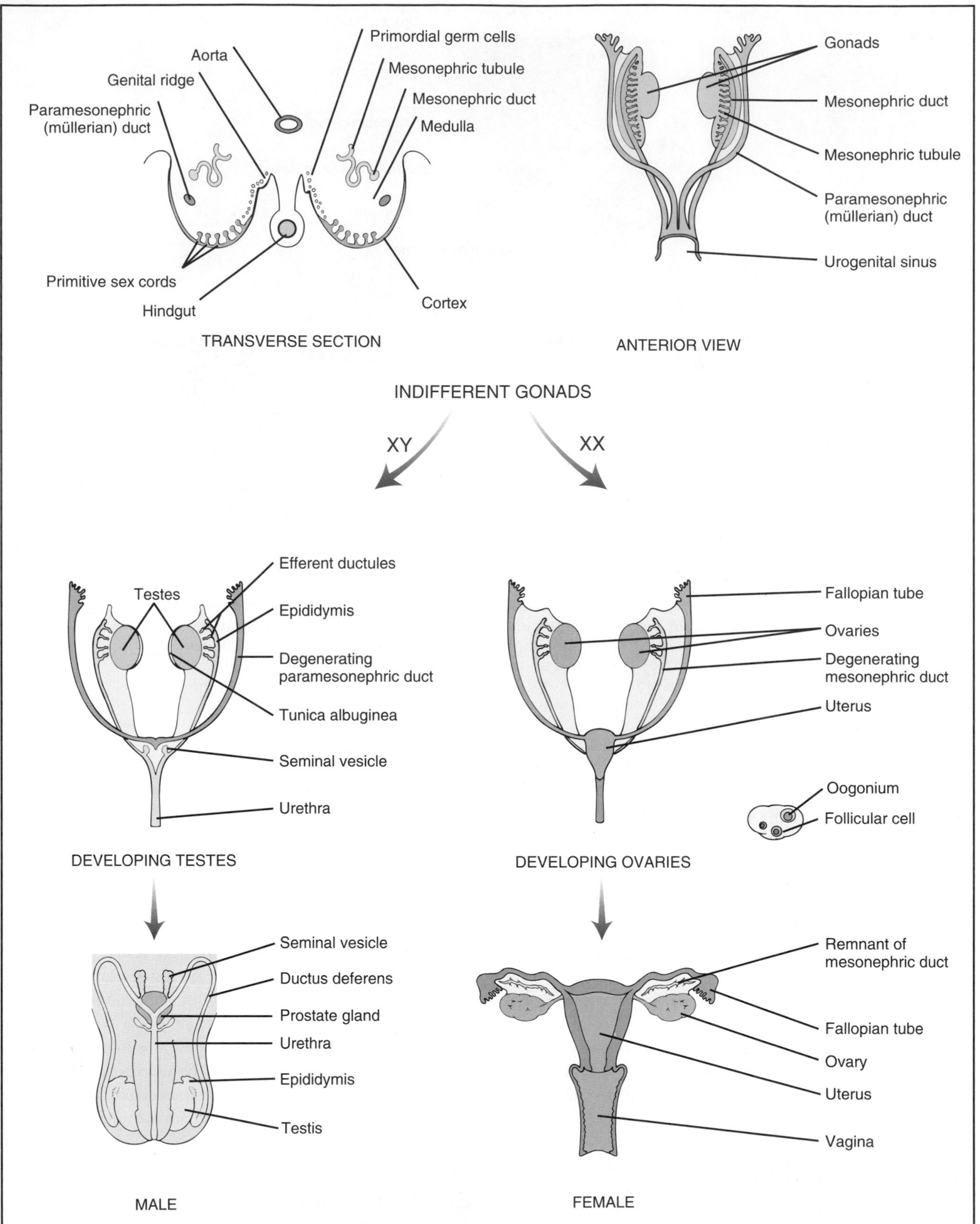

FIGURE 30-12 ■ Transformation of the undifferentiated genital system into the definitive male and female systems. (From Nichols FH, Zwelling E: *Maternal-newborn nursing: theory and practice,* Philadelphia, 1997, Saunders, p 174.)

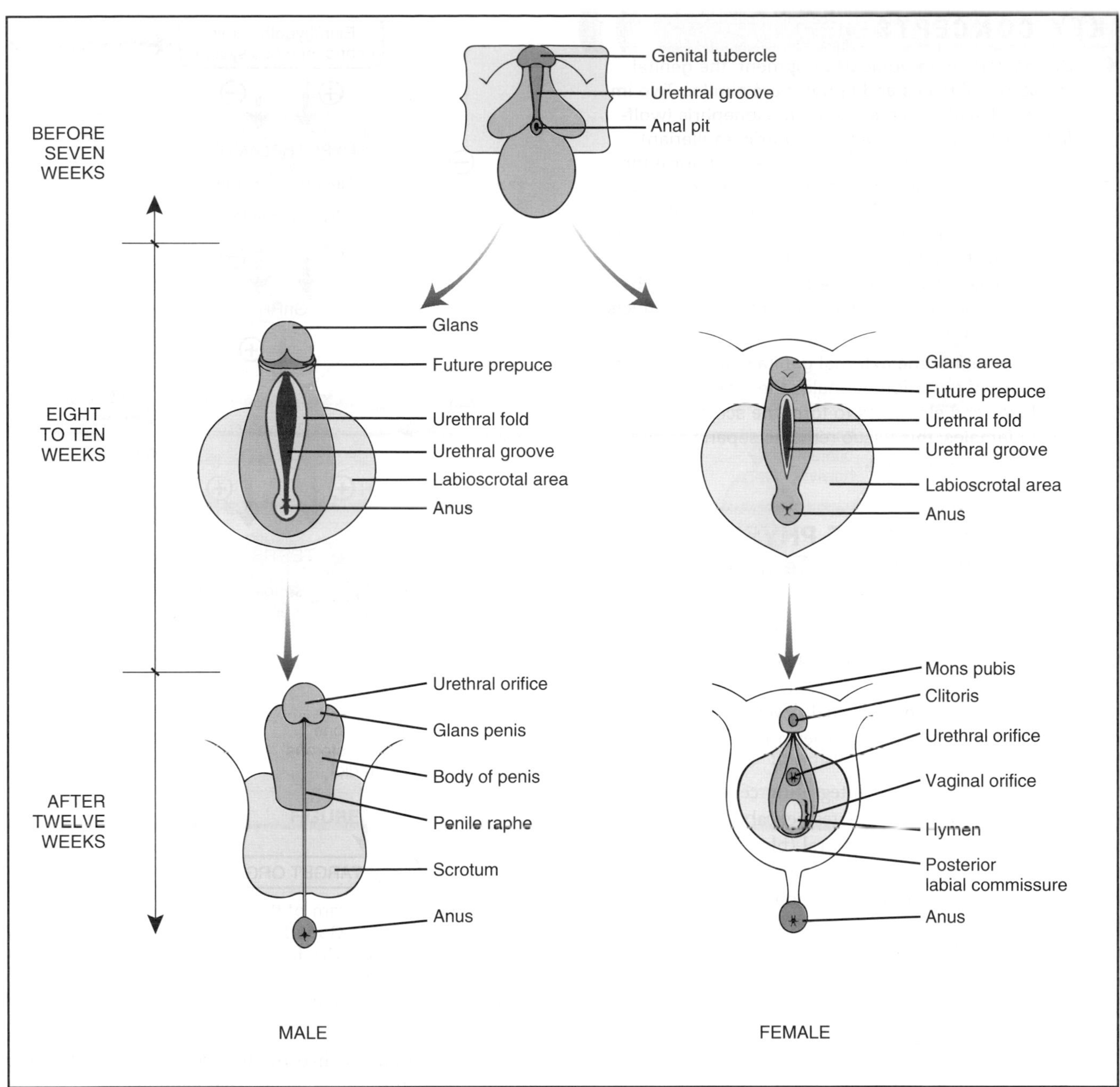

FIGURE 30-13 ■ Development of the external genitalia from the indifferent stage (before 7 weeks) to fully differentiated stages (after 12 weeks of gestation). (From Nichols FH, Zwelling E: *Maternal-newborn nursing: theory and practice,* Philadelphia, 1997, Saunders, p 175.)

The genital tubercle is located anteriorly and the genital swellings are situated on either side of the membrane. In the seventh week, rupture of the urogenital membrane gives the urogenital sinus a separate opening on the undersurface of the genital tubercle.

In males, the genital or labioscrotal swellings migrate and fuse centrally to form the scrotum. The fused genital tubercles elongate. The elongated fused tubercles form a cylindric shape with a ventral groove communicating with the urogenital sinus. This groove subsequently becomes covered by folds of tissue and forms the penile urethra (Figure 30-13).

The female external genitalia closely resemble those of the male until about the eighth intrauterine week. At this time the genital tubercle lags behind in growth and becomes the clitoris. The urogenital sinus shortens and widens somewhat to form the vaginal vestibule, and the genital swellings form the labia majora. The urethral folds become the labia minora.

mature sperm cell, or spermatozoon, within each tubule are spermatozoa in all stages of development. This characteristic allows new spermatozoa to be continuously produced across the male life span. The effects of aging on the male reproductive system are described in the Geriatric Considerations section on p. 788.

Anatomy of Spermatozoa

The human spermatozoon is approximately 60 μm in length. The oval head contains a nucleus that is highly condensed and stabilized by cross-links between its molecules, which makes it very resistant to physical injury during its passage and storage in the epididymis. An outer membrane, the acrosome, contains the enzymes required for penetration of the female egg before fertilization.

The tail accounts for 90% of the length of the spermatozoon and is divided into a middle piece, principal piece, and end piece. The spermatozoon derives its motile ability from the motor apparatus of the tail, which is called the **axoneme.** The axoneme, which runs the length of the tail, is composed of a central pair of tubules surrounded by a ring of nine pairs of tubules (the 9 + 2 pattern). This ring of tubules is surrounded by a supporting structure of nine noncontractile dense fibers. Within the middle piece, a circular sheath of mitochondria[9] (Figure 30-16) surrounds these outer dense fibers.

The mitochondria contain the enzymes required for the production of adenosine triphosphate, the energy source for the cell. Within the axoneme are enzymes and structural proteins. These enzymes convert chemical energy from adenosine triphosphate to the mechanical energy of sperm cell movement to aid in fertilization of the egg.

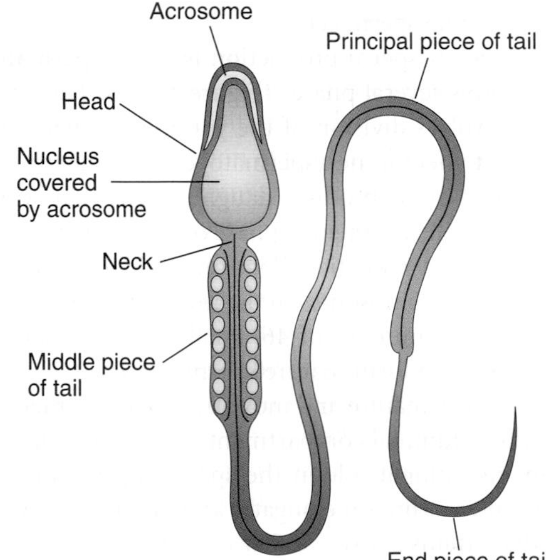

FIGURE 30-16 ■ Anatomy of a mature sperm cell. (From Moore KL, Persaud TVN, editors: *The developing human: clinically oriented embryology,* ed 7, Philadelphia, 2003, Saunders, p 21.)

Transport of Spermatozoa

Once mature spermatozoa are released from the Sertoli cells into the seminiferous tubules, they must pass through approximately 6 m of duct in the male reproductive tract before leaving the urethral meatus and being deposited in the vagina during sexual intercourse. From the seminiferous tubules, the spermatozoa are deposited into the rete testis, a collecting chamber for all the seminiferous tubules. From the rete testis, the sperm travel through the efferent ductules, 12 to 20 channels that pass into a single compact duct, the epididymis. The epididymis is a tightly convoluted duct that is divided into three regions: the caput (globus major), the corpus (body), and the cauda epididymis (tail, or globus minor). Unfolded and stretched, the epididymis would measure 12 to 15 feet.

After leaving the epididymis, the sperm enter the ductus or vas deferens. Embryologically, this duct is derived from the mesonephric duct. It passes through the scrotum, traverses the inguinal canal into the pelvis, and then passes behind the bladder to enter the prostatic urethra at the ejaculatory ducts of the verumontanum. The terminal portion of the vas deferens is known as the **ampulla.** It is joined by the ducts of the seminal vesicle before entering the ejaculatory ducts.

As one passes in a proximal-to-distal direction from the efferent ducts to the vas deferens, the thickness of the muscle gradually increases. In the vas deferens, three interconnected smooth muscle layers form a thick muscular wall, with the ratio of wall thickness to lumen being the greatest in any human structure.[7] This thick muscular wall facilitates rapid sperm transport at the time of ejaculation.

Aside from serving as a conduit and storage depot for spermatozoa, the epididymis probably sustains maturational processes. Most studies have demonstrated that sperm taken directly from the testes are incapable of fertilizing eggs. It appears that the development of motility and increased fertility are acquired during transit through the epididymis.[7]

Because epididymal sperm are probably immotile, other mechanisms must be involved in their transport. Initially, spermatozoa are carried into the efferent ducts by fluid from the rete testis. Within the efferent ducts, motile cilia within the lumen function to reabsorb testicular fluid and help move spermatozoa into the epididymis. Within the epididymis, the spermatozoa are probably transported by rhythmic contraction of the smooth muscle cells.[7]

Ejaculation accelerates the passage of spermatozoa through the vas deferens and distal end of the epididymis. In young men, approximately 200 million sperm can be found in the reservoir of the epididymis. About 50% are found in the cauda region. With ejaculation, sperm from the distal part of the epididymis and vas deferens are deposited into the prostatic urethra, where they account for less than 10% of the normal ejaculate.[10]

Erection, Emission, and Ejaculation

To penetrate the vagina and deposit sperm, the penis must be erect. The physiology of **erection** is a complicated interaction of vascular, neurologic, and hormonal factors. Although erection has classically been thought of as a parasympathetic function, it is more complex. Erection may be mediated by either local stimulation, which causes a reflexogenic erection through the sacral spinal cord, or psychological stimulation, which causes a psychogenic erection through cerebral centers. The presence of erections in patients with spinal cord injuries attests to the presence of reflex erections. Such patients have an intact sacral spinal cord and its reflex arc of afferent and efferent nerves below the site of spinal cord injury.

The penis receives sensory innervation from the pudendal sensory nerves entering the sacral spinal cord. The pudendal nerve is a mixed nerve that provides motor innervation to the pelvic floor musculature and penile sensory fibers. The motor supply to the penis appears to be provided by sacral parasympathetic fibers. Although erection is possible in patients with spinal cord injuries, in intact men it is a much more controlled process influenced to a great extent by the cerebral cortex. Impulses may traverse the spinal cord from the cerebral cortex in the lateral columns and exit the spinal cord through sacral parasympathetic and possibly the thoracolumbar sympathetic nerves as well.[7]

During erection, the vascular spaces that make up the spongy vacuous tissues of the corpora cavernosa and corpus spongiosum fill with blood. The relaxation of smooth muscle tone in these structures that allows filling and subsequent penile erection is modulated by an undetermined neurotransmitter. Research indicates that erectile function cannot be fully explained by parasympathetic or sympathetic mechanisms; this observation has led to consideration that nonadrenergic and noncholinergic neuromodulators may be involved in such function.[11] For example, penile injection of certain prostaglandins has been shown to induce smooth muscle relaxation and has been used to induce erections in some men experiencing erectile dysfunction.[12]

Ejaculation may be divided into two phases: *emission* and *ejaculation*. During **emission,** secretions from the periurethral glands, seminal vesicles, and prostate are deposited with sperm from the vasa deferentia and the cauda epididymis into the prostatic urethra. Control of emission is mediated primarily through the sympathetic nerves, which stimulate contraction of smooth muscle in these genital structures.

With **ejaculation,** the bladder neck or internal sphincter closes. This closure is also mediated through the sympathetic nervous system. Next, the external sphincter relaxes and the perineal and bulbourethral muscles surrounding the bulb of the corpus spongiosum contract and expel the ejaculate from the posterior urethra and through the urethral meatus.

The physiologic function of the secretory products of the accessory sex glands is uncertain. These secretions make up most of the seminal plasma, with the sperm and testicular fluid probably composing less than 10% of the final ejaculated semen volume. Although some investigators have demonstrated that sperm removed directly from the epididymis are capable of fertilization, these secretions most likely optimize conditions for sperm motility, survival, and transport in both the female and male reproductive tracts.

Capacitation

Capacitation of the spermatozoa refers to the multiple changes that activate the sperm and enhance their ability to participate in the final process of fertilization. Although sperm are anatomically complete and highly motile when ejaculated, the complex process of capacitation is necessary before the sperm are actually capable of fertilizing the egg. The capacitation process occurs over a period of 1 to 10 hours and occurs in sperm only after they have been introduced into the vagina of the female. Once the sperm are inside the female, the uterine and fallopian tube fluids wash away the various inhibitory factors that had suppressed sperm activity in the male genital ducts. During the time that the spermatozoa were in the fluid of the male genital ducts, they were continually exposed to many floating vesicles from the seminiferous tubules containing large amounts of cholesterol. This cholesterol, continually donated to the cellular membrane covering the sperm acrosome, toughens the outside membrane and prevents release of its enzymes. After ejaculation, the sperm that are deposited in the vagina swim away from the cholesterol vesicles upward into the uterine fluid, and they gradually lose much of their excess cholesterol during the next few hours. As the cholesterol is lost, the membrane at the head of the sperm becomes much weaker.

The membrane of the sperm head also becomes much more permeable to calcium ions. Large amounts of calcium enter the sperm to increase the powerful whiplike motion of the flagellum beyond its previously weak, undulating motion. In addition, the calcium ions probably also alter the intracellular membrane covering the leading edge of the acrosome, thus making it possible for the acrosome to release its enzymes very rapidly and easily as the sperm penetrates the granulosa cell mass surrounding the ovum. These enzymes are released even more rapidly and easily as the sperm attempts to penetrate the zona pellucida of the ovum itself.[13]

Acrosome Reaction

The head of a sperm is essentially a highly compact package of genetic chromatin material covered by a specialized **acrosome** and acrosomal (head) cap. Stored in the acrosome of the sperm are large quantities of hydrolytic (water-splitting) enzymes that are released during capacitation. The specialized acrosomal enzymes first break down cervical mucus to allow sperm to pass into the uterus and uterine tubes. If an ovum is present in the female reproductive tract when semen is introduced, continued release of acrosomal enzymes results in digestion of proteins in the structural elements of the outer covering of the egg. A high sperm count is essential for male fertility because the female ovum, once it is expelled from the ovarian follicle into the abdominal cavity and fallopian tube, contains multiple layers of granulosa cells. Before a sperm can fertilize the ovum, it must first pass through the granulosa cell layer, and then it must penetrate the thick covering of the ovum itself, the **zona pellucida.** It is believed that the acrosomal enzyme hyaluronidase plays an important role in opening pathways between the granulosa cells so that the sperm can reach the ovum.

On reaching the zona pellucida of the ovum, the anterior membrane of the sperm binds specifically with a receptor protein in the zona pellucida. Then the entire anterior membrane of the acrosome rapidly dissolves, and all the acrosomal enzymes are immediately released. Within minutes, these open a penetrating pathway for passage of the sperm head through the zona pellucida.

The head at first enters the perivitelline space lying beneath the zona pellucida but outside the membrane of the underlying oocyte. Within 30 minutes, the membranes of the sperm head and the oocyte fuse; the sperm genetic material enters the oocyte to cause fertilization, and the embryo begins to develop.

Geriatric Considerations

A decline in male fertility and reproductive organ function usually occurs with aging. However, the magnitude of functional decline of the male reproductive organs is variable. For example, some elderly men maintain their fertility into their 70s and 80s.

Male reproductive organ variability is due to organ-specific tissue changes. Active male germinal cells continue to produce spermatozoa (spermatogenesis), although the number of sperm produced declines proportionally over time. The testes become smaller as a result of increased connective tissue, fibrosis of the tubules, and decreased numbers of capillaries. The number of active seminiferous tubules declines with aging. The number of Leydig cells that produce testosterone decreases, leading to a decrease in testosterone with aging.

After age 50, the prostate gland undergoes changes with an increase in connective tissue, collagen, and smooth muscle fibers and a decreasing vascular supply. The acini may atrophy but often become hyperplastic. Secretions within the gland may become calcified.

The arteries and veins in the penis become increasingly sclerotic. The penis itself becomes smaller, with an increase in fibroelastic tissue. Penile sensation is decreased. Sexually, the aging male has a longer refractory period after orgasm and decreased force of ejaculation.

KEY CONCEPTS

- Normal male sexual development and spermatogenesis depend on the appropriate secretion of reproductive hormones. GnRH, secreted by the hypothalamus, induces the anterior pituitary gland to secrete LH and FSH. The blood stream receives these hormones, which then travel to the testes where they bind to testicular cells.
- Leydig cells in the testes possess LH receptors and respond by increasing production of testosterone. Testosterone and related androgens are necessary for maturation of the male external genitalia. The function of FSH is less well understood, but it may be necessary for spermatogenesis.
- Spermatogenesis occurs when germinal cells within the seminiferous tubules undergo meiosis to form haploid (23 chromosomes) spermatids. Spermatids then develop into mature spermatozoa with the assistance of Sertoli cells. Sperm require 70 days to mature, and they are continuously produced and released into the epididymis.
- Sperm are well formed to perform their function in that they have a highly stabilized nucleus that is resistant to physical trauma, a mobile tail (axoneme) for swimming, and specialized enzymes to enhance penetration of the egg.
- Sperm traveling from their site of origin in the testes must travel through approximately 6 m of tubules before arriving at the penile meatus. This tubular system includes the seminiferous tubules in the testes, epididymis, vas deferens, and urethra. About 200 million sperm may be stored in the epididymal reservoir. Increased motility and fertility appear to be acquired by sperm as they pass through the epididymis. Sperm account for less than 10% of the ejaculate volume.
- The physiologic process of erection is a complex interplay of vascular, neurologic, and hormonal factors. The sacral parasympathetic nerves provide important innervation to the penis. Acetylcholine from parasympathetic nerves causes relaxation of penile smooth muscle with subsequent engorgement. Injected prostaglandins may also induce penile erections.
- The sympathetic nervous system mediates the process of ejaculation. Sympathetic actions include contraction of the internal sphincter to prevent retrograde ejaculation and relaxation of the external sphincter to allow emission.
- Sperm deposited in the vagina undergo further changes in a process known as capacitation. This process improves the chances of sperm successfully producing fertilization of an egg. Enzymes are released (acrosome reaction) to facilitate penetration of the ovum, a process that further increases the chances of successful fertilization.

SUMMARY

The male genitourinary tract may be divided into upper and lower tracts, with the upper tract composed of the kidneys and ureters and the lower tract composed of the bladder and urethra. Auxiliary genital glands that lie adjacent to or surround the urethra include the prostate, seminal vesicles, and bulbourethral glands. The external genitalia of the male consist of the scrotum, testis, epididymis, and penis.

Embryologic development of the male and female genital and urinary systems is closely related. The nephric system develops progressively through three distinct phases: the pronephros, mesonephros, and metanephros. The gonads are derived from the urogenital ridge, from which the primitive kidney also forms. Finally, the genital duct systems develop from two different but related ducts adjacent to the undifferentiated gonads, the müllerian ducts and the mesonephric, or wolffian, ducts.

Male reproductive function depends on an intact hypothalamic-pituitary-testicular endocrine axis. Spermatogenesis takes place in the seminiferous tubules. Spermatozoa mature in their transit through the male reproductive tract. Through erection, emission, and ejaculation, sperm enter the vagina. Through capacitation and the acrosome reaction, spermatozoa acquire the ability to fertilize ova residing in the female reproductive tract.

MEDIA RESOURCES

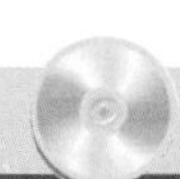

evolve

Remember to check out the ***CD Companion*** included with this book for Review Questions, Key Concepts Review, Glossary (with audio for selected terms), Disease Profiles, and Animations.

PLUS, visit the ***Evolve website*** at http://evolve.elsevier.com/Copstead/ for Case Studies, Disease Profiles, and WebLinks.

References

1. Bullock N, Sibley G, Whitaker R: *Essential urology,* ed 2, Edinburgh, 1994, Churchill Livingstone, pp 1-2.
2. Zderic SA, Levin RM, Wein AJ: Voiding function and dysfunction. In Gillenwater JY et al, editors: *Adult and pediatric urology,* vol 2, ed 3, St Louis, 1996, Mosby, pp 1159-1219.
3. Redman JF: Anatomy of the genitourinary system. In Gillenwater JY et al, editors: *Adult and pediatric urology,* vol 1, ed 3, St Louis, 1996, Mosby, pp 3-61.
4. Kissane JM: Development and structure of the urogenital system. In Murphy WM, editor: *Urological pathology,* ed 2, Philadelphia, 1997, Saunders, pp 1-3.
5. Hoffman GE, Berghorn KA: Gonadotrophin-releasing hormone neurons: their structure and function, *Semin Reprod Endocrinol* 15(1):5-17, 1997.
6. Grayhack JT, Kozlowski JM: Benign prostatic hyperplasia. In Gillenwater JY et al, editors: *Adult and pediatric urology,* vol 2, ed 3, St Louis, 1996, Mosby, pp 1501-1574.
7. Meacham RB, Lipschultz LI, Howards SS: Male infertility. In Gillenwater JY et al, editors: *Adult and pediatric urology,* vol 2, ed 3, St Louis, 1996, Mosby, pp 1747-1802.
8. Pyror JP: Male infertility. In Sant GR, editor: *Pathophysiologic principles of urology,* Oxford, 1994, Blackwell, pp 155-179.
9. Gondos B, Wong T-W: Non-neoplastic diseases of the testis and epididymis. In Murphy WM, editor: *Urological pathology,* ed 2, Philadelphia, 1997, Saunders, pp 277-341.
10. Pabst RZ: Investigations of the construction and function of the human ductus deferens, *Z Anat Entwicklungsgesch* 129(20):154-176, 1969.
11. Lerner SE, Melman A, Christ G: A review of an erectile dysfunction: new insights and more questions, *J Urol* 149(5):1246-1255, 1993.
12. O'Leary MP, Lue TF: Penile function. In Sant GR: *Pathophysiologic principles of urology,* Oxford, 1994, Blackwell, pp 181 207.
13. Guyton AC, Hall JE: Reproductive and hormonal functions of the male (and the pineal gland). In Guyton AC, Hall JE, editors: *Textbook of medical physiology,* ed 9, Philadelphia, 1996, Saunders, pp 1003-1016.

chapter 31

Alterations in Male Genital and Reproductive Function

Marvin Van Every • David Mikkelsen • Donna W. Bailey

MEDIA RESOURCES

Additional Material for Study, Review, and Further Exploration

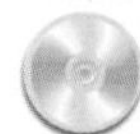

CD Companion ◆ Review Questions and Answers ◆ Key Concepts Review
◆ Glossary *(with audio pronunciations for selected terms)*
◆ Disease Profiles ◆ Animations

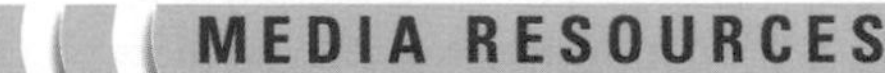

evolve Website at http://evolve.elsevier.com/Copstead/
◆ Case Studies ◆ Disease Profiles ◆ WebLinks

KEY QUESTIONS

- What are the common causes of and clinical findings in priapism?
- What are the common causes of primary and secondary impotence?
- What are the usual clinical manifestations and significance of testicular cancer, testicular torsion, cryptorchidism, and hydrocele or spermatocele?
- What clinical manifestations would lead to a suspicion of prostatitis, and how would confirmed prostatitis be treated?
- How can benign prostatic hyperplasia be distinguished from prostate cancer?
- What clinical manifestations are indicative of prostatic enlargement?

CHAPTER OUTLINE

The male genital system is susceptible to numerous congenital, acquired, and infectious conditions and, to a lesser extent, neoplasms. These disorders may interrupt the normal functions of urinary excretion and sexual function and fertility and directly affect the quality of life. This chapter will identify and explain the most common conditions that come to the attention of practitioners.

DISORDERS OF THE PENIS AND MALE URETHRA

CONGENITAL ANOMALIES

Micropenis

Micropenis is defined as a small, normally formed penis with a stretched length more than two standard deviations below the mean.[1] The normal range in newborns is 2.0 to 3.5 cm, so micropenis may be defined as a stretched length of less than 1.9 cm.[2]

Etiology and Pathogenesis. Penile development and growth are both testosterone dependent. Therefore, micropenis may result from defects in testosterone production or a deficiency that results in poor growth of the organs that are targets of this hormone.

Diagnoses and Treatment. Patients with micropenis must be evaluated for endocrine abnormalities. To check for these one should measure serum levels of testosterone, luteinizing hormone, and follicle-stimulating hormone. Depending on what these measurements show, the problem may be determined to involve the hypothalamic-pituitary axis (Prader-Willi and Kallmann syndromes) or testicular disorders (Klinefelter syndrome).[3]

Treatment depends on providing testosterone, either intramuscularly or topically, to stimulate penile growth. Such treatment requires caution because growth may be altered by premature closure of the epiphyseal growth plates in the long bones. In rare cases, when micropenis fails to respond to testosterone, a female sex assignment is indicated.[3]

Urethral Valves

The vast majority of **urethral valves** are posterior in location and occur in the distal prostatic urethra. They are the most common cause of urinary obstruction in male newborns and

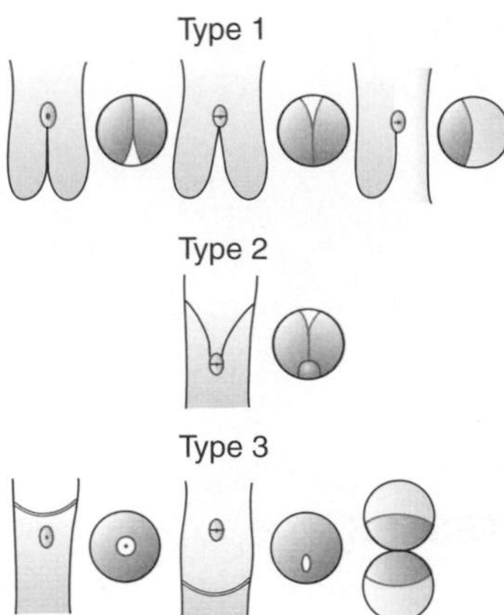

FIGURE 31-1 ■ Posterior urethral valves. (Redrawn from Young HH, Frontz WA, Baldwin JC: Congenital obstruction of the posterior urethra, *J Urol* 3:289, 1919.)

infants. These valves are mucosal folds that resemble thin membranes and cause obstruction when the child attempts to void (Figure 31-1).

Etiology. Many theories have been given to explain how valves develop. It has been suggested that several different processes may occur to form different posterior valves. Most commonly, posterior valves may result from abnormal insertion and persistence of the distal wolffian ducts. Less frequently, a persistent urogenital membrane may result in valves and obstruction.[4]

Clinical Manifestations. Children with posterior valves may have variable degrees of obstruction. In the most severe cases, intrauterine renal failure may cause oligohydramnios (decreased amniotic fluid), pulmonary hypoplasia (incomplete lung development), and either stillbirth or extreme distress at the time of delivery. More frequently, inability to void is noted shortly after birth (normal voiding occurs within 48 hours after birth), or the infant has abdominal masses representing a thickened palpable bladder or hydronephrotic kidneys. Varying degrees of azotemia and renal failure occur with this scenario. Finally, urinary ascites (extravasated urine in the peritoneum) may result from a urinary leak that is usually difficult to localize. In an infant with abdominal distention, the diagnosis of urethral valves is confirmed by a plain abdominal radiograph showing the bowel "floating" in the center of the abdomen.

Older infants with a urethral valve are less likely to have a palpable kidney or ascites. Rather, urinary infection, poor stream with straining to void, or occasionally hematuria may be present. Urethral valves in these older male infants may not produce much obstruction, thus making the diagnosis more difficult.[5]

Treatment. Management of posterior valves involves initial management of the metabolic abnormalities with appropriate fluid management and electrolyte replacement. In patients with a urinary tract infection, drainage of urine with a urethral or occasionally a suprapubic catheter is necessary. Finally, ablation of the valves with an endoscopic resectoscope should be performed. In infants, this step may be delayed and a cutaneous vesicostomy made to temporarily divert and drain the urine. This approach reduces the risk of traumatizing the infant's delicate urethra, which may create urethral stricture disease.

Rarely, urethral valves are located anteriorly in the penile urethra. Valves in this location are a very rare congenital anomaly and most likely represent urethral dilation or a diverticulum proximal to the valve.[6] Endoscopic resection will correct the problem.

Urethrorectal and Vesicourethral Fistulas

Etiology. **Urethrorectal** and **vesicourethral fistulas** are rare and almost always associated with an imperforate anus. Failure of the urorectal septum to develop completely leads to persistent communication between the rectum posteriorly and the urogenital tract anteriorly.

Clinical Manifestations and Treatment. Children with a urethrorectal or vesicourethral fistula may pass fecal material and gas through the urethra. If the anus has formed normally with an external opening, urine may drain through the rectum. The diagnosis is made with cystoscopy and contrast-enhanced radiography to delineate a blind rectal pouch or communication. Surgery is needed to resect the fistula and open the imperforate anus.

Hypospadias

In **hypospadias** the urethral meatus is located on the ventral undersurface of the penis or on the perineum (Figure 31-2). The condition may occur with varying degrees of severity. In the least severe cases, the meatus is located distally on the penis, either at the corona or on the undersurface of the glans. With increasing severity of the condition, the meatus assumes a more proximal location and is more often associated with chordee, or curvature of the penile shaft (Figure 31-3).

Etiology and Treatment. Hypospadias is the result of incomplete fusion of the urethral folds, so the meatus may be found anywhere along the phallus from the perineum to the glans. In the majority of cases hypospadias occurs distally, with about 85% of all cases involving the glans or corona.[7] Because incomplete fusion of urethral folds may indicate insufficient masculinization, it is recommended that the more severe penoscrotal and perineal openings be evaluated for conditions of intersex.[8]

Management of hypospadias involves surgical repair. Many procedures are available, with several repairs indicated for

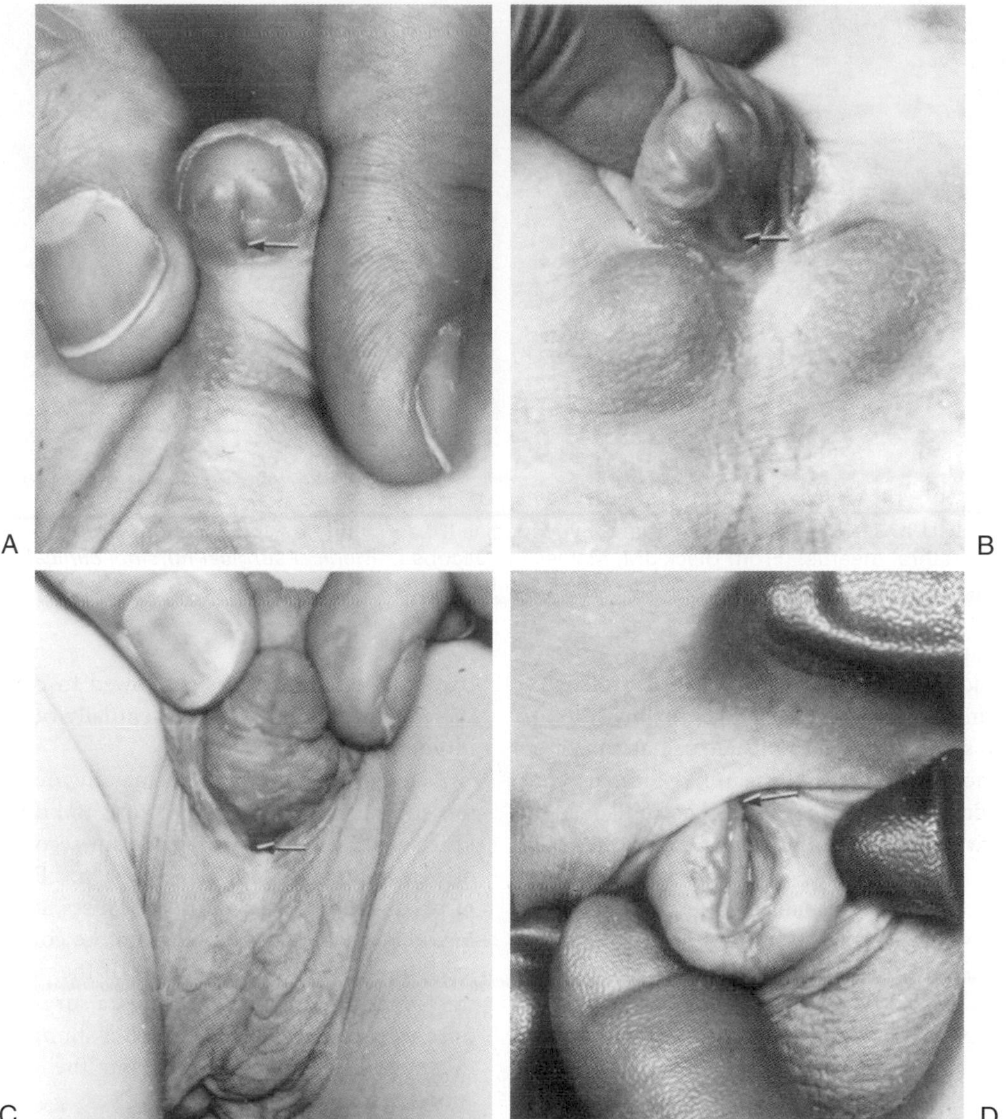

FIGURE 31-2 ■ Penile anomalies. **A,** Glandular hypospadias, the most common form of hypospadias. The external urethral orifice (meatus) is on the ventral aspect of the glans *(arrow).* A shallow pit in the glans penis is at the usual site of the urethral orifice. Note the moderate degree of chordee (ventral curvature of the penis). **B,** Penile hypospadias. The penis is short and curved (chordee). The external urethral orifice *(arrow)* is near the penoscrotal junction. **C,** Penoscrotal hypospadias. The external urethral orifice *(arrow)* is located at the penoscrotal junction. **D,** Epispadias. The external urethral orifice *(arrow)* is on the dorsal surface of the penis. (**A,** From Jolly H: *Diseases of children,* ed 2, Oxford, 1968, Blackwell. **D,** Courtesy Mr. Innes Williams, Genitourinary Surgeon, The Hospital for Sick Children, London.)

each type of hypospadias. The goal of surgery is a good overall cosmetic appearance that will allow the patient to stand and direct his urinary stream and will also allow normal sexual function.

Epispadias

In **epispadias** the urethra opens on the dorsal aspect of the penis at a point proximal to the glans (see Figure 31-2). Although much less common than hypospadias, it can be considerably more disabling.

Etiology and Treatment. The embryogenesis of epispadias is related to another congenital condition, exstrophy of the bladder. In this condition, the abdominal wall fails to form below the level of the umbilicus. At birth, the back wall of the bladder is exposed to the external environment.[9] The development of epispadias is simply a mild degree of exstro-

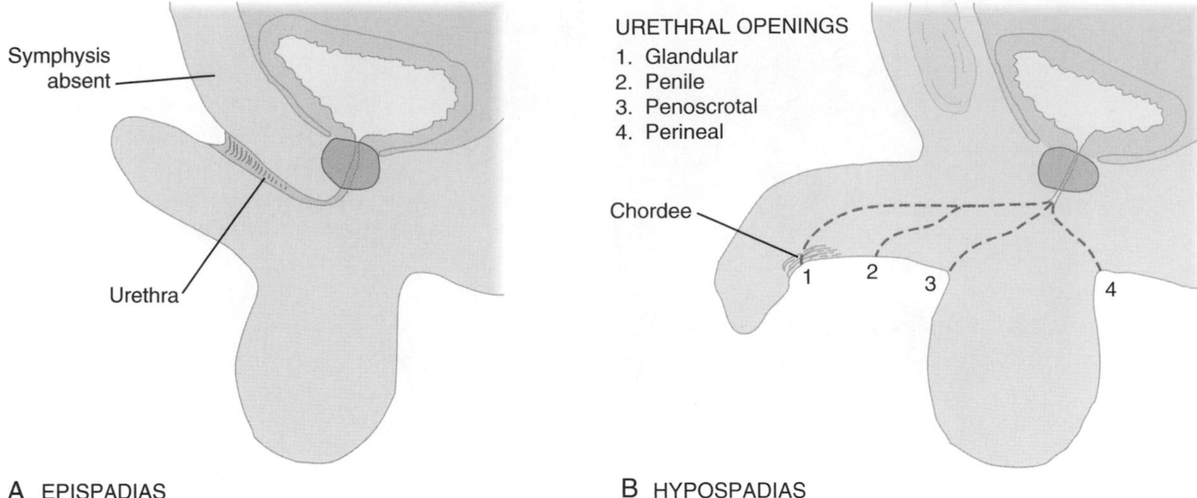

FIGURE 31-3 ■ Epispadias **(A)** and hypospadias **(B)** showing possible locations of the urethral meatus. (From Black JM, Matassarin-Jacobs E: *Medical-surgical nursing: clinical management for continuity of care,* ed 6, Philadelphia, 2001, Saunders, p 971.)

phy, with a deficiency of abdominal wall formation present inferiorly. Most commonly, the defect extends proximally to involve the urinary sphincter and results in urinary incontinence. Less commonly, the urethral meatus is located more distally along the dorsum of the penis and is accompanied by urinary continence because the sphincter is not affected (see Figure 31-3).

Management of proximal epispadias with incontinence is difficult and involves staged surgical procedures to reconstruct a continent bladder neck and a functional urethra. The less common distal epispadias is usually managed with tubular reconstruction procedures similar to those used for repair of hypospadias.

ACQUIRED DISORDERS

Priapism

Priapism may be defined as a painful, persistent erection. The patient usually reports several hours of painful erection in which the corpora cavernosa are tense with congested blood. The corpus spongiosum and glans are characteristically soft and uninvolved.

Etiology and Treatment. The causes of priapism are multiple. Most cases are idiopathic, with the next most common cause being sickle cell disease. Other etiologic factors include anticoagulant therapy, diabetes mellitus, leukemia, and the use of certain antidepressant medications.[10] Recently, intracavernosal injection of vasoactive substances for the management of impotence has been noted to cause priapism. Although multiple causes exist, the common abnormality is probably an obstruction of venous drainage resulting in the buildup of viscous, poorly oxygenated blood in the corpora.[11] If the process is allowed to continue, fibrosis of the corpora cavernosa will eventually occur and may cause impotence.

Management of priapism may involve a combination of measures, depending on the cause and duration of the condition. Initial therapy for priapism secondary to sickle cell disease includes sedation and oxygen.[12] For the management of priapism secondary to other causes, initial measures may include aspiration of blood from the corpora, as well as injection of α-adrenergic agents.[13] If the priapism remains refractory to these initial measures, a surgical shunting procedure may be necessary in which a shunt is created between the erect corpora cavernosa and the detumesced corpus spongiosum.

Phimosis and Paraphimosis

Etiology, Clinical Manifestations, and Treatment. **Phimosis** occurs when the uncircumcised foreskin cannot be retracted over the glans of the penis (Figure 31-4, *A*). Phimosis is usually the result of chronic inflammation and infection from poor hygiene. Calculi and squamous cell carcinoma may occur, although it is usually the presence of erythema, tenderness of the phimotic foreskin, or a discharge that prompts the patient to seek medical attention.[14] Management involves treating the infection with antibiotics, followed by circumcision.

Paraphimosis, on the other hand, occurs when a foreskin that has been retracted over the glans cannot be replaced in its normal position (see Figure 31-4, *B*). In this condition, which is usually secondary to chronic inflammation under the foreskin, a constricting ring of skin forms around the base of the retracted glans. The constriction causes venous

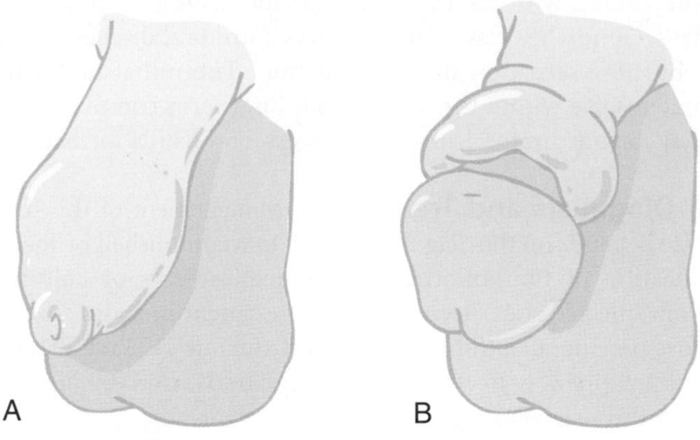

FIGURE 31-4 ■ **A,** Phimosis. **B,** Paraphimosis.

congestion of the glans, with further swelling and edema making the condition worse. Treatment entails reducing the paraphimotic foreskin back over the glans, which can usually be accomplished by compressing the glans to reduce the edema. Occasionally, a slit or formal circumcision is needed to manage the problem.

Peyronie Disease

Etiology and Treatment. **Peyronie disease** refers to the formation of palpable, fibrous plaque on the surface of the corpora cavernosa. This plaque subsequently causes curvature of the penis with painful, incomplete erections. No satisfactory treatment for this disease is available, although some cases may remit with time. Conservative therapies that have had limited success include the use of vitamin E or aminobenzoate potassium (Potaba). In addition, several operative procedures have been developed. These procedures involve excising the plaque and repairing the corporal defect with a graft.[15]

Urethral Strictures

Etiology. **Urethral strictures** are fibrotic narrowings of the urethra and are usually composed of scar tissue. Most acquired strictures are due to a prior infection such as gonorrhea or trauma. Traumatic causes can be both iatrogenic, such as large urethral catheters and instrumentation, and noniatrogenic, such as straddle injuries.

Clinical Manifestations and Treatment. A decreased urinary stream is the most common complaint. Other common complaints include urethral discharge, bladder infection, and urine retention. Urethral strictures are usually diagnosed by cystoscopy or retrograde urethrography, which would demonstrate a narrowing of the urethra. Management of urethral strictures involves procedures to dilate, incise, or reconstruct the urethra, depending on the extent and duration of the stricture.

Erectile Dysfunction

The physiologic process of penile erection is a complex interaction of the vascular, hormonal, and neurologic systems. **Impotence,** or the inability to attain an erection, may be primary or secondary. Primary impotence refers to the inability to attain an erection throughout life and is often related to deep-seated psychiatric problems of some duration. Occasionally, vascular trauma sustained during early childhood or adolescence may account for primary impotence.[16]

Etiology. Far more common than primary impotence is secondary impotence. An individual with secondary impotence is no longer able to achieve normal erections but did have normal erections in the past. The causes of secondary impotence are multiple and may be discovered by examining the patient's medical history. Common causes of secondary impotence are peripheral vascular disease, the use of certain medications, endocrine problems, trauma, iatrogenic causes, and psychological causes. To differentiate organic causes from psychogenic impotence, one relies on the history, physical, and basic laboratory testing such as serum glucose and testosterone. Penile tumescence testing can also be utilized to make this distinction.

Arterial insufficiency of the penis may occur from obstruction of the arterial supply. Several processes may account for this obstructive arteriosclerosis. Stenosis of the arteries secondary to atheromatous plaque may be the most common etiologic factor. Diabetes mellitus may not only result in occlusion of arterial vessels but may also cause a neuropathy of the pudendal nerve that might result in erectile dysfunction.[17] Finally, some investigators have suggested that erectile dysfunction may result from excessive venous drainage from the penis.

The list of medications that may cause erectile dysfunction is long. Several antihypertensive agents, including propranolol, monoamine oxidase inhibitors, and thiazides, have been associated with varying degrees of impotence. Other medications linked to erectile dysfunction include phenothiazines, antihistamines, and some antidepressants.[18]

Endocrinopathy accounts for a small percentage of impotence cases.[19] Pituitary dysfunction resulting in decreased or no secretion of luteinizing hormone may result in decreased secretion of testosterone. Primary failure of the testes may also occur, resulting in decreased secretion of testosterone. Finally, excessive secretion of the hormone prolactin by the pituitary may result in low testosterone levels.

Trauma to the penis resulting in penile fractures and damage to penile erectile tissue may occasionally lead to partial or complete impotence. More common injuries include pelvic fractures with subsequent damage to the penile vascular and nervous supply. Iatrogenic trauma secondary to several commonly performed operations, including aortoiliac vascular surgery, and to radical pelvic cancer operations may also result in impotence.

Finally, it must be remembered that successful sexual function depends not only on intact vascular, hormonal, and neurologic systems but also on intact psychological and social responses. Several psychological factors may be manifested as problems of low desire, erectile failure, or premature ejaculation. A discussion of the psychological contribution to impotence is beyond the scope of this chapter.

Treatment. Management of erectile dysfunction requires an initial evaluation to differentiate organic causes from psychogenic causes. Further evaluation to distinguish among the various organic causes may then be needed. Once a psychogenic cause has been ruled out, several therapeutic options exist. Surgical options include the insertion of an inflatable or semirigid prosthetic device into the corpora cavernosa. In the past few years, several investigators have discovered that intracavernous injection of various vasoactive substances can cause an erection. Several of these substances, including papaverine, phentolamine, and prostaglandin E_1, are commonly used and afford a nonsurgical treatment option.

Viagra, an oral therapy for erectile dysfunction, is the citrate salt of sildenafil, a selective inhibitor of cyclic guanosine monophosphate (cGMP)–specific phosphodiesterase type 5 (PDE5). To understand its clinical pharmacology, a review of some of the physiologic mechanisms of erection follows. Briefly, erection of the penis involves release of nitric oxide in the corpus cavernosum during sexual stimulation. Nitric oxide then activates the enzyme guanylate cyclase, and the subsequently increased levels cGMP produce smooth muscle relaxation in the corpus cavernosum and allow inflow of blood. Sildenafil has no direct relaxant effect on isolated human corpus cavernosum, but it enhances the effect of nitric oxide by inhibiting PDE5, which is responsible for degradation of cGMP in the corpus cavernosum. When sexual stimulation causes local release of nitric oxide, inhibition of PDE5 by sildenafil causes increased levels of cGMP in the corpus cavernosum, smooth muscle relaxation, and inflow of blood to the corpus cavernosum, which results in erection. Sildenafil citrate at the recommended doses appears to have no effect in the absence of sexual stimulation and affords another nonsurgical treatment option.

Another nonsurgical alternative entails the use of a vacuum device to sustain an erection. Finally, in very specific cases of erectile dysfunction, surgical procedures may be done to revascularize the arterial supply of the penis or ligate the penile venous drainage.

INFECTIOUS DISORDERS

Gonococcal Urethritis

Etiology and Clinical Manifestations. Gonococcal urethritis is associated with a gram-negative diplococcus, *Neisseria gonorrhoeae.* Most cases are acquired during sexual intercourse, with the incubation period lasting from 3 to 10 days. Gonorrhea classically produces a urethral discharge and a burning sensation during urination. The initial urethritis may resolve without treatment, but long-term complications may include urethral stricture, abscess, and fistula formation.

Diagnosis and Treatment. Management of this disease depends on the diagnosis, which is accomplished by identification of the gonococcus in stained smears or cultures from infected sites. Recommended treatment includes single-dose parenteral administration of ceftriaxone (125 mg IM) or oral treatment with cefixime (400 mg), ofloxacin (400 mg), or ciprofloxacin (500 mg).[20]

All persons with gonorrhea should receive appropriate follow-up care and evaluation and treatment for other sexually transmitted diseases. The potential presence of coexisting chlamydial infection is an important consideration.

Nongonococcal Urethritis

Etiology, Diagnosis, and Treatment. Nongonococcal urethritis has several specific causes. The organism most responsible is probably *Chlamydia trachomatis.* Chlamydia is an intracellular organism that usually causes a urethral discharge and dysuria. A second organism, *Ureaplasma urealyticum,* has also been implicated as a causative agent of nongonococcal urethritis. Urethral swabs can be used to culture the urethra and determine the causative organism. Treatment of nongonococcal urethritis involves oral antibiotics, either tetracycline or erythromycin, 500 mg four times daily for 7 days.[21]

Syphilis

Etiology and Diagnosis. Syphilis is caused by the organism *Treponema pallidum,* a spirochete that gains entrance to the body through the skin or mucous membranes. The initial site of involvement in males is usually the penis, where a characteristic painless, shallow ulcer (chancre) is formed. This primary chancre often becomes associated with enlarged inguinal lymph nodes.

The diagnosis of syphilis may be made by microscopic dark-field examination of serous drainage from the ulcer. In the absence of a dark-field microscope, the diagnosis may be made by either of two serologic tests, the rapid plasma reagin test or the Venereal Disease Research Laboratory (VDRL) test. Management of early or primary syphilis involves an intramuscular injection of benzathine penicillin G, 2.4 million units. For patients allergic to penicillin, tetracycline, or erythromycin, 500 mg four times a day for 15 days is the treatment of choice.[22]

Genital Herpes

Etiology, Pathogenesis, Clinical Manifestations, and Treatment. Herpes simplex virus is a double-stranded DNA virus that may cause persistent or latent infections. Two subtypes are recognized. The majority of patients with genital herpes have type 2 virus, whereas type 1 infections usually involve the oral cavity. Vesicles grouped together on an erythematous base constitute the typical lesion seen in genital herpes. Symptoms of herpes usually arise several days after the sexual contact. They include local discomfort, neuralgic pain, and malaise.[23] Occasionally patients develop meningitis, encephalitis, or disseminated infections. Usually after 5 to 10 days the symptoms resolve, but the virus then travels up the nerves and settles into the basal ganglia of the spinal cord where it resides forever. Periodically it can spread back down the nerves and cause recurrent disease. Both forms of the virus (type 1 and type 2) can cause the disease.[23] To confirm the diagnosis, smears of the lesions to demonstrate intranuclear inclusions may be performed. In addition, viral cultures or tests to measure serum antibody to herpes simplex virus may also be obtained. Acyclovir is one of the few drugs that have demonstrated efficacy in managing this disease. Given orally or intravenously, acyclovir stops the formation of viral DNA chains by inhibiting viral DNA polymerase.

Genital Warts

Etiology, Clinical Manifestations, and Treatment. Genital warts, or **condylomata acuminata** (singular: condyloma acuminatum), are caused by various strains of papillomavirus. The disease may be transmitted when viral particles from lesions come in contact with another person during sexual intercourse. The relationship between genital warts and cervical carcinoma in women has received considerable attention.[24]

Male patients may have warts anywhere on the external genitalia, but commonly on the penile shaft or glans. Warts may also be found in the urethra, as well as around or within the anus. Treatment involves the topical application of podophyllin. The warts may also be removed with electrocautery or a carbon dioxide laser.

NEOPLASTIC DISORDERS

Neoplasms of the Penis

Etiology. Although cancer of the penis is rare in the United States and accounts for fewer than 0.2% of cancer deaths, its prevalence fluctuates widely among various locations. The causes are poorly understood, but phimosis of the foreskin accompanied by chronic inflammation has been thought to be the primary etiologic factor. The incidence of penile cancer among circumcised men is extremely low.[25]

The majority of penile cancer cases are squamous cell carcinoma (97%). They usually occur on the glans or the inner surface of the foreskin. Metastasis occurs by lymphatic dissemination, with initial involvement of the palpable inguinal lymph nodes. Death from penile carcinoma is a result of uncontrolled lymphatic spread and subsequent necrosis of the overlying skin, debilitation, and sepsis.

Penile carcinoma is staged as follows[26]:

Stage I: The lesion is limited to the glans or foreskin.
Stage II: The tumor involves the shaft of the penis.
Stage III: The inguinal nodes are involved but the lesion is operable.
Stage IV: Disseminated disease.

The lesion of penile cancer is usually ulcerative and fungating in appearance and may be associated with pain, bleeding, and urethral discharge. Inguinal adenopathy is present in more than 50% of patients at the time of diagnosis, although frequently the adenopathy represents an inflammatory response secondary to the lesion rather than metastasis.

Treatment. Therapy for penile carcinoma depends on the stage of the lesion. Topical chemotherapy and radiation therapy may be considered for certain small superficial lesions. Larger distal penile lesions usually require partial penectomy, whereas proximal lesions may require total penectomy with creation of a perineal urethrostomy. Finally, removal of the involved inguinal lymph nodes by inguinal lymphadenectomy may be performed in cases of suspected stage III disease.

The prognosis of penile carcinoma depends on the stage of disease. The 5-year survival rate for men with tumors localized to the penis is 65% to 90%. With inguinal node involvement, 5-year survival rates drop to about 30% to 50%, and if distant metastases are present, the 5-year survival rate is virtually zero.[26]

KEY CONCEPTS

- Congenital disorders of the penis may result from hormonal deficiencies or abnormalities in embryonic development. Micropenis, for example, is usually a result of testosterone deficiency. Urethral valves, fistulas, and malpositioning of the urinary meatus (hypospadias, epispadias) are related to abnormal embryonic development.
- Priapism is a persistent, painful erection, most commonly of unknown cause. Priapism may occur in conditions that cause obstruction of venous drainage, including sickle cell anemia, anticoagulant therapy, diabetes mellitus, and certain antidepressant medications.
- Phimosis and paraphimosis are disorders of the foreskin. Phimosis is associated with chronic inflammation and poor hygiene and results in a foreskin that cannot be retracted. Paraphimosis refers to a foreskin that remains retracted and cannot be returned to its normal position.
- Urethral strictures may be congenital or acquired. Most acquired strictures are secondary to gonorrheal infection or urethral trauma. Poor stream,

bladder infections, and retained urine are common manifestations.

- Impotence is the inability to achieve a sustained erection. Causes of impotence are categorized as primary and secondary. Primary impotence is rare and usually related to adolescent vascular trauma or psychiatric problems. Secondary impotence may be due to a variety of factors, including vascular disease, medications, endocrine disorders, trauma, and psychological distress.
- A number of infections are sexually transmitted and affect the penis and urethra, including gonococcal urethritis, nongonococcal urethritis, syphilis, herpes, and genital warts. Gonococcal and nongonococcal urethritis and syphilis are effectively managed with antibiotics. Herpes and genital warts are associated with viruses and tend to be chronic, with intermittent recurrence.
- Penile neoplasms are rare, particularly in circumcised males. Phimosis and chronic inflammation may be important etiologic factors. Like other neoplasms, penile cancer has a better prognosis if managed before dissemination.

DISORDERS OF THE SCROTUM AND TESTES

CONGENITAL DISORDERS

Cryptorchidism

Cryptorchidism means "hidden testis" and refers to any testis that occupies an extrascrotal position. The cryptorchid testis may be incompletely descended and as such be located intraabdominally, within the inguinal canal, or just external to the canal but above the scrotum. Occasionally the testis may emerge from the external ring of the inguinal canal and be misdirected into an abnormal extrascrotal position. In this situation the testis may be called ectopic. An ectopic testis may be located in any of several locations but is most commonly found in a superficial inguinal pouch[27] (Figure 31-5).

The incidence of cryptorchidism is about 0.7% to 1.0% of male infants at 1 year of age. The cause of the condition is uncertain but may be related to an intrinsic testicular defect or a subtle hormonal deficiency.[27]

The incompletely descended, cryptorchid testis undergoes deleterious changes. The tubules become fibrotic, with a deficiency of spermatogenesis and subsequent infertility. More important is the increased incidence of testicular malignancy in cryptorchid testes.[28] Several studies have revealed an increased prevalence of testicular tumors in subjects with a history of cryptorchidism.

Treatment. Because of the increased risk of malignancy and infertility, treatment at an early age to bring the testis into

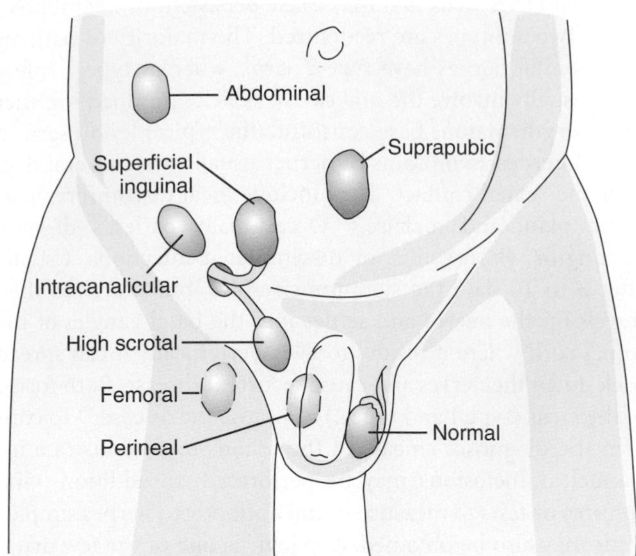

FIGURE 31-5 ■ Sites of ectopic testes.

a normal scrotal position is recommended. An operative procedure *(orchiopexy)* is usually required, although in certain situations descent may be stimulated by the administration of human chorionic gonadotropin, which is given in a series of intramuscular injections.[29]

ACQUIRED DISORDERS

Hydrocele

Etiology and Clinical Manifestations. A **hydrocele** consists of a fluid collection surrounding the testicle or spermatic cord and contained within the tunica or processus vaginalis (Figure 31-6). Scrotal swelling in infants or young boys may indicate a hydrocele. These congenital hydroceles exist because of communication between the abdominal cavity and scrotum through the processus vaginalis. The scrotum is characteristically small and soft in the morning but larger and tense at night as it fills with fluid from the abdominal cavity.

Hydroceles may also develop secondary to scrotal injury, radiation therapy, infection of the epididymis, or testicular neoplasms. More commonly, however, the cause is uncertain, with the hydrocele developing slowly over time and occurring in middle-aged or elderly men. These acquired hydroceles may vary in size and consistency from small and soft to large and tense. The fluid is usually clear and yellow.

Treatment. Because hydrocele is a benign condition, treatment is required only if the fluid collection becomes uncomfortable for the patient. Occasionally, a tense hydrocele might restrict circulation to the testicle. Management usually involves a surgical procedure to drain the fluid with either resection or plication of the hydrocele sac to prevent reaccumulation of the fluid. Aspiration of the hydrocele may be performed, although fluid often reaccumulates.

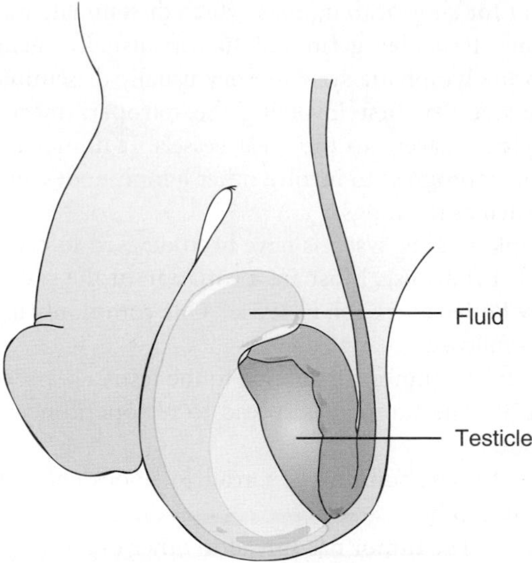

FIGURE 31-6 ■ Hydrocele.

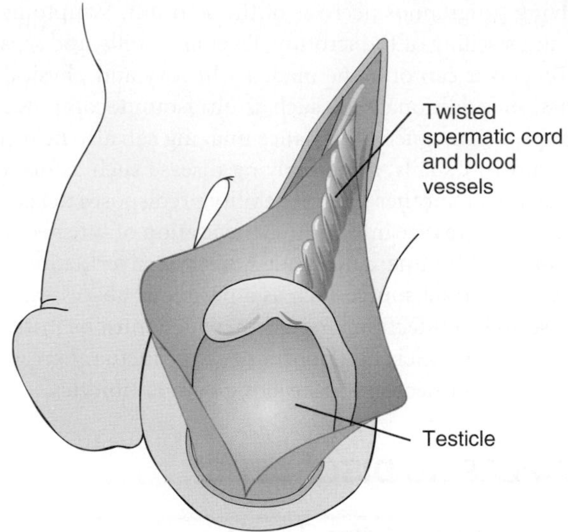

FIGURE 31-7 ■ Testicular torsion.

Spermatocele

Etiology and Treatment. **Spermatoceles** are painless, cystic masses containing sperm. Although they are usually small, they may be quite large and difficult to distinguish from a hydrocele. The cause of spermatoceles is uncertain; they may arise from the tiny tubules that connect the epididymis to the testis (vasa efferentia) or from the epididymis itself. Like hydroceles, spermatoceles need not be treated unless they become large enough to trouble the patient, in which case an operative procedure to excise the spermatocele may be performed.

Testicular Torsion

Torsion of the testicle is described as a twisting of the spermatic cord with subsequent compromise of the testicular vascular supply and testicular ischemia, followed by infarction (Figure 31-7). Although torsion may occur in the neonatal period, the majority of cases occur in prepubertal boys.

Clinical Manifestations. The diagnosis is suggested by the onset of severe pain in one testis, followed by swelling of the scrotum. Lower abdominal pain accompanied by nausea and vomiting may also occur. The condition may be differentiated from epididymitis (inflammation of the epididymis), which is also associated with scrotal swelling, by the presence of vascular echoes detected with a Doppler ultrasound stethoscope. A testis made ischemic by torsion will not echo sound, whereas the inflammation of epididymitis and its hypervascularity increase sound emission. Testicular nuclear scanning is the most definitive test, with torsion making the testis avascular.

Treatment. Management of torsion involves an operation to open the scrotum, untwist the testis, and "pex" (secure) it to the scrotal wall. Because the chance of torsion also involving the contralateral testis is increased, the contralateral testicle is "pexed" to the scrotal wall as well. If detorsion is accomplished within 12 hours of the event, the prognosis for testicular viability is usually good. If torsion has been present for more than 24 hours, viability of the testis is doubtful.

INFECTIOUS DISORDERS

Epididymitis

Etiology. **Epididymitis,** or inflammation of the testis, has several causes. It may occur as a result of trauma or the reflux of sterile urine up the vas deferens. However, the majority of cases are probably secondary to a bacterial cause, with both sexually transmitted organisms (*N. gonorrhoeae* and *C. trachomatis*) and non–sexually transmitted organisms (*Pseudomonas* and *Escherichia coli*) involved.

Clinical Manifestations and Treatment. With epididymitis the scrotum may be enlarged, reddened, and tender. The pain may radiate along the spermatic cord into the inguinal area. Fever may also occur, as may urethral discharge, cystitis, and cloudy urine. Laboratory testing usually reveals an elevated white blood cell (WBC) count, and urine culture may reveal the infecting organism.

Treatment for the condition involves bed rest, scrotal support, and administration of antibiotics. In advanced cases, incision and drainage with the intravenous administration of antibiotics may be needed to effectively manage a resulting scrotal abscess.

Fournier Gangrene

Etiology, Clinical Manifestations, and Treatment. **Fournier gangrene** is a severe but rare condition involving gangrenous necrosis of the scrotum. Symptoms are pain and swelling of the scrotum, fever and chills, and sepsis.[30] The diagnosis can often be made by history and physical examination. Additional tests such as ultrasound, computed tomography, or magnetic resonance imaging can also be helpful in diagnosis. Usually, an underlying disease such as diabetes, alcoholism, or another general debility predisposes the patient to such an aggressive infection. Extravasation of infected urine from urethral trauma, a perforated urethral diverticulum, or a non–urinary tract source such as a perirectal abscess may act as the source of infection. Treatment, which must be instituted swiftly, includes incision and drainage of fluctuant areas and debridement of necrotic tissue along with antibiotics.

NEOPLASTIC DISORDERS

Neoplasms of the Testis

Although testicular tumors are rare, with a prevalence of 3.7 cases per 100,000 population, their peak incidence is in late adolescence to early adulthood. These neoplasms therefore represent the most common solid tumors of men aged 20 to 34 years in the United States.[31] Testicular self-examination is an important tool for early detection because prompt treatment is associated with a higher success rate.

Etiology. Although the cause of testicular tumors is uncertain, a strong association is seen between cryptorchidism and the subsequent development of malignancy. Nevertheless, the majority of patients with testicular tumors have no history of cryptorchidism, which suggests that several unrecognized factors may be contributing to the pathogenesis.

Histologically, testicular tumors may be considered in two groups. In the first group are nongerminal neoplasms, including tumors that originate from either the Leydig cells or other stromal tissue cells of the testis. In the second group are germinal neoplasms, which are derived from the germinal cells of the testis. This group accounts for the vast majority (95%) of testicular tumors. Germinal neoplasms may be further subdivided into five groups: seminomas, embryonal carcinomas, teratomas, choriocarcinomas, and yolk sac tumors.[31]

Treatment. Although germinal tumors may consist entirely of one histologic subtype, many contain elements of more than one subtype. Treatment and prognosis vary according to the subtype of germinal tumor. For example, seminoma in its early stages is exquisitely sensitive to and easily cured with radiation therapy. On the other hand, nonseminomatous germ cell tumors in the early stage are usually successfully managed with surgery. The prognosis is also variable. Pure choriocarcinomas are usually first seen at an advanced stage with distant metastases. Treatment is usually less effective for this aggressive lesion. However, the majority of germ cell tumors may be effectively managed even if lymph node metastases are present.

Except for choriocarcinomas, which disseminate by vascular means, testicular germ cell tumors usually metastasize through the lymphatic system. They usually disseminate in a stepwise manner, first involving the retroperitoneal lymph nodes lying adjacent to the great vessels. If unmanaged, the disease may progress to involve other lymph nodes and other organs such as the lungs.

Multiple staging systems have been devised to classify the extent of this disease. Most are a variation of the system proposed by Boden and Gibb in 1951.[31] One commonly used system is as follows:

Stage I: The tumor is confined to the testis.
Stage II: The tumor has spread to retroperitoneal lymph nodes.
Stage III: The tumor has spread to nodes above the diaphragm
Stage IV: The tumor has spread to other organs.

Because the management of testicular tumors is complicated and somewhat controversial, a complete discussion is not possible here; however, several issues can be pointed out. After diagnosis of a testicular tumor, an operation to remove the testicle is performed. This procedure involves an inguinal incision with removal of the testis from the scrotum, followed by ligation and removal of the spermatic cord and testicle together. Histologic classification, additional staging studies, and other factors then determine further treatment. This treatment may involve close observation with frequent radiologic studies to determine new progression, surgery to remove the retroperitoneal lymph nodes (retroperitoneal lymphadenectomy), chemotherapy, or radiation therapy. Some situations may call for a combination of these measures.

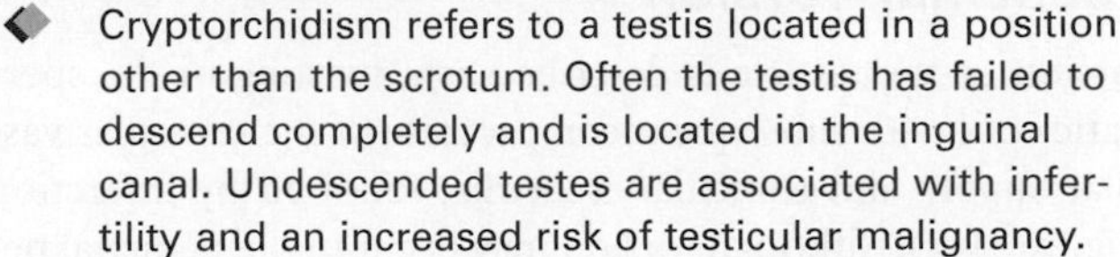

KEY CONCEPTS

- Cryptorchidism refers to a testis located in a position other than the scrotum. Often the testis has failed to descend completely and is located in the inguinal canal. Undescended testes are associated with infertility and an increased risk of testicular malignancy.
- A hydrocele is a collection of fluid in the testicle or spermatic cord, commonly associated with communication between the abdominal cavity and the scrotum (hernia). Hydroceles are benign and treated only if they become uncomfortable. A spermatocele is a cyst that contains sperm. Like hydroceles, they are benign and do not require treatment unless they cause discomfort.
- Testicular torsion refers to a twisting of the spermatic cord with subsequent testicular ischemia and infarction. Sudden onset of severe testicular pain is common. If the torsion is reduced within 12 hours, the testicle may be viable.
- Inflammation of the epididymis, called epididymitis, is most commonly associated with infectious agents. Manifestations include a swollen, tender, reddened

scrotum with associated bladder infection and cloudy urine. Antibiotics are indicated. Aggressive infections of the scrotum may result in Fournier gangrene manifested by gangrenous necrosis of the scrotum.

- Although rare in the population, testicular cancer is the most common solid tumor in men aged 20 to 34 years. The great majority of testicular neoplasms originate in the germ cells. Most germ cell tumors can be effectively managed even after lymph node metastasis. Management includes surgical removal of the testis and spermatic cord, with irradiation and chemotherapy as indicated.

DISORDERS OF THE PROSTATE

Benign Prostatic Hyperplasia

Benign prostatic hyperplasia, also referred to as benign prostatic hypertrophy (BPH), is a very common disorder. An estimated 80% of men older than 60 years experience some degree of BPH. It is important to recognize that BPH and prostate cancer are not related entities, and no study has conclusively demonstrated that BPH predisposes to the development of prostate cancer.[32]

Etiology. Although the exact cause of BPH is unknown, the occurrence of the disease with aging suggests a relationship to changes in the aging male endocrine system. The process involves hyperplasia of the glands surrounding the prostatic urethra (Figure 31-8). As this tissue increases in size, it compresses the urethra and produces symptoms of bladder outlet obstruction.

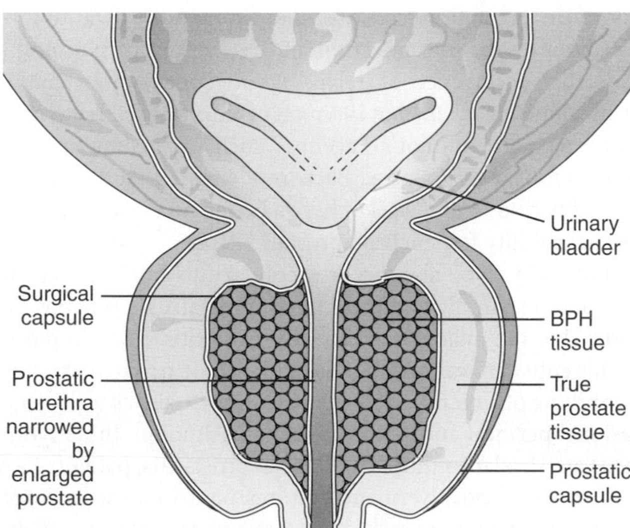

FIGURE 31-8 ■ Gross appearance of hyperplastic prostatic tissue obstructing the prostatic urethra. *BPH,* Benign prostatic hypertrophy.

Clinical Manifestations. Symptoms of obstruction may be minimal at first but may eventually progress to complete obstruction and urinary retention. A decrease in the force of the urinary stream, hesitancy or difficulty in initiating a urinary stream, and interruption of the stream may occur. Because the bladder may fail to empty completely, infection associated with residual urine may occur. Figure 31-9 illustrates possible complications of benign prostatic enlargement.

The diagnosis of BPH usually involves recognition of the characteristic symptoms. Rectal examination disclosing an enlarged prostate, urethral catheterization to document a postvoiding urinary residual, and intravenous pyelography to provide radiographic evidence of hypertrophy and obstruction are some of the measures that may be used to confirm the diagnosis.

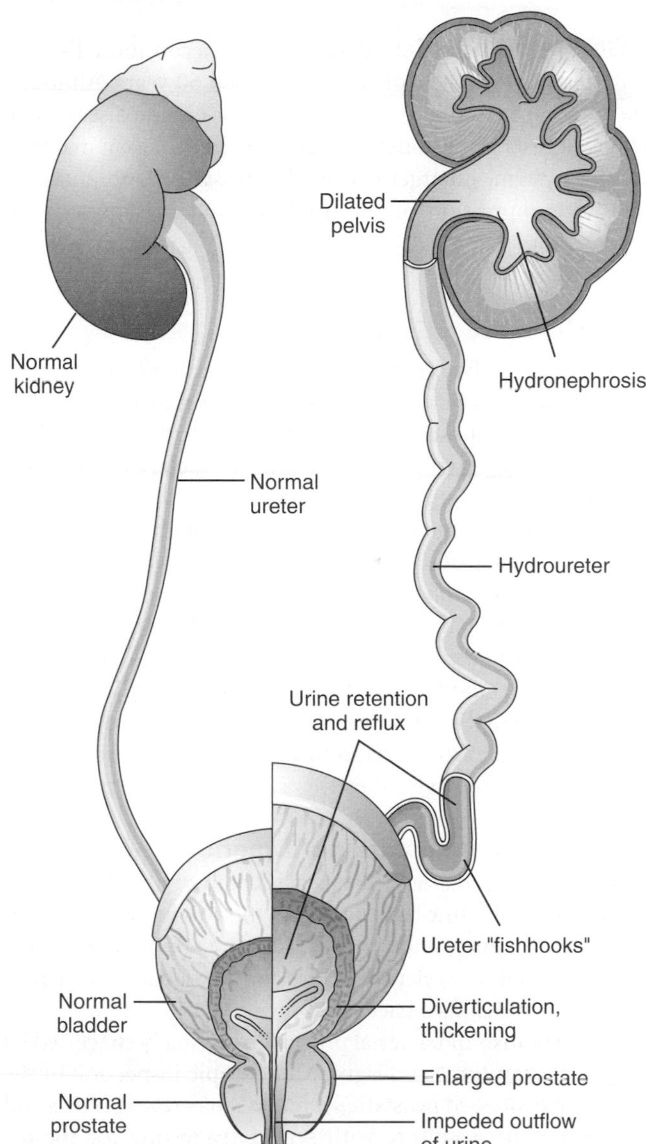

FIGURE 31-9 ■ Sites for potential complications caused by benign prostatic enlargement *(right)* are compared with a normal kidney, ureter, bladder, and prostate *(left).*

Treatment. Treatment often involves a surgical procedure to remove the obstructing prostatic tissue. The operation may be performed transurethrally with an endoscopic resectoscope. The resectoscope uses a wire filament that cuts by means of an electrical current. If the prostate is greatly enlarged, an open operation may be required. Endoscopic incision of the bladder neck, treating the prostate with lasers, microwave, or thermal therapies are other options available for this problem.[33]

Medications are playing a bigger role in management of BPH. Several drugs are used to decrease the tension in the urethra by blocking sympathetic α receptors in the gland. In addition, the gland can actually be decreased in size by drugs that prevent the conversion of testosterone to dihydrotestosterone. By using these medications, many patients can avoid an invasive procedure.[33]

Geriatric Considerations. BPH is a common disorder that affects about 80% of men older than 60 years. Although the exact cause is unknown, the occurrence of the disease with aging suggests a relationship to changes in the aging male endocrine system. Enlargement of the prostate gland and progressive compression of the urethra result in symptoms of obstruction.

Prostatitis

Prostatitis, or inflammation of the prostate, has several causes and encompasses several syndromes. A common classification of prostatitis proposed by Drach et al[32] in 1978 considers four types: acute bacterial prostatitis, chronic bacterial prostatitis, nonbacterial prostatitis, and prostatodynia.[34]

The causative organism in bacterial prostatitis is usually *E. coli,* with species of *Proteus, Klebsiella, Enterobacter, Pseudomonas,* and *Serratia* occurring less commonly.[35] Possible routes of infection include ascending infection up the urethra, reflux of infected urine into the prostatic ducts, hematogenous infection, and invasion of rectal bacteria by direct extension or lymphogenous spread (Figure 31-10). Many cases of prostatitis result from periurethral infection associated with an indwelling urethral catheter.[36]

Clinical Manifestations, Diagnosis, and Treatment. Acute bacterial prostatitis is characterized by the onset of fever, chills, low back pain, and the voiding symptoms of frequency, urgency, and dysurea. Rectal examination usually reveals a tender, swollen prostate, and subsequent urinalysis may reveal WBCs and bacteria.

The diagnosis of bacterial prostatitis is usually suggested by the initial symptoms and signs. Microscopic inspection of the urine and expressed prostatic secretions may reveal WBCs and bacteria. A urine culture with sensitivity testing for the offending organism is recommended to direct therapy with an appropriate antibiotic. In the event of high fever and an elevated WBC count, intravenous antibiotics are recommended.

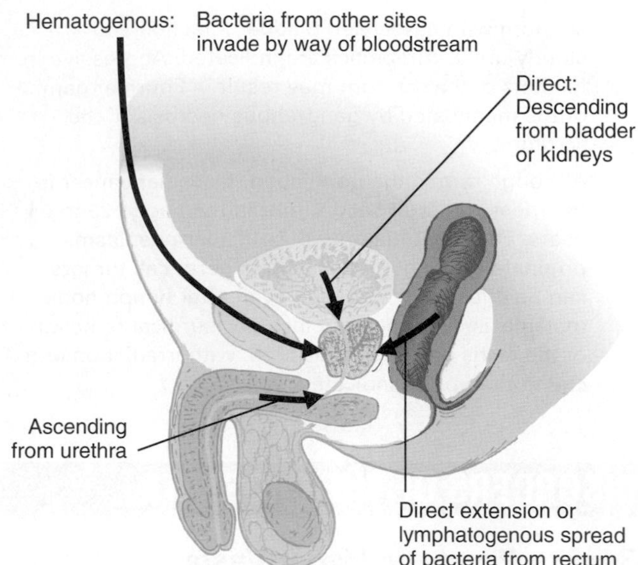

FIGURE 31-10 ■ Postulated pathways of infection to the prostate gland. (From Black JM, Matassarin-Jacobs E: *Medical-surgical nursing: clinical management for continuity of care,* ed 6, Philadelphia, 2001, Saunders, p 963.)

Chronic bacterial prostatitis may be associated with variable symptoms. Although some men with chronic bacterial prostatitis may report a history of acute bacterial prostatitis, many have no history of this problem. Most men complain of voiding symptoms with pain localized to various areas, including the perineum, back, suprapubic area, and occasionally, the testis. High-grade fever and chills are uncommon with this entity, as opposed to acute bacterial prostatitis.

In chronic bacterial prostatitis, pathogenic organisms may persist in prostatic tissues unaltered by the administration of several antibiotics. Because most antibiotics accumulate poorly in prostatic secretions, discontinuation of antibiotic use often results in reinfection and recurrence of symptoms. It is this occurrence of relapsing infections, often caused by the same organism, that is typical of chronic bacterial prostatitis. Several antibiotic agents, such as trimethoprim-sulfamethoxazole (Septra, Bactrim), when used for a prolonged period (4 to 6 weeks) have a better cure rate because of their capability to penetrate prostatic tissue.

Prostatitis may also occur secondary to nonbacterial inflammation. In fact, nonbacterial prostatitis probably accounts for the majority of cases of prostatitis. The symptoms of this entity are variable but usually include irritative voiding, symptoms of urgency, frequency, and nocturia, as well as occasional perineal and suprapubic pain. Although these symptoms are similar to those of bacterial prostatitis, patients have no history of positive urine cultures or urinary tract infections. Treatment may include a course of antibiotics, oral antiinflammatory agents (e.g., ibuprofen), prostatic massage, and occasionally, sitz baths. Symptoms are often intermittent, and patients should be reassured that the disease is not contagious and does not predispose to the development of cancer or other serious disease.

The final classification of prostatitis, **prostatodynia,** is typified by symptoms of prostatitis but no history of urinary tract infection and no evidence of inflammation in prostatic secretions. The cause of this entity is uncertain and may involve spasm of the pelvic floor musculature. Treatment may involve the use of α-adrenergic receptor–blocking agents and occasionally diazepam (Valium).[36]

Prostate Cancer

Other than skin cancers, prostate cancer is now recognized as the most prevalent form of cancer in men. About 200,000 cases are diagnosed annually in the United States, with approximately 35,000 deaths annually attributed to the disease. Prostate cancer ranks as the second leading cause of cancer death among men. Cancer of the prostate rarely occurs in men younger than 50 years, and its incidence increases with age. The majority (95%) of prostate cancers are adenocarcinomas with abnormal proliferation of prostatic glandular structures.[37]

Etiology. The precise cause of prostate cancer is undetermined, although genetic, hormonal, dietary, and viral factors have all been suggested. Varying degrees of aggressiveness of prostate cancer have been recognized, with different tumors expressing different malignant potential and ultimately carrying a different prognosis. Attempts to classify prostate cancer into separate groups of cancer have been made, with different tumors expressing different malignant potential and ultimately carrying a different prognosis. Such attempts to classify prostate cancer into different groups consider the structure and internal architecture of tumor cells and their pattern of proliferation. For example, cells of the more aggressive or poorly differentiated prostate cancers have more indistinct cell borders, larger nuclei, and loss of acinar (gland) formation.

Prostate cancer is staged as follows:

Stage A: The tumor is microscopic and intracapsular.
Stage B: The tumor is palpable on rectal examination but confined to the prostate.
Stage C: The tumor has extended beyond the capsule of the prostate.
Stage D: The tumor has metastasized to distant organs.

Diagnosis. The diagnosis of prostate cancer may involve several clinical scenarios. The disease may be diagnosed after microscopic inspection of prostate tissue removed for the management of presumed BPH. Prostate cancer may also be detected on rectal examination in patients with or without voiding symptoms. Occasionally, patients have urinary retention or even azotemia and renal failure secondary to obstructive nephropathy. Much interest has focused on the search for effective measures to detect prostate cancer in its early and most easily manageable stages. Two new techniques, a blood test for serum prostate-specific antigen and transrectal ultrasonography, have generated considerable excitement within the field of urology. Several initial investigations have shown efficacy in the early detection of prostate cancer.

Once the diagnosis of prostate cancer is made, the lesion must be staged. Staging usually involves a bone scan to rule out bone metastases, chest radiography to rule out lung metastases, and occasionally abdominal and pelvic computed tomography to rule out abdominal lymphadenopathy.

Treatment. Management of prostate cancer depends on several factors, including the stage of the tumor, as well as the age and health of the patient. Debate exists over treatment for men with localized disease, with options ranging from aggressive therapy to "watchful waiting." Watchful waiting may be an option for older men with asymptomatic stage A prostate cancer. Younger men may be candidates for the more aggressive approach, which includes surgery to remove the prostate and surrounding tissue (radical prostatectomy) or radiation therapy. It is important to note that approximately 70% to 90% of men who undergo radical prostatectomy will experience impotence. Urinary incontinence may also occur. Given the effects of surgical intervention, it is important that patients have access to preoperative and postoperative counseling about issues arising from their diagnosis and the effect of various treatments and potential complications.

In addition to radical prostatectomy or radiation therapy, in most cases some of the lymph nodes in the pelvis are also removed (pelvic lymph node dissection). Advanced lesions may respond to hormonal manipulation. Orchiectomy, oral administration of estrogens, or intramuscular injection of luteinizing hormone–releasing hormone agonists may reduce the patient's serum testosterone level. Many prostate cancers are androgen sensitive and may be temporarily controlled with androgen ablation. In more advanced cases that are no longer hormonally responsive, palliative measures such as spot radiation treatment of painful areas of bone metastasis and analgesics may be required.

Geriatric Considerations. Cancer of the prostate rarely occurs in men younger than 50 years, and its incidence increases with age. The majority (95%) of prostate cancers are adenocarcinomas with abnormal proliferation of prostatic glandular structures. Symptoms vary depending on the stage of the disease. Men who are older and have stage A prostate cancer may be monitored closely without any treatment. Men with more advanced stage disease may be treated more aggressively.

KEY CONCEPTS

- Symptoms of BPH include diminished force of the urinary stream, hesitancy, and poor bladder emptying. Transurethral resection of the obstructing prostatic tissue is the usual treatment.
- Inflammation of the prostate, or prostatitis, is characterized by low back pain, urinary frequency, urgency,

and dysuria. Fever and chills may also be present with acute bacterial prostatitis. *E. coli* is the most commonly associated organism. Prostatitis may also occur in the absence of infection.

- Prostate cancer is usually detected as a lump or enlargement of the prostate gland. As with other cancers, early, accurate diagnosis is important for effective therapy. Surgical resection, radiation therapy, and hormone therapy (to reduce androgens) may be used. The choice of treatment depends on the grade and stage of the disease and the individual's age, general health, and life expectancy.

SUMMARY

Disorders of the penis and male urethra may be grouped into congenital and acquired anomalies, infections, and neoplasms. Common congenital anomalies include urethral valves and hypospadias. Common acquired disorders involve phimosis, urethral strictures, and impotence. Sexually transmitted diseases are some of the most common infections involving the penis and urethra; they include gonococcal urethritis, nongonococcal urethritis, syphilis, genital herpes, and genital warts. Neoplasms of the penis and urethra are relatively rare.

Congenital disorders of the scrotum and testes include cryptorchidism. This condition is one of the most common problems seen by pediatric urologists. Testicular torsion and Fournier gangrene are two of the more immediate urologic emergencies. Finally, neoplasms of the testes, although rare, may afflict younger men in the prime of life.

Disorders of the prostate account for a majority of the visits to a practicing urologist. Briefly, these disorders can be divided into problems of benign prostatic hyperplasia, prostatitis, and prostatic cancer. Prostate cancer is the most frequently diagnosed cancer in men, with more than 100,000 cases diagnosed and 35,000 deaths yearly.

MEDIA RESOURCES evolve

Remember to check out the ***CD Companion*** included with this book for Review Questions, Key Concepts Review, Glossary (with audio for selected terms), Disease Profiles, and Animations.

PLUS, visit the ***Evolve website*** at http://evolve.elsevier.com/Copstead/ for Case Studies, Disease Profiles, and WebLinks.

References

1. Underwood LE, Van Wyk JJ: Normal and aberrant growth. In Wilson JD, Foster DW, editors: *Williams textbook of endocrinology,* ed 9, Philadelphia, 1998, Saunders, pp 1117-1124.
2. Feldman KW, Smith DW: Fetal phallic growth and penile standards for newborn male infants, *J Pediatr* 86(3):395-398, 1975.
3. Kogan SJ, Williams DI: The micropenis syndrome: clinical observations and expectations for growth, *J Urol* 118(2):311-313, 1977.
4. Greenfield SP: Posterior urethral valves: new concepts. *J Urol* 157(3):996-997, 1997.
5. King LR: Posterior urethra. In Kelalis PP, King LR, editors: *Clinical pediatric urology,* ed 3, Philadelphia, 1992, Saunders.
6. Van Savage JG et al: An algorithm for the management of anterior urethral valves, *J Urol* 158(3 pt 2):1030-1032, 1997.
7. Zaontz MR, Packer MG: Abnormalities of the external genitalia, *Pediatr Clin North Am* 44(5):1267-1297, 1997.
8. Albers N et al: Etiologic classification of severe hypospadias: implications for prognosis and management, *J Pediatr* 131(3):344-346, 1997.
9. Beaudoin S, Simon L, Bargy F: Anatomical basis of a common embryological origin for epispadias and bladder or cloacal exstrophies, *Surg Radiol Anat* 19(1):11-16, 1997.
10. Mulhall JP, Honig SC: Priapism: etiology and management, *Acad Emerg Med* 3(8):810-816, 1996.
11. Powars DR, Johnson CS: Priapism, *Hematol Oncol Clin North Am* 10(6):1363-1372, 1996.
12. Fitzpatrick TJ: Spongiograms and cavernosograms: a study of their value in priapism, *J Urol* 109(5):843-846, 1973.
13. deHoll JD et al: Alternative approaches to the management of priapism, *Int J Impot Res* 10(1):11-14, 1998.
14. Golubovic Z et al: The conservative treatment of phimosis in boys, *Br J Urol* 78(5):786-788, 1996.
15. Licht MR, Lewis RW: Modified Nesbit procedure for the treatment of Peyronie's disease: a comparative outcome analysis, *J Urol* 158(2):460-463, 1997.
16. Bortolotti A et al: The epidemiology of erectile dysfunction and its risk factors, *Int J Androl* 20(6):323-334, 1997.
17. McMillan DE: Development of vascular complications in diabetes, *Vasc Med* 2(2):132-142, 1997.
18. Fabbri A, Aversa A, Isidori A: Erectile dysfunction: an overview, *Hum Reprod Update* 3(5):455-466, 1997.
19. Roy JB: Advances in the management of impotence, *J Okla State Med Assoc* 91(1):14-16, 1998.
20. Jones RB et al: Randomized trial of trovafloxacin and ofloxacin for single-dose therapy of gonorrhea. Trovafloxacin Gonorrhea Study Group, *Am J Med* 104(1):28-32, 1998.
21. Martin SJ et al: Levofloxacin and sparfloxacin: new quinolone antibiotics, *Ann Pharmacother* 32(3):320-336, 1998.
22. Centers for Disease Control and Prevention: 1998 guidelines for treatment of sexually transmitted diseases, *MMWR Morb Mortal Wkly Rep* 47(RR-1):1-111, 1998.
23. Patel R: Progress in meeting today's demands in genital herpes: an overview of current management, *J Infect Dis* 186:547-556, 2002.
24. Jablonska S, Majewski S: Human papillomavirus infection in women. Special aspects of infectious diseases in women, *Clin Dermatol* 15(1):67-79, 1997.
25. Micali G et al: Squamous cell carcinoma of the penis, *J Am Acad Dermatol* 35(3 pt 1):432-451, 1996.
26. Schellhammer PF, Grabstald H: Tumors of the penis. In Walsh PC et al, editors: *Campbell's urology,* ed 7, Philadelphia, 1997, Saunders.
27. Kogan SJ: Cryptorchidism. In Kelalis PP, King LR, editors: *Clinical pediatric urology,* ed 3, Philadelphia, 1992, Saunders.

28. Cortes D: Cryptorchidism: aspects of pathogenesis, histology and treatment, *Scand J Urol Nephrol Suppl* 196:1-54, 1998.
29. Gill B, Kogan S: Cryptorchidism. Current concepts, *Pediatr Clin North Am* 44(5):1211-1227, 1997.
30. Morpurgo E, Galandiuk S: Fournier's gangrene, *Surg Clin North Am* 82(6):1213-1224, 2002.
31. Morse MJ, Whitmore WF: Neoplasms of the testis. In Walsh PC et al, editors: *Campbell's urology,* ed 7, Philadelphia, 1997, Saunders.
32. Drach GW et al: Classification of benign diseases associated with prostatic pain: prostatitis or prostatodynia (letter)? *J Urol* 120(2):266, 1978.
33. Roehrborn CG et al: Guidelines for the diagnosis and treatment of benign prostatic hyperplasia: a comparative, international overview, *Urology* 58(5):642-650, 2001.
34. Nickel JC: Prostatitis: myths and realities, *Urology* 51(3):362-366, 1998.
35. Meares EM: Prostatitis and related disorders. In Walsh PC et al, editors: *Campbell's urology,* ed 7, Philadelphia, 1997, Saunders.
36. Walsh PC: Benign prostatic hyperplasia. In Walsh PC et al, editors: *Campbell's urology,* ed 7, Philadelphia, 1997, Saunders.
37. Catalona WJ: Carcinoma of the prostate. In Walsh PC et al, editors: *Campbell's urology,* ed 7, Philadelphia, 1997, Saunders.

chapter 32

Female Genital and Reproductive Function

Paul D. Silva • Jane M. Georges

MEDIA RESOURCES

Additional Material for Study, Review, and Further Exploration

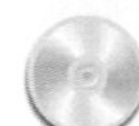

CD Companion ◆ Review Questions and Answers ◆ Key Concepts Review
◆ Glossary *(with audio pronunciations for selected terms)*
◆ Disease Profiles ◆ Animations

evolve ***Website*** at http://evolve.elsevier.com/Copstead/
◆ Case Studies ◆ Disease Profiles ◆ WebLinks

KEY QUESTIONS

- What are the major structures of the internal and external female reproductive tract?
- What are the major hormonal events of the female reproductive cycle?
- Which hormones are involved in breast development during pregnancy and lactation, and what are their specific functions?
- What are the physiologic changes associated with pregnancy?
- What gestational events occur in the fetus during each of the three trimesters of pregnancy?
- What hormonal changes lead to menopause?
- What physiologic changes and complications may result from menopausal hormone deficiencies?

CHAPTER OUTLINE

The female reproductive system is complex both in structure and in function. From birth to senescence, the organs of the female reproductive system function in concert with each other, with the brain, and with other endocrine organs. This integrated functioning constitutes some of the most intricate and elegant processes of the human body. This chapter presents an overview of these functions, beginning with the development of the female reproductive tract.

The major processes related to the reproductive tract throughout life, including the menstrual cycle, pregnancy, lactation, and menopause, are then described with an emphasis on recent research findings. Because the functioning of the female reproductive system has an enormous impact on the life of the individual woman, increased importance has been placed on the active involvement of women in understanding their own health care needs. Health care professionals are encouraged to include women as collaborators in decisions about their reproductive health.[1,2]

REPRODUCTIVE STRUCTURES

Embryology

Until the sixth week of gestation, the gonads in both sexes are bipotential, which means that the gonads present in the embryo may become either testes or ovaries. Beginning about the seventh week, the so-called indifferent gonad begins to develop into either a male or a female derivative.[3] Recent research has demonstrated that SRY (sex-determining region of the Y chromosome) is the gene that influences the indifferent gonad to organize into a testis.[4] In a genetically female embryo, the gonad organizes into an ovary under the influence of one or more ovary-determining genes, which have not yet been well characterized. The cortex of the gonad accumulates nests of cells that differentiate into ovarian follicles, each containing a primary oocyte. The wolffian ducts, the primordial structures that are precursors to the male internal reproductive organs, begin to disappear, and the müllerian ducts, the structures that will develop into the female internal reproductive organs, become dominant.[3]

The external genitalia of both the male and female are identical until the eighth week of gestation. Like the gonads, the genitalia are bipotential until this time, with the capability of developing into organs of either sex. In a genetically male embryo, dihydrotestosterone, a metabolite of testosterone, binds to androgen receptors in the external genitalia and effects the differentiation of these structures into the male external genitalia. Without the influence of dihydrotestosterone, the bipotential external genitalia will spontaneously develop into female external genitalia.[3]

During the later period of fetal development, maternal hormones may have some influence on reproductive structures.

Estrogens and progestins from the mother cause cervical enlargement, hypertrophy of the vaginal epithelium, and enlargement of the mammary gland of the female fetus. These alterations may be present at birth but usually subside during the first 1 to 2 months.[5]

Organization of the Female Reproductive Organs

The internal organs of the female reproductive system include the ovaries, **oviducts** (fallopian tubes), uterus, cervix, and vagina (Figure 32-1). These organs are situated in the pelvic cavity and are supported and anchored in place by a series of ligaments (Figure 32-2).

Ovaries

The two ovaries, which are the female gonads, are located close to the lateral walls of the pelvic cavity. When the ovary is in its normal position, its long axis is nearly vertical with respect to the horizontal axis of the body. The size of the ovary varies with age and with the stage of the menstrual cycle. It is somewhat larger before than after pregnancy and further reduces in size with the aging process.[6]

The ovary is covered with a single layer of epithelium. Underneath the epithelium is a layer of dense fibrous connective tissue called the tunica albuginea. The tunica albuginea constitutes the outer portion of the cortex of the ovary. The remainder of the cortex consists of connective tissue called the stroma, which contains ova in various stages of maturation. The innermost part of the ovary, the medulla, consists of loose connective tissue that is richly supplied with blood and lymph vessels and nerve fibers.[7]

Before birth, hundreds of thousands of **oogonia** (cells that develop into ova) are present in the ovaries. Thus the entire lifetime supply of ova is established during embryonic development; no new oogonia arise after birth. Each oogonium is surrounded by a cluster of granulosa cells. The oogonium and its granulosa cells constitute a follicle. During prenatal development, the oogonia increase in size and become primary oocytes. By the time of full gestational development, the primary oocytes are in the prophase of the first meiotic division (Figure 32-3). During childhood and into adult life, the oocytes enter a nonactive phase. After puberty, a few of the oocytes develop in follicles each month in response to follicle-stimulating hormone (FSH) secreted by the anterior pituitary gland. The vast majority of follicles and their oocytes die by atresia. Generally, each month, only one mature follicle will develop to eject an oocyte through the wall of the ovary in the process of ovulation, which is described in more detail under the Menstrual Cycle section.

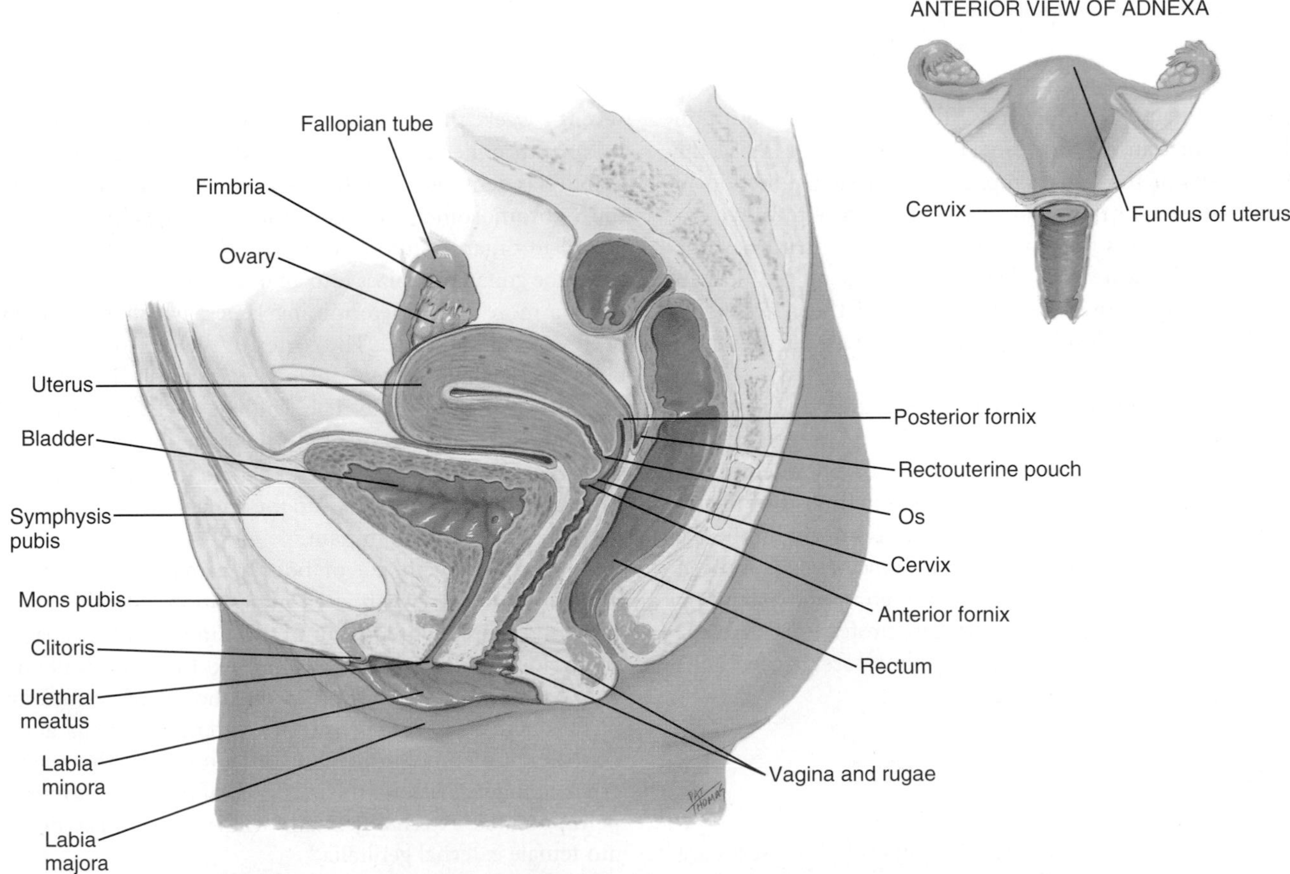

FIGURE 32-1 ■ Cross-sectional view of the female reproductive system. (From Jarvis C: *Physical examination and health assessment,* ed 4, Philadelphia, 2004, Saunders, p 767.)

Oviducts

The two **oviducts,** also called the fallopian or uterine tubes, are each about 10 cm long and located in the upper margin of the broad ligament. Each oviduct runs laterally from the uterus to the uterine end of the ovary. The free end of the oviduct adjacent to the ovary is called the *infundibulum.* It is shaped like a funnel with long, fingerlike projections termed *fimbriae.* The ampulla, the longest part of the oviduct, has an inner lining consisting of ciliated mucous membrane arranged in longitudinal folds. Beneath this ciliated lining is a double layer of smooth muscle with a thick outer layer of peritoneal serosa. The oviduct has an active role in propelling the ovum toward the uterus; the current created by the beating cilia and the peristaltic contractions of the muscular wall are powerful forces that move ova along the oviduct. Once inside the oviduct, the ovum is moved through the ampulla to the isthmus (the short, narrow portion near the uterus) and finally through the intramural passageway to the uterus. Fertilization of the ovum occurs in the upper third of the oviduct, and the **zygote** (fertilized ovum) begins developing as it moves through the oviduct. If no fertilization occurs, the ovum undergoes degeneration in the oviduct.[7]

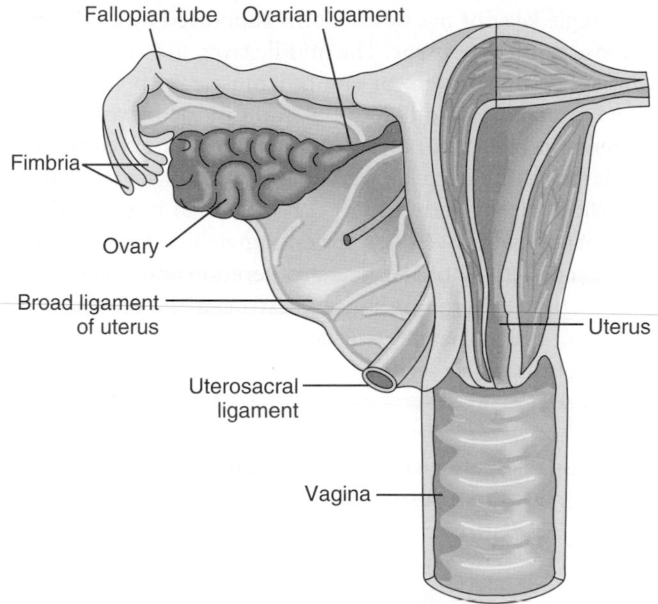

FIGURE 32-2 ■ View of the female pelvis showing the ovarian and uterine ligaments.

Uterus

The uterus varies in size, shape, location, and structure during various phases of a woman's life and reproductive status. In the nonpregnant state, the uterus is about 8 cm long, 4 cm wide in its upper part, and 2 cm thick. The rounded part of the uterus, which lies above and in front of the openings of the oviducts, is called the fundus; the main portion of the uterus is the corpus, or body. The lower, narrow portion of the uterus is the cervix,

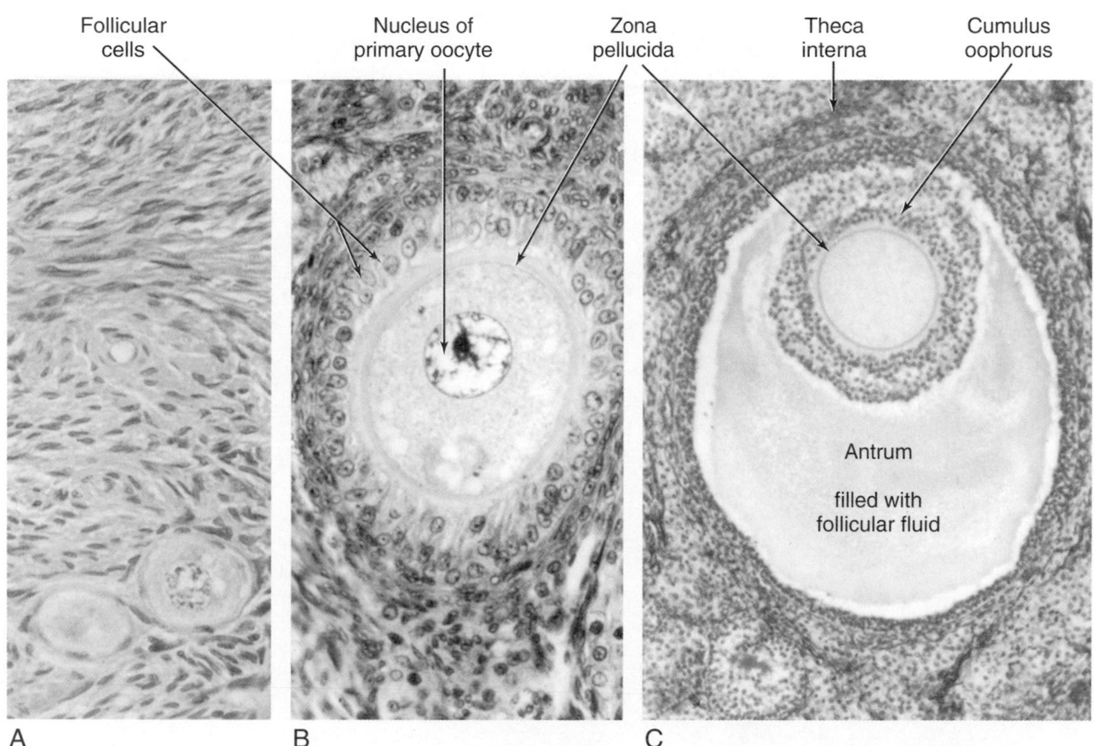

FIGURE 32-3 ■ Photomicrographs of sections from adult human ovaries. **A,** Ovarian cortex showing two primordial follicles containing primary oocytes that have completed the prophase of the first meiotic division. **B,** Growing follicle containing a primary oocyte. **C,** An almost mature follicle. (From Leeson CR, Leeson TS, Paparo AA: *Text/atlas of histology,* Philadelphia, 1988, Saunders.)

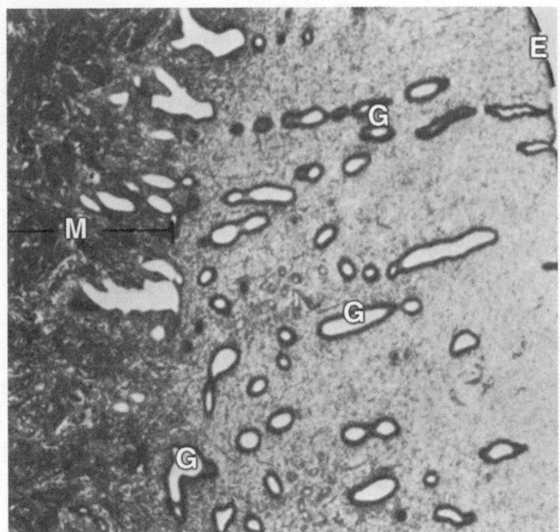

FIGURE 32-4 ■ The uterine wall consists of an epithelial lining *(E)* from which uterine glands *(G)* extend through the full thickness of the mucosa. Beneath the endometrium, a small portion of myometrium *(M)* is shown. (From Leeson CR, Leeson TS, Paparo AA: *Atlas of histology,* ed 2, Philadelphia, 1985, Saunders, p 261.)

which extends downward to the opening within the vagina. The cervix contains a narrow canal that joins the uterine cavity at the internal os and opens into the vagina at the external os.

The wall of the body and fundus of the uterus consists of three layers: endometrium, myometrium, and serosa (Figure 32-4). The outermost layer of the uterus, the serosa, consists of a single layer of mesothelial cells supported by a thin layer of loose connective tissue. The middle layer, the myometrium, consists of three layers of smooth muscle with the muscle fibers arranged in a different direction in each layer. The innermost lining of the uterus, the **endometrium,** consists of two layers: a thin deep layer called the basilar layer and a thick superficial layer referred to as the functional layer. During a woman's reproductive years, the endometrium displays a constant cyclic activity of alternate proliferation and sloughing of the functional layer in response to **estrogen** and **progesterone** secretion. These changes will be discussed in more detail in the Menstrual Cycle section.[7]

Vagina

The vagina is the sexual organ that enfolds the penis during sexual intercourse, serves as an exit for discarded en-

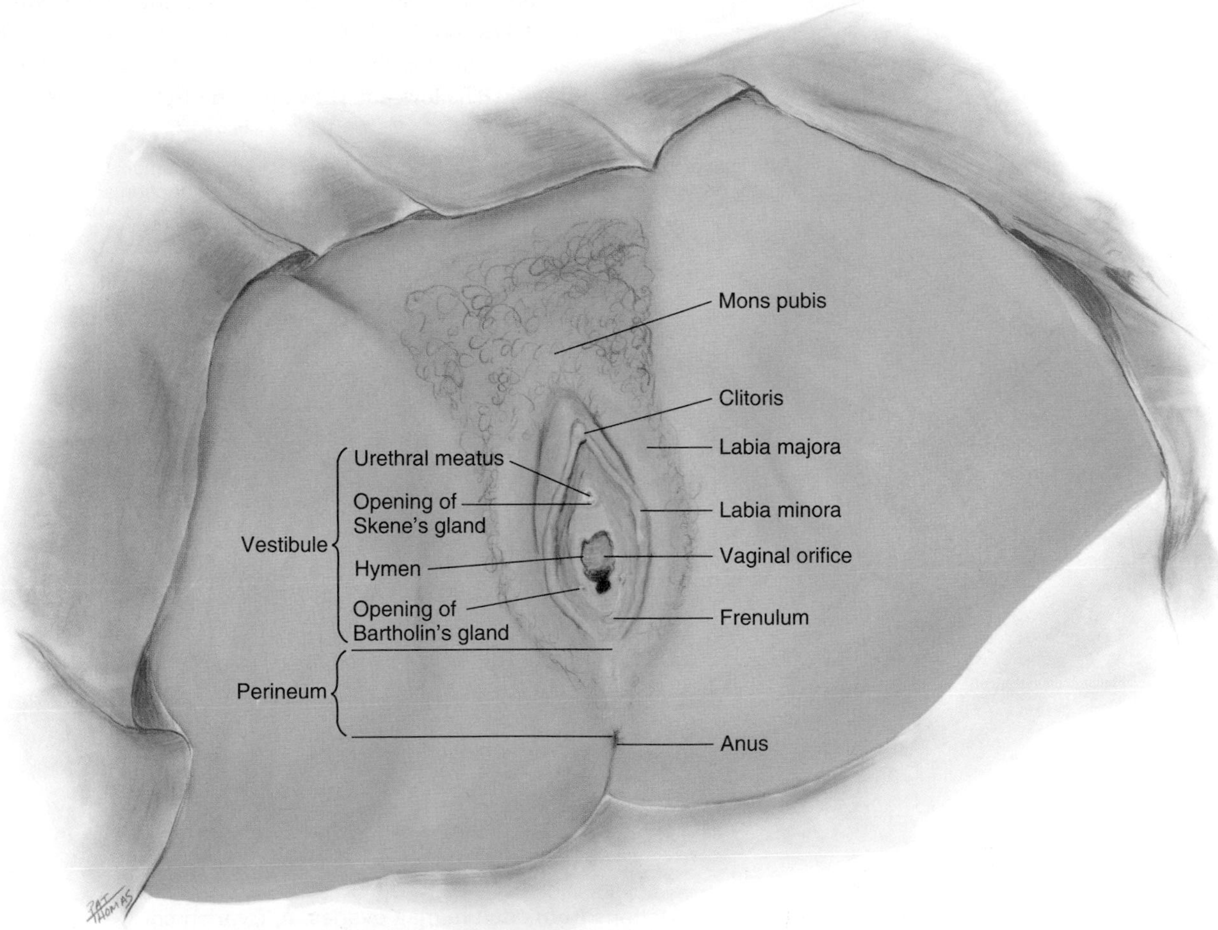

FIGURE 32-5 ■ External female genitalia. (From Jarvis C: *Physical examination and health assessment,* ed 4, Philadelphia, 2004, Saunders, p 766.)

dometrium, and forms the lower end of the birth canal. It is located anterior to the rectum and posterior to the urethra and urinary bladder. The vagina surrounds the cervix at one end and opens to the vestibule at its other end. The vagina is a highly elastic muscle that is capable of considerable distention. Two longitudinal ridges run along the anterior and posterior walls, with numerous transverse folds called rugae. The vagina is lined by a mucous membrane of stratified squamous epithelium overlying a layer of connective tissue.[7] The vaginal wall is subject to thinning with aging; this and other age-related changes in the female sexual organs are described in the Menopause section.

External Genitalia

The external female genital structures include the mons pubis, labia majora, labia minora, clitoris, and vestibule of the vagina (Figure 32-5). The mons pubis is a rounded elevation in front of the pubis symphysis. It consists primarily of an accumulation of fat. After puberty, the skin over it is covered by coarse hair. The labia majora, which are **homologous** (i.e., corresponding in structure) with the scrotum of the male, are folds of skin that run downward and backward from the mons pubis to the area behind the vaginal opening. After puberty, the labia majora become pigmented and covered with hair. The labia minora are two small folds of skin located between the labia majora on either side of the vaginal opening. The vestibule of the vagina is the cleft between the labia minora and contains the openings of the vagina, the urethra, and the ducts of the greater vestibular glands (also called Bartholin glands). These glands, along with the lesser vestibular or Skene glands, secrete mucus to provide lubrication during sexual intercourse.[6,7]

The clitoris is a body of erectile tissue that projects from the anterior end of the vulva at the anterior junction of the labia minora. It is about 2 cm long and 0.5 cm in diameter and is covered by a fold of tissue called the prepuce, which is formed by the merging of labial tissue. The glans of the clitoris is the rounded elevation on the free end of the body and is highly sensitive to stimulation. During sexual arousal, the erectile tissue of the clitoris becomes engorged with blood.[6,7]

KEY CONCEPTS

- Organs of the female reproductive tract include the ovaries, oviducts, uterus, cervix, and vagina. Ovaries contain a lifetime supply of ova at birth. After puberty, a few of the ovarian follicles develop about every 28 days in response to secretion of FSH.
- The oviducts (fallopian tubes) actively propel the ovum toward the uterus by ciliary action and peristaltic contractions. The uterine lining undergoes a cyclic process of proliferation and then sloughing in response to estrogen and progesterone.
- External genitalia in the female include the mons pubis, labia majora, labia minora, clitoris, and vestibule of the vagina. The urinary meatus, vaginal opening, and vestibular gland ducts are located in the vaginal vestibule.

MENSTRUAL CYCLE

From **menarche** onward, the normal reproductive years of the female are characterized by rhythmic changes in hormonal secretion and corresponding changes in the sexual organs, which are called the target organs of the female hormones. This rhythmic pattern is called the **menstrual cycle.** Two significant results of the menstrual cycle are stimulation of the production of an ovum and preparation of the uterine endometrium for the implantation of a fertilized ovum at the appropriate phase of the cycle.[8]

Although considerable variation can be found in human females, an average menstrual cycle is 28 days long, with cycles as short as 20 days or as long as 45 days occurring in normal women. The first day of menstruation is considered the first day of the menstrual cycle. Ovulation occurs approximately 14 days before the next cycle begins; thus in a 28-day cycle, ovulation occurs on about day 14 of the cycle.

The release of hormones and accompanying response of the female sexual target organs are depicted in Figure 32-6. The principal female reproductive hormones are summarized in Table 32-1. As shown in Figure 32-6, the events of the menstrual cycle require precise synchronization between the activities of the pituitary, ovary, and uterus. Beginning at the first day of the menstrual cycle, or the first day of menstruation, these events can be summarized as follows. The thickened functional layer of the endometrium of the uterus is gradually sloughed off, and about 35 ml of blood is lost. During this phase of the menstrual cycle, FSH is released by the pituitary gland and stimulates a group of follicles to develop in the ovary.

In the preovulatory phase, also called the proliferative phase, theca and granulosa cells in the developing follicles in the ovary secrete estrogen, which stimulates growth of the uterine endometrium once again. At about the midpoint of the cycle, an increase in estrogen secretion from the follicles occurs. This increase in estrogen is thought to render the anterior pituitary more responsive to luteinizing hormone–releasing hormone secreted by the hypothalamus. The anterior pituitary then produces a burst of luteinizing hormone. FSH also increases about twofold at the same time, and these two hormones act synergistically to cause the extremely rapid swelling of the follicle that culminates in ovulation.[9] During the process of ovulation, the secondary oocyte is ejected through the wall of the ovary into the peritoneal cavity. The free end of the oviduct is strategically located so that the ovum enters its fimbriated end almost immediately.[7]

After ovulation, the postovulatory phase (also called the luteal phase) begins. During the luteal phase the site of the ruptured follicle becomes a **corpus luteum** (Latin for "yellow

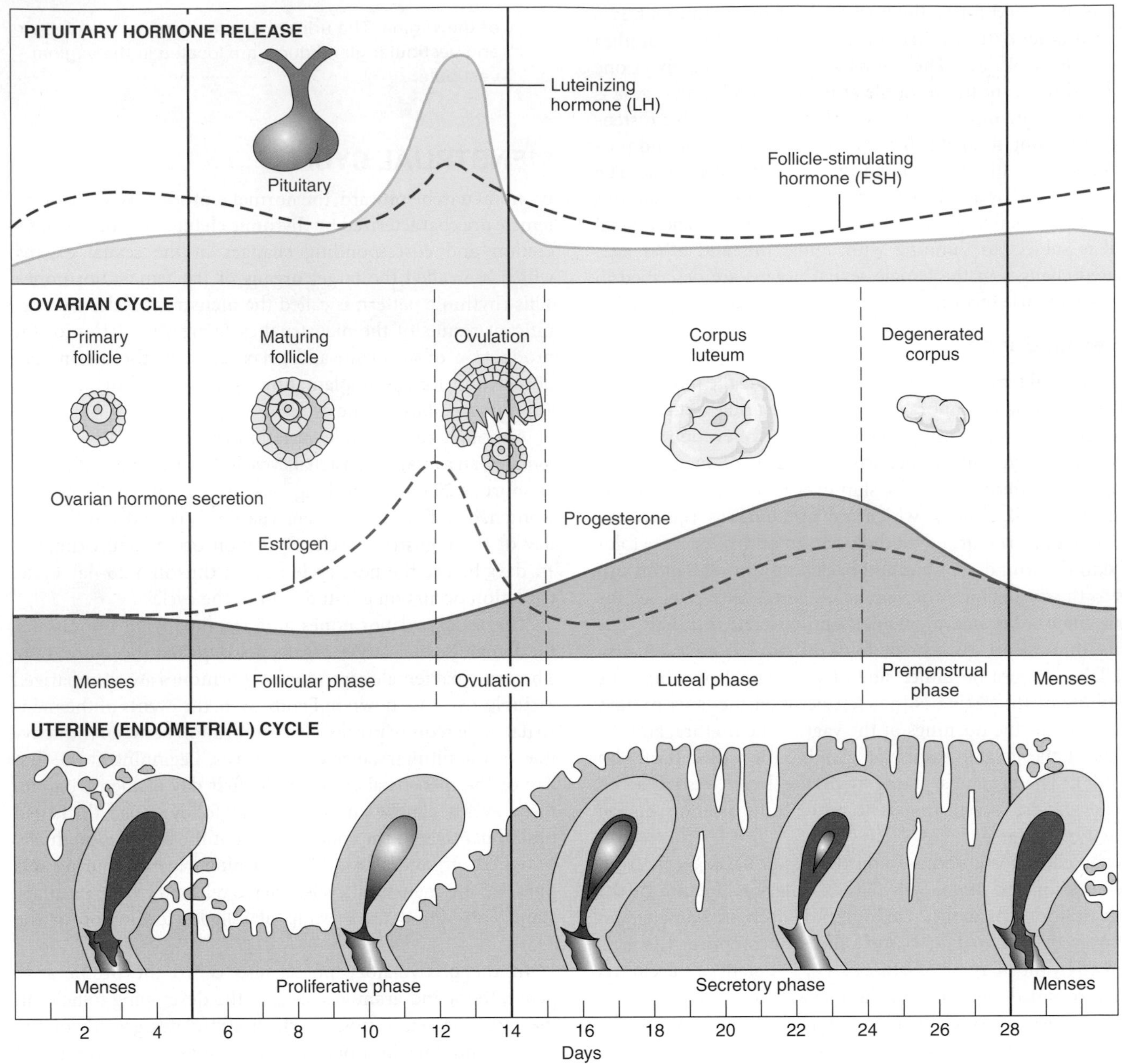

FIGURE 32-6 ■ The menstrual cycle. The events that take place within the pituitary, ovary, and uterus are precisely synchronized. When fertilization does not occur, the cycle repeats itself about every 28 days.

body"), which secretes estrogen and progesterone. These hormones stimulate continued thickening of the uterine endometrium. The cells of the corpus luteum become greatly enlarged and develop lipid, or fatty, areas that give the cells a distinctive yellow color. In a normal cycle, the corpus luteum grows to approximately 1.5 cm, with maximal development attained about 7 to 8 days after ovulation. If pregnancy does not occur, the corpus luteum begins to degenerate, and progesterone and estrogen levels in the blood fall markedly. Constriction of the spiral arteries located in the uterine wall occurs, and the portion of the endometrium supplied by these arteries becomes ischemic. As the cells in the endometrium die, tissue is sloughed off and menstruation begins again. It is presently thought that prostaglandins liberated in the endometrium may have a role in stimulating the sloughing of endometrial tissue.[7,10]

If fertilization of the ovum occurs, the embryo arrives in the uterus on about the fourth day of development. Small glands in the endometrium stimulated by progesterone produce a nutritive fluid for the developing embryo. On approximately the seventh day after fertilization, the embryo implants itself in the thick endometrium of the uterus, and development of the **placenta** occurs. The placenta secretes the hormone human chorionic gonadotropin (hCG), which in turn signals the corpus lu-

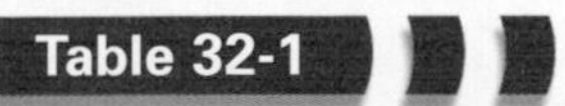

Principal Female Reproductive Hormones

Hormone	Target Organs	Significant Actions
Estrogen	Multiple sites throughout the body, including reproductive structures, bone, fat, and muscle tissues	Development of reproductive organs during puberty Development of secondary sex characteristics, including breast maturation, widening of the pelvis, and distribution of fat and muscle tissues in a distinctively female pattern Cyclic preparation of the endometrium for implantation of an ovum
Progesterone	Primarily uterus and breasts	Cyclic preparation and maintenance of the endometrium for implantation of an ovum Stimulation of development of breast lobes and alveoli
Follicle-stimulating hormone	Ovary	Stimulates ovarian follicle development; with luteinizing hormone, stimulates secretion of estrogen and ovulation
Luteinizing hormone	Ovary	Stimulates final development of the ovarian follicle, ovulation, and development of the corpus luteum

teum to continue to function. Subsequent events in pregnancy are described later in this chapter.

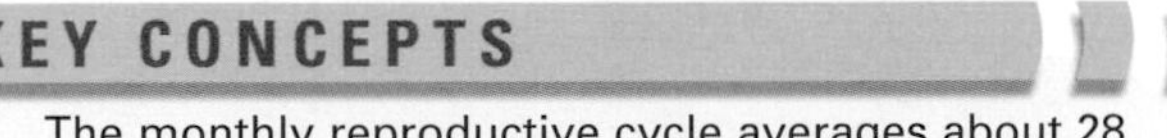

- The monthly reproductive cycle averages about 28 days. Beginning on the first day of menses, the important events of the cycle are as follows:
  1. The endometrial layer is sloughed off.
  2. The ovarian follicles are stimulated by pituitary FSH.
  3. Estrogen is secreted from the developing follicles.
  4. Proliferation of the endometrium occurs in response to estrogen.
  5. At the midpoint of the cycle, a burst of luteinizing hormone and a doubling of FSH secretion from the pituitary stimulate ovulation.
  6. The ruptured follicle changes into a corpus luteum and secretes estrogen and progesterone.
  7. In the absence of pregnancy, secretion of estrogen and progesterone drops rapidly and the endometrial lining sloughs off again to complete the cycle.
- With fertilization and implantation of the ovum, the developing placenta secretes hCG, which in turn stimulates the corpus luteum to continue to secrete estrogen and progesterone and thus prevent endometrial sloughing.

BREAST

The breast is an important accessory organ in sexual function and human reproduction. Although its primary physiologic function is **lactation** (production of milk) to nourish the human infant, the significance of the breast as a symbol of feminine sexuality in contemporary Western culture must also be recognized.

Structure of the Breast

The breasts are located anterior to the pectoralis major muscle and are separated from it by a layer of fat. The position of the breasts is maintained by fibrous bands called Cooper ligaments, which are easily stretched, especially if the breasts are large. Lymph drainage from the breasts is mainly toward the axillary lymph nodes, with some drainage toward the substernal and diaphragmatic lymph nodes.[11]

Each breast consists of 15 to 20 lobes of glandular epithelial tissue and a duct system embedded in interstitial tissue and fat. The secretory cells that constitute the glandular epithelium are arranged in grapelike clusters called alveoli (Figure 32-7). Ducts or openings from each alveolus unite to form a single duct from each lobe. These main ducts then enlarge slightly into ampullae immediately before opening onto the surface of the nipple. The nipple, located at the center of the adult female breast, is composed of bundles of smooth muscle fiber with erectile properties. The areola that surrounds the nipple has a diameter of 1.5 to 2.5 cm. The openings from the lactiferous ducts are arranged radially under the areola; thus 15 to 20 small openings are located on the surface of each nipple through which milk flows in a lactating female.[7]

Breast Development

The stages of development of the female breast are depicted in Figure 32-8. As shown in this figure, the breasts contain only rudimentary glands during childhood. At puberty, estrogen and progesterone, in the presence of growth hormone and

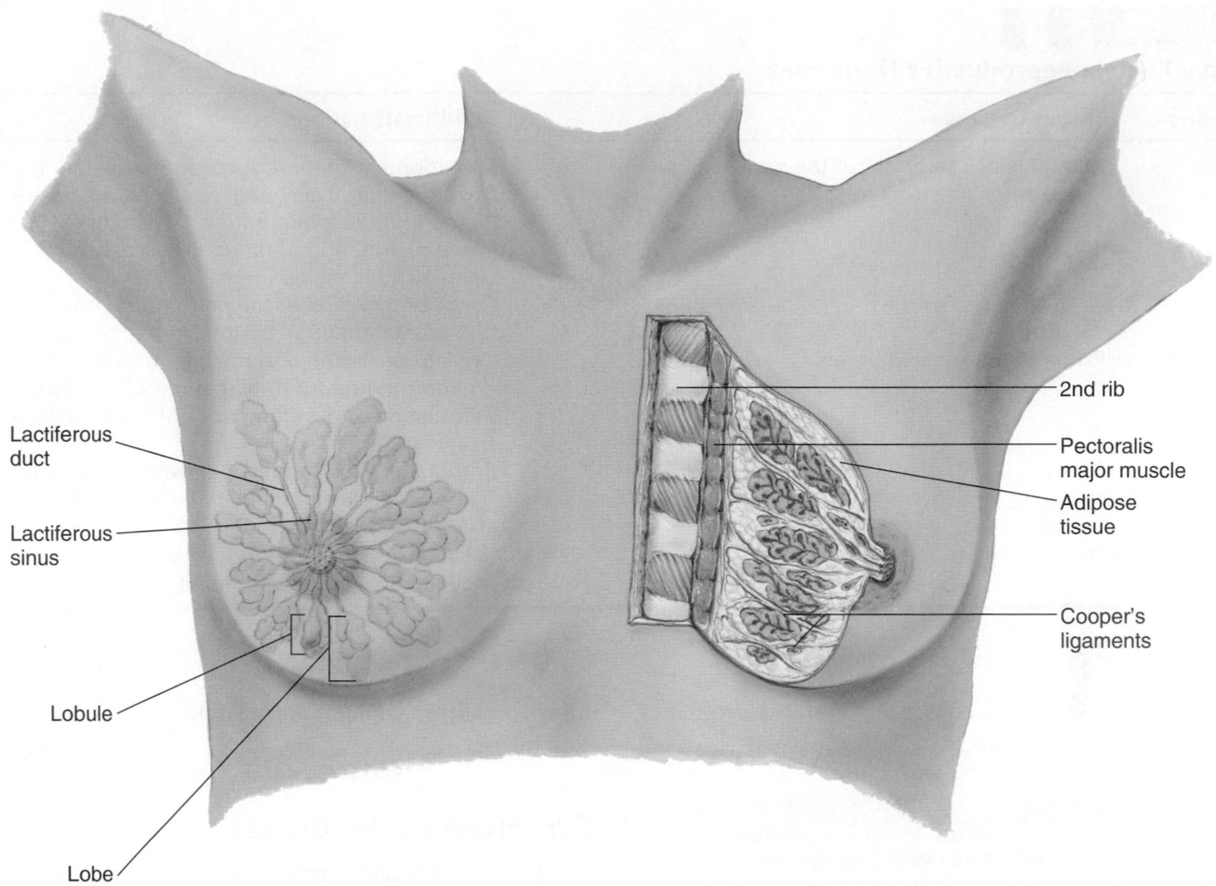

FIGURE 32-7 ■ The mature female breast. (From Jarvis C: *Physical examination and health assessment,* ed 4, Philadelphia, 2004, Saunders, p 409.)

prolactin, promote the development of glandular tissue and ducts and the deposition of fat characteristic of the adult female breast. Throughout the reproductive years, some women note swelling of the breast around the latter part of each menstrual cycle before the onset of menstruation. The water retention and subsequent swelling of breast tissue during this phase of the menstrual cycle are thought to be due to high levels of circulating progesterone stimulating the secretory cells of the breast.[11]

Lactation

During pregnancy, high concentrations of estrogen and progesterone produced by the corpus luteum and the placenta stimulate the development of glands and ducts in the breast. During the first trimester of pregnancy, the ducts proliferate; in the second trimester, the ducts group together to form large lobules with new alveoli formation. In the third trimester, the existing alveoli dilate in preparation for lactation. Toward the end of pregnancy and until 1 to 3 days after childbirth, the mammary glands form colostrum, which contains protein and lactose but little fat. After birth of the infant, the hormone **prolactin** secreted by the mother's anterior pituitary stimulates milk production, and milk is produced by the third day after delivery. The initiation and maintenance of lactation are a complex neuroendocrine process involving sensory nerves in the nipples and breast tissue, the spinal cord and hypothalamus, and the pituitary gland. The suckling movements of the infant on the breast stimulate the release of prolactin from the anterior pituitary gland and **oxytocin** from the posterior pituitary gland. These hormones in turn stimulate lactation and ejection of milk from the alveoli into the ducts, where it is accessible to the infant. Oxytocin then promotes the actual release of milk, called the "milk ejection reflex."[7,12]

KEY CONCEPTS

- At puberty, breast development occurs in response to estrogen and progesterone in cooperation with growth hormone and prolactin. During pregnancy, high estrogen and progesterone levels stimulate further development of the mammary glands and ducts.
- Milk production and release are stimulated by the pituitary hormones prolactin and oxytocin in response to suckling.

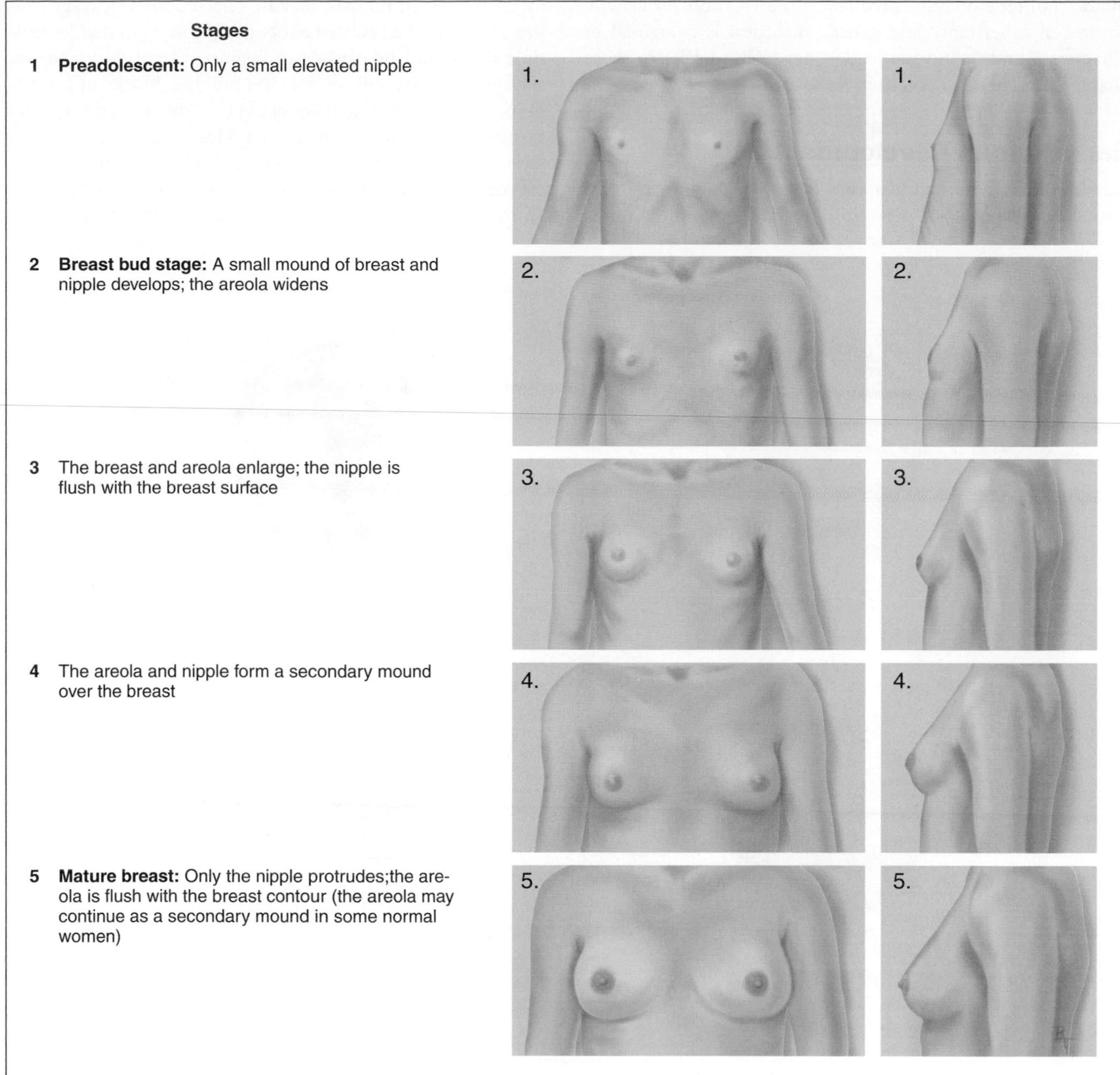

Stages
1 **Preadolescent:** Only a small elevated nipple
2 **Breast bud stage:** A small mound of breast and nipple develops; the areola widens
3 The breast and areola enlarge; the nipple is flush with the breast surface
4 The areola and nipple form a secondary mound over the breast
5 **Mature breast:** Only the nipple protrudes;the areola is flush with the breast contour (the areola may continue as a secondary mound in some normal women)
1.
1.
2.
2.
3.
3.
4.
4.
5.
5.

FIGURE 32-8 ■ The five Tanner stages of development of the female breast. (From Jarvis C: *Physical examination and health assessment,* ed 4, Philadelphia, 2004, Saunders, p 411.)

PREGNANCY

During the 9 months of human gestation, the single-celled zygote gives rise to an infant with a complex set of physiologic systems. The fertilized ovum contains the entire genetic complement—or encoded genetic instructions—to develop into a fully functioning term infant, given adequate nutrition and time. Three basic developmental processes—growth, **morphogenesis,** and cellular differentiation—are involved in this transformation.[7] Growth denotes the proliferation of new cells by mitosis, a necessary but not sufficient process for development. The arrangement of cells in a particular order is called morphogenesis and is essential to the elaboration of higher forms of life. In addition to growth and morphogenesis, cellular differentiation is needed for cells to specialize structurally and biochemically in a myriad of ways. This section describes the sequence of events in which growth, morphogenesis, and cellular differentiation function to transform a human zygote with encoded genetic information into a human infant. In addition, this section will describe the response of the mother's body to pregnancy. Information on genetic control of inheritance and genetic disorders is contained in Chapters 5 and 6, and the reader may wish to refer to these chapters for specific content in these areas.

Early Human Development

Fertilization of the ovum occurs in the oviduct. Within 24 hours after fertilization, the zygote begins a series of divisions, by the process of mitosis, that are referred to as cleavage (Figure 32-9). From a two-cell entity the zygote soon divides multiple times, and its cytoplasm begins to be partitioned into specific cells that will serve as the building blocks of the embryo. As more cleavage takes place, the embryo is transported through the oviduct to the uterus. This process takes about 4 days. The embryo receives nutrition during this time from secretions released by the epithelial cells lining the oviduct. After the embryo enters the uterus, the zona pellucida, the mem-

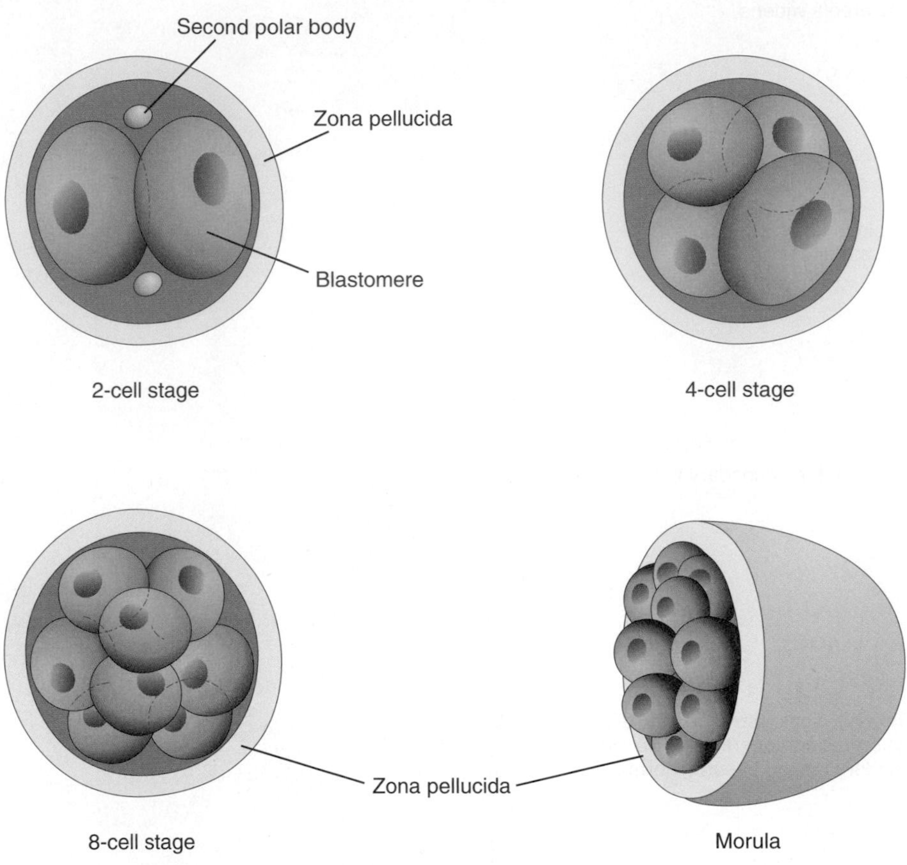

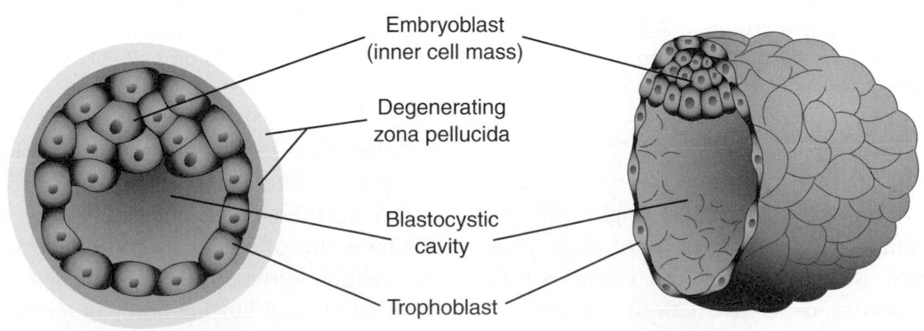

FIGURE 32-9 ■ Early human development. Drawings illustrate cleavage of the zygote and formation of the blastocyst. (From Moore KL, Persaud TVN: *The developing human: clinically oriented embryology,* ed 7, Philadelphia, 2003, Saunders, p 38.)

brane surrounding the embryo, dissolves. At about day 4, the embryo arrives in the uterus and floats freely while receiving nutrition from secretions from the endometrial glands stimulated by progesterone.

At this point the cells of the embryo have arranged themselves into a hollow spherical structure called the blastocyst (Figure 32-10). The outer cells of the blastocyst, called the trophoblast, will ultimately become the protective and nutritive membranes (chorion and placenta) that surround the developing embryo. The inner cell mass, a small cluster of cells that projects into the cavity of the blastocyst, will develop into the structures of the embryo itself. If at this point the inner cell mass divides into two separate groups of cells, identical twins with an identical genetic complement will result. Fraternal twins develop when two ova are fertilized by two sperm cells and do not have an identical genetic complement.[5]

Implantation

On approximately day 7 after fertilization, the embryo attaches to the uterine lining and then implants itself in the endometrium. Enzymes secreted by the trophoblast erode a small portion of the uterine lining, and by day 10 of development the embryo has worked its way down into the endometrium completely. The opening in the uterine lining is closed, initially by a blood clot and then by regeneration of uterine epithelium; all subsequent development of the embryo takes place in the wall of the uterus.[7]

Fetal Membranes and Placenta

Fetal membranes protect the developing embryo or fetus and provide needed substrates for growth and development, particularly oxygen and nutrition. In addition, they serve the purpose of elimination of waste products of metabolism. All terrestrial vertebrates have four fetal membranes: amnion, yolk sac, chorion, and allantois.[7] In the developing human, the yolk sac is usually thought to be a vestigial structure, although it serves as an important temporary center for the formation of blood cells between the second and sixth weeks. The allantois is also considered vestigial, although its blood supply contributes to formation of the umbilical vessels.

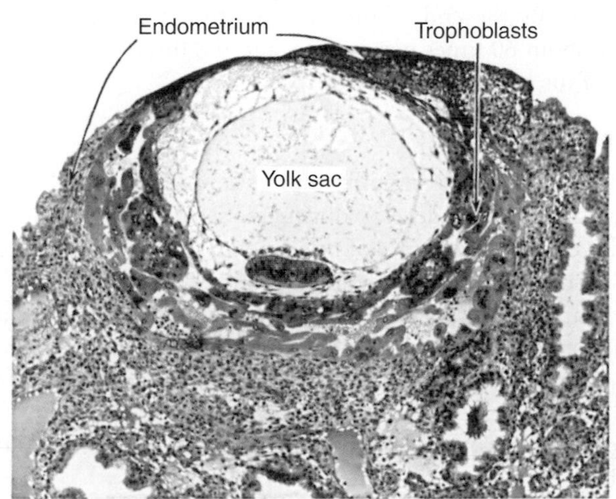

FIGURE 32-10 ■ Implantation of the early human embryo. (From Guyton AC, Hall JE: *Textbook of medical physiology,* ed 9, Philadelphia, 2000, Saunders, p 945. Courtesy Arthur Hertig, MD.)

The amnion begins to develop at a very early stage and eventually expands to surround the entire embryo. The space between the amnion and the embryo is called the **amniotic cavity**. It is filled with a clear amniotic fluid that keeps the embryo moist and provides a measure of protection against mechanical injury.

The **placenta** serves two basic functions. It is the organ of exchange between the developing fetus and the mother; nutrients are provided to the fetus and wastes removed. It is also an endocrine organ and produces several hormones, most notably hCG. The placenta develops from both the chorion and maternal uterine tissue. After implantation, the chorion develops rapidly and forms highly vascularized villi as the embryonic circulation develops. The umbilical cord develops and connects the embryo with the placenta. Two umbilical arteries arise in the umbilical cord and connect with a rapidly proliferating network of capillaries in the villi. The umbilical vein, also located in the umbilical cord, carries blood from the villi back to the fetus.

The placenta eventually consists of the portion of the chorion in which villi develop, along with the uterine tissue between the villi that contains maternal capillaries and small pools of maternal blood. The placenta brings maternal blood adjacent to fetal blood, although the two circulatory systems are completely separate from each other. Thus oxygen and nutrient substrates pass from the maternal blood through the placental tissue and diffuse into the blood of the fetus, where these substances can be used for growth and development of various body tissues. Waste products of fetal metabolism from fetal blood then pass through the placenta into the maternal blood supply and are eventually transported to the maternal kidneys for disposal.[7]

The placenta, like the corpus luteum, secretes both estrogen and progesterone during pregnancy. These hormones serve a variety of purposes in pregnancy. Estrogen promotes enlargement of the uterus and growth of the ductal structure of the breast, as well as alters the elasticity of various pelvic ligaments and the symphysis pubis to allow passage of the infant through the pelvic structures during delivery. In addition to its role in providing early nutrition for the embryo, progesterone has the special effect of decreasing contractility of the gravid uterus, thus preventing spontaneous abortion. In addition, progesterone may have a role in preparing the breasts for lactation, as described in an earlier section.

Of major importance in the role of the placenta as an endocrine gland is its production of hCG. From the time of implantation, the trophoblastic cells begin to secrete hCG, which sends a signal to the corpus luteum that a pregnancy has

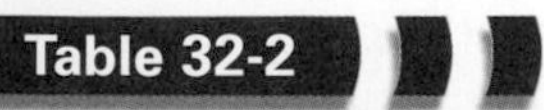

Summary of Developmental Events in Human Fetal Life

Time from Fertilization	Key Events
36 hr	Embryo has achieved two-cell stage
4th day	Embryo reaches the uterus
7th day	Implantation of the embryo in the uterine wall
2.5 wk	Differentiation of heart tissue
	Blood cell formation in the yolk sac and chorion
	Formation of the notochord and neural plate
3.5 wk	Formation of the neural tube
	Heart tubes begin to beat
	Primordial eye and ear visible
	Respiratory system begins development
	Liver bud differentiates
	Blood vessels established
4 wk	Formation of three primary brain vesicles
	Limb buds appear
2nd mo	Embryo capable of movement
	Cerebral cortex differentiating
	Gonad identifiable as testis or ovary
	Bones begin ossification and muscles are differentiating
	Major blood vessels in final positions
3rd mo	Fetus performs breathing and sucking movements
	Sex is clearly identifiable
5th mo	Heartbeat is audible with a stethoscope
	Fetus moves freely through the amniotic cavity
6th-9th mo	Rapid growth with final differentiation of tissues and ogans
266 days	Birth

begun. The corpus luteum responds by increasing its size and its secretion of estrogen and progesterone, which then promote continued development of the endometrium and the placenta. In the absence of hCG, the corpus luteum would disintegrate, as it does in a nonfertilized menstrual cycle, and the endometrium would deteriorate and be sloughed off along with the embryo. Thus, hCG is an essential element in continuation of the pregnant state.[7]

Development of the Human Embryo and Fetus

From fertilization to the end of the eighth week, the developing organism is referred to as an embryo; from the ninth week until birth, the developing baby is referred to as a fetus. Development of the fetus proceeds in an orderly sequence of complex events. With recent developments in fetal physiology, it is possible to predict which structures will begin their development or function on a particular day of development after conception. Table 32-2 depicts some important developmental events from the time of fertilization to birth. Detailed information on the development of organ systems during fetal life is contained in the chapters in this book that focus on these organ systems; for example, Chapter 35 contains a description of the development of the gastrointestinal tract.

First Month

Rapid growth, morphogenesis, and cell differentiation occur early in development of the human embryo. By 2½ weeks of development, the notochord and neural plate are formed; these structures eventually give rise to the central nervous system. In addition, the tissue that will form the heart has differentiated. By the end of the first month, an S-shaped heart beats about 60 times per minute, and the three primary vesicles of the brain have formed.

Second Month

Figure 32-11 shows an embryo in its seventh week. All of the organs continue to develop during the second month, and the embryo becomes capable of movement. The major blood vessels assume their final positions, and the heart assumes its final shape. The brain begins to transmit impulses to regulate function of the organ systems, and a few reflexes are now present. Although sex cannot be distinguished externally, either an ovary or testis has begun to form internally. At the end of the second month, the rudiments of all organs are present and the embryo is referred to as a fetus.[7]

Third Month

During the third month, the ears and eyes approach their final positions, and some of the bones become distinct. The fe-

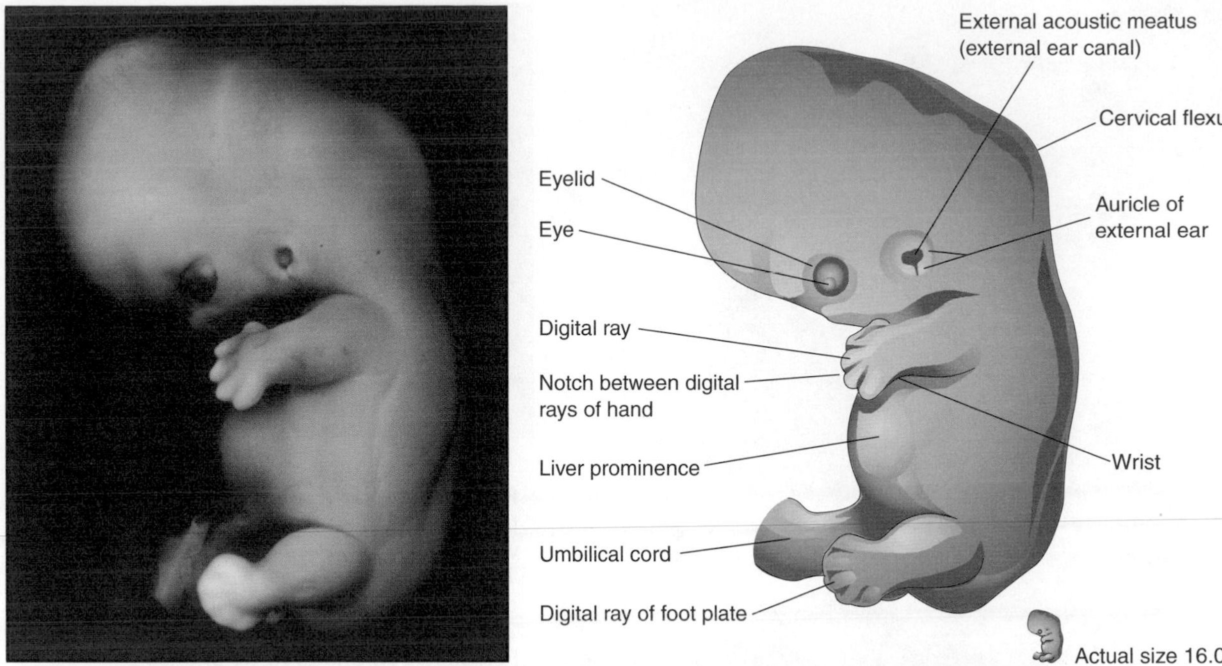

FIGURE 32-11 ■ **A** and **B,** Human embryo in the seventh week of development. (In Moore KL: *The developing human: clinically oriented embryology,* ed 7, Philadelphia, 2003, Saunders, p 93. **A,** Courtesy Kazumasa Hoshino, MD, former Professor of Anatomy and Director of the Congenital Anomaly Center, Faculty of Medicine, Kyoto University, Japan. **B,** From Moore KL, Persaud TVN: *The developing human: clinically oriented embryology,* ed 7, Philadelphia, 2003, Saunders, p 93.)

tus performs breathing movements consisting of moving amniotic fluid in and out of the lungs and can carry on sucking movements. By the end of the third month, the fetus is almost 56 mm in length and weighs about 14 g (Figure 32-12).

Second Trimester

A trimester refers to a period of 3 months during pregnancy. During the second trimester, or months 4 through 6 of development, the fetus achieves independent mobility and can move freely through the amniotic cavity. The heartbeat of the fetus is now audible through a stethoscope and averages 150 beats per minute. By the fifth month of development, the fetus measures 250 mm (10 inches) in length, which is half its total length at birth.[7] Figure 32-13 shows a fetus in the second trimester at 17 weeks of development.

Third Trimester

By far the greatest growth of the fetus occurs during the third trimester. The weight of the fetus almost doubles during the

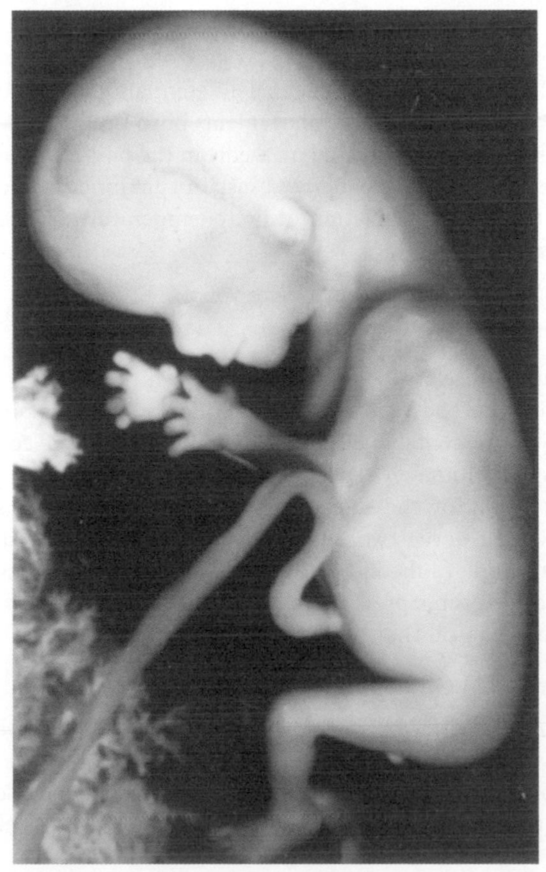

FIGURE 32-12 ■ Photograph of the human fetus at 11 weeks of development. (From Moore KL, Persaud TVN: *The developing human: clinically oriented embryology,* ed 7, Philadelphia, 2003, Saunders, p 106. Courtesy Professor Jean Hay [Retired], Department of Anatomy, University of Manitoba, Winnipeg, Canada.)

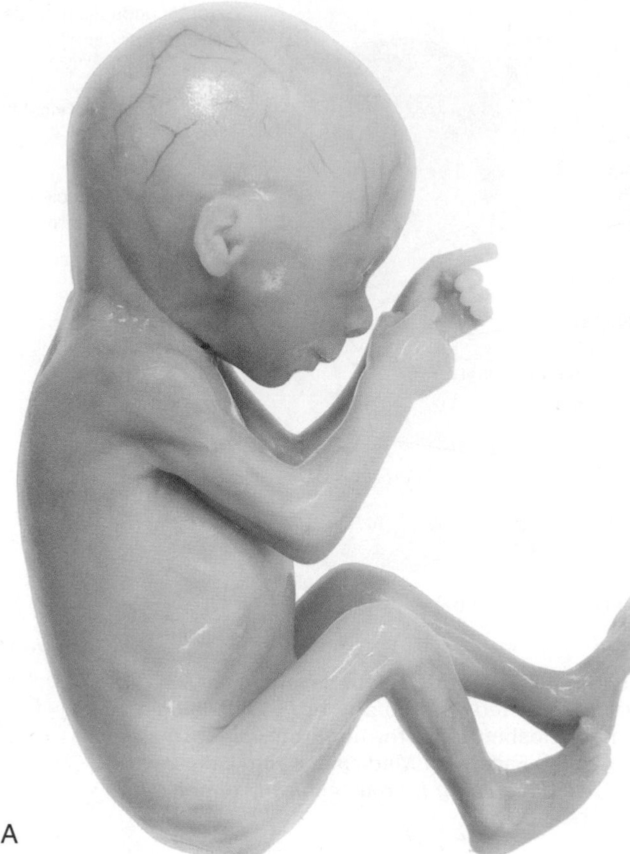

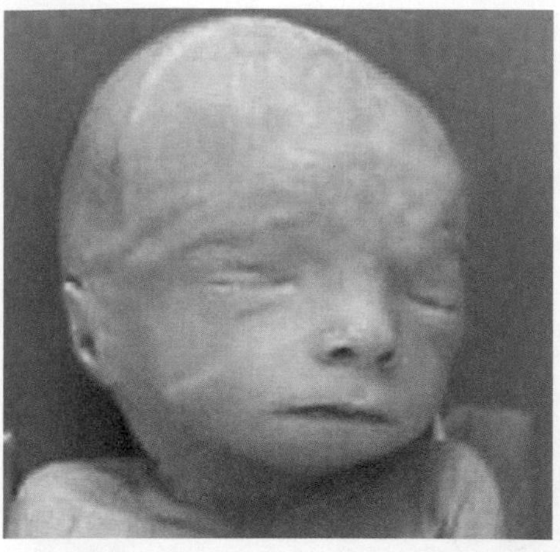

FIGURE 32-13 ■ **A,** Side view of human fetus at 17 weeks. **B,** Frontal view of 17-week fetus. (In Moore KL, Persaud TVN: *The developing human: clinically oriented embryology,* ed 7, Philadelphia, 2003, Saunders. **A,** From Moore KL, Persaud TVN, Shiota K: *Color atlas of clinical embryology,* ed 2, Philadelphia, 2000, Saunders. **B,** Courtesy Dr. Robert Jordan, St. Georges University Medical School, Grenada.)

last 2 months.[11] In addition, final differentiation of tissues and organs takes place. Survival of infants born prematurely during this time has increased markedly in the past few years because of an enhanced ability to sustain vital functions such as respiration and regulation of body temperature in neonatal intensive care settings.

Parturition

Parturition refers to the process by which the infant is born. Toward the end of pregnancy, the uterus becomes progressively more excitable until it begins strong rhythmic contractions that ultimately expel the infant.[11] At the present time, the exact cause of the increased uterine activity remains unknown. However, two sets of effects have been suggested as contributing to the increased excitability of uterine musculature at this time: progressive hormonal changes and progressive mechanical changes.[11,13]

Hormonal Changes

During the latter part of pregnancy, large amounts of estrogen, which has a definite tendency to increase uterine contractility, are secreted. Concurrent with this enhanced estrogen release, the secretion of progesterone, which inhibits uterine contractility, remains constant or may decrease slightly. Thus it is hypothesized that the increased ratio of estrogen to progesterone secretion in the latter part of pregnancy may promote the increased contractility of the uterus.[11]

Oxytocin is a hormone secreted by the posterior pituitary that specifically causes uterine contraction and is thought to have a major role in promoting increased uterine contractility during parturition. The rate of oxytocin secretion is considerably increased at the time of labor (see the following discussion of mechanical changes), and the uterus displays increased responsiveness to a given dose of oxytocin at this time.[11,13]

Mechanical Changes

Stretching smooth muscle organs increases their contractility; in addition, intermittent stretching of smooth muscle can elicit contraction. Thus it is hypothesized that the stretch or irritation of the fetal head against the cervix begins a reflex action that causes the uterus to contract. As the cycle of stretching and contraction is repeated again and again, increased contractions result. In addition, stretching of the cervix causes the release of oxytocin from the posterior pituitary. Oxytocin then stimulates additional uterine contractions, thus initiating another feedback cycle of stretching and contraction.[11,14]

Response of the Mother's Body to Pregnancy

The presence of a developing fetus in the uterus creates an extra physiologic load for the pregnant woman, with resulting effects on her basal metabolism and specific organ systems. Normal physiologic responses to pregnancy are described here; complications of pregnancy are discussed in Chapter 33.

Metabolism During Pregnancy

As a result of increased secretion of many hormones, including thyroxine, adrenocortical hormones, and the sex hormones, the basal metabolic rate increases by about 15% during the latter half of pregnancy.[11] This increase in metabolism results in alterations in many organ systems, including the circulatory, respiratory, and urinary systems.

Changes in the Female Reproductive Organs

The hormones secreted during pregnancy, either by the placenta or the endocrine glands, directly promote alterations in body structures. In particular, the organs of the female reproductive tract increase markedly in size, with the uterus increasing from 30 to 1100 g and the breasts approximately doubling in size. Concurrently, the vagina enlarges with a widening of the vaginal introitus.

Changes in the Circulatory System

In the latter stages of pregnancy, about 625 ml of blood flows through the maternal circulation of the placenta each minute. This factor, along with a general increase in metabolism, causes an increase in maternal cardiac output to 30% to 40% above normal by the 27th week of pregnancy. However, for reasons not understood at the present time, cardiac output decreases to a little above normal during the last 8 weeks of pregnancy, although the high uterine blood flow continues.[11]

As shown in Figure 32-14, an increase in maternal blood volume occurs mainly during the latter half of pregnancy. This increase is mainly due to hormonal factors. Both aldosterone and estrogens, which are greatly increased in pregnancy, promote increased fluid retention by the kidneys. In addition, bone marrow increases its activity to produce an excess of red blood cells to accompany the excess vascular volume. At the time of parturition, the mother has an additional 1 to 2 extra liters of blood in her circulatory system.[11]

Changes in the Respiratory System

The increased basal metabolic rate and size of the pregnant woman result in an increase in oxygen utilization, with utilization of oxygen being 20% above normal at the time of birth. Concurrently, a commensurate amount of carbon dioxide is formed. In addition, the growing uterus is pressing upward against the abdominal organs, which in turn press against the diaphragm and cause a decrease in diaphragmatic excursion. The net result of these changes is an increase in minute ventilation of approximately 50% and a decrease in arterial P_{CO_2} to slightly below normal.[11]

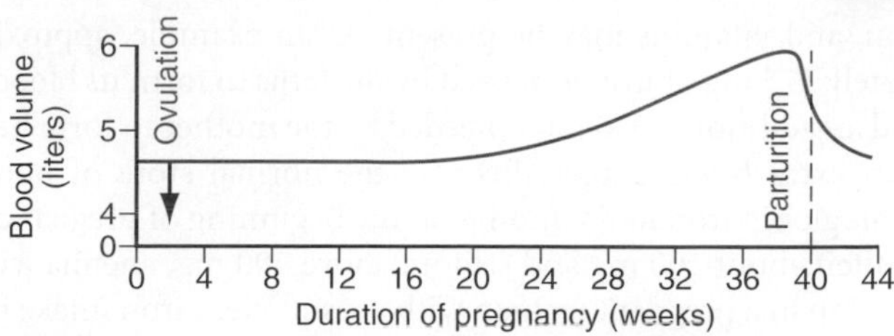

FIGURE 32-14 ■ Effect of pregnancy on blood volume. (From Guyton AC, Hall JE: *Textbook of medical physiology,* ed 10, Philadelphia, 2000, Saunders, p 951.)

Changes in the Urinary System

Because of an increased load of excretory products, the rate of urine formation in pregnancy is usually slightly increased. In addition, other alterations in urinary function occur. Renal tubule reabsorption of sodium, chloride, and water is increased as a result of increased production of steroidal hormones by the placenta and adrenal cortex. Concurrently, the glomerular filtration rate often increases by as much as 50%, a change that serves to increase the rate of water and electrolyte loss in the urine. These two events tend to balance each other out, with the result that only a moderate excess of water and salt accumulation occurs under normal circumstances.[11] However, in the condition of toxemia of pregnancy, excess water and salt accumulation may occur with life-threatening consequences.

Weight Gain and Nutrition During Pregnancy

The average weight gain during pregnancy is about 24 lb, with most of this gain occurring during the last two trimesters. Approximately 7 lb of this weight gain is the fetus; 4 lb of the increased weight is amniotic fluid, placenta, and fetal membranes; 2 lb represents an increase in uterine tissue; and another 2 lb of the weight gain is an increase in breast tissue. Thus an average 9-lb increase in weight occurs in the remainder of the woman's body. Approximately 6 lb of fluid may be excreted during the days following birth, after loss of the fluid-retaining hormones of the placenta.[11]

Appetite may be greatly increased during the latter part of pregnancy, in part because of fetal removal of food substrates from the mother's blood and partly because of hormonal factors. The developing fetus assumes priority in regard to many of the nutritional substrates of the mother's body fluids and will continue to grow even when maternal nutrition is inadequate. However, although fetal length may increase normally in the absence of adequate maternal nutrition, fetal weight will be considerably decreased, and abnormal bone formation and decreased size of many bodily organs of the fetus may result.[11]

If the intake of nutritional elements during pregnancy is inadequate, a number of deficiencies can be present in the mother. In particular, deficiencies of calcium, phosphates, iron, and vitamins may be present. As an example, approximately 375 mg of iron is needed by the fetus to form its blood, and an additional 600 mg is needed by the mother to form her own extra blood supply. Because the normal store of nonhemoglobin iron in the mother at the beginning of pregnancy is often about 100 mg and seldom above 700 mg, anemia will develop in a pregnant woman without sufficient iron intake in her food.[11] Important also is adequate folic acid intake, which has been shown to help prevent neural tube defects.[15]

KEY CONCEPTS

- At about the seventh day after fertilization, the embryo attaches to the uterine lining. The placenta is the fetal lifeline that provides nutrients and oxygen and eliminates wastes. The placenta also secretes hCG, which is important in maintaining pregnancy.
- Normal gestation is about 9 months. Each 3-month period is called a trimester. By the end of the first trimester, fetal structures and organ systems are present. During the second and third trimesters, the fetus grows in size and weight.
- Near the end of the third trimester, an increase in estrogen production and mechanical stretching of the uterus and cervix are thought to induce parturition. Cervical stretching stimulates the release of oxytocin from the pituitary. Oxytocin stimulates uterine contractions.
- Pregnancy is associated with many physiologic changes, including an increased basal metabolic rate (15%), increased cardiac output (30% to 40%) and blood volume (1 to 2 L), increased oxygen consumption (20%) and minute ventilation (50%), increased glomerular filtration rate and tubular reabsorption of sodium and water, and increased body weight (24 lb).

MENOPAUSE

Although **menopause** is defined specifically as the last menstrual period in a woman's reproductive life, the term is often used to denote the entire period of years before and after this event in which the function of the ovaries is in transition. The terms *climacteric* and *perimenopause* are used in the health care literature to describe this transitional period. At about 45 to 52 years of age the supply of ovarian follicles declines, with the majority becoming atretic or degenerated. With the depletion of ovarian follicles, secretion of estrogen and progesterone by the ovaries declines, and the menstrual cycle becomes irregular. When too little estrogen is secreted to cause endometrial growth, menstrual periods stop permanently.[11]

The decline in ovarian hormone production that occurs in the perimenopausal period causes important physiologic changes in a woman's body. The decline in plasma estrogen levels may result in a number of distressing symptoms, although some women experience no symptoms during this time. Hot flashes, described by women as an unpleasant sensation of sudden warmth sweeping upward over the abdomen, chest, neck, and face, are experienced by nearly 75% of postmenopausal women. Although the precise cause of hot flashes is unknown, it is thought that decreased estrogen levels have an effect on the temperature-regulating center in the hypothalamus. Hot flashes are often accompanied by other symptoms of autonomic nervous system instability such as tachycardia, palpitations, and feelings of faintness. Other distressing symptoms, including pain and stiffness in the joints, sleep pattern disturbances, and changes in gastrointestinal function, have been noted by women in the perimenopausal period. These symptoms are presently the focus of many nursing research projects examining the health of aging women. Although such psychological symptoms as increased nervousness have been reported in the medical literature as being related to hormonal imbalance in menopause, it has been established that psychological symptoms are not directly related to estrogen deficiency.[16,17]

With the decline in estrogen associated with perimenopause, many structural changes occur in various organs. These changes are summarized in The Aging Process: Changes in the Female Reproductive System. The epidermis of the skin becomes thinner and less elastic throughout the entire body. The breasts may decrease in size; the labia may also lose their underlying fat and become thinner.[18] The vaginal epithelium may become thin and atrophied, with the result that sexual intercourse may be painful. The decline in estrogen also leads to osteoporosis and decreased bone density, particularly in white women, with resulting bone fractures. Exercise and supplemental calcium and vitamin D are recommended for postmenopausal women to prevent accelerated bone loss. At present, some authorities recommend estrogen therapy during the perimenopausal period to prevent osteoporosis and relieve symptoms such as hot flashes and vaginal atrophy. However, supplemental estrogen and progestin therapy has been associated with an increased risk of breast cancer and cardiovascular disease.[19] Newer treatments that have been developed for osteoporosis include bisphosphonates, calcitonin nasal spray, and raloxiphene.[20] Work continues on the development of selective estrogen receptor modulators that may retain some of the beneficial effects of estrogen while avoiding the bad effects.[21] Women in perimenopause may wish to discuss the risks and potential benefits of hormone replacement therapy and other menopausal therapies with their health care providers before making an informed decision about these medications.

KEY CONCEPTS

- Menopause begins at 45 to 52 years of age and denotes the cessation of menstruation. A declining supply of ovarian follicles with decreased estrogen and progesterone production results in irregular menses and then complete cessation of menstruation.

THE AGING PROCESS

Changes in the Female Reproductive System

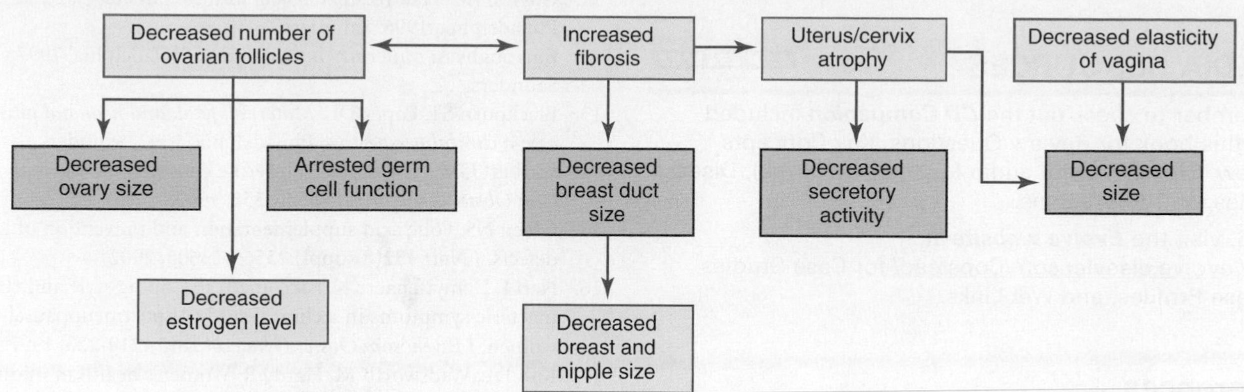

Female reproductive system function declines with organ-specific tissue changes. Active female germ cells decline over time with variable function before they are arrested in menopause. The ovaries become smaller and increasingly fibrotic and have fewer ovarian follicles.

The secretion of estrogen by the ovaries stops at menopause, resulting in a marked estrogen level decrease. The ovarian follicles become insensitive to gonadotropins (FSH and luteinizing hormone). However, the peripheral conversion of androgens to estrogen causes a small maintenance level of estrogen to persist at 10% to 30% of previous levels. The androgen-producing ovarian cells (hilar and thecal) continue to secrete testosterone in postmenopausal women.

The follicles, uterus, and cervix undergo atrophy with a decrease in size and secretory action. The vagina is reduced in size with a loss of elasticity and atrophy of the vaginal epithelium. The vascular supply to the vaginal walls decreases with reduced glycogen and mucopolysaccharide. The pH of Bartholin gland secretions is increased or alkaline due to the loss of estrogen.

The breasts decrease in size. Breast ducts become smaller and are replaced by fat tissue. Some fibrosis and calcification may occur within the ducts. The nipples are smaller with less nipple pigmentation. The aging female nipple may be normal or retracted.

◆ Declines in estrogen production are associated with hot flashes, tachycardia, palpitations, faintness, joint pain, and sleep disturbance. Structural changes associated with menopause include osteoporosis, thinning of the skin, and atrophy of the vaginal structures and breast tissue.

SUMMARY

This chapter has described the major processes related to the human female reproductive tract, including the menstrual cycle, pregnancy, lactation, and menopause. In approaching this material, the reader must view the information presented within the current context of social change in which women are taking an active role in meeting their health care needs. In addition, recent research in the area of reproductive endocrinology has yielded a rapidly expanding understanding of the reproductive structures and their function.

The female reproductive structures are a complex set of organs with multiple, integrated functions. Careful review of the section on reproductive structures, including their embryologic development, will assist the reader in understanding the various alterations in these structures that occur throughout a woman's life. Although the hormonal and structural changes occurring in the female reproductive organs may at first seem overwhelmingly complex to the student, some basic concepts will help in organizing this material. First, the menstrual cycle has two significant results: production of an ovum and preparation of the uterus for implantation of the fertilized ovum. Second, the fertilized ovum contains the entire encoded genetic instructions to produce a unique human individual. Third, pregnancy consists of three basic developmental processes—growth, morphogenesis, and cellular differentiation—to bring about this transformation, which will also result in multiple changes in the body of the mother. The breast, with its function of lactation, is also a component of the reproductive system and is subject to alterations throughout a woman's life span. Finally, menopause is not a discrete event but rather a process during which the supply of ovarian follicles declines. A review of these concepts will prepare the student for a better understanding of women's health concerns and provide a basis for approaching the next chapter, which considers alterations in reproductive functioning.

MEDIA RESOURCES

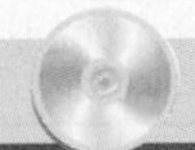

evolve

Remember to check out the ***CD Companion*** included with this book for Review Questions, Key Concepts Review, Glossary (with audio for selected terms), Disease Profiles, and Animations.

PLUS, visit the ***Evolve website*** at http://evolve.elsevier.com/Copstead/ for Case Studies, Disease Profiles, and WebLinks.

References

1. Wilmoth MC: The middle years: women, sexuality, and the self, *J Obstet Gynecol Neonatal Nurs* 25(7):615-621, 1996.
2. Sulak PJ: The perimenopause: a critical time in a woman's life, *Int J Fertil Menopausal Stud* 41(2):85-89, 1996.
3. Josso N: Anatomy and endocrinology of fetal sex differentiation. In DeGroot LJ, Jameson JL, editor: *Endocrinology,* ed 4, Philadelphia, 2001, Saunders.
4. Capel B: Sex in the 90s: SRY and the switch to the male pathway, *Annu Rev Physiol* 69:497-523, 1998.
5. Nichols FH, Zwelling E: *Maternal-newborn nursing,* Philadelphia, 1997, Saunders.
6. Black JM, Matassarin-Jacobs E: *Medical-surgical nursing,* ed 5, Philadelphia, 1997, Saunders.
7. Solomon EP: *Introduction to human anatomy and physiology,* Philadelphia, 1992, Saunders.
8. Apter D: Development of the hypothalamic-pituitary-ovarian axis, *Ann N Y Acad Sci* 17(816):9-21, 1997.
9. Guyton AC, Hall JE: *Human physiology and mechanisms of disease,* ed 6, Philadelphia, 1996, Saunders.
10. Genazzani AR et al: Neuroendocrinology of the menstrual cycle, *Ann N Y Acad Sci* 17(816):143-150, 1997.
11. Guyton AC, Hall JE: *Textbook of medical physiology,* ed 9, Philadelphia, 1996, Saunders.
12. Burroughs A: *Maternity nursing,* ed 9, Philadelphia, 1997, Saunders.
13. Blackburn ST, Loper DL: *Maternal, fetal, and neonatal physiology: a clinical perspective,* Philadelphia, 1992, Saunders.
14. Harbert GM: Assessment of uterine contractility and activity, *Clin Obstet Gynecol* 35(3):546-558, 1992.
15. Green NS: Folic acid supplementation and prevention of birth defects, *J Nutr* 132(8 suppl):23565-23605, 2002.
16. Neri I, Demyttenaere K, Facchinetti F: Coping style and climacteric symptoms in a clinical study of postmenopausal women, *J Psychosom Obstet Gynaecol* 18(3):219-223, 1997.
17. Kuh DL, Wadsworth M, Hardy R: Women's health in midlife: the influence of the menopause, social factors and health in earlier life, *Br J Obstet Gynaecol* 104(8):923-933, 1997.
18. Barhan S, Ezenagu L: Vulvar problems in elderly women, *Postgrad Med* 1102(3):121-125, 1997.
19. Writing Group for the Women's Health Initiative Investigators: Risks and benefits of estrogen plus progestin in healthy postmenopausal women: principal results from the Women's Health Initiative randomized controlled trial, *JAMA* 288:321-333, 2002.
20. Johnell O et al: Additive effects of raloxifene and alendronate on bone density and biochemical markers of bone remodeling in postmenopausal women with osteoporosis, *J Clin Endocrinol Metab* 87:985-992, 2002.
21. Riggs BL, Hartmann LC: Selective estrogen-receptor modulators: mechanisms of action and application to clinical practice, *N Engl J Med* 348:618-629, 2003.

Alterations in Female Genital and Reproductive Function

chapter 33

Paul D. Silva • Jane M. Georges

MEDIA RESOURCES

Additional Material for Study, Review, and Further Exploration

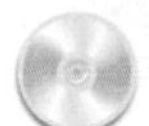

CD Companion ◆ Review Questions and Answers ◆ Key Concepts Review
◆ Glossary *(with audio pronunciations for selected terms)*
◆ Disease Profiles ◆ Animations

evolve ***Website*** at http://evolve.elsevier.com/Copstead/
◆ Case Studies ◆ Disease Profiles ◆ WebLinks

KEY QUESTIONS

- What are the differentiating factors of the common menstrual disorders?
- What are the common etiologic factors leading to uterine prolapse, uterine retrodisplacement, cystocele, and rectocele?
- How can the pain of endometriosis be differentiated from that of dysmenorrhea?
- What is the rationale for routine Papanicolaou testing for cervical cancer?
- What factors contribute to the high mortality rate of ovarian cancer?
- What clinical findings would indicate the development of pregnancy-induced hypertension, placenta previa, and abruptio placentae in a pregnant woman?
- How can benign and malignant breast lumps be clinically differentiated?

CHAPTER OUTLINE

The complex functioning of the female reproductive system described in Chapter 32 may be subject to alterations in structure and function throughout a woman's life that can have far-reaching effects on her health and well-being. This chapter is a survey of these alterations and describes the pathophysiologic basis of the most common disorders of the female reproductive system. In addition, current therapeutics for these alterations, including pharmacologic therapy, will be summarized. The information presented here is an introduction to these complex areas, and the reader may wish to consult in-depth gynecology and obstetrics texts for more detailed information.

Perhaps no other function of the human body is so closely linked to psychological, social, and spiritual concerns as reproductive function. Any alteration in reproductive status (or the perceived threat of such an alteration) may have profound effects on an individual. Clinicians caring for women experiencing alterations in functioning of the reproductive system should bear in mind the profundity of such alterations for the individual woman and must also maintain an awareness of the context in which women seek help for such problems. A clinical approach in which information is freely shared between caregiver and client and in which mutual decision making is an integral part of the therapeutic environment is a necessary component of care for women seeking help for reproductive concerns. Previous clinical approaches in which women's concerns were labeled as unimportant or merely psychogenic often resulted in anger, frustration with health care providers, and withdrawal from the health care delivery system. Women consumers of health care are now seeking active involvement in their own care, and clinicians who care for women experiencing the alterations described in this chapter need to approach women's health concerns with sensitivity and openness.

MENSTRUAL DISORDERS

Alterations in the normal functioning of the menstrual cycle include amenorrhea (no menses), abnormal uterine bleeding patterns, and dysmenorrhea (painful menstruation). Although many pathologic conditions can cause these alterations, an obvious cause is often not found.

Amenorrhea

Etiology and Pathogenesis. Amenorrhea is the absence or suppression of menstruation. Amenorrhea is normal before menarche (the first menstrual period at the time of puberty), after menopause, and during pregnancy and lactation.[1] At other times it is considered pathologic and may result from a wide range of pathophysiologic causes (Figure 33-1). In the majority of cases, amenorrhea is due to an abnormal pattern of hormonal functioning that interrupts the normal sequence of events in which the endometrial tissue lining the uterus proliferates and then sloughs off. The endometrial tissue must be stimulated and regulated by the correct quantity and sequence of the female sex hormones estrogen and progesterone and the gonadotropic hormones follicle-stimulating hormone (FSH) and luteinizing hormone (LH). As described in Chapter 32, the menstrual cycle is dependent on the sequential changes in estrogen and progesterone levels. The initial rise in LH and FSH in the menstrual cycle occurs in response to a decline in estrogen and progesterone; estrogen levels then rise again in response to actions of the gonadotropic hormones, and the endometrium proliferates again in response to estrogen secretion. Thus events that prevent estrogen production, interfere with the normal fluctuations in estrogen levels, or block the action of estrogen on the endometrium will result in abnormal or absent menstrual flow.[2] Such events may include physical or emotional stress, which can interfere with normal production of the gonadotropic hormones and alter the

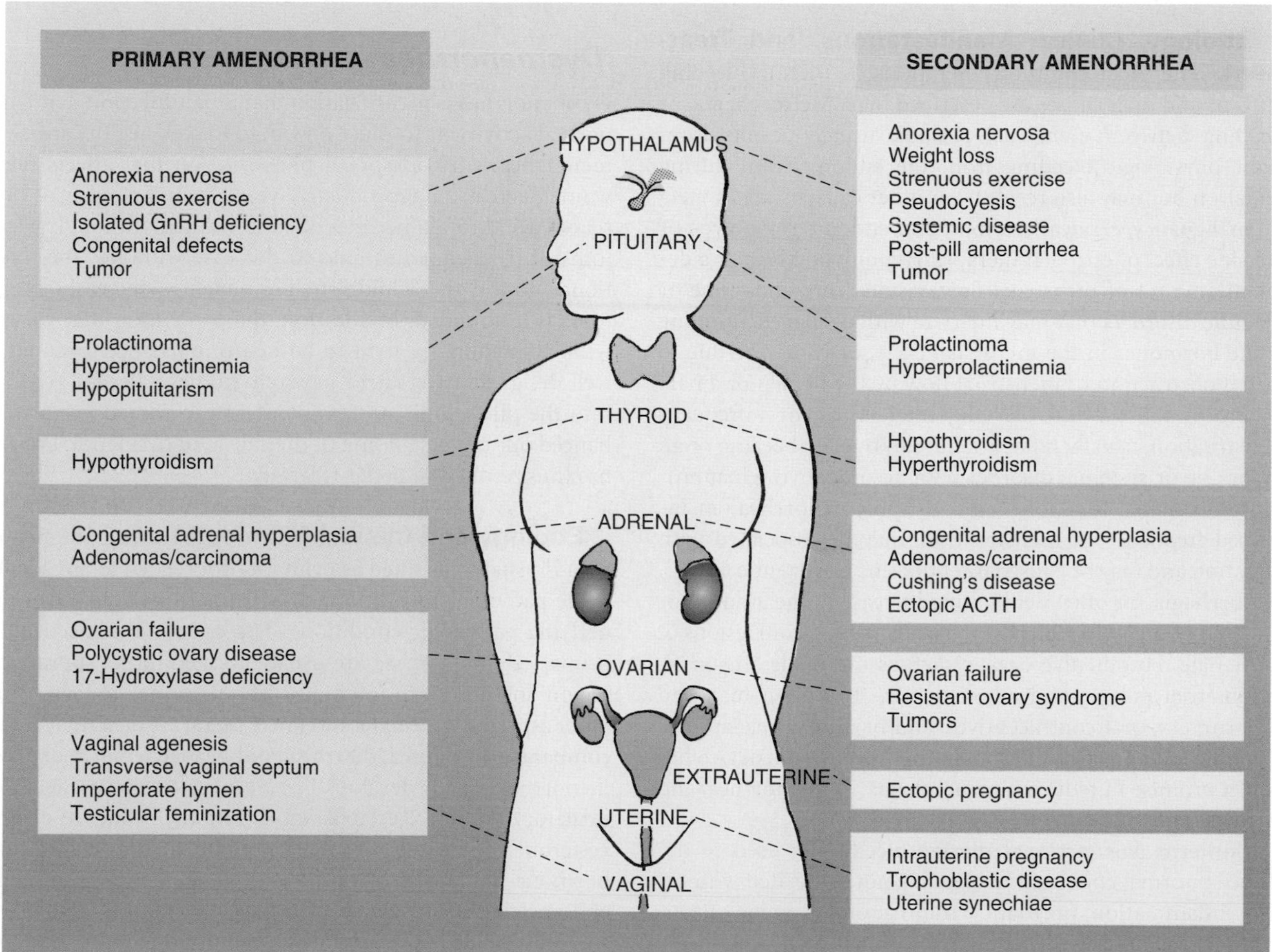

FIGURE 33-1 ■ Causes of amenorrhea. *GnRH,* Gonadotropin-releasing hormone; *ACTH,* adrenocorticotropic hormone. (From Black JM, Hawks JH: *Medical-surgical nursing: clinical management for positive outcomes,* ed 7, Philadelphia, 2005, Saunders, p 1058.)

pattern of estrogen functioning. In addition, ovarian, adrenal, or pituitary tumors may interfere with the normal production of female sex hormones or LH and FSH. Neoplasms of the ovaries or adrenal and pituitary glands may result in excess or deficient production of these hormones, with a consequent interruption in normal menstrual flow.

Treatment. Therapeutic strategies for amenorrhea are directed to correcting the cause of the interruption in hormonal functioning and may include the use of hormonal supplementation to reinstate a normal sequence of events in the menstrual cycle. If amenorrhea is the result of a neoplastic process, surgery may be indicated for tumor removal.

Abnormal Uterine Bleeding Patterns

Irregular or excessive bleeding from the uterus is one of the most common alterations in the female reproductive system. Uterine bleeding that varies from a woman's normal pattern either in quantity or in frequency may occur at any age and for a variety of reasons.

Etiology, Clinical Manifestations, and Treatment. The most common alterations in uterine bleeding patterns and their causes are described here. **Metrorrhagia,** or bleeding between menstrual periods, usually results from slight physiologic bleeding from the endometrium during ovulation but may also result from other causes such as uterine malignancy, cervical erosions, and endometrial polyps or as a side effect of estrogen therapy.[1] **Hypomenorrhea,** or a deficient amount of menstrual flow, results from endocrine or systemic disorders that may interfere with proper functioning of the hormones in the menstrual cycle, or it may be due to partial obstruction of menstrual flow by the hymen or a narrowing of the cervical os. **Oligomenorrhea,** or infrequent menstruation, usually reflects failure to ovulate because of an endocrine or systemic disorder with accompanying inappropriate hormonal function. Similarly, **polymenorrhea,** an increased frequency of menstruation, may be associated with ovulation and may be caused by endocrine or systemic factors. **Menorrhagia,** an often debilitating increase in the amount or duration of menstrual bleeding, usually results from lesions of the female reproductive organs such as uterine leiomyomas, endometrial polyps, and adenomyosis. It is often managed with surgery, oral contraceptives, and/or antiprostaglandins. More recently, a progestin-containing intrauterine device has shown promise in reducing menorrhagia, dysmenorrhea, and anemia.[3]

The term **dysfunctional uterine bleeding** is used to describe abnormal endometrial bleeding not associated with tumor, inflammation, pregnancy, trauma, or hormonal effects. Dysfunctional uterine bleeding is most common around the time of menarche and menopause and not as common in women between the ages of 20 and 35.[2,4] In adolescents, dysfunctional uterine bleeding is most often due to immaturity in functioning of the pituitary and ovary, which have not yet properly orchestrated their activities.[5] Thus an imbalance may be present in the ratio of estrogen to progesterone. Absent or diminished levels of progesterone will result in a thick and extremely vascular endometrium that lacks structural support. As a result of this fragile structure, spontaneous and superficial hemorrhage occurs randomly throughout the endometrium. In addition, the blood vessels in the endometrium fail to constrict to limit the extent and duration of bleeding.[2] Uterine bleeding that is abnormal in both quantity and frequency can therefore occur in a noncyclic pattern.

In perimenopausal women, dysfunctional uterine bleeding may be the result of progressive degeneration and failure of the ovary to produce estrogen. As the number of ovarian follicles diminishes, the production of estrogen by the ovary becomes unpredictable, and the secretion of LH and FSH may also assume an unpredictable pattern. As in adolescents with dysfunctional uterine bleeding, diminished or absent production of progesterone may result in unopposed stimulation of the endometrium by estrogen, with subsequent unpredictable bleeding from a fragile endometrium.[2]

Dysmenorrhea

Dysmenorrhea is menstruation that is painful enough to limit normal activity or to cause a woman to seek health care. Dysmenorrhea is a widespread phenomenon that affects many women across the reproductive years, including girls of high school age through perimenopausal women. Although symptoms of dysmenorrhea tend to decrease with age, the traditional notion that childbirth permanently decreases symptoms is unfounded. In addition, the contention that women with dysmenorrhea tend to be neurotic has been refuted in well-designed psychiatric research studies.[2] Recent research into the physiologic process of uterine contractions has enhanced our understanding of the causes of dysmenorrhea and has thus resulted in better treatment.

Etiology and Clinical Manifestations. Dysmenorrhea is usually classified as primary (not related to any identifiable pathologic condition) or secondary (related to an underlying pathologic condition). The cramps that occur with primary dysmenorrhea are usually located in the suprapubic region and are sharp in quality. The pain may radiate to the inner aspect of the thighs and lower sacral area and may be accompanied by nausea, diarrhea, and headache.[2] Primary dysmenorrhea usually develops 1 or 2 years after menarche, when ovulatory cycles are established. Under the influence of progesterone, increased amounts of prostaglandins, potent hormone-like unsaturated fatty acids, are released from the endometrium. Prostaglandins have significant effects on smooth muscle and vasomotor tone; when released from the endometrium, prostaglandins promote uterine contractions and ischemia of the endometrial capillaries and thereby cause the cramping pain of dysmenorrhea.[3]

Secondary dysmenorrhea is characterized more often by dull pain that may increase with age. It is associated with pelvic disorders such as endometriosis, leiomyomas, or pelvic adhesions.[5]

Treatment. Recent therapeutic strategies for the management of primary dysmenorrhea have focused on the phenomenon of prostaglandin-induced enhanced uterine contractility. The use of prostaglandin synthetase inhibitors such as ibuprofen and naproxen, which inhibit the formation of prostaglandins, has been very effective in many women experiencing dysmenorrhea.[2] Other approaches that use steroid hormones, such as progestins or combined high-progestin/low-estrogen oral contraceptives, have also been advocated. The rationale is that production of the high menstrual levels of prostaglandins needed to produce dysmenorrhea requires high levels of estrogen without progesterone in the proliferative phase of the menstrual cycle. Progestin administration therefore inhibits the production of prostaglandins and relieves the symptoms of dysmenorrhea.[2] However, the use of steroid hormones may involve significant risks, which the individual client must weigh against the benefits of such therapy.

Therapeutic strategies for secondary dysmenorrhea may involve diagnostic operative procedures such as laparoscopy, as well as medical and surgical therapy for the underlying condition.[3]

KEY CONCEPTS

- Amenorrhea, the absence of menstruation, is most commonly due to hormonal disturbances. Stress and neoplasms (ovarian, adrenal, or pituitary tumors) may interfere with the normal patterns of hormone secretion. Treatment is aimed at the underlying cause of the hormonal imbalance.
- Irregular or excessive uterine bleeding is a common problem. Metrorrhagia is bleeding between periods, hypomenorrhea is reduced menstrual flow, oligomenorrhea is infrequent menstruation, polymenorrhea is an increased frequency of menstruation, and menorrhagia is prolonged and heavy bleeding during menstruation. These disorders may be associated with hormonal imbalances or primary lesions of the reproductive tract.
- Dysfunctional uterine bleeding is common at menarche and menopause and is due to irregular secretion of reproductive hormones. Other causes of abnormal bleeding, such as tumor, trauma, inflammation, and endocrine diseases, are ruled out before a diagnosis of dysfunctional uterine bleeding is made.
- Dysmenorrhea is painful menstruation, generally described as sharp suprapubic cramping severe enough to limit activity. Dysmenorrhea may be treated with prostaglandin inhibitors. Dysmenorrhea secondary to pelvic disorders (endometriosis, adhesions) generally has a dull quality and may increase with age.

ALTERATIONS IN UTERINE POSITION AND PELVIC SUPPORT

Alterations in uterine position and pelvic support may occur anytime during a woman's reproductive years. The major support for the uterus and upper part of the vagina is provided by the thickenings of the endopelvic fascia known as the cardinal ligaments. Although tearing of the cardinal ligaments during labor and delivery is rare, they can be stretched abnormally during a difficult or prolonged delivery and subsequently fail to support the pelvic organs adequately.[4] In addition, congenital defects in the muscles of the pelvic floor may promote alterations in position of the uterus and other pelvic structures. The two most common alterations in uterine position are **uterine prolapse** and **retrodisplacement** of the uterus. Other commonly occurring alterations resulting from a weakening of the vaginal and pelvic floor musculature are **cystocele** and **rectocele.**

Uterine Prolapse

Etiology. The axis of the uterus normally forms an acute angle with the axis of the vagina. This anatomic feature itself tends to prevent a prolapse, or sinking, of the uterus from its normal position. Descent of the uterus occurs when supporting structures, such as the uterosacral ligaments and the cardinal ligaments, relax and allow the relationship of the uterus to the vaginal axis to be altered. This relaxation permits the cervix to sag downward into the vagina. If the support of the vaginal wall is also compromised, the pressure of the abdominal organs on the uterus will gradually force it downward through the vagina into the introitus.[4] Uterine prolapse may occur at any age. In female infants and in women who have never given birth, congenital defects in the basic integrity of the pelvic supporting structures are usually responsible. Trauma to the ligaments during childbirth is the cause of uterine prolapse in women who have given birth, particularly if multiple deliveries have occurred. Uterine prolapse is classified as first, second, or third degree according to the level to which the uterus has descended (Figure 33-2). In first-degree prolapse, the uterus is approximately halfway between the vaginal introitus and the level of the ischial spines. In second-degree prolapse, the end of the cervix has begun to protrude through the introitus. In third-degree or complete prolapse, the body of the uterus is outside the vaginal introitus. Figure 33-3 shows a third-degree, or complete, uterine prolapse.

Clinical Manifestations. The symptoms of uterine prolapse depend on the degree of severity of prolapse. The woman may become increasingly aware of a sensation of bearing down and discomfort in the vagina. If the prolapse has advanced to the second or third degree, she may note discomfort while walking or sitting and have difficulty urinating. In addition, as the end of the cervix begins to protrude outside the

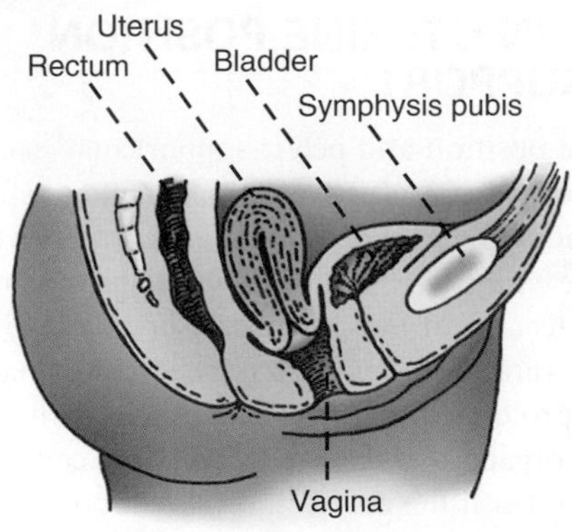

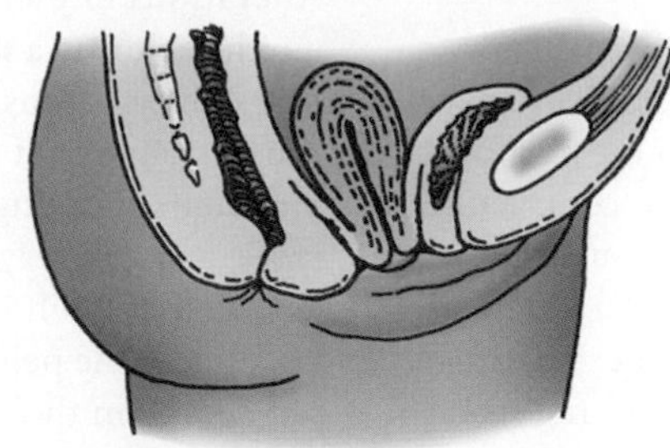

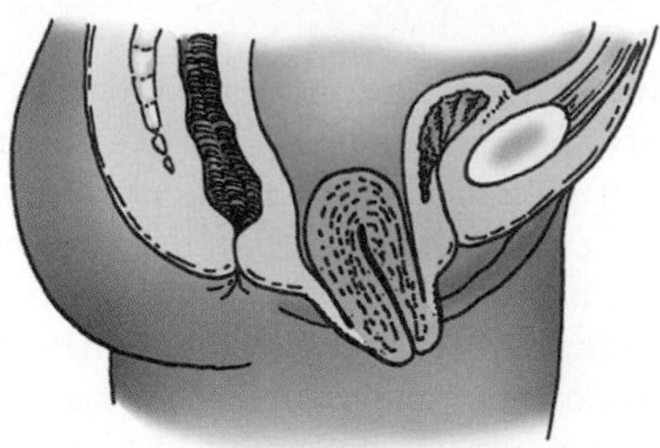

FIGURE 33-2 ■ Degrees of uterine prolapse. (From Black JM, Hawks JH: *Medical-surgical nursing: clinical management for positive outcomes,* ed 7, Philadelphia, 2005, Saunders, p 1078.)

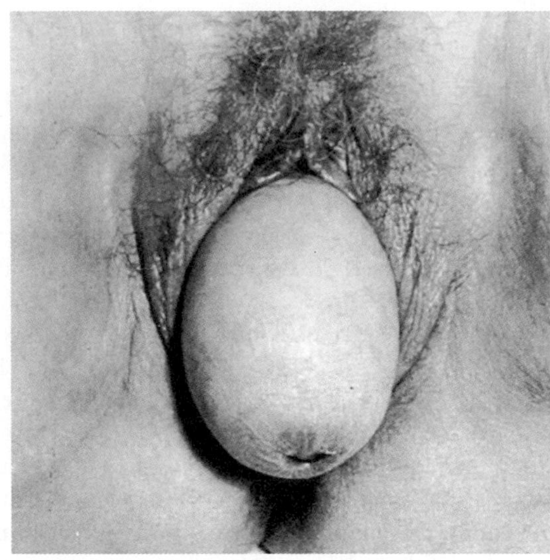

FIGURE 33-3 ■ Complete uterine prolapse. (From Parsons L, Sommers SC: *Gynecology,* ed 2, Philadelphia, 1978, Saunders, p 1443.)

body, it may be subject to trauma from friction and ulceration. Bleeding and ulceration of the cervix may be present.

Treatment. Uterine prolapse is one of the most common reasons for hysterectomy usually from the vaginal approach.[6] In patients who are at poor risk for surgery, a pessary, which is a small supportive device, is inserted to hold the uterus in place.[4]

Retrodisplacement of the Uterus

The term **retrodisplacement** refers to situations in which the body of the uterus is displaced from its usual location overlying the bladder to a position in the posterior of the pelvis.[4] As shown in Figure 33-4, the uterus may be in one of five positions: anteverted, midposition, anteflexed, retroflexed, or retroverted.

Etiology, and Clinical Manifestations. Retrodisplacement can be detected in 20% to 30% of all women.[4] It may be a normal variation and therefore be present throughout a woman's entire life, or it may develop after childbirth when the supporting structures are injured.

In many women, no symptoms occur from uterine retrodisplacement. In some women, symptoms of pelvic pain or pressure, dysmenorrhea, and dyspareunia (painful intercourse) may be present. In addition, infertility has been associated with retrodisplacement.[4]

Treatment. If the woman has no symptoms, no treatment is indicated. The use of a pessary to support the uterus in a normal position may relieve the symptoms, but surgical correction is sometimes indicated when symptoms are severe.[4]

Cystocele

Etiology. A cystocele is a protrusion of a portion of the urinary bladder into the anterior of the vagina at a weakened part of the vaginal musculature (Figure 33-5, *A*). The defect in the vaginal wall is usually caused by injury during childbirth or surgery but may also result from the aging process or as an inherent weakness. Other predisposing factors include obesity and a history of lifting heavy objects. The pressure created by this protrusion causes the anterior vaginal wall to bulge in a downward direction.

Clinical Manifestations and Treatment. A wide range of symptoms may be present, depending on the degree of severity of the cystocele. A mild degree of protrusion of the bladder may result in no symptoms. In moderate to severe cases, a sensation of pressure is felt in the vagina, along with dysuria and back pain. Fullness at the vaginal opening may be observed, as may a soft, reducible mucosal mass bulging into the anterior of the vaginal introitus.

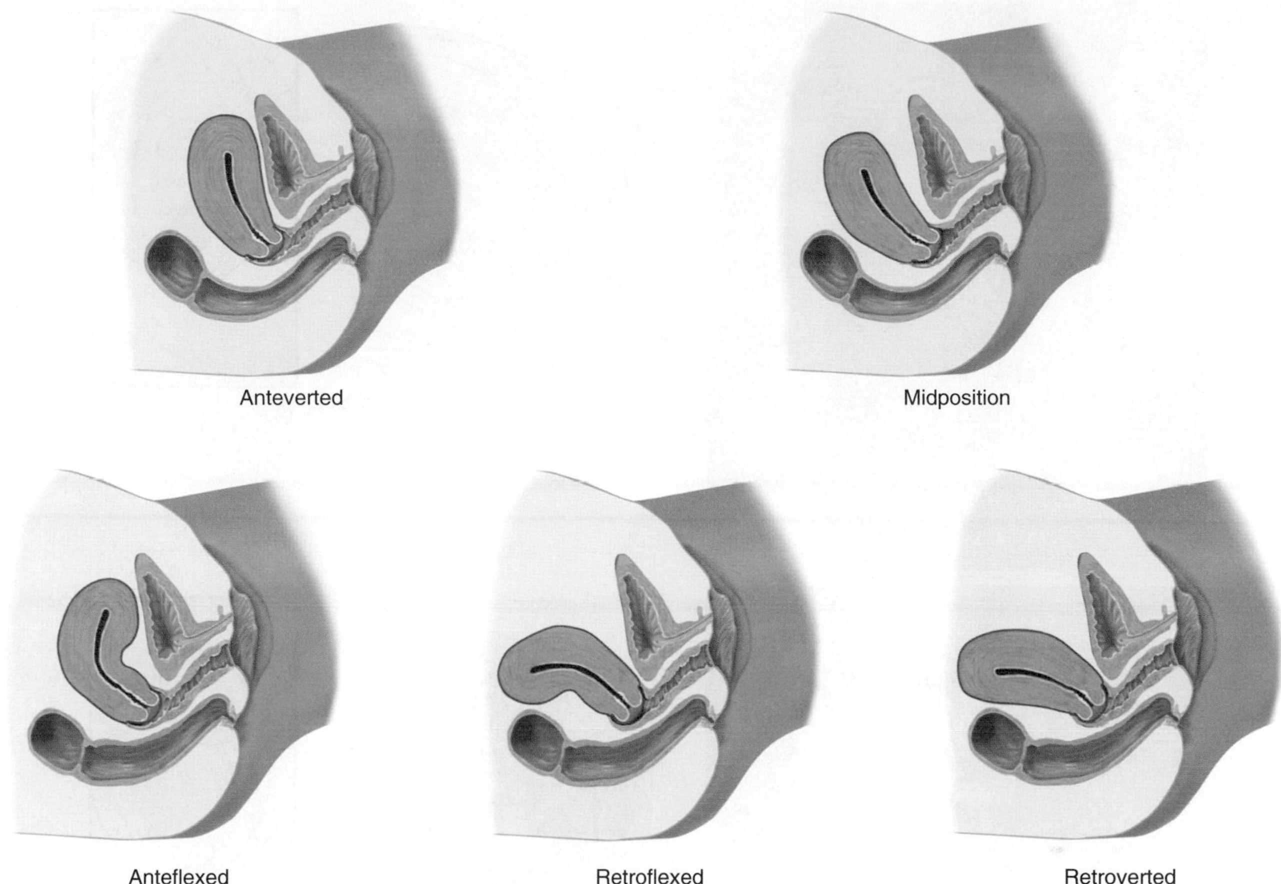

FIGURE 33-4 ■ The various positions of the uterus. Note that the classifications describe the position of the long axis of the uterus with respect to the long axis of the body. (From Jarvis C: *Physical examination and health assessment,* ed 4, Philadelphia, 2004, Saunders, p 785.)

Surgical repair of the vagina is done to correct the cystocele and reestablish support of the anterior vaginal wall. The bladder is restored to a normal position by reinforcement of the weakened portion of the anterior vaginal wall.

Rectocele

Etiology. A **rectocele** (also called proctocele) is a protrusion of the anterior rectal wall into the posterior of the vagina at a weakened part of the vaginal musculature (see Figure 33-5, *B*). As for a cystocele, the defect in the vaginal wall is usually caused by injury during childbirth or surgery but may also occur with aging or as an inherent weakness. Other predisposing factors for a rectocele include multiparity, obesity, and postmenopausal status. The rectocele forms a bulging mass beneath the posterior vaginal mucosa and pushes downward into the lower vaginal canal. Gradually, the rectum may be torn from its fascial and muscular attachments to the pelvic wall. The levator ani muscles may also become stretched or torn.

Clinical Manifestations and Treatment. A wide range of symptoms may be present, depending on the degree of severity of the rectocele. The client may report a history of difficulty in bowel evacuation and may have experienced chronic constipation with laxative and enema dependency. A feeling of pressure may also be reported, along with painful sexual intercourse. Physical examination reveals a mass bulging into the posterior of the vaginal introitus.[6]

Surgical repair of the vagina is done to correct the rectocele and reestablish support of the posterior vaginal wall. The rectum is restored to its normal location, and the levator ani muscles are brought together in proper position.

KEY CONCEPTS

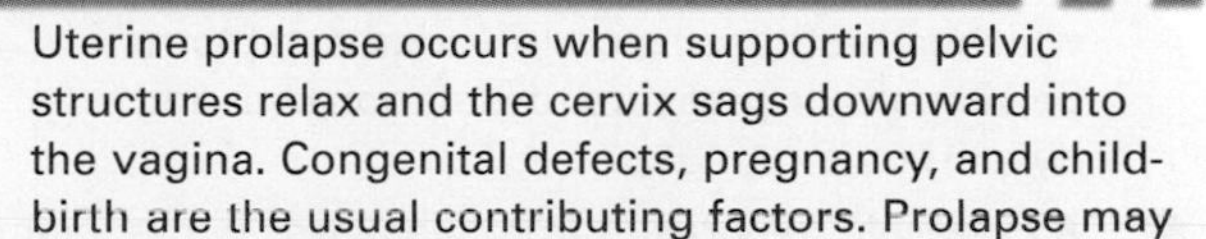

- Uterine prolapse occurs when supporting pelvic structures relax and the cervix sags downward into the vagina. Congenital defects, pregnancy, and childbirth are the usual contributing factors. Prolapse may be accompanied by a sensation of pelvic fullness and vaginal discomfort.
- Retrodisplacement of the uterus is common (20% to 30% of women) and may be congenital or due to

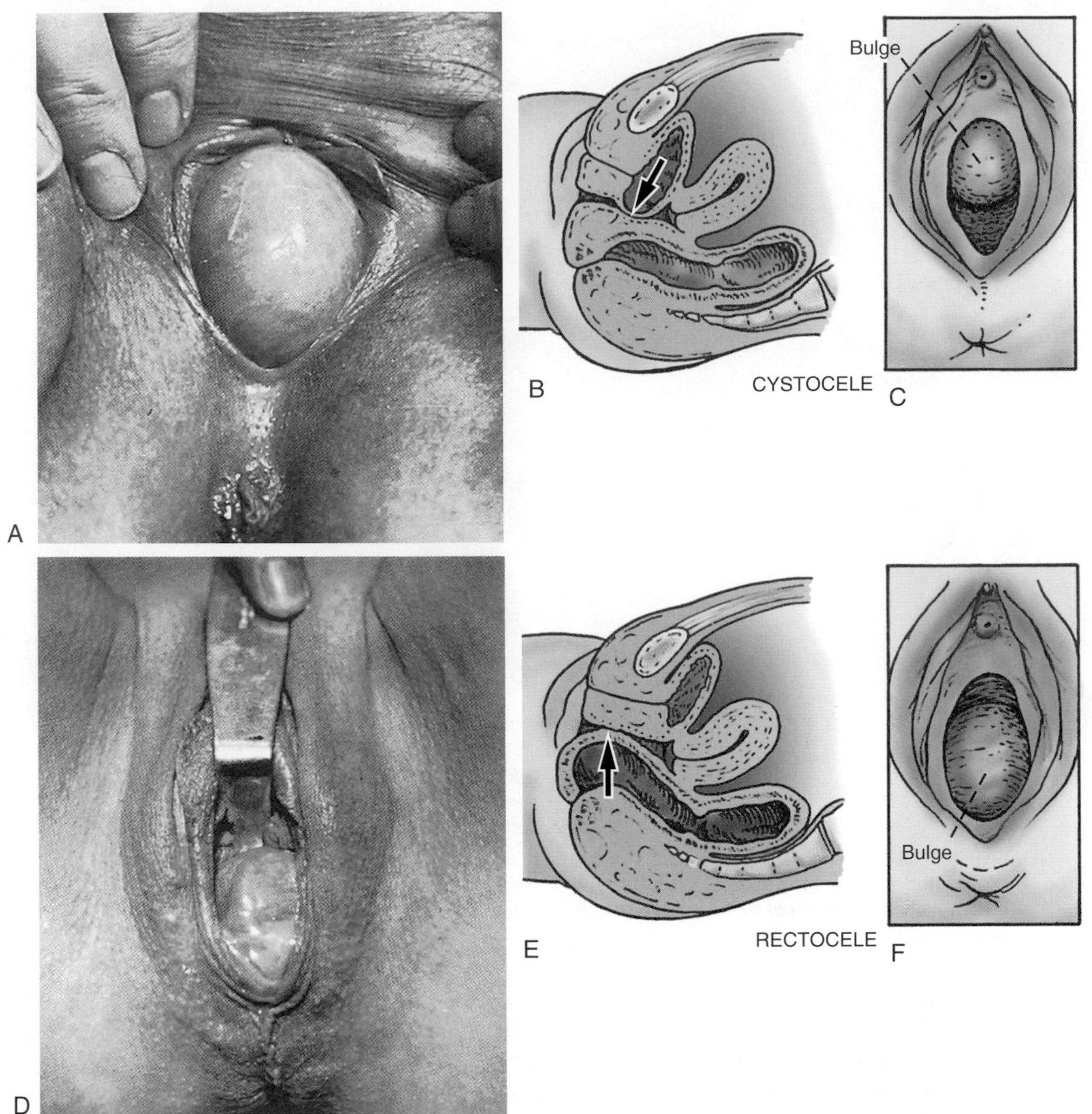

FIGURE 33-5 ■ **A, B,** and **C,** Cystocele. **B,** Note the bulging of the anterior vaginal wall. The urinary bladder is displaced downward. **C,** The cystocele pushes the anterior wall downward into the vagina. **D, E,** and **F,** Rectocele. **E,** Note the bulging of the posterior vaginal wall. (**A** and **D,** From Huffman JW: *Gynecology and obstetrics,* Philadelphia, 1962, Saunders. **B, C, E,** and **F,** From Black JM, Hawks JH: *Medical-surgical nursing: clinical management for positive outcomes,* ed 7, Philadelphia, 2005, Saunders, p 1077.)

pregnancy and childbirth. The body of the uterus is flexed or rotated into the posterior of the pelvis, which sometimes leads to varied symptoms of pelvic pain or pressure, dysmenorrhea, and dyspareunia.

- A cystocele may result from weakness in the vaginal musculature that allows the urinary bladder to protrude into the anterior of the vagina. Contributing factors include childbirth, surgery, aging, obesity, and heavy lifting. Vaginal pressure, dysuria, and back pain may be present.
- A rectocele may result from weakness in the posterior vaginal musculature that allows the rectum to protrude into the vagina. Contributing factors are similar to those for cystocele. Symptoms include constipation, painful bowel evacuation, and painful intercourse.

INFLAMMATION AND INFECTION OF THE FEMALE REPRODUCTIVE TRACT

Inflammatory and infectious processes of the female reproductive tract may have effects that range from discomfort to

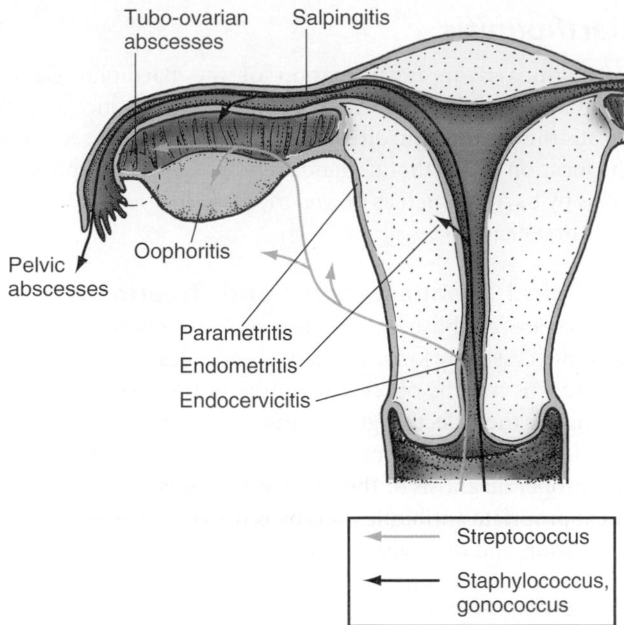

FIGURE 33-6 ■ The spread of pelvic inflammatory disease. (From Ignatavicius DD, Workman ML: *Medical-surgical nursing,* ed 4, Philadelphia, 2002, Saunders, p 1817.)

life-threatening situations. Because the infectious agents responsible for inflammation and infection of the female genital tract may be sexually transmitted, some overlap in the discussion of these processes and sexually transmitted diseases is necessary. This chapter will describe the two principal inflammatory and infectious processes of the upper and lower female reproductive tract: pelvic inflammatory disease (PID) and vulvovaginitis. The reader may wish to refer to Chapter 34 for additional information on sexually transmitted infections.

Pelvic Inflammatory Disease

Pelvic inflammatory disease is any acute, subacute, recurrent, or chronic infection of the oviducts and ovaries with involvement of the adjacent reproductive organs (Figure 33-6). It includes inflammation of the cervix (cervicitis), uterus (endometritis), oviducts (salpingitis), and ovaries (oophoritis). When the connective tissue underlying these structures between the broad ligaments is also involved, the condition is called **parametritis.**[1]

Approximately 1 million women are treated for PID each year in the United States.[2] In addition, significant reproductive health problems may occur as a result of PID. Twenty-five percent of all women who have had PID eventually experience one or more long-term health problems. Infertility is present in 20% of women who have had PID, and the incidence of ectopic pregnancy is increased six to ten times. Chronic pelvic pain, dyspareunia, pelvic adhesions, and chronic inflammation and abscesses of the oviducts and ovaries may all occur in women after PID.[2]

Etiology. Normally, cervical secretions provide protective and defensive functions for the reproductive organs. By providing a bacteriostatic barrier, cervical mucus prevents bacterial agents present in the cervix or vagina from ascending into the uterus. Therefore, conditions or surgical procedures that alter or destroy cervical mucus may impair this bacteriostatic mechanism. PID may follow the insertion of an intrauterine device, pelvic surgery, abortion procedures, and infection during or after pregnancy. Bacteria may also enter the uterine cavity through the blood stream or from drainage from other foci of infection such as a pelvic abscess, ruptured appendix, or diverticulitis of the sigmoid colon.[1]

PID can result from infection with aerobic and anaerobic organisms. *Neisseria gonorrhoeae* and *Chlamydia trachomatis* are the most common causative agents because they readily penetrate the bacteriostatic barrier of cervical mucus. However, a variety of bacterial organisms may contribute to the development of PID, including staphylococci, streptococci, diphtheroids, and coliforms such as *Pseudomonas* and *Escherichia coli.* These bacteria are commonly found in cervical mucus, and PID can result from infection by one or several of these bacteria. In addition, PID may occur after multiplication of bacteria in the endometrium that are normally nonpathogenic. During parturition, the traumatized endometrium favors the multiplication of bacteria.[1]

Clinical Manifestations. The associated signs and symptoms of PID vary with the affected part of the reproductive tract but generally include abdominal tenderness and tenderness or pain of the cervix or adnexa on palpation. In addition, the temperature may be elevated above 38° C and the white blood cell count elevated above 10,000/mm^3. A pelvic abscess or inflammatory mass may be present on physical examination or ultrasound, and purulent vaginal discharge may be noted.[1,2]

Treatment. Early and aggressive use of antibiotic agents best suited for the causative organisms is essential in preventing the progression of PID. Various antibiotic regimens involving the use of multiple antimicrobial agents have been suggested by the Centers for Disease Control and Prevention for use in PID.[2] Inpatient hospitalization may be indicated for patients with rapidly progressing PID and those requiring surgical drainage of pelvic abscesses. Rupture of a pelvic abscess is a potentially life-threatening condition, and a total abdominal hysterectomy (removal of the uterus) with bilateral salpingo-oophorectomy (removal of both oviducts and ovaries) may be indicated in this situation.

Vulvovaginitis

Vulvovaginitis is an inflammation of the vulva (vulvitis) and vagina (vaginitis). Because the vulva and vagina are anatomically close to each other, inflammation of one location usually precipitates inflammation of the other. Vulvovaginitis may occur at any time during a girl's or woman's life and affects most females at some point in life.[1]

Etiology. Infection by *Candida albicans* (formerly called *Monilia*) accounts for approximately half of all reported cases of vulvovaginitis. (Infection by *Candida* is referred to as candidiasis.[2]) *C. albicans* is a fungus that requires glucose for growth; thus its growth may be promoted during the secretory phase of the menstrual cycle when glycogen levels increase in the vaginal environment. In addition, other conditions in which the glycogen content of the vagina is enhanced may favor candidiasis, such as pregnancy and the use of oral contraceptives. Other factors predisposing to the development of vulvovaginitis from *Candida* infection include the use of estrogen supplementation and antibiotics. Women using estrogen supplementation in the perimenopausal period may be at greater risk for candidal infection of the vagina inasmuch as the glycogen content of the vagina may increase with these therapies. The mechanism by which antibiotic use promotes candidiasis is presently unclear, but it is thought that destruction of the bacteria that normally exert the protective effect of consuming *Candida* results in overgrowth of the *Candida* population with subsequent infection.[1,2]

Other infectious agents that may result in vulvovaginitis include *Trichomonas vaginalis, Haemophilus vaginalis,* and *N. gonorrhoeae.* Viral agents that may cause vulvovaginitis include human papillomavirus (venereal warts, condylomata acuminata) or herpesvirus type 2. These organisms can be transmitted during sexual intercourse and are discussed in more detail in Chapter 34.

In addition to infectious processes, vulvovaginitis may be promoted by conditions or agents that irritate the vulva and vagina. Chemical irritation or allergic reactions to detergents, feminine hygiene products, and toilet paper may be a causative factor. Trauma to the vulva or vagina or the atrophy of the vaginal wall that occurs postmenopausally may predispose to vulvovaginitis as well.[1]

Clinical Manifestations. Vulvovaginitis from candidiasis results in a thick, white discharge and red, edematous mucous membranes with white flecks adhering to the vaginal wall. Intense itching usually accompanies this discharge. The vaginal pH is usually normal (less than 4.5), and fungal organisms are often seen on microscopy. Vulvovaginitis from other infectious agents may involve a malodorous, purulent discharge. Irritation and subsequent inflammation of the vulva and vagina may be manifested by red, swollen labia, pain on urination and intercourse, and itching.

Treatment. Appropriate medical therapy for the causative organisms is usually instituted, including local antifungal preparations for vaginal candidiasis and local and systemic antibiotic therapy for vulvovaginitis caused by bacterial agents. Cool compresses and sitz baths provide relief of itching and burning of inflamed tissues. Avoidance of factors that promote irritation of the vulva, such as drying soaps and tight clothing, is also of therapeutic benefit.[1]

Bartholinitis

Bartholinitis is an inflammation of the Bartholin glands, which are located on either side of the vaginal orifice and lubricate the vaginal introitus with a clear, viscous secretion. The location of Bartholin glands renders them susceptible to access by bacteria such as *N. gonorrhoeae, C. trachomatis,* and other organisms.

Clinical Manifestations and Treatment. Once bacteria are established, an abscess (also referred to as a Bartholin cyst) may form and cause tenderness and swelling at the site. Pus may be observed coming out of the duct orifice leading to the affected gland, and symptoms of fever and malaise are present in some individuals. Laboratory culture with proper diagnosis of the causative organism is performed, and appropriate antibiotic therapy is usually instituted. Surgical incision and drainage of the abscess may be necessary for effective management.

KEY CONCEPTS

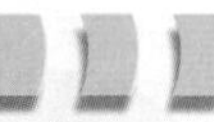

- PID refers to any infection of the oviducts, ovaries, and adjacent reproductive organs. It includes cervicitis, endometritis, salpingitis, and oophoritis. Manifestations and complications of PID include infertility, ectopic pregnancy, pelvic pain, dyspareunia, and abscesses.
- Intrauterine devices, abortion, and pelvic surgery predispose to PID. *N. gonorrhoeae* and *C. trachomatis* are the most common causative organisms, and treatment centers on aggressive antibiotic therapy.
- Inflammation of the vulva and vagina, or vulvovaginitis, is a common problem in women. Most cases are associated with fungal infection by *C. albicans* and are manifested as a white vaginal discharge and an irritated, itchy mucosa. Predisposing factors include chemical irritation from feminine hygiene products, trauma, allergic reactions, and antibiotic therapy that inhibits the growth of normal flora.
- Inflammation of the Bartholin glands, or bartholinitis, is typically a result of the entry and subsequent infection of the glands by *N. gonorrhoeae* or *C. trachomatis.* Tenderness, swelling, and pus may be present and signify the formation of an abscess within one of the Bartholin glands. Antibiotic therapy and surgical drainage are used to manage the abscess.

BENIGN GROWTHS AND ABERRANT TISSUE OF THE FEMALE REPRODUCTIVE TRACT

Benign growths and aberrant tissue in the female reproductive tract are not uncommon; for example, uterine leiomyomas develop in 20% of all women older than 35 years.[3] The presence of benign growths or aberrant tissue in the reproductive tract may cause no symptoms and go entirely unnoticed, or symptoms ranging from debilitating to life threatening may be present. The diagnosis of these growths or tissue may cause anxiety in the woman experiencing them; in spite of their benign classification, their presence can have devastating effects on the underlying reproductive structures.[7] This section focuses on three of the most common forms of benign growths and aberrant tissue in the female reproductive organs: uterine leiomyomas, ovarian cysts, and endometriosis.

Uterine Leiomyomas

Uterine **leiomyomas,** which are also called myomas or fibroids, are the most common form of uterine growths that appear in women. Their actual incidence is difficult to establish because many myomas are either too small or inaccessibly placed to be palpated. Uterine leiomyomas occur in approximately 20% of all women older than 35 years and affect black women three times more often than white women. Age appears to be a factor in their development inasmuch as myomas are not found before the onset of puberty and rarely exhibit growth activity after menopause.

Etiology. Uterine leiomyomas make their appearance and exhibit growth activity during the reproductive years. Therefore, although the actual cause of myomas is presently unknown, it is thought that estrogen and human growth hormone may influence tumor formation by stimulating susceptible fibromuscular elements in the uterine wall. This theory is supported by the finding that tumor growth is enhanced by large doses of estrogen and the later stages of pregnancy, when human growth hormone and estrogen levels are high. In addition, uterine leiomyomas usually shrink or disappear after menopause, when estrogen levels decrease.[1]

Clinical Manifestations. Uterine leiomyomas can grow to a large size (Figure 33-7). Obviously, the presence of such a large mass within the uterus will cause symptoms of abdominal pain and pressure, but smaller myomas can result in such symptoms as well. Other symptoms associated with leiomyomas may include abnormal vaginal bleeding and discharge, depending on the location of the mass. If the myoma is sufficiently large to cause pressure on surrounding abdominal organs, backache, constipation, and urinary frequency or urgency may also be present.

Treatment. Treatment for uterine leiomyomas depends on such factors as the severity of symptoms, size and location of the leiomyoma, and the patient's age. Small myomas that cause no health problems are generally monitored carefully for growth patterns. Large or multiple masses that promote severe uterine bleeding or interfere with functioning of the gastrointestinal or urinary tract are surgically removed, and hysterectomy may be indicated.[1]

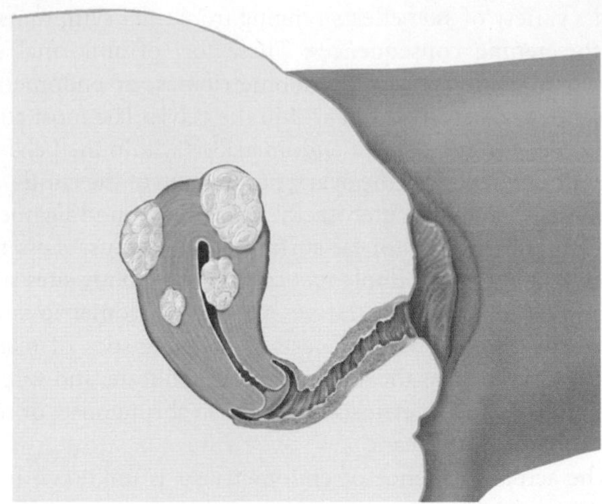

FIGURE 33-7 ■ Uterine leiomyomas. (From Jarvis C: *Physical examination and health assessment,* ed 4, Philadelphia, 2004, Saunders, p 799.)

Ovarian Cysts

Ovarian cysts are sacs on an ovary that contain fluid or semisolid material. Ovarian cysts can develop at any time between puberty and menopause, including during pregnancy.

Etiology. The cause of the formation of ovarian cysts is presently unknown. They can arise in several locations in the ovaries:

1. Follicular cysts result when a maturing ovarian follicle fails to release an ovum; instead, the follicle continues to enlarge and produce estrogen.
2. Corpus luteum cysts occur when the corpus luteum fails to degenerate normally; the cyst continues to grow and produce progesterone.
3. Theca-lutein cysts are commonly bilateral and filled with clear, straw-colored fluid. Often their development is associated with hydatidiform mole, choriocarcinoma, or hormone therapy.[4]

Clinical Manifestations and Treatment. Normally, ovarian cysts produce no symptoms. They may be noted on periodic examination and may increase and decrease in size with the menstrual cycle. However, when an ovarian cyst ruptures, an ovarian vessel may tear, with variable amounts of intraperitoneal hemorrhage and abdominal pain. Occasionally, immediate surgical intervention is indicated to control the hemorrhage and repair the site of rupture.[3]

Endometriosis

Endometriosis is the presence of endometrial tissue outside the lining of the uterine cavity. Because the only normal location for endometrial tissue is the endometrial lining of the uterus, the presence of this abnormal growth is associated with a variety of side effects ranging from mild symptoms to life-threatening consequences. These foci of abnormal endometrial tissue are called **endometriomas,** or endometrial implants, and usually occur within the pelvis. The most common sites of occurrence of endometriosis within the pelvis in order of frequency are the ovary, peritoneum of the cul-de-sac or pouch of Douglas, uterosacral ligaments, round ligament, oviduct, and the peritoneal surface of the uterus.[3] Less frequently, endometrial implants occur in other body sites such as the bladder or large intestine. Although endometriosis is a benign disease, it possesses certain characteristics of malignant disease, such as the ability to grow, infiltrate, and spread. Symptoms of endometriosis may have an abrupt onset or may develop over many years.

The actual incidence of endometriosis is unknown inasmuch as it exists in many women without any significant symptoms. Endometrial implants have been identified in at least 20% of women undergoing gynecologic surgery.[3,8] Active endometriosis usually occurs between 30 and 40 years of age, particularly in women who have never given birth. Endometriosis is rare in women younger than 20 years or after menopause. Although some authorities report a higher incidence of endometriosis in white women of higher socioeconomic levels,[3] these impressions may not be accurate given the tendency of this group to delay childbearing and to have enhanced access to health care. The fertility rate for women in whom endometriosis is diagnosed is about 66% as compared with 88% for the general population.[3]

Etiology. At the present time, three major theories on the etiology of endometriosis have been proposed:

1. *Transportation.* Endometrial tissue flows backward through the oviducts during a normal menstrual period. After this retrograde flow, endometrial fragments implant on the ovary, peritoneal surfaces, and other areas.
2. *Metaplasia.* Inflammation or a hormonal change triggers metaplasia (conversion of one kind of tissue to a form that is not normal for that tissue). Thus, coelomic epithelium at certain sites converts to endometrial epithelium.
3. *Induction.* In this theory, a combination of transportation and metaplasia takes place, and regurgitated endometrium chemically induces mesenchyma to form endometrial epithelium. (At present, this theory is thought to be the most likely.[1,3])

Once the endometrial implants arise in their abnormal locations, they continue to be under hormonal influence, just as the endometrial lining of the uterus responds to hormonal influence. Thus they periodically proliferate and bleed in response to hormonal stimulation. In some instances they may rupture, usually immediately before or after a menstrual period. Endometriomas are filled with brown blood debris; when they rupture, their contents spill onto the sensitive pelvic peritoneum. This irritative discharge sets up a local chemical peritonitis, followed by the formation of fibrous tissue in the injured location. Dense tissue adhesions in the pelvis may result as the pelvic peritoneum undergoes repeated irritation by the cyclic activities of the endometrial implants.

Clinical Manifestations. The most prominent symptom of endometriosis is acquired dysmenorrhea, which produces pain in the lower part of the abdomen and in the vagina, posterior of the pelvis, and back. The pain usually begins 5 to 7 days before menses reach their peak and lasts for 2 to 3 days. It differs from the pain of primary dysmenorrhea, which is more cramplike and concentrated in the abdominal midline. Pain may be extremely severe, although the degree of pain does not necessarily indicate the extent of disease. Dyspareunia and pain with defecation may also be present.[1] Significant changes in the pattern of menstrual flow may occur, with excessive bleeding that may progress to anemia and fatigue.

Treatment. Treatment varies according to the extent of disease. Many women with endometrial implants never experience symptoms and require no treatment; others experience a rapidly progressive set of severe symptoms requiring immediate intervention. Both medical and surgical treatment modalities may be used. Hormonal agents, including progestational steroids and antigonadotropic agents, may be used to produce a hormonal state similar to pregnancy or menopause. Because endometriosis responds to cyclic hormonal functioning, it is thought that the use of hormones to interrupt this cyclic pattern may result in atrophy of the endometrial implants. Surgical intervention includes removal or destruction of the endometriosis. If damage to the pelvic organs is widespread and the disease is progressing rapidly, total abdominal hysterectomy with removal of the oviducts and ovaries is performed.[3]

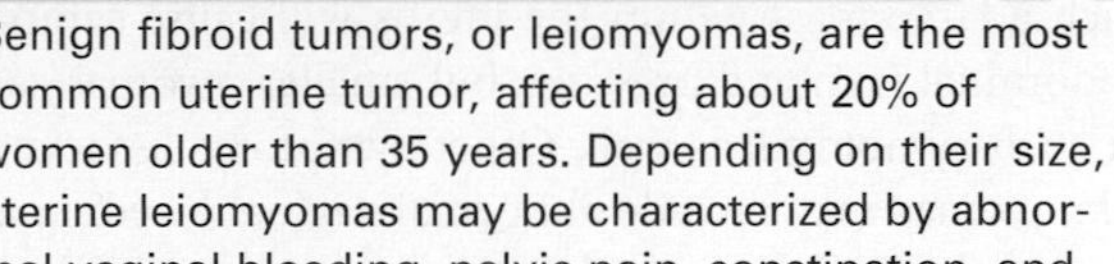

- Benign fibroid tumors, or leiomyomas, are the most common uterine tumor, affecting about 20% of women older than 35 years. Depending on their size, uterine leiomyomas may be characterized by abnormal vaginal bleeding, pelvic pain, constipation, and urinary frequency.
- Ovarian cysts are usually asymptomatic and may change in size with the menstrual cycle. Rupture of an ovarian cyst may result in severe abdominal pain and hemorrhage, which occasionally necessitates immediate surgical intervention.
- Endometriosis occurs when endometrial tissue grows in areas other than the uterine lining. Endometriosis may involve the ovary, peritoneum, oviduct, outer layer of the uterus, bladder, and intestine. Although considered benign, endometriosis tends to infiltrate and spread to adjacent tissues. En-

dometriosis may be initiated by reflux of the uterine lining through the oviducts into the abdominal cavity during menses.

- Ectopic endometrial tissues periodically proliferate and bleed in response to fluctuations of reproductive hormones. Dysmenorrhea, with pelvic, back, and lower abdominal pain, usually begins 5 to 7 days before the peak of menses and lasts for 2 to 3 days. The pain is more diffuse than that of primary dysmenorrhea. Treatment may include induction of a menopause-like state with hormone administration or the surgical excision of affected structures.

CANCER OF THE FEMALE GENITAL STRUCTURES

Malignant neoplasms occur in every part of the female reproductive system. This section describes the incidence and pathophysiologic aspects of the most common types of malignancies in female genital structures. For further information about the process of neoplasm development, the reader may wish to refer to Chapter 7 of this text.

Cancer of the Cervix

Etiology. Cancer of the uterine cervix is a neoplasm that can be detected in the early, curable stage by the Papanicolaou (Pap) test.[3] There are approximately one quarter of a million deaths worldwide per year from cervical cancer.[9] The main cause of cervical cancer appears to be certain human papillomavirus types. Other factors include intercourse at a young age, multiple sexual partners, multiple pregnancies, and herpesvirus type 2 and other venereal infections.[1] Widespread screening with a yearly Pap test in women at risk has continued to decrease the mortality of cervical cancer. The American Cancer Society now recommends that after three consecutive negative Pap tests, women older than 30 years who are not at high risk can be tested every 2 to 3 years. Sexually active women younger than 21 years should also be tested within three years of first coitus. For women who have had a hysterectomy unrelated to cervical neoplasia, the Centers for Disease Control and Prevention no longer recommends Pap screening.[10] Low-risk women who have been screened regularly may also stop screening at age 70.

Clinical Manifestations. Preinvasive cervical cancer produces no symptoms, although the Pap test can detect changes in cells of the cervical epithelium, which may be present for 10 years before invasive cancer develops.[1,3] Early invasive cancer causes abnormal vaginal bleeding, persistent vaginal discharge, and pain and bleeding after intercourse.[1] When symptoms appear, the cancer has usually progressed beyond its early stages. Squamous cell carcinoma accounts for 95% of all invasive cervical cancers diagnosed, and adenocarcinomas account for most of the rest. Invasive carcinoma of the cervix spreads by direct extension to the vaginal wall, laterally into the parametrium toward the pelvic wall, and anteroposteriorly into the bladder and rectum. Metastasis to the pelvic lymph nodes is more common than spread to distant lymph nodes.[3]

Treatment. The treatment strategy depends on the clinical stage of the tumor at the time of diagnosis. Surgery—including cryotherapy, excision, and laser surgery for precancer and hysterectomy for invasive carcinoma—may be indicated. Chemotherapy and radiation therapy may be used in invasive disease. More than 55% of treated patients live 5 years or longer. Radical surgery, including *pelvic exenteration,* or removal of all the pelvic organs, can now be performed with limited morbidity. The overall cure rate for cervical cancer is 29%.[3] Initial testing of a vaccine against human papillomavirus type 16 allows great hope for reducing the incidence of cervical cancer.[11]

Endometrial Cancer

Cancer of the endometrial lining of the uterus is less common than cervical cancer in young women, but both types of cancer occur with equal frequency in postmenopausal women.[3] Related factors include infertility, late menopause (older than 55 years), obesity, diabetes, and hypertension. Unopposed estrogen therapy also increases the frequency.

Clinical Manifestations and Treatment. The most common initial symptom is bleeding between menstrual periods or postmenopausal bleeding. The diagnosis of endometrial cancer is based on histologic tissue examination. Treatment strategies for endometrial cancer include radiation therapy and total hysterectomy with removal of the ovaries and oviducts. The 5-year survival rate for patients in whom early endometrial cancer is diagnosed is greater than 85%. The cure rate drops to 50% if the cancer has metastasized before diagnosis.[3]

Ovarian Cancer

Ovarian cancer has replaced cervical cancer as the leading cause of death from genital cancer. The peak incidence is between 60 and 80 years of age.[3] Because no symptoms are noted until late in the disease, the mortality is high, with only a 34% long-term survival rate.[3]

Clinical Manifestations and Treatment. When symptoms occur, they are related to intraabdominal metastasis and include increasing abdominal girth, weight loss, abdominal pain, dysuria or urinary frequency, and constipation. Management of ovarian cancer includes removal of the uterus, ovaries, and oviducts. Radiation therapy and chemotherapy may be used in conjunction with surgery. Increasingly, prophylactic oophorectomy or salpingo-oophorectomy is being recommended in high-risk women.[12]

Vaginal Cancer

Cancer of the vagina generally occurs in women in their early to mid-50s, although it has an increased incidence in young women whose mothers took diethylstilbestrol during pregnancy.[1] Because the vagina is a thin-walled structure with rich lymphatic drainage, vaginal cancer may metastasize to the bladder, rectum, vulva, pubic bone, and other surrounding structures.

Clinical Manifestations and Treatment. The primary signs and symptoms of vaginal cancer are vaginal spotting and discharge, pain, groin masses, and changes in urinary pattern.[3] Early-stage therapy is designed to treat the malignant area while preserving normal parts of the vagina. Radiation therapy or surgery varies based on the size, depth, and location of the tumor.[1] Preservation of a functional vagina is generally possible only in the early stages, although grafting from other body sites may be performed to avoid vaginal stenosis, particularly in younger women.[3]

Cancer of the Vulva

Clinical Manifestations and Treatment. Cancer of the vulva accounts for approximately 5% of all gynecologic malignancies. It can occur at any age, including infancy, but has a peak incidence in the mid-60s. Factors that seem to predispose to the disease include venereal disease, chronic pruritus of the vulva with swelling and dryness, obesity, hypertension, diabetes, and never having been pregnant.[1]

Leukoplakic changes (the presence of whitish plaque-like or ulcerated lesions) in the vulva may precede the development of carcinoma. Once the carcinoma develops, vulvar masses may be present, with groin masses and abnormal urination and defecation later in the disease.[1] Management of vulvar cancer includes partial excision of the vulva to remove precancerous leukoplakic lesions and total vulvar excision for advanced disease.[3] Local relapse is common whether conservative or radical procedures are undertaken.[13]

KEY CONCEPTS

- Cervical cancer may be detected by evaluation of cervical cells (Pap test). Early-stage cervical cancer may be asymptomatic. When they appear, symptoms include abnormal vaginal bleeding and discharge. Cervical cancer may spread to the vaginal wall, pelvis, bladder, rectum, and pelvic lymph nodes. The overall cure rate is about 29%.
- Other cancers of the female reproductive tract include endometrial, ovarian, vaginal, and vulvar cancers. No routine screening tests are available for these cancers. Ovarian cancer has a high mortality rate because it is usually diagnosed after it has metastasized.

DISORDERS OF PREGNANCY

Pregnancy results in a number of physiologic alterations in the mother that are usually well tolerated, particularly if adequate prenatal care is available. However, pregnancy can result in a number of conditions that may be life threatening to the mother and the developing fetus. The most common pregnancy-related disorders are described here; in addition, for information concerning diabetes in pregnancy, the reader may wish to consult Chapter 41, which covers the topic of diabetes in depth.

Pregnancy-Induced Hypertension

Pregnancy-induced hypertension (PIH) is known by other names such as toxemia and preeclampsia-eclampsia. Hypertension complicates 0.5% to 10% of pregnancies in the United States.[4] PIH is characterized by a rapid rise in arterial blood pressure associated with the loss of large amounts of protein in the urine. Women at risk for the development of PIH include teenagers and women in their late 30s and early 40s. In addition, the presence of multiple fetuses and the preexistence of hypertension, renal and cardiovascular disease, and diabetes may predispose to the development of PIH.[4]

Etiology, Clinical Manifestations, and Treatment. The exact causes of PIH are presently unknown, although poor nutrition and genetic and immunologic factors have been suggested. PIH is characterized by salt and water retention by the kidneys, weight gain, and edema. In addition, arterial spasm occurs in many parts of the body, most significantly in the kidneys, brain, and liver. Both renal flow and the glomerular filtration rate are decreased, a condition exactly opposite the normal changes in pregnancy. The renal effects are caused by thickening of the glomerular tufts, which contain a fibrinoid deposit in the basement membranes.[14]

The severity of symptoms of PIH is closely related to the retention of salt and water and the degree of the increase in arterial pressure. The increasing arterial pressure seems to promote a vicious cycle in which arterial spasm and other pathologic effects give rise to further increases in arterial pressure. Milder forms of the disease are managed with bed rest. Fetal well-being is periodically assessed and the infant is delivered if conditions deteriorate or maturity is achieved.

In its severe form, PIH is characterized by extreme vascular spasticity throughout the body, clonic convulsions followed by coma, renal failure, liver malfunction, and extreme hypertension. Usually, this severe form occurs shortly before parturition. The mortality rate in women with severe PIH who are left untreated is high. However, the immediate use of rapidly acting vasodilating drugs, seizure prophylaxis, and rapid delivery have reduced the mortality rate from PIH to less than 1%.[14]

Hyperemesis Gravidarum

Hyperemesis gravidarum is a Latin term for excess of vomiting in pregnant women. Although transient nausea and vomiting occur in about half of women in the first trimester of pregnancy, in a few women these symptoms continue throughout the entire course of pregnancy. Intractable vomiting, or hyperemesis gravidarum, occurs in about 1 in 1000 pregnancies, sometimes with life-threatening consequences.[14] Severe dehydration and electrolyte imbalance, hepatic and renal damage, encephalopathy, and ultimately death may ensue if the vomiting cannot be controlled.

Clinical Manifestations and Treatment. The causes of hyperemesis gravidarum are unknown, but it is thought that an abnormal response to the production of large amounts of human chorionic gonadotropin by the placenta may be implicated. Intravenous therapy to correct metabolic and nutritional abnormalities, antiemetic agents, and supportive care in a hospital environment may be needed to resolve the symptoms.

Placenta Previa and Abruptio Placentae

Etiology and Clinical Manifestations. **Placenta previa** is a condition in which the placenta is implanted abnormally over the internal cervical os. **Abruptio placentae** is premature separation of the placenta before delivery of the fetus. Placenta previa occurs in approximately 1 in 200 deliveries and is more common in women with multiple pregnancies and previous cesarean section; its cause is unknown. Placenta previa may occur in varying degrees of severity ranging from partial to entire coverage of the internal cervical os. Abruptio placentae, or premature separation of the placenta, occurs after 20 weeks of gestation in about 1% of deliveries. The detachment may be partial or complete and may cause overt or concealed hemorrhage.[4] Abruptio placentae can be caused by trauma, a short umbilical cord, occlusion of the inferior vena cava, PIH, or abnormal uterine anatomy.

Treatment. Therapeutic strategies for placenta previa and abruptio placentae include cesarean section for fetal distress or hemorrhage control. Medications designed to control preterm labor may also be administered.

Spontaneous Abortion

Spontaneous abortion is expulsion of the products of conception from the uterus before the period of fetal viability. It is usually called a miscarriage by laypersons, and it is differentiated from elective abortion. Although the precise incidence is unknown, it is estimated that 15% to 25% of pregnancies end in spontaneous abortion.

Etiology. Abnormal development accounts for a large percentage of aborted pregnancies. Some 61% of abortuses expelled in the first trimester demonstrate chromosomal abnormalities.[4] In addition, abnormal development may result from faulty implantation of the fertilized ovum or from an abnormality in the uterine environment. Maternal factors responsible for spontaneous abortion include both systemic and localized conditions. Infectious processes that may contribute to spontaneous abortion include cytomegalovirus, herpesvirus, and rubella infections. Abnormalities of the reproductive organs, immune disorders, endocrine malfunction, and physical and psychic trauma may all contribute to spontaneous abortion.[4]

Clinical Manifestations and Treatment. Associated signs and symptoms of spontaneous abortion include vaginal bleeding and abdominal cramps. The cramps may intensify as the cervix dilates for expulsion of the uterine contents. If the entire contents are expelled, the bleeding and cramps subside. However, if any contents remain, an incomplete abortion has occurred and intervention may be needed to control bleeding and to surgically remove the remaining uterine contents.[15]

KEY CONCEPTS

- PIH is characterized by a rapid rise in blood pressure and proteinuria. Renal blood flow and the glomerular filtration rate are reduced, and the kidneys retain salt and water. When severe, PIH may be associated with convulsions and coma. Antihypertensive therapy may be indicated.
- Excessive vomiting during pregnancy is termed hyperemesis gravidarum. Dehydration, electrolyte imbalance, hepatic and renal damage, and death may ensue. An excessive response to human chorionic gonadotropin may be responsible for hyperemesis.
- Placenta previa occurs when the placenta is implanted over the cervical os. Abruptio placentae is premature separation of the placenta. Both conditions may interrupt fetal oxygen supply and cause maternal hemorrhage. Cesarean section is indicated.
- It is estimated that 10% to 15% of pregnancies end in spontaneous abortion. Fetal abnormalities, faulty implantation, infections, and trauma increase the risk of spontaneous abortion.

DISORDERS OF THE BREAST

The breast is considered an accessory organ of the female reproductive tract and is affected by many of the same factors that promote alterations in the other reproductive organs. Women's breast health has become a critical concern in the United States because the breast is the most common site of cancer in women between 25 and 75 years of age.[16] In addition, women are playing an increasingly important role in recognizing the symptoms of breast disease and are seeking earlier intervention with improved outcomes. It is essential that health care professionals continue to encourage this enhanced role and provide accurate information about breast health to their clients. This section includes information on specific breast disorders involving reactive-inflammatory breast disorders, benign breast disorders, and carcinoma of the breast. Before reading this information, the reader may wish to review the section on the structure and function of the breast in Chapter 32 of this text and the specific information on neoplasm development in Chapter 7.

REACTIVE-INFLAMMATORY BREAST DISORDERS

Breast disorders in which an inflammatory response occurs in reaction to irritation, injury, or infection include mammary duct ectasia, breast abscess, fat necrosis, and reactions to injections or implantation of foreign materials in the breast.

Mammary Duct Ectasia

Mammary duct ectasia is a chronic inflammatory process occurring in and around the terminal subareolar ducts of the breast (it is also referred to as periductal mastitis). It is more prevalent in older women, primarily postmenopausal women.[16] The Latin word **ectasia** means dilation, and in mammary duct ectasia the collecting ducts beneath the nipple and areola become dilated, thinned, and filled with secretions.

Pathogenesis. Over time, the ducts become distended with cellular debris, and the debris begins to have an irritating effect on the duct walls. The inflammatory response is initiated, and a zone of granulation tissue is created around a small cavity filled with thick yellowish or brownish material. This area will be palpable as a mass in the central area of the breast, beneath or near the areola. By the time the duct ectasia has grown into a palpable mass, a reactive fibrosis will also have formed in the tissue around the mass. This fibrous thickening of the surrounding breast tissue causes dimpling and distortion of the breast and nipple inversion (Figure 33-8). However, a congenital inverted nipple is already present in some women with mammary duct ectasia, and it is thought that the presence of this nipple anomaly may in some way contribute to ductal wall irritation.[16]

Clinical Manifestations and Treatment. In addition to a palpable mass and dimpling or distortion of the breast or areola, women with mammary duct ectasia may have a persistent nipple discharge. These signs must be evaluated carefully because they may also be indicative of a malignant breast mass. A biopsy is usually performed to rule out the presence of a malignancy. After confirmation of the diagnosis of mammary ductal ectasia, surgical excision of the dilated subareolar ducts is performed.[16]

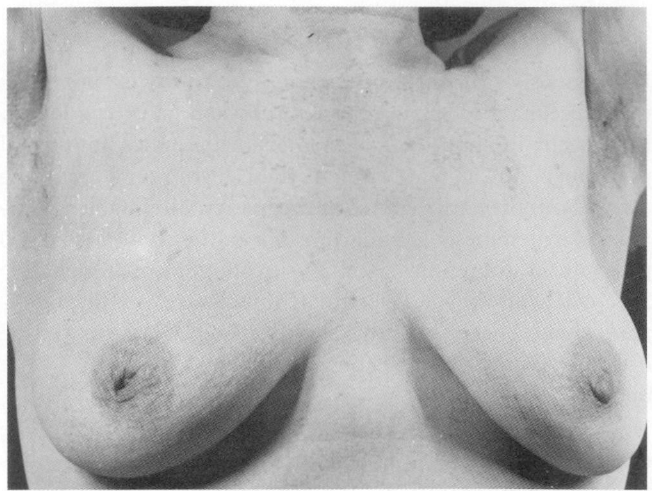

FIGURE 33-8 ■ Nipple retraction in the right breast as a result of mammary duct ectasia. (From Haagensen CD: *Diseases of the breast,* ed 3, Philadelphia, 1986, Saunders, p 359.)

Breast Abscess

The majority of abscesses occurring in the breast are not associated with breast-feeding and are referred to as nonlactational breast abscesses (for a complete description of abscesses or mastitis related to lactation, the reader may wish to refer to an obstetric or maternity nursing text). Nonlactational breast abscesses are most often a recurring problem and usually affect persons with conditions that predispose to infections, such as diabetes, steroid therapy, or other skin lesions.

Etiology. Multiple factors may contribute to the formation of nonlactational breast abscesses. In some women, the presence of a congenital inverted nipple may predispose to abscess formation. Abscesses may also be part of the syndrome of mammary duct ectasia; in addition, women with the aforementioned preexisting conditions that predispose to infections may be at increased risk for the development of an infectious process in the breast tissue. Unlike breast abscesses occurring during breast-feeding, in which *Staphylococcus aureus* is the most common causative organism, nonlactational breast abscesses usually yield multiple organisms when cultured.

Clinical Manifestations and Treatment. Signs and symptoms of these abscesses include an area of tenderness, redness, and induration under the periareolar skin.[16] Unfortunately, nonlactational breast abscesses do not respond well to antibiotic therapy and often recur, and it is sometimes necessary to excise the major duct system beneath the areola to prevent further recurrence.[16]

Fat Necrosis

Necrosis refers to the death of a portion of tissue, and fat necrosis in the breast is the death of fat tissue after trauma or injury to the breast. The position of the breasts makes them vulnerable to trauma, particularly in larger women with pendulous breasts. This phenomenon is important for health care professionals to assess because fat necrosis may mimic or obscure carcinoma of the breast.

Clinical Manifestations and Diagnoses. Fat necrosis of the breast may have many of the same clinical signs as breast malignancy, including a painless mass in the breast that is firm, ill defined, and poorly mobile. Skin thickening and retraction may also be present. In addition, a mammogram may not provide a clear diagnosis.[16] Unfortunately, many women with pendulous breasts frequently sustain injuries to the breast and may be unable to recall any specific trauma; thus a diagnosis of fat necrosis may be difficult to make. If fat necrosis cannot be reliably distinguished from carcinoma based on clinical observation or mammography, excisional biopsy must be performed.[16]

Reactions to Foreign Material

Surgery to enlarge the female breast has become one of the most popular of all cosmetic surgical procedures in the past 25 years.[16] Since the early 20th century, a variety of materials have been used for breast augmentation. Silicone implants, which consist of silicone gel encased in polyurethane or other materials, have been the most widely used devices for breast enlargement and have been implanted in more than 1 million women.[16] At present, controversy surrounds the use of silicone breast implants because some side effects, including irritation at the implantation area and other symptoms suggestive of an immune system response, have been reported. Currently, the use of silicone implants for routine cosmetic breast augmentation is specifically controlled in the United States, and implants filled with a saline solution are now being used for this purpose. Health care professionals should be aware of the reported side effects of silicone breast implants inasmuch as a substantial segment of the female population in the United States and western Europe has undergone breast augmentation with these devices. In addition, persons with silicone implants who sustain blunt trauma to the chest are at risk for rupture of the implant, with subsequent leakage of the silicone gel into surrounding tissue. After chest trauma, the communication of information regarding the presence of silicone breast implants to other health care professionals is an important consideration in planning care and preventing further tissue exposure to silicone.

BENIGN BREAST DISORDERS

The term **benign breast disorders** encompasses a group of lesions affecting the breast. These disorders are usually divided into two categories: (1) fibrocystic breast disease and (2) specific benign neoplasms of the breast such as fibroadenomas, adenomas, and papillomas. It is important for health care professionals to understand the clinical significance of these benign disorders. Although these entities are "benign" in the sense of being differentiated from malignant breast neoplasms, clients experiencing them may be at risk for experiencing a psychological crisis and may need to be educated regarding their potential risk for breast malignancy.

Fibrocystic Breast Disease

Although the term **fibrocystic breast disease** is frequently used by health care professionals, it is important to understand that it is not a distinct disease entity.[16] Instead, it is a diagnosis classification that is applied to a condition in which the presence of palpable breast masses fluctuates with the menstrual cycle and may be associated with pain or tenderness. Laboratory examination of this breast tissue shows macroscopic and microscopic cysts, along with a variety of alterations in tissue structure such as fibrosis or overgrowth of stromal fibrous tissue. However, these alterations in breast tissue are present to some degree in all female breasts, which has led some authorities to question use of the term "disease" for such a widespread condition.[16] Until a more precise system for classifying this type of benign breast disorder is widely adopted, fibrocystic breast disease will probably continue to be used to describe this phenomenon of tender breast masses that occur on a cyclic basis.

Etiology and Clinical Manifestations. Hormonal imbalance in the reproductive years is thought to contribute to fibrocystic breast disease. Fibrocystic breast disease is more common in women aged 30 to 50 years. It is usually characterized by tenderness or pain in one or both breasts immediately before onset of the menstrual period. On palpation, the cysts tend to be firm, regular in shape, and mobile. They are located most often in the upper outer quadrant of the breasts, and their size may fluctuate throughout the menstrual cycle.[16]

Although it was previously thought that all women with fibrocystic breast disease were at increased risk for breast cancer, recent research has disproved this theory.[16] It is now known that only certain types of tissue changes may predispose a woman with fibrocystic breast disease to the development of breast malignancy. The vast majority of women with fibrocystic disease do not have these alterations in breast tissue and therefore are not at a substantially increased risk for breast cancer.[15]

Diagnoses and Treatment. Diagnostic studies, including needle aspiration of a cyst for histologic analysis, may be performed (Figure 33-9). Danazol, a weak androgen, has shown efficacy in the treatment of fibrocystic breast disease. Other supportive measures include the application of local heat and use of a support bra. Nutritional therapies have

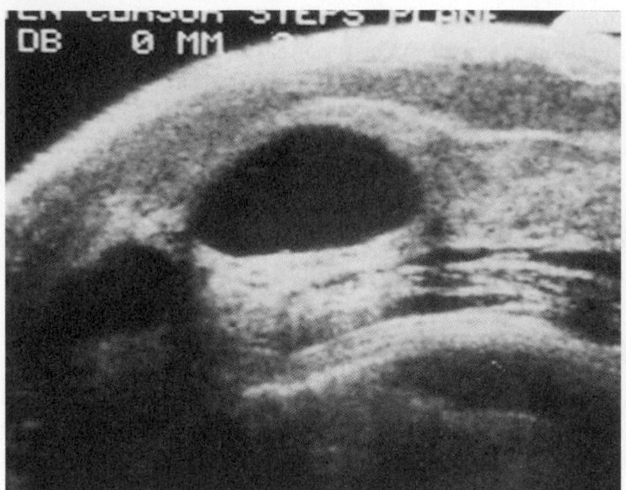

FIGURE 33-9 ■ Ultrasonic image of a cyst showing typical smooth margins, dark center, edge shadows, and a bright posterior wall. (From Donegan WL, Spratt JS: *Cancer of the breast,* ed 5, Philadelphia, 2002, Saunders, p 331.)

shown success in some women, particularly avoidance of foods with methylxanthines such as tea, coffee, cola, and chocolate. It is thought that methylxanthines tend to stimulate cyclic adenosine monophosphate and thus increase metabolic activity in the breast.[16] A low-fat, high-carbohydrate diet has been shown to decrease breast swelling and tenderness.

Specific Benign Neoplasms

Specific benign neoplasms of the breast, such as fibroadenomas, adenomas, and papillomas, may occur at any time during a woman's life from childhood through old age. These neoplasms behave in a clinically "benign" fashion; that is, they do not invade the surrounding tissue or metastasize to other sites. They generally appear as freely movable, encapsulated masses that are sharply delineated from the surrounding breast tissue.[16] However, it is important to have any breast mass evaluated because biopsy and histologic examination may be needed to differentiate these benign neoplasms from breast carcinoma.

MALIGNANT DISORDER OF THE BREAST

Cancer of the Breast

Carcinoma of the breast remains the most common form of cancer in women between the ages of 25 and 75 years, although lung cancer is increasing in prevalence in this group.[16] In the United States it is the leading cause of death from all causes in women between the ages of 40 and 44 years. The incidence of breast carcinoma appears to be increasing in the United States, and the prevalence (the number of women with breast cancer in a given year) is approximately 100 per 100,000 women.[16] Although the disease is more common in white women, its incidence in blacks and Asians is rising.[16] Breast cancer does occur in males but is 100 times less common.[16] Even though recent advances in early detection and treatment have afforded longer survival after diagnosis, invasive breast carcinoma remains an incurable disease that continues to take the lives of a large segment of the population.

Etiology. A substantial number of studies conducted in the past 20 years have begun to establish the risk factors and possible causes of breast cancer. Some factors that may place a woman at risk for breast cancer include hormonal influences, reproductive factors, dietary factors, family history, age, radiation exposure, and a history of cancer.[17] It should be noted that helping a client understand and interpret her personal breast cancer risk is a difficult task for a health care professional. The public media has given much attention to some of the risk factors for breast cancer but has not provided much context in which to interpret evaluations for individual risk factors.[15]

Risk factors are characteristics related to the probability of a certain outcome—in this case, breast cancer. These risk factors may be either causally or correlatively associated with an outcome. For example, a factor may directly *cause* an outcome (as the smallpox virus causes smallpox) or may be *correlated* with an outcome (as not wearing a seat belt is correlated with an increased degree of injury in a motor vehicle accident). The distinction between causality and correlation is an important concept to impart to clients when discussing risk factors. A client may express concern, for example, that a certain risk factor will directly cause breast cancer to develop in her. The ability of a health care professional to describe and discuss risk factors in a knowledgeable way will greatly enhance the client's ability to make decisions regarding such issues as hormonal replacement therapy after menopause.

Hormonal Factors. Hormones are now thought to be a major factor in the development of breast cancer.[16] Length of exposure to the hormones secreted by the ovary (estrogen and progesterone) has been shown to affect the risk for breast cancer in the following way. If a woman has had an early (younger than 12 years) onset of menses and a late (older than 55 years) menopause, her risk is increased. Put another way, women with 40 or more years of menstrual activity have twice the breast cancer risk as women with fewer than 30 years of menstrual activity.[16] Postmenopausal hormone replacement therapy may increase the risk of breast cancer.[18] For some women, the known benefits of these medications may outweigh effects on cancer risk. Future research is needed to clarify the way in which hormonal exposure may foster breast cancer development and the many interactive factors associated with taking hormonal medications.

Reproductive Factors. It has been observed in many research studies that giving birth at a young age (less than 18 years) is associated with a decreased risk of breast cancer and that giving birth for the first time at 35 years or older increases the risk.[16] In addition, parity (the number of children a woman has given birth to) has been associated with risk, with

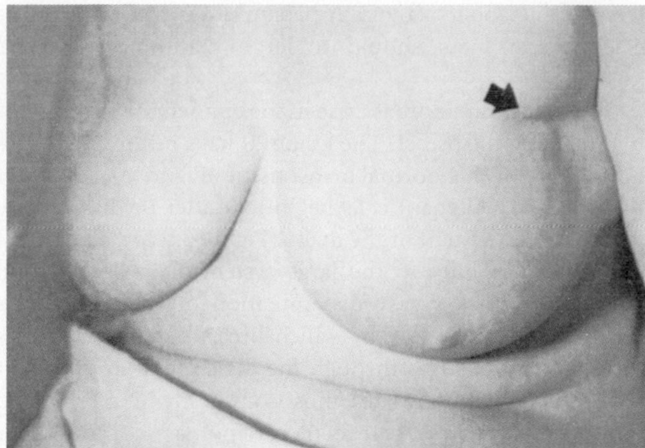

FIGURE 33-10 ■ Skin dimpling caused by an underlying malignant tumor. (From Donegan WL, Spratt JS: *Cancer of the breast,* ed 5, Philadelphia, 2002, Saunders, p 321.)

low parity increasing risk and high parity having a protective effect.[16] Breast-feeding is also associated with a decrease in breast cancer.[19]

Dietary Factors. It has been suggested that the amount of fat in the diet is a risk factor for breast cancer.[16] Researchers who favor this theory point to the relatively low rates of dietary fat ingestion in countries with low rates of breast cancer. Although the media has given a great deal of attention to this issue, scientific data have been inconclusive thus far.[16] Countries in which low-fat diets are widespread are typically nonindustrialized countries in which other factors, such as age at first delivery or parity, differ from those in westernized countries. No single dietary pattern or food has been shown to "cause" cancer, just as no specific food has been shown to prevent or cure it.

Family History. The role of heredity in contributing to breast cancer has long been recognized. Most recently, specific gene mutations such as *BRCA1* and *BRCA2* have been identified in high-risk families. Women with these mutations are at risk for breast and ovarian cancer and may benefit from prophylactic salpingo-oophorectomy to reduce their risk of both cancers.[20] Research studies have also indicated that women with a mother or sister with breast cancer have an increased risk of breast cancer, even if specific gene mutations are not identified. Increasingly, chemoprevention with tamoxifen, an estrogen antagonist in the breast, is being recommended in such high-risk women.[21] Tamoxifen is not recommended in low- to average-risk women because it has its own adverse effects such as thromboembolic events and endometrial cancer.

Age. Breast cancer is extremely rare in young women. The incidence of breast cancer begins to increase by 25 to 30 years of age and continues to increase with advancing age.[16]

Other Factors. Other factors, such as radiation exposure and a history of cancer, have been shown to be risk factors for the development of breast cancer.[16] Several potential factors have been suggested, such as exposure to low-frequency electric or magnetic fields and a virus transmitted through lactation. More research is required to establish the role of these potential factors.[21]

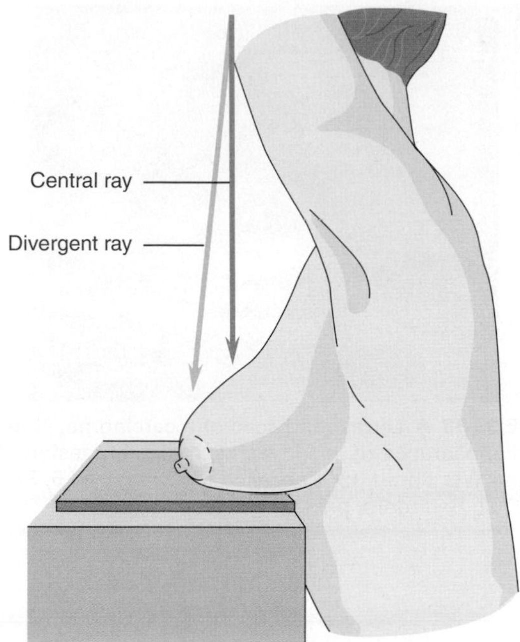

FIGURE 33-11 ■ Placement of the breast for mammography, along with the direction of the x-rays.

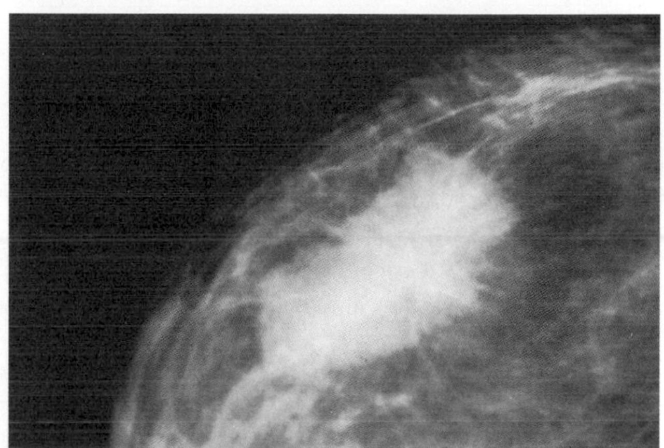

FIGURE 33-12 ■ Mammographic image of a typical cancer. (From Donegan WL, Spratt JS: *Cancer of the breast,* ed 5, Philadelphia, 2002, Saunders, p 328.)

Clinical Manifestations. Breast cancer is usually discovered by the woman herself. She usually finds a single lump that is painless, hard, and poorly movable. Half of malignant tumors occur in the upper outer quadrant of the breast.[16] Other signs of advanced tumor development include dimpling of the skin (Figure 33-10), nipple retraction, changes in breast contour, and bloody discharge from the nipple. Breast cancer is diagnosed by a number of techniques that use films (mammography, xerography) (Figures 33-11 and 33-12) and by thermography, a technique in which "hot spots" indicate

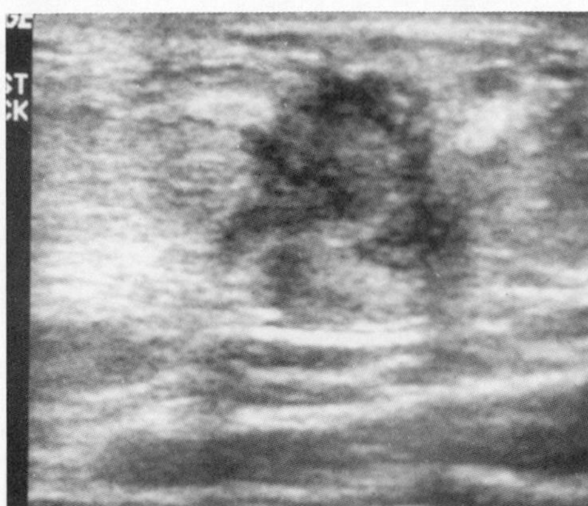

FIGURE 33-13 ■ Ultrasound scan of a carcinoma. Note the ragged appearance of this invasive, malignant lesion. (From Donegan WL, Spratt JS: *Cancer of the breast,* ed 5, Philadelphia, 2002, Saunders, p 332.)

increased metabolic activity. A person of any age with a suspected breast mass should undergo mammography and biopsy.

Most breast carcinomas arise in the epithelium of the glandular ducts of the breast. The lesion(s) have infiltrating edges that begin to invade normal breast tissue (Figure 33-13). After this invasion, malignant cells begin to scatter or disseminate into the lymph system of the axilla (Figure 33-14). The breast is in close proximity to the large system of axillary lymph nodes, which makes easy dissemination of malignant cells possible. The major way by which breast carcinoma causes morbidity and death is through the dissemination of malignant cells to other body sites, most commonly lung, liver, and bone.[16] **Metastasis** (or spread of carcinoma) to these other body sites signifies an extremely poor prognosis. The prognosis is vastly better for persons with no evidence of spread of malignant cells to the regional lymph nodes. The 5-year sur-

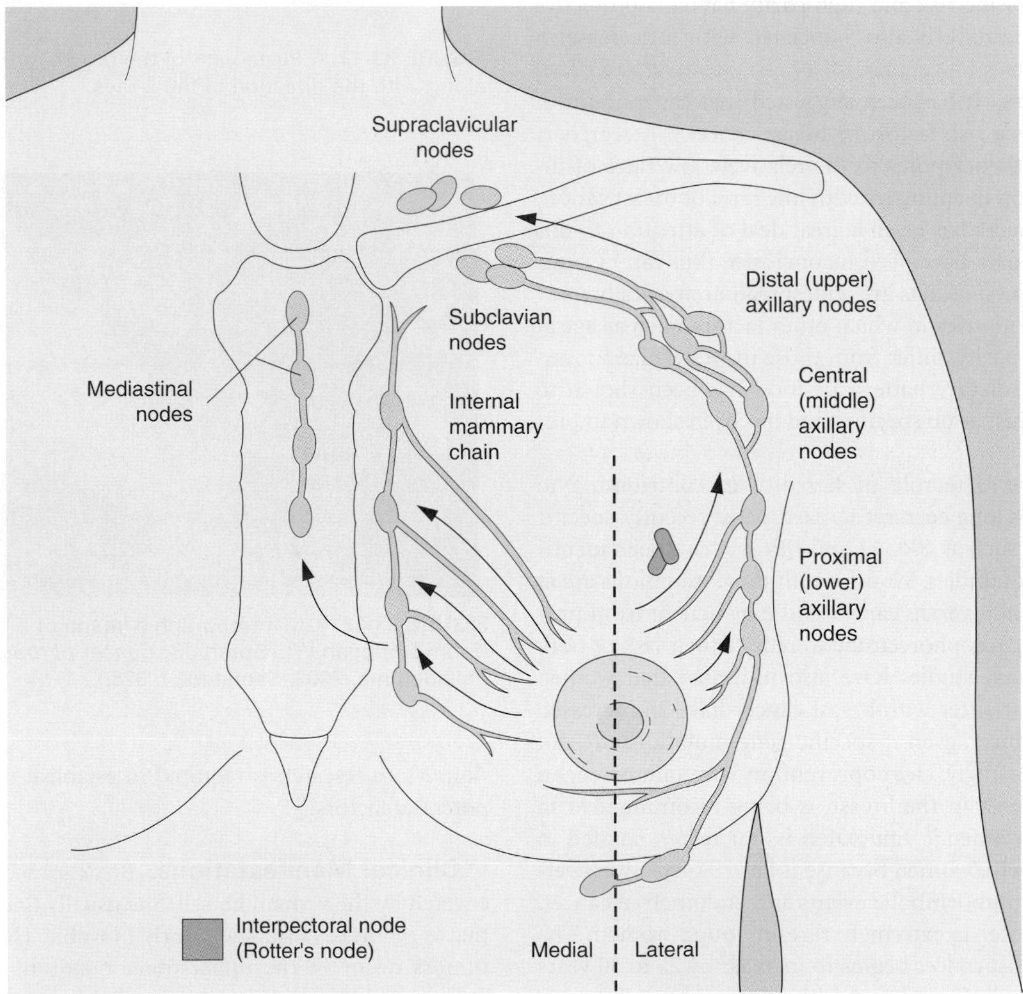

FIGURE 33-14 ■ Lymphatic spread of breast cancer. In general, lateral lesions in the breast metastasize to axillary and supraclavicular nodes, whereas medial tumors tend to metastasize to the internal mammary and mediastinal lymph nodes, as well as the supraclavicular nodes. (From Skarin AT, editor: *Atlas of diagnostic oncology,* ed 3, St Louis, 2003, Mosby, p 260.)

vival rate is 84% when no lymph node involvement is found at surgery but averages 56% when lymph node involvement is present.[15] The more positive lymph nodes (nodes with malignant cells) that are found at surgery, the less favorable is the prognosis.

Treatment. Treatment for breast cancer includes surgery, chemotherapy, radiation therapy, and supportive measures. Surgical therapy is a controversial area, and various options are available. Removal of only the lesion is called a **lumpectomy;** removal of only the breast is a simple **mastectomy.** Other surgical interventions include a **modified radical mastectomy,** in which the breast is removed and a portion of the axillary lymphatic system is dissected, and a **radical mastectomy,** in which the breast, lymphatic drainage, and underlying pectoral muscles are removed.[15]

Chemotherapy entailing a variety of hormonal and antineoplastic agents is also used. Malignant cells appear to have cytoplasmic hormone receptors that bind to hormone molecules and promote cellular division and growth. Tamoxifen, an estrogen antagonist, is the most common agent used. Antineoplastic agents are given to control the spread of malignant cells.[16]

Radiation therapy may be used as an adjunct to the aforementioned therapy and to control pain by shrinking large tumor masses. Other supportive measures in advanced disease include operations to reduce the bulk of tumors.[15]

Continuum of Care. Breast cancer is characterized by a wide variation in clinical course. Many patients who undergo therapy for breast carcinoma are able to achieve a satisfying quality of life. Educational and support programs for breast cancer patients and their families, both preoperatively and postoperatively, have been an important means of providing emotional support. Programs for continuing care after mastectomy have helped patients and families face the adaptive challenges of living with breast cancer. Follow-up care includes early detection of recurrent disease, with an emphasis on breast self-examination, yearly mammography, and regular examination by health care professionals.

KEY CONCEPTS

- Chronic inflammation of the subareolar ducts may result in mammary duct ectasia. Fibrous thickening results in a palpable central mass, breast distortion and dimpling, and nipple inversion. Persistent nipple discharge may occur. These signs are similar to those of malignancy and are carefully evaluated by biopsy. Surgical excision may be performed.
- Breast abscesses in nonlactating women are commonly associated with chronic infection, diabetes, and steroid therapy. These abscesses respond poorly to antibiotics and tend to recur.
- Fibrocystic breast disease is a condition in which palpable breast masses are present and fluctuate with the menstrual cycle. Breast cysts are firm, mobile, and tender, and are usually located in the upper outer quadrant. There is no evidence that women with fibrocystic breasts are at higher risk for breast cancer. A low-fat, high-carbohydrate diet; danazol; heat therapy; and avoidance of methylxanthines may be recommended.
- Breast cancer is the most common cancer in women between 25 and 75 years of age. Malignant tumors tend to be painless, hard, and fixed in place, in contrast to benign breast tumors, which are mobile and encapsulated. Risk factors for breast cancer include a high-fat diet, a first-degree relative with breast cancer, increasing age, radiation exposure, and a previous malignancy. In addition, reproductive factors such as the age at first pregnancy and the number of pregnancies may be associated with altered cancer risk.
- Breast cancer may spread to the regional lymphatics and disseminate to other sites. Localized breast cancer, without lymph node involvement, has an 84% 5-year survival rate. The survival rate falls to 56% when lymph nodes are cancerous. Depending on the extent of tumor spread, surgery may be performed to remove the tumor only (lumpectomy), the affected breast only (simple mastectomy), the affected breast and involved lymph nodes (modified radical mastectomy), or the breast, lymphatics, and underlying muscle (radical mastectomy). In addition, radiation therapy and chemotherapy may be initiated.

SUMMARY

This chapter has described the most prevalent women's reproductive health problems at the present time. Any alteration in reproductive status may have profound implications for the individual; thus the reader should review this material carefully to acquire the ability to distinguish the differences and similarities in these alterations.

Commonly occurring alterations in reproductive health for women may have serious consequences and require immediate intervention. Menstrual disorders may have multiple manifestations, and such disorders as amenorrhea and abnormal uterine bleeding may occur at any time throughout a woman's life. Alterations in uterine position and pelvic support, including uterine prolapse, retrodisplacement of the uterus, cystocele, and rectocele, may result in severe symptoms and require surgical correction. Inflammation and infection of the female reproductive tract, including PID and vulvovaginitis, may have far-reaching effects for the individual experiencing them.

The reader should pay particular attention to the section on benign growths and aberrant tissue of the female reproductive tract given the widespread nature and potentially serious consequences of these lesions. A thorough understanding of uterine leiomyomas, ovarian cysts, and endometriosis includes the ability to define these syndromes as described in this book, as well as an ability to explain them to clients. In addition, the reader is urged to review the material regarding the efficacy of the Pap smear in detecting cervical cancer at an early stage.

The section on disorders of pregnancy highlighted the most important aspects of this topic; the reader will probably wish to use this information as a basis for a more in-depth study of this area in a specialized course in maternal-child nursing. Finally, because of the widespread threat to women's health posed by disorders of the breast, particular attention should be paid to the final section. Specifically, the reader must be able to compare and contrast the differences between benign breast disorders and carcinoma of the breast and discuss the meaning and importance of various risk factors for breast carcinoma in a knowledgeable way.

MEDIA RESOURCES

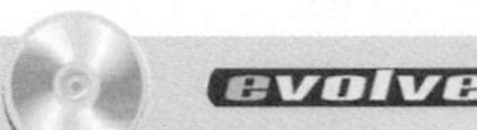

evolve

Remember to check out the ***CD Companion*** included with this book for Review Questions, Key Concepts Review, Glossary (with audio for selected terms), Disease Profiles, and Animations.

PLUS, visit the ***Evolve website*** at http://evolve.elsevier.com/Copstead/ for Case Studies, Disease Profiles, and WebLinks.

References

1. Hacker NF, Moore JG: *Essentials of obstetrics and gynecology,* ed 2, Philadelphia, 1992, Saunders.
2. Glass RH: *Office gynecology,* ed 4, Baltimore, 1992, Williams & Wilkins.
3. Hubasher D, Grimes DA: Noncontraceptive health benefits of intrauterine devices: a systematic review, *Obstet Gynecol Surv* 57:120-128, 2002.
4. Wilson RJ, Carrington ER: *Obstetrics and gynecology,* ed 9, St Louis, 1991, Mosby.
5. Diamond MP, Freeman ML: Clinical implications of postsurgical adhesions, *Hum Reprod Update* 7:567-576, 2001.
6. Keshavarz H et al: Hysterectomy surveillance—United States, 1994-1999, *MMWR Morb Mortal Wkly Rep* 51(ss-5):1-8, 2002.
7. Kimura I et al: Ovarian torsion: CT and MR imaging appearances, *Radiology* 190(2):337-341, 1994.
8. Mahmood TA, Templeton A: Prevalence and genesis of endometriosis, *Hum Reprod* 6(4):544-549, 1991.
9. Parkin DM, Bray FI, Devesa SS: Cancer burden in the year 2000: the global picture, *Eur J Cancer* 37(suppl 8):S4-S66, 2001.
10. Saraiya M et al: Observations from the CDC. An assessment of Pap smears and hysterectomies among women in the United States, *J Women's Health Gend Based Med* 11:103-109, 2002.
11. Koutsky LA et al: A controlled trial of a human papillomavirus type 16 vaccine, *N Engl J Med* 347:1645-1651, 2002.
12. Rebbeck TR et al: Prophylactic oophorectomy in carriers of BRCA1 or BRCA2 mutations, *N Engl J Med* 346:1616-1622, 2002.
13. Rouzier R et al: Local relapse in patients treated for squamous cell vulvar carcinoma: incidence and prognostic value, *Obstet Gynecol* 100:1159-1167, 2002.
14. American College of Obstetricians and Gynecologists: *Diagnosis and management of preeclampsia and eclampsia,* ACOG Practice Bulletin No 33, Washington, DC, 2002, The College.
15. American College of Obstetricians and Gynecologists: *Management of early pregnancy loss,* ACOG Practice Bulletin No 24, Washington, DC, 2001, The College.
16. Harris JR et al: *Diseases of the breast,* Philadelphia, 1995, Lippincott-Raven.
17. Haile RW et al: A case-control study of reproductive variables, alcohol, and smoking in premenopausal bilateral breast cancer, *Breast Cancer Res Treat* 37(1):49-56, 1996.
18. Writing Group for the Women's Health Initiative Investigators: Risks and benefits of estrogen plus progestin in healthy postmenopausal women: principal results from the Women's Health Initiative randomized controlled trial, *JAMA* 288:321-333, 2002.
19. Breast cancer and breastfeeding: collaborative reanalysis of individual data from 47 epidemiological studies in 30 countries, including 50,302 women with breast cancer and 96,973 women without the disease, *Lancet* 360:187-195, 2002.
20. Kauff ND et al: Risk-reducing salpingo-oophorectomy in women with a BRCA1 or BRCA2 mutation, *N Engl Med* 346:1609-1615, 2002.
21. US Preventative Services Task Force: Chemoprevention of breast cancer: recommendations and rationale, *Ann Intern Med* 137:56-58, 2002.

Sexually Transmitted Diseases

chapter 34

Paul D. Silva • Jane M. Georges

MEDIA RESOURCES

Additional Material for Study, Review, and Further Exploration

CD Companion ◆ Review Questions and Answers ◆ Key Concepts Review
◆ Glossary *(with audio pronunciations for selected terms)*
◆ Disease Profiles ◆ Animations

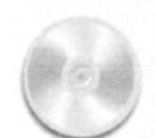

evolve ***Website*** at http://evolve.elsevier.com/Copstead/
◆ Case Studies ◆ Disease Profiles ◆ WebLinks

KEY QUESTIONS

- What are the characteristic clinical manifestations and lesions of gonorrhea and chlamydial infection?
- How do the pathologic changes and clinical manifestations of syphilis differ during the incubation, primary, secondary, and tertiary phases?
- How do the lesions of herpes simplex, syphilis, and lymphogranuloma venereum differ?
- Which sexually transmitted diseases remain localized and which have systemic consequences?
- What are the causative organisms and characteristic lesions of the following localized sexually transmitted diseases: chancroid, granuloma inguinale, molluscum contagiosum, and condylomata acuminata (genital warts)?

CHAPTER OUTLINE

An epidemic of sexually transmitted diseases (STDs) currently exists in the United States.[1,2] About one million gonococcal infections are reported each year to the Public Health Service, and it is estimated that 3 million to 4 million chlamydial infections occur each year.[1,3] The true incidence of these infections is likely to be significantly higher inasmuch as many sexually transmitted infections go unreported. The cost of STDs, in both economic and personal terms, is extremely high. It is estimated that the annual total cost associated with managing acute pelvic inflammatory disease associated with STDs in women amounts to more than $3 billion.[1] In addition, the personal costs to the individual experiencing an STD may include pain, disfigurement, and permanent sterility. It has been estimated that about 15 million persons acquire a new STD each year in the United States.[3] Because of the epidemic status of these diseases and the enormous costs associated with them, it is imperative that health care providers become sufficiently knowledgeable to assess their clients' STD status and educate them about STDs in an accurate and compassionate manner.

The term **sexually transmitted diseases** refers to a large group of disease syndromes that can be transmitted sexually, regardless of whether the disease has manifestations in genital structures.[1] In older texts, STDs are referred to as venereal diseases. Although STDs are more prevalent in the 15- to 25-year-old age group, they can occur at any age. These diseases are sometimes contracted by nonsexual transmission, as when a newborn infant contracts an STD from an infected mother during passage through the birth canal.[1]

A list of sexually transmitted organisms grouped according to type of pathogen is found in Box 34-1. As the box shows, the list of pathogens that can be transmitted sexually is quite extensive, and the diseases that these pathogens can produce are equally extensive. Many pathogens produce multiple diseases, and many diseases may be caused by more than one pathogen. A useful approach to learning the complex pathophysiologic processes of STDs is to group STDs according to the disease manifestations that the client is most likely to exhibit when first seen by the care provider. These categories of STDs and the disease manifestations associated with them are listed in Table 34-1. This chapter describes each of these categories and the pathophysiologic processes associated with each relevant STD.

Box 34-1

Sexually Transmitted Organisms

Bacterial Pathogens
Calymmatobacterium granulomatis
Chlamydia trachomatis
Gardnerella vaginalis
Haemophilus ducreyi
Mycoplasma hominis
Neisseria gonorrhoeae
Shigella
Group B streptococci
Ureaplasma urealyticum
Treponema pallidum

Fungal Pathogens
Candida albicans
Candida glabrata

Viral Pathogens
AIDS-related viruses
Cytomegalovirus
Herpes simplex virus
Hepatitis virus
Human papillomavirus
Molluscum contagiosum virus

Protozoan Pathogens
Entamoeba histolytica
Giardia lamblia
Trichomonas vaginalis

Some diseases listed in Table 34-1 are discussed elsewhere in this volume but have been included here for completeness. In particular, the reader may wish to refer to Chapter 33 for more detailed information on pelvic inflammatory disease and vulvovaginitis. Also, certain systemic infections are potentially transmitted by sexual contact. Cytomegalovirus infection, hepatitis A and B, and acquired immunodeficiency syndrome (AIDS) have the potential for sexual transmission. These diseases are covered in detail in Units III and X, along with more in-depth information concerning infectious processes and immune responses. Before studying this chapter, the reader may wish to refer to Chapters 8 and 9 for a review of basic terminology such as *incubation period* and *period of*

Table 34-1

Sexually Transmitted Diseases Categorized According to Disease Manifestations

Disease Manifestations	Disease
Urethritis, cervicitis, and salpingitis	Gonorrhea Nongonococcal urethritis Pelvic inflammatory disease
Ulcerative lesions with systemic involvement	Syphilis Lymphogranuloma venereum Herpes
Ulcerative lesions only	Chancroid Granuloma inguinale (donovanosis)
Nonulcerative lesions	Molluscum contagiosum Condylomata acuminata
Vulvovaginitis	Trichomoniasis Candidiasis *Gardnerella vaginalis* vaginitis
Systemic infections	Cytomegalovirus Hepatitis AIDS
Enteric infections	Giardiasis *Campylobacter* enteritis Shigellosis Amebic dysentery

communicability. Health care providers caring for persons at risk for STDs should be aware of the potential for acquisition of systemic diseases by sexual contact and include assessment of these diseases as part of their overall clinical evaluation.

URETHRITIS, CERVICITIS, SALPINGITIS, AND PELVIC INFLAMMATORY DISEASE

Three types of STD are manifested by *urethritis* (inflammation of the urethra), *cervicitis* (inflammation of the uterine cervix), and/or *salpingitis* (inflammation of the oviduct or fallopian tube). **Gonorrhea** is an inflammation of epithelial tissue by the organism *Neisseria gonorrhoeae.* Nongonococcal urethritis refers to urethritis resulting from a pathogen other than the gonococcus, which is usually *Chlamydia trachomatis. Pelvic inflammatory disease,* which was described in Chapter 33, is usually the result of acute salpingitis caused by gonococcal or chlamydial infection that has extended into nearby pelvic tissue.[1,4]

Gonococcal Infection

Etiology and Clinical Manifestations. In gonorrhea, disease transmission occurs through contact with exudates from the mucous membranes of infected persons, usually by direct contact. The gonococcus then attaches to and penetrates columnar epithelium and produces a patchy inflammatory response in the submucosa with a polymorphonuclear exudate.[1] Although usually asymptomatic in women, gonorrhea may produce purulent vaginal discharge, dysuria, and abnormal vaginal bleeding. The most commonly affected areas in women are the cervix, the urethra, the Skene and Bartholin glands, and the anus. Adolescents (age 15 to 19 years) now have the highest rates of gonorrhea.[5] In men, symptoms of urethritis, including dysuria and a purulent urethral discharge accompanied by redness and swelling at the site of infection, usually occur after a 3- to 6-day incubation period. In both sexes, infection and inflammation of the pharynx, conjunctivae, and anus may be present. Direct extension of the infection with gonococci occurs by way of the lymphatic system. In the female, extension may spread unilaterally or bilaterally to the oviducts, with subsequent salpingitis. In the male, direct extension of the infection most frequently occurs to the epididymis.[1,6]

Once gonococcal infection has spread to other areas, localized infection occurs and may cause the formation of cysts and abscesses. Purulent exudate containing the organism causes damage to tissue, and fibrous tissue replaces inflamed tissue. This hardened, fibrous tissue may result in scarring and narrowing of the urethra, epididymis, or oviducts. In women, partial or complete closure of the oviducts results in sterility. Infection of the oviducts may also result in pelvic inflammatory disease if exudate is released into the peritoneal cavity.[1,7,8] As described in Chapter 33, pelvic inflammatory disease may be an acute or chronic condition causing widespread damage to the pelvic organs in the female.

Nongonococcal Infection

Etiology. Nongonococcal urethritis and cervicitis are often caused by strains of *C. trachomatis* that act on columnar epithelium in a manner similar to that noted for the gonococcus. The symptoms of infection with *Chlamydia* are generally less severe than those of gonorrhea. As with gonorrhea, the infection may spread by extension to the oviducts, and pelvic inflammatory disease may eventually result. Upper reproductive tract infection, whether symptomatic or subclinical, is an important cause of infertility and ectopic pregnancy.[9] Transmission of *Chlamydia* during birth may result in **ophthalmia neonatorum,** or infection of the eyes in the newborn.[2]

Treatment. Resistance of *N. gonorrhoeae* to antimicrobial agents continues to spread and intensify. Newer antimicrobial agents such as ceftriaxone, cefixime, ciprofloxacin, ofloxacin, and levofloxacin are now being used to manage uncomplicated gonococcal infections.[9] Unless chlamydial infection is ruled out, dual therapy for gonococcal and chlamydial infection consisting of azithromycin or doxycycline added to one of the above agents is recommended.[9] Pelvic inflammatory disease is also generally managed with two agents to cover potential chlamydial and gonorrheal infection. A number of organizations now recommend *Chlamydia* (as well as gonorrhea) screening for sexually active adolescents and women through age 25 who have no symptoms in order to reduce the sequelae of infection.[10]

KEY CONCEPTS

- Urethritis, cervicitis, salpingitis, and pelvic inflammatory disease are commonly due to gonorrhea or chlamydial infection. Transmission is usually by direct contact with infected mucous membranes. The symptoms of chlamydial infection are usually less severe than those of gonorrhea.
- Gonorrhea may produce purulent discharge, dysuria, and abnormal vaginal bleeding. Cysts and abscesses may form in localized areas of infection, followed by scarring and fibrosis. Inflammation of the pharynx, conjunctivae, and anus may be present. Antibiotic therapy is indicated.

DISEASES WITH SYSTEMIC INVOLVEMENT

Several STDs cause a distinctive ulcerative lesion and disseminate throughout the body to affect multiple organ systems. Most prominent of this type of STD are syphilis, herpesvirus infections, and lymphogranuloma venereum (LGV).

Syphilis

Syphilis is a systemic infection of the vascular system consisting of five distinct stages: incubation, primary and secondary stages, latency, and late syphilis.[1] Syphilis is communicable by persons with primary, secondary, or early latent syphilis.[1] The incidence of syphilis has been on the rise in the United States since 1958. An estimated 136,000 cases of primary and secondary syphilis occur annually. Although much of the increase in cases has occurred in the male homosexual population, an increasing rate has also been observed in heterosexual women.[3]

Etiology. Syphilis is caused by *Treponema pallidum,* an anaerobic spirochete. Syphilis is acquired when *T. pallidum* penetrates intact mucous membrane or abraded skin during sexual contact. (The process of transmission of congenital syphilis is described later.) Some of the *T. pallidum* pathogens remain at the original invasion site, whereas others migrate to regional lymph nodes within hours. During this incubation phase, *T. pallidum* is disseminated throughout the body and can invade and multiply in any organ system.[1]

Pathogenesis. During all stages of syphilis, invasion of tissue by *T. pallidum* results in pathologic changes in the vascular system. The inflammatory response in endothelial tissue causes the infiltration of lymphocytes and plasma cells, with subsequent endothelial swelling. The terminal arterioles and small arteries may become obliterated and no longer functional. Finally, long-term inflammation of vascular tissue results in the formation of hardened, fibrous thickening in the blood vessels and eventually tissue necrosis.[2]

After the initial incubation period of 10 to 90 days, the primary phase begins with the formation of a **chancre,** a painless, ulcerative lesion that arises at the original spirochete portal of entry (Figure 34-1). The chancre may go unnoticed in a female if it occurs on the cervix or in the vagina; in fact, most cases of syphilis in women go undiagnosed until recognized by positive testing of the blood in the latent phase. In males, the chancre may form on the genitalia; in both sexes, chancres may erupt on the anus, fingers, lips, tongue, nipples, tonsils, or eyelids.[4]

Untreated chancres will resolve spontaneously within 3 to 6 weeks and are followed by the secondary stage of syphilis, which is characterized by a low-grade fever, malaise, sore throat, headache, lymphadenopathy, and mucosal or cutaneous rash (Figure 34-2). This secondary stage occurs as *T. pallidum* is spread throughout the blood stream and lymphatic system. The secondary stage is also self-limiting and is followed by a latent phase in which no symptoms are present. During the latent stage, the affected person will test positive for syphilis on serologic assays and may still experience infectious mucocutaneous lesions during the early latent stage. Thus, the early latent stage is considered contagious. The latent stage is of variable length and may last more than 40 years.[2] In approximately two thirds of patients the infection remains asymptomatic and never causes a recurrence of symptoms. If syphilis remains untreated, then late syphilis—the final, destructive phase of the disease—will eventually develop in approximately one third of affected people.[4] The manifestations of late syphilis depend on the area of arterial lesions and the extent of circulatory insufficiency.[2] Body sys-

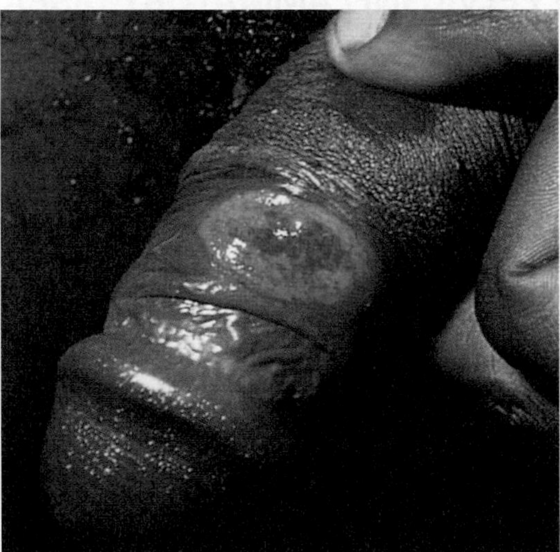

FIGURE 34-1 ■ Typical syphilitic chancre, a painless, ulcerative lesion that arises at the original spirochete portal of entry. (From Morse SA et al: *Atlas of sexually transmitted diseases and AIDS,* ed 3, St Louis, 2003, Mosby, p 28.)

tems particularly at risk are the cardiovascular and central nervous systems. Damage to the cardiovascular system may include aortic necrosis and subsequent aortic insufficiency; damage to the central nervous system may be progressively widespread, with degeneration of the cortical neurons and, eventually, paresis, blindness, and mental deterioration.[4]

Transmission of *T. pallidum* from the mother to the fetus may occur transplacentally at any point during pregnancy, but an inflammatory response to the pathogen does not develop in the fetus until around the 15th week of gestation. Therefore, treatment of infected women before the 15th week may prevent damage to the fetus. Infection with syphilis before birth may result in physical deformities and developmental disabilities in the infant. Infants born to untreated or inadequately treated mothers will have active infection and must be treated.[1] A presumptive diagnosis of syphilis is generally based on a positive result of a serologic screening test, such as the Venereal Disease Research Laboratory (VDRL) or rapid plasmid reagin (RPR) test, followed by a positive result of a treponemal serologic test.[2] Dark-field examination of tissue and exudates or direct fluorescent antibody tests may also be useful.

Treatment. Penicillin is the first choice for the management of syphilis. If the affected person is allergic to penicillin, tetracycline or doxycycline is given. Treatment is administered to all individuals with positive evidence of syphilis on laboratory testing and to people who have had sexual contact with infected individuals.[1] Response to antibiotic treatment is monitored by repeating laboratory testing for evidence of syphilis at regular intervals up to 24 months after therapy.[4] Management during pregnancy is complex, but it focuses on maternal cure and prevention of congenital syphilis.[11]

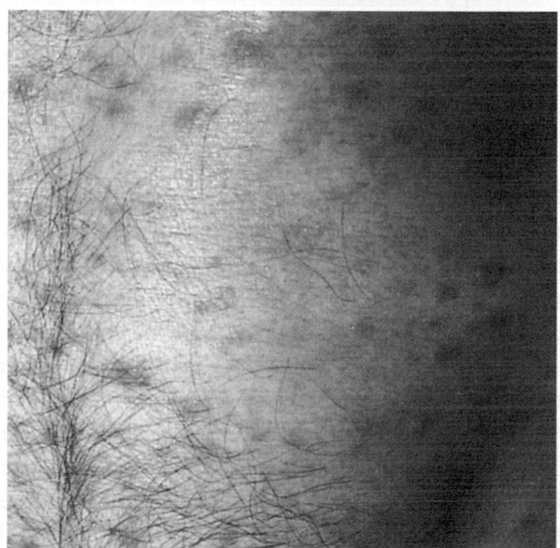

FIGURE 34-2 ■ Typical generalized skin rash of secondary syphilis. (From Morse SA et al: *Atlas of sexually transmitted diseases and AIDS*, ed 3, St Louis, 2003, Mosby, p 29.)

Lymphogranuloma Venereum

Lymphogranuloma venereum is a highly contagious systemic infection caused by a number of closely related strains of ***Chlamydia.*** The disease occurs more commonly in the tropics but has been reported with some frequency in the southeastern United States.[4] LGV develops more often in males than in females and has a higher incidence among sexually active young adults.

Etiology and Pathogenesis. Like syphilis, LGV has stages of development in which an initial lesion forms and systemic disease occurs after dissemination via the lymphatic system. Three stages occur in LGV: (1) a primary lesion; (2) regional inflammation of the lymphatic system (also called lymphadenitis); and (3) late complications resulting from progression of the lymphadenitis.[1]

After invasion of the mucosa by *Chlamydia* during sexual contact, a painless lesion appears on the genitalia after a 1- to 3-week incubation period. The lesion may range from a slight erosion to a small papule and often goes undetected (Figure 34-3). This lesion heals spontaneously in a few days. During this period, the pathogens are disseminated to regional lymph nodes, primarily the inguinal lymph nodes.

About 2 weeks after appearance of the primary lesion, the inguinal lymph nodes begin to swell, and the systemic symptoms of fever and malaise develop. The nodal swelling is a manifestation of inflammation of the lymphatic system in which lesions filled with polymorphonuclear leukocytes are forming in the lymph nodes. Spread of the inflammation throughout adjacent lymph nodes causes multiple nodes to become matted together and form a large abscess. These abscesses are said to be regional because they develop in one or more areas along the lymphatic system. If a person with LGV remains untreated, the abscesses rupture through the skin and other body cavities to create chronic fistulas. Thus, as the regional lymphadenitis progresses, complications such as perianal and rectovaginal fistulas develop, along with strictures of the rectum. Other complications include extreme swelling of the genitalia; this occurs because the normal lymph drainage of this area is impeded.[4] The diagnosis is usually made by serologic testing (antibody titers).

Treatment. Doxycycline is the recommended antibiotic with erythromycin being the alternative. Surgical treatment may include aspiration of lymph nodes as needed; rectal strictures and fistulas may require surgical correction.[2]

Herpesvirus Infections

Herpesviruses are an important group of viral agents that produce infection in humans. Two types of herpes simplex virus (HSV)—type 1 and type 2—may be sexually transmitted and are discussed in this section. HSV type 1 is most often associated with herpetic infections above the waist, typically

called soft chancre) and **granuloma inguinale** are both manifested by ulcerative lesions, although their pathophysiologic courses differ.

Chancroid

Etiology. Chancroid is an ulcerative, infectious disease of the genital tract caused by the sexually transmitted anaerobic bacillus *Haemophilus ducreyi.* Chancroid was relatively rare in the United States until the past decade. Since 1981, small epidemic outbreaks of chancroid have been reported in the United States. In terms of outbreaks in Western countries there is an approximately 10:1 male-to-female ratio.[1] Chancroid is a cofactor for human immunodeficiency virus infection.

Pathogenesis and Clinical Manifestations. *Haemophilus ducreyi* initially invades the genital skin or mucous membranes at sites traumatized by sexual contact. The patient generally has one or more painful genital ulcers, unlike the chancre in syphilis, which is generally solitary and painless. Fresh lesions may occur from autoinoculation (self-infection). The ulcerated lesions may enlarge, continue to erode (Figure 34-6), and produce destruction of surrounding tissue. In addition, inguinal lymph nodes may become tender and painful as the infection is disseminated to this region. If the infection goes untreated, the enlarged lymph gland (called a *bubo*) may rupture, draining pus and leaving a large inguinal ulcer. The infection is communicable until the lesions heal, which may be a period of weeks.[18,19] Scarring may occur in advanced cases. Diagnosis is usually made by culture for *H. ducreyi.*

Treatment. Antiinfective agents recommended for management of chancroid include azithromycin, erythromycin, ceftriaxone, and ciprofloxacin.[9] Large ulcers may not heal for more than 2 weeks. As with all STDs, sexual partners should be treated simultaneously and reexposure avoided until therapy is completed. Aspiration of enlarged inguinal lymph nodes may also be indicated.[1]

Granuloma Inguinale

Etiology. *Calymmatobacterium granulomatis* is the causative agent of granuloma inguinale. This intracellular bacterium is also referred to as a Donovan body and the disease as donovanosis. Granuloma inguinale is rare in the United States, with the highest incidence in homosexual males.[1,2]

Pathogenesis and Clinical Manifestations. Transmission of granuloma inguinale is not clearly understood. It is generally thought to be an STD, but the disease is also seen in adults who are not sexually active and in young children, possibly as a result of autoinoculation. The causative bacterium is found in the rectum of nondiseased persons, which suggests that the organism may be part of the normal gastrointestinal flora in some persons.[2] The communicability of the disease is relatively low, and it is generally believed that repeated exposure is necessary.[1]

The incubation period is variable and ranges from a few days to months. The initial sign of the disease may be a painless papule or nodule that subsequently ulcerates into an enlarging, granulomatous, red velvety ulcer. The raised mass of granulation tissue may look more like a tumor than an ulcer. The lesions are highly vascular and bleed easily with minor contact. Single or multiple lesions may coalesce, or lesions may spread to nearby tissue.[2] Secondary infection of the ulcers and expanding tissue necrosis in lesions may lead to erosion of

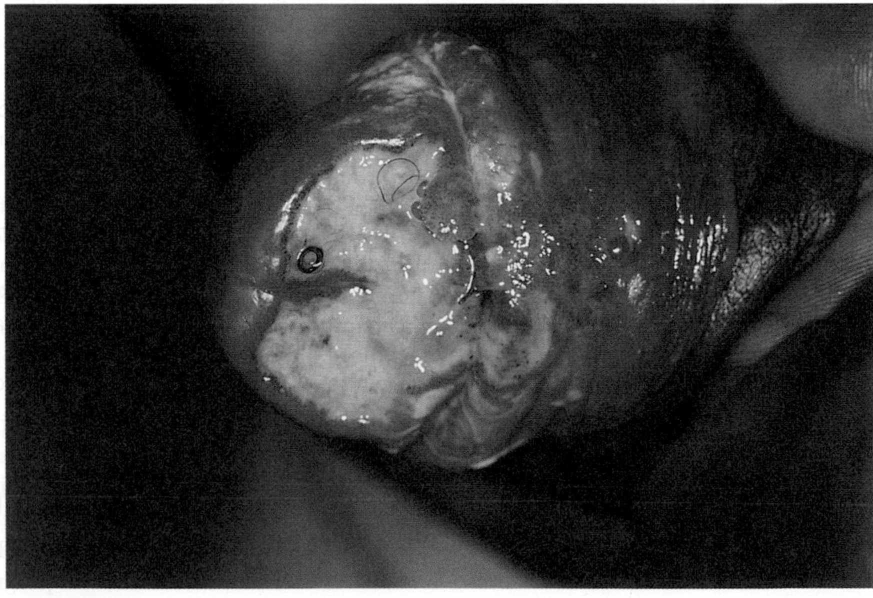

FIGURE 34-6 ■ The eroded, purulent ulcer of chancroid. (From Morse SA et al: *Atlas of sexually transmitted diseases and AIDS,* ed 3, St Louis, 2003, Mosby, p 56.)

the genitals. In addition, the formation of scar tissue on genital structures during the healing process may produce urethral occlusion.[2] Lymph node involvement is minimal, and inguinal swelling is usually due to the presence of subcutaneous granulomas.[1,20] Diagnosis is by identification of the dark-staining Donovan bodies on biopsy or tissue crush preparations.

Treatment. Doxycycline or trimethoprim-sulfamethoxazole is given for at least 3 weeks or until all lesions are healed.[9] Alternative agents include ciprofloxacin, erythromycin, and azithromycin.[9] Long-term follow-up should be provided because this disease may recur.[1]

Nonulcerative Lesions

Molluscum contagiosum and condylomata acuminata (also called genital warts) are two prevalent types of STDs that produce nonulcerative lesions. Both are caused by viral agents that invade superficial layers of the epidermis during sexual contact.

Molluscum Contagiosum

Etiology. **Molluscum contagiosum** is a viral skin disease caused by a member of the poxvirus family.[2] (The term "poxvirus" refers to a viral agent that causes an eruption, or "pox," on the skin.) The manifestations are much milder than those of smallpox or chickenpox. Two forms of the disease exist. One affects children and is transmitted by skin-to-skin contact and indirect contact; the other affects young adults and is transmitted during sexual contact.[1]

Pathogenesis and Clinical Manifestations. After invasion of the epidermis by the virus, pink to white lesions with an exudative core appear on the genitalia. The lesions are multiple, are slow to develop, and remain stable for long periods. The disease is usually asymptomatic, tends to be self-limiting, and lasts on average 2 years.[1,2]

Treatment. The goal of treatment is primarily to prevent spread of the infection for cosmetic reasons. The lesions can be removed by minor surgery or frozen with liquid nitrogen. Sexual contacts of affected persons should be examined to prevent further spread.[1]

Condylomata Acuminata

Etiology. **Condylomata acuminata** (singular: condyloma acuminatum) are benign epithelial tumors of the anogenital region.[1] The wartlike appearance of these lesions has caused them to be referred to as genital or venereal warts. Condylomata acuminata are caused by strains of the human papillomavirus. Condylomata acuminata are predominantly transmitted sexually in young adults, with the highest prevalence in the 16- to 25-year-old age group.[1] The risk of contracting the disease by sexual contact with an infected person is high; lesions will develop in up to two thirds of the sexual contacts of affected persons. Nonsexual transmission has also been documented, and lesions have been found in infants.[1] The period of communicability is unknown but is thought to last as long as the lesions persist.[1]

Pathogenesis and Clinical Manifestations. After invasion of the epidermis by human papillomavirus, an incubation period of 1 to 20 months (usually about 4 months) precedes the appearance of lesions. It is thought that the virus infects single epithelial cells and stimulates the cells to divide and proliferate into the wartlike lesions. The lesions are single or multiple, soft pink to brown, and usually elongated. They may occur in clusters and sometimes as large cauliflower-like masses (Figure 34-7). The lesions are generally asymptomatic but may be pruritic (itchy), painful, or friable (bleed easily). In females, condylomata acuminata may be found in the vagina

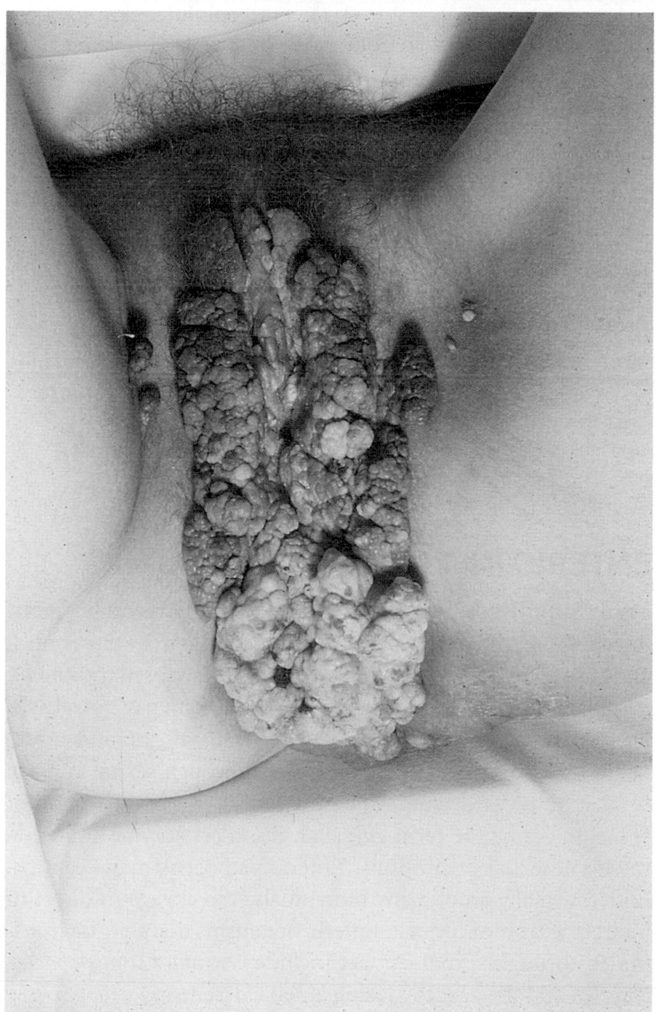

FIGURE 34-7 ■ Clusters of condylomata acuminata form large, cauliflower-like masses on the vulva. (From Morse SA et al: *Atlas of sexually transmitted diseases and AIDS,* ed 3, St Louis, 2003, Mosby, p 268.)

and cervix, as well as in the anogenital area.[1] In males, they may occur in the anterior urethra and anogenital area.

Treatment. External genital warts may be treated with patient applied podofilox or imiquimod topical preparations.[9] Providers can administer cryotherapy, podophyllin, trichloroacetic acid, bichloroacetic acid, or surgery.[9] Alternative regimens include intralesional interferon and laser surgery. Because malignant transformation to invasive carcinoma has been observed with some types of condylomata acuminata, it is generally agreed that affected persons should be treated or monitored carefully.[9] A number of strains of human papillomavirus have been associated with cervical cancer, and there has been an increasing use of human papillomavirus testing in evaluating abnormal Papanicolaou smears.[20]

KEY CONCEPTS

- Chancroid is caused by infection with an anaerobic bacillus. Initially the lesion is a small erythematous papule, and after 2 to 3 days the painful lesion ulcerates. Lesions resemble those of syphilis; however, the lesions of syphilis are painless.
- Granuloma inguinale is caused by an intracellular bacterium. The initial papule is painless and subsequently ulcerates into a growing granulomatous ulcer resembling a tumor.
- Molluscum contagiosum is associated with infection by a poxvirus. Genital lesions are pink to white with an exudative core. The disease is usually asymptomatic and self-limiting.
- Condylomata acuminata, or genital warts, are associated with infection by human papillomavirus. Warts are pink to brown and painless and may occur in clusters. Human papillomavirus infection is an important risk factor for cervical cancer.

ENTERIC INFECTIONS

Until recently, information regarding the transmission of enteric infections of the gastrointestinal tract through sexual contact was limited. Recent research in this area has increased the knowledge base of health care providers, and the term **gay bowel syndrome** has been coined to describe the transmission and subsequent infection with enteric pathogens through sexual contact. It must be stressed that despite the specific reference to homosexual males by the term *gay,* such disorders are *not* limited to the homosexual community. Enteric pathogens may be transmitted sexually among any individuals who engage in direct or indirect fecal-oral contact. Enteric organisms that may be transmitted through sexual contact include *Giardia, Campylobacter, Shigella,* and the agents causing amebic dysentery.[4]

The pathophysiologic process of enteric infections of the gastrointestinal tract is described in Chapter 36, and the reader may wish to refer to this material. In general, persons who have acquired enteric infections by sexual contact will have variable manifestations. Some individuals may experience no symptoms, whereas others will have marked symptoms of enteritis or proctitis. All individuals who engage in oral-anal sexual practices should be monitored for the presence of enteric infections with laboratory studies and diagnostic examinations. Education for persons at risk for sexually transmitted enteric infections includes an emphasis on protective hygienic practices. Infected persons should avoid all sexual contact until all partners are examined and treated if necessary. After completion of appropriate therapy for enteric infections, affected individuals should be retested for assessment of therapeutic effectiveness.[4]

SUMMARY

Because of the epidemic nature of STDs, it is essential for readers preparing for careers in the health sciences to have a complete grasp of the material in this chapter. The STDs considered in the chapter are grouped according to the disease manifestations that the client is most likely to exhibit. Gonorrhea, most chlamydial infections, and pelvic inflammatory disease are manifested by urethritis, cervicitis, or salpingitis. A second group of STDs cause ulcerative lesions with systemic involvement. Syphilis, herpes, and LGV all cause a distinctive ulcerative lesion and may disseminate throughout the body to affect multiple organ systems.

In reviewing the material on STDs related to ulcerative and nonulcerative lesions, the reader should compare and contrast the appearance of these lesions and consider the differing pathophysiologic characteristics of each type. Finally, the reader should consider how he or she would incorporate this material into an overall assessment process. Nurses and other health care providers caring for persons at risk for STDs should be aware of the potential for acquisition of these diseases as well. The overall goal in learning the material in this chapter is to be able to assess and educate clients with STDs in a comfortable and accurate manner.

MEDIA RESOURCES

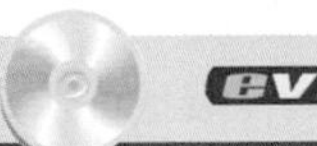

Remember to check out the ***CD Companion*** included with this book for Review Questions, Key Concepts Review, Glossary (with audio for selected terms), Disease Profiles, and Animations.

PLUS, visit the ***Evolve website*** at http://evolve.elsevier.com/Copstead/ for Case Studies, Disease Profiles, and WebLinks.

References

1. Holmes KK et al, editors: *Sexually transmitted diseases,* ed 3, New York, 1999, McGraw-Hill.
2. Borchardt KA, Noble MA, editors: *Sexually transmitted diseases: epidemiology, pathology, diagnosis, and treatment,* Boca Raton, Fla, 1997, CRC Press.

3. Cates W, the American Social Health Association Panel: estimates of the incidence and prevalence of STDs in the United States, *Sex Transm Dis* 26(suppl 4):S2-S7, 1999.
4. Gorbach SL, Bartlett JG, Blacklow NR, editors: *Infectious diseases,* ed 2, Philadelphia, 1998, Saunders.
5. Division of STD Prevention: *Sexually transmitted disease surveillance, 1999,* Atlanta, 2000, Centers for Disease Control and Prevention.
6. Horner PJ et al: Gonorrhoea: signs, symptoms, and serogroups, *Int J STD AIDS* 3(6):430-433, 1992.
7. Copeland LJ, editor: *Textbook of gynecology,* Philadelphia, 1993, Saunders.
8. Jossens MO, Schacter J, Sweet RL: Risk factors associated with pelvic inflammatory disease of differing microbial etiologies, *Obstet Gynecol* 83(6):989-997, 1994.
9. Centers for Disease Control and Prevention: Sexually transmitted diseases treatment guidelines 2002, *MMWR Morb Mortal Wkly Rep* 51(No. RR-6):1-80, 2002.
10. U.S. Preventive Services Task Force: Screening for chlamydial infection: recommendations and rationale, *Am J Prev Med* 20(3S):90-94, 2001.
11. Wendel GD et al: Treatment of syphilis in pregnancy and prevention of congenital syphilis, *Clin Infect Dis* 35(suppl 2):S200-S209, 2002.
12. Fleming DT et al: Herpes simplex virus type 2 in the United States, 1976 to 1994, *N Engl J Med* 337:1105-1111, 1997.
13. Schacker T et al: Frequency of symptomatic and asymptomatic herpes simplex type 2 reactivations among human immunodeficiency virus-infected men, *J Infect Dis* 178:1616-1622, 1998.
14. Mostad MB et al: Cervical shedding of herpes simplex virus in human immunodeficiency virus–infected women: effects of hormonal contraception, pregnancy, and vitamin A deficiency, *J Infect Dis* 181:58-63, 2000.
15. Corey L: Challenges in genital herpes simplex virus management, *J Infect Dis* 186(suppl 1):S29-S33, 2002.
16. Wald A et al: Effect of condoms on reducing the transmission of herpes simplex virus type-2 from men to women, *JAMA* 285:3100-3106, 2001.
17. Brown ZA et al: The acquisition of herpes simplex virus during pregnancy, *N Engl J Med* 337:509-515, 1997.
18. Robin MC: *The handbook of sexually transmitted diseases: a clinical approach,* San Diego, 1995, KW Publications.
19. Quinn TE: *Sexually transmitted diseases,* vol 8, *Advances in host defense mechanisms,* New York, 1992, Raven Press.
20. Solomon D, Schiffman M, Tarone R. Comparison of three management strategies for patients with atypical squamous cells of undetermined significance: baseline results from a randomized trial, *J Natl Cancer Inst* 93:293-299, 2001.

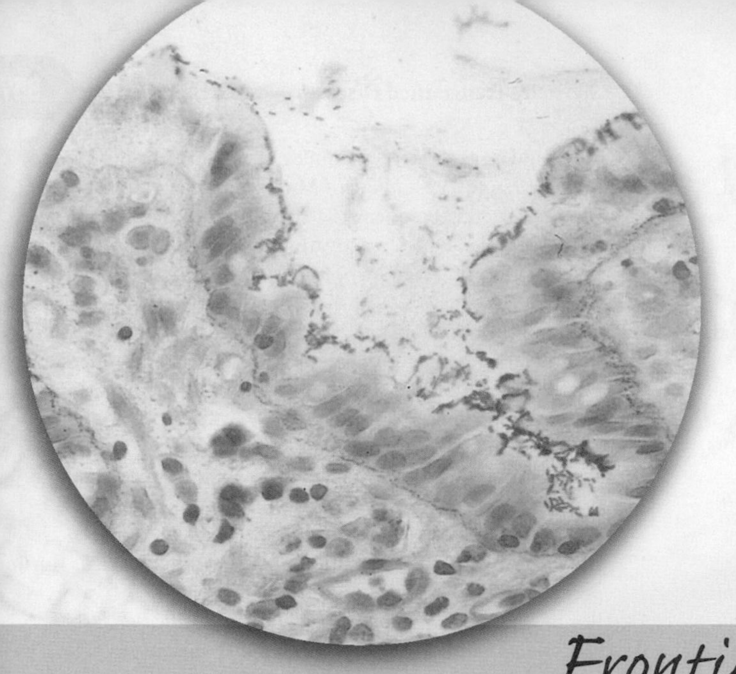

Frontiers of Research

Advances in Treatment of Gastrointestinal Disorders

Jacquelyn L. Banasik and Michael J. Kirkhorn

When the gastrointestinal (GI) system is working properly, we are happy not to have to think about it. When it shows signs of stress or disease, we think about it only reluctantly. It seems so complicated—its coilings, its odd junctures, its paradoxical purposes—in nourishing the body and disposing of wastes, processes sustaining life in two invaluable but seemingly contradictory ways. It is vitally important that the system work properly in both of its essential functions. The standard textbook listing of GI disorders is unappetizing: gastritis, peptic ulcer, pancreatitis, sprue, constipation, megacolon, diarrhea, vomiting, GI disruption, and cancer.

Fortunately, research on a variety of fronts is leading to greater knowledge about some of the more significant GI disorders. Researchers are confronting a paradigm shift in their understanding of many of the causes of GI distress. As with other medical conditions, disorders of the GI tract are increasingly understood as an interplay between lifestyle, genetic constitution, and environmental factors. The symptom experience itself or the outcome may have reciprocal effects on its determinants.

The role of *Helicobacter pylori* in the biology of peptic ulcer disease and gastric cancer is an important example of this interplay. Its presence alone does not explain why some individuals are susceptible to these conditions. *H. pylori* is a factor in nearly all cases of ulcer formation in patients who are not taking nonsteroidal antiinflammatory agents. However, a large proportion of the population has *H. pylori* as a component of their normal flora, and these individuals never develop peptic ulcer disease or cancer. Perhaps psychoneuroendocrine or psychoimmune factors (i.e., stress) will be shown to affect host resistance or the clinical expression of gastric cancer and peptic ulcer, as has occurred with other diseases.

Colorectal cancer, the most common GI malignancy, is common in the United States and is a major source of concern throughout the world. Colorectal cancer accounts for about 11% of all cancers in both men and women, as well as about 11% of cancer-related deaths. Each year more than 150,000 new cases occur in the United States, and more than 55,000 persons die from the disease.

Scientists are encouraged by their ability to cure colon cancer if the malignant polyps are detected

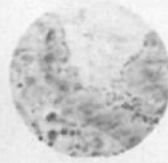

Helicobacter pylori *gastritis. Numerous darkly stained* Helicobacter *organisms along the luminal surface of the gastric epithelial cells with no tissue invasion by bacteria. (From Kumar V, Cotran RS, Robbins ST:* Robbins basic pathology, *ed 7, Philadelphia, 2003, Saunders.)*

Gastrointestinal Function

UNIT X

early. They have also identified noncancerous lesions that are responsible for colon cancers and provide early warning because they often appear years before the cancer itself. Early screening even of individuals without symptoms will help detect the neoplastic polyps that precede cancer. The polyps may then be removed to reduce the possibility of colon cancer. Only 6% of colon cancers are inherited; for those individuals, genetic studies promise an effective screening test.

The liver is another target of intense interest. A British researcher reports that about 60% of patients suffering from severe, acute alcoholic hepatitis die during the first 6 weeks after hospitalization. Alcoholic hepatitis is frequently found in patients in whom cirrhosis, an often fatal liver disease, eventually develops.

Chronic hepatitis C is the most common cause of nonalcoholic liver disease. The Centers for Disease Control and Prevention estimate that there are 38,000 new cases of acute hepatitis C in the United States annually. Very few of these are diagnosed. In studies approximately 60% to 70% of patients with acute hepatitis C virus cleared the infection spontaneously.

Clinicians are encouraged by their improved ability to diagnose, treat, and manage a variety of liver diseases. Among these improvements are new developments in liver transplantation, including the possibility of grafting transplanted tissue onto the diseased liver to allow it to recover.

In industrialized nations where advanced technology is available, new treatment strategies are aiding in the diagnosis of GI diseases. Computed tomography can be used to diagnose pancreatitis and help pinpoint the cause and aid in the diagnosis of fatty infiltration of the liver or liver metastases in cases of cancer.

Recent innovations have also led to far less painful recovery for surgical patients. Each year more than 500,000 Americans undergo surgical treatment of gallbladder disease—a formerly excruciatingly painful condition. Laparoscopic cholecystectomy affords a minimally invasive surgical approach. Rather than making a single large incision, surgeons remove the gallbladder and stones through four small abdominal incisions. Usually the patient is able to go home in a day or two, at a significant cost savings.

Gastrointestinal Function

Jeffrey S. Sartin

MEDIA RESOURCES

Additional Material for Study, Review, and Further Exploration

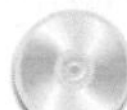

CD Companion ◆ Review Questions and Answers ◆ Key Concepts Review ◆ Glossary *(with audio pronunciations for selected terms)* ◆ Disease Profiles ◆ Animations

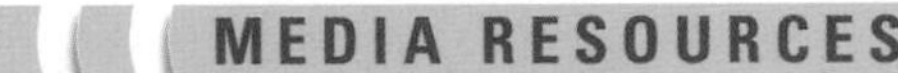

Website at http://evolve.elsevier.com/Copstead/
◆ Case Studies ◆ Disease Profiles ◆ WebLinks

KEY QUESTIONS

- What are the major structures of the gastrointestinal tract and their corresponding functions?
- How does the autonomic nervous system influence gastrointestinal motility?
- How do segmental and propulsive movements influence the digestive and absorptive functions of the small intestine?
- What are the major secretions of each of the following secretory cells and glands: salivary, gastric, intestinal epithelium, pancreas, and gallbladder?
- How and where are complex carbohydrates, proteins, and lipids digested and absorbed?
- How and where are water and electrolytes absorbed?
- What alterations in gastrointestinal function occur in association with very young or very old age?

CHAPTER OUTLINE

The gastrointestinal (GI) system consists of the GI tract and the related solid organs of digestion. Beginning with the mouth and pharynx, the GI tract includes the esophagus, stomach, and small and large intestines (Figure 35-1). These components can be thought of as a continuous tube about 7 m in length running from the mouth to the anus. Other parts of the GI system that are located outside the GI tract include the salivary glands, the pancreas, and the biliary system (liver, gallbladder, and bile ducts).

The function of the GI system is to provide nutrients for the body. The process of ingesting nutrients, propelling them through the GI tract, and transforming them into a form capable of absorption into the body's internal milieu constitutes a remarkable interface of the human organism with the external environment. The general functions of the GI tract in providing nutrients for the body can be divided into (1) GI motility, including propulsive and mixing movements; (2) secretion of digestive juices; (3) digestion of nutrients; and (4) absorption of nutrients.[1,2] This chapter describes each of these functions in detail and provides an overview of the structure and organization of the GI tract and its growth and alteration across the life span.

STRUCTURE AND ORGANIZATION OF THE GASTROINTESTINAL TRACT

Embryology

As early as the fourth week of gestation, the GI system begins to form from the primitive gut structures of the foregut, midgut, and hindgut.[3] The foregut gives rise to the pharynx, esophagus,

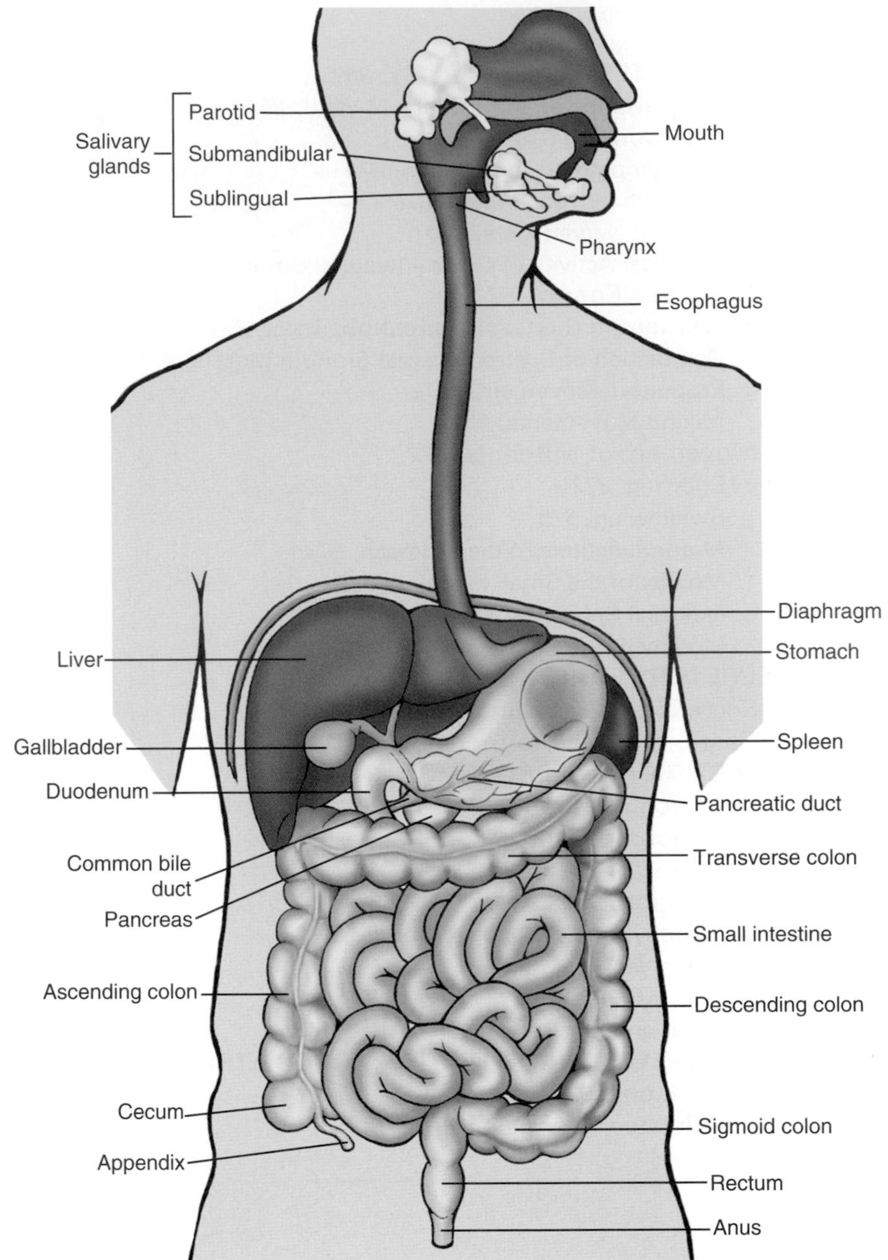

FIGURE 35-1 ■ The gastrointestinal system. (From Monahan FD, Neighbors M: *Medical surgical nursing, foundations for clinical practice,* ed 2, Philadelphia, 1998, Saunders, p 950.)

stomach, the duodenum proximal to the opening of the common bile duct, the hepatobiliary system, and the pancreas. The trachea and esophagus share a common developmental origin, and incomplete partitioning of these structures may lead to **tracheoesophageal fistula,** a developmental anomaly characterized by an abnormal connection between the trachea and esophagus. This anomaly may be accompanied by **esophageal atresia,** a condition in which the esophagus is closed off in a blind pouch at some point. These disorders are two of the most serious surgical emergencies in newborns and require immediate diagnosis and correction.[4] Esophageal atresia occurs in about 1 of every 4000 live births, and about one-third of the infants affected by this anomaly are born prematurely.

The midgut gives rise to the small intestine (below the opening of the common bile duct), the cecum, the appendix, the ascending colon, and the proximal portion of the transverse colon. Failure of normal partitioning between the foregut and midgut can lead to duodenal atresia, a condition in which the lumen of the small intestine is obliterated. This anomaly is the most common cause of intestinal obstruction in the newborn.[4] Failure of the midgut to develop or rotate properly with respect to the umbilical cord can result in **om-**

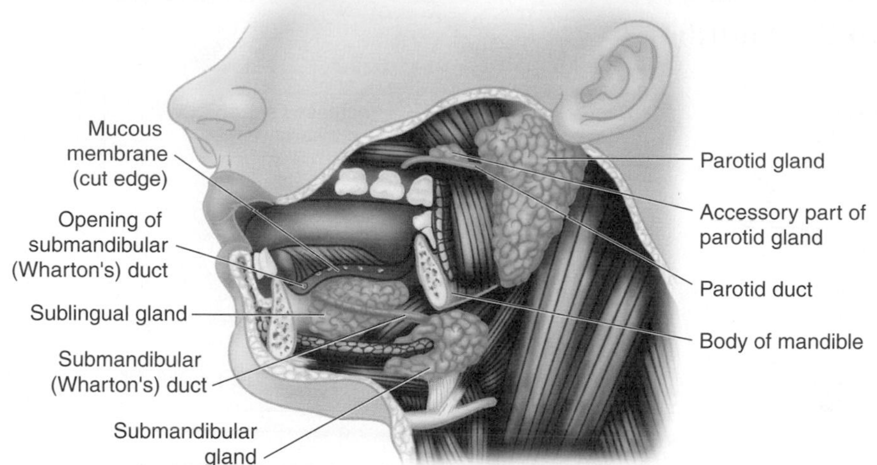

FIGURE 35-2 ■ Oral cavity. Structures of the mouth and location of the salivary glands. (From O'Toole M, editor: *Miller-Keane encyclopedia and dictionary of medicine, nursing, and allied health,* ed 7, Philadelphia, 2003, Saunders.)

phalocele, a congenital herniation of viscera into the base of the umbilical cord.

The hindgut gives rise to the distal part of the transverse colon, the descending and sigmoid colon, the rectum, and the superior portion of the anal canal. Congenital malformations resulting from inappropriate development of the anorectal portion of the GI tract include anal agenesis, a condition in which the rectal pouch ends blindly above the surface of the perineum. Other developmental anomalies of this portion of the GI tract include anal stenosis, in which the anal aperture is small, and anal membrane atresia, in which the anal membrane covers the aperture and creates an obstruction.

After its initial embryologic development, the GI tract continues to grow in length and caliber until somatic growth ends after puberty. The degree of growth and development of the GI tract during childhood appears to depend on the same general factors as growth of the rest of the body. Such general factors as nutritional adequacy, insulin, growth hormone, thyroid hormone, cortisol, androgens, and estrogens may play a role in its development, as well as such specific factors as the direct effect of ingested nutrients, GI hormones, and secretions.[5]

Physiologic Anatomy

Each part of the GI tract is uniquely adapted for a specific function in the process of providing nutrients for the body—a process that continues from birth to senescence. Each major component of the GI tract is described as a basis for understanding the overall structure and innervation of the GI tract.

Oral Cavity and Pharynx

The mouth, or oral cavity, is the usual point of entry for nutrients and is the site of the initial breakdown of nutrient substances into a usable form. Food is pushed toward the side of the mouth by the tongue to facilitate chewing and grinding on the surfaces of the molar and premolar teeth. As the food is manipulated and broken down, it is moistened by saliva secreted by three major pairs of salivary glands: the parotid, submandibular, and sublingual glands (Figure 35-2). Saliva serves three major functions that are important in the ingestion of nutrients: (1) by its moistening action, saliva allows the tongue to convert a mouthful of food into a bolus, or semisolid mass, that can be swallowed easily; (2) by its moistening action, saliva changes dry foods into a solute form and allows for taste perception by the papillae on the surface of the tongue, which are sensitive to chemical differences among food molecules; and (3) the digestive enzyme contained in saliva, **salivary amylase** (also called ptyalin), initiates carbohydrate digestion by effecting the breakdown of polysaccharides (also called starch) into the simpler molecular structures of dextrin and maltose.[6,7] Important changes in oral structure and function that occur during aging are detailed in The Aging Process: Changes in the Mouth.

The pharynx, or throat, is a muscular tube about 12 cm long that serves as the entryway for both the respiratory and the GI systems. The oropharynx is the portion of the pharynx posterior to the mouth and is separated from the nasopharynx, the portion of the pharynx posterior to the nose, by the soft palate. The laryngopharynx is the portion of the pharynx that opens into the larynx and the esophagus. During swallowing, the soft palate is pulled upward to close off the nasopharynx. The bolus of food being swallowed is propelled by reflex movements of muscles in the pharynx through the laryngopharynx and into the esophagus. Simultaneously, the opening to the larynx is closed by the epiglottis. This coordinated set of actions prevents food substances and liquids from inadvertently entering the respiratory system, a potentially life-threatening occurrence referred to as aspiration.

THE AGING PROCESS

Changes in the Mouth

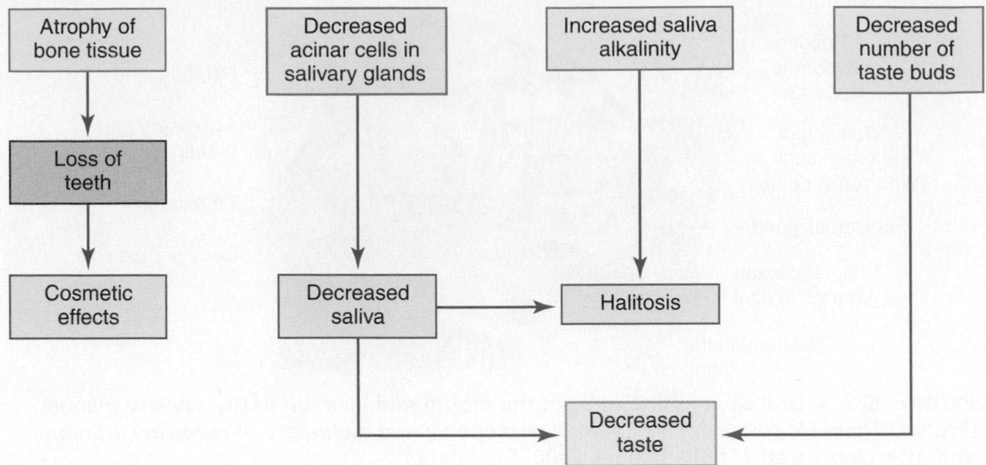

Elderly people experience a decline in taste. This decline is due to both an increase in the sensation threshold for all four tastes and a decrease in the number of papilla. For example, children have more than 200 taste buds, whereas the elderly have fewer than 100. Of the four basic tastes, the elderly experience a particular decrease in salt and sugar tastes.

The elderly also experience a decrease in the number of acinar cells in the salivary glands, leading to a reduction in the amount and secretory rate of saliva. The saliva becomes more alkaline as well. The decrease in the amount of saliva and the increased alkalinity contribute to halitosis (bad breath).

Loss of teeth in the elderly is due to atrophy of gum and bone tissue as well as actual tooth wear and tear. The enamel of the teeth may wear away, exposing dentin. As a result of secondary dentin deposition with aging, the size of the pulp chamber is decreased and the pulp is limited to the root cavity only. There is controversy as to whether the loss of gingival epithelial tissue is pathologic or a normal part of aging.

Esophagus

The esophagus is a muscular tube approximately 25 cm in length. Passage of food through the esophagus is greatly facilitated by mucus secreted by cells in the epithelial lining. Extremely rough or fibrous foods may potentially penetrate the mucous lining of the esophagus and cause damage. The stratified squamous epithelium lining the esophagus is constantly renewed by cells moving to the surface from below, thus providing a means of renewal for such damage. The esophagus propels nutrients to the stomach by means of strong muscular contractions (a capability that may be affected by aging). **Presbyesophagus,** or an abnormal esophageal motility pattern occurring with advanced age, is described in detail in a later section. When the body is in an upright position, gravity assists in the downward movement of food to the stomach. However, the muscular contractions of the esophagus are extremely strong and are sufficient to transport nutrients to the stomach even in the absence of gravity, just as persons living (and eating) in the weightless conditions of space have demonstrated.[1,3]

At the lower end of the esophagus, about 2 to 5 cm above its juncture with the stomach, the circular muscle of the esophagus functions as a sphincter; this region is referred to as the **lower esophageal sphincter** (LES). Although anatomically this sphincter is no different from the remainder of the esophagus, it remains tonically constricted, in contrast to the mid- and upper portions of the esophagus, which are completely relaxed under normal conditions.[2] Thus the LES serves to prevent the highly acidic gastric contents from moving in a retrograde motion back into the esophagus. Under certain conditions the LES does not function properly, and reflux of gastric contents into the esophagus may occur. The resulting subjective sensation of irritation and spasms of the distal portion of the esophagus is often referred to as heartburn.

Stomach

The stomach (Figure 35-3) is essentially a food reservoir and is the site of the start of the digestive process. Under normal circumstances its capacity is 1000 to 1500 ml, although a capacity of as much as 6000 ml is possible.[2] The portion of the stomach immediately below the LES is called the cardia. The fundus is the part of the stomach that continues lateral to and above the cardia; the body of the stomach extends from the cardia to the antrum, which stretches from the angulus to the pylorus. The antrum differs markedly from the rest of the stomach in function and is distinguished by the absence of ru-

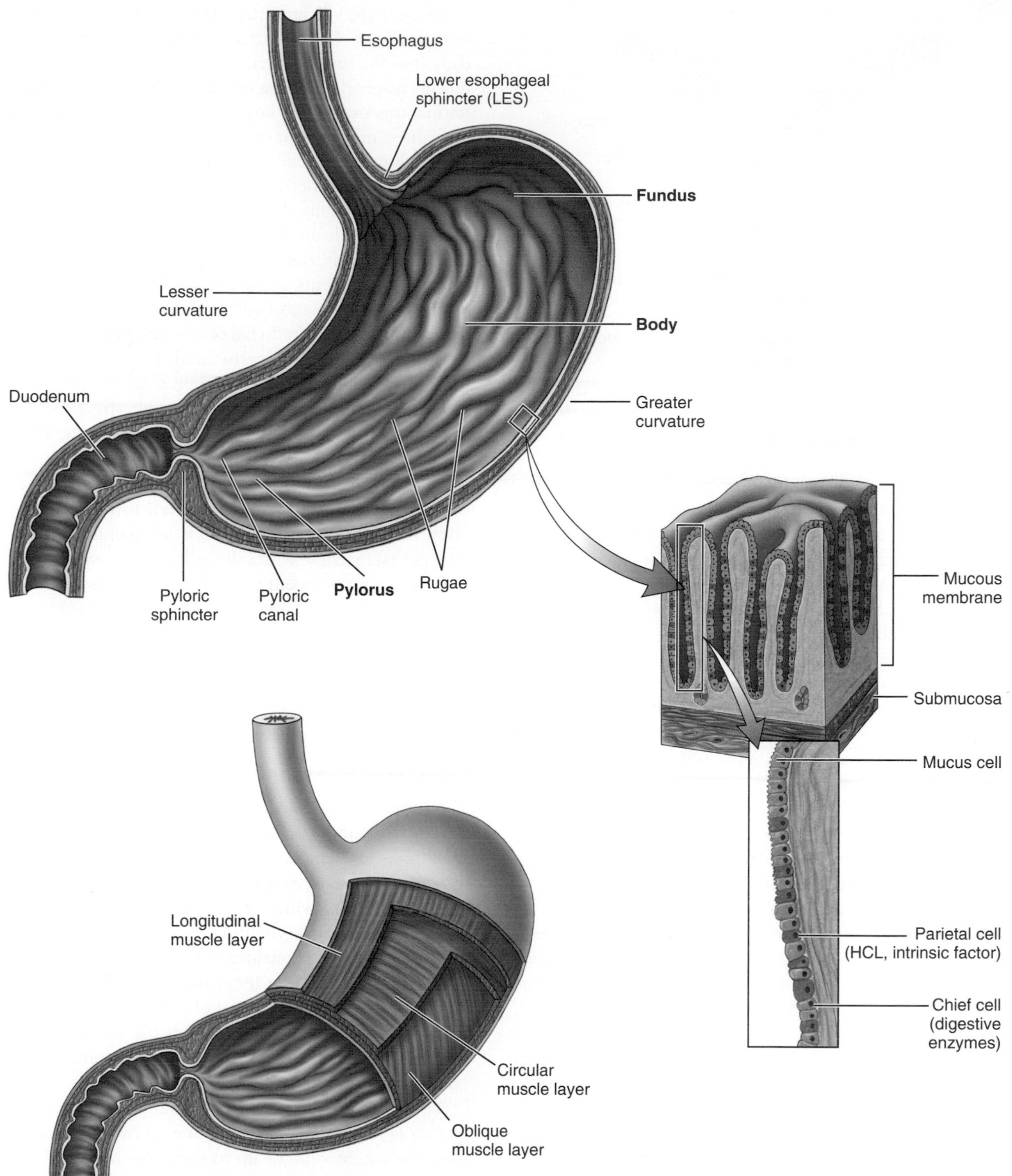

FIGURE 35-3 ■ Physiologic anatomy of the stomach. *HCL,* Hydrochloric acid. (From Herlihy B, Maebius NK: *The human body in health and illness,* Philadelphia, 2000, Saunders, p 394.)

gae, the folds present in the mucous membrane of the other areas of the stomach. The **pylorus** is a muscular sphincter between the stomach and duodenum that serves to control gastric emptying and limit the reflux of bile from the small intestine.

The stomach is lined with simple columnar epithelium containing millions of gastric glands that extend down to the mucosa. A typical gastric gland is shown in Figure 35-4. As shown in this illustration, gastric glands are lined by several types of specialized cells. Chief cells produce pepsinogen, the

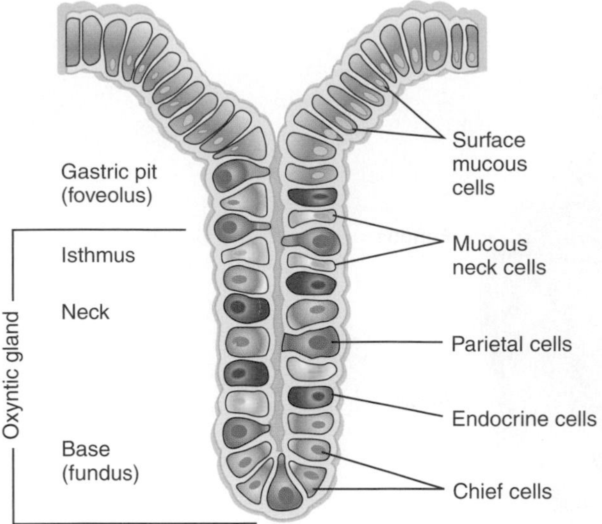

FIGURE 35-4 ■ Gastric mucosa and gastric glands.

inactive form of the enzyme pepsin; parietal cells produce hydrochloric acid and also a substance called intrinsic factor that is needed for adequate intestinal absorption of vitamin B_{12}.[8] Mucous cells produce an alkaline mucus that serves to shield the stomach wall and neutralize the acidity in the immediate area of the lining. A layer of mucus more than 1 mm thick continuously bathes the free surfaces of the gastric epithelial lining. In addition to these cells, gastrin cells are located in the antral epithelium and have surface microvilli that monitor intragastric pH. The role of these cells and the substances they secrete in the digestion of nutrients are described in detail in a later section of this chapter.

Small Intestine

The small intestine of a living adult is approximately 5 to 6 m long (the longest portion of the GI tract). The first 22 cm of the small intestine is called the duodenum; the jejunum constitutes the next 2 m, and the ileum forms the remainder. The entire inner wall of the small intestine is marked by circular folds of a mucous membrane called the plicae circulares; these permanent ridges do not stretch out when the intestine is distended.

On microscopic examination, the lining of the small intestine contains millions of fingerlike projections called **intestinal villi** (Figure 35-5). Like the circular folds just described, these villi serve to increase the surface area of the intestine for digestion and absorption of nutrients. Each villus has its own microscopic projections called microvilli, which in turn are covered by a fuzzy coat (called the **brush border** because of its brushlike appearance when viewed with an electron microscope) containing many digestive enzymes. The combined effect of the circular folds, villi, and microvilli is to increase the surface area of the small intestine by about 600 times, thereby creating a remarkably efficient milieu for nutrient digestion and absorption. Figure 35-6 shows a microscopic section of the small intestine.

Between the villi are situated the intestinal glands, or crypts of Lieberkühn. The intestinal glands secrete about 2 L of fluid daily into the lumen of the intestine, but most of the fluid is quickly reabsorbed by the villi. Goblet cells throughout the intestinal mucosa secrete large amounts of mucus. In addition, specialized mucous glands located in the first few centimeters of the duodenum, called Brunner glands, release the thick coating of mucus needed in that area to protect the mucosa from the potentially damaging effects of acidic gastric juice that may enter through the pylorus.

Although the details of the process of digestion and absorption of nutrients in the intestinal mucosa will be covered in greater detail in subsequent sections, a unique and salient feature of the villus epithelial cells is described here. Villus epithelial cells have both digestive and absorptive functions, apparently dependent on their current stage of maturation. The rapidly dividing cells at the base of the intestinal glands are responsible for secretion, but as they migrate to the villus, they mature into absorptive cells and are eventually pushed out of the villus tip. Turnover of cells in the small intestine occurs in 48 to 72 hours, one of the fastest cell turnover rates in the body. Therefore, conditions such as malnutrition or substances that interfere with cell replication or protein synthesis, such as chemotherapeutic agents, may adversely affect intestinal function.

The **ileocecal valve,** a sphincter between the small and large intestines, is normally closed so that the contents of the large intestine cannot move in a retrograde fashion back into the small intestine. In response to a peristaltic contraction bringing intestinal contents toward it, the ileocecal valve opens.

Large Intestine

The large intestine (Figure 35-7) is so termed because of its 6.5-cm diameter, which is greater than the diameter of the small intestine. The large intestine is a 1.5-m-long muscular tube that forms a frame around the small intestine. The vermiform appendix, which is attached to the cecum, is a worm-shaped blind tube containing specialized lymphatic structures. It is generally considered a vestigial structure that may have served a role as an incubator for bacteria that digested cellulose in the vegetarian past of the human species. Inflammation of the appendix, or appendicitis, is a potentially life-threatening occurrence that can lead to peritonitis if not diagnosed and managed promptly.

The portion of the large intestine from the cecum to the rectum is known as the colon. The ascending colon extends from the cecum straight up to the lower border of the liver; the transverse colon then extends across the abdomen, anterior to the small intestine. The descending colon then turns downward on the left side of the abdomen, finally becoming the S-shaped sigmoid colon, which empties into the rectum. The rectum has its outlet at the anus, the opening for elimination of feces (see Figure 35-7).

The mucosa of the large intestine has no villi and does not produce digestive enzymes (Figure 35-8). The epithelial sur-

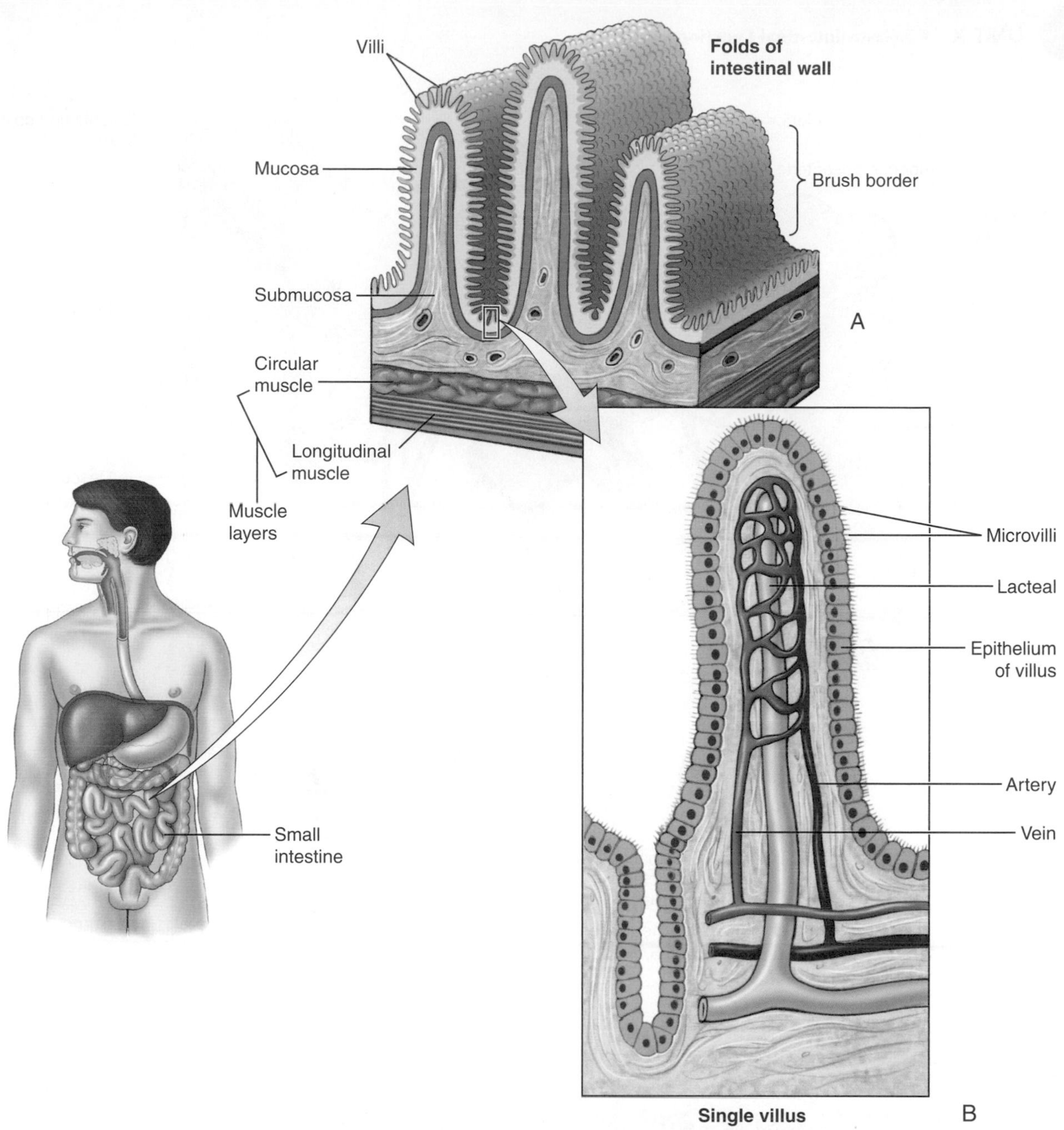

Villi
Folds of intestinal wall
Mucosa
Brush border
Submucosa
A
Circular muscle
Longitudinal muscle
Muscle layers
Microvilli
Lacteal
Epithelium of villus
Artery
Vein
Small intestine
Single villus
B

FIGURE 35-5 ■ Villi of the small intestine. **A,** Folds of the intestinal wall showing the layers of the wall and the brush border (villi). **B,** Single villus showing the blood capillaries, the lacteal (lymph capillary), and the microvilli. (From Herlihy B, Maebius NK: *The human body in health and illness,* Philadelphia, 2000, Saunders, p 398.)

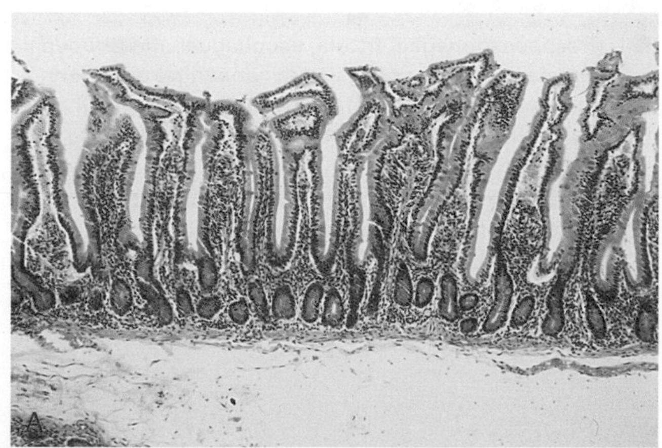

FIGURE 35-6 ■ Microscopic section of the small intestine. (From Kumar V, Cotran RS, Robbins ST: *Robbins basic pathology,* ed 7, Philadelphia, 2003, Saunders, p 803.)

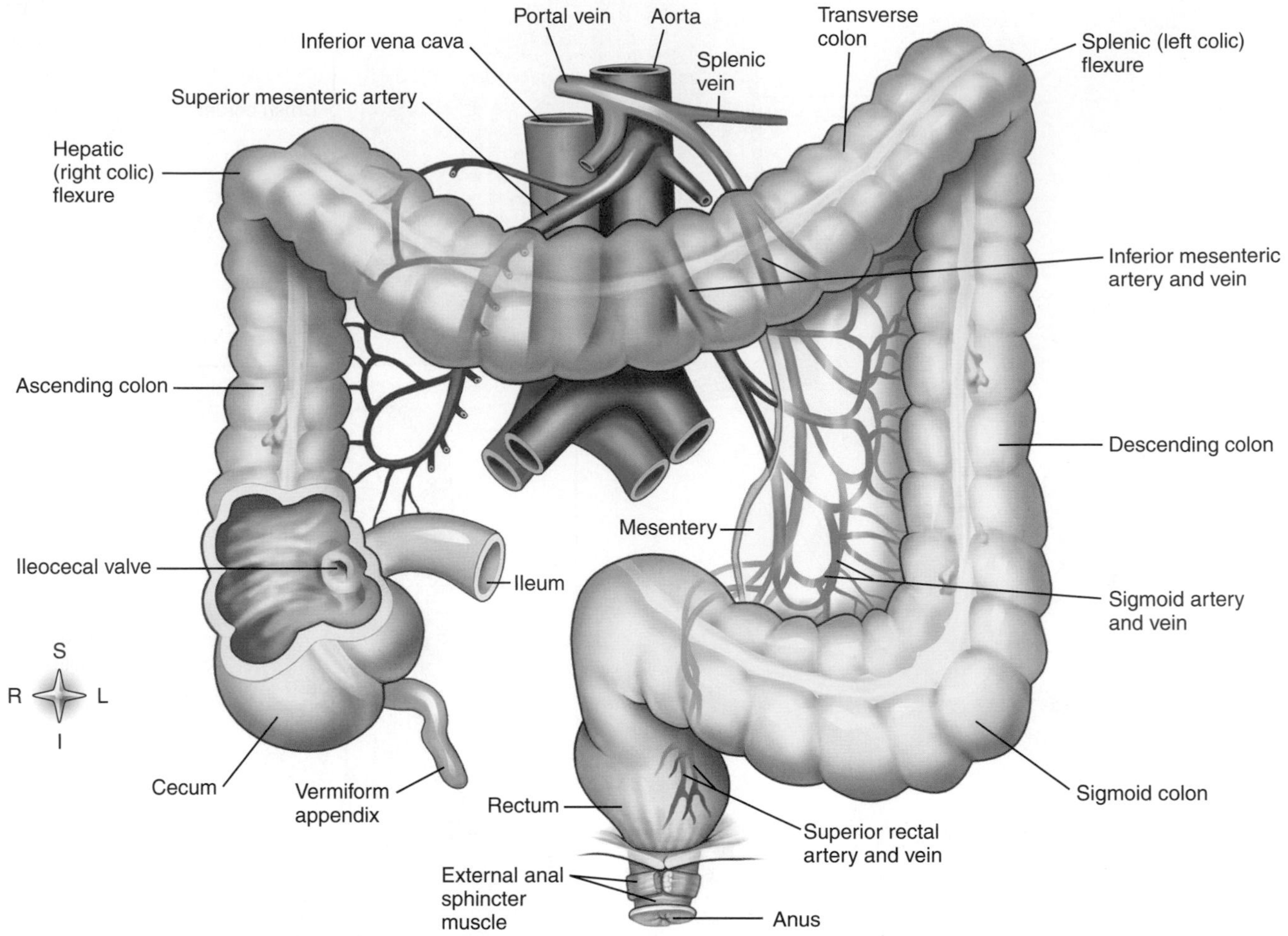

FIGURE 35-7 ■ Divisions of the large intestine. (From Thibodeau GA, Patton KT: *Anatomy and physiology,* ed 5, St Louis, 2003, Mosby, p 754.)

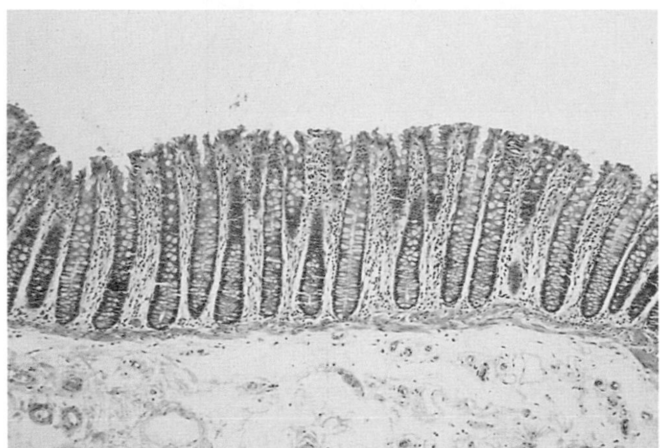

FIGURE 35-8 ■ Normal colon histology showing a flat mucosal surface and abundant vertically oriented crypts. (From Kumar V, Cotran RS, Robbins ST: *Robbins basic pathology,* ed 7, Philadelphia, 2003, Saunders, p 803.)

face of the colon consists of absorptive cells that predominantly absorb water and electrolytes.[9] Mucus-producing goblet cells line the glandular crypts present in the surface epithelium. Endocrine cells are also present, but the function of hormones in the large intestine is presently not well understood. The turnover time of cells in the colonic mucosa is 3 to 8 days, comparatively longer than that of cells in the small intestine.

KEY CONCEPTS

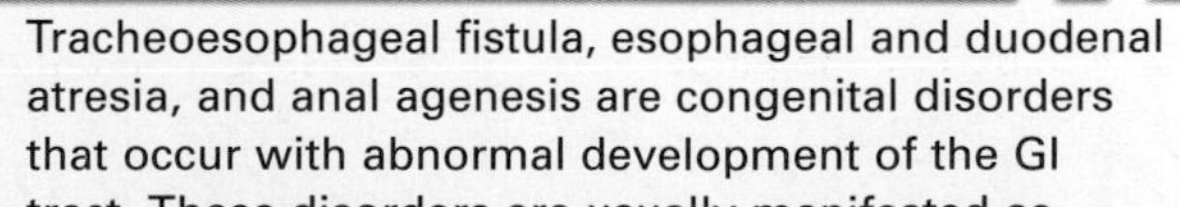

- Tracheoesophageal fistula, esophageal and duodenal atresia, and anal agenesis are congenital disorders that occur with abnormal development of the GI tract. These disorders are usually manifested as obstructions.
- The major structures and corresponding functions of the GI tract can be summarized as follows:
  Mouth and salivary glands: Mastication, moistening, and the beginning of starch digestion (by the enzyme salivary amylase) of foodstuff.

Pharynx: Transport of food to the esophagus and protection of the airway from aspiration of food particles.
Esophagus: Movement of food to the stomach by peristaltic waves. The LES prevents reflux of stomach contents.
Stomach: Reservoir for food, mixing, and initial digestion of proteins (by the enzyme pepsin); secretion of hydrochloric acid, intrinsic factor, and gastrin. The pyloric sphincter prevents reflux of intestinal contents.
Small intestine: Digestion and absorption of nearly all nutrients in the duodenum and jejunum; absorption of bile salts in the terminal ileum. The brush border contains numerous digestive enzymes. The enzymes secretin and cholecystokinin are secreted by intestinal mucosa.
Pancreas and gallbladder: The pancreas delivers digestive enzymes and bicarbonate to the duodenum. The gallbladder delivers bile salts to the duodenum.
Large intestine: Reabsorption of water and storage of feces. Feces are delivered to the rectum for defecation.

GASTROINTESTINAL MOTILITY

The way in which nutrients and their eventual waste products are propelled through the GI tract is a complex and fascinating process involving an exquisitely timed set of autoregulatory actions and responses. A summary of the characteristics of the intestinal wall, innervation of the gut, and hormonal control of GI motility is presented as a basis for a description of the path taken by nutrients moving through the GI tract.

Characteristics of the Intestinal Wall

A typical cross-section of the intestinal wall is depicted in Figure 35-9. From the outer surface inward are five main layers: the serosa, a longitudinal muscle layer, a circular muscle layer, the submucosa, and the mucosa. A small layer, the muscularis mucosa, is located between the mucosa and submucosa. The muscular movements of the GI tract are performed mostly by the different layers of the smooth muscle, which extends from the distal end of the esophagus through most of the large intestine. However, skeletal muscle has a key role in motility at both ends of the GI tract; motility from the mouth through the proximal portion of the esophagus at the upper end and through the external anal sphincter at the lower end is mediated by the action of skeletal muscle.[2,10]

The general characteristics of smooth muscle are covered in Chapter 5. Specific characteristics of smooth muscle in the gut that render its function possible include the close proximity of these smooth muscle fibers to each other. In most areas of the GI tract, smooth muscle fibers are extremely close; about 12% of their membrane surfaces are actually fused with the membranes of other adjacent muscle fibers to form a nexus, or junction. This close proximity of smooth muscle fibers in the GI tract allows intracellular current to travel very easily from one muscle fiber to another. Electrical signals originating in one smooth muscle fiber in the GI tract are generally propagated from fiber to fiber; the GI tract is said to be a **functional syncytium,** which means that separate cells have

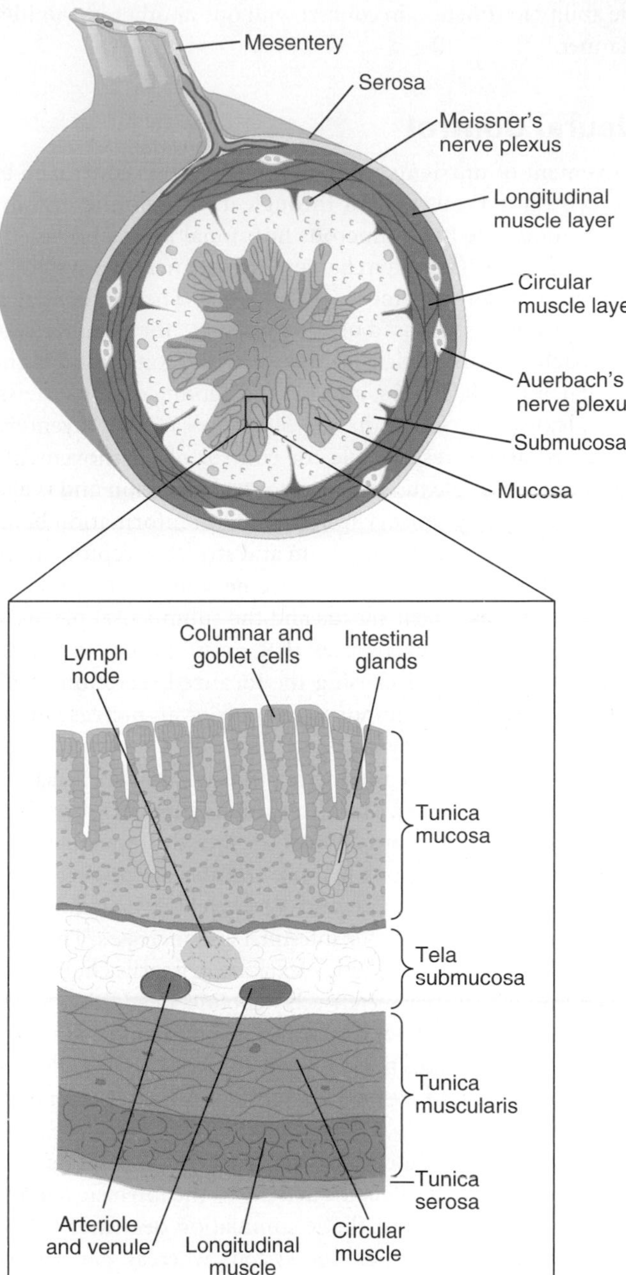

FIGURE 35-9 ■ Typical cross-section of the intestinal wall. *Inset* shows enlargement of a cross-section of the intestine. (From Black JM, Hawks JH, Keene AM: *Medical-surgical nursing: clinical management for positive outcomes,* ed 7, Philadelphia, 2005, Saunders, p 658.)

the ability to function in concert with one another in a unified manner.[1]

Neural Control

Movement of nutrients through the GI tract is controlled by the central nervous system through its autonomic division and is modulated by numerous hormonal interactions.[2,3,8,11] In addition, the GI system has an intrinsic nervous system of its own that controls most GI functions. The **intrinsic nervous system** is composed of two layers: (1) the myenteric, or Auerbach, plexus, which lies between the longitudinal and circular muscular layers; and (2) the submucosal, or Meissner, plexus, which lies in the submucosa. The myenteric plexus is largely responsible for control of GI movements; the submucosal plexus serves to control secretion and is also involved in many sensory functions, with information being received from the gut epithelium and stretch receptors in the intestinal wall. The entire intrinsic nervous system, including both the myenteric plexus and the submucosal plexus, is responsible for many reflexes that occur locally in the GI tract, such as reflexes causing the localized secretion of digestive juices by the submucosal glands or an increase in gut smooth muscle activity.

In general, when the myenteric plexus is stimulated, activity in the GI tract increases. This stimulation results in four principal effects: (1) tonic contraction of the intestinal wall increases; (2) rhythmic contractions increase in intensity; (3) rhythmic contractions increase in rate; and (4) the velocity of conduction of excitatory waves along the intestinal wall increases. These excitatory fibers of the myenteric plexus are primarily cholinergic, which means that they secrete acetylcholine, in addition to one or more other excitatory transmitter substances. However, some myenteric plexus fibers have an inhibitory effect and may secrete purine-based transmitter substances such as adenosine triphosphate.[12]

Input from the sympathetic and parasympathetic nervous systems can strongly affect the activity of the intrinsic nervous system. In general, sympathetic stimulation decreases the activity of the intrinsic nervous system whereas parasympathetic stimulation increases its activity.

Parasympathetic Innervation

The parasympathetic supply to the GI tract is divided into cranial and sacral divisions. Cranial parasympathetic stimulation is transmitted almost entirely in the vagus nerves, which provide extensive innervation to the esophagus, stomach, pancreas, and the first half of the large intestine (with little innervation of the small intestine). The sacral parasympathetic division originates in the second, third, and fourth sacral segments of the spinal cord and innervates the distal half of the large intestine. The sigmoid, rectal, and anal regions of the large intestine are especially well supplied with parasympathetic fibers; these fibers have a key role in the defecation reflex.

Sympathetic Innervation

The sympathetic fibers that innervate the GI tract have their origin in the spinal cord between T8 and L3. After exiting the cord, the preganglionic fibers enter the sympathetic chains and then pass through these chains to various ganglia located adjacent to the GI tract, such as the celiac ganglion and the mesenteric ganglia. From these locations, postganglionic fibers radiate out to all parts of the gut. The sympathetics supply essentially all parts of the GI tract, in contrast to the concentration of parasympathetic innervation at locations close to the entry and exit points of the gut.[2,12] The sympathetic nerve endings in the GI tract secrete norepinephrine, which promotes the inhibitory effect of the sympathetic nervous system on the GI tract in the following ways. Norepinephrine acts directly on smooth muscle in the GI tract to inhibit activity; in addition, norepinephrine has an inhibitory effect on the neurons of the intrinsic nervous system of the GI tract. Strong stimulation of the sympathetic nervous system can effectively shut down motility in the gut and can block the movement of nutrients through the GI tract.

Afferent Nerve Fibers

The GI tract is richly supplied with afferent nerve fibers arising from the gut that can transmit important information about the status of the GI tract. Afferent fibers that have their cell bodies in the submucosal plexus and terminate in the myenteric plexus transmit signals in response to irritation of the gut mucosa, excessive distention, or the presence of specific chemical substances. These signals can result in excitation or, in some circumstances, inhibition of intestinal motility or secretion. Other afferent fibers with cell bodies in the dorsal root ganglia of the spinal cord or cranial nerve ganglia can transmit signals to higher levels of the central nervous system by traveling along sympathetic or parasympathetic pathways. For example, the vagus nerves contain many afferent fibers that transmit signals to the medulla; this information is then used to initiate and modulate vagal signals that control many important functions of the GI tract.

Electrical Activity of Gastrointestinal Smooth Muscle

Electrical activity is almost constantly present in the smooth muscle layers of the GI tract. Two basic types of electrical wave activity have been identified in the gut: slow waves and spikes (the latter named for the spiking appearance of these sudden increases in membrane potential).[1,2] These two types of electrical wave patterns are shown in Figure 35-10. **Slow-wave electrical activity** represents an ongoing basic oscillation in membrane potential that occurs in the smooth muscle of the GI tract, especially in the muscle in the longitudinal layer. Normally, between 3 and 12 slow waves occur per minute. Slow waves can be any degree of intensity and are not the "all-or-nothing" type of action potential seen in other smooth muscle fibers in the body. In contrast to these nearly continuous slow waves, spikes occur under certain circumstances. When the muscle layer in the GI tract is stimulated by being stretched or by the effects of acetylcholine or parasympathetic excitation, the intracellular resting membrane potential of the muscle fibers becomes more positive. The entire potential level of the slow waves is raised—an effect called depolarization.[1,13,14] As shown in Figure 35-10, when the depolarization rises above a certain level (around 40 mV), spikes, or sudden increases in the membrane potential, start to appear on the peaks of the slow waves. If the resting potential rises further, spikes appear more frequently. With very strong stimulation, the spikes generally disappear because the membrane now remains entirely depolarized. Figure 35-10 also illustrates the response of smooth muscle fibers to stimulation by norepinephrine or sympathetic excitation. In this situation, the resting membrane potential is decreased, or hyperpolarized, and electrical activity is almost abolished.

Hormonal Control

The following section on secretory function of the GI tract describes in detail the role of hormones in controlling GI secretion. It is important to note that many of these same hormones are involved in controlling motility in different portions of the GI tract. Gastrin, which is secreted by the mucosa of the stomach antrum in response to food entering the stomach, increases stomach motility. In addition, it promotes increased constriction of the LES, which serves to prevent reflux of stomach contents into the esophagus. Gastrin may also have a small effect in increasing motility of the small intestine and gallbladder.[2,3,15]

Cholecystokinin, which is secreted mainly by the mucosa of the jejunum in response to the entry of fatty substances, has an extremely strong effect in increasing contractility of the gallbladder. This stimulation of gallbladder activity results in an outpouring into the small intestine of bile, which plays an important role in promoting fat digestion and absorption. Secretin, which is secreted by the mucosa of the duodenum in response to the entry of acidic gastric juice from the stomach, has a mild inhibitory effect on motility in most of the GI tract.[2,3]

Gastric inhibitory peptide, which is secreted by the mucosa of the upper portion of the small intestine primarily in response to the presence of fat but also carbohydrate, has a moderate effect in decreasing stomach motility. Thus it serves to slow the emptying of stomach contents into the duodenum in circumstances in which the upper part of the small intestine already contains an oversupply of nutrient substances.

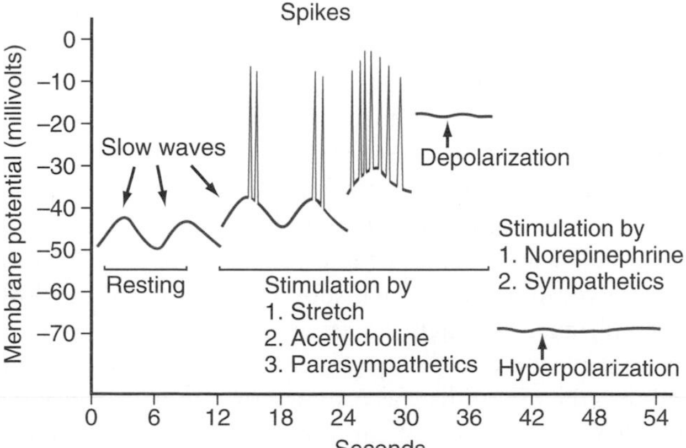

FIGURE 35-10 ■ Membrane potentials in intestinal smooth muscle. (From Guyton AC, Hall JE: *Textbook of medical physiology,* ed 10, Philadelphia, 2000, Saunders, p 801.)

Movement in the Gastrointestinal Tract

Contraction of Gastrointestinal Smooth Muscle

In general, most contraction in the GI tract occurs in response to **spike potentials;** slow waves without superimposed spikes ordinarily do not give rise to contraction. Spike potentials occurring in GI smooth muscle are analogous to action potentials in skeletal muscle and are responsible for the membrane changes that initiate contraction. As calcium enters the cell membrane and passes to the interior of the smooth muscle, it initiates a reaction between actin and myosin,[1] a process described in detail in Chapter 50.

The electrical activity occurring in the smooth muscle of the gut gives rise to tonic contractions and rhythmic contractions, both of which occur in most types of smooth muscle. Tonic contraction is continuous, instigated by pacemaker cells that are believed to reside at the interface between the longitudinal and circular muscle layers.[16] The intensity of tonic contraction may vary with the frequency of spike potentials. In turn, the intensity of tonic contraction in a specific segment of the gut will determine the amount of pressure in that segment. The degree of tonic contraction in the sphincters of the GI tract determines the amount of resistance to the movement of intestinal contents along the tract. Thus the degree of contraction exerted by the pyloric, ileocecal, and anal sphincters serves to regulate the movement of nutrients through the GI tract.

The degree of rhythmic contraction varies in different parts of the GI tract. These differing rhythmic frequencies are dependent on the rate of slow-wave activity in a particular segment and may occur at rates of 3 to 12 times per minute. These slow wave–dependent contractions are responsible for the mixing and peristaltic propulsive movements present in the GI tract.

Two types of muscular activity are involved in the digestive and absorptive functions of the GI tract: mixing movements and propulsive movements. In different portions of the GI tract these movements may serve different functions to achieve proper digestion and absorption of nutrients. For example, mixing movements in the stomach and small intestine promote digestion by mixing the digestive juices with the food that enters from above. In the small intestine and proximal segment of the large intestine, mixing movements facilitate absorption by bringing newly arrived intestinal contents into contact with absorbing surfaces. In the case of propulsion, the rate at which nutrients are propelled through the GI tract depends on the function of the different organs of the tract. For example, the passageway for nutrients from the mouth through the pharynx and esophagus is simply a conduit; essentially no digestive or absorptive function occurs here. Thus the transit of nutrients through these regions is quite rapid. In contrast, transit from the stomach and through the small and large intestines is quite slow. This slow rate of passage allows for completion of the digestive and absorptive processes that occur in these portions of the GI tract.

Although the characteristics of mixing and propulsive movements differ in various parts of the GI tract and will be described separately in the next section, a description of the general characteristics of these movements is presented here.

Propulsive Movements

The basic propulsive movement of the GI tract is peristalsis (Figure 35-11). Nutrients are propelled by the slow advancement of a circular constriction that squeezes the materials in front of the constricted area forward. Peristalsis is an inherent property of any smooth muscle tube that, like the intestine, is a functional syncytium. However, effective intestinal peristalsis requires the presence of an intact myenteric nerve plexus. The usual stimulus for peristalsis is distention of the intestinal walls. The entry and subsequent stretching of the intestinal wall by a bolus of food will have the effect of stimulating the gut wall 2 to 3 cm above this point, and a circular constriction will then occur and propel the food with a peristaltic movement. Although peristalsis can move in both directions in the gut (either toward the mouth or toward the anus), it normally moves toward the anus. The exact cause of this generally anal direction of peristalsis is still being debated by physiologists; it is thought that the myenteric plexus may be organized in such a way that preferential transmission of signals downward occurs simultaneously with relaxation of the portion of the intestine below the distended stimulus point. This posited ability of the GI tract to propel nutrients downward while relaxing an adjacent lower portion to receive these nutrients is sometimes referred to as the "law of the gut."[1,2]

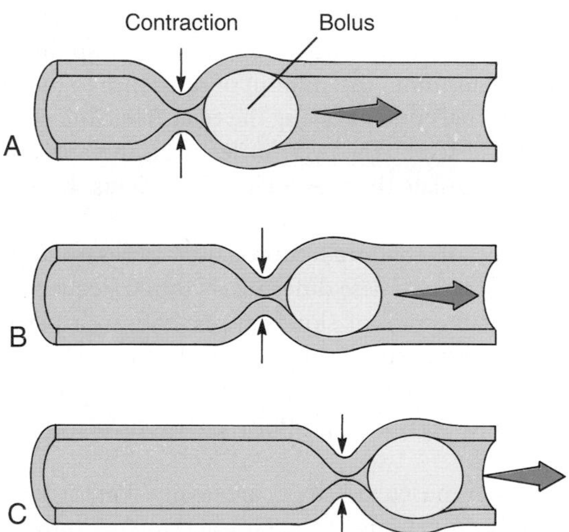

FIGURE 35-11 ■ Peristalsis. Peristalsis is a progressive type of movement, propelling material from point to point along the GI tract. **A,** A ring of contraction occurs where the GI wall is stretched, pushing the bolus forward. **B,** The moving bolus triggers a ring of contraction in the next region, which pushes the bolus even farther along. **C,** The ring of contraction moves like a wave along the GI tract, pushing the bolus forward. (From Thibodeau GA, Patton KT: *Anatomy and physiology,* ed 5, St Louis, 2003, Mosby, p 773.)

Mixing Movements

Mixing movements that serve to keep the intestinal contents thoroughly mixed on a constant basis are caused by either peristaltic contractions or local constrictive contractions of small segments of the gut wall. These movements may vary according to the specific function of each portion of the GI tract (see the discussion under Secretory Function).

Movement of Nutrients

The path taken by foods ingested into the GI tract as these nutrients travel down the tract and are digested and absorbed and their waste products eventually excreted will be traced beginning with the mouth. Although this process is described here as a linear sequence, it is important to note that several steps may occur simultaneously. The individual steps involved in nutrient ingestion constitute a synergistic process, and an inability to perform one phase of the process will ultimately have a profound effect on the entire GI tract. In addition, different individuals may manifest a great deal of variability in such aspects of digestive function as tolerance of certain nutrients and defecation patterns. Such variations may represent age-related differences or conditioned responses to environmental cues.

Chewing

The entry of solid food into the mouth results in the action of chewing, an important first step in the process of nutrient digestion. The process of moving the food around in the mouth and mixing it with saliva results in stimulation of the taste buds and olfactory epithelia; this sensory input greatly increases the subjective enjoyment of eating. As the food is mixed with saliva, it becomes softened and formed into a mass of appropriate size (bolus) that can be swallowed. The action of the molars and premolars in crushing more rigid forms of foods serves to prepare rough substances for transport down the esophagus. Although the act of chewing is under voluntary control, it is also partly reflexive in nature. The entry of food into the mouth has been shown to stimulate chewing in animals in the absence of full cerebral function. The movements of the skeletal muscles responsible for chewing are coordinated by impulses traveling through cranial nerves V, VII, IX, X, XI, and XII. Interruption of the proper transmission of impulses through these nerve tracts places an individual at risk for decreased voluntary control of the chewing function, with a resultant risk of aspiration.

Swallowing

Swallowing is the transport of material from the mouth to the stomach. The process of swallowing has been divided into three stages that describe the regions through which the bolus of nutrients passes on its way to the stomach: (1) the oral stage, (2) the pharyngeal stage, and (3) the esophageal stage.[2,3,8]

During the oral stage, the bolus is passed from the mouth to the pharynx through the space called the *fauces.* The bolus, either solid or liquid, is rolled toward the back of the tongue, and the front of the tongue is then pushed up against the hard palate. Respiration is inhibited briefly in this phase, as the pharyngeal muscles constrict to force the bolus of food into the pharynx. In the pharyngeal stage the bolus is passed through the pharynx into the esophagus, a process taking about one-fifth of a second. Continued contraction of the pharyngeal muscles and the position of the tongue prevent reentry of the bolus into the oral cavity. The soft palate is pulled upward to close off the nasopharynx; simultaneously, food is prevented from entering the larynx by elevation of the larynx and approximation of the vocal cords, both of which actions serve to close the glottis. As these openings are closed off, the pharyngeal constrictors contract and force the bolus of food into the esophagus. Respiration is now resumed, and pressure in the pharynx rises as a result of the muscular activities that have occurred.

The muscular characteristics of the esophagus are of particular importance in effecting the third, or esophageal, stage of swallowing. The upper one-third of the esophagus consists of skeletal muscle, whereas the lower two-thirds is composed of predominantly smooth muscle. In the normal resting stage, the upper part of the esophagus is closed by the tonic contraction of a band of skeletal muscle that serves as the pharyngoesophageal sphincter. The pressure exerted by the pharyngoesophageal sphincter in this region is normally about 20 to 40 cm H_2O above atmospheric pressure; this zone of high pressure keeps air from entering the esophagus during inspiration. Almost immediately after initiation of a swallow, the sphincter relaxes and pressure in the region drops to atmospheric pressure, thus allowing the bolus to be forced into the esophagus by the pressure generated in the pharynx. Pressure in the pharyngoesophageal junction region then rises as a result of contraction of skeletal muscle in this area, thus preventing reflux of food from the esophagus back to the pharynx. Pressure in this region then gradually subsides to a resting level as muscular relaxation occurs.

If the bolus being swallowed is a liquid, it is propelled through the esophagus by the initial force of swallowing and travels by gravity to the stomach in about 1 second. If the bolus is a semisolid mass, it is propelled down the esophagus by means of a peristaltic wave. This esophageal peristalsis is caused by a contraction of circular muscle that forces the bolus ahead of it toward the stomach, with a transit time of about 4 to 6 seconds.

Although no well-differentiated muscular structure is located in the area where the esophagus joins the stomach, the region approximately 2 to 5 cm above the juncture with the stomach is referred to as the LES and was described in a previous section. Almost immediately after initiation of a swallow, pressure at the LES drops and remains low during the time that a peristaltic wave is passing down through the lower end of the esophagus. Once the bolus has passed through the lower esophageal region and pressure in the lower portion of the esophagus has fallen to a resting level, the pressure in the LES rises and remains elevated for about 10 seconds before falling to a resting level once again.[2]

Neural Control of Swallowing. Figure 35-12 illustrates the neural pathways involved in the swallowing mechanism. Swallowing receptors in the posterior of the mouth and throat transmit impulses in response to a stimulus to the mucous membranes in the mouth, such as the presence of a moderate amount of fluid. These impulses travel mainly through the trigeminal nerve into the reticular substance of the medulla oblongata, where the swallowing center is located. Once this center has been activated, the sequence of muscular reactions described earlier occurs automatically and usually cannot be voluntarily stopped. The swallowing center then sends impulses over a number of efferent nerves to the numerous skeletal and smooth muscles involved in the swallowing

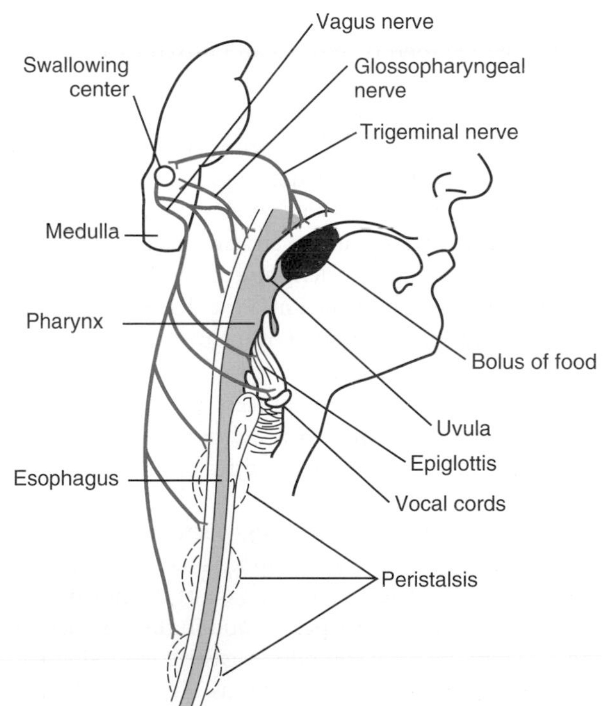

FIGURE 35-12 ■ Neural pathways of the swallowing mechanism. (From Guyton AC, Hall JE: *Textbook of medical physiology,* ed 10, Philadelphia, 2000, Saunders, p 729.)

process to allow the complete act of swallowing to occur in the appropriate sequence. The glossopharyngeal and hypoglossal nerves are primarily concerned with the oral and pharyngeal stages, whereas the vagus nerve is important in activating the esophageal stage.

Motor Functions of the Stomach

The motor functions of the stomach include the storage of ingested nutrients for variable lengths of time and the discharge of gastric contents into the small intestine at an appropriate rate for optimal digestion and absorption. The stomach also aids in the digestive process by its mixing movements, which convert large pieces of food to a finer, liquid consistency.

Gastric Filling and Storage. Upon entering the stomach from the esophagus, newly arrived food forms concentric circles in the body and fundus of the stomach, with the newest food lying closest to the esophagus and older food lying closer to the stomach wall. The smooth muscle in the fundus and body of the stomach can adapt to the volume of contents so that relatively large contents can be introduced with little increase in intragastric pressure. The fundus and body of the stomach maintain a certain pressure at all times. This tonic contraction continually presses on the food mass and aids in its delivery to the pyloric antrum.

Peristaltic contractions occur in the stomach once every 20 seconds. These rippling peristaltic waves begin in the corpus and move at a velocity of about 1 to 2 cm/sec. When they reach the more thickly walled pyloric antrum, they become much more vigorous and also increase in speed. These strong peristaltic contractions in the pyloric antrum are largely responsible for mixing ingested nutrients with gastric secretions. As ingested food is churned and mixed to a greater degree of fluidity, the mixture takes on a milky white sludge appearance and is then called **chyme.**

Emptying. As pressure in the antrum rises momentarily as the result of peristaltic contraction, a pressure differential exists between pressure in the antral pylorus and the duodenal bulb. The higher pressure in the antrum is sufficient to overcome resistance of the pyloric sphincter, and the contents of the stomach are then propelled into the duodenum. Concurrently, the degree of constriction of the pyloric sphincter may increase or decrease, depending on several factors discussed in the next section. Because this process is dependent on the muscular activity of the antrum as well as pyloric muscle tone, gastric emptying is largely regulated by mechanisms that affect each of these regions.

Regulation of Gastric Emptying. Factors that may affect the rate at which the stomach empties include the degree of distention of the gastric wall and release of the hormone **gastrin** in response to certain types of food in the stomach. Both of these factors increase the rate of gastric emptying by increasing the force of antral contractions while simultaneously inhibiting pyloric constriction. Distention of the gastric wall results in stimulation of mechanoreceptors in the stomach with subsequent activation of reflexes over the vagus and the intrinsic nerve plexuses. These neural influences, along with contractile activity (which is a direct response to the stretch of gastric muscle), constitute a major mechanism in providing the stimulus for gastric emptying.

Gastrin is a hormone released from the antral mucosa in response to stretching of the gastric wall, as well as the presence of certain foods, particularly meat. The role of gastrin in promoting the secretion of highly acidic gastric juices will be discussed later. With respect to stomach emptying, gastrin has a key role by enhancing peristalsis while at the same time relaxing the pylorus.[17]

In addition to these influences, many of the mechanisms that affect gastric emptying are initiated in the duodenum. Reflex nervous signals are transmitted from the duodenum back to the stomach in response to intraluminal stimuli; these signals probably have a key role in controlling both peristaltic activity and the degree of pyloric constriction. Stimulation of the duodenum in a variety of ways has the effect of slowing gastric emptying; both the chemical and physical properties of chyme entering the duodenum may affect the rate of gastric emptying. A variety of both duodenal cells and receptors, including osmoreceptors, mechanoreceptors, and chemoreceptors, respond to intraluminal stimuli to produce hormonal and reflex inhibition of gastric motor activity and enhancement of pyloric tone. The presence in the duodenum of chyme containing the breakdown products of proteins and, to a lesser extent, fats may impede gastric emptying. Also, the presence of highly acidic or highly hypertonic or hypotonic chyme in the duodenum may inhibit the rate of gastric emptying. The degree of distention of the duodenum, as well as the presence of any degree of irritation of the duodenum, may serve to impede stomach emptying. These inhibitory mechanisms have a protective function and are effective in preventing the intestinal mucosa from overloading its digestive and absorptive abilities and potentially being damaged by chemical or mechanical sources.

Although regulation of gastric emptying is largely dependent on factors in the stomach and duodenum, gastric motility may be stimulated or inhibited reflexively from a variety of regions of the body. For example, stomach emptying is inhibited when the ileum is full and when the anus is mechanically distended. Stimulation of visceral and somatic pain receptors may result in inhibition of gastric motility. Various strong emotions such as anger, fear, and anxiety may produce changes in motility of the stomach, but whether these states tend to predispose an individual to inhibition or excitation of gastric motility is not always predictable.[3,18]

Vomiting. Vomiting is rapid emptying of the contents of the stomach into the esophagus through the pharyngoesophageal sphincter and into the mouth. The major force for vomiting is supplied by the skeletal muscle of the diaphragm and abdomen rather than by contraction of the muscle of the stomach wall. Vomiting is the result of an extremely complex set of neural events coordinated by a center located in the medulla. Afferent impulses from receptors in various regions of the body, including the sensory nerve endings of the pharynx, abdominal viscera, and the labyrinths, arrive at this center and the vomiting reflex is initiated. This reflex causes closure of the glottis and trachea, relaxation of the gastroesophageal sphincter, and contraction of the diaphragm and the abdominal muscles, which forcibly expels the contents of the stomach.

Motility of the Small Intestine

What began as intact food entering the mouth has now been liquefied and partially digested in the stomach. It enters the small intestine, where the major part of digestion and absorption occurs. As in other parts of the GI tract, movements of the small intestine can be described as propulsive and mixing movements. Although this separation of types of movement is somewhat arbitrary in the small intestine because all its movements may cause both propulsion and mixing simultaneously, these processes are usually described separately.

Propulsion. Chyme is propelled through the small intestine by peristaltic waves that move at a rate of 0.5 to 2 cm/sec, with a faster rate at the proximal part of the intestine and a slower rate in the terminal portion. Approximately 3 to 5 hours is normally needed for the passage of chyme from the pyloric sphincter to the ileocecal valve, but this period may vary in some disease states. Peristaltic activity in the small intestine is greatly increased after the ingestion of a meal. The increase in contractile activity in the stomach caused by distention of the stomach wall is conducted principally through the myenteric plexus down along the wall of the small intestine. This so-called gastroenteric reflex serves to increase the activity of the small intestine, with an enhancement of both intestinal motility and secretion.

The usual stimulus for peristalsis in the small intestine is distention of the intestinal walls; stretch receptors in the gut wall are sensitive to circumferential stretch and initiate a local myenteric reflex in response to this stimulation. The resulting contraction of longitudinal muscle, followed by the contraction of circular muscle, spreads downward in a peristaltic motion.

The peristaltic waves in the small intestine not only propel chyme downward toward the ileocecal valve but also spread out the chyme along the intestinal mucosa, thus facilitating the process of absorption of nutrients (Figure 35-13). As ad-

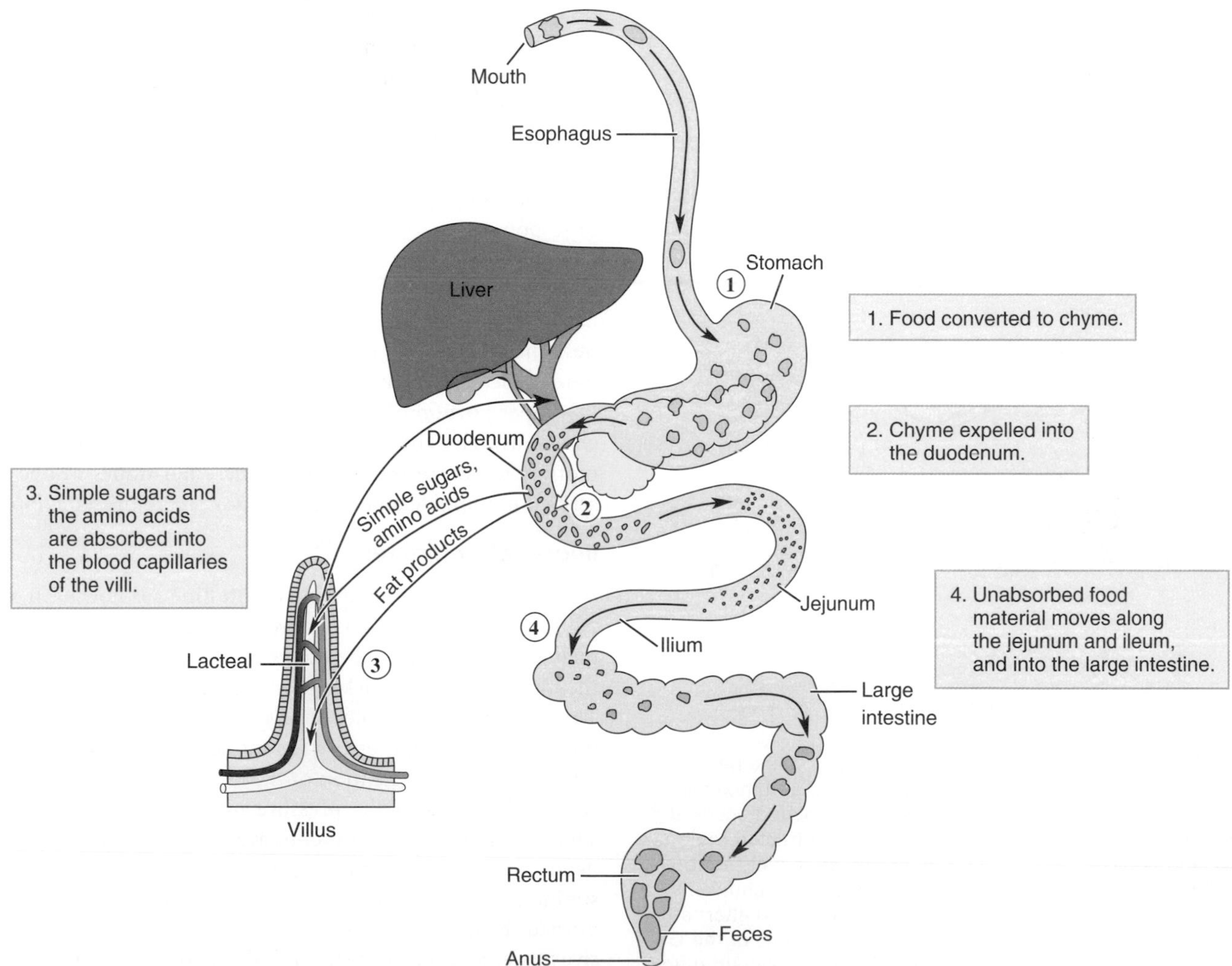

FIGURE 35-13 ■ Chyme and the process of absorption of nutrients. (From Herlihy B, Maebius NK: *The human body in health and illness,* Philadelphia, 2000, Saunders, p 408.)

ditional chyme enters the small intestine, this spreading process intensifies as peristalsis increases. When chyme reaches the ileocecal valve, it is sometimes stationary for several hours until the individual eats another meal and a new gastroenteric reflex intensifies the peristaltic process and propels the remaining chyme through the ileocecal valve.

Certain disease states, particularly those that involve intense irritation of the intestinal mucosa, may result in a peristaltic rush, a powerful peristaltic wave that travels long distances in the small intestine in a short period. The peristaltic rush clears the contents of the small intestine into the colon, thus relieving the small intestine of either irritating substances or excessive distention.[2,8]

Mixing. In addition to propulsive peristaltic movements, a set of movements characterized as **segmentation contractions** also occur in the small intestine. The primary effect of these contractions is progressive mixing of solid chyme particles with secretions of the small intestine. As their name implies, segmentation contractions involve contraction of the small intestine in regularly spaced segments that have the appearance of sausages (Figure 35-14). As one set of segmentation contractions is completed, a new set begins, with contractile points located at different locations along the small intestine. Segmentation contractions occur at a rate of 7 to 12 times per minute and effectively chop and mix the chyme, as well as assist in propelling the chyme toward the ileocecal valve (see Figure 35-14).

Control of Motility. The electrical and mechanical activities of the small intestine are closely associated. Slow waves, as described previously in this chapter, occur at the membranes of the longitudinal smooth muscle, with frequencies of 11 to 12 per minute in the duodenum decreasing to 7 to 9 per minute in the terminal ileum. Slow waves do not directly produce muscular contractions in the small intestine but provide the conditions under which contractions can occur. Although slow waves determine the velocity and direction of peristalsis, other factors determine whether action potentials and thus contraction will occur. Local mechanical and chemical stimulation by chyme is probably largely responsible for the initiation and continuance of contraction in the small intestine. Thus when the intestinal tract becomes overly distended or when the mucosa becomes irritated, myenteric reflexes enhance the electrical activity of the gut and spike potentials are superimposed on the slow waves. These spike potentials then spread through both longitudinal and circular muscle, and contraction results.

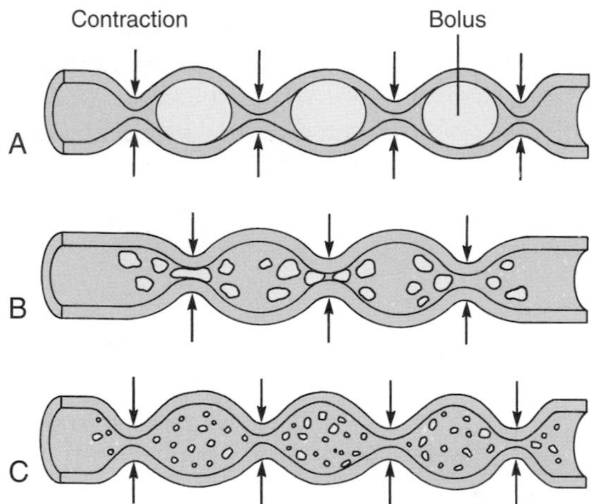

FIGURE 35-14 ■ Segmentation. Segmentation is a back-and-forth action that breaks apart chunks of food and mixes in digestive juices. **A,** Ringlike regions of contraction occur at intervals along the GI tract. **B,** Previously contracted regions relax and adjacent regions now contract, effectively "chopping" the contents of each segment into smaller chunks. **C,** Locations of the contracted regions continue to alternate back and forth, chopping and mixing the contents of the GI lumen. (From Thibodeau GA, Patton KT: *Anatomy and physiology,* ed 5, St Louis, 2003, Mosby, p 774.)

Intestinal motility may also be influenced by stimulation from extrinsic sources. Stimulation of the vagus nerve generally causes increased intestinal motility, with sympathetic stimulation resulting in inhibition. Intestinal motility can be altered reflexively by stimulation of many sensory areas. For example, trauma to organs outside the GI tract, such as irritation of the peritoneum or urinary tract, may cause intestinal inhibition. A condition called paralytic ileus, in which intestinal motility is inhibited as the result of reflex inhibition, may occur after surgery on these areas.[3,19]

Much current research is focused on the involvement of GI hormones in the regulation of GI tract motility.[18] Cholecystokinin, a hormone released from the mucosa of the jejunum in response to fatty substances in chyme, has been shown to block the increased gastric motility caused by gastrin. Another hormone, secretin, which is released mainly from the duodenal mucosa in response to gastric acid entering the duodenum, has the general effect of decreasing GI motility. A hormone called gastric inhibitory peptide, which is released from the upper portion of the small intestine in response to fat in chyme, as well as to carbohydrates, is known to inhibit gastric motility under some conditions. These hormones will be described in more detail in the section on secretory function.

Ileocecal Sphincter

The chyme that entered the small intestine has now been propelled downward and has arrived at the terminal ileum immediately proximal to the cecum, where the last 2 to 3 cm of the muscular coat is thicker than that in the rest of the ileum. This region, called the ileocecal sphincter, is normally closed; it is an area of high pressure (about 20 cm H_2O above atmospheric pressure). Distention of the lower part of the ileum results in lowering of the pressure in the ileocecal sphincter. Thus when intestinal contents are present in the terminal ileum and are ready to be propelled into the cecum, the sphincter reflexly relaxes and the intestinal contents are pushed through the sphincter into the cecum by the propulsive movements of the distal end of the small intestine. Subsequently, distention of the cecum after it is filled with contents passing through the ileocecal valve results in increased pressure in the sphincter, which prevents reflux flow back into the ileum (Figure 35-15).

Motility of the Colon

The movements of the colon are effective in promoting the two major functions of the colon: (1) absorption of water and electrolytes from chyme and (2) storage of the fecal mass until it can be expelled from the body by defecation.

Colonic Movements. For most of the time, the large intestine in humans is inactive. However, the presence of material in the proximal end of the colon results in a type of mixing movement in the haustra (the outpouchings in the colon wall), termed **haustral churning,** that is similar to the segmenting movements in the small intestine. This movement is the major type of motility in the large intestine. Haustral churning exposes the contents of the large intestine to the mucosa, thus promoting the absorption of water. Normally, about 500 ml of chyme enters the proximal part of the colon each day. Out of this total volume, 400 ml—mostly water and electrolytes—is reabsorbed before defecation takes place, with an average volume of 100 ml of feces remaining for eventual disposal from the body.[1,19]

At infrequent intervals of about three to four times a day, a strong peristaltic movement termed a *mass movement* occurs and propels the fecal material long distances. These strong contractions may reach a peak of 100 cm H_2O pressure in the segment undergoing the contraction. Fecal material may be transported all the way from the ascending colon to the descending colon by a mass movement. Feces are then stored in the distal end of the colon until defecation takes place.

Defecation. Under normal conditions, it takes about 18 hours for intestinal contents to reach the distal end of the colon after leaving the small intestine. Fecal material is stored in the distal part of the colon for varying lengths of time; defecation may take place 24 hours or longer after the ingestion of food. Ordinarily the rectum is empty, but fecal material is occasionally shifted into it after one of the mass movements, and the resulting distention of the rectum initiates the urge to defecate. The act of defecation is a combination of voluntary and involuntary movements. Contraction of the distal end of the colon and relaxation of the internal anal sphincter, which are regions composed of smooth muscle, are involuntary movements. Relaxation of the external anal sphincter, which consists of striated muscle, is a voluntary movement. Other voluntary movements that may assist in the act of defecation are contraction of the abdominal muscles and forcible expiration with closure of the glottis (bearing down).

Regulation of Colonic Motility. Movements in the proximal portion of the colon are largely initiated by distention in the colonic walls, which stimulates contractile activity by triggering short reflexes through the intrinsic nerve plexuses. Although the proximal part of the colon receives extrinsic innervation via the vagus nerve, it functions in a relatively normal manner in the absence of extrinsic motor innervation and is thus a somewhat self-regulating structure. Extrinsic nerves may occasionally modify proximal colonic activity, however; for example, entry of food into the stomach or duodenum may result in a mass contraction in the proximal end of the colon. Sometimes termed the gastrocolic or duodenocolic reflexes, these strong mass movements are most evident after the first intake of nutrients in the morning and are often followed by a strong need to defecate.

In contrast, the distal part of the colon is somewhat more dependent on its extrinsic nerve supply, so movements in this region, including the act of defecation, may be entirely abolished after injury to these nerves. However, weak movements return eventually, and defecation can still occur without voluntary control after the initial response to injury has passed.[3]

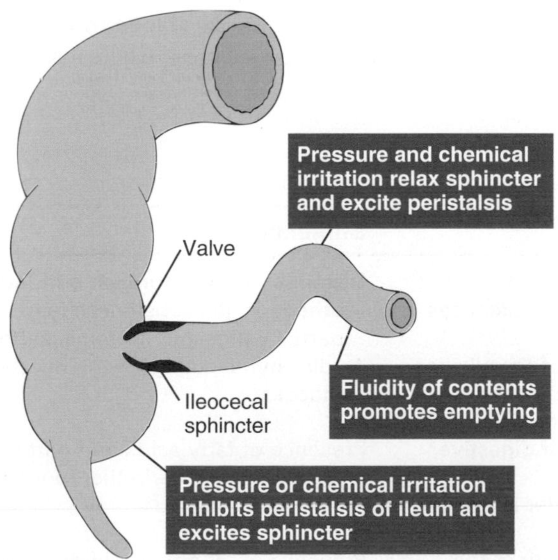
Pressure and chemical irritation relax sphincter and excite peristalsis
Valve
Ileocecal sphincter
Fluidity of contents promotes emptying
Pressure or chemical irritation inhibits peristalsis of ileum and excites sphincter

FIGURE 35-15 ■ Emptying of the ileocecal valve. (From Guyton AC, Hall JE: *Textbook of medical physiology,* ed 10, Philadelphia, 2000, Saunders, p 735.)

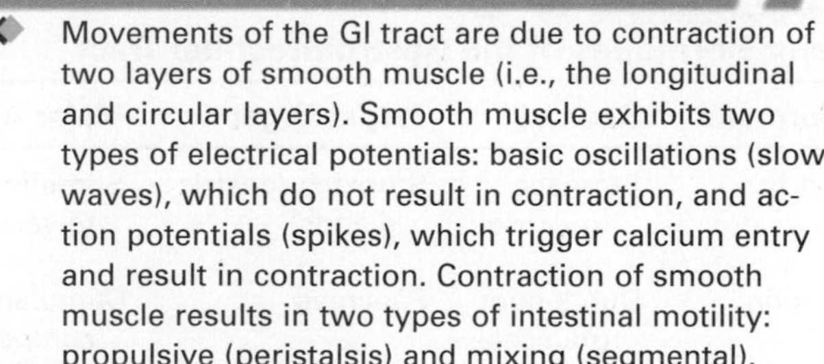

KEY CONCEPTS

- Movements of the GI tract are due to contraction of two layers of smooth muscle (i.e., the longitudinal and circular layers). Smooth muscle exhibits two types of electrical potentials: basic oscillations (slow waves), which do not result in contraction, and action potentials (spikes), which trigger calcium entry and result in contraction. Contraction of smooth muscle results in two types of intestinal motility: propulsive (peristalsis) and mixing (segmental).
- GI motility is regulated by the enteric nervous system, the autonomic nervous system, and hormonal mediators. The enteric nervous system has two branches—myenteric and submucosal—that coordinate reflexive contraction and relaxation along the entire GI tract. Luminal distention is an important stimulus for reflexive motility. Sympathetic nervous

system activity is generally inhibitory to GI motility (and secretion). Parasympathetic nervous system activity generally enhances motility. Regulatory hormones include gastrin (increases gastric motility), gastric inhibitory peptide (decreases gastric motility), cholecystokinin (gallbladder contraction), and secretin (decreases GI motility).

- Swallowing is a complex function coordinated by a swallowing center in the medulla. Swallowing is partially voluntary and partially involuntary. Cranial nerves IX, X, and XI mediate the various stages of swallowing.
- Regulation of gastric emptying involves gastric and duodenal factors. Gastric distention and the release of gastrin from gastric mucosa promote gastric emptying. Duodenal distention, acidity, hypertonicity, and high protein and fat concentrations inhibit gastric emptying.
- Chyme remains in the small intestine for 3 to 5 hours. There it is continually mixed by segmental contractions and slowly propelled toward the ileocecal valve by peristalsis. Distention of the terminal ileum results in relaxation of the ileocecal sphincter, which allows contents to enter the large bowel.
- Segmental contractions (haustra) in the large intestine promote water absorption. About 18 hours is required for the contents to traverse the large intestine and reach the distal end of the colon. Three to four times a day a peristaltic mass movement sweeps fecal material along the colon. Mass movements may be initiated by entry of food into the stomach and duodenum (gastrocolic reflex).
- An urge to defecate occurs when feces enters the rectum. Contraction of the distal end of the colon and relaxation of the internal anal sphincter occur involuntarily as feces enters the rectum. The external anal sphincter is under voluntary control and inhibits defecation until voluntarily relaxed.

SECRETORY FUNCTION

Secretion of Gastrointestinal Juices

The many glands associated with the GI tract generally produce enzymes that participate in the digestive process to break down the major nutrient components of carbohydrates, fats, and proteins. The somewhat archaic term "juices" is still used to describe the fluids secreted in the GI tract, which contain a complex mixture of salts and protein enzymes. Thus the glands located in the stomach are said to produce gastric juice and the glands of the intestinal wall produce intestinal juice. Secretion of these digestive juices is stimulated by various factors, including mechanical and chemical stimulation by chyme, parasympathetic stimulation (in certain regions of the GI tract), and various hormones.

Gastrointestinal Hormones

Table 35-1 lists the major hormones of the GI tract and their sources, target organs, major actions, and factors that stimulate release. These hormones are released from the GI mucosa in response to distention or the presence of certain nutrient substances. They are then absorbed into the blood and carried to glands in target tissues (i.e., tissues on which they exert their effects), where they stimulate secretion. Chemically, GI hormones are polypeptides or polypeptide derivatives.

Gastrin, secretin, cholecystokinin, and gastric inhibitory peptide have been mentioned previously in this chapter as having additional roles in motility of the GI tract. Gastrin is secreted by the stomach mucosa and stimulates the gastric glands to secrete the specific substances produced by the different specialized cells of these glands. Secretin was one of the first of the many hormones of the body to be discovered. The most potent stimulus for secretin release is hydrochloric acid, and the presence of acidic chyme acting on the mucosa of the duodenum promotes its release into the blood from the duodenal mucosa. It is carried to the pancreas, where it stimulates

Table 35-1

Major Hormones of the Gastrointestinal Tract

Hormone	Source	Target Organ	Major Actions	Stimulated By
Gastrin	Stomach (mucosa)	Stomach (gastric glands)	Stimulates gastric glands to secrete specific substances	Distention of the stomach by food; other specific substances (e.g., partially digested proteins, caffeine)
Secretin	Duodenum (mucosa)	Pancreas	Stimulates release of the alkaline component of pancreatic juice	Acidic chyme acting on the duodenal mucosa
		Liver	Increases bile secretion rate	
Cholecystokinin	Duodenum (mucosa)	Pancreas	Stimulates release of digestive enzymes	Presence of fatty acids and partially digested proteins in the duodenum
		Gallbladder	Stimulates gallbladder contraction and emptying	
Gastric inhibitory peptide	Duodenum (mucosa)	Stomach	Reduces motor activity of the stomach; slows rate of gastric emptying	Presence of fat or carbohydrate in the duodenum

the secretion of a large volume of bicarbonate-rich juice, or the alkaline component of pancreatic juice. In the duodenum, sodium bicarbonate then neutralizes the HCl of the chyme, thus protecting the duodenal mucosa from potential damage and creating a slightly alkaline medium that is optimal for chemical digestion by pancreatic intestinal enzymes. Although the liver produces bile continuously, secretin is effective in increasing the rate of bile secretion. Hormonal regulation is the most important mechanism governing the activity of the pancreas, and cholecystokinin has a key role in stimulating the release of large amounts of digestive enzymes from the pancreas. Cholecystokinin also stimulates the gallbladder to release the bile it stores. Gastric inhibitory peptide acts to slow stomach emptying by decreasing gastric motor activity.[1,17]

Recent research has shown that histamine is a powerful stimulant of gastric acid secretion.[20] Histamine, an amine with multiple roles in human physiologic processes, including an ability to constrict bronchial smooth muscle, is abundant in mastlike cells of the gastric mucosa and is released during an antigen-antibody reaction. After its release, histamine diffuses readily into nearby parietal cells. Although less potent than gastrin, it causes the parietal cells to produce large amounts of gastric secretions. The exact mechanism by which histamine controls acid secretion is presently uncertain, although it is known that physical or emotional stress increases its release. The administration of certain medications that block its action (H_2 antagonists) is effective in reducing gastric acid secretions, and it is posited that histamine has an important role in acid secretion.

Stimulation of the parasympathetic nerves to certain regions of the GI tract will also increase the rates of glandular secretion. Those glands in the upper portion of the GI tract that are innervated by the vagus and other cranial parasympathetic nerves, particularly the salivary, esophageal, and gastric glands, the pancreas, and some duodenal glands, are especially subject to parasympathetic stimulation. Glands in the distal portion of the large intestine are also affected by parasympathetic stimulation because this region is innervated by the pelvic parasympathetic nerves. In the small intestine, the major stimulus for intestinal secretion is local and mechanical stimulation of the intestinal wall, which initiates the excitation of local myenteric reflexes and subsequent release of secretions.

KEY CONCEPTS

- Major secreting glands and secretions in the GI tract can be summarized as follows:
  Salivary gland: Salivary amylase.
  Gastric glands: Chief cells secrete pepsinogen; parietal cells secrete HCl and intrinsic factor. HCl activates pepsinogen to pepsin, and intrinsic factor enhances vitamin B_{12} absorption. Parietal cell secretion is stimulated by acetylcholine, histamine, and gastrin. G cells secrete gastrin into the blood stream. Gastrin increases gastric motility and stimulates chief and parietal cell secretion.
  Intestinal epithelium: Secretes brush border enzymes (peptidases, lipases, sucrase, lactase), secretin, which stimulates pancreatic secretion, and cholecystokinin, which stimulates gallbladder contraction.
  Pancreas: Secretes bicarbonate-rich fluid containing amylase, trypsin, chymotrypsin, and lipase into the duodenum when stimulated by secretin.
  Gallbladder: Secretes concentrated bile salts into the duodenum when stimulated by cholecystokinin.

DIGESTION AND ABSORPTION

Substances contained in foods that are important to maintenance of the body include carbohydrates, fats (also called lipids) proteins, vitamins, inorganic salts, and water. Many of the nutrient constituents that make up intact food substances are structurally complex and cannot be easily absorbed from the GI tract in their original forms. During the process of digestion, digestive juices and the enzymes contained in these secretions convert these complex organic molecules to smaller molecules (Figure 35-16). These simpler compounds are then capable of absorption, or transfer across the wall of the small intestine into the blood and lymph, which in turn transport them to the cells. This complex task of digestion and absorption of nutrients is the primary task of the GI tract. An inability to perform this function can compromise the health and existence of individuals experiencing interruptions in proper nutrient digestion and absorption. This section describes the mechanisms of digestion of the three major groups of nutrients—carbohydrates, lipids, and proteins—and then considers the absorption of these substances.

Digestion of Carbohydrates

In terms of calories, carbohydrates account for approximately half of the American diet. The major digestible carbohydrate in food is the polysaccharide plant starch, a large molecule composed of straight and branched chains of glucose. A summary of carbohydrate digestion is presented in Table 35-2.

Digestion of starch begins in the mouth as the enzyme salivary amylase breaks down polysaccharides to the much smaller disaccharide molecules maltose and dextrin. In the stomach, this action of salivary amylase continues until the enzyme is eventually inactivated by the acidic gastric juice. In the duodenum, the enzyme pancreatic amylase completes the task of splitting any remaining undigested polysaccharides and dextrins to small maltose units. Then maltase, an enzyme located in the brush border of the epithelial cells lining the duodenum, hydrolyzes each maltose molecule to two molecules of glucose. Other carbohydrates that are present in the diet in smaller quantities are the disaccharides sucrose, which

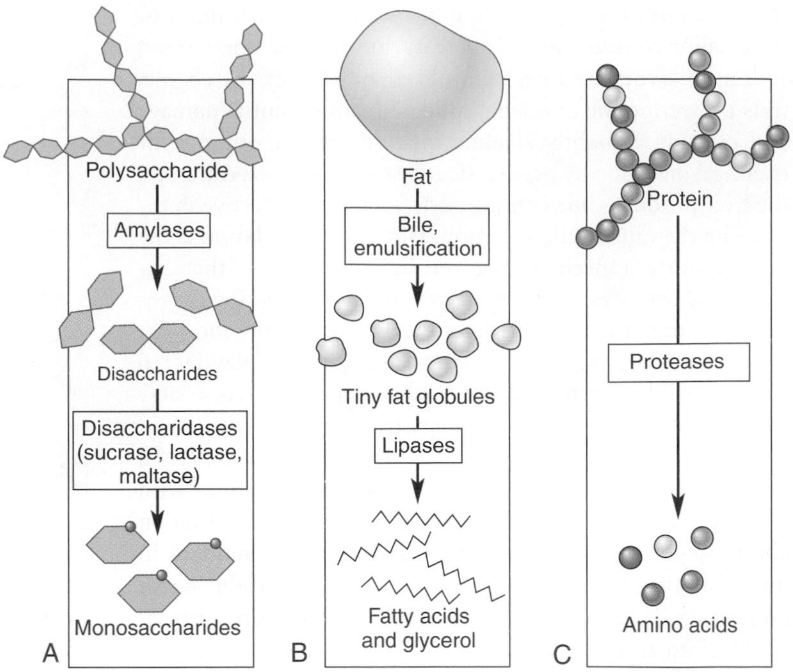

A
Polysaccharide
Amylases
Disaccharides
Disaccharidases (sucrase, lactase, maltase)
Monosaccharides

B
Fat
Bile, emulsification
Tiny fat globules
Lipases
Fatty acids and glycerol

C
Protein
Proteases
Amino acids

FIGURE 35-16 ■ Chemical digestion. **A,** Amylases and disaccharidases break carbohydrates down into monosaccharides. **B,** Lipases break fats down to fatty acids and glycerol. The large fat globule must first be emulsified by bile. **C,** Proteases and peptidases break proteins down into amino acids. (From Herlihy B, Maebius NK: *The human body in health and illness,* Philadelphia, 2000, Saunders, p 407.)

Table 35-2

Summary of Carbohydrate, Protein, and Lipid Digestion

Location of Digestive Process	Source of Digestive Enzyme or Substance	Basic Digestive Process
Carbohydrates		
Mouth, stomach	Salivary glands (salivary amylase)	Polysaccharides $\xrightarrow{\text{salivary amylase}}$ maltose + dextrin
Small intestine lumen	Pancreas (pancreatic amylase)	Undigested polysaccharides/dextrins $\xrightarrow{\text{pancreatic amylase}}$ maltose
Brush borders	Intestine (maltase, sucrase, lactase)	Maltose $\xrightarrow{\text{maltase}}$ glucose + glucose Sucrose $\xrightarrow{\text{sucrase}}$ glucose + fructose Lactose $\xrightarrow{\text{lactase}}$ glucose + galactose
Lipids		
Small intestine	Liver Pancreas	Lipid particle $\xrightarrow{\text{bile salts}}$ emulsified fat (triglycerides) Triglyceride $\xrightarrow{\text{lipase}}$ fatty acids + glycerol
Proteins		
Stomach	Stomach (gastric glands)	Protein $\xrightarrow{\text{pepsin}}$ polypeptides
Small intestine lumen	Pancreas	Polypeptides $\xrightarrow{\text{trypsin, chymotrysin}}$ tripeptides + dipeptides $\xrightarrow{\text{carboxypeptidase}}$ free amino acids
Brush borders (and within cytoplasm of epithelial cells)	Small intestine	Tripeptides and dipeptides $\xrightarrow{\text{peptidase}}$ free amino acids

is table sugar (glucose-fructose), and lactose, which is milk sugar (glucose-galactose). These two carbohydrates remain chemically unaltered until they reach the duodenum. There the enzyme sucrase in the brush border converts the sucrose to the monosaccharides glucose and fructose. Lactose is acted on by lactase, which splits it into the monosaccharides glucose and galactose.[5,21]

Glucose, the major product of carbohydrate digestion, accounts for about 80% of the monosaccharides obtained from food, whereas fructose and galactose account for the other 20%. Humans do not secrete an enzyme capable of digesting cellulose, a plant polysaccharide found in the cell walls of plants and present in large amounts in fibrous vegetables. Although cellulose consists of glucose molecules, it contains molecular linkages different from those of starch. Thus much of this complex carbohydrate passes through the digestive tract without being digested and is excreted in the feces.

Digestion of Lipids

The lipids of the diet are mostly in the form of triglycerides but also include phospholipids, cholesterol, and fat-soluble vitamins A, D, E, and K. Digestion of lipids occurs in the small intestine, where fats are emulsified by the action of bile; neither salivary nor gastric enzymes appear to have any effect on triglycerides. As the lipid particles enter the duodenum from the stomach, bile exerts a detergent action on them in which the surface tension of the particles is decreased. This decrease in surface tension promotes breakup of the particles into smaller particles as they are pushed around by the mixing movements of the small intestine. The emulsification process is an entirely mechanical action inasmuch as bile contains no enzymes and thus performs no chemical digestion.

Eventually, the detergent action of bile salts reduces the particles of fat to tiny droplets so that their surface area is greatly increased. This enhancement of surface area allows for maximal exposure to pancreatic lipase, an enzyme, which (along with intestinal lipase, to a lesser extent) hydrolyzes the triglycerides to free fatty acids and glycerol. Some monoglycerides (glycerol with one fatty acid still attached) may remain; in fact, some fat may escape digestion entirely or be reduced only to diglycerides (glycerol with two fatty acids attached).[22] A summary of triglyceride digestion is present in Table 35-2.

Cholesterol, a steroid type of lipid, is ingested in the form of cholesterol esters. These ester compounds cannot be directly absorbed. An esterase in pancreatic juice degrades cholesterol esters to cholesterol and fatty acid, which then undergo absorption.

Digestion of Proteins

Proteins are composed of molecular subunits called amino acids that are linked together by peptide bonds. Protein that undergoes digestion in the small intestine includes both protein from food and protein from desquamated cells and the many enzymes of the GI tract. This protein of endogenous origin constitutes a sizable portion of the total protein subjected to digestion and absorption.[23]

Protein digestion involves breakage of the peptide bonds by hydrolysis and release of free amino acids. Protein digestion begins in the stomach with the action of the enzyme pepsin, which is secreted by the gastric glands. By its action on peptide bonds, pepsin reduces most protein to intermediate-sized polypeptides. Pepsin is also capable of breaking down collagen, a protein component of intercellular connective tissue, thus rendering cellular proteins more accessible to enzymatic action in the GI tract. In the duodenum, the trypsin and chymotrypsin contained in pancreatic juice reduce the polypeptides to small peptides (tripeptides and dipeptides). Carboxypeptidase, which has its source in the pancreas, and peptidases in the brush borders of the intestinal epithelial cells split some of these peptides into free amino acids. Free amino acids, in addition to dipeptides and tripeptides, are absorbed into the intestinal epithelial cells. Within the cytoplasm of epithelial cells the small peptides are then hydrolyzed by various peptidases into free amino acids before their passage into the circulation. Numerous proteolytic enzymes are involved in protein digestion, and each enzyme acts on a slightly different type of peptide linkage. Protein digestion is summarized in Table 35-2.

Absorption

Intestinal absorption is the movement of water and dissolved materials, such as the products of nutrient digestion, vitamins, and inorganic salts, from the inside of the small intestine through the semipermeable intestinal membrane and into the blood and lymph. A major feature of the intestinal absorptive surface is the villus, the small fingerlike projection lined with epithelial cells that was described earlier in this chapter. Within each villus is a network of capillaries that branch from a miniscule artery and empty into a miniscule vein. A central lymph vessel called a lacteal is also located in the villus. In the process of absorption, nutrient molecules must pass through the single layer of epithelial cells lining the villus and through the single layer of cells forming the wall of the capillary or lacteal. A number of transport systems specific to certain nutrient components function in the intestinal epithelium to promote this process of absorption.[4]

Energy for operation of the intestinal transport systems is provided by certain chemical reactions occurring in the epithelial cells. These systems are capable of moving the products of nutrient digestion and inorganic salts from the intestinal lumen into the blood against electrochemical gradients (active transport). If the oxidative metabolism of mucosal cells becomes inhibited, these active transport systems will be impeded. In addition to active transport, some molecules may move across the intestinal epithelium when a difference in concentration on the two sides of the epithelium exists. The rate of molecular transfer based on diffusion gradients is dependent not only on the magnitude of the difference in concentration but also on the size of the molecules and the lipid solubility of the substances involved.

Almost all substances capable of intestinal absorption disappear from the lumen of the small intestine by the time that the intestinal contents reach the mid-jejunum. The ileum is not involved in absorption to any significant degree inasmuch as the proximal regions of the small intestine have usually done the work of absorption before the intestinal contents reach the ileal region. Nevertheless, the distal end of the small intestine has the capability of absorption and may do so in situations in which absorption has not taken place in the proximal part of the small intestine. Thus about 50% of the small intestine can be surgically removed without compromising absorptive ability. However, it is important to note that vitamin B_{12} and bile salts are absorbed specifically in the terminal ileum and that surgical removal of this portion of the small intestine will result in impaired absorption of these substances.[5]

The intestinal contents arriving at the terminal ileum contain no digestible carbohydrate, very little fat, and only 15% to 17% nitrogen-containing substances. Most of the contents of the terminal ileum consist of bacteria, desquamated epithelial cells, digestive secretions, and the residue of foods that are undigested and therefore unabsorbed, such as the cellulose walls of fibrous plants and connective tissue from animal sources.

Carbohydrates

Carbohydrates are absorbed in the form of monosaccharides. Polysaccharides and disaccharides lack the capacity for absorption; apparently the intestinal epithelium is impermeable to carbohydrates of such high molecular weight, and no transport systems exist for these types of carbohydrate molecules. The monosaccharides glucose and galactose are absorbed by an active, energy-requiring process in which a carrier molecule located on the luminal border of epithelial cells transports glucose and galactose across the border. It is theorized that the same carrier molecule that ferries glucose and galactose also carries sodium and that the carrier affinity for sugar is greatest when sodium is bound to the carrier. In contrast to the other monosaccharides, the monosaccharide fructose is absorbed passively by means of a diffusion gradient.[5]

Lipids

Absorption of lipids occurs by a highly complex, unique process. As fatty acids and monoglycerides are freed during digestion, they become dissolved in bile salt micelles, which are colloidal particles composed of many molecules. Within the micelles, the products of lipid digestion are now soluble and can be absorbed far more efficiently. The bile salt micelles transport the lipid products to the epithelial brush borders, where the monoglycerides or fatty acids, which are highly soluble in the lipid cell membrane, diffuse into the epithelial cells and leave the micelle behind. The micelle is now emptied of its cargo and can pick up more fatty acids and monoglycerides and transport them to the cell membrane.

Bile salts, which are required for micelle formation, are absorbed mostly in the terminal ileum and then recycled in the liver. In the absence of bile, the amount of lipid absorbed in this manner is reduced by more than 25%. In this situation, the absorption of fat-soluble vitamins (vitamins A, D, E, and K), which are absorbed with fat, is compromised. Several cholestatic conditions, such as primary biliary cirrhosis, may be associated with deficiencies of fat-soluble vitamins.[24,25]

Monoglycerides may be further degraded into glycerol and fatty acids by the enzyme lipase within the epithelial cell. Short-chain fatty acids (those with fewer than 12 carbon atoms) can be absorbed directly into the blood at this point. Longer chain fatty acids and glycerol, however, are reassembled into triglycerides by the endoplasmic reticulum. These newly synthesized triglycerides are aggregated into droplets that become progressively larger during passage through the cell. These lipid droplets are stabilized by enclosure with absorbed cholesterol and phospholipids and encased by a protein coat. The final product, called a chylomicron, passes out of the cell and into the lacteal of the villus. From the lacteal, chylomicrons pass through a series of lymph vessels that eventually drain into the general circulation.

Proteins

Amino acids are transported across the epithelial membrane by means of an active transport carrier system in much the same way as monosaccharides are. It is currently thought that different carrier systems exist to carry the different chemical classes of amino acids (i.e., neutral, basic, dicarboxylic, and imino acids). As is the case for the transport of sugars, brush border membrane carriers are involved in the transfer of amino acids across the intestinal epithelial cell; these carriers require energy and are coupled to the transport of sodium. After being transported to the epithelial cells of the villi, amino acids diffuse through the base of the cell and into the blood. Both amino acids and monosaccharides are transported directly to the liver by the hepatic portal vein.

Water and Electrolytes

Water and inorganic ions, which are in the GI tract as a result of ingestion and secretion, are absorbed mainly from the small intestine and, to a lesser extent, from the colon. The process of absorption of water and ions is the same in both the small and large intestine: sodium is actively transported to the blood, and water follows passively in response to the osmotic gradient created by the removal of sodium from the intraluminal fluid. About 8000 ml of water is absorbed every day by the small intestine and about 300 to 400 ml by the colon. Frequently, diarrhea is the result of failure of the small intestine to absorb water appropriately. If large quantities of water are allowed to enter the colon from the small intestine because of some malfunction of the small intestine's absorptive ability, the colonic absorptive mechanism may be overwhelmed, and diarrhea is the result (Figure 35-17).

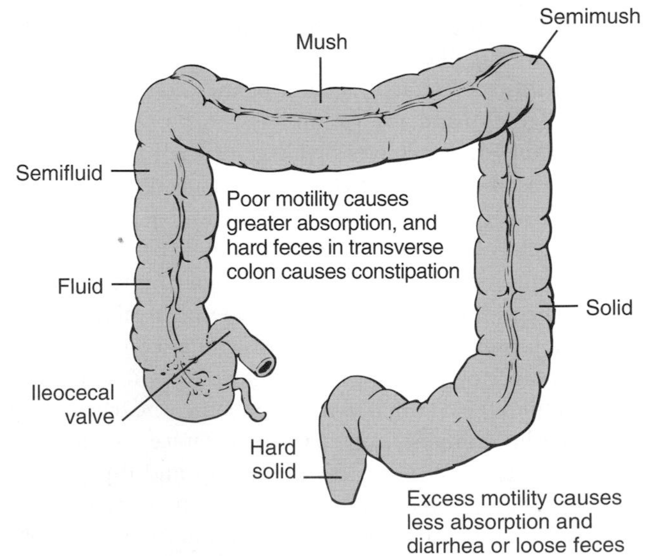

FIGURE 35-17 ■ Absorptive function of the large intestine. (From Guyton AC, Hall JE: *Textbook of medical physiology,* ed 10, Philadelphia, Saunders, 2000, p 735.)

KEY CONCEPTS

- Digestion, the process of converting large molecules to simpler forms, is accomplished by mechanical and enzymatic processes. Digestion is a necessary prelude to absorption because only simple molecules can cross the intestinal epithelia.
- Digestion of complex carbohydrates is initiated in the mouth, where salivary amylase begins to cleave large molecules into disaccharides. Pancreatic amylase continues this process in the small intestine. Disaccharides (maltose, sucrose, lactose) are cleaved into monosaccharides (glucose, fructose, galactose) by brush border enzymes (maltase, sucrase, lactase) on the intestinal epithelia. Glucose and galactose are absorbed across the intestinal epithelia by a sodium-dependent cotransporter. Fructose is absorbed passively by facilitated diffusion. Monosaccharides then travel via the blood stream to the liver.
- Lipid digestion begins in the small intestine, where bile salts from the gallbladder mix and emulsify the fatty substances. Emulsification mechanically separates the lipids into small drops that are more accessible to enzymatic digestion. Pancreatic lipase and brush border lipases digest the fats into free fatty acids and glycerol, which remain associated with the bile salts and form micelles. Cholesterol is digested by pancreatic esterase. Fatty acids are transported to the intestinal epithelia by micelles. Free fatty acids diffuse out of the micelle and into the epithelial cell passively. Epithelial cells synthesize large protein-lipid complexes (chylomicrons) that enter the lymphatic system.
- Protein digestion begins in the stomach, where HCl from parietal cells activates pepsinogen to pepsin. Pepsin cleaves proteins into smaller polypeptides. Pepsin is neutralized in the duodenum, and pancreatic trypsin, chymotrypsin, and carboxypeptidase take over protein digestion. Brush border peptidases split tripeptides and dipeptides into single amino acids. Amino acid transport into intestinal epithelial cells is mediated by a sodium-dependent cotransport system similar to monosaccharide transport. Small peptides may also undergo endocytosis and be cleaved into amino acids within the epithelial cells.
- Amino acids pass into the blood stream and travel to the liver.
- Absorption of water occurs passively by osmosis. An osmotic gradient for water absorption is created as electrolytes are absorbed.

GASTROINTESTINAL FUNCTION ACROSS THE LIFE SPAN

Maturation

During the first months of life, the newborn's GI tract undergoes many maturational changes. In the first 3 to 4 months of life, sucking reflexes are present, and extrusion reflexes protect against the ingestion of solids that the immature GI tract is still unable to digest. The pressure in the LES remains low during this time, and "spitting up" of gastric contents is common because intragastric pressure often exceeds LES pressure. Gastric motility is not well coordinated for the first 3 to 4 months, so antral mixing is inadequate for the digestion of solid foods. At about 12 weeks of age, intestinal peristalsis similar to that in adults begins to develop, but it is one-third slower. This slower transit in infants may serve to improve nutrient digestion and absorption by increasing the exposure of nutrients to the intestinal mucosa. The motor function of the large intestine appears to be fully developed at birth. During the first 2 years of life, the secretory and absorptive functions of the intestine mature and begin a pattern of functioning that continues into senescence.[5,9]

Age-Related Changes

Changes in GI function in older adults occur simultaneously with other age-related changes such as a decrease in lean body mass and impaired homeostasis of multiple body systems. Within the GI tract, a variety of changes occur that may place an aging individual at risk for health problems related to GI functioning and nutrition. Important elements of this process are summarized in The Aging Process: Changes in the Gastrointestinal System.

Loss of dentition and reduced taste and smell acuity may promote a decreased interest in food intake as chewing becomes difficult and the sensory enjoyment associated with food becomes impaired. A condition called **presbyesophagus,** in which esophageal motility is slowed or disorganized, may develop in older adults. Presbyesophagus may be manifested as difficulty in swallowing and may cause discomfort as food passes through the esophagus. The incidence of hiatal hernia is also increased in the aging population, affecting 69% of persons over 70 years. The transit time for intestinal contents to pass through the GI tract is decreased in older persons; this factor, coupled with a decreased perception of the sensory stimuli that produce the urge to defecate, may promote constipation in the aging population. Conversely, a confused or neurologically impaired older individual may experience fecal incontinence because the sensation and tone of the rectum diminish with aging.[5,26]

KEY CONCEPTS

- Infants may experience GI dysfunction because of immaturity of the GI tract. Motility is not well coordinated until 3 to 4 months of age, making digestion of solids difficult in infancy. Pressure in the LES is low, which leads to "spitting up" and gastric distention. Maturation of the GI tract is complete by about 2 years of age.
- Elderly individuals may experience GI dysfunction for a number of reasons. Poor dentition, loss of taste and smell acuity, and reduced esophageal motility may lead to poor intake of nutrients. Hiatal hernia and constipation are common in the elderly.

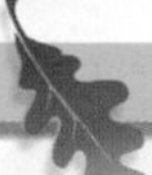

THE AGING PROCESS

Changes in the Gastrointestinal System

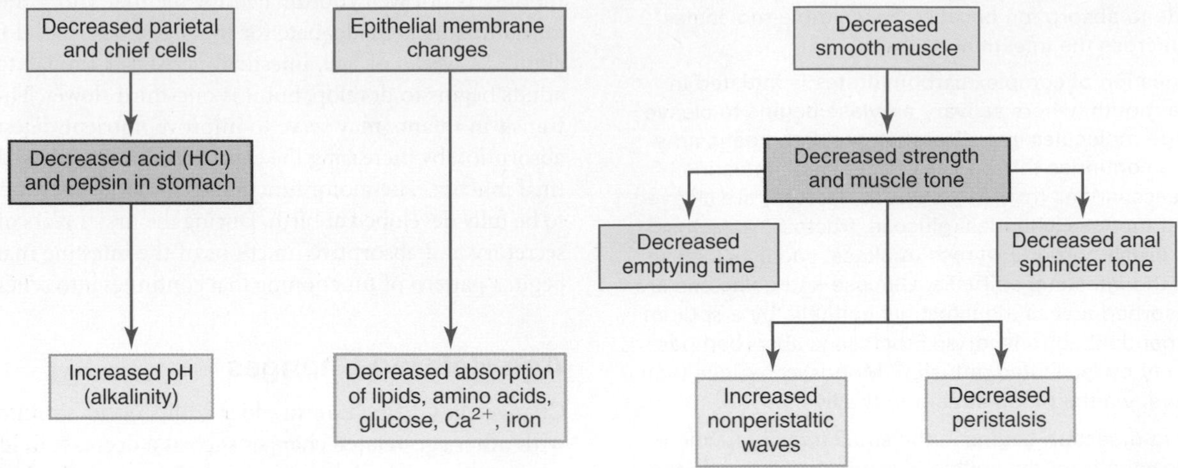

As a person ages, gastrointestinal muscle strength and movement decrease, leading to reduced peristalsis and decreased gastrointestinal motility throughout the system.

In the esophagus the elderly person experiences greater numbers of muscle movements that do not propel the contents onward. These nonperistaltic waves are common in the lower esophagus. The phenomenon of presbyesophagus—in which the esophageal sphincter fails to relax and the lower esophagus becomes dilated—may not necessarily be normal to the elderly.

In the stomach, decreased numbers of parietal and chief cells result in diminished acid (HCl) and pepsin secretion. This leads to increased pH and a more alkaline secretion. The protective alkaline viscous mucus in the stomach is also decreased. The loss of smooth muscle in the stomach can delay emptying time, which increases and prolongs the exposure of gastric epithelial cells to the gastric contents.

The small intestinal smooth muscle, Peyer patches, and lymphatic follicles are decreased. Normal intestinal absorption in the elderly is not well understood and may be influenced by a number of factors, including bowel motility, epithelial membranes, vascular perfusion, and gastrointestinal membrane transport. However, absorption of lipids, amino acids, glucose, calcium, and iron is known to be decreased. Normal changes in the large intestine have been difficult to determine. As a result of smooth muscle changes, anal sphincter tone decreases.

SUMMARY

This chapter describes the structure of the human GI system and the process by which it provides nutrients for the body. A thorough understanding of the structure of the GI tract, GI motility, secretion of digestive juices, digestion of nutrients, and absorption of nutrients is needed as a basis for understanding other principles of health and disease.

GI motility is a complex process involving a set of carefully timed autoregulatory action responses (Figure 35-18). You may wish to trace the path and destiny of the apple you ate for lunch as an example of this process. As you track the movement of nutrients through the GI tract, consider the ways in which secretion of digestive juices occurs in response to the ingestion of your apple, which contains a great deal of carbohydrate (fructose), small amounts of protein, and minimal lipid. Consider also how digestion and absorption of these nutrients are occurring. What part of the apple will you use, for example, for energy to study this text? What part of the apple will your body "throw away," and how will this be accomplished? Finally, will your GI tract respond the same way to eating an apple when you are 85 years old? A careful review of the elegant and nearly automatic function of the human GI tract will prepare you to care for individuals experiencing interruptions in proper nutrient digestion and absorption.

MEDIA RESOURCES

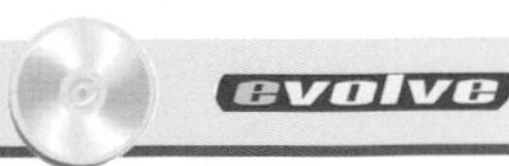

Remember to check out the ***CD Companion*** included with this book for Review Questions, Key Concepts Review, Glossary (with audio for selected terms), Disease Profiles, and Animations.

PLUS, visit the ***Evolve website*** at http://evolve.elsevier.com/Copstead/ for Case Studies, Disease Profiles, and WebLinks.

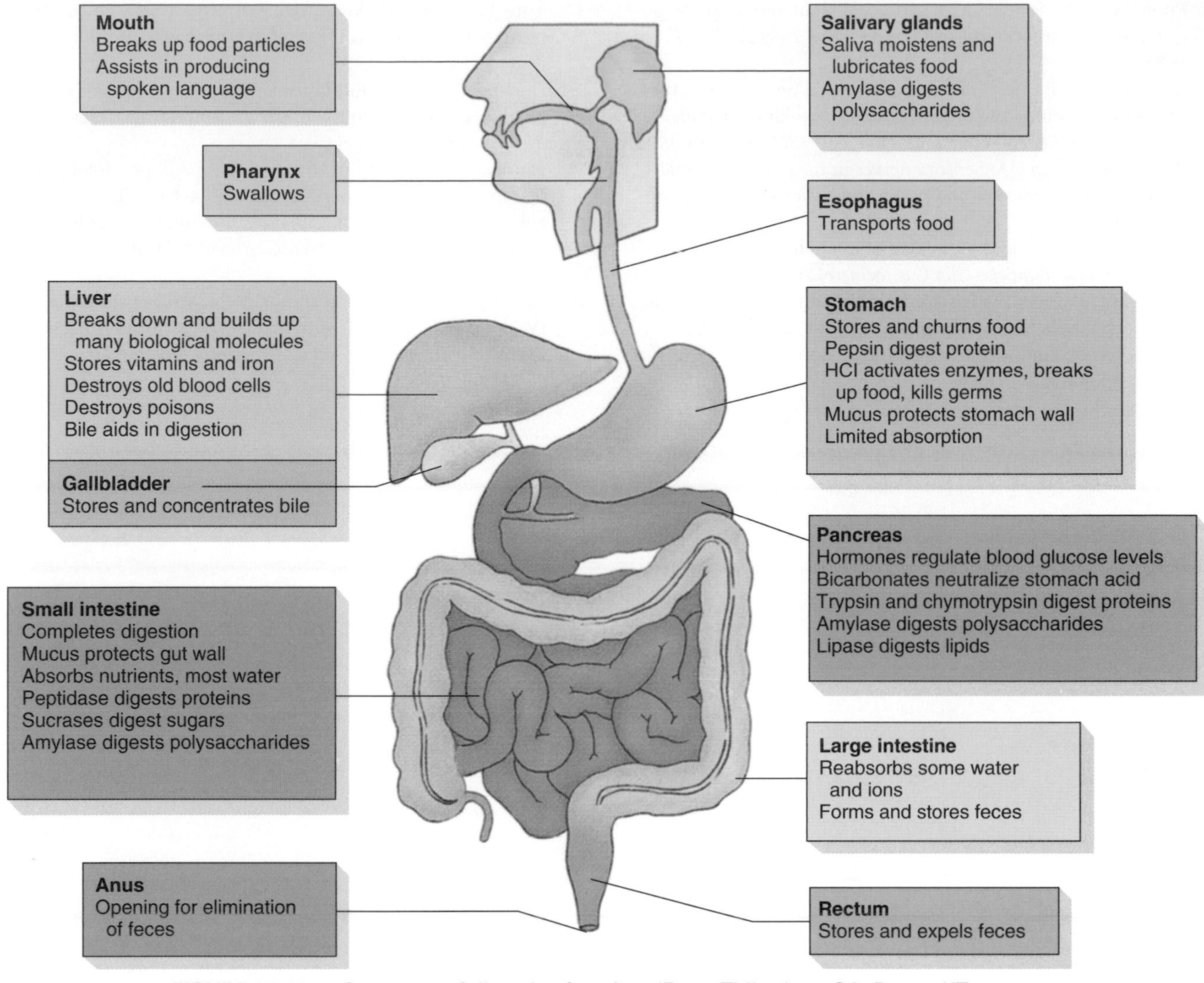

FIGURE 35-18 ■ Summary of digestive function. (From Thibodeau GA, Patton KT: *Anatomy and physiology,* ed 5, St Louis, 2003, Mosby, p 788.)

References

1. Guyton AC, Hall JE: *Textbook of medical physiology,* ed 10, Philadelphia, 2000, Saunders.
2. Johnson LR, Gerwin TA: *Gastrointestinal physiology,* ed 6, St Louis, 2001, Mosby.
3. Feldman M, Friedman LS, Sleisenger MH: *Sleisenger and Fordtran's gastrointestinal and liver disease: pathophysiology, diagnosis, management,* ed 7, Philadelphia, 2002, Saunders.
4. Yazbeck S: Gastrointestinal emergencies of the neonate. In Roy CC, Siverman A, Alagille D, editors: *Pediatric clinical gastroenterology,* ed 4, St Louis, 1995, Mosby.
5. Shils ME, Olson JA: *Modern nutrition in health and disease,* ed 8, Philadelphia, 1994, Lea & Febiger.
6. Pedersen AM et al: Saliva and gastrointestinal functions of taste, mastication, swallowing and digestion, *Oral Dis* 8(3):117-129, 2002.
7. Herrera JL, Lyons MF 2nd, Johnson LF: Saliva: its role in health and disease, *J Clin Gastroenterol* 10(5):569-578, 1988.
8. Yamada T et al: *Textbook of gastroenterology,* ed 3, Philadelphia, 1999, Lippincott Williams & Wilkins.
9. Gebruers EM, Hall WJ: Role of the gastrointestinal tract in the regulation of hydration in man, *Dig Dis* 10(2):112-120, 1992.
10. Current concepts in research of gastrointestinal motility: international symposium, Aarhus, Denmark, July 18-20, 1991, *Dig Dis* 9(6):321-443, 1991.
11. Thomson AB et al: Small bowel review: normal physiology part 2, *Dig Dis Sci* 46(12):2588-2607, 2001.
12. McIntyre AS, Thompson DG: Review article: adrenergic control of motor and secretory function in the gastrointestinal tract, *Aliment Pharmacol Ther* 6(2):125-142, 1992.
13. Huizinga JD: Action potentials in gastrointestinal smooth muscle, *Can J Physiol Pharmacol* 69(8):1133-1142, 1991.
14. Sanders KM: Ionic mechanisms of electrical rhythmicity in gastrointestinal smooth muscles, *Annu Rev Physiol* 54:439-453, 1992.
15. Thulin L, Johansson C: Gastrointestinal hormones, *Acta Chir Scand Suppl* 482:69-72, 1978.

16. Publicover NG, Sanders KM: Myogenic regulation of propagation in gastric smooth muscle, *Am J Physiol* 248:G512-G520, 1985.
17. Jenkins AP et al: Effects of bolus doses of fat on small intestinal structure and on release of gastrin, cholecystokinin, peptide tyrosine-tyrosine, and enteroglucagon, *Gut* 33(2):218-223, 1992.
18. Surrenti C, Maggi CA: Sensory nerves in the gastrointestinal tract: changing concepts and perspectives, *Ital J Gastroenterol* 23(2):94-99, 1991.
19. Karaus M, Wienbeck M: Colonic motility in humans: a growing understanding, *Baillieres Clin Gastroenterol* 5(2):453-478, 1991.
20. Barocelli E, Ballabeni V: Histamine in the control of gastric acid secretion: a topic review, *Pharmacol Res* 47(4):299-304, 2003.
21. Marks V et al: Gut hormones in glucose homeostasis, *Proc Nutr Soc* 50(3):545-552, 1991.
22. Titus E, Ahearn GA: Vertebrate gastrointestinal fermentation: transport mechanisms for volatile fatty acids, *Am J Physiol* 262(4):R547-R553, 1992.
23. Dockray GJ, Forster ER, Louis SM: Peptides and their receptors on afferent neurons to the upper gastrointestinal tract, *Adv Exp Med Biol* 298:53-62, 1991.
24. Hofmann AF: Cholestatic liver disease: pathophysiology and therapeutic options, *Liver* 22(suppl 2):14-19, 2002.
25. Sokol RJ: Fat-soluble vitamins and their importance in patients with cholestatic liver diseases, *Gastroenterol Clin North Am* 23(4):673-705, 1994.
26. Orr WC, Chen CL: Aging and neural control of the GI tract, IV: clinical and physiological aspects of gastrointestinal motility and aging, *Am J Physiol Gastrointest Liver Physiol* 283(6):G1226-G1231, 2002.

chapter 36

Gastrointestinal Disorders

Jeffrey S. Sartin

MEDIA RESOURCES

Additional Material for Study, Review, and Further Exploration

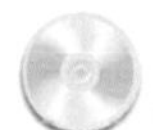

CD Companion ◆ Review Questions and Answers ◆ Key Concepts Review
◆ Glossary *(with audio pronunciations for selected terms)*
◆ Disease Profiles ◆ Animations

evolve ***Website*** at http://evolve.elsevier.com/Copstead/
◆ Case Studies ◆ Disease Profiles ◆ WebLinks

KEY QUESTIONS

- What are the common causes of the following general manifestations of gastrointestinal disorders: pain, nausea, vomiting, diarrhea, and constipation?
- What are the predisposing factors and characteristic manifestations common to inflammatory disorders of the gastrointestinal tract?
- What are the common causes of and clinical findings in functional and mechanical bowel obstructions?
- What are the common causes of and clinical findings in malabsorption?
- What warning signs may indicate cancer of the gastrointestinal tract?

CHAPTER OUTLINE

Alterations in function of the gastrointestinal (GI) tract may have far-reaching consequences in an individual's life. The ability to take in nutrients, convert them to usable forms for body functions, and dispose of their waste products goes beyond physiologic function and is intimately associated with social and psychological functioning. A person with an alteration in GI function may experience great emotional distress and be unable to participate fully in social activities, which in American society are largely centered on food consumption. Certain symptoms that may accompany GI disorders, such as chronic diarrhea and abdominal pain, may severely limit an individual's ability to maintain employment. It has been estimated that 200,000 people miss work daily because of GI-related problems.[1] In addition, GI diseases account for more hospital admissions in the United States than any other category of disease. Because many chronic GI conditions begin in midlife and continue into old age, their prevalence will increase as the U.S. population continues to age.

This chapter describes the pathophysiologic process of the most common disorders of the GI tract and summarizes current treatment for these conditions. Because knowledge about many GI disorders is expanding rapidly, some current research on selected GI conditions is described. Finally, because of the intimate relationship between GI function and the integrity and well-being of the person, a discussion of the psychological and emotional aspects of GI disorders across the life span is included.

MANIFESTATIONS OF GASTROINTESTINAL TRACT DISORDERS

As a basis for discussing individual types of GI disorders, a description of some common manifestations of these disorders and their pathophysiologic mechanisms is presented. Common manifestations include dysphagia, esophageal and abdominal pain, intestinal gas, vomiting, and alterations in bowel patterns.

Dysphagia

Dysphagia is difficulty in swallowing (Figure 36-1) as perceived by the individual. It may include the inability to initiate swallowing or the sensation that the swallowed solids or liquids "stick" in the esophagus. In certain disorders, **odynophagia,** or pain with swallowing, may accompany dysphagia. The physiologic mechanism of normal swallowing is described in Chapter 35; the reader may wish to refer to this information.

Categories

The pathophysiologic basis for dysphagia usually falls into three major categories: (1) problems in delivery of the bolus of food or fluid into the esophagus as a result of neuromuscular incoordination; (2) problems in transport of the bolus down the body of the esophagus as a result of altered esophageal peristaltic activity; and (3) problems in bolus entry into the stomach as a result of lower esophageal sphincter (LES) dysfunction or obstructing lesions.[2]

In the first category of dysphagia, individuals have a decreased ability to accomplish the initial steps of swallowing in an orderly sequence. The normal sequence of pharyngeal contraction, closure of the epiglottis, upper esophageal sphincter relaxation, and initiation of peristalsis by contraction of the striated muscle in the upper portion of the esophagus is altered, or certain steps in the sequence may be absent. Persons experiencing this type of dysphagia may cough and expel the ingested food or fluids through their mouth and nose or aspirate when they attempt to swallow. These symptoms are usually worse with liquids than with solids in this type of swallowing dysfunction.

The second type of dysphagia may be the result of any disorder, structural or neuromuscular, in which the peristaltic activity of the body of the esophagus is altered. The presence of (1) esophageal **diverticula,** or outpouchings of one or more layers of the esophageal wall, (2) **achalasia,** a disorder of esophageal smooth muscle function, or (3) structural disorders such as neoplasms or strictures may interfere with proper peristaltic activity in the esophagus.[3,4] This alteration in peristalsis may be simply weak peristaltic activity, aperistalsis (the absence of all peristaltic activity), or disorganized and therefore ineffective peristalsis. With this type of dysphagia the individual may have the sensation that food is "stuck" behind the sternum. Initially, dysphagia may be noted with solid foods; if the underlying pathologic process fosters a worsening of peristaltic ability, the passage of liquids may also become impaired.

The third category of dysphagia, which results from problems of bolus entry into the stomach, is secondary to any condition in which the LES functions improperly or is obstructed by a lesion. Tumors of the mediastinum, lower part of the esophagus, and gastroesophageal junction may invade the myenteric plexus or produce an obstruction at the LES, thus interrupting normal LES function by neural invasion or direct obstruction. In addition, motor disorders resulting from neuromuscular diseases or chronic lower esophageal inflammation from the reflux of acidic gastric contents may limit the ability of the LES to function properly. This type of dysphagia may be manifested as tightness or pain in the substernal area during the swallowing process.

Esophageal Pain

Two types of pain occur in the esophagus: (1) heartburn (also called **pyrosis**) and (2) pain located in the middle of the chest, which may mimic the pain of angina pectoris. Heartburn is caused by the reflux of gastric contents into the esophagus and is a substernal burning sensation that may radiate to the neck or throat. Two probable mechanisms contribute to the development of heartburn.[2] First, the highly acidic gastric contents may be a noxious stimulant to sensory afferent nerve endings in the esophageal mucosa. Second, heartburn may be

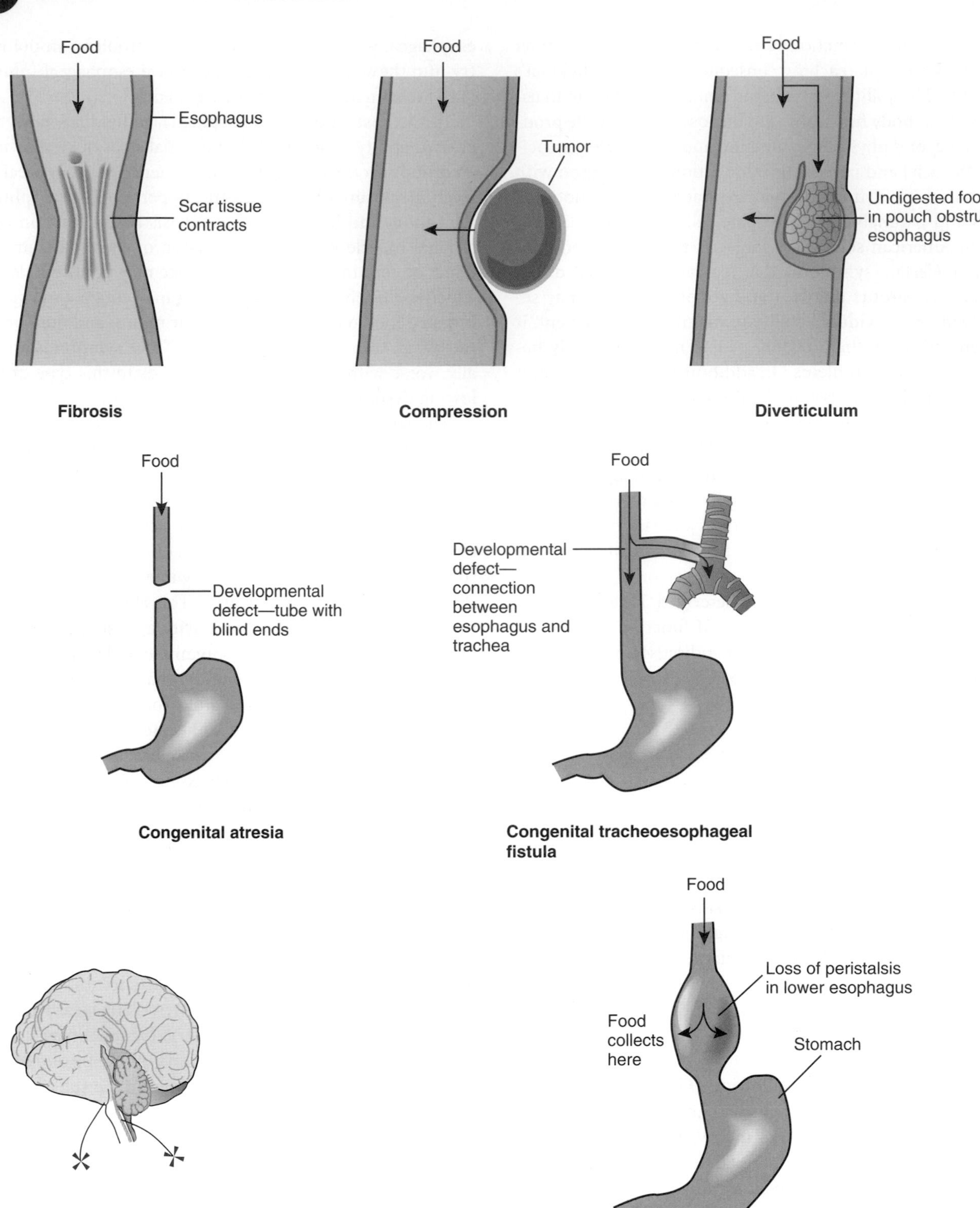

FIGURE 36-1 ■ Causes of dysphagia. (From Gould BE: *Pathophysiology for the health professions*, ed 2, Philadelphia, 2002, Saunders, p 382.)

produced by a spasm of the esophageal muscle brought on by acid stimulation.

Chest pain other than heartburn may be the result of esophageal distention or powerful esophageal contractions. These stimuli may arise from esophageal obstruction or a condition called diffuse esophageal spasm, in which high-amplitude, simultaneous contractions in the smooth muscle portion of the esophagus may be randomly interspersed with normal-appearing peristalsis.[1]

This type of esophageal pain is similar to that of angina pectoris, particularly in its pattern of radiation into the neck, shoulder, arm, and jaw. Odynophagia may accompany diffuse esophageal spasm and be indistinguishable from esophageal chest pain except that it is brought on specifically by swallowing.

Persons with herpetic or monilial **esophagitis,** infections of the esophagus that may be present in an immunocompromised state, may also experience a dull, aching chest pain. Swallowing may worsen the pain sensation and cause symptoms such as heartburn or chest pain.

Abdominal Pain

Pain in the abdominal region may be the first sign of a disorder of the GI tract and is often an important impetus for seeking medical care. Although abdominal pain may result from GI tract disorders, it may also be the result of reproductive, genitourinary, musculoskeletal, and vascular disorders, as well as presence of toxins or drug use. Abdominal pain is usually categorized into three types, although persons experiencing abdominal pain may manifest a combination of these types. (1) Visceral pain develops from stretching or distending an abdominal organ or from inflammation. The pain is diffuse and poorly localized and has a gnawing, burning, or cramping quality. (2) Somatic pain arises from injury to the abdominal wall, the parietal peritoneum, the root of the mesentery, or the diaphragm. In contrast to visceral pain, it is sharper, more intense, and generally well localized to the area of irritation. (3) Referred pain is felt at a location distant from the source of the pain but in the same dermatome or neurosegment. Referred pain is usually sharp and well localized and may be felt in the skin or deeper tissues.

Abdominal pain may be acute, with an instantaneous onset, and signal such events as a perforated ulcer or a ruptured internal organ. A more gradual development of abdominal pain may accompany such chronic states as diverticulitis or ulcerative colitis. Abdominal pain seldom occurs as a solitary manifestation of GI disorders but is usually accompanied by other manifestations such as vomiting or alteration in bowel patterns to a variable degree.

Vomiting

Vomiting is the forceful expulsion of gastric contents through the mouth. Usually accompanied by a feeling of nausea, vomiting results from a coordinated sequence of abdominal muscle contractions and reverse esophageal peristalsis. Although vomiting is a common sign of GI disorders, it may also occur with metabolic, endocrine, labyrinthine, and cardiac disorders, as well as with infection and fluid and electrolyte imbalances. It is also associated with such nonpathologic causes as pharmacologic agents, surgery, and the first trimester of pregnancy.

Vomiting associated with GI disorders may be the result of alterations in the integrity of the GI tract wall, such as gastroenteritis, or alterations in the motility of the GI tract, such as intestinal obstruction. The characteristics of the vomitus, such as the presence of blood or fecal matter, may suggest the nature of the GI disorder that is promoting vomiting and the level of the GI tract at which the disorder is located.

Intestinal Gas

Gas normally occurs in the GI tract and is the result of swallowed air, bacterial and digestive action on intestinal contents, diffusion from the blood, and the neutralization of acids by bicarbonate within the upper GI tract. The manifestations of excess intestinal gas may include excessive belching, distention of the abdomen, and excessive flatus. These manifestations may occur singly or in combination and may stem from a variety of causes. Belching is caused by the eructation of swallowed air and may be the result of a motility disorder or gastric outlet obstruction that prevents the passage of air from the stomach into the proximal end of the small intestine. Abdominal distention may be due to failure to adequately digest some particular nutrient such as the sugar lactose. In the absence of adequate lactase (the digestive enzyme that breaks down lactose into glucose and galactose in the intestine), lactose undergoes bacterial fermentation, which results in gas production in the intestinal lumen. In some individuals, abdominal distention from excess gas may result from a defect in intestinal motility in which the intestinal contents are not propelled in a regular fashion, rather than from the production of too much gas. Excessive flatus may have causes similar to those of abdominal distention. Usually it is the result of increased amounts of gas produced by the action of bacteria on nutritional substrates that are particularly gas producing, such as certain vegetables and legumes.

Alterations in Bowel Patterns

Both constipation and diarrhea are difficult to define with precision inasmuch as a wide variation in bowel pattern can be found in different individuals. In addition, cultural and family socialization may play a role in the way in which an individual perceives bowel patterns. Alterations in bowel patterns may be the result of a change in GI tract motility or may be a component of a functional GI disorder such as irritable bowel syndrome (IBS).

Constipation

Constipation may be defined as small, infrequent, and difficult bowel movements.[3,5] Authorities have agreed on a norm of fewer than three stools per week as a guideline for defining constipation.[1] Dietary factors, particularly a diet low in fiber, have been shown to contribute to constipation. The presence of cellulose, the carbohydrate component of dietary fiber that is indigestible in the human intestine, may be effective in promoting regular peristaltic movement in the GI tract by forming bulk within the intestinal lumen to stimulate propulsion. In addition, because exercise stimulates intestinal peristalsis, a lack of exercise has been implicated in the development of constipation. In elderly persons the slowed rate of peristalsis that occurs with the aging process, coupled with a decreased level of physical activity, may promote chronic constipation. These factors may eventually contribute to the development of fecal impaction, a condition in which a firm, immovable mass of stool becomes stationary in the lower GI tract. Constipation may also be the result of pathologic conditions, including processes that alter the motility of the GI tract such as intestinal obstruction or processes that alter the integrity of the GI tract wall such as diverticulitis.

Diarrhea

Diarrhea is defined as an increase in the frequency and fluidity of bowel movements and is usually a primary sign of GI tract disorders. Stool weight in excess of 200 g/24 h is one easily obtainable, objective definition of diarrhea.[4] Diarrhea may be present as an acute or chronic manifestation. Acute diarrhea may be the result of an acute infection, emotional stress, or leakage of stool around impacted feces. Chronic diarrhea may be the result of a chronic GI tract infection (often associated with immune system compromise), alterations in the motility or integrity of the GI tract, malabsorption, and certain endocrine disorders.[6] Diarrhea that occurs on an episodic basis may be related to a food allergy or may be due to the ingestion of irritants to the GI tract or caffeine. Diarrhea in children frequently results from infection, although malabsorption, anatomic defects, and allergy may also be causative factors.[7]

Pathophysiologic Mechanisms. Four major pathophysiologic mechanisms have been identified in the development of diarrhea. (1) In osmotic diarrhea, increased amounts of poorly absorbable, osmotically active solutes such as a carbohydrate or magnesium sulfate cause sodium and water influx into the bowel lumen, resulting in diarrhea. (2) In secretory diarrhea, a pathophysiologic event such as the presence of a bacterial toxin causes enhanced secretion of chloride ion and water in the small intestine by simultaneously stimulating active secretion and inhibiting resorption. Diarrhea of 1 L or more per day may result from this inappropriate secretion of fluid across the intestinal mucosa.[3] Causes of secretory diarrhea include enterotoxins produced by such organisms as *Vibrio cholerae* and *Staphylococcus aureus*. (3) Exudative diarrhea is the result of exudation of mucus, blood, and protein from sites of active inflammation into the bowel lumen. This creates an increased osmotic load and a subsequent shift of water across the epithelium. In addition, if a large surface area of the bowel has an alteration in its integrity, intestinal absorption will be severely impaired, further compounding the diarrhea produced. Diarrhea associated with Crohn disease and ulcerative colitis may be the result of this exudative process.[3,6] (4) Diarrhea related to motility disturbances is a result of the decreased contact time of chyme with the absorptive surfaces of the intestinal lumen. If inadequate absorption takes place in the small intestine, large amounts of fluid will be delivered to the colon and may overwhelm the absorptive capability of the colon and cause diarrhea. In addition, if the fatty acids and bile salts present in chyme have not been adequately absorbed in the small intestine, they may induce a secretory diarrhea once they reach the colon, further compounding the process of diarrhea formation. Diarrhea associated with the postgastrectomy dumping syndrome and IBS are examples of this type of diarrhea.[5,6]

KEY CONCEPTS

- Dysphagia is the perception of difficulty in swallowing. Dysphagia caused by neuromuscular disorders may be accompanied by coughing and aspiration, particularly with liquid ingestion. Altered esophageal peristalsis is associated with the sensation that food has become "stuck" behind the sternum. LES dysfunction may be manifested as substernal pain.
- Pain is a common symptom of GI disorders. A heartburn type of pain is associated with esophageal reflux. Chest pain similar to anginal pain may result from esophageal distention and obstruction. Abdominal pain may be visceral (diffuse, poorly localized), somatic (sharp, well localized), or referred (at a distance from the source but in the same dermatome).

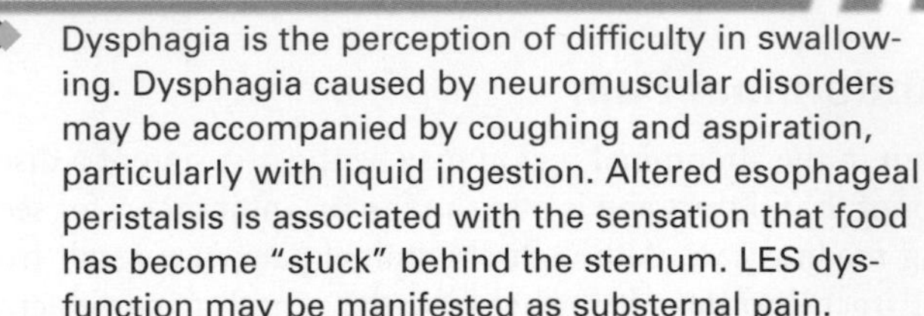

- Nausea and vomiting are manifestations of many GI and other disorders. Alterations in bowel motility or integrity are causative factors. Excess gas may result from altered motility or lack of digestive enzymes. Gas is generated by swallowed air and bacterial action on nutritional substrates.
- Constipation is defined as small, infrequent (less than three per week), or difficult bowel movements. Lack of exercise, lack of dietary fiber, slowed peristalsis, and pathologic conditions that alter motility (e.g., obstruction) may produce constipation.
- Diarrhea is defined as an increased frequency and fluidity of bowel movements. Acute infection, stress, fecal impaction, malabsorption, and ingestion of bowel irritants may produce diarrhea. Osmotic diarrhea is due to increased amounts of poorly absorbed solutes in the intestine. Secretory diarrhea is usually due to toxins that stimulate intestinal fluid secretion and impair absorption. Exudative diarrhea (mucus, blood, protein) results from inflammatory processes. A decreased transit time in the small intestine results in diarrhea because the absorptive capacity of the large intestine is exceeded.

DISORDERS OF THE MOUTH AND ESOPHAGUS

The mouth and the esophagus are the portals of entry for nutrients into the GI tract. An impairment in the proper functioning of these structures may have a profound effect on the ability of the individual to ingest adequate nutrients and begin the initial steps of the digestive process. Although disorders of the mouth and esophagus may not be acute, life-threatening emergencies, they may have severe long-term consequences for the well-being of the individual experiencing them.

ORAL INFECTIONS

Stomatitis

Etiology. **Stomatitis** is defined as an inflammation of the oral mucosa that may extend to the buccal mucosa, lips, and palate. Stomatitis may be caused by many factors or conditions. Among its causes are pathogenic organisms, including bacteria and viruses; mechanical trauma; exposure to such irritants as alcohol, tobacco, and other chemical substances; certain medications, particularly chemotherapeutic agents; radiation therapy; nutritional deficiencies, especially vitamin deficiencies; and such systemic inflammatory diseases as measles and syphilis. Stomatitis is a common manifestation of human immunodeficiency syndrome.[8] Stomatitis may also occur with no identifiable cause.[9]

Acute Herpetic Stomatitis

Etiology and Clinical Manifestations. One of the most commonly encountered types of stomatitis is acute herpetic stomatitis, also called herpetic gingivostomatitis or "cold sores." It is caused by infection with herpes simplex virus, which has an affinity for the skin and nervous system. This type of stomatitis is common in children between the ages of 1 and 3 years, although it may occur at any age. In primary infection, a brief period of prodromal tingling and itching may be present along with fever and pharyngitis. Vesicles may erupt on any part of the oral mucosa, particularly the tongue, gums, and cheeks. Vesicles form on an erythematous base, eventually rupture, and leave a painful ulcer. Once herpes simplex virus is acquired, it tends to remain latent in the skin or tissues of the nervous system and may be reactivated by the presence of physical or emotional stressors.

Treatment. The pharmacologic therapy used for stomatitis will depend on its cause. The antiviral drugs famciclovir and valacyclovir have been approved for treating acute herpetic stomatitis in immunocompromised patients (e.g., those with AIDS). Unfortunately, in a large number of cases stomatitis is idiopathic or not amenable to specific therapy (e.g., stomatitis due to chemotherapy). In all types of stomatitis, measures designed to provide adequate oral hygiene and increase comfort in the oral cavity will be helpful in preventing decreased nutritional intake during the period of inflammation and assist in promoting the healing process. Topical mucosal barriers and corticosteroids may be of some benefit.[8]

ESOPHAGEAL DISORDERS

Gastroesophageal Reflux

Gastroesophageal reflux disease (GERD) is the backflow of gastric contents into the esophagus through the LES. GERD may or may not produce symptoms.

Pathogenesis. The extent and severity of damage to the esophagus from GERD reflect the frequency and duration of exposure to refluxed material, as well as the volume and acidity of the gastric juices being refluxed.[3,4,10,11] The production of GERD is a multifactorial process. Any condition or agent that alters the closure strength and efficacy of the LES or increases intraabdominal pressure may predispose an individual to GERD. For example, the closure strength of the LES may be adversely affected by the intake of fatty foods, caffeine, and large amounts of ethanol; cigarette smoking; a side-lying position; or sitting. In addition, pharmacologic agents such as progesterone-containing medications (e.g., birth control pills), morphine, and theophylline may also decrease the pressure of the LES. Certain anatomic features, especially hiatal hernia, have also been associated with GERD. The role of *Helicobacter pylori*, a cause of gastric and duodenal ulceration, in GERD is poorly understood and controversial.[12]

Clinical Manifestations. The most common manifestations of GERD are heartburn, regurgitation, chest pain, and dysphagia. Persistent GERD can result in reflux **esophagitis,** which is esophageal inflammation caused by the highly acidic refluxed material.

Treatment. Appropriate therapy is directed to increasing LES pressure, enhancing esophageal clearance, improving gastric emptying, and suppressing gastric acidity. Dietary and behavioral changes, such as avoiding tobacco and aggravating food and drink, are indicated for all patients, while over-the-counter antacid medications may be effective for occasional GERD. If reflux esophagitis has progressed in severity, tissue damage, including ulceration, fibrotic scarring, and strictures, may be present in the distal third of the esophagus. Newer potent gastric acid inhibitors, such as histamine (H_2) blockers and especially proton pump inhibitors, have been very successful in halting and even reversing the changes of chronic GERD. Endoscopic dilatation is necessary in some patients with stricture. Surgical intervention, such as thoracoscopic Nissan fundoplication, may be helpful for intractable GERD.[13]

Complication. **Barrett esophagus** is a complication of chronic GERD and represents columnar tissue replacing the normal squamous epithelium of the distal esophagus. It carries a significant risk for esophageal cancer, and patients with Barrett esophagus should undergo regular endoscopic screening for cancer, along with pharmacologic control of their reflux.[14]

Hiatal Hernia

A **hiatal hernia** is a defect in the diaphragm that allows a portion of the stomach to pass through the diaphragmatic opening into the thorax. Two types of hiatal hernia are commonly recognized: (1) a sliding hernia, in which both a portion of the stomach and the gastroesophageal junction slip up into the thorax so that the gastroesophageal junction is above the diaphragmatic opening, and (2) a paraesophageal hernia, in which a part of the greater curvature of the stomach rolls through the diaphragmatic defect (Figure 36-2). "Mixed" hiatal hernias with features of both of these types may also occur. Sliding hernias are three to ten times more common than paraesophageal and mixed hernias combined. The incidence of hiatal hernia increases with age, and this form of hernia occurs more often in women than in men.

Etiology. Although the cause of the anatomic deformity leading to hiatal hernia is not well understood, certain conditions seem to predispose to loosening of the muscular band around the esophageal and diaphragmatic junction. Conditions in which intraabdominal pressure increases, such as ascites, pregnancy, obesity, and chronic straining or coughing, have been associated with the development of hiatal hernia.

Clinical Manifestations and Treatment. Individuals with hiatal hernia may experience symptoms similar to those of GERD, such as heartburn, chest pain, and dysphagia, and GERD often accompanies hiatal hernia. Hiatal hernia can be a potentially life-threatening situation if a large portion of the stomach becomes caught above the diaphragm and is incarcerated, although this is extremely rare. Medical therapy for hiatal hernia is exactly the same as that for GERD, detailed above. Indications for surgery would be acute incarceration or intractable reflux.

Mallory-Weiss Syndrome

Etiology. **Mallory-Weiss syndrome** is bleeding caused by a tear in the mucosa or submucosa of the cardia or lower portion of the esophagus. The tear is usually longitudinal and is primarily caused by forceful or prolonged vomiting in which the upper esophageal sphincter fails to relax during the vomiting process. Approximately 75% of individuals with Mallory-Weiss syndrome are men with a history of excessive ingestion of alcohol or salicylates.[2] Other factors and conditions that may contribute to the development of esophageal tearing in Mallory-Weiss syndrome are coughing, straining during bowel movements, trauma, hiatal hernia, esophagitis, and gastritis.

Clinical Manifestations and Treatment. Manifestations of Mallory-Weiss syndrome include vomiting of blood and passing of large amounts of blood rectally after an episode of forceful vomiting. Epigastric or back pain may also be present. Bleeding may range in severity from mild to massive. It is often profuse when the tear is near the cardia of the stomach and may proceed to fatal shock in this circumstance. Identification is made by endoscopic examination during an episode of acute upper GI bleeding. Control of active bleeding may be achieved through endoscopic multipolar electric coagulation or similar techniques, or through interventional radiologic procedures (vasopressin infusion, Gelfoam embolization, etc.).[6,15] In selected cases surgical intervention may be necessary.

Esophageal Varices

Esophageal varices result from portal hypertension, which in Western society is generally the result of alcoholic or posthepatitis cirrhosis. In developing tropical countries, chronic infection with *Schistosoma* species is a major cause of portal

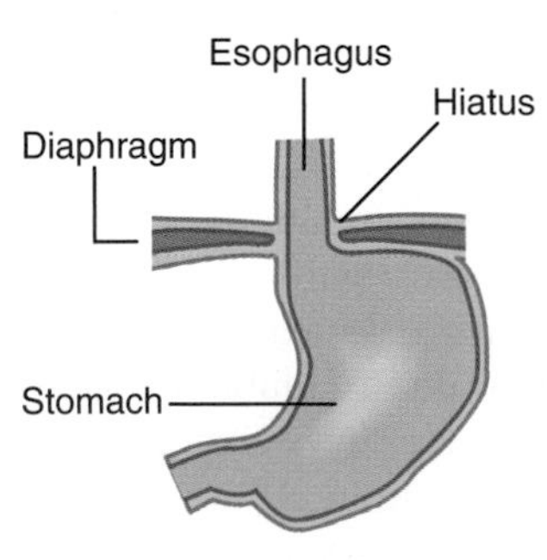

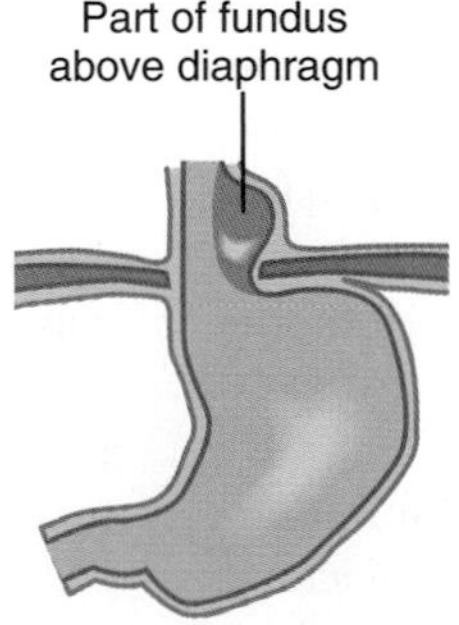

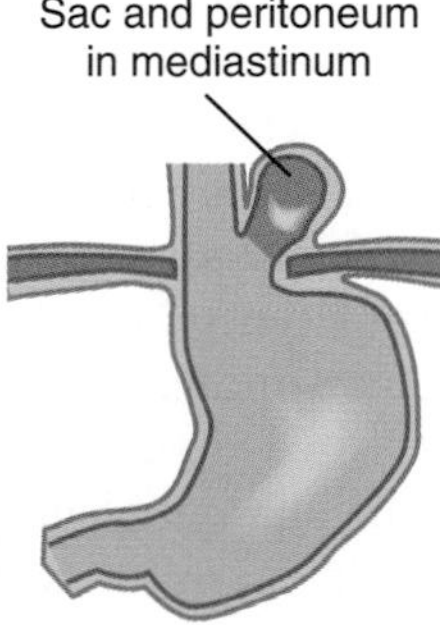

FIGURE 36-2 ■ Types of hiatal hernia. (From Gould BE: *Pathophysiology for the health professions*, ed 2, Philadelphia, 2002, Saunders, p 383.)

hypertension. Varices will affect more than half of cirrhotic patients, and approximately 30% of them experience an episode of variceal hemorrhage within 2 years of the diagnosis of varices.[16] The diagnosis and management of varices is discussed in detail in Chapter 38.

KEY CONCEPTS

- Stomatitis is inflammation of the oral mucosa. It may result from pathogenic organisms, trauma, chemical irritants, chemotherapy, radiation therapy, or nutritional deficiencies.
- Common esophageal disorders are GERD with esophagitis, hiatal hernia, and bleeding. Reflux esophagitis is manifested as heartburn, chest pain, and dysphagia and may be precipitated by gastric overdistention or poor LES tone. Fatty foods, cigarettes, morphine, theophylline, and progesterone may inhibit LES tone.
- Hiatal hernias may be sliding or rolling (paraesophageal). Conditions that increase intraabdominal pressure predispose to the development of hiatal hernia. Esophageal reflux often accompanies hiatal hernia, and the manifestations are similar: heartburn, chest pain, dysphagia.
- Bleeding from the esophagus may pose a life-threatening situation. Mallory-Weiss syndrome is bleeding caused by tears in the lower end of the esophagus or upper part of the stomach. Alcohol and salicylate ingestion appear to be factors. Esophageal bleeding may also be precipitated by coughing, straining, or esophagitis. Rupture of esophageal varices is a dreaded complication of cirrhosis with portal hypertension and carries a high mortality rate.

ALTERATIONS IN INTEGRITY OF THE GASTROINTESTINAL TRACT WALL

Alterations in the integrity of the GI tract wall may occur at any location along the GI tract and may result from an infection, inflammatory process, or weakness in a structure of the GI tract wall. Such alterations may present a life-threatening situation or induce a chronic, disabling condition. When the integrity of the GI tract wall is compromised, the ability of the GI tract to perform its digestive and absorptive functions may also be compromised because the surface area or the motility (or both) of the GI tract may be altered.

INFLAMMATION OF THE STOMACH AND INTESTINES

Gastritis

Etiology. **Gastritis** is defined as an inflammation of the stomach lining. Acute inflammation of the stomach lining may occur after the ingestion of alcohol, aspirin, or irritating substances, as well as in the presence of viral, bacterial, or chemical toxins. In Western countries overuse of nonsteroidal antiinflammatory drugs (NSAIDs) and overindulgence in alcohol and tobacco are preeminent causes of acute gastritis.

Clinical Manifestations. The symptoms of acute gastritis may include anorexia, nausea, vomiting, and postprandial discomfort. Occasionally, **hematemesis** may occur in response to damage to the gastric epithelial mucosa. These manifestations usually disappear when the causative agent is removed and the gastric epithelium undergoes a process of renewal by sloughing off the layer of damaged cells.

Research. Chronic gastritis is currently the focus of rapidly developing research. The factors promoting chronic gastritis have always been poorly understood. However, in 1983, identification of the bacterium *Helicobacter pylori* proved to be a landmark event.[17] Since that time, *H. pylori* has generated worldwide attention for its role in the promotion of chronic gastritis, peptic ulcer disease (PUD), and gastric carcinoma. Circumstantial evidence suggests that the mode of transmission of *H. pylori* is primarily person to person.[18] Some studies suggest a fecal-oral route, and the possibility of a reservoir in water sources has been investigated.

It is now known that *H. pylori* causes chronic active, nonatrophic, superficial gastritis in virtually all infected persons.[3] Once established as a colony in the gastric mucosa, *H. pylori* sets up a destructive pattern of persistent inflammation. This persistent inflammation may resolve spontaneously, and clearance of the organism occurs regularly over time, leading to a decreased prevalence of *H. pylori* infection among older individuals. Consequences of *H. pylori* gastritis include PUD (discussed below), atrophic gastritis, gastric adenocarcinoma, and mucosa-associated lymphoid tissue (MALT) lymphoma. The diagnosis and management of *H. pylori* infection will be discussed below.

Gastroenteritis

Etiology. **Gastroenteritis** refers to inflammation of the stomach and small intestine, and may occur on an acute or chronic basis. Chronic gastroenteritis is usually the result of another GI disorder, such as ulcerative colitis, and is discussed in a later section. Acute gastroenteritis is the result of direct infection of the GI tract lining by a pathogenic organism such as Norwalk virus; or by the ingestion of preformed bacterial toxins (e.g., *Staphylococcus aureus, Bacillus cereus*); or by the ingestion of bacteria that produce toxins (*Clostridium perfringens*). Acute gastroenteritis may also be caused by an imbalance in the normal bacterial flora of the GI tract precipitated by the introduction of an unusual bacterial strain, as may occur during travel.

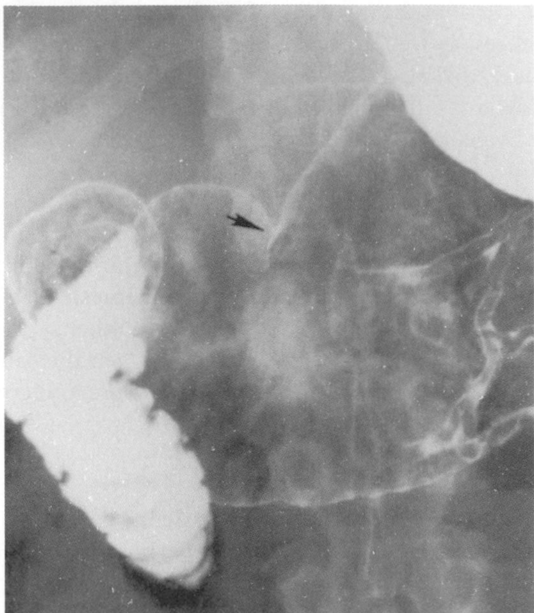

FIGURE 36-3 ■ Radiograph of an ulcer in the lesser curvature of the stomach *(arrow)*. (From Laufer I: *Double contrast gastrointestinal radiology with endoscopic correlation,* Philadelphia, 1979, Saunders.)

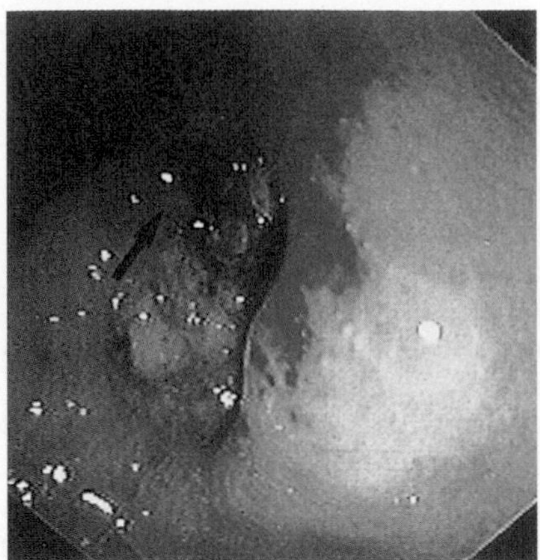

FIGURE 36-4 ■ Photograph of an ulcer. (From Sleisenger MH, Fordtran JS, editors: *Gastrointestinal disease,* ed 5, Philadelphia, 1993, Saunders.)

Clinical Manifestations and Treatment. Acute gastroenteritis in adults is usually a self-limiting, nonfatal disease with manifestations of diarrhea, abdominal discomfort and pain, nausea, and vomiting. An elevated temperature and malaise may also be present. The manifestations vary according to the type of causative pathologic organism and the region of the GI tract affected. Many pathogenic organisms induce a severe secretory type of diarrhea (see the earlier discussion on the pathophysiologic mechanism of secretory diarrhea). In children and elderly people, fluid losses from diarrhea and vomiting can have serious consequences and may be life threatening, particularly in underdeveloped countries. Supportive treatment designed to provide fluid and electrolyte replacement may be required by these high-risk groups experiencing severe acute gastroenteritis.

Peptic Ulcer Disease

The term **peptic ulcer disease** refers to disorders of the upper GI tract caused by the action of acid and pepsin. These disorders may include injury to the mucosa of the esophagus, stomach, or duodenum and may range from a slight mucosal injury to severe ulceration (Figures 36-3 and 36-4). Peptic disease seems to be the result of an increase in factors that tend to injure the mucosa relative to factors that tend to protect it. Factors such as the gastric mucosal barrier and the ability of the mucosa to renew epithelium serve to protect it against injury. On the other hand, the presence of acid, which potentiates the actions of pepsin and other injurious substances such as aspirin and NSAIDs, will promote injury to the mucosa.

Previously, PUD was attributed to stress and an irritative diet, and treatment revolved around removing any hint of spice in diet and lifestyle. In recent years, however, research has suggested that the organism *H. pylori* is a major precipitant of PUD, along with NSAIDs. A brief review of the current understanding of the pathogenesis of PUD is presented as a basis for further discussion of the manifestations and management of PUD.

Etiology and Pathogenesis. Most peptic ulcers arise in the stomach and duodenum. Although the precise mechanisms of ulcer formation remain incompletely understood, the process involves the interplay of mucosal defense mechanisms, pepsin, and acid.[3] In the stomach, it is thought that a breakdown in the normally protective epithelial lining occurs (Figure 36-5). In the formation of a gastric peptic ulcer, the barrier of the epithelial layer and the slightly alkaline layer of mucus may be interrupted by the chronic presence of such injurious substances as aspirin, NSAIDs, alcohol, and bile acids, which may be regurgitated from the duodenum. These substances apparently strip away the surface mucus and cause degeneration of the epithelial cell membranes, with diffusion of acid into the gastric epithelial wall.

Inappropriate excess secretion of acid is a major factor in the development of PUD in the duodenum (Figure 36-6). Studies have documented that the basal activity of the vagus nerve is increased in persons with PUD of the duodenum, particularly during a fasting state and at night. This stimulates the pyloric antrum cells to release gastrin, which travels via the blood stream and acts on the gastric parietal cells to release HCl. The result is an inappropriately high level of HCl in the duodenum.

H. pylori has a key role in promoting both gastric and duodenal ulcer formation (Figure 36-7). It has been reported that

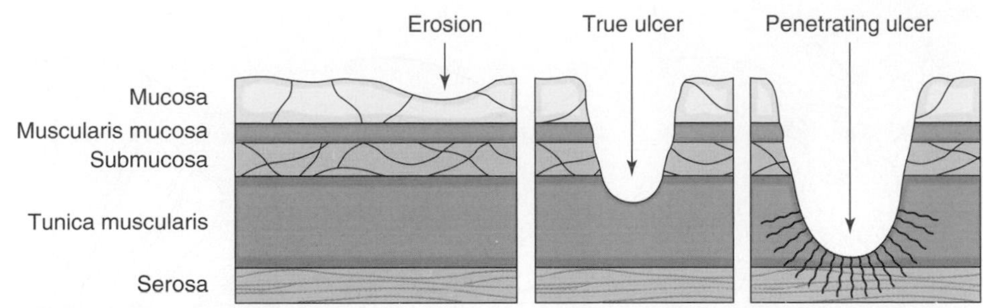

FIGURE 36-5 ■ Lesions caused by peptic ulcer disease. (From Phipps WJ et al: *Medical-surgical nursing: health and illness perspectives*, ed 7, St Louis, 2003, Mosby, p 1027.)

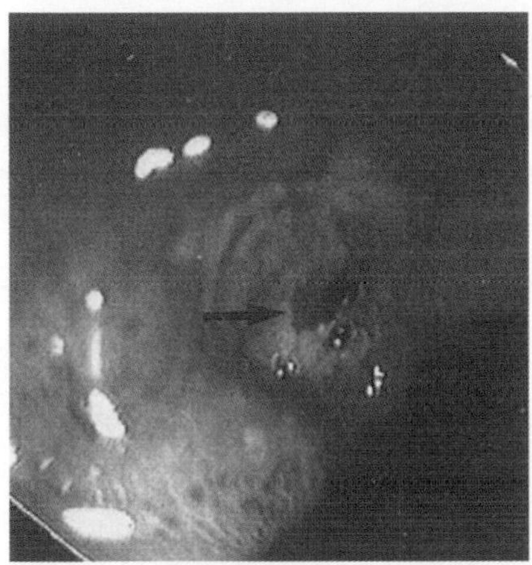

FIGURE 36-6 ■ Duodenal bulbar ulcer. (From Sleisenger MH, Fordtran JS, editors: *Gastrointestinal disease*, ed 5, Philadelphia, 1993, Saunders.)

up to 80% of persons with duodenal ulcers and 60% of persons with gastric ulcers have *H. pylori* infection.[3] Although the precise mechanisms of the development of PUD remain complex and poorly understood, *H. pylori* virulence seems to be associated with the presence of unique, lengthy DNA sequences known as *pathogenicity islands*, particularly the *CagA* gene.[19] *H. pylori* thrives in acidic conditions; thus, infection with *H. pylori* renders a person with PUD subject to a slow rate of ulcer healing and a high rate of recurrence, and clearance of *H. pylori* promotes ulcer healing.[20]

Other cofactors in the development of PUD have been investigated. Stress has long been considered a key factor in PUD. Substances called glucocorticoids that are released in response to stress may have a role in the promotion of excess acid production or the destruction of gastric mucosal defenses. Smoking is an important risk factor, as identified by epidemiologic studies showing that PUD is twice as likely to develop in smokers as in nonsmokers.[21] In addition, smoking is related to poor ulcer healing and high rates of ulcer recurrence. Heredity is thought to have a role in the development of PUD. Certain patterns of gastrin release and pepsin secretion have been identified as genetic traits in families with an increased incidence of PUD.[13] Somewhat surprisingly, there is little evidence of a pathogenic role for alcohol, spicy foods, and caffeine.[3]

Clinical Manifestations and Diagnoses. Manifestations of PUD include epigastric burning pain that is usually relieved by the intake of food (especially dairy products) or antacids. The pain of gastric ulcers typically occurs on an empty stomach but may present soon after a meal. Duodenal ulcer pain classically occurs 2 to 3 hours after a meal and is relieved by further food ingestion. Other manifestations that may occur in individuals with PUD include nausea, abdominal upset, and chest discomfort. A significant proportion of ulcers are asymptomatic, and life-threatening complications, such as GI bleeding, may occur in patients with no warning. The symptoms of PUD are not specific enough to allow for a diagnosis, and malignant conditions can mimic benign PUD.

Diagnosis can be accomplished by upper GI barium contrast radiography or by endoscopy. The finding of a duodenal ulcer indicates a high probability of *H. pylori* and a low probability of malignancy, and the condition can be managed on this basis. All gastric ulcers should be visualized with endoscopy and biopsied to rule out malignancy and confirm the presence of *H. pylori*.[3]

Treatment. The major treatment objectives for PUD are to encourage healing of the injured mucosa by reducing gastric acidity and to prevent recurrence. H_2 receptor antagonists or proton pump inhibitors are generally given to block acid secretion. Agents such as sucralfate form a protective coating over the injured mucosa and may be useful under some circumstances. Eradication of *H. pylori* infection with antibiotics has led to a marked reduction in the recurrence rate of PUD.[20,22,23]

In addition to these pharmacologic strategies, such measures as smoking cessation, avoidance of aspirin and NSAIDs, and stress reduction are all part of a comprehensive program to manage PUD. At the present time, no conclusive research has demonstrated that any specific diet has a therapeutic effect. Susceptible people are generally advised to avoid foods that seem to exacerbate symptoms, including caffeinated beverages and alcohol.

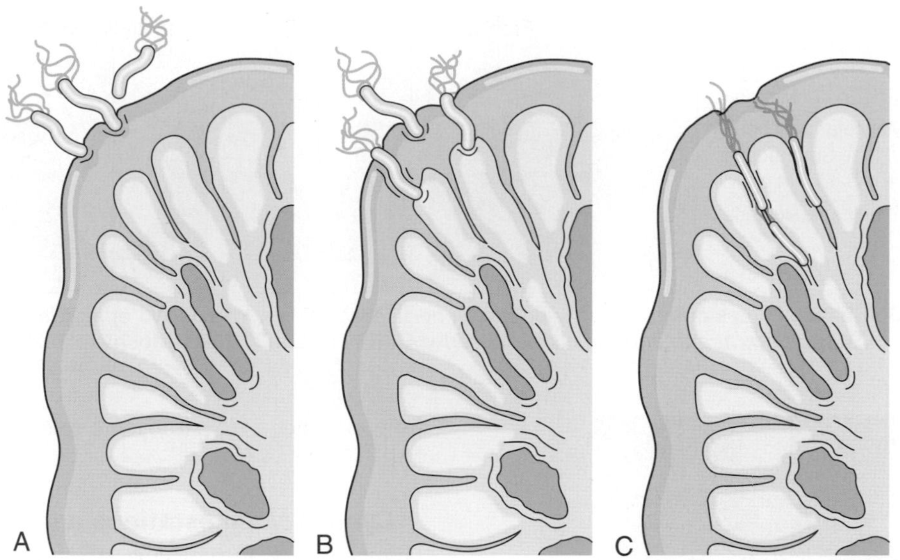

FIGURE 36-7 ■ Penetration of the mucosal layer by *Helicobacter pylori*. **A**, After penetration, *H. pylori* forms clusters near membranes of surface epithelial cells. **B**, Some attach to the cell membrane. **C**, Others lodge between the epithelial cell.

INFLAMMATORY BOWEL DISEASE

The term **inflammatory bowel disease (IBD)** refers to the two separate disease entities of ulcerative colitis and Crohn disease. (The term is somewhat misleading because many conditions may cause inflammation of the bowel, such as bacterial enterocolitis.) IBD is generally a life-altering chronic illness with serious consequences for people and their families who must cope with it. Both ulcerative colitis and Crohn disease have their onset most commonly in childhood and young adulthood, with obviously profound implications. This section describes the pathophysiologic aspects of ulcerative colitis and Crohn disease separately; a later section in this chapter discusses the psychosocial aspects of IBD.

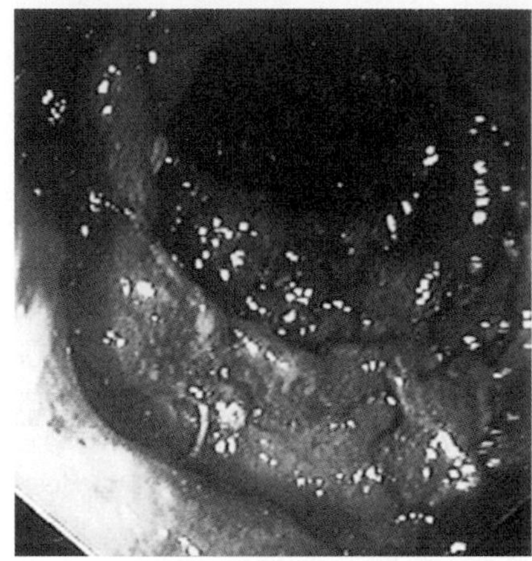

FIGURE 36-8 ■ Ulcerative colitis. (From Sleisenger MH, Fordtran JS, editors: *Gastrointestinal disease,* ed 5, Philadelphia, 1993, Saunders.)

Ulcerative Colitis

Ulcerative colitis (Figure 36-8) is an inflammatory disease of the mucosa of the rectum and colon. Approximately one-fifth of patients have total colitis, one-third have subtotal disease extending beyond the sigmoid, and one-half have disease limited to the rectum and rectosigmoid.[3] The changes are usually most severe in the rectum and extend for a variable extent around the colon, although there are several exceptions to this general rule. IBD is typically characterized by exacerbations and remissions; the disease is alternately active and inactive. The manifestations of ulcerative colitis are abdominal pain, diarrhea, and rectal bleeding. Its causes are poorly understood, but recent research has focused on genetic, environmental, and immunologic factors.[24] The immunologic basis for the disease is supported by the fact that ulcerative colitis frequently accompanies other autoimmune conditions such as thyroid disease and pernicious anemia.

Etiology and Clinical Manifestations. Ulcerative colitis begins as an inflammation at the base of the crypts of Lieberkühn. Damage to the crypt epithelium results, with eventual invasion of leukocytes and the formation of abscesses in the crypts. When multiple abscesses form in close proximity and begin to coalesce, large areas of ulcerations develop in the epithelium. Concurrent with this destructive process are attempts at repair of damaged tissue, along with the development of fragile and highly vascularized granulation tissue. The manifestations of ulcerative colitis are the result of these processes. Bleeding occurs as a result of mucosal destruction and ulceration, as well as damage to newly developed granulation tissue. Diarrhea is a result of the mucosal destruction in the colon, which leads to a decreased ability of the bowel to absorb water and sodium and thus to an increased volume of fluid in the intestinal contents.

The progression of ulcerative colitis may be highly variable. In some individuals it may have very mild manifestations; in others it may rapidly progress to a life-threatening disorder. Five percent to 10% of persons with ulcerative colitis have only one attack, with no further recurrence. However, 65% to 75% of those with ulcerative colitis experience an intermittent series of exacerbations and remissions. A number of conditions in other organ systems complicate ulcerative colitis, the most devastating of which is the relentlessly progressive liver condition primary sclerosing cholangitis, which occurs in 3% of ulcerative colitis patients.

An additional concern is increased risk for the development of colon cancer in persons who have had ulcerative colitis for more than 7 to 10 years. Authorities recommend monitoring these individuals carefully with regular endoscopy and biopsy. The presence of high-grade dysplasia should necessitate consideration of prophylactic complete colectomy. Recent surgical advances, such as the ileoanal pouch, have allowed colectomy patients to avoid colostomy and have close to normal bowel function.

Treatment. Management of ulcerative colitis is complex and ever evolving. Corticosteroids have long been the mainstay of treatment of acute exacerbations, but side effects limit their long-term use. Important categories of disease-modifying agents include the salicylate analogs and immunomodulating agents, such as azathioprine and mercaptopurine.

Crohn Disease

Crohn disease, also called regional enteritis and granulomatous colitis, is an inflammation of the GI tract that extends through all layers of the intestinal wall (Figure 36-9). It most commonly affects the proximal portion of the colon and, less often, the terminal ileum. It may affect multiple portions of the colon, with intervening normal areas left in between the affected regions. The manifestations of Crohn disease differ in some respects from those of ulcerative colitis, although some overlap may occur and distinction may be difficult. In Crohn disease, abdominal pain is often constant and is usually in the right lower quadrant of the abdomen. A palpable abdominal mass may be present in the right lower quadrant. The stool may be bloody, although not to the extent that it often is in ulcerative colitis. The cause of Crohn disease is unknown at the present time. There are fascinating parallels with ulcerative colitis as well as unexpected distinctions. For instance, smoking has been shown to protect against ulcerative colitis but to increase the risk of Crohn disease.[25] Up to 5% of people with Crohn disease have one or more affected relatives.

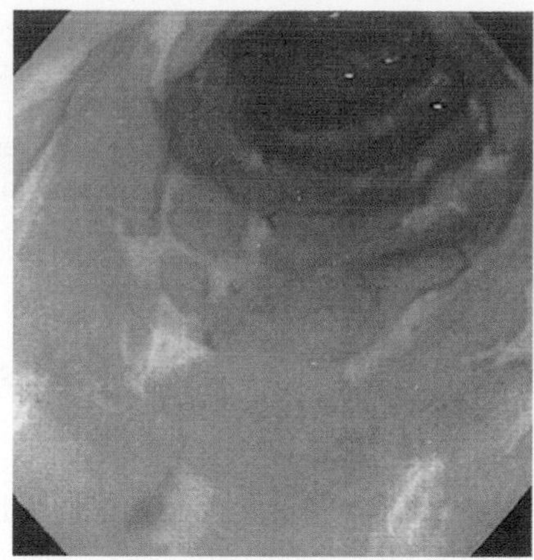

FIGURE 36-9 ■ Crohn disease. (From Sleisenger MH, Fordtran JS, editors: *Gastrointestinal disease,* ed 5, Philadelphia, 1993, Saunders.)

Etiology and Pathogenesis. Certain features of the pathogenesis of Crohn disease differ from those of ulcerative colitis. Crohn disease appears to be the result of a process in which the lymphoid and lymphatic structures of the GI tract become blocked. Subsequent engorgement and inflammation of surrounding tissue leads to the development of deep linear ulcers in the bowel wall. Eventually, all layers of the GI tract wall may become involved, and the portion of intestine that is affected may become thickened by fibrous scar tissue. Deep fissures may develop into fistulas, which may extend into adjacent tissue of other organs such as the bladder wall or even the skin.[2]

Clinical Manifestations. The manifestations of Crohn disease are the result of the pathologic changes described above, and the bowel becomes incapable of adequately absorbing the intestinal contents. Complications such as perianal fissures, fistulas, and abscesses are common in Crohn disease and may be the symptoms that lead individuals to seek health care. The onset and course of Crohn disease may vary a great deal; unlike in ulcerative colitis, the symptoms present during a period of Crohn exacerbation may be subtle but persistent. At the present time it is unclear whether a significantly increased incidence of intestinal cancer occurs in persons with Crohn disease. However, when Crohn disease involves the large bowel, the risk of colorectal cancer appears to be similar to that of ulcerative colitis of similar extent.[26]

Treatment. Because the cause of IBD is unknown, therapeutic strategies are focused on alleviating and reducing inflammation. Therapeutic drug categories are similar to those for ulcerative colitis. The antibiotic metronidazole is particularly useful for colonic Crohn disease. New types of treatments include the anti–tumor necrosis factor agent infliximab, which has shown particular success, as well as other investigational anticytokine treatments.[24] Despite these advances, there is no cure for this challenging condition.

ENTEROCOLITIS

Pseudomembranous Enterocolitis

Etiology. **Pseudomembranous enterocolitis** is an acute inflammation and necrosis of the small and large intestines caused by *Clostridium difficile*, usually affecting the mucosa but sometimes extending to other layers.[27] Exposure to antibiotics is the major factor predisposing to the development of this disorder, and patients with cancer or who have undergone abdominal surgery are at particular risk. The disease is mediated by bacterial toxins, leading to mucosal necrosis and the characteristic pseudomembrane composed of leukocytes, mucus, fibrin, and inflammatory cells.

Clinical Manifestations and Treatment. Resulting manifestations include diarrhea (often bloody), abdominal pain, fever, and rarely, colonic perforation. Treatment involves stopping the offending antibiotic, if possible, treating ischemia and other contributing conditions, and using antibiotics such as oral metronidazole or vancomycin. Recurrences are relatively common and may necessitate retreatment.

Necrotizing Enterocolitis

Etiology. **Necrotizing enterocolitis** is a disorder occurring most often in premature infants (less than 34 weeks gestation) and infants with low birth weight (less than 5 lb or 2.25 kg). This disorder is characterized by diffuse or patchy intestinal necrosis accompanied by sepsis.

Clinical Manifestations and Treatment. Early manifestations include a distended abdomen and stomach. The major complication of necrotizing enterocolitis is intestinal perforation, which may necessitate surgery. Various theories regarding the etiologic progression of necrotizing enterocolitis include perinatal oxygen deficit with insufficient blood flow to the viscera, and the use of hypertonic feeding formulas in newborn infants. A special form of necrotizing enterocolitis, called typhlitis, may afflict neutropenic cancer patients and carries a grave prognosis. Management is surgical, with appropriate antibiotics.

Appendicitis

Etiology. The most common cause of emergency surgery on the abdomen, **appendicitis** is an inflammation of the vermiform appendix. The classic hypothesis suggests that obstruction of the appendiceal lumen, usually by a fecalith or, less commonly, lymphoid hyperplasia or parasitic worms, causes most cases of appendiceal inflammation. However, more than 100 years of experience with this condition has failed to provide a single hypothesis that explains the etiologic progression of appendicitis in all cases.[3] In an unknown number of cases appendiceal inflammation may be self-limited and may remit (e.g., with relief of the obstruction). If left unchecked, inflammation generally leads to necrosis of the appendix, with subsequent abscess formation and life-threatening peritonitis. Rarely appendicitis may occur in a subacute or stuttering fashion over several days or weeks.

Clinical Manifestations and Treatment. Appendicitis is twice as common before age 45 as after, and affects men somewhat more often than women. The earliest manifestation of appendicitis is generalized periumbilical pain accompanied by nausea and, occasionally, diarrhea. The pain is often described as "migrating" or localizing to the lower right abdomen (**McBurney point**) due to distention of the serosa from inflammatory edema, at which time fever usually manifests. Experienced surgeons generally operate in suspicious cases. Less typical cases should be assessed with computed tomography (CT), or ultrasound, if the patient is a child or pregnant women or if CT is not readily available. Such an approach yields a relatively low false-positive surgical rate of around 5%.[3] Surgical removal of the appendix, either through an open procedure or laparoscopically, is the treatment of choice for appendicitis. Administration of antibiotics with replacement of fluid and electrolytes may be necessary. Localized abscesses secondary to perforation may be managed with percutaneous tube drainage and antibiotics alone, if there are no signs of peritonitis.[28]

Diverticular Disease

Etiology. The term diverticular disease generally refers to **diverticulosis**, or the presence of diverticula in the colon. Diverticula are acquired herniations of the mucosa and submucosa through the muscular coat of the colon (Figure 36-10) that probably result from a combination of structural and functional factors. In particular, areas of weakness in the bowel wall, particularly where blood vessels enter, are subject to damage from high intraluminal pressures. Colonic diverticulosis is very common in westernized countries and is associated with a diet low in fiber; this lack of fiber presumably fails to provide enough bulk to dampen pressure variations in the intestine. The prevalence of diverticulosis increases with age; about 30% of the general population at 60 years of age and about 80% at 80 years will have diverticula in the colon.[1] Most persons experience no manifestations of diverticulosis, and by itself diverticulosis is not considered a pathologic condition. However, when diverticula become inflamed, the condition is referred to as **diverticulitis** (see Box 36-1 for the terminology of diverticulosis).

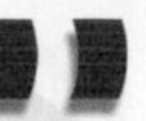

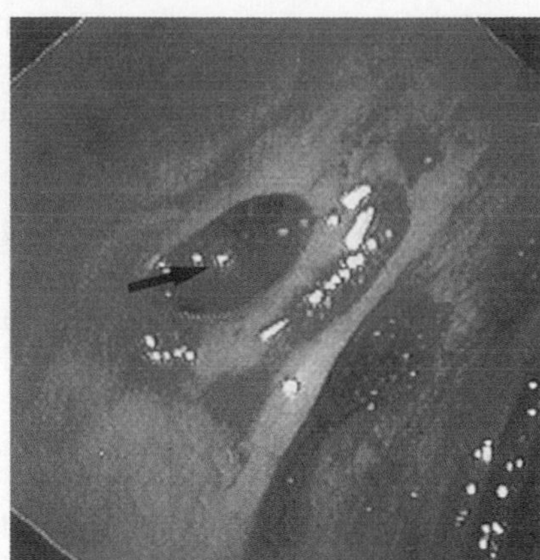

FIGURE 36-10 ■ Colonic diverticula. Small outpouchings of colonic mucosa are evident *(arrow).* (From Sleisenger MH, Fordtran JS, editors: *Gastrointestinal disease,* ed 5, Philadelphia, 1993, Saunders.)

Clinical Manifestations and Treatment. Inflammation of the diverticula can lead to serious consequences such as the development of abscesses in the bowel wall, peritonitis, and intestinal obstruction. Manifestations of diverticulitis include acute lower abdominal pain, fever, and tachycardia. During an acute episode of diverticulitis, the administration of broad-spectrum antibiotics is indicated, and on occasion intravenous fluid and electrolyte support is necessary. Recurrence of diverticulitis is common. Long-term complications include colonic strictures and fistulae, which may necessitate surgery.

Box 36-1

Terminology of Diverticulosis

Diverticulum: A single pouchlike herniation through the muscular layer of the colon
Diverticula: More than one diverticulum (Latin plural form)
Diverticulosis: The presence of one or more diverticula
Diverticulitis: Inflammation of one or more diverticula
Diverticular disease: Complications related to the presence of diverticula

KEY CONCEPTS

- Alterations in intestinal wall integrity are generally a result of infection, inflammation, or weakness of the muscular layers. General symptoms include pain, bleeding, and diarrhea.
- Gastritis may be acute or chronic. Acute gastritis is generally precipitated by the ingestion of irritating substances, including alcohol and aspirin. Chronic gastritis may lead to atrophy of the gastric mucosa and the subsequent decreased production of HCl and intrinsic factor. Acute gastroenteritis is usually due to the ingestion of pathogenic organisms or preformed bacterial toxins and is characterized by self-limited vomiting, diarrhea, and abdominal pain.
- PUD may affect the esophagus, stomach, and duodenum. Gastric ulcers are thought to be due to breakdown of the protective mucus layer that normally prevents the diffusion of acids into gastric epithelia. Duodenal ulcers are caused by excessive acid secretion that is mediated by increased vagal activity. The organism *H. pylori* has been implicated in the pathogenesis of both gastric and duodenal ulcers. PUD is characterized by epigastric pain that is relieved by food or antacids. Perforation and bleeding are the major complications of PUD. Management of PUD is aimed at minimizing acid secretion and eradicating *H. pylori.*
- Ulcerative colitis and Crohn disease are chronic inflammatory disorders of the bowel. Ulcerative colitis (inflammation and ulceration of the colon and rectal mucosa) is manifested as bloody diarrhea and abdominal pain. There is an increased risk for colon cancer in persons who have had ulcerative colitis for more than 7 to 10 years. Crohn disease generally affects the proximal portion of the colon or the terminal ileum. Involvement of all layers of the intestinal wall predisposes to fistula formation and malabsorption. Crohn disease may result from blockage and subsequent inflammation of lymphatic vessels. Chronic abdominal pain and diarrhea are common. Management of ulcerative colitis and Crohn disease is aimed at reducing inflammation.
- Acute inflammation of the intestinal wall may manifest as pseudomembranous enterocolitis or necrotizing enterocolitis. Abdominal pain, diarrhea, fever, and sepsis may result. The use of broad-spectrum antibiotics has been implicated in the etiologic development of pseudomembranous enterocolitis. Necrotizing enterocolitis, which occurs most often in infants, is thought to be due to bowel ischemia.
- Appendicitis is characterized by right lower quadrant pain, nausea and vomiting, and systemic signs of inflammation. Surgical removal of the appendix is necessary. Untreated appendicitis may result in rupture of the appendix and subsequent peritonitis; localized abscesses may be managed with tube drainage and antibiotics alone.
- Diverticula of the colon are very common in Western society because of a low intake of dietary fiber. Low-bulk stools result in the development of high intraluminal pressure, which predisposes to diverticula formation. Diverticulosis is generally asymptomatic. Inflammation of the diverticula, or diverticulitis, is manifested as fever and lower abdominal pain. Antibiotics and surgery may be required for management of complicated diverticulitis.

ALTERATIONS IN MOTILITY OF THE GASTROINTESTINAL TRACT

Disorders of the GI tract that primarily alter its regular propulsive ability may have a negative effect on its ability to absorb nutrients. In these alterations in motility, the transit time of substances passing through the GI tract may be too fast to allow for adequate absorption. Conversely, a blockage or impedance of the GI tract may result in slowed or absent motility, which also prevents normal ingestion and processing of nutrient substances. As with alterations in the integrity of the GI tract wall, these alterations in GI motility may represent a chronic condition, with many implications for the person experiencing altered GI motility, or may be a life-threatening, acute situation requiring immediate intervention.

MOTILITY DISORDERS

Irritable Bowel Syndrome

Irritable bowel syndrome is a complex entity that has been the focus of much recent research. A clear definition of this syndrome has not been agreed on by all authorities; nevertheless, certain defining characteristics have been established. Typically, IBS is the presence of alternating diarrhea and constipation accompanied by abdominal cramping pain in the absence of any identifiable pathologic process in the GI tract.[3] (Other terms that have been used for this syndrome include spastic colitis and irritable colon syndrome.) Many authorities point out that the quantity of symptoms is not as important as their effect of the normal lifestyle of an individual. Persons with IBS may miss work, curtail their social life, and avoid sexual intercourse. This is an extremely common disorder affecting up to 20% of the U.S. population.[6] It is important to differentiate IBS, in which no pathologic process of the GI tract has been identified, from IBD, in which a pathologic process is identifiable.

Etiology and Pathogenesis. The etiologic factors and pathogenesis of IBS are presently obscure. Most evidence seems to show that IBS is primarily a disorder of bowel motility. Research studies have demonstrated that the myoelectric activity of the colon of persons with IBS is altered. In particular, the slow wave activity of the colon, which usually occurs at a rate of three to six times per minute, is markedly increased in IBS.[1,3] Whether this altered pattern is the result of genetic factors or such environmental factors as episodic infection, the level of stress or dietary patterns remains unknown.

Clinical Manifestations and Treatment. The manifestations of IBS may vary greatly, with some persons experiencing only diarrhea or constipation and others experiencing an alternating pattern of both. In addition to the abdominal cramping pain, other manifestations, such as mucus in the stool and nausea, may also be present. The severity of manifestations may range from barely noticeable to incapacitating. Current therapy focuses on the use of antidiarrheal agents and antispasmodic medications as appropriate. No study has shown a clearly demonstrable benefit for a particular agent.[29] Ingestion of a diet with increased amounts of fiber has proved useful in many cases and is thought to promote a more normal pattern of myoelectric activity by providing a regular propulsive stimulus in the gut.[30] Perhaps with IBS more than with most GI disorders patients may benefit from support groups, internet-based resources, and alternative therapies.

Intestinal Obstruction

Intestinal obstruction is partial or complete blockage of the intestinal lumen of the small or large bowel. Mechanical obstructions are caused by blockage of the intestine by adhesions, hernia, tumor, inflammation and resulting stricture (as in Crohn disease), impacted feces, volvulus, or intussusception. (Volvulus and intussusception are covered in more detail in the following section.) Functional obstruction refers to the loss of propulsive ability by the bowel and may occur after abdominal surgery or in association with hypokalemia, peritonitis, severe trauma, spinal fractures, ureteral distention, and the administration of some narcotic medications.

Etiology and Pathogenesis. Obstruction of the small bowel occurs most often (90% of cases). Intestinal obstruction is most common in persons who have previously undergone abdominal surgery and have adhesions or who have congenital abnormalities of the bowel. Metastatic carcinoma, particularly cancers of the intestines and female reproductive organs, is an important cause of obstruction and should be considered in patients with obstruction who have never had abdominal surgery. The severity and types of symptoms initially accompanying an intestinal obstruction vary with its cause and location.

With obstruction of the bowel lumen, fluid and gas begin to accumulate proximal to the obstructed location. The distention produced by trapped fluid and gas causes water and electrolytes to be secreted into the obstructed lumen of the small bowel. Distention also results in the impedance of venous return, and the bowel wall becomes edematous. The absorptive ability of the bowel wall is compromised, and fluid and gas continue to accumulate as additional water and electrolytes are secreted into the lumen. The pressure on the bowel wall exerted by the excess fluid and gas may result in leakage of fluid through the wall into the peritoneum, as well as necrosis of the bowel wall.

In addition to the process just described, other complications may be present with blockage of the intestinal lumen. Bacteria may translocate across the bowel wall into the blood stream to produce fever and other signs of sepsis. Impairment of bowel circulation (referred to as strangulation obstruction) leads to ischemia and a resultant increased peristalsis. As blood escapes from the engorged veins, significant loss of blood and plasma from the affected segment may result in the rapid development of shock. In addition, the strangulated segment may become gangrenous, with resulting peritonitis, or become perforated, with the leakage of highly toxic bacterial material into the peritoneal cavity.[3] If left untreated, a person with an intestinal obstruction has a high risk of death from shock and vascular collapse.

Clinical Manifestations and Treatment. The manifestations of an intestinal obstruction depend on its site and duration. Obstructions in the upper jejunal area usually result in vomiting, dehydration, and electrolyte depletion. In obstruction of the distal portion of the small bowel or ileus, constipation may be an early manifestation, with massive accumulation of fluid in the lumen occurring later. Dehydration may progress to hypovolemic shock if the obstruction is left untreated. In obstructions of the colon, massive gas distention may be present. The fluid and electrolyte losses associated with colonic obstruction may not be as severe as those seen in obstruction of the small bowel. Blockage of the colon by a tumor is the most common cause of colonic obstruction, and perforation of the bowel wall adjacent to the tumor may occur in association with an obstruction.

Therapeutic strategies for intestinal obstruction include surgical intervention to correct or remove the source of a mechanical obstruction. Supportive therapy, including decompression of the bowel with specialized tubes or endoscopy, and fluid and electrolyte replacement therapy may be needed during an acute obstructive episode.

Volvulus

Etiology, Clinical Manifestations, and Treatment. **Volvulus** is twisting of the bowel on itself, causing intestinal obstruction and blood vessel compression (Figure 36-11). The two most common sites for the development of volvulus are the cecum and the sigmoid colon.[3] A volvulus may be the result of an anomaly of rotation, an ingested foreign body, or an adhesion; however, the cause cannot always be determined. Volvulus tends to occur in elderly individuals with coexistent medical conditions. With the sudden tight twisting of the bowel on its mesentery, blood flow to the bowel is impeded. Gangrene, necrosis, and perforation may develop, resulting in a life-threatening situation. If both ends of a bowel segment are twisted, a closed-loop obstruction results, with the manifestations described earlier for intestinal obstruction. Treatment varies according to the severity and location of the volvulus and includes the therapeutic approaches described for intestinal obstruction.[3,6]

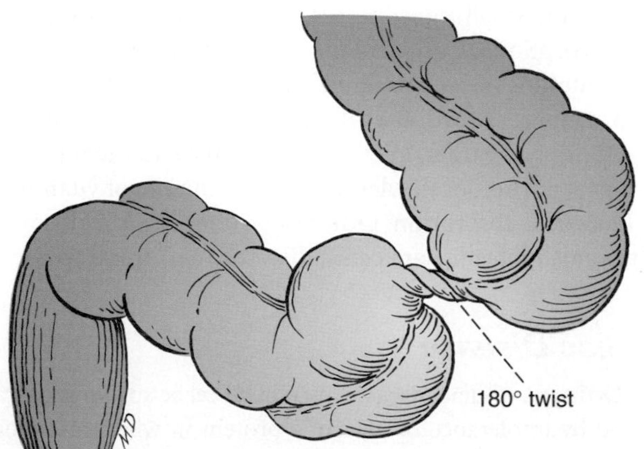

FIGURE 36-11 ■ Volvulus. Intestine twists at least 180 degrees, causing obstruction and ischemia. (From Black JM, Hawks JH, Keene AM: *Medical-surgical nursing: clinical management for positive outcomes,* ed 7, Philadelphia, 2005, Saunders, p 843.)

Intussusception

Etiology, Clinical Manifestations, and Treatment. **Intussusception** is a telescoping or invagination of a portion of the bowel into an adjacent distal portion (Figure 36-12). It is most common in infants and occurs three times more often in males than in females.[3] Intussusception may be linked to viral infections because its occurrence seems to coincide with the peak incidence of enteritis and respiratory tract infections. In most cases involving infants, the actual cause is unknown, although in older children it may be associated with alterations in intestinal motility or a condition called Meckel diverticulum, in which a congenital abnormality consisting of a blind tube is present in the distal end of the ileum. In adults, intussusception usually results from the presence of benign or malignant tumors.

As a bowel segment undergoes intussusception, peristalsis acts to pull more bowel along with it. The resulting area of tightened, invaginated bowel becomes edematous; venous engorgement with hemorrhage may occur. Intestinal obstruction of the bowel may develop, with eventual gangrene, shock, and perforation of the bowel if surgical treatment is delayed.[6]

Megacolon

Megacolon can be congenital or acquired at any age. Perhaps the most common cause in westernized countries is prolonged constipation/obstipation, usually chronic in nature.

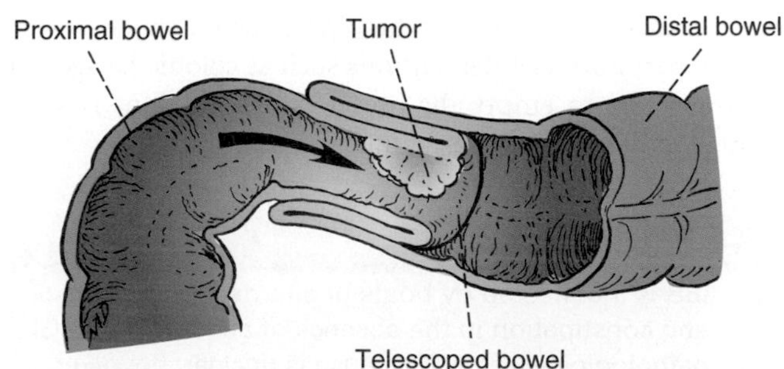

FIGURE 36-12 ■ Intussusception. A portion of bowel telescopes into adjacent (usually distal) bowel. (From Black JM, Hawks JH, Keene AM: *Medical-surgical nursing: clinical management for positive outcomes,* ed 7, Philadelphia, 2005, Saunders, 843.)

This is particularly common in younger children who are dealing with the psychological aspects of toilet training and bowel control. Although most of these children are psychologically normal, a small number of children with **encopresis** have experienced sexual abuse, and its presence should be considered.[31] Significant voiding issues also plague the other end of the age spectrum, and constipation/obstipation in the elderly may lead to megacolon, particularly when the sufferer has relied on regular enemas or laxatives for many years.

Hirschprung disease (see below) is characterized by the congenital absence of autonomic smooth muscle ganglia. The aganglionic bowel segment contracts but without the reciprocal relaxation needed to propel the intestinal contents forward. Stasis of stool and dilation of the proximal end of the colon result in megacolon, or massive dilation of the colon. **Chagas disease** caused by *Trypanosoma cruzii* is a common cause of acquired colon neuronal dysfunction and megacolon in Central and South America but is rarely seen in the United States. As discussed in Chapter 35, antibiotic-associated colitis may result in acute megacolon, which is a surgical emergency. Finally, the idiopathic syndrome of intestinal pseudoobstruction (**Ogilvie syndrome**) may rarely result in megacolon.

Hirschsprung Disease

Hirschsprung disease is a congenital disorder of the large intestine in which the autonomic nerve ganglia in the smooth muscle are absent or markedly reduced. In 90% of individuals with Hirschsprung disease, the aganglionic segment is in the rectosigmoid area, but occasionally the entire colon may be affected.[3] Hirschsprung disease is believed to be familial and occurs in approximately 1 in 5000 live births. It is more common in males than females, with a ratio of 3.8:1.[3] The disease often coexists with other anomalies, particularly Down syndrome. Although Hirschsprung disease is most commonly identified in infants and children, it may be present in adults as a longstanding undiagnosed condition.

Clinical Manifestations and Treatment. In infants, Hirschsprung disease may have severe, life-threatening effects. Fecal stagnation may result in enterocolitis with bacterial overgrowth, profuse diarrhea, hypovolemic shock, and intestinal perforation. Interventions such as colonic lavage may be performed to empty the bowel until the infant is stable enough to withstand surgical intervention.

KEY CONCEPTS

- IBS is manifested by bouts of alternating diarrhea and constipation in the absence of an identifiable GI pathologic process. The cause is unclear; however, the slow wave activity of the bowel is markedly increased. A high-fiber diet and antidiarrheal agents may be recommended.
- Intestinal obstructions may be mechanical or functional. Mechanical obstructions are due to adhesions, hernia, tumors, impacted feces, volvulus (twisting), or intussusception (telescoping). Mechanical obstructions are characterized by increased bowel sounds initially, accompanied by abdominal pain, nausea, and vomiting. Functional obstructions are due to conditions that inhibit peristalsis, such as narcotics, anesthesia, surgical manipulation, peritonitis, hypokalemia, and spinal cord injuries. Functional obstructions are characterized by the absence of bowel sounds. Uncorrected obstruction may lead to intestinal wall edema, ischemia, and necrosis. Bowel gangrene, sepsis, and shock can result. Surgical intervention or decompression with an intestinal tube is often required.
- Hirschsprung disease is a familial, congenital disorder of the large intestine in which the autonomic ganglia are reduced or absent. Stasis of stool and megacolon may occur in the abnormally innervated section of bowel. Megacolon can also be acquired as an adult.

MALABSORPTION

Malabsorption refers to failure of the GI tract to absorb or normally digest one or more dietary constituents.[1] It is typically manifested as diarrhea, with the passage of inappropriately processed intestinal contents resulting in impaired fluid absorption. A variety of pathologic processes produce malabsorption syndromes, including intestinal enzyme abnormalities (e.g., lactase deficiency), infection (e.g., AIDS enteritis), and radiation enteritis, among others. The types of malabsorption syndromes discussed here result from a mucosal disorder of the small bowel or from the surgical removal of portions of the stomach or small bowel.

MUCOSAL DISORDERS

Myriad disorders may affect the mucosa of the small intestine. Because the small intestine is the principal site of digestion and absorption of nutrients, a defect in the mucosa of the small intestine has the potential for causing malabsorption of fat, protein, carbohydrate, vitamins, and minerals. Crohn disease, described earlier, may result in damage to the mucosa of the distal portion of the ileum, which is the site of vitamin B_{12} and bile acid absorption. Other important mucosal disorders of the small intestine are celiac disease and tropical sprue.

Celiac Disease

Etiology. **Celiac disease** (also called celiac sprue) is characterized by intolerance of gluten, a protein in wheat and wheat products. Current research suggests that celiac sprue is an immune disorder triggered by exposure to gliadin (a specific wheat gluten) in genetically predisposed persons.[3] Environmental, genetic, and immune factors play pivotal roles in determining the nature of symptoms. The main pathologic finding is villus atrophy, with a decrease in the activity and amount of surface epithelial enzymes. The resulting malabsorption of ingested nutrients may promote malnutrition and severe debilitation.

Celiac disease affects twice as many females as males and may have a familial inheritance pattern. The incidence in the general population is 1 in 3000, and those affected are primarily of northwestern European ancestry. The onset of celiac disease may present in infancy, when gluten-containing products are first introduced into the diet, but is more common in the fourth and fifth decades.[32]

Diagnosis and Treatment. In the past the diagnosis of celiac disease relied on intestinal biopsy showing the typical pathologic manifestations. New blood tests assay for anti–tissue transglutaminase antibody (anti-ttG) and the more specific immunoglobulin A (IgA) endomysial antibody, although in general biopsy is still recommended for confirmation. Effective treatment includes the elimination of all gluten from the diet, which results in significant improvement in the intestinal mucosa, and the administration of supplemental iron, folate, and in specific cases B_{12} and fat-soluble vitamins (A, D, E, K). Importantly, the incidence of intestinal malignancy, especially lymphoma, is two times higher among sprue patients than among the general population.

Tropical Sprue

Etiology. A malabsorptive syndrome of unknown cause is prevalent in equatorial countries. In **tropical sprue**, the mucosa of the small intestine atrophies, with resulting malabsorption, malnutrition, and B_{12} and folic acid deficiency. Although tropical enteropathy often seems to occur in epidemics, no single organism has been implicated in its development. Its incidence is high in persons living in or visiting tropical climates, and it appears to affect adults more often than children.[5] While environmental factors seem preeminent, a genetic component may be present in some cases.

Clinical Manifestations and Treatment. The atrophy of the small intestinal mucosa may have severe effects. Massive malabsorption may result from failure of the mucosa to produce the enzymes needed for digestion. Manifestations include severe diarrhea with blood-tinged stools, abdominal distention, and steatorrhea (the presence of excess fat in the stool). In the Caribbean, tropical sprue is strongly linked to the presence of enterotoxin-producing coliforms and responds well to broad-spectrum antibiotics.[3] The response of patients from other areas (e.g., India) to treatment is less predictable than that of patients with Caribbean sprue. Treatment includes antidiarrheal medication and prolonged antimicrobial therapy.

MALABSORPTION DISORDERS AFTER SURGICAL INTERVENTION

Surgical procedures in which a portion of the stomach or small bowel is removed may result in loss of the ability to absorb nutrients properly, either through a loss of appropriate motility patterns or through a loss of the surface area of the small bowel needed for adequate absorption. Two types of disorders of malabsorption may occur after surgical intervention on the stomach or small bowel: dumping syndrome and short-bowel syndrome.

Dumping Syndrome

Etiology, Pathogenesis, and Clinical Manifestations. **Dumping syndrome** is a term used to describe the literal dumping of stomach contents into the proximal portion of the small intestine because of impaired gastric emptying (Figure 36-13). This loss of normal, gradual pyloric emptying may occur after removal of all or part of the stomach (gastrectomy), a procedure performed commonly for PUD in previous years, but more recently especially for control of obesity. With the normal reservoir function of the stomach now impaired, a large volume of hyperosmolar food is dumped rapidly into the small intestine, with consequences that may be severe. The hyperosmolar contents of the small intestine draw water into the lumen and stimulate bowel motility, with manifestations of diarrhea and abdominal pain. In addition, the rapid absorption of a large amount of glucose and a subsequent rise in blood glucose levels promotes an excessive rise in plasma insulin. The elevated insulin level then causes a rapid fall in blood glucose levels 1 to 3 hours after a meal. This sudden reversal is referred to as "rebound hypoglycemia."[3]

Treatment. Persons who have undergone a gastrectomy procedure will require specific instruction regarding eating small meals six to eight times a day rather than three large meals. Restriction of carbohydrate intake may be needed to limit glucose absorption. Medications to reduce bowel motility have been helpful in promoting a more normal pattern of bowel function in this population.

Short-Bowel Syndrome

Clinical Manifestations. **Short-bowel syndrome** refers to the severe diarrhea and significant malabsorption that develop after the surgical removal of large portions of the small intestine. The severity of the manifestations depends on the amount and location of the bowel resected. In particular, removal of the distal two-thirds of the ileum and the ileocecal valve may result in severe malabsorption. Because the ileocecal valve serves to regulate the transit time of intestinal contents, its removal may promote a transit time that is too rapid for adequate absorption of nutrients. In addition, loss of large portions of the small intestine will result in a diminished ability to absorb water, electrolytes, protein, fat, carbohydrates, vitamins, and trace elements.

Recovery. The small intestine displays an amazing ability to adapt after bowel resection. The remaining villi may enlarge and lengthen, thus increasing the absorptive surface area of the bowel. The presence of orally ingested nutrients is needed for this adaptive process to occur, and a gradual

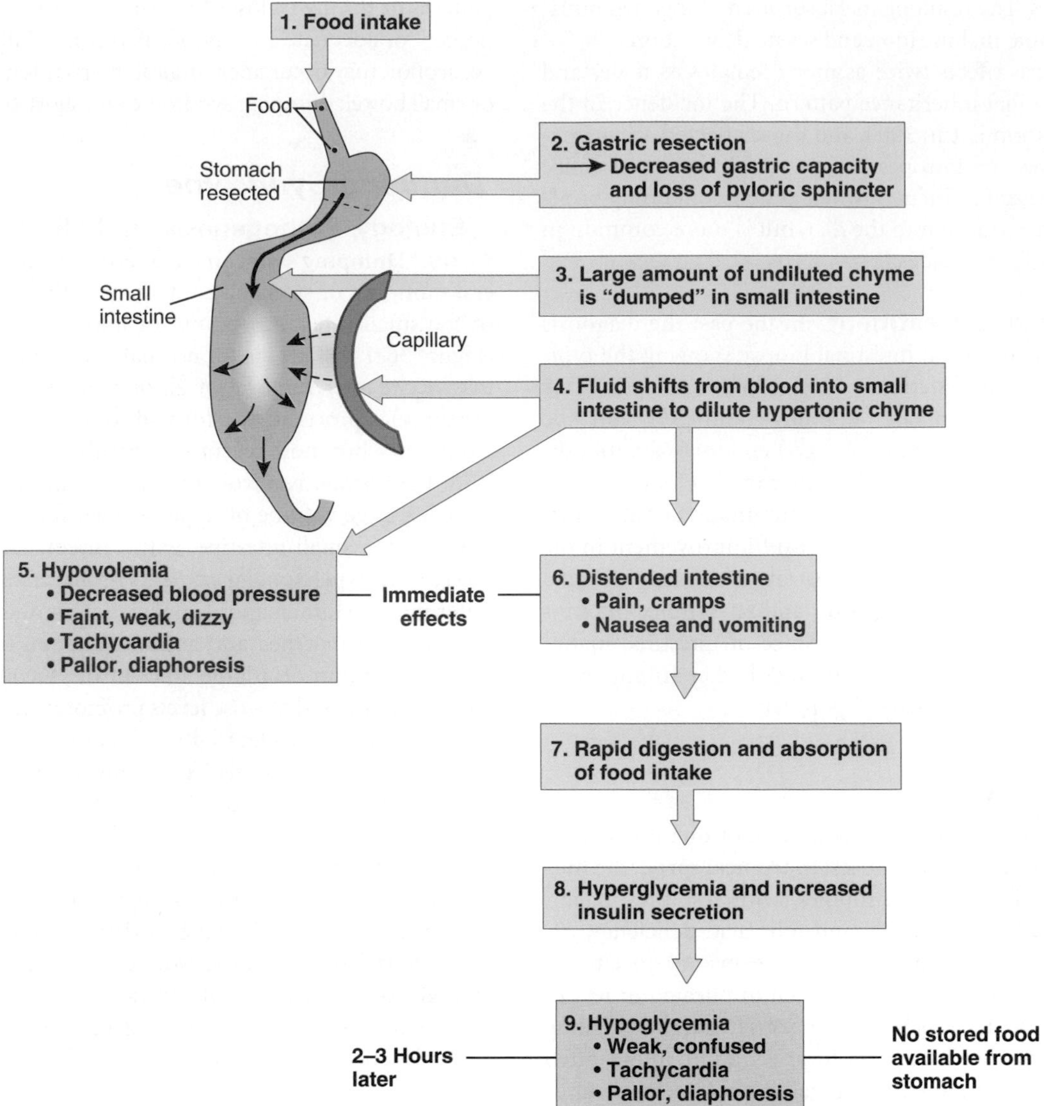

FIGURE 36-13 ■ Dumping syndrome (postgastrectomy). (From Gould BE: *Pathophysiology for the health professions*, ed 2, Philadelphia, 2002, Saunders, p 390.)

increase in oral intake after bowel resection may promote gradual improvement in absorptive ability.[30] Intravenous nutritional support may be required temporarily or indefinitely following surgical foreshortening of the gut.

KEY CONCEPTS

- Malabsorption occurs when the small bowel fails to absorb one or more dietary components. Diarrhea and abdominal discomfort are the usual manifestations. Malabsorption may occur because of mucosal dysfunction (Crohn disease, celiac disease, tropical sprue), enzyme deficiencies, or surgical alterations that affect transit time and absorptive surface area.
- Celiac disease appears to be caused by a familial intolerance of gluten-containing foods. Ingestion of gluten leads to inflammation and atrophy of the intestinal villi. A reduced surface area and decreased brush border enzymes impair nutrient absorption.
- Dumping syndrome occurs with loss of pyloric sphincter regulation, generally after gastric surgery for ulcers or cancer. Rapid dumping of chyme into the duodenum causes an osmotic shift of water into the lumen and diarrhea. Glucose absorption may be rapid and lead to overshoot of insulin secretion and rebound hypoglycemia.
- Short-bowel syndrome follows surgical procedures involving removal of large sections of the small intestine. Rapid transit time and reduced surface area for absorption lead to diarrhea and malabsorption.

NEOPLASMS OF THE GASTROINTESTINAL TRACT

Neoplasms may develop in every region of the GI tract. They vary in their severity and in their ability to disrupt normal GI functioning. The most common neoplastic processes of the GI tract are summarized here; the reader may wish to refer to the chapter on neoplasms as a background for understanding these specific types of neoplasms occurring in the GI tract.

ESOPHAGEAL, GASTRIC, AND SMALL INTESTINAL CANCERS

Esophageal Cancer

Etiology. Esophageal cancer accounts for 1% to 2% of all cancers and affects men three times more often than women.[1] It usually develops in men older than 60 years, with a 1-year survival rate of less than 20%.[33] Although the cause of esophageal cancer is presently unknown, several predisposing factors have been identified, including genetic predisposition, dietary habits (especially ingestion of foods high in nitrosamine content), environmental exposures, and chronic irritation of the esophagus from heavy smoking and alcohol use. Chronic severe reflux, especially that associated with **achalasia**, is a prominent risk factor as well.

Most esophageal tumors are squamous cell carcinomas; fewer than 10% are adenocarcinomas. The incidence of adenocarcinoma of the gastroesophageal junction is increasing and seems to reflect an increased prevalence of **Barrett esophagus** (see Chapter 35). Interestingly, infection with *H. pylori* seems to protect against development of this form of esophageal cancer.[3,34]

Pathogenesis. Regardless of the cell type, the prognosis is extremely poor. Tumors of the esophagus are usually infiltrating, and the disease may spread extensively to surrounding organs by way of the esophageal lymphatics at an early stage. Invasion of surrounding structures may lead to the formation of esophagobronchial or esophagopleural fistulas, with subsequent pneumonia or abscess. The tumor may partially constrict the lumen of the esophagus, and surgery, radiation therapy, and other measures may be considered to maintain a patent esophagus. Endoscopic procedures of benefit include stent placement and ablation of the tumor through heat probe and laser techniques. If the individual survives the initial extension of the tumor, the liver and lungs are the usual sites of distant metastasis.[33]

Gastric Carcinoma

Gastric carcinoma is common throughout the world; however, certain population groups appear to be at higher risk than others.[1,33] In Japan, the prevalence of gastric adenocarcinoma is about 10 times the prevalence in the United States. The incidence is higher in men older than 30 years than in other age and sex groups. The overall 5-year survival rate is approximately 10%, although the prognosis depends on the stage of the disease at the time of diagnosis.[33] Early stage gastric cancer has not penetrated the major muscle layer of the stomach wall and is associated with a more favorable survival rate than seen in more advanced disease.

Etiology. Research into the etiologic development of gastric cancer is a rapidly expanding area. A recent consensus Committee of the World Health Organization concluded that sufficient evidence has amassed that *H. pylori* has a role in promoting gastric cancer, with a twofold increased risk compared with that in uninfected individuals.[3] In particular, the development of multifocal atrophic gastritis induced by persistent *H. pylori* infection is a critical step in the development of gastric cancer.[12] Other risk factors are similar to those for esophageal cancer, with the exception that alcohol is not a significant contributor to gastric carcinoma.[3] Aspirin use seems to be protective against stomach cancer.[35] Small numbers of gastric neoplasms may have different histologic characteristics, including lymphoma and carcinoid tumors, and have distinct clinical courses.

Gastric carcinoma extends rapidly to the regional lymph nodes and surrounding organs by way of the lymphatic system, the blood stream, and direct extension through the wall of the stomach.

Clinical Manifestations and Treatment. Unfortunately, early gastric cancer typically has no manifestations and may not be identified. Advanced gastric cancer (Figure 36-14) is gastric cancer that has penetrated the muscle layer of the stomach. Most people in North America identified with gastric cancer already have the advanced form and have manifestations such as anorexia and GI bleeding.

Surgical resection of the tumor with appropriate surrounding margins of tissue remains the only effective treatment for this cancer.

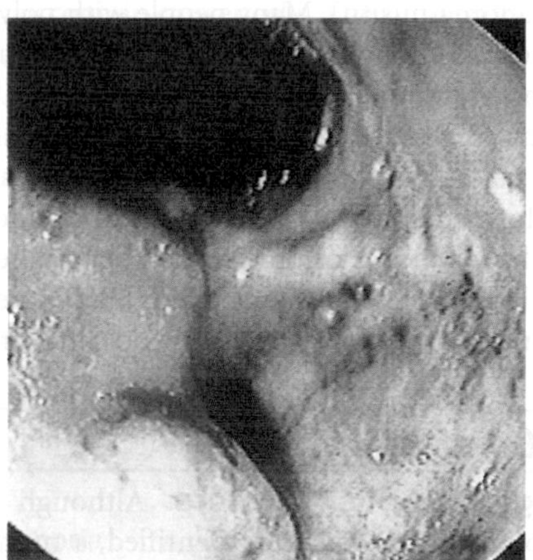

FIGURE 36-14 ■ Ulcerating gastric cancer. (From Sleisenger MH, Fordtran JS, editors: *Gastrointestinal disease,* ed 5, Philadelphia, 1993, Saunders.)

Chemotherapy in particular has advanced rapidly over the last two decades and has significantly improved the prognosis for moderately advanced (i.e., with nodal metastases) colon cancer.[37]

KEY CONCEPTS

- Warning signs for cancer of the GI tract include black, tarry, bloody, or pencil-shaped stool and a change in bowel habits. Risk factors for GI cancer include a low-fiber, high-fat diet, polyps, and chronic irritation or inflammation.
- The prognosis for GI cancer is related to the extent of spread in the body. Surgical removal of tumors followed by chemotherapy, radiation therapy, or both is the usual treatment. Early detection is associated with a better prognosis.

PSYCHOSOCIAL ASPECTS OF GASTROINTESTINAL DISORDERS

STRESS OF LIFESTYLE CHANGES

GI disorders may have profound effects on the psychosocial functioning of the affected individual. Moreover, these disorders may place great stress on the family who are attempting to cope with the demands of that person's illness. A teenager affected by a chronic GI disorder such as Crohn disease may be unable to participate in social eating activities and thus may feel isolated from peers. IBS in a young adult who is beginning the most productive years of life may curtail the ability to function fully in the roles of spouse, parent, and wage earner. Finally, the onset of GI disorders, particularly a neoplastic process, in a middle-aged or older individual may not only limit that person's ability to perform activities of daily living but may also bring about an increased awareness of aging and mortality. However, the meaning of a disorder of the GI tract, or any health problem, to a particular person will be highly individualized. Nutrition and bowel elimination are behaviors that are dependent on cultural norms; changes in these basic areas of human activity brought about by a GI disorder may have a variety of meanings to different individuals.

In the past, much of the health care literature, including nursing texts, tended to stereotype individuals experiencing chronic disorders of the GI tract as having abnormal mental functioning. Aberrant psychological characteristics, it was thought, were somehow associated with or even responsible for certain diseases of the GI tract, such as Crohn disease and ulcerative colitis. It is now recognized that although some chronic diseases of the GI tract may be aggravated by emotional factors, the pathogenic process is almost never the result of primarily psychological causes.[1,3] The stress of coping with a chronic, disabling illness may result in psychological trauma; in addition, any type of illness represents a threat to the integrity of the person. Individuals experiencing a chronic GI disorder may exhibit the psychological effects of such threats and will benefit from a sensitive approach to meeting their needs.

SUMMARY

This chapter has described the major alterations in the GI tract that may occur across the human life span. Because of the strong links between cultural and psychological functioning and activities associated with the GI tract, an in-depth understanding of these alterations is essential for health care professionals.

Disorders of the GI tract may have many manifestations, including dysphagia, pain, vomiting, gas, and alterations in bowel elimination patterns. Disorders may occur in any portion of the GI tract, from the mouth to the anus, and may be the result of alterations in the integrity of the GI tract wall (as in ulcerative colitis) or alterations in motility (as in IBS). Disorders of malabsorption, such as celiac disease, may seriously limit the individual's ability to utilize dietary nutrients and are therefore potentially life threatening. Patients who have undergone surgery on the GI tract may also be at risk for malabsorption. Neoplasms of the GI tract are prevalent in the U.S. population, and the reader will want to review the associated risk factors for these neoplasms very carefully. Finally, readers who are preparing for a career in health care should carefully consider the information provided on the psychosocial aspects of GI disorders and identify ways to provide optimal care for patients with these disorders.

MEDIA RESOURCES

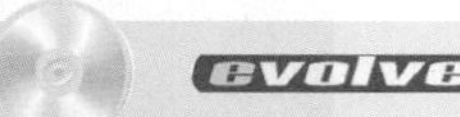

Remember to check out the ***CD Companion*** included with this book for Review Questions, Key Concepts Review, Glossary (with audio for selected terms), Disease Profiles, and Animations.

PLUS, visit the ***Evolve website*** at http://evolve.elsevier.com/Copstead/ for Case Studies, Disease Profiles, and WebLinks.

References

1. Avunduk C: *Manual of gastroenterology*, ed 3, Philadelphia, 2002, Lippincott Williams & Wilkins.
2. Gitnick G: *Current gastroenterology*, vol 14, St Louis, 1994, Mosby.
3. Feldman M, Friedman LS, Sleisenger MH: *Sleisenger and Fordtran's gastrointestinal and liver disease: pathophysiology, diagnosis, management*, ed 7, Philadelphia, 2002, Saunders.
4. Yamada T et al: *Textbook of gastroenterology*, ed 3, Philadelphia, 1999, Lippincott Williams & Wilkins.
5. Haubrich WS, Schaffner F, Berk JE: *Bockus gastroenterology*, ed 5, Philadelphia, 1995, Saunders.
6. Barrett KE: Mechanisms of inflammatory diarrhea, *Gastroenterology* 103(2):710-711, 1992.

7. Kneepkens CM, Hoekstra JH: Chronic nonspecific diarrhea of childhood: pathophysiology and management, *Pediatr Clin North Am* 43(2):375-390, 1996.
8. Scully C, Gorsky M, Lozada-Nur F: The diagnosis and management of recurrent aphthous stomatitis: a consensus approach, *J Am Dent Assoc* 134(2):200-207, 2003.
9. Perry HO: Idiopathic gingivostomatitis, *Dermatol Clin* 5(4):719-722, 1987.
10. Hillemeier AC: Gastroesophageal reflux: diagnostic and therapeutic approaches, *Pediatr Clin North Am* 43(1):197-212, 1996.
11. Weinberg DS, Kadish SL: The diagnosis and management of gastroesophageal reflux disease, *Med Clin North Am* 1996;80(2):411-429.
12. Vakil N: Gastroesophageal reflux disease and *Helicobacter pylori* infection, *Rev Gastroenterol Disord* 3(1):1-7, 2003.
13. Liu JY et al: Determining an appropriate threshold for referral to surgery for gastroesophageal reflux disease, *Surgery* 133(1):5-12, 2003.
14. Spechler SJ: Barrett's esophagus and esophageal adenocarcinoma: pathogenesis, diagnosis, and therapy, *Med Clin North Am* 86(6):1423-1445, vii, 2002.
15. Morales P, Baum AE: Therapeutic alternatives for the Mallory-Weiss tear, *Curr Treat Options Gastroenterol* 6(1):75-83, 2003.
16. Navarro VJ, Garcia-Tsao G: Variceal hemorrhage, *Crit Care Clin* 11(2):391-414, 1995.
17. Marshall B: Unidentified curved bacilli on gastric epithelium in active chronic gastritis, *Lancet* 1:1273-1274, 1983 (letter).
18. Malaty HM et al: Transmission of *Helicobacter pylori* infection: studies in families of healthy individuals, *Scand J Gastroenterol* 26:927-932, 1991.
19. Atherton JC: CagA, the cag pathogenicity island and *Helicobacter pylori* virulence, *Gut* 44:307-308, 1999.
20. Walsh JH, Peterson WL: The treatment of *Helicobacter pylori* infection in the management of peptic ulcer disease, *N Engl J Med* 333:984-991, 1995.
21. Kurata JH, Nogawa AN: Meta-analysis of risk factors for peptic ulcers: nonsteroidal anti-inflammatory drugs, *Helicobacter pylori,* and smoking, *J Clin Gastroenterol* 24:2-17, 1997.
22. Suerbaum S, Michetti P: Medical progress: *Helicobacter pylori* infection, *N Engl J Med* 347:1175-1186, 2002.
23. Shiotani A, Graham DY: Pathogenesis and therapy of gastric and duodenal ulcer disease, *Med Clin North Am* 86(6): 1447-1466, 2002.
24. Podolsky DK: Medical progress: inflammatory bowel disease, *N Engl J Med* 347:417-429, 2002.
25. Cosnes J et al: Smoking cessation and the course of Crohn's disease: an intervention study, *Gastroenterology* 120:1093-1099, 2001.
26. Lewis JD, Deren JJ, Lichtenstein GR: Cancer risk in patients with inflammatory bowel disease, *Gastroenterol Clin North Am* 28(2):459-477, 1999.
27. Hurley BW, Nguyen CC: The spectrum of pseudomembranous enterocolitis and antibiotic-associated diarrhea, *Arch Intern Med* 162(19):2177-2184, 2002.
28. Oliak D et al: Initial nonoperative management for periappendiceal abscess, *Dis Colon Rectum* 44(7):936-941, 2001.
29. Klein KB: Controlled treatment trails in irritable bowel syndrome: a critique, *Gastroenterology* 95:232-241, 1988.
30. Shils ME, Olson JA: *Modern nutrition in health and disease*, ed 8, Philadelphia, 1994, Lea & Febiger.
31. Loening-Baucke V: Encopresis, *Curr Opin Pediatr* 14(5): 570-575, 2002.
32. Kagnoff MF: Celiac disease: a gastrointestinal disease with environmental, genetic, and immunologic components, *Gastroenterol Clin North Am* 21(2):405-425, 1992.
33. Daly JM et al: *Gastrointestinal oncology*, Philadelphia, 2001, Lippincott Williams & Wilkins.
34. Chow WH et al: An inverse relation between cagA$^+$ strains of *Helicobacter pylori* infection and risk of esophageal and gastric cardia adenocarcinoma, *Cancer Res* 58:589-590, 1998.
35. Thun MJ et al: Aspirin use and risk of fatal cancer, *Cancer Res* 53(6):1322-1327, 1993.
36. Trowbridge B: Colorectal cancer screening, *Surg Clin North Am* 82(5):943-945, 2002.
37. Skibber JM, Minsky BD, Hoff PM: Cancer of the colon. In DeVita DT, Hellman S, Rosenberg SA, editors: *Cancer: principles and practice of oncology,* Philadelphia, 2001, Lippincott Williams & Wilkins.

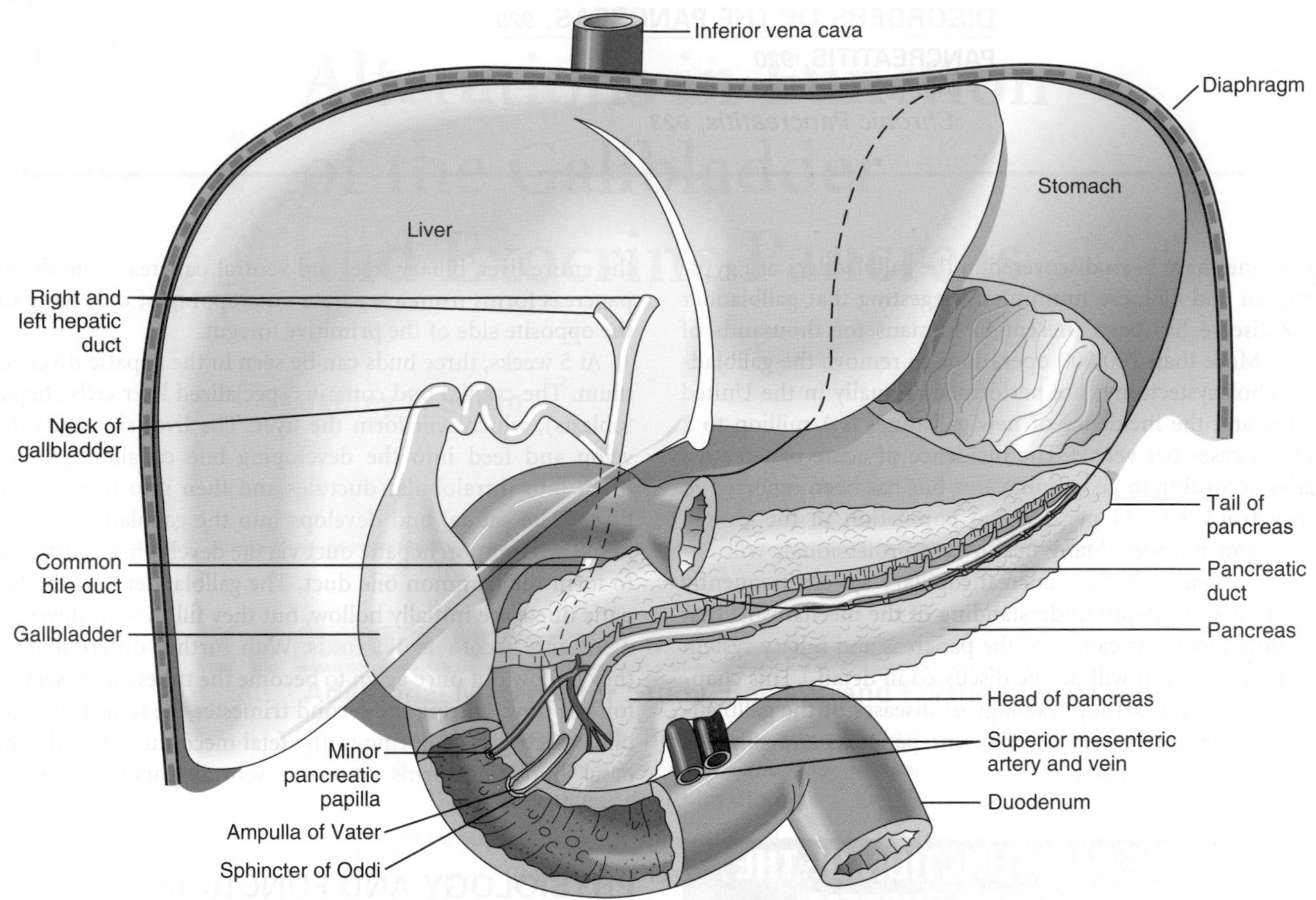

FIGURE 37-1 ■ Detailed physiology of the pancreaticobiliary system showing the anatomic placement of the gallbladder and pancreas, the junction of the common bile duct and the pancreatic duct in the ampulla, and the ampulla of Vater.

With the first morning meal, a hormonally and neurally regulated contraction of the gallbladder occurs, releasing the concentrated bile into the duodenum. Bile acids eventually will be absorbed again in the terminal ileum and travel by the portal circulation to be secreted again into the bile. (Bile acids are reabsorbed on average two or three times.) A small amount of the bile acid pool (less than 5%) enters the colon, where primary bile salts undergo bacterial transformation into secondary bile salts (Figure 37-3).[7]

After secretion into the bile, bile salts have dual properties, being **hydrophilic** (soluble in water) at one end and **hydrophobic** (insoluble in water) at the other. Thus, these molecules tend to aggregate into clusters called *micelles,* which surround lipids such as cholesterol and allow them to go into solution (Figure 37-4). Micelles are not good stabilizers of cholesterol alone, but another molecule, lecithin, also secreted in large amounts in the bile, is readily incorporated in the core of the micelle to greatly enhance the solubility of cholesterol. In this way, bile keeps cholesterol partly solubilized. Precipitation of cholesterol from bile occurs at high concentrations, predisposing to formation of gallstones.[7]

FUNCTIONAL ANATOMY OF THE PANCREAS

The pancreas is really two organs in one: it functions as both an endocrine and an exocrine organ. On the one hand, hormones such as insulin, glucagon, and somatostatin are produced and secreted into the vascular system (characteristic of an endocrine organ). On the other hand, every 24 hours the pancreas secretes more than 1 L of digestive juice into the digestive tract (characteristic of an exocrine organ).[6]

Embryologically, the pancreas is composed of two fused organs: a dorsal and a ventral pancreas (Figure 37-5). Microscopically, the pancreas is somewhat lobular and arranged into exocrine glands. The pancreatic juices are secreted into the glandular acini, which eventually drain into the main pancreatic duct and then enter the intestinal tract. The juices themselves are composed of both active digestive enzymes (e.g., amylase, lipase) and precursor or proenzymes (e.g., trypsinogen). Their release during a meal is controlled by hormones secreted from the small intestinal mucosa: **cholecystokinin** (CCK) and **secretin.** When this regulation is de-

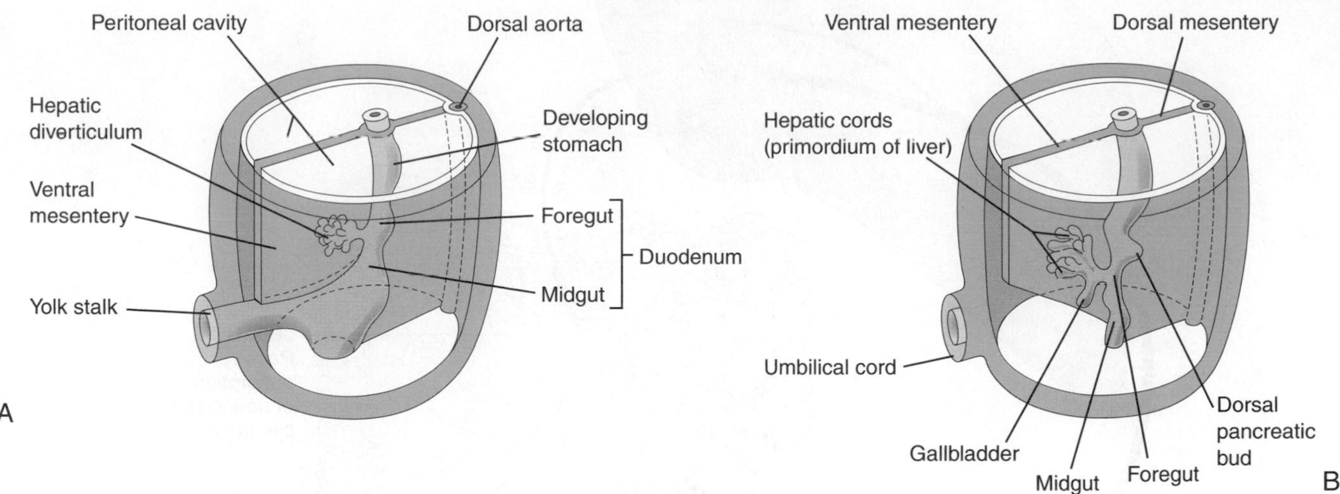

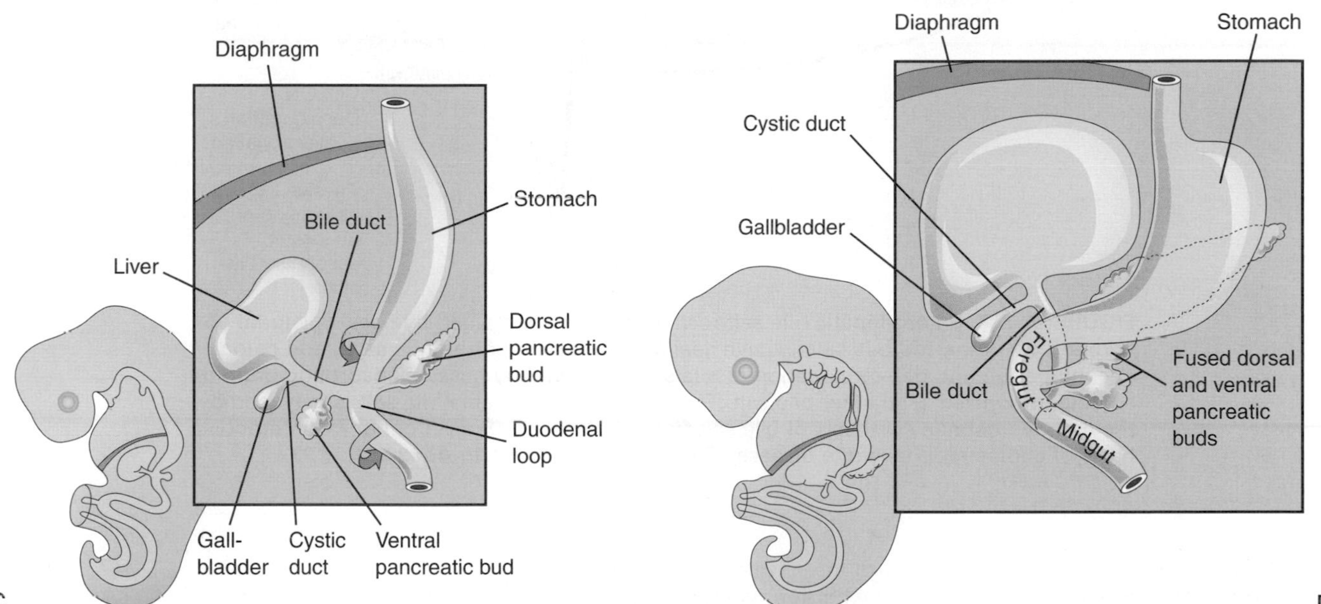

FIGURE 37-2 ■ Stages in the embryonic development of the liver, pancreas, and duodenum at 4 weeks **(A)**, 5 weeks **(B** and **C)**, and 6 weeks **(D)**. (From Moore KL, Persaud TVN: *The developing human: clinically oriented embryology*, ed 7, Philadelphia, 2003, Saunders, p 262.)

ranged, enzymes may be released within the gland and produce **acute pancreatitis.**

KEY CONCEPTS

- Bile is produced by hepatocytes in the liver and stored in the gallbladder. The main components of bile are bile acids, pigment, cholesterol, and phospholipids. Bile salts are important for digestion and absorption of fats from the small bowel. Bile is an important route for excretion of waste products, particularly bilirubin. The gallbladder receives bile from the liver, concentrates bile by absorbing water, and then contracts to expel stored bile into the common bile duct, which terminates in the duodenum.
- The pancreas is both an endocrine organ, secreting insulin, glucagon, and somatostatin into the blood stream, and an exocrine gland, secreting digestive juice into the duodenum. Some pancreatic enzymes are secreted in active form (amylase, lipase), whereas others are proenzymes that are activated in the duodenum (trypsinogen). Release of pancreatic enzymes is stimulated by cholecystokinin and secretin.

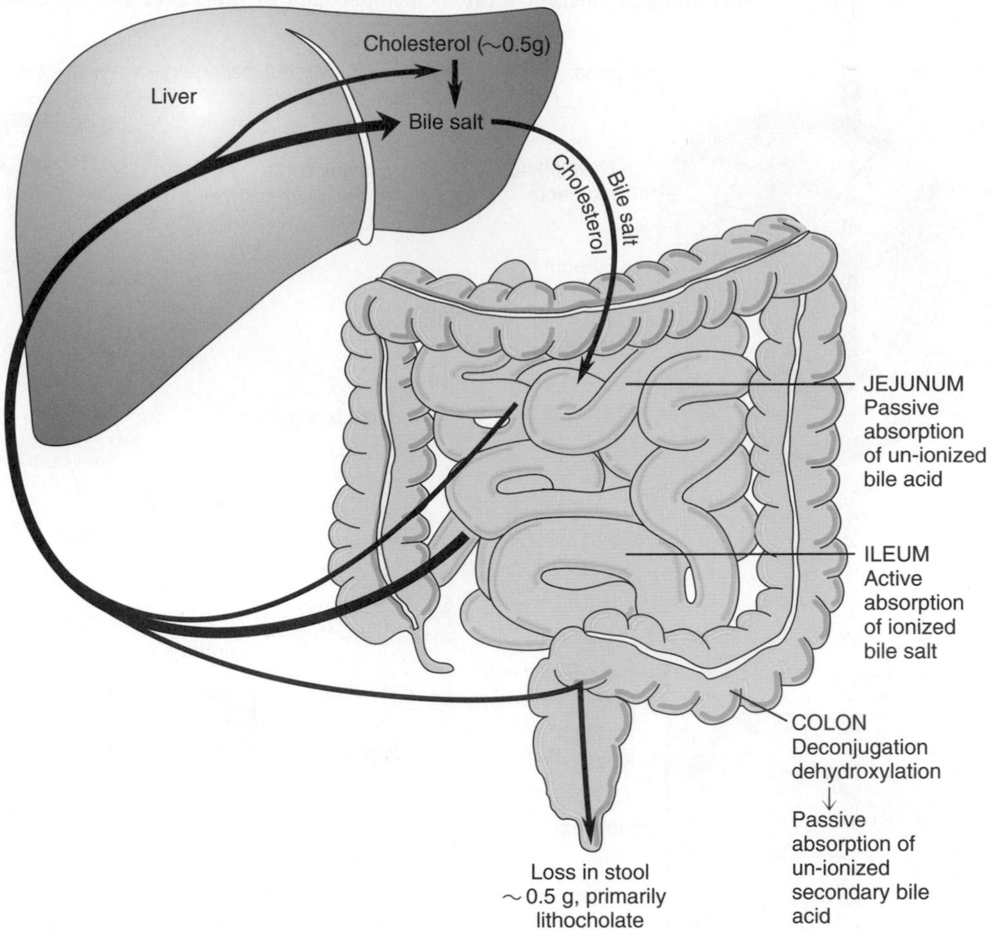

FIGURE 37-3 ■ Enterohepatic bile salt recirculation is maintained by passive jejunal absorption of un-ionized bile salts, active ileal absorption of ionized bile salts, and colonic deconjugation and dehydroxylation of bile salts followed by passive absorption of lipid-soluble un-ionized secondary bile salt. The loss of unabsorbable bile salt is balanced by the de novo hepatic synthesis of bile salt from cholesterol. (From Cooper AD: Metabolic basis of cholesterol gallstone disease, *Gastroenterol Clin North Am* 20:34, 1991.)

FIGURE 37-4 ■ Bile acid–lecithin–cholesterol mixed micelle. Polar ends of bile acid and lecithin are oriented outward, whereas hydrophobic, nonpolar portions make up the interior. Cholesterol is solubilized within the hydrophobic, nonpolar center. (From Saunders KD, Cates JA, Roslyn JJ: Pathogenesis of gallstones, *Surg Clin North Am* 70:1197-1216, 1990.)

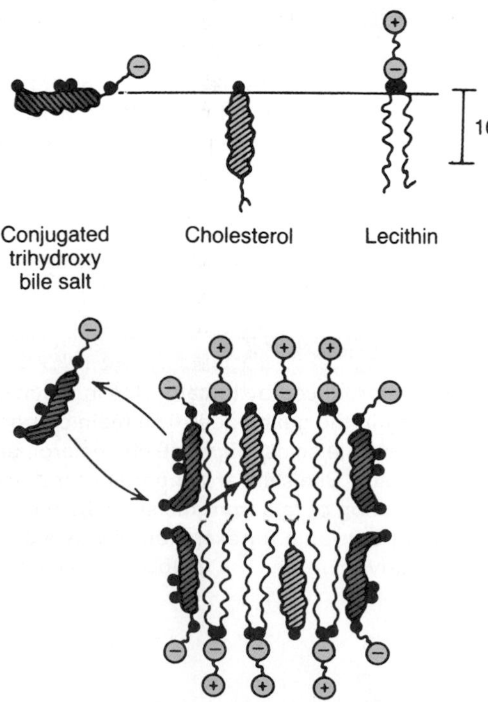

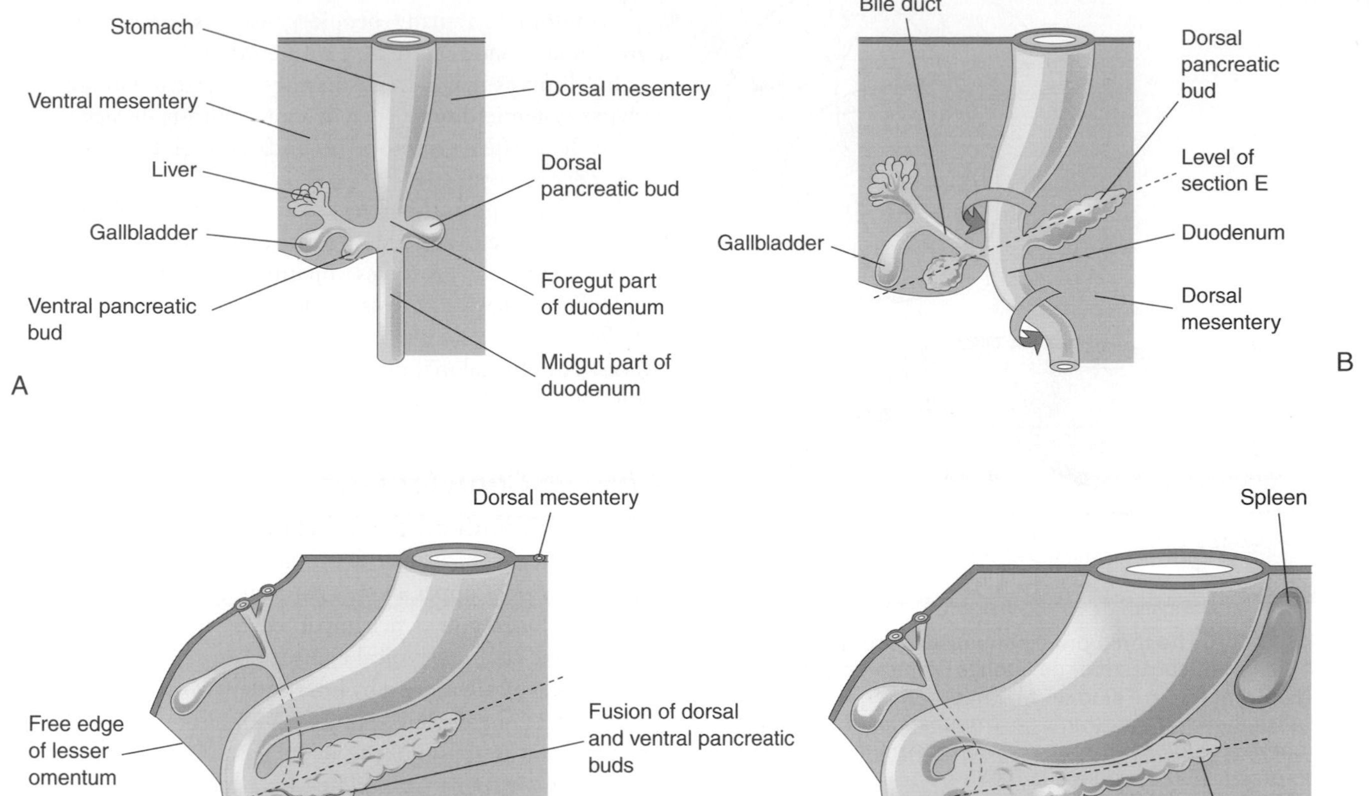

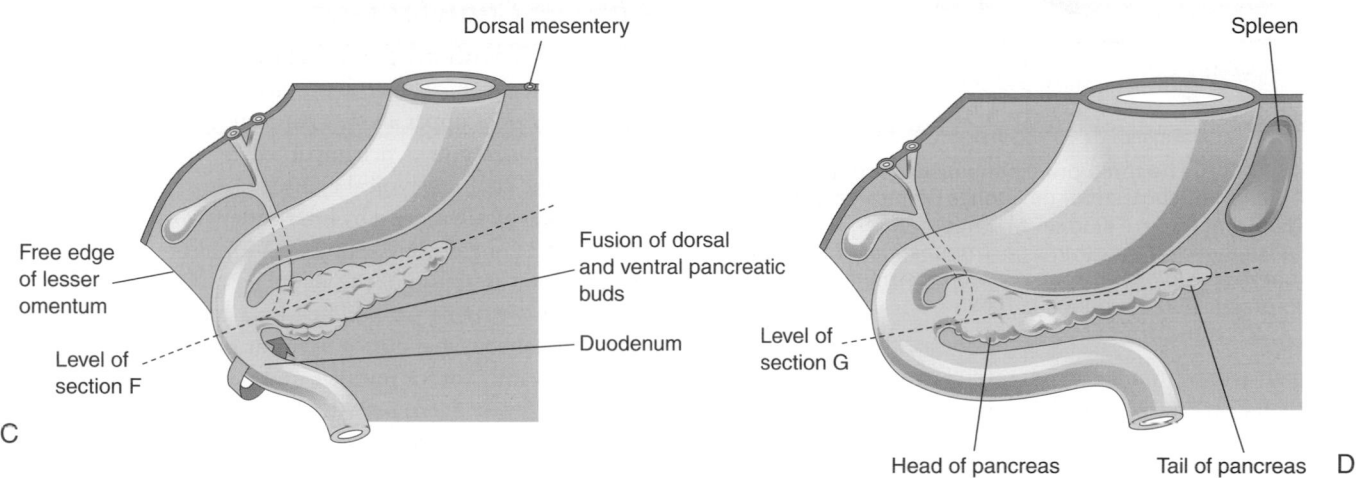

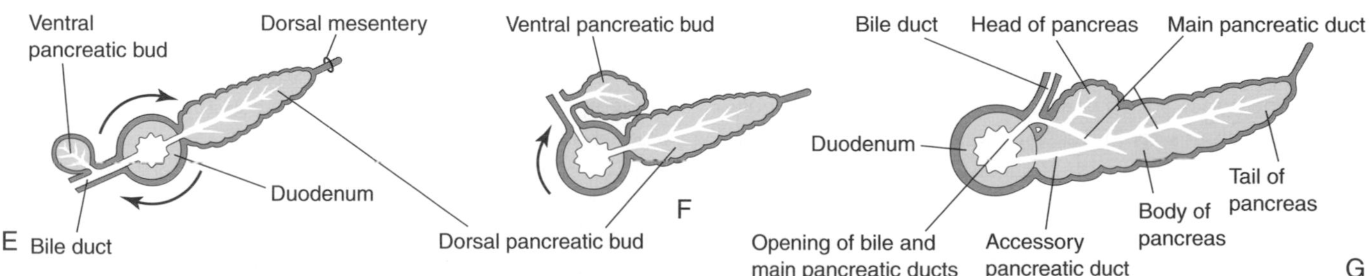

FIGURE 37-5 ■ Stages in the embryonic development of the pancreas from the fifth to eighth week **(A-D)** and a diagram of the progressive development of the bile duct and main pancreatic duct **(E-G)**. (From Moore KL, Persaud TVN: *The developing human: clinically oriented embryology,* ed 7, Philadelphia, 2003, Saunders, p 267.)

DISORDERS OF THE GALLBLADDER

PATHOPHYSIOLOGY OF CHOLESTEROL GALLSTONE FORMATION

The majority of gallstones among patients in the United States are cholesterol stones.[1] In general, the formation of cholesterol stones in the gallbladder (**cholelithiasis**) can be broken down into three phases: (1) supersaturation of bile with cholesterol; (2) nucleation of crystals; and (3) hypomotility allowing stone growth (Figure 37-6).

As described previously, cholesterol eventually precipitates from supersaturated bile. If conditions are right for the formation of cholesterol gallstones, nucleation occurs in which the cholesterol crystals aggregate together. Continued growth of the crystals then becomes a balance between cholesterol growth–promoting factors and factors that tend to cause stone dissolution. A significant factor that promotes the con-

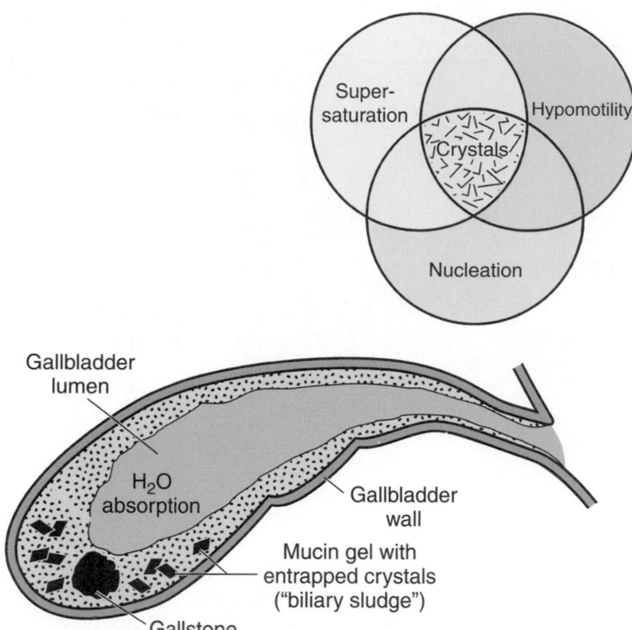

FIGURE 37-6 ■ The three principal phases responsible for the formation of cholesterol gallstones illustrated with a Venn diagram. (From Feldman M, Friedman LS, Sleisenger MH: *Sleisenger and Fordtran's gastrointestinal and liver disease: pathophysiology, diagnosis, management,* ed 7, Philadelphia, 2002, Saunders, p 1069.)

tinued growth of stones is hypomotility or stasis of bile within the gallbladder. **Stasis** in this context means a condition of inactivity or staying. Patients with high spinal cord injuries are at particular risk for development of cholesterol gallstones. Pregnancy, oral contraceptives, obesity, diabetes mellitus, and octreotide therapy are also associated with impaired emptying and cholelithiasis.[1]

About 25% of gallstones in westernized countries are due to pigment stones, which contain a mixture of pigment polymers and calcium salts. "Black" pigment stones are most common and are associated with cirrhosis and hemolysis, or they may be idiopathic. "Brown" pigment stones differ in their composition and are much more common in developing countries, where they are associated with biliary parasitosis and bacterial colonization and infection.[1]

CHOLELITHIASIS AND CHOLECYSTITIS

Currently, about 20 million people in the United States have gallstones (cholelithiasis). The incidence of gallstones is related to age, sex, and a variety of medical factors. Gallstones are twice as common in women as in men. Native Americans, particularly the Pima Indians of North America, are markedly susceptible to gallstones, American Caucasians somewhat less so. European Caucasians are intermediate in prevalence, and persons of Asian descent are at lowest risk. Obesity correlates with the development of gallstones, but so does rapid weight loss in an obese individual. However, the presence of gallstones does not necessarily mean that an individual will have any symptoms. In many people gallstones are completely asymptomatic and require no treatment.[8]

Cholelithiasis in children is usually associated with an underlying systemic disease such as cystic fibrosis or sickle cell disease. It is often symptomatic and requires treatment by gallbladder removal.

The term **cholecystitis** refers to inflammation of the gallbladder wall. The continued presence of gallstones in the gallbladder ultimately promotes inflammatory changes in the gallbladder wall, with fibrosis and thickening.[9] Cholecystitis is classified as acute or chronic, according to its clinical manifestations. The clinical manifestations of each are described, followed by diagnostic and treatment methods.

Chronic Cholelithiasis

Clinical Manifestations. The chief complaint of most patients with chronic cholelithiasis is biliary colic, a persistent epigastric or right upper abdominal pain. Often the pain radiates to the back and is accompanied by nausea, vomiting, sweating, and flatus. A typical episode lasts several hours. Biliary colic is typically caused by intermittent obstruction of the cystic duct by a gallstone (Figure 37-7), although some authorities point to spasm of the sphincter of Oddi as etiologic.

Symptoms may be precipitated by a meal, but they often occur spontaneously and may occur at night. The pain often increases steadily for 15 minutes and persists for an hour or more, then slowly decreases. Attacks may recur on a frequent or infrequent schedule. Patients often describe additional symptoms, including fatty food intolerance, belching, flatus, bloating, and epigastric burning.[8]

Diagnosis and Treatment. The diagnosis of chronic cholelithiasis depends on imaging studies, particularly ultrasonography, and is essentially the same as that described for acute cholecystitis.

In cases of chronic cholelithiasis with no or very few recurrent symptoms, "watchful waiting" may be considered.[8,9] However, patients with significant recurrences of biliary colic are candidates for one of the three current modes of treatment for cholecystitis: cholecystectomy (surgical removal of the gallbladder), chemical dissolution of gallstones, or lithotripsy (mechanical breaking up of gallstones within the gallbladder). These will be discussed in more detail in the section on acute cholecystitis.

Acute Cholecystitis

Clinical Manifestations. Acute cholecystitis is defined as acute inflammation of the gallbladder wall. It is characterized by severe right upper abdominal pain that may radiate to the back. Abdominal tenderness and fever are often present. The pathogenesis of acute cholecystitis is not well understood. Cholelithiasis is present in about 90% of patients. Obstruction of the cystic duct is present in almost all cases, suggesting that

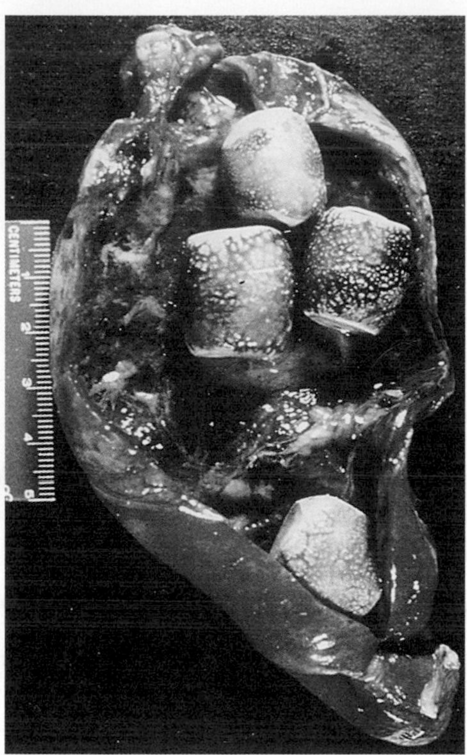

FIGURE 37-7 ■ Chronic cholecystitis demonstrated by a thickened gallbladder wall and luminal cholesterol stones. (From Cotran RS, Kumar V, Collins T: *Robbins pathologic basis of disease,* ed 6, Philadelphia, 1999, Saunders, p 897.)

stasis of bile in the gallbladder is important in the pathogenesis of the disease. Bacterial infection may also be present in acute cholecystitis, although it is not thought to be the direct cause of the inflammatory process. If left untreated, the inflammatory process will escalate, and rupture of the gallbladder may occur. Laboratory evaluation may reveal leukocytosis, mild jaundice, and, occasionally, elevated amylase levels.[9,10]

Acalculous cholecystitis is an important subgroup of acute cholecystitis. It tends to occur in the setting of major surgery, critical illness, trauma, or burn-related injury. The patients tend to be predominantly male and older than 50 years, and total parenteral nutrition (TPN) is a common cofactor. It carries a somewhat more serious implication than stone-associated cholecystitis, in part because of the associated medical conditions. In fact, gangrene of the gallbladder wall and perforation, emphysematous cholecystitis, and **empyema** all develop more rapidly than in calculous cholecystitis.[1]

Diagnosis. Evaluation for possible cholecystitis includes an appropriate history and physical examination, laboratory studies, and an imaging study designed to evaluate the gallbladder and biliary tree. Ultrasound of the abdomen is the procedure of choice early in the diagnostic evaluation. Typically, the ultrasound scan reveals the presence of stones, occasionally in the cystic duct, as well as thickening of the gallbladder wall and distention of the lumen. It may also point to another diagnosis of right upper quadrant pain, such as a liver neoplasm or hydronephrosis of the kidney. The sensitivity and specificity of ultrasound for stones larger than 2 mm in diameter approach 95%.[10] Sensitivity rates for acalculous cholecystitis are somewhat lower.[11]

However, the presence of cholelithiasis and a thickened gallbladder wall are not definitive evidence of cholecystitis, and other diagnostic tests are used on occasion. Hepatobiliary scintigraphy by hydroxyiminodiacetic acid (HIDA) provides a good functional assessment of gallbladder excretion, which is markedly impaired with cholecystitis. Computed tomography (CT) and endoscopic retrograde cholangiopancreatography (ERCP) are useful for selected cases. The latter carries a risk of perforation and pancreatitis, and so is reserved for cases requiring intervention (stent placement, etc.), biopsy, or special contrast studies.

Treatment. Treatment for cholecystitis depends on the severity of symptoms and the patient's clinical status. Acute cholecystitis may necessitate intervention, but surgeons generally prefer to allow a "hot" gallbladder to "cool down" before performing surgery. Percutaneous catheter drainage or endoscopic drainage with stent placement may be performed to relieve obstruction, particularly if infection is involved. If the patient's condition precludes surgery, these may be the main treatments, and drains can be left in place indefinitely. Advanced acute cholecystitis complicated by empyema, gangrene, or emphysematous change is a surgical emergency.

Laparoscopic cholecystectomy was first performed in 1987 and since then has been popularized by the rapid development of video **laparoscopy** instrumentation. The procedure is usually performed with four small incisions through which instruments are inserted. The gallbladder is freed either by electrosurgical or by laser excision and is then withdrawn through one of the small incisions. Advantages of the laparoscopic technique include less postoperative pain than after laparotomy and small incision size, which allows rapid return to daily activities. In addition, patients do not require a lengthy hospital stay following the procedure.[12] Laparoscopic cholecystectomy is now the treatment of choice for symptomatic gallstones.

Open cholecystectomy was first performed in the 19th century and remains an extremely safe operation with low morbidity and mortality. However, the length of the incision and accompanying postoperative pain render many patients extremely immobile after the procedure. Altered anatomy or scarring from previous surgery or the presence of common bile duct stones may necessitate a traditional cholecystectomy. A laparoscopic procedure may be converted to an open one intraoperatively if necessary (e.g., upon finding a malignant tumor in the vicinity of the gallbladder). Complications of cholecystectomy can include infection, inadvertent transection of the common bile duct, and the rare but debilitating syndrome of recurrent sclerosing cholangitis.

Some patients, such as elderly or debilitated persons, may be poor surgical risks and cannot undergo the stress of surgery.[13] Nonoperative methods to manage gallstones, such as **chemodissolution** with a variety of bile acids or organic solvents and **lithotripsy,** have been tried as alternatives to surgery. Chemodissolution is the use of chemical substances, such as bile acids or organic solvents, to dissolve gallstones. Such agents as chenodeoxycholic acid (CDCA), a secondary bile salt, are administered orally. However, this approach has several major drawbacks, including diarrhea in about 50% of patients and a low overall efficacy. Extracorporeal shock wave lithotripsy (ESWL), which involves the breaking up of gallstones using shock waves, is another nonsurgical approach. The objective is to fragment stones into pieces small enough to be passed through the cystic duct, or small enough to allow dissolving agents to work. ESWL is safe and relatively effective, under proper circumstances. The disadvantages include strict selection criteria (e.g., stones less than 2 cm in diameter), resulting in a low percentage of eligible patients. The gallbladder also is left in place, allowing for possible recurrence of gallstones and necessitating the concurrent use of dissolving agents such as CDCA to prevent new stone formation.

For the most part, in the near future the management of gallstone disease is likely to remain surgical, with traditional or laparoscopic cholecystectomy being the major forms of intervention.

Chronic Cholecystitis

Clinical Manifestations. Chronic cholecystitis is defined as chronic inflammation of the gallbladder wall due to persistent low-grade irritation from gallstones or to recurrent attacks of acute cholecystitis. Diabetes mellitus and obesity are important predisposing factors. Although many patients suffer from intermittent biliary colic or have symptomatic acute attacks, a surprising number of patients experience no symptoms. Chronic cholecystitis may lead to many of the complications described above for acute cholecystitis, including biliary sepsis, as well as a specific type of scarring known as a calcified or "porcelain" gallbladder, which is associated with a higher risk of cancer.[1]

KEY CONCEPTS

- Lecithin is an important component of bile that helps keep cholesterol from precipitating into crystals. Crystals of cholesterol may initiate gallstone formation. The relative concentrations of cholesterol, lecithin, and bile acids appear to determine the likelihood of cholesterol gallstone formation. Bile hypomotility or stasis contributes to growth of cholesterol stones.
- Gallstones occur more frequently in women than in men. Ethnicity, obesity, and rapid weight loss are predisposing factors. Gallstones may be asymptomatic or associated with symptomatic cholecystitis. Colicky pain due to intermittent obstruction of the cystic duct by a stone is the chief complaint. Symptoms of chronic cholecystitis include epigastric or right upper quadrant pain radiating to the back, nausea, vomiting, sweating, fat intolerance, bloating, and flatus.
- Acute cholecystitis is acute inflammation of the gallbladder associated with abdominal pain, leukocytosis, and fever. Cholelithiasis is present in about 90% of patients; obstruction of the cystic duct is present in nearly all patients.
- Treatment for cholecystitis includes surgical removal of the gallbladder (cholecystectomy), chemodissolution, ESWL (lithotripsy) for stones, antibiotics if indicated, and management of pain. Cholecystectomy is the mainstay of therapy.

DISORDERS OF THE PANCREAS

PANCREATITIS

Acute Pancreatitis

Etiology and Pathogenesis. Acute **pancreatitis** is an inflammatory process involving the pancreas that may range from mild to severe and life-threatening. After an attack, the exocrine and endocrine functions of the pancreas may remain impaired for a variable period. Pancreatitis affects between 1 and 5 per 10,000 persons in the United States annually. Predisposing factors for pancreatitis have been well known for more than 100 years (Box 37-1); in the United States the most

Box 37-1

Conditions Predisposing to Acute Pancreatitis

Gallstones
Biliary sludge and microlithiasis
Other causes of mechanical ampullary obstruction
Alcohol
Hypertriglyceridemia
Hypercalcemia
Drugs
Infections and toxins
Trauma
Pancreas divisum
Vascular disease
Pregnancy
Post-ERCP
Postoperative pancreatitis
Hereditary pancreatitis
Structural abnormalities
- Duodenum/ampullary region
- Bile duct
- Sphincter of Oddi dysfunction
- Main pancreatic duct

From Feldman M, Friedman LS, Sleisenger MH: *Sleisenger and Fordtran's gastrointestinal and liver disease: pathophysiology, diagnosis, management*, ed 7, Philadelphia, 2002, Saunders, p 914.
ERCP, Endoscopic retrograde cholangiopancreatography.

common causes are biliary tract disease and ethanol-associated pancreatitis.[1] Although the exact mechanisms leading to pancreatitis are not fully understood, three possible pathways are known (Figure 37-8). The most prominent factor is obstruction of the pancreatic duct by a stone or other cause (usually unknown), with release of digestive enzymes within the parenchyma, followed by enzyme activation and then autodigestion of the pancreas.[14] Edema leading to vascular insufficiency and ischemic injury is a contributing factor. Other possible mechanisms include acinar cell injury from alcohol or drugs, trauma, or viral infection; and defective intracellular transport of proenzymes within acinar cells.

Up to 66% of first cases of pancreatitis are associated with alcoholism.[15] While there is clearly an association of alcohol with pancreatitis, the causal mechanism has not been determined. Transient increases in pancreatic exocrine secretion, contraction of the sphincter of Oddi, and direct toxic effects on acinar cells have all been postulated from experimental studies. Many authorities now think that most cases of alcoholic pancreatitis are sudden exacerbations of chronic pancreatitis, presenting as apparent de novo acute pancreatitis.[14] According to this view, chronic alcohol ingestion causes secretion of protein-rich pancreatic fluid, leading to deposition of inspissated protein plugs and obstruction of small pancreatic ducts, followed by the train of events described above. However, other pathologic studies show no evidence of chronic pancreatitis in up to 40% of acute alcoholic pancreatitis patients.[16]

Clinical Manifestations. The presentation of acute pancreatitis usually begins with steady, boring pain in the epigastrium or left upper quadrant, which gradually increases in intensity. It often radiates or penetrates through to the back and is accompanied by nausea and vomiting. Tenderness on palpation may be exquisite. Bowel sounds are reduced but not absent. Abdominal distention may be present. Fever is common but is usually low grade initially. In more severe pancreatitis, this clinical picture is accompanied by signs of circulatory instability, respiratory insufficiency, and, occasionally, shock.[17]

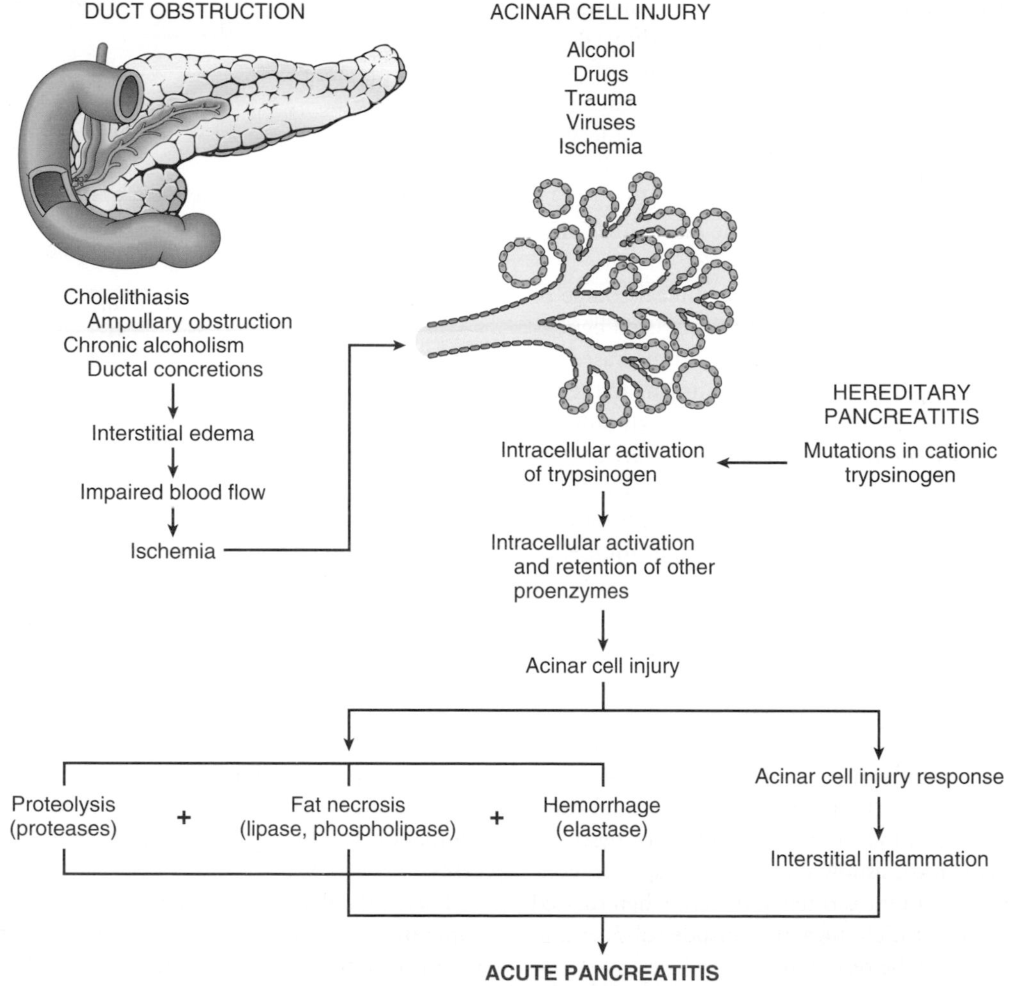

FIGURE 37-8 ■ Three proposed pathways in the pathogenesis of acute pancreatitis. (From Kumar V, Cotran RS, Robbins SL: *Basic pathology,* ed 7, Philadelphia, 2003, Saunders, p 638.)

Diagnosis. The laboratory evaluation of acute pancreatitis begins with measurements of serum pancreatic enzymes. Serum lipase and amylase levels rise more or less in tandem during the first 12 hours and remain elevated for several days. Lipase is more specific and persists longer, and therefore has become the preferred test for most clinicians. Serum aminotransferases (aspartate aminotransferase, alanine aminotransferase) may also be elevated. Marked elevation of the alkaline phosphatase and bilirubin levels also suggest the possibility of biliary disease or obstruction, particularly by gallstones. Associated laboratory findings include leukocytosis, hyperlipidemia (which may be marked), and hypocalcemia.[1,9]

The diagnosis of acute pancreatitis is based on the signs and symptoms, laboratory data, and imaging studies of the pancreas and surrounding organs. Radiographs of the abdomen may reveal an ileus pattern or the "sentinel loop" (a distended loop of small bowel in the area of the pancreas). Ultrasound can provide a bedside technique to visualize the pancreas, gallbladder, common bile duct, and other abdominal structures, but is limited by poor image resolution due to bowel gas. Computed tomography (CT) of the abdomen is the gold standard for evaluation of the pancreas and allows depiction of the pancreas in remarkable detail, including edema and abscess or cyst formation as well as the degree of peripancreatic involvement. The differential diagnosis of acute pancreatitis includes perforated peptic ulcer, acute cholecystitis, mesenteric vascular disease, and a variety of other illnesses (some associated with elevated amylase levels) (Box 37-2), most of which may be differentiated on the basis of CT and other radiographic tests.

Grading systems allow prediction of the clinical course of acute pancreatitis. Ranson's criteria are a widely used benchmark for prognostic assessment, but modifications based on CT scoring may be more reliable.[18] Early monitoring in the intensive care unit is indicated for patients with a high number of risk factors. One particularly important finding on contrast CT is the presence of significant pancreatic necrosis. Acute necrotizing pancreatitis carries a high risk for progression to infected pancreatic necrosis, a devastating complication with a high morbidity and mortality.

Box 37-2

Causes of Increased Serum Amylase Activity

Pancreatic diseases
- Acute pancreatitis
- Complications of pancreatitis
- Acute exacerbation of chronic pancreatitis
- Pancreatic tumors, cysts

Other serious intraabdominal diseases
- Acute cholecystitis
- Common bile duct obstruction
- Perforation of esophagus, stomach, small bowel, or colon
- Intestinal ischemia or infarction
- Intestinal obstruction
- Acute appendicitis
- Acute gynecologic conditions such as ruptured ectopic pregnancy and acute salpingitis

Diseases of salivary glands
- Mumps
- Effects of alcohol

Tumors
- Ovarian cysts
- Papillary cystadenocarcinoma of ovary
- Carcinoma of lung

Renal insufficiency

Macroamylasemia

Miscellaneous
- Morphine
- Endoscopy
- Sphincter of Oddi stenosis or spasm
- Anorexia nervosa
- Head trauma with intracranial bleeding
- Diabetic ketoacidosis
- Human immunodeficiency virus

From Feldman M, Friedman LS, Sleisenger MH: *Sleisenger and Fordtran's gastrointestinal and liver disease: pathophysiology, diagnosis, management,* ed 7, Philadelphia, 2002, Saunders, p 914.

Treatment. Conservative management is indicated for mild to moderate cases of acute pancreatitis. In general, withholding oral feedings, providing nasogastric suction for significant adynamic ileus, and providing careful volume replacement with IV fluids are indicated. Analgesics are administered parenterally. All narcotics should be used carefully because of the potential of sphincter of Oddi dysfunction, although recent studies show that no single agent is contraindicated.[19] This treatment is often sufficient when carried out for 3 to 7 days, after which the acute episode subsides and oral intake may gradually be resumed.

Severe pancreatitis, particularly in the setting of acute necrotizing pancreatitis, may result in multisystem organ dysfunction, requiring aggressive support in the intensive care unit setting. Nutritional deficits develop rapidly with extensive catabolism (tissue breakdown) and lack of caloric intake; total parenteral nutrition is usually indicated with pancreatitis of more than a few days duration or if complications arise.[7] Additional supportive measures include calcium administration to reverse severe hypocalcemia, correction of magnesium deficiency, and control of hyperglycemia. Causes of death from severe pancreatitis include respiratory failure (usually associated with the adult respiratory distress syndrome), acute renal failure, and acute intraabdominal sepsis. Mechanical ventilation and hemodialysis may be required in complicated cases.

Bacterial infection is a critical determinant of poor outcome in acute necrotizing pancreatitis. Some authorities advocate prophylactic broad-spectrum antibiotics directed to common pathogens such as *Escherichia* and *Klebsiella* species, although definitive studies are lacking.[1] In the patient with fever and signs of sepsis, empiric antibiotics should be begun, and any significant fluid collections found on CT should be aspirated for culture and sensitivity.

Abscess or hemorrhage may complicate pancreatitis with or without significant pancreatic necrosis and may necessitate surgical intervention. Open laparotomy with debridement of devitalized tissue and major pancreatic resection (pancreatectomy) are the main surgical options.[20] Drains are typically left in place postoperatively, and repeated debridement may be needed to remove infective debris and necrotic tissue.

Localized complications of acute pancreatitis may result in prolonged morbidity for the patient. The most common localized complication is pancreatic **pseudocyst.** This is a collection of fluid within or adjacent to the pancreas that often has a direct communication to the pancreatic duct. It is called a pseudocyst because, unlike a true cyst, it contains no epithelial lining. A pseudocyst can develop rather acutely or more subacutely, as the patient recuperates from the acute illness. The presentation often includes fever, tachycardia, and an abdominal mass and tenderness. Complications of pseudocysts include infection (usually termed an "infected pseudocyst," as opposed to the pancreatic abscess described above), spontaneous rupture, or hemorrhage. Management of pseudocyst includes endoscopic or surgical drainage of the cyst, either externally or internally, usually into the stomach or bowel.[1,20]

Pancreatic ascites may occur and may represent a persistent leak in the main pancreatic duct. It is usually painless and often massive. The fluid may find its way into unusual places, including the pleural space and mediastinum.[21] Pancreatic ascites may be detected by ultrasonography or CT, and diagnosis is confirmed by analysis of fluid obtained by aspiration, in particular the amylase level. Management is often conservative, with prolonged parenteral nutrition. Improvement may occur following the endoscopic placement of a stent (a thin-walled tube) into the main pancreatic duct.

Other complications of acute pancreatitis include common bile duct obstruction, portal or splenic vein thrombosis, peptic ulcer disease, and chronic fistula formation.

Endoscopic treatment may be carried out for gallstone pancreatitis in selected cases. Indications for *urgent* ERCP with ampullotomy (incision of the ampulla) include biliary sepsis, recalcitrant severe pancreatitis, and jaundice.[1] In milder cases, traditional conservative therapy followed by elective ERCP is acceptable. The risks of ERCP include exacerbation of pancreatitis, and so the need for this procedure must be carefully considered.

Chronic Pancreatitis

Etiology and Pathogenesis. Chronic pancreatitis is defined histologically as the presence of chronic inflammatory lesions in the pancreas, and in practice is persistence of symptoms secondary to pancreatic dysfunction over weeks and months. Destruction of exocrine parenchyma and fibrosis precedes the destruction of endocrine parenchyma. After a variable time most patients with chronic pancreatitis develop calcifications that become visible on radiologic films of the abdomen or CT. Chronic pancreatitis is most often associated with alcohol consumption, although a small percentage of cases are idiopathic, hereditary, or associated with hyperparathyroidism (hypercalcemia), trauma, or various other factors.[1,14]

The association of alcohol ingestion with chronic pancreatitis is profound. Autopsy studies have shown that the changes of chronic pancreatitis are present in 45% of alcoholics, even those without symptoms, and that this rate is 40 to 50 times higher than that in nondrinkers.[1,9] Exactly how alcohol causes chronic pancreatitis is not known (see the previous discussion of alcohol and acute pancreatitis). One recent theory suggests that the initial factors include an increase in the protein concentration in pancreatic juice coupled with reduction in a specific "pancreatic stone protein" that inhibits the formation of pancreatic protein plugs.[22] This biochemical situation allows the formation of protein plugs that can later calcify, in addition to causing obstruction to the flow of pancreatic juice. A key element seems to be necrosis, followed by fibrosis, perhaps analogous to cirrhosis of the liver. Another facet of alcohol-associated pancreatitis is its tendency to progress after alcohol consumption is stopped.

Clinical Manifestations. The presentation of chronic pancreatitis often includes bouts of acute pancreatitis with progressive signs of persistent pancreatic dysfunction. Alternatively, an insidious onset of pain in the epigastrium that radiates to the back may be the first symptom. About 10% to 15% of patients will not present with pain but rather with the sequelae of chronic pancreatitis, including diabetes mellitus, malabsorption, and weight loss.[23] The mortality is 3% to 4% per year. Interestingly, the incidence of pancreatic carcinoma does not appear to be substantially increased in patients with chronic pancreatitis.

The pain of chronic pancreatitis is often the major form of debility. Nerve fibers from the pancreas pass to the celiac plexus and then to spinal sympathetic ganglia. The events that actually trigger the pain are not well understood. There may be a relation to ductal pressures or possibly to ischemia in the pancreas. The pain is often accompanied by nausea and is steady and boring in nature. The pain is usually located in the upper abdomen, particularly in the epigastrium, and radiates to the back in more than half of cases. In alcoholic pancreatitis, continued drinking affords temporary anesthesia but may foster recurrences of pain. Cessation of drinking may allow for a better long-term prognosis. After about 5 years of continual pain, many patients note a decrease in the symptoms (i.e., the pain "burns out").

Endocrine and exocrine pancreatic insufficiency lead to diabetes mellitus, malabsorption, and weight loss. Diabetes mellitus arises from progressive loss of acinar cells and usually requires exogenous insulin administration; diabetic ketoacidosis and nephropathy are unusual findings. Weight loss may be aggravated by poor intake as a result of pancreatic pain.

Malabsorption of fat does not occur until pancreatic enzyme output drops to 10% of normal. Along with the malabsorption of fat, the absorption of fat-soluble vitamins (A, D, E, and K) may be impaired, leading to coagulopathy and night vision problems.

Further complications of chronic pancreatitis are similar to those of acute pancreatitis and include pseudocyst, pancreatic ascites, and obstruction of the common bile duct. Obstruction of the bile duct may lead to elevated values on liver function tests and the need to intervene either surgically or endoscopically. Alkaline phosphatase and bilirubin levels may become markedly elevated if obstruction is severe. Unusual complications include thrombosis of the portal and splenic veins. This may lead to gastrointestinal hemorrhage from gastric varices.[17] Peptic ulcer disease is also increased in patients with chronic pancreatitis, although a definite causal relationship has not been established.

Diagnosis. The diagnosis of chronic pancreatitis is usually suggested by the clinical history, physical examination findings, and routine blood chemical analyses. Biochemical studies of pancreatic function may be helpful. Confirmation of the diagnosis is aided by plain radiographs showing calcifications in the area of the pancreas. Abdominal ultrasound or CT is usually performed with reasonable sensitivities and specificities. ERCP is reserved for suspicious cases that cannot be confirmed by other techniques, or for cases in which biopsy or cytologic examination are necessary to rule out malignancy.[1] It shows the pancreatic duct to range from almost normal in early cases, to markedly dilated or beaded—the "chain of lakes" appearance (Figure 37-9). A common finding is truncation of the secondary branches of the pancreatic duct.

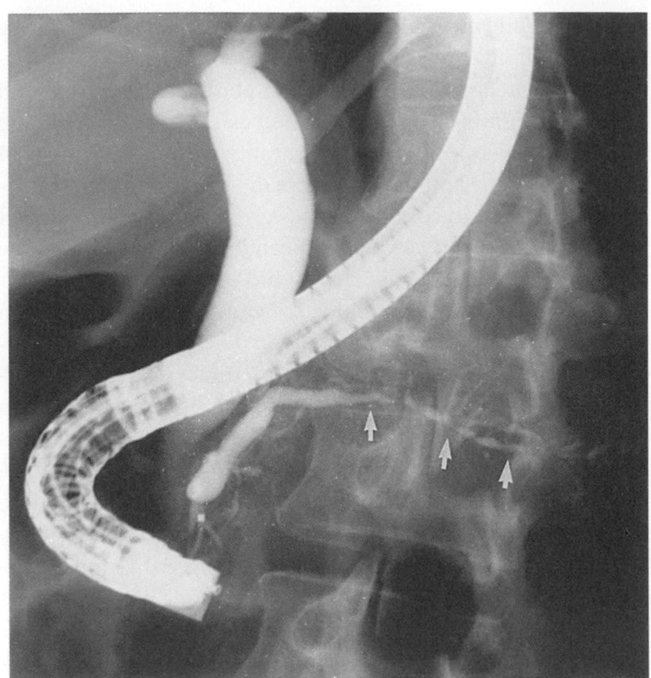

FIGURE 37-9 ■ Endoscopic retrograde cholangiopancreatogram in a patient with chronic pancreatitis shows marked narrowing and irregularity of the main pancreatic duct body and tail. (From Feldman M, Scharschmidt BF, Sleisenger MH: *Sleisenger and Fordtran's gastrointestinal and liver disease: pathophysiology, diagnosis, management,* ed 6, Philadelphia, 1998, Saunders, p 952.)

Treatment. The treatment for chronic pancreatitis is directed toward pain control, exocrine and endocrine insufficiency, and management of complications. By far the most challenging is the management of pain. Absolute abstention from alcohol is paramount to prevent worsening of symptoms. For almost 40 years, analgesics and surgical intervention have been the mainstay of pain control, and celiac plexus block is helpful for some patients. With the advent of ERCP, less drastic forms of intervention are now possible. Pancreatic sphincterotomy is indicated for the management of single or multiple stones. Endoscopic drains may be placed for pseudocysts of the pancreas if they are adjacent to the stomach or duodenum. Obstruction of the common bile duct can be managed with endoscopically placed biliary stents. Strictures of the main pancreatic duct can be managed with indwelling pancreatic stents.[24]

If endoscopic management fails or is not appropriate in a given patient, surgery may be indicated. A Puestow procedure, which allows drainage of the pancreas, involves opening the main pancreatic duct and reducing intraluminal pressure and pain. Distal pancreatectomy may be helpful if there is a large midduct stricture that will not stay open after pancreatic stenting. As with management of acute pancreatitis, the judgment of the surgeon is paramount to prevent the catastrophic complications that can result from surgery on the pancreas.

Pancreatic enzyme therapy has been used for the management of chronic pain based upon hypothetical grounds and a series of favorable reports.[1] As proteases (e.g., trypsin, chymotrypsin, and elastase) exert a controlling influence on pancreatic secretion, feedback regulation should result in relief of pain following oral administration of pancreatic enzymes. Unfortunately, only 20% to 30% of patients with the typical alcohol-induced type of disease respond to such therapy. Responses seem to be higher in patients with small-duct disease. Pancreatic enzyme replacement has become a standard therapy for chronic pancreatitis. Research has also been undertaken on octreotide, a synthetic long-acting analog of somatostatin that has been shown to inhibit CCK release and both basal and neural-stimulated pancreatic secretion.[1] Disappointingly, controlled trials of treatment with pancreatic supplements and with octreotide show mixed results, and further work is clearly needed.

Management of exocrine insufficiency can usually be accomplished with low-fat diets and pancreatic enzyme supplementation. Likewise, endocrine insufficiency in the form of diabetes mellitus is managed with diet and either oral hypoglycemic agents or insulin.[7]

KEY CONCEPTS

- Acute pancreatitis is commonly associated with biliary tract disease and excessive ethanol ingestion. Activation of pancreatic proenzymes to active forms within the pancreas leads to autodigestion and inflammation of the gland. The manifestations of acute pancreatitis may be mild or severe and include a steady, boring pain in the epigastrium or left upper quadrant, nausea, vomiting, a tender abdomen, reduced bowel sounds, and fever. In severe cases, circulatory shock may occur. Elevated serum amylase and lipase levels are indicative of pancreatitis.
- Management of acute pancreatitis is aimed at reducing pancreatic secretion. Because chyme entering the duodenum is the primary stimulus for pancreatic secretion, food is withheld and nasogastric suctioning may be instituted. Complications of acute pancreatitis include hyperglycemia, nutritional deficit, and pancreatic hemorrhage, infection, abscess formation, or necrosis. Antibiotics, fluid management, total parenteral nutrition, and insulin may be indicated to manage complications.
- Chronic pancreatitis is closely associated with alcohol use. Acute pancreatitis due to biliary obstruction rarely progresses to chronic pancreatitis. Chronic pancreatitis results in progressive destruction of endocrine and exocrine function. Manifestations of chronic pancreatitis are more insidious than those of acute pancreatitis. Epigastric pain, diabetes mellitus, malabsorption, and weight loss may be the presenting problems.
- The complications of chronic pancreatitis are similar to those of acute pancreatitis. Therapy is directed to pain control, amelioration of endocrine and exocrine deficiency, and monitoring for and management of complications. Surgery to correct obstruction of the pancreatic duct may be performed. Pancreatic enzyme therapy may be helpful in reducing pain by providing negative feedback, which reduces pancreatic secretion.

SUMMARY

The pancreaticobiliary system is central to the digestion of food because it provides necessary digestive enzymes and lipid-emulsifying agents that allow the intestine to absorb nutrients. This chapter has considered alterations in the function of the gallbladder and exocrine pancreas. A major disease of the pancreaticobiliary system is the formation of cholesterol gallstones, which can lead to acute and chronic cholecystitis and acute and chronic pancreatitis. New forms of surgical and nonsurgical interventions for the management of gallstone disease have become available in the past few years, with conventional open surgery remaining a useful option. These interventions, as well as interventions for acute and chronic pancreatitis, are currently the focus of much clinical research.

MEDIA RESOURCES

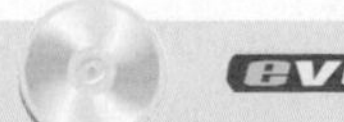

Remember to check out the ***CD Companion*** included with this book for Review Questions, Key Concepts Review, Glossary (with audio for selected terms), Disease Profiles, and Animations.

PLUS, visit the ***Evolve website*** at http://evolve.elsevier.com/Copstead/ for Case Studies, Disease Profiles, and WebLinks.

References

1. Yamada T et al: *Textbook of gastroenterology,* ed 3, Philadelphia, 1999, Lippincott Williams & Wilkins.
2. Avunduk C: *Manual of gastroenterology,* ed 3, Philadelphia, 2002, Lippincott Williams & Wilkins.
3. Go VLW, Everhart JE: Pancreatitis. In Everhart JE, editor: *Digestive diseases in the United States: epidemiology and impact,* NIH Publication No. 94-1447, Washington, DC, 1994, US Department of Health and Human Services.
4. Moore KL, Persaud TVN, Chabner DE: *The developing human: clinically oriented embryology,* Philadelphia, 2003, Saunders.
5. Moore KL, Persaud TVN, Shiota K: *Color atlas of clinical embryology,* ed 2, Philadelphia, 2000, Saunders.
6. Guyton AC, Hall JE: *Textbook of medical physiology,* ed 10, Philadelphia, 2000, Saunders.
7. Shils ME, Olson JA: *Modern nutrition in health and disease,* ed 8, Philadelphia, 1994, Lea and Febiger.
8. Goroll AH, Mulley AG: *Primary care medicine,* ed 3, Philadelphia, 2000, Lippincott Williams & Wilkins.
9. Feldman M, Friedman LS, Sleisenger MH: *Sleisenger and Fordtran's gastrointestinal and liver disease: pathophysiology, diagnosis, management,* ed 7, Philadelphia, 2002, Saunders.
10. Shea JA et al: Revised estimates of diagnostic test sensitivity and specificity in suspected biliary tract disease, *Arch Intern Med* 154(22):2573-2581, 1994.
11. Mirvis SE et al: The diagnosis of acute acalculous cholecystitis: a comparison of sonography, scintigraphy, and CT, *AJR Am J Roentgenol* 147(6):1171-1175, 1986.
12. Orlando R, Russell JC: Managing gallbladder disease in a cost-effective manner, *Surg Clin North Am* 76:117-128, 1996.
13. Behrman SW et al: Laparoscopic cholecystectomy in the geriatric population, *Am Surg* 62:386-390, 1996.
14. Cotran RS, Kumar V, Collins T: Robbins pathologic basis of disease, ed 6, Philadelphia, 1999, Saunders.
15. Laoser C, Faolsch UR: A concept of treatment in acute pancreatitis: results of controlled trials and future developments, *Hepatogastroenterology* 40:569-573, 1993.
16. Renner IG, Savage WE, Pantoja JL, Renner VJ. Death due to acute pancreatitis: a retrospective analysis of 405 autopsy cases, *Dig Dis Sci* 30(10):1005-1018, 1985.
17. Clochesy JM et al: *Critical care nursing,* Philadelphia, 1996, Saunders.
18. Chatzicostas C et al. Computed tomography severity index is superior to Ranson criteria and Apache II and III scoring systems in predicting acute pancreatitis outcome, *J Clin Gastroenterol* 36(3):253-260, 2003.

19. Thompson DR: Narcotic analgesic effects on the sphincter of Oddi: a review of the data and therapeutic implications in treating pancreatitis, *Am J Gastroenterol* 96(4):1266-1272, 2001.
20. Townsend CM et al: *Sabiston textbook of surgery: the biological basis of modern surgical practice,* ed 15, Philadelphia, 2001, Saunders.
21. Maringhini A, Ciambra M, Patti R: Ascites, pleural, and pericardial effusions in acute pancreatitis, *Dig Dis Sci* 41:848-852, 1996.
22. Yamedera K, Moriyama T, Makino I: Identification of immunoreactive pancreatic stone protein in pancreatic stone, pancreatic tissue and pancreatic juice, *Pancreas* 5(3):255-260, 1990.
23. Haubrich WS, Schaffner F, Berk JE: *Bockus gastroenterology,* ed 5, Philadelphia, 1995, Saunders.
24. Treacy PJ, Worthley CS: Pancreatic stents in the management of chronic pancreatitis, *Aust N Z J Surg* 66:210-213, 1996.

chapter 38

Liver Diseases

Jeffrey S. Sartin

MEDIA RESOURCES

Additional Material for Study, Review, and Further Exploration

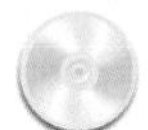

CD Companion ◆ Review Questions and Answers ◆ Key Concepts Review
◆ Glossary *(with audio pronunciations for selected terms)*
◆ Disease Profiles ◆ Animations

evolve *Website* at http://evolve.elsevier.com/Copstead/
◆ Case Studies ◆ Disease Profiles ◆ WebLinks

KEY QUESTIONS

- What role does the liver play in nutrient metabolism, bile synthesis, storage of vitamins and minerals, urea synthesis, clotting factor synthesis, and detoxification?
- Which manifestations of liver disease are due to hepatocellular failure and which are due to portal hypertension?
- How do the different types of viral hepatitis vary with regard to mode of transmission and severity of symptoms?
- What clinical and laboratory findings would lead to a diagnosis of liver cirrhosis?
- What treatment modalities are available to patients with end-stage liver failure?

CHAPTER OUTLINE

The liver is a vital but vulnerable organ. Its role in digestion of fats, storage of sugars, blood detoxification, and protein production makes it indispensable; in contrast to the kidney and heart, there are no "artificial livers." Nevertheless, the liver is susceptible to a wide variety of metabolic, circulatory, toxic, microbial, and neoplastic insults. In some instances the disease is primary to the liver, as in viral hepatitis and hepatocellular carcinoma (HCC). More often the hepatic involvement is secondary, a consequence of some of the more common diseases of humans, such as cardiac decompensation, metastatic cancer, alcoholism, and infections. This chapter will focus on primary diseases of the liver.

STRUCTURE AND FUNCTION OF THE LIVER

The liver, the largest parenchymal organ of the body, averages 1500 g. It is located in the right upper quadrant of the abdomen, beneath the diaphragm, and is commonly divided into a right and left lobe but may be further subdivided according to the pattern of its blood supply and biliary drainage. It is covered by a connective tissue capsule, the Glisson capsule, which in turn is covered by visceral peritoneum, reflections of which form the various suspensory hepatic ligaments. These structures demarcate the bare area of the liver directly in contact with the diaphragm (Figure 38-1).[1-3]

The liver has a dual blood supply. Arterial inflow from the aorta via the celiac trunk and hepatic artery provides 25% of the organ's blood supply. The remainder comes from the portal vein, which drains the capillary bed of the alimentary canal and pancreas (Figure 38-2). This oxygen-depleted venous blood is rich in substances absorbed and secreted by the gut. These afferent blood vessels then branch throughout the liver in association with the bile ducts and form the portal triads (consisting of the portal veins, hepatic arteries, and bile ducts). Eventually, blood from both the hepatic artery and the

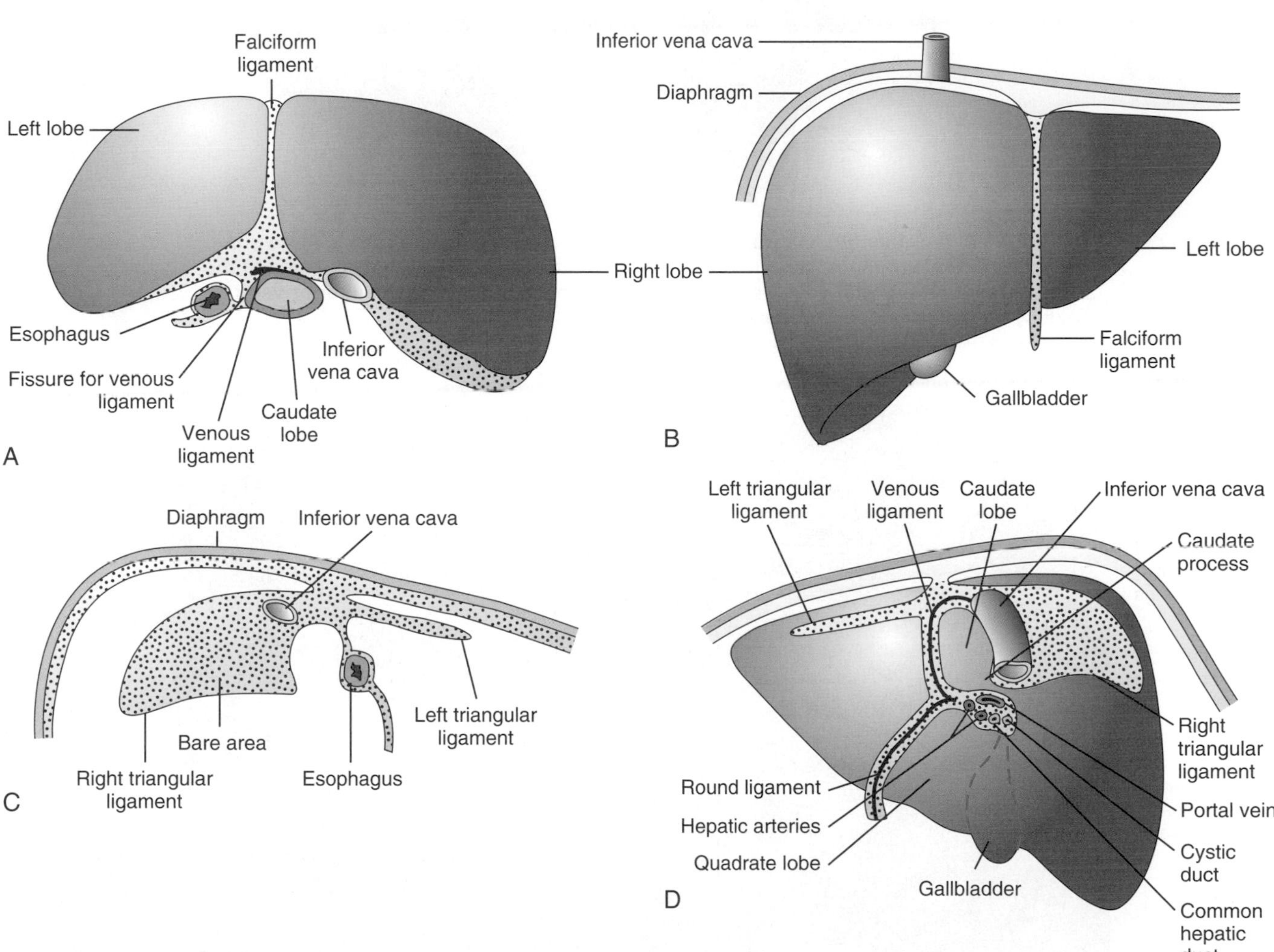

FIGURE 38-1 ■ The liver and its peritoneal relations. *Stippled areas* represent surfaces not covered with peritoneum. **A,** Superior view. **B,** Anterior view. **C,** The diaphragm, viewed from in front, showing the position of the bare area of the liver. **D,** Visceral surface of the liver, viewed from behind. (Redrawn from Gardner E, Gray DJ, O'Rahilly R: *Anatomy: a regional study of human structure,* ed 3, Philadelphia, 1969, Saunders, p 414.)

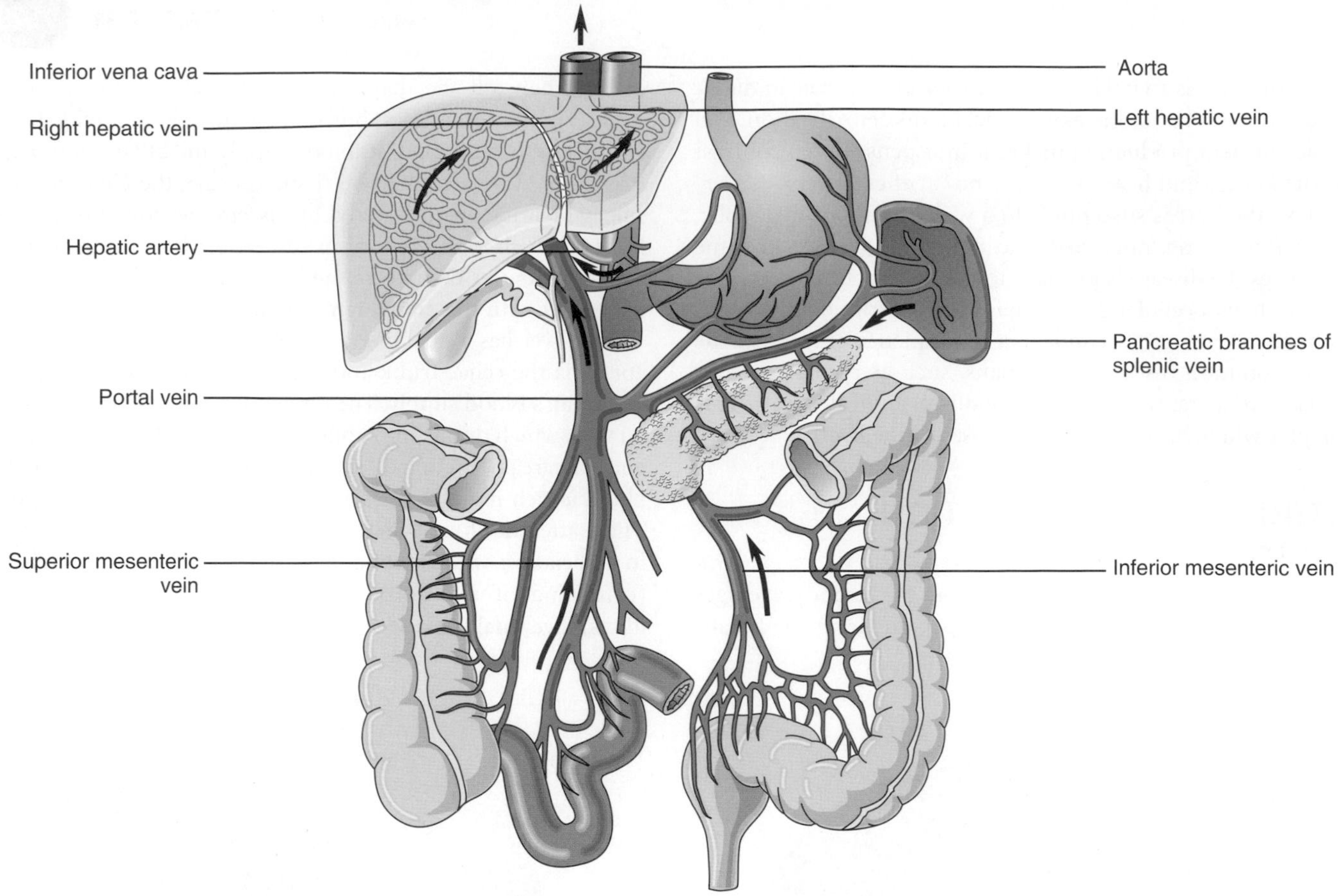

FIGURE 38-2 ■ Schematic diagram of the portal circulation. Blood from the aorta supplies the alimentary canal. Venous blood from the intestine reaches the sinusoids of the liver by way of the portal vein. Venous blood from the liver reaches the inferior vena cava by way of the hepatic veins.

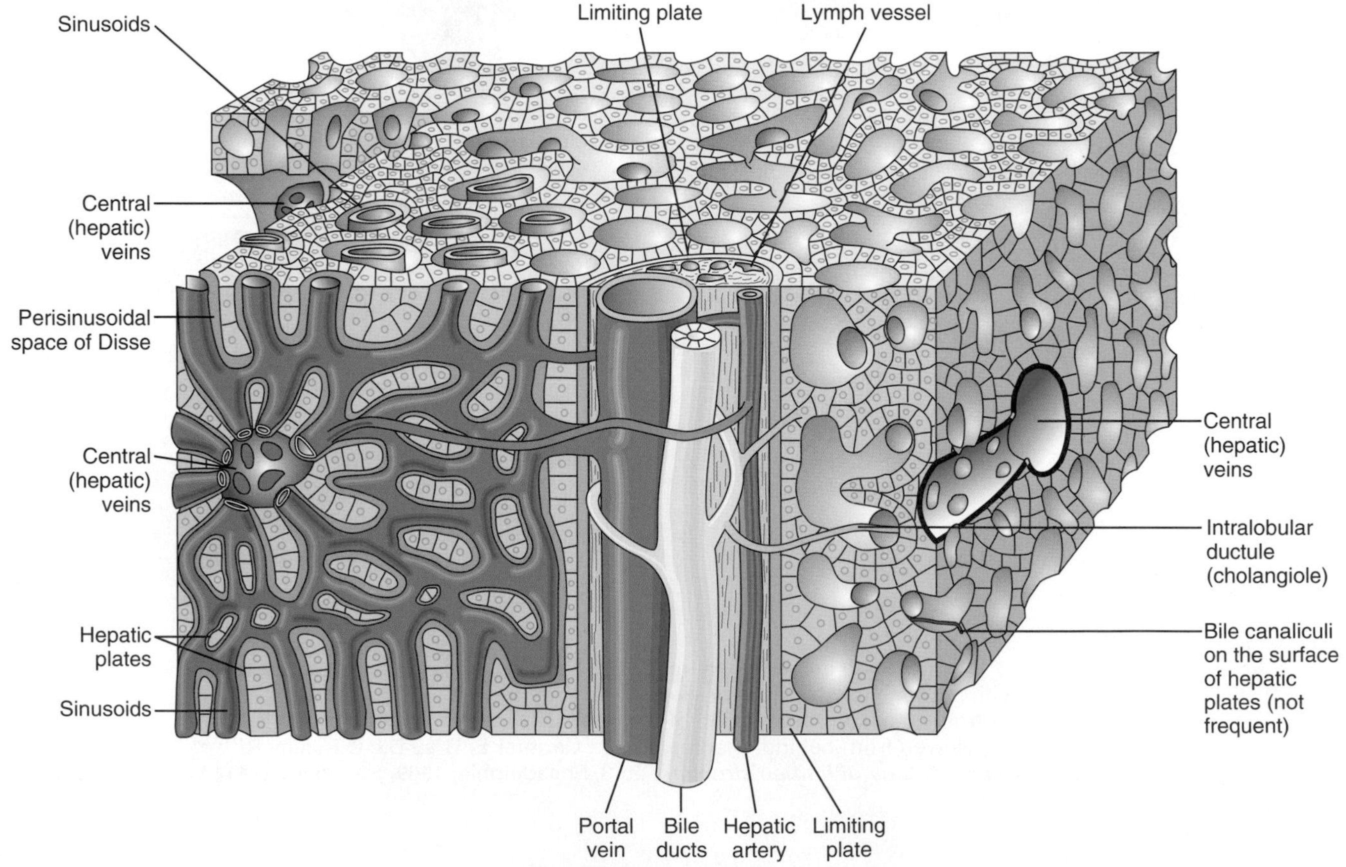

FIGURE 38-3 ■ Liver lobule.

portal vein drains into the hepatic sinusoids, which surround sheets of liver cells, or hepatic plates (Figure 38-3). The sinusoids are lined by endothelial cells and Kupffer cells (a type of phagocytic macrophage). This blood drains into the central veins, which finally coalesce into the hepatic vein and empty into the inferior vena cava. Any obstruction to the flow of blood may result in a rise in portal venous pressure proximal to the level of blockage. This condition is called **portal hypertension** and is a central pathophysiologic event in many liver diseases. The liver also has a rich and complex lymphatic drainage system.

The liver is one of the most metabolically active organs in the body and functions simultaneously as a digestive organ, an endocrine organ, a hematologic organ, and an excretory organ (Box 38-1). All of these functions are elegantly interwoven with such redundancy that more than 80% of the liver may be destroyed before life is threatened.

GENERAL MANIFESTATIONS OF LIVER DISEASE

Whether primary or secondary, all hepatic derangements tend to cause similar signs and symptoms that are directly attributable to loss of hepatocellular function or disruption of blood flow through the liver. Because of the liver's considerable reserve, however, manifestations appear only when the injury is significant and diffuse or so strategically located that it obstructs biliary outflow.

Box 38-1

Summary of Normal Liver Function

The Liver as Digestive Organ
- Bile salt secretion for fat digestion
- Processing and storage of fats, carbohydrates, and proteins absorbed by the intestines
- Processing and storage of vitamins and minerals

The Liver as Endocrine Organ
- Metabolism of glucocorticoids, mineralocorticoids, and sex hormones
- Regulation of carbohydrate, fat, and protein metabolism

The Liver as Hematologic Organ
- Temporary storage of blood
- Synthesis of bilirubin from blood breakdown products
- Hematopoiesis in certain disease states
- Synthesis of blood clotting factors

The Liver as Excretory Organ
- Excretion of bile pigment
- Excretion of cholesterol via bile
- Urea synthesis
- Detoxification of drugs and other foreign substances

Hepatocellular Failure

Hepatocellular failure results in a number of typical manifestations, including jaundice, muscle wasting, bleeding, hypoalbuminemia, glucose imbalance, osteomalacia, and feminization (Table 38-1). At its most basic the liver is a sophisticated biochemical factory, and these conditions all derive from problems with processing the essential molecules of the body. Inadequate protein metabolism leads to decreased production of clotting factors and hypoalbuminemia. Decreased serum albumin in turn leads to generalized edema as a result of low serum oncotic pressure. Abnormal storage and release of glucose in the form of glycogen may result in bouts of either hyperglycemia or hypoglycemia. Reduced production of bile salts by the liver impairs absorption of the fat-soluble vitamins A, D, E, and K from the gastrointestinal (GI) tract. Lack of vitamin D may lead to osteomalacia; lack of vitamin K contributes to poor blood clotting factor production. Altered lipoprotein processing leads to dyslipidemias, particularly hypertriglyceridemia.

Hepatocellular failure is associated with impaired processing of endogenous steroid hormones and the byproducts of protein metabolism, as well as decreased clearance of exogenous drugs and toxins. Impaired metabolism of estrogen leads to feminization in men (gynecomastia, impotence, testicular atrophy, female hair distribution), irregular menses in women, palmar erythema, and spider telangiectasia. Impaired conversion of ammonia to urea may lead to hepatic encephalopathy, which will be discussed further later in this chapter.

Jaundice

Etiology and Pathogenesis. Jaundice, the green-yellow staining of tissues by bilirubin, results from impaired bilirubin metabolism and is one of the most characteristic signs of liver disease. A study of the pathophysiologic mechanism of bilirubin metabolism is essential to an understanding of liver disease and may serve as a paradigm for other hepatic processes (Figure 38-4).[4-6]

As red blood cells age or are damaged by disease, they lyse and release the oxygen-carrying hemoglobin molecule. They are taken up by the reticuloendothelial system, which separates heme from globin and through the action of heme oxygenase opens the heme ring to release the central iron atom. This process yields biliverdin, which in turn is converted by the enzyme bilirubin reductase to bilirubin. (A small percentage of bilirubin is derived from immature cells in the bone marrow and spleen and from heme proteins such as myoglobin and the cytochromes in the liver.) Bilirubin is released into the plasma and transported to the liver tightly bound to the plasma protein albumin. The free unconjugated bilirubin is lipid soluble and can be displaced from albumin by fatty acids and certain organic anions (e.g., sulfonamides, salicylates). The neonate is particularly sensitive to free unconjugated

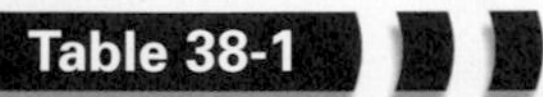

Pathophysiology Underlying the Symptoms and Signs of Liver Disease

Symptoms/Signs	Pathophysiologic Mechanism
Weakness, fatigue, anorexia, weight loss, muscle wasting	Failure of multiple metabolic functions
Fever	Liver inflammation, decreased reticuloendothelial function with increased risk of infection
Bruising, increased bleeding	Thrombocytopenia secondary to splenic enlargement; decreased synthesis of clotting factors I, II, V, VII, VIII, IX, X
Palmar erythema, cutaneous spider telangiectases, irregular menses, gynecomastia, impotence, female body hair distribution in men, testicular atrophy	Altered metabolism of sex hormones, chronic debilitation
Hepatic encephalopathy	Abnormal protein metabolism
Fetor hepaticus	Decreased detoxification
Pruritus	Decreased bile salt excretion
Cyanosis	Arteriovenous shunts in lungs, liver
Jaundice	Biliary obstruction, decreased bilirubin synthesis, decreased bilirubin excretion
Hyperdynamic circulation, wide pulse pressure, tachycardia	Generalized vasodilation (? Hormonally mediated)
Ascites, peripheral edema	Portal hypertension, sodium and water retention, low serum albumin secondary to decreased hepatic synthesis
Splenomegaly	Portal hypertension
Hepatomegaly	Cirrhosis (liver may be small), hepatitis, vascular congestion, bile duct obstruction, infection, benign infiltrative disease (e.g., fatty liver, amyloid, hemochromatosis), malignant infiltrative disease (e.g., metastatic cancer, lymphoma, large space-occupying lesions such as neoplasm, abscess)
Varices (esophageal, gastric, rectal, ectopic) or abnormal abdominal vascular pattern (caput medusae, umbilical bruit)	Portal hypertension with collateral blood flow around hepatic block
Osteomalacia, hypocalcemia, night blindness, coagulopathy	Fat-soluble vitamin malabsorption and loss of fat-soluble vitamin reserves A, D, and K; loss of vitamin K metabolism (a cofactor for I, II, VII, VIII, IX, and X)
Anemia	Multifactorial: blood loss, chronic disease, vitamin B_{12} deficiency, splenic sequestration
Leukopenia	Hypersplenism secondary to portal hypertension
Hypoglycemia	Altered glycogenolysis, gluconeogenesis
Hyperglycemia	Portosystemic shunting with delayed hepatic uptake of absorbed glucose
Hypercholesterolemia	Obstructive jaundice with decreased cholesterol excretion

bilirubin, which can diffuse into the brain and cause a type of encephalopathy known as **kernicterus** (see Liver Diseases and Pediatric Considerations).

Liver cells are able to extract unconjugated bilirubin from the plasma with special transport proteins. In the cytosol, bilirubin is quickly bound, or conjugated, to water-soluble derivatives of glucuronic acid by action of the enzyme uridine diphosphate glucuronosyltransferase (UDPGT) located in the endoplasmic reticulum. This process yields water-soluble bilirubin monoglucuronide and diglucuronide, which is then actively excreted into microscopic bile ducts (canaliculi). Bilirubin is then transported through the biliary system as a component of bile to the small intestine. Because it cannot be absorbed in the small intestine, it passes to the colon where bacterial β-glucuronidase enzymes break it down to urobilinogen. A small fraction of urobilinogen is absorbed from the colon and reexcreted by the kidneys and the liver. In the presence of liver disease, the hepatic fraction decreases and the urinary fraction increases, thus accounting for the rise in urinary urobilinogen seen with liver dysfunction. With complete obstruction to bile flow or with intestinal obstruction above the colonic level, urinary urobilinogen falls to zero, as no bilirubin reaches the colon. (The function of bile salts and the other components of bile flow are discussed in Chapter 37.)

Therefore, jaundice may result from dysfunction anywhere along this complex pathway. Classically, it is divided into prehepatic, hepatic, and posthepatic or cholestatic, but much overlap occurs.

Prehepatic. The most common causes of prehepatic jaundice are hemolysis and ineffective erythropoiesis. The resorp-

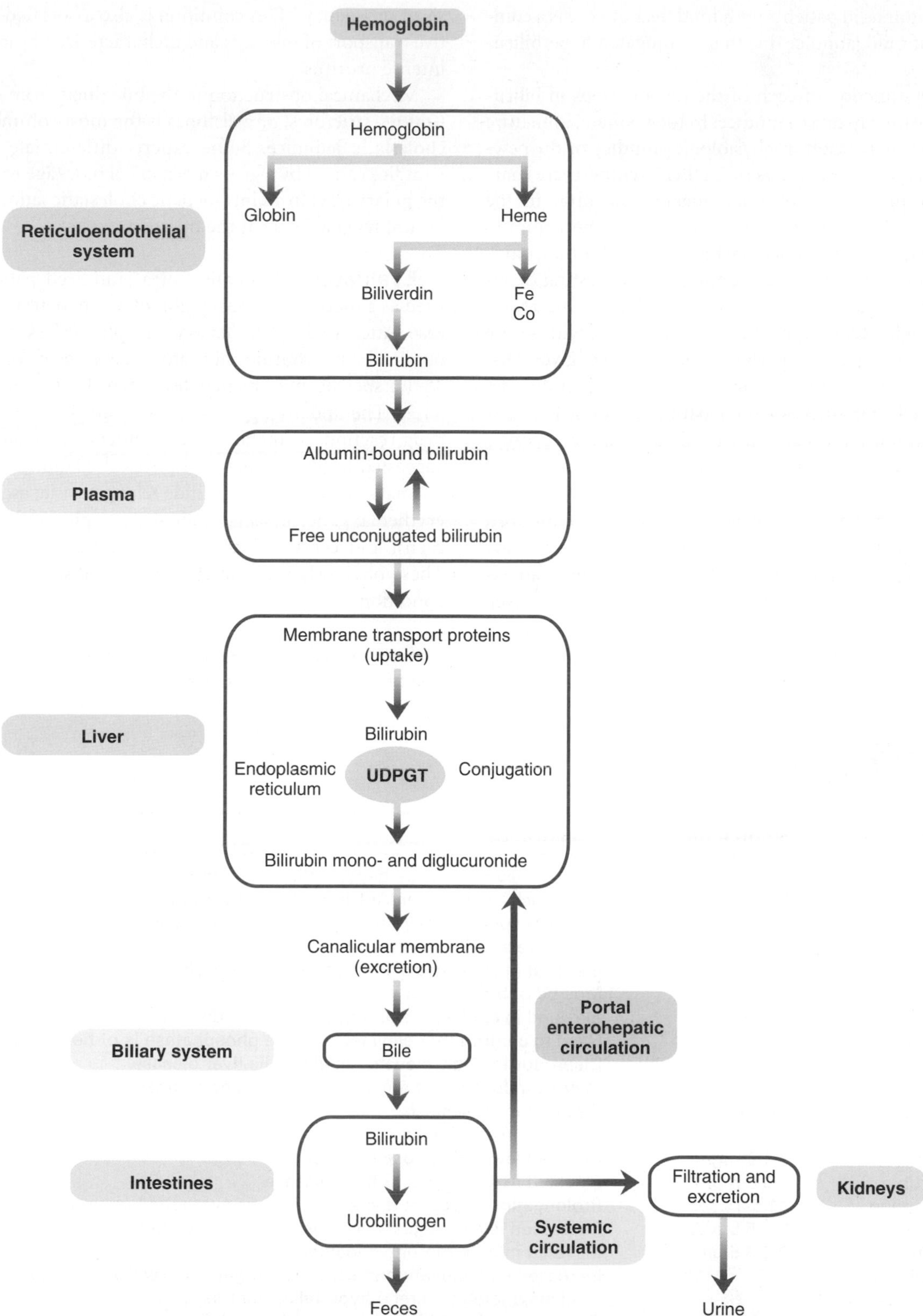

FIGURE 38-4 ■ Summary of bilirubin metabolism (see the text for an explanation). *UDPGT,* Uridine diphosphate glucuronyltransferase.

tion of hematomas in patients with mild liver disease is a common cause of mild jaundice due to unconjugated hyperbilirubinemia.

Hepatic. Dysfunction of each of the hepatic steps in bilirubin metabolism may cause jaundice. In the neonate, immature UDPGT levels may result in physiologic jaundice of the newborn. Various genetic disorders of UDPGT synthesis are characterized by high levels of unconjugated bilirubin in the blood. Mutant UDPGT enzymes can produce the common and benign Gilbert syndrome, in which low levels of unconjugated hyperbilirubinemia may be increased by fasting or illness (e.g., viral gastroenteritis). Other UDPGT mutations cause the Crigler-Najjar type 1 and 2 syndromes with severe neonatal unconjugated hyperbilirubinemia (see Liver Diseases and Pediatric Considerations). Most of the liver diseases to be discussed later, such as viral hepatitis, alcoholic liver disease, and autoimmune hepatitis, result in jaundice because dysfunction within the liver cell results in elevated levels of conjugated bilirubin.

Posthepatic. At the level of canalicular bilirubin transport, the rare inherited Dubin-Johnson and Rotor syndromes cause conjugated hyperbilirubinemia. Both conditions have an excellent prognosis. At the canalicular post-hepatocytic level, many drugs such as the phenothiazines and the sex hormones may cause jaundice.[7] In susceptible women, the high sex hormone levels of normal pregnancy can cause benign cholestasis of pregnancy.[8] This condition is also associated with defective transport of bile salts and is characterized by jaundice and intense pruritus.

Mechanical obstruction to the bile ducts from obstructing tumors, strictures, or gallstones is the most common cause of cholestatic jaundice. Some experts differentiate obstructive jaundice caused by a gross mechanical blockage to bile flow in the biliary tract from intrahepatic cholestatic jaundice, the latter implying a defect at the microscopic level.

Evaluation. Evaluation of a jaundiced patient may be used as a model for investigation of any patient with liver disease. After a complete history and physical examination are obtained and routine laboratory data reviewed (see Table 38-1), specific liver-related tests may be performed (Table 38-2). The underlying cause, such as alcoholic liver disease, a drug reaction, or metastatic or primary malignancy, is often suggested by the history and physical examination. Physical stigmata of liver disease include telangiectasia; ascites; palmar erythema; gynecomastia, testicular atrophy, and hair loss (in men); and central obesity with peripheral muscle wasting. These obviously indicate chronic liver disease, not an acute condition.

Diagnostic Tests. Biochemical tests usually fall into one of several categories. A significant elevation in transami-

Table 38-2

Common Laboratory Tests in Liver Disease

Test	Normal Range	Significance
AST/SGOT	5-40 U/ml	Elevated levels indicate hepatocellular inflammation or necrosis
ALT/SGPT	5-35 U/ml	AST much greater than ALT in alcoholic liver disease AST less specific; may be of skeletal muscle, myocardial, kidney, or liver origin ALT more specific for liver disease
Alkaline phosphatase	35-150 U/ml	Elevated in cholestasis, infiltrative liver disease (cancer, granulomas, etc.) May be of bone origin
γ-Glutamyl transpeptidase	10-48 U/ml	Elevated in cholestasis and hepatocellular disease Used to confirm that elevated alkaline phosphatase is of hepatic origin Disproportionately elevated in alcoholic liver disease May be induced by many drugs (e.g., phenobarbital)
5'-Nucleotidase	2-11 U/ml	Elevated in cholestasis Very specific to the liver
Total bilirubin	$<$1.0 mg/dl	Elevated levels diagnose jaundice
Indirect bilirubin	$<$0.8 mg/dl	Elevated in hemolysis, Gilbert disease
Prothrombin time	11.5-14 sec	Prolongation suggests decreased hepatic synthetic function
Serum albumin	3.5-5.5 g/dl	Decreased level suggests decreased hepatic synthesis
Serum globulin	2.5-3.5 g/dl	Elevated in autoimmune hepatitis
Urine bilirubin	0	Increased with elevation of serum conjugated (direct) bilirubin, zero in unconjugated (indirect) hyperbilirubinemia
Urinary urobilinogen	0-4 mg/24 hr; spot test ± on urine dipstick	Zero in complete biliary or proximal bowel obstruction Increase may suggest liver disease Nonspecifically insensitive Primary utility because its presence on urine dipsticks allows simple office/bedside testing or screening with one-time urinalysis

nases out of proportion to the other liver enzymes indicates a hepatocellular disorder (i.e., hepatitis). Alcoholic and other toxic hepatitides virtually always show the aspartate aminotransferase (AST) markedly elevated in comparison with the alanine aminotransferase (ALT), whereas in viral hepatitis the reverse is usually true. Predominant elevations of alkaline phosphatase (ALP) indicate intrahepatic cholestasis and are often due to an infiltrative process (e.g., metastatic carcinoma, sarcoidosis). Predominant bilirubin elevations point to so-called extrahepatic cholestasis due to biliary obstruction. It is noteworthy that jaundice in patients with cirrhosis often shows elevations in all parameters, reflecting the widespread liver dysfunction and obstruction of the bile canals and small vessels because of scarring. Elevated bilirubin can be either direct (conjugated) or indirect (unconjugated). Although an overwhelming liver process in an adult will produce elevations of both, as a practical matter unconjugated hyperbilirubinemia points to significant hemolysis.

Hepatocellular and cholestatic disorders may warrant evaluation for viral hepatitis markers (Table 38-3), various biochemical assays (see the specific disorders discussed later), or needle biopsy of the liver. Needle biopsies may be carried out "blind" or may be directed by ultrasound or computed tomography (CT), the latter allowing examination of a specific target such as a mass lesion.

Radiologic imaging with ultrasonography is helpful in significant disease. This is particularly true given the fact that structural liver abnormalities such as tumors may present with any of the above enzyme patterns or with a mixed picture. CT provides more information and is especially useful for evaluating the content of iron in the liver in cases of suspected hemochromatosis. Specific visualization of the bile ducts may necessitate percutaneous transhepatic cholangiography or endoscopic retrograde cholangiopancreatography (see Chapter 37).

Portal Hypertension

Manifestations of liver disease not attributed to hepatocellular failure are mainly due to impaired blood flow through the liver as a result of increased resistance from fibrosis and degeneration of liver tissue. Sluggish blood flow through the liver results in increased pressure in the portal circulation (**portal hypertension**) (Figure 38-5). In this condition, venous drainage of much of the GI tract is congested. Symptoms are surprisingly few early in the course, but as abnormal vascular patterns progress anorexia may result. The end result of elevated venous pressure are varices, particularly esophageal, but also gastric and hemorrhoidal. A pathognomic feature of advanced liver disease is superficial periumbilical varices, known as "caput medusae," or the head of Medusa. Portal hypertension contributes to the accumulation of peritoneal fluid, or **ascites.** A serious consequence of portal hypertension is uncontrolled bleeding from esophageal varices, which are prone to rupture.

Gastroesophageal Varices

Etiology. Esophageal varices result mainly from portal hypertension, which in Western society is generally the result of alcoholic or post-hepatitis cirrhosis. In developing tropical countries, chronic infection with *Schistosoma* species is a major cause of portal hypertension. Recently, it has been recognized that vasoactive hormones, as well as increased splanchnic blood flow and increased vascular resistance in the liver, have a prominent role in the formation of variceal esophageal veins.[1] Gastric varices may occur in connection with or independently from esophageal varices.

Pathogenesis. Gastroesophageal varices are merely one of a number of collateral venous pathways that dilate in response to elevated portal pressure in an attempt to transport blood from the splanchnic bed around the cirrhotic liver and back to the heart. Other common pathways include spontaneous splenorenal shunts, a variety of deep and usually entirely asymptomatic portosystemic shunts; dilated veins in the small intestine, colon, and rectum are also not uncommon.[1] Unfortunately, part of the very complex venous network that surrounds the proximal part of the stomach and esophagus lies just beneath the mucosa, rendering it especially liable to rupture when portal pressures reach a critical level. Rupture results in massive, often life-threatening upper GI bleeding (Figure 38-6).

Clinical Features. Varices will affect more than half of cirrhotic patients, and approximately 30% of them experience an episode of variceal hemorrhage within 2 years of the diagnosis of varices.[1] Variceal size is the main determinant of risk for bleeding, which is often catastrophic and is one of the main causes of death (20% to 33%) in persons with long-standing cirrhosis. The mortality after an episode of significant variceal bleeding is as high as 50%. The diagnosis is made mainly endoscopically, but varices may be seen on upper GI barium examinations as well, and occasionally on CT scans of the abdomen.

Bleeding from gastroesophageal varices is one of the most dreaded complications of portal hypertension. The initial symptoms and signs are those of major upper GI hemorrhage and include hematemesis, melena, and rapid intestinal transit and vigorous bleeding, even bright red rectal bleeding. These characteristics may be associated with profound anemia and symptoms and signs of shock. In most cases, concomitant evidence of chronic liver disease and portal hypertension is seen.

Treatment. Initial treatment is directed at volume repletion and blood replacement. Primary acute pharmacologic management rests on drugs that can effectively lower portal pressure by dilating alternative collateral pathways, reducing splanchnic blood flow, or both. Traditionally, in the United States the agent of choice has been vasopressin, an analog of

Table 38-3

Immunologic Markers in Viral Hepatitis

Marker	Description
Hepatitis A	
Anti-HAV IgM	Acute infection with HAV, but may persist for months
Anti-HAV IgG	Past infection with HAV Implies immunity to the virus
Hepatitis B	
Hepatitis B surface antigen (HBsAg)	Surface protein coat of HBV Implies active infection Detectable 2-6 wk after infection Remains present as long as infection is active
Hepatitis B surface antibody IgM (HBsAb)	Antibody to surface protein of HBV Detectable shortly after or with clearance of HBsAg Implies resolution of infection and immunity to HBV
Hepatitis B core antibody IgM (HBcAb IgM)	Antibody to inner core protein of HBV Detectable 3-5 wk after infection Implies recent infection
Hepatitis B core antibody IgG (HBcAb IgG)	As for HBcAb IgM, but implies past infection
Hepatitis e antigen (HBeAg)	Soluble fraction of HBV Detectable 2-6 wk after infection Implies ongoing infection with high infectivity May resolve independently of HBsAg
Hepatitis B e antibody (HBeAb)	Antibody to soluble fraction of HBV Detectable when HBeAg clears Implies decreased infectivity
HBV DNA polymerase activity	Same significance as HBV DNA
Hepatitis C	
Anti-HCV	Antibody to HCV antigens May not be detectable early in infection Does *not* indicate immunity to the virus Rapidly evolving area; many commercially available assays of different sensitivity and specificity Many false-positive and false-negative results
HCV RNA by PCR	Assay for level of viremia Correlates positively with activity of infection Clears with resolution of infection Technically difficult; available through reference laboratories
Hepatitis D (Delta)	
Hepatitis delta antigen (HDAg)	Assay for 35-nm RNA virus Detectable 2-10 wk after infection Implies early infection
Anti-HDV	Implies past or chronic infection Does not indicate immunity to the virus
Hepatitis E	
HEV RNA by PCR	Detects presence of virus
HEV antibody IgG and IgM	Not well standardized
Hepatitis G	
HGV by PCR	Measures level of viremia

PCR, Polymerase chain reaction.

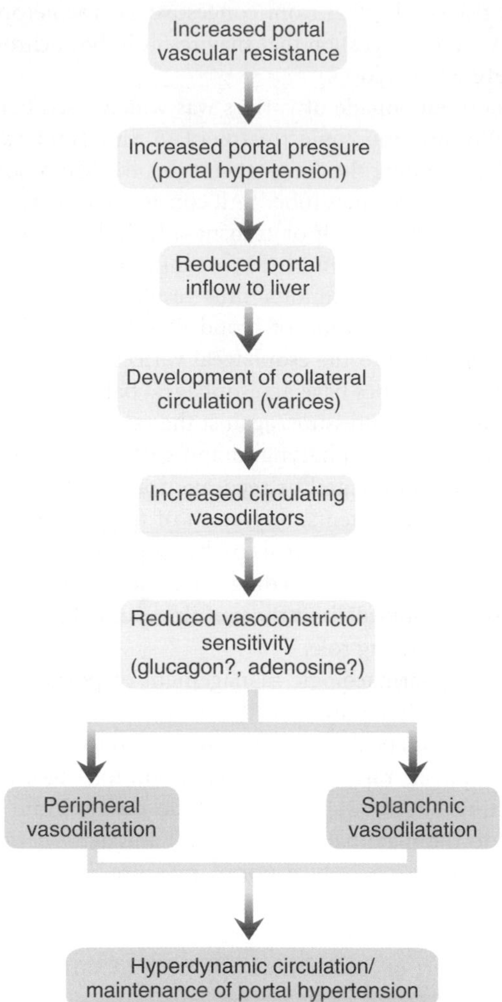

FIGURE 38-5 ■ Pathophysiologic process of portal hypertension. (Redrawn from MacMathuna P: The pathogenesis of variceal rupture, *Gastrointest Endosc Clin North Am* 2[1]:1-8, 1992.)

antidiuretic hormone, administered by continuous intravenous infusion. Although effective in controlling variceal bleeding, its use may be associated with angina pectoris, severe abdominal cramping, and, with long-term infusion, hyponatremia. These side effects often limit both the dose administered and the duration of therapy. Nitroglycerin, itself is very effective in lowering portal pressure, counteracts some of these side effects and is generally given concomitantly with vasopressin by the intravenous route.[3]

In recent years, octreotide acetate, a synthetic analog of the naturally occurring hormone somatostatin, has been effectively used as a replacement for vasopressin.[9] It is administered as an initial intravenous bolus followed by continuous infusion, which may be administered for as long as 3 to 5 days. In the doses used, the drug is remarkably free of side effects and more effective than vasopressin. However, it should be noted that no drug treatment has shown a mortality benefit for this condition.

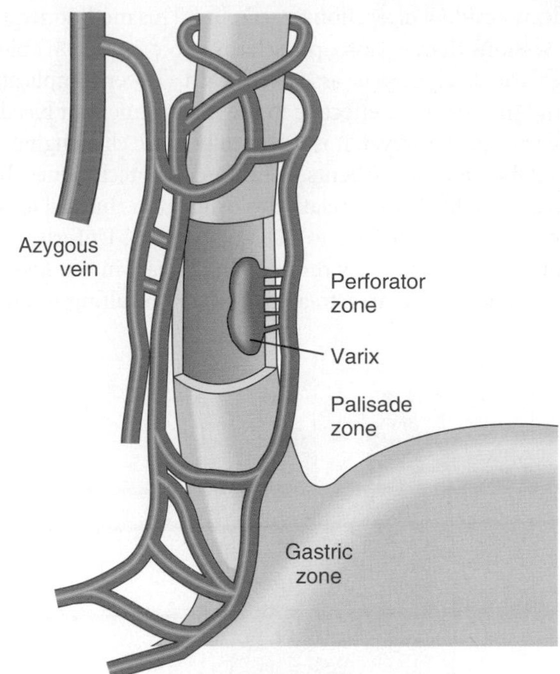

FIGURE 38-6 ■ Gastroesophageal venous anatomy. (Redrawn from MacMathuna P: The pathogenesis of variceal rupture, *Gastrointest Endosc Clin North Am* 2[1]:1-8, 1992.)

Metoclopramide and β-blockers have been used as ancillary treatments in the past and may be considered for selected patients. Intravenous H_2 blockers or proton pump inhibitors are also often administered. Any coagulopathy may necessitate administration of parenteral vitamin K, fresh frozen plasma, and platelet infusions if profound thrombocytopenia is present.

Emergency esophagogastroduodenoscopy (EGD) is crucial in determining the site of bleeding, as well as excluding other causes of upper GI bleeding. In addition to its diagnostic role, EGD actively addresses bleeding varices. **Endoscopic sclerosis** of esophageal varices is accomplished by passing a flexible needle through the gastroscope and injecting various sclerosant solutions into and around the bleeding varix (Figure 38-7). Such treatment results in initial thrombosis of the vein with hemostasis. Repeated injections cause fibrosis and obliteration of the varix and fibrosis of the overlying mucosa. This process can effectively obliterate all of the varices at risk of bleeding. Unfortunately, this treatment may be associated with a variety of acute and chronic complications, including drug reactions to the sclerosing solutions, exacerbation of bleeding, perforation, ulceration, infection, and stricture formation.[5]

An alternative treatment method is endoscopic ligation of esophageal varices (Figure 38-8). In this technique, a special apparatus is preloaded onto the gastroscope so that the endoscopist can suction a varix into a special chamber at the end of the gastroscope and then ligate the varix with a small rubber band. This technique also results in immediate loss of flow in the varix and eventually leads to thrombosis and fibrosis. The area ligated simply sloughs off over the next week or so without significant residual ulceration or scarring. This method requires fewer sessions than endoscopic sclerosis to completely obliterate the varices, seems to be associated with a lower complication rate, and may be more effective in the management of bleeding gastric varices.[6] However, it is technically more challenging and not suitable for all patients.[10] Endoscopic techniques have shown a mortality benefit relative to drugs alone but fail to control acute bleeding in 10% to 20% of patients. Unfortunately, both of these methods may result in an increase in venous pressure proximal to the area treated, perhaps resulting in an increased risk of bleeding from congestive gastroenteropathy (a diffuse venous congestion that may result in both chronic and acute severe blood loss).

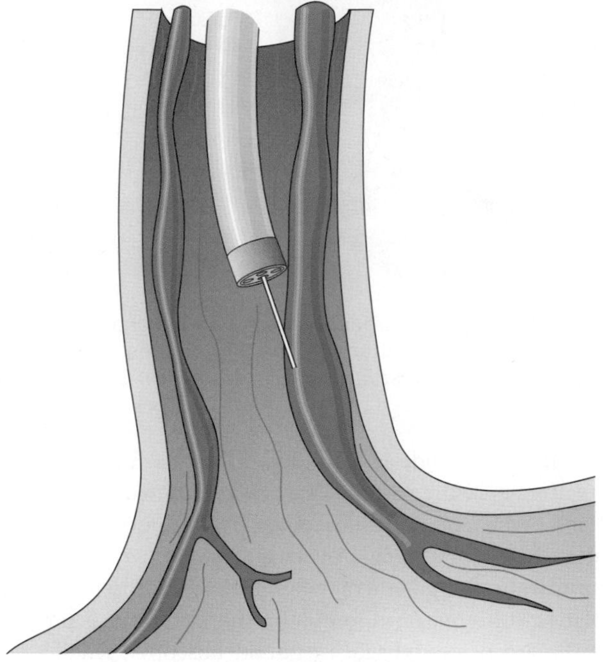

FIGURE 38-7 ■ Endoscopic sclerosis of varices.

Balloon tamponade of varices was widely used before the availability of endoscopic treatment. A variety of tubes are available, including the Sengstaken tube, the Minnesota tube, and the Linton-Nachlas tube.[11] All consist of a gastric balloon that is passed by mouth or transnasally, inflated to volumes specific to each tube, and held in gentle traction against the gastric varices in the fundus, thus resulting in compression hemostasis and occlusion of blood flow from the fundus of the stomach up into the esophageal varices (Figure 38-9). In addition, some tubes have an esophageal balloon that may be inflated to specific pressures against the esophageal varices directly. Suction of oropharyngeal and gastric secretions is accomplished with integral or separate drainage tubes. Aspiration of stomach contents, migration of the tube with airway compression, pressure necrosis of the esophagus and stomach, balloon rupture, and rebleeding after the maximal inflation period of 24 hours all limit the usefulness of balloon tamponade to a temporizing role.

Chronic pharmacologic management of portal hypertension is frequently successful with nonselective β-blockers such as propranolol. The drug is carefully titrated to reduce the initial resting heart rate by 25%. In addition to β-blockers, oral long-acting nitrates such as isosorbide mononitrate may be titrated to the maximal tolerated dose and act synergistically with β-blockers to reduce portal pressure.[12,13] These drugs may be used prophylactically in patients with known portal hypertension and are often prescribed following endoscopic therapy as part of a combined approach to variceal bleeding prevention.

If the aforementioned measures are ineffective, a number of surgical and radiologic procedures are possible. Although

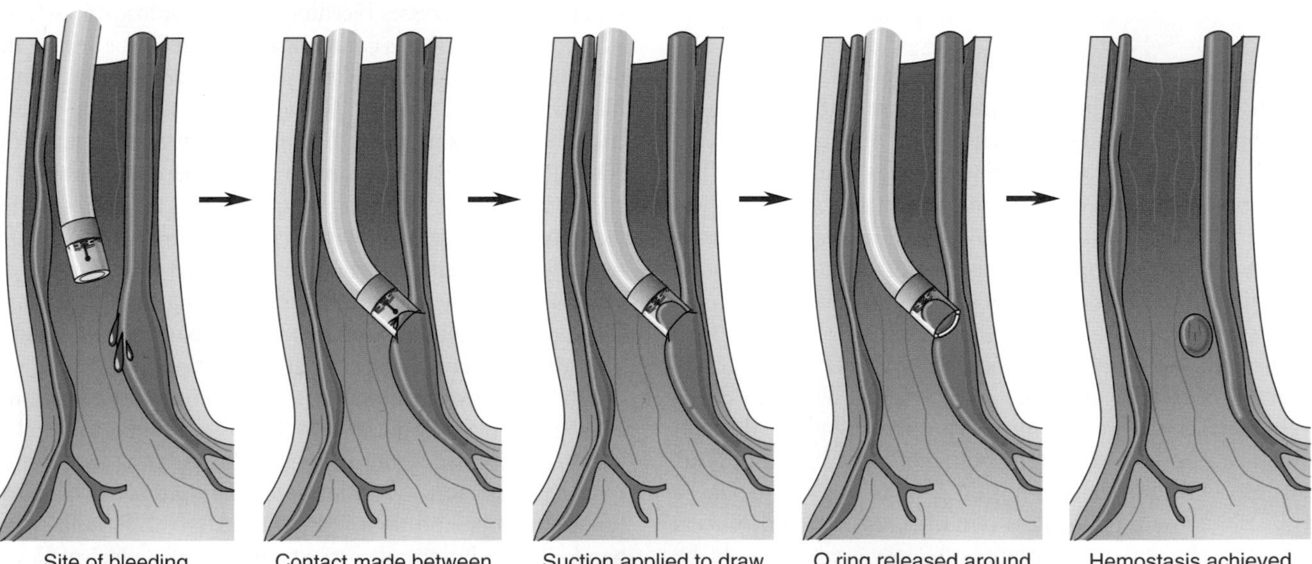
Site of bleeding identified
Contact made between ligator and varix
Suction applied to draw varix into ligator lumen
O ring released around neck of varix
Hemostasis achieved

FIGURE 38-8 ■ Endoscopic band ligation of varices.

rarely used in the United States, esophageal transection and reanastomosis with ligation of other collateral channels has been used in other countries.[1] Surgery to reduce portal pressure is very effective in decreasing the rate of rebleeding, but it may not alter overall survival. A variety of surgical techniques are used, all of which create an alternative connection between the splanchnic and systemic circulation. These techniques include portacaval, mesocaval, splenorenal, and distal splenorenal shunts (Figure 38-10). A discussion of the specific indications and technical aspects of these shunts is beyond the scope of this text, but each has certain specific indications, advantages, and disadvantages.[14]

In recent years a radiographic procedure called transjugular intrahepatic portosystemic shunting (TIPS) has been developed that combines angiographic and ultrasonographic techniques.[1] The hepatic vein is cannulated by the transjugular route. A needle is then passed into a main portal vein branch. Catheters are passed over this guidewire along with balloon dilation of the tract so created. This step is then followed by placement of an expandable metallic stent, thus creating a portosystemic shunt (portal vein to hepatic vein) within the liver itself. This procedure is technically very demanding and may be complicated by hemorrhage, infection, stent migration, stent stenosis, and occlusion, both acute and chronic. In addition, hepatic encephalopathy and congestive heart failure may result. The primary use of this modality is as a bridge to allow stabilization of patients who are candidates for liver transplantation.[15]

Treatment of esophageal varices is often unsatisfactory. Ideally, the underlying condition for varices (i.e., portal hypertension) should be reversed. The only consistently effective way to accomplish this goal is by liver transplantation (see below), which is limited in its application to a select group of patients.

Portal Systemic Encephalopathy

Hepatic Encephalopathy

Pathogenesis. Hepatic encephalopathy is a complex neuropsychiatric syndrome characterized by symptoms ranging from mild confusion and lethargy with altered personality to stupor and coma. Some patients exhibit dementia, psychotic symptoms, spastic myelopathy, and cerebellar or extrapyramidal signs. The classic physical finding is asterixis, or "liver flap," a spastic jerking of the hands held in forced extension. Hepatic encephalopathy is associated with fulminant hepatic failure or severe chronic liver disease, conditions in which liver function is severely depressed and blood is shunted around the liver. The arterial ammonia

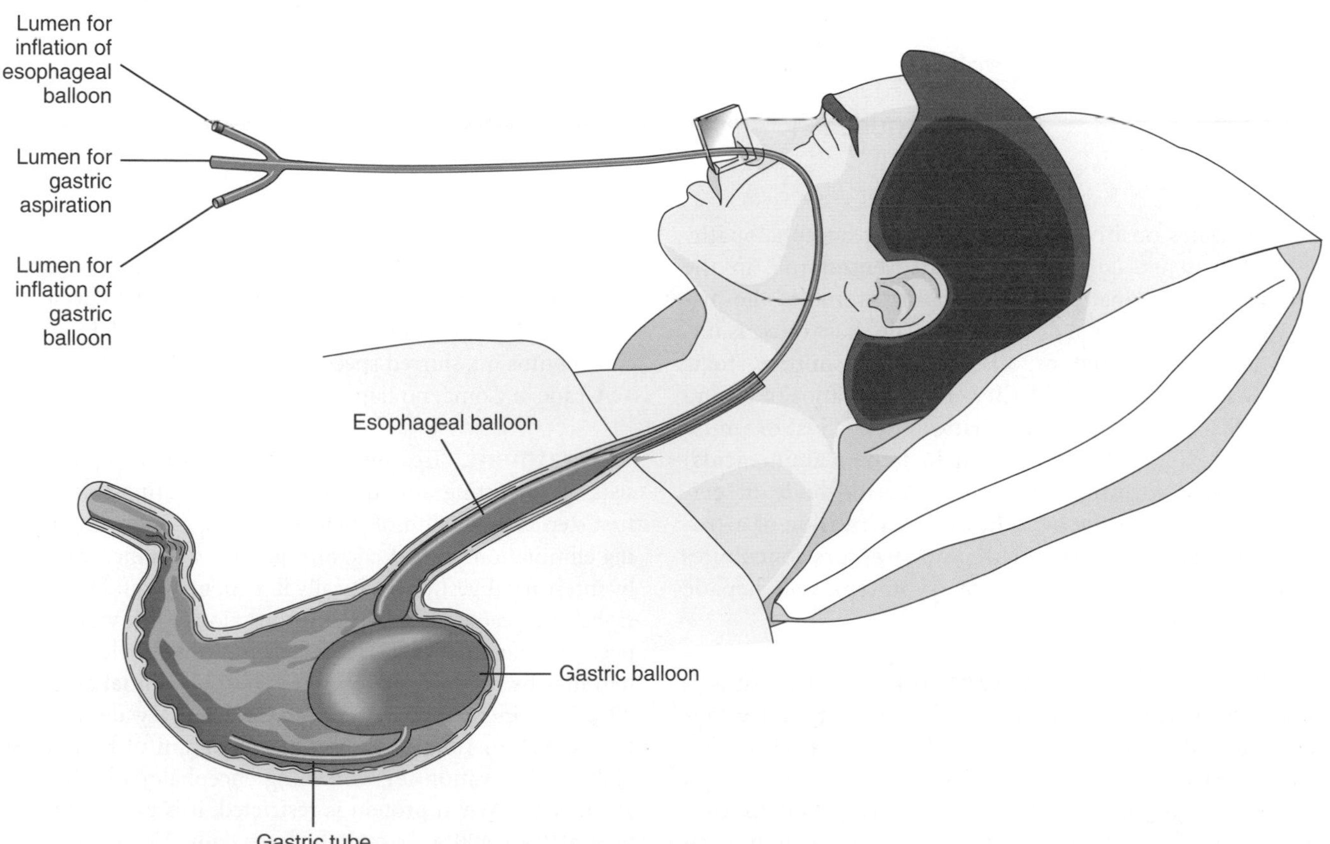

FIGURE 38-9 ■ Sengstaken-Blakemore tube.

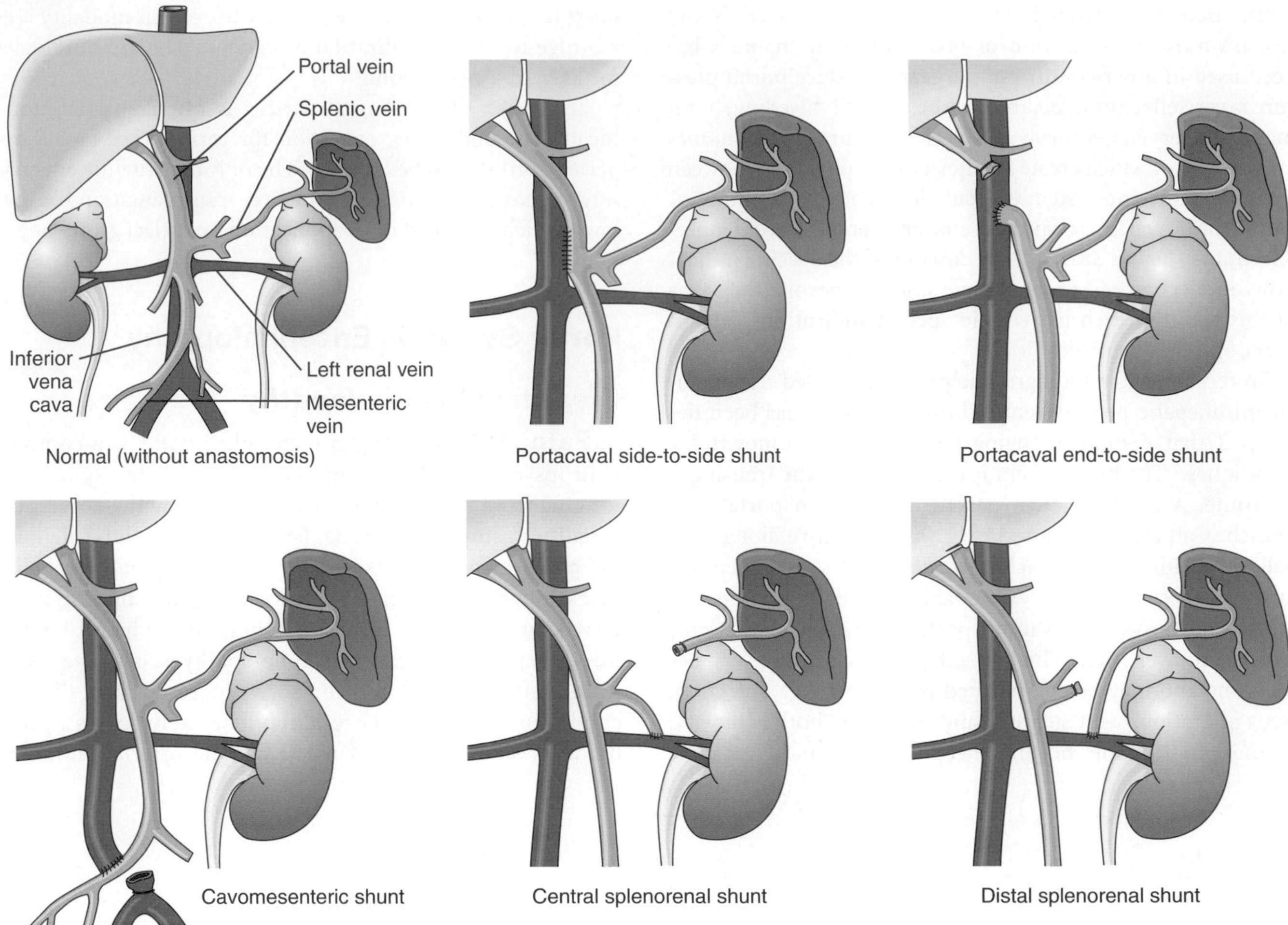

FIGURE 38-10 ■ Portosystemic shunt operations.

level correlates positively with the level of encephalopathy in most patients, consistent with its central role in the pathogenesis of hepatic encephalopathy as one of the primary causes of neuronal dysfunction. The exact cause is unclear, although altered or false neurotransmitters, toxic short-chain fatty acids, and altered plasma ratios of amino acids with a ring structure (aromatic amino acids) to amino acids with a linear structure (branched-chain amino acids) remain under investigation.[1] An increasing body of evidence also supports the hypothesis that activation of astrocytic peripheral-type benzodiazepine receptors contributes to the central nervous system symptoms of hepatic encephalopathy.[16]

Clinical Manifestations. Hepatic encephalopathy is usually precipitated by certain well-defined clinical developments, including hypokalemia, hyponatremia, alkalosis, hypoxia, hypercarbia, infection, use of sedatives, GI hemorrhage, protein meal gorging, renal failure, and constipation. In some patients, progressive liver failure leads to chronic encephalopathy without other exacerbating factors.

Hepatic encephalopathy is graded 1 to 4:

Grade 1: Confusion, subtle behavioral changes, no flap
Grade 2: Drowsy, clear behavioral changes, flap present
Grade 3: Stuporous but can follow commands, marked confusion, slurred speech, flap present
Grade 4: Coma, no flap

Treatment. Treatment of hepatic encephalopathy consists of correcting any identifiable precipitating factors. The first step is restriction of dietary protein, along with enhancing elimination of the toxic nitrogenous substances produced by intestinal digestion. Critically ill patients should receive peripheral or central glucose infusions along with vitamins, especially thiamine. As the patient's ammonia levels drop, protein may be reintroduced into the diet. The initial amount of 20 g/day is increased by 10 or 20 g/day every few days to an ultimate 0.75 to 1.0 g of protein per kilogram of body weight daily.[17] Observation for worsening encephalopathy is crucial at this time. When protein is restricted, it is essential to provide at least 400 g of carbohydrate daily. Vegetable protein may be better tolerated than animal protein. High dietary fiber intake may help by decreasing constipation. If dietary measures fail, oral defined-formula feedings containing essential amino acids and enriched with branched-chain amino acids may be indicated.

Osmotic diuretics or antibiotics are used to enhance elimination of nitrogenous wastes. Lactulose is the standard osmotic cathartic and may be given orally or by enema. (Standard precautions must be taken before any cathartic is administered, including ruling out bowel obstruction and monitoring electrolytes, particularly in patients with renal insufficiency.) Some evidence suggests that a lactulose-related change in pH also inhibits ammonia production by the gut flora, possibly by selecting for bacterial populations that are less ammoniagenic. No serious adverse reactions have been reported with lactulose therapy, although flatulence and abdominal cramping may occur. The dosage should be individually titrated so that two soft, acidic stools are passed daily.

Oral neomycin sulfate has been used for many years to suppress the intestinal flora that break down dietary protein and release ammonia. Oral paromomycin, metronidazole, and vancomycin are other alternatives. Ototoxicity, nephrotoxicity, and bacterial overgrowth are among the complications that limit the long-term use of antibiotics; therefore, this treatment is reserved for persons who cannot tolerate lactulose.

Cerebral Edema

Pathogenesis. Swelling of the brain (cerebral edema) often develops in patients with grade 3 or 4 hepatic encephalopathy and results in an increase in intracranial pressure. Both vascular and toxic mechanisms have been implicated as etiologic factors. With increasing intracranial pressure, blood perfusion of the brain is decreased (cerebral perfusion pressure = carotid artery pressure − intracranial pressure) with resulting cerebral hypoxia. Cerebral edema is a major cause of death in patients with acute hepatic failure.[18,19]

Clinical Manifestations. Clinically, cerebral edema is suggested by deepening coma, systolic hypertension, and extensor rigidity (decerebrate posture), followed by pupillary dilation and, if brainstem herniation occurs, respiratory arrest. Some highly specialized referral centers monitor patients with advanced hepatic encephalopathy by extradural pressure monitors to permit early detection. Unfortunately, complications of extradural monitors occur up to 20% of the time and include infection and intracranial bleeding.[1,20]

Treatment. Cerebral edema is managed by the intravenous infusion of mannitol, which by increasing serum osmolarity draws water from the brain and thus reduces the swelling. Patients should be kept in the semi-Fowler position (head and trunk elevated 30 degrees). The barbiturate sodium pentothal is used as a second-line agent for patients with recalcitrant intracranial hypertension and those who cannot tolerate the fluid volume component of mannitol therapy

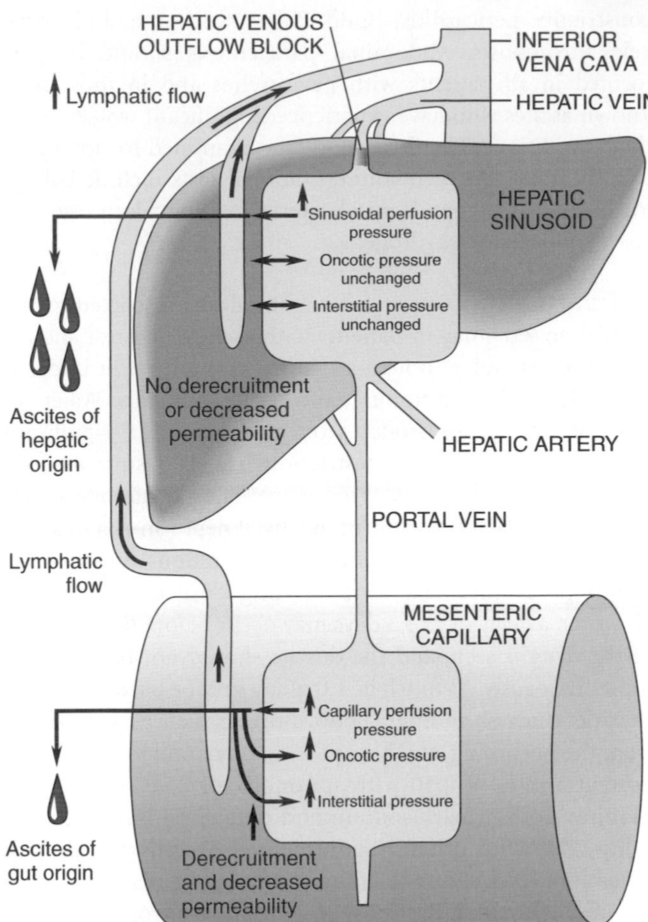

FIGURE 38-11 ■ Pathophysiologic process of ascites. (Redrawn from Dudley FJ: Pathophysiology of ascites formation, *Gastroenterol Clin North Am* 21:215-235, 1992.)

(e.g., those in heart or kidney failure). Aggressive treatment allows patient survival in 60% of cases, until liver failure resolves or liver transplantation can be accomplished.

Conditions of Advanced Liver Disease

Ascites

Etiology, Pathogenesis, and Clinical Manifestations. Ascites, or the pathologic accumulation of fluid in the peritoneal cavity, can occur in patients with advanced liver disease complicated by portal hypertension and hypoalbuminemia (Figure 38-11). Abdominal distention results from an inappropriate osmotic gradient across the pleura, with the intraabdominal accumulation of sodium, water, and protein.[1,21] A small amount of ascites may not require specific therapy. However, with increasing volumes, abdominal discomfort, respiratory embarrassment, abdominal or umbilical herniation, or infection may occur. The specific chemical and cellular composition of the ascites varies with its cause.

Other causes of ascites are malignancy, infection, pancreatitis, hypothyroidism, vasculitis, nephrosis, cardiac failure, constrictive pericarditis, Budd-Chiari syndrome, and portal vein thrombosis. Abdominal paracentesis should be performed in all patients with new ascites and in those with known ascites who have experienced significant worsening of their condition.[1] The fluid should be examined for total protein, albumin, and cell count. Optional tests include culture for bacteria, fungi and mycobacteria; cytology; amylase; glucose; and lactate dehydrogenase.

Treatment. Dietary sodium should be restricted to 500 mg/day to 2.0 g/day in patients with ascites. Bed rest and diuretics are useful, although strict bed rest can result in decubitus ulcers, deconditioning, and other problems. Water restriction is recommended for patients with significant hyponatremia, but strict restriction usually results in noncompliance and is counterproductive. The aldosterone antagonist spironolactone works in the distal nephron as a weak diuretic that also inhibits potassium secretion, thus sparing serum potassium. The usual starting dose is 100 mg/day. However, a delay of 2 to 3 days may occur before the full effect of the drug is seen, and the dosage should not be increased more frequently. As much as 1.0 g/day may be used. Many authorities suggest adding a loop diuretic such as furosemide from the beginning, at a dose of 40 mg/day, and increasing the dose at a ratio of 4:10 with spironolactone.[1] It is helpful to monitor both urinary sodium and potassium levels periodically. When the urinary sodium level exceeds the urinary potassium level, spironolactone is exerting its maximal effect. Serum potassium levels must be carefully controlled.

The goal is the loss of approximately 0.5 kg of body weight daily, although in patients with peripheral edema, slightly more rapid weight loss is tolerable. More rapid losses may result in diuretic-induced renal impairment, intravascular volume depletion and severe electrolyte abnormalities, and hepatic encephalopathy. Diuresis should be continued until the ascites is barely detectable. Free water restriction is prescribed if hyponatremia is present or develops during treatment.

In patients who do not respond to both diuretic therapy and sodium restriction, the use of 25% albumin infusions may help initiate diuresis. However, the effect of this treatment is often short lived and not without a risk of overexpansion of the intravascular volume, with congestive heart failure, pulmonary edema, and precipitation of variceal hemorrhage all possible.[22] Alternatively, large volumes of ascitic fluid can be removed from the peritoneal space through paracentesis. This "large-volume therapeutic paracentesis" is a very rapid and effective treatment that can be safely instituted if the intravascular volume is maintained by appropriate measures.[22] Diuretic and dietary treatment should be continued, but in severe cases, large-volume paracentesis may be repeated as needed.

Shunting procedures such as the LeVeen (Figure 38-12) and Denver shunts have been used. These one-way valves connect the peritoneal space with the venous system, usually at the jugular vein. These shunting procedures, although useful, carry significant risks and are best reserved for a small subset of ascites patients who have refractory ascites and are not candidates for liver transplantation.[23]

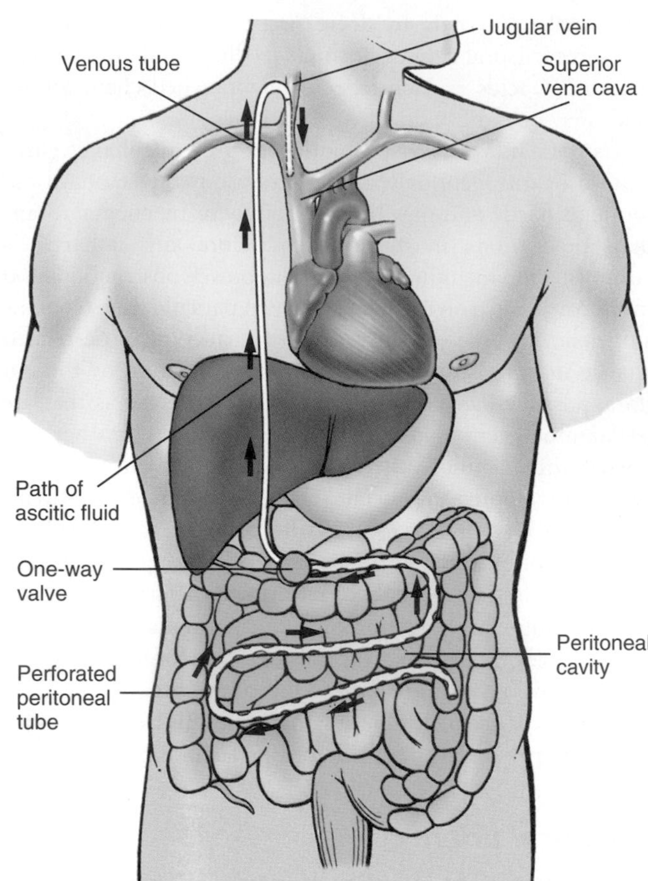

FIGURE 38-12 ■ LeVeen shunt. *Arrows* show direction of flow of ascitic fluid out of the peritoneal cavity, through the shunt, into the superior vena cava. (From Monahan FD, Neighbors M: *Medical-surgical nursing: foundations for clinical practice,* ed 2, Philadelphia, 1998, Saunders, p 1146.)

Spontaneous Bacterial Peritonitis

Pathogenesis and Clinical Manifestations. Patients with cirrhosis and ascites suffer from a variety of defects in host defense. This observation is especially true in patients who have ascites with a low protein concentration. These defects include diminished opsonic activity of the ascitic fluid, diminished reticuloendothelial function, and transmigration of gut bacteria across the intestinal wall and into the ascites (so-called monomicrobial non-neutrocytic bacterascites).[1,24] Chronic alcoholics demonstrate abnormal white blood cell function as well (Figure 38-13).

Typically, patients with spontaneous bacterial peritonitis have a single infecting organism of gut origin in the fluid. This pattern is in marked distinction to patients with secondary infection of the ascites, as may occur after traumatic paracentesis with gut perforation or the usual variety of other GI tract

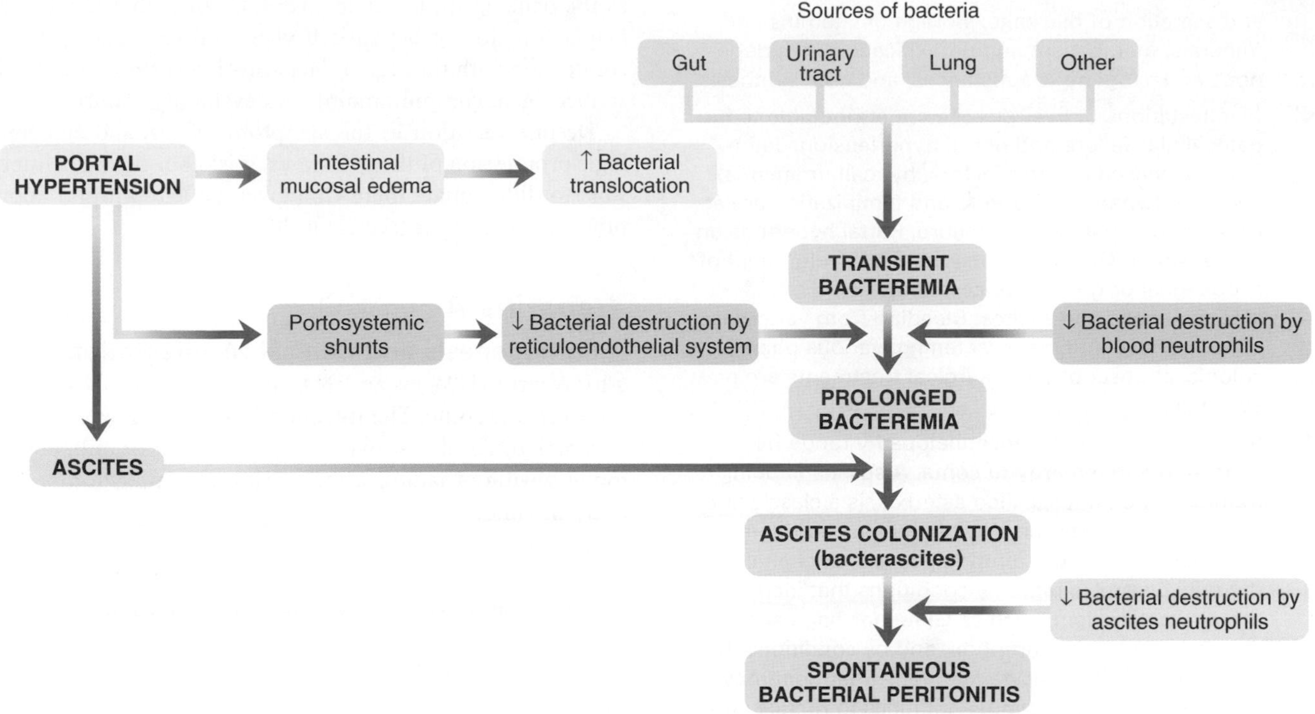

FIGURE 38-13 ■ Pathophysiologic process of spontaneous bacterial peritonitis. (Redrawn from Garcia-Tsao G: Spontaneous bacterial peritonitis, *Gastroenterol Clin North Am* 21:257-275, 1992.)

perforations, in which a polymicrobial infection is typical. The onset of spontaneous bacterial peritonitis may be subtle, with only mild abdominal discomfort or general clinical deterioration, including worsening hepatic encephalopathy, renal failure, or a nonspecific "septic" picture. Significant fever may be lacking. The most important diagnostic study is abdominal paracentesis. An ascitic polymorphonuclear leukocyte count greater than $250/cm^3$ and positive ascitic fluid cultures confirms the diagnosis.

Treatment. Antimicrobial therapy should be initiated promptly in suspected cases of spontaneous bacterial peritonitis pending culture results. Third-generation cephalosporins and quinoline antibiotics are effective empirical therapy. Use of long-term oral antibiotics for prophylaxis in at-risk patients with cirrhosis is controversial but may be considered for selected patients. Use of a narrow-spectrum agent such as sulfamethoxazole-trimethoprim therapy (e.g., Bactrim DS, 1 tablet orally daily) is preferable to agents of the quinolone class.[25] Overall, the occurrence of spontaneous bacterial peritonitis is a poor prognostic sign, as it is typically associated with end-stage liver disease.

Hepatorenal Syndrome

Etiology and Pathogenesis. Patients with liver failure may experience acute kidney failure with rising serum creatinine levels and oliguria. The kidney itself is normal, but intrarenal blood flow is seriously disturbed. This disturbance in blood flow appears to be due to an imbalance between vasoconstricting and vasodilating mechanisms related to the liver disease.[1,26] The course is usually acute and progressive, but chronic cases are occasionally seen. Differentiation from reversible causes of renal failure is essential. Hepatorenal syndrome may be precipitated by overly vigorous diuretic therapy, severe diarrhea, nonsteroidal antiinflammatory drugs, variceal bleeding, and sepsis.

Prognosis and Treatment. The prognosis depends on the severity of the liver disease and is generally poor.[27] Treatment is primarily preventive and supportive; hemodialysis should be considered only as a bridge to definitive therapy. Fortunately, liver transplantation generally results in return of normal renal function, providing no undue delay has occurred.

KEY CONCEPTS

- The liver is a vital, multifunctional organ located in the right upper quadrant beneath the diaphragm. Blood is supplied to the liver by the hepatic artery and the portal vein. The portal vein drains the capillaries of the alimentary canal and pancreas. Arterial and portal blood flows into the hepatic sinusoids, which have direct contact with hepatic cells.
- The functions of the liver are multiple and include metabolism of fats, proteins, and glucose; synthesis

and secretion of bile salts; storage of vitamins and minerals; metabolism and detoxification of endogenous and exogenous substances; and urea synthesis.

- Manifestations of liver disease are attributable to hepatocellular failure and portal hypertension. Jaundice, decreased clotting factors, hypoalbuminemia, decreased vitamins D and K, and feminization are attributed to hepatocellular failure. Portal hypertension may result in GI congestion with the development of esophageal or gastric varices, hemorrhoids, splenomegaly, and ascites. Bleeding from varices is often massive and life threatening; various pharmacologic, endoscopic, and surgical treatments are now available.
- Symptoms of hepatic encephalopathy range from confusion and lethargy to coma. A spastic flapping tremor of the hands, called asterixis, is a classic finding. The severity of the encephalopathy correlates positively with serum ammonia levels. Encephalopathy may be precipitated by conditions that increase protein metabolism, such as GI hemorrhage and increased protein consumption, and by conditions that further impair hepatocyte function. Treatment may include protein restriction, antibiotics to reduce ammonia production by intestinal organisms, and lactulose to enhance ammonia excretion in the stool. Cerebral edema is a common cause of death in patients in deep hepatic coma.
- Ascites is a pathologic accumulation of fluid in the peritoneal cavity. It occurs commonly in liver disease because of the increased fluid transudation that occurs with portal hypertension and hypoalbuminemia. In severe ascites, treatment may be instituted to ameliorate pain and respiratory difficulty. Sodium restriction, diuretics, and intermittent paracentesis are commonly prescribed. Surgical shunting procedures that allow accumulated peritoneal fluid to flow back into the circulation through a one-way valve may be effective.
- Spontaneous bacterial peritonitis is infection of ascites by a single organism unrelated to bowel perforation or surgical procedures. Antibiotic therapy alone is usually curative.
- Hepatorenal syndrome is a type of functional renal failure caused by severe liver disease. The prognosis is poor and is contingent on the outcome of the liver disease.

DISORDERS OF THE LIVER

HEPATITIS

Acute Viral Hepatitis

Hepatitis is inflammation of the liver parenchyma. Acute hepatitis may be caused by many viruses, among them cytomegalovirus and Epstein-Barr virus. However, the term viral hepatitis is usually applied to illnesses caused by hepatitis A, hepatitis B, and hepatitis C viruses. A fourth virus, known as the delta agent, is a defective RNA virus that requires the helper function of hepatitis B virus and so occurs only as a coinfection with that agent. Hepatitis E virus is a recently described agent common mainly in developing countries.

Despite variation in the symptoms, signs, and epidemiologic progression of these diseases, it is often clinically impossible to differentiate them in a given patient without appropriate serologic tests (see Table 38-2).

Hepatitis A

Pathogenesis and Clinical Manifestations. Hepatitis A virus (HAV) is an RNA virus that is usually spread by the fecal-oral route. The infection has a 2- to 7-week incubation period. The illness may be asymptomatic or mildly symptomatic without jaundice (anicteric); the latter occurs especially in children, with the patient exhibiting nonspecific GI symptoms. The majority of adults develop hepatitis with jaundice. The prodromal symptoms of icteric hepatitis consist of malaise, anorexia, nausea, low-grade fever, and right upper quadrant pain. This is followed by jaundice lasting 2 weeks on average. The clinical course is generally self-limited, although fulminant and fatal attacks occur rarely, particularly in patients with preexisting chronic active hepatitis B or C infection. Two uncommon prolonged syndromes are recognized: prolonged cholestasis and relapsing hepatitis.[1]

Diagnosis, Treatment, and Prevention. HAV infection is diagnosed through serologic testing. Presence of anti-HAV immune globulin G (IgG) indicates previous infection, and presence of immune globulin M (IgM) indicates acute infection. The test is highly reliable within several weeks of exposure.

Treatment does not change the course of acute HAV infection. Supportive management includes rest and a nutritious diet. Alcohol, acetaminophen, and other potential hepatotoxins should be avoided. HAV is a common infection control concern, particularly in the community setting.[28] The usual fecal-oral precautions, such as careful hand washing, segregation, and cleaning of laundry and personal items, should be undertaken by patients and contacts.

Active immunization is indicated for risk groups (e.g., foreign travelers, persons in institutions) using an inactivated whole-virus vaccine that is highly immunogenic and effective in preventing acute hepatitis A.[29] An intramuscular dose is followed by a booster 6 months later, providing lifelong immunity in at least 98% of recipients.[30] The vaccine is ideally administered at least 2 weeks preexposure (e.g., before travel to a developing country) but can also be administered in the setting of a community outbreak. It is effective even among persons with advanced chronic liver disease.

Patients exposed to HAV who are anti–HAV antibody negative should receive passive immunization with pooled human immune globulin, in addition to active vaccination. An intramuscular dose of 0.02 ml per kilogram of body weight should be given within 2 weeks of exposure. Passive immunity lasts 4 to 6 months and does not diminish vaccine effectiveness. However, subclinical infections may develop in some exposed patients, whereas other patients have a clinically evident but attenuated illness.

Hepatitis B

Pathogenesis and Clinical Manifestations. Hepatitis B virus (HBV) is a partially double-stranded DNA virus that is highly prevalent worldwide. Probably 300 million persons, or 5% of the world population, have chronic HBV infection. Chronic infection in the United States affects approximately 1 to 1.25 million people, most of them immigrants from endemic countries. In contrast to HAV, HBV is spread by parenteral contact with infected blood or blood products, including contaminated needles, and by sexual contact. Perinatal infection is a major route in endemic (mainly developing) countries. Other risk factors for HBV infection include working in a health care setting (3% of cases in the United States), transfusions and dialysis (1% each), acupuncture, tattooing, extended overseas travel, and residence in an institution.[1]

HBV has an incubation period of 2 to 6 months. The prodrome of HBV infection is often longer and more insidious than that of HAV infection and may involve a variety of immune complex–related phenomena, including urticaria and other rashes, arthralgia and arthritis, angioedema, serum sickness, and glomerulonephritis. Severity of illness ranges from no symptoms to moderate illness to fulminant hepatitis (1% of cases). The jaundice phase for most HBV infections is similar in degree and duration to that of HAV infections, although serious extrahepatic illness occurs more frequently.

Diagnosis. The serologic diagnosis is somewhat complicated. In brief, with acute infection HBV core antigen (HBcAg) appears first, followed by seroconversion to core antibody (HBcAb). Presence of HBV surface antigen (HBsAg) shows up early and may persist, indicating *active infection;* development of surface antibody (HBsAb) points to resolution and immunity. It should be noted that conversion from surface antigen to surface antibody positivity can take as long as 1 year after acute infection, so treatment should not be considered right after infection. In chronic infection, hepatitis B e antigen (HBeAg) is associated with viral replication and infectivity, whereas hepatitis B e antibody (HBeAb) indicates no significant replication or infective potential. A typical screening panel for HBV infection includes HBsAg, HbsAb, and HBcAb.

Chronic infection is indicated by HBsAg positivity. There are two important features of chronic infection: ongoing liver inflammation and active viral replication. Liver damage may be deduced from persistently elevated liver enzymes and confirmed by liver biopsy. Viral replication can be measured by molecular testing (HBV DNA by hybridization) and is associated with a positive HBeAg. Persons who have detectable virus and are HBeAg positive can transmit virus to their contacts, and should be counseled regarding appropriate sexual and blood exposure precautions (including no blood donation). Patients with chronic HBV and cirrhosis are at risk for development of hepatocellular carcinoma, and periodic screening (e.g., at least every 2 years) with ultrasound and α-fetoprotein determinations should be considered.

Treatment. Fulminant hepatitis is a life-threatening illness with high mortality. Care for patients with acute hepatitis is largely supportive, and those with fulminant hepatitis may require aggressive treatment for coagulopathy, encephalopathy, cerebral edema, and other manifestations. Liver transplantation is the only definitive treatment for progressive liver failure in acute hepatitis. Most nonfulminant HBV infections resolve spontaneously, although about 5% of acute hepatitis cases progress to chronic infection. Management of acute HBV infection is similar to that of HAV infection in terms of supportive care.

Management of chronic HBV infection has advanced dramatically over the last decade.[31,32] The two currently indicated therapies are interferon-α and lamivudine. Interferon-α_{2B} is given as 5 million units daily for 16 weeks. Lamivudine is a nucleoside analog also used in human immunodeficiency virus (HIV) therapy given as 100 mg daily for a minimum of 1 year, until loss of HbeAg occurs. About one-third of patients respond to interferon therapy; a somewhat smaller number respond to lamivudine, but treatment for longer than 1 year increases the chance of a favorable response. Adefovir is a nucleoside analog that is currently under investigation for management of chronic HBV infection.[31]

Patients with chronic active hepatitis B infection are considered at risk of fulminant hepatitis with a superimposed hepatitis A infection and should be vaccinated against hepatitis A using the killed, two-dose vaccine.

Prevention. HBV vaccine is a recombinant vaccine that is highly immunogenic with no material of human origin. (Thus, there is no risk of transmission of other agents such as HIV.) Adults are vaccinated intramuscularly with three doses of HBV vaccine given at 0, 1, and 6 months. Simultaneous administration of hepatitis B immune globulin (HBIG) and other vaccines has no effect on efficacy. After the full course, the antibody response rate is 95%.[1] The duration of protection is at least 5 years; postvaccination testing is not recommended but could be considered for certain high-risk groups (e.g., sexual partners of chronic carriers).

Universal immunization is suggested for individuals of any age, but especially recommended for the following high-risk groups: male homosexuals, Alaskan Eskimos, immigrants from highly endemic areas, users of illicit drugs, household contacts of HBV carriers, hemodialysis patients, residents of institutions, medical and dental personnel, patients needing frequent transfusions, and those planning to reside in high-risk areas (e.g., the Far East and sub-Saharan Africa).[29] If exposed to HBV, a susceptible person should receive one dose of HBIG and HBV vaccine as soon as possible after exposure and then complete the vaccination program. Many states require HBV vaccine for all children as a routine vaccination. The issue of how to deal with persistent nonresponders, especially health care workers, is unsettled, but most authorities recommend a full three-shot course according to the usual schedule.[33]

The administration of immune globulin containing high levels of hepatitis B surface antibody (HBIG) affords effective postinoculation prophylaxis if given within 7 days of exposure. The indications for HBIG are as follows: (1) neonates born to HBsAg-positive mothers; (2) prophylaxis after needlestick or sexual exposure in nonimmune persons; (3) after liver transplantation in patients who are HBsAg positive prior to transplantation.[1,34] The usual dose is 0.05 to 0.07 ml/kg given intramuscularly, with the same dose repeated 25 to 30 days later. (See reference for dosing recommendations for perinatal vaccination.[34]) The immune status of the recipient may be determined before treatment to avoid unnecessary administration. HBV vaccine should be given concomitantly with HBIG in most cases.

Hepatitis C

Pathogenesis and Clinical Manifestations. Hepatitis C virus (HCV; previously categorized as non-A, non-B hepatitis virus) is a relatively recently described single-stranded RNA virus that belongs to the Flavivirus family. Our knowledge of HCV is evolving rapidly but has lagged behind that of HAV and HBV for two important reasons: lack of a suitable cell line for replication in the laboratory and an extremely high mutation rate. Worldwide about 3% of the population is chronically infected, with a somewhat lower rate in the United States. The mode of transmission of HCV closely resembles that of HBV, although sexual and perinatal transmission are much less likely. The main pool of infected individuals in the United States acquired HCV through intravenous drug use or blood transfusions prior to availability of the screening test in 1990. HCV remains an important occupational risk for health care workers, with the risk after a single needlestick being about 3%, as opposed to 30% for HBV or 0.3% for HIV. A significant number of seropositive persons have no known risk factors for HCV.

Acute HCV infection is usually asymptomatic. Clinical illness, when it occurs, is usually mild, with transaminase levels rarely exceeding 1000 IU/L. Only 15% of acute infections resolve, with the remainder progressing to chronic active infection. The course is erratic, with wide fluctuations on liver enzymes (primarily ALT). A number of extrahepatic manifestations occur, the most prominent of which are a medium-vessel vasculitis (polyarteritis nodosa), essential mixed cryoglobulinemia, and membranoproliferative glomerulonephritis.[1] Chronic infection seems to progress to significant liver disease about 20% of the time, although there are no reliable noninvasive ways to predict who will progress. HCV infection is currently one of the most common causes of end-stage liver disease with cirrhosis in the United States. If untreated, chronic active HCV infection with cirrhosis predisposes to HCC.

Treatment. Management of acute HCV infection is the same as for other acute viral strains (i.e., supportive and expectant unless complications or subacute hepatic failure develop). Management of acute HCV infections with antiviral agents is not currently recommended, and immune globulin is not helpful in preventing infection in the acute exposure setting. Between 20% and 40% of acute seropositive patients will convert to seronegativity and an undetectable viral load during the first 6 months after infection, so early treatment is not recommended. Chronic infections should be assessed by a viral load and viral genotype, and a liver biopsy to stage disease activity should be strongly considered.[1] The current standard of treatment for chronic HCV infection is pegylated interferon-α, given intramuscularly once weekly, and ribavirin orally twice daily.[1,35] The response rate overall is about 60%; for the more common type 1 infection (85% of cases) it is 45%, and for the less common types 2 and 3 it is 85%. Side effects are significant and include cytopenias, malaise, and flulike symptoms, as well as induction or aggravation of depression and anxiety. In fact, the latter side effects are severe and have resulted in suicides. About 5% to 10% of recipients drop out of treatment because of side effects. The expense is considerable, about $15,000 per year, and insurance coverage is inconsistent. Treatment for type 1 virus lasts 12 months, and for other types 6 months. New treatments for HCV infection are currently a burgeoning area of research.

Patients with chronic active hepatitis C infection should be vaccinated against hepatitis A and B and counseled regarding blood-borne precautions. Although the issue of sexual transmission is controversial, the Centers for Disease Control and Prevention does not currently recommend barrier methods for patients with long-term sexual partners because of the apparent low risk of infection.

Hepatitis D (Delta)

Pathogenesis and Clinical Manifestations. Hepatitis D virus (HDV) infection may coincide with or succeed HBV infection and requires its presence for replication. The disease is primarily transmitted by parenteral routes and by intimate personal contact.[1] In the United States and northern Europe, HDV infection is most prevalent in persons exposed to blood and blood products (e.g., drug addicts and hemophiliacs). HDV infection tends to accelerate the progress of liver disease associated with HBV infection. In fact, fulminant hepatitis may result from HDV infection superimposed on chronic HBV infection. The duration of HDV infection is determined by the duration of the HBV infection. Chronic HDV infection also appears to cause additional damage to a liver that has already been compromised by HBV infection. Diagnosis is by anti-HDV IgM and IgG enzyme-linked immunosorbent assays (ELISAs).

Treatment and Control. HDV infection is controlled through the same measures used to prevent transmission of other hepatitis viruses: safe sexual practices, screening of blood products, avoidance of intravenous drug use, and vaccination of susceptible persons with the HBV vaccine.

Hepatitis E

Pathogenesis and Clinical Manifestations. Hepatitis E virus (HEV) may be the most common cause of acute hepatitis in the developing countries. Cases in developed countries are usually related to recent travel. HEV is an RNA virus spread via the fecal-oral route, especially through contaminated water. Parenteral transmission may occur.

The incubation period is 2 to 9 weeks. The prodrome and icteric illness are similar to those of HAV infection but usually last only 2 weeks. It is assumed that many subclinical cases occur, but in the absence of widely available serologic testing, subclinical infection is difficult to determine. Fulminant hepatic failure may occur, especially in pregnant woman (see the section Liver Diseases and Pediatric Considerations).

Treatment. Treatment is supportive. Because no vaccine is available, the only prophylaxis is avoidance of undercooked foods, careful hand washing, and drinking of safe water and beverages (i.e., canned, bottled, or purified through the usual means).

Chronic Hepatitis

Chronic hepatitis encompasses a group of diseases characterized by inflammation of the liver that lasts 6 months or longer. The condition may be idiopathic, autoimmune, or metabolic. It may also follow acute viral hepatitis or may be caused by hepatotoxic drugs or toxins.

Chronic Persistent Hepatitis

Chronic persistent hepatitis, often called triaditis or transaminitis, is an archaic term for a chronic, low-grade liver inflammation of any cause. The inflammation is confined to the portal triads without destruction of normal liver structures, but serum transaminase levels are elevated. The condition may be asymptomatic or may be associated with mild, nonspecific symptoms. Progressive liver disease does not usually develop, and no drug treatment is indicated. The illness has an excellent prognosis. However, other more serious liver diseases may pass through a phase that is histologically indistinguishable from chronic persistent hepatitis and may progress (e.g., chronic viral hepatitis).

Current classification schemes emphasize (1) etiologic factor, (2) histologic grade, and (3) stage in terms of fibrosis. Therefore, chronic persistent hepatitis would generally correspond to a liver condition with mild disease activity and minimal or no fibrosis by biopsy.

Chronic Active Hepatitis

Pathogenesis and Clinical Manifestations. On the other hand, **chronic active hepatitis** is a progressive, destructive inflammatory disease that extends beyond the portal triad to the hepatic lobule (piecemeal necrosis). In the new nomenclature, grade and stage span the spectrum from mild to severe. The disease could spontaneously arrest with any degree of fibrosis or could progress to macronodular or micronodular cirrhosis. Symptoms typical of acute hepatitis are often seen. Eventually chronic active hepatitis often culminates in cirrhosis and end-stage liver disease.

Four main subgroups of patients with chronic active hepatitis are identified. First, as discussed above, a minority of newly infected HBV patients but a majority of those with HCV will go on to have chronic active hepatitis. The second subgroup (mainly young women) manifest autoimmune hepatitis and exhibit a variety of immunologic markers, including antinuclear antibodies and anti–smooth muscle antibodies. In addition, these patients frequently suffer from a second autoimmune disease such as Hashimoto thyroiditis. In the third subgroup are patients with chronic hepatitis induced by therapeutic agents such as minocycline or nitrofurantoin. In the fourth subgroup are patients with a metabolic liver disorder such as Wilson disease or hemochromatosis. A small number of patients have neither a suggestive history nor any detectable markers that would place them in any of the four main groups; advanced liver disease in this group is usually termed **cryptogenic cirrhosis.**

Diagnosis. The diagnosis of chronic hepatitis is made on the basis of the clinical setting and abnormal liver enzymes. Several serologic studies are indicated for presumed autoimmune hepatitis. Serum iron and ferritin studies are performed to diagnose hemochromatosis, and a serum ceruloplasmin is used to screen for Wilson disease. A liver biopsy may be performed to confirm the diagnosis and to exclude specific causes. Biopsy also allows for grading and staging, as discussed above.

Management of Autoimmune Hepatitis. Corticosteroids and immunosuppressive drugs have been used since the early 1960s for the management of autoimmune chronic active hepatitis. Their use is based on the assumption that immunologic mechanisms either cause or maintain ongoing hepatic inflammation. Corticosteroids alone or in combination clearly lower mortality in chronic active hepatitis, most noticeably in symptomatic patients and those with very severe pathologic lesions demonstrated on liver biopsy. Patients with autoimmune chronic active hepatitis should be treated until a remission is induced (indicated by significant improvement in liver function test results and sometimes confirmed by liver biopsy). After 6 months in remission, corticosteroid use should be tapered to the lowest effective dose and stopped if possible. Treatment with corticosteroids may be accompanied by well-known complications: arterial hypertension and fluid retention, hypokalemia, glucose intolerance, mental status changes, cataracts, thinning of skin and bones, suppression of the adrenal gland, avascular necrosis of the joints, rounding of the face (moon facies), loss of muscle mass, and central adiposity, as well as increased risk for certain infections. Suddenly stopping long-term treatment with corticosteroids may result in acute adrenal insufficiency with hypotension and shock.

The current standard is medium-dose corticosteroids (e.g., prednisone 0.5 mg/kg per day) in combination with the immunosuppressive drug azathioprine (50 mg/day).[1] Allergic reactions, pancreatitis, cholestatic hepatitis, and bone marrow suppression with lowered white blood cell and platelet counts are complications of azathioprine and should be watched for. Alternatively, higher dose corticosteroids, such as prednisone 1 mg/kg per day, can be used initially as monotherapy, with the dose tapered over time. Short-term results are generally excellent, although it may take more than 1 year to achieve a clinical remission. Patients are generally treated for 2 to 3 years, then weaned off medication. Relapse is common, and patients who relapse should generally be maintained after achieving remission on the lowest dose of prednisone possible to prevent future relapse. Other therapies are available for nonresponders, and liver transplantation remains a fallback for persons with advanced liver decompensation.

Management of drug-induced chronic active hepatitis involves stopping the offending drug. Specific antidotes or treatments are available for certain of these conditions.[1] Specific treatments for Wilson disease and hemochromatosis are discussed below.

KEY CONCEPTS

- Acute viral hepatitis is generally classified as hepatitis A, B, C, D (delta), and E infection. Modes of transmission and severity of symptoms differ among types.
- HAV infection is also known as enteric hepatitis because it is generally transmitted by ingestion of contaminated substances. Symptoms are flulike and tend to be less severe than those of HBV infection. Early treatment with γ-globulin and vaccination after exposure may be effective in preventing disease.
- HBV infection is also known as serum hepatitis because its usual route of transmission is through infected blood. The incubation period is longer and the severity of symptoms (particularly jaundice) greater than in HAV infection. Hepatitis B immune globulin (HBIG) is effective after inoculation if given within 7 days of exposure. HBV vaccine is recommended as part of the childhood vaccination regimen and for high-risk individuals, and after exposure. Treatment is with intramuscular interferon-α for 4 months, or with oral lamivudine for 1 to 2 years.
- HCV, also known as non-A, non-B hepatitis virus, resembles HBV in its routes of transmission. Chronic HCV infection develops in 85% of cases and is usually asymptomatic until advanced liver disease intervenes. Immune globulin does not protect against HCV infection. Treatment is with intramuscular pegylated interferon and oral ribavirin for 6 to 12 months.
- HDV coinfects with HBV and requires the presence of HBV to be active. Infection appears to accelerate and worsen HBV infection symptoms. Prevention of HBV infection also prevents HDV infection.
- HEV is a common virus in the developing world that causes an illness similar to HAV infection but has a high mortality rate in pregnant women.
- Chronic hepatitis is characterized by persistent inflammation of the liver lasting 6 months or more. Autoimmune disease, viral hepatitis (B and C), toxins, and metabolic diseases may result in chronic hepatitis. Chronic active hepatitis may progress to cirrhosis. Corticosteroids (prednisone) and immunosuppressants (azathioprine) are common therapeutics for autoimmune hepatitis.

CIRRHOSIS

Cirrhosis represents the irreversible end stage of many different hepatic injuries, including severe acute hepatitis, chronic hepatitis, the metal storage diseases, alcoholism, and toxic hepatitis. It is characterized by diffuse hepatic fibrosis surrounding nodules of liver tissue and results in permanent alteration in hepatic blood flow and liver function. We will discuss briefly the sequelae of chronic biliary disease and alcoholic liver disease.

Biliary Cirrhosis

Etiology and Pathogenesis. **Biliary cirrhosis** is initiated by damage to the bile ducts, which may be due to macroscopic or microscopic biliary obstruction. Persistent biliary obstruction results in inflammation and scarring of the liver, with obliteration of the bile ductules. The end result is diffuse and widespread fibrosis with regenerative nodule formation (nodules are islands of liver cell regeneration within the fibrosis), and the consequences of portal hypertension described above. Examples of large-duct obstruction include gallstone disease, chronic biliary fluke infestation, and primary sclerosing cholangitis (PSC). The biliary flukes endemic in Asia, *Opisthorchis* and *Clonorchis* species, are acquired by eating raw fish that carry the larval cyst forms.[36] *Fasciola hepatica* is found in all sheep- and cattle-producing areas of the world and infects humans as accidental hosts; it is acquired by eating fecally contaminated watercress and other aquatic plants that harbor the immature cysts.

Diagnosis and Treatment. Diagnosis of biliary flukes in immigrants and foreign travelers can usually be made by serial stool examinations for parasitic ova, but serologic examination may at times be necessary. Treatment with antiparasitic agents will eliminate the live worms but will not necessarily prevent recurrent episodes of cholangitis and other consequences.

Primary Sclerosing Cholangitis

Etiology and Pathogenesis. PSC is an autoimmune condition generally seen in patients with ulcerative colitis;

80% of PSC patients have coexistent ulcerative colitis, whereas 3% to 5% of ulcerative colitis patients develop PSC.[1] It is characterized by recurrent episodes of cholangitis, with progressive biliary scarring and obstruction. Secondary forms of sclerosing cholangitis, such as that following bile duct injury during surgery, behave in a similar fashion.

Diagnosis and Treatment. Diagnosis is primarily by means of endoscopic retrograde cholangiopancreatography showing the typical beaded and atrophic appearance of the biliary tree; liver biopsy is often performed for staging reasons. Medical and endoscopic treatments are merely palliative, and the only effective recourse is liver transplantation.[37] The end result of recurrent cholangitis of any cause is cirrhosis, and such patients are predisposed to cholangiocarcinoma.

A microscopic form of biliary obstruction is seen in primary biliary cirrhosis.[38] Primary biliary cirrhosis is an autoimmune disease with an epidemiologic development similar to that of autoimmune hepatitis, and in fact often coexists with this condition. The site of pathologic activity is the intrahepatic bile ductule in the portal triad, which is attacked by immune cells in a relentless fashion. Antimitochondrial antibodies are pathognomonic for this condition. Treatment is supportive, as corticosteroids are not helpful for this condition. Ultimately, liver transplantation is usually required.

Alcoholic Liver Disease

Alcoholic liver disease is manifested by fatty liver, hepatitis, and cirrhosis. One or more of these manifestations may be found in alcoholic patients.

Alcoholic Fatty Liver

Etiology. Alcoholic fatty liver *(alcoholic hepatosteatosis)* is an accumulation of fat in the liver cells. It is caused by more fat being delivered to the hepatocyte than it can normally metabolize or by a defect in fat metabolism within the cell.

Diagnosis and Treatment. Hepatosteatosis is not exclusively alcohol related. Indeed, diabetes mellitus, obesity, protein malnutrition, total parenteral nutrition, drugs, and many other factors may result in a similar pathologic process. It is usually mild and asymptomatic, and is often diagnosed incidentally on ultrasound or CT examination or by liver biopsy for another reason. Liver enzymes are often mildly abnormal. Hypertriglyceridemia is commonly found and at times may be dramatically elevated (e.g., greater than 1500 mg/dl). Occasionally, there is significant liver enlargement, abdominal discomfort, and even portal hypertension. Treatment involves stopping alcohol intake and providing appropriate nutrition. Nonalcoholic steatosis may be managed with weight reduction, control of diabetes and hyperlipidemia, or other treatment directed at the underlying cause.

Alcoholic Hepatitis

Pathogenesis and Clinical Manifestations. Alcoholic hepatitis is an active inflammation of the centrilobular region of the liver. The liver cells show pathologic changes of necrosis, with an infiltrate of polymorphonuclear cells and lymphocytes. This form of liver disease often occurs in chronic alcoholics who "go on a bender" and binge on quantities much greater than their usual intake. Clinically the illness ranges from mild to very severe, with the worst cases characterized by hepatomegaly, fever, and encephalopathy. Hepatitis may be complicated by acute alcohol withdrawal and delirium tremens. Mortality rates as high as 33% are seen with this condition.[1]

Diagnosis and Treatment. The diagnosis is supported by the history, if the patient is reliable. The finding of a serum AST (SGOT) markedly higher than ALT (SGPT) strongly suggests a toxic etiology, rather than acute viral hepatitis. Viral serologies, serum acetaminophen levels, and tests for certain metabolic disorders (e.g., serum ceruloplasmin for Wilson's disease) may help sort out diagnostic dilemmas.

As one of the pathogenetic factors in alcoholic hepatitis is malnutrition and vitamin deficiencies, special attention should be given to nutrition. Thiamine 100 mg daily and a multivitamin should be administered routinely, and B_{12} and folate levels should be measured and replenished as necessary. Corticosteroid therapy is recommended for seriously ill patients, especially those with declining liver function and coma.[39]

KEY CONCEPTS

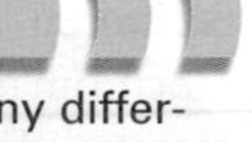

- Cirrhosis is the irreversible end stage of many different hepatic injuries. The liver is fibrotic, scarred, and nodular. Symptoms of cirrhosis are due to hepatocellular failure and portal hypertension.
- Biliary cirrhosis is associated with chronic bile duct obstruction with resultant backup of bile in the liver. Gallstones and extra- and intrahepatic bile duct inflammation are common causes.
- Alcoholic cirrhosis is associated with chronic alcohol ingestion, which may precipitate fatty liver, hepatitis, and, finally, cirrhosis.

TOXIC LIVER DISORDERS
Metal Storage Diseases

Hereditary Hemochromatosis

Pathogenesis and Diagnosis. Hereditary hemochromatosis is one of the most common autosomal recessive disorders in the world. In European populations, approximately 1 in 10 persons is a heterozygous carrier, and 0.3% are homozygous persons with disease.[40] The disease is caused by the activity of a mutant gene called *HFE*, which allows excessive and uncontrolled iron absorption by the GI tract. This results in deposition in numerous organs; in advanced disease, the body may contain 20 g or more of iron, mainly in the liver, pancreas, and heart. Because of menstruation and perhaps endocrinologic factors, hemochromatosis is much less common in women than in men (ratio of 1:5-10).[40]

The liver is usually the first organ to show evidence of involvement, with hepatomegaly and elevated liver enzymes. Specific manifestations in organ systems other than the liver include heart failure, diabetes mellitus, hyperpigmentation, polyarthritis, hypogonadism, and heart failure. (In previous times the condition was often known as "bronze diabetes" because of the association of diabetes and bronze discoloration of the skin.) In advanced disease fibrosis and macronodular cirrhosis of the liver develop insidiously and represent the major cause of death. Splenomegaly is common, although portal hypertension and its complications (see discussion above) occur less frequently than with other forms of liver disease. HCC develops in about 30% of persons with hemochromatosis, exclusively in the setting of cirrhosis.[40] Therefore, early diagnosis and treatment are critical.

Clinical Manifestations and Diagnosis. The diagnosis is suggested by clinical features and family history. Plasma iron and transferrin saturation are increased, and serum ferritin is dramatically elevated, often to several thousand micrograms per liter (normal 10 to 200). The diagnosis of hereditary hemochromatosis is confirmed by genetic analysis for the *HFE* gene. In selected cases liver biopsy may be performed, with Perls Prussian blue stain for the determination and localization of storage iron, which is generally confined to hepatocytes in a periportal distribution.[1] The diagnosis of hereditary hemochromatosis should prompt investigation of other family members for carriage and expression of the *HFE* gene.

It should be noted that a second large category of iron overload syndromes exists, that of *secondary* hemochromatosis. This may occur with chronic hereditary dyserythropoietic states (e.g., sideroblastic anemia and thalassemia), in alcoholic patients with liver disease, and in patients with excessive iron ingestion over a period of many years. Hemochromatosis related to anemias is generally the result of repeated blood transfusions and iron intake. An interesting condition called Bantu siderosis occurred in the past among South African tribesmen who imbibed beer fermented in iron pots. All of these secondary forms of hemosiderosis are not associated with the *HFE* gene.

Treatment. The mainstay of treatment for hemochromatosis is repeated phlebotomy. The typical protocol is weekly phlebotomy of 500 mL (1 unit) of whole blood until the hematocrit drops below 37%, at which time maintenance phlebotomy of 1 unit is carried out every 2 to 3 months. Patients who do not tolerate phlebotomy may be treated with subcutaneous or intramuscular deferoxamine, a drug that chelates iron and facilitates its renal excretion. Deferoxamine is much less efficient than phlebotomy and requires adequate renal function. If identified early, hereditary and acquired hemochromatosis carries an excellent prognosis in terms of preventing heart failure and liver disease. Diabetes may still develop, however, and iron removal does not change hypogonadism or arthritis. Liver transplantation is available for patients with irreversible cirrhosis whose heart involvement does not preclude surgery.

Wilson Disease (Hepatolenticular Degeneration)

Etiology. **Wilson disease,** or hepatolenticular degeneration, is a rare autosomal recessive disorder in which excessive amounts of copper accumulate in the liver and other organs. As with hereditary hemochromatosis, it has now been linked to a specific abnormal gene, *ATP7B*, which results in retention of copper in the liver as well as impaired incorporation of copper into ceruloplasmin. The condition may present at any time before age 50, generally as one of three syndromes: intravascular hemolytic anemia, hepatic dysfunction, or neuropsychiatric illness.

Clinical Manifestations. Hepatic disease is more common in children than adults and begins as hepatomegaly, fatty infiltration of the liver, and elevated liver enzymes. Great variability in liver disease is seen, and Wilson disease may manifest as acute hepatitis progressing to fulminant hepatic failure, a condition very similar to autoimmune hepatitis with numerous extrahepatic symptoms, or insidious development of macronodular cirrhosis with portal hypertension. Neurologic involvement presents as a movement disorder or rigid dystonia, or occasionally as primarily psychiatric symptoms. Other manifestations include renal tubular acidosis with a Fanconi-like syndrome, cardiomyopathy, hypogonadism, metabolic bone disease (i.e., vitamin D–resistant rickets), and arthritis.

Diagnosis. Clinical signs and symptoms suggest the diagnosis, in particular the finding on slit-lamp examination of the brownish Kayser-Fleischer rings at the margin of the cornea. However, lack of Kayser-Fleischer rings does not exclude the diagnosis. Unlike hereditary hemochromatosis, genetic analysis is not the primary diagnostic pathway; it should be reserved for those with proven metabolic abnormalities because of variability in the genetic mutations that cause copper overload syndromes. The combination of low serum ceruloplasmin and elevated 24-hour urinary copper excretion is highly suggestive of Wilson disease.[1] Results of 24-hour urinary copper excretion after penicillamine administration provide additional diagnostic proof in ambiguous cases. The liver biopsy technique for copper determination is technically demanding and is not routinely performed. As with hereditary hemochromatosis, genetic screening of close relatives should be carried out.

Treatment. Treatment involves dietary modification and copper removal therapy. Patients should try to eliminate copper-rich foods from their diet, including organ meats, shellfish, nuts, chocolate, and mushrooms.[1,17] (Vegetarians require specific dietary counseling.) Dietary measures include testing home water sources and filtering water with a high copper content. The primary oral chelation treatment is penicillamine, and patients receiving this medication early in the course of the disease will show marked improvement and protection against liver and neurologic disease.[1] Even patients with advanced Wilson disease may expect some functional recovery. The usual starting dosage is 1 to 1.5 g/day (adults) or 20 mg/kg per day (children), divided 2 or 3 times daily to a target 24-hr urinary copper of 500 to 800 μg/day. Then maintenance is carried out at a dosage of 0.75 to 1 g/day as needed. Treatment is lifelong, and noncompliance leads to definite progression.

Unfortunately, penicillamine commonly causes serious side effects and must be carefully monitored. Hypersensitivity reactions such as rashes and drug fever may be treated by temporarily withdrawing treatment with the drug and instituting systemic corticosteroid therapy. Other adverse reactions include a lupus-like syndrome, chronic skin effects, aplastic anemia, nephrotic syndrome, Goodpasture nephropathy, and myasthenia gravis. Trientine, or Trien, is a second-line copper chelator with fewer side effects. Oral zinc is another therapy that works not by chelation, but by inhibiting copper absorption and enhancing excretion. Finally, ammonium tetrathiomolybdate is occasionally used for severe neurologic Wilson disease because, unlike penicillamine, it is not associated with early transient neurologic deterioration.[41] As with hemochromatosis, liver transplantation has a limited but useful role.

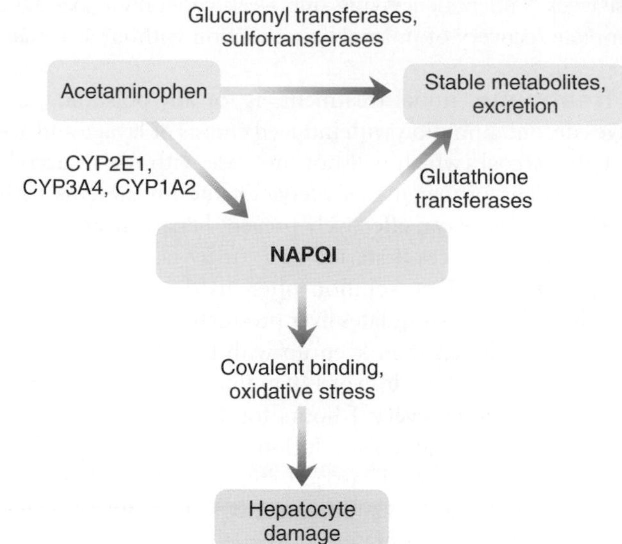

FIGURE 38-14 ■ Mechanism of acetaminophen toxicity. The majority of an administered dose of acetaminophen is conjugated with sulfate or glucuronic acid to form stable metabolites that are promptly excreted in urine. Under most circumstances, only a minority of the total acetaminophen dose undergoes bioactivation to the reactive intermediate *N*-acetyl-*p*-benzoquinone imine *(NAPQI)*. This species is capable of binding to intracellular proteins and mediating cell injury or death. The liver enzymes capable of bioactivating acetaminophen to NAPQI are CYP2E1, CYP3A4, and CYP1A2. Accumulation of NAPQI in the liver does not generally occur because the liver has sufficient ability to detoxify this metabolite through glutathione conjugation. (Redrawn from Fontana RJ, Watkins PB: Genetic predisposition to drug-induced liver disease, *Gastroenterol Clin North Am* 24: 811-823, 1995.)

Toxic Metabolic Agent

Acetaminophen Poisoning

Etiology. Many drugs and toxins cause liver damage. Unfortunately, treatment is often limited to withdrawal of the offending agent and administration of supportive care. Standard measures, including gastric lavage, induced emesis, and activated charcoal, are used in cases of acute ingestive poisoning. Specific antidotes are few, although heavy metal intoxication may be managed with chelating drugs. Acetaminophen overdose is an important exception that bears further discussion.

Pathogenesis and Clinical Manifestations. Acetaminophen (paracetamol, in Britain and Europe) is a widely used, nonprescription analgesic and antipyretic that is frequently implicated in suicide attempts and accidental poisonings. In fact, a multicenter study recently showed that acetaminophen overdose was responsible for 39% of cases of acute hepatic failure in the United States.[42] Oral acetaminophen is rapidly absorbed and metabolized (Figure 38-14). A toxic metabolite, *N*-acetyl-*p*-benzoquinone imine, is formed and rapidly detoxified by reaction with glutathione. However, acute ingestion of at least 140 mg of acetaminophen per kilogram of body weight may expose the liver to high levels of the toxic metabolite with resultant hepatic necrosis. Importantly, repeated ingestion of smaller amounts may cause harm in children, the elderly, patients with preexisting liver disease, persons abusing alcohol, and persons on other possibly hepatotoxic drugs. Significant liver damage is rare if serum acetaminophen levels are less than 150 and 37 g/ml, respectively, 4 and 12 hours after ingestion. Given the many variables affecting acetaminophen toxicity, it is imperative for clinicians evaluating a suspected case to refer to a published nomogram and obtain periodic drug levels of acetaminophen.[43] (Screening for ingestion of other drugs, such as tricyclic antidepressants, should also be done.)

Within several hours of ingestion, the patient generally experiences nausea, vomiting, and diarrhea. After these symptoms, there is often a temporary "window" period, in which the patient feels well and may wish to withdraw from medical care. Within 24 to 48 hours, signs of hepatic injury occur, including abnormal liver enzyme levels. If untreated, progressive liver failure with jaundice, encephalopathy, hypoglycemia, coagulopathy, and even death may occur, generally within the first week. Patients surviving one week generally experience complete recovery of normal liver function without sequelae.

Treatment. Initial treatment, as for any poisoning, involves decontamination with induced emesis or lavage and activated charcoal (which will not interfere with use of acetylcysteine). The proper use of acetylcysteine for patients with clearly toxic levels can effectively prevent hepatic necrosis and its fatal consequences if started in a timely fashion.[44] Acetylcysteine, a mucorlytic solution often used in patients with bronchial diseases, stimulates liver production of reduced glutathione, which can then keep up with blood levels of toxic metabolites. A loading dose of 140 mg/kg is administered, followed by 70 mg/kg every 4 hours for 17 additional doses.[43] The drug is diluted to a 5% solution in a soft drink, juice, or water, given orally or by gastric tube. Acetylcysteine is nontoxic but may cause rash and frequently induces vomiting because of its foul odor and taste.

KEY CONCEPTS

- The liver is subject to damage because of its role in storing and detoxifying potentially injurious substances. Metal storage diseases are genetic disorders in which excessive minerals are absorbed and subsequently deposited in the liver. Hemochromatosis is characterized by excessive iron absorption and is manifested by elevated serum ferritin and iron levels. Phlebotomy is the usual treatment. Wilson disease is due to excessive accumulation of copper in the liver and other organs. Copper chelators are effective in preventing liver damage.
- Acetaminophen is converted to a toxic metabolite in the liver that is normally rapidly detoxified by liver enzymes. In acetaminophen overdose, the detoxification reaction may be overwhelmed and liver necrosis results. Treatment is with acetylcysteine.

OTHER STRUCTURAL LIVER CONDITIONS

Liver Abscess

Pathogenesis, Clinical Manifestations, and Diagnosis. Pyogenic liver abscess is a very common condition worldwide. In the United States it represents most commonly a complication of ascending cholangitis with or without gallstones, "upstream" seeding from a distal intestinal infection (e.g., appendicitis, through the portal vein), or hematogenous seeding from an endovascular infection.

Liver abscess should be considered in any patient with fever and right upper abdominal pain. Nausea and vomiting are common, and jaundice from biliary obstruction may rarely be present. Frequently, tender hepatosplenomegaly and sometimes a palpable mass are noted. Typical signs of pyogenic infection are usually present, including leukocytosis, an elevated erythrocyte sedimentation rate, and elevated liver enzymes, usually in a "mixed" pattern. As the primary diagnostic considerations include acute cholecystitis and cholangitis, imaging of the liver with ultrasonography or CT is usually carried out. Ultrasound- or CT-guided thin-needle aspiration of abscesses is recommended to provide the necessary material for Gram stain and cultures; blood cultures should also be obtained.

Pyogenic liver abscess from abdominal sources generally contains enteric aerobic and anaerobic gram-negative bacteria. *Escherichia coli, Klebsiella* species, and *Bacteroides fragilis* are particularly important. Abscesses of hematogenous origin are more heterogeneous. *Streptococcus viridans* and related streptococcal species are commonly seen. *Staphylococcus aureus* is seen in the setting of endocarditis or widespread bacteremia.

Other uncommon causes of cystic liver abnormalities should be considered, in particular hydatid liver cysts secondary to *Echinococcus* species and amebic liver abscess. These conditions are virtually always seen among persons who have lived in developing countries for many years. Their appearance on ultrasound and CT is usually characteristic, and serologies are available to assist with diagnosis. (Aspiration of echinococcal cysts is contraindicated because of the possibility of anaphylactic shock due to leakage of immunogenic cyst material.) Fungal and mycobacterial infections of the liver are usually granulomatous and diffuse, but in certain settings, such as in neutropenic patients, localized infection with an organism such as *Aspergillus* may be seen.

Treatment. Large (2.0 cm) solitary or multiple liver abscesses require drainage, formerly a surgical procedure. However, at present CT- and ultrasound-guided percutaneous drainage tubes are the standard of care and may be placed with minimal morbidity and discomfort. These should be kept in place until drainage has essentially resolved.

Antibiotic coverage should be directed at likely organisms. A third-generation cephalosporin such as ceftriaxone can be used alone or in combination with metronidazole, if anaerobic bacteria are likely. A β-lactam with β-lactamase inhibitor (e.g., ampicillin/sulbactam) is an excellent choice, but it must be given four times daily. Ertapenem is a new, once-daily carbapenem with broad aerobic and anaerobic coverage and is a good choice for outpatient administration. As 3 to 4 weeks of antibiotic administration is generally required, the latter part of the treatment course could be given orally, using an oral quinolone such as levofloxacin with or without oral metronidazole. Therapy should be adjusted depending on culture results.

Trauma

Etiology and Clinical Manifestations. The liver is the most common solid organ to be injured by penetrating abdominal trauma (such as gunshot wounds, stab wounds, or rib fractures) and the second most commonly injured organ in blunt trauma. Damage or injury to the liver should be suspected when any upper abdominal or lower chest trauma is sustained. The liver is frequently injured by steering wheels in vehicular accidents. Common injuries to the liver include simple lacerations, multiple lacerations, avulsions, and crush injuries.

The gravity of liver wounds arises from the fact that the liver is a highly vascular organ receiving approximately 29% of the body's cardiac output. When hepatic trauma occurs, blood loss can be massive. The patient generally exhibits the typical signs of hemorrhagic shock: hypotension, tachycardia, tachypnea, pallor, diaphoresis, and confusion. Hemoglobin/hematocrit may be normal early on but eventually will reflect significant blood loss. Clinical manifestations include right upper quadrant pain with abdominal tenderness, distention, guarding, and rigidity. Abdominal pain exaggerated by deep breathing and referred to the shoulder may indicate diaphragmatic irritation.

Treatment. Treatment entails the administration of fresh whole blood or packed red blood cells and fresh frozen plasma, as well as massive fluid infusion to maintain adequate intravascular volume and hematocrit.[45] Most patients require surgical management, although some may be treated angiographically or expectantly with medical support. Postoperatively, a patient with hepatic trauma is usually admitted to a critical care unit and monitored for persistent bleeding. The complete blood cell count and coagulation parameters must be closely monitored for trends in changes.

Malignancy

Etiology. Malignancy in the liver usually develops as a metastatic process. Because of the vascularity and lymphatic drainage of the liver, the organ is a common site for metastasis from primary cancers of the esophagus, stomach, colon, rectum, breast, and lung—among many other possibilities.

Primary hepatic malignancy (cancer originating within the liver) is rare in the United States. However, in other parts of the world such as Africa, it is one of the most common sites of malignancy because of a high prevalence of chronic hepatitis B virus infection. Primary liver tumors include hepatocellular carcinoma (discussed below), cholangiocarcinoma, and angiosarcoma. Hepatoblastoma is the most common malignant tumor in children. Lymphoma, especially T-cell lymphoma, may occasionally arise primarily in the liver. Benign liver tumors are much less common, with the exception of cavernous hemangioma.

Clinical Manifestations and Diagnosis. The most common form of primary hepatic malignancy is **hepatocellular carcinoma** (HCC), often referred to as hepatoma. HCC is an uncommon malignancy of middle-aged persons, more frequent in men than in women. The incidence may be increasing in the United States as a result of increasing HBV and HCV prevalence; it is always preceded in these situations by cirrhosis. Signs and symptoms of HCC include hepatomegaly, abdominal pain, weight loss, nausea, and, in advanced cases, jaundice and ascites. HCC has an extraordinary number of paraneoplastic syndromes, including hypercalcemia, erythrocytosis, hypoglycemia, thyrotoxicosis, and hypertrophic osteoarthropathy (finger clubbing).[1]

Space-occupying masses of the liver may first be suggested by abnormal liver-related enzymes, especially alkaline phosphatase. α-Fetoprotein is often dramatically elevated in cases of HCC, although some false-positive results can occur. Definitive diagnosis requires imaging of the liver with ultrasonography, CT, or magnetic resonance imaging, although on occasion the tumor may be diffuse and not diagnostic. These studies also allow guided needle biopsy of the liver lesion.

Treatment. The only treatment for HCC is hepatic resection. Unfortunately, because of advanced diffuse liver disease or multifocal tumors, such treatment is not usually possible. Partial resection is preferred, but complete hepatectomy followed by liver transplantation is a radical option for tumor localized to the liver. Other treatments include systemic chemotherapy and chemotherapy directed selectively to the liver via portal vein or hepatic artery cannulation.[46] Other novel palliative treatments include hepatic artery ligation, direct percutaneous injection of alcohol into hepatic tumors, cryotherapy, and other thermal techniques.

KEY CONCEPTS

- Liver abscesses are suspected in patients with fever, nausea, vomiting, and right upper quadrant pain. Ascending biliary infection, abdominal infections transported by the portal vein, and direct extension of infection from neighboring structures are usual sources of infection. Antibiotics and drainage are commonly prescribed.
- The liver commonly sustains injury during penetrating and blunt trauma to the abdomen. Because the liver is highly vascular, trauma may produce extreme blood loss and hemorrhagic shock. Liver trauma is manifested by abdominal tenderness, distention, guarding, and rigidity.
- In the United States, cancer of the liver is usually metastatic and rarely primary. Tumors of the esophagus, stomach, colon, rectum, breast, and lung commonly seed in the liver. HCC is more common in other parts of the world but its incidence is increasing in the United States, with HBV and HCV as important contributing factors.

TRANSPLANTATION

Patients with end-stage liver disease that has not responded to conventional medical or surgical intervention are potential candidates for **liver transplantation** (Boxes 38-2, 38-3, and 38-4). In adults, diseases currently managed by orthotopic (in-place) liver transplantation (OLT) include end-stage cirrhosis from chronic active hepatitis, alcoholic liver disease, primary biliary cirrhosis, and PSC; and hepatic metabolic diseases such as hemochromatosis and Wilson disease.[1,47] Liver transplantation is rarely performed for patients with malignant neoplasms, although there is clearly a subset of patients with HCC who are candidates for this procedure.[48] The major indication for pediatric OLT is biliary atresia following a failed Kasai procedure (portoenterostomy) or delayed recognition of the diagnosis. Other major pediatric indications include α_1-antitrypsin deficiency and other metabolic disorders. Currently about 5000 liver transplantations are performed yearly, although the waiting list contains about three times that number.

Evaluation of the Transplantation Patient

Potential transplantation patients undergo extensive physiologic and psychological evaluation by physicians, nurses, psychologists, and social workers to identify potential contraindications to the procedure. Conditions that would normally preclude OLT include uncontrolled bacterial sepsis, failure of other major organ systems, extrahepatic malignancy, and more. Additional identified risk factors include portal vein thrombosis, previous portosystemic shunt operations, current alcohol or drug addiction, a poor psychosocial support system, and psychological instability. Many of these conditions are relative contraindications that diminish the chance of a successful outcome, but they do not always preclude transplantation. One group whose numbers are growing is patients with HIV and end-stage liver disease, and this group is increasingly being considered for OLT.[49]

Patients with viral hepatitis are particularly susceptible to recurrence in the transplanted organ and must be managed with care. Recent data show that patients transplanted for HBV who are treated indefinitely with high-dose HBIG have low recurrence rates, with acceptable survival and quality of life.[50] In contrast to HBV, it has not been possible to develop an effective regimen to prevent recurrent HCV infection.[51] A promising approach is preemptive antiviral therapy started shortly after OLT but before histologic recurrence is established; in particular, the use of long-acting pegylated interferons is currently the focus of ongoing clinical trials.[52]

After the patient has been identified as a candidate and a donor organ has been procured, the actual surgical procedure can take 8 to 22 hours to complete. The procedure involves five anastomoses between recipient and donor organs, including the following vascular anastomosis sites: suprahepatic inferior vena cava, infrahepatic vena cava, portal vein, hepatic

Box 38-2

Conditions Treated with Liver Transplantation

Cirrhosis Secondary To
Viral hepatitis
Alcoholic hepatitis
Autoimmune hepatitis
Cryptogenic source (no cause determinable)

Metabolic Liver Diseases
Wilson disease
α_1-Antitrypsin deficiency
Hemochromatosis, neonatal
Glycogen storage disease
Tyrosinemia
Byler disease
Crigler-Najjar syndrome
Miscellaneous others

Cholestatic Liver Diseases
Primary biliary cirrhosis
Sclerosing cholangitis
Biliary atresia
Miscellaneous others

Acute Liver Failure
Drug reactions
Toxins (e.g., mushroom poisoning)
Viral hepatitis
Acute Budd-Chiari syndrome, other ischemic insult

Box 38-3

Indications for Liver Transplantation

Acute Liver Disease
Fulminant liver failure with progressive encephalopathy
Prothrombin time >10 sec above control
Bilirubin <15 mg/dl and rising

Chronic Liver Disease
Bilirubin >15 mg/dl
Intractable hepatic encephalopathy
Intractable ascites
Serum albumin <2.5 mg/dl
Prothrombin time ≥20 sec
Hepatorenal syndrome

Box 38-4

Contraindications to Liver Transplantation

Absolute Contraindications
End-stage cardiopulmonary disease
Metastatic cancer
Active sepsis
Acquired immunodeficiency syndrome
Psychiatric illness preventing compliance with treatment

Relative Contraindications (Vary Greatly Among Transplant Centers)
Renal failure
Hepatitis B infection
Liver cancer
Portal vein thrombosis
Active alcoholism

artery, and biliary tract. The biliary anastomosis site varies, depending on the patient's extrahepatic biliary tract.

Posttransplantation Management

A cornerstone of posttransplantation management is immunosuppression to prevent rejection of the transplant graft. The rejection response after liver transplantation most often occurs between postoperative days 4 and 10. Clinical manifestations of acute rejection include tachycardia, fever, right upper quadrant or flank pain, diminished bile flow through the T tube or a change in bile color, and increasing jaundice. Laboratory findings include elevated serum bilirubin, transaminase, and alkaline phosphatase levels and increased prothrombin time. Following the successful use of cyclosporine, a number of immunosuppressive drugs have appeared and provide several choices for improving outcome. Immunosuppressives may be broadly categorized into three groups: initial immunosuppression, maintenance immunosuppression, and management of acute cellular rejection.[1] Prednisone is the primary posttransplantation immunosuppressive and is steadily tapered off in favor of maintenance drugs. The calcineurin inhibitors cyclosporine and tacrolimus are begun during induction and represent the mainstays of maintenance therapy. In many centers, tacrolimus has supplanted cyclosporine as the preferred immunosuppressive. Adjunctive maintenance agents include either mycophenolate mofetil or the older drug azathioprine. Acute rejection is managed with infusion of either muromonab-CD3 (OKT3) or an interleukin-2 receptor blocker (e.g., basiliximab).

Side effects limit the usefulness of all these drugs and are a main source of morbidity and mortality among transplant recipients. The main nonimmunologic side effects of cyclosporine and tacrolimus are hypertension and renal insufficiency. Blood levels must be carefully monitored. Side effects of mycophenolate mofetil and azathioprine include bone marrow suppression with cytopenias. Problems with the acute antirejection infusions include hypersensitivity and cytokine reactions, and a heightened risk of opportunistic infection, especially cytomegalovirus, immediately after use. Among the many side effects of prednisone are hypertension and hyperglycemia. The main consequence of all these treatments is immune suppression and increased risk for infection.

Early infections are generally due to issues surrounding surgical technique and preexisting infection (e.g., cholangitis) and have declined significantly in recent years.[1] They usually represent nosocomially acquired pathogens. Infections in the middle period from 1 to 6 months often represent viral infection or reactivation. Trimethoprim-sulfamethoxazole (TMP-SMX) is usually prescribed for prophylaxis against bacterial infection and *Pneumocystis carinii* for the first year. Of particular concern and the focus of several prophylactic strategies is cytomegalovirus. Cytomegalovirus occurs at a high rate among seronegative recipients who receive a liver from a seropositive recipient, and reactivation rates are significant as well. In the middle and late periods fungal infection is important, especially *Aspergillus* species, and lymphoproliferative disorder due to Epstein-Barr virus is seen. OLT recipients should be instructed to avoid exposure to environmental or food-borne mold, which could increase their risk for fungal infection. Another important preventive strategy is appropriate vaccinations, particularly annual influenza shots. (Live virus vaccinations, such as varicella, yellow fever, and so forth, should be avoided.)

Critical issues in the posttransplantation period include the following: hypertension, renal dysfunction, hyperlipidemia and cardiovascular disease, obesity, osteoporosis, and increased risk for cancer. Psychological issues are especially prominent, and caregivers and family should be alert for signs of depression and anxiety. Many of the antirejection medications exacerbate these symptoms. With careful follow-up, OLT recipients can live productive lives for many years after transplantation. Chronic rejection, often in the setting of progressive ductopenia, and recurrence of primary pretransplantation liver disease tend to cause graft failure with time. Actuarial survival at 5 years is approximately 88% for persons with cholestatic liver disease, 78% for patients with noncholestatic liver disease who are HCV negative, and 70% for persons with HCV.[53]

AGE-RELATED LIVER DISORDERS

LIVER DISEASES AND PEDIATRIC CONSIDERATIONS

Liver disease in infants and children not only encompasses pediatric variations of adult liver diseases but also incudes conditions unique to that age group. Many of these conditions present at birth or shortly thereafter, although several may appear in later life.

Abnormal Bilirubin Metabolism in the Neonatal Period

Physiologic jaundice of the newborn is a harmless condition lasting no longer than 2 weeks after delivery. (Bilirubin metabolism in the neonatal period has already been discussed; see above section on jaundice.) Immature bilirubin conjugation and transport mechanisms are the primary causes, along with increased gut absorption of bilirubin. Hyperbilirubinemia is not considered physiologic or normal if the bilirubin is greater than 5 mg/dl on the first postpartum day, 10 mg/dl on the second, or 13 mg/dl at any time.[54] It should be noted that breast-fed babies have a higher incidence of hyperbilirubinemia than do bottle-fed babies because the β-glucuronidase in breast milk results in increased unconjugated bilirubin in the gut, which can be absorbed. If significant hyperbilirubinemia occurs, breast-feeding can be stopped.

Pathologic bilirubin levels should lead to an immediate evaluation to exclude congenital hemolytic disorders,

Crigler-Najjar syndrome, hypothyroidism, congenital pyloric stenosis, sepsis, resorbing hematomas, and other conditions associated with an elevated serum bilirubin level. Treatment should be undertaken.

Kernicterus refers to brain injury as a result of hyperbilirubinemia. It is a serious complication of the neonatal period, generally occurring in the setting of premature birth, neonatal jaundice, and especially hemolytic disease of the newborn.[55] In brief, the immature blood-brain barrier allows free unconjugated bilirubin to enter the brain, leading to encephalopathy. The term *kernicterus* refers to yellowish staining of permanently damaged brain tissue, primarily in the basal ganglia and thalamus. Despite decades of research, the exact pathophysiologic mechanisms by which elevated bilirubin causes brain damage have not been elucidated. Unfortunately, most infants die of this condition, and survivors often suffer from cerebral palsy, movement disorders, and mental retardation. Drugs that displace bilirubin from albumin seriously worsen the condition.

If recognized early, treatment with exchange transfusions, phenobarbital (to increase the levels of UDPGT; see previous discussion), and phototherapy ("bili-lights") may prevent these catastrophic consequences.[56] Phototherapy with light in the 450-nm-wavelength band is used to treat unconjugated hyperbilirubinemia in infants. Light at this wavelength converts unconjugated lipid-soluble bilirubin into water-soluble photoisomers that can be excreted by the kidneys, thus lowering the bilirubin level.

Infectious and Acquired Hepatitides in Children

Acute hepatitis A virus infection is often mild or asymptomatic in children. The prevalence of childhood infection correlates inversely with the quality of sanitation and hygiene. Treatment is supportive, and prevention guidelines parallel those for adults. The utility of universal childhood vaccination is being studied.

Globally, **hepatitis B virus infection** is a common childhood disease, with vertical transmission from an HBsAg-positive mother to the infant being the most common mechanism of spread. Infected blood products and drugs are modes of infection in less developed areas. Features suggesting immune complex disease such as arthritis, fever, papular acrodermatitis (a rash not seen in adults), renal disease, and hematologic complications are more common in children. The incidence of chronic infection is also much higher after neonatal or childhood infection, which has grave long-term consequences because of the late sequelae of liver failure and HCC.

Passive immunization with HBIG should be given within 12 hours of birth to children of HBsAg-positive mothers. Active immunization with HBV vaccine should be given as a series of intramuscular injections at birth and at 1 and 6 months of age. Identical prophylaxis should be given to children of high-risk mothers even if not screened for HBsAg and to children otherwise exposed to HBV. In 1991, the Public Health Service recommended universal childhood HBV vaccination.[33] Strategies include infant vaccination, possibly with a booster dose in young adulthood, or adolescent vaccination.

Unlike HBV, **hepatitis C virus** is less commonly spread vertically, and effective screening of blood products has greatly reduced the risk of childhood infection. **hepatitis delta virus** may be spread by the intrafamily route as a coinfector with hepatitis B.

Acute **hepatitis E virus** is especially virulent in adolescents and young adults, with a very high mortality rate in pregnant women. In endemic regions it is the most common cause of childhood hepatitis and is indirectly a cause of infant mortality.

Many systemic viruses may cause biochemical or clinical hepatitis in the pediatric population, including Epstein-Barr virus, cytomegalovirus, herpesvirus, adenovirus, coxsackievirus, varicella virus, HIV, yellow fever virus, and rubella virus. Neonatal hepatitis may be caused by a variety of congenital infections, including cytomegalovirus, herpesvirus, varicella, *Toxoplasma*, and syphilis. Encephalitis and retinitis may accompany these conditions, with lifelong sequelae. The finding of an enlarged liver and elevated transaminases in the newborn should necessitate a search for congenital infection.

Reye syndrome is primarily a disease of children, although adult cases are reported. The syndrome usually occurs shortly after a viral illness such as influenza or chickenpox, and begins with nausea and vomiting rapidly progressing to coma. The exact pathophysiologic mechanism is unknown, but significant mitochondrial dysfunction of hepatocytes occurs.[57] Reye syndrome is characterized by fatty infiltration of the liver with severe hepatic dysfunction, including encephalopathy, coagulopathy, and elevated levels of hepatocellular enzymes. Mortality may be as high as 40%. A strong association with aspirin use during the preceding viral illness has been noted, but other drugs may be causative as well.[57] (Because of the risk of Reye syndrome, aspirin is contraindicated for childhood viral illnesses.) Treatment of Reye syndrome is supportive, and if the child survives, recovery is complete. As with other toxic hepatitides, liver transplantation is reserved for irreversible disease.

Congenital Liver Disease

Many heritable diseases of the liver occur in childhood. These may be broadly characterized as enzyme deficiencies affecting multiple organ systems including the liver (e.g., α_1-antitrypsin deficiency), disorders of bilirubin metabolism (e.g., Crigler-Najjar syndrome), inborn errors affecting other metabolic pathways, intrahepatic ductopenic conditions, and extrahepatic ductopenia (biliary atresia).

Multisystem Enzyme Deficiencies

α_1-Antitrypsin deficiency is an autosomal recessive condition that commonly affects children and young adults, although it may become obvious later in life. α_1-Antitrypsin is an enzyme inhibitor found in many tissues that prevents normal enzymes, such as elastase and collagenase, from causing damage to those tissues. Production of this enzyme is genetically controlled by a gene that has many allelic variations (gene types). Although numerous abnormal alleles have been identified, the most common pathologic form, which causes both liver and lung disease, is the protease inhibitor Z variant *PiZZ,* which produces α_1-ATZ protein.[1] This defective α_1-antitrypsin protein accumulates in the liver and produces the diagnostic granules seen microscopically, although the exact mechanism of liver damage is unclear. A characteristic centrilobular emphysema, pancreatic insufficiency, and cirrhosis may occur. Treatment by liver transplantation is often precluded by these other problems. Gene therapy for α_1-antitrypsin deficiency is an area of very active investigation.[1]

Cystic fibrosis is an autosomal recessive condition primarily known as a cause of lung disease in children. However, this relatively common genetic disease may also cause pancreatic insufficiency, intestinal obstruction, gallstone disease, neonatal giant cell hepatitis, bile duct obstruction, and biliary cirrhosis. Treatment is directed at complications.[58] Ursodeoxycholic acid improves the biochemical indices of liver injury; however, conclusive evidence that the drug halts the progression to cirrhosis is lacking. Gene therapy for the pulmonary disease is in the experimental phase.

Wilson disease and **hemochromatosis** are single-gene-mutation illnesses with significant liver involvement and were discussed previously.

Disorders of Bilirubin Metabolism

Inherited defects in bile acid metabolism can manifest as impaired synthesis or transport. The first group includes **cerebrotendinous xanthomatosis,** a steroid hydroxylase deficiency that leads to premature atherosclerosis and encephalopathy. However, manifestations do not generally include liver disease. Children treated with chenodeoxycholic acid have shown marked improvement. Peroxisomes are responsible for β oxidation in the final steps of bile acid synthesis, and numerous hereditary peroxisomopathies have been described. The most well known of these conditions is X-linked adrenal leukodystrophy, which is manifested by progressive neurologic dysfunction and adrenal insufficiency. Treatments for this and related conditions remain generally ineffective, but investigational therapies are frequently tried.[59] X-linked adrenal leukodystrophy was recently the subject of a major movie focusing on the experimental "Lorenzo's oil."[60]

Disorders of bile acid transport include **Gilbert syndrome,** a very common (about 10% of the Caucasian population in the United States), entirely benign, autosomal dominant condition that results in mild unconjugated (indirect) hyperbilirubinemia. It is caused by decreased bilirubin glucuronidation. Awareness of this disorder is important to avoid inappropriate evaluation of these patients.

Crigler-Najjar syndrome is a rare autosomal recessive disorder marked by significant unconjugated hyperbilirubinemia.[61] In type I Crigler-Najjar syndrome, the near-total absence of bilirubin conjugation results in high levels of unconjugated bilirubin crossing the immature blood-brain barrier. This condition presents shortly after birth, and neonates usually die of kernicterus or suffer irreversible neurologic damage. Liver transplantation following phototherapy and plasma exchange transfusion has been lifesaving in rare instances. In type II Crigler-Najjar syndrome, some conjugating capability exists and is enhanced by the administration of phenobarbital. These patients rarely experience bilirubin encephalopathy and can lead normal lives. Treatment consists of phototherapy, phenobarbital, and liver transplantation.

Progressive familial intrahepatic cholestasis (PFIC) is a rare autosomal recessive disorder involving severe jaundice, pruritus, and malabsorption due to a defect in bile salt excretion. PFIC type I, or **Byler syndrome,** is caused by a single-gene mutation and traces back to an Amish kindred descended from Jacob Byler. Other genetic defects cause different types of PFIC with similar manifestations. Medical therapy with ursodeoxycholic acid is helpful in some children, and biliary diversion procedures have given symptomatic relief to some patients by decreasing the bile acid pool.[1] In the past the disease was uniformly fatal, but liver transplantation has been shown to normalize bile acid synthesis and growth in selected patients.[62]

Other rare disorders of bile salt transport exist and are generally fatal in infancy. These chronic cholestatic diseases, such as North American Indian childhood cirrhosis and cholestasis-lymphedema syndrome (Aagenaes syndrome), are undergoing investigation at the molecular genetic level and are generally linked to single-gene mutations.

Inborn Errors of Metabolism

A very broad range of enzyme abnormalities resulting from single-gene mutations, generally autosomally recessive, may show up in children. These result in abnormal processing of lipids, glycogen, amino acids and proteins, lipopolysaccharides, and other substances. The pathologic process generally results from excessive accumulation of precursor substances in target organs, such as the brain and spinal cord. The liver is often the primary site of processing and may be the target of toxic accumulation as well. The latter may result in signs of liver disease, including hepatomegaly, liver enzyme elevation, and jaundice. Inborn errors that show up in the neonatal period are usually fatal unless immediate treatment is undertaken. Inborn errors presenting in infancy and later years may be amenable to specific therapies. Liver or bone marrow transplantation[63] may be effective for some of these conditions, and many of them are foci of intense research regarding gene therapy. The diagnosis of any inborn error of metabolism should prompt a thorough investigation of family history and appropriate genetic counseling and testing of family members.

As noted above, given the heterogeneity and rarity of these conditions, they will not be discussed further in this chapter, and the interested reader is referred to a standard text on the subject.[64]

Intrahepatic Cholestatic Conditions

Intrahepatic cholestasis may be defined as cholestatic liver disease in which the pathologic process is confined to the liver (i.e., the extrahepatic biliary system is normal).[65] One cause of this condition is neonatal hepatitis, which can be idiopathic, viral, or secondary to an inborn error of metabolism. (Viral hepatitis and inborn errors were discussed previously.) The second category of these illnesses includes conditions in which the number of bile ducts is decreased and inadequate to accommodate normal bile metabolism and transport.

Alagille syndrome, or arteriohepatic dysplasia, is the most common form of inherited intrahepatic cholestasis. This autosomal dominant condition has incomplete penetrance and expressivity, and is associated with typical bony and cardiovascular malformations, as well as a paucity of intrahepatic bile ducts. The disease generally progresses slowly; pruritus, hypercholesterolemia, xanthomas, and neurologic complications due to vitamin E deficiency may occur if untreated. Patients may be maintained on ursodeoxycholic acid until liver transplantation, which is the current treatment of choice.[66]

Several other conditions manifest a paucity of intrahepatic bile ducts. Some of these arise from defective bile transport mechanisms and are discussed under Inborn Errors of Bilirubin Metabolism.

Extrahepatic Cholestatic Conditions (Biliary Atresia)

Extrahepatic ductopenia is often referred to as **biliary atresia.** Biliary atresia or, as some authors prefer, *progressive obliterative cholangiopathy,* can be either congenital or acquired. The latter occurs in the setting of certain autoimmune illnesses and is one of the principle forms of chronic rejection of a transplanted liver allograft. Biliary atresia is a rather common birth defect, occurring in 1/10,000 to 1/15,000 live births (and is therefore much more common than intrahepatic cholestatic conditions).[1] Distinguishing between this disorder and idiopathic neonatal hepatitis can be challenging, but the liver biopsy findings are usually characteristic. Infants and children with biliary atresia have progressive cholestasis with all the usual concomitant features: pruritus, malabsorption with growth retardation, fat-soluble vitamin deficiencies, hyperlipidemia, and eventually cirrhosis with portal hypertension. Some children have recurrent episodes of bacterial cholangitis as well. A cholangiogram should be obtained to assess the possibility of a correctable obstruction. The Kasai procedure is often performed to create a hepatoportoenteric connection, which may allow adequate bile drainage. This procedure is not usually curative but ideally does "buy time" until the child can achieve growth and undergo liver transplantation.

LIVER DISEASES AND GERIATRIC CONSIDERATIONS

Liver size and blood flow decrease with aging, but this observation has little functional significance. Drugs whose metabolism is primarily related to hepatic blood flow and drugs processed by the mixed-function oxidase system (cytochromes) may have a prolonged serum half-life requiring careful monitoring and dose adjustment. Routine blood test results of liver-related enzymes are not changed by aging.

In the United States, **hepatocellular carcinoma** is usually the result of years of injury from alcohol or chronic viral hepatitis and is therefore more often seen in older people. The prognosis is unfortunately dismal.

Ischemic hepatitis is usually associated with underlying cardiovascular disease and episodes of hypotension, as during surgery or sepsis, and is more common in older patients. Typically, serum transaminases rise rapidly and the prothrombin time is prolonged. Recovery may be rapid, but the prognosis depends on the severity of the underlying disorder. Ischemic hepatitis alone is rarely a cause of death in such patients. Right-sided heart failure may result in passive hepatic congestion with ascites and (rarely) liver failure. In developing countries, constrictive pericarditis and uncorrected valvular heart disease due to rheumatic fever are still significant causes of intractable ascites and should be considered in the differential diagnosis.

Metabolic liver diseases rarely present in the geriatric population. **Hemochromatosis** in women often presents after menopause and may present as new-onset diabetes mellitus, heart failure, arthritis, cirrhosis, or HCC. Typically, **autoimmune liver diseases** are seen in young to middle-aged people. However, autoimmune chronic active hepatitis may be a cause of "cryptogenic" cirrhosis in older women. **Primary biliary cirrhosis** is uncommon in later life. **PSC** may afflict older persons with long-standing ulcerative colitis, even those who had colectomies many years, even decades, earlier.

Because **alcohol abuse** generally starts early in life, older patients bear the cumulative injury of years of exposure and are likely to show signs of advanced liver disease. Treatment is the same as in younger patients, but attention must be given to the older patients' social circumstances and intercurrent medical problems. Symptoms and signs of alcohol intoxication and hepatic encephalopathy may be confused with senile dementia and made worse by concomitant drug use (e.g., minor tranquilizers, opiates).

The diagnosis of **acute viral hepatitis** may be more difficult in older people because of nonspecific symptoms in mild cases and decreased clinical suspicion. Acute HAV infection is less common as a result of the higher incidence of immunity, but it may be more severe with higher mortality rates in the elderly. The end results of HBV and HCV infection often become evident in elderly persons, and in the United States the increased prevalence of persons living with these viruses will mean more elderly patients with liver disease in coming decades.

Older patients with chronic HBV and HCV infection may be treated with the standard treatments, but comorbid medical problems, intolerance to the side effects of treatment, and advanced liver disease may preclude treatment in many persons. The indications for **liver transplantation** do not change with advancing years, and no arbitrary age limits have been set on transplantation. However, there may be subtle barriers in effect, and the allocation of organs remains a highly controversial issue. Each patient must be evaluated individually regarding the propriety of transplantation and the likelihood of success.

SUMMARY

Disorders of the liver are diverse and complex. Because the liver is vital to most life processes, even mild disorders can cause life-threatening alterations. Health care professionals need a good understanding of hepatobiliary anatomy and physiology to appreciate the effects of these disorders on patients.

Many liver disorders are the consequence of lifestyle choices such as alcoholism and drug abuse. Health care professionals are in a position to explain the risks of detrimental lifestyles and their relationship to liver diseases so as to prevent occurrence of these diseases.

Medical treatment entails the use of drugs from many different classes. Because the liver is central to the metabolism of many of these drugs, their use requires special attention. Before any drug is given to a patient with liver disease, it is essential to become completely familiar with it by consulting a good pharmacology text or drug information source.

MEDIA RESOURCES

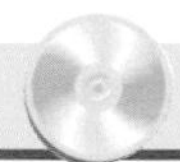

evolve

Remember to check out the ***CD Companion*** included with this book for Review Questions, Key Concepts Review, Glossary (with audio for selected terms), Disease Profiles, and Animations.

PLUS, visit the ***Evolve website*** at http://evolve.elsevier.com/Copstead/ for Case Studies, Disease Profiles, and WebLinks.

References

1. Feldman M, Friedman LS, Sleisenger MH: *Sleisenger and Fordtran's gastrointestinal and liver disease: pathophysiology, diagnosis, management,* ed 7, Philadelphia, 2002, Saunders.
2. Moore KL, Persaud TVN, Chabner DE: *The developing human: clinically oriented embryology,* Philadelphia, 2003, Saunders.
3. Moore KL, Persaud TVN, Shiota K: *Color atlas of clinical embryology,* Philadelphia, 2000, Saunders.
4. Guyton AC, Hall JE: *Textbook of medical physiology,* ed 10, Philadelphia, 2000, Saunders.
5. Johnson LR, Gerwin TA: *Gastrointestinal physiology,* ed 6, St Louis, 2001, Mosby.
6. Kamisako T et al: Recent advances in bilirubin metabolism research: the molecular mechanism of hepatocyte bilirubin transport and its clinical relevance, *J Gastroenterol* 35(9): 659-664, 2000.
7. Gurakar A et al: Androgenic/anabolic steroid–induced intrahepatic cholestasis: a review with four additional case reports, *J Okla State Med Assoc* 87:399-404, 1994.
8. Davies MH et al: The adverse influence of pregnancy upon sulphation: a clue to the pathogenesis of intrahepatic cholestasis of pregnancy, *J Hepatol* 21:1127-1134, 1994.
9. Imperiale TF, Teran JC, McCullough AJ: A meta-analysis of somatostatin versus vasopressin in the management of acute esophageal variceal hemorrhage, *Gastroenterology* 109(4): 1289-1294, 1995.
10. Laine L, Cook D: Endoscopic ligation compared with sclerotherapy for treatment of esophageal variceal bleeding: a meta-analysis, *Ann Intern Med* 123(4):280-287, 1995.
11. D'Amico G, Pagliaro L, Bosch J: The treatment of portal hypertension: a meta-analytic review, *Hepatology* 22(1):332-354, 1995.
12. Gournay J et al: Isosorbide mononitrate and propranolol compared with propranolol alone for the prevention of variceal rebleeding, *Hepatology* 31(6):1239-1245, 2000.
13. Bosch J, Garcia-Pagan JC: Prevention of variceal rebleeding, *Lancet* 361(9361):952-954, 2003.
14. Rikkers LF, Sorrell WT, Gongliang J: Which portosystemic shunt is best? *Gastroenterol Clin North Am* 21:179-196, 1992.
15. Escorsell A et al: TIPS versus drug therapy in preventing variceal rebleeding in advanced cirrhosis: a randomized controlled trial, *Hepatology* 35(2):385-392, 2002.
16. Butterworth RF: The astrocytic ("peripheral-type") benzodiazepine receptor: role in the pathogenesis of portal-systemic encephalopathy, *Neurochem Int* 36(4-5):411-416, 2000.
17. Shils ME, Olson JA: *Modern nutrition in health and disease,* ed 8, Philadelphia, 1994, Lea and Febiger.
18. Crippin JS, Gross JB Sr, Lindor KD: Increased intracranial pressure and hepatic encephalopathy in chronic liver disease, *Am J Gastroenterol* 87:879-882, 1992.
19. Blei AT, Larsen FS: Pathophysiology of cerebral edema in fulminant hepatic failure, *J Hepatol* 31(4):771-776, 1999.
20. Blei AT et al: Complications of intracranial pressure monitoring in fulminant hepatic failure, *Lancet* 341:157-158, 1993.
21. Schrier RW, Gurevich AK, Cadnapaphornchai MA: Pathogenesis and management of sodium and water retention in cardiac failure and cirrhosis, *Semin Nephrol* 21(2):157-172, 2001.
22. Runyon BA: Management of adult patients with ascites caused by cirrhosis, *Hepatology* 27(1):264-272, 1998.
23. Stanley MM et al: Peritoneovenous shunting as compared with medical treatment in patients with alcoholic cirrhosis and massive ascites: Veterans Administration Cooperative Study on Treatment of Alcoholic Cirrhosis with Ascites, *N Engl J Med* 321(24):1632-1638, 1989.
24. Runyon BA et al: A rodent model of cirrhosis, ascites, and bacterial peritonitis, *Gastroenterology* 100(2):189-193, 1991.
25. Singh N et al: Trimethoprim-sulfamethoxazole for the prevention of spontaneous bacterial peritonitis in cirrhosis: a randomized trial, *Ann Intern Med* 122(8):595-598, 1995.
26. Watt K, Uhanova J, Minuk GY: Hepatorenal syndrome: diagnostic accuracy, clinical features, and outcome in a tertiary care center, *Am J Gastroenterol* 97(8):2046-2050, 2002.
27. Arroyo V, Guevara M, Gines P: Hepatorenal syndrome in cirrhosis. Pathogenesis and treatment, *Gastroenterology* 122(6):1658-1676, 2002.
28. Alexander IM: Viral hepatitis: primary care diagnosis and management, *Nurse Pract* 23(10):13-26, 1998.

29. General recommendations on immunization: recommendations of the Advisory Committee on Immunization Practices (ACIP) and the American Academy of Family Physicians (AAFP), *MMWR Morb Mortal Wkly Rep* 51(RR02):1-36, 2002.
30. Braconier JH, Wennerholm S, Norrby SR: Comparative immunogenicity and tolerance of Vaqta and Havrix, *Vaccine* 17(17):2181-2184, 1999.
31. Marcellin P: Advances in therapy for chronic hepatitis B, *Semin Liver Dis* 22(suppl 1):33-36, 2002.
32. Wai CT, Lok AS: Treatment of hepatitis B, *J Gastroenterol* 37(10):771-778, 2002.
33. Hepatitis B virus: A comprehensive strategy for eliminating transmission in the United States through universal childhood vaccination: recommendations of the Immunization Practices Advisory Committee (ACIP), *MMWR Morb Mortal Wkly Rep* 40(RR13):1-19, 1991.
34. Updated U.S. Public Health Service guidelines for the management of occupational exposures to HBV, HCV, and HIV and recommendations for postexposure prophylaxis, *MMWR Morb Mortal Wkly Rep* 50(RR11):1-42, 2001.
35. McHutchison JG, Fried MW: Current therapy for hepatitis C: pegylated interferon and ribavirin, *Clin Liver Dis* 7(1):149-161, 2003.
36. Gorbach SL, Bartlett JG, Blacklow NR: *Infectious diseases,* ed 3, Philadelphia, 2004, Lippincott Williams & Wilkins.
37. Lee YM, Kaplan MM: Management of primary sclerosing cholangitis, *Am J Gastroenterol* 97(3):528-534, 2002.
38. Burt AD: Primary biliary cirrhosis and other ductopenic diseases, *Clin Liver Dis* 6(2):363-380, 2002.
39. Crosse KI, Anania FA: Alcoholic hepatitis, *Curr Treat Options Gastroenterol* 5(6):417-423, 2002.
40. Braunwald E et al: *Harrison's principles of internal medicine,* ed 15, New York, 2001, McGraw-Hill.
41. Brewer GJ et al: Treatment of Wilson disease with ammonium tetrathiomolybdate, III: Initial therapy in a total of 55 neurologically affected patients and follow-up with zinc therapy, *Arch Neurol* 60(3):379-385, 2003.
42. Ostapowicz G et al: Results of a prospective study of acute liver failure at 17 tertiary care centers in the United States, *Ann Intern Med* 137(12):947-954, 2002.
43. Ahya SN et al: *The Washington manual of medical therapeutics,* ed 30, Philadelphia, 2001, Lippincott Williams & Wilkins.
44. Makin AJ, Wendow J, Williams R: A 7-year experience of severe acetaminophen-induced hepatotoxicity (1987-1993), *Gastroenterology* 109:1907-1916, 1995.
45. Clochesy JM et al: *Critical care nursing,* Philadelphia, 1996, Saunders.
46. Ravoet C, Bleiberg H, Gerard B: Non-surgical treatment of hepatocarcinoma, *J Surg Oncol* (suppl)13:104-111, 1993.

47. Keeffe EB: Liver transplantation: current status and novel approaches to liver replacement, *Gastroenterology* 120(3):749-762, 2001.
48. Yu AS, Keeffe EB: Management of hepatocellular carcinoma, *Rev Gastroenterol Disord* 3(1):8-24, 2003.
49. Boyd AE et al: Liver transplantation and HIV: a case series of 7 patients, *Conf Retroviruses Opportunistic Infect* 8(Feb 4-8):217 (abstract 578), 2001.
50. Shouval D, Samuel D: Hepatitis B immune globulin to prevent hepatitis B virus graft reinfection following liver transplantation: a concise review, *Hepatology* 32:1189-1195, 2000.
51. Sheiner P: The efficacy of prophylactic interferon alfa-2b in preventing recurrent hepatitis C after liver transplantation, *Hepatology* 28:831-838, 1999.
52. Samuel D et al: Interferon-alpha 2b plus ribavirin in patients with chronic hepatitis C after liver transplantation: a randomized study, *Gastroenterology* 124(3):642-650, 2003.
53. Wiesner RH et al: Recent advances in liver transplantation, *Mayo Clin Proc* 78(2):197-210, 2003.
54. Sherlock S, Dooley J: The liver in infancy and childhood. In *Diseases of the liver and biliary system,* ed 10, Oxford, 1997, Blackwell.
55. Hansen TW: Mechanisms of bilirubin toxicity: clinical implications, *Clin Perinatol* 29(4):765-778, 2002.
56. Bratlid D: Criteria for treatment of neonatal jaundice, *J Perinatol* 21(suppl)1:S88-S92, 2001; discussion S104-S107.
57. Casteels-Van Daele M et al: Reye syndrome revisited: a descriptive term covering a group of heterogeneous disorders, *Eur J Pediatr* 159(9):641-648, 2000.
58. Sokol RJ, Durie PR: Recommendation for management of liver and biliary tract disease in cystic fibrosis, *J Pediatr Gastroenterol Nutr* 28:S1-S13, 1999.
59. McGuinness MC, Wei H, Smith KD: Therapeutic developments in peroxisome biogenesis disorders, *Expert Opin Investig Drugs* 9(9):1985-1992, 2000.
60. Suzuki Y et al: The clinical course of childhood and adolescent adrenoleukodystrophy before and after Lorenzo's oil, *Brain Dev* 23(1):30-33, 2001.
61. Ishak KG: Inherited metabolic diseases of the liver, *Clin Liver Dis* 6(2):455-479, 2002.
62. Ismail H et al: Treatment of progressive familial intrahepatic cholestasis: liver transplantation or partial external biliary diversion, *Pediatr Transplant* 3(3):219-224, 1999.
63. Yeager AM: Allogeneic hematopoietic cell transplantation for inborn metabolic diseases, *Ann Hematol* 81 (suppl 2):S16-S19, 2002.
64. Behrman RE, Kliegman RM, Jenson HB: *Nelson textbook of pediatrics,* ed 16, Philadelphia, 2000, Saunders.
65. Bezerra JA, Balistreri WF: Cholestatic syndromes of infancy and childhood, *Semin Gastrointest Dis* 12(2):54-65, 2001.
66. Balistreri WF: Intrahepatic cholestasis, *J Pediatr Gastroenterol Nutr* 35(suppl 1):S17-S23, 2002.

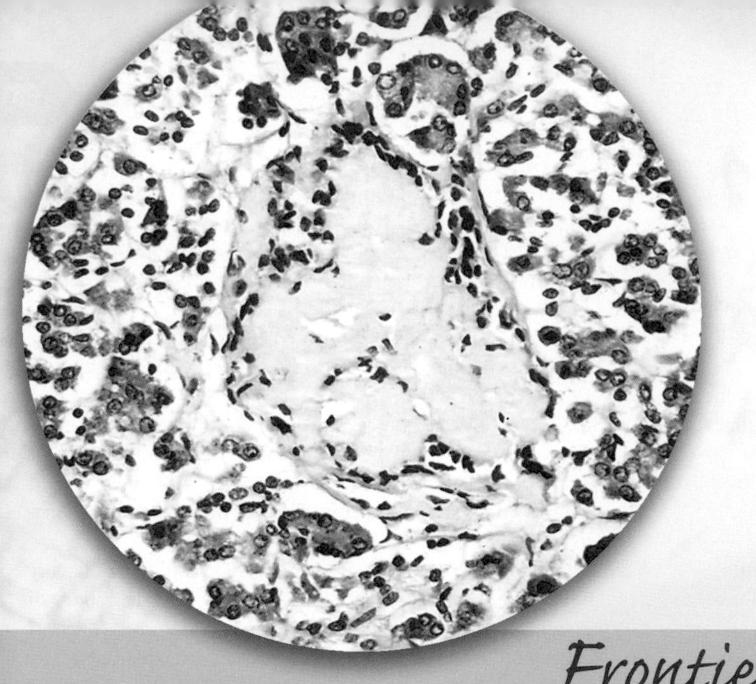

Frontiers of Research

Diabetes Mellitus

Arnold A. Asp and Michael J. Kirkhorn

Diabetes mellitus refers to a group of clinical syndromes characterized by excessive glucose in the blood, causing abnormal thirst, increased fluid consumption, and frequent urination. Excessive blood glucose is caused by either a lack of insulin or resistance to the insulin produced by β cells of the pancreas. Insulin acts at the cellular level to activate "transporters," which facilitate movement of glucose molecules from the blood across cell membranes into the cells hungry for an energy source. Excess glucose that has not moved into cells is eventually passed through the kidneys, causing the "polyuria and polydipsia" classically ascribed to diabetes mellitus.

Diabetes mellitus type 1 (DM1), sometimes referred to as *childhood-onset diabetes,* results from complete loss of insulin production. Patients with DM1 experience rapid, permanent autoimmune destruction of pancreatic β cells. The trigger for this destruction is unknown; although genetic predisposition would seem likely, only 50% of identical twins both develop the disease. Viral infection and/or exposure to unknown environmental toxins may be responsible for stimulating the immune system to attack the pancreas. Therapy for DM1 patients revolves around replacement of the insulin their pancreas formerly produced in response to meals. To date, no effective therapy has been discerned that can prevent the development of DM1 in susceptible individuals.

Diabetes mellitus type 2 (DM2), also referred to as *adult-onset diabetes,* has a more heterogeneous clinical course than DM1. Patients with DM2 usually have insulin production by the pancreatic β cells, but the amount released may be insufficient for the patient's body mass. The patient's cells may also be resistant to the action of insulin. This predisposition to produce too little insulin or to be resistant to the insulin produced appears to be genetically determined; nearly 100% of identical twins will develop the disorder, even if raised apart.

Regardless of the type of diabetes mellitus causing hyperglycemia, prolonged excessive blood glucose eventually leads to devastating multisystem damage. Microvascular complications predominantly affect the retina, glomerulus, and peripheral nervous system, resulting in impaired vision, renal failure, and loss of tactile sensation, respectively. Macrovascular complications include accelerated atherosclerosis in the coronary arteries, the systemic arteries, and the central nervous system. It is not surprising, then, to find that in the developed world, diabetes mellitus is the leading cause of blindness and renal failure leading to hemodialysis. Diabetes mellitus is the leading cause of lower extremity amputation in Europe and North America. Diabetes mellitus and its associated cholesterol abnormalities are major comorbid conditions contributing to the epidemic of atherosclerosis afflicting the world population.

Basic research into cellular and molecular pathophysiology has revealed the mechanism of diabetic complications, and clinical research into diabetic therapy has offered promising insights into prevention of these complications. There had

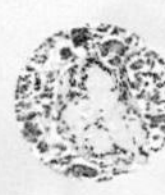

Amyloidosis of a pancreatic islet in type 2 diabetes. (From Kumar V, Abbas AK, Fausto N: Robins and Cotran pathologic basis of disease, *ed 7, Philadelphia, 2005, Saunders, p 1200.)*

Endocrine Function, Metabolism, and Nutrition

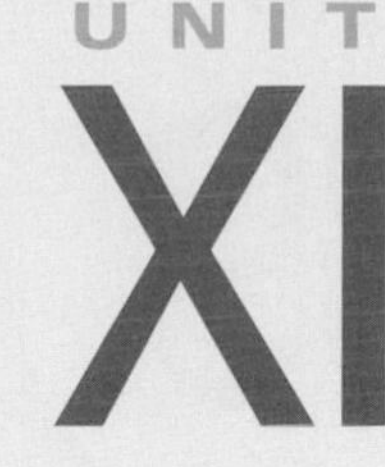

been longstanding controversy as to whether near-normal blood glucose values were sufficient to prevent complications. Skeptics suspected genetic predisposition toward diabetes mellitus made development of retinopathy, neuropathy, and nephropathy inevitable. In the Diabetes Control and Complication Trial (DCCT), 1440 subjects with DM1 were randomly selected to receive either "conventional therapy" with one to two injections of intermediate and short-acting insulin daily or "intensive treatment" with an insulin infusion pump or insulin injections at least three times daily. Subjects treated with intensive therapy experienced more hypoglycemia but noted a 76% decrease in the incidence of retinopathy over conventionally treated subjects. Intensive-therapy subjects with mild retinopathy on enrollment noted a 54% reduction in disease progression over their conventionally treated counterparts. Early diabetic nephropathy, causing renal excretion of miniscule amounts of albumin, called *microalbuminuria,* was reduced by 39% in the intensive-therapy group. Finally, diabetic neuropathy was reduced by 60% in the intensive-therapy group during the 10 years of intervention. The results of the DCCT indicate that the goal of therapy for all patients with DM1 should be reduction of blood glucose to values as near normal as possible without causing frequent hypoglycemia.

Diabetic control in patients with DM2 was also the subject of a recent large clinical trial that confirmed the benefit of near-normal blood glucose levels. As mentioned earlier, DM2 has a stronger genetic predisposition and heterogeneous defects that may require several forms of pharmacotherapy to maintain glycemic control. In the United Kingdom Prospective Diabetes Study (UKPDS), "conventional therapy" was compared with "intensive therapy" using sulfonylureas, insulin, and metformin. Subjects whose HgA1c levels were reduced to 7% or less had a statistically significant decrease in microvascular complications, as compared with those whose control levels were less stringently managed. Recent advances in pharmacotherapy for DM2 have permitted a "tailored approach" to the treatment of the metabolic disorder that was impossible 5 years ago. Aside from insulin therapy used to supplement failing β cells, sulfonylureas can stimulate insulin release in response to glucose absorption from the intestine. Metformin, a type of drug called a *biguanide,* enhances the sensitivity of the muscle cells to endogenous insulin. Metformin also inhibits hepatic gluconeogenesis and glycogenolysis, decreasing inappropriate glucose release from stores in the liver. Another class of drugs called the *thiazoladinediones* (or *glitazones*) stimulates a unique set of cellular receptors called the peroxisome proliferator-activated receptor (PPAR). PPAR activation causes cellular expression of glucose transporters, which efficiently move glucose from the blood stream to the cytoplasm. Blood glucose control is vital to the prevention of microvascular and macrovascular complication in DM2, and several complementary classes of medications are available to effect this control.

chapter 39

Mechanisms of Endocrine Control

Arnold A. Asp

MEDIA RESOURCES

Additional Material for Study, Review, and Further Exploration

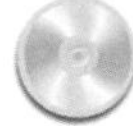

CD Companion ◆ Review Questions and Answers ◆ Key Concepts Review ◆ Glossary *(with audio pronunciations for selected terms)* ◆ Disease Profiles ◆ Animations

evolve ***Website*** at http://evolve.elsevier.com/Copstead/
◆ Case Studies ◆ Disease Profiles ◆ WebLinks

KEY QUESTIONS

- Which hormones act at intracellular receptors and which act through extracellular receptors?
- Which hormones circulate freely and which require transport proteins?
- How do target cells regulate their responsiveness to endocrine hormones?
- How do feedback mechanisms control the secretion of hormones?
- What are the anterior and posterior pituitary hormones, their target tissues, and their negative-feedback mechanisms?

CHAPTER OUTLINE

Communication between organs, tissues, and individual cells is maintained by the actions of and interactions between the nervous and endocrine systems. Whereas the nervous system consists of anatomically connected elements, the **endocrine** system has a more loosely organized structure. It is composed of cells and organs that manufacture and secrete hormones that act at distant target organs. Thus the endocrine system is a functional rather than an anatomic system. The nervous and endocrine systems are closely coupled in that they affect each other's functions and share some of the same chemical messengers, such as epinephrine and norepinephrine. Their actions are coordinated at the level of the hypothalamus. Anatomically part of the central nervous system, the hypothalamus produces and secretes hormones that determine the function of the pituitary gland, long considered a major coordinator for the endocrine system.

Although the nervous and endocrine systems are closely related, they are traditionally studied separately. This chapter covers general mechanisms of endocrine control and provides an overview of endocrine pathology. In the latter part of the chapter, integration of the nervous and endocrine systems at the hypothalamus and pituitary gland is described.

HORMONE PRODUCTION, SECRETION, AND ACTION

Hormone Function and Classification

A **hormone** may be defined as a blood-borne chemical messenger that has an effect on **target cells** anatomically distant from the secreting cell. An **endocrine organ** or gland manufactures and secretes hormones. Major hormones, their primary gland of origin, and their major physiologic effects are listed in Table 39-1. Figure 39-1 illustrates the locations of the major endocrine glands. Some hormone-producing organs have predominantly nonendocrine functions. The atria of the heart secrete the sodium-controlling hormone atrial natriuretic peptide, although the primary activity of the atrium is to transfer blood from the venous circulation to the ventricle.[1] As noted in Table 39-1, more than one organ may secrete a particular hormone, and more than one hormone may be secreted by a particular organ.

Hormones usually travel through the circulatory system to exert their actions in distant locations. Hormones may also act in a **paracrine** fashion; the hormone molecule is secreted by one cell but affects adjacent cells. Hormones may also act in an **autocrine** fashion, directly influencing the cellular function of the secreting cell. Paracrine and autocrine actions of hormones are not traditionally included in endocrine discussions; however, the reader should be aware that the same molecule can have autocrine, paracrine, and hormonal actions.[2] As an example, estrogen acts locally within the ovary potentiating maturation of ova but is required systemically for outward female sexual differentiation.

Function

Hormones control four broad categories of body function: reproduction; growth and development; maintenance of the internal environment; and energy production, utilization, and storage.[3] Endocrine control of reproduction is described in Chapters 30 and 32, regulation of growth and development in Chapter 40, and hormonal impact on general systemic homeostasis in Chapter 2. Hormonal control of energy production, storage, and use is discussed in Chapter 42.

Hormonal function may be complicated; most hormones have an effect on several body systems and functions. For example, among the effects of testosterone are growth and differentiation of the male genitourinary tract, growth of facial and body hair, promotion of muscle growth, erythropoietin production, and, unfortunately, male pattern baldness.

Another characteristic of endocrine control is that one body function may require the interaction of several complementary hormones. The plasma level of glucose is kept in a relatively narrow normal range by the complex interactions of at least six hormones (insulin, glucagon, epinephrine, norepi-

Table 39-1

Major Hormones and Their Functions

Major Function	Hormone	Primary Endocrine Gland
Anterior pituitary "tropic" hormones	Adrenocorticotropic hormone	Anterior pituitary
	Follicle-stimulating hormone	Anterior pituitary
	Luteinizing hormone	Anterior pituitary
	Thyroid-stimulating hormone	Anterior pituitary
Blood pressure control	Renin (angiotensin II)	Kidneys
Fluid and electrolyte balance	Aldosterone	Adrenal cortex
	Atrial natriuretic hormone	Atria of the heart
	Calcitonin	Thyroid
	Parathyroid hormone	Parathyroid
	Vasopressin/antidiuretic hormone	Posterior pituitary
	Vitamin D	Kidneys
Gastrointestinal function	Cholecystokinin	Gastrointestinal tract
	Gastrin	Gastrointestinal tract
	Secretin	Gastrointestinal tract
Growth and metabolism	Cortisol	Adrenal cortex
	Epinephrine	Adrenal medulla
	Glucagon	Pancreas
	Growth hormone	Anterior pituitary
	Insulin	Pancreas
	Norepinephrine	Adrenal medulla
	Thyroid hormones	Thyroid
Hypothalamic-releasing hormones	Corticotrophin-releasing hormone	Hypothalamus
	Gonadotropin-releasing hormone	Hypothalamus
	Growth hormone–releasing hormone	Hypothalamus
	Prolactin-inhibiting hormone (dopamine)	Hypothalamus
	Prolactin-releasing hormone (TRH)	Hypothalamus
	Somatostatin	
	Thyrotropin-releasing hormone (TRH)	
Immune response	Cortisol	Adrenal cortex
	Thymosin	Thymus
Red blood cell production	Erythropoietin	Kidneys
Reproduction and lactation	Chorionic gonadotropin	Placenta
	Estrogens	Ovaries and placenta
	Oxytocin	Posterior pituitary
	Progesterone	Ovaries and placenta
	Prolactin	Anterior pituitary
	Testosterone	Testes
Stress response	Cortisol	Adrenal cortex
	Epinephrine	Adrenal medulla
	Norepinephrine	Adrenal medulla

nephrine, growth hormone, and cortisol). In addition, other hormones may exert indirect effects on glucose levels by influencing appetite and nutrient absorption. The homeostatic implication of this redundancy is that backup systems and fine-tuning mechanisms maintain blood glucose levels within normal or nearly normal limits, even when portions of the system are dysfunctional.

Cellular Receptors and Transport

Hormones may be classified according to chemical structure as amines, peptides, or steroids (Box 39-1). A functional classification of hormones is made according to their site of action at the cellular level. Amine and peptide hormones, including the catecholamines, are water soluble and easily transported through the circulation to target cells.[2] They influence intracellular activity by activating receptors located on cell membranes.[4,5]

Steroids are lipid-soluble molecules derived from cholesterol. Steroids dissolve poorly in blood and require a transport protein (globulin) to convey them through the circulation. At the target cell, the steroid detaches from the transport protein and diffuses through the lipid-containing cell membrane to activate intracellular receptors in the cytoplasm or nucleus.[4,6] Not all hormones requiring transport proteins are steroids; the thyroid hormone thyroxine is a small lipid-soluble dipeptide that is transported on thyroxine-binding globulin. Other examples of transport proteins include sex hormone–binding globulin and cortisol-binding globulin. Hormones can also be carried by "nonspecific proteins," such as albumin.[6]

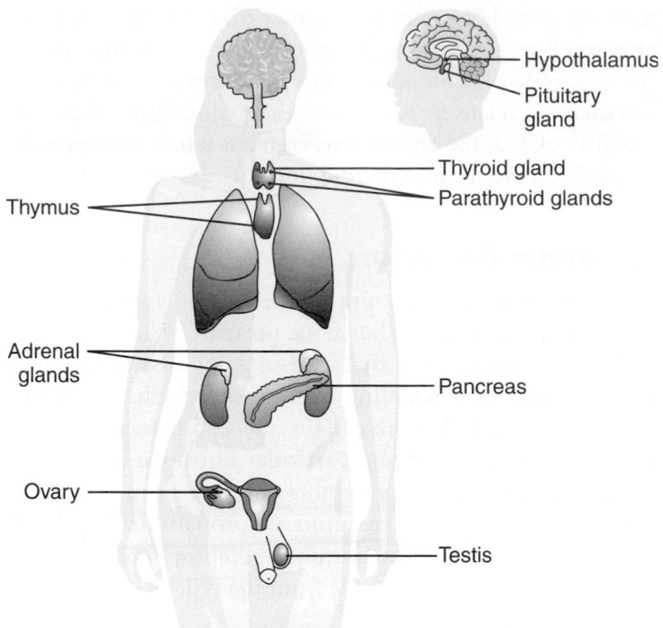

FIGURE 39-1 ■ The major endocrine glands.

Box 39-1

Chemical Classification of Hormones

Peptides
Anterior pituitary tropic hormones
Atrial natriuretic hormone
Follicle-stimulating hormone
Growth hormone
Glucagon
Hypothalamic-releasing hormones
Insulin
Luteinizing hormone
Oxytocin
Vasopressin

Amines
Dopamine
Epinephrine
Norepinephrine
Triiodothyronine
Thyroxine

Steroids
Aldosterone
Cortisol
Corticosterone
Estrogen
Progesterone
Testosterone
Vitamin D

Hormone Synthesis, Secretion, and Metabolism

Hormone synthesis occurs in the cell organelles. Usually one organ produces the majority of the circulating hormone and is considered the endocrine organ source for that hormone, although hormone synthesis and secretion may take place in other organs or cell types. One organ may produce and release a variety of hormones.

The stimulus for hormone synthesis and secretion may be closely controlled. Steroid hormones are not stored in large quantities, and once synthesized, they simply diffuse out through the cell membrane into the circulation. When a steroid hormone is needed, increased production of the hormone closely precedes hormone release into the circulation.[2]

Hormone synthesis may also precede secretion by weeks or months, as is the case with thyroid hormones. Triiodothyronine (T_3) and thyroxine (T_4) are synthesized in the thyroid follicle, then bound to a protein called thyroglobulin. Secretion occurs via cleavage of the thyroid hormone from thyroglobulin in response to systemic needs determined by the hypothalamus and pituitary.

Polypeptide hormones are not stored for long periods after synthesis. The initial forms of the polypeptide hormones are usually large molecules called *prohormones* or *pre-prohormones.* When needed, these large molecules are cleaved by specific enzymes to release the active form of the hormone.[2] Parathyroid hormone is an example of a polypeptide formed as a preprohormone when calcium levels are adjusted in the blood.

Factors Affecting Hormone Secretion

Secretion of hormone is dependent on the interplay of many factors. Some hormones are secreted in cyclic patterns. These cycles may occur over several minutes, several hours, or in a 24-hour (circadian) period. Cycles also occur over longer periods (e.g., the 28-day menstrual cycle) or over years (e.g., the hormones that control reproductive differentiation and maturity).[3] Immediate systemic needs or stressors can override cyclic patterns and modify hormone secretion. An example of this is that activation of the stress response alters the normal circadian pattern of cortisol secretion.

Feedback Mechanisms

The most common process regulating hormone production and secretion is feedback control.[3] An excellent example of **negative feedback** is provided by the interaction between the hypothalamic-pituitary system and the respective hormone-releasing organs controlled by this system. Figure 39-2 illustrates negative feedback control of thyroid hormone synthesis. Thyroid-releasing hormone (TRH) is secreted by the hypothalamus when the central nervous system senses an inadequate supply of thyroid hormones in the circulation. TRH stimulates the release of thyroid-stimulating hormone (TSH) from specific cells in the anterior pituitary; TSH then stimulates release of the thyroid hormones T_3 and T_4 from the thyroid follicle. The resulting increase in plasma thyroid hormone concentration exerts an inhibitory effect, or negative feedback, on the release of TSH by the anterior pituitary. Negative feedback from an increased concentration of thyroid hormones also affects, but to a lesser extent, the hypothalamic release of TRH.[3] The prevalence of feedback systems explains why the diagnosis of endocrine disorders is complex. In the case of T_3 and T_4 an elevated thyroid hormone concentration may be related to a disease process of the thyroid gland or to pathologically elevated levels of TSH or TRH. Assessment of the plasma concentrations of several hormones may be necessary to determine the cause of the clinical pathologic process.

Feedback loops may be complicated and involve actions of several organ systems. Generally, hormones change body functions; these changes then provide a negative feedback so that hormone secretion is decreased. For example, increased insulin is released when blood glucose levels rise following meals. As insulin causes glucose to move into cells, the resultant decline in blood glucose creates a negative feedback at the pancreatic β cells, decreasing insulin secretion. Ionic changes in the extracellular fluid, increased or decreased amounts of the products of metabolism, osmolality, and extracellular fluid volume all act by feedback mechanisms to regulate circulating hormone levels.[3] Box 39-2 summarizes factors that may affect hormone secretion.

Hormone Metabolism and Excretion

The plasma concentration of hormone depends not only on the rate of synthesis and release of the hormone but also on how rapidly the hormone is metabolized and excreted. Like other compounds, hormones are frequently degraded and excreted by the liver and kidneys. Lipid-soluble hormones, which are bound to plasma proteins and stored in adipose tissue, are less readily metabolized and remain in the circulation for a more prolonged period.[2] In addition to metabolism by the kidneys and liver, hormones are often degraded by the target cell after binding to receptors.[5] Metabolism of a hormone may actually activate a hormone. An example of this is thyroxine (T_4). Thyroxine is relatively less potent than triiodothyronine; metabolism of T_4 at the cellular level converts it to T_3, the more biologically active form of thyroid hormone.[2]

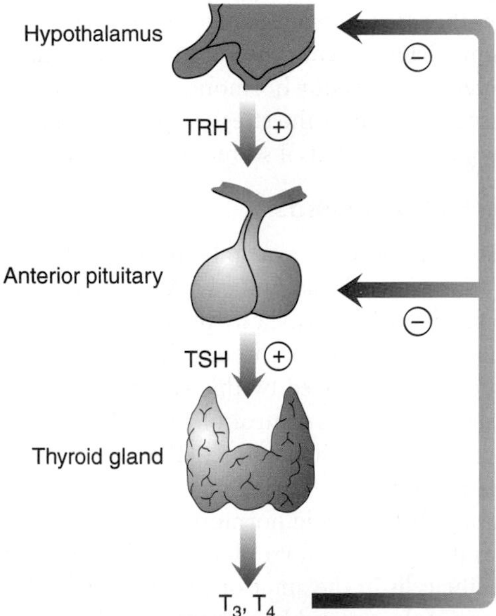

FIGURE 39-2 ■ Negative-feedback loop. Secretion of the thyroid hormones (triiodothyronine *[T₃]*, thyroxine *[T₄]*) inhibits the release of thyroid-releasing hormone *(TRH)* from the hypothalamus and thyroid-stimulating hormone *(TSH)* from the anterior pituitary gland.

Hormone Receptors

Tissue response to circulating hormone is only partially controlled by the amount of hormone present in the circulation. Although virtually all body tissues are exposed to the same concentration of circulating hormones, specific hormones elicit a response only from certain cells and tissues. The ability of a cell to respond to a particular hormone depends on the presence of specific receptors for that hormone on or in the cell. Cell **hormone** receptors are proteins that bind with the circulating hormone; hormone-receptor binding is the first step in eliciting a response from the cell.[5,6]

Receptor Specificity and Affinity

The concept of **receptor specificity** is an important one for understanding the endocrine system. As indicated in Figure 39-3, cells respond only to hormones for which they have receptors. Specificity refers to the "fit" of a hormone within a receptor. Specificity cannot easily be separated from the concept of **affinity.** Affinity describes the degree of "tightness" of the hormone-receptor bond, or the inclination of the hormone to remain bound to the receptor. Specificity and affinity determine whether a cell with a receptor will respond to a hormonal stimulus and the degree of that response. The potency of the hormone, or the amount of hormone required to elicit a cellular response, is dependent on the affinity of the receptor for a particular hormone. The higher the affinity of the receptor for a hormone, the less hormone needed to produce a response.[5,6] Therefore, hormones that circulate in very minute amounts may have a disproportionately large effect on cellular activity because of the tightness of the hormone-receptor bond.

"Cross-specificity" between hormones of similar structure may occur. For example, growth hormone and the lactation-stimulating hormone, prolactin, both may bind to the prolactin receptor. Under normal circumstances, the plasma con-

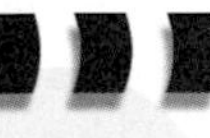

Box 39-2

Factors Affecting Hormone Secretion

Extracellular ion concentration
Cyclic rhythms
Stress (nervous system input)
Feedback mechanisms
- Hormonal feedback
- Extracellular ion concentration
- Metabolic byproducts
- Osmolality
- Extracellular fluid volume

centration of growth hormone is not adequate to bind a significant number of prolactin receptors. However, in the condition called acromegaly, in which excessive concentrations of growth hormone lead to massive bone and tissue overgrowth, milk may be secreted from the mammary glands secondary to growth hormone stimulation of prolactin receptors.[5]

Down-Regulation and Up-Regulation

As mentioned earlier, another factor determining the degree of response to a circulating hormone is the number of cell receptors available for hormone binding. When cells are exposed to high concentrations of hormone for a prolonged period, a common result is that the cell decreases the number of receptors. This phenomenon is known as **down-regulation.** An example of down-regulation occurs with insulin receptors in the obese. An increase in the plasma insulin level commonly occurs in obese individuals. This increased concentration of insulin does not result in an increase in cellular activities in most cells because the number of insulin receptors is down-regulated in response to the high plasma insulin concentration.[5] Down-regulation probably serves a protective function: the cells are protected against excessive activity despite pathologic processes that cause excessive hormone levels.

Up-regulation, or an increase in the number of receptors in response to chronically low hormone concentrations, may also occur. Up-regulation would make the cell more sensitive to the hormone, and hormone-dependent cellular activity could occur at normal or nearly normal levels despite a lower than normal hormone concentration.[5]

Permissiveness

Down-regulation and up-regulation are not the only means by which hormone receptors are controlled. One effect that hormones may have on target cells is to increase the number of receptors for other hormones, thus enhancing the effect of the second hormone. This phenomenon is known as **permissiveness.** For example, the effect of thyroid hormone on adipose cells is to increase the number of receptors for epinephrine. When the adipose tissue is subsequently exposed to epinephrine, a greater release of fatty acids (used in providing energy for cellular processes) takes place than would occur in the absence of thyroid hormone.[2] Permissiveness also allows cellular events to occur in sequence. One effect of estrogen, secreted early in the menstrual cycle, is to increase the number of uterine receptors for progesterone. The uterus is therefore sensitive to progesterone when it is present during the last part of the menstrual cycle, and normal proliferative changes take place.[2,5,7]

In addition to receptor specificity, affinity, and concentration, other factors also affect hormone-receptor binding, including pH, ion concentration, and temperature.

Hormone Agonists and Antagonists

To produce a cellular effect, a hormone must bind to the receptor and initiate a series of events that lead to a change in cellular activity. A chemical may bind to (and block) a receptor without initiating the typical intracellular changes; this chemical is described as a hormone **antagonist. Agonists,** on the other hand, bind hormone receptors and cause the same intracellular events that would occur with hormone-receptor binding. The use of agonists and antagonists has important pharmacologic implications.[8] For example, hormone antagonists that compete with epinephrine and norepinephrine for receptor sites are frequently used to block the cardiac stimulatory properties of these hormones and thus decrease cardiac workload. Conversely, medications that bind to the receptor sites for these catecholamines may be used to increase cardiac output and blood pressure in patients who have severe hypotension.

Mechanisms of Hormone Action

Binding of hormone to receptor, or **receptor activation,** is only the first step in changing cellular activity. Because the events after receptor activation vary according to whether the hormone receptor is located on the cell membrane or internally, the postbinding activity of these different categories will be described separately.

Hormones with Cell Membrane Receptors

Catecholamine and peptide hormones are incapable of independently crossing the lipid-containing cell membranes; recep-

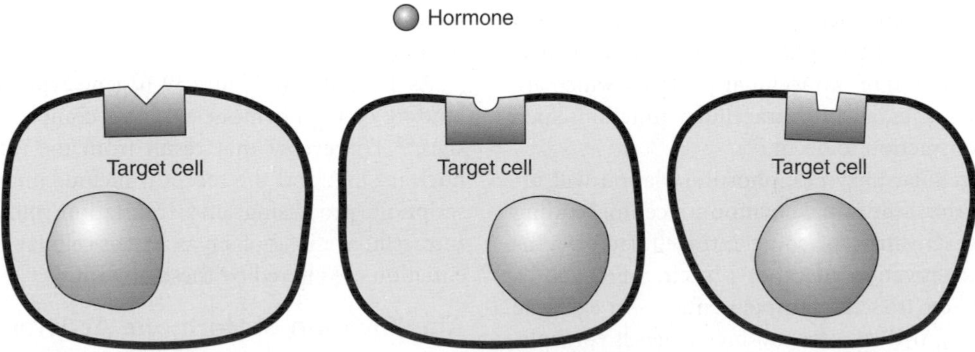

FIGURE 39-3 ■ Receptor specificity. Although many cells may be exposed to a particular hormone, the hormone binds only to cells with appropriate receptors.

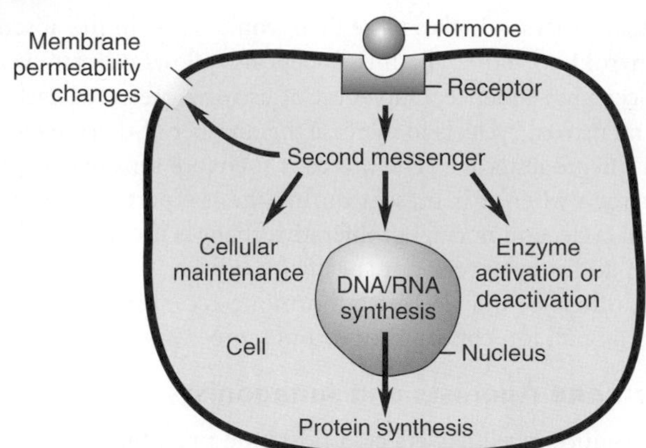

FIGURE 39-4 ■ Some types of intracellular activity after receptor activation.

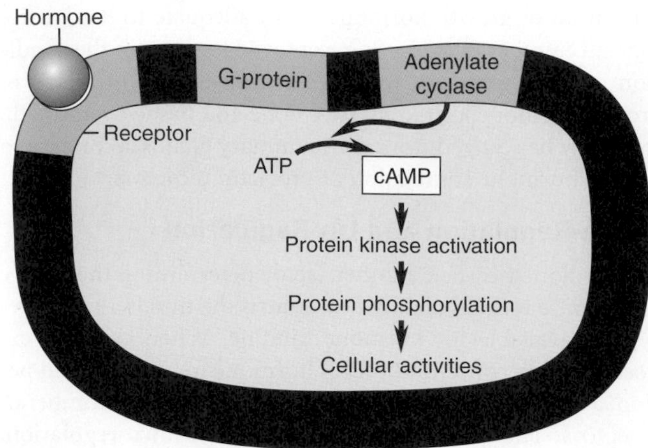

FIGURE 39-5 ■ Cyclic adenosine monophosphate *(cAMP)* as a second messenger. Receptors are located in the cell membrane. *ATP,* Adenosine triphosphate.

tors for these hormones are located at the cell surface. Once hormone-receptor binding takes place, postreceptor activity varies according to cell type. Intracellular activity after binding of the receptor to circulating hormone is dependent on the activation of secondary messengers or secondary signals within the cell. As illustrated in Figure 39-4, a variety of intracellular events can take place once receptor activation occurs. The intracellular activities occurring after hormone-receptor binding may include changes in cell membrane permeability; activation or inactivation of enzymes; cellular maintenance, growth, and differentiation; protein synthesis; and genetic expression via RNA and DNA synthesis in the cell nucleus.[5]

Second Messenger. Hormones can be described as "first messengers"; the hormone carries a message from the secreting cell to the target cell. A **second messenger** (or sometimes a secondary change or signal) must be activated for the needed intracellular response to occur. A variety of second messengers have been identified.

The best-researched second messenger is cyclic adenosine monophosphate (cAMP). As illustrated in Figure 39-5, hormone receptors, through the intermediation of an intramembrane protein known as a G protein, activate the enzyme adenylate cyclase. Adenylate cyclase then allows the conversion of intracellular adenosine triphosphate (ATP) to cAMP. cAMP activates cAMP-dependent protein kinase, which then catalyzes the attachment of phosphate groups to intracellular proteins. Phosphorylation of intracellular proteins, which are most commonly enzymes, allows intracellular functions such as secretion and contraction to occur.[2,5]

For some intracellular enzymes, phosphorylation will inhibit activity. Thus the same initial hormone-receptor binding that results in the activation of some intracellular proteins may lead to the inactivation of other proteins. Frequently, these intracellular activities are complementary. An example of a hormone using cAMP as a second messenger is epinephrine. Epinephrine causes both the activation of intracellular enzymes that allow the conversion of glycogen to glucose and the inactivation of other enzymes that promote the intracellular synthesis of glycogen from glucose. The result of these combined effects is to free more glucose for energy needs.[2]

Box 39-3

Second Messengers

Cyclic adenosine monophosphate
Cyclic guanosine monophosphate
Calcium and other ions
Arachidonic acid
Inositol triphosphate
Diacylglycerol

Other second messengers currently identified are listed in Box 39-3. In some cases, rather than using a classic second messenger, the hormone-receptor complex itself acts directly as a secondary signal and effects changes in protein phosphorylation or cell membrane channels.[5]

Hormones with Intracellular Receptors

Thyroid and steroid hormones diffuse easily through the lipid-containing cell membrane. Receptors for these hormones are located in the cytoplasm or, more frequently, the nucleus of the target cell. Binding of the hormone causes an increase in affinity of the receptor for binding sites on DNA in the cell nucleus.[6]

As illustrated in Figure 39-6, gene expression is changed by binding of the hormone-receptor complex to DNA acceptor sites.[6,9] The events that result from the interaction between nuclear DNA and the receptor include messenger RNA transcription, processing, and translation into specific proteins. Intracellular metabolism as well as cellular growth and differentiation are altered by these proteins.[6]

Amplification of Hormone Activity

The process of intracellular activation by secondary signals occurs via a cascade effect. Progressively larger numbers of chemical reactions occur at each step, so that activation of one

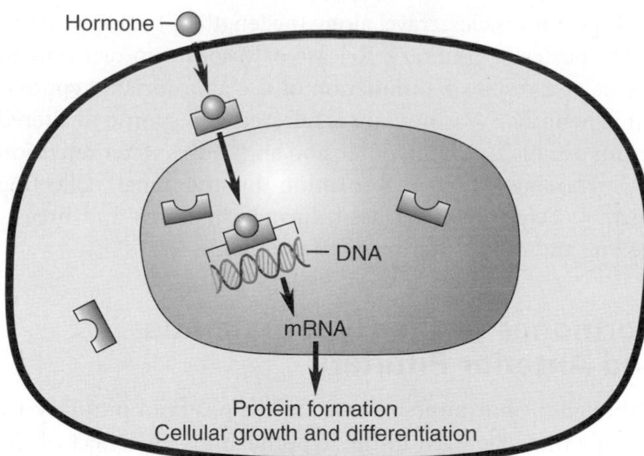

FIGURE 39-6 ■ Lipid-soluble hormone activation. Binding of the hormone initiates messenger RNA transcription, processing, and translation into proteins. Receptors are intracellular.

molecule of adenylate cyclase (or another enzyme) leads to activation of many molecules of cAMP (or another second messenger), each molecule of cAMP activates many molecules of protein kinase, and so forth. This mechanism of signal amplification explains why minute amounts of circulating hormone cause disproportionate cellular and systemic effects.

Pharmacologic Hormone Concentrations

It is important to differentiate between physiologic and pharmacologic hormone concentrations. Pharmacologic levels of hormones can be defined as plasma hormone concentrations much greater than would normally be secreted by endocrine organs. Pharmacologic levels occur as a consequence of either pathologic processes or the administration of large doses of hormones. The kinds and amounts of cellular activity created by pharmacologic hormone concentrations may be radically different from those caused by physiologic levels of hormones.[2]

KEY CONCEPTS

- Hormones are chemical messengers that travel via the blood stream to exert effects on target cells distant from the secreting glands. Hormones regulate four major body functions: reproduction, growth and development, homeostasis, and metabolism.
- Hormones may be classified according to chemical structure as amines, peptides, and steroids and by whether cell receptors are located on the cell surface (catecholamines, peptides) or intracellularly (thyroid hormones, steroids).
- Hormone concentration depends on the rate of secretion and degradation by the liver, kidneys, and target tissues. Lipid-soluble hormones are less readily metabolized.
- Only target cells displaying the corresponding receptor will respond to a particular hormone.
- The number of hormone receptors on a cell's surface may adapt to changes in cell environment. Down-regulation refers to a decrease in the number of receptors in response to excessive hormone. Up-regulation refers to an increase in receptor number in response to low hormone concentration.
- Permissiveness: receptor number and responsiveness may be enhanced by the presence of other hormones.
- Chemicals other than the usual hormone may be able to bind to the hormone's receptors. Chemicals that bind receptors and block activity are antagonists; those that bind receptors and activate them are agonists.
- The secretion of most hormones is regulated by negative-feedback mechanisms. Target gland hormones feed back to inhibit secretion of the initial hormone.
- Peptide and catecholamine hormones exert their effects by binding with receptors on the target cell membrane.
- Receptor activation leads to the production of second messengers or secondary activity within the cell and alteration in intracellular functions. These include: changes in membrane permeability, enzyme activation/inactivation, protein synthesis, and genetic expression.
- Steroid and thyroid hormones are carried in the circulation by transport proteins. Their receptors are in the cytoplasm or nucleus. Hormone-receptor complexes bind to specific targets on nuclear DNA and alter gene expression.

HYPOTHALAMIC-PITUITARY CONTROL OF THE ENDOCRINE SYSTEM

The central nervous system and endocrine system are coordinated at the level of the hypothalamus and pituitary. Understanding of hypothalamic-pituitary function is critical to basic knowledge of the endocrine system. The hypothalamus is a collection of nerve centers clustered about the third ventricle at the base of the brain. A series of neurons and capillaries pass inferiorly from the hypothalamus to the pituitary, carrying nervous and chemical signals from the hypothalamus.

The pituitary is located in the sella turcica, a pocket of bone at the base of the skull (Figure 39-7). In adults, the pituitary is composed of distinct anterior and posterior lobes. Synthesis and secretion of the various pituitary hormones are controlled, directly or indirectly, by the hypothalamus.

Hormones of the Posterior Pituitary

The posterior pituitary gland consists of nerve axons whose neurons originate in the hypothalamus. In some respects, the posterior pituitary can be considered an anatomic extension of the hypothalamus. Two major hormones, oxytocin and vasopressin (also known as antidiuretic hormone), are secreted from the posterior pituitary into the circulation. These hormones are produced in the neurons of the hypothalamus and,

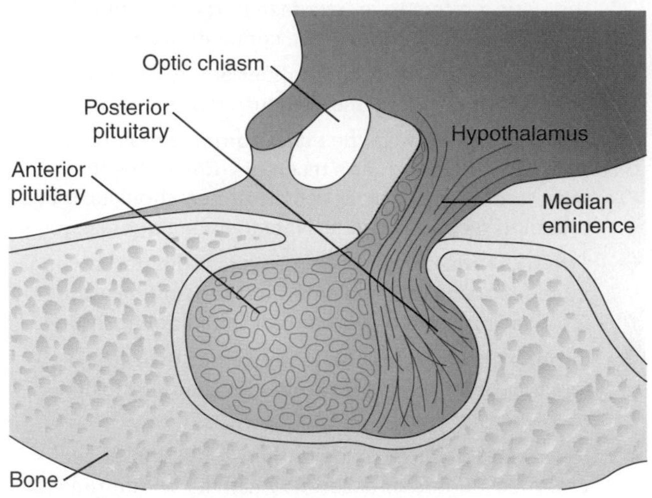

FIGURE 39-7 ■ Anatomic relationship of the hypothalamus and pituitary gland.

packaged in vesicles, travel along the length of the nerve axons to the posterior pituitary. Release of vasopressin or oxytocin occurs as a result of stimulation of the appropriate hypothalamic neurons.[10] Vasopressin is released in response to altered serum osmolality and hypotension and causes water retention by increasing water reabsorption by the renal collecting duct.[11,12] Oxytocin is released during childbirth and breastfeeding and causes uterine contractions.[13]

Hormones of the Hypothalamus and Anterior Pituitary

Although the hormones released by the posterior pituitary are actually manufactured in the hypothalamus, the effect of the hypothalamus on the anterior pituitary is less direct. Hypothalamic hormones are released into a capillary bed that is connected to the anterior pituitary gland. The hormones secreted by the hypothalamus are called **releasing hormones** because they affect the release of other hormones from the anterior pituitary gland.[2,10]

Figure 39-8 illustrates the interactions between hypothalamic and anterior pituitary hormones and their target or-

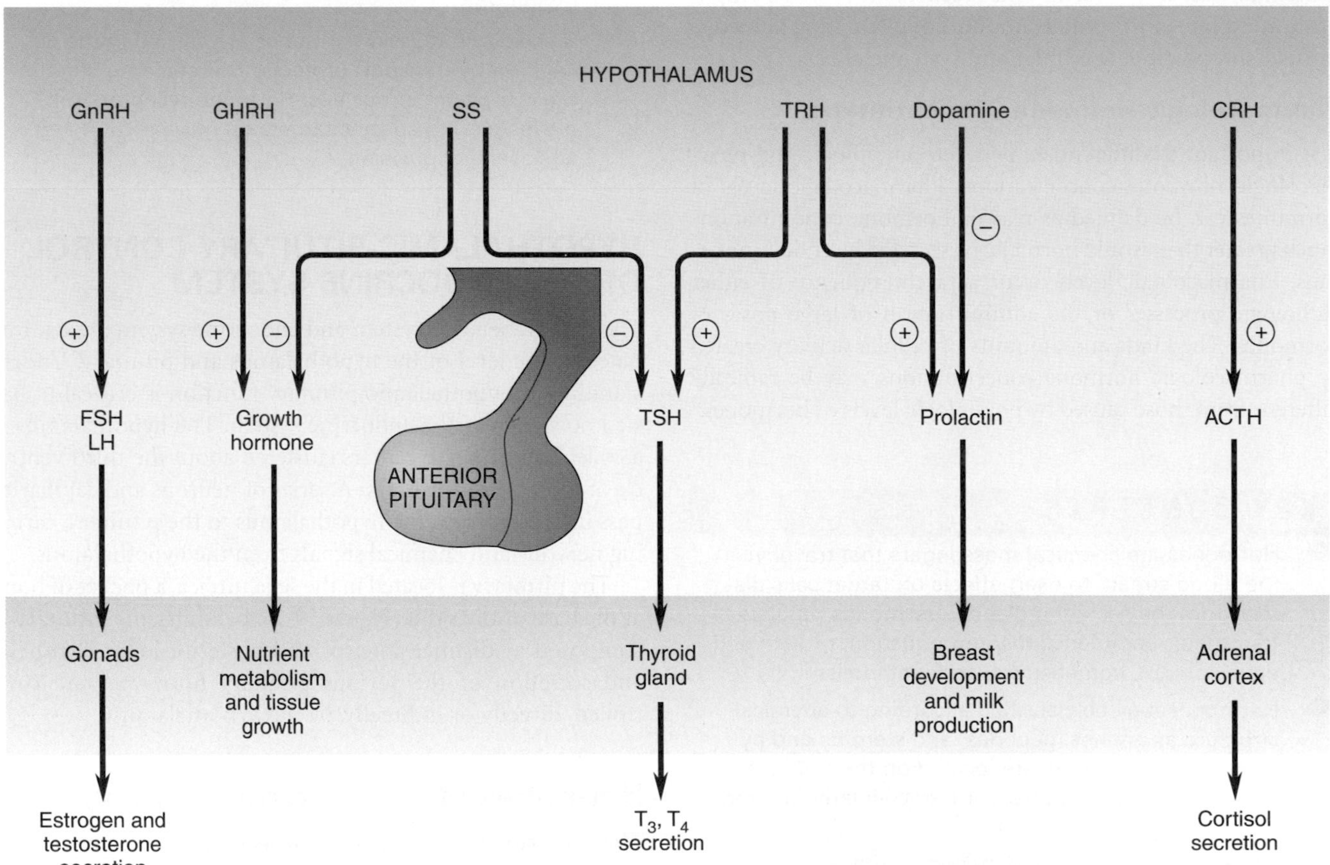

FIGURE 39-8 ■ Relationship of the hypothalamic and pituitary hormones. *GnRH,* Gonadotropin-releasing hormone; *GHRH,* growth hormone–releasing hormone; *SS,* somatostatin; *TRH,* thyroid-releasing hormone; *PIH,* prolactin-inhibiting hormone dopamine; *CRH,* corticotropin-releasing hormone; *FSH,* follicle-stimulating hormone; *LH,* luteinizing hormone; *TSH,* thyroid-stimulating hormone; *ACTH,* adrenocorticotropic hormone.

gans. As illustrated in the diagram, some anterior pituitary hormones act directly on target cells. Other anterior pituitary hormones, termed **tropic hormones,** stimulate the secretion of yet other hormones that finally act on target cells.

This multistep process provides a great deal of fine modulation of hormone action on target organs. Further modulation of target cell activity comes from inhibition of anterior pituitary hormone release by some hypothalamic hormones. As seen in Figure 39-8, hypothalamic hormones may either inhibit or stimulate the release of hormones from the anterior pituitary gland. Secretion of anterior pituitary hormones is obviously dependent on whether inhibitory or stimulatory impulses predominate.

Hormone cross-sensitivity is also illustrated in Figure 39-8. Some hypothalamic hormones affect the secretion of more than one type of anterior pituitary hormone. For example, TRH stimulates the anterior pituitary release of both TSH and prolactin. Thus, in situations in which TRH is released, the potential for prolactin release is also present.

The hypothalamic and pituitary hormones exemplify some of the complexity of endocrine interactions. In addition to interactions between various hormones, other influences such as neuron activity, circadian rhythm, ion and metabolite concentrations, and temperature also affect endocrine function profoundly.[2]

CATEGORIES OF ENDOCRINE DISEASE

Endocrine pathologic processes can be divided into three general categories: disorders of hyposecretion, hypersecretion, and target cell hyporesponsiveness.

Hyposecretion

Primary hyposecretion occurs when an endocrine organ such as the thyroid gland releases an inadequate amount of hormone to meet physiologic needs. Secondary hyposecretion occurs when secretion of a tropic hormone such as TSH is inadequate to cause the thyroid gland to secrete adequate amounts of thyroid hormone. The diagnosis of hormone deficiency is complex inasmuch as knowledge of tropic and releasing hormone levels, as well as the deficient hormone level, is necessary. In a primary thyroid hormone deficiency, thyroid hormone would be low but TSH levels would be high because the anterior pituitary would not be receiving negative feedback from thyroid hormone. However, in secondary thyroid hormone deficiency, thyroid hormone and TSH concentrations would both be abnormally low.

Hypersecretion

Hypersecretion disorders can also be either primary or secondary.[14] When a diseased endocrine gland is secreting an abnormally high amount of a hormone, the tropic hormone will be at unusually low plasma levels because of excessive negative feedback. If hypersecretion is secondary to elevated tropic hormone levels, the plasma concentration of both the hormone in question and its tropic hormone will be elevated. Excessive plasma hormone levels can also occur secondary to hormone secretion by an ectopic source, as sometimes occurs with malignancies.[15]

Hyporesponsiveness

Finally, hyporesponsiveness (hormone resistance) of the target organ will cause the same set of clinical symptoms as hyposecretion. The usual reason for hyporesponsiveness is lack of or a deficiency in receptors, although postreceptor mechanisms such as second-messenger dysfunction can also cause decreased cellular response. If the target cell does not have appropriate receptors for a hormone, the clinical symptoms will be the same as if inadequate hormone levels were reaching the target cells. However, plasma concentrations of hormone would be expected to be normal or high because of the lack of negative feedback to hormone-secreting organs.

KEY CONCEPTS

- Oxytocin and vasopressin (antidiuretic hormone), hormones of the posterior pituitary, are synthesized in hypothalamic neurons that send axons to the posterior pituitary. Oxytocin is released during childbirth and suckling. Vasopressin is released in response to increased serum osmolality and decreased blood pressure.
- Major hormones of the anterior pituitary are growth hormone, TSH, prolactin, adrenocorticotropic hormone, and gonadotropins (luteinizing and follicle-stimulating hormones). The release of anterior pituitary hormones is regulated by releasing and inhibiting hormones secreted into pituitary portal blood by the hypothalamus. Many factors influence the release of releasing and inhibiting hormones, including circadian rhythms, hormone release from target cells, emotions, and pain.
- Endocrine disorders occur because of hyposecretion, hypersecretion, or lack of responsiveness by target cells. Hyporesponsiveness is clinically similar to hyposecretion and usually results from a lack of functional receptors.
- Endocrine disorders may be due to abnormal tropic signals from the pituitary or to dysfunction of target glands (e.g., thyroid, adrenal cortex). Secondary disorders are due to abnormalities in pituitary hormone secretion. Primary disorders are due to abnormalities of the target gland. With secondary hypersecretion, pituitary hormone levels are high; with primary hypersecretion, pituitary hormone levels are low because of excessive negative feedback. With secondary hyposecretion, pituitary hormone levels are low; with primary hyposecretion, pituitary levels are high due to lack of negative feedback.

SUMMARY

The endocrine system, together with the nervous system, is responsible for coordination of cellular activity between many body systems and organs. Hormone secretion occurs in response to a variety of stimuli, including psychological or physiologic stress, electrolyte and metabolite levels, and normal circadian cycles. Increases or decreases in the quantity of a particular circulating hormone tend to regulate levels of that hormone through feedback mechanisms.

The cellular response to hormones is controlled through other factors in addition to the circulating hormone level. Receptor availability to hormones allows the hormones to stimulate the cell. Intracellular processes also help control cell and tissue responses.

MEDIA RESOURCES

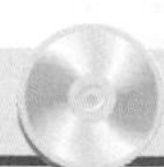

evolve

Remember to check out the ***CD Companion*** included with this book for Review Questions, Key Concepts Review, Glossary (with audio for selected terms), Disease Profiles, and Animations.

PLUS, visit the ***Evolve website*** at http://evolve.elsevier.com/Copstead/ for Case Studies, Disease Profiles, and WebLinks.

References

1. Wilson JD et al: Introduction. In Wilson JD et al, editors: *Williams textbook of endocrinology,* ed 9, Philadelphia, 1998, Saunders, pp 1-10.
2. Chin WW: Molecular and cellular biology. In Lavin N, editor: *Manual of endocrinology and metabolism,* ed 3, Philadelphia, 2002, Lippincott Williams & Wilkins, pp 44-49.
3. Vander AJ, Sherman JH, Luciano DJ: *Human physiology: the mechanisms of body function,* ed 7, New York, 1998, McGraw-Hill.
4. Gill GN: Principles of endocrinology. In Bennett JC, Plum F, editors: *Cecil textbook of medicine,* ed 20, Philadelphia, 1996, Saunders, pp 1176-1185.
5. Kahn CR, Smith RJ, Chin WW: Mechanism of action of hormones that act at the cell surface. In Wilson JD et al, editors: *Williams textbook of endocrinology,* ed 9, Philadelphia, 1998, Saunders, pp 95-143.
6. Tsai MJ et al: Mechanisms of action of hormones that act as transcription-regulatory factors. In Wilson JD et al, editors: *Williams textbook of endocrinology,* ed 9, Philadelphia, 1998, Saunders, pp 55-94.
7. Carr BR: Disorders of the ovaries and female reproductive tract. In Wilson JD et al, editors: *Williams textbook of endocrinology,* ed 9, Philadelphia, 1998, Saunders, pp 751-818.
8. Ross EM: Pharmacodynamics: Mechanisms of drug action and the relationship between drug concentration and effect. In Gilman AG et al, editors: *Goodman and Gilman's the pharmacological basis of therapeutics,* ed 8, New York, 1993, McGraw-Hill, pp 33-48.
9. Biondi B et al: Effects of thyroid hormone on cardiac function: the relative importance of heart rate, loading conditions, and myocardial contractility in the regulation of cardiac performance in human hyperthyroidism, *J Clin Endocrinol Metab* 37(3):968-974, 2002.
10. Reichlin S: Neuroendocrinology. In Wilson JD et al, editors: *Williams textbook of endocrinology,* ed 9, Philadelphia, 1998, Saunders, pp 165-248.
11. Cooper MS, Stewart PM: Corticosteroid insufficiency in acutely ill patients, *N Engl J Med* 348:727-734, 2003.
12. Victorina WM, Rydstedt LL, Sowers JR: Clinical disorders of vasopressin. In *Manual of endocrinology and metabolism,* ed 3, Philadelphia, 2002, Lippincott Williams & Wilkins, pp 68-82.
13. Ladewig PW, London ML, Olds SB: *Essentials of maternal-newborn nursing,* ed 3, Redwood City, Calif, 1994, Addison-Wesley.
14. Tannenbaum C et al: Yield of laboratory testing to identify secondary contributors to osteoporosis in otherwise healthy women, *J Clin Endocrinol Metab* 87:4431-4438, 2003.
15. Women's Health Initiative Investigators: Risks and benefits of estrogen plus progestin in healthy postmenopausal women, *JAMA* 288:321-333, 2002.

Alterations in Endocrine Control

chapter 40

Arnold A. Asp

MEDIA RESOURCES

Additional Material for Study, Review, and Further Exploration

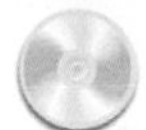

CD Companion ◆ Review Questions and Answers ◆ Key Concepts Review
◆ Glossary *(with audio pronunciations for selected terms)*
◆ Disease Profiles ◆ Animations

evolve ***Website*** at http://evolve.elsevier.com/Copstead/
◆ Case Studies ◆ Disease Profiles ◆ WebLinks

KEY QUESTIONS

- How can primary and secondary endocrine disorders be differentiated?
- What etiologic factors would lead to clinical manifestations of hormone excess or deficiency?
- What are the etiologic factors, clinical findings, and management of growth hormone excess and deficiency?
- What are the etiologic factors, clinical findings, and management of antidiuretic hormone (ADH) excess and deficiency?
- What are the etiologic factors, clinical findings, and management of thyroid hormone excess and deficiency?
- What are the etiologic factors, clinical findings, and management of parathyroid excess and deficiency?
- What are the etiologic factors, clinical findings, and management of adrenocortical hormone excess and deficiency?
- What are the etiologic factors, clinical findings, and management of medullary adrenal hormone excess and deficiency?

CHAPTER OUTLINE

Together with the nervous system, the endocrine system (the glands and the hormones they secrete) regulates body processes involving growth, maturation, metabolic functions, and reproduction. This regulation is carried out through the actions of the hormones produced and secreted by the endocrine glands. Endocrine glands release hormones directly into the blood stream. **Hormones** are potent chemical messengers that exert a physiologic effect on specific target cells and tissues. In the healthy state, hormones are released by the glands when their action is needed and inhibited when their effect is attained. Endocrine disease is marked by either hyperfunction (excessively high blood concentrations of a hormone, or conditions that mimic high hormone levels) or hypofunction (depressed levels, or conditions that mimic low hormone levels).

This chapter discusses the anterior pituitary gland and alterations in growth hormone; the posterior pituitary gland and alterations in antidiuretic hormone; the thyroid gland and alterations in thyroid hormone; the parathyroid glands and alterations in parathyroid hormone; and, finally, the adrenal glands and alterations in hormones secreted by the adrenal cortex and adrenal medulla.[1,2] Table 40-1 lists the glands discussed in this chapter, the hormones produced by those glands, and the major actions of those hormones.

BASIC CONCEPTS OF ENDOCRINE DISORDERS

Hypothalamic-Pituitary Function

The hypothalamus regulates endocrine function by secreting "releasing hormones," which stimulate the anterior pituitary gland. The **pituitary gland,** or ***hypophysis,*** is often called the *master gland,* owing to its important role in regulation of other endocrine glands. The pituitary gland consists of an anterior lobe and a posterior lobe, sometimes referred to as the *adenohypophysis* and the *neurohypophysis,* respectively. The anterior lobe of the pituitary is made up of five main types of cells: (1) somatotropes, which secrete growth hormone (GH); (2) gonadotropes, which secrete gonadotropins (luteinizing hormone [LH], follicle-stimulating hormone [FSH]); (3) thyrotropes, which secrete thyroid-stimulating hormone (TSH, thyrotropin); (4) corticotropes, which secrete adrenocorticotropic hormone (ACTH); and finally (5) lactotropes, which secrete prolactin (PRL).

The hormones produced by the anterior pituitary gland have direct actions on other endocrine glands in the body, with the exception of GH (Figure 40-1). The posterior pituitary is composed of the axons and synaptic ends of hypothalamic neurons. The hormones of the posterior pituitary are released directly in response to hypothalamic stimulation.

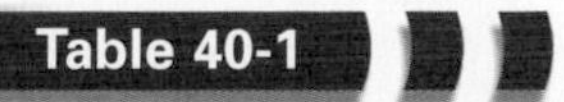

Endocrine Glands, Hormones, and Major Actions

Gland	Hormone	Action
Pituitary Gland		
Anterior lobe	Growth hormone, somatotropin	Promotes growth of all tissues of the body capable of growing, increases rate of protein synthesis, decreases rate of carbohydrate utilization, increases mobilization of fats and use of fats for energy
	Thyroid-stimulating hormone	Controls the rate of secretion of thyroxine by the thyroid gland
	Adrenocorticotropic hormone	Controls the secretion of some of the adrenocortical hormones
	Gonadotropins	
	Luteinizing hormone and follicle-stimulating hormone	Controls growth and reproductive activities of the gonads
	Prolactin	Promotes mammary gland development, and initiation and maintenance of lactation
Posterior lobe	Antidiuretic hormone (vasopressin)	Important role in water conservation and maintenance of body fluid osmolality, blood volume, and blood pressure
	Oxytocin	Stimulates the flow of breast milk
Thyroid gland	Thyroxine (T_4), triiodothyronine (T_3)	Regulate the body's metabolic rate
	Calcitonin	Can decrease blood calcium concentration
Parathyroid gland	Parathyroid hormone	Maintains normal calcium levels in the blood
Adrenal Glands		
Cortex	Glucocorticoids	
	Cortisol (major glucocorticoid)	Promotes gluconeogenesis by the liver, and storage of carbohydrate as glycogen
	Mineralocorticoids	
	Aldosterone (major mineralocorticoid)	Regulates electrolyte concentrations (Na^+, K^+) in the extracellular fluid
	Androgens	
	Dehydroepiandrosterone sulfate	
	Androstenedione (major androgens)	Produce and maintain secondary sexual characteristics
Medulla	Catecholamines	
	Epinephrine	Actions are primarily excitatory and metabolic: ◆ Increases excitability/contractility of the heart muscle ◆ Increases blood flow to muscle, brain ◆ Increases blood glucose levels ◆ Inhibits gastrointestinal smooth muscle contraction
	Norepinephrine	Actions are excitatory: vasoconstriction, increased blood pressure

Dysfunction, either hyposecretion or hypersecretion, may originate in the hypothalamus/pituitary, the hormone-producing gland, or the target organ (Figure 40-2). The source of endocrine disorders may be congenital, infectious, neoplastic, autoimmune, or idiopathic. The onset of the disorders can be slow and insidious or abrupt and life threatening. The age at onset may range from infancy to old age.

Classification of Endocrine Disorders

Endocrine disorders can be classified as **primary** (direct malfunction of the hormone-producing gland) or **secondary** (malfunction of the hypothalamus/pituitary cells that control the hormone-producing gland). Measurement of pituitary and endocrine gland hormones allows differentiation between primary and secondary endocrine failure. When the primary gland fails, inadequate hormone is produced, low levels of hormone are present in the circulation, but blood levels of the corresponding trophic pituitary hormone levels become very elevated. For example, in primary hypothyroidism, the thyroid fails and serum levels of thyroxine become very low. TSH levels rise as the pituitary attempts to stimulate the malfunctioning thyroid. In secondary hypothyroidism, the pituitary fails to elaborate TSH, so both thyroxine and TSH levels are abnormally low in the circulation.

Endocrine disorders can also be classified as **functional** disorders caused by nonendocrine disease such as chronic renal failure, liver disease, or heart failure. Dysfunction may arise if the end organ fails to respond to the hormones. The presence of normal or elevated hormone levels without normal hor-

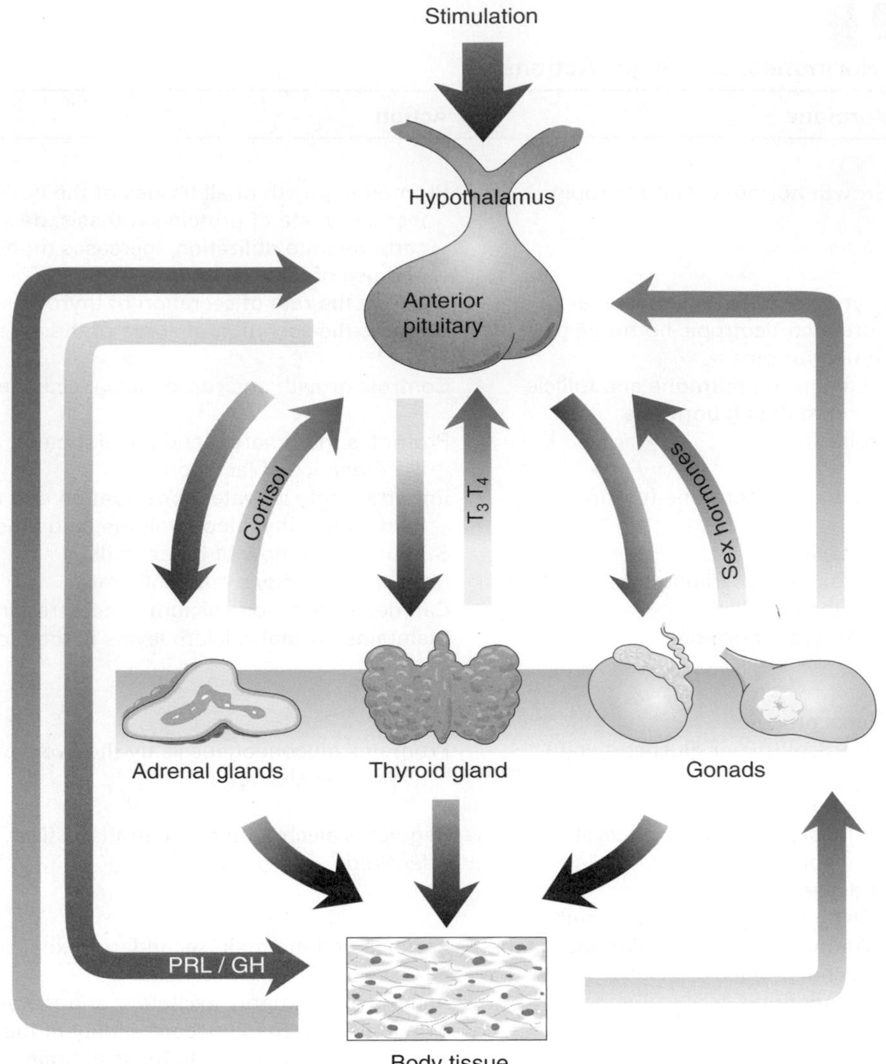

FIGURE 40-1 ■ The hypothalamic-pituitary axis, including hormones, target glands and tissues, and negative-feedback loops. T_3, Triiodothyronine; T_4, thyroxine; *ACTH,* adrenocorticotropic hormone; *TSH,* thyroid-stimulating hormone; *FSH,* follicle-stimulating hormone; *LH,* luteinizing hormone; *PRL,* prolactin; *GH,* growth hormone.

monal action indicates hormone resistance. This problem is also illustrated by diminished or absent response to the administration of exogenous hormones. The mechanisms of hormone resistance may be genetic or acquired and may include defects at receptor sites, antibody reaction to hormone receptors, and defective postreceptor hormone action.

Abnormal hormone production occasionally results from an inborn error of metabolism. Such defects include excessive production of hormone precursors due to an enzymatic block in the synthetic pathway, and enzyme deficiencies that impair hormone synthesis. If such defects are not complete, increased pituitary stimulus may compensate by causing glandular hyperplasia, resulting in near-normal hormone levels.

In addition, hormones may be produced by normally "nonendocrine" tissue. Such ectopic hormone production is usually caused by a malignant tumor. Although different tumors can produce hormones, some cell types are more commonly associated with specific tumors. For example, some lung tumors produce vasopressin, leading to water intoxication and hyponatremia.

Finally, some endocrine disorders may be induced by medical treatments, such as therapy for a nonendocrine disorder. These iatrogenic disorders can also be caused by chemotherapy, radiation therapy, or surgical removal of glands.

Some endocrine disorders have such striking characteristics that recognition is obvious. Other symptoms of endocrine disease may be nonspecific and more difficult to detect. Observing and interviewing skills are important because, with the exception of the thyroid and testicles, the endocrine glands cannot be directly examined. Laboratory diagnostic

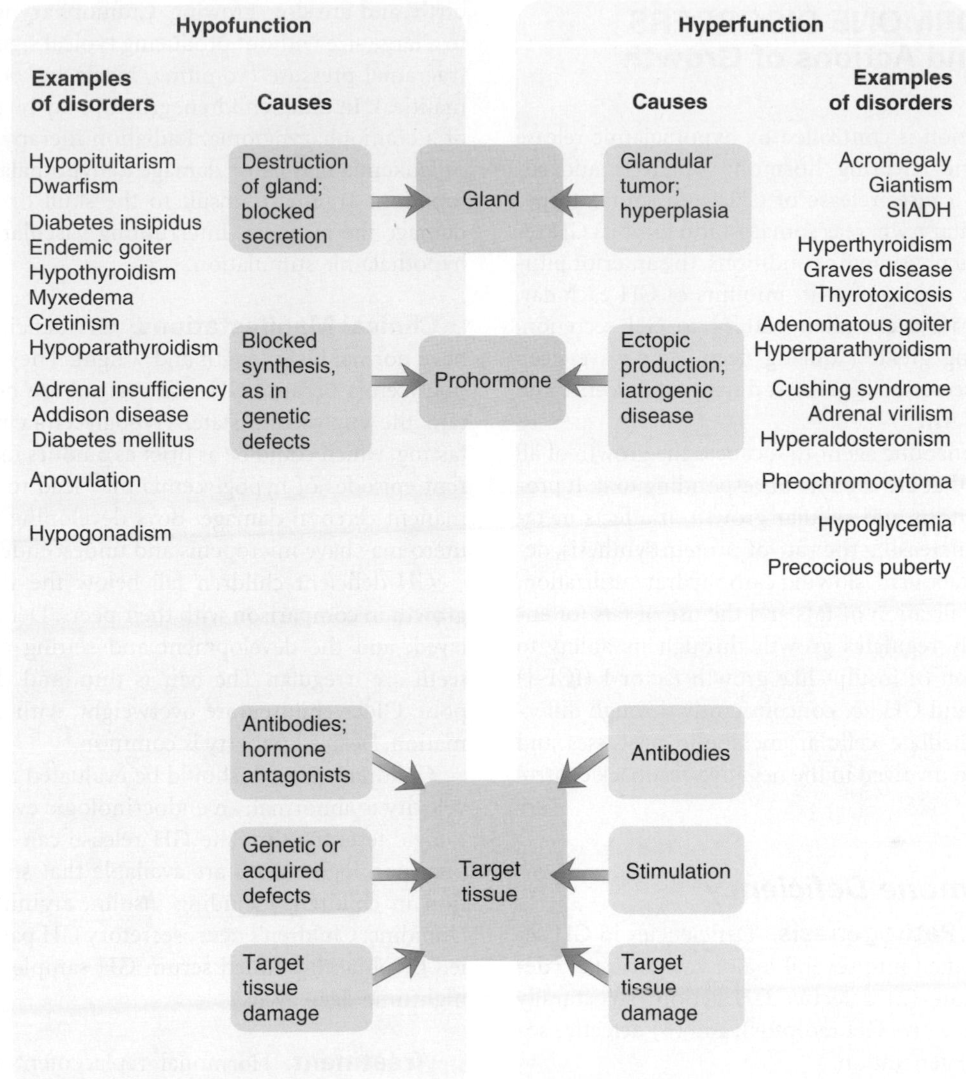

FIGURE 40-2 ■ Examples of endocrine disorders and their causes. *SIADH,* Syndrome of inappropriate antidiuretic hormone secretion.

tests are especially important in assessing the endocrine system.

The treatment for endocrine disorders is varied and depends on the cause and classification of the problem. Methods such as surgical excision of tumor, radiation therapy, and hormone replacement therapy may be employed.

KEY CONCEPTS

- Endocrine disorders occur because of hypersecretion, hyposecretion, or nonresponsiveness by target cells.
- *Hypersecretion* is usually due to secreting tumors or excessive stimulation of the gland by trophic signals.
- *Hyposecretion* may be due to failure or congenital absence of glandular tissue, surgical removal of the gland, or lack of normal trophic signals.
- *Hyporesponsiveness* is clinically similar to hyposecretion and is due to hormone receptor dysfunction.
- Endocrine disorders involving the hypothalamic-pituitary system are often classified as primary and secondary.
- Primary endocrine disorders result from intrinsic defects within the hormone-secreting gland.
- Secondary disorders result from abnormal pituitary secretion of trophic signals. Manifestations of an endocrine disorder are due to abnormal target gland function and are therefore similar whether the etiologic classification is primary or secondary.

GROWTH HORMONE DISORDERS

Regulation and Actions of Growth Hormone

Pituitary GH secretion is controlled by hypothalamic release of growth hormone–releasing hormone (GHRH) and somatostatin. GHRH causes release of GH from somatotropes in the anterior pituitary, whereas somatostatin inhibits GH release. Under normal physiologic conditions, the anterior pituitary gland secretes small pulsatile amounts of GH each day. Sleep studies indicate a circadian pattern to GH secretion, with secretion being greatest during deep, slow-wave sleep (stage 3 or 4). GH secretion is greatest during adolescence and decreases in the elderly.[3]

GH is a potent anabolic agent that causes the growth of all tissues of the body that are capable of responding to it. It promotes increased mitosis and cellular growth. It affects metabolic processes by increasing the rate of protein synthesis, decreasing protein catabolism, slowing carbohydrate utilization, and increasing mobilization of fats and the use of fats for energy.[4] GH indirectly regulates growth through its ability to stimulate production of insulin-like growth factor I (IGF-I) by the liver. IGF-I and GH act concomitantly through different receptors to mediate cellular metabolic processes and growth. IGF-I is also involved in the negative-feedback control of GH secretion.

Growth Hormone Deficiency

Etiology and Pathogenesis. Deficiencies in GH secretion can be classified into several major categories: (1) decreased GH secretion, (2) defective GH action (structurally abnormal GH or defective GH receptor), and (3) defective somatomedin (IGF-I) generation.

Growth hormone deficiency is most clinically relevant in children. A birth history of prolonged labor or breech delivery is common, but GH deficiency may also be present in children who are born with midline craniocerebral defects, most likely due to congenital malformations or as sequelae of a chromosomal anomaly. Deficiencies in GH and other pituitary hormones should be considered in any child with nystagmus, retinal abnormalities, and other midline or midfacial abnormalities, such as cleft lip or palate.

Classic Growth Hormone Deficiency. Children with GH deficiency have a variety of presentations, depending on the cause of the deficiency, the age at onset, and the severity of the disorder. The basis for this defect may be failure of the hypothalamus to stimulate pituitary GH secretion or failure of the pituitary to produce GH.

The most common tumors to influence hypothalamic-pituitary function are midline brain tumors. These include gliomas of the optic nerve and craniopharyngiomas. Craniopharyngiomas arise from cells at the junction of the anterior and posterior pituitary gland, are believed to be present at birth, and are slow growing. Craniopharyngiomas may grow to a large size without producing typical signs of increased intracranial pressure (vomiting, headache, oculomotor abnormalities). In older children, growth may be the first symptom of a craniopharyngioma. Radiation therapy for brain tumors or leukemia may cause damage to hypothalamic and pituitary function. Traumatic insult to the skull or sella turcica may damage the pituitary, interrupting vascular connections and hypothalamic stimulation.

Clinical Manifestations. GH-deficient infants usually have normal birth length and weight. They may manifest hypoglycemia because GH and cortisol are necessary to maintain the euglycemic state. Hypoglycemia may present after fasting, which could be as brief as 3 hours in an infant. Recurrent episodes of hypoglycemia may lead to seizures and permanent cerebral damage. Boys developing GH deficiency in utero may have micropenis and undescended testicles.

GH-deficient children fall below the third percentile of growth in comparison with their peers. Dental eruption is delayed, and the development and setting of the permanent teeth are irregular. The hair is thin, and the nail growth is poor. Older children are overweight, with delayed bone formation. Delayed puberty is common.[3]

Children's growth should be evaluated annually. If growth velocity is abnormal, an endocrinologic evaluation and physiologic tests to stimulate GH release can be planned. Many pharmacologic agents are available that stimulate GH secretion in children, including insulin, arginine, levodopa, and clonidine. Children's neurosecretory GH patterns can be studied by obtaining timed serum GH samples during a normal nighttime sleep cycle.

Treatment. Hormonal replacement therapy for GH-deficient children has been available for about 30 years. The most obvious effect of GH replacement is stimulation of growth in children whose bones have not fused. With treatment, children experience an increase in growth velocity as well as depletion of the fat stores noted in GH-deficient children. GH injections are given subcutaneously 3 to 7 days a week.[1] The greatest response occurs during the first year of treatment. Side effects of GH replacement have been minor compared with the benefit of attaining full adult height.

Adults. Acquired GH deficiency in adults has only recently been recognized and treatment approved by the Food and Drug Administration.[5] Adults may become GH deficient after resection of pituitary tumors or after traumatic head injuries, but these patients are usually evaluated for deficiency of pituitary hormones other than GH. There is controversy regarding the manifestations of GH deficiency acquired in adulthood. There appears to be increased mortality due to cardiovascular causes when adults do not receive GH replacement following pituitary damage. GH-deficient adults have diminished lean body mass, hypercholesterolemia, and de-

Table 40-2

Signs and Symptoms of Growth Hormone Imbalance

Growth Hormone Excess	Growth Hormone Deficiency
Children	
Increased linear growth and tall stature	Delayed growth Fine features Short stature, proportionate
Adults	
Soft-tissue hypertrophy Increased bone density Large hands, feet Coarse facial features Thick, leathery skin Weight gain Glucose intolerance	May be associated with hyposecretion of other pituitary hormones

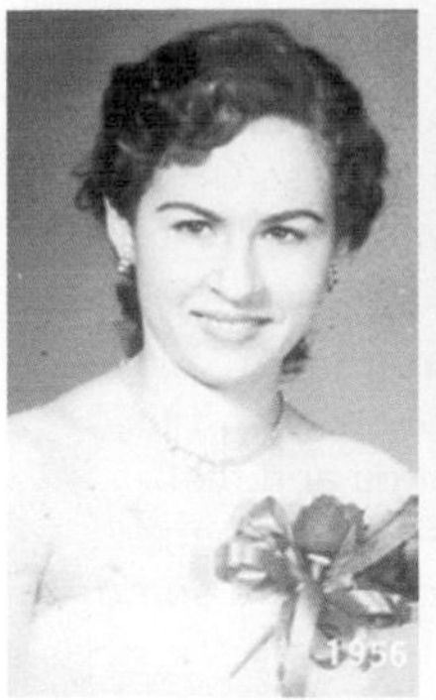
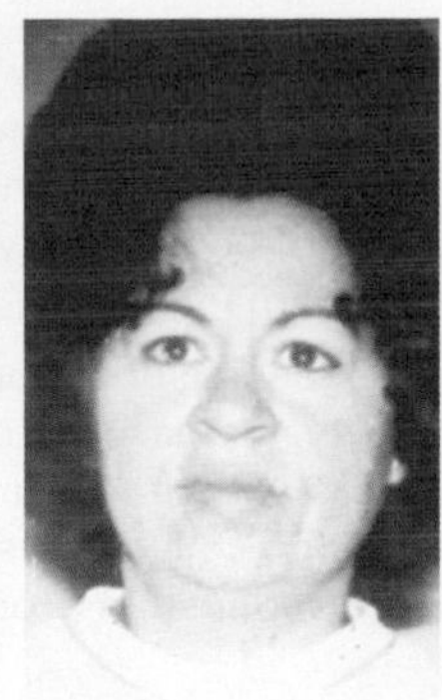
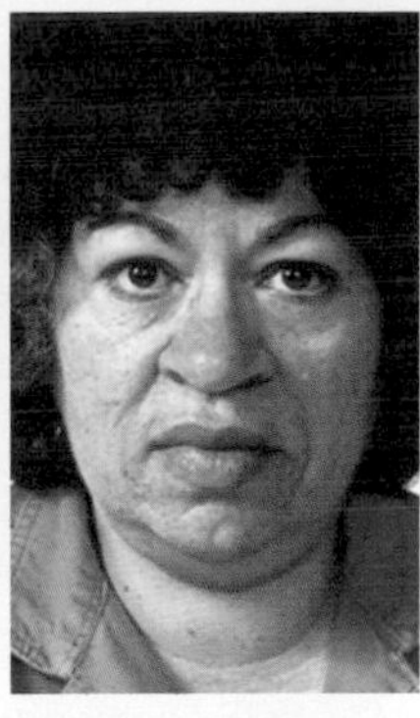

FIGURE 40-3 ■ Progressive development of facial features of acromegaly. (From Lewis SM, Heitkemper MM, Dirksen SR: *Medical-surgical nursing,* ed 6, St Louis, 2004, Mosby, p 1304.)

creased bone density.[6] The latest research seems to indicate that individualized therapy for GH-deficient adults is beneficial.[7] Table 40-2 summarizes the major signs and symptoms of GH imbalance.

Growth Hormone Excess

Etiology and Pathogenesis. GH excess is nearly always due to uncontrolled production of the hormone by a benign somatotropic tumor in the pituitary. GH stimulates the liver to produce IGF-I, and these two hormones act in concert to cause unregulated growth of soft and bony tissues. If the tumor presents in childhood before the skeletal epiphyses are closed, rapid growth results in "pituitary gigantism." Those children experience markedly accelerated growth velocity and quickly exceed the 95th percentile on pediatric growth charts. When the disorder is allowed to progress untreated, some of these children grow to 8 feet in height and usually suffer an early cardiovascular death.

In adults, GH excess is called acromegaly and may be clinically subtle.[1] Acromegaly occurs with equal frequency in men and women during the fourth and fifth decades of life. After the skeletal epiphyses close, bony growth occurs at the short bones, such as the hands and feet.

Clinical Manifestations. Patients will notice increased ring and shoe size, which progressively advances over several years. Enlargement of the frontal sinus causes a prominent brow, and growth of the mandible results in progressive underbite (prognathism) (Figure 40-3). Soft tissues also slowly hypertrophy, causing coarsening of facial features and skin tags. Internal organs increase in size, resulting in goiter (thyroid enlargement) and cardiomegaly. Other manifestations include deepening of the voice secondary to vocal cord thickening and enlargement of the tongue, resulting in sleep apnea. Colonic polyps become more common, with the potential for malignant degeneration. It is estimated that the average patient with acromegaly has an active tumor for 7 or more years before seeking evaluation. Most often the changes are attributed by the patient and his or her family as "just growing older."

Treatment. Effective therapy for acromegaly involves surgically removing the tumor while counteracting the effects of excess GH.[8] Octreotide, a synthetic form of somatostatin, suppresses production of GH. Octreotide is administered subcutaneously three times daily or in a long-acting form every 4 weeks. GH and IGF-I levels decrease and soft-tissue changes described above partially reverse. Unfortunately, octreotide frequently causes diarrhea and cholelithiasis. In 20% of cases, bromocriptine used in conjunction with octreotide may reduce GH levels further. Surgery is usually performed using a transsphenoidal approach, but often the tumor is too large to completely resect. Radiation may be used postoperatively in these cases.[9]

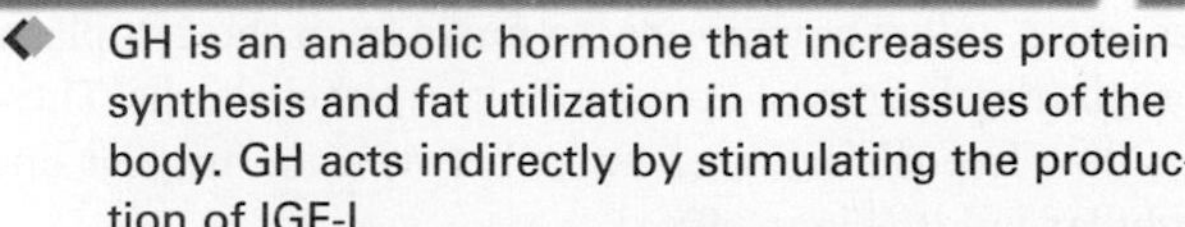

KEY CONCEPTS

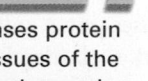

- GH is an anabolic hormone that increases protein synthesis and fat utilization in most tissues of the body. GH acts indirectly by stimulating the production of IGF-I.
- Hyposecretion of GH results in decreased linear growth in children. In some cases decreased linear growth occurs despite normal GH levels, and abnormalities of IGF-I generation or responsiveness are suspected.
- GH deficiency may be idiopathic or related to tumors, radiation, or trauma. The diagnosis is confirmed by a finding of decreased GH levels in the blood and deficient GH release in response to hypoglycemia or other stimulants.

- Excessive GH production is usually due to pituitary adenoma. Excess GH during childhood results in increased linear growth and giantism. Excess GH secretion after closure of bone epiphyses results in increased bulk and acromegaly.
- Features of acromegaly include a protruding jaw, increased bone density, increased growth of soft tissues (e.g., nose, ears), and large hands and feet. Excessive GH secretion causes persistent hyperglycemia and increased insulin production in some individuals.
- IGF-I screening is the best test for acromegaly. An elevated GH level that is not suppressed by administration of oral glucose aids in the diagnosis. Treatment entails surgical removal or pharmacologic palliation of the pituitary tumor.

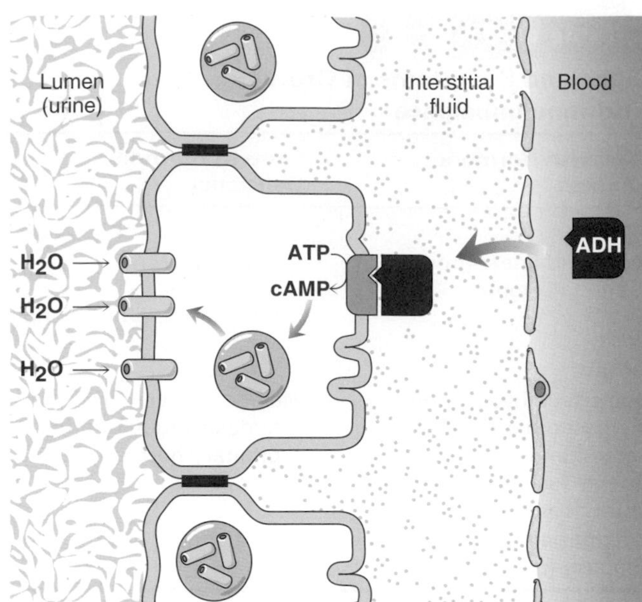

FIGURE 40-4 ■ The current hypothesis for the action of antidiuretic hormone *(ADH)* on the water permeability of collecting-duct epithelial cells. *ATP,* Adenosine triphosphate; *cAMP,* cyclic adenosine monophosphate.

ANTIDIURETIC HORMONE DISORDERS

Regulation and Actions of Antidiuretic Hormone

The posterior pituitary lobe consists of pituicytes (nervelike cells) that originate in the hypothalamus. Arginine vasopressin (antidiuretic hormone, ADH) is synthesized primarily in the supraoptic and paraventricular nuclei of the hypothalamus. ADH is transported in neurosecretory granules through nerve fibers for storage in the posterior pituitary.

The most significant regulator of ADH release is the osmotic pressure of plasma, mediated by specialized neurons called osmoreceptors that are found in the hypothalamus. The osmoreceptors have a set point that influences the stimulation and suppression of ADH. Therefore, when body fluids become too concentrated, ADH is released, leading to increased reabsorption of water in the kidneys.[2]

In the presence of ADH, the permeability of the renal collecting ducts and tubules to water increases greatly and allows most of the water to be reabsorbed from the urine filtrate. The enhanced reabsorption conserves water in the body.

The precise mechanism by which ADH acts on the ducts to increase their permeability has recently been elucidated. ADH causes pores, called aquaporins, to move from the cytoplasm to the cell membranes of apical tubular epithelial cells. These pores allow free diffusion of water between the tubular and peritubular fluids (Figure 40-4).

Antidiuretic Hormone Deficiency (Diabetes Insipidus)

Etiology and Pathogenesis. ADH acts directly on the renal collecting ducts and distal tubules, increasing membrane permeability to water. Damage to the ADH-producing cells in the hypothalamus can occur with closed head trauma, intracranial tumors, and neurosurgery.[10] Some pharmacologic agents can lead to abnormalities in ADH secretion (Table 40-3). For example, the diuresis that follows alcohol ingestion occurs because of decreased ADH secretion.[11]

The most common entity seen when there is damage to the posterior pituitary is **diabetes insipidus** (DI), a large diuresis of very dilute urine. In adults with DI, 30% of cases are idiopathic, 20% are caused by the surgical treatment of brain tumors, 16% result from nonsurgical brain trauma, 25% are secondary to brain tumors, and 9% follow a hypophysectomy.[2] ADH deficiency may be accompanied by other hypothalamic-pituitary hormone deficiencies. Damage to the posterior pituitary may cause temporary or permanent deficiency of ADH. With insufficient amounts of ADH, urine cannot be concentrated and free water is lost, causing hyperosmolality. This is called "central DI" because the ability to produce and release ADH is lost. "Nephrogenic" DI occurs when chronic renal disease prevents the renal tubules from responding to ADH. Central DI may be confused clinically with nephrogenic DI. With nephrogenic DI, the kidney is unable to respond to ADH because of chronic renal disease, serum electrolyte abnormalities, or drugs (e.g., lithium).

The regulation of osmolality is based on control of water balance. Water balance is dependent on the interplay between the amount of water brought into the system (control of thirst) and renal conservation of water controlled through ADH. ADH secretion is triggered by changes in osmolality detected by hypothalamic osmoreceptors. In the absence of ADH, the permeability to water is diminished, resulting in the excretion of large volumes of hypotonic fluid.

Although ADH is a pressor agent, at physiologic levels it does not typically elevate blood pressure. ADH secretion is

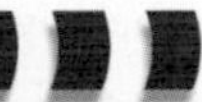

Table 40-3

Agents Causing Alterations in Antidiuretic Hormone Secretion

Agents That Enhance Release	Agents That Suppress Release
Vincristine	Phenytoin
Cyclophosphamide	Alcohol
Prostaglandin E_2	α-Adrenergic agents
β-Adrenergic agents	
Histamine	
Hypercapnia	
Morphine and narcotic analogs	
Nicotine	
Clofibrate	
Carbamazepine	
Barbiturates	
Hypoxia	

triggered by changes in osmolality; volume status has a weak effect on ADH secretion. (Changes in the renin-angiotensin-aldosterone system, however, are sensitive to changes in volume and less responsive to changes in osmolality.)

Clinical Manifestations and Diagnosis. The development of **polyuria** (excessive urination) and **polydipsia** (excessive drinking) is the hallmark of DI. The patient may void as much as 15 L of urine daily. Specific gravity of the urine will be greatly decreased. If the thirst center of the hypothalamus is functional, the patient will consume up to 15 L of water (preferably cold) to maintain osmolar balance. Symptoms persist at night (nocturia), interrupting normal sleep patterns. Usual patterns of behavior and work habits can be affected by the need to frequently drink and urinate. Inability to ingest adequate water to replenish losses leads to dehydration, with clinical manifestations such as dry mucous membranes, poor skin turgor, and decreased saliva and sweat production.[11] If the thirst center has been damaged, DI becomes a life-threatening illness because increased water losses from the kidneys (due to the absence of ADH) are not counteracted by increased thirst and hydration.

DI results in hypernatremia, due to loss of water without concurrent loss of sodium. Hypernatremia is associated with serum sodium concentrations in excess of 145 mEq/L. It usually indicates a body water deficit relative to sodium; signs and symptoms are similar to those of dehydration and include thirst, disorientation, lethargy, and seizures. The neurologic symptoms are thought to be due to shrinkage and dehydration of cells.

Most sudden, critical presentations will be straightforward, with documented hypotonic polyuria, hypernatremia, and hypertonicity indicating a defect in secretion of ADH. Individuals presenting with the sudden onset of polyuria and polydipsia should undergo laboratory studies, including tests for glucose, urine and serum electrolytes, serum creatinine, and blood urea nitrogen (BUN) levels. The results of these tests should exclude diabetes mellitus and kidney disease as the basis for the presenting complaints. A comparison of serum and urine osmolality is needed, as is a urine specific gravity measurement. Dilute urine in the presence of dehydration and hypernatremia along with (if possible) abnormally low ADH levels are diagnostic of DI.

A water deprivation test confirms the diagnosis. When water intake is restricted, the individual becomes dehydrated quickly, as the urine output is not diminished because of the inadequate ADH release by the pituitary. The osmolality of urine decreases as serum osmolality increases rapidly. Urine osmolality is measured hourly, and once a plateau is reached, vasopressin is injected subcutaneously. With neurogenic DI, urine osmolality increases following vasopressin administration. Polyuria and polydipsia also resolve. In the case of nephrogenic DI, no response to vasopressin occurs.[2]

Magnetic resonance imaging (MRI) or computed tomography (CT) of the hypothalamic-pituitary region should be performed to uncover possible causes of DI.

Treatment. Daily replacement of ADH is needed for the management of DI. DDAVP (1-deamino-8-D-arginine vasopressin), a synthetic analog of ADH, can be given by nasal insufflation.[10] One dose lasts between 8 and 24 hours. Free access to fluids is necessary, and home testing of urine specific gravity may be useful for some individuals to allow them to adjust their dose of DDAVP independently. Careful education and follow-up of these individuals are needed.

Antidiuretic Hormone Excess (Syndrome of Inappropriate Antidiuretic Hormone Secretion)

Etiology and Pathogenesis. The ectopic production of ADH has been noted in association with several types of tumors, the most common of which are primary lung malignancies. Nonmalignant lung disorders are also capable of ADH synthesis, or stimulation of central ADH production, especially pulmonary tuberculosis. Drug-induced ADH secretion occurs with the administration of a number of medications, including (but not limited to) chlorpropamide, carbamazepine, morphine, and barbiturates. This inappropriate secretion of ADH is referred to as **syndrome of inappropriate antidiuretic hormone** secretion (SIADH).[11]

SIADH results in hyponatremia when free water is inappropriately conserved and "dilutes" the serum to a sodium concentration below the normal range (<136 mEq/L). In hyponatremia there is an excess of water relative to solute. Cells swell, and the effects of cellular swelling on neurons can be profound. Adrenal insufficiency and hypothyroidism may also cause decreased cardiac output, increased ADH secretion, and hyponatremia. Both of these hormonal deficiencies must be excluded before SIADH is diagnosed.

Clinical Manifestations. Clinical manifestations are due to the hypotonicity of body fluids.[12] SIADH is characterized by hyponatremia. Urine osmolality is inappropriately high because of increased water reabsorption in the renal tubules and collecting ducts. Serum osmolality is low because of dilution by the reabsorbed water (Figure 40-5). Despite the increased water retention (without sodium), the patient does not become edematous.

The symptoms of SIADH include weakness, muscle cramps, nausea and vomiting, postural blood pressure changes, poor skin turgor, fatigue, anorexia, and lethargy. In very severe cases, confusion, hemiparesis (motor weakness on one side of the body), seizures, and coma may occur. Laboratory findings include low serum sodium, hematocrit, and BUN levels as a result of expansion of the extracellular fluid volume.

Treatment. Fluid restriction should be implemented for individuals with SIADH. Fluid restriction should result in a slow, steady rise in serum sodium levels and osmolality. If severe symptoms develop, intravenous (IV) administration of saline, combined with furosemide therapy, may cause loss of free water. Hyponatremia should be corrected slowly. If hyponatremia is persistent, demeclocycline or lithium may be used to block the effects of ADH.

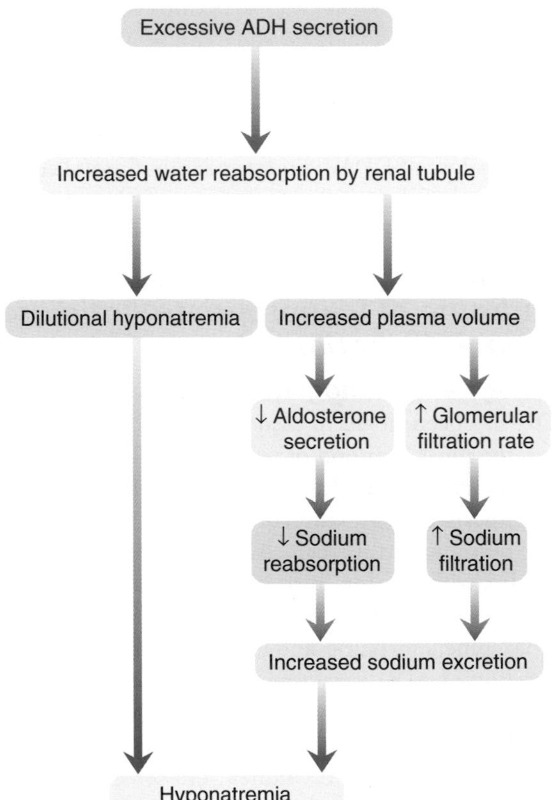

FIGURE 40-5 ■ The syndrome of inappropriate antidiuretic hormone secretion leads to hyponatremia by two mechanisms: (1) dilution of plasma and (2) increased excretion of sodium by the kidneys. Sodium excretion is increased because of the expanded plasma volume, which enhances sodium filtration and reduces sodium reabsorption. *ADH,* Antidiuretic hormone.

KEY CONCEPTS

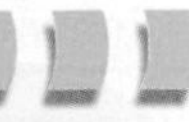

- ADH secretion is primarily regulated by osmoreceptors in the hypothalamus that respond to changes in extracellular osmolality. An increase in osmolality stimulates secretion of ADH. Renal distal and collecting tubules respond to ADH by becoming more permeable to water. In the presence of ADH, water is reabsorbed from the urine filtrate, resulting in a concentrated urine.
- Central DI is due to lack of production of ADH by the hypothalamus or release by the posterior pituitary. Central DI may be idiopathic or related to brain surgery, trauma, or tumor.
- Nephrogenic DI is caused by lack of renal collecting tubule responsiveness to ADH. Nephrogenic DI may be caused by medications or electrolyte abnormalities.
- Most commonly, DI causes polydipsia accompanied by thirst, polyuria, and increased serum sodium and osmolality. Increased osmolality may cause cellular shrinkage with neurologic signs and symptoms. The diagnosis is confirmed when dilute urine is formed during water deprivation, which is promptly corrected with administration of vasopressin.
- DI is treated with ADH hormone replacement therapy (DDAVP) and fluid therapy.
- SIADH is associated with pulmonary tumors, central nervous system disease, and certain drugs. Excess ADH stimulates the renal tubules to reabsorb water despite decreased blood osmolality.
- Clinical manifestations of hyponatremia are associated with cellular swelling and neurologic dysfunction (e.g., confusion, coma). Fluid restriction and diuretics may be administered to manage hyponatremia. Detection and management of the underlying cause are paramount.

THYROID HORMONE DISORDERS

Regulation and Actions of Thyroid Hormone

The thyroid gland, a two-lobed gland, lies in the neck region on either side of and anterior to the trachea. It secretes the thyroid hormones **thyroxine** (T_4) and **triiodothyronine** (T_3). The secretion of thyroid hormone is regulated by the hypothalamic-pituitary-thyroid feedback system. The effect of this system is to maintain an appropriate concentration of free thyroid hormones in the circulating body fluid. The amount of thyroid hormone released by the thyroid gland is controlled by TSH released by the anterior lobe of the pituitary gland.

TSH, in turn, is regulated by thyrotropin-releasing hormone (TRH) produced by the hypothalamus.

Thyroid hormones influence the metabolic rate of the body. A well-vascularized gland, the thyroid is composed of microscopic follicles surrounded by follicular and parafollicular cells. Follicular cells trap dietary iodine, oxidize it to iodide, and couple it to molecules of the amino acid, tyrosine. These iodotyrosines are then combined to form T_4 and T_3. Thyroid hormones are then coupled to thyroglobulin, a storage protein, which accumulates in the thyroid follicles. When stimulated by TSH, the follicular cells release T_4, T_3, and thyroglobulin into the circulation.[13]

Iodine is essential for the formation of T_4 and T_3, the two thyroid hormones that are necessary for maintenance of normal metabolic rates in all of the cells. Lack of iodine prevents production of both T_4 and T_3 but does not stop the formation of thyroglobulin. As a result, insufficient hormone is available to inhibit production of TSH by the anterior pituitary. This imbalance allows the pituitary gland to secrete excessively large quantities of TSH. The TSH then causes the thyroid cells to secrete tremendous amounts of thyroglobulin (colloid) into the follicles, and the gland grows larger and larger, producing a **goiter** (Figure 40-6).

Hypothyroidism

Etiology and Pathogenesis. **Hypothyroidism** may be congenital in origin or acquired later in life. The majority of cases of hypothyroidism are primary, due to direct dysfunction of the thyroid. Congenital hypothyroidism (cretinism) may result from a variety of causes. Thyroid dysgenesis (lack of thyroid gland development) accounts for most congenital hypothyroidism. Blocking of TSH receptors and defective synthesis of thyroid hormone are other mechanisms causing congenital hypothyroidism.[14]

Lymphocytic thyroiditis (Hashimoto thyroiditis, or autoimmune thyroiditis) is the most common cause of acquired hypothyroidism. Lymphocytic thyroiditis is characterized by an enlarged thyroid gland (see Figure 40-6) caused by lymphocytic infiltration. Thyroid hormone production decreases, stimulating the release of TSH from the pituitary, indicating a hypoactive thyroid gland. Hypothyroidism and its clinical symptoms progress as the gland becomes fibrotic.

Other causes of acquired hypothyroidism include irradiation of the thyroid gland, surgical removal of thyroid tissue, and iodine deficiency.[15] Some foods contain "goitrogenic" substances that interfere with thyroid hormone synthesis. Such goitrogenic substances occur in some varieties of turnips and cabbage, but the clinical significance of these goitrogens is considered to be minimal. The drug lithium inhibits thyroid hormone synthesis and secretion and causes hypothyroidism in up to 20% of patients treated for bipolar disease.[13]

Secondary hypothyroidism is caused by defects in TSH production. Individuals who have been exposed to severe head trauma, cranial neoplasms, brain infections, cranial irradiation, and neurosurgery can be left with secondary hy-

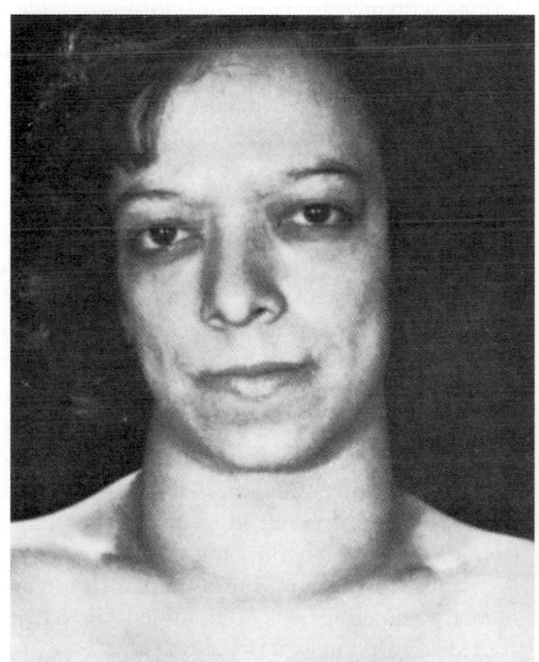
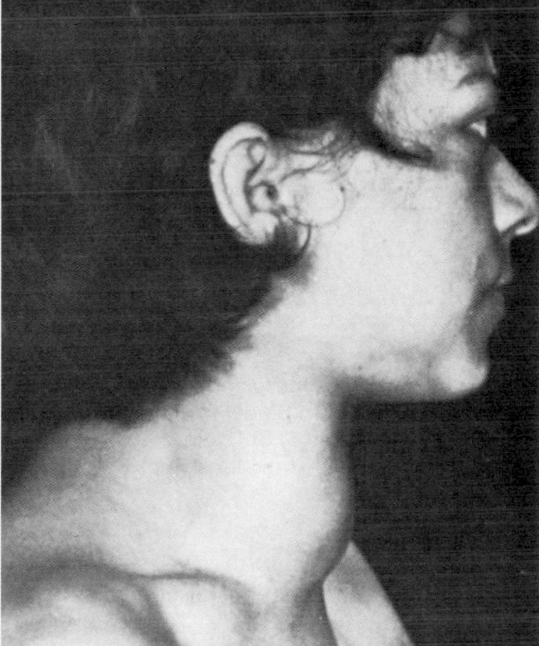

FIGURE 40-6 ■ An enlarged thyroid gland (goiter) can be present in both hypothyroid and hyperthyroid states. Note enlargement at the base of the neck. (From Wilson JD, Foster DW, editors: *Williams textbook of endocrinology,* ed 8, Philadelphia, 1992, Saunders, p 425.)

Table 40-4

Signs and Symptoms of Thyroid Imbalance

Hyperthyroidism	Hypothyroidism
Sleeplessness, nervousness	Lethargy
Muscle weakness, fatigue	Weakness
Susceptibility to infection	
Skin texture warm, silky, damp	Dry, pale, cool, coarse skin
Heat intolerance	Cold intolerance
Increased appetite with weight loss	Weight gain
Increased gastric motility	Constipation
Tachycardia, narrow pulse pressure, palpitations, angina	Bradycardia, wide pulse pressure
Dyspnea	Dyspnea, chest pain
Goiter	Thyroid shows diffuse enlargement or is not palpable
Hair silky, nail loose or detached from nail bed	Hair coarse
Hyperreflexia	Sluggish return of reflexes; mental impairment: slowed cognitive ability, poor memory, forgetfulness, depressed affect; deafness (in one-third of population)
Eye symptoms: burning, tearing, diplopia, lid lag, prominent eyes (exophthalmia), stare, eyelid tremors when closed	Facial edema (especially periorbital); thinned lateral aspect of eyebrows
Absence of forehead wrinkling on upward gaze	
Decreased or absent menses	Heavy, prolonged menses; infertility

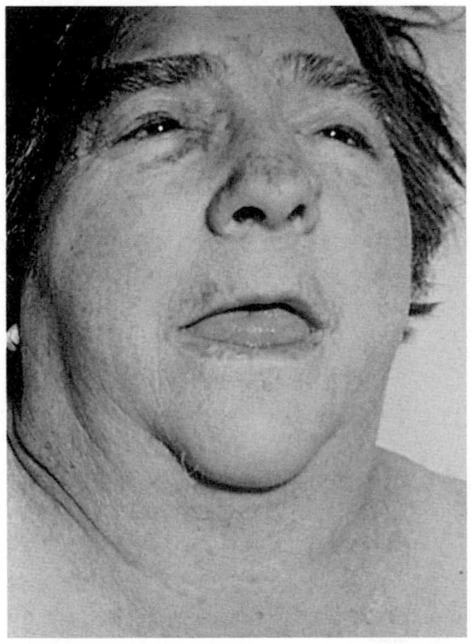

FIGURE 40-7 ■ Typical facial puffiness and dull expression of patients with myxedema. (From Seidel HM et al: *Mosby's guide to physical examination,* ed 5, St Louis, 2003, Mosby. Courtesy Paul W. Ladenson, MD, The Johns Hopkins University and Hospital, Baltimore, Md.)

pothyroidism.[15] Acquired hypothyroidism can be iatrogenic in origin, as a result of surgery or irradiation, or, although rare in the United States, may be due to dietary deficiencies of iodine.

Clinical Manifestations. Individuals with hypothyroidism have decreased basal metabolic rates. The thyroid gland may become enlarged (goitrous), the skin may be cool and dry, and constipation may be present. Patients report the subjective feelings of weakness, lethargy, cold intolerance, and decreased appetite. Bradycardia, narrowed pulse pressure, and mild to moderate weight gain may occur. Depression and difficulties with concentration and memory occur. Women with acquired hypothyroidism may experience menstrual irregularities, with increased flow and clotting.[13] Table 40-4 summarizes the signs and symptoms of thyroid imbalance.

Myxedema refers to severe or prolonged thyroid deficiency. Individuals with myxedema usually present in an altered mental state, with alterations in thermoregulation and a history of a precipitating event such as sepsis, trauma, or the use of certain medications.[14] Without medical intervention, patients may lapse into myxedema coma, a medical emergency with upward of 60% mortality. Figure 40-7 shows the typical features of patients with myxedema.

Routine screening of newborns has resulted in early treatment of most infants with congenital hypothyroidism. Few clinical manifestations are present at birth. In untreated infants, symptoms appear in the first months of life and include a dull appearance; a thick, protuberant tongue; and thick lips (leading to feeding difficulties). Other signs include prolonged neonatal jaundice, poor muscle tone, bradycardia, mottled extremities, umbilical hernia, and a hoarse cry. Thyroid hormone is essential for normal central nervous system development; mental retardation will occur unless thyroid replacement is started early in infancy.

Children with acquired hypothyroidism have essentially the same clinical manifestations as adults. In addition, growth retardation, delayed bone development, and delayed or precocious puberty may occur.[13]

Table 40-5

Thyroid Hormone Levels in Various States

State	Serum T_4 (μg/dl), Range	Serum T_3 (ng/dl), Range	Serum TSH (μU/ml), Range
Euthyroid	4.5-11.5	60-180	0.5-4.5
Infants (<2 wk)	8.0-15.0	—	0.5-4.5
Children (prepubertal)	6.5-11.5	80-220	0.5-4.5
Hyperthyroid	>11.5	—	<0.15
Hypothyroid	<1.0-5.0	—	>10

In individuals with typical presentations of hypothyroidism, the diagnosis can be confirmed by thyroid hormone levels. Since the most common cause of hypothyroidism is thyroid failure (primary hypothyroidism), nearly all patients will have elevated TSH levels.[15] TSH is the most sensitive indicator of thyroid hypoactivity and is detectable long before many symptoms develop. T_4 and T_3 levels decline later in the course of disease. In the rare case of hypothalamic-pituitary dysfunction, both TSH and T_4 will be inappropriately low (Table 40-5).

Treatment. The goal of treatment is to return the individual with congenital or acquired hypothyroidism and thyroiditis to a euthyroid state. When serum thyroid levels are replaced too quickly, patients may experience insomnia, anxiety, and mood lability. Once treatment has begun, those individuals with a goiter usually experience a regression in glandular enlargement.[16]

Oral levothyroxine is used to replace or supplement hormone production from an underactive thyroid. Patients notice an increase in exercise tolerance, decreased fatigue, and improved mentation with therapy. Resolution of symptoms occurs gradually over weeks; too rapid replacement can cause anxiety and insomnia. Rarely, adrenal insufficiency may coexist with hypothyroidism, and patients may develop symptoms of nausea and vomiting as their thyroid disorder is treated (see the section on adrenocortical insufficiency). Intravenous levothyroxine may be used in myxedema coma. The goal of therapy is to return patients to a "euthyroid" (normal thyroid balance) state, marked by a TSH level in the normal range.

Hyperthyroidism

Etiology and Pathogenesis. Mechanisms that can produce hyperthyroidism and thyrotoxicosis include thyroid follicular cell hyperfunction with increased synthesis and secretion of T_4 and T_3, thyroid follicular cell destruction with release of preformed T_4 and T_3, and ingestion of excessive thyroid hormone or iodide preparations. The increased serum levels of thyroid hormones increase the metabolic rate (see Table 40-5).

Hyperfunction of thyroid follicular cells can be either autonomous or mediated through stimulation of TSH receptors by substances such as TSH or TSH receptor antibodies (TRAb). The basic abnormalities underlying autonomous hyperfunction are unknown. Autonomous hyperfunction can be caused by adenomas and, rarely, thyroid carcinoma. Stimulation of TSH receptors by TRAb leads to the diffuse toxic goiter of **Graves disease.**[13]

Graves disease is the most common cause of hyperthyroidism.[14] The hyperthyroidism of Graves disease is mediated through an autoimmune process. Immunoglobulins bind to TSH receptors on the plasma membrane, resulting in thyroid overgrowth and hyperthyroidism. This is more common in women than men, with increased incidence during the second and third decades of life.

Inflammation of thyroid follicular cells, with release of preformed thyroid hormone, can be associated with viral or autoimmune processes. Examples are the toxic thyroiditis of Hashimoto disease and subacute thyroiditis.

Acute or chronic ingestion of thyroid hormone preparations can produce excess levels of thyroid hormones. Excessive intake of iodides may also result in thyrotoxicosis. Iodine is not usually ingested in toxic amounts, but some medications (such as amiodarone) have a high iodine content.

Clinical Manifestations. Individuals with Graves disease present with thyromegaly (diffusely enlarged thyroid), thyrotoxicosis, and, often, **exophthalmos** (enlargement of retroorbital muscles causing protrusion of the eyes) (Figure 40-8). A diffuse toxic goiter or thyroid enlargement is the most common manifestation. Symptoms include changes in behavior, insomnia, restlessness, tremor, irritability, palpitations, heat intolerance, diaphoresis, and an inability to concentrate that interferes with work performance (see Table 40-4). Increased basal metabolic rate may result in weight loss, although appetite and dietary intake increase. In women, amenorrhea or scant menses is a frequent finding.[13]

Spasm and retraction of the eyelids leads to widening of the palpebral fissure, resulting in exposed sclera. Lid lag develops, and severe, progressive exophthalmos may occur. Eye complaints may include vision changes and photophobia.

Thyroid storm is a form of life-threatening thyrotoxicosis that occurs when an individual is not able to maintain adequate metabolic balances through compensatory mechanisms. Thyroid storm presents with the clinical features of thyrotoxicosis in a more exaggerated state. Most individuals have a goiter and, possibly, ophthalmopathy. Exceedingly elevated temperatures, significant tachycardia, cardiac arrhythmias, and congestive heart failure are common findings at presentation. Extreme restlessness, agitation, and psychosis may occur. The patient may also experience vomiting, nausea, and diarrhea; jaundice may develop due to hepatic dysfunction.[17]

Undetectable TSH levels are the best indicator of primary hyperthyroidism. Serum T_4 and T_3 levels are elevated. A 24-hour radioactive iodine uptake study can confirm the diagno-

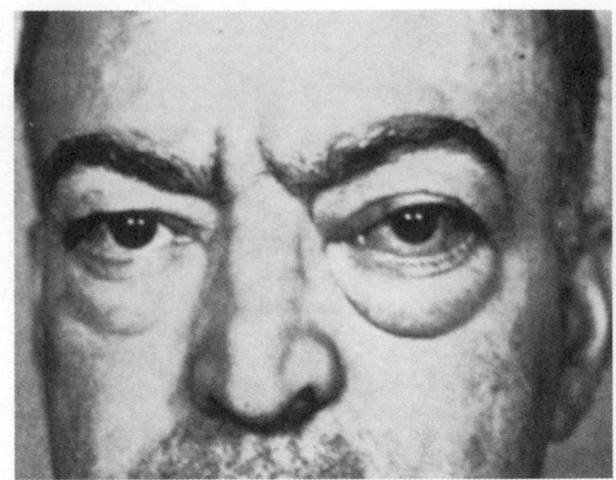

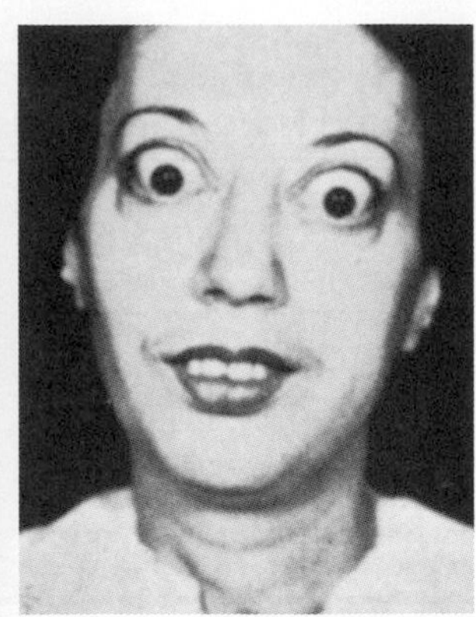

FIGURE 40-8 ■ Patients with the usual ophthalmopathy found in Graves disease. **A,** Patient with periorbital swelling, exophthalmos, and chemosis (edema). **B,** Woman with widening of the palpebral fissures owing to lid retraction and proptosis. (From Larsen PR, Ingbar SH: The thyroid gland. In Wilson JD, Foster DW, editors: *Williams textbook of endocrinology,* ed 8, Philadelphia, 1992, Saunders, p 426.)

sis of Graves disease when the scan shows diffuse homogeneous uptake of tracer and can exclude the presence of thyroid neoplasms.

Treatment. Once hyperthyroidism is diagnosed, thyroid hormone production is decreased with a class of antithyroid drugs called thionamides (propylthiouracil, methimazole). Thionamides decrease the production of thyroid hormone by follicular cells. Administration of β-adrenergic blockers decreases tachycardia and tremor. Patients with Graves disease may receive these medications for months to years, depending on their response to the drugs and patient preferences. Appropriate dosages of thionamides can produce a gradual reduction in the basal metabolic rate and the disappearance of symptoms (decreased size of the gland). The exophthalmos that is present at diagnosis may not reverse. Possible toxic reactions to these drugs include urticaria and agranulocytosis. At least 18 months of treatment may be required, and relapse frequently occurs once medications are stopped.

Radioactive iodine treatment to ablate the gland, thereby curtailing its ability to produce excess thyroid hormones, is now the treatment of choice. Hypothyroidism occurs following radioactive iodine therapy in 50% to 80% of patients, so patients should be prepared for the likelihood of lifelong thyroid replacement therapy.

Surgical removal of the thyroid gland, now rarely practiced, may result in hypoparathyroidism due to inadvertent resection of one or more parathyroids. In addition, the recurrent laryngeal nerve controlling vocal cord function may be damaged during thyroidectomy, resulting in hoarseness.

Thyroid Storm. Because thyroid storm is a life-threatening form of thyrotoxicosis, aggressive management to achieve metabolic balance is mandated. All measures should be taken to block the production and binding of thyroid pathways. Antithyroid drugs, such as propylthiouracil, must be given orally or through a nasogastric tube because parenteral preparations are not available. Inorganic iodine may be given to further inhibit release of T_3 and T_4 only after an effective blockade of new hormone synthesis (with propylthiouracil) has been initiated. β-Blockers used for their antiadrenergic effects also inhibit the peripheral conversion of T_4 to T_3. β-Blockers are available in both oral and parenteral forms. Extremely careful monitoring of individuals receiving treatment for thyroid storm must be provided. Antipyretic therapy (cooling blankets, ice packs, acetaminophen) must be started to achieve peripheral cooling. Fluid replacement with dextrose and electrolytes must be provided and the cardiovascular status diligently monitored during stabilization of the individual's condition. The addition of glucocorticoids to the pharmacologic regimen improves survival. Thyroid storm is fatal if untreated. With treatment, the mortality is between 20% and 30%; therefore, aggressive, multifocused preventive measures must be implemented early in individuals who present with thyroid storm.[17]

KEY CONCEPTS

- Thyroid hormone (T_3, T_4) is produced in follicular cells of the thyroid gland. The synthesis and secretion of thyroid hormone are stimulated by TSH from the pituitary. Thyroid hormone is an important stimulator of growth and cellular metabolism.
- Hypothyroidism may be primary (due to congenital agenesis, autoimmune destruction, irradiation, trauma, surgical removal of the gland, or iodine deficiency) or secondary to pituitary hyposecretion of TSH.
- TSH level is helpful in differentiating between primary (high TSH) and secondary (low TSH) causes of hypothyroidism. Low serum T_3 and T_4 levels confirm the diagnosis of hypothyroidism.
- Manifestations of hypothyroidism (myxedema) are attributable to a generalized decrease in metabolism. Untreated congenital hypothyroidism results in profound mental and physical retardation (cretinism).
- Manifestations of hypothyroidism include nonpitting edema, slowed mentation, weight gain, dry skin, constipation, decreased heart rate, decreased pulse pressure, lethargy, and loss of the outer third of the eyebrow. Severe hypothyroidism may lead to myxedema coma, characterized by bradycardia, hypothermia, hypotension, and decreased level of con-

sciousness. Treatment centers on hormone replacement therapy.

- Hyperthyroidism may be primary (Graves disease, autoimmune, tumor related, inflammatory) or secondary to pituitary hypersecretion of TSH. The blood level of TSH is helpful in differentiating primary (low TSH) from secondary (high TSH). High levels of T_3 and T_4 confirm the diagnosis of hyperthyroidism.
- The manifestations of hyperthyroidism result from a generalized increase in metabolism. Hyperactivity, irritability, insomnia, weight loss, increased appetite, heat intolerance, diarrhea, and palpitations are common. Most individuals have a detectably enlarged thyroid gland. Exophthalmos occurs with Graves disease.
- Thyroid storm may be precipitated by stress or manipulation of the gland. It is characterized by tachycardia, hypertension, high temperature, and cardiac dysrhythmias. Treatment includes β-blockers to control cardiovascular symptoms, antithyroid drugs to reduce thyroid production, radioactive iodine to ablate the gland, and surgical removal of tumors.

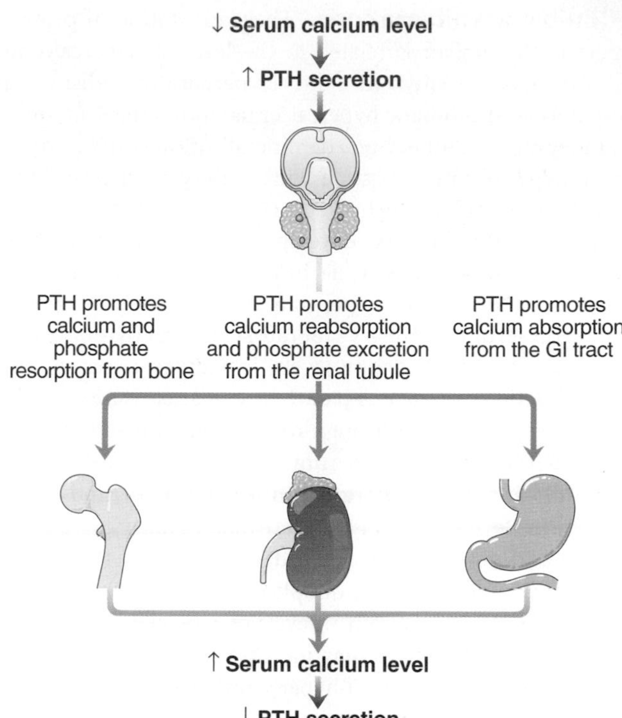

FIGURE 40-9 ■ Parathyroid hormone *(PTH)* increases serum calcium level through its effects on bone, renal tubules, and intestine. *GI,* Gastrointestinal.

PARATHYROID GLAND DISORDERS

Regulation and Actions of Parathyroid Hormone

The parathyroid glands are small glands located at the upper and lower poles of the thyroid. There are usually four parathyroid glands, although there are reports of fewer or more than four being found during surgery. The parathyroid glands help maintain homeostasis through the regulation of calcium concentrations in the blood (Figure 40-9). Parathyroid hormone (PTH) is released and acts on bones and renal tubules. The effect of PTH is to increase serum calcium levels.

In the bone, PTH increases osteoclastic activity, resulting in the release of calcium from bone into extracellular fluid. Renal calcium reabsorption increases under the effect of PTH, thus decreasing urinary calcium excretion. PTH stimulates the activation of vitamin D; vitamin D then increases intestinal calcium absorption.

Serum calcium levels provide the feedback necessary to regulate PTH secretion. A decrease in serum calcium causes a release of PTH. An elevated serum calcium level leads to suppression of PTH secretion.[18] A marked increase or decrease in serum PTH levels can have severe, often fatal consequences.[19] PTH is not part of the hypothalamic-pituitary feedback system.

Calcitonin, produced by thyroid parafollicular cells, also influences the processing of calcium by bone cells. Calcitonin controls the calcium content of the blood by increasing bone formation by osteoblasts and inhibiting bone breakdown by osteoclasts. Although the role of calcitonin in calcium homeostasis is not entirely clear, calcitonin tends to decrease blood calcium levels and promote conservation of hard bone matrix. PTH is an antagonist to calcitonin, as it has the opposite effects. Together, calcitonin and PTH help maintain calcium homeostasis.

Hyperparathyroidism

Etiology and Pathogenesis. The causes of primary hyperparathyroidism remain unclear. Despite an elevated serum calcium level, PTH continues to be secreted. Some forms of hyperparathyroidism can have a genetic origin. Hyperparathyroidism from a single parathyroid adenoma occurs in 80% of surgically proven cases. Hyperplasia of the parathyroid is found in the remainder of the cases.

In hyperparathyroidism, bone resorption and formation rates are increased. Serum calcium levels do not rise uncontrollably; indeed, excessive parathyroid gland secretion rarely causes hypercalcemic crisis. Malignant tumors elsewhere in the body can also release PTH and are a more frequent cause of extreme hypercalcemia and hypercalcemic crisis.[20]

A hyperparathyroid state during pregnancy leads to perinatal and neonatal complications. The newborn's PTH production will be suppressed by maternal hypercalcemia, and neonatal hypocalcemia and tetany can develop. This presentation in a newborn may be the first indication of the need for investigative studies in the mother if the disorder was asymptomatic during pregnancy.[21] In chronic renal failure, secondary hyperparathyroidism may result from abnormal levels of phosphate and calcium.

Clinical Manifestations. The presentation of primary hyperparathyroidism is related to the level of hypercalcemia and the hyperparathyroid state. Hyperparathyroidism may present as asymptomatic hypercalcemia. Individuals are prone to kidney stones and to bone demineralization (osteoporosis). Severe hypercalcemia causes a wide variety of effects, dominated by polyuria and dehydration. Anorexia, nausea, vomiting, and constipation may develop. Various cardiac problems can arise including bradycardia, heart block, and cardiac arrest.

Often, mild cases of hyperparathyroidism are recognized on general serum chemistry laboratory reports that note mild elevations in serum calcium levels. In fact, an apparent current rise in the incidence of parathyroid disease is actually due to improved detection through routine calcium screening on blood chemistry surveys. Serum calcium levels are elevated (1 mg/dl above the laboratory normal range) and serum phosphorus levels are low to low-normal. Urinary excretion of calcium and phosphate is elevated, as are serum PTH levels. Urinary cyclic adenosine monophosphate (cAMP) levels are increased, and 1,25-vitamin D levels may be elevated.[22]

Lithium and thiazides may increase serum calcium levels, leading to a misdiagnosis of hyperparathyroidism.

Treatment. Surgical removal of the abnormal parathyroid gland is the treatment of choice. Individuals with asymptomatic hyperparathyroidism may defer or refuse surgery. In such cases, medical management may work for a time. Medical management includes hydration (to prevent kidney stone formation) and ambulation. Also, alendronate may prevent bone loss.[23]

For hypercalcemic crisis, rapid volume expansion with normal saline reverses dehydration. Volume replacement also results in improved glomerular filtration rate and increased calcium excretion.

Hypoparathyroidism

Etiology and Pathogenesis. Hypoparathyroidism most frequently occurs as a consequence of parathyroid or thyroid surgery or surgery in the area of these glands. The resulting hypoparathyroidism may be temporary or permanent. In some cases it may take years to develop.

Hypoparathyroidism can occur following the removal of one hyperfunctioning parathyroid gland. The hyperfunctioning gland suppresses the function of the other parathyroid glands, creating a temporary state of deficiency. Permanent hypoparathyroidism rarely follows initial surgery. Permanent hypoparathyroidism may develop following thyroidectomy because of damage to parathyroid gland blood supply, postsurgical swelling, or fibrosis.[20]

Congenital lack of parathyroid tissue and idiopathic hypoparathyroidism are causes of hypoparathyroidism in infants and children. Autoimmune processes may also target and damage the parathyroid gland.[19]

Clinical Manifestations. Clinical manifestations of hypoparathyroidism occur as a result of low serum calcium levels. The manifestations of acute hypocalcemia include circumoral numbness, paresthesias of the distal extremities, muscle cramps, fatigue, hyperirritability, anxiety, depression, nonspecific electroencephalographic changes, increases in intracranial pressure, and prolongation of corrected Q-T intervals on the electrocardiogram. Severe manifestations of hypocalcemia include carpopedal spasm, laryngospasm, and seizures. The clinical signs of hypocalcemia include neuromuscular irritability associated with tetany. Tetany is indicated by the Chvostek sign (ipsilateral contraction of the facial muscles that is elicited by tapping the facial nerve anterior to the ear) or Trousseau sign (carpal spasm produced by pressure ischemia of the nerves in the upper arm during inflation of a blood pressure cuff for 3 to 5 minutes above the systolic blood pressure).[19]

The serum calcium level is low (5 to 7 mg/d) and the phosphorus level is high (7 to 12 mg/dl). Levels of antibodies to the parathyroid gland are high if an autoimmune mechanism is operant.

Treatment. Emergency treatment with IV calcium is needed if an individual presents in acute hypocalcemic crisis (tetany, laryngospasm, and convulsions). Calcitriol, an activated form of vitamin D, should also be given in the emergent phase. Long-term treatment includes oral calcium supplement and vitamin D.[20] Serum calcium levels should be maintained in the low-normal range in an attempt to avoid hypercalciuria.

KEY CONCEPTS

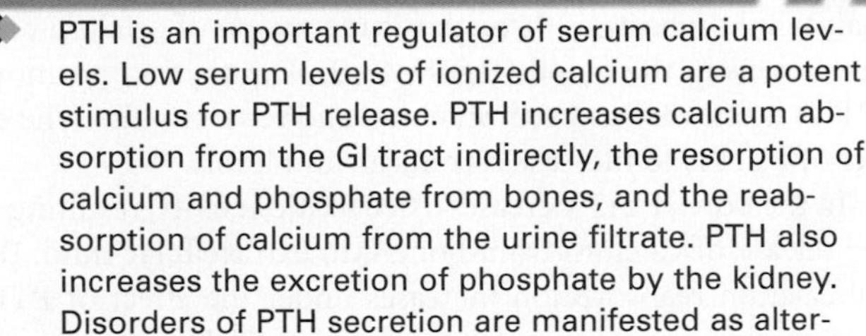

- PTH is an important regulator of serum calcium levels. Low serum levels of ionized calcium are a potent stimulus for PTH release. PTH increases calcium absorption from the GI tract indirectly, the resorption of calcium and phosphate from bones, and the reabsorption of calcium from the urine filtrate. PTH also increases the excretion of phosphate by the kidney. Disorders of PTH secretion are manifested as alterations in serum Ca^{2+} levels.
- Hyperparathyroidism may be idiopathic or may be due to a parathyroid adenoma. Its manifestations result from high serum calcium levels and bone demineralization. High serum calcium levels decrease neuromuscular excitability. Treatment entails removing the abnormal glands. Adequate hydration may help prevent the formation of kidney stones.
- Hypoparathyroidism may be idiopathic, autoimmune, or secondary to surgical removal of the parathyroid gland. The manifestations result from low serum calcium levels, which increase neuromuscular excitability. Paresthesias, cramps, spasms, tetany, and seizures may result. Elicitation of Chvostek and Trousseau signs indicates neuromuscular hyperexcitability. Treatment entails calcium (and vitamin D) supplementation rather than hormone replacement.

ADRENOCORTICAL HORMONE DISORDERS

Regulation and Actions of Adrenocortical Hormones

The secretion of adrenocortical hormones is regulated by hypothalamic secretion of corticotropin-releasing hormone (CRH) and pituitary secretion of ACTH. As with most of the other hormones of the hypothalamic-pituitary axis, negative feedback serves to modulate the release of the adrenocortical hormone. The hormones produced by the adrenal cortex are called **steroids** and include (1) glucocorticoids (cortisol), (2) mineralocorticoids (aldosterone), and (3) sex steroids (androgens) (Figure 40-10). Changes in the levels of any of these hormones cause a dysfunction in many body tissues and organs. The synthesis and secretion of these hormones, especially cortisol, are considered essential for life, regulating the body's response to normal and abnormal levels of physiologic and psychological stress. The activities of these three hormones can be remembered as regulating the "three S's": sugar, salt, and sex.

Glucocorticoids, principally cortisol, are named for their primary effect on glucose metabolism. They also influence the way proteins and fats are utilized. Glucocorticoids are antiinsulin hormones whose overall effect is to raise blood sugar, making glucose immediately available. This is accomplished by decreasing glucose uptake by many body cells (decreased glycogenesis), and increasing glucose synthesis in the liver from glycogen and amino acid and glycerol substrates in protein and fat stores (glycogenolysis, **gluconeogenesis**). Glucocorticoids also contribute to protein catabolism by releasing muscle stores of proteins, providing amino acids for glucose production in the liver. Glucocorticoids promote lipolysis and increased blood cholesterol. Finally, glucocorticoids protect against the damaging physiologic effects of stress and suppress the inflammatory and immune responses (which may sometimes have detrimental effects).[18]

Mineralocorticoids, principally aldosterone, function to maintain normal salt and water balance by promoting sodium retention and potassium excretion at the distal renal tubules. Aldosterone, however, is not dependent on pituitary ACTH control. Its production is regulated primarily by the renin-angiotensin system associated with the juxtaglomerular cells of the kidney in response to a reduction in renal perfusion, and by a high serum potassium level (Figure 40-11).

Androgenic hormone secretion by the adrenal cortex plays a relatively minor role in the development and maintenance of secondary sex characteristics, except in children with adrenogenital syndromes, which produce virilization in the female and precocious sexual development in the male. Physiologically, adrenal androgens are the main source of androgens in the female. As with mineralocorticoids, there is no known feedback mechanism to suppress ACTH production associated with adrenal sex hormone plasma levels, but in-

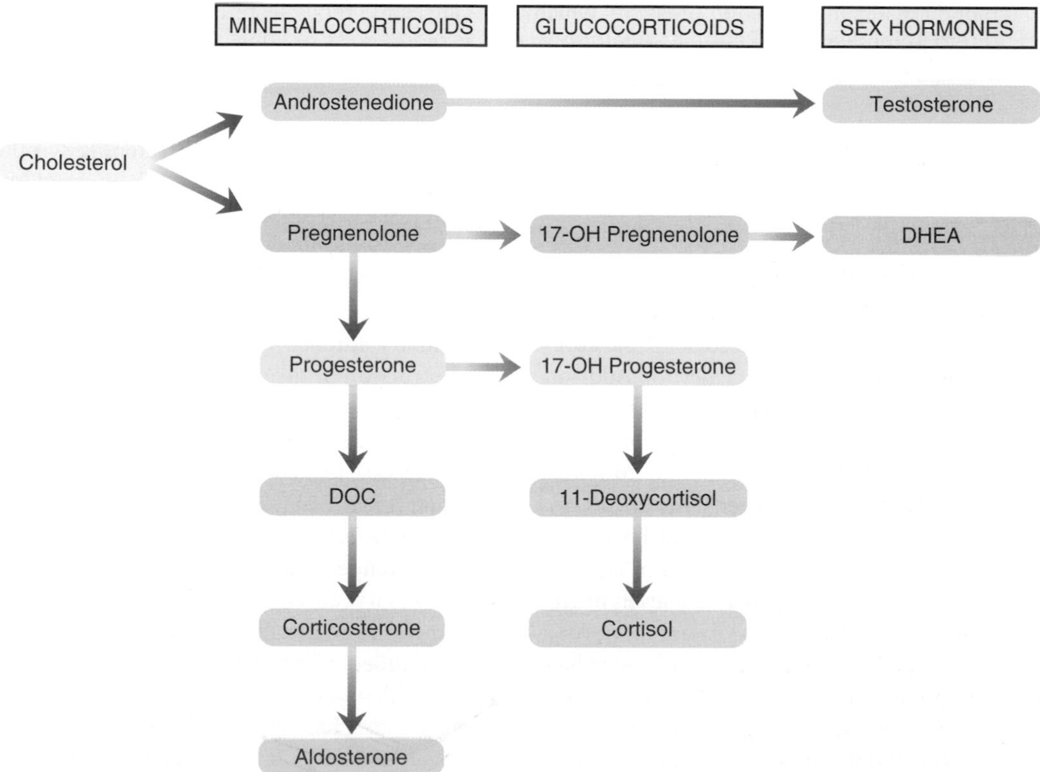

FIGURE 40-10 ■ Adrenal cortex hormone production. *DOC,* Deoxycorticosterone; *DHEA,* dehydroepiandrosterone. (Redrawn from Betz CL, Hunsberger M, Wright S, editors: *Family-centered nursing care of children,* ed 2, Philadelphia, 1994, Saunders, p 1957.)

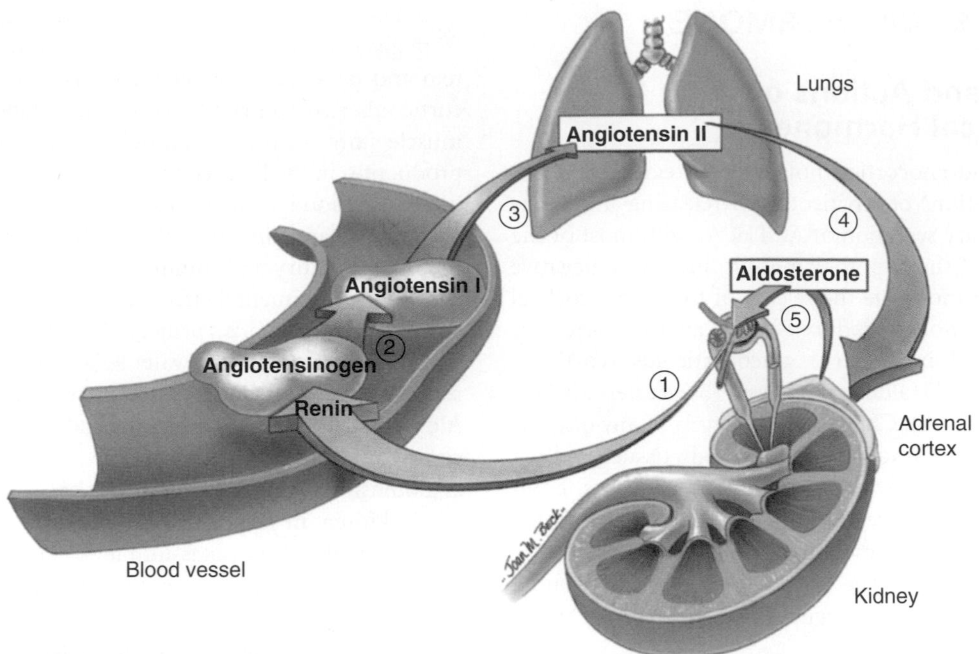

FIGURE 40-11 ■ Renin-angiotensin mechanism for regulating aldosterone secretion. *(1)* When the incoming blood pressure in the kidneys drops below a certain level, a piece of tissue near the vessels (the juxtaglomerular apparatus) secretes **renin** into the blood. *(2)* Renin, an enzyme, causes angiotensinogen (a normal constituent of blood) to be converted to angiotensin I. *(3)* Angiotensin I circulates to the lungs, where converting enzymes in the capillaries split the molecule, forming angiotensin II. *(4)* Angiotensin II circulates to the adrenal cortex, where it stimulates the secretion of aldosterone. *(5)* Aldosterone causes increased reabsorption of sodium, which causes increased water retention. As water is retained, the volume of blood increases. The increased volume of blood creates higher blood pressure, which then causes the renin secretion to stop. (From Thibodeau GA, Patton K: *Anatomy and physiology,* ed 5, St Louis, 2003, Mosby, p 509.)

creased ACTH or adrenal hyperplasia may cause excessive production of these hormones.

Adrenocortical Insufficiency

Etiology and Pathogenesis. Hyposecretion of adrenocortical hormones can result from disease of the adrenal cortex (primary adrenocortical insufficiency, or **Addison disease**) or from the inadequate secretion of ACTH from the anterior pituitary (secondary adrenal insufficiency), or from a lack of CRH secretion from the hypothalamus due to hypothalamic malfunction or injury (tertiary adrenal insufficiency). Although hyposecretion of all the adrenocortical hormones may occur, the most severe clinical manifestations of adrenocortical insufficiency occur because of inadequate levels of circulating cortisol. Aldosterone is necessary to maintain normal blood pressure levels and sodium, potassium, and water balance, but its release, although stimulated by ACTH, is mainly controlled by the renin-angiotensin regulatory system.[24]

The syndrome of **congenital adrenal hyperplasia,** a rare cause of adrenal insufficiency in pediatric populations, is due to specific enzymatic defects in the biosynthesis of cortisol by the adrenal. Severe and life-threatening symptoms of adrenal insufficiency occur because of lack of circulating cortisol. The lack of negative feedback results in overproduction of ACTH, leading to hyperplasia of the adrenal glands and excessive androgen secretion.[25,26] Congenital adrenal hyperplasia is discussed at the end of the section on adrenal insufficiency.

Primary adrenal insufficiency (Addison disease) is caused by destruction of the adrenal gland through idiopathic or autoimmune mechanisms, tuberculosis, trauma or hemorrhage of the adrenals (often associated with anticoagulant therapy), fungal disease (e.g., histoplasmosis), and neoplasia. Because of the high functional reserve, symptoms of adrenal insufficiency may or may not be recognized until 90% of the cortical tissue has been rendered nonfunctional.

Secondary adrenal insufficiency (hypothalamic-pituitary dysfunction) is usually iatrogenic in origin because of the large numbers of patients receiving corticosteroid therapy for chronic illnesses (rheumatoid arthritis, asthma). Prolonged exposure to pharmacologic doses of exogenous corticosteroids suppresses ACTH and CRH stimulation of the adrenal gland through negative feedback. If corticosteroid administration is suddenly halted, or if the individual experiences a sudden stress-induced increase in need for cortisol, the adrenal gland will be unable to respond by increasing cortisol secretion. Acute and severe manifestations of adrenal insufficiency ensue.

Adrenal insufficiency can also occur because of surgical removal of the anterior pituitary (secondary adrenal insufficiency). Damage to the anterior pituitary or hypothalamus by tumors, infection, radiation, postpartum necrosis, trauma, or surgery may lead to adrenal insufficiency.[25] In primary insufficiency, cortisol, aldosterone, and androgen secretion are all decreased. In secondary insufficiency, only glucocorticoids are diminished (since decreased ACTH stimulation is the etiologic factor), with aldosterone and androgens continuing to be produced by other mechanisms.

Addisonian crisis or acute adrenal insufficiency represents a true medical emergency caused by inadequate levels of glucocorticoids and mineralocorticoids in the circulation. This may occur as the result of a slowly developing and unrecognized ACTH or cortisol deficiency in which secretion is adequate for the normal demands of life but inadequate for increased stress or trauma. Individuals who are taking corticosteroids on an ongoing basis may also develop acute life-threatening adrenal insufficiency if the corticosteroid is suddenly withdrawn.

Clinical Manifestations. The clinical manifestations of adrenal insufficiency (Table 40-6) occur because of inadequate levels of circulating cortisol and aldosterone (Figure 40-12). Diminished vascular tone, reduced cardiac output, and inadequate circulating blood volume all contribute to potentially lethal vascular collapse. Clinical manifestations may appear gradually, especially if adrenal destruction is slow and incremental, such as in autoimmune adrenal insufficiency. Symptoms are more dramatic if adrenal destruction is sudden (hemorrhage) or if a stressor, such as trauma, causes sudden decompensation in a patient with chronic adrenal insufficiency.

Table 40-6

Signs and Symptoms of Adrenocortical Hormone Imbalance

Cushing Syndrome	Adrenocortical Insufficiency
Truncal obesity	Weakness
Moon face	Hypotension
Buffalo hump	Hypoglycemia
Hirsutism	Hyperpigmentation (Addison disease)
Muscle wasting	Hyperkalemia
Striae	Weight loss
Petechiae	
Glucose intolerance	
Hypertension	
Hypokalemia	

Early signs of adrenal insufficiency include anorexia, weight loss, weakness, malaise, apathy, electrolyte imbalances, and hyperpigmentation of the skin caused by unsuppressed ACTH production (Figure 40-13). Salt craving may be present as a result of sodium deficit. If the condition is unrecognized or left untreated, gastrointestinal symptoms can develop, including nausea, vomiting, diarrhea, and dehydration. The patient may be hypotensive or tachycardic. The sudden onset of nausea, vomiting, anorexia, and hypotension suggests acute adrenal insufficiency, which is a medical emergency.[24]

Diagnosis. The diagnosis of adrenal insufficiency is made on clinical grounds, taking into account the patient's medical history (use of steroids, trauma, anticoagulation), physical examination, and biochemical findings. Decreased plasma cortisol levels assist in the diagnosis; however, since acute decompensation progresses to death so rapidly, levels are often drawn and therapy is initiated presumptively. Resolution of symptoms may be remarkably rapid with therapy.

In cases of chronic adrenal insufficiency, an ACTH test should be given. Cosyntropin, synthetic ACTH, is given IV, and serum samples of cortisol are measured 30 and 60 minutes after administration. Serum cortisol levels should increase following this stimulus if the adrenal cortex is functioning normally. Abdominal CT should be performed to determine the size of the adrenal glands. Small adrenals occur with autoimmune destruction, whereas tuberculous glands are large and calcified, and hemorrhagic glands are large, smooth, and hyperintense.

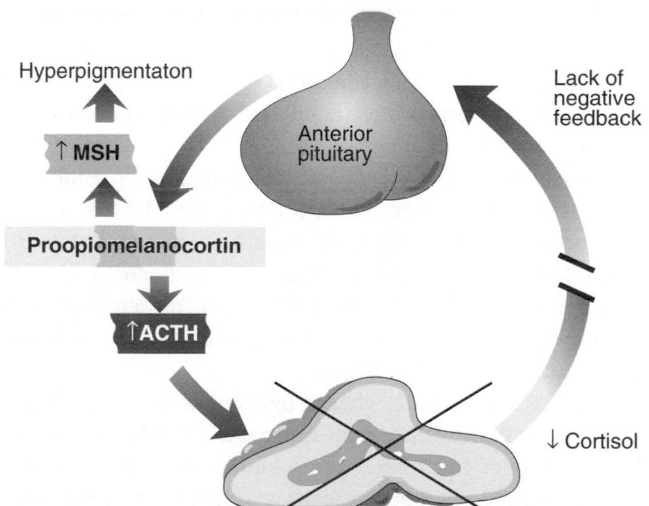

FIGURE 40-12 ■ Primary adrenocortical insufficiency (decreased cortisol production) leads to hypersecretion of melanocyte-stimulating hormone *(MSH)* and adrenocorticotropin hormone *(ACTH)* because of lack of negative feedback. MSH and ACTH are derived from the same precursor molecule, pro-opiomelanocortin. Even though ACTH levels are high, the adrenal gland is unable to produce adequate levels of cortisol.

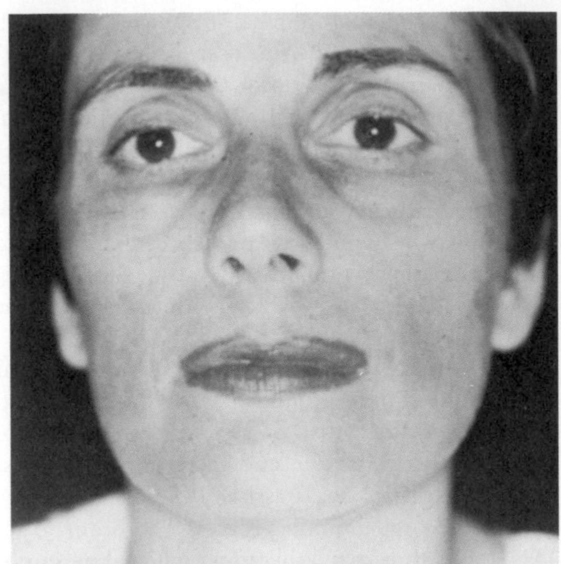

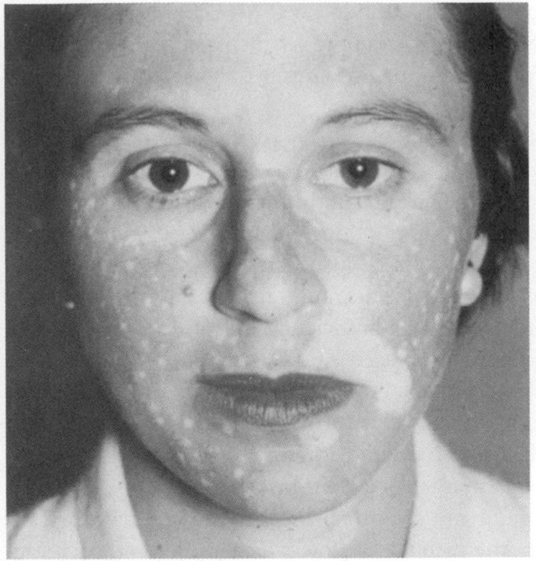

FIGURE 40-13 ■ Altered pigmentation in adrenocortical insufficiency. **A,** Increased pigmentation across the bridge of the nose. **B,** Generalized hyperpigmentation with vitiligo. (From Bondy PK, Rosenberg LE: *Metabolic control and disease,* ed 8, Philadelphia, 1980, Saunders, p 1462.)

Treatment. The treatment for adrenal insufficiency entails replacing the absent or deficient hormones usually produced by the adrenal cortex: glucocorticoids and, frequently, mineralocorticoids (aldosterone). Glucocorticoid replacement is given in the form of hydrocortisone; the daily dosage may be given in morning and evening doses to more closely mimic physiologic adrenal cortical function. In the case of adrenal crisis, large doses of IV hydrocortisone are administered at 6-hour intervals until the symptoms (hypotension, hypoglycemia) resolve; the dose is then titrated downward. In addition, volume replacement is needed to replace the increased urine output associated with renal sodium excretion.[26]

Aldosterone replacement, when needed, is in oral form (fludrocortisone acetate, Florinef) and must be taken daily. Fludrocortisone is basically equivalent to aldosterone and is available only as an oral formulation. If the glucocorticoid replacement given does not have significant mineralocorticoid action (e.g., prednisone, dexamethasone), the dose of fludrocortisone needed will be higher.

Cortisol is released when physiologic or psychological stress is experienced, and it is frequently referred to as a "flight-or-fight" hormone.[25] Stress situations include acute illness (increased temperature causes an increase in metabolic rate), injury (e.g., trauma, surgery, burns), and psychological episodes that affect an individual's ability to function normally (death of a significant relative). During these episodes of stress, an individual may need double or triple the usual daily corticosteroid dose. If illness or injury restricts the patient's ability to tolerate oral intake, hydrocortisone must be given IM or IV.[26]

Congenital Adrenal Hyperplasia

Adrenal hyperplasia occurs when enzymes needed for cortisol production are lacking. Because circulating cortisol levels are inadequate to provide negative feedback to the anterior pituitary gland, ACTH secretion continues unabated. This leads to adrenal hypertrophy and overproduction of androgens. In the newborn, classic congenital adrenal hyperplasia is a life-threatening condition because of inadequate cortisol and (sometimes) aldosterone.

Infants are frequently diagnosed at birth because of the effects of excessive androgens on the genitals of the newborn. Virilization of a female fetus's genitalia occurs. The female infant may be born with an enlarged clitoris and fused labia, resembling a scrotal sac (Figure 40-14). Male infants with congenital adrenal hyperplasia may have an enlarged penis and hyperpigmented scrotum, but the examiner may not recognize these signs.

Depending on the enzymes affected, androgen overproduction may occur at any time from birth to early adult life. If it occurs in an adult female, she develops such virile characteristics as a beard, a much deeper voice, baldness (if she has inherited that genetic trait), masculine distribution of pubic hair, growth of the clitoris to resemble a penis, and deposition of proteins in the skin and muscles to yield typical masculine characteristics.

In adult men, the virilizing characteristics of the adrenogenital syndrome are less obvious because male virilizing characteristics are normally associated with testosterone, which is secreted by the testes. Therefore, the diagnosis is difficult to make.[27] In the prepubertal male,

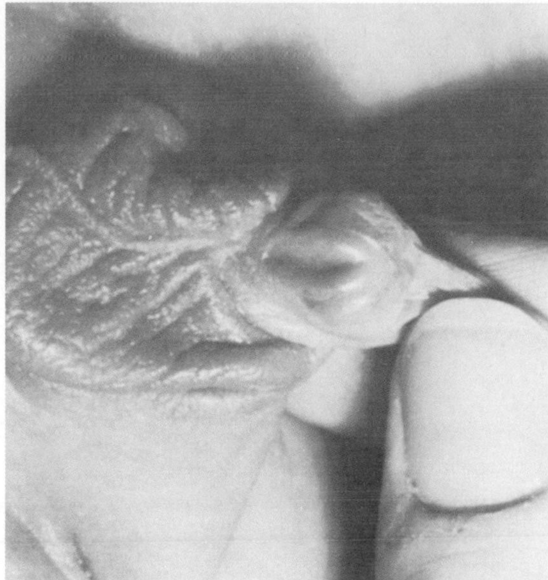

FIGURE 40-14 ■ Female infant with congenital adrenal hyperplasia demonstrating virilization of the genitalia. Note the enlarged clitoris and the fused labia, which resemble a scrotal sac. (From Hurwitz LS: Nursing implications of selected endocrine disorders, *Nursing Clin North Am* 15:528, 1980.)

adrenogenital syndrome may cause either precocious or delayed sexual maturity.

Hypercortisolism

Etiology and Pathogenesis. Hyperfunction of a portion of the hypothalamic-pituitary-adrenal axis results in conditions characterized by **hypercortisolism.** Primary adrenocortical hyperfunction is caused by disease of the adrenal cortex (adrenal adenoma). Secondary disease is caused by hyperfunction of the anterior pituitary ACTH-secreting cells, and tertiary disease is caused by hypothalamic dysfunction or injury. The term **Cushing syndrome** is used to describe the clinical features of hypercortisolism, regardless of cause. **Cushing disease** is the diagnosis reserved for pituitary-dependent conditions.[25]

In pediatric and adult populations, hypercortisolism is frequently caused by the excessive production of pituitary ACTH by microadenomas or adenomas. Ectopic ACTH production by nonpituitary tumors can also stimulate the adrenal glands. Exogenous steroids used in the management of various diseases, such as asthma and connective tissue diseases, can also lead to Cushing syndrome.[24]

Clinical Manifestations. An individual with excess circulating glucocorticoids will develop a round face with prominent, flushed cheeks, often referred to as "moon facies" (see Table 40-6). There is a noticeable weight gain with increasing total body fat, especially in the abdomen. A cervical fat pad, capillary friability, and thinning of the skin with the formation of purple striae and ecchymoses over the abdomen, arms, and thighs develop. Muscle mass decreases and muscle weakness develops. Figure 40-15 shows the common clinical manifestations of Cushing syndrome.

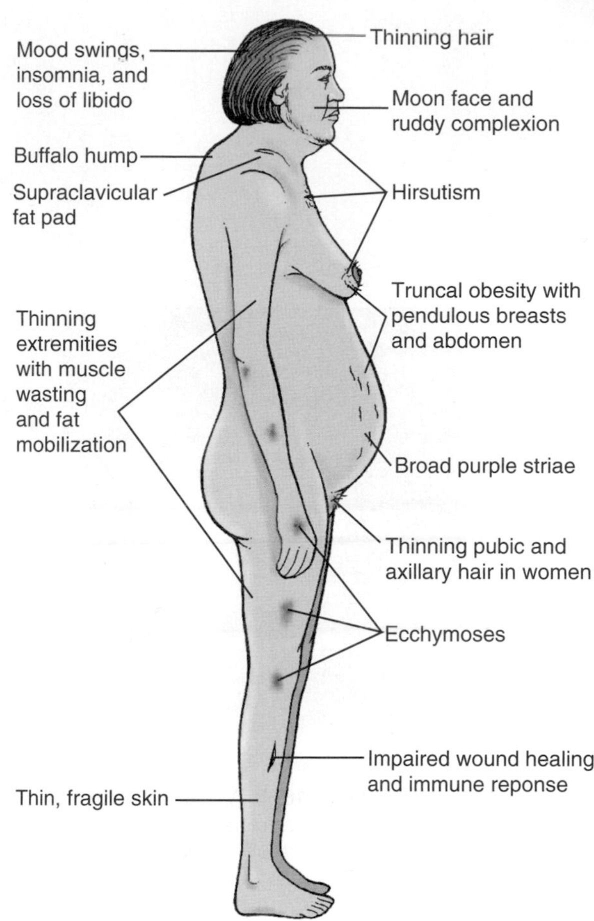

FIGURE 40-15 ■ Common clinical manifestations of Cushing syndrome. (From Monahan FD, Neighbors M: *Medical-surgical nursing: foundations for clinical practice,* ed 2, Philadelphia, 1998, Saunders, p 1286.)

Hypertension may develop as a consequence of the salt-retaining activity of cortisol and of the increased blood volume. With chronic Cushing syndrome, demineralization of the bones (osteoporosis) and resulting fractures may occur. The cortisol excess may be accompanied by increased androgen production (excessive hair production, acne, menstrual irregularities).

Emotional changes include depression, emotional lability, anxiety, and irritability. Rarely, euphoria is noted. Decreases in short-term memory, concentration, and attention span may be present.

The diagnosis of adrenocortical disease depends on reliable, accurate laboratory measurements. Urinary free cortisol levels will be elevated; the upper normal range is laboratory dependent. Complete collections of urine are needed to ex-

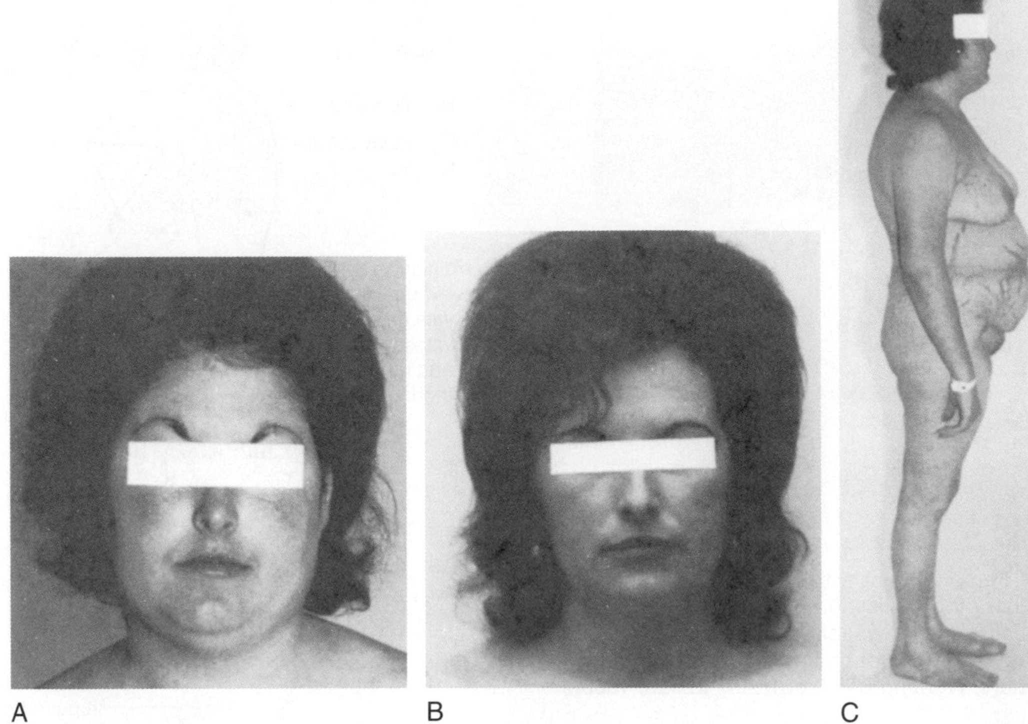

FIGURE 40-16 ■ A woman with Cushing syndrome before (**A** and **C**) and after (**B**) removal of an adrenal adenoma. (From Wyngaarden JB, Smith LH, Bennett JC, editors: *Cecil textbook of medicine,* ed 19, Philadelphia, 1992, Saunders, p 1285.)

clude inappropriate diagnoses due to diurnal variations in cortisol production. If 24-hour urinary free cortisol is found to be elevated, a series of dexamethasone suppression tests may be used to confirm the diagnosis. The interpretation of these tests is beyond the scope of this text.

Treatment. The choice of treatment for Cushing syndrome is based on its cause. For pituitary disease (Cushing disease), transsphenoidal hypophysectomy has become the surgical treatment of choice. Figure 40-16 shows a woman before and after treatment for Cushing syndrome.

Unilateral adrenalectomy is used if the cause of the hypercortisolism is an adrenal tumor. Bilateral removal of the adrenal glands is rarely performed today; lifelong glucocorticoid and mineralocorticoid replacement is essential following this surgery. Radiation therapy may be an option if surgery is contraindicated.[25]

Chemotherapeutic agents that block cortisol production can also be utilized either alone or in conjunction with surgery and radiation. When any of these therapies is used, the patient should be assessed for adrenal insufficiency.

Hyperaldosteronism

Both primary hyperaldosteronism (excess production of aldosterone by the adrenal cortex) and excess levels of glucocorticoids (Cushing disease or syndrome) raise blood pressure. Aldosterone and glucocorticoids facilitate salt and water retention by the kidney; the hypertension that accompanies excessive levels of either hormone is probably due to this mechanism. Because aldosterone acts on the distal renal tubule to promote sodium exchange for the potassium lost in the urine, persons with hyperaldosteronism usually have decreased potassium levels (Figure 40-17). The drug spironolactone is an aldosterone antagonist and therefore is useful in the medical management of aldosterone excess. Spironolactone increases sodium excretion and potassium retention. Sodium restriction and potassium replacement are also necessary.[25]

KEY CONCEPTS

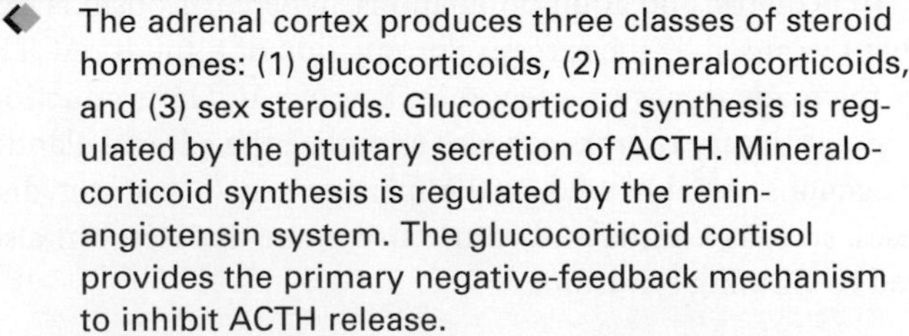

- The adrenal cortex produces three classes of steroid hormones: (1) glucocorticoids, (2) mineralocorticoids, and (3) sex steroids. Glucocorticoid synthesis is regulated by the pituitary secretion of ACTH. Mineralocorticoid synthesis is regulated by the renin-angiotensin system. The glucocorticoid cortisol provides the primary negative-feedback mechanism to inhibit ACTH release.
- Adrenocortical insufficiency may be primary (Addison disease), in which case it is characterized by high ACTH levels in the blood and hyperpigmentation of skin related to excessive pituitary secretion, or it may be secondary, in which case it is characterized by low ACTH levels.

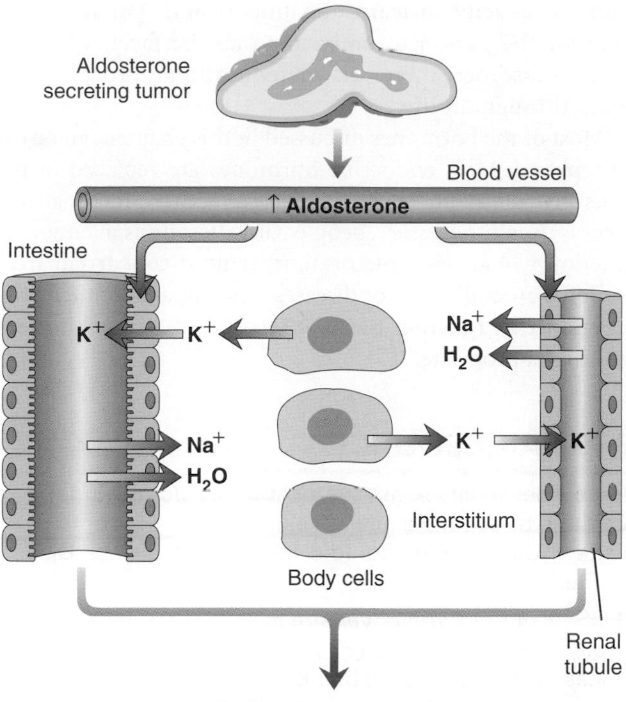

FIGURE 40-17 ■ Hyperaldosteronism, regardless of the cause, results in sodium and water retention and potassium excretion.

- Primary adrenal insufficiency may follow autoimmune destruction of, surgical removal of, or trauma to the gland. Exogenous administration of steroids suppresses ACTH, resulting in adrenocortical atrophy. Sudden withdrawal of exogenous steroids may result in adrenal insufficiency.
- Inherited defects in biosynthetic enzymes necessary for cortisol production may affect one or more of the steroid hormone synthesis pathways. Cortisol deficiency stimulates pituitary release of ACTH, stimulating the adrenal gland to enlarge (congenital adrenal hyperplasia). Excess androgens may be synthesized, leading to masculinization of females and precocious puberty in males.
- Manifestations of primary adrenocortical insufficiency include weight loss, salt wasting, volume depletion, low blood pressure, hypoglycemia, and hyperkalemia. Stress may lead to severe symptoms (Addisonian crisis), including circulatory collapse (hypotension). Treatment includes hormone replacement therapy. Dosages are generally increased during periods of stress (e.g., surgery).
- Excess cortisol production due to pituitary hyperstimulation of the adrenal cortex is termed Cushing disease. Hypercortisolism of any other cause is termed Cushing syndrome. ACTH excess may be due to pituitary adenoma or exogenous production by nonpituitary tumors. Cushing syndrome is commonly due to administration of exogenous steroids.
- Clinical manifestations of Cushing disease and syndrome include moon facies, cervical fat pad, central obesity, thin extremities, weight gain, thin skin, striae, hypertension, and hyperglycemia. Plasma cortisol levels and the urinary excretion of cortisol metabolites are increased. Surgical removal of ACTH-producing tumors or removal of the adrenal gland is the usual treatment.
- Primary hyperaldosteronism is usually due to adrenal tumor. Aldosterone enhances sodium and water reabsorption and potassium excretion from the kidney, leading to hypervolemia, hypertension, and hypokalemia.

ADRENAL MEDULLA

Hormone Disorders of the Adrenal Medulla (Pheochromocytoma)

Etiology and Pathogenesis. The adrenal medulla secretes two important catecholamine hormones in response to stimulation by the sympathetic nervous system. Epinephrine, or adrenaline, accounts for about 80% of the adrenal medulla's secretion; norepinephrine accounts for the other 20%. Norepinephrine is also the neurotransmitter produced by the postganglionic sympathetic fibers. Sympathetic effectors such as the heart, smooth muscle, and glands have receptors for norepinephrine. Both epinephrine and norepinephrine can bind to the receptors of sympathetic effectors to prolong and enhance the effects of sympathetic stimulation.

Pheochromocytoma is an uncommon disease that results in the excessive production of catecholamines. A pheochromocytoma is a tumor of chromaffin tissue. It is usually found in the adrenal medulla, but it may also arise in other sites where there is chromaffin tissue, such as the sympathetic ganglia. Like adrenal medullary cells, the tumor cells of a pheochromocytoma produce and secrete the catecholamines epinephrine and norepinephrine in response to sympathetic stimulation. The massive release of these catecholamines results in severe hypertension.[28] The hypertension in individuals with pheochromocytoma is influenced by the level of sympathetic nervous system stimulation, the circulating catecholamine levels, and the cardiovascular response to these changes.

Clinical Manifestations. The most common symptom experienced by an individual with a pheochromocytoma is persistent hypertension. The presence of the classic triad of headache, tachycardia, and diaphoresis (caused by massive circulating catecholamine levels) strongly suggests the diagnosis of pheochromocytoma. Sporadic hypertensive episodes may occur secondary to stress, excitement, physical activity, ingestion of certain drugs, and the smoking of tobacco products. Other symptoms may include tremor, nervousness, emotional lability, pallor, fatigue, generalized gastrointestinal complaints, and orthostatic hypotension. Signs of a hypermetabolic state may be present, such as fever, weight loss, polyuria, and polydipsia.[29] Many other manifestations are experienced by these individuals, but the presenting complaints frequently resemble those of other conditions, such as renal disease, thyrotoxicosis, or psychological problems, if hypertension is intermittent. The final diagnosis may be delayed until symptoms worsen.

Because most pheochromocytomas are located on the adrenal glands, CT is the most common diagnostic tool. Uncontrolled hypertension can lead to end-organ damage and death, so prompt diagnosis and aggressive therapy are necessary.[30]

Treatment. The usual treatment for this condition is surgical removal of the tumor. Before surgery, α-adrenergic, then β-adrenergic blocking medications are prescribed to manage blood pressure and relieve some of the symptoms related to this factor.

If surgery is contraindicated, treatment with metyrosine is used. Metyrosine decreases catecholamine production by inhibiting an enzyme necessary for the synthesis of catecholamines. However, surgery is the only curative therapy.

If both adrenal glands are removed, lifetime treatment for adrenocorticoid insufficiency is necessary. Because there is an increased risk of recurrence of the tumor in later years, annual follow-up by an endocrinologist should be planned.[30]

KEY CONCEPTS

- The adrenal medulla releases catecholamines into the blood stream when stimulated by the sympathetic nervous system. Catecholamines increase heart rate, blood pressure, and glucose release from the liver.
- A pheochromocytoma is a catecholamine-secreting tumor that is usually located in the adrenal medulla. Excessive catecholamine release from the tumor causes intermittent or persistent hypertension, headache, tachycardia, tremor, and irritability. Most tumors are benign, and surgical removal relieves the disorder. Adrenergic blocking agents may be used to manage the hypertension until surgical treatment is accomplished.

SUMMARY

Education is the key to maintaining an adequate state of health in individuals with an endocrine dysfunction. The individual with an alteration in endocrine function needs to understand the etiologic process, pathogenesis, clinical manifestations, treatment plan, prognosis, and consequences of proper as well as inadequate hormone replacement. The educational plan should be tailored to the individual's capacity to learn and understand. Often, it takes time for the person to understand all the facets of an endocrine disorder; therefore, the educational process is ongoing throughout life.

Most of the hormones discussed in this chapter can be easily replaced. Most endocrine hormones are replaced in patterns that mimic their natural release. Because lifelong treatment is usually necessary, people with alterations in endocrine function will at one time or another need concurrent treatment for other illnesses or diseases. The impact of other drugs on endocrine function must be recognized and adjustments made as appropriate.

MEDIA RESOURCES

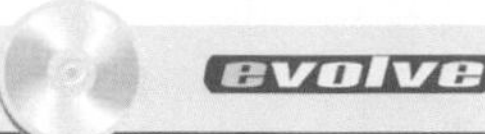

Remember to check out the ***CD Companion*** included with this book for Review Questions, Key Concepts Review, Glossary (with audio for selected terms), Disease Profiles, and Animations.

PLUS, visit the ***Evolve website*** at http://evolve.elsevier.com/Copstead/ for Case Studies, Disease Profiles, and WebLinks.

References

1. Thorner MD et al: The anterior pituitary. In Wilson JD, Foster DW, editors: *Williams textbook of endocrinology,* ed 9, Philadelphia, 1998, Saunders.
2. Reeves WB, Bichet DG, Andreoli TE: Posterior pituitary and water metabolism. In Wilson JD, Foster DW, editors: *Williams textbook of endocrinology,* ed 9, Philadelphia, 1998, Saunders.
3. Hintz RL: The pituitary gland and growth failure. In Lavin N, editor: *Manual of endocrinology and metabolism,* ed 3, Philadelphia, 2002, Lippincott Williams & Wilkins.
4. Cuneo RC: Efficacy of growth hormone replacement therapy: lipid and cardiovascular effects, *Endocrinologist* 8:22S-30S, 1998.
5. Kleinberg DL, Melmed S: The adult growth hormone deficiency syndrome: signs, symptoms, and diagnosis, *Endocrinologist* 8:8S-14S, 1998.
6. Colao A et al: Effect of growth hormone (GH) and/or testosterone on the prostate in GH-deficient adult patients, *J Clin Endocrinol Metab* 88:88-94, 2003.
7. Murray RD, Shalet SM: Adult growth hormone replacement: lessons learned and future direction, *J Clin Endocrinol Metab* 87:4427-4428, 2002.
8. Melmed S et al for the Acromegaly Treatment Consensus Workshop participants: Guidelines for acromegaly management, *J Clin Endocrinol Metab* 87:4054-4058, 2002.
9. Lipscombe L, Asa SL, Ezzat S: Management of lesions of the pituitary stalk and hypothalamus, *Endocrinologist* 13:38-51, 2003.
10. Victorina WM, Rystedt LL, Sowers RJ: Disorders of vasopressin. In Lavin N, editor: *Manual of endocrinology and metabolism,* ed 3, Philadelphia, 2002, Lippincott Williams & Wilkins.
11. Davies P: Caring for patients with diabetes insipidus, *Nursing* 26(5):62-63, 1996.

12. Moses AM et al: Central diabetes insipidus due to cytomegalovirus infection of the hypothalamus in a patient with acquired immunodeficiency syndrome: a clinical, pathological and immunohistochemical case study, *J Clin Endocrinol Metab* 88:51-54, 2003.
13. Larsen PR, Davies TF, Hay ID: The thyroid gland. In Wilson JD, Foster DW, editors: *Williams textbook of endocrinology,* ed 9, Philadelphia, 1998, Saunders.
14. Hershman JM: Hypothyroidism and hyperthyroidism. In Lavin N, editor: *Manual of endocrinology and metabolism,* ed 3, Philadelphia, 2002, Lippincott Williams & Wilkins.
15. Gudmundsdottir A, Schlecte JA: Central hypothyroidism, *Endocrinologist* 12:218-223, 2002.
16. Nieuwlaat WA, Hermus AR, Huysmans DA: Nontoxic, nodular goiter: new management paradigms, *Endocrinologist* 13:31-37, 2003.
17. Tietgens ST, Leinung MC: Thyroid storm, *Med Clin North Am* 79:169-184, 1995.
18. Vander A, Sherman J, Luciano D: *Human physiology: the mechanisms of body function,* ed 7, New York, 1998, McGraw-Hill.
19. Bringhurst FR, Demay MB, Kronenberg HM: Hormones and disorders of mineral metabolism. In Wilson JD, Foster DW, editors: *Williams textbook of endocrinology,* ed 9, Philadelphia, 1998, Saunders.
20. Brickman AS: Disorders of calcitropic hormones in adults. In Lavin N, editor: *Manual of endocrinology and metabolism,* ed 3, Philadelphia, 2002, Lippincott Williams & Wilkins.
21. Recker BF: Pregnancy at risk: metabolic and renal alterations. In Dickason EJ, Silverman BL, Schult MO, editors: *Maternal-infant nursing care,* ed 2, St Louis, 1994, Mosby.
22. Tannenbaum C et al: Yield of laboratory testing to identify secondary contributors to osteoporosis in otherwise healthy women, *J Clin Endocrinol Metab* 87:4431-4437, 2002.
23. Parker C et al: Alendronate in the treatment of primary hyperparathyroid-related osteoporosis: a 2-year study, *J Clin Endocrinol Metab* 87:4482-4489, 2002.
24. Stern N, Tuck ML: The adrenal cortex and mineralocorticoid hypertension. In Lavin N, editor: *Manual of endocrinology and metabolism,* ed 3, Philadelphia, 2002, Lippincott Williams & Wilkins.
25. Orth DN, Kovacs WJ: The adrenal cortex. In Wilson JD, Foster DW, editors: *Williams textbook of endocrinology,* ed 9, Philadelphia, 1998, Saunders.
26. Cooper MS, Stewart PM: Corticosteroid insufficiency in acutely ill patients, *N Engl J Med* 348:727-734, 2003.
27. Azziz R: Polycystic ovary syndrome, insulin resistance, and molecular defects of insulin signaling, *J Clin Endocrinol Metab* 87:4085-4087, 2002.
28. Yu J, Pacak K: Management of malignant pheochromocytoma, *Endocrinologist* 12:291-299, 2002.
29. Landberg L, Young JB: Catecholamines and the adrenal medulla. In Wilson JD, Foster DW, editors: *Williams textbook of endocrinology,* ed 9, Philadelphia, 1998, Saunders.
30. Sowers KM, Sowers JR: Pheochromocytoma. In Lavin N, editor: *Manual of endocrinology and metabolism,* ed 3, Philadelphia, 2002, Lippincott Williams & Wilkins.

chapter 41

Diabetes Mellitus

Arnold A. Asp

MEDIA RESOURCES

Additional Material for Study, Review, and Further Exploration

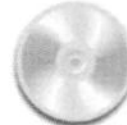

CD Companion ◆ Review Questions and Answers ◆ Key Concepts Review ◆ Glossary *(with audio pronunciations for selected terms)* ◆ Disease Profiles ◆ Animations

evolve ***Website*** at http://evolve.elsevier.com/Copstead/
◆ Case Studies ◆ Disease Profiles ◆ WebLinks

KEY QUESTIONS

- Which hormones are involved in regulation of serum glucose, and under what physiologic conditions would each be secreted?
- What are the differentiating characteristics of type 1 and type 2 diabetes?
- How do the pathophysiologic processes differ among the various types of diabetes?
- What clinical findings are associated with hyperglycemia, and how do they differ from those of hypoglycemia?
- How is diabetes mellitus diagnosed, monitored, and managed?
- What are the acute and chronic complications of diabetes mellitus?

CHAPTER OUTLINE

The public health impact of diabetes mellitus is enormous. In the United States, more than 18 million persons (>6% of the population) have diabetes mellitus, although it is estimated that only 60% are aware of their diagnosis. Should this trend continue unabated, worldwide the number of persons with diabetes will exceed 250 million by 2010. The annual cost of diabetes to the U.S. medical care system is more than $135 billion, with annual increases expected to exceed 11%. Diabetes mellitus is a leading cause of death and disability in the United States. It increases the risk for heart disease, end-stage renal disease, blindness, amputation, and complications of pregnancy and is ranked as the sixth leading cause of death. Diabetes mellitus disproportionately affects non-Caucasian and elderly individuals; its complications strain health care resources.[1]

REGULATION OF GLUCOSE METABOLISM

Because diabetes mellitus affects the utilization of all energy nutrients, it is helpful to review energy nutrient metabolism to understand the disease process of diabetes mellitus. The energy requirements of humans are predominantly met by glucose and fats. Produced from endogenous glycogen stores in the muscles and liver or manufactured from such substrates as amino acids and lactate, glucose is supplied to the blood stream from the gastrointestinal tract and liver. Glucose is typically present in greater quantities in extracellular fluid than within cells.

The plasma membranes of cells are variously permeable to glucose, and the diffusion of glucose into some cells is controlled by glucose transporters (GLUT 1-7) specific to each tissue. The glucose transporters of neural tissue and erythrocytes (GLUT 2) do not require activation with the hormone **insulin.** Adipose and muscle cells possess insulin receptors on the cell membrane that bind to insulin and activate glucose transporters (GLUT 4). Activated glucose transporters translocate to the cell membrane and facilitate the diffusion of glucose. Insulin may have additional, as yet undefined, roles in glucose uptake.[2]

Hormonal Regulation

Protein and fat metabolism are regulated by the anabolic effects of insulin. Insulin appears to increase the uptake and decrease the release of amino acids by skeletal muscle, thus inducing protein synthesis and preventing muscle breakdown. The amount of stored fats in the form of triglyceride is potentiated by the action of insulin in preventing fat breakdown and inducing lipid formation. Insulin also appears to have a role in growth by stimulating the secretion of somatomedin.

Normal glucose metabolism is usually described in reference to the fed and fasting, or absorptive and postabsorptive, states. The fed state occurs after ingestion of a meal and is characterized by utilization and storage of ingested energy nutrients. The fasting state is characterized by utilization of stored nutrients for the energy needs of the body.

In the fed state, glucose from ingested food provides the primary energy source (Figure 41-1). The post-meal rise in blood glucose and the presence of certain gastrointestinal hormones stimulate the production of insulin. Initial stimulation produces a brief rise in insulin secretion, termed the *first phase.* The continued presence of increased glucose produces the second phase of insulin secretion, a state characterized by insulin synthesis.

Insulin is synthesized in the **pancreas** by the β cells of the islets of Langerhans. The islets are groups of cells dispersed throughout the pancreas. Within the islets can be found β cells that produce insulin in the form of **proinsulin,** α cells that produce **glucagon,** δ cells that produce somatostatin, and F cells that produce pancreatic polypeptide.

Proinsulin is produced and packaged into granules. Enzymes within the granules cleave proinsulin into insulin and C-peptide, with some remaining proinsulin. Granules release their contents into the blood stream by exocytosis.

The presence of insulin stimulates the diffusion of glucose into adipose and muscle tissue and inhibits the production of glucose by the liver. After diffusion into the cell, glucose may be oxidized for the energy needs of the cell, a process termed **glycolysis.** Most ingested glucose is utilized in **glycogenesis** (production of glycogen in the muscle and the liver).

In the fasting state, glucose is produced by **glycogenolysis** (breakdown of stored glycogen) in the liver and muscles and by **gluconeogenesis** (production of glucose from amino acids and other substrates) in the liver (Figure 41-2). Insulin levels, no longer stimulated by an influx of ingested glucose, fall to a basal level. The catabolic effects of the absence of insulin are evident in the stimulation of glycogenolysis and are accompanied by a rise in glucagon levels. If insulin is the hormone that dominates the fed state, glucagon dominates the fasting state. Glucagon-stimulated glycogenolysis and gluconeogenesis are responsible for up to 75% of glucose production in the fasting state.

The primary source of energy to muscle tissue in the fasting state is free fatty acids produced by **lipolysis** (breakdown of fat from adipose tissue). Lipolysis is stimulated by the fall in plasma insulin. Neural tissue preferentially uses glucose.

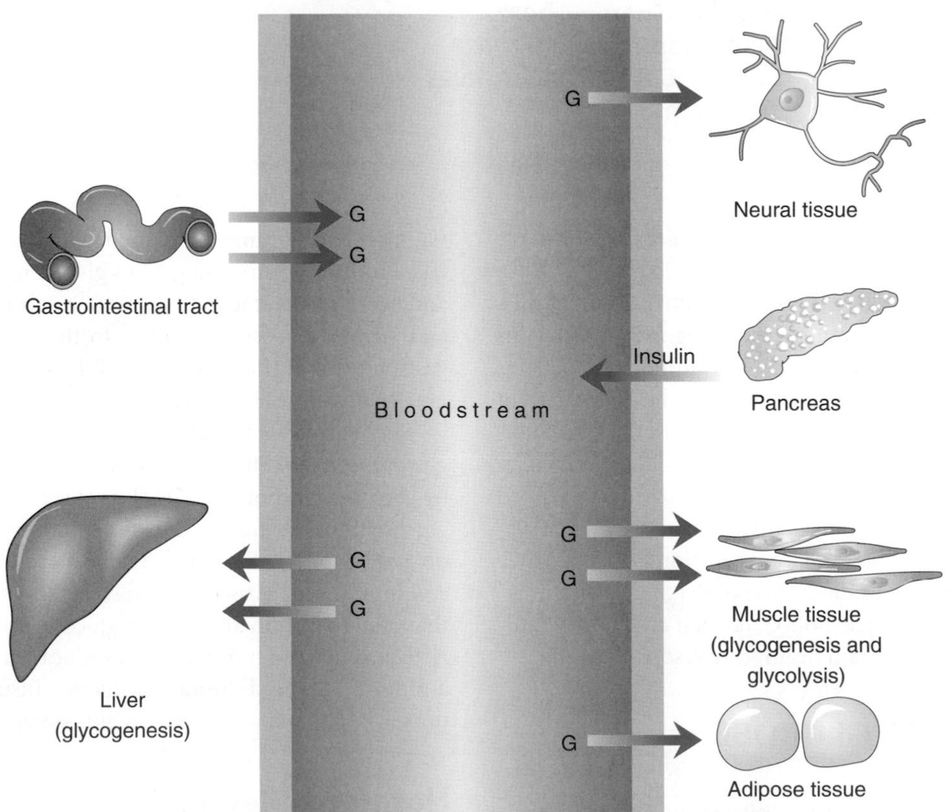

FIGURE 41-1 ■ Energy metabolism in the fed state. *G,* Glucose.

Other hormones referred to as *counterregulatory hormones* have a role in glucose metabolism in the fasting state. **Corticosteroids** stimulate gluconeogenesis and counteract the hypoglycemic action of insulin. **Growth hormone** increases peripheral **insulin resistance** and prevents insulin from suppressing hepatic glucose production. **Catecholamines** augment glucose production by prompting hepatic glycogenolysis and gluconeogenesis.[3]

Exercise

Increasing activity requires increased fuel for muscle tissue. At the onset of exercise, insulin levels drop and glucagon and catecholamine levels initially rise and increase the production of free fatty acids, the primary energy source of resting muscle (Figure 41-3). Falling insulin levels and increased glucagon levels stimulate glycogenolysis. Under the influence of catecholamines, muscle tissue shifts from using primarily fatty acids for fuel to using stored glycogen. The relative absence of insulin and increased production of glucagon also stimulate hepatic glycogenolysis. Glucose released by the liver increasingly meets the energy needs of muscle tissue as exercise continues. After 10 to 40 minutes of exercise, blood glucose use by muscle tissue increases 7 to 20 times. The interactions of hormones thus produce the mixture of glucose and free fatty acids used by muscle tissue during exercise.

Muscle tissue is affected not only by the influence of hormones but also by exercise itself. The postreceptor activities of glucose transporters are enhanced by muscular contraction. The resulting increase in insulin sensitivity can last as long as 16 hours. Thus in normal metabolism, increased insulin sensitivity allows normal blood glucose values in the presence of lower levels of circulating insulin.

Stress

During stress such as injury, illness, and pain, stress hormones, including corticosteroids and catecholamines, interact to ensure continuous supplies of glucose. Corticosteroids increase the production of glucose in the liver and elevate the production of glucagon. Glucocorticoids also decrease the utilization of glucose by muscle tissue by diminishing the effect of insulin on glucose transporters and by generating a decline in the number of insulin receptors and their function.

Catecholamines increase serum glucagon levels, increase glucose production by the liver, and decrease the use of glucose by muscle and fat tissue. The production of fatty acids that is triggered by the action of catecholamines further inhibits glucose uptake in the periphery. The series of events produced by traumatic stress is referred to as *stress hyperglycemia.*

Psychological stress can produce metabolic changes comparable with those of physical stress. Deterioration in

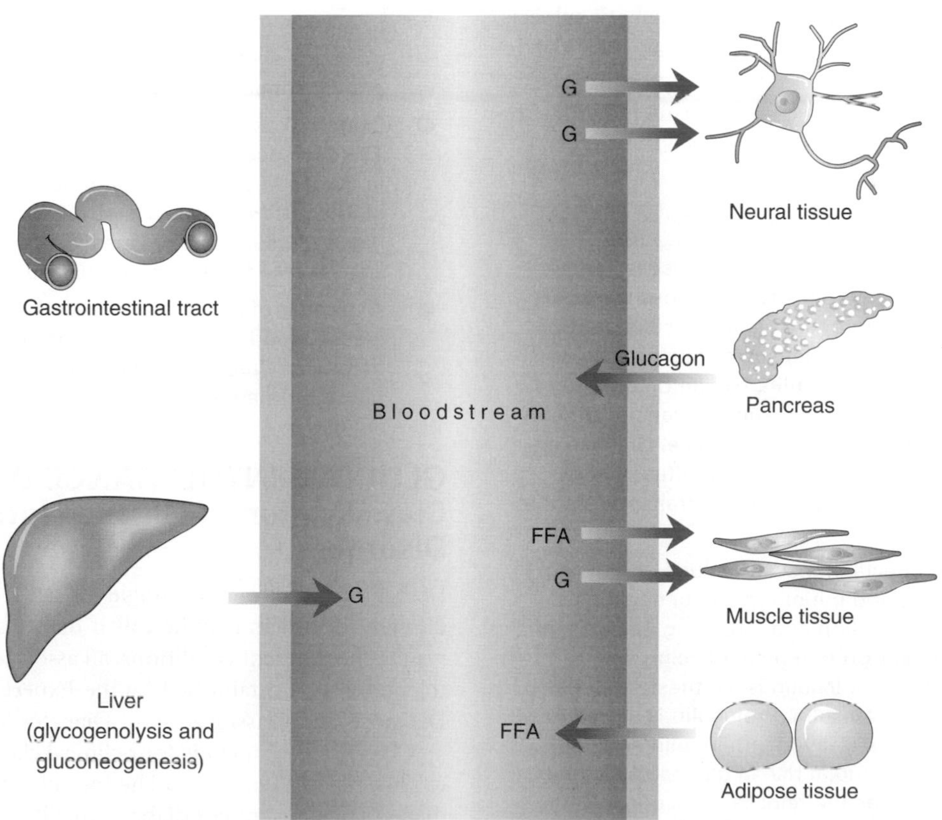

FIGURE 41-2 ■ Energy metabolism in the fasting state. *G,* Glucose; *FFA,* free fatty acids.

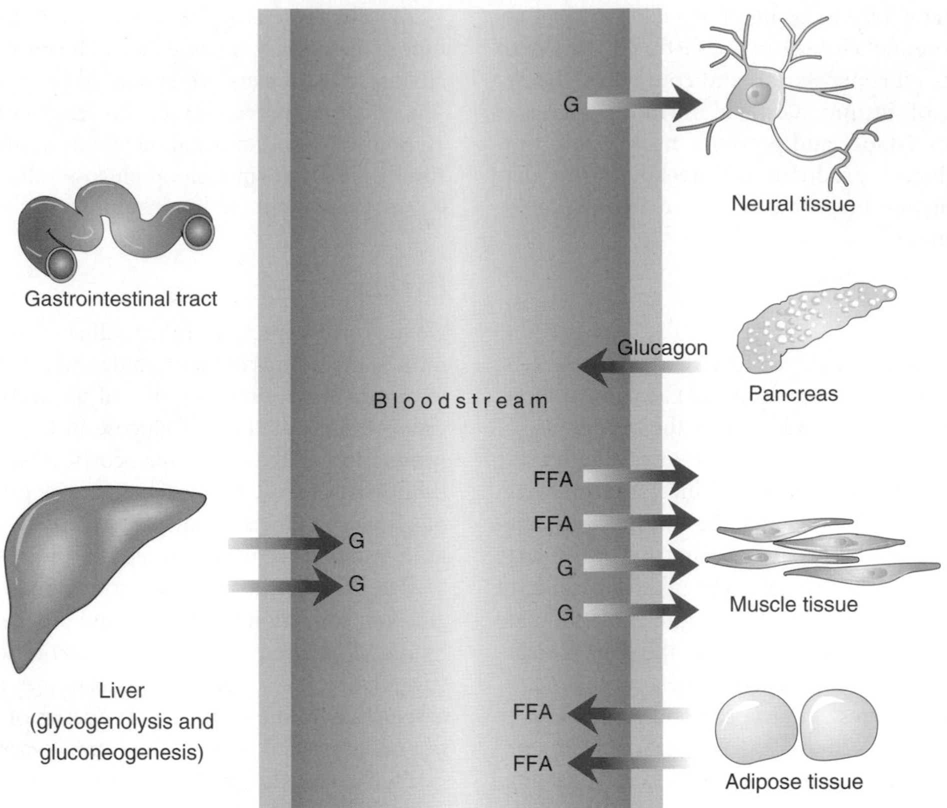

FIGURE 41-3 ■ Energy metabolism during exercise. *G,* Glucose; *FFA,* free fatty acids.

metabolic control has been noted in stressed diabetic subjects. However, the response is by no means universal. An actual decrease in blood glucose levels has frequently been observed during acute stress, perhaps reflecting differing individual responses to psychological stress (e.g., disordered eating).

KEY CONCEPTS

- Plasma membrane permeability to glucose is determined by the type and density of glucose transport proteins in the membrane. In some tissues, particularly muscle and fat, the density of glucose transporters is regulated by insulin. Insulin binding to receptors on the cell surface results in translocation of glucose transporters to the cell surface. Glucose enters the cell passively by facilitated diffusion. Neurons and erythrocytes have glucose transporters that do not require insulin.
- The metabolic effects of insulin include enhancing protein synthesis and inhibiting gluconeogenesis, enhancing fat deposition and inhibiting lipolysis, and stimulating cellular growth by enhancing somatomedin secretion. Insulin is synthesized in pancreatic β cells as proinsulin. Proinsulin is stored in granules, where it is cleaved into insulin and C-peptide. A postprandial rise in glucose and other substrates stimulates the release of insulin into the blood stream. During fasting, when blood glucose levels fall, the decrease in insulin and the increase in glucagon secretion lead to lipolysis, glycogenolysis, and gluconeogenesis.
- Exercise has complex effects on glucose metabolism. The decrease in insulin production and the increase in glucagon and catecholamines lead to elevated blood glucose levels. However, exercising muscle has increased insulin sensitivity, which facilitates glucose uptake for as long as 16 hours after exercise.
- A number of hormones released during stress increase blood glucose levels and oppose the effects of insulin. Catecholamines, glucocorticoids, and glucagon may precipitate *stress hyperglycemia.*

GLUCOSE INTOLERANCE DISORDERS

Classification of Glucose Intolerance Disorders

Diabetes mellitus is not a single disease entity; as many as 30 different disorders may be called diabetes. Criteria for diagnosing the different conditions, all associated with glucose intolerance, were established by the Expert Committee on the Diagnosis and Classification of Diabetes Mellitus in 1997.

Classifications include four clinical classes and two statistical risk classes (Box 41-1). The four clinical classes are type 1 diabetes mellitus, type 2 diabetes mellitus, other specific types of diabetes mellitus, and gestational diabetes mellitus. Statisti-

Box 41-1

Classifications of Glucose Metabolism Disorders

Type 1 Diabetes Mellitus
- Immune mediated
- Idiopathic

Type 2 Diabetes Mellitus

Other Specific Types of Diabetes

Genetic Defects of β-Cell Function
Chromosome 12, *HNF1A* (formerly *MODY3*)
Chromosome 7, glucokinase (formerly *MODY2*)
Chromosome 20, *HNF4A* (formerly *MODY1*)
Mitochondrial DNA
Others

Genetic Defects in Insulin Action
Type A insulin resistance
Leprechaunism
Rabson-Mendenhall syndrome
Lipoatrophic diabetes
Others

Diseases of the Exocrine Pancreas
Pancreatitis
Trauma pancreatectomy
Neoplasia
Cystic fibrosis
Hemochromatosis
Fibrocalculous pancreatopathy
Others

Endocrinopathies
Acromegaly
Cushing syndrome
Glucagonoma
Pheochromocytoma
Hyperthyroidism
Somatostatinoma
Aldosteronoma
Others

Drug or Chemical Induced
Pyriminil (Vacor)
Pentamidine
Nicotinic acid
Glucocorticoids
Thyroid hormone
Diazoxide
β-Adrenergic agonists
Thiazides
Phenytoin (Dilantin)
Interferon-α
Others

Infections
Congenital rubella
Cytomegalovirus
Others

Uncommon Forms of Immune-Mediated Diabetes
Stiff-man syndrome
Antiinsulin receptor antibodies
Others

Other Genetic Syndromes Sometimes Associated With Diabetes
Down syndrome
Klinefelter syndrome
Turner syndrome
Friedreich ataxia
Huntington chorea
Laurence-Moon-Beidl syndrome
Myotonic dystrophy
Porphyria
Prader-Willi syndrome
Others

Gestational Diabetes Mellitus

Statistical Risk of Diabetes Mellitus
Impaired glucose tolerance
Impaired fasting glucose tolerance

Data from American Diabetes Association: Report of the Expert Committee on the Diagnosis and Classification of Diabetes Mellitus, *Diabetes Care* 20(7):1183-1197, 1997.

cal risk classes are impaired glucose tolerance and impaired fasting glucose tolerance.

Diabetes Mellitus

Guidelines for the diagnosis of diabetes mellitus have been developed by the Expert Committee for the Classification of Diabetes Mellitus (Box 41-2).[1] The diagnostic criteria were revised in 1997 to more accurately reflect the degree of hyperglycemia associated with the onset of diabetic complications. The same diagnostic criteria apply in type 1, type 2, and other specific types of diabetes mellitus, and some of the same pathophysiologic process is present in these disorders. The pathophysiologic and etiologic mechanisms of type 1 and type 2 diabetes mellitus are different, with resulting differences in sequelae.

Type 1 Diabetes Mellitus

Type 1 diabetes mellitus is, by definition, characterized by destruction of the β cells of the pancreas. Type 1 diabetes can occur at any age but is most commonly diagnosed in persons between the ages of 5 and 20 years. Type 1 diabetes affects about 10% of individuals with diabetes mellitus in the United States. The prevalence is 1.7 per 1000 individuals younger than 20 years. Caucasian populations are more susceptible to type 1 diabetes mellitus than are African-American, Hispanic, Asian, or Native American populations. Little difference is noted in

Box 41-2

Diagnosis of Diabetes

Classic symptoms of the disease (polydipsia, polyuria, polyphagia, and weight loss) and a random plasma glucose value of 200 mg/dl or greater

or

Fasting plasma glucose value of 126 mg/dl or greater

or

Two-hour postprandial plasma glucose value of 200 mg/dl or greater during an oral glucose tolerance test

Diagnosis of Impaired Glucose Tolerance

Two-hour post–glucose ingestion value of ≥140 <200 mg/dl

Impaired Fasting Glucose Tolerance

Fasting plasma glucose value of >100 <126 mg/dl

Data from American Diabetes Association: Report of the Expert Committee on the Diagnosis and Classification of Diabetes Mellitus, *Diabetes Care* 20(7):1183-1197, 1997.

The criteria must be confirmed by repeat testing on a different day unless acute metabolic decompensation is present. The oral glucose tolerance test is not recommended for routine screening for diabetes.

the incidence of type 1 diabetes mellitus between men and women.[3]

Etiology. The two forms of type 1 diabetes mellitus are immune mediated and idiopathic. Immune-mediated type 1 diabetes is the result of an autoimmune attack on the β cells of the pancreas. A strong association with the presence of a gene or genes in the major histocompatibility complex on chromosome 6 has been observed. Genes in the major histocompatibility complex are responsible for the creation of cell surface proteins (human leukocyte antigens, or HLAs) that interact with lymphocytes to stimulate or suppress antibody production. DR3 and DR4 are associated with the development of type 1 diabetes mellitus.

Environment and heredity are factors in the development of immune-mediated type 1 diabetes mellitus. The incidence of immune-mediated diabetes in identical twins when one twin is affected is only 33%. Viral infection or exposure to a toxic agent may be the responsible environmental influence.

Antibodies against the islet cells of the pancreas, against insulin, or against both frequently appear early in the onset of immune-mediated diabetes. Antibodies may be present for as long as 9 years before diagnosis. The presence of hyperglycemia indicates that autoimmune destruction of β cells has reached the point at which insulin secretion is inadequate.

Recognition of the autoimmune component in the pathogenesis of immune-mediated type 1 diabetes has led to varying attempts to prevent the disease. Immunosuppressive agents such as cyclosporine and azathioprine have been effective in some human studies. Oral delivery of insulin from animal species to reduce the reaction to islet cell antibodies has been proposed as a preventive measure, as has nicotinamide.

The etiologic progression of idiopathic type 1 diabetes mellitus is not known. Idiopathic diabetes is associated with β-cell destruction without autoimmune markers or HLA association.

Pathogenesis and Clinical Manifestations. Type 1 diabetes mellitus is characterized by an absolute insulin deficiency, and thus glucose cannot enter muscle and adipose tissue (Figure 41-4). Production of glucose by the liver is no longer opposed by insulin. Overproduction of glucagon by pancreatic α cells stimulates glycogenolysis and gluconeogenesis. Plasma blood glucose levels rise. When the maximal tubular absorptive capacity of the kidney is exceeded, glucose is lost in the urine, and the resulting glycosuria and osmotic fluid loss eventually lead to profound hypovolemia. Tissues dependent on insulin for glucose transport do not have glucose available as a substrate. Neural tissue in the brain responds to this emergency by promoting eating behavior. The thirst, increased urination, and hunger resulting from the aforementioned processes are the classic symptoms of diabetes: polydipsia, polyuria, and polyphagia.

Continued insulin deficiency and other hormonal influences (increased levels of catecholamines, cortisol, glucagon, and growth hormone, in part caused by hypovolemia, physical stress, or insulin deficiency itself) lead to lipolysis in body tissues. As the catabolic process continues, metabolism of fats stored in adipose tissue leads to the production of fatty acids. The resulting fatty acids undergo transformation to keto acids in the liver. Hepatic gluconeogenesis in response to tissue glucose deprivation is also responsible for the increased production of keto acids. Under normal circumstances, keto acids can be used by neural and muscle tissue in energy metabolism. When the normal pathway is saturated, the pH falls (6.8 to 7.3) and ketone bodies are present in the urine, thus sharply increasing osmotic fluid loss. Metabolic acidosis ensues as the bicarbonate concentration decreases, and diabetic ketoacidosis results. In response to the metabolic acidosis, extracellular hydrogen ions are exchanged for intracellular potassium ions. Serum potassium levels rise (transient hyperkalemia) and excess potassium is excreted into the urine, eventually leading to a net potassium loss. Losses of sodium, magnesium, and phosphorus also occur as total body water decreases. Serum levels of the ions may be normal or elevated owing to hypovolemia. Hypovolemia also accounts for an increased hematocrit, hemoglobin (Hb), protein, white blood cell count, creatinine, and serum osmolality (Table 41-1). Lactic acidosis, or an excessive amount of lactate, a product of metabolism, can also be present because of hypovolemia and possibly reduced uptake of lactate by the liver as a result of acidosis. Hypovolemia and muscle catabolism are responsible for the significant weight loss present in persons with ketoacidosis and often at diagnosis of type 1 diabetes. Hypovolemic shock can lead to death if the patient is not promptly treated.

Respiratory compensation for the metabolic acidosis in the form of deep, labored respirations that are "fruity" in odor

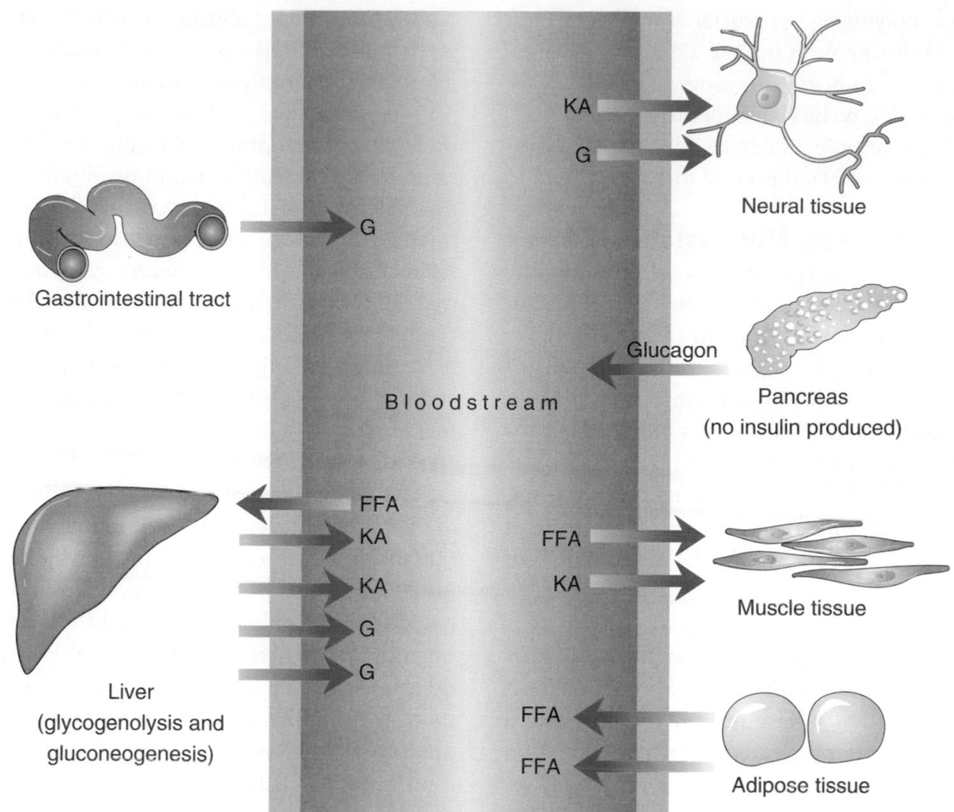

FIGURE 41-4 ■ Pathophysiology of energy metabolism in diabetes mellitus type 1. *G,* Glucose; *FFA,* free fatty acids; *KA,* keto acids.

Table 41-1

Diabetic Ketoacidosis and Nonketotic Hyperglycemic Hyperosmolar Coma

Parameter	Diabetic Ketoacidosis	Nonketotic Hyperglycemic Hyperosmolar Coma
Glucose	>300 mg/dl	>600 mg/dl
Urine ketones	Moderate to high	None
pH	6.8-7.3	Normal
Na^+, K^+	Low, normal, or high	Low, normal, or high
Hct, Hb, protein, WBC, Cr, BUN, serum osmolality	High	High

BUN, Blood urea nitrogen; *Cr,* creatinine; *Hb,* hemoglobin; *Hct,* hematocrit; *WBC,* white blood cell count.

(Kussmaul respirations) results in lowered P_{CO_2} values (compensatory respiratory alkalosis). Ketoacidosis may be the initial symptom of a new diagnosis of type 1 diabetes. Other factors that may precipitate ketoacidosis are intercurrent illness and inadequate treatment. Fourteen percent of individuals with type 1 diabetes mellitus are hospitalized with ketoacidosis every year.[3]

Type 2 Diabetes Mellitus

Etiology. Individuals with **type 2 diabetes mellitus** are resistant to the action of insulin on peripheral tissues and have a secretory defect in insulin production. Type 2 diabetes mellitus affects 90% to 95% of individuals with diabetes in the United States. Non-Caucasian and elderly populations are disproportionately affected. The prevalence of diabetes is 5.9% in the American Caucasian population, 10.1% in African-Americans, and 14.3% in Hispanic-Americans. The prevalence of diabetes in Native American populations can be as high as 50%. Overall, close to 11% of American individuals older than 65 years have diabetes mellitus. The prevalence of diabetes mellitus is usually higher in women than men.[3]

Risk factors include aging and a sedentary lifestyle, but the most powerful predictor is obesity. Excessive abdominal (visceral) fat introduces a greater threat of diabetes mellitus (and cardiovascular disease) than does lower body obesity. The initial symptoms of polydipsia, polyuria, polyphagia, and weight loss may be subtle or absent in type 2 diabetic patients.

Epidemiologic studies indicate a strong genetic component, but no specific HLA type has been identified. Studies indicate that the incidence of type 2 diabetes mellitus in identical twins when one twin is affected is close to 100%.[4]

Pathogenesis and Clinical Manifestations. Type 2 diabetes is characterized by a relative lack of insulin. The processes instrumental in producing the relative lack of insulin are insulin resistance and β-cell dysfunction (Figure 41-5).

The insulin resistance of type 2 diabetes mellitus is defined as a requirement for more insulin for the same biological action, along with lowered glucose utilization at all levels of insulin concentration. A decreased number of insulin receptors and such postreceptor defects as decreased action of glucose transporters are associated with insulin resistance. Impaired glycogen synthesis may also be a factor in the development of type 2 diabetes.[5]

Impaired production of insulin by the pancreatic β cells that intensifies as the disease progresses is also present in type 2 diabetes mellitus. Individuals with type 2 diabetes mellitus ultimately have an absent first-phase insulin response and a diminished second-phase response. Basal insulin secretion may be higher than normal in type 2 diabetes. Glucagon secretion is increased absolutely or relatively (relative to insulin levels). Individuals with type 2 diabetes may be predominantly insulin resistant or predominantly insulin deficient.

Type 2 diabetes mellitus is a progressive disease characterized by the development of insulin resistance, at first compensated for by increased insulin production and hyperinsulinemia. Decompensation occurs as the impaired β cells are unable to produce sufficient insulin to overcome insulin resistance. Insulin levels, however, remain elevated above normal until later in progression of the disease. Relatively decreased insulin levels, continued insulin resistance, and hyperglucagonemia result in the hyperglycemia of diabetes. Hyperglycemia itself may then increase insulin resistance and further diminish insulin secretion. The latter process has been termed *glucose toxicity*.

The relative lack of insulin seen in individuals with type 2 diabetes mellitus leads to similar but not identical sequelae as the absolute lack of insulin of type 1 diabetes mellitus. The initial symptoms of polyuria, polydipsia, and polyphagia may be present, possibly in a more subtle form. Ketoacidosis is an uncommon occurrence in type 2 diabetes. The presence of endogenous insulin in type 2 diabetes suppresses the lipolysis that leads to the production of ketone bodies and subsequently ketoacidosis in type 1 diabetes mellitus. More common in type 2 diabetes mellitus, especially in older individu-

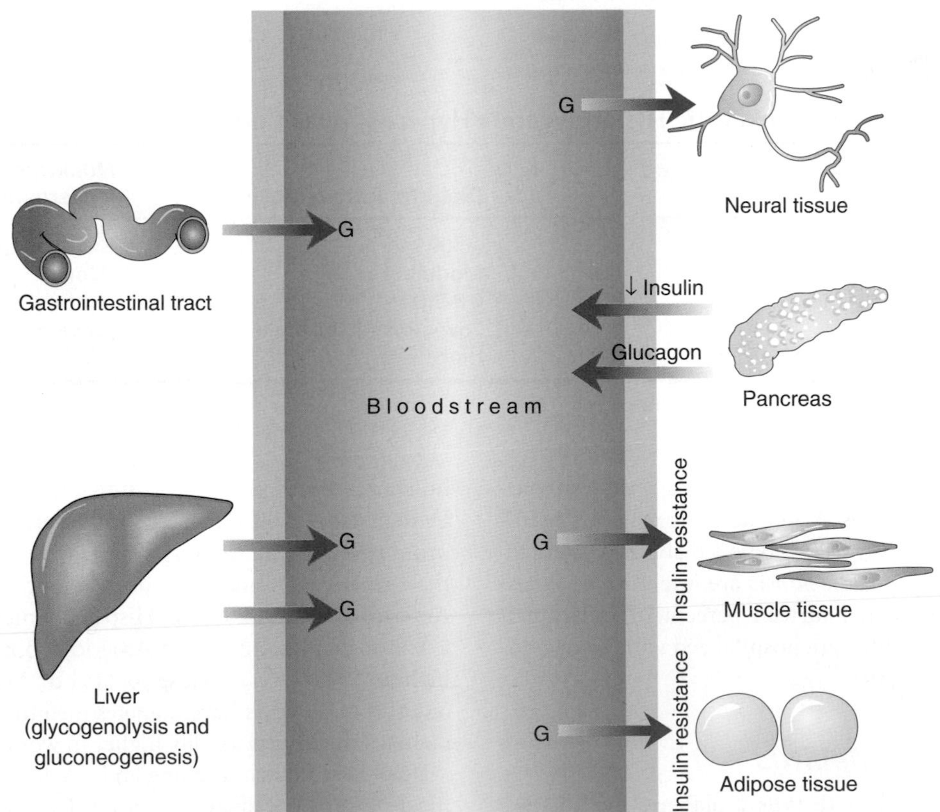

FIGURE 41-5 ■ Pathophysiology of energy metabolism in diabetes mellitus type 2. *G*, Glucose.

als, is nonketotic hyperglycemic hyperosmolar coma, characterized by severe hyperglycemia with no or slight ketosis and striking dehydration. Nonketotic hyperglycemic hyperosmolar coma is more likely to occur in institutionalized patients, especially patients unable to recognize or respond appropriately to thirst. Diabetic ketoacidosis and nonketotic hyperosmolar coma can be life-threatening events, especially in the elderly. Seventy percent of all cases of nonketotic hyperglycemic hyperosmolar coma occur in individuals older than 64 years. The mortality rate is 10% to 50%.[3]

Other Specific Types of Diabetes

- Genetic defects of β cells: The genetic defects of β cells follow an autosomal dominant pattern of inheritance and are characterized by a defect in the production of insulin. Affected individuals are identified before they reach 25 years of age, respond to oral sulfonylureas, and are nonketotic. The disorder is also referred to as "mature-onset diabetes of the young" (MODY).
- Genetic defects in insulin action: The disorders listed in Box 41-1 result in relatively rare, genetically determined defects of the insulin receptor.
- Diseases of the exocrine pancreas: Diseases of the pancreas can affect the insulin-producing capability of the organ (see Box 41-1).
- Endocrinopathies: Excessive production of insulin antagonists (e.g., cortisol, growth hormone, glucagon, epinephrine) affects glucose metabolism (see Box 41-1).
- Drug- or chemical-induced diabetes: Many chemicals can affect the ability of the pancreas to produce insulin (see Box 41-1).
- Infections: Destruction of the β cells of the pancreas has been linked to various infectious agents (see Box 41-1).
- Uncommon forms of immune-mediated diabetes.
- Certain autoimmune disorders are linked to glucose intolerance (see Table 41-1).
- Other genetic syndromes sometimes associated with diabetes: Certain genetic syndromes are linked to glucose intolerance (see Table 41-1).

Gestational Diabetes Mellitus

Gestational diabetes mellitus is by definition a disorder of glucose tolerance of variable severity with onset or first recognition during pregnancy. Between 2% and 5% of pregnancies are affected by gestational diabetes.[3,6]

Etiology. In its pathophysiologic characteristics, gestational diabetes mellitus closely resembles type 2 diabetes mellitus. As in type 2 diabetes, tissue insulin resistance is present during normal pregnancy. Insulin resistance in normal pregnancy is most likely precipitated by the presence of placental hormones: human chorionic somatomammotropin, estrogen, and cortisol. The weight gain of pregnancy is also responsible for an increase in insulin resistance. During pregnancy, women require two to three times as much insulin as they do in the nonpregnant state. Women with gestational diabetes are unable to produce sufficient insulin to meet their needs during pregnancy.

Risk factors for gestational diabetes mellitus include obesity, history of gestational diabetes or offspring weighing more than 9 lb at birth, age older than 40 years, and a family history of type 2 diabetes. Because insulin needs rise sharply in the 24th to 28th weeks of pregnancy, it is recommended that all pregnant women older than 25 years be screened for gestational diabetes during the 24th to 28th weeks with 50 g of oral glucose. Younger pregnant women who are obese, have a first-degree relative with diabetes, or are members of an ethnic/racial group with a high prevalence of diabetes (e.g., African-American, Hispanic, Asian, Native American) should also be screened. If the venous plasma glucose concentration is 140 mg/dl or greater, an oral glucose tolerance test is performed (Table 41-2).[6]

Untreated gestational diabetes can result in metabolic abnormalities and stillbirth. However, the most common complications of gestational diabetes are macrosomia and neonatal hypoglycemia. Macrosomia (birth weight greater than 4000 g) is a result of increased glucose, free fatty acids, and amino acids delivered to the fetus. Neonatal hypoglycemia is due to increased production of insulin by the fetal pancreas in response to the chronic stimulation of hyperglycemia while in utero.

Treatment. Management of gestational diabetes mellitus includes dietary counseling, exercise, and blood glucose and urine ketone monitoring. If hyperglycemia persists, insulin therapy should be initiated. Only glyburide does not cross the placenta to cause fetal hypoglycemia; this sulfonylurea may be used in gestational diabetes mellitus.

Glucose tolerance will return to normal after parturition in 97% of women with gestational diabetes mellitus. Women with gestational diabetes mellitus have a markedly increased risk for the development of type 2 diabetes mellitus or an impairment in glucose tolerance later in life. In subsequent pregnancies, 90% of women with a history of gestational diabetes mellitus will have a recurrence.

Table 41-2

Oral Glucose Tolerance Test Criteria for the Diagnosis of Gestational Diabetes

Determination Time	Blood Glucose (mg/dl)
Fasting	105
1 hr	190
2 hr	165
3 hr	145

Two or more blood glucose determinations must be equal to or greater than these values to establish the diagnosis.

Statistical Risk Factors

Impaired Glucose Tolerance and Impaired Fasting Glucose Tolerance

Guidelines for diagnosing the categories of **impaired glucose tolerance** and **impaired fasting glucose tolerance** (IFG) are listed in Box 41-2. Impaired glucose tolerance and IFG are intermediate stages between normal glucose metabolism and the onset of diabetes. They represent risk factors for the development of diabetes and are also risk factors for the onset of cardiovascular disease. The latter association is not fully understood.

Screening for Diabetes

Because of the high prevalence of undiagnosed type 2 diabetes mellitus, current recommendations are to screen all adults over the age of 45 for diabetes every 3 years. There is some controversy regarding screening individuals with asymptomatic disease. Individuals with risk factors should be screened at more frequent intervals (Box 41-3).[1] Although the results of a glucose tolerance test can be used to screen for diabetes, a fasting blood glucose test is preferable. The glucose tolerance test is inconvenient, more expensive, and less reliable than tests of fasting glucose. No diagnostic criteria use HbA_{1c} as yet because of a lack of standardization of methods of measurement.

Screening for gestational diabetes is discussed in the section on gestational diabetes. It is not recommended that routine screening for type 1 diabetes mellitus be performed. No agreement has been reached on the blood level of immune markers that represents a risk for type 1 diabetes or on treatment after identification of the presence of such markers.

Box 41-3

Screening for Diabetes

All individuals over the age of 45 should be screened for diabetes every 3 years.

Screening should be performed at an earlier age in individuals who

- Are obese
- Have a first-degree relative with diabetes
- Are members of a high-risk population (African-American, Asian, Native American, Hispanic)
- Have delivered a macrosomic baby
- Have high blood pressure
- Have an HDL cholesterol level of 35 mg/dl or less, a triglyceride level of 250 mg/dl or more, or both
- Have a history of IGT or IFG

Data from American Diabetes Association: Report of the Expert Committee on the Diagnosis and Classification of Diabetes Mellitus, *Diabetes Care* 20(7):1183-1197, 1997.
HDL, High-density lipoprotein; *IGT,* impaired glucose tolerance; *IFG,* impaired fasting glucose tolerance.

KEY CONCEPTS

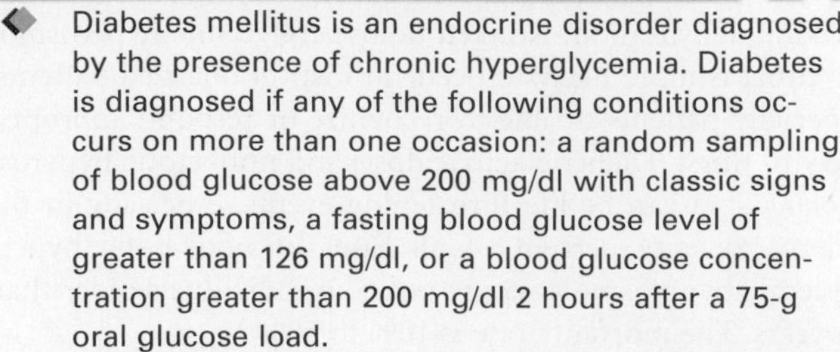

- Diabetes mellitus is an endocrine disorder diagnosed by the presence of chronic hyperglycemia. Diabetes is diagnosed if any of the following conditions occurs on more than one occasion: a random sampling of blood glucose above 200 mg/dl with classic signs and symptoms, a fasting blood glucose level of greater than 126 mg/dl, or a blood glucose concentration greater than 200 mg/dl 2 hours after a 75-g oral glucose load.
- The classification of diabetes mellitus includes two broad categories: (1) actual glucose intolerance and (2) the risk of glucose intolerance. Disorders of actual glucose intolerance include type 1, type 2, other specific types, and gestational diabetes. Statistical risk categories include individuals with impaired glucose tolerance and those with impaired fasting glucose tolerance. Individuals at risk for glucose intolerance include those with a history of glucose intolerance and those with a positive family history, obesity, or other risk factors.
- Persons with type 1 diabetes have an absolute insulin deficiency caused by pancreatic β-cell failure. Immune-mediated type 1 diabetes is associated with a specific HLA genetic makeup and may be autoimmune. Idiopathic type 1 diabetes is not an autoimmune process. Type 1 diabetes may affect people of any age. Classic manifestations include polyuria, polydipsia, polyphagia, and weight loss. Persons with type 1 diabetes are more prone to the development of ketoacidosis because of lipolysis associated with absolute insulin deficiency.
- Persons with type 2 diabetes have a relative insulin deficiency caused by decreased tissue sensitivity and decreased responsiveness to insulin. A decreased number of insulin receptors or abnormal translocation of glucose transporters is suspected. As the disease progresses, pancreatic insulin production may become impaired. Obesity, female sex, family history, older age, and lack of exercise are risk factors. Individuals with type 2 diabetes are prone to the development of nonketotic hyperglycemic hyperosmolar coma.
- Gestational diabetes is a disorder of glucose tolerance that is diagnosed during pregnancy. Placental hormones and weight gain are contributing factors. High infant birth weight and neonatal hypoglycemia are common complications. Gestational diabetes is a risk factor for the later development of type 2 diabetes.
- Ketoacidosis occurs primarily in type 1 diabetes mellitus as a result of increased lipolysis and conversion to ketone bodies. Excessive ketones result in metabolic acidosis, which is recognized by a fall in pH and bicarbonate levels. Ketoacidosis may occur in patients with type 2 diabetes mellitus under severe stress, such as concomitant sepsis, stroke, or myocardial infarction. Acidosis-induced hyper-

kalemia and compensatory hyperventilation (Kussmaul respirations) resulting in reduced arterial carbon dioxide are associated findings.

- Hyperosmolar coma is more common in type 2 diabetes because endogenous insulin suppresses ketone formation and thus prevents ketoacidosis. Hyperglycemia may go untreated for a time and result in persistent glycosuria with osmotic diuresis. Dehydration may be manifested as high osmolality and hemoconcentration of erythrocytes, proteins, and creatinine.

CLINICAL MANIFESTATIONS AND COMPLICATIONS

Acute Hyperglycemia

Etiology. Acute hyperglycemia is most commonly caused by alterations in nutrition, inactivity, inadequate use of antidiabetic medications, or any combination of these factors. Persistent fasting hyperglycemia can occasionally be attributed to the dawn phenomenon, or a rise in blood glucose concentration in the early morning hours attributed to increased levels of growth hormone.

Complications. A primary concern of individuals with diabetes and their health care providers is avoiding the acute and chronic complications of diabetes. Acute complications of diabetes include the signs and symptoms of hyperglycemia—polydipsia, polyphagia, and polyuria—and concomitant metabolic and fluid problems. Prolonged insulinopenia can result in ketoacidosis and nonketotic hyperglycemic coma with the accompanying more severe electrolyte and fluid derangements.

Acute complications of diabetes also include infections, most commonly of the skin, urinary tract, and vagina. Infections that particularly affect elderly diabetic patients include malignant otitis externa, necrotizing fasciitis, and persistent candidal infections. Tuberculosis infection and reactivation can be a particular problem in diabetic residents of extended care facilities.

Nausea, fatigue, and a generally decreased sense of well-being frequently accompany hyperglycemia. Blurred vision is a common short-term problem of acute hyperglycemia. These symptoms can be quite distressing and uncomfortable. Acute complications are directly linked to hyperglycemia and recede as euglycemia is approached.

Chronic Hyperglycemia

Chronic complications associated with diabetes are extensive and are generally placed into two categories, vascular and neuropathic. The vascular complications are further subdivided into macrovascular and microvascular components. Microvascular complications affect the capillaries, and macrovascular complications involve damage to blood vessels further up the cardiovascular tree.

Vascular Complications

Macrovascular Complications. Macrovascular complications of diabetes mellitus are defined as damage to the large blood vessels providing circulation to the brain, heart, and extremities. These complications include cardiovascular disease and stroke (7.5% to 20% of all individuals with diabetes mellitus), as well as peripheral vascular disease (as high as 45%). The presence of heart and blood vessel disease is increased twofold to fourfold in individuals with diabetes and is responsible for more than half of all deaths.[7] Ischemic cerebrovascular accidents (strokes) are more prevalent in individuals with diabetes and are associated with poorer outcomes. Cerebrovascular accidents are responsible for 11% of hospitalizations of individuals with diabetes mellitus.[3]

Diabetes is an independent risk factor for coronary artery disease. However, several important risk factors for coronary artery disease—dyslipidemia, hypertension, and impaired fibrinolysis—are present in uncontrolled diabetes and decrease with improved blood glucose control. The latter risk factor may be linked to the presence of the compensatory hyperinsulinemia of type 2 diabetes mellitus.[7]

Reduction of insulin resistance by such hygienic measures as caloric restriction and exercise and possibly by pharmacologic means may be of principal importance in reducing the incidence of macrovascular complications. Conventional measures of risk reduction, including measures to control dyslipidemia and hypertension, continue to be considered essential. Improved glycemic control is thought to affect the microvasculature rather than the macrovascular complications.

Microvascular Complications. The microvascular complications of diabetes, retinopathy and nephropathy, are thought to result from abnormal thickening of the basement membrane in muscle capillaries. Capillary basement membrane thickening has been shown to increase with the length of time after diagnosis and with persistent hyperglycemia.[8]

Hyperglycemia has been shown to disrupt platelet function and growth of the basement membrane. The presence of proteins altered by high glucose levels (advanced glycosylation end products) is also believed to play a part in the pathogenesis of microvascular complications. Thickening of capillary basement membranes has actually been shown to decrease with improved glycemic control.[9] Other risk factors for microvascular disease include hypertension and smoking.

Diabetic retinopathy affects 80% of all individuals with diabetes mellitus 15 years after diagnosis. Because of the prevalence of long-standing undiagnosed diabetes mellitus, as many as 21% of individuals with newly diagnosed type 2 diabetes are affected by retinopathy.[3]

Retinopathy is the primary cause of new cases of blindness in adults in the United States. The incidence of diabetic retinopathy appears to correlate with the duration of diabetes. Retinopathy is a progressive disease involving three stages: background retinopathy, preproliferative retinopathy, and proliferative retinopathy. Background retinopathy is characterized by microaneurysms and small hemorrhages in the retinal capillaries. Background retinopathy usually does not affect visual acuity. Preproliferative and proliferative retinopathy involves further damage to retinal capillaries, with the latter condition characterized by capillary neovascularization. The small new capillaries are particularly prone to hemorrhage. Proliferative retinopathy is managed with laser photocoagulation.

Nephropathy affects 30% of individuals with type 1 diabetes mellitus and 4% to 20% of individuals with type 2 diabetes mellitus. Diabetic nephropathy accounts for 36% of cases of end-stage renal disease. Ethnic origin is a risk factor in the development of diabetic nephropathy, with African-American and Native American diabetic individuals experiencing an increased rate of end-stage renal disease as compared with Caucasians. The characteristic lesion of diabetic nephropathy is glomerulosclerosis, or thickening and hardening of the basement membrane of capillaries in the glomeruli. Filtration, an essential component of kidney function, occurs in the glomerulus. The first stage of diabetic nephropathy is an increase in the glomerular flow rate, or the rate of blood flow through the glomerulus. This increased flow rate leads to hyperfiltration in the glomerulus, or a rise in the rate at which blood is filtered. The mechanisms leading to the increase in glomerular flow rate are unclear but are evidently related to poor glycemic control. As hyperfiltration progresses, the glomeruli become damaged. The resulting glomerulosclerosis leads to blockage and leaking of the capillaries. Protein is characteristically seen in the urine, at first in small amounts (microalbuminuria) and then grossly. As diabetic nephropathy advances, the glomerular filtration rate drops and renal failure ensues.[10] Hypertension is an important contributing factor to diabetic nephropathy. Management of hypertension with medications that inhibit angiotensin-converting enzyme has been shown to reduce the rate of renal failure, end-stage renal disease, and mortality.[10]

Neuropathic Complications. Diabetic neuropathy produces symptoms in 60% to 70% of individuals with diabetes and is responsible for 6% of hospitalizations.[3] Neuropathic complications are divided into autonomic dysfunction and sensory dysfunction. Autonomic complications include gastrointestinal disturbances, bladder dysfunction, postural hypotension, and sexual dysfunction. Approximately half of all men with diabetes who are older than 50 years experience erectile dysfunction. Sensory disturbances include carpal tunnel syndrome and paresthesias or lack of sensation in the feet. Neuropathy is largely responsible for the increased risk of serious foot problems in individuals with diabetes. The rate of lower extremity amputation in individuals with diabetes is 15 to 40 times higher than in nondiabetic individuals. Approximately half of all nontraumatic amputations in the United States are performed on individuals with diabetes.

Diabetes in humans and experimentally induced diabetes in animals are associated with decreased levels of myoinositol in peripheral nerves. Myoinositol is a cell membrane component normally found in abundance in nerve tissue. Several theoretical explanations have been proposed for the myoinositol link to neuropathy. Glucose appears to compete with myoinositol in transport into the cell. Degradation of glucose to sorbitol and fructose (the polyol pathway) occurs in the nerves in the presence of hyperglycemia and insulinopenia. Increased activity of the polyol pathway also appears to be linked to reduced myoinositol in the peripheral nerves. Focal ischemic lesions of the nerves may also have a role in diabetic neuropathy. Pathologic findings include degeneration or loss of nerve fibers resulting in decreased nerve function.[3]

Glycemic control has been shown to improve nerve function in animals and in humans and to decrease perceived pain. In addition to hyperglycemia, cigarette smoking, excessive alcohol use, male sex, and older age are risk factors for the development of neuropathy. Race also appears to be a risk factor, with higher amputation rates in African-American and Native American populations.[3]

Strong evidence linking prolonged hyperglycemia to neuropathy and the microvascular complications of diabetes was provided by the Diabetes Control and Complications Trial, a 9-year multicenter prospective study designed to examine the effect of intensive insulin therapy on the development of retinopathy. Renal and neurologic indices were also examined. Subjects in this trial were individuals with type 1 diabetes and no or mild retinopathy at baseline.[11] The experimental group was intensively treated with three or more insulin injections daily or with insulin delivered by a pump. The incidence of initial retinopathy was reduced by 76%, and progression of existing retinopathy was reduced by 54% in the experimental group. Indices of beginning nephropathy such as microalbuminuria and albuminuria were reduced in the experimental group by 39% and 54%, respectively. Symptomatic neuropathy was reduced by 60% in the experimental group. Dilemmas presented by the Diabetes Control and Complications Trial include the presence of a significant increase in severe hypoglycemia in the experimental group and some question about the validity of extrapolating all results to individuals with type 2 diabetes. As cited in the *Frontiers of Research* for this unit, a large study of the effect of lowering blood glucose in type 2 diabetes has also yielded data on decreased morbidity and mortality with improved glycemic control (United Kingdom Prospective Diabetes Study).[12]

Complications in Pregnancy. Pregnancy in women with type 1 diabetes has been complicated by an increased risk for perinatal infant mortality and congenital anomalies. Metabolic control during pregnancy reduces the risk of perinatal mortality to a rate approximating that of the general population. An increased rate of congenital malformations continues to attend pregnancies in women with type 1 diabetes. Because the affected organs develop early in the first trimester, excellent glycemic control before conception is recommended.[13]

Infants of women with gestational diabetes are at risk for macrosomia, perinatal hypoglycemia, respiratory distress, and cardiac arrhythmias. Untreated maternal hyperglycemia can result in spontaneous abortion or increased neonatal mortality.[6]

KEY CONCEPTS

- The acute complications of hyperglycemia are hyperosmolar coma, ketoacidosis, and infection. Hyperglycemia may be associated with nausea, fatigue, and blurred vision.
- The chronic complications of hyperglycemia are primarily caused by vascular and neuropathic dysfunction. People with diabetes are prone to vascular complications, including coronary artery disease, stroke, and peripheral vascular disease. These complications are related to dyslipidemia, hypertension, and impaired fibrinolysis. Retinopathy and nephropathy are thought to be due to hyperglycemia-induced thickening of retinal and glomerular basement membranes. Neuropathy is manifested as pain and loss of sensation. Excessive glucose is thought to interfere with myoinositol in neurons.

Box 41-4

American Diabetes Association Recommendations for Nutritional Therapy

Maintenance of as nearly normal blood glucose levels as possible by balancing food intake with insulin (either endogenous or exogenous) or oral glucose-lowering medications and activity levels

Achievement of optimal serum lipid levels

Provision of adequate calories for maintaining or attaining reasonable weights for adults, normal growth and development rates in children and adolescents, and increased metabolic needs during pregnancy and lactation or recovery from catabolic illnesses. Reasonable weight is defined as the weight an individual and health care provider acknowledges as achievable and maintainable in both the short and long term, which may not be the same as the traditionally defined desirable or ideal body weight

Prevention and *management* of the acute complications of insulin-managed diabetes such as hypoglycemia, short-term illnesses, and exercise-related problems and the long-term complications of diabetes such as renal disease, autonomic neuropathy, hypertension, and cardiovascular disease

Improvement of overall health through optimal nutrition

TREATMENT AND EDUCATION

The usual treatment goals in diabetes are achieving metabolic control of blood glucose levels and preventing acute and chronic complications. The American Diabetes Association recommends as goals a fasting blood glucose level less than 140 mg/dl and a postprandial blood glucose level less than 160 mg/dl in type 2 diabetes.[14] For type 1 diabetes, these goals are a fasting blood glucose level less than 120 mg/dl and a postprandial blood glucose level less than 180 mg/dl.[15] The goals of treatment are accomplished by diet, exercise, medication, and such hygiene practices as daily foot care and smoking cessation. Each treatment involves lifestyle changes that are difficult to accomplish initially and challenging to maintain. Treatment must be individualized to the type of diabetes and the individual patient.

Nutrition

Nutrition has often been called the cornerstone of diabetes therapy. Ideas about the optimal dietary prescription have been far from constant throughout recorded history. From wheat, fruit, and beer in ancient Egypt through blood pudding and rancid meats in 19th century France to more recent investigations of fiber and fat, nutritional controversies are far from over.

In a position statement the American Diabetes Association has listed five recommendations for nutritional therapy in patients with diabetes (Box 41-4).[16] Accomplishing the goals can involve changes in composition of the diet, meal patterns and timing, and caloric consumption. All the energy nutrients—carbohydrates, fats, and protein—have an essential role in optimal nutrition. Obesity and such eating disorders as bulimia have an important impact on nutritional status.

Protein

Protein is used in the repair and growth of tissues. Proteins are composed of amino acids and contain 4 calories/g. The addition of protein to a meal will stimulate the secretion of insulin and blunt the postprandial rise in blood glucose levels in diabetic patients. Growth, development, and maintenance, as well as glycemic control, are considered to occur optimally at the recommended daily allowance of 0.8 g protein per kilogram of body weight. Most Americans exceed this guideline.

Chronic high-protein intake is linked to heightened glomerular flow rates and renal hypertrophy. It is thought that continued renal hyperfunction can lead to nephropathy in diabetic patients. Restriction of dietary protein has been shown to improve renal function in patients with diabetes without adversely affecting metabolic control.[17]

Present recommendations call for not exceeding the recommended daily allowance for protein (10% to 20% of calories) except in cases of increased need, as in gestation, childhood, and adolescence.

Fat

Fats are composed of fatty acids and other substances. Fats contain 9 cal/g. Dietary fats are classified as saturated, monounsaturated, and unsaturated based on their molecular structure. Dietary saturated fat and dietary cholesterol may contribute to hypercholesterolemia. Elevated serum cholesterol levels have been identified as an important risk factor for cardiovascular disease. Hypertriglyceridemia, or an elevated level of fatty acids in the blood stream, is linked to hyperglycemia and is an independent risk factor for cardiovascular disease in diabetes.

Fat metabolism is dependent on the appropriate presence of insulin. Untreated diabetes is associated with hypertriglyceridemia, elevated levels of very low density lipoprotein, and lowered high-density lipoprotein levels. Although effective treatment reduces the incidence of dyslipidemia, the risk of cardiovascular disease may not be affected.

A lower incidence of cardiovascular lesions has been noted when serum cholesterol is lowered by drugs or by diet. The ideal diet for control of serum lipids continues to be a source of controversy. A diet high in carbohydrates and low in all sources of fat has been shown to reduce total and low-density lipoprotein cholesterol but contribute to hypertriglyceridemia, reduced high-density lipoprotein cholesterol, and a deterioration in glycemic control.[18] A diet high in monounsaturated fat has been shown to lower serum triglycerides and very low density lipoprotein cholesterol, raise high-density lipoprotein cholesterol, and promote euglycemia in patients with diabetes.[18]

Current recommendations include a diet composed of not more than 10% of calories as saturated fat and not more than 10% of calories as polyunsaturated fat; 60% to 70% of calories would then be distributed between monounsaturated fats and carbohydrates. It is recommended that not more than 300 mg of cholesterol be consumed daily.

Carbohydrates

Carbohydrates are categorized as monosaccharides (simple sugars) and polysaccharides (complex carbohydrates or starches). Carbohydrates contain 4 cal/g. For many years the American Diabetes Association recommended restriction of carbohydrate, especially sucrose. The atherogenic potential of the resulting high-fat diet became a cause of concern.

Current recommendations are for an individualized diet with 60% to 70% of calories distributed between monounsaturated fats and carbohydrate. Lower fat diets would be appropriate for individuals attempting to lose weight. Sucrose-containing foods can be included in moderation and should be substituted for other carbohydrate-containing foods. The use of artificial sweeteners is condoned at levels lower than the acceptable daily intake established by the FDA.

Alcohol

Alcohol contains 7 cal/g. Moderate alcohol intake does not appear to have a deleterious effect on glycemic control. Alcohol intake increases the risk of sulfonylurea- or insulin-induced hypoglycemia because of the ability of alcohol to suppress gluconeogenesis. For this reason, alcohol intake should always be accompanied by food intake. Alcohol should not replace food intake in individuals with type 1 diabetes. In those with type 2 diabetes, where weight reduction is desirable, alcohol calories can be exchanged for fat calories. It is recommended that alcohol be avoided in the presence of poor glycemic control, pancreatic or liver disease, triglyceridemia, neuropathy, pregnancy, and alcoholism.[19]

Obesity and Eating Disorders

Obesity is the strongest risk factor for type 2 diabetes, in addition to being a risk factor for cardiovascular disease in women. Obesity is defined as a **body mass index** (weight in kilograms divided by the square of the height in meters) of 25 or greater.[20] Increased risk for health problems occurs at a body mass index of greater than 25.[21] A body mass index of 20 to 24 is considered ideal. Weight management is a chronic and difficult problem for many individuals. No single strategy has been shown to be effective for all individuals. Current recommendations for management of obesity include the use of a nutritionally complete diet, a program of maintenance, and exercise. Consult Chapter 42 for additional nutritional risk factors related to obesity.

Eating disorders such as bulimia and anorexia may be more common in women with type 1 diabetes. Inducing weight loss by reducing insulin has also been noted. In order for clinicians to be aware of eating disorders in their patients, careful patient assessment is necessary.

Exercise

Exercise, one of the oldest treatments for diabetes, was prescribed in India in 500 BC. Exercise can have a role in both type 1 and type 2 diabetes in terms of lowering blood glucose levels and promoting health maintenance. Exercise lowers such cardiovascular risk factors as high blood pressure and dyslipidemia, increases work capacity, reduces stress, prevents bone loss, and improves reaction time. Exercise may also be beneficial in weight reduction.

The effects of exercise on fuel utilization and insulin sensitivity are comparable to exercise-induced changes in normal metabolism. As glucose production increases and plasma insulin levels drop, the reduction in tissue insulin resistance can result in a net fall in blood glucose. Exercise has the potential to decrease insulin requirements in type 1 diabetes, decrease and possibly eliminate the need for pharmacologic agents in type 2 diabetes, and reduce the risk for heart disease in all persons with diabetes. It has been shown to actually prevent the onset of type 2 diabetes in persons who are genetically at risk.[22]

Although the benefits of exercise are numerous, there are associated risks. Individuals with type 1 diabetes are at risk for hypoglycemia and ketoacidosis. Exercise in individuals with type 2 diabetes can be associated with hypoglycemia, cardiac dysfunction, orthopedic injury, and worsening of some complications.

When insulin or an oral hypoglycemic agent is used in the management of diabetes, the usual fuel metabolism of exercise is disturbed. Inappropriately high insulin levels result in decreased hepatic glucose production and increased tissue insulin sensitivity. The latter processes can lead to hypoglycemia. Replacement of expended glycogen and continued insulin sensitivity can result in hypoglycemia as long as 24 hours after activity.

When insulin levels are inappropriately low, hepatic glucose production is increased and tissue insulin sensitivity is decreased. The production of free fatty acids increases, probably because of the influence of exercise-stimulated production of catecholamines. Hyperglycemia and ketosis may be a result of exercise under insulinopenic conditions. Safeguards must be built into exercise programs to prevent hypoglycemia, ketoacidosis, injury, cardiac compromise, and exacerbation of diabetic complications.

The exercise prescription is as essential in diabetes management as the medication or nutrition prescription. To achieve maximal metabolic and cardiovascular benefit, exercise must be performed for 20 to 45 minutes at least 3 days a week and must incorporate aerobic activity at 50% to 70% $\dot{V}O_{2max}$ (maximal aerobic capacity), which approximates 65% to 80% of the maximal heart rate. The maximal heart rate is often estimated as 220 minus age (in years). However, even rather small increases in activity have been associated with improved metabolic profile. Patients with autonomic neuropathy should be taught a method of judging exercise intensity by perceived exertion.[23] The Centers for Disease Control and Prevention recommend an exercise program of moderate intensity for 30 minutes, continuously or intermittently, preferably daily for all individuals.[24]

Before an exercise program is begun, a physical examination should rule out the presence of such limiting diabetic complications as retinopathy and neuropathic foot ulcers or malformations. Screening for cardiovascular problems should include exercise-stress electrocardiography in diabetic patients older than 35 years. To avoid orthopedic injury, the exercise session should be preceded by a warm-up period involving mild activity or stretching. Exercise should be initiated at a low intensity and duration and gradually increased. Patients must be counseled to wear appropriate clothing and footwear and to carefully inspect their feet after the exercise session.

Individuals with type 1 diabetes are encouraged to eat additional carbohydrates or to reduce the dose of injected insulin when exercise is anticipated. A consistent exercise program can facilitate such adjustments. Additional food is not often necessary in type 2 diabetes; however, patients should be encouraged to have rapidly acting carbohydrate available should it become needed. Exercise should be avoided if the blood glucose level is less than 100 mg/dl or greater than 250 mg/dl when ketosis is present. The presence of ketosis in individuals with type 1 diabetes can indicate an acute shortage of insulin. Exercise under the latter conditions can actually lead to increased hyperglycemia. Exercise when blood glucose values are greater than 250 mg/dl is safe if ketosis is not present.

Pharmacologic Agents

Oral Antidiabetic Agents

When diet and exercise have been ineffective in controlling hyperglycemia in individuals with type 2 diabetes, an oral agent is usually the next treatment chosen. Sulfonylurea drugs have been used in the management of type 2 diabetes for more than 40 years. These drugs have been joined by other agents with different mechanisms of action.

Sulfonylureas exert their hypoglycemic effect by inducing insulin release by β cells, augmenting the action of insulin in glucose disposal, diminishing insulin clearance by the liver, and reducing hepatic glucose production. Because sulfonylureas are ineffective in the management of type 1 diabetes, stimulation of β cells is a crucial factor in the action of these oral agents. Enhanced insulin secretion appears to be a short-term effect, possibly caused by a reduction in insulin requirements as a result of the other hypoglycemic activities of sulfonylurea agents.

The so-called first-generation agents (those formulated earliest) are tolbutamide, chlorpropamide, acetohexamide, and tolazamide. Second-generation agents include glyburide, glipizide, and glimepiride. Differences exist between the sulfonylureas in duration of action and excretion[25,26] (Table 41-3). Second-generation agents are more potent than first-

Table 41-3

Oral Antidiabetic Agents

Oral Antidiabetic Agent	Onset (hr)	Duration (hr)	Comment
Tolbutamide	0.3	8-12	Useful in renal disease
Chlorpropamide	1	24-70	Antidiuretic action
Acetohexamide	1	12-24	Uricosuric agent Contraindicated in renal disease
Tolazamide	3-4	14	Useful in renal disease
Glyburide	1	24	No disulfiram effect
Glipizide	1	Up to 24	No disulfiram effect
Glimepiride	1	24	Extrapancreatic action
Metformin	1-2	24	Diarrhea, slight risk of lactic acidosis
Acarbose	1	14-24	Decreases intestinal absorption of carbohydrate
Troglitazone	2-3	16-34	Increased absorption when taken with a meal

generation agents, possibly because of increased capacity to bind to the plasma membrane of the β cell. Glyburide appears to characteristically increase basal secretion of insulin and glipizide to heighten postprandial insulin production. Glimepiride appears to selectively exert extrapancreatic hypoglycemic effects. However, no second-generation agent has been shown to be effective after a first-generation agent has failed.

The side effects of sulfonylureas include hypoglycemia, nausea, dizziness, headache, allergic reactions, flushing with alcohol use (disulfiram effect), and other rarer blood disorders. Sulfonylureas that are metabolized to inactive compounds by the liver are considered safer for use in renal disease. Duration of action is another safety issue. Sulfonylureas are the major cause of severe hypoglycemia caused by a drug. The longer acting sulfonylureas chlorpropamide and glyburide are responsible for the majority of cases of severe hypoglycemia and fatal hypoglycemic coma.

Metformin, classified as a biguanide, suppresses hepatic gluconeogenesis and enhances glucose uptake by peripheral tissues without causing hypoglycemia. Metformin has been used alone and in combination with a sulfonylurea drug. Metformin is associated with improvement in dyslipidemia and weight loss. Side effects include nausea and diarrhea. A rare side effect, lactic acidosis, is one-tenth as likely to occur with metformin as with the related phenformin.[27] Because of the possibility of lactic acidosis, metformin is contraindicated in individuals with liver or renal disease. Metformin should be withheld for 24 hours before surgery or radiologic studies involving dyes.

Acarbose, an α-glucosidase inhibitor, diminishes postprandial hyperglycemia by delaying carbohydrate absorption. It can be used alone and in combination with sulfonylurea drugs. Side effects include symptoms related to decreased gastrointestinal absorption (e.g., flatulence and diarrhea). It does not cause hypoglycemia but can complicate management of hypoglycemia if used in combination with a sulfonylurea. Sulfonylurea-induced hypoglycemia cannot be managed with sucrose when acarbose is being used because of drug-induced delayed sucrose absorption.

Rosiglitazone and piaglitazone, two thiazolidinedione drugs, increase tissue sensitivity to insulin and inhibit hepatic gluconeogenesis. Thiazolidinediones are thought to lower blood pressure, insulin levels, and triglycerides, as well as blood glucose levels.[28] Thiazolidinediones were initially approved for use only in individuals with type 2 diabetes mellitus who require the use of insulin. Because thiazolidinediones do not increase pancreatic production of insulin, they cannot by themselves cause hypoglycemia. However, the improvement in insulin sensitivity can result in hypoglycemia in individuals treated with another hypoglycemic drug. Troglitazone, the first marketed thiazolidinedione, caused hepatic failure and was withdrawn from use. Evidence of rare liver damage with thiazolidinediones has led to the recommendation that liver enzymes be checked regularly.

After an initial trial of diet and exercise, any of the oral antidiabetic agents may be chosen as an initial pharmacologic agent for type 2 diabetes. If euglycemia does not occur, an additional oral agent may be prescribed. If the resulting combination therapy is ineffective, insulin therapy is initiated.

When prescribed along with an appropriate meal plan, oral antidiabetic agents can be very effective in the management of type 2 diabetes mellitus. Primary failure of the drug is considered to have occurred when initiation of oral agent therapy does not result in a significant decline in blood glucose levels. Primary failure can be due to misdiagnosis of type 1 diabetes mellitus or inadequate adherence to the diet and exercise regimen. Secondary failure, or hyperglycemia after an effective initial response to the drug, is often due to dietary nonadherence but may also be due to the progressive β-cell dysfunction of type 2 diabetes mellitus.

Insulin

Insulin therapy is required in 100% of persons with type 1 diabetes mellitus and 35% with type 2 diabetes mellitus. Persons with type 1 diabetes mellitus require replacement of the deficient hormone in as physiologic a manner as possible. The role of insulin in type 2 diabetes mellitus is more complex.

Because type 2 diabetes mellitus is a progressive disease, many if not most individuals will need insulin at some time, either because of increasing insulin resistance or because of β-cell dysfunction. Glucose toxicity, a phenomenon in which insulin resistance and decreased production of insulin are worsened by hyperglycemia, may respond to insulin therapy. Insulin may be necessary in type 2 diabetes intermittently during times of physiologic stress that increase insulin requirements (e.g., intercurrent illness, surgery, inactivity, weight gain). However, with resolution of the stress, the individual may be able to discontinue insulin use.

Bioengineered human insulin is the only insulin available for use in the United States. Human insulin contains fewer noninsulin proteins than does the previously available beef or pork insulin.[29]

Table 41-4

Action of Insulin

Type of Insulin	Onset (hr)	Peak (hr)	Duration (hr)
Rapid Acting			
Aspart	0.16-0.33	1-3	3-5
Lispro	0-0.25	0.5-1.5	5
Regular	0.3-0.7	2-4	5-8
Semilente	0-1.0	2-8	12-16
Intermediate Acting			
NPH	1-2	6-12	11-16
Long Acting			
Glargine	5	None	≥24
Ultralente	4-6	14-20	24-36

Types of insulin are classified into three groups according to their duration of action: rapid acting, intermediate acting, and long acting (Table 41-4). The most commonly used insulins in the rapid-acting category are regular and semilente; in the intermediate category, NPH and lente; and in the long-acting category, ultralente and Lantus. Lispro and aspart insulins, both insulin analogs, are very rapidly acting insulins that are used within 15 minutes of eating.

Patterns of insulin use vary with the type of diabetes and the degree of desired metabolic control (Figure 41-6). For patients with type 1 diabetes mellitus, a minimum of two or more daily injections of a mixture of rapid- and intermediate-acting insulins has been used to control postprandial and fasting hyperglycemia. If hypoglycemia occurs during the night, the intermediate-acting insulin can be shifted to bedtime to produce a more intensive schedule. Ultralente insulin can be substituted for NPH before breakfast and the evening meal to produce longer insulin action. NPH and regular insulin may be mixed in the same syringe and given as one injection. Insulin mixtures are stable if given within 15 minutes of preparation. Another popular regimen includes use of long-acting Lantus with preprandial injections of aspart or lispro insulin.

Intensive insulin schedules are an attempt to mimic normal insulin secretion closely and are considered important for optimal control. One such schedule calls for the use of regular or lispro insulin before meals and intermediate- or long-acting insulin at bedtime. Other schedules use longer acting insulin twice daily: at breakfast and before supper or at

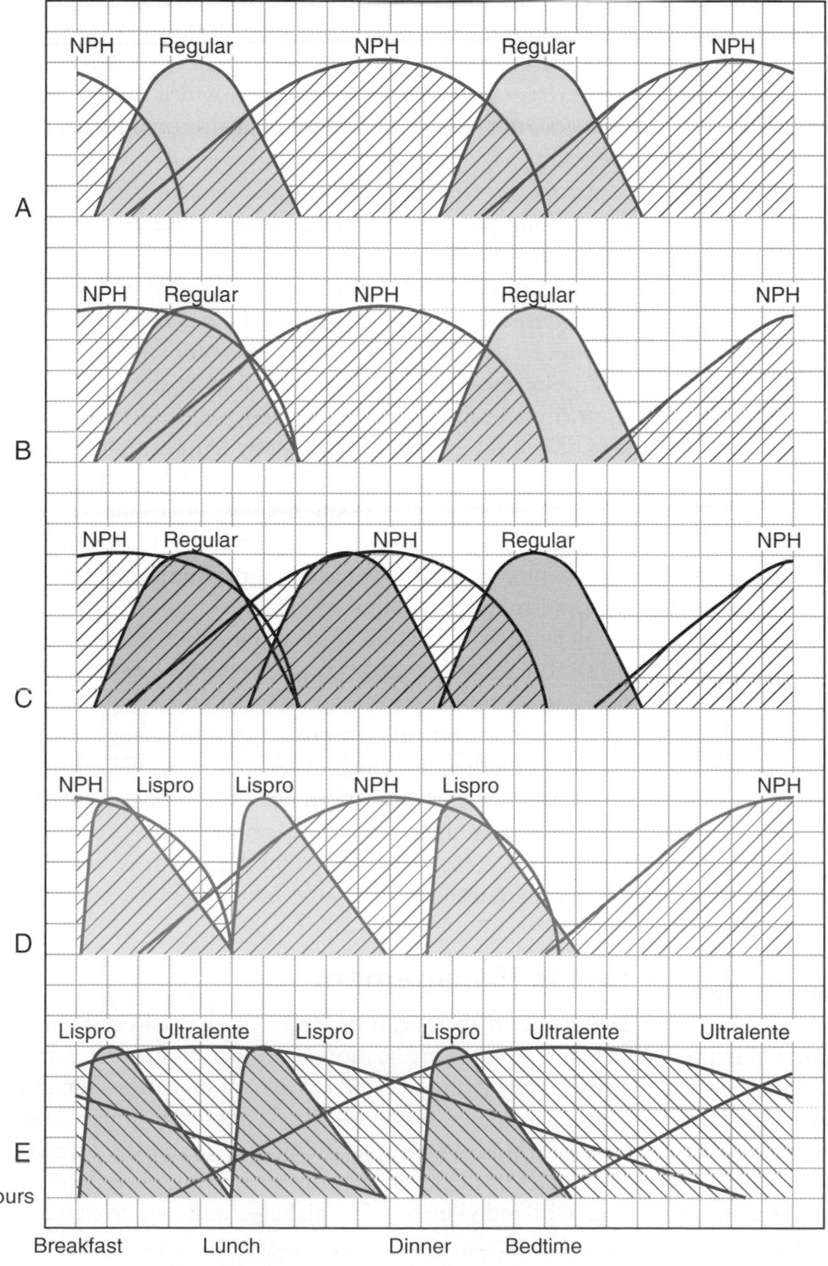

FIGURE 41-6 ■ Typical patterns of insulin use. **A,** A mixture of regular (rapid-acting) and NPH (intermediate-acting) insulin taken twice daily. **B,** A mixture of regular and NPH insulin taken before breakfast, regular taken before dinner, and NPH taken at bedtime. **C,** NPH insulin taken twice daily, regular taken before each meal. **D,** NPH insulin taken before breakfast and dinner, lispro taken before each meal. **E,** Ultralente taken before breakfast and dinner, lispro taken before each meal. (Designed by Lisa Siegel.)

breakfast and bedtime. In the latter schedule, the long- or intermediate-acting insulin stands in for basal insulin secretion. Insulin doses can be adjusted by the use of an algorithm based on capillary blood glucose monitoring or by an estimate of the carbohydrate content of the next meal.

Continuous subcutaneous insulin infusion (CSII) by means of an insulin pump has been used to approximate nondiabetic insulin secretion in situations in which intensive insulin therapy has not been effective. CSII technology supplies a constant infusion of regular or lispro insulin and delivers a premeal bolus dose programmed by the user. Improvement in glycemic control has been noted with CSII. Complications associated with CSII therapy (infected infusion sites, ketoacidosis, and hypoglycemic coma) have resulted in a 34.5% rate of discontinuation of pump use.[30]

Other insulin delivery devices include jet injectors and insulin pens. Jet injectors, mechanisms that deliver a spray of insulin under the skin, increase the rate of insulin absorption. Insulin pens include the insulin, measuring device, and needle in one pen-sized instrument. Delivery of inhaled insulin is under study.

Pancreas transplantation has been performed in individuals with diabetes since 1966 and has shown consistent improvement in patient outcomes. Pancreas transplantation restores normal metabolism but must be accompanied by lifelong treatment with immunosuppressive agents.

In the management of type 2 diabetes, insulin is prescribed when a management plan that includes an oral antidiabetic agent no longer produces acceptable glycemic control. Two injections of rapid- and intermediate-acting insulins can be used. Nocturnal doses of NPH or Lantus may be added to oral hypoglycemic medications. Premixed preparations of NPH and regular insulin facilitate the use of mixed doses, especially in the elderly. A mixture containing 70% NPH insulin and 30% regular insulin (70:30 insulin) is widely used in the United States, and 50:50 insulin (50% NPH and regular) has been introduced. Certain individuals with type 2 diabetes benefit from more intensive therapy. A select group of individuals may benefit from a bedtime dose of intermediate-acting insulin added to daytime sulfonylurea therapy. The use of an oral sulfonylurea in addition to insulin may improve metabolic control.[26,31]

The action of insulin is affected by many elements, including climate, alteration in blood flow, tobacco use, and the injection site. Insulin is absorbed most rapidly from the abdomen, less rapidly from the arm, and most slowly from the leg. Insulin is absorbed more rapidly from areas that are exercised or massaged after injection.

Hypoglycemia is the most common complication of hypoglycemic therapy and the most hazardous. The incidence of hypoglycemia has been estimated at 20% in individuals treated with sulfonylureas, 35% in individuals with type 2 diabetes treated with insulin, and 100% in individuals with type 1 diabetes mellitus. Severe hypoglycemia occurs in as many as 44% of insulin-treated individuals. Hypoglycemia may cause or be a factor in 2% to 13% of deaths in individuals with type 1 diabetes mellitus.[32]

Neural tissue depends on a constant supply of glucose for normal function. When insufficient food intake, unplanned activity, or an inappropriate insulin or sulfonylurea dose lowers the blood glucose concentration excessively, counterregulatory mechanisms are activated to ensure a continued supply of glucose to the brain. The production of glucagon, catecholamines, corticosteroids, and growth hormone is increased. The latter hormones increase glucose production by mechanisms outlined earlier in this chapter.

Symptoms of hypoglycemia produced by counterregulatory mechanisms include pallor, tremor, diaphoresis, palpitation, and anxiety. Neuroglycopenic symptoms noted in hypoglycemia are hunger, visual disturbance, weakness, paresthesias, confusion, agitation, coma, and death. In long-standing diabetes, neuropathy can alter the counterregulatory mechanisms. Hypoglycemic unawareness, in which the diabetic patient does not experience counterregulatory symptoms, can be the result.

Alcohol interferes with counterregulatory processes by suppressing gluconeogenesis. Alcohol intake has resulted in fatal hypoglycemic coma even in the absence of other hypoglycemic drugs. The combination of alcohol and insulin or sulfonylurea drugs can be particularly dangerous.

Another typical complication of insulin therapy is lipodystrophy. Lipoatrophy has been linked to the use of insulin from animal sources and is manifested as hollows in the surface of the skin caused by the destruction of subcutaneous adipose tissue. Lipohypertrophy is characterized by an increase in subcutaneous tissue because of insulin-stimulated growth of adipose tissue at the injection sites. Avoiding repeated injections at the same site is recommended to prevent lipodystrophy.

An acute complication of insulin use can be insulin edema, or a localized or generalized accumulation of fluid. Weight gain can accompany initiation of insulin therapy, especially when glycemic control is improved. A third complicating factor in insulin therapy is insulin resistance. Insulin resistance is exacerbated by obesity and can necessitate the use of large insulin doses. An appropriate diet and exercise program is as important to insulin-treated individuals as it is to other patients with diabetes.

Stress Management

Living with diabetes can be stressful. The tasks of blood glucose monitoring, medication administration, meal planning, and preventive care to avoid complications can be demanding. Fearing the onset of complications and their impact in addition to living with complications are parts of the psychological impact of diabetes. Depression is more likely to be diagnosed in individuals with diabetes and is correlated with deterioration of glycemic control.[33] Stress management can have an important role in diabetes care by improving quality of life and reducing the possible impact of stress on glycemic control.

Assessment of Efficacy

Several measures are used by clinicians to determine the adequacy of glycemic control. One indirect but very useful indication of blood glucose levels is the level of **glycosylated hemoglobin.** Hemoglobin becomes glycosylated when glucose is nonenzymatically attached to one of its terminal amino acids. Four glycosylated hemoglobin products are formed: HbA_{1a1}, HbA_{1a2}, HbA_{1b}, and HbA_{1c}. The latter is produced in the largest quantity and is used in most assays.

Because erythrocytes are freely permeable to glucose, the quantities of glycosylated hemoglobin formed are proportional to the quantity of glucose in the blood plasma. Glycosylated hemoglobin values will reflect mean blood glucose levels for the life of the average erythrocyte (100 to 120 days). Highly significant correlations have been found between HbA_{1c} levels and mean blood glucose.[34] The presence of abnormal hemoglobins or hemolytic anemia can skew results. The normal value for Hb A_{1c} varies with the laboratory technique but is usually less than 7%.

HbA_{1c} values are used clinically to estimate long-term control and to set and evaluate therapeutic goals. Values of less than 7% are considered desirable. An HbA_{1c} value of greater than 8% indicates a need for change in the therapeutic regimen. However, HbA_{1c} values cannot be used for day-to-day management of therapy.

Assessment of glycemia on a daily basis was attempted in the past by the use of testing for glycosuria. However, the blood glucose level at which glucose is measurable in the urine, the glycemic threshold, varies from individual to individual, is usually unacceptably high, and cannot be used to establish the presence of hypoglycemia.

Venous blood can be drawn in a clinic or office and analyzed for glucose content. Office laboratory evaluation is inconvenient and expensive. The advent of capillary blood glucose monitoring in the late 1970s provided a solution to the problem of short-term evaluation of glycemic control. Individuals with diabetes and health professionals can use a drop of capillary blood applied to a glucose oxidase reagent strip to measure the blood glucose level. The treated strips are generally read in 1 or 2 minutes. Test strips are read visually or by a meter. Some test strips can be read both ways.

The First and Second Consensus Development Conference on Self-Monitoring of Blood Glucose, convened by the American Diabetes Association and other involved agencies, formulated several goals for the use of capillary blood glucose monitoring. The goals included use of capillary blood glucose monitoring to achieve and maintain a specific level of glycemic control, prevent and manage hypoglycemia, avoid severe hypoglycemia, adjust care in response to changes in lifestyle in individuals requiring pharmacologic therapy, and determine the need for initiating insulin therapy in women with gestational diabetes mellitus.[35]

Capillary blood glucose monitoring has been shown to be an accurate reflection of venous blood glucose when performed by health professionals and by individuals with diabetes. However, unacceptable variation has been found in some studies. Hematocrit, altitude, temperature, humidity, hypotension, hypoxia, and hypertriglyceridemia can affect results. Accuracy can be affected by such performance errors as underloading or overloading the strip, incorrect placement of the sample, and improper sample handling. Training improves performance.

Diabetic individuals using capillary blood glucose monitoring have frequently reported enthusiasm and increased insight into the relationship between blood glucose and such factors as diet, exercise, and stress or have reported increased feelings of well-being. Capillary blood glucose monitoring has been associated with improved glycemic control. Monitoring of capillary blood glucose levels is simply a biofeedback technique that can provide immediate information on the effects of a change in therapy.

Hazards are associated with the use of capillary blood glucose monitoring. Institutional use of capillary blood glucose monitoring involves potential handling of blood, with the concomitant risk of transmission of such blood-borne diseases as hepatitis B and human immunodeficiency virus infection. The American Association of Diabetes Educators has published guidelines for the safe use of capillary blood glucose monitoring in institutional[36] and home[37] settings. Patient use of capillary blood glucose monitoring has also been associated with such hazards as hand infection and improper disposal of used medical waste. Hand washing and use of a fresh lancet for every test have been recommended to prevent finger infection. Proper disposal of lancets and insulin syringes to avoid injury to household members and waste disposal personnel is essential and mandated by law in many municipalities.

In the replacement of testing for glycosuria with capillary blood glucose monitoring, testing for ketonuria should not be neglected. The presence of ketones in the urine can be an indication of diabetic ketoacidosis and may be harmful to a developing fetus in diabetes complicated by pregnancy. All individuals with diabetes should be tested for ketonuria when blood glucose values are greater than 300 mg/dl, during intercurrent illness, during pregnancy, and in the presence of symptoms of diabetic ketoacidosis (nausea, vomiting, abdominal pain).[38]

Education

Individuals with diabetes must meet physical and financial challenges and uncertainty about the future. They must also learn a variety of skills, some relatively easy to master, others more demanding. Persons with diabetes must learn to perform biological tests and interpret results correctly, measure and administer medication (often injectable medication), manage the side effects of medications, plan meals, design an exercise program, perform foot inspection and care, and accomplish other difficult tasks. Many of these tasks would require a license if performed on another person.

Few other chronic diseases make so many demands on patients. For this reason, diabetes education is considered an essential component of diabetes treatment. Participation in a diabetes education program has been shown to increase patient knowledge about diabetes and improve performance of self-care procedures and psychological outlook. Benefit has been shown in such biochemical indices as blood glucose, HbA_{1c}, and serum lipids. Hospitalization rates have been decreased by 19% to 87%, and the rate of diabetic ketoacidosis decreased by 86% after educational intervention. A reduction in the incidence of foot lesions, amputation, and congenital malformations has been demonstrated and has led to health care cost savings. The efficacy of education programs is increased when behavior change approaches are emphasized.[39]

Many individuals with diabetes lack essential skills for performing diabetes self-care. More than half of all individuals with diabetes have never attended a diabetes education program.[38] It is the position of the American Diabetes Association that diabetes education is a critical constituent of diabetes care and should be a benefit included in third-party reimbursement.[40]

Individuals with diabetes are a diverse group with wide variations in age, ethnic background, disease duration, education, and intellectual abilities. For this reason, diabetes education must be tailored to the individual's needs. Individuals with newly diagnosed diabetes will need education in such survival skills as medication administration and the management of hypoglycemia. More comprehensive education is best provided after the initial disturbance of the diagnosis has receded. Individuals with low literacy skills will benefit from educational materials designed for their special needs. The education of elderly individuals must take sensory deficits into consideration. The short attention spans of children necessitate special guidelines for educating the young.

To ensure quality in diabetes education programs, national standards have been established by the American Diabetes Association. The standards define key content areas and provide guidelines for assessment, setting of objectives, follow-up, and other areas (Box 41-5). Diabetes education programs that can demonstrate adherence to the national standards are officially recognized by the American Diabetes Association.

Box 41-5

Content Areas Stipulated by National Standards for Diabetes Patient Education

- Diabetes overview
- Stress and psychosocial adjustment
- Family involvement and social support
- Nutrition
- Exercise and activity
- Medications
- Monitoring and use of results
- Relationships among nutrition, exercise, medication, and blood glucose levels
- Prevention, detection, and management of acute complications
- Prevention, detection, and management of chronic complications
- Foot, skin, and dental care
- Behavior change strategies, goal setting, risk factor reduction, and problem solving
- Benefits, risks, and management options for improving glucose control
- Preconception care, pregnancy, and gestational diabetes
- Use of health care systems and community resources

KEY CONCEPTS

- The mainstays of diabetic treatment are diet, exercise, and drug therapy. Education is an integral part of treatment, enabling individuals with diabetes to follow the diabetic regimen and avoid complications. The efficacy of therapy can be assessed by monitoring blood glucose and HbA_{1c} levels. Blood glucose monitoring is useful for assessing short-term efficacy. HbA_{1c} is a better measure of the long-term efficacy of therapy. A mean blood glucose level less than 155 mg/dl (HbA_{1c} level of 7% or less) is desirable.
- The recommended diabetic diet includes 10% to 20% of calories from protein sources, 60% to 70% of calories distributed between carbohydrate and monounsaturated fat, and fewer than 10% of calories as saturated and polyunsaturated fat. High-protein intake may hasten the development of nephropathy. For individuals with type 2 diabetes, a diet geared toward weight loss may be beneficial. Even modest weight loss usually improves glycemic control.
- Exercise has several benefits for an individual with diabetes. Insulin requirements may be reduced, weight loss facilitated, and the risk of cardiovascular complications decreased. Exercise may precipitate hypoglycemia, so insulin injections or dietary intake may have to be adjusted. Oral antidiabetic agents may be successfully used in type 2 diabetes. The sulfonylureas exert their effects primarily by stimulating the release of endogenous insulin. They also reduce insulin degradation and suppress the release of glucose from the liver. Metformin suppresses hepatic gluconeogenesis and enhances glucose uptake by peripheral tissue; thiazolidinediones enhance glucose uptake by peripheral tissue; and acarbose delays absorption of ingested carbohydrate.
- Insulin replacement therapy is required in patients with type 1 and in about one-third of patients with

type 2 diabetes mellitus. Insulin is classified according to its onset, peak, and duration of action. A combination of insulins may be given to produce optimal control. Regular and NPH insulin are commonly used. Regular insulin is rapid acting. NPH is intermediate acting and may be given in combination with regular insulin.

◆ Hypoglycemia is the most common complication of pharmacologic therapy. Symptoms are mediated primarily by activation of the sympathetic nervous system stress response. Secretion of catecholamines, glucagon, corticosteroids, and growth hormone rises in an attempt to increase blood glucose levels. Pallor, tremor, diaphoresis, weakness, and decreased consciousness are the usual manifestations of hypoglycemia.

PEDIATRIC CONSIDERATIONS

Diabetes has been diagnosed in approximately 127,000 children and adolescents younger than 20 years. Eighteen new cases per population of 100,000 are diagnosed yearly. The overwhelming majority have type 1 diabetes, with an approximately 5% prevalence of genetic defects in the β cell.

Type 1 diabetes is characterized by destruction of the β cells of the pancreas with resulting insulinopenia. Type 1 diabetes in children is often manifested acutely as diabetic ketoacidosis when insulin secretion falls below insulin needs. A condition termed the "honeymoon period" can occur if the diagnosis occurs during a time of increased insulin needs, such as during a viral illness. When the illness is resolved, insulin needs can fall below residual insulin production and normoglycemia results without the use of exogenous insulin. The honeymoon period rarely lasts more than 1 year and is usually shorter.

Goals of Therapy

Goals of therapy for children include achieving normal growth and development, avoiding acute and chronic complications of diabetes, addressing psychosocial issues, and educating children regarding self-care.

Acute Complications

Whenever children with type 1 diabetes mellitus experience hyperglycemia, the resulting glycosuria can precipitate dehydration. The threat of dehydration is especially severe during episodes of diabetic ketoacidosis. Supplemental fluids and insulin may be necessary during these times.

Diabetic ketoacidosis can occur when insulin administration is inadequate for needs. Diabetic ketoacidosis frequently accompanies the diagnosis of type 1 diabetes mellitus. Avoiding diabetic ketoacidosis involves knowledge of appropriate care during times of increased insulin need, such as during intercurrent illness. To ensure early detection of incipient diabetic ketoacidosis, children and adolescents should be tested for ketonuria when the blood glucose concentration is greater than 240 mg/dl and during intercurrent illness.

Hypoglycemia can be difficult to detect in very young children. Caregivers should be alert for behavioral changes such as lethargy, pallor, and sleep disturbances.

Chronic Complications

Chronic complications of diabetes are rarely manifested during adolescence. Screening for neuropathy and nephropathy and determinations of serum lipid levels should occur on a regular basis. Adolescent girls must be counseled on the importance of excellent metabolic control before initiation of pregnancy.

Treatment

Insulin requirements are usually 0.7 to 1.0 U/kg per day. An intensive regimen of at least three injections per day is recommended to prevent chronic complications. The administration of very small doses of insulin in infants and children may necessitate the use of a diluent.

Insulin needs increase during times of physiologic stress, such as during intercurrent illness or puberty. Children who are inadequately treated with insulin will not grow or mature normally.

Children are usually able to begin administering insulin and performing capillary blood glucose monitoring with supervision when they are of school age. The age may vary with different children. When administering insulin, the abdomen is the least preferred site because of insufficient abdominal subcutaneous fat.

Diabetic teaching of such self-management skills as insulin injection, capillary blood glucose monitoring, and recognition and treatment of hypoglycemia should include all caregivers. Baby sitters and teachers will need information on prevention, recognition, and management of hypoglycemia. All educational materials used with children should be age appropriate.

Children must be provided with a caloric intake adequate to meet needs for energy expenditure, growth, and maturation. Calorie intake is usually calculated as 1000 cal/day plus 100 added calories for each year until age 11 years. From age 11 to age 18 years, an additional 100 calories is added for girls and an additional 200 calories for boys. Growth should be plotted at each medical appointment to assess adequate nutrition and adequate insulinization. After the age of 2 years, recommended dietary guidelines for percentage of fat, carbohydrate, and protein are the same as for adults.

Exercise is encouraged, with careful attention to adequate nutritional intake. Insulin doses may have to be adjusted to plan for unusual levels of activity, such as during long-distance bike riding or hiking.

Following a regimen designed to prevent acute and chronic complications of diabetes is difficult under the best of conditions. The goals of treatment are best accomplished when meals, medication, exercise, and blood glucose monitoring are consistent. Achieving consistency while also achieving developmental goals of separation and independence is very difficult. Peer pressure during adolescence can lead to poor adherence to therapeutic regimens. Concern regarding weight can lead to omission of insulin injections or other forms of eating disorders.

The child and family need support and counseling to develop effective strategies for achieving desired goals. Disturbed family functioning can have an impact on children and adolescents with diabetes and can lead to an increased frequency of hospitalization for diabetic ketoacidosis.

Genetic defects of the β cell are usually diagnosed in individuals younger than 25 years. These individuals are not likely to become ketotic. Management is identical to that of type 2 diabetes in young adults.

KEY CONCEPTS

- Children and adolescents with diabetes overwhelmingly have type 1 diabetes mellitus (5% have genetic defects of the β cell). In type 1 diabetes, insulin is required at diagnosis or shortly after.
- Goals of therapy for children include achieving normal growth and development, avoiding acute and chronic complications of diabetes, addressing psychosocial issues, and educating children regarding self-care.
- Acute complications of diabetes in children and adolescents include hyperglycemia leading to dehydration, possible diabetic ketoacidosis, and hypoglycemia. Hypoglycemia may manifest differently in children than in adults.
- Chronic complications in children and adolescents are rare. Screening for complications should nevertheless be initiated. Adolescent girls should be counseled on issues regarding diabetes and pregnancy.
- Insulin needs will vary according to growth stages, exercise, and intercurrent illness. Regular capillary blood glucose monitoring is crucial for determining the efficacy of treatment. The age at which children will perform insulin measurement and administration and capillary blood glucose monitoring independently will vary. Nutritional needs are calculated at 1000 cal/day, with 100 added calories per year until age 11 and an additional 100 calories for girls and an additional 200 calories for boys until age 18.
- Education in self-care activities should be appropriate for age and include other family members. Support for the person with diabetes and the family is important. Counseling may be helpful in some circumstances.

GERIATRIC CONSIDERATIONS

The prevalence of type 2 diabetes mellitus increases with age. Adults older than 65 years constitute 41% of the diabetic population of the United States. The prevalence of diabetes in the elderly is 18.4% for individuals age 65 or older and more than double that of younger adults age 45 to 64.

The increase in risk for type 2 diabetes in older adults is multifactorial. Aging often involves increased adiposity and a decrease in lean body mass and activity levels. The latter factors contribute to insulin resistance. Insulin secretion also diminishes with age. The risk of diabetes in the elderly is likewise increased by surgery, illness, and the use of such medications as steroids and diuretics.

Diabetes in the elderly can be difficult to diagnose because of fluctuating blood glucose values in response to food intake and activity and because of inconsistent or absent symptoms of hyperglycemia. Chronic complications of diabetes such as neuropathy and retinopathy are frequently present at diagnosis and indicate glucose intolerance of long duration.

Goals of Therapy

Goals of treatment for the elderly include prevention of acute complications, prevention and management of chronic complications, attention to psychosocial issues, and education regarding self-care.

Acute Complications

Uncontrolled hyperglycemia in the elderly may be asymptomatic or may produce such classic symptoms as polyuria and fatigue. Polydipsia is less common because of decreased thirst perception. Hyperglycemia can result in increased perception of pain and slowing of intellectual processes. The risk of infection is greater when blood glucose values are over 200 mg/dl. Such infectious disease processes as malignant otitis externa and reactivation of chronic tuberculosis are linked to hyperglycemia. Elderly individuals with diabetes are two times as likely to be hospitalized for kidney infections as individuals without diabetes.

Chronic hyperglycemia can cause mild to moderate dehydration in the elderly that can be exacerbated by age-related changes in kidney function and water conservation. The resulting electrolyte imbalances can increase the risk of falls.

Elderly people with type 2 diabetes mellitus are not prone to ketosis, but they are at risk for nonketotic hyperglycemic hyperosmolar coma. Particular risk factors include impaired thirst recognition, polypharmacy, dementia, and intercurrent illness. Profound dehydration can occur and lead to a significant mortality rate for this complication (10% to 50%).

Older individuals with type 2 diabetes mellitus must be instructed in care during intercurrent illness and advised to perform capillary blood glucose monitoring on a regular basis to avoid undetected hyperglycemia.

Hypoglycemia can occur when an elderly individual with diabetes is treated with a sulfonylurea or insulin. Hyperglycemia can occur atypically with symptoms of lethargy or focal neurologic dysfunction. Elderly individuals may have age-related decreases in counterregulatory function or an inability to report hypoglycemic symptoms. Glycemic targets for these individuals may be higher. The risk of injury during a hypoglycemic episode warrants careful observation of blood glucose values and regular evaluation of treatment of all elderly individuals with diabetes.

Chronic Complications

The increased prevalence of heart and blood vessel disease, kidney disease, eye disease, and foot disease in patients with diabetes overlaps with the increased prevalence of these conditions in the general elderly population. Diabetes increases the incidence and severity of these diseases.

Aging-related changes can present a particular problem in the performance of diabetic foot care. Orthopedic deformity, loss of protective subcutaneous fat, and atherosclerotic changes are all common problems of the elderly. Inspection of the feet and nail care can be compromised by changes in visual acuity and joint function. Assistance with foot care is often necessary to minimize the risk of diabetic complications involving the feet.

Treatment

Oral antidiabetic agents must be chosen carefully to avoid age-related adverse effects. Oral agents with a shorter duration of action are preferable. Elderly individuals with diabetes should be evaluated for changes in renal and hepatic function. Oral agents metabolized in an impaired system should be avoided. Metformin is not appropriate for individuals with decreased liver and renal function because of the increased risk of lactic acidosis.

Insulin is safe to use with caution in the elderly. Thin elderly individuals can be highly sensitive to insulin and may require very small amounts to control hyperglycemia. Some elderly are quite sensitive to regular insulin. Daily or twice-daily dosing of NPH or lente insulin may be preferable.

Age- or illness-related changes in vision, manual dexterity, and cognition can diminish the ability to measure and administer insulin. Magnification devices and the use of prefilled syringes can be of assistance.

Exercise is of benefit to individuals of all ages. Exercise plans must often be modified to account for orthopedic or other mobility problems. Armchair exercise can be an excellent way for elderly individuals to stay active.

Appropriate food intake can help control hyperglycemia and reduce the risk of chronic complications in the elderly, as in all individuals with diabetes. The quality and quantity of nutrients must be assessed carefully in the elderly. Elderly individuals may be obese, malnourished, or both. Increasing the nutritional value of a meal plan that is low in calories because of choice or a desire to lose weight is an important and difficult goal. Dental and other oral disease or dysfunction can have an impact on nutritional intake.

Education of the elderly in diabetic self-care practices can be challenged by age-related changes in vision, hearing, and cognition. Simple, clearly written educational materials and less complex therapeutic regimens can be of assistance. Caretakers and family members should be included in education sessions if possible. Family or other assistance can ensure safe performance of diabetic self-care activities while maintaining as much independence as possible.

KEY CONCEPTS

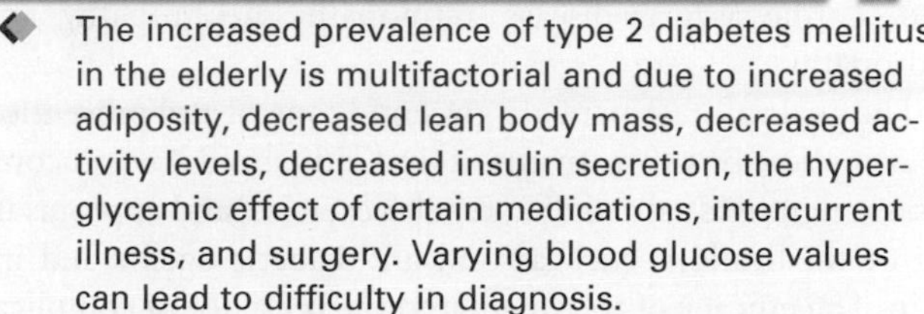

- The increased prevalence of type 2 diabetes mellitus in the elderly is multifactorial and due to increased adiposity, decreased lean body mass, decreased activity levels, decreased insulin secretion, the hyperglycemic effect of certain medications, intercurrent illness, and surgery. Varying blood glucose values can lead to difficulty in diagnosis.
- Goals of treatment for the elderly include prevention of acute complications, prevention and management of chronic complications, attention to psychosocial issues, and education regarding self-care.
- Acute complications of diabetes in the elderly include hyperglycemia, often asymptomatic, which can lead to dehydration, increased risk of infection, and nonketotic hyperglycemic hyperosmolar coma. Hypoglycemia can occur atypically and may lead to injury.
- Heart and blood vessel disease, foot problems, visual disabilities, and kidney disease have a significant presence in the aging population in general, as well as being chronic complications of diabetes. Avoiding foot problems can be particularly challenging given the frequent presence of orthopedic deformity and other common aging-related changes, as well as the decreased ability to perform appropriate foot care.
- Oral antidiabetic agents should be carefully chosen with consideration of renal and hepatic function. Short-acting agents are preferable. When insulin treatment is necessary, visual or orthopedic and other changes may hinder measurement of insulin. Adaptive devices can be helpful. Exercise should be encouraged and may have to be modified for people with limited mobility or other limiting factors. Meal planning for elderly individuals should emphasize appropriate amounts of foods with high nutritional value.
- Simple, clearly written educational material can be helpful for individuals with visual or cognitive impairments. Caretakers or family members should be included in education sessions if necessary.

SUMMARY

Diabetes mellitus, the most common endocrine disorder, affects millions of Americans. Diabetes is characterized and diagnosed by chronic hyperglycemia, the result of a relative or absolute deficiency of insulin; however, the metabolism of all energy nutrients is altered. Of the four clinical classes of diabetes, the most common are type 1 and type 2. Type 1 diabetes is the result of destruction of the insulin-producing β cells of the pancreas because of an autoimmune or idiopathic process. Type 2 diabetes is characterized by insulin resistance and a reduction in insulin production leading to a relative insulin deficiency.

Sequelae of insulin deficiency include the acute and chronic complications of diabetes. Acute complications include diabetic ketoacidosis in type 1 and nonketotic hyperglycemic hyperosmolar coma in type 2 diabetes. Chronic complications include cardiovascular disease, retinopathy, nephropathy, and neuropathy.

The goals of treatment are glycemic control and prevention of complications. Treatment is individualized and encompasses an individualized diet, regular exercise, and appropriate use of medications such as oral antidiabetic agents and insulin. The efficacy of treatment and the presence of complications of therapy are evaluated by capillary blood glucose monitoring. Patient education is an essential component in teaching skills associated with treatment.

Special considerations attend the treatment and education of individuals with diabetes in the pediatric and geriatric age groups. Children and adolescents require careful monitoring to adjust insulin levels for variations in maturation, exercise, and intercurrent illness. The elderly may have chronic complications of diabetes or other impairments of mobility, vision, or cognition that affect treatment.

Educational materials must be appropriate for age in children and be accessible for elderly individuals with visual or cognitive impairments.

MEDIA RESOURCES

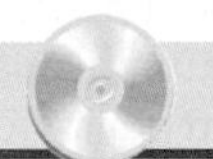

evolve

Remember to check out the ***CD Companion*** included with this book for Review Questions, Key Concepts Review, Glossary (with audio for selected terms), Disease Profiles, and Animations.

PLUS, visit the ***Evolve website*** at http://evolve.elsevier.com/Copstead/ for Case Studies, Disease Profiles, and WebLinks.

References

1. American Diabetes Association: Report of the expert committee on the diagnosis and classification of diabetes mellitus, *Diabetes Care* 26:5-20, 2003.
2. Kahn CR, Smith RJ, Chin WM: Mechanism of action of hormones that act at the cell surface. In Wilson RH et al, editors: *Williams textbook of endocrinology,* ed 9, Philadelphia, 1998, Saunders, pp 95-144.
3. Unger RH, Foster DW: Diabetes mellitus. In Wilson RH et al, editors: *Williams textbook of endocrinology,* ed 9, Philadelphia, 1998, Saunders, pp 973-1060.
4. Elbein SC et al: The genetics of NIDDM, *Diabetes Care* 17:1523-1533, 1994.
5. Polonsky KS, Sturis J, Bell GI: Non–insulin-dependent diabetes mellitus: a genetically programmed failure of the beta cell to compensate for insulin resistance, *N Engl J Med* 334:777-783, 1996.
6. Jovanic-Peterson L: The diagnosis and management of gestational diabetes mellitus, *Clin Diabetes* 13(2):32-39, 1995.
7. Després JP et al: Hyperinsulinemia as an independent risk factor for ischemic heart disease, *N Engl J Med* 334:952-957, 1996.
8. Clark CM, Lee DAL: Prevention and treatment of the complication of diabetes mellitus, *N Engl J Med* 332:1210-1217, 1995.
9. American Diabetes Association: Diabetic nephropathy, *Diabetes Care* 26:94-98, 2003.
10. Vijan S, Hayward RA: Treatment of hypertension in type 2 diabetes mellitus: blood pressure goals, choice of agents, and setting priorities in diabetic care, *Ann Intern Med* 138:593-602, 2003.
11. American Diabetes Association: Implications of the Diabetes Control and Complications Trial, *Diabetes Care* 26:25-27, 2003.
12. American Diabetes Association: Implications of the United Kingdom Prospective Diabetes Study, *Diabetes Care* 26:28-32, 2003.
13. Kitzmiller JL et al: Pre-conception care of diabetes, congenital malformations, and spontaneous abortions, *Diabetes Care* 19:514-541, 1996.
14. Weinstock RS: Treating type 2 diabetes mellitus: a growing epidemic, *Mayo Clin Proc* 78:411-413, 2003.
15. American Diabetes Association: *Medical management of insulin dependent (type I) diabetes,* ed 2, Alexandria, Va, 1994, American Diabetes Association.
16. American Diabetes Association: Translation of the diabetes nutrition recommendations for health care institutions, *Diabetes Care* 26:70-72, 2003.
17. Franz MJ et al: Technical review: nutrition principles for the management of diabetes and related complications, *Diabetes Care* 17:490-518, 1994.
18. Garg A: High–monounsaturated fat diet for diabetic patients, *Diabetes Care* 17:242-246, 1994.
19. Bell DSH: Alcohol and the NIDDM patient, *Diabetes Care* 19:509-513, 1996.
20. Kuczmarski RJ et al: Increasing prevalence of overweight among US adults, *JAMA* 272:205-211, 1994.
21. Wolf AM, Colditz GA: Social and economic effects of body weight in the United States, *Am J Clin Nutr* 63(suppl):S466-S469, 1996.
22. Perseghin G: Increased glucose transport-phosphorylation and muscle glycogen synthesis after exercise training in insulin-resistant subjects, *N Engl J Med* 335:1357-1362, 1996.
23. American Diabetes Association: Physical activity/exercise and diabetes mellitus, *Diabetes Care* 26:73-77, 2003.
24. Pate RR et al: Physical activity and public health: a recommendation from the Centers for Disease Control and Prevention and the American College of Sports Medicine, *JAMA* 273:402-407, 1995.

25. Gerich JE: Contributions of insulin-resistance and insulin-secretory defects to the pathogenesis of type 2 diabetes mellitus, *Mayo Clin Proc* 78:447-458, 2003.
26. Chan JL, Abrahamson MJ: Pharmacological management of type 2 diabetes mellitus: rationale for use of insulin, *Mayo Clin Proc* 78:459-471, 2003.
27. Bloomgarden ZT: Metformin, *Diabetes Care* 18:1078-1080, 1995.
28. Zanfgenech F, Kudva YC, Basu A: Insulin sensitizers, *Mayo Clin Proc* 78:472-480, 2003.
29. Howey DC et al: [Lys(B28), Pro(B29)]-human insulin: a rapidly absorbed analogue of human insulin, *Diabetes* 43:396-402, 1994.
30. Weissberg-Benchall J, Antisdel-Lomaglio J, Seehadri R: Insulin pump therapy: a meta-analysis, *Diabetes Care* 26:1079-1087, 2003.
31. Chow CC et al: Comparison of insulin with or without continuation of oral hypoglycemic agents in the treatment of secondary failure in NIDDM patients, *Diabetes Care* 18:307-314, 1995.
32. Cryer PE, Fisher JN, Shamoon H: Hypoglycemia, *Diabetes Care* 17:734-755, 1994.
33. Jacobson AM: The psychological care of patients with insulin-dependent diabetes mellitus, *N Engl J Med* 334:1249-1253, 1996.
34. Goldstein DE et al: Tests of glycemia in diabetes, *Diabetes Care* 18:896-909, 1995.
35. American Diabetes Association: Tests of glycemia in diabetes, *Diabetes Care* 26:106-108, 2003.
36. American Association of Diabetes Educators: Position statement: prevention of transmission of blood-borne infectious agents during blood glucose monitoring, *Diabetes Educ* 14:425-426, 1988.
37. American Association of Diabetes Educators: Infection control guidelines for patient education as a means of preventing blood-borne disease transmission during diabetes self-care procedures, *Diabetes Educ* 17:321-325, 1991.
38. Clement S: Diabetes self-management education, *Diabetes Care* 18:1204-1214, 1995.
39. American Diabetes Association: Third-party reimbursement of diabetes care, self-management education, and supplies, *Diabetes Care* 19(suppl 1):S48-S49, 1996.
40. American Diabetes Association: National standards for diabetes self-management education, *Diabetes Care* 26:149-156, 2003.

chapter 42

Alterations in Metabolism and Nutrition

Arnold A. Asp

MEDIA RESOURCES

Additional Material for Study, Review, and Further Exploration

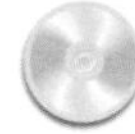

CD Companion ◆ Review Questions and Answers ◆ Key Concepts Review ◆ Glossary *(with audio pronunciations for selected terms)* ◆ Disease Profiles ◆ Animations

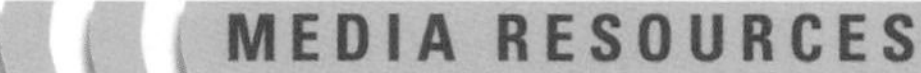

evolve Website at http://evolve.elsevier.com/Copstead/ ◆ Case Studies ◆ Disease Profiles ◆ WebLinks

KEY QUESTIONS

- How does acute physiologic stress affect body metabolism?
- What information about nutritional status can be gained from each of the following biochemical tests: serum albumin, transferrin, prealbumin, red and white blood cell counts, blood urea nitrogen, serum creatinine, and urinary nitrogen excretion?
- What anthropometric measurements are used to assess nutritional status?
- What information gained from a nutritional assessment would indicate potential or actual nutritional problems?
- How do insulin, glucagon, catecholamines, thyroid hormone, cortisol, and growth hormone affect the metabolism of fats, sugars, and proteins?

CHAPTER OUTLINE

Each moment, millions of chemical reactions occur within the body to create or expend energy to meet physiologic needs. The process, known as **metabolism,** uses energy to sustain the body's vital functions.[1] Metabolism converts energy by synthesizing and breaking down molecules. These interrelated and dynamic reactions meet the requirements of each body cell.[2] Adequate nutrition is needed for growth and metabolism, organ function, activity, repair of injury, and resistance to infection.

Many hospitalized patients experience a significant degree of physiologic stress and multiple organ dysfunction, both of which increase specific and general nutritional needs. Treatment modalities, altered intake, and restricted mobility may also increase nutritional problems. In many cases these problems could be averted if nutritional assessment and therapy were started early. This chapter reviews normal nutrient metabolism and nutritional assessment. The chapter concludes with a comprehensive discussion of nutritional and metabolic alterations.

METABOLIC PROCESSES

Anabolism and Catabolism

Anabolism refers to the constructive phase of metabolism and involves the creation of organic molecules by cells. Larger molecules are built from smaller ones, and in the process energy is used. Anabolism occurs during times of rest, healing, pregnancy, lactation, and growth. Hormonal secretions such as insulin and sex hormones may also trigger anabolism. Obesity, with the accumulation of adipose tissue, is a form of anabolism.[3] Conversely, **catabolism** is the degradative phase of metabolism. Complex molecules are broken down into simpler substances with the concurrent release or production of energy. During times of disease, stress, fever, or starvation or during the release of certain hormones such as thyroid hormone and cortisol, catabolism dominates the body's metabolic processes. The resultant tissue wasting may lead to cellular injury or death if excessive catabolism is left unresolved.[4] Anabolism and catabolism occur simultaneously and together create the dynamic balance of substance and energy known as metabolism.

The metabolic process requires nutrients in the form of carbohydrates, fats, and proteins. Each of these three nutrients is altered or broken down into simpler substances. Enzymes, or their coenzymes derived from vitamins and hormones, may accomplish the process of producing glucose, fatty acids, and amino acids. In this fashion the body's continual cellular energy requirements are met.[4] Energy produced by metabolic processes is used to create the energy currency of the body known as **adenosine** triphosphate (ATP). ATP consists of adenine, ribose, and three phosphate radicals. Loss of one phosphate radical produces adenosine diphosphate, whereas loss of two phosphates produces adenosine monophosphate. Energy is produced with hydrolysis of the phosphate bonds. Located in the cytoplasm and nucleoplasm of all cells, ATP or other high-energy compounds provide the energy necessary for normal cellular function. Cells use ATP to release energy for the performance of work such as muscle contraction, transport of chemicals across cell membranes, and synthesis of chemical compounds. Continual cellular consumption of energy is enabled by the release of high-energy phosphate bonds from ATP and by the recreation of ATP through cellular oxidation of food.[4]

Cells use energy to perform essential body processes. **Energy** is measured in kilocalories; 1 kcal represents the amount of energy required to raise the temperature of 1 kg of water from 15° C to 16° C. During catabolism of fuel molecules, approximately 40% of the available energy is converted to ATP, with the remaining 60% being used for the production of heat.[2] The energy released as heat is important for maintaining body temperature.

Metabolic Rate

Several factors determine the body's energy requirements or metabolic needs, including the basal metabolic rate (BMR), activity level, and the energy necessary for digestion.[4]

The **basal metabolic rate** refers to the rate of energy use by resting tissue. It is a measurement of the energy used in maintenance of the body at rest after a 12-hour fast.[4] It represents the energy used in maintaining basic body processes such as respiration, cellular metabolism, circulation, glandular activity, and the maintenance of body temperature.[4] The body's BMR is determined by calculating oxygen use during a specific period. The normal range for BMR is generally between 0.8 and 1.43 kcal/min.[4] Several factors that affect an individual's BMR are described in Table 42-1. Body stature and size affect BMR by the amount of heat lost from the body surface. Age is also an important determinant of BMR. A growing child's BMR is significantly higher than an adult's, primarily because of an increased rate of cellular reactions and the generation of new tissue.[4] Conversely, as one ages, the BMR gradually declines by about 2% per decade. Body composition, determined by the amount of fat and lean tissue, also affects BMR. Muscle tissue requires more oxygen than adipose tissue does, which explains why athletes have an approximately 5% higher BMR than nonathletes.[2] Women typically have a metabolic rate 5% to 10% less than that of men, probably because of differences in body mass. Women also tend to have more adipose tissue than men, and fat is less metabolically active than muscle.[3] Pregnancy increases the BMR by about 20% to 28%, or 300 kcal/day, as a consequence of increased uterine and mammary gland size, fetal development, and additional cardiopulmonary workload.[4] Other factors affecting BMR include nutritional status, muscle tone, sleep, fever, environmental temperature, and stress.[2]

Almost any alteration in the body's normal homeostatic state will alter its energy requirements and BMR. Many diseases are known to dramatically increase the body's energy requirements; examples include chronic obstructive and restrictive pulmonary disease, hyperthermia, burns, cancer, diabetes, and Graves disease (hyperthyroidism).

Table 42-1

Factors Affecting Basal Metabolic Rate

Increasing Metabolism	Decreasing Metabolism
Childhood growth	Aging process
Exercise	End-stage illness
Sympathetic stimulation	Starvation
Shivering	Sleep
Fever	Tropical climates
Thyroid hormone	
Muscle tissue	
Pregnancy	
Stress	
Male sex hormone	

KEY CONCEPTS

- Anabolism refers to energy-requiring processes involving synthesis of biomolecules. Catabolism refers to energy-producing processes during which biomolecules are broken down into simpler forms. Metabolism refers to the dynamic state of simultaneously occurring anabolism and catabolism.
- The BMR is the rate of energy utilization when the body is at rest. Factors affecting the BMR include body size and composition, age, nutritional status, muscle mass, fever, stress, and pregnancy.

NUTRIENT METABOLISM

Energy for the body is supplied by three classifications of nutrients: **carbohydrates, fats,** and **proteins.** These three groups of food sources supply the body with energy for ATP formation, but each acts in its own way. Metabolism in general is controlled by both the nervous system and the endocrine system. Four major hormones involved in substrate metabolism are insulin, glucagon, catecholamines, and cortisol. The effects of these four hormones on carbohydrate, fat, and protein metabolism are summarized in Tables 42-2 through 42-4. Both the nervous system and the endocrine system directly affect metabolism by release of the catecholamines epinephrine and norepinephrine, which during times of stress inhibit insulin secretion. The pancreatic hormones insulin and glucagon have a crucial role in the metabolic processes that govern the body's energy requirements. These hormones function antithetically, with insulin lowering blood glucose levels and glucagon ultimately increasing blood glucose levels.[2] Growth hormone affects metabolism by decreasing cellular uptake and use of glucose. High levels of growth hormone tend to decrease affinity for insulin at the receptor site such that even increased secretion of insulin by the pancreas has diminutive effects on blood glucose levels. Glucocorticoid hormones, primarily cortisol, stimulate gluconeogenesis by the liver. Blood glucose levels six to ten times normal may occur with significant cortisol secretion. Left uncorrected, diabetes mellitus may develop (see Chapter 41).[3]

Carbohydrates

Carbohydrates are the main energy source for the body and must be supplied in a fairly constant manner to meet the energy requirements for normal body functioning. Approximately 45% of the typical American diet consists of carbohydrates, with almost half of that supplied in the form of simple sugars.[5] Dietary carbohydrates are starches or sugars and are composed of carbon, hydrogen, and oxygen molecules. Carbohydrates are classified into the three categories of **monosaccharides** (simple sugars), **oligosaccharides** (2 to 10 joined monosaccharide units), and **polysaccharides** (10 to 10,000 monosaccharide units). They range from very simple sugars consisting of three to seven carbons to incredibly complex polymers made up of repeating units of thousands of monosaccharides.[4]

Monosaccharides are the simplest form of carbohydrate. The most common in this category are the six-carbon sugars of glucose, mannose, fructose, and galactose. Glucose, the most physiologically important of the group, is the form of sugar normally found in the blood stream. Glucose is derived from the catabolism of more complex carbohydrates during the process of digestion. Fructose and galactose are also eventually converted to glucose by the liver. Once in the blood stream, glucose is either oxidized to provide cellular energy or stored in the liver and muscles as glycogen. Blood sugar levels then reflect the difference between the amount of glucose released into the blood stream by the liver and the amount of glucose taken up by the cells for energy.[3]

Table 42-2

Hormonal Actions on Carbohydrate Metabolism

Hormone	Actions
Insulin	Stimulates glucose uptake by cells Stimulates glycolysis Inhibits gluconeogenesis
Glucagon	Stimulates glycogen breakdown Increases gluconeogenesis
Catecholamines	Maintain blood glucose level during stress Diminish glucose uptake by cells Increase glycogen breakdown
Cortisol	Stimulates gluconeogenesis Diminishes glucose uptake by cells

Table 42-3

Hormonal Actions on Fat Metabolism

Hormone	Actions
Insulin	Increases fatty acid uptake by fat cells Promotes glucose uptake by fat cells
Glucagon	Promotes lipolysis in fat cells
Catecholamines	Increases fat mobilization Increase serum free fatty acid levels
Cortisol	Increases fat cell membrane permeability

Intracellular Glucose Metabolism

Once in the cell, glucose undergoes additional breakdown called **glycolysis,** which is the metabolic sequence that converts glucose to pyruvate and eventually yields the end products of carbon dioxide and water.[4] Catabolism of glucose may occur anaerobically along the Embden-Meyerhof pathway, which in a 10-step process alters the chemical composition of glucose to pyruvic acid and results in a net gain of two ATP molecules for each molecule of glucose that enters the pathway. Pyruvic acid has two important roles in the catabolic process of carbohydrates. It provides the body with acetyl coenzyme A, which is required for conversion of fatty acids to energy, and it is the initial step for the second stage of carbohydrate metabolism, the Krebs cycle and oxidative phosphorylation. The Krebs or citric acid cycle occurs in the mitochondria of the cell. Oxidative phosphorylation (see Chapter 3) produces a total of 30 to 36 molecules of ATP for each molecule of glucose. Although other pathways exist, the interrelated Embden-Meyerhof pathway, Krebs cycle, and respiratory chain enzymes produce nearly all of the energy required for cellular functioning.[4] Figure 42-1 illustrates the metabolism of carbohydrate, fat, and protein through the anaerobic Embden-Meyerhof and the Krebs pathways. The respiratory chain requires molecular oxygen (aerobic).

Just as glucose is constantly catabolized for the production of energy, it is also continuously created. **Gluconeogenesis** refers to the process by which glucose is formed from noncarbohydrate sources, including amino acids supplied by muscle tissue and glycerol supplied from fat breakdown.[5] The glucose created through this mechanism may either be stored in the liver as glycogen or released into the blood stream. During periods of fasting, gluconeogenesis and glycogenolysis provide the necessary glucose to meet the metabolic requirements of the brain and other glucose-dependent tissues.[3]

Hormonal Control of Glucose Metabolism

Many hormones affect glucose levels by either increasing or decreasing carbohydrate metabolism. The only hormone known to lower blood glucose levels is insulin. Hormones that tend to raise blood glucose levels include glucagon, growth hormone, glucocorticoid hormones, epinephrine and

Table 42-4

Hormonal Actions on Protein Metabolism

Hormone	Actions
Insulin	Actively transports amino acids into cells Accelerates cellular protein synthesis
Glucagon	Stimulates protein breakdown into amino acids Increases amino acids movement into hepatic cells
Cortisol	Increases protein catabolism

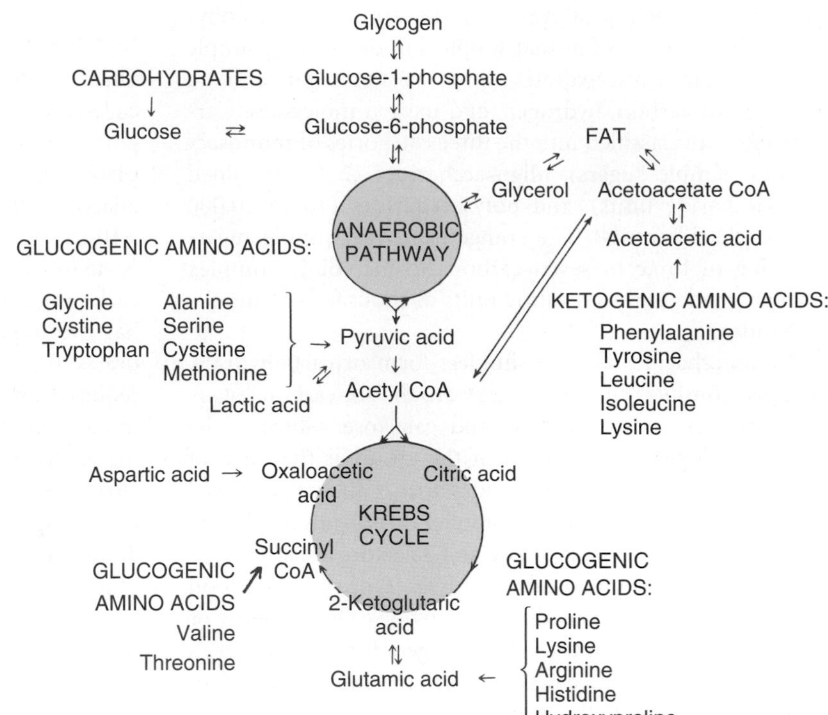

FIGURE 42-1 ■ Metabolic integration of carbohydrate, fat, and protein metabolism. *CoA,* Coenzyme A. (From Mahan LK, Arlin MT: *Krause's food, nutrition and diet therapy,* ed 8, Philadelphia, 1992, Saunders, p 345.)

norepinephrine, and thyroid hormone. Table 42-2 describes the major hormonal effects on glucose metabolism.

Insulin. Formed from its precursor proinsulin and synthesized by β cells in the pancreas, insulin is secreted in response to increased blood glucose levels. Minutes after ingestion of a meal, insulin levels in the blood rise significantly, peak in 30 minutes, and level off in about 3 hours. Between meals, when blood glucose levels tend to drop, insulin levels also remain low. At that time, glucose and amino acid stores are used for cellular energy requirements.[3]

Insulin directly affects glucose metabolism by promoting glucose uptake by the liver, which then favors the synthesis of glycogen. Glucose formation (**gluconeogenesis**) and the breakdown of glycogen to form glucose (**glycogenolysis**) are inhibited by insulin. The active transport of glucose across cellular membranes into muscle and adipose tissue is facilitated by insulin and has a direct lowering effect on blood glucose levels.[6] Individuals with diabetes mellitus have either insulin hyposecretion or cellular hyporesponsiveness to insulin as a consequence of receptor down-regulation. Obese and elderly persons are especially at risk for insulin receptor down-regulation with resultant diabetes. Diabetes mellitus is discussed in Chapter 41.

Glucagon. The protein hormone glucagon is secreted by α cells in the pancreas and also by some cells lining the gastrointestinal tract. Acting in a fashion opposite that of insulin, glucagon increases blood glucose levels.[7] As blood glucose levels begin to drop, plasma glucagon levels begin to rise. The two primary effects of glucagon, then, are to promote the breakdown of liver glycogen with subsequent release of glucose into the blood stream and to promote liver gluconeogenesis. These actions tend to bring serum glucose levels back to normal. Conversely, as glucose levels rise, glucagon secretion is diminished and serum glucose levels drop toward normal. The diametric actions of insulin and glucagon partially explain why increased glucagon secretion may also have a role in the elevated blood glucose levels seen in people with diabetes mellitus.[2]

Catecholamines. In carbohydrate metabolism, the primary role of the catecholamines epinephrine and norepinephrine is to maintain blood glucose levels during times of stress. As the stress response occurs, catecholamines stimulate the conversion of glycogen to glucose in the muscles and liver. Although muscles, unlike the liver, cannot release glucose into the general circulation, mobilization of muscle glycogen frees up unused blood glucose for other tissues such as the brain and the peripheral nervous system. The second primary action of epinephrine during the stress response is to stimulate glucagon secretion and prevent insulin release from the pancreas, thereby preventing glucose movement into muscle cells. Epinephrine also promotes glycogenolysis by the liver and muscles and reduces glucose uptake by muscle tissue. The role of catecholamines in glucose metabolism is very similar to that of glucagon and opposite that of insulin.[2]

Glucocorticoids. Cortisol, the primary glucocorticoid hormone secreted from the adrenal cortex, acts as an insulin antagonist to maintain serum glucose levels. During fasting, cortisol permissively enables other hormonal changes to occur, such as decreased insulin production and increased glucagon and epinephrine secretion. The end result is promotion of gluconeogenesis and lipolysis. If cortisol deficiency occurs simultaneously with fasting, hypoglycemic reactions significant enough to alter brain functioning can occur. A recent study indicated that cortisol deficiency may be a significant cause of morbidity and mortality in critically ill surgical patients, who frequently are poorly nourished.[8]

Growth Hormone. Although the role of growth hormone in carbohydrate metabolism is minor in comparison with its role in growth regulation and protein anabolism, it can have a significant impact under certain circumstances. Growth hormone's effects parallel those of cortisol: growth hormone increases gluconeogenesis in the liver and inhibits glucose uptake by muscle cells.[2] Elevated serum growth hormone levels tend to increase blood glucose levels. As a result, the insulin-secreting β cells in the pancreas are stimulated. If this process is not corrected, the β cells will eventually be exhausted. It is for this reason that diabetes mellitus eventually develops in people with excessive growth hormone, as in acromegaly.[3]

Thyroid Hormone. The major physiologically active thyroid hormone is triiodothyronine. Thyroid hormone tends to raise blood glucose levels. In carbohydrate metabolism, the primary mode of action is to increase glucose absorption from the intestines and stimulate the release of epinephrine. Thyroid hormone also promotes the rate of insulin destruction. Ultimately, thyroid hormone causes an increase in cellular oxygen consumption and the basal metabolic rate of tissues.

Fats

Fats, the most concentrated form of energy, are derived from animal fats and vegetable oils. Fats supply 9 kcal of energy per gram, as compared with 4 kcal from glucose and 4 kcal from protein. Fats are 98% **triglycerides.** Like carbohydrates, fats are made up of carbon, hydrogen, and oxygen. The bulk of each triglyceride molecule consists of fatty acids containing 4 to 30 carbon atoms. Fats are frequently categorized as **saturated** or **unsaturated.** Figure 42-2 gives the chemical composition of some common saturated and unsaturated fatty acids. The degree of hydrogen **saturation** refers to the number of double bonds between the carbon atoms in the chain. If a fatty acid chain contains all the hydrogen molecules possible with no double bonds, it is called a **saturated fatty acid.** Those fatty acids with one double bond are typed as **monounsaturated,** and those with several double bonds are **polyunsaturated.**[4]

Fats in the form of triglycerides supply approximately two thirds of the cell's total energy requirements. Whereas the human body is able to economically store approximately 140,000 kcal of usable fats in adipose tissue, it can store only 24,000 kcal of protein and a mere 800 kcal of carbohydrate in an adult man.[7] Carbohydrates and amino acids not immediately used by the tissues are converted to fat and stored, along with ingested fat, as adipose tissue. Fat deposits are extremely important in the economical use of metabolites. If intake exceeds expenditure, obesity results. During times of fasting, the body quickly reverts to the breakdown and use of fats as its energy source.[8] All tissues in the body, with the exception of brain cells, can metabolize and use fats as an energy source as effectively as glucose.[7]

18-Carbon Fatty Acids	
Stearic acid	$CH_3(CH_2)_{16}COOH$ (saturated)
Oleic acid	$CH_3(CH_2)_7CH{=}CH(CH_2)_7COOH$ (monounsaturated)
Linoleic acid	$CH_3(CH_2)_4CH{=}CHCH_2CH{=}CH(CH_7)COOH$ (polyunsaturated)

FIGURE 42-2 ■ Chemical composition of some fatty acids.

Almost all fats are absorbed into the lymph system from the intestinal mucosa. They are then converted to a chylomicron consisting of 80% triglyceride, 9% cholesterol, 7% phospholipid, and 4% lipoprotein coat.[9] Chylomicrons empty into the venous blood at the thoracic duct and are carried to the liver for metabolism or assimilated into adipose tissue. Once in the liver, triglycerides are generally hydrolyzed into glycerol and fatty acids in a process known as **lipolysis.** When released, the fatty acids, bound to albumin, are quickly assimilated into tissue. Oxidation in tissue begins when acetyl coenzyme A binds to the end of a fatty acid. Progressing through a series of reactions known as β oxidation, the fatty acid chain is shortened by two carbon atoms until all the carbon atoms have been transferred to coenzyme A. Acetyl coenzyme A then enters the Krebs cycle, with each 2-carbon segment producing 2 molecules of carbon dioxide and 12 molecules of ATP. The average fatty acid contains approximately 18 carbon molecules, with 146 ATP molecules being produced during catabolism.[2] Unlike fatty acids, glycerol (the other component of triglycerides) can only be metabolized by a few tissues. Glycerol is generally carried to the liver, where it is either oxidized for energy or used to generate new triglycerides.

Within the liver, fatty acids are generally transformed to acetyl coenzyme A, which is further processed into one of three compounds collectively known as **ketone bodies.** Once released into the blood stream, ketones have a critical role as an energy source for tissues able to oxidize them in the Krebs cycle. During the fasting state, tissues use ketones as a primary energy source, with glucose reserved for brain metabolism. If the fasting state continues, many areas of the brain begin to use ketone bodies as an energy source. As the brain begins to use ketones, less protein is broken down to provide glucose. For this reason the body is able to withstand periods of fasting with minimal protein breakdown and tissue disruption.[2]

The liver is the major organ responsible for lipid metabolism and regulation of serum lipid levels. The four primary functions of the hepatic system in regard to lipid metabolism are (1) synthesis of triglycerides from carbohydrates and protein, (2) synthesis of phospholipids and cholesterol from triglycerides, (3) desaturation of fatty acids, and (4) utilization of triglycerides as an energy source.[4] Liver disease can significantly alter any of these processes and cause serious metabolic disturbances. A fatty liver is characterized by fat deposits in the liver cells caused either by ingestion of hepatotoxic substances such as alcohol or halocarbons or by diets significantly low in protein for a prolonged period. Infections managed with protein synthesis–inhibiting antibiotics such as tetracycline and malignancies may also lead to increased fat deposits within the liver by adversely affecting the hepatic cells or biliary tract. Increased mobilization of fatty acids from adipose tissue to the liver occurs in certain conditions, such as diabetes mellitus, starvation, and obesity, where lipogenesis exceeds the ability of the liver to export the fat as lipoproteins.[10] Metabolic studies of critically ill patients indicate that fatty acid breakdown occurs at a much higher rate than patient caloric needs require. This excess lipolysis may cause fatty liver.[11]

Hormonal Control of Lipid Metabolism

Because carbohydrates and lipids may both be metabolized along the anaerobic Embden-Meyerhof pathway, hormones that affect carbohydrate metabolism also affect lipid metabolism. Table 42-3 describes the hormones considered to have the greatest effect on lipid metabolism. These hormones include insulin, thyroid hormone, glucocorticoids, mineralocorticoids, growth hormone, epinephrine, and norepinephrine. Insulin prevents fat utilization by indirectly causing fatty acids to be taken up by adipose tissue and by decreasing the activity of hormone-sensitive lipase, which promotes the movement of fat out of adipose tissue. Glucocorticoids increase fat cell membrane permeability, whereas mineralocorticoids increase the activity of hormone-sensitive lipase. Epinephrine and norepinephrine increase fat mobilization by stimulating the activity of hormone-sensitive lipase, thus increasing the serum free fatty acid level. Growth hormone increases fatty acid mobilization and use by tissues as an energy source.[4]

Proteins

Proteins are composed of nitrogen, carbon, hydrogen, oxygen, and, occasionally, sulfur. When hydrolyzed, they yield amino acids. Twenty-two amino acids have been identified in protein, 8 of which are essential—meaning that they must be supplied through the diet.[9] Muscle tissue, bones, teeth, skin, and hair are made up primarily of protein. To function properly, most body processes require an adequate supply of proteins, many of which must be obtained through a balanced diet. Children, because of their rapid growth, require more protein per kilogram of body weight than adults do. In addition, when compared with adults, children also need a larger percentage of their dietary intake of protein to contain essential amino acids.

Once ingested, proteins are broken down into amino acids or peptides and are absorbed through the intestinal lumen. They are then carried to the liver through the portal vein. The liver regulates protein metabolism through enzymatic breakdown of amino acids, formation of nonessential amino acids from simple precursors, and detoxification of ammonia, urea, uric acid, and other catabolic end products. Proteins are quickly synthesized and broken down by the liver, which enables a quick response to changing metabolic demands. Amino acids supplied in excess of metabolic requirements are degraded to byproducts such as urea, uric acid, or creatinine, and the remaining carbon molecules are converted to carbohydrate and fat or oxidized for energy.[12] Of particular importance is the conversion of amino acids to fatty acids, which are carbohydrate-like in structure and created by removal of the amino group during deamination. These keto acids may then enter the Krebs cycle, where they provide energy for liver metabolism, or they may be converted to fatty acids by the liver.

Protein metabolism can be measured in terms of **nitrogen balance.** If nitrogen intake approximates output, an equal nitrogen balance exists. If dietary intake of proteins exceeds output, a **positive nitrogen balance** occurs. Protein anabolism exceeds catabolism during periods of rapid growth, pregnancy, and the formation of new tissue. Experimentally, positive nitrogen balance has been induced in malnourished patients through the administration of growth hormone.[13] A **negative nitrogen balance** occurs when protein breakdown exceeds daily protein intake and synthesis. If the daily caloric intake is insufficient, the body catabolizes dietary and tissue protein for energy, as is the case after severe burns and during fever, illness, or stress.[2]

Hormonal Control of Protein Metabolism

Anabolic and catabolic protein metabolism is controlled by various hormones. Table 42-4 lists the major hormonal effects on protein metabolism. Hormones that also promote protein synthesis include growth hormone, especially during growth spurts; testosterone in specific reproductive organs during puberty; and thyroid hormone indirectly, by increasing the metabolic rate. Insulin also promotes the active transport of amino acids across cell membranes and accelerates protein synthesis within the cell. Insulin, in concert with growth hormone, is required for normal growth and development of children and adolescents. Glucagon, whose actions diametrically oppose those of insulin, promotes gluconeogenesis by stimulating the breakdown of protein into amino acids and increasing their transport into hepatic cells. Glucagon also enables the conversion of amino acids into glucose precursors.

KEY CONCEPTS

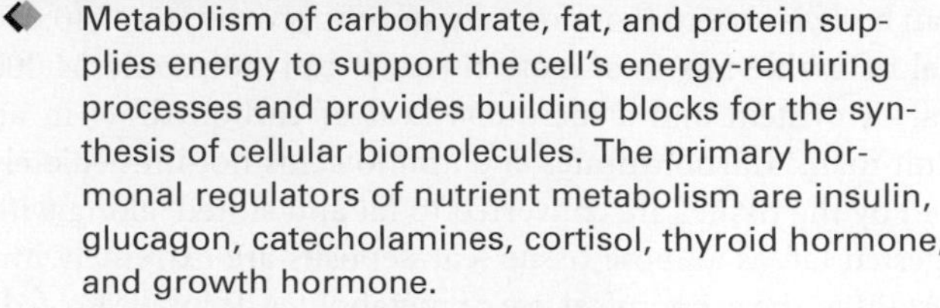

- Metabolism of carbohydrate, fat, and protein supplies energy to support the cell's energy-requiring processes and provides building blocks for the synthesis of cellular biomolecules. The primary hormonal regulators of nutrient metabolism are insulin, glucagon, catecholamines, cortisol, thyroid hormone, and growth hormone.

- Insulin is secreted from pancreatic β cells in response to elevated serum glucose levels. Binding of insulin to receptors on target cells (muscle, adipose tissue) facilitates the transport of glucose into cells and reduces blood glucose levels. Insulin inhibits lipolysis and gluconeogenesis.
- Glucagon is secreted from pancreatic β cells in response to low blood glucose levels. Glucagon promotes glycogenolysis and gluconeogenesis (from protein and glycerol) by the liver, thereby increasing blood glucose levels.
- Catecholamines increase glycogenolysis and gluconeogenesis by the liver, thereby increasing blood glucose levels. Catecholamines also stimulate lipolysis in adipose cells by enhancing the action of hormone-sensitive lipase. Glucagon secretion is enhanced and insulin secretion is inhibited by catecholamines.
- Cortisol enhances the actions of glucagon and catecholamines and promotes glycogenolysis, gluconeogenesis, and lipolysis, thus raising blood levels of glucose and fatty acids.
- Thyroid hormone tends to raise blood glucose levels. In carbohydrate metabolism, the primary mode of action is to increase glucose absorption from the intestines and stimulate the release of epinephrine. Thyroid hormone also enhances the rate of insulin destruction. Ultimately, thyroid hormone causes an increase in cellular oxygen consumption and the general metabolic rate of tissues.
- Growth hormone increases blood glucose by inhibiting uptake by muscle cells and by stimulating gluconeogenesis in the liver. Growth hormone enhances the cellular uptake of amino acids and stimulates protein synthesis.
- The main sources of cellular energy are glucose and fatty acids. Glucose is the primary energy source for the brain, although the brain can use ketones. Ketones are produced from fatty acids by the liver, particularly under conditions of decreased carbohydrate intake.

AGING AND METABOLIC FUNCTION

Without doubt, the aging process has an effect on normal metabolism. It is sometimes difficult, however, to distinguish the effects of aging from the effects of chronic illness, drug therapy, or obesity.

There seems to be little difference in the ability of healthy people, young or old, to metabolize glucose and little difference in insulin secretion by the β cells in the pancreas. What does appear to occur with the aging process is a change in tissue sensitivity to insulin. Although many possible causes for this phenomenon have been proposed, such as reduced carbohydrate intake, decreased muscle mass, and lowered activity levels, the reason appears to lie in an alteration in the molecular makeup of insulin. The elderly have higher levels of circulating serum proinsulin than younger adults do. It is also believed that the aging process alters insulin receptor sites and thus renders insulin less effective.[14]

The aging process may also affect lipid metabolism as proportionate body fat increases. Although caloric intake generally decreases, a concurrent loss of lean body mass and a decline in energy expenditure begin with adulthood. A decline in the resting metabolic rate also occurs with the aging process. This change is related to several factors, such as reduced lean body mass, reduced lipogenic enzyme response to glucose, and decreased catecholamine secretion after a meal. Although cross-sectional studies demonstrate that cholesterol and triglyceride serum levels tend to rise with age, evidence is increasing that this change may be due more to obesity than to the aging process itself. As a risk factor, hyperlipidemia poses less threat for coronary artery disease and atherosclerosis with the aging process.[14]

A decrease in the quantity of skeletal muscle normally occurs with aging. Although this decrease in muscle is associated with factors such as physical inactivity and a decrease in the number of neurons to muscle cells, endocrine factors also influence the loss of muscle mass. The decreased growth hormone secretion noted in elderly individuals leads to decreased protein synthesis.[14]

Box 42-1 summarizes some of the effects that the aging process has on normal metabolism.

Box 42-1

Geriatric Variations Associated with Aging and Metabolic Function

- With aging comes a change in tissue sensitivity to insulin because of an alteration in the molecular makeup of insulin. Elderly persons have higher levels of circulating serum proinsulin than younger adults do. The aging process may also alter insulin receptor sites and thereby render insulin less effective.
- The aging process may affect lipid metabolism as proportionate body fat increases. Although caloric intake generally decreases, a concurrent loss of lean body mass and decline in energy expenditure begin with adulthood.
- A decline in the resting metabolic rate also occurs with aging. This change is related to several factors, such as reduced lean body mass, reduced lipogenic enzyme response to glucose, and decreased catecholamine secretion after a meal.

KEY CONCEPTS

- Aging is associated with a change in tissue sensitivity to insulin and altered insulin receptor sites, factors hypothesized to render insulin less effective.
- As proportionate body fat increases with aging, lipid metabolism may be affected.
- The resting metabolic rate slows with aging.

NUTRITIONAL ALTERATIONS OF PHYSIOLOGIC STRESS

Metabolic Response

The response of the body to starvation is different from the response to physiologic stress.[15] Starvation is a gradual process in which the metabolic rate decreases and carbohydrate reserves are exhausted. As insulin levels dwindle, free fatty acids are released for energy use. Despite the available free fatty acids, protein is used for energy by means of gluconeogenesis because the body's tissues prefer glucose as an energy source. This preference creates a negative nitrogen balance. As starvation continues, overall energy needs are reduced and the tissues that usually require glucose for function adapt by using ketones for energy. Then lipolysis provides the source of needed energy, and the use of protein as an energy source decreases. This change is an adaptive response through which the body strives to conserve lean body mass. Overall, the result is minimal depletion of the body's protein. Decreased serum glucose and urinary nitrogen excretion, along with elevation in ketones and free fatty acids, characterizes starvation. Fasting (voluntary starving) alone is not associated with a high mortality unless it is prolonged, as it is in anorexia nervosa. Figure 42-3 provides a summary of the physiologic effect of starvation.

With physiologic stress, conservation of lean body mass does not occur. The metabolic rate increases rather than decreases, and a high sustained rate of catabolism (breakdown of protein to meet energy needs) results. Protein is used as an energy source by gluconeogenesis through release of muscle stores of amino acids. This adaptation quickly results in a negative nitrogen balance. Cell mass is redistributed in response to the stressor, with an increase in the production of acute phase proteins. The degree of hypermetabolism, hypercatabolism, and negative nitrogen balance associated with a physiologic stress depends on the type, duration, and severity of the stressor present.

Phases of Catabolic Response

Typically, the catabolic response to stress occurs in two phases: the immediate phase, lasting 5 to 8 days, and the subsequent adaptive phase. The physiologic effects of each phase are summarized in Figures 42-4 and 42-5.

The immediate phase of **catabolism** is characterized by high sympathetic nervous system stimulation with release of glucagon, glucocorticoids, and catecholamines. The resultant decreased production and circulation of insulin cause a pseudodiabetic state. Hyperglycemia develops from decreased circulating insulin and decreased utilization of glucose by muscle and other tissues (insulin resistance).

An energy deficit is created, and alternative mechanisms of glucose production are needed. The oxidation of branched-chain amino acids occurs for two reasons: to meet energy requirements and for the amino acids to provide the liver a substrate for the synthesis of acute phase proteins (immuno-

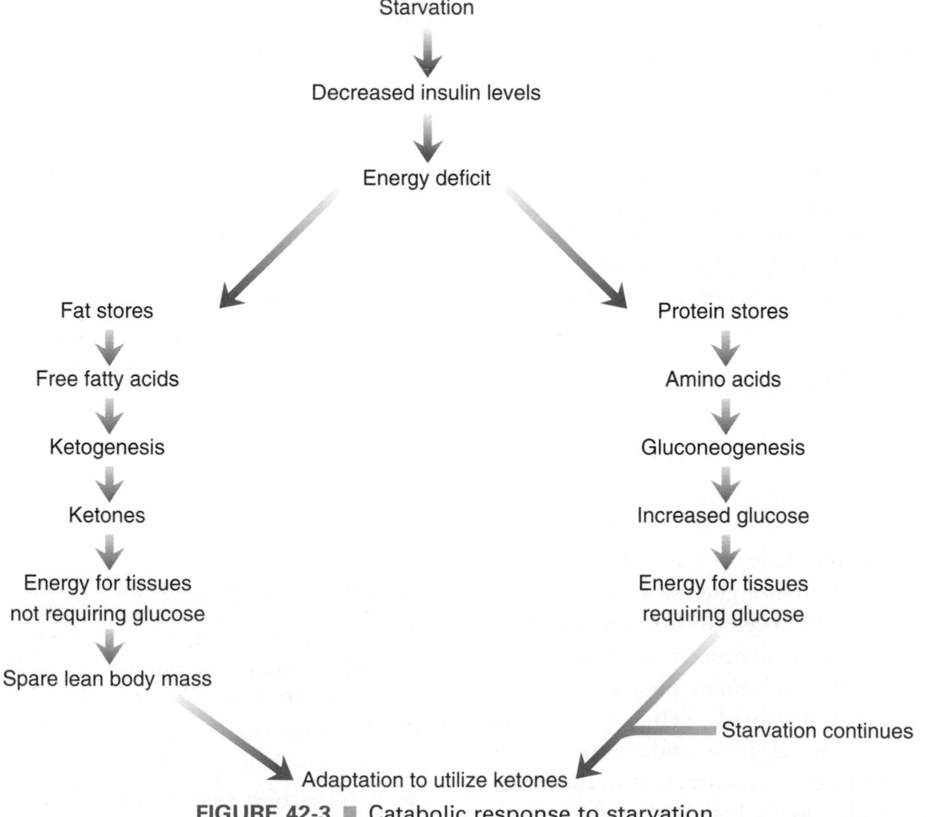

FIGURE 42-3 ■ Catabolic response to starvation.

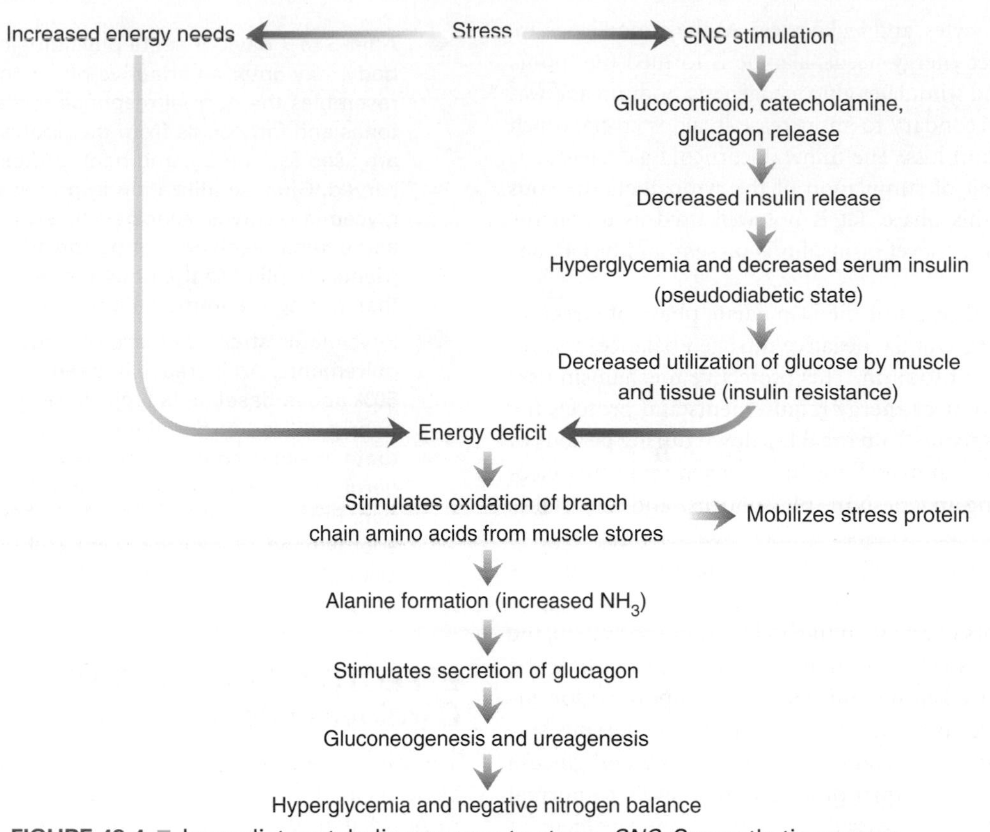

FIGURE 42-4 ■ Immediate catabolic response to stress. *SNS,* Sympathetic nervous system.

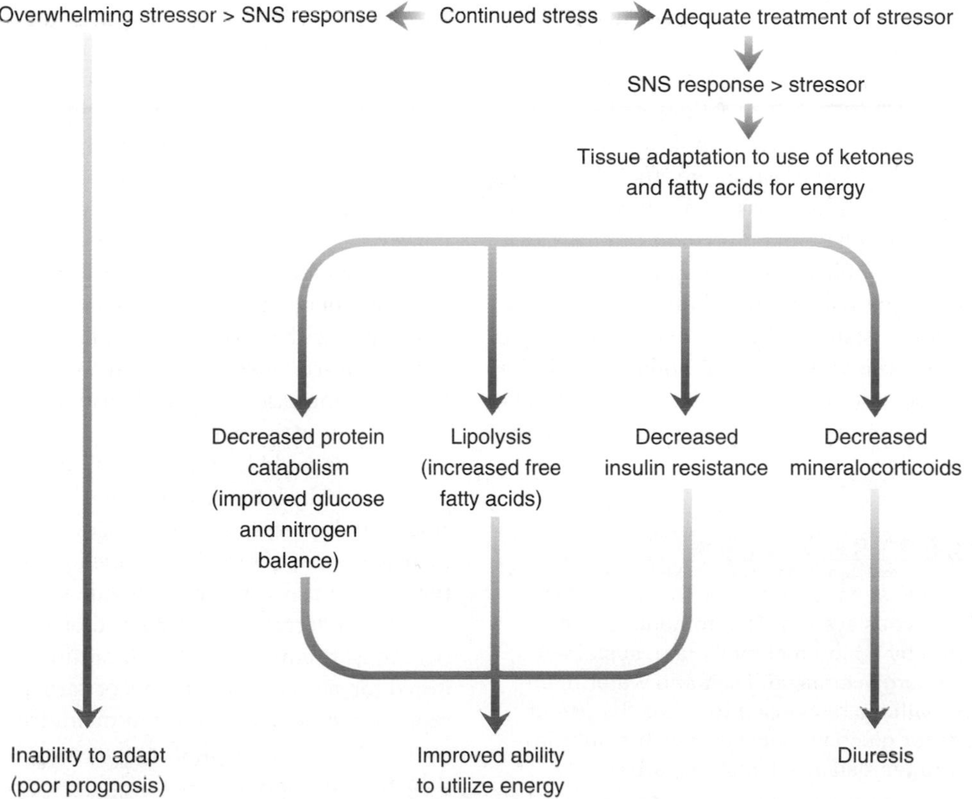

FIGURE 42-5 ■ Adaptive phase of the catabolic response to stress. *SNS,* Sympathetic nervous system.

globulins, lymphocytes, and leukocytes). As the amino acids are mobilized to meet energy needs, alanine is formed (ammonia plus pyruvate) and stimulates gluconeogenesis. Sodium and water are retained secondary to an increase in aldosterone, which results in potassium loss. The mineralocorticoid aldosterone is released as a result of stimulation of the sympathetic nervous system. During this phase, fat is not well used as an energy source because some level of insulin is present and has an antilipolytic action.

The nutritional result of the immediate phase of stress on the body is hyperglycemia, negative nitrogen balance, and retention of fluid and sodium. This protective mechanism uses skeletal muscle to meet energy requirements and protects the rest of the body's tissue from breaking down during periods of high-energy need. An overall loss of nitrogen and other electrolytes, including magnesium, phosphorus, and zinc, takes place.

The adaptive phase occurs if the sympathetic nervous system response can selectively keep up with the stressors present. If the stressors overwhelm the body's response system, the effect on prognosis will be negative. In the adaptive phase the body begins to use ketones and fatty acids (lipolysis) for energy and conserves proteins. As the sympathetic nervous system response lessens, insulin resistance decreases and glucose utilization improves. Return of aldosterone levels to normal results in diuresis. The overall result is an improvement in negative nitrogen balance as the serum glucose level improves. This phase is similar to the response of the body during starvation, when fat is used to meet energy requirements. Chronic conditions such as diabetes, liver disease, or renal disease restrict the body's ability to move into the adaptive phase during physiologic stress. Chronic system failure or inadequate support of the current disease process complicates the course of recovery. Nutritional support is used more efficiently by the body's tissue during the adaptive phase than during the immediate phase. It is in this phase that nutrition can have a vital role in recovery. The combination of starvation and a physiologic stress increases the risk for morbidity and mortality. When poor nutritional status coincides with physiologic stress, the body's response is weakened. The ability to mobilize the immune response also decreases with impaired cell-mediated immunity, humoral immunity, and alteration of the tissue barriers to infection.

KEY CONCEPTS

- Acute physiologic stress results in activation of the sympathetic nervous system. The immediate phase is characterized by a high metabolic rate, sustained catabolism, hyperglycemia, and salt and water retention. The sympathetic response promotes the use of protein stores for gluconeogenesis, which results in a negative nitrogen balance. Fat stores are poorly utilized.
- After 5 to 7 days of acute physiologic stress, the body may enter an adaptive phase that more closely resembles the normal response to starvation. Ketones and fatty acids from the lipolysis of fat stores are used for energy, and body proteins are conserved. Glucose utilization improves and hyperglycemia resolves. Aldosterone secretion diminishes and edema resolves. During the adaptive phase, nutrients supplied to the body are used more efficiently than during the immediate phase.
- Physiologic stress increases energy and protein requirements. An increase in needed calories of 20% to 50% above baseline is typical. Because glucose is poorly utilized during the immediate phase, carbohydrate intake is controlled to avoid exacerbation of hyperglycemia and excessive carbon dioxide production. Protein should supply about 16% of the total energy needs. Fats are given to fill the remaining caloric requirements. Vitamin and mineral replacement may also be required.

EFFECTS OF MALNUTRITION

Cardiovascular System

The cardiovascular system may be injured by malnutrition. Deficiencies in thiamine and selenium can cause primary myocardial disease. Protein-energy malnutrition as seen in an acutely ill patient can result in visceral protein loss and decreases in myocardial function.[16] A decrease in heart size and atrophy of cardiac muscle could result in decreased cardiac output. The increase in extracellular fluid commonly associated with physiologic stress could further compromise cardiac output. In compensation, the cardiac muscle fibers lengthen in response to increased workload. This compensation, together with a decreased oxygen demand secondary to decreased intake, curtails the development of cardiac failure. However, if the cardiac muscle is diseased, malnutrition will contribute to uncompensated heart failure.

Even though the body compensates to prevent heart failure in a malnourished patient, heart failure is common even in a healthy heart when starvation is corrected by refeeding. Refeeding increases the metabolism of the stressed state, and cardiac output is increased to meet oxygen demands. This added stress could lead to heart failure. In addition, providing a high-carbohydrate diet (RQ = 1) during the refeeding period would increase carbon dioxide production and result in increased work of breathing, which places further demand on the heart. It is necessary to provide some of the energy needs with fat to decrease the carbon dioxide production. The patient must resume feeding with caution and be carefully monitored for signs and symptoms of cardiac failure. In addition, rapid weight loss secondary to malnutrition has been associated with ventricular dysfunction and dysrhythmias, so cardiac monitoring is an essential component in the care of such patients.

Cardiac cachexia associated with chronic congestive heart failure promotes malnutrition. The mechanisms involved in cardiac cachexia are shown in Figure 42-6. A vicious cycle exists, with congestive heart failure causing malnutrition and malnutrition further contributing to the congestive heart failure.

Respiratory System

Malnutrition affects the functioning of the lungs. It decreases the structure of the lung parenchyma because the use of protein for energy reduces protein synthesis. This structural alteration can cause increased lung compliance and result in increased work of breathing.[17] Respiratory muscle function is decreased as a result of visceral protein loss, and both endurance and contractility are affected.

Malnourished patients often suffer from decreased vital capacity and respiratory muscle strength. If vital capacity and muscle strength fall below 50% of predicted norms, respiratory failure is probable owing to retention of carbon dioxide. Malnutrition also decreases the immune response in the lung. Surfactant stability is decreased, contributing to decreased lung compliance and microatelectasis. The result of an alteration in immune function and structural changes is an increase in respiratory infections. Infections develop easily and are not controlled by the protein-deficient immune system. The consequences of energy deficit in lung disease are summarized in Figure 42-7. When a patient has respiratory distress and must work harder to breathe, the caloric requirement for breathing alone can increase to 10 times normal levels. Inadequate intake and increased utilization further contribute to the effects of malnutrition on the respiratory system.

Immune System

Increased rates of infection in malnourished patients secondary to depression of the immune system and defense mechanisms are caused by nutrient deficiency. Changes in the immune system vary according to the type of nutrient lacking (Table 42-5). For example, lack of protein can impair the immune response differently from lack of other nutrients.[18] As previously mentioned, cellular immunity (delayed cutaneous hypersensitivity), which is needed for reaction to an antigen in skin testing, is often depressed in undernourished patients. In addition, the total lymphocyte count decreases. Thus the normal reaction that occurs with antigen stimulation is absent or decreased in malnutrition secondary to both decreased synthesis of immune system cells and a decrease in antibody response to stimulation (humoral immunity).

Malnutrition also causes a decrease in lymphoid mass, a decrease in circulating T and B lymphocytes, depression of phagocytic function, and a decrease in complement activity. The overall result is a decrease in resistance and an increased infection rate. In the critical care setting, the high number of invasive procedures and indwelling lines increases the potential for infection and complicates the patient's recovery.

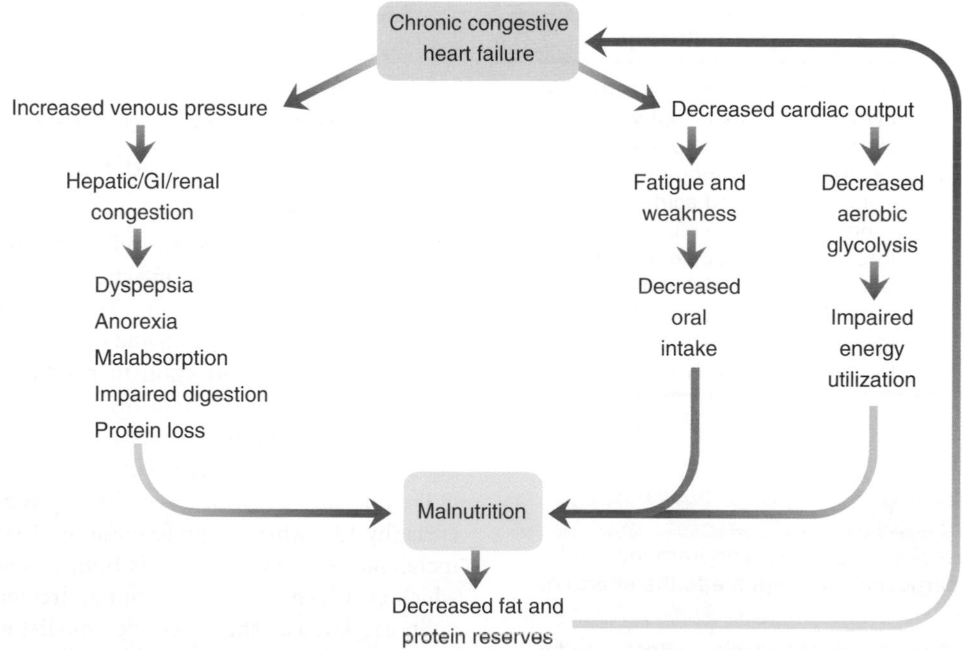

FIGURE 42-6 ■ Cyclic effect of malnutrition on chronic congestive heart failure. *GI,* Gastrointestinal.

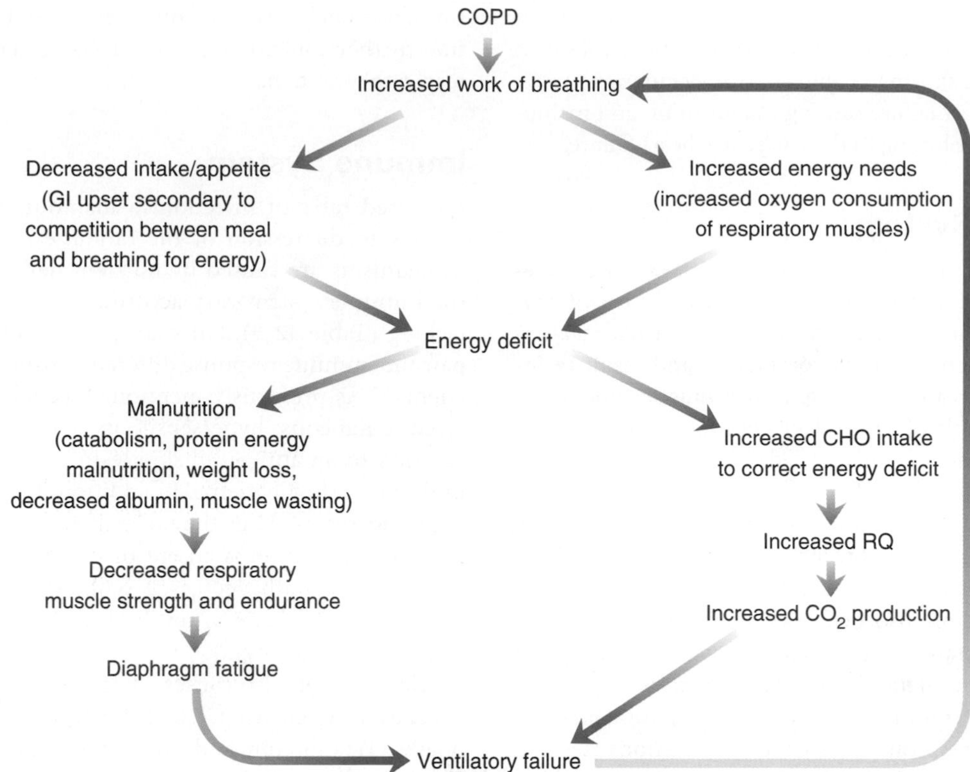

FIGURE 42-7 ■ The increased work of breathing with chronic obstructive pulmonary disease *(COPD)*. *CHO,* Carbohydrate; *RQ,* respiratory quotient; *GI,* gastrointestinal.

Table 42-5

Effects of Deficiency of Selected Nutrients on Immunity

Deficient Nutrient	Immune System Change
Vitamin C	Decreased mobility of neutrophils
Vitamin A	Lymphoid tissue atrophy
Vitamin B group	Lymphoid tissue atrophy
Amino acids	Decreased immunoglobulins, interferons, and acute phase proteins
Fatty acids	Impaired lymphocyte function
Iron	Decreased bacterial activity of phagocytes
Zinc	Lymphoid tissue atrophy
Selenium	Decreased antibody production

KEY CONCEPTS

- The cardiovascular, respiratory, and immune systems are particularly susceptible to the effects of malnutrition.
- Cardiac atrophy and reduced cardiac output may be associated with heart failure, particularly during refeeding, which increases the myocardial workload.
- Respiratory muscle atrophy and fatigue and deficient surfactant production impair effective respiration.
- Immune system depression is associated with an increased risk of infection.

NUTRITIONAL REQUIREMENTS OF ALTERED HEALTH STATES

Infection, Sepsis, and Fever

A complex interaction exists between the development of infection, the immune system, and nutritional intake.[19] Malnutrition contributes to the infectious process by directly depressing the immune system. This depression impairs the patient's defense mechanism and opens a path for infection to develop unchecked. Infection then potentiates malnutrition through a variety of mechanisms.

Fever is a common symptom accompanying infection. Fever increases metabolic needs by 7% for each 1° F increase (13% for each 1° C increase). Energy requirements can increase by 40% when a high fever (above 104° F) is present. The metabolic response to fever is both anabolic and catabolic, which greatly increases nutrient requirements.

It is known that peptide mediators stimulated by macrophages initiate the metabolic alterations associated with infection. The mediator-stimulated response is summarized in Figure 42-8. This process is complex, with the need for pro-

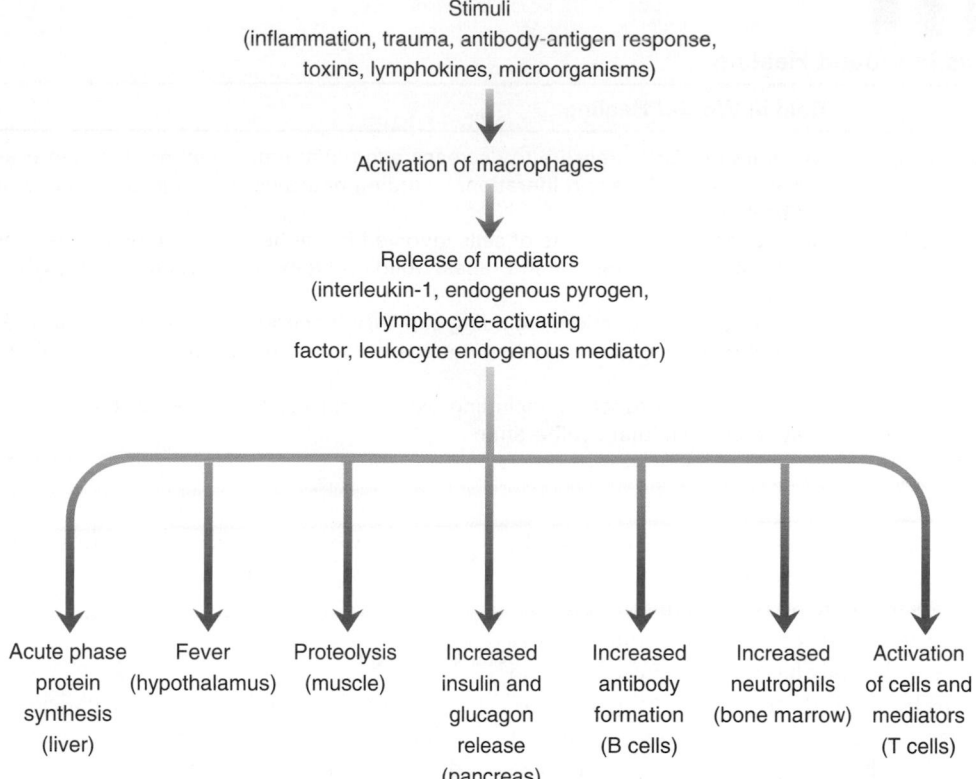

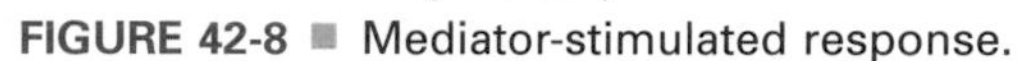
Stimuli
(inflammation, trauma, antibody-antigen response, toxins, lymphokines, microorganisms)
Activation of macrophages
Release of mediators
(interleukin-1, endogenous pyrogen, lymphocyte-activating factor, leukocyte endogenous mediator)
Acute phase protein synthesis (liver)
Fever (hypothalamus)
Proteolysis (muscle)
Increased insulin and glucagon release (pancreas)
Increased antibody formation (B cells)
Increased neutrophils (bone marrow)
Activation of cells and mediators (T cells)

FIGURE 42-8 ■ Mediator-stimulated response.

tein synthesis requiring the availability of amino acids.[20] Although catabolism may be detrimental in some aspects, it is also a protective mechanism that provides needed substrates for activation of the immune response to infection. Nutritional support is often aimed at decreasing catabolism, but it is also important to provide substrate (amino acids) for the protective mechanisms that catabolism supports.

Infection is a stressor that increases energy expenditure as a result of fever, increased immune cell demand, and catabolism. The body's metabolic response to the infection is to increase available glucose. Often the demand is too great for the body to manage; for example, sepsis can increase energy expenditure 20% to 60% above basal energy requirements. Nutritional support is needed to supply additional energy and the necessary substrates so that body stores are not totally depleted.

Surgery

Adequate nutrition before and after surgery promotes wound healing, prevents infection, and decreases complications and mortality. A patient should be in the best nutritional condition possible before surgery.[21] A common cause of malnutrition in postoperative patients is starvation. The combination of poor presurgical nutrition and postoperative starvation may increase complications after surgery, such as separation of the layers of the surgical wound. Obesity, malnutrition, and dehydration are among the causes of this serious postoperative problem.

Nutritional needs in the postoperative period depend on the extent and type of surgery, as well as the presurgical nutritional status. The postoperative energy requirement can increase from 10% to 35% above BMR. Frequently, postoperative oral intake is delayed in critically ill patients well beyond the return of bowel function. This combination of increased need with decreased intake can have a major impact on wound healing. The functions of various nutrients in wound healing have long been established and are listed in Table 42-6. In addition, nitrogen loss through wounds can be large and create a greater need for increased protein intake. Protein intake sufficient to replace losses and promote anabolism will be required, together with nonprotein calories for energy requirements. As with every patient, individual assessment and determination of exact needs are required.

Trauma

The general catabolic response to stress is also seen in trauma patients.[22] Energy expenditure is increased by 15% to 30%. Increased carbohydrate intake will be needed, but nurses must watch for complications of high carbohydrate intake. Nitrogen loss secondary to catabolism and to cellular damage can be high. Circulating hormones in the immediate phase have an antiinsulin effect that decreases glucose utilization;

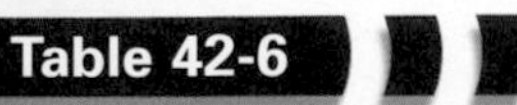

Role of Nutrients in Wound Healing

Nutrient	Role in Wound Healing
Proteins (amino acids and albumin)	Maintain osmotic pressure to decrease edema; maintain cell-mediated immune responses; cellular proliferation, including neurovascular components, lymphocytes, and fibroblasts
Carbohydrates (glucose)	Meet energy requirements of cells involved in the healing process and prevention of infection
Fats (essential fatty acids)	Components of cellular membranes; building blocks for prostaglandins, which regulate cellular function
Vitamins	Roles in cellular function, including capillary function and formation, enzyme cofactors, immune cell function, clotting mechanism, calcium and phosphorus metabolism, collagen synthesis
Minerals	Roles in cellular function, including oxygen transport, immune cell function, collagen synthesis, cellular proliferation

therefore, gluconeogenesis is increased to meet energy needs. As with other stress states, the catabolism of protein provides a source of amino acids for acute phase protein synthesis. Because trauma is a sudden stress, catabolism is much greater than anabolism because the body has not had enough time to replenish the proteins lost. This dominance of catabolism results in excessive negative nitrogen balance and significant loss of skeletal muscle, which is a problem in posttrauma rehabilitation.

With other forms of physiologic stress, fatty acids cannot be used as a source of energy. In trauma patients, however, it is thought that fatty acids can be used because of extremely high levels of catecholamines, which mobilize fat through the stimulation of lipases. In addition, if glycogen stores are intact, an initial source of glucose and free fatty acids is available. Glucose utilization is maintained in trauma patients, so glucose is an effective source of energy during the immediate phase. These differences in the nutritional effect of physiologic stress on trauma patients stem from both the suddenness of the stress and the usually healthy state of such patients before admission.

Burns

A burn is an extreme physiologic stressor that results in significant hypermetabolism.[23] In addition, the destruction of skin increases energy expenditure through evaporative heat loss. The energy needs of a burn patient increase 50% to 100% from the basal metabolic requirement. Because of individual variations such as preburn nutritional status, other physiologic stresses present, activity level, stage of burn, and age, indirect calorimetry is the best method for determination of individual needs.

As with other stressors, negative nitrogen balance is increased by catabolism and by the use of amino acids to form stress proteins. In addition, burn wounds directly contribute to protein loss. Fatty acids are also increased in response to the release of stress hormones and breakdown of lipoproteins. The ability of burn patients to use this available energy source in the immediate phase is unclear.

Cancer

An increasing number of cancer patients receive support in critical care units over periods of marked physiologic stress during treatment. The nutritional effects of cancer can be severe and result in what is commonly termed **cancer cachexia.**[24] Cachexia is associated with the end stage of cancer but can also develop earlier. The cause of cachexia is a decrease in nutritional intake relative to energy requirements. It results in significant weight loss, muscle weakness, and anorexia. A major cause of cachexia is anorexia associated with the malignancy and with the treatment. Sensory changes such as changes in smell or taste may be associated with cancer treatment and malnutrition. These changes can contribute significantly to the anorexia experienced during cancer treatment. Thus cancer patients often enter the critical care environment with mild to severe malnutrition.

Beyond the anorexia and sensory changes, abnormalities of intermediate metabolism in cancer promote tissue loss. The normal response to decreased intake is a decreased resting metabolic rate. Abnormalities in substrate metabolism in cancer patients increase total energy expenditure and raise the resting metabolic rate. The tumor also requires energy for growth, often using anaerobic metabolism, which increases lactic acid production and promotes an increase in gluconeogenesis. The metabolism of vitamins, minerals, and enzymes is also thought to be altered. Because both nutrient intake and substrate metabolism are altered, nutritional support is difficult to achieve and frequently ineffective in reversing the existing cachexia.

Immobility

The main nutritional effect of partial or total immobility is loss of calcium from nonstressed bone, a process that can elevate serum calcium and phosphorus levels. This demineralization is best managed with weight-bearing as early as possible rather than calcium supplementation. A physical therapist should be consulted early to assist in prevention of demineralization. Because negative calcium balance can increase in a catabolic state, serum calcium levels must be monitored and abnormalities treated.

A second effect of immobilization is nitrogen loss as tissue mass is decreased from disuse atrophy. This loss can total 2 to 3 g/kg per day and require up to 10 to 15 g of protein to replenish the daily loss, which further emphasizes the need for early physical therapy and aggressive range-of-motion exercises.

KEY CONCEPTS

- Infection is associated with fever and an increased metabolic rate. For each 1° F increase in body temperature, metabolic needs increase 7%. The synthesis of acute phase proteins and immune factors requires sufficient amino acid substrates.
- A major nutritional problem in postoperative patients is starvation. In addition, nitrogen loss through wounds may be significant.
- Major trauma is associated with a 15% to 30% increase in energy expenditure. Glucose utilization is maintained. Trauma victims are usually in good nutritional health before admission.
- Major burns are extreme physiologic stressors that result in an increase in energy expenditure of 50% to 100% above baseline. Protein loss from burned areas is high.
- Cancer cachexia is a result of several factors, including anorexia, poor intake, and nutrient utilization by tumor cells.
- Immobility is associated with muscle atrophy and bone demineralization.

SUMMARY

Metabolism is a dynamic and continuous process affecting every organ and physiologic process in the human system. The building phase of anabolic metabolism occurs concurrently with the energy-consuming and tearing-down phase of catabolic metabolism. Phases of metabolism either release or require energy in the form of ATP. The rate at which metabolism occurs in the resting human system is referred to as the basal metabolic rate, and the process releases both heat and energy. The metabolic fate of carbohydrate, protein, and fat depends on cellular needs and systemic regulatory functions. The endocrine system greatly affects metabolism. Only one hormone, insulin, is known to lower serum glucose levels by decreasing liver glucose production and promoting the transfer of glucose into cells. Although each works in a unique manner, growth hormone, cortisol, epinephrine, thyroid hormone, and glucagon all work in concert to maintain or raise blood glucose levels.

Physiologic stress is accompanied by changes in metabolism that alter nutrient utilization and increase nutrient requirements. The degree to which these changes occur varies with the type and severity of the particular stress. If the patient is not provided with adequate nutrition when one or more stressors are present, the hypermetabolism, hypercatabolism, and negative nitrogen balance associated with the physiologic stress will have detrimental effects on recovery.

Health care professionals must be aware of the impact of stressors on the nutritional status of the body, as well as the impact of nutrition on the well-being of body systems. If this point is well understood, appropriate interventions can be taken to prevent some of the complications that can develop when nutritional support is inadequate. Most well-nourished patients can tolerate a short period of inadequate intake (about 5 days) without untoward effects. However, critically ill patients require early nutritional support because of the magnitude and intensity of the stressors. Identification of the various risk factors and the nutritional needs of patients is an essential part of nursing care for critically ill patients. Overfeeding of patients is also to be avoided because specific complications can develop with inappropriate nutritional support. Nurses must also understand nutritional interventions in critical care so that decisions regarding nutritional support for the patient can be based on specific nutritional assessments and knowledge of individual needs.

MEDIA RESOURCES

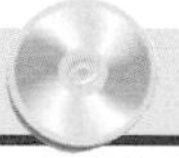

evolve

Remember to check out the ***CD Companion*** included with this book for Review Questions, Key Concepts Review, Glossary (with audio for selected terms), Disease Profiles, and Animations.

PLUS, visit the ***Evolve website*** at http://evolve.elsevier.com/Copstead/ for Case Studies, Disease Profiles, and WebLinks.

References

1. Keesey RE: Physiological regulation of body weight and the issue of obesity, *Med Clin North Am* 73(1):15-27, 1989.
2. Vander AJ, Sherman JH, Luciano DJ: *Human physiology: the mechanisms of body function,* ed 7, New York, 1998, McGraw-Hill.
3. Mahan LK, Escott-Stump S, Mahan K: *Krause's food, nutrition, and diet therapy,* ed 9, Philadelphia, 1996, Saunders.
4. Guyton AC, Hall JE: *Textbook of medical physiology,* ed 9, Philadelphia, 1996, Saunders.
5. Hershman JM: *Endocrine pathophysiology: a patient-oriented approach,* ed 3, Philadelphia, 1987, Lea & Febiger.
6. Ignatavicius DD, Workman ML, Mishler MA: *Medical-surgical nursing: a nursing process approach,* ed 2, Philadelphia, 1995, Saunders.
7. Bray GA: Nutrient balance and obesity: an approach to control of food intake in humans, *Med Clin North Am* 73(1):29-45, 1989.

8. Tepperman J, Tepperman HM: *Metabolic and endocrine physiology,* ed 5, Chicago, 1987, Year Book.
9. Mirtallo JM: Nutrient metabolism in health and disease. In DiPiro JT, Talbert RL, Yee GC, editors: *Pharmacotherapy: a pathophysiologic approach,* ed 3, Stanford, Conn, 1996, Appleton & Lange, pp 1151-1570.
10. Griffin JE, Ojeda SR: *Textbook of endocrine physiology,* ed 3, Oxford, 1996, Oxford University Press.
11. Klein S et al: Lipolytic response to metabolic stress in critically ill patients, *Crit Care Med* 19(6):776-779, 1991.
12. Bennett JC, Plum F: *Cecil textbook of medicine,* ed 20, Philadelphia, 1996, WB Saunders.
13. Ziegler TR et al: Metabolic effects of recombinant human growth hormone in patients receiving parenteral nutrition, *Ann Surg* 208(1):6-16, 1988.
14. MacLennan WJ, Peden NR: *Metabolic and endocrine problems in the elderly,* London, 1989, Springer-Verlag.
15. Kinney J, Weissman C: Forms of malnutrition in stressed and unstressed patients, *Clin Chest Med* 7(1):19-28, 1986.
16. Webb JG, Kiess MC, Chan-Yan CC: Malnutrition and the heart, *Can Med Assoc J* 135(7):753-758, 1986.

17. Openbrier D, Covey M: Ineffective breathing pattern related to malnutrition, *Nurs Clin North Am* 22(1):225-247, 1987.
18. Beisel W: Role of nutrition in immune system diseases, *Compr Ther* 13(1):13-19, 1987.
19. Keusch G, Farthing M: Nutrition and infection, *Annu Rev Nutr* 6:131-154, 1986.
20. Pomposelli J: Role of biochemical mediators in clinical nutrition and surgical metabolism, *JPEN J Parenter Enteral Nutr* 12(2):212-218, 1988.
21. Bellanton R: Preoperative parenteral nutrition in the high risk surgical patient, *JPEN J Parenter Enteral Nutr* 12(2):115-121, 1988.
22. Anderson B: The metabolic needs of head trauma victims, *J Neurosci Nurs* 19(4):211-215, 1987.
23. Lang CE: *Nutritional support in critical care,* Gaithersburg, MD, 1987, Aspen.
24. Kern K, Norton J: Cancer cachexia, *JPEN J Parenter Enteral Nutr* 12(3):286-298, 1988.

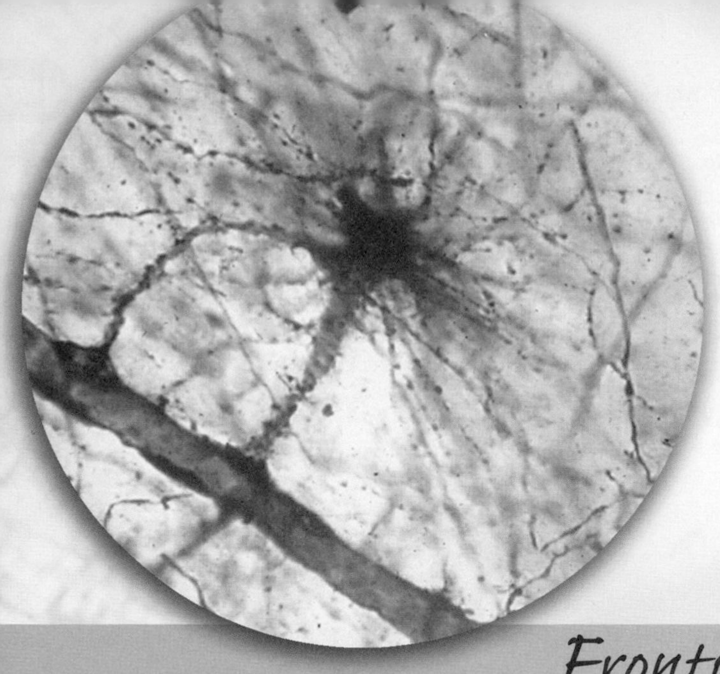

Frontiers of Research

Pain and Its Control

Timothy A. Harbst and Michael J. Kirkhorn

Through the sensation of pain, the brain monitors the body's organs and sounds the alarm when something goes wrong. Responding to complicated signaling processes, the brain also provides relief from pain.

Pain is pervasive in the United States. One estimate suggests that nearly one third of the population has some form of chronic pain not associated with malignancy. Cancer offers its own peculiar challenges because it often causes sharp and lasting pain. As cancer advances in the body, pain becomes more severe. Cancer patients are not the only ones who suffer pain that is difficult or impossible to endure without assistance. Women experience intense pain during childbirth, and burn patients nearly always experience severe pain. More than half of a sample of medical-surgical patients said that they experienced "excruciating" pain.

When Dr. Hans A. Kosterlitz was living the last years of his life in Aberdeen, Scotland, he might have found satisfaction in a great accomplishment paralleled in few careers: he had helped untold millions of people in coming generations find relief from pain.

Kosterlitz, who died in 1996 at the age of 93 years, was working in relative obscurity when in 1975, with colleague John Hughes, he identified the small opiatelike proteins in the brain that suggested the possibility that pain might be controlled through natural processes without resort to potentially addictive opiates.

Kosterlitz and Hughes were building on a foundation laid by discoveries made by other researchers. Only 2 years before, researchers at Johns Hopkins University, New York University, and Uppsala University had reported that brain cells had receptors that might accommodate opiates like morphine. Why would the brain have these receptors? How had they evolved? Researchers had to assume that the receptors were there to interact with endogenous molecules.

From earlier work, Kosterlitz already knew that the potency of opiatelike chemicals depended on their ability to inhibit the contractions of muscle tissues. The University of Aberdeen scientists studied pig brains for opiate activity and isolated two enkephalins, small pain-reducing proteins. The larger brain chemical molecules, or endorphins, which have since been found in humans and other mammals, all contain one of the enkephalins found in Kosterlitz's laboratory. Kosterlitz also learned that there are different kinds of opiate receptors. One might relieve pain and another cause addiction.

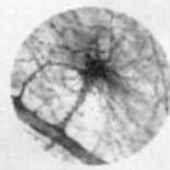

Astrocytes. Glia cells found throughout the central nervous system in both gray and white matter. (From Kumar V, Abbas AK, Fausto N: Robins and Cotran pathologic basis of disease, *ed 7, Philadelphia, 2005, Saunders, p 1350. Courtesy Dr. J. Corbo, Brigham and Women's Hospital, Boston.)*

Neural Function

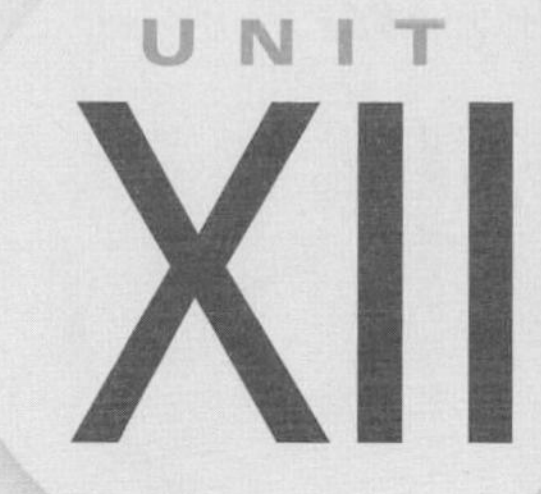

Researchers study pain not only to relieve it but also because it is a useful diagnostic tool. The body senses danger in its external as well as internal environment with a network of pain receptors—free nerve endings—in the skin and in certain internal tissues. When they are stimulated, pain impulses move along two separate paths from the dorsal spinal roots into the spinal cord to various destinations in the brain. When the signals reach their destinations, the outcome is clear: we hurt, we know how much, and except in the case of "referred pain," we know precisely where and when the pain occurs. However, the brain's response is more than an alarm: the brain controls pain as well.

Pain control resides in the brain's analgesia system—a complex network capable of controlling the input of pain signals to the nervous system by blocking pain signals at their entry point to the spinal cord and by blocking other reflexes triggered by pain signals. The analgesia system and other areas of the brain have opiate receptors, which also dull pain. Researchers do not entirely understand the brain's intricate opiate system, but it is clear that activation of the analgesia system either by nervous signals entering the periaqueductal gray area of the brainstem or by the administration of morphinelike drugs suppresses many pain signals.

The study of pain management is a relatively new science and, as yet, not far advanced. In the past, health care professionals were at times unable to control pain. Today, thanks to improved understanding, all or nearly all pain is treatable.

Unfortunately, pain management continues to be hindered by a number of common misconceptions that prevent health care professionals from doing all they can to relieve pain. One recent study demonstrated that more than half of nurses surveyed did not know that the patient's report of pain is the single most reliable indicator of pain, and many nurses failed to increase the dose of opioid analgesic when a weaker dose had failed to relieve pain and caused no side effects.

Other studies indicate that physicians and nurses are misinformed about pharmacologic pain controllers and are needlessly anxious over the possibility that a patient given pain control drugs might become addicted. A survey of 2459 nurses attending pain programs revealed that only about 1 in 4 knew that the incidence of addiction to opioid analgesics was less than 1%. About the same number thought that addiction would occur in more than 25% of all cases.

chapter 43

Structure and Function of the Nervous System

Jacquelyn L. Banasik

MEDIA RESOURCES

Additional Material for Study, Review, and Further Exploration

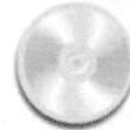

CD Companion ◆ Review Questions and Answers ◆ Key Concepts Review ◆ Glossary *(with audio pronunciations for selected terms)* ◆ Disease Profiles ◆ Animations

evolve ***Website*** at http://evolve.elsevier.com/Copstead/
◆ Case Studies ◆ Disease Profiles ◆ WebLinks

KEY QUESTIONS

- How do the central nervous system (CNS), peripheral nervous system, and autonomic nervous system interrelate?
- How is the CNS protected and supported?
- What structures are located in each of the four principal areas of the brain: cerebrum, diencephalon, cerebellum, and brainstem?
- What neurologic functions have been mapped to particular locations in the brain?
- How do the properties of neuronal action potentials and neuronal communication through synapses relate to the functions of the nervous system?
- How is the somatotopic organization of sensory receptors and muscles maintained in the CNS?
- How do the properties of the mind, including, thought, memory, learning, consciousness, and sleep, relate to the physiologic substance of the nervous system?

CHAPTER OUTLINE

The nervous system is a complex network of neurons and supportive cells that enables rapid communication between sensory receptors, central processing neurons, and functional responses. Much has been discovered about the mechanisms of sensory input and motor output, but the physiologic bases of thought, consciousness, emotion, and learning remain elusive. The idea that the mind is within the biological realm has only recently been generally accepted, although the effects of mind-altering drugs on emotions, appetite, sleep, thought, and sensory perception have long been recognized. Research continues to reveal the great complexity of neurologic function. A bewildering array of neurotransmitter signaling molecules and an even greater number of neurotransmitter receptors have been identified. Recently, the long-held notion that neurons cannot regenerate in the mature brain has been disproved and neuronal stem cells have been identified in certain areas. Each discovery brings us closer to understanding neural physiologic processes and gives hope for finding effective therapies for the devastating diseases that affect them. This chapter provides an overview of neural structure and function and is the basis for understanding the neurologic disorders in the chapters that follow.

STRUCTURAL ORGANIZATION

The nervous system is traditionally divided into three principal anatomic units: the central nervous system (CNS), the peripheral nervous system (PNS), and the autonomic nervous system (ANS). These systems are not anatomically or functionally distinct, and they work together as an integrated whole. Therefore, when function, rather than anatomy, is the topic of concern, the nervous system is more conveniently divided into the sensory, motor, and higher brain functions. This chapter begins with a review of the major anatomic features of the nervous system, then addresses neurologic function at the cellular and synaptic level, and concludes with a summary of sensory, motor, and cognitive functions.

CENTRAL NERVOUS SYSTEM

The CNS includes the brain and spinal cord. Its primary functions are receiving and processing sensory information and creating appropriate responses to be relayed to muscles and glands. It is the site of emotion, memory, cognition, and learning. The CNS is bathed in cerebrospinal fluid (CSF) and shielded from the periphery by the blood-brain barrier. The CNS interacts with the neurons of the PNS through synapses in the spinal cord and cranial nerve **ganglia.** The cranial and spinal nerves constitute the PNS.

Support and Protection of the Central Nervous System

Nervous tissue has the consistency of gelatin, so measures to support and protect its fragile structure are necessary. In addition, the CNS must be shielded from circulating substances that would interfere with neurotransmission. These protective functions are provided by the skull and vertebral column, meninges, CSF, and blood-brain barriers. The bony structures of the skull and vertebral column encase the brain and cord and protect them from external trauma, whereas the CSF and meninges provide buoyancy and shock-absorbing capacity.

The meninges are composed of three layers that serve to suspend and maintain the shape and position of the nervous tissue during head and body movements. The brain is suspended within layers of meninges that are fixed to the skull. In this manner, the brain turns with the movement of the skull. The CSF circulates within the subarachnoid space, giving buoyancy to the brain and making an average 1500-g structure effectively weigh 50 g.[1] The brain is thus more resistant to distortion, which could occur from gravity alone were it not for the buoyancy effect. The three meningeal layers are the *dura mater, arachnoid,* and *pia mater* (Figure 43-1).

The dura mater, the outermost meningeal layer, is a thick, tough, collagenous membrane. It is composed of two layers, one contiguous with the periosteum of the skull and the other, which is adherent to the first, covering the surface of the brain. The tough dura protects the soft tissue of the brain. Support and stability are also provided by dural septa that invaginate into the cranial cavity. The falx cerebri is a thin wall of dura that folds down the cortical midline, separating the two hemispheres (see Figure 43-1). The tentorium cerebelli is a septum

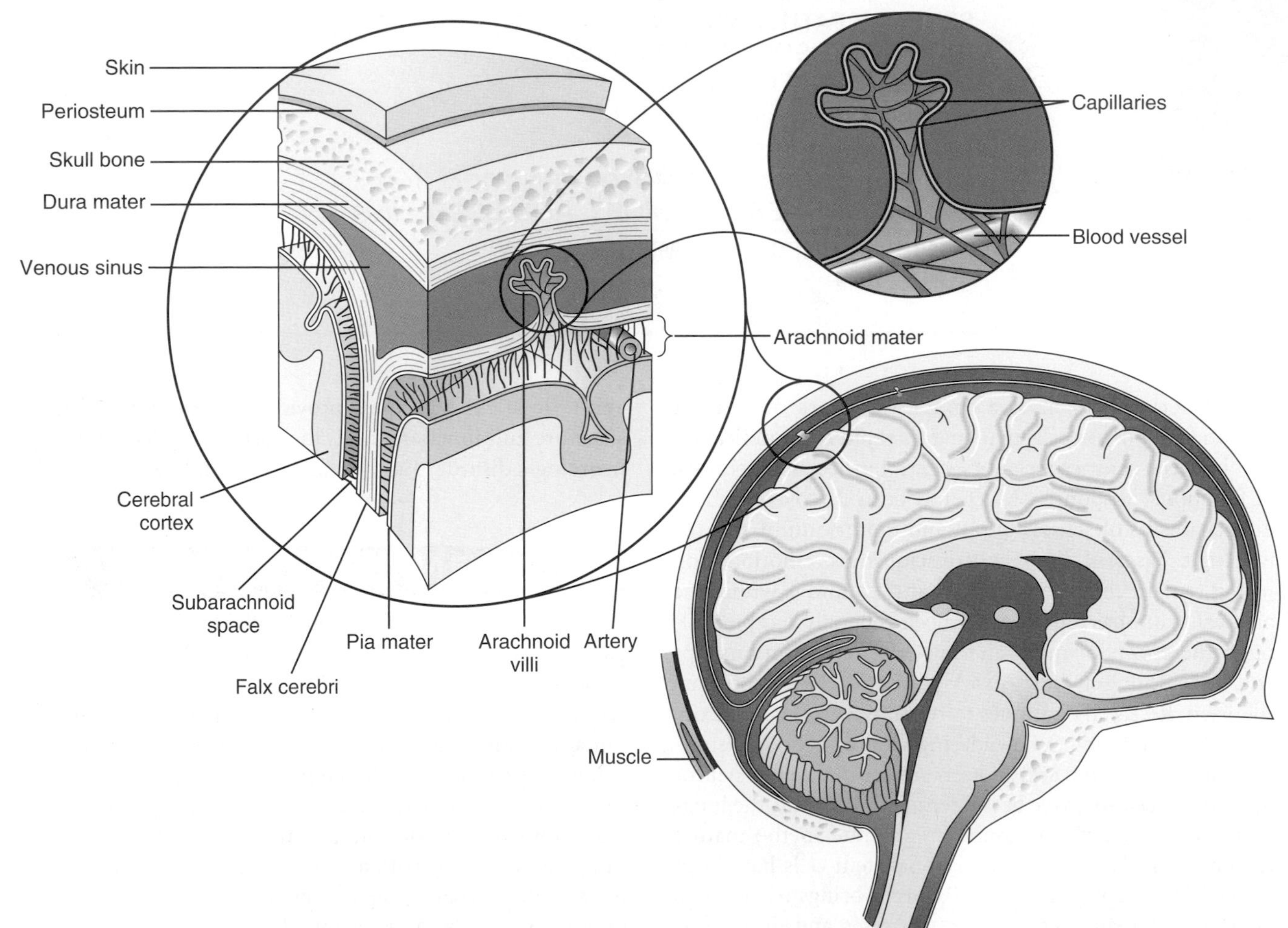

FIGURE 43-1 ■ Principal membranes of the cranial meninges. Cerebrospinal fluid flows in the subarachnoid space and is reabsorbed by arachnoid villi within the dural sinuses.

that separates the cerebellum and brainstem from the rest of the cerebrum. The dural septa fix the brain in place by their tentlike structure and limit its movement within the skull. Venous sinuses that collect venous blood from cerebral veins are located between the two layers of the dura at the base of the septum.

Beneath, and continuous with, the dura is the arachnoid layer. The spaces between the dura and the skull and between the dura mater and the arachnoid are potential spaces. Only in the presence of pathologic processes, notably epidural and subdural hemorrhages, do these spaces become evident (see Chapter 44). Unlike the dura mater, the arachnoid is a thin, delicate membrane. It is semitransparent and weblike in appearance; hence its name. From the arachnoid layer come strands of collagenous connective tissue, called *trabeculae,* that extend down to the pia mater, forming a subarachnoid space. The CSF flows in this space.

Pia mater, the third meningeal layer, is also very thin. However, unlike the other meningeal layers, the pia is attached to the brain and closely follows its contours over every **sulcus** and into every **gyrus.** Consequently, the subarachnoid space between the arachnoid and the pia mater is not evenly distributed. The arachnoid meshes with the pia via the trabeculae in such a subtle manner that it is often difficult to differentiate one from the other. Consequently, the two layers together are often referred to as the *leptomeninges.*

The meninges that cover and provide protection to the spinal cord are similar to those of the brain, with a few variations (Figure 43-2). The spinal dura, for example, has no periosteal layer, so it is a single rather than a double layer. It is

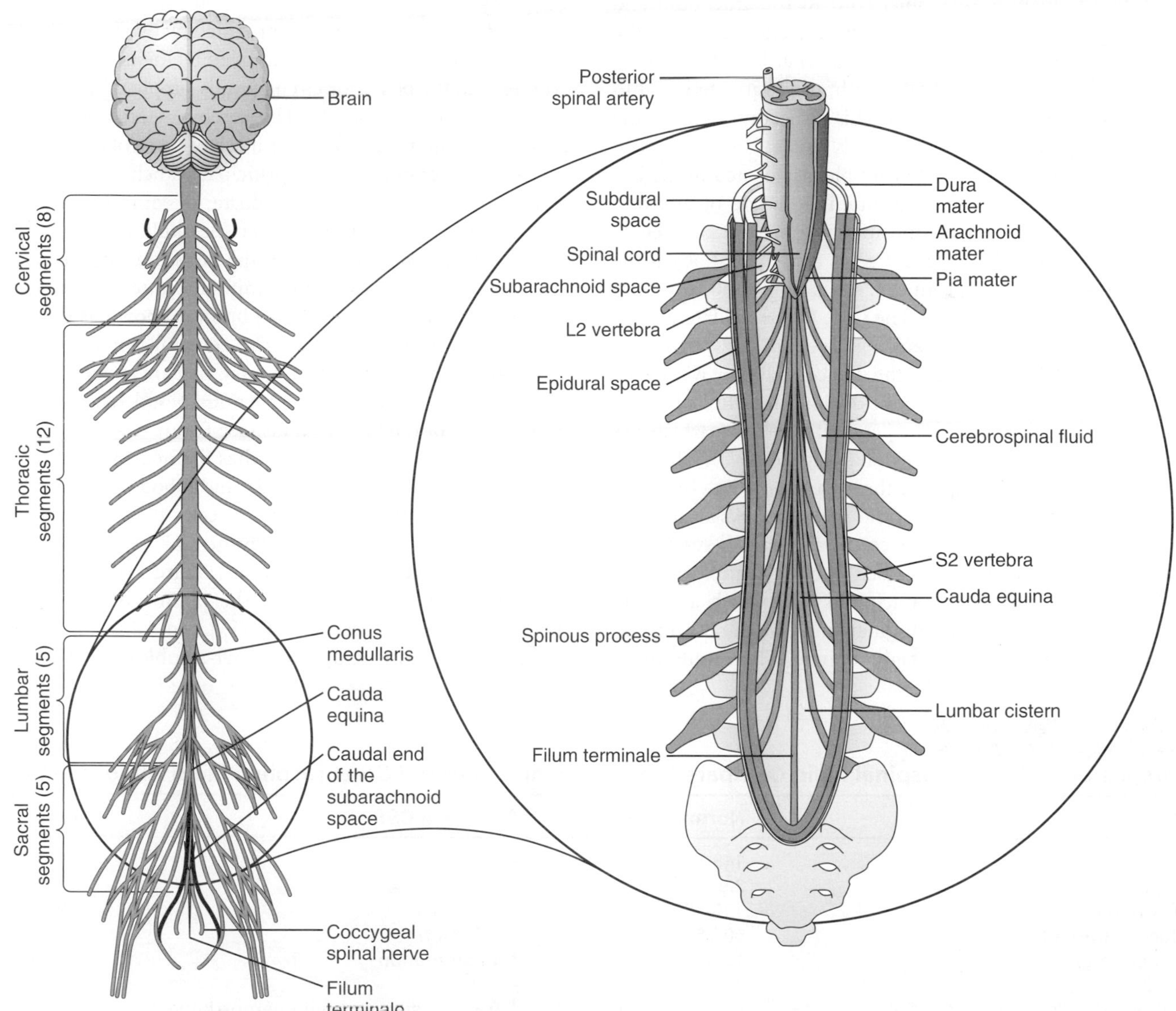

FIGURE 43-2 ■ The spinal cord, spinal nerves, and meninges. Spinal meninges are similar to cranial membranes. Spinal meninges end at S2, creating a CSF-filled cistern below the spinal cord. The cauda equina (horse tail) is formed by the lumbar and sacral nerves, which protrude from the end of the spinal cord.

continuous with the foramen magnum at the base of the skull and is separated from the spinal vertebral periosteum by an epidural space. Thus, in the spinal cord, the epidural space is a true space, unlike its counterpart in the cranium, which is only a potential space. Within this space lie fatty connective tissue and a vertebral venous plexus.

The spinal arachnoid, much like that covering the cerebrum, is closely adherent to the spinal dura. Between the arachnoid layer and the pial lining is the CSF-filled subarachnoid space. The spinal meninges end at approximately the second sacral vertebra. However, the spinal cord ends between the first and second lumbar vertebrae (L1-2). This results in a large subarachnoid cistern, called the *lumbar cistern,* which is a favored place to obtain CSF samples (see Figure 43-2). The spinal pia is much tougher and thicker than the cerebral pia. Projecting along the length of each side is the dentate ligament, which anchors the spinal cord to the arachnoid and through it to the dura. Another pial projection connects the tail of the spinal cord (the cauda equina) at level L1-2 to the **caudal** end of the spinal dural sheath, where it is tethered to the end of the vertebral column. This projection is called the *filum terminale.*

CSF is produced by the choroid plexus, located in the lateral and third ventricles of the brain, at a rate of approximately 500 ml/day.[2] The composition of normal CSF is compared to plasma in Table 43-1. CSF is absorbed at about the same rate at which it is produced, so that only 150 to 175 ml is in circulation at any time.[2] The large C-shaped lateral ventricles occupy the center of each hemisphere. They communicate with the third ventricle in the diencephalon by way of the intraventricular foramen. The third ventricle is linked to the fourth ventricle by way of the cerebral aqueduct, which lies between the pons and the medulla (Figure 43-3). The CSF flows from the fourth ventricle through the median or lateral aperture and into the subarachnoid space. It flows around the spinal cord and up over the cerebral hemispheres to the arachnoid villi, where it is absorbed into the venous system.

CSF is absorbed by the arachnoid villi, which are small tufts of the arachnoid that invaginate into the dural sinus, especially along the superior sagittal sinus. These tufts bring CSF into close approximation with venous blood. CSF flows into the venous system through one-way valves as a consequence of bulk flow or pressure gradient differences. Although the CSF flows readily into the venous sinus, flow in the opposite direction cannot occur[2]; that is, the fluid in the venous sinus cannot flow into the subarachnoid space. This mechanism is part of a system of barriers between the extracellular space in the nervous system and the rest of the body.

The rate of production of CSF is independent of blood pressure or intraventricular pressure.[2] Thus, CSF will continue to be produced even when its path of circulation or absorption is blocked. If this occurs, the amount of CSF increases, as does the size of the ventricles. This pathologic process is called **hydrocephalus.** Although hydrocephalus is usually caused by blockage of CSF pathways, it can also be caused by overproduction and malabsorption of CSF (see Chapter 45).

Blood supply to the brain is provided by two pairs of arteries; the anterior circulation is supplied by the internal carotid arteries, and the posterior circulation is supplied by the vertebral arteries (Figure 43-4). The cerebral circulation is discussed in detail in Chapter 44 as it relates to stroke. The internal carotid arteries have three principal branches: the anterior and middle cerebral arteries and posterior communicating arteries. The vertebral arteries enter the skull at the foramen magnum and join at the level of the pons to form the basilar arteries. The ring of vessels that unites the anterior and posterior circulation at the base of the brain is known as the *circle of Willis* (see Figure 43-4, *B*). The cerebral veins drain into large vascular channels, called *sinuses,* that are formed by folds in the dura. From the sinuses, venous blood returns to the heart by way of the jugular veins (see Figure 43-4, *C*).

The extracellular fluid that bathes the neurons is carefully shielded from elements in the CSF and blood by cellular barriers. Tight junctions between the cells that line the CSF spaces and brain capillaries prevent leakage of molecules through the spaces between the cells (Figure 43-5). Therefore, substances must move through the plasma membranes of these barrier cells to access the CNS. Lipid-soluble molecules move through more easily than water-soluble ones. Thus, the

Table 43-1

Composition of Cerebrospinal Fluid Compared to Plasma and Selected Cerebrospinal Fluid Abnormalities

Substance	Normal CSF	Abnormal CSF	Plasma
Na^+ (mEq/L)	148	—	136-145
K^+ (mEq/L)	2.9	—	3.5-5.0
Cl^- (mEq/L)	120-130	—	100-106
Glucose (mg/dl)	50-75	↓ Infection	70-100
Protein (mg/dl)	15-45	↑ Inflammation	6800
pH	7.3	—	7.4
Red blood cells (high-power field)	None	↑ Trauma, subarachnoid hemorrhage	—
White blood cells (high-power field)	<5	↑ Infection (e.g., meningitis)	—
Pressure (mm H_2O)	70-180	↑ Mass lesions	—

flow of ions, nutrients, drugs, proteins, and other charged or polar substances is highly restricted.[2] The blood-brain barrier is a crucial structure for protecting the brain, but it may also restrict access of beneficial molecules, such as antibiotics and cancer drugs, making treatment more difficult.

The integrity of the blood-brain barrier is maintained in part by CNS cells called astrocytes. These specialized **glial** cells have foot processes that contact the brain capillaries and are thought to help regulate transport across the capillary endothelium[3] (see Figure 43-5). The blood-brain barrier is less effective in infancy and can also be compromised by ischemia and chemical injury in adults.

A similar barrier exists between the circulating CSF and the interstitial fluid of the CNS, the CSF-brain barrier. The ependymal cells that line the ventricles are tightly joined and regulate the movement of water-soluble elements between the CSF and neurons. In addition, these cells serve the important function of removing unwanted substances from the CNS and secreting them into the CSF for eventual removal by the venous system.

Some areas of the brain have need to sample the contents of the blood or CSF more directly to make regulatory adjustments in respiratory, autonomic, or endocrine functions, and these areas therefore have more permeable barriers. These areas include the hypothalamus, pituitary, and other circumventricular organs (around the ventricles).

The Brain

Various schemes have been used to subdivide the structures of the brain using embryologic, evolutionary, and anatomic frameworks (Table 43-2). In this section, an anatomic framework is used that includes the cerebrum, diencephalon, cerebellum, and brainstem (Figure 43-6).

Cerebrum

The cerebrum is divided into left and right hemispheres by the longitudinal fissure and is the largest part of the brain. The cerebral cortex is the outermost layer of the cerebrum and is composed of gray matter arranged in six histologically distinct layers[4] (Figure 43-7). Each of the six layers makes connections with other parts of the brain. The cortex is characterized by its convoluted exterior having ridges (gyri), grooves

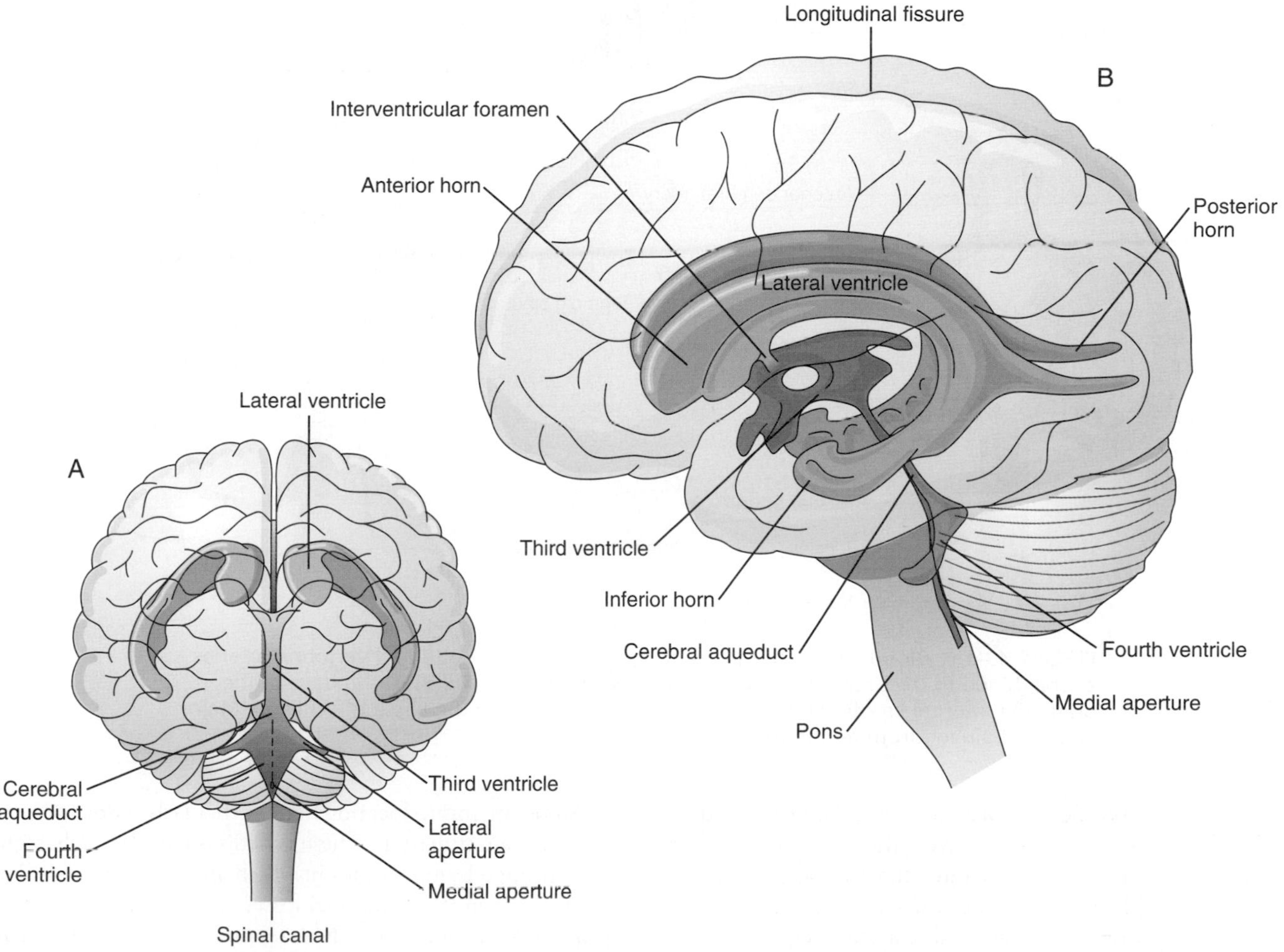

FIGURE 43-3 ■ The ventricles within the brain from frontal **(A)** and lateral **(B)** views.

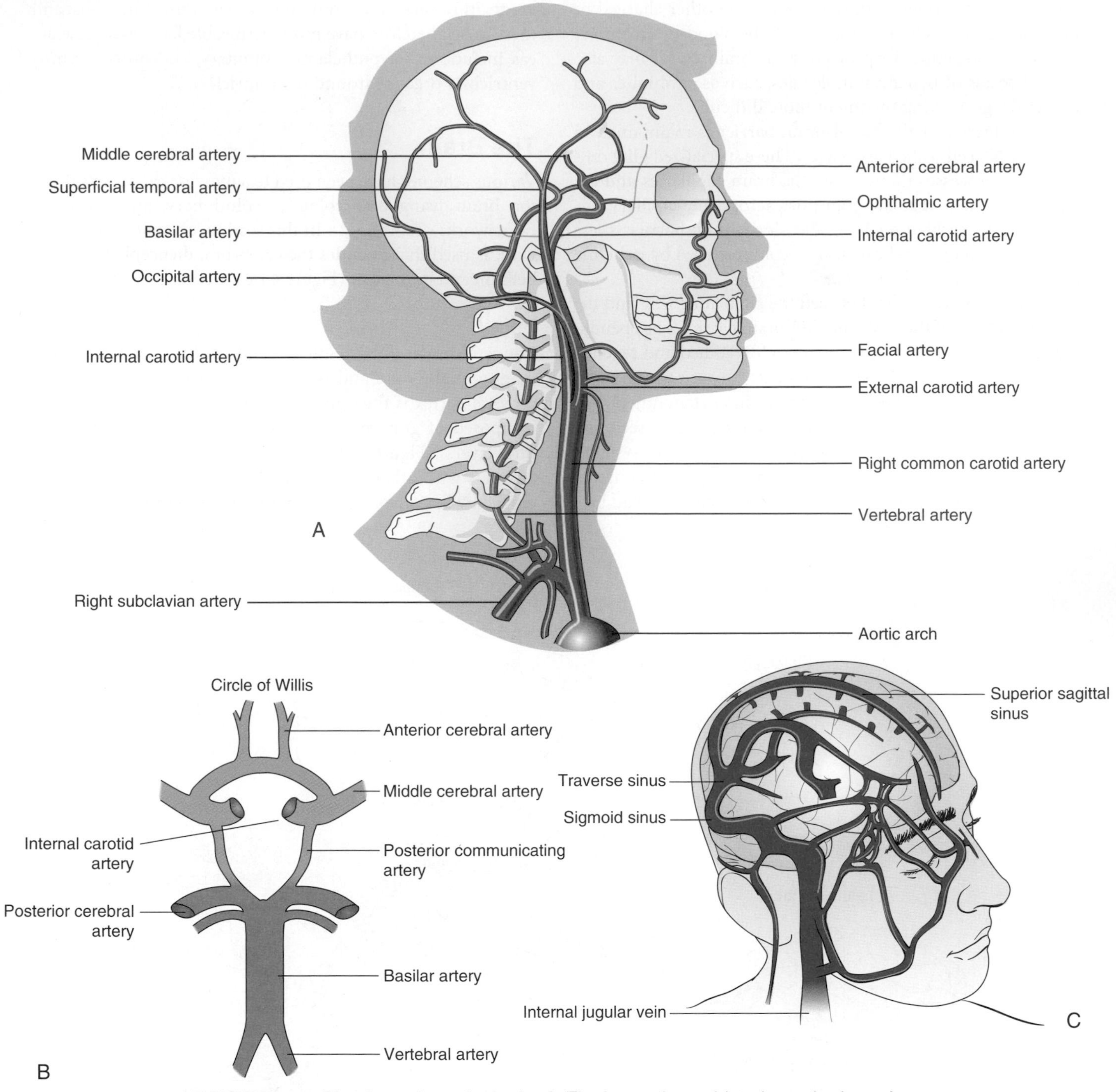

FIGURE 43-4 ■ Blood supply to the brain. **A,** The internal carotid and vertebral arteries supply blood to the anterior and posterior aspects of the brain. **B,** At the base of the brain, the internal carotid and vertebral arteries join to form the circle of Willis. **C,** Major venous drainage from the brain.

(sulci), and deeper depressions (fissures). The sulci and fissures are used as landmarks to divide the cerebral cortex into lobes. The central sulcus separates the frontal and parietal lobes, the lateral sulcus separates the temporal lobe from the parietal and frontal lobes, and the parieto-occipital line defines the occipital lobe (Figure 43-8).

Some anatomic locations are particularly associated with certain brain functions. These functions have been characterized through lesion studies in which an area of brain is damaged and then the functional losses studied, and by mapping procedures during which the cerebral cortex is stimulated and responses are recorded. Functional specialization of brain loci

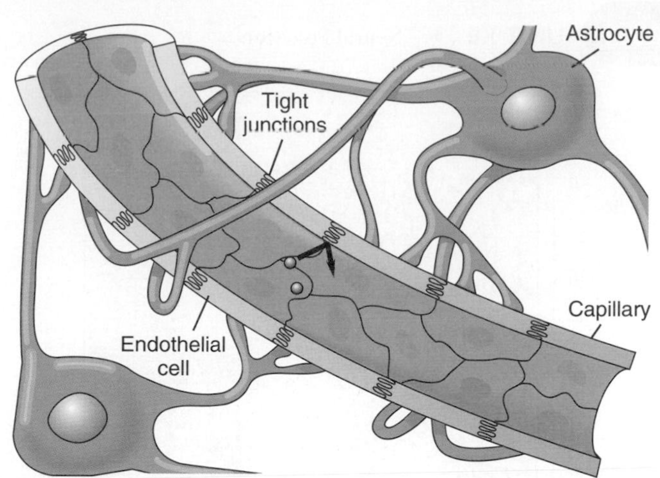

FIGURE 43-5 ■ Tight junctions between brain capillary endothelial cells prevent polar and charged molecules from passing between cells. Astrocytes have foot processes on the capillary that help to maintain integrity of the blood-brain barrier.

Table 43-2

Subdivisions of the Brain Using Embryologic, Evolutionary, and Anatomic Frameworks

	Framework		
Structure	**Embryologic**	**Evolutionary**	**Anatomic**
Cerebral hemisphere	Telencephalon	Forebrain (includes diencephalon)	Cerebrum
Thalamus, hypothalamus	Diencephalon	—	Diencephalon
Midbrain	Mesencephalon	Midbrain	—
Cerebellum	Metencephalon (includes pons)	Cerebellum	Cerebellum
Medulla	Myelencephalon	Hindbrain	Brainstem (includes midbrain, pons)

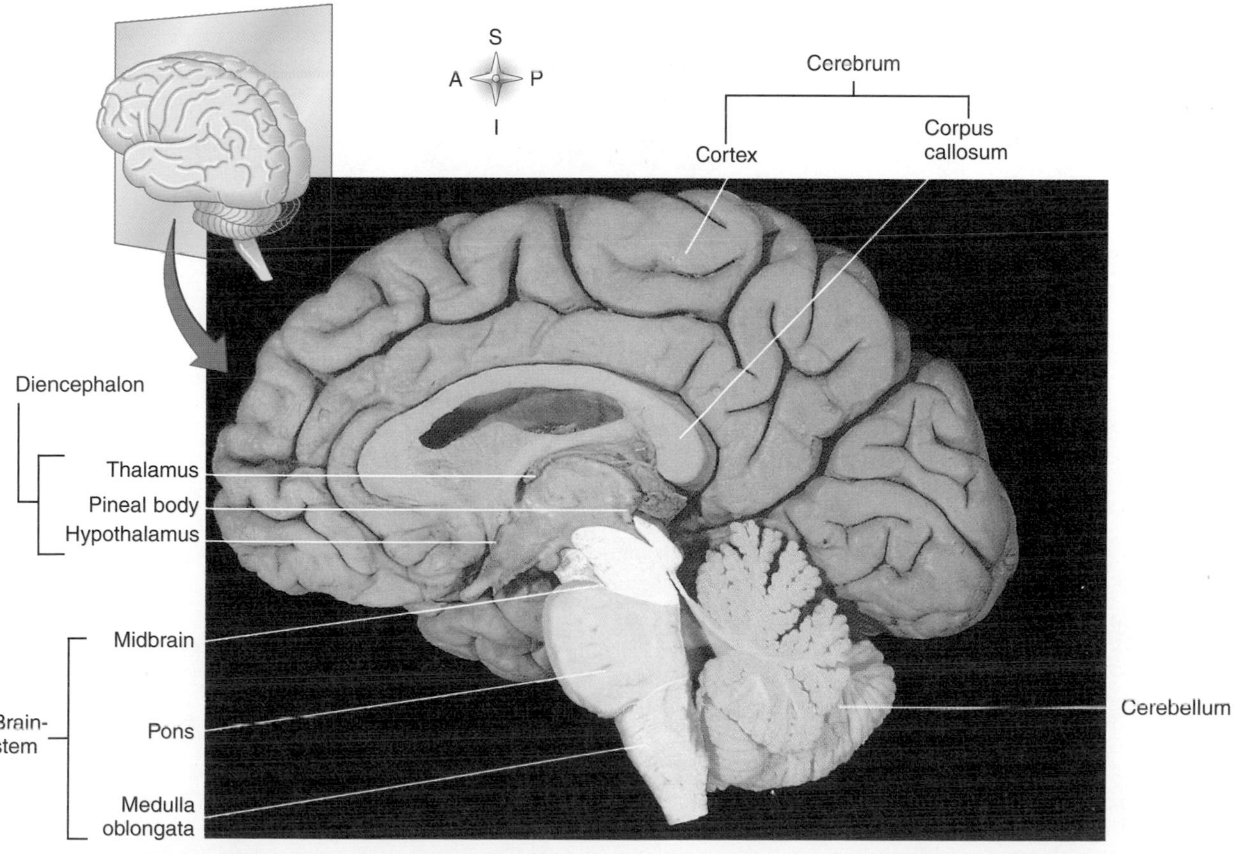

FIGURE 43-6 ■ The four principal anatomic areas of the brain. (From Thibodeau GA, Patton KT: *Anatomy and physiology,* ed 5, St Louis, 2003, Mosby, p 384.)

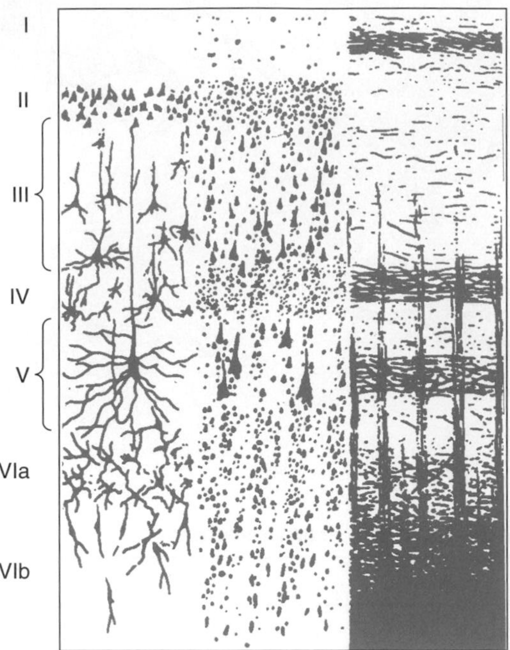

FIGURE 43-7 ■ The cortex of the brain is histologically divided into six layers, which differ in their connections to other parts of the nervous system. (From Ransom and Clark [after Brodmann]: *Anatomy of the nervous system,* Philadelphia, 1959, Saunders.)

are listed in Table 43-3. A partial map of Brodmann areas is shown in Figure 43-9. Although the concept of functional anatomic areas is clinically useful, one should realize that even though an area may be critical for a particular function, it is not wholly responsible for that function, and many brain areas may be involved. A certain degree of reassignment of brain function from one area to another can occur, allowing the brain to adapt to loss of normal neural function.

Functional areas of the cortex that can be mapped to specific sensory receptors or muscles are called *primary* areas. Primary areas are surrounded by secondary areas that provide greater character to sensations and greater complexity to movements. In addition to primary and secondary cortical areas, there are large areas of association cortex that add interpretive and learned responses. The organization of primary and secondary cortex is best characterized for the somatosensory and motor cortex (to be discussed later in the chapter).

Cortical areas involved in visual perception are located in the occipital lobe. Brodmann area 17 is the primary visual cortex, and areas 18 and 19 are secondary visual cortex. Interpretive association areas for vision are found in the adjacent temporal and parietal lobes. The primary auditory cortex is located on the superior temporal lobe, whereas vestibular information projects to the inferior temporal lobe.

Language expression and interpretation have been mapped to areas in the temporal lobe, particularly the Wernicke area (Brodmann areas 39, 40, and 22). One hemisphere, usually the left, is dominant for language. Lesions in this area lead to difficulty recognizing written words (alexia) and spoken lan-

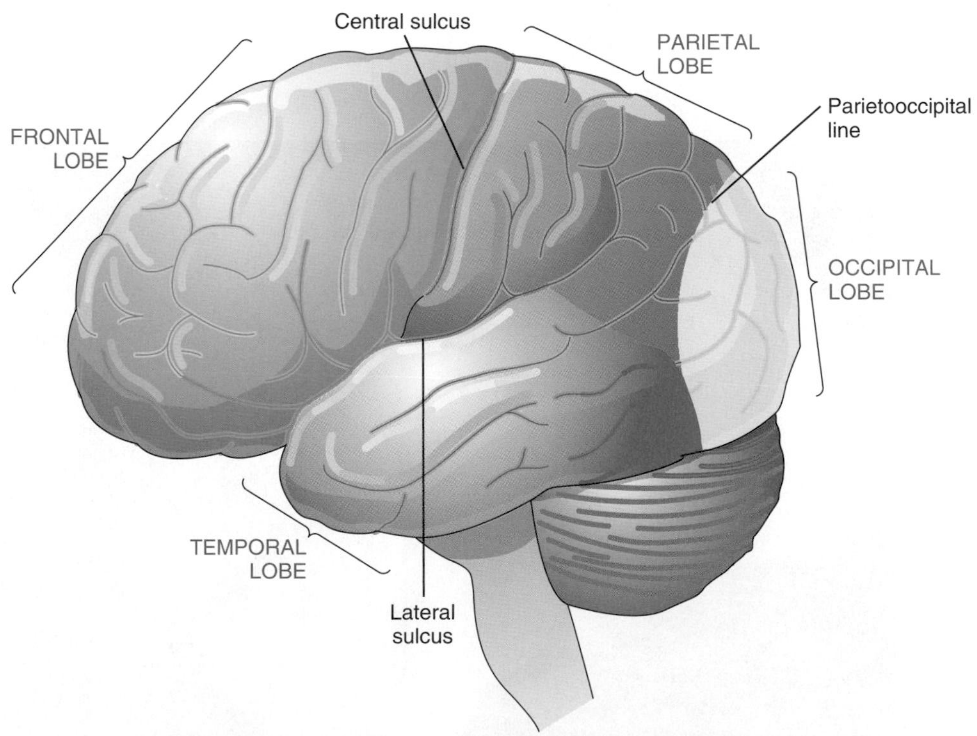

FIGURE 43-8 ■ The four principal lobes of the cerebral cortex.

guage (receptive aphasia). Another area closely associated with speech is the Broca area (Brodmann area 44) in the frontal lobe. Damage to this region interferes with the ability to use language (expressive aphasia) (see Chapter 44).

The frontal lobe is usually credited with control over emotional responses, ethical behavior, and morality. It is also the site of initiative and motivation. Patients with lesions of the frontal lobe may fail to conform to societal behavioral norms.

Another small cortical lobe, the central lobe or insula, lies deep in the lateral cerebral fissure under the junction of the frontal, parietal, and temporal lobes. Little is known about its specific functions, although it is thought to regulate visceral and intestinal functions.

The limbic lobe and **limbic system** are the parts of the cerebrum most closely associated with memory and emotion. The limbic lobe is a ring of cortex on the medial surface of each hemisphere containing the cingulate gyrus, isthmus, and parahippocampal gyrus (Figure 43-10). Olfaction (the perception of smell) occurs within the limbic cortex. The limbic system is a group of structures that encircle the brainstem. Some of these lie within the anatomic division of the cerebrum, whereas others are within the diencephalon and upper brainstem. In addition to the limbic lobe, the limbic system includes the amygdala, fornix, hippocampus, and portions of the thalamus (see Figure 43-10). Lesions of the limbic system, particularly the hippocampus, cause impairment of short-term memory.

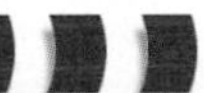

Table 43-3

Functional Areas of Brain Specialization

Area	Specialized Function
Occipital lobe	Visual cortex and association areas
Parietal lobe	Somatosensory cortex and association areas
Temporal lobe	Hearing and equilibrium, emotion, and memory
Frontal lobe	Motor cortex and association areas; prefrontal cortex involved in complex thought, ethical behavior, and morality
Limbic structures	Emotions, short-term memory, olfaction
Basal ganglia	Initiation and planning of learned motor activities

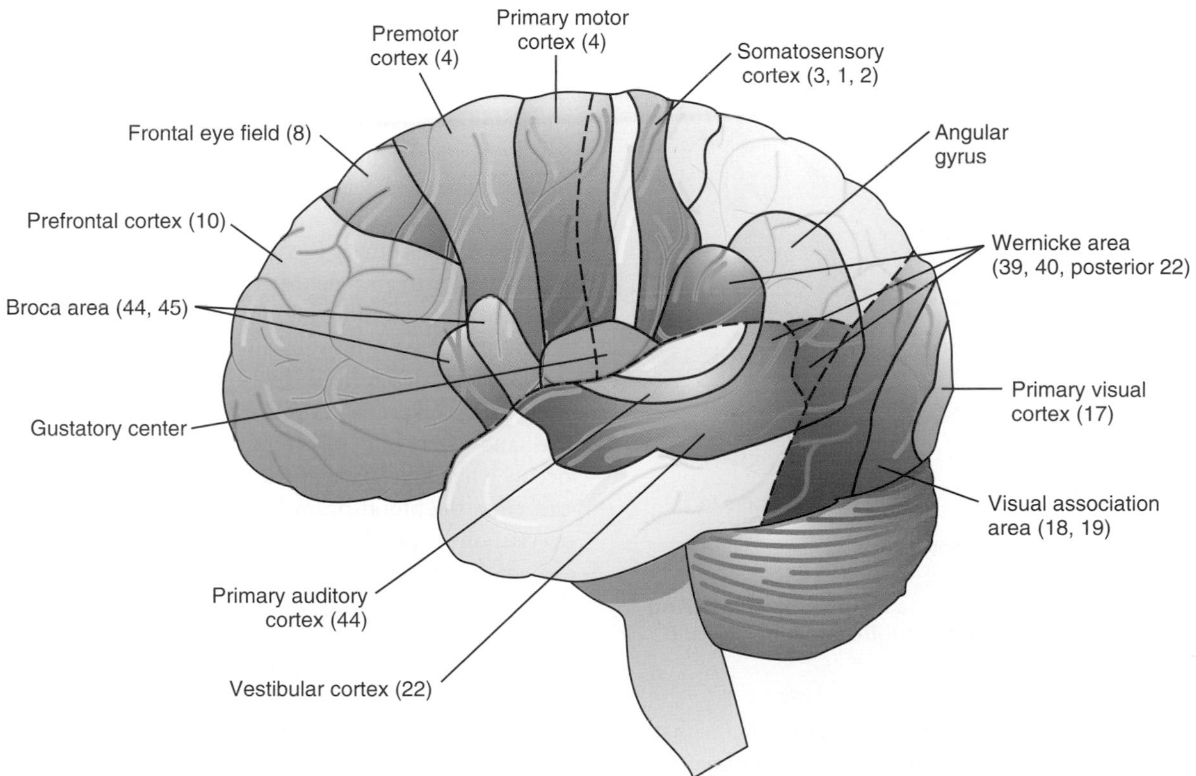

FIGURE 43-9 ■ A partial Brodmann map of the cerebral cortex. Note the locations of Broca and Wernicke areas, which are important in the expression and understanding of language.

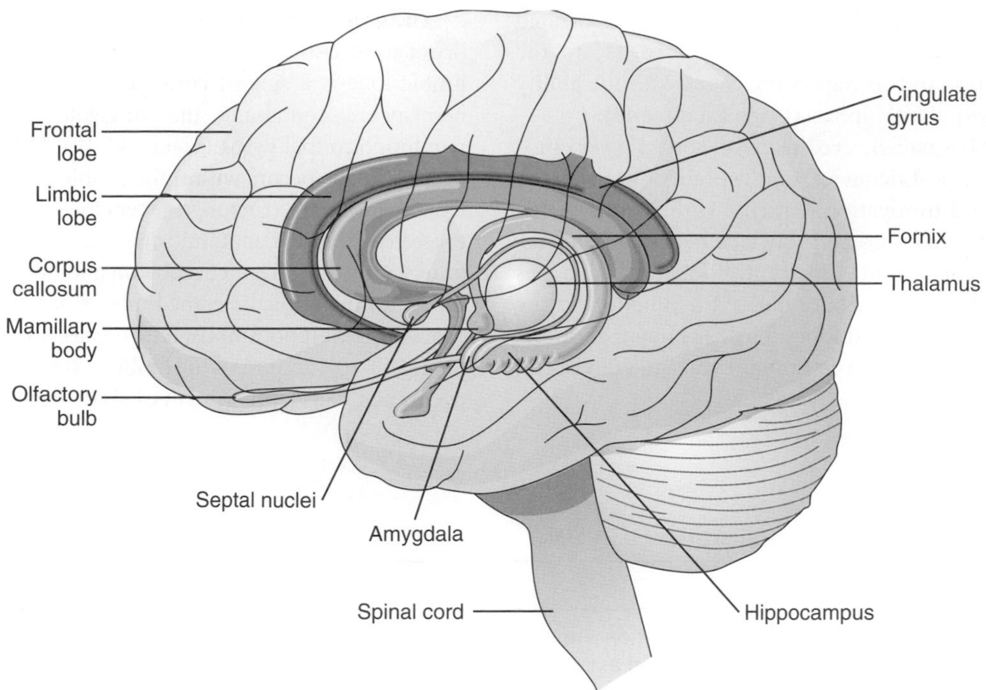

FIGURE 43-10 ■ The limbic system is composed of a group of structures deep in the brain that are important in memory and emotion. These structures include the limbic lobe, amygdala, fornix, hippocampus, olfactory cortex, and portions of the thalamus.

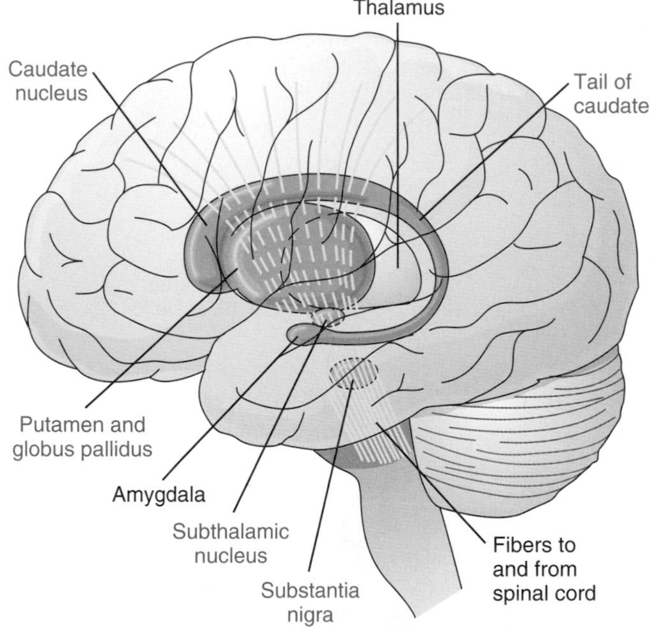

FIGURE 43-11 ■ The basal ganglia include the caudate nucleus, putamen, globus pallidus, subthalamic nuclei, and substantia nigra.

The **basal ganglia** are large masses of gray matter that lie deep within the cerebral hemispheres. They are intimately involved in the initiation, coordination, and execution of movement.[5,6] The basal ganglia include the caudate nucleus, putamen, globus pallidus, subthalamus, and substantia nigra (Figure 43-11). The caudate nucleus and putamen together are called the *striatum.* The five basal ganglia structures occur in pairs, with each cerebral hemisphere containing a set.

The basal ganglia are connected by complex neural circuits that incorporate sensory information about the current muscle conditions, cortical input about desired motor activities, and cerebellar signals about timing and coordination. The basal ganglia then relay motor signals to the thalamus, which projects to areas of the motor cortex. Finally, the program of desired muscle activity is conveyed to the primary motor cortex, which activates neurons projecting to muscle groups. Much of what is known about the function of basal ganglia has been learned from studying Parkinson disease. Parkinson disease is characterized by difficulty initiating voluntary movements (akinesia), stiff muscles (rigidity), and a tremor of the hands when idle (rest tremor). Improvement in symptoms occurs when a precursor of dopamine (DA, levodopa), which can cross the blood-brain barrier, is given. Drugs that block acetylcholine are also effective. Studies of these patients revealed degeneration of DA-secreting neurons that project from the substantia nigra to the striatum. As these neurons slowly degenerate over many years, the amount of DA secreted decreases, and the relative activity of acetylcholine-secreting neurons in the basal ganglia is increased.[7] We do not know what causes Parkinson disease, but a number of drugs (those that block DA) are known to produce a similar clinical syndrome (see Chapter 45).

In addition to the gray matter of the cerebral cortex and the basal ganglia, the cerebrum contains thick layers of white mat-

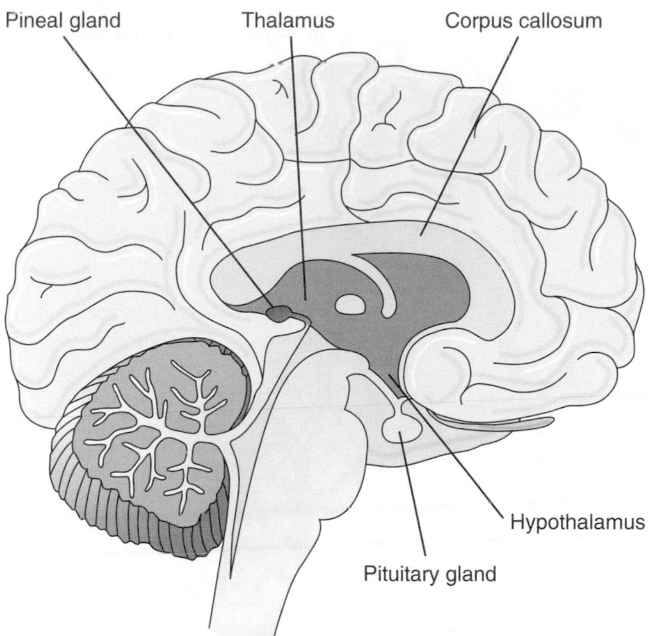

FIGURE 43-12 ■ The diencephalon includes the thalamus, hypothalamus, pineal gland, and hypothalamic extension to the pituitary gland.

ter that consist of myelinated axons. Some of these axons connect the two cerebral hemispheres (commissural fibers), some connect one area of cortex to another within the same hemisphere (association fibers), and others connect the cortex with lower brain centers, including the thalamus, basal ganglia, brainstem, and spinal cord (projection fibers). The corpus callosum and the anterior commissure connect the two hemispheres. The corpus callosum is a massive bundle of fibers crossing the brain just above the lateral ventricles and is the principal means of communication between the hemispheres.

In summary, the cerebrum is the largest brain structure, garnering about 70% of the neurons and supporting cells of the brain to accomplish its diverse and complex functions. Each of the 100 billion neurons in the brain may make hundreds of synaptic connections with other neurons, providing an incomprehensible number of potential interactions. Discovering the ways in which the substance of the cerebrum relates to the workings of the mind is truly one of the great remaining mysteries of science.

Diencephalon

The diencephalon lies deep in the brain, forming a connecting structure between the upper brainstem (midbrain) and the cerebral hemispheres. The four principal structures of the diencephalon are the thalamus, hypothalamus, epithalamus, and ventral thalamus (Figure 43-12). The third ventricle also traverses the diencephalon.

The thalamus is the principal receiving site and relay center for impulses traveling to the cerebral cortex from the spinal cord, cerebellum, and basal ganglia. In addition to processing and relaying sensory information, the thalamus is integrally involved in executing motor activities through its projections to the motor cortex. The thalamus also is involved in propagating the constant background electrical activity of the brain, which can be detected by electroencephalography. Large groups of neurons sending impulses between the thalamus and cortex are responsible for the typical waveforms noted on the electroencephalogram during sleep, rest, and wakeful activities. Connections between the brainstem reticular activating system and thalamus are necessary to maintain consciousness.

Thalamic connections, including the limbic and association cortex, are integral to the expression of those qualities considered to be human: emotion, language, creativity, and complex thought. Indeed, the thalamus is much more than a relay station; it is a complex integrative center that makes possible the functioning of higher brain centers.[8]

The hypothalamus is located just beneath the thalamus on the floor of the diencephalon. The inferior aspect of the hypothalamus extends downward to form the pituitary gland (hypophysis). The posterior pituitary is an extension of the neuronal tissue of the hypothalamus, whereas the anterior pituitary is derived from glandular tissue (Figure 43-13). Hormones secreted by the pituitary gland enter the systemic circulation and influence target cells at a distance. Neurons in the hypothalamus regulate the secretion of anterior pituitary hormones by releasing and inhibiting hormones (see Chapter 39 for a discussion of the endocrine system).

The hypothalamus is also an important regulatory center for the ANS and for vegetative functions, such as sleep, body temperature, appetite, and sex drive. Input from sensors of blood pressure, osmolarity, blood oxygen, carbon dioxide and pH, and temperature is received and integrated into appropriate regulatory responses. Perhaps more than any other structure, the hypothalamus is responsible for homeostasis of life-sustaining functions, including cardiovascular, respiratory, metabolic, fluid and electrolyte, and stress responses.

The epithalamus contains the pineal gland, thought to be important in regulating circadian rhythms in response to light-dark cycles. The ventral thalamus contains the basal ganglia structure called the *subthalamic nucleus.*

Cerebellum

The cerebellum is located in the posterior fossa behind the pons. It is separated from the cerebrum by the tentorium cerebelli. The main roles of the cerebellum are to coordinate and smooth movements and to maintain posture and balance. The cerebellum compares the desired motor program with the moment-to-moment execution of the movement and makes instantaneous adjustments to improve the match.[9] The cerebellum receives information from proprioceptors in muscles and joints and from the vestibular apparatus in the inner ear about the position of the head in space. Some of the fastest-conducting neurons in the nervous system are involved in relaying sensory information to the cerebellum.

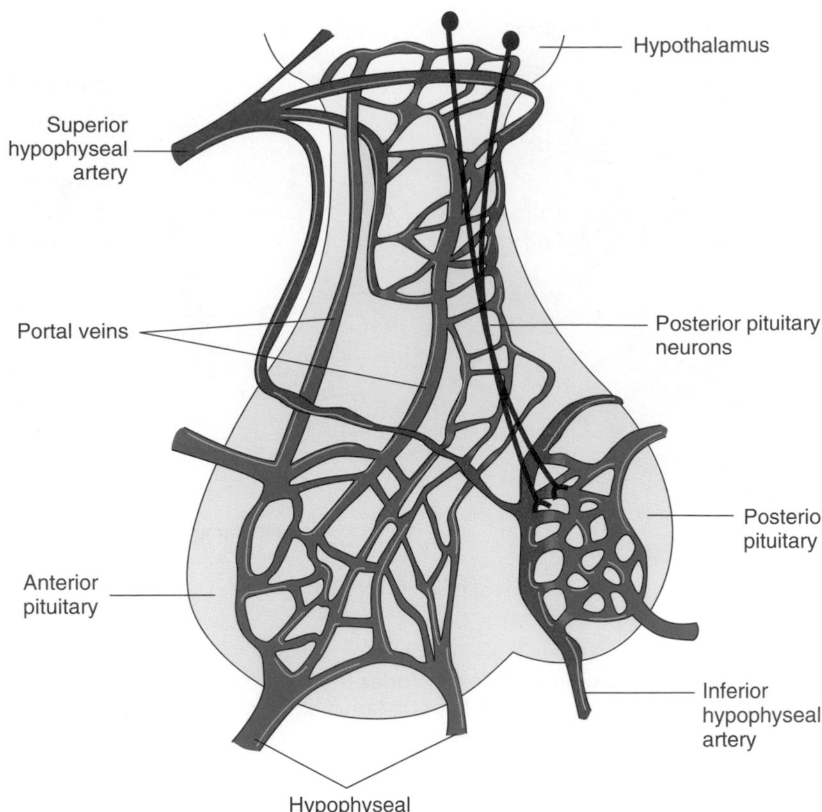

FIGURE 43-13 ■ Anatomy of the hypothalamus and pituitary gland. Note that the posterior pituitary is connected to the hypothalamus by neuronal axons, whereas the anterior pituitary receives signals by way of a portal vein system. The portal veins drain blood from the capillaries of the hypothalamus and take it to the capillaries of the anterior pituitary.

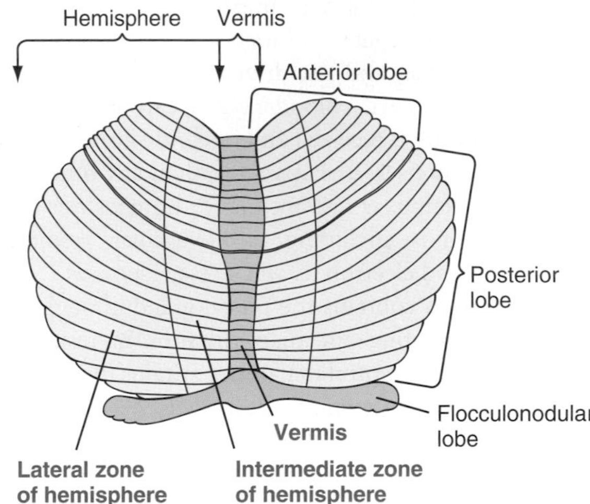

FIGURE 43-14 ■ Lobes of the cerebellum from the posteroinferior view. (Adapted from Guyton AC, Hall JE, editors: *Textbook of medical physiology,* ed 10, Philadelphia, 2000, Saunders, p 648.)

The cerebellar cortex is folded much as the cerebral cortex is folded, in a way that significantly increases surface area. Its tightly folded shape gives it a banded appearance. The cortical ridges on the surface of the cerebellum are called *folia.* The white matter beneath is called the *medullary center* and is made up of fibers running to and from the cerebellar cortex.

The cerebellum is divided anatomically, first by the posterolateral fissure, which separates the flocculonodular lobe (the region immediately inferior to the middle cerebellar peduncles) from the main body, the corpus cerebelli (Figure 43-14). Another prominent landmark is the primary fissure, which subdivides the corpus cerebelli into the anterior and posterior lobes. The midline body is called the *vermis,* and it is straddled on either side by the cerebellar hemispheres. The portion of the hemisphere that is adjacent to the vermis is called the *paravermal* zone.

The prominent tracts that attach the cerebellum to the brainstem are called the *inferior, middle,* and *superior* cerebellar peduncles. The inferior cerebellar peduncle is composed primarily of afferent fibers coming from the spinal cord and the brainstem. The middle peduncle contains afferent fibers from the contralateral pontine **nuclei.** The superior cerebellar peduncle is composed of major efferent pathways leaving the cerebellum.

Deep within the medullary center in each cerebellar hemisphere are the cerebellar nuclei. These include the dentate nuclei, the interposed nuclei, and the fastigial nuclei. The deep cerebellar nuclei are the final pathway of cerebellar output.

The lateral hemispheres form the biggest part of the cerebellum. Their major neural activity involves a feedback loop in which input from several areas of the cerebral cortex is received by the cerebellar hemispheres and dentate nuclei, then sent back to the motor and premotor cortex. This circuit is believed to influence the planning and programming of voluntary movements, especially learned, skilled movements (those that become more rapid, precise, and automatic with practice).

The major input to the paravermal region, also called the intermediate cortex, consists of somatotopically arranged projections from the motor cortex and spinal cord. The primary output from this region is through the interposed nucleus to the red nucleus and also back to the motor cortex by way of the thalamus. The intermediate cerebellum therefore can influence spinal cord and motor neurons through the corticospinal tract and the rubrospinal tract, where it is involved in interpreting and responding to the position and velocity of the moving body.

The vermis receives input and contains representation of the trunk as conveyed by the spinocerebellar tracts. It sends output to the vestibular nuclei and the reticular formation by way of the fastigial nucleus and through direct projections to the vestibular nuclei. The vestibulospinal and reticulospinal tracts in turn influence spinal motor neurons. This area of the cerebellum, then, is most involved with regulation of posture and stereotyped movements that are programmed in the brainstem and spinal cord.

The flocculonodular lobe receives most of its transmissions by way of the inferior cerebellar peduncle from the vestibular nerve and nuclei. Because of this primary source of input, this lobe is often referred to as the vestibulocerebellum. Its role is to maintain equilibrium and mediate the eye movements needed for visual tracking.

Lesions of the cerebellum result in ataxia (impaired balance), intention tremor, past pointing (failure of finger-to-nose test), and dysdiadochokinesia (failure of rapid movements).

Brainstem

The brainstem is a stalk of neural tissue that lies between the upper spinal cord and the diencephalon. It has three parts; from top to bottom these are the midbrain, pons, and medulla oblongata. The brainstem is critical for transmission of impulses between the brain and spinal cord. Vital centers for regulating respiratory and cardiovascular function are located in the medulla and pons. In addition, the reticular activating neurons that maintain consciousness and alertness traverse the brainstem to reach the thalamus. Ten of the 12 pairs of cranial nerves originate from nuclei in the brainstem; only cranial nerves I (olfactory) and II (optic) originate elsewhere (diencephalon).

The midbrain or mesencephalon contains the cerebral peduncles, consisting of motor tracts to the spinal cord; the superior and inferior colliculi, which control head and eye movements; and the red nucleus, part of a major motor tract. Cranial nerve III (oculomotor) emerges from the midbrain and is prone to compression when pressure in one of the cerebral hemispheres is elevated. Increased intracranial pressure (e.g., from tumor, ischemia, edema, bleeding) is commonly manifested by dysfunction of cranial nerve III resulting in abnormal pupil size and poor reactivity to light (see Chapter 44). Cranial nerve IV (trochlear) also emerges at the level of the midbrain.

The pons (Latin for *bridge*) connects the midbrain above to the medulla below. The dorsal pons consists of reticular formation fibers, ascending sensory tracts and descending motor tracts. Two respiratory centers, pneumotaxic and apneustic, located in the dorsal pons work in coordination with the principal respiratory centers in the medulla. The ventral pons contains the relay nuclei (pontine nuclei) for fibers projecting from the cortex to the cerebellum. The major pathway of voluntary motor control, the corticospinal tract, also passes through the ventral pons on its way from the motor cortex to the spinal cord.

The medulla oblongata makes up the lower third of the brainstem and is continuous with the spinal cord. Nuclei within the reticular formation of the medulla form the vital centers that regulate cardiac, vascular, and respiratory function. The medulla also contains centers that coordinate swallowing, vomiting, coughing, and sneezing. The medulla is the site of decussation (crossing over) of the major sensory (dorsal column) and motor (corticospinal) tracts such that innervation of one side of the body is connected to the opposite (contralateral) cerebral hemisphere. The corticospinal tract neurons decussate within ridges on the ventral surface of the medulla called medullary pyramids. Motor tracts that do not cross over within the pyramids (e.g., tectospinal, vestibulospinal) are sometimes referred to as extrapyramidal tracts and disorders associated with function of these tracts (balance, posture, gait) may be called *extrapyramidal disorders* (e.g., Parkinson disease). Although the anatomic correlation is not quite accurate, use of the term persists in a clinical context.

All of the remaining cranial nerves (VI, VII, VIII, IX, X, XI, and XII) originate in the medulla. The cranial nerves themselves are part of the PNS and are discussed in that section. The name, origin, and function of the 12 cranial nerves are included in Table 43-4.

The Spinal Cord

The spinal cord conveys nervous impulses between the brain and 31 pairs of spinal nerves that innervate sensory organs and muscle cells of the body. The spinal cord mediates spinal reflexes involved in maintenance of posture, protective responses to pain, urination, and muscle tone. A great deal of integration and processing occurs in the gray matter of the spinal cord, whereas the white matter contains bundles of myelinated axons forming tracts that run up and down the cord. Tracts in the spinal cord are **somatotopically** organized such that the innervation of a particular body region is connected to a specific region in the cerebral cortex.

The typical adult spinal cord is about 18 inches long, extending from the base of the skull (foramen magnum) to the first or second lumbar vertebra (L1-2).[10] The vertebral column extends for several more inches, providing a reservoir for CSF and exit points for the lumbar and sacral spinal nerves. The vertebral column is formed by interlocking sections of bone

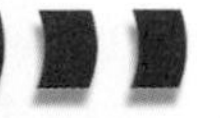

Table 43-4

Cranial Nerves

Cranial Nerve	Origin	Function
I (Olfactory)	Nasal mucous membrane	Olfaction
II (Optic)	Retina	Vision
III (Oculomotor)	Midbrain	Movement of eyeball, eyelid, constriction of pupil
IV (Trochlear)	Lower midbrain	Lateral eye movements
V (Trigeminal)		
Ophthalmic	Forehead, eyes	Sensation from forehead, eye, scalp
Maxillary	Upper jaw, lip	Sensation from cheek, upper lip
Mandibular	Lower jaw area	Sensation from chin and lower jaw, motor chewing
VI (Abducens)	Lower pons	Lateral eye movements
VII (Facial)	Pons	Taste from anterior tongue, control of muscles of face
VIII (Vestibulocochlear)	Cochlea	Hearing
	Inner ear	Equilibrium
IX (Glossopharyngeal)	Medulla	Taste from posterior tongue, secretion of saliva, swallowing
X (Vagus)	Medulla	Monitors oxygen, carbon dioxide, and pH levels in the blood; senses blood pressure; inhibits cardiac action and extensive gastrointestinal activities
XI (Spinal accessory)	Medulla and cervical cord	Voice production, movement of head and shoulders
XII (Hypoglossal)	Medulla	Movements of tongue during speech and swallowing

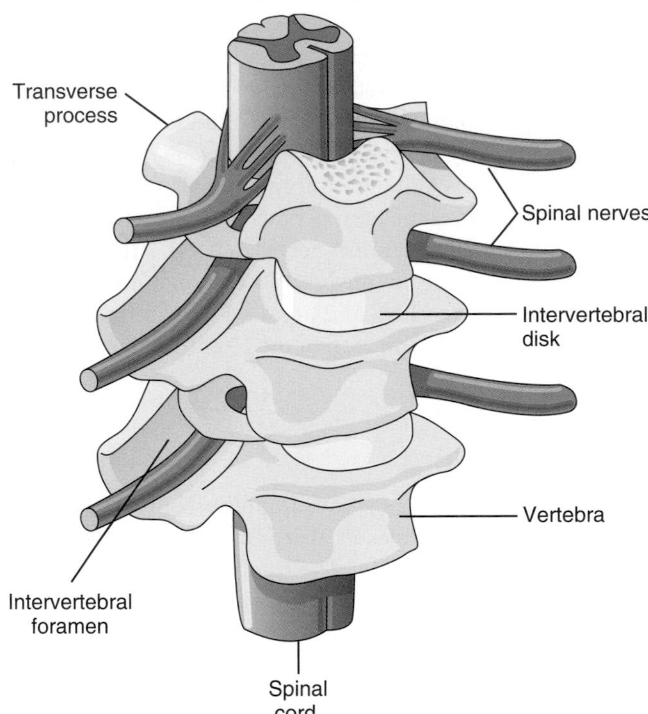

FIGURE 43-15 ■ The spinal cord travels down the center of the vertebral column. A foramen at the intersection of two vertebrae forms an exit point for the spinal nerves.

separated and cushioned by intervertebral disks. At the lateral aspect of the intersection of two vertebrae is an opening (intervertebral foramen) that provides a passageway for spinal nerves to exit the cord. The spinal cord travels in a small lumen (1 cm) in the center of the vertebral column and is itself only slightly larger than the diameter of a pencil[10] (Figure 43-15).

On cross-section the spinal cord has a butterfly pattern of gray matter surrounded by white matter (Figure 43-16). Three bumps on the butterfly wings are called horns: the ventral horn (motor neurons), the dorsal horn (sensory neurons), and the lateral horn (sympathetic neurons). The horns consist of neuron cell bodies, synapses, and small unmyelinated interneurons. The white matter is divided into columns that contain tracts of nerve fibers traveling to and from the brain. These are the posterior (dorsal) columns, anterior columns, and lateral columns. Some of the neurons in the columns convey signals from one level of the cord to another and are important in reflex and postural adjustments. The principal ascending sensory tracts include the dorsal column–lemniscal and the anterolateral (spinothalamic) tracts, which send **afferent** signals to the brain. The principal descending motor tracts include the corticospinal, rubrospinal, reticulospinal, and vestibulospinal tracts. These tracts are located in specific regions of the cord (Figure 43-17). Sensory and motor pathways are discussed in later sections of this chapter.

Spinal nerves divide into two sections as they make contact with the spinal cord: the ventral and dorsal roots (Figure 43-18). Ventral roots contain motor neurons that originate in the anterior horn and travel in the spinal nerve to skeletal muscles. Dorsal roots carry sensory information from somatic receptors to neurons in the posterior horn. The cell bodies of sensory afferents collect together in the dorsal root ganglion. Autonomic nerves also travel in the spinal cord and exit and enter the cord by way of the ventral and dorsal roots.

The points at which sensory neurons enter the cord and at which motor neurons exit represents the separation of the CNS and PNS.

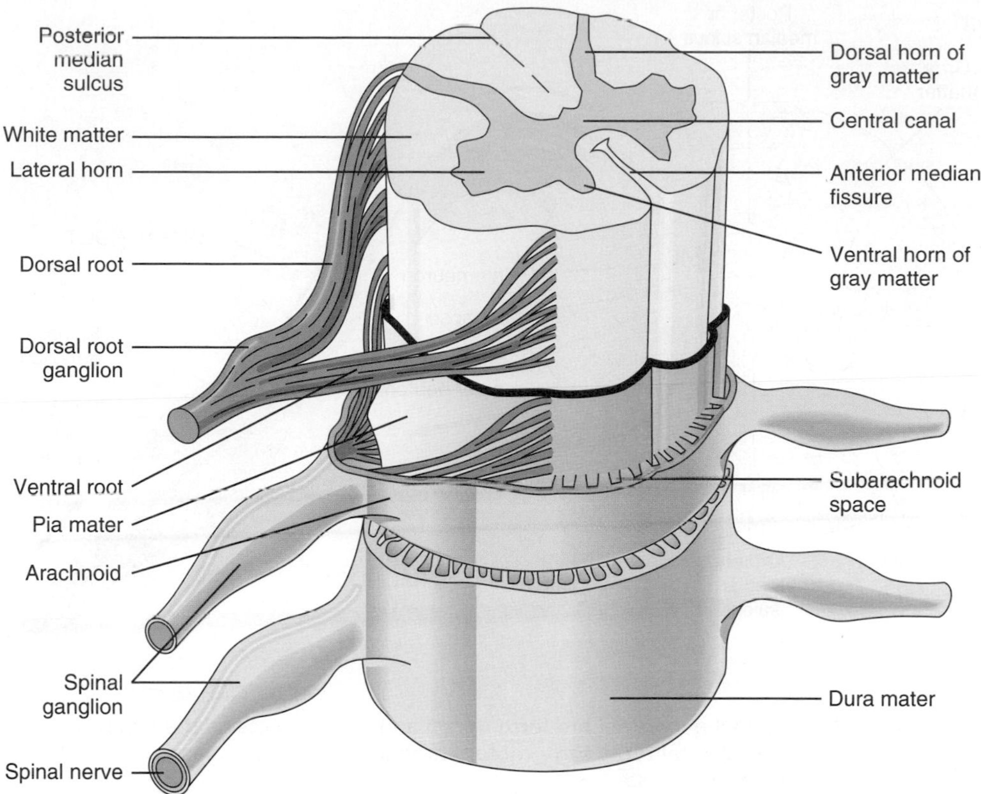

FIGURE 43-16 ■ The spinal cord in cross-section, showing the butterfly pattern of white and gray matter.

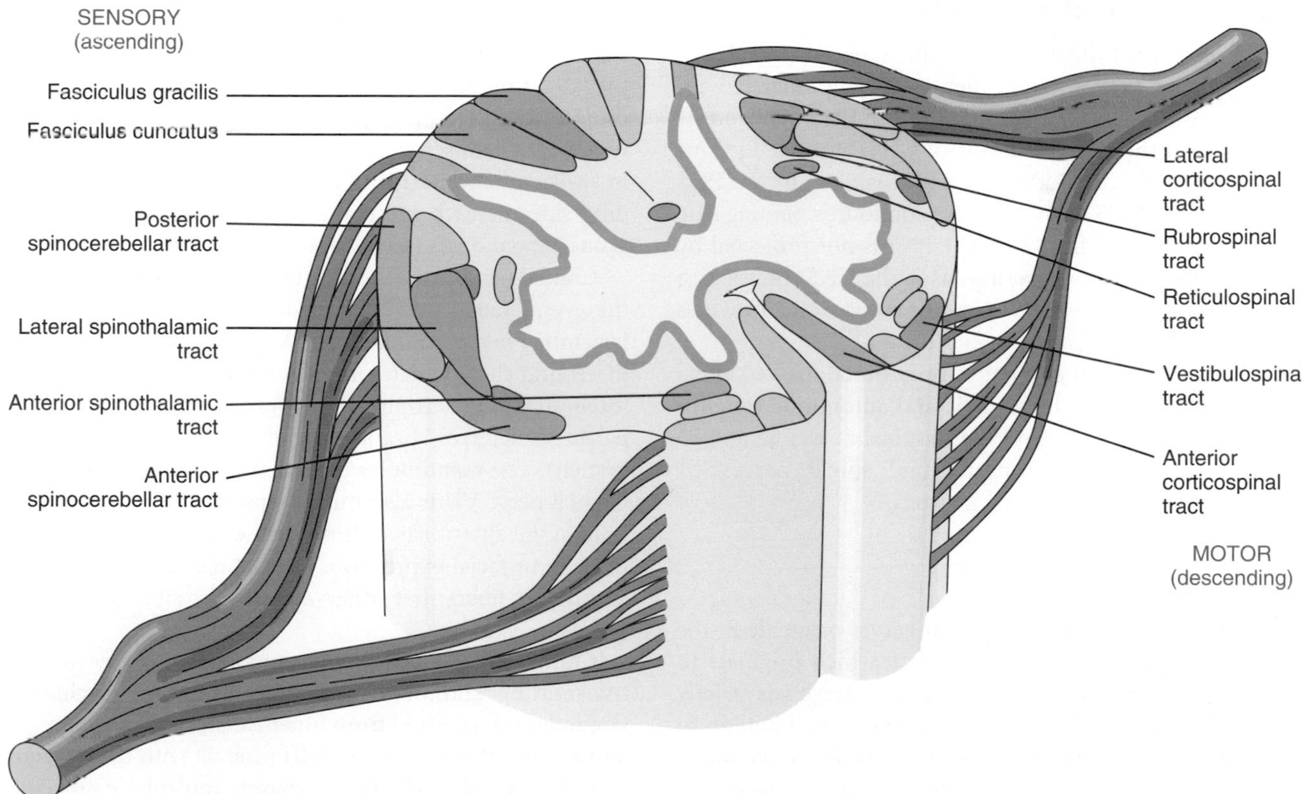

FIGURE 43-17 ■ The main ascending *(left)* and descending *(right)* tracts of the spinal cord.

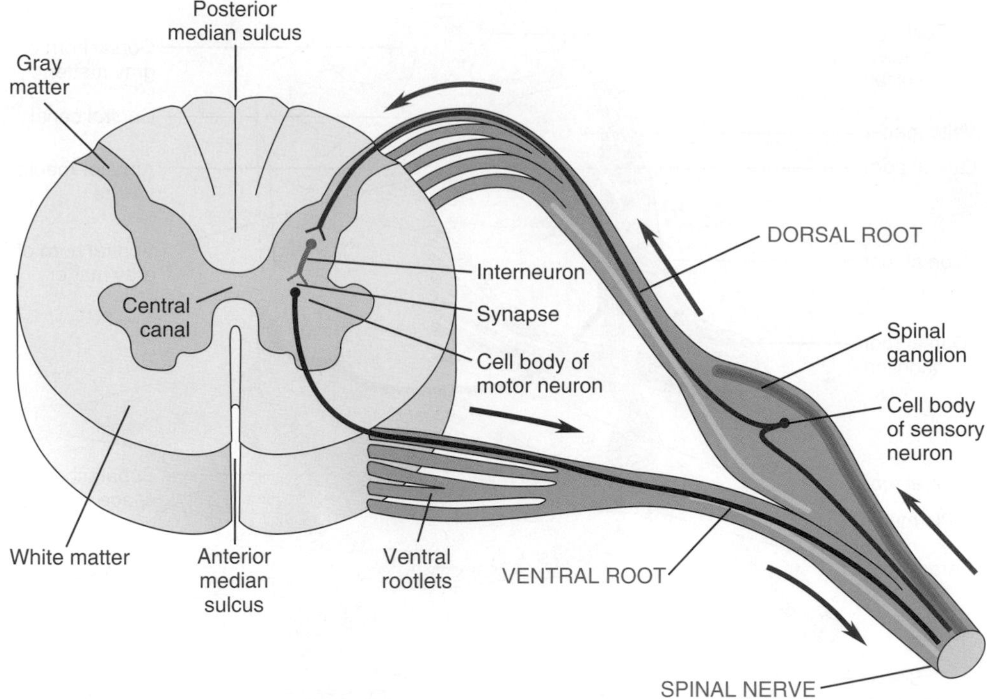

FIGURE 43-18 ■ Spinal nerves split to form dorsal and ventral roots as they emerge from the spinal cord. Ventral roots carry motor efferent neurons, whereas dorsal roots carry sensory afferent neurons.

PERIPHERAL NERVOUS SYSTEM

The PNS consists of the 31 pairs of spinal nerves and the 12 pairs of cranial nerves. These nerves are myelinated with Schwann cells, which differ somewhat from the oligodendrocytes that form the myelin sheaths of CNS neurons. By convention, groups of cell bodies are called *ganglia* in the PNS and *nuclei* in the CNS. A major exception to this naming rule is the basal ganglia of the CNS. The PNS is not protected by CSF, meninges, or bony coverings as is the CNS; however, a sheath of connective tissue covers the nerves and provides support.

The PNS serves both afferent sensory functions and efferent motor functions of the somatic and autonomic systems. Cranial nerves III, VII, IX, and X and spinal nerves S2 and S3 contain parasympathetic neurons, and spinal nerves T1 through L2 contain sympathetic neurons.[11]

Cranial Nerves

As previously noted, all of the cranial nerves originate in the brainstem except cranial nerves I and II, which originate in the diencephalon[12] (Figure 43-19). Cranial nerve I is strictly sensory, transmitting olfactory signals from the 10 million to 20 million olfactory neurons in the nasal cavities to the olfactory bulbs. The olfactory bulb neurons then project to the olfactory cortex. Cranial nerve II is also sensory, conveying visual information from the retina to the brain. The optic nerve is unusual in that it is an extension of the CNS, myelinated by oligodendrocytes rather than Schwann cells. The neurons from the medial retina decussate in the optic chiasm, whereas the lateral retina neurons do not. Thus, the right visual field projects to the left hemisphere and the left visual field projects to the right hemisphere. Damage to one hemisphere, as occurs in stroke, often interrupts visual signals from the corresponding sides of each retina—a condition known as homonymous hemianopsia (see Chapters 44 and 46).

Cranial nerves III, IV, and VI innervate motor structures in the eyes. Cranial nerve III mediates pupil constriction. The trigeminal nerve (cranial nerve V) is so named because it has three branches, which provide sensory innervation of the forehead and eyes (ophthalmic branch), upper lip, teeth, and palate (maxillary branch), and lower jaw (mandibular branch). The mandibular branch is both sensory and motor. Cranial nerve VII is also mixed sensory and motor, detecting taste in the anterior two thirds of the tongue and innervating muscles of facial expression. Cranial nerve VII also contains autonomic fibers that innervate salivary and lacrimal (tear) glands.

Cranial nerve VIII has two important sensory functions: transmitting auditory information from the cochlea and vestibular information from inner ear structures. The vestibular neurons of cranial nerve VIII interact with the neurons of cranial nerves III and VI to reflexively control eye movements during head rotation such that a visual image can remain fixed on the retina. This reflex, the oculovestibular reflex, is com-

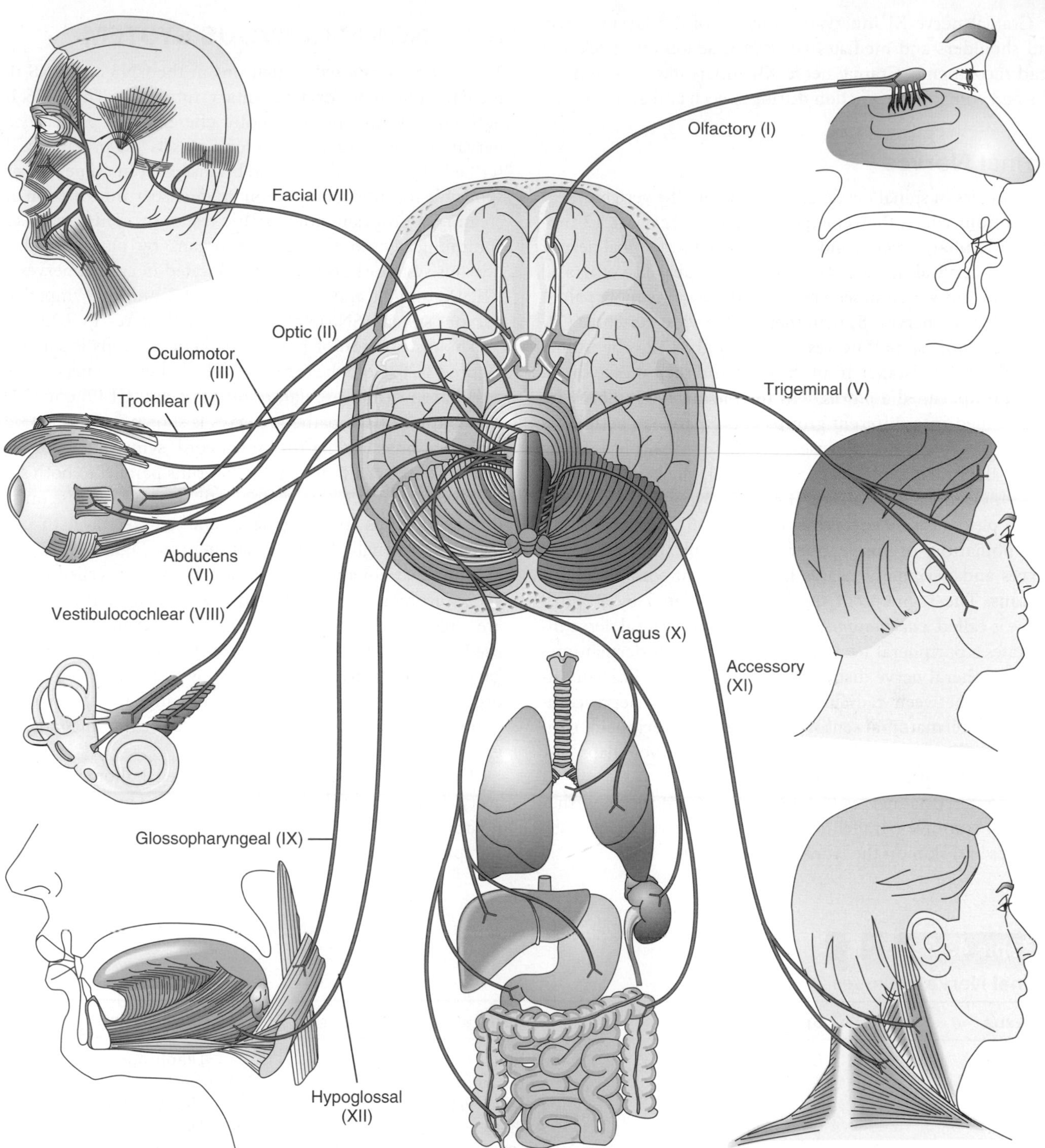

FIGURE 43-19 ■ View of the inferior aspect of the brain showing the origin and distribution of the 12 cranial nerves. Only one of each pair is shown.

monly assessed in the unconscious patient to evaluate brainstem function (see Chapter 44).

Cranial nerve IX innervates tongue and pharyngeal muscles, conveying taste from the posterior tongue and controlling pharyngeal motion during swallowing. Cranial nerve IX also has autonomic functions and transmits sensory information from the carotid baroreceptors and carotid bodies to the brainstem. Cranial nerve X, the vagus nerve, contains parasympathetic afferent and efferent fibers that innervate many visceral structures, including heart, lungs, and gastrointestinal (GI) tract from pharynx to anus. Sensory information from aortic baroreceptors and aortic bodies is conveyed to the brainstem by the vagus nerve.

Cranial nerve XI innervates muscles of the larynx, neck, and shoulders and mediates voice production and neck and head movements. Cranial nerve XII innervates tongue muscles and controls their action during speech and swallowing.

Spinal Nerves

The 31 pairs of spinal nerves are named after the vertebral segments from which they emerge. There are 8 cervical, 12 thoracic, 5 lumbar, 5 sacral, and 1 coccygeal pair of spinal nerves. The first cervical nerve exits above C1, whereas the others all exit below the vertebral segment; thus there is one more pair of cervical spinal nerves (8) than there are cervical vertebrae (7).

Except for spinal nerves T2 through T12, the spinal nerves travel a distance from the cord and then merge into a large group, called a *plexus.*[12] In the plexus, nerve fibers are recombined into different groups and emerge as peripheral nerves. There are five plexuses: (1) the cervical plexus (C1-4), (2) the brachial plexus (C5-8, T1), (3) the lumbar plexus (L1-4), (4) the sacral plexus (L4-5, S1-3), and (5) the coccygeal plexus (S4-5, coccygeal) (Table 43-5). Because of this recombination of nerve fibers in the plexus, the spinal nerves and peripheral nerves have different somatic distributions. The segment of the body innervated by a spinal nerve is called a *dermatome,* whereas the peripheral nerve innervates a peripheral nerve field. Knowledge of dermatomes and peripheral nerve distribution can help the clinician differentiate between radiculopathy from spinal nerve compression (dermatomal sensory changes) and peripheral neuropathy. (Dermatomal and peripheral nerve maps are located in Chapter 47.)

The intercostal nerves (T2-12) do not form plexuses; they travel in a course parallel to the ribs to innervate intercostal muscles and skin on the trunk and abdomen.

AUTONOMIC NERVOUS SYSTEM

The ANS is composed of neurons in the CNS and PNS that mediate automatic or involuntary functions. The ANS has both sensory afferents and motor efferents that primarily innervate visceral organs and blood vessels. As previously described, the hypothalamus and brainstem contain neurons responsible for integrating autonomic sensory information and creating appropriate homeostatic responses. This response is communicated to the effector organs by parasympathetic nervous system (PSNS) efferents located in cranial nerves III, VII, IX, and X, and spinal nerves S2-3 and by sympathetic nervous system (SNS) neurons in spinal nerves T1-L2.[11]

The distribution of parasympathetic neurons is shown in Figure 43-20. Note the extensive role that cranial nerve X (vagus) has in cardiovascular, respiratory, and GI function. The distribution of sympathetic nerves is shown in Figure 43-21. Note that after leaving the spinal cord, sympathetic neurons converge on a chain of ganglia that runs parallel to both sides of the spinal cord. Some sympathetic neurons synapse on secondary neurons in the ganglia, and others travel to other plexuses or ganglia before synapsing (see Figure 43-21). The neurons that emerge from the spinal cord are called *preganglionic neurons,* whereas the neurons traveling to the target cell are called *postganglionic neurons.* This terminology is also used for the PSNS system; however the parasympathetic preganglionic neurons are long, traveling all the way to the target organ, and they do not terminate in ganglia.[11] The postganglionic neurons are short and are located within the target organ (see Figure 43-20).

The neurotransmitter secreted by preganglionic neurons is acetylcholine for both the SNS and PSNS. The postganglionic neurotransmitters differ (Figure 43-22). The SNS secretes norepinephrine (NE) in most cases, although sweat glands

Table 43-5
Spinal Nerve Plexuses

Plexus	Spinal Nerves	Peripheral Nerves	Distribution
Cervical	C1-4	Phrenic	Diaphragm
		Cutaneous	Neck
		Ansa cervicalis	Hyoid bone
Brachial	C5-8, T1	Axillary	Upper arm
		Ulnar	Forearm, wrist, 5th digit
		Median	2nd-4th digits
		Radial	Thumb
		Musculocutaneous	Upper arm
Lumbar	L1-4	Femoral (saphenous)	Hip, knee (lower leg)
		Obturator	Inner thigh
Sacral	L4-5, S1-3	Superior gluteal	Gluteus medius, minimus
		Inferior gluteal	Gluteus maximus
		Sciatic (tibial, peroneal)	Thigh, leg, foot
		Pudendal	Perineum
Coccygeal	S4-5, coccygeal	Coccygeal fibers	Skin on coccyx

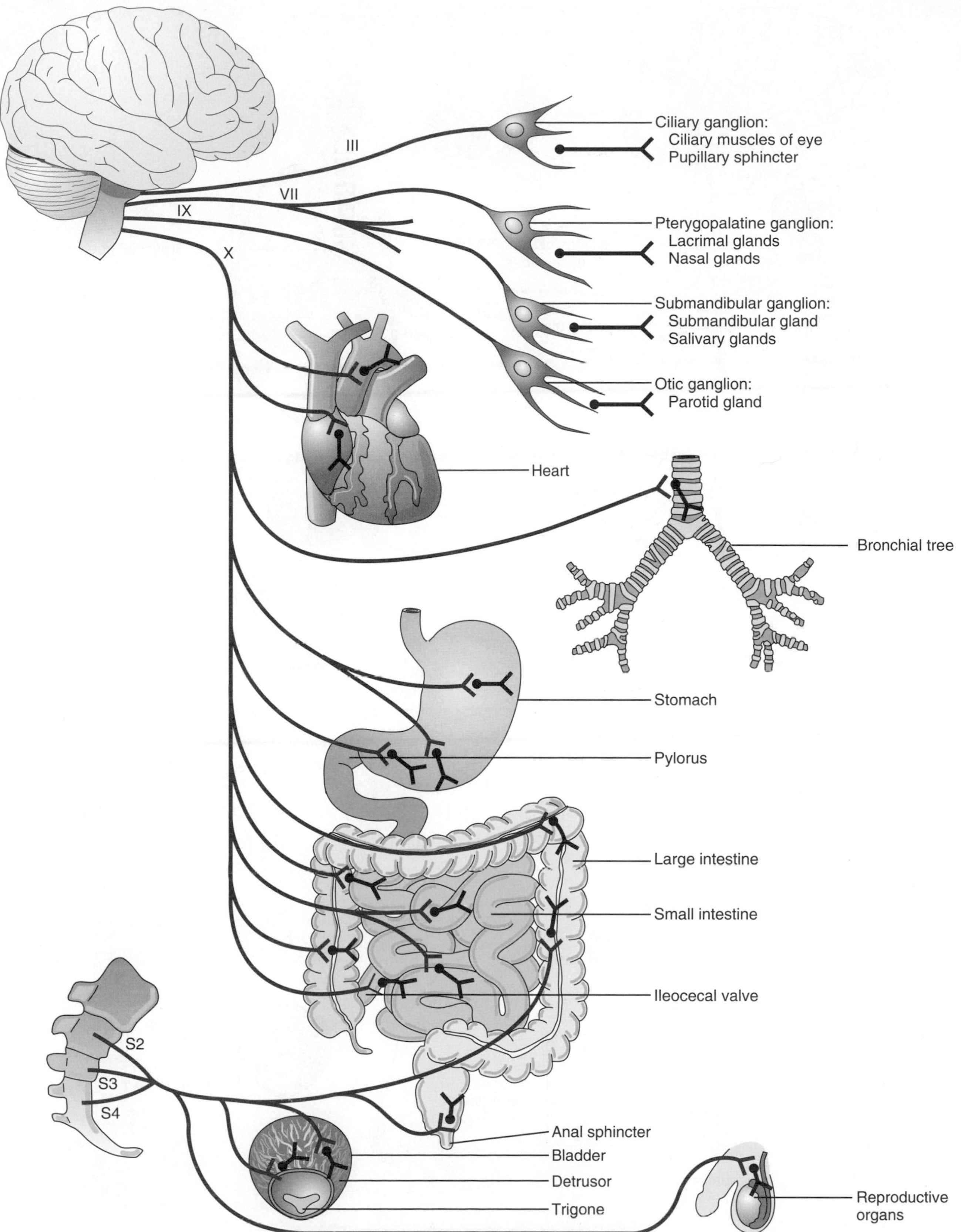

FIGURE 43-20 ■ Distribution of parasympathetic nerves.

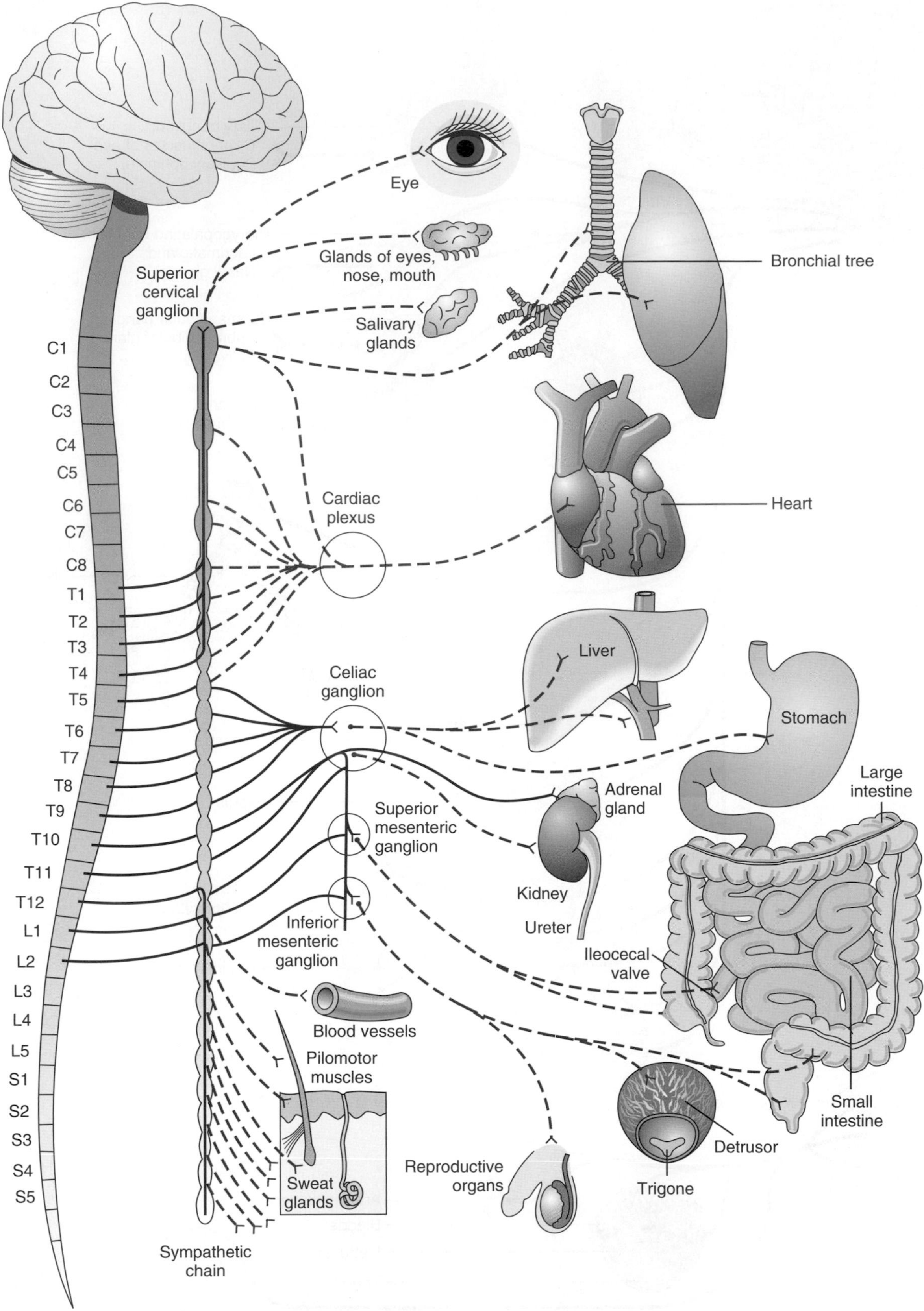

FIGURE 43-21 ■ Distribution of sympathetic nerves.

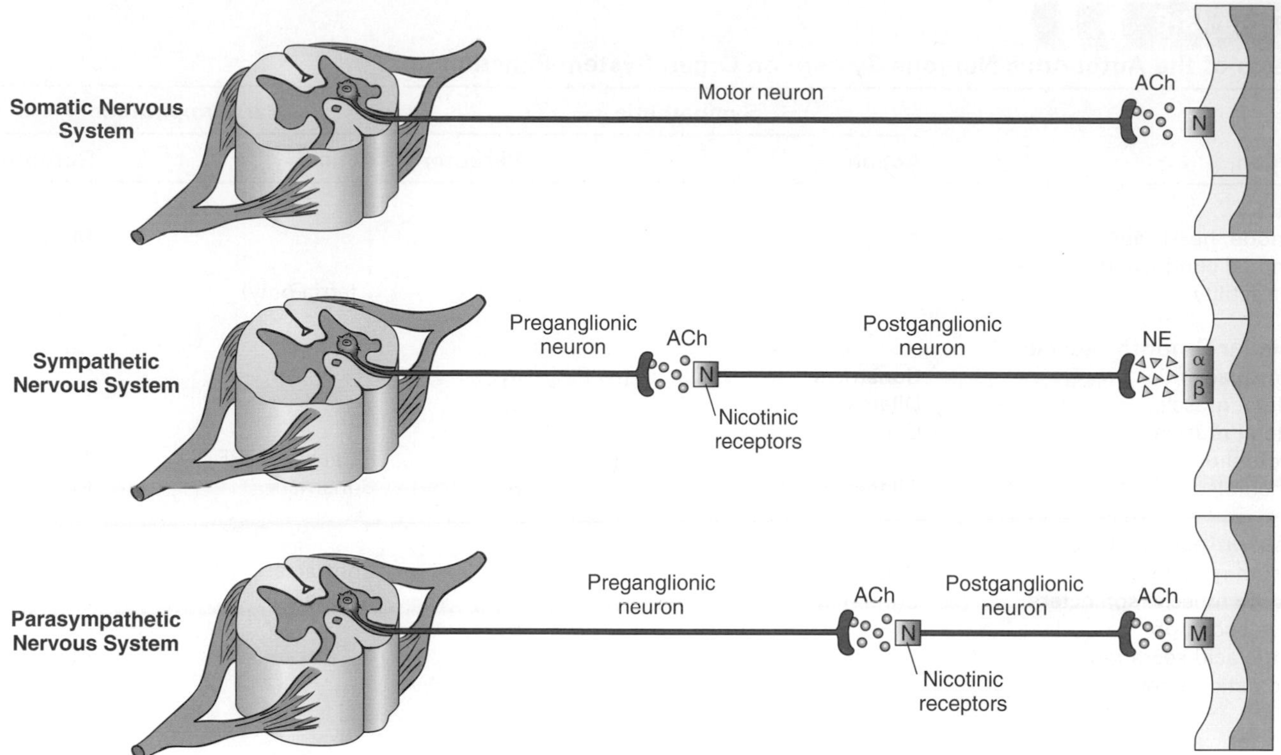

FIGURE 43-22 ■ Comparison of preganglionic and postganglionic neurotransmitters in the sympathetic and parasympathetic systems. Acetylcholine *(ACh)* is the neurotransmitter of the motor neuron, but its receptor differs from that of the parasympathetic terminations. *NE,* Norepinephrine; *N,* nicotinic receptors; *M,* muscarinic receptors.

and skeletal muscle vessels are innervated by acetylcholine secreting SNS neurons. The PSNS secretes acetylcholine as the postganglionic neurotransmitter. Acetylcholine is also the neurotransmitter of the motor neurons that innervate skeletal muscle; however, the target cell receptors differ. Skeletal muscle contains nicotinic acetylcholine receptors whereas autonomic organs contain muscarinic acetylcholine receptors (see Figure 43-22).

The effect of the SNS and PSNS on target organs is nearly always antagonistic. If one contracts smooth muscle, the other relaxes it; if one stimulates glandular secretion, the other inhibits it; if one speeds up a process, the other slows it down. The effects of SNS and PSNS stimulation on major target organs are shown in Table 43-6.

A specialized extension of the SNS is found in the adrenal gland. The adrenal medulla receives preganglionic neurons from SNS neurons emerging from the spinal cord, which stimulate the gland to secrete NE and epinephrine into the bloodstream. These hormones have effects similar to those of direct SNS stimulation.

The manner in which target cells respond to SNS stimulation depends on the types of receptors they possess. Several subtypes of receptors bind and respond to NE and epinephrine; these include α_1, α_2, β_1, β_2, β_3, and several DA receptors (see Table 43-6). (The details of autonomic regulation of cardiac, GI, and genitourinary function can be found in Chapters 17, 35, and 29, respectively.)

The coordination of SNS and PSNS activity within a target organ is accomplished by centers in the brainstem and hypothalamus with input from sensory neurons and cortical neurons. Most of these systems work on a negative-feedback principle to achieve homeostasis. Negative feedback requires accurate sensory input about the conditions being regulated. Much of this feedback is provided by the vagus nerves, which obtain extensive sensory information from receptors in the GI tract and aorta. This sensory input is processed in lower brain centers and does not reach the level of perception.

KEY CONCEPTS

- The nervous system can be divided into three principal systems: (1) the central nervous system (CNS), consisting of the brain and spinal cord; (2) the peripheral nervous system (PNS), consisting of 31 pairs of spinal nerves and 12 pairs of cranial nerves; and (3) the autonomic nervous system (ANS), consisting of the sympathetic and parasympathetic branches.
- Meninges affix the brain to the skull so that the brain is suspended and supported. Meninges have three layers: (1) The dura mater is the tough outer layer at-

Table 43-6

Effects of the Autonomic Nervous System on Organ System Function

Organ	Sympathetic Action	Sympathetic Receptor	Parasympathetic Action	Parasympathetic Receptor
Heart				
SA node, heart rate	↑	β_1	↓	M
AV nodal conduction	↑	β_1	↓	M
Contractility	↑	β_1	↓ (atria only)	M
Vascular Smooth Muscle				
Skin; splanchnic	Constricts	α_1		
Skeletal muscle	Dilates	β_2		
Skeletal muscle	Constricts	α_1		
Endothelium			Releases EDRF	M
Bronchioles	Dilates	β_2	Constricts	M
Gastrointestinal Tract				
Smooth muscle, walls	Relaxes	α_2, β_2	Contracts	M
Smooth muscle, sphincters	Contracts	α_1	Relaxes	M
Saliva secretion	↑	β_1	↑	M
Gastric acid secretion			↑	M
Pancreatic secretion			↑	M
Bladder				
Wall, detrusor muscle	Relaxes	β_2	Contracts	M
Sphincter	Contracts	α_1	Relaxes	M
Male genitalia	Ejaculation	α	Erection	M
Eye				
Radial muscle, iris	Dilates pupil (mydriasis)	α_1		
Circular sphincter muscle, iris			Constricts pupil (miosis)	M
Ciliary muscle	Dilates (far vision)	β	Contracts (near vision)	M
Skin				
Sweat glands, thermoregulatory	↑	M*		
Sweat glands, stress	↑	α		
Pilomotor muscle (goose bumps)	Contracts	α		
Lacrimal glands			Secretion	M
Liver	Gluconeogenesis; glycogenolysis	α, β_2		
Adipose tissue	Lipolysis	β_1		
Kidney	Renin secretion	β_1		

From Constanzo LS: *Physiology*, Philadelphia, 2002, Saunders, p 46.
AV, Atrioventricular; *EDRF*, endothelial-derived relaxing factor; *M*, muscarinic receptor; *SA*, sinoatrial.
*Sympathetic cholinergic neurons.

tached to the periosteum of the skull. (2) The arachnoid is a delicate weblike membrane spanning the space between the dura and the pia mater. (3) The pia mater covers the contours of the brain surface. The spinal cord has a similar arrangement of meningeal coverings.

- Cerebrospinal fluid (CSF) is produced in the brain ventricles and circulates in the subarachnoid spaces, providing cushioning and nutritive functions.
- The brain is protected by specialized tight junctions between the cells of the capillary endothelium (blood-brain barrier) and between the ependymal cells that line the ventricles (CSF-brain barrier).
- The brain can be anatomically divided into four principal structures: (1) the cerebrum (cerebral cortex, basal ganglia, limbic cortex, and corpus callosum); (2) the diencephalon (thalamus and hypothalamus); (3) the cerebellum; and (4) the brainstem (midbrain, pons, and medulla).
- Certain cortical areas are closely associated with specific functions: the frontal lobe contains the motor cortex and is involved in complex thought, motivation, and morality; the temporal lobe contains the auditory

and vestibular centers and parts of the language center; the occipital lobe contains the visual cortex; the parietal lobe contains the somatosensory cortex; the limbic area is involved in memory and emotion.

- Basal ganglia are located deep within the cerebral hemispheres and are important in the control of skeletal muscles. Parkinson disease is an important example of basal ganglia dysfunction characterized by akinesia, rigidity, and rest tremor.
- The thalamus is a centrally located structure that processes and relays most of the signals traveling to and from the cortex and lower centers. Connections between the thalamus and the brainstem and cortex are needed to maintain consciousness and allow higher brain functions.
- The hypothalamus and brainstem are important structures regulating the ANS. The sympathetic nerves originate in spinal cord segments T1 to L2. The parasympathetic nerves emerge from the sacral segments and also travel in cranial nerves III, VII, IX, and X.

NEURONAL STRUCTURE AND FUNCTION

The ways in which the nervous system achieves its rapid communication function can be understood by examining the structure and behavior of neurons and neuronal synapses.

NEURONS AND SUPPORTIVE CELLS

The nervous system is composed of two principal cell types: neurons, which generate and transmit nerve impulses, and glial cells, which provide supportive functions to neurons but do not transmit impulses. There are approximately 10 glial cells per neuron and about 100 billion neurons in the CNS.[13]

Neurons

A neuron has three basic components: (1) the cell body containing cellular organelles, (2) the dendrites that receive signals and conduct them to the cell body, and (3) the axon that generates and conducts action potentials. Neurons can be categorized according to their structure or by the neurotransmitters they secrete. Neurons come in three basic configurations based on the location of the cell body and the relative length and number of dendrites and axons[13] (Figure 43-23).

Multipolar neurons have a large number of dendrites extending from the cell body and one axon. Most neurons are of this type. Bipolar neurons have only one dendrite and one axon extending from the cell body. These neurons are prevalent in the retina, cochlea, and olfactory structures but are rare elsewhere. Unipolar neurons have a single process protruding from the cell body, which splits to form a dendrite and axon. This arrangement makes the cell body appear to be off-center. Unipolar neurons are prevalent in the somatosensory nerves in which the cell bodies are grouped in the dorsal root ganglia.

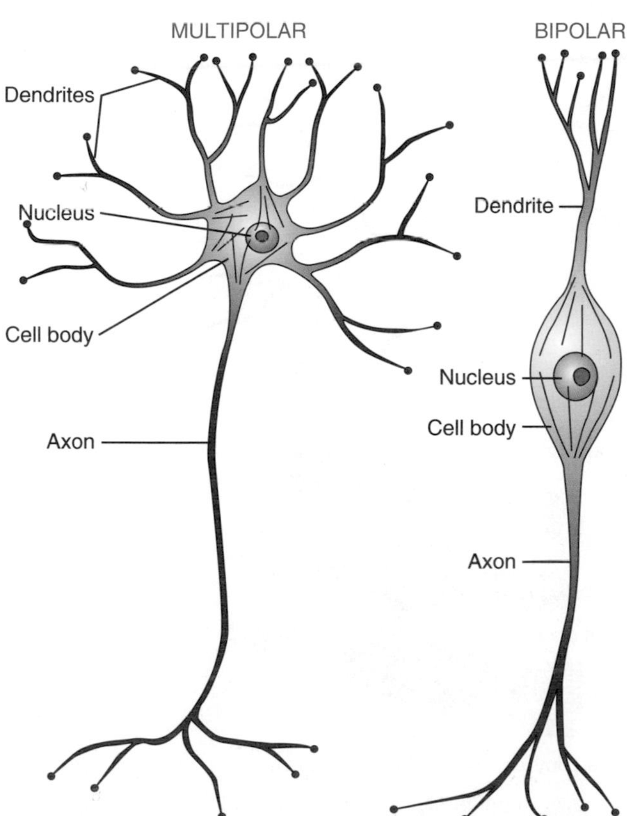

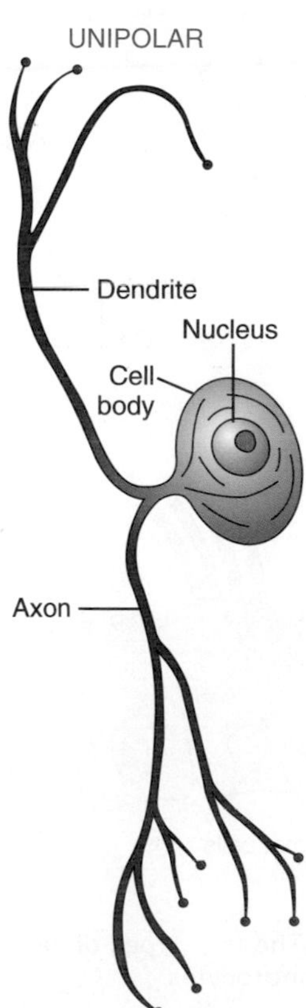

FIGURE 43-23 ■ The three basic types of neurons: multipolar, bipolar, and unipolar.

The dendrites extend to the sensory receptors and the axons enter the spinal cord.

Neurons also can be grouped as excitatory or inhibitory based on the nature of the neurotransmitter they secrete. Each neuron secretes one principal neurotransmitter, which is excitatory if it depolarizes the target neuron or inhibitory if it results in hyperpolarization.

Glia

Glial cells in the nervous system (neuroglia) serve a number of supportive functions, but they are not capable of generating action potentials. Four types of neuroglia are recognized: oligodendrocytes, astrocytes, microglia, and ependymal cells (Figure 43-24). The Schwann cells of the PNS are similar to oligodendrocytes. Both of these cell types form the myelin sheath that wraps around nerve axons to insulate and speed the rate of action potential conduction (Figure 43-25). Myelin gives the white matter its color.

Astrocytes serve many functions in the CNS. Some astrocytes have foot processes that contact the brain capillaries and help maintain integrity of the blood-brain barrier. Astrocytes regulate ionic balance of the interstitial fluid and may influence the transfer of nutrients from capillaries to neurons. Astrocytes also participate in nervous system signaling and have been shown to release molecules such as D-serine, which binds to neuron receptors and modulates neurotransmission.[14]

Microglia are derived from the monocyte-macrophage cell type and provide phagocytic functions within the CNS.[15] Ependymal cells line the ventricles and central canal of the spinal cord, producing CSF and maintaining the CSF-brain barrier.

Terminally differentiated neurons are not capable of cell division and cannot replace themselves if they die. However, certain areas of the brain, particularly the hippocampus and ventricles, are populated by neural stem cells. These cells are capable of cell division to produce two daughter cells, one of which retains stem cell characteristics while the other may differentiate into a neuron or glial cell (Figure 43-26). Specific signals are thought to guide the new cell as it migrates to the brain tissue and begins differentiation. Approximately half of the newborn cells will not find a suitable place and undergo apoptosis (programmed cell suicide).[16] The discovery that neural stem cells provide a reservoir for producing new neurons has numerous implications for treating neurodegenerative disorders such as Alzheimer disease, Parkinson disease, as well as brain damage after stroke and trauma. However, the methods for stimulating proliferation and coaching the neurons to migrate to the right places to make the correct synaptic connections have not been elucidated.

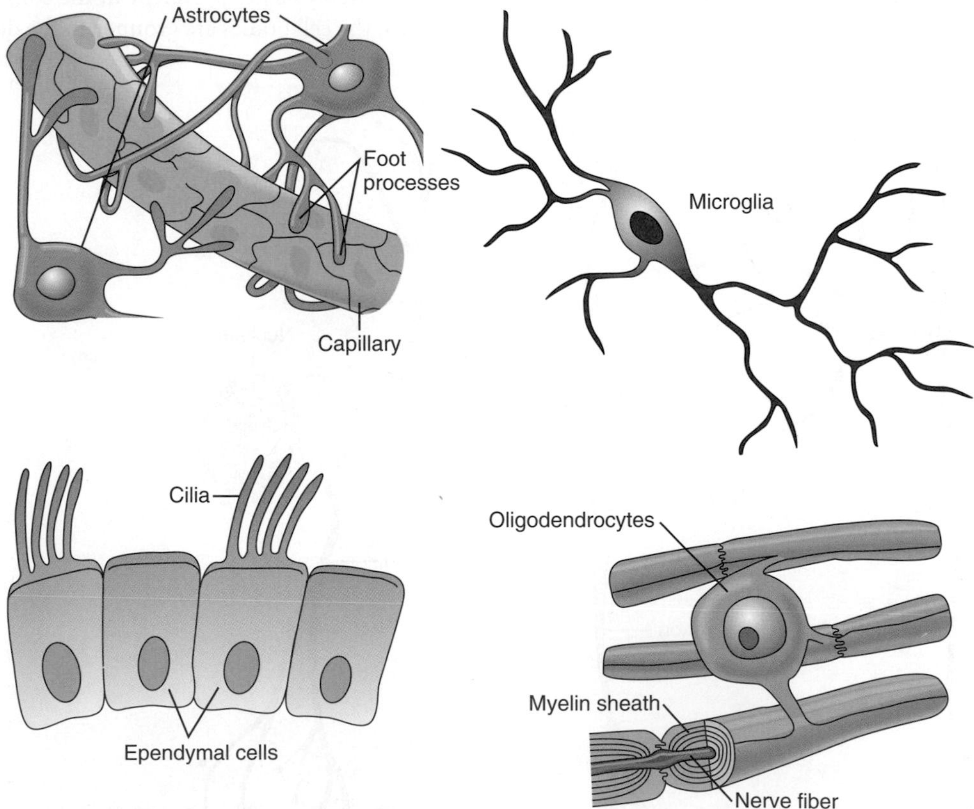

FIGURE 43-24 ■ The four types of neuroglial cells: astrocytes, microglia, ependymal cells, and oligodendrocytes.

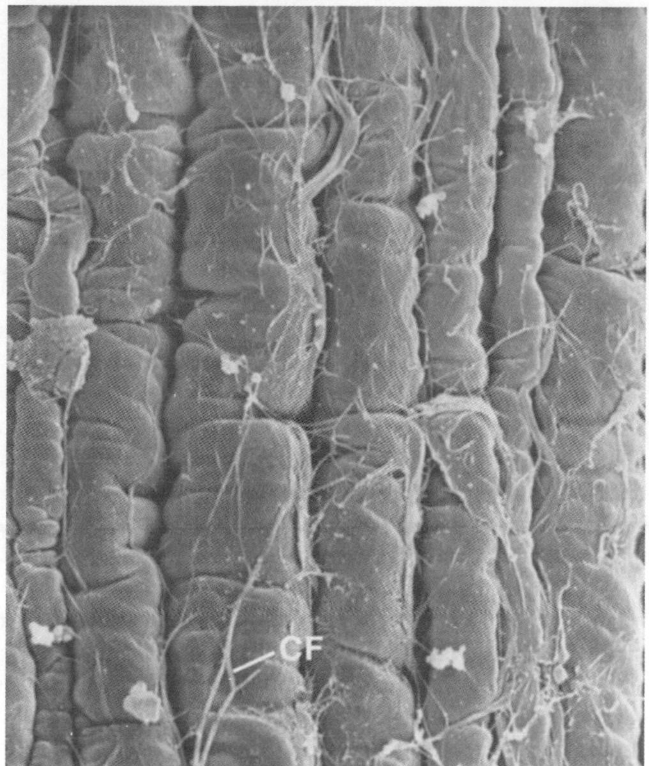

FIGURE 43-25 ■ Oligodendrocytes wrap around nerve axons to form a myelin sheath. The nodes of Ranvier are the small spaces between the oligodendrocytes. *CF,* C-fiber (unmyelinated). (From Kessel RG, Kardon RH: *Tissues and organs: a text-atlas of scanning electron microscopy,* San Francisco, 1979, Freeman, p 80.)

The term *neural plasticity* is used to describe the potential for the brain to change its structure and function. Traditionally, neural plasticity was thought to be a result of recruitment of formed neurons into new functional networks. With the discovery of neural stem cells, plasticity in some regions of the brain is likely to include the addition of new neurons as well as reassignment of the participants in the neuronal circuits. Neural plasticity is used to advantage to train different brain areas to assume new functions. For example, when a person suffers a stroke causing destruction of neurons in the motor cortex, it is possible to train nearby cortical neurons to take over some of the lost motor functions. Persistent attempts to use the muscles in an affected area may recruit cortical neurons into the neuronal circuit and improve motor strength and coordination over time. Neural plasticity is a fundamental process that endows the brain with the potential for memory and learning. Within certain boundaries, it appears that greater exposure to a particular stimulus prompts the brain to dedicate more neurons to that stimulus (and a lack of stimulation allows the brain to reassign neurons to a different function). And so the old adage "use it or lose it" appears to hold true for the brain. However, with significant effort, it is possible to reclaim at least some of what was lost.

NEURONAL COMMUNICATION

Neurons communicate through the release of neurotransmitters into the synapses adjacent to target neurons. Postsynaptic neurons have receptors for these neurotransmitters and

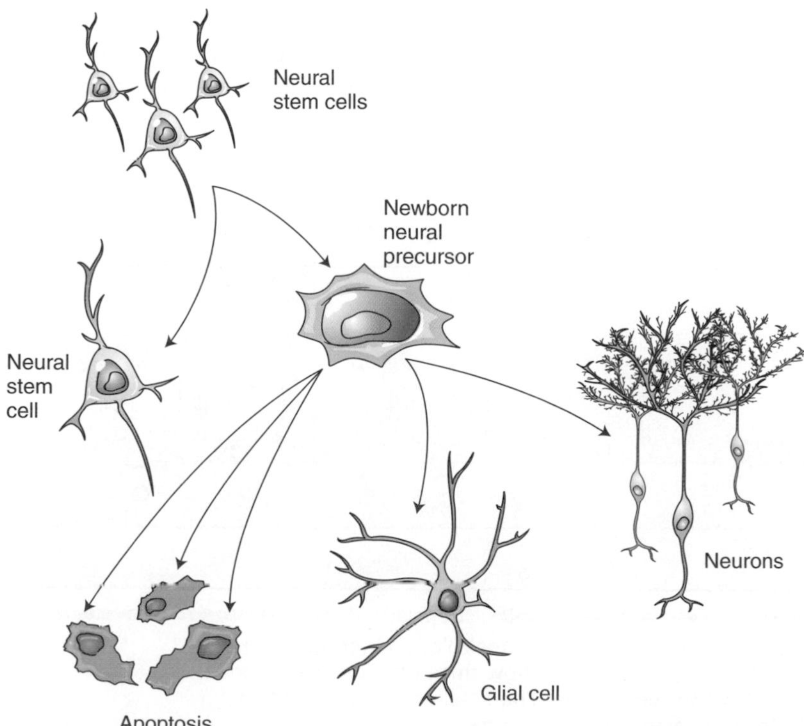

FIGURE 43-26 ■ Schematic drawing of neural stem cell proliferation. Stem cells can differentiate into glial cells or neurons under the right conditions, but half fail to find a home and undergo apoptosis (programmed cell death).

respond by changing the flow of ions through channels in the cell membrane.

Sufficient depolarization of the membrane results in the generation of action potentials, which transmit signals quickly from one end of the axon to the other. Action potentials reaching the axon terminal open voltage-gated Ca^{2+} channels and stimulate the release of neurotransmitter into the next synapse. Not all neurotransmitters are excitatory; some are inhibitory and suppress the formation of action potentials in the postsynaptic neuron. Most neurons have many contacts, some inhibitory and some excitatory, such that the response of the postsynaptic neuron is a summation of all the input.

Membrane Potentials

A detailed discussion of membrane potentials can be found in Chapter 3, and the major points are reviewed here. All cells of the body contain slightly more negatively charged molecules than positively charged ones. These negative ions are trapped intracellularly because they cannot pass through the plasma membrane. Positive ions are attracted to the cell membrane by the negatively charged cellular ions. Because the cell membrane is permeable at rest to K^+ ions, but not to Ca^{2+} or Na^+ ions, potassium accumulates in the cell to neutralize the intracellular anions. The unequal distribution of K^+ across the cell membrane creates a concentration gradient, pulling K^+ back out of the cell. At equilibrium, the electrical gradient pulling K^+ into the cell and the chemical gradient pulling it out are balanced. This equilibrium point leaves a few extra negatively charged ions inside the cell with no positive ion to neutralize them. The negative ions line up on the inside of the cell membrane to interact with positive ions on the other side (Na^+, K^+, Ca^{2+}). This separation of charge across the membrane at rest creates a membrane potential that can be measured and is about –65 to –90 mV.[17] The membrane potential changes when the concentration of K^+ changes and when the permeability of the membrane to other ions changes.

Excitable cell types, like nerve and muscle, have ion channels in their cell membranes that open and close in response to fluctuations in membrane voltage. The most important voltage-gated ion channels in nerves are the fast Na^+ channels and the K^+ channels. Fast sodium channels allow Na^+ influx during the upstroke of the action potential, whereas potassium channels allow K^+ to leave the cell and help repolarize the membrane (Figure 43-27).

An action potential is initiated when neurotransmitters bind to receptors on the dendrite and cell body and allow cations, especially Na^+, to leak in. These channels are not voltage-gated channels; they are ligand-gated channels that open in response to a neurotransmitter binding to their receptor domain. If sufficient Na^+ leaks into the cell to raise the membrane potential to threshold, the fast voltage-gated Na^+ channels open and an action potential results. Opening of fast Na^+ channels in one section of the membrane allows Na^+ to flow in and bring the next section to threshold, thus opening the fast Na^+ channels in that section. This pattern repeats over and over again down the length of the axon. Threshold represents the amount of membrane depolarization required to cause fast Na^+ channels to flip into their open conformation (see Chapter 3). The axon hillock, the point at which the axon emerges from the cell body, is the usual site of action potential initiation because it has a high density of fast Na^+ channels and, therefore, a lower threshold.

Voltage-gated K^+ channels assist with repolarization because K^+ is allowed to flow out of the cell. During an action potential, the electrical gradient holding K^+ in the cell temporarily disappears as the membrane voltage moves toward zero. Potassium flows out of the cell passively down its concentration gradient. The Na^+-K^+ pumps work continuously to remove Na^+ from the cell interior and bring K^+ back in.

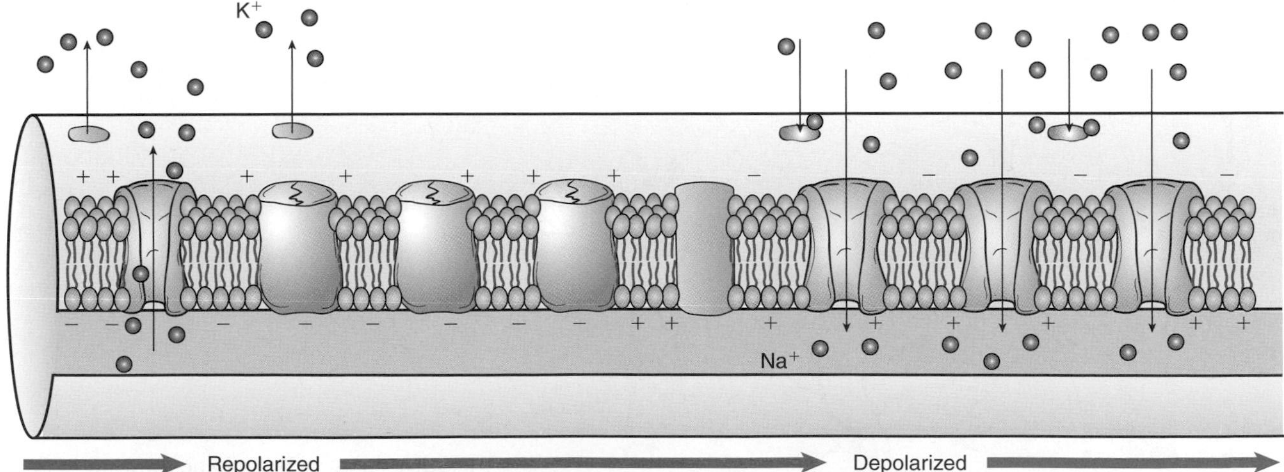

FIGURE 43-27 ■ When the voltage in the neuron reaches threshold, voltage-gated Na^+ and K^+ channels open in the membrane, allowing ions to flow through. Fast Na^+ channels stay open very briefly and allow Na^+ to rush inside. The K^+ channels allow K^+ to leak out of the cell, which contributes to a faster repolarization.

The majority of a nerve cell's energy expenditure is used to power the Na^+-K^+ pumps.

The speed at which an action potential travels is determined by axonal diameter and myelination. Larger and myelinated neurons conduct impulses more quickly (Figure 43-28). In myelinated neurons, action potentials are generated only at the nodes of Ranvier, allowing the impulse to hop quickly from node to node down the axon. This is called *saltatory conduction.*

Synaptic Transmission

The great majority of synapses responsible for signal transmission in the CNS function by using neurotransmitters. A neurotransmitter is released from the synaptic terminal of one neuron, proceeds across the synaptic cleft, and acts on the receptor proteins in the membrane of the second neuron to excite, inhibit, or modify its activity. The response at the postsynaptic membrane depends on the type of ion channel that is opened or closed when the neurotransmitter binds to the receptor. The neurotransmitter is therefore a chemical messenger that stimulates a response that is built into the postsynaptic cell. Once neurotransmitters are released into the synaptic cleft, their potential to activate the postsynaptic receptors is limited by deactivation processes. Neurotransmitters are either actively transported back into the axon terminals for reuse or destroyed by enzyme activity.

An *excitatory postsynaptic potential* (EPSP) results when a neurotransmitter has a depolarizing effect on the postsynaptic membrane. The EPSP may be too small to bring the axon hillock to threshold, and EPSPs from several presynaptic neurons may be required to generate an action potential. Thus postsynaptic potentials are not all-or-none phenomena, as are action potentials. Neurotransmitters that produce EPSPs do so by opening channels in the membrane that allow Na^+ influx. In some cases, the receptor itself is a channel *(ionotropic receptor);* in others, the receptor is linked to the channel through a second messenger cascade *(metabotropic receptor)* (Figure 43-29). In general, the ionotropic receptors are concerned with producing changes in membrane potential, whereas the metabotropic receptors influence complex cytoplasmic signaling cascades that affect synthesis, metabolism, gene expression, and ion channels. The ion channels regulated by metabotropic receptors may participate in action potential generation, but receptor activation also exerts more long-lasting effects on cell structure and behavior.

Some neurotransmitters inhibit depolarization and may produce hyperpolarization of the postsynaptic membrane by

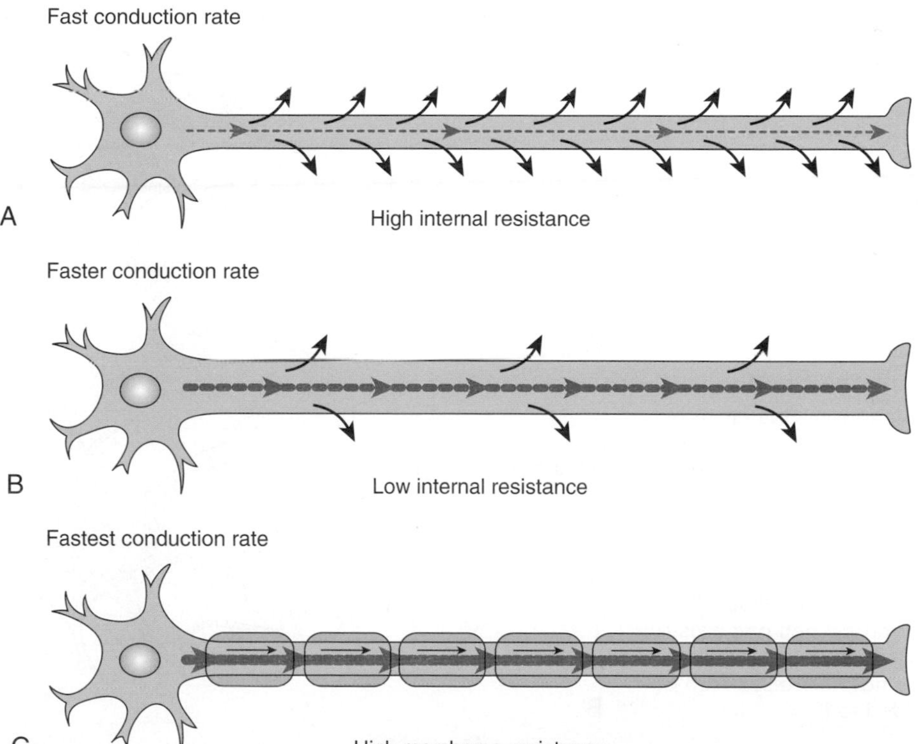

FIGURE 43-28 ■ The rate of action potential conduction down an axon depends on the relative degree of internal resistance to current flow. When the diameter is small **(A)**, there is high internal resistance and slower conduction. A larger diameter **(B)** reduces internal resistance and speeds up the rate of conduction. Myelination **(C)** produces the fastest rate of conduction by increasing membrane resistance and decreasing internal resistance.

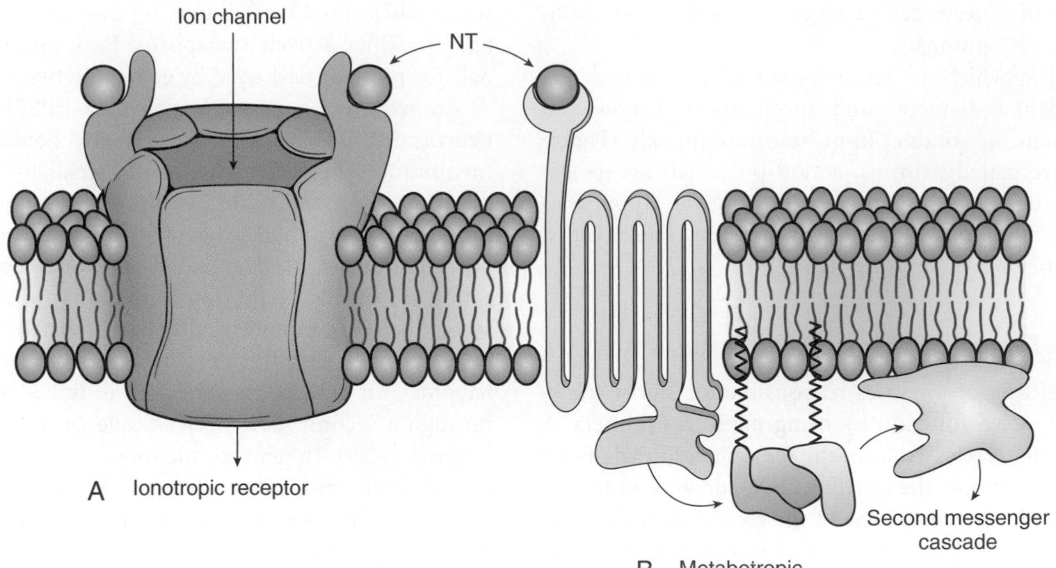

FIGURE 43-29 ■ Neurotransmitter *(NT)* receptor classes. **A,** Ionotropic receptors are channel proteins that open when a neurotransmitter binds to them. **B,** Metabotropic receptors activate intracellular signaling cascades that generate second messengers in the cell when the neurotransmitter binds.

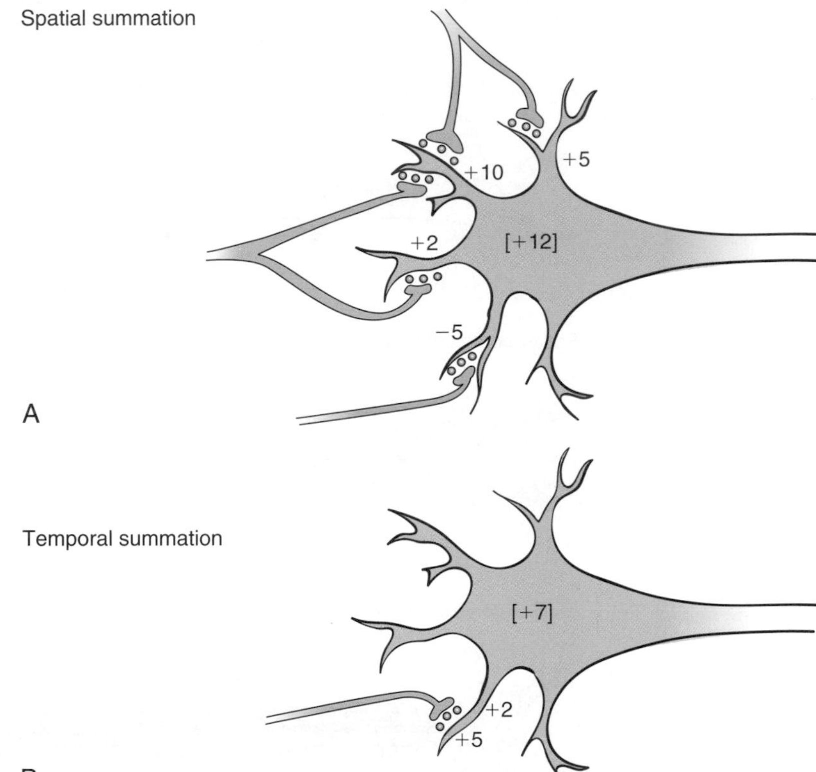

FIGURE 43-30 ■ Summation. **A,** Spatial summation occurs when two or more presynaptic neurons release neurotransmitter onto one postsynaptic cell at the same time. The various excitatory postsynaptic potentials and inhibitory postsynaptic potentials add algebraically to determine the overall postsynaptic potential (PSP) reaching the axon hillock. **B,** Temporal summation occurs when one presynaptic neuron fires in rapid succession such that a previous PSP has not fully dissipated before the next PSP is added to it.

opening Cl^- or K^+ channels. Chloride ions leaking into the cell or potassium ions leaking out of the cell serve to short-circuit the effect of sodium ion influx, thus making it more difficult to reach threshold. This effect is called an *inhibitory postsynaptic potential* (IPSP). Neurotransmitters that result in IPSPs include γ-aminobutyric acid (GABA) and glycine.

Most synapses in the CNS have many presynaptic neurons, some producing EPSP and some producing IPSP. The membrane potential of the postsynaptic membrane is an algebraic sum of all the IPSP and EPSP occurring at any one moment in time. This is called *summation* and is the basis of neuronal processing and integration (Figure 43-30). The term *spatial*

Box 43-1

Six Major Classes of Neurotransmitters

Acetylcholine

Amines
Dopamine
Norepinephrine
Epinephrine
Serotonin
Histamine

Amino Acids

Excitatory
Glutamate
Aspartate

Inhibitory
Glycine
γ-Aminobutyric acid

Polypeptides
Substance P, other tachykinins
Vasopressin
Oxytocin
Corticotropin-releasing hormone
Thyrotropin-releasing hormone
Growth hormone–releasing hormone
Somatostatin
Gonadotropin-releasing hormone
Endothelins
Enkephalins
β-Endorphin, other derivatives of pro-opiomelanocortin
Cholecystokinin
Vasoactive intestinal polypeptide
Neurotensin
Gastrin-releasing peptide
Gastrin
Glucagon
Motilin
Secretin
Calcitonin gene–related peptide α
Neuropeptide Y
Activins
Inhibins
Angiotensin II
Galanin
Atrial natriuretic peptide
Brain natriuretic peptide

Purines
Adenosine
Adenosine triphosphate

Gases
Nitric oxide
Carbon monoxide

summation is applied when multiple presynaptic neurons release their neurotransmitters onto one postsynaptic neuron at the same time. The IPSPs and EPSPs sum algebraically to produce the overall postsynaptic potential. *Temporal summation* occurs when one presynaptic neuron fires in rapid succession so that it releases more neurotransmitter onto the postsynaptic cell before the postsynaptic neuron has completely recovered from a previous dose.

Neurotransmitters

Neurotransmitters are grouped according to their chemical structure into six principal categories[15,17] (Box 43-1). *Acetylcholine* is the sole neurotransmitter in its class and is prevalent in numerous areas in the CNS. It is the neurotransmitter in autonomic ganglia, postganglionic parasympathetic synapses, and neuromuscular junctions. There are two major types of acetylcholine receptors; the nicotinic receptors (N) are of the ionotropic variety and the muscarinic receptors (M) are metabotropic (Table 43-7). When acetylcholine is released into the synapse it is quickly degraded by acetylcholinesterase to limit the duration of action (Figure 43-31). Choline is actively taken back up into the presynaptic membrane for resynthesis. Acetylcholine receptors located on the presynaptic membrane provide a negative feedback loop, whereby the presynaptic neuron monitors the amount of acetylcholine in the synapse. Acetylcholinesterase inhibitor drugs are used for diseases, such as Alzheimer disease and myasthenia gravis, in which there is a deficiency of acetylcholine in the synapse and for reversing the effect of neuromuscular blocking drugs.

The *amines* include DA, NE, epinephrine, serotonin (5-hydoxytryptamine, 5HT), and histamine. Amines are particularly involved in the limbic system, hypothalamus, and basal ganglia. NE is the neurotransmitter released at SNS postganglionic nerve endings. DA, NE, and serotonin are important in regulating thought processes and mood. Antipsychotic and mood-altering drugs change the activity of one or more of these amines in the brain (see Chapters 48 and 49). DA-secreting neurons project to the striatum (basal ganglia), pituitary, limbic system, and frontal cortex (Figure 43-32, *A*). DA can be degraded by enzymes in the extracellular fluid (catechol-*O*-methyltransferase, COMT) or by enzymes in the presynaptic nerve (monoamine oxidase, MAO). The primary means of clearing DA from the synapse is by active reuptake into the presynaptic membrane (see Figure 43-32, *B*). There are at least five DA receptor subtypes all of which are metabotropic and linked to the production of second messengers (see Table 43-7). Abnormality of DA metabolism is apparent in various diseases, including Parkinson disease and schizophrenia.

Some neurons have an enzyme for the hydroxylation of DA to form NE. The NE-secreting neurons originate in the brainstem (locus coeruleus) and project widely throughout the brain including the cerebral cortex, cerebellum, limbic structures, brainstem, and spinal cord (see Figure 43-32, *C*). Most

Table 43-7

Mechanism of Action of Selected Nonpeptide Neurotransmitters

Transmitter	Receptor	Second Messenger	Net Channel Effects
Acetylcholine	Nicotinic	—	↑ Na^+, other small ions
	M_1	↑ IP_3, DAG	↑ Ca^{2+}
	M_2 (cardiac)	↓ cAMP	↑ K^+
	M_3	↓ cAMP	
	M_4 (glandular)	↑ IP_3, DAG	
	M_5	↑ IP_3, DAG	
Dopamine	D_1,D_5	↑ cAMP	
	D_2	↓ cAMP	↑ K^+, ↓ Ca^{2+}
	D_3,D_4	↓ cAMP	
Norepinephrine	α_{1A}, α_{1B}, α_{1D}	↑ IP_3, DAG	↓ K^+
	α_{2A}, α_{2B}, α_{2C}	↓ cAMP	↑ K^+, ↓ Ca^{2+}
	β_1	↑ cAMP	
	β_2	↑ cAMP	
	β_3	↑ cAMP	
5HT*	$5HT_{1A}$	↓ cAMP	↑ K^+
	$5HT_{1B}$	↓ cAMP	
	$5HT_{1D}$	↓ cAMP	↓ K^+
	$5HT_{2A}$	↑ IP_3, DAG	↓ K^+
	$5HT_{2C}$	↑ IP_3, DAG	
	$5HT_3$	—	↑ Na^+
	$5HT_4$	↑ cAMP	
Adenosine	A_1	↓ cAMP	
	A_2	↑ cAMP	
Glutamate	Metabotropic†		
	Ionotropic		
	AMPA, Kainate	—	↑ Na^+
	NMDA	—	↑ Na^+, Ca^{2+}
GABA	$GABA_A$	—	↑ $C1^-$
	$GABA_B$	↑ IP_3, DAG	↑ K^+, ↓ Ca^{2+}

From Ganong WF: *Review of medical physiology,* ed 21, New York, 2003, Lange/McGraw-Hill, p 99.

AMPA, α-Amino-3-hydroxy-5-methyl-4-isoxazolepropionate; *cAMP,* cyclic adenosine monophosphate; *DAG,* diacylglycerol; GABA, γ-aminobutyric acid; *5HT,* serotonin; *IP_3,* inositol triphosphate; *NMDA, N*-methyl-D-aspartate.

*$5HT_{1E}$, $5HT_{1F}$, $5HT_{2B}$, $5HT_{5A}$, $5HT_{5B}$, $5HT_6$, and $5HT_7$ receptors also cloned.

†Eleven subtypes identified; all decrease cAMP or increase IP_3 and DAG, except one, which increases cAMP.

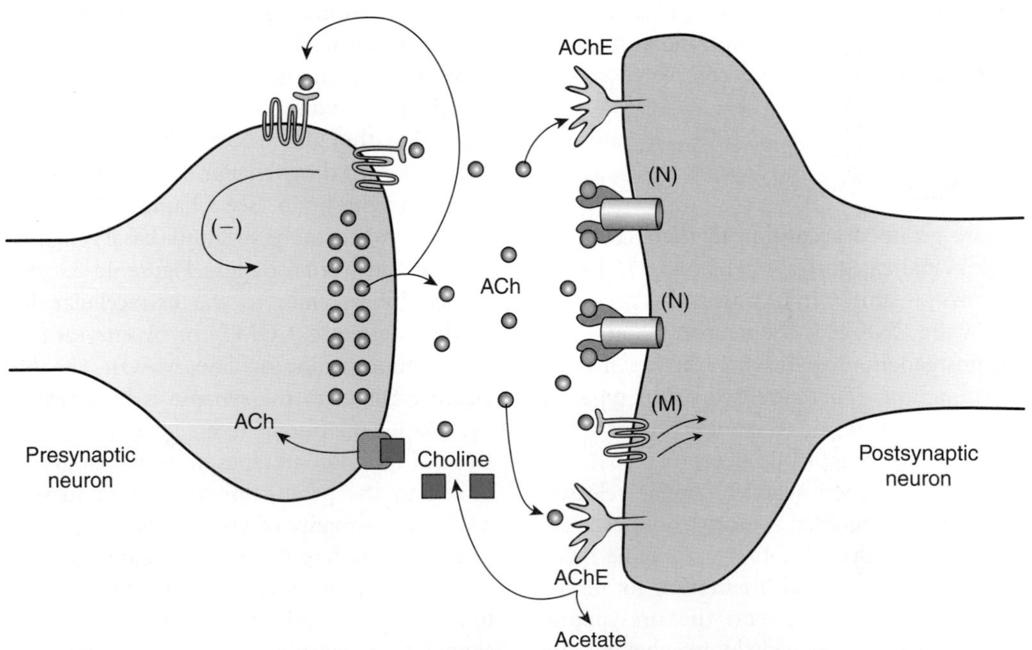

FIGURE 43-31 ■ The acetylcholine synapse. Acetylcholine *(ACh)* released into the synapse binds to nicotinic *(N)* or muscarinic *(M)* receptors on the postsynaptic membrane. ACh also can bind to presynaptic receptors that are linked to a decrease in ACh release (negative feedback). Acetylcholinesterase *(AChE)* quickly degrades the ACh into acetate and choline. Choline is actively taken back into the presynaptic neuron for resynthesis.

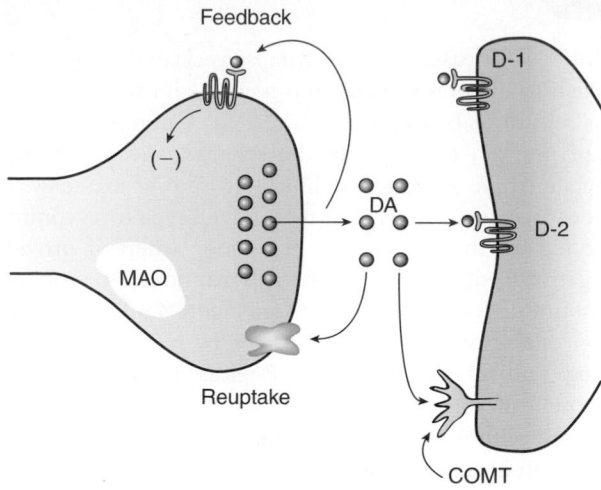

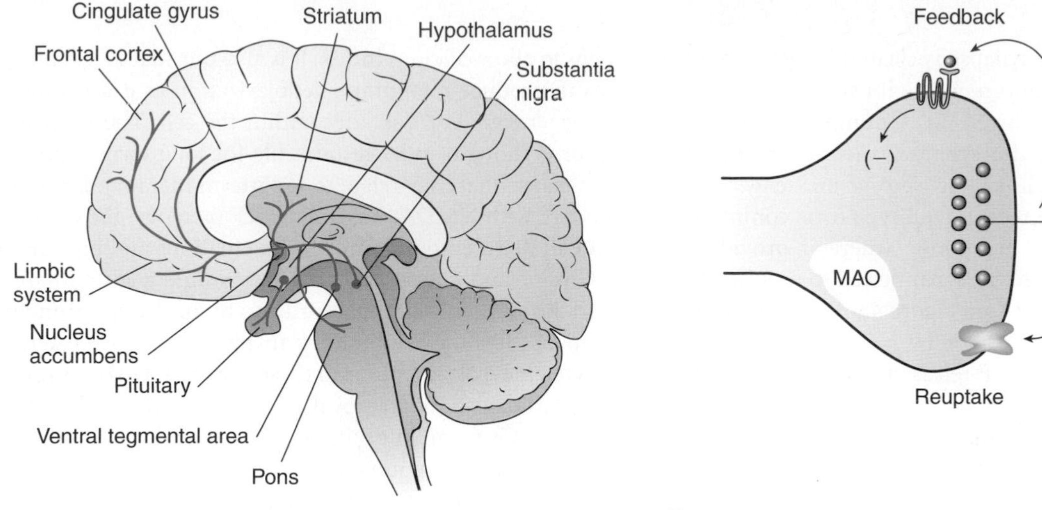

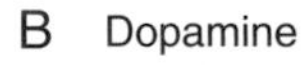

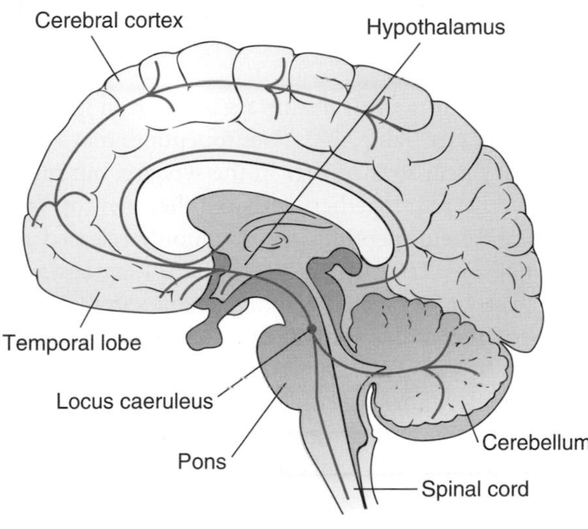

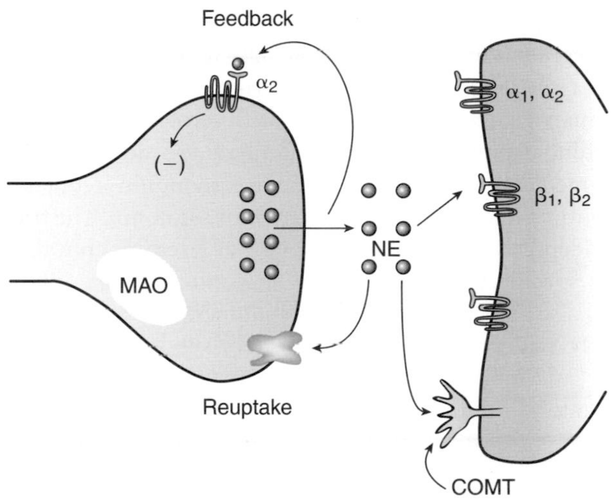

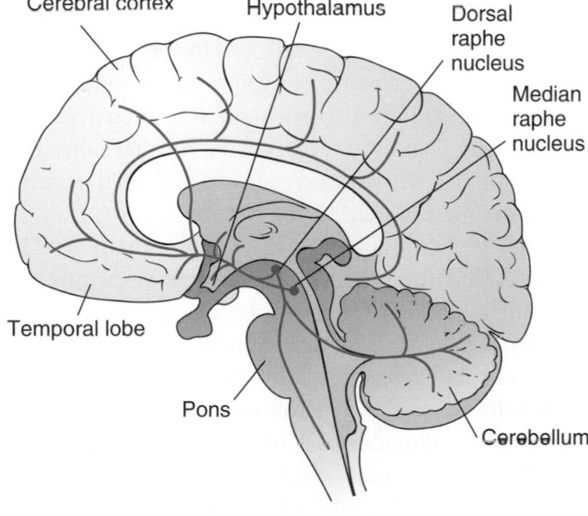

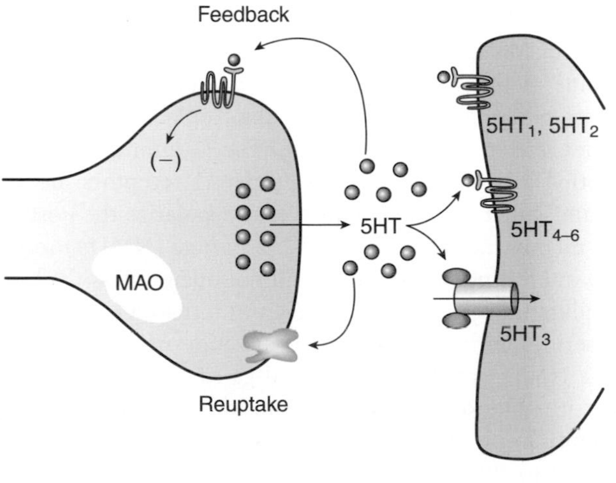

FIGURE 43-32 ■ Amine synapses. **A,** Dopamine *(DA)* distribution in the brain. **B,** The DA synapse. **C,** Norepinephrine *(NE)* distribution in the brain. **D,** The NE synapse. **E,** Serotonin *(5HT)* distribution in the brain. **F,** The 5HT synapse. *COMT,* Catechol-*O*-methyl transferase; *MAO,* monoamine oxidase.

of the NE released into the synapse is cleared by active reuptake into the presynaptic neuron, where it can be repackaged for release or broken down by MAO. A number of receptor subtypes can bind NE in the synapse, and all are of the metabotropic variety and linked to second-messenger cascades (see Table 43-7). The receptor subtype α_2 is commonly located on the presynaptic membrane where it provides a negative-feedback loop for the presynaptic cell to monitor the amount of NE in the synapse (see Figure 43-32, *D*). Stimulation of the presynaptic α_2 receptor by NE or by α_2-agonist drugs reduces the amount of NE released into the synapse by the neuron.

Serotonin is another amine that affects numerous areas of the brain in a pattern similar to that of NE (see Figure 43-32, *E*). Numerous serotonin receptor subtypes have been identified, including one ionotropic ($5HT_3$) and several metabotropic (see Table 43-7). Like NE and DA, serotonin is cleared from the synapse by an active reuptake carrier on the presynaptic membrane (see Figure 43-32, *F*). It is also subject to degradation by MAO and can bind to presynaptic receptors that regulate its release. Numerous drugs have been developed to manage disorders associated with serotonin pathways, including depression, anxiety, and migraine headache. The class of medications known as selective serotonin reuptake inhibitors blocks the reuptake carrier for serotonin. The tricyclic antidepressants also block reuptake of serotonin, but they are less specific than the selective serotonin reuptake inhibitors and also affect reuptake of other amines.

The category of *amino acids* can be subdivided into excitatory and inhibitory mechanisms of action. Glutamate and aspartate are the principal excitatory amino acids. Glutamate neurons are widely distributed throughout the brain, and it is considered to be the primary excitatory neurotransmitter. Glutamate is involved in memory and has been implicated as a neurotoxin when released in excessive amounts (Chapter 44). Glutamate is removed from the synapse by active reuptake transporters on the presynaptic membrane. When energy stores are low because of interrupted blood supply or hypoxia, the transporters do not function effectively and glutamate remains in the synapse where it can behave as a neurotoxin. Most glutamate receptors are ionotropic; the metabotropic types are poorly understood. The α-amino-3-hydroxy-5-methyl-4-isoxazolepropionate (AMPA) receptors are classic ligand-gated sodium channels that depolarize the postsynaptic membrane. The *N*-methyl-D-aspartate (NMDA) receptors are interesting because they will not open unless the binding of glutamate is paired with a cotransmitter (such as glycine or D-serine) and concurrent depolarization of the membrane.[15] The NMDA receptor is a ligand-gated calcium ion channel, but it is blocked by a magnesium ion when the postsynaptic membrane is polarized (Figure 43-33). It only opens in response to glutamate binding if a depolarization is produced at the same time by another neurotransmitter-receptor interaction. The depolarization releases the blocking magnesium ion from the channel, so that when glutamate binds, the channel opens to allow calcium influx. It is also unusual to use calcium ions to produce membrane depolarization as it can function to trigger signaling cascades within the cell. The NMDA receptor is thought to be responsible for long-term changes in the synapse that may relate to long-term memory. Drugs that interfere with NMDA receptors block memory; those that activate these receptors produce hallucinations and nightmares.

Glycine and GABA are inhibitory amino acids and are located throughout the spinal cord and brain. A large number of synapses (30%) are inhibitory in nature, and GABA is the principal neurotransmitter in these synapses. GABA is formed by decarboxylation (removal of CO_2) of glutamate, which transforms it from an excitatory amino acid to an inhibitory one. The GABA receptors are of two types: $GABA_A$ is a classic ligand-gated chloride channel that produces an IPSP when activated. The $GABA_B$ receptor is a metabotropic receptor that also produces an IPSP and is linked to cytoplasmic signaling cascades within the cell. Barbiturates and benzodiazepines are thought to exert their depressive effects by increasing GABA activity.

A long list of neurotransmitters is found in the *neuropeptide* category (see Table 43-7). Neuropeptides may function as the primary neurotransmitter in the synapse, but more often they are released together with another neurotransmitter. Amines and neuropeptides are commonly released together into synapses.[18] The neuropeptides have long-lasting effects on the postsynaptic cell, mediating changes in receptor number or structure and altering the responses of intracellular signaling pathways. Well-known neuropeptides include substance P, endorphins, and enkephalins, which are involved in the transmission and perception of pain. Neuropeptides are synthesized in the neuronal cell body and not in the nerve terminal like other neurotransmitters. The amount produced depends on the degree of gene activity that produces messenger RNA to direct the synthesis of the neuropeptide. Once synthesized and packaged into vesicles, the neuropeptides must be actively transported along the axon to the nerve terminal. All neuropeptide receptors are linked to second messenger cascades. Neuropeptides are released in very small quantity in comparison to other neurotransmitters, and reuptake mechanisms are not required to turn off their activity. The neuropeptide with its bound receptor may be internalized into the postsynaptic cell, where the receptor is degraded or recycled to the synaptic membrane.

Purines, including adenosine triphosphate (ATP) and adenosine, function as neurotransmitters in various brain regions. Adenosine is thought to be continuously released by most neurons and modulates neurotransmission by blocking neurotransmitter release. Adenosine may be important in preventing seizure activity. The role of ATP as a neurotransmitter continues to be elucidated. There are at least two ATP receptor subtypes, one metabotropic and one an ionotropic-type cation channel. Little is known about either type.

Nitric oxide (NO) is a gas that can diffuse through cell membranes and therefore does not require a synaptic receptor

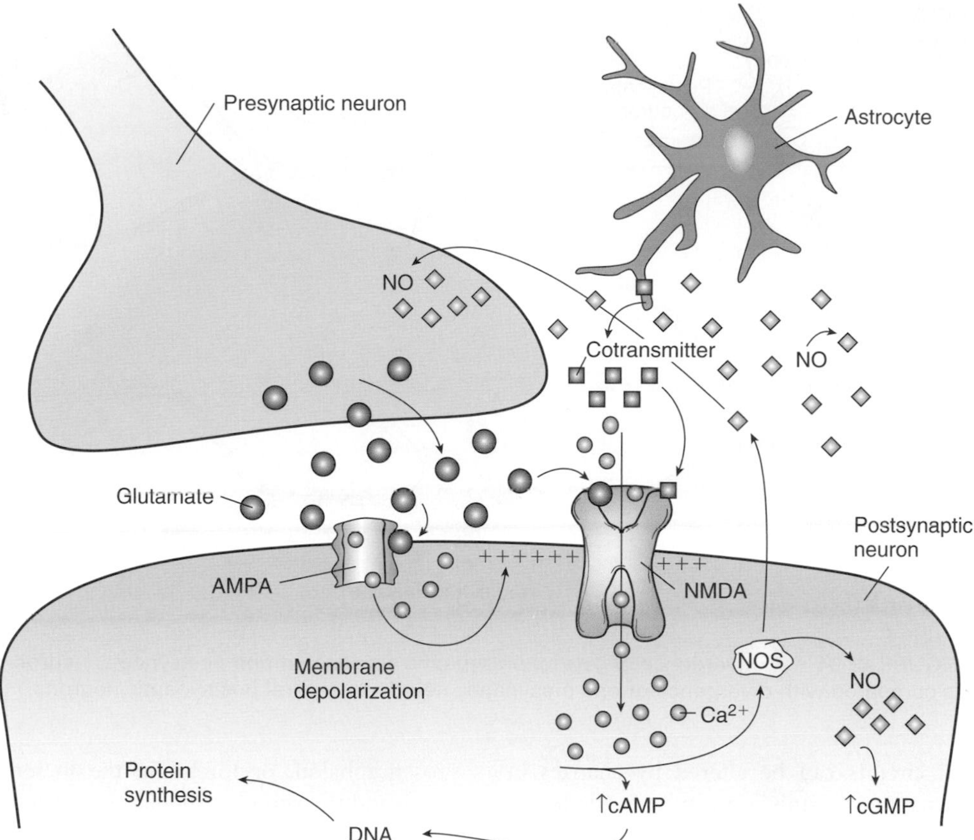

FIGURE 43-33 ■ The glutamate synapse. Glutamate signaling is complex, having several receptor subtypes and costimulating molecules. The *N*-methyl-D-aspartate *(NMDA)* receptor is of special interest because it requires binding of glutamate and a cotransmitter (glycine or D-serine). In addition, the NMDA ion channel is blocked by Mg^{2+} and cannot open unless the postsynaptic membrane is already depolarized. Glutamate binding to its α-amino-3-hydroxy-5-methyl-4-isoxazolepropionate *(AMPA)* receptors can provide this depolarization. When the NMDA channel opens, it allows calcium ions to flow in, triggering intracellular signaling cascades that produce nitric oxide *(NO)*. Nitric oxide is a gas that can diffuse throughout the synapse. NMDA receptor activation has been linked to long-term changes in synaptic efficiency; *NOS,* nitric oxide synthase.

for its activity. NO has several different potential targets within cells. For example, NO can bind and stimulate guanylyl cyclase, an enzyme that produces cyclic guanosine monophosphate (cGMP), a second messenger in the cell, or it can alter the activity of ion pumps, metabolic enzymes, and DNA transcription factors.[15] Unlike other neurotransmitters that are produced and released by presynaptic neurons, NO can be synthesized in the postsynaptic neuron and diffuse locally to affect presynaptic neurons. The functions of NO are not completely known, but it is thought to be important in memory and pain perception. One trigger known to stimulate NO is activation of the previously described NMDA receptor. The calcium ions that flow in through the open NMDA receptor cause activation of an enzyme called nitric oxide synthase (NOS), which produces NO. NO may be the messenger that alerts the presynaptic membrane that the paired stimuli required to open the NMDA receptor were received.[18]

Neuronal Circuits

Patterns of neuronal synaptic connections are called *neuronal circuits.* Activity in particular groups of neurons in one or more circuits is the basis of nervous system function: thoughts, memories, sensations, movements, and learning.

Divergence is a term used to describe neuronal circuits in which one presynaptic neuron makes contact with more than one postsynaptic neuron (Figure 43-34). Divergence is a strategy used to send sensory input to a large number of receiving neurons. *Convergence* occurs when many presynaptic neurons synapse with one postsynaptic neuron (see Figure 43-34). This arrangement is typical in the motor pathways, in which sensory, reflex, and voluntary inputs must be integrated into a response by the motor neurons that innervate skeletal muscle. Convergence is a mechanism of processing and integration of input.

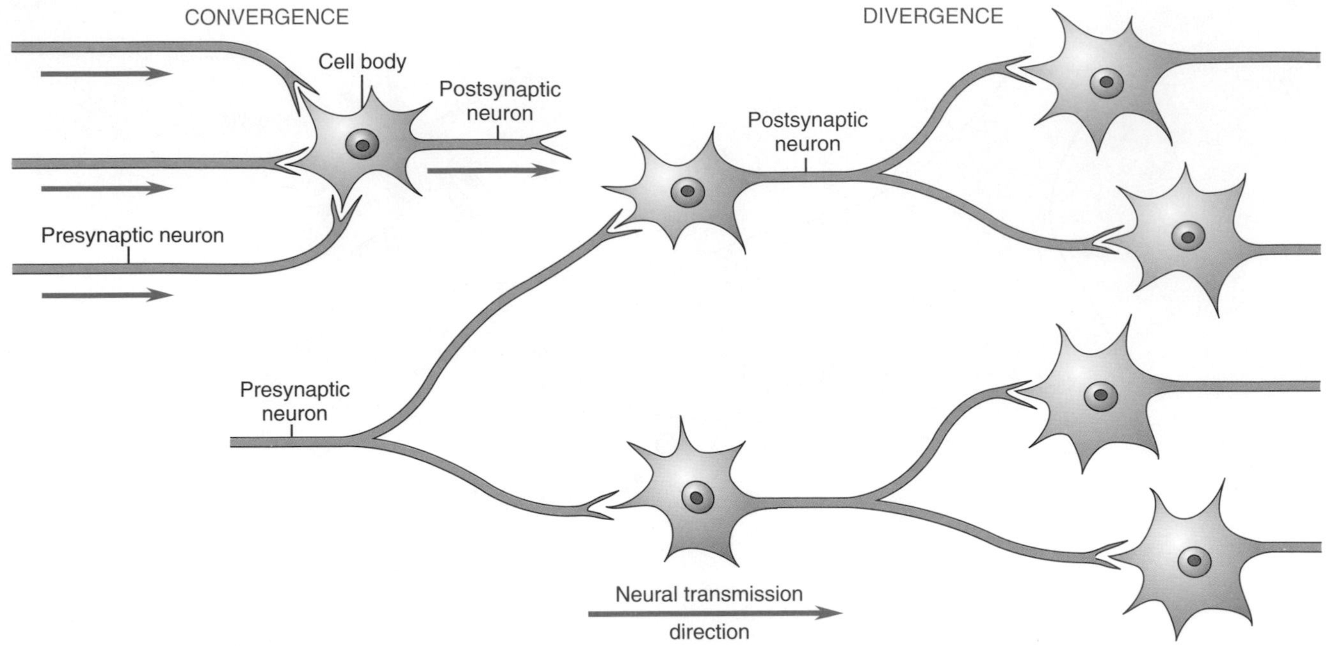

FIGURE 43-34 ■ Convergence of several presynaptic neurons on one postsynaptic neuron is compared with divergence of one presynaptic neuron to several postsynaptic neurons.

The efficiency of circuits can be altered by changes in synaptic function. Synaptic transmission can be facilitated or inhibited in various ways. Alteration in the ease of synaptic transmission is the basis of memory and is discussed in more detail in the last section of this chapter.

NEURAL DEVELOPMENT, AGING, AND INJURY

Development

The nervous system starts to take shape during the third week of embryonic development. At this time, three primary tissues of the embryo are distinguishable: the ectoderm, endoderm, and mesoderm. A thickened plate of ectoderm, running longitudinally on the dorsal surface of the embryo (neural plate), gives rise to the CNS and PNS. By the end of the third week, the neural plate folds to form a neural tube. Openings at either end of the neural tube are called *neuropores.* The neural tube is the precursor of the future brain and spinal cord.

Fusion of cells and formation of the neural tube starts in the cervical region of the future spinal cord and then progresses rapidly in a **rostral** direction toward the future brain. Failure of the neural tube to close properly is a cause of congenital malformation of the nervous system. Anencephaly (absent brain) results from failure of the rostral portion to close, whereas failure of the caudal portion results in myelomeningocele. In this defect, the spinal cord and meninges are displaced into a sac on the back (see Chapter 45). A reduction in neural tube defects has been achieved through prenatal maternal supplementation with folic acid.[19]

At the end of the fourth week of gestation, three primary vesicles are evident at the rostral end of the neural tube: the prosencephalon, or forebrain; the mesencephalon, or midbrain; and the rhombencephalon, or hindbrain.[20] The mature brain develops from these three primary structures. The prosencephalon divides to form the cerebral hemispheres and diencephalon; the mesencephalon forms the upper part of the brainstem (midbrain); and the rhombencephalon divides to form the cerebellum and lower brainstem (pons and medulla).

Neurons grow and divide at an incredible rate during embryologic development and make primitive synaptic connections according to a basic architecture that is genetically programmed. The number of neurons and synapses ultimately dedicated to particular functions is determined in large part by their use. For example, if no visual sensory input is relayed to the primary visual cortex (as occurs with congenital cataracts), the cortical neurons will be reassigned to other functions. Similarly, a person born without arms will lack representation of these structures in the primary somatosensory cortex. In contrast, greater stimulation appears to increase the number of neurons dedicated to a particular function. Critical periods in the early neonatal period have been identified when neuronal assignment to specific functions is determined.[21] In recent years it has been recognized that a significant degree of neural plasticity exists throughout life; however, it is much less than that during early childhood. The brain continues to increase in size until puberty and remains stable until middle age.

Aging

A gradual loss of neurons in later adulthood does not result in significant alteration in brain function during the usual life span. However, the older one gets, the greater the neurologic

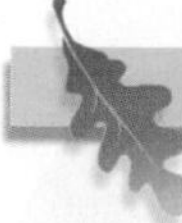

THE AGING PROCESS

Changes in the Nervous System

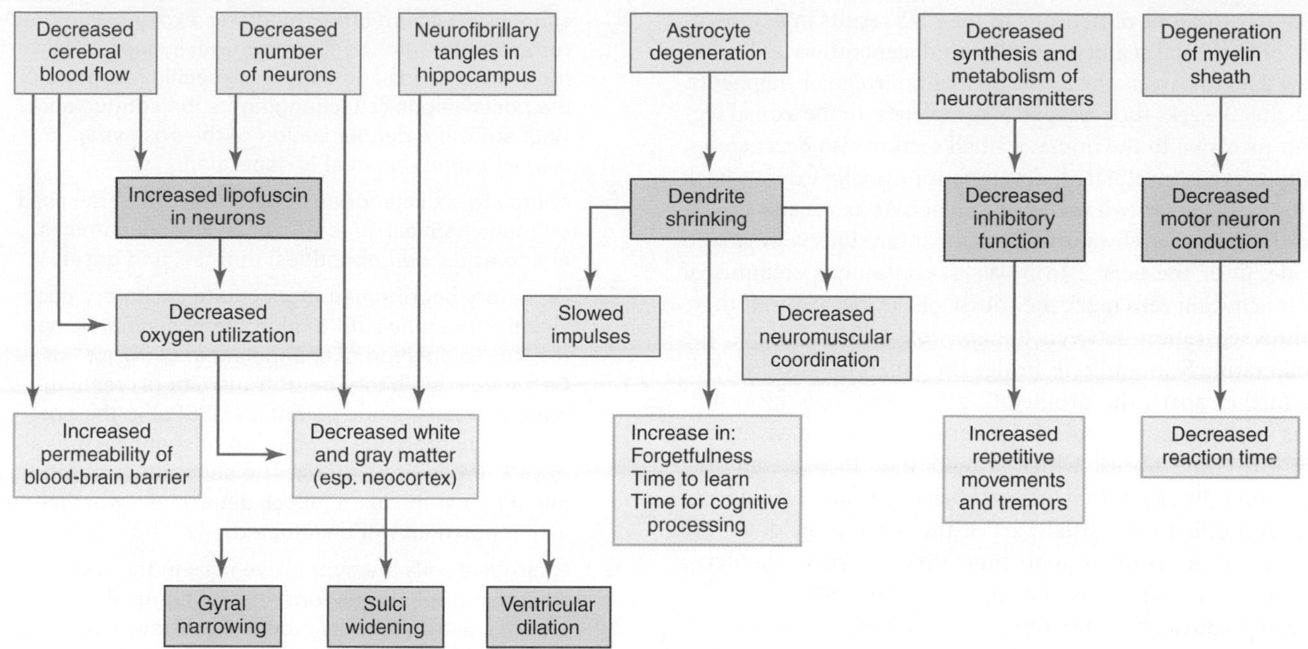

With aging, brain atrophy and a decrease in brain weight occur. This is evidenced by a decrease in white matter and gray matter up to 0.5% per year, with gyral narrowing, sulci widening, and ventricular dilation. There is a gradual atrophy and loss of neurons in the brain and spinal cord over time; but neuron loss is not uniform within the brain. Most of the neuron loss is in the neocortex (20%), Purkinje cells of the cerebellum, substantia nigra, and locus coeruleus. Some parts of the brain, such as the vestibular nucleus, have no neuron loss. Blood supply to the brain is decreased owing to the decreased metabolic demands and brain atrophy. There is also increased permeability of the blood-brain barrier.

Intracellularly there is an increase in lipofuscin, which hampers cellular oxygen use, crowds intracellular organelles, and reduces the number of mitochondria. There are also neurofibrillary tangles in the hippocampus and neuritic plaques that are found only in the elderly.

Nerve fibers in the brain decrease in number and show signs of splitting or fragmentation. The cortex, subcortex, and cerebellar astrocytes degenerate. Nerve axons develop swellings near their ends called *neuroaxonal dystrophy.* The relevance of these swellings is unknown. Dendrites shrink decreasing the number of messages received from other cells and synaptic linkages. This causes slowing of impulses and decreases neuromuscular coordination. These changes result in decreased short-term memory, reduced speed of learning, prolonged new information processing, increased reaction time, diminished abstract reasoning, and impaired perception.

Changes in the secretion and metabolism of neurotransmitters also impact the aging brain. There is a decrease in norepinephrine and dopamine secretion with an increase in monoamine oxidase. The reduction of dopamine leads to decreased inhibitory functions.

In the spinal cord, posterior root fibers and sympathetic nerve fibers of the autonomic nervous system decline in number. Peripherally, there is degeneration of the motor nerve fibers and myelin sheath. Motor neuron axons remain intact. Decreasing motor neuron conduction velocity and prolonged muscle action potentials lead to decreased reaction times. Reflexes may be decreased or absent.

impairment. Excessive neuronal degeneration in adulthood is called Alzheimer disease or senile dementia, and is distinguished from the normal changes of aging. The effects of aging on nervous system function are summarized in The Aging Process: Changes in the Nervous System.

Injury

Mature neurons are terminally differentiated cells that are unable to undergo mitosis. Injury to neurons usually results in neuronal cell death and loss of function; however, some regrowth is possible in peripheral nerves if the injury is not severe. Stem cells in the brain are capable of producing new, immature neurons; however, the likelihood that they will find and repair a site of injury and make appropriate synaptic connections is uncertain.

Injury to axons of neurons in the PNS results in degeneration of the distal segment (**wallerian degeneration**).[19] Within a few days to a week, the axons break into irregular fragments, and after 3 weeks they disappear completely. In the axonal segment proximal to the injury, a small section also degenerates. If the nerve is myelinated, degeneration usually extends back to the next one or two nodes of Ranvier. As axons and myelin sheaths degrade, Schwann cells of the injured nerve swell and divide. Over the next 2 to 3 weeks, continuous columns of short Schwann cells mark the course of the lost axons. If there is little separation between the ends of a divided nerve, the proliferating Schwann cells bridge the gap. If the divided ends are further apart, the proliferating Schwann cells form bulbous swellings at the end of the nerves and the surviving axons form fine fibrils, which extend into the surrounding Schwann cells at random. Those fibrils that find a column of Schwann cells in the distal part of the nerve grow down the column. There is often good functional return to the nerve secondary to this process. If continuity is not restored, the distal end gradually becomes replaced by collagenous scar tissue.

Damaged axons in the CNS show a pattern of degeneration that is similar to that of peripheral neurons. Damaged axons become irregular and beaded, break up, and disappear, but the process is significantly slower. Methods using stains for β-amyloid precursor protein to identify axonal injury in the CNS have revealed that axonal injury is a common event even in mild concussion.[22] Axonal damage impairs axonal streaming and causes a buildup of β-amyloid precursor protein proximal to the injury. This buildup is taken as evidence of axonal injury. Contrary to previously held notions, a significant degree of axonal repair appears to occur in CNS neurons when the injury is not too severe.[22] If neurons that were the principal source of stimulation to some other group of neurons are damaged and die, that other group of neurons may also degenerate because of the loss of trophic (growth and survival) signals. Researchers continue to discover new nerve growth and survival factors. Eventually they may find ways to minimize neuronal degeneration after injury and encourage repair or replacement.

KEY CONCEPTS

- The fundamental unit of the nervous system is the neuron. Neurons have three basic parts: cell body, dendrites, and axon. The dendrites receive signals and transmit them to the cell body. The axon generates and conducts action potentials. Conduction of action potentials is faster in large and myelinated axons.
- Neuronal communication through chemical synapses can be summarized as follows: Stimulation from other neurons occurs primarily at the dendrite and cell body. Action potentials are initiated at the axon hillock and conducted down the axon to the axon terminal, where neurotransmitter is stored. Depolarization of the terminal opens voltage-gated calcium channels. Calcium influx mediates exocytosis of neurotransmitter into the interneuronal synapse. Neurotransmitter binds and activates specific receptors on the postsynaptic cell, changing its ion conductance. With sufficient depolarization of the postsynaptic cell, an action potential is generated.
- There are six categories of neurotransmitters based on their chemical structure: acetylcholine, amines, amino acids, neuropeptides, purines, and gases.
- Excitatory neurotransmitters create excitatory postsynaptic potentials (EPSPs) in the postsynaptic neuron due to opening of channels that allow Na^+ or Ca^{2+} influx. Inhibitory neurotransmitters create inhibitory postsynaptic potentials (IPSPs) in the postsynaptic neuron due to opening of channels that allow Cl^- influx or K^+ efflux. The summation of EPSPs and IPSPs at the axon hillock determines whether an action potential will be initiated.
- Neuroglial cells are supportive cells in the CNS. Oligodendroglial cells form insulating myelin sheaths, astroglial cells moderate extracellular fluid composition, microglial cells are derived from circulating monocytes and destroy foreign materials, and ependymal cells form CSF.
- Development of the nervous system follows a basic architecture that is genetically programmed. However, the brain is quite plastic, especially during infancy, and alters the assignment of neurons to certain functions based on the degree of stimulation.
- Neurons in the CNS that are severely injured generally do not regenerate. Peripheral neurons may regenerate if the Schwann cells provide a pathway for growth. Neural stem cells in the ventricles and hippocampus of the brain can proliferate to produce either glial or neuronal cells depending on specific cues, most of which have yet to be elucidated.

SENSORY FUNCTION

The discussion of sensory function in this chapter is restricted to the somatosensory system. The special senses of hearing, vision, taste, and olfaction are discussed in Chapter 46. Neural pathways related to pain transmission are discussed in detail in Chapter 47.

Transmission of sensory signals begins with activation of specialized dendritic processes, called *sensory receptors,* at the ends of sensory afferents that project to the spinal cord (or brainstem in the case of some cranial nerves). Secondary neurons in the cord are activated and carry the signals up the cord to the brain. The thalamus is the principal receiving site for

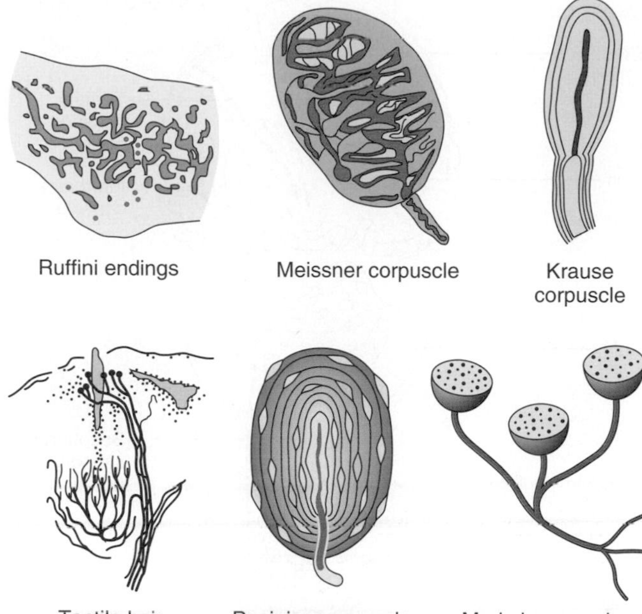

FIGURE 43-35 ■ Common types of somatosensory receptors. Sensory receptors are specialized to respond to particular types of stimuli.

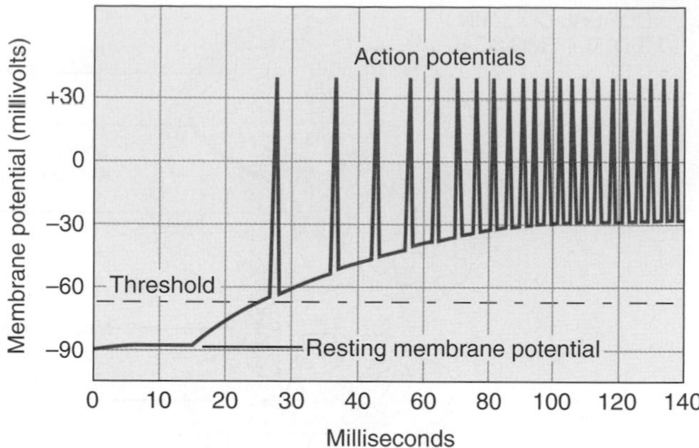

FIGURE 43-36 ■ Relationship between stimulus intensity and action potential generation. As the stimulus increases, the receptor potential is greater, and action potentials are generated at a faster rate. (From Guyton AC, Hall JE, editors: *Textbook of medical physiology,* ed 10, Philadelphia, 2000, Saunders, p 530.)

somatosensory signals, which are then relayed to various brain areas, including the somatosensory cortex in the parietal lobe.

An important principle of sensory transmission is that somatotopic organization is maintained from receptor to somatosensory cortex. This property allows for precise localization of the origin of sensory signals. The somatosensory system conveys a number of different sensory modalities, including fine touch, vibration sense, pressure, temperature, itch, crude touch, and pain. In general, different modalities are sensed by different types of sensory receptors.

SENSORY RECEPTORS

Sensory receptors are specialized terminations of the dendrites of primary sensory neurons. The receptor may be a free nerve ending or may have various connective tissue elaborations that affect its responsiveness (Figure 43-35). All types of receptors respond to stimuli by altering their membrane permeability to ions, thus creating a change in the membrane voltage. These receptor potentials are similar to the EPSPs generated in postsynaptic neurons, except that the stimulus is not a neurotransmitter. Different receptor types respond to different kinds of stimuli: mechanical stretch, changes in temperature, or the binding of chemicals. When a stimulus depolarizes the receptor sufficiently, voltage-gated fast Na^+ channels in the membrane open and an action potential is generated. The rate of action potential generation by the receptor depends on the intensity of the stimulus (Figure 43-36).

Some receptors are rapidly adapting and generate action potentials only when a change in the stimulus intensity occurs. The pacinian corpuscle is a classic example of a rapidly adapting receptor that is well suited to transmitting the sense of vibration. Tonic receptors adapt slowly and are good for conveying information about stimulus intensity over time. Free nerve endings, such as pain receptors, are usually tonic receptors.

Impulses generated by receptors are transmitted to the dorsal root of the spinal nerve. Depending on the sensory modality, the nerve impulses may travel up the **ipsilateral** side of the cord or may cross the spinal cord to travel up the **contralateral** side. In general, the well-localized sensations of touch, pressure, and vibration travel up the ipsilateral side of the cord, whereas the sensations of pain, itch, and temperature usually cross over and travel to the brain on the contralateral side.

SENSORY PATHWAYS

Two major tracts, the dorsal column–medial lemniscal tracts and the anterolateral tracts, carry information from the spinal segments to the brain[23] (Figure 43-37). The dorsal column–medial lemniscal tract carries fine touch, vibration sense, and proprioception and remains ipsilateral until the level of the medulla. As the fibers progress upward, they gradually move toward the midline, so that those corresponding to the lower extremities occupy the medial white column and those representing the arm are more lateral. From the nuclei in the medulla, neurons of the dorsal column pathway cross to the opposite side and travel up the brainstem, where they form the medial lemniscus, and then on to the thalamus. In the thalamus, fibers synapse with tertiary neurons, which in turn pass upward in a great band of fibers known as the *internal capsule,* and then travel on to primary sensory cortex.

The anterolateral tract (previously called the spinothalamic tract) carries impulses for sensations of pain, itch, and temperature from small myelinated (Aδ) and unmyelinated

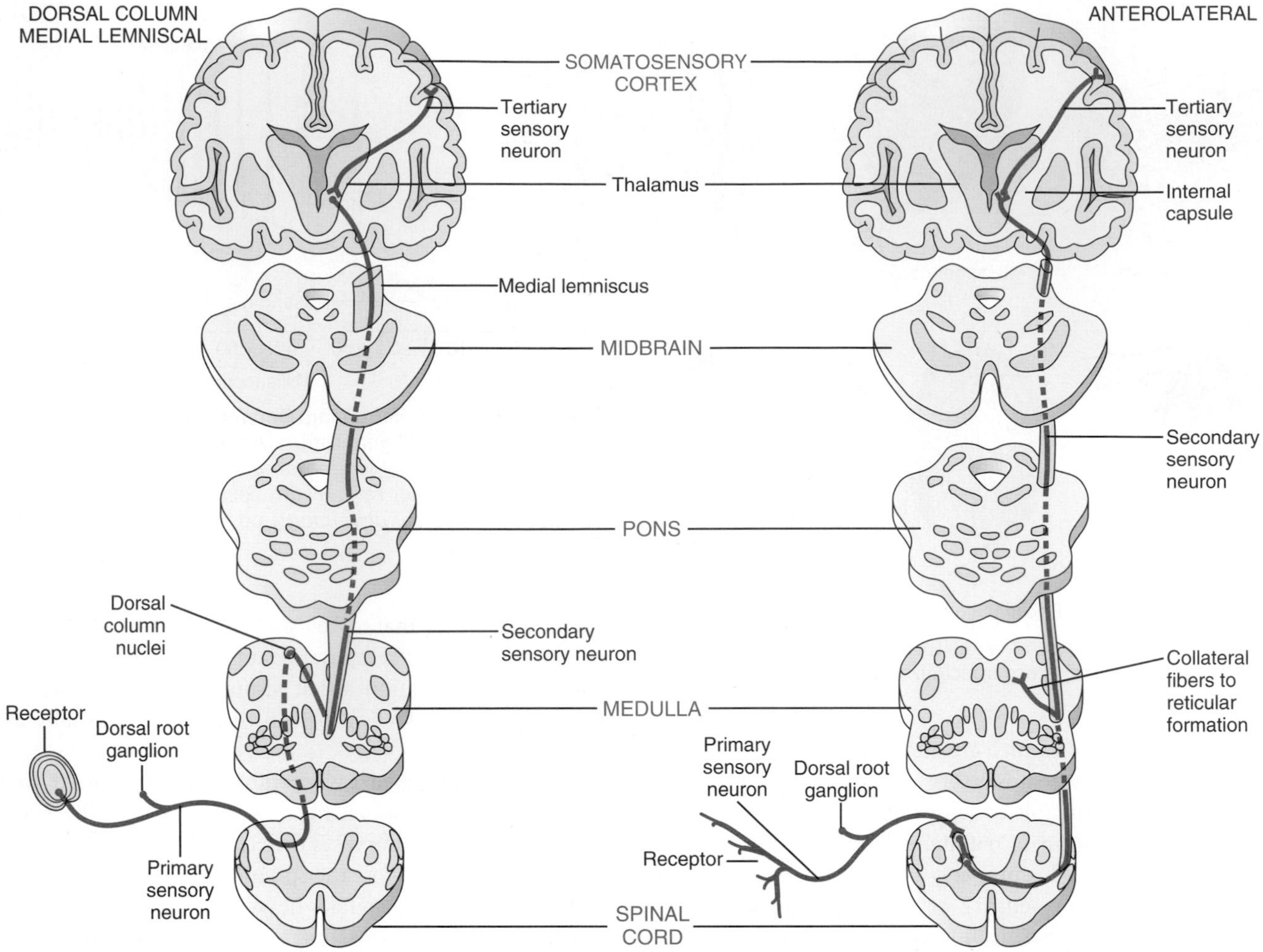

FIGURE 43-37 ■ Comparison of the two major ascending somatosensory tracts. *Left,* Dorsal column–medial lemniscal tract. *Right,* Anterolateral tract. Note that the dorsal column tracts do not cross the midline until the level of the medulla, whereas the anterolateral tracts cross at the spinal cord level.

(C-fiber) neurons. These neurons ascend one or more spinal segments before entering the posterior horn and synapsing with their secondary neuron. A few secondary fibers ascend ipsilaterally in the Lissauer fasciculus all the way to the thalamus. However, the majority of fibers cross the midline and ascend as the anterolateral tract. Fibers from the lower extremities and trunk are pushed laterally as they ascend in the spinal cord by the addition of fibers from the upper extremities and upper body, which enter medially.

On their way to the thalamus, these fibers give off collaterals to the reticular formation of the brainstem and the periaqueductal gray matter in the midbrain, where it is believed that one of their functions is pain inhibition (see Chapter 47). Secondary fibers of the anterolateral tract terminate in several thalamic regions. Tertiary neurons project from the thalamus to the somatosensory cortex. Thus, although the sensations of fine touch and pain are separated in the cord, they reunite in the somatosensory cortex that lies in the cerebral hemisphere opposite the site of sensory receptor origin.

SOMATOSENSORY CORTEX

The primary somatosensory cortex is organized in columns of gray matter that correspond to specific body locations. All modalities of sensation are grouped together in adjacent sections. The somatotopic representation of the body along a strip of cortex creates a distorted picture of the human body, called a homunculus map[23] (Figure 43-38). Body areas with a greater density of receptors garner a larger part of the homunculus map. The homunculus map was created by stimulating discrete areas of the cortex in awake subjects and recording the sensations that they reported. The *perception* of sensation from the body occurs at the level of the somatosensory cortex.

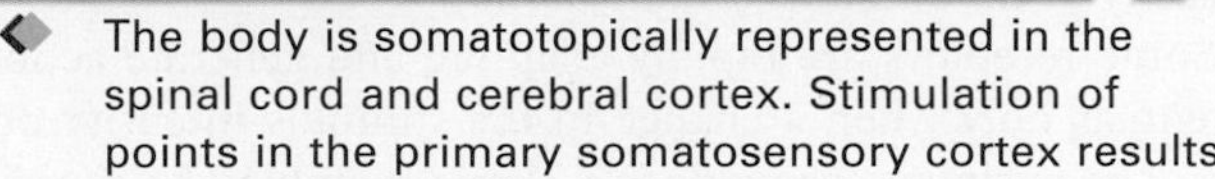

- The body is somatotopically represented in the spinal cord and cerebral cortex. Stimulation of points in the primary somatosensory cortex results

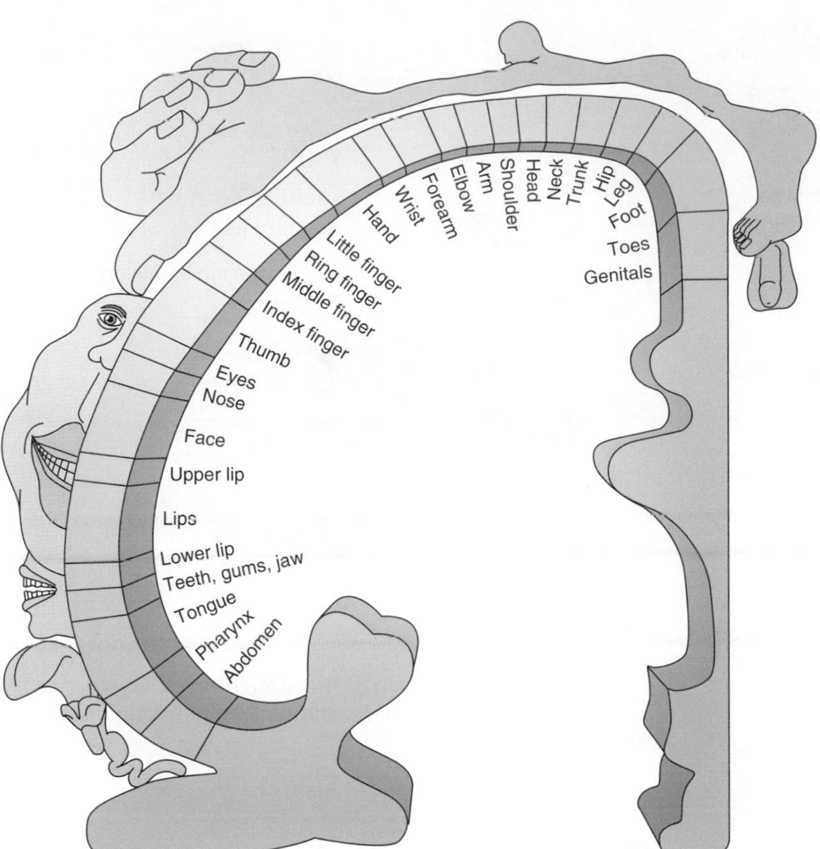

FIGURE 43-38 ■ Topographic organization of the body on the somatosensory cortex, forming a homunculus map.

in discrete sensations in the contralateral side of the body.

- Projections to the somatosensory cortex begin in sensory receptors throughout the body. Receptors send axons to the spinal cord through the dorsal root. Stimulation of receptors by mechanical deformation, temperature, or chemicals alters membrane permeability, resulting in receptor potentials. The intensity of the stimulus is reflected in the rate of action potentials generated.
- Sensations of touch and proprioception (dorsal column–medial lemniscal tract) project up to the medulla on the ipsilateral side, then cross over and terminate in the thalamus.
- Sensations of pain, temperature, and itch (anterolateral tract) usually cross the cord near the level of entry and travel to the brain on the contralateral side.
- Sensory information from both tracts is transmitted from the thalamus to the same areas of the somatosensory cortex by way of the internal capsule.

MOTOR FUNCTION

The execution of voluntary movement requires interaction among basal ganglia, cerebellum, and several regions of the cortex. The final program of voluntary muscle activity is transmitted from the primary motor cortex down the spinal cord by way of the corticospinal tract. As previously noted, the corticospinal tract decussates in the medullary pyramids and travels down the spinal cord to control muscles on the contralateral side of the body (Figure 43-39). The corticospinal tract primarily controls distal muscles of the arms, wrists, fingers, lower legs, feet, and toes. These are the muscles capable of fine motor control. Another group of motor tracts innervate large proximal muscle groups and axial muscles that control posture and balance. These tracts include the vestibulospinal, reticulospinal, and tectospinal tracts. Motor tracts descending from the brain synapse on the cell bodies of motor neurons that lie in the anterior horn of the spinal cord and project to skeletal muscles.

MOTOR NEURONS

Motor neurons travel from the anterior horn of the spinal cord through the ventral root and within the spinal and peripheral nerves to finally innervate target muscles. Alpha motor neurons release acetylcholine into neuromuscular junctions, depolarizing skeletal muscle cells and contracting all the fibers in the *motor unit.* A motor unit consists of a single motor neuron and all of the muscle fibers under its control. Some motor units are large, containing hundreds of muscle cells, whereas others may contain only one muscle cell per motor

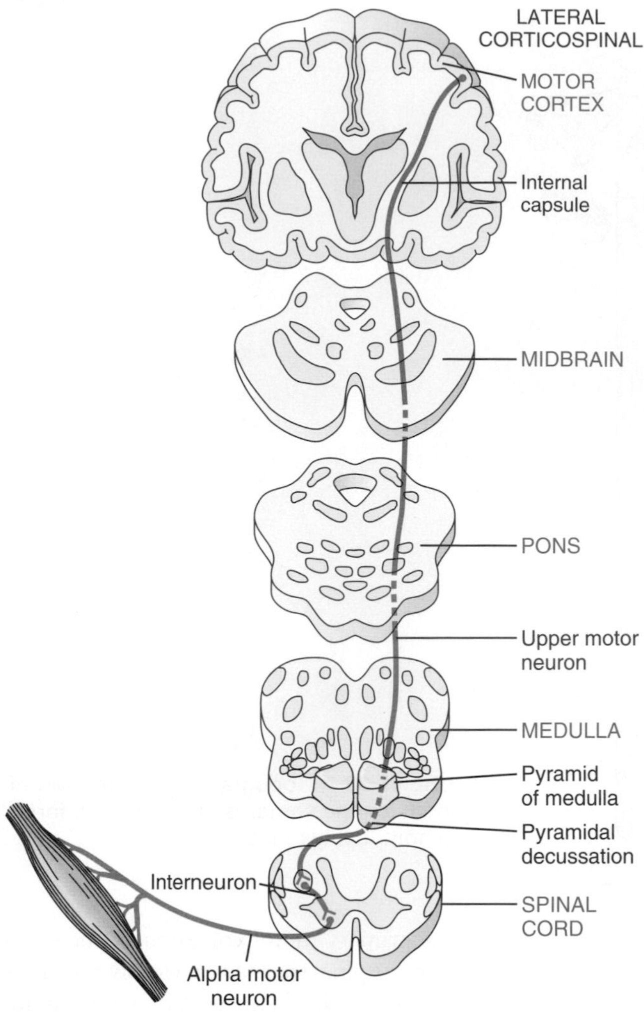

FIGURE 43-39 ■ The corticospinal tract showing decussation at the level of the medulla.

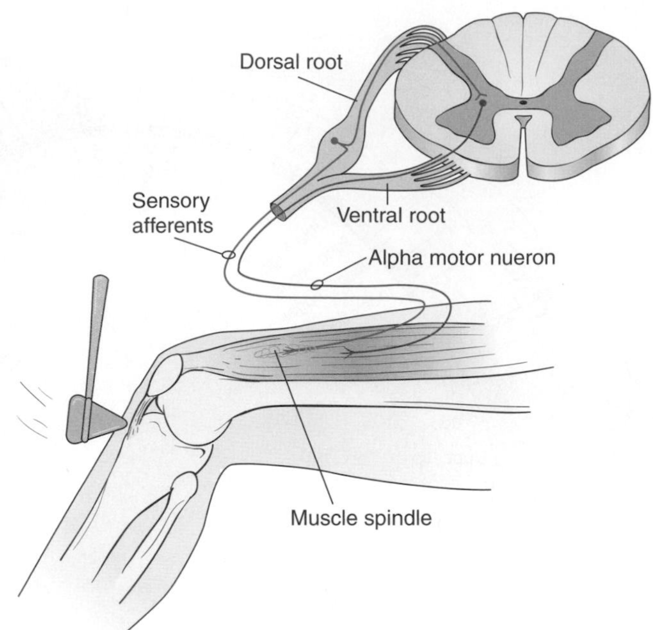

FIGURE 43-40 ■ Diagram of the stretch reflex in which activation of the muscle spindle stimulates contraction of the stretched muscle.

neuron. Smaller motor units produce finer gradations of muscle control.

A single action potential in the α motor neuron is sufficient to release enough neurotransmitter to contract the motor unit. Therefore, the point of control of muscle contraction is at the cell body of the α motor neuron that lies within the anterior horn. A typical motor neuron receives hundreds of synaptic inputs, which summate to control the generation of action potentials. Some presynaptic inputs are from corticospinal neurons, others are sensory inputs from primary sensory afferents and spinal cord interneurons.

Gamma motor neurons are small fibers that innervate structures within the body of the muscles, called *muscle spindles.* Muscle spindles are specialized sensory receptors that sense the length or stretch within the muscle and relay the information to the spinal cord. The γ motor neurons contract muscle fibers within the muscle spindle and regulate the spindle sensitivity. Excessive γ motor neuron activity occurs in some types of brain coma, making the spindles hypersensitive and the muscles stiff and resistant to stretch (see discussions of decerebrate and decorticate rigidity in Chapter 44).

SPINAL REFLEXES

A great deal of motor coordination is exerted in the spinal cord through complex reflex pathways. These pathways allow upper motor neurons from the brain to initiate preprogrammed movements, rather than having to excite and inhibit each and every lower motor neuron individually. For example, experiments in lower animals have demonstrated that pressure on the pads of the feet initiates complex walking movements even when the brain is no longer functional.

Spinal reflexes allow sensory information from pain receptors, proprioceptors, and muscle spindles to alter muscle contraction very quickly, even before the information reaches the brain. The stretch reflex and withdrawal reflex are illustrative examples.

The stretch reflex can be demonstrated by tapping the patellar tendon (below the knee) with a rubber hammer, which results in contraction of the quadriceps muscle and elevation of the lower leg. Evaluation of deep tendon reflexes is helpful in localizing a motor abnormality to the PNS or CNS. The deep tendon reflex tests the reflex arc between the sensory muscle spindles and the α motor neurons. Tapping the tendon produces a quick stretch in the muscle fibers of the quadriceps muscle and stimulates the muscle spindles. The muscle spindle sends action potentials along neurons (group Ia) that enter the dorsal horn of the spinal cord and then synapse directly on α motor neurons in the anterior horn that activate the muscle in which the spindles lie (Figure 43-40). Other branches of the group Ia neurons make connections with antagonistic muscle groups and inhibit their contraction. The stretch reflex makes only one synapse (monosynaptic) and

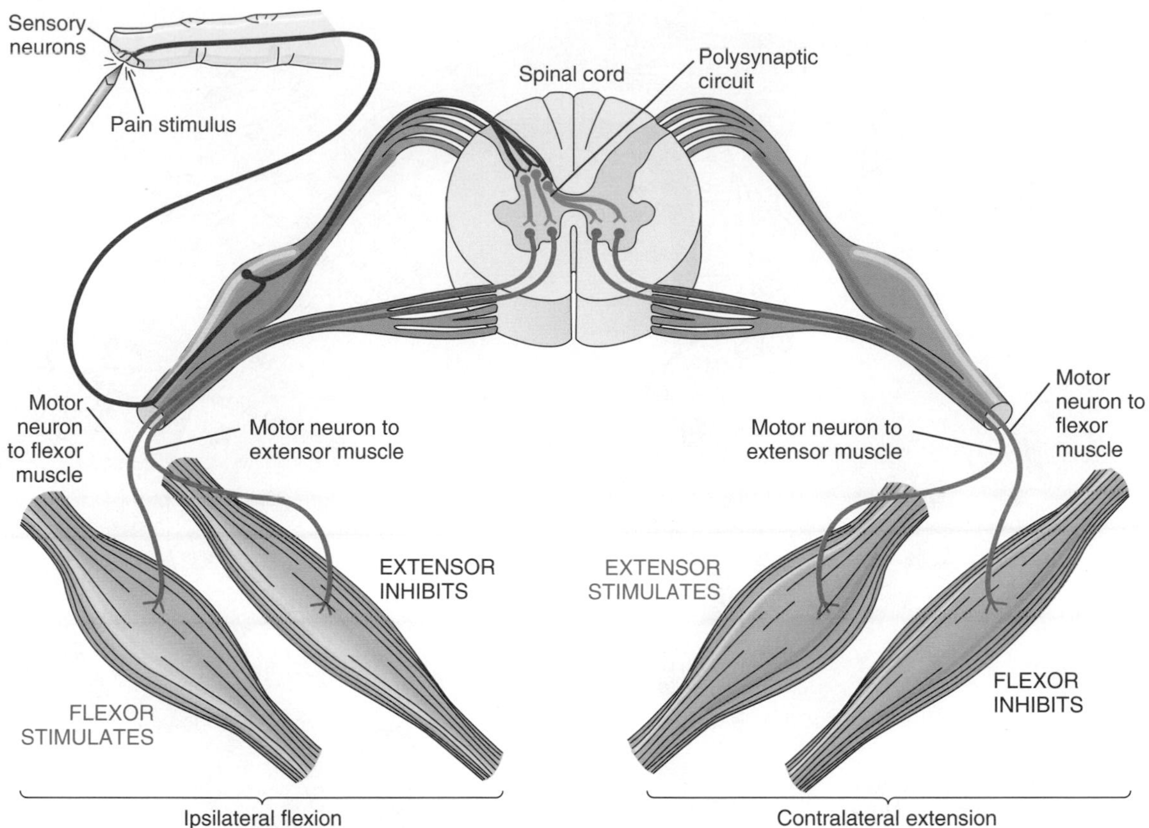

FIGURE 43-41 ■ Neural connections mediating the flexor-withdrawal reflex.

produces a very quick response in the muscle. The physiologic function of the muscle spindle stretch reflex is to provide feedback to α and γ motor neurons to adjust the strength of muscle contraction to match the load on the muscle.

The withdrawal reflex is an important protective mechanism that allows reflexive withdrawal of a body part from a physical threat while simultaneously making postural adjustments to avoid loss of balance. The withdrawal reflex is polysynaptic, making connections with interneurons in the cord to affect muscles on both sides of the body. A simplified model of the withdrawal reflex is shown in Figure 43-41. Note that a painful stimulus to one extremity results in activation of flexor muscles and inhibition of extensor muscles on the ipsilateral side. This allows quick withdrawal of the extremity from the source of injury. Connections with muscle groups on the opposite side of the cord stimulate extensors and inhibit flexors to stabilize posture.

CENTRAL CONTROL OF MOTOR FUNCTION

Corticospinal tract neurons originate in the primary motor cortex, which is arranged in a similar manner to the somatosensory cortex. The motor homunculus map (Figure 43-42) shows that muscles of the face, lips, tongue, and hands occupy most of the cortical neurons. These areas have small motor units and produce fine motor control. Activation of corticospinal neurons from the primary motor cortex is the last CNS step in executing a voluntary motor command. A great deal of neural activity occurs before the primary motor cortex is activated.

First, a motivation to move is needed to spur an individual to action. Little is known about motivation; however, signals from the limbic system are thought to be important. Circuits between the basal ganglia and association areas of the cerebral cortex plan the intended movement. Somewhat different circuits are involved in new situations, such as first learning to type, than are involved in the execution of learned, but subconscious, patterns of movement (e.g., typing 100 words per minute).[5] An important part of the planning process involves the somatosensory cortex, which provides information about the spatial coordinates of all body parts in relation to the physical surroundings (e.g., placement of the fingers on the keyboard).

The cerebellum serves to adjust the timing and intensity of movements to improve the similarity between the intended and actual movements. Neurons in the cerebellum learn with practice. Visual, proprioceptive, and vestibular information are used by the cerebellum to make adjustments in the execution phase of the movement. In addition, the cerebellum functions with the cerebral cortex to make muscle adjustments in advance of the movement. For example, if a person is asked to lift what appears to be a pile of bricks, but the bricks are made of lightweight Styrofoam, the unsuspecting subject will throw

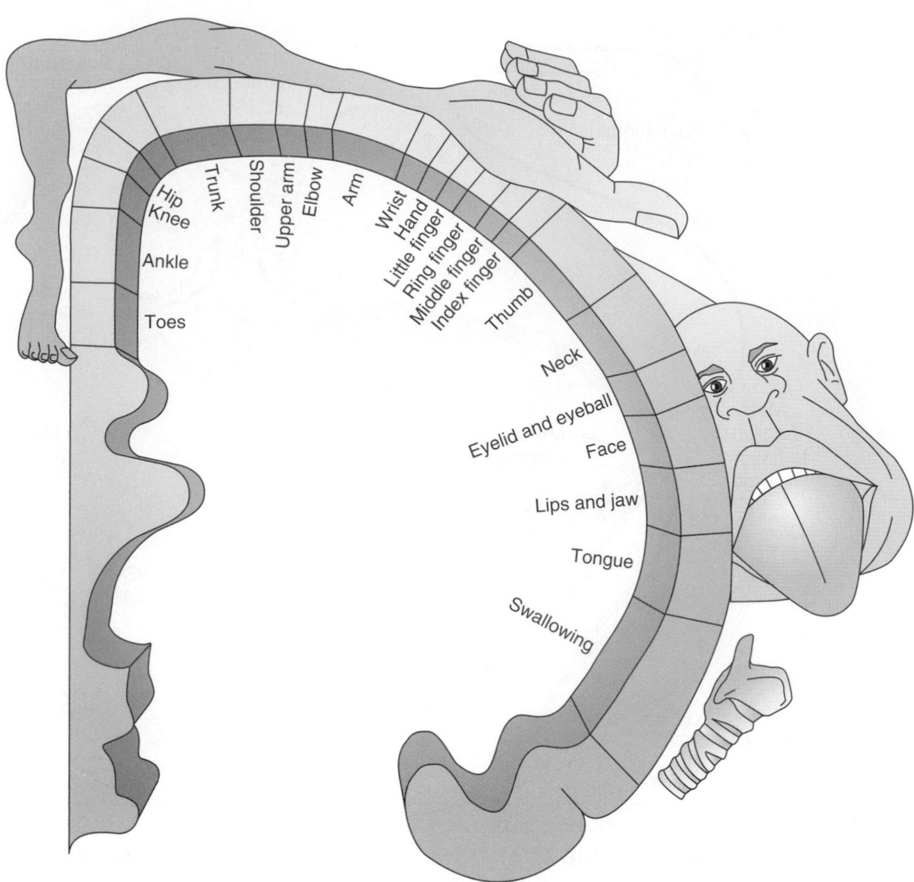

FIGURE 43-42 ■ Cortical representation of the muscles of the body. Note the large area devoted to control of the hands and face.

the pile up into the air. Visual cues and past learned experiences are used to gauge the intensity of muscle contraction. The brain learns quickly, however, and if the subject is asked to repeat the maneuver, the intensity of muscle contraction will exactly match that needed to lift the load smoothly. Once a motor activity is well learned and can be performed "automatically," the cerebellum participates less and the basal ganglia and cortical neurons are most active.[5]

KEY CONCEPTS

- The body is somatotopically represented in the motor cortex. Simulation of points in the primary motor cortex results in discrete movements in the contralateral side of the body.
- Projections from the motor cortex (corticospinal tract) travel by way of the internal capsule, cross over at the medulla, and travel down the contralateral spinal cord to synapse on α motor neurons in the anterior horn. The α motor neurons innervate skeletal muscle.
- Extrapyramidal tracts (tectospinal, vestibulospinal, reticulospinal) from subcortical nuclei innervate antigravity muscles and are primarily involved in balance, posture, and movement of large proximal muscle groups.
- A great deal of motor activity is preprogrammed into neuronal connections in the spinal cord. These connections produce reflexive alterations in muscle contraction in response to sensory information about the tension on the muscle or the need to move a body part away from a painful stimulus.
- The planning and execution of movements is accomplished through neuronal circuits between the basal ganglia and association areas of the motor cortex. The cerebellum contributes primarily to the learning phase of motor skill by making instantaneous adjustments in muscle force and timing to improve the match between the intended and the actual movement.

CONSCIOUSNESS, MEMORY, AND SLEEP

That the cerebral cortex is integral to the elaboration of complex thought, learning, memory, and so-called higher brain functions is well supported by lesion studies, yet little is known about the ways in which these higher functions are accomplished. Each thought involves neuronal circuits in portions of the cerebral cortex, thalamus, limbic system, and reticular formation of the brainstem. A thought or memory is not stored in any one place; rather it is the outcome of a pattern or circuit of neuronal activation.[24] Neurons in the limbic system, especially the amygdala, are thought to determine the general emotional value of the thought as being pleasant, painful, or neutral, whereas neurons in the cerebral cortex add the specific details, including remembered sensations and visual and auditory images. Consciousness and memory are prerequisites to thinking.

CONSCIOUSNESS AND MEMORY

Consciousness can be defined as awareness of the surroundings and of one's own thoughts and sensations. The neural correlates of consciousness are not known; however, continuous activation of neuronal circuits between the thalamus and cortex and thalamus and brainstem are believed to be necessary.[25] Consciousness is assessed by the expression of motor behaviors, such as speech, response to questions, and body movements. However, behavioral responses are not necessarily an outcome of consciousness. A person completely paralyzed with neuromuscular blocking agents is still conscious even though all outward behaviors are suppressed. It is difficult to know the level of brain activity in an individual who cannot move. Brain waves are frequently measured in an attempt to assess brain activity, and a correlation with consciousness is assumed. Alpha waves are thought to reflect search and retrieval functions and θ waves are associated with memory encoding tasks. Groups of neurons firing synchronously produce the regular oscillations of brain waves that seem to underlie consciousness. Much remains to be discovered before the phenomenon of consciousness and its counterpart, unconsciousness, are understood.

To think and learn one must be able to remember past events and link them to current circumstances. Memory is a synaptic phenomenon in which neurons in the memory trace or circuit alter the efficiency of synaptic transmission. Greater stimulation of neurons in the memory circuit results in longer lasting effects. Once the memory trace is established, it can be reactivated by the thinking mind to reproduce the memory. Reactivation by the mind is called *retrieval* and may be enhanced by rehearsal or strategies to link the memory trace with associated circuits that are already established. Experiences that have important consequences, such as pain or pleasure, are usually enhanced and stored as memory traces, whereas experiences of little consequence may be suppressed. The value of a memory is determined primarily by the limbic system, which helps the brain learn to ignore information of little consequence (which can be construed as a form of negative memory, or remembering to ignore). This is an important function, as it prevents preoccupation and overload of brain circuits with useless stimuli.

Some memories last for a short time and others persist for a lifetime. The mechanisms for different types of memory are mostly unknown; however, it is believed that short-term alteration of *presynaptic* neurons in the memory trace is responsible for short-term memory, whereas long-term memory requires more permanent changes in the *postsynaptic* neurons.[24] A certain time period is required for memories to be consolidated into long-term memory. An interruption of the consolidation phase, by head trauma, for example, results in loss of memory for events occurring just prior to the injury.

Some examples of presynaptic modulation are shown in Figure 43-43. The interaction between the presynaptic and postsynaptic neurons is modified by activity of the modulating neuron. For example, the modulating neuron could send a signal from the limbic system to indicate that the incoming signal was important. The modulating neuron would then enhance neurotransmitter release from the presynaptic neuron to facilitate transmission to the postsynaptic cell. Presynaptic inhibition could suppress synaptic transmission by preventing or reducing the amount of neurotransmitter released from the presynaptic neuron.

Longer term memory is thought to occur because of long-term changes in synaptic efficiency. In some cases memory may incorporate new neurons into the memory circuit. The hippocampus is an important limbic structure that must be intact for memory to be consolidated. It is also a site of neural stem cell proliferation, leading some to conclude that memory involves the growth of new neurons.[16] Changes in synaptic efficiency could include alterations in receptor number or structure and changes in the components of second-messenger cascades. Protein synthesis in the involved neurons is necessary to consolidate long-term changes in synaptic efficiency.[24] Memories are thought to be stored in the brain in association with memories of similar qualities that share some of the same neuronal circuits. Information is added to the memory circuit that is already in place. This makes it easier to learn information that is connected to previously learned material. Learning something completely new, such as a foreign language, requires a great deal of rehearsal.

SLEEP

Sleep is a state of decreased arousal from which a person is easily awakened. Different levels of brain activity from wakefulness to deep sleep are characterized by different electroencephalographic waveforms. Brain waves become progressively slower and more synchronized with deeper levels of sleep. These waveforms are called α, β, θ, and δ waves (Figure 43-44). The α and β waves are found in awake individuals. Alpha waves predominate during a relaxed state with the eyes closed; β waves occur during visual stimulation and with active problem solving. Beta waves are also apparent during a stage of sleep called rapid eye movement (REM) sleep. Both θ and δ waves occur during sleep.

Most sleep is of the restful, slow-wave type of deep sleep. Interspersed at about 90-minute intervals are episodes of REM sleep, which last 5 to 30 minutes. REM sleep is

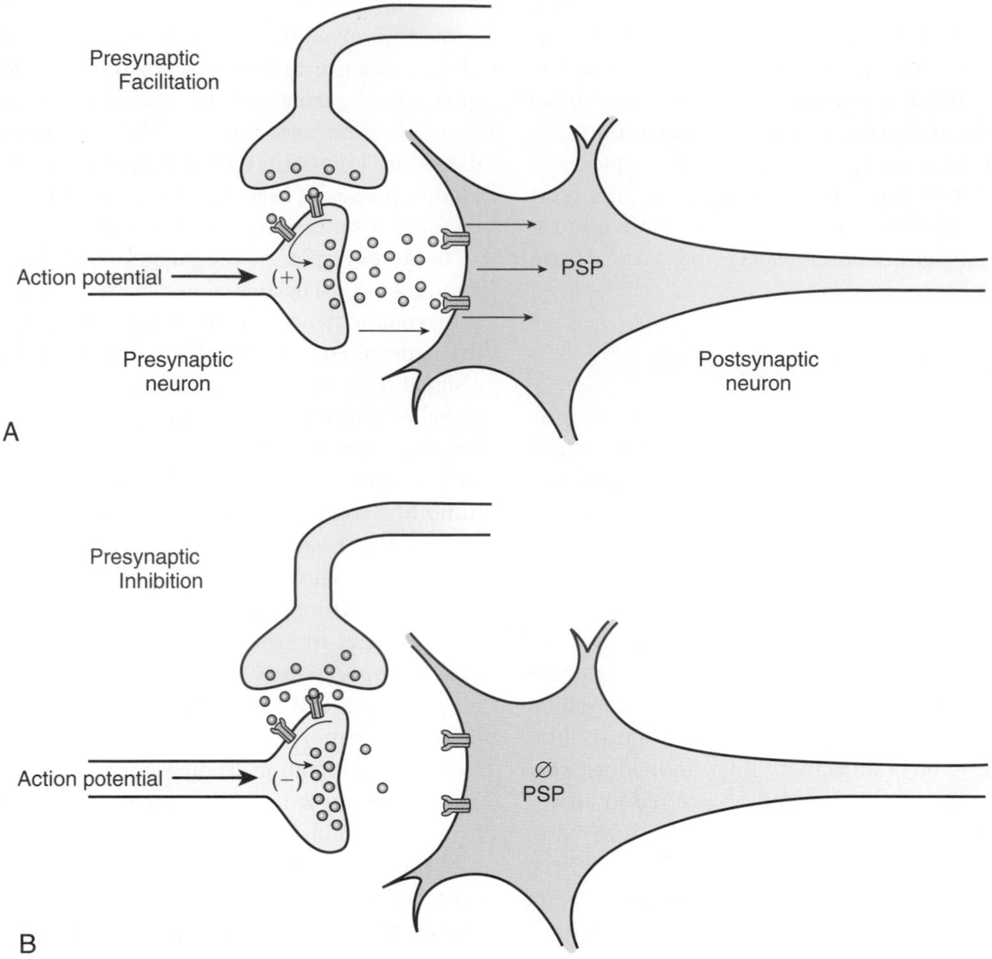

FIGURE 43-43 ■ Example of a modulating neuron that terminates on the presynaptic cell and alters its response. **A,** Facilitation: The presynaptic neuron releases more neurotransmitter into the synapse when an action potential arrives. **B,** Inhibition: The presynaptic neuron releases less neurotransmitter into the synapse with each action potential. *PSP,* Postsynaptic potential.

characterized by irregular breathing and heartbeat, rapid eye movements, depressed muscle tone, and active dreaming.[26] The number and length of REM episodes usually increases over the course of the night. Individuals who have been awake for a prolonged period spend more time in deep sleep at the beginning of sleep and begin to have more REM sleep as the brain becomes more rested.[26] Dreams occur in both types of sleep but are more likely to be remembered when they occur during REM sleep.

The mechanisms of the sleep-wake cycle and the reason the brain needs to sleep are not well understood. Experiments in animals have demonstrated that sleep is an active process initiated by sleep-inducing substances within the brain. CSF removed from sleep-deprived animals promptly produces sleep when injected into another animal. Production of sleep-inducing substances within the brain occurs during wakefulness; they gradually accumulate, producing a desire to sleep. A period of sleep is thought to inhibit production of sleep-inducing chemicals, and they are cleared from the CNS.

The physiologic significance of sleep to neural functioning is unknown, although the behavioral consequences of sleep deprivation are well characterized. Prolonged sleep deprivation produces hallucinations, disordered thought processes, and personality changes. It has been noted that the smaller the animal and the higher the metabolic rate, the greater the sleep requirement. Non-REM sleep is associated with lowering of metabolism and body temperature and may provide an opportunity to avoid or repair metabolism-induced brain damage.[26] REM sleep is associated with an active brain; however, certain types of neurons—those that secrete amines—are turned off during REM sleep. The younger and more immature brain spends more time in REM sleep, and some have speculated that the brain is laying down circuits for genetically programmed or instinctive neural pathways.[26] Less time is spent in REM sleep with aging.

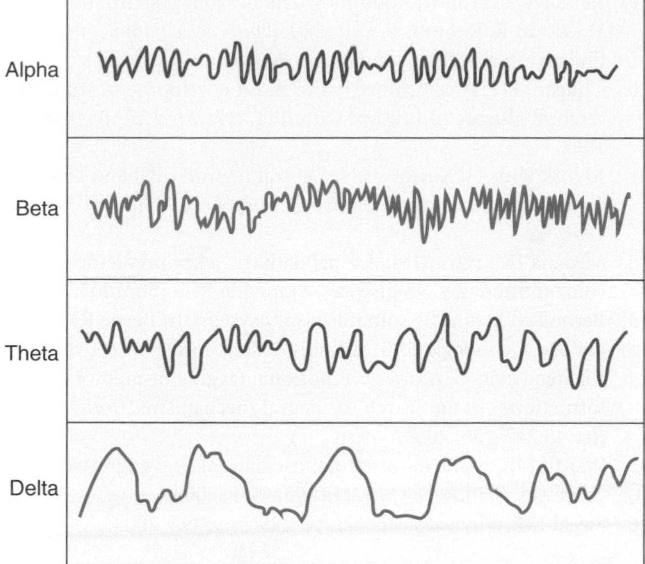

FIGURE 43-44 ■ Brain waves are categorized according to frequency and synchrony as α, β, σ, and δ.

KEY CONCEPTS

- Thoughts and memories are not stored in a particular location in the brain; rather, they are the outcome of activation of neurons in a neuronal circuit.
- Memories are stored by altering the synaptic efficiency of neurons in the memory trace. Short-term memory is thought to result from presynaptic mechanisms, whereas long-term memory is consolidated by more permanent changes in the postsynaptic neurons.
- Sleep is characterized as REM sleep (β waves) and deep sleep (σ and δ waves). Most sleep is of the deep-sleep variety, interspersed with periods of REM activity at about 90-minute intervals. Sleep is an active process produced by sleep-inducing chemicals in the brain. The nature of these chemicals and the reason that the brain requires sleep remain unknown.

SUMMARY

The nervous system is a complex network of neurons and supporting cells that provides the body with a rapid means of communication. The anatomy of the nervous system has been extensively studied, but the functional mechanisms of thought, memory, emotion, and sleep are poorly understood. The nervous system can be partially understood by examining the function of individual neurons and their synaptic connections. Neural communication occurs primarily through the secretion of neurotransmitters into synapses between neurons. Neurotransmitters bind to specific receptors to exert their effects on the membrane potential of the target cell.

Activation of groups of neurons in a particular circuit is the basis for neuronal processing of information, thoughts, and memories and for learning. Although certain brain locations have been associated with particular functions, most brain activities require participation by neurons in widespread locations. The ability of the nervous system to learn and adapt is remarkable in the early childhood period, and a significant degree of neural plasticity is maintained throughout life. However, damage to large numbers of neurons in a particular location usually results in significant disability because mature neurons cannot regenerate and neural stem cells may not survive or establish appropriate connections.

MEDIA RESOURCES

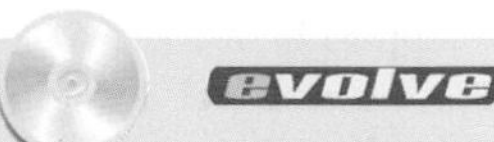

Remember to check out the ***CD Companion*** included with this book for Review Questions, Key Concepts Review, Glossary (with audio for selected terms), Disease Profiles, and Animations.

PLUS, visit the ***Evolve website*** at http://evolve.elsevier.com/Copstead/ for Case Studies, Disease Profiles, and WebLinks.

References

1. Nolte J, Sundsten JW: *The human brain: an introduction to its functional anatomy,* ed 5, St Louis, 2002, Mosby.
2. Guyton AC, Hall JE: Cerebral blood flow, the cerebrospinal fluid, and brain metabolism. In Guyton AC, Hall JE, editors: *Textbook of medical physiology,* ed 10, Philadelphia, 2000, Saunders, pp 709-715.
3. Britta E: Development of the blood-brain barrier, *Cell Tissue Res* 314:119-129, 2003.
4. Guyton AC, Hall JE: Somatic sensations: I. General organization, the tactile and position senses. In Guyton AC, Hall JE, editors: *Textbook of medical physiology,* ed 10, Philadelphia, 2000, Saunders, pp 540-551.
5. Doyon J, Penhune V, Ungerleider LG: Distinct contribution of the cortico-striatal and cortico-cerebellar systems to motor skill learning, *Neuropsychologia* 41:252-262, 2003.
6. Brown P, Marsden CD: What do the basal ganglia do? *Lancet* 351:1801-1804, 1998.
7. Nelson MV, Berchou RC, LeWitt PA: Parkinson's disease. In Dipiro J et al, editors: *Pharmacotherapy: a pathophysiologic approach,* ed 5, New York, 2002, McGraw-Hill, pp 1089-1102.
8. Steriade M: Corticothalamic networks, oscillations, and plasticity, *Adv Neurol* 77:105-134, 1998.
9. Salman MS: The cerebellum: it's about time! But timing is not everything—new insights into the role of the cerebellum in timing motor and cognitive tasks, *J Child Neurol* 17(1):1-9, 2002.
10. Thibodeau GA, Patton KT: Central nervous system. In Thibodeau GA, Patton KT: *Anatomy and physiology,* ed 5, St Louis, 2003, Mosby, pp 374-412.
11. Guyton AC, Hall JE: The autonomic nervous system and the adrenal medulla. In Guyton AC, Hall JE, editors: *Textbook of medical physiology,* ed 10, Philadelphia, 2000, Saunders, pp 697-708.

12. Thibodeau GA, Patton KT: Peripheral nervous system. In Thibodeau GA, Patton KT: *Anatomy and physiology,* ed 5, St Louis, 2003, Mosby, pp 413-447.
13. Thibodeau GA, Patton KT: Nervous system cells. In Thibodeau GA, Patton KT: *Anatomy and physiology,* ed 5, St Louis, 2003, Mosby, pp 342-373.
14. Boehning D, Snyder SH: Novel neural modulators, *Annu Rev Neurosci* 26:105-131, 2003.
15. Kaur C et al: Origin of microglia, *Microsc Res Tech* 54(1):2-9, 2001.
16. Gage FH: Brain, repair yourself, *Sci Am* 289(3):46-53, 2003.
17. Guyton AC, Hall JE: The nervous system: general principles and sensory physiology. In Guyton AC, Hall JE, editors: *Textbook of medical physiology,* ed 10, Philadelphia, 2000, Saunders, pp 512-527.
18. Swanson TH: Synaptic transmission. In Levin KH, Luders HO, editors: *Comprehensive clinical neurophysiology,* Philadelphia, 2000, Saunders, pp 57-68.
19. Kumar V, Cotran R, Robbins S: The nervous system. In Kumar V, Cotran R, Robbins S, editors: *Robbins basic pathology,* ed 7, Philadelphia, 2003, Saunders, pp 809-850.
20. Chugani HT: A critical period of brain development: studies of cerebral glucose utilization with PET, *Prev Med* 27:184-188, 1998.
21. Aldoskogius H, Kozlova EN: Central neuron-glial and glial-glial interactions following axon injury, *Prog Neurobiol* 55:1-26, 1998.
22. Medana IM, Esiri MM: Axonal damage: a key predictor of outcome in human CNS diseases, *Brain* 126:515-530, 2003.
23. Berne RM et al: The somatosensory system. In Berne RM et al, editors: *Physiology,* ed 5, St Louis, 2004, Mosby, pp 100-117.
24. Richter-Levin G, Akirav I: Emotional tagging of memory formation—in the search for neural mechanisms, *Brain Res Rev* 43:247-256, 2003.
25. Ward LM: Synchronous neural oscillations and cognitive processes, *Trends Cog Sci* 7(12):553-559, 2003.
26. Siegel JM: Why we sleep, *Sci Am* 289(5):92-97, 2003.

Acute Disorders of Brain Function

chapter 44

Jacquelyn L. Banasik

MEDIA RESOURCES

Additional Material for Study, Review, and Further Exploration

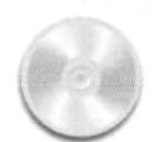

CD Companion ◆ Review Questions and Answers ◆ Key Concepts Review
◆ Glossary *(with audio pronunciations for selected terms)*
◆ Disease Profiles ◆ Animations

evolve ***Website*** at http://evolve.elsevier.com/Copstead/
◆ Case Studies ◆ Disease Profiles ◆ WebLinks

KEY QUESTIONS

- What are the proposed mechanisms and potential consequences of secondary brain injury?
- What brain components determine intracranial pressure and under what conditions might each contribute to elevated intracranial pressure?
- How are level of consciousness and cranial nerve reflexes used to assess changes in neurologic status in the brain-injured patient?
- What are the common manifestations of types of traumatic brain injury (focal, polar, diffuse) and hemorrhage (epidural, subdural, subarachnoid)?
- How do the three most common causes of stroke (thrombi, emboli, and hemorrhage) differ as regards risk factors, prevention strategies, and acute management?
- How do the clinical manifestations of ischemic stroke vary depending on the location of cerebral artery obstruction?
- What are the common long-term sequelae of stroke and how are they managed?
- What is the cause and usual presentation of cerebral aneurysm and arteriovenous malformation?
- How do meningitis and encephalitis differ with regard to usual infective organisms, cerebrospinal fluid analysis findings, clinical manifestations, and treatment?

CHAPTER OUTLINE

Disorders of brain function can result from a wide variety of pathophysiologic processes. The focus of this chapter is on primary causes of acute brain injury including brain trauma, cerebrovascular disease, brain hemorrhage, and central nervous system (CNS) infections. These conditions are considered to be acute because they generally have a sudden onset and progress rapidly. Thus, early detection and prompt management are necessary to prevent death and minimize morbidity. However, the majority of patients who survive acute injury to brain structures will be left with some degree of permanent neurologic damage and chronic dysfunction. The designation of acute and chronic disorders is, therefore, somewhat arbitrary. The chronic aspects of neurologic diseases, including seizure disorders and dementias, are discussed in the following chapter. Acute neurologic dysfunction often is a complication of diseases primarily affecting other systems. Hypoglycemia, renal failure, liver failure, human immunodeficiency virus infection, drug overdoses, fluid imbalances, and many others may cause acute brain dysfunction. Accurate determination of the source of acute alterations in brain function is an important step in developing an appropriate treatment plan. However, there are many common elements in the pathogenesis of acute brain injuries, regardless of etiologic factors. These cellular aspects are presented as a foundation for understanding the specific disorders that follow.

MECHANISMS OF BRAIN INJURY

The mechanisms of brain injury are varied, complex, and incompletely understood. Mechanical trauma, ischemia, cellular energy failure, reperfusion injury, excitotoxins, edema, vascular failure, and injury-induced apoptosis (programmed cell death) are all factors thought to be operative in most kinds of acute brain injury. These mechanisms are often separated into two categories: primary injury and secondary injury. The primary injury is that which occurs immediately at the onset of brain injury. This definition implies that there is little that can be done to reverse the process once it has occurred. For example, in the case of head trauma, some tissues will be irreversibly damaged at the time of impact owing to mechanical forces. This damage represents the primary injury. Similarly, with the sudden cessation of blood flow to an area of brain tissue, as occurs in stroke, an area of irreversible ischemia in cells may develop quickly, and this constitutes the primary injury. The rapid cell death that accompanies the primary injury is necrotic because the injury is so severe that cells lose membrane integrity, rupture, and release their intracellular contents into the extracellular space. Necrosis can initiate inflammatory responses that trigger additional cell damage.

Secondary injury refers to the development of further neurologic damage subsequent to the primary injury, and this may progress over days or weeks. Delayed cell death may involve necrosis from further acute injury or may be a delayed consequence of the primary injury. Cells that die slowly after injury are said to undergo apoptosis or programmed cell death. Apoptosis requires energy and protein synthesis, and the cells shrink and die in a tidy fashion without releasing their internal contents. Necrosis follows severe ischemic injury whereas apoptosis is associated with moderate injury. A critical factor in determining the neuronal cell fate after injury is the degree of adenosine triphosphate (ATP) depletion. If ATP levels fall profoundly, increased membrane permeability and necrosis ensue. If the ATP level is partially maintained for a period of time after the injury, apoptosis is the likely consequence. Mild reductions in ATP are associated with reversible injury and cellular recovery.[1] ATP reduction is a consequence of ischemia and hypoxia, which accompany many types of acute brain injury including trauma and stroke.

Mechanisms of secondary injury are the subject of much interest because of the potential to effectively intervene to limit brain damage. Unfortunately, effective means of preventing secondary damage have remained elusive, leading to high rates of mortality and morbidity. The effort to elucidate mechanisms of secondary injury and develop effective treatments would seem worthwhile because the degree of primary injury is thought to be small in most cases.[2] Thus, the high rates of mortality and morbidity may be attributed in large part to mechanisms of secondary injury.

Ischemia and Hypoxia

Ischemia occurs when the delivery of oxygenated blood is below the level needed to meet metabolic demands of the brain tissue. Ischemia is a contributing factor in most forms of acute brain injury, either as the primary insult (e.g., stroke) or as part of the secondary response to injury (e.g., vasospasm, vascular compression, or abnormal autoregulation). Hypoxia is a deficiency of oxygen at the cellular level, which may occur as a result of decreased blood flow (ischemia) or decreased blood oxygenation (hypoxemia). In practice, ischemia and hypoxia usually occur together and are considered together in this discussion. Ischemia results in immediate neurologic dysfunction because of the inability of neurons to generate the ATP needed for energy-requiring processes. In addition, ischemia sets the stage for secondary injury by oxygen free radicals, excitatory amino acids, and inflammatory cells.

Cellular Energy Failure

Neuronal tissue is highly sensitive to oxygen deprivation because it has great ATP requirements and limited capacity for anaerobic metabolism during ischemia. The normal brain receives about 15% of the total cardiac output and garners 20% of the body's oxygen consumption (750 ml/min), despite contributing only 2% of the body weight.[3] Neurons are dependent on glucose for production of ATP; however, they store little in the form of glycogen. Thus, when oxygen supply is decreased, not only is oxidative phosphorylation impaired, but the low supply of stored glucose restricts anaerobic production of ATP as well.

Most of the ATP used by neurons is for maintenance of ion gradients across the plasma membrane. The sodium-potassium (Na^+-K^+) pump consumes three fourths of the ATP in a typical neuron.[4] Energy also is required to maintain calcium balance and regulate neurotransmitter synthesis and reuptake. Not surprisingly, energy failure results in neuronal dysfunction, injury, and, if severe or prolonged, necrotic cell death. Ischemia also is the probable inciting factor for apoptosis.

A general sequence of events following acute brain ischemia has been proposed (Figure 44-1).[5,6] The critical event is

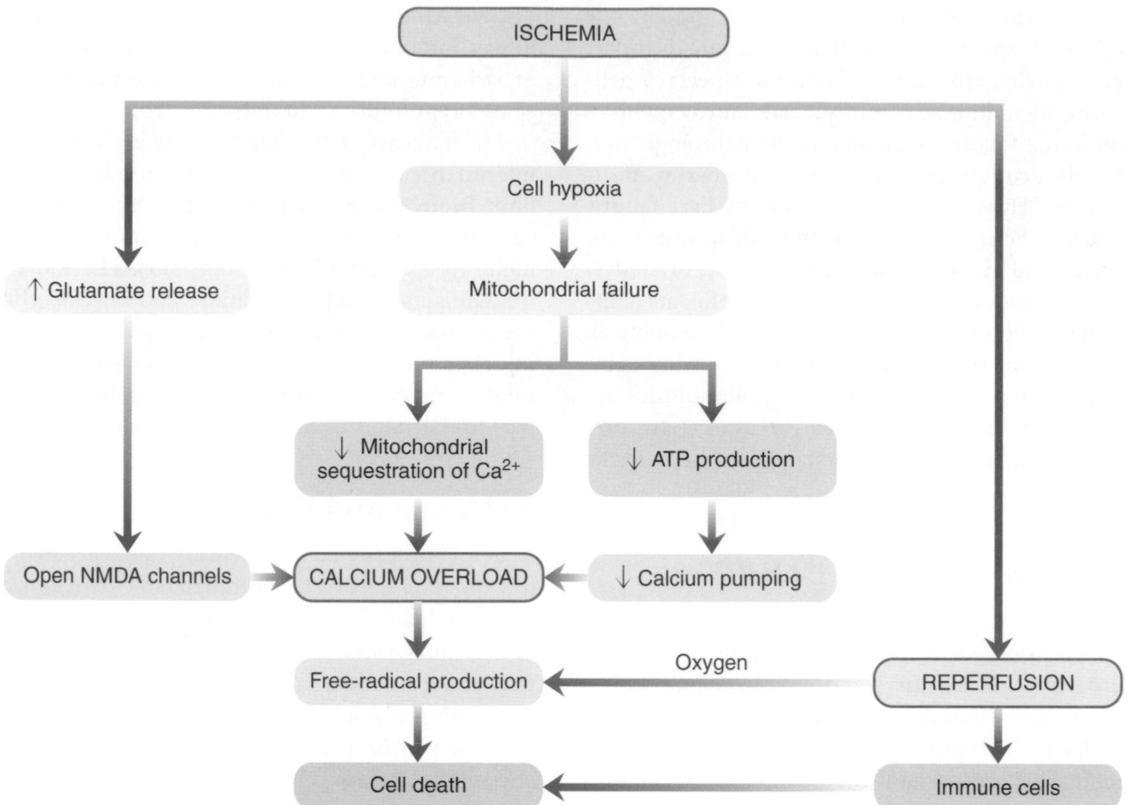

FIGURE 44-1 ■ Sequence of neuronal cell injury following acute ischemia. Calcium overload is a key event in producing cellular damage.

mitochondrial dysfunction owing to lack of cellular oxygen.[5] Recall that oxygen is required to accept electrons from the mitochondrial electron transport chain. In the absence of oxygen, the transport proteins and cytochromes remain reduced and unable to accept any more electrons from the Krebs cycle (tricarboxylic acid cycle). ATP production falls rapidly. Glycolysis may continue for a short time, producing pyruvate, which is converted to lactate. This conversion releases H^+ and contributes to cellular acidosis. The lack of ATP results in failure of energy-requiring processes throughout the cell.

The mitochondria are also important regulators of calcium ion concentration in the cell. The mitochondrial membrane contains calcium transporters that sequester calcium ions within the mitochondria when cytoplasmic calcium levels are elevated. Mitochondrial energy failure impairs the ability of mitochondria to perform this sequestering function. Even so, the mitochondria may become severely overloaded with calcium, which activates enzymes (phospholipases) that can damage mitochondrial membrane structures. Ischemic cells are prone to calcium overload because pumps that move calcium out of the cell are energy dependent. Calcium ions have a large electrochemical gradient for diffusion into the neuron and tend to accumulate intracellularly.

Unfortunately, the activity of many intracellular enzymes is regulated by intracellular calcium. Calcium overload is thought to be a critical factor leading to activation of enzyme cascades, which disrupt function and cause irreversible damage to cell membranes (lipid peroxidation). One might speculate that measures to inhibit calcium entry into damaged cells would be of therapeutic benefit. One way to reduce calcium influx is by administration of calcium channel–blocking agents. These drugs block voltage-gated calcium channels. Unfortunately, clinical trials with calcium channel–blocking agents have failed to show benefit.[7] Other avenues for inhibiting calcium overload are being investigated, including those that block the effect of glutamate receptors described below.

Excitatory Amino Acids

Calcium may gain entry into cells by portals other than voltage-gated channels. Glutamate is an excitatory amino acid neurotransmitter thought to be important in learning and memory. Overstimulation of neurons by glutamate is associated with cell injury, leading to its designation as an *excitotoxin.* Glutamate binds two kinds of receptors that are linked to the opening of ion channels in the plasma membrane of neurons. *N*-Methyl-D-aspartate (NMDA) receptors have received the most attention, but α-amino-3-hydroxy-5-methylisoxazolepropionic acid (AMPA) channels are also thought to contribute to the neurotoxic effects of glutamate. Activation of AMPA receptors results in opening of Na^+ channels in the membrane, which leads to depolarization. Depolarization then affects the NMDA channels by removing a

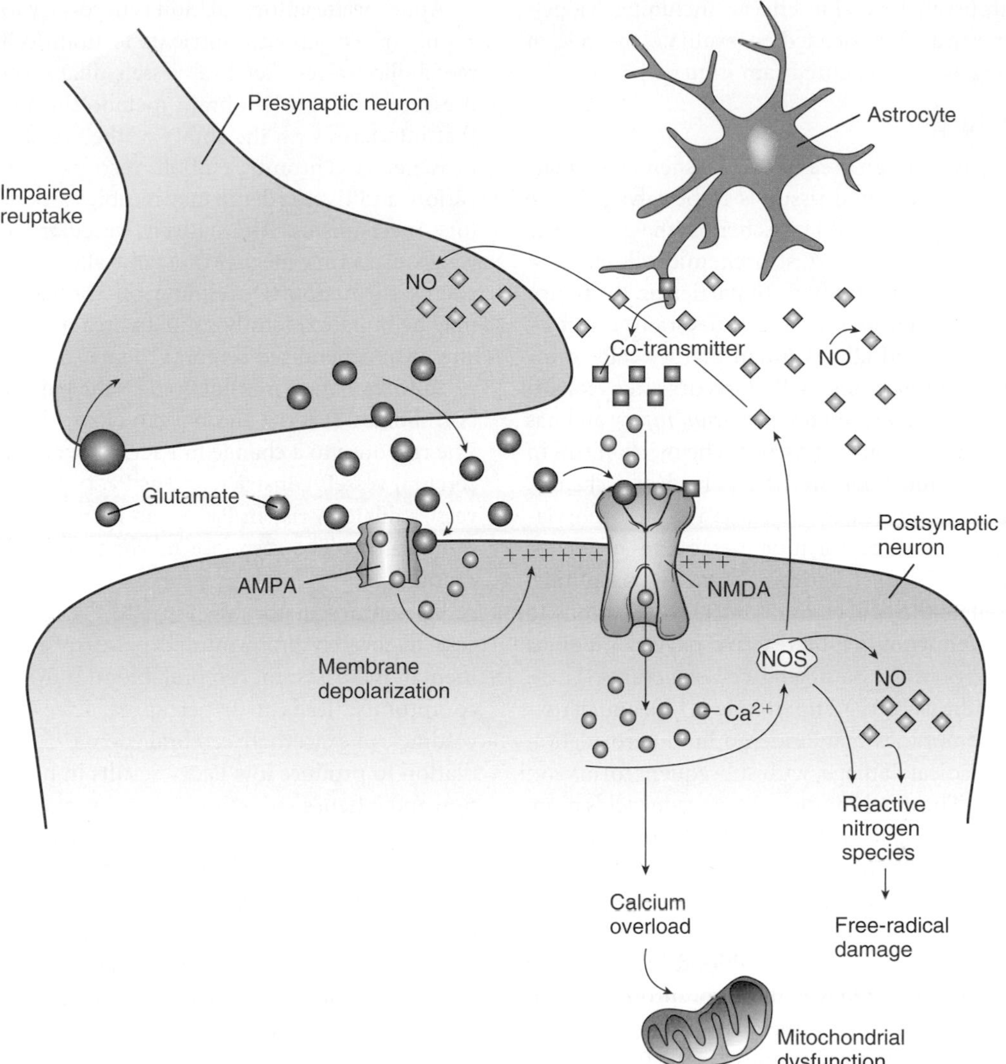

FIGURE 44-2 ■ Mechanism of glutamate-mediated calcium influx. Impaired removal of glutamate from the synapse by energy-requiring reuptake mechanisms on the presynaptic membrane contributes to excessive glutamate in the synapse. Glutamate binds to the *N*-methyl-D-aspartate *(NMDA)* channel, causing it to open and allow calcium influx. A previous depolarization is necessary to remove the Mg^{2+} that normally blocks the channel. Excessive calcium entry impairs mitochondrial function and triggers nitric oxide production. Excessive nitric oxide can increase cell damage through free radical production. *AMPA,* α-Amino-3-hydroxy-5-methyl-4-isoxazolepropionate; *NO,* nitric oxide; *NOS,* Nitric oxide synthase.

Mg^{2+} ion that usually blocks the NMDA channel (Figure 44-2). Subsequent binding of glutamate to the NMDA receptor opens it and allows Ca^{2+} to enter the cell. As previously described, calcium overload mediates a cascade of events leading to cell injury.

The amount of glutamate in the synapses is usually tightly regulated by release and reuptake controls. In the presence of neuronal injury, excessive glutamate may be released because of impaired membrane integrity. With concomitant ischemia, reuptake mechanisms fail to remove excess glutamate from the synapse because they are energy-dependent processes. Excess glutamate stimulates nearby neurons, which take up large amounts of injurious calcium ions. Small neurons in the cerebral cortex and hippocampus are particularly prone to glutamate excitotoxicity, and selective damage in these areas may occur. In addition to the calcium overload mechanism of injury, NMDA receptor activation stimulates nitric oxide (NO) production in neurons. NO is a neurotransmitter, but in excess it may increase the production of reactive nitrogen species (RNS), which function as free radicals to damage cellular components. The potential neuroprotective effects of controlling glutamate release or activity has been investigated. Studies with NMDA receptor–blocking agents have indicated benefit in some patients; however, conscious patients have experienced neuropsychiatric side effects, including hallucinations.[7] Further research is needed to evaluate the role of glutamate-blocking agents in acute brain injury.

Reperfusion Injury

Reestablishing perfusion to an area of prior ischemia is a matter of great urgency if neuronal tissue is to be salvaged. The longer and more severe the period of ischemia, the greater the extent of necrosis. However, previously ischemic cells face new dangers with the return of blood flow. In particular, the return of oxygen brings the potential for oxygen free radical formation, and the flow of blood allows inflammatory cells to invade the area. The secondary injury that occurs after reestablishing blood flow has been termed *reperfusion injury* and has been studied extensively in cardiac tissues. The mechanisms in brain appear to be similar. During the period of ischemia, brain cells accumulate substrates for oxidative phosphorylation, including the free radical–forming metabolites of adenosine monophosphate (AMP), xanthine, and hypoxanthine. When oxygen reenters the cell, erratic transfer of electrons to oxygen can produce a number of reactive oxygen products that behave as free radicals, damaging cell structures. These include hydroxyl radicals ($OH^{\cdot}$), superoxide (O_2^-), and peroxide (H_2O_2). Cell membranes may undergo lipid peroxidation in response to free radical damage, with subsequent formation of arachidonic acid. The arachidonic acid cascade yields more oxygen free radicals as well as mediators of inflammation.[1]

The role of immune mechanisms in reperfusion injury of brain tissue is only partially understood. Previously, the CNS was thought to be relatively shielded from immune cells because of the low permeability of the blood-brain barrier (BBB). However, the BBB is believed to be compromised with ischemia because the capillary endothelial cells are injured. Inflammatory cytokines, including interleukin-1 (IL-1), interleukin-6 (IL-6), and tumor necrosis factor (TNF), increase in the brain during ischemic injury and are thought to attract neutrophils to the area and contribute to brain inflammation.[8] The importance of neutrophil recruitment to secondary injury remains controversial, but it may contribute further free radical generation and vascular obstruction by aggregated neutrophils. Trauma and inflammation also promote platelet aggregation in cerebral vessels with subsequent reduction in perfusion and worsening of ischemia.

Abnormal Autoregulation

Under normal conditions, blood flow through brain tissue is controlled primarily by autoregulation. Cerebral vessels respond to metabolic factors including pH, carbon dioxide, and oxygen levels. Cerebral blood flow is closely matched to metabolic needs despite wide fluctuations in perfusion pressure. Blood flow is maintained at a fairly constant rate over a range of mean arterial pressure (MAP) from about 50 to 150 mm Hg.[4] Above and below these levels, autoregulation fails. Hypotension predisposes to ischemia, whereas severe hypertension may lead to vascular damage and brain edema.

Appropriate autoregulation is necessary to provide a steady supply of oxygen and nutrients to brain cells and to remove metabolic wastes. Cerebral vessels dilate when arterial blood pressure falls or when brain metabolism increases. Anything that interferes with the ability of the vessels to dilate can lead to ischemia. Thrombi, emboli, vasospasm, neutrophil aggregation, and tissue edema may inhibit vasodilating autoregulatory mechanisms. Alternatively, vascular injury may impair vasoconstricting mechanisms and allow hyperperfusion and edema formation. Depending on the cause, autoregulation may be impaired locally, as in an area of thrombosis, or globally, as in generalized cerebral edema.

Autoregulation is influenced by the partial pressures of carbon dioxide ($Paco_2$) and oxygen (Pao_2) in the arterial blood. The response to a change in $Paco_2$ is very brisk: as $Paco_2$ falls, cerebral vessels constrict, and as $Paco_2$ levels rise, the cerebral vessels dilate. A rise in $Paco_2$ can increase cerebral blood flow significantly. The response to changes in Pao_2 is much less dramatic.

The autoregulatory response to $Paco_2$ remains robust, except in severely brain-injured patients, and can cause detrimental increases in cerebral blood flow when respiratory compromise leads to hypercapnia. Excessive cerebral blood volume can exacerbate cerebral edema. Conversely, hyperventilation to produce low $Paco_2$ results in prompt vasoconstriction and, often, a reduction in intracranial pressure (ICP). Hyperventilation had been used for many years as standard therapy in the treatment of patients with increased ICP. However, excessive hyperventilation may do more harm than good because it critically reduces cerebral blood flow to responsive vessels and triggers tissue ischemia in these areas.

Loss of matching between oxygen supply and demand occurs when autoregulatory mechanisms fail. Cerebral oxygen demand is correlated with the degree of neuronal activity and may vary widely from region to region. Excessive catecholamine or excitatory amino acids can significantly increase cerebral metabolism. In the context of impaired blood flow, these neurotransmitters may contribute to ischemia by increasing cerebral oxygen demand. Likewise, seizure activity greatly increases neuronal metabolism and can precipitate ischemia.[9] Efforts to reduce release of excitatory neurotransmitters through hypothermia, rest, and pain control may be beneficial. Pharmacologic suppression of brain seizures is imperative in the patient with cerebral ischemia. Drug-induced coma, with agents such as barbiturates, has been advocated to reduce brain metabolism.[10]

Hypothermia is a strategy for reducing brain metabolism and protecting the brain from ischemic injury. A number of animal and human studies suggest that cerebral injury can be delayed, and possibly avoided, by cooling the brain.[6] Possible mechanisms include inhibition of glutamate release, inhibition of IL-1 release, reduced cerebral metabolic rate, and suppression of inflammation. The effects of hypothermia on patient outcomes and the optimal degree of hypothermia remain controversial. Moderate degrees of cooling (28° C to

32° C) are associated with platelet dysfunction and coagulopathy.[6] Shivering negates the usefulness of hypothermia and must be suppressed, usually by pharmacologic means. Further research is ongoing to determine the therapeutic window for effectiveness, appropriate duration, and safe rewarming protocols.[6]

Two related concepts important to the discussion of autoregulation are cerebral edema and increased ICP. Swelling and space-occupying lesions (mass lesions), such as tumors or hematomas, may increase the pressure within the cranium such that blood supply is compromised. Measures to reduce cerebral edema, remove mass lesions, and prevent elevations of ICP help to maintain functional autoregulation.

Increased Intracranial Pressure

ICP is the pressure exerted by the contents of the cranium, and it normally ranges from 0 to 15 mm Hg.[11] Elevated ICP may occur in most types of acute brain injury and is associated with impaired neurologic function due to compression of brain structures. In all but very young children, the skull is a rigid, closed system with a set volume and a finite ability to accommodate changes in volume before elevations in ICP occur.

The volume of the cranium is made up of three components: brain tissue, cerebrospinal fluid (CSF), and blood. A relationship known as the Monro-Kellie hypothesis describes the compensatory responses to a change in volume in any of the three components.[12] A slight increase in one component can be offset by a reduction in the volume of the other two. An increase in brain volume, as might occur with cerebral edema, can be offset by a reduction in the CSF space and the space occupied by the cerebral vasculature. The ability to accommodate changes in volume without significant increases in pressure is called *compliance.* Intracranial compliance is limited because of the rigid skull; although small increases in intracranial volume may be absorbed, moderate changes result in significant increases in ICP (Figure 44-3).

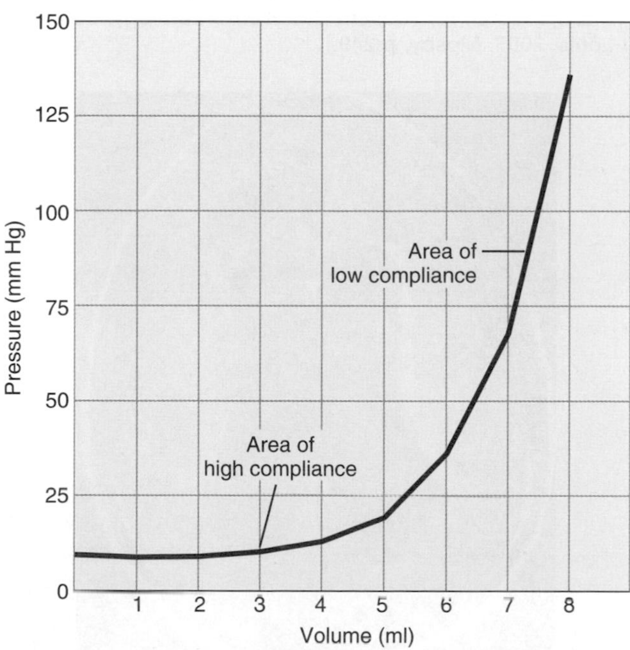

FIGURE 44-3 ■ A volume-pressure curve showing intracranial compliance. Small increases in volume have little effect on pressure, but larger increases exceed the ability to compensate, and pressure rises dramatically.

Each of the cranial components has a varying capability to compensate for the others. Cerebral blood vessels can reduce their volume through vasoconstriction. The CSF compartment is capable of significant reduction in volume by shunting CSF to the spinal cord or into the venous system via the arachnoid villi. The brain parenchyma has little ability to reduce its volume to compensate for CSF or blood volume expansion. In young children, an increase in ICP may manifest as an increase in head circumference. This occurs because the cranial bones have not yet fused, and the skull can expand to accommodate the increased intracranial volume.

In the healthy brain, transient changes in ICP are common and well tolerated. Sneezing, coughing, straining, and head-dependent positions all cause elevated ICP, but they are without consequence because ICP quickly returns to normal. In the brain-injured person, however, elevations in ICP can be very dangerous and poorly tolerated.

Etiology. The most common causes of increased ICP include stroke, trauma, and tumors, but many other primary and secondary disorders can cause significant elevations in ICP (Box 44-1). These disorders have common features in that they all affect the volume of CSF, blood, or brain tissue. An increase in brain tissue volume commonly occurs from diseases that cause cerebral edema. Edema of brain tissues is due to accumulation of fluid in interstitial or intracellular spaces.

Box 44-1

Common Causes of Increased Intracranial Pressure

Increased Brain Tissue Volume
Tumor
Hemorrhage
Infection
Cytotoxic edema
Vasogenic edema
Ischemia and necrosis

Increased Cerebrospinal Fluid Volume
Obstructive hydrocephalus
Nonobstructive hydrocephalus
Pseudotumor cerebri

Increased Blood Volume
Increased right atrial pressure
Dural sinus thrombosis
High arterial $Pa{CO_2}$
Acidosis

Interstitial edema is usually secondary to increased capillary pressure or damage to the capillary endothelium from a chemical injury or sudden increase in vascular pressure beyond autoregulatory limits. This type of edema has been termed *vasogenic,* and it results in extravasation of electrolytes, proteins, and fluid into the intercellular space. Vasogenic edema is a consequence of stroke, ischemia, and severe hypertension. The edema is often localized to a particular brain region where the BBB has been disrupted. Thus the swelling may be unilateral, occurring in one brain hemisphere or the other. Unilateral swelling often is poorly tolerated because midbrain structures are compressed and shifted, which produces life-threatening brain dysfunction.

Intracellular edema, called *cytotoxic edema,* occurs when ischemic tissue swells because of cellular energy failure. A lack of ATP allows Na^+ to accumulate in the cell, creating an osmotic force to draw in water. Cytotoxic edema predominates in cases of global ischemia. Global ischemia occurs when oxygenation of the whole brain is impaired, as would occur with cardiac arrest or severe hypoxemia. Generalized brain edema flattens the gyri and reduces the spaces between them (Figure 44-4).

In many cases of acute brain injury, vasogenic and cytotoxic edema occur together. Cerebral edema, when severe, can start a feedback cycle that promotes further edema of increasing severity and contributes to increased ICP. As edema fluid collects, it compresses local vessels, preventing adequate blood and oxygen from reaching the cells. This results in ischemia, which in turn triggers vasodilation and increased capillary pressure, further fluid leakage into the injured tissue, and increased edema. Vasogenic edema tends to be a delayed process in terms of the secondary effects of brain injury, progressively worsening during the first several days after injury. Clearance of brain edema occurs primarily by bulk flow into the CSF.[3]

In addition to edema, a number of space-occupying processes, such as tumors, hematomas, and abscesses, can increase intracranial volume and contribute to elevated ICP. These mass lesions are often unilateral and may result in severe compression of vital brain structures.[13] Attempts by the brain to accommodate the expanding mass result in typical findings on computed tomography (CT) scans (Figure 44-5). The ventricles are reduced in size and midline structures are displaced.

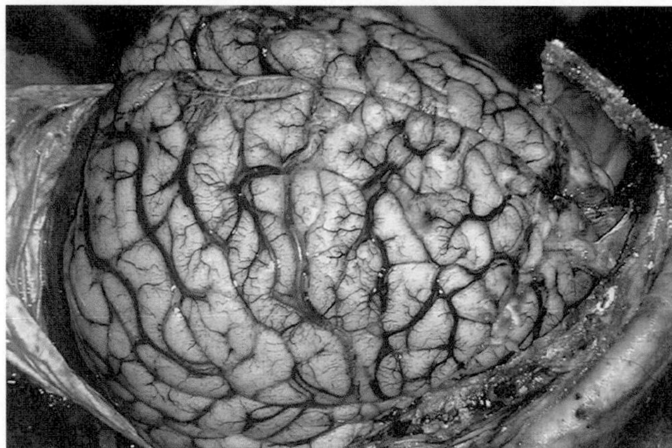

FIGURE 44-4 ■ Generalized brain edema with increased intracranial pressure. The convolutions of the brain surface (gyri) are flattened and the space between them is reduced. (From Kumar V, Cotran R, Robbins S: *Robbins basic pathology,* ed 7, Philadelphia, 2003, Saunders, p 812.)

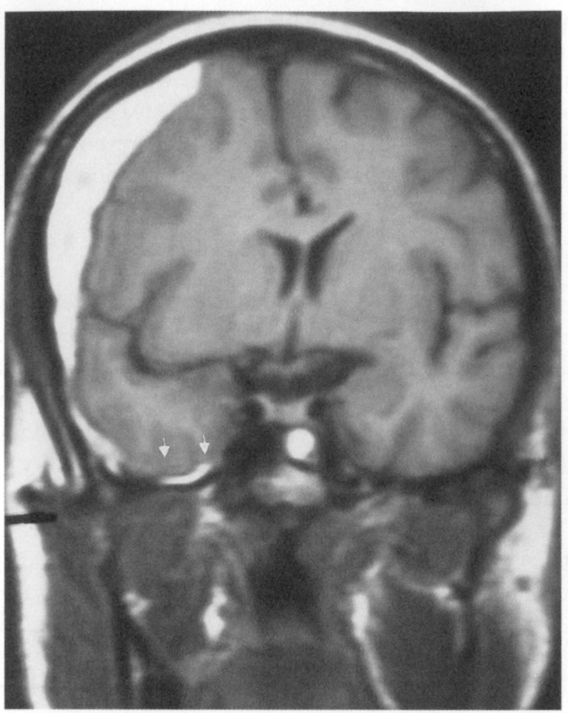

FIGURE 44-5 ■ Right subacute subdural hematoma on weighted CT scan. Note the shift in midline structures. (From Grossman RI, Yousem DM: *Neuroradiology,* ed 2, St Louis, 2003, Mosby, p 249.)

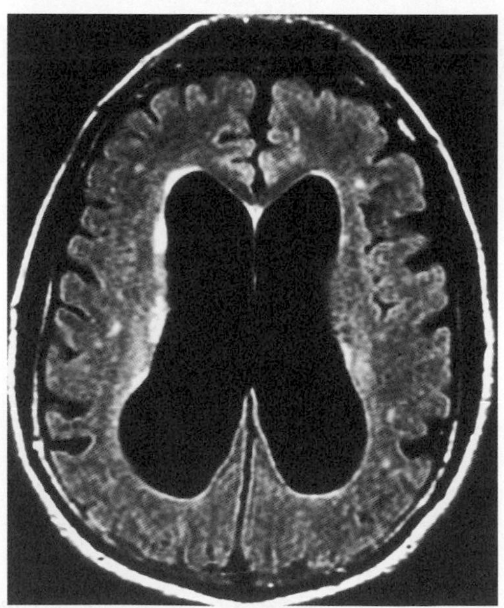

FIGURE 44-6 ■ Normal-pressure hydrocephalus. (From Grossman RI, Yousem DM: *Neuroradiology,* ed 2, St Louis, 2003, Mosby, p 377.)

Excessive accumulation of CSF (hydrocephalus) is another important cause of increased ICP. Elevated CSF volume causes the ventricles to enlarge and press on cerebral brain structures (Figure 44-6). Hydrocephalus may be a primary disorder or may develop as a consequence of brain swelling due to compression and obstruction of the outflow tract from the brain to the spinal cord.

Increased intravascular cerebral blood volume is unlikely to be a primary cause of high ICP, but it may contribute to pressure elevations initiated by ischemia or trauma. High Pa_{CO_2} or loss of autoregulatory controls can lead to vasodilation and increased cerebral blood volume.

Manifestations. Manifestations of elevated ICP include headache, vomiting, and altered level of consciousness (drowsiness). The patient may complain of blurry vision, and evaluation of the fundi may reveal edema of the optic disk (papilledema). As ICP rises to higher levels, the degree of alertness decreases and pupil responsiveness to light may be impaired. Eventually the patient may become unresponsive to stimulation and be unable to move, verbalize, or open the eyes. Prolonged elevations of ICP are thought to damage brain structures by compressing the blood supply and causing ischemia.

Patients exhibiting manifestations of elevated ICP, or those with significant risk for elevated ICP, may be monitored with a pressure device inserted into the brain parenchyma through an opening in the skull (burr hole). The pressure device is connected to an electrical transducer and the ICP waveforms can be monitored continuously (Figure 44-7). In general, a high ICP is associated with poor outcome. Different ICP waveforms are thought to carry different prognoses. The normal ICP waveform is characterized by three pressure peaks called P1, P2, and P3. These waves are reflections of changes in ICP associated with each arterial pulsation. Normally, P1 is higher than P2 and P2 is higher than P3 (see Figure 44-7). As ICP begins to increase, the pattern of waves remains normal, but the peak and mean pressure are higher. Further increases in ICP are characterized by a P2 wave that exceeds P1 and a dampening of the individual waveforms (plateau waves).[14]

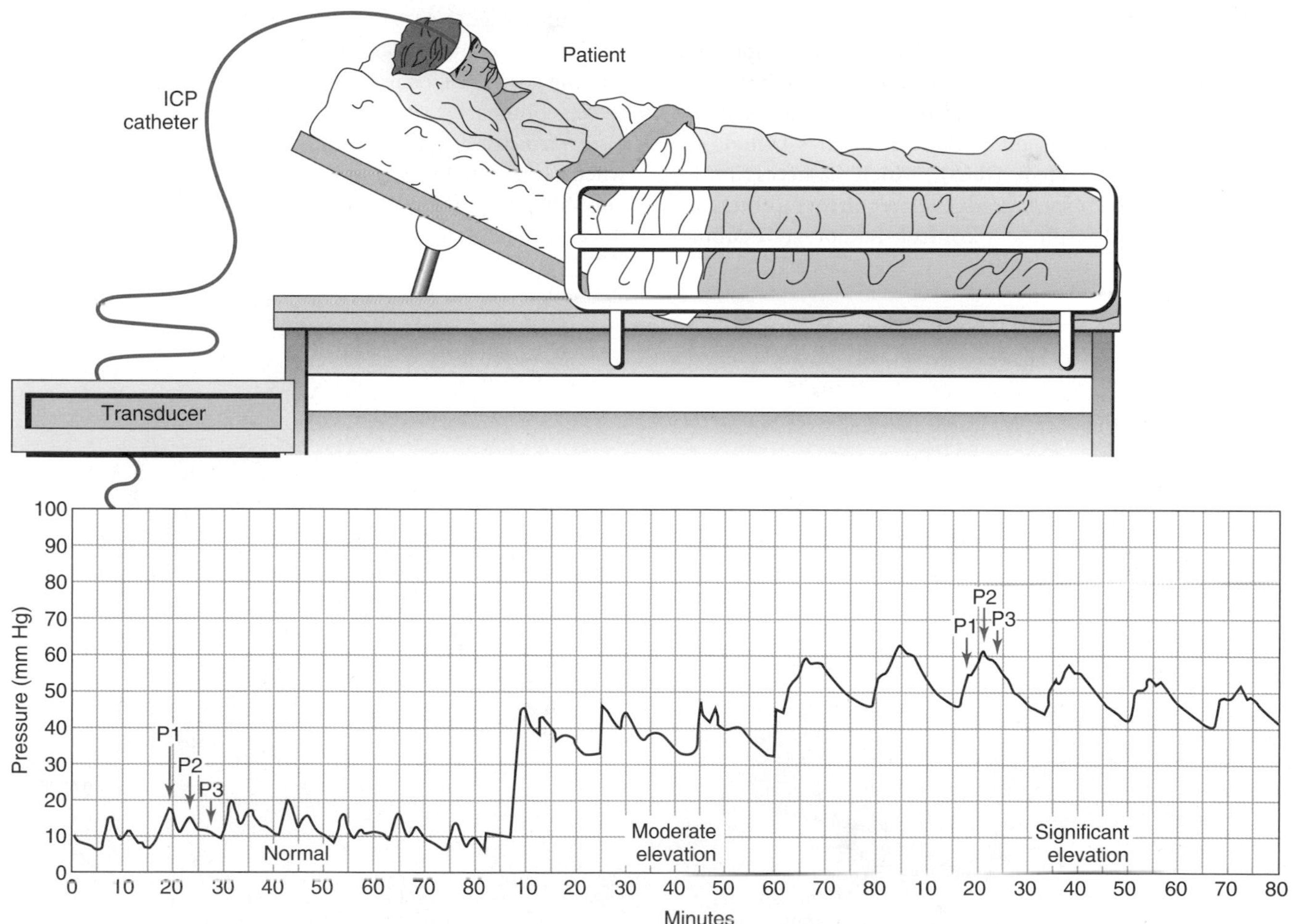

FIGURE 44-7 ■ Intracranial pressure *(ICP)* monitoring can be used to continuously measure ICP. The ICP tracing shows normal, elevated, and plateau waves. At high ICP the P2 peak is higher than the P1 peak, and the peaks become less distinct and plateau.

Plateau waves reflect severe pathologic increases in ICP due to changes in cerebral volume. Plateau waves can reach 50 to 100 mm Hg. After the plateau period the ICP slowly decreases, but it usually remains elevated above baseline. These waves reflect a potentially life-threatening situation, and if the pathologic process is not stopped, a cycle of increased ICP followed by vasodilation to maintain constant blood flow through swollen tissues continues, which in turn further increases ICP. Plateau waves are associated with ischemia and brain damage and are frequently accompanied by neurologic symptoms, including changes in level of consciousness, alteration in respiratory patterns, headache, nausea, vomiting, pupillary changes, and motor paresis. An extreme increase in ICP can precipitate an intense reaction by the sympathetic nervous system as it attempts to maintain cerebral perfusion through the compressed blood vessels. This has been termed an *ischemic* response or *Cushing reflex.* The systolic blood pressure can jump to values exceeding 200 mm Hg, accompanied by bradycardia and a widening pulse pressure. The Cushing reflex generally is viewed as a "last ditch" effort by the brain to reestablish cerebral perfusion.[12]

Brain Compression and Herniation

A dreaded complication of elevated ICP is brain compression and herniation. Compression of midbrain and brainstem structures is associated with rapid neurologic demise unless corrected quickly. Important midline structures include the reticular activating system (RAS), which is necessary for maintaining consciousness, and vital regulatory centers for cardiovascular and respiratory control. Radiologic examination by CT scan or other means (e.g., magnetic resonance imaging [MRI]) is useful in evaluating the patient with increased ICP who exhibits a change in neurologic status. CT scans may show midline shifts and herniations when ICP is sufficiently elevated.

Herniation refers to the protrusion of brain tissue through an opening in the supporting dura of the brain. Brain herniations have long been considered the harbinger of serious neurologic demise. Some researchers, however, suggest that herniations are markers of high ICP rather than initiators of demise, and that midbrain compression and shifting are more closely linked with altered neurologic function.[15] In either scenario, the finding of brain herniation carries a significant risk of severe morbidity and mortality.

Several types of brain herniation have been described according to their anatomic locations. The brain parenchyma is divided into compartments by the supporting structure of the dura. The dura folds into the space between the cerebral hemispheres to form the falx cerebri and folds in from the lateral aspects to form the tentorium, which separates the cerebellum from the cerebral hemispheres (Figure 44-8). The most common herniations occur through openings in these structures (Figure 44-9).

There is a small space between the tip of the falx cerebri and the corpus callosum through which the cingulate lobe of the cerebral cortex can herniate (Figure 44-10). This is called a *subfalcine* or *cingulate hernia.* Subfalcine herniation occurs when a lesion in one hemisphere is large enough to cause a lateral shift across the midline of the intracranial cavity, forcing the cingulate gyrus under the falx cerebri. This results in dis-

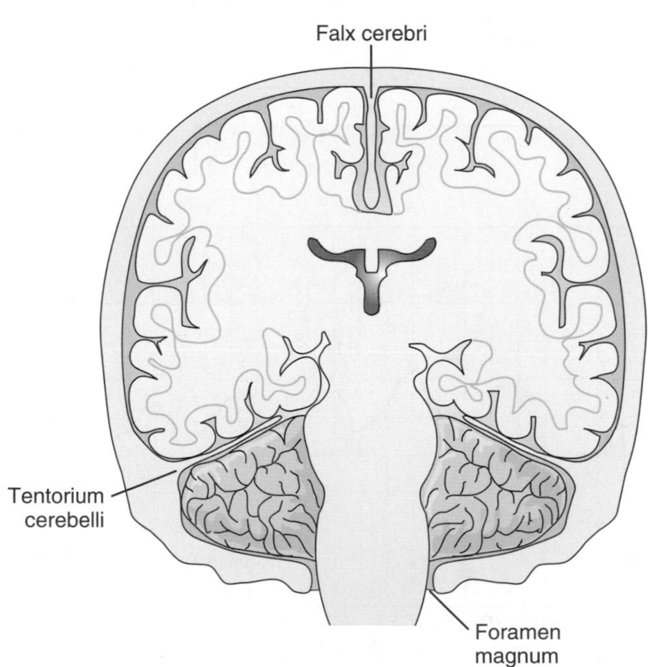

FIGURE 44-8 ■ Schematic drawing of the normal brain compartments showing the dural folds that form the falx cerebri and the tentorium.

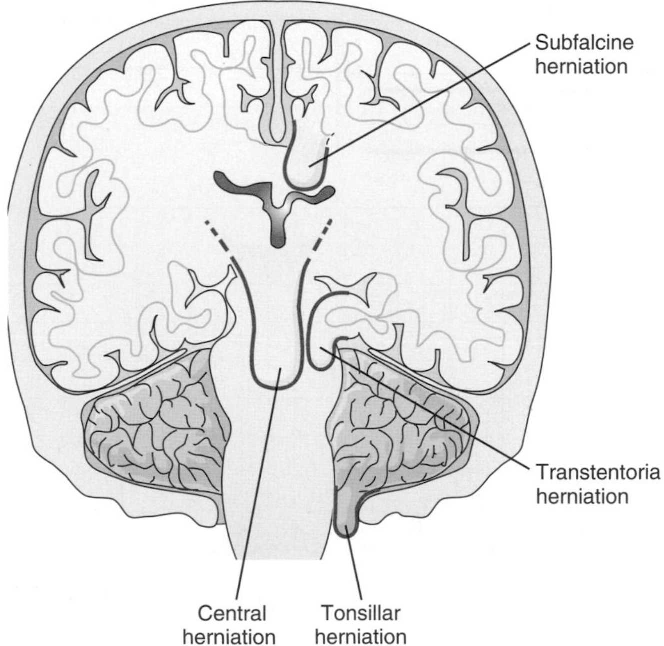

FIGURE 44-9 ■ Herniations occur when brain tissue is pushed through openings beside the dural folds or the foramen magnum.

tortion and compression of the internal cerebral vein. Subfalcine herniation can be asymptomatic and generally carries a better prognosis than other types of brain herniation. The greatest danger results from compression of blood vessels, particularly the ipsilateral anterior cerebral artery, which can cause cerebral ischemia and edema and contribute to the ICP elevation.

The tentorium is a rigid dural fold that separates the cerebellum and cerebral hemispheres. Midbrain structures pass between the infoldings of the dura in a structure called the *incisura.* With transtentorial herniations, a part of the brain protrudes through this space. Tentorial herniations are of two types: (1) bilateral herniations, which cause central transtentorial herniation, and (2) lateral herniations, in which one hemisphere compresses midbrain structures to the side and herniates through the tentorial opening (see Figure 44-9).

Central tentorial herniation results from expanding lesions in the frontal, parietal, and occipital lobes that force a downward displacement of the hemispheres and basal nuclei with compression of the diencephalon and adjoining midbrain. Transtentorial herniation can occur rapidly or slowly, depending on the type of lesion. The speed with which the process is recognized is a critical factor in patient survival. Slowly dilating or odd-shaped pupils is an ominous sign that indicates compression of the third cranial nerve and midbrain. Transtentorial herniations are associated with significant intracranial hypertension and may initiate vascular compression and CSF obstruction, which then contribute to the existing problem of ischemia and hypertension.

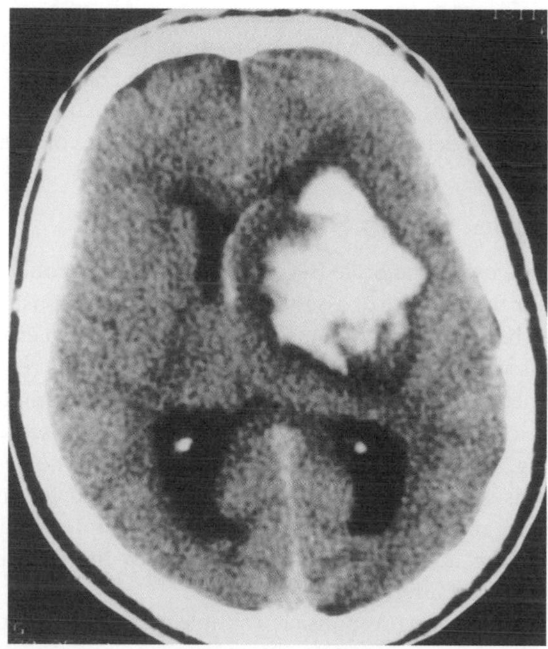

FIGURE 44-10 ■ CT scan of acute hemorrhage with mass effect and subfalcine herniation and shift of the lateral ventricle. (From Grossman RI, Yousem DM: *Neuroradiology,* ed 2, St Louis, 2003, Mosby, p. 263.)

Uncal herniation is a type of tentorial herniation that typically occurs with expanding lesions in the temporal lobe. As the lobe shifts, the basal edge of the uncus and the hippocampal gyrus bulge over the edge of the incisura (see Figure 44-9). In the process, the third cranial nerve and the posterior cerebral artery are compressed. The pupil on the same side (ipsilateral) as the lesion often becomes dilated an unresponsive to light (fixed). Flattening of the midbrain interferes with the ascending RAS and depresses the level of consciousness. The ipsilateral cerebral peduncle is also compressed, resulting in contralateral motor dysfunction. Compression of the contralateral cerebral peduncle is also common, leading to the confusing symptom of ipsilateral motor dysfunction.

Tonsillar herniation is less common than the other herniation syndromes and involves the shift of the cerebellar tonsils through the foramen magnum and compression of the medulla and upper cervical cord (see Figure 44-9). This typically occurs in patients with cerebellar lesions. Because of the proximity of the cerebellum to the brainstem, tonsillar herniation evolves very rapidly and can result in death in a matter of minutes. Signs usually include precipitous changes in blood pressure and heart rate, small pupils, disturbances in conjugate gaze, ataxic breathing, and quadriparesis.

Management

Management of increased ICP is often based on the results of CT or MRI. Processes amenable to surgical intervention can be detected and treated. Removal of excess CSF, tumors, abscesses, and hematomas can dramatically improve ICP. Nonsurgical processes such as cerebral edema, intracerebral bleeding, and infections are managed medically.

Traditionally, ICP measurements and determinations of cerebral perfusion pressure (CPP) have been used to guide therapy. A CPP of greater than 60 mm Hg is generally thought to be sufficient to ensure adequate blood flow and to prevent ischemia. CPP is calculated by subtracting the ICP from the MAP. Thus, as ICP increases, a higher MAP is required to maintain CPP. More recently, the value of assessing more direct measures of cerebral oxygenation has been recognized. Measures of oxygen utilization by the brain are thought to provide a better assessment of brain ischemia. The oxygen level of jugular venous blood can be intermittently or continuously monitored and compared with arterial oxygen levels. An increasing difference between arterial and venous oxygen (A-VDO_2) is thought to indicate inadequate delivery of blood to the brain.

With these new assessment tools, it became obvious that measures to reduce ICP were not always associated with improvement in brain oxygenation, and in some cases they were detrimental. Controversy regarding the appropriate treatment of increased ICP continues, and the focus of management has shifted from ICP control to management of cerebral oxygenation. The roles of previously established therapies such as hyperventilation, brain dehydration with diuretics, head-up positions, and administration of corticosteroids have been called into question. Previously discarded therapies, such as hypothermia, hypertonic saline infusion, and drug-induced comas, are being reintroduced. Despite these controversies in medical management, the value of careful observation and assessment of neurologic function are unquestioned. Many times subtle changes in neurologic function are detectable early in the process of evolving brain injury. Several tools have been developed to help standardize neurologic examination and are discussed in the following section.

KEY CONCEPTS

- Primary brain injury occurs as a direct result of the initial insult. Secondary injury refers to progressive damage resulting from the body's physiologic response to the initial insult.
- Ischemia is an important mechanism of brain injury that occurs when the blood supply is inadequate to meet metabolic needs. A lack of oxygen results in mitochondrial failure, ATP depletion, and accumulation of intracellular calcium ions.
- Excessive release of excitatory amino acids, like glutamate, is thought to contribute to calcium overload during acute brain injury. Calcium overload is a critical event leading to cell dysfunction, membrane damage, and cell necrosis.
- Reperfusion injury occurs when blood flow is reintroduced to previously ischemic but viable cells. Free radicals are generated, which damage cell structures. Inflammatory cells are recruited to the area and may increase edema, block vessels, and contribute to free radical production.
- Autoregulation of cerebral blood flow achieves appropriate flow to meet metabolic needs despite changes in blood pressure and metabolism. Autoregulation is effective over a range of MAP from 50 to 150 mm Hg. Hypoxia and high $Paco_2$ result in dilation of cerebral vessels. Hyperventilation with low $Paco_2$ results in cerebral vasoconstriction.
- Pressure in the cranium is a product of the volume of brain tissue, blood, and CSF. Increases in any one component are partially offset by reductions in the others to maintain ICP.
- Brain swelling is a common cause of increased ICP. Edema may result from changes in vascular competency that lead to transudation of fluid into intercellular spaces (vasogenic), or from cellular swelling (cytotoxic) owing to a deficiency in cellular ATP.
- Normal ICP ranges from 0 to 15 mm Hg. Transient increases are well tolerated, but chronically increased ICP results in compression of vessels and brain tissue, leading to cellular ischemia and brain damage. High ICP may precipitate herniation of brain tissue through dural compartments.

MANIFESTATIONS OF BRAIN INJURY

Depending on the severity and location of brain injury, a wide variety of clinical manifestations may occur. Patients may present with symptoms ranging from minor headache and visual disturbances to complete loss of consciousness. Patients with significant acute injuries require frequent neurologic assessments to detect changes that may evolve rapidly. Level of consciousness, cranial nerve reflexes, and brain hemodynamics provide important clues to neurologic status.

Level of Consciousness

A change in level of consciousness is one of the most sensitive indicators of altered brain function. Efforts have been made to standardize the terms used to describe level of consciousness (Table 44-1). Consciousness is a state of alertness and attentiveness to one's environment and situation. A fully conscious individual is awake, alert, and oriented to time, person, place, and current circumstances. Consciousness is thought to be dependent on activity in the RAS neurons, which project to the thalamus, and in tracts between the thalamus and cortex.[16] Although consciousness may be suddenly and completely lost, the decline is usually progressive. Cortical neurons are most sensitive, and cognitive and memory functions are impaired early, leading to confusion.

Delirium may follow, characterized by severe confusion and hallucinations. As RAS function is compromised, the patient becomes difficult to arouse and requires increasingly noxious stimuli to produce verbal or motor responses. Eventually complete loss of consciousness may occur, a condition called coma. The **Glasgow Coma Scale** can be used to assess levels of consciousness with greater reliability among different observers (Box 44-2). Sudden or progressive changes in level of consciousness should prompt a thorough neurologic examination to determine the cause and best course of therapy.

Glasgow Coma Scale

The Glasgow Coma Scale (GCS) is a standardized tool developed for the purpose of assessing the level of consciousness in acutely brain-injured patients. It can also be used to evaluate patients with an altered level of consciousness as a result of other neurologic insults such as hemorrhage or craniotomy. Numeric scores are given to arousal-directed responses of eye opening, verbal utterances, and motor reactions. The best response is scored, bilateral responses are recorded for motor reactions, and consistent application of a painful stimulus is required for accuracy. When used correctly, the GCS has a high degree of interrater reliability.

The eye opening response is a simple measure of alertness. Normally, the eyes open spontaneously in response to verbal stimuli. If the eyes do not open in response to verbal stimuli, noxious stimuli, such as compression of the nail beds, may be

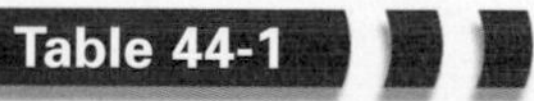

Table 44-1

Terms Used to Describe Altered Level of Consciousness

Term	Description
Confused	Unable to think clearly or engage in effective problem solving; orientation to time, place, person impaired; easily aroused by verbal stimuli
Delirious	Restless and disoriented, may have hallucinations; easily aroused, but may have difficulty with attention
Lethargic	Uninterested in surroundings or events; sluggish in thought and motor activities; does not engage spontaneously in activities
Obtunded	Falls asleep unless stimulated; arousable with voice or touch, but quickly returns to sleep
Stuporous	In a deep state of sleep; vigorous stimulation is required to arouse and a wakeful state is not maintained
Comatose	Unable to be aroused, even with vigorous painful stimuli; motor responses, such as withdrawal or posturing, may occur

Box 44-2

Glasgow Coma Scale

Eye Opening

4. Spontaneously (eyes open, does not imply awareness)
3. To speech (any speech, not necessarily a command)
2. To pain
1. Never

Verbal Response

5. Oriented (to time, person, place)
4. Confused speech (disoriented)
3. Inappropriate (swearing, yelling)
2. Incomprehensible sounds (moaning, groaning)
1. None

Motor Response

6. Obeys commands
5. Localizes pain (deliberate or purposeful movement)
4. Withdrawal (moves away from stimulus)
3. Abnormal flexion (decortication)
2. Extension (decerebration)
1. None (flaccidity)

applied. It is important to be consistent and vigorous enough to achieve the best response from the patient. In patients with acute mass lesions, eye opening is usually depressed in conjunction with impaired response to pain and motor function. Spontaneous eye opening in the acute phase is an encouraging sign, as it implies that the arousal mechanism in the brainstem is intact.

The verbal response on the GCS measures orientation. A full score in this category indicates that the patient is alert and fully oriented: the patient knows his or her name, current location, and the time of day. In the next level down the patient is awake and can pay attention to a certain degree, but is confused as to who he or she is and does not know the time or the location. If attention is poor and the verbal responses consist of yelling and swearing, it is scored as an inappropriate response. Incomprehensible verbalizations are unintelligible sounds or mumbling. Absence of verbalization is given a score of 1. As in the eye opening category, noxious stimuli are applied to achieve the best verbal response from the patient.

Motor response is a powerful predictor of outcome. Motor response is scored as the best level of response the patient is able to perform. Each extremity is evaluated to avoid misinterpretation secondary to muscle paralysis. At the highest level, the patient can obey a command to move. At the next level down, the patient does not obey commands, but when a painful stimulus is applied, the patient moves in a purposeful manner to avoid the stimulus; the patient is able to localize the source of pain. As status deteriorates, the patient withdraws only the extremity from the painful stimulus. This is not considered a purposeful response. Further deterioration results in abnormal posturing movements. *Decorticate* posturing is characterized by an abnormal flexor response of the arms and wrists. The legs and feet extend and internally rotate (Figure 44-11). The level below decorticate posturing is called *decerebrate* or *abnormal extension.* The arms extend with external rotation of the wrists. The legs and feet extend and rotate internally (see Figure 44-11). The lowest level of motor response is no response to painful stimuli (i.e., flaccidity in all four limbs). It is important to emphasize that all limbs must be tested separately, as motor responses may be preserved on one side only, and levels of involvement may vary from side to side. Level of coma occurs on a continuum from mild (GCS score >12), to moderate (GCS score 9-12), to severe (GCS score <8).[17]

Cranial Nerve Reflexes

The GCS score alone is not sufficient to accurately determine the status of the patient with an acute insult to the brain. Assessment of the integrity of brainstem function is also important and is indicated by various brainstem reflexes including the pupil light reflex, oculovestibular reflex, and corneal reflex.

Pupil Reflex

Pupillary assessment provides important information about the function of the brainstem and cranial nerves II and III.

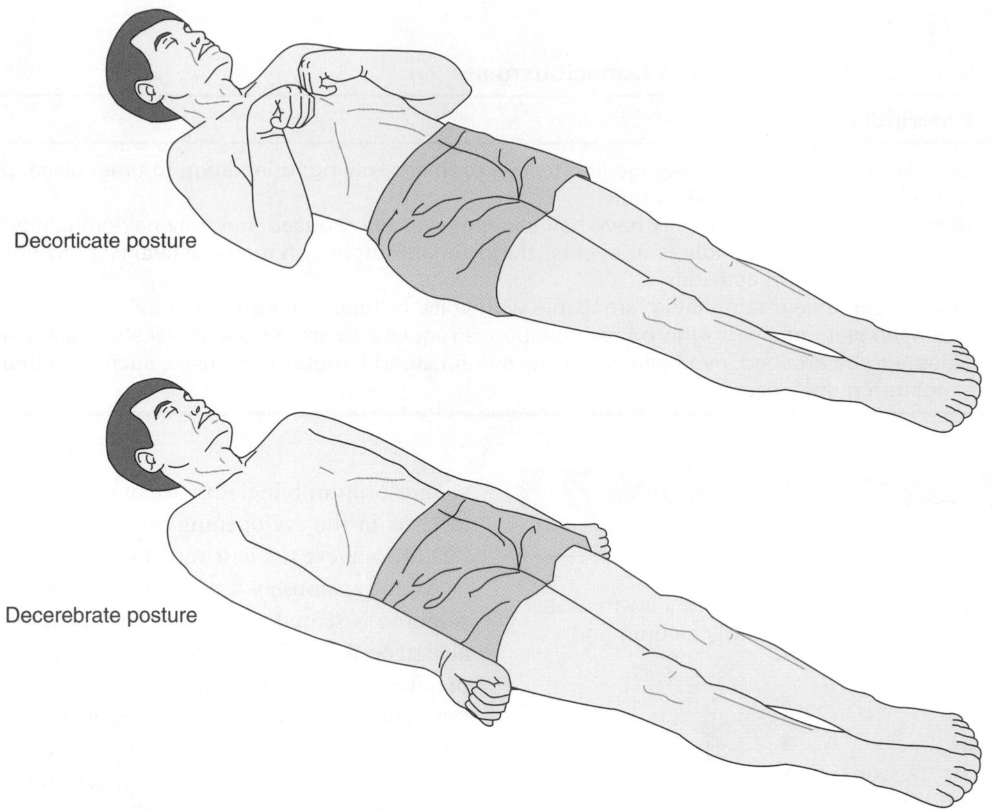

FIGURE 44-11 ■ Abnormal motor activity with coma. Decorticate posturing is indicated by flexed wrist and arm and extended legs and feet. Decerebrate posturing is indicated by arm and leg extension.

The normal pupillary response to light results from an intact afferent cranial nerve II (optic) detecting the light and stimulating the intact efferent cranial nerve III (oculomotor) to constrict the pupils. The response of the pupil to light, in terms of both its shape and the speed of reaction, is a function of cranial nerve III.

The pupillary response is recorded by noting pupil size in millimeters, shape, and reactivity to light. Careful monitoring of the pupillary response to light during the acute phase is critical, as a failing response may be the first indication of brain compression. Mild dilation of a pupil with sluggish or absent light response is ominous. This phenomenon results from pressure on the oculomotor nerve (cranial nerve III) by lateral displacement of midbrain structures. An oval pupil may be an early indicator of dangerously poor compliance and transtentorial herniation. The oval pupil represents a transitional pupil that can return to normal responsiveness if ICP is controlled.

Other pupillary responses indicate damage to the optic nerve. The afferent pupillary defect is a paradoxical response that is detected with the swinging-light test. As the examiner swings a light from the normal eye to the abnormal eye, the abnormal pupil responds by dilating instead of constricting. This occurs because the light signals transmitted to the Edinger-Westphal nucleus in the midbrain through the injured optic nerve are insufficient to maintain constriction brought on by stimulation of the normal eye.

Bilaterally small pupils suggest a destructive lesion in the pons or the presence of certain drugs. Bilaterally fixed and dilated pupils suggest inadequate cerebral perfusion. This could be related to hypotension or increased ICP. If perfusion is not interrupted for too long, a normal pupillary response returns with adequate flow.

Eye movements are important indicators of brainstem function. Cranial nerves III, IV, and VI are responsible for normal eye movements. Abnormalities of eye movement are useful in localizing the site of brain dysfunction. Abnormal eye movements seen in the brain-injured patient can include nystagmus, dysconjugate eye movements, and ocular palsies. **Nystagmus** is a persistent rhythmic or jerky movement in one or both eyes. **Dysconjugate movements** occur when the eyes do not move together in the same direction. Ocular palsies occur when one or more cranial nerves are dysfunctional such that motor paralysis of the eye muscles impairs movements in one or more directions.

Oculovestibular Reflex

The oculovestibular reflex normally detects head movements (via receptors in the semicircular canals) and causes appropriate adjustments of eye position such that an object can remain fixed on the retina even though the head is moving. An impaired oculovestibular reflex implies brainstem dysfunction. Two tests can be performed to evaluate this reflex in the unconscious patient: the doll's-eyes test and cold calorics.

The oculocephalic or doll's-eyes test is performed only in patients in whom a lateral spine radiograph has been obtained to rule out spinal injury. The test is performed by holding open the patient's eyelids and rotating the head from one side to the other (Figure 44-12). If the brainstem is intact, the eyes will turn in a direction opposite to the direction of head rotation. If the eyes do not move in conjugate fashion or are asymmetrical, the response is abnormal and brainstem function is impaired. If the eyes remain fixed at the midline and do not move, the response is said to be absent. An absent response indicates severe brainstem impairment.

The oculovestibular response or cold calorics is a similar test of brainstem function using cold water instillation into the ear. Cold against the tympanic membrane causes action potentials from the vestibular apparatus to change and simulates the neuronal response to head rotation. If the brainstem is intact, the normal response will be a tonic deviation of both eyes toward the side that is irrigated. Dysconjugate or asymmetrical eye movement is abnormal. If there is no eye movement, the response is absent. Testing of the oculovestibular response is one of the essential examinations performed in patients thought to be brain dead. It is not performed on conscious individuals. Patients with depression of brain function due to metabolic abnormalities usually retain an intact oculovestibular response. Certain drugs, such as barbiturates and high doses of phenytoin, can severely depress the oculovestibular response. In the absence of drug effect, an absent response to cold calorics is a poor prognostic sign indicating minimal chance of brain recovery.

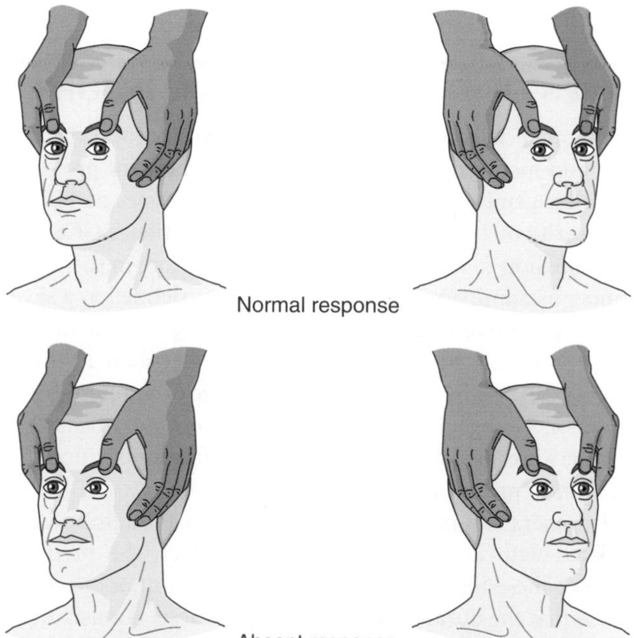

FIGURE 44-12 ■ Doll's eyes response is indicated by an absent (abnormal) response to the oculocephalic head turning test and indicates brainstem damage. In the normal response the eyes turn in a direction opposite to head rotation. In the absent response the eyes stay midline and do not turn when the head is rotated.

Corneal Reflex

A simple test of cranial nerve function is the corneal reflex. A wisp of cotton is touched to the cornea of the eye to elicit a blink response. Absence of blink is another indicator of severely impaired brain function.

Brain Hemodynamics and Metabolism

Monitoring of hemodynamic and metabolic parameters commonly is done in the patient with acute brain injury. Hypotension is poorly tolerated and must be promptly detected and managed to prevent further ischemia. Blood pressure can be monitored continuously by an indwelling arterial catheter. In general, the MAP should not fall below about 70 mm Hg. However, this may be too low in patients with chronic hypertension or elevated ICP. In patients with ICP monitors, CPP should not fall below 60 mm Hg:

$$\text{CPP} = \text{MAP} - \text{ICP}$$

Elevated temperature increases the metabolic rate of neuronal tissue and is poorly tolerated. Measures to keep body temperature at 37° C or lower are usually employed, and in some cases hypothermia may be purposefully induced to reduce brain metabolism. The adequacy of brain perfusion in meeting metabolic demands of the brain can be estimated by the arteriovenous oxygen difference (A-VDO_2). An arterial oxygen level (PaO_2) and a jugular vein oxygen level (PjvO_2) are obtained simultaneously and used to calculate the A-VDO_2:

$$\text{A-VDO}_2 = \text{PaO}_2 - \text{PjvO}_2$$

Alternatively, oxygen saturation can be used to derive similar information. Monitoring devices can be applied for continuous measurement of arterial (SaO_2) and venous saturation (SjvO_2). The A-V difference can then be calculated and expressed as a percentage:

$$(\text{SaO}_2 - \text{SjvO}_2) \div \text{SaO}_2 \times 100$$

This value reflects the degree of cerebral extraction of oxygen. An increase in the cerebral extraction is thought to reflect an inadequate rate of cerebral blood flow. It has been suggested that the percent extraction should not exceed a critical value of 40% and the SjvO_2 should remain greater than 50%.[18] Measures such as less aggressive hyperventilation, volume replacement, and blood pressure support may help return the extraction ratio back toward normal. Treating potential sources of increased brain metabolism, such as fever, seizures, agitation, and pain, can be helpful in restoring the balance between cerebral oxygen demand and supply.

KEY CONCEPTS

- A change in level of consciousness often is an early indicator of compromised neurologic status. Normal consciousness is apparent as alertness and orientation to time, person, place, and situation.
- The Glasgow Coma Scale is used to assess level of coma by scoring alertness (eye opening response), orientation (verbal response), and motor control (movements). The highest score is given to demonstration of spontaneous eye opening, full orientation, and obeying of motor commands.
- Pupillary responses indicate the function of the brainstem and cranial nerves II and III. Changes in size, shape, and reactivity of the pupil may be an early indicator of impending brain herniation. Eye movements controlled by cranial nerves III, IV, and VI may be impaired with increased ICP. Nystagmus, dysconjugate gaze, and ocular palsies may be evident.
- An absent doll's-eyes response when the subject's head is turned and an abnormal response to activation of the oculovestibular reflex upon installation of cold water in the ear are very poor prognostic signs.
- Hemodynamic and metabolic assessments are helpful in maintaining adequate balance between cerebral oxygen supply and demand. Measures to restore the balance should be taken if cerebral oxygen extraction exceeds 40%.

TRAUMATIC BRAIN INJURY

Traumatic brain injury (TBI) refers to injuries of brain tissues sustained as a consequence of trauma. The term is sometimes used interchangeably with head injury; however, injuries to the cranium do not always result in brain injury. Confusion in terms has led to difficulty in determining actual rates of traumatic brain injury, but there is no doubt that it is a major public health concern.

EPIDEMIOLOGY

It is estimated that 7 million to 10 million new cases of head injury occur each year in the United States[19] and that as many as 85% of these go unreported.[20] Among the 1.5 million cases diagnosed annually, about 50,000 result in death. In the United States, an estimated 5.3 million persons are living with permanent TBI-related disability.[6] Falls, sports injuries, and transportation-related trauma are important causes of TBI. The great majority of traumatic brain injuries in the United States are sustained in automobile accidents, whereas other forms of transportation are more significant contributors in other countries. The worldwide incidence of TBI may approach 500 million annually.[20]

Certain age, gender, and ethnic groups are at higher risk for sustaining TBI. In the United States, 15- to 24-year-olds are at highest risk. Males are twice as likely as females to sustain TBI and are more than three times more likely to die from their injuries. African-Americans have a slightly higher risk than white and Hispanic Americans. Individuals at the lowest socioeconomic levels have the highest per capita rates of brain injury.[20]

It is difficult to quantify the social, medical, and economic impact of TBI. The cost of acute hospital care for a moderately to severely brain-injured patient is substantial, and the long-term care, rehabilitation, and loss of productivity for survivors add significantly to the cost. One in five patients who are hospitalized for TBI and survive will have a substantial long-term disability.

Prevention of TBI is an important initiative for public health. Because most TBI is associated with automobile accidents, efforts to prevent driving while under the influence of alcohol and other drugs, driver education, seatbelt use laws, and safer roads and automobiles may be most helpful. Helmet use by motorcyclists significantly reduces crash mortality. It is interesting to note that public concern does not seem to reflect the magnitude of the problem, and TBI is likely to continue to have a major impact on the health care system for years to come.

Early rescue from the trauma scene and immediate emergency management are important in the effort to reduce morbidity and mortality after TBI. Half of TBI fatalities occur within 10 minutes of the traumatic event.[20] Victims who survive until hospitalization require expert monitoring and intervention.

TYPES OF TRAUMATIC BRAIN INJURY

TBI is often characterized according to severity, location of injury, and mechanism of injury. There are different prognoses and management strategies for the different types of TBI.

Severity of TBI usually is based on the patient's GCS score on admission to the hospital or the lowest score in the first 48 hours postadmission. A GCS of 8 or less is defined as a severe injury; moderate injury is defined by a GCS of 9 to 12; mild injury is associated with a GCS score greater than 12. Injury severity can also be estimated by the degree of brain injury detected on CT examination. The Traumatic Coma Data Bank Criteria (Box 44-3) use the degree of diffuse injury noted on CT scan to predict injury severity.

In general, an increased severity score is thought to be associated with a poorer prognosis; however, the predictive value of these tools is not very high. Some authors have suggested that the duration of postinjury amnesia is a useful predictor of outcome,[19] but this measure often cannot be made early in the course of treatment and may not be timely enough to be helpful.

Injury severity and outcome are dependent on the physiologic state of the brain prior to the trauma. Physical factors

Box 44-3

Trauma Code Data Bank Diagnostic Categories of Abnormalities Visualized on Computed Tomography Scanning

Diffuse Injury I
No visible intracranial pathology seen on CT scan

Diffuse Injury II
Cisterns are present with a shift 0 to 5 mm and/or lesion densities present
No high- or mixed-density lesion greater than 25 ml
May include bone fragments and foreign bodies

Diffuse Injury III (with Swelling)
Cisterns compressed or absent
Shift 0 to 5 mm
No high- or mixed-density lesion greater than 25 ml

Diffuse Injury IV (with Shift)
Shift greater than 5 mm
No high- or mixed-density lesion greater than 25 ml

Evacuated Mass Lesion
Any lesion surgically evacuated

Nonevacuated Mass Lesion
High- or mixed-density lesion greater than 25 ml, not surgically evacuated

such as bone thickness, dural stability, brain atrophy, drug effects, previous brain damage, preexisting dementia, and cerebral atherosclerosis have an impact on the outcome of TBI. There is so much individual variation in brain response to injury that making a prognosis statement is often guesswork. After 48 to 72 hours following the injury, a better guess at outcome is possible because the degree of secondary injury will be manifest.

PRIMARY INJURY

Primary injury is the result of the initial trauma on neural tissue. Primary injuries are commonly described as focal, polar, or diffuse. Although such injuries rarely occur in pure form, they are discussed separately for the sake of simplicity.

Focal injuries (coup) are those that are localized to the site of impact to the skull. The extent of the damage is quite variable. They may be superficial or extend deep into the brain matter. Local injury to the brain can result in specific neurologic symptoms, depending on the site. An injury over the motor cortex may result in contralateral weakness of the face and arm, whereas an injury to the frontal lobe can lead to apraxia, impulsive behavior, and poor judgment. However, localized hemorrhages or significant edema may act as space-occupying lesions and result in increased ICP, brain shifting, and herniation. In such cases symptoms may include a decreased level of consciousness, cranial nerve dysfunction, and contralateral muscle weakness.

Polar injuries (coup contracoup) occur as a consequence of the brain shifting within the skull and meninges during the course of an acceleration-deceleration movement resulting in local injury at two opposite poles of the brain. This is commonly the case in motor vehicle accidents in which the head, traveling at the same high speed as the motor vehicle, is abruptly stopped by an obstacle such as the windshield. As a result, the frontal and temporal poles are crushed against the anterior and middle cranial fossae, damaging the tips and inferior surface of the temporal and frontal lobes. Damage may cause bruising or bleeding and, in combination with edema, may result in significant intracerebral mass lesions. Most forces to the head have a lateral rotational component; thus, one side of the brain typically is more severely injured than the other. Patients with polar injuries may or may not need significant acute care, depending on the severity of the injury. Polar injuries can, however, be a significant factor in the extent of subsequent cognitive impairment, affecting rehabilitation and long-term recovery.

Diffuse injuries occur when movement of the brain within the cranial cavity causes widespread neuronal damage. The brain is often subject to shifting and rotational forces during injury. The combined force causes stretching and shearing of the axonal white matter, known as *diffuse axonal injury.* Patients with severe diffuse axonal injury frequently are comatose from the time of injury. Coma is a consequence of axonal damage in the cerebral cortex or reticular activating center in the brainstem and can be prolonged. Recovery may be limited to a severely disabled or vegetative state. In addition to falls and motor vehicle accidents, diffuse injury is an unfortunate consequence of vigorous shaking, particularly of babies and the elderly, who have greater mobility of the brain within the skull.

In addition to categorizing primary injuries according to location as focal, polar, or diffuse, they can be differentiated by the mechanism of injury: concussion, contusion, and intracranial hematoma. *Concussion* is the term applied when head injury produces an alteration in consciousness, but no evidence of brain damage is found on physical or radiologic examination. Concussion is a common consequence of sports-related head trauma. Concussion is graded according to severity (Box 44-4), and management differs depending on the grade of concussion (Box 44-5).[21] *Contusion* is said to be present when CT or MRI reveals an area of brain tissue damage (necrosis, laceration, bruising). An intracranial hematoma is a localized collection of blood within the cranium resulting from vascular damage.

Intracranial Hematomas

Three types of hematoma are common after traumatic head injury: epidural (extradural), subdural, and subarachnoid

Box 44-4

Grades of Concussion

Grade 1

Transient confusion (inattentiveness, inability to maintain a coherent stream of thought and carry out goal-directed movements)

No loss of consciousness

Concussion symptoms or mental status abnormalities on examination resolve in less than 15 minutes

Grade 2

Transient confusion

No loss of consciousness

Concussion symptoms or mental status abnormalities (including amnesia) on examination last more than 15 minutes

Grade 3

Any loss of consciousness

- Brief (seconds)
- Prolonged (minutes)

Box 44-5

Management Recommendations

Grade 1

1. Remove from contest
2. Examine immediately and at 5-minute intervals for the development of mental status abnormalities or postconcussive symptoms at rest and with exertion
3. May return to contest if mental status abnormalities or postconcussive symptoms clear within 15 minutes

Grade 2

1. Remove from contest and disallow return that day
2. Examine on-site frequently for signs of evolving intracranial pathologic process
3. A trained person should reexamine the athlete the following day
4. A physician should perform a neurologic examination to clear the athlete for return to play after one full asymptomatic week at rest and with exertion

Grade 3

1. Transport the athlete from the field to the nearest emergency department by ambulance if still unconscious or if worrisome signs are detected (with cervical spine immobilization, if indicated)
2. A thorough neurologic evaluation should be performed emergently, including appropriate neuroimaging procedures when indicated
3. Hospital admission is indicated if any signs of pathologic process are detected or if the mental status of the athlete remains abnormal

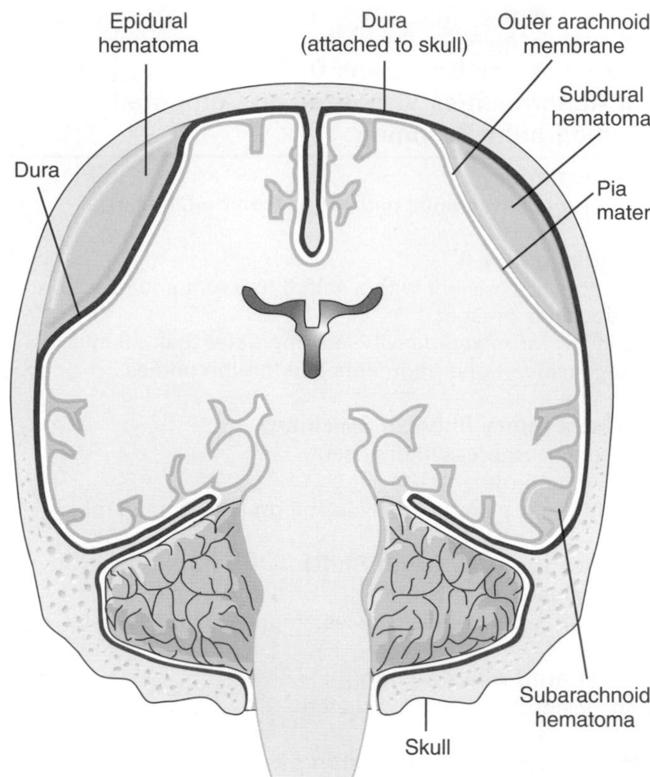

FIGURE 44-13 ■ Locations of epidural, subdural, and subarachnoid hematomas.

(Figure 44-13). Hematomas may expand slowly or rapidly, progressively compressing brain structures and increasing ICP. The types of hematoma differ in their clinical presentation and significance. Recognition and prompt management of intracranial hematomas can significantly improve outcome in the patient with TBI.

Epidural Hematoma

Epidural hematomas are collections of blood in the epidural space, which lies between the inner surface of the skull and the dura mater (extradural). Vessels that travel within the dura are susceptible to injury in conjunction with skull fractures. Fracture of the temporal bone commonly disrupts the middle meningeal artery, resulting in an acute epidural hemorrhage. Because the source of bleeding in most epidural hematomas is arterial, the hematoma can expand rapidly, causing acute deterioration of neurologic function. Often, the severity of the primary injury is minor, and the patient may suffer only a brief period of disturbed consciousness followed by a period of normal cognition (lucid interval). Then consciousness rapidly deteriorates as the epidural hematoma expands and compresses brain structures.

Rapid evaluation by CT is recommended to detect the hematoma, and surgical intervention to evacuate the hematoma is necessary. Patients with promptly managed epidural hematomas usually have an excellent prognosis because the associated primary injury is minimal.

Subdural Hematoma

Subdural hematomas form in the space between the dura and the outer arachnoid membrane (see Figure 44-5). The vessels traversing this area are called *bridging veins.* Bridging veins drain venous blood from the surface of the brain, crossing the arachnoid and subdural spaces before emptying into the venous sinuses. Venous sinuses are relatively fixed to the dura and are immobile, whereas the brain, which floats in the CSF, is quite mobile. With a sudden change in head velocity, as occurs with falls and vehicular accidents, the brain moves, the venous sinuses remain stationary, and the bridging veins between the two are stretched and sheared apart.

Because venous blood is under low pressure in the head, the rate of hematoma formation is usually slower than that of an epidural bleed. When subdural bleeds do produce an acute deterioration in neurologic status, the severity of the primary injury is likely to be high. Acute subdural hematomas produce symptoms within 24 hours of injury and have a worse prognosis than epidural or subacute subdural bleeds.

Subacute subdural hematomas can present a diagnostic challenge because the symptoms may be so delayed that the patient does not associate them with a head injury event. Venous bleeding is usually self-limited but may slowly progress and produce symptoms of increased ICP (headache, vomiting, blurred vision) 2 to 10 days after the primary event.

When subdural hematomas are large and sufficiently localized, they are amenable to surgical evacuation. If the subdural hematoma has been present for some time, it enters a chronic stage in which fibroblasts infiltrate the area and granulation tissue forms. Hematomas at this chronic stage are prone to rebleeding from thin-walled capillaries in the new granulation tissue. The risk of rebleeding is highest in the first few months.[3] Chronic subdural hematomas are a common finding at autopsy of elderly individuals. In addition to the increased incidence of falls, the elderly usually have some cerebral atrophy, which makes the brain more mobile within the skull. In the elderly, the likelihood of damage to bridging veins is high even with minor trauma.

The manifestations of chronic subdural hematoma may be subtle and go undiagnosed. In the elderly, changes in mentation may be erroneously attributed to dementia. Chronic subdural hematomas are detectable by CT and MRI, and if they are symptomatic they may be managed by surgical removal of the clot and surrounding reactive tissue.

Subarachnoid Hemorrhage

The space between the outer arachnoid membrane and the pia mater is the subarachnoid space. The pia mater is tightly bound to the surface of the brain. The subarachnoid space is filled with CSF. Traumatic subarachnoid bleeding is due to rupture of the bridging veins that pass through the space, in a manner similar to subdural bleeding. Although trauma is an important cause of subarachnoid hemorrhage, it is more commonly associated with rupture of cerebral aneurysms or arteriovenous malformations (AVMs). In that case, bleeding is arterial in origin.

Blood in the CSF manifests with meningeal irritation and a bloody spinal tap. Blood in the subarachnoid space can spread throughout the CSF spaces and may not organize into a confined hematoma. Blood in the CSF produces severe headache in the conscious person and predisposes to secondary vasospasm and ischemia. It also predisposes to clogging of ventricular drainage, which leads to hydrocephalus. Further discussion of manifestations and management of subarachnoid hemorrhage is included in the section on cerebral aneurysms.

SECONDARY INJURY

Mechanisms of secondary injury are initiated by TBI, resulting in ischemia, increased ICP, and altered vascular regulation. Most of the research on secondary mechanisms of injury has been conducted in the TBI model. Often the damage done by secondary mechanisms far exceeds that of the primary trauma.

In contrast to other types of brain injury, patients with TBI must be carefully evaluated for skull fractures, epidural and subdural hematomas, and injuries to other body systems. Concomitant trauma may compound the brain injury. For example, uncontrolled hemorrhage can lead to hypovolemia and hypotension, which contributes to brain ischemia. Injuries to the chest can compromise ventilation and produce hypoxemia and hypercarbia, which contribute to cerebral dilation and increased ICP. Attention to other life-threatening injuries may extend the time until radiologic examination of the head can be accomplished, thus delaying management of surgical lesions.

Once the TBI patient's condition is stabilized, many other sources of secondary injury still loom. Brain swelling from both cytotoxic and vasogenic edema may increase for 48 to 72 hours after injury. Ruptured vessels may rebleed, and CSF drainage can become clogged. Open skull fractures predispose to CNS infections, as do ICP monitors, burr holes, and surgical incisions. Seizures and fevers may develop, significantly increasing the brain's metabolic rate and further contributing to brain ischemia. Inflammation and free radical damage continue to cause injury to cells even after ischemia has resolved. Monitoring and managing a patient's course through the myriad perils of secondary injury requires expert knowledge and skill.

TREATMENT

After cardiopulmonary stabilization, the first priority in the TBI patient is radiologic screening of the brain for surgically correctable lesions. Hematomas, depressed skull fractures, and bleeding vessels require prompt surgical intervention. Surgical decompression by craniectomy, ICP monitors, and CSF drainage devices also may be done during surgery.

Further therapy is individualized, seeking to maintain ICP, cerebral blood flow, and cerebral oxygen utilization within optimal ranges. Treatment recommendations are controversial, but in patients with acceptable cerebral blood flow, maintenance of normal body temperature or mild hypothermia, normal $Pa\text{CO}_2$, normal serum glucose level, and normal intravascular volume is suggested.[17] Acutely elevated ICP can be managed with administration of mannitol (osmotic diuretic), sedation, hypothermia, and mild hyperventilation. Repeat radiologic examination is indicated to determine if a new surgical lesion has developed. If it has not and the patient continues to exhibit high ICP, more aggressive measures, including diuretics, hypertonic saline, moderate hyperventilation, and barbiturate coma, may be tried, but the outcome is likely to be poor.

Patients with open head injuries may be treated with prophylactic antibiotics to prevent CNS infection. Sometimes fractures at the base of the skull are not visible on the routine CT scan but allow drainage of CSF into the nasal sinuses. Head-injured patients who have drainage of clear fluid from the ears or nose should be evaluated for basilar skull fracture. CSF drainage fluid can be differentiated from normal nasal mucus because it has a high glucose content and tends to separate into layers (halo) on tissue paper. Other findings with basilar skull fracture are bilateral periorbital hematomas (black eyes, "raccoon sign") and bruising under the ear. The presence of basilar skull fracture increases the risk of CNS infection.

Although morbidity and mortality after acute TBI remain high, significant advances in prehospital, hospital, and rehabilitative care continue to occur. The care received during the first hour of injury can dramatically affect outcome. Efforts to improve prehospital management are likely to have the greatest impact on patient outcomes.

KEY CONCEPTS

- Most head injuries are incurred in motor vehicle accidents, falls, and sports accidents. Young males aged 15 to 24 years are the most common victims. The seriousness of head injury can be classified according to Glasgow Coma Scale scores as severe (<8), moderate (9 to 12), or mild (>12).
- Injury that is directly due to the initial impact is called primary injury. Primary injuries are classified as focal, polar, or diffuse. Focal injuries are localized to the site of skull impact. Polar injuries are due to acceleration-deceleration movement of the brain within the skull, resulting in double injury. Diffuse injury is due to movement of the brain within the skull, resulting in widespread axonal injury.
- Disruption of the vasculature can result in intracranial hemorrhage. Epidural hematomas are associated with skull fracture and progress rapidly because they are arterial in origin. Subdural hematomas are associated with shearing of bridging veins and may develop slowly. Traumatic subarachnoid hemorrhage is also due to trauma to bridging veins.
- Secondary injury is a consequence of the body's response to the primary injury. Mechanisms are similar to those described for nontraumatic brain injury. In addition, concomitant injuries and cardiopulmonary impairment may contribute.
- The management of head injury is directed primarily to detecting and managing surgical lesions and reducing brain damage from secondary injury. Normovolemia, normothermia (or mild hypothermia), normal glucose level, and normal $Pa\text{O}_2$ and $Pa\text{CO}_2$ values are recommended for most patients. In those with high ICP, diuretics, hyperventilation, and drug-induced coma may be tried. Open head injuries constitute a risk for CNS infections, and prophylactic antibiotics may be used.

CEREBROVASCULAR DISEASE AND STROKE

Cerebrovascular diseases cause abnormalities of cerebral perfusion including transient ischemic attacks (TIA), ischemic stroke, and hemorrhagic stroke. *Stroke* is a term applied to cerebrovascular events that result in a localized area of brain infarction. The term "brain attack" has been popularized to educate the public about the importance of seeking care early, as is recommended for heart attack.

The symptoms of stroke usually are sudden in onset and may include the following: (1) numbness or weakness of face, arm, or leg, especially affecting only one side of the body; (2) confusion, trouble in speaking or in understanding others; (3) visual disturbances in one or both eyes; (4) dizziness, loss of balance, and difficulty with walking; and (5) severe headache. Persons experiencing any of these symptoms, even temporarily, should seek medical care immediately.

EPIDEMIOLOGY

More than 700,000 new and recurrent strokes occur each year in the United States, making stroke the third leading cause of death.[22] The majority of these victims survive, with most requiring long-term care and rehabilitation. Currently, there are about 5 million stroke survivors living in the United States. Stroke is the leading cause of serious disability. Among long-term survivors (>6 months), 50% have **hemiparesis,** 30% cannot walk, 26% are unable to independently perform activities of daily living, 19% are aphasic, 35% are clinically depressed, and 26% are institutionalized in a nursing home.[22] Females account for 61% of all stroke fatalities. Seventy-eight percent of stroke victims are older than 65 years. Stroke death rates are significantly higher for black males and females than for their white counterparts.

Risk factors for stroke are similar to those for other atherosclerotic vascular diseases and include hypertension, diabetes, hyperlipidemia, cigarette smoking, advancing age, and family history. A previous stroke significantly increases the risk for suffering a subsequent stroke. Cardiac disease complicated by atrial fibrillation is an important risk factor for embolic types of strokes. Strokes can be categorized according to cause as ischemic and hemorrhagic strokes. Ischemic strokes are by far the most common (88%) and include thrombotic and embolic types.[22]

ISCHEMIC STROKE

Ischemic strokes result from sudden occlusion of a cerebral artery secondary to thrombus formation or embolization. Thrombotic and embolic strokes are grouped together because the clinical presentation and treatment are similar. However, etiologic risk factors and preventive measures are different and are discussed separately.

Thrombotic strokes are associated with atherosclerosis and hypercoagulable states. Risk reduction strategies for thrombotic stroke are those aimed at reducing atherosclerosis and platelet aggregation. Significant atherosclerotic plaques in the carotid arteries are sometimes evident as carotid bruits. Assessment for the presence of carotid bruits in all individuals older than 50 years may help identify persons at risk so that prevention strategies can be initiated early.

Emboli usually are from a cardiac source, although disruptions in carotid artery plaques may lead to downstream embolization. Cardiac sources include thrombi formed in the cardiac chambers (mural thrombi) and thrombi or vegetations on valve leaflets. Because atrial fibrillation allows stagnation of blood in the left atrium, it is associated with a high risk of mural thrombi, which can dislodge and travel to the cerebral circulation. Patients with chronic atrial fibrillation commonly receive anticoagulant medications to prevent this occurrence.

Sudden blockage of a cerebral artery by a thrombus or embolus produces acute ischemia in the territory served by the artery. Insufficient blood flow to brain tissue results in oxygen deprivation and rapid cerebral deterioration. Neurologic deficits become evident after just 1 minute of insufficient oxygen. If the ischemia continues for several minutes, irreversible cellular damage can occur. With further progression the local area becomes infarcted and necrotic. Surrounding the infarct is a much larger area of ischemic but viable cells, called the **penumbra.** The penumbra receives some partial or collateral flow and may recover if the ischemia is mild or perfusion is restored in a timely manner. Salvaging the penumbra is the aim of early thrombolytic therapy; however, treatment must be instituted within 3 hours of stroke onset to be maximally effective.

In some cases, the obstructing clot is efficiently lysed by the endogenous fibrinolytic system before permanent tissue damage occurs. If the associated neurologic deficits completely resolve, the episode is called a *transient ischemic attack* (TIA). The neurologic symptoms of a TIA typically last only minutes, but they may last as long as 24 hours. Symptoms resolve completely without evidence of neurologic dysfunction. TIAs are important warning signs of thrombotic disease and carry a significant risk for subsequent stroke. The occurrence of one or more TIA episodes increases the risk of stroke by about 10-fold.[23]

Patients who present with TIAs should undergo evaluation to determine the origin of their symptoms. Unless contraindicated, these patients are started on daily aspirin therapy to prevent thrombus formation. Carotid endarterectomy or angioplasty may prevent stroke in a subset of patients experiencing TIAs who have carotid artery plaques occluding more than 70% of the arterial lumen.[24]

Manifestations of ischemic stroke are related to the cerebral vasculature involved (Figure 44-14). The middle cerebral artery is most commonly occluded, resulting in damage to the lateral hemisphere. Contralateral **hemiplegia,** hemisensory loss, and contralateral visual field blindness are usual. If the dominant hemisphere is affected, global aphasia will occur. Occlusion of smaller branches of the middle cerebral artery produce more limited neurologic findings. Occlusions of the other cerebral arteries have different neurologic manifestations depending on the brain area they normally perfuse (Table 44-2).

Occlusion of the small penetrating arterioles can produce small lesions called *lacunar infarcts.* The basal ganglia, pons, cerebellum, and internal capsule are common sites of lacunar infarcts. These lesions are sometimes not observable on CT scan. The prognosis for recovery from a lacunar infarct is usually good, and neurologic manifestations are more circumscribed, often affecting purely motor or sensory functions.

HEMORRHAGIC STROKE

Intracerebral hemorrhage usually occurs in the context of severe and often long-standing hypertension. It carries a 38% mortality, with death usually occurring within minutes to hours.[22] Most hemorrhagic strokes occur in the basal ganglia or thalamus (see Figure 44-10). If the hemorrhage is large, it may significantly increase ICP, which can lead to herniation and death. The prognosis for hemorrhagic stroke depends on the patient's age, the location and size of the hemorrhage, and how rapidly the hemorrhage produces brain distortion and shift. The degree of secondary injury and associated morbidity and mortality is higher for hemorrhagic stroke than for ischemic stroke.

TREATMENT

Initially, an assessment of stroke severity and associated neurologic deficits is made and adequacy of the patient's airway and respiratory and cardiovascular function are assured. Patients who have experienced a hemorrhagic stroke secondary to hypertensive disease often have extremely high blood pressure. Bringing their blood pressure into normotensive ranges

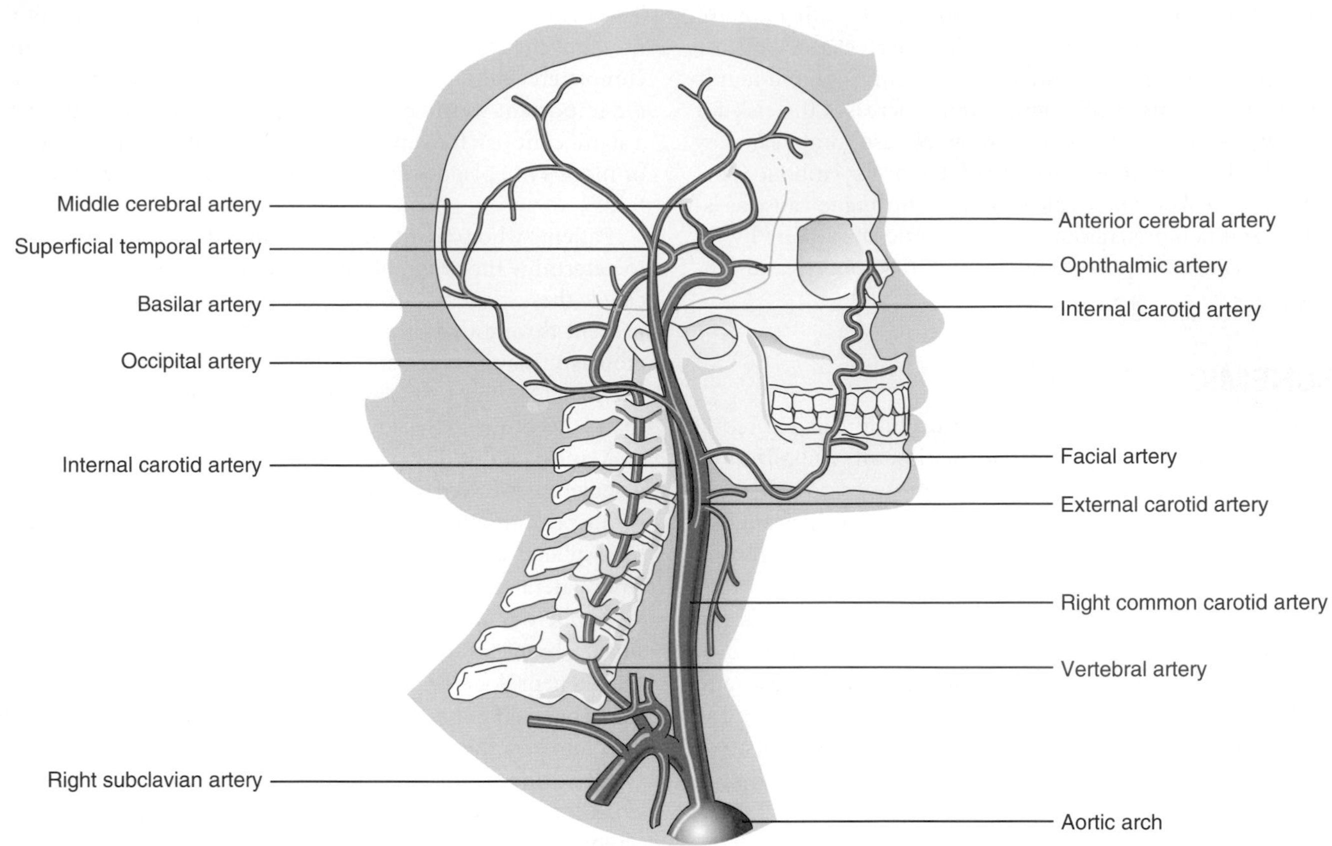

FIGURE 44-14 ■ Cerebral vasculature showing fields of perfusion.

Table 44-2

Manifestations of Ischemic Stroke According to Location of Arterial Blockage

Cerebral Artery	Territory of Perfusion	Clinical Manifestations
Anterior cerebral	Medial aspect of frontal lobes	Contralateral hemiparesis; contralateral sensory loss; impaired cognition and decision making, aphasia (left-sided stroke); incontinence
Middle cerebral	Most of lateral cerebral hemisphere, internal capsule, and basal ganglia	Contralateral hemiplegia; contralateral sensory loss; aphasia (left-sided stroke); homonymous hemianopsia; altered consciousness; neglect syndrome
Posterior cerebral	Occipital lobe and medial aspect of temporal lobe	Visual defects including homonymous hemianopsia, central blindness, color blindness; memory impairment
	Thalamus	Sensory loss, mild hemiparesis
Basilar and vertebral	Cerebellum and brainstem	Disturbances of gait, speech, swallowing, and vision

could result in ischemia. In these circumstances it is best to keep the patient mildly hypertensive with the goal of normalizing the blood pressure once the patient is medically stable.[7,10] Patients who have experienced cerebral hemorrhage are at risk for increased intracranial hypertension and are treated and assessed much as patients with a traumatic head injury.

The goals of therapy for acute ischemic stroke are to minimize infarct size and preserve neurologic function. The administration of 325 mg of aspirin as soon as ischemic stroke is suspected immediately affects platelet aggregation and may help inhibit thrombus size. Patients who are considered candidates for thrombolytic therapy undergo CT to rule out a hemorrhagic source. Thrombolytic therapy is most effective in limiting infarct size if it is initiated early. The American Heart Association guidelines for thrombolytic therapy in stroke are shown in Box 44-6.

It is critical to prevent further cerebral hypoxia or ischemia after ischemic stroke. Thus, volume depletion, hemo-

Box 44-6

American Heart Association Guidelines for Administration of Thrombolytic Therapy in Ischemic Stroke

Intravenous recombinant tissue plasminogen activator (0.9 mg/kg) with 10% given as a bolus followed by a 1-hour infusion is recommended for ischemic strokes presenting within 3 hours of symptom onset.

Inclusion Criteria (All *Yes* Boxes Must Be Checked Before Treatment)

Yes

- ☐ Age 18 years or older
- ☐ Clinical diagnosis of ischemic stroke causing a measurable neurologic deficit
- ☐ Time of symptom onset well established to be less than 180 minutes before treatment would begin

Exclusion Criteria (All *No* Boxes Must Be Checked Before Treatment)

No

- ☐ Evidence of intracranial hemorrhage on noncontrast head CT scan
- ☐ Only minor or rapidly improving stroke symptoms
- ☐ High clinical suspicion of subarachnoid hemorrhage even with normal CT scan
- ☐ Active internal bleeding (e.g., gastrointestinal/genitourinary bleeding within 21 days)
- ☐ Known bleeding diathesis, including but not limited to platelet count less than 100,000/mm^3
- ☐ Patient has received heparin within 48 hours and had an elevated aPTT
- ☐ Recent use of anticoagulant (e.g., warfarin) and elevated PT (more than 15 seconds)/INR
- ☐ Intracranial surgery, serious head trauma, or previous stroke within 3 months
- ☐ Major surgery or serious trauma within 14 days
- ☐ Recent arterial puncture at noncompressible site
- ☐ Lumbar puncture within 7 days
- ☐ History of intracranial hemorrhage, arteriovenous malformation, or aneurysm
- ☐ Witnessed seizure at stroke onset
- ☐ Recent acute myocardial infarction
- ☐ Systolic blood pressure greater than 185 mm Hg or diastolic blood pressure greater than 110 mm Hg at time of treatment

aPTT, Activated partial thromboplastin time; *CT,* computed tomography; *INR,* international normalized ratio; *PT,* prothrombin time.

concentration, hypotension, and arterial obstruction must be avoided. As with the hemorrhagic stroke patient, careful blood pressure management is critical. Overhydration can result in cerebral edema in the ischemic area of the brain and raise ICP. Patients who are taking fluids by mouth should have their ability to swallow evaluated *before* they take any food or liquids orally. Injury to cranial nerves V, VII, IX, X, or XII can place a patient at risk for respiratory aspiration and further compromise the individual's health and potential for recovery.

Anticoagulation therapy may be used in ischemic stroke, especially if the event is progressive. A stroke is termed *progressive* if an initial focal deficit worsened or fluctuated before hospital admission or deteriorated on serial examinations after admission. Patients who receive thrombolytic therapy should not receive anticoagulation therapy because the risk of bleeding is high. Throughout the course of therapy, it is essential to monitor clotting parameters and recognize the potential for hemorrhage into the ischemic area. Even in the absence of thrombolytic or anticoagulant therapy, a significant number of ischemic strokes convert to hemorrhagic lesions. A sudden change in neurologic function should prompt reevaluation by CT. Numerous clinical studies on antioxidants, glutamate blockers, and calcium channel blockers have failed to show benefit, and early fibrinolytic therapy remains the cornerstone of treatment.[7]

Management of the stroke patient also must include efforts to prevent stroke recurrence. Evaluation and management of risk factors is an essential part of prevention. The survivor of a stroke is at high risk for a subsequent stroke if precipitating factors are still present. Patients who have experienced thrombotic strokes are also at significant risk for other vascular events, such as myocardial infarctions. Secondary prevention varies according to the cause of the stroke. For hemorrhagic strokes, careful monitoring and control of blood pressure is essential. For ischemic strokes of embolic origin, efforts are made to identify and remove the source of emboli. Usually the source is the heart, and therapy includes control of dysrhythmias, anticoagulation therapy, and antiplatelet drugs such as aspirin. The most common cause of embolic stroke is atrial fibrillation. Conversion of this dysrhythmia to normal sinus rhythm can sometimes be accomplished with antiarrhythmic agents or electrical cardioversion. Measures to improve left ventricular function may help to reduce atrial pressure and correct atrial fibrillation. Patients with long-standing atrial fibrillation require anticoagulation therapy. When abnormal valves are suspected to be the source of emboli, evaluation for surgical replacement may be indicated.

Secondary prevention for thrombotic stroke includes lifestyle modifications to address modifiable risk factors, including smoking cessation and lowering of serum lipid levels. In addition, the long-term daily use of aspirin or other antiplatelet agents (e.g., ticlopidine) has been recommended. Some patients may benefit from surgical removal of carotid artery plaque by endarterectomy or angioplasty. Placement of rigid tubes, called *stents,* in the area of plaque removal may be helpful in preventing reocclusion.

STROKE SEQUELAE

Recovery after stroke depends on the size and location of the cerebral infarct, comorbid conditions, and rehabilitative efforts. Stroke rehabilitation begins during the acute hospitaliza-

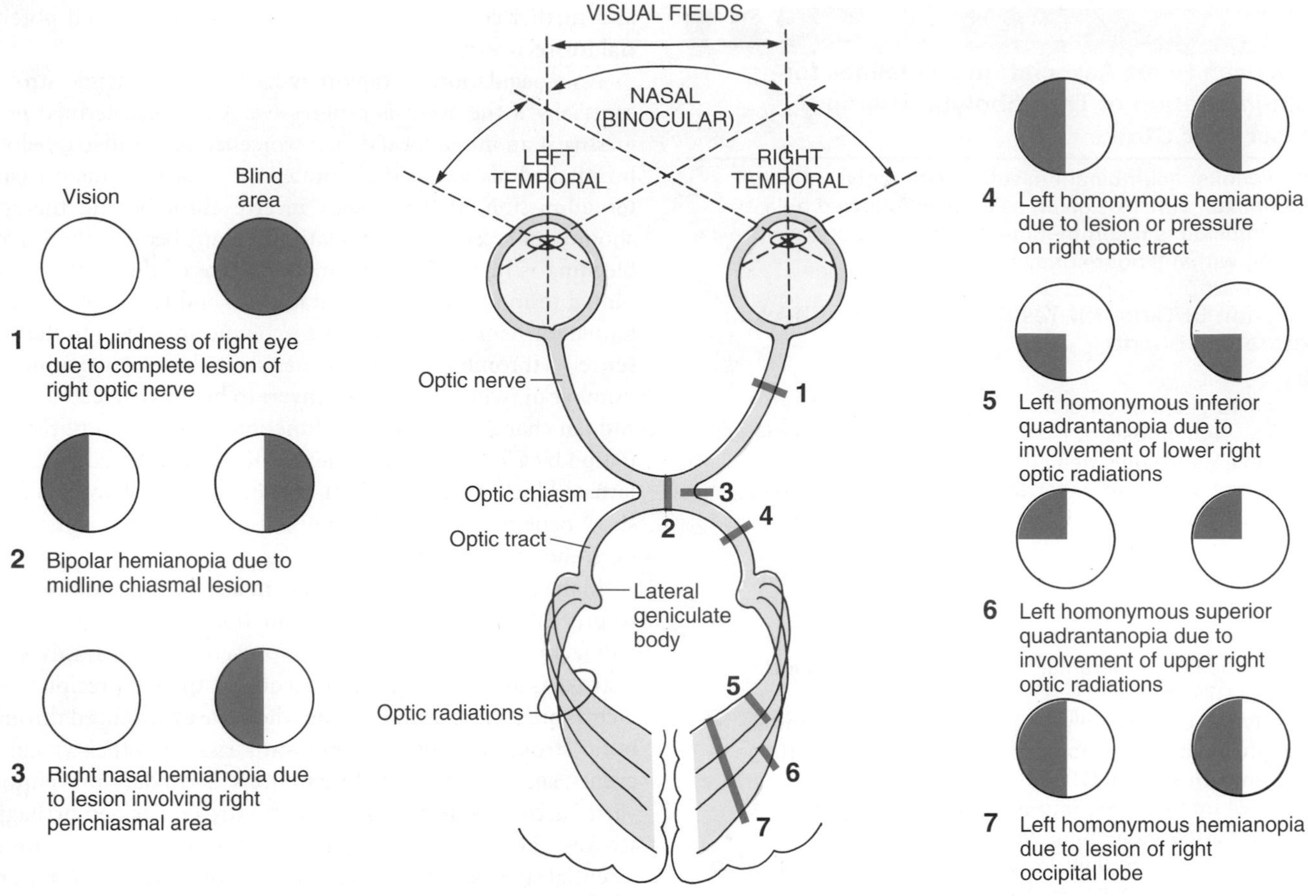

FIGURE 44-15 ■ Homonymous hemianopsia. A right-sided brain stroke may cause lesions that disturb visual fibers and result in blindness in the left visual field. The optic pathway from the other side remains intact. (From Black JM, Hawks JH, Keene AM: *Medical-surgical nursing: clinical management for positive outcomes,* ed 6, Philadelphia, 2001, Saunders, p 1959.)

tion phase and continues after the patient has returned to the community. Many patients have residual deficits in motor, sensory, language, and cognitive functions that necessitate intensive strategies to maximize return to a productive life.

Motor and Sensory Deficits

Motor impairment from a stroke is initially characterized by flaccidity, which is a decrease in or absence of muscle tone in the affected extremities. Most commonly, motor paralysis is contralateral to the side of the brain in which the stroke occurs. Thus a stroke on the right side of the brain results in left-sided body paralysis, whereas left brain strokes result in right-sided body paralysis. Footdrop, outward rotation of the leg, and dependent edema are common features in the lower extremity. In the upper extremity, the arm may separate from the shoulder if not supported. Muscles in the affected limbs tend to atrophy from lack of tone and use. Many of the complications can be limited with therapeutic interventions, including frequent range-of-motion exercises, elevation of edematous limbs, use of elastic stockings, and maintenance of body alignment.

Starting at about 6 weeks after the stroke, recovery of motor function is evident by the onset of spasticity. Spasticity is the resistance of muscle groups to passive stretch with an increase in tone. Increased flexor tone is usually seen in the upper extremities and increased extensor tone in the lower extremities. Passive or active range-of-motion exercises and positioning are critical to maintenance of function, as uncontrolled spasticity can result in contractures of the limbs, including adduction of the shoulder, pronation of the forearm, and finger flexion. In the lower extremity the patient may have problems with hip and knee extension. If spasticity is not evident within 3 months, function is not likely to return to the affected limb.

Sensory impairment occurs in the same locations as the motor paralysis. A lack of sensory information from the paralyzed side contributes to the phenomenon of *neglect* (also called *hemiattention*). The patient seems not to realize that the affected body parts belong to him. Loss of the visual field on the paralyzed side also contributes to neglect. Contralateral field blindness is called *homonymous hemianopsia* because the same side of the retina in each eye is blinded (Figure 44-15). Patients with neglect may crush, burn, or otherwise injure the neglected body parts without realizing it. Poor hygiene of affected extremities may be apparent. Neuropsychological studies have shown that objects in the field of neglect are usually ignored. When asked to draw the numbers on the face of a clock, all 12 are drawn on one side. Self-portraits may be conspicuous for the distortion or omission of structures on the neglected side. Neglect is associated with a high risk for falls and other injuries.

Language Deficits

Aphasia is an integrative language disorder that occurs with brain damage to the dominant cerebral hemisphere (usually left) and involves all language modalities. Characteristics of aphasia include a reduced vocabulary, reduced verbal attention span, and reduced ability to use learned linguistic rules. Aphasia is associated with lesions in the primary language centers (Broca and Wernicke areas) as well as in adjacent cortical areas. Aphasia is categorized according to the location of the lesion and the linguistic deficit. The following is a brief description of those categories.

Broca aphasia, also known as verbal motor or expressive aphasia, results from a lesion in the third frontal convolution of the left hemisphere in most persons. Patients speak with poorly articulated and sparse vocabulary and in the simplest grammatic constructions.

Wernicke aphasia, also known as sensory, acoustic, or receptive aphasia, is characterized by impaired auditory comprehension and speech that is fluent but empty of content. This form of aphasia is caused by lesions in the posterior portion of the first temporal gyrus of the left hemisphere. Speech is frequently circumlocutory or tangential and contains paraphasic errors and jargon. Word finding and naming difficulties are a prominent feature of this disorder. Patients with Wernicke aphasia are unable to monitor their own language production and cannot comprehend or monitor the language production of others.

Anomic aphasia results from lesions in the parietotemporal area in proximity to the angular gyrus. This is a fluent aphasia with intact grammatic structure. Patients have greater word-finding difficulties than those with Wernicke aphasia but do not make paraphasic errors and have intact comprehension. However, their speech is typically constructed of simple words.

Conduction or central aphasia is associated with increased paraphasic errors and a reduced ability to repeat words. It is associated with a lesion in the arcuate fasciculus in the left hemisphere. Patients are well aware that they are making language errors. However, the more they struggle to find the correct words, the more likely they are to repeat paraphasic errors.

Cognitive Deficits

Patients experience impairments of cognition owing to diffuse cortical or subcortical injuries that affect the ability to be alert, to concentrate or attend to stimuli, to remember, and to reason. Cognitive impairment varies according to the area of brain affected and the severity of the injury. Injuries that disturb an individual's ability to maintain an alert status are the most severe. Increasing cognitive skill is necessary for the function of memory and the ability to learn and associate, to discriminate, to separate, and to categorize various stimuli. The highest levels of cognitive function include analysis, synthesis, and reasoning abilities.

Cognitive impairment is commonly evidenced as language deficit, impaired spatial relationship skills, short-term memory impairment, and poor judgment. Patients who do not retain the ability to learn are unlikely to benefit from rehabilitative services.

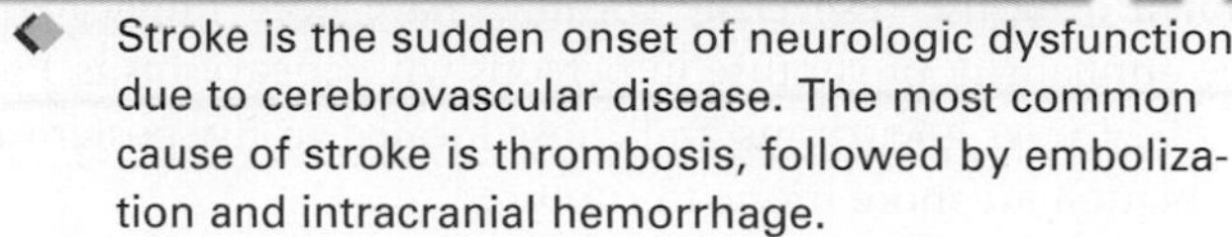

- Stroke is the sudden onset of neurologic dysfunction due to cerebrovascular disease. The most common cause of stroke is thrombosis, followed by embolization and intracranial hemorrhage.
- Thrombi form at atherosclerotic plaques, causing sudden occlusion of an already narrowed vessel. If the clot is quickly lysed, the deficits may completely disappear, a phenomenon associated with a TIA. Emboli are usually a consequence of clots from within the heart chambers due to disease or dysrhythmia. Hemorrhagic stroke is usually associated with uncontrolled hypertension.
- Stroke symptoms depend on the area of brain affected, which in turn depends on the vessel occluded: internal carotid, anterior cerebral, middle cerebral, or posterior cerebral artery. Common manifestations include contralateral motor and sensory loss, aphasia, and contralateral visual field loss.
- Treatment is aimed at limiting the size of the brain infarction, supporting bodily functions, and initiating aggressive rehabilitation strategies. Acute therapy with thrombolytic agents may limit infarct size in patients with ischemic stroke.
- Stroke is associated with long-term deficits in motor, sensory, language, and cognitive abilities. Initially, affected muscles are flaccid, with spasticity occurring after about 6 weeks. Prevention of contractures is a major concern. Aphasia may be described as expressive or receptive. Most individuals with aphasia have impaired integrative ability involving all language modalities. Concentration, memory, and reasoning may be impaired.

CEREBRAL ANEURYSM AND ARTERIOVENOUS MALFORMATION

Structural abnormalities of the cerebral arteries predispose to intracerebral bleeding and hemorrhagic stroke. Cerebral aneurysms and AVMs are the two most common causes of subarachnoid hemorrhage. Early recognition and surgical management of these conditions are necessary to prevent significant mortality and morbidity associated with rupture.

Cerebral Aneurysm

Etiology. An aneurysm is a lesion of an artery that results in dilation and ballooning of a segment of the vessel. Aneurysm rupture occurs in about 15,000 Americans each year, or 6 per 1,000,000.[25] The prevalence is higher in women than in men, and rupture most often occurs between the ages of 30 and 60 years. Intracerebral aneurysms are found in about 6% of the general population, and more than half remain unruptured and undiagnosed.[25] Thus, other factors are likely to be important in precipitating aneurysm rupture. High blood pressure, acute alcohol intoxication, and recreational drug use (especially cocaine) have been implicated. The annual risk of rupture in persons with aneurysms is 1% to 2%. Larger aneurysms and those located in the posterior circulation are more prone to rupture.[25]

Approximately 15% of patients with ruptured cerebral aneurysms die before they receive medical attention. Of those who do receive hospital care, 25% to 50% die during the acute phase.[26]

Pathogenesis and Manifestations. Although the exact pathogenesis is not understood, saccular aneurysms are believed to result from congenital defects of the medial layer of the artery. This structural weakness permits gradual ballooning at the site as a consequence of arterial pressure effects over years. A common location for saccular aneurysms is the arterial bifurcations, where turbulent blood flow might have a greater impact on a weakened vessel wall. Ninety-five percent of cerebral aneurysms are located in the circle of Willis. Ten percent to 20% of affected individuals have more than one aneurysm.

Saccular aneurysms (berry aneurysms) are round and are the most common (Figure 44-16). The aneurysmal sac is composed of thickened intima and adventitia, the media layer having abruptly ended at the sac edge (Figure 44-17). Rupture of the aneurysm generally occurs from the dome of the sac or at the edge of the atheromatous plaque.

Warning leaks may occur before an aneurysm ruptures and often produce severe headache, which is typically described by the patient as "the worst headache I have ever had," and if recognized as such can significantly improve the morbidity.[26] Patients may also complain of photophobia (visual sensitivity to light) and stiff neck. A stiff and painful neck results from meningismus caused by the irritating properties of blood in the CSF. After rupture, the onset of symptoms is very rapid. Sudden injection of blood into the subarachnoid space raises ICP and distorts intracranial structures. Secondary cerebral vasospasm, a pathologic narrowing of the major vessels around the area of rupture, typically occurs from day 4 to day 14. This process significantly reduces cerebral blood flow and results in increased cerebral ischemia and possibly infarction. Vasospasm is due to the presence of blood in the CSF. The next most serious consequence of the initial rupture is rebleeding. The risk for rebleeding is highest in the first 14 days. Patients are also at risk for developing hydrocephalus from clogging and obstruction of CSF flow through the ventricular system.

Diagnostic procedures for detecting ruptured aneurysm include CT or MRI to confirm a subarachnoid hemorrhage. If the scan is negative but suspicion of subarachnoid hemor-

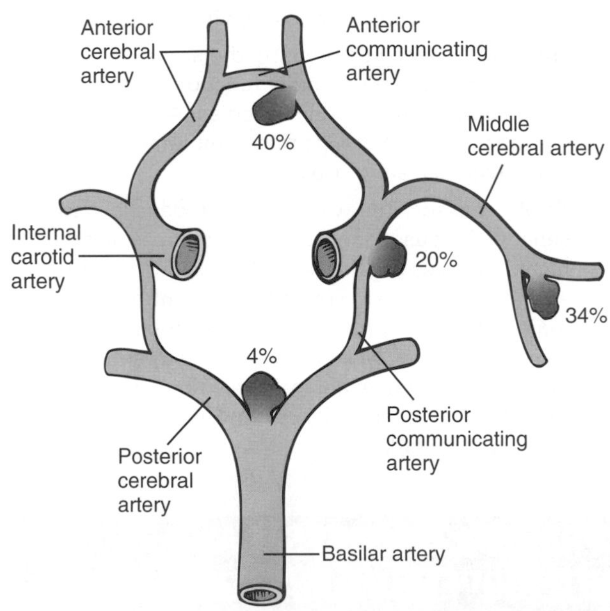

FIGURE 44-16 ■ Saccular (berry) aneurysms are most commonly found in the circle of Willis, particularly at arterial bifurcations. (From Kumar V, Cotran R, Robbins S, editors: *Robbins basic pathology,* ed 7, Philadelphia, 2003, Saunders, p 817.)

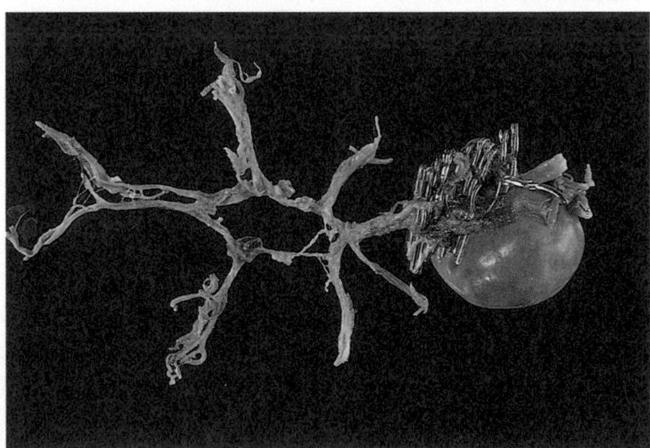

FIGURE 44-17 ■ Gross view of a massive saccular aneurysm arising at the junction of the basilar and vertebral arteries. Surgical clips are visible at the base of the aneurysm. (From Kumar V, Cotran R, Robbins S, editors: *Robbins basic pathology,* ed 7, Philadelphia, 2003, Saunders, p 817.)

rhage is high, a lumbar puncture for CSF analysis can be done. Blood in the CSF is indicative of subarachnoid hemorrhage. A cerebral angiogram is obtained to demonstrate the location of aneurysms in preparation for surgical management.

Treatment. The primary treatments for aneurysms are surgical stabilization by clipping or placement of endovascular coils for embolization. Prognosis is favorable if the aneurysm is detected and managed before significant rupture occurs. In most cases, the aneurysm is not diagnosed until after subarachnoid hemorrhage has occurred, and mortality is higher. Early surgery in stable patients with subarachnoid hemorrhage is associated with a lower overall mortality. Aneurysm clipping is accomplished by placement of a permanent vascular clip at the neck of the aneurysm. Coil devices may be inserted under radiographic guidance to thrombose or sclerose the area. The 1-year mortality of aneurysm clipping or coil placement in unruptured aneurysm is 10% to 12%.[25]

In patients experiencing subarachnoid hemorrhage as a consequence of ruptured aneurysm, the complications of cerebral vasospasm and hydrocephalus must be monitored and managed. Vasospasm can be managed by keeping blood volume and blood pressure at normal to high levels. Calcium channel blockers may be used to reduce vasospasm. In addition to hemodynamic monitoring, careful and frequent neurologic assessments are essential to monitor stability and indicate the first signs of deterioration so that rapid intervention can be undertaken.

Arteriovenous Malformation

Etiology. AVMs are the second most common cause of spontaneous subarachnoid hemorrhage. The majority of AVMs are diagnosed in patients between 20 and 40 years.[27] Ninety percent of AVMs are found in the cerebral hemispheres and only about 10% in the posterior fossa. AVMs are vascular lesions thought to be congenital; however, they are rarely diagnosed in the pediatric population.[27]

The risk of clinically recognizable hemorrhage from an AVM is 2% to 3% per year.[27] The risk of rebleeding within the first year after an initial hemorrhage is 6%. The mortality associated with AVM rupture is 10% to 15%, much lower than with aneurysm rupture.[26]

Pathogenesis and Manifestations. In the normal vascular system, the capillaries are situated between the arterioles and the venules. In an AVM, the capillary system fails to develop appropriately, and arterial blood is shunted directly into the venous system. Exposure of the high-capacitance venous system to the high pressure of the arteries causes the vessels to progressively enlarge, as do the arteries and veins that feed and drain the lesion. Eventually the AVM becomes a congested mass of enlarged vessels.

Because of their abnormal structure and the high vascular pressure, AVMs are vulnerable to hemorrhage. Hemorrhage is the initial manifestation in 50% of cases of AVM; 25% are manifested by seizures and the rest by varying degrees of vascular steal syndrome, which is progressive neurologic dysfunction as a result of ischemia in normal tissue caused by abnormal shunting of blood into the AVM.

Treatment. If possible, the AVM is surgically removed. For deep or very large AVMs, other approaches (e.g., irradiation and glue embolization) may be used.[27] Supportive therapy for AVMs that rupture and cause subarachnoid hemorrhage is similar to that described for ruptured cerebral aneurysms.

KEY CONCEPTS

- Cerebral aneurysms and arteriovenous malformations are the two most common causes of subarachnoid hemorrhage. Aneurysm is most common and has a higher mortality rate.
- Blood in the subarachnoid space is associated with headache, stiff neck, and secondary cerebral vasospasm. Vasospasm, which leads to cerebral ischemia, is an important cause of morbidity and mortality.
- Aneurysms are congenital weaknesses in the arterial walls that lead to dilation and ballooning of the wall. Treatment includes surgical stabilization by clip ligation and aggressive management of secondary vasospasm.
- AVMs are congenital malformations in which arterial blood is shunted directly into the venous system, causing high venous pressure. The AVM enlarges and may compress adjacent structures or rupture. Surgical management, radiation, or glue embolization to occlude the AVM may be done to prevent bleeding.

CENTRAL NERVOUS SYSTEM INFECTIONS

Infections of the CNS include meningitis, encephalitis, and abscesses. A frequent consequence of bacterial infections is obstructive hydrocephalus, as the bacteria, white blood cells, and cellular debris block CSF reabsorption in the arachnoid villi.

Organisms gain access to the CNS by various portals of entry. These include the blood stream, by direct extension from a primary site (e.g., sinuses), by extension along peripheral and cranial nerves, and through maternal-fetal exchange. Factors contributing to infections include such conditions as immunocompromise, debilitation, poor nutrition, radiation therapy, steroid therapy, and contact with vectors. Meningitis and cerebral abscess are most commonly associated with bacterial infections, whereas encephalitis is usually viral.

Meningitis

Meningitis is the most common sequela to microbial invasion of the CNS. Most frequently, meningitis is bacterial in origin, but it can also be viral or fungal. Persons with acquired immunodeficiency syndrome (AIDS) have an increased susceptibility to infection and have an increased prevalence of meningitis of viral, fungal, or parasitic origin.

Etiology. The bacteria most frequently involved in causing meningitis in adults are *Streptococcus pneumoniae* and *Neisseria meningitidis.*[28] *Haemophilus influenzae* type B (HIB) is a causative agent in children; however, the incidence has fallen dramatically since the introduction of the HIB vaccines.[28] The bacteria that cause meningitis usually reach the CNS by way of the blood stream or by extension from cranial structures, such as the paranasal sinuses or ears. Some of the organisms responsible for causing meningitis may be normal inhabitants of the nasopharynx. Pathogens can also gain access to the CNS through breaks in the barrier system, as occur with penetrating head wounds or skull fractures or following neurosurgery in which the dura is penetrated. The overall mortality rate for meningitis is approximately 10% for *N. meningitidis* and 26% for *S. pneumoniae* infection.[28]

Pathogenesis and Clinical Manifestations. Bacterial meningitis is a pyogenic infection that invades the **leptomeninges** and the subarachnoid space. Because of its involvement in the subarachnoid space, the infection travels readily around the brain and spinal cord. The accumulation of inflammatory exudate frequently results in obstructive hydrocephalus and exudative invasion into the sheaths of the blood vessels and spinal and cranial nerves.

The combination of headache, fever, stiff neck (meningismus), and signs of cerebral dysfunction (confusion, delirium) is the classic presentation of meningitis. Deterioration in level of consciousness is progressive and often rapid. Patients who deteriorate rapidly often demonstrate dramatic tachypnea. About one third of patients experience seizures. Cranial nerve involvement is also common and is most often seen as ocular palsies, facial weakness and/or deafness, and vertigo.

The diagnosis of meningitis is usually made by lumbar puncture. Typical CSF findings are shown in Table 44-3. Gram stain of the CSF will reveal the causative organism in most patients. In addition to the causative organism, classic CSF findings include white blood cell counts between 1000 and 10,000/mm^3 with a predominance of neutrophils. The CSF glucose level is reduced and often extremely low, and patients with bacterial or fungal meningitis have increased protein levels.

Treatment. Recovery from bacterial meningitis depends largely on how quickly effective treatment is started. Treatment includes general supportive care, intravenous antibacterial drug therapy targeting the specific pathogen, and management of any complications. Complications from meningitis can include visual impairment, optic neuritis, deafness, headache, seizures, personality changes, motor weakness, hydrocephalus, endocarditis, and pneumonia. Much of the damage to CNS structures is not a direct result of the pathogen; rather, it is the immune response that is injurious. Antibiotic therapy, with resultant bacterial cell wall lysis, can increase the immune-mediated injury. This has led some investigators to recommend the use of corticosteroids during the antibiotic treatment phase. A significant reduction in mortality was achieved in some studies in adults receiving dexamethasone beginning with the initiation of antibiotics.[28]

Prevention strategies include public education promoting prompt and appropriate management of sinusitis, mastoiditis, ear infections, and pneumonia. Strict aseptic techniques for all procedures involving a break in the CNS barrier system may help prevent nosocomial CNS infections. Vaccination against *N. meningitidis* provides short-term protection (a few years) and may be useful prior to situations in which exposure is more likely, such as during the college years.

Encephalitis

Etiology. Encephalitis, an inflammation of the brain, can be caused by the same infectious agents as meningitis, although viruses are most often the pathogen. There are no well-established diagnostic criteria for acute encephalitis, and

Table 44-3

Typical Cerebrospinal Fluid Findings in Bacterial Meningitis

CSF Variable	Typical Findings	Normal
White blood cell count	1000-5000 cells/mm^3 (up to 10,000) (high)	<5
Neutrophils	$\geq$90% (high)	60%-80%
Protein	80-500 mg/dl (high)	30 mg/dl
Glucose	$\leq$40 mg/dl (low)	50-80 mg/dl
Gram stain	Positive (60%-90% of cases)	Negative
Culture	Positive (70%-85% of cases)	Negative
CSF opening pressure	$>$20 cm H_2O (high)	$<$15 cm H_2O

CSF, Cerebrospinal fluid.

the manifestations mimic other brain injuries. The diagnosis of acute viral encephalitis is often a diagnosis of exclusion.

The most common types of viral encephalitis in the United States include West Nile virus, western equine encephalitis, and herpes simplex encephalitis. In 2002, the largest encephalitis outbreak in U.S. history, with more than 3800 cases and 225 deaths, was attributed to the West Nile virus.[29] West Nile is transmitted by infected mosquitoes (*Culex* species) during summer months in the United States. Previously, West Nile virus was confined to more tropical areas and considered to be fairly benign. Its usual hosts are birds, and it may affect horses and humans. Dogs and cats do not appear to be affected.[30]

Western equine encephalitis is transmitted by the mosquito *Culex tarsalis,* which breeds in sunlit grassy marshes, ground pools, and streams. Birds are the preferred host, and humans are not usually infected unless the population of *C. tarsalis* far outnumbers the bird host population. In the eastern United States, western equine encephalitis is carried by the mosquito vector *Culiseta melanura* and rarely infects humans. Western equine encephalitis is primarily a disease of the summer months, typically May to September. It most often infects the very young and those older than 50 years.

Herpes simplex encephalitis is an important cause of sporadic and often fatal (70%) encephalitis in the United States. It results from spread of the herpes simplex virus type 1 to the CNS. This can occur as a primary or secondary infection or as a reactivation of latent virus. There is no seasonal incidence of this disease.

Pathogenesis and Manifestations. The incubation period for West Nile ranges from 3 to 14 days and symptoms usually last 3 to 6 days. Most infections are mild and asymptomatic. Twenty percent of infected individuals develop a febrile illness with headache, malaise, muscle pain, or rash. Approximately 1 in 150 infections results in severe neurologic disease, most commonly encephalitis, but some cases of meningitis have been reported. Advanced age is a significant risk factor for developing a more severe infection. The manifestations of severe infection include fever, muscle weakness or flaccid paralysis, headache, and changes in mental status.[30]

The incubation period for western equine encephalitis is 5 to 15 days. Onset of symptoms is typically rapid, and symptoms include general malaise, mild headache, and, often, nausea and vomiting. A moderately elevated temperature develops and the headache usually becomes severe. Lethargy and irritability are often present after a few days. In an uncomplicated infection symptoms persist for about 10 days and then gradually subside. In severe cases, lethargy progresses to stupor alternating with extreme restlessness. In fatal cases the progression of disease is rapid, culminating in coma and death.

The manifestations of herpes simplex encephalitis are variable. The patient may initially complain of flulike symptoms. Subsequent lethargy, confusion, and delirium are common and may evolve into coma. Some patients may experience a much more rapid course with acute necrotizing encephalitis and widespread destruction of white matter and extensive brain edema. Herpes simplex encephalitis is typically associated with a profound memory impairment and changes in personality.

The diagnosis of encephalitis is usually made from the history, clinical findings, and lumbar puncture in which there is a normal or mildly elevated white blood cell count, a small increase in protein, and a normal glucose. Viral serology may detect the virus in a minority of cases. Some viral infections can be diagnosed by detecting antibodies in serum or cerebrospinal fluid. Since IgM does not cross the BBB, an elevated IgM antiviral antibody titer in CSF is highly suggestive of CNS infection by the virus. In many cases of acute encephalitis, no causative organisms can be identified. A brain biopsy may be the only means to confirm the diagnosis.

Treatment. In general, the management of encephalitis is supportive and symptomatic. As with all severe illnesses, respiratory and cardiovascular support is imperative. Patients with encephalitis must be carefully hydrated as they frequently show signs and symptoms of excessive antidiuretic hormone secretion and water retention. Those with moderate to severe disease require careful and ongoing neurologic assessment. Seizures are a common complication in encephalitis secondary to hypoxia, tissue destruction, toxic encephalopathy, inflammatory vasculitis, and hyponatremia. All patients with moderate to severe illness should be monitored for intracranial hypertension. Although there is no definitive drug treatment, steroids may be given to control edema, anticonvulsants to prevent seizures, analgesics for headache, and antipyretics for hyperthermia. Patients in whom herpes simplex encephalitis has been diagnosed should be treated with antiviral medications such as acyclovir. Intravenous immunoglobulin, interferon-α, and ribavirin have been tried in some forms of viral encephalitis, but their efficacy is not yet proven.[29]

Brain Abscess

Etiology. A brain abscess is a localized collection of pus within the brain parenchyma. **Pyogenic** (pus producing) pathogens reach the brain by a number of routes, including (1) penetrating wounds, (2) direct extension or retrograde thrombophlebitis of an infected neighboring structure (e.g., mastoiditis, sinusitis), or (3) blood-borne dissemination from a distant infected site (e.g., lungs). Most brain abscesses are bacterial. The most common infective organisms are streptococci, staphylococci, and anaerobes.[31]

Pathogenesis and Manifestations. Brain abscess presents as a space-occupying lesion in the brain. Most patients experience symptoms 1 to 4 weeks after the initial infection. The abscess has a focal infected core in which the central portion contains an abundance of neutrophils and tissue

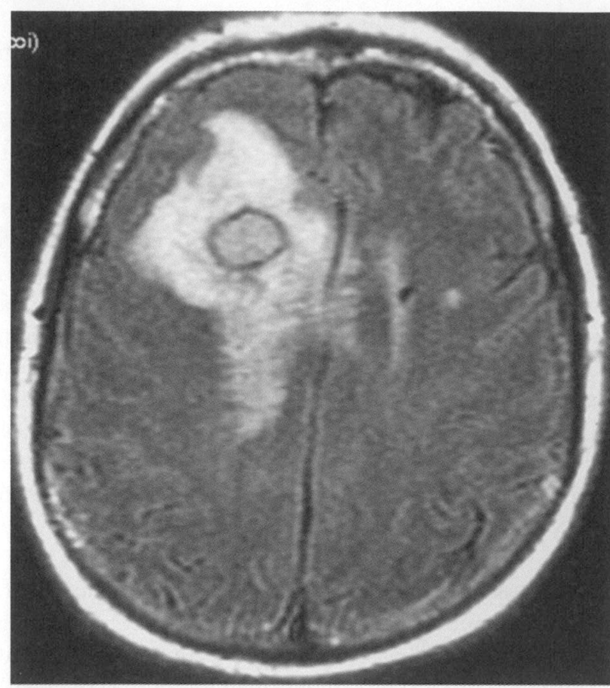

FIGURE 44-18 ■ CT scan of a cerebral abscess showing typical ring with decreased core density and an edematous area surrounding the abscess. (From Grossman RI, Yousem DM: *Neuroradiology,* ed 2, St Louis, 2003, Mosby, p 285.)

debris (pus). The peripheral portion of the abscess is made up of inflammatory granulation tissue. Around the abscess is perifocal edema with proliferation of surviving astrocytes. In the chronic phase the core of the abscess is liquefied and the peripheral portion forms a collagenous capsule that in turn is surrounded by fibrous gliosis. A CT scan typically shows an outer ring surrounding a low-density core (Figure 44-18).

Treatment. Management of a brain abscess depends on its location and accessibility, and usually involves drainage or excision. A critical feature in management is the administration of intravenous antibiotics, which is required for several weeks. Recently, the treatment of patients with brain abscess has become increasingly challenging because of the increase in unusual bacterial, fungal, and parasitic infections, particularly in immunosuppressed patients. Postinfection care must address residual neurologic deficits of cognitive, motor, or sensory function.

KEY CONCEPTS

- Meningitis is usually a consequence of bacterial infection in the CNS. Infection may be introduced through the blood stream or by invasion from infected sinuses or ears. Fever, stiff neck, and headache are common. Seizures may occur. The diagnosis is based on an elevated CSF white cell count and the presence of bacteria in the CSF.
- Obstructive hydrocephalus is a serious complication of meningitis that leads to increased ICP. Antibiotics are used for treatment.
- Encephalitis is inflammation of the brain that is most commonly due to viral infection. Common causes of viral encephalitis in the United States include West Nile virus, western equine encephalitis, and herpes simplex virus. Management is based on symptoms and may include steroids, anticonvulsants, analgesics, and antipyretics. Antiviral agents (e.g., acyclovir) are helpful in the treatment of herpes simplex encephalitis. Other antivirals are under investigation.
- Brain abscesses are usually due to pus-forming bacteria. Abscesses may be asymptomatic at first, later showing manifestations of a progressive space-occupying lesion. Drainage or excision and antibiotics are indicated.

SUMMARY

Acute disorders of brain function are characterized by rapidly progressing neurologic deficits and life-threatening complications. The cellular pathophysiologic process is similar for most types of brain injury and includes mechanisms of ischemia, cellular calcium overload, and free radical and immune-mediated damage. The development of increased ICP with compression of vital brain structures is a potential complication of all types of brain injury.

Efforts to minimize brain damage are focused on recognizing and managing secondary brain damage. Careful monitoring and management of body temperature, blood pressure, volume status, and respiratory function are essential. Efforts to reduce brain ischemia are important because it is thought to be a critical factor in acute brain injury.

The acute brain injury disorders presented in this chapter, including TBI, stroke, vascular rupture, and CNS infections, are all largely preventable. Efforts at prevention are paramount because often the outcome of acute brain injury is poor.

MEDIA RESOURCES

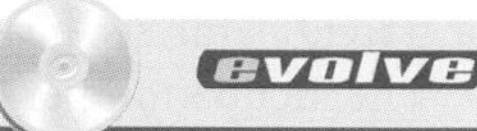

Remember to check out the ***CD Companion*** included with this book for Review Questions, Key Concepts Review, Glossary (with audio for selected terms), Disease Profiles, and Animations.

PLUS, visit the ***Evolve website*** at http://evolve.elsevier.com/Copstead/ for Case Studies, Disease Profiles, and WebLinks.

References

1. Phillis JW, O'Regan MH: A potentially critical role of phospholipases in central nervous system ischemic, traumatic, and neurodegenerative disorders, *Brain Res Rev* 44:13-47, 2004.

2. Povlishock JT, Christman CW: The pathobiology of traumatically induced axonal injury in animals and humans: a review of current thoughts, *J Neurotrauma* 12:555-563, 1995.
3. Burns DK, Kumar V: The nervous system. In Kumar V, Cotran R, Robbins S, editors: *Robbins basic pathology,* ed 7, Philadelphia, 2003, Saunders, pp 809-850.
4. Guyton AC, Hall JE, editors: *Textbook of medical physiology,* ed 10, Philadelphia, 2000, Saunders, pp 40-67.
5. Gaetz M: The neurophysiology of brain injury, *Clin Neurophysiol* 115:4-18, 2004.
6. Bramlett HM, Dietrich WD: Pathophysiology of cerebral ischemia and brain trauma: similarities and differences, *J Cereb Blood Flow Metab* 24:133-150, 2004.
7. Smith WS: Pathophysiology of focal cerebral ischemia: a therapeutic perspective, *J Vasc Interv Radiol* 15:S3-S12, 2004.
8. Wang CX, Shuaib A: Involvement of inflammatory cytokines in central nervous system injury, *Prog Neurobiol* 67(2):161-172, 2002.
9. Dutton RP, McCunn M: Traumatic brain injury, *Curr Opin Crit Care* 9:503-509, 2003.
10. Singh V: Critical care assessment and management of acute ischemic stroke, *J Vasc Interv Radiol* 15:S21-S27, 2004.
11. Natham BR: Cerebrospinal fluid and intracranial pressure. In Goetz CG, Pappert EJ, editors: *Textbook of clinical neurology,* Philadelphia, 1999, Saunders, pp 475-490.
12. Cushing H: *Studies in intracranial physiology and surgery,* London, 1926, Oxford University Press, pp 19-23.
13. Grossman RI, Yousem DM: *Neuroradiology,* ed 2, St Louis, 2003, Mosby.
14. Kirkness CJ et al: Intracranial pressure waveform analysis: clinical and research implications, *J Neurosci Nurs* 32(5):271-277, 2000.
15. Fisher CM: Brain herniation: a revision of classical concepts, *Can J Neurol Sci* 22:83-91, 1995.
16. Guyton AC, Hall JE: The cerebral cortex; intellectual functions of the brain; and learning and memory. In Guyton AC, Hall JE, editors: *Textbook of medical physiology,* ed 10, Philadelphia, 2000, Saunders, pp 663-677.
17. American Association of Neurological Surgeons, Joint Section on Neurotrauma and Critical Care: *Management and prognosis of severe traumatic brain injury,* New York, 2000, Brain Trauma Foundation.
18. Gopinath SP et al: Comparison of jugular venous oxygen saturation and brain tissue Po_2 as monitors of cerebral ischemia after head injury, *Crit Care Med* 27(11):2337-2345, 1999.
19. Berker E: Diagnosis, physiology, pathophysiology and rehabilitation of traumatic brain injuries, *Int J Neurosci* 85:195-220, 1996.
20. Kraus JF, McArthur DL: Epidemiologic aspects of brain injury, *Neuroepidemiology* 14:435-451, 1996.
21. Centers for Disease Control and Prevention: *Heads up for physicians about mild traumatic brain injury (MTBI),* Bethesda, Md, 2003, Department of Health and Human Services.
22. American Heart Association: *Heart disease and stroke statistics—2004 update,* Dallas, 2003, American Heart Association.
23. American Heart Association: Stroke symptoms—warning signs. Available at http://www.american heart.org.
24. Johnson DCC, Hill MD: The patient with transient cerebral ischemia: a golden opportunity for stroke prevention, *Can Med Assoc J* 170(7):1134-1137, 2004.
25. White PM, Wardlaw JM: Unruptured intracranial aneurysms, *J Neuroradiol* 30(5):336-350, 2003.
26. Sawin PD, Loftus CM: Diagnosis of spontaneous subarachnoid hemorrhage, *Am Fam Physician* 55:145-156, 1997.
27. Soderman M et al: Management of patients with brain arteriovenous malformations, *Eur J Radiol* 46:195-205, 2003.
28. van de Beek D et al: Steroids in adults with acute bacterial meningitis: a systematic review, *Lancet* 4:139-143, 2004.
29. Solomon T: Exotic and emerging viral encephalitides, *Curr Opin Neurol* 16:411-418, 2003.
30. Petersen LR, Marfin AA: West Nile virus: a primer for the clinician, *Ann Intern Med* 137:173-179, 2002.
31. Yogev R, Bar-Meir M: Management of brain abscesses in children, *Pediatr Infect Dis J* 23:157-160, 2004.

chapter 45

Chronic Disorders of Neurologic Function

Joni D. Nelsen-Marsh

MEDIA RESOURCES

Additional Material for Study, Review, and Further Exploration

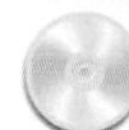

CD Companion ◆ Review Questions and Answers ◆ Key Concepts Review
◆ Glossary *(with audio pronunciations for selected terms)*
◆ Disease Profiles ◆ Animations

evolve ***Website*** at http://evolve.elsevier.com/Copstead/
◆ Case Studies ◆ Disease Profiles ◆ WebLinks

KEY QUESTIONS

- How are the various types of seizures recognized, classified, and treated?
- How is Alzheimer dementia diagnosed and managed?
- What are the proposed neurotransmitter alterations in Parkinson disease and how are drugs used to restore balance?
- What are the similarities and differences between multiple sclerosis and amyotrophic lateral sclerosis?
- How are congenital disorders, such as cerebral palsy, hydrocephalus, and spina bifida, manifested in the newborn?
- How does the level of spinal cord injury relate to expected functional losses and clinical manifestations?
- What is the role of immune mechanisms in Guillain-Barré syndrome and multiple sclerosis?
- What are the causes of facial paralysis in Bell palsy, and how is this condition different from other chronic disorders of neurologic function?

CHAPTER OUTLINE

Patients experiencing neurologic dysfunction from chronic disease states present a challenge to health care professionals, who must strive to maximize the patient's function and quality of life. This chapter focuses on common chronic disabilities of neuraxis I through IV. Disorders primarily affecting the brain are called axis I disorders; these include seizures, dementia, Parkinson disease, cerebral palsy, and hydrocephalus. Cerebellar disorders are axis II disorders. Disorders of the spinal cord are axis III disorders and include multiple sclerosis (MS), spina bifida, and spinal cord injury. Guillain-Barré syndrome and Bell palsy are axis IV disorders, which involve the spinal and cranial nerves of the peripheral nervous system.

BRAIN AND CEREBELLAR DISORDERS

Seizure Disorder

Seizures are a transient neurologic event of paroxysmal abnormal or excessive cortical electrical discharges that are manifested by disturbances of skeletal motor function, sensation, autonomic visceral function, behavior, or consciousness. Symptoms are not constant, and the length of time between seizure episodes is extremely variable. Epilepsy refers to the disorder of recurrent seizures. Seizures are a component of many diseases.

It is believed that approximately 1.4 million Americans have a seizure disorder, the vast majority of which are younger than 45 years.[1] With appropriate treatment 50% to 80% of people with a seizure disorder can achieve control of symptoms.[2]

Etiology. Seizures have many causes, and under the right circumstances anyone can experience one. A seizure disorder can be acquired as a consequence of cerebral injury or other pathologic process, including structural lesions such as tumors, blood clots, or infection. Other causes are metabolic and nutritional disorders such as electrolyte and water imbalance, hypoxia, acidosis, pyridoxine deficiency, acute withdrawal from alcohol, therapeutic medication overdose, and toxins such as heavy metals or street drugs. If seizures develop as a result of a structural change, the onset is not predictable. In some cases, seizures may not develop for months or years after the structural change has occurred. In some cases, no explanation for the seizure disorder can be found. These individuals are classified as having **idiopathic** seizures.

A seizure event is often triggered by specific stimuli, usually unique for each individual. Physical inducements include specific sensory stimuli such as flashing lights, loud noises, and rhythmic music. Fever, physical exhaustion, inadequate nutrition, menses, hyperventilation, injury, and drugs can also prompt seizure activity. Psychosocial factors include family and environmental stress, shock, and emotional stress.

Pathogenesis. Seizures are due to an alteration in membrane potential that makes certain neurons abnormally hyperactive and hypersensitive to changes in their environment. These physiologically abnormal neurons form an **epileptogenic focus,** i.e., an area of the brain from which the seizure emanates. The epileptogenic focus functions autonomously, emitting excessively large numbers of paroxysmal electrical discharges. Nerve cells in this area can recruit neurons in adjacent areas as well as synaptically related neurons in distant areas of the brain, greatly increasing the number of neurons involved in the seizure activity. Recruitment can also incorporate neurons in the opposite hemisphere. Clinical symptoms become evident when a sufficient number of neurons have been excited. Seizures are classified according to clinical symptoms and the electroencephalographic features. Clinical manifestations depend on the area of the brain involved, the area of origin, and the areas to which the seizure spreads.

Clinical Manifestations. Seizures may be classified as partial, in which only part of the brain surface is affected in each seizure (also known as focal seizures), or generalized, in which the whole brain surface is affected during the seizure (Box 45-1).

Generalized Seizures. Episodes in which the entire brain is involved from the onset of the seizure are referred to as **generalized seizures.** Spread to the thalamus and reticular activating system results in loss of consciousness. This category includes the following: absence (petite mal), atypical absence,

Box 45-1

Classifications of Seizures

Generalized Seizures: The Entire Brain Surface Is Affected During the Seizure

Absence (petit mal)
Atypical absence
Myoclonic
Atonic (drop attack)
Clonic
Tonic
Generalized tonic-clonic (grand mal)

Partial Seizures: Part of the Brain Surface Is Affected in Each Seizure

Simple partial: There is no impairment of consciousness during the seizure.
Complex partial: There is impairment of consciousness during the seizure.
With secondary generalization: Onset begins as simple partial, then progresses to impairment of consciousness.

myoclonic, atonic (drop attack), clonic, tonic, or tonic-clonic (grand mal) seizures. Metabolic or toxin-induced seizures tend to be generalized.

Absence or petit mal seizures usually occur only in children and are sometimes identified in children manifesting poor academic performance. They are very brief (2 to 10 seconds) and are characterized by staring spells that last only seconds. Onset and termination of attacks are abrupt. During the spell, the individual is unaware of the surrounding environment and is usually motionless; however, it is not unusual for the person to continue walking or performing a routine motor task. If the seizure activity occurs during conversation, the individual may pause or miss a few words. About 10% of children with absence seizures develop tonic-clonic seizures.[3]

Atypical absence seizures have accompanying myoclonic jerks and automatisms with the staring spell. The electroencephalographic patterns are unique to each syndrome. Myoclonic seizures are extremely brief and are characterized by a single jerk or multiple jerks of one or more muscle groups. Atonic seizures or drop attacks are characterized by a sudden and complete loss of muscle tone. Falls and injuries are common with this type of seizure activity. Myoclonic episodes may also be associated with atonic seizures. Clonic seizures involve jerking of muscle groups, whereas tonic seizures result in stiffening of muscle groups.

Tonic-clonic or grand mal seizures are characterized by a sudden loss of consciousness followed by muscle rigidity (tonic phase). The individual falls, and initial motor signs include opening of the mouth and eyes, extension of the legs, and adduction of the arms. There may be tongue biting or a high-pitched cry as the whole musculature is in spasm and air is forced out of the lungs through closed vocal cords. Respiration is arrested, and cyanosis may occur. Bowel and bladder incontinence frequently occurs. The tonic phase may last 10 to 15 seconds and is followed by clonic activity. There is often violent but rhythmic muscular contractions. During this phase the eyes roll, the face grimaces, and the pulse accelerates. Salivation increases and the patient may become diaphoretic. The clonic phase usually lasts 1 to 2 minutes with a gradual decline in the amplitude of the clonic jerks. The individual remains apneic until the end of the clonic phase that is marked by a deep inspiration.

During the terminal or postictal phase, the individual may regain consciousness or drift into a deep comalike state. Disorientation and confusion are common. If allowed, the individual may sleep for several hours. Other findings include headache, drowsiness, nausea, muscle soreness, and no memory of the seizure event. During the seizure, the person is at risk for injury from the initial fall as well as from the muscle contractions of the clonic phase.

A potentially life-threatening situation known as **status epilepticus** occurs in some seizure disorders. Status epilepticus is a continuing series of seizures without a period of recovery between seizure episodes. It can occur with all types of seizures but is somewhat common in generalized seizures. Irreversible brain damage and possible death from hypoxia, cardiac arrhythmias, or lactic acidosis can occur if the airway is not maintained and seizure activity is not halted. Studies in animals have revealed that the increased metabolic activity that occurs during status epilepticus results in ischemic brain damage if a patient in this state receives no treatment for 30 to 40 minutes.[4]

Partial Seizures. Partial seizures are those in which activity is restricted to one brain hemisphere. They are further divided into three categories: simple partial, complex partial, and partial seizures that are secondarily generalized.

In simple partial seizures, the individual does not lose consciousness. The symptoms may be motor, sensory, autonomic, or any combination of the three. Motor symptoms may be limited to one part of the body. Sensory seizures may result in tingling or numbness that spreads or "marches" to different parts of the limb or body depending on the location of the seizure activity in the brain or may involve the special senses, producing auditory (buzzing sounds), olfactory, or visual manifestations (flashing lights). Autonomic symptoms may include pupillary (pupil dilation), skin (diaphoresis, flushing), or respiratory changes.

Complex partial seizures have many different cognitive, affective, and psychomotor symptoms. Either loss or alteration of consciousness may occur when the seizure begins. After the attack, the individual may feel drowsy or confused. At the onset of impairment of consciousness, the individual often displays automatisms such as lip smacking or repetitive or semipurposeful movements. Aggressive behavior may be displayed as well, especially if bystanders attempt to restrain the individual. Complex partial seizures often last several minutes and may be followed by a postictal state.

Partial seizures that are secondarily generalized are the third subtype of partial seizures. This category comprises seizures that begin as simple partial seizures then progress to involve both brain hemispheres. Once generalized, these seizures are clinically similar to primary generalized seizures.

Aura/Prodrome. Some people may have a subjective sense of an impending seizure. This **prodromal period** may be characterized by any one of several phenomena such as a type of myoclonic jerking, headache, lethargy, mood alterations, palpitations, or epigastric sensations, which may precede the actual seizure by several hours. In about half of cases there is some type of movement or odd sensory experience that occurs seconds before consciousness is lost and that is remembered by the individual after recovery from the seizure. This experience is known as an aura. Although the individual may interpret the aura as an indication that a seizure is about to occur, in fact it is the beginning of the seizure episode. Auras can be significant, as they may be a clue to the location of the epileptogenic focus.

Diagnosis and Treatment. The diagnosis and management of seizure disorders is based on patient history, physical and neurologic examination results, and electroencephalographic studies. Electroencephalograms (EEGs) may be normal between seizures, so activation techniques (sleep deprivation, hyperventilation) may be used to elicit the pathologic mechanism. Laboratory studies are frequently used to investigate metabolic abnormalities as well as therapeutic serum levels in those already using anticonvulsant drugs. Initial studies ruling out structural causes may include computed tomography (CT) or magnetic resonance imaging (MRI).

Treatment of an individual experiencing a seizure is concentrated on maintaining an airway and protecting the individual from injury. Recording the course of the seizure episode is useful for identifying the location of the epileptogenic focus and for noting any change in the patient's seizure pattern. This data is useful in treatment planning. The information recorded should include the time of onset and duration of the seizure, precipitating factors, presence of a prodrome or aura, sequence of seizure activity, autonomic signs, level of consciousness, and postictal state.

Long-term treatment depends on the cause of the seizure disorder. In seizures resulting from a metabolic abnormality, infection, or tumor, the precipitating source is removed. If the seizures are due to irreversible or unidentifiable factors, anticonvulsant medications specific to the type of seizure are the best management. The objective of therapy is to achieve seizure control with a minimum of side effects. Medication is continued until there have been no seizures for at least 3 years.[5] If seizures continue despite treatment at a maximal dose of a single medication, a second agent is added and the dosage increased depending on patient tolerance. The first drug is then gradually withdrawn. Anticonvulsant medication is a form of control, not a cure.

Treatment also includes patient education in the avoidance of activating factors (e.g., stress, loud noise, alcohol). Patients should be advised to avoid situations that could be dangerous or life threatening if seizures should reoccur (e.g., driving or swimming). Compliance to the treatment plan is sometimes difficult due to side effects of pharmacologic interventions. However, most patients are able to achieve optimal seizure control and lead active and productive lives.

For some patients with uncontrolled seizure disorder, surgical excision of the seizure focus may be an option. Vagal nerve stimulation for adults and adolescents with partial-onset seizures may provide an alternative approach to treatment. The mechanism of action is unknown, but intermittent stimulation of the left vagus nerve in the neck has been shown to decrease the frequency and intensity of seizure activity.[5,6]

KEY CONCEPTS

- Seizure disorder is characterized by recurrent episodes of abnormal electrical impulses in the brain. Some individuals appear to have a lower-than-normal threshold for seizure activity. Seizure activity may occur in anyone, given the right conditions. Head injury, meningitis, brain tumors, and metabolic disorders (electrolyte imbalance, fever, acidosis) may predispose an individual to having seizures.
- Initiation of seizure activity may occur in a particular brain area (the epileptogenic focus). Nearby and distant neurons may then be recruited into the seizure. When sufficient neurons are involved, the seizure becomes clinically evident as involuntary movement or unusual sensations.
- Seizures are classified as partial or generalized. Partial seizures involve a part of the brain; generalized seizures involve the entire brain at the onset. Partial seizures are further classified as simple, in which consciousness is retained, and complex, in which consciousness is impaired. Seizures may begin as partial and then generalize to affect the entire brain. Generalized seizures include absence, myoclonic, atonic, and tonic-clonic types. Consciousness is always impaired in generalized seizures.
- Status epilepticus is a serious condition in which seizures occur continuously, resulting in intense brain metabolism. Ischemic brain damage may result. Management of a seizure in progress is aimed at maintaining the individual's airway and protecting the person from trauma. Close attention is given to the quality and progression of seizure activity. Anticonvulsant medications are used to suppress seizure activity.

Dementia

Dementia is not a specific disease but rather a syndrome associated with many pathologic processes. It is characterized by progressive deterioration of memory and other cognitive changes. Personality and behavior changes accompany the cognitive deterioration. The onset of dementia may be insidious (as in the case of Alzheimer type), and the affected

THE AGING PROCESS

Changes in Sleep Patterns

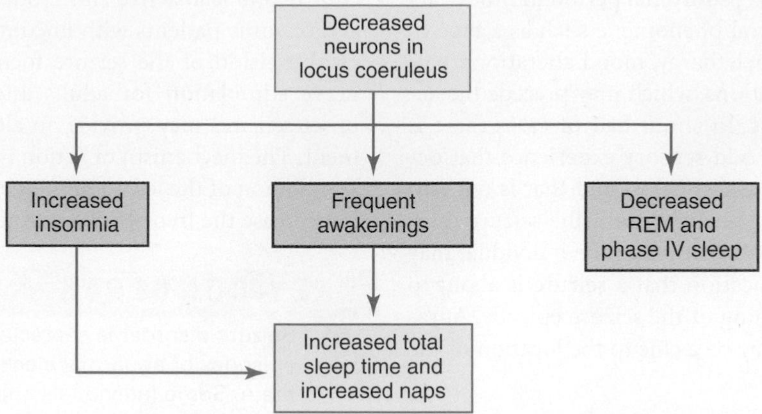

Aging affects the patterns of sleep. The locus coeruleus, the part of the brain that controls sleep, undergoes a loss of neurons. The decrease in neurons from this center is hypothesized to increase insomnia and cause frequent awakenings in the elderly. There is also a decrease in rapid eye movement (REM) and slow-wave (phase IV) sleep, as well as variability in all sleep stages. There is an increased total daily sleep time, with an increased number of naps.

individual may initially appear uninterested or lacking initiative. Many demented patients have **anosognosia** or lack of insight into their cognitive deficiencies.[7] Disruption of sleep patterns may also be present as described in The Aging Process: Changes in Sleep Patterns.

Dementia is the fourth leading cause of death in the United States and affects 30% to 50% of individuals aged 85 and over. Women are affected more often than men.[5] The typical age of onset is older than 65 years.[8] Alzheimer disease is the most common cause of dementia, constituting 60% to 70% of all cases—and the number of people with Alzheimer disease doubles every 5 years after age 65.[9] Approximately 4 million Americans suffer from Alzheimer disease and 14 million may have it by 2050.[10]

Etiology. Multiple types of dementia exist, and a full discussion of each is beyond the scope of this chapter. Some examples of dementia-causing illness include alcoholism, intracranial tumor, normal-pressure hydrocephalus, Parkinson disease, Lewy body disease, Huntington disease, multiple sclerosis, Pick disease, Creutzfeldt-Jakob disease, and bovine spongiform encephalopathy (mad cow disease). Because Alzheimer- and vascular-type dementias are the first and second most common causes of dementia, they will be discussed in detail. The subsequent discussion of treatment of persons with dementia will be more general because the care issues are similar regardless of type of dementia.

It is important to consider other causes of cognitive change when dealing with patients with mental status change. Both delirium and depression in the elderly can cause signs and symptoms that resemble those of Alzheimer disease. Delirium is a global mental dysfunction that includes disturbed consciousness, decreased awareness of the environment, inability to maintain attention, disrupted sleep-wake cycles, drowsiness, restlessness, emotional lability, incoherence, and hallucinations.[11] Symptoms of delirium tend to have an abrupt onset and may fluctuate often, becoming worse at night. Delirium can result from numerous causes such as medication/polypharmacy, metabolic abnormalities, nutritional deficiencies, and infection, among others. Delirium may occur more frequently in individuals with an underlying dementing illness.

Pathogenesis. Structural lesions of the cerebral hemisphere and diencephalon are associated with dementia. Although the neuronal damage may be diffuse, the temporal and frontal lobes are frequently involved.[11] At autopsy, the brain of the patient with Alzheimer disease reveals two major neuropathophysiologic lesions: neurofibrillary tangles and amyloid deposits in the form of senile plaques and cerebrovascular accumulations (Figure 45-1).

A main component of tangles is a ***tau* protein,** also known as **neural thread protein.**[8] In the central nervous system (CNS), neural thread proteins bind and help stabilize microtubules (the cell's internal support structure or skeleton). But in Alzheimer disease, chemically altered tau twists into paired helical filaments known as **neurofibrillary tangles.**

It is not known whether amyloid plaques cause Alzheimer disease or result from it. The number of senile plaques seems

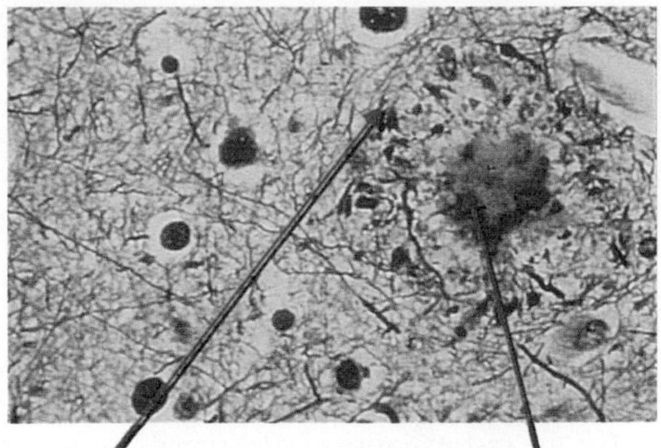

FIGURE 45-1 ■ Amyloid plaques and neurofibrillary tangles. (Courtesy James King-Holmes and Science Photo Library.)

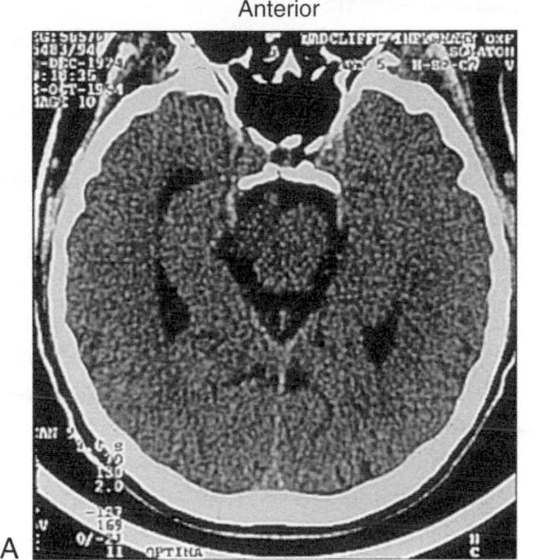

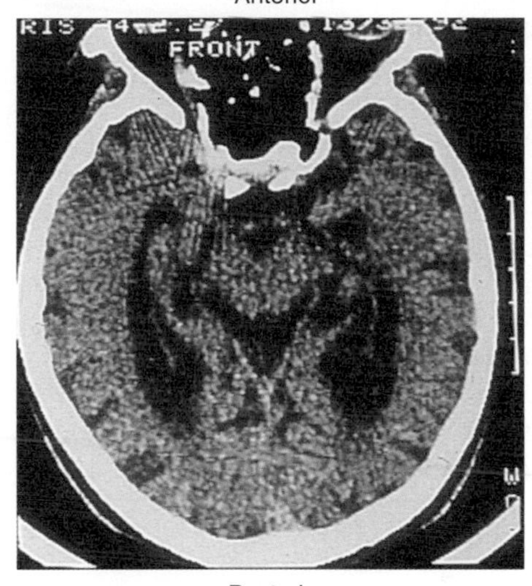

FIGURE 45-2 ■ Axial (horizontal) CT scan section through the temporal lobes. **A,** Normal. **B,** Alzheimer disease. (Courtesy James King-Holmes and Science Photo Library.)

to correlate with the severity of disease. Beta protein is a major component of the amyloid fibrils of the plaques and cerebral vessels as well as the neurofibrillary tangles.[8] In plaques, β-amyloid is a protein fragment snipped from a bigger protein—**amyloid precursor protein (APP)**—during metabolism.[11] APP is a member of a large family of proteins that are associated with cell membranes. During metabolism, APP becomes embedded in the membrane of the nerve cell, partly inside and partly outside the cell. While APP is embedded in the cell membrane, proteases cleave APP apart. β-Amyloid is produced only when the cleavage happens at the wrong place in APP.

After β-amyloid is formed it is not known how it moves through or around the nerve cells. In the final stages of its journey, it joins with other β-amyloid filaments and fragments of dead and dying neurons to form the dense, insoluble plaques that are a hallmark of Alzheimer disease in brain tissue. Inflammatory processes including acute phase response, complement activation, and accumulation of activated microglia and astrocytes accompany the amyloid deposition and neurofibrillary tangle formation.[12] The accumulation of β-amyloid also causes oxidation of lipids, activation of apoptotic genes, disruption of cell membranes, and excitotoxicity from the neurotransmitter glutamate.[13,14] Gross examination of the brain of the Alzheimer disease patient after death finds that it is atrophic, often weighing less than 1000 g, compared with a normal brain weight of 1380 g. The temporoparietal and anterior frontal regions of the brains are chiefly affected, exhibiting enlarged sulci and atrophic gyri (Figure 45-2).

Much interest exists in the neurotransmitter systems in relation to Alzheimer disease. Damage in Alzheimer disease involves changes in three mechanisms: nerve cell communication, metabolism, and repair. Several studies have found abnormalities in the cholinergic system, including reduced activity of choline acetyltransferase (the enzyme necessary for acetylcholine synthesis) and decreased acetylcholine synthesis

(Figure 45-3). Some researchers believe that β-amyloid may be responsible for lower choline levels in nerve cells and decreased acetylcholine levels. The degeneration of cells in the nucleus basalis, a band of gray matter in the ventral portion of the medulla oblongata, has also been linked to diminished levels of acetylcholine in the cerebral cortex, a finding that provides further evidence for the significant role of the cholinergic system in Alzheimer disease.[13,15]

The primary risk factors for the development of Alzheimer disease include age and family history. Epidemiologic studies show that individuals who have an affected first-degree relative with Alzheimer disease have a fourfold greater risk of developing the disease. The risk is greater if there are individuals in more than one generation with the disease.[8] Genetic factors have been found to have a role in come cases of Alzheimer disease. Two types of Alzheimer disease exist: familial and sporadic. Familial Alzheimer disease follows a certain inheritance pattern whereas sporadic occurs without any obvious inheritance pattern. Because of the differences in age at onset, familial Alzheimer disease is further described as early onset (symptoms apparent before age 65) and late onset (symptoms appearing later than age 65). However, the clinical manifestations of these various classifications of Alzheimer disease are indistinguishable. Although genetics accounts for 1% to 2% of all cases of Alzheimer disease, the mutations have been the foundation of all Alzheimer disease pathophysiologic study. Thus far, three causative genes have been found in early-onset families.[8,16]

Genetic mutations of chromosomes 1 (presenilin-2), 14 (presenilin-1), and 21 (β-APP) cause rare, early-onset forms of Alzheimer disease. Late-onset Alzheimer disease has been linked to chromosome 19.[8] Presenilin-1 mutations are associated with the earliest age of onset of symptoms and cause the most rapidly progressing disease.[8] Presenilin-2 mutations were found linking familial Alzheimer disease with individuals who descended from a group of Germans living in the Volga Valley of the former Soviet Union (called Volga Germans). This is the least common form of genetically associated Alzheimer disease. Abnormalities of chromosome 21 cause early-onset Alzheimer disease due to abnormal coding for β-APP. The β-amyloid is formed when APP is abnormally cleaved.[8,13]

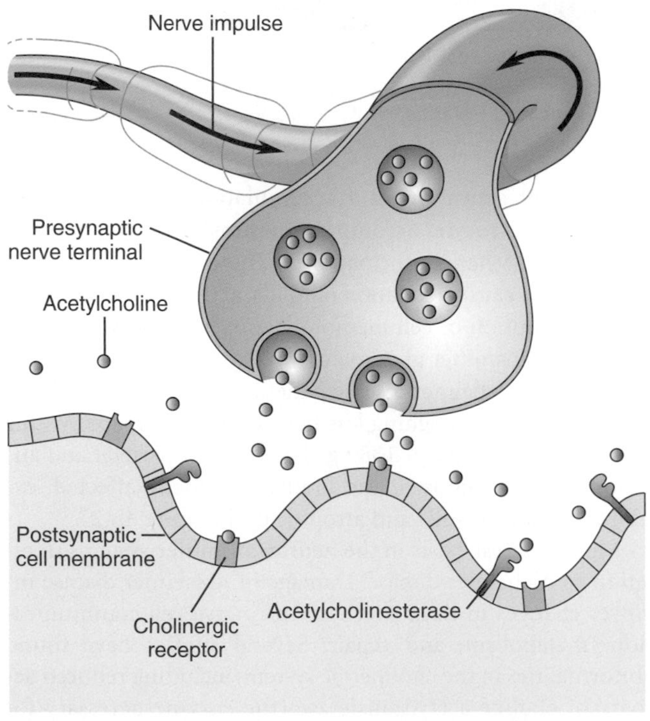

FIGURE 45-3 ■ The cholinergic synapse.

For the vast majority of Alzheimer disease patients, aside from age and family history, the only other risk factor is the presence of apolipoprotein E4 (apoE4) allele on chromosome 19.[13] ApoE4 is a protein that rests on the surface of the cholesterol molecule and helps carry blood cholesterol through the body.[9] It is found in neurons of healthy brains but is also found in amyloid plaques and neurofibrillary tangles.[8] Carrying the ApoE4 allele has been associated with increased incidence of Alzheimer disease. Having two copies of the gene even further increases the risk.[17] However, this genetic pattern also occurs in individuals without Alzheimer disease.

Other risk factors for the development of Alzheimer disease are common also to the development of other types of dementia, such as vascular dementia. This type of dementia is responsible for up to 15% of all dementia.[13] Histologic changes of Alzheimer disease often coexist with vascular dementia. Elderly patients who have suffered from cerebral damage from vascular causes seem to require fewer plaques and tangles to have severe disease. Hypertension, peripheral vascular disease, lower education, lower estrogen levels, and history of a traumatic brain injury have been associated with an increased risk of developing Alzheimer disease.[13] An elevated serum level of homocysteine is also a modest independent risk factor.[18]

Clinical Manifestations. Regardless of when patients first present with dementia or Alzheimer disease, it is likely that brain disease has been present for quite some time.[13] Most patients experience a gradual onset with a chronic progressive decline in cognitive functioning. There is memory loss, especially in short-term memory whereas long-term memory may be preserved. Thinking ability declines and there is a decreasing ability to function at work and in social settings. Anxiety and agitation are common. As the disease progresses, individuals have increasing difficulty with judgment, problem solving, and communication. Assistance may be necessary for completing activities of daily living (ADLs). Difficulty with eating, swallowing, and weight loss are common. Loss of bladder and bowel control and eventual complete loss of the ability to ambulate occurs in the late stages. Accidents and infection are common causes of death.[15]

Diagnosis and Treatment. The initial evaluation of a patient thought to have dementia of any type begins with a complete history and physical examination. This should address the patient's overall general health and any coexisting medical conditions. All manageable causes for dementia and delirium should be ruled out. It is recommended by the American Academy of Neurology that the evaluation should include complete blood cell count, chemistry panel, thyroid function, vitamin B_{12} levels, syphilis serology, and neuroimaging. Other evaluations such as a chest x-ray, urinalysis, and lumbar puncture may also be helpful.[5,7] Mental status examinations, the clock drawing test, and tests of functional status are recommended.[10] A current list of the patient's medications, including over-the-counter medications, must also be reviewed. Medications with anticholinergic actions/side effects are a common cause of changes in cognitive functioning in the elderly. These include antihistamines such as diphenhydramine (Benadryl), H_2 blockers (Zantac, Cimetidine), some pain medications and narcotics, oxybutynin (Ditropan, Ditropan XL), and hyoscyamine (Levsin, Anaspaz).[9]

Early diagnosis and intervention is key in the management of dementias. The financial and legal ramifications of dementia can be devastating to patients and their families and caregivers. If the diagnosis is made before the onset of severe cognitive disability, the patient can be involved in decisions regarding long-term care, power of attorney, and living will issues. Early diagnosis is also vital in terms of initiating therapy as early as possible. Some research suggests that delay in the initiation of therapy may result in a less than maximal response to therapy.[10]

Functional brain imaging studies such as positron emission tomography (PET) scanning show promise in the early diagnosis of Alzheimer disease. PET measures of glucose metabolism in patients with Alzheimer dementia show a consistent pattern of decreased cerebral glucose. When this information is combined with genetic risk, a diagnosis of Alzheimer disease may be made sooner.[13]

Currently, two classes of drugs are approved by the Food and Drug Administration for the treatment of Alzheimer disease (Table 45-1). The first class is the acetylcholinesterase inhibitors: tacrine (Cognex), donepezil (Aricept), rivastigmine (Exelon), and galantamine (Reminyl).[19] These agents are indicated for use in patients with mild to moderate Alzheimer disease. Although not a cure, the acetylcholinesterase inhibitors have been shown to stabilize cognitive function and slow progression of the illness.[15,20] Acetylcholinesterase inhibitors have also been shown to improve cognitive functioning in patients with vascular dementia.[15,21]

The second class of drugs used in the treatment of Alzheimer disease is known as the *N*-methyl-D-aspartate (NMDA) receptor antagonists. Currently only one drug in this class is available in the United States. Memantine (Namenda)

Table 45-1

Drug Therapies for Alzheimer Disease

Drug	Dosing	Mechanism of Action	Side Effects
Donepezil (Aricept)	Initial dose 5 mg daily; after 4-6 weeks may increase to 10 mg daily	Acetylcholinesterase inhibition	Nausea, vomiting, diarrhea; initial agitation; possible drug interactions: cimetidine, theophylline, warfarin, digoxin
Rivastigmine (Exelon)	Initial dose 1.5 mg bid; may be increased by 1.5 mg bid every 4 weeks; maximum dose 6 mg bid	Acetylcholinesterase inhibition; butyryl cholinesterase inhibition	Nausea, vomiting, diarrhea, weight loss, fatigue, malaise, anxiety, agitation; drug interactions with aminoglycosides, procainamide
Galantamine (Reminyl)	Initial dose 4 mg bid; after 4 weeks dosage increased to 8 mg bid; dosage may be increased to maximum of 12 mg bid with 4 weeks between dosage changes	Acetylcholinesterase inhibition; nicotinic modulation	Nausea, vomiting, diarrhea; contraindicated in hepatic/renal impairment
Tacrine (Cognex) First drug in this class; rarely used now	Initial dose 10 mg qid; may be increased by 10 mg qid increments every 4 weeks to a maximum dosage of 40 mg qid	Acetylcholinesterase inhibition	Hepatotoxicity; liver function test monitoring; drug interactions with theophylline, procainamide
Memantine (Namenda)	Initial dose 5 mg qd; may be increased by 5 mg/day weekly until 10 mg bid is reached	Inhibits glutamate excitation at NMDA receptors	Dizziness, headache, constipation, confusion, caution in renal impairment

Adapted from Bonner LT, Peskind EP: Pharmacologic treatments of dementia, *Med Clin North Am* 86(3):656-671, 2002; Cummings JL et al: Guidelines for managing Alzheimer's disease: part II, *Am Fam Physician* 67(12):2525-2534, 2002; Geldmacher DS, editor: Summation of Proceedings of the First Annual Dementia Congress, *Treatment of dementia in the new millennium,* New York, 2002, Academy for Healthcare Education; Griffith VT: Diagnose and treat mild to moderate Alzheimer's disease, *Nurse Pract* 27(12):3-25, 2002; and Guthrie EW: The use of memantine (Namenda) in patients with mild to moderate Alzheimer disease, Document No. 200202, 2002, Prescriber's Letter website. Available at http://www.prescribersletter.com.

is indicated for the treatment of moderate to severe Alzheimer-type dementia. This drug blocks stimulation by the neuroexcitatory transmitter glutamate. Again, this medication is not a cure, but slows progression of the disease.[22] Early studies using combination therapy of acetylcholinesterase inhibitors and NMDA antagonists are showing modest improvement in cognitive functioning.[23]

Many other medications, although not approved for use in treating Alzheimer disease, are used to manage the symptoms, such as depression, sleep disturbance, agitation, and psychosis. These medications include antidepressants, anxiolytics, antipsychotics, and mood stabilizers.[5,20]

A variety of alternative medications have been used in the management of Alzheimer disease, including estrogen; gingko biloba; antioxidants such as vitamin E, vitamin C, and β-carotene; vitamin B; folate; nonsteroidal antiinflammatory drugs (NSAIDs); and steroids. The data regarding estrogen therapy are mixed but for the most part show no benefit in slowing disease progression or improving cognitive functioning.[24] Early research is showing reduced occurrence of Alzheimer disease in patients using NSAIDs and aspirin.[25] However, randomized controlled trials using prednisone in Alzheimer patients failed to show any improvement in symptoms.[12,26] Studies also do not conclusively support the use of gingko biloba.[27] Research is currently underway exploring the role of oxidative stress and homocysteine levels and Alzheimer disease. Use of antioxidants, vitamin B, and folate may prove useful in the prevention of the disease. Early research on the use of 3-hydroxy-3-methylglutaryl coenzyme A (HMG-CoA) reductase inhibitors, the lipid-lowering medications also known as the *statins*, is showing promise in reducing the risk of the developing Alzheimer disease.[28,29]

Other treatments for dementia include optimal management of other coexisting illnesses, interventions aimed at wellness, nutritional management, and protection from injury. In early stages of the disease, most patients are cared for at home, often by family members. It is important that the home environment be safe and that there be measures in place to control wandering. Consistent routines and familiar surroundings allow the patient to feel more comfortable and experience less confusion. As the disease progresses, the individual with dementia may have to be placed in an alternative living situation such as a nursing home or assisted-living program. Caring for the caregivers of patients with dementia is important.

KEY CONCEPTS

- Dementia refers to progressive degeneration of cognitive function due to organic causes. In many instances the cause is unknown. There is no definitive treatment for dementia, and it is important to first rule out manageable causes of mental impairment.
- The dementia of Alzheimer disease is characterized by degeneration of neurons in temporal and frontal lobes, brain atrophy, amyloid plaques, and neurofibrillary tangles. The synthesis of brain acetylcholine is deficient. The cause of Alzheimer disease remains unknown, although genetic factors and environmental triggers are suspected.
- The behavioral problems of people with Alzheimer disease progresses from forgetfulness to total inability for self-care. Depression and psychosis may be significant.

Parkinson Disease

Parkinson disease is a disorder of mobility that affects nearly 1% of the U.S. population older than 50 years. The disease has highest incidence in persons 45 to 65 years of age and occurs in all ethnic groups with an approximately equal gender distribution.[5]

Etiology. Parkinson disease may be idiopathic or acquired. Idiopathic Parkinson disease is that in which no demonstrable cause is identified. Common causes of acquired **parkinsonism** include infection, intoxication, and trauma.[5] Typically, parkinsonism due to drug toxicity evolves rapidly, unlike the slow insidious onset of the idiopathic disease. Side effects of drugs of the phenothiazine class (e.g., chlorpromazine, prochlorperazine, and thioridazine) and butyrophenone class (e.g., haloperidol) may manifest in a parkinsonian syndrome at toxic levels. Discontinuing the medication generally results in improvement in the symptoms. However, use of the anticholinergic antiparkinsonian drugs may aid in more rapid recovery.

Pathogenesis. Parkinson disease results from degeneration of the pigmented dopaminergic neurons found in the substantia nigra (Figure 45-4) and, to a lesser extent, neurons elsewhere in the brain. Eosinophilic cytoplasmic inclusions known as Lewy bodies may be found in the surviving neurons. Incidentally, Lewy bodies are found along with amyloid plaques at autopsy in the brains of some patients with a severe form of dementia. This suggests a possible link with Alzheimer disease. The exact cause of this degeneration is unknown, but oxidative stress, genetics, and environmental toxins have been implicated.[30,31]

A number of genes have been identified as having a role in the development of Parkinson disease. In particular, identification of a mutation in the α-synuclein gene has become the focus of much interest. Although mutations in the gene are a rare cause of Parkinson disease, α-synuclein is abundant in neurons, specifically in presynaptic terminals, and is a major component of Lewy bodies.[32] Another gene identified in the development of Parkinson disease is *parkin*. This gene is thought to have a role in protein degradation and clearance. Mutations in this gene may be associated with abnormal protein accumulations within the neuron.[32] Although genetics has received much attention in Parkinson disease research, en-

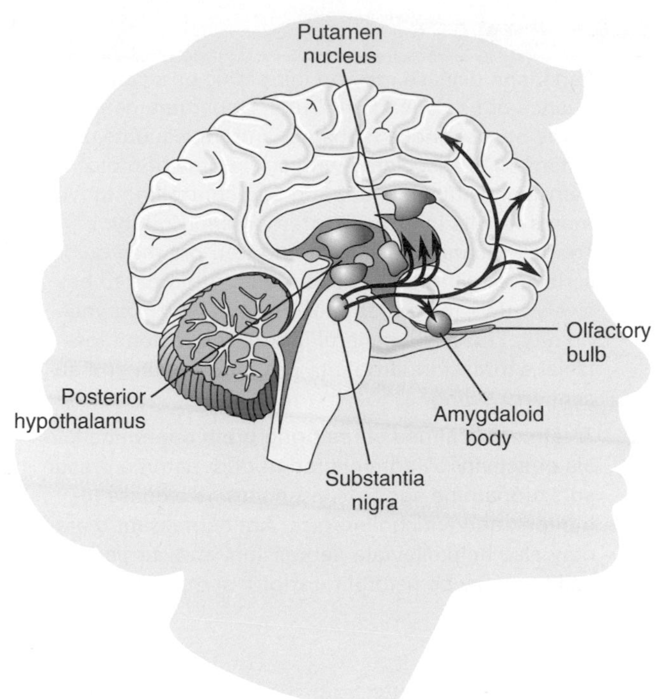

FIGURE 45-4 ■ Dopamine neurons and their pathways in the human brain.

vironmental factors have also been studied. High caffeine intake has been found to have an inverse relationship to the risk of developing the disorder. Long-term exposure to the pesticide rotenone has been linked to increasing risk for Parkinson disease.[32] Whatever the cause of the degeneration of the dopaminergic cells, 75% to 80% of the neurons have died before any symptoms of the disease become apparent.[31]

Clinical Manifestations and Treatment. Because of the insidious onset, earlier evidence of Parkinson disease may be discovered in a thorough health history. Frequently, the very early signs of the disorder (loss of flexibility, aching and fatigue) are overlooked by the patient or are attributed to the aging process. Initially, symptoms are usually worse on one side of the body and then progress to involve both sides. Tremor is often the first symptom recognized that prompts patients to seek treatment and is apparent in 70% of those with the disease.[11] Additional early signs of the disease include bradykinesia, rigidity, hypokinesia, loss of facial expression, and infrequent eye blinking (Figure 45-5). Again, these symptoms may be overlooked by patients but are usually apparent to observant family members.

As the disease progresses, additional functional changes are noted. The patient's handwriting may become small (micrographia) and cramped, with evidence of tremor. Speech may become low in volume, monotonous, and dysarthric. There may be a mumbling quality to the speech. The effects of bradykinesia are evident in the patients' swallowing function, ability to initiate activity, and mobility. Swallowing becomes delayed so much so that the individual may drool, and patients are at risk for aspiration. The effect of the disease on the ability to initiate activity is evident when the individual rises from a chair or begins to walk from a standing-still position. However, many people with Parkinson disease are able to act quickly in times of emergency, such as fire. This phenomenon is known as paradoxical kinesia.

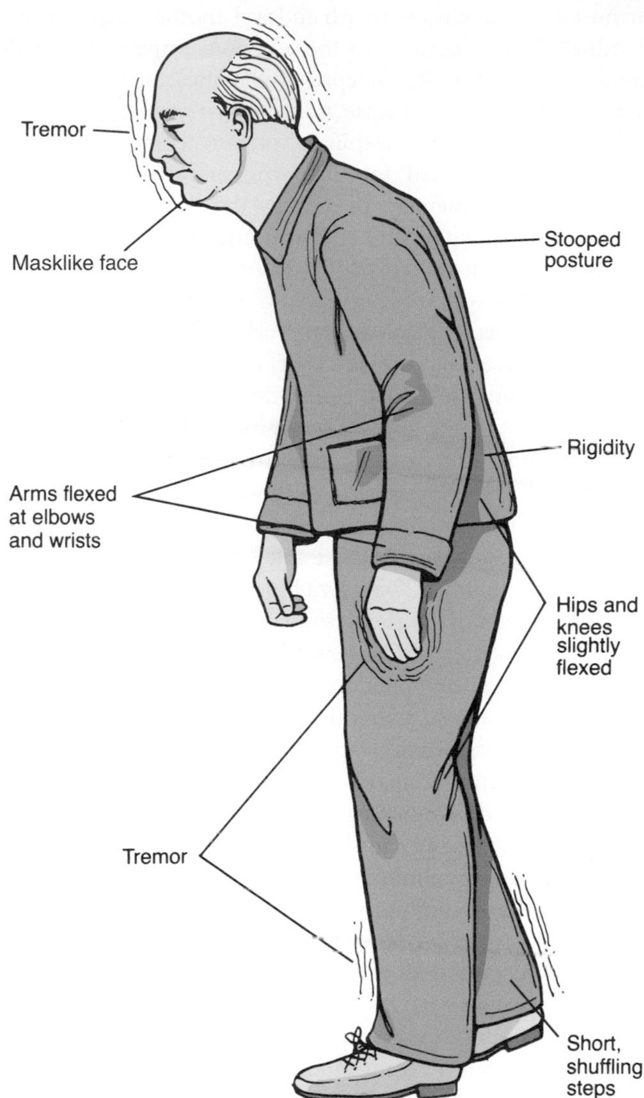

FIGURE 45-5 ■ Clinical manifestations of Parkinson disease. (From Monahan FD, Neighbors M: *Medical-surgical nursing: foundations for clinical practice,* Philadelphia, 1998, Saunders, p 787.)

Additional difficulties in mobility are evident from the lack of spontaneous position changes while the individual is sitting in one position, from the decreased or absent arm swing while the individual is walking, and from the shuffling gait. Impairment of postural reflexes presents particular safety problems for the individual with Parkinson disease in maintaining balance, as evidenced by propulsive or retropulsive gaits. Involvement of the autonomic nervous system may result in orthostatic hypotension, which adds yet another risk to the individual's health. Because of these various impairments, falls are a common problem. Depression is present in many patients with Parkinson disease, occurring in more than 50% of individuals. Daytime sleepiness is also common and is thought to be related to underlying pathologic processes rather than treatment as previously thought.[30] Dementia is prevalent in patients with Parkinson disease.

There is no known cure for Parkinson disease. Treatments are aimed at slowing the progression of the disease and managing symptoms. The mainstay of Parkinson therapy has been aimed at increasing the level of dopamine in the CNS. Dopamine precursors such as levodopa are one approach to increasing dopamine levels. Dopamine itself cannot be used because it does not cross the blood-brain barrier efficiently. Outside the CNS, levodopa is metabolized to dopamine and then to adrenaline and noradrenaline, which cause nausea and hypotension. To minimize these side effects, levodopa is combined with carbidopa. This agent blocks the conversion of levodopa to dopamine in the periphery, allowing it to cross the blood-brain barrier.[30] Long-term use of levodopa has been associated with "on-off" phenomena (in which the action of the drug suddenly stops, leaving the patient with sudden onset of symptoms) or abnormal movements called dyskinesias. Other medications aimed at increasing the level of dopamine in the CNS include dopamine agonists (pergolide, pramipexole, ropinirole), medications to slow the metabolism of dopamine (monoamine oxidase inhibitors such as selegiline, catechol-*O*-methyltransferase inhibitors), and others, such as amantadine, which enhance the release of dopamine from neuronal storage sites.[31] Anticholinergic medications may help with tremor, rigidity, or drooling.

Surgical options for the management of Parkinson disease have received much recent attention. Ablative surgical techniques of thalamotomy and pallidotomy create small lesions in the pallidum or thalamus; this can improve rigidity, tremor, and bradykinesia.[31,32] Symptoms are also better controlled with medication following the surgery. These surgical techniques are considered for patients who have been unresponsive to the medical treatments or who are unable to tolerate the side effects. Deep brain stimulation involves the surgical implantation of a high frequency thalamic electrical stimulator that interrupts the tremor-causing nerve impulses. Deep brain stimulation can decrease the need for Parkinson medication.[32] Tissue transplantation of adrenal tissue or fetal brain tissue in an attempt to increase the level of dopamine in the CNS are very controversial and have not been consistently shown to improve the symptoms of Parkinson disease.[5,32]

Treatment therapies on the horizon for Parkinson disease may include the implantation of encapsulated dopaminergic cells from animals into the brain in an attempt to avoid host immune rejection of the grafted cells and to avoid controversy over the use of fetal cells.[33] Early antioxidant research shows modest improvement in symptoms in patients taking coenzyme Q_{10} supplements.[34] Genetic research on Parkinson disease continues.

KEY CONCEPTS

- Parkinson disease may be idiopathic or a consequence of use of certain drugs. Dopamine deficiency in the basal ganglia (substantia nigra, caudate, and putamen) is associated with symptoms of motor impairment. Difficulty initiating and controlling movements results in akinesia, tremor, and rigidity. Tremor occurs at rest and hand tremors may be described as pill-rolling movements. Attempts to passively move the extremities are met with cogwheel rigidity. There is a general lack of movement, loss of facial expression, drooling, propulsive gait, and absent arm swing.
- Treatment is aimed at restoring brain dopamine levels or activity by administration of dopamine precursors, dopamine agonists, monoamine oxidase inhibitors, and anticholinergics. Antidepressant therapy may also help alleviate depression, and surgical procedures may be helpful for motor symptoms.

Cerebral Palsy

Etiology and Pathogenesis. **Cerebral palsy** refers to a diverse group of crippling syndromes that appears during childhood and involves permanent, nonprogressive encephalopathic damage to the developing brain.[3] Such damage is present at birth or occurs shortly after birth and remains throughout life. It may be classified on the basis of neurologic signs and symptoms, with the major types involving spasticity, ataxia, dyskinesia, or a mix of one or more of the three. Cerebral palsy is one of the most common crippling disorders of childhood, with an incidence of between 2 and 5 of 1000 births.[3] Etiologic factors include prenatal infections or diseases of the mother; mechanical trauma to the head before, during, or after birth; nerve-damaging poisons; or reduced oxygen supply to the brain. Neonatal hypoglycemia, **kernicterus,** prematurity, and low birth weight are also risk factors.[3,35]

Clinical Manifestations. Spastic cerebral palsy manifests with hypertonia, prolonged primitive reflexes, exaggerated deep tendon reflexes, clonus, rigidity of the extremities, scoliosis, and contractures. This type of cerebral palsy is the most common and accounts for approximately 65% to 75% of cases.[3] Spastic paralysis often affects one entire side of the body (hemiplegia), both legs (paraplegia), both legs and one arm (triplegia), or all four extremities (quadriplegia). Dyskinetic cerebral palsy caused by neonatal hyperbilirubinemia or severe anoxia manifests with extreme difficulty in purposeful movement and fine motor coordination.[11] Movements are jerky, uncontrolled, and abrupt, resulting from injury to the **basal ganglia** or **extrapyramidal tracts.** This is the second most common form of cerebral palsy and accounts for approximately 20% to 25% of cases.[36] Ataxic cerebral palsy is associated with gait disturbances and instability. The infant with this type of cerebral palsy may have hypotonia at birth, but stiffness of the trunk muscles develops by late infancy. Persistence of truncal stiffness affects the child's gait and ability to maintain equilibrium. Pure ataxic cerebral palsy is rare. This palsy denotes maldevelopment of the cerebrum or its pathways, which if severe may be associated with significant cognitive impairment.[11] More typically, a child will have a mixed disorder with clinical manifestations of each of the types. Mixed disorder accounts for approximately 13% of cases.[36]

Children with cerebral palsy often have neurologic complications such as seizures (35% to 50%), intellectual difficulties ranging from mild to severe (50% to 75%), and visual problems (50%).[36] Other associated clinical manifestations include hearing impairment, communication disorders, respiratory problems, bowel and bladder problems, and orthopedic disabilities.

Treatment. Treatment varies according to the nature and extent of brain damage. Muscle relaxants may help reduce spasms. Anticonvulsant drugs are necessary when seizures are among the symptoms of the disorder. Orthopedic surgery, casts, braces, and traction may be useful to correct some types of associated disability. A comprehensive rehabilitation program including early muscle training and special exercises may help the child with cerebral palsy lead a more useful, productive life.

KEY CONCEPTS

- Cerebral palsy refers to a diverse group of crippling syndromes that appear during childhood and involve permanent, nonprogressive damage to motor control areas of the brain.
- Cerebral palsy may be classified on the basis of neurologic signs and symptoms, with the major types involving spasticity, ataxia, dyskinesia, or a mix of one or more of the three.
- Etiologic factors include prenatal infections or diseases of the mother; mechanical trauma to the head before, during, or after birth; exposure to nerve-damaging poisons; or reduced oxygen supply to the brain.
- Treatment varies according to the nature and extent of brain damage. Muscle relaxants, anticonvulsant drugs, orthopedic surgery, casts, braces, and traction are among the therapies used.

Hydrocephalus

Etiology. **Hydrocephalus** is a condition caused by abnormal accumulation of cerebrospinal fluid (CSF) in the cerebral ventricular system. Figure 45-6 illustrates the normal flow of CSF. Hydrocephalus is generally associated with a congenital defect, usually a neural tube defect. Although hydrocephalus is typically a congenital disorder, it occurs occasionally in adults and elderly persons as a consequence of mass lesions or after hemorrhage. There are three types of hydrocephalus: (1) normal-pressure hydrocephalus; (2) obstructive hydrocephalus; and (3) communicating hydrocephalus. Normal-pressure hydrocephalus is a condition in which CSF volume increases without change in CSF pressure because brain tissue has been lost, as in Alzheimer disease. Current research with elderly adults suggests that arterial hypertension might be a vascular risk factor for normal-pressure hydrocephalus.[37] Viral infections or other neurotoxic agents acquired during pregnancy have been implicated with the congenital forms. Besides normal-pressure hydrocephalus, classification of the remaining two types of hydrocephalus is based on whether there is abnormal absorption of the CSF or an obstruction to its flow.

In obstructive hydrocephalus, there is an obstruction at some point in either the intraventricular or extraventricular pathways of the ventricular system.[11] The cause of obstructive hydrocephalus usually is a congenital abnormality, such as stenosis of the foramina of the fourth ventricle or spina bifida cystica. Other etiologic factors include intraventricular hemorrhage, which is a common complication in premature infants.[11]

Communicating hydrocephalus (sometimes referred to as acquired communicating hydrocephalus) is identified by an abnormality in the capacity to absorb fluid from the subarachnoid space. There is no obstruction to the flow of fluid between the ventricles. Infections, trauma, and tumors have been identified as etiologic factors.[11] Because the most common types of hydrocephalus are either obstructive or communicating, the remainder of this section will focus on these conditions. The reader is referred to a textbook of neurology for additional information about hydrocephalus, including normal-pressure hydrocephalus.

Pathogenesis and Clinical Manifestations. Usually the obstructive type of hydrocephalus is caused by a block in the aqueduct of Sylvius, resulting from premature closure before birth in affected babies or from a brain tumor at any age (Figure 45-7). As fluid is formed by the choroid plexus in the two lateral and the third ventricles, the volumes of these three ventricles increase greatly. This flattens the brain into a thin shell against the skull. In neonates, the increased pressure also causes the whole head to swell because the skull bones have not fused.

The communicating type of hydrocephalus is usually caused by blockage of fluid flow in the **subarachnoid space** around the basal regions of the brain or blockage of the **arachnoid villi** themselves. Fluid therefore collects both inside the ventricles and on the outside of the brain. If it occurs in infants when the skull is still pliable and can be stretched, the head swells tremendously.

Treatment. Medical treatment has been used with only limited success in controlling the secretion of CSF and

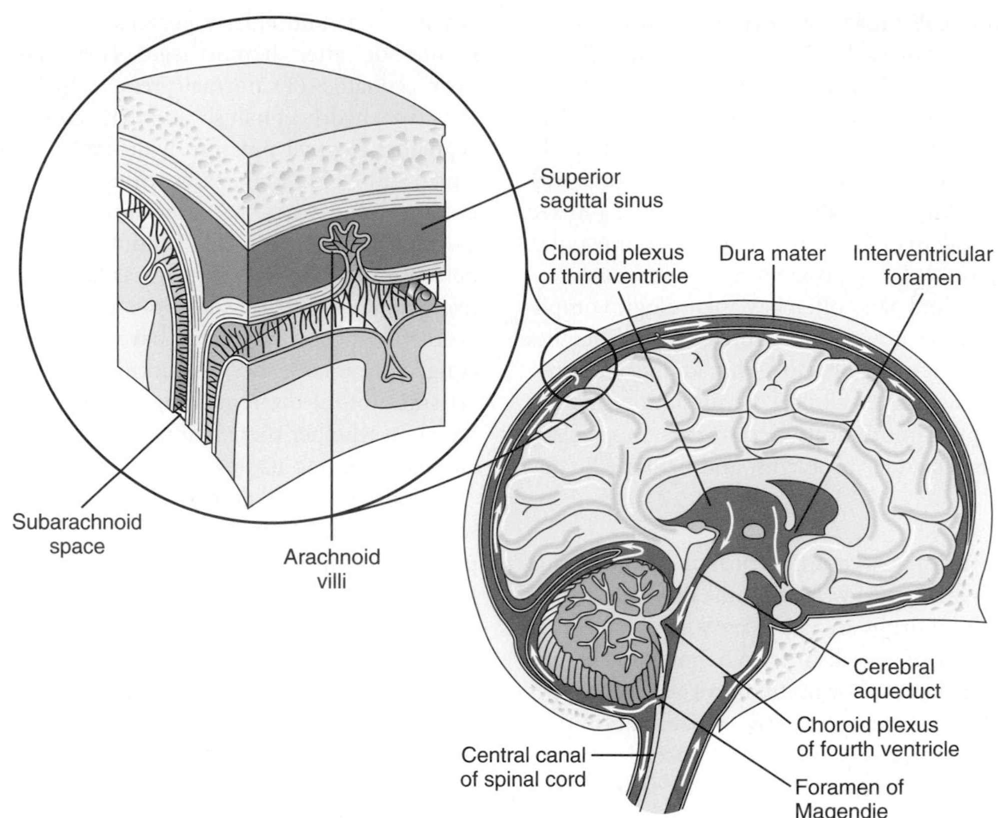

FIGURE 45-6 ■ The ventricular system of the brain and the distribution of the cerebrospinal fluid (CSF). CSF is formed in the ventricles, passes to the subarachnoid space outside the brain and spinal cord, and moves through small valvelike structures into the large veins of the head.

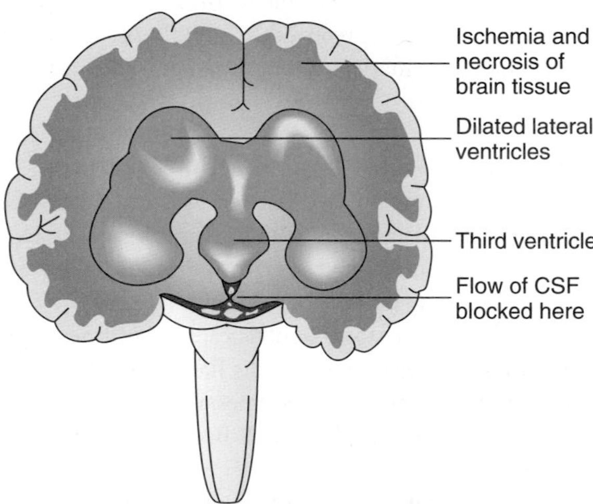

FIGURE 45-7 ■ Hydrocephalus. *CSF,* Cerebrospinal fluid. (From Gould BE: *Pathophysiology for the health professions,* ed 2, Philadelphia, 2002, Saunders, p 490.)

relieving hydrocephalus. The most effective treatment is surgical correction employing a shunting technique. The basic components of the shunt are a ventricular catheter, a valve, and a distal catheter. Multiple perforations along the ventricular catheter permit the drainage of fluid from the ventricle. The valve is constructed so that fluid will flow in one direction only, and some valves have a pumping chamber to facilitate drainage. The distal catheter may be positioned at any of a number of sites, the most common being the peritoneal cavity (ventriculoperitoneal shunt) (Figure 45-8). The shunt thus extends all the way from one of the ventricles to the peritoneal cavity where the fluid can then be absorbed and excreted.

It should be emphasized that the correlation between degree of hydrocephalus and impaired cognitive function often results from additional complications, such as severe congenital malformations, acute or chronic infections, or progressive brain tumors. Current research suggests that when treated successfully with shunting, two thirds of children with uncomplicated congenital hydrocephalus may have normal or nearly normal intellect.[38]

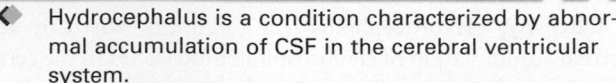

KEY CONCEPTS

- Hydrocephalus is a condition characterized by abnormal accumulation of CSF in the cerebral ventricular system.
- There are three types of hydrocephalus: normal-pressure hydrocephalus, due to an increased volume of CSF without change in CSF pressure; obstructive

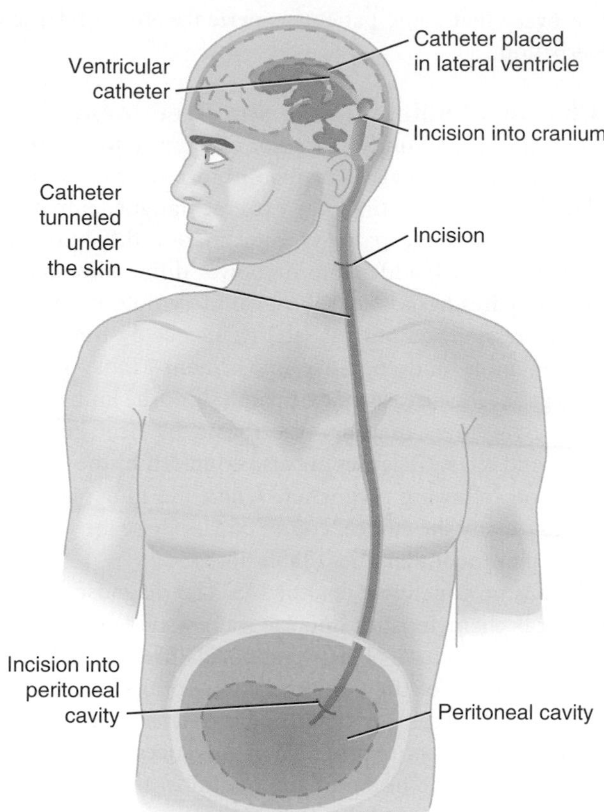

FIGURE 45-8 ■ Ventriculoperitoneal shunt placed for chronic hydrocephalus. (From Black JM, Hawks JH, Keene AM: *Medical-surgical nursing: clinical management for positive outcomes,* ed 6, Philadelphia, 2001, Saunders, p 2039.)

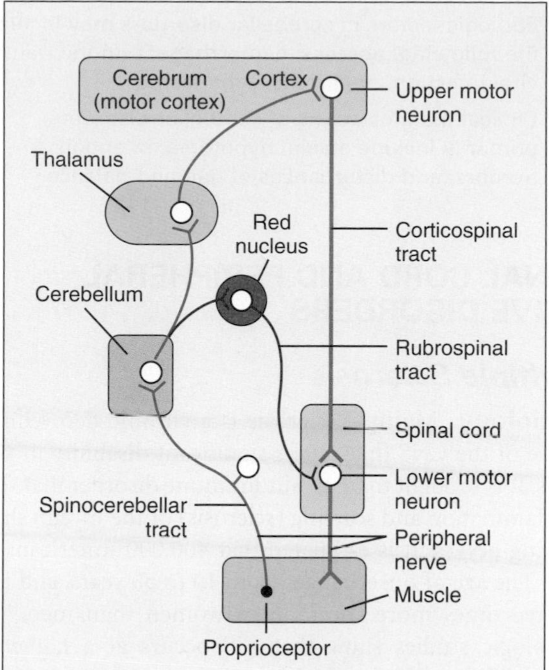

FIGURE 45-9 ■ The cerebrum and the cerebellum work together to control muscles. Impulses from the cerebrum travel simultaneously to skeletal muscle and to the cerebellum. The cerebellum compares the intended movement with the actual movement and sends impulses to both the cerebrum and the muscle tissue, coordinating and smoothing muscle activity. (From Thibodeau GA, Patton KT: Mechanisms of disease. In *Anatomy and physiology,* ed 4, St Louis, 2003, Mosby, p 388.)

hydrocephalus, due to an obstruction to the flow of CSF; and communicating hydrocephalus, in which absorption of CSF is abnormal.

- The most effective treatment for the latter two types of hydrocephalus is surgical correction employing a shunt.

Cerebellar Disorders

The cerebellum performs three general functions in the control of skeletal muscles: (1) together with activity of the cerebral cortex, it coordinates the activities of muscle groups to produce skilled movement; (2) it functions below the level of consciousness to maintain posture and make movements smooth, steady, efficient, and coordinated; and (3) it controls skeletal muscles to maintain balance (see Chapter 43). Figure 45-9 illustrates the cerebrum and cerebellum working together to coordinate muscle movement. Impulses from the motor control areas of the cerebrum travel down the corticospinal tract and through peripheral nerves to skeletal muscle tissue. Simultaneously, the impulses go to the cerebellum. The cerebellum compares the motor commands of the cerebrum to information coming from receptors in the muscle. In effect, the cerebellum compares the intended movement to the actual movement. Impulses then travel from the cerebellum to both the cerebrum and the muscle tissue to adjust or coordinate the movements to produce the intended action.[11]

Etiology and Clinical Manifestations. Cerebellar disorders may have myriad causes. Abscess, hemorrhage, tumors, trauma, viral infection, and chronic alcoholism have been implicated. Identification and eradication of the causal agent determines treatment and prognosis. The clinical manifestations of cerebellar disorders primarily include **ataxia** (muscle incoordination), hypotonia, intention tremors, and disturbances of gait and balance.[11] Disturbances of gait and balance vary, depending on the muscle groups involved. The walk, for instance, is often characterized by staggering or lurching and by a clumsy manner of raising the foot too high and bringing it down with a clap. Loss of cerebellar function does not result in paralysis.[11]

KEY CONCEPTS

- The cerebellum is responsible for coordinated control of muscle action, excitation and inhibition of postural reflexes, and maintenance of balance.

- Etiologic factors in cerebellar disorders may include the following: abscess, hemorrhage, tumors, trauma, viral infection, or chronic alcoholism.
- Clinical manifestations of cerebellar disorders primarily include ataxia, hypotonia, intention tremors, and disturbances of gait and balance.

SPINAL CORD AND PERIPHERAL NERVE DISORDERS

Multiple Sclerosis

Etiology. **Multiple sclerosis** is a chronic demyelinating disease of the CNS that causes significant disability in young adults. It is thought to be an autoimmune disorder that results in inflammation and scarring (sclerosis) of the myelin sheaths covering nerves. It is estimated that 400,000 Americans have MS.[39] The age of onset ranges from 10 to 50 years, and is two to three times more common in women than men.[11] Epidemiologic studies show that MS occurs at a higher rate among individuals from white northern European descent and those who live in northern latitudes (above the 37th parallel). Several studies indicate that those who were born and spent the early years of life (first 15 years) in northern areas carry an increased risk of MS even if they migrate south at some time later in their life.[40]

MS is an unpredictable disease with a wide variety of clinical presentations. Symptoms can vary from day to day, and the disease may cause only mild disability with occasional exacerbations. In some individuals, however, MS may cause extreme progressive disability. Despite great advances in research, the exact cause of MS is unknown. Genetics may have a role. About 15% of MS patients have an affected relative.[40] Certain histocompatibility antigens (human leukocyte antigens) are more prevalent in patients with MS.[37]

Pathogenesis. In MS, the **demyelination** of nerves can occur anywhere in the CNS. However, structures most frequently affected are the optic nerves, the oculomotor nerves, and the corticospinal, cerebellar, and posterior column systems. Figure 45-10 illustrates demyelination. Myelin facilitates nerve conduction; the inflammation and scarring that occurs with MS slows or interrupts the conduction of nerve impulses. The triggering event for this process is not understood. It is theorized, that an exposure to a viral infection or environmental toxin initiates the autoimmune attack in a genetically predisposed individual. Both humoral and cellular immune factors have been implicated in demyelination. Antibodies to specific myelin proteins have been found in both the serum and CSF of MS patients. T-cell lymphocyte–mediated damage to the myelin has also been implicated in causing the autoimmune damage and sustaining inflammation.[40] Some remyelination of the nerves may occur, but it is a slow process and provides only partial repair at best. This explains the partial recovery that some patients experience after a relapse or exacerbation.

Clinical Manifestations and Treatment. Symptoms of MS depend on the location of damage to the myelin but include impaired visual acuity or blurred vision, diplopia weakness, numbness, tingling, extreme fatigue, imbalance, movement disorders, spasticity, coordination difficulties and gait disturbance, bladder and/or bowel difficulties, vertigo, pain, and paresthesia. Neurobehavioral symptoms may include depression, emotional lability, sexual dysfunction, as well as memory and cognitive impairment (Table 45-2). In later stages of the disease, spastic paralysis of the limbs may be present. Symptoms may be exacerbated by heat, infection, trauma, and stress. Relapses are also common in the postpartum period following pregnancy.[5] There are four main categories to classify the clinical course of MS; these are also used to guide treatment therapies (Table 45-3).

There is no conclusive test for MS. The diagnosis is based on clinical characteristics and laboratory evidence. Clinical characteristics include objective abnormalities of CNS function in two parts of the CNS and a temporal sequence of at least two attacks that were remitting or relapsing in nature or followed a slow stepwise progression. Advances in neuroimaging techniques have become quite useful in the diagnosis of MS. MRI of the brain and spinal cord may show presence of

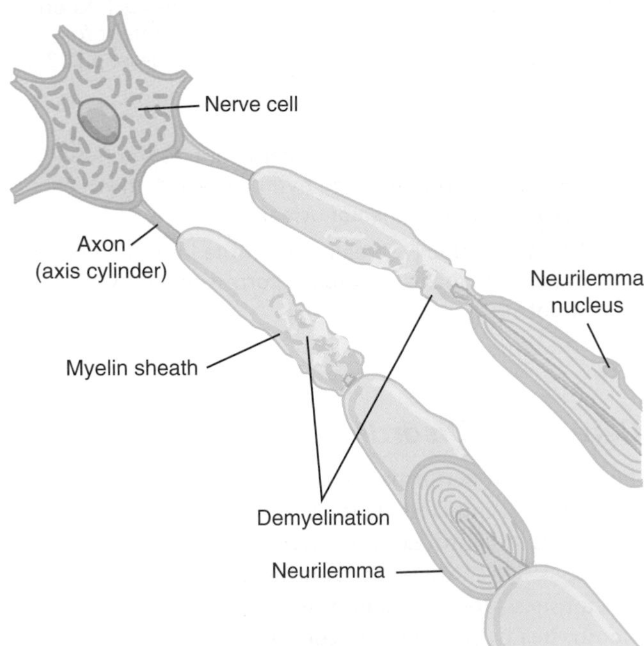

FIGURE 45-10 ■ Changes in the nerve sheath, as seen in multiple sclerosis. Myelin is made by the oligodendrocyte and coats nerves, facilitating nervous impulse. In clients with multiple sclerosis, the myelin degenerates in patches, causing nerve transmission to become erratic. (From Black JM, Hawks JH, Keene AM: *Medical-surgical nursing: clinical management for positive outcomes,* ed 6, Philadelphia, 2001, Saunders, p 2013.)

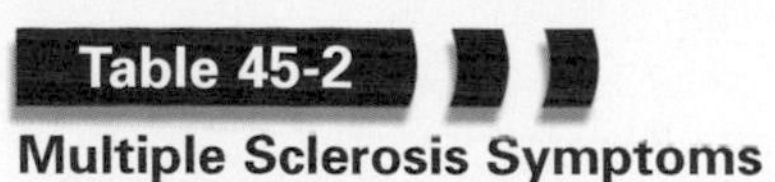

Multiple Sclerosis Symptoms

Area of Dysfunction	Symptoms
Cranial nerve dysfunction	Blurred central vision; faded colors; blind spots (optic neuritis)
	Diplopia
	Dysphagia
	Facial weakness, numbness, pain
Motor dysfunction	Weakness
	Paralysis
	Spasticity
	Abnormal gait
Sensory dysfunction	Paresthesias
	Lhermitte sign (electric shock–like sensation radiating down spine into extremities)
	Decreased proprioception
	Decreased temperature perception
Cerebellar dysfunction	Dysarthria
	Tremor
	Incoordination
	Ataxia
	Vertigo
Bowel and bladder dysfunction	Fecal urgency, constipation, incontinence
	Urinary frequency, urgency, hesitancy, nocturia, retention, incontinence
Cognitive dysfunction	Decreased short-term memory
	Difficulty learning new information
	Word-finding trouble
	Short attention span
	Decreased concentration
	Mood alterations (depression, euphoria)
Sexual dysfunction	Women: decreased libido, decreased orgasmic ability, decreased genital sensation
	Men: erectile, orgasmic, and ejaculatory dysfunction
Fatigue	Overwhelming weakness not overcome with increased physical effort

From Beare PG, Myers J: *Principles and practice of adult health nursing,* ed 3, St Louis, 1998, Mosby.

Table 45-3

Clinical Course and Treatments for Multiple Sclerosis

Course	Characteristics	Treatments
Relapsing-remitting		
Most common form; approximately 85% of MS patients have this form	Clearly defined exacerbations (relapses) with acute decline in neurologic function; followed by periods of partial/complete recovery and remissions; remissions may last months to years	Acute relapses: Methylprednisolone Interferon β1b (Betaseron) Interferon β1a (Avonex, Rebif) Glatiramer acetate (Copaxone) Immunoglobulin*
Primary-progressive		
Relatively rare; approximately 10% of MS patients have this form	Slow but almost continuous decline in neurologic function; plateaus or temporary minor improvements may occur; relapses/remissions not present; severe disability develops early	Interferon β1b (Betaseron)* Interferon β1a (Avonex, Rebif)* Bone marrow/stem cell transplantation*
Secondary-progressive		
Prior to use of disease-modifying drugs, approximately 50% of relapsing-remitting patients developed this form	Begins as relapsing-remitting followed by steady decline in neurologic function with or without occasional relapses, remissions, or plateaus	Mitoxantrone (Novantrone) Interferon β1a (Avonex, Rebif)* Bone marrow/stem cell transplantation*
Progressive-relapsing		
Relatively rare; approximately 5% of patients are affected by this form of MS	Progressive from the outset but with clear exacerbations with or without recovery	Mitoxantrone* (Novantrone) Cyclophosphamide (Cytoxan)* Methotrexate (Rheumatrex)* Azathioprine (Imuran)

Adapted from Rakel RE, Bope ET, editors: *Conn's current therapy,* Philadelphia, 2003, Elsevier; Tierney LM, McPhee SJ, Papadakis MA, editors: *Current medical diagnosis and treatment,* ed 42, New York, 2003, Lange; and 2003 National Multiple Sclerosis Society. *About MS.* Available at: www.nationalmssociety.org/What%20is%20MS.asp.
MS, Multiple sclerosis.
*Treatment not currently approved by the FDA for this indication; or currently in clinical trials.

demyelination (plaques). Evoked potential recording of nerve stimulation in the visual and other nerve pathways may be helpful. Laboratory tests may show mild lymphocytosis and elevated serum protein, especially following an acute relapse. Elevated immunoglobulin G (IgG) in the CSF with the presence of discrete bands of IgG (oligoclonal bands) may also be present.[5]

There is no cure for MS. Treatment centers not only on managing the symptoms of the disease but also at minimizing the damage inflicted by the autoimmune attack on myelin. Corticosteroids such as prednisone are used to reduce edema and the inflammatory response in acute exacerbations. Recovery may be hastened by the use of these agents; however, the extent of recovery is unchanged.[5] The use of immune-modulating medications such as interferon, glatiramer acetate (Copaxone), and immunosuppressive agents such as cyclophosphamide (Cytoxan) and methotrexate (Rheumatrex) may slow the progression of the disease.[5,41]

Management of symptoms frequently requires participation from multiple disciplines, including medicine, nursing, speech pathology, neuropsychiatry, social services, and vocational services. Treatment with an array of medications such as antispasmodics, anticholinergics, antidepressants, and antimicrobials helps to manage symptoms. Treatment also includes avoidance of complications such as urinary tract infections, constipation/impactions, respiratory infections, and pressure sores.

Research in MS continues to examine the immune system role. The lipid-lowering medications HMG-CoA inhibitors, otherwise known as statins, have been shown to decrease the number and size of plaques in patients with MS. These agents have some action against the immune cells responsible for demyelination.[42]

KEY CONCEPTS

- MS is a demyelinating disease of the CNS that primarily affects young adults. The risk of contracting MS is greater for persons living above the 37th parallel. The cause of MS is unknown, but immunologic abnormalities and environmental factors are suspected.
- Demyelination can occur throughout the CNS but most frequently affects the optic and oculomotor nerves and spinal nerve tracts.
- In most cases symptoms are slowly progressive, and the disease is marked by exacerbations and remissions.
- Symptoms include double vision, weakness, poor coordination, and sensory deficits. Bowel and bladder control may be lost. Memory impairment is common.
- Management is symptomatic. Short-term steroid therapy may be helpful during acute exacerbations, and immune-modifying drugs may slow the progression of symptoms.

Spina Bifida

Etiology and Pathogenesis. **Spina bifida** is a developmental anomaly characterized by defective closure of the bony encasement of the spinal cord (neural tube) through which the spinal cord and meninges may or may not protrude. If the anomaly is not visible, the condition is called *spina bifida occulta.* If there is an external protrusion of the saclike structure, the condition is called *spina bifida cystica* and is further classified according to the extent of neural involvement (e.g., meningocele, meningomyelocele, or myelomeningocele) (Figure 45-11).

Both environmental factors and genetics appear to be a factor in the etiologic development of neural tube defects.[11] However, in more than 50% of cases, the cause is unknown.[11] Known genetic and environmental factors include congenital rubella, the anticonvulsant drug valproic acid, and chromosomal abnormalities.[35] Substituting another anticonvulsant drug may be recommended for pregnant women or for those considering pregnancy. Supplementation of folic acid prior to conception also appears to decrease the prevalence of neural tube defects.

Clinical Manifestations. In spina bifida occulta, the posterior vertebral laminae have failed to fuse. The defect is extremely common and occurs to some degree in 10% to 25% of infants.[36] Approximately 80% of these vertebral defects are located in the lumbosacral regions, most commonly in the fifth lumbar vertebra and the first sacral vertebra, and may be detected prenatally through ultrasound and α-fetoprotein testing.

Spina bifida occulta may be manifested by changes in the skin and body hair: either very coarse or silky hair along the spine; a midline dimple with or without a sinus tract; a cutaneous port-wine angioma; and/or a subcutaneous mass typically representing a lipoma or dermoid cyst.[43] Spina bifida occulta usually causes no serious neurologic problems. Common lumbosacral defects can cause gait disturbances, positional deformities of the feet, or bladder/bowel dysfunction. These symptoms become evident in childhood during periods of rapid growth.

In the **meningocele** form of spina bifida cystica, a saclike cyst filled with CSF protrudes through the spinal defect but does not involve the spinal cord. Meningoceles occur with equal frequency in the cervical, thoracic, and lumbar areas. A **myelomeningocele** or **meningomyelocele** deformity contains meninges, CSF, and a portion of the spinal cord that protrudes from the vertebral defect in a cystlike sac. These defects most often occur in the lumbar or lumbosacral region of the spine as these are the last areas of the neural tube to close during fetal development.[43] These defects may be detected in prenatal ultrasound and with α-fetoprotein testing.[11] The bony prominences of the unfused neural arches are palpable at the lateral borders of the defect. The sac includes a transparent membranous covering that may have neural tissue attached to its inner surface. This membrane may be intact at birth or leak CSF,

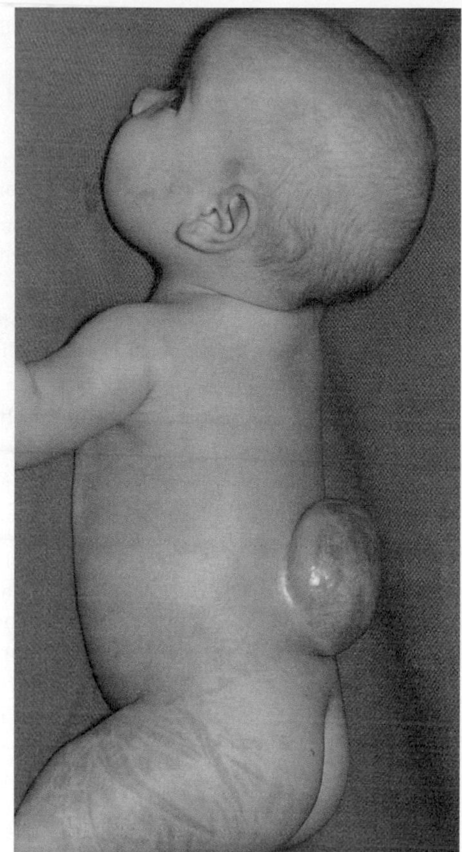

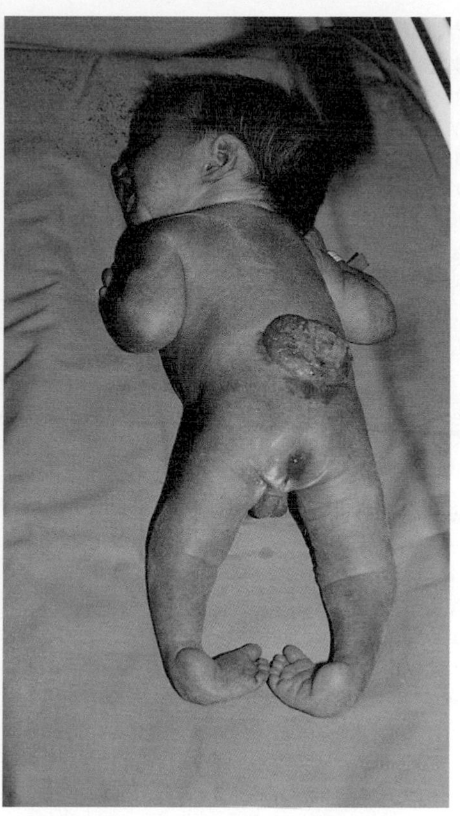

FIGURE 45-11 ■ Photographs of infants with spina bifida cystica. **A,** Spina bifida with meningomyelocele in the lumbar region. **B,** Spina bifida with myeloschisis in the lumbar region. Note that the nerve involvement has affected the lower limbs. (Courtesy Dr. Dwight Parkinson, Department of Surgery and Department of Human Anatomy and Cell Science, University of Manitoba, Winnipeg, Manitoba, Canada. In Moore KL, Persaud TVN: *The developing human: clinically oriented embryology,* ed 7, Philadelphia, 2003, Saunders, p 439.)

thereby increasing the risk of infection and neural damage. These infants are delivered via caesarean section to decrease the trauma to the exposed neural tissue, and surgical closure is attempted soon after delivery.[36] They often suffer from permanent neurologic damage resulting in motor weakness or paralysis and sensory deficit below the level of the spinal defect, bowel and bladder dysfunction, scoliosis, hydrocephalus, and seizures. Often the problems worsen as the child grows and the cord ascends within the vertebral canal, pulling primary scar tissue and thereby tethering the cord.[38]

Treatment. Treatment for this common disorder is based on the severity of the defect and neurologic dysfunction. The use of folic acid during the period prior to conception has been shown to significantly decrease the risk of having a child with a neural tube defect. It is recommended that all women of childbearing age take 0.4 mg folic acid daily for prevention. In fact, in the United States common foods are being supplemented with folic acid to decrease the incidence of this deformity.

KEY CONCEPTS

- Spina bifida is a developmental anomaly characterized by defective closure of the bony encasement of the spinal cord (neural tube) through which the spinal cord and meninges may or may not protrude.
- If the anomaly is not visible, the condition is called *spina bifida occulta.* If there is an external protrusion of the saclike structure, the condition is called spina *bifida cystica,* and is further classified according to extent of neural involvement (e.g., meningocele, myelomeningocele).
- The natural history of myelomeningocele supports an early and aggressive operative approach before significant clinical deterioration begins. A cesarean section before rupture of amniotic membranes and onset of labor may decrease the degree of paralysis.
- Folic acid supplementation taken before conception and during pregnancy appears to decrease the prevalence of neural tube defects.

Amyotrophic Lateral Sclerosis

Etiology and Pathogenesis. **Amyotrophic lateral sclerosis (ALS)** is a progressive degenerative disease affecting both the upper and lower motor neurons characterized by muscle wasting and atrophy of the hands, arms, and legs. ALS is also known as Lou Gehrig disease after the famed "Iron Man" of the New York Yankees who died from the disease. ALS is diagnosed in an estimated 5000 Americans each year. It most commonly strikes between the ages of 40 and 60 with a higher incidence in men than women. The majority of ALS cases occur at random; however, 5% to 10% of cases are familial.[44] Genetic research has determined at least four different genetic mutations responsible for causing ALS. One in particular involves a gene responsible for coding a free-radical–scavenging enzyme superoxide dismutase 1 (SOD1).[45] SOD1 is the basis for much ALS research, and there seems to be multiple intracellular enzymatic pathways affected causing premature programmed cell death, or **apoptosis** (see Chapter 4) of the neurons.[45] Like Alzheimer and Parkinson diseases, ALS has been linked with oxidative stress and cellular damage. Neurons are highly susceptible to damage from oxygen-free radicals and the activation of immune cells that propagate further cellular injury.[46] High levels of the neurotransmitter glutamate have also been found in the CSF of ALS patients and are thought to be associated with the neuronal degeneration.[44]

Clinical Manifestations and Treatment. Most patients with ALS demonstrate muscle weakness and atrophy. The earliest symptoms may be muscle twitching, cramping, and stiffness. Often the hands or upper extremities are affected first. The weakness is progressive and eventually affects the muscles that control speech, swallowing, and breathing. Most people die from respiratory failure within 3 to 5 years from the onset of symptoms.[44] Despite the marked physical disability, most patients maintain their sensory and cognitive functions.

ALS is a diagnosis of exclusion, based on the patient's clinical signs and symptoms. Electromyography (EMG), nerve conduction studies, MRI, and serum laboratory testing may be used to rule out other causes of weakness, such as MS, brain and spinal tumors, human immunodeficiency virus, and Lyme disease.

The only treatment for ALS is riluzole (Rilutek), a glutamate inhibitor. This medication is not a cure, but its use can prolong life for several months and may delay the need for mechanical ventilation.[11] Patients with ALS benefit from a multidisciplinary approach to care to prevent complications from immobility as well as to address both the physical and psychological needs of these patients.

KEY CONCEPTS

- ALS is a progressive disease affecting both the upper and lower motor neurons.
- The cause of ALS remains unknown. Weakness and wasting of the upper extremities usually occur, followed by impaired speech, swallowing, and respiration.
- The mean survival time is about 3 years from the time of diagnosis.
- ALS usually strikes between the ages of 40 and 60, and it is more common in men than women.
- Clinical manifestations include weakness, atrophy, cramps, stiffness, and irregular twitchings of muscle fibers.
- Diagnosis is based on clinical signs and symptoms, EMG, nerve conduction studies, MRI, and serum laboratory testing.
- Riluzole (Rilutek) is a glutamate inhibitor, which may be helpful in management of ALS.

Spinal Cord Injury

Spinal cord injuries are among the most devastating and costly problems faced by patients and their families. Marked changes in lifestyle are required for survivors. Medical advances in the emergent management of spinal cord injuries and their associated complications have been responsible for increasing survival rates. Continuing research is focused on minimizing the incidence of injury and the mortality/morbidity of spinal cord injury.

Etiology. Spinal cord injury is primarily a problem of the young. Sixty-five percent of patients are younger than 35, with the greatest incidence between the ages of 20 and 24. Males are three to four times more likely to have suffered a spinal cord injury, and these injuries are most common on the weekends and during the summer months.[11]

Motor vehicle crashes contribute the highest number of spinal cord injuries, followed by violence (primarily gunshot wounds), followed by falls and recreational accidents.[11] Other

Box 45-2

ASIA Impairment Scale

- ☐ **A** = Complete: No motor or sensory function is preserved in the sacral segments S4-S5.
- ☐ **B** = Incomplete: Sensory but not motor function is preserved below the neurological level and includes the sacral segments S4-S5.
- ☐ **C** = Incomplete: Motor function is preserved below the neurological level, and more than half of key muscles below the neurological level have a muscle grade less than 3.
- ☐ **D** = Incomplete: Motor function is preserved below the neurological level, and at least half of key muscles below the neurological level have a muscle grade of 3 or more.
- ☐ **E** = Normal: Motor and sensory function are normal.

From American Spinal Injury Association: http://www.asia-spinalinjury.org/publications/2001_Classif_worksheet.pdf.

causes of spinal cord injuries include birth injuries, herniated intravertebral disk, or bone spurs related to degenerative changes of aging and osteoporosis. Injuries to the spinal cord are classified by level, degree (complete or incomplete), and mechanism of injury (Box 45-2).

Pathogenesis. Spinal cord injury results from compression (tumor, hematoma, or bony encroachment) and from blunt trauma causing contusion or penetration/transection of neural tissue. The major mechanisms of injury are hyperflexion, hyperextension, and compression (Figure 45-12). Flexion

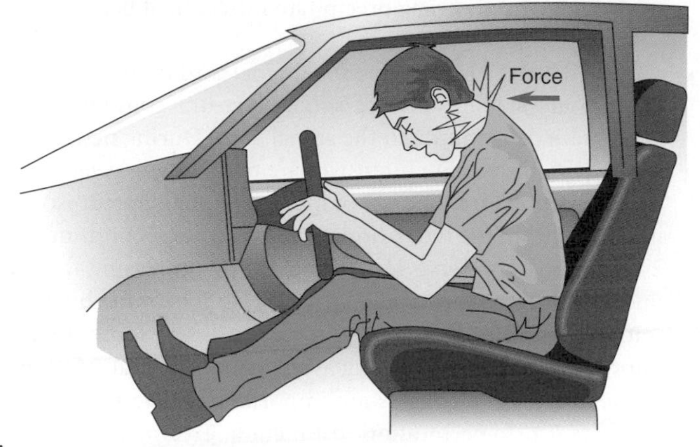

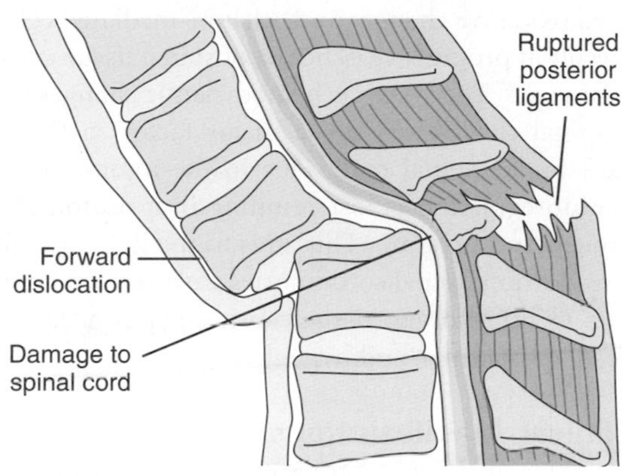

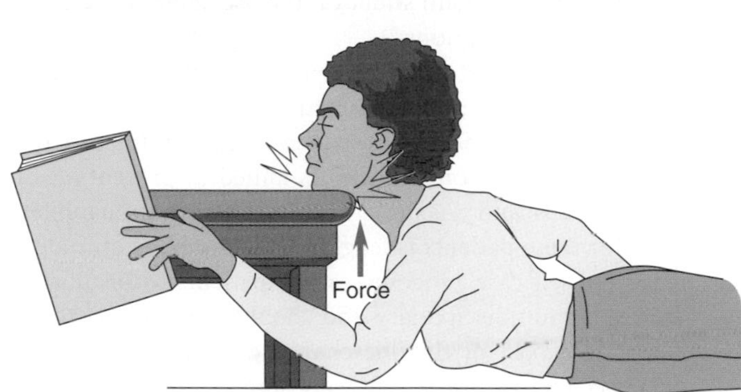

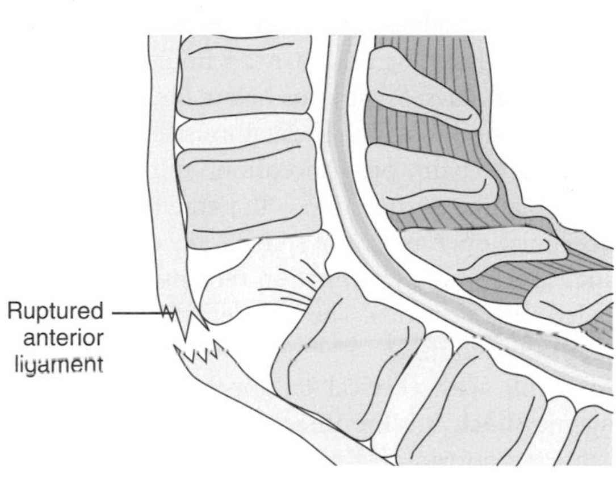

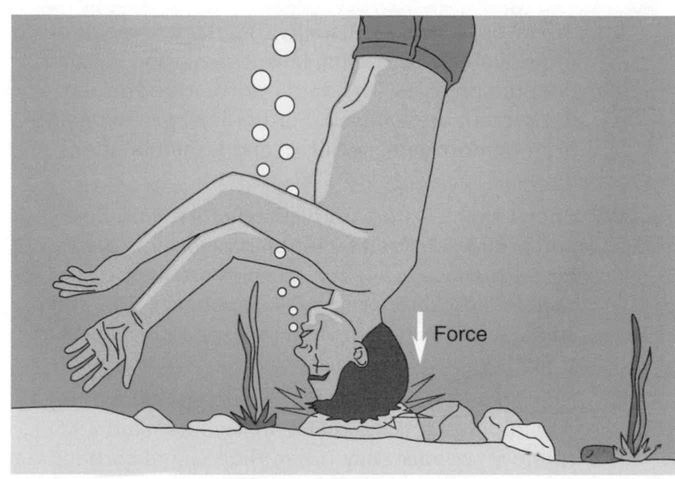

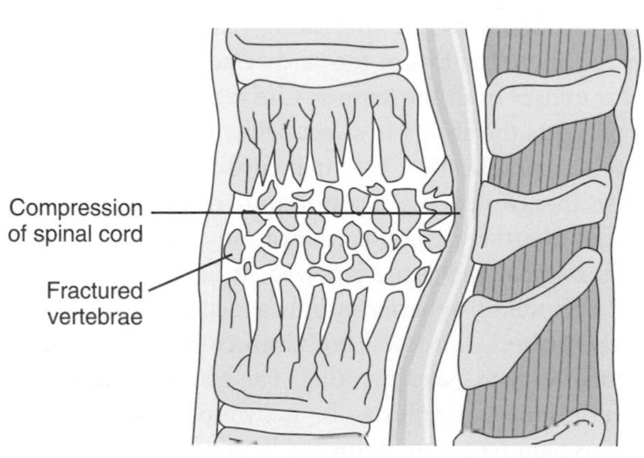

FIGURE 45-12 ■ Mechanisms of spinal cord injury. Many situations may produce these consequences. This figure shows examples only. **A,** Flexion injury of the cervical spine ruptures the posterior ligaments. **B,** Hyperextension injury of the cervical spine ruptures the anterior ligaments. **C,** Compression fractures crush the vertebrae and force bony fragments into the spinal canal.

injury with tearing of the posterior ligaments and dislocation is the most unstable injury and is often associated with severe neurologic deficits. Hyperextension injury is the most common. Aside from the primary injury to the spinal cord, damage also results from secondary injury. The primary trauma triggers a complex cascade of events involving free-radical–induced oxidative changes and calcium-mediated cell changes that result in progressive ischemia of spinal tissue causing further damage.[47] The systemic hemodynamic changes that occur after spinal cord injury are a major factor in the resulting damage to the spinal cord. Due to the injury to the spinal cord, autoregulation is lost resulting in a profound drop in systemic blood pressure. This adds to the ischemia of the tissue. In addition, spinal cord injuries are often accompanied by trauma to other organ tissue causing hypoxia, hypotension, hyper-/hypothermia, and hypoglycemia.

Clinical Manifestations. Immediately following injury to the spinal cord, there is complete loss of function below the level of injury. This may occur even in incomplete injuries to the spinal cord, causing the injury to appear more severe than it actually is. This phenomenon, known as **spinal shock,** usually lasts for less than 24 hours but occasionally lasts for several days. Symptoms below the level of injury include flaccid paralysis of all skeletal muscles; loss of all spinal reflexes; loss of pain, proprioception, and other sensations; bowel and bladder dysfunction with paralytic ileus; and loss of thermoregulation. A return of spinal reflexes indicates the end of spinal shock. As reflex function returns, spastic paraplegia or quadriplegia develops. The bladder and bowel may regain some reflex function.[5]

In patients with cervical or upper thoracic cord injury, **neurogenic shock** is a life-threatening complication. Neurogenic shock is a form of distributive shock caused by the loss of brainstem and higher center control of the sympathetic nervous system. The loss of sympathetic outflow results in hypotension caused by peripheral vasodilation. Bradycardia occurs (secondary to the overriding parasympathetic influence), and there is a loss of the cardiac accelerator reflex. The loss of impulses from the temperature regulatory center in the brain prevents the ability to sweat below the level of injury.

Another complication of spinal cord injuries occurring at or above the T6 vertebra is **autonomic dysreflexia.** This is a potentially life-threatening complication that may occur any time after spinal shock has resolved. It is characterized by a sudden episode of hypertension, headache, bradycardia, upper body flushing and lower body vasoconstriction, piloerection (goose bumps), and sweating. The usual stimulus initiating autonomic dysreflexia is activation of visceral or cutaneous pain receptors below the level of injury. A full bladder or constipation is a common cause.

Stimulation of afferent pain receptors causes activation of sympathetic efferents in the cord and reflex vasoconstriction. Sustained activation of sympathetic neurons below the level of cord injury increases blood pressure significantly. The hypertension initiates the baroreceptor response. Baroreceptors mediate inhibition of heart rate and vasodilation of vessels above the level of injury. This is responsible for the upper body flushing. Descending signals from the brain cannot pass the cord injury, so inhibition of sympathetic neurons below the level of injury does not occur. Blood pressure may be dangerously high, and this may precipitate intracranial hemorrhage.

Treatment. Management of spinal cord injuries includes appropriate stabilization of spinal vertebra components to prevent further trauma to the spinal cord. During neurogenic shock, patients require intensive care to maintain oxygenation and blood pressure. The use of high-dose methylprednisolone initiated within the first 8 hours after injury and continued for 24 hours may preserve some function by decreasing the secondary injury to the spinal cord.[5,48] The benefit of this medication is modest at best, but at least it offers some hope of improving function. Ongoing assessment is critical. Methodical neurologic evaluations are important in determining improvement or deterioration in function. Treatment for autonomic dysreflexia includes removing or alleviating the painful stimulus, and in certain situation the use of adrenergic receptor blocking medications.

Individuals suffering from spinal cord injuries are at high risk for respiratory and urinary tract infection, skin pressure sores, septicemia, and fecal impaction. Much of the care of patients with spinal cord injuries is aimed at preventing these complications and maximizing function. The rehabilitation phase for these patients is lengthy with emphasis on independence and self-care. Ongoing care of patients with spinal cord injuries is multidisciplinary and should also address the psychosocial impact of this life-changing event. Level of injury and expected functional ability are summarized in Table 45-4.

KEY CONCEPTS

- Spinal cord injury is usually traumatic, a result of motor vehicle accidents, falls, penetrating wounds, or sports injuries. The cord may be compressed, transected, or contused. Further injury may result from hemorrhage, swelling, and ischemia after injury.
- Spinal shock occurs immediately following injury and is characterized by temporary loss of reflexes below the level of injury. Muscles are flaccid, and skeletal and autonomic reflexes are lost. The end of spinal shock is noted when reflexes return and flaccidity is replaced by spasticity.
- Neurogenic shock may occur after spinal cord injury due to peripheral vasodilation. Hypotension and circulatory collapse may occur. High spinal cord injuries may also affect respiratory muscles, leading to ventilatory failure.
- Autonomic dysreflexia is an acute reflexive response to sympathetic activation below the level of injury.

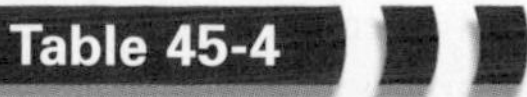

Table 45-4

Levels of Injury and Expected Functional Ability

Level	Normal Activity	Functional Expectation
C4	Head control Mouth control Shoulder/scapular movement Diaphragm movement	Adaptive devices (i.e., mouthstick) for phone, reading/computer Total dependence for transfers/ADLs Pulmonary toileting concerns; skin care issues
C5	Shoulder flexion Elbow flexion Increased scapular motion	Self feeding with adaptive devices; able to move wheelchair short distances, electric wheelchair preferred; ADLs and bed mobility with assistance; pulmonary toileting assistance
C6	Good elbow flexion Wrist extension Shoulder rotation and abduction	Independent with grooming/feeding with adaptive devices; weak hand grasp; can roll over in bed; drive with car adaptations; transfers with assistance; self propel wheelchair
C7	Elbow extension Strong wrist extension Good shoulder movement	Transfers to wheelchair independently; most ADLs independently, excellent bed mobility
T1	Normal hand strength Normal upper body strength	Bed and wheel chair independent; performs self catheterization
T10	Normal strength/motion above umbilicus	May stand for exercise with braces; still wheelchair dependent for ambulation
L2-5	Some leg and thigh movement	Ambulate indoors with braces/canes
Sacral segments	Mild weakness in lower extremities	Ambulation with braces/canes; still significant bowel/bladder dysfunction

ADLs, Activities of daily living.

Visceral stimulation (full bladder or bowel) and activation of pain receptors below the injury are common initiating stimuli. Manifestations include hypertension, bradycardia, flushing above the level of injury, and clammy skin below the level of injury. Prompt removal of the offending stimulus is indicated.

Guillain-Barré Syndrome

Etiology and Pathogenesis. **Guillain-Barré syndrome,** also known as acute idiopathic polyneuropathy or polyradiculoneuropathy, is an inflammatory demyelinating disease of the *peripheral* nervous system. Between 0.6 and 1.9 cases per 100,000 population occur annually, with an increasing incidence in the aging population.[11] It is one of the most common causes of nontraumatic paralysis in the Western world.[30] There is an equal gender distribution.[11]

The cause of Guillain-Barré syndrome is not well understood, but it sometimes follows an infection, inoculation, or surgical procedure 1 to 8 weeks prior to the onset of signs and symptoms.[37] *Campylobacter jejuni* enteritis has been associated with the syndrome.[5] The basis for Guillain-Barré syndrome is probably immunologic, but the exact mechanism is unknown. There is segmental demyelination, and most evidence suggests that this damage is T cell and B cell mediated. Aggregates of lymphocytes are found at the sites of demyelination. This process slows or stops nerve conduction. Primarily motor neurons are affected, but sensory nerves may also be involved.

Clinical Manifestations and Treatment. Patients with Guillain-Barré syndrome have progressive ascending weakness or paralysis. It usually begins in the legs, spreading often to the arms and face. The respiratory muscles may also be affected. The severity and extent of neurologic deficit may vary greatly between patients. Most patients reach the peak of disability in 10 to 14 days. Sensory nerves may also be affected but to a lesser extent than motor neurons. Patients often experience paresthesia or dysesthesia; neuropathic pain may also be present. During this time, patients may demonstrate loss of autonomic regulation, with consequent changes in blood pressure and heart rhythm, and may require intensive care for ventilatory and circulatory support.

Diagnosis of Guillain-Barré syndrome is made through patient history, physical examination, and nerve conduction studies. The CSF characteristically contains high protein concentrations. Other laboratory studies and imaging are used to rule out other causes for neurologic dysfunction.

The majority of patients experience spontaneous recovery; however, 10% to 20% of patients may be left with a mild disability.[30] Gradually, neurologic function returns, often in a descending pattern. Treatment within 14 days of onset of symptoms with plasmapheresis, especially in those with severe or rapidly progressing symptoms, has been shown to have some value. Intravenous immunoglobulin is also helpful.[5] Nursing care of these patients is aimed at preventing complications of immobility.

KEY CONCEPTS

- Guillain-Barré syndrome is characterized by muscle weakness that begins in the lower extremities and spreads to the proximal spinal neurons.
- The cause is unknown; however, a postinfectious immunologic mechanism is suspected.
- Treatment is supportive, and spontaneous recovery usually occurs.

Bell Palsy

Etiology and Pathogenesis. **Bell palsy** is an acute idiopathic paresis or paralysis of the facial nerve involving an inflammatory reaction at or near the stylomastoid foramen or in the bony facial canal.[5] The incidence peaks at age 60.[49] There is mounting evidence that Bell palsy is caused by viral infection. Antibodies to the herpes simplex and herpes zoster virus have been found in patients with Bell palsy.[49]

Clinical Manifestations and Treatment. Symptoms of Bell palsy develop rapidly over 24 to 48 hours. Physical examination shows unilateral facial weakness with facial droop and diminished eye blink, **hyperacusis,** and decreased lacrimation (Figure 45-13). Patients may complain of a heavy sensation in their face as well as a decreased sense of taste, but sensation of the face is generally intact. Posterior auricular pain may be present.[49] In the diagnosis of Bell palsy, other causes of facial paralysis, such as bacterial infection (otitis media), tumor, trauma, and cerebrovascular accident (stroke), must be ruled out. MRI, CT, and EMG can be helpful in certain situations. Laboratory testing is of limited value.

Management of Bell palsy is controversial. Most patients recover complete facial nerve function spontaneously within approximately 3 weeks. However, approximately 15% of patients are left with some level of residual disability.[49] Patients with the poorest prognosis for complete recovery are those older than 60, those with diabetes, and individuals who have had symptoms lasting longer than 3 months.[30] Prevention of corneal damage due to the inability of the eye to close is vital. Lubricating drops, ointments, and nighttime eye patching may be necessary. The use of corticosteroids has been shown to improve the likelihood of complete recovery. Due to the association of viruses with Bell palsy, some sources recommend the use of antiviral medications such as acyclovir. Studies regarding the use of these medications have shown inconsistent results.[49] Surgical decompression of the nerve has not been shown to confer great benefit.[30]

KEY CONCEPTS

- Bell palsy, or neuropathy of the facial nerve, results in paralysis of the muscles on one side of the face. Often a self-limiting condition with unknown cause, Bell palsy may last only a few days or weeks.
- Treatment is supportive, and spontaneous recovery usually occurs.

SUMMARY

A traumatic event, such as a spinal cord injury, or a chronic neurologic disease, such as dementia, can transform an individual from a relatively healthy state to one of almost complete dependence. At best, some of the neurologic states described in this chapter may resolve spontaneously or require

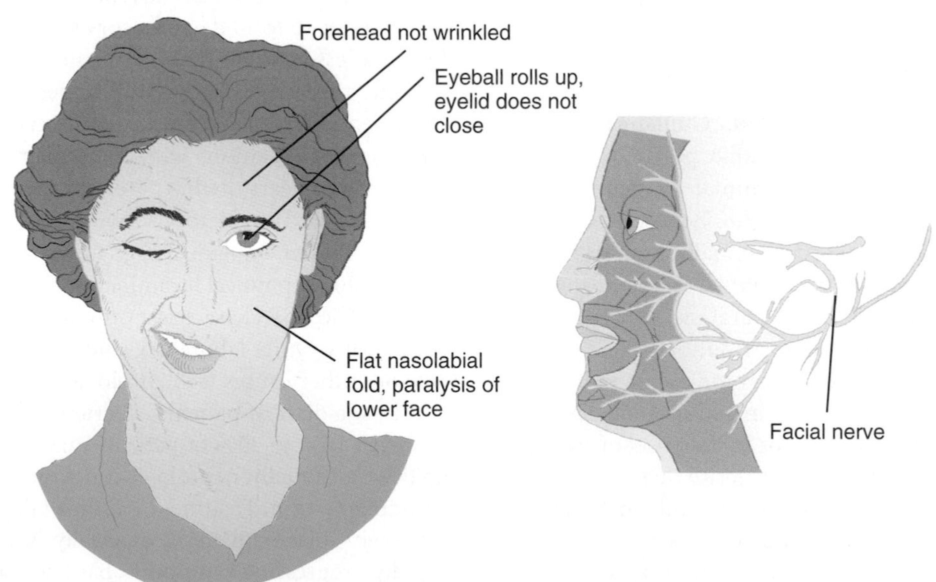

FIGURE 45-13 ■ Bell palsy. Location of the branches of the facial nerve (cranial nerve VII) corresponds to the areas of peripheral facial paralysis. (From Black JM, Hawks JH, Keene AM: *Medical-surgical nursing: clinical management for positive outcomes,* ed 6, Philadelphia, 2001, Saunders, p 1996.)

only minor lifestyle adjustment, but more commonly, chronic neurologic conditions require lifetime rehabilitation.

The process of life care planning includes taking stock of current health status, future health care concerns, appropriate resources, and associated costs to address lifelong disability and illness management.

In general, the goal of rehabilitation is to increase self-care and promote a meaningful lifestyle that incorporates the neurologic disability. The primary goal of such tertiary prevention is to help the affected individual maintain the highest possible level of wellness.

MEDIA RESOURCES

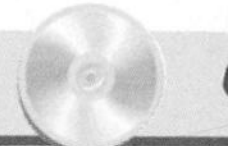

evolve

Remember to check out the ***CD Companion*** included with this book for Review Questions, Key Concepts Review, Glossary (with audio for selected terms), Disease Profiles, and Animations.

PLUS, visit the ***Evolve website*** at http://evolve.elsevier.com/Copstead/ for Case Studies, Disease Profiles, and WebLinks.

References

1. 2003 National Vital Statistics Report website. Available at: http://www.cdc.gov/nchs/data/nvsr/nvsr50.nvsr50_/5.pdf.
2. National Institute of Neurological Disorders and Stroke Epilepsy Information Page website. Available at: http://www.ninds.gov/health_and_medical/disorders/epilepsy.htm.
3. Green-Hernandez C, Singleton JK, editors: *Primary care pediatrics,* Philadelphia, 2001, Lippincott.
4. Marshall S et al: *Neuroscience critical care,* Philadelphia, 1990, Saunders.
5. Tierney LM, McPhee SJ, Papadakis MA, editors: *Current medical diagnosis and treatment,* ed 42, New York, 2003, Lange.
6. Fisher RS, Handforth A: Reassessment: vagus nerve stimulation for epilepsy, *Neurology* 52:666-669, 1999.
7. Bolla LR, Filley CM, Palmer RM: Dementia DDx: office diagnosis of the four major types of dementia, *Geriatrics* 55(1): 34-46, 2000.
8. Tsuang DW, Bird TD: Genetics in dementia, *Med Clin North Am* 86:591-614, 2002.
9. Glaser V: Alzheimer's disease: strategies for early diagnosis, *Patient Care Nurse Pract* 4(2):12-22, 2001.
10. Blackwell J: Alzheimer's disease management, *J Am Acad Nurse Pract* 14(8):338-340, 2002.
11. Rowland LP, editor: *Merritt's neurology,* ed 10, Philadelphia, 2000, Lippincott Williams & Wilkins.
12. Aisen PS et al: A randomized controlled trial of prednisone in Alzheimer's disease, *Neurology* 54:588-592, 2000.
13. Geldmacher DS, editor: *Treatment of dementia in the new millennium, summation of proceedings of the First Annual Dementia Congress,* New York, 2002, Academy for Healthcare Education.
14. Cummings JL: Alzheimer's disease, *N Engl J Med* 351(1):56-67, 2004.
15. Bonner LT, Peskind ER: Pharmacologic treatments of dementia, *Med Clin North Am* 86:657-674, 2002.
16. Kukall WA, Bowen JD: Dementia epidemiology, *Med Clin North Am* 86:573-590, 2002.
17. Green RC et al: Risk of dementia among white and African-American relatives of patients with Alzheimer disease, *JAMA* 287(3):329-335, 2002.
18. Seshari S et al: Plasma homocysteine as a risk factor for dementia and Alzheimer's disease, *N Engl J Med* 346(7):476-483, 2002.
19. Hines SE: Alzheimer's disease: contemporary drug treatment, *Patient Care Nurse Pract* 4(2):23-34, 2001.
20. Cummings JL et al: Guidelines for managing Alzheimer's disease: part II, *Am Fam Physician* 67(12):2525-2534, 2002.
21. Román GC: Vascular dementia revisited: diagnosis, pathogenesis, treatment and prevention, *Med Clin North Am* 86:477-499, 2002.
22. Tariot PN et al: Memantine treatment in patients with moderate to severe Alzheimer disease already receiving donepezil, *JAMA* 291(3):317-324, 2004.
23. Reisberg BR et al: Memantine in moderate-to-severe Alzheimer's disease, *N Engl J Med* 348(14):1333-1341, 2003.
24. Mulnard RA et al: Estrogen replacement therapy for the treatment of mild to moderate Alzheimer's disease: a randomized trial, *JAMA* 283(8):1007-1015, 2000.
25. Anthony JC et al: Reduced prevalence of AD in users of NSAIDs and H_2 receptor antagonists: the Cache County study, *Neurology* 54:2066-2071, 2000.
26. Mackenzie I: Anti-inflammatory drugs and Alzheimer's type pathology in aging, *Neurology* 54:732-734, 2000.
27. Solomon PR et al: Ginkgo for memory enhancement: a randomized controlled trial, *JAMA* 288(7):835-840, 2002.
28. Fassbender K et al: Effects of statins on human cerebral cholesterol metabolism and secretion of Alzheimer amyloid protein, *Neurology* 59(8):1257-1258, 2002.
29. Jick H et al: Statins and the risk of dementia, *Lancet* 356: 1627-1631, 2000.
30. Rakel RE, Bope ET: *Conn's current therapy,* Philadelphia, 2003, Saunders.
31. Chapuis T: Parkinson's disease manifestations and management, *Clin Rev* 12(2):63-69, 2002.
32. Siderowf A, Stern M: Update on Parkinson disease, *Ann Intern Med* 138(8):651-657, 2003.
33. Yoshida H et al: Stereotactic transplantation of dopamine-producing capsule in the striatum for treatment of Parkinson's disease: a preclinical primate study, *J Neurosurg* 98(4):874-881, 2003.
34. Muller T et al: Coenzyme Q_{10} supplement provides mild symptomatic benefit in patients with Parkinson's disease. *Neurosci Lett* 341(3):201-204, 2003.
35. Hay WW et al, editors: *Current pediatric diagnosis and treatment,* ed 15, New York, 2001, Lange/McGraw-Hill.
36. McCance KL, Huether SE, editors: *Pathophysiology: the biologic basis for disease in adults and children,* ed 4, St Louis, 2002, Mosby.
37. Ignatavicius DD, Workman ML, editors: *Medical-surgical nursing: critical thinking for collaborative care,* ed 4, Philadelphia, 2002, Saunders.
38. Jackson PL, Vessey JA, editors: *Primary care of a child with a chronic condition,* ed 3, St Louis, 2000, Mosby.
39. Multiple sclerosis: an overview website. Available at: http://www.mayoclinic.com/invoke.cfm?id=DS00188.
40. Victor M, Ropper AH, editors: *Adams and Victor's principles of neurology,* ed 7, New York, 2001, McGraw-Hill.

41. Halper J: Multiple sclerosis care: meeting the patient's clinical needs, *Clin Rev* 12(5):65-72, 2002.
42. Neuhaus O et al: Statins as immune modulators: comparison with interferon β1b in MS, *Neurology* 59:990-997, 2002.
43. Behrman RE, Kliegman RM, Jenson HB, editors: *Nelson's textbook of pediatrics,* ed 16, Philadelphia, 2000, Saunders.
44. National Institute of Neurological Disorders and Stroke Amyotrophic Lateral Sclerosis website. Available at http://www.ninds.nih.gov/health_and_medical/pubs/als.htm.
45. Guegan C, Przedborski S: Programmed cell death in amyotrophic lateral sclerosis, *J Clin Invest* 111:153-161, 2003.
46. Ischiropoulos H, Beckman JS: Oxidative stress and nitration in neurodegeneration: cause, effect or association, *J Clin Invest* 111:163-169, 2003.
47. Hockberger RS, Hirshenbaum KJ: Spine. In Marx JA et al, editors: *Rosen's emergency medicine: concepts and clinical practice,* vol 1, St Louis, 2002, Mosby.
48. Hugenholtz H: Commentary: methylprednisolone for acute spinal cord injury—not a standard of care, *Can Med Assoc J* 168(9):1145, 2003.
49. Karnath B: Bell's palsy: update on causes, recognition, management, *Consultant* 43(5):601-605, 2003.

Alterations in Special Sensory Function

chapter 46

Joni D. Nelsen-Marsh

MEDIA RESOURCES

Additional Material for Study, Review, and Further Exploration

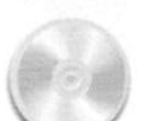

CD Companion ◆ Review Questions and Answers ◆ Key Concepts Review
◆ Glossary *(with audio pronunciations for selected terms)*
◆ Disease Profiles ◆ Animations

evolve ***Website*** at http://evolve.elsevier.com/Copstead/
◆ Case Studies ◆ Disease Profiles ◆ WebLinks

KEY QUESTIONS

- What are the general manifestations of hearing impairment?
- How do conductive and sensorineural mechanisms of hearing loss differ in cause and treatment?
- What are the predisposing factors, clinical manifestations, and management of otitis media?
- What are the general manifestations of visual impairment?
- What are the causes, clinical manifestations, and management of common visual disorders, including errors of refraction, strabismus, cataract, and retinopathies?
- How do open-angle and closed-angle glaucoma differ?
- How do the two forms of macular degeneration differ?

CHAPTER OUTLINE

The human body has countless sense organs that fall into two main categories: general sense organs and special sense organs. By far the most numerous are the general sense organs or receptors. The receptors function to produce the general or somatic senses. Examples of these senses are touch, temperature, and pain, and the receptors initiate various reflexes necessary for maintaining homeostasis (see Chapter 43). The largest general sense organ in the body is the skin.

Special sense organs, by comparison, function to produce the unique sensations of hearing, balance, vision, smell, and taste. These senses allow humans to interact with their environment in a meaningful way.

Alterations in sensory function may be acute or progressive and may result from such factors as genetics, disease, infection, trauma, and normal aging. Alterations in special sensory function require prompt assessment, evaluation, and treatment from appropriate health professionals. Equally important is an assessment of how the sensory impairment affects the individual's daily functioning. This chapter discusses special sensory function with regard to physiologic process, sensory impairment, and the diagnosis and management of such impairment.

HEARING AND BALANCE

STRUCTURE AND FUNCTION OF THE EAR

External Ear

Hearing results from normal functioning of several complex structures both external and internal to the body. Sound consists of waves of vibrations in the air produced in the environment. These vibrations travel much like ripples in a pool of water. Externally, these vibrations are caught and funneled into the ear canal by the auricles (Figure 46-1). Even though the auricles are in a fixed position and lie close to the head, they concentrate sound waves, especially high-frequency waves. The auricles also have an important role in sound localization.

The ear canal has a somewhat "S" shape from its opening to its termination at the tympanic membrane. This configuration affords both protection from airborne foreign objects and access to sound. The outer portion of the ear canal grows hair to filter out unwanted substances. Along the ear canal are also glands that secrete cerumen. This brown, waxlike substance coats the hairs in the canal to help prevent the entrance of foreign bodies into the ear canal. After entering the ear canal, sound waves strike the tympanic membrane (eardrum) and cause it to vibrate. The tympanic membrane is a thin, elastic membrane that is very sensitive to changes in pressure.

Middle Ear

The middle ear functions primarily as a structure by which sound energy is transmitted from the air to the fluids of the inner ear. The tympanic membrane is connected to the first of the **ossicles,** the malleus (hammer), followed by the incus (anvil) and stapes (stirrup). The middle ear is a bony, air-containing space. The ossicles further amplify the sound waves and then, along with the tympanic membrane, transfer airborne sound waves to the fluid-filled inner ear at the oval window.

The eustachian tube is also part of the middle ear, and although it does not contribute directly to the transmission of sound through the ear, absence of proper function can greatly affect hearing. This tube has a mucosal lining and extends downward, forward, and inward from the middle ear cavity to the nasopharynx. It makes equalization of pressure against the inner and outer surfaces of the tympanic membrane possible and therefore prevents the membrane rupture and discomfort that marked pressure differences produce.[1]

Inner Ear

The inner ear is composed of the oval window, the cochlea, and the semicircular canals. Within the cochlea are three parallel tubes: the scala vestibuli, the scala media, and the scala tympani. Movement of perilymph through the scala vestibuli and the scala tympani is eventually dissipated by movement of the round window (Figure 46-2). The scala tympani and the scala vestibuli are continuous with one another at the apex of the cochlea through an opening called the *helicotrema.* Perilymph, the fluid contained in the scala tympani and the scala vestibuli, is much like cerebrospinal fluid.

Transmission of the sound stimulus from the scala vestibuli to the vestibular membrane results in displacement of the endolymph, the fluid contained in the membranous labyrinth of the scala media and the basilar membrane. The organ of Corti, which contains the receptors for hearing, lies on the basilar membrane. Perilymph and endolymph transmit the mechanical vibrations from the footplate of the stapes to the organ of Corti. Endolymph also transports nutrients to the organ of Corti. No direct communication between endolymph and perilymph is normally present.

The organ of Corti consists of a series of sensory hair cells and supporting cells. The hair cells are innervated by the sensory fibers from the vestibulocochlear nerve (cranial nerve VIII). Overhanging the organ of Corti is a flexible flap of tissue called the *tectorial membrane* (Figure 46-3). Hairs of the sensory cells of the organs of Corti are in contact with the tec-

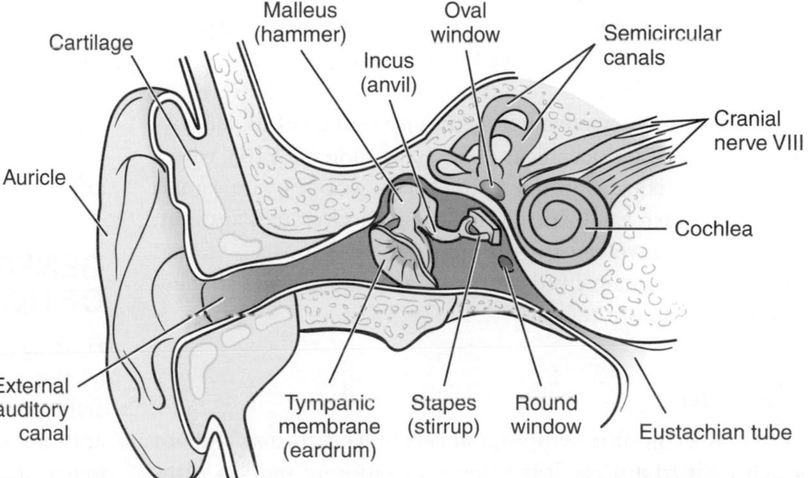

FIGURE 46-1 ■ Anatomic structures of the ear.

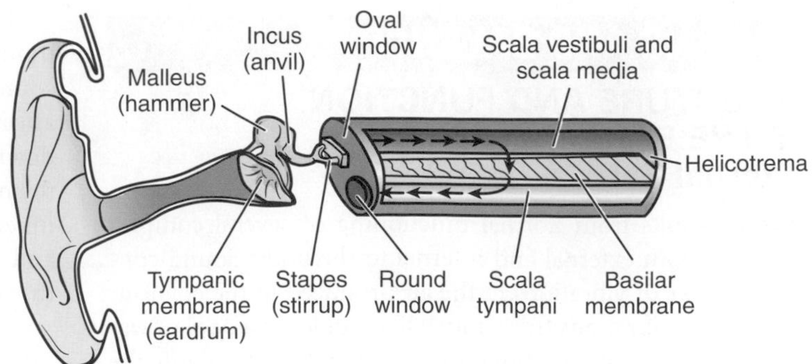

FIGURE 46-2 ■ Movement of fluid in the cochlea after forward thrust of the stapes.

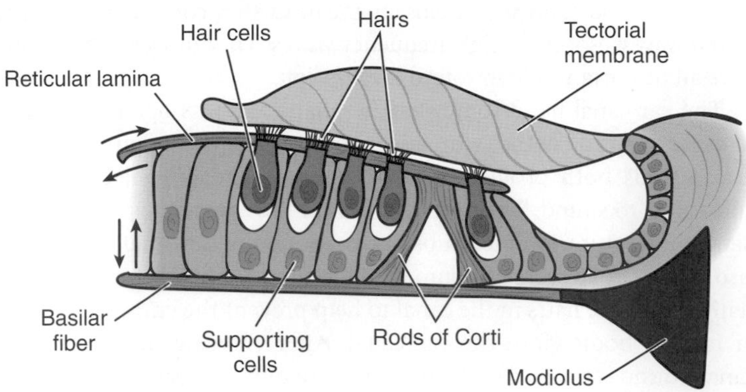

FIGURE 46-3 ■ Stimulation of hair cells by the back-and-forth movement of the hair cells in the tectorial membrane.

torial membrane. The wave of perilymph induces movement of the basilar membrane, which causes a pull or shearing force on the hair cells in contact with the tectorial membrane. This action transforms the mechanical energy of sound into electrical impulses stimulating the vestibulocochlear nerve. Before reaching the auditory area of the temporal lobe, impulses are relayed through nuclei in the medulla, pons, midbrain, and thalamus.

Balance

The ear has dual sensory functions. In addition to its role in hearing, it also functions as the sense organ of **equilibrium.** The stimulation or "trigger" responsible for balance involves activation of receptor hair cells contained in the semicircular canals. Movement of the head causes movement of the endolymph contained in the semicircular canals. The receptor hair cells in turn create a nerve impulse in the vestibular portion of the vestibulocochlear nerve (cranial nerve VIII), where the stimulus is transmitted to the brain. Not only are signals from the inner ear involved in keeping individuals upright; they are also involved in controlling the eye muscles so that the eyes can remain fixed on the same point despite changes in the position of the head.

Vertigo

Vertigo is a common symptom of vestibular disorders and not a well-defined disease. It is either a sensation of motion without any actual motion or an exaggerated sense of motion; it is not simply a sensation of "spinning." Accompanying symptoms may include nausea, vomiting, pallor, and sweating. **Nystagmus** often is also noted. Objective vertigo involves the perception that the surroundings are moving while the body remains still. Subjective vertigo involves the feeling that the surroundings remain still while the body is moving.[2] The clinical significance of this difference is doubtful. Vertigo is caused by a problem with the inner ear, the cochlear nerve, or the connection of the cochlear nerve with the central portion of the brain. In the case of Meniere disease (discussed later in this chapter), a disorder in which vertigo is common, the cause is unknown.

Disorders of the brainstem or cerebellum that may also cause vertigo include tissue ischemia secondary to atherosclerosis, tumors, or diseases such as multiple sclerosis. However, in these cases, additional neurologic signs and symptoms are typically present. Management of vertigo is usually aimed at the cause if known. Medications such as antihistamines and anticholinergics can be helpful.

GENERAL MANIFESTATIONS OF HEARING IMPAIRMENT

Hearing impairment is a very common disorder and the third leading chronic health problem in the United States following arthritis and hypertension.[3] One in three adults older than 60 and one half of those older than 85 have some hearing impairment.[4]

Hearing may be impaired in many ways, and impairments occur across the age spectrum. Disorders may affect the outer ear, such as impacted cerumen and foreign bodies in the ear canal. The middle ear may be affected by fluid **effusion,** infection (otitis media), tumors, or diseases such as otosclerosis. Hearing loss may also be caused by repeated exposure to loud sounds and **ototoxic** medications such as aminoglycoside antibiotics, chemotherapeutic agents, and rapidly infused high-dose loop diuretics.[5] Other causes of hearing loss, especially in children, include environmental teratogens (radiation), intrauterine infections (cytomegalovirus, herpes simplex virus, human immunodeficiency virus, and *Toxoplasma*), maternal metabolic disorders (diabetes, hypothyroidism), and exposure to industrial chemicals (solvents or pesticides).[6,7] By whatever mechanism hearing impairment occurs, the signs and symptoms are similar.

Symptoms of hearing impairment may be manifested in behavior such as inattentiveness, speaking out of turn in conversations, withdrawal from social situations, increased volume of voice when speaking, increased volume of radio or television, confusion, postural changes, loss of reaction to loud sounds, and emotional outbursts. Children with hearing impairment may demonstrate inattentiveness and difficulty with articulation and the development of speech. Alterations in hearing function can generally be classified into two categories, conductive and sensorineural, depending on the cause of the impairment. Some hearing impairments have a component of both. The following alterations in hearing function are categorized according to the primary cause of dysfunction.

HEARING IMPAIRMENT DISORDERS

Conductive Hearing Impairment

Conductive hearing loss occurs when sound cannot reach the cochlea. Individuals with conductive hearing impairment have a decreased sensitivity to sound. This type of hearing impairment is caused by dysfunction in the external or middle ear. Four mechanisms, each resulting in impairment of the passage of sound vibrations to the inner ear, lead to conductive hearing impairment: (1) obstruction (cerumen impaction), (2) mass loading (middle ear effusion), (3) stiffness effect (otosclerosis), and (4) discontinuity (ossicular disruption). Conductive hearing loss is generally correctable with medical or surgical therapy—or in some cases both.[6]

Loss Caused by Cerumen Impaction and Foreign Body Occlusion

Etiology. Cerumen impaction is a common and frequently overlooked cause of conductive hearing loss, especially in the elderly. In most cases, cerumen impaction is self-induced through attempts at cleaning the ear with objects such as cotton swabs. Treatment most commonly consists of removing the excess cerumen with gentle irrigation.

Foreign bodies in the ear canal occur most frequently in children. Objects such as small stones, pieces of wood, peas, beans, and paper are fairly common. Sometimes no symptoms are present and the foreign body is discovered on routine examination. If the foreign body is an insect, beating of its wings and movement may cause distress. When symptomatic, however, foreign bodies can cause pain or drainage of pus from the ear.

Clinical Manifestations and Treatment. The external ear canal is very sensitive to touch and bleeds easily, which increases the risk for subepithelial hematomas from minor trauma. Therefore, removal of solid foreign bodies carries a risk of additional trauma to the ear canal, as well as tympanic membrane rupture, if the individual is not completely cooperative or removal is difficult. Light anesthesia may be necessary to aid in removal of the foreign body.[5] Firm materials may be removed from the canal with a loop or hook, taking care not to push the object further into the canal. Irrigation should not be performed on organic foreign bodies (beans, peas) because water may cause them to swell. Living insects may be immobilized with lidocaine before removal.[5]

Otosclerosis

Etiology. Otosclerosis is a progressive conductive sensorineural or mixed hearing impairment caused most often by stapedial fixation. Resorption of bone is followed by the formation of new spongelike bony lesions usually occurring on and around the ossicles of the middle ear. Lesions involving the footplate of the stapes cause decreased transmission of sound waves to the oval window. However, when otosclerotic lesions impinge on the cochlea, permanent sensorineural hearing loss can occur. The basic initiating factors are unknown, but many individuals with clinical otosclerosis have a history of the disease in the family.[5] The disease is most common in white middle-aged women. It is theorized that there may be a relationship of otosclerosis and the hormones of pregnancy. Viral infections are also thought to be a cause. New research is being done to examine the presence of monoclonal antibodies to the measles virus in patients with otosclerosis.[8,9] The age of onset is variable due to the insidious progression of the disorder, but the most common ages are between 15 and 45. There may be periods of symptom worsening, followed by times of little apparent change.[9]

Diagnosis and Treatment. The diagnosis of otosclerosis is made through careful history taking and radiologic studies, along with audiometric studies. Although hearing loss may be severe, speech discrimination is preserved except in the rare instance of cochlear involvement. The individual may report being able to hear better in a noisy environment than in a quiet one.[8] **Tinnitus** is often present. Hearing tests reveal a conductive loss of varying severity. Otosclerosis generally affects both ears.

Management of otosclerosis at this point is generally surgical, in efforts to prevent the conductive hearing loss. The limitation on treatment options for otosclerosis is related largely to the lack of exact knowledge regarding the cause and pathogenesis of the disease. The universally accepted operation for otosclerosis is stapedectomy, or removal of the focus of the disease by removing the stapes and inserting a prosthesis. In the case of otosclerosis involving the cochlea, treatment with oral sodium fluoride, vitamin D, and calcium supplements is associated with some decrease in development of the sensorineural hearing loss.[5,9]

Sensorineural Hearing Impairment

In sensorineural hearing impairment, the hearing mechanism is disturbed in the inner ear in the cochlea or the vestibulocochlear nerve to the brain. Long-term exposure to loud sounds, ototoxic medication, trauma, metabolic causes, aging, and certain disease states cause sensorineural hearing impairment. Sensorineural hearing loss is usually irreversible.[5]

Loss Caused by Ototoxic Medications

Drug toxicity is an increasingly important cause of sensorineural hearing loss. The drugs most well known for this effect are the aminoglycoside antibiotics, salicylates, quinine and related antimalarials, and antineoplastic drugs. Most ototoxic drugs affect the hair cells of the cochlea. Unfortunately, these ototoxic effects may not become apparent during drug administration but may occur days to weeks after the therapy has been terminated. Ototoxicity may also be unilateral. Aspirin can produce a temporary hearing loss and tinnitus in individuals receiving high doses. In most cases, however, the hearing loss and tinnitus disappear after aspirin use is terminated.

Loss Caused by Trauma

Etiology. Acquired sensorineural hearing loss caused by chronic, repeated exposure to loud sounds is common in the U.S. population. Noise-induced hearing loss is one of the most common occupational diseases and the second most self-reported occupational illness or injury. Approximately 30 million workers are exposed to hazardous noise on the job.[7] Noise-induced hearing loss can be associated with the use of firearms, personal stereo systems, and power tools and with occupations such as firefighting, construction, agriculture, manufacturing, transportation, and the military.

The loudness of sound/noise is measured in the logarithmic units of decibels (dB). A normal whisper is measured at approximately 20 dB, a conversation at 3 feet at 50 to 60 dB. In contrast, rock concerts have been measured at 140 dB, lawnmowers and motorcycles at 90 dB. Sounds exceeding 85 dB are considered potentially injurious, and chronic noise exposure is the most damaging.[5] If exposure is severe enough, most structures of the inner ear can be damaged, including the organ of Corti. Sensory hair cells and supporting cells are lost because of overexposure. Noise-induced hearing loss typically is bilateral and affects higher (speech) frequencies first.

Noise exposure has two phases: the first is a temporary *threshold* shift. When the ear is exposed to a loud sound, it will show a loss of sensitivity (a rise in the threshold for sound). If the hearing returns to normal after the sound has been removed, the shift was temporary and no permanent damage has occurred. If hearing does not return to normal, damage has occurred and the hearing impairment is permanent. Such a permanent threshold shift is the second phase of the damage.[9] The ears of some individuals are more easily affected by noise, and considerable damage may occur before individuals are aware of the hearing loss.

Clinical Manifestations. Individuals with hearing loss caused by noise trauma report that they are unable to discriminate words, particularly in noisy environments. Complaints about tinnitus are expressed more often than complaints about hearing loss. A diagnosis of noise-induced hearing loss is made through careful history and audiometric testing. Because noise-induced hearing loss is irreversible, no medical therapy can help once the problem has been established. Prevention is presently the only treatment for this type of hearing impairment.

Sensorineural hearing impairment can also occur with head trauma and subsequent damage to the structures of the inner ear. If blood is coming from the ear or the temporal bone is fractured, damage should be suspected. As a rule, hearing loss from trauma or head injury is permanent if the cochlea is damaged.

Presbycusis

Presbycusis is a sensorineural hearing loss and the most common form of hearing loss in older adults. Approximately 25% of people age 65 to 75 and 50% of those older than 75 suffer from age-related hearing loss.[5] Typically, the hearing impairment is of gradual onset, is bilateral, and results in difficulty hearing high-pitched tones and conversational speech. Presbycusis can progress to involve the middle and lower tones. Frequently, individuals complain that people are mumbling to them but deny any other type of hearing loss.

Etiology. Four categories of presbycusis have been theorized: (1) sensory, characterized by atrophy and degeneration of the sensory and supporting cells; (2) neural, typified by loss of neurons in the cochlea and central nervous system; (3) metabolic, characterized by atrophy of the wall of the cochlea; and (4) mechanical, in which the middle ear undergoes changes in properties with a resulting conductive hearing loss.[3,10] Some of these age-related changes are shown in The Aging Process: Changes in Hearing. However, these theories have not been consistently supported by audiometric studies

THE AGING PROCESS

Changes in Hearing

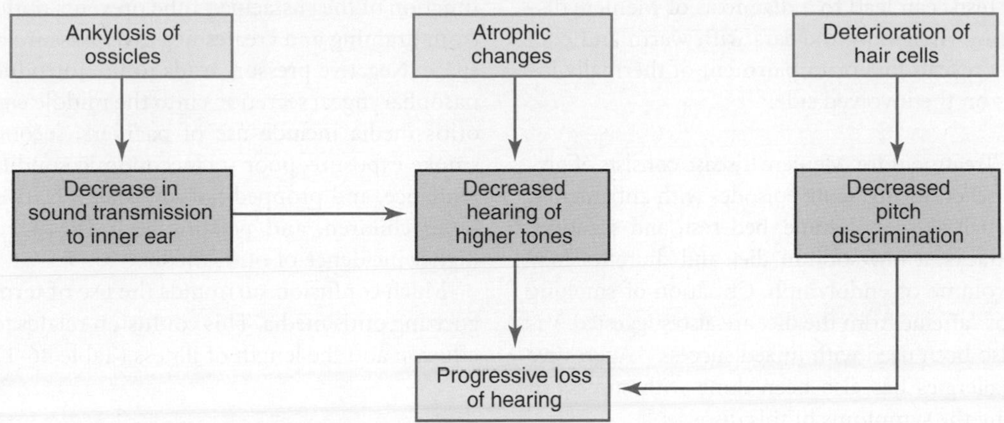

Presbycusis, or age-related hearing problems, occurs after age 50 and is thought to be caused by structural changes in the organs of hearing. Ankylosis of the ossicles can lead to a functional decrease in transmission of sound to the inner ear.

In the inner ear or cochlea, degeneration of hair cells, changes in the basilar membrane, or atrophic changes can lead to decreased hearing of higher tones. With these changes is also noted a decline in pitch discrimination. As hearing is progressively lost, even lower pitch tones will be more difficult to hear.

or clinical observations. An endless list of genetic, environmental, and disease states can also cause hearing loss in an older adult, many of which may occur concurrently. Thus controversy and uncertainty remain regarding the exact cause of presbycusis. Recent animal research findings suggest that vitamin/nutritional deficiencies and oxidative stress contribute to hearing loss.[3,11]

Diagnosis. Assessment of an individual with suspected presbycusis should begin with exclusion of all other causes of hearing impairment. Diseases such as diabetes, stroke, and heart disease may produce effects similar to those seen with hearing loss and must be ruled out. The diagnosis is made with a careful history and audiometric studies. Individuals with presbycusis respond well to hearing aids that amplify sound. Many simple lifestyle adjustments that will be mentioned at the end of this section can dramatically improve the quality of life for an individual experiencing presbycusis.

Meniere Disease

Etiology and Pathogenesis. Meniere disease is an excessive accumulation of endolymph in the membranous labyrinth. The volume of endolymph increases with distention of the scala media until the membrane ruptures. Consequently, the neural end organs of the cochlea degenerate. Meniere disease is thought to be caused by many conditions including allergies, viral and bacterial infections (such as syphilis), head trauma, metabolic derangements, and chronic stress. The precise cause cannot be established in most cases.[5] Men and women are equally affected by this disorder, and the onset of symptoms occurs frequently in the fifth decade.[12]

Clinical Manifestations. Clinical manifestations of Meniere disease include tinnitus, fluctuating sensorineural hearing loss, vertigo, and sensations of ear fullness. In the early stages, hearing loss fluctuates, with return to normal after the rupture heals. This hearing loss is usually in the low tones. As the disease progresses, hearing loss becomes permanent. Hearing loss also usually precedes the first attack of vertigo.[12]

Episodes of vertigo may be immediately preceded by the sensation of pressure in the ear, increased hearing loss, increased tinnitus, or an alteration in the quality of these symptoms. The onset of vertigo is usually sudden, reaches maximal intensity within a few minutes, usually lasts for an hour or more, and either subsides completely or continues as a sensation of unsteadiness for several hours or days. The tinnitus is typically a low buzzing or blowing sound and is frequently louder before the attack of vertigo. The attacks are not precipitated by positional changes and may be several weeks or months apart. In the initial stages of the disease they may be years apart. If not treated, the episodes may become more frequent and severe. Nystagmus, which occurs only during acute attacks, may be directed to the side opposite the involved ear.

Physical examination, including neurologic and otolaryngologic examination, is generally normal in those with

Meniere disease. Radiologic studies are often used to rule out other causes of the symptoms of Meniere disease such as acoustic neuroma. Electrophysiologic studies, such as auditory brainstem response testing and electrocochleography[13] and audiometric tests, can lead to a diagnosis of Meniere disease. Caloric testing (irrigating the ears with warm and cool water) commonly reveals loss or impairment of thermally induced nystagmus on the involved side.[5]

Treatment. Treatment for Meniere disease consists of giving symptomatic relief during acute episodes with antiemetics, anticholinergics such as scopolamine, bed rest, and sedation. Between acute attacks, a low-sodium diet and diuretics may help reduce the volume of endolymph. Cessation of smoking and elimination of caffeine from the diet are also suggested. Vasodilators have also been used with mixed success.[12] Aggressive management of allergies has also been done with success in terms of decreasing the symptoms of this disorder.[14]

Several surgical interventions are used to manage Meniere disease. Shunts can be placed to drain excess endolymph, and ablation of portions of the eighth cranial nerve and destruction of the labyrinth are the options at this time. These interventions have different indications, risks, and benefits associated with them. Almost all patients who choose surgical intervention have failed to respond to medical treatment.[5]

OTITIS MEDIA

Otitis media is inflammation of the middle ear. It is almost always due to poor functioning of the eustachian tube and is often diagnosed by the presence of **effusion.** It is the most common reason for a child to require medical attention.[6]

Otitis media is more common in the winter months when viral and bacterial infections are most common. Upper respiratory tract infections affect eustachian tube function and predispose individuals to middle ear inflammation. Children are especially susceptible because of shorter, more flexible, and more horizontally positioned eustachian tubes. The dysfunction of the eustachian tube prevents middle ear secretions from draining and creates negative pressure in the middle ear space. Negative pressure leads to the introduction of infected nasopharyngeal secretions into the middle ear. Risk factors for otitis media include use of pacifiers, second-hand cigarette smoke exposure, poor socioeconomic conditions, daycare attendance, and propped bottles. Males, Native Americans, Eskimo children, and persons with Down syndrome have a higher incidence of otitis media.[6]

Much confusion surrounds the use of terminology in categorizing otitis media. This confusion relates to the presence of effusion and the length of illness (Table 46-1).

Acute Otitis Media

Acute otitis media is characterized by sudden onset of ear pain in association with symptoms of upper respiratory tract infection and is usually of short duration (less than 3 weeks).[9] Although older children and adults complain of pain, younger children may demonstrate irritability as well as difficulty eating and sleeping, or tug at the affected ear.

Physical examination reveals a reddened tympanic membrane that has poor mobility. Bulging or rupture of the tympanic membrane may also be present.

Management of acute otitis media generally includes a 10- to 14-day course of antibiotics effective against *Streptococcus pneumoniae* and *Haemophilus influenzae* (the bacteria commonly involved).[6] Most individuals receiving antibiotic therapy should have significant improvement in symptoms within 48 hours. Additional therapy such as analgesics, antipyretics,

Table 46-1

Comparison of Otitis Media Types

Type	Onset/Duration	Symptoms	Treatment Options
Acute otitis media	Sudden onset, associated with upper respiratory infections	Reddened tympanic membrane with poor mobility, may be bulging or ruptured, ear pain	Antibiotics, analgesics, antipyretics, decongestants, or "watch and see"
Recurrent acute otitis media	3 or more episodes in 6 months	Same as above	Daily doses of prophylactic antibiotics, ventilation tube placement
Chronic otitis media	Duration of more than 12 wk, may develop as consequence of acute otitis media	Thick immobile tympanic membrane, purulent drainage from ear, may have conductive hearing loss, pain is rare	Removal of debris from middle ear, ventilation tube placement
Otitis media with effusion	May precede or follow any type of otitis media	Ear popping, feeling of pressure in middle ear, hearing loss, retraction of tympanic membrane, fluid line or bubbles	Treat acute otitis media, decongestants, "watch and see"

and decongestants may assist with symptom management. Follow-up examination is extremely important to determine that appropriate antibiotic selection and resolution have occurred. However, recent concern relating to antibiotic-resistant strains of bacteria has stimulated controversy regarding the use of antibiotics to manage acute otitis media. Some research suggests that antibiotics do not reduce pain, episodes of distress, or absence from school. Practitioners may choose a "watch and see" approach, waiting 72 hours before prescribing antibiotics.[15]

Recurrent acute otitis media, defined as three or more episodes of acute otitis media in 6 months, is managed with daily doses of prophylactic antibiotics.[6] Surgical placement of ventilation tubes in the tympanic membrane is also done in cases of recurrent otitis media. Complications of unresolved otitis media include mastoiditis, meningitis, osteomyelitis of the skull bones, and facial paralysis.

Chronic Otitis Media

Chronic otitis media is inflammation in the middle ear lasting longer than 12 weeks.[6] Irreversible damage has occurred to structures in the middle ear. This damage comes in many forms, including atrophy or perforation of the tympanic membrane or adhesions in the middle ear causing tympanic membrane retraction. Calcification of the ossicles may occur, as may the formation of cholesteatomas (benign, slowly growing collections of skin tissue) within the middle ear space. The hallmark clinical sign of chronic otitis media is purulent drainage from the ear. Pain is an uncommon finding, and conductive hearing loss may occur. Chronic otitis media generally develops as a consequence of acute otitis media, but it may follow other diseases or trauma. Management of chronic otitis media generally includes surgical removal of debris in the middle ear, placement of ventilation tubes in the tympanic membrane, and adenoidectomy to assist with eustachian tube function.

INTERVENTIONS FOR INDIVIDUALS WITH HEARING IMPAIRMENT

In general, interventions for individuals with hearing loss are aimed at maximizing whatever hearing ability the individuals possess and allowing for compensation with other senses. To improve communication, adequate visual contact should be made. Lighting and positioning should be such that the individual can see the speaker's lips. Reductions should be made in background noise. Speech should be at a normal rate and rhythm and at normal volume. Shouting can distort sounds and actually make them more difficult to hear. The speaker should use shorter sentences and gestures such as pointing when appropriate.

Devices that amplify sound or transform sounds into tactile or visual signals may be helpful. Amplifiers for the telephone, television, or radio, closed-captioned television, and teletypewriters are examples of these devices. Others include doorbells and telephones that light up as well as ring, and flashing smoke detectors and alarm clocks.

Implanted hearing devices such as cochlear implants may be helpful for patients over the age of 2 years with profound hearing loss. Surgically implanted cochlear electrodes work together with an external processor that converts sound waves to electrical signals that can be recognized by the brain. This device can improve communication and provide psychosocial benefits.[3]

KEY CONCEPTS

- Perception of sound requires that sound waves be transmitted through the outer ear canal, across the tympanic membrane, and through the ossicles to the oval window. Movement of the oval window initiates movement of perilymph, which causes movement of endolymph through the vestibular membrane. This fluid's motion stimulates the neurosensory organs of hearing, the hair cells. Bending of the hair cells induces action potentials in the cochlear nerve, which projects to the brainstem. Neural projections to the auditory area in the temporal lobe result in sound perception.
- Balance is controlled by hair cells contained in the semicircular canals. Stimulation of these cells by head movement causes nerve impulses to be transmitted to the brain to keep individuals upright and control eye movement.
- Vertigo, the sensation of motion or aggravation of motion, is a cardinal symptom of disorders of the vestibular system. Vertigo is often associated with nystagmus and nausea.
- Hearing loss may result from interruptions in any part of the sound transmission pathway. Disorders of the outer and middle ear are generally termed conductive because sound waves are not reliably conducted to sensory organs of hearing. Accumulation of wax in the outer ear, ossification of bones, and middle ear infections and edema may result in conductive hearing loss. Conductive hearing loss is amenable to treatment.
- Sensorineural hearing loss is due to dysfunction of the hair cells or neural pathways to the brain. Chronic exposure to loud noise, ototoxic drugs, head trauma, and aging changes may lead to sensorineural hearing loss. Sensorineural hearing loss is not amenable to treatment.
- Otosclerosis is a disorder characterized by resorption of healthy bone and deposition of weak, spongelike bone in the ossicles of the middle ear, most frequently the stapes. These bony lesions lead to progressive conductive hearing loss.
- Presbycusis is a gradual sensorineural hearing loss common in older adults. Its cause is unclear and dif-

ficult to distinguish from other types of hearing loss, especially noise trauma.

- Meniere disease is a chronic inner ear disease of unknown cause characterized by vertigo and progressive unilateral sensorineural hearing loss.
- Otitis media, or inflammation of the middle ear, is most frequently seen in children and commonly results from eustachian tube dysfunction after upper respiratory infections. Otitis media can be both acute and chronic.

VISION

Healthy vision requires three basic processes: formation of an image on the retina, stimulation of rods and cones, and conduction of nerve impulses to the brain. Malfunction of any of these processes can disrupt normal vision.

STRUCTURE OF THE EYE

The eye is essentially a spherical structure contained in the bony cavity of the eye socket. It is composed of three basic layers: the sclera, the choroid, and the retina (Figure 46-4). The sclera is white and opaque. It is made up of dense connective tissue, aids in protecting the inner structures of the eye, and helps maintain the shape of the eye. The sclera merges with the coverings of the optic nerve on the posterior of the eye. The clear front window of the sclera is the cornea. The cornea is also composed of dense connective tissue and has a greater curvature than the sclera that causes it to protrude from the sclera. No blood vessels are located in the cornea. Deep within the anterior portion of the sclera at its conjunction with the cornea lies a ring-shaped venous sinus, the canal of Schlemm. Affixed to the sclera are the **extraocular** muscles that control eye movement.

The choroid layer of the eye is highly vascularized and darkly pigmented. Attached to this layer is the iris. The iris is a muscular diaphragm whose pigments are responsible for eye color. The iris controls the size of the pupil, the opening through which light stimuli enter the posterior portion of the eye. Behind the pupil is a clear lens. The lens is a transparent, avascular elastic membrane. This elasticity assists in focusing light stimuli on the retina.

The eye is composed of anterior and posterior chambers separated by the lens and iris. The anterior chamber is filled with aqueous humor, the transparent protein-free liquid that is formed in the ciliary body and drained through the canal of Schlemm (Figure 46-5). Aqueous humor provides oxygen and nutrients to the lens and cornea and is continually being formed and reabsorbed. The balance between formation and reabsorption of aqueous humor regulates the total volume and pressure of the **intraocular fluid.**[1] The posterior chamber is the portion of the eye behind the lens that contains a thicker fluid, vitreous humor.

VISUAL PATHWAYS

The innermost layer of the eye is the retinal layer. It is here that light waves are transformed into nerve impulses. Three layers of neurons make up the major portion of the retina (Figure 46-6). The outermost layer is composed of **photoreceptor** neurons, the rods and cones. Cones are responsible for daylight vision, color vision, and visual acuity. The greatest concentration of cones occurs in the macula. This area is devoid of retinal vessels and is responsible for the most detailed vision. Rods are important for nighttime and peripheral vi-

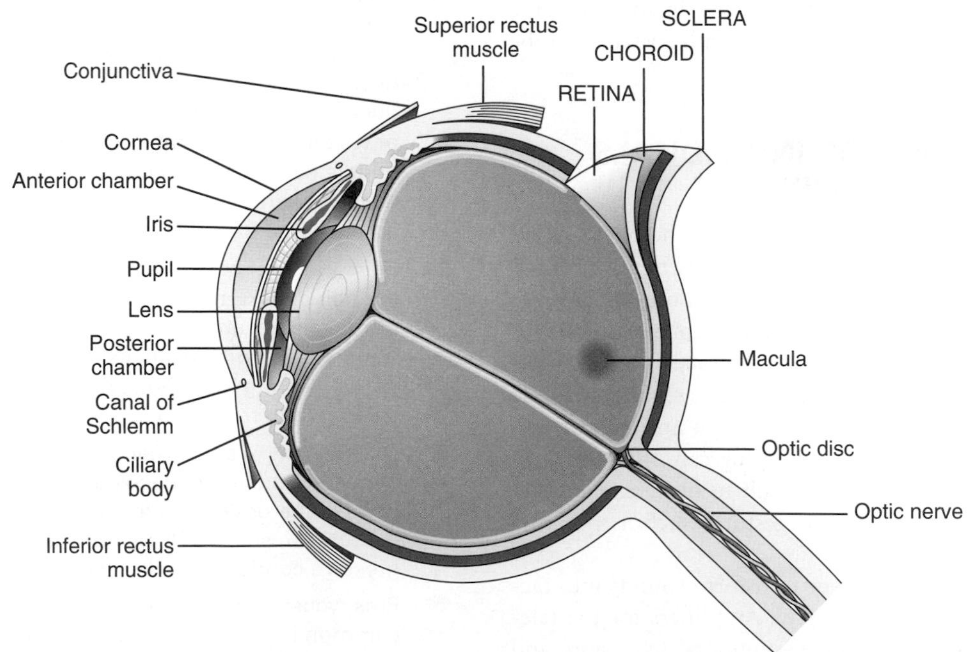

FIGURE 46-4 ■ Anatomic structures of the eye.

sion and outnumber cones by nearly 20 to 1. The pigmented layer of the retina or the retinal pigment epithelium is one cell thick. It functions to protect and nourish the retina. The retinal pigment epithelium also removes metabolic cellular debris from the photoreceptor cells, prevents new blood vessel growth into the retina, and absorbs light to diminish scattering and thereby enhance vision.[16]

Action potentials from the rods and cones are communicated throughout the other layers of the retina. All axons of the ganglion neuron extend back to a small circular area in the posterior of the eye, the optic disk, where the optic nerve passes through the sclera. When an image is focused on the retina, it is projected upside down and reversed left to right. An object in the upper temporal visual field of the right eye reflects its image on the lower nasal area of the retina. The optic disk is a blind spot because it does not contain any rods or cones. The optic nerve maintains the spatial arrangement of upside-down and reversed images, and at the optic chiasm just anterior to the pituitary gland half of the nerve fibers cross over to the other side of the brain (Figure 46-7). The left optic tract contains fibers from the left half of each retina and the right optic tract contains fibers from the right half of each retina. The nerve impulse travels through the optic nerves to connections in the thalamus and finally connects with the neurons of the occipital cortex.

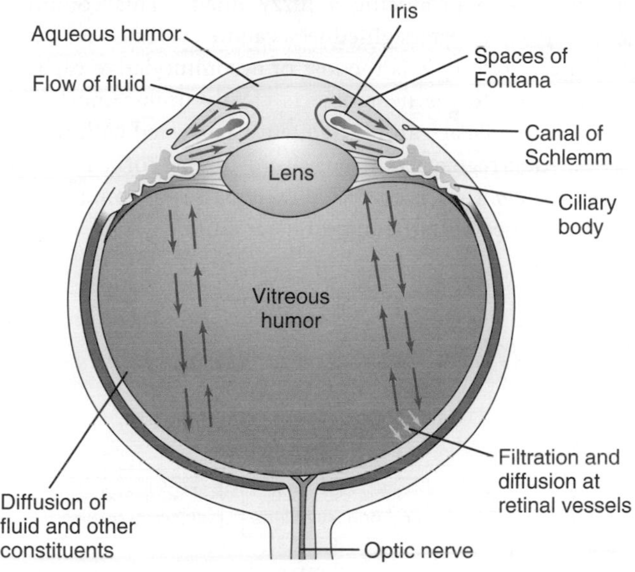

FIGURE 46-5 ■ Circulation of the aqueous and vitreous humor of the eye.

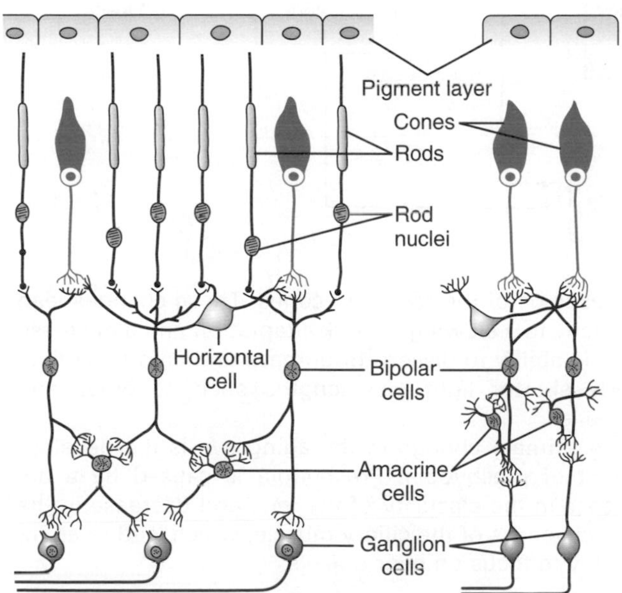

FIGURE 46-6 ■ Three-neuron organization of the retina. (Redrawn from Guyton AC, Hall JE: *Textbook of medical physiology,* ed 9, Philadelphia, 1996, Saunders, p 646.)

GENERAL MANIFESTATIONS OF VISUAL IMPAIRMENT

Visual impairment may occur or become evident at any time during the life span. If these impairments occur during infancy or early childhood and are not immediately detected and managed, vision may not develop normally. In older children, academic performance may suffer. In adults and elderly

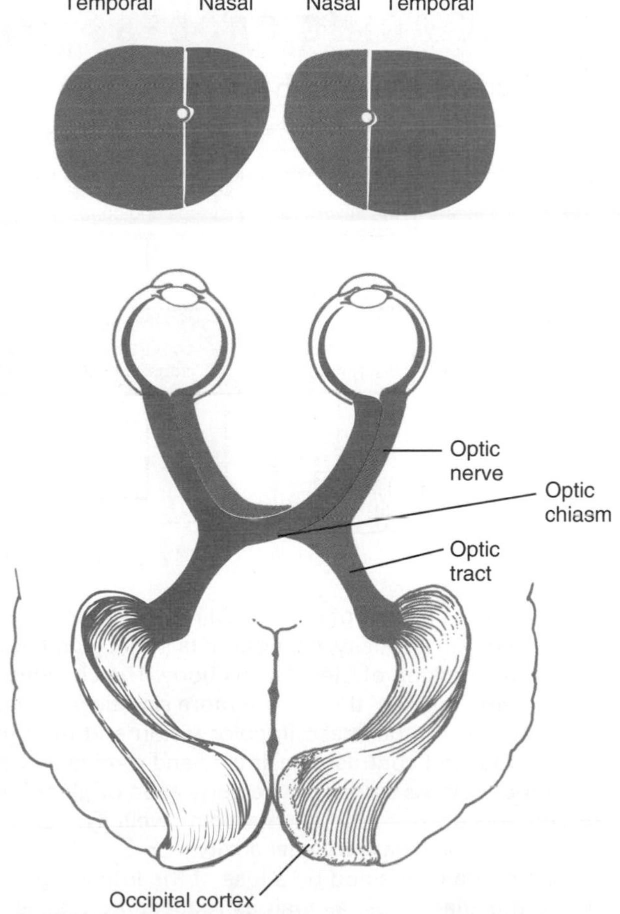

FIGURE 46-7 ■ Visual pathways. (From Jarvis C: *Physical examination and health assessment,* ed 4, Philadelphia, 2004, Saunders, p 301.)

individuals, poor eyesight affects activities of daily living and can limit a person's ability to function normally and meaningfully in the environment. The various effects of aging on the eye can be seen in The Aging Process: Changes in the Eyes.

Clues that may indicate a visual impairment include squinting, closing one eye, tilting the head, redness of the eye, excessive tearing, and eye rubbing. These signs are especially helpful in identifying children who may be unable to verbalize visual difficulties. In older children and adults, complaints of blurred vision, halos, "floaters" in the visual fields, headaches, and eye pain may indicate a visual impairment. A thorough health history and physical examination along with *visual acuity testing* and *ophthalmoscopic examination* will provide health care providers with the necessary information to appropriately treat or refer individuals with visual impairment.

DISORDERS OF THE EYE

Errors of Refraction

Focusing a clear image on the retina is essential for good vision. In a normal eye, light rays enter the eye and are focused into a clear, upside-down image on the retina. The brain can easily "right" the upside-down image in conscious perception but cannot correct an image that is not sharply focused (Figure 46-8).

Myopia, Hyperopia, Presbyopia, and Astigmatism

If the eye is elongated, the image focuses in front of the retina rather than on it. The retina receives only a fuzzy image. This condition, called *myopia* or nearsightedness, can be corrected with concave contact lenses or glasses. Frequently seen in late childhood or early adolescence, individuals with myopia are unable to see distant objects clearly.

If the eye is shorter than normal, the image focuses behind the retina, also producing a fuzzy image. This condition, called *hyperopia* or farsightedness, can be corrected with convex lenses. *Presbyopia* is the loss of **accommodative capacity.** This inability to see near objects clearly occurs most commonly in middle age and is frequently corrected with reading glasses. An irregularity in curvature of the cornea or lens, termed *astigmatism*, is corrected with glasses or contact lenses that are formed with the opposite curvature.

THE AGING PROCESS

Changes in the Eyes

Decreased function of lacrimal glands → Dryness, burning

Loss of luteal pigment in macular area → Decreased color vision/discrimination → Increased need for light; Decreased dynamic visual acuity

Decreased light sensing thresholds of rods and cones → Decreased contrast sensitivity → Increased need for light; Decreased dynamic visual acuity

Decreased lens elasticity → Decreased accommodation (presbyopia) → Decreased dynamic visual acuity

Decreased pupil size → Decreased dynamic visual acuity

Increased size and density of lens → Yellowing of lens → Decreased dynamic visual acuity

Decreased skin elasticity of eyelid → Ptosis

Aging affects all parts of the eye. Minor changes include decreased skin elasticity, changes in lacrimal gland function, and shrinking of the vitreous body. The changes in the lens and retina of the eye are more significant. These changes cause a decrease in color vision and discrimination, reduced contrast sensitivity, and diminished accommodation. As a result, the elderly need brighter light to see and do not differentiate color well. The elderly also have less dynamic visual acuity.

The retina is affected by a loss of the luteal pigment in the macular areas, as well as reduced light-sensing thresholds of the rods and cones. These changes lead directly to a slowing of dark adaptation and a decrease in the ability to discern brightness and colors, particularly shorter light wavelengths such as blues and greens.

A primary change in the aging eye is the development of presbyopia. Presbyopia is caused by a decrease in the elasticity of the lens and decrease in the effectiveness of the ciliary muscle, which lead to an inability to focus on near objects.

Age-Related Disorders

Strabismus

To make visual perceptions meaningful, the visual images in the two eyes normally fuse with each other on corresponding points of the two retinas. Strabismus, also called "squint" or "cross-eyedness," means a lack of fusion of the eyes. The eyes appear misaligned on examination. Symptoms include squinting and frowning when reading, closing one eye to see, having trouble picking up objects, dizziness, and headache. Strabismus is often caused by an abnormal "set" of the fusion mechanism of the visual system and is most commonly found in children. Strabismus affects approximately 4% of children younger than 6 years.[6]

In the early efforts of the child to fixate the two eyes on the same object, one of the eyes fixates satisfactorily but the other fails to fixate, or both eyes fixate satisfactorily but never simultaneously. Soon the patterns of conjugate movements of the eyes become abnormally set so that the eyes never fuse.

Treatment of strabismus includes occlusion therapy, or patching of the good eye to force use of the weak eye, corrective lenses, surgery on the eye muscles, use of prisms, and eye exercises. If management of strabismus is begun before 24 months of age, amblyopia may be prevented.

Amblyopia

Amblyopia is poor vision, even with the proper optical correction, in one or both eyes and is the most common cause of decreased vision in children.[17] It results from altered visual development despite normal-appearing retinal and optic nerve pathways.[15] Amblyopia occurs when the normal course of visual development is interrupted, such as when visual images do not fuse as in the case of untreated strabismus.

The diagnosis of amblyopia is confirmed when a complete ophthalmologic examination reveals a decrease in visual acuity that cannot be explained by organic causes. Amblyopia is generally asymptomatic. Although screening for it is much easier in older children, at this point treatment is more diffi-

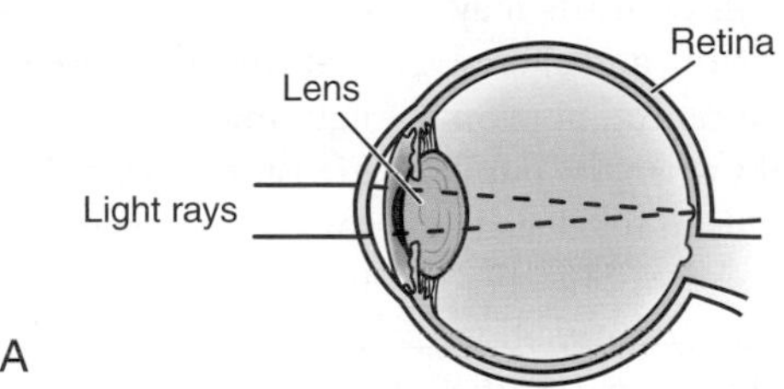

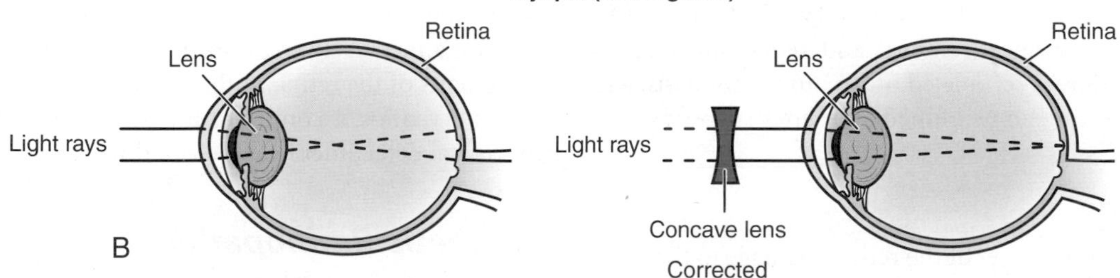

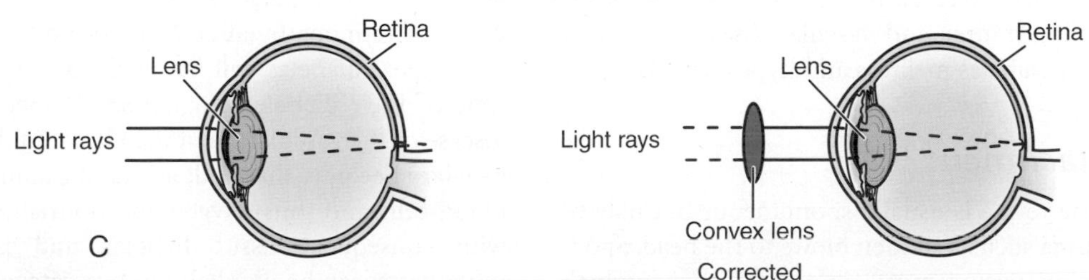

FIGURE 46-8 ■ **A,** Light rays are focused to produce a clear visual image (emmetropia). **B,** In myopia, light rays are focused in front of the retina. A concave lens moves the focus back onto the retina and results in a clear image. **C,** In hyperopia, light rays are focused behind the retina. A convex lens moves the focus forward so that the light rays fall directly on the retina.

cult. Therefore, screening must take place at an early age. Successful management of amblyopia depends on several factors. The most important is the age of onset and the length of time between onset and the commencement of treatment.[18] Management of amblyopia includes the use of atropine to blur vision or patching of the "stronger" eye. This forces the brain and weaker eye to work together to stimulate vision.[17,18]

Cataracts

Cataracts are a clouding or opacity of the lens that leads to gradual, painless blurring of vision and eventual loss of sight. More than half of all Americans age 65 and older have a cataract.[19] Cataracts result from the process of aging (senile), trauma (causing lens rupture and swelling), congenital factors (Down syndrome, intrauterine rubella infection), metabolic disease (diabetes mellitus, hypoparathyroidism), and certain medications (systemic corticosteroids). Cigarette smoking and heavy alcohol consumption may also increase the risk of cataract formation.[20]

Oxidative stress and exposure to ultraviolet light are factors contributing to the development of cataracts.[20] Both eyes may be affected, but at different rates. Patients with cataracts may experience increased glare at night, blurred vision, and altered color perception. Persons with opacity in the central portion of the lens can generally see better in dim light when the pupil is dilated. The degree of visual loss corresponds to the density of the cataract.

A diagnosis of cataracts can be made through examination of the eye with an ophthalmoscope or slit lamp. As the cataract worsens or "matures," visualization of the retina becomes increasingly difficult until finally the pupil appears white and the retina cannot be visualized at all. Treatment for cataracts involves surgical removal and replacement of the lens. This procedure is completed on an outpatient basis, with individuals returning home immediately after surgery.

Retinopathy

Retinopathy is any disorder of the retina. Damage to the retina impairs vision because even a well-focused image cannot be perceived if some or all of the light receptors do not function properly. Retinopathies can result from a variety of causes, the most common being trauma and vascular disease, especially in individuals with diabetes mellitus and hypertension.

Retinal Detachment

Detachment of the retina is usually spontaneous but may be secondary to trauma such as sudden blows to the head. Spontaneous detachment occurs most frequently in individuals older than 50 years.[5] Eye tumors, myopia, and cataract extraction are other common predisposing factors.

Tearing of the retina allows vitreous fluid to flow behind the retina and cause traction and progressive detachment

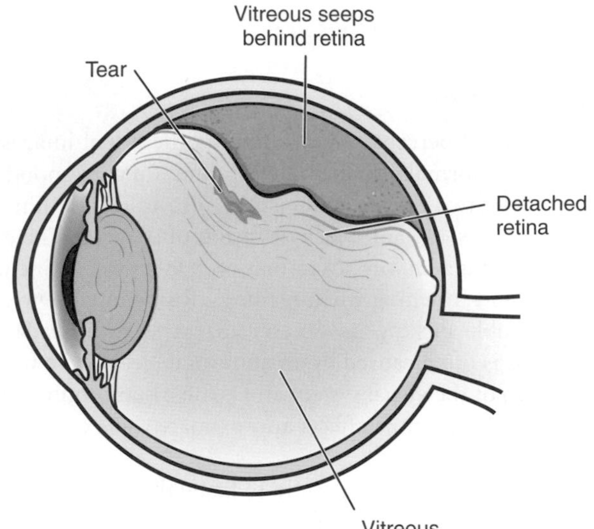

FIGURE 46-9 ■ Retinal detachment.

(Figure 46-9). The area of detachment increases rapidly, and visual loss is progressive. Common manifestations of retinal detachment include the sudden appearance of floating spots that may decrease over a period of weeks and odd flashes of light that appear when the eye moves. Others include blurring of vision in a single eye that appears as though "a curtain is being pulled down over the eye." If untreated, the retina may detach entirely and result in total blindness in the affected eye. Retinal detachments may also cause vitreous hemorrhage.

Retinal detachments are diagnosed through ophthalmoscopic examination. The retina appears to hang in the vitreous like a gray cloud. One or more retinal tears, generally crescent shaped, are usually present. Management of retinal detachment is aimed at closing tears in the retina and positioning the fragments of the retina so that reattachment can occur. Surgical intervention is common, and 80% of uncomplicated cases of retinal detachment can be cured with one operation.[5]

Diabetic Retinopathy

Etiology and Pathogenesis. Diabetic retinopathy is the leading cause of new cases of blindness in the United States. Nearly all persons with type 1 diabetes will have evidence of retinopathy after 20 years, and up to 21% of those with type 2 diabetes will have evidence of retinopathy at the time of their diabetes diagnosis.[21] Diabetic retinopathy is a disease of the vasculature of the retina. In diabetes, the retinal capillary becomes diseased; it loses the ability to transport red blood cells and thus oxygen and nourishment to the retina, with consequent tissue hypoxia and ischemia. Diabetic retinopathy can be divided into two categories: nonproliferative and proliferative.

In nonproliferative diabetic retinopathy, retinal veins become dilated and microaneurysms develop. This effect is a result of damaged vascular epithelium. Small retinal hemorrhages and cotton-wool spots (infarctions in the nerve fibers) occur. Early in the process, visual changes may be minimal or resolve after a few days. As the disease progresses, retinal edema occurs. If the edema involves the macular area, visual acuity is noticeably affected.

Proliferative diabetic retinopathy is characterized by the development of new but abnormal blood vessels (neovascularization) caused by the loss of retinal blood flow and ischemia. These new vessels affect vision in two ways: first, because they are abnormal, they are prone to leakage of blood into the vitreous cavity and may thus result in vitreous hemorrhage. Second, the vessels firmly attach themselves to the retina and grow out into the vitreous. The subsequent traction on the retina increases the risk for retinal detachment.[5]

Clinical Manifestations. Diabetic retinopathy is associated with complaints of blurred, darkened, and distorted vision. Visual changes may fluctuate in severity. Some individuals complain of being unable to read or have vague changes in vision.

Diagnosis and Treatment. The diagnosis of diabetic retinopathy is made through careful history taking, visual acuity testing, ophthalmologic examination, and retinal angiography. Management of nonproliferative diabetic retinopathy is aimed at controlling blood glucose levels and managing other systemic diseases such as hypertension. Laser treatments are also used to prevent further vision loss. Because the retina is nervous system tissue, it does not regenerate efficiently. Therefore, treatment may prevent any further injury to eye tissue, but it cannot restore vision.

Management of proliferative diabetic retinopathy must be instituted as soon as possible to prevent blindness. Surgical intervention and laser procedures are used in conjunction with the measures used for nonproliferative retinopathy. Because of the risk of diabetic retinopathy, it is recommended that individuals with diabetes mellitus have annual ophthalmologic examinations.

Age-Related Macular Degeneration

Etiology and Pathogenesis. Age-related macular degeneration (AMD) is the leading cause of permanent visual loss in the elderly.[5] Approximately 2% of people in their 50s and 30% of individuals older than 75 are affected.[22] The cause of macular degeneration is unknown, but the outcome is bilateral progressive macular deterioration with central vision loss. Risk factors for developing AMD include gender (incidence is higher in females than in males), smoking, family history of AMD, increased serum cholesterol, cardiovascular disease, hypertension, and significant cumulative sunlight exposure.[16,22] There is also a strong relationship between AMD and nutrition.[23] AMD includes a wide spectrum of findings that can be divided into two subgroups. Manifestations, diagnosis, and management of each subgroup differ.

"Dry" or atrophic AMD is the most common form, affecting approximately 90% of patients with AMD.[22] Atrophic AMD causes visual loss due to degeneration of the outer retina, the pigmented layer, and the choroidal layer. There are subretinal accumulations of cellular debris known as drusen, along with metabolic dysfunction of the retina. Hard drusen may be seen during ophthalmologic examination and appear as discrete yellow deposits on the retina. Atrophic AMD often affects just one eye initially but later develops in the unaffected eye.

In "wet" or exudative AMD, visual loss is usually more rapid in onset and causes more severe visual disruption. Impairment of barrier function allows for subretinal fluid collections, which may cause retinal detachments and/or neovascularizations. These fluid buildups may be visualized on retinal examination.

Clinical Manifestations. AMD is generally painless. In the atrophic form, the initial symptom is slightly blurred vision and decreased ability to see fine detail. Often patients need more light for completing fine tasks such as reading and needlework. As the disorder progresses, the area of central vision loss becomes larger and darker.

Exudative AMD may also be manifested by a progressive blurring of vision. A hallmark of this form of AMD is the wavy appearance of straight lines. This occurs due to distortion of the retina from fluid accumulations behind it. Vision may be lost rapidly or occur suddenly in previously undiagnosed patients due to retinal detachment or hemorrhage.

Diagnosis and Treatment. AMD is diagnosed with thorough history and physical examination to rule out other causes of visual loss, visual acuity testing, dilated retinal examination, and use of the Amsler grid (Figure 46-10). If AMD is suspected, fluorescein angiography may be completed by the ophthalmologist. In this examination, fluorescein dye is injected into the patient. Photos of the retina show characteristic changes of the choroidal vascular layer.

Management of AMD depends on the type and severity of the disease. Antioxidant/zinc vitamin supplementation has been shown to slow/delay the progression of AMD.[23] Other treatment modalities are aimed at correcting the vascular changes and include laser photocoagulation and photodynamic therapy. As with all progressive diseases, patients with AMD should have regular comprehensive eye examinations and daily self-evaluation using the Amsler grid.

Glaucoma

Glaucoma is characterized by increased intraocular pressure and progressive loss of vision. As fluid pressure inside the eye and against the retina increases, blood flow through the retina slows. Reduced blood flow causes degeneration of the retina and thus loss of vision. Glaucoma can be catagorized into two main types: open angle and closed (narrow) angle (Figure 46-11).

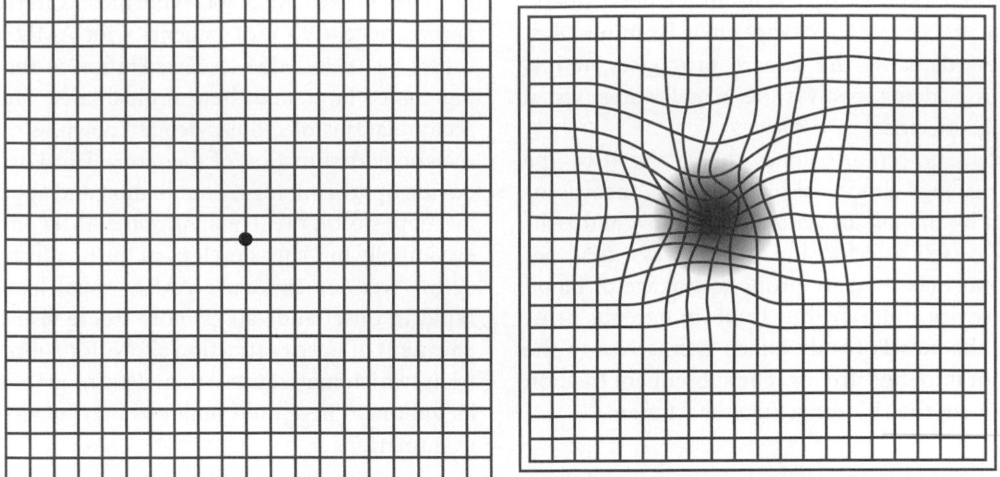

FIGURE 46-10 ■ *Left,* What an Amsler grid looks like to a person with normal vision. *Right,* What an Amsler grid might look like to a person with macular degeneration. (From National Eye Institute, National Institutes of Health: Age-related macular degeneration: what you should know, website: http://www.nei.nih.gov/health/maculardegen/armd_facts.asp#agrid.)

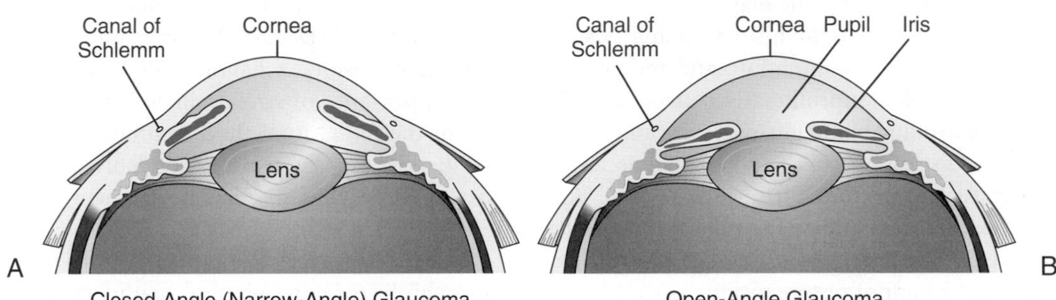

FIGURE 46-11 ■ Closed-angle (narrow-angle) glaucoma compared with open-angle glaucoma. **A,** In closed-angle glaucoma, the outflow of aqueous humor is obstructed by the iris root of the dilated pupil. **B,** In open-angle glaucoma, the obstruction to outflow of aqueous humor is in the drainage canals.

Glaucoma is more common in the elderly, African-Americans, those with a family history, those with myopia, and persons with diabetes. There is also a weak association between systemic hypertension, migraine with vasospasm, and the development of glaucoma.[20]

Open-Angle Glaucoma

Etiology and Pathogenesis. The cause of open-angle glaucoma is not clear. The drainage channels for aqueous humor appear normal. The disease is often bilateral and has a genetic component. Open-angle glaucoma accounts for 90% of all cases of glaucoma.[5]

Open-angle glaucoma has an insidious onset with no symptoms in the early stages. However, the intraocular pressure is consistently elevated and over a period of months or years symptoms appear, including gradual loss of vision in the periphery resulting in tunnel vision. Affected individuals may have complaints of vague but persistent dull eye pain or an inability to distinguish colors. Halos may appear around lights if the intraocular pressure is markedly elevated.

Diagnosis and Treatment. The diagnosis of open-angle glaucoma is made through intraocular pressure measurement, ophthalmoscopic examination of the optic disk, and central visual field testing. Because of the insidious nature of the disorder, it is recommended that all persons older than 40 years have an intraocular pressure measurement and ophthalmoscopic examination every 3 to 5 years. If a family history of glaucoma is present, more frequent examination is recommended.

Management of open-angle glaucoma is aimed at increasing drainage of aqueous humor and decreasing intraocular pressure. β-Adrenergic blocking eyedrops, such as timolol, are used to help decrease intraocular pressure by decreasing aqueous humor production. Miotics such as pilocarpine are also useful in that they constrict the pupil and thereby stimulate the ciliary muscles to pull on the trabecular meshwork surrounding the canal of Schlemm to increase the flow of aqueous humor. If the intraocular pressure elevation persists or the optic nerve damage progresses despite treatment, laser surgery aimed at the trabecular meshwork may be done to lower intraocular pressure.[20]

Closed-Angle (Narrow-Angle) Glaucoma

Etiology and Pathogenesis. Closed-angle (narrow-angle) glaucoma is caused by abnormality of the angle between the pupil and lateral cornea. This angle is narrow and blocks outflow of aqueous humor when the pupil is dilated. Closed-angle glaucoma is much less common than open-angle glaucoma but is more prevalent in the elderly, hyperopes, and Asian populations.[18] This form of glaucoma has a rapid onset and is treated as an emergency. Closed-angle glaucoma is associated with pupillary dilation and thus might occur when an individual is sitting in a darkened room or during times of stress. Forward displacement of the iris toward the cornea with dilation narrows or closes the chamber angle, obstructing the outflow of aqueous humor (see Figure 46-11).[20]

Manifestations of closed-angle glaucoma include severe eye pain, nausea and vomiting, blurred vision with halos around lights, redness of the eye, a steamy cornea, and a dilated pupil that is nonreactive to light. Closed-angle glaucoma is an emergency situation because permanent blindness can occur 2 to 5 days after onset of symptoms.[5]

Diagnosis and Treatment. Diagnosis of closed-angle glaucoma involves the same tests as used for diagnosis of open-angle glaucoma. Treatment again in this case is aimed at decreasing intraocular pressure. Acutely, carbonic anhydrase inhibitors such as acetazolamide and miotics may be used to decrease aqueous humor production and blockage. Laser iridectomy usually results in a permanent cure.

Visual Field Deficits

Visual Field Loss

Etiology and Pathogenesis. Visual field loss can be caused by changes in the eye itself, as is the case in cataracts, or result from tumors, vascular lesions, and demyelinating lesions near or in the neural pathways of the retina, optic nerve, or the visual cortex of the brain.

Damage to the visual pathway does not always result in a total loss of vision. Depending on where the damage occurs, only part of the visual field may be affected (Figure 46-12). Monocular field loss indicates disease of the retina or optic nerve. For example, a certain form of neuritis often associated with multiple sclerosis can cause loss of only the center of the visual field, called a scotoma.

Damage or lesions may also cause bilateral visual field losses or loss of half of the visual field, called **hemianopsia.** Lesions of the optic chiasm, usually caused by pituitary tumors, characteristically produce a bitemporal hemianopsia. Lesions occurring behind the optic chiasm cause a homonymous hemianopsia, which is a visual field loss involving the same side in both eyes. The more posterior the lesion in the visual pathway, the more congruous (similar size, shape, location) are the defects in the two eyes. Cerebrovascular accidents (strokes) and tumors are responsible for most of these lesions.

Diagnosis and Treatment. Visual field deficits are easily and rapidly assessed through confrontation (i.e., comparison of a person's vision to the examiner's own). Visual field deficits should be suspected if patients demonstrate one-sided neglect of their environment or eye deviation toward the side of the lesion. Treatment for visual field loss includes managing the underlying cause (tumor removal) and adapting the patient's environment.

INTERVENTIONS FOR INDIVIDUALS WITH VISION IMPAIRMENT

Once the visual impairment of an individual has been thoroughly investigated, specific interventions may be prescribed. Interventions may be thought of in three general categories: assistive devices, environment, and behavior. Proper care and cleaning of contact lenses and eyeglasses directly influences the effectiveness of the prosthesis. Tinted lenses are generally available and may be effective in reducing glare for some individuals. Pocket magnifiers are frequently useful for persons with an acuity impairment. Large print is now available on many household items (e.g., watches, playing cards, telephones, books), and various textures are used in further modifications for the visually impaired.

An unchanging, structured environment where items are kept in fixed locations familiar to the visually impaired person promotes safety and independence. Attempts to structure temporary environments, such as by introducing personal items into a hospital room, might yield positive results if consistently considered by the staff. Attention to adequate lighting, glare reduction, and appropriate use of contrasting colors enhances safety and independent function of those with visual impairment.

Behavioral techniques for the health care professional and visually impaired individuals can promote client comfort, safety, and independence. Such techniques for the professional include announcing oneself at all interactions and explaining sensory occurrences. Encouraging independence and social interaction often benefits individuals inasmuch as they may experience anger, frustration, or changes in self-concept as a result of their visual deficit.

Visually impaired individuals may be taught to wait several minutes for changes in dark-light adaptation and avoid abrupt changes in lighting. Individuals should be discouraged from looking directly into bright lights to reduce glare. As-

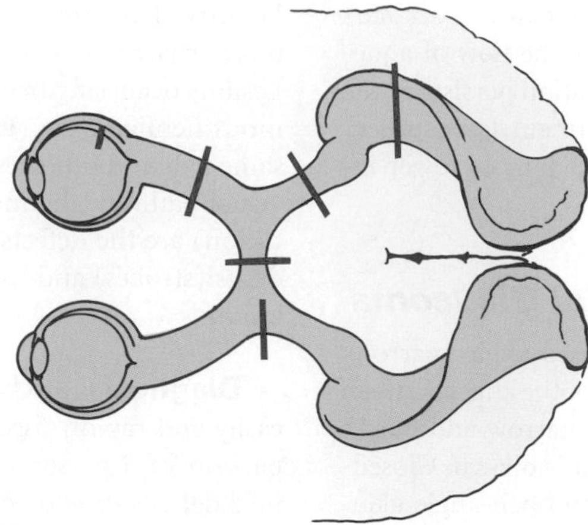

1. Retinal damage
   - Macula—central blind area (e.g., diabetes):

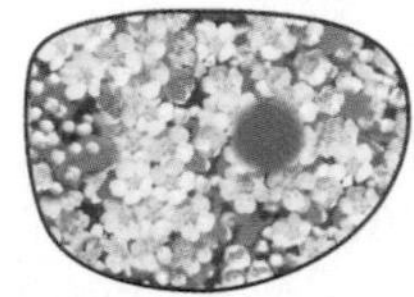
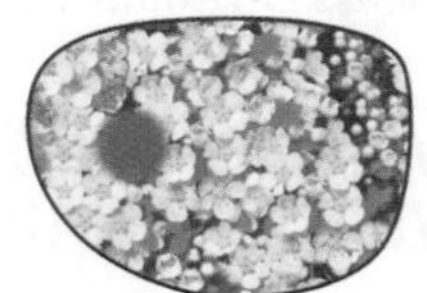

   - Localized damage—blind spot (scotoma) corresponding to particular area:

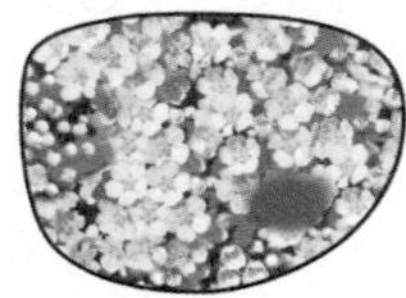
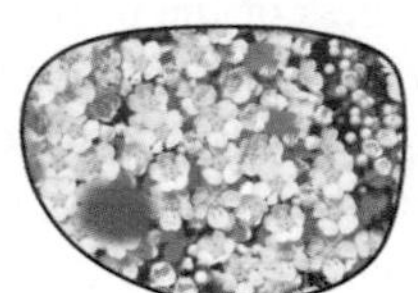

   - Increasing intraocular pressure—decrease in peripheral vision (e.g., glaucoma). Starts with paracentral scotoma in early stage:

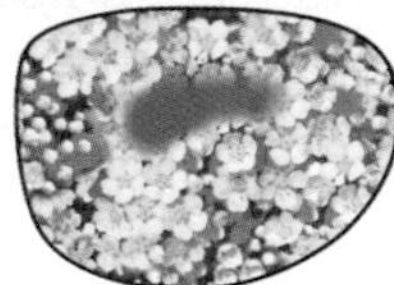
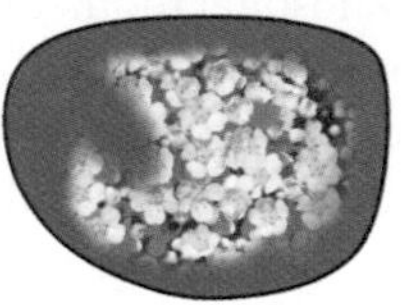

   - Retinal detachment. Person has shadow or diminished vision in one quadrant or one half of visual field:

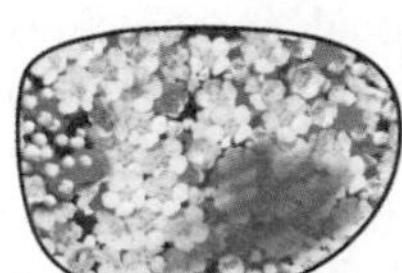
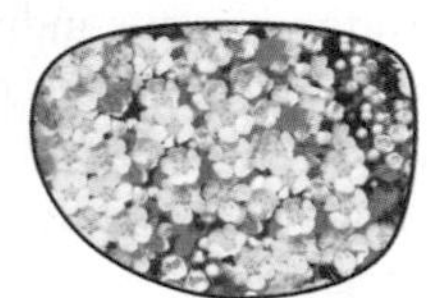

2. Lesion in globe or optic nerve. Injury here yields one blind eye, or unilateral blindness:

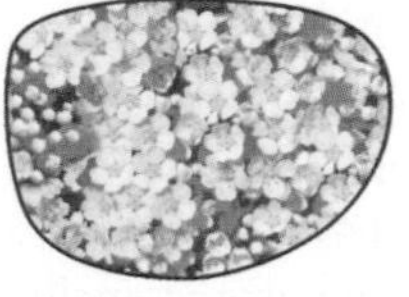

3. Lesion at optic chiasm (e.g., pituitary tumor)—injury to crossing fibers only yields a loss of the nasal part of each retina and a loss of both temporal visual fields. Bitemporal (heteronymous) hemianopsia:

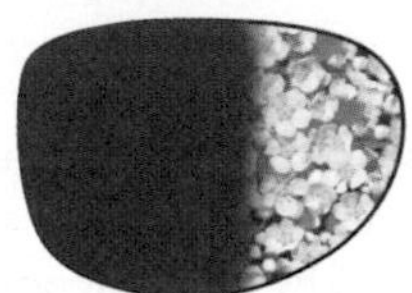
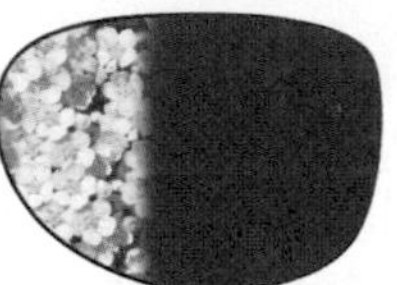

4. Lesion of outer uncrossed fibers at optic chiasm (e.g., aneurysm of left internal carotid artery exerts pressure on uncrossed fibers). Injury yields left nasal hemianopsia:

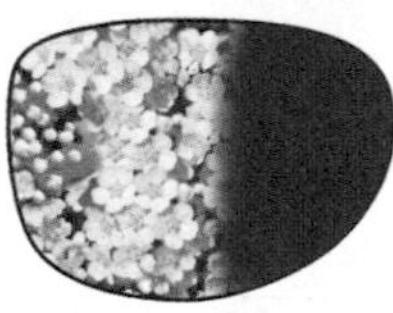
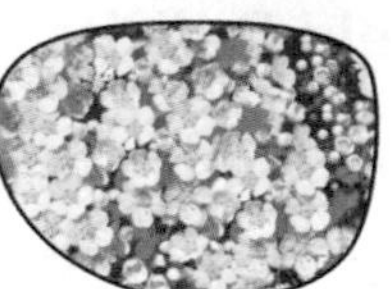

5. Lesion of right optic tract or right optic radiation. Visual field loss in right nasal and left temporal fields. Loss of same half of visual field in both eyes is homonymous hemianopsia:

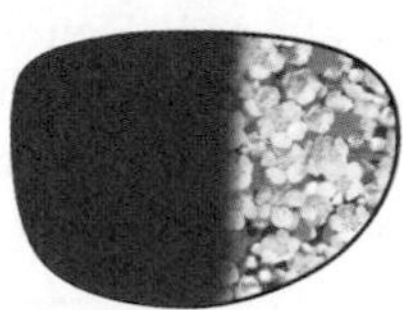
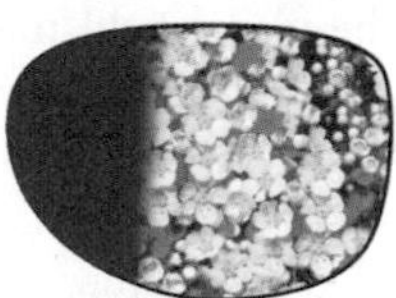

FIGURE 46-12 ■ Visual field losses. (From Jarvis C: *Physical examination and health assessment,* ed 4, Philadelphia, 2004, Saunders, p 330.)

sessment of the visually impaired person's ability to summon help in the health care and home settings is advised.

KEY CONCEPTS

- Visual acuity depends on the formation of discrete patterns of light on the retina. Errors of refraction such as myopia and hyperopia cause light to focus in front of or behind the retina. Irregular curvature of the cornea results in astigmatism. These disorders are correctable with lenses to refract the light to the appropriate retinal location.
- Strabismus occurs when both eyes do not focus together to form a single image. If this is not corrected, the brain may ignore the image from one eye in an attempt to avoid double imaging; eventually, amblyopia can result.
- Cataracts are due to opacification of the lens that blocks and scatters light. Cataracts may be congenital, traumatic, or associated with aging.
- Retinopathy is any disorder affecting the retina. Trauma and systemic disorders such as diabetes mellitus, hypertension, and vascular disease are the most common causes of retinopathy.
- Retinal detachment is characterized by tearing of the retina away from the choroid layer of the eye, with seepage of vitreous humor behind the retina causing further detachment.
- Diabetic retinopathy is a disorder of the retinal vessels characterized by the formation of microaneurysms and hemorrhage (nonproliferative) or neovascularization and subsequent leakage and retinal detachment (proliferative).
- Macular degeneration is an age-related, progressive loss of central vision due to atrophic or exudative changes to the macula of the retina.
- Glaucoma occurs when intraocular pressure is increased by a decrease in the outflow of aqueous humor from the anterior chamber of the eye. Open-angle glaucoma has an unclear cause because no clear obstruction impedes the outflow of aqueous humor. Closed-angle (narrow-angle) glaucoma occurs when the angle between the pupil and lateral aspect of the cornea is narrow and blocks outflow when the pupil is dilated.
- Visual field losses are caused by lesions anywhere along the visual pathways. The location of the lesion determines monocular or binocular involvement and the portion of vision lost.

SMELL AND TASTE

The senses of smell and taste allow separation of noxious or even lethal agents from those that are desirable. The sense of smell has a protective function in signaling danger: animals use smell to recognize the proximity of other animals, and humans use smell to sense harmful substances, such as smoke or spoiled food items, in the environment. The sense of taste allows a person to select food in accordance with desire and perhaps also in accordance with tissue needs. Both senses are strongly tied to primitive emotional and behavioral functions of the nervous system. These chemical senses are interrelated and will be discussed together.

Nerve fibers of the **olfactory** system have their cells of origin in the mucous membrane of the upper and posterior parts of the nasal cavity. The sense of smell begins with chemical stimulation of these cells. Axons of these receptor cells pass through the cribriform plate and travel to the olfactory area of the cortex through the first cranial nerve. These nerves lie under the frontal lobes of the brain. Olfactory impulses reach the cerebral cortex without relay through the thalamus; in this respect, olfaction is unique among the sensory systems.[12]

Like stimuli for smell, stimuli for taste are chemical. Food particles dissolved in fluid stimulate sensory receptors (taste buds) located on the surface of the tongue and in lesser density on the palate, pharynx, and larynx.[12] Stimulation from the sensory receptors is conducted through the cranial nerves of taste (VII, IX, X) to connections in the brainstem and thalamus with eventual termination in the **gustatory** cortex in the parietal lobe. The gustatory sensory receptors have a heightened sensitivity for one of the primary taste sensations (sweet, salty, sour, or bitter); however, they can respond to a variety of stimuli. The number of sensory receptors for taste diminishes with age.

Disorders of Smell and Taste

Etiology and Pathogenesis. Olfactory disorders range from loss or reduction in the sense of smell to distortions and olfactory hallucinations. Commonly the sense of smell is diminished because of smoking and conditions involving congestion and swelling of the nasal mucosa, such as allergies and sinusitis. Head trauma often results in the loss of smell because of actual shearing of the neuronal fibers as they traverse the cribriform plate. Tumors and large cerebral aneurysms of the anterior cerebral and anterior communicating arteries are lesions capable of diminishing olfactory sense. Epilepsy and psychiatric disorders may be associated with olfactory hallucinations.[12]

A decreased gustatory sense can also result from heavy smoking, as well as extreme dryness of the tongue and mucous membranes. A variety of medications are known to alter the sense of taste, including certain antidepressant, antithyroid, antirheumatic, and anticancer medications. In addition, influenza-like illnesses and lesions on the thalamus and parietal lobe may impair taste sensation.

Clinical Manifestations. Individuals with smell dysfunction frequently complain of a diminished ability to taste. They may experience a decreased appetite and use excessive amounts of salt, sugar, or other seasonings on their foods. These individuals may stop reacting to strong smells and not notice their own body odor. Smell dysfunction increases the risk of accidents in that these individuals may not detect signs of imminent danger such as gas or smoke. In addition, spoiled food may be ingested, and excessive use of salt is associated with health risks.

Diagnosis and Treatment. Assessment of the sense of smell is done by asking the individual to smell different known odors while keeping the eyes closed. Irritating substances such as ammonia should be avoided because they stimulate the trigeminal nerve. Assessment of gustatory sense should include the primary taste sensations in appropriate areas of the tongue, with the surface of the tongue wiped clean between substances. Questions regarding weight loss and appetite add valuable information to the assessment data.

Interventions for those with smell and taste dysfunction focus on augmenting the stimulus, teaching the individual to rely on other senses, and changing the environment. Because their senses of smell and taste are unreliable in identifying spoiled foods, people with these dysfunctions are encouraged to adhere to a strict schedule for discarding leftovers and be aware of expiration dates on food products. Because significant nutritional problems may occur, it is important to educate and monitor the individual's diet. The creative use of seasonings and spices along with variations in the texture and presentation of food may enhance appetite. Individuals with taste impairments are encouraged to avoid blended foods and to practice frequent oral hygiene. Smoke detectors should be installed in all rooms where smell-impaired individuals sleep and fire safety emphasized.

KEY CONCEPTS

- The senses of smell and taste result from chemical stimulation of specialized nerve fibers located in the nose and the tongue and are closely related to each other. Nerve impulses travel through the cranial nerves to separate areas of the brain.
- Changes in smell and taste most commonly result from smoking and inflammation caused by colds, sinusitis, or allergies. A change in smell or taste sensation in the absence of an obvious cause may indicate a brain tumor and should prompt a thorough neurologic evaluation.

SUMMARY

Humans interact with their environment by means of the special senses of hearing, vision, smell, and taste. Through a variety of stimuli including chemicals, light, and sound, individuals are able to enjoy everything from a symphony performance to a hot fudge sundae. The special senses also protect individuals from harm by allowing the perception of smoke or alarms. Only when these special senses are impaired does their importance become apparent.

Loss of these senses may result from congenital conditions, trauma, tumors, illness, or unknown causes. Loss may also be a consequence of aging. The mechanism of impairment may be a disruption of the mechanical aspect of the special sense, as in the obstruction of sound waves from cerumen impaction in the ears, or may be a neurologic event, as in the occurrence of homonymous hemianopsia after a stroke.

Regardless of the cause of loss of the sense of hearing, vision, smell, or taste, prompt intervention and treatment can make tremendous differences in outcome. The loss may be totally corrected, or its progression may be slowed. Treatment may be aimed at the underlying cause of the sensory impairment or at altering the individual's behavior or environment to maximize the remaining function. In working with individuals who have alterations in special sensory function, health care professionals have the opportunity to make a great difference in that person's quality of life.

MEDIA RESOURCES

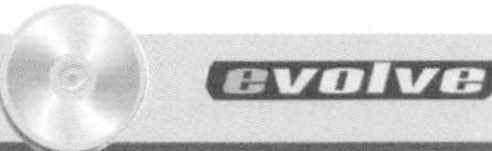

Remember to check out the ***CD Companion*** included with this book for Review Questions, Key Concepts Review, Glossary (with audio for selected terms), Disease Profiles, and Animations.

PLUS, visit the ***Evolve website*** at http://evolve.elsevier.com/Copstead/ for Case Studies, Disease Profiles, and WebLinks.

References

1. Ignatavicius DD, Workman M, editors: *Medical-surgical nursing: critical thinking for collaborative care,* ed 4, Philadelphia, 2002, Saunders.
2. Saundhaus S: Stop the spinning: diagnosing and managing vertigo, *Nurse Pract* 27(8):11-23, 2002.
3. Dean WA, Davison M: Hearing loss in adults: physical limitations, psychosocial barrier, *Clin Rev* 12(6):62-67, 2002.
4. National Institutes on Deafness and Other Communication Disorders: Hearing loss in adults. Available at http://www.nidcd.nih.gov/health/hearing/older.asp.
5. Tierney LM, McPhee SJ, Papadakis MA, editors: *Current medical diagnosis and treatment,* ed 43, New York, 2004, Lange/McGraw-Hill.
6. Green-Hernandez C, Singleton K, Aronzon P, editors: *Primary care pediatrics,* Philadelphia, 2001, Lippincott.
7. Centers for Disease Control and Prevention: Work related hearing loss. Available at http://www.cdc.gov.noish/hp-workrel.html.
8. National Institute on Deafness and Other Communication Disorders: Otosclerosis. Available at http://www.nidcd.nih.gov/health/hearing/otosclerosis.asp.
9. Bailey BJ, Calhoun K, Healy GB, editors: *Head and neck surgery: otolaryngology,* ed 3, Philadelphia, 2001, Lippincott Williams & Wilkins.
10. Mazelova J, Popelar J, Syka J: Auditory function in presbycusis: peripheral vs central changes, *Exp Gerontol* 38(1-2):87-94, 2003.

11. Hosokawa M: A higher oxidative status accelerates senescence and aggravates age-dependent disorders in SAMP strains of mice, *Mech Ageing Dev* 123(12):553-561, 2002.
12. Victor M, Ropper AH: *Adams and Victor's principles of neurology,* ed 7, New York, 2001, McGraw-Hill.
13. National Institute on Deafness and Other Communication Disorders: Meniere's disease. Available at http://www.nidcd.nih.gov/health/balance.meniere.asp.
14. Derebery MJ: Allergic management of Meniere's disease: an outcome study, *Otolaryngol Head Neck Surg* 122(2):174-182, 2000.
15. Little P et al: Pragmatic randomized controlled trial of two prescribing strategies for childhood acute otitis media, *BMJ* 322(7282):336-342, 2001.
16. Frock TL: Gaining insight into age-related macular degeneration, *J Am Acad Nurse Pract* 14(5):207-213, 2002.
17. National Eye Institute: Amblyopia. Available at http://www.nei.nih.gov/health/amblyopia/index.htm.
18. Behman RE, Kleigman RM, Jenson HP: *Nelson textbook of pediatrics,* ed 16, Philadelphia, 2000, Saunders.
19. National Eye Institute: Facts about cataracts. Available at http://www.nei.nih.gov/health/cataract_facts.htm.
20. Silverstone B et al, editors: *Lighthouse handbook on vision impairment and vision rehabilitation,* vol 1, New York, 2000, Oxford University Press.
21. American Diabetes Association: Diabetes and eye conditions. Available at http://www.diabetes.org.
22. National Eye Institute: Facts about age-related macular degeneration. Available at http://www.nei.nih.gov/health/maculardegen/armd_facts.htm.
23. Kassoff A, Kassoff J, for the Age-Related Eye Disease Study Research Group: A randomized, placebo-controlled, clinical trial of high-dose supplementation with vitamins C and E, beta carotene, and zinc for age-related macular degeneration and vision loss, *Arch Ophthalmol* 119(10):1417-1436, 2001.

chapter 47

Pain

Joni D. Nelsen-Marsh • Jacquelyn L. Banasik

MEDIA RESOURCES

Additional Material for Study, Review, and Further Exploration

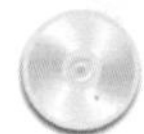

CD Companion ◆ Review Questions and Answers ◆ Key Concepts Review ◆ Glossary *(with audio pronunciations for selected terms)* ◆ Disease Profiles ◆ Animations

evolve ***Website*** at http://evolve.elsevier.com/Copstead/ ◆ Case Studies ◆ Disease Profiles ◆ WebLinks

KEY QUESTIONS

- How do the processes of transduction, transmission, perception, and modulation relate to the phenomenon of nociception?
- How is neurotransmission of pain signals modulated at the receptor, spinal cord, and brain?
- How do acute and chronic pain differ with regard to cause and clinical manifestations?
- Why are some painful sensations perceived at a distance from the site of injury (referred)?
- Why is it important to adequately manage pain?

CHAPTER OUTLINE

Pain is a complex physiologic and perceptual phenomenon. Because pain is very much a subjective experience, defining and assessing it are difficult. Merskey defined pain as "an unpleasant sensory and emotional experience associated with actual or potential tissue damage or described in terms of such damage."[1] McCaffery offered a clinically useful definition: "Pain is whatever the experiencing person says it is, existing whenever the experiencing person says it does."[2] Accurate assessment and optimal management of pain are extremely important not only because relief of pain and suffering is ethically desirable but also because unrelieved pain is physiologically harmful. Studies have documented the benefits of adequate pain control on the rate of recovery, health care costs, and postoperative morbidity. In fact, the Joint Commission on Accreditation of Healthcare Organizations (JCAHO) has developed standards of care regarding the assessment and management of pain that must be followed by all accredited agencies. Pain is often referred to as the fifth vital sign.[3]

PHYSIOLOGY OF PAIN

The physiologic mechanisms involved in the pain phenomenon are termed **nociception.** Nociception can be divided into four stages: transduction, transmission, perception, and modulation. Transduction is the process of converting painful stimuli to neuronal action potentials at the sensory receptor. Transmission refers to the movement of action potentials along neurons that make their way from the peripheral receptor to the spinal cord and then centrally to the brain. Perception occurs when the brain becomes aware of pain signals and interprets them as painful. The complex mechanisms whereby synaptic transmission of pain signals is modified is called modulation. It is clinically useful to conceptualize pain physiology according to these four processes because each stage provides an opportunity for intervention in the pain experience (Figure 47-1).

Transduction

Pain normally begins in the periphery when free nerve endings called **nociceptors** are stimulated. Nociceptors transduce noxious stimuli into neuronal action potentials that flow centrally to the spinal cord and then the brain. Nociceptors are found in skin, muscle, connective tissue, the circulatory system, and abdominal, pelvic, and thoracic viscera. Stimulation can be the result of direct damage to nerve endings, or it can result from release of chemicals at the site of injury.

Numerous substances participate in the initiation of nociceptive impulses.[4] Some of these substances are released as a direct result of tissue injury, whereas others may be produced as part of the inflammatory response to the injury. Important chemical mediators of pain include K^+, H^+, lactate, histamine, serotonin, bradykinins, and prostaglandins. These chemicals influence the membrane potential of the pain receptor, and if depolarization is sufficient, the nociceptor produces action potentials. When these impulses are conducted centrally, the second step, transmission, is initiated.

Prostaglandin involvement in the process of nociceptor stimulation is of particular interest because prostaglandin inhibitors such as aspirin and other nonsteroidal antiinflammatory drugs (NSAIDs) are commonly used to manage pain. Prostaglandins are formed when cells are damaged and an enzyme, phospholipase A, breaks down phospholipids in the cell membrane and converts them to arachidonic acid[5] (Figure 47-2). Arachidonic acid undergoes further breakdown by the enzyme cyclooxygenase to form prostaglandins. Sensitization by prostaglandins lowers the threshold of nociceptive fibers so that stimuli that would not cause pain under normal circumstances are now pain producing. NSAIDs prevent

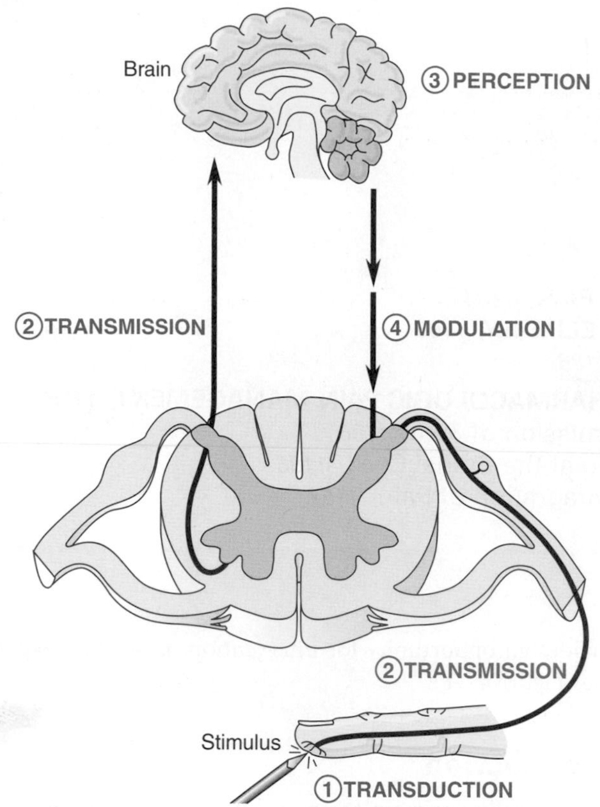

FIGURE 47-1 ■ The four processes of pain signaling: transduction, transmission, perception, and modulation.

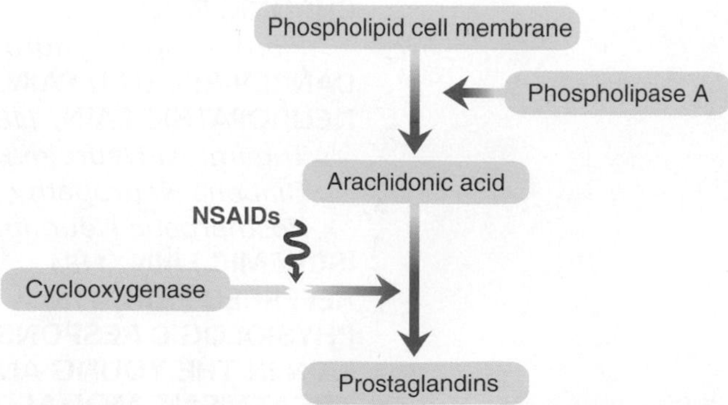

FIGURE 47-2 ■ Tissue injury results in the release of prostaglandins from the breakdown of phospholipid cell membranes. Nonsteroidal antiinflammatory agents *(NSAIDs)* inhibit the cyclooxygenase enzyme and block the production of prostaglandins.

prostaglandin production by inhibiting the action of cyclooxygenase.

Transmission

Stimulated nociceptors transmit impulses to the central nervous system (CNS) by means of specialized sensory fibers. The primary sensory fibers involved in the transmission of nociceptive impulses are the Aδ and C fibers.[4,6,7] The characteristics and functions of these fibers are summarized in Table 47-1. In general, the larger, myelinated Aδ fibers transmit the nociceptive impulses very quickly as an initial response to tissue injury. The nature of the pain carried by the fast-traveling Aδ fibers is characterized as sharp, stinging, and highly localized. In contrast, unmyelinated C fibers transmit pain more slowly. Pain transmitted by C fibers is poorly localized and has a dull or aching quality that lingers long after the initial sharp pain abates. The majority of pain sensations travel via C fibers and project to areas of the brain that evoke emotional responses such as displeasure and anxiety.

Most sensory afferent pain fibers enter the spinal cord by way of the posterior nerve roots (Figure 47-3). The cell bodies of pain neurons are located in the dorsal root ganglion. As the afferent neurons enter the dorsal horn, collateral branches spread up and down the spinal cord for two to three segments by way of the tract of Lissauer. These spinal connections are important for reflex postural adjustments when a painful body part is suddenly withdrawn from the painful stimulus.

Sensory afferent neurons synapse with interneurons, anterior motor neurons, and sympathetic preganglionic neurons in specific regions of the spinal cord (see Figure 47-3). Aδ and C fibers carry excitatory impulses from cutaneous pain receptors in small, localized areas of the skin to interneurons in lamina I. Many of the neurons originating in lamina I cross the spinal cord to activate neurons in the anterolateral tract.

Laminae II and III represent a key anatomic region of the cord involved in pain transmission known as the **substantia gelatinosa.** The substantia gelatinosa is characterized by multiple synaptic connections among primary sensory afferent neurons, interneurons, and anterolateral ascending fibers. There is much opportunity at this point for pain signal transmission to be modulated by other sensory input or from CNS activity. Pain signals can be either enhanced or blocked at these synapses.

Another key synaptic area involved in nociception is lamina V. Numerous Aδ and C fibers deliver somatic input from mechanical, thermal, and chemical receptors in the periphery to lamina V. Sensory afferent neurons from visceral receptors also terminate in lamina V. The convergence of both somatic and visceral fibers in lamina V may help explain the phenomenon of referred pain, in which pain from a visceral organ is perceived at the body surface.[6] The remaining, deeper laminae VI through VIII receive sensory input from muscles, joints, and visceral afferent fibers.

A number of neurotransmitters and neuropeptides are involved in synaptic transmission in the spinal cord. Substance P is a well-known example. Others include excitatory amino acids (glutamate), cholecystokinin, and calcitonin gene–related peptide. These neurotransmitters bind to the next neurons in the pathway and thereby initiate action potentials. The pain signal is propelled along its pathway toward the brain. Interruption of these synaptic processes can inhibit pain transmission. The synapses in the spinal cord are extremely important points of pain modulation by both endogenous and exogenous means.

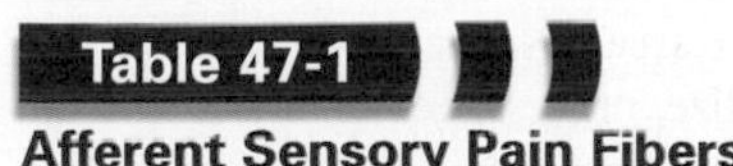

Table 47-1

Afferent Sensory Pain Fibers

Feature	Aδ Fibers	C Fibers
Structure	Myelinated	Unmyelinated
Amount	10%	90%
Source	Mechanical stimuli	Polymodal stimuli (mechanical, thermal, chemical)
Speed	Fast traveling, 5-10 m/sec	Slower traveling, 0.6-2 m/sec
Sensory quality of pain mediated	Sharp, stinging, cutting, pinching	Dull, burning, aching

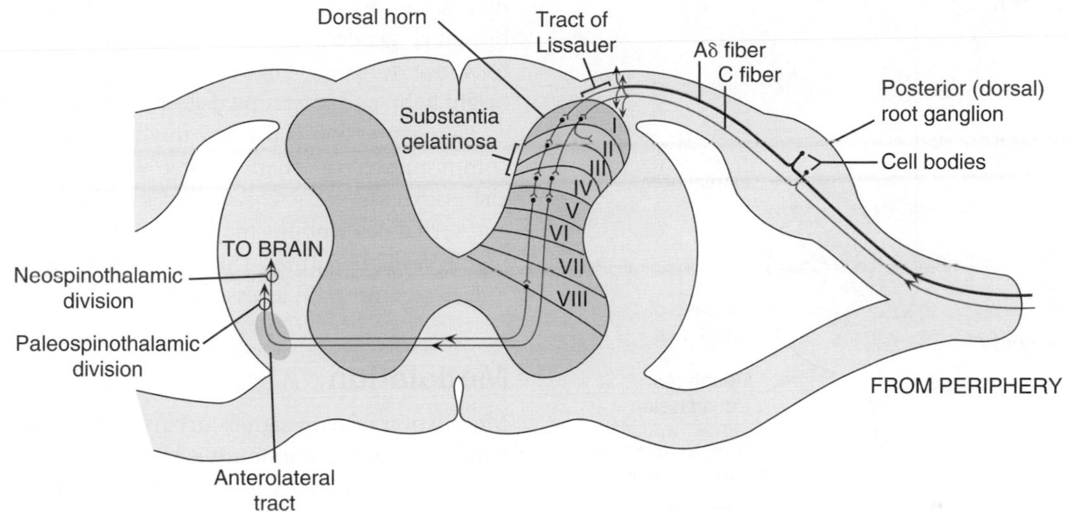

FIGURE 47-3 ■ A spinal cord segment showing primary afferent pain fibers, Aδ and C fibers, entering the dorsal horn, synapsing on interneurons, crossing to the opposite side, and traveling to the brain in the anterolateral tract.

The excitatory neurotransmitter glutamate is involved in carrying the nociceptive message from primary afferent fibers to secondary neurons. Glutamate binding to its *N*-methyl-D-aspartate (NMDA) receptors on the postsynaptic neuron is thought to induce a kind of synaptic memory in the pain pathway. Excessive or repeated stimulation of C fibers sensitizes the spinal cord neurons so that even mild stimulation may be perceived as painful.[5] This phenomenon has been termed "wind-up" and may be an important mechanism in the development of chronic pain syndromes. Drugs that inhibit glutamate production may impede the wind-up response, thereby controlling pain before synaptic memory of the pain develops in the pain pathways.

Pain signals transmitted by the spinal interneurons are then conducted to the brain by ascending spinal pathways (Figure 47-4). The major pathway for pain signal transmission up the spinal cord is the anterolateral tract, so named because it travels in the anterolateral portion of the white matter of the spinal column. This tract is also called the spinothalamic tract in some texts and has two divisions: the neospinothalamic tract and the paleospinothalamic tract. Both divisions cross at the spinal segment and carry pain signals up the contralateral (opposite) side of the cord. Thus nociceptor input from the right side of the body travels in the anterolateral tracts on the left side of the cord, whereas signals from the left side of the body travel on the right side of the cord.

The neospinothalamic division has fewer synapses in the cord and projects first to the thalamus and then to the primary somatosensory cortex. Aδ fiber signals are transmitted in this tract and reach the brain quickly to provide specific information about pain location with little emotional connotation. C fiber impulses travel mainly in the paleospinothalamic division, which makes a greater number of synapses and reaches the brain more slowly. The paleospinothalamic tract projects to widespread brain areas and stirs aversive emotional responses. The paleospinothalamic tract travels with the neospinothalamic tract in the anterolateral portion of the spinal cord to the level of the medulla and then sends diffuse projections to the reticular formation, the mesencephalon, and, finally, the thalamus. From the thalamus, further projections to the cerebral cortex, limbic system, and basal ganglia occur. The pain sensation from C fibers is poorly localized, longer lasting, and more distressing than Aδ fiber pain.

The brain can localize a pain sensation to a particular part of the body because nociceptor pathways are kept in specific anatomic order in the cord and somatosensory cortex. Each

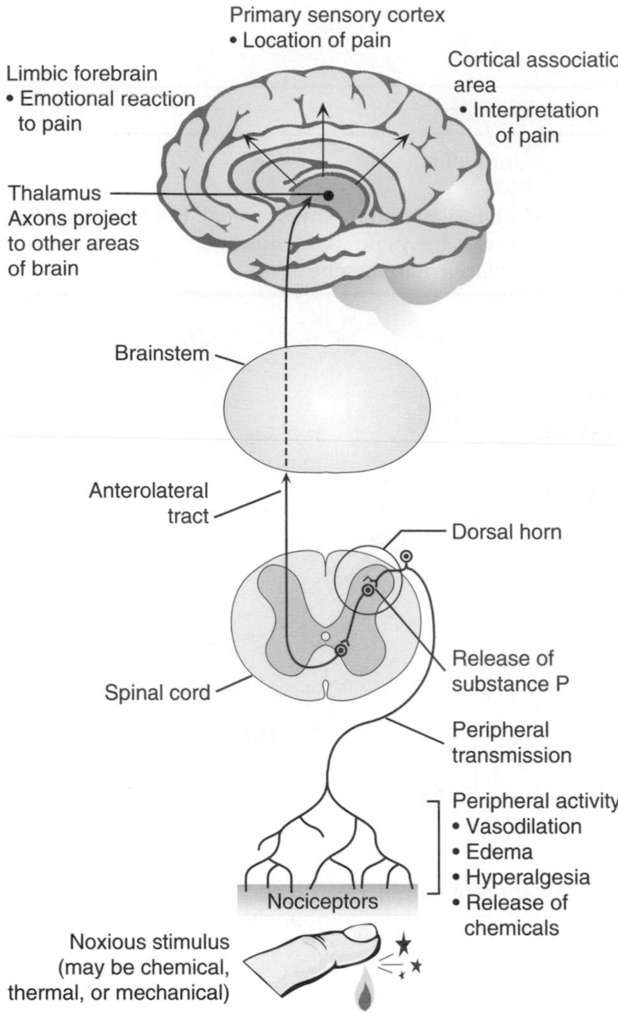

FIGURE 47-4 ■ The anterolateral nociceptive pathways travel up the spinal cord and project to the thalamus, somatosensory cortex, cortical association areas, and limbic structures.

spinal nerve contains the nociceptor fibers for a particular area of the body surface, called a sensory dermatome (Figure 47-5). Dermatomal maps are useful for locating a source of neurologic pain. Pain that follows a dermatomal distribution is due to spinal nerve compression or trauma and is called a radiculopathy. Vertebral disk disease is a common cause of radiculopathy. Peripheral neuropathies, in contrast, do not follow a dermatomal pattern. Examples of peripheral neuropathies are carpal tunnel syndrome (median nerve) and diabetic neuropathy, which often affects both legs in a stocking-like pattern.

Perception

Perception is the result of neural processing of pain sensations in the brain. Perception includes an awareness and interpretation of the meaning of the sensation. Pain perception is influenced by attention, distraction, anxiety, fear, fatigue, and previous experience and expectations. Pain perception is not localized to a specific brain area.[5] Numerous neuronal networks are necessary to localize, process, and interpret painful sensations. The primary somatosensory cortex, association cortex, frontal lobe, and limbic structures all participate in this processing.

Pain perception can be described in terms of pain threshold and pain tolerance. Pain threshold is the level of painful stimulation required to be perceived and is remarkably similar from one individual to another. Pain tolerance is the degree of pain that one is willing to bear before seeking relief. Pain tolerance varies widely among individuals and within the same individual under differing conditions. Age, culture, family upbringing, gender, and previous pain experience influence tolerance to pain. Environmental factors, including noise, bright light, and interrupted sleep, may affect pain tolerance.

Pain expression is the way in which the pain experience is communicated to others. Pacing, writhing, jaw clenching, facial grimacing, muscle guarding, crying, moaning, groaning, and verbal descriptions may be used to express pain. Thus the highly variable nature of pain expression among individuals makes accurate pain assessment difficult.

Modulation

Modulation of pain signals occurs at multiple sites along the pain pathway. A fair amount is known about pain modulation at the spinal cord, where neurons from nociceptors, somatosensory receptors, and descending neurons from the CNS all converge and interact. Modulation also occurs at the peripheral nociceptor ending and within the brain; however, these mechanisms are less well understood.

Attempts to decrease the perception of painful stimuli may be initiated spontaneously by the person experiencing pain. Rubbing, pressing, or shaking the painful area may reduce the intensity of pain. In 1965, Melzack and Wall proposed the gate control theory to explain how stimulation of large "touch" neurons could inhibit the transmission of nociceptor impulses.[8] This theory was very useful in focusing efforts to understand pain signal processing at the spinal cord level.

Central to the gate control theory is the capacity for interneurons in the spinal cord to modify the transmission of nociceptor impulses. The original gate control theory suggested that impulses carried by large myelinated cutaneous fibers (Aβ) could "close the gate" on nociceptor impulses so that pain signals would be blocked in the spinal cord and not allowed to progress centrally to the brain. The physiologic process underlying the closing-the-gate mechanisms has been the subject of much study. Numerous interneurons, neurotransmitters, and neuropeptides have been implicated in this complex gating mechanism.

Descending pathways from the brain to the dorsal horn region of the spinal cord are important modulators of the pain response (Figure 47-6). These descending pathways originate in a brainstem nucleus called the raphe magnus and project to the dorsal horn regions of laminae I, II, and IV.[5] Neurotrans-

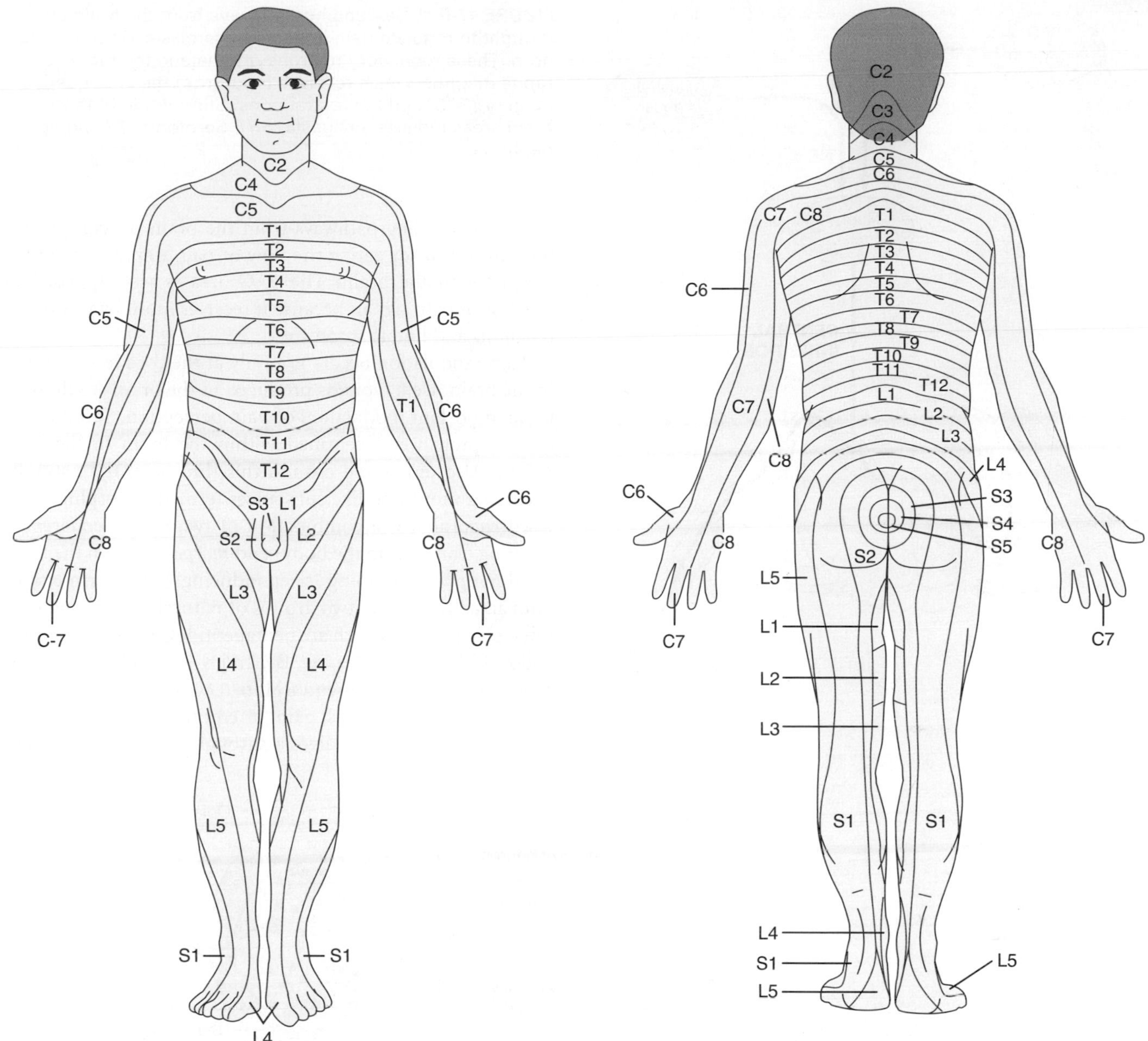

FIGURE 47-5 ■ Sensory dermatomes. Pain located in the pattern of a dermatome occurs with spinal nerve injury and is referred to as radiculopathy.

mitters released by these neurons can inhibit synaptic transmission of pain signals. One way to inhibit synaptic transmission is through presynaptic inhibition of substance P release from nociceptor neurons (Figure 47-7). **Opioids** such as **endorphins** are thought to be the mediators of presynaptic inhibition. A similar inhibitory effect can be achieved by administering opioid drugs, such as morphine, that bind to opioid receptors and mimic the effect of endorphins.

The raphe magnus receives input from two other brain areas important in the pain response: the periaqueductal gray (PAG) area in the midbrain and the rostral pons in the brainstem. The PAG area has a high concentration of endogenous opioids (endorphins and enkephalins) that are known to produce analgesic effects similar to narcotic drugs. Stimulation of the PAG area causes release of these endogenous opioids and also sends nerve impulses to the raphe magnus. Serotonin (5-hydroxytryptamine, 5HT) is the neurotransmitter that conveys analgesic signals from the PAG area to the raphe magnus. This finding helps explain the pain-relieving action of drugs that enhance serotonin activity in the brain, such as tricyclic antidepressants.

The neurons projecting to the raphe magnus from the rostral pons secrete norepinephrine as the neurotransmitter. Stimulation of these neurons also produces an analgesic effect. Clonidine, a drug that mimics the effect of norepinephrine in the brain, has been shown to have pain-relieving properties.

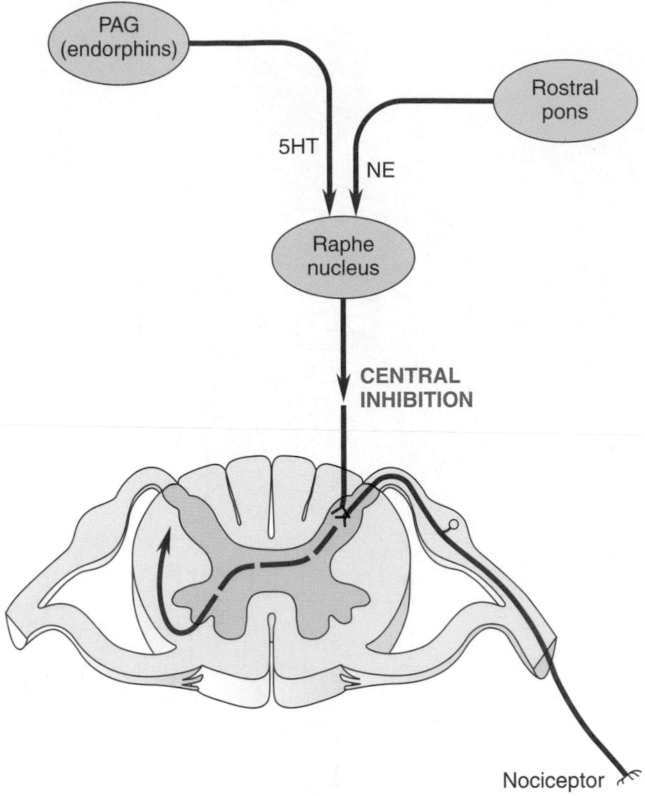

FIGURE 47-6 ■ Descending pathways from the brain are thought to regulate pain impulse transmission in the dorsal horn. These regulatory neurons originate in the brainstem raphe magnus, which receives input from the periaqueductal gray *(PAG)* and the rostral pons. Stimulation of these brain areas induces analgesia. *5HT,* Serotonin; *NE,* norepinephrine.

The descending pathways from the brain provide an important means for gating the flow of pain impulses from the periphery to the brain. The PAG area is well apprised of the flow of pain signals because it receives input by way of the thalamus and limbic structures.

Pain modulation occurs not only at the cord level but also in the brain itself. Opioids produced in the brain are thought to be important modulators of pain perception. Specific opioid receptors were identified within the brain in the early 1970s.[9] Also discovered around this time were the naturally occurring morphine-like substances termed endorphins. The word *endorphin* is a combination of two words, *endogenous* (coming from within the body) and *morphine* (from the Latin word *morpheus,* meaning "sleep inducing"). The term endorphin actually refers to two groups of naturally occurring peptides: enkephalins, which are pentapeptides, and three types of endorphin polypeptides, α-, β-, and γ-endorphin. Of these, most is known about β-endorphin.

During times of stress, pain, or emotion, the brain apparently creates its own analgesia through the secretion of en-

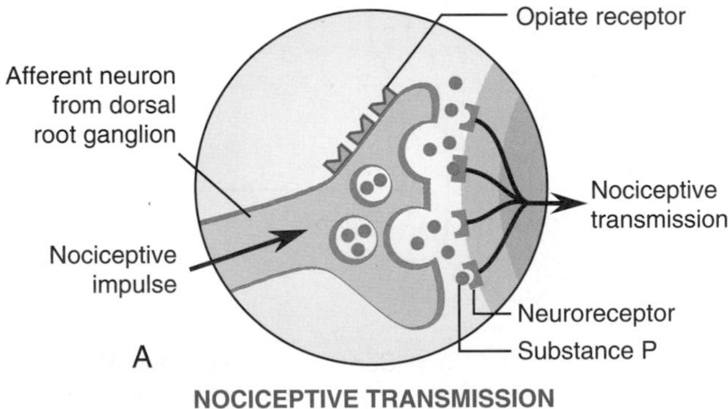

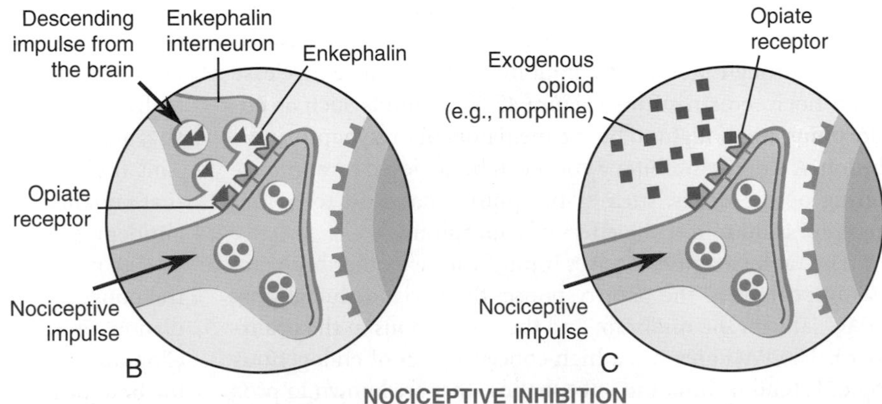

FIGURE 47-7 ■ Pain transmission and inhibition at the molecular level. **A,** Nociceptive transmission to higher levels of the central nervous system. **B,** Nociception inhibited through binding of endogenous opioids (e.g., enkephalin). The release of substance P is prevented. **C,** Nociception inhibited through binding of exogenous opioid (e.g., morphine). Release of substance P is prevented.

Table 47-2

Opioid Receptor Activity

Opioid Receptor	Activity
Mu (μ)	Analgesia Sedation Respiratory depression Pupil constriction Nausea and vomiting Constipation Urine retention Pruritus
Kappa (κ)	Analgesia Sedation Respiratory depression Pupil constriction Diuresis
Sigma (σ)	No analgesia Vasomotor stimulation Tachypnea Pupil dilation Psychotomimetic effects (hallucinations, paranoia, delirium)
Delta (δ)	No analgesia Respiratory depression Nausea and vomiting Pruritus

dogenous opioids—a process known as stress-induced analgesia. Stress-induced analgesia is reversed by naloxone, a drug that blocks opioid receptors, thus supporting the role of endogenous opioids in the process.[5] As previously described, the PAG area produces large quantities of endogenous opioids that are thought to inhibit pain signal perception within the brain. High concentrations of β-endorphin are also found in the pituitary gland, and it is likely that release of pituitary stress hormones (adrenocorticotropic hormone) is accompanied by the release of endorphins. The adrenal glands also produce endogenous opioids as a sympathetic response to stress. Endorphins released into the blood stream by the pituitary and adrenals have their effects in the periphery because they cannot effectively cross the blood-brain barrier.

Opioids have different effects depending on the types of receptors they activate. Four types of opioid receptors have been identified: mu (μ), kappa (κ), sigma (σ), and delta (δ) (Table 47-2). The distribution of the specific opioid receptors varies throughout the body. The μ and κ receptors have analgesic activities. The μ receptors are found in high concentration in the brain, where they are thought to modulate pain perception. The κ receptors are concentrated primarily in the spinal cord, where they contribute to pain modulation by CNS descending pathways. Each opioid receptor subtype is associated with a number of undesirable side effects. Depending on the affinity for certain receptors, different drugs may have differing analgesic potency and side effect profiles[10] (Table 47-3).

Table 47-3

Receptor Affinity of Commonly Used Opioids

		Agonist		Antagonist	
Drug	**Receptor Affinity**	**Pure**	**Partial**	**Pure**	**Partial**
Morphine, meperidine, hydromorphone, methadone, fentanyl	mu (μ)	X			
	kappa (κ) (*morphine only*)		X		
	delta (δ)		X		
Buprenorphine	mu (μ)		X		
	kappa (κ)	X			
Butorphanol	mu (μ)				X
	kappa (κ)	X			
	sigma (σ)	X			
Nalbuphine	mu (μ)				X
	kappa (κ)	X			
	sigma (σ)		X		
Pentazocine	mu (μ)	X			X
	kappa (κ)	X			
	sigma (σ)				
Naloxone	mu (μ)			X	
	kappa (κ)			X	
	sigma (σ)				
	delta (δ)				
Naltrexone	mu (μ)			X	
	kappa (κ)			X	

KEY CONCEPTS

- Nociception can be conceptualized as four interdependent processes: stimulus transduction, signal transmission, pain perception, and pain modulation.
- Nociceptor activity is transmitted to the spinal cord by two types of neurons: large, myelinated Aδ fibers, which transmit sharp, localized sensations; and small, unmyelinated C fibers, which transmit dull, aching, poorly localized sensations.
- Pain signals are transmitted by afferent fibers that enter the cord through the dorsal horn, synapse on interneurons, and then cross the cord and project centrally in the anterolateral tract.
- The anterolateral tract has two divisions: the neospinothalamic tract, which carries Aδ fiber input and projects to the thalamus and then the sensory cortex; and the paleospinothalamic tract, which carries C fiber input and projects diffusely to the reticular formation, mesencephalon, and thalamus.
- Perception of painful stimuli involves several brain structures, including the primary somatosensory cortex, association areas, and limbic structures. Pain perception is influenced by culture, environment, and physical status and varies widely among individuals.
- Afferent pain signals can be modulated at several levels. Descending pathways project from the PAG area and rostral pons by way of the raphe magnus to inhibit pain neurons in the dorsal aspect of the spinal cord. Pain is also modulated within the brain by endogenous opioids (enkephalins, endorphins).

TYPES OF PAIN

Pain can be classified according to duration (acute, chronic), source (cancer, neuropathic, ischemic), or location and referral pattern. Pain is a symptom of an underlying problem rather than a primary disorder; attempts to alleviate pain should be accompanied by efforts to locate and manage the underlying etiology. The character, location, and duration of pain can provide helpful clues to aid the diagnostic process.

ACUTE PAIN

Pain is often categorized as being acute or chronic, depending on the duration of symptoms. Acute pain results from tissue injury and resolves when the injury heals, usually in less than 3 months. Acute pain is typically accompanied by clinical signs and symptoms of pain that result from stimulation of the sympathetic nervous system. These signs and symptoms include an elevated heart rate, respiratory rate, and blood pressure, as well as pallor, sweating, and nausea (Table 47-4). Persons experiencing acute pain may express pain behavior such as pacing, grimacing, crying, or moaning. Short-term therapy with nonopioid and opioid agents is often helpful. The risk of becoming dependent on pain medications is small in persons experiencing acute pain. Adequate management of pain during an acute episode may help prevent the development of some types of chronic pain syndromes.

Headache

Etiology and Pathogenesis. Headache is one of the most common causes of acute pain. An estimated 80 million Americans suffer from headaches, and women are more commonly affected than men.[11] Headaches have historically been classified according to strict etiologic categories (e.g., tension, migraine, sinus). However, new research into the pathogenesis of headaches indicates that these may not be separate entities but rather categories along the same spectrum sharing a common pathophysiologic process.

Migraine remains one of the most common yet underdiagnosed headache types. An estimated 1 million Americans have

Table 47-4

Physiologic Responses to Pain

Criteria	Response
Signs and symptoms	↑ Heart rate ↑ Blood pressure ↑ Respiratory rate Dilated pupils Pallor and perspiration Nausea and vomiting Urine retention
Physiologic response	Blood shifts from superficial vessels to striated muscle, heart, lungs, and brain Bronchioles dilated to ↑ oxygenation ↓ Gastric secretions ↓ Gastrointestinal motility ↑ Circulating blood sugar Hypomotility of the bladder and ureters

Adapted from Wild L: Pain management, *Crit Care Clin North Am* 2(4):538, 1990.

a migraine on any given day; 150,000 will require bed rest.[11] Previous theories of migraine included simply a vascular causation. It was thought that cerebral vessel spasm and then vasodilation caused the throbbing pain typical of migraine. Current theories involve stimulation of the trigeminal nerve in combination with changes in neurotransmitter levels in the CNS and blood vessel tone.

An individual headache is thought to be initiated by a drop in plasma serotonin (5HT), which acts at the $5HT_1$ inhibitory receptor. This decrease in inhibitory activity allows the brain to become more sensitive to triggering stimuli such as changes in level of hormones (menstrual cycle, menopause, hormonal contraceptives), chemicals, stress, fasting, and sleep deprivation, among others. In response to the decrease in $5HT_1$ inhibition, the dorsal raphae nucleus releases additional 5HT that binds to the $5HT_2$ receptor. This causes vasodilation in the intracerebral vessels and stretching of the perivascular neurons. Inflammatory cytokines are released. This activates the trigeminal nerve, sending pain signals to the hypothalamus (Figure 47-8).[12,13]

Clinical Manifestations. Typical signs of a migraine headache include severe unilateral pounding or throbbing pain that may be accompanied by nausea, vomiting, photophobia, phonophobia, and lacrimation. The pain is increased by any routine physical activity. Some migraines may be preceded by an aura such as flashing lights or other visual disturbances, and unilateral paresthesias. Other symptoms may include sinus/nasal congestion, neck muscle stiffness and pain, vertigo, and changes in bowel pattern.[14]

Diagnosis and Treatment. Headaches are diagnosed through careful history and physical examination. Brain tumors, infection, hydrocephalus, and increased intracranial pressure must be ruled out. Physical assessment should include ears, nose and throat, sinuses, temporomandibular joint, neck musculature, cranial nerves, and retinal examination. General cognitive, neurologic, and motor function should also be examined. Headaches caused by trauma, following a worsening pattern, accompanied by other neurologic symptoms, or those of sudden onset that are the worst experienced by an individual require neuroimaging. In 1988, the International Headache Society established criteria for a migraine diagnosis, and this has been adopted by many health care providers (Box 47-1). However, many whose migraines do not meet the criteria have been diagnosed with sinus (a relatively rare cause of headaches, according to ear-nose-throat experts) or tension-type headaches.[15,16] As a result, patients have received at times inadequate control of their headache pain, creating disability for the patients and an economic burden resulting from sick days and lost work productivity.

It has since been discovered that some of the "nonmigraine" headaches have responded well to treatment with medications that alter the level of serotonin in the CNS (medications once reserved only for migraines).[15,16] This result

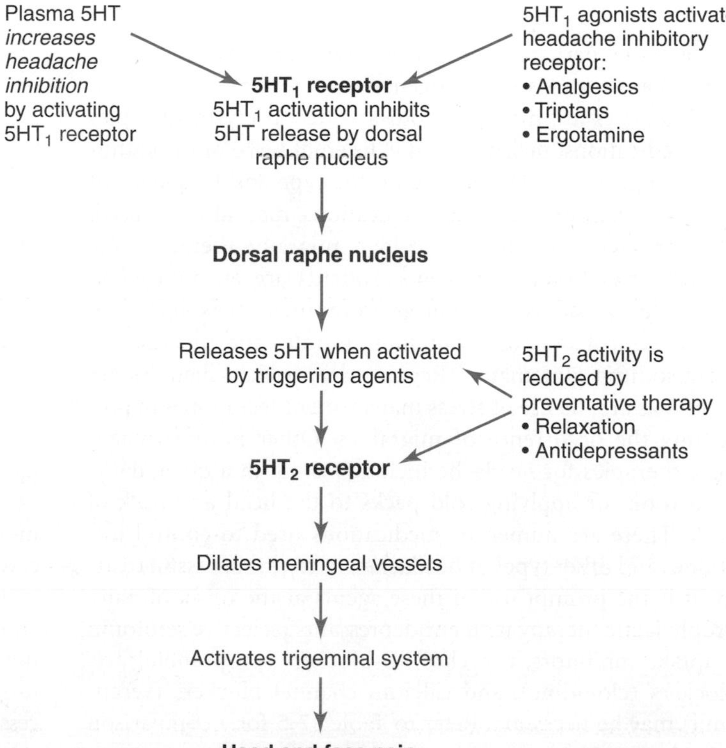

Plasma 5HT *increases headache inhibition* by activating $5HT_1$ receptor
$5HT_1$ receptor
$5HT_1$ activation inhibits 5HT release by dorsal raphe nucleus
$5HT_1$ agonists activate headache inhibitory receptor:
• Analgesics
• Triptans
• Ergotamine
Dorsal raphe nucleus
Releases 5HT when activated by triggering agents
$5HT_2$ activity is reduced by preventative therapy
• Relaxation
• Antidepressants
$5HT_2$ receptor
Dilates meningeal vessels
Activates trigeminal system
Head and face pain

FIGURE 47-8 ■ Headache pathogenesis. *5HT,* Serotonin. (From Rakel RE, Bope ET, editors: *Conn's current therapy,* Philadelphia, 2003, Elsevier.)

Box 47-1

International Headache Society Diagnosis Criteria for Migraine

Migraine Without Aura

1. At least five attacks that fulfill criteria 2 to 4
2. Headache attacks lasting 4 to 72 hours (untreated or unsuccessfully treated)
3. Headaches has at least two of the following characteristics:
   - Unilateral location
   - Pulsating quality
   - Moderate or severe intensity that inhibits or prohibits daily activities
   - Aggravated by climbing stairs or similar routine physical activity
4. During a headache at least one of the following two symptoms occurs:
   - Nausea and/or vomiting
   - Photophobia and phonophobia
5. At least one of the following characteristics is present:
   - History and physical and neurologic exams do not suggest any of the following: head trauma, vascular disorders; nonvascular intracranial disorders; substance abuse or withdrawal; noncephalic infection; metabolic disorders; cranial neuralgias; disorders of the cranium, neck, eyes, ears, nose, sinuses, teeth, mouth, or other facial or cranial structures
   - History and/or physical and/or neurologic examination do suggest one of the above disorders, but it is ruled out by appropriate investigations
   - One of the above disorders is present, but migraine attacks do not occur for the first time in close temporal relationship to the disorder

Migraine with Aura

1. At least two attacks that fulfill the second criteria
2. Headache has at least three of the following four characteristics:
   - One or more fully reversible aura symptoms indicating focal cerebral, cortical, and/or brainstem dysfunction
   - At least one aura symptom develops gradually over more than 4 minutes, or two or more symptoms occur in succession
   - No aura symptoms last more than 60 minutes; if more than one aura symptom is present, accepted duration is proportionately increased
   - Headache follows aura with a free interval of less than 60 minutes (it may also begin before or simultaneously with the aura)
3. At least one of the following characteristics is present:
   - History and physical and neurologic examinations do not suggest any of the following: head trauma, vascular disorders; nonvascular intracranial disorders; substance abuse or withdrawal; noncephalic infection; metabolic disorders; cranial neuralgias; disorders of the cranium, neck, eyes, ears, nose, sinuses, teeth, mouth, or other facial or cranial structures
   - History and/or physical and/or neurologic examination do suggest one of the above disorders, but it is ruled out by appropriate investigations
   - One of the above disorders is present, but migraine attacks do not occur for the first time in close temporal relationship to the disorder

Data from Diamond ML: Migraine: still underdiagnosed, still undertreated; *Consultant Suppl* 42(13):56-59, 2002.

suggests that perhaps sinus, tension-type, and migraine headaches share a common pathogenesis.

Headaches are managed with a wide variety of therapies and medications, each aimed at a different piece of the pathophysiologic puzzle. Depending on the type and frequency of the headache, prophylactic medications may also be used. One mainstay of nonpharmacologic migraine therapy is the avoidance of headache triggers. Patients are encouraged to eliminate vasoactive substances from their diets including cheese, chocolate, foods containing nitrates and nitrites, and monosodium glutamate.[13] Regular sleep-wake schedules are helpful as are the use of stress management techniques in preventing the occurrence of migraines. Other nonpharmacologic therapies for headache include resting in a quiet, darkened room or applying cold packs to the head and back of neck. There are numerous medications used to control migraines and other types of headaches. A key to successful treatment is the prompt use of these agents at the onset of pain. Prophylactic therapy with antidepressants (selective serotonin reuptake inhibitors, tricyclics), β-blockers (propranolol), α-blockers (clonidine), and calcium channel blockers (verapamil) may be necessary. Refer to Table 47-5 for a comparison of pharmacologic therapies for the acute management of headache.

CHRONIC PAIN

Pain is considered chronic when it lasts more than several months beyond the expected healing time (more than 6 months). When chronic pain is not due to a malignancy, its cause is often difficult to ascertain. Chronic pain is not always manifested by signs and symptoms of sympathetic activity. As the body becomes accustomed to pain, the nervous system desensitizes itself to the noxious input; therefore, symptoms are more often psychological. Lack of sleep because of pain causes fatigue and irritability. Loss of a job or loss of body image because of pain causes personal and family difficulties. Treatment failures may create a sense of hopelessness or distrust of caregivers.

Depression is a common finding in persons experiencing chronic pain. In many cases the cause of the chronic pain cannot be determined, and therefore treatment is difficult. The use of narcotic pain relievers is discouraged because of the necessity of long-term therapy. Satisfactory treatment may re-

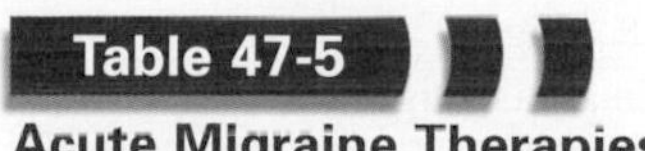

Acute Migraine Therapies

Drug	Route of Administration	Comments
Serotonin Receptor Agonists (Triptans)		
Sumatriptan (Imitrex) Zolmitriptan (Zomig) Rizatriptan (Maxalt) Naratriptan (Amerge) Eletriptan (Relpax)	PO, nasal spray, SC injection, dissolvable tablet	Increases serotonin; cannot be given with monoamine oxidase inhibitors, contraindicated in renal/hepatic failure, risk of serotonin syndrome if given with selective serotonin reuptake inhibitors
Ergot Alkaloids		
Ergotamine with caffeine (Wigraine, Ercaf, Cafergot) Dihydroergotamine mesylate (DHE, Migranal)	IV, IM, SC, PO, rectal suppository, inhaler	Increases serotonin; intracerebral vasoconstriction; best if given early after onset; contraindicated in patients with cardiovascular disease and pregnancy, may cause nausea/vomiting
Nonsteroidal Antiinflammatories and Nonopiates		
Acetaminophen (Tylenol) Ketorolac (Toradol) Naproxen Sodium (Naprosyn, Aleve) Ibuprofen (Motrin, Advil) Aspirin	PO, IV, IM	May cause gastrointestinal upset/bleeding; frequent use may cause "rebound" headache
Barbiturate-Hypnotic Combinations		
Butalbital with aspirin and caffeine (Fioricet, Fioricet with codeine)	PO	High abuse/addictive potential; may cause sedation; rebound headache with frequent use, withdrawal potential
Opiates/Combinations		
Acetaminophen with codeine, oxycodone, or hydrocodone (Tylenol no. 3/4, Percocet, Lorcet) Butorphanol (Stadol)	PO, nasal spray (Stadol only)	High abuse/addictive potential; may cause sedation, considered "rescue medications"

Adapted from Moloney MF et al: Caring for the woman with migraine headache, *Nurse Pract* 25(1):17-36, 2000; and Aminoff MJ: Nervous system. In Tierney LM, McPhee SJ, Papadakis MA, editors: *Current medical diagnosis and treatment,* ed 43, New York, 2004, Lange.

quire numerous coordinated approaches, and the patient may benefit from the services of a pain clinic that specializes in multimodal therapies.

Fibromyalgia Syndrome

Etiology and Pathogenesis. Fibromyalgia syndrome (FMS) is a chronic pain syndrome affecting 3% to 10% of the population.[17] Women are affected more frequently than men, with a ratio of 9:1, and the syndrome usually occurs between the ages of 20 and 50.[17,18] FMS is a collection of symptoms without a clear physiologic cause. Patients have a history of chronic widespread pain affecting all four extremities. FMS is a controversial diagnosis; some classify it as a rheumatologic disorder whereas others believe it is more of a psychiatric disorder.

The cause of FMS is unknown. However, etiologic studies have identified several risk factors for the development of the syndrome. Individuals with a medical history of excessive stress, trauma (both physical and emotional), sexual abuse, infections (parvovirus, hepatitis C, Epstein-Barr), and endocrine disorders (hypothyroid) are more commonly affected.[7] Disordered pain mechanisms in the CNS are a suspected factor in FMS. Patients with FMS have a lower threshold for pain than those without the disorder. However, there is no difference in the ability to perceive pain.[19] Pain maintenance and modulation mechanisms in the brain and spinal cord are also suspect. Studies have demonstrated a higher level of substance P in the cerebrospinal fluid of FMS patients. Lower levels of pain-inhibitory neurochemicals are also found.[18] Other theories include growth hormone deficiency, abnormalities in the hypothalamic-pituitary-adrenal axis, and abnormal activation of the sympathetic stress response. Arnold-Chiari malformations are also thought to be linked to FMS.

Clinical Manifestations. Patients complain of pain that waxes and wanes, and does not follow a dermatomal pattern. The pain tends to be exacerbated by physical exertion.[7] **Hyperalgesia** and **allodynia** are common. Allodynia is a condition in which a mild stimulus such as soft touch causes pain. Hyperalgesia is a lower threshold for nociceptor stimulation. Musculoskeletal examinations are generally normal. Other symptoms commonly seen associated with FMS include sleep disturbance/insomnia and irritable bowel syndrome. Fatigue is a hallmark of the syndrome. Depression and anxiety are also common along with cognitive difficulties such as problems with attention and short-term memory, thus suggesting the psychiatric theory of pathogenesis.[19]

Diagnosis and Treatment. FMS is a diagnosis of exclusion. Thyroid disorders, myopathies, rheumatoid arthritis, and chronic viral infections (e.g., human immunodeficiency virus) must be ruled out. In FMS there is a lack of objective or laboratory findings. However, the American College of Rheumatology has established criteria to assist in the diagnosis of FMS. An individual must complain of widespread pain in all four extremities that has been present for 3 months or more and have pain in 11 of 18 "trigger" or "tender" points when pressure is applied to these areas (Figure 47-9).

Management of FMS begins with patient education. Although sometimes disabling, FMS is not a fatal illness and does not affect life span. Treatment includes a variety of medications including antidepressants, such as the selective serotonin reuptake inhibitors and the tricyclic antidepressants.[18] Restoration of sleep patterns seems to be a key factor of successful treatment. NSAIDs and muscle-relaxing agents are also helpful. Opioid medications and corticosteroids are generally avoided as these are not effective long-term therapies.[17] Nonpharmacologic therapies include regular physical exercise, good nutrition, and psychological counseling.

CANCER-RELATED PAIN

Cancer pain is a subcategory of chronic pain, although it may be associated with acute pain episodes. Malignant pain differs from nonmalignant chronic pain in that it often has an identifiable cause. Pain associated with cancer may result from infiltration of organs or compression of structures by an expanding tumor, or it may occur as a result of treatments that damage tissue such as radiation therapy or chemotherapy.[5] In patients with cancer pain, clinical signs and symptoms are often a mixture of sympathetic nervous system activation and behavioral changes. Unremitting cancer pain requires a multifaceted approach and use of potent medications. Often the quality of life is a larger consideration than the length of life, and adequate pain control is a major factor affecting the quality of life.

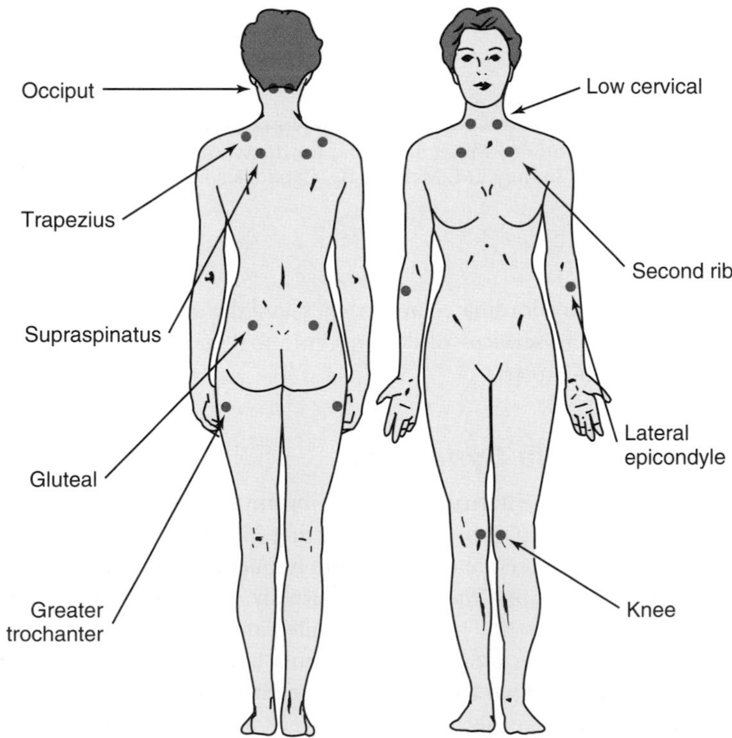

FIGURE 47-9 ■ Posterior and anterior trigger points. (From Lewis SM, Heitkemper MM, Dirksen SR: *Medical surgical nursing*, ed 6, St Louis, 2004, Mosby, p 1750. Redrawn from Freundlich B, Leventhal L: The fibromyalgia syndrome. In Schumacher HR Jr, Klippel JH, Koopman WJ, editors: *Primer on the rheumatic diseases,* ed 11, Atlanta, 1997, Arthritis Foundation. Reprinted with permission from the Arthritis Foundation, Atlanta, Ga.)

NEUROPATHIC PAIN

Neuropathic pain results from abnormalities of the nervous system.[7] Nerve injury from surgery, tumor growth, metastasis, radiation therapy, chemotherapy, elevated blood glucose, viral infection, or trauma often causes neuropathic pain. It is characterized by constant aching sensations that may be interrupted by bursts of burning or shock-like pain in the affected area. Allodynia is common. Neuropathic pain may not occur immediately after an injury. Days, weeks, or even months after the tissue-damaging source of pain has resolved, the onset of neuropathic pain can initiate a new and complex pain state.

Neuropathic pain is thought to result from altered central processing of nociceptive input. In some cases, excessive responsiveness to ongoing stimulation of afferent pain fibers appears to be important; however, central perception of pain may occur in the absence of any nociceptor input.[5] The mechanisms of centrally maintained pain remain poorly understood. Examples of neuropathic pain include postherpetic neuralgia, diabetic neuropathy, trigeminal neuralgia, epidural spinal cord compression, cauda equina compression, plexus injuries, neuropathy, and phantom limb pain.[5] Sympathetically maintained pain is a unique type of neuropathic pain that may occur in the absence of nerve injury.[7] Sympathetically maintained pain is attributed to hyperactivity of the sympathetic nervous system. Release of norepinephrine from sympathetic nerve endings sensitizes nociceptors such that they respond to a lower level of nociceptor stimuli.[5] The diagnosis is made on the basis of improved analgesia with sympathetic blockade or aggravation of pain with sympathetic nerve stimulation. Not all sufferers exhibit the same symptoms, but most prevalent are allodynia, hyperalgesia, atrophy of the affected extremity, coldness in the affected area, and dystrophic changes, most often manifested as hair loss and a shiny appearance of the skin. Neuropathic pain is difficult to manage. It is frequently unresponsive to opioid or other pharmacologic therapy.

Trigeminal Neuralgia

Etiology and Pathogenesis. Trigeminal neuralgia is a form of neuropathic pain that can be quite disabling for patients. It is sudden, momentary, but excruciating pains along the second and third divisions of the trigeminal nerve. Trigeminal neuralgia is more common in women than in men, and occurs more frequently in middle-aged or older individuals.[17] If trigeminal neuralgia occurs at an earlier age, multiple sclerosis should be ruled out.[17] Other causes of trigeminal neuralgia include lesions or tumors of the brainstem. Chronic compression of the trigeminal nerve by a vessel is suspected in most cases. This causes demyelination of the trigeminal nerve and interruption and alteration in nerve signaling.[12]

Clinical Manifestations. The pain of trigeminal neuralgia is often described as sharp or shooting; some have compared it to the pain of an electrical shock. Patients may be pain free between episodes or complain of a dull ache in the affected area. Sometimes patients may only have a few episodes of pain followed by a long remission. However, others may unfortunately experience an increase in frequency and duration of the pain. Anxiety is common as patients worry about when their next attack may occur.

Diagnosis and Treatment. Diagnosis of neuralgia is most frequently based on the clinical history. The result of neurologic evaluation is normal if there is no underlying lesion. Management of trigeminal neuralgia includes antiseizure medications such as carbamazepine (Tegretol), phenytoin (Dilantin), or gabapentin (Neurontin). Surgical nerve decompression has been used successfully for trigeminal neuralgia in patients who do not respond to or cannot tolerate the medications. Gamma radiosurgery is the newest treatment for this condition, and early results appear promising.[17]

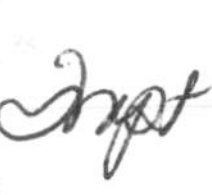

Diabetic Neuropathy

Etiology and Pathogenesis. One of the most common complications of diabetes, diabetic neuropathy affects approximately 50% of all persons with diabetes, both type 1 and type 2.[20] Diabetic neuropathy is caused by damage to the peripheral nerves. The exact pathogenetic mechanism is unknown, but this damage is thought to be mediated by occult inflammation and demyelination of the larger peripheral nerves, leaving an excess of smaller myelinated fibers. This causes a loss of inhibitory input from the spinal cord with unopposed nociceptive afferent bombardment.[5] Ischemic damage to nerves is also a contributing factor. Some also hypothesize that hyperglycemia and related biochemical changes in the nerve microenvironment cause nerve malfunction and injury.[12]

Clinical Manifestations. Although pain is the most common feature, patients also complain of numbness and tingling, mild weakness, and loss of vibratory sense and proprioception. Fine touch and vibratory sensation are decreased. Patients complain of burning pain in the distal bilateral lower extremities, often with a symmetric distribution. Pain is frequently worse at night.

Diagnosis and Treatment. Diabetic neuropathy is confirmed through careful physical examination. Diabetic patients are encouraged to keep tight control of their blood sugars to prevent neuropathy. Studies have shown that this is true for many people with type 1 diabetes; however, close blood sugar monitoring and control has not been shown to decrease the incidence of neuropathy in those with type 2 diabetes.[12] Management of this disorder includes the use of a wide variety of topical and systemic pain medications. Systemic therapeutic agents include tricyclic antidepressants and anticonvulsants. Although opioids can help with pain relief of diabetic neuropathy, their use has been limited due to tolerance issues.[20] Side effects of all of these medications can limit their usefulness, especially in elderly patients or those with other comorbid conditions. The use of transcutaneous electrical nerve stimulation (TENS) is promising. TENS is moderately beneficial while lacking major side effects.[20] Many patients use a combination of topical and systemic therapies. An important nonpharmacologic treatment for diabetic neuropathy is the prevention of further complications. Diabetic patients are strongly encouraged to perform daily foot examinations, taking precautions against the development of foot sores and ingrown toenails. The combination of numbness and impaired circulation make diabetic patients at high risk for undetected injuries that do not heal and become easily infected. Amputation is a common outcome.

Postherpetic Neuralgia

Etiology and Pathogenesis. A common but disabling complication of the varicella virus is herpes zoster. Years after an individual has recovered from the chickenpox virus, herpes zoster (shingles) may occur. This is a reactivation of the latent virus that has lain dormant along the nerve roots. The painful blisters erupt along dermatomal pathways.

Postherpetic neuropathy is persistent pain that lasts for more than 8 weeks after the onset of skin lesions. Approximately 10% to 15% of patients with herpes zoster develop postherpetic neuralgia.[20] Risk factors for the development of this neuralgia are advanced age and history of immune compromise.

Clinical Manifestations. Herpes zoster is characterized by a burning pain that follows along a dermatomal pathway and is accompanied by a blistering rash. It occurs in individuals who have a history of varicella infection (chickenpox). Frequently the pain is present prior to the eruption of the blisters.

Diagnosis and Treatment. The diagnosis is most often made clinically; however, cultures can be used to determine the presence of the virus. The early use (within 72 hours of eruption of rash) of antiviral medications such as acyclovir (Zovirax) can decrease the risk of developing postherpetic neuralgia.[12]

Management of the neuralgia includes both topical and systemic therapies. Transdermal lidocaine and capsaicin cream may be helpful in mild cases.[20] Anticonvulsants and tricyclic antidepressants are also useful. NSAIDs and opioids may be mildly helpful as well.

ISCHEMIC PAIN

Pain resulting from a sudden or profound loss of blood flow to the tissues in a particular part of the body may result in ischemic pain. Decreased perfusion leads to tissue hypoxia and injury, with release of inflammatory and pain-producing chemicals. Ischemic pain is described as aching, burning, or prickling (paresthesia). The symptoms of ischemic pain depend on the origin of the ischemia. For example, pain of cardiac origin is visceral and radiates to the arm or jaw. This pain is perceived as being deep, aching, diffuse, and pressing. Ischemia resulting from acute deep venous occlusion is also aching and has a deep quality and gradual onset. Acute arterial occlusion may be felt as either burning or aching but has a sudden onset.[5]

Chronic ischemic pain can occur in atherosclerotic syndromes. Arteriosclerosis obliterans occurs gradually as plaque develops in the intima of the arteries, most often arteries of the lower extremities. In the early stages, the pain is intermittent and has a cramping quality. In severe cases, ischemic neuropathy may ensue and cause a burning, shooting pain in the leg or foot.

Management of ischemic pain is directed at improving blood flow and reducing tissue hypoxia. Acute ischemia is usually associated with a thrombus or embolus and can be managed with drugs to dissolve the clot or surgery to remove it. Chronic ischemia is most often associated with atherosclerosis and may be improved through lifestyle changes, including smoking cessation, weight loss, lipid lowering, and regular exercise.

REFERRED PAIN

Referred pain is perceived in an area other than the site of the injury. It is often felt at some distance from the point of nociceptor activation. A familiar example is the pain of myocardial infarction that is felt in the jaw or left arm. Other examples of referred pain include shoulder pain after pelvic procedures and cutaneous abdominal pain experienced with visceral irritation or tension. Common patterns of referral are shown in Figure 47-10. Pain is generally referred to other structures in the same sensory dermatome. Convergence of nociceptors from internal organs with somatic afferents from the body surface occurs in the dorsal horn of the spinal cord.[7] The brain cannot differentiate the two sources of pain signals and tends to attribute the visceral pain to a body surface location. Patterns of referred pain are fairly uniform and can be used to help locate a source of visceral pathologic process.[5]

PHYSIOLOGIC RESPONSES TO PAIN

The autonomic nervous system, which is responsible for much of the physiologic response to pain, includes both the sympathetic and parasympathetic divisions. Activation of the sympathetic nervous system results in a predictable cluster of physical signs and symptoms, including an elevated heart rate, blood pressure, and respiratory rate, as well as dilated pupils, perspiration, and pallor[4] (see Table 47-4). Sympathetic stimulation results in constriction of superficial vessels to divert blood to striated muscle, heart, and lungs; bronchodilation; increased cardiac contractility; and increased circulating

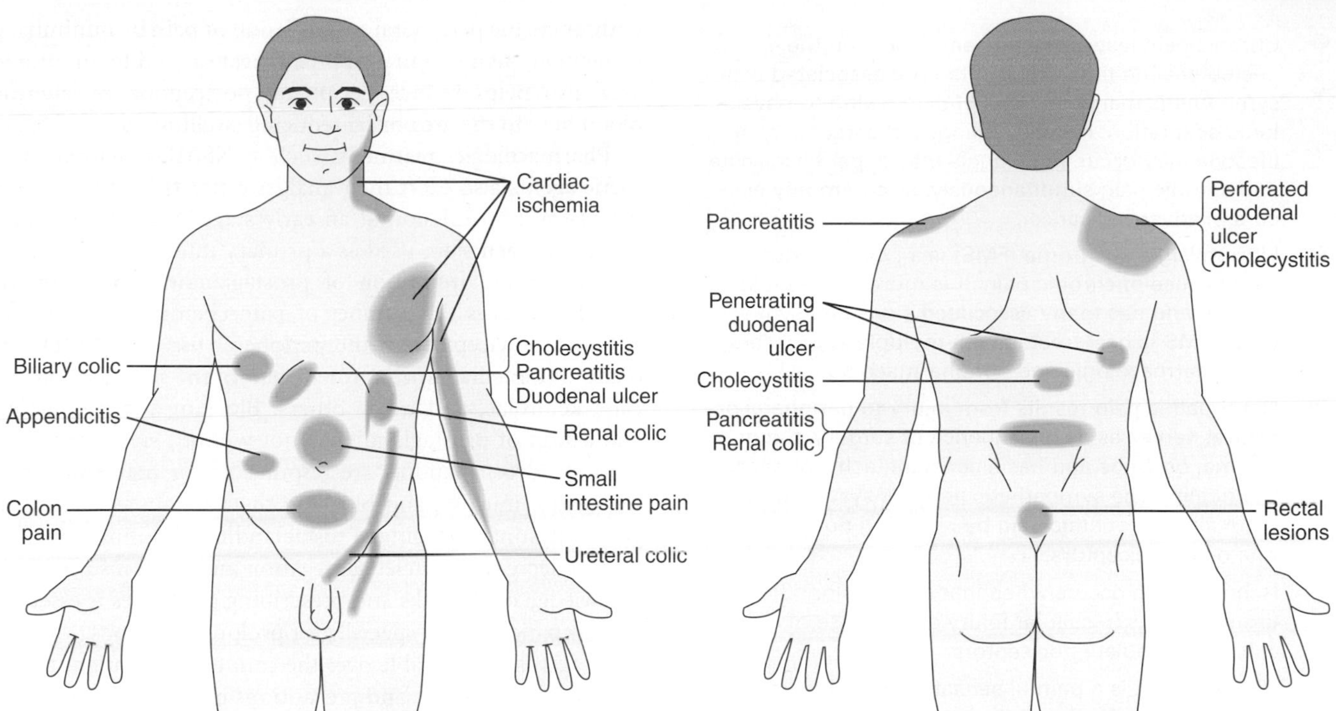

FIGURE 47-10 ■ Areas of referred pain.

blood glucose. In addition, although gastrointestinal motility and secretion decrease, sphincter tone increases. Nausea, vomiting, and even paralytic ileus may develop. Hypomotility of the bladder and ureters can also result from sympathetic activation and lead to urine retention. Pain stimulates the release of numerous stress hormones, including antidiuretic hormone, aldosterone, and cortisol. These hormones help the kidneys conserve fluid and stimulate the release of glucose from the liver.

The sympathetic responses to pain may be physiologically helpful in the short term but become deleterious if excessive or prolonged. The body cannot sustain this level of activation for long periods. Eventually, physiologic adaptation occurs and the observed sympathetic response to pain abates. Thus the heart rate, blood pressure, and respiratory rate return toward normal or baseline. Signs and symptoms of sympathetic nervous system activation may be an important clue in pain assessment when present, but their absence does not guarantee the absence of pain sensations.

PAIN IN THE YOUNG AND THE ELDERLY

Many myths and misconceptions surround the issue of pain, especially in the very young and the elderly. As a result, often the young and the old receive inadequate treatment of their pain. It was previously thought that neonates were unable to perceive pain. Because their CNS had not yet fully developed and they were unable to remember painful events, neonates often did not receive pain medication or anesthesia for surgery.[21] It has since been found that infants do indeed have pain perception and that inadequate pain control may lead to hemodynamic instability, catabolism, and poor surgical outcomes, especially for premature infants.[5]

In the elderly, it has also been theorized that pain perception is decreased. Research in this area has been inconclusive.[5] Social expectations interfere with the adequacy of pain control in the elderly, as pain is often an expected part of aging. Cognitive factors also hinder pain treatment especially in patients with dementia who are unable to communicate their need for pain medication. However, it has been found that pain has a huge effect on an elderly person's quality of life.[5] No matter what the age of the patient, adequate pain control is important to his or her care.

KEY CONCEPTS

- Acute pain results from tissue injury and generally resolves when the injury resolves. The clinical manifestations result from activation of the sympathetic nervous system (elevated heart rate, blood pressure, and respiratory rate; dilated pupils; perspiration; and pallor).
- Headaches are a common but disabling cause of acute pain. Migraine headaches are caused by an interaction between neurotransmitters and cerebrovascular mechanisms and may be triggered by factors such as stress, foods, and sleep deprivation. There are a variety of treatments for headaches, but all must be initiated early in the course of the headache.

- Chronic pain lasts several months beyond the expected healing time and is often not associated with sympathetic manifestations of pain owing to physiologic adaptation. Instead, changes in personality or lifestyle may occur. Individuals may experience acute and chronic pain simultaneously, as commonly occurs in advanced cancer.
- Fibromyalgia syndrome (FMS) is a poorly understood cause of chronic pain. It is more common in women and has many associated signs and symptoms. FMS is best treated with multiple approaches, both pharmacologic and nonpharmacologic.
- Neuropathic pain results from injury to peripheral or central nerves as a consequence of surgery, tumor, trauma, or drugs and has a constant, achy, or shock-like quality. The sympathetic nervous system may maintain neuropathic pain by releasing norepinephrine onto nociceptors.
- Ischemic pain occurs when inadequate blood flow to tissues results in cellular injury and release of chemicals that stimulate nociceptors.
- Referred pain is a painful sensation perceived at some distance from an injury but generally within the same dermatome. Referred pain is thought to occur because of the convergence of visceral nociceptor activity with primary somatic afferents in the posterior horn of the cord.

TREATMENT MODALITIES

PHARMACOLOGIC AND NONPHARMACOLOGIC PAIN MANAGEMENT

Many pain management strategies are available. By understanding the basic mechanisms of pain transmission, one can readily identify potential sites where various types of treatment modalities could interrupt pain transmission and perception. Pain management interventions can be directed at three points: (1) interrupting peripheral transmission of nociception; (2) modulating pain transmission at the spinal cord level; and (3) altering the perception and integration of nociceptive impulses in the brain. Recently, the terms "balanced analgesia" and "preemptive analgesia" have been used to describe approaches to pain management aimed at multiple sites and applied before stimulation of pain receptors when possible.[5] These approaches are based on the idea that pain memory and hyperalgesia are not prevented by drugs that affect only perception in the brain.

Interrupting Peripheral Transmission of Pain

Modalities that interrupt the peripheral transmission of nociceptive impulses are often the first step in controlling pain. The basic action of splinting an injured limb or area of the body alters the peripheral transmission of pain by minimizing or reducing tissue injury. Applying heat or cold to an injured area also helps reduce peripheral nociception by altering blood flow to the area or by reducing swelling.

Pharmacologic treatments such as NSAIDs or local anesthetic agents also exert their analgesic effects by interrupting peripheral transmission at an early stage. NSAIDs and local anesthetic agents are used as a primary intervention for pain management.[5,7] Inhibition of prostaglandin production by NSAIDs reduces the number of pain chemicals available to stimulate nociceptors in the peripheral tissues. NSAIDs include indomethacin, ibuprofen, naproxen, sulindac, piroxicam, ketorolac, and many others. Blocking the production and action of prostaglandins is not without side effects. For example, prostaglandins are responsible for maintenance of the gastric mucosa, and blocking their actions can result in gastrointestinal bleeding. Prostaglandin inhibition can also lead to decreased platelet aggregation and renal insufficiency. Knowledge of the risks and prescribing guidelines is essential for safe patient care, especially for prolonged periods. Many of these agents are available over the counter, and patient teaching regarding benefits and precautions may be needed.

Local anesthetic agents can be applied either to nerve endings at the site of injury or to the nerve plexus supplying the area. By providing localized or regional blockade, peripheral pain transmission is interrupted. Local anesthetic agents diminish or block conduction of the nociceptive impulses by blocking sodium influx during phase 0 of the action potential. The degree of blockade achieved with local agents depends on the amount of drug applied and hence the extent of sodium channel blockade. Local infiltration of a wound or surgical site with local anesthetic agents such as bupivacaine or lidocaine is common practice even when the patient is also receiving a general anesthetic.

Modulating Pain Transmission at the Spinal Cord

Numerous procedures and agents are used to modulate pain transmission at the level of the spinal cord. Nonpharmacologic techniques that inhibit pain transmission include several types of cutaneous stimulation. Cutaneous stimulation activates and recruits large sensory fibers that can block the central progression of nociceptive transmission at the interneurons. Examples of cutaneous stimulation include TENS, massage, acupuncture, application of heat or cold, and therapeutic touch.

Pharmacologic measures that act at the level of the spinal cord include epidural and intrathecal analgesia. Spinal analgesia can be achieved with opioids, local anesthetics, and α-adrenergic blocking agents. Intraspinal opioids work by binding with opioid receptors in the posterior horn of the spinal cord, thereby decreasing the release of neurotransmitters such as substance P. Intraspinal local anesthetic agents block nerve conduction at the posterior nerve root. Epidural administration of an α-adrenergic blocking agent such as clonidine is

Table 47-6

Equianalgesic Table for Common Opioid Analgesics

Drug	Approximate Equianalgesic Dose	
	Oral	Parenteral
Morphine	30 mg q3-4h	10 mg q3-4h
Codeine	30-60 mg	—
Controlled-release morphine (MS Contin)	90-120 mg q12h	—
Hydrocodone	5 mg q4-6h	—
Hydromorphone (Dilaudid)	7.5 mg q3-4h	1.5 mg q3-4h
Meperidine (Demerol)	300 mg q2-3h	100 mg q3h
Methadone	20 mg q6-8h	10 mg q6-8h

Data from Keck JK, Baker S: Clients with pain. In Black JM, Hawks JH, Keen AM, editors: *Medical-surgical nursing: clinical management for promoting positive outcomes*, ed 6, Philadelphia, 2001, Saunders, pp 489-490.

thought to achieve analgesic effects by blocking sympathetically mediated pain transmission.

Dorsal column stimulators, sometimes used in chronic pain management, also work at the level of the spinal cord to "close the pain gate" by modulating descending input from the brain to the spinal cord.

Altering the Perception and Integration of Pain

The traditional modality for managing moderate to severe pain is the administration of systemic opioids. This pharmacologic intervention has stood the test of time. Opioids work at specific receptor sites that are located throughout the body but are highly concentrated in the brain. Opioid analgesic agents such as morphine and other derivatives alter the perception of pain by the brain. Opioid analgesics have similar mechanisms of action but vary widely in potency. This difference in potency has led to the development of equianalgesic tables to help clinicians prescribe these drugs appropriately (Table 47-6).

Systemic opioids work best for suppressing pain at rest and are less effective during function (moving, coughing).[10] Opioid administration is associated with numerous side effects that may limit effectiveness (nausea, vomiting, respiratory depression, constipation). Long-term use of opioids leads to physical dependence and tolerance.[5] Although the incidence of opioid addiction in persons experiencing acute pain is very low, fears about addiction contribute to inadequate pain therapy. Physical dependence is characterized by withdrawal symptoms if treatment is stopped abruptly. Tolerance to opioids is characterized by the need for increasing dosages to achieve the same analgesic effect. Dependence and tolerance are expected responses to long-term opioid therapy. Drug addiction is a behavioral pattern characterized by craving and preoccupation with obtaining the drug.

Nonpharmacologic techniques of pain management include such activities and procedures as distraction, imagery, relaxation, biofeedback, and hypnosis. With distraction, the number of generalized stimuli reaching the brain increases. Because the brain has a limited capacity to sort and attend to multiple and varied stimuli, it is less able to integrate the pain experience when other competition is present. Imagery may alter the perception of painful stimuli in the higher centers of the brain and produce relaxation as well as analgesia. Biofeedback is a conditioned response that can be learned as a pain control strategy. Biofeedback is thought to control pain by increasing blood flow (usually as a consequence of relaxation) to targeted body areas. The increased blood flow decreases the concentration of pain-inducing chemicals in the area. Biofeedback may also increase the amount of endorphins produced and released.

A combination of nonpharmacologic and pharmacologic strategies may help reduce the need for high doses of medications. The choice of drug therapy should correspond to the severity of the pain. It has been recommended that mild pain be managed with nonopioid analgesics such as NSAIDs or acetaminophen, whereas moderate pain may require low-potency opioids such as codeine.[10] Severe pain requires larger and more potent doses of opioids like morphine and fentanyl. Recently, the value of combination therapy in blocking pain transmission at multiple sites has been recognized.

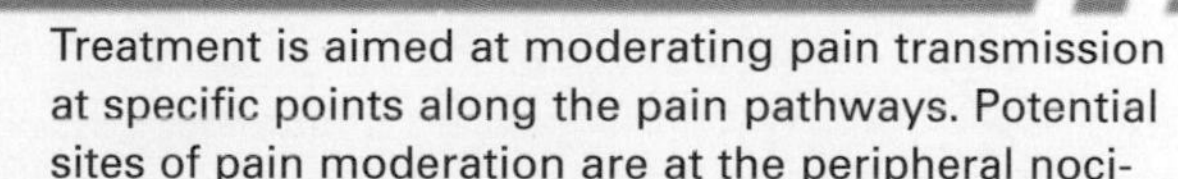

- Treatment is aimed at moderating pain transmission at specific points along the pain pathways. Potential sites of pain moderation are at the peripheral nociceptor, spinal cord, and brain.
- Nociceptor activation can be altered by prostaglandin inhibitors (NSAIDs), heat and cold, and local anesthetics that block sodium influx through fast channels.
- Spinal cord transmission can be altered by cutaneous stimulation (gate control theory), intraspinal

analgesics (opioids, local anesthetics, α-adrenergic blockers), and dorsal column stimulators.

- The perception of pain can be altered within the brain by systemic opioids and by nonpharmacologic means such as hypnosis, distraction, and biofeedback.

SUMMARY

The human experience of pain, although unpleasant, is a normal and expected phenomenon in response to injury. Pain sensations alert the individual to a physiologic problem and help ensure that timely treatment is sought. However, prolonged severe pain serves no good purpose and can be physiologically and psychologically harmful. Appropriate efforts to alleviate pain may enhance recovery from illness and prevent the development of some types of chronic pain syndromes. As understanding of pain physiologic mechanisms grows, treatment strategies can more effectively combine the best of pharmacologic and nonpharmacologic therapies.

MEDIA RESOURCES

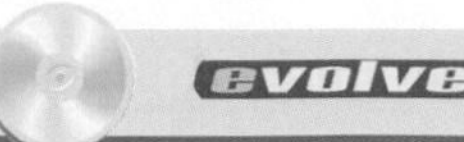

Remember to check out the ***CD Companion*** included with this book for Review Questions, Key Concepts Review, Glossary (with audio for selected terms), Disease Profiles, and Animations.

PLUS, visit the ***Evolve website*** at http://evolve.elsevier.com/Copstead/ for Case Studies, Disease Profiles, and WebLinks.

References

1. Pain terms: a list with definitions and notes on usage. Recommended by the IASP Subcommittee on Taxonomy, *Pain* 6(3):249, 1979.
2. McCaffery M: *Nursing practice theories related to cognition, bodily pain and man-environment interactions,* Los Angeles, 1968, University of California, Los Angeles (master's thesis).
3. Berry PH, Dahl JL: The new JCAHO pain standards: implications for pain management nurses, *Pain Manage Nurs* 1(1): 3-12, 2000.

4. Keane A, McMenamin EM, Polomano RC: Pain: the fifth vital sign. In Ignatavicius DD, Workman ML, editors: *Medical-surgical nursing: critical thinking for collaborative care,* ed 4, Philadelphia, 2002, Saunders.
5. Loeser JD, editor: *Bonica's management of pain,* ed 3, Philadelphia, 2000, Lippincott Williams & Wilkins.
6. Victor M: Pain. In Victor M, Ropper AH, editors: *Adams and Victor's principles of neurology,* ed 7, New York, 2001, McGraw-Hill.
7. Braunwald E et al, editors: *Harrison's principles of internal medicine,* ed 15, New York, 2001, McGraw-Hill.
8. Melzack R, Wall PD: Pain mechanisms: a new theory, *Science* 150:971-974, 1965.
9. Melzack R, Wall PD, editors: *The challenge of pain,* ed 2, Harmondworth, UK, 1988, Penguin.
10. Hardman JG, Limbird LE, editors: *Goodman and Gilman's the pharmacologic basis of therapeutics,* ed 10, New York, 2001, McGraw-Hill.
11. Cady RK: Headache: why the "default diagnosis" needs to be migraine, *Consultant Suppl* 42(13):54-55, 2002.
12. Rakel RE, Bope ET, editors: *Conn's current therapy,* Philadelphia, 2003, Elsevier.
13. Moriarty-Sheehan M, Jamieson DG, Russell DD: Managing migraine: strategies for successful patient outcomes, *Nurse Pract* 26(4):1-11, 2001.
14. Moloney MF et al: Caring for the woman with migraine headaches, *Nurse Pract* 25(2):17-36, 2000.
15. Cady RK, Schreiber CP: Sinus headache or migraine: considerations in making a differential diagnosis, *Neurology* 59(suppl 6):S10-S14, 2002.
16. Kaniecki RG: Migraine and tension-type headache: an assessment of challenges in diagnosis, *Neurology* 59(suppl 6): S15-S19, 2002.
17. Tierney LM, McPhee SJ, Papadakis MA: *Current medical diagnosis and treatment,* ed 43, New York, 2004, Lange.
18. Staud R, Domingo M: New insights into the pain mechanisms of fibromyalgia syndrome, *Med Aspects Hum Sexuality* 1(15):51-57, 2001.
19. Clauw DJ: Fibromyalgia. In Harris ED, Sledge CB, editors: *Kelly's textbook of rheumatology,* ed 6, Philadelphia, 2001, Saunders.
20. Perkins FM: Coping with post-herpetic neuralgia and painful diabetic neuropathy: treatment similarities and differences, *Consultant* 42(7):936-942, 2002.
21. Rouzan A: An analysis of research and clinical practice in neonatal pain management, *J Am Acad Nurse Pract* 3(2):57-60, 2000.

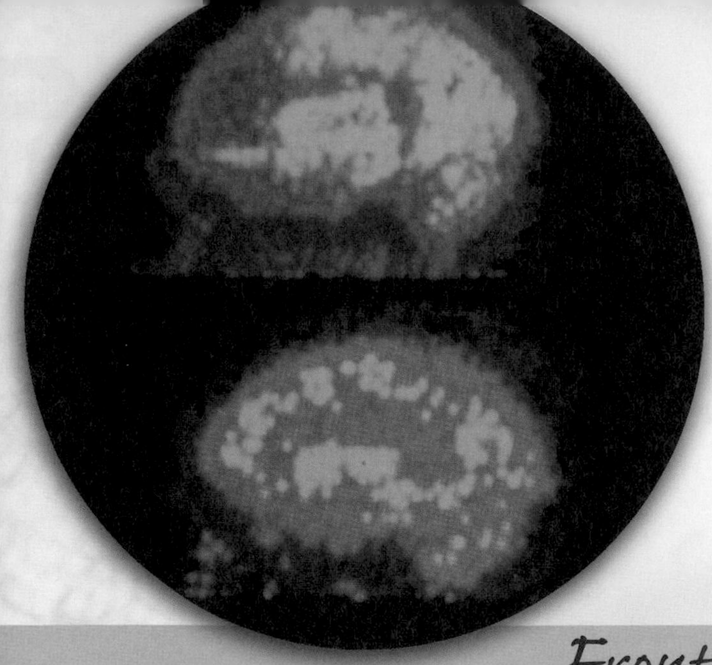

Frontiers of Research

Biological Markers of Depression and Schizophrenia

David W. Metzler and Michael J. Kirkhorn

Depression occurs in the lives of most people. It can be described as a temporary sadness, the blues, loneliness, or part of normal life, or it can result in a very deep sadness called a major depression. Major depression is a syndrome resulting in lack of sleep, lack of desire to do things, depressed mood, poor appetite, anxious feelings, and suicidal thoughts. It may end in a completed suicide, devastating a person's family and ending a once-promising life.

Researchers have identified categories of people who are most likely to develop depression. The number and variety of these categories suggest that depression is a common problem. As many as 8% of Americans may suffer serious depression at any one time.

Recent epidemiologic studies have demonstrated that young women are more than twice as likely to suffer depression as young men. Depression among the elderly is common, especially if they suffer other illnesses, as many elderly people do. However, health care professionals who have infrequent contact with individual patients may overlook it, or if they do diagnose depression, they are likely to undertreat it, resulting in significant morbidity.

People with chronic illnesses may also have chronic depression. Depression has been found increasingly among persons with multiple sclerosis, in which depression is studied both as a possible symptom and as a precipitating factor in the disease. Depression is also commonly found in persons suffering from dementia of the Alzheimer type, which is characterized by memory loss and intellectual disabilities.

Researchers have noted differences in the emotional outlook of persons who have suffered single ischemic strokes to their right and left hemispheres. Those with right hemisphere damage were found to have less anxiety than those with left hemisphere stroke, leading researchers to speculate that this decreased anxiety in patients with right hemisphere damage was misunderstood and described in clinical notes as indifference and failure to recover as expected. Research also indicates a relationship between depression and immunity. One study argues that indices of immunocompetence are lower among depressed people.

The use of biological markers in depression may one day prove to be important, but to this point, they have proved unhelpful in the diagnosis and treatment of depression. Biological depression is likely to be a syndrome with multiple genetic causes that will continue to be elusive.

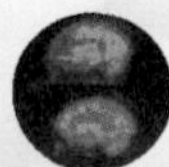

Top, *PET scan of glucose use in a depressed subject showing frontal hypometabolism on left side.* Bottom, *Improvement after treatment with antidepressant medication. Note increased glucose metabolism in frontal lobe. (From Stuart GW, Laraia MT:* Principles and practice of psychiatric nursing, *ed 7, St Louis, 2001, Mosby, p 109.)*

Neuropsychological Function

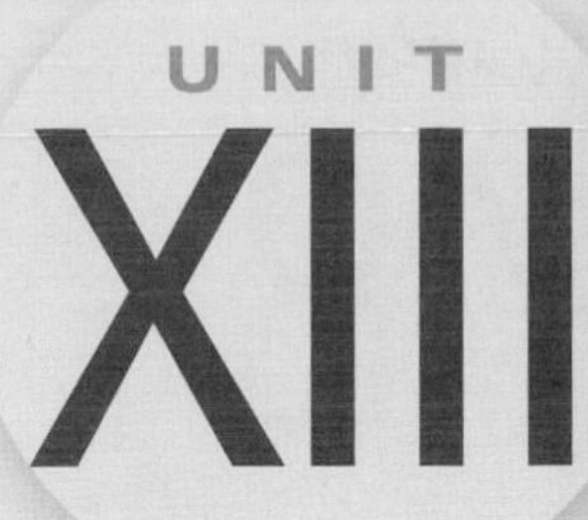

The greater availability of newer antidepressant agents has also noticeably influenced mental health care, in which the use of these agents and other psychotropic medications has increased dramatically during the past decade.

Like depression, schizophrenia can be a severely disabling disease characterized by serious brain chemistry dysfunction in many areas of the brain. Schizophrenia is a chronic disease that typically affects the young. More than three fourths of sufferers become ill before the age of 25 years, are unlikely to return to normal function without treatment, and may suffer continued decline after repeated episodes. More than 2 million Americans have been diagnosed with schizophrenia, and 200,000 new cases are diagnosed every year.

Over nearly two generations, researchers have followed a hypothesis suggesting that schizophrenia patients suffer from functional changes in the central dopaminergic systems of their brains. This hypothesis is being refined, given the evolution of new antipsychotic medications that affect both the dopamine and the serotonin systems.

Although researchers agree that schizophrenia produces brain dysfunctions, there is still no clear agreement on exactly how and where the brain harbors the disease. For many decades, scientists have suspected that they might find a genetic explanation for schizophrenia, but attempts to identify genes linked with the disease have been disappointing. Researchers now hope that searches of the entire genome will be more revealing.

New diagnostic examinations such as functional brain imaging have confirmed abnormal frontal cortex functioning in schizophrenia, but subcortical pathology also seems to be involved, and this process is not clearly understood.

Recently, several new drugs have been introduced in a strenuous regulatory context required by the Food and Drug Administration. Risperdal (risperidone), Zyprexa (olanzapine), Abilify (aripiprazole), and Seroquel (quetiapine fumarate) all have been shown to be effective in the treatment of psychosis associated with schizophrenia. These drugs, along with Clozaril (clozapine, which was first introduced in 1989 and subjected to unusual Food and Drug Administration restrictions because of the deaths of European patients using the drug and because it is associated with agranulocytosis), promise treatment with fewer of the side effects that can cause many sufferers to give up and refuse treatment with medication.

chapter 48

Neurobiology of Psychotic Illnesses

Linda Denise Oakley

MEDIA RESOURCES

Additional Material for Study, Review, and Further Exploration

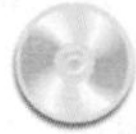

CD Companion ◆ Review Questions and Answers ◆ Key Concepts Review ◆ Glossary *(with audio pronunciations for selected terms)* ◆ Disease Profiles ◆ Animations

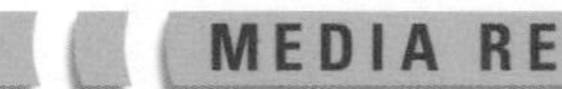

Website at http://evolve.elsevier.com/Copstead/ ◆ Case Studies ◆ Disease Profiles ◆ WebLinks

KEY QUESTIONS

- What genetic, gestational, and neurologic risk factors are related to schizophrenia?
- What are the "positive" and "negative" symptoms of schizophrenia?
- How are dopamine D_1 and D_2 receptors related to positive and negative symptoms of schizophrenia?
- How is schizophrenia managed?
- What is the neurobiology of major depression?
- What are the hallmark symptoms of major depression?
- What are the subtypes of bipolar disorder?
- How are major depression and bipolar disorder managed?

CHAPTER OUTLINE

Psychosis is a term used to describe a serious and debilitating mental state. The hallmark symptoms of psychosis are delusions, hallucinations, cognitive disorganization, and altered reality. These symptoms characterize a small number of specific mental disorders; however, a wide range of different physical and mental conditions can produce psychotic symptoms. The neurobiological basis of psychosis can be summarized as acute or chronic alterations in neuron anatomy and physiology and cellular biochemical processes. Thought disorders and mood disorders are only two categories of mental disorders with symptom profiles that may include psychosis. Symptoms of psychosis may also occur with substance disorders, delirium, dementia, and acute stress disorder. Groundbreaking research in brain imaging techniques and psychopharmacology now allow highly precise definitions of the various biochemical pathways associated with psychosis. This chapter addresses four disorders: schizophrenia, delusional disorder, major depression, and bipolar disorder.

Schizophrenia

Disturbance and deterioration of cognitive, social, and emotional functioning characterize **schizophrenia.** Schizophrenia appears to be more a syndrome with unique symptoms then a single disease. Reports of persons described as suffering from these unique symptoms have been recorded for thousands of years in all cultures. The global incidence rate of schizophrenia has consistently been estimated to be about 1% of the world population.[1] The term schizophrenia literally is defined as "split mind." Once believed to be a disorder that caused the personality to split into multiple subtypes that communicated with each other, thanks to Eugene Bleuler, who first coined the term, schizophrenia now is correctly understood as a split or separation among normally well-synchronized brain functions. This loss of synchronized brain functioning leads to thoughts, behaviors, and feelings that are disordered, disorganized, and disconnected from reality—a condition generally referred to as psychosis.

Etiology and Neurobiology. Most persons first diagnosed with schizophrenia are 15 to 54 years old. The most common age of symptom onset and clinical diagnosis is between 25 and 35 years for women and 15 and 25 years for men. Psychiatrists once disagreed over the likelihood that schizophrenia could first emerge after the age of 45. Most experts now place far less emphasis on first age of symptom onset and focus instead on the presenting symptoms regardless of age.

Antipsychotic medications, first discovered in the 1950s, were the first interventions to truly relieve many of the common symptoms of schizophrenia. Although far from being universally effective and often causing profound side effects, that first generation of antipsychotic medications, also known as neuroleptics, eased suffering, made discharge possible for long-term and seriously ill patients, and radically shifted the focus of treatment from inpatient to outpatient care. The effectiveness of the first generation of antipsychotic medications primarily was attributed to their effectiveness in blocking specific dopamine receptor activity in the brain. This observation was confirmation that schizophrenia was a neurophysiologic illness with complex biopsychosocial symptoms that could be managed pharmacologically. This advance made it possible to more accurately describe the illness, but the exact cause of schizophrenia remains unknown.[2]

Dopamine Effects. Because dopamine antagonists (competitive) reduce symptoms of schizophrenia and dopamine agonists (complementary) produce them, abnormalities in dopaminergic pathways in specific regions of the brain were hypothesized as the etiologic key to schizophrenia. Dopamine-specific neurons in the brain primarily are located in the ventral tegmentum of the mesencephalon, medial and superior to the substantia nigra. These regions, as a whole, are referred to as the *mesolimbic dopaminergic system.* The long nerve fibers leaving this system mainly project into the medial and anterior portions of the limbic system. The limbic system contains three powerful centers of behavior control: the nucleus accumbens, the amygdala, and the anterior caudate nucleus (Figure 48-1).

Generally speaking, decreased neurotransmission and connectivity appear to be the neurobiological basis of schizophrenia. This conclusion, reported in findings from an international conference on synaptic dysfunction and schizophrenia,[3] represents the core biochemical process of schizophrenia. As summarized by these experts, the two core neurochemical processes involved are an excess of subcortical dopaminergic transmission at dopamine D_2 receptors and a deficit of glutamate transmission at *N*-methyl-D-aspartate (NMDA) receptors. The dopamine pathogenesis of schizophrenia can be thought of as disordered synaptic organization. In the brain, normal synaptic organization implies the provision for normal brain cell–to–brain cell communication.

That said, dopamine receptor activity and synaptic transmission are subject to a variety of mediators such as brain-derived neurotrophic factor (BDNF), a neurotrophin that increases synaptic activity and neurotransmitter output.[4] Dopamine synaptic activity also has been closely linked with stress-related cortisol activity and drugs of abuse (cocaine, amphetamine, morphine, nicotine, and ethanol).[5] Although dopamine dysregulation clearly is the driving force[6] behind the neurochemical processes of psychosis, other experts caution against this purely biological model of illness. If schizophrenia were merely a biochemical process, the correct biochemical intervention would be expected to reverse the process instantly. Since this is not the case, critics note that the affected person's cognitive, psychodynamic, and cultural contexts shape the expression of biochemical dysregulation.[6]

Positron emission tomography (PET) brain images have enabled researchers to further examine the overall role of dopamine activity in psychosis and schizophrenia. PET studies have demonstrated low glucose metabolism rates in the

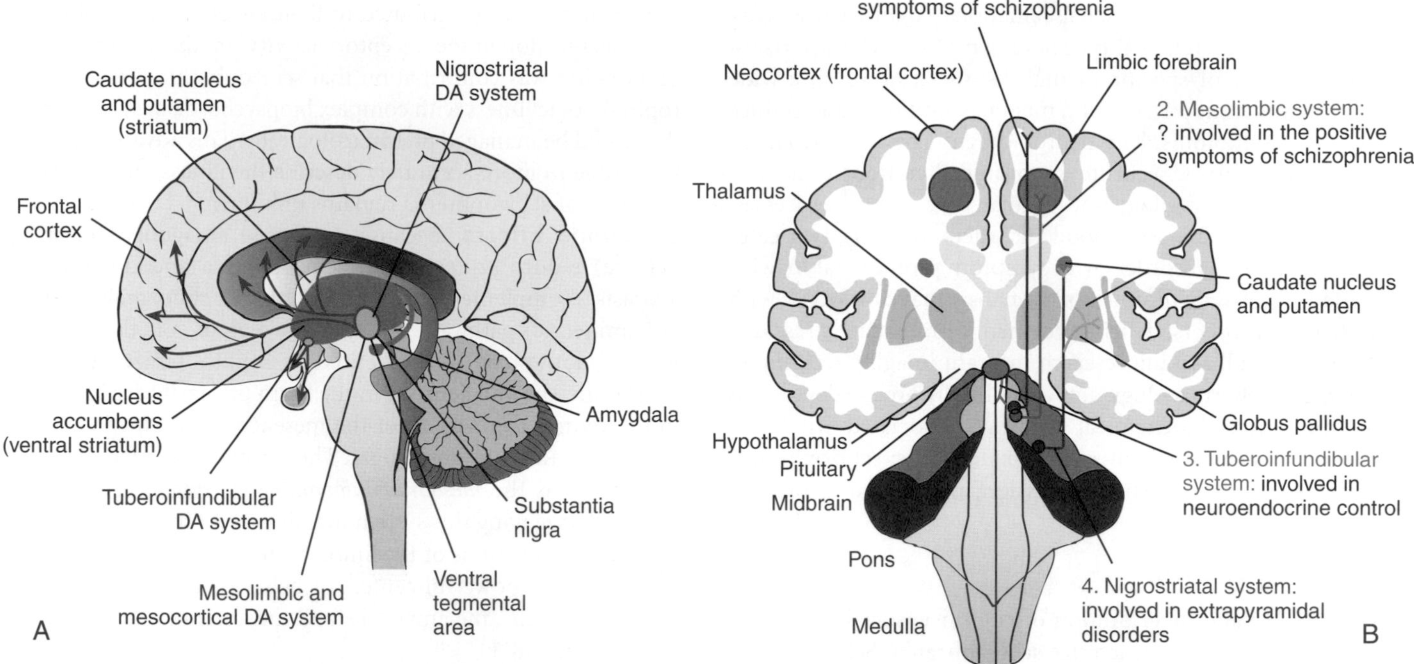

FIGURE 48-1 ■ **A,** A midsagittal section shows the approximate anatomic routes of the four dopamine *(DA)* tracts. **B,** A coronal section shows the sites of origin and the targets of all four tracts. (Modified from Kandel E, Schwartz J, Jessell T: *Principles of neural science,* ed 3, New York, 1991, Elsevier. In Stuart GW, Laraia MT: *Principles and practice of psychiatric nursing,* ed 7, St Louis, 2001, Mosby, p 414.)

frontal cortex and dopamine regions[7] of the brains of persons with schizophrenia (Figure 48-2). Of the many different types of dopamine brain cell receptors identified, dopamine D_2 receptors once again were found to be strongly associated with symptoms of schizophrenia. Similar research has shown that dopamine D_2 receptors are particularly responsive to antipsychotic drugs.

Thus, the **dopamine hypothesis,** which postulates that schizophrenia symptoms result from presynaptic dysregulation of dopamine transmission, continues to be the focus of neurobiological studies. The specific neuropathologic mechanism of schizophrenia appears to be a functional excess of postsynaptic dopamine receptor activity and dopamine receptor hypersensitivity, either alone or in combination.

Genetic Effects. The onset of schizophrenia symptoms largely is determined by the biopsychosocial characteristics of persons who genetically are predisposed[8] to the illness. Researchers continue to study the actual versus potential genetic risks of schizophrenia. For example, it was once thought that individual genetic predisposition to schizophrenia was triggered by severe stress. For example, severe physical or sexual abuse during vulnerable periods of growth and development might trigger symptoms in persons who are genetically vulnerable. In other words, what factors appear to be most reliably associated with symptom onset? Absent any other condition, having a family history of schizophrenia does not alone lead to schizophrenia. Schizophrenia can and often does develop in persons with no family history of psychopathology. Nevertheless, significant genetic factors have been identified.

Initial interest in identifying possible genetic contributions to schizophrenia was based on early research on monozygotic (identical) and dizygotic twins. In identical twins born to parents with schizophrenia but reared apart from their parents, the percentage of offspring who do and who do not develop schizophrenia is about equal.[9] Children of two parents with schizophrenia have a 40% to 68% risk of developing the illness, whereas children with one parent with schizophrenia have a 9% to 16% risk.[9] At 8% to 14%, the risk in a nontwin sibling of a brother or sister with schizophrenia is slightly less. The obvious limitation of these findings is that they do not explain why an at-risk offspring does not develop schizophrenia.

Several additional conditions are thought to be involved in the transformation from genetic risk to actual illness. Factors such as prenatal infections, malnutrition, birth complications, and brain injury have been associated with the development of schizophrenia in persons who have increased genetic risk.[10] Moreover, different gene locations appear to also be relevant to the illness onset. Experts question whether inherited genetic risk for schizophrenia could explain observed differences in incidence and prevalence rates based on gender and race.

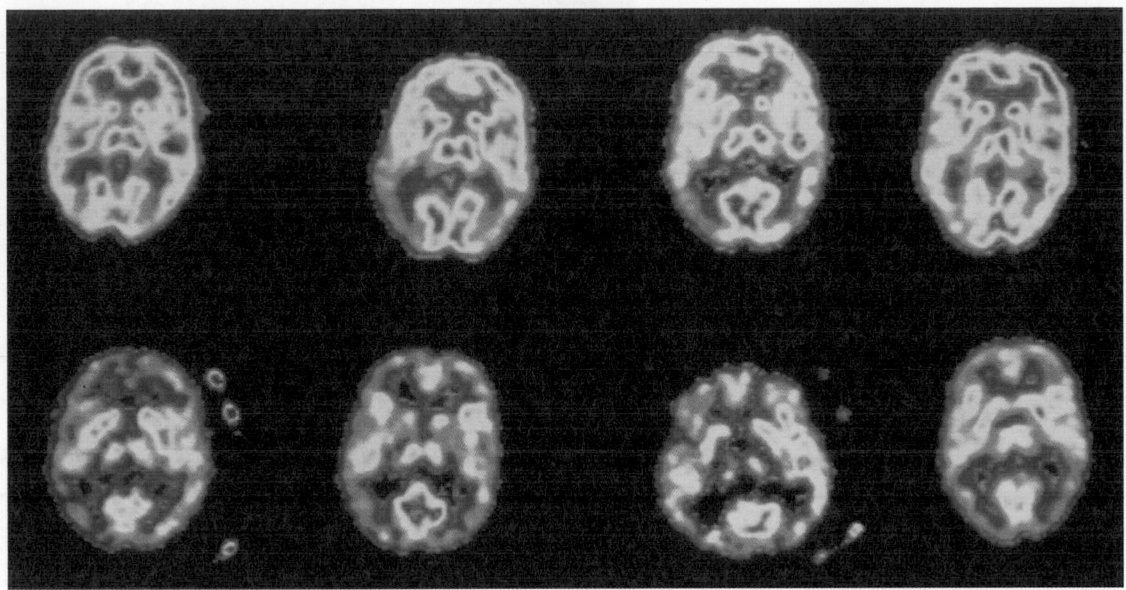

FIGURE 48-2 ■ Individual variation in positron emission tomography (PET) scans. Four normal individuals *(top row)* and four schizophrenics *(bottom row)* show range of hypofrontality and diminished basal ganglia metabolism. (From Buchsbaum MS, Haier RJ: Functional and anatomical brain imaging: impact on schizophrenia research, *Schizophr Bull* 13(1):115-132, 1987. Reproduced by permission of Monte S. Buchsbaum, MD.)

Lastly, genetic models of schizophrenia typically do not address risk in terms of the subtype of schizophrenia, such as symptoms with versus symptoms without paranoia. Given the high standards of proof required for gene typing, a purely genetic explanation of an illness as complex as schizophrenia seems unlikely. Increased genetic risk of schizophrenia appears to be a critical part of a puzzle composed of many pieces.

Gestational Effects. Early findings noted that in persons with schizophrenia pyramidal cells in the hippocampus were not lined up like a "picket fence," as they were in control subjects (Figure 48-3). Instead, the cells appeared to be rotated at 70- to 90-degree angles.[11] Pyramidal cells migrate during the second trimester of gestation and later become fastened by neuronal cell adhesion molecules (N-CAMs). Researchers focused on the possibility of pyramidal cell misalignment and lost N-CAM adhesive effects as links between gestation and schizophrenia. Researchers noted that in pregnant women living in Scandinavia and England who were exposed to the 1957 flu epidemic during their second trimester, 300% more of their children were diagnosed with schizophrenia than those of women who experienced flu during the first or third trimester.

These findings were considered significant for two reasons: (1) neuronal migration peaks during the second trimester, and (2) the influenza virus is one of a very few viruses that produce capsular neuraminidase, an enzyme that can change the adhesive properties of N-CAMs.[12] Hippocampus, parahippocampal gyrus, and amygdala neurons process information and emotional expression. Researchers speculated that the symptoms of schizophrenia might be due to failed neuronal connections and distorted interpretation of incoming messages to the brain that reduce the brain's ability to filter out extraneous stimuli.

In an effort to explain why gestational exposure to influenza might manifest years later in young adults, a 29-year longitudinal study, conducted by the University of Southern California and Danish researchers,[13] followed 207 Danish children born to mothers with severe schizophrenia. The teams examined reports of elementary school behavior in an attempt to identify children with early behavioral dysfunctions. The study revealed that children who later developed negative symptoms of schizophrenia as young adults had been described by their elementary teachers as withdrawn, isolated, and passive. The children who later developed more positive symptoms of schizophrenia, including hallucinations, delusions, and inappropriate behavior, had been described as high-strung and aggressive with behavior problems. These findings indicate that although the full onset of the illness may not occur at early stages of growth and development, related alterations can be observed.

More recent studies of gestational abnormalities focused on specific brain regions and stages of prenatal neurodevelopment.[14] This research is exemplified in a well-controlled Canadian study that examined the association of hippocampus formation abnormalities and first adult episode of schizophrenia.

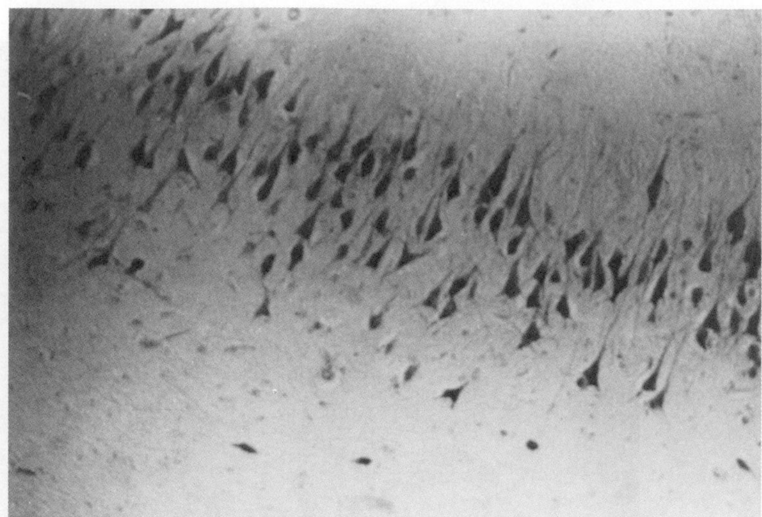

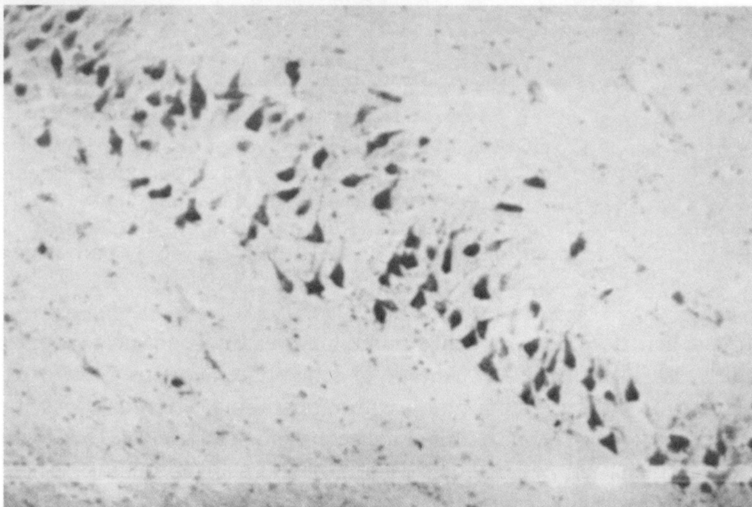

FIGURE 48-3 ■ Photographic comparison of hippocampal tissue at CA 2/3 interface in a control *(top)* and in a person with chronic schizophrenia *(bottom)*. (Original magnification of the Nissl-stained tissue, × 100.) (From Kovelman JA, Scheibel AB: A neurohistological correlate of schizophrenia, *Biol Psychiatry* 19:1601-1621, 1984.)

The main functions of the hippocampus are learning and new-memory formation. Both abilities may be lost when hippocampal functioning is impaired. Macroscopic cell abnormalities, such as fewer synapse connections and diminished synapse activity, result in reduced hippocampal volume. Reduced hippocampal volume has been associated with severe stress, mood disorders, and schizophrenia.[15] The Canadian researchers hypothesized that schizophrenia was associated with incomplete formation of the hippocampus during the second trimester of development. They used magnetic resonance images to compare the brains of newly diagnosed patients with healthy matched controls. Although the number of participants in the study was too small to allow for generalizations to be drawn, the magnetic resonance images of the newly diagnosed patients clearly showed enlarged hippocampal fissures or disrupted hippocampal formation. Interestingly, obstetric complications during pregnancy were not significant factors.

Neurologic Effects. Observed neuroanatomic differences in persons with schizophrenia led researchers to study anatomic and functional abnormalities in the limbic and frontal brain. Structural abnormalities in these brain regions would suggest that abnormal functioning might contribute to the disrupted cognitive processes or symptoms of schizophrenia. Beginning in 1976, computed tomography (CT) studies revealed enlarged brain ventricles in persons with schizophrenia. A groundbreaking 1980 study showed that the neurochemical basis of schizophrenia might involve two processes: dopamine neurotransmission dysregulation and abnormal cerebral structure.[16]

Magnetic resonance imaging (MRI) studies of persons with chronic schizophrenia indicated larger-than-normal lateral and third ventricles and reduced temporal lobe gray matter[17] (Figure 48-4). MRI findings also showed reduced frontal lobe blood flow and relative decreases in frontal lobe metabolic activity. Prefrontal cortex structure and functioning deficits were consistently observed when the subject was simultaneously placed under stress (Figure 48-5). The stress used in the study was primarily psychological, such as contingency planning exercises or divergent thinking during per-

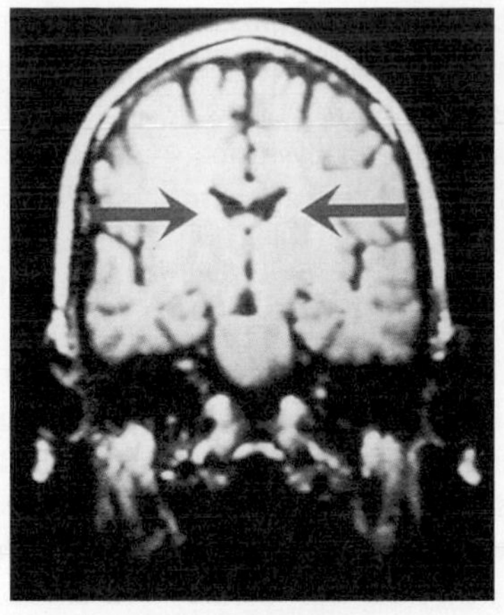

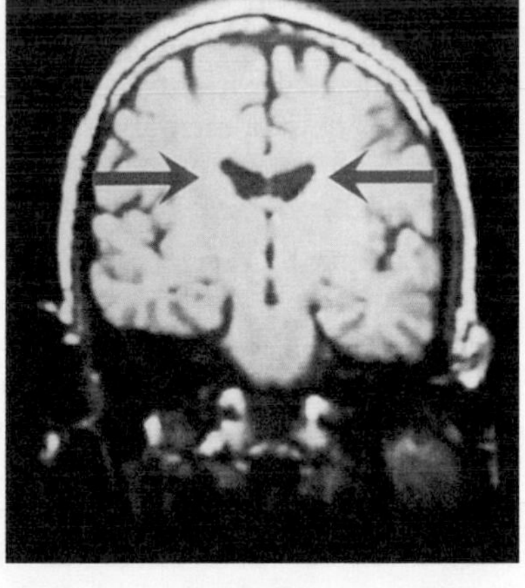

FIGURE 48-4 ■ Loss of brain volume associated with schizophrenia is clearly shown by magnetic resonance images comparing the size of ventricles (butterfly-shaped, fluid-filled spaces in the midbrain) of 44-year-old male identical twins, one of whom has schizophrenia *(right).* The ventricles of the person with schizophrenia are larger, suggesting structural brain changes associated with the illness. Note that such magnetic resonance images cannot be used to diagnose schizophrenia in the general population because of normal genetic variation in ventricle size; many unaffected people have large ventricles. (From Fortinash KM, Worret PA: *Psychiatric mental health nursing,* ed 3, St Louis, 2004, Mosby, p 240. Courtesy Daniel Weinberger, MD, Clinical Brain Disorders Branch, Division of Intramural Research Program, NIMH, 1990. Updated December 11, 2000.)

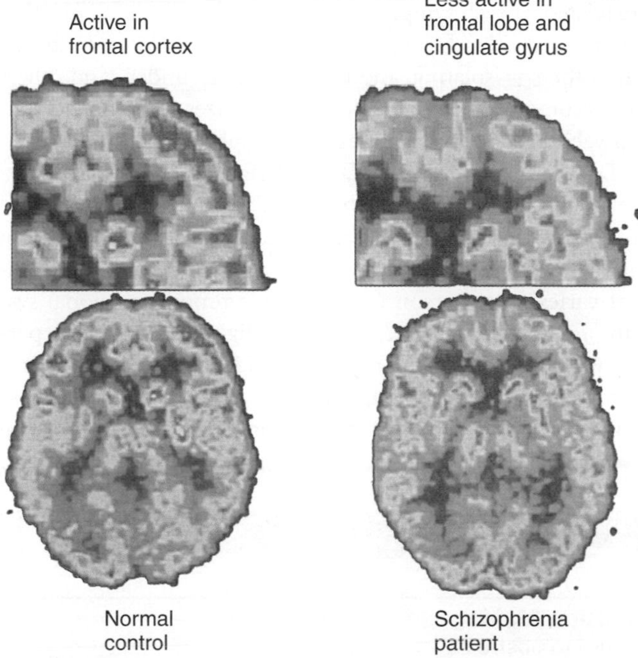

FIGURE 48-5 ■ Positron emission tomography (PET) scan with ^{18}F-deoxygluose shows metabolic activity in a horizontal section of the brain in a control subject *(left)* and in an unmedicated client with schizophrenia *(right).* Red and yellow indicate lower activity in the white matter areas of the brain. The frontal lobe is magnified to show reduced frontal activity in the prefrontal cortex of the client with schizophrenia. (From Fortinash KM, Worret PA: *Psychiatric mental health nursing,* ed 3, St Louis, 2004, Mosby, p 259. Courtesy Monte S. Buchsbaum, MD, Mt. Sinai School of Medicine, New York.)

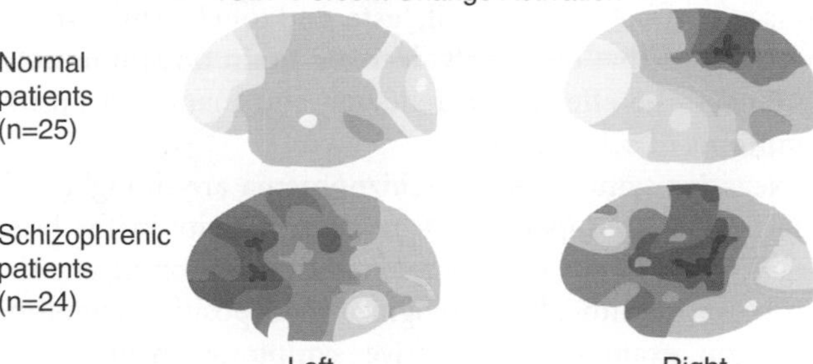

FIGURE 48-6 ■ Regional cerebral blood flow *(rCBF)* maps showing lateral views of cerebral cortex with frontal pole at *left,* occipital pole at *right.* Lateral view of percent change in rCBF in left and right hemisphere during the Wisconsin Card Sorting (WCS)/number matching tasks. Data are for 25 normal subjects *(top)* and 24 patients with schizophrenia treated with neuroleptic agents *(bottom).* Note that the normal subjects show striking rCBF increases during WCS/number matching tasks. (Redrawn from Berman KF, Zec RF, Weinberger DR: Physiologic dysfunction of dorsolateral prefrontal cortex in schizophrenia II, *Arch Gen Psychiatry* 43:126-135, 1986.)

formance of a cognitive task that utilized specific regions of the prefrontal cortex[18] (Figure 48-6).

Subsequent studies of brain structure with persons with severe schizophrenia replicated the earlier findings of abnormal limbic-cortical structures and smaller, misarranged hippocampal pyramidal cells. This includes replication of MRI findings of reduced bilateral temporal lobe volume, decreased hippocampal volume, and reduced volume in the parahippocampal gyrus region of the brain. Studies of brain regions other than the limbic system revealed frontal lobe structural alterations in the dorsolateral area of the prefrontal cortex and in the cingulate and motor cortices. The finding of decreased frontal lobe glucose metabolism associated with schizophrenia also has been replicated.[19]

Postmortem brain tissue studies of deceased patients indicated fewer nicotinic receptors present in the hippocampus. Tobacco dependence is a common secondary disorder with schizophrenia. The finding of fewer nicotinic receptors was of particular interest to researchers in that previous studies had shown that smoking could temporarily normalize auditory sensory gating that typically becomes impaired with schizophrenia.[20] Since then, researchers found that a neurophysiologic deficit at chromosome 15, at the OC7-nicotinic receptor gene, may partially explain the inheritance of this neurophysiologic symptom.[21] Although the development of schizophrenia is associated with any number of specific abnormalities, early neurodevelopmental alterations that result in dysfunction of the limbic and prefrontal regions of the brain appear to be critical.

Clinical Manifestations. **Positive symptoms**[22] of schizophrenia are thought to result from excessive dopamine D_2 receptor activity in the brain. Positive symptoms are more apparent to the casual observer than negative symptoms. Common symptoms include disorganized thinking (inability to logically connect thoughts), unusual speech (e.g., invented words, tangential ideas), odd behavior, delusions (systematic fixed false beliefs), and hallucinations (sensory perceptions with no apparent stimulus). Delusions often are persecutory, grandiose, or religious in nature. Auditory hallucinations are most common, but hallucinations may affect vision, smell, taste, and touch. Antipsychotic medications that effectively decrease brain dopamine activity tend to be effective in relieving and managing positive symptoms of schizophrenia.

Negative symptoms[22] of schizophrenia are thought to be associated with dopamine D_1 receptor activity in the brain. Negative symptoms represent deficits in functioning and thus can be more difficult to recognize than positive symptoms. Common examples of negative symptoms include social withdrawal and isolation, dull or blunted emotional affect, poverty of speech (limited verbal communication), posturing or remaining in one position for prolonged periods, and autism. Antipsychotic medications that effectively block dopamine D_1 receptors tend to be effective in relieving and managing negative symptoms of schizophrenia.

Disorganization, in comparison with previous functioning, is generally accepted as a behavioral hallmark of schizophrenia. This includes some degree of impairment in work or academic performance, interpersonal relating, and self-care. Disorganization and disturbance in language and communication may be the most common observation made of persons with schizophrenia. The person finds it difficult if not impossible to conform to accepted rules governing behavior, appearance, and speech, and these discrepancies cannot be attributed to intelligence, education, or cultural background.

Speech manifestations of schizophrenia include tangential ideas, words with private or approximate rather than generally accepted meanings, and neologisms. Neologisms are invented words with invented, special, or private meanings. Loose associations are seemingly unrelated ideas presented as though they are related. Speech symptoms are a serious source of frustration for persons with schizophrenia. Loss of ability to communicate with others is isolating, and the inability to understand others can become alarming. Box 48-1 summarizes some of the neuropsychological abnormalities in schizophrenia.

Delusions are systematic false beliefs that persist despite evidence to the contrary. The beliefs or ideas have meaning and are true to the individual rather than to reality and are not merely reflections of cultural values or ideals. Delusional content varies from person to person. Common delusional systems are grandiose, persecutory, or religious in nature. A person with delusions of persecution might believe he or she is being poisoned, watched, harassed, cheated, or otherwise plotted against by a powerful group or individual. Fearful

Box 48-1

Problems in Cognitive Functioning

Memory
Difficulty retrieving and using stored memory
Impaired short-term/long-term memory

Attention
Difficulty maintaining attention
Poor concentration
Distractibility
Inability to use selective attention

Form and Organization of Speech (Formal Thought Disorder)
Loose associations
Tangentiality
Incoherence/word salad/neologism
Illogicality
Circumstantiality
Pressured/distractible speech
Poverty of speech

Decision Making
Failure to abstract
Indecisiveness
Lack of insight
Impaired concept formation
Impaired judgment
Illogical or concrete thinking
Lack of planning and problem solving skills
Difficulty initiating tasks

Thought Content
Delusions
Paranoid
Grandiose
Religious
Somatic
Nihilistic
Thought broadcasting
Thought insertion
Thought control

From Stuart GW, Laraia MT: *Principles and practice of psychiatric nursing,* ed 7, St Louis, 2001, Mosby, p 406.

convictions that one's thoughts, feelings, or actions are under the control of others can occur. Thought broadcasting is the belief that one's thoughts are being broadcasted and made audible to others. Inversely, thought insertion is the belief that others are able to place thoughts into one's mind. Believing that one can control the thoughts, feelings, and actions of others also occurs. Delusions generally have themes of control and passivity and have been referred to as *first-rank symptoms.*

Hallucinations indicate the breakdown of perceptual selectivity. The ability to sort and process sensory information is lost. Perceptions (vision, hearing, taste, smell, touch) occur without objectively discernible stimuli. Hallucinations usually are auditory, but any or all of the five senses can be affected. Clear conscious awareness of hearing one's own thoughts or hearing voices, known or unknown, argue, comment, comfort, threaten, or appraise is not uncommon. Command hallucinations are the least predictable form of auditory hallucinations with the tremendous potential for tragic effects. Command hallucinations are experienced as impulses that the person has no choice but to carry out.

Affect, or emotional tone, may become blunted, shallow, flat, inappropriate, or silly. Loss of emotional tone is characterized by an unchanging, inexpressive facial expression, lack of eye contact, few gestures, and little to no tone or inflection in speech.

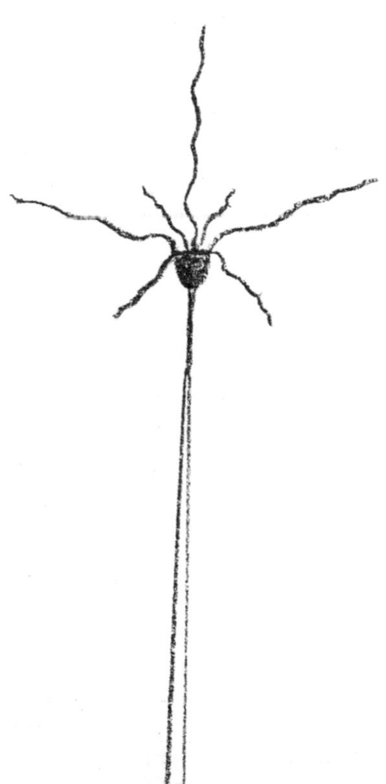

FIGURE 48-7 ■ An actively psychotic person was asked to draw a tree. Black was chosen from a selection of colors. The slender, tapered tree trunk may represent the instability of the ego. The branching structure is reminiscent of religious symbolism and poverty of hope. (Courtesy Chris Rost, RNC, MN, Spokane, Wash.)

Anhedonia, or the absence of pleasure or interest, is observed with many disorders, including schizophrenia. The affected individual may feel little pleasure from pleasurable experiences or may no longer engage in pleasurable experiences.

Self-identity disturbances with schizophrenia can be profound. Generally, having a sense of oneself means being able to differentiate one's physical self from the physical environment (Figure 48-7). This can take the form of a cosmic feeling of being one with the universe or being limitless. The disturbance is related to impaired perceptual and cognitive recognition of boundaries (Figure 48-8). Self-identity disturbances also are psychological. Identity requires discernment of self as distinct from others. Without this, people can feel exposed and defenseless.

Autism is a term used to indicate profound detachment. In autism, the external world becomes inaccessible, leaving the person alone in a separate world. Behavior, communication, and mood may reflect this separate world and thus, to casual observers, appear inappropriate.

Motor behavior is affected by schizophrenia. Posturing, mannerisms, pacing, bizarre rituals, clumsiness, grimacing, and aimless activity are examples of impaired psychomotor behavior (Figure 48-9). These behavioral symptoms of schizophrenia can be confused with extrapyramidal side effects of antipsychotic medications.

Sleep disturbance with acute schizophrenia generally takes the form of being unable to sleep. Tension, anxiety, psychomotor hyperactivity, active delusions, and hallucinations literally keep people awake. Those who are able to find sleep may spend close to the normal amount of time sleeping but their sleep is not restful, including less deep sleep or rapid eye movement (REM) sleep, frequent awakenings, nightmares, and early-morning awakening. As a result, the normal wake-up time tends to shift from morning to early afternoon.

Pharmacologic Treatment. Newer antipsychotic medications are intended to generally manage psychosis as well as both the positive and negative schizophrenia symptoms. Older antipsychotic medications were less effective in managing negative schizophrenia symptoms. They mainly acted as dopamine antagonists, blocking the dopamine receptors (D_2). This action diminishes the amount of dopamine received by the receptor sites (Figure 48-10). Specific schizophrenia symptoms have been associated with neurotransmission dysregulation that diminished or elevated dopamine activity. Hyperdopaminergic states have primarily been associated with positive symptoms of schizophrenia such as hallucinations, delusions, and psychosis. Hypodopaminergic states have primarily been associated with negative symptoms of schizophrenia such as cognitive difficulties, lack of energy and motivation, and depression.[23] Dopamine D_2 receptors have been associated with positive symptoms and psychosis, whereas dopamine D_1 receptors have been associated with

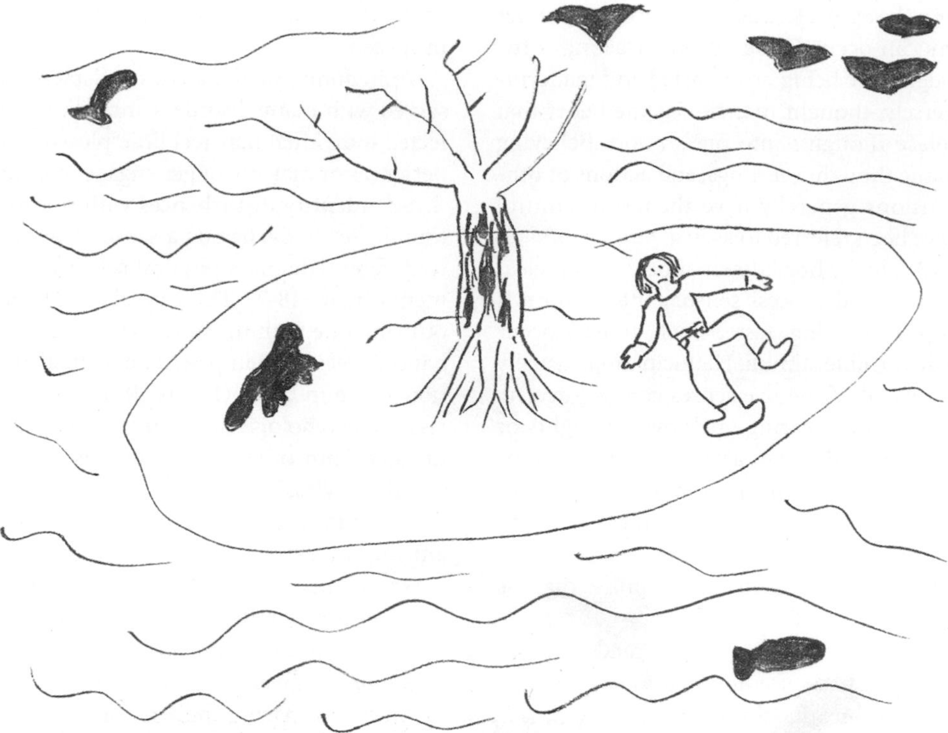

FIGURE 48-8 ■ This "schizophrenic drawing" (created by a thought-disordered person) demonstrates absence of boundaries between sky and sea. The isolation and powerlessness are underscored by the island and body position of the person. Negation of vital life is represented by the decaying tree. The fish and birds and squirrel maintain a menacing quality. Although a full color range of markers was available, the person used only black. (Courtesy Chris Rost, RNC, MN, Spokane, Wash.)

negative symptoms. Effective antipsychotic medications have significant dopamine effects; however, schizophrenia symptoms are highly complex and likely to involve other neurotransmitters, particularly serotonin and norepinephrine (Table 48-1).

When effective, antipsychotic medications[24] can be expected to diminish or remit hallucinations or reduce their impact on functioning. The ability to reason should improve; ambivalence, delusions, and suspiciousness should be greatly reduced; agitation and confusion should be relieved; and social behavior should improve. Antipsychotic medications are designed to have specific effects on targeted neurotransmitters. Dopamine and serotonin have been the most important neurotransmitters associated with the symptoms of schizophrenia. Antipsychotic medications employ different biochemical methods to achieve similar objectives, the primary objective being the reduction of dopamine activity in the limbic system and the frontal cortex.

Newer antipsychotic medications are equally effective in this regard but they vary in their side effect profiles and their potential for interacting with other medications. First-generation antipsychotic medications (e.g., chlorpromazine) had relatively nonspecific neurotransmitter effects and numerous side effects. Haloperidol was the first high-potency antipsychotic medication that had significantly less anticholinergic and hypotensive side effects. By 1990, atypical antipsychotics became widely available. The first atypical antipsychotic, clozapine, was quickly followed by a generation of new atypical antipsychotics (risperidone, olanzapine, and quetiapine), each promising still fewer side effects, better relief of both positive and negative schizophrenia symptoms, and minimal risk of tardive dyskinesia (the one antipsychotic medication side effect that can become irreversible).

Dopamine D_2 remains the lead neurotransmitter target of the atypical antipsychotics.[24] Researchers found that the most common side effects of antipsychotic medication could be reduced if the drugs impact on dopamine D_2 receptors was not excessive. Lower receptor occupancy, less receptor affinity, and faster release[25] of the receptor were methods shown to be associated with fewer side effects. More recently, the aim for effective antipsychotic medication is to stabilize rather than reduce dopamine activity. These medications, such as aripiprazole and ziprasidone, show greater affinity for serotonin receptors (negative symptoms) and moderate affinity for dopamine and norepinephrine receptors (positive symptoms).[25]

Pharmacologic Side Effects. Metabolic side effects of the new atypical antipsychotic medications can be significant. The two most worrisome side effects are weight gain,[26] typically 40 to 60 pounds, and hyperglycemia.[27] Experts have speculated that hyperglycemia may have to do with dopamine receptor involvement in the regulation of insulin secretion. Numerous explanations for weight gain as a major side effect of antipsychotic medication continue to be developed and tested. The glutamate neurobiological model[28] of psychosis and schizophrenia, an alternative to the dopamine model, may be the basis for the next new generation of antipsychotic medications.

FIGURE 48-9 ■ Model exhibiting catatonic posturing. (Photographer: Kathleen Kelly, Spokane, Wash.)

The *glutamate deficit*[28] model attempts to focus attention on the cause of excessive dopamine receptor activity rather than the excessive activity itself. γ-Aminobutyric acid (GABA) is the most important inhibitory brain neurotransmitter. GABA synthesis depends on and is controlled by the enzyme glutamic acid decarboxylase (GAD). GAD activity is modulated by the glutamate receptor NMDA. GAD dysregulation is thought to lead to insufficient GABA activity and, consequently, excessive dopamine activity. Reduced GAD activity has been observed in the dorsolateral prefrontal cortex and hippocampus of patients with schizophrenia. The interesting observation for pharmacological researchers is that a broad range of different drugs has been shown to be capable of affecting GAD activity. Although the glutamate deficit model is not new, the model might yet lead to a class of antipsychotic medications unlike any generation before.

KEY CONCEPTS

- Schizophrenia is characterized by altered perceptions of reality and disordered thinking. Genetic predisposition and environmental factors are thought to interact to produce biological changes in the brain, particularly in the hippocampus, temporal lobes, and dopaminergic pathways that project to the limbic system. Exposure to influenza virus during the fifth to sixth months of gestation appears to predispose to schizophrenia. The age at onset is 15 to 25 years for men and 25 to 35 years for women. There is a higher incidence in industrialized societies. Stress and childhood experiences may affect the expression of schizophrenia. Lack of safety, security, order, and predictability and low self-worth are probable contributing factors in relation to increased stress.
- Neurologic abnormalities found in those with schizophrenia and children who later develop schizophre-

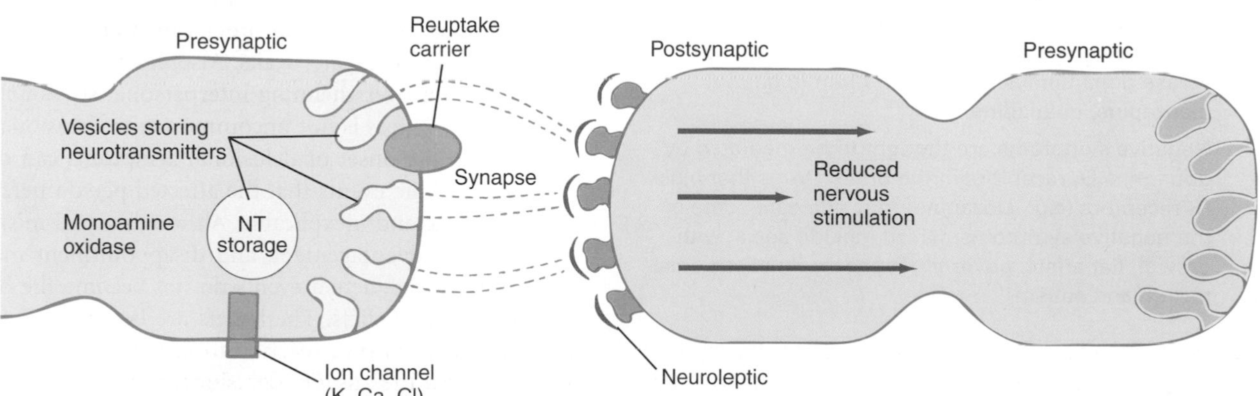

FIGURE 48-10 ■ Neuroleptic (antipsychotic) action. Neurotransmitter *(NT)* action at the synapse is modified by neuroleptics, which block postsynaptic receptor sites to reduce nervous stimulation (reducing symptoms of schizophrenia). (From Fortinash KM, Worret PA: *Psychiatric mental health nursing,* ed 3, St Louis, 2004, Mosby, p 241.)

Table 48-1

Neurotransmitters in Schizophrenia: Type and Function

Neurotransmitter	Type	Function
Dopamine	Catecholamine	Regulates motor behavior in extrapyramidal nerve tracts and also transmits in the cortex. Increases vigilance and may increase aggression. Too much may produce psychosis; too little may cause movement disorders (EPS).
Serotonin	Indolamine	Brainstem transmitter; modulates mood; lowers aggressive tendencies. A deficiency may be responsible for some forms of schizophrenia.
Acetylcholine	Cholinergic	Transmits at nerve-muscle connections (central nervous system and autonomic nervous system). A deficiency may increase confusion and acting out behavior. Controls EPS.
Norepinephrine	Catecholamine	Transmits in the sympathetic nervous system. Induces the "flight or fight" syndrome (hypervigilance). May be insufficient in clients with schizophrenia who display anhedonia (loss of pleasure).
Cholecystokinin	Peptide	Excites the limbic neurons. A deficiency is related to avolition (lack of motivation) and a flat affect.
Glutamate	Amino acid	Excitatory neurotransmitter. Impairment in the *N*-methyl-D-aspartate affects glutamate metabolism, which can lead to problems with cognition, delusions, and possibly some negative symptoms of schizophrenia.[55]
γ-Aminobutyric acid (GABA)	Amino acid	Inhibitory neurotransmitter; predominantly a brain transmitter. Promotes a balance between dopamine and glutamate and thus inhibits impulsive behaviors.

From Fortinash KM, Worret PA: *Psychiatric mental health nursing,* ed 3, St Louis, 2004, Mosby, p 241.
EPS, Extrapyramidal symptoms.

nia include abnormal blinking and blink reflex, abnormal pupil reflex and facial movements, enlarged lateral and third ventricles, reduced temporal gray matter, decreased blood flow, and decreased glucose metabolism in frontal lobes.

- The positive symptoms of schizophrenia are thought to be due to excessive dopamine D_2 receptor activation in the brain. Disorganized thinking (inability to connect thoughts logically), disorganized speech (rambling, tangentiality), delusions (fixed system of false beliefs), and hallucinations (sensory perceptions when no apparent stimulus exists) are typical positive symptoms. Delusions are often persecutory, grandiose, or controlling. Hallucinations are most often auditory but may also be visual, olfactory, or tactile. Positive symptoms respond to drugs that decrease dopamine activity in the brain (e.g., olanzapine, quetiapine).
- Negative symptoms are thought to be mediated by dopamine D_1 receptors in the brain. Drugs that block D_1 receptors (e.g., clozapine) may alleviate some of the negative symptoms, which include social withdrawal, flat affect, poverty of speech, ritualistic posturing, and autism.

Delusional Disorder

Delusional disorder does not present a clear clinical picture. The disorder is characterized by behaviors that are dominated by systematic false beliefs that persist despite objective contradictory evidence. Unlike the delusions typically associated with schizophrenia, the delusions are highly systematic with very limited themes. The actual content and process of the delusions remain constant. Usually other symptoms of disordered thinking are absent or are rare. Systematic delusions are persistent and pervasive and may impact several aspects of daily life. Delusional disorder is similar to schizophrenia in that acute psychosis can occur.

Etiology and Neurobiology. Delusional disorder may eventually prove to be a form of schizophrenia or schizophrenia spectrum disorder.[29] Presently most experts consider delusional disorder a separate disorder with neurophysiological properties that overlap with those of schizophrenia. Unlike schizophrenia, delusional disorder can dramatically reshape personality and character traits. Also, learned suspiciousness resulting from overwhelming interpersonal stress and negative life experiences is not uncommon with delusional disorder. In fact, the onset of delusional symptoms can coincide with stressful life events that the affected person perceives as overwhelming and inexplicable. Although actual misfortune, suffering, disadvantagement, and disappointment may have been experienced, actual events do not become the basis for systematic false beliefs. The beliefs are better understood as cognitive symptoms in reaction to actual events, which does not imply that the onset of delusional disorder is triggered by the experience of disturbing life events. The etiologic progression of delusional disorder continues to be studied.

A key characteristic of delusional disorder is the readiness and ease with which new, neutral, and coincidental life experiences become incorporated into the system of delusional beliefs. Once a delusional system has been developed, actual life experiences are likely to be viewed through the lens of the delusional system. In this way, life seems always to confirm rather than challenge the delusions. Life experiences thought to be associated with the onset of delusional disorder tend to be profound experiences that generate intense feelings of failure or personal inadequacy. In effect, the delusions appear to function as a massive psychological defense against further injury or damage to self-esteem. Given its low incidence, believed to be 3 to 4 cases per 100,000, and low prevalence, believed to be less than 0.10%, delusional disorder is a relatively rare condition. That said, low incidence and prevalence rates also could be explained by the observation that few persons with delusional disorder are likely to recognize their condition and seek mental health care.

Clinical Manifestations. **Delusions**[30] are the hallmark or defining symptom of delusional disorder. With this disorder, delusions typically take the form of false beliefs that are systematic without being bizarre. The core feature of these false beliefs is that the beliefs *in theory* could be true but are nevertheless highly unlikely. Mental and cognitive functions that are not directly involved in the delusions remain intact. Two common delusional systems are the belief that one is having a secret relationship with a famous person and the belief that one is being pursued by a powerful government agency intent on destroying the individual. Grandiose delusions also are extremely common. In this case the person believes she or he possesses great attributes or is in some way extraordinary. Jealousy delusions often have to do with a sexual partner who is perceived as unfaithful or untrustworthy. Less obvious delusions involve litigation and persistent legal actions to seek redress for perceived wrongs or slights. Retaliation or the unpredictable use of aggression or violence is a constant concern with any person who is delusional and feels unfairly wronged or slighted.

Reality testing[30] or the ability to evaluate and appreciate the difference between internal experiences and external experiences is, by definition, impaired by delusions. Delusional beliefs are unaffected by the lack of objective evidence. Normal reality testing implies that, in the face of compelling evidence to the contrary, the belief no longer is accepted as valid. With delusional disorder, impaired reality testing maintains the delusions. In other words, impaired reality testing indicates that the person is unable, rather than unwilling, to perceive reality.

KEY CONCEPTS

- Delusional disorder is a psychotic illness dominated by a tenacious system of false beliefs. It is a slowly developing disorder that may begin with a "grain of truth" and then escalate to delusional proportions as the person assigns false meaning to life experiences. Delusional beliefs often have themes of jealousy, secret love, grandiosity, persecution, and legal retaliation for perceived wrongs (litigiousness).
- The biochemical and structural basis of delusional disorder is unknown. Some commonality with schizophrenia is suspected.

Major Depression

Once referred to as endogenous depression, or depression that arises from characteristics of the person, major depression now is understood to be a complex illness involving inherited genetic susceptibility and symptoms associated with specific alterations in brain structures and functioning. According to the *Diagnostic and Statistical Manual of Mental Disorders,*[31] the American Psychiatric Association reference guide that is updated every 10 years, a diagnosis of major depression requires the presence of multiple symptoms that are intense enough to cause distress and to persistently impair psychosocial functioning. Depression with one or two symptoms that last 2 years or more is commonly referred to as minor depression or **dysthymia.**

Major depression is a leading cause of suicide. This illness frequently occurs as a comorbid disorder with serious physical illness as well as other mental disorders. Major depression also can develop as a serious secondary illness or illness complication. For example, as early as 1937, researchers were able to show that cardiac patients with severe depression had higher cardiac death rates than their counterparts. More recent studies of depression and mortality during the first year following myocardial infarction showed significantly greater risk for 1-year mortality in patients who were depressed.[32]

Evidence of a possible genetic susceptibility to major depression partially explains why female rates consistently are twice the rates observed in males, but significant rates of major depression are observed in all age, race, education, and income groups.[33] The complexity of managing severe depression in adolescents[34] and older adults[35] has made these population groups particularly concerning. As a result of the potentially serious disability, morbidity, and mortality risks directly associated with the illness, the World Health Organization (WHO) ranks major depression among the top five global health problems.

Etiology and Neurobiology. Improved neurobiological research techniques have made possible the accomplishment of basic scientific advances in determining the neurobiological mechanisms of major depression. Nevertheless, the specific cause of major depression remains unknown. Table 48-2 summarizes key mood disorder risk factors.

Cognitive-behavioral[33] models of depression, particularly learned helplessness,[34] have been shown to correlate with the basic neurobiology of depression. Avoidant persons, when faced with a highly stressful situation, anxiously withdraw from or avoid confronting the situation, despite opportunities

Table 48-2

Risk Factors for Major Depressive and Bipolar Disorders

Risk Factor	Major Depression	Bipolar Disorder
Lifetime prevalence (%)	F: 5-9	0.6-0.9
M/F ratio	1:2	1:1.2
Age at onset (yr)	Mid to late 30s	Late teens to early 20s
Social class	No relationship	Slight increase in upper classes
Race	No relationship	No relationship
Family history		
Major depression in relatives (%)	17	15
Bipolar depression in relatives (%)	2-3	8

From Hirschfeld RMA, Goodwin PR: Mood disorders. In Talbott JA, Hales RE, Yudofsky SC, editors: *The American Psychiatric Press textbook of psychiatry,* Washington, DC, 1988, American Psychiatric Press, p 410.

Table 48-3

Prefrontal Cortex and Serotonin Interconnections: Implications in Depression

Interconnected Brain Structures	Hypothesized Role of These Interconnections in Depression
Prefrontal cortex	Covering the frontal lobes, it is unique within the central nervous system for its strong interconnections with all other areas of the brain; it receives information that has already been processed by other sensory areas and then merges this information with other emotional, historical, or relevant information, thus attending to both feelings and intellect.
Limbic system structures	The prefrontal cortex modulates limbic system activities (emotional and instinctive) by way of these three structures: Hippocampus — Major importance in cognitive function, including memory. Amygdala — Major importance in modulating feelings such as aggression, anger, love, and shyness. Cingulated gyrus — Involved in motivation and interest.
Brainstem	Responsible for regulating the general state of arousal and tone of brain function; also the location of structures that manufacture various neurotransmitters, such as serotonin, norepinephrine, and dopamine.
Raphe nuclei	Located in the brainstem, they manufacture serotonin; they also modulate excessive stimuli, as well as the organization and coordination of appropriate responses to these stimuli.
Hypothalamus	This interconnection allows for direct prefrontal input into neuroendocrine function via the hypothalamic-pituitary axis.
Suprachiasmatic nucleus	Located in the hypothalamus, it regulates circadian (24-hr) rhythms and circannual rhythms; thus it is also implicated in seasonal affective disorder.

From Stuart GW, Laraia MT: *Principles and practice of psychiatric nursing,* ed 7, St Louis, 2001, Mosby, p 406.

to do so. Persistent avoidance eventually conditions the person to automatically respond to stressful situations with strong feelings of helplessness. Helpless response to a stressful situation exposes the person to the full negative impact of the stress, which in turn promotes more withdrawal, more avoidance, more helplessness, and, most importantly, higher levels of stress.

Neurobiological changes associated with major depression are thought to involve neurotransmission dysregulation,[35] altered hippocampal and prefrontal cortex cell structure and functioning,[36] and hypothalamic-pituitary-adrenal (HPA) system activation[37] (Table 48-3). Based on observations of low central nervous system levels of serotonin (Figure 48-11) in persons with severe symptoms of depression, the basic neurobiology of depression has been hypothesized to be reduced brain serotonin neurotransmission activity either through excessive presynaptic uptake or through stress-related down-regulation of postsynaptic receptors (Figure 48-12). Chronic or persistent vulnerability to depression is thought to be related to decreased hippocampal volume or capacity[38] and suppressed hippocampal neurogenesis.[39]

Research focused on the biological model supports a biological basis for mood disorders. Some of the biological factors associated with depression are illustrated in Figure 48-13.

HPA axis dysfunction has been associated with depression. Genetic susceptibility to depression appears to mediate the link between stress and depression.[40] Comparison studies of

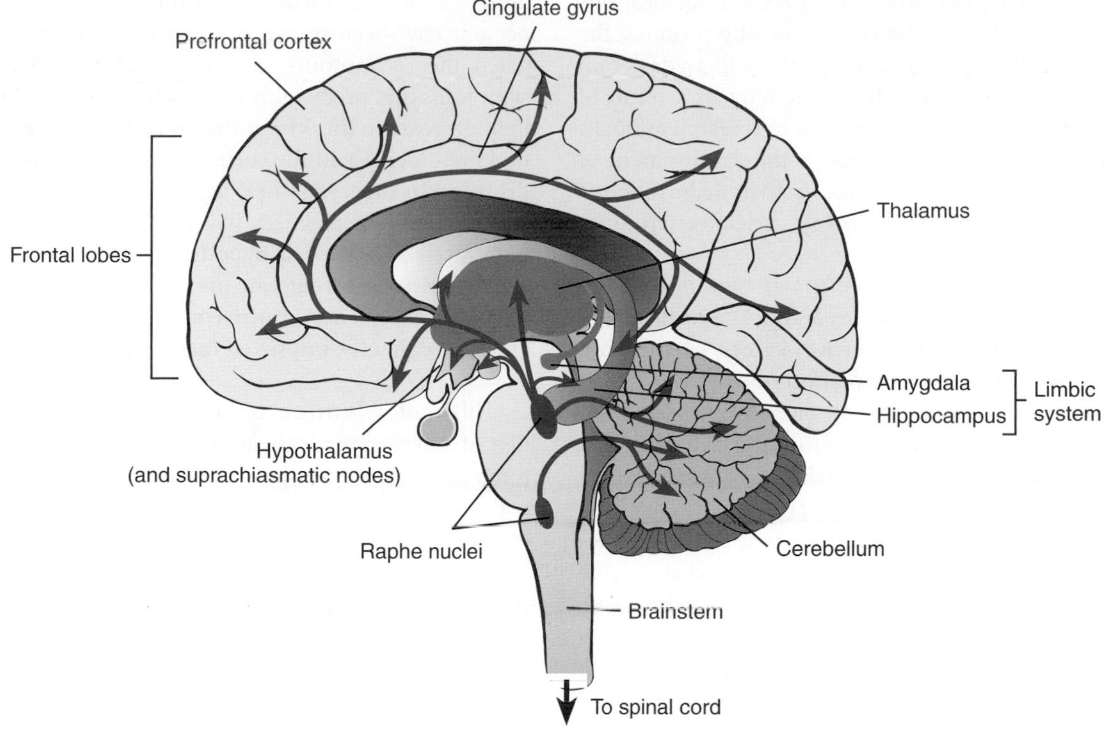

FIGURE 48-11 ■ The serotonin neurotransmitter system implicated in depression. (From Stuart GW, Laraia MT: *Principles and practice of psychiatric nursing,* ed 7, St Louis, 2001, Mosby, p 356.)

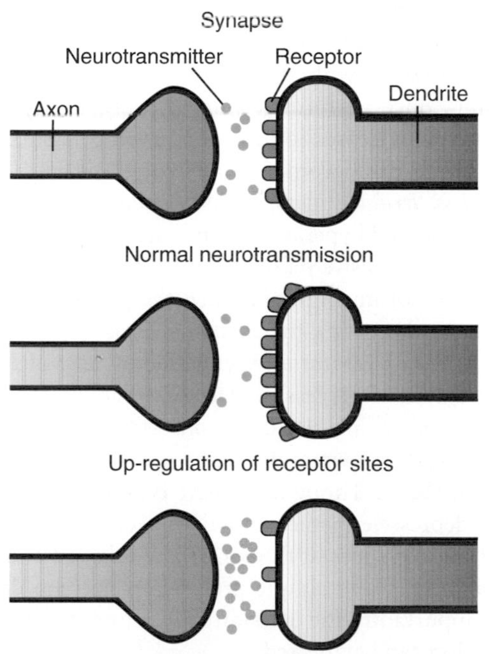

FIGURE 48-12 ■ Levels of postsynaptic serotonin (5-HT) receptors. There are more receptors when there is too little serotonin (up-regulation) and fewer receptors when there is too much serotonin (down-regulation). (From Stuart GW, Laraia MT: *Principles and practice of psychiatric nursing,* ed 7, St Louis, 2001, Mosby, p 388.)

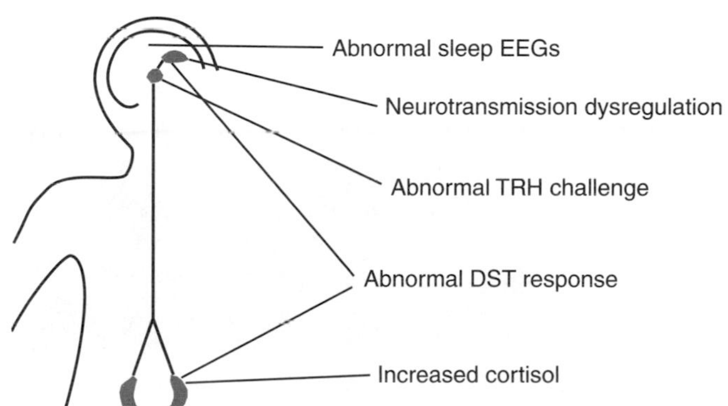

FIGURE 48-13 ■ Biological factors related to depression. *EEGs,* Electroencephalograms; *DST,* dexamethasone suppression test; *TRH,* thyroid-releasing hormone. (From Stuart GW, Laraia MT: *Principles and practice of psychiatric nursing,* ed 7, St Louis, 2001, Mosby, p 357.)

stress-induced cortisol levels in depressed persons and healthy control subjects showed significant links between stress hormones and depression, but far more information is needed before the precise nature of the link can be understood.[41]

One of a number of stress and depression theories proposes that increased stress hormone levels can lead to significant decreases in the expression of brain-derived neurotrophic factor (BDNF). Reduced BDNF has been shown to lead to hippocampal cell atrophy and, consequently, reduced neurotransmission activity in this area of the brain.[42] According to the researchers, effective antidepressant medications seemed to improve BDNF activity and thereby promote the growth and survival of serotonin neurons in this vital brain region. Significant reduction in BDNF activity, as a result of severe stress, has also been demonstrated in research animals. The HPA model of depression supports the development of novel treatments that can target cortisol activity (e.g., mifepristone) rather than serotonin activity (e.g., selective serotonin reuptake inhibitors, SSRIs).[43]

Sleep studies of depression have shown significantly reduced slow-wave (delta) sleep (stages 3 and 4) and increased light sleep (stage 1). The periods of REM sleep latency with depression are shortened but the total number of REM periods does not decrease (Figure 48-14). Sleep is restorative for brain cells. Among the numerous restoration activities that occur, mood-related hormone activity during sleep appears to decrease although severe reductions in serotonin activity have been associated with less restful sleep. Because of the link between fluctuations in mood-related hormones and sleep, disturbed sleep is a hallmark symptom of depression. The classic sleep disturbances include difficulty falling asleep, early-morning waking, and decreased total sleep time.[44]

Circadian rhythms (synchronizing cycles) are closely associated with symptoms of major depression. The pineal gland in the brain produces the hormone melatonin. Brain melatonin levels can fluctuate significantly, with annual and daily increases and decreases in light and dark periods. Melatonin helps regulate circadian rhythms; in turn, these cycles govern body temperature changes and the urge to sleep. Depressed persons have been shown to suffer from low melatonin levels when their symptoms include disturbed sleep. Depression symptoms that predictably occur when the daily hours of daylight decrease in the winter then remit when the hours of natural light increase in the spring is known as **seasonal affective disorder**. In theory, natural light acts as a *zeitgeber*, or a biological clock synchronizer that is based on the 24-hour day-night cycle. It has been hypothesized that persons with seasonal affective disorder who are exposed to additional natural light will experience improvement in their sleep-wake cycle and, consequently, improved mental health.

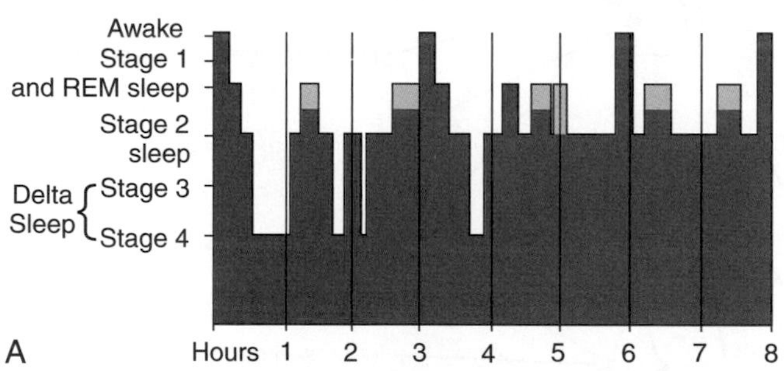

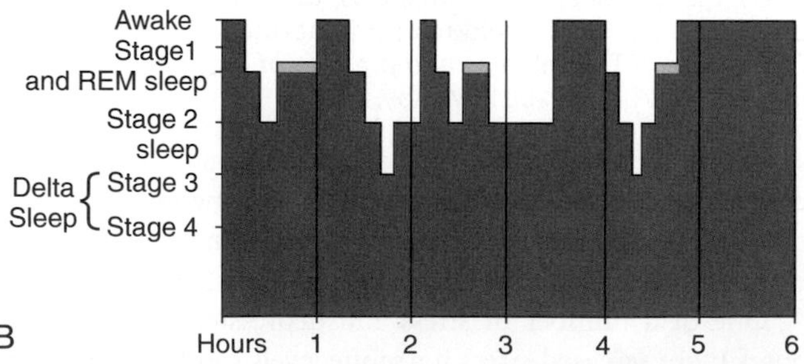

FIGURE 48-14 ■ **A,** Normal sleep architecture. **B,** Depressed sleep architecture. Green areas indicate rapid eye movement *(REM)* sleep. (From Stuart GW, Laraia MT: *Principles and practice of psychiatric nursing,* ed 7, St Louis, 2001, Mosby, p 357.)

Clinical Manifestations. **Depressed mood** and the loss of interest or pleasure (anhedonia) are hallmark symptoms of major depression. This change in mood is relatively constant and is recognized both by the depressed person and by others. Depressed mood associated with major depression is qualitatively different from the normal sadness or grief associated with loss. Depressed mood typically is experienced as painful, numbing, and bottomless. Loss of interest or pleasure can be more difficult to recognize. Others may notice this change before the depressed person does but the loss may be absolute, meaning that if the person engages in such activities, interest and pleasure are not experienced. In effect, the capacity for interest and pleasure appears to be lost.

Fatigue or loss of energy is a common yet somewhat alarming symptom of depression. Depressed people may associate their severe or sudden fatigue with serious physical illness such as cancer, diabetes, or cardiovascular disease. The fatigue associated with depression can make ordinary daily activities, once performed automatically, nearly impossible. The fatigue of depression is not relieved by rest or sleep and, when severe, can become immobilizing.

Restless, irritable agitation associated with depression can range from mild hyperactivity and sarcasm to hostility and aggression. Compulsive yet meaningless physical activities such as pacing are not uncommon. Often the person attempts to engage the restlessness with activities such as "organizing" papers.

Impaired concentration is experienced as a highly disturbing symptom of depression. Decreased ability to concentrate, attend, and think is common with severe depression. Thoughts slow down and the process of thinking literally becomes difficult. Thought content typically is dominated by highly depressive themes. Impaired decision making is one of many consequences of thinking that is slowed and narrowed. Minor choices and simple preferences become difficult, but more importantly, the decision to seek or accept treatment for depression can be affected.

Low self-esteem is the psychological hallmark of depression. Negative self-appraisals range from pointless guilt to self-hate. In some cases, the guilt reaches delusional proportions or is markedly disproportionate to actual misdeeds or perceived failings. Loss of self-esteem with depression differs from the ordinary day-to-day waxing and waning of self-esteem. People generally find ways to protect their self-esteem from the normal assaults of daily life. With severe depression, self-esteem can be absent and only rarely is the loss related to actual life events.

Negative thinking, expressed as negative views of self, life, and the future, is a symptom of severe depression that is common but often misunderstood. Severe depression is an empty experience that makes life itself seem futile. Expressions of negative thinking essentially reflect this deep psychological experience. Negative thinking associated with depression can be mistaken as willful or so unpleasant that others avoid contact with the depressed person.

Vegetative states associated with depression manifest as slowed or reduced physical activity. Normal daily activities, particularly bathing and dressing, may not be performed. Vegetative symptoms typically are described as feeling as though one is sleep walking, living in slow motion, or has become a robot.

Sleep disturbances of depression follow the neurobiological and cognitive-behavioral symptoms of depression. Insomnia is most common, but some people may sleep more or shift their sleep hours from nighttime to daytime. Sleep symptoms include difficulty falling asleep, early-morning awakening, frequent awakenings, and waking tired. The cognitive activity generated by obsessive negative thinking disturbs sleep essentially by preventing it or by literally waking the person.

Appetite disturbance associated with depression ranges from increased to decreased appetite to marked change in food preferences. Severely depressed persons can become unaware of their hunger or thirst. Diminished salivary and gastric activity can dampen appetite. Weight loss of 10 to 20 pounds over relatively short periods is not uncommon. Overeating also occurs, but this disturbance appears to be related more to restlessness than to appetite. People who normally use food for emotional comfort may, when depressed, increase their consumption of high-fat, high-sugar, high-salt foods.

Psychosis associated with major depression is thought to result from extreme symptom severity, prolonged symptom duration, or comorbid illness complications. Hallucinations, delusions, and disorganization may become prominent and require treatment with antipsychotic medications. Severely depressed older adults are at increased risk of depression-associated psychosis.

Pharmacologic Treatment. Most antidepressants currently available act by improving brain norepinephrine and serotonin activity. Earlier generations of antidepressants had less specific effects on these neurotransmitters and significantly more side effects. Monoamine oxidase inhibitors (MAOIs) blocked the destruction of norepinephrine and serotonin once it was released into the synaptic cleft. Tricyclic antidepressants (TCAs) blocked the reuptake of norepinephrine and serotonin, thereby allowing more neurotransmitter activity. SSRIs became widely available in the 1990s and were the first antidepressants with selective serotonin effects. SSRIs such as fluoxetine, paroxetine, and sertraline have been shown to relieve depression symptoms three times faster than earlier medications with far fewer side effects.

SSRIs quickly became the primary class of antidepressants; some have multiple treatment indications for additional disorders. Although the side-effect profile of SSRIs represents real improvement over earlier antidepressants, SSRIs are not side effect free.[45] Serotonin syndrome[46] is a serious side effect that results from excessive serotonin activity. This side effect can be caused by drug-drug interactions or individual sensitivity to serotonergic drugs. Symptoms of serotonin syndrome include altered mental status, restless agitation, myoclonus, hyperreflexia, sweating, shivering, tremor, gastrointestinal upset, ataxia, and headache.

Sexual dysfunction also is thought to result from SSRI-induced excessive serotonin activity. Onset can be immediate or gradual, with effects ranging from loss of interest, to impaired arousal, to anorgasmia. Less severe but equally troublesome side effects include gastrointestinal upset, headache, allergy, dry mouth, constipation, urination difficulties, sweating, and significant weight gain.

SSRI cellular and neurochemical mechanisms continue to be the subject of a great deal of basic and clinical research. It would appear that the SSRIs share the basic action of boosting neurotransmission activity of mood-related monoamines. More recent research findings suggest that SSRIs may also alter the genetics-based expression of BDNF and cell neurogenesis in the hippocampus.[47]

Bipolar Disorder

Etiology and Neurobiology. Bipolar disorder is a highly complex mood disorder characterized by recurring symptoms of depression and elation that can become severe enough to produce psychosis. Decades of clinical and genetic research findings indicate that the increased risk of developing the illness is both inherited and acquired (Figure 48-15). Symptom onset leading to the initial diagnosis of bipolar disorder typically does not occur before late adolescence or early young adulthood. However, childhood onset and older age onset also can occur. The most recognizable course of illness with bipolar disorder is the sudden onset of severe mania lasting from weeks to months. Mania is the hallmark symptom of bipolar disorder; however, when the initial symptoms of mania are severe enough to produce psychosis, bipolar disorder can be mistaken for schizophrenia. Accurate diagnosis of bipolar disorder when the initial symptom profile is depression can be quite difficult or long delayed.

Efforts to identify the neurobiological factors that characterize bipolar disorder have yielded mixed results. First, the similarities between psychosis associated with mania, psychosis associated with depression, and psychosis associated with schizophrenia are a major hurdle. Second, the depression associated with bipolar disorder differs very little from the depression that characterizes major depression. Third,

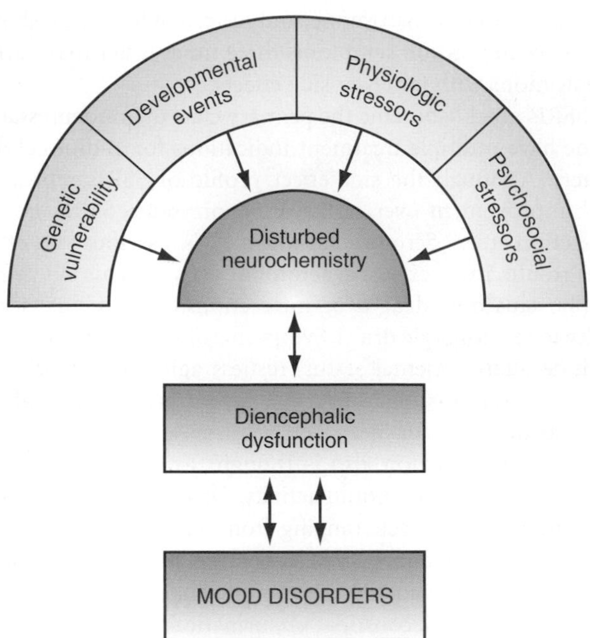

FIGURE 48-15 ■ Unified model of mood disorders. (Redrawn from Stuart GW, Sundeen SJ: Disturbances of mood. In Stuart GW, Sundeen SJ, editors: *Principles and practice of psychiatric nursing,* ed 4, St Louis, 1991, Mosby, p 429.)

when bipolar symptom onset is gradual, changes in behavior can be mistaken for personality disorder or substance use disorder.

Thus far there is little evidence of a stable genetic or biochemical distinction between bipolar disorder, schizophrenia, and major depression. However, as with schizophrenia and major depression, the significant inherited risks of bipolar disorder have been documented. The findings of twin studies and parent-child studies show significant inherited risk of bipolar disorder.[48] The risk in monozygotic twins of a parent with bipolar disorder is 75%. The risk in a person with two parents with bipolar disorder is 60%. The risk in first-degree relatives is 20%, and the risk in the general population is 1%.

The neurotransmission model of bipolar disorder follows the basic *catecholamine hypothesis* for major depression and schizophrenia. Neurotransmission activity deficits are thought to promote depression symptoms associated with bipolar disorder whereas excessive activity is thought to promote symptoms of mania and psychosis. The assumption is that the depression and mania of bipolar disorder are the result of two different neurobiological processes. The alternative hypothesis is that bipolar disorder is the result of a specific form of neurotransmission dysregulation that results in the loss of mood stabilization. Given the fact that with bipolar disorder a mixed mood state that includes symptoms of both mania and depression is not uncommon, the mood destabilization hypothesis is of great interest. Both models focus on serotonin, norepinephrine, and dopamine as the neurotransmitters involved.[49]

Neuroimaging studies of brain structural changes associated with bipolar disorder indicate findings potentially similar to those of major depression. For example, ventricular enlargement, increased numbers of T2 signal hyperintensities, and tissue loss in the basal ganglia, lateral and mesial temporal structures, and cortical regions have been observed. At the same time, other researchers have reported no significant tissue changes associated with bipolar disorder. Experts suggest that tissue changes probably are linked with greater mania symptom severity and duration. For example, symptom onset in older age has been related to greater tissue changes.[49] Neurobiological studies of the evidence of tissue changes associated with bipolar disorder thus far have not linked specific changes with depression, elation, or mania. Nevertheless, impaired functioning has consistently been associated with tissue changes. Findings such as these lend important support to the hypothesis of impaired emotion processing and impaired regulation of emotional behavior as the probable neurobiological mechanism of bipolar disorder.[49]

Clinical Manifestations. The two basic forms of bipolar disorder are bipolar I and bipolar II. Multiple subtypes of bipolar II disorder, a subtler but equaling distressing condition, have been proposed. A diagnosis of bipolar I disorder requires at least one episode of mania as well as major depression. A diagnosis of bipolar II disorder requires no episodes of mania and at least one episode of hypomania and major depression. Numerous subtypes of bipolar II have been proposed and defined based on the nature of psychosocial functioning impairment involved.

The subtyping of bipolar II symptoms, also referred to as bipolar spectrum disorders, allows for earlier and more accurate diagnosis and treatment of persons who clearly suffer from mood dysregulation but who do not meet the symptom criteria for bipolar I or bipolar II disorder. Some experts have suggested that these subtypes should be classified as bipolar III disorder.[50] Examples of potential bipolar III symptoms include years of repeated episodes of depression before the initial episode of mania; protracted hypomania causing psychosocial disturbance without psychosocial impairment; rapid cycling of moods presenting with significant interpersonal instability more typically associated with personality disorder; spontaneous hypomania or mania associated with use of antidepressant medication, drugs, or alcohol; and disinhibited or hyperthymic mood disorder.[51]

Mania or full mania is characterized by apparent symptoms and marked impairment. Overwhelming increase in energy and drive manifest as nonstop activity, grandiose thinking, impulsivity, euphoria, impaired judgment, acting-out behaviors, and hypersexuality. Changes in thinking, appearance, speech, personality, and emotions can be dramatic and last weeks to months with or without evidence of psychosis. Anger, belligerence, and aggression can develop quickly when others attempt to set limits or interfere. The person sleeps very little if at all and may believe that he or she either is too busy to eat or no longer requires food. Highly inappropriate phone calls, attempts to contact public officials or famous persons, excessive spending, and "schemes" can result in very serious financial and legal consequences.

Hypomania or partial mania can include any symptoms of mania but without the loss of reality testing, without psychosis (e.g., hallucinations, delusions), and without impaired functioning. The person who is hypomania may insist that the sudden onset of increased energy, expanded self-esteem, and decreased anxiety has improved his or her productivity or that it is an acceptable *natural high.* Unlike mania, it is possible for an episode of hypomania to run its course without being recognized as hypomania.

Depression or dysphoria can have a sudden onset and include symptoms similar in number and intensity to those of major depression (see the Major Depression section).

Euphoria or expanded mood is a hallmark symptom of both mania and hypomania. Extreme cheerfulness, enthusiasm, and optimism are present, but the joyful, buoyant mood is disproportionate to events and surroundings.

Racing thoughts, also referred to as "flights of ideas," grossly impair cognitive ability and speech. People who experience racing thoughts typically describe having thoughts "flying through my mind" at such a volume and speed that they cannot talk fast enough or move fast enough to keep up.

Irritable mood occurs with both mania and hypomania, particular after prolonged symptom duration. Sarcasm, hurtful criticism, fault finding, and general unpleasantness predominate. Attempts to limit the activities of a person who is hypomanic or fully manic can quickly be met with dramatic displays of aggressive irritability.

Grandiosity or wildly inflated self-esteem is expressed through self-appraised importance, claims of limitless expertise, and insulting put-downs. When grandiose, the person with bipolar disorder has little or no tolerance for being criticized, questioned, or contradicted. This perceived self-importance can reach delusional proportions resulting in the person's attempting to act on his or her importance, genius, and infallibility. Serious negative consequences of grandiose actions as well as financial and criminal schemes are not uncommon.

Energy level with mania and hypomania can appear to be limitless. At lower levels, increased energy can be productive. But more often, increased energy produces aimless hyperactivity with constantly shifting interests and distractions. Signs of physical fatigue become obvious but the hyperactivity continues. Dangerously low sensitivity to fatigue as well as increased risk of injury and self-harm can occur. At extremely high levels of energy, the person becomes disorganized if not psychotic. Compulsive collecting and hoarding of meaningless objects is common.

Speech disturbance with bipolar disorder can become dramatic. The most common disturbance with mania is loud, rapid, constant, pressured, or explosive speech that may not be interpretable. At early stages, pressured speech may seem an adroit and humorous play with words. Entertaining jokes, rhymes, and puns are common. At later stages, clang associations, runaway thoughts, and invented words make communication extremely difficult. Untreated, eventually speech becomes incoherent.

Hallucinations and **delusions** can occur with the psychosis that typically develops with severe, prolonged mania. Unlike the hallucinations and delusions associated with schizophrenia, the alterations in perceptions and thinking that occur with mania generally are mood congruent. In other words, grandiose mood is likely to be mirrored by grandiose delusions and hallucinations.

Impulsive action is a hallmark symptom of mania and hypomania. This mood state typically is characterized by behavior with little to no consideration of effects or consequences. People who become impulsive when manic or hypomanic are truly unable to explain or predict their actions and may be unable to appreciate the consequences of their actions. Impulsivity can make the affected person a potential danger to self or others.

Impaired judgment with bipolar disorder can lead to significant deviancy. Socialized behavior is behavior that conforms to the social rules defining right and wrong. Without this internal switch governing behavior, primitive drives can take over. The more common examples of impaired judgment associated with mania and hypomania have to do with inappropriate sexual behavior, substance abuse, inappropriate and excessive spending, thrill seeking, and rule breaking.

Appetite is indirectly affected by mania and hypomania in that food intake can decrease dramatically, resulting in significant weight loss and loss of appetite. No single explanation holds true for all cases, but typically the person either is too busy with other activities to stop or insists that food and water are no longer necessary. In effect, loss of weight and appetite occurs as a secondary effect of mania and hypomania. True loss of appetite, as with major depression, is rare, meaning that the person may be hungry but is too distracted or busy to eat.

Sleep disturbance with mania and, in some cases, with hypomania takes the form of little or no sleep. Sleeping can become difficult and, as with food, the person may insist that sleep is unnecessary. Days without sleep may force the person to take brief naps but, without treatment, restorative sleep can become unattainable.

Hypersexuality associated with mania and hypomania creates high-risk situations and potentially serious consequences. Combined with impulsivity and impaired judgment, a sudden increase in the drive for sex can lead to highly uncharacteristic and unpredictable behavior. This includes serious risk of the patient being victimized or exploited by others as well as carrying out harmful behaviors toward others. Marriages and long-term relationships can suffer greatly from indiscriminate sexual behavior that the person cannot explain. The risk of atypical sexual behaviors or activity involving persons with whom the patient might normally not have contact is a serious source of concern.

Pharmacologic Treatment. Medications presently indicated for use as mood stabilizers include lithium, anticonvulsants, and atypical antipsychotics. Appropriate pharmacologic treatment for bipolar disorder requires accurate diagnosis. Before bipolar disorder diagnosis and treatment are considered, the possibility of a primary medical condition or drug reaction as the cause of depression, elation, mania, or psychosis must be considered (Table 48-4). Because of the

Table 48-4

Selected Physical Illnesses and Drug Reactions Associated with Psychiatric Conditions

	Psychiatric Symptoms Associated with Specific Disorders			
Cause	**Depression**	**Mania**	**Paranoia**	**Anxiety**
Infectious processes	Influenza; viral hepatitis; infectious mononucleosis; general paresis (tertiary syphilis); tuberculosis	Influenza; St. Louis encephalitis; Q fever; general paresis (tertiary syphilis)		
Endocrine disorders	Myxedema; Cushing disease; Addison disease	Hyperthyroidism	Addison disease; Cushing disease; hypothyroidism; hypoparathyroidism; hyperparathyroidism	Hyperadrenalism (Cushing disease); hyperthyroidism; hypothyroidism
Neoplastic disorders	Occult abdominal malignancies (e.g., carcinoma of head of pancreas)			Secreting tumors (carcinoid, insulinoma, pheochromocytoma)
Collagen disorders	Systemic lupus erythematosus	Systemic lupus erythematosus; rheumatic chorea	Systemic lupus erythematosus	Systemic lupus erythematosus
Neurologic disorders	Multiple sclerosis; cerebral tumors; sleep apnea; dementia; Parkinson disease; non-dominant temporal lobe lesions	Multiple sclerosis; diencephalic and third ventricular tumors	Brain tumors; temporal lobe epilepsy; Alzheimer disease; Pick disease; Huntington disease; Parkinson disease; multiple sclerosis, cerebral atherosclerosis; hypertensive encephalopathy; multi-infarct dementia	Encephalopathies (infectious, metabolic, toxic); essential tremor; intracranial mass lesions; postconcussional syndrome; complex partial seizures; vertigo
Nutritional states	Pellagra; pernicious anemia		Vitamin B_{12} deficiency	Caffeine; monosodium glutamate; vitamin deficiency diseases; anemias
Reactions to drugs	Steroidal contraceptives, reserpine; methyldopa; physostigmine; alcohol; sedative-hypnotics; amphetamine withdrawal	Steroids; levodopa; amphetamines; methylphenidate; cocaine; monoamine oxidase inhibitors; tricyclic antidepressants; thyroid hormones	Amphetamines; cocaine; hallucinogens (LSD, PCP); marijuana; mescaline; withdrawal syndromes (alcohol, sedative-hypnotics, barbiturates, benzodiazepines)	Akathisia (secondary to antipsychotic drugs); anticholinergic toxicity; digitalis toxicity; hallucinogens; hypotensive agents; stimulants (cocaine, amphetamines, related drugs); withdrawal syndromes (alcohol, sedative-hypnotics); bronchodilators (theophylline)
Metabolic disorders			Hypoglycemia; liver failure; uremia	Hyperthermia; hyponatremia; hyperkalemia; hypocalcemia; hypoglycemia; menopause; porphyria (acute intermittent)

Table 48-4

Selected Physical Illnesses and Drug Reactions Associated with Psychiatric Conditions—cont'd

Cause	Psychiatric Symptoms Associated with Specific Disorders			
	Depression	**Mania**	**Paranoia**	**Anxiety**
Cardiovascular disorders				Angina pectoris, arrhythmias; congestive heart failure; hypertensive; hypovolemia; myocardial infarction; syncope (of multiple causes); valvular disease; vascular collapse (shock)
Respiratory disorders				Asthma; chronic obstructive pulmonary disease; pneumonia; pneumothorax; pulmonary edema; pulmonary embolism

Data from Whybrow P, Akiskal H, McKinney W: *Mood disorders: toward a new psychology,* New York, 1984, Plenum Press; Hyman SE, Jenike MA: *Manual of clinical problems in psychiatry,* Boston, 1990, Little, Brown; Rosenbaum JF: The drug treatment of anxiety, *N Engl J Med* 306:401-404, 1982.

many overlapping symptoms, it is not uncommon for persons with bipolar disorder to be misdiagnosed as depressed or schizophrenic.[52]

Lithium is the standard mood stabilization medication used to manage bipolar disorder. Recent, well-controlled clinical treatment studies confirm lithium's effectiveness in the management of bipolar I and bipolar II disorders.[53] That said, many individuals with severe bipolar disorder symptoms nonetheless require additional antidepressant and antipsychotic medications to achieve optimal symptom management. Antipsychotic medications have been found to be effective in remitting symptoms of psychosis as well as in preventing their recurrence. Managing the depression symptoms of bipolar disorder can prove more complicated. In some cases antidepressant medications can trigger mood switching or destabilize mood.

Growing numbers of anticonvulsants now are being considered for use as mood stabilizers. These include various reformulations of carbamazepine, divalproex, and lamotrigine. Many of the pharmacodynamic and pharmacokinetic properties of the commonly used mood-stabilizing medications have been well defined.[54] A variety of potential mechanisms have been proposed for lithium. The neurotransmission effects of lithium have been attributed to calcium-dependent cell wall depolarization. Through this process, dopamine and norepinephrine are released, and major secondary messenger neurotransmitter signals are released.

Lithium is absorbed in the gastrointestinal tract but is not metabolized; more than 90% is excreted by the renal system. Any interference with the excretion of lithium (e.g., fluid volume depletion, angiotensin-converting enzyme inhibitors, diuretics) can lead to rapidly increasing plasma lithium levels and toxicity. Continuous patient education and routine plasma lithium level checks help to reduce the risk of toxicity. Early symptoms of lithium toxicity include confusion, nausea, and fatigue. Prelithium assessment of liver, renal, and thyroid functioning is required. In some cases, lithium leads to hypothyroidism that requires treatment. Lastly, lithium treatment for bipolar disorder requires multiple daily doses, generally twice a day or more often. Multiple daily doses can exacerbate patient ambivalence about taking lithium. Euphoria, mania, and long symptom-free periods typically are misperceived as signs that lithium no longer is needed.

Divalproex often is the next best choice when lithium cannot be taken. This anticonvulsant has been found to have neuroprotective effects similar to those of lithium.[54] Unlike lithium, divalproex is highly bioavailable, is metabolized by the liver, produces an active metabolite, has a long half-life, and can be used to manage acute mania. Persons with impaired liver functioning or liver disease cannot take divalproex, and the routine evaluation of plasma levels is required to reduce the risk of toxicity.

Several atypical antipsychotic medications show promise as potentially effective mood-stabilizing medications. Of these, olanzapine, risperidone, quetiapine, and ziprasidone have received considerable attention. These medications exhibit a range of dopaminergic, serotonergic, and norepinephrinergic effects that improve many bipolar symptoms, particularly when the symptoms include full mania rather than hypomania. Once-daily dosing is an important advantage.

KEY CONCEPTS

- Affective disorders are due to disordered emotions or affect. Included in this category of psychoses are bipolar disorder (periods of mania and depression) and unipolar depression. The average age at onset is 30 years for bipolar disorder and 40 years for unipolar depression. Depression affects women twice as often as men.
- A biochemical basis for **bipolar disorder** is supported by observations that brain monoamines (norepinephrine, serotonin) are below normal or the ratio of norepinephrine to serotonin is altered. Depression is thought to occur when serotonin and norepinephrine activity in the brain is low. Mania may be due to a relative excess of norepinephrine in the context of low serotonin or acetylcholine activity. Plasma membrane transport of small molecules such as lithium also is different. Bipolar disorder has a familial pattern of expression, suggesting a genetic cause.
- Psychosocial factors that may affect the development and expression of mood disorders include loss (real, anticipated, or perceived) and low self-esteem. Sleep disorders accompany both extremes of mood. Depression is associated with altered REM sleep and decreased slow-wave sleep. Mania is associated with short sleep and reduced fatigue.
- **Depression** is manifested by low energy, inability to experience joy, difficulty initiating tasks, reduced decision making ability, difficulty sleeping, poor appetite, weight loss, and decreased libido. Thoughts may focus on guilt, futility, emptiness, hopelessness, helplessness, and suicide. The management of unipolar depression is aimed at increasing norepinephrine and serotonin activity in the brain. MAOIs reduce the rate of neurotransmitter destruction; TCIs inhibit reuptake; newer agents (fluoxetine) selectively prevent serotonin reuptake.
- **Mania** is manifested by high energy; inflated self-esteem; hyperactivity; inability to focus or concentrate; low sensitivity to fatigue, injury, or pain; rapid or incoherent speech; hallucinations; delusions; increased appetite and libido; decreased sleep; poor judgment; and poor impulse control. Mania is managed with lithium, a compound that inhibits the action of norepinephrine and serotonin in the brain.

Elderly Considerations

- Schizophrenia and delusional disorder may continue into old age or may appear later in life. Late-onset schizophrenia, which emerges after age 45 years, occurs more often in women than in men.
- Psychiatric admissions of older individuals are characterized by significantly more major depression and less dysthymia than that seen in younger adults. The incidence of bipolar disorder in the geriatric age group should approach that of lifetime risk. It is extremely rare for bipolar disorder to emerge after age 60 years, and all bipolar disorder patients who survive to old age continue to be vulnerable to that illness.
- Mood disorders in the elderly are likely to be associated with concomitant illnesses or their treatments.
- Management of late-appearing psychoses is complicated by a number of factors. Older patients are more sensitive to medication than younger patients, and their response varies more than that of younger patients; they may suffer cognitive impairment; they may have visual or auditory impairment; they may be taking drugs for other chronic disorders; and they may forget to take their medications or take wrong doses. In addition, older patients may suffer side effects such as tardive dyskinesia, a disorder related to antipsychotic drug dosage and duration and characterized by involuntary chewing motions and darting of the tongue.

SUMMARY

The clinical symptoms, causes, and neurobiological mechanisms of schizophrenia, major depression, and bipolar disorder have been presented. Significant risk of psychosis is a common characteristic shared among these seemingly unrelated disorders. Brief overviews of the neurobiological basis of medications used to manage the symptoms of these disorders reflect the tremendous neurobiological advances that have been accomplished. Nevertheless, these three illnesses are potentially disabling conditions that all too often rob the affected person of academic goals, meaningful work, close relationships, self-actualization, and, in some circumstances, survival. Psychosis is associated with a wide range of illnesses and disorders; this chapter has covered three of the most common mental disorders.

MEDIA RESOURCES

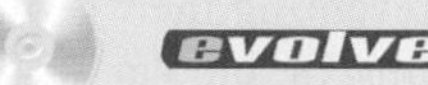

Remember to check out the ***CD Companion*** included with this book for Review Questions, Key Concepts Review, Glossary (with audio for selected terms), Disease Profiles, and Animations.

PLUS, visit the ***Evolve website*** at http://evolve.elsevier.com/Copstead/ for Case Studies, Disease Profiles, and WebLinks.

References

1. Keltner NL et al: *Psychobiological foundations of psychiatric care*, St Louis, 1998, Mosby.
2. Csernansky JG, Grace AA: New models of the pathophysiology of schizophrenia: editors' introduction, *Schizophr Bull* 24(2):185-187, 1998.

3. Frankle WG, Lerma J, Laruell M: The synaptic hypothesis of schizophrenia, *Neuron* 39:205-216, 2003.
4. Goggi J et al: Signalling pathways involved in the short-term potentiation of dopamine release by BDNF, *Brain Res* 968:156-161, 2003.
5. Saal D et al: Drugs of abuse and stress trigger a common synaptic adaptation in dopamine neurons, *Neuron* 37:577-582, 2003.
6. Kapur S: Psychosis as a state of aberrant salience: a framework linking biology, phenomenology, and pharmacology in schizophrenia, *Am J Psychiatry* 160(1):13-23, 2003.
7. Portin P, Alanen YO: A critical review of genetic studies of schizophrenia: II. Molecular genetic studies, *Acta Psychiatr Scand* 95:73-80, 1997.
8. Moldin SO: The maddening hunt for madness genes, *Nature Genet* 17:127-129, 1997.
9. Rinomhota AS, Marshall P: *Biological aspects of mental health nursing*, Edinburgh, 2000, Churchill Livingstone.
10. Javitt DC, Coyle JT: Decoding schizophrenia, *Sci Am* 290(1):48-55, 2004.
11. Weinberger D: Implications of normal brain development for the pathogenesis of schizophrenia, *Arch Gen Psychiatry* 44:660-669, 1987.
12. Susser E et al: No relation between risk of schizophrenia and prenatal exposure to influenza in Holland, *Am J Psychiatry* 151:922-924, 1994.
13. Baxter RD, Liddle PF: Neuropsychological deficits associated with schizophrenic syndromes, *Schizophr Res* 30:239-249, 1998.
14. Nasralla HA, Smeltzer DJ: *Contemporary diagnosis and management of the patient with schizophrenia*, Newtown, Pa, 2002, Handbooks in Health Care.
15. Smith GN et al: Developmental abnormalities of the hippocampus in first-episode schizophrenia, *Society Biol Psychiatry* 53:555-561, 2003.
16. Jampala VC, Taylor MA, Abrams R: The diagnostic implica tions of formal thought disorder in mania and schizophrenia: a reassessment, *Am J Psychiatry* 146:459-471, 1989.
17. Milev P et al: Initial magnetic resonance imaging volumetric brain measurements and outcome in schizophrenia: a prospective longitudinal study with 5-year follow-up, *Society Biol Psychiatry* 54:608-615, 2003.
18. Jessen F et al: Reduced hippocampal activation during encoding and recognition of words in schizophrenia patients, *Am J Psychiatry* 160(7):1305-1312, 2003.
19. Holden C: Deconstructing schizophrenia, *Science* 299: 333-335, 2003.
20. Schmitz Y et al: Presynaptic regulation of dopaminergic neurotransmission, *J Neurochemistry* 87:273-289, 2003.
21. Evans JD et al: The relationship of neuropsychological abilities to specific domains of functional capacity in older schizophrenia patients, *Society Biol Psychiatry* 53:422-430, 2003.
22. Fadem B: *High-yield behavioral science,* ed 2, Philadelphia, 2001, Lippincott Williams & Wilkins.
23. Keltner NL: Neuroreceptor function and psychopharmacologic response, *Issues Ment Health Nurs* 21:21-31, 2000.
24. Kapur S, Seeman P: Does fast dissociation from the dopamine D_2 receptor explain the action of atypical antipsychotics? A new hypothesis, *Am J Psychiatry* 158:360-369, 2001.
25. Keltner NL, Folks DG: *Psychotropic drugs,* ed 3, St Louis, 2001, Mosby.
26. Jibson MD, Tandon R: New atypical antipsychotic medications, *J Psychiatr Res* 32:215-228, 1998.
27. Aquila R: Management of weight gain in patients with schizophrenia, *J Clin Psychiatry* 63(suppl 4):33-36, 2002.
28. Kalkman HO, Loetscher E: GAD: the link between the GABA-deficit hypothesis and the dopaminergic and glutamatergic theories of psychosis, *J Neural Transm* 110:803-812, 2003.
29. Winokur G, Clayton P, editors: *The medical basis of psychiatry,* ed 2, Philadelphia, 1994, Saunders.
30. Kaplan HI, Sadock BJ, Grebb JA: *Kaplan and Sadock's synopsis of psychiatry,* ed 7, Baltimore, 1994, Williams & Wilkins.
31. American Psychiatric Association: *Diagnostic and statistical manual of mental disorders,* ed 4, Washington, DC, 1994, The Association.
32. Frasure-Smith N et al: Social support, depression, and mortality during the first year after myocardial infarction, *Circulation* 101:1919-1924, 2000.
33. Zubenko GS et al: D2S2944 identifies a likely susceptibility locus for recurrent, early-onset, major depression in women, *Mol Psychiatry* 7:460-467, 2002.
34. Brent DA, Birmaher B: Adolescent depression, *N Engl J Med* 347(9):667-671, 2002.
35. Blumenthal JA et al: Effects of exercise training on older patients with major depression, *Arch Intern Med* 1159(19):2349-2356, 1999.
36. Racagni G, Brunell N: Physiology to functionality: the brain and neurotransmitter activity, *Int Clin Psychopharmacol* 14(suppl 1):S3-S7, 1999.
37. Stockmeir CA et al: Neurokinin-I receptors are decreased in major depressive disorder, *Clin Neurosci* 13(9):1223-1227, 2002.
38. Young E, Korszun A: Psychoneuroendocrinology of depression hypothalamic-pituitary-gonadal axis, *Psychoneuroendocrinology* 21(2):309-325, 1998.
39. Jacobs BL, van Praag H, Gage FH: Depression and the birth and death of brain cells, *Am Sci Online* 88(4):340-347, 2000.
40. Caspi A et al: Influence of life stress on depression: moderation by a polymorphism in the 5-HTT gene, *Science* 01:386-389, 2003.
41. Posener JA et al: 24-hour monitoring of cortisol and corticotropin secretion in psychotic and nonpsychotic major depression, *Arch Gen Psychiatry* 57:755-760, 2000.
42. Shimizu E et al: Alterations of serum levels of brain derived neurotrophic factor (BDNF) in depressed patients with or without antidepressants, *Soc Biol Psychiatry* 54:70-75, 2002.
43. Manji HK et al: Enhancing neuronal plasticity and cellular resilience to develop novel improved therapeutics for difficult to treat depression, *Soc Biol Psychiatry* 53:707-742, 2003.
44. Phillips ML, Drevets WC, Rauch SL, Lane R: Neurobiology of emotion perception II: implications for major psychiatric disorders, *Soc Biol Psychiatry* 54:515-528, 2003.
45. Preskorn SH: Comparison of the tolerability of bupropion, fluoxetine, imipramine, nefazodone, paroxetine, sertraline and venlafaxine, *J Clin Psychiatry* 56(suppl 6):12-21, 1995.
46. Gillman PK: Serotonin syndrome: history and risk, *Fundam Clin Pharmacol* 12:482-491, 1998.
47. Sheline YI: Neuroimaging studies of mood disorder effects on the brain, *Soc Biol Psychiatry* 54:338-352, 2003.
48. Fadem B, Simring S: *High yield psychiatry*, Philadelphia, 1998, Lippincott Williams & Wilkins.

49. Stahl SM: *Essential psychopharmacology: neuroscientific basis and practical applications,* ed 2, Cambridge, UK, 2000, Cambridge University Press.
50. Akiskal HS, Pinto O: The evolving bipolar spectrum: prototypes I, II, III, IV, *Psychiatr Clin North Am* 22(3):517-535, 1999.
51. Perugi G, Akiskal HS: The soft bipolar spectrum redefined: focus on the cyclothymic, anxious-sensitive, impulse-dyscontrol, and binge-eating connection in bipolar II and related conditions. *Psychiatr Clin North Am* 25:713-737, 2002.
52. Tugrul K: The nurse's role in the assessment and treatment of bipolar disorder, *J Am Psychiatr Nurs Assoc* 9(6):180-186, 2003.
53. Suppes T, Dennehy EB: Evidence based long-term treatment of bipolar II disorder, *J Clin Psychiatry* 63(suppl 10):29-33, 2002.
54. Keck PE, McElroy SL: Clinical pharmacodynamics and pharmacokinetics of antimanic and mood stabilizing medications, *J Clin Psychiatry* 63(suppl 4):3-11, 2002.
55. Maguire GA: Comprehensive understanding of schizophrenia and its treatment, *Am J Health Syst Pharm* vol 58, 2002.

Neurobiology of Nonpsychotic Illnesses

chapter 49

Linda Denise Oakley

MEDIA RESOURCES

Additional Material for Study, Review, and Further Exploration

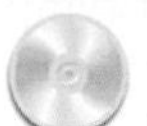

CD Companion ◆ Review Questions and Answers ◆ Key Concepts Review
◆ Glossary *(with audio pronunciations for selected terms)*
◆ Disease Profiles ◆ Animations

evolve ***Website*** at http://evolve.elsevier.com/Copstead/
◆ Case Studies ◆ Disease Profiles ◆ WebLinks

KEY QUESTIONS

- What neurobiological alterations have been associated with anxiety symptoms?
- What neurobiological alterations have been associated with personality disorders?
- What neurobiological alterations have been associated with anorexia?

CHAPTER OUTLINE

Eventually, the neurobiological mechanisms of mental disorders that do not cause psychosis may prove to be more similar than different from those of mental disorders associated with psychosis. These conditions already show similarity in that altered neuronal structures and functioning, genetic risk factors, and neurotransmission dysregulation characterize them. A major difference between them is that individual variations in nonpsychotic conditions can be extensive. Greater individual variations increase the difficulty of defining the hallmark symptomatology and neurobiological basis of the condition. In addition, much has been learned about the neurobiological impact of stress response systems in psychotic illnesses whereas the impact of stress response systems in nonpsychotic illnesses is less well understood. In the past, simple comparisons, such as comparing schizophrenia with eating disorders, invited the false assumption that one disorder may be more or less serious than another. For the affected person, such comparisons are unhelpful. Any mental disorder has the potential of causing profound suffering and disability.

The purpose of this chapter is to briefly demonstrate the complexity of nonpsychotic illnesses. Three representative illnesses—anxiety disorders, personality disorders, and eating disorders—are described. **Anxiety disorders** are characterized by highly distressing physical and emotional symptoms that are difficult to control. The three anxiety disorders reviewed are panic disorder, generalized anxiety disorder, and obsessive-compulsive disorder. **Personality disorders** are characterized by rigid patterns of thinking and behaving that are highly maladaptive, negatively impact all aspects of daily life, and expose the affected person to increased risk for comorbid substance disorders. The two disorders reviewed are border-line personality disorder and antisocial personality disorder. **Eating disorders** are characterized by food and weight obsessions and compulsions and gravely distorted body image. The two disorders reviewed are anorexia nervosa and bulimia nervosa.

ANXIETY DISORDERS

This section presents three anxiety disorders: panic disorder, generalized anxiety disorder (GAD), and obsessive-compulsive disorder (OCD). Anxiety disorders are characterized by similar physical symptoms but they differ greatly in terms of symptom onset triggers, symptom duration, and symptom management. Because anxiety disorders primarily are characterized by physical symptoms, physical illnesses (e.g., hyperthyroidism) and medication reactions (e.g., antidepressants, steroids, anticholinergic medications) must be ruled out before a diagnosis of anxiety disorder can be made.

Panic Disorder

Panic disorder is characterized by acute episodes of anxiety symptoms that are unexpected, sudden, recurrent, and generate intense feelings of fear. Sudden symptom onset can cause affected persons to seek emergency health care for what they believe is a cardiac arrest, respiratory arrest, or "nervous breakdown."

Panic anxiety or panic disorder is diagnosed more often in women (1.6% to 2.9%) than in men (0.4% to 1.7%).[1] Initial illness onset usually is in late adolescence or young adulthood, with a mean age of onset of 26.6 years. Initial symptom onset in older age adults is less typical. Persons diagnosed with panic disorder typically report that their first panic episode occurred relatively early in life. Panic disorder is characterized by two important psychological symptoms: anticipatory anxiety and avoidance anxiety.

Anticipatory anxiety refers to fearful expectation of panic anxiety onset. With panic disorder, no single experience consistently triggers symptom onset. People with the disorder tend to develop a morbid dread of events or experiences that they come to believe *might* trigger panic anxiety. In short, they try to anticipate their anxiety.

Avoidance refers to personal strategies used to increase feelings of control and thereby decrease the risk of panic anxiety. True panic disorder without avoidance anxiety is unlikely. Persons with panic disorder strive to avoid situations and circumstances they associate with their symptoms. For example, panic disorder and agoraphobia, the phobic avoidance of public spaces beyond personal control (e.g., airports, shopping mall), often coexist.

Etiology and Neurobiology. The risk of anxiety disorder symptom onset has been associated with significant genetic, psychological, and biological system alterations.[2] Family, twin, and adoptive family studies have consistently shown a strong genetic liability for these disorders. However, experts now speculate that the etiology question no longer is nature versus nurture. Current models seek to explain the *interactions* of nature and nurture that can create susceptibility to anxiety. Brain regions that underpin the experiences of fear, anxiety, and stress are thought of as circuits that can be shaped and altered by a wide range of forces. Neurobiological conditioning is one force shown to impact such circuits and thus is of particular importance to understanding the development of anxiety disorders.

Brain serotonin activity has been shown to interact with both genes and environment, and these interactions contribute to what has come to be referred to as *synaptic plasticity*.[2] In this way, genes are linked with brain cell neurochemistry and psychological characteristics such as temperament. More specifically, evidence of genetic variability in negative emotions, such as anxiety, has been found in studies of serotonin transporter cells. In this research, gene variability is in gene allele length. For example, family studies have shown that siblings with serotonin transporter cells with the short-form gene allele had higher neuroticism scores than their siblings with the long-form gene allele. Research aimed at gene typing mental disorders clearly is in its infancy and findings such as these are inconclusive, but they demonstrate the possibility of genetics-based neurobiological models of anxiety.

Susceptible persons who breathe air with high levels of carbon dioxide will experience an acute onset of panic anxiety symptoms.[3] A small study of persons with panic anxiety disorder, using an infusion of doxapram (respiratory stimulant) to cause profound hyperventilation, examined the effectiveness of cognitive interventions to reduce respiratory anxiety symptoms.[4] Cognitive interventions were designed to minimize misinterpretation of drug-induced hyperventilation as a sign of danger and thereby reduce the odds of the respiratory stimulant triggering panic anxiety. Breath-by-breath analyses of the patients and healthy controls were performed. The researchers[4] hypothesized that if the respiration anxiety symptoms were the result of dysregulation within the brain respiratory control center, cognitive interventions would not be particularly effective. They found that less fearful thinking did reduce panic but some respiratory anxiety symptoms persisted despite less fearful thinking. In other words, respiratory anxiety symptoms appeared to result both from anticipatory anxiety and from dysregulation within the brain respiratory center.

Surges of physiologic activation and physiologic instability are thought to be the hallmark neurobiological processes underlying panic anxiety disorder.[5] Multiple organ systems, including the cardiovascular and respiratory systems, are thought to be involved. Observations such as these help to explain why, for example, caffeine triggers panic anxiety symptoms in susceptible persons. All anxiety disorders are thought to share key symptom characteristics, but physiologic instability appears to be unique to panic. Physiologic instability may prove to be the key to identifying a genetics-based marker for susceptibility to panic. However, the biopsychological marker for the disorder is likely to be the overinterpretation of physical anxiety symptoms (e.g., sudden increase in heart rate) as life threatening. This thinking, referred to as *learned panic,* is thought to result from inordinately high levels of life stress in early childhood.

Overwhelming life stress can increase the level of circulating glucocorticoids (stress hormones) and stimulate the release of glutamate (which inhibits neurogenesis).[6] Early-childhood life stress, specifically abuse and neglect, have been studied as possibly predictors of various adult-onset anxiety disorders. These models are based on altered serotonin, norepinephrine, and dopamine neurotransmission, glutamate release, and physiologic instability. Repeated and prolonged childhood exposure to overwhelming stress is thought to create adult susceptibility to anxiety disorders. The leading theory is that early life stress leads to *overspecialized* or excessive stress response.

Early life stress is thought to produce adult susceptibility to anxiety by altering critical neuron structures and functioning during this critical stage of human growth and development. Brain regions most vulnerable to alteration as a result of early life stress include the hippocampus (glucocorticoid receptors), amygdala (γ-aminobutyric acid [GABA] and benzodiazepine receptors), corpus callosum (glial cells critical to myelination), cerebellar vermis (glucocorticoid receptors), and the prefrontal cortex (glucocorticoid receptors, dopamine projections, and inhibition of hypothalamic-pituitary-adrenal axis [HPA] activation).[6,7] When the developing brain of a young child is exposed to overwhelming life stress, the stress response system appears to adapt by overbuilding or building additional brain stress-response pathways. Later, under less stressful adult circumstances, this overbuilt stress response system becomes maladaptive. Like a very large overpowered car on a small, winding road, the overbuild stress response system could become the source of physiologic instability that has come to be associated with panic anxiety.[8]

Clinical Manifestations. Physical symptoms include respiratory distress, heart palpitations, tachycardia, pounding heart, chest pain, smothering or choking sensation, dizziness, light-headedness, faintness, sweating, trembling, shaking, hot flushes, chills, numbness, tingling, nausea, abdominal distress, and urinary frequency.[9]

Psychological and *cognitive* symptoms include expressed fears of dying, fear of cardiac arrest, fear of losing control, fear of nervous breakdown, derealization, depersonalization, and perceptual distortions.

Behavioral symptoms include hyperkinesis, pressured speech, and exaggerated startle response.

Pharmacologic Treatment. Panic anxiety disorder can be effectively managed with cognitive-behavior therapy aimed at reducing fearful thinking and desensitization of cognitive and physical stress responses. When panic symptoms are disabling, medication for symptom management is recommended. Long-acting benzodiazepines, such as clonazepam, are the sedatives of choice when short-term calming and symptom relief are mandatory. Tolerance to benzodiazepines develops with continuous use regardless of dosage. Misuse of benzodiazepines represents a serious health hazard. Many atypical psychiatric medications that can target serotonin, dopamine, or norepinephrine receptors have been clinically tested and shown to be effective treatment for anxiety symptoms. Examples of such medications found to be helpful include paroxetine, sertraline, citalopram, and fluoxetine. Unless contraindicated, β-blocker medications that dampen physical anxiety symptoms may also be helpful.

Generalized Anxiety Disorder

Generalized anxiety disorder is characterized by worry that is chronic and persistent, as well as physical anxiety symptoms. Persistent worry that is difficult to control typically leads to multiple anxiety symptoms including restlessness, fatigue, impaired concentration, irritability, muscle tension, muscle pain, and disturbed sleep. Lacking clear symptom onset patterns, GAD is easily overlooked or misdiagnosed.

Etiology and Neurobiology. Generalized anxiety disorder[10] differs from other anxiety disorders in that the cognitive, psychological, and behavioral symptoms of GAD are relatively constant. Psychoanalysts developed most of the original etiology theories concerning persistent worry. What now is referred to as persistent worry was then described as anxious expectation. Even at that early stage of discovery it was apparent that generalized anxiety rarely occurred without comorbid conditions such as depression. This *psychodynamic* view of generalized anxiety prevailed until the late 1980s and early 1990s. At that time, the disorder still was so poorly understood that the diagnosis was used to refer to what was then thought to be leftover or residual anxiety symptoms from other disorders. Technologically advanced research methods have now made it possible to precisely define GAD symptoms in terms of their actual qualities, intensity, and duration, but physical GAD symptoms continue to be viewed as *somatic* expressions of psychological problems.[10]

Unlike other anxiety disorders, GAD onset typically is gradual with symptom duration measured in years. As has been observed with other anxiety disorders, vulnerability to GAD likely is inherited. Twin and family study findings indicate a 30% increase in risk of GAD among the relatives of persons with the disorder. Efforts to describe the neurobiological basis of GAD will no doubt be greatly advanced by theoretical models of inherited vulnerability as well as improved understanding of GAD symptoms, but critical questions remain unanswered. The most important unanswered question likely will have to do with the fact that the alterations in brain structure and functioning shown to be associated with GAD also are consistent with alterations observed with other disorders.

Preliminary positron emission tomography (PET) studies measuring brain glucose metabolism rates in GAD have shown higher than normal rates in patients at rest.[11] With GAD, apparently some brain regions undergo both increases and deceases in glucose metabolism rates. This mixed response is most apparent in the frontal and cingulate areas of the cortex, the brain region associated with worry and hypervigilance. Findings such as these lend support to the basic GAD explanatory hypothesis of anxiety symptoms as manifestations of hyperactive brain circuits. Just the opposite condition (hypoactive brain circuits) is thought to be the fundamental basis of depressive disorders.[11]

Neurotransmitter findings with GAD, as with other disorders that produce mood, thinking, and behavior symptoms, point to alterations in GABA receptors, benzodiazepine receptors, norepinephrine systems, serotonin systems, HPA axis activation, and plasma cortisol. Thus far, no specific alterations that can consistently explain GAD symptoms have been identified.[11] Nevertheless, one interesting observation shows considerable promise. At rest, no obvious alterations in neurotransmission are noted in GAD patients. Only when subjected to laboratory activities designed to induce stress responses is significant neurotransmitter overactivity observed. Evidence of norepinephrine receptor down-regulation lends additional support to this stress response model. Attempting to modulate overactive responses, receptor down-regulation is thought to occur automatically when subjected to prolonged, recurrent, excessive, or hyperactive neurotransmitter activity.

Whereas norepinephrine activity is thought to be associated with physical symptoms of GAD, anticipatory and avoidance symptoms are thought to be associated with activity along a key serotonin pathway linking the amygdala and frontal cortex. As might be expected, insufficient serotonin activity in specific brain regions is thought to be associated with GAD. Given the obvious symptom overlap between stress and anxiety, hyperactivity within the HPA axis and high plasma cortisol levels continue to be leading models in GAD research. Much of the difficulty in defining the neurobiological basis of GAD has to do with significant individual variations in GAD symptomatology. Uncontrollable worry (frontal cortex) is the only symptom likely to show meaningful consistency over time and from person to person. A second major research difficulty has to do with the frequency with which GAD symptoms co-occur with depression symptoms—so much so that some experts now view mixed depression-anxiety as a specific disorder.

Clinical Manifestations. **Physical** symptoms vary too greatly to allow for a meaningful listing, but common GAD symptoms include muscle tension, light-headedness, sweating, palpitation, dizziness, and stomach distress.

Psychological symptoms also vary over time and from person to person, but a few symptoms are essential for a diagnosis of GAD. These are uncontrollable worry with no areas of life excluded, fearfulness, and foreboding. Worry is not limited to any single area of concern (e.g., children). Concentration typically is severely impaired and irritability is common. Diffuse anticipatory anxiety, avoidance anxiety, and dysphoria are common.

Behavioral symptoms include severe sleep disturbance and fatigue. Although much of the behavior associated with GAD is likely to be the result of maladaptive methods of coping with physical and psychological GAD symptoms, impaired social and academic/employment functioning are common.

Pharmacologic Treatment. Effective psychological and drug treatments for GAD can be relatively complex. Comorbid conditions such as alcohol abuse are not uncommon and, when present, may extend the duration of needed treatment. Duration of treatment also is likely to be prolonged when GAD symptoms are long-standing and highly disabling. Lastly, neurobiological research findings indicate that effective drug treatment is likely to require one or more medications that are reliable modulators of multiple neurotransmission systems across multiple brain regions. Medications shown to relieve and in some cases remit GAD symptoms include long-acting benzodiazepines (e.g., clonazepam), partial serotonin (5-HT_{1A}) agonists (e.g., buspirone), tricyclic antidepressants (e.g., imipramine), selective serotonin reuptake inhibitors (e.g., sertraline), serotonin-norepinephrine reuptake inhibitors (e.g., venlafaxine), and long-acting β-blockers (e.g., propranolol).[12]

Obsessive-Compulsive Disorder

Obsessive-compulsive disorder is one of the most severe anxiety disorders. Even modest OCD symptomatology can become disabling. The disorder is characterized by persistent involuntary thoughts that then provoke anxiety and involuntary anxiety management rituals. Unlike the acute onset and short duration of panic anxiety symptoms or the chronic symptoms of GAD, the obsessions and compulsions that characterize OCD are localized but nevertheless impact all areas of functioning.

People with OCD strive to avoid disclosing their symptoms to relatives, friends, and health professionals, so that accurate incidence and prevalence statistics are nearly impossible to determine. The lifetime OCD prevalence rate for the general population is 2.2%, whereas the risk in first-degree relatives is 9.2%. Some experts consider this general-population estimate to be an underestimate, but disabling OCD is not thought to be common. The median age of symptom onset is about 23 years, with 15 to 39 being the peak-onset age range.

Etiology and Neurobiology. True OCD symptoms cause a great deal of emotional distress, are very time consuming, and significantly interfere with normal functioning. Neurobiological research findings indicate strong genetic or inherited risks of OCD. Family studies show that when an adult family member is diagnosed with the disorder, child relatives also may be diagnosed. Depression, anorexia, and Tourette's syndrome are common OCD comorbid disorders. Close links between OCD and the hereditary neurologic disorder Tourette's syndrome have been reported, but it is not clear whether this link represents an increased risk of OCD or if Tourette's syndrome and OCD are related in some other way.

OCD studies using PET brain scans have shown significant increases in glucose metabolism rates in the frontal lobes, caudate nucleus, and cingulate gyrus regions of the brain (Figure 49-1). These brain regions are directly associated with response to strong emotions. However, several OCD models of altered brain functioning have been hypothesized. One model proposes that a causal pathway for OCD exists between the frontal cortex region and basal ganglia region of the brain. This model draws on the observation that similar illnesses with well-defined etiologic factors have been shown to involve both cognitive and motor brain regions. Predictably, serotonin activity dysregulation and dysfunction also represent possible OCD models.

As shown in Figure 49-1, PET scans of the brain of a person with OCD reveal significant increases in glucose metabolism activity in the prefrontal cortex brain region. Magnetic resonance imaging (MRI) findings have suggested widely distributed cellular abnormalities such as significantly lower amounts of total white matter (connection fibers) and greater cortex cell volume. More recent models of OCD focus on the possibility of deficient serotonin inhibitory action in the basal ganglia region of the brain, which then permits excessive release of dopamine, a stimulating neurotransmitter.

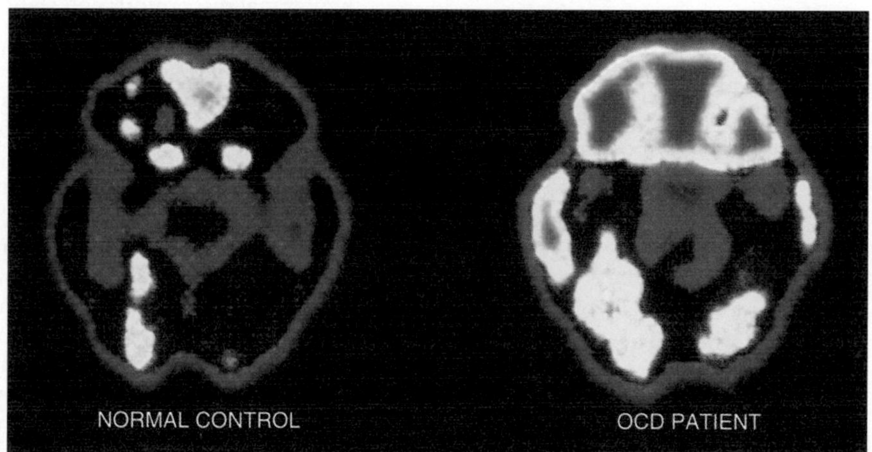

FIGURE 49-1 ■ Hyperactivity of the orbitofrontal cortex has been a consistent finding in more than a decade of brain imaging research on patients with obsessive-compulsive disorder *(OCD)*. These positron emission tomographic images are from the initial report of this finding by a UCLA group. This excessive metabolic activity could generate spurious "error detection" signals that result in patients with obsessive-compulsive disorder experiencing repetitive adventitious feelings that "something is wrong." (Originally adapted from Baxter LR Jr et al: Local cerebral glucose metabolic rates in obsessive compulsive disorder: a comparison with rates in unipolar depression and in normal controls, *Arch Gen Psychiatry* 44:211-218, 1987. As published in Schwartz JM: Obsessive-compulsive disorder, *Sci Med* 4:16, 1997.)

PET, functional MRI (fMRI), and single-photon emission computed tomography (SPECT) studies of persons with OCD have confirmed the correlation between OCD symptoms and abnormal brain circuit activity in the orbitofrontal cortex, caudate nucleus, anterior cingulate cortex, and thalamus.[13] An fMRI study of medicated OCD patients and comparison subjects explored the possibility of meaningful links between anterior cingulate cortex activity and the severity of OCD symptoms by observing this activity under laboratory stress designed to trigger symptom onset. Patients attempted to successfully perform the computer-based tasks quickly without error, but the program had been designed to increase their error rate and generate doubt. Comparison subjects were faster than OCD patients; otherwise few group behavior differences were noted. Hyperactivity was observed only in one brain region (anterior cingulate cortex) and was significantly related to error making and expressed doubt. That study showed the possibility of developing a neurobiological model of disabling self-correction urges associated with OCD.[13]

Clinical Manifestations. **Obsessions** are strong, persistent, intrusive, uncontrollable thoughts. Obsessive thoughts manifest as ideas, images, and urges that dominate normal thinking and functioning. Affected persons recognize that their obsessions are products of their own mind and may judge them as senseless. Nevertheless, they are unable to stop, govern, or resist their obsessions.

Compulsions are repetitive, ritualistic actions performed with urgency. Compulsions typically are content related to obsessions. Performance of compulsions neutralizes or prevents the anxiety triggered by obsessions. True compulsions absorb inordinate amounts of time daily and are performed despite negative consequences. Realization that a compulsion is unreasonable, senseless, and excessive has little impact on the urge to perform the action. Examples of common compulsions are counting, symmetry, touching, checking, cleaning, and picking. Hoarding (inability to dispossess meaningless, worthless objects) is one example of more complex compulsions.[14] A case study of 20 people noted the onset of severe anxiety associated with the thought of discarding hoarded objects. In that study, the items most commonly hoarded were newspapers/magazines, junk mail, old clothing, receipts, lists, food, and gifts for others. The magnitude of hoarding ranged from clutter in all closets and one or two rooms to all closets filled, garage filled, and more than one room filled. These hoarding compulsions were in addition to primary OCD compulsions (e.g., symmetry, checking, cleaning). Ninety percent of the study patients had one or more relatives with OCD symptoms.[14]

Pharmacologic Treatment. Cognitive-behavioral therapy with effective medication treatment can effectively diminish OCD obsessions and compulsions. Nevertheless, the disorder itself makes entering treatment extremely difficult if not impossible. To be successful, cognitive-behavioral therapy must target the person's obsessions and compulsions. This would require full disclosure, and disclosure is very difficult. Higher doses of antianxiety and antidepressant (fluvoxamine, paroxetine, sertraline, venlafaxine, fluoxetine) medications have generally proved effective in reducing OCD symptoms. Atypical antipsychotics, such as risperidone, in combination with antidepressants and β-blockers may be considered when OCD symptoms are disabling. Effective OCD symptom relief has been reported with the tricyclic antidepressant clomipramine, and some experts recommend the seizure medication gabapentin.[15]

KEY CONCEPTS

- Anxiety disorders are characterized by irrational and debilitating fears. The three major categories of anxiety disorders are panic disorder, generalized anxiety disorder, and obsessive-compulsive disorder. These disorders show some evidence of heritability, and biochemical correlates are suspected. Defects in serotonin pathways have been proposed as etiologic factors.
- Panic disorder is characterized by acute episodes of severe anxiety accompanied by dyspnea, chest pain, and a sense of impending doom. Palpitations, hyperventilation, dizziness, paresthesias, and diaphoresis may occur during an attack, which may last 5 to 30 minutes. Anticipatory anxiety and phobic avoidance may develop in people with panic disorder. Efforts to avoid future episodes may result in agoraphobia.
- Generalized anxiety disorder is characterized by a continuous but moderate degree of anxiety without discrete periods of acute attacks. Agoraphobia rarely develops, but chronic headaches, muscle tension, abdominal discomfort, and sleep disturbances are common.
- Obsessive-compulsive disorder is characterized by obsessive thoughts and compulsive behavior. Obsessions (persistent, intrusive, compelling thoughts) commonly have themes of committing violent acts, being a victim of violence, or fear of contamination. In contrast to schizophrenia, such persons realize that the obsessive thoughts are from their own minds but are helpless to control them. Compulsions (repetitive, ritualistic behavior) include such actions as excessive washing and grooming, repeated checking to ensure safety, and elaborate measures to avoid contact with dirt or bodily wastes. If the individual is prevented from performing compulsive rituals, a high state of anxiety ensues.
- Benzodiazepines and antidepressants may be used to manage anxiety disorders.

PERSONALITY DISORDERS

Personality disorder refers to pervasive and persistent disturbance of emotions and behavior. The disturbance is stable and sufficiently predictable that emotions and behaviors appear to be rigid. Given that personality dramatically influences how individuals interact with others, personality disorder symptoms significantly impact all areas of interpersonal functioning. It is not unusual for affected persons to fully deny any link between their emotions and behaviors and problems in their life. More often, they believe their disturbed emotions and behaviors are acceptable.[15]

Persons with personality disorder maintain global views of self, others, and the world that can be extremely maladaptive. Evidence of maladaptive life views, if not actual disturbances in emotions and behavior, may be recognized in early childhood but rarely is the formal diagnosis of personality disorder made before late adolescence or young adulthood. Hallmark symptoms make it possible to group specific personality disorders into general groups. Cluster A disorders are characterized by unusual behavior (schizotypal, schizoid, paranoid). Cluster B disorders are characterized by instability (antisocial, borderline, histrionic, narcissistic). Cluster C disorders are characterized by anxiety (avoidant, dependent, obsessive compulsive).[16] Additional diagnoses, such as depressive personality disorder[17] and further subtyping, such as treatment seeker and treatment rejector[18] continue to be explored. Comparative studies of monozygotic versus dizygotic twins confirm the common observation that personality disorder attributes, rather than personality disorder per se, show significant genetic inheritability.

Borderline Personality Disorder

The term **borderline** originally was intended to suggest a condition that bordered both psychosis and neurosis. Now the term refers to instability as the hallmark characteristic of the disorder. With borderline personality disorder, dramatic lack of stability is evident in mood, behavior, interpersonal relationships, and self-esteem. Behavior can become highly unpredictable and impulsive. Mood states, whether positive or negative, tend to be extreme and labile, but the disorder actually is characterized by persistent feelings of alienation and emotional emptiness. These characteristics result in a basic lifestyle that is dominated by crisis.[19]

Etiology and Neurobiology. Biological models of borderline personality disorder are used to determine the underlying basis of extreme symptoms such as impulsive aggression. Both self-directed and other-directed impulsive aggression has been shown to be associated with serotonin activity in brain regions that process emotions.[20] Findings such as these support apparent links between trauma, as the most consistent antecedent to diagnosis, and borderline personality disorder. Sexual and physical abuse are among the most commonly observed forms of trauma. One theory holds that undergoing trauma of this magnitude contributes to the overdevelopment of brain stress response systems that lead to altered serotonin activity. Yet brief increases in dopamine activity also have been observed and linked with impulsive aggression that, in extreme cases, can produce psychotic-like symptoms. Family studies have yielded mixed results, leading researchers to speculate that specific traits may be inherited and that in susceptible individuals these traits may lead to the development of borderline personality disorder.[20] In other words, borderline personality disorder may reflect selective interaction of high-risk genetic, family, and environmental characteristics.

Possible models of neurotransmission dysregulation that might explain the instability and impulsive aggressive behavior of borderline personality disorder have focused on hyperresponsive HPA axis activity as a biological linkage between the stress and trauma of childhood abuse and adult illness onset.[20] Comparisons of abused and nonabused persons with borderline personality disorder and healthy controls showed hyperresponsiveness of corticotropin and cortisol activity in women with a history of sustained childhood abuse. However, these links did not appear to be exclusive to borderline personality disorder. For example, as might be expected, links also were observed between childhood abuse and adult posttraumatic stress disorder.

Other neurobiological models focus on alterations in brain structure and functioning using advanced electrophysiologic tools such as electroencephalograms. A review of that line of research[21] showed inconclusive findings. In some studies, electroencephalographic abnormalities such as slowing and spikes were observed but no consistent abnormalities were noted. The lack of clear findings might have to do with the high rate of comorbid conditions found with borderline personality disorder. Nevertheless, electroencephalographic findings are promising enough to represent a third line of research in addition to fMRI and PET studies. The implication here being that the development of a biological model of borderline personality disorder that is useful is likely to require the combined application of these technologies.[21]

Although somewhat more difficult to interpret, models that address specific borderline personality disorder traits also show promise. For example, one of the many interpersonal instability characteristics of borderline personality disorder has come to be referred to as *abandonment issues.* A study of women diagnosed with borderline personality disorder who had a history of childhood sexual or physical abuse asked the women to prepare narratives of personal experiences of abandonment.[22] Brain scans were performed as each woman's narrative was read back to her and during the reading of neutral experiences. Compared with healthy controls, the women with borderline personality disorder showed increased blood flow in the right dorsolateral prefrontal cortex region of the brain and decreased blood flow in the anterior cingulate and in the hippocampus-amygdala regions as they listened to the abandonment narratives. These three brain regions process strong emotions. Similar alterations in volume measures have been reported for the same brain regions. Volume refers to brain structures rather than the neurobiological functions of the brain structure. Significant reduction in hippocampus and amygdala volumes have been observed in women with borderline personality disorder.[23] Findings such as these help demonstrate the complex structural and functional neurobiological alterations thought to underlie the defining characteristics of the disorder.

Clinical Manifestations. *Interpersonal instability* is evident in relationships and interactions with others.

Splitting refers to a predictable pattern of alternately devaluing and idealizing others. Devaluation appears to be unpredictably triggered by sudden angry responses to perceived or actual interpersonal loss.

Manipulation refers to the relating to others as objects for the purpose of achieving unstated goals. Manipulation may be covert or overt, but the aim almost always is to obtain caretaking responses from others.

Self-harm and *suicidal ideation* refer to impulsive harmful behaviors toward self that vary widely in severity. Self-harm sometimes is intended to elicit a rescue response from others but also may be used to relieve severe feelings of emptiness, numbness, frustration, anger, or interpersonal tension. Common self-harm behaviors include cutting and burning, hitting objects, and drug overdose. Suicidal thoughts and attempted suicide in response to perceived or actual trauma or crisis characterizes severe forms of the disorder.

Anger and **dysphoria** are commonly experienced or chronic negative mood states. Displays of negative emotions can vary greatly but can reach levels of intensity that simply overwhelm the affected person. Negative emotions also include loneliness and boredom. Complaints of never experiencing good or happy emotions may not be an overstatement.

Derealization refers to transient experiences in which nothing seems real. When derealization also includes depersonalization the affected person does not feel *real* and instead feels like a disembodied observer. Although short lived the experience is highly disturbing to the affected person. Bizarre activities intended to regain a sense of realness are not uncommon.

Impulsive aggression is common. This propensity may manifest as alarming episodes of substance abuse, promiscuity, fighting, and self-harm. Flight or escape in response to impulsive aggression can be anticipated.

Pharmacologic Treatment. Medications used to manage symptoms of borderline personality disorder are determined by the person's immediate treatment needs. Persons with this disorder are at increased risk for depression, anxiety, stress, panic, and substance abuse. In some cases of borderline personality disorder, long-term use of antidepressants may prove helpful. Severe impulsive aggression may require short-term treatment with an atypical antipsychotic medication (e.g., risperidone, olanzapine) that produces multiple neurotransmitter effects. Mood stabilization medications (e.g., gabapentin) might improve severe mood instability. Given the somewhat unpredictable mixture of clinical symptoms that can be associated with a diagnosis of borderline personality disorder, psychotherapy treatment must be emphasized. The primary psychotherapeutic goals for borderline personality disorder include crisis prevention and management and stabilization of object relations. In effect, therapy provides opportunities for the patient to explore and experience success and stability and to learn how to safely manage overwhelming emotions. Treatment effectiveness is associated with treatment duration, but both long-term psychodynamic and cognitive-behavioral therapy have been shown to be effective.[24,25]

Antisocial Personality Disorder

Psychopath and *sociopath* are early terms once used to describe the condition now referred to as antisocial personality disorder. The term literally refers to patterns of mood, thinking, and behaviors that consistently show absolute disregard for others. In effect, persons with antisocial personality disorder are against and separate from the people, norms, rules, and laws that define society.

Etiology and Neurobiology. No single psychological, social, or neurobiological factor explains the onset of antisocial personality disorder. That said, a great deal of useful information has been generated. Males with antisocial personality disorder typically are the sons of antisocial fathers. This parental link is less apparent in females with antisocial personality disorder. Horrific experiences found to be associated with the onset of this disorder include childhood traumatic loss; physically or emotionally absent parents; childhood abuse and neglect; rigid, punishing childrearing practices; overwhelming childhood stress; and emotional trauma. Absent such experiences, childhood identification with an antisocial adult also significantly increases the risk of developing this highly disturbing disorder.

Persons with antisocial personality disorder can appear dangerous but are far more likely to be charismatic and charming. The many damaging effects of antisocial personality disorder include the ability to design and *wear* a public face that bears no relationship to the person's actual antisocial thoughts, feelings, and actions. Many characteristics of the disorder actually are personality characteristics that are absent. Antisocial personality disorder is not associated with feelings of anxiety, depression, remorse, concern, or empathy. Delusions or evidence of thought disorder are highly uncommon. Evidence of apparent intelligence and calculated cleverness are common. Dishonesty and deceit are hallmark characteristics of antisocial personality disorder. Antisocial personality disorder is distinct from sadistic personality disorder, a proposed diagnosis under consideration; however, persons with antisocial personality disorder can behave in a highly sadistic manner.

It should be noted that considerable disagreement exists among experts who study antisocial personality disorder. For example, traditionally the disorder has been viewed as a specific diagnosis, but many experts note that the presence of many overlapping characteristics of the cluster B disorders argues against this framework. They propose that rather than being a diagnostic category, antisocial personality disorder should be viewed in terms of behavior on a continuum that ranges from histrionic, narcissistic, and borderline to antisocial and sadistic.[26] The continuum model emphasizes specific characteristics, such as intelligence, that might better predict antisocial behavior. For example, extremely low intelligence has been shown to be associated with more frequent impulsive aggression.[27]

The debate regarding the proper classification of various antisocial behaviors speaks volumes in terms of the confounding nature of this inexplicable disorder. Others argue that difficulty comprehending antisocial behavior is a hallmark characteristic of the disorder. That said, researchers interested in developing causal models of antisocial personality disorder have attempted to apply various continuum models. For example, researchers have noted that substance dependence, antisocial behaviors, and disinhibition typically cooccurred. *Externalization* was identified as key factor predicting advancement along the continuum of increasingly dangerous behaviors.[27] Progressive externalization appeared to be inherited. If this turns out to be a generalizable finding, externalization might reliably predict antisocial behavior.

Biosocial models of violent antisocial personality disorder have strived to understand the interactions of genetics, biological, environmental, and social risk factors.[28] Relying both on family studies and on PET and fMRI findings, and attempting to account for potentially protective biological and environmental factors, researchers have identified biological and environmental interactions that may prove more predictive of antisocial behavior than any single risk factor. Nevertheless, models that attempt to explain antisocial personality disorder based on the interactions of multiple factors, such as birth complications and negative home environments, are likely to be exceedingly complex. National programs designed to reduce the risk of prenatal and negative home environment as lifelong risk factors have long been in operation.

Strictly neurobiological models of antisocial personality disorder attempt to rely solely on brain scan findings to more fully characterize the disorder rather than to predict behavior. For example, in an fMRI study that compared prison inmates with and without an antisocial diagnosis,[29] researchers hypothesized that antisocial inmates would show less brain activation than healthy controls or criminals not diagnosed with an antisocial disorder. Inmates were asked to respond to emotionally neutral and emotionally negative words. No group differences were observed with neutral words, but antisocial inmates showed significantly less emotional limbic and frontal cortex activation.[29] Less activation suggested that the antisocial inmates used different, nonemotional ways of processing negative emotional experiences. In other words, their emotions did not influence their thinking. This finding is consistent with the "cold" lack of emotion associated with antisocial personality disorder.

Clinical Manifestations. *Disregard for others* is a hallmark symptom of antisocial personality disorder. Although persons with this disorder are likely to be described as predators, indifference to others is more accurate.

Charm ironically is a common characteristic among persons with antisocial personality disorder. Possibly as a result of their indifference to others, they are able to project charm and may even be charismatic. These normally positive attributes tend to be little more than masks used to disarm or to create opportunities to manipulate and exploit others.

Blaming is a hallmark symptom of antisocial personality disorder. Others consistently are blamed for the person's actions and consequences of their actions. Often rather than a calculated ploy, blaming reflects the lack of self-awareness. When confronted with their actions they automatically look to explanations outside of themselves.

Impulsivity is observed with all cluster B personality disorders; however, with antisocial personality disorder, impulsivity frequently takes the form of thoughtless, harmful, or dangerous actions toward others.

Rule breaking refers to the ease with which norms, rules, and laws are disregarded. Calm contempt for others practically ensures recurrent antisocial behavior despite society's efforts to discourage such behavior. Few persons with this disorder are without a history of criminal activity. However, criminal activity should be distinguished from a criminal record of arrest, conviction, and incarceration. Large portions of prison inmate populations are persons with antisocial personality disorder. But antisocial personality disorder also can be observed among people of wealth, power, and standing who have the resources to avoid the legal system or successfully defend themselves in a legal action.

Deceitfulness and *deceptiveness* are hallmark symptoms of antisocial personality disorder.

Aggression and *assault* with antisocial personality disorder can occur on impulse or may reflect coldly calculated planning. This behavior is viewed as natural, appropriate, or "just the way it is." A matter-of-fact manner is typical.

Irresponsibility with antisocial personality disorder is evidenced by disregard for the expectations of others. Family members, employers, and others are likely to expect responsible actions, but from the perspective of the person with antisocial personality disorder, the expectations of others are not his or her concern.

Pharmacologic Treatment. As with other personality disorders, treatment for antisocial personality disorder typically is determined by the presenting symptomatology. Substance disorders are common comorbid disorders; however, when these disorders are present all too often they dominate treatment with too little emphasis given to the antisocial personality disorder diagnosis. When specific antisocial personality disorder symptoms are the focus of treatment, the symptoms commonly include impulsivity, anger, and aggression. Serotonin-activating medications, including antidepressants (e.g., paroxetine) and atypical antipsychotics (e.g., quetiapine) may be helpful in reducing chronic negative mood states. In some cases, atypical antipsychotic medications such as olanzapine may reduce agitation and impulsivity. Symptom-focused treatment may improve behavior management, but long-term adaptive improvements can require extensive care. Psychotherapy using cognitive-behavioral methods and behavior contracts can be useful when development of insight and behavior alternative training are needed. However, much of the promised effectiveness of these therapies is based on involuntary inmate populations. Until reliable neurobiological findings can be used to inform medication treatment for antisocial personality disorder, limited symptom remission methods are a reasonable treatment alternative.

KEY CONCEPTS

- Personality disorders are characterized by behavior deemed "inappropriate" or deviant within the cultural context. Behavioral patterns are recognizable by adolescence and include paranoid, schizophrenia-like, narcissistic, self-absorbed, antisocial, and compulsive, passive-aggressive, and dependent.
- Borderline personality disorder is characterized by unstable and dependent interpersonal relationships. Exclusive possession of another person is desired. To this end the individual may exhibit clinging, manipulation (complaints of illness, threatened suicide), self-destruction, and lying. Fear of abandonment may be ever present. Impulsiveness, substance abuse, loneliness, and lack of life goals are common. Psychosocial and biochemical factors are thought to be contributory; poor early mother-child relationships, child abuse, separation, or abandonment are significant contributing factors. Biological deficits in mood regulation could contribute to poor child-parent bonding.
- Antisocial personality disorder is characterized by failure to internalize moral and ethical values consistent with societal norms. Lack of anxiety and guilt, cold-bloodedness, and careless indifference or contempt for others are hallmarks of the disorder. The diagnosis of antisocial personality disorder is based on repeated antisocial behavior before age 15, along with failure to establish an occupational history after age 18. Psychosocial and biological factors are thought to be contributory and include lack of adequate parental role models, child abuse, inconsistent parenting, emotional deprivation, and having an alcoholic parent. A genetic component has been proposed.

EATING DISORDERS

Eating disorders can be subtyped as conditions characterized either by undereating (anorexia), overeating (bulimia), or compulsive eating (binge eating). Although extremely common, eating disorders are profoundly complex conditions manifested by dysregulation of psychological, behavioral, metabolic, and neurobiological systems. The exemplar disorder presented in this section is anorexia nervosa (AN). Once primarily observed in well-educated, very young women from middle- and high-income households, anorexia increasingly is observed in all age, income, educational, and ethnic groups.

Dieting has long been assumed to be a possible trigger of eating disorder onset, but this assumption may not be supported by research. Ordinary weight loss dieting has not been shown to be related to eating disorder onset unless the eating disorder preceded dieting; reliable evidence of a relationship between "yo-yo" weight loss and eating disorder onset has not been found; and the risk of negative psychological outcomes related to dieting is unknown.[30] Whatever the relationship between dieting and eating disorder onset, adolescents appear to be highly vulnerable.

The incidence of eating disorders in a sample of high school girls up to age 18 was found to be 2.8%; for ages 19 to 24 the incidence was 1.3%.[31] However, the incidence of psychological disorders, particularly depression, was 89.5%, and evidence of impaired functioning and increased risk of adult-onset mental disorders well exceeded expectations.[31] The age of onset for anorexia tends to be much younger than the age of onset for bulimia. But a finding of unique interest is that, in addition to low incidence rates, in young girls, these eating disorders may be transient and short lived.

Nevertheless, the high incidence of depression demands that experts continue to strive to determine what, if any, relationship exists between depression and anorexia. Are young depressed women more likely to explore disordered eating? Or are young eating-disordered women significantly more likely to become seriously depressed? Longitudinal studies of eating disorder risk transference from childhood to adolescence to adulthood suggest that the greatest risk is from adolescence to young adulthood.[32] Findings such as these would suggest that, although severe eating disorders in young females are less common than depression, early age onset might predict adult disordered eating.

Genetic studies of anorexia and major depression have shown a 58% concordance rate of anorexia in female twins.[33] Findings such as these indicate substantial heritability for anorexia. PET studies have shown a connection between emotionality and dopamine activity in areas of the brain associated with appetite and the risk of anorexia, but completely different neurobiological factors appear to underlie eating for survival and eating for emotional reward.[34] Neurobiological alterations affecting survival eating may be more closely related to anorexia. However, PET studies showing significant brain glucose hypometabolism in the parietal cortex of underweight patients with anorexia further complicate the model.[35] As yet, it is unclear whether less brain glucose metabolism and altered survival appetite drive characterize anorexia or are the result of excessive weight loss. Clear discernment of the direction of such findings is likely to remain difficult. Currently, cause-and-effect associations are absolutely clear only in studies such as the measurement of anorexia affects on bone reabsorption rates (serum osteocalcin levels) in severely underweight patients.[36]

Anorexia Nervosa

Anorexia nervosa is characterized by severe restriction of total calorie intake, refusal to maintain a healthy body weight, fear of weight gain, and fear of obesity.[37] Calorie restriction methods can include compulsive rituals that are dangerous, peculiar, or irrational. Normal dieting and successful weight loss may precede the onset of anorexia. Obsessive body dysmorphic thoughts and severe body image disturbance are hallmark symptoms of the disorder. This obsessive thinking in dangerously underweight persons can maintain the drive for calorie restriction and weight loss without consideration for actual hunger or body weight. That said, anorexia starts out as volitional behavior, but severe undereating can become compulsive. Loss of voluntary control of calorie intake can make it difficult for even dangerously emaciated persons to stop restricting their calorie intake.

Etiology and Neurobiology. Phobic avoidance anxiety associated with weight, neurotransmitters (serotonin, norepinephrine, dopamine, dysregulation), altered hunger-satiety signals, and psychological, physiologic, and autoimmune mechanisms have been studied as possible models of AN. Early AN models focused on the loss of secondary sex characteristics that accompanied extreme weight loss. Those models generally attributed anorexia to psychological fears of impregnation. Later models focused on intense struggles for power and control between very young women with anorexia and their parents. These psychodynamic models seemed only to explain a very small portion of the illness experience. More recent psychodynamic models focus on attributes such as obsessive-compulsive perfectionism.[38]

Researchers now are exploring neurobiological models of anorexia that involve hypothalamic dysfunction, metabolic dysfunction, comorbid psychological disorders, stress response dysregulation, and altered norepinephrine, serotonin, and dopamine neurotransmission systems. The findings of long-term survival studies make plain the need for more sophisticated biological models of anorexia. A 30-year study found that 93% of 208 persons survived anorexia.[39] In addition to malnutrition, the causes of death were liver failure, cardiac arrest, pneumonia, suicide, convulsion, and acute alcohol toxicity. Of these causes, the incidence of alcohol-related deaths far exceeded expectations. Similar findings were observed in a 21-year study.[40]

The search for strong causal models of anorexia has been underway for decades, yet the most convincing findings continue to describe survival analysis and comorbid illnesses. In other words, although currently understood to be an eating disorder that can persist, the disorder may be far more complicated. For example, early stages appear to be far less complex than later stages, and anorexia with depression or alcohol abuse appears to be more dangerous than anorexia alone. Neurobiological findings for these comorbid disorders would suggest that alterations in brain structures and functioning associated with anorexia are likely to be related to age of illness onset and symptom duration.

Clinical Manifestations. *Calorie restriction* is the hallmark symptom of AN. These restrictions can take the form of elaborate rituals and rules that govern all calorie intake. Weight loss is viewed as evidence of successful calorie restriction.

Appetite suppression may go unnoticed but AN does not produce true loss of appetite until dangerously low body weight is reached. Persons with AN must battle against their hunger, a battle that of course is not always successful. Any lapse is likely to be met with redoubled efforts.

Bingeing and *purging* can occur with AN when the disorder essentially includes both anorexia and bulimia.

Physical symptoms of AN in younger adolescent girls and boys include delayed psychosexual development, hypothermia, dependent edema, bradycardia, hypotension, and languor. Amenorrhea is predictable when young girls maintain a body weight insufficient for reproductive health. Severe, potentially life-threatening physical symptoms include hypokalemia and QRS rhythm changes. Cardiac arrhythmias typically are the actual cause of death in severe cases of AN. These physical symptoms are reversed by adequate calorie intake and normal weight. However, remission of physical symptoms of AN does not necessarily lead to remission of the psychological symptoms that may have triggered the disorder.

Pharmacologic Treatment. Recovery from AN is considered to be a long and costly process, with fewer than 50% of patients achieving recovery in less than 6 years.[41] Severity is clearly a factor. The more severe the weight loss at the outset, the more difficult and more prolonged recovery will be. Persons with anorexia may have a host of treatment needs and remain vulnerable to serious health crisis for years. Treatment is further complicated by the existence of profound comorbid disorders such as alcoholism, depression, anxiety, bipolar disorder, and personality disorder. For profoundly low-weight persons, the process of *refeeding* for weight gain is in itself slow and difficult, and other treatment goals may have to be secondary. With these concerns in mind, recent treatment guidelines for anorexia recommend a comprehensive care plan that includes medication treatments, psychosocial interventions, medical, and nutritional interventions.[42] Selective serotonin reuptake inhibitors are the medications of choice when depression is a comorbid disorder. In some cases, antidepressant medications may exert central effects on appetite that may prove helpful. Severely underweight patients must be closely monitored for medication side effects such as dizziness.

KEY CONCEPTS

- AN is an eating disorder characterized by excessive dietary restriction, significant weight loss (>15%), irrational fears of gaining weight, and disturbed body image. The disorder appears to have a genetic predisposition and affects females almost exclusively. The average age at onset is 13 to 15 years. Afflicted individuals tend to be secretive about their food restrictions. Self-induced vomiting and laxative abuse may also occur. Manifestations of AN include amenorrhea, hypothermia, edema, hypotension, and fluid and electrolyte imbalance. Potassium imbalance may lead to the serious consequence of cardiac dysrhythmias.

SUMMARY

Hypotheses regarding the cause and pathogenesis, clinical manifestations, and implications for management of representative subsets of three large categories of illnesses have been presented. It is important to recognize that these illnesses represent mixtures of biological, psychological, social, and environmental factors. Researchers have yet to unlock the mysteries surrounding the neurobiological mechanisms of nonpsychotic illnesses.

MEDIA RESOURCES

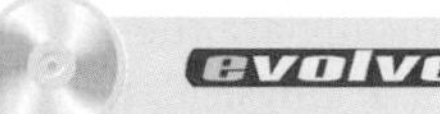

evolve

Remember to check out the ***CD Companion*** included with this book for Review Questions, Key Concepts Review, Glossary (with audio for selected terms), Disease Profiles, and Animations.

PLUS, visit the ***Evolve website*** at http://evolve.elsevier.com/Copstead/ for Case Studies, Disease Profiles, and WebLinks.

References

1. Stahl S: *Essential psychopharmacology: neuroscientific basis and clinical applications,* New York, 1996, University of Cambridge Press.
2. Lesch KP: Molecular foundation of anxiety disorders, *J Neural Transm* 108:717-746, 2002.
3. Gorman JM et al: Physiological changes during carbon dioxide inhalation in patients with panic disorder, major depression, and premenstrual dysphoric disorder: evidence for a central fear mechanism, *Arch Gen Psychiatry* 58(2):125-131, 2001.
4. Abelson JL et al: Persistent respiratory irregularity in patients with panic disorder, *Soc Biol Psychiatry* 49:588-595, 2001.
5. Wilhelm FH, Trabert W, Roth WT: Physiologic instability in panic disorder and generalized anxiety disorder, *Soc Biol Psychiatry* 49:596-605, 2002.
6. Mathew SJ, Coplan JD, Gorman JM: Neurobiological mechanisms of social anxiety disorder, *Am J Psychiatry* 158(10):1558-1567, 2001.
7. Heim C et al: Altered pituitary-adrenal axis responses to provocative challenge tests in adult survivors of childhood abuse, *Am J Psychiatry* 158(4):575-581, 2001.
8. Teicher MH et al: The neurobiological consequences of early stress and childhood maltreatment, *Neurosci Biobehav Rev* 27:33-44, 2003.
9. Sheikh J: Anxiety in older adults: assessment and management of three common presentations, *Geriatrics* 58(5):44-45, 2003.
10. Rickels K, Rynn MA: What is generalized anxiety disorder? *J Clin Psychiatry* 62(suppl 11):4-12, 2001.
11. Nutt DJ: Neurobiological mechanisms in generalized anxiety disorder, *J Clin Psychiatry* 62(suppl 11):22-27, 2001.
12. Davidson JRT: Pharmacotherapy of generalized anxiety disorder, *J Clin Psychiatry* 62(suppl 11):46-50, 2001.
13. Ursu S et al: Overactive action monitoring in obsessive-compulsive disorder: evidence from functional magnetic resonance imaging, *Am Psychol Soc* 14(4):347-353, 2003.
14. Winsber ME, Cassic KS, Koran LM: Hoarding in obsessive-compulsive disorder: a report of 20 cases, *J Clin Psychiatry* 60(9):591-597, 1999.
15. Endler NS, Kocovski NL: Personality disorders at the crossroads, *J Pers Disord* 16(6):487-502, 2002.
16. McDermut W, Zimmerman M, Chelminski I: The construct validity of depressive personality disorder, *J Abnorm Psychol* 112(1):49-60, 2003.
17. Tyrer P et al: Treatment rejecting and treatment seeking personality disorders: type R and type S, *J Pers Disord* 17(3):263-268, 2003.
18. Coolidge FL, Thede LL, Jang KL: Heritability of personality disorders in childhood: a preliminary investigation, *J Pers Disord* 15(1):33-40, 2001.
19. Skodol AE et al: The borderline diagnosis II: biology, genetics, and clinical course, *Soc Biol Psychiatry* 51:951-963, 2002.
20. Rinne T et al: Hyperresponsiveness of hypothalamic-pituitary-adrenal axis to combine dexamethasone/corticotropin-releasing hormone challenge in female borderline personality disorder subjects with a history of sustained childhood abuse, *Soc Biol Psychiatry* 52:1102-1112, 2002.
21. Boutros NN, Torello M, McGlashan TH: Electrophysiological aberrations in borderline personality disorder: state of the evidence, *J Neuropsychiatry Clin Neurosci* 15(2):145-154, 2003.
22. Schmahl CG et al: Neural correlates of memories of abandonment in women with and without borderline personality disorder, *Soc Bio Psychiatry* 54:142-151, 2003.
23. van Elst LT et al: Frontolimbic brain abnormalities in patients with borderline personality disorder: a volumetric magnetic resonance imaging study, *Soc Biol Psychiatry* 54:163-171, 2003.
24. Gabbard GO: Psychotherapy of personality disorders, *J Psychother Pract Res* 9(1):1-6, 2000.
25. Leichsenring F, Leibing E: The effectiveness of psychodynamic therapy and cognitive behavior therapy in the treatment of personality disorders: a meta analysis, *Am J Psychiatry* 160(7):1223-1232, 2003.
26. Murphy C, Vess J: Subtypes of psychopathy: proposed differences between narcissistic, borderline, sadistic, and antisocial psychopaths, *Psychiatr Q* 74(1):11-29, 2003.
27. Krueger RF et al: Etiologic connections among substance dependence, antisocial behavior, and personality: modeling the externalizing spectrum, *J Abnorm Psychol* 111(3):411-424, 2002.

28. Raine A: Biosocial studies of antisocial and violent behavior in children and adults: a review, *J Abnorm Child Psychol* 30(4):311-326, 2002.
29. Kiehl KA et al: Limbic abnormalities in affective processing by criminal psychopaths as revealed by functional magnetic resonance imaging, *Soc Biol Psychiatry* 50:677-684, 2001.
30. National Task Force on the Prevention and Treatment of Obesity: Dieting and the development of eating disorders in overweight and obese adults, *Arch Intern Med* 160(17):1581-2589, 2000.
31. Lewinsohn PM, Striegel-Moore RH, Seeley JR: Epidemiology and natural course of eating disorders in young women from adolescence to young adulthood, *J Am Acad Child Adolesc Psychiatry* 39(10):1284-1292, 2000.
32. Kotler LA et al: Longitudinal relationships between childhood, adolescent, and adult eating disorders, *J Am Acad Child Adolesc Psychiatry* 40(12):1434-1440, 2001.
33. Wade TD et al: Anorexia nervosa and major depression: shared genetic and environmental risk factors, *Am J Psychiatry* 157(3):469-471, 2000.
34. Volkow ND et al: Brain dopamine is associated with eating behaviors in humans, *Int J Eat Disord* 33:136-142, 2003.
35. Delvenne V et al: Brain glucose metabolism in eating disorders assessed by positron emission tomography, *Int J Eat Disord* 25:29-37, 1996.
36. Hotta M et al: The relationship between bone turnover and body weight, serum insulin-like growth factor (IGF) I, and serum IGF-binding protein levels in patients with anorexia nervosa, *J Clin Endocrinol Metab* 85(1):200-206, 2000.
37. Meehler PS: Diagnosis and care of patients with anorexia nervosa in primary care settings, *Ann Intern Med* 134:1048-1059, 2001.
38. Halmi KA et al: Perfectionism in anorexia nervosa: variation by clinical subtype, obsessionality and pathological eating behavior, *Am J Psychiatry* 157(11):1799-1805, 2000.
39. Korndorfer SR et al: Long term survival of patients with anorexia nervosa: a population based study in Rochester, Minn, *Mayo Clin Proc* 78(3):278-284, 2003.
40. Zipfel S et al: Long term prognosis in anorexia nervosa: lessons from a 21-year follow-up study, *Lancet* 355:721-722, 2000.
41. Finfgeld DL: Anorexia nervosa: analysis of long-term outcomes and clinical implications, *Arch Psychiatr Nurs* 16(4):176-186, 2002.
42. American Psychiatric Association: Practice guidelines for the treatment of patients with eating disorders (revision), *Am J Psychiatry* 157(1 suppl):1-39, 2000.

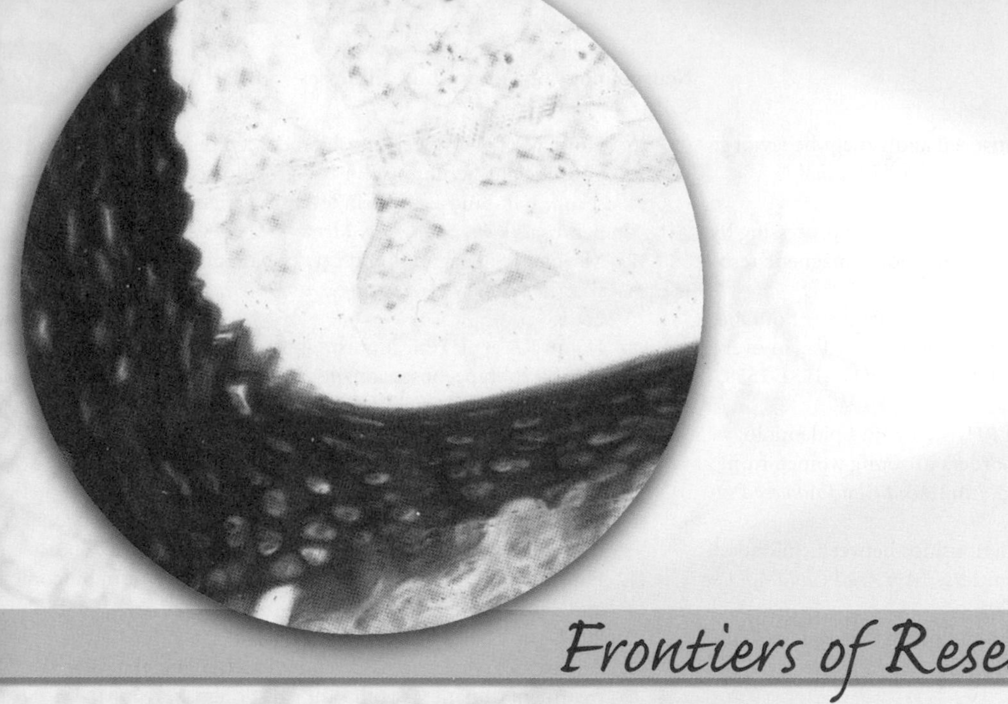

Frontiers of Research

Advances in Treatment of Musculoskeletal Disorders

Robert H. Caplan and Michael J. Kirkhorn

When health care providers find themselves caring for one of the 2 million Americans who each year suffer fractures, they are concerned with the patient's comfort, with alignment of the healing bones, and with the patient's rehabilitation. If the fracture is due to osteoporosis, which occurs most commonly without a severe injury, they are also concerned with preventing further fractures.

Perhaps because our boniness is always with us conspicuously, whether we are walking, sitting, stretching, or rapping our "funny bone," we tend to take the skeleton for granted—for the wrong reasons.

We may notice one person's cheekbones or say that another has a "raw-boned" look. However, we are not much aware of the bones' processes, of their life, as we are bound to be, for example, when the gastrointestinal or the genitourinary system reminds us of its processes. Most of the time, bones live quietly in the body.

For some fairly obvious reasons, we regard our connected armature of bones as a durable but lifeless framework for the body. Bones' durability reminds us that they are strong. One writer observes that bones are constructed like reinforced concrete, a combination of fibers and crystals with a compressed strength greater than that of reinforced concrete and a tensile strength nearly as great.

However, there is much more to the bone than its "boniness."

The skeleton is the sturdy framework of each human body. As long as humans have walked, they have been supported by this armature, and as they watch their children grow, they take special pleasure in the straight, strong growth of the bones.

The skeleton supports the muscular system and protects the internal organs. When women enter menopause and the female hormone estrogen decreases, bone breaks down excessively. The delicate balance between bone formation and resorption is disrupted, and the bone becomes weaker and susceptible to fracture. This disorder, osteoporosis, or *brittle bone disease,* also develops with the aging process in men, albeit about 10 years later than in women.

Some scientists interested in helping people resist brittle bone disease might be drawn to the other end of the spectrum, where bones are formed. Age-related osteoporosis has been increasing in Western nations, and this fact—the brittleness of aging bones—has led to research on how diet, exercise, and modern lifestyles affect bone growth and condition. Researchers assume that high peak bone mass may be a defense against the eventual development of osteoporosis. Scientists assume that calcium intake during childhood is a major determi-

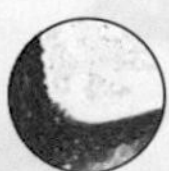

Fibrocartilage of intervertebral disk. (From Thibodeau GA, Patton KT: Anatomy & physiology, *ed 5, St Louis, 2003, Mosby, p 203.)*

Musculoskeletal Support and Movement

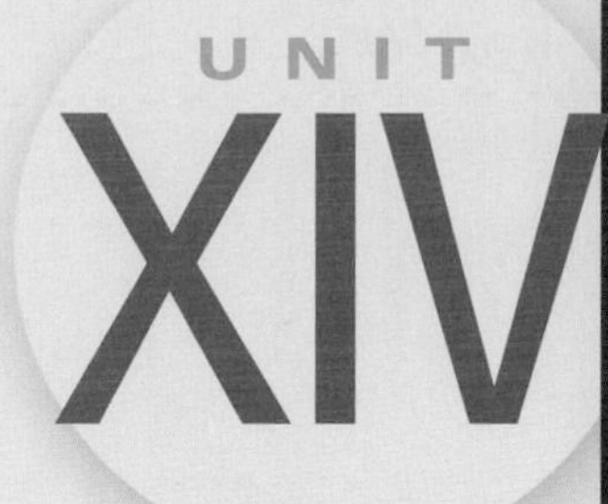

nant of bone development. Exercise, hormonal levels, avoiding phosphorus-containing sodas, and avoiding smoking and excessive alcohol intake are also probably important factors. Although a heavy body weight is blamed for many medical problems, it is good insurance against osteoporosis.

New technology has allowed researchers to understand important factors. Dual-energy x-ray absorptiometry and its low-radiation exposure has helped in the development of studies that are needed to determine peak bone mass and enables providers to identify patients with or at high risk for developing osteoporosis. This is important because potent drugs are now available that increase bone density and prevent fractures.

The skeleton moves through contraction of the muscles that adorn the armature and give it power and mobility. Stripped of its musculature and therefore of its mobility and power, the skeleton becomes a reminder of the final immobility, death.

As genetic research progresses, gene therapy offers promising directions for some muscle diseases, as it does for many other diseases.

Duchenne-type muscular dystrophy is a degenerative disorder that first attacks skeletal muscle and proceeds to loss of ambulation, respiratory and cardiac dysfunction, and early death. It also affects the brain. It is the most common form of muscular dystrophy in children. The Duchenne type is the first muscular dystrophy for which the defective gene was cloned and characterized and the corresponding protein identified. Therefore it is a model for muscle gene therapy research. Experimental gene therapies are currently under evaluation.

Among the most intractable disorders associated with the musculoskeletal system is back pain. Backache is nagging and sometimes chronic and debilitating. Millions of people would welcome its alleviation as enthusiastically as they would the cure of other unglamorous disorders such as the common cold. That development is not yet in sight, unfortunately. A survey of 475 family physicians revealed that many feel more or less helpless when it comes to the treatment of back pain. They know that their patients are not satisfied with the care they receive. Only 22% of patients surveyed about the treatment of back pain said that they were "very satisfied" with the treatment.

Research suggests that for treatment of lower back pain, which tends to be recurrent, the best advice is for patients to continue or resume normal activity. One study shows that patients encouraged to engage in light activity and walk as soon as possible were less likely to continue on sick leave than those who were advised to rest in bed or accept another form of immobility.

Structure and Function of the Musculoskeletal System

Carol L. Danning

MEDIA RESOURCES

Additional Material for Study, Review, and Further Exploration

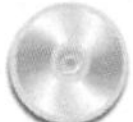

CD Companion ◆ Review Questions and Answers ◆ Key Concepts Review ◆ Glossary *(with audio pronunciations for selected terms)* ◆ Disease Profiles ◆ Animations

evolve ***Website*** at http://evolve.elsevier.com/Copstead/ ◆ Case Studies ◆ Disease Profiles ◆ WebLinks

KEY QUESTIONS

- What are the functions of osteoblasts and osteoclasts in bone remodeling?
- What is the relationship between joint structure and joint mobility?
- Why is articular cartilage particularly susceptible to degenerative changes?
- What factors determine tendon strength and compliance?
- How does the striated structure of skeletal muscle relate to its contractile function?
- How does an action potential in the α motor neuron lead to a contraction in the muscle cells of the motor unit?

CHAPTER OUTLINE

Movement is one of the most characteristic and visible aspects of human life. Ease of movement adds to self-worth and well-being because the ability to move is closely connected to independence. A working knowledge of the system responsible for body movement is imperative to the health care provider. This chapter examines the basic characteristics of the firm support of bone and joint structures that make motion possible and the properties of skeletal muscles that are responsible for actually moving the body's framework.

STRUCTURE AND FUNCTION OF BONE

The primary purposes of the skeletal system are to protect internal organs, provide bony attachments for muscles and ligaments, present rigid levers to allow functional movement of the body and its separate parts, and store mineral and marrow elements for forming new blood cells. Bone is highly vascular and is metabolically active from birth to death.

Composition

The organic component of bone is 90% to 95% collagen fibers, which extend along lines of tension and give bone its great tensile strength.[1] Bone can remodel itself throughout life in response to external forces (or loads) such as the pull of tendons and body weight during activities. Bone is the hardest connective tissue in the body. A specialized connective tissue, bone has a high content of inorganic material (mineral salts) that combines with an organic matrix. This combination provides for a hard, rigid structure that is both flexible and resilient.

Similar to other connective tissue, bone consists of a cellular component, ground substance, and fibrous component. The cellular component consists of fibroblasts, fibrocytes, osteoblasts, osteocytes, osteoclasts, and osteoprogenitor cells. **Fibroblasts** and **fibrocytes** are needed for collagen production. **Osteoblasts,** which lay down bone, are formed from **osteoprogenitor** cells, which are bone stem cells lining bone surfaces. **Osteocytes** are mature bone cells. **Osteoclasts** are responsible for bone resorption. **Ground substance** is a homogeneous gelatinous substance composed of extracellular fluid and proteoglycans, chondroitin sulfate, and hyaluronic acid, which help control the deposition of calcium salts.[2]

The mineral portions of bone, mainly calcium and phosphate, account for 65% to 75% of the dry weight of bone and give bone its solid structure. Bone is also a source of essential minerals, especially calcium. Bone mineral is embedded in fibers of protein collagen, the fibrous aspect of the extracellular matrix. Collagen fibers are tough, pliable, and resistant to stretching. Collagen composes approximately 95% of the extracellular matrix and accounts for 25% to 35% of the dry weight of bone. Collagen is the chief fibrous component of the musculoskeletal system.

A ground substance surrounds collagen fibers in bone. Ground substance consists of protein polysaccharides, or **glycosaminoglycans,** mainly in a molecule called **proteoglycan.** Glycosaminoglycans serve as cement between layers of collagen fibers.

Water accounts for approximately 25% of the weight of live bone. Most of the water is located in the organic matrix surrounding collagen fibers and ground substance. Another 15% of the water is located in canals that carry nutrition to bone tissue.

Microscopically, the basic unit of bone is the **osteon** or the **haversian system** (Figure 50-1). The haversian canal lies at the center of each osteon and contains blood vessels and nerve fibers. A concentric series of lamellae of mineralized matrix surrounds the central canal. Bordering the lamellae are small cavities (lacunae) that contain a bone cell, the **osteocyte.** Many small channels, the canaliculi, connect adjacent lamellae with each other and eventually with the main haversian canal. This canal system allows nutrients from blood vessels in the haversian canal to reach osteocytes. Collagen fibers connect one lamella to another within the osteon and increase the mechanical strength of bone.

At the tissue level, bones are classified as two types: **cancellous** or **trabecular** bone and **compact** or **cortical** bone (Figure 50-2). **Cancellous bone** is formed in thin plates called **trabeculae.** Trabeculae are laid down in response to stress and shape to accommodate loads placed on the bone. Cancellous bone is covered by compact bone. **Compact bone** is quite resistant to compression and is dense in structure. Compact bone is laid down in concentric layers. A tough fibrous membrane called the periosteum covers all bones. The periosteum is highly vascularized and provides nutrition for bone via Volkmann canals (see Figure 50-1). An inner layer of the periosteum contains **osteoblasts,** which are responsible for bone growth and repair. The periosteum covers the entire bone except for the ends, which are covered by hyaline cartilage.

In longer bones, a central cavity (**medullary cavity**) is present (see Figure 50-2). A thin membrane called the **endosteum** covers this cavity. The central cavity is filled with fatty marrow. Osteogenic cells are located in the endosteum.[3]

Blood vessels are distributed through the haversian canals. Living cells in bone communicate with each other and the haversian system via threadlike processes.

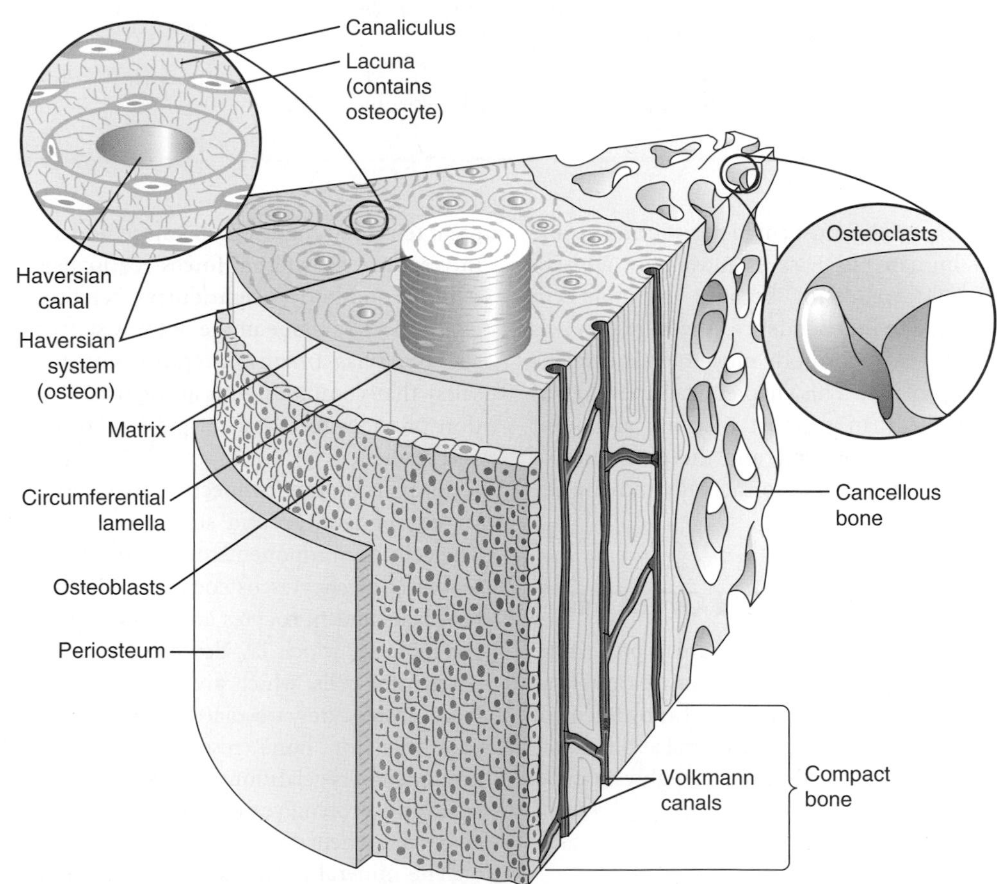

FIGURE 50-1 ■ Microscopic anatomy of bone. The section has been enlarged to show periosteum, osteoblasts, the haversian system, lacunae, and osteoclasts.

Functional Properties

Growth and Ossification

The process of longitudinal bone growth involves endochondral ossification. In this type of growth, cartilage is replaced by bone as in embryonic development, fracture healing, and some bone tumor growth. In children, fracture through the shaft of a long bone stimulates bone growth, possibly because of increased nutrition to growth cartilage from the hyperemia associated with fracture healing. Particular attention to bone alignment or overlapping of fracture ends must be paid when managing a fracture in a child between 2 and 10 years of age since predictable bone overgrowth can lead to limb length discrepancies.[4]

Circumferential bone growth occurs via intramembranous ossification. In this case, connective tissue is transformed into bone. Interstitial growth is not possible in bone. Bone can grow in length only by a process of growth within cartilage, followed by endochondral ossification (Figure 50-3). Two sites of cartilage growth are available in a long bone: articular cartilage and epiphyseal plate cartilage. In longer bones, the epiphysis provides the only growth plate for the entire bone.

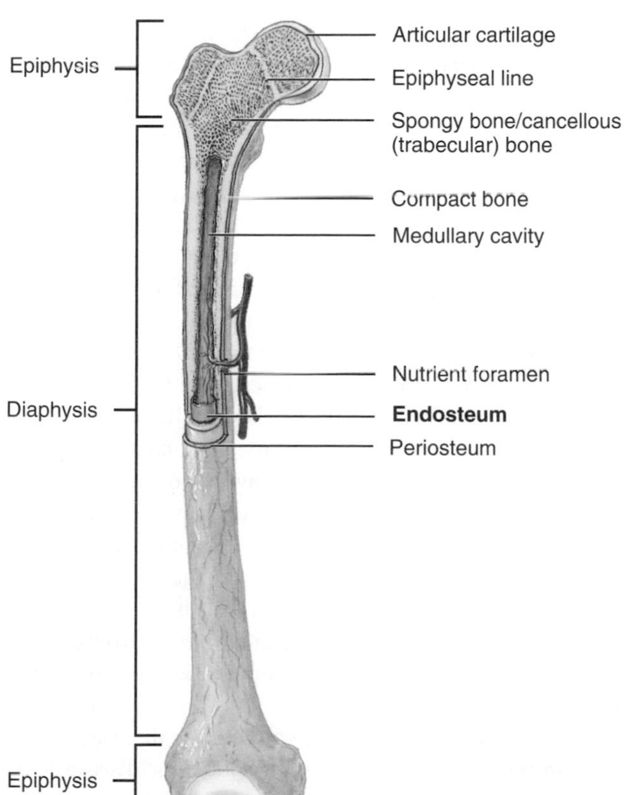

FIGURE 50-2 ■ Structure and composition of a typical long bone. (From Applegate E: *The anatomy and physiology learning system*, 2nd ed, Philadelphia, 2000, Saunders, p 93.)

Continuous Growth

The **epiphyseal plate** (see Figure 50-3) allows for lengthening of the metaphysis and diaphysis of a long bone. Injuries to this growth plate in children may lead to limb length discrepancies. The plate is the site of continuous growth. Growth and thickening of cartilage cells of the plate move the epiphysis away from the metaphysis. Calcification and replacement of cartilage occur on the metaphyseal surface (endochondral ossification).

The function of the epiphyseal plate in the growth process may be illustrated by examining the specific zones (Figure 50-4) of the plate and how they contribute to the growth process. The **zone of resting cartilage** maintains adherence of the plate to the epiphysis. Immature chondrocytes and vessels penetrate this first zone from the epiphysis and nourish the plate. The **zone of young proliferating cartilage** demonstrates the most active cartilage cell growth. The **zone of maturing cartilage** contains the enlarged and mature cartilage cells as they migrate toward the metaphysis. The final zone is the **zone of calcifying cartilage,** which is a very thin line of chondrocytes and the weakest segment of the epiphyseal plate. These chondrocytes are no longer living because of calcification of the matrix.

Bone is also deposited quite actively on the metaphyseal side of the plate. With the addition of new bone, the metaphysis becomes longer.

Osteoblasts in the inner layer of the periosteum are responsible for growth in the width of bones. This process is called **intermembranous ossification.** Resorption of bone, through a process of osteoclastic resorption, causes the medullary cavity to enlarge, causing additional widening of bone.

Hormones influence bone growth. Too little secretion of thyroxine by the thyroid or too little growth hormone from the pituitary gland results in dwarfism. Oversecretion of growth hormone results in giantism. Sex hormones, such as estradiol, are produced in higher amounts during and after puberty and can cause more rapid maturation and fusion of the epiphyseal plates. These hormones may limit the growth spurts of puberty, and early sexual maturity, especially in girls, can lead to shorter stature.[3]

Response to Injury, Stress, and Aging

The ability of bone to remodel after injury is important. Although remodeling of bone continues throughout life, death of the osteon or removal of calcium from bone requires that new bone be deposited to retain strength and function. (See Chapter 51 for further discussion.) Physical stresses lead to the realignment of bone trabecular systems and the deposition of additional bone at the site of increased stress. The response of bone to stress is summarized by **Wolff's law,** which states that bone is laid down where it is needed and resorbed where it is not needed.[5] If bone is immobilized or not subjected to mechanical stress, as occurs with prolonged bed rest,

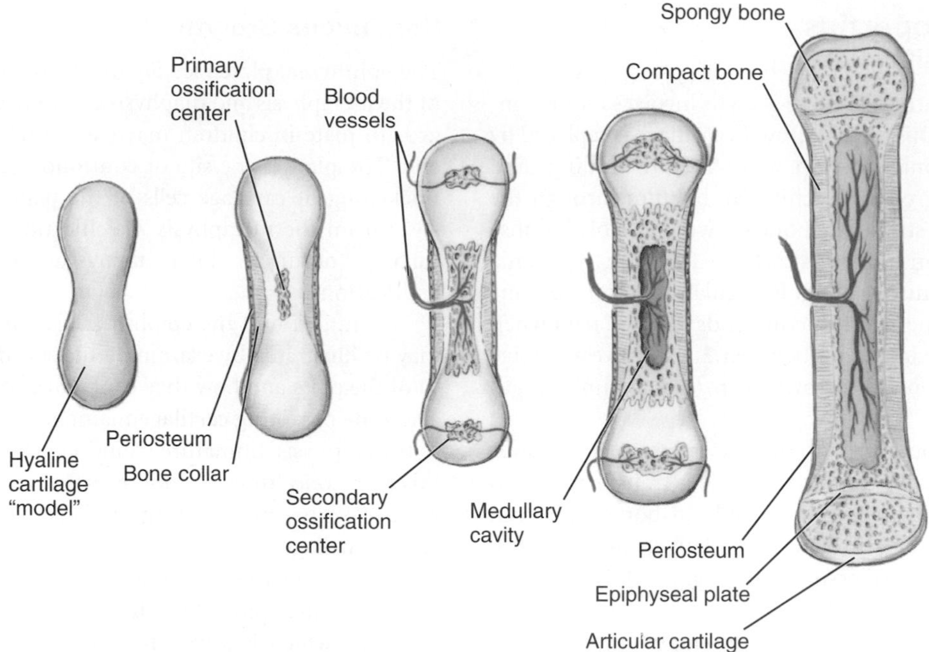

FIGURE 50-3 ■ Events in endochondral ossification. (From Applegate E: *The anatomy and physiology learning system*, 2nd ed, Philadelphia, 2000, Saunders, p 95.)

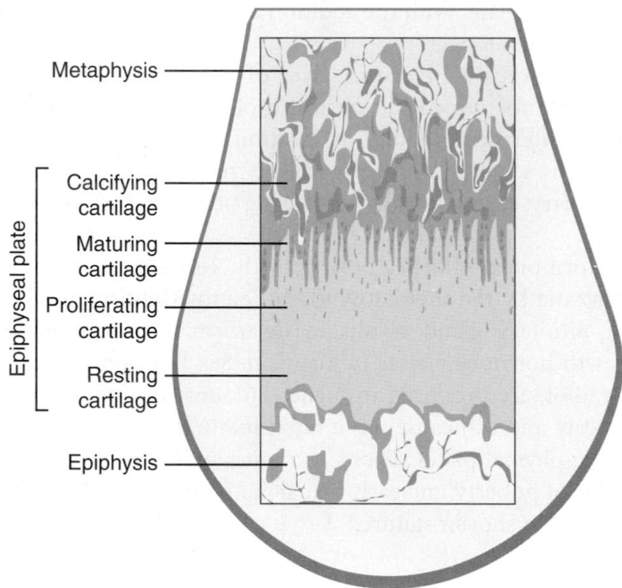

FIGURE 50-4 ■ Zones of the epiphyseal plate.

the activity of bone-resorbing cells increases.[6] Without external forces (or loads), osteoclast activity is greater than osteoblast activity and bone mass decreases. It is probable that during bed rest, age-related bone loss might be temporarily accelerated and may result in a greater decline in bone mass over time. Patients becoming mobile after prolonged bed rest are at risk for fractures because of a combined loss of muscle and bone strength. With loss of muscle, gait becomes unsteady and patients are more prone to falls.

Internal fixation of a fracture may also cause decreased bone strength. With metal implants, mechanical stress is dispersed from bone and carried by the implant. Bone under the plate is resorbed, and "stress relief" osteoporosis may occur. Care must be taken once implants are removed, and the bone must be protected until strength returns. Some implants are designed to compress fracture fragments to aid healing.

Bone mass decreases with age. Studies have shown that elderly individuals express higher levels of certain markers associated with bone resorption whereas bone formation markers are much more variable. One common cause of increased bone resorption is calcium and vitamin D deficiency, which causes more rapid mobilization of calcium from bone. A secondary hyperparathyroidism can also result. Decreased levels of estrogen in elderly women and men can contribute to age-related bone loss since osteoblasts have estrogen receptors and their ability to increase bone formation may be affected by the estrogen deficiency. An increase in local production of cytokines that influence bone resorption may also occur with decreased estrogen levels. The end result is an imbalance between osteoblast and osteoclast function and progressive decline in bone mass.[3] See The Aging Process: Changes in the Skeletal System.

Bone mass can also decrease with certain disease processes. For example, osteoporosis is a metabolic bone disease characterized by a severe general reduction in skeletal bone mass and thus a susceptibility to fractures. In short, bone resorption is more rapid than bone formation. (See Chapter 51 for further discussion.)

THE AGING PROCESS

Changes in the Skeletal System

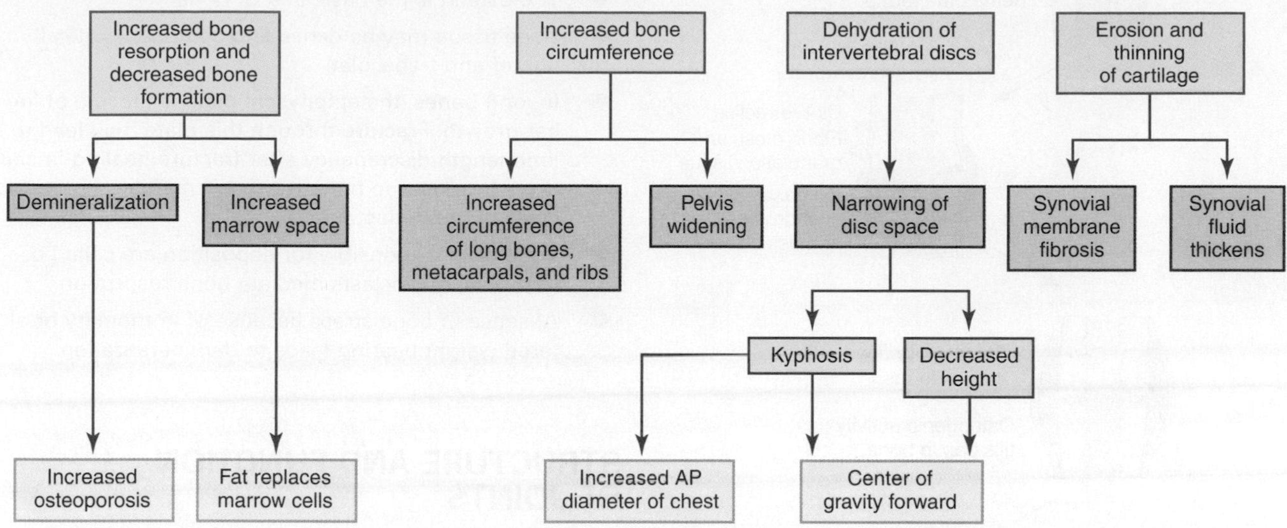

With aging, bone absorption exceeds bone formation. There is a net loss of bone mass and bone protein matrix. The interior of the long and the flat bones is absorbed faster than that of other bones. Trabecular bone destruction is greater than cortical bone loss. Aging women have a greater amount of bone loss than aging men do. The bone marrow space is decreased, with fat replacing marrow cells.

Although interior bone is lost, the circumference of the bones increases because osteoblasts on the exterior bone beneath the periosteum continue bone formation. The long bones, metacarpals, and ribs become bigger in circumference, whereas the pelvis becomes wider and the skull thicker.

The intervertebral disks become dehydrated, with narrowing of the disk space leading to a decrease in height of 3 to 5 cm. An increase in the thoracic curve occurs, resulting in kyphosis and anterior scapular displacement. This change leads to an increase in the anteroposterior diameter of the chest. A decrease in the lordotic curve results in lumbar flattening and a decrease in lumbar flexibility. Greater flexion of the knees and hips is noted. The relationship between the pelvis and the femoral head and neck also changes.

Fissuring, erosion, and thinning of cartilage occur. With the loss of cartilage, the greater pressure that subchondral bone must withstand results in increased density and the formation of joint margin osteophytes. The synovial membrane undergoes fibrosis and the synovial fluid thickens.

Fracture Healing

Bone may heal in one of two ways after a fracture. A periosteal or external callus forms in fractures managed by closed methods. The blood supply to surrounding soft tissue and motion at the fracture site contribute to healing. Medullary callus formation takes place with rigid immobilization at the fracture site. The process of bone turnover contributes to healing.

The five stages of fracture healing are (1) hematoma formation, 1 to 3 days; (2) fibrocartilage formation, 3 days to 2 weeks; (3) callus formation, 2 to 6 weeks; (4) ossification, 3 weeks to 6 months; and (5) consolidation/remodeling, 6 weeks to 1 year (Figure 50-5). These five stages can be grouped into three phases: (1) inflammatory phase, (2) reparative phase (stages 2 to 4), and (3) remodeling phase.

Stage 1 begins when a hematoma forms at the fracture site. The size of the hematoma depends on the amount of damage at the fracture site. The hematoma offers some stability to fracture ends. Aseptic inflammation occurs at the fracture site.

Healing continues during *stage 2* with the formation of granular tissue containing blood vessels, fibroblasts, and osteoblasts. The hematoma provides the foundation for reparative tissue and bone healing. Vascular and mechanical factors such as motion and distraction of fragments influence stage 2.

Callus formation occurs during *stage 3* after the granulation tissue matures. If this stage is delayed or interrupted, the final stages cannot occur.

Stage 4, or ossification, occurs as the space in the bone is bridged and the fracture ends are united. The callus is slowly

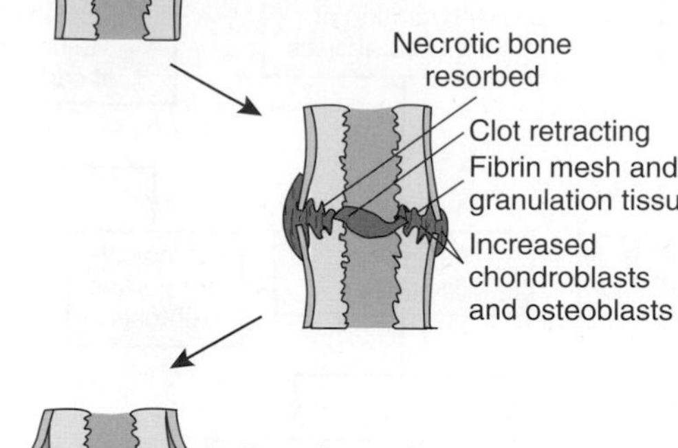

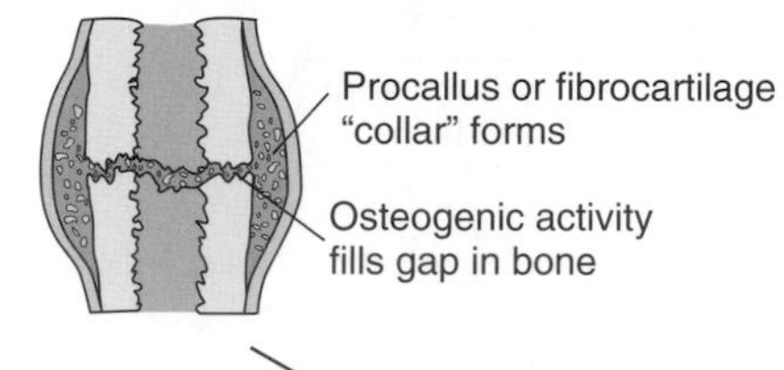

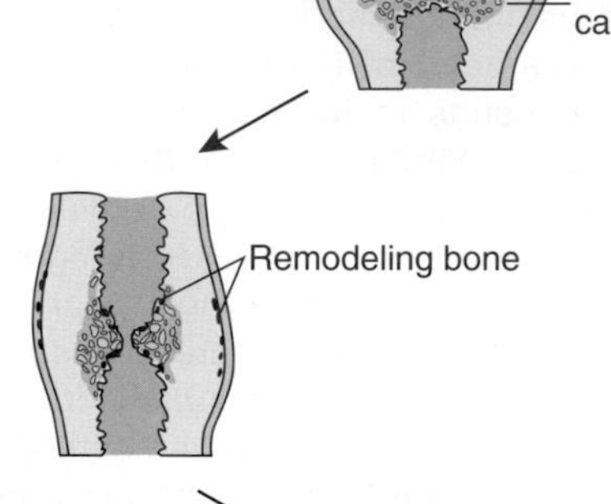

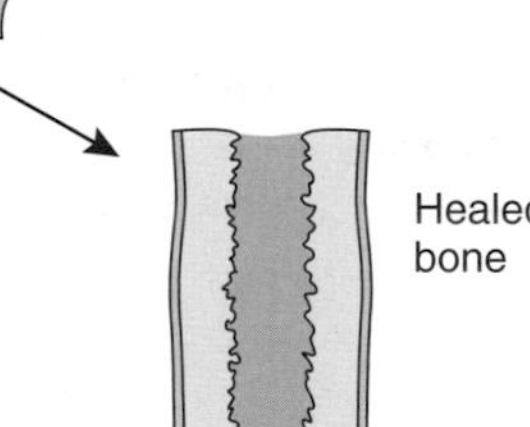

FIGURE 50-5 ■ Healing of a fracture. (From Gould BE: *Pathophysiology for the health professions,* 2nd ed, Philadelphia, 2002, Saunders, p 559.)

replaced by trabecular bone along the lines of stress and unnecessary callus is reabsorbed.

During *stage 5,* consolidation and remodeling occur as the medullary canal is reestablished. Bone is resorbed and deposited along stress lines as bone reshapes to meet its mechanical requirements.

Fractures are usually considered healed when clinical healing is achieved. Clinical healing occurs when the fracture is stable and strong enough to resume its function, the fracture site is free of pain, no gross movement is seen across the fracture site, and radiographs show bone crossing the fracture site.

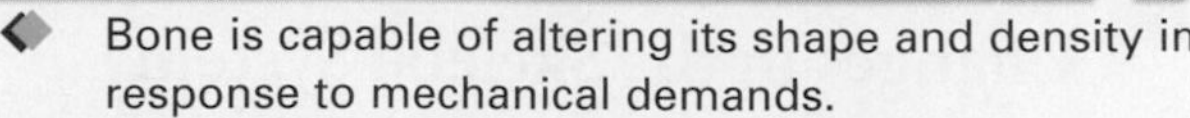

KEY CONCEPTS

- Bone is capable of altering its shape and density in response to mechanical demands.
- The osteon is the basic unit of bone.
- Bone tissue may be dense and compact (cortical) or lighter and trabecular.
- In long bones, the epiphyseal plate is the site of linear growth. Fracture through this plate may lead to limb length discrepancy after fracture healing in children. Increases in bone width are mediated by osteocytes in the periosteum.
- Bone cells responsible for deposition are called osteoblasts; osteoclasts mediate bone resorption.
- Absence of bone stress because of immobility or altered weight bearing leads to demineralization.

STRUCTURE AND FUNCTION OF JOINTS

Coordinated movement is only possible because of joint, bone, and muscle structure. Joints permit complex, highly coordinated, and purposeful movements. A **joint,** also called an **articulation,** is a point of contact between bones. Functional articulations between bones in extremities such as the shoulder, elbow, hip, and knee contribute to controlled and graceful movement.

The type and configuration of a joint depend on the functional demands placed on that joint. As is the case with all aspects of the musculoskeletal system, structure determines function (Figure 50-6). When considering the human joint, or articulation, it is also important to remember that once the articulation has developed, the configuration of the joint surface will determine the movement of the joint. Any aberrant joint movement has the potential to disrupt function and cause a breakdown in joint integrity.

Articulations can provide more than a single function, such as flexion and extension. Flexion, extension, adduction, abduction, rotation, opposition, and circumduction may all be functional movements of a joint. The more complex the movements, the more complex is the joint structure.

Broadly speaking, articulations, or arthroses, in the human body may be divided into two categories based on the makeup of the joint and the method in which the joints unite the body components. The two categories are **synarthroses,** or fibrous and cartilaginous (nonsynovial) joints, and **diarthroses,** or synovial joints.

Synarthroses

Synarthroses have two subdivisions based on the type of connective tissue used to form the joint. Fibrous and cartilaginous tissues give these joints their names.

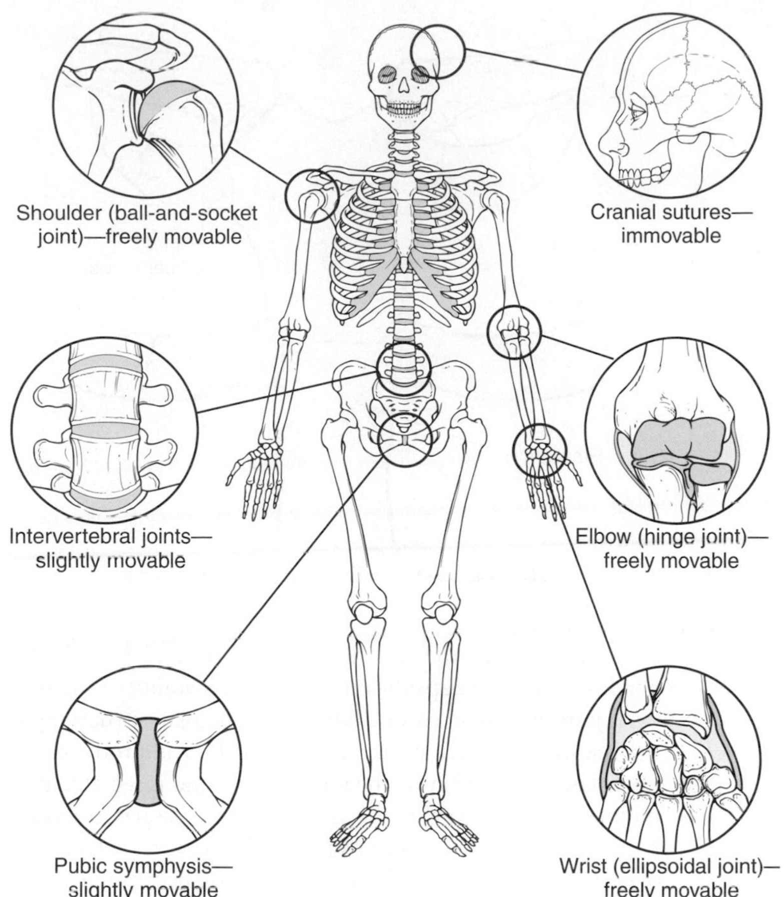

FIGURE 50-6 ■ Examples of types of joints. (From Frazier MS, Drzymkowski JW: *Essentials of human diseases and conditions,* 2nd ed, Philadelphia, 2000, Saunders, p 184.)

Fibrous Structure

In a fibrous joint, bones are united by fibrous tissue. Three types of fibrous joints are found in the human body: suture joints, gomphosis joints, and syndesmosis joints. A suture joint unites bones with a thin but dense layer of fibrous tissue. Interlocking bony ends overlap and increase stability. Suture joints are found only in the skull (Figure 50-7). Fusion of the joint occurs later in life. This bony union is called a synostosis.[2]

The joint that is found between a tooth and the mandible or maxilla is the only gomphosis joint in the human body. The best description of a gomphosis joint is that of a peg implanted into a hole. Fibrous tissue stabilizes the two bony structures and permits little movement.

A syndesmosis joint is a joint in which the two bony components are joined by a ligament or interosseous membrane. These joints normally allow slight movement and are quite functional. The interosseous membrane joining the fibula and the tibia is an example of a syndesmosis joint (Figure 50-8).

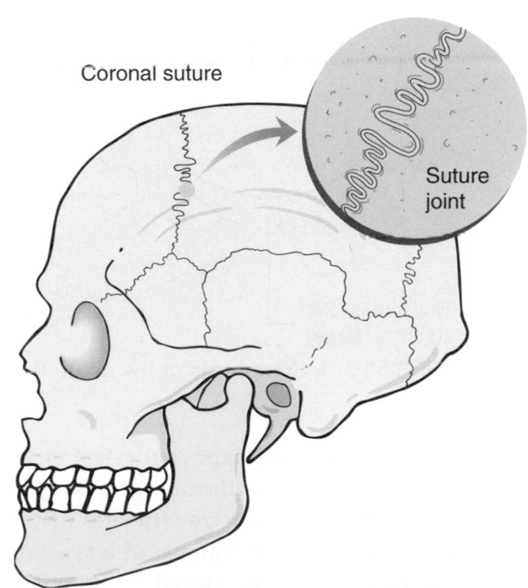

FIGURE 50-7 ■ A suture joint is found only in the skull.

Cartilaginous Structure

Bony segments connected by fibrocartilage or hyaline growth cartilage are classified as **cartilaginous joints.** Symphysis joints and synchondrosis joints are the two types of cartilaginous joints in the body.

A **symphysis joint** connects bony segments by a fibrocartilaginous plate or disk. The symphysis pubis joint (Figure 50-9) joins the two pubic bones of the pelvis. This joint is a weight-bearing structure and is important in transmitting stress and providing stability. Little or no motion is permitted or desired.

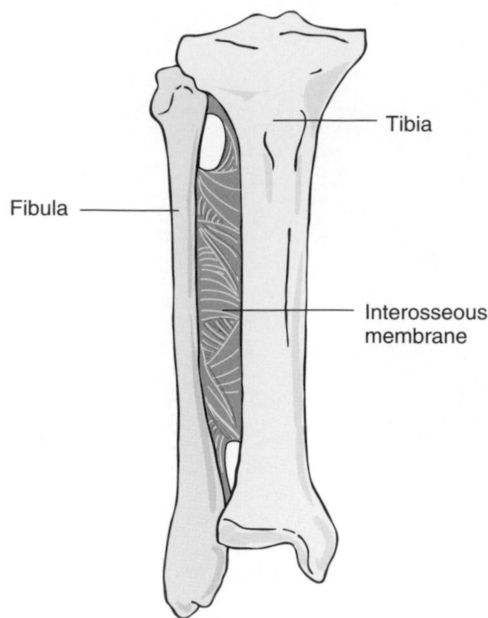

FIGURE 50-8 ■ The interosseous membrane joining the fibula and the tibia is an example of a syndesmosis joint.

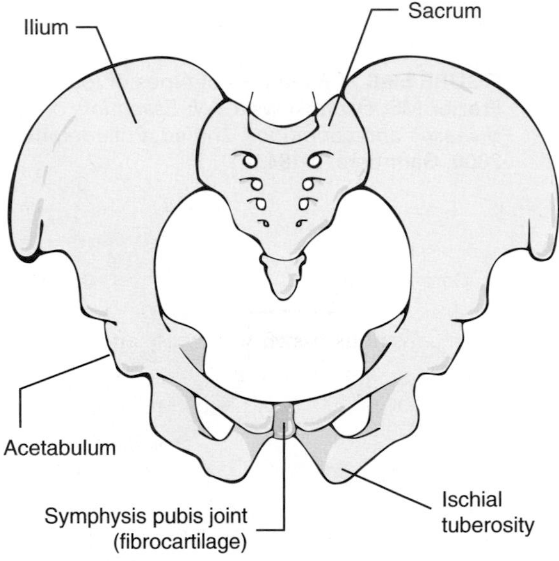

FIGURE 50-9 ■ Symphysis pubis joint.

In a **synchondrosis joint,** cartilage connects bony components. This joint allows bone growth while providing stability. This type of joint can be found at growth sites of the body. The first sternocostal joint is an example of a synchondrosis joint (Figure 50-10). When bone growth is complete, these joints ossify and become unions (synostoses).

Diarthroses

Joints designed to allow mobility are classified as **diarthroses,** or **synovial joints.** These joints are covered with a **joint capsule,** or **synovial sheath.** Movement in these joints is provided by contraction of the muscle-tendon unit, and control depends on the joint capsule and ligaments. Stability of the synovial joint is enhanced by additional soft tissue structures—the menisci, disks, and labra. Synovial fluid is produced by fibroblast-like cells lining the joint capsule and is secreted into mobile joints to provide the lubrication necessary to reduce friction between articulating surfaces. In diarthrodial, or synovial, joints, the bony ends are free to move because no cartilaginous tissue connects the adjacent bony surfaces. The synovial joint connects adjacent bony surfaces through a joint capsule that surrounds the joint.

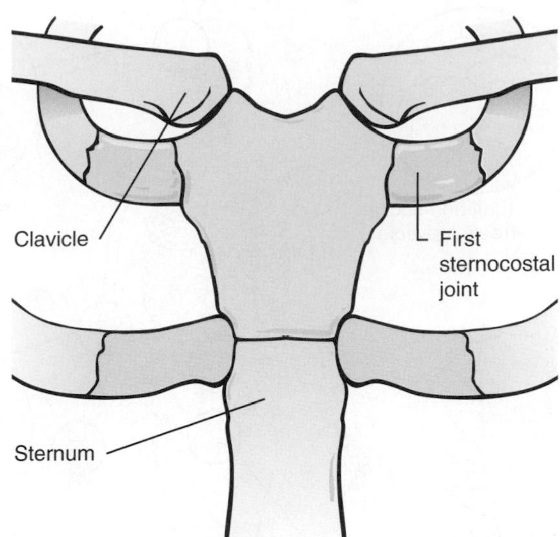

FIGURE 50-10 ■ First sternocostal joint.

Synovial Structure

Features common to all synovial joints include (1) a fibrous joint capsule, (2) a joint cavity enclosed by a joint capsule, (3) a synovial membrane that lines the inner surface of the capsule, (4) lubricating synovial fluid that coats joint surfaces, and (5) hyaline cartilage, which covers the joint surface (Figure 50-11).

Many synovial joints also have accessory structures within the joint capsule. Ligaments, fat pads, disks, and menisci are a few of the structures situated in the capsule that are important to proper function of the joint. Ligaments and tendons keep joint surfaces together and aid in joint motion. Menisci, disks, and synovial fluid limit excessive compression of articulating surfaces.

The lateral and medial menisci of the knee are located on top of the tibia between the tibia and femur (Figure 50-12). These semilunar fibrocartilaginous structures function as shock absorbers in the knee. In cross-section, these wedge-shaped cartilages are thinnest on the inner edge. Around the inner edge, the area of the synovial cavity between a femoral condyle and a meniscus is continuous with that between the meniscus and corresponding tibial condyle. On the outer edge, the cartilages are attached to both the synovial and retic-

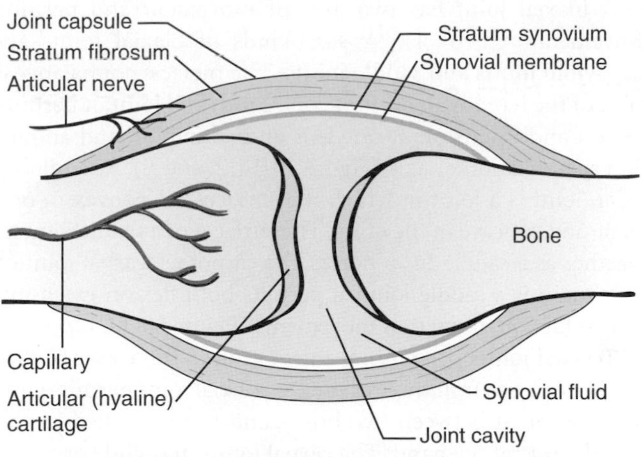

FIGURE 50-11 ■ Typical synovial joint.

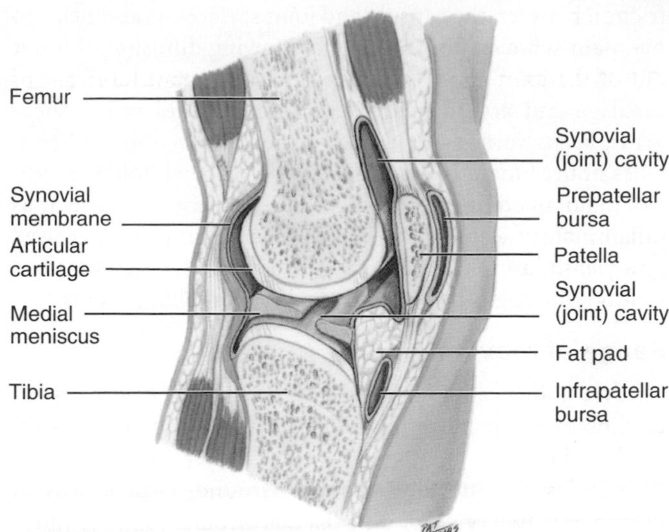

FIGURE 50-12 ■ Schematic drawing of a typical diarthrodial (synovial) joint. (From Applegate E: *The anatomy and physiology learning system,* 2nd ed, Philadelphia, 2000, Saunders, p 115.)

ular capsule. The medial meniscus is attached to the collateral ligament. The lateral meniscus has weak attachments to the lateral area of the capsule, from which it is in part separated by the tendon of the popliteal muscle. It is possible that because the medial cartilage is more firmly attached, it is torn more often than the lateral meniscus, which has no attachment to the fibular collateral ligament and is thus more mobile. Both menisci are anchored to the tibia via strong fibrous bands.

Menisci facilitate rotation at the knee by allowing better contact of the tibial surfaces with the femoral condyles. They function to evenly distribute load bearing on the tibial plateau. Menisci are often torn by rotation of the femur when the knee is flexed.[2] The torn portion of the meniscus locks the joint, with accompanying pain and edema in the knee. If torn, the menisci can be removed; however, weight-bearing areas on the femur and tibia may then decrease by almost 50%.[2]

Intervertebral disks are padlike structures between vertebrae that help bind vertebrae together and act as shock absorbers between adjacent vertebrae. These disks allow slight movement between any two adjacent vertebral bodies. Disks contribute to the natural curves of the spine in the cervical and lower lumbar areas.

Each intervertebral disk consists of an outer annulus fibrosus, or outer fibrous layer, and a nucleus pulposus, or soft center.[7] The annulus fibrosus consists of many layers of fibrous tissue and fibrocartilage that are strongly attached to the ends of the bodies adjoining the disks.

The nucleus pulposus is semigelatinous, containing 70% to 80% water, and is located closer to the posterior edge of the disk. Because of its high water content, the intervertebral disk is prone to dehydration. Even when the vertebral column is not supporting the weight of the body, as in the supine position, intervertebral disks are maintained under pressure by ligaments connecting the arches.[7]

Although the nucleus pulposus is incompressible, its softness allows it to change shape easily. As the vertebral column bends, the nucleus pulposus becomes wedge shaped, with the thin edge in the direction of bending. The annulus fibrosus on this side bulges out and on the opposite side is stretched by its attachment to the adjoining vertebrae.[7]

Pain caused by the pressure of a protruded disk on a nerve root or spinal nerve leads to pain in the area innervated by compressed nerve fibers and is called radicular pain.[7]

Standing and moving causes water to be squeezed out of disks into the blood stream. Bed rest reduces the pressure on disks and water is reabsorbed from the blood stream by the disks.

Joint Capsule. The **joint capsule** is composed of two layers of connective tissue. The outer layer is the fibrous membrane composed of collagenous tissue. It is dense and encapsulates the entire joint. This dense tissue is solidly attached to the periosteum of the adjacent bony components. The fibrous membrane is poorly vascularized and innervated by joint receptors. Joint receptors are able to detect motion, compression, tension, vibration, proprioception, and pain.[2]

The inner layer, or synovial membrane, is highly vascularized and often only one or two cell layers thick. It is minimally innervated and less pain sensitive than other joint components. Since the outer joint capsule as well as ligaments have more abundant nerve endings, pain can be caused by swelling and stretch of the capsule, as in arthritis or infection, or by injury to the ligaments, as in a strain.[2] Articular cartilage has no nerve fibers. A general rule notes that a joint is innervated by the major nerves that cross it. Specialized cells in the synovial membrane, called synoviocytes, synthesize the hyaluronic acid component of synovial fluid. The inner layer of the joint capsule is the entry point for nutrients and the exit point for waste material.

Synovial Fluid. Synovial fluid contains hyaluronic acid, a high molecular weight polysaccharide, and lubricin, a glycoprotein. Hyaluronic acid provides for viscosity and reduces friction between the capsule and joint surfaces. It also helps to maintain synovial fluid volume by slowing diffusion of water out of the joint space. Lubricin is an important lubricant of cartilage and articular surfaces. Synovial fluid resists shear loads, keeps surfaces lubricated to reduce friction, and provides nourishment for cartilage. While synovial fluid is generally maintained at a constant volume, disease states, such as inflammatory arthritis or infection, can stimulate increased synovial fluid production by synoviocytes. The accumulation of fluid outweighs its clearance and joint swelling results.[2]

Range of Movement

Synovial joints can be divided into three main categories according to visible movement allowed at the joint: uniaxial, biaxial, and triaxial.

A **uniaxial joint** allows motion around a single axis of movement. Two types of uniaxial diarthrodial joint are **hinge joints** and **pivot joints.** A hinge, or **ginglymus,** joint permits flexion and extension; an example is the interphalangeal joint of the finger, the elbow, or the knee (Figure 50-13, *A*). A pivot, or trochoid, joint allows rotation as its single axis movement. The superior radioulnar joint of the elbow and the union between the first and second vertebrae are examples of a pivot joint (Figure 50-13, *B*).

A **biaxial joint** has two axes of movement and permits movement in two planes. Two kinds of biaxial joints are **condyloid joints** and **saddle joints.** The metacarpophalangeal joint of the hand is an example of a condyloid joint; it permits flexion and extension at one axis and adduction and abduction around another axis (Figure 50-14, *A* and *B*). A saddle, or sellar, joint is a joint in which the surfaces are convex in one plane and concave in the other. The surfaces of a saddle joint fit together as a saddle fits a horse. The carpometacarpal joint of the thumb is a saddle joint; it permits both flexion-extension and adduction-abduction movements (Figure 50-14, *C*).

Triaxial joints permit movement around three axes so that motion can occur in three planes. A triaxial joint permits gliding movement between two bones and is exemplified by the carpal joints of the hand. The **carpal** joints may glide or rotate relative to the adjacent surfaces. A **ball-and-socket joint** is formed by a ball-like surface fitting into a concave socket. Ball-and-socket joints permit flexion-extension, adduction-abduction, and rotational movements. The hip and shoulder are examples of a ball-and-socket joint (Figure 50-15).

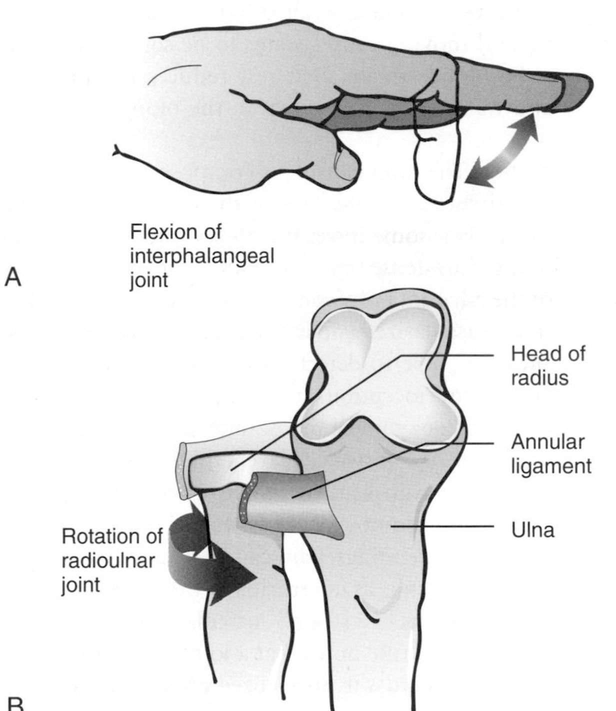

FIGURE 50-13 ■ A hinge joint permits flexion and extension and is represented by the interphalangeal joint of the finger **(A)**. A pivot joint allows rotation and is represented by the superior radioulnar joint of the elbow **(B)**. Both the hinge joint and the pivot joint are considered uniaxial joints because they allow motion around a single axis.

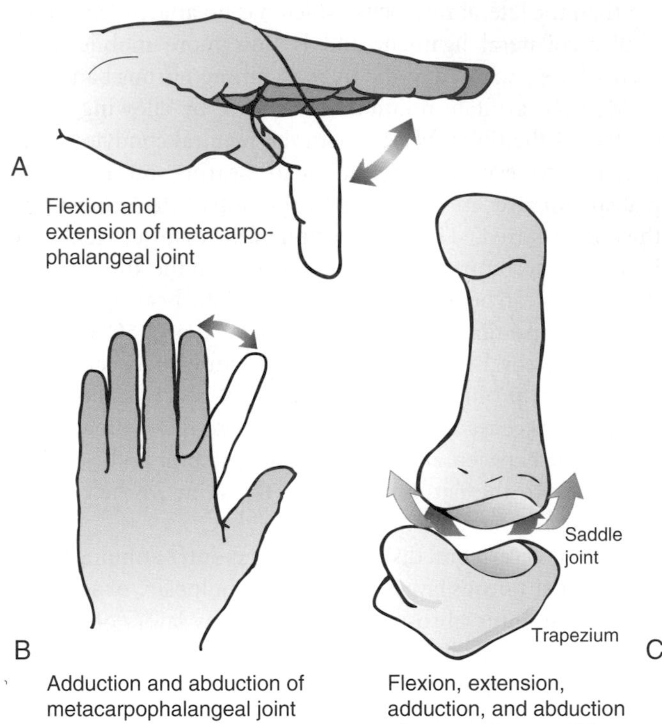

FIGURE 50-14 ■ A condyloid joint permits flexion and extension at one axis and adduction and abduction around another axis; it is represented by the metacarpophalangeal joint of the hand **(A and B)**. Because of its convex and concave surfaces, a saddle joint allows for flexion and extension, as well as adduction and abduction; it is represented by the carpometacarpal joint of the thumb **(C)**. Both the condyloid joint and the saddle joint are considered biaxial joints because they have two axes of movement and permit movement in two planes.

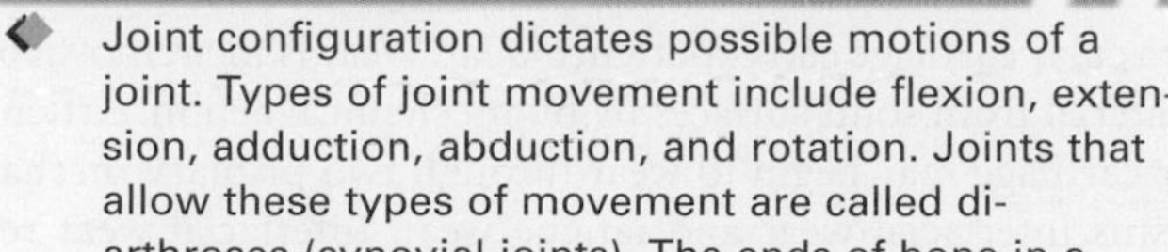

KEY CONCEPTS

- Joint configuration dictates possible motions of a joint. Types of joint movement include flexion, extension, adduction, abduction, and rotation. Joints that allow these types of movement are called diarthroses (synovial joints). The ends of bone in a synovial joint are held together by a joint capsule composed of two layers of connective tissue.
- The lateral and medial menisci in the knee serve as shock absorbers between the femur and tibia. The medial meniscus has strong attachments to the collateral ligaments, whereas the lateral meniscus has weak attachments to the lateral area of the joint capsule. Thus because of its strong attachment the medial meniscus is more likely to be torn than the lateral meniscus.
- Intervertebral disks are padlike structures that act as cushions between vertebrae. A strong annulus fibrosus surrounds a gelatinous, high-water-content nucleus pulposus that can herniate and press on spinal nerves.
- The joint capsule is composed of two layers of connective tissue: an outer fibrous membrane and an inner synovial membrane.
- Synovial fluid provides nourishment and lubrication for cartilage. It becomes more viscous with slow movement and low temperatures and less viscous with fast joint movement and high temperatures.
- Synovial joints are classified according to the visible movements that they allow:
  - Uniaxial: Movement in one plane only (e.g., distal hinge joints of the fingers)
  - Biaxial: Movement in two planes (e.g., thumb saddle joint)
  - Triaxial: Movement in three planes (e.g., ball-and-socket hip joint)
- Some bones are held together by joints that allow little or no movement. These joints are called synarthroses (nonsynovial joints). Examples include sutures between skull bones, tooth-jawbone joints, and the symphysis pubis joint.

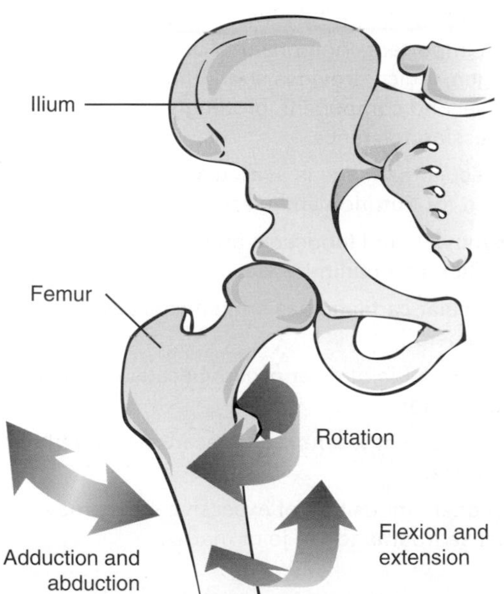

FIGURE 50-15 ■ A ball-and-socket joint permits flexion and extension, adduction and abduction, and rotation; it is represented by the hip joint. A ball-and-socket joint is considered a triaxial joint because it permits movement around three axes; motion can occur in three planes.

STRUCTURE AND FUNCTION OF ARTICULAR CARTILAGE

Articular cartilage appears smooth, shiny, and white on gross inspection. It is a specialized tissue designed to withstand stress imposed by the movement of bony structures. Articular (hyaline) cartilage covers the ends of bone. It functions to distribute joint loads over a wide area, to decrease the stress of prolonged compression from contracting joint surfaces, and to allow movement of joint surfaces with minimal friction and deterioration. Articular cartilage is devoid of blood vessels, lymph channels, and nerves. If a mechanical defect is present, however, this avascular structure can cause major disruption of joint movement.

Composition

Cartilage is hydrophilic in nature, with 65% to 80% of it being primarily water with some inorganic salts, proteins, glycoproteins, and lipids. Its intracellular matrix, which consists mostly of collagen fibers, accounts for almost all of the remaining weight. The cellular component of cartilage, chondrocytes, represents less than 2% of its weight.[2] Although sparsely distributed, chondrocytes manufacture the organic component of the matrix. This organic matrix, or ground substance, is composed of a network of collagen fibrils encased in a solution of **proteoglycans.** The extracellular matrix of cartilage is composed of a fibrous component that includes elastin and different types of collagen. Articular cartilage is primarily avascular and is limited to how much it can regenerate and repair itself.

Functional Properties

Articular cartilage has a biomechanical function. It spreads loads applied to articulating bone ends over a large area to decrease contact stress and limit wear and friction in the joint during movement.[2]

Collagen fibers in articular cartilage are highly structured to provide stability (Figure 50-16). The most important

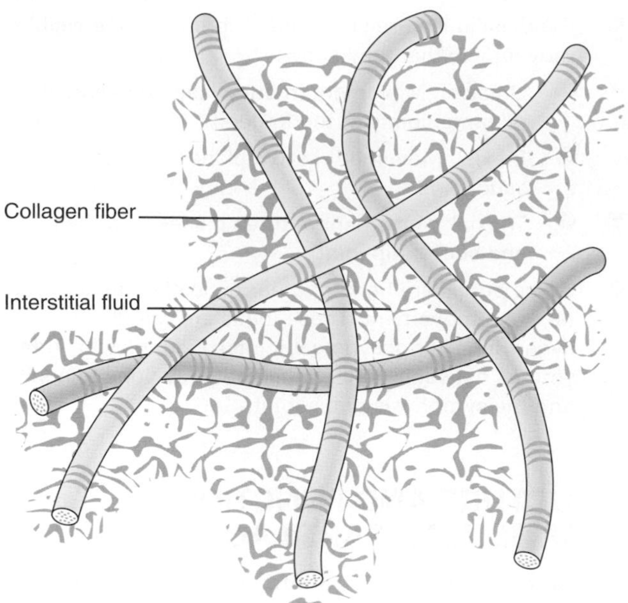

FIGURE 50-16 ■ Collagen fiber in articular cartilage.

mechanical properties of collagen fibers are strength and tensile stiffness. By themselves, collagen fibrils tolerate tension but not compression.

To improve tolerance to compression, cartilage proteoglycan works with hyaluronate to form proteoglycan aggregates. This proteoglycan aggregation fosters immobilization of the proteoglycans within the collagen meshwork, which adds structural rigidity and better compression tolerance to the extracellular matrix.

The importance of proteoglycans and interaction with collagen does not end with an increase in tolerance to compression. Proteoglycans also associate with collagen as a bonding agent to stabilize cross-links between collagen fibers. By maintaining ordered structure and the mechanical properties of collagen fibers, proteoglycans assist in increasing strength.

Articular cartilage requires a sophisticated lubrication process to ensure a decrease in friction between joint surfaces. Without correct lubrication by synovial fluid, articular cartilage will begin to break down as a result of mechanical action of the joint.

Joints are lubricated by two methods. One method is by mechanics of joint physiology. A lubricating coating is formed between the joint surfaces when a weight-bearing force or load is applied to the cartilage and fluid is abstracted from the matrix. The movement of fluid under pressure acts as a self-lubricating mechanism. When the load is removed, liquid from the matrix is reabsorbed by the cartilage.[2] The second method is assisted by glycoproteins covering cartilage and providing a lubricated surface. Lubrication of cartilage from a combination of these two methods decreases friction in the joint. Weight-bearing and joint motion are essential for healthy cartilage. Cartilage will atrophy if joints are not used because cells cannot be nourished by the synovial fluid.[2]

Response to Injury, Stress, and Aging

Articular cartilage can experience wear. Wear is the removal of material from solid surfaces by biomechanical action. Articular cartilage may begin to wear through two primary mechanisms interfacial wear and fatigue wear. Interfacial wear results from the interaction of weight-bearing surfaces by either adhesive or abrasive action. Interfacial wear occurs when joint surfaces come into direct contact as a result of a lack of lubricating film. The non-lubricated surfaces are quite abrasive to each other, and joint surfaces may wear down. Fatigue wear results from repeated deformation secondary to weight bearing. Fatigue wear occurs as a result of the accumulation of microscopic injuries from repeated stress.

Due to the changes in the nature of glycoproteins with aging, cartilage becomes less able to retain water. This "drying out" effect can change the biomechanics of cartilage and lead to increased stress fractures or cracks in the collagen network. Over time and with joint wear, microcracks can accumulate and fragments of cartilage can detach into the joint space creating "loose bodies." The resulting cartilage surface is rough and irregular and subject to further mechanical wear and degeneration. This process can form the basis of osteoarthritis or degenerative joint disease.[8] The effects of aging on the skeletal system are described in The Aging Process: Changes in the Skeletal System.

KEY CONCEPTS

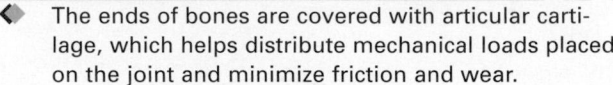

- The ends of bones are covered with articular cartilage, which helps distribute mechanical loads placed on the joint and minimize friction and wear.
- An important component of articular cartilage is collagen, which provides strength and tensile stiffness. A second component, proteoglycan, increases compression tolerance.
- Articular cartilage is avascular and relies on synovial fluid for nutrition and waste removal.
- Synovial fluid lubricates articular surfaces to reduce friction and minimize wear.
- Articular cartilage has limited capacity for repair and regeneration.
- Interfacial joint wear occurs because of insufficient lubrication.
- Fatigue joint wear occurs because of repetitive stress injuries.
- Sudden imposition of excessive stress may also cause trauma to the joint matrix.

STRUCTURE AND FUNCTION OF TENDONS AND LIGAMENTS

Approximately 200 bones in the human skeleton are connected by joints that provide movement and dynamic stability. Ligaments, tendons, and joint capsules provide joint sta-

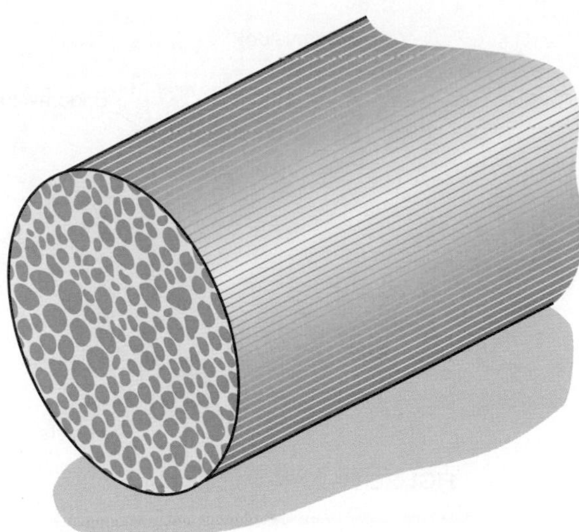

FIGURE 50-17 ■ Parallel bundles of collagen fiber in tendons.

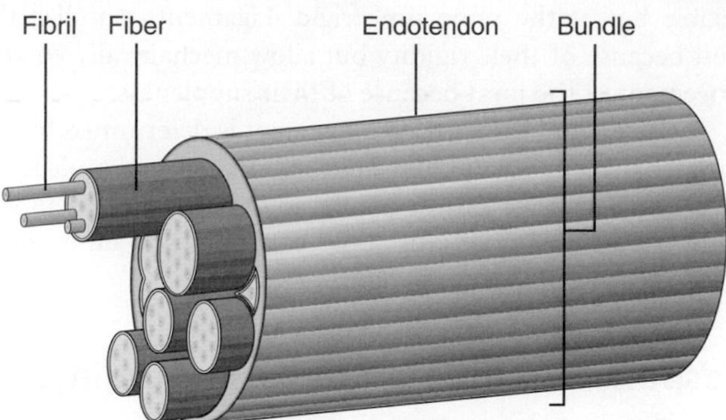

FIGURE 50-18 ■ Schematic representation of a tendon.

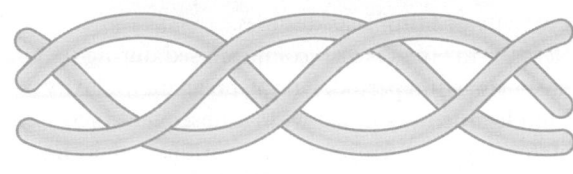

FIGURE 50-19 ■ Triple helix formation of collagen molecules.

bility but not movement because they are not contractile structures. Without joint stability, no movement of the limbs would be possible.

Ligaments and joint capsules connect bone to bone, provide mechanical stability to joints, and guide joint motion. Tendons, through attachment to a contractile structure (muscle) and a rigid object (bone), assist in the generation of movement. Injuries to ligaments and tendons are common, so an understanding of their function and properties is important.

Composition

Tendons and ligaments are dense connective tissue in which collagen fibers are positioned in generally parallel alignment (Figure 50-17). The arrangement of fibers provides greater tensile strength to these tissues. It has been noted that although most collagenous fibers of a tendon run in the same direction, they are not solely parallel. They intertwine to form small bundles, which again intertwine to form the larger parallel bundles that give tendons their unique appearance. As tendons near the bony attachments, larger tendon bundles also intertwine with each other. As a result, pull of any part of the muscle, instead of being limited to a tendon bundle, is spread widely through the tendon. Collagen fibers of the tendon nearest the bone blend into fibrocartilage and then become mineralized, merging into bone and forming a firm attachment.

Ligaments are similar in appearance to tendons, but they unite bone to bone rather than muscle to bone. Most ligaments are composed of dense collagenous tissue, whereas a few consist of almost pure elastic tissue.

Figure 50-18 shows a schematic representation of a tendon. Tendon and ligament tissue is composed of few cells (fibroblasts) and large amounts of extracellular matrix. Approximately 20% of the total tissue is fibroblastic and 80% of the structure consists of extracellular matrix. Of the matrix, 70% is water and 30% is solid material. The solids consist of collagen (75%), ground substance, and small amounts of elastin. Tendons contain more collagen than ligaments do.

Collagen molecules are in a triple-helix formation (Figure 50-19), with hydrogen-bonded water bridges or cross-links providing molecular stability. Cross-links give strength to tissue and increase tolerance to mechanical stress.

The protein **elastin** is found in tendons and ligaments. Elastin provides for some elasticity or extensibility. With the exception of the ligamentum flavum, the majority of tendons and ligaments contain very little elastin, and minimal stretch is allowed. Unlike these stiffer tendons and ligaments, the ligamentum flavum connects laminae of adjacent vertebrae and provides stretch and stability to the spine. The ratio of elastin to collagen fibers in the ligamentum flavum is 2:1.

Ground substance in ligaments and tendons consists of a large amount of proteoglycans, as well as glycoproteins and plasma proteins. The proteoglycan aggregate binds extracellular water in the matrix and acts to stabilize collagen fibers and strengthen ligaments and tendons.

Functional Properties

Tendons and ligaments are quite interesting relative to function. Tendons are extremely strong but can angulate around bony prominences. This capability enables the pull of muscle to change direction and thus improve mechanical leverage. The smooth movement of tendons across bony prominences is facilitated by the presence of bursae. A bursa is a closed sac, lined with mesenchymal cells, which is located where one tissue must glide over another.[2] Ligaments are supple and flexible but at the same time rigid. Ligaments stabilize the joint because of their rigidity but allow mechanically correct movement of the joint because of their suppleness.

The strength of a tendon or ligament is determined by the number and quality of cross-links within collagen molecules. As a child matures into a young adult, the increase in the number and quality of cross-links contributes to an increase in tendon and ligament strength.

Response to Injury, Stress, and Aging

With disuse of muscle, ligaments and tendons lose elasticity and resiliency. With aging, the tensile strength and stiffness of ligaments and tendons decrease as the proliferative and synthetic activity of fibroblasts declines.[9]

Tolerance to stress is also compromised during pregnancy and the postpartum period. During pregnancy, a laxity of tendons and ligaments is noted with a subsequent increased potential for injury. Estrogens relax various pelvic ligaments during pregnancy, and the sacroiliac joint and symphysis pubis become elastic. These alterations allow easier passage of the fetus through the birth canal.

Similar to bone, ligaments and tendons respond to mechanical demands placed on them. Increased stress causes these structures to become stronger and tolerate higher mechanical loads. With a decrease in stress, ligaments and tendons become less stiff and weaker. Immobilization may also decrease the tensile strength of ligaments.

KEY CONCEPTS

- Ligaments and joint capsules connect bones to bones and provide stability to joints.
- Tendons attach bones to muscles to allow movement.
- Tendons and ligaments are composed of dense connective tissue formed by fibroblasts.
- Collagen and elastin are the primary protein components in tendons and ligaments. Most tendons and ligaments have little elastin, which makes them strong but not very compliant. An exception is ligaments that connect adjacent vertebrae, which have more elastin than collagen.
- Tendons are composed of many very fine fibers, each of which originates on endomysium.
- Ligament and tendon strength is determined by the quantity and quality of collagen cross-links.
- Maximal strength is achieved in young adulthood; pregnancy and aging reduce collagen strength.
- Ligaments and tendons respond to increased functional demand by increasing strength. Disuse results in weakened structures.

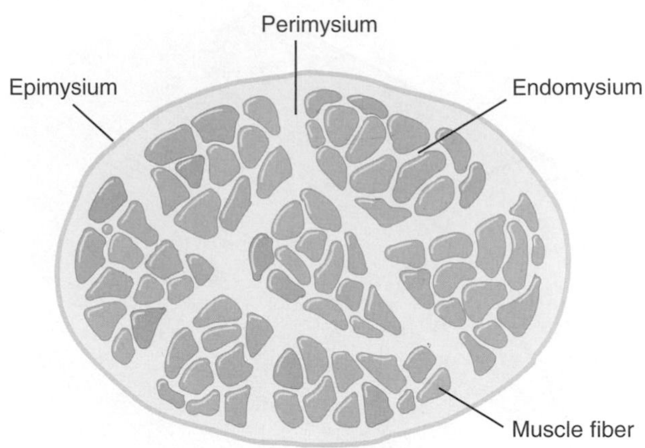

FIGURE 50-20 ■ Muscle fiber.

STRUCTURE AND FUNCTION OF SKELETAL MUSCLE

Approximately 40% of the total body weight is composed of skeletal muscle.[2] Nearly another 10% is smooth and cardiac muscle. Although many of the same principles of contraction apply to these various muscle types, skeletal muscle will be the focus here. Skeletal muscle not only enables bones to move at the joint but also provides strength, stability, and protection to the skeleton by distributing loads and absorbing shock.

Composition

The structural unit of skeletal muscle is the muscle fiber (Figure 50-20). A skeletal muscle is composed of thousands of muscle fibers. Each fiber is a single muscle cell, or myofibril, enclosed in a membrane called the **sarcolemma.** Muscle fibers are grouped together in bundles called **fasciculi.** Individual muscles are composed of many fasciculi. The sarcolemma of individual muscle fiber is surrounded by connective tissue called the **endomysium.** Connective tissue surrounding the fasciculi is called the **perimysium.** Connective tissue surrounding the entire muscle is called the **epimysium.** The epimysium runs continuously with the endomysium and the perimysium (Figure 50-21, *A*). Tendons are attached to bones by Sharpey fibers, which are continuous with the perimysium.

The arrangement of fasciculi varies among muscles and can present a specific visual effect of the muscle (Figure 50-21, *B*). Fasciculi that lie parallel to each other are often found in muscles that function to generate larger range of motion of joints. Muscles, designated as strap or spiral, have fibers situated in parallel arrangements. Fibers situated in an oblique pattern relative to the long axis of the muscle are called **unipennate, bipennate,** or **multipennate** muscles. Pennate (Latin for "feather") muscles usually contain a large number of muscle fibers and can transmit a large amount of force to the muscle tendon. Examples of pennate muscles include the gastrocnemius (a bipennate muscle), the deltoid (a multipen-

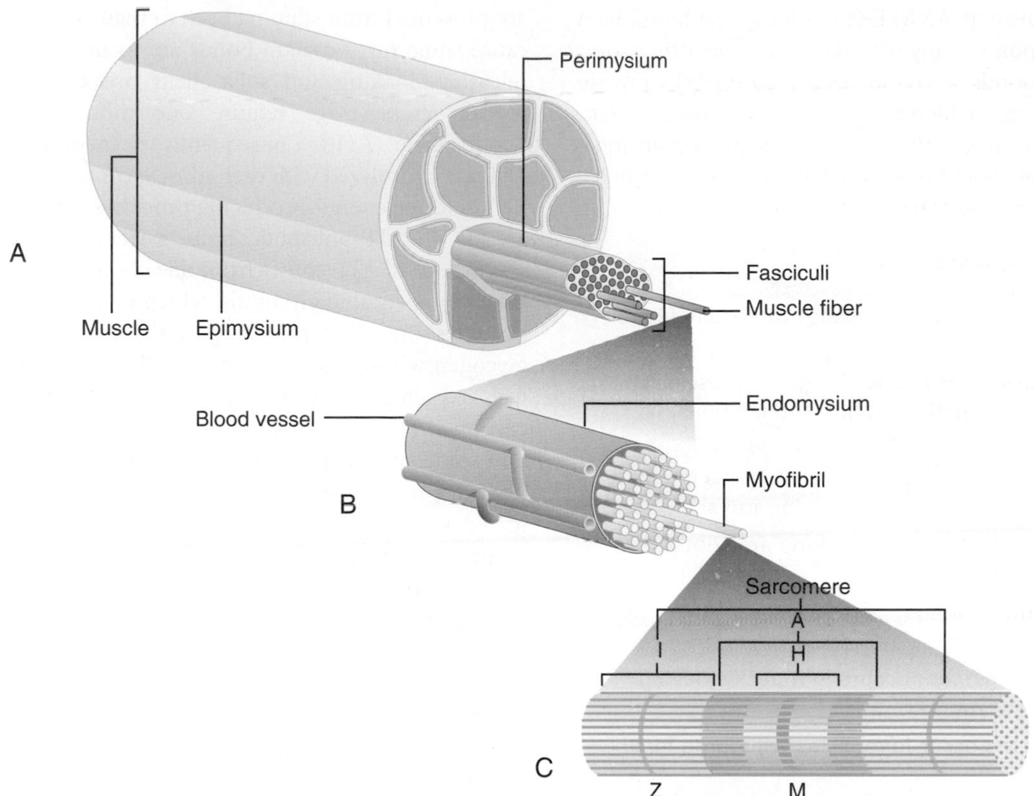

FIGURE 50-21 ■ Muscle fiber. **A,** The epimysium runs continuously with the endomysium and the perimysium. **B,** The arrangement of fasciculi varies among muscles. **C,** The banding pattern apparent on microscopic inspection of a muscle cell results from the organized structure of the proteins (myofibrils) of the contractile apparatus.

nate muscle), and the flexor pollicis longus found in the forearm and serving the thumb (a unipennate muscle).

The cytoplasm of the muscle fiber is called the **sarcoplasm.** Structures composing the sarcoplasm include ribosomes, glycogen, and mitochondria, which are required for cell metabolism. Muscle contraction is accomplished by protein filaments of the contractile apparatus.

Contractile Apparatus

Microscopic inspection of a skeletal muscle cell reveals a typical pattern of banding called **striation.** This striated appearance is due to an organized structure of proteins (myofibrils) of the contractile apparatus (Figure 50-21, *C*). The contractile proteins actin and myosin are called filaments because they are long and narrow. **Myosin** filaments are larger and are referred to as thick filaments. Thin filaments are actually composed of three different types of proteins bundled together. **Actin** is the primary constituent of thin filament, with smaller amounts of the proteins tropomyosin and troponin bound to it.

Thick and thin filaments are specifically arranged in contractile units called **sarcomeres** (Figure 50-22). Sarcomeres are defined by dark bands called **Z lines** that lie perpendicular to actin and myosin filaments. A sarcomere extends from one Z line to the next. Thin actin filaments are attached to Z lines and extend from them. The **I bands** (isotropic) are light in

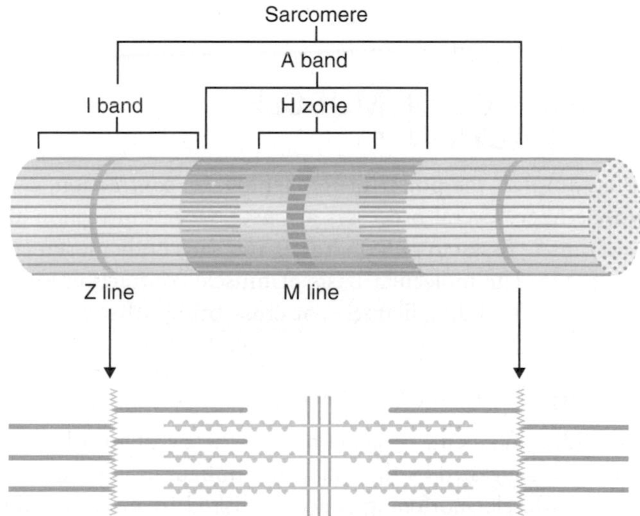

FIGURE 50-22 ■ Thick and thin filaments are organized into contractile units called sarcomeres.

color and correspond to the position of thin actin filaments extending in both directions from the Z line. Thick myosin filaments lie parallel to and between the thin filaments. Each myosin filament is actually surrounded by six thin filaments. The dark **A band** corresponds to an area where actin and myosin filaments overlap. An **M line** marks the center of the A band and the midpoint of myosin filaments. One other zone, the **H zone,** corresponds to a region occupied solely by myosin filaments with no actin filament overlap. An efficient, synchronized contraction is enhanced by this precise arrangement of contractile elements. (See Chapter 17 for a detailed description of contractile filament structure.)

KEY CONCEPTS

- Muscles are composed of bundles of muscle fibers called fasciculi.
- A single muscle fiber is one elongated muscle cell packed with contractile proteins and cytoplasmic organelles.
- Connective tissue encases each fasciculus (endomysium) and the muscle as a whole (perimysium).
- Tendons that attach muscle to bone are continuous with the perimysium.
- The arrangement of fibers within a muscle may be parallel or oblique.
- A parallel arrangement occurs in muscles having greater range of motion.
- Oblique patterns occur in muscles with large force potential.
- Skeletal muscle is striated because of an orderly arrangement of contractile proteins in muscle cells.
- Myosin is the primary component of the thick filament. Thin filaments are composed mainly of actin, with smaller amounts of the regulatory proteins troponin and tropomyosin.

MECHANICS OF MUSCLE CONTRACTION

To accomplish the powerful shortening, or contraction, of a muscle fiber, several processes are necessary. Contraction allows muscle tissue to pull on bones and thus body movement is possible. The molecular basis of muscle contraction is described by the sliding filament, or cross-bridge, theory.

Sliding Filament Theory

The **sliding filament,** or **cross-bridge,** theory of muscle contraction is suggested by the anatomic configuration of the sarcomere. Muscle shortening is accomplished by increasing the amount of overlap of actin and myosin filaments. The Z lines at the ends of the sarcomere move closer together as interdigitating actin and myosin filaments slide past one another. Myosin head groups grip binding sites on actin filaments and pull the thin filaments toward the sarcomere's center. Each time a myosin head binds an actin bead, it forms a **cross-bridge.** Flexible myosin heads move in a ratchet-like manner to tug on actin filaments. Myosin heads bend back and forth, binding and pulling on actin filaments in a steplike fashion. Actin filaments are prevented from slipping back to their original position because some myosin-actin bonds are forming while others are releasing. Making and subsequent breaking of each actin-myosin cross-bridge require one molecule of adenosine triphosphate (ATP). Consequently, tremendous quantities of ATP are hydrolyzed with each muscle contraction.

The three energy-producing processes for ATP production are (1) the ATP-phosphocreatine system in which energy for resynthesis of ATP comes from one compound, phosphocreatine; (2) anaerobic glycolysis, which generates lactic acid but provides some ATP from the partial degradation of glucose or glycogen without oxygen; and (3) the aerobic system, which uses oxygen and has two parts: part A, in which oxidation of carbohydrates is completed, and part B, in which fatty acids and some amino acids are oxidized. The Krebs cycle is the final route of oxidation in both parts. Some protein can be oxidized via the Krebs cycle; thus it is referred to as the final common pathway.[10]

ATP is the immediate source of energy for muscle contraction. Glucose, obtained from glycogen in the muscles and liver, is the primary source of energy for muscle contraction. When enough oxygen is present, glucose is oxidized to carbon dioxide and water. The energy released is partly used to form more ATP. Some energy is wasted in heat. When enough oxygen cannot be supplied via the respiratory and vascular systems, as during intense exercise, glucose is converted to lactic acid. The lesser energy liberated by the reaction contributes to the formation of additional ATP. Lactic acid is basically a poison to muscle and oxygen is needed to remove it, so the muscle is said to have accumulated an oxygen debt. Resting muscle receiving enough oxygen uses the oxygen to re-form glucose and glycogen from lactic acid and oxidize the lactic acid to carbon dioxide and water.[1]

Role of Calcium

Muscle contraction depends on an adequate amount of calcium ion in the cytoplasm. In the absence of free intracellular calcium, no muscle contraction will take place even though myosin head groups have high affinity for actin binding sites. This phenomenon can be explained in the following way. Myosin heads are prevented from binding to actin by **tropomyosin proteins,** which lie on top of actin binding sites. The position of tropomyosin protein is controlled by **troponin.** When calcium is absent, troponin induces tropomyosin to cover the actin binding sites. When calcium is present, troponin allows tropomyosin to move over and uncover the binding sites (Figure 50-23). Cross-bridge formation immediately ensues because myosin heads have a high affinity for these sites in the relaxed state.

Electromechanical Coupling

The nerve impulse that a muscle fiber receives to begin contraction is transmitted through the α motor neuron (Figure

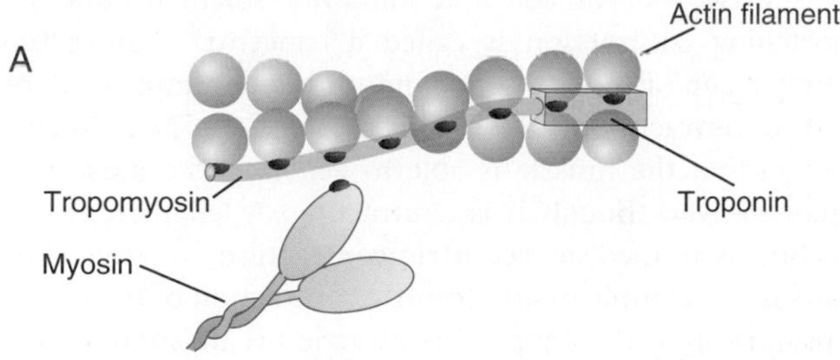

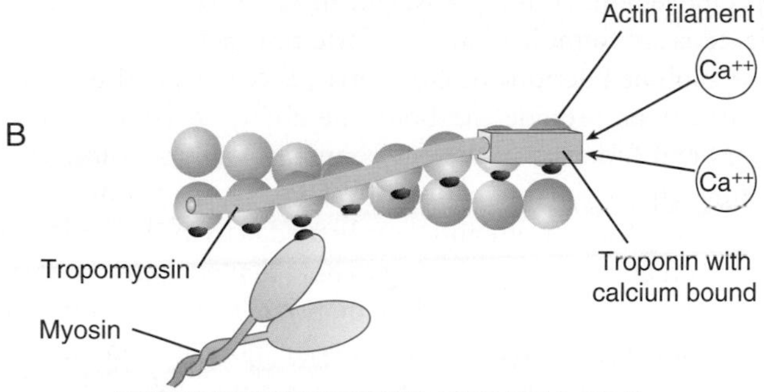

FIGURE 50-23 ■ The proteins troponin and tropomyosin regulate the ability of actin and myosin to form cross-bridges. **A,** In the absence of calcium, tropomyosin covers the binding sites on actin and inhibits cross-bridge formation. **B,** In the presence of calcium, troponin induces the tropomyosin to uncover the actin binding sites and allows cross-bridge formation.

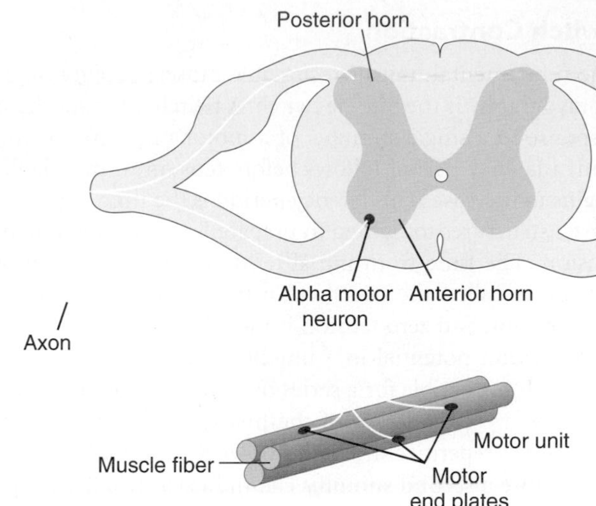

FIGURE 50-24 ■ Relationship of the α motor neuron to the motor unit of muscle. The nerve impulse that a muscle fiber receives to begin contraction is transmitted through the α motor neuron. All muscle fibers innervated by a single motor neuron are part of one motor unit.

50-24). The neuron's cell body is located in the anterior horn of the spinal cord. The axon extends from the cell body to the muscle and divides into many small branches. Each branch ends in a structure called a **motor end-plate.** The end-plate is positioned near the sarcolemma of a single muscle fiber. All muscle fibers innervated by a single motor neuron are part of one motor unit (see Figure 50-24).

After the nerve impulse is transmitted from the cell body, it passes along the axon to the motor end-plate. Acetylcholine is released into the neuromuscular synapse and diffuses across to bind with receptors on the skeletal muscle cell. More than enough acetylcholine is released with a single action potential to ensure depolarization of the muscle cell. Acetylcholine binding opens channels in the membrane that allow Na^+ to flow into the cell. Depolarization of the motor end-plate area to threshold then opens voltage-gated channels and produces an action potential. An enzyme (acetylcholinesterase) in the synapse quickly degrades acetylcholine to stop receptor activation. The sarcolemma is depolarized and an action potential spreads along the surface of the sarcolemma and into the interior of the fiber through the transverse tubules (T tubules). The **sarcoplasmic reticulum,** a calcium-storing structure, fills the space between myofibrils and forms sacs. The sacs, the terminal cisternae, are positioned close to the T tubules. When the action potential passes down the T tubules, free calcium from the terminal cisternae is released into the myofibrils. Release of the calcium ions stimulates the actin-myosin cross-bridge thereby causing muscle tension. After depolarization, or when the sarcolemma becomes electrically stable, calcium ions rebind in the sarcoplasmic reticulum and the muscle fiber relaxes.

The motor unit is the functional unit of skeletal muscle and consists of the α motor neuron and all of the muscle fibers that it innervates. When stimulated, all of the muscle fibers innervated by a motor unit will respond as one. This response is called the **all-or-none response,** which means that the motor unit will contract to its maximum or it will not contract. The size of the contraction of the muscle depends on the number of motor units recruited. The greater the demand placed on the muscle or the more stimuli provided, the greater the number of motor units firing. Fibers of each motor unit are not in contact with each other but are dispersed throughout muscle and intermixed with other fibers. If a single motor unit is stimulated, a large section of muscle visibly contracts. If additional motor units of the nerve are stimulated, the muscle can contract with greater force. **Recruitment** is the term used for calling in more motor units in response to an increase in stimulation of the motor nerves.

Types of Muscle Contraction

Electromyography is used to evaluate muscle contraction. With electromyography, aspects of the contractile process such as time relationships between the beginning of electrical activity and the actual contraction of the muscle may be studied. The mechanical response of a muscle to electrical stimulation causes movement in the joint, control of joint motion, or joint stabilization.

Twitch Contraction

The fundamental unit of recordable muscle activity on electromyography is the muscle twitch. A **twitch** is the mechanical response to a single stimulus of a motor unit. After stimulation, a latency period follows before tension in muscle fibers begins to increase. This **latency period** is the time required for elastic structures to tighten to prepare for the development of tension. The time from initial tension development to peak tension is called the **contraction time.** The period between peak tension and zero tension is the **relaxation time.**

An action potential in a muscle lasts only a fraction of a second. It is possible for a series of action potentials to be initiated before completion of the first twitch. The mechanical response to repetitive stimuli is known as **summation.** The period before a second stimulus can induce a twitch during the latency period of the first muscle twitch so no additional response of the muscle occurs is termed the **refractory period.**

The frequency of motor unit stimulation is quite variable. The greater the frequency of stimulation, the greater the tension produced in the muscle. A muscle may achieve higher levels of work when it shortens right after being stretched. The elastic components of muscle do not entirely account for this phenomenon. Some energy must be stored in the contractile component of muscle. If the stimulus is so great that the ability of the muscle to increase tension is exceeded, the muscle is said to be in tetanus. In this situation, the speed of stimulation is faster than the contraction-relaxation time of the muscle. Little relaxation occurs before the next contraction.

The variable grade of contraction demonstrated by muscles is important. Repetitive twitching of all recruited motor units develops as a summation of contractions of the muscle, which is responsible for the smooth movements of skeletal muscle.

Based on the mechanical activity that they exhibit, muscles can be divided into two groups: **slow twitch** (type I, red) and **fast twitch** (type II, white). Slow-twitch fibers contract and relax more slowly. They support high levels of oxidative metabolism instead of using glycolytic processes to produce energy. Continual energy is provided by large amounts of myoglobin, which potentiates the action of stored oxygen. Slow fibers are modified for either prolonged or continuous muscle activity such as in the case of endurance marathon running and posture. These muscles have a high content of myoglobin and are thus red.[1]

Fast-twitch muscle fibers depend on energy released from the glycolytic process. Type II fibers are used for fast muscle contractions such as in distance sprinting, blinking of an eye, or jumping. Because of the lack of myoglobin in their fibers, they are white. Fast-twitch fibers fatigue more easily than slow-twitch fibers.[1]

Concentric, Eccentric, and Isometric Contractions

Contraction of a muscle exerts a force that causes a torque, or turning, effect on the joint involved. When muscle force generates sufficient tension to overcome the resistance of a limb, the muscle will shorten and joint movement occurs. This shortening contraction is called a **concentric contraction.** Lifting a cup of water to one's mouth is an example of a concentric contraction. If the load is greater than the amount of tension that the muscle is able to generate, the muscle will lengthen even though it is contracting. A lengthening contraction is termed an **eccentric contraction.** Walking down stairs is an example of an eccentric contraction of the quadriceps muscles. A third type of contraction is an **isometric contraction.** No movement occurs, and the muscle maintains its specific length. Holding a weight in the hand with the elbow flexed is an example of an isometric contraction.

Combined actions of concentric, eccentric, and isometric contractions provide the body the ability to control movement and function in the environment. Walking, eating, and lifting require the interaction of various types of contractions to provide for smooth and coordinated activity. In a rehabilitative situation, it is interesting to note that isometric contractions generate greater tension than concentric contractions do. Eccentric contraction may generate more tension than isometric contractions do. When using strengthening programs in rehabilitation settings, a working knowledge of strengthening and tolerance of traumatized tissue is imperative to ensure safe reconditioning.

Mechanical Principles

The amount of tension that a muscle can generate is dictated by a number of mechanical concepts or principles of relationship. These principles include the length-tension relationship, load-velocity relationship, force-time relationship, and effects of muscle temperature and muscle fatigue. Muscle tension, fatigue, and prestretching are other important factors in muscle force production. A brief review follows.

Length-Tension Relationship

Maximal tension is produced when muscle is at its usual resting length because this position allows actin and myosin filaments to overlap and provide the maximal number of cross-bridges between filaments. At a short resting length, little tension or muscle shortening is possible inasmuch as myosin filaments abut the Z line. If muscle fiber is held at lengths beyond the resting length, tension decreases because actin and myosin do not overlap and therefore no active tension is present.

Load-Velocity Relationship

The velocity of the shortening of a muscle contracting concentrically is inversely related to the load applied. The lower the weight, the higher the velocity is. The greater the weight, the slower the contraction of the muscle is. An isometric contraction occurs when the load equals the amount of force that the muscle exerts. If the load exceeds the force generated by the muscle, an eccentric contraction occurs. The greater the load, the faster the eccentric lengthening.

Force-Time Relationship

The longer the time of contraction, the greater the force that the muscle can generate until the muscle reaches its point of maximal tension. An increase in the duration of force allows higher levels of tension to be produced by the contractile structures.

Effects of Temperature Change

Conduction velocity across the sarcolemma increases with a rise in muscle temperature. Temperature elevation increases the enzymatic activity of muscle metabolism and the elasticity of collagen in elastic components. Muscle temperature increases when athletes warm up as a result of the increased blood flow and heat generated by metabolism. Both changes increase the amount of force that a muscle can produce.

Effects of Prestretching

A muscle can do more work when it shortens immediately after being stretched in a concentrically contracted state from a state of isometric contraction because of the elastic energy stored in the series elastic component and energy stored in the contractile component.

Effects of Fatigue

The availability of ATP determines muscles' ability to contract and relax. Prolonged activity of muscles can be sustained only when the muscle has an adequate supply of nutrients and oxygen to synthesize ATP. If the activity is of sufficient intensity to deplete ATP faster than it can be replaced, muscle tension will gradually weaken and at some point drop to zero. When muscle returns to its original state, creatine phosphate, a major storage form of energy in muscle, must be resynthesized and glycogen stores replaced. This revitalization process requires energy, so the muscle will continue to consume oxygen at high rates even after termination of activity. Heavy, rapid breathing continues after a period of strenuous exercise to provide adequate oxygen for ATP synthesis. This oxygen is also essential for removing lactic acid from muscle. Resting muscle uses oxygen to re-form glucose and glycogen from lactic acid and to oxidize the lactic acid to carbon dioxide and water.[1]

Response to Movement and Exercise

Early mobilization may prevent muscle atrophy after surgery or injury. With early motion, muscle fibers position themselves in a more parallel alignment as opposed to the fibers in an immobilized individual. With movement, capillarization occurs more rapidly and tensile strength improves more quickly. With immobilization, the cross-sectional area of muscles decreases and oxidative enzyme activity is reduced. Early mobility prevents atrophy. Afferent impulses from the muscle spindles are increased, thus improving the stimulation of some muscle fibers.

Physical training and conditioning increase the cross-sectional area of muscle fibers. An increase in area coincides with an increase in muscle bulk and strength. In addition, stretching exercises are effective in preventing injury and improving performance, as well as increasing muscle flexibility, maintaining and improving joint motion, and enhancing the elasticity and length of the musculoskeletal unit.

KEY CONCEPTS

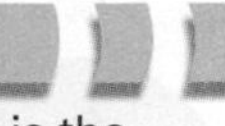

- The fundamental unit of muscle contraction is the sarcomere.
- A sarcomere extends from one Z line to the next and consists of interdigitating thick and thin filaments.
- Muscle contraction occurs when myosin head regions bind to sites on the actin filament to form cross-bridges.
  - After binding, myosin tugs on the actin filament, which causes thick and thin filaments to overlap more.
  - Myosin then releases and proceeds to bind at another point farther along the actin filament. Each cross-bridge cycle requires one molecule of ATP.
- For contraction to occur, the cytoplasm must have sufficient calcium ions.
  - In the absence of calcium, tropomyosin covers binding sites on the actin filament and prevents cross-bridge formation.
  - Another regulatory protein, troponin, controls the position of tropomyosin.
  - When calcium is bound to troponin, tropomyosin is moved to expose binding sites on actin and cross-bridge formation ensues.
- Calcium ions are stored in the sarcoplasmic reticulum and released into the cytoplasm when the muscle cell depolarizes during an action potential.
- A group of skeletal muscle cells innervated by a single motor neuron is called a motor unit. All of the cells in the unit contract simultaneously when the motor neuron depolarizes.
  - An action potential in the α motor neuron releases acetylcholine at the motor end-plate. Acetylcholine binds to receptors on the muscle cell membrane and triggers an action potential in the cell. To generate more force in the muscle, a greater number of motor units can be activated, a process termed recruitment.
- Activation of a motor unit by a single action potential results in a brief twitch contraction.
- A train of action potentials in the motor neuron results in a sustained contraction, in which calcium is released into the cytoplasm faster than it is removed.

- Sustained contraction in response to repetitive stimulation is termed summation.
- Muscle contraction does not always result in muscle shortening.
  - Isometric contraction refers to contraction with no change in muscle length.
  - Eccentric contraction occurs when the muscle lengthens while contracting (because of a high load).
  - Muscle shortening with contraction is termed concentric.
  - Isometric contraction generates greater tension than concentric contraction does; eccentric contraction may generate the highest tension.
- The behavior of contracting muscle is governed by several mechanical principles:
  - Length-tension relationship: Up to a point, a greater resting length of the muscle generates a greater force of contraction. Optimal actin-myosin overlap occurs at about the usual resting muscle length.
  - Load-velocity relationship: The velocity of muscle shortening is inversely related to the applied load.
  - Force-time relationship: A longer contraction is associated with a greater force of contraction.
- Creatine phosphate is a storage form of energy that is quickly converted to ATP when cellular ATP levels fall.

THE AGING PROCESS

Changes in the Muscular System

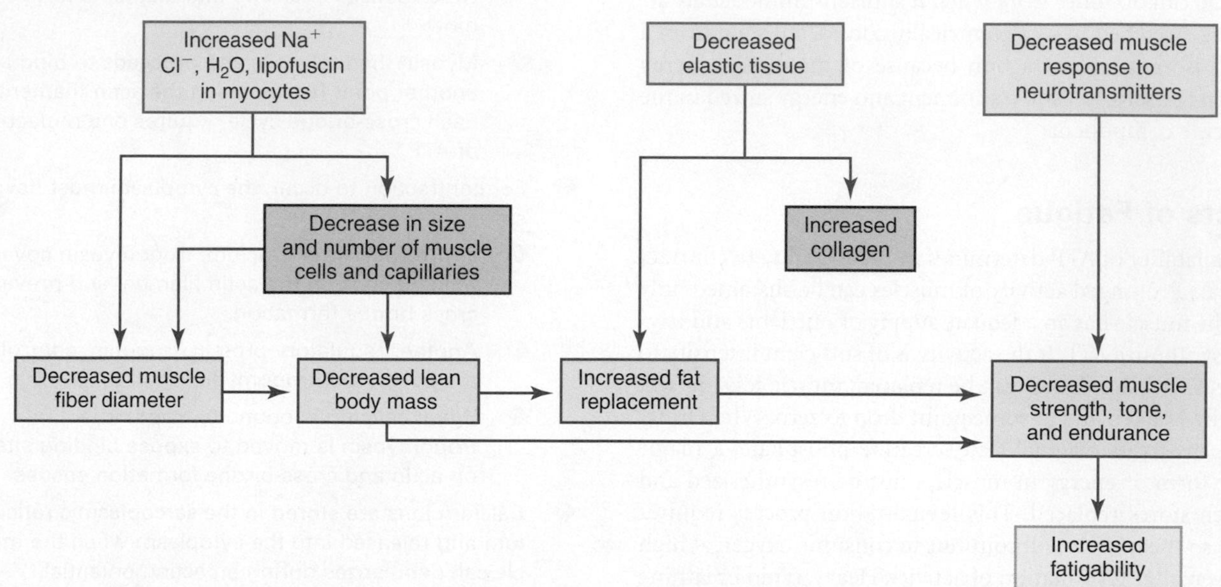

With aging, the size and number of muscle cells decrease. The remaining muscle cells undergo atrophy, decreased muscle fiber diameter, and reduced elastic tissue. These changes result in reduced muscle mass. Within muscle cells, extracellular sodium, chloride, water, and lipofuscin pigment increase, with diminished intracellular potassium. The loss of muscle protein may not be obvious because of increased collagen and fat replacement.

Because fewer capillaries are available to supply the muscles, removal of metabolites is decreased. Hormonal stimulation of muscle by testosterone, somatotropin, and thyrotropin is decreased, in addition to reduced muscle uptake of glucose during exercise.

Muscle response to nervous system stimulation is decreased with decreased muscle norepinephrine. Muscles are also less responsive to neurotransmitters, including acetylcholine at the myoneural junction, and cholinesterase activity is decreased as well.

The muscle, neural, and hormonal changes of aging that affect the muscular system lead to a functional decrease in muscle strength of 30% to 50%, reduced muscle endurance, diminished muscle tone, and increased fatigability. Muscular decline rises with increasing age and usually occurs earlier in men; however, the extent of muscular system decline varies. An elderly individual with good nutritional balance and protein intake combined with adequate active exercise maintains muscle function and strength.

- Fatigue results when energy and nutrient supply are insufficient.
- A higher rate of muscle oxygen consumption occurs during and for a period after muscle activity.
- Lack of muscle use (disuse) leads to a reduction in muscle mass and slowing of oxidative enzyme activity.
- Early activity after injury is associated with quicker recovery of tensile strength, less atrophy, and better circulation.

SUMMARY

The musculoskeletal system provides movement for the body. Alterations in function of the musculoskeletal system that decrease the efficiency of movement can often magnify the stress placed on uninvolved structures and increase the potential for degeneration, joint laxity, and pain.

A sound knowledge base of the anatomy, physiology, and mechanics of movement makes the diagnosis of aberrant movement and function easier and thus aids in planning the necessary care and education of patients. Too often, in attempts to provide relief for patients with musculoskeletal dysfunction, the tissue involved or the mechanism of activity causing the injury is not properly identified. Short-lived relief of pain may be provided through the use of analgesics. However, return to activity exacerbates pain and the restriction of movement present before medical care.

Familiarity with the musculoskeletal system also allows health care providers to identify basic tissues involved in injury or disease. Such awareness empowers the clinician to provide relief of pain as well as address quality-of-life issues. Determination of the type of activity that creates the problem and identification of segments of the musculoskeletal system affected provide the basis to achieve positive long-lasting improvement. Weakness, instability, or decreased motion of structures involved in the dysfunction must be identified. Analysis of physical limitations can lead to patient education and referral to sources that can reduce the impact of physical limitations. In addition, the use of tested exercise, modification of living and working environments, and education of family members will help affected individuals achieve optimal motor function and prevent further injury. The effects of aging on the muscular system are described in The Aging Process: Changes in the Muscular System.

MEDIA RESOURCES

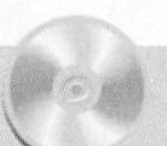

evolve

Remember to check out the ***CD Companion*** included with this book for Review Questions, Key Concepts Review, Glossary (with audio for selected terms), Disease Profiles, and Animations.

PLUS, visit the ***Evolve website*** at http://evolve.elsevier.com/Copstead/ for Case Studies, Disease Profiles, and WebLinks.

References

1. Guyton AC, Hall JE: *Human physiology and mechanisms of disease,* ed 10, Philadelphia, 2000, Saunders.
2. Ruddy S, Harris ED, Sledge CB, editors: *Kelley's textbook of rheumatology,* ed 6, Philadelphia, 2001, Saunders.
3. Favus MJ, editor: *Primer on the metabolic bone diseases and disorders of mineral metabolism,* ed 4, Philadelphia, 1999, Lippincott-Raven.
4. Chapman MW et al, editors: *Chapman's orthopaedic surgery,* ed 3, Philadelphia, 2001, Lippincott Williams & Wilkins.
5. Wolff J: *Des Gesetz der Transformation der Knochen,* Berlin, 1892, Hirschwold.
6. Giangregorio L, Blimkie CJ: Skeletal adaptations to alterations in weight-bearing activity: a comparison of models of disuse osteoporosis, *Sports Med* 32(7):459-476, 2002.
7. Koopman WJ, editor: *Arthritis and allied conditions,* ed 14, Philadelphia, 2001, Lippincott Williams & Wilkins.
8. Klippel JH, editor: *Primer on the rheumatic diseases,* ed 12, Atlanta, 2001, Arthritis Foundation.
9. Beers MH, Berkow R, editors: *The Merck manual of geriatrics,* Rahway, NJ, 2000, Merck.
10. Foss ML, Keteyian SJ: *Fox's physiological basis for exercise and sport,* ed 6, Boston, 1997, WCB/McGraw-Hill.

chapter 51

Alterations in Musculoskeletal Function: Trauma, Infection, and Disease

Carol L. Danning

MEDIA RESOURCES

Additional Material for Study, Review, and Further Exploration

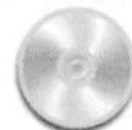

CD Companion ◆ Review Questions and Answers ◆ Key Concepts Review
◆ Glossary *(with audio pronunciations for selected terms)*
◆ Disease Profiles ◆ Animations

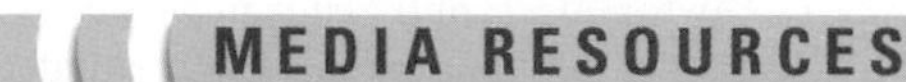

evolve ***Website*** at http://evolve.elsevier.com/Copstead/
◆ Case Studies ◆ Disease Profiles ◆ WebLinks

KEY QUESTIONS

- What is the process and duration of normal bone healing after a fracture?
- How are osteoporosis, osteomalacia, and rickets similar and how do they differ?
- What are the clinical findings and management of bone infections?
- What terminology is used to describe primary bone tumors?
- How can clinical manifestations of soft tissue injuries be used to differentiate noncontractile and contractile injuries?
- What are the manifestations and management of compartment syndrome?
- What are the cause and pathogenesis of muscular dystrophy and myasthenia gravis?

CHAPTER OUTLINE

A smoothly functioning musculoskeletal system facilitates a complete range of human actions, including walking, talking, running, breathing, and a myriad of voluntary physical activities. Any abnormality in the musculoskeletal system decreases the efficiency of movement and increases mechanical stress. Ballistic requirements of many sports and occupations, such as skiing and driving an automobile, have increased the potential for trauma. Diseases also disrupt the integrity of the musculoskeletal system. Infectious processes, genetic abnormalities, and nutritional deficiencies may all affect movement.

Clinicians who work with patients experiencing dysfunctions of the musculoskeletal system must have a solid background in evaluation and management of such disorders. Without this preparation, interventions will not be sufficient to promote maximal functional return. This chapter discusses lesions particular to the musculoskeletal system as they affect the skeletal frame, soft tissue, and muscles.

BONE AND JOINT TRAUMA

The skeletal system is subject to alterations in function from mechanical stress and infection. The purposes of the skeletal system are to protect internal organs, contribute to mineral homeostasis, produce blood cells, and provide muscle attachment sites and thus facilitate body movement. Bone is one of the body's hardest structures, as well as one of its most dynamic and metabolically active tissues. Bone is vascular with a capacity for repair. It adapts to mechanical demands placed on it and alters its configuration in response to those mechanical stresses.

Types of Bone

Two basic forms of bone are present in the human body: cortical bone and cancellous bone. **Cortical bone** forms the cortex, or outer shell, of the bone. Cortical bone is designed to tolerate compression and shearing forces, but tension forces may exceed the tolerance of cortical bone. Most fractures are due to tension failures in which bone is pulled apart. With bending, twisting, or straight tension, stress may exceed the bone's tolerance, and a fracture occurs on the convex side of the bend. **Cancellous bone,** which has a spongy or lattice-like appearance, is found in the interior of bones. Unlike cortical bone, cancellous bone does not tolerate compression stress. Cancellous bone provides structural support to cortical bone and increases a bone's potential to withstand stress.

Fracture

A **fracture** is a break in continuity of a bone, an epiphyseal plate, or a cartilaginous joint surface. Trauma generating enough energy to fracture a bone also produces force sufficient to traumatize adjacent soft tissue. With that concept in mind, the remainder of this section will address injury to the bony component of the musculoskeletal system.

Types of Fracture

Fracture type reflects the type of tension stress placed on bone (Figure 51-1). A **transverse** fracture occurs in a straight line at approximately a 90-degree angle to the longitudinal axis of the bone. **Spiral** fractures are the result of rotational forces and cause bone to separate in the form of an S around the bone. **Longitudinal** fractures split bone along its length. **Oblique** fractures result from a rotational force, but unlike spiral fractures, the break is along an oblique course (45-degree angle) and does not rotate around the entire bone. **Comminuted** fractures consist of more than one fracture line and more than two bone fragments. These fragments may be shattered or crushed. Comminuted fractures often present considerable treatment problems because of associated soft tissue damage and multiple bone fragments. An **impacted** fracture is caused by excessive force that telescopes or drives one fragment into another. A **greenstick** fracture is an incomplete break in the bone with the intact side of the cortex flexed. It is usually seen in children. A **stress** fracture is a failure of one cortical surface of the bone, often caused by repetitive activity such as running. Without proper treatment, a stress fracture can become a complete fracture with two distinct fragments. An **avulsion** fracture is separation of a small fragment of bone at the site of attachment of a ligament or tendon.

Of special concern are fractures at or near a joint line in children. This location of a fracture may suggest an epiphyseal growth plate fracture (Figure 51-2). With epiphyseal injuries, the potential for disruption of growth of the long bones is present. Proper reduction and fixation are necessary to avoid growth disturbance in fractures through the growth plate. Crush injury to the epiphyseal plate commonly leads to premature growth cessation. Cancellous bone does not tolerate compression stress; it buckles and then cracks. Therefore, **crush** or **compression** fractures (Figure 51-3) are consistent with cancellous bone trauma. In children, a compression injury to cancellous bone of the metaphysis of a long bone is identified as a **buckle** fracture, where bone buckles and eventually cracks. In adults, compression fractures are often found in a vertebral body of the spine, especially in older people with osteoporosis.

Extent of Fracture

Fractures can be classified according to extent and depth. A **displaced** fracture is one in which the ends of fracture fragments are separated. In a **nondisplaced** fracture, the fracture

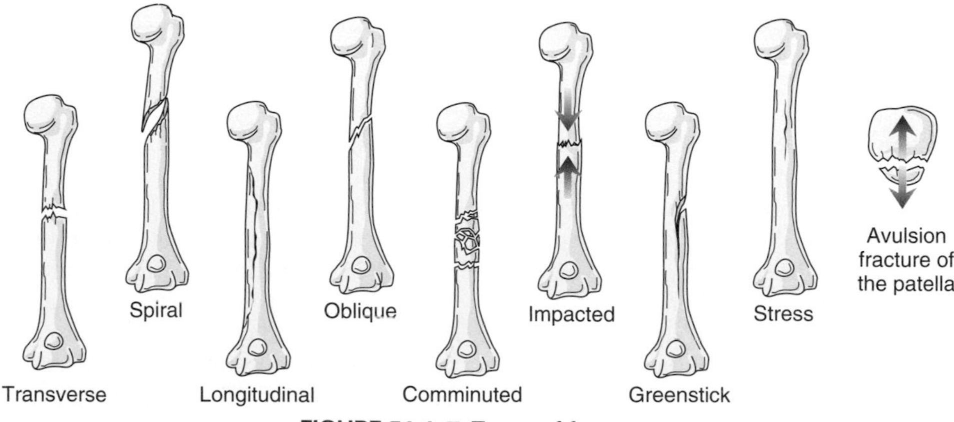

FIGURE 51-1 ■ Types of fracture.

fragments remain in alignment and position. With a **depressed** fracture, the fragment is displaced below the level of the surface of the bone, usually in the skull. A **complete** fracture is one in which the fracture line disrupts bone continuity through the whole thickness of the bone, including the cortex (Figure 51-4). In an **incomplete** fracture, the cortex of the bone buckles or cracks; however, bone continuity is not disrupted. Incomplete fractures tend to occur in the more flexible, growing bones of children. Fractures can also be classified as **open** (compound) or **closed** (simple) (Figure 51-5). An open fracture occurs when bone is broken and an external wound leads to the fracture site. These fractures present an increased risk of infection and are therefore difficult to manage.

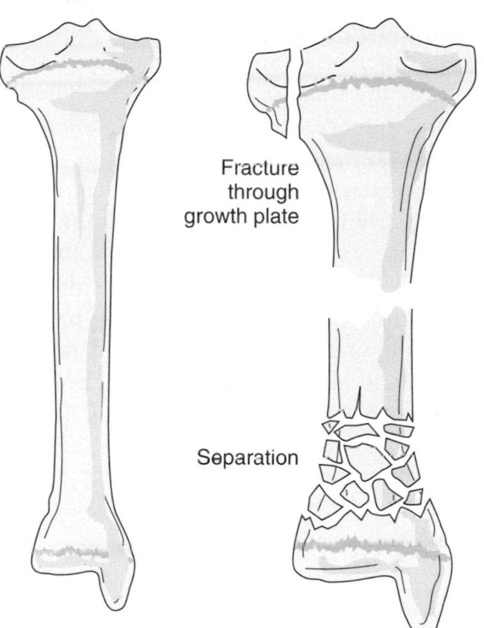

FIGURE 51-2 ■ Epiphyseal injury.

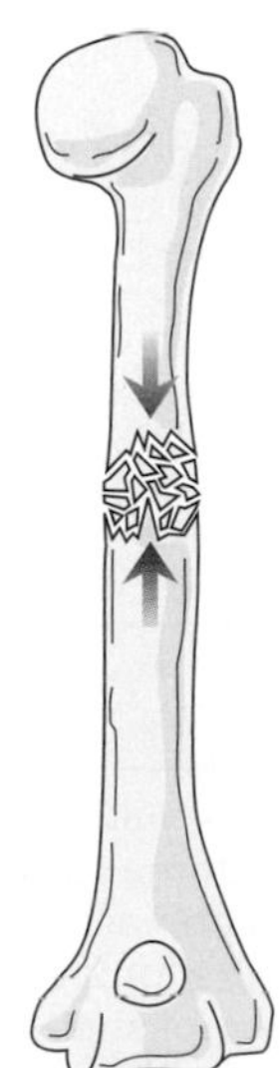

FIGURE 51-3 ■ Compression fracture.

A closed fracture is a fracture in which the fragments do not extend through mucous membrane or skin and skin is not broken.

In cases of open fractures, a wound classification system may be used that ranges from type I to type IIIC in increasing degree of severity. Type I is a wound smaller than 1 cm, moderately clean with minimal contamination. The fracture is simple transverse or oblique fracture with a bone spike piercing the skin. Soft tissue damage is minimal. Type II wounds are larger than 1 cm with moderate contamination.

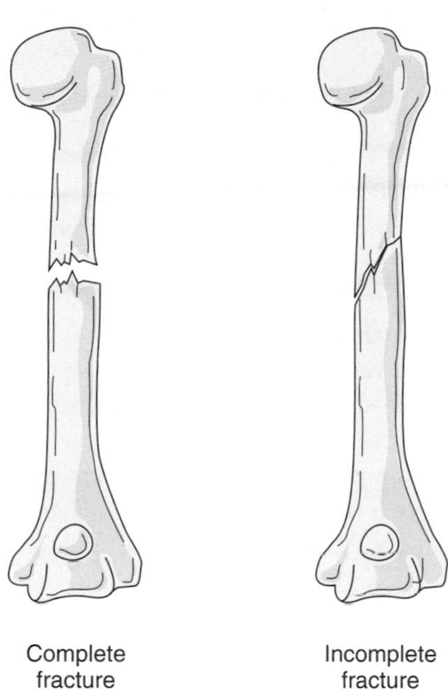

FIGURE 51-4 ■ Comparison of complete and incomplete fractures.

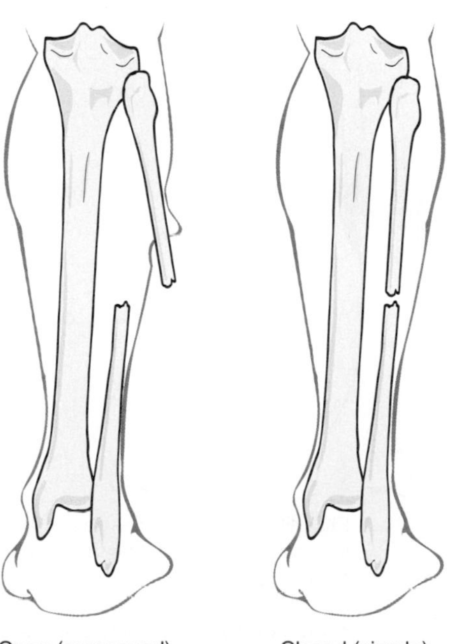

FIGURE 51-5 ■ Comparison of open and closed fractures.

The fracture might be a moderate comminution or crush injury with moderate soft tissue damage. Type III wounds have a high degree of contamination. The fracture is severely comminuted and unstable. It is accompanied by much soft tissue damage involving muscle, skin, and neurovascular structures. Traumatic amputations would be classified here. With type IIIA wounds, soft tissue coverage of the fracture is sufficient. Segmental or severely comminuted fractures occur with these wounds. Type IIIB wounds with open fractures include extensive injury or loss of soft tissue, as well as periosteal stripping and bone exposure. Fractures are severely comminuted. Massive contamination is found with such wounds. Type IIIC wounds include any open fracture associated with arterial injury requiring repair regardless of the extent of soft tissue injury.[1]

Healing Process

When a fracture occurs, the continuity of both cortical and cancellous bone is usually compromised. The five stages of fracture healing are described in Chapter 50.

Healing in a Cortical Bone. At the time of fracture in a cortical bone, blood vessels in the haversian systems are torn. After a period of bleeding, clotting occurs at the fracture site and for a short distance on both sides of the fracture. Because of lack of circulation, a small section of bone distal to the fracture site undergoes necrosis (Figure 51-6). The avascular bone eventually is replaced by living bone through resorption and bone deposition. The majority of bleeding occurs from arteries in the periosteal sleeve.

The hematoma that forms becomes the medium for early stages of healing. Osteogenic cells, which develop from the periosteum, form the external and internal callus. If the periosteum is severely torn, healing cells must proliferate from the mesenchymal cells of surrounding soft tissue. During the early stages of repair, the amount of osteogenic tissue is extensive. Within the first few weeks, the thick mass of osteogenic tissue has formed a fracture callus.

During the initial stages of **callus formation,** no bone cells are present within the matrix. The callus is quite soft but becomes progressively firmer. With consolidation of the fracture callus, new bone formation begins. Initially, new bone forms at the edges of the periosteum, where the blood supply is more substantial. Where blood supply is sufficient, osteogenic cells differentiate into osteoblasts and primary woven bone. Near the fracture site, where the blood supply is less adequate, osteogenic cells initially differentiate into chondroblasts (cartilage).

As both the external callus (which unites cortical bone) and the internal callus (which unites cancellous bone) harden from the cartilage stage through ossification, the fracture site becomes firm and stable. No movement is detected by the medical evaluator or client. At this point the fracture is clinically united. Although stable, cartilage and primary woven bone may be found intermixed at the site of healing.

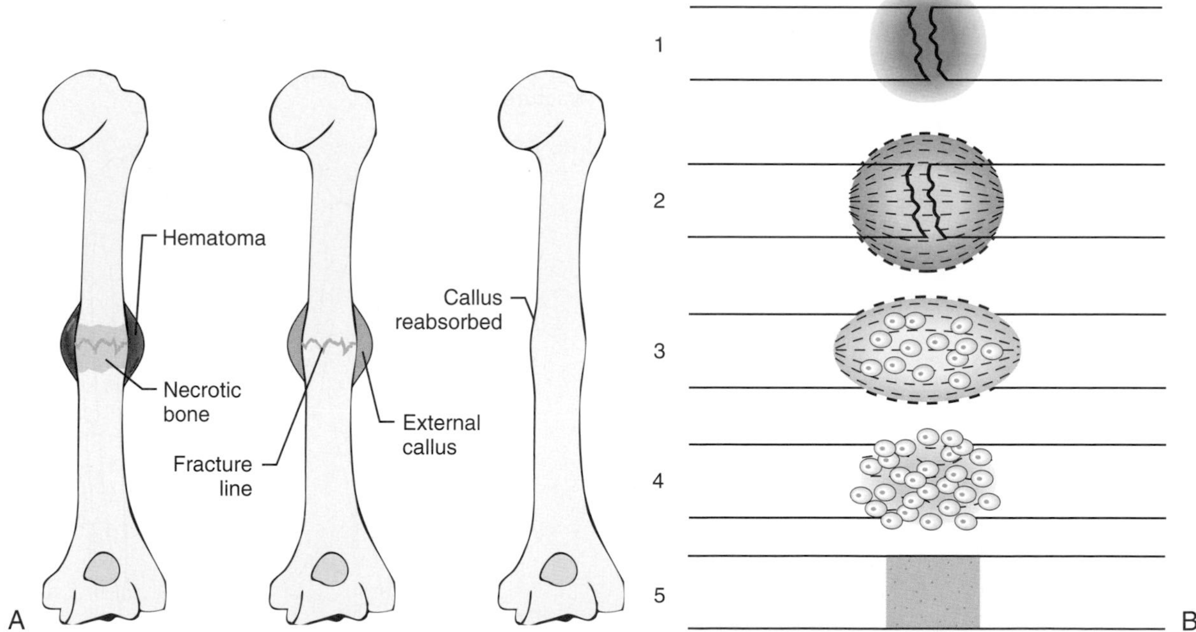

FIGURE 51-6 ■ **A,** Stages of healing of cortical bone. **B,** Bone healing (schematic representation). *1,* Bleeding at broken ends of the bone with subsequent hematoma formation. *2,* organization of hematoma into fibrous network. *3,* Invasion of osteoblasts, lengthening of collagen strands, and deposition of calcium. *4,* Callus formation: New bone is built up as osteoclasts destroy dead bone. *5,* Remodeling is accomplished as excess callus is reabsorbed and trabecular bone is laid down. (**B,** From Lewis SM, Heitkemper MM, Dirksen SR: *Medical-surgical nursing,* ed 6, St Louis, 2004, Mosby, p 1658.)

With time, the primary callus is replaced by mature bone, and any excess callus is reabsorbed. This phase is the remodeling (last) stage of bone healing. When all immature bone cells have been replaced by mature lamellar bone, the fracture is said to be consolidated (radiographic union).

Healing in a Cancellous Bone. Cancellous fracture healing occurs mainly through development of an internal callus. The rich blood supply present in cancellous bone prevents necrosis of bone at the fracture site. If the fracture is nondisplaced, the healing process is much more rapid than that of cortical bone. Osteogenic cells in the trabeculae form the primary woven bone in the internal fracture hematoma (Figure 51-7). The internal callus fills the open space of cancellous bone and crosses the fracture site. Woven bone develops and is eventually replaced by lamellar bone. As noted earlier, cancellous bone is susceptible to compression forces, and the majority of injuries incurred are compression-type fractures. With a compression fracture, fragments of bone are impacted together, which provides a more suitable environment for healing of cancellous bone. Rapid union occurs because fracture fragments move in unison.

Treatment. Medical treatment for a fracture consists of stabilization of the fracture site until healing is sufficient to allow stress to be placed on the structure. Rehabilitation of a patient with a fracture really begins at the time of release from treatment, when the fracture has had time to heal.

Complications in Bone Healing

Delayed Healing. Fracture healing may not always progress smoothly without complications. Delayed union, malunion, and nonunion of the fracture are all complications that might occur. Delayed union is usually identified anywhere from 3 months to 1 year after the fracture, when bone pain and tenderness are continuously increasing beyond the expected healing period for the wound type. Healing is slowed. The cause of delayed union might be either distraction of fracture fragments or systemic causes such as infection. Bone healing can be delayed by additional factors such as smoking, malnutrition, use of corticosteroids, and poor vascular circulation to the area.[1]

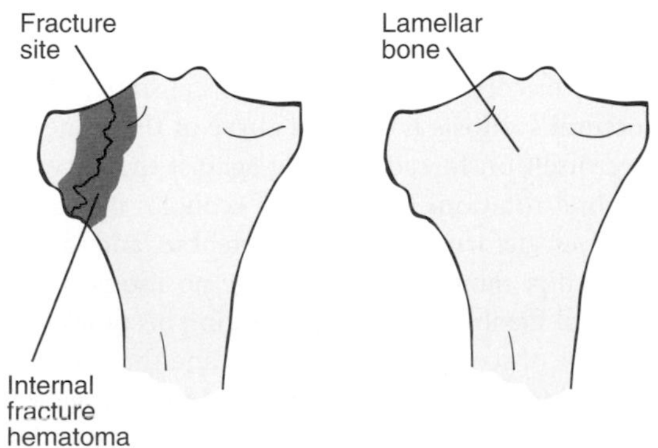

FIGURE 51-7 ■ Healing of cancellous bone.

Malunion results when unequal stresses of muscle pull and gravity lead to improper alignment of fracture fragments. It often happens in the case of fractures managed with cast immobilization after skeletal traction. Malunion may also happen if an ambulatory device is applied before the fracture is firm or if the extremity is subjected to weight bearing too early in the healing process. Primary features of malunion are external deformity and radiographic evidence of internal derangement. Prevention is adequate reduction and immobilization of the fracture and adherence to specific activity and positioning restrictions.[1]

Nonunion occurs when a fracture has not healed by 4 to 6 months after a fracture. Failure to heal is due to poor blood supply and repetitive stress on the fracture site, and can be the result of interposition of muscle, tendon, or soft tissue between fracture pieces; prolonged or excessive traction; poor immobilization that allows motion at the fracture site; poor internal fixation; or wound infection after internal fixation.

Treatment. Treatment includes bone grafting, internal/external fixation, electrical bone stimulation, or any combination of these methods.[1] Bone grafts bridge gaps in bone. In normal bone healing, when bone is compressed, it becomes electronegative, thus stimulating bone formation. Negative current applied through the use of a bone stimulator is believed to induce bone formation similar to that stimulated by bone compression.[1]

Soft Tissue Complications in Bone Healing. Soft tissue as well as bone is subjected to insult when the stress is of sufficient magnitude to cause a fracture. Soft tissue is also stressed with the immobilization requirements of a healing fracture. Rehabilitation of a fracture site is, in reality, rehabilitation of soft tissue surrounding the site. Although soft tissue injuries are discussed in more depth later in this chapter, compartment syndrome and neurovascular injuries are discussed here.

Although bone may heal without complication, surrounding tissues may have complications. Compartment syndrome and neurovascular injuries are two examples. A compartment is an area in the body where muscles, nerves, and blood vessels are enclosed within tissue such as fasciae. **Compartment syndrome** is a result of high pressure in a muscle compartment in the closed fascial space. Capillary pressure is reduced below what is essential for tissue viability. Compartment syndrome may be classified as acute, chronic, or crush. In the case of a fracture, the acute classification is of concern because it is the most severe form and often requires surgery urgently.

Compartment syndrome can be triggered by injury to the tissues surrounding bone with soft tissue inflammation, swelling, and, in some cases, hemorrhage into the area. Decreased blood flow from arterial damage can also occur, which leads to hypoxia of the cells of capillary walls. Capillary integrity is diminished, and colloid proteins and fluid escape into the extravascular tissues causing further swelling. Intracompartment pressures increase because the fasciae enclosing the compartment are restrictive. If the tissue pressure exceeds the intravascular pressure, blood vessels will collapse impeding blood flow and leading to further hypoxia and worsening edema. Intracompartment pressures of 30 to 40 mm Hg can compromise microcirculation in muscle. The excessive compartment pressures lead to hypoxia, damage, and eventual necrosis of the soft tissue, especially muscles and nerves. Emergent decompression is needed to preserve limb viability. Compartment syndrome can also occur due to extrinsic compression, such as that of a cast on an injured, swollen limb.[1] Symptoms of compartment syndrome are pain out of proportion to the injury, paralysis, paresthesia, pallor, and pulselessness.

Neurovascular injury after a fracture may be due to either the fracture or the treatment for the fracture. Neurovascular damage occurring at the time of fracture may be the result of either the force causing the fracture, fracture fragments, hemorrhage, joint dislocation, or the body position assumed after trauma. Neurovascular damage related to treatment may be due to moving or splinting the fracture, manipulation at the time of reduction of the fracture, application of stabilizing devices such as a cast or splint, or hemorrhage or edema.

Dislocations and Subluxations

Two additional mechanical alterations in the musculoskeletal system are dislocations and subluxations. A **dislocation** is displacement of a bone from its normal position to the extent that articulating surfaces lose contact.[1] A **subluxation** is displacement of a bone from its normal joint position to the extent that articulating surfaces partially lose contact.[1] A dislocation or subluxation can occur when forces cause one aspect of the joint complex to move beyond its normal anatomic limit. A considerable amount of tissue damage occurs in dislocation and subluxation, including possible ligament tear or rupture. With any dislocation, especially first-time dislocation, evaluation for a fracture is necessary. Although almost any joint may dislocate, some joints are more prone to dislocation than others. Joints most commonly dislocated are small joints of the fingers, the patella, and the shoulder. Symptoms of dislocation are pain, alteration in the normal contour of the joint, change in extremity length, and loss of normal mobility. Treatment must include consideration of local soft tissue trauma and healing.

KEY CONCEPTS

- Bones are subject to different types of fracture, depending on the type of tension stress imposed.
- Fractures can be classified according to the orientation of the break as transverse, longitudinal, oblique, or spiral.
- A comminuted fracture consists of more than one fracture line and more than two bone fragments.
- A greenstick fracture is an incomplete break.
- Fractures are classified as open or compound when the skin is penetrated and as closed or simple when the skin is not broken.
- Healing of fractured cancellous bone occurs more quickly than healing of cortical bone.
- Trauma causes hematoma formation, followed by callus formation.
- The callus is initially soft and cartilaginous; then it progressively ossifies to become firm and stable.
- The fracture is clinically stable when no movement at the break is detectable.
- Radiographically apparent union occurs when the callus has been completely replaced by mature bone.
- Healing of fractured bone is contingent on stabilization and time.
- Complete separation of joint articulating surfaces is termed dislocation. Subluxation refers to partial separation. Soft tissue damage is the primary problem.

ALTERATIONS IN BONE MASS AND STRUCTURE

Scoliosis

Etiology and Pathogenesis. **Scoliosis** is a lateral curvature of the spine resulting in an S- or a C-shaped spinal column with vertebral rotation. Scoliosis can be a consequence of numerous congenital, connective tissue, and neuromuscular disorders. Seventy-five percent to 85% of all cases of scoliosis are classified as idiopathic.[1] Scoliosis occurs in approximately 5% of children screened for scoliosis. About half of the children, in whom scoliosis is diagnosed, require treatment, with the majority being female.

Clinical Manifestations. Scoliosis may be described as either structural or nonstructural. Nonstructural scoliosis resolves when the patient bends to the affected side. No vertebral rotation or bony deformity of the vertebrae is present, and the condition is not progressive. When the patient bends laterally, the spine usually appears symmetric. The scoliotic curve will disappear on forward flexion. Nonstructural scoliosis may be related to postural problems, hysteria, nerve root irritation, inflammation, or compensation caused by leg length discrepancy or contracture (in the cervical spine).[1]

Structural scoliosis is a lateral curve of the spine that fails to correct itself on forced bending against the curvature and has vertebral rotation. This type of scoliosis is more serious and involves deformity of the vertebrae and asymmetric changes in hip, shoulder, and rib cage positions. The patient lacks normal flexibility, and side bending becomes asymmetric. This type of scoliosis is progressive and the curve does not disappear on forward flexion. Structural scoliosis generally requires intensive therapy or surgical intervention to halt progression and correct deformities.

Scoliosis is detected by typical asymmetric changes (Figure 51-8), including (1) uneven shoulders or hips, (2) shoulder or scapular prominence, (3) rib or chest hump when bending over, and (4) a C- or S-shaped spine. Scoliosis is usually diagnosed after puberty because of a tendency for the curve to be accentuated during periods of rapid skeletal growth. The diagnosis is confirmed by radiographic examination of the spine. The degree of curvature is determined from radiographs and is classified as right or left, depending on the direction of convexity. Surgery is indicated for curvatures of 40 degrees or greater. Less significant degrees of curvature may be managed conservatively with exercise and frequent reevaluation to assess progression to more significant deformity.

In addition to body image disturbances, scoliosis predisposes a patient to a number of physiologic problems. Respiratory difficulties from restricted expansion of the lungs may occur. Severe forms may be associated with significant pain. Gastrointestinal dysfunction can result from compression of abdominal organs. If uncorrected, scoliosis may progressively worsen with age owing to increased upper body weight and gravitational forces exacerbating the vertebral deformity.

Treatment. Treatment for structural scoliosis is aimed at correcting spinal malalignment. Nonsurgical measures include primarily braces and exercises. Bracing applies constant pressure to the spinal convexity to straighten the curve. Braces must be worn for prolonged periods each day to be effective. Compliance is a major difficulty because the braces are stiff and uncomfortable. Spinal muscle strengthening should accompany brace therapy because trunk musculature loses tone after prolonged bracing.[1] Surgical intervention includes spinal realignment, fusion, and bracing with internal appliances, and most surgical procedures require prolonged body immobilization postoperatively.

Conditioning exercises to strengthen muscles and correct posture are used to treat nonstructural, or postural, scoliosis.

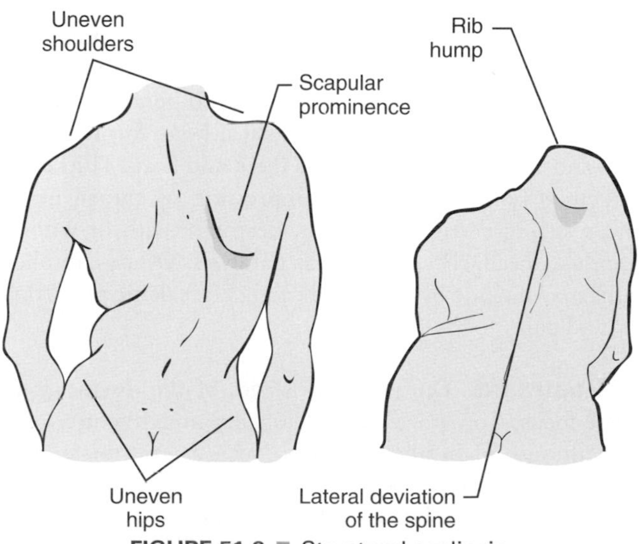

FIGURE 51-8 ■ Structural scoliosis.

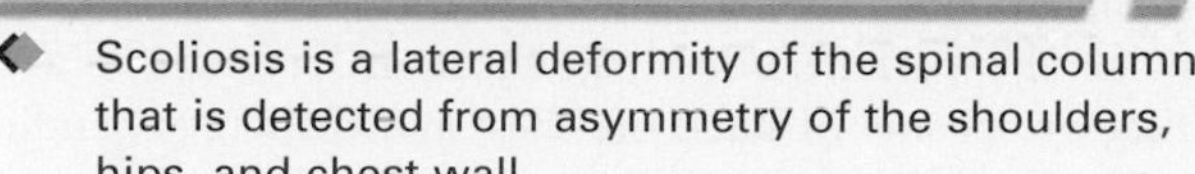

KEY CONCEPTS

- Scoliosis is a lateral deformity of the spinal column that is detected from asymmetry of the shoulders, hips, and chest wall.
- Scoliosis may be described as structural or nonstructural.
- Severe scoliosis can compromise lung expansion and lead to a restrictive respiratory disorder.

Osteoporosis

Etiology and Pathogenesis. **Osteoporosis,** the most common metabolic bone disease, affects approximately one in two women and one in five men older than 60 years. It occurs when the rate of bone resorption is greater than that of bone formation. The normal osteoblastic and osteoclastic balance is disrupted, and mineral and protein matrix components are decreased. Trabeculae are decreased in amount, and width and bone mass is decreased. This process leads to fragile bone and thus fractures. Cancellous bone is lost faster than cortical bone, with fractures happening sooner in cancellous bone (vertebrae) than in cortical bone (femoral neck). A current definition of osteoporosis is based on gradations of low bone mass. The World Health Organization defines osteoporosis as "bone mineral density (BMD) more than 2.5 standard deviations below the peak BMD of gender- and ethnicity-matched 30-year-old healthy Caucasian women."[2]

The specific cause of osteoporosis is not known. However, the rate of bone loss is influenced greatly by age, genetics, estrogen, and risk factors. A family history of osteoporosis is a major risk factor. The normal bone loss that occurs with aging is accelerated during menopause, with the most rapid phase of loss occurring in the first 5 years due to the sudden decrease in estrogen. The exact mechanisms of estrogen action are unclear, but estrogen derivatives may influence osteoblast activity and the production of local cytokines and growth factors that modulate the balance of bone resorption and formation. Estrogen deficiency increases the risk of osteoporosis by stimulating bone resorption over formation.[3] Other risk factors include small frame, Caucasian or Asian race, early surgically induced menopause, high doses of thyroid medication, use of corticosteroid drugs (such as prednisone), a diet low in sources of calcium and vitamin D, physical inactivity, and excessive smoking or increased alcohol intake. Patients with chronic renal disease often have abnormal parathyroid function, as well as altered calcium and vitamin D metabolism, which can lead to a decline in bone mass. Furthermore, chronic inflammatory diseases, such as rheumatoid arthritis or systemic lupus erythematosus, can be associated with increased risk of osteoporosis, even independent of corticosteroid use.[3]

Clinical Manifestations. On physical examination the patient may have a Colles fracture, femoral or hip fractures, or vertebral compression fractures. Obvious kyphosis of the thoracic spine (dowager's hump) may be present. The patient often has shortened stature, muscle wasting or spasms of back muscles, and difficulty bending over. The patient may complain of impaired breathing (because of deformities of the spine and rib cage) and poor dentition. Laboratory tests may show normal urinary and serum calcium, phosphorus, and alkaline phosphatase but elevated serum osteocalcin levels. Radiographic and computed tomographic findings may show diffuse radiolucency of bones, sparse transverse trabeculae, normal vertical trabeculae, indistinct articular cortices, wedge-shaped thoracic vertebrae, biconcave lumbar vertebral bodies, and possibly old or new compression fractures.

Treatment. Treatment varies depending on the cause. Adequate dietary intake of calcium is required and vitamins, especially vitamin D, may be prescribed. Estrogen replacement therapy may be indicated for postmenopausal osteoporosis. For women not wishing to use estrogen replacement therapy, alendronate sodium (Fosamax), etidronate disodium (Didronel), or risedronate sodium (Actonel) may be prescribed. Moderate exercise such as walking, swimming, or riding a stationary bicycle is best. Physical therapy exercises for persons who are immobilized or paralyzed are necessary. For pain and muscle spasms, analgesics and muscle relaxants may be necessary.

Other Causes of Osteoporosis. **Disuse osteoporosis** may occur with prolonged bed rest, which leads to an increase in osteoclastic activity and resorption of bone greater than osteoblastic buildup. Stress placed on bone as a result of weight bearing is necessary for osteoblast function. The stress of exercise stimulates new bone growth as a result of changes in electrical charges on the bone surface.

The loss of bone density following a period of reduced weight bearing may be restored upon return to normal activity, although recovery may not be complete.[4] Osteoporosis may also occur when collagen formation is impaired in such conditions as scurvy, protein deficiency, or Cushing syndrome.

Rickets and Osteomalacia

Clinical Manifestations. **Rickets** and **osteomalacia** are characterized by deficits in mineralization of newly formed bone matrix with resulting soft osteopenic bone. Vitamin D deficiency prevents maintenance of normal levels of calcium and phosphorus. Children may have either vitamin D–resistant rickets or congenital hypophosphatasia. In rickets, cartilage that occurs in the growing epiphyses fails to calcify. Cartilage is not replaced by bone and continues to enlarge. Bone is poorly calcified and less rigid. Kyphosis, genu valgum ("knock knee"), and genu varum ("bowleg") are common deformities.

Osteomalacia is the adult counterpart of rickets. Osteomalacia is always due to an inadequate concentration of calcium or phosphorus in the body as a result of either decreased intestinal absorption of calcium, increased urinary excretion of calcium, loss of calcium or phosphorus during pregnancy or lactation, malabsorption syndrome, or any combination of these conditions.[2] In the case of vitamin D deficiency, calcification fails to occur and the bone is soft. All bones are affected, but weight-bearing structures may collapse and cause compression-type fractures.

Treatment. Treatment involves taking vitamin D supplements and adding vitamin D, calcium, and calcitonin to the diet. Exposure to sunlight increases vitamin D metabolism and absorption, especially for elderly persons.

Paget Disease

Paget disease of bone (osteitis deformans) is a slowly progressive metabolic bone disease characterized by an initial phase of excessive bone resorption, mediated by osteoclasts, followed by excessive bone formation (Figure 51-9). The end product is a disorganized mosaic of bone matrix made up of woven and lamellar bone at affected sites of the skeleton. This new bone is less compact, more vascular, and more fragile, which accounts for the deformities and fractures of Paget disease.[3]

Etiology and Pathogenesis. The specific cause of Paget disease is unknown, but the disease has a familial tendency suggesting a genetic component. It has also been theorized that a viral infection may affect osteoclastic function leading to aberrant bone remodeling. Changes in certain cytokines produced in the local bone marrow environment may also influence the bone formation/resorption balance.[3] In the United States, about 3% of people older than 50 years have Paget disease, with males being affected slightly more than females. It also tends to be more prevalent in persons of northern European descent.

Clinical Manifestations. In the early stages the disease may not cause any symptoms; however, when pain develops, it is severe and persistent. In the initial stages of Paget disease, affected bones soften and tend to bend. As the disease progresses, irregular subperiosteal bone formation occurs and causes bone to become thick and hard. Thickening of cranial bones may cause compression of cranial nerves and result in vertigo, blindness, deafness (with or without tinnitus), headaches, and facial paralysis. Other complications may include hypertension, arthritis, calcific periarthritis, and pain.

Treatment. During active stages of the disease, treatment focuses on preventing deformity and fracture, often with the use of bisphosphonates (such as etidronate, alendronate, or pamidronate, among many others.) These medications have been shown to decrease bone resorption, stabilize the fragile bone lesions, and reduce pain and the risk of fractures.[3]

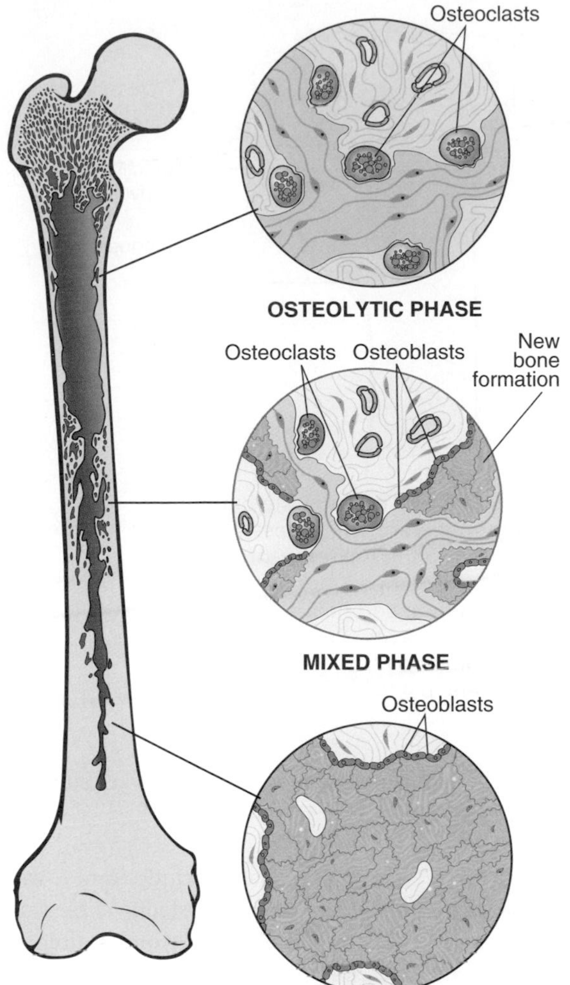

FIGURE 51-9 ■ Diagrammatic representation of Paget disease of bone demonstrating the three phases in the evolution of the disease. (From Kumar V, Cotran RS, Robbins ST: *Robbins basic pathology,* ed 7, Philadelphia, 2003, Saunders, p 764.)

KEY CONCEPTS

- Bone density is a product of the rate of bone resorption and bone deposition.
- Osteoporosis occurs when the rate of bone resorption is greater than that of bone formation. A reduction in bone mass predisposes to fractures.
- Hormone deficiencies (estrogen, androgen), poor calcium intake, and lack of use are common factors in the development of osteoporosis.
- The rate of bone loss is influenced by genetics, estrogen levels, calcium intake, and lack of activity.
- Vitamin D deficiency is associated with rickets and osteomalacia, disorders characterized by soft, weak bones.
- Paget disease may be genetic. It has also been theorized that a viral infection may affect osteoclastic function leading to aberrant bone remodeling. Painful deformities or bone fractures may result.

INFECTIONS OF THE BONE

Osteomyelitis

Osteomyelitis is a severe pyogenic infection of bone and local tissue that requires immediate treatment. Organisms may reach bone by one of three routes: (1) via the blood stream (hematogenous osteomyelitis), (2) from adjacent soft tissue (contiguous focus), and (3) by direct introduction of the organism into the bone.[1]

Etiology and Pathogenesis. *Hematogenous osteomyelitis,* in which the infectious agent may be introduced by blood from infection elsewhere in the body, is the most common type of osteomyelitis. It occurs most often in children younger than 16 years (mean age of 6 years old) and adults older than 50 years.[1] It involves bone rich in red marrow. In children as well as infants, these are long bones and the infection usually begins acutely in the metaphyseal region of the bone. Blood-borne bacteria reach the marrow space via the nutrient artery, or after blunt trauma a hematoma develops; thus a pathway for the organism to reach the bone is present (Figure 51-10).

Clinical Manifestations. In children, acute hematogenous osteomyelitis manifests as a high fever and pain at the site of bone involvement. The infection may remain localized if it becomes walled off by fibrotic tissue reaction, a condition referred to as a Brodie abscess. Muscle spasms, redness, and swelling are common, and the child may refuse to move the limb. In adults, hematogenous osteomyelitis is more difficult to detect. Symptoms are vague and may include fever, malaise, anorexia, night sweats, and weight loss. Pain at rest is common. The diagnosis may be supported by radiographic signs of bone destruction. The most common causative organism is *S. aureus,* with gram-negative bacillary infections increasing in frequency. In children between 2 months and 3 years of age, *Haemophilus influenzae* can also be a cause.[1]

Osteomyelitis secondary to an introduced or contiguous focus of infection can occur after burns, sinus disease, trauma, malignant tumor necrosis, periodontal infection, or an infected pressure ulcer. Again, *S. aureus* is the most common pathogen; however, some infections are polymicrobial and include gram-negative and anaerobic agents.[1]

Direct invasion of the organism into bone can occur as a result of open fractures, penetrating wounds, surgical contamination, or insertion of prostheses, metal plates, or screws. The latter three can act as a focus for bacterial reproduction.

During the acute stage of osteomyelitis, bacteria remain in bone and proliferate where the circulation is not optimal. Before puberty the bacteria grow in the metaphyseal sinusoidal vein, which leads to infection of the metaphysis near the growth plate. The loose attachment of overlying periosteum permits exudate to accumulate in the subperiosteal area. Uncontrolled infection can disrupt the cortex and lead to joint infection or septic arthritis, which can lead to osteoarthritis

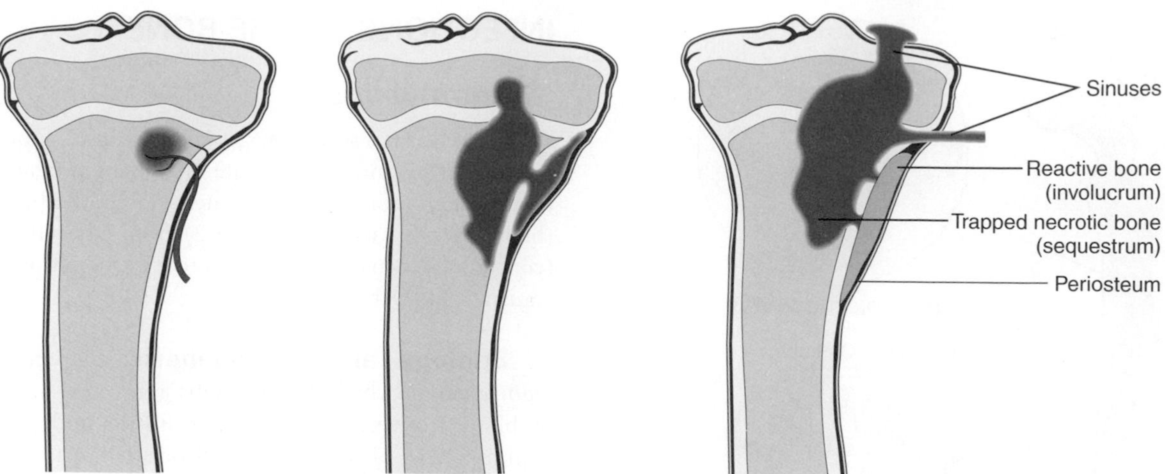

FIGURE 51-10 ■ Osteomyelitis. The bacteria reach the metaphysis through the nutrient artery. Bacterial growth results in bone destruction and formation of an abscess. From the abscess cavity, the pus spreads between the trabeculae into the medulla, through the cartilage into the joint, through the haversian canals of the compact bones to the outside. These sinuses traversing the bone persist for a long time and heal slowly. The pus destroys the bone and sequesters parts of it in the abscess cavity. Reactive new bone is formed around the focus of inflammation. (From Damjanov I: *Pathology for the health-related professions,* ed 2, Philadelphia, 2000, Saunders, p 444.)

later in life. In infants, medullary infection can reach the epiphysis and joint surfaces via capillaries crossing the growth plate, and stunted growth and angular deformities can result. The growth plate in children is avascular, so infection is limited. The inflammatory reaction leads to pus formation, edema, and vascular congestion. Pus collects and is confined within bone, thus increasing pressure and adding to vascular occlusion, ischemia, and, finally, necrosis of bone. Volkmann and haversian canals allow a route for release of pus and thus spread of bacteria. Blood and therefore antibiotics cannot reach bone tissue when vascular system pressure equals arteriolar pressure. As a result, the course and virulence of the osteomyelitis are affected. Even after meticulous treatment, the organism can reappear years later in a context of trauma or immunosuppression.

Healing Complications. If osteomyelitis is not managed or if the treatment is not sufficient, the resulting necrotic bone can separate from healthy bone into dead segments called sequestra. A sequestrum is then a medium for the continued bacterial proliferation described as chronic osteomyelitis. Sequestra can enlarge and extrude through bone into soft tissue, where it is possible that it might revascularize and resolve as a result of the body's defense mechanisms.

Osteoblasts may try to heal infected bone by isolating the dead tissue and forming an involucrum (a layer of new bone around old bone). Involucrum formation prevents successful effects of antibiotics and phagocytosis and leads to chronic infection.[1]

Any type of osteomyelitis may become chronic, especially if the treatment was inadequate during the acute phase. It may be manifested months or years after assumed cure, especially after acute hematogenous disease. Drainage via a sinus tract to the skin can occur.

Treatment. Treatment usually includes 4 to 6 weeks of parenteral antibiotic therapy for acute osteomyelitis. A shorter period of parenteral therapy followed by oral antibiotics can be effective if the infection is under control and a therapeutic blood level of the antibiotic can be maintained. Antibiotic choice is based on culture and sensitivity results.

If acute osteomyelitis is complicated by an abscess or extensive necrosis, the involved area is debrided and antibiotic therapy is instituted. If a prosthesis is involved, it is usually removed. After debridement, dead space is usually filled with packing, bone grafts, muscle pedicles, or skin grafts. In osteomyelitis associated with peripheral vascular disease, amputation is performed if antibiotic therapy is unsuccessful.[1]

Tuberculosis

Etiology and Pathogenesis. Bone and joint tuberculosis (TB) is an extrapulmonary form of TB that occurs after lymphohematogenous spread from a primary lung lesion. As the incidence of TB increases in the United States, one can expect to see more cases of skeletal TB. Persons with skeletal TB may have a history of pulmonary TB, drug abuse, crowded and poor living conditions, diseases that depress the immune system, and immigration to the United States after 1991. Musculoskeletal TB is not communicable to others unless an open wound exists. *Mycobacterium tuberculosis,* the organism responsible for the destruction of bone and joint, is transmitted via the air-borne route. Initially, infectious droplets are inhaled and infect lungs; then *M. tuberculosis* spreads hematogenously from lungs or lymphatic drainage to bone. The bacterium may lie dormant for a long while before it is detected.

Clinical Manifestations. When involving the bone or joint, *M. tuberculosis* likely first infects bone where the blood supply is richest after which the infection spreads into the bone and possibly joint spaces (tuberculous arthritis). The most common site of skeletal TB is the vertebral column, particularly the lower thoracic and lumbar vertebrae (often called Potts disease). Vertebral infection results in destruction of the bone, anterior wedging, and collapse. On x-ray, the appearance is of a lytic lesion in the bone without local sclerotic (new bone formation) reaction. When the infection spreads to adjacent disks, paraspinal fluid may accumulate as a "cold abscess."[5] Symptoms may include local pain, low-grade fever, and possible neurologic symptoms due to impingement.

Other common sites of skeletal TB or tuberculous arthritis include weight-bearing joints such as hips, knees, and ankles, although any joint or bone could be involved.[5]

Risk Factors. Persons most at risk for TB are those at extremes of age or individuals who are immunosuppressed or undernourished. Children are at higher risk for skeletal TB because of extreme vascularity. In acquired immunodeficiency syndrome, knowledge of the patient's human immunodeficiency virus status is critical to optimize the therapeutic plan for the patient.[5]

Treatment. Treatment for skeletal TB requires long-term combination antibiotic therapy. Agents such as isoniazid, rifampin, pyrazinamide, ethambutol, and others are used in combinations for 9 to 12 months. Therapeutic response can be complicated by development of drug resistance. Surgical intervention may be indicated in cases of spinal TB when severe deformities or neurologic deficits are seen.

KEY CONCEPTS

- Bone infections may be from blood-borne organisms or direct traumatic infection.
- Osteomyelitis—organisms reach the bone by one of three routes: blood stream (hematogenous osteomyelitis), adjacent soft tissue (contiguous focus), and direct introduction of the organism into the bone.
- TB of the bone—infection is spread via lung or lymphohematogenous drainage.
- Antibiotic therapy can help to reduce the progression of bone infection and is the main treatment; however, abscess formation and chronic infection may occur.

BONE TUMORS

Neoplasms occurring in the musculoskeletal system can be benign or malignant. Benign tumors often go undiagnosed because they cause no pain. The most common benign bone tumor is a fibrous cortical defect often referred to as a developmental anomaly. An osteochondroma (exostosis) can occur in multiple locations such as the femur, pelvis, and shoulder. The tumor grows with skeletal growth. Malignant neoplasms are referred to as sarcomas. More common than sarcomas are metastatic lesions, which have spread to bone from primary carcinomas. These metastatic tumors usually occur when patients are in their 60s or 70s. Primary carcinomas that most commonly metastasize to bone are breast, prostate, lung, and kidney carcinomas. Other malignancies that can metastasize to bone include thyroid, bladder, uterine, colorectal, and vaginal cancer. Common sites of bone metastases are the vertebral bodies, pelvis, proximal ends of the femur and humerus, and ribs. Metastases occur via direct spread within a body cavity or by hematogenous or lymphatic spread.

Thus although the majority of bone tumors are metastatic, a number of primary tumors of bone can be identified. Some bone tumors are benign (Figure 51-11).

Osteochondroma

Etiology, Pathogenesis, and Clinical Manifestations. **Osteochondroma,** the most common bone tumor, is a cartilage-forming benign tumor that accounts for 35% to 50% of all benign bone tumors and 10% to 15% of all primary bone tumors.[1] Osteochondroma is hereditary and usually occurs in persons 30 years or younger.

Bony projections on the external surface of the bone are capped with cartilage. Exostoses are usually asymptomatic and found by chance. Pressure on surrounding soft tissue may cause pain. These tumors are usually located on the metaphyses of long bones such as the proximal end of the tibia and distal part of the femur, the shoulder, and the pelvis (see Figure 51-11).

Chondroma

Chondroma or enchondroma is a cartilage-forming tumor in bone that can be located in the medullary cavity or in the subperiosteal layers of bone.[1] It is believed to arise from remnants of epiphyseal cartilage. Chondromas arise most often in the small bones of the hands and feet but can develop in other areas. Tumor growth may erode the cortex of bone and expand the contour. Chondroma usually occurs in persons 30 to 40 years of age.

Osteoid Osteoma

Osteoid osteoma is a painful but benign bone-forming tumor that accounts for approximately 10% to 13% of symptomatic benign tumors.[1] Sharp or dull pain can be felt, often worse at night and alleviated by aspirin or other nonsteroidal antiinflammatory drugs. This small lesion is often found in the cortex of the tibia and femur, but any bone may be involved. Radiographs show the lesion enclosed in a sclerotic shell. This tumor usually occurs in persons 10 to 20 years old.

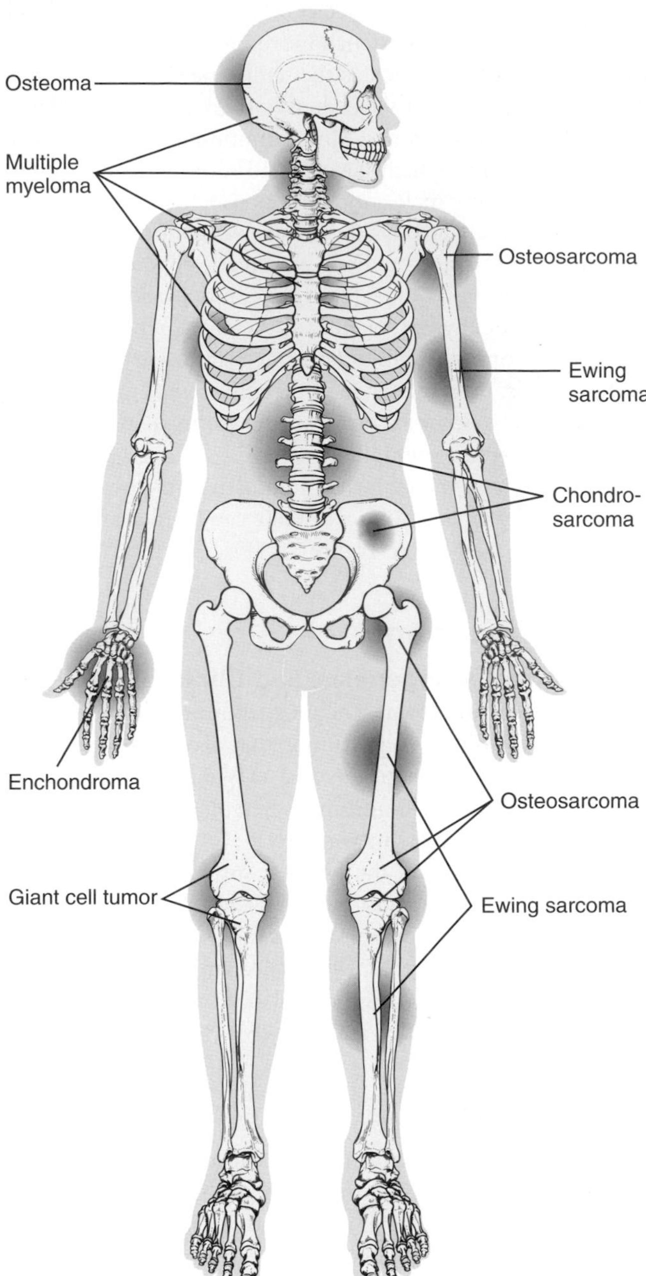

FIGURE 51-11 ■ Schematic presentation of the most common sites of origin of bone tumors. Most often, osteosarcomas originate in the metaphyses of long bones, chondrosarcomas arise in the axial skeleton, Ewing sarcomas develop in the diaphyses of long bones, and giant cell tumors originate in the epiphyses of long bones. Osteomas occur most often in the skull and enchondromas in the small bones of the hand. Multiple myelomas involve the calvaria, vertebrae, and ribs, but also other bones that contain hematopoietic bone marrow. (From Damjanov I: *Pathology for the health-related professions,* ed 2, Philadelphia, 2000, Saunders, p 453.)

Giant Cell Tumor

A **giant cell tumor,** or osteoclastoma, is benign but aggressive with richly vascularized tissue consisting of plump spindle-shaped cells and numerous giant cells. These lesions account for about 4% to 5% of all primary bone tumors.[1] In some cases, giant cell tumors undergo transformation to sarcomas. The cells can metastasize without malignant transformation. Giant cell tumors commonly occur between the ages of 20 and 40 years and do not have any gender predilection. The area of development includes the distal end of the femur, proximal part of the tibia, distal part of the radius, and proximal end of the humerus (see Figure 51-11). Pain is the initial complaint.

Osteosarcoma

Etiology and Pathogenesis. **Osteosarcoma,** an extremely malignant bone-forming tumor, is the most common primary malignant bone tumor that develops in the metaphyseal region of long bones. It is characterized by the formation of bone or osteoid by tumor cells. The majority of victims are children, adolescents, and young adults 10 to 30 years of age, although a second peak in incidence can be seen in adults 60 to 70 years old.[6] The most active epiphyseal growth areas—the distal end of the femur, proximal end of the tibia, fibula, and proximal end of the humerus—are common sites of involvement (see Figure 51-11). Lesions can also be seen in flat bones of the pelvis, skull, scapula, ribs, or spine.[6]

Clinical Manifestations. Osteosarcoma grows rapidly and is quite destructive; destruction of the cortex of the metaphyseal region predisposes it to pathologic fracture. Metastasis to lungs is noted early in disease development. Pain is consistent and progressively more intense. Joint function may be compromised as a result of the proximity of the metaphysis.

Treatment. Although amputation may be necessary, conservative surgery, radiation therapy, and chemotherapy have provided positive results, with studies showing 5-year disease-free survival of nonmetastatic disease between 41% and 87%.[6]

Chondrosarcoma

Pathogenesis. A **chondrosarcoma** is a malignant cartilage-forming tumor. These tumors usually develop slowly, so pain is not a prominent clinical symptom. Even with a slow rate of development the tumor will eventually metastasize, typically to the lung. Chondrosarcomas tend to develop in the pelvic and shoulder girdles and the proximal ends of long bones (see Figure 51-11).

Secondary chondrosarcoma is a benign lesion, like osteochondroma or multiple enchondromatosis, that undergoes malignant transformation. It occurs in the pelvis and proximal ends of the femur and humerus in persons between the ages of 20 and 40 years. Evidence of malignant transformation may include pain, an irregular border, or an increase in cap size after patient growth is complete.[6]

Clinical Manifestations. Primary chondrosarcoma is characterized by the formation of cartilage by tumor cells. This tumor has a higher cellularity and greater pleomorphism than a chondroma. It usually occurs in the femur, pelvis, ribs, and scapula in persons between 30 and 60 years of age.

Ewing Sarcoma

Pathogenesis. **Ewing sarcoma** is the third most common primary sarcoma of bone and is characterized as a rapidly growing malignant round cell tumor. This tumor most often develops in the long bones of children between the ages of 10 and 15 years. Ewing tumor is composed of densely packed small cells with round nuclei. It arises in the medullary canal of bone and perforates the cortex of the shaft producing a painful soft tissue mass overlying the involved bone. The tumor favors long tubular bones, such as the femur, tibia, proximal fibula, or humerus (see Figure 51-11); however, it can arise in the pelvis and flat bones where it may be more difficult to diagnose.[6]

Clinical Manifestations and Treatment. Ewing sarcoma metastasizes quite early in its development to the lungs and other bones. Because of the rapid rate of growth, pain is a dominant symptom that increases in severity. Ewing sarcoma is often confused with osteomyelitis because patients often appear systemically ill and may develop fever, anemia, leukocytosis, and an increased sedimentation rate.[6] Treatment includes radiotherapy and possible adjunct surgical therapy.

Multiple Myeloma

Etiology and Pathogenesis. **Multiple myeloma** is a slowly growing bone marrow malignancy with neoplastic proliferation of a single clone of plasma cells. The annual incidence is approximately 4 per 100,000 and represents about 1% of all malignant cancers.[6]

Clinical Manifestations and Treatment. Although multiple myeloma is not a sarcoma, its symptoms and radiographic findings are similar. On radiographs, evidence of bone destruction by a lytic, or bone-destroying, process and bone marrow involvement can be seen. Homogeneous immunoglobulin is also present in urine or serum. Because multiple myeloma is a slow-growing lesion, it takes a long time to become symptomatic. Bone pain is the most common symptom, particularly of the chest and back, and is related to excessive accumulation of abnormal plasma cells in the bone marrow. Although it can affect any bone, multiple myeloma most commonly occurs in the thoracic and lumbar vertebrae. Patients experience hypercalcemia and pathologic fractures where bone has been destroyed. This disease can also cause kidney dysfunction, lung or pleural involvement, and neurologic symptoms due to nerve compression.[6] Treatment often requires aggressive combination chemotherapy, although at times local radiation may be useful for refractory bone pain.

KEY CONCEPTS 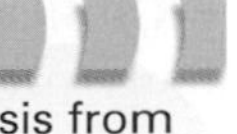

- Most bone tumors are secondary to metastasis from other sites. Osteochondroma, chondroma, osteoid osteoma, and giant cell tumors are benign, primary bone tumors.
- Malignant bone tumors include osteosarcoma, chondrosarcoma, and Ewing sarcoma.
- Multiple myeloma is a slow-growing bone marrow malignancy in which plasma cells proliferate. This disease affects the kidneys and the immune and circulatory systems.

SOFT TISSUE INJURIES

In addition to injuries of the bony skeleton, soft tissue may also be traumatized. At times it is difficult to differentiate among the types of soft tissue. In an attempt to differentiate the exact site of a lesion, Cyriax[7] described two types of soft tissue: contractile and inert. **Contractile** tissue is composed of structures involved in the contraction of muscle and includes not only the muscle belly but also the tendon and bony insertion. Although not involved in a pure contraction, as is the muscle belly, the tendon and its insertion into bone are mechanically linked to tension generated by the muscle. According to Cyriax, pain may be elicited by active contraction and by passive stretching in the opposite direction.[7] Pain with resisted contraction may also occur at a fracture site near a muscular insertion, lymphatic gland, or bursa, or an abscess situated under a muscle.

INERT SOFT TISSUE INJURIES

Inert, or **noncontractile,** tissue possesses no ability to contract or relax. Inert soft tissues include joint capsules, ligaments, bursae, fasciae, dura mater, and nerve roots. Passive stretching provokes pain from inert tissue. Evaluation of inert tissue lesions requires identification of all structures involved: the capsule of a joint, a section of a ligament or a nerve, or mechanical displacement of the meniscus.

Ligament Injuries

A **ligament** is a dense connective tissue with parallel-fibered collagenous tissues designed to connect bone to bone. Ligaments contribute to mechanical stability of the joint, guide motion, and prevent excessive motion. Injuries to ligaments occur when loading exceeds the physiologic range of motion. Microfailure precedes total failure of the ligament. With total failure of a ligament, damage to surrounding soft tissue occurs. Ligament injuries are classified by the extent of tear and may be described as mild, moderate, or severe. With a mild injury, a few ligament fibers are damaged, but ligament strength is not lost.

Clinical Manifestations. A common site of ligament injury, particularly among athletes, is the knee with the anterior cruciate ligament (Figure 51-12). Symptoms may include a sudden "tearing" sensation or "popping" in the knee followed by pain with weight bearing and often acute swelling of the knee. Another common site for ligament injury is the anterior ankle (talofibular ligament).[8]

Treatment. Treatment is geared primarily toward relief of symptoms, and recovery is usually complete. A moderate ligament injury is a definite tear in some component of the ligament with loss of strength. The fibers are not widely separated. Treatment is primarily protection of the ligament. With a severe ligament injury, the ligament is completely torn and no longer functions. Potentially the fragments are widely separated. Treatment is restoration of ligament continuity.

Joint Capsule Injuries

Another inert structure that is intimately involved in stabilization of a synovial joint is the **joint capsule** (Figure 51-13). The joint capsule is composed of an inner and outer layer. The inner layer is highly vascularized but has minimal innervation. It synthesizes the hyaluronic acid component of synovial fluid, produces matrix collagen, and is essential for joint nutrition.[9] The outer layer of the capsule is attached to the periosteum of the bones through Sharpey fibers. The capsule is reinforced by ligaments and musculotendinous structures. The outer layer of the capsule is poorly vascularized but richly innervated by joint receptors. Joint receptors are able to detect the rate and direction of motion, proprioception, compression and tension, vibration, and pain.[9]

After injury to the joint capsule, the ensuing increase in vascularity and development of fibrous tissue lead to a thick capsule. Any effusion into the joint cavity may lead to stretching of the capsule and its associated ligaments. The joint capsule, like ligaments, provides joint stability. The capsule, however, has an interesting mechanical adaptation: capsular redundancy. An example of the importance of the redundancy has been identified by Hettinga[10]: "The inferior medial portion of the shoulder joint capsule is a loose, redundant sac that becomes tense only when the shoulder is fully abducted or flexed. The posterior capsule of the knee is loose in flexion but so tight in extension that it becomes an important stabilizer."

Capsular redundancy provides for a stable joint at the end ranges of movement. Any injury or edema in the joint that causes scarring in the lax section of the capsule prevents full range of motion. Prolonged immobilization of a joint causes loss of mobility and extensibility of the capsule, with subsequent loss of motion. Immobilization of a joint causes an alteration in the flow of synovial fluid and contracture of the joint capsule and periarticular muscle. The altered flow of synovial fluid prevents fluid diffusion into and out of cartilage and causes compression and distention of cartilage. Nutrition of the joint components stagnates, leading to degenerative changes in the joint that become permanent. Contracture of the joint capsule and periarticular muscle results when fatty tissue proliferates in the joint space. This increase in connective tissue leads to adhesions that limit joint motion. The increase in connective tissue is due to failure to keep the lattice-

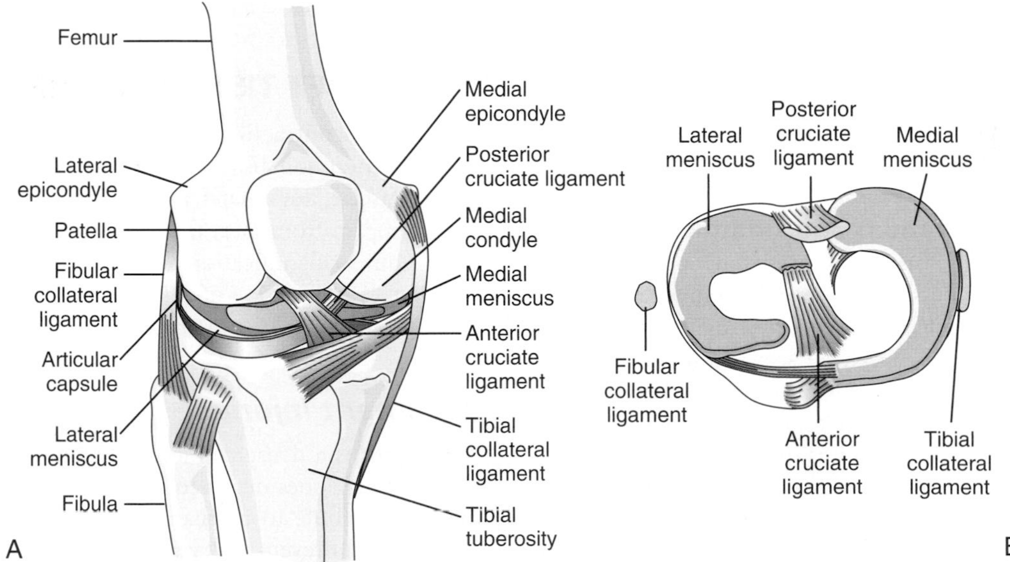

FIGURE 51-12 ■ The principal structures of the interior of the knee joint. **A,** From the front. **B,** From above with the femur removed.

work of tissue stretched open, which is usually kept open by normal flexion and extension of muscle. The muscles bridging the immobilized joint also shorten.

Frozen Shoulder. An example of such a restriction is loss of function in the shoulder after even a minor injury leading to a "frozen shoulder," also called adhesive capsulitis. With an injury to any component of the shoulder complex, inflammation occurs in the joint along with swelling and distention of the joint capsule. With prolonged immobilization, thickening of the capsule may ensue possibly due to proliferation of fibroblasts and capsular contraction. Capsular tightness leads to a loss of movement and an increase in pain especially at night. Excessive joint motion may cause a tearing of the capsule, similar to a ligamentous tear, and render the joint unstable. Conservative treatment of the frozen shoulder is usually recommended with intraarticular corticosteroid injections, gentle stretching and physical therapy, and antiinflammatory medication. Prevention of adhesive capsulitis involves avoiding prolonged or excessive immobilization of the shoulder after minor injuries and early gentle stretching.[9]

Internal Joint Derangement

Internal joint derangement may be caused by injury to inert soft tissue structures. Meniscal tears at the knee, labrum tears at the glenohumeral joint, and disk tears in the temporomandibular joint all cause restrictions of the joint and may lead to soft tissue dysfunction in the form of weakness, loss of motion, or pain. Tears of the medial and lateral menisci in the knee are common causes of knee pain, with the medial meniscus being torn more often. A meniscal tear is usually the result of a twisting motion.

The anterior and posterior cruciate ligaments prevent anterior and posterior displacement of the tibia relative to the femur, respectively (see Figure 51-12). These ligaments can be torn in varying degrees of severity. Injury to either ligament leads to some degree of instability in the knee joint.

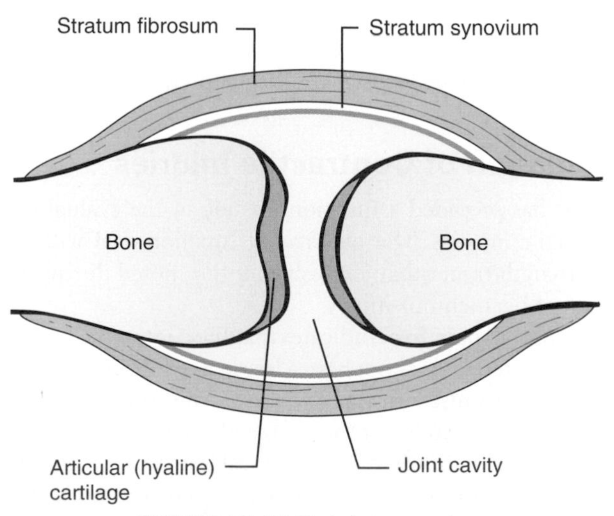

FIGURE 51-13 ■ Joint capsule.

Injuries to Fasciae and Bursae

Fasciae and **bursae** may also be causes of pain and restriction of movement of the musculoskeletal system.

Fasciae. When connective tissues of the body are arranged in sheaths that envelop muscles, they are designated **fasciae.** Individual muscles are surrounded by a thin fascia called the **perimysium.** Trauma to fascia, as with any soft tissue, may cause edema and scarring. Restrictions in fascia movement cause a restriction in joint function.

Bursae. In many locations between muscles or between muscle or tendon and bone, connective tissue forms a pocket lined with synovium that contains fluid. These pockets are identified as **bursae.** Bursae are located in areas of high friction and are designed to dissipate some of the stress. With faulty mechanics of the joint, repetitive movement, or direct trauma, the bursal sac may become inflamed (bursitis) and extremely painful. Bursitis, because of its strategic position at stress points of muscle function, causes major disruption of movement. An inflamed bursa may restrict any movement of the joint and lead to restriction in capsular function or muscle dysfunction as a result of edema. Some of the more common sites of bursitis include the trochanteric bursa (lateral hip), the subacromial bursa (shoulder), the pes anserine bursa (medial knee), and the olecranon bursa (elbow).

Injuries to Nerves, Nerve Roots, or Dura Mater

Trauma to any soft tissue may lead to adhesive restriction in movement of the nerve, nerve root, or dura mater. Irritation or entrapment of a nerve causes pain that radiates along the structures innervated by that nerve. Pain, altered sensation (numbness and tingling), motor weakness, and diminished reflexes may result from trauma to these essential soft tissue components of the musculoskeletal system.[2]

An example is trauma to vertebrae in the lumbosacral area with nerve root impingement. Components of the intervertebral disk can herniate and cause pressure on nerve roots (Figure 51-14). The intervertebral disk is a shock absorber located between vertebrae. The center is a gelatinous-like material, the nucleus pulposus, that has a high water content. The nucleus pulposus is surrounded by the fibrous annulus fibrosus. Trauma to the back can cause unequal pressure on the disk leading to herniation. Common sites of disk problems are at L3-4, which affects the L4 nerve root; L4-5, which affects the L5 nerve root; and L5-S1, which affects the S1 nerve root.

CONTRACTILE SOFT TISSUE INJURIES

Injury to Tendons

Injury to tendons occurs along a continuum from minor strain, in which a few fibers of the tendon are torn, to a complete tear or rupture. The sheath in which a tendon slides may

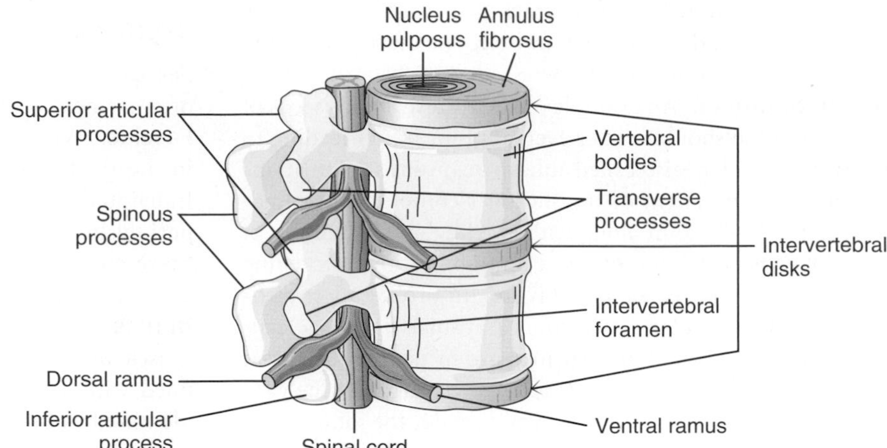

FIGURE 51-14 ■ Lateral view (somewhat superior) of a segment of the lumbar part of the vertebral column.

also be traumatized. Inflammation of the tendon within the sheath is called **tendinitis.** This inflammation may be due to infection, direct injury, or injury from repetitive motion. Tendons are injured when the stress placed on them is greater than the fibers can tolerate. Muscle tendons that are subjected to high tensile stress or compression are more prone to injury. Frequently injured tendons include the following: extensor pollicis brevis and abductor pollicis longus of the thumb (de Quervain syndrome), rotator cuff of the shoulder, biceps brachii tendon, tendons of the patellar complex, quadriceps tendon, hamstring tendon, Achilles tendon, and posterior tibialis tendon.

Muscle and Tendon Strains

Muscle trauma compromises the contractile unit. As in the case of injury to a tendon, tears in a muscle may range from a minor tear to complete rupture. Most injuries to muscle are due to abnormal muscle contraction. Muscle and tendon strains are often categorized by the severity of injury[11]:

Grade I: Minute tear of connective tissue and muscle fiber.

Grade II: Tear of a large portion of the contractile unit, with a segment still intact.

Grade III: Total rupture or loss of continuity of the contractile structure.

Blunt Trauma

A soft tissue contusion or crush injury also compromises the contractile structure. Any blunt trauma that causes bleeding into the muscle belly may lead to an inability to contract the muscle. Hemorrhage in a muscle belly has the potential to coagulate and calcify. This abnormal calcification in a muscle results in a painful condition called **myositis ossificans.** Calcification prevents a normal and strong contraction of the muscle involved.

Compartment Syndrome

Compartment syndrome is due to trauma to soft tissue caused by the unyielding structure of inert tissue. Causes of compartment syndrome may be divided into three categories: decreased compartment size, increased compartment content, or externally applied pressure. With an injury, edema causes an increase in pressure within the compartment. Because volume is expanding in a confined area, pressure reduces capillary flow. Muscle and nerves become ischemic, with a resultant excruciating pain. Besides pain, the skin looks pale, the pulse may be absent, and sensation is diminished. Compartment syndrome is a medical emergency requiring immediate decompression. Nerves can survive only 2 to 4 hours of ischemia and muscles approximately 6 to 8 hours. However, muscles do not have the ability to regenerate, and if the muscle becomes necrotic, it will be replaced by fibrous connective tissue and fat. Compartment syndromes are noted most often in the leg (anterior, deep posterior, superficial posterior, and lateral), forearm (dorsal and volar), upper arm (deltoid and biceps), hand (interosseous), buttock (gluteal), and thigh (quadriceps). For additional discussion of compartment syndrome, see "Complications in Bone Healing" in this chapter.

Evaluation of Contractile Injuries

Cyriax[7] has provided a functional guide to the evaluation of contractile injuries. The patterns of function deal with pain and strength rather than excessive motion noted during evaluation of ligamentous injury.

Strong and pain free: Indicates that the contractile structure being tested does not have a lesion, regardless of how tender the muscle is on palpation. The muscle functions painlessly and is not the source of the patient's pain.

Strong and painful: Indicates a local lesion of the muscle or tendon, previously listed as a grade I or II muscle strain.

No limitation of passive movement is noted unless secondary joint restriction from disuse is present. Stiffness in the joint would then take precedence in treatment.

Weak and painful: Indicates a severe lesion around the joint, such as a fracture. Weakness is usually due to reflex inhibition of the muscles around the joint.

Weak and pain free: Indicates rupture of a muscle or involvement of the nerve supplying the muscle.

If all movements are painful, pain may be due to fatigue, emotional hypersensitivity, or emotional problems.

Soft Tissue Healing After Trauma

Trauma to soft tissue results in disruption of the circulatory and lymphatic systems. Hemorrhage, fluid loss, and cell death result. Blood vessels at the site of trauma constrict, which limits blood loss from the affected area. Norepinephrine mediates this initial constriction response, which may last a few minutes. Serotonin (from mast cells of connective tissue) and platelets prolong vasoconstriction. It may also contribute to vasodilation in inflamed tissue.

Platelets adhere to collagen fibers and release serotonin and adenosine diphosphate, which causes platelets to adhere to the traumatized endothelial wall and form a platelet plug that temporarily decreases bleeding. Trauma to the endothelial surface triggers release of an enzyme that initiates clotting by converting prothrombin to thrombin, which converts fibrinogen to fibrin. The endothelial surfaces of small vessels are also compressed, thereby ensuring that vessels remain closed after vasoconstriction has ceased. In the early stages of inflammation, the endothelial margins of the venules may be covered with neutrophilic leukocytes, a process called neutrophilic margination. At this point the release of histamine from mast cells, basophils, and platelets causes vasodilation and increased permeability of venules. With the increase in permeability, serous fluid containing cells and plasma proteins accumulates as edema in tissue spaces (Figure 51-15). This edema fluid contains fibrinogen, which forms fibrin through an interaction with thrombin. Fibrin seals damaged lymphatics and confines the inflammatory reaction to an area immediately surrounding the injury.

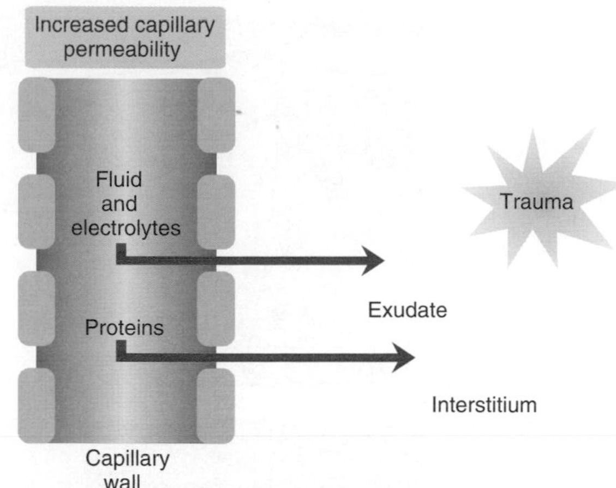

FIGURE 51-15 ■ Edema formation. With trauma, increased capillary permeability and dilation cause leaking into tissue space. Initially clear, the exudate in the tissue space becomes more viscous with an increase in plasma protein.

Wound Repair

The inflammatory response prepares injured tissue to progress to the healing process of repair and reorganization. Figures 51-16 and 51-17 provide a summary of the phases of wound repair. The acute response lasts about 2 weeks and the subacute phase another 2 weeks. When the wound is clear of foreign substances, an infiltrate of macrophages and fibroblasts is noted. A matrix of collagen, hyaluronic acid, and fibronectin develops. Lymphatics form in the matrix, prevent additional edema, and assist in preventing infection. This granulation tissue develops in the wound space. Macrophages have an important role in wound repair.

Next in the process of wound repair is reepithelialization of the wound surface. Epidermal cells migrate over established epidermal cells until the defect is closed. The formation of basement membrane follows. This membrane is first laid down at the wound periphery and then progresses to the center of the wound. A strong bond forms between epidermal cells and the newly formed basement membrane to complete reepithelialization (granulation tissue formation).

Wound tensile strength is a result of the deposition of collagen. Collagen production begins approximately 5 days after myofibroblast migration into the wound space. Hyaluronic acid, found in the extracellular matrix, assists glycosaminoglycans to stimulate fibroplasia. Myofibroblasts secrete an extracellular matrix, which induces cell migration and proliferation, and synthesize proteoglycans, which stimulate collagen formation and increase tissue resilience and tensile strength. By the end of the first month, tensile strength begins to increase, but several months is required to achieve the maximal level. Collagen reaches its maximal strength approximately 3 months after injury. Maximal tensile strength is only 70% to 80% of preinjury levels.

Revascularization (angiogenesis or growth of new blood vessels) must take place to ensure survival of the new tissue. Vascularization occurs through the development of new circulatory networks in the wound and reattachment of existing vessels. Extracellular matrix, endothelial cell development, lactic acid, and heparin are a few of the factors that stimulate revascularization.

Wound closure or contraction is the final phase of healing in soft tissue injuries. Contraction begins soon after injury and is completed in approximately 2 weeks. Myofibrils assist in wound closure. Interaction between extracellular matrix and granulation tissue results in a contractile unit called a fibronexus. Cytoplasmic actin binds to the fibronexus and

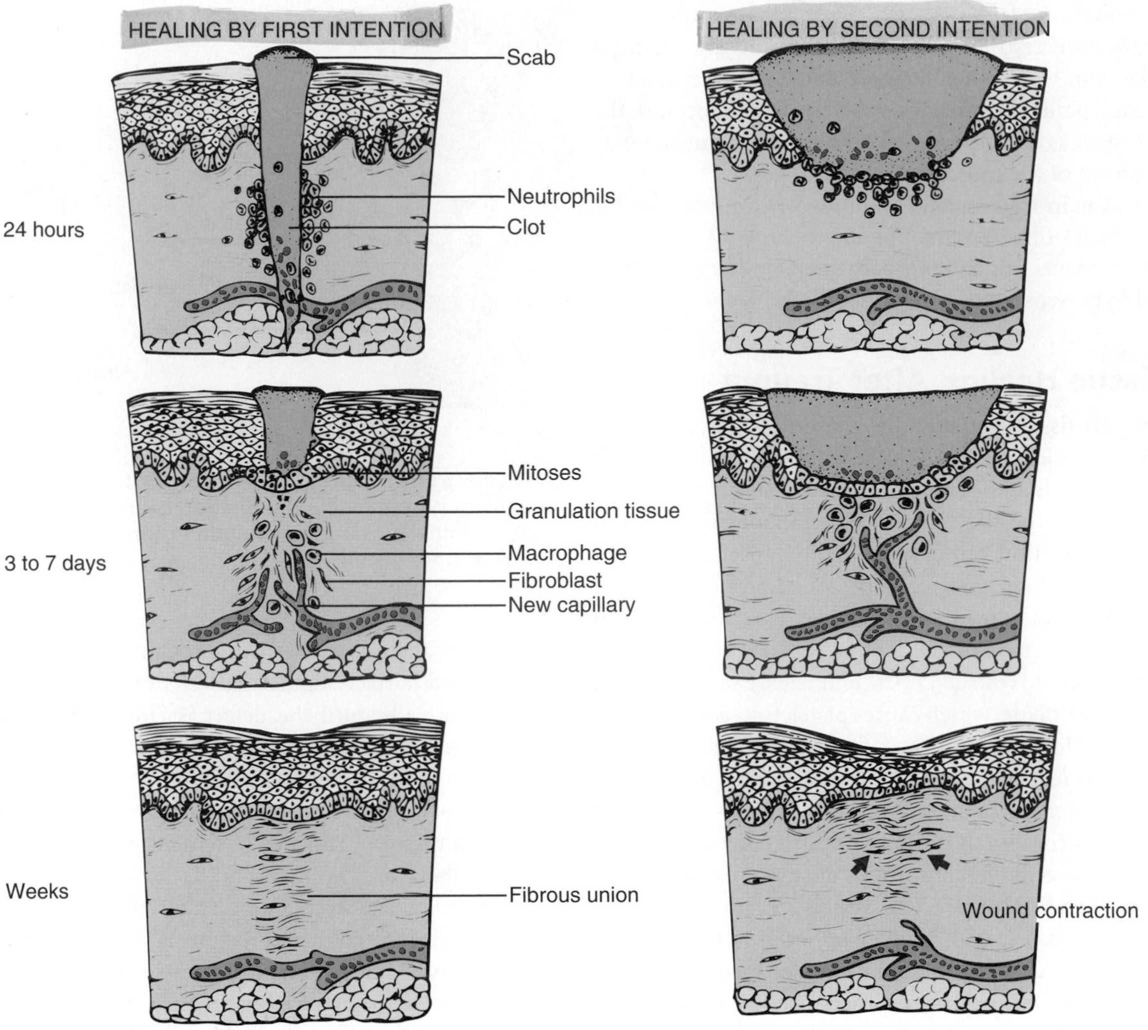

HEALING BY FIRST INTENTION
HEALING BY SECOND INTENTION
Scab
Neutrophils
Clot
24 hours
Mitoses
Granulation tissue
Macrophage
Fibroblast
New capillary
3 to 7 days
Fibrous union
Weeks
Wound contraction

FIGURE 51-16 ■ Steps in wound healing by first intention and second intention. In the latter, the resultant scar is much smaller than the original wound because of wound contraction. (From Kumar V, Cotran RS, Robbins ST: *Robbins basic pathology,* ed 7, Philadelphia, 2003, Saunders, p 75.)

Wound contraction
Granulation tissue
Inflammation
Collagen accumulation
Remodeling
0.1
0.3
1
3
10
30
100
Days

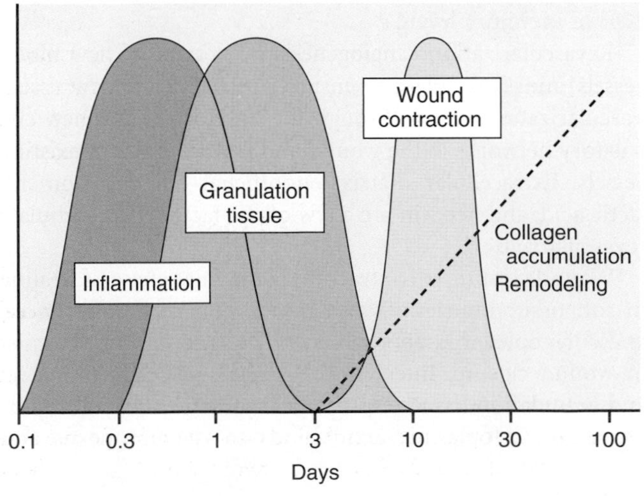

FIGURE 51-17 ■ Orderly phases of wound healing. (Modified from Clark RA: In Goldsmith LA, editor: *Physiology, biochemistry and molecular biology of the skin,* ed 2, vol 1, New York, 1991, Oxford University Press, p 577. In Kumar V, Cotran RS, Robbins ST: *Robbins basic pathology,* ed 7, Philadelphia, 2003, Saunders, p 74.)

draws tissue together to ensure a stable wound. As tension increases across the wound, collagen fibers are reoriented and collagen phagocytosis increases. Complete organization and concentration of collagen may require more than 40 weeks. In the case of rupture of soft tissue structures, surgical intervention may be necessary to ensure that the traumatized tissue is in close enough proximity to allow healing.

KEY CONCEPTS

- Soft tissue injury refers to injuries of noncontractile elements (joint capsule, ligament, bursa, fascia, dura mater, and nerve root) and contractile elements (muscle and tendons).
- Passive stretching causes pain in noncontractile tissue injury, whereas active contraction is painful in contractile injury.
- Noncontractile tissue injuries generally cause altered range of motion around a joint as a result of pain, edema, adhesion, or fibrosis.
- Contractile tissue injuries are characterized by decreased muscle strength.
- Compartment syndrome is a dangerous complication of soft tissue injury that results from swelling of injured tissue within a restrictive fascia. Unless pressure is quickly reduced, compressed tissue may become ischemic and necrotic.
- Manifestations of compartment syndrome include severe pain, pallor, pulselessness, paralysis, and paresthesia.
- Soft tissue injury results in local inflammation and initiates the process of wound healing. Strength of the injured tissue is improved by the deposition of collagen. Normalization of collagen may require more than 40 weeks.

DISEASES OF SKELETAL MUSCLE

Skeletal muscle, the most abundant tissue in the human body, accounts for approximately 40% of total body weight.[9] Skeletal muscle performs dynamic work (locomotion) and static work (posture). As with other tissue of the musculoskeletal system, muscle atrophies in response to disuse and immobilization, and hypertrophies when subjected to increased stress.

MUSCULAR DYSTROPHY

Muscular dystrophy comprises a group of genetically determined myopathies characterized by progressive muscle weakness and degeneration as muscle tissue is replaced by fat and fibrous connective tissue. The dystrophies are classified by their pattern of inheritance, age on onset, and distribution of muscular weakness.

Duchenne Muscular Dystrophy

Etiology and Pathogenesis. **Duchenne muscular dystrophy,** the most common and most severe form of muscular dystrophy, is inherited as an X-linked trait and therefore afflicts only males. The incidence is 1 in 3500 male births. Due to a genetic mutation, muscle cells are deficient in the protein dystrophin, a deficiency that weakens the cell membrane and allows extracellular fluid to leak into the cell. Proteases and inflammatory processes are activated leading to muscle fiber necrosis and muscle degeneration.[12]

The disease begins at birth and is usually apparent by the age of 3 years, with initial involvement of the pelvic girdle and progression to the shoulder girdle.

Clinical Manifestations. The calf muscles of an individual with Duchenne muscular dystrophy are noticeably enlarged because of the infiltration of fat cells and degeneration of muscle fibers. Distal muscle involvement leads to frequent falling by the age of 5 or 6 years, and by age 12 to 14 years most children are confined to a wheelchair. Some muscles, such as those in the hands, face, jaw, pharynx, larynx, and eyes, are spared to the end. Survival to age 20 is rare. Cardiac failure or pulmonary infection is the usual cause of death.[12]

Treatment. Treatment in muscular dystrophy is focused on appropriate education for the patient and family, preservation of physical function as long as possible, and prevention of contractures. In some cases, corticosteroid therapy may be useful for temporary improvement in muscle strength and function. Immunosuppressive therapies have also been tried but with limited success.

Becker Muscular Dystrophy

Etiology, Pathogenesis, and Clinical Manifestations. **Becker dystrophy** is a milder form of inherited muscle degeneration, somewhat less common than the Duchenne type with an annual incidence of 5 per 100,000. The genetic mutation leads to production of a reduced amount of an abnormal dystrophin protein and a slower muscular degeneration. Calf hypertrophy is still prominent and often painful with progressive loss of strength and ability to ambulate. The mean age of symptom onset is somewhat later (5 to 15 years) with patients requiring a wheelchair by the age of 30 years.[12]

Facioscapulohumeral Muscular Dystrophy

Etiology and Pathogenesis. **Facioscapulohumeral muscular dystrophy** is an inherited autosomal dominant trait that affects the muscles of the shoulder girdle and the face. It is rare with an annual incidence of 1 in 20,000. The onset of disease can occur at any age, but it usually begins in the second decade. Facial muscles are involved early, with later involvement of scapular and upper arm musculature. It progresses slowly with periods of arrest and can ultimately involve more distal muscles of the upper and lower extremities. Both males and females are affected, and most live to a normal age, although approximately 20% of these patients require a wheelchair eventually.[12]

OTHER DISORDERS OF MUSCLE

Myasthenia Gravis

Myasthenia gravis is a chronic autoimmune disease affecting the neuromuscular function of voluntary muscles and characterized by profound muscle weakness and fatigability. Its peak onset in females occurs at 20 to 30 years of age. Men may experience it after 40 years of age. Women are affected more often than men. Characteristically, weakness begins with ocular and cranial muscles, and then limb muscles can also be involved. During times of emotional stress, respiratory muscles may be included.

In myasthenia gravis, acetylcholine receptor antibodies are produced that destroy or block acetylcholine receptors of the muscle end-plate of the neuromuscular junction. These antibodies impair the transmission of acetylcholine across the junction. The result is the muscle weakness and fatigability so prevalent in this disease.[12]

Treatment. Anticholinesterase agents (e.g., neostigmine) may be used to inhibit breakdown of acetylcholine in the neuromuscular synapse. Increased synaptic acetylcholine enhances the activation of postsynaptic receptors and improves skeletal muscle contraction force. Because myasthenia gravis is an autoimmune disorder, steroids, plasmapheresis, and cytotoxic agents may be used to suppress the immune system. In severe cases, respiratory muscle fatigue may necessitate mechanical ventilation.

Myasthenia crisis can be due to insufficient medication, emotional stress, trauma, infection, or surgery. A sudden increase in blood pressure and pulse is noted. Other symptoms include cyanosis from hypoxia, absent cough and gag reflexes, restlessness, increased secretions and lacrimation, diaphoresis, decreased urine output, bowel and bladder incontinence, dysarthria, and respiratory distress.

Cholinergic crisis is usually due to excessive medication. Patients experiencing such a crisis will have fasciculations, especially around the mouth; difficulty chewing, swallowing, and speaking; advancing muscle weakness approximately 1 hour after anticholinesterase medication; nausea and vomiting; cramps and diarrhea; increased secretions (salivary, perspiration, lacrimal, bronchial); headache; confusion; irritability and anxiety; syncope; and respiratory distress leading to respiratory arrest.

Thymectomy for hyperplasia, which is often apparent in 85% of patients, is often recommended. If done within the first 2 years of the disease, thymectomy induces remission of symptoms in about 40% of patients. Women seem to achieve greatest benefit from thymectomy.[12]

CHRONIC MUSCLE PAIN

Fibromyalgia Syndrome

Etiology and Pathogenesis. The cause of **fibromyalgia syndrome** (FMS) is unknown. No laboratory abnormalities have been found, muscle biopsy findings are nonspecific, and patients are normal on psychological testing. The condition is not an inflammatory process but rather a "pain syndrome," with recent studies suggesting that changes in the central nervous system may lead to amplification of pain fiber impulses, a so-called "central sensitization." This generalized increase in pain sensitivity may involve both ascending and descending neural pathways and a variety of neurotransmitters and neuropeptides.[13]

FMS is characterized by chronic pain in muscles and surrounding structures often of months or years duration. Additional symptoms include fatigue, sleep dysfunction, headache, numbness and tingling, joint pain, memory and concentration difficulties, irritable bowel syndrome, depression, edema of the hands, and sensitivity to cold.[8] Patients may either have no disease or have rheumatoid arthritis, osteoarthritis, Lyme disease, or sleep apnea. FMS is characterized by a strong female preponderance (more than 75% in most epidemiology studies), with a peak incidence between 20 and 60 years of age.

Clinical Manifestations. Patients with FMS complain of musculoskeletal pain, stiffness, and fatigability. Generalized pain is a common complaint. Joint pain and swelling are perceived by the patient, but the swelling cannot be documented. Complaints of muscle pain and weakness are expressed without objective demonstration. In addition to stiffness and fatigue, sleep disturbances are a common complaint. The examination of a patient with FMS is characterized by an excessive number of reported symptoms with minimal objective findings other than muscular tenderness. Proposed criteria for the diagnosis of FMS established by the American College of Rheumatology include widespread pain in combination with tenderness of at least 11 of 18 (9 bilateral sites) specific tender point sites.[8]

1. Occiput—bilaterally at suboccipital muscle insertions
2. Low cervical—bilaterally at anterior aspects of the intertransverse spaces at C5-7
3. Trapezius—bilaterally at the midpoint of the upper border
4. Supraspinatus—bilaterally at the origins above the scapular spine near the medial border
5. Second rib—bilaterally at the second costochondral junctions, just lateral to junctions on the upper surfaces
6. Lateral epicondyle—bilaterally, 2 cm distal to the epicondyles

7 Gluteal—bilaterally in the upper outer quadrants of the buttocks in the anterior fold of the muscle
8 Greater trochanter—bilaterally, posterior to the trochanteric prominence
9 Knee—bilaterally at the medial fat pad proximal to the joint line

Although these tender points are the most common and are included in the criteria for fibromyalgia, in actuality, nearly any muscle in the human body could contain a tender point.

Treatment. FMS is neither a psychiatric condition nor life threatening. Because the cause of FMS is unknown, treatment focuses on maintaining functionality and reducing symptoms. Patient education is important and may be associated with improved outcomes and better prognosis. An exercise regimen is also useful and should include regular stretching, improvement in physical conditioning via low-impact aerobic exercise (biking, swimming, walking), and measures of pacing, muscle protection, and relaxation. Because pain and fatigue may be aggravated by stress and other psychological factors, counseling may be helpful.[14]

Blinded, randomized, placebo-controlled studies of amitriptyline, cyclobenzaprine, zolpidem, and alprazolam administered at bedtime have indicated that all are effective FMS therapy. Treatment begins at the lowest possible doses and increases as tolerated, with the goal being to improve quality of sleep without drug side effects, such as daytime somnolence or excessive dry mouth. Other medications under investigation in FMS are meant to lower pain sensitivity. The selective serotonin reuptake inhibitors that have been studied in FMS include fluoxetine, sertraline, and citalopram. Although their efficacy as monotherapy is modest at best, they may prove beneficial in combination with other agents. Additional medications that may have a role include venlafaxine, pregabalin (an antiepileptic agent), and tramadol (an opioid-like analgesic) among many other agents being investigated.[13]

KEY CONCEPTS

- Muscular dystrophy comprises a group of genetic disorders characterized by degeneration of skeletal muscle.
- Duchenne muscular dystrophy is inherited as an X-linked disorder and affects only males.
- Facioscapulohumeral muscular dystrophy is an autosomal dominant disorder in which degenerating muscle fibers are replaced by connective tissue such that muscles may gain in bulk even though muscle strength is lost.
- Myasthenia gravis is an autoimmune disorder characterized by progressive weakness as the muscles are used. Antibodies against acetylcholine receptors in the motor end-plate interrupt neuromuscular transmission.
- FMS is a poorly characterized chronic disorder associated with generalized pain, stiffness, sleep dysfunction, and fatigability.

SUMMARY

A solid working knowledge of the anatomy, physiology, and biomechanics of movement is extremely important when dealing with any type of alteration in the musculoskeletal system. With a grasp of the mechanics involved in function, the clinician is able to approach each aberration with an awareness of the time requirements for healing, stress tolerances, and expected management outcomes.

The injuries and diseases discussed in this chapter are a small representation of the many dysfunctions that may afflict the musculoskeletal system. An ability to determine the specific type of tissue involved (contractile or inert) allows the clinician to be cognizant of activities that would aggravate trauma, types of injury that require supportive devices, and injuries that respond to medical intervention.

An awareness of the tissue response to healing enhances the clinician's evaluative skills and provides a signal regarding when intervention has achieved the expected results within an appropriate time frame. It is the responsibility of the practitioner to become knowledgeable about the variety of dysfunctions that occur. This knowledge base must continue to expand as technological advancements provide increasingly complex levels of information and new diagnostic tools become available.

MEDIA RESOURCES

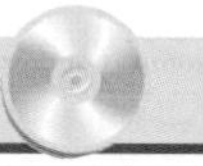

evolve

Remember to check out the ***CD Companion*** included with this book for Review Questions, Key Concepts Review, Glossary (with audio for selected terms), Disease Profiles, and Animations.

PLUS, visit the ***Evolve website*** at http://evolve.elsevier.com/Copstead/ for Case Studies, Disease Profiles, and WebLinks.

References

1. Chapman MW et al, editors: *Chapman's orthopaedic surgery,* ed 3, Philadelphia, 2001, Lippincott Williams & Wilkins.
2. Koopman WJ: *Arthritis and allied conditions,* ed 14, Philadelphia, 2001, Lippincott Williams & Wilkins.
3. Favus MJ, editor: *Primer on the metabolic bone diseases and disorders of mineral metabolism,* ed 4, Philadelphia, 1999, Lippincott-Raven.
4. Giangregorio L, Blimkie CJ: Skeletal adaptations to alterations in weight-bearing activity: a comparison of models of disuse osteoporosis, *Sports Med* 32(7):459-476, 2002.
5. Iseman MD: *A clinician's guide to tuberculosis,* Philadelphia, 2000, Lippincott Williams & Wilkins, pp 162-167.

6. Abeloff MD et al, editors: *Clinical oncology,* ed 2, New York, 2000, Churchill Livingstone.
7. Cyriax J: *Textbook of orthopedic medicine: diagnosis of soft tissue lesions,* ed 8, London, 1982, Bailliere Tindall.
8. Klippel JH: *Primer on the rheumatic diseases,* ed 12, Atlanta, 2001, Arthritis Foundation.
9. Ruddy S, Harris ED, Sledge CB: *Kelley's textbook of rheumatology,* ed 6, Philadelphia, 2001, Saunders.
10. Hettinga DL: Inflammatory response of synovial joint structures. In Gould J, editor: *Orthopedic and sports physical therapy,* ed 2, St Louis, 1990, Mosby, p 100.
11. Richardson JK, Iglarsh ZA: *Clinical orthopedic physical therapy,* Philadelphia, 1993, Saunders.
12. Goldman L, Bennett JC, editors: *Cecil textbook of medicine,* ed 21, Philadelphia, 2000, Saunders.
13. Rao SG: The neuropharmacology of centrally-acting analgesic medications in fibromyalgia, *Rheum Dis Clin North Am* 28(2):235-259, 2002.
14. Bennett RM: The rational management of fibromyalgia patients, *Rheum Dis Clin North Am* 28(2):181-199, 2002.

Alterations in Musculoskeletal Function: Rheumatic Disorders

chapter 52

Carol L. Danning

MEDIA RESOURCES

Additional Material for Study, Review, and Further Exploration

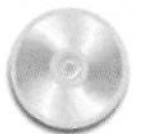

CD Companion ◆ Review Questions and Answers ◆ Key Concepts Review
◆ Glossary *(with audio pronunciations for selected terms)*
◆ Disease Profiles ◆ Animations

evolve ***Website*** at http://evolve.elsevier.com/Copstead/
◆ Case Studies ◆ Disease Profiles ◆ WebLinks

KEY QUESTIONS

- How are osteoarthritis and rheumatoid arthritis differentiated on the basis of cause, clinical findings, and treatment?
- What are the similarities and differences among rheumatoid arthritis, systemic lupus erythematosus, and scleroderma?
- What are the infective organisms leading to rheumatic joint disease and Lyme disease?
- What is the pathogenesis of gouty arthritis?
- How do the three subtypes of juvenile rheumatoid arthritis differ?

CHAPTER OUTLINE

Arthritis is the most common disabling musculoskeletal condition in the United States. The National Arthritis Foundation estimates that more than 40 million people have arthritis and 125,000 are newly diagnosed with arthritis each year. More than 150 defined rheumatologic diseases have been identified. This chapter discusses the more common rheumatologic diseases.[1]

LOCAL DISORDERS OF JOINT FUNCTION

Osteoarthritis

Osteoarthritis (degenerative joint disease) is the most common arthritis worldwide. It is a progressive, noninflammatory disease of diarthrodial joints, especially those that bear weight. It is characterized by a progressive loss of articular cartilage and by formation of thick subchondral bone and new bone at the joint margins.[1] Osteoarthritis (OA) becomes more prevalent with increasing age. Individuals older than 65 years have the highest incidence. In women older than 50 years, the knee is the joint most frequently effected by OA.[1] It is difficult to estimate the exact prevalence of OA due to difficulties associated with diagnosis, lack of longitudinal data, and difficulty defining disease onset.

Etiology and Pathogenesis. The etiologic progression of OA varies widely. Development of OA may be related to factors that increase the likelihood of abnormal "wear and tear" on joints such as obesity, joint trauma, joint sepsis, and congenital disorders (i.e., hip dysplasia, leg length discrepancy). Other predisposing conditions include lifestyle factors (stress to joints), primary diseases affecting joints (Paget disease, diabetes mellitus), genetic predisposition, and hormonal status (postmenopausal).[1]

Biomechanical, biochemical, inflammatory, and immunologic factors may all be involved in the development of OA (Figure 52-1). An initial injury causes release of proteolytic and collagenolytic enzymes from chondrocytes. A breakdown of the matrix of proteoglycan and collagen occurs. The decreased hydration of cartilage that occurs with aging can increase the likelihood of wear and damage. Collagen fatigue and microfracture occur with the stress of weight bearing. The ability of the structure to absorb shock is decreased due to subcortical bone and cartilage microfractures. Breakdown of joint integrity overloads the capacity for repair, with resultant degenerative changes.

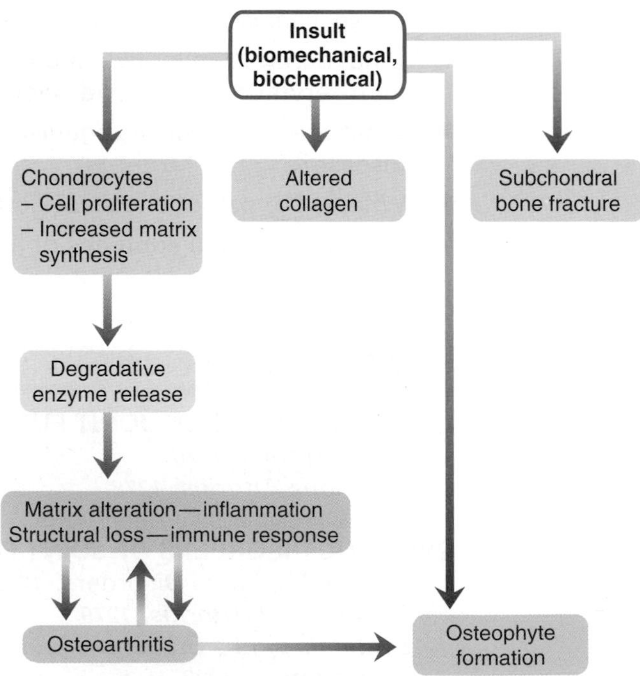

FIGURE 52-1 ■ Pathogenesis of osteoarthritis.

Structural breakdown of the cartilage involves fissuring, pitting, and erosion. Erosion can become so extensive that the articular surface denudes the full thickness of the cartilage. Osteophyte spur formation, sclerosis of subchondral bone, and cyst formation are also examples of structural changes present in OA. Cartilage fragments may break off into joints and form "loose bodies" (Figure 52-2). Joint effusions are common in advanced cases. Synovium becomes inflamed and secretes an increased amount of synovial fluid, which causes the joint to distend.

Clinical Manifestations. Bony enlargement of joints, crepitus with movement, morning stiffness lasting less than 30 minutes (that improves with joint mobility), and pain with function are typical clinical manifestations of OA. These signs and symptoms are usually local. Although any joint may be affected, weight-bearing joints such as the hips and knees, cervical and lumbosacral joints, and interphalangeal joints are most frequently involved. Rheumatoid arthritis (RA) has symmetric distribution in peripheral joints and is inflammatory in nature. Degenerative arthritis or OA usually occurs in an isolated joint, although multiple joints can be involved especially in hands. Mechanical dysfunction, anatomic anomalies, or trauma may cause breakdown of joint surface. It is imperative to establish a differential diagnosis and to rule out a systemic or medical problem. OA is localized, whereas RA is systemic.

Radiologic abnormalities are normally consistent with clinical symptoms. Classic findings include bony proliferation at the joint margins (i.e., osteophytes or bone spurs), asymmetric narrowing of the joint space, and subchondral bone sclerosis. Later, malalignment of the joints and cyst formation in subchondral bone can also be seen. When significant synovial fluid accumulates in the joint, it is usually noninflammatory fluid containing less than 2000 white blood cells per cubic millimeter.[1]

The most common deformity of the hands occurs in the distal interphalangeal (DIP) joints (Figure 52-3). Enlargement is caused by spurs *(Heberden nodes)* that form on the dorsolateral and medial aspects of the joint. Similar enlargements in the proximal interphalangeal (PIP) joints are called *Bouchard nodes.* The knees and hips are also common locations for OA. Local pain over joint margins, tenderness, crepitus, and muscle atrophy are common findings. Loss of cartilage in medial or lateral compartments of the knee may lead to such structural changes as genu valgus or varus (Figure 52-4).

Pain is relieved by rest during initial stages. Because cartilage does not contain nociceptors (pain receptors), pain originates from intraarticular and periarticular structures.

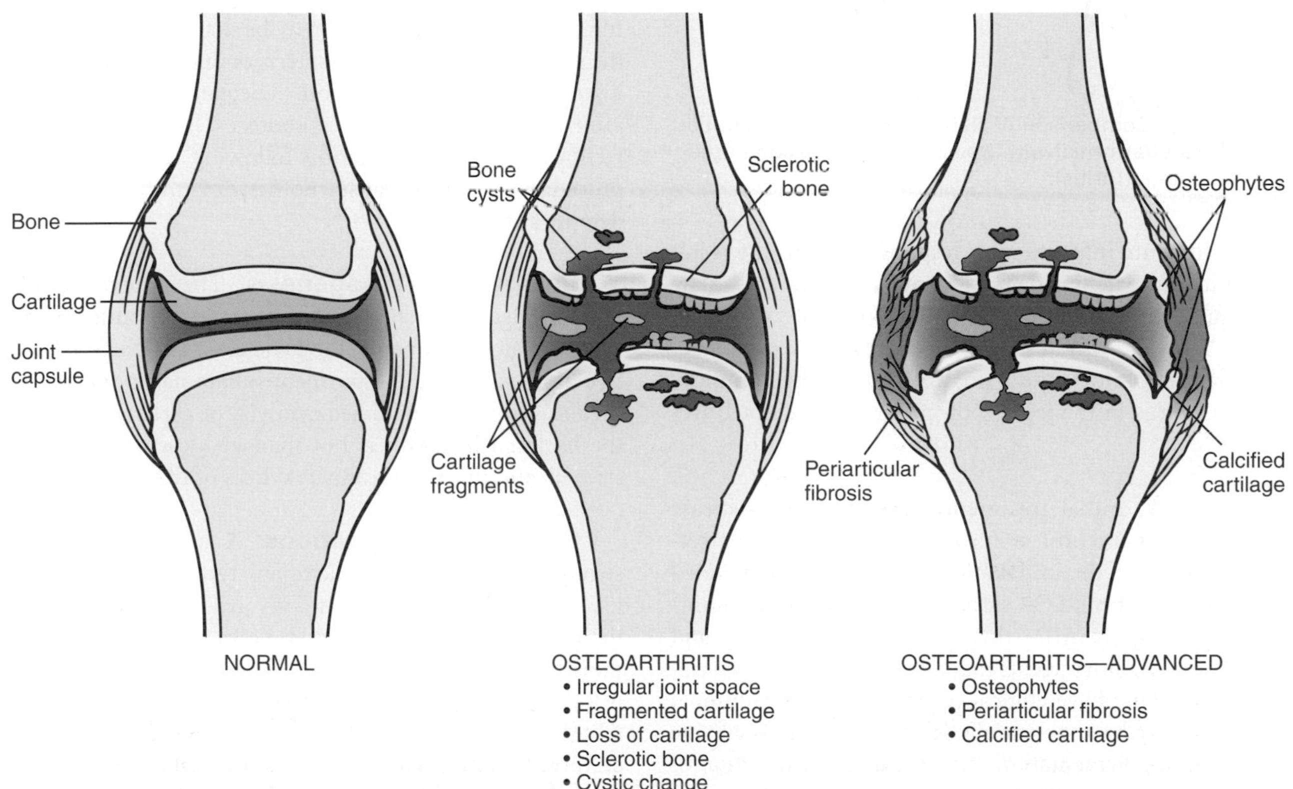

FIGURE 52-2 ■ Schematic presentation of the pathologic changes in osteoarthritis. Fragmentation and loss of cartilage denude the subchondral bone, which undergoes sclerosis and cystic change. Osteophytes form on the lateral side and protrude into the adjacent soft tissues, causing irritation, inflammation, and fibrosis. (From Damjanov I: *Pathology for the health-related professions,* ed 2, Philadelphia, 2000, Saunders, p 455.)

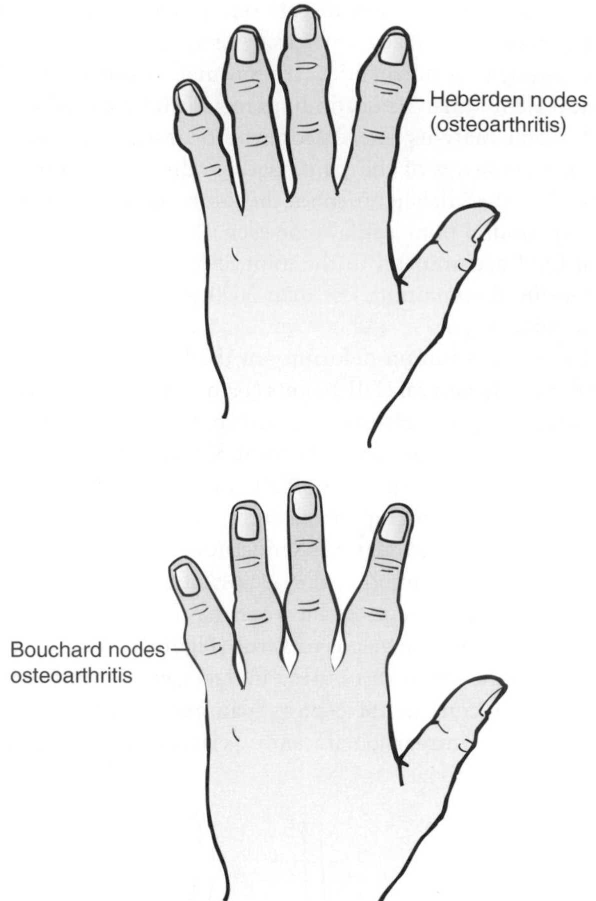

FIGURE 52-3 ■ Comparison of Heberden nodes (seen in patients with osteoarthritis) with Bouchard nodes (seen in patients with osteoarthritis).

Although an acute inflammatory response is often the result of a specific traumatic incident and may cause synovitis in the joint capsule, acute inflammation is not commonly associated with OA. As breakdown in structure progresses, even light activity elicits discomfort, and pain at night is quite common. Pain and crepitus in the joint with movement are noted frequently.

Treatment. Initial treatment is designed to decrease stress on the joint and protect it from additional trauma. Acetaminophen is often the initial analgesic agent recommended for management of mild OA symptoms. Nonsteroidal antiinflammatory drug (NSAID) therapy decreases swelling and pain. Antiinflammatory agents that target the cyclooxygenase-2 (COX-2) enzyme have clinical benefit equal to traditional NSAIDs but may have potentially fewer gastrointestinal side effects. Visco-supplementation, the intraarticular injection of hyaluronan or its derivatives, may increase joint lubrication, reduce inflammation, and alleviate pain. These agents are currently only available for use in knee OA.

Physical therapy to improve range of motion, muscle strength, and joint conditioning as well as weight reduction can improve symptoms and prevent loss of function. Assistive devices, such as a cane or walker, afford mechanical relief of weight-bearing stress. Surgical intervention may be necessary if the joint surface loses enough integrity to prevent joint function. OA is the most common cause for total hip and total knee replacement.

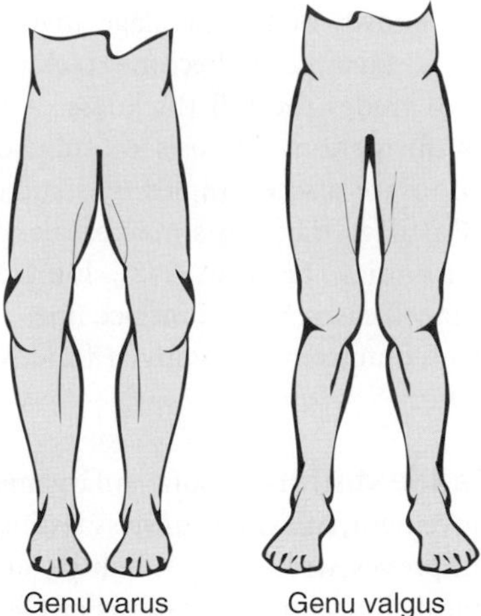

FIGURE 52-4 ■ Genu varus and genu valgus.

Infectious Arthritis

Infectious or septic arthritis may be defined as an invasion of the synovial membrane by bacteria or another pathogen, leading to a closed-space infection.[1] The pathogen can invade the joint space via hematogenous route, extension of adjacent infection, or direct inoculation following trauma or invasive procedure. Infection causes both synovium and cartilage to deteriorate.

Etiology and Pathogenesis. The basic cause of bone and cartilage destruction is the interaction of antigenic bacterial cell wall components, the toxic effects of bacteria, the destruction caused by the purulent inflammatory exudate, and the local immune-mediated synovial or cartilage response. If the bacterial infection is not managed, cartilage can be destroyed, and this can lead to ankylosis of the joint.

Clinical Manifestations. A singular, warm, very swollen joint is symptomatic of any type of infectious arthritis. Usually only a single joint is involved, but sometimes more than one joint may be infected. Polyarticular involvement is more common in debilitated or immunosuppressed persons. A low-grade fever is present in most patients. Diagnosis is established by recovery of bacteria from synovial fluid. Blood cultures are also used to provide a medical diagnosis.

The patient with septic arthritis presents with joint pain, fever, chills, and leukocytosis. Fever may range from mild to high fever with shaking chills. In neonates, children older than 4 years, and adults, *Staphylococcus aureus* is the most common causative organism. In children 6 months to 5 years of age,

Haemophilus influenza type B is most common. *Neisseria gonorrhoeae* is a causative organism in some adults younger than 30 years.[2]

Treatment. Treatment of a septic joint should include appropriate antibiotic therapy (often initially intravenous and then oral) with the average duration required being 4 to 6 weeks. This therapy is most effective when the bacteria can be isolated and identified from the synovial fluid and antibiotic sensitivities can be used to determine the most effective antibiotic to be used. In addition, the infected joint usually requires drainage to facilitate bacterial clearance, decrease pain, and prevent loss of function. This can be done either through repeated joint aspiration or open surgical drainage.

Joint Prosthesis Infection

Anaerobic bacterial arthritis may be found in patients after total joint replacement or fracture or in patients with RA. Generally, a prosthetic joint infection requires removal of the prosthesis followed by a rigorous course of intravenous antibiotic therapy, often for 6 weeks or longer. Antibiotic beads may also be placed in the wound. The prosthesis is replaced when cultures from the wound show no growth.[2]

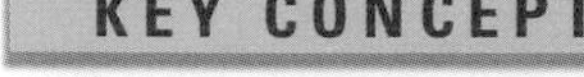

KEY CONCEPTS

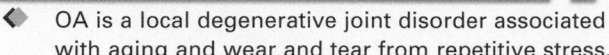

- OA is a local degenerative joint disorder associated with aging and wear and tear from repetitive stress.
- OA is characterized by loss of articular cartilage, wear of underlying bone, and the formation of bone spurs. The process is noninflammatory. Weight-bearing joints are often affected.
- Signs and symptoms of OA are localized (not systemic) and include joint pain and crepitus with movement.
- Joint infection may be due to a variety of infectious agents, but bacteria are most problematic. The route of infection is usually by way of the blood stream. Signs and symptoms are due to localized infection and the systemic manifestation of inflammation.

SYSTEMIC DISORDERS OF JOINT FUNCTION

Immune-Mediated Disorders

Rheumatoid Arthritis

Rheumatoid arthritis is a systemic inflammatory disease. In the United States, approximately 1% to 2% of the population is affected.[1] Women are two to three times more likely to develop RA than men, with a ratio of 3:1 and a peak incidence between the fourth and sixth decades. Gender difference disappears in older age. RA affects all races, and its prevalence is not affected by climate. Eighty percent of RA patients test rheumatoid factor (RF) positive.

Etiology and Pathogenesis. The specific cause of RA is unknown. There are two basic theories. One is that RA has an infectious cause; however, an infectious organism has not been isolated from any joint. A more likely theory is that it is due to an abnormal autoimmune response that occurs in individuals who have a genetic predisposition to the disease. RA occurs two to three times more often in women with a familial history of RA.[3]

Current research suggests that susceptibility to RA is determined by gene products of the major histocompatibility system. β-Lymphocyte alloantigen human leukocyte antigen DR4 (HLA-DR4) has been noted in 60% to 70% of adult Caucasian patients with RA although it is likely that several genes are involved.[3] These genes possibly control humoral and cell-mediated immune mechanisms believed to contribute to the pathogenesis of RA. The cause and type of stimulus of immunologic abnormalities are not known, but they might be due to an infectious agent, environmental influences, or other lifestyle factors. Trauma to the joint is also a possible cause. An increase in physical and/or psychological stress has also been associated with precipitating acute exacerbation of the disease.

Initially, pathologic changes in RA occur when the immune response localizes in synovial tissue. Here lymphocytes (T and B) and macrophages are activated by an unknown antigen trigger. B cells produce RF antibodies against immunoglobulin G (IgG) to form immune complexes. Although immunoglobulins are natural human antibodies, the body produces an antibody (RF) against its own antibody (IgG). Activated lymphocytes, macrophages, and antigen-antibody complexes activate the complement system, stimulate recruitment of other immune cells into the synovium, and produce an extensive array of inflammatory cytokines, metalloproteinases, and other mediators. These products of macrophages and lymphocytes are believed to be critical in RA pathogenesis because they stimulate and perpetuate the inflammation in the joint. Key proinflammatory cytokines demonstrated in the synovium include tumor necrosis factor α (TNF-α), and interleukins-1β (IL-1β), 8, 15, and 18, although many other are also being studied. Newer biological therapies are designed to target these cytokines.

The escalating inflammatory response in the rheumatoid joint leads to accumulation of dense aggregates of immune cells and infiltration of the synovium. The cells produce more cytokines and growth factors, which also stimulate edema, neovascularization, and proliferation of the synovium (which expands in a tumorlike manner.) This hypertrophied synovium invades such surrounding tissue as cartilage, ligaments, joint capsule, and tendons. Granulation tissue forms, covering articular cartilage and leading to pannus formation. Pannus is vascularized scar tissue made up of lymphocytes, macrophages, histiocytes, fibroblasts, and mast cells. Pannus can erode and destroy articular cartilage, resulting in bone erosion, bone cysts, and fissures (Figure 52-5). The expansion and destruction of joint structures can lead to inflammation, shortening, and even rupture of tendons as well as ligament laxity, joint subluxations, contractures, and deformities.[1]

Clinical Manifestations. RA has a number of clinical features. In 1987, the American Rheumatism Association revised the then 30-year-old criteria for classification of RA. There are seven criteria, and RA is defined by the presence of four or more criteria. Criteria 1 through 4 must present for a minimum of 6 weeks. The criteria are as follows:

1. Morning stiffness in and around joints lasting at least 1 hour before maximal improvement.
2. Soft tissue swelling (arthritis) of three or more joint areas (including the right and left proximal PIP, metacarpophalangeal [MCP], wrist, elbow, knee, ankle, and metatarsophalangeal [MTP] joints).
3. Swelling of at least one wrist, MCP, or PIP joint.
4. Simultaneous symmetric swelling in joints listed in criterion 2.
5. Subcutaneous rheumatoid nodules.
6. Presence of rheumatoid factor.
7. Radiographic erosions and/or periarticular osteopenia in hand and/or wrist joints.[4]

Malaise, fatigue, and diffuse musculoskeletal pain are common manifestations during acute flare-ups of the disease. It is interesting to note that symmetric patterns involving the joints of the hands, wrists, elbows, and shoulders are evident. DIP joints are usually spared. This symmetry and the noninvolvement of the DIP joint assist in making the diagnosis of RA.

The hands, wrists, knees, and feet are most commonly involved. In the spine, the upper cervical area is most often af-

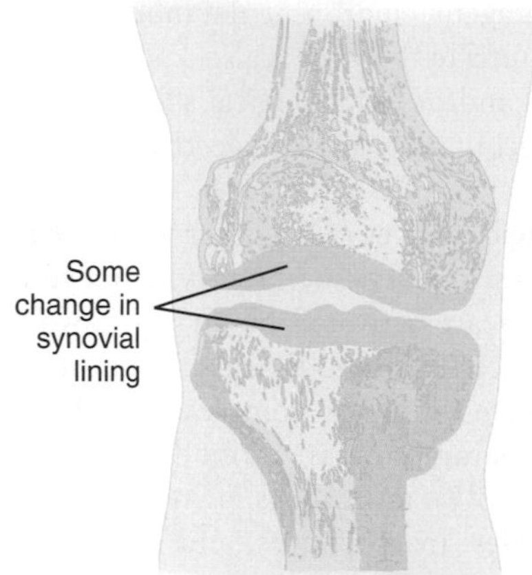

INITIATION PHASE

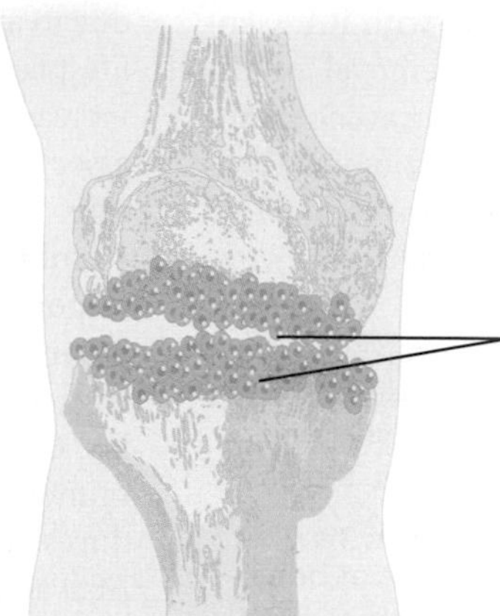

IMMUNE RESPONSE PHASE
Hyperplasia of synovium

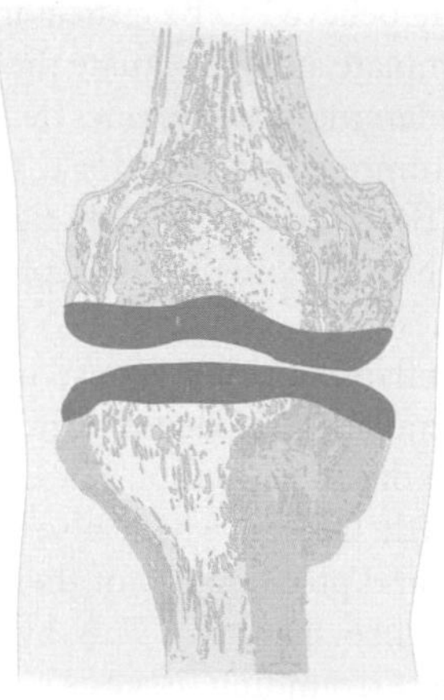

INFLAMMATORY PHASE
Oxygen radicals, arachidonic acid radicals, and lysosomes destroy synovial tissue

Pannus

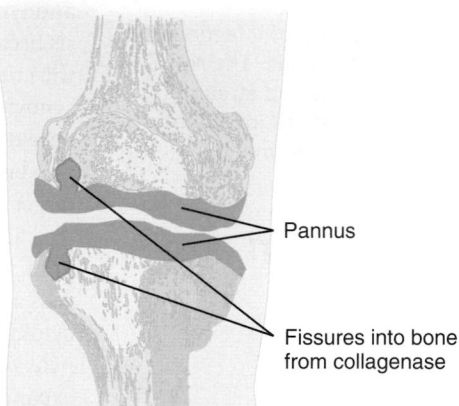

Fissures into bone from collagenase

DESTRUCTION PHASE

FIGURE 52-5 ■ Schematic presentation of the pathologic changes in rheumatoid arthritis. The inflammation (synovitis) leads to pannus formation, obliteration of the articular space, and finally, ankylosis. The periarticular bone shows disuse atrophy in the form of osteoporosis. (From Black JM, Hawks JH, Keene AM, *Medical-surgical nursing, clinical management for positive outcomes,* ed 6, Philadelphia, 2001, Saunders.)

fected. However, any diarthrodial joint is potentially at risk. The development of pannus followed by inflammatory destruction of the soft tissue leads to laxity of the ligaments and tendons and results in biomechanical dysfunction. This mechanical stress causes the typical deformities of RA.

Swelling in the hands is a typical sign of PIP joint involvement, as is swelling of the MCP joints. Pain is elicited on palpation of the joints. Gradually, progressive synovial damage leads to characteristic ulnar deviation in the MCP joint (Figure 52-6). In advanced situations, a swan-neck deformity develops in the fingers. Swan-neck deformity is a hyperextension of the PIP joint with flexion of the MCP and DIP joints due to contractures of intrinsic muscles and tendons.[5] A boutonnière deformity, consisting of flexion of the PIP joints and hyperextension of the DIP joints, is also a common dysfunctional position due to rupture of extensor tendons over the fingers (Figure 52-7). Loss of strength and the ability to achieve a strong pinch is frequently noted in the hand affected by RA. A rupture of tendons and loss of the ability to extend the fingers are common findings in later stages of the disease.

The wrist is commonly involved. The synovium around the wrist becomes boggy and affects the tendon sheaths. Limitation of movement, especially dorsiflexion of the wrist, is often noted. Proliferation of the synovium on the volar or palmar aspect of the wrist may cause compression of the median nerve and development of carpal tunnel syndrome. Flexion contractures and swelling of the elbow are other common manifestations; in later stages of the disease, shoulder involvement may occur. Typical signs of shoulder involvement are limitations of movement and pain on palpation in the area of the coracoid process. Dislocation, subluxation, or rupture of the joint capsule may occur as the disease progresses.

Involvement of the upper cervical vertebrae is another common finding. Destruction of structures of the atlantoaxial vertebrae creates the potential for subluxation of this joint and endangerment of the spinal cord. Laxity in the cervical region may also allow compression of the vertebral artery, leading to vertebrobasilar insufficiency. Limitation of motion (especially rotation), pain on palpation, and headache in the occipital region are common.

Abnormalities in gait and limitations of movement are signs noted when RA affects the hip. Groin pain due to capsular involvement may be present. If synovitis of the hip becomes extensive, severe pain may be noted on evaluation. RA involvement in the knee is often extensive. Effusion, quadriceps atrophy, contractures, and synovitis of the semimembranous bursa (Baker cyst) may be observed. Destruction of the articular surface, bone, and soft tissue may result from joint instability. One common clinical sign of involvement of the foot is retrocalcaneal bursitis. Other features of foot involvement include swelling of joints, a cocking-up of the toes due to subluxation of the metatarsal heads (claw toes), and lateral deviation of the first through fourth toes.

These clinical manifestations may develop rapidly or progress over many years. Usually symptoms develop over weeks and months. Initially, the patient may feel fatigued or chronically tired and may complain of systemic aching in the musculoskeletal system. Specific joint pain, tenderness, swelling, redness, and nodules are quite common.

Prolonged inactivity, such as sitting, initiates complaints of stiffness and swelling. As the disease progresses, walking,

Ulnar drift

FIGURE 52-6 ■ Typical deformity of the hand seen in patients with rheumatoid arthritis. Note ulnar deviation. (From Black JM, Hawks JH: *Medical-surgical nursing, clinical management for positive outcomes,* ed 7, Philadelphia, 2005, Saunders.)

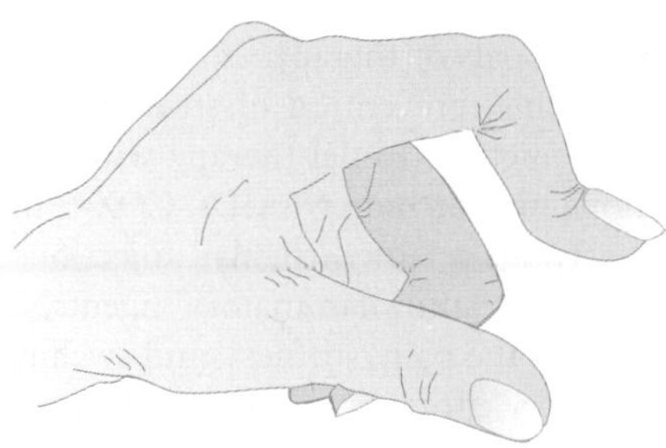

Boutonnière deformity

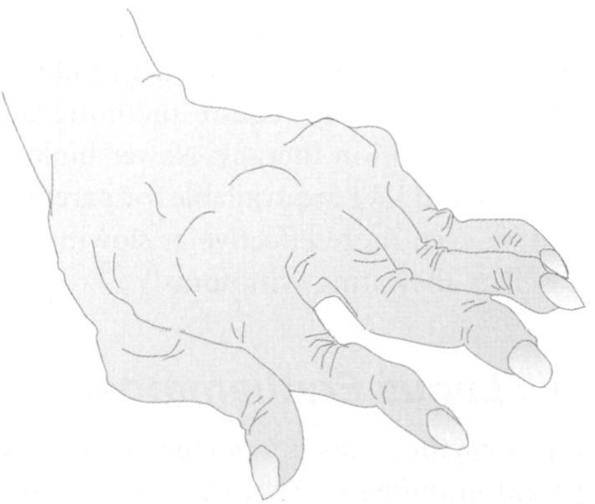

Swan-neck deformity

FIGURE 52-7 ■ Swan-neck and boutonnière deformities. (From Black JM, Hawks JH: *Medical-surgical nursing, clinical management for positive outcomes,* ed 7, Philadelphia, 2005, Saunders, p 2335.)

climbing stairs, opening jars or doors, and precise movement of the digits become quite difficult. Weight loss, depression, and a low-grade fever often are noted in these patients.

Unlike OA, RA is a systemic connective tissue disease. It is imperative that a definitive differential diagnosis be developed. RA may be confused with a number of disease entities such as Lyme disease, systemic lupus erythematosus (SLE), or gout. RA may also cause subcutaneous nodules and present with cardiac, pulmonary, and ophthalmologic manifestations.

Cardiac manifestations may include pericarditis, myocarditis, mitral valve disease, and conduction system disease or complete heart block. Pulmonary manifestations may occur as pleuritis, pulmonary fibrosis, pleural effusions, or pulmonary nodules. Ophthalmic manifestations might include episcleritis, scleritis, or secondary Sjögren syndrome (dry eyes and mouth.)

A positive RF is found in the sera of approximately 85% patients with RA. The titer of the RF does not fluctuate with disease activity and is not essential for the diagnosis of RA. Inflammatory markers (sedimentation rate, C-reactive protein) are often elevated. Other laboratory features may include hypergammaglobulinemia, thrombocytosis, and hypochromic microcytic anemia.[1]

Radiography may demonstrate structural damage due to RA. Typical findings include erosions on the margins of bone, joint space narrowing, osteopenia, and eventual malalignment and subluxation of the bones.

Treatment. Goals of therapy should include alleviation of pain and swelling, prevention of structural damage, and preservation of function. Initial therapy with antiinflammatory medications may include NSAIDs, COX-2 inhibitors, or corticosteroids (oral or intraarticular injections.) Corticosteroids are potent antiinflammatory agents, effective at quickly controlling the pain, stiffness, and swelling of RA activity; however every effort is made to avoid long-term steroid use due to adverse consequences such as steroid-induced osteoporosis, diabetes mellitus, cataracts, and more. Disease-modifying antirheumatic drugs are used to achieve long-term control of RA activity and are recommended early in the course of disease. Medications such as antimalarial agents, sulfasalazine, and oral gold can be used in milder cases, but more aggressive disease may require methotrexate, leflunomide, or even combination therapy. Newer biological agents that target TNF-α and IL-1 are available for parenteral use and may prove to be even more effective at slowing disease progression as well as alleviating symptoms.[1]

Systemic Lupus Erythematosus

Systemic lupus erythematosus is a chronic, multisystem, inflammatory, autoimmune disease. It is characterized by periods of exacerbations and remission, with multiple organs systems being affected at different times.

Etiology and Pathogenesis. Genetic involvement has been demonstrated in familial occurrences of SLE.[6] Although SLE occurs in all races, it occurs more often in the United States among African-Americans than Caucasians and yet is uncommon in Africa.[6] Environmental factors such as sunlight, thermal burns, and other types of physical stress may initiate the development of SLE. SLE is more common in women, with peak incidence between 15 and 40 years of age, suggesting hormonal involvement.

SLE is the result of an abnormal reaction of the body against its own tissues, cells, and serum proteins—the body has a decreased tolerance to itself. One of the main mechanisms is B-lymphocyte overactivity leading to excessive autoantibody production. SLE patients can express a myriad of antibodies directed against many self-molecules and antigens located in cell nuclei and cytoplasm. Among these antibodies, those directed against nuclear antigens (antinuclear antibodies, or ANAs) are found in more than 95% of SLE patients.[1] As antigen-antibody complexes form, they enter the basement membranes of capillaries specifically in the kidneys, heart, skin, brain, and joints. Immune complexes then activate complement and trigger the inflammatory responses, which are responsible for tissue destruction.

Clinical Manifestations. SLE typically affects multiple organ systems such as the kidneys, heart, skin, brain, joints, lungs, and gastrointestinal tract. Not all systems are affected simultaneously. The characteristic clinical course is one of exacerbation and remission. A remission may last for many years.

In the joints, tendons, and bones, arthralgias and synovitis are common features of SLE. Most patients complain of joint pain at some time during the course of the disease. Swelling, tenderness, pain on movement, and morning stiffness are noted. Involvement of the capsule, ligaments, and tendons can be extensive, causing reducible deformities in hands and feet. Deformities range from contractures of the fingers, to hyperextension of the interphalangeal joint of the thumb, to subluxation of the MCP joint of the thumb. With steroid therapy, tendon rupture is not uncommon.

Skin lesions may be quite extensive in SLE. Acute cutaneous lupus erythematosus often manifests with a classic butterfly (malar) rash present in 40% of patients. The skin lesion may be exacerbated during systemic flare-up. Swelling and redness are noted, and sunlight or artificial ultraviolet light may initiate a response. Skin involvement may occur on the shoulders, upper arms, upper back, chest, and neck. Scales or plaques develop on the scalp, ears, face, and neck. A latticelike venular skin change (livedo reticularis) is a very common skin manifestation. Alopecia may also occur.

A number of systemic manifestations may also be present. Cardiac complications include pericarditis, myocarditis, and congestive heart failure. Lung and pleural involvement includes pleuritis or pleural effusion. Renal involvement is common and can vary in severity. Glomerulonephritis (inflammation in the glomeruli of the kidneys) can be associated with proteinuria, hematuria, and progressive renal failure. Necrosis may develop on the fingertips, elbows, toes, and surfaces of the arms. Central nervous system involvement has also been recognized (ptosis, diplopia, ataxia, seizures, psychosis).[6] Lymphadenopathy may also be noted at some time in the course of the illness.

When SLE involves autoantibodies against blood elements, laboratory testing can reveal hemolytic anemia, leukopenia, lymphopenia, or thrombocytopenia. Renal disease often causes proteinuria, hematuria, or cellular casts on microscopic urinalysis. While many autoantibodies cannot be measured by conventional laboratory methods, testing for the ANA class of antibodies is most important in screening for SLE, although a positive ANA test result can be seen in about 2% healthy young women and an even higher number of elderly individuals.[1] Also found in the sera of some SLE patients are autoantibodies against double-stranded DNA and other extractable nuclear antigens such as SSA (Ro), SSB (La), Smith (Sm), and RNP. Complement levels (C3 and C4) can be low in the setting of active SLE since the complement proteins are "consumed" in the antigen-antibody–mediated immune activation.

Treatment. The choice of therapeutic agents often depends on disease manifestations. Topical corticosteroids, avoidance of sun, and use of sun block can help control skin disease. NSAIDs are useful for the management of arthritis and serositis. For more aggressive disease, including renal, hematologic, or neural involvement, oral or parenteral corticosteroids may be needed for initial control followed by immunosuppressive medications.

Scleroderma

Scleroderma is a multisystem inflammatory connective tissue disease characterized by skin thickening and a deposition of large quantities of connective tissue, which results in severe fibrosis.[3] Skin, blood vessels, synovium, skeletal muscle, and microvasculature of internal organs are all affected. Two major types of systemic scleroderma are limited systemic sclerosis (LSS) and diffuse systemic sclerosis (DSS). It affects women three to four times more frequently than men. Onset is most common between the ages of 50 and 60 years.

Etiology and Pathogenesis. The cause of scleroderma is unknown. Early in the disease, inflammation and immune cell infiltration can be found in skin, lungs, and other tissues. Widespread vasculopathy is seen with proliferation of smooth muscle cells within vessels causing vascular wall thickening and eventual obliteration, especially of small arteries, arterioles, and capillaries. Tissue ischemia can result. Diffuse tissue fibrosis occurs with increased production of collagen and other connective tissue components by fibroblasts that are stimulated by local cytokines and mediators.[1]

Clinical Manifestations. Clinical manifestations include Raynaud phenomenon (blanching of the digits in response to cold) and puffiness of the fingers. Polyarthritis involving small joints of the hands is common. A few months after the initial complaints, thickening of the skin may be noted. Evaluation of the skin discloses initial bilateral swelling of the fingers, hands, and, periodically, feet. After a few weeks or months, edema is replaced by thick, tight skin. Skin folds are lost and a shiny appearance is noted. Hyperpigmentation or hypopigmentation may occur. Thickening of the skin can spread to arms, face, and trunk.

Joints and tendons become involved, with polyarthralgia or arthritis affecting small and large joints. Tenosynovial involvement may be seen with tendon friction rubs, carpal tunnel syndrome, and very severe flexion contractures.

Patients with scleroderma may present with disuse atrophy of muscle since muscular motion is limited by involvement of skin and joints; atrophy and overall weakness are common. Gastrointestinal involvement is present in a majority of patients. Musculature of the esophagus is involved, with dysmotility leading to difficulties in swallowing. Involvement of the esophageal sphincter musculature may result in reflux of gastric contents and development of peptic esophagitis. Malabsorption problems may also result from intestinal dysfunction.

Pulmonary involvement may cause reduced vital capacity and pulmonary arterial hypertension. Manifestations of myocardial involvement include congestive heart failure and a variety of atrial and ventricular arrhythmias. Renal involvement is the predominant cause of death. In scleroderma *renal crisis,* malignant arterial hypertension may rapidly progress to oliguric renal failure without immediate treatment.

DSS appears with symmetrical thickening of the skin on extremities, face, and trunk, with distal thickening more prominent than proximal thickening. Problems with gastrointestinal, heart, lung, and kidneys develop rapidly, with the esophagus being affected. Progression of this type of scleroderma is often rapid.[6] With LSS, skin changes are usually confined to fingers, extremities, and face. Skin changes occur more slowly than with DSS, but these patients are still at risk of pulmonary and other organ involvement, especially pulmonary hypertension.[1]

A syndrome, abbreviated CREST, refers to *c*alcinosis (deposits of calcium in tissues); *R*aynaud phenomenon (intermittent vasospasm of the fingertips); *e*sophageal hardening and dysmotility; *s*clerodactyly or scleroderma of digits; and *t*elangiectasias or capillary dilation, which causes formation of vascular lesions on the face, lips, and fingers. Some patients with CREST syndrome develop pulmonary hypertension and intestinal malabsorption, often resulting in death. Survival rates in LSS are reported to be about 85% at 5 years after diagnosis and about 74% at 10 years.[6]

Treatment. Treatment for scleroderma is largely organ specific since systemic disease–modifying agents have had disappointing results. Raynaud phenomenon is managed with avoidance of cold exposure and use of vasodilator medications. Symptoms from gastrointestinal disease may be controlled with antacids, H_2 antagonists, proton pump inhibitors, and promotility agents. Previously associated with very high mortality, acute renal crisis (renal failure with malignant hypertension) can now be successfully managed with angiotensin-converting enzyme inhibitors.

Ankylosing Spondylitis

Ankylosing spondylitis (AS) literally means fusion (ankylosis) of inflamed vertebra (spondylitis). It is arthritis of the sacroiliac joints that often involves the entire axial skeleton and, to some extent, peripheral joints. The disease often begins in the spine of young males in their late teens or early 20s. The male-to-female incidence ratio is 5:1, with symptoms being mild in women.[1] The disease in women tends to manifest more prominently in peripheral joints and less severely in the spine, whereas in men there is equal spinal and peripheral joint involvement.

Etiology and Pathogenesis. A strong genetic component likely plays a role in the development of AS since 90% to 95% patients are positive for the HLA-B27 marker and the frequency of the arthritis in different ethnic groups roughly parallels the frequency of HLA-B27 presence.[5] The role of the HLA molecule in the pathogenesis of the arthritis is not clear, although antigen-presenting cells (expressing these HLA markers) may interact with certain bacterial or environmental factors and cross-react with self-antigens found in joint tissues. Activation of immune-mediated inflammation occurs within the sacroiliac joints of the pelvis and the ligaments supporting the vertebral column. This leads to persistent back pain, stiffness, and gradual loss of mobility.

Clinical Manifestations. Clinical features include the insidious onset of low back pain that improves with exercise and is not relieved by rest and severe morning stiffness for more than 3 months. Evaluation of the spine suggests an increase in muscle tone and a loss of normal lumbar lordosis. Marked limitation of mobility is noted in both anterior and lateral planes. With limitation of movement and a position of spinal flexion, the hips and knees must compensate, creating lower extremity joint degeneration and deformities. Because of restricted postural position and decreased chest expansion, tidal volume may be diminished. A typical postural position for advanced ankylosing spondylitis is shown in Figure 52-8.

Peripheral arthritis with swelling of knees, ankles, or toes can also occur along with enthesitis (inflammation at the sites of ligament attachment to bone), with the plantar fascia and Achilles tendon being the most common sites. Other organ systems that may be affected include the eyes (anterior uveitis, iritis), the heart (aortitis, aortic valve insufficiency), and nervous system (nerve root or spinal cord impingement related to spinal deformities or fractures.)

Treatment. The primary objectives of treatment are to relieve pain, decrease inflammation, and strengthen and maintain posture and function. Regular stretching and range-of-motion exercises are often recommended. Medication options include NSAIDs to reduce pain and swelling and disease-modifying agents, possibly soon to include the new TNF-α antagonists, to slow disease progression if possible.

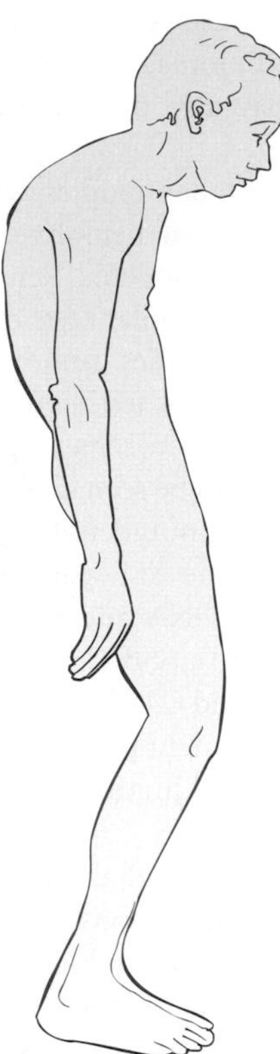

FIGURE 52-8 ■ Typical posture of patient with ankylosing spondylitis.

Polymyositis and Dermatomyositis

Polymyositis and **dermatomyositis** are idiopathic inflammatory myopathies. With these diseases there is focal or extensive degeneration of muscle fibers due to inflammatory infiltrates of lymphocytes and macrophages.[3] Necrosis of muscle fibers can occur. Possible causative agents include viruses, bacteria, parasitic organisms, neoplasms, drugs, vaccinations, and stress. A viral cause has been proposed since various researchers have noted viruslike inclusion bodies in muscle tissue of dermatomyositis patients.[3]

Proximal limb and neck weakness and associated muscle stiffness are clinical signs of these illnesses. Muscle pain is often mild. Most patients initially complain of hip and leg weakness and difficulty with climbing stairs and rising from a chair. Later in the progression of the disease, weakness in the arms prevents functional overhead activity. Anterior neck weakness makes lifting the head from the pillow very difficult. When classic skin changes occur with polymyositis, the disease is classified as dermatomyositis.

Clinical Manifestations. During the physical examination, manual muscle testing reveals weakness in the proximal limb muscles. Contractures are not usually present, but they may develop later. Facial and ocular muscle weakness seldom occurs, distinguishing myositis from myasthenia gravis.

In dermatomyositis, cutaneous manifestations may develop with muscle involvement. Common findings are flat-topped papules overlying the dorsal surface of the interphalangeal joints of the hands (Gottron papules). These areas atrophy, and hypopigmentation develops. A more common finding is development of an erythematous smooth or scaly patch over the DIP or MCP joints of the elbow, knees, or medial malleoli areas.

Cardiac involvement is often noted. Dysrhythmias, congestive heart failure, conduction defects, ventricular hypertrophy, or pericarditis is typical. Weakness of the respiratory muscles and lung pathologic changes can cause pulmonary disease.

Treatment. Initial therapy with corticosteroids is usually used to decrease muscle inflammation and preserve function. Immunosuppressive agents may be helpful in severe cases. Physical therapy is also important and should include passive range-of-motion activities, followed by assisted and then active strengthening exercises.

Postinfectious Systemic Disorders

Reiter Syndrome (Reactive Arthritis)

Historically, **Reiter syndrome** consisted of three types of clinical problems: arthritis, urethritis, and conjunctivitis. Currently, it is defined as a seronegative arthritis preceded by urethritis, cervicitis, or dysentery. Additional problems may include inflammatory lesions, oral ulcers, and keratoderma. The male-to-female ratio is approximately 9:1, with young white males experiencing the disorder most frequently. Reiter syndrome is linked to the greater prevalence of HLA-B27 antigen in the young white male population.[1] Reiter syndrome occurs in persons who are genetically susceptible following an infection by bacteria such as *Chlamydia trachomatis* in the genitourinary tract or *Salmonella, Shigella, Yersinia,* or *Campylobacter* in the gastrointestinal tract. It is thought that persistence of bacterial antigens and cross-reactivity of immune cells with these antigens trigger the inflammation seen in joints and tendons of this syndrome.

Clinical Manifestations. Clinically, arthritis typically appears 2 to 6 weeks after the onset of the infectious episode. This acute arthritis onset predominantly affects knees and ankles. Three additional features of musculoskeletal manifestations are typical: diffuse swelling of entire fingers or toes (sausage digits or dactylitis); swelling at the Achilles tendon insertion or plantar fascia (enthesitis); and low back pain, especially in the sacroiliac region.

Involvement of the genitourinary system is not uncommon in Reiter syndrome. Prostatitis and clinical cystitis have been noted. The most common eye involvement is noninfectious conjunctivitis. Iritis, uveitis, episcleritis, and corneal ulceration could lead to impairment of vision.

Cutaneous lesions related to Reiter syndrome include development of small, shallow, painless ulcers on the glans penis and urethral meatus. A hyperkeratotic skin lesion (keratoderma blennorrhagicum) may form on the soles of the feet and palms of the hands. Hyperkeratosis (extreme thickening beneath the nails) can occur.

Reiter patients may have elevated inflammatory markers (sedimentation rate, C-reactive protein) as well as a mild normocytic anemia, transient leukocytosis, and thrombocytosis. RF test results are usually negative.

Treatment. Antiinflammatory medications, particularly NSAIDs, are usually effective at controlling pain and swelling, although intraarticular corticosteroid injections may also help. Second-line agents can be used in refractory cases.

Acute Rheumatic Fever

Acute rheumatic fever (ARF) is an inflammatory disease that follows a β-hemolytic group A streptococcal pharyngeal infection. The incubation period, or latent period from infection to onset of the disease, ranges from 2 to 6 weeks. Streptococcal infections have been on the rise since the 1980s, with pockets of ARF reappearing even in affluent populations.[1] This might be due to the reappearance of heavily encapsulated, highly virulent rheumatogenic streptococcal strains and/or to the decrease in awareness of the disease and less stringent adherence to disease control measures, especially prevention.

Etiology and Pathogenesis. One theory of disease occurrence is the cross-reactivity of a patient's immune cells within the lymphoid tissue of the pharynx. Lymphocyte activity and antibody production are stimulated by streptococcal antigens, and then these cells cross-react with proteins in the target organs such as joints, heart, skin, and nervous system leading to inflammatory reactions in these areas.[1]

Clinical Manifestations. The clinical aspects of ARF depend on the age of the affected individual. Peak incidence is between ages 5 and 20 years. Children and teenagers present with polyarthritis and carditis. Polyarthritis is usually the only manifestation in the adult. Fever is present in most patients.

Polyarthritis is the most common symptom noted in patients with ARF. Pain may be quite severe and usually reaches its maximum in 12 to 24 hours. Synovial effusion, inflammation, and erythema may be noted. The knees, ankles, elbows, and shoulders are affected most often. Hips, wrists, and small joints of the hands and feet may also be compromised. Numerous joints (average of seven joints) may be involved. Joint symptoms usually respond rapidly to treatment with antiinflammatory medications.

Children and teenagers with ARF are more likely than adults to develop carditis. The signs of carditis include murmurs, cardiomegaly, congestive heart failure, and pericarditis. Mitral valve regurgitation is the most common murmur, followed by aortic regurgitation. Evidence of rheumatic heart disease may not be apparent for many years after the acute incident.

A rash is noted in approximately 10% to 20% of the children affected by ARF. The rash begins as small, pink, blanching macules over the trunk and proximal regions of the extremities. Painless nodules may cover the extensor surfaces.

Throat cultures may be negative by the time the symptoms of ARF are recognized, but certain antibody tests (antistreptolysin O, anti-DNAse B) can be useful to aid in diagnosis.

Treatment. The most common therapy is NSAIDs, especially aspirin, and response can be rapid. Corticosteroids may be required in cases of severe cardiac involvement. Antibiotic therapy, including long-term prophylaxis in some cases, is generally recommended.

Postparasitic Disorders

Lyme Disease

Lyme disease is a complex illness caused by the *Borrelia burgdorferi* tick-borne spirochete. It is commonly carried by the deer tick, although other species serve as vectors as well. How presence of the spirochete leads to the later clinical features of Lyme disease is unclear. One theory is that persistent antigenic fragments of the dead or inactivated organism trigger the inflammatory responses seen within the synovium of joints and tissues of nervous or cardiac systems.[1]

Clinical Manifestations and Treatment. The tick bite produces a red macule or papule that may expand to form an annular lesion. The lesion may expand and become quite red. The lesion is warm to the touch but not painful and is often accompanied by severe headache, neck stiffness, fever, chills, myalgia, arthralgia, malaise, and fatigue. Systemic involvement may consist of lymphadenopathy, splenomegaly, hepatitis, nonproductive cough, testicular swelling, and conjunctivitis.

Musculoskeletal symptoms occur early in the illness and follow a pattern of migratory pain in joints, tendons, bursae, muscles, or bones. More than half of patients develop frank arthritis with involvement of the large joints. The knee is a particularly common site of Lyme arthritis and can be associated with large effusions. Cartilage can erode, and joints are chronically involved in about 10% of patients.

Neurologic abnormalities suggest meningeal irritation. Neurologic abnormalities may include meningitis, cranial neuritis, motor and sensory radiculoneuritis, and chorea.

Cardiac involvement may be noted, including atrioventricular blocks, left ventricular dysfunction, or cardiomegaly. Although cardiac involvement lasts only a few weeks, it can be fatal.

Treatment is with oral or parenteral antibiotics.

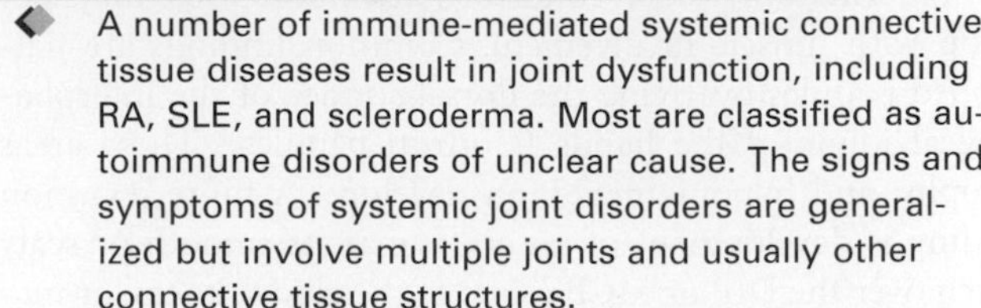

KEY CONCEPTS

- A number of immune-mediated systemic connective tissue diseases result in joint dysfunction, including RA, SLE, and scleroderma. Most are classified as autoimmune disorders of unclear cause. The signs and symptoms of systemic joint disorders are generalized but involve multiple joints and usually other connective tissue structures.
- Differentiation among types of systemic joint disorders is based on patterns of joint dysfunction, immunologic factors (e.g., rheumatoid factor), and related lesions (e.g., the butterfly rash of SLE).
- Joint destruction in systemic joint disorders is inflammatory in nature and involves synovial membrane, cartilage, joint capsule, and surrounding ligaments and tendons.
- Rheumatic fever and Lyme disease are inflammatory joint disorders associated with a known organism.
- Rheumatic joint disease is a sequela of group A streptococcal infection. Lyme disease is associated with a spirochete carried by ticks.

JOINT DYSFUNCTION SECONDARY TO OTHER DISEASES

Psoriatic Arthritis

Psoriatic arthritis (PA) is an inflammatory arthritis associated with psoriasis occurring in approximately 0.1% population in the United States. Peak age of onset is 30 to 55 years of age, and the arthritis can occur in patients who have had psoriasis for many years.[1]

Etiology and Pathogenesis. Studies have shown a strong familial tendency for psoriatic arthritis, suggesting genetic factors may cause an increased predisposition to the disease. Environmental factors, such as infection or physical trauma, may trigger the onset of the arthritis. Immunologic features also have a role, with activated T lymphocytes and macrophages infiltrating skin and joint tissue and producing multiple inflammatory cytokines (TNF-α, IL-1, and IL-15, among others). These immune reactions cause proliferation of synoviocytes within joints, angiogenesis (new blood vessel formation), and expansion of inflammatory tissue. In the skin, keratinocytes are stimulated and will proliferate extensively.

Clinical Manifestations. The pattern of joint involvement seen clinically varies. The majority of patients have peripheral joint involvement in the form of asymmetric arthritis. Fewer patients have a polyarthritis that is difficult to distinguish from RA. In some PA patients, the DIP joints of the hands can be affected, which is different from RA. Sacroiliac and spinal involvement can also occur.

Commonly, PA is characterized by a combination of soft tissue and peripheral joint disease. Inflammation occurs in the joints as well as the periosteum, along the tendons, and at tendon insertions in bone. Fusiform swelling of the digits (called dactylitis) is common.

Evidence of skin or nail changes, typical of psoriasis, is noted in psoriatic arthritis. These skin changes include macular or papular lesions with characteristic scales. Nail involvement includes pitting and transverse or longitudinal ridging. Subungual hyperkeratosis and oil droplet discoloration suggest psoriasis.

Inflammatory markers may be elevated, and the rheumatoid factor is usually negative. Radiographs may show minimal changes; however, some cases involve aggressive disease with bone erosion, fluffy new bone formation (periostitis), and marked loss of joint spaces.

Treatment. Psoriasis may respond to topical corticosteroids, emollients, and keratolytic agents. Light therapy, utilizing ultraviolet A radiation, can also be effective. Management of the arthritis centers on NSAIDs or corticosteroids to control pain and swelling, but in many cases, more aggressive immunosuppressive therapy is needed, including methotrexate, cyclosporine, or possibly TNF-α antagonists.

Enteropathic Arthritis

Enteropathic arthritis refers to articular manifestations of two inflammatory bowel diseases (IBDs): **ulcerative colitis** and **Crohn disease.** A peripheral or axial arthritis can occur in 10% to 20% patients with IBD, and in some cases the arthritis can precede the onset of gastrointestinal symptoms.[1]

As in the case of the other spondyloarthropathies, the cause of enteropathic arthritis is unclear, but it is postulated to be associated with immune cross-reactivity with bacterial antigens. In the setting of IBD, inflammation of the gut lining may permit entrance of bacteria from the bowel lumen into the lymphoid tissue and blood stream.

Clinical Manifestations. Articular manifestations include peripheral arthritis, spondylitis, and involvement of muscle and bone. Peripheral arthritis is most commonly noted in the knees and ankles. Synovial inflammation may be mild to severe. The development of granuloma in patients with Crohn disease may cause destruction of the articular surfaces of the joint. Spondylitis can cause extensive spinal involvement, similar to features seen in patients with ankylosing spondylitis.

Various cutaneous, mucosal, serosal, and ocular manifestations can occur in IBD. Skin lesions, leg ulcers, and thrombophlebitis may also be associated with the disease. Ocular manifestations such as uveitis, conjunctivitis, and episcleritis, as well as pericarditis, have been noted to occur. Amyloidosis with involvement of major organs can be observed in Crohn disease.

Anemia is common in IBD as well as leukocytosis. In the setting of arthritis, elevated inflammatory markers are often seen and the HLA-B27, when positive, may identify patients at higher risk of developing spondylitis.[1]

Treatment. Treatment focuses on management of the gastrointestinal disease with antiinflammatory agents. Control of the arthritis can be sought with use of NSAIDs (when tolerated by the gut), COX-2 inhibitors, or corticosteroids. In severe cases, immunosuppressive medications may be required, particularly the use of TNF-α antagonists as in the setting of Crohn disease.

Neuropathic Osteoarthropathy

Commonly called *Charcot joint,* **neuropathic osteoarthropathy** is a neurologic disease that leads to bone abnormalities and joint involvement. There is damage to the joint due to loss of position and pain sensation. The mechanics of disease development are probably a combination of neurovascular and neurotraumatic processes. Neurovascular changes desensitize the joint. With repetitive trauma, injury to the joint causes a breakdown in structure. Peripheral nerve injuries, diabetes mellitus, pernicious anemia, alcoholism, and multiple sclerosis can lead to a Charcot joint.[1] Motor neuron involvement can affect both upper and lower motor neurons. Diabetes, tabes dorsalis, and syringomyelia are the three most prevalent disease processes that lead to neuropathic osteoarthropathy.

Clinical Manifestations and Treatment. Clinically, the patient presents with a swollen, deformed, and unstable joint. Radiographs reveal advanced joint destruction and pathologic fractures. Management requires protection of involved joint through immobilization and less weight bearing. Surgical intervention has had poor results due to nonunion, dislocation, or infection.

Hemophilic Arthropathy

Bleeding into joints, as noted in hemophilia, causes extension of the joint capsule and a limitation of movement. Hemorrhage stimulates a synovial proliferative response, chronic inflammation with a release of degradative proteinase, and changes in cartilage composition with less resistance to stress.[6] Chronic synovitis alters the synovial lining and eventually leads to joint destruction.

Clinical Manifestations. Three stages of hemophilic arthropathy are described. Muscle hemorrhage (iliopsoas, forearms, gastrocnemius), muscle cysts, and pseudotumors (due to osseous hemorrhage) may develop.[3] The acute stage manifests with bleeding in the joint and occurs as the child begins to walk. Bleeding into the confined area of the capsule causes the joint to be positioned in flexion and increases stress to articular structures. Atrophy of muscles around the joint predisposes it to further hemarthrosis. The second stage is due to repetitive hemorrhages into the joint, resulting in chronic synovitis. The joint is edematous and warm but painless. The third stage is characterized by destruction of joint integrity.[3]

Larger joints are affected more frequently than smaller joints. Seldom are structures of the wrist involved. Elbow, hip, and knee are subject to major destruction. Medical treatment to enhance clotting is imperative. Education and prevention of joint deformity are essential in the management of hemophilia.

Gout

Gout is a heterogeneous disorder in which disturbance of uric acid metabolism leads to deposition of monosodium urate salts in articular, periarticular, and subcutaneous tissue (Figure 52-9). It is also characterized by hyperuricemia and urate crystal–induced arthritis. Gout arises in humans because of a lack of the enzyme uricase and subsequent inability to oxidize uric acid to a soluble compound. Uric acid is a normal waste product of purine metabolism and therefore must be filtered primarily by the kidneys. When production of uric acid exceeds removal, hyperuricemia results and the possibility of deposition of crystalline sodium urate increases. The acute attack is often triggered by a traumatic event, a surgical procedure, an acute illness, or use of alcohol or drugs.

Clinical Manifestations. Prevalence of gout in the United States is approximately 275 cases per 100,000 persons. Risk of developing gout increases with age and with an increase in serum urate concentrations. Clinically, acute gouty arthritis is the form most frequently observed. Gouty arthritis is common in middle-aged men and postmenopausal women. A familial tendency is often noted.

Manifestations of gout include recurrent attacks of articular and periarticular inflammation (acute gouty arthritis), accumulation of tophi (crystalline deposits) in bony and connective tissue, renal impairment, and uric acid calculi. There are four phases in gout: asymptomatic hyperuricemia, acute gouty arthritis, intercritical gout, and chronic tophaceous gout.

Asymptomatic Hyperuricemia. Hyperuricemia has been reported in approximately 5% of Americans with asymptomatic gout. In this phase there are no clinical signs; however, the serum urate level is elevated. In the male, hyperuricemia can begin at puberty. In women, hyperuricemia usually does not appear before menopause.[1]

Acute Gouty Arthritis. Gouty arthritis is the most common early clinical sign. Weight-bearing joints are usually affected and are warm, red, and tender to palpation. The MTP joint of the great toe is most often involved. Ankle, tarsal, and knee joints are often affected although attacks can occur in hands, wrists, and elbows also. The first attack of acute gouty

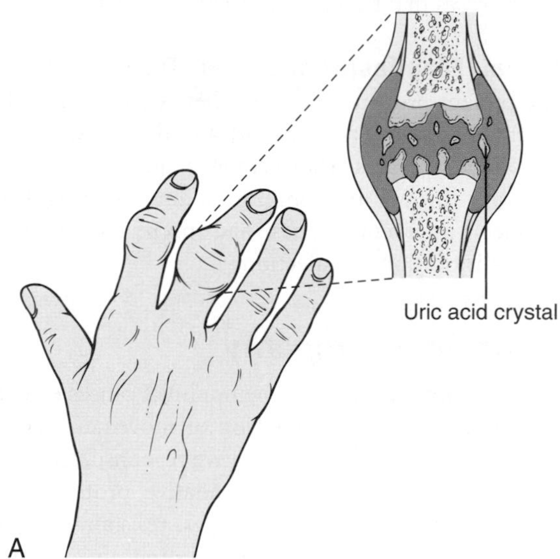

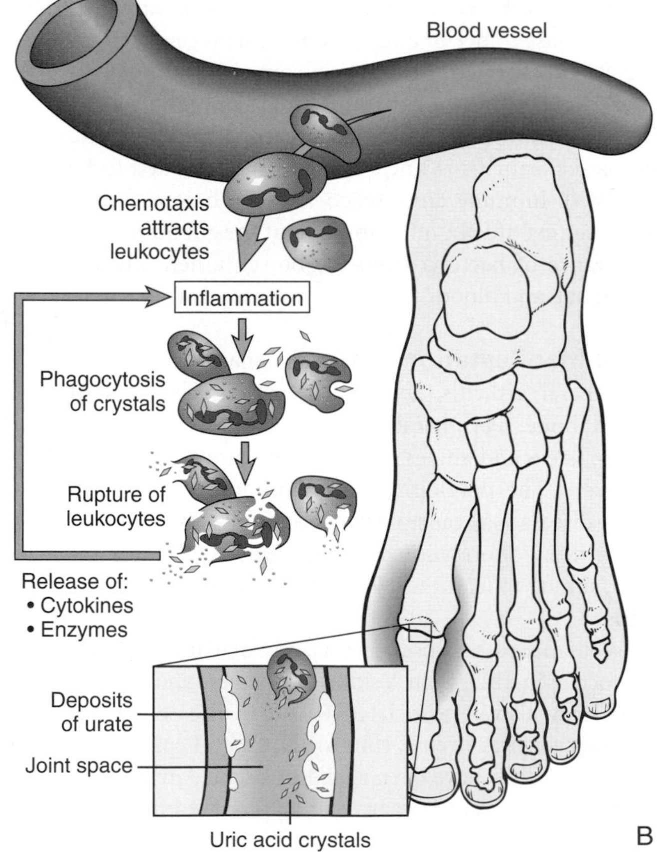

FIGURE 52-9 ■ **A,** Gout. **B,** Gouty arthritis. Deposits of uric acid crystals in the connective tissue have a chemotactic effect and cause exudation of leukocytes into the joint. The inflammation most often affects the metatarsophalangeal joint. (**A,** From Frazier MS, Drzymkowski JW: *Essentials of human diseases and conditions,* ed 2, Philadelphia, 2000, Saunders, p 194. **B,** From Damjanov I: *Pathology for the health-related professions,* ed 2, Philadelphia, 2000, Saunders, p 459.)

arthritis is often sudden and quick with an intense pain that wakens the patient from a sound sleep. Diffuse periarticular erythema often accompanies the attack.[1] Diagnosis relies on classic clinical presentation, hyperuricemia, and the demonstration of urate crystals in synovial fluid of the involved joint.

Initial attacks subside within a day or may last 1 to 2 weeks after which the patient is symptom free until the next episode. Later attacks tend to become more frequent, and mild arthralgia may occur between episodes.[1]

Intercritical Gout. Intercritical gout, the name for the disease in the intervals between acute attacks, presents no symptoms. Even during asymptomatic periods, urate crystals can be aspirated from involved joints.[1]

Chronic Tophaceous Gout. This is an advanced stage of gout. Tophi begin to appear approximately 10 years after initial onset of gout. Tophi occur commonly in the synovium, subchondral bone, olecranon bursa, and infrapatellar and Achilles tendons. Tophi have been noted in walls of the aorta, valves of the heart, ear cartilage (pinna), cornea, sclerae, and kidneys.[1]

As a result of deposition of crystals and chronic inflammation, deforming arthritis can develop. Development of tophi in tendon sheaths of the hand and wrist can cause a trigger finger or carpal tunnel syndrome.

Patients with gout may have involvement of kidneys and develop renal malfunction. These individuals have a higher incidence of arterial hypertension, diabetes mellitus, and cardiac and cerebral atherosclerosis. Hypertriglyceridemia occurs more frequently in the patient diagnosed with gout.

Treatment. Management of an acute gouty attack usually requires aggressive antiinflammatory medication such as NSAIDs or corticosteroids (oral, parenteral, or intraarticular). Colchicine may also be used early in the course of an attack or in lower doses as a prophylactic agent. Medications to correct hyperuricemia and prevent gout flares may target uric acid excretion by the kidneys (uricosuric agents) or uric acid production (allopurinol).

Adult-Onset Still Disease

Adult-onset Still disease is a form of seronegative (i.e., negative RF) polyarthritis with a number of symptoms similar to those of systemic onset JRA in children (see discussion under "Pediatric Joint Disorders" in this chapter). Adult-onset Still disease may follow diagnosis of RA. Its cause is unknown.

Clinical Manifestations and Treatment. Clinical features include high-spiking fever, a rash on the trunk and extremities, and, possibly, a sore throat. Polyarthritis usually affects the PIP and MCP joints of the hands. Arthritic changes are noted in wrist, knees, hips, and shoulders, and fusion of the carpometacarpal and intercarpal joints is seen. Visceral involvement includes hepatic insufficiency, chronic respiratory failure, cardiac tamponade, congestive heart failure, and splenomegaly. Laboratory features may include anemia, leukocytosis, elevated sedimentation rate, thrombocytosis, and elevated liver enzymes.

Some patients respond well to high-dose aspirin or NSAIDs during the acute illness, although in severe cases corticosteroids are used.

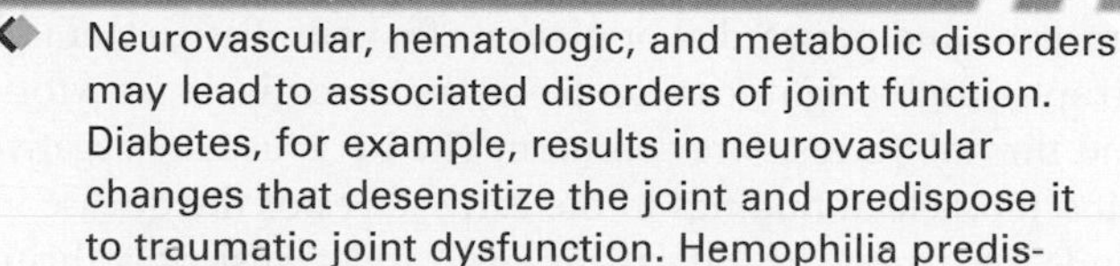

KEY CONCEPTS

- Neurovascular, hematologic, and metabolic disorders may lead to associated disorders of joint function. Diabetes, for example, results in neurovascular changes that desensitize the joint and predispose it to traumatic joint dysfunction. Hemophilia predisposes to intraarticular bleeding.
- Altered uric acid metabolism leads to deposition of uric acid crystals in joints, causing inflammation and gouty arthritis.

PEDIATRIC JOINT DISORDERS

Pediatric rheumatic diseases include more than 100 illnesses associated with arthritis and musculoskeletal syndromes. Soft tissue pain and restrictions constitute a major proportion of the complaints brought to pediatric rheumatologists.

Nonarticular Rheumatism

"Growing pain" or **nonarticular rheumatism** is a common soft tissue syndrome in children. Nocturnal pain, usually occurring in the calves, shins, and thighs, is the most common symptom. Although this problem seems to be benign, medical consultation and education concerning the problem is essential.

Hypermobility of Joints

Hypermobility of joints is a common cause of complaints of pain in the joints. Mobility may be excessive in any joint, but it is most apparent in passive apposition of the thumb to the forearm, hyperextension of the fingers parallel to the forearm, and excessive extension (greater than 10 degrees) of the knees and elbows.

Juvenile Rheumatoid Arthritis

Juvenile rheumatoid arthritis (JRA) is a chronic, inflammatory childhood disease that sometimes resolves by the time the child reaches adulthood. However, residual joint damage remains. JRA begins with synovial inflammation of unknown cause and affects approximately 57 to 113 per 100,000 children in the United States.[1] JRA may be defined as arthritis in one or more joints (pain, redness, swelling, warmth, and limited range of motion). Onset is usually in children 16 years or younger. The duration of the arthritis is at least 6 weeks. JRA may present with one of three types of onset, which is classified during the first 6 months of the disease: (1) systemic (Still disease), (2) polyarticular, and (3) pauciarticular (oligoarticular).[1]

Clinical Manifestations. Systemic onset (**Still disease**) JRA is noted in approximately 10% of children with JRA with peak onset at 1 to 6 years old. Clinical manifestations include spiking fevers (103° F to 104° F), daily or twice daily, usually in the afternoon, with return to baseline without antipyretics; transient, pale pink rash; lymphadenopathy; hepatosplenomegaly; and pericardial or pleural effusions. Fatigue, muscle atrophy, and weight loss can be severe. Anemia, leukocytosis, and thrombocytosis are common. The RF is usually negative. Musculoskeletal findings in the early stages of the disease include recurrent arthralgia, myalgia, and transient arthritis, which are concurrent with fever spikes. Polyarthritis can develop weeks to months after the onset of the disease. Severe chronic arthritis may continue after the systemic symptoms subside.[1]

A **polyarticular onset (oligoarticular)** of JRA (i.e., involving five or more joints) is seen in approximately 40% of patients with peak onset at age 8 to 16 years. The female-to-male ratio is 3:1.[1] RF positivity is also more common in girls with later onset of disease that can resemble adult RA. These patients are at a higher risk of developing progressive bone erosions, nodules, and poor functional outcome.[1] Malaise, growth retardation or weight loss, low-grade fever, organomegaly, adenopathy, and anemia are other clinical manifestations.

By definition, a child with **pauciarticular onset** of JRA has arthritis in four or fewer joints. One subset of this form of JRA includes patients who are very young at disease onset (1 to 5 years old), can have a positive ANA test result, and are most often girls (female-to-male ratio is 4:1). Patients with a positive ANA test result are at highest risk for developing inflammatory ocular disease, a complication that may start with minimal or no symptoms yet can lead to severe irreversible vision impairment. A second group of patients with pauciarticular JRA have later disease onset. These children are more commonly boys, may be HLA-B27 positive (50%), and often develop large joint disease (hips, knees, shoulders, or spine). These patients may also develop eye inflammation, but this is less likely than in the early-onset group.

Treatment. All forms of JRA can cause general growth retardation, although it is more of a risk in people with systemic or polyarticular onset of disease. Inflammation close to the epiphyseal plates can result in altered growth of long bones. It is therefore imperative to achieve early diagnosis and apply appropriate treatment to minimize deformity and disability. Education and counseling are also important. Relief of symptoms and maintenance of joint position and muscle function are immediate goals of treatment.

Pharmacologic intervention is an important component of the treatment regimen. Drug therapy is instituted to decrease pain and arrest progression of the disease. The following categories of drugs are used: (1) antiinflammatory analgesics (aspirin), (2) NSAIDs, (3) corticosteroids, and (4) disease-modifying drugs.[1] Physical and occupational therapy assessment and treatment plans are important, and daily activity should be an integral part of the child's lifestyle. Joint support and physical activity help prevent joint contracture.

KEY CONCEPTS

- JRA has three subtypes: Systemic onset (which has more systemic manifestations, including rash, high fever, lymphadenopathy, splenomegaly, fatigue, and polyarthritis), polyarticular arthritis (in which symptoms are primarily localized to five or more joints), and pauciarticular arthritis (which involves four or fewer joints).

SUMMARY

This chapter has provided an overview of major rheumatic disorders. Broadly speaking, interventions must assist in controlling disease activity, managing pain, minimizing deformity, and maintaining or restoring function. Depending on the stage of the disease, correct intervention must be implemented using knowledge of joint physiology biomechanics and pathologic changes resulting from the disease.

The challenge to the health professional is to ensure that an inflammatory response is not exacerbated while the body structures are being stimulated to increase strength, enhance nutrition, and improve tolerance to stress. Long periods of immobilization, bed rest, and sedentary behavior are counterproductive in the patient with arthritis. Lack of activity poses particular problems in people with arthritis. Deleterious effects on muscle strength, reflexes, connective tissue extensibility, and cardiovascular fitness are identifiable in the immobilized arthritic patient. It is imperative that the health professional look beyond disease-specific interventions and prescribe a well-developed exercise program for people with arthritis. Achievement or retention of as much function as possible is the ultimate goal for an individual with arthritis. Every level of intervention must be directed to achievement of specific performance goals cooperatively developed by clinician and patient.

MEDIA RESOURCES

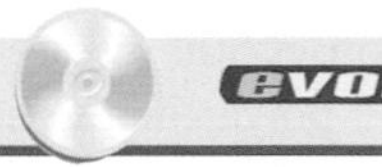

Remember to check out the ***CD Companion*** included with this book for Review Questions, Key Concepts Review, Glossary (with audio for selected terms), Disease Profiles, and Animations.

PLUS, visit the ***Evolve website*** at http://evolve.elsevier.com/Copstead/ for Case Studies, Disease Profiles, and WebLinks.

References

1. Klippel JH, editor: *Primer on the rheumatic diseases,* ed 12, Atlanta, 2001, Arthritis Foundation.

2. Chapman MW et al, editor: *Chapman's orthopaedic surgery,* ed 3, Philadelphia, 2001, Saunders.
3. Ruddy S, Harris ED, Sledge CB, editor: *Kelley's textbook of rheumatology,* ed 6, Philadelphia, 2001, Saunders.
4. Arnett FC et al: The American Rheumatism Association 1987 revised criteria for the classification of rheumatoid arthritis, *Arthritis Rheum* 31:315-324, 1988.
5. Hunder GG, editor: *Atlas of rheumatology,* ed 2, Philadelphia, 2001, Current Medicine.
6. Koopman WJ: *Arthritis and allied conditions,* ed 14, Philadelphia, 2001, Lippincott Williams & Wilkins.

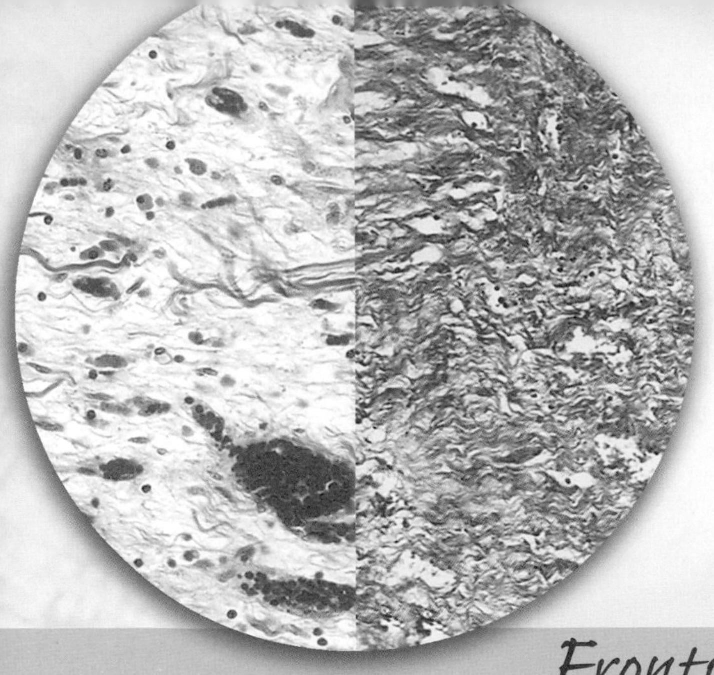

Frontiers of Research

Wounds and Wound Healing

Paul D. Silva and Michael J. Kirkhorn

Through accidents, surgery, war, and violence, millions are inflicted with wounds each year. Unfortunately, many of these wounds become chronic. Even with modern treatment chronic wounds may not heal quickly and may leave a scarred reminder of the previous accident, violent act, or surgery. In the United States chronic wounds are usually the painful and dangerous afflictions of cancer patients, patients with diabetes, patients confined to bed for long periods, the elderly, or those whose immune and vascular systems have been compromised and whose wounds may be prone to serious infection. The debilitated, chronically ill patient undergoing major surgery is particularly susceptible to developing a slow-healing wound.

The majority of wounds heal by themselves, perhaps with some timely help from medical professionals. After a wound occurs, almost immediately the specialized cells that contribute to healing rush to the site, attracted by chemical signals. Unusually rapid cell proliferation begins, and the process of healing starts. For patients troubled by slowly healing or nonhealing wounds, physicians and nurses have been able to provide some relief through treatment and watchful care. However, researchers assume that additional help is needed, and they are finding that the understanding of growth factors provides a direction for better therapy in healing.

For some time researchers have known that endogenous growth factors released at the location of the wound are conducive to wound healing. Multiple molecules involved in local intercellular communication and/or chemoattraction have been identified and are being intensively studied. It appears that some growth factors are active at every stage of wound healing. The process of wound healing is incredibly complex, and it has been hard to affect it favorably by simple manipulations of individual factors. However, in some pathologic states individual growth factors have shown success in clinical trials. For example, topical platelet-derived growth factor has shown significant benefit in certain cases of diabetic foot ulcers.

The first response to a surgical wound is the formation of a fibrin clot by a protein called fibrinogen, which circulates in the blood stream and in an emergency seals damaged blood vessels. Platelets also adhere to the damaged blood vessels. Next, inflammatory changes occur as release of local chemical mediators attracts leukocytes to the damaged area. Polymorphonuclear leukocytes and activated macrophages digest damaged tissue components, modify the extracellular matrix, and kill bacteria. They also release growth factors and other soluble products that magnify and extend the healing process. Soon comes a migratory and proliferative process. On the surface of the wound, locally produced growth factors encourage epidermal migration with reepithelialization. Beneath this, vascular endothelial budding and migrating fibroblasts form the new vessels and collagen of granulation tissue.

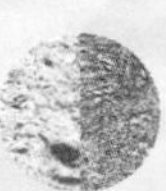

Left, *Granulation tissue showing numerous blood vessels, edema, and a loose extracellular matrix containing occasional inflammatory cells; minimal mature collagen* (blue) *can be seen at this point.* Right, *Mature scar, showing dense collagen, with only scattered vascular channels. (From Kumar V, Abbas AK, Fausto N:* Robbins and Cotran: pathologic basis of disease, *ed 7, Philadelphia, 2005, Saunders, p 107.)*

Integumentary System

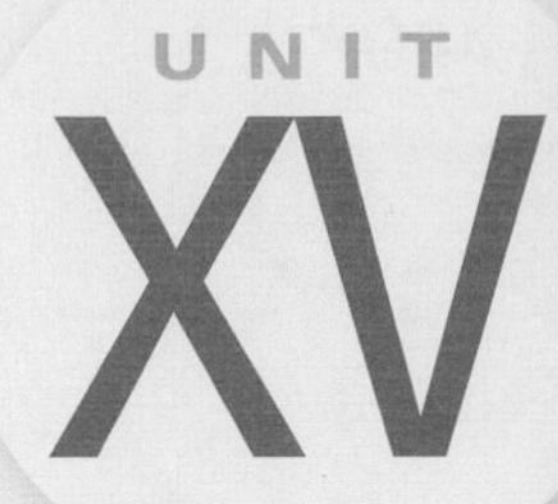

Under normal postoperative circumstances, by the fifth day the processes of reepithelialization, neovascularization, and fibroblast migration have formed a wound that can maintain its integrity to minor tension. Over the ensuing months the extracellular matrix consisting of proteins and mucopolysaccharides is extensively remodeled to further strengthen the wound. The final product is a relatively acellular scar made up primarily of strong collagen bundles that affords about 70% of the strength of normal skin.

Wound healing is strongly affected by the age, nutritional status, immunocompetence, cardiopulmonary condition, and habits of the patient seeking care. Age is a major consideration in wound healing. Older patients heal more slowly than younger patients, but the outcome is likely to be the same if the requirements of age are taken into account. Aged skin is more fragile, and the elderly are less able to defend themselves against infection. They may be poorly nourished, and decreased perfusion may slow down the healing process. Chronic disease, medications, motivation, and social habits are other factors that nurses take into account as they observe the healing process. They often help with wound healing and recovery in the debilitated patient by encouraging early postoperative nutrition and ambulation. The attitudes and behaviors of nurses are of vital importance to a good recovery.

Partly because it decreases capillary and arteriolar flow to the skin, perhaps damaging connective tissues, cigarette smoking retards wound healing. Health care professionals find that cigarette smoke, which contains nicotine, carbon monoxide, and hydrogen cyanide, reduces healing. Nicotine reduces blood flow to the skin and may also directly inhibit fibroblast function, carbon monoxide reduces oxygen transport and metabolism, and hydrogen cyanide inhibits metabolism and oxygen transport at the cellular level. Smokers heal less satisfactorily and have more complications after a variety of surgeries.

Wounds caused by violence and aggravated by poverty are attracting the attention of dermatologists, who see patients with injuries or unhealed lesions caused by physical abuse, intravenous drug use, and sexually transmitted diseases.

The wounds suffered by children who have been subjected to abuse by parents, guardians, or others provide a depressing example of cruelty and a reminder that although the body is sturdy and capably defended against diseases, it is often not so well protected against those who through uncontrollable anger, frustration, immaturity, or other imbalances would harm the helpless. Here consideration of the pathophysiology of wounds must involve psychiatry, psychology, social work, and other professional disciplines, including law enforcement, that are concerned with reducing the disease of violence that continues in even some of the most advanced societies.

chapter 53

Alterations in the Integumentary System

Lee-Ellen C. Copstead • Kurt K. Mueller

MEDIA RESOURCES

Additional Material for Study, Review, and Further Exploration

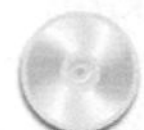

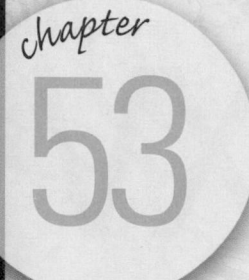

CD Companion ◆ Review Questions and Answers ◆ Key Concepts Review
◆ Glossary *(with audio pronunciations for selected terms)*
◆ Disease Profiles ◆ Animations

evolve ***Website*** at http://evolve.elsevier.com/Copstead/
◆ Case Studies ◆ Disease Profiles ◆ WebLinks

KEY QUESTIONS

- How does the aging process affect the integumentary system?
- Why is it important to differentiate primary from secondary skin lesions?
- What lesion characteristics are assessed to aid in determination of the lesion's cause?
- How do systemic disorders affect nail and hair growth?
- Which skin disorders are more likely to occur more commonly in certain age groups, including infants, children, adolescents, and the elderly?
- How does ultraviolet radiation affect the skin?
- How do superficial and deep pressure ulcers differ in clinical and etiologic features?
- How can malignant melanoma be differentiated from other skin lesions?

CHAPTER OUTLINE

This chapter focuses on altered structure and function of the integumentary system. The etiologic factors, pathogenesis, and clinical manifestations of selected skin disorders, as well as general considerations regarding treatment modalities and their therapeutic application are described.

AGE-RELATED CHANGES

The skin undergoes dramatic changes from birth through the mature years. Healthy infants and young children have relatively smooth and unwrinkled skin characterized by elasticity and flexibility. Because skin tissues are in an active phase of new growth, healing of skin injuries is often rapid and efficient. Young children and elderly persons have fewer sweat glands than adults do, so their bodies rely more on increased blood flow to maintain a normal body temperature.

As adulthood begins at puberty, hormones stimulate the development and activation of sebaceous glands and sweat glands. After the sebaceous glands become active, especially during the initial years, they may overproduce sebum and thus give the skin an unusually oily appearance. Sebaceous ducts may become clogged or infected and form acne pimples or other blemishes on the skin. Activation of apocrine sweat glands during puberty causes increased sweat production, an ability needed to maintain an adult body properly, and also the possibility of increased "body odor." Body odor is caused by wastes produced by bacteria that feed on the organic compounds found in apocrine sweat and on the surface of the skin.

Past early adulthood and into middle age, the sebaceous and sweat glands become less active. Although this can provide relief to those who suffer from acne or other problems associated with overactivity of these glands, it can affect the normal function of the body. For example, the reduction in sebum production can cause the skin and hair to become less resilient.

Changes in the appearance and function of the skin, perhaps more than in any other organ, reflect the continual aging process (The Aging Process: Changes in the Integumentary System). One need only look at a person to determine an approximate age. Evidence of advancing age includes wrinkling and sagging skin, gray hair, and baldness. Aging changes are also linked to environmental influences, genetic makeup, and other bodily changes (Figure 53-1).

Exposure to sunlight is one of the greatest factors in age-related skin changes. The result of such exposure can be seen in people who work outdoors in sunlight. Results are also evident when skin exposed to sunlight is compared with unexposed skin. Skin that is usually covered shows little change with age. Blue-eyed, fair-skinned individuals are more susceptible to solar skin damage than are people with darker, more heavily pigmented skin.

Epidermis

The epidermis shows a generalized thinning with advancing age, although there may be some thickening in sun-exposed areas. Although there is an increased variation in epidermal

THE AGING PROCESS

Changes in the Integumentary System

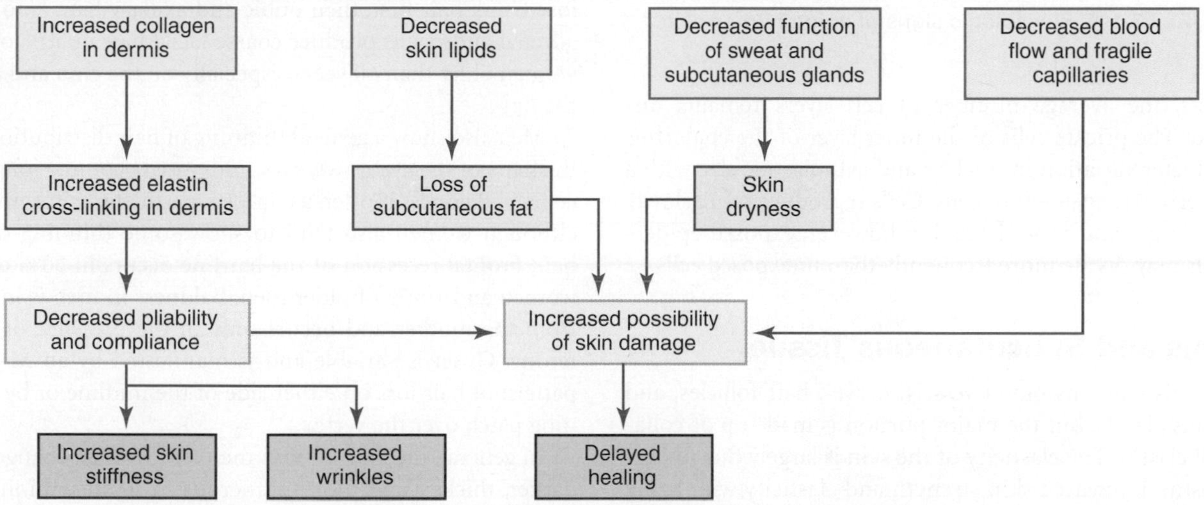

With aging, the skin's protective functions decline. The function of the water and chemical barriers in the stratum corneum is reduced, although the thickness of the stratum corneum remains the same. In the epidermis, mitosis decreases and cellular variation increases. The thickness of the epidermis is unchanged. Melanocytes decrease in whites, with declining function. The melanocytes are less efficient and lack uniformity in pigment production with sun exposure.

In the dermis, there is a decrease in thickness and subcutaneous fat. There is an increase in collagen and elastin with cross-linking and calcification of elastin fibers. These changes cause a loss of skin pliability, compliance, and resiliency. There is an accompanying rise in skin stiffness and an increase in skin wrinkles.

Sebaceous and sweat gland function declines, resulting in drier, less oily skin. The number of sensory nerves and blood vessels in the skin declines, resulting in decreased sensation and loss of effective vasoactivity by dermal arterioles.

Nail and hair growth declines. The nails may become yellowed and thickened. Graying of the hair is due to the loss of melanocytes at the hair follicle base. The degree and pattern of hair loss are affected by genetic and endocrine factors. Body hair patterns change, with thinning of leg, axillary, and pubic hair.

The cumulative effect of these skin changes is loss of the regulatory, secretory, and excretory properties of the skin. The skin becomes injured more easily, and, once injured, heals more slowly.

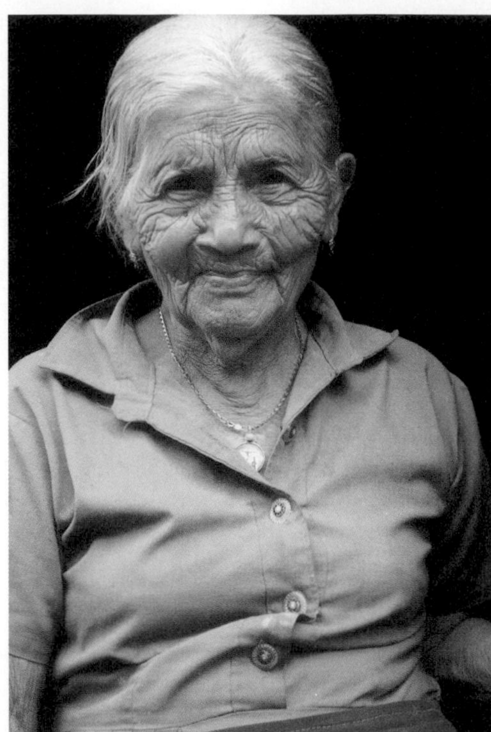

FIGURE 53-1 ■ Physiologic signs of aging human skin.

thickness, the average number of cell layers remains unchanged. The prickle cells of the inner layer of the epidermis show greater variation in nuclear and cytoplasmic size with a less orderly arrangement of cells. Cells reproduce more slowly and are larger and more irregular; however, exposed epidermal cells may divide more frequently than unexposed cells.

Dermis and Subcutaneous Tissue

The dermis contains blood vessels, nerves, hair follicles, and sebaceous glands, but the major portion is made up of collagen and elastin. The elasticity of the skin is largely due to dermal elastin. Decreased skin strength and elasticity with aging are attributed to a decreased amount of elastin and a proportionate increase in the collagen-to-elastin ratio. Collagen fibers change with age, becoming cross-linked and rearranged into thicker bundles. This condition is called **elastosis** and is closely associated with exposure to sunlight (**solar elastosis**). It produces a weather-beaten or tanned appearance.

Aging also produces a decrease in the vascularity of the dermal skin, as evidenced by decreasing numbers of epithelial cells and blood vessels. There is greater vascular fragility, leading to the frequent appearance of hemorrhages (senile purpura), cherry angiomas, venous stasis, and venous lakes on the ears, face, lips, and neck. The decreased vascularity and circulation in the dermis and the underlying subcutaneous tissue also have an effect on drug absorption. Drugs administered subcutaneously are absorbed more slowly, thus prolonging their half-life. The amount of subcutaneous fat tissue also decreases, especially in the extremities, so that arms and legs appear to be thinner.

Appendages

Hair

The most obvious change in aging hair is its color. Half of the population over age 50 years has at least 50% gray body hair, regardless of sex or hair color. Gray hair is determined by an autosomal dominant gene and results from a decreased rate of melanin production by the hair follicle. Hair color generally darkens with age, but this process is reversed with the onset of graying. Graying usually begins at the temples of the head and extends to the vertex of the scalp. It may not occur in the axilla, especially in women, and occurs to a lesser extent in the presternum, or pubis.

Changes in hair growth and distribution are also associated with aging. The amount and distribution of hair are determined by racial, genetic, and sex-linked factors; however, almost all older people have a diminution of body hair except on the face. Adults develop a full terminal hair pattern by age 40 years, and this is followed by a progressive loss of hair in reverse order of development. Postmenopausal white women lose trunk hair first, then pubic and axillary hair. Unopposed adrenal androgens produce coarse facial hair in 50% of white women older than 60 years, especially on the chin and around the lips.

Men also show a general thinning of hair distribution, with the hairs of the eyebrows, ears, and nose becoming longer and coarser. Baldness is often a concern, particularly in aging men, although women also tend to show some thinning of scalp hair. Frontal recession of the hairline occurs in 80% of older women and 100% of older men. Baldness in men is inherited from the mother and occurs only in the presence of testosterone. Onset is variable and is manifested by an M-shaped pattern of hair loss on either side of the midline or by a thinning patch over the vertex.

In general, the hair of both men and women changes from darker, thicker, and more numerous to lighter, thinner, and less numerous with aging. Hair changes begin in midlife and become highly noticeable in later life, especially after age 60 years. Women seem to manifest more hair loss on the trunk and extremities, whereas men have greater hair loss on the head.

Nails

With aging, nails become dull, brittle, hard, and thick. Most nail changes are due to a diminished vascular supply to the nail bed. There is approximately a 30% to 50% decrease in the growth rate of fingernails, from 0.1 mm/day in 30 year olds to 0.07 mm/day in 90 year olds. Aging nails show an increase in longitudinal striations, which can cause splitting of the nail surface.

Toenails are particularly prone to hyperkeratosis and resultant thickening. Pressure and trauma from poorly fitting footwear may be a significant factor but onychomycosis, which affects approximately 20% of individuals over age 60, is the primary factor.[1]

Glands

Sebaceous glands show little atrophy or histologic change with age; however, their function tends to diminish, as evidenced by a decrease in sebum secretion. In men the decrease is minimal, but in women there is a gradual diminution in sebum secretion after menopause, with no significant changes after the seventh decade. There are fewer sebaceous glands in older people, which appears related to the loss of hair follicles. The decrease in sebum secretion and in the number of sebaceous glands results in the drier, coarser skin associated with aging.

Sweat glands generally decrease in size, number, and function with age. In the eccrine glands, the secretory epithelial cells become uneven in size, ranging from normal to small, and there is a progressive accumulation of lipofuscin in the cytoplasm. In the very old, the secretory coils of many eccrine glands are replaced by fibrous tissue, which drastically diminishes their capacity to produce sweat. The thermal threshold for sweating is raised, so that the amount of sweat output at a body temperature of 38°C decreases. This may be due to the fact that there are fewer blood vessels and nerve cells around the glands that enable the body to respond to temperature changes. Apocrine glands do not decrease in number or size, but they do decrease in function. An accumulation of lipofuscin has also been noted in apocrine glands. The diminished functioning of sweat glands in the elderly greatly impairs the ability to maintain body temperature homeostasis.

Table 53-1 summarizes the morphologic features of aging human skin, and Figure 53-2 summarizes the histologic changes associated with aging in normal human skin.

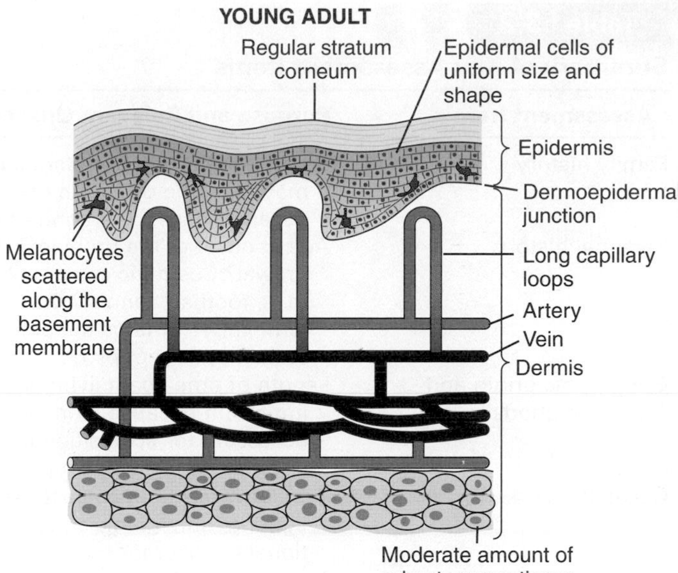

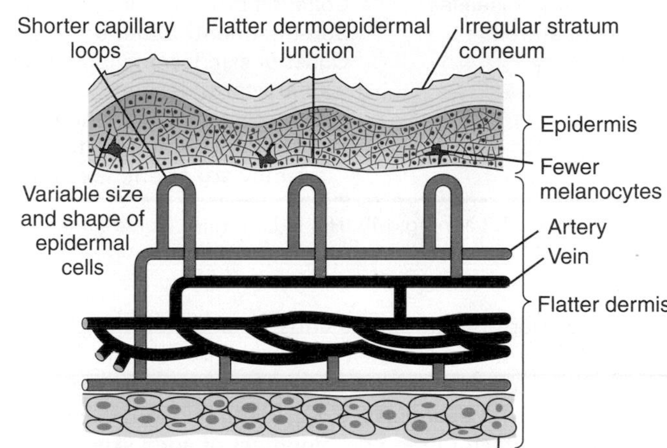

FIGURE 53-2 ■ Histologic changes associated with aging in normal human skin. Note flattening of the dermoepidermal junction and shortening of capillary loops in older skin. Variability in size and shape of epidermal cells, irregular stratum corneum, and loss of melanocytes are also apparent. Age-associated loss of dermal thickness and subcutaneous fat is also illustrated.

KEY CONCEPTS

- The glandular function of skin varies considerably with age. Young children and elderly adults have fewer functional sweat glands and therefore less efficient evaporative heat loss capabilities. Sebaceous glands are particularly active during puberty, causing a predisposition to acne; they become less active with age, causing a predisposition to dry skin.

Table 53-1 Morphologic Features of Aging Human Skin

Epidermis	Dermis	Appendages
Flat dermoepidermal junction	Atrophy	Graying of hair
Variable thickness	Fewer fibroblasts	Loss of hair
Variable cell size and shape	Fewer blood vessels	Conversion of terminal to vellus hair
Occasional nuclear atypia	Shortened capillary loops	Abnormal nail plates
Loss of melanocytes	Abnormal nerve endings	Fewer glands

From Gilchrest BA: Skin. In Rowe JW, Besdine RW, editors: *Health and disease in old age,* Boston, 1982, Little, Brown, p 383.

Table 53-2

Summary of Key Assessment Items

Assessment Item	Purpose and Relevant Questions to Ask
Family history	Some skin diseases are familial or hereditary. When hereditary skin disease is ascertained, one may have the opportunity to both correct misconceptions and allay fears about the presence, absence, or prognosis of disease. What are the current familial dermatologic diseases?
Personal history	Age at onset of the problem? How has the patient adjusted to the problem? By social withdrawal? Cosmetic cover-up? Withdrawal from school athletic activities that require showers (e.g., football, tennis)? Does the problem threaten the patient's self-image of masculinity or femininity? What is the patient's ethnic origin? (Some skin diseases are more common in certain ethic groups.)
Geographic origin and present abode	Length of time spent living in each area? Some skin diseases are indigenous, which may be important because of increased exposure. Occasionally, a contact of only 5 min is all that is necessary for acquisition of a disease.
Season	Seasonal occurrence of a problem? Pollen? Sunlight?
Occupation	Type of work? Skin contact material (e.g., chemicals, dust, gas), excessive heat and abnormal lighting, unhygienic surroundings, possible infective insects, other family members' occupational exposures?
Leisure activities	Does the problem occur only on weekends? After yard activities? Painting? Woodworking? Camping? Fishing? Hiking? In association with children's play?
Accompanying diseases	Collagen disease? Drug therapy for collagen disease? Other diseases and their drug therapy?
Previous treatment	Self-treatment? Other drugs prescribed?
Special history	Onset of skin lesions (abnormality)? Remissions, exacerbations, or recurrences? Site of onset? Character of lesions? Original character and subsequent changes? Course or extension? Symptoms? Itching? Ability to perform duties? Topical therapy? Self-treatment? Psychological factor? What does the patient associate with exacerbations of the problem (e.g., stress of a family argument, tax time, report time)?

Data from Rosen T, Lanning, MB, Hill MJ, editors: *Nurse's atlas of dermatology,* Boston, 1983, Little, Brown.

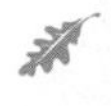

◆ The epidermis and dermis undergo degenerative changes with aging. The epidermis thins, and the dermis becomes less elastic and less vascular. Subcutaneous fat decreases. Exposure to sunlight is an important factor in the development of aged skin.

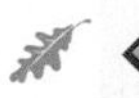

◆ Graying of hair results from decreased melanin production by the hair follicle. After age 40 years, progressive hair loss occurs. Male pattern baldness is an inherited trait that is mediated by testosterone.

EVALUATION OF THE INTEGUMENTARY SYSTEM

A careful examination of the skin yields valuable information that may aid in identifying a systemic disease or a specific problem of the skin or appendages. Diagnostic evaluations include a careful history, and Table 53-2 provides a general guide. A proper skin examination also describes the objective signs of dermatologic disease, including all types of lesions and their distribution.

Primary and Secondary Lesions

Physical descriptions should include the lesions and their classification, generally **primary** (original appearance) or **secondary** (appearance modified by normal progress over time or by such external agents as scratching). Figure 53-3 shows clinical examples of primary and secondary lesions.

Lesion Descriptors

After a skin lesion has been classified as primary or secondary, other features should be noted, particularly size, symmetry of color and shape, and distribution if more than one lesion is present. Skin lesions may assume a wide range of colors—red–salmon pink, brown-black, blue-purple, bone white–slate gray, and yellow, to name a few. Each color suggests certain diagnoses. Skin lesions may be solitary, few, or profuse. When more than one lesion is present, the distribution pattern may be important in suggesting the diagnosis. Look for the following common patterns: symmetric (affecting mirror-image portions of the body), sun exposed (affecting skin sites that routinely receive solar irradiation), intertriginous (affecting warm, moist, apposed skin sites), acral (affecting the distal extremities, ears, and nose), genital, and flexor or extensor predominance. Additional descriptors are often used to further characterize and describe a skin lesion or the relationship between various skin lesions such as confluent or clustered. Table 53-3 lists common morphologic and configurational terms.

NONPALPABLE

PRIMARY LESIONS (Original Appearance)

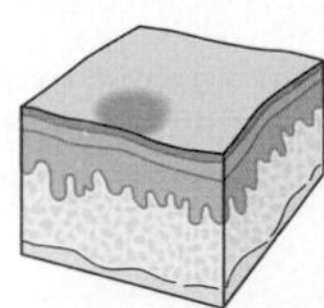

Macule: A spot, circumscribed, up to 1 cm; not palpable; not elevated above or depressed below surrounding skin surface; hypopigmented, hyperpigmented, or erythematous. **Example:** Freckles. Referred to as **patch** if greater than 1 cm. **Examples:** Café au lait spots, mongolian spots.

PALPABLE, SOLID

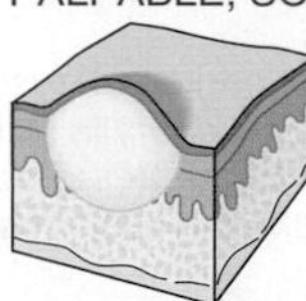

Papule: A bump, palpable and circumscribed, elevated and less than 5 mm in diameter; may be pigmented, erythematous, or flesh-toned. **Example:** Elevated nevus (mole).

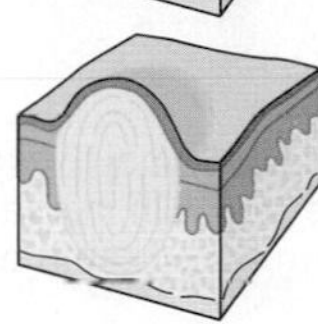

Nodule: A lesion similar to a papule, with a diameter of 5 mm to 2 cm; may have a significant palpable dermal component. **Examples:** Fibroma, xanthoma, intradermal nevi.

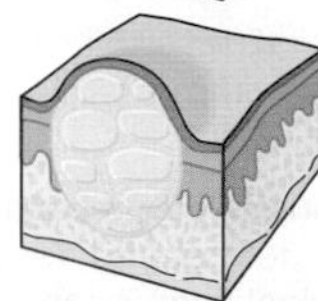

Tumor: Any mass lesion; generally larger than a nodule; may be either malignant or benign. **Example:** Lipoma.

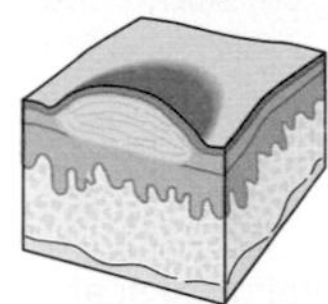

Plaque: Usually well-circumscribed lesion with large surface area and slight elevation. **Examples:** Psoriasis, lichen planus.

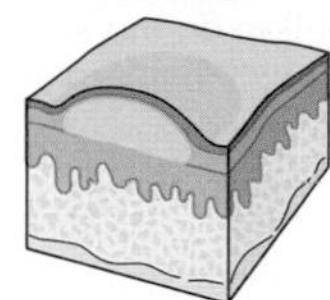

Wheal: An elevation in the skin, with a smooth surface, sloping borders, and (usually) light pink color; caused by acute areas of edema in the skin; may appear, disappear, or change form abruptly within minutes or hours; size ranges from 3 mm to 20 cm. **Example:** Mosquito bite.

PALPABLE, FLUID-FILLED

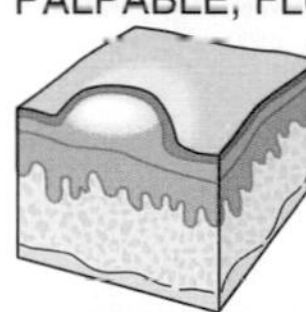

Vesicle: A small blister (up to 5 mm in diameter); fluid collection may be subcorneal, intraepidermal, or subepidermal. **Example:** Herpes simplex (early stages).

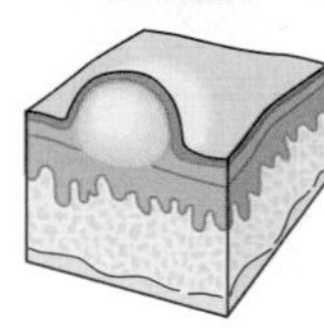

Bulla: A blister larger than 5 mm; fluid may be located at various levels. **Examples:** Pemphigus, pemphigoid.

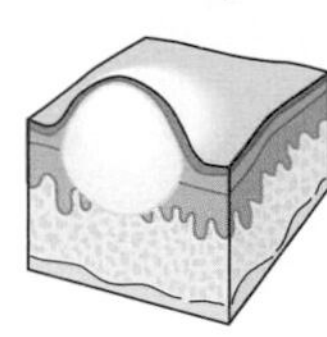

Pustule: An elevated, well-circumscribed lesion containing purulent exudate. **Example:** Acne vulgaris.

FIGURE 53-3 ■ Characteristics of common skin lesions.

Continued

SECONDARY LESIONS (Modification of Original Appearance)

DAMAGED OR DIMINISHED SKIN SURFACE

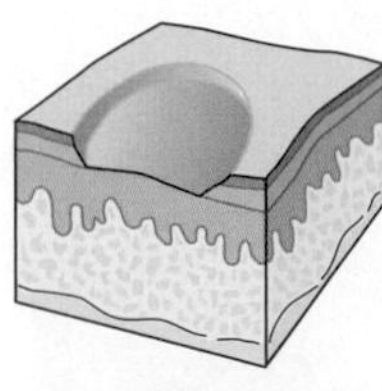

Erosion: Loss of epidermis that does not extend into dermis. **Example:** Ruptured chickenpox vesicle.

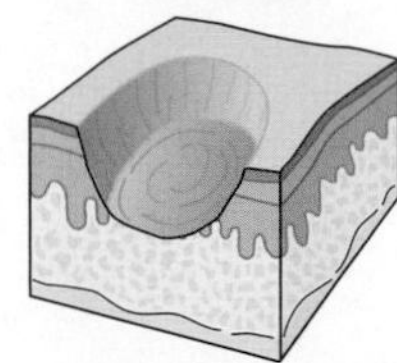

Ulcer: Loss of skin through the epidermis; healing results in scar formation. **Example:** Stasis ulcer.

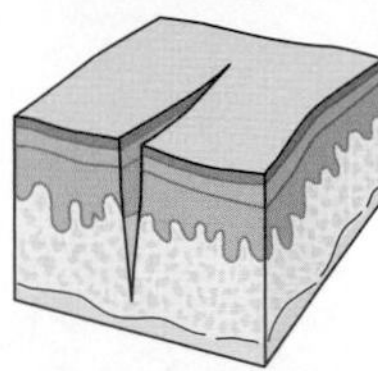

Fissure: A split in all epidermal layers of skin. **Example:** Athlete's foot.

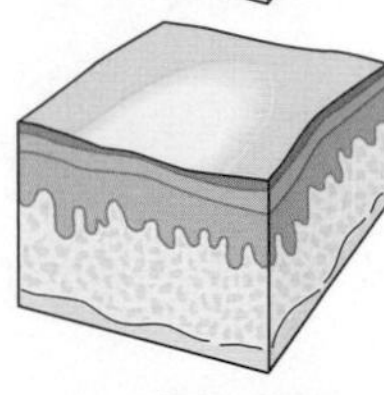

Atrophy: Diminution of epidermal surface; skin looks thinner and more translucent than normal; atrophy of the dermal layers may result in wasting or depression of the skin surface. **Example:** Arterial insufficiency.

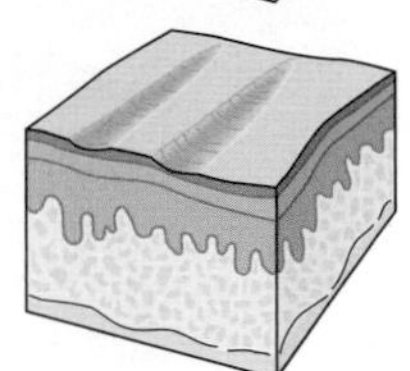

Excoriation: Loss of outer skin layers from scratching or rubbing. **Example:** Scratched insect bite.

AUGMENTED OR INCREASED SKIN SURFACE

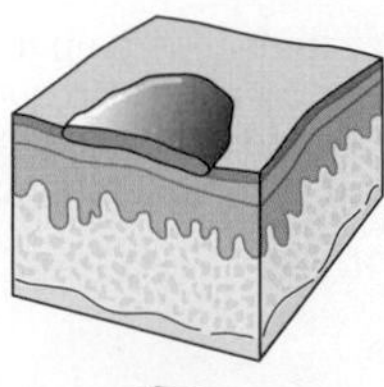

Crust: A collection of serous exudate and debris on the surface of damaged or absent outer skin layers. **Example:** Impetigo.

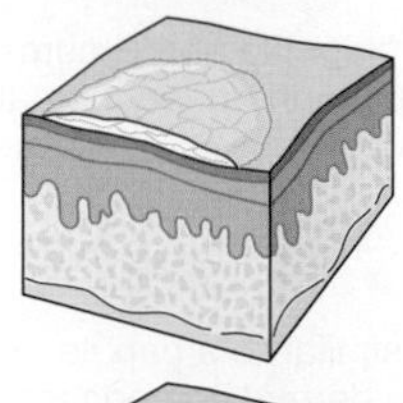

Scale: A compact portion of desquamating stratum corneum; may vary in size, thickness, and consistency. **Examples:** Psoriasis scale (compact and thick), pityriasis rosea scale (thin and small).

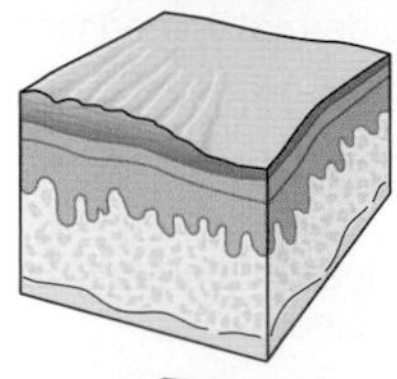

Lichenification: Epidermal thickening and roughening of the skin with increased visibility of skin surface furrows. **Example:** Chronic atopic dermatitis.

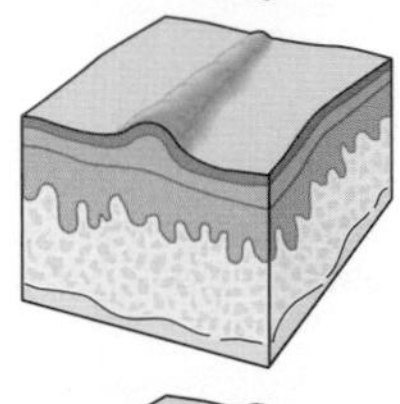

Scar: A collection of fibrous tissue that forms to replace lost epidermal and dermal tissue. **Examples:** Surgical scar, acne scar.

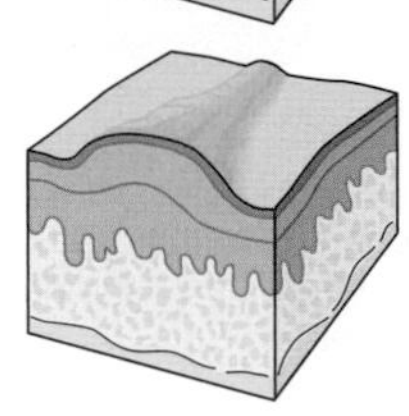

Keloid: Augmentation of scar tissue, creating a significant elevation on the skin surface after healing. **Examples:** Postsurgical scar, postacne scar.

FIGURE 53-3—cont'd ■ Characteristics of common skin lesions.

Table 53-3

Lesion Descriptors

Term	Definition
Confluent	Blending together
Discrete	Remaining separate although close together
Diffuse	Generalized or widespread
Eczematous	Vesicles with an oozing crust
Herpetiform	Closely grouped vesicles (herpeslike)
Linear	Set in a straight line
Localized	Found only in one area
Pedunculated	On a stalk
Reticulated	Netlike array
Round lesions	Annular (ring shaped, active edge, clear center)
	Arcuate (arc shaped, incomplete circle)
	Circinate (circular)
	Guttate (small droplet–like)
	Iris (concentric circles such as a bull's eye)
	Nummular (coin shaped)
	Ovoid (oval shaped)
Serpiginous	Wandering, snakelike
Telangiectatic	Characterized by dilated surface vessels
Verrucous	Rough, wartlike surface
Zosteriform	Similar to shingles, following along a nerve root dermatome

Data from Sauer GC: *Manual of skin diseases,* ed 6, Philadelphia, 1991, Lippincott.

KEY CONCEPTS

- Skin lesions may be categorized as primary or secondary.
- Primary lesions retain their original appearance, unmodified by time and external processes such as scratching.
- Secondary lesions are those whose appearance has been modified over time; they may look quite dissimilar to the original lesion. The differentiation of primary from secondary lesions aids in establishing a correct diagnosis.
- A description of lesion color, shape, number, and distribution is helpful in determining the cause of a lesion.

SELECTED SKIN DISORDERS

Diseases of the skin are divisible into two broad etiologic categories: inflammatory/infectious and proliferative/neoplastic. Inflammatory disorders of the skin often occur in individuals who have hypersensitivity reactions to substances in the environment. Infectious agents ranging from viruses to insects may infect the skin. Proliferative conditions include psoriasis, seborrheic keratosis, cysts, warts, and papillomas. Other benign tumors arise from other cells in the skin: nevi, lipomas, dermatofibromas, neuromas, and hemangiomas. Kaposi sarcoma is a malignant, opportunistic neoplasm that occurs in persons with preexisting immunodeficiency.

Skin cancer is the most common malignancy in the United States, but except for malignant melanoma and a few squamous carcinomas, skin cancers are not life threatening. Ultraviolet light damages sun-exposed skin and is a major factor in development of skin cancer. Although many of the disorders described in the following section are not life threatening, they can affect the quality of life.

INFECTIOUS PROCESSES
Viral Infections

Verrucae

Etiology and Pathogenesis. **Verrucae,** or warts (Figure 53-4), are common benign papillomas caused by DNA-containing papillomaviruses. Although warts vary in appearance depending on their location, the histologic characteristics of all lesions are similar. A wart is actually an exaggeration of normal skin composition, with the stratum corneum being irregularly thickened. The human papillomaviruses, the subgroup of papovaviruses that causes human warts, are not found in other animals and invade only the skin and mucous membranes of humans.

Warts may resolve spontaneously if immunity to the virus develops, but the immune response can be delayed for years and is not reliably activated in every case. In 95% of cases, untreated warts will resolve within 5 years,[2] but they may multiply into hundreds of lesions and can involve any body site. Current surgical treatment may be directed at removal of the wart by laser. Liquid nitrogen or acid chemicals, cryotherapy, and salicylic acid paint or plasters have also been effective medical treatments.

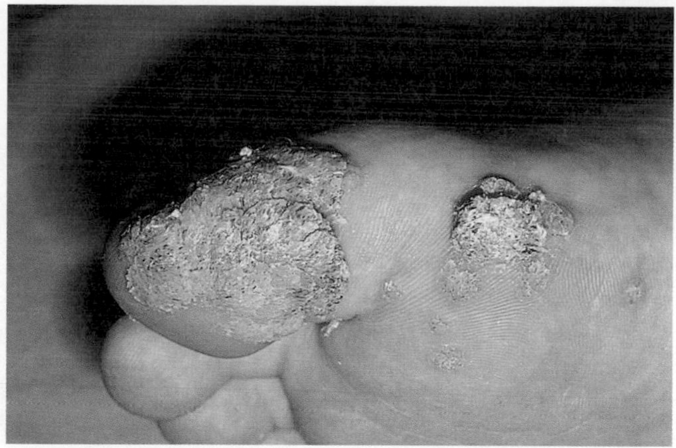

FIGURE 53-4 ■ Plantar warts. (From Callen JP et al: *Color atlas of dermatology,* ed 2, Philadelphia, 2000, Saunders, p 92.)

Herpes Simplex Virus

Etiology and Pathogenesis. **Herpes simplex virus** (HSV) infections of the skin and mucous membranes are common (Figure 53-5). Two types of herpesviruses infect humans: type 1 and type 2. Most HSV 1 infections occur above the waist.[3] HSV-1 may result when external infection is spread to the other parts of the body through the occupational hazards that exist in professions such as dentistry and medicine and some athletics. HSV-2 is responsible for most infections in the genital region.[3]

Herpesvirus lesions usually begin with a burning or tingling sensation. Vesicles and erythema follow and progress to pustules, ulcers, and crusts before healing. The lesion is most common on the lips, face, and mouth. Pain is common, and healing takes place in 10 to 14 days.[4] After the initial infection, the herpesvirus persists in latent form in the trigeminal and other ganglia. Recurrent lesions are common and may be precipitated by stress, sunlight exposure, menses, or injury.[5,6] The vast majority of patients have at least one episode of herpesvirus reactivation, and some individuals may have 10 or more outbreaks per year. Recently, concern has arisen over the identification of infectious viral shedding in the absence of symptomatic lesions.[5]

Treatment. No cure for herpes simplex is known, and most treatment measures are palliative. Lidocaine (Xylocaine) or diphenhydramine (Benadryl) application and aspirin help relieve pain. Cold compresses help in the acute stages.

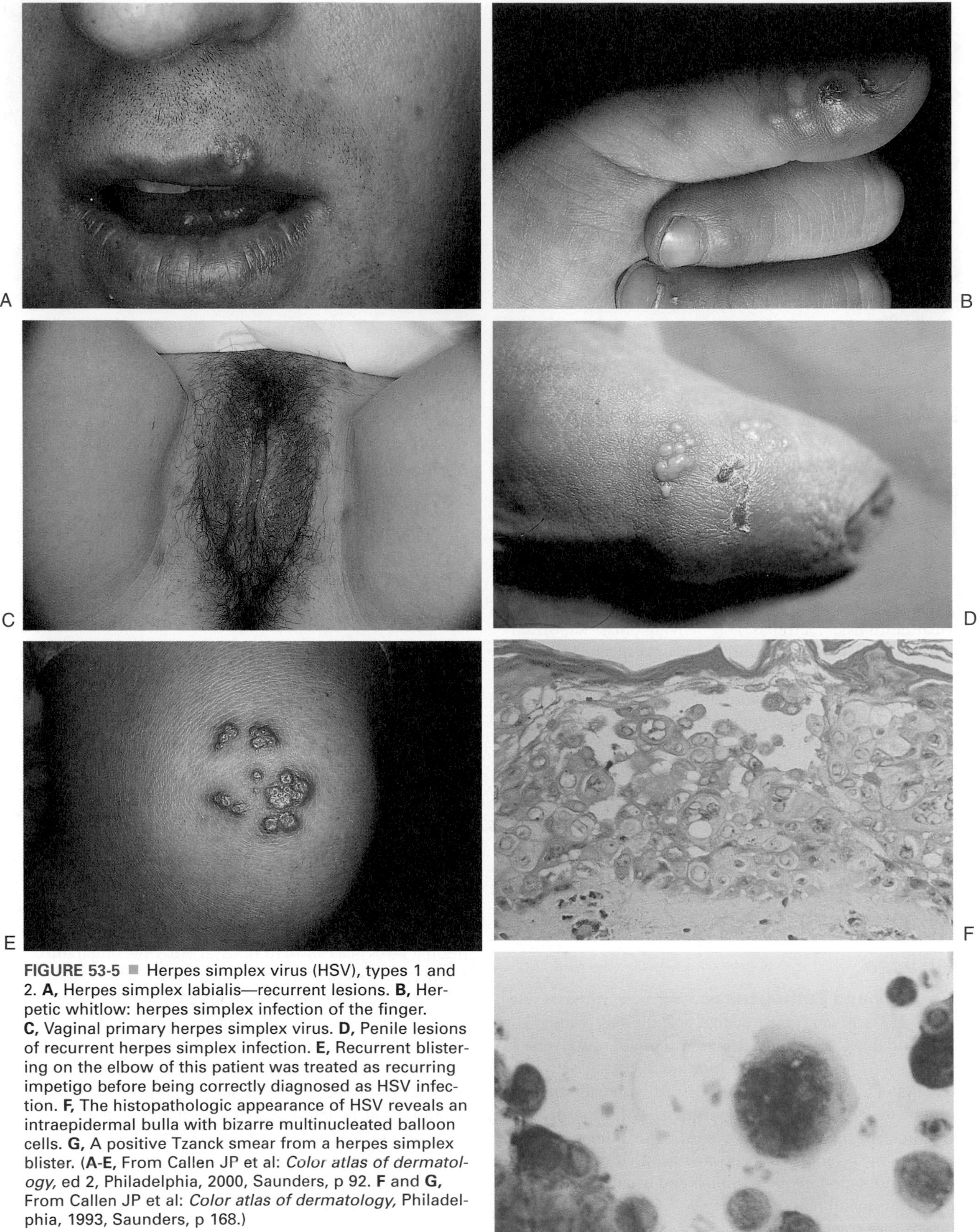

FIGURE 53-5 ■ Herpes simplex virus (HSV), types 1 and 2. **A,** Herpes simplex labialis—recurrent lesions. **B,** Herpetic whitlow: herpes simplex infection of the finger. **C,** Vaginal primary herpes simplex virus. **D,** Penile lesions of recurrent herpes simplex infection. **E,** Recurrent blistering on the elbow of this patient was treated as recurring impetigo before being correctly diagnosed as HSV infection. **F,** The histopathologic appearance of HSV reveals an intraepidermal bulla with bizarre multinucleated balloon cells. **G,** A positive Tzanck smear from a herpes simplex blister. (**A-E,** From Callen JP et al: *Color atlas of dermatology,* ed 2, Philadelphia, 2000, Saunders, p 92. **F** and **G,** From Callen JP et al: *Color atlas of dermatology,* Philadelphia, 1993, Saunders, p 168.)

Acyclovir, famciclovir, or valacyclovir are recommended to shorten the duration of active disease outbreaks; in certain situations, these drugs may be used for daily prophylaxis.

Herpes Zoster

Etiology and Pathogenesis. Herpes zoster *(shingles)* is an acute localized inflammatory disease of a dermatomal segment of the skin (Figure 53-6). It is caused by the same herpesvirus that causes chickenpox (varicella-zoster). It is believed to be the result of reactivation of a latent varicella-zoster virus that has been present in the sensory dorsal ganglia since childhood infection. During an attack of shingles, the reactivated virus travels from the ganglia to the skin of the corresponding dermatome.

Clinical Manifestations and Treatment. The clinical manifestations of shingles include the eruption of vesicles with erythematous bases that are restricted to skin areas supplied by sensory neurons of a single or associated group of

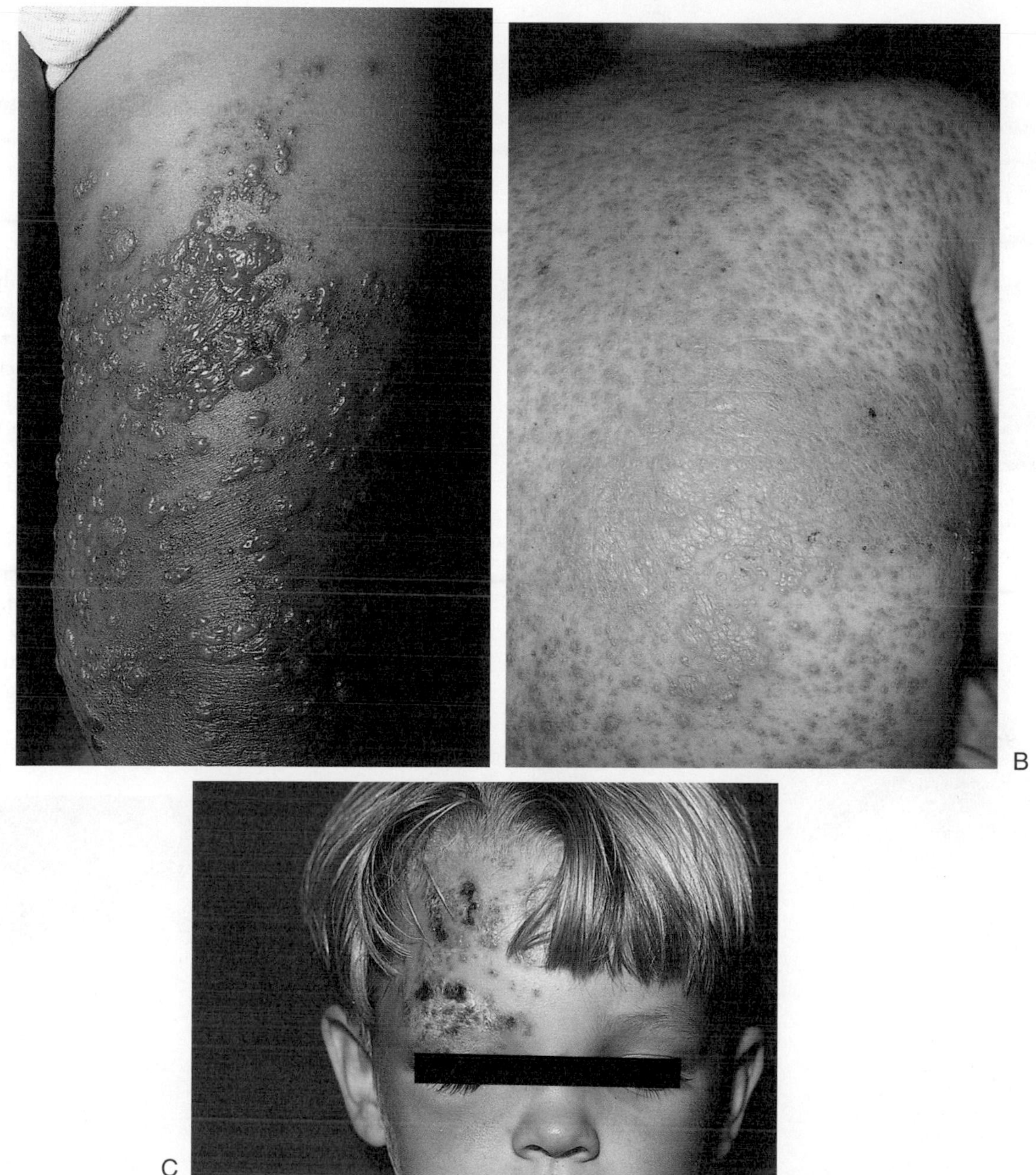

FIGURE 53-6 ■ Herpes zoster. **A,** Recurrent infection with the varicella-zoster virus. The eruption is usually dermatomal but can become generalized. **B,** Disseminated herpes zoster. **C,** Herpes zoster ophthalmicus. (From Callen JP et al: *Color atlas of dermatology,* ed 2, Philadelphia, 2000, Saunders, p 92.)

dorsal root ganglia. Eruptions generally follow a unilateral dermatomal distribution and most often occur on the thorax, trunk, and face. In immunosuppressed persons, the lesions may extend beyond the dermatome. New crops of vesicles erupt for 3 to 5 days along the nerve pathway.[3] Lesions are deeper and more confluent than those of chickenpox. The vesicles dry, form crusts, and eventually fall off. Lesions usually clear in 2 to 3 weeks.[3] Severe pain and paresthesias are common. In the elderly, herpes-zoster is a particularly serious condition that may be long lasting. Pain reports from elderly individuals indicate an increased severity and lengthy episodes of up to 1 year.[3] Systemic treatment with acyclovir, famciclovir, or valacyclovir should be initiated as soon as possible, preferably within the first 48 to 72 hours.

Postherpetic neuralgia is the most important complication occurring in people older than 50 years.[3] Eye involvement can result in permanent blindness.

Treatment. Management of shingles includes acyclovir (Zovirax). Topical agents such as Burrow compresses or aqueous alcohol shake lotions may also be used. Pain medication may be indicated in severe cases. Systemic corticosteroids have also been effective in healthy persons older than 50 years with severe pain, but their use remains controversial. High doses of interferon, an antiviral glycoprotein, have been used in persons with cancer when the herpetic lesions are limited to the dermatome.[7]

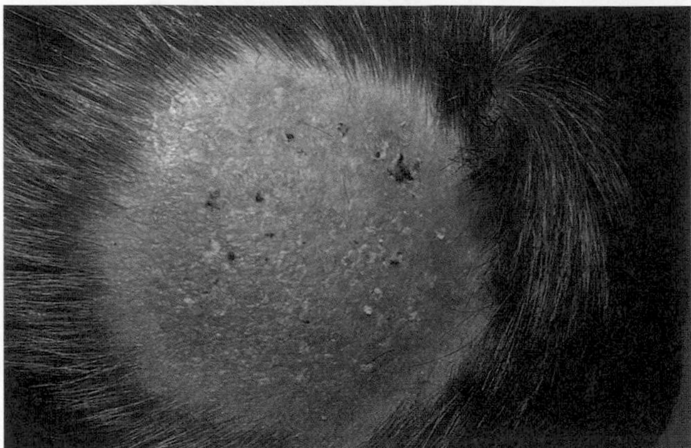

FIGURE 53-7 ■ Tinea capitis, localized patch. (From Callen JP et al: *Color atlas of dermatology,* Philadelphia, 1993, Saunders, p 106.)

Fungal Infections

Superficial Fungal Infections

Three genera of **fungi (dermatophytes)** commonly infect human skin: *Microsporum, Trichophyton,* and *Epidermophyton.* These organisms can cause an infection termed **tinea** in any cutaneous area, including the hair and nails. Infections in different locations are named after the location: tinea capitis (scalp) (Figure 53-7), tinea barbae (beard), tinea faciei (face) (Figure 53-8), tinea corporis (trunk) (Figure 53-9), tinea manus (hand), tinea cruris (groin), and tinea pedis (foot).

Clinical Manifestations. The clinical signs of superficial fungal infection vary depending on the physical location and the host's response to the invading organism. Often fungal infections are manifested as erythematous macules or plaques with peripheral scaling and some central clearing. Vesicular lesions often accompany the dry scaling on the feet.

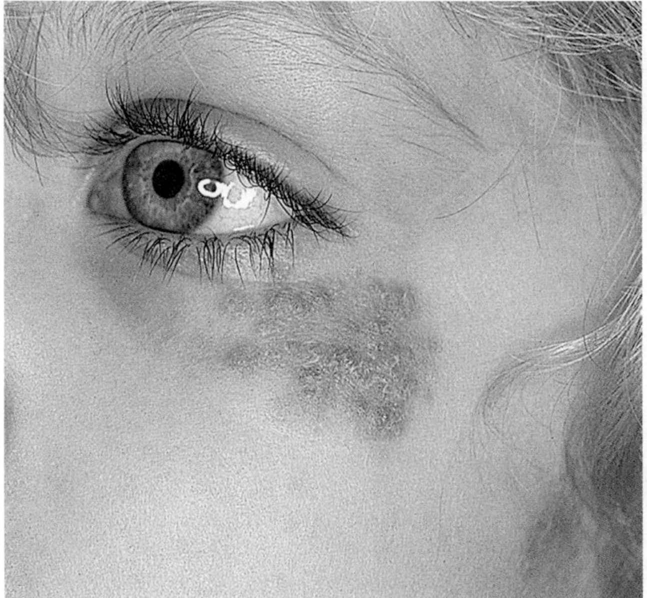

FIGURE 53-8 ■ Tinea faciei. (From Callen JP et al: *Color atlas of dermatology,* ed 2, Philadelphia, 2000, Saunders, p 89.)

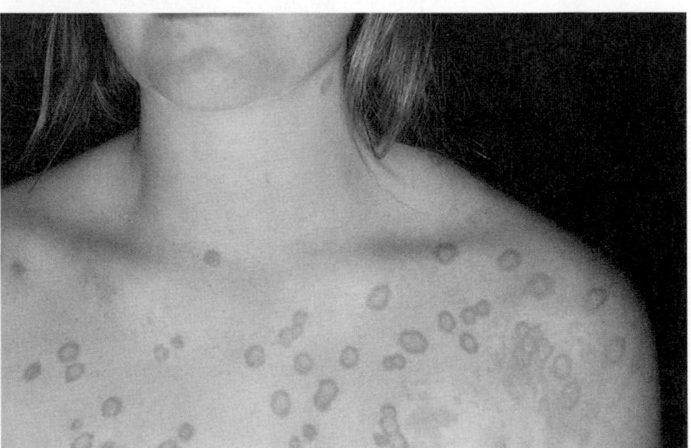

FIGURE 53-9 ■ Tinea corporis. Annular scaly plaques in superficial basal cell epithelioma. (From Callen JP et al: *Color atlas of dermatology,* Philadelphia, 1993, Saunders, p 106.)

Because of the variability of signs and symptoms, superficial dermatophytosis must be considered when evaluating even a weeping, crusted area more suggestive of eczema or impetigo. Dermatophyte infection of the nails, or onychomycosis, is usually seen as a white or yellow opaque discoloration that often progresses to a thickened, crumbed, or deformed nail (Figure 53-10).

Treatment. Topical management of localized superficial dermatophyte infections is very effective. Among the topical antifungal preparations available in cream and solution form are miconazole nitrate, clotrimazole, econazole nitrate, ciclopirox olamine, and terbinafine; a 4-week course of twice-daily applications will usually clear the symptoms. For more extensive infections involving the hair, nails, or resistant organisms, systemic therapy (e.g., griseofulvin or intraconazole and terbinafine) is required. Treatment duration ranges from 3 to 4 weeks (tinea corporis) to 12 months (onychomycosis).

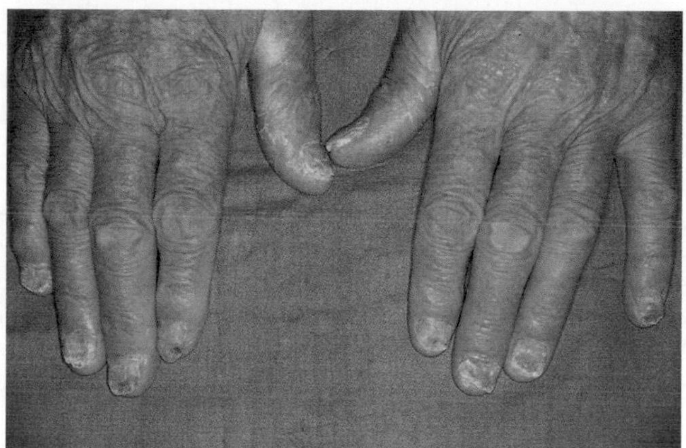

FIGURE 53-10 ■ Dermatophyte infection of the nails resulting in onycholysis. (From Callen JP et al: *Color atlas of dermatology,* Philadelphia, 1993, Saunders, p 347.)

Yeast Infections

The yeast *Candida albicans* is another common source of superficial infection (Figure 53-11). It is manifested in newborns as the white lesions of **thrush,** in infants and bedridden patients as **intertrigo,** and in immunoimpaired persons as the systemic disorder **mucocutaneous candidiasis.** Mucocutaneous candidiasis may actually be the presenting sign in an individual with a previously undiagnosed immunodeficiency disorder.

Localized yeast infections such as oral candidiasis (thrush) may be managed with nystatin mouth rinse or clotrimazole troches (throat lozenges). The topical antifungal medications mentioned earlier may also be used in the management of localized yeast infections. Widespread or systemic infections respond well to oral ketoconazole or fluconazole (Diflucan).

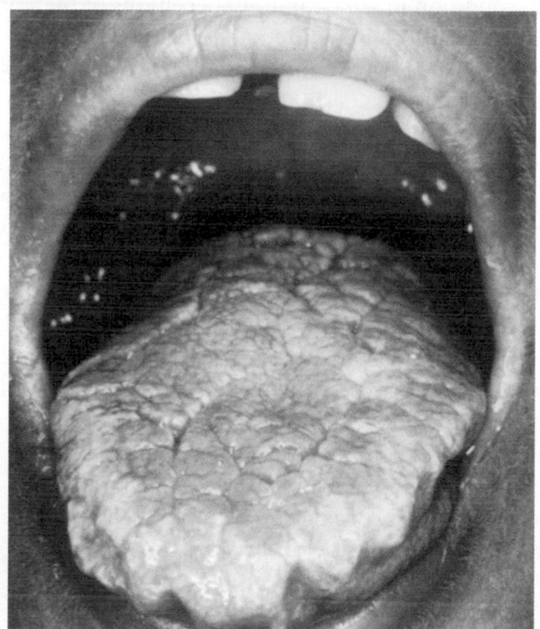

FIGURE 53-11 ■ *Candida albicans* infection of the tongue in chronic mucocutaneous candidiasis. (From Arnold HL, Odom RB, James WD: *Andrews' diseases of the skin: clinical dermatology,* ed 8, Philadelphia, 1990, Saunders, p 341.)

Bacterial Infections

Impetigo

Etiology and Clinical Manifestations. **Impetigo** is an acute, contagious skin disease characterized by the formation of vesicles, pustules, and yellowish crusts (Figure 53-12). The most common cause of infection of the skin, impetigo is caused by staphylococci or streptococci. Approximately 5% of

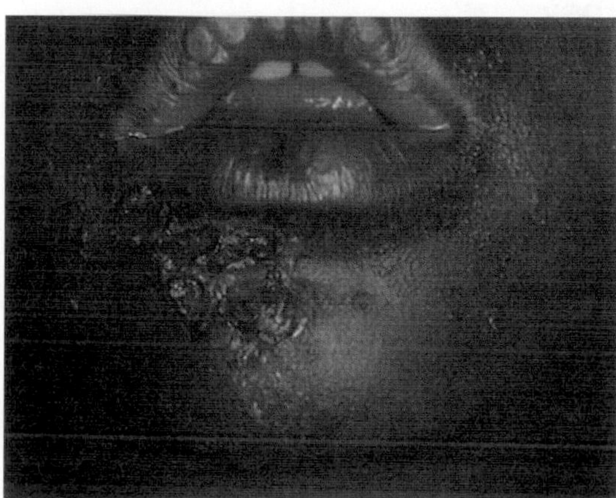

FIGURE 53-12 ■ Impetigo. (From Swartz MH: *Physical diagnosis, history and examination,* ed 4, Philadelphia, 2002, Saunders, p 713.)

the population each year sustains *Staphylococcus* infections of a severity sufficient to require medical attention.[8] Approximately 20% of adults are chronic carriers of the bacterium *Staphylococcus aureus,* and another 60% are intermittent carriers.[8] The bacterium is carried in the nasal area and may pass onto the skin and produce disease. Staphylococcal infections are a special problem for hospitalized patients, who may become infected from the infected staff of the hospital.

Treatment. Treatment for impetigo includes topical application of 2% mupirocin ointment (Bactroban). If a large area of skin is involved or if the person is febrile, impetigo may be managed systemically with oral dicloxacillin, cephalexin, or erythromycin.

Syphilis

Etiology and Clinical Manifestations. A variety of sexually transmitted diseases caused by bacteria can infect the genitalia. The most serious is **syphilis,** which is caused by *Treponema pallidum.* If the person remains untreated, three stages can occur. In primary syphilis, a chancre (ulcer) generally occurs as a single lesion on the genitalia; the spirochetal microorganism that causes syphilis can be seen in a scraping of the chancre. Secondary syphilis is characterized by a disseminated rash that cannot be clearly distinguished from other rashes. Both the primary and secondary stages of syphilis are contagious.

Treatment. Studies to detect serum antibodies against syphilis (such as the Venereal Disease Research Laboratory, VDRL) and examination of the pustules for the spirochete are required to achieve a diagnosis. Penicillin is very effective in eradicating syphilis in the primary and secondary stages, but unfortunately damage caused by tertiary syphilis to the cardiovascular and central nervous systems is permanent.

Leprosy

Leprosy is a chronic infectious disease of the skin caused by the intracellular bacillus *Mycobacterium leprae.* Approximately 11 million people worldwide have leprosy.[8] The diagnosis is made with a skin biopsy. Leprosy has a low rate of infectivity and is usually responsive to sulfone drugs like dapsone. For chronic deformities, corrective orthopedic surgery may be required.

INFLAMMATORY CONDITIONS

Lupus Erythematosus

Lupus erythematosus (LE) is an inflammatory disease that has cutaneous manifestations. Systemic LE and chronic discoid LE are clinically dissimilar but basically related diseases. The two diseases differ with regard to characteristic skin lesions, subjective complaints, other organ involvement, LE cell test findings, response to treatment, and eventual prognosis. Discoid lupus presents with scaly red plaques with scarring that involve sun-exposed skin. Classically, systemic lupus presents with a butterfly-shaped erythema involving the cheeks and nose; discoid lesions may be seen as well. A comparison of the two conditions is found in Table 53-4. Figure 53-13 illustrates characteristic skin lesions of both conditions.

Seborrheic Dermatitis

Clinical Manifestations and Treatment. Seborrheic dermatitis (Figure 53-14) is a papulosquamous skin disease manifested by various degrees of scaling and erythema in areas of high oil gland concentration such as the scalp, eyebrows, glabellae, eyelids, nasolabial folds, pinna and posterior sulcus of the ears, sternum, axillae, umbilicus, and anogenital area. Common manifestations of this disease are cradle cap in newborns and dandruff in adolescents and adults.

Although seborrheic dermatitis is not curable, it may be controlled with topical medication. The regular use of tar shampoos often clears the symptoms and signs of seborrheic dermatitis in the scalp; mild topical corticosteroids (e.g., 1% hydrocortisone) clear lesions on the face and ears.

Psoriasis

Etiology and Clinical Manifestations. **Psoriasis** is a common chronic skin disease characterized by papules and plaques with an overlying silvery scale. The specific cause of psoriasis is unknown, but it appears to be a multifactorial inherited condition in which minor aberrations of the immune system promote inflammation and hyperproliferation within the skin. The disease may affect, with varying degrees of severity, people of all ages. Lesions can appear on any area of the body; however, they seem to have a predilection for the knees, elbows, lower part of the back, scalp, and nails (Figure 53-15). Disease progression is unpredictable, and the patient may periodically experience spontaneous exacerbations or remission.

Treatment. No cure for psoriasis is known. Treatments, both topical and systemic, are directed at clearing and controlling the lesions. Therapies include topical corticosteroids (most commonly used), a vitamin D derivative (calcipotriene ointment [Dovonex]), ultraviolet light exposure, topical tar preparations, and combinations of ultraviolet light with topical tar or systemic psoralen. Systemic therapies with methotrexate and hydroxyurea are also effective in clearing psoriasis but carry considerable risk of toxicity.

Lichen Planus

Etiology and Pathogenesis. **Lichen planus** is a relatively common, chronic, pruritic disease involving inflammation and papular eruption of the skin and mucous membranes. Idiopathic lichen planus is of unknown cause but can be stimulated by a variety of drugs and chemicals in suscepti-

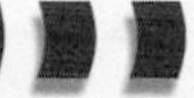

Table 53-4

Comparison of Chronic Discoid with Systemic Lupus Erythematosus

Parameter	Chronic Discoid LE	Systemic LE
Primary lesions	Red, scaly, thickened, well-circumscribed patches with enlarged follicles and elevated border	Red, mildly scaly, diffuse, puffy lesions Purpura also seen
Secondary lesions	Atrophy, scarring, and pigmentary changes	No scarring Mild hyperpigmentation
Distribution	Face, mainly in the "butterfly" area, but also on the scalp, ears, arms, and chest May not be symmetric	Face in the "butterfly" area, arms, fingers, and legs Usually symmetric
Course	Very chronic with gradual progression; slow healing under therapy; no effect on life	Acute onset with fever, rash, malaise, and joint pains Most cases respond rather rapidly to steroid and supportive therapy, but the prognosis for life is poor
Season	Aggravated by intense sun exposure or radiation therapy	Same
Sex incidence	Almost twice as common in females	Same
Systemic pathology	None obvious	Nephritis, arthritis, epilepsy, pancarditis, hepatitis, etc.
Laboratory findings	Biopsy characteristic in classic case LE cell test negative, as are other laboratory tests	Biopsy less useful LE cell test usually positive Leukopenia, anemia, albuminuria, increased sedimentation rate, positive antinuclear antibody test, and biological false-positive serologic test for syphilis

From Sauer GC: *Manual of skin diseases*, ed 6, Philadelphia, 1991, Lippincott, p 253.
LE, Lupus erythematosus.

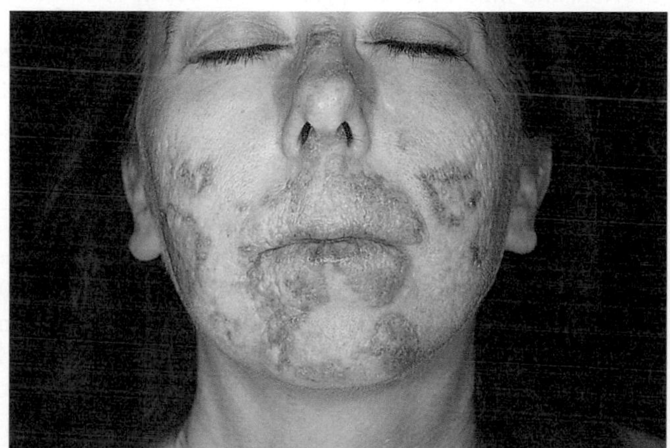

A

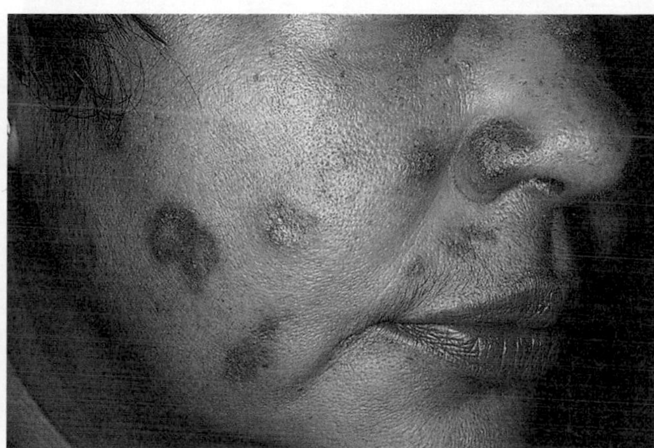

B

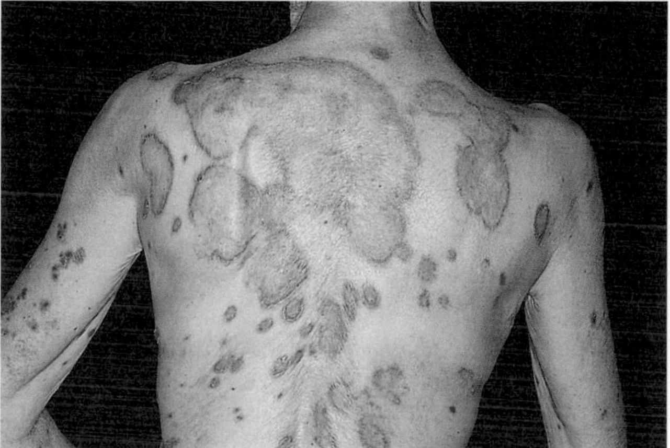

C

FIGURE 53-13 ■ **A** and **B**, Discoid lupus erythematosus. Round or oval cutaneous lesions occurring in patients with lupus erythematosus. **C**, Subacute cutaneous lupus erythematosus. (From Callen JP et al: *Color atlas of dermatology*, ed 2, Philadelphia, 2000, Saunders, pp 15, 16.)

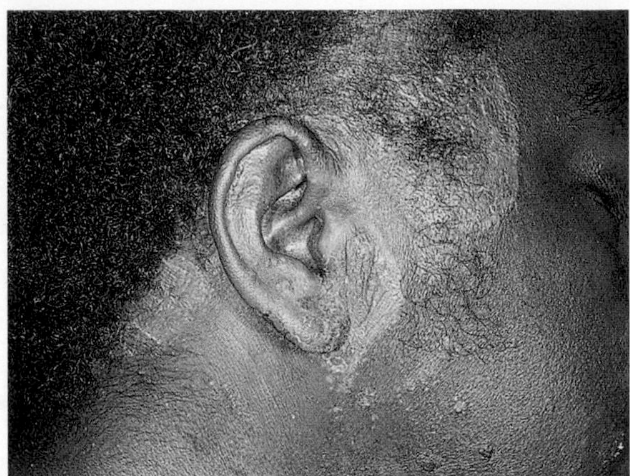

FIGURE 53-14 ■ Annular seborrheic dermatitis of the ear. (From Callen JP et al: *Color atlas of dermatology,* ed 2, Philadelphia, 2000, Saunders, p 246.)

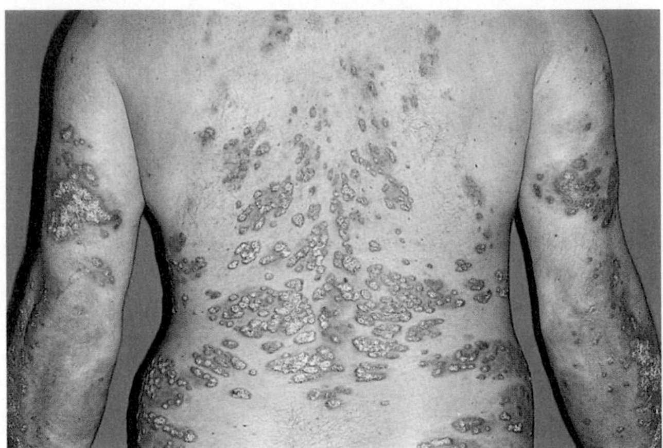

FIGURE 53-15 ■ Psoriasis vulgaris. (From Callen JP et al: *Color atlas of dermatology,* ed 2, Philadelphia, 2000, Saunders, p 280.)

ble persons. The characteristic lesion is a shiny, white-topped, purplish, polygonal papule. Lesions appear on the wrists, ankles, and trunk (Figure 53-16). Mucous membrane lesions are white and lacy and may become bullous. Pruritus is severe, and new lesions develop as a result of scratching (Koebner phenomenon). Nails are affected in approximately 10% of people with lichen planus.[9]

Treatment. In the majority of people, lichen planus is a self-limiting disease. Treatment measures include discontinuing all medications, followed by the administration of topical corticosteroids and occlusive dressings. Systemic corticosteroids may be indicated in severe cases, and antipruritic agents are helpful in reducing the itch.

Pityriasis Rosea

Etiology, Pathogenesis, and Treatment. **Pityriasis rosea** is a rash of unknown origin that primarily affects

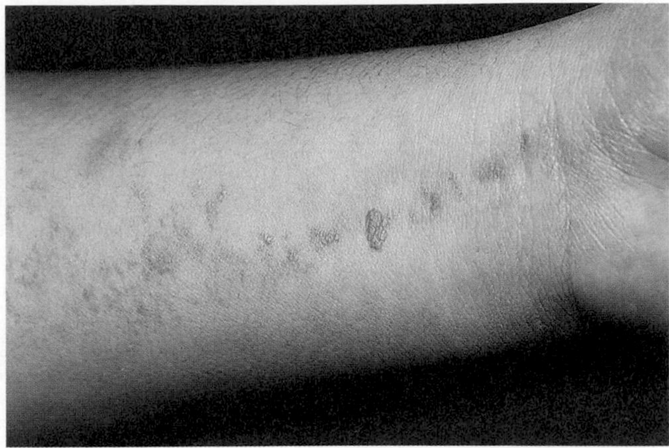

FIGURE 53-16 ■ Linear lichen planus as a result of Koebner phenomenon. (From Callen JP et al: *Color atlas of dermatology,* ed 2, Philadelphia, 2000, Saunders, p 249.)

young adults. The incidence is highest in spring and fall. It has been speculated to be viral in origin, but to date no virus has been isolated. The characteristic lesion is a macule or papule with surrounding erythema. The lesion spreads with central clearing, much like tinea corporis. This initial lesion is a solitary lesion, called the herald patch, and is usually located on the trunk or neck. As the lesion enlarges and begins to fade away (2 to 10 days), successive crops of lesions appear on the trunk and neck.[10] The extremities, face, and scalp may be involved, and mild to severe pruritis may occur. The disease is self-limiting and usually disappears within 2 to 10 weeks.[10] Treatment is palliative and includes topical steroids, antihistamines, and colloid baths. Systemic corticosteroids may be indicated in severe cases.

Acne Vulgaris

Etiology and Pathogenesis. Acne, an extremely common disease of the pilosebaceous unit, affects up to 90% of all individuals and produces unsightly lesions and sometimes permanent scarring and disfigurement[11] (Figure 53-17). Etiologically, acne involves multiple factors such as sex hormones, heredity, bacterial flora of the skin, stress, mechanical occlusion, and cosmetics use. Acne arises when sludging of sebaceous oils and deposition of loose epithelial cells cause an obstruction of the follicular canal. Continued oil production and bacterial growth in this obstructed follicle may cause rupture of the wall or sebaceous gland and result in an inflamed lesion.

Treatment. No cure for acne is known. Treatment modalities are directed to clearing the lesions and maintaining a clear complexion. Topical therapy works for most patients. Such medications are designed to cause increased peeling of the stratum corneum and loosening of the follicular plugs.

Many products are available to achieve this goal. Soaps, lotions, and gels containing sulfur, resorcinol, salicylic acid, or

A

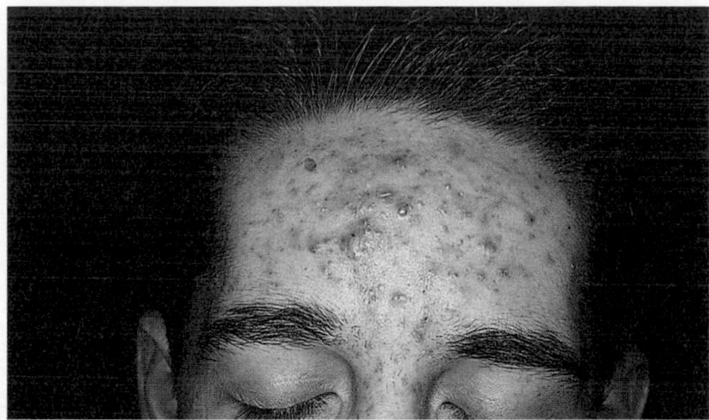

B

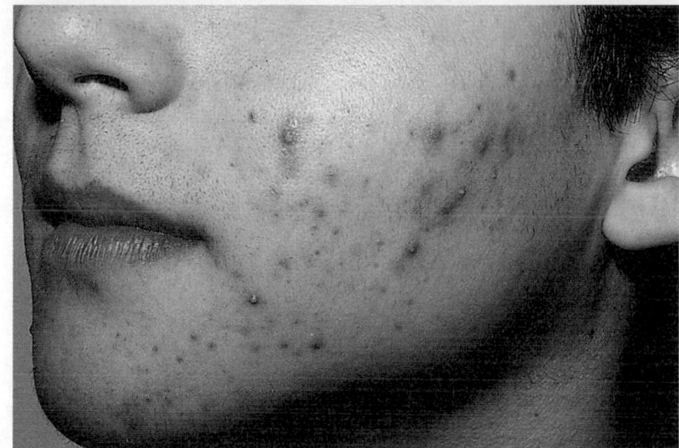

FIGURE 53-17 ■ **A** and **B,** Acne vulgaris with papules and pustules. (From Callen JP et al: *Color atlas of dermatology,* ed 2, Philadelphia, 2000, Saunders, p 151.)

benzoyl peroxide all enhance drying and peeling. Astringents, which are liquids primarily composed of alcohol with acetone, are used as solvents to remove the surface lipid and loose skin cells, as well as to enhance drying. Another effective topical preparation is retinoic acid, a derivative of vitamin A.[4] A peeling agent, it is very useful in dealing with open comedones and papules. Topical antibiotics are also available, the most effective being liquid preparations of erythromycin and clindamycin (Cleocin T) with an alcohol base.

For cases characterized by inflammatory lesions, pustules, or nodules, systemic therapy can be useful. Antibiotics, especially tetracycline and erythromycin, have long been used in such treatments. In cases that are resistant, minocycline, sulfamethoxazole-trimethoprim, and sulfones are occasionally used. Isotretinoin, a vitamin A derivative, is effective in the management of nodular and cystic acne.[12] Birth control pills, especially the estrogen-dominant type, can be of value in managing severe recalcitrant acne in females. However, androgen-dominant contraceptives can aggravate or precipitate acne.

As with any medication regimen, both systemic and topical acne treatments can produce unwanted side effects in sensitive patients. Systemic tetracycline may cause gastrointestinal upset, nausea, diarrhea, and vaginal *Monilia* overgrowth. Tetracycline should not be used in children because their unerupted teeth may be severely and permanently discolored. Topical antibiotics can cause irritant or allergic contact dermatitis.

Other useful acne treatments include corticosteroid injection into cysts and nodules and surgery, which involves extraction of the comedones and drainage of fluctuant cystic lesions.[6]

Pemphigus

A group of related disorders (**pemphigus group** of vulgaris, vegetans, foliaceus, and erythematosus) is characterized by bullous eruptions (blisters). These disorders are thought to be caused by autoimmune reactions. Patients show antibodies against keratinocytes and basement membranes. The autoantibodies perhaps cause the keratinocytes to separate from one another to form blisters. Of the group of related diseases, **pemphigus vulgaris** has the worst prognosis (Figure 53-18). Bullae can erupt on the skin and mucous membranes (e.g., esophagus), and toxemia and infection can cause death if proper treatment (cortisone) is not administered.

ALLERGIC SKIN RESPONSES

Atopic Dermatitis

Etiology and Clinical Manifestations. **Atopy,** or **allergy,** is indicated by a personal and sometimes family history of asthma, allergic rhinitis, or the most commonly seen manifestation, eczematous dermatitis (Figures 53-19 to 53-21). The highest incidence of atopic dermatitis occurs in children, with most cases developing in those younger than 5 years.[13] The characteristic features depend on the age at onset, but pruritus is always present. In infants, the disease characteristically appears on the face, scalp, or extensor surfaces of the extremities; the predominant lesion is an oozing, crusting, coalescent papule. The disease in children is most often seen as erythema, papules, and lichenification of the flexor surfaces of the extremities, especially the antecubital and popliteal areas, the wrists, and the nape of the neck. Older children and young adults have thickening of the skin, or lichenification, along with fine, dry scaling and some papules. These changes are again seen on the flexor surfaces of the extremities and the scalp, face, and upper chest. Retrospective studies show that in nearly half of all patients with childhood atopic dermatitis, the disease improves or clears with age.[14]

Treatment. Treatment of atopic dermatitis is usually carried out on an outpatient basis. The most important considerations are moisturization of the skin and prevention of continued drying and water loss. The drying and scaling that are characteristic features of atopic dermatitis impair the skin's ability not only to retain moisture but also to repel such external invaders as chemical irritants and surface bacteria. Milder cases of atopic eczema can be managed conservatively

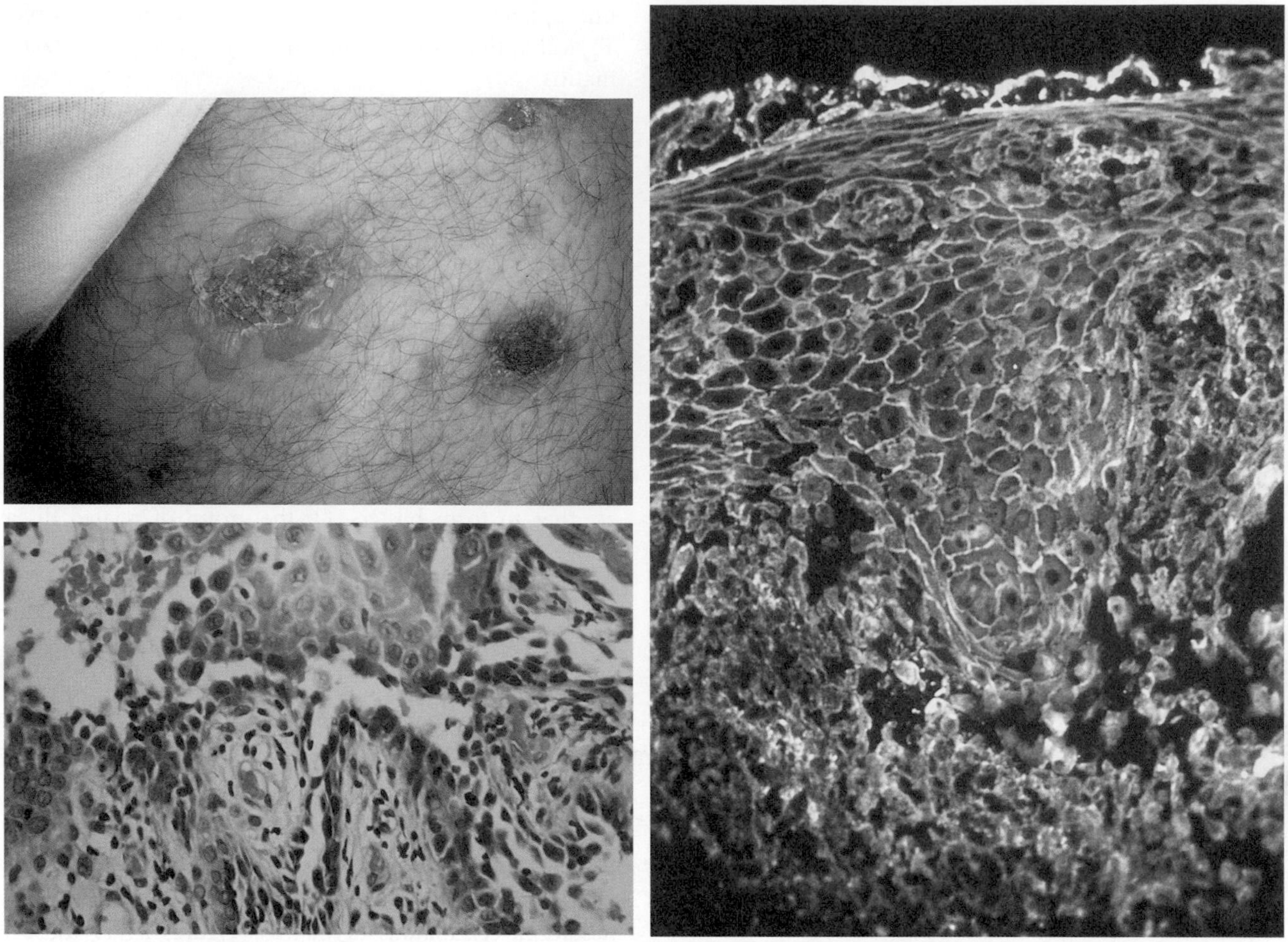

FIGURE 53-18 ■ Pemphigus vulgaris. **A,** Bullae are transient in this disorder; erosion is more characteristic. **B,** The blister is suprabasilar within the epidermis. Individual cells are unattached within the bulla (acantholytic cells). **C,** Deposition of IgG in the intercellular areas of the epidermis is characteristic of pemphigus. (From Callen JP et al: *Color atlas of dermatology,* Philadelphia, 1993, Saunders, p 163.)

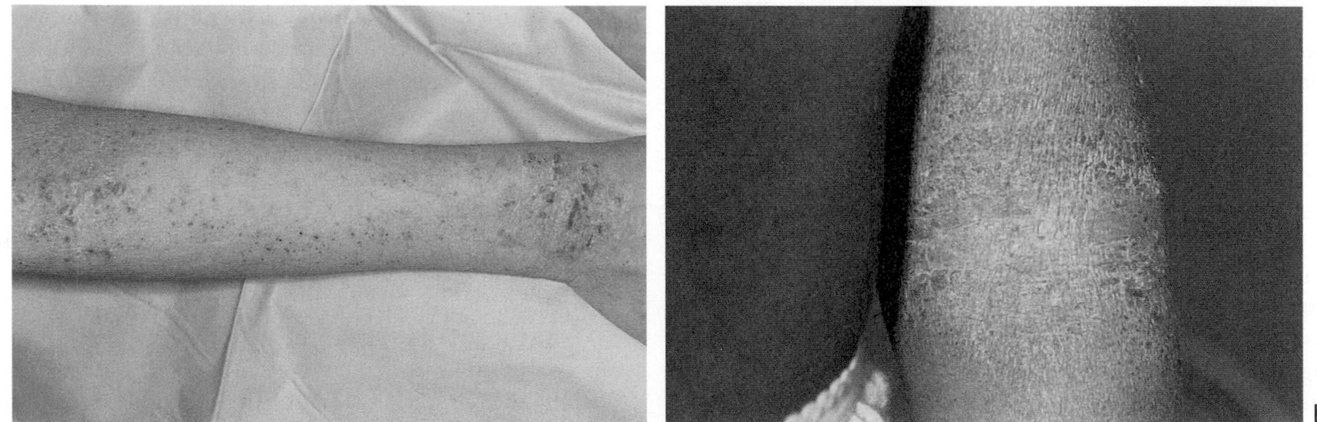

FIGURE 53-19 ■ Atopic dermatitis. An extremely pruritic condition. **A,** Multiple excoriations, vesiculation, and marked lichenification are seen in this patient. **B,** Minute excoriations with marked lichenification in the antecubital fossa. (From Callen JP et al: *Color atlas of dermatology,* Philadelphia, 1993, Saunders, p 192.)

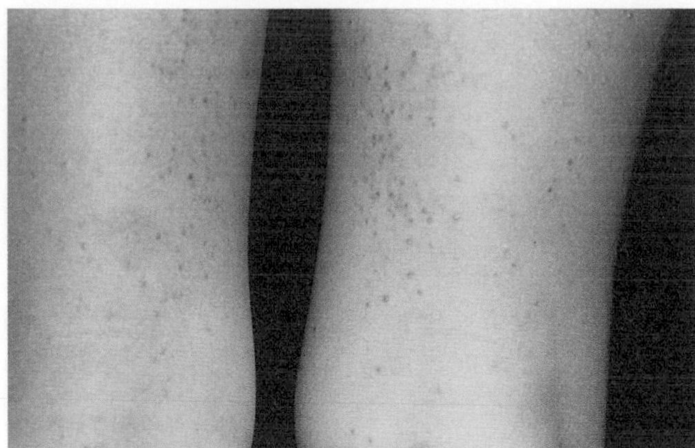

FIGURE 53-20 ■ Papular eczema. (From Callen JP et al: *Color atlas of dermatology,* Philadelphia, 1993, Saunders, p 192.)

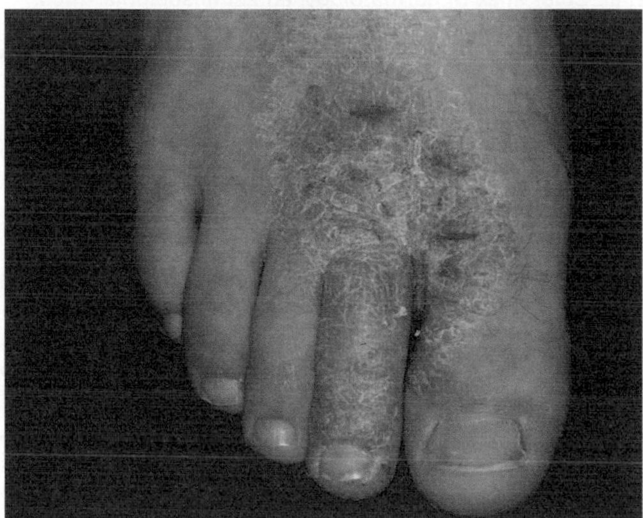

FIGURE 53-21 ■ Chronic eczema of the feet (and hands). (From Callen JP et al: *Color atlas of dermatology,* Philadelphia, 1993, Saunders, p 192.)

by decreasing the frequency of bathing, using tepid water in baths, eliminating alkaline soaps, and using moisturizing creams (especially after baths and washing). In more severe cases that involve an inflammatory response to skin breakdown, topical steroids are an important part of therapy. Short courses of systemic antibiotics such as erythromycin have also been helpful in controlling the severity of atopic eczema by reducing the concentration of cutaneous bacterial flora. Even after all these measures have been executed, some patients with severe atopic dermatitis are hospitalized for continuous wet dressings and topical steroids.

An important feature of all atopic dermatitis that must be dealt with is pruritus. The topical treatments mentioned previously are helpful in reducing itch. If additional measures are needed, systemic antihistamines (e.g., hydroxyzine and diphenhydramine) are effective.

Contact Dermatitis

Etiologies and Clinical Manifestations. **Contact dermatitis** is a cutaneous reaction to topical irritation or allergy. Irritant contact dermatitis develops in any person exposed to a sufficiently high concentration of the irritating agent. Some of the more active irritants are acids, alkalis, and hydrocarbons.

Allergic contact dermatitis indicates delayed acquired hypersensitivity to a specific allergen. Dermatologic problems may appear after years of asymptomatic exposure to the precipitating agent. Chromates, nickel, ethylenediamine, paraphenylenediamine, neomycin, formaldehyde, and lanolin components may cause allergic contact dermatitis.

Aside from reactions to various industrial chemicals, the most common type of allergic contact dermatitis reaction is to plants. **Rhus dermatitis** encompasses allergy to poison ivy, poison oak, and poison sumac. Clinically, rhus dermatitis begins within 48 hours of contact. The first symptom is pruritus, followed by erythema and vesicle formation, sometimes in linear fashion (Figure 53-22). As long as the allergen remains on the surface of the skin, it can be spread to nonexposed areas. Therefore, thorough washing can help prevent spread by hand contact. Exposure to blister fluid does not spread poison ivy lesions.

Treatment. Contact dermatitis from exposure to poison ivy can range from mild to severe. For the mildest cases, application of topical steroids or cooling shake lotions of camphor and menthol may effectively decrease discomfort. Severe cases may require hospitalization for cooling baths and wet dressings, which dry the lesions and decrease the tense, pruritic blisters. Discomfort and generalized edema often respond to systemic steroids administered over a 10- to 14-day period.

Drug Eruptions

Etiology and Clinical Manifestations. Adverse or undesirable reactions to medically administered drugs are common, yet cutaneous reactions are uncommon (0.1%) within the overall prescription-taking population.[15] Cutaneous reactions to medication usually begin within a week of drug exposure, although reactions to penicillins may occur later. Women experience more cutaneous drug eruptions than men do. The drugs that most frequently result in adverse cutaneous eruptions are ampicillin, penicillin, cephalosporins, and barbiturates. Blood transfusions also occasionally produce cutaneous reactions identical to a drug eruption.

The most common type of adverse cutaneous drug eruption is an erythematous maculopapular exanthem (rash). These often pruritic lesions are usually widely dispersed, and clearing is gradual and continues for several weeks after the drug has been discontinued. Other common drug reactions

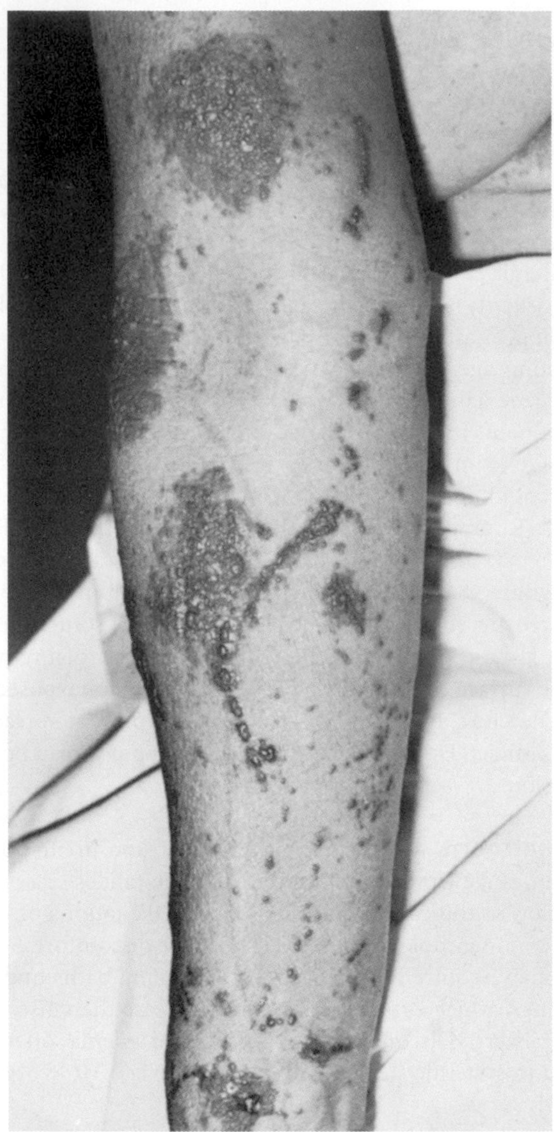

FIGURE 53-22 ■ Rhus dermatitis with the characteristic linear groups of vesicles. (From Arnold HL, Odom RB, James WD: *Andrews' diseases of the skin: clinical dermatology,* ed 8, Philadelphia, 1990, Saunders, p 95.)

include urticaria, erythema multiforme (including Stevens-Johnson syndrome), exfoliative dermatitis, photosensitivity, vasculitis, and fixed-drug eruption.

Exanthem-type eruptions can be caused by such medications as barbiturates, griseofulvin, penicillin, thiazides, and sulfonamides. Urticarial eruptions may result from the use of barbiturates, penicillin, chloramphenicol, phenolphthalein, salicylates, sulfonamides, or tetracycline. Erythema multiforme is seen with erythromycin, penicillin, phenolphthalein, salicylate, diphenylhydantoin, and thiazide. Exfoliative dermatitis can be caused by barbiturates, gold, penicillin, phenothiazides, and sulfonamides, and photosensitivity is seen with chlordiazepoxide, fluoroquinolones, griseofulvin, phenothiazines, sulfonamides, tetracycline, and thiazides. Cutaneous vasculitis may be triggered by iodines, erythromycin, penicillin, quinidine, sulfonamides, and thiazides. Fixed-drug eruption (Figure 53-23) is a round to oval, violaceous macule or slightly palpable plaque that is often recurrent, especially in previously affected sites, on reexposure to the irritating medication. This effect can be caused by barbiturates, gold, phenolphthalein, sulfonamides, and tetracycline. These drug lists are not inclusive, and several substances are known to cause multiple adverse cutaneous reactions.[16]

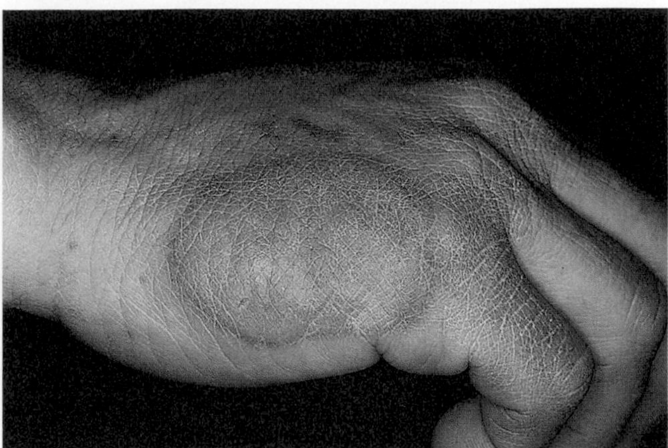

FIGURE 53-23 ■ Fixed-drug eruption. An early lesion may be manifested as an urticarial plaque. This lesion frequently resolves with macular hyperpigmentation. (From Callen JP et al: *Color atlas of dermatology,* ed 2, Philadelphia, 2000, Saunders, p 217.)

Treatment. Management of drug eruptions includes discontinuation of the offending drug and administration of oral antihistamines and antipruritic lotions of hydrocortisone, menthol, camphor, or other proven substances for relief of pruritus. For more severe eruptions, a 2- to 3-week course of systemic corticosteroids should be considered. In addition, the patient should be counseled regarding use of the offending medication and an appropriate notation placed in the patient's medical record.

Vasculitis

Etiology. When antigen and antibody react in blood vessels in the skin, severe **necrotizing inflammation (vasculitis)** can appear. This condition can be caused by drug allergies; disorders such as systemic LE, rheumatoid arthritis, and glomerulonephritis; and certain infectious diseases such as hepatitis B. **Polyarteritis nodosa** is a form of systemic vasculitis that can cause inflamed arteries in visceral organs, brain, and skin.

Treatment. Immunofluorescent studies reveal antigens and serum immunoglobulins trapped in the wall of the blood vessel that is inflamed by neutrophils. Acute vasculitis can

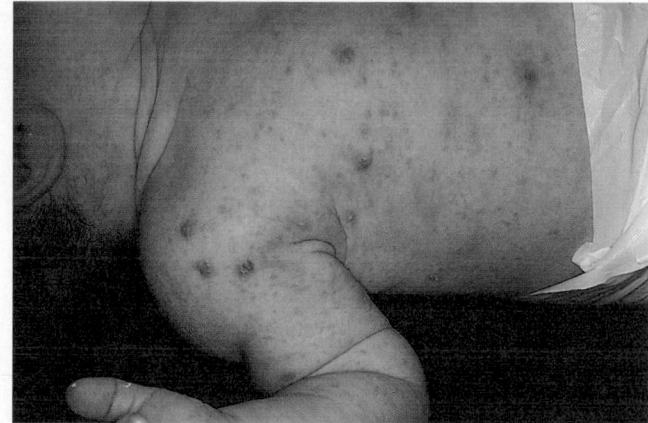

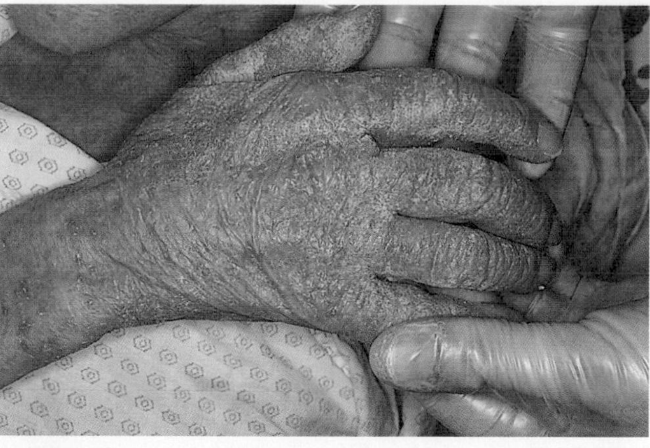

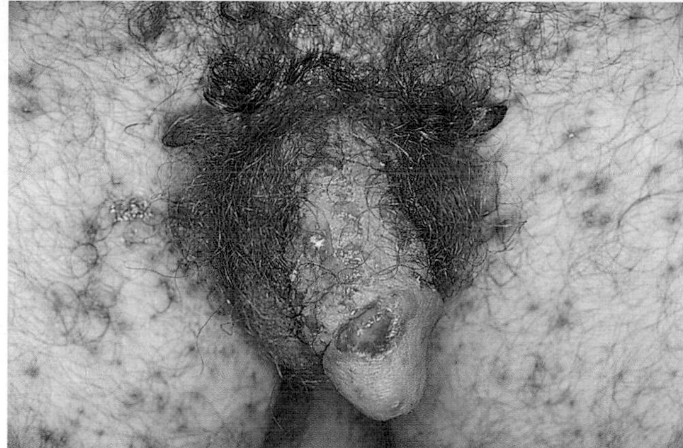

FIGURE 53-24 ■ **A,** Scabies. **B,** An extremely pruritic infestation. **C,** Crusted (Norwegian) scabies. (**A,** From Callen JP et al: *Color atlas of dermatology,* ed 2, Philadelphia, 2000, Saunders, pp 170, 283.)

cause damage not only to skin but also to the brain and visceral organs. When the vasculitis is severe, systemic corticosteroids may be administered in high doses.

PARASITIC INFESTATIONS

Scabies

Sarcoptes scabiei is a mite, and infestation with this mite in humans is called **scabies.** Scabies begins with eggs laid in the stratum corneum. These eggs hatch into larvae within 3 to 4 days and grow to adulthood within 2 months. Scabies is usually contracted after close personal contact with an infested individual.

Clinically, scabies lesions are small (1 to 4 mm) erythematous papules, some with an overlying dry scale or crust (Figure 53-24). In some cases, linear burrows are seen. Scabies mites have a predilection for the finger webs, wrists, umbilicus, and groin area. The history related by most patients is an intensely pruritic eruption that spreads over a period of weeks from a single area of the body to other areas.

Scabies treatment consists of topical permethrin cream (Elimite), γ-benzene hexachloride (Lindane), or crotamiton (Eurax). For infants, 5% to 6% precipitated sulfur in petrolatum applied twice daily for a week is usually adequate.

Fleas

Three types of flea commonly bite and cause cutaneous reactions in humans: the human flea *(Pulex irritans),* the cat flea *(Ctenocephalides felis),* and the dog flea *(Ctenocephalides canis).* Flea bites may appear as small erythematous macules, erythematous papules, wheals, or a vesicle (Figure 53-25).

Diethyltoluamide or pyrethrin insect repellents are effective in preventing flea infestation. Indoor carpeting, an ideal environment for fleas, should be treated with an appropriate insecticide.

The milder papular form of flea bites can be managed with soothing shake lotions of menthol and camphor or with topical steroids. More severe reactions (e.g., vesicles or bullae) may require a course of systemic steroids.

Lice

Phthirus pubis (crab lice), *Pediculus humanus* var. *capitis* (head lice), and *Pediculus humanus* var. *corporis* (body lice) are the types of lice most often found on human beings. They are surface dwelling, unlike the burrowing scabies mite, and they usually can be seen without magnification. Control and eradication are possible with one of the following: permethrin

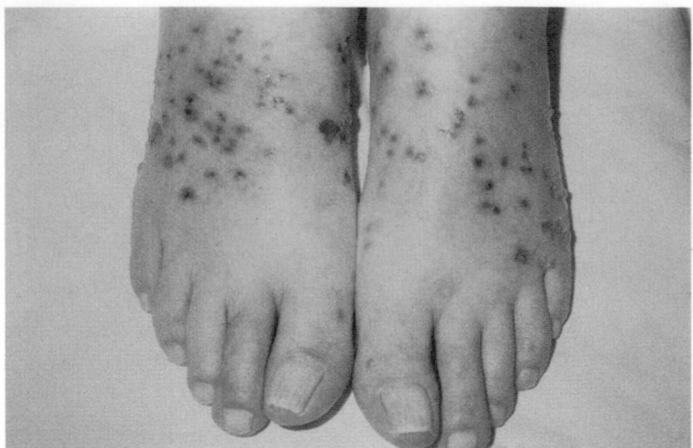

FIGURE 53-25 ■ Insect bites (fleas) led this patient to scratch. (From Swartz MH: *Physical diagnosis, history and examination,* ed 4, Philadelphia, 2002, Saunders, p 163.)

cream rinse or pyrethrin and piperonyl butoxide liquid, gel, or shampoo.

Chiggers

Chiggers are mites that reside in grass and bushes. They are common in the southern United States but can be found as far north as Canada. Puncture of the skin by the mite to obtain nourishment produces pruritic papules commonly seen wherever it encounters resistance, such as the top of socks, at the belt line, or around the neckband area (Figure 53-26). Secondary lesions are excoriations from scratching that have become infected by bacteria. Treatment is palliative, and the use of insect repellent is encouraged for prevention.

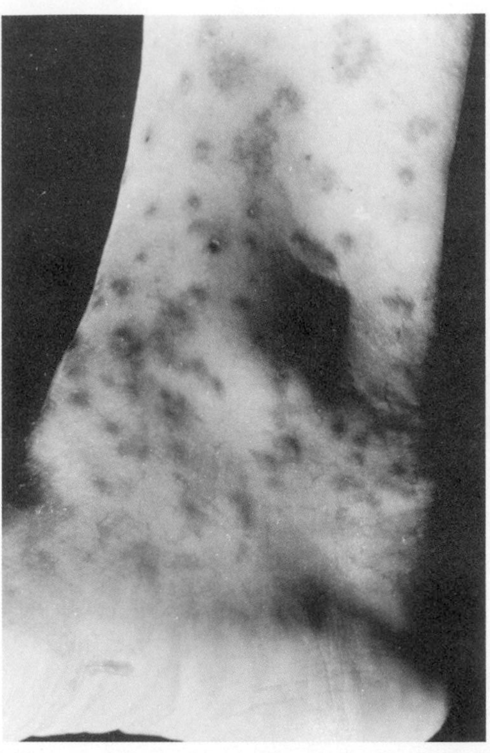

FIGURE 53-26 ■ Chigger bites. (From Arnold HL, Odom RB, James WD: *Andrews' diseases of the skin: clinical dermatology,* ed 8, Philadelphia, 1990, Saunders, p 529.)

Bedbugs

The common bedbug, *Cimex lectularius,* is a reddish brown insect 3 to 6 mm long that turns purple after feeding. Like most parasites, bedbugs feed on human blood. Importantly, they can also alternate between human and animal hosts, and they live up to and sometimes beyond 1 year.[8] When not feeding, bedbugs stay hidden in the cracks and crevices of furniture, mattresses, wallpaper, picture frames, baseboards, flooring, door locks, or any darkened area. Unless their source is eliminated, recurrence is inevitable. Professional extermination is advised because of their many hiding places. Bedbugs have been known to feed on animal populations when forced from their living quarters. On rehabitation in the same quarters, the bedbug can easily return to human hosts.

They are nocturnal feeders, and, when crushed, they emit a foul odor. The bedbug bite is painless and produces a pruritic oval or oblong wheal with a small hemorrhagic punctum at the center. Bullous lesions are not uncommon. Usually, lesions are multiple and arranged in rows or clusters on the face, neck, hands, and arms. No area is exempt. The wheal is probably a type 1 sensitivity reaction to the anticoagulant saliva of the bedbug. Secondary excoriation and bacterial infections may occur.

The diagnosis depends on the time of the day when the lesions appear. Because of the painless bite, it is not uncommon for the victim to awake with one or several pruritic papules. Topical antipruritics are used as treatment.

Mosquitoes

Most people have experienced mosquitoes and are familiar with their bites. The typical lesion is a raised wheal on an erythematous base, accompanied by pruritus within 45 minutes of the bite. A second type of reaction is the delayed response. Eight to 12 hours after the bite, the lesion becomes raised, erythematous, and indurated, with extensive pruritus or pain. This reaction peaks 24 hours to 72 hours after the bite.[9] The saliva of the mosquito is believed to be the source of the skin reaction. Although severe skin reactions are possible, they are rare. Insect repellents are recommended for prevention; local antipruritics are used for treatment.

Blood Flukes

Bathers in the freshwater lakes of Wisconsin, Michigan, and Minnesota are prone to periodic attacks of inflammatory, papular, urticarial, and vesicular eruptions on the uncovered areas of the body, mainly the legs. This pruritic eruption, commonly called "swimmer's itch," usually subsides within a week and is caused by invasion of the skin by cercariae (larvae) of the schistosomes (worms) of ducks and mammals. The life cycle of these various species of schistosomes includes the snail as an intermediate host. On invasion of the abnormal definitive host, the human skin, the cercariae die, and the resulting skin eruption is the skin's reaction in ridding itself of the foreign bodies. Repeated attacks are met with stronger resistance, and the dermatitis becomes increasingly severe. Secondary infection, edema, and lymphangitis can occur.

Swimmer's itch is best prevented by destruction of the snails through careful addition of a combination of copper sulfate and hydrated lime to the lake water. Rapid drying of the swimmer with a towel apparently prevents penetration of the cercariae. Active therapy is directed to relief of the itching and prevention of secondary infection.

Ticks

Ticks are insects that live in woods and underbrush. They attach to human and animal hosts and burrow in the epidermis, where they feed on blood. The tick bite itself is not problematic, but the infectious bacteria or viruses that ticks carry to human hosts create problems. Many tick-borne illnesses are known, including Central European encephalitis, Q fever, babesiasis, relapsing fever, Rocky Mountain spotted fever (RMSF), and Lyme disease. Both RMSF and Lyme disease are relatively common in the United States.

Rocky Mountain Spotted Fever

Etiology, Pathogenesis, Clinical Manifestations. **Rocky Mountain spotted fever** is caused by a tick that carries *Rickettsia rickettsii.* In the past RMSF was localized to the Rocky Mountain area, but by 1982 most states had reported a case of RMSF.[8]

The initial tick bite appears as a papule or macule, with or without a central punctate area. The tick burrows in and enlarges as it feeds. The tick must be attached to the human host for 4 to 6 hours before the rickettsiae are activated by the blood.[8] Rickettsiae are found in the tick feces and body parts. The rickettsiae then enter the blood stream and multiply in body tissues. Within 4 to 8 days the patient experiences fever, headache, muscle aches, nausea, and vomiting.[8] A rash then appears on the wrist or ankle. The characteristic rash is a macular or maculopapular one that spreads to the rest of the body. Other symptoms include generalized edema, conjunctivitis, petechial lesions, photophobia, lethargy, confusion, and cranial nerve deficits.

Treatment. Treatment for RMSF requires hospitalization and antibiotic therapy. The most important measure is to prevent tick bites by using insect repellents while engaged in activities in the woods. Once a tick has attached itself, it is important to remove all the body parts to limit the possibility of infection. One can remove ticks by dousing them with mineral oil or alcohol before slowly pulling them out with tweezers. The practice of applying a hot match to the end of the tick is not an effective method for removal because the tick may regurgitate into the open wound.[8]

Lyme Disease

Etiology. **Lyme disease** is caused by the bite of a tick that carries the spirochete *Borrelia burgdorferi.* White-tailed deer and white-footed mice are the main reservoirs of this disease-causing spirochete. Lyme disease causes multiple symptoms affecting the skin, nervous system, heart, and musculoskeletal system.

Pathogenesis, Clinical Manifestations, and Treatment. The disease has three clinical stages. Stage I usually occurs in the summer and early fall with single or multiple erythematous papules that may itch, sting, or burn. The thighs, groin, and axillae are particularly common sites of involvement. This disease is often accompanied by flulike symptoms (fatigue, headache, chills, fever, sore throat, stiff neck, nausea, myalgias, and arthralgias). If the patient remains untreated, stage II Lyme disease appears weeks to months later. This stage is characterized by meningitis, cranial nerve palsies, and peripheral neuropathy; occasionally, cardiac involvement is noted. In stage III, oligoarticular arthritis occurs. In early Lyme disease, treatment includes antibiotic therapy such as doxycycline, amoxicillin, or erythromycin for 10 to 21 days. Neurologic disease, arthritis, or cardiac disease is managed with doxycycline or amoxicillin for 1 month or with intravenous penicillin for 10 to 14 days.

OTHER DISORDERS OF THE DERMIS

Scleroderma

Scleroderma is characterized by massive collagen deposition with fibrosis accompanied by inflammatory reactions and vascular changes in the capillary network. The process by which these changes occur is not known but may represent an autoimmune mechanism or primary vasculopathy.

The two forms of scleroderma, localized and diffuse, are clinically dissimilar except for some common skin histopathologic features. Localized scleroderma (morphea) is a benign disease; diffuse scleroderma (progressive systemic sclerosis) is serious, progressive, and fatal.

Localized Scleroderma. Localized scleroderma has an unknown etiology, no systemic involvement, and no known treatment. Disability is confined to the area involved. Lesions tend to involute (shrivel) slowly and spontaneously. Relapses are rare. Primary skin lesions are single or multiple, violet colored, firm, inelastic macules and plaques that enlarge slowly. The progressing border retains a violet hue while the center becomes whitish and slightly depressed beneath the skin surface. Bizarre lesions occur, such as long linear bands on extremities, "saber cut" lesions in scalp, or lesions involving one side of the face or the body. Secondary lesions include mild or severe scarring after healing, permanent hair loss from the scalp lesions, and, rarely, ulceration. The trunk, extremities, and head are most frequently involved (Figure 53-27).

Diffuse Scleroderma. Diffuse scleroderma is a rare systemic collagen disease of unknown cause characterized by a long course of progressive disability resulting from lack of mobility of the areas and the organs affected. The skin becomes hardened like hide, the esophagus and the gastrointestinal tract semirigid, the lungs and the heart fibrosed, the bones resorbed, and the overlying tissue calcified. Figure 53-28 illustrates the "hidelike" skin on the face of a woman with diffuse scleroderma.

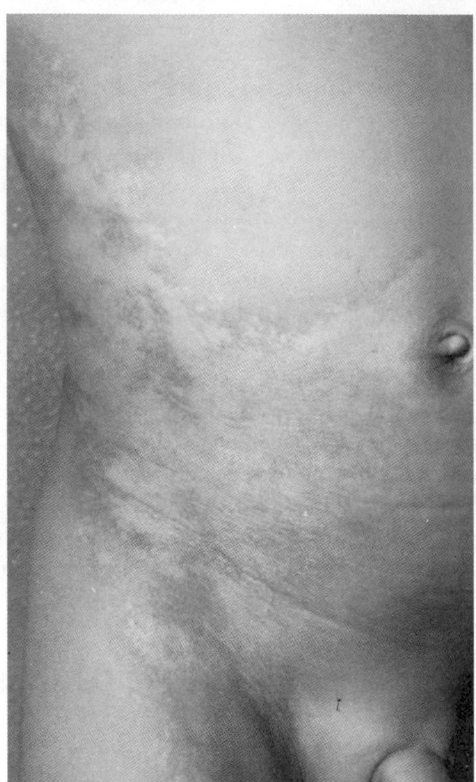

FIGURE 53-27 ■ Extensive morphea (localized scleroderma). (From Arnold HL, Odom RB, James WD: *Andrews' diseases of the skin: clinical dermatology,* ed 8, Philadelphia, 1990, Saunders, p 177.)

Another rare collagen disorder, **dermatomyositis,** is characterized by the acute or insidious onset of muscle pain, weakness, fever, arthralgia, and, in some cases, a puffy erythematous eruption that is usually confined to the face and the eyelids. Progression of the disease results in muscle atrophy and contractures, skin telangiectasias (vascular lesions formed by blood vessel dilation) and atrophy, and generalized organ involvement. Death occurs in 50% of cases.[12,17]

Sunburn and Photosensitivity

Effects of Sunlight

Sunlight is an extremely harmful environmental agent because it produces the short ultraviolet wavelength that is responsible for sunburn, thickening of the stratum corneum, suntan, and increased melanin production. Sunlight produces direct local effects on the skin in the form of elastotic syndromes, keratoacanthomas, premalignant diseases, basal cell epitheliomas, and squamous cell epitheliomas. Both indirect and direct effects can produce malignant melanomas.[18]

Sunburn is initially manifested as erythema, pain, heat, and occasionally blistering, edema, and tenderness. In severe sunburn, these symptoms may also be accompanied by the constitutional symptoms of chills, fever, nausea, and generalized discomfort.

The most effective treatment is to avoid or limit exposure to sunlight. Wearing protective clothing is effective; sunscreens are also quite useful in preventing sunburn and the chronic solar changes of the skin. Para-aminobenzoic acid is the most widely used sunscreen. People sensitive to para-aminobenzoic acid may use cinnamates and benzophenones as substitutes. Opaque screens such as zinc oxide and titanium dioxide also work well. However, these white preparations are not cosmetically elegant. Recently, titanium dioxide has been incorporated into foundation makeup for women.

Sunburn can be managed symptomatically with cold water baths or compresses; topical steroids are often effective in re-

FIGURE 53-28 ■ Hidelike skin on the face of a woman with diffuse scleroderma (progressive systemic sclerosis). (From Arnold HL, Odom RB, James WD: *Andrews' diseases of the skin: clinical dermatology,* ed 8, Philadelphia, 1990, Saunders, p 176.)

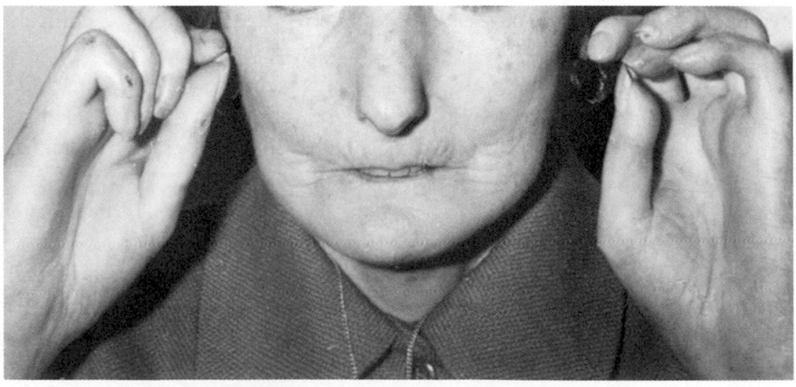

lieving the discomfort of localized severe burns. For widespread sunburn, a 10- to 14-day course of systemic steroids may suppress the symptoms.

Ulcers

An unfortunate problem for a bedridden person may be the development of **pressure sores,** or **decubitus ulcers.** Because thinning epithelial cells and blood vessels have a slower rate of repair, the incidence of decubitus ulcers is higher and the ulcer more severe in the elderly, and healing of damaged skin is slower.

Pressure sores are localized areas of cellular necrosis resulting from prolonged pressure between any bony prominence and an external object such as a bed or wheelchair. The tissues are deprived of blood supply and eventually die. Areas frequently affected in older persons include the heels, greater trochanter, sacrum, dorsal (especially in thin kyphotic persons) and scapular regions of the spine, and elbows. Long-term pressure increases vulnerability to decubitus ulcer development. High pressure maintained for a short time is less dangerous than low pressure continued for a long time. Predisposing factors include poor nutrition, aging, immobility, superficial sensory loss, and disturbed autonomic function (loss of bowel and bladder control).[19] Older people with dementia are particularly prone to the development of pressure sores because of arteriosclerotic changes in the vessels, loss of subcutaneous tissue and tissue elasticity, and clouding of the sensorium.[19]

Pressure sores can be evaluated clinically using the staging system described in Table 53-5. Pressure sores are superficial (benign) or deep (malignant). Superficial sores are reddened areas involving only the outer skin layers. They are less dangerous than deep sores and are caused by friction, shearing stresses, trauma, infection, and saturation with urine or other wet agents. The lesions are frequently painful but are easily treated and prevented. Treatment consists of keeping the area clean, dry, and free from infection or further pressure; a covering with a nonstick dressing also promotes healing. Measures such as frequent turning (every 2 hours), getting the person out of bed and into a chair, keeping the vulnerable areas clean and dry, and keeping the weight of the bed coverings off the feet are most effective in warding off superficial pressure sores.

Deep sores develop quickly as a result of thrombosis of the vessels in deep tissue overlying bony prominences. Muscle and fat layers are more vulnerable than the dermis, and involvement of these layers causes deep, large ulcers. The sore begins as a reddening of the skin with unobservable necrosis in the deep underlying tissue. In 1 to 2 days the lesion bursts through the skin like an abscess to reveal a deep cavity full of black or infected slough, which may go through to the bone.[19] Skin loss from such a large area results in extensive scarring. The appearance of deep pressure sores with an illness can delay recovery and may even be fatal.

Prevention is more difficult with deep pressure sores, especially in the elderly. The risk of these lesions developing is greatest during the 10 days after the onset of illness or admission to the hospital, which coincides with the period of greatest immobility.[19] A deep sore that develops early and penetrates deeply is most dangerous to an older person. Early signs of deterioration include apathy, loss of appetite, and

Table 53-5

Clinical Description of Decubitus Ulcers

Grade/Stage	Description
1	Acute inflammatory response primarily in the epidermis with minimal soft tissue swelling and warmth; erythema of intact skin; it is erythematous and, unless abraded, the erythema will blanch; blanchable erythema (reactive hyperemia) can be expected to be present for 30-45 minutes following exposure to pressure; it is usually very discretely bordered; the heralding lesion of skin ulceration, but reversible with intervention
2	Pressure sore representing an inflammatory and fibroblastic response extending through the epidermis into the dermis; there is partial thickness or superficial skin loss involving the epidermis and/or the dermis; it may present as blistering with erythema and/or induration; the ulcer may also present as an abrasion of shallow crater; the wound base is moist and pink; the wound is painful but free of necrotic tissue
3	Pressure sore clearly penetrating the subcutaneous layers; often there is exposed muscle, fat, and tendons; the full-thickness tissue loss extends through the dermis to involve the subcutaneous tissue; damage or necrosis of dermis may extend down to, but not through, underlying fascia; the ulcer presents clinically as a deep crater with or without undermining of adjacent tissue; this stage may also include sinus tract formation, exudates, and/or infection; the wound base is usually painful
4	Pressure sore extending beyond the deep fascia, almost always to the bone; deep tissue destruction occurs, extending through the subcutaneous tissue and fascia; there is full-thickness skin loss with extensive tissue necrosis and damage to muscle, bone, and supporting structures (tendons and joint capsules); undermining sinus infection may be present; the wound base is usually not painful

Box 53-1

Prevention of Deep Pressure Sores

1. Change position every 2 hours.
2. Do not oversedate or undersedate.
3. Avoid or correct malnutrition.
4. Avoid dehydration; maintain blood pressure and cardiac output.
5. Use an alternating-pressure airbed or waterbed.

Data from Rosen T, Lanning MB, Hill MJ, editors: *Nurse's atlas of dermatology,* Boston, 1983, Little, Brown.

incontinence. Some measures that can help prevent deep pressure sores are described in Box 53-1.

Treatment consists primarily of reinforcing preventive measures, including maintenance of fluid and protein stores that are lost through serous and purulent discharge, repair of tissues by giving vitamin supplements, avoidance of general infections such as pneumonia or cystitis, and remediation of anemia. The lesions should be cleaned and dressed, with care taken to manage local infection. To promote granulation and healing, the wound should be irrigated with warm saline every day. Irrigation washes out the debris, reduces the growth of anaerobes, promotes separation of the slough, and decreases the pocketing of infection in deeper tissues. Infection must be eradicated and the slough must separate before healing can take place.

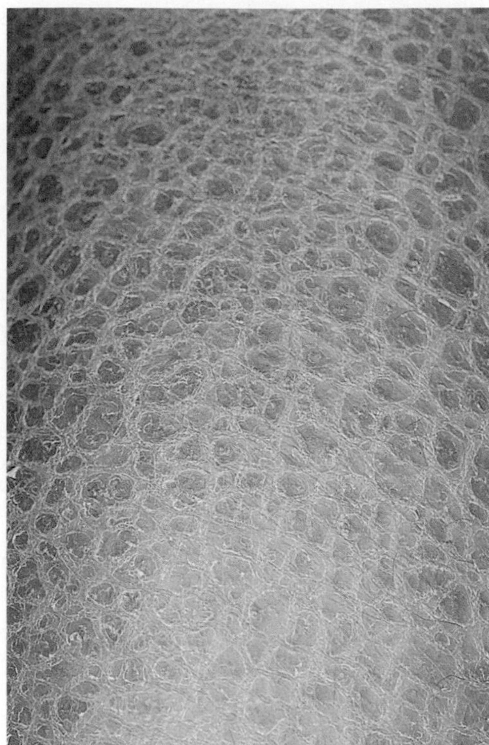

FIGURE 53-29 ■ Ichthyosis. (From Callen JP et al: *Color atlas of dermatology,* ed 2, Philadelphia, 2000, Saunders, p 14. Courtesy Donald Hazelrigg, MD, Evansville, Ind.)

Altered Cell Growth

Epidermal Proliferation

Keratinocytes produce keratin. Rare, inherited defects in keratinocytes can occur, and the inherited disease **congenital ichthyosis** is characterized by an excessive growth of keratinocytes and keratin, which gives the skin a fish scale appearance (Figure 53-29).

Corns and **calluses** result from **hyperkeratosis.** Stimulation of the epidermis by intermittent pressure elicits hyperkeratosis (corn and callus formation). By contrast, *atrophy* of the epidermis can arise from a decreased blood supply.

Benign or malignant **neoplasms** commonly arise from keratinocytes. **Warts** (verrucae), for instance, are caused by a virus that provokes a benign proliferation of keratinocytes. **Squamous cell carcinomas** (arising from keratinocytes) often occur in areas of skin excessively exposed to sunlight.

Tumors

Each cell type of the skin can give rise to either benign or malignant tumors. Benign tumors, including squamous papillomas, arise from keratinocytes, common moles (**nevi**) arise from melanocytes, lipomas from adipose cells, vascular tumors (hemangiomas) from blood vessels, dermatofibromas from fibroblasts, and neuromas from nerves.

Kaposi sarcoma arises from reticulocytes and is multifocal, metastasizing, and malignant. Kaposi sarcoma is classified as an opportunistic neoplasm because it occurs in persons with preexisting immunodeficiency: for example, in persons with primary immunodeficiency, in those who undergo therapeutic immunosuppression, and in persons with human immunodeficiency virus (HIV) infection. Figures 53-30 and 53-31 show some of the cutaneous diseases associated with HIV infection.

Cancer

Cancer of the skin is common. Most skin cancers are slowly progressive, but certain types can be rapidly lethal. Excessive exposure to sunlight by a person with fair skin often leads to skin cancer. In addition to sunlight, exposure to irritating chemicals, recurrent trauma, and irradiation are associated with a high risk of skin cancer.

Basal cell carcinomas are the most common skin tumors and the most benign[20] (Figure 53-32). Squamous cell carcinomas are the next most common malignancy[20] (Figure 53-33). They can occasionally metastasize. By contrast, melanoma is rare but can be highly malignant (Figure 53-34). Melanoma is notoriously unpredictable; however, the prognosis is based on size, depth of invasion of the tumor, and the presence of metastasis.[21] Lumps that increase rapidly in size, change color, ulcerate, or bleed should undergo biopsy and be examined microscopically to rule out malignancy. Complete surgical excision is the treatment of choice for skin cancers.

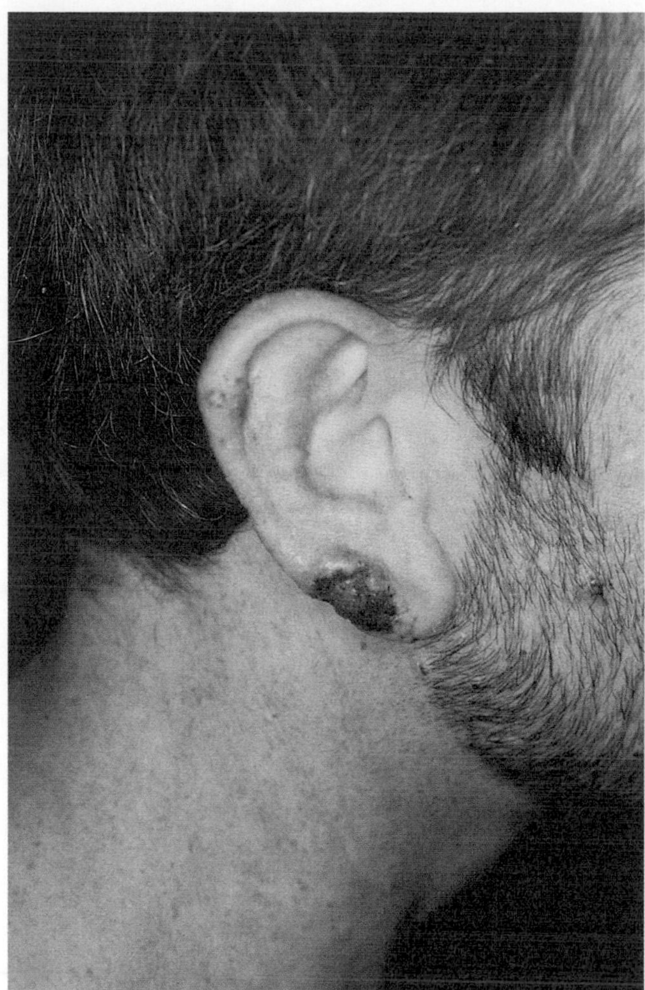

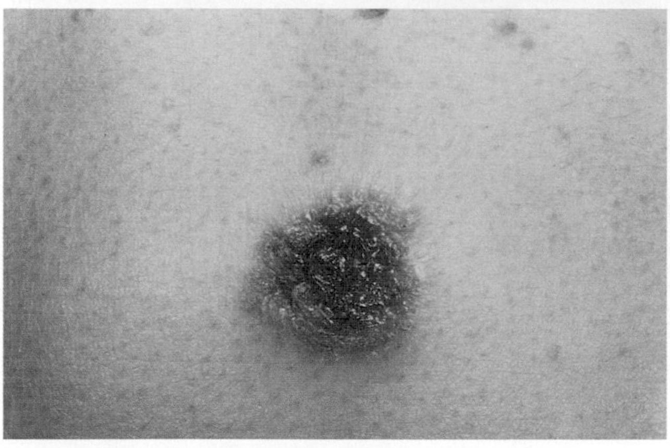

FIGURE 53-30 ■ Cryptococcosis associated with HIV infection. (From Callen JP et al: *Color atlas of dermatology,* Philadelphia, 1993, Saunders, p 229.)

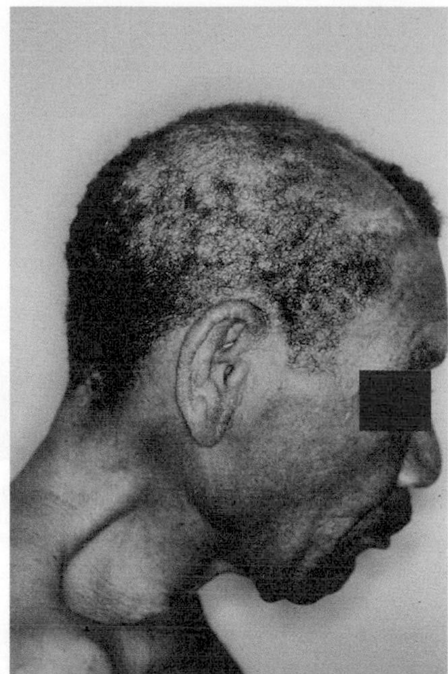

FIGURE 53-31 ■ Seborrheic dermatitis associated with HIV infection. (From Callen JP et al: *Color atlas of dermatology,* Philadelphia, 1993, Saunders, p 372.)

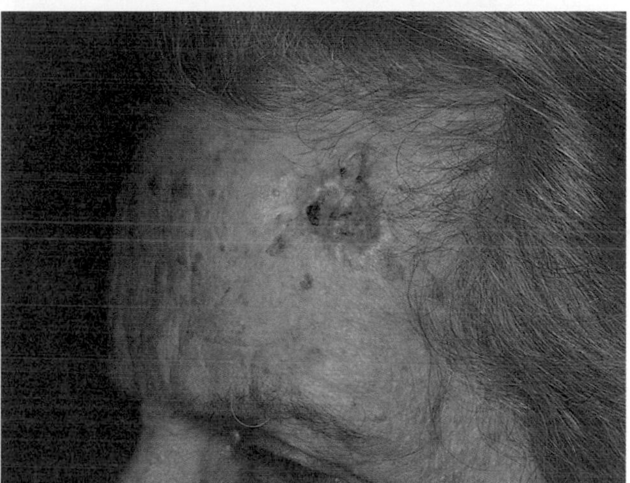

FIGURE 53-32 ■ Basal cell carcinoma. Notice the rolled, well-defined margin. (From Swartz MH: *Physical diagnosis, history and examination,* ed 4, Philadelphia, 2002, Saunders, p 144.)

Pigmentation Alterations

Vitiligo

Vitiligo (leukoderma) is a condition in which pigment disappears from a patch of skin. The onset is sudden and may be associated with pernicious anemia, hyperthyroidism, and diabetes mellitus.

Vitiligo is a concern to darkly pigmented people of all races. It also affects light-skinned persons, but not as often. The lesion is a depigmented patch with definite borders on the face, axillae, neck, or extremities (Figure 53-35). The borders are smooth. Size varies from small to large macules involving large areas of the skin surface. The large macular type is much more common. Depigmented areas, which burn in sunlight, appear bone colored or grayish blue.

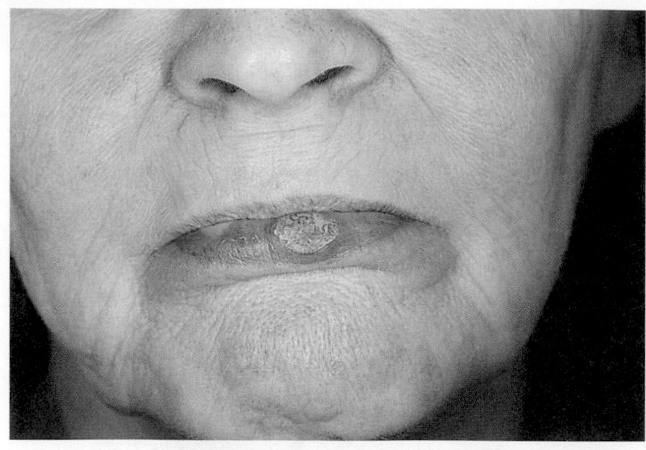

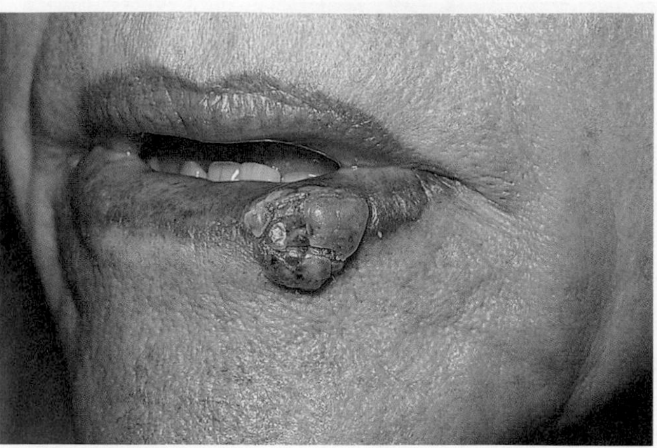

FIGURE 53-33 ■ **A** and **B,** Squamous cell carcinomas. (From Callen JP et al: *Color atlas of dermatology,* ed 2, Philadelphia, 2000, Saunders, p 367.)

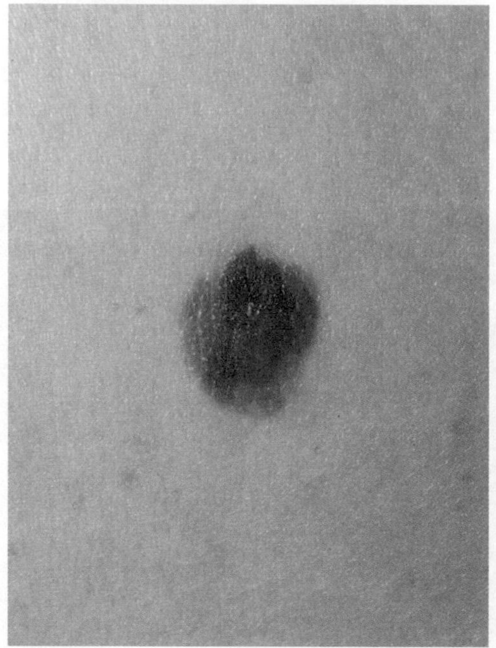

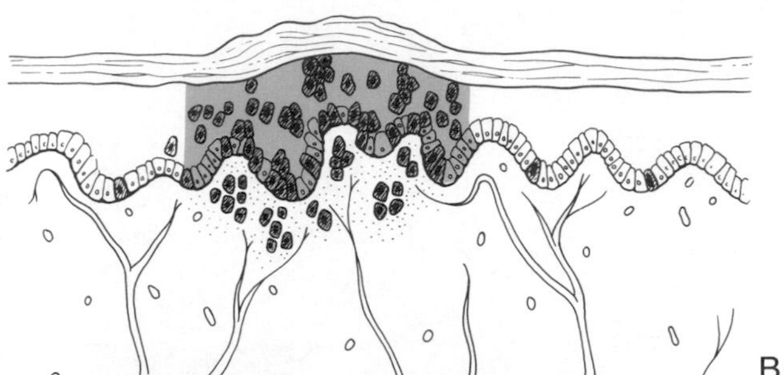

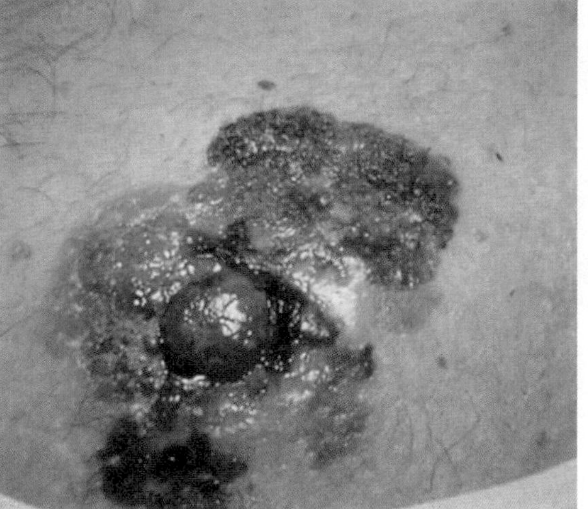

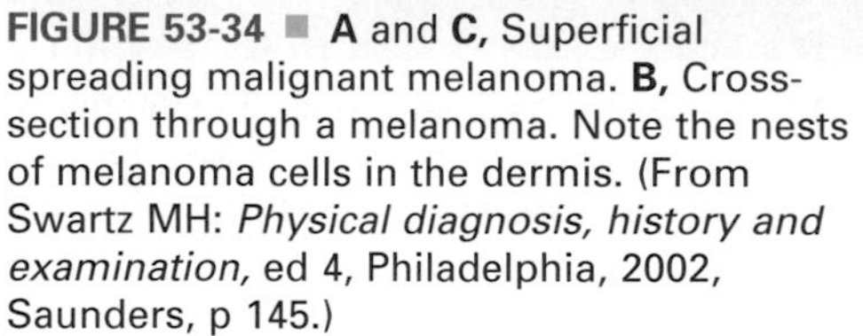

FIGURE 53-34 ■ **A** and **C,** Superficial spreading malignant melanoma. **B,** Cross-section through a melanoma. Note the nests of melanoma cells in the dermis. (From Swartz MH: *Physical diagnosis, history and examination,* ed 4, Philadelphia, 2002, Saunders, p 145.)

Vitiligo appears at any age, in men and women alike, and usually occurs before the age of 21.[22] Its incidence has been increasing in India, Pakistan, and Far Eastern countries.[22] Although the cause is unknown, inheritance and autoimmune factors have been implicated. Affected areas spread over time.

Treatment is experimental and consists of psoralen administration in conjunction with ultraviolet radiation. Cosmetics such as Derma Blend may be used to camouflage the areas of depigmentation.

Albinism

Etiology and Pathogenesis. Melanocytes produce melanin. A partial or total absence of melanin arises as an inborn error in metabolism in persons with **albinism.** Albinism,

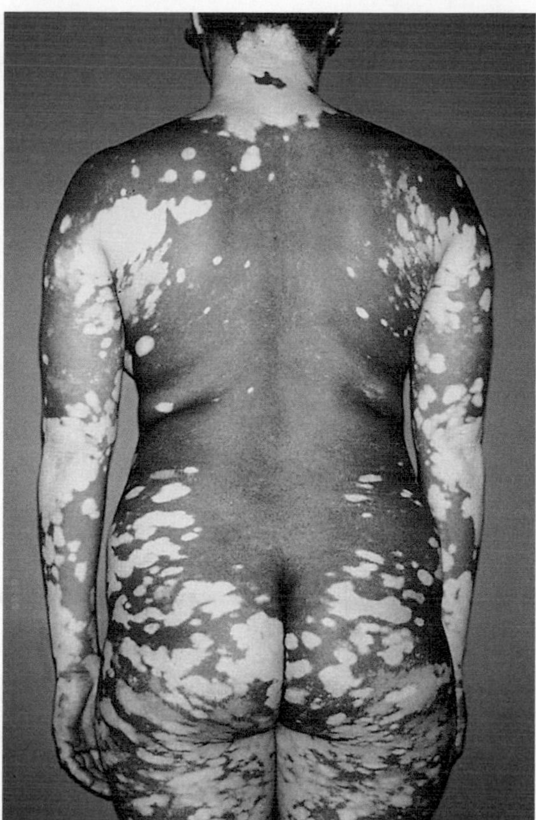

FIGURE 53-35 ■ Vitiligo. (From Callen JP et al: *Color atlas of dermatology,* ed 2, Philadelphia, 2000, Saunders, p 282.)

also termed oculocutaneous albinism, is characterized by a generalized lack of pigmentation of the skin and the hair. In addition, the eyes may show nystagmus and a lack of pigmentation of the fundi and translucent irises. The condition is recessively inherited. Biochemically, albinism occurs because of impaired or absent melanin synthesis. The long-term consequences of albinism may include solar keratoses and basal and squamous cell cancers.

Education regarding the use of sunscreens and clothing for protection against ultraviolet light–induced damage is indicated. Sunglasses and magnifiers are beneficial for the ocular symptoms.

KEY CONCEPTS

- Skin infections may be caused by viral, fungal, or bacterial organisms.
- Viruses are associated with warts (human papillomavirus), cold sores (herpes simplex), and shingles (herpes zoster). Warts are painless. They may be surgically removed but often resolve spontaneously. Herpes simplex lesions are painful, may be managed symptomatically, and often recur in times of stress. Herpes zoster inhabits sensory dorsal ganglia neurons and causes pain along a dermatome.
- Superficial fungal infections (tinea, ringworm) are often characterized by central clearing and peripheral scaling. They may be effectively managed with topical antifungals. Yeast infections tend to occur in moist areas such as mucous membranes and are managed with systemic or topical drugs.
- Impetigo is caused by staphylococcal or streptococcal infection and is characterized by yellowish pustules and crusts. It responds to antibiotic therapy.
- The cause of noninfectious inflammatory diseases is usually unknown. Lupus erythematosus, seborrheic dermatitis, psoriasis, lichen planus, pityriasis rosea, and acne are in this category. Treatment is aimed at reducing inflammation rather than cure. Antibiotics may be used to prevent or manage lesion superinfections.
- Skin allergies are associated with substances that cause erythema and itching. Atopic dermatitis (eczema), commonly seen in young children, may be aggravated by substances to which the individual is allergic. Contact dermatitis occurs in anyone coming in contact with a certain substance. Drug reactions are allergic responses manifested as widely dispersed, often pruritic rashes. Antigen-antibody reactions within cutaneous blood vessels can result in severe necrotizing vasculitis.
- The skin is subject to invasion by a number of different bugs, ticks, and parasites. Lesions tend to be singular or grouped and in areas exposed to the particular pest. Scabies commonly occurs on the hands and wrists and may appear as linear burrows. Bites from fleas, mites, bedbugs, and mosquitoes often induce pruritic macules or papules. Tick bites are usually painless but may be problematic because ticks may carry diseases such as RMSF and Lyme disease.
- Scleroderma is a collagen disease of unknown cause. It may be localized to the skin or produce systemic involvement. The skin is discolored, thick, and hardened.
- Ultraviolet rays in sunlight are associated with acute damage to the skin (sunburn) and also increase the long-term risk of skin cancer.
- Pressure ulcer is a significant problem of immobility caused by prolonged pressure on bony prominences. Superficial sores are reddened areas involving the outer skin layers. Deep sores are due to thrombosis of vessels deep in tissue. Deep sores may be unnoticed initially and then burst through the skin like an abscess.
- Abnormalities of skin cell growth may result in such benign processes as corns and calluses or the more serious consequence of cancer. Basal cell and squamous cell carcinomas are slowly progressive and generally amenable to surgical excision. Malignant melanoma is more prone to metastasis and carries a poorer prognosis.

◆ Abnormal pigmentation may occur in response to skin injury, infection, or inflammation or may be genetically determined. Albinism is due to lack of melanin production. Vitiligo is a depigmented patch of skin that is most noticeable in dark-skinned persons. The cause of vitiligo is unknown.

SPECIAL CHARACTERISTICS OF DARK SKIN

A number of disorders of the skin exclusively affect people with dark skin. Pigmentary disturbances from many causes, both hypopigmentation and hyperpigmentation, are common. Postinflammatory hyperpigmentation, for example, may occur in African-American individuals when melanocytes are stimulated by inflammation. Hyperpigmentation in any person with dark skin can occur after traumatic injury, skin infection, or inflammatory skin disease. Patchy areas of depigmentation (vitiligo), described earlier, are more noticeable in persons with dark skin because of the color contrast. Some lesions, such as those causing erythema, may show no visible color change in darkly pigmented individuals. For example, petechiae, which cause pinpoint purplish red lesions, are usually observable only on the oral mucosa or conjunctiva.

Disorders such as seborrheic dermatitis and keloids are seen with greater frequency in African-Americans.[23] The custom of tightly plaiting the hair or using hot oil and tension on the scalp leads to gradual damage to hair follicles, hair thinning, and, eventually, hair loss. Known as **traumatic alopecia,** this condition is also seen with greater frequency in African-Americans (Figures 53-36 and 53-37).

Conversely, many skin disorders that affect light-skinned people, such as squamous cell or basal cell carcinoma, senile keratoses, and psoriasis, only rarely affect darker skinned persons.

Psoriasis is rare among the African-American population. If present, it may be difficult to detect. The typical bright red color is not present. The plaques assume a blue or violet hue because of stimulation of melanocytes. The characteristic silvery scale is often absent.

Literature related specifically to abnormalities of dark skin is also rare. Normal variants such as the mongolian spot in infants, Futcher or Voigt lines, and linear nail pigmentation are

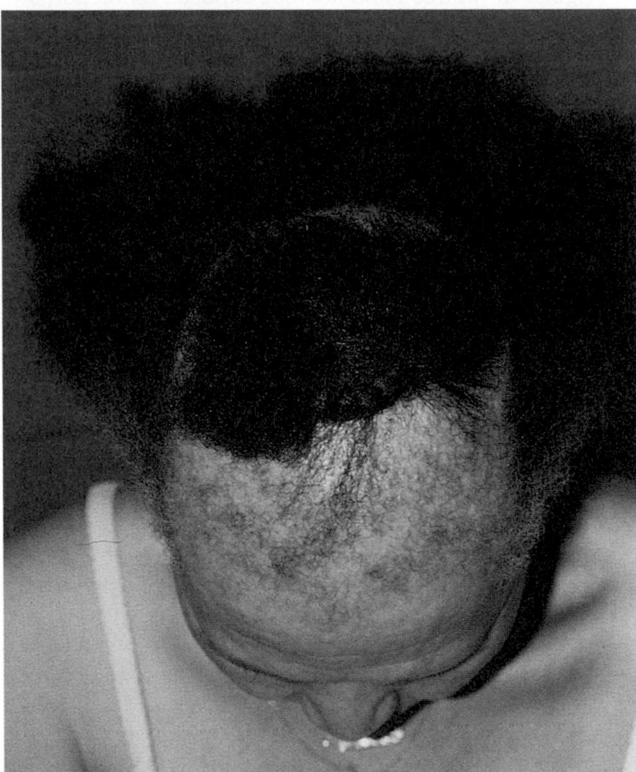

FIGURE 53-36 ■ Traction alopecia from tight braiding and use of a hot comb. (From Callen JP et al: *Color atlas of dermatology,* Philadelphia, 1993, Saunders, p 363.)

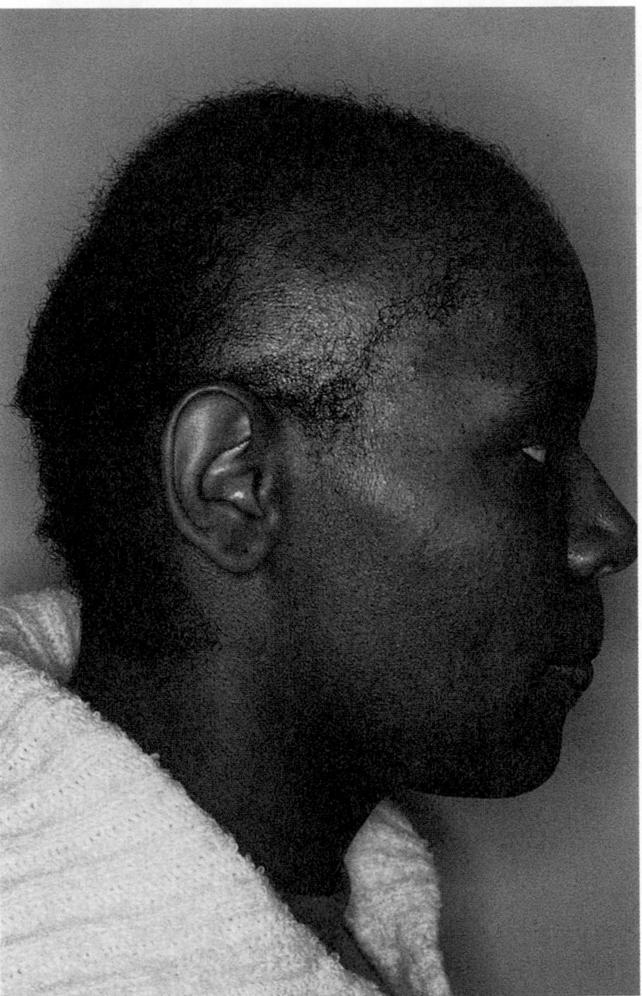

FIGURE 53-37 ■ Hot comb damage resulting in scarring alopecia. (From Callen JP et al: *Color atlas of dermatology,* Philadelphia, 1993, Saunders, p 366.)

frequently mistaken for disorders. Box 53-2 presents tips for assessing dark skin.

KEY CONCEPTS

- Certain skin disorders are manifested differently or appear in greater or lesser frequency in persons with dark skin. Normal variants such as the mongolian spot in infants, Futcher or Voigt lines, and linear nail pigmentation are frequently mistaken for disorders.
- Disorders such as seborrheic dermatitis and keloids are seen more often in African-Americans.
- Traumatic alopecia occurs more often in African-Americans because of tight plaiting of the hair or the use of hot oil and tension on the scalp.
- Squamous cell or basal cell carcinoma, senile keratoses, and psoriasis only rarely affect darker skinned persons.

INTEGUMENTARY MANIFESTATIONS OF SYSTEMIC DISEASE

The skin reflects the status of many organ systems. For example, the endocrine, cardiovascular, renal, respiratory, and hepatic systems all have possible dermal manifestations. Metabolic disorders and internal malignancies also cause cutaneous alterations. Certainly, skin manifestations of internal malignancy can be obvious. The late-appearing features of **cachexia** (wasting), pallor, and cutaneous metastases are obvious signs of malignancy. Abnormalities in endocrine function also produce a myriad of cutaneous changes. In general, systemic disease states are expressed through altered color, sensation, texture, and temperature of the skin; altered growth, texture, color, and lubrication of the hair; and changes in nail shape, color, and texture.

Skin

Color

Color changes in the skin can signal the presence of systemic disease. The entire color spectrum (red, orange, yellow, green, blue, indigo, and violet) is represented through possible coloration changes in the skin.

Redness (**erythema**) may be generalized, as with carbon monoxide poisoning, or may be generalized or localized, as with rashes or on the palms. Although erythema is often visible in lighter skinned persons, it may be less apparent in those whose skin is dark; however, the affected part may become an even deeper shade of brown. Redness may accompany inflammation.

Box 53-2

Tips for Assessing Dark Skin

1. Skin color should be observed in the sclerae, conjunctivae, buccal mucosa, tongue, lips, nail beds, palms, and soles.
2. Inspection should be accompanied by palpation, especially if inflammation or edema is suspected.
3. Findings should always be correlated with the patient's history to arrive at a diagnosis.
4. ***Pallor*** in brown-skinned patients may appear as a yellowish brown tinge to the skin. In a black-skinned patient the skin will appear ash gray. Pallor can be difficult to determine. In dark-skinned individuals it is characterized by absence of the underlying red tones in the skin.
5. ***Jaundice*** may be observed in the sclera but should not be confused with the normal yellow-pigmented sclera of a dark-skinned black patient. The best place to inspect is in the portion of the sclera that is observable when the eye is open. If jaundice is suspected, the posterior portion of the hard palate should also be observed for a yellowish cast, which is most effective when done in bright daylight.
6. The ***oral mucosa*** of dark-skinned individuals may have a normal freckling of pigmentation that may also be evident on the gums, the borders of the tongue, and the lining of the cheeks.
7. The gingiva may normally have a dark blue color that may appear blotchy or be evenly distributed.
8. ***Petechiae*** are best observed over areas of lighter pigmentation—the abdomen, gluteal areas, and volar aspect of the forearm. They may also be seen in the palpebral conjunctiva and buccal mucosa.
9. To differentiate petechiae and ecchymosis from erythema, remember that pressure over the area will cause erythema to blanch but will not affect either petechiae or ecchymosis.
10. ***Erythema*** is usually associated with increased skin temperature, so palpation should also be used if an inflammatory condition is suspected.
11. ***Edema*** may reduce the intensity of the color of an area of skin because of the increased distance between the external epithelium and the pigmented layers. Therefore, darker skin would appear lighter. On palpation the skin may feel "tight."
12. ***Cyanosis*** can be difficult to determine in dark-skinned individuals. Familiarity with the precyanotic color is often helpful. However, if it is not possible to determine cyanosis from the skin, close inspection of the nail beds, lips, palpebral conjunctiva, palms, and soles should show evidence of cyanosis.
13. ***Rashes*** may be assessed by palpating for changes in skin texture.

Data from Rosen T, Martin S: *Atlas of black dermatology,* Boston, 1981, Little, Brown.

When inflammation is suspected in a dark-skinned person, other parameters can be assessed by palpation, among them increased skin temperature, tight skin suggestive of edema, induration of deep tissue or blood vessels, and tenderness. Because the dorsal skin surface of the fingers is more sensitive to subtle skin temperature differences than the palmar surface is, the examiner should use the dorsal portion of the fingers to move from one skin area to another for comparison. The patient's family and friends are also helpful in validating color change, particularly when it has occurred gradually.

Orange discoloration can occur from the deposition of carotene. Protein-calorie malnutrition can cause hypopigmentation in African-American children, with the hair and skin appearing orange.

Yellow discoloration can occur locally when lipids are deposited in skin secondary to a metabolic defect in blood lipids. More commonly, a generalized yellow (jaundiced) appearance arises because of liver disease. Bilirubin accumulates in blood and saturates the tissues. **Jaundice** is observed in the usual sites (e.g., mucous membranes, nail beds). Because many factors can alter these findings, one single positive finding should not be held as conclusive. Other parameters, such as environmental temperature, drugs, smoking, amount of hemoglobin, and the color of urine or stool, can support a description of cyanosis or jaundice. In both dark-skinned and light-skinned persons, yellow sclerae may indicate jaundice, but other factors can cause yellow scleral pigmentation; fatty deposits that contain carotene are a common finding in dark-skinned people. To determine whether the yellow sclerae signify jaundice, observe the hard palate in bright daylight. Jaundice can be detected there quite early (i.e., when serum bilirubin is 2 to 4 mg/100 ml) if the palate does not have heavy melanin pigmentation.[24] If the hard palate does not show jaundice when the sclerae are yellow, the pigmentation may be due to some other factor, such as carotene accumulation. All these factors support the importance of repeated observation and accurate description of what is seen. As often as possible, the same person should perform the entire examination and confirm specific findings in one area with additional data from other areas.

When jaundice is severe, **biliverdin** also accumulates. A person with obstructed bile ducts can become green-yellow because of biliverdin.

Blueness of the skin (**cyanosis**) often occurs on the tips of the fingers, toes, nose, and lips in people with cardiac or respiratory problems that prevent oxygenation of blood. Localized blueness with pain of the fingers on exposure to cold is termed Raynaud disease. It frequently arises from cryoglobulins, which solidify in the cold, and is also associated with disorders of the immune system, such as lymphoma and acquired immunodeficiency syndrome.[25]

Indigo discoloration occurs locally, as in gangrene of the toes from severe generalized arteriosclerosis. The skin can darken from increased melanin synthesis, as in chronic adrenal insufficiency. Also, silver poisoning can make the skin dusky. Violet-colored palms (palmar erythema) can be seen in some persons with liver disease and occasionally in pregnant women as a response to hyperestrogenism.

Shades of violet occur on the legs as a result of vascular insufficiency or when cardiopulmonary function is compromised.

The primary sites for assessing skin **pallor** are the nail beds, lips, and conjunctivae. When observing the lower eyelid (inferior palpebral conjunctiva) for pallor, the examiner should lower the lid sufficiently to see the conjunctiva near not only the outer canthus but also the inner canthus because the former is often darker. Greater perception is necessary when assessing a darkly pigmented individual for pallor because the changes are subtle. Red tones may be absent; a brown-skinned person may appear more yellowish brown, and a black-skinned person may appear ash gray. This variability supports the need for accurate baseline data for comparison.

Sensation

Sensory innervation is generally responsible for the itching (**pruritis**) and **pain** that accompany most skin diseases. *Itching* is often the initial symptom in such conditions as atopic eczema, allergic contact dermatitis, scabies, dermatophytosis, psoriasis, and varicella. It can also be associated with systemic disorders, including carcinoma, diabetes, thyroid disease, uremia, and obstructive biliary disease. Other dermatologic conditions, such as herpes simplex, aphthous stomatitis, herpes zoster, furuncles, and cellulitis, produce considerable *pain.*

Texture

Normal aging produces an alteration in the texture of skin. Loose and wrinkled skin that lacks tone may also indicate **dehydration** (an abnormal finding). Dehydration may also be apparent through inspection of the oral cavity. On inspection, a dry, leathery appearance of the tongue is *not* a reliable indicator of dehydration inasmuch as mouth breathing frequently makes the tongue look dry even when the individual is well hydrated. A more reliable method of assessing hydration of the oral cavity is to palpate the mucous membranes along the area of the gum and cheek where the membranes approximate. If the membranes are dry and the finger does not slide easily, dehydration is evident.

To evaluate **fluid excess,** palpate the skin over the hands, feet, ankles, and sacrum. If the skin is firm and indents easily (pitting edema) on moderate pressure from the fingertips, fluid excess is present.

Feeling the deeper portions of the skin may reveal areas of **induration** (hardness) such as those resulting from multiple intramuscular or subcutaneous injections of medication. **Lipodystrophies** consist of smooth, large depressions in the skin that indicate atrophy of the subcutaneous fat layer, which has a spongy consistency. Both induration and lipodystrophy are often seen at sites of repeated insulin injections.

Temperature

If the skin feels warm and dry in a person who is febrile (feverish), the blood temperature is probably rising, an indication that the thermoregulatory mechanism of sweating may not be functioning. Likewise, if the skin is warm and wet, the temperature can be expected to fall owing to the cooling mechanism of sweating.

Sweating can also occur when the blood glucose concentration falls rapidly with a resultant rise in the blood epinephrine level. Hypoglycemic sweating can usually be distinguished from other causes of sweating because of the additional symptoms of weakness, tachycardia, hunger, headache, and "inward nervousness" manifested as mental irritability and confusion.

Because skin temperature depends on the amount of blood circulating through the dermis, decreased localized blood flow (resulting in coolness), often to the feet, may indicate a peripheral vascular dysfunction. Generalized skin coolness may indicate decreased metabolism such as that occurring after general anesthesia. If the temperature is very low, signs of shock may be evident.

On the other hand, an increase in skin temperature may indicate a **hypermetabolic state,** such as that occurring in hyperthyroidism and after sun exposure or sunburn.

Hair

Disturbances in body function are often reflected in changes in growth pattern, amount, texture, color, and lubrication of the hair.

Growth

The high speed of growth of the scalp hair makes it more susceptible to damage from systemic disease, toxic drugs, radiation, and stress. The rate of growth varies with general health and age, and hair growth is dependent on circulating hormonal factors (primarily testicular or adrenal androgens). Thus hormonal imbalances or shifts (e.g., those accompanying childbirth) may also result in disturbances in the hair growth cycle. Nutritional factors, although often promoted in the nonmedical literature, have little effect on hair growth except in cases of severe malnutrition.

Amount

Alterations in the amount of body hair can be extremely anxiety provoking for both males and females. In females with hypertrichosis, or **hirsutism,** hair growth is intensified on the upper lip, chin, cheeks, and chest, around the nipples, and from the pubic crest to the umbilicus (along the linea alba); the downy hair on the arms, legs, and back becomes coarse. The pubic hair often takes on the upright triangular distribution typical of the male as opposed to the female's usual inverted triangle. An endocrine malfunction such as excess androgen production may sometimes be associated with hirsutism, but the ethnic background (Mediterranean groups predominantly) may also be responsible for the excessive hair growth. This propensity is especially true of the hair on the arms, legs, back, and face. Other ethnic group members such as full-blooded African-American females and male Native Americans rarely have facial hair. Distribution of the hair in family members and ethnic background are thus important considerations in ascertaining hair growth.

Hypertrichosis lanuginosa is typically a congenital, autosomal dominant disorder in which excessive hair is distributed over the entire body throughout life. The condition is usually associated with other congenital anomalies such as spina bifida.[26] In some cases, such as with certain internal carcinomas, hypertrichosis lanuginosa is an acquired disorder; the degree of hairiness is variable and usually involves the face.

Color

Perhaps the most common color change in the hair is the generalized graying that accompanies the aging process.

Texture

Normal aging also produces a decrease in hair thickness.

Disturbances of the thickness of scalp hair are common. Baldness (**alopecia**) or thinning of the hair that is generalized or creates a receding hairline is often genetically determined (Figure 53-38). Some rare genetic defects in the hair shaft itself may produce breaking of the hairs and be erroneously diagnosed as alopecia. Generalized and localized baldness may result from treatment modalities such as radiation therapy or chemotherapy. In addition, various types of scalp diseases (e.g., fungal, lupus) and telogen effluvium (transient hair loss occurring 2 to 3 months after general anesthesia, febrile illness, or giving birth) can cause hair loss. Other traumatic types of hair loss may result from pulling of the hair because of a nervous habit, hair styles such as tight braids or ponytails, or wearing of constrictive apparel such as a hat.

Lubrication

Hyperfunction of the sebaceous glands is associated with androgen stimulation such as occurs with the excessive scalp oiliness and facial acne in adolescence. Dry, brittle hair is commonly the result of excessive washing or the application of

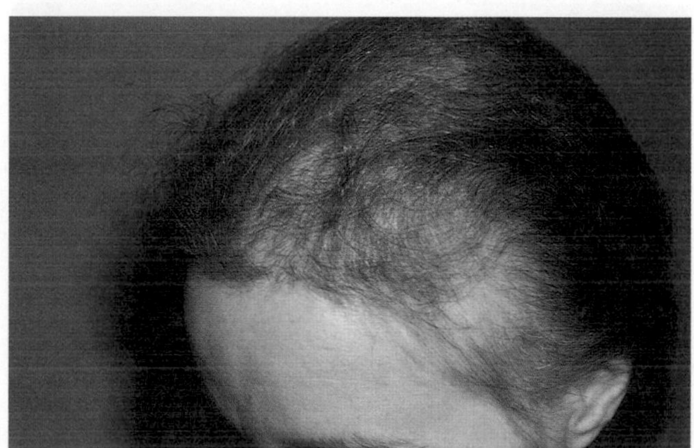

FIGURE 53-38 ■ Male pattern baldness (androgenetic alopecia) in a woman. (From Callen JP et al: *Color atlas of dermatology,* Philadelphia, 1993, Saunders, p 365.)

chemical agents (coloring, bleach, or detergent shampoos) to the hair.

In addition to direct observation of the scalp and face, correlation of the findings with data from the patient history helps determine dysfunctional states of health.

Nails

Because nails are derived from a highly active tissue, they may be affected by any serious systemic illness. Moreover, any local skin disease that affects the epidermis may also affect the nail matrix (epidermal cells that give rise to the nail plate) and lead to an abnormal (**dystrophic**) nail. By measuring the distance between abnormalities (pits, grooves, and lines) and the proximal nail border, one may estimate the time of initial illness.

Shape

Transverse furrows (**Beau lines**) in the nail indicate that nail growth has been disturbed (Figure 53-39). These furrows can result from infection, systemic disease, or injury. Nails with a concave curve are known as spoon nails, or **koilonychia.** This may signal a form of iron deficiency anemia and is also associated with other disorders such as coronary disease, syphilis, or the use of strong soaps. Destruction of the nails (**onycholysis**) may accompany a great variety of unrelated conditions ranging from the application of false nails to hyperthyroidism, fungal nail infection, or psoriasis (Figures 53-40 to 53-42). Certain medications may also cause onycholysis (Figure 53-43). **Splinter hemorrhages** may be linked to bacterial endocarditis and trichinosis. These red or brown splinters or streaks run parallel to the finger in the nail bed (Figure 53-44). **Clubbing** of the fingers is characterized by a flattening of the angle of the base of the nail. It may occur in association with cardiovascular disease, subacute bacterial endocarditis, and pulmonary disease.

Color

Nail color indicates the amount of blood oxygenation. Bluish or purplish discoloration of the nail beds occurs with

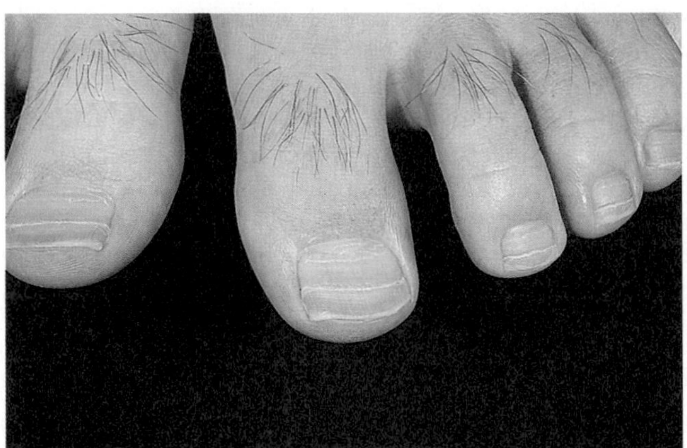

FIGURE 53-39 ■ Beau lines. This patient had major surgery 5 months previously. (From Callen JP et al: *Color atlas of dermatology,* ed 2, Philadelphia, 2000, Saunders, p 334.)

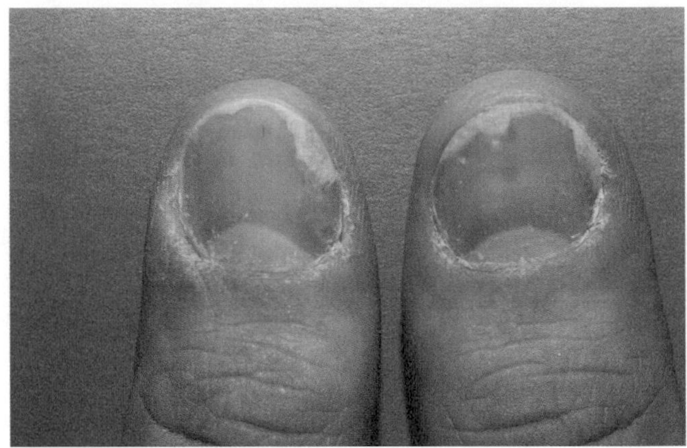

FIGURE 53-41 ■ Psoriasis resulting in onycholysis. (From Callen JP et al: *Color atlas of dermatology,* Philadelphia, 1993, Saunders, p 347.)

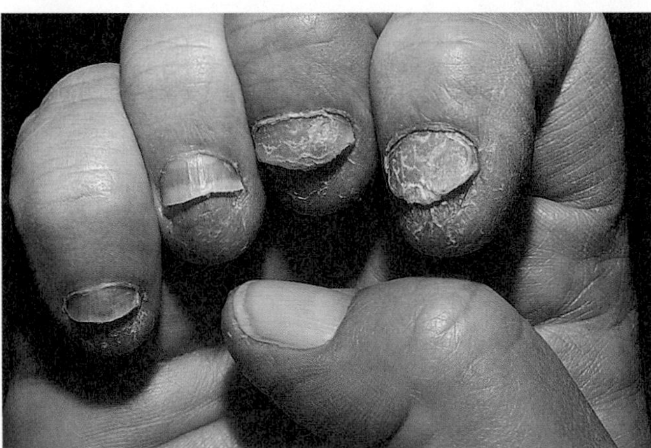

FIGURE 53-40 ■ *Candida albicans* infection resulting in onycholysis. (From Callen JP et al: *Color atlas of dermatology,* ed 2, Philadelphia, 2000, Saunders, p 333.)

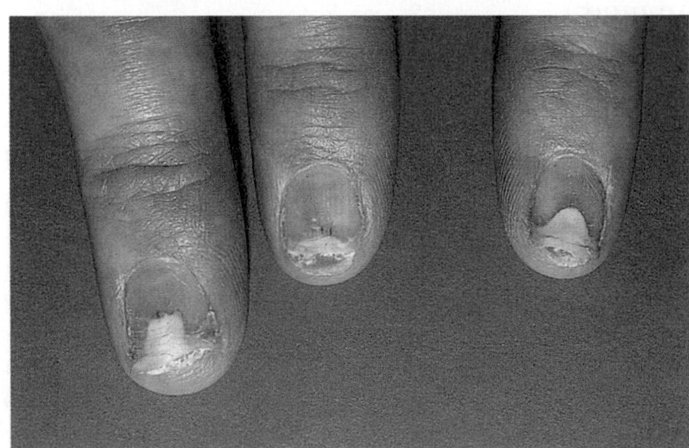

FIGURE 53-42 ■ Onycholysis secondary to false "sculptured" nails. (From Callen JP et al: *Color atlas of dermatology,* ed 2, Philadelphia, 2000, Saunders, p 367.)

cyanosis, whereas pallor often indicates anemia. To compare color of the nail beds, apply slight pressure on the free edge of the second or third fingernail. The blanching that results is then compared with the normal color of the nail. The rate of color return also indicates the quality of peripheral vasomotor function.

Texture

Thickening of the nail may result from nutritional disturbances, repeated trauma, inflammation, and local infection. Along with thickening, toenails may become discolored and grooved, and debris may accumulate under the nail. This condition may be exacerbated as the distal portion of the nail works free from the underlying nail bed and more debris is accumulated; fungal infections may also follow. Treatment usually consists of periodic debridement of the nail plate; however, a return to normal nail structure rarely occurs after thickening.

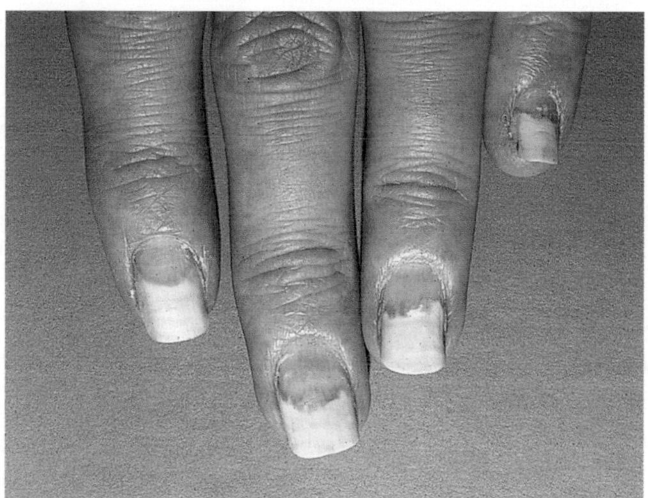

FIGURE 53-43 ■ Drug-induced onycholysis. (From Callen JP et al: *Color atlas of dermatology,* ed 2, Philadelphia, 2000, Saunders, p 334.)

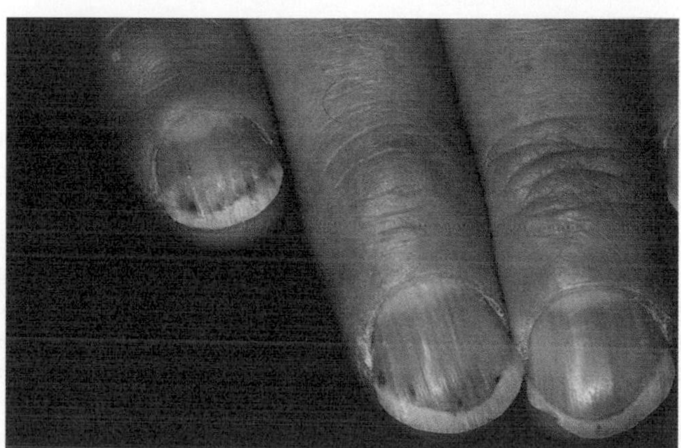

FIGURE 53-44 ■ Splinter hemorrhages in a patient with leukocytoclastic vasculitis. (From Callen JP et al: *Color atlas of dermatology,* ed 2, Philadelphia, 2000, Saunders, p 337.)

KEY CONCEPTS

- Many systemic diseases are associated with alterations in skin, hair, and nails. Skin reflects systemic inflammation and fever as erythema. A rising fever is manifested as warm, dry skin, whereas warm, moist skin indicates a fever beginning to decline. Poor oxygenation and circulation may be manifested by cyanosis, pallor, or coolness. Jaundice indicates altered bilirubin metabolism, usually caused by liver or biliary disease. Fluid balance may be manifested in the skin as decreased turgor or edema. Sympathetic activation may be indicated by cool, pale, diaphoretic skin.
- Hair growth, strength, texture, and color are affected by systemic diseases such as endocrine abnormalities, extreme malnutrition, and drugs. Excessive androgen may result in hirsutism. Alopecia may result from chemotherapeutic drugs or radiation therapy.
- Abnormalities of nail growth (pits, grooves, lines) occur as a result of nearly any serious systemic illness. Certain nail defects are characteristic of particular diseases: spoon nails may indicate iron deficiency anemia; clubbing is associated with cardiopulmonary disease. Nail color is commonly assessed to determine the adequacy of oxygenation and perfusion.

TREATMENT IMPLICATIONS

A distinct advantage in treating the skin is the ease of direct observation of the pathologic process and the effects of treatment. Culture, macroscopic examination of skin scrapings, and biopsy also facilitate diagnosis. A correct diagnosis can help prevent complications from improper therapy but does not lessen the importance of choosing an appropriate delivery system.

Topical Treatment

Wet Dressings

Wet dressings, the application of a liquid in compress form, are a very important part of the dermatologic therapy delivery system. The applied liquid can be plain water or water with additives (e.g., sodium, magnesium, or aluminum salts).

Wet dressings are a versatile, even paradoxical therapeutic approach in that they can dry or hydrate as necessary. Intermittently applied, they serve as an effective astringent for the weeping, oozing lesions that accompany stasis and decubitus ulcers and impetigo. Vesicular lesions, including those seen in dyshidrotic eczema, herpes zoster, and pemphigus, also respond nicely to treatment with intermittent wet dressings. By drying disease-related lesions, intermittent dressings help speed recovery.

Continuous wet dressings, on the other hand, are effective in rapidly hydrating the skin. This technique, used most often in severe cases of atopic eczema, normally requires hospitalization. Wet dressings of gauze soaked in tap water are applied directly to the skin and covered with an insulating agent such as towels, large thick gauze pads, or even long underwear to prevent evaporation. It is very important that the dressings remain moist. Therefore, they must be resoaked and changed every 3 hours around the clock throughout the course of treatment. Once the desired state of hydration has been achieved, the dressings can be discontinued and emollient creams used to prevent redrying of the treated area.

Lotions

Shake lotions are mixtures of small suspended particles in a liquid vehicle such as water or alcohol. These are especially useful for application directly to moist or exudative processes such as rhus dermatitis. As the liquid phase dissipates, the evaporative effect cools and dries the skin.[27]

Emollient lotions are a mixture of oil in water and have a slightly greasy consistency. These preparations are useful when skin moisturization is needed such as in xerotic conditions. Lotions are often used as a vehicle for other medications such as topical steroids that must be applied over large areas of skin.[27]

Gels

Most gels are clear, colorless, volatile substances. They generally penetrate better than creams. Gels are very convenient to use on wet lesions because of their astringent tendencies. Because they do not leave the white or oily residue of creams and ointments, they are appropriate for use on scalp lesions.

Creams

Creams are the most widely used dermatologic delivery system. Many different bases are used in creams, but the "vanishing" type is most common and allows application with no surface residue. Creams penetrate well and have some moisturizing capability. They are used most frequently in the management of dry to slightly moist dermatoses.

Ointments

The medication in most ointments is carried in a petrolatum-type base, which facilitates penetration into the upper skin layers. Ointments are frequently used on skin lesions that have overlying dry scaling and crusting, but they are also very effective on severe dermatoses requiring an increased medication dosage. Ointments are semiocclusive and often not appropriate for use on lesions that are oozing and discharging a transudate or exudate.

Aerosols

Aerosols, fine particle sprays of medication usually delivered by gas under pressure, are a cosmetically elegant way of treating dermatoses, especially on hairy areas of the body.

Intralesional Injection

Intralesional injection, or the deposition of medication directly into the lesion, can be done with a conventional needle and syringe or with an instrument (Dermajet) that injects fine particles of medication through the skin with air pressure. This delivery form is especially useful in delivering higher concentrations of corticosteroids to lesions (usually with deep dermal components) that do not respond to topical medication.

Selection of a Delivery System

Delivery system selection depends on the disease being treated, the type of lesions clinically present, and the practitioner's preferred medication routine. For instance, weeping exudative lesions require drying (wet dressings) and perhaps corticosteroids. Initial delivery as a gel would increase the drying tendency; as the lesion dries, a cream may be used to prevent overdrying and fissure formation.

In a disease state such as chronic atopic eczema with lichenoid or thickened skin, the prescriber may choose an ointment to enhance penetration of the medication into the lesion. The ointment's occlusive nature reduces moisture loss from the skin.

Seborrhea and psoriasis in the scalp may be treated with aerosols, which are quick and easy to use and are associated with a high degree of patient compliance. Patients often find them cosmetically superior to the identical medication in cream form. Keloids, which require highly concentrated medication to be delivered to a small area, are ideal candidates for intralesional injection of corticosteroids.

Corticosteroids

Corticosteroids are a very important tool in the practice of dermatology. Dermatologists administer steroids systemically and topically. Steroids may be characterized as short acting (cortisone or hydrocortisone), intermediate acting (prednisone, prednisolone, methylprednisolone, or triamcinolone), or long acting (dexamethasone or betamethasone).

Systemic Steroids

Administration of systemic steroids in dermatologic disease is usually oral. Intermediate-acting steroids (prednisone, prednisolone, methylprednisolone) are used most often. The greatest benefit of oral administration is the ability to adjust dosage schedules quickly if required. Once-daily doses, divided daily dosage, or alternate-day regimens are all effective.

Intramuscular administration of corticosteroids is also common. Preparations such as triamcinolone acetonide are used most often. These drugs, which may reduce inflammation for more than 4 weeks, ensure that an unreliable patient will receive appropriate doses of medication.

Systemic corticosteroids are generally used for relatively short periods. Therefore, the complications commonly associated with corticosteroid use are not usually seen in dermatologic treatment. However, the long-term use of corticosteroids in dis-cases such as pemphigus and LE often results in cushingoid features such as a round, puffy face and a "buffalo hump." Additional adverse effects include fatiguing, weakness, and acne.

Topical Steroids

Corticosteroids can also be applied topically to suppress inflammation. Although this approach does not cure the disease, the reduction in erythema, edema, and pruritis promotes healing. Topical steroids are available in a variety of forms. Based on their capacity to cause cutaneous vasoconstriction, topical steroids are divided into seven groups, with group 1 being the most potent (augmented betamethasone dipropionate [Diprolene AF] and clobetasol dipropionate [Temovate]) and group 7 being the least potent (1% hydrocortisone).

KEY CONCEPTS

- Selection of topical treatment depends largely on whether the goal is to moisturize or dry the affected area. Continuous wet dressings, lotions, creams, and ointments tend to be moisturizing. Intermittent wet dressings and gels tend to be astringents for weeping, oozing lesions.
- Corticosteroids are commonly administered to reduce inflammation. They may be given topically, intralesionally, or systemically.

DEVELOPMENTAL CONSIDERATIONS

The skin and the skin problems of special groups warrant consideration. Certain skin problems are seen only in infants and children (e.g., cradle cap and diaper rash) (Figure 53-45). Other dermatoses are seen in both children and adults, but in children these dermatoses may appear different from the adult counterpart. Still other dermatoses affect primarily older persons.

INFANCY

Infancy connotes soft, flawless skin. In general, this is a true image. Several congenital skin lesions, such as mongolian spots, hemangiomas, and nevi (moles), are nevertheless associated with the early neonatal period.

Mongolian spots are caused by selective pigmentation. They usually occur on the buttocks or sacral area and are commonly seen in Asian-Americans or African-Americans.

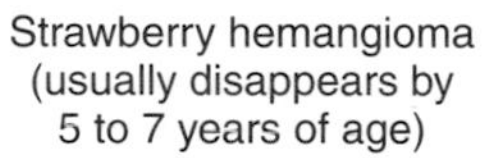

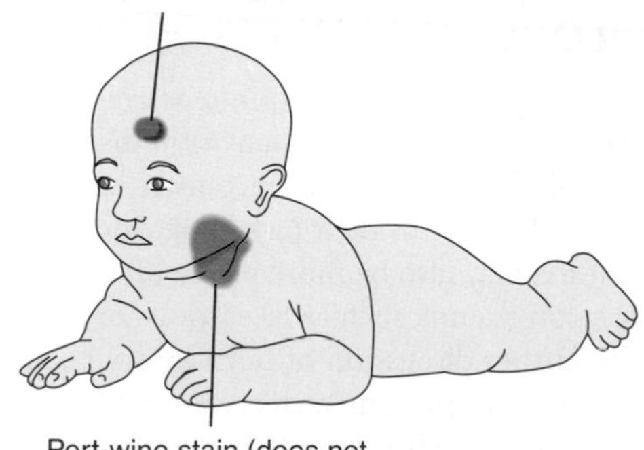

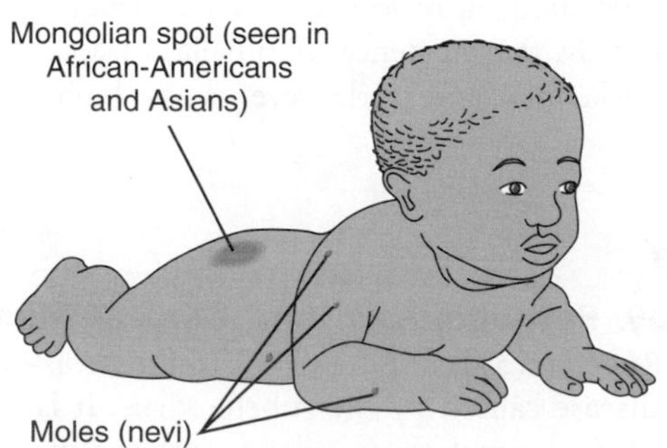

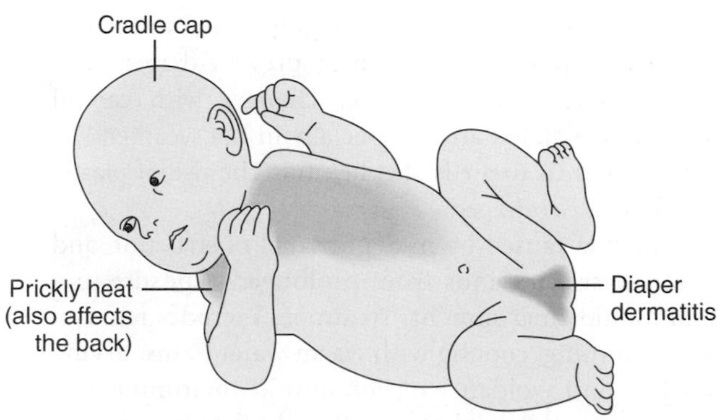

FIGURE 53-45 ■ Sites of common dermatoses in infants and small children.

Hemangiomas are vascular disorders of the skin. Two types of hemangiomas are commonly seen in infants and small children: bright red, raised *strawberry hemangiomas* and flat, reddish purple *port-wine stain hemangiomas.* Strawberry hemangiomas begin as small red lesions shortly after birth. They may remain as small superficial lesions or extend to involve subcutaneous tissue. Strawberry hemangiomas usually disappear before the child reaches 5 to 7 years of age without leaving an appreciable scar.[28] Port-wine stain hemangiomas are rare, usually occur on the face and neck, and can be quite disfiguring. They do not disappear with age and no satisfactory medical treatment is available, although laser surgery may be effective in some cases. Coverage using cosmetic makeup such as Derma Blend may sufficiently conceal their disfiguring effects.

Nevi may vary in shape or size, and they may be present at birth or develop later in life.

Infant skin is also exquisitely sensitive to irritation, injury, and extremes of temperature. Prolonged exposure to a warm humid environment can lead to **prickly heat,** and too frequent bathing can cause excessive dryness. Soiled diapers, left unchanged, can lead to **contact dermatitis** and bacterial infections. **Cradle cap** is a harmless and usually self-limited scaly condition of the scalp. Figure 53-45 illustrates common skin problems of infants and small children.

The primary factor in preventing infant skin disorders is careful and meticulous skin care. Baby lotions are helpful in maintaining skin moisture, whereas baby powder acts as a drying agent. Both are helpful aids when used selectively and according to the nature of the skin problem (excessive moisture or dryness).

Baby powders containing talc can cause serious respiratory problems if inhaled; therefore, containers should be kept out of the reach of small children. Corn starch is preferable to talc, and baby powders containing corn starch are readily available. Unnecessary bathing should be avoided, and clothing should be comfortable and appropriate for environmental conditions.

Diaper rash results from the ammonia and alkali byproducts of urine breakdown. Disposable diapers or diapers washed in gentle detergent and thoroughly rinsed to remove all traces of ammonia and alkali help prevent diaper rash. Treatment includes frequent diaper changes with careful cleansing of any irritated areas, especially in hot weather. Exposing irritated areas to air is also helpful. The use of plastic pants should be discouraged.

Prickly heat is caused by midepidermal obstruction and rupture of the sweat glands from prolonged exposure to a warm and humid environment. Treatment includes removal of excessive clothing, cooling with warm water baths, drying with powders, and avoidance of hot, humid environments.

Cradle cap is usually managed with mild shampooing and gentle combing to remove the scales.

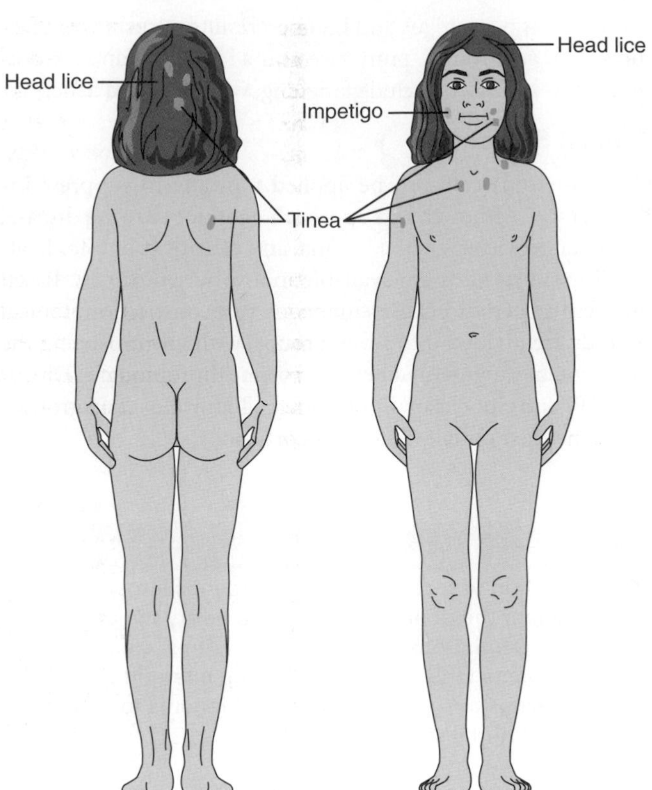

FIGURE 53-46 ■ Sites of selected common communicable dermatoses affecting children.

CHILDHOOD SKIN DISORDERS

As infants grow and develop into active young children, they become susceptible to the many skin disorders affecting people of all age groups who encounter environmental agents. Children, because of their physiologic development and playful nature, may also be more prone to accidents that result in major skin trauma such as lacerations or burns. (See Chapter 54 for further discussion of burn injury.) Careful activity supervision helps prevent such accidental trauma.

Besides interacting with the environment, children are frequently in close contact with other children. As a result, communicable diseases such as head lice, tinea capitis, and impetigo are more frequently seen in children (Figure 53-46). Epidemiologically, the incidence of rubella, roseola, rubeola (measles), chickenpox, and scarlet fever is also highest in this age group.

Rubella

Etiology, Pathogenesis, and Clinical Manifestations. **Rubella** (3-day measles, German measles) is a childhood disease caused by the rubella virus. It is characterized by a diffuse punctate, macular rash that begins on the trunk and spreads to the arms and legs. Mild febrile states occur; generally the temperature is less than 100° F.[28] Postauricular, suboccipital, and cervical lymph node adenopathy is common. Coldlike symptoms usually accompany the disease in the form of cough, congestion, and coryza (profuse nasal mucous membrane discharge). Treatment is based on symptoms.

Rubella generally has no long-lasting sequelae; however, transmission of the disease to pregnant women early in the gestation period may result in severe teratogenic effects in the unborn fetus. Among the teratogenic effects are cataracts, microcephaly, mental retardation, deafness, patent ductus arteriosus, glaucoma, purpura, and bone defects.[25]

Prevention. Most states require immunization to prevent the transmission of rubella to pregnant women. Immunization is with a live virus vaccine called measles-mumps-rubella (MMR). One injection during infancy is followed by one booster dose as the child enters kindergarten or first grade or as the child enters middle school or junior high school. Administration of these two injections is considered adequate to prevent rubella. Cases of rubella in immunized children are rare.

Roseola Infantum

Pathogenesis and Clinical Manifestations. **Roseola infantum** is a contagious viral disease that generally affects children younger than 4 years and usually children about 1 year of age.[28] It produces a characteristic maculopapular rash covering the trunk and spreading to the appendages. A rapid rise in temperature to 105°F and coldlike symptoms accompany the disease.[28] Unlike rubella, no cervical or postauricular lymph node adenopathy occurs. The symptoms usually subside within 3 to 5 days.[28] Roseola infantum is frequently mistaken for rubella, which can usually be ruled out by the age of the child, as well as by the absence of lymph node adenopathy. Generally, rubella does not develop in children younger than 6 to 9 months because of maternal antibodies.[28] Blood antibody titers may be assayed to determine the actual diagnosis. In most cases, no long-term effects from this disease are noted.

Treatment. Management of roseola infantum is palliative. As with rubella, antipyretic drugs such as acetaminophen (Tylenol) and cooling baths are used to reduce the fever. Rest and fluids are recommended for recuperation and body rehydration. Pruritus may rarely accompany the other symptoms. If severe, pruritis can be managed with topical lotions such as Caladryl.

Measles

Etiology, Pathogenesis, and Clinical Manifestations. Hard **measles,** or 7-day measles (rubeola), is a communicable viral disease caused by the Morbillivirus. The characteristic rash is macular and blotchy; sometimes the macules become confluent. The rubeola rash usually begins on the face and spreads to the appendages. Accompanying symptoms are a temperature of 100° F or greater, Koplik spots (small irregular red spots with a bluish white speck in the center) on the buccal mucosa, and mild to severe photosensitivity.[29] Coldlike symptoms and general malaise and myalgia are often present. In severe cases the macule may hemorrhage into the skin tissue or to another body surface, a condition called *hemorrhagic* measles. Measles is more severe in malnourished children. Complications include otitis media, pneumonia, and encephalitis. For a positive diagnosis, most states require antibody titer determination. Blood titers are usually determined during the disease process and 6 weeks after disappearance of the symptoms.

Prevention and Treatment. Measles is preventable by vaccine (MMR), and immunization is required by law in most states. Immunization is accomplished by the MMR schedule (see discussion under "Rubella").

Management of measles is based on symptoms. Children are kept in darkened rooms. Antipyretic medications are given to reduce the fever, and rest and fluids are recommended.

Chickenpox

Etiology, Pathogenesis, and Clinical Manifestations. **Chickenpox** (varicella) is a common communicable childhood disease. It is caused by the varicella zoster virus, which is also the causative agent in shingles. The characteristic skin lesion occurs in three stages: macule, vesicle, and granular scab (Figure 53-47). The macular stage is characterized by the rapid development (within hours) of macules over the trunk of the body that spread to the limbs, buccal mucosa, scalp, axillae, upper respiratory tract, and conjunctivae. During the second stage, the macules vesiculate (blister) and may become depressed or umbilicated (raised blisters with depressed centers). The vesicles break open, and a scab forms during the third stage. Crops of lesions occur successively, so all three forms of the lesion are usually visible by the third day of illness. Mild to extreme pruritus accompanies these lesions and can be a complicating factor by leading to scratching and the subsequent development of secondary bacterial infection. Other symptoms that accompany chickenpox are coldlike symptoms, including cough, coryza, and sometimes photosensitivity. Mild febrile states usually occur. Complications such as pneumonia, sepsis, and encephalitis may occur but are rare among healthy children. Disease severity is age dependent and risk of visceral involvement is considerably higher in adults.

Prevention and Treatment. Treatment is based on symptoms. Antipyretic drugs such as acetaminophen are

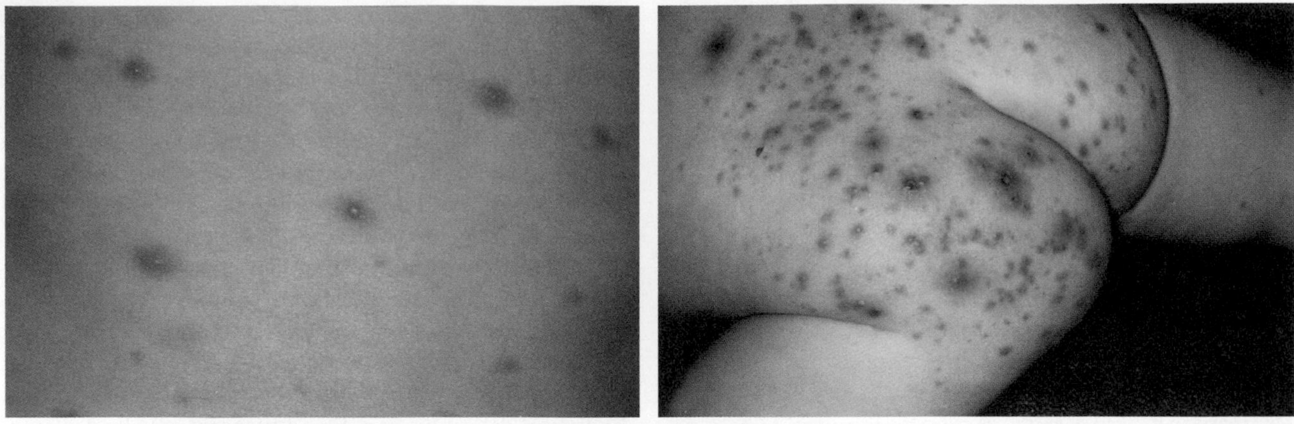

FIGURE 53-47 ■ Varicella (chickenpox). **A,** Typical "dewdrop on a rose petal." **B,** Multiple stages of lesions exist. (From Callen JP et al: *Color atlas of dermatology,* Philadelphia, 1993, Saunders, p 170.)

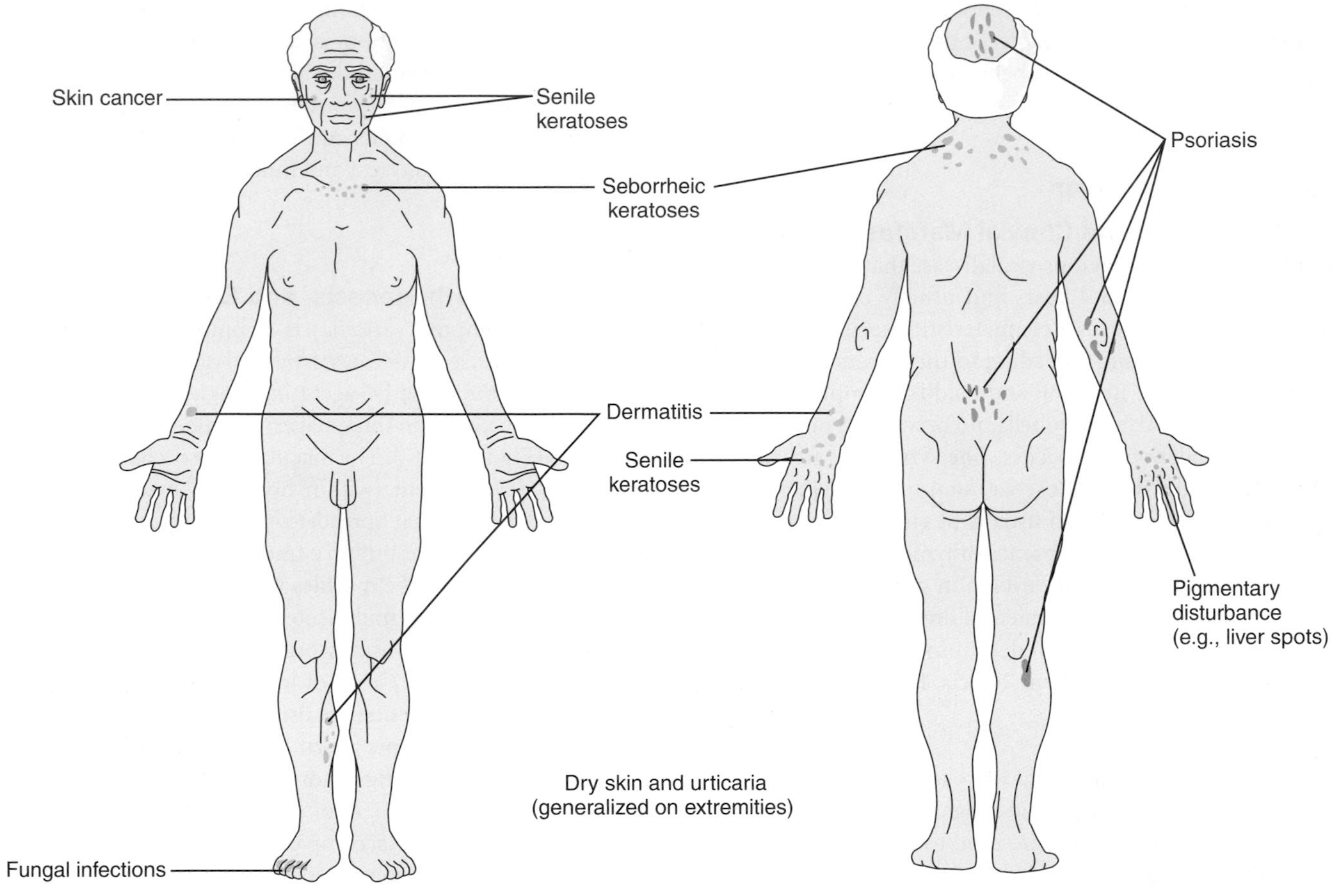

Skin cancer
Senile keratoses
Seborrheic keratoses
Dermatitis
Senile keratoses
Psoriasis
Pigmentary disturbance (e.g., liver spots)
Dry skin and urticaria (generalized on extremities)
Fungal infections

FIGURE 53-48 ■ Sites of common dermatoses of the elderly.

given for fever reduction; they may also relieve local discomfort. Pruritus is relieved with lukewarm baths. Oral administration of diphenhydramine (Benadryl) or other antihistamines may be prescribed to alleviate itching. Application of topical antipruritics such as Caladryl lotion is also helpful. However, in young children, care must be taken to avoid topical preparations of Caladryl containing diphenhydramine to avoid possible overdose of this agent through systemic absorption. (This consideration is especially important if the young child is also taking oral Benadryl.) Home remedies such as baking soda baths also relieve itching, and rest and fluids are important in recuperation and rehydration. Some authorities recommend acyclovir, an antiviral agent, for the management of chickenpox.[30,31]

Varicella-zoster immune globulin provides passive immunity against chickenpox and is recommended after exposure, especially for high-risk groups. A vaccine against chickenpox that will provide active immunity is also available. Vaccination is currently recommended for all children and sometimes required for school entrance.

Scarlet Fever

Etiology, Clinical Manifestations, and Treatment. **Scarlet fever** is a systemic reaction to the toxins produced by group A β-hemolytic streptococci. It occurs when the person is sensitized to the toxin-producing variety of streptococci. Scarlet fever frequently occurs in association with streptococcal sore throat (strep throat), but it may also be associated with a wound, skin infection, or puerperal infection. Scarlet fever is characterized by a pink punctate skin rash on the neck, chest, axillae, groin, and thighs. When palpated, the rash feels like fine sandpaper. Flushing of the face with circumoral pallor is evident. Other symptoms include high fever, nausea and vomiting, strawberry tongue, raspberry tongue, and skin desquamation. Complications of scarlet fever include otitis media, peritonsillar abscess, rheumatic fever, acute glomerulonephritis, and cholera. Penicillin is the treatment of choice.

ADOLESCENCE AND YOUNG ADULTHOOD

The most common disorder of adolescence and young adulthood is **acne vulgaris.** The increased production of sex hormones and oils contributes to the development of acne. Childhood diseases are less common in adolescence; however, chronic skin diseases may be exacerbated.

GERIATRIC CONSIDERATIONS

Skin disorders are so common in elderly people that it is difficult to distinguish normal from abnormal. More than 90% of elderly people have some kind of skin disorder[32,33] (Figure 53-48). The most common skin disorders in the elderly are keratoses and skin cancers, followed by fungal infections, dermatitis, pigmentary disturbances, psoriasis, and urticaria. Other skin disorders frequently seen in the elderly are comedones (blackheads), asteatoses (scaling), cherry angiomas (small, red, benign tumors), nevi (moles), skin tags (pedunculated fleshy growths), and lentigines ("liver spots"). In addition, the incidence of senile purpura and senile warts (papillomas) significantly increases, especially among the very old. Senile purpura is related to loss of the subcutaneous tissue that supports the skin capillaries. Minor trauma can cause small bruises or ecchymotic lesions, which largely occur on the extensor surface of the forearms. Forty percent of older men and 77% of older women show evidence of senile purpura.[34] Senile papillomas are small yellow, brown, or black warts located on the trunk, limbs, and face. Sixty-three percent of all older people have some senile papillomas.[35]

Figure 53-49 illustrates several of the common skin lesions associated with aging. Most of these lesions are considered normal concomitants of aging and cause little discomfort. The greatest concern regarding body image is the appearance of the skin, which tends to look mottled and spotty. Disorders of the skin that tend to cause the most physical discomfort are pruritus, keratoses, epitheliomas, malignant melanomas, herpes zoster, psoriasis, and pressure sores.

KEY CONCEPTS

- Certain skin disorders are more common in particular age groups.
- Infants are prone to irritating lesions, including prickly heat, contact dermatitis, and cradle cap. Altered areas of pigmentation are first noticed in infancy, including mongolian spots, hemangiomas, and nevi.
- Children are prone to skin injuries and communicable diseases. A number of viral infections, including rubella, roseola, measles, and chickenpox, are associated with characteristic skin rashes. Fever and malaise are usually present. Treatment is symptomatic. Vaccinations are available to prevent rubella, measles, and chickenpox. Scarlet fever is due to a bacterial infection and is managed with antibiotics. Children are often exposed to superficial infections and infestations, including head lice, ringworm, scabies, and impetigo.
- Acne is the most common skin disorder of adolescents.
- Elderly skin is prone to a number of problems, including psoriasis, angiomas, and skin tags. Cancerous and precancerous lesions are common and require careful screening examination.

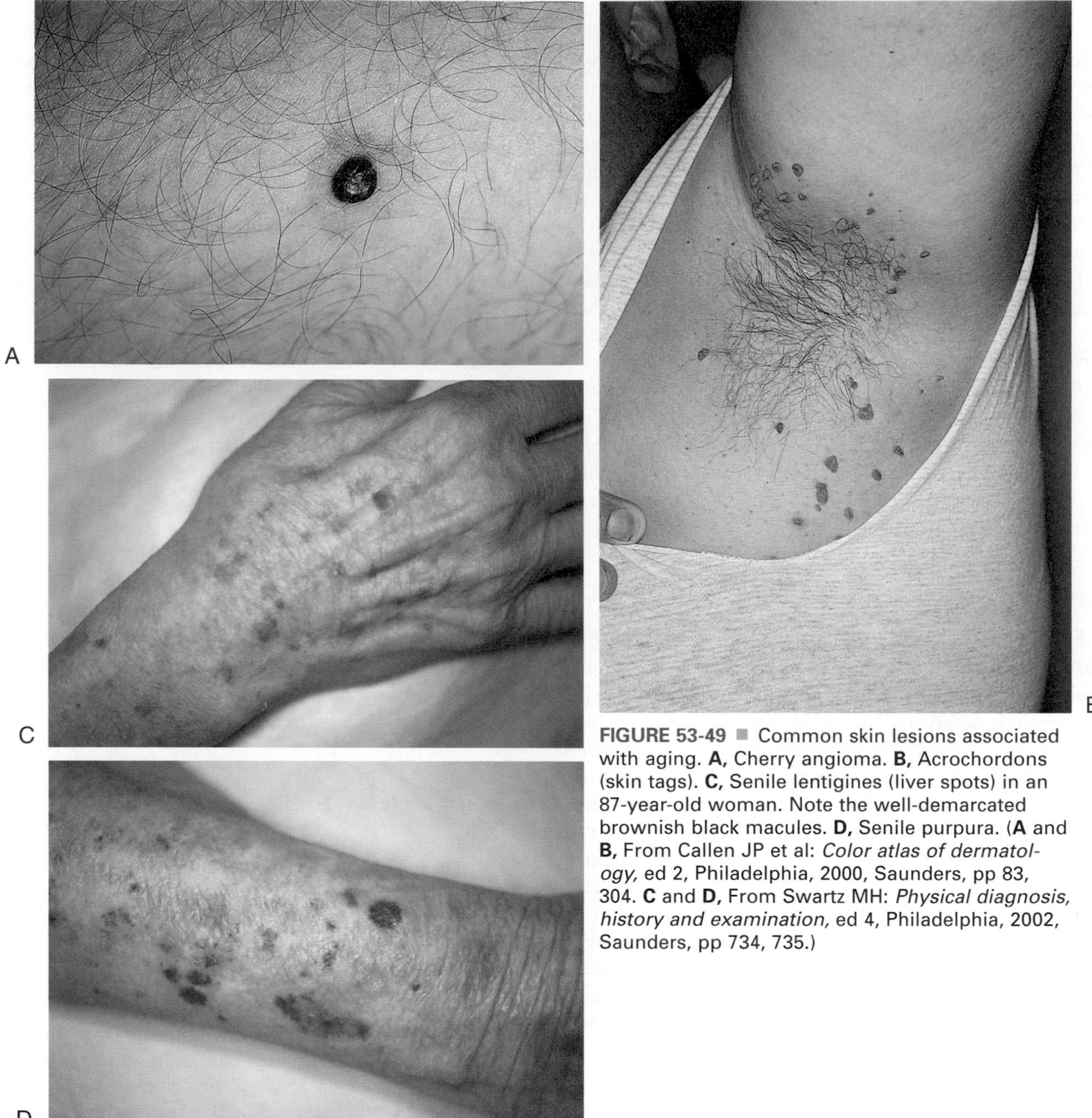

FIGURE 53-49 ■ Common skin lesions associated with aging. **A,** Cherry angioma. **B,** Acrochordons (skin tags). **C,** Senile lentigines (liver spots) in an 87-year-old woman. Note the well-demarcated brownish black macules. **D,** Senile purpura. (**A** and **B,** From Callen JP et al: *Color atlas of dermatology,* ed 2, Philadelphia, 2000, Saunders, pp 83, 304. **C** and **D,** From Swartz MH: *Physical diagnosis, history and examination,* ed 4, Philadelphia, 2002, Saunders, pp 734, 735.)

SUMMARY

In systemic diseases, the color, texture, and composition of the skin mirror and participate in widespread pathophysiologic events. For example, internal disease states such as acquired immunodeficiency syndrome, collagen diseases such as scleroderma and dermatomyositis, diabetes, gout, malignancies, neurologic diseases, liver disease, muscle weakness, and vascular, inflammatory, and metabolic disorders all exhibit cutaneous manifestations. Because the skin mirrors the interior condition of the body, it is important in the diagnosis of disease. Cutaneous manifestations may be caused by bodily changes such as pregnancy or obesity. They may also be caused by external factors such as climate, industrial contamination, indoor heating systems, clothing, plant life, and toxic or allergic reactions to drugs and cosmetics.

A distinct advantage in treating individuals with skin disease is the ability to observe the pathology and the effects of treatment. In addition to a careful history, a culture, skin scraping, or biopsy provides good diagnostic information. A correct diagnosis can help prevent complications from improper therapy, but it does not lessen the importance of choosing an appropriate delivery system.

MEDIA RESOURCES

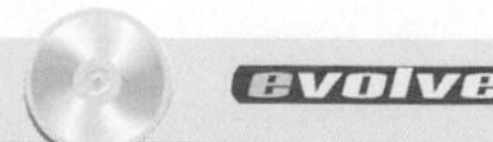

Remember to check out the ***CD Companion*** included with this book for Review Questions, Key Concepts Review, Glossary (with audio for selected terms), Disease Profiles, and Animations.

PLUS, visit the ***Evolve website*** at http://evolve.elsevier.com/Copstead/ for Case Studies, Disease Profiles, and WebLinks.

References

1. Gupta AK et al: Prevalence and epidemiology of onychomycosis in patients visiting physicians' offices: a multicenter Canadian survey of 15,000 patients, *J Am Acad Dermatol* 43(2 pt 1):244-248, 2000.
2. Spanos NP, Williams V, Gwynn MI: Effects of hypnotic, placebo, and salicylic acid treatments on wart regression, *Psychosom Med* 52(1):109-114, 1990.
3. Gulick R: Herpes virus infections. In Arndt KA et al, editors: *Cutaneous medicine and surgery: an integrated program in dermatology,* vol 1, Philadelphia, 1996, Saunders, pp 1074-1092.
4. Dicken CH: Retinoids: a review, *J Am Acad Dermatol* 11(4):541-552, 1984.
5. Yeung-Yue KA et al: Herpes simplex viruses 1 and 2, *Dermatol Clin* 20:249-266, 2002.
6. Epstein JH: Phototherapy and photochemotherapy, *N Engl J Med* 322(16):1149-1151, 1990.
7. Groopman J: Neoplasms in the acquired immune deficiency syndrome: the multidisciplinary approach, *Semin Oncol* 14(2 suppl 3):S1-S6, 1987.
8. Benenson AS, editor: *Control of communicable diseases manual,* ed 16, Washington, DC, 1995, American Public Health Association.
9. Ackerman AB, Cockerell CJ: Papules, *Cutis* 37(4):242-245, 1986.
10. Gonzalez E: Pityriasis rosea. In Arndt KA et al, editors: *Cutaneous medicine and surgery: an integrated program in dermatology,* vol 1, Philadelphia, 1996, Saunders, pp 218-220.
11. Strauss JS: Biology of the sebaceous gland and the pathophysiology of acne vulgaris. In Soter NA, Baden HP, editors: *Pathophysiology of dermatologic diseases,* New York, 1991, McGraw-Hill, pp 195-210.
12. Callen JP: The value of malignancy evaluation in patients with dermatomyositis, *J Am Acad Dermatol* 6(2):253-259, 1982.
13. Kristal L, Clark RAF: Atopic dermatitis. In Arndt KA et al, editors: *Cutaneous medicine and surgery: an integrated program in dermatology,* vol 1, Philadelphia, 1996, Saunders, pp 195-202.
14. Roth H, Kierland R: The natural history of atopic dermatitis, *Arch Dermatol* 89:209-214, 1964.
15. Shear B, Stern RS: Cutaneous reactions to drugs and biologic response modifiers. In Arndt KA et al, editors: *Cutaneous medicine and surgery: an integrated program in dermatology,* vol 1, Philadelphia, 1996, Saunders, pp 412-425.
16. Sober AJ, Fitzpatrick TB: Adverse drug reactions. In Sober AJ, Fitzpatrick TB, editors: *Year book of dermatology,* St Louis, 1990, Mosby, pp 109-120.
17. Rockerbie NR et al: Cutaneous changes of dermatomyositis precede muscle weakness, *J Am Acad Dermatol* 20(4):629-632, 1989.
18. Gilchrest BA, Yaar M: Ageing and photoageing of the skin: observations at the cellular and molecular level, *Br J Dermatol* 127(suppl 41):25-30, 1992.
19. Bryant RA et al: Pressure ulcers. In Bryant RA, editor: *Acute and chronic wounds,* St Louis, 1992, Mosby, pp 105-163.
20. Friedman RJ et al: Skin cancer: basal cell and squamous cell carcinoma. In Holleb AI, Fink DJ, Murphy GP, editors: *Clinical oncology,* ed 7, New York, 1991, American Cancer Society, pp 290-303.
21. Sherman CD et al: Malignant melanomas. In Rubin P, editor: *Clinical oncology: a multidisciplinary approach for physicians and students,* ed 7, Philadelphia, 1993, Saunders, pp 667-675.
22. Boissy RE, Nordlund JJ: Vitiligo. In Arndt KA et al, editors: *Cutaneous medicine and surgery: an integrated program in dermatology,* vol 1, Philadelphia, 1996, Saunders, pp 1210-1218.
23. Berardesca E, Maibach HI: Sensitive and ethnic skin: a need for special skin-care agents? *Dermatol Clin* 9(1):89-92, 1991.
24. Martin S: Variants of normal skin in blacks. In Rosen T, Martin S, editors: *Atlas of black dermatology,* Boston, 1981, Little, Brown, pp 1-16.
25. Ackerman AB, Cockerell CJ: Cutaneous lesions: correlations from microscopic to gross morphologic features, *Cutis* 37(2):137-138, 1986.
26. Arnold HL, Odom RB, James WD: Diseases of the skin appendages. In Arnold HL, Odom RB, James WD, editors: *Andrew's diseases of the skin: clinical dermatology,* ed 8, Philadelphia, 1990, Saunders, pp 879-924.
27. Leyden JJ, Rawlings AV: *Skin moisturization,* New York, 2002, Marcel Dekker.
28. Cohen S: Programmed instruction: skin rashes in infants and children. *Am J Nurs* 78(suppl):S1-S32, 1978.
29. Johnson ML: Skin diseases. In Wyngaarden JB, Smith LH Jr, Bennett CJ, editors: *Cecil textbook of medicine,* vol 2, ed 19, Philadelphia, 1992, Saunders, pp 2280-2330.
30. Dunkle LM et al: A controlled trial of acyclovir for chickenpox in normal children, *N Engl J Med* 325(22):1539-1544, 1991.
31. Arvin AM: Varicella-zoster virus. *Clin Microbiol Rev* 9(3):361-381, 1996.
32. Gilchrest BA: Dermatologic disorders in the elderly. In Rossman I, editor: *Clinical geriatrics,* ed 3, Philadelphia, 1986, Lippincott, pp 375-387.
33. Goldman R: Decline in organ function with aging. In Rossman I, editor: *Clinical geriatrics,* ed 2, Philadelphia, 1979, Lippincott, pp 23-52.
34. Smith L: Histopathologic characteristics and ultrastructure of aging skin, *Cutis* 43(S):414-424, 1989.
35. Cerimele D, Celleno L, Serri F: Physiological changes in ageing skin, *Br J Dermatol* 122(suppl 35):S13-S20, 1990.

chapter 54

Burn Injuries

Nirav Patel • K. John Hartman

MEDIA RESOURCES

Additional Material for Study, Review, and Further Exploration

CD Companion ◆ Review Questions and Answers ◆ Key Concepts Review ◆ Glossary *(with audio pronunciations for selected terms)* ◆ Disease Profiles ◆ Animations

evolve ***Website*** at http://evolve.elsevier.com/Copstead/ ◆ Case Studies ◆ Disease Profiles ◆ WebLinks

KEY QUESTIONS

- What are the most common causes of burn injuries?
- How are burn degree and severity determined?
- What are the principles that guide the management of burn injuries?
- What are the potential complications associated with burn injuries?
- What are the outcomes following burn injuries?

CHAPTER OUTLINE

Burns are injuries to tissues caused by contact with dry heat (flame or hot surfaces), moist heat (steam or hot liquids), electricity (current or lightning), chemicals (corrosive substances), friction, or radiant and electromagnetic energy. Approximately 2.5 million burn injuries occur annually in the United States, of which approximately 50,000 necessitate acute hospitalization. In recent decades, burn mortality rates have decreased significantly, with most patients enjoying excellent functional and cosmetic outcomes. Improved outcomes have clearly been related to an improved understanding of the pathophysiologic mechanism of burns, advances in burn care management, and the development of a comprehensive, treatment-oriented approach to care.[1,2,3a] The American Burn Association in conjunction with the American College of Surgeons Committee on Trauma has been instrumental in promoting the development of burn centers, of which there are now 139 in the United States.[3] Advanced burn life support prehospital and provider courses have also been developed to provide emergency care personnel the skills and information to facilitate rapid assessment, stabilization, and transport of burn victims to appropriate emergency facilities, and providing hospital caregivers guidelines in the assessment and treatment of burn patients during the first 24 hours after injury. The priorities for assessment and treatment of burn victims irrespective of etiologic factors are no different from that of other trauma patients. However, depending on the cause, burn injuries influence a variety of systemic, circulatory, and metabolic changes. As a result, in order to make appropriate treatment decisions and recognize potential complications such as compartment syndrome, rhabdomyolysis, inhalation injuries, and cardiac arrhythmias, a clear understanding of the pathophysiologic processes associated with the burn injury is necessary.

THERMAL INJURY

Etiology

Thermal injuries are burns caused by contact with or exposure to extremes of temperature. Thermal injuries from dry heat result most commonly from exposure to flames or hot surfaces and are often associated with absence of any clear external stigmata such as with inhalation injuries. This also applies to injuries resulting from contact with or exposure to moist heat on one end of the spectrum, and hypothermia and frostbite on the other.

Incidence and Mortality

According to the American Burn Association's 2000 fact sheet, more than 1 million thermal burn injuries occur in the United States each year. This incidence has declined significantly from the 2 million annual injuries estimated in the first report of the National Health Interview Survey (NIHS), drawn from 1957 to 1961 data. As of the early 1990s, the rate of reportable burn injuries in the United States had declined from about 10 per 10,000 to 4.2 per 10,000.[4] Thermal injuries result in approximately 45,000 hospitalizations per year, of which approximately half are to specialized burn treatment centers, and the other half to the nation's approximately 5000 other hospitals.[4] According to the U.S. Centers for Disease Control and Prevention (CDC), in the year 2000 there were 3907 deaths as a result of fire/burn injuries in the United States.[4]

Eighty-five percent of all fire deaths occurred in residential fires, with most of the victims succumbing to smoke inhalation. Although cooking remains the leading cause of residential fires, smoking-related fires remain the leading cause of mortality.[5,6] Dramatic decline in mortality rates has been observed with thermal injuries as a result of advances in our understanding of the pathophysiologic mechanisms, a multidisciplinary team-oriented approach, improved fluid resuscitation strategies, improved infection control, early surgical excision, improved skin grafting techniques, advances in skin substitute development, and overall improved rehabilitation techniques.[7-11]

The fire loss record in the United States is the worst in the industrialized world, with the fire-related mortality double that of most countries on a per capita basis. In the year 2000, residential fires in the United States caused more than $5 billion in property damage.[5] Ignition of upholstered furniture and mattresses by cigarettes was the single leading cause of fire-related mortality. In addition, approximately 200 deaths per year were associated with fires resulting from the use of cigarette lighters, with 125 of these victims being younger than 5 years.[6]

A half century ago, burns over 50% total body surface area (TBSA) resulted in a greater than 50% mortality in pediatric patients.[12] Currently, most children survive burns of this size, and more than half survive burns of more than 90% of their TBSA.[13] Early mortality generally occurred as a result of inadequate initial resuscitation. As vigorous resuscitation protocols were developed, a significant reduction in mortality occurred. Unfortunately, the reduction in mortality was replaced by an increased incidence of wound sepsis. With the advent of topical and systemic antimicrobials, recognition of the importance of maintaining nutrition, early wound excision, and grafting again resulted in a significant reduction in mortality. As a result of these advances, acute mortality in patients with thermal injuries remains relatively low. The primary cause of death in this population now occurs in the subacute setting as a result of pulmonary sepsis, often occurring secondary to inhalation injury. More than 80% of patients sustaining burns have involvement of less than 20% of their TBSA and are treated on an outpatient basis. Despite burn degree, the associated physical and emotional sequelae are often extensive and prolonged. As a result, this unique population requires vigilant follow-up.

Risk Factors

The CDC has identified the following groups as being at high risk for fire-related injuries and deaths: children younger than 4 years; adults 65 years and older; Native Americans and African-Americans; economically challenged individuals; people living in rural areas; and those residing in manufactured homes or substandard housing. Children younger than 15 years account for one third of all admissions to burn units and one third of all deaths from burns and burn-related injuries.[5] Each year, 250,000 children sustain burns severe enough to necessitate medical attention. 15,000 (0.06%) subsequently require acute hospitalization. Scald injuries are the most common in this population and account for up to 60% of all burn injuries. In 1998, nearly 24,000 children were treated for scald injuries, with 20% or more involving an element of abuse or neglect (Figure 54-1).[3a,14] Other causes of pediatric burns include flame injuries (30%), contact with hot surfaces (10%), and chemical and electrical burns (2%) (Table 54-1).[12,14]

Approximately 3000 seniors are injured in home fires annually. The population over 65 years of age accounts for approximately 25% of all burn/fire-related deaths in the United States. Burns in the elderly carry a high mortality rate as a result of preinjury disability, age-related immunosuppression, and impaired healing responses (see Table 54-1).[5]

Environmental and lifestyle factors influence the frequency and magnitude of thermal burn injuries. Alcohol and drug abuse contributes to approximately 40% of all residential fire-related deaths. Neurologic and psychiatric disorders have also been found to increase the risk of accidental burn injury, with one study finding that approximately 3% of patients admitted to the burn unit had thermal injuries associated with neurologic disorders.

Integument Effects

The skin is the largest organ of the body and constitutes approximately 20% of the total body weight. It consists of two layers, the epidermis and dermis, which rest on the hypodermis (or subcutaneous layer). The epidermis contains two main cell types, melanocytes and keratinocytes, as well as

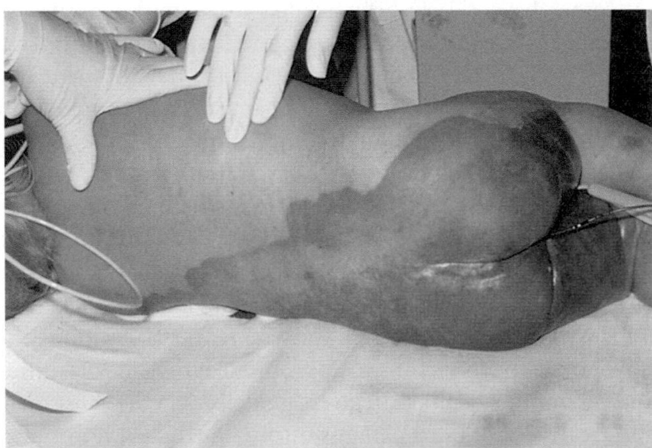

FIGURE 54-1 ■ All burns in children must be carefully evaluated with a consideration for nonaccidental or intentional injury. This 2-year-old boy was immersed by his father in a bathtub of hot water and sustained burns over 55% of his total body surface area. One feature that characterizes abuse burns is a clear demarcation between burned and unburned skin and the absence of drip, spill, or splatter marks. (Courtesy Michael Peck, MD, University of North Carolina Burn Center, Chapel Hill.)

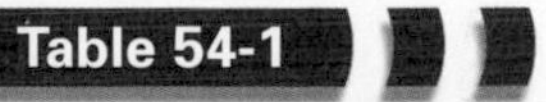

Physiologic Changes Associated with Age

Body System	Pediatric	Elderly
Cardiovascular	Symptoms of shock: Increased heart rate Decreased blood pressure Decreased urine output Cardiac output dependent on heart rate Decreased myocardial compliance Stroke volume plateaus at lower filling pressures Peripheral cyanosis: Neonates: a normal finding Children: decreased cardiac output	Increased chronic disease processes Decreased vascular elasticity results in increased systolic blood pressure Decreased cardiac output Decreased β-adrenergic responsiveness Decreased cardiac stress response Decreased intrinsic heart rate Decreased blood flow Decreased vascular permeability Increased myocardial irritability Decreased myocardial perfusion Increased dysrhythmias Conduction system changes
Pulmonary	Small trachea is easily obstructed Neck hyperextension leads to epiglottal or tracheal obstruction At <8 yr, cricoid cartilage is narrowest airway point At <8 yr, no cuff is needed on endotracheal tube Hypoxemia leads to decreased heart rate in neonates Hypoxemia leads to increased heart rate in children Diaphragmatic breathing Lower airways are easily obstructed Decreased O_2 reserve	Increased need for ventilatory support Increased incidence of inhalation injury Increased pneumonia Decreased lung elasticity Decreased chest wall muscle Decreased oxygen saturation Decreased tidal volume Decreased vital capacity Decreased pulmonary capillary circulation
Thermoregulation and metabolism	Increased resting metabolic rate Increased resting O_2 consumption Increased BSA in relation to body weight Increased hypothermia Increased heat loss from evaporation and convection At <6 mo, inability to shiver to increase body heat Stress leads to hypoglycemia Glycosuria is a sign of infection At <2 yr, buffering capacity is decreased Increased metabolic demands of growth	Increased burn wound infection Increased sepsis Poor or delayed wound healing Increased preexisting malnutrition Decreased febrile response Increased hypothermia
Gastrointestinal and renal	Decreased endogenous calorie stores Increased diarrhea with fluid and calorie deficits At <2 yr, gastric emptying is delayed At <2 yr, increased gastric distention At <30% TBSA burn, can take sufficient calories by mouth At >30% TBSA burn, requires caloric supplementation At <12 mo, poor renal filtration and absorption	Increased volume sensitivity Decreased nutritional status Increased likelihood of hypotensive or hypertensive renal damage Increased incidence of type 2 diabetes mellitus Decreased creatinine clearance

Continued

Table 54-1

Physiologic Changes Associated with Age—cont'd

Body System	Pediatric	Elderly
Neurocognitive	Increased incidence of cerebral edema with fluid resuscitation Increased irritability Increased regressive behavior Increased risk taking behavior Immature judgment	Decreased brain mass Decreased cerebral nerve cells Decreased brain cortex layer Decreased cerebellar cortical cells Decreased nerve conduction velocity Decreased memory Decreased electroencephalographic activity Slower reaction time Decreased taste Decreased smell Decreased vision Decreased hearing Increased pain threshold Decreased judgment and cognitive abilities
Immune	Immature immune system Decreased immunocompetence	Decreased number of leukocytes Decreased immunocompetence Decreased T-cell response

From Carrougher GJ, editor: *Burn care and therapy,* St Louis, 1998, Mosby, p 100.
BSA, Body surface area; *TBSA,* total body surface area.

multiple appendages such as hair, nails, and glands (sweat and sebaceous). The appendages, although originating from the epidermal layer, are anatomically located in both the epidermis and the dermis. Keratinocytes constitute 95% of the epidural binary cell system and synthesize keratin. The melanocytes are scattered throughout the basal layer (stratum germinativum) and produce melanin, a pigment that shields deeper structures of the skin from sunlight. Two types of sweat glands are found in the skin. Apocrine glands, the large sweat glands, are rudimentary structures with no known useful purpose. They respond to autonomic nerve stimulation rather than thermal stimulation to produce an odorless, viscous, milk-like droplet from the hair shaft. Apocrine glands are more numerous in women and are located in the axilla, areola of nipples, groin, perineum, and perianal and periumbilical regions. Eccrine glands are small sweat glands distributed over the body that act as true secretory glands and produce the sweat responsible for heat regulation. At environmental temperatures above 31° C or 32° C (90° F), sweating occurs over the entire body; at lower temperatures, microscopically visible droplets are secreted periodically as part of the total insensible water loss from the body. Sweat normally provides skin with an acid mantle (average pH, 5.7 to 6.4) that retards growth of the many bacteria that reside in the keratin layer, glands, and hair follicles. The function of sweat glands is severely altered in areas of thermal injury after healing, and they become hypersecretory (Box 54-1).

Sebaceous glands secrete sebum, a complex mixture of lipids that is emptied into the hair shaft. The rate of production of sebum and its location depend on androgens, which initiate and continue production. During the hypermetabolic state that follows major thermal injury, production of sebum is decreased, leading to the dry skin conditions commonly found after recovery.

Thermal injury to the integument occurs in two phases. The first is immediate and is a result of direct cellular injury. The second is delayed and occurs as a result of the associated progressive dermal ischemia.

The degree of tissue destruction is related to the duration of exposure and the temperature, or the amount of energy, to which the skin is exposed. The cellular damage is the product of protein denaturation. There are three zones of injury described in the burn wound. The first is the zone of necrosis and is the area in the burn wound where coagulation necrosis has occurred. This area is surrounded by the zone of stasis, a region with decreased blood flow, which can be returned to normal with appropriate resuscitation or converted to necrosis in the case of dehydration, infection, or decreased perfusion. The zone of hyperemia surrounds the zone of stasis and is comprised of minimally injured tissue that usually recovers normal function within 1 week.[15]

In response to thermal injury, keratinocytes develop from cells in the basal layer of the epidermis and progress upward from the stratum germinativum to the stratum corneum over a 14-day period. Over this time the wound develops a light pink or reddish coloration, with normal skin color restored in a delayed fashion by the melanocytes. Regeneration of hair and nails is dependent on viability of the hair follicle and nail

Box 54-1

Normal Physiologic Functions of the Skin Altered or Lost After Thermal Injury

Protection

Barrier between the internal organs and the external environment

Continuous with the mucous membrane at the external openings of organs of the digestive, respiratory, and urogenital systems

Acidic skin (pH 4.2 to 5.6) and perspiration protect against bacterial invasion

Thickened skin of palms and soles provides padding

Percutaneous Absorption

Epidermis is relatively impermeable to most chemical substances; some may be absorbed through the epidermis or the orifices of hair follicles

Sensory Processing

Receptor skin nerve endings allow constant monitoring of the environment by sensing warm and cold temperature, pain, touch, and pressure

Production

Endogenous production of vitamin D_3, which is necessary for synthesis of vitamin D

Barrier

Skin prevents water and electrolyte loss, maintains moist subcutaneous tissues, and prevents water absorption during immersion

Thermoregulation

The body continuously produces heat as a byproduct of cellular metabolism; heat is dissipated through skin

Internal body temperature is regulated by radiation, conduction, or convection

Rate of heat loss depends primarily on the surface temperature of skin, which is a function of skin blood flow

Immunologic

The major site of immune complexes is the dermal-epidermal junction and the dermal vessels of skin

Monocyte/macrophage system is mobilized by local tissue mediators

Circulatory

Skin temperature depends on the rate of blood flow through the skin

Circulatory system distributes pharmacologic agents to local tissues

Aesthetic

Provides the individual identity of a person

matrix. With intact follicles, hair generally grows back at approximately 1 cm per month. New nail formation is often irregular and of abnormal thickness as regrowth occurs.

Major burns produce a chain of pathophysiologic changes characterized by the onset of shock and related hypoperfusion, acid-base imbalance, erosion of tissues, bacterial infection, and organ dysfunction or failure. The body responds to serious burns with increases in energy expenditure, enhanced catabolism, and accelerated loss of lean body mass. Patients with severe burns are susceptible to systemic inflammatory response syndrome, adult respiratory distress syndrome, and multiple organ dysfunction syndromes.[16]

Burn injury activates the immune system. The body responds to burn injury by producing inflammation, which might be seen as a summoning of the forces that are needed to repair damaged tissue. After the injury occurs, blood vessels constrict to reduce blood loss, clots form, and healing cells migrate to the wound. Edema, a potentially dangerous condition, may begin to emerge almost immediately and continue for several days. The inflammatory period lasts about 2 weeks.[16]

As the inflammatory period progresses, fiber-producing cells called fibroblasts contribute to wound repair by producing the structural protein collagen, which strengthens the damaged dermis. Fibroblasts also produce elastin, a protein that adds elasticity to the wound, but its contribution is considerably less significant than that of collagen. As these proteins and other elements begin the healing process, macrophages respond to the inflammation by attacking bacteria and other foreign substances.

New vascular networks begin to form during the inflammatory period and continue their development in the subsequent proliferative stage. New epithelial cells move inward from the edges of the injury and wound contraction begins, although deeper burns require wound excision and skin grafting to facilitate healing.

Depth Classification

Depth of burn injury is divided into five classifications: first degree, second degree (superficial partial thickness and deep partial thickness), third degree, and fourth degree, based on criteria established by the American Burn Association (Table 54-2).[17]

First-Degree Burns

First-degree burns involve only superficial tissue destruction in the outermost layers of the epidermis, with no associated compromise of the function of the skin (see Table 54-2). These burns are often associated with local discomfort,

Table 54-2
Burn Wound Classification

Degree of Burn	Cause of Injury	Depth of Injury	Wound Characteristics	Treatment Course
First-degree burn	Prolonged ultraviolet light exposure, brief exposure to hot liquids	Limited damage to epithelium, skin intact	Erythematous, hypersensitive, no blister formation	Complete healing within 3-5 days without scarring
Superficial partial-thickness burn: second degree	Brief exposure to flash, flame, or hot liquids	Epidermis destroyed, minimal damage to superficial layers of dermis, epidermal appendages remain intact	Moist and weepy, pink or red, blisters, blanching, hypersensitive	Complete healing within 21 days with minimal or no scarring
Deep partial-thickness burn: second degree	Intense radiant energy; scalding liquids or hot semiliquids (e.g., tar) or solids; flame	Epidermis destroyed, underlying dermis damaged, some epidermal appendages remain intact	Pale, decreased moistness, blanching absent or prolonged; intact sensation to deep pressure but not to pin-prick	Prolonged healing (often longer than 21 days), may require skin grafting to achieve complete healing with better functional outcome
Full-thickness burn: third degree	Prolonged contact with flame, scalding liquids, steam; hot objects; chemicals; electrical current	Epidermis, dermis, and epidermal appendages destroyed; injury through dermis	Dry, leatherlike; pale, mottled brown, or red; thrombosed vessels visible; insensate	Requires skin grafting
Full-thickness burn: fourth degree	Electrical current, prolonged contact with flame (e.g., unconscious victim)	Epidermis, dermis, and epidermal appendages destroyed; injury involves connective tissue, muscle, and possibly bone	Dry; charred, mottled brown, white, or red; no sensation; limited or no movement of involved extremities or digits	Requires skin grafting, amputation of involved extremities or digits likely

From Carrougher GJ, editor: *Burn care therapy,* St Louis, 1998, Mosby, p 138.

erythema, and mild systemic responses such as headache, chills, nausea, and vomiting. Erythema, a thermovascular response that occurs in first-degree burns in the absence of direct trauma to the dermis, is probably related to the release of tissue contents in the superficial circulation. First-degree burns are generally self-limiting, require no fluid resuscitation, and are therefore not included in estimates of the percentage of TBSA burned. However, in infants and elderly, first-degree burns may lead to systemic dehydration, necessitating intravenous resuscitation. Therapy generally includes simple analgesia. These injuries typically heal in 3 to 5 days without scarring or pigmentation changes.

Second-Degree Burns

Superficial Partial-Thickness Burns. Superficial partial-thickness burns involve the epidermis and dermis and appear red to pale ivory. Moist, thin-walled blisters often form within minutes of the injury (Figure 54-2). Pain is a major clinical feature of this depth of injury as tactile and pain sensors remain intact (see Table 54-2). Injuries typically heal in 21 to 28 days in the absence of wound infection. The amount of scarring that follows is a genetically determined trait, with some groups of people tending to scar excessively (African-Americans and Caucasians with red hair) or minimally (Native American and Asian groups). Hair follicles remain intact and will regrow hair in the area of injury. Hair usually reappears 7 to 10 days after injury.

Deep Partial-Thickness Burns. Deep partial-thickness burns may involve the entire dermis and leave only the epidermal skin appendages located in the hair follicles. The area of injury has a mottled appearance, with large areas of waxy-white tissue surrounded by light pink or red tissue. The surface is generally dry, and blisters tend to resemble flat, dry tissue paper rather than the fluid-filled raised areas seen with superficial partial-thickness injury. Tactile and pain sensors are either absent or greatly diminished in the area of deepest

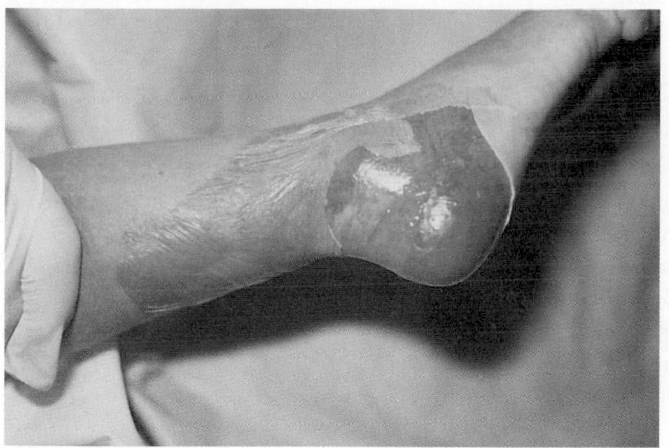

FIGURE 54-2 ■ This young child sustained a hot water scald burn on the heel of the right foot that resulted in a superficial second-degree burn. A superficial second-degree (partial-thickness) burn will reepithelialize within 3 weeks. These burns are characterized by loss of epidermis (blistering) and by a shiny, sensate, vascularized dermis. (Courtesy Michael Peck, MD, University of North Carolina Burn Center, Chapel Hill.)

tissue destruction, but this area is usually surrounded by margins of lesser depth of injury in which pain and tactile sensors remain intact. Deep partial-thickness injury is visually and clinically indistinguishable from full-thickness injury at the time of injury. These wounds heal spontaneously in previously healthy people in about 4 weeks in the absence of secondary infection. The longer the time to healing, the more significant the scarring and depigmentation is observed. As a result, these burns are often excised early and subsequently skin grafted in an effort to diminish scarring and achieve early wound closure.

Third-Degree Burns

Third-degree burns involve the entire epidermis, the dermis, and the underlying subcutaneous tissue. Immediately following injury, these areas appear white, cherry red, or black. Deep blisters may be present under a dry layer of dehydrated skin. Superficial blood vessels coagulated by the heat of injury may be visible through the skin as thrombosed veins. One of the physiologic characteristics of the skin that is lost (see Box 54-1) is the elasticity of the dermis, resulting in a wound with a dry, hard, leathery texture. The massive edema that accompanies major burn injury combined with the loss of elasticity may result in a tourniquet-like effect when the injury occurs circumferentially around a limb or torso. This often necessitates escharotomies or, rarely, fasciotomies to restore distal circulation.

Full-thickness burns are painless to touch, as all superficial nerve endings in the skin have been destroyed. However, as with partial-thickness injuries, rarely are burn injuries totally uniform, and an area of lesser injury in which pain and tactile sensors are intact is usually located on the periphery. Areas of full-thickness injury require skin grafting with the patient's own skin as all dermal elements have been destroyed, leaving no residual tissue for regeneration. However, small injuries often heal by secondary intention as a result of ingrowth of dermal elements from the margins of the wound.

Fourth-Degree Burns

Full-thickness injuries that extend beyond the dermis and involve muscle, bone, or both are often classified as fourth degree. These injuries often occur in victims of high-voltage electrical injury or those who have had prolonged exposure to intense heat, such as unconscious fire victims.

Extent of Injury

Extent of injury refers to the percentage of TBSA burned. Estimates can be calculated with the rule of nines (Figure 54-3) or the Lund and Browder chart (Figure 54-4). The rule of nines is commonly used in prehospital settings and emergency departments, and provides a rough estimate of TBSA involved. The Lund and Browder chart, or a variation of it, is generally used in burn centers and is more precise particularly in assessing TBSA in children under the age of 10 years (see Figure 54-4).

Severity Classification

The severity of a burn injury is determined by the extent to which the physiologic functions of the skin are disrupted beyond the body's normal ability to respond with compensatory mechanisms. The American Burn Association[17] classifies burn injury as minor, moderate, and major (Table 54-3). The severity of the burn injury and the eventual morbidity and mortality associated with it are related to a combination of factors: the patient's medical history, the extent and depth of the burn, the body area involved, the presence of concomitant trauma sustained at the time of the burn, and the patient's age.

Acute Management

The first priority in burn management is the elimination of the source of burn. People whose clothing has caught fire tend to run, thereby increasing exposure time and extent of the injury. This is compounded by inhalation injury from the flaming gases from the burning garments. A national campaign to educate the public, the "stop, drop, and roll" campaign, has had a significant impact in decreasing the severity and extent of flame burns associated with clothing fires. The physical rolling helps extinguish flames from the mechanical standpoint, whereas the supine position also serves to keep the flames away from the face and airway. People familiar with the "stop, drop, and roll" concept often acutely tend, as a natural instinct, to run, and hearing somebody repeat the phrase often may initiate the action. If despite reinforcing the concept the appropriate action is not seen, attempts should be made to assist the individual in accomplishing it. However, extreme

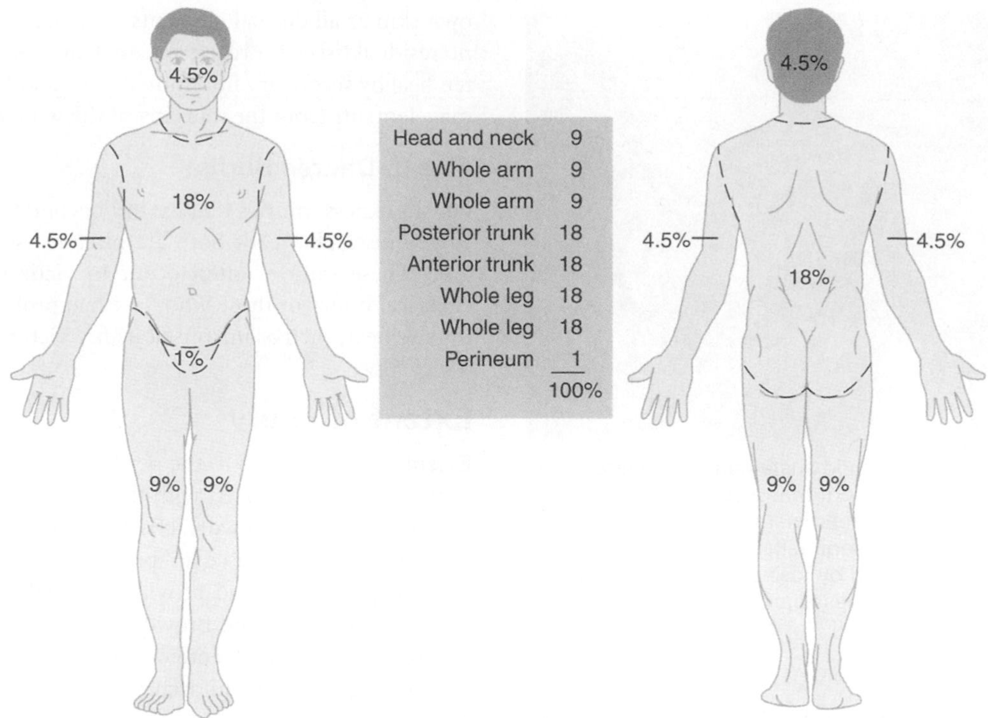

FIGURE 54-3 ■ The rule of nines is a commonly used assessment tool that permits a timely and useful estimate of the percentage of total body surface area burned.

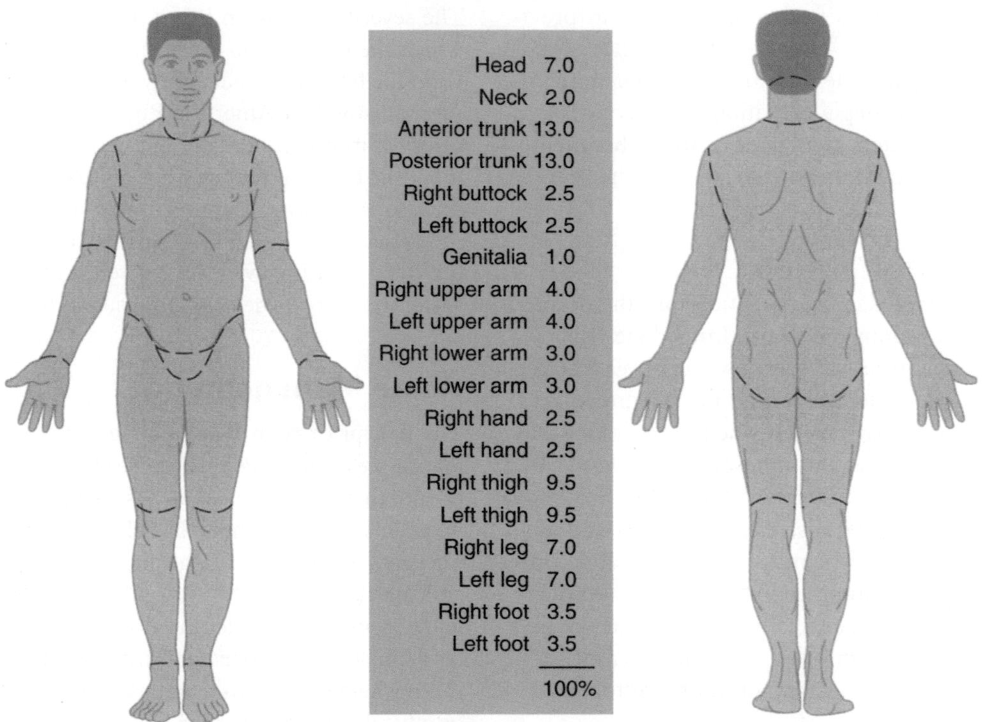

Head 7.0
Neck 2.0
Anterior trunk 13.0
Posterior trunk 13.0
Right buttock 2.5
Left buttock 2.5
Genitalia 1.0
Right upper arm 4.0
Left upper arm 4.0
Right lower arm 3.0
Left lower arm 3.0
Right hand 2.5
Left hand 2.5
Right thigh 9.5
Left thigh 9.5
Right leg 7.0
Left leg 7.0
Right foot 3.5
Left foot 3.5
100%

FIGURE 54-4 ■ The Lund and Browder chart. The areas of the body are presented in section, which permits a more accurate estimation of burn size.

Table 54-3

American Burn Association Burn Severity Classification Schedule

Classification	Assessment Criteria
Minor burn injury	<15% TBSA burn in adults <40 yr old <10% TBSA burn in adults >40 yr old <10% TBSA burn in children <10 yr old *and* <2% TBSA full-thickness burn without risk of cosmetic or functional impairment or disability
Moderate burn injury	12%-25% TBSA burn in adults <40 yr old 10%-20% TBSA burn in adults >40 yr old 10%-20% TBSA burn in children <10 yr old *and* 10% TBSA full-thickness burn without cosmetic or functional risk to burned area involving the face, eyes, ears, hands, feet, or perineum
Major burn injury	>25% TBSA burn in adults <40 yr old >20% TBSA burn in adults >40 yr old >20% TBSA burn in children <10 yr old *or* >10% TBSA full-thickness burn (any age) *or* Injuries involving the face, eyes, ears, hands, feet, or perineum likely to result in functional or cosmetic disability *or* High-voltage electrical burn injury *or* All burn injuries with concomitant inhalation injury or major trauma

Modified from American Burn Association guidelines. In Carrougher GJ, editor: *Burn care and therapy,* St Louis, 1998, Mosby, p 94.
TBSA, Total body surface area.

caution must be exercised to ensure that the rescuer does not become a victim. If available, water should be used to put out the fire, as it not only eliminates the source of the heat but also enables cooling of the underlying skin. The water need not be sterile or even clean, as the primary objective is elimination of the source. In the absence of any available water, flames may be smothered with a blanket, coat, or any other nonflammable covering that will aid in deprivation of oxygen required for combustion. Once the flames are eliminated, the cover should be promptly removed to enable escape of the underlying heat, thereby minimizing injury depth. Scald injuries are best treated initially with cool water, which allows cooling of the scalding liquid as well as the underlying skin. Contact burns from chemicals are managed by removing the clothing; dusting off any powdered chemicals; and subsequent dilution of the chemicals by copious flushing with water.[18] No attempts, however, should be made to neutralize chemicals on the skin, as neutralization is a heat-producing chemical reaction resulting in a compounding thermal injury component. Burns from tar, asphalt, or melted plastics are also initially treated with water. If no water is available, the material is allowed to cool to room temperature, which generally occurs within 2 to 3 minutes. However, the increased exposure duration often results in significant increase in burn extent. Once cooled, the material acts as a sterile dressing; therefore no attempt should be made to remove it unless it is causing in a life-threatening airway compromise.

Assessment

Patients with thermal burn injuries are trauma patients, and clinicians should treat them as such by following the ABCs (airway-breathing-circulation) of trauma resuscitation.[3a] During the course of resuscitation, the possibility of associated inhalation injury suggested by history or physical findings such as facial hair singeing or carbonaceous sputum should be recognized. Inhalation injuries generally evolve over time; therefore in the presence of findings highly suggestive of inhalation injury, consideration should be given early to bronchoscopy and possible intubation.[19] Compromise of breathing in burn patients is often attributed to underlying inhalation injury or circumferential full-thickness burns resulting in impaired chest excursion. Although such injuries do occur, burn patients, like other trauma patients, are also at risk of developing pneumo- or hemothoraces, as well as chest wall instability from multiple segmental fractures (flail chest). These should be sought and, if identified, appropriately treated. Vascular access is preferentially obtained peripherally through unburned tissue if possible. If no such sites are available, access may be established through burned skin. The patient is then evaluated for any other associated traumatic injuries, which are identified and managed as required. TBSA is then determined using a standardized chart such as the Lund-Browder (see Figure 54-4). Fluid resuscitation requirements are subsequently determined and initiated while the patient is placed on clean sheets and the burned areas are wrapped in sterile dressings. The wounds, however, should not be treated with any topical agent such as Silvadene in the acute setting. Burns should not be covered with cool wet sheets as these quickly become cold wet sheets, and with the loss of the burned skin's ability to regulate body temperature, hypothermia quickly ensues. A Foley catheter is also placed to monitor urine output during resuscitation, and in patients with burns greater than 20% TBSA, if possible, a nasogastric tube should be placed to allow for gastric decompression to minimize risk of aspiration and gas bloat. Transfer of patients to burn units or other facilities with appropriate resources is initiated during the course of the initial assessment. The American College of Surgeons Committee on Trauma has developed a set of burn unit referral criteria to assist initial evaluators in triage (Box 54-2).

Box 54-2

Burn Unit Referral Criteria

- Partial-thickness burns greater than 10% TBSA
- Burns that involve the face, hands, feet, genitalia, perineum, or major joints
- Third-degree burns in any age group
- Electrical burns, including lightning injury
- Chemical burns
- Inhalation injury
- Burn injury in patients with preexisting medical disorders that could complicate management, prolong recovery, or affect mortality
- Any patients with burns and concomitant trauma (such as fractures) in which the burn injury poses the greatest risk of morbidity or mortality; in such cases, if the trauma poses the greater immediate risk, the patient may be initially stabilized in a trauma center before being transferred to a burn unit; physician judgment will be necessary in such situations and should be in concert with the regional medical control plan and triage protocols
- Burned children in hospitals without qualified personnel or equipment for the care of children
- Burn injury in patients who will require special social, emotional, or long-term rehabilitative intervention

From American College of Surgeons Committee on Trauma: *Resources for optimal care of the injured patient,* Chicago, 1999, The College, p 55.
TBSA, Total body surface area.

Burn Shock and Acute Resuscitation

Two different but simultaneous mechanisms occur in cases of major burns: local wound pathophysiologic processes related to the loss of skin integrity and systemic pathophysiologic processes related to sequelae of the burn injury. The most immediate systemic change identified is burn shock and includes pathophysiologic changes in the cardiovascular system that are profound, systemic, and lethal without timely and appropriate medical intervention to support the patient's failing cardiovascular system.

Within minutes of a burn injury, the cardiovascular system, which is normally a closed, semipermeable system, becomes an open system through which the patient's circulating volume leaves the circulatory system. This phenomenon, known as "capillary leak," occurs within a few minutes of injury and persists for 24 hours. Burn shock is not confined to the burn area but, rather, is a systemic process. As the capillary system throughout the body becomes leaky, fluid lost in the

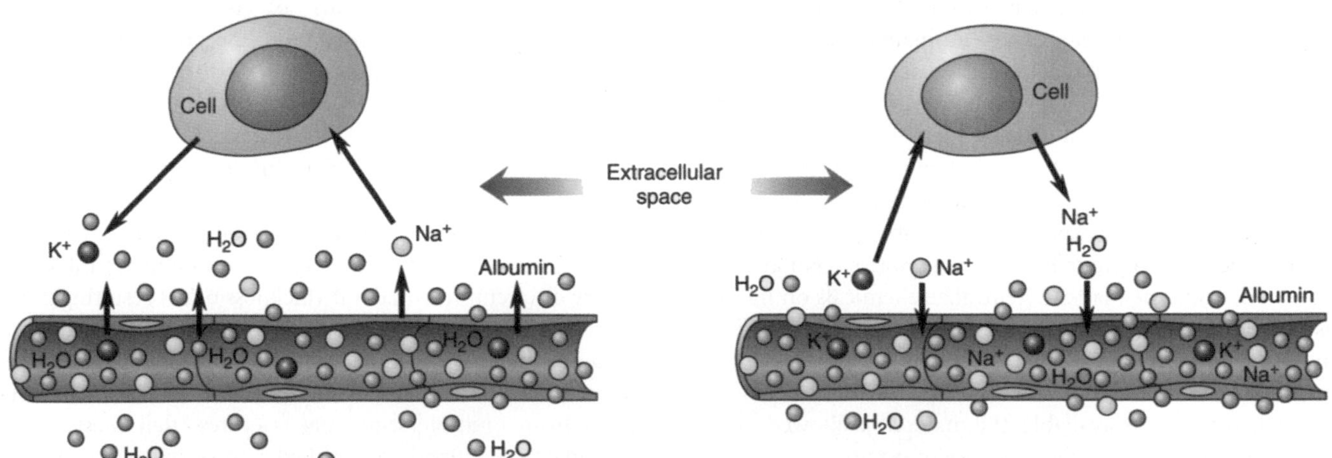

FIGURE 54-5 ■ Direction of fluid and electrolyte shifts associated with burn shock. During burn shock, K^+ is moving out of the cell, and Na^+ and H_2O are moving in. After burn shock, K^+ moves in, and Na^+ and H_2O move out.

area of the burn leaks through the burn into the environment in an evaporative fashion, whereas fluid loss internally collects in the nearby soft tissues, producing extensive edema (Figure 54-5).

Restoration of the patient's circulating volume is an essential part of acute burn management. The rate and volume of fluids lost are related directly to the severity of burn. Therefore, the extent and depth of the burn injury must be ascertained during the initial clinical assessment.

The most widely used formula to guide fluid resuscitation within the first 24 hours of burn injury is the Parkland formula (Box 54-3). The formula utilizes lactated Ringer solution as the resuscitation fluid, as it most closely approximates the fluid it is replacing and thereby minimizes the profound electrolyte imbalances often seen with large-volume resuscitation. Colloid is rarely used in the acute phase of fluid resuscitation (Box 54-4). The standardized formulas provide an excellent guideline for initiating fluid resuscitation but do not ensure adequacy of resuscitation. Depending on the underlying pathophysiologic state and degree of burn, few patients will require less than the predicted 5 ml/kg/% TBSA. Patients with accompanying inhalation injury, burns extending into muscle, and those in whom fluid resuscitation is delayed often require more. In Carotto's series, 30 patients with mean TBSA of burns of 27% received 6.7 ± 2.8 ml/kg/% TBSA burn to ensure adequate resuscitation.[20] Adequacy of resuscitation is as determined by the global response of the patient to the fluid administration and not by one single variable.[21] Markers commonly used to reflect adequacy of resuscitation include normalization of mental status, blood pressure, pulse, capillary refill, arterial pH, base deficit, and maintenance of urine output at 0.5 tol ml/kg per hour for adults and 1 to 1.5 ml/kg per hour for children. In addition to the fluid volumes calculated by the standardized formulas, the patient should also receive appropriate maintenance fluid over the first 24-hour period.

Approximately 24 hours following the acute burn injury, the capillary leak syndrome begins to resolve as cardiovascular integrity is restored. At this time, collagen solution such as albumin may be administered according to a formula (see Box 54-4) in an effort to replace the protein lost during the acute burn shock phase.

One of the major functions of intact skin is to serve as a barrier to water evaporation. With major burn injury, this ability of the skin to regulate evaporative loss is totally disrupted. In a classic study done in 1962, Moncrief and Mason[22] attempted to determine the magnitude of such a loss and found that daily evaporative loss was in the range of 20 times normal in the early phase of burn injury, with gradual decreases as wound closure was achieved. Further studies revealed that the insensible water loss through burned skin is not caused by evaporation of water from sweat glands but rather by water vapor formed within the body and lost through the skin.[23,24] The amount of evaporative water loss through the burn wound per hour may be calculated using the following formula: (25 + % TBSA burn)m^2 of body surface area. Thus, a 70-kg patient with a 50% TBSA burn requires an additional 3 L of free water per day to replace evaporative losses. As the patient progresses to the subacute phase of re-

Box 54-3

Parkland Formula for Fluid Resuscitation in Burn Shock

During the first 24 hours after a burn, administer intravenous LRS at the following rate:

4 ml LRS/% TBSA burn/kg body weight

where

- Time is calculated from the time of burn injury
- TBSA is total body surface area
- Half of the total fluid is administered in the first 8 hours after burn
- One fourth of the total is administered in the second 8 hours
- One fourth of the total is administered in the third 8 hours or in quantities to maintain adult urine output at 30 ml/hr or child urine output at 1 ml/kg/hr

Example of formula calculation in a 70-kg patient with a 50% TBSA burn:

4 ml × 70 kg × 50% TBSA burn = 14,000 ml (14 L) LRS in 24 hr

- Administer 7000 ml in the first 8 hours at 875 ml/hr
- Administer 3500 ml in the second 8 hours at 437 ml/hr
- Administer 3500 ml in the third 8 hours at 437 ml/hr

Data from Baxter CR: Guidelines for fluid resuscitation, *J Burn Care Rehabil* 2:279-286, 1981.
LRS, Lactated Ringer solution; *TBSA,* total body surface area.

Box 54-4

Plasma Requirements and Evaporative Water Loss After Burn Injury

Colloid Replacement

Twenty percent of blood volume given as fresh-frozen plasma or plasma expander
Adult males: 20% = 5 ml/kg body weight
Adult females and children: 20% = 8 ml/kg

Maintenance Fluids Until Wound Closure Is Achieved

Basal fluid requirements
1500 ml fluid/m^2 TBSA = 24-hour requirement
Evaporative water loss from burn wound until healed
Adults: (25 + % TBSA burn) × m^2 BSA = ml/hr requirement
Children: (35 + % TBSA burn) × m^2 BSA = ml/hr requirement
Maintenance fluids equal basal fluid requirements plus evaporative water loss and may be administered intravenously, orally, or by nasogastric or jejunal tube, according to patient need

BSA, Body surface area; *TBSA,* total body surface area burned.

suscitation, it is imperative that attention be paid to these unaccountable losses.

Children and older patients require special care. Older patients are more likely to have cardiopulmonary disease, chronic illnesses, and weakened immune systems, all of which complicate fluid resuscitation. Children are also sensitive to resuscitation volumes that are insufficient or exceed requirements. Table 54-1 summarizes the physiologic changes associated with age that increase the vulnerability of children and elderly persons.[25-27]

Organ Dysfunction

Cardiovascular Dysfunction

Burn shock is often accompanied by a precipitous drop in cardiac output that does not parallel the gradual reduction in blood volume and is refractory to restoration of the circulating volume. This finding of low cardiac output in the presence of vigorous intravenous fluid resuscitation and massive catecholamine release has led to the suggestion of a specific myocardial depressant factor.[28-31] The pathophysiologic mechanism behind this myocardial dysfunction is poorly understood. There appears to be no simple, specific myocardial depressant factor but rather a cascade of events involving metabolic and immunologic factors (Figure 54-6).[14]

Respiratory Dysfunction

Respiratory dysfunction following burn injury generally is the result of obstruction, interstitial alterations, and metabolic changes. Obstruction generally occurs as a result of edema of the upper airway secondary to direct injury, but more often the generalized edema that occurs following fluid resuscitation in the face of an ongoing capillary leak syndrome that often accompanies burn injuries. On occasion, burns of the oral cavity and upper airway occur as superheated air is inhaled or hot water enters the mouth. The pulmonary system is extremely efficient at dissipating heat and prevents the inhalation of superheated air beyond the bronchi, but steam may permeate further into the lung parenchyma (Figure 54-6).[15,19]

Airway obstruction secondary to edema generally has its onset within the first few hours following burn injury but tends to manifest clinically 2 to 4 hours later as resuscitation is undertaken. Endotracheal intubation is recommended prophylactically when impending airway obstruction is identified. The endotracheal tube is preferably secured with cotton twill tape that enables readjustment to allow for the increase in head and face circumference related to increasing facial and soft tissue edema.[32]

Smoke or fume inhalation often leads to acute hypoxia that is refractory to oxygen administration. Inhalation injury di-

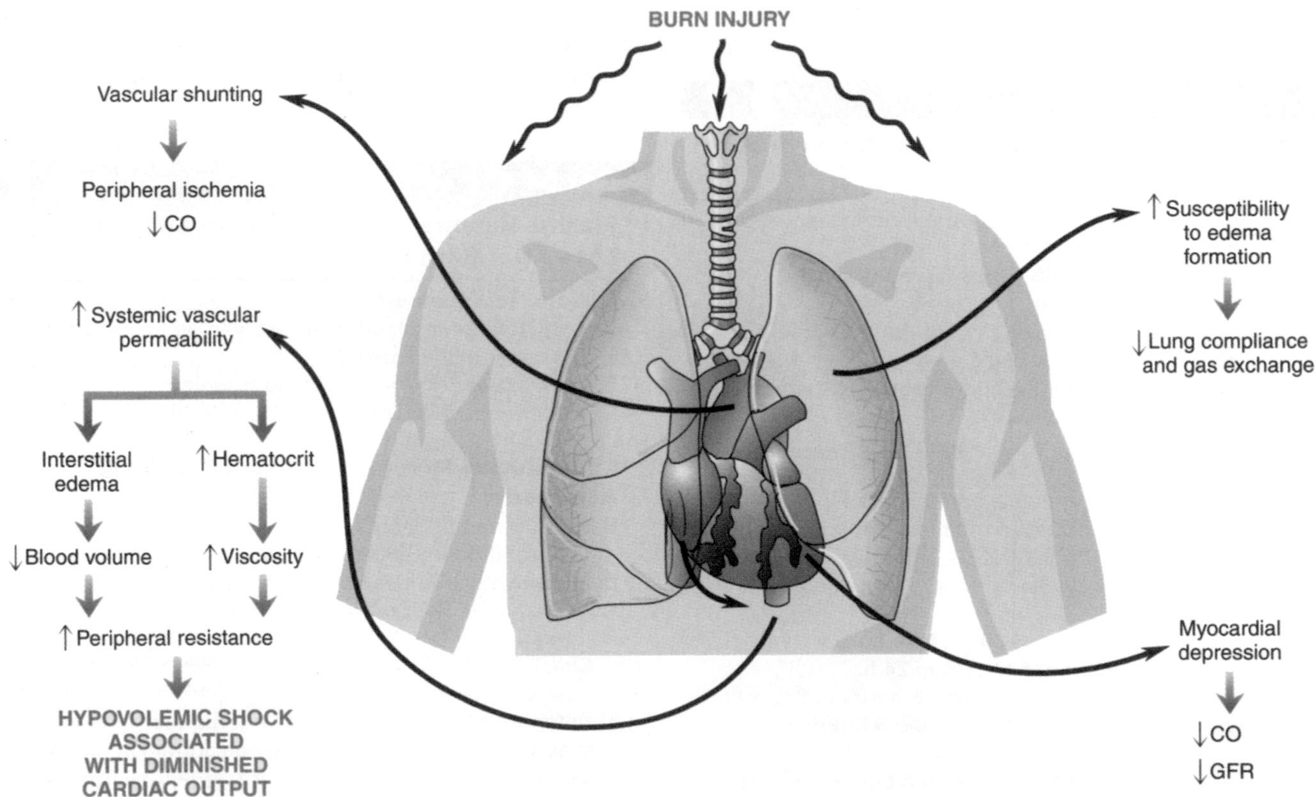

FIGURE 54-6 ■ Cardiovascular and pulmonary effects of major burn injury within the first 24 hours after burn injury, during burn shock. *CO,* Cardiac output; *GFR,* glomerular filtration rate.

rectly results in the chemical denaturing of pulmonary tissue, and the subsequent edema results in increased distances over which oxygen must diffuse to the capillaries. This often progresses to adult respiratory distress syndrome. Treatment consists primarily of ventilatory support.[32]

Carbon monoxide poisoning often accompanies smoke inhalation. The other toxic components of smoke vary depending on the products of combustion produced in a particular fire. The initial treatment of all patients with suspected smoke inhalation injury is the administration of oxygen, as this results in dilution of the carbon monoxide and accelerates its elimination.[3a]

Metabolic Changes

Acute burn injury results in changes in the body's metabolism related to the massive release of catecholamines into the general circulation as part of the "fight-or-flight" reaction that accompanies major trauma. The metabolic response to the stress of a major burn injury involves the response of the sympathetic nervous system and other homeostatic regulators. Hypermetabolism is manifest as a sustained heart rate in the 120 to 140 beats/min range and oxygen consumption increased to about 150% of normal. The hypermetabolism of burn injury generally persists until the burn wound is reduced to less than approximately 20% TBSA. This burn-related hypermetabolism poses a major challenge in the treatment of these patients. A number of modalities for ameliorating this hypermetabolism have been tried, including reduction of metabolic rate using propranolol, administration of counter-regulatory hormones such as insulin and insulin-like growth factor, and stimulation of anabolism using growth hormones and steroids (natural or synthetic). A study from Shriner's Burns Institute in Galveston, Texas, randomized 56 children with major burns to receive supplemental growth hormone, propranolol, or both. Propranolol markedly reduced resting heart rate and energy expenditure measured by indirect calorimetry and improved net muscle protein synthesis. Interestingly, the addition of growth hormone did not increase these effects.[26] Muscle protein wasting appears to be caused primarily by accelerated protein breakdown. Although protein synthesis is also increased, it fails to keep pace with proteolysis and amino acid mobilization. Thomas et al. evaluated the effect of continuous infusions of insulin (to maintain blood glucose levels between 100 and 140 mg/dl) on preservation of muscle mass in a randomized controlled clinical trial in 18 children with major burns. Evaluation of each patient when 95% healed showed that insulin-treated patients had improved lean body mass, less muscle wasting, and reduced length of hospital stay in comparison with controls.[33]

Gianotti and colleagues studied temporal fluctuations in insulin-like growth factor type I and its binding protein in a group of burn patients, and demonstrated that both decline for the first 14 days after the burn, paralleling decreases in prealbumin and transferrin.[34] However, plasma levels of growth hormone remained unchanged. In a small trial in children, administration of insulin-like growth factor type I and insulin growth factor binding protein appeared to exert widespread effects in ameliorating acute inflammation by reducing the synthesis of type 1 and 2 acute phase proteins and interleukin 6 (IL-6) while increasing synthesis of constituted protein such as prealbumin and transferrin. Anabolic steroids, including testosterone and analogs like oxandrolone, are widely used to ameliorate muscle wasting in patients with cancer and acquired immunodeficiency syndrome. However, studies have suggested limited benefits associated with their use in burn patients.

Cellular Changes

Major burn injury affects the entire body, but survival ultimately depends on its effect at the cellular level. The cellular response to burn injury occurs as a metabolic and an immunologic pathophysiologic process. The basic pathologic condition, named the "sick cell syndrome" by Welt [35] in 1967, is a cell membrane transport defect related to an alteration in the steady-state composition, characterized by high intracellular concentrations of sodium. Entry of sodium into the intracellular space occurs simultaneously with entry of water, which leads to cellular edema and, possibly, rupture of the cell wall. Trunkey et al.[36] found a marked decrease in primate muscle extracellular water and an increase in intracellular sodium and water during burn shock. An associated decrease in resting membrane potential occurs as the transmembrane potential is disrupted and results in a decrease in amplitude of the action potential and prolongation of the repolarization and depolarization time.[37,38] As sodium and water enter the cell, the sodium-potassium pump is disrupted and potassium moves out, thus further exacerbating the electrolyte imbalance intracellularly.[39] Calcium channel transport is disrupted, along with a loss of intracellular magnesium and phosphate[31] and an increase in serum lactate dehydrogenase levels.[40] The cascade of events that occurs at the level of the cell membrane suggests impairments of basic cellular function as the underlying cause of the diminished membrane potentials. Although the pathophysiologic mechanism has not been completely described, data suggest a decrease in the efficiency of the sodium-potassium pump, a change that can be reversed over time with adequate fluid resuscitation.

Evidence suggests that the burn wound itself at least partially mediates the physiologic response to burn injury at both the local and systemic level. Burn tissue inflammation can lead to vasodilation, increased capillary permeability, and edema, which would be normal conditions that promote wound healing. Despite profound redistribution of the peripheral circulation after burn injury, both heat and glucose are preferentially transported to the wound. Massive injury results in increased metabolic demands and consumption of inflammatory mediators by the wound when the priority for survival should be transport of these mediators to healthy tissue.

The extensive evaporative water loss that accompanies burn injury is a heat-consuming process, with the energy need met in part by increased visceral heat production. This hypermetabolic state persists during rest, sleep, and external cooling. The increased oxygen consumption cannot be accounted for on the basis of elevated body temperature alone; thus, an increased basal metabolic rate, not a thermoregulatory drive, is responsible for the increased heat production.

Immune Response

The immune system normally protects the body from disease by recognizing foreign material and mobilizing the body's defenses to maintain homeostasis. When the body is burned, the immune response is immediate and extensive. Burn, which upsets homeostasis more than any other injury, can profoundly suppress the immune system and thereby increase the risk of infection. The result in individuals surviving burn shock is immunosuppression with increased susceptibility to potentially fatal system burn wounds, pulmonary sepsis, or both.

Local and systemic physiologic changes are caused by the release of cytokines from burn wounds.[41] Cytokines act directly on the burn wound and also activate other agents, including those that release oxidants, arachidonic acid metabolites, and proteases, thereby contributing to further local and systemic inflammation and, potentially, multisystem organ dysfunction. Recent studies have shown a relationship between decreased cellular cytotoxicity in burned patients and increased production of the cytokines IL-4 and IL-10. Research also shows that the administration of immunopotentiators such as IL-12 improves mortality rates and resistance to bacterial infection.[42]

A host of chemicals found in altered concentrations in burn plasma may also play a role in burn shock. These substances include vasoactive amines (histamine, serotonin), products of complement activation (C3a, C5a), prostaglandins, kinins, endotoxin, and metabolic hormones (catecholamines, glucocorticoids). A decrease in the complement components C3a and C5a in the circulation after burn injury suggests nonspecific activation of the complement system. Activation of the complement system in injured tissue results in an inflammatory response caused by the release of histamine and serotonin by C3a and C5a. Because both histamine and serotonin alter capillary permeability, some investigators propose this mechanism as a cause for burn shock inasmuch as these vasoactive amines initiate the inflammatory response along with kinin polypeptides and other chemical mediators. As a result of these vascular changes, fluid and fibrinogen leave the dilated, permeable vessels.

The emergent phase of burn care refers to the time between the end of burn shock and closure of the burn wound to less than 20% TBSA. Three elements are essential for survival after a major burn injury: meticulous wound management, adequate nutritional support to establish positive nitrogen balance, and early surgical excision and grafting of full-thickness wounds. The goal of burn management is wound closure in a manner to promote survival.

Elements of Burn Injury Survival

Management of Wounds

Meticulous wound management consists of measures to limit bacterial proliferation on the wound and adjacent tissue as a result of the loss of the first line of defense—the skin. Burn wounds are sterile initially as a result of thermal decontamination. However, bacterial flora soon reestablish colonies on the burned skin, or eschar. This medium is favorable for pathogenic growth because of the necrotic tissue and warm environment that exist within the burn wound dressing. Benign microorganisms normally found on skin, in the gastrointestinal tract, and in the pulmonary system become lethal as they colonize the burn wound, often resulting in burn progression, invasive sepsis, and death.

The most common source of burn wound bacteria is the patient's own hair follicles, sweat glands, pulmonary tract, and gastrointestinal system, although poor hand-washing technique by staff members can contribute to infection through cross-contamination from other patients.

The goals of wound care are to cleanse and debride the wound of necrotic tissue and debris that promote bacterial growth, minimize further destruction of viable tissue, prevent cross-contamination, preserve body heat and energy, and promote patient comfort. Initial care of the burn wound involves debridement with soap and water. The excision of blisters is controversial and varies from institution to institution. Wound care requires daily observation and management, which includes bathing the patient at least once each day with mild soap and water. Burn wounds are washed to remove accumulated bacteria and previously applied ointments and to debride necrotic tissue. Cleansing of wounds is the most stressful and painful experience that burn patients endure. Pain medication diminishes the pain only marginally because the most effective analgesics work best on visceral or deep pain rather than pain at superficial skin nerve endings. Benzodiazepines are often added to decrease anxiety and provide a degree of amnesia.

After the wound is clean, topical antibacterial agents are applied and covered with a light dressing (Table 54-4). Systemic antibiotics are not helpful in controlling burn wound flora because the burn eschar has no blood supply, limiting local antibiotic bioavailability. Topical burn agents penetrate the eschar, thereby inhibiting bacterial invasion of the wound. Systemic antibiotics are administered when the patient demonstrates signs of systemic infection and are used prophylactically at times of surgical procedures. Appropriate antibiotic selection is based on laboratory cultures of the patient's wound tissue to identify and deliver antibiotics to which the bacteria are sensitive.

Healing of burn wounds begins when white blood cells have surrounded the burn wound and phagocytosis begins.

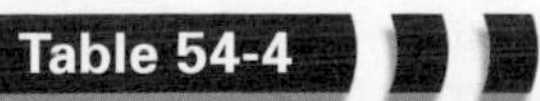

Topical Antibiotic Therapy for Thermal Injury Wounds

Drug	Indications for Use	Advantages	Disadvantages	Method of Use
Bacitracin	Bland ointment with minimal antibiotic properties used to promote comfort in patients with minor injury (<25% TBSA)	Prevents drying of wounds, keeps eschar soft and pliable, economical, works well on facial burns to promote healing and patient comfort without facial dressings, painless upon application	No major antibiotic properties; oil based, so it is difficult to wash away	1. Apply to cleansed wound twice daily, cover with Adaptic and Kerlix 2. Apply to facial burns twice daily 3. Apply to recently grafted or healed areas twice daily, wrap with Adaptic and Kerlix
Silver sulfadiazine (Silvadene)	Partial- and/or full-thickness thermal injury (>25% TBSA); small wounds that require topical antibiotic therapy such as frostbite	Wide-spectrum bacteriostatic action and painless on application; organisms resistant to silver nitrate are usually sensitive to silver sulfadiazine; eschar remains soft and pliable; water-miscible base promotes ease of removal	Not effective against fungal organisms, can cause leukopenia, expensive; sulfa component can produce allergic reactions in sensitive patients; resistance can emerge with prolonged use	Apply to cleansed wound 1-3 times daily; may leave wound open or cover with light dressing
Silver nitrate	Partial- and/or full-thickness burns (>25% TBSA), fungal infections, patients with sulfa allergy	Wide-spectrum bacteriostatic action, effective against fungal infections, comfortable, economical, no sensitivity reported, painless on application, no resistant organisms	Can cause severe electrolyte imbalances (hyponatremia and hypochloremia), which are corrected with oral and intravenous NaCl; poor penetration into wound; requires bulky dressing, thereby severely limiting motion; messy and time consuming to use	0.5% solution in distilled water applied to wet dressing every 2 hr; dressing changes twice daily
Mafenide acetate (Sulfamylon)	Electrical injury, ear burns, wounds colonized with organisms resistant to other topical agents because it penetrates eschar more deeply	Wide-spectrum bacteriostatic action; active penetration allows delayed therapy to be effective; requires no dressing, thereby promoting motion; resistant organisms do not develop with prolonged use; drug of choice for all	Causes severe metabolic alterations within 72 hr when used on >20% TBSA wounds; carbonic anhydrase inhibition with HCO_3^- excretion and chloride retention; compensation is by hyperventilation with subsequent CO_2 decreased or depletion	Apply to cleansed wound 1-2 times daily. Leave open because wrapping produces maceration

From Kravitz M: Thermal injuries. In Cardona VD et al, editors: *Trauma nursing: from resuscitation through rehabilitation,* Philadelphia, 1988, Saunders, p 723.
TBSA, Total body surface area.

Necrotic tissue begins to slough. Fibroblasts begin to lay down matrices of the collagen precursors that eventually form granulation tissue. Kept free from infection, a partial-thickness burn will heal from the edges and from below in a process that occurs over a 14- to 21-day period. Full-thickness burns require autografting to achieve wound closure because no dermal elements are available to form new skin.

Burn Surgery

The third element essential to survival after major burn injury is surgical excision of dead skin, or burn eschar, followed by skin grafting with the patient's own skin (autograft). Areas of full-thickness burn are excised. In some cases it is difficult to assess the depth of the burn. In these cases it may be appropriate to wait 7 to 10 days to allow the area to declare its depth. This is especially true in young children with scald burns. In burns involving the face, scalp, and ears, it may be appropriate to wait as long as 3 weeks for the area to declare itself. These sites are particularly dense areas of dermal appendages and may heal without grafting if given time. Current medical management of burn wounds involves early removal of the necrotic tissue followed by split-thickness autografts. This therapy has changed the management of burn care in the past 20 years from one of daily bathing and mechanical debridement of necrotic tissue for months after burn injury to one of early surgical removal of the burn wound and a dramatic reduction in hospitalization time. In the past, patients with major burns had low rates of survival because healing and wound coverage took so long that death from infection usually occurred before healing. Now, mortality and morbidity are greatly decreased as a result of early surgical intervention.

Excision and Grafting. The two types of surgical excision are *tangential excision* and *full-thickness excision*. With tangential excision, eschar is removed in thin layers with an instrument called a dermatome until viable tissue is visible. The procedure is usually done 2 to 7 days after injury. Full-thickness excision using surgical knives removes eschar to fascia. Full-thickness excision often leaves an uneven contour postexcision, which is difficult to graft, with resultant poor cosmetic effects. After bleeding has been controlled in the area of excision, application of an autograft, skin substitute, or dressing follows. To establish optimal conditions for autografting, the area is often covered with wet dressings soaked in antibiotic solutions for 24 hours, with delayed autografting. Both tangential and full-thickness excision procedures involve massive blood loss often requiring red blood cell transfusion.

Skin Substitutes. Several temporary biological dressings are available for patients with extensive burns that do not permit initial autografting. Products available for temporary coverage include homograft (skin harvested from cadavers), xenograft (skin harvested from pigs), synthetic skin (a variety of products for temporary coverage), and amnion (amniotic lining of human placenta harvested from afterbirth following human delivery). Integra is a bilayer membrane that provides a dermal matrix of bovine collagen and an epidermal layer of silicone to prevent desiccation (drying). The matrix allows ingrowth of capillaries and fibroblasts. The matrix is slowly degraded as a neodermis develops. The silicone layer is then removed and allograft is applied over the neodermis.[43]

These dressings promote patient comfort while partially restoring the water vapor barrier and some antibacterial properties to the wound until an autograft is available. The unburned area of the patient from which skin is harvested in a paper-thin sheet is referred to as the donor site. Donor sites heal in about 5 to 7 days in the presence of adequate nutritional support and the absence of infection and can be reharvested at that time. Donor sites can be repeatedly harvested depending on graft thickness, enabling increased wound coverage, which thereby permits survival in some patients with TBSA injury as large as 90%. To expand the surface area that a sheet of autograft will cover, skin is cut in a manner that resembles a net or mesh by using an instrument called a skin mesher. The skin may then be expanded, depending on the size of the mesh, to cover two, three, four, or more times its original size. This combination of repeated harvesting and meshing allows autografting of massive burn injuries over a period of a few weeks. After grafting, the areas must be protected from infection, pressure, shearing, and trauma that produce bruising or bleeding under the graft. Bulky dressings are used the first few days, followed by the use of wraps and elastic bandages to protect extremity or trunk grafts. Patients are returned to the operating room about once a week until the grafting procedures are complete.[44]

The greatest risk of infection is after postoperative day 3, as the bacteria begin to recolonize the area. Grafts are usually stable by postoperative day 4 at which time physical and occupational therapy can begin.[6,45]

Surgical wound management of elderly burn patients is determined by the philosophy of the burn center. Elderly patients do not generally tolerate any surgical procedure as well as younger patients; this knowledge has been applied to the management of burn wounds in some patients, and conservative, nonsurgical wound management for weeks after injury has produced acceptable survival rates in elderly patients.[46] Others report that early excision of eschar and early wound closure are associated with increased survival and decreased length of stay for older patients with burns.[47] Children younger than 2 years have a high mortality rate with major burn injury, but older children recover at a high rate with proper medical management.[9,11,26] Table 54-5 summarizes physiologic changes related to the aging process that can affect surgical outcome.

Nutritional Support for Positive Nitrogen Balance

Healing occurs only in a state of positive nitrogen balance. Hypermetabolism characterizes the metabolic response to thermal injury; with the magnitude of the physiologic alteration related to the extent of the burn injury. One of the most significant advances in recent burn management is recognition of the critical importance of nutrition to the wound healing process. The magnitude of nutritional support required by burn patients depends on two factors: the patient's preburn nutritional status and the extent of the TBSA burn. Patients with minor burns require no nutritional support beyond a regular diet, whereas those with moderate and large burns require additional carbohydrate and protein supplementation. Patients with poor preburn nutritional status are classified as having a critical injury regardless of the burn size due to the associated immune deficiencies and limited metabolic reserves. The most easily recognized and documented finding in the absence of adequate nutritional support after burn injury is massive loss of body weight. Maintenance of body protein appears to be critical for survival. Loss of one fourth to one third of the protein mass from the body is predictably fatal; this degree of negative nitrogen balance in humans is associated with a 40% to 50% body weight loss.

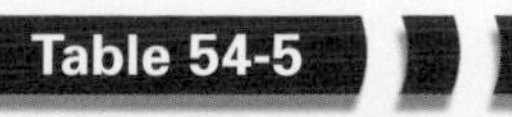

Table 54-5

Physiologic Changes Related to the Aging Process That Can Affect Surgery

Physiologic Changes	Effects	Potential Postoperative Complication
Cardiovascular		
↓ Elasticity of blood vessels ↓ Cardiac output ↓ Peripheral circulation	↓ Circulation to vital organs Slower blood flow	Shock (hypotension), thrombosis with pulmonary emboli, delayed wound healing, postoperative confusion, hypervolemia, decreased response to stress
Respiratory		
↓ Elasticity of lungs and chest wall ↑ Residual lung volume ↓ Forced expiratory volume ↓ Ciliary action Fewer alveolar capillaries	↓ Vital capacity ↓ Alveolar volume ↓ Gas exchange ↓ Cough reflex	Atelectasis, pneumonia, postoperative confusion
Urinary		
↓ Glomerular filtration rate ↓ Bladder muscle tone Weakened perineal muscles	↓ Kidney function Stasis of urine in bladder Loss of urinary control	Prolonged response to anesthesia and drugs, overhydration with intravenous fluids, hyperkalemia, urinary tract infection, urinary retention
Musculoskeletal		
↓ Muscle strength Limitation of motion	↓ Activity	Atelectasis, pneumonia, thrombophlebitis, constipation or fecal impaction
Gastrointestinal		
↓ Intestinal motility	Retention of feces	Constipation or fecal impaction
Metabolic		
↓ γ-Globulin level ↓ Plasma proteins	↓ Inflammatory response	Delayed wound healing, wound dehiscence or evisceration
Immune System		
Fewer killer T cells ↓ Response to foreign antigens	↓ Ability to protect against invasion by pathogenic microorganisms	Wound infection, wound dehiscence, pneumonia, urinary tract infection

From Keeling AW, Muro GA, Long BC: Preoperative nursing. In Phipps WJ et al, editors: *Medical-surgical nursing: concepts and clinical practice,* ed 5, St Louis, 1995, Mosby.

Patients with greater than a 40% TBSA burn demonstrate the maximal stress response within predictable ranges of body mass. In these hypermetabolic patients, providing early protein and caloric support of at least the predicted energy requirement is necessary for optimal outcome and may be essential for survival. Weight loss after thermal injury is not an obligatory component of the response to trauma but rather a reflection of the difference between the total energy requirements and the ability to supply them in the form of adequate caloric intake.[13] Kao et al. demonstrated that enteral feeding should begin within 18 hours of admission with a Dobhoff feeding tube.[48] These feedings should be continuous and should not be stopped when the patient goes to the operating room. With early initiation of vigorous nutritional support, initiated within this time frame, erosion of total body mass and subsequent starvation leading to immunologic alteration are not inevitable in a massively burned patient.[39,49,50]

General formulas are used to estimate the caloric requirements of burn patients, all of which are based on either preburn body weight and % TBSA burn or square meters of body surface area and % TBSA burn. The two most widely used formulas are the Curreri formula for adults and the Polk formula for children. Curreri et al.[51] demonstrated that caloric requirements in adult burn patients could be expressed by the following formula:

(25% body weight [kg]) + (40% TBSA burn) = 24-hour caloric needs

The requirements in children[52] are predicted as follows:

(60% body weight [kg]) + (36% TBSA burn) = 24-hour caloric needs

It is important to emphasize that these formulas represent more than just total caloric intake; they are used to predict positive nitrogen balance for each patient. Thus if the patient is losing tremendous amounts of nitrogen or is not absorbing glucose, the net caloric utilization will be much less than the intake, even though the adult patient may be receiving as much as 5000 kcal/day. Monitoring of daily nitrogen balance by indirect calorimetry is essential throughout the course of burn treatment to ensure a positive nitrogen balance (nonprotein kilocalorie to nitrogen ratio of 100:1 and at least 2 g of protein per kilogram per day). The prealbumin concentration is a useful indicator of nutritional progress.

The routes for initiating caloric support after major burn injury are either enteral or parenteral. Any patient with a functioning gastrointestinal tract should receive enteral nutrition orally, by tube feeding, or by a combination of both. In some burn patients, enteral feeding may not be possible, and intravenous hyperalimentation may become the only method available for providing nutritional support. The possibility of infection may be increased when hyperalimentation is used.

Hart et al. demonstrated that the catabolic response may continue for 4 to 6 months in adults and as long as 9 months in children.[53] Given this information, the nutritional status and dietary habits of burn patients should be continually evaluated for many months after their discharge from the burn unit.

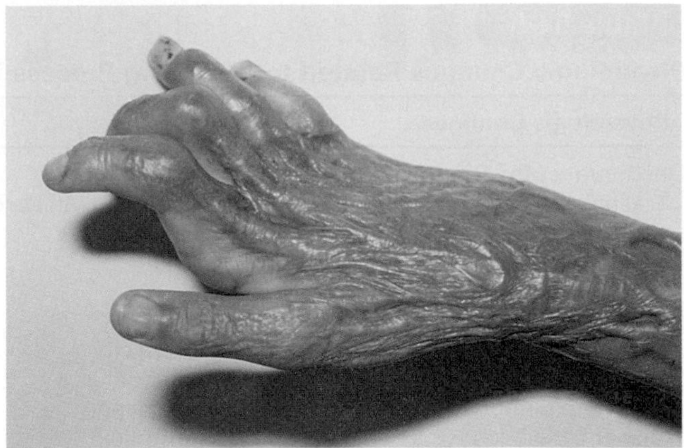

FIGURE 54-7 ■ Physical and occupational therapy is necessary from the time of injury. This 8-year-old girl was burned 4 years previously in a house fire. Inadequate follow-up because of parental neglect led to severe scar contractures and hand disability. (Courtesy Michael Peck, MD, University of North Carolina Burn Center, Chapel Hill.)

Rehabilitation Phase

The rehabilitation phase begins when the burn size is reduced to less than 20% TBSA and the patient is capable of assuming some self-care. This phase may occur as early as 2 weeks or as long as 2 to 3 months after the burn and, in the case of a major debilitating or disfiguring injury, may last many years. Goals for this period are to assist the patient in resuming a functional role in society and to accomplish functional and cosmetic reconstruction.[6,8,10]

Wound Healing

During the rehabilitation phase the pathophysiologic mechanism of hypermetabolism and the impaired immune function have begun to be restored to normal, although some changes will persist beyond discharge from the hospital. The major pathophysiologic process of this phase is related to the dysfunctional results of wounds healing in a manner that causes flexor contractures, excessive scarring, and keloid formation. The burn wounds have healed either by primary intention or by autografting. Layers of epithelialization begin building back the tissue structure destroyed by the burn injury. Collagen fibers present in the new scar tissue help healing and add strength to weakened areas. After healing, the new skin appears flat and pink, even in dark-skinned people.

In approximately 4 to 6 weeks the area becomes raised and hyperemic. If adequate range-of-motion exercises are not instituted early in the hospital course, the new tissue will shorten and a contracture will result (Figure 54-7).[6,8] Mature healing is reached in 6 to 12 months, when suppleness has returned and the pink or red color has faded to a slightly lighter hue than the surrounding unburned tissue. It takes longer for darker skin to regain its color because many of the melanocytes were destroyed, and often the skin never regains its original color. The mesh pattern in meshed autograft fades with time, but in larger expansions such as 4:1 or greater the pattern may persist.

Scarring has two components: discoloration and contour. The discoloration of scars fades with time and can be covered with makeup on visible body surface areas. However, scar tissue tends to develop altered contours; that is, the skin is no longer flat but becomes raised above the contour of the surrounding area (also known as hypertrophic scarring). Areas of the face tend to scar in an even plane—a process that deletes the natural contours around the nose, chin, and mouth and thus greatly alters a patient's appearance. Scarring on the cheeks can contract and pull the lower eyelid down sufficiently to prevent closure and protection of the eye normally afforded by the eyelid—a condition called ectropion. Burns on the eyelid can also result in ectropion and must be corrected by reconstructive surgery. Pressure can help keep a scar flat if the pressure is slightly greater than capillary pressure and is continuous during the healing process. This knowledge led to the development of burn garments, which are custom made for each patient to contour with pressure over the area of burn for about 12 to 18 months after burn injury. Except for bath times, the garments must be worn continuously; patient compliance often becomes an issue (Figure 54-8).

Excessive and sometimes debilitating discomfort from itching occurs in the healing burn wound and persists for many months. The exact pathophysiologic process is not known but is related to the absence of sebaceous glands in the area and to the hyperactivity of sweat glands. Topical lotions and orally administered antihistamines give partial relief of symptoms, but tolerance to the drugs develops and patients often require a series of different medications over time. The newly formed skin is extremely sensitive to trauma, and blisters form after very slight pressure or friction. The newly healed areas may be hypersensitive or hyposensitive to cold, heat, or touch. Ward et al.[54] studied loss of cutaneous sen-

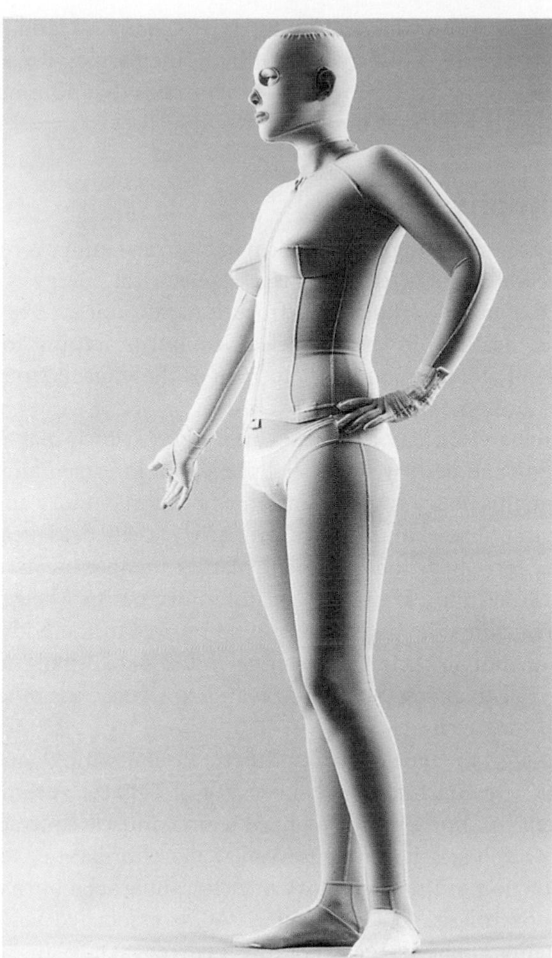

FIGURE 54-8 ■ The custom-fitted antiscar support garment modeled here effectively provides pressure therapy over wounds, which helps to minimize the development of hypertrophic scarring. (From Black JM, Matassarin-Jacobs E, editors: *Medical-surgical nursing: clinical management for continuity of care,* ed 6, Philadelphia, 2001, Saunders, p 1356. Courtesy Medical Z Corp., San Antonio, Tx.)

sibility after grafting in 60 patients and found that 97% demonstrated markedly diminished or absent responses to sharp/dull, hot/cold, and light touch stimuli over the grafted areas. Grafted areas are more likely to be hyposensitive until peripheral nerve regeneration occurs, although donor sites harvested several times will show all the same healing pathologic process as healed burn wounds.

Scarring is a genetically inherited trait. Some people will have minimal scarring whereas others, especially African-Americans and Caucasians with red hair, tend to have significant scarring and keloid formation in which the scar tissue actually outgrows the bounds of the original wound. Healed burn wounds must be protected from direct sunlight for 1 year to prevent hyperpigmentation.

The most common complications during the rehabilitation phase are related to the formation of skin and joint contractures. Because of pain associated with movement, the patient will want to assume the position of comfort, which is with all extremities flexed, but this position predisposes to contracture formation. To minimize contracture formation, postioning in extension, splinting in the position of function, and active range-of-motion exercises are initiated on admission and continue throughout the course of treatment. The areas most subject to contracture formation include the anterior and lateral neck areas, axillae, antecubital fossae, fingers, groin areas, popliteal fossae, and ankles. Not only do contractures develop in the skin, but the underlying tissues such as ligaments and tendons also have a tendency to shorten during the healing process. Therapy is aimed at extension of body parts to ensure that the flexors are longer than the extensors.[6]

KEY CONCEPTS

- The emergent phase is the time between the end of burn shock and closure of the wound to less than 20% TBSA. Wound management, nutritional support, and surgical grafting of full-thickness wounds are the priorities of treatment during the emergent phase.
- Wound management is necessary to prevent bacterial colonization of the wound and subsequent septicemia. Early surgical wound management is essential. Topical antibiotics are used because systemic antibiotics cannot reach the wound because of a lack of blood supply.
- Nutritional requirements after burn injury are high. A high-calorie, high-protein diet is needed. Persons with major burns usually cannot ingest sufficient nutrients and require parenteral and enteral supplementation. A positive nitrogen balance is essential for healing.
- Early surgical excision and skin grafting are the treatment of choice for deep burns. Excision procedures result in significant blood loss requiring blood transfusions. Skin grafts are taken from a healthy portion of the patient's skin. Temporary grafts (e.g., cadaver skin, synthetics, pig skin) may be used to cover the wound until an autograft can be obtained.
- The rehabilitation phase begins when the burn is reduced to less than 20% TBSA. Problems during this phase include skin contracture and excessive scarring. Healing is complete at 6 to 12 months. Positioning in extension and range-of-motion exercises are important to prevent contracture.

Factors That Increase Risk

Environmental and lifestyle factors influence the frequency and magnitude of burn injury. Certain factors increase the risk of accidental burn injury, among them alcohol or drug abuse, neurologic or psychiatric disorders, and immobilizing physical disabilities. Alcohol use contributes to an estimated 40% of residential fire deaths. One study found that 3.25% of patients admitted to a burn unit had both thermal injury and neurologic disorders. The occurrence of burns during pregnancy is rare but often results in fetal death, even with relatively small maternal

TBSA burns. In cases of electrical burns the fetal mortality rate is 15% to 73%, and in the case of lightning strike 50%. The high fetal death rate is caused by adaptive mechanisms that identify the gravid uterus and fetal-placental circulation as low priority in the presence of diminished circulating blood volume such as occurs with burn injury.[55]

Between 1980 and 1995 there were 1587 deaths related to fires in the occupational setting in the United States civilian work force.[56] Quinney et al. reported 1189 fatal burns in the workplace from 1992 to 1999.[57]

ELECTRICAL INJURY

Incidence and Mortality

Electrical injury accounts for fewer than 2% of admissions to burn facilities, but injury from electricity has been increasing in the United States.[58] Electrical injuries are classified as high voltage (1000 volts or greater) or low-voltage. Household currents of 120 and 220 volts typically cause low-voltage electrical injury. High-voltage injuries are frequently due to high-tension sources, which commonly carry from 7200 to 19,000 volts (Figure 54-9) but may involve 100,000 to 1 million volts.[59]

Burn facilities serving rural areas tend to have a higher percentage of electrical injury admissions than do facilities serving urban areas.[58] Few of these injuries are the result of household accidents, although toddlers are occasionally injured when they insert metal objects into electrical outlets. Teething infants may sustain electrical burns to the mouth by chewing on electrical cords,[60-62] but electrical current rarely passes through the body.

Lightning injuries kill between 150 and 300 people per year in the United States.[62] Lightning carries a direct current of 100 million or more volts and up to 200,000 amperes, and it can injure either by a direct strike or by a side flash as a result of the flow of current between the victim's body and a nearby object struck by lightning.[62]

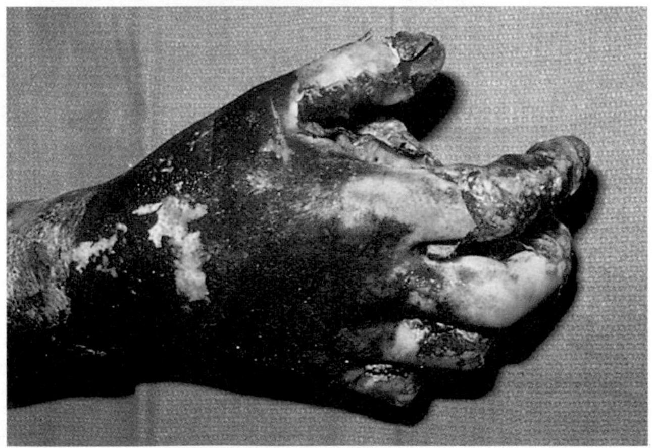

FIGURE 54-9 ■ High-voltage electrical injuries produce devastating injuries, such as the damage to the right hand of this electrician who inadvertently contacted a 17,000-V line. The underlying muscle damage is often greater than the thermal skin burn. Myoglobinuria, if inadequately managed, can lead to acute tubular necrosis. Early fasciotomies are mandatory, and amputation may be necessary to control rhabdomyolysis. (Courtesy Michael Peck, MD, University of North Carolina Burn Center, Chapel Hill.)

Pathophysiology

The pathophysiologic mechanism of electrical injury is related to the subsequent tissue damage as electrical energy is converted to heat. Workplace electrocutions account for 5% of all worker deaths.[63] In children, electrical burns account for 2% to 3% of all burns, and 60% to 70% of these result from biting extension cords.

Arcing electricity produces surface heat, which may ignite clothing and destroy superficial tissue, but internal damage is absent; this injury is actually a flame or thermal injury and not electrical. These injuries are properly classified as heat injuries, for which the treatment plan is identical to that for other heat injuries.[58] True electrical injury occurs as electrical current enters the body, traverses some area of the body, and exits at another body site. Electrical injuries are usually deeper than full-thickness skin injury and are often classified as fourth-degree injury.

Voltage, the type of current (direct or alternating), and the length of contact influence the extent of damage. Alternating current (AC) produces prolonged tetanic muscle contraction. At low voltages it can cause ventricular fibrillation, tetanic contraction of the respiratory muscles, superficial burns, and rhabdomyolysis. At lower voltage AC is associated with low mortality. High-voltage AC or direct current (DC) causes ventricular fibrillation, a single sustained contraction, rhabdomyolysis, and higher overall mortality.[64]

Each true electrical injury produces an entrance wound and at least one exit wound, with the most extensive damage commonly occurring at the exit point. Electrical current follows the path of least resistance: in humans, this path is through blood vessels, nerves, tendons, and bone. Skin has high resistance; thus the current enters through the skin but goes deeper to travel the path of least resistance until it exits the body. The current rarely produces direct visceral damage, but severe injuries to the extremities are common. The amputation rate after severe electrical injury exceeds 90%. The pathophysiologic process, in addition to direct tissue destruction, involves heat coagulation of blood vessels, which leaves distal areas without blood supply. Electrical injuries produce both systemic and local alterations. The systemic changes produce three common complications during the acute period: arrhythmias or cardiac arrest, metabolic acidosis, and myoglobinuria. Electrical injury may also cause direct myocardial necrosis. Arrhythmias are exacerbated by any given voltage of AC. Higher voltage may also cause asystole. Locally, electrical injury produces direct cellular denaturation; areas of healthy tissue are devascularized as a result of heat coagulation of arteries and veins. These events are followed 48 to 72 hours after injury by gross tissue necrosis and subsequent gangrene resulting from lack of blood flow. Amputation is required early in electrical injury to prevent the development of clinical gangrene and sepsis leading to death.

Management, Treatment, and Complications

Once the patient is in the health care system, airway management is the primary focus of concern; patients with major electrical injury often require endotracheal intubation to ensure a patent airway. A condition similar to burn shock develops within a few minutes of major electrical injury and requires similar fluid resuscitation measures. No formula exists to predict fluid requirements for patients with electrical injury shock because often the only apparent damage is the entrance and exit wounds and no assessment of internal damage is possible. An adult patient is given a 1-L bolus of Ringer lactate solution intravenously within the first 15 minutes after intravenous line placement; children are given a smaller, size-appropriate amount. Thereafter, fluid is infused at a rate to produce a urine volume of 100 ml/hr in adults and 1 to 2 ml/kg per hour in children. Adult patients frequently require 1 to 2 L of fluid per hour to support the cardiovascular system.

Patients have traditionally been on cardiac monitoring for the first 24 hours after injury. Bailey et al. determined that this is unnecessary if the initial electrocardiogram (ECG) is normal, there was no loss of consciousness at the scene, and the patient is an adult. Twenty-four-hour monitoring is indicated in adult patients with an abnormal initial ECG, a history of cardiac disease, positive loss of consciousness at the scene, and/or voltage greater than 240 volts.[64] Measurement of cardiac enzymes initially reveals elevated values, also suggesting acute myocardial damage, but in such patients these findings are not indicative of a cardiac pathologic process.

Electrical injury also produces a profound, potentially lethal metabolic acidosis. These patients often have initial serum pH values of 6.8 to 7.2 on admission; pH levels of less than 7.0 are incompatible with survival. Treatment consists of intravenous administration of sodium bicarbonate in amounts to return the values toward normal. Metabolic acidosis is a recurring problem requiring ongoing treatment until the problem resolves 24 to 48 hours after injury. The pathophysiologic mechanism is related to the release of intracellular contents into the general circulation from areas of tissue damage and to the lactic acidosis that accompanies hypotensive shock states.

Myoglobinuria follows electrical injury as myoglobin, a component of muscle tissue, is released from muscles damaged by electrical current and enters the systemic circulation.[65] Myoglobin is a large protein that precipitates in the tubules and leads to cast formation. Subsequently the tubules become obstructed and tubular acidosis develops. This accumulation is prevented by maintaining urine output at 100 to 200 ml/hr in adults and 2 ml/kg per hour in children until the urine clears. Mannitol, an osmotic diuretic, is administered along with large volumes of intravenous fluids to prevent the development of acute tubular necrosis, a totally preventable sequela of electrical injury with proper management. Sodium bicarbonate is often administered to alkalinize the urine, thereby increasing the solubility of myoglobin. Its efficacy in preventing renal failure or dysfunction remains controversial.

Local effects of electrical injury are related to alterations in tissue perfusion. Surgical decompression of areas of electrical burn is performed for the purpose of releasing any increased compartment pressures that may be compromising blood flow. Amputation may be required during the initial surgery for devascularized areas. Because of the continued presence of necrotic tissue, areas of surgical decompression or initial amputation are not closed surgically.[66]

Central nervous system alterations will be noted in all patients with major electrical injury. The typical patient has no short-term memory: events before the injury are remembered clearly, but hour-to-hour memory deficits occur for many weeks. The condition improves gradually and usually resolves 4 to 6 weeks after injury. The patient may not remember the initial hospital course and may experience daily emotional distress because the visual impact of the extensive physical damage is perceived as *new* information with each dressing change. Rarely does the patient have immediate perceptions of altered body image; thus an abrupt crisis may occur as the extent of change is eventually realized. Another complication of short-term memory loss is the patient's inability to remember visitors, which may lead to anger and charges of abandonment toward family members and health care personnel because the patient does not remember who was present earlier. Other central nervous system deficits after electrical injury include ataxia and gait alterations accompanied by sensory deficits. These alterations may improve or remain constant over time.

Electrically injured patients have all the problems of rehabilitation plus possible adjustments to amputation and gait instability related to central nervous system impairment. Skin grafting in areas adjacent to amputation presents challenging prosthetic problems that may delay independent ambulation and restoration of self-care abilities.[67] In general, patients with major electrical injury experience longer rehabilitation periods than do thermally injured patients.

A unique complication of electrical injury is the formation of corneal cataracts,[68] the cause of which is unknown. The cataracts may be detected on ophthalmic examination as early as 1 month or as late as 12 months after injury and may occur in one or both eyes. The electrical injury does not have to be on or near the head for the condition to develop. Progression is rapid, with the cornea becoming completely opaque within months. Ophthalmic examinations should be performed monthly for the first year and then every 3 months during the second year after injury to identify this pathologic process early. The patient will usually complain of blurring vision, but young children may not mention blurring because they do not know the concept. Treatment consists of corneal transplantation.[68]

MEDIA RESOURCES

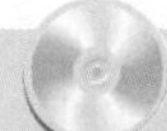

evolve

Remember to check out the ***CD Companion*** included with this book for Review Questions, Key Concepts Review, Glossary (with audio for selected terms), Disease Profiles, and Animations.

PLUS, visit the ***Evolve website*** at http://evolve.elsevier.com/Copstead/ for Case Studies, Disease Profiles, and WebLinks.

References

1. Arturson G: Pathophysiology of the burn wound and pharmacological treatment, *Burns* 22(4):255-274, 1996.
2. Nguyen TT et al: Current treatment of severely burned patients, *Ann Surg* 223(1):14-25, 1996.

3a. Sheridan RL: Burns, *Crit Care Med* 30(11 suppl):S500-S514, 2002.

3. American College of Surgeons Committee on Trauma: *Resources for optimal care of the injured patient,* Chicago, 1999, The College, p 55.
4. National Center for Injury Prevention and Control. Fire Deaths and Injuries: [cited 3 October 2002]. Available from: URL:http://www.cdc.gov/ncipc/factsheets/fire.htm.
5. Istre GR et al: Residential fire related deaths and injuries among children: fireplay, smoke alarms, and prevention, *Inj Prev* 8(2):128-132, 2002.
6. Richard R: OT/PT forum, *J Burn Care Rehabil* 23(3):220, 2002.
7. Ho WS, Ying SY, Burd A: Outcome analysis of 286 severely burned patients: retrospective study, *Hong Kong Med J* 8(4):235-239, 2002.
8. Young A: Rehabilitation of burn injuries (review), *Phys Med Rehabil Clin North Am* 13(1):85-108, 2002.
9. Stoddard FJ et al: Treatment of pain in acutely burned children, *J Burn Care Rehabil* 23(2):135-136, 2002.
10. Partridge J: Psychosocial rehabilitation after burn injuries, *Nurs Times* 97(48):47, 2001.
11. Sheridan RL et al: Long-term outcome of children surviving massive burns, *JAMA* 283(1):69-73, 2000.
12. Muller MJ, Pegg SP, Rule MR: Determinants of death following burn injury, *Br J Surg* 88(4):583-587, 2001.
13. Gore DC et al: Hyperglycemia exacerbates muscle protein catabolism in burn-injured patients, *Crit Care Med* 30(11): 2348-2342, 2002.
14. Gibran NS, Heimbach DM: Current status of burn wound pathophysiology, *Clin Plast Surg* 27(1):11-22, 2000.
15. Arturson G: Forty years in burns research—the postburn inflammatory response, *Burns* 26(7):599-604, 2000.
16. Nebraska Burn Institute: *Advanced burn life support provider's manual,* Lincoln, Nebraska, 1994, Burn Institute.
17. American Burn Association [cited 3 October 2002]. Available from: URL:http://www.ameriburn.org.
18. Berkowitz Z et al: Hazardous substances emergency events in the agriculture industry and related services in four mid-western states, *J Occup Environ Med* 44(8):714-723, 2002.
19. Holm C et al: The relationship between oxygen delivery and oxygen consumption during fluid resuscitation of burn-related shock, *J Burn Care Rehabil* 21(4):391-393, 2000.
20. Cartotto RC et al: How well does the Parkland formula estimate actual fluid resuscitation volumes? *J Burn Care Rehabil* 23:258-265, 2002.
21. Tompkins RG: ABA 2002 presidential address: The American Burn Association in the new millennium, *J Burn Care Rehabil* 22:369-374, 2001.
22. Moncrief JA, Mason AD: Water vapor loss in the burned patient, *Surg Forum* 1962;13:38-41, 1962.
23. Moncrief JA: Burns. In Schwartz SI et al, editors: *Principles of Surgery,* ed 2, New York, 1974, McGraw-Hill, pp 253-274.
24. Roe CF, Kinney JM: Water and heat exchange in third-degree burns, *Surgery* 56:212-220, 1964.
25. White DJ et al: Calcium and cardiac dysfunction after burn trauma, *Crit Care Med* 30(1):14-22, 2002.
26. Sheridan RL, Schnitzer JJ: Management of the high-risk pediatric burn patient, *J Pediatr Surg* 36(8):1308-1312, 2001.
27. Wibbenmeyer LA et al: Predicting survival in an elderly burn patient population, *Burns* 27(6):583-590, 2001.
28. Baxter CR, Cook WA, Shires GT: Serum myocardial depressant factor of burn shock, *Surg Forum* 17:1-2, 1996.
29. Lefer AM, Martin J: Origin of myocardial depressant factor in shock, *Am J Physiol* 218(5):1423-1427, 1970.
30. Ribeiro CA et al: Association between early detection of soluble TNF-receptors and mortality in burn patients, *Intens Care Med* 28(4):474-478, 2002.
31. Sukuki M et al: Correlation between QT dispersion and burn severity, *Burns* 28(5):481-485, 2002.
32. Turnage RH et al: Mechanisms of pulmonary microvascular dysfunction during severe burn injury (review), *World J Surg* 26(7):848-853, 2002.
33. Thomas JA et al: IRAK contributes to burn-triggered myocardial contractile dysfunction, *Am J Physiol Heart Circ Physiol* 283:H829-H836, 2002.
34. Gianotti L et al: Activity of GH/IGF-1 axis in burn patients: comparison with normal subjects and patients with GH deficiency, *J Endocrinol Invest* 25(2):116-124, 2002.
35. Welt LG: Membrane transport defect: the sick cell, *Trans Assoc Am Physicians* 80:217-226, 1967.
36. Trunkey DD et al: The effect of hemorrhagic shock on intracellular muscle action potentials in the primates, *Surgery* 74(2):241-250, 1973.
37. Cunningham JN Jr, Shires GT, Wagner Y: Changes in intracellular sodium and potassium content of red blood cells in trauma and shock, *Am J Surg* 122(5):650-654, 1971.
38. Rosenthal SM, Tabor H: Electrolyte changes and chemotherapy in experimental burn and traumatic shock and hemorrhage, *Arch Surg* 51:244-252, 1945.
39. Turinsky J, Gonnerman WA, Loose LD: Impaired mineral metabolism in post-burn muscle, *J Trauma* 21(6):417-423, 1981.
40. Deets DK, Glaviano VV: Plasma and cardiac lactic dehydrogenase activity in burn shock, *Proc Soc Exp Biol Med* 142(2): 412-416, 1973.
41. Ogura H et al: Long-term enhanced expression of heat shock proteins and decelerated apoptosis in polymorphonuclear leukocytes from major burn patients, *J Burn Care Rehabil* 23(2):103-109, 2002.
42. Rose JK, Herndon DN: Advances in the treatment of burn patients, *Burns* 23(suppl 1):S19-S26, 1997.
43. Boyce ST et al: The 1999 clinical research award: cultured skin substitutes combined with Integra artificial skin to replace na-

tive skin autograft and allograft for the closure of excised full-thickness burns, *J Burn Care Rehabil* 20:453-461, 1999.

44. Minn R et al: Prospective trial of thick vs. standard split-thickness skin grafts in burns of the hand, *J Burn Care Rehabil* 22:390-392, 2001.
45. Latenser BA, Kowal-Vern A: Paediatric burn rehabilitation (review), *Pediatr Rehabil* 5(1):3-10, 2002.
46. Housinger T et al: Conservative approach to the elderly patient with burns, *Am J Surg* 148(6):817-820, 1984.
47. Slater AL, Slater H, Goldfarb IW: Effect of aggressive surgical treatment in older patients with burns, *J Burn Care Rehabil* 10(6):527-530, 1989.
48. Kao CC, Garner WL: Acute burns, *Plast Reconstr Surg* 105(7):2482-2492, 2000.
49. Deveci M et al: Comparison of lymphocyte populations in cutaneous and electrical burn patients: a clinical study, *Burns* 26(3):229-232, 2000.
50. Pratt VC et al: Alterations in lymphocyte function and relation to phospholipid composition after burn injury in humans, *Crit Care Med* 30(8):1753-1761, 2002.
51. Curreri PW et al: Dietary requirements of patient with major burns, *J Am Diet Assoc* 65(4):415-417, 1974.
52. Haynes BW Jr: The management of burns in children, *J Trauma* 12:267-277, 1965.
53. Hart DW et al: Persistence of muscle catabolism after severe burn, *Surgery* 128(2):12-19, 2000.
54. Ward RS et al: Sensory loss over grafted areas in patients with burns, *J Burn Care Rehabil* 10(6):536-538, 1989.
55. Deitch EA et al: Management of burns in pregnant women, *Surg Gynecol Obstet* 161(1):1-4, 1985.
56. Biddle ED, Hartley D: Fire and flame related events with multiple occupational injury fatalities in the United States, 1980-1995, *Inj Control Saf Promot* 9(1):9-18, 2002.
57. Quinney B et al: Thermal burn fatalities in the workplace, United States, 1992 to 1999, *J Burn Care Rehabil* 23(5):305-310, 2002.
58. Artz CP: Electrical injury. In Artz CP, Moncrief JA, Pruitt BA Jr, editors: *Burns: a team approach,* Philadelphia, 1979, Saunders, pp 351-362.
59. Luce EA, Gottlieb SE: "True" high-tension electrical injuries, *Ann Plast Surg* 12(4):321-326, 1984.
60. Leake JE, Curtin JW: Electrical burns of the mouth in children, *Clin Plast Surg* 11:669-683, 1984.
61. Port RM, Cooley RO: Treatment of electrical burns of the oral and perioral tissues in children, *J Am Dent Assoc* 112(3): 352-354, 1986.
62. Jain S, Bandi V: Electrical and lightning injuries, *Crit Care Clin* 15(2):319-331, 1999.
63. American Burn Association: *American Burn Association Committee on Specific Optimal Criteria for Hospital Resources for Care of Patients With Burn Injury,* San Antonio, Tx., 1976, The Association.
64. Bailey B, Gaudreault P, Thivierge RL: Experience with guidelines for cardiac monitoring after electrical injury in children, *Am J Emerg Med* 18(6):671-675, 2000.
65. David WS: Myoglobinuria, *Neurol Clin* 18(1):215-243, 2000.
66. Holliman CJ et al: Early surgical decompression in the management of electrical injuries, *Am J Surg* 144(6):733-739, 1982.
67. Ward RS et al: Prosthetic use in patients with burns and associated limb amputations, *J Burn Care Rehabil* 11(4):361-364, 1990.
68. Saffle JR, Crandall A, Warden GD: Cataracts: a long-term complication of electrical injury, *J Trauma* 25(1):17-21, 1985.

APPENDIX

Clinical and Laboratory Values

Table A-1

Blood, Plasma, and Serum Values

Test	Normal Values*	Significance of a Change
Acid phosphatase	*Women:* 0.01-0.56 sigma U/ml *Men:* 0.13-0.63 sigma U/ml	↑ in kidney disease ↑ in prostate cancer ↑ after trauma and in fever
Alanine aminotransferase (ALT, SGPT)	7-56 U/L	↑ in liver damage
Albumin	3.5-5.0 g/dl	↓ in liver disease ↓ in malnutrition
Alkaline phosphatase	*Adult:* 38-110 IU/L *Child:* up to 104 IU/L	↑ in bone disorders ↑ in liver disease ↑ during pregnancy ↑ in hypothyroidism
Amylase	20-110 U/L	↑ in pancreatitis
α_1-Antitrypsin	110-270 mg/dl	↓ in genetic emphysema
Aspartate aminotransferase (AST, SGOT)	0-35 U/L	↑ in liver damage
Bicarbonate (arterial)	22-26 mEq/L	↑ in metabolic alkalosis ↓ in respiratory alkalosis ↓ in metabolic acidosis ↑ in respiratory acidosis
Blood urea nitrogen (BUN)	5-25 mg/dl	↑ with increased protein intake ↑ in kidney failure
Blood volume	*Women:* 65 ml/kg body weight *Men:* 69 ml/kg body weight	↓ during hemorrhage
Calcium		
Total	8.4-10.5 mg/dl (2.1-2.6 mmol/L)	↑ in hypervitaminosis D ↑ in hyperparathyroidism ↑ in bone cancer and other bone diseases ↓ in hypoparathyroidism ↓ in avitaminosis D (rickets and osteomalacia)
Ionized	4.6-5.3 mg/dl	

Continued

Table A-1

Blood, Plasma, and Serum Values—cont'd

Test	Normal Values*	Significance of a Change
Carbon dioxide content (venous bicarbonate)	24-32 mEq/L	↑ in severe vomiting ↑ in hypoventilation disorders ↑ in obstruction of intestines ↓ in metabolic acidosis ↓ in severe diarrhea ↓ in kidney disease
Chloride	98-110 mEq/L	↑ in hyperventilation ↑ in kidney disease ↑ in Cushing syndrome ↓ in severe diarrhea ↓ in severe burns ↓ in Addison disease
Cholesterol		
Total	<200 mg/dl	↑ in chronic hepatitis ↑ in hyperthyroidism ↑ in atherosclerosis ↓ in acute hepatitis ↓ in hypothyroidism
High-density lipoprotein (HDL)	>40 mg/dl	↑ with regular exercise
Low-density lipoprotein (LDL)	<130 mg/dl	↑ with high-fat diet ↑ in diabetes mellitus ↓ in chronic obstructive pulmonary disease
Triglycerides	<165 mg/dl	↑ in cardiovascular disease ↑ in diabetes mellitus ↓ in hyperthyroidism ↓ with exercise
Clotting time (bleeding time)	5-10 min	↓ in hemophilia ↓ in platelet deficiency or defects
Copper	100-200 μg/dl	↑ in some liver disorders
Cortisol (at 8 AM)	5-20 μg/dl	↑ in Cushing disease ↓ in Addison disease
Creatine phosphokinase (CK)	32-260 U/L	↑ in Duchenne muscular dystrophy ↑ during myocardial infarction ↑ in muscle trauma
Creatinine	0.6-1.5 mg/dl	↑ in some kidney disorders
Ferritin	*Women:* 4-161 ng/ml *Men:* 16-300 ng/ml	↑ in hemochromatosis ↓ in iron deficiency
α-Fetoprotein	0-15 ng/ml	↑ in neural tube defects
Fibrinogen	175-433 mg/dl	↑ may increase risk of thrombus ↓ in disseminated intravascular coagulation
Folic acid (RBC)	165-760 ng/dl	↓ in macrocytic anemia
Glucose	60-100 mg/dl (fasting)	↑ in diabetes mellitus ↑ in liver disease ↑ during pregnancy ↑ in hyperthyroidism ↓ in hypothyroidism ↓ in Addison disease ↓ in hyperinsulinism
Glycolated hemoglobin (HbA_1c)	3.9%-6.9%	↑ in hyperglycemia
Hematocrit (packed cell volume)	*Women:* 38%-47% *Men:* 40%-54%	↑ in polycythemia ↑ in severe dehydration ↓ in anemia ↓ in leukemia ↓ in hyperthyroidism ↓ in cirrhosis of liver

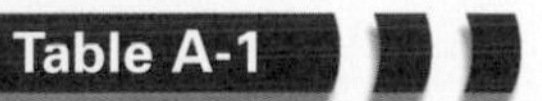

Blood, Plasma, and Serum Values—cont'd

Test	Normal Values*	Significance of a Change
Hemoglobin	*Women:* 12-16 g/dl *Men:* 13-18 g/dl *Newborn:* 14-20 g/dl	↑ in polycythemia ↑ in chronic obstructive pulmonary disease ↑ in congestive heart failure ↓ in anemia ↓ in hyperthyroidism ↓ in cirrhosis of liver
Iron	50-150 μg/dl (can be higher in men)	↑ in liver disease ↓ in iron-deficiency anemia
Iron-binding capacity (TIBC)	250-460 μg/dl	↑ in iron deficiency
Lactic dehydrogenase (LDH)	88-230 U/L	↑ during myocardial infarction ↑ in anemia (several forms) ↑ in liver disease ↑ in acute leukemia and other cancers
Lipase	0-160 U/L	↑ in pancreatitis
Magnesium	1.8-3.0 mg/dl	↑ in excessive intake ↓ in alcoholism, renal disease
Mean corpuscular hemoglobin concentration	31%-36%	↓ in iron-deficiency anemia
Mean corpuscular volume (RBC)	82-98 fl	↑ or ↓ in various forms of anemia
Osmolality	285-295 mOsm/L	↑ or ↓ in fluid and electrolyte imbalances
Pa_{CO_2}	35-43 mm Hg	↑ in severe vomiting ↑ in hypoventilation disorders ↑ in obstruction of intestines ↓ in metabolic acidosis ↓ in severe diarrhea ↓ in kidney disease
Pa_{O_2}	75-100 mm Hg (breathing standard air)	↓ in cyanotic heart defects ↓ in chronic obstructive pulmonary disease
Partial thromboplastin time (activated PTT)	25-35 sec	↑ in intrinsic pathway defects
pH	7.35-7.45	↑ during hyperventilation ↑ in Cushing syndrome ↓ during hypoventilation ↓ in acidosis ↓ in Addison disease
Phosphorus	2.5-4.5 mg/dl	↑ in hypervitaminosis D ↑ in kidney disease ↑ in hypoparathyroidism ↑ in acromegaly ↓ hyperparathyroidism ↓ in hypovitaminosis D (rickets and osteomalacia)
Plasma volume	*Women:* 40 ml/kg body weight *Men:* 39 ml/kg body weight	↑ or ↓ in fluid and electrolyte imbalances ↓ during hemorrhage
Platelet count	150,000-400,000/μl	↑ in heart disease ↑ in some forms of cancer ↑ in cirrhosis of liver ↑ after trauma ↓ in anemia (some forms) ↓ during chemotherapy ↓ in some allergies
Potassium	3.5-5.1 mEq/L	↑ in hypoaldosteronism ↑ in acute kidney failure ↓ in vomiting or diarrhea ↓ in starvation

Continued

Table A-1

Blood, Plasma, and Serum Values—cont'd

Test	Normal Values*	Significance of a Change
Prostate-specific antigen	0-4 ng/ml	↑ in prostate cancer
Protein		
Total	6-8.4 g/dl	↑ (total) in severe dehydration
Albumin	3.5-5 g/dl	↓ (total) during hemorrhage
Globulin	2.3-3.5 g/dl	↓ (total) in starvation
Prothrombin time (PT)	11-15 sec	↑ in extrinsic pathway defects
Red blood cell count	*Women:* 4.2-5.4 million/μl *Men:* 4.5-6.2 million/μl	↑ in polycythemia ↑ in dehydration ↓ in anemia (several forms) ↓ in systemic lupus erythematosus
Reticulocyte count	33,000-135,000/μl (0.5%-1.5% of RBC count)	↑ in hemolytic anemia ↑ in leukemia and metastatic carcinoma ↓ in pernicious anemia ↓ in iron-deficiency anemia ↓ during radiation therapy
Sodium	135-145 mEq/L	↑ in dehydration ↑ in trauma or disease of the central nervous system ↑ or ↓ in kidney disorders ↓ in excessive sweating, vomiting, diarrhea ↓ in burns (sodium shift into cells)
Specific gravity	1.058	↑ or ↓ in fluid imbalances
Thyroid–stimulating hormone (TSH)	0.4-6 μU/ml	↑ in hypothyroidism (primary) ↓ in hyperthyroidism (primary)
Thyroxin (T_4)—total	5-11 μg/dl	↑ in hyperthyroidism ↓ in hypothyroidism
Transferrin	190-375 mg/dl	↓ in certain anemias
Troponin I	<0.05 ng/ml	↑ in myocardial infarction
Uric acid	*Women:* 1.5-6.0 mg/dl *Men:* 3-9 mg/dl	↑ in gout ↑ in toxemia of pregnancy ↑ during trauma
Viscosity	1.4-1.8 times the viscosity of water	↑ in polycythemia ↑ in dehydration
Vitamin B_{12}	140-820 pg/ml	↓ in pernicious anemia
White blood cell count		
Total	4,500-11,000/μl	↑ in acute infections ↑ in trauma ↑ in some cancers ↓ in anemia (some forms) ↓ during chemotherapy
Basophils	0.5%-1% of total	↓ in severe allergies
Eosinophils	2%-4% of total	↑ in allergies
Lymphocytes	20%-25% of total	↑ during antibody reactions
Monocytes	3%-8% of total	↑ in chronic infections
Neutrophils	60%-70% of total	↑ in acute infection

Adapted from Thibodeau GA, Patton KT: *Anatomy & physiology,* ed 5, St Louis, 2003, Mosby, p 1023-1026.
*Values vary with the analysis method used.

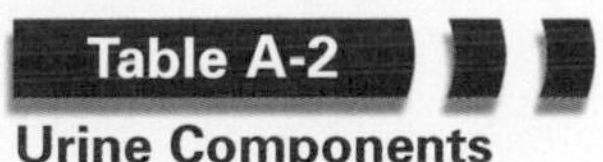

Table A-2
Urine Components

Test	Normal Values*	Significance of a Change
Routine Urinalysis		
Acetone and acetoacetate	0	↑ during fasting ↑ in diabetic acidosis
Albumin	0-trace	↑ in hypertension ↑ in kidney disease ↑ after strenuous exercise (temporary)
Ammonia	20-70 mEq/L	↑ in liver disease ↑ in diabetes mellitus
Bile and bilirubin	—	↑ during obstruction of the bile ducts
Calcium	<150 mg/day	↑ in hyperparathyroidism ↓ in hypoparathyroidism
Color	Transparent yellow, straw-colored, or amber	Abnormal color or cloudiness may indicate blood in urine, bile, bacteria, drugs, food pigments, or high solute concentration
Odor	Characteristic slight odor	Acetone odor in diabetes mellitus (diabetic ketosis)
Osmolality	500-800 mOsm/L	↑ in dehydration ↑ in heart failure ↓ in diabetes insipidus ↓ in aldosteronism
pH	4.6-8.0	↑ in alkalosis ↑ during urinary infections ↓ in acidosis ↓ in dehydration ↓ in emphysema
Potassium	25-100 mEq/L	↑ in dehydration ↑ in chronic kidney failure ↓ in diarrhea or vomiting ↓ in adrenal insufficiency
Sodium	75-200 mg/day	↑ in starvation ↑ in dehydration ↓ in acute kidney failure ↓ in Cushing syndrome
Creatinine	1-2 g/day	↑ in infections ↓ in some kidney diseases ↓ in anemia (some forms)
Creatinine clearance	100-140 ml/min	↑ in kidney disease
Glucose	0	↑ in diabetes mellitus ↑ in hyperthyroidism ↑ in hypersecretion of adrenal cortex
Urea	25-35 g/day	↑ in some liver diseases ↑ in hemolytic anemia ↓ during obstruction of bile ducts ↓ in severe diarrhea
Urea clearance	>40 ml blood cleared per min	↑ in some kidney diseases
Uric acid	0.6-1.0 g/day	↑ in gout ↓ in some kidney diseases
Microscopic Examination		
Bacteria	<10,000/ml	↑ during urinary infections
Blood cells (RBC)	0-trace	↑ in pyelonephritis ↑ from damage by calculi ↑ in infection ↑ in cancer
Blood cells (WBC)	0-trace	↑ in infection
Blood cell casts (RBC)	0	↑ in pyelonephritis
Blood cell casts (WBC)	0	↑ in infection

Table A-2

Urine Components—cont'd

Test	Normal Values*	Significance of a Change
Microscopic Examination—cont'd		
Crystals	0-trace	↑ in urinary retention Very large crystalline masses are calculi
Epithelial casts	0-trace	↑ in some kidney disorders ↑ in heavy metal toxicity
Granular casts	0-trace	↑ in some kidney disorders
Hyaline casts	0-trace	↑ in some kidney disorders ↑ in fever

Adapted from Thibodeau GA, Patton KT: *Anatomy & physiology,* ed 5, St Louis, 2003, Mosby, p 1027-1028.
*Values vary with the analysis method used.

GLOSSARY

■ **Audio pronunciation available on the CD-ROM included with this book.**

A

A band A dark band corresponding to an area where actin and myosin filaments overlap in skeletal or cardiac muscle.

Abruptio placentae Premature separation of the placenta prior to delivery; the separation may be partial or complete and may result in overt or concealed hemorrhage.

Absolute anemia Anemia involving a decrease in the number of red cells (as opposed to a decrease in the percent of cells).

Acalculous cholecystitis An important subgroup of acute cholecystitis. It tends to occur in the setting of major surgery, critical illness, trauma, or burn-related injury and does not occur in association with gallstones.

Accelerated (malignant) high blood pressure Rapidly progressing, potentially fatal form of hypertension in which diastolic blood pressure exceeds 120 mm Hg.

Acclimatization A normal adaptive response to environmental changes, such as changes in altitude. For example, the red blood cell count increases when a person moves to a high altitude.

Accommodative capacity Ability of the eye to adjust to see objects at changing distances. This is a function of the ciliary muscle's ability to flatten or thicken the lens, thereby focusing the image on the retina.

Achalasia A disorder of esophageal smooth muscle function resulting in difficulty in swallowing both liquids and solids.

Acid A substance that releases hydrogen ions in solution and from which hydrogen may be displaced by a metal to form a salt. An increase in acid concentration produces a decrease in pH.

Acidemia The state in which the blood is overly acidic; usually defined as a pH <7.35.

Acidosis Presence of a condition that tends to make body fluids overly acidic.

Acne vulgaris A disease of the skin common where sebaceous glands are numerous (face, upper back, and chest). Characteristic lesions include open (blackhead) and closed (whitehead) comedo, inflammatory papules, pustules, nodules, and cysts.

Acquired immunodeficiency syndrome (AIDS) A syndrome caused by the human immunodeficiency virus (HIV) in which the CD4 lymphocyte count is <200/μl or an AIDS-indicator condition is present.

Acquired or secondary immunodeficiency An immunodeficiency that develops after birth and is the result of an illness rather than a genetic defect. Examples include impaired immune function secondary to poor nutrition or medication. This type of immunodeficiency may be reversible.

Acromegaly Excessive growth of bone, soft tissues, and organs in adults due to abnormally high levels of growth hormone.

Acrosome Covering on the head of the sperm that contains large quantities of hydrolytic (water-splitting) enzymes that are released during capacitation.

Actin A cytoskeletal protein that makes up the thin filament of the muscle sarcomere in skeletal and cardiac muscle. It is also present in nonmuscle cells and is an important component of cell movement.

Actinic keratosis A horny premalignancy of skin epithelium caused by excessive exposure to sunlight.

Acute Relatively severe but running a short course.

Acute HAV infection A viral hepatitis infection caused by the hepatitis A virus characterized by jaundice and fatigue.

Acute renal failure An abrupt reduction of renal function that is potentially reversible.

Acute rheumatic fever An inflammatory disease following a β-hemolytic group A streptococcal pharyngeal infection.

Acute viral hepatitis Inflammatory liver disease usually caused by hepatitis A virus, hepatitis B virus, and hepatitis C virus.

Adaptation An alteration in structure or function in response to a changed environment, which enhances or promotes survival.

Adapting Making an adjustment to a change in internal or external conditions or circumstances.

Addison disease Primary adrenocortical insufficiency thought to be autoimmune in etiology.

Adenosine triphosphate (ATP) A nucleoside with three phosphate groups and an adenine base, which functions as the principal source of energy in cells.

Affect The outward expression of emotion associated with a mental state or in response to a stimulus.

Afferent neuron A neuron that transmits impulses from the periphery (sensory receptors) to the central nervous system.

Affinity The "tightness" of a ligand-receptor bond; the tendency of ligand and receptor to remain bound at low ligand concentration.

Afterload The impedance or resistance that must be overcome in order to eject blood from a cardiac chamber. Systemic vascular resistance is the primary determinant of left ventricular afterload.

Agoraphobia Irrational fear of open spaces. In panic disorder, agoraphobia is a fear of any place or situation in which assistance would be unavailable in case of an unexpected panic attack. Agoraphobia is also known as *phobic avoidance.*

Airway resistance Relationship between pressure and flow of gas, as determined by the radius of the airway.

Alagille syndrome Also called *arteriohepatic dysplasia;* this autosomal dominant condition is associated with typical bony and vascular malformations and paucity of intrahepatic bile ducts.

Alarm The initial response to stress. The major features of the alarm reaction are attributable to activation of the sympathetic nervous system.

Albinism Partial or total absence of pigment in skin, hair, and eyes.

Alcohol abuse Overingestion of alcohol to the point of a person's being dependent on the substance.

Alcoholic fatty liver An accumulation of fat in the liver cells resulting from chronic alcohol consumption; also called *steatosis.*

Alcoholic hepatitis An active inflammation, especially of the centrilobular region of the liver, resulting from acute or chronic alcohol consumption.

Alcoholic liver disease Manifested by fatty liver, hepatitis, and cirrhosis. One or more of these manifestations may be found in alcoholic patients.

Aldosterone A mineralocorticoid synthesized by the adrenal cortex in response to angiotensin II that conserves sodium, producing increased water retention and consequently increased blood volume.

Alkalemia The state in which the blood is overly alkaline; usually defined as a pH >7.45.

Alkalosis Presence of a condition in which body fluids are overly alkaline.

Allele One of two or more alternative forms of a gene located at the same site on homologous chromosomes.

Allergic contact dermatitis Indicates delayed acquired hypersensitivity to a specific allergen on the skin. Chromates, nickel, ethylenediamine, paraphenylenediamine, neomycin, formaldehyde, and lanolin components may cause allergic contact dermatitis.

Allergy Type I hypersensitivity of the immune system to environmental agents. Antigens that trigger an allergic response are often called *allergens.*

Allodynia Perception of pain in response to normally nonpainful sensory stimuli.

Allogenic Referring to transplanted tissue that was obtained from a closely matched donor, usually a sibling, parent, or child.

All-or-none response In a skeletal muscle, all of the muscle fibers innervated by a motor unit will respond as one to its maximum or they will not contract at all. In a nerve, a depolarization will result in either a full amplitude action potential or none at all.

Alopecia Loss of hair, usually referring to the scalp.

α_1-Antitrypsin A plasma protein produced primarily in the liver; it is an acute phase reactant that inhibits the activity of elastase, cathepsin G, trypsin, and other proteolytic enzymes.

Alveolar period The last stage in fetal lung development when alveolar ducts form from terminal sacs and alveoli mature by increasing in size and in number.

Amenorrhea Absence or suppression of menstrual bleeding, usually due to an altered pattern of hormonal functioning that interrupts the normal sequence of endometrial proliferation and sloughing.

Amniocentesis A procedure in which fluid is obtained from the amniotic cavity by an ultrasound-guided needle. The fluid contains fetal cells that can be used to screen for chromosomal and other defects.

Amniotic cavity The space between the amniotic sac and the developing embryo. It is filled with a clear amniotic fluid that keeps the embryo moist and provides a measure of protection against mechanical injury.

Amphipathic Having different characteristics. For example, membrane lipids are partly hydrophobic and partly hydrophilic, and hence are amphipathic.

Ampulla A flasklike cavity or dilatation of a tubular structure.

Amyloid plaque A microscopic lesion in the cerebral cortex composed of fragmented axon terminals and dendrites surrounding a core of β-amyloid as found in Alzheimer disease.

Amyloid precursor protein A member of a large family of proteins that are associated with cell membranes and a precursor to β-amyloid, a component of brain plaques in Alzheimer disease.

Amyotrophic lateral sclerosis A progressive degenerative disease affecting both the upper and lower motor neurons characterized by muscle wasting and atrophy of the hands, arms, and legs; also called *Lou Gehrig disease.*

Anabolism The energy-requiring phase of metabolism through which molecules, cells, and tissues are created.

Anagen The growing phase of the hair cycle.

Anaplasia A lack of differentiated features in a tumor cell as evidenced by variations in cell size and shape and presence of abnormal nuclei.

Androgenic Producing masculine characteristics such as the androgenic hormone testosterone.

Anemia A decrease in the quantity of hemoglobin, hematocrit, and/or red blood cells.

Anergy Diminished immune responsiveness to antigens.

Aneuploidy An abnormal number of chromosomes—either too few (hypoploidy) or too many (hyperploidy, polyploidy).

Aneurysm Local dilation of arterial wall or muscular chamber (e.g., cardiac ventricle).

Angina pectoris A paroxysmal chest pain most often due to cardiac ischemia associated with atherosclerotic coronary artery disease.

Anhedonia Loss of interest in and withdrawal from all regular and pleasurable activities, often associated with depression.

Ankylosing spondylitis An arthritis of the axial skeleton including the sacroiliac joints, spine, hips, and shoulders. Marked limitation of motion develops, and a flexed spinal posture with flexed hips and knees may predominate.

Anorexia Loss of appetite.

Anorexia nervosa A refusal to eat or an aberration in eating patterns to the point of danger. The clinical syndrome may be due to an intense fear of becoming obese or to emotional states such as anxiety, irritation, or anger. Affected individuals become obsessed with the desire to become thin, and food intake is restricted even as weight falls well below minimal normal value for age and height. Periods of fasting may alternate with periods of bingeing.

Anosognosia Lack of insight into one's own cognitive deficiencies.

Anthropometric Pertaining to measurements of the body or body parts such as height and weight.

Antibody Protein produced by B cells that destroys or inactivates a specific antigen.

Anticipatory anxiety Anxious anticipation of an anxiety-provoking event.

Anticodon Sequence of three nucleotides in a transfer RNA molecule that is complementary to the messenger RNA codon.

Antigen Macromolecule that provokes an immune system response.

Antimicrobial A chemical or agent that inhibits microbial growth, as in "antimicrobial resistance"; this is conferred to microorganisms that have developed mechanisms to evade antimicrobial actions.

Antisocial personality disorder A mental disorder characterized by failure to acquire the conditioned responses that are necessary for the learning of avoidance behaviors, conventional morality, and socialized positive responses to others. Also known as *character disorder.*

Anuria Severe decrease or lack of urine output.

Anxiety disorders General group that comprises three major diagnoses: panic disorder, generalized anxiety disorder, and obsessive-compulsive disorder. Anxiety disorders are characterized by irrational fears and have great potential to cause disability in affected persons.

Aortic valve The cardiac valve that lies between the left ventricle and the aorta. It is open during ventricular systole and closed during ventricular diastole. Aortic valve closure contributes to heart sound S_2.

Aphasia A global disorder of language involving impaired speech (expressive aphasia) and impaired ability to understand the spoken word (receptive aphasia).

Apocrine sweat gland A sweat gland that discharges its products onto the skin through the hair follicle (hair pore).

Apoprotein The protein component of lipoproteins, which differ among the various types of lipoproteins and contribute to their function.

Apoptosis Programmed cell death, characterized by DNA degradation and cell dissolution, but without necrosis.

Appendicitis Inflammation of the vermiform appendix due to an obstruction. This inflammation may lead to necrosis of the appendix, with subsequent abscess formation and peritonitis.

Apraxia An inability to execute previously learned skills, usually following a stroke.

Arachnoidal villi Fingerlike projections in the delicate membrane between the dura mater and the pia mater of the brain.

Arnold-Chiari II malformation A congenital anomaly associated with meningomyelocele and hydrocephalus in which the cerebellum and medulla oblongata protrude into the cervical spinal canal through the foramen magnum.

Arterial pulse pressure The difference between systolic and diastolic blood pressure.

Arteriosclerosis Generalized term for pathologic conditions resulting in decreased distensibility of arteries; also known as *hardening of the arteries.*

Arteriovenous fistula Abnormal communication between an artery and a vein.

Arteriovenous malformation A type of arteriovenous fistula resulting in a tangle of vessels in the vasculature of the brain.

Arteritis Inflammation of an artery. May be associated with an autoimmune reaction.

Articular (hyaline) cartilage Connective tissue that forms a smooth, resilient, low-friction surface for articulation of two bones. It is without nerves, is avascular in adults, and derives nourishment from synovial fluid. It tolerates extreme compression stress.

Articulation A point of contact between bones. Also called *joint.*

Ascites Abnormal accumulation of fluid in the peritoneal cavity. Causes include liver disease, heart failure, constrictive pericarditis, infection, malnutrition, pancreatitis, lymphatic obstruction or leakage, renal disease, hypothyroidism, collagen vascular diseases, and malignancy.

Aspiration Inadvertent entry of food substances, liquids, or gastric content into the respiratory system. This potentially life-threatening occurrence is normally prevented by the coordinated set of actions performed by the muscles in the pharynx during swallowing.

Asthenia The lack or loss of strength or energy; weakness.

Asthma A respiratory condition characterized by increased responsiveness of the trachea and bronchi to various stimuli and manifested by widespread narrowing of the airways and inflammation.

Ataxia Failure of muscular coordination, resulting in incoordination and disturbances in posture and gait.

Atelectasis Full or partial collapse of the lung alveoli.

Atherosclerosis A type of arteriosclerosis characterized by proliferation of smooth muscle cells and lipid collection within the walls of arteries, resulting in narrowed lumina and impaired ability to dilate.

Atopic 1. Displaced, ectopic. 2. Pertaining to atopy.

Atopy A genetic predisposition to allergies.

Atresia Congenital failure to develop (absence) or abnormal closure of a normally open passage.

Atrial fibrillation A completely disorganized and irregular atrial rhythm accompanied by an irregular ventricular rhythm of variable rate.

Atrophy A reduction in size and function of a cell or tissue; wasting.

Aura A peculiar sensation preceding the appearance of more definite symptoms, as in migraine and seizure.

Auscultatory gap The time during cuff deflation after systolic blood pressure when the Korotkoff sounds disappear.

Autism A mental disorder primarily characterized by abnormal development of social interaction and communicative skills. Affected individuals may manifest an inability to perceive or understand others' feelings or to express their own feelings, and may adhere to rigid, nonfunctional behaviors or rituals.

Autocrine Relating to hormone-like chemicals in which the target cell is the same cell that secretes the chemical.

Autocrine signaling The secretion of factors that feed back onto the cell that secreted them. Usually used in reference to growth factors.

Autografting Surgical procedure to move skin from one area of the body to an area of injury. The purpose is to provide permanent skin coverage to the injured area.

Autoimmune liver disease Hepatic injury from self-reactive antibodies produced by errant B lymphocytes.

Autoimmunity An inappropriate and excessive response of the immune system to self antigens causing disease. Disorders that result from an autoimmune response are called *autoimmune diseases.*

Autonomic dysreflexia Hyperreflexia; an uninhibited and exaggerated reflex of the autonomic nervous system in response to stimulation in spinal cord patients.

Autoregulation The intrinsic tendency of an organ or tissue to maintain adequate blood flow despite changes in metabolism or blood pressure.

Autosomal dominant polycystic kidney disease Hereditary disorder associated with defects on chromosome 16 (95% of cases) or chromosome 4 (5% of cases), resulting in dilation of all collecting ducts and impaired renal function.

Autosomal recessive polycystic kidney disease Congenital disorder linked to a defect on chromosome 6 that results in dilations of the renal collecting ducts and hepatic fibrosis.

Autosome Any ordinary paired chromosome, as distinguished from a sex chromosome.

Avoidance Refers to conscious or subconscious defensive reactions used to increase feelings of control and decrease the risk of anxiety.

Avulsion fracture A separation of a small fragment of bone at the site of attachment of a ligament or tendon.

Axoneme 1. Central core of a cilium or flagellum, consisting of two central fibrils surrounded by nine peripheral fibrils. 2. Motor apparatus of the sperm's tail.

Azotemia Increased levels of nitrogenous waste products, especially urea nitrogen, in the blood indicative of impaired renal clearance.

B

B cell A type of lymphocyte that can produce antibodies that attack pathogens or directs other cells to attack them. B cells that are actively producing antibodies are called *plasma cells.*

Bacillus Rod-shaped bacterium that may or may not be motile.

Bacterial enzyme An enzyme that aids in the microorganism's ability to spread or invade tissues, such as fibrinolysin, coagulase, and hyaluronidase.

Ball-and-socket joint Formed by a ball-like surface fitting into a concave socket. Ball-and-socket joints permit flexion-extension, adduction-abduction, and rotational movements, such as those of the hip and shoulder.

Barrett esophagus A complication of chronic gastroesophageal reflux disease that represents replacement of the normal squamous epithelium of the distal esophagus by columnar tissue. Considered to be a preneoplastic condition.

Basal energy expenditure A term used to describe the calculated basal metabolic rate, metabolic rate at rest.

Basal ganglia Groups of cell bodies (nuclei) located deep within the cerebral hemispheres that help plan and execute motor activities, including the caudate, putamen, globus pallidus, substantia nigra, and subthalamus.

Basal metabolic rate The amount of energy required for an individual to maintain vital processes such as respiration, digestion, and circulation at rest.

Base 1. The nonacid part of a salt. 2. A substance that accepts hydrogen ions in solution to form salts and increases pH.

Basophil/basophilic granulocyte A leukocyte that is functionally and chemically related to the mast cell and has a kidney-shaped nucleus and large deep basophilic granules, which contain vasoactive amine and heparin and are important in IgE binding.

Beau line Transverse furrow in the nail that indicates a disturbance in nail growth.

Becker dystrophy A milder form of inherited muscle degeneration than the Duchenne type and somewhat less common with an annual incidence of 5 per 100,000. The genetic mutation leads to production of a reduced amount of an abnormal dystrophin protein and slower muscular degeneration.

Bell palsy An acute idiopathic paresis or paralysis of the facial nerve involving an inflammatory reaction at or near the stylomastoid foramen or in the bony facial canal.

Bence Jones proteins Proteins found in the urine of patients with plasma cell (multiple) myeloma. They are derived from overproduction of light chain fragments of antibodies by malignant plasma cells. Bence Jones proteins are nephrotoxic and may contribute to development of kidney disease.

Benign breast disorders A group of lesions affecting the breast, which are usually divided into two categories: fibrocystic breast disease and benign neoplasms of the breast.

Benign prostatic hyperplasia/hypertrophy (BPH) A noncancerous enlargement of the prostate gland.

Benign tumor A type of tumor that is strictly local, usually well differentiated, and does not metastasize.

β-Amyloid Protein fragment snipped from a larger molecule—called *amyloid precursor protein*—during metabolism. Abnormal β-amyloid is a component of neuritic plaques found in Alzheimer disease.

Biaxial joint A joint that has two axes of movement and permits movement in two planes.

Bile A substance produced by hepatocytes in the liver and stored in the gallbladder. It is composed primarily of water, electrolytes, bile salts, cholesterol, and phospholipids. The major functions of bile are to aid in the digestion of dietary lipids through emulsification and to transport waste products, particularly bilirubin, into the intestine for disposal or reabsorption.

Biliary atresia Also called *extrahepatic ductopenia* or *progressive obliterative cholangiopathy;* biliary atresia can be either congenital or acquired. The latter occurs in the setting of certain autoimmune illnesses and is one of the principal forms of chronic rejection of a transplanted liver allograft. Biliary atresia is a rather common birth defect, occurring in 1 in 10,000 to 1 in 15,000 live births.

Biliary cirrhosis A disease initiated by damage to the bile ducts, which may be due to microscopic or microscopic biliary obstruction. Persistent biliary obstruction results in inflammation and scarring of the liver, with obliteration of the bile ductules.

Biliary colic Persistent epigastric pain related to intermittent obstruction of the cystic duct, usually by a gallstone. A typical episode lasts several hours.

Bilirubin A substance formed from the degradation of hemoglobin from erythrocytes by the reticuloendothelial cells.

Biliverdin A greenish bile pigment formed in the breakdown of hemoglobin and converted to bilirubin.

Bipennate Pertaining to a muscle with a central tendon toward which the fibers converge on either side like the barbs of a feather.

Bipolar disorder A mood disorder characterized by alternating periods of mania and depression.

Bladder calculus A solid mass (stone) formed from debris within the bladder.

Blast An immature precursor of a lymphoid or myeloid white blood cell. Blasts are not normally found in the peripheral blood because they are retained in the marrow until mature. Blasts in the peripheral blood indicate leukemia.

Blood urea nitrogen (BUN) Urea is an end product of amino acid metabolism, measured in the blood as BUN and excreted primarily by the kidney.

Blunted affect A severe reduction in the intensity of externalized feelings.

Body fluid The water contained in the body plus the substances dissolved in it.

Body mass index (BMI) A weight reference standard. The formula for BMI is weight (kg) divided by height squared (m^2).

Body water All of the water contained in the body.

Bolus 1. A round mass of food that has been softened and formed into an appropriate size for swallowing by the action of chewing. 2. A concentrated mass of pharmaceutical preparation.

Bone and joint tuberculosis An extrapulmonary form of tuberculosis that occurs after lymphohematogenous spread from a primary lung lesion.

Borderline personality disorder Personality disorder that represents a pervasive and persistent disturbance in ways of handling events and situations. Personalities influenced by this disorder are unstable, unpredictable, impulsive, and often moody and self-deprecating. Some overlap with depression is suggested.

Brainstem Portion of the brain made up of the midbrain, pons, and medulla oblongata.

Branched-chain amino acids A group of amino acids that includes valine, leucine, and isoleucine, which are mainly metabolized in the muscle.

Bronchiectasis A disorder characterized by destruction of the elastic and muscular structures leading to dilation of the bronchi.

Bronchiolitis Inflammation of small bronchi.

Bronchitis Widespread inflammation of bronchi and bronchioles due to infectious agents or allergic reactions.

Bronchospasm Narrowing of the bronchi and bronchioles because of an abnormal contraction of the smooth muscles of the bronchial walls.

Bruit Sound generated by turbulent blood flow auscultated over a blood vessel.

Brush border Covering of the microvilli projecting from the intestinal villi. This fuzzy coating contains many digestive enzymes.

Buck fascia or fascia of Buck Thick fibrous envelope surrounding the tunica albuginea, which encloses each of the erectile bodies of the penis.

Buckle fracture A fracture in children whereby the bone buckles and eventually cracks as a result of a compression injury to cancellous bone of the metaphysis of a long bone.

Buffer A chemical that releases hydrogen ions when a fluid is too alkaline and takes up hydrogen ions when a fluid is too acidic.

Bulbourethral glands Also called Cowper glands, these two glands produce viscous fluid that is secreted into the urethra near the base of the penis.

Bulbous urethra The proximal portion of the penile urethra. The bulbous urethra is surrounded by the bulb of the urethra and bulbospongiosus muscle.

Bulimia nervosa Recurrent episodes of binge eating followed by self-induced vomiting or diarrhea, excessive exercise, strict dieting or fasting, and an exaggerated concern about body shape and weight.

Bulla Large, thin-walled cyst. Commonly used in reference to lung or skin.

Bursa Pocket of connective tissue lined with liquid-containing synovium, located between muscles or between muscle or tendon and bone.

Byler syndrome A rare autosomal recessive disorder involving severe jaundice, pruritus, and malabsorption caused by an error in bile salt metabolism. Also called *progressive intrahepatic cholestasis* and *progressive familial intrahepatic cholestasis.*

C

Cachexia A combination of symptoms, including anorexia, weight loss, muscle wasting, and weakness, that is associated with the severe malnutrition of chronic diseases such as cancer.

Calcitonin A hormone produced by thyroid parafollicular cells, it influences the processing of calcium by bone cells.

Calculus A mass of solid mineral or metabolic substance. A stone.

Callus (bone) The bony deposit formed between and around the broken ends of a fractured bone during healing. Also called *keratoma.*

Calluses (skin) Common, usually painless thickenings of the stratum corneum at locations of external pressure or friction.

Cancellous bone Bone with a spongy or lattice-like appearance, found in the interior of bones. Cancellous bone does not tolerate compression stress.

Cancer cachexia The severe nutritional effects of cancer. See *cachexia.*

Capacitation The multiple changes that activate sperm and enhance their ability to participate in the final process of fertilization.

Capillary hydrostatic pressure The outward push of the vascular fluid against the capillary walls from blood pressure.

Capillary osmotic pressure The inward pull of particles in the vascular fluid from dissolved proteins in the blood.

Carbohydrates The main energy source for the body consisting of simple or complex sugars. They must be supplied in a fairly constant manner to meet the energy requirements for normal body functioning. Provides 4 kcal/g.

Carbonic anhydrase The enzyme that catalyzes the reversible conversion of carbon dioxide and water to carbonic acid.

Carcinogen A substance that initiates or promotes the development of cancers. Most carcinogens cause cancer by damaging DNA to produce mutations.

Cardiac asthma Results from bronchospasm precipitated by congestive heart failure.

Cardiac cycle A cardiac cycle includes one diastolic and one systolic phase.

Cardiac index A measure of the heart's pumping ability taking into account body surface area. The cardiac index is calculated by dividing cardiac output by body surface area. A cardiac index less than 2.0 L/min/m^2 is considered to be insufficient for adequate peripheral perfusion.

Cardiac output A measure of the amount of blood pumped by the heart in 1 minute, usually expressed in liters per minute.

Cardiac tamponade Abnormal external pressure on the heart resulting in poor cardiac filling and decreased cardiac output.

Cardiomyopathy Diseases that primarily affect myocardial cells, often of unknown cause. Three common types of cardiomyopathy are dilated, hypertrophic, and restrictive.

Carina A ridgelike structure at the base of the trachea that projects from the area that separates the left and right bronchi.

Carpal joint A synovial joint between the carpal bones.

Carrier A person who harbors a recessive gene for a particular trait. A recessive heterozygote.

Carrier proteins Proteins located in lipid bilayers that transport ions and small molecules through the membrane by first binding on one side and then moving to the other side by changing conformation.

Cartilaginous joint A joint that connects bony segments by fibrocartilage or hyaline growth cartilage.

Casts White or red blood cells that collect in a nephron tubule and conform to the shape of the tubule; their presence indicates infection or inflammation of the kidney.

Catabolism The process of converting large molecules of carbohydrate, protein, and fat to smaller molecules to be utilized for energy.

Catecholamine A hormone (e.g., epinephrine and norepinephrine) that stimulates glycogenolysis and gluconeogenesis. An amine neurotransmitter (e.g., norepinephrine, dopamine).

Catecholamine hypothesis A hypothesis that abnormally low catecholaminergic neurotransmission leads to depression and abnormally high catecholaminergic neurotransmission leads to mania.

Caudal A positional term referring to the tail end.

Caudate nuclei Portion of each cerebral hemisphere that, together with the lentiform nuclei, forms the corpus striatum of the basal ganglia.

Celiac disease Also called *celiac sprue;* this disease is characterized by intolerance of gluten, a protein in wheat and wheat products that causes bowel inflammation and malabsorption.

Cell cycle The phases through which a cell progresses during cellular reproduction, including gap 1, synthesis, gap 2, and mitosis.

Centromere Constricted region that holds two sister chromatids together. The centromere is the site of attachment to the microtubules, which pull the chromatids apart during mitosis.

Centrosome A centrally located organelle that organizes microtubules in the cell. It acts as the spindle pole during mitosis.

Cerebellum Portion of the brain, attached to the brainstem, that has an essential role in maintaining muscle tone, posture, and coordinating normal movements.

Cerebral dysrhythmia An abnormality in an otherwise normal rhythmic pattern, as seen on electroencephalography.

Cerebral palsy Refers to a diverse group of crippling syndromes that appears during childhood and involves permanent, nonprogressive encephalopathic damage to the developing brain.

Cerebrospinal fluid Fluid found in the cavities and canals of the brain and spinal cord.

Cerebrotendinous xanthomatosis A steroid hydroxylase deficiency that leads to premature atherosclerosis and encephalopathy.

Cerebrum Portion of the brain that controls consciousness, memory, sensations, emotions, and voluntary movements. The largest part of the brain, it consists of two hemispheres.

Ceruminous gland A special variety or modification of apocrine sweat gland. The mixed secretions of sebaceous and ceruminous glands form a brown waxy substance called *cerumen,* which protects the ear canal from dehydration.

Chagas disease Caused by *Trypanosoma cruzii,* it is a common cause of acquired myocarditis and megacolon in Central and South America but is rarely seen in the United States.

Chancre Painless, ulcerative lesion arising at the original port of entry of the spirochete that causes syphilis.

Chancroid An ulcerative, infectious disease of the genital tract caused by the sexually transmitted bacillus *Haemophilus ducreyi.* Unlike the chancre in syphilis, the lesion in chancroid is painful, tender, and often multiple.

Channel proteins Proteins located in lipid bilayers, which form porelike structures that allow ions to pass through by diffusion when appropriately stimulated.

Chemodissolution Use of chemical substances, such as bile acids or organic solvents, to dissolve gallstones. Used as a nonoperative method to treat gallstones.

Chemotaxis The movement of cells according to chemical gradients (chemotaxins) that attract them.

Chest physiotherapy Use of percussion and postural drainage to mobilize secretions from specific segments of the lungs.

Chickenpox Also called *varicella.* Chickenpox is a common communicable childhood disease. It is caused by the varicella zoster virus, which is also the causative agent in shingles. The characteristic skin lesion occurs in three stages: macule, vesicle, and granular scab.

Chlamydia Genus of a microorganism that lives as an intracellular bacterium. *Chlamydia trachomatis* inhabits the epithelium of the urethra and cervix and is responsible for the highly contagious systemic infection lymphogranuloma venereum.

Chloride shift An exchange of chloride ions for HCO_3^- in red blood cells in peripheral tissues in response to changes in P_{CO_2} of blood.

Cholecalciferol Precursor substance of active vitamin D.

Cholecystectomy Surgical removal of the gallbladder.

Cholecystitis Inflammation of the gallbladder wall; may be acute or chronic and usually is associated with cholelithiasis.

Cholecystokinin Hormone secreted from the small intestinal mucosa; two of its chief functions are stimulation of the release of pancreatic enzymes during a meal and contraction of the gallbladder.

Cholelithiasis Formation of stones in the gallbladder.

Cholinergic-noradrenergic imbalance hypothesis A hypothesis that suggests that a relative increase in the ratio of acetylcholine activity to norepinephrine activity produces depression and that mania is the result of a relative increase in the ratio of norepinephrine activity to acetylcholine activity.

Chondroma Also called *enchondroma;* a cartilage-forming tumor located within bone that accounts for about 15% of benign bone tumors.

Chondrosarcoma A malignant cartilage-forming tumor; chondrosarcomas tend to develop in the pelvic and shoulder girdles and the proximal ends of long bones.

Chordae tendineae Bands of fibrous connective tissue that anchor the atrioventricular valves to the papillary muscles of the ventricular chambers.

Chorionic villus sampling A procedure in which tissue is obtained from the placenta by ultrasound-guided biopsy. Chorionic villus sampling can be performed earlier in pregnancy (9 to 11 weeks) than amniocentesis (16 weeks).

Chromatid One copy of a chromosome formed by DNA replication that may be joined to the other copy (sister chromatid) at the centromere.

Chromosome A linear thread of nuclear DNA that becomes visible under the microscope during cell mitosis.

Chronic Refers to a condition that lasts for a long time, months to years.

Chronic active hepatitis A progressive, destructive inflammatory disease that extends beyond the portal triad to the hepatic lobule (piecemeal necrosis).

Chronic bronchitis A condition characterized by excessive secretion of bronchial mucus and manifested by productive cough for 3 or more months in at least 2 consecutive years in the absence of any other disease process that may cause this symptom.

Chronic hepatitis Ongoing inflammation of the liver, usually of more than 6 months duration, following viral hepatitis or due to autoimmune disease.

Chronic persistent hepatitis Also called *triaditis* or *transaminitis.* A benign disease in which the inflammation is confined to the portal triads without destruction of normal liver functions despite elevated serum transaminase levels.

Chronic renal failure Gradual loss of renal function that is progressive and irreversible.

Chronic venous insufficiency Varicosity of the deep veins that prevents effective return of blood from the periphery. Usually manifests as edema.

Chylothorax An accumulation of chylous fluid attributable to leakage of chyle (lymph fluid) from the thoracic duct or to rheumatoid pleural effusion or tuberculous pleuritis. Also called *chylous pleural effusion.*

Chyme Viscous, semifluid contents of the stomach following the mixture of ingested nutrients with gastric secretions. Chyme then passes through the pylorus into the duodenum, where further digestion occurs.

Cilia Motile hairlike processes on the surface of some cells.

Circadian rhythm The regular recurrence of certain biological phenomena in approximately 24-hour cycles, regardless of constant darkness or other conditions of illumination.

Circumferential burn A burn injury that wraps completely around an extremity or the trunk. Loss of elasticity of skin results in a tourniquet effect, compromising circulation to distal tissues or respiratory expansion of chest. Escharotomy or fasciotomy is necessary.

Cirrhosis A diffuse, irreversible scarring of the liver resulting in abnormal nodules of liver cells surrounded by fibrosis.

Clang association Association of words similar in sound but not in meaning, or words having no logical connection; may include rhyming and punning.

Clinical dehydration The combination of extracellular fluid volume deficit and hypernatremia.

Clinical manifestations The functional consequences of the structural and associated alterations in cells or tissues that are either characteristic of the disease or diagnostic of the process.

Clonic Characterized by alternating periods of involuntary muscular contraction and relaxation in rapid succession.

Closed fracture A type of fracture that occurs when fragments of a fracture do not extend through mucous membranes or skin and skin is not broken.

Closing volume Lung volume at which airways in the lower lung zones collapse and ventilation ceases.

Clubbing A process characterized by flattening of the angle of the base of the nail. It may occur in association with cardiovascular disease, subacute bacterial endocarditis, and pulmonary disease.

CO_2 Carbon dioxide; this gas is produced by cells during metabolism, is carried in the blood as carbonic acid, and is excreted by the lungs.

Coagulation The process of blood clot formation.

Coagulopathy An abnormality in blood clot formation.

Cocci Round nonmotile bacteria.

Codon Sequence of three nucleotides in DNA or messenger RNA that represents the instruction for a particular amino acid in a polypeptide chain.

Collagen Most abundant protein in the body. The major protein of the white fibers of connective tissue. Has tensile strength similar to that of steel and is responsible for functional integrity of connective tissue.

Colloid osmotic pressure Pressure produced by passage of fluid from an area of less concentration to an area of higher concentration of colloids (large charged molecules such as proteins).

Colonization Harmless inhabitation of the skin or mucous membranes by microorganisms.

Colostomy Establishment of an artificial opening of the colon on the abdominal wall; usually performed following removal of a diseased or injured bowel segment.

Comminuted fracture A fracture consisting of more than one fracture line and more than two bone fragments.

Compact bone Hard, dense bone that is usually found at the periphery of skeletal structures.

Compartment syndrome A syndrome resulting from trauma to soft tissue caused by swelling within the unyielding structure of a nonelastic tissue or device (e.g., a cast).

Compensation The counterbalancing of any defect of structure or function. For example, a process that tends to restore pH to normal by making other blood chemistry values abnormal.

Complement A protein that participates in a cascade of reactions resulting in inflammation and cell lysis. Complement activation can occur by the classical or the alternative pathways.

Complete fracture A fracture whose line disrupts bone continuity through the whole thickness of the bone, including the cortex.

Compliance A measure of the ease of elastic distensibility of a hollow organ.

Complication A new or separate process that may arise secondarily because of some change produced by the original entity. For example, bacterial pneumonia may be a complication of viral infection of the respiratory tract.

Compression fracture Consistent with cancellous bone trauma. Also called a *crush fracture.*

Compulsion Repetitive ritualistic behavior that has a driven quality.

Concentric contraction The shortening contraction of a muscle when the muscle force generates sufficient tension to overcome the resistance of limb. One example is lifting a cup of water to one's mouth.

Condyloid joint A joint that permits flexion and extension at one axis and adduction and abduction around another axis, like the metacarpophalangeal joint of the hand.

Condylomata acuminatum; condylomata acuminata Genital wart(s) caused by papillomavirus forms.

Conformational change A movement or alteration in the three-dimensional formation of a protein without any change in amino acid structure.

Congenital adrenal hyperplasia Overproduction of adrenal androgens due to a lack of an enzyme needed for cortisol production. Symptoms include virilization of the female infant's genitalia.

Congenital ichthyosis An inherited disease characterized by an excessive growth of keratinocytes and keratin, which gives the skin a fish-scale appearance.

Congenital immunodeficiency Rare condition that results from improper development of immune system components before birth.

Congenital malformation A general term meaning a defect in form or function that is present at birth.

Congestive heart failure Dysfunctional cardiac pumping that results in congestion of blood behind the dysfunctional cardiac pump. Right-sided heart failure is associated with systemic venous congestion. Left-sided heart failure is associated with pulmonary congestion.

Consanguinity Mating of blood-related individuals.

Consolidation The process of tissues becoming firm and solid, as when the lung alveoli become firm as air spaces are filled with exudate in pneumonia.

Constipation A condition of having small, infrequent, and difficult bowel movements. Authorities have established a norm of fewer than three stools per week as a guideline for defining constipation.

Contact dermatitis A cutaneous reaction to topical irritation or allergy. Irritant contact dermatitis can develop in any person exposed to a sufficiently high concentration of the irritating agent. Some of the more active irritants are acids, alkalis, and hydrocarbons.

Contractile tissue Tissues involved in the contraction of muscle, including not only the muscle belly but also the tendon and bony insertion.

Contractility The force and velocity of cardiac muscle shortening in response to stimuli that increase cytoplasmic free calcium ion levels.

Contraction time The time from initial tension development to peak tension.

Contralateral Referring to the opposite side of the body.

Convalescence The stage of recovery after a disease, injury, or surgical operation.

Coombs antiglobulin test The direct test is an assay for antibody that is attached to red cells; the indirect test is an assay for antibody circulating in serum.

Coping A measure of the individual's resourcefulness and ability to deal with stress and stressors.

Corns Horny masses of condensed epithelial cells overlying bony prominences. Corns result from chronic friction and pressure.

Cor pulmonale Right ventricular hypertrophy secondary to pulmonary diseases that increase right ventricular afterload.

Corpora cavernosa Two paired erectile bodies that lie dorsally in the penis.

Corpus luteum Anatomic structure on the surface of the ovary that grows in the ruptured ovarian follicle following ovulation and acts as a temporary endocrine organ that secretes progesterone.

Corpus spongiosum Erectile body in the penis containing the urethra.

Correction A process whereby normal values are restored when the underlying cause is addressed. An example would be restoring pH to normal by addressing the underlying cause of an acid-base imbalance.

Cortical bone The dense cortex or outer shell of bone, designed to tolerate compression and shearing forces.

Corticosteroid A hormone produced by the adrenal gland that stimulates gluconeogenesis and contributes to insulin resistance (e.g., cortisol) or a drug that has similar effects.

Cortisol A glucocorticoid (steroid hormone) released by the adrenal gland that causes an increase in blood glucose level by promoting liver gluconeogenesis.

Coryza A head cold with profuse nasal drainage.

Costovertebral angle Area lateral to the sacrospinalis muscle and beneath the 12th rib used as an external landmark for the kidneys.

Cowper glands Also called bulbourethral glands, these two glands produce viscous fluid that is secreted into the urethra near the base of the penis.

Crackles Rales (pronounced "rahls"); discontinuous fine crackling sounds, usually heard on inspiration, that are indicative of air moving through fluid.

Cradle cap A seborrheic condition in infants characterized by scaling of the scalp. Occurs as a result of infrequent or inadequate washing of the scalp.

Creatine kinase An enzyme that catalyzes the transfer of a phosphate group between adenosine triphosphate and creatine. The isoenzyme found in cardiac muscle is called *CK-MB* (the MB fraction of creatine kinase).

Creatinine End product of muscle metabolism that is filtered freely through the glomeruli and excreted by the kidney only. Creatinine clearance is used as a measure of glomerular filtration rate.

Cretinism Extreme hypothyroidism during infancy and childhood that causes mental and physical abnormalities.

Cricothyroidotomy Incision through the site below the thyroid cartilage for emergency opening of the tracheal passageway.

Crigler-Najjar syndrome A rare autosomal recessive disorder marked by severe unconjugated hyperbilirubinemia seen shortly after birth.

Crohn disease An inflammation of the gastrointestinal tract that extends through all layers of the intestinal wall, most commonly affecting the terminal ileum. It may affect multiple portions of the intestine, leaving intervening normal areas in between the affected regions. The manifestations of Crohn disease differ in some respects from those of *ulcerative colitis,* although some overlap may occur. In Crohn disease, abdominal pain is the predominant symptom.

Cross-bridge The interaction between thick and thin filaments of the contractile apparatus when myosin heads bind to actin.

Cross-bridge theory This theory of muscle contraction is suggested by the anatomic configuration of the sarcomere. Muscle shortening is accomplished by increasing the amount of overlap of actin and myosin filaments. Also called the *sliding filament theory.*

Crush fracture A fracture that is consistent with cancellous bone trauma. Also called *compression fracture.*

Cryptogenic cirrhosis Advanced liver disease in a small number of patients with neither a suggestive history nor any detectable markers that would place them in any of the four main groups of cirrhosis.

Cryptorchidism Undescended testes.

Culture An integrated pattern of customs, attitudes, values, and shared beliefs that bind people together to form a society.

Cushing disease Hyperfunctioning of the adrenal cortex with increased glucocorticoid (cortisol) secretion because of excessive secretion of adrenocorticotropic hormone (ACTH) from the anterior pituitary.

Cushing syndrome The clinical features of hypercortisolism, regardless of cause.

Cutaneous membrane Thin, flat organ, also known as *skin.* It is composed of two main layers: an outer, thinner layer, termed the *epidermis;* and an inner, thicker layer, termed the *dermis.*

Cyanosis A blue coloration of the skin as a result of poor saturation of hemoglobin with oxygen. Cyanosis is usually not evident until saturation falls below 75%.

Cystic fibrosis An autosomal recessive condition with abnormal chloride channel function, producing lung and pancreatic disease in children.

Cystitis Inflammation of the urothelium (lining of the bladder) resulting from infection, irritation, presence of foreign body, or trauma.

Cystocele Protrusion of a portion of the urinary bladder into the anterior vagina at a weakened part of the vaginal musculature. Predisposing factors include obesity, aging, inherent weakness, history of heavy-object lifting, or injury during childbirth or surgery.

Cytokine A peptide factor released by cells to influence the behavior of target cells. Cytokines have signaling, inflammatory, growth, and inhibitory functions.

Cytopathic Pertaining to significant cellular injury or death.

Cytoskeleton System of protein filaments in the cytoplasm of a cell that give the cell its shape and the capacity for purposeful movement.

D

Decubitus ulcer Localized area of cellular necrosis resulting from prolonged pressure between a bony prominence and an external object such as a bed or wheelchair. The tissues are deprived of blood supply and eventually die. Also called *pressure sore.*

Deep partial-thickness burn Second-degree burn characterized by destruction of entire dermis, leaving only epidermal skin appendages. All physiologic functions of skin are absent.

Degranulate The release of granules by mast cells and basophils; the granules contain proinflammatory chemicals.

Degranulation Exocytosis of stored molecules contained in cytoplasmic vesicles.

Delusion A fixed, false belief that is held despite considerable contradictory evidence.

Delusional disorder A behavioral constellation dominated by a system of fixed, false beliefs that are tenacious and typically refractory to contrary evidence.

Dementia Syndrome characterized by a general loss of intellectual abilities caused by either reversible or progressive disorders, most typically Alzheimer disease or multi-infarct dementia.

Demyelination Destruction, removal, or loss of the myelin sheath of a nerve or nerves.

Deoxyribonucleic acid (DNA) The biomolecule that carries genetic information in the cell. DNA is composed of covalently linked nucleotides that form long polymers.

Depressed fracture A fracture in which the fragment is displaced below the level of the surface of the bone, usually in the skull.

Depressed mood A hallmark symptom of major depression. This change in mood is relatively constant and is recognized both by the depressed person and by others.

Depression Also called *dysphoria,* can have a sudden onset and include symptoms similar in number and intensity to those of major depression.

Dermatitis Inflammation of the skin.

Dermatome An area of skin that is innervated by a specific spinal cord segment.

Dermatomyositis A rare collagen disorder characterized by the acute or insidious onset of muscle pain, weakness, fever, arthralgia, and, in some cases, a puffy erythematous eruption that is usually confined to the face and the eyelids.

Dermatophyte A fungus that causes infection of the skin. The most common dermatophytes are *Microsporum, Trichophyton,* and *Epidermophyton.*

Dermatosis Any disorder of the skin.

Dermis Inner, thicker layer of the cutaneous membrane.

Dermoepidermal junction The specialized area where the cells of the epidermis meet the connective tissue cells of the dermis.

Desensitization The process of manipulating or "training" the hypothalamus to react less forcefully to a perceived threat or stressor. This technique works by changing the predominant brain waves of the individual from beta waves to alpha waves that are slower and more normal.

Desquamation The shedding of epithelial elements from the skin surface.

Detrusor muscle Smooth muscle of the bladder body.

Diabetes insipidus An endocrine deficiency of antidiuretic hormone manifesting as excretion of large quantities of very dilute urine.

Diabetes mellitus An endocrine disorder characterized by impaired glucose entry into insulin-sensitive cells due to an absolute or relative deficiency of insulin.

Dialysate fluid Prepared solution with varying concentrations of glucose and electrolytes used to aid dialysis.

Dialysis An artificial process that replaces the renal functions of diffusion and filtration necessary to maintain homeostasis.

Diaper rash A skin irritation resulting from the ammonia and alkali byproducts of urine breakdown.

Diarrhea An increase in the frequency and fluidity of bowel movements. It is usually a primary sign of gastrointestinal tract disorders.

Diarthrosis Also called *synovial joint;* a freely movable joint in which a contiguous bony surface is covered by articular cartilage and connected by a fibrous connective tissue capsule lined with a synovial membrane.

Diastole A phase of the cardiac cycle in which the ventricles are relaxing and filling with blood.

Diastolic blood pressure The lowest measured pressure in the arteries just prior to the next ventricular ejection.

Diencephalon "Between" brain; part of the brain between cerebral hemispheres and the midbrain.

Diffusion Movement of a gas from an area of high concentration to low concentration, or the process by which solutes move across a semipermeable membrane from an area of greater concentration to one of lesser concentration.

Diffusion coefficient A constant that depends on the properties of the tissue and the solute; the rate of movement of a solute is proportional to the diffusion coefficient.

Diploid Containing two sets of homologous chromosomes and, therefore, two copies of each gene, one from each parent.

Disconjugate An abnormal positioning of the eyes such that they deviate from one another in the direction of gaze.

Disease Sum of the deviations from normal structure or function of any part, organ, or system (or combination thereof) of the body manifested by a characteristic set of symptoms and/or signs and whose cause, pathogenesis, and prognosis may be known or unknown.

Dislocation Displacement of a bone from its normal position in a joint to the degree that the articulating surfaces lose contact.

Displaced fracture A fracture in which the ends of fragments are separated.

Disuse atrophy The tendency of cells and tissues to reduce size and function in response to lack of trophic stimuli.

Disuse osteoporosis Reduction in quantity of bone or atrophy of skeletal tissue in response to lack of weight-bearing activity. May occur with prolonged bed rest.

Diuresis Excretion of large amounts of urine as a result of the actions of a diuretic.

Diurnal variation The regular (24-hour) recurrence of certain biological phenomena under conditions of illumination; recurring during the daytime, or period of light.

Diverticulitis Inflammation of one or more diverticula, or outpouchings, in the intestinal wall.

Diverticulosis The presence of diverticula, or outpouchings, in the wall of the colon.

Diverticulum Outpouching of one or more layers of the wall of a structure in the gastrointestinal tract, especially in the colon or esophagus.

DNA polymerase An enzyme complex that binds to DNA, using it as a template for synthesis of a complementary DNA strand.

Dominant Referring to the gene allele that is overtly expressed in the cell's phenotype. Opposite of recessive.

Dopamine hypothesis A hypothesis that postulates that schizophrenia is the result of neuronal overactivity dependent on dopamine.

Down-regulation A decrease in the number of cell receptors for a specific hormone resulting from the cell's prolonged exposure to high concentrations of the hormone. Down-regulation results in a decrease in the target cell response to a hormone.

Drug-induced asthma Asthma related to an ingested drug. An attack may occur within minutes of ingestion or may be delayed up to 12 hours. Nonsteroidal antiinflammatory drugs including indomethacin (Indocin) and ibuprofen (Motrin, Advil) are common causes.

Duchenne muscular dystrophy The most common and most severe form of muscular dystrophy, inherited as an X-linked trait and therefore afflicting only males.

Ductus deferens Thick, muscular tube that is continuous with the epididymis. The ductus deferens travels along the pelvic wall and joins with the seminal vesicle duct at the prostate to form the ejaculatory duct. Also called *vas deferens.*

Dumping syndrome The rapid emptying or "dumping" of stomach contents into the proximal small intestine due to loss of pyloric regulation of gastric emptying. This loss of function may occur following a gastrectomy.

Dysconjugate See *disconjugate.*

Dysfunctional uterine bleeding Abnormal endometrial bleeding not associated with tumor, inflammation, pregnancy, or trauma. It is most common around the time of menarche and menopause.

Dysmenorrhea Pain associated with menstruation, usually classified as primary (unrelated to an identifiable disease) or secondary (related to the presence of an underlying disease).

Dysphagia Difficulty in swallowing as perceived by the individual. It may include the inability to initiate swallowing and/or the sensation of ingested substances sticking in the esophagus.

Dysphoria The constant experience of unpleasant emotions.

Dysplasia An alteration in cellular growth in which cell morphologic characteristics are variable and disorderly. Dysplastic cells may become cancerous and therefore are often termed *preneoplastic.*

Dyspnea Breathlessness or difficulty breathing.

Dysrhythmia An abnormality of heart rhythm, including altered rates or sites of impulse initiation and abnormal conduction pathways.

Dysthymia A state of chronic depression.

Dystrophic Abnormal tissue growth that impairs function. May result from disordered growth (trophic) signals.

E

Eating disorder *Anorexia nervosa* or *bulimia nervosa.* See definitions of *anorexia* and *bulimia.*

Eccentric contraction A lengthening contraction that occurs when the load is greater than the amount of tension that the muscle is able to generate, such as walking down stairs (eccentric contraction of the quadriceps muscles).

Ecchymosis Discoloration of the skin (bruise) caused by escape of blood into the tissues.

Eccrine sweat gland A sweat gland that opens directly onto the skin surface.

Ectasia Dilation of a tubular structure, as in mammary duct ectasia (in which the collecting ducts beneath the nipple and areola become dilated, thinned, and filled with secretions).

Ectopic In an abnormal location.

Ectopic ureter A single ureter that implants during fetal growth in any position other than normal, or an additional ureter.

Ectopy (cardiac) A cardiac impulse initiated at a site other than the sinoatrial node.

Edema An excess of fluid in the interstitial compartment.

Efferent neuron A neuron that carries information away from the central nervous system to the muscle cells, glands, or postganglionic neurons.

Effusion Presence of fluid in a contained space, causing pressure on structures within the space.

Ejaculation Expulsion of the ejaculate from the posterior urethra through the urethral meatus.

Ejection fraction Stroke volume divided by end-diastolic volume; indicates pumping efficiency of the ventricle.

Elastin A protein found in tendons and ligaments that provides some elasticity or extensibility.

Elastosis Skin wrinkling due to changes in collagen with fibers becoming cross-linked and rearranged in thicker bundles.

Electrochemical gradient A difference in concentration of charged particles across a membrane. Driving force that moves charged particles across a membrane due to the combined influences of concentration gradient and electrical charge gradient.

Electroencephalogram Graphic tracing of brain's action potentials; used to evaluate nervous tissue function.

Electrolyte Substance that releases charged particles (ions) when dissolved.

Electromyography A technique for evaluating muscle contraction; using electromyography, aspects of the contractile process such as time relationships between the beginning of electrical activity and the actual contraction of the muscle can be studied.

Electron transport chain A series of proteins on the inner mitochondrial membrane that move an electron from a higher to a lower energy level and create a proton gradient.

Embolus A collection of material (thrombus, air, fat, tumor cells, bacteria, amniotic fluid) propelled by blood flow to another site, where it lodges and causes obstruction of flow.

Embryoscopy A procedure in which a scope is passed through the cervix and into the uterus to visualize and sample embryonic tissues.

Emission One of the two phases of ejaculation. During emission, secretions from the periurethral glands, seminal vesicles, and prostate are deposited with sperm into the prostatic urethra.

Emphysema A chronic obstructive respiratory condition characterized by abnormal, permanent enlargement of air spaces distal to the terminal bronchiole with destruction of their walls and without obvious fibrosis.

Empyema Accumulation of pus in the pleural space.

Encapsulation Physiologic process of enclosure in a sheath composed of a substance not normal to the part. Prevents opsonization (recognition and binding) by antibodies and thus prevents the microorganism from being phagocytized.

Encopresis Fecal holding with constipation and fecal soiling.

Endocardium A layer of endothelial cells that lines the chambers of the heart. The layer of heart muscle just under the endocardium is called the *subendocardium.*

Endocrine organ Any organ that manufactures and secretes hormones into the bloodstream.

Endocrine system The cells and organs that produce and secrete hormones into the bloodstream.

Endocytosis Cellular ingestion of extracellular molecules.

Endogenous depression Major depression arising from characteristics within the person as opposed to depression resulting from external events.

Endometrioma A mass of endometrial tissue that grows outside the lining of the uterine cavity in the condition known as *endometriosis.*

Endometriosis Growth of endometrial tissue outside the lining of the uterine cavity; an abnormal condition with potentially destructive effects on the pelvic organs.

Endometrium The innermost lining of the uterus, consisting of two layers: a thin deep layer, called the *basilar layer,* and a thick superficial layer, referred to as the *functional layer.* During a woman's reproductive years, the endometrium displays a constant cyclic activity of alternate proliferation and sloughing of the functional layer in response to hormonal secretion.

Endomysium The connective tissue that surrounds the sarcolemma of individual muscle fiber.

Endorphin One of a group of potent endogenous opioid peptides derived from cells in the hypothalamus, also found in the periaqueductal gray matter of the brain. β-Endorphin has been found to have analgesic properties.

Endoscopic retrograde cholangiopancreatography (ERCP) A procedure whereby an optical scope is passed through the mouth, esophagus, stomach, and duodenum, and then guided in a retrograde fashion into the pancreaticobiliary system. Using this technique, physicians can perform a number of therapeutic procedures without performing a laparotomy.

Endoscopic sclerosis A procedure of the esophageal varices that is accomplished by passing a flexible needle through the gastroscope and injecting various sclerosant solutions into and around the bleeding varix.

Endosteum The thin membrane that covers the medullary cavity in longer bones.

Endotoxin A heat-stable lipopolysaccharide derived from the cell wall of gram-negative bacteria that induces the release of pyrogens and inflammatory mediators from immune cells.

Energy The capacity to operate or work, measured in kilocalories (kcal); 1 kcal represents the amount of energy required to raise the temperature of 1 kg of water from 15° C to 16° C.

Enteropathic arthritis Refers to joint manifestations of inflammatory bowel diseases such as ulcerative colitis and Crohn disease.

Enuresis Involuntary voiding; the term is generally used when referring to inappropriate wetting in children.

Eosinophil A leukocyte that is the same size as a neutrophil but contains a two-lobed nucleus and large, coarse, eosinophilic granules that fill the cell; these participate in allergic and inflammatory responses.

Epicardium A layer of epithelial cells that covers the outer surface of the heart and forms the inner (visceral) layer of the pericardial sac.

Epidemic An outbreak of a disease that occurs suddenly and affects numbers of people clearly in excess of normal expectancy.

Epidemiology The study of patterns of disease among human populations for the purpose of establishing programs to prevent and control their spread.

Epidermal proliferating unit Group of active basal cells, together with vertical columns of migrating keratinocytes, that are undergoing mitosis.

Epidermis Outer, thinner layer of the cutaneous membrane.

Epididymis Tightly coiled tube in which sperm mature and develop the ability to swim; lies along the top of and behind the testes.

Epididymitis Inflammation of the epididymis.

Epileptogenic focus Cellular focus in the brain with the capacity to induce epilepsy.

Epimysium The connective tissue surrounding a muscle.

Epinephrine A neurotransmitter that produces some of the same effects as norepinephrine but has a greater influence on cardiac action. Epinephrine enhances myocardial contractility, increases heart rate, and increases venous return to the heart, thus increasing cardiac output and blood pressure.

Epiphyseal plate A segment of a long bone between metaphysis and epiphysis developed from a center of ossification and distinct from the shaft. An area of growth in a bone.

Epispadias A congenital anomaly in which the urethra opens on the dorsal aspect of the penis at a point proximal to the glans.

Epistaxis Hemorrhage from the nose; nosebleed.

Epitope A site on the surface of an antigen that is specifically recognized by an immune cell, thus stimulating an immune response.

Equilibrium Sense of balance.

Erection A complicated interaction of vascular, neurologic, and hormonal factors that enables the penis to achieve penetration and deposit sperm.

Erythema Diffuse redness of skin.

Erythroblastosis Presence of erythroblasts in the blood due to premature release from the bone marrow.

Erythromelalgia Painful erythema (redness of the skin) of the palms and soles due to congestion of the capillaries.

Erythron The blood as a single body system.

Erythropoiesis The process of red blood cell production.

Erythropoietin Hormone produced primarily by the kidney that stimulates bone marrow to produce erythrocytes.

Eschar Burn tissue.

Escharotomy A surgical incision through eschar of a circumferential extremity burn for the purpose of restoring distal blood flow, or through eschar of the chest to restore respiratory expansion.

Esophageal atresia Congenital anomaly in which the esophagus is closed off in a blind pouch at some point. It occurs in about 1 of every 4000 live births and requires immediate surgical correction.

Esophageal varix Abnormally dilated blood vessel lying just below the mucous membrane of the esophagus that connects the hypertensive portal system with the systemic circulation. Esophageal varices may rupture, causing massive hemorrhage.

Esophagitis Inflammation or infection of the esophagus.

Essential amino acids Amino acids that must be supplied in the diet because the body cannot manufacture them.

Estrogen One of a group of ovarian hormones that promote the development of female secondary sex characteristics. During the menstrual cycle, estrogen renders the female reproductive tract suitable for fertilization of the ovum, implantation of the zygote, and nutrition of the early embryo.

Etiology Study of the assignment of causes or reasons for phenomena.

Euchromatin Chromatin that is less densely packed and potentially open to transcription, as opposed to heterochromatin that is condensed and not open to transcription. "Normal" chromatin.

Eukaryote A cell that has a true nucleus bounded by a nuclear membrane.

Euphoria Also called *expanded mood,* is a hallmark symptom of both mania and hypomania. Extreme cheerfulness, enthusiasm, and optimism are present, but the joyful, buoyant mood is disproportionate to events and surroundings.

Ewing sarcoma A malignant round cell tumor (marrow tumor) that is relatively uncommon but rapidly growing.

Exacerbation A relatively sudden increase in the severity of a disease or any of its signs and symptoms.

Exercise-induced asthma Asthma that manifests 5 to 10 minutes after the exercise period begins. The increased rate and depth of respiration during exercise, especially in cold air, leads to cooling and dehydration of the lower airways.

Exhaustion A stage in the stress response that occurs when the stressor is too great or prolonged, resulting in depletion of energy reserves.

Exocytosis The process of cellular secretion.

Exon The portion of an RNA transcript that remains after unwanted sections (introns) have been removed from the primary transcript. A linear section of DNA that serves as a template for synthesis of a particular RNA sequence.

Exophthalmos Protrusion of the eyeball.

Exotoxin Toxins, such as enzymes or pore-forming proteins, produced by bacteria that cause physiologic dysfunction in the host.

Extracellular fluid Body fluid that is not inside the cells; includes vascular, interstitial, and transcellular fluids.

Extraocular Outside the globe of the eyeball.

Extrapyramidal system Part of the brain that includes the corpus striatum, subthalamic nucleus, substantia nigra, and red nucleus, and the interconnections with the reticular formation, cerebellum, and cerebrum.

Extrapyramidal tract Outside the pyramidal tract of the brain. Comprised of the nuclei and fibers involved in motor activities, extrapyramidal tracts control and coordinate postural, static, support, and locomotor mechanisms. Do not crossover in the medullary pyramid.

Extrinsic Originating from sources outside of the individual.

Extrinsic asthma Also called *allergic asthma,* it commonly affects children and young adults. Attacks are related to specific antigens and are immunoglobulin E mediated.

Extrinsic pathway of clotting The mechanism that produces fibrin following tissue injury, beginning with formation of an activated complex between tissue factor and activated factor VII and leading to activation of factor X, which induces the reactions of the common pathway of coagulation.

Exudate Fluid of high protein content that moves into tissues or cavities as part of a reaction to inflammation or injury.

F

Fascia A sheath of connective tissue that envelops muscles or other parts of the body.

Fasciculus Bundle of muscle fibers that compose individual muscles.

Fascioscapulohumeral muscular dystrophy A rare inherited autosomal dominant trait that affects the muscles of the shoulder girdle and the face.

Fast twitch (type II, white) A muscle fiber that can develop high tension rapidly. It is usually innervated by a single α motor neuron and has low fatigue resistance, low capillary density, low levels of aerobic enzymes, and low oxygen availability.

Fat The most concentrated dietary source of energy, derived from either animals or vegetables. Provides 9 kcal/g.

Fatigue A lack of physical or emotional energy or power.

Fatty acid An organic acid with a long, straight hydrocarbon chain that is a fundamental component of lipids. Some fatty acids are manufactured by the body, others are essential and must be supplied in the diet.

Fetotoxic Referring to a substance that is damaging to a developing fetus.

Fibrillation Cardiac dysrhythmia characterized by rapid, random myocardial contractions and discoordinated pumping action.

Fibrinolysis Dissolution or breakup of a fibrin clot.

Fibroblast A component of collagen fibers, which compose the bulk of the dermis.

Fibrocystic breast disease A condition in which palpable breast masses correspond to fluctuations in the menstrual cycle; the masses may be associated with pain and tenderness.

Fibromyalgia syndrome A painful, noninflammatory musculoskeletal disorder associated with fatigue and multiple somatic complaints.

Fibrosis Condition of decreased elasticity because of excessive deposition of fibrin and collagen in the tissue (e.g., restrictive process characterized by thickening of the alveolar interstitium).

Filtration Movement of fluid across capillary walls, as a net result of opposing forces.

First-degree burn Superficial tissue destruction in the outermost layers of the epidermis. All physiologic functions of the skin remain intact.

Fistula An abnormal tubelike passage between two organs or between an internal organ and the body surface.

Flagellum Motile (whiplike) appendage that allows a cell to move or swim.

Flat affect Lack of appropriate emotional expression.

Fomite An inanimate object that transmits a pathogen to a new host.

Foreskin Also called *prepuce;* penile skin that overlies the glans and is removed in circumcision.

Fossa navicularis Area of widening near the end of the penile urethra.

Fournier gangrene A rare condition involving a gangrenous necrosis of the scrotum, penis, or perineum.

Fourth-degree burn A full-thickness burn that penetrates the dermis to reach muscle or bone.

Fracture A break or disruption in continuity of a bone, an epiphyseal plate, or cartilage.

Frank-Starling law of the heart Describes the relationship between diastolic stretch and subsequent increased strength of contraction. Also called the *length-tension relationship.*

Free-living bacteria Bacteria that can live outside the host cell.

Free radical An extremely reactive compound that avidly makes molecular bonds with other compounds.

Full-thickness burn Also called a *third-degree burn,* this type of burn is marked by destruction of epidermis, dermis, and underlying tissue. All physiologic functions of the skin are absent. This burn will not heal and requires autografting.

Full-thickness excision Removal by surgical knife of complete eschar to fascia. Full-thickness excision often leaves an uneven contour, which presents difficulty with grafting, resulting in poor cosmesis.

Functional disorder of the endocrine system An endocrine disorder caused by a nonendocrine disease (e.g., chronic renal failure, liver disease, or heart failure).

Functional incontinence Loss of urine or feces as a result of factors external to the urinary or digestive tract, such as physical or cognitive impairment.

Functional syncytium A multinucleate mass of protoplasm that results from the merging of cells. It is characteristic of the gastrointestinal tract and heart, meaning that its separate cells have the ability to function in concert with one another in a unified manner.

Fungal infection Any inflammatory condition caused by a fungus.

Fungus A nonphotosynthetic, eukaryotic protist that is disseminated throughout the environment.

G

Gallbladder A distensible sac of about 30 to 50 ml capacity that connects the common hepatic duct to the common bile duct via the cystic duct.

Ganglion A group of neuronal cell bodies located outside of the central nervous system.

Gangrene Cellular death involving a large area of tissue; may be characterized as wet, dry, or gaseous.

Gap junction A cell-to-cell communication pore that allows small biomolecules to flow from the cytoplasm of one cell to the cytoplasm of an adjacent cell.

Gastrectomy Surgical removal of all or, more commonly, part of the stomach. This procedure may be used to remove a chronic peptic ulcer, to stop hemorrhage in a perforating ulcer, or to remove a malignancy.

Gastrin A stomach hormone that is released in response to certain types of food. Gastrin increases acid secretion by stomach parietal cells.

Gastritis Inflammation of the stomach lining. It may occur following the ingestion of irritating substances or in the presence of viral, bacterial, or chemical toxins.

Gastroenteritis Inflammation of the stomach and intestines, which may occur on an acute or chronic basis and is commonly caused by viruses.

Gastroesophageal reflux disease (GERD) Backflow of gastric contents into the esophagus through the lower esophageal sphincter. GERD may or may not produce symptoms. The most common manifestations of GERD are heartburn, regurgitation, chest pain, and dysphagia.

Gay bowel syndrome Transmission of and subsequent infection with enteric pathogens through sexual contact. These disorders are not limited to the homosexual community and may be transmitted among any individuals who engage in direct or indirect fecal-oral contact.

Gene A unit of heredity made up of a segment of DNA nucleotides that encodes a messenger RNA capable of being translated into a protein.

General adaptation syndrome The total organism's nonspecific response to stress. Term was coined by Hans Selye.

Generalized anxiety disorder (GAD) Characterized by the continual presence of a moderate degree of anxiety without discrete periods of acute attacks. GAD symptoms include chronic anxiety and tension accompanied by headaches, abdominal problems, or sleep disturbances. Agoraphobia is rarely seen in GAD.

Generalized seizure A seizure that involves the whole brain surface and impairs consciousness.

Genome The entire complement of genes located on chromosomes in the nucleus of a cell.

Genotype The genetic constitution of an individual, often described by listing the allele types at a certain gene locus.

Gestational diabetes mellitus A disorder of glucose tolerance first diagnosed in the mother during pregnancy.

Ghon tubercle A nodule or swelling containing *Mycobacterium tuberculosis.*

Giant cell tumor Also called *osteoclastoma;* a benign but aggressive tumor with richly vascularized tissue consisting of plump spindle-shaped cells and numerous giant cells.

Gilbert syndrome A common, benign autosomal dominant condition that results in mild unconjugated (indirect) hyperbilirubinemia.

Ginglymus A type of joint that permits flexion and extension like the interphalangeal joint of the finger, the elbow, or the knee. Also called a *hinge joint.*

Glasgow Coma Scale Scale developed by G. Teasdale and B. Jennett for the purpose of objectively assessing coma and impaired consciousness.

Glomerular filtration rate The rate of fluid filtration through the glomeruli into Bowman capsule per minute; normally 125 ml/min.

Glomerulonephritis Inflammation of the glomerular capillary walls causing impaired filtration and renal function.

Glucagon Hormone produced by the α cells of the pancreas that stimulates glycogenolysis and gluconeogenesis in the liver.

Glucocorticoid resistance model This model proposes a specific link between stress, immunity, and disease. Rather than viewing disease as a result of increased vulnerability due to stress, this model proposes that overwhelming stress reduces the sensitivity of the immune system to cortisol.

Glucocorticoids A class of steroid hormones secreted by the adrenal cortex, necessary for use of sugars, fats, and proteins and for the body's normal response to stress.

Gluconeogenesis The production of glucose from amino acids and other substrates in the liver.

Glycogen A carbohydrate consisting of branched chains of glucose produced by the muscle and liver as a storage form of glucose.

Glycogenesis Production of glycogen from glucose in hepatic and muscle tissue.

Glycogenolysis Production of glucose from the breakdown of glycogen in hepatic and muscle tissue.

Glycolysis The anaerobic process of breaking down sugars into simpler molecules, with the net production of two adenosine triphosphate and two pyruvate molecules per glucose molecule.

Glycosaminoglycan A protein polysaccharide contained in ground substances surrounded by collagen fibers in bone.

Glycosylated hemoglobin An index of glycemic control; the quantity of glucose attached to hemoglobin molecules, reflecting mean blood glucose values for a period of 120 days.

Goiter Enlargement of the thyroid gland.

Golgi apparatus A membrane-bound organelle in which the proteins and lipids that are synthesized in the endoplasmic reticulum are modified and sorted in preparation for transport to the lysosomes or plasma membrane.

Gomphosis joint An articulation created by the insertion of a conical process into a socket, such as the insertion of a root of a tooth into an alveolus of the mandible or the maxilla. Gomphosis is not a connection between true bones but is considered a type of fibrous joint.

Gonad An organ that produces sex cells. Derived from the urogenital ridge, the undifferentiated and primitive gonads become the testes in males and the ovaries in females.

Gonorrhea Common sexually transmitted disease involving the inflammation of epithelial tissue by the organism *Neisseria gonorrhoeae.* Characteristic symptoms include urethritis, dysuria, purulent urethral discharge, and redness and swelling at the site of the infection.

Gout A condition caused by lack of the enzyme uricase and inability to oxidize uric acid into a soluble compound; characterized by recurrent attacks of articular and periarticular inflammation, accumulation of tophi (crystalline deposits) in bony and connective tissue, renal impairment, and uric acid calculi.

Grading Assignment of degree of differentiation of tumor cells by histologic examination. The degree of anaplasia usually correlates with the degree of malignancy.

Gram stain A process by which it is determined whether a bacteria can retain a basic dye after iodine fixation. This ability is the basis for classifying bacteria into gram-negative and gram-positive organisms.

Granulocyte A leukocyte with polymorphic nuclei and cytoplasmic granules. Neutrophils, basophils, and eosinophils are types of granulocytes.

Granulocytopenia An abnormal decrease in the total number of granulocytes in the blood.

Granuloma Tissue that forms into a nodular mass as a result of inflammation, infection, or injury.

Granuloma inguinale An ulcerative disease of the genital tract caused by the bacterium *Calymmatobacterium granulomatis.* The communicability of the disease is relatively low, and it is generally believed that repeated exposure is necessary for infection.

Granulomatous Relating to granulomas, chronic inflammatory lesions characterized by an accumulation of macrophages; epithelioid macrophages, with or without lymphocytes; and giant cells into a discrete granule.

Graves disease Hyperthyroid state characterized by exophthalmos and goiter from autoimmune stimulation of the thyroid.

Greenstick fracture An incomplete break in the bone with the intact side of the cortex flexed; this is usually seen in children.

Ground substance A material composed of hydrated network of proteins, mainly glycoproteins and proteoglycans, that serves as the "cement" between layers of collagen fibers.

Growing pain A common soft tissue syndrome in children. The most common symptom is nocturnal pain that usually occurs in the calves, shins, and thighs. Also called *nonarticular rheumatism.*

Growth hormone A hormone secreted by the anterior pituitary gland with wide-ranging action, including effects on energy metabolism and increasing lean body mass.

Guillain-Barré syndrome Also called *acute idiopathic polyneuropathy* or *polyradiculoneuropathy;* Guillain-Barré syndrome is an inflammatory demyelinating disease of the peripheral nervous system.

Gustatory Pertaining to the sense of taste.

Gyrus A raised ridge or convolution on the surface of a structure (e.g., cerebral cortex).

H

H^+ Hydrogen ion; released by acids; determines pH; also called a *proton.*

HCO_3^- Bicarbonate ion; a base that binds and buffers H^+.

H_2CO_3 Carbonic acid; this acid is removed from the body in the form of carbon dioxide and water during exhalation.

H zone Corresponds to a region occupied solely by myosin filaments with no actin filament overlap in cardiac and skeletal muscle.

Hair Keratinized, threadlike outgrowth of the skin that covers most of the body.

Hair follicle Slender, cylindrical tube in which hair grows.

Hallucination A perception for which there are no real sensory data.

Haploid Containing only one set of chromosomes (as distinct from diploid), as in a sperm cell or egg cell.

Hapten Incomplete, lipid-soluble particle that is incapable of being an antigen by itself, but that becomes an antigen inside the body when it binds with a host protein called a carrier. When a hapten penetrates the epidermis and binds to a carrier, it can cause contact hypersensitivity.

Haustral churning The mixing movement of the haustra (the outpouchings in the colon wall) when material is in the proximal end of the colon.

Haversian system The basic unit of bone; also called *osteon.*

HBV infection Hepatitis B virus infection. Vertical transmission from an HBsAg-positive mother to the infant is a common mechanism of spread. Features suggesting immune complex disease such as arthritis, fever, papular acrodermatitis (a rash not seen in adults), renal disease, and hematologic complications are more common in children.

HCV infection Hepatitis C virus infection. A type of hepatitis transmitted most commonly by blood transfusion or percutaneous inoculation.

HDV infection Hepatitis D virus infection. A form of hepatitis that occurs only in patients coinfected with hepatitis B. HDV relies on HBV replication and cannot replicate independently. The disease usually progresses to a chronic state.

Heimlich maneuver An emergency procedure for dislodging an obstruction from the trachea. It consists of grasping the choking person from behind and placing the hands around the victim's waist just below the sternum, in a fist, and pulling inward and upward with force to dislodge the obstruction.

Helicobacter pylori An infectious gastrointestinal tract bacterium first identified in 1982. Since then, *H. pylori* has generated worldwide attention for its role in the promotion of chronic gastritis, peptic ulcer disease, and gastric carcinoma. The mode of transmission of *H. pylori* is still unclear, although person-to-person, fecal-oral spread is suspected because of the tendency of *H. pylori* infections to cluster in families.

Hemarthrosis Blood in a joint cavity.

Hematemesis Blood in vomitus.

Hematochezia Feces containing bright red blood.

Hematoma A mass caused by extravasation of blood into a tissue or cavity.

Hematopoiesis Production of cells in the bone marrow, including red cells, white cells, and platelets.

Hematuria Blood in the urine.

Hemianopsia Partial loss of vision.

Hemiparesis Motor weakness affecting one side of the body, usually occurring with lateral cerebral injuries.

Hemiplegia Paralysis of one side of the body.

Hemochromatosis A disorder (usually genetic) of iron metabolism characterized by excess absorption of iron and deposition in organs such as the liver.

Hemodynamics Principles of blood flow.

Hemoglobin Oxygen-carrying protein in the red blood cells.

Hemolysis Separation of hemoglobin from red blood cells and its appearance in the fluid in which the corpuscles are suspended; red cell lysis.

Hemoptysis Spitting up of blood, the origin of which is the lungs or bronchial tubes.

Hemostasis Arrest of bleeding; prevention of blood loss.

Hemothorax Accumulation of blood in the pleural space.

Hepatitis An inflammatory condition of the liver. Potential causes include viral, bacterial, fungal, and protozoal infections; drugs and toxins; autoimmune disorders; and metabolic disorders.

Hepatocellular carcinoma A common form of primary hepatic malignancy. Signs and symptoms include hepatomegaly, abdominal pain, weight loss, nausea, and, in advanced cases, jaundice and ascites. Also called *hepatoma.*

Hepatocellular failure Acute or chronic loss of essential liver function resulting in portal systemic encephalopathy and a variety of other problems, including coagulopathy, renal failure, bleeding, infection, hypoglycemia, respiratory failure, and death.

Hepatoma A primary liver cancer arising from cells normally found in the liver, not to be confused with cancer metastatic to the liver from a distant site.

Hereditary hemochromatosis An autosomal recessive disorder caused by the activity of a mutant gene called *HFE,* which allows excessive and uncontrolled iron absorption by the GI tract.

Herpesviruses Important group of viral agents producing infections in humans. Two types of herpes simplex viruses, referred to as types 1 and 2, may be sexually transmitted.

Herpes zoster (shingles) An acute localized inflammatory disease of a dermatomal segment of the skin caused by the same herpesvirus that causes chickenpox.

Heterochromatin A type of chromatin (DNA) that is tightly compacted and genetically inactive.

Heterozygous Having two different alleles for a specific gene product.

HEV infection Hepatitis E virus infection. A self-limited type of hepatitis acquired by ingestion of fecally contaminated water or food.

Hiatal hernia A defect in the diaphragm that allows a portion of the stomach to protrude through the diaphragmatic opening into the thorax.

High blood pressure Elevation of blood pressure above 140 mm Hg systolic and/or 90 mm Hg diastolic.

Hilum Concave portion of the kidney that faces the vertebral column through which nerves, blood vessels, and ureter enter and exit the kidney.

Hinge joint A joint that permits flexion and extension like the interphalangeal joint of the finger, the elbow, or the knee. Also called a *ginglymus joint.*

Hirschsprung disease A congenital disorder of the large intestine in which the autonomic nerve ganglia in the smooth muscle are absent or markedly reduced in number.

Hirsutism Excessive growth of the hair or presence of hair in unusual places.

Histiocyte A type of cell normally present in small numbers around blood vessels, but in pathologic conditions it can migrate in the dermis as a tissue monocyte. It can also form abundant reticulum fibers. When it phagocytizes bacteria and particulate matter, it is referred to as a *macrophage.*

Histone A protein around which linear DNA is wrapped.

Histrionic Theatrical, dramatic.

Hodgkin disease A progressive malignancy of the lymph node characterized by the presence of Reed-Sternberg cells and slow, predictable spread through the lymphatic vessels.

Homeostasis A dynamic steady state, representing the net effect of all the turnover reactions.

Homologous Corresponding in structure. For example, the labia majora are *homologous* with the scrotum of the male.

Homologous chromosomes A pair of chromosomes in a diploid cell that contain similar gene loci, each being derived from a different parent.

Homozygous Having two identical alleles for a specific gene product.

Hormone A blood-borne chemical messenger that affects target cells anatomically distant from the secreting cells.

Hormone agonist A chemical that binds to a hormone receptor and initiates intracellular activities identical to those caused by hormones. Some medications exert their therapeutic effects through this process.

Hormone antagonist A chemical that competes with hormones for cell receptors. Antagonists bind to cell receptors and prevent the occurrence of intracellular activities associated with hormone-receptor binding. Some medications produce their therapeutic effects through this process.

Hormone receptor A protein on or within a target cell that binds to circulating hormones and allows the cellular response to a specific hormone. Hormone-receptor binding is the first step in the cellular response to a particular hormone.

Host-parasite relationship The interaction between the host and the microorganisms that reside on or in it.

Human immunodeficiency virus (HIV) A general term for several types of retroviruses that affect the immune system, causing a defect in cell-mediated immunity and failure of the immune system to function properly.

Human leukocyte antigen (HLA) complex The major histocompatibility complex (MHC) in human leukocytes.

Hyaline membranes Membranes in alveolar tissue that look like glass. The alveoli are filled with proteinaceous fluid and epithelial cells.

Hydrocele Accumulation of fluid in the tunica vaginalis testis; one of the most common causes of scrotal swelling.

Hydrocephalus Increase in the amount of cerebrospinal fluid due to blocked circulation or absorption and the consequent enlargement of the ventricles.

Hydrophilic Soluble in water but not in lipid.

Hydrophobic Insoluble in water but soluble in lipid.

Hydropic swelling An increase in intracellular fluid volume and changes in intracellular organelles in association with cell injury. Also termed *oncosis.*

Hydrostatic pressure Pressure exerted by a liquid.

Hydroureter Distention of a ureter with urine, usually resulting from an obstruction process.

Hyperacusis Exceptionally acute hearing, the hearing threshold being unusually low. It may or may not be accompanied by pain.

Hyperalgesia An increased sensitivity to painful stimuli characterized by a lower than normal pain threshold.

Hypercalcemia Serum calcium concentration above normal.

Hypercapnia An abnormally high amount of carbon dioxide in the blood.

Hypercortisolism Elevated serum level of cortisol.

Hyperemesis gravidarum A Latin term meaning "excess vomiting in pregnant women." Unlike the transient nausea and vomiting that occurs in about half of women in the first trimester of pregnancy, hyperemesis gravidarum continues throughout the entire pregnancy. It is often severe and can have life-threatening consequences.

Hyperemia Localized redness produced by increased blood flow.

Hyperkalemia Serum potassium concentration above normal.

Hyperkeratosis Horny overgrowth of epidermis, such as callus formation.

Hypermagnesemia Serum magnesium concentration above normal.

Hypermetabolic state A condition of abnormally high basal metabolic rate. May be indicated by an increase in skin temperature, such as that occurring in hyperthyroidism and after sun exposure or sunburn.

Hypernatremia Serum sodium concentration above normal; results from gain of salt relative to water or loss of water relative to salt; water deficit.

Hyperphosphatemia Serum phosphate concentration above normal.

Hyperplasia Abnormal multiplication or increase in the number of normal cells in normal arrangement in a tissue.

Hypersensitivity An abnormal excessive response to a sensitizing antigen.

Hypertension Elevation of blood pressure above 140 mm Hg systolic and/or 90 mm Hg diastolic.

Hyperthyroidism Overactivity of the thyroid gland.

Hypertonic fluid Fluid that has a higher particle concentration (osmolality) than normal body fluid; causes a net flow of water across cell membranes out of cells.

Hypertrichosis lanuginosa Excessive hair growth over the entire body.

Hypertrophy An increase in cell or tissue size and function.

Hypocalcemia Serum calcium concentration below normal.

Hypochromia An abnormal decrease in the hemoglobin content of the erythrocytes.

Hypodermis Loose subcutaneous layer rich in fat and areolar tissue lying beneath the dermis. Also known as *superficial fascia.*

Hypoglycemic sweating Sweating caused by low blood glucose. Usually distinguishable from other causes of sweating due to the additional symptoms of weakness, tachycardia, hunger, headache, and "inward nervousness" manifested as mental irritability and confusion.

Hypokalemia Serum potassium concentration below normal.

Hypomagnesemia Serum magnesium concentration below normal.

Hypomania Also called *partial mania,* can include any symptoms of mania but without the loss of reality testing, without psychosis (e.g., hallucinations, delusions), and without impaired functioning.

Hypomenorrhea A deficient amount of menstrual flow, usually the result of an endocrine or systemic disorder that interferes with hormonal function. It may also result from partial obstruction of the menstrual flow by the hymen or a narrowing of the cervical os.

Hyponatremia Serum sodium concentration below normal; results from gain of water relative to salt or loss of salt relative to water; water intoxication.

Hypophosphatemia Serum phosphate concentration below normal.

Hypophysis The pituitary gland, which consists of anterior and posterior lobes.

Hyposensitization Reduction in sensitivity to an allergen, accomplished by administering low doses of the allergen, which binds with immunoglobulin G.

Hypospadias A congenital anomaly in which the urethral meatus is located on the undersurface of the penis or on the perineum.

Hypothalamic-pituitary-adrenal (HPA) axis Refers to a hierarchy of control mechanisms whereby the hypothalamus regulates the anterior pituitary and the pituitary regulates the secretion of hormones from the adrenal cortex.

Hypothalamus A group of nuclei at the base of the brain concerned with regulation of body processes: temperature, thirst, hunger, satiety, and adaptive sexual behaviors.

Hypothyroidism Underactivity of the thyroid gland.

Hypotonic fluid Fluid that has a lower particle concentration (osmolality) than normal body fluid; causes a net flow of water across cell membranes into cells.

Hypoventilation Decreased exchange of air in the alveoli in relation to oxygen consumption, influenced by a decreased rate and depth of respiration.

Hypoxemia An abnormally low amount of oxygen in the blood.

Hypoxia A reduction in oxygen at the tissue level that may lead to failure of aerobic production of adenosine triphosphate.

I

I bands "I" for "isotropic"; these bands are light in color and correspond to the position of thin actin filaments extending in both directions from the Z line in striated muscle.

Iatrogenic Resulting from the activity of a physician.

Icterus Also called *jaundice.* A yellow discoloration of the skin, mucous membranes, and sclerae of the eyes, caused by greater than normal amounts of bilirubin in the blood.

Idiopathic Without known cause.

Idiopathic hypertension High blood pressure of unknown cause; also called *primary hypertension.*

Ileocecal valve Sphincter between the small and large intestines that is normally closed, so that the contents of the large intestine cannot move in a retrograde fashion back into the small intestine. It opens in response to a peristaltic contraction, bringing intestinal contents toward it.

Illusion The misperception of a real sensory stimulus.

Immobilization A mechanical action of limiting or preventing movement at a joint. Prolonged immobilization may cause a shortening of connective tissue, a breakdown of cartilage, a weakening of ligaments, and a decrease in the muscles' ability to contract, as well as increased bone resorption.

Immunity A state of active resistance to a particular pathogen, which requires functional T- and B-cell memory cells.

Immunization Exposure of a susceptible host to an altered pathogen that does not cause disease but causes the host to create antibodies to that pathogen.

Immunodeficiency Failure of immune system mechanisms to defend against pathogens. There are two broad categories of immunodeficiencies, based on the mechanism of lymphocyte dysfunction: primary and acquired.

Immunogen Foreign substance, cell, toxin, or protein that causes the components of the immune system to react and respond, inducing the formation of antibodies. Also known as *antigen.*

Immunogenicity The ability to stimulate an immune response.

Immunosuppression The inability to produce an immune response to an antigen, resulting in reduced resistance to infection.

Impacted fracture A fracture caused by excessive force that telescopes or drives one fragment into another.

Impaired fasting glucose A disorder of glucose tolerance, not diagnostic of diabetes, that is characterized by a fasting blood glucose value between 100 and 126 mg/dl.

Impaired glucose tolerance A disorder of glucose tolerance, not diagnostic of diabetes, that is characterized by a 2-hour postprandial blood glucose value of between 140 and 200 mg/dl.

Impetigo An acute, contagious skin disease characterized by the formation of vesicles, pustules, and yellowish crusts.

Impotence Failure to achieve and maintain an erection of the penis.

Impulsivity Spontaneous acting out of impulses accompanied by failure to plan ahead, predict consequences, or consider other possibilities.

Incomplete fracture A fracture in which the cortex of the bone buckles or cracks without disrupting bone continuity.

Induration Hardness, such as that resulting from multiple intramuscular or subcutaneous injections of medication.

Inert tissue Soft tissue that possesses no ability to contract or relax; this includes the joint capsule, ligament, bursa, fascia, dura mater, and nerve root.

Infectious disease A pathologic process caused by a microorganism that is transmissible from one host to another.

Infiltrate Fluid or material that has moved into tissues.

Inflammation The body's protective response at the site of injury or tissue destruction. It is important to recognize that although infectious agents can produce inflammation, infection is not synonymous with inflammation.

Inflammatory bowel disease A general term for inflammatory diseases of the bowel of uncertain cause, such as ulcerative colitis and Crohn disease.

Inhalation injury Cellular injury to lung tissue as a result of inhalation of a toxic substance such as smoke. Smoke inhalation significantly increases the morbidity and mortality from burn injury.

Innate immune response Part of the host defense system that is composed of mechanical and biochemical barriers, phagocytes, and chemical mediators.

Inotropy The force or energy of cardiac contraction; similar to contractility.

Insulin Hormone produced by the β cells of the pancreas; has wide-ranging effects on energy metabolism and protein synthesis.

Insulin resistance The condition of requiring an increased amount of insulin for the same level of tissue glucose utilization combined with lowered glucose utilization at all levels.

Integrins A large family of transmembrane proteins that mediate adhesion of cells to the extracellular matrix.

Integument Covering; refers to the skin.

Integumentary system The skin and its appendages, including the hair and nails.

Intercurrent Occurring during the course of an already existing disease.

Intermembranous ossification The process in which osteoblasts in the inner layer of the periosteum are responsible for the increase in the width of bones.

Interstitial fluid Fluid that lies between the cells; a component of extracellular fluid.

Interstitial space The space between cells.

Intertrigo An erythematous irritation of opposing skin surfaces caused by friction.

Intestinal villi Fingerlike projections, numbering in the millions, that line the small intestine and serve to increase the surface area of the intestine for digestion and absorption of nutrients.

Intraaortic Within the aorta. For example, in intraaortic balloon counterpulsation, a catheter with a balloon at the distal segment is inserted through the femoral artery and positioned in the aorta just distal to the left subclavian artery.

Intracellular fluid Fluid that is inside the cells.

Intracellular obligate parasites Bacteria that must live inside a living cell.

Intraocular Inside the globe of the eyeball.

Intravenous pyelography A diagnostic procedure in which an iodine-based contrast material is injected into the vascular system to allow visualization of the kidneys and urinary tract.

Intrinsic Originating from within the individual.

Intrinsic asthma Asthma caused by pathophysiologic disturbances that do not involve IgE-mediated mechanisms. This type of asthma frequently develops in middle age. Psychological stress factors, pulmonary irritants, and exercise may precipitate an asthma attack.

Intrinsic nervous system Neural structures belonging entirely to the gastrointestinal (GI) system that control most GI functions and are responsible for many reflexes occurring locally in the GI tract. It is composed of two layers: the myenteric plexus and the submucosal plexus.

Intrinsic pathway of coagulation A sequence of reactions leading to fibrin formation, beginning with the contact activation of factor XII, followed by the sequential activation of factors XI and IX and resulting in the activation of factor X, which in activated form initiates the common pathway of coagulation.

Intron The portion of a primary RNA transcript that is removed prior to translation of the RNA message.

Intussusception A telescoping of a portion of the bowel into an adjacent distal portion. It is most common in infants and occurs three times more often in males than in females.

Ipsilateral Referring to the same side of the body.

Irritable bowel syndrome The presence of alternating diarrhea and constipation accompanied by abdominal cramping in the absence of any identifiable pathologic process in the gastrointestinal tract.

Ischemia Inadequate flow through the arterial system, producing tissue hypoxia.

Ischemic hepatitis A lack of blood or oxygen supply to the liver that causes injury to liver cells.

Isoimmunity The condition occurring when an individual's immune system reacts against antigens on tissues from other members of the same species, such as a blood transfusion reaction in which a person with type A blood reacts against a transfusion with type B blood.

Isolated systolic hypertension An elevation in systolic blood pressure above 140 mm Hg without an increase in diastolic blood pressure. Most commonly occurs in the elderly.

Isolated urinary tract infection A first infection or an infection that occurs more than 6 months after a previous infection.

Isometric contraction A contraction in which no movement takes place and the muscle maintains its specific length. For example, holding a weight in the hand with elbow flexed produces an isometric contraction.

Isotonic fluid Fluid that has the same particle concentration (osmolality) as normal body fluid.

J

Jaundice Yellowness of skin.

Joint A point of contact between bones. Also called *articulation.*

Joint capsule A dense layer of connective tissue surrounding a synovial joint. The capsule is solidly attached to the periosteum of the adjacent bony components. The joint capsule provides strength to the joint and, through its neural receptors, detects motion, compression, tension, vibration, and pain.

Juxtaglomerular apparatus The collection of macula densa cells in the distal convoluted tubule, afferent and efferent arterioles, and the juxtaglomerular cells located around the arterioles, which work together to control glomerular filtration rate.

Juxtamedullary nephron A nephron with long loops of Henle that extend deep into the medulla and create a concentrated interstitium via the countercurrent mechanism.

K

Keratin Tough, water-repellent protein produced by keratinocytes and found in hair, nails, and horny tissue.

Keratinocyte One of several types of epithelial cells. Keratinocytes are able to synthesize DNA and produce keratin.

Keratosis Any skin lesion in which there is overgrowth and thickening of the cornified epithelium.

Kernicterus An abnormal toxic accumulation of bilirubin in central nervous system tissues caused by hyperbilirubinemia.

Ketone bodies The result of fatty acids in the liver that are transformed to acetyl coenzyme A, which is then processed into one of three compounds known as ketone bodies.

Kilocalorie The unit of measure for energy value of foods.

Kinin A vasoactive peptide produced during inflammation and injury.

Koilonychia Dystrophy of the fingernails, in which the nails are concave; also known as *spoon nail.*

Korotkoff sounds Sounds heard during auscultation of arterial blood pressure. As the pressure in the blood pressure cuff is released, blood begins to flow turbulently through the artery, producing Korotkoff sounds.

L

Lactation Formation and secretion of milk from the breasts for the nourishment of the infant.

Lactic acidosis An increase in the anaerobic production of lactate, which, when released into the blood stream, creates a condition of metabolic acidosis.

Laminar flow Flow of air or fluid in which there is no turbulence and the direction of flow is linear and parabolic.

Langerhans cell One of several types of epithelial cell. Langerhans cells are thought to have a role in immunologic reactions that affect the skin and may serve as a defense mechanism for the body.

Laparoscopic cholecystectomy Surgical removal of the gallbladder using an optical scope and instruments inserted through four small abdominal incisions.

Laparoscopy Examination of the abdominal cavity via a small incision to permit the insertion of a variety of optical scopes for diagnosis or therapy.

Latency period A period of time when there is no apparent change in status. The time required for elastic structures to tighten to prepare for the development of tension.

Leiomyoma Benign neoplasm of the smooth muscle of the uterus that is characteristically firm, well circumscribed, and round. Uterine leiomyomas usually appear and exhibit growth activity during the reproductive years.

Leprosy A chronic infectious disease of the skin caused by the intracellular bacillus *Mycobacterium leprae.*

Leptomeninges The combined structures of the pia mater and arachnoid mater.

Lesion A demonstrable structural change produced in the course of a disease. Lesions may be evident at a gross or microscopic level.

Leukemia A malignant disease of bone marrow stem cells, with accumulation of immature blasts in the marrow and peripheral blood.

Leukocyte A cell that mediates immune function. Leukocytes protect the body by phagocytosis of microorganisms and production of antibodies and memory cells. Also called *white blood cell.*

Leukoderma Patch of depigmentation, also called *vitiligo.*

Leukopenia A deficiency of white blood cells in the peripheral circulation, which is usually indicative of bone marrow failure.

Leydig cell An interstitial cell in the testes that produces and secretes testosterone.

Libido Sexual drive; feeling of sexual desire.

Lichen planus A relatively common, chronic, pruritic disease involving inflammation and papular eruption of the skin and mucous membranes.

Ligament A dense connective tissue with parallel-fibered collagenous tissues designed to connect bone to bone.

Limbic system A group of structures surrounding the corpus callosum that produce various emotional feelings.

Lipid bilayer A double layer of lipid molecules that forms cellular membranes, including the plasma membrane, organelle membranes, and vesicles.

Lipodystrophy A group of conditions due to defective metabolism of fat, resulting in atrophy of subcutaneous fat.

Lipolysis Production of free fatty acids resulting from the breakdown of fat in adipose tissue.

Lipoproteins A group of biomolecules composed of differing amounts of cholesterol, triglyceride, and protein, such as high-density lipoprotein (HDLs) and low-density lipoprotein (LDLs).

Lithotripsy Mechanical or chemical fragmentation of a calculus.

Liver transplantation Surgical transfer of an appropriately matched donor liver into a host who has inadequate liver function to sustain life.

Longitudinal fracture Fracture in which a bone is split along its length.

Loose association Flow of thought in which ideas shift from one subject to another in a completely unrelated or noncohesive way. When severe, speech may be unintelligible.

Lower esophageal sphincter The circular band of muscular tissue at the lower end of the esophagus. It serves to prevent the highly acidic gastric contents from moving in a retrograde motion back into the esophagus.

Lumpectomy Surgical removal of only the malignant tumor or "lump" from an affected breast.

Lunula "Little moon"; the crescent-shaped white area nearest the root of the nail body.

Lusitropy Relaxation of cardiac muscle and chambers.

Lyme disease An infectious, immune-mediated multisystem disease caused by a tick-borne spirochete. It is characterized by an erythema migrans rash in which the area of redness begins at the site of the tick bite. The site is generally flat, warm, and indurated, but not painful. Headache, neck stiffness, fever, chills, myalgia, arthralgia, malaise, and fatigue accompany skin involvement, and arthritis of the large joints may develop.

Lymphadenopathy A pathologic lymph node enlargement, which is usually painless and may be associated with malignancy, especially lymphoma. Lymphadenopathy must be distinguished from normal reactive lymph node enlargement in response to infection. Reactive nodes are usually tender and are situated "downstream" from a site of infection.

Lymphedema Swelling produced by an obstruction of lymphatic flow.

Lymphocyte A white blood cell derived from the lymphoid stem cell that is not affected by diseases of the myeloid stem cell. Lymphocytes are of three basic types: T, B, and natural killer cells.

Lymphogranuloma venereum Highly contagious systemic infection caused by a number of strains of *Chlamydia.* It has progressive stages of development in which an initial lesion forms, and systemic disease occurs following dissemination via the lymphatic system.

Lymphoid group Dermal cells consisting of lymphocytes commonly found in inflammatory lesions of the skin.

Lymphopoiesis Formation of lymphocytes.

Lysosome An organelle containing hydrolytic enzymes that function to digest intracellular materials.

Lysozyme An enzyme secreted by macrophages and neutrophils to control foreign particle activity.

M

M line Marks the center of the A band and the midpoint of myosin filaments in striated muscle.

Macrocyte An abnormally large erythrocyte.

Macrophage A mature monocyte that migrates from the blood vessels to sites in the lymphoid tissues. Macrophages are powerful phagocytes and secrete a number of cytokines that stimulate inflammation.

Major histocompatibility complex (MHC) The gene regions on chromosome 6 that contain the genes for MHC proteins. Class I proteins are present on virtually all nucleated cells. Class II proteins are found mainly on antigen-presenting cells: B cells, macrophages, and dendritic cells.

Malabsorption Failure of the gastrointestinal tract to absorb or normally digest one or more dietary constituents.

Maladaptation Ineffective, inadequate, or inappropriate change in response to new or altered circumstances.

Malignant tumor A type of tumor that has a tendency to invade local tissues and spread to distant sites (metastasis). Malignant tumors are generally poorly differentiated and are associated with a poor prognosis if not promptly managed.

Mallory-Weiss syndrome Mild to massive bleeding due to a tear in the mucosa or submucosa of the cardia or lower esophagus. The tear is usually longitudinal and is caused by forceful or prolonged vomiting during which the upper esophageal sphincter fails to relax.

Mania Also called *full mania,* it is characterized by an overwhelming increase in energy and drive manifest as nonstop activity, grandiose thinking, impulsivity, euphoria, impaired judgment, acting-out behaviors, and hypersexuality.

Mass lesion Any lesion in the cranium that behaves like a space-occupying mass. Mass lesions tend to progress and cause signs and symptoms of increased intracranial pressure.

Mast cell Also called *histiocytic cell.* Mast cells have intracytoplasmic basophilic metachromatic granules containing heparin and histamine. The normal skin contains relatively few mast cells, but their number is increased in many different skin conditions, particularly the itching dermatoses.

Mastectomy Surgical removal of a breast. See *modified radical mastectomy* and *radical mastectomy.*

McBurney point Located in the lower right quadrant of the abdomen situated in the normal area of the appendix midway between the umbilicus and the anterior iliac crest.

Mean arterial pressure The average pressure in the arterial system through the cardiac cycle; estimated clinically as diastolic pressure plus one third of the pulse pressure.

Measles Known as *hard measles, 7-day measles,* or *rubeola.* This is a communicable viral disease caused by Morbillivirus with a characteristic macular and blotchy rash; sometimes the macules become confluent.

Mediastinum The area of the chest between the sternum and vertebral column and between the lungs. Mediastinal structures include the trachea, esophagus, aorta, heart, and lymph nodes.

Medullary cavity Central cavity in longer bones.

Megakaryocyte A large bone marrow cell that sheds platelets from its cytoplasm.

Megaloblastic dysplasia Abnormal development of large red cells and nonlymphocytic bone marrow cells.

Megaloblasts Large abnormal hematopoietic bone marrow cells.

Meiosis A type of cell division that results in daughter cells with one half the normal number of chromosomes. Meiosis occurs in gonadal germ cells.

Melanin Dark pigment found in melanocytes that gives color to hair and skin.

Melanocyte One of several types of epithelial cells. Melanocytes contribute color to the skin and serve to filter ultraviolet light.

Melena Tarry, black feces due to the action of gastrointestinal secretions on blood in the intestine.

Membranous urethra The urethral segment that passes through the muscular layers of the urogenital diaphragm.

Menarche The first menstrual period at the time of puberty, usually occurring around age 12 years in North America.

Meninges Membranes surrounding the brain and spinal cord, which include the dura mater, arachnoid, and pia mater.

Meningocele Hernial protrusion of meninges through a neural tube defect in the vertebral column.

Meniscus Curved, fibrous cartilage located in the knee and other joints. Menisci facilitate rotation at the knee by allowing better contact of the tibial surfaces with the femoral condyles.

Menopause A process by which the supply of ovarian follicles and estrogen hormones declines, usually beginning between the ages of 45 and 52 years.

Menorrhagia An increase in the amount or duration of menstrual bleeding, usually resulting from a lesion of the female reproductive organs.

Menstrual cycle The rhythmic pattern of changes in hormonal secretions and in sexual organs occurring approximately every 28 days during a female's reproductive years. The cycle culminates in the production of an ovum and the preparation of the uterus for implantation of a fertilized ovum.

Merkel cells One of several types of epithelial cells. Merkel cells consist of free nerve endings attached to modified epidermal cells. It is generally agreed that Merkel cells function as touch receptors.

Mesoblastic nephroma Benign congenital renal tumor.

Mesonephros One of three distinct stages in the development of the renal system. Mesonephros, which is the middle stage, corresponds to the mature excretory organ of some amphibians. In humans, it begins developing at about the fourth to fifth week of gestation.

Metabolic acidosis Any of the types of acidosis resulting from accumulation in the blood of noncarbonic, nonvolatile acids; characterized by a low HCO_3^- concentration.

Metabolic alkalosis A disturbance in which the acid-base balance shifts to the alkaline because of uncompensated loss of acids, ingestion or retention of excess base, or potassium depletion.

Metabolism Synthesis and breakdown of molecules in a living organism. Metabolism involves both the use and the release of energy.

Metanephros The final stage of development of the renal system. The metanephros begins in the fourth week when the ureteral bud grows out of the mesonephric duct.

Metaplasia Transformation of one kind of tissue to another fully differentiated tissue.

Metastasis Dissemination of cancer cells from the location of origin to other distant areas in the body.

Methemoglobin A transformation product of oxyhemoglobin, formed when the iron of the hemoglobin molecule is oxidized to the ferric state (Fe^{3+}).

Metrorrhagia Bleeding between menstrual periods, usually the result of slight physiologic bleeding from the endometrium during ovulation. It may also result from other causes such as uterine malignancy, cervical erosions, endometrial polyps, or estrogen therapy.

Microbial adherence The ability of the microorganism to latch onto and gain entrance into the host.

Microcytic Referring to an abnormally small erythrocyte.

Micropenis A small, normally formed penis with a stretched length more than 2 standard deviations below the mean, or a stretched length less than 2.5 cm.

Mineralocorticoids A class of steroid hormones, secreted by the adrenal cortex, that regulate the mineral salts (electrolytes) and water balance in the body.

Mitochondrion A membrane-bounded organelle that carries out oxidative phosphorylation to synthesize most of the adenosine triphosphate in a eukaryotic cell.

Mitosis A type of cell division that results in daughter cells with chromosomes that are identical to the parent cell. Mitosis occurs in somatic cells.

Mitral valve The cardiac valve that lies between the left atrium and left ventricle. The valve is normally closed during ventricular systole and open during ventricular diastole. Mitral valve closure contributes to heart sound S_1. Also called the *bicuspid atrioventricular valve.*

Mixed acid-base imbalance A combined disturbance of acid-base balance in which a primary respiratory disorder and primary metabolic disorder coexist.

Mixed incontinence Loss of bladder control with symptoms of both stress and urge incontinence.

Modified radical mastectomy Surgical removal of the breast accompanied by dissection of a portion of the axillary lymphatic system.

Molluscum contagiosum A viral skin disease with two forms. One form affects children and is spread through indirect contact; the other is sexually transmitted and occurs in young adults. It is characterized by pink and white lesions on the genitalia with an exudative core.

Mongolian spots Caused by selective pigmentation. They usually occur on the buttocks or sacral area and are commonly seen in Asian-Americans and African-Americans.

Monocyte An immature circulating macrophage.

Monosaccharide A simple sugar (e.g., glucose, fructose).

Monosomy Having only one member of a homologous chromosome pair, as in monosomy X, also called *Turner syndrome.*

Monounsaturated fatty acid A fatty acid with one double bond.

Mood Sustained expression of an emotion that affects one's outlook.

Mood disorder A disturbance of mood that may be caused by either organic damage to the brain or chemical alterations in neurotransmission. Mood disorders may also have no known biological basis.

Mood swings Oscillation between periods of euphoria (elevated mood) and depression or anxiety.

Morphogen A substance that triggers growth, proliferation, and differentiation of cells in a concentration-dependent manner.

Morphogenesis Arrangement of cells in a particular order during the development of complex organisms.

Morphologic changes Structural and associated functional alterations in cells or tissues that are either characteristic of the disease or diagnostic of the etiologic process.

Motor end-plate The points of contact between an α motor neuron and the muscle cells it innervates.

Mucocutaneous candidiasis Candidal infection of the mucous membrane and the skin.

Mucosal edema Also called *myxedema;* a dry, waxy swelling of the skin with abnormal deposits of glycosaminoglycans in skin and other tissues, associated with primary hypothyroidism.

Müllerian ducts Genital structures, also called *paramesonephric ducts* because they develop alongside the mesonephric ducts.

Multipennate muscle A muscle with several central tendons toward which the muscle fibers converge like the barbs of feathers.

Multiple myeloma (plasma cell myeloma) A malignant disorder of antibody-secreting plasma cells that produce large quantities of monoclonal antibodies and have a predilection to settle in the skeleton, where osteoclastic bone lesions are produced.

Multiple sclerosis A chronic demyelinating disease of the central nervous system that causes significant disability in young adults. It is thought to be an autoimmune disorder that results in inflammation and scarring (sclerosis) of the myelin sheaths covering nerves.

Muscular dystrophy Term referring to a group of genetically determined myopathies characterized by progressive degeneration of muscle fibers.

Mutagen A physical or chemical agent capable of causing alterations in an organism's DNA by inducing mutations.

Mutation A heritable change in the nucleotide sequence of a chromosome, which is passed on to daughter cells when the cell divides.

Myasthenia gravis A chronic autoimmune disease affecting the neuromuscular function of voluntary muscles and characterized by profound muscle weakness and fatigability.

Mycosis Infection caused by a fungus.

Myeloid group Cells of the dermis consisting of polymorphonuclear leukocytes and eosinophilic leukocytes. These cells occur commonly with allergic dermatoses.

Myelomeningocele or meningomyelocele Hernial protrusion of meninges, spinal fluid, and a portion of the spinal cord with its nerves through a defect in the vertebral column.

Myocardial infarction Localized area of cardiac necrosis most often associated with coronary heart disease.

Myocardium The middle layer of the heart, composed of cardiac muscle tissue.

Myosin A cytoskeletal protein that makes up the thick filament of the muscle sarcomere in skeletal and cardiac muscle. It is also present as a contractile filament in other types of cells. Myosin binds with actin during muscular contraction.

Myositis ossificans An abnormal calcification within a muscle.

Myxedema Nonpitting edema caused by advanced hypothyroidism in adulthood.

N

Narcissism Self-absorption; excessive self-love.

Necrosis Death and degradation of body cells or tissues in response to injurious events.

Necrotizing enterocolitis A disorder occurring most often in premature infants (less than 34 weeks gestation) and infants with low birth weight (less than 5 lb or 2.25 kg). This disorder is characterized by diffuse or patchy intestinal necrosis accompanied by sepsis.

Necrotizing inflammation Also called *vasculitis.* This response can occur when antigen and antibody react in blood vessels in the skin. Necrotizing inflammation can be caused by drug allergies; disorders such as systemic lupus erythematosus, rheumatoid arthritis, and glomerulonephritis; and certain infectious diseases such as hepatitis B.

Negative feedback A term used to explain homeostatic mechanisms. Negative feedback causes the controller to respond in a manner that opposes or negates deviation from normal level (set point). Most body systems operate on the principle of negative feedback.

Negative nitrogen balance The condition of protein breakdown exceeding daily protein intake and synthesis.

Negative symptoms (schizophrenia) Symptoms of schizophrenia that are thought to be mediated by dopamine D_1 receptors in the brain. Drugs that block D_1 receptors may alleviate some of the negative symptoms, which include social withdrawal, flat affect, poverty of speech, ritualistic posturing, and autism.

Neologism New word, often created by combining syllables of other words; or a word given special or private significance.

Neoplasia New growth. The term implies an *abnormality* of cellular growth and may be used interchangeably with the term *tumor.*

Neoplasm A new and abnormal proliferation of cells. If malignant, the growth infiltrates tissue, metastasizes, and often recurs, even after attempts at surgical removal.

Nephralgia Renal pain.

Nephroblastoma (Wilms tumor) The most common childhood malignant kidney tumor, result from a defect on chromosome 13.

Nephrolithiasis The presence of a stone or calculus anywhere in the urinary tract.

Nephron Functional unit of the kidney composed of epithelial cells forming the glomerulus, proximal convoluted tubule, loop of Henle, distal convoluted tubule, and collecting duct.

Nephropathy A pathologic process in the kidney. Many disorders can lead to nephropathy, as in diabetic nephropathy, toxic nephropathy, ischemic nephropathy, and obstructive nephropathy.

Nephrotic syndrome A common set of symptoms caused by damage to the glomeruli, in which proteins cross the glomerulus and are lost in the urine at a rate of >3.5 g/day.

Nephrotoxic Poisonous to the kidney.

Neural thread protein Microscopic protein thread that binds and helps stabilize microtubules (the cell's internal support structure or skeleton). In Alzheimer disease, the threads become chemically altered and twist into paired helical filaments, known as *neurofibrillary tangles.* See *tau protein.*

Neurofibrillary tangle Abnormal bundle of twisted threads inside a nerve cell that is the collapsed remains of the neuron's microtubules, which normally provide structural support.

Neurogenic bladder Bladder dysfunction caused by a lesion at any level in the nervous system.

Neurogenic shock Often called "fainting," neurogenic shock may be caused by severe pain, fear, an unpleasant sight, or other strong stimuli that overwhelm the usual regulatory capacity of the nervous system.

Neuroglia, glia A group of cell types, including astrocytes, microglia, ependymal cells, and oligodendrocytes, that support nerve cells and do not themselves conduct action potentials.

Neuropathic osteoarthropathy A neurologic disease that leads to bone abnormalities and joint involvement. The mechanics of disease development are probably a combination of neurovascular and neurotraumatic processes.

Neurovascular injury An injury that affects the nerves that control the caliber of blood vessels.

Neutropenia A type of leukopenia in which the absolute neutrophil count is below 500 cells/μl. Neutropenia is associated with a high risk of bacterial sepsis.

Neutrophilia A high blood neutrophil count.

Neutrophil/neutrophilic granulocyte A cell that contains small lysosomal granules and a segmented nucleus with two to five lobes. These cells compose 57% to 67% of leukocytes.

Nevus Congenital discoloration of a circumscribed area of the skin, commonly called *mole* or *birthmark.*

Nociception Activation of nociceptors by potentially tissue-damaging stimuli, resulting in the perception of pain by the central nervous system. Nociception includes the processes of receptor transduction, signal transmission, perception, and signal modulation.

Nociceptor Pain receptor.

Nonarticular rheumatism A common soft tissue syndrome in children. The most common symptom is nocturnal pain that usually occurs in the calves, shins, and thighs. Also called *growing pain.*

Noncontractile tissue Soft tissue that possesses no ability to contract or relax; this includes the joint capsule, ligament, bursa, fascia, dura mater, and nerve root. Also called *inert tissue.*

Nondisjunction The failure of homologous chromosomes to separate normally during meiosis or mitosis, resulting in unequal distribution of chromosomes to daughter cells.

Nondisplaced fracture A fracture in which the fragments remain in alignment and position.

Non-Hodgkin lymphoma A varied group of malignant disorders of lymph node cells involving B cells, T cells, and natural killer cells. In comparison with Hodgkin disease, these lymphomas tend to spread unpredictably and metastasize early, and thus carry an overall worse prognosis.

Non–Q-wave infarct A subendocardial infarct affecting only the inner third to half of the ventricular wall and generally associated with less severe symptoms.

Nonspecific immune response Referring to a series of mechanical, biochemical, and phagocytic barriers to infection; also called the *innate immune system..*

Norepinephrine A major monoamine neurotransmitter involved in the etiologic development of mood disorders. See *serotonin.*

Nuclei A cluster of neuronal cell bodies located in the central nervous system.

Nucleocapsid The core of the human immunodeficiency virus (HIV), which contains two strands or chains of RNA, protein, and enzymes.

Nucleotide A biomolecule composed of a purine or pyrimidine base linked to a ribose or deoxyribose sugar, with one or more phosphate groups attached to the sugar. DNA and RNA are polymers of nucleotides.

Nucleus A cellular organelle that contains chromosomal DNA.

Nutritional screening A method for quickly determining the nutritional status of an individual from a selected group of anthropometric and biochemical tests.

Nutritional status The state of an individual's nutrition, resulting from the consumption and utilization of nutrients.

Nystagmus Involuntary, rapid, rhythmic movements of the eyeball; these occur commonly in a horizontal direction, but can also occur in a vertical or a rotational direction.

O

Oblique fracture Fracture resulting from a rotational force; however, unlike a spiral fracture, the break is along an oblique course (45-degree angle) and does not rotate around the entire bone.

Obsession A powerful, persistent, intrusive thought, impulse, or image that dominates the mental life of the individual to the extent of seriously interfering with normal living.

Obstruction Refers to an anomaly that compromises or prevents flow because of abnormal narrowings. Stenosis or atresia (failure to develop) of valves and coarctation of the aorta are the most common cardiac obstructive defects.

Occupational asthma Resembles allergic asthma and may be accompanied by positive skin test reactions to protein allergens in the work environment.

Odynophagia Pain with swallowing; may accompany *dysphagia,* or difficulty with swallowing.

Ogilvie syndrome The idiopathic syndrome of intestinal pseudoobstruction; may result in megacolon.

Olfactory Pertaining to the sense of smell.

Oligomenorrhea Infrequent menstruation, usually the result of failure to ovulate due to inappropriate hormonal function.

Oligosaccharide A compound consisting of 2 to 10 joined monosaccharide units.

Oliguria Urine output of less than 400 to 500 ml/day.

Omphalocele Congenital anomaly in which a herniation of viscera at the base of the umbilical cord is present; requires surgical correction.

Oncocytoma Benign renal tumor consisting of large eosinophilic cells that have granular cytoplasm and round, uniform nuclei.

Oncogene A gene associated with the initiation of cancerous behavior in a cell.

Onycholysis Separation of the nail from its bed.

Oogonia The cells present in the female ovaries during prenatal development that ultimately develop into ova. The entire lifetime supply of ova is established prenatally; no new oogonia arise after birth.

Open fracture Fracture occurring when bone is broken and an external wound leads to the fracture site.

Ophthalmia neonatorum Purulent gonococcal conjunctivitis and keratitis in the newborn resulting from exposure of the infant's eyes to infected maternal secretions during the passage through the vagina at birth.

Ophthalmoscopic examination Examination of the structures of the eye, both extraocular and intraocular, using an ophthalmoscope.

Opioid Any of a group of drugs with an affinity for opioid receptors in the central nervous system. Morphine is the standard opioid with which others are compared for characteristics and potency.

Opportunistic infection An infection caused by organisms that are usually nonpathogenic but that become pathogenic because of decreased function of the immune system.

Opsonization The process of proteins, usually antibodies or complement fragments, binding to an antigen in order to make the antigen easier for phagocytic cells to locate. Phagocytic cells have receptors for opsonins.

Organelles The membrane-bound structures in the cell cytoplasm, including nucleus, mitochondria, endoplasmic reticulum, and Golgi apparatus.

Orthopnea Difficulty with breathing that is brought on or exacerbated by lying horizontal.

Orthostatic (postural) hypotension A form of low blood pressure that occurs after positional change from supine to standing. Diagnosed by an increase in heart rate of more than 15% and a decrease in either systolic blood pressure, by more than 15 mm Hg, or diastolic blood pressure, by more than 10 mm Hg.

Osmolality A measure of degree of concentration; number of particles per kilogram of solvent.

Osmosis Movement of water across a semipermeable membrane to equalize the particle concentration of the fluid on both sides of the membrane.

Ossicle One of several small bones in the middle ear responsible for transmitting sound waves to the inner ear.

Osteoarthritis A common degenerative joint disease characterized by progressive loss of articular cartilage and by formation of new bone from subchondral bone at joint margins.

Osteoblast A bone-forming cell that is derived from the embryonic mesenchyme and, during the early development of the skeleton, differentiates from a fibroblast to function in the formation of bone tissue.

Osteochondroma A benign bone tumor consisting of bone and cartilage.

Osteoclast A cell responsible for bone resorption.

Osteocyte A mature bone cell.

Osteoid osteoma A painful but benign bone-forming tumor that is often found in the cortex of the tibia and femur.

Osteomalacia An abnormal condition of lamellar bone, characterized by a loss of calcification of the matrix and consequent softening of the bone. The condition is the result of an inadequate amount of phosphorus and calcium available in the blood for mineralization of the bones.

Osteomyelitis A severe pyogenic infection of bone and local tissue that requires immediate management.

Osteon The basic unit of bone; also called the *haversian system.*

Osteoporosis A common metabolic bone disease in which reduction in bone mass results from bone resorption proceeding at a rate faster than that of new bone formation.

Osteoprogenitor A type of bone stem cell that lines bone surfaces.

Osteosarcoma A malignant bone-forming tumor and the most common primary malignant bone tumor that develops in the metaphyseal region of long bones.

Ototoxic Damaging to the structures of the inner ear.

Ovarian cyst A sac on an ovary that contains fluid or semisolid material. It may develop at any time between puberty and menopause; the cause is presently unknown.

Overflow incontinence Loss of bladder control associated with urinary retention and a bladder distention due to obstruction, detrusor underactivity or inactivity, or sphincteric malfunction.

Oviduct Another term for *fallopian tube.* Each oviduct runs laterally from the uterus to the uterine end of the ovary. The free end of the oviduct adjacent to the ovary is called the *infundibulum.*

Oxygen consumption The amount of oxygen used by the tissues in 1 minute, usually expressed as V_{O_2}.

Oxygen delivery The amount of oxygen delivered to the tissues each minute. Oxygen delivery (D_{O_2}) is calculated by multiplying cardiac output and arterial oxygen content.

Oxytocin Hormone secreted by the mother's posterior pituitary. It causes uterine contraction and is thought to have a major role in promoting increased uterine contractility during parturition. After birth, it is secreted in response to suckling by the infant and stimulates the release of milk, called the *milk ejection reflex.*

P

Paco$_2$ Partial pressure of carbon dioxide in arterial blood; an indicator of the effectiveness of respiratory excretion of carbonic acid.

Paget disease Also called *osteitis deformans;* a slowly progressive metabolic bone disease characterized by an initial phase of excessive bone resorption followed by a reactive phase of abnormal excessive bone formation.

Pain An unpleasant sensation caused by noxious stimulation of the sensory nerve endings, or perceived as such.

Pallor Paleness of skin; primarily assess skin pallor of the nail beds, lips, and conjunctivae. A possible symptom of anemia.

Pancreas Gland located in the abdomen; has both endocrine and exocrine functions. The endocrine pancreas produces insulin, glucagon, and somatostatin.

Pancreatitis Inflammation of the pancreas.

Pancytopenia Decreased production of red cells, white cells, and platelets.

Pandemic An epidemic that affects large geographic regions, possibly spreading worldwide.

Panhypopituitarism A condition of deficiency in all pituitary hormones.

Panic disorder Psychiatric disorder characterized by recurrent, unexpected episodes of acute anxiety, fear, and panic, often accompanied by the subject's belief that he or she may be having a heart attack, is unable to breathe, is losing control, or that death is imminent.

Panmyelosis Overproduction of normal red cells, white cells, and platelets.

Papillary layer One of two layers of the dermis. The papillary layer consists of bumps (papillae) that project into the epidermis.

Papillary muscles Muscles within the ventricles that connect the chordae tendineae to the ventricular wall. Papillary muscles contract during ventricular systole to place tension on the valves and prevent backflow through them.

Paracrine Referring to hormone-like chemicals, the target cell of which is located next to the cell secreting the chemical.

Parametritis An infection of the connective tissue between the broad ligaments underlying the female reproductive organs.

Paraneoplastic syndrome A cluster of systemic conditions associated with cancer, such as hypercalcemia, hyponatremia, or Cushing syndrome.

Paraphimosis Painful constriction of the glans penis by foreskin, which has been retracted behind the corona.

Parasite One of a variety of protozoa (single-celled animals), nemathelminths (roundworms), platyhelminths (flatworms), and arthropods (invertebrate animals with jointed appendages). Parasites depend on another organism for survival.

Parkinsonism Parkinson disease symptoms; a neurologic disorder characterized by tremor, muscle rigidity, hypokinesia, a slow shuffling gait, and difficulty in chewing, swallowing, and speaking caused by various lesions in the extrapyramidal motor system.

Paroxysm A sudden outburst or change from the norm, as in a sudden burst of electrical activity seen on electroencephalography, as occurs with seizure activity.

Paroxysmal nocturnal dyspnea A sudden severe feeling of suffocation, which usually occurs at night and wakes the person from sleep.

Partial seizure A seizure in which part of the brain surface is involved in the seizure.

Parturition The process by which an infant is born.

Pathogen An agent that causes disease.

Pathogenesis Development or evolution of disease. A description of the pathogenesis includes everything that happens in the body from the initial stimulus to the ultimate expression of manifestations of the disease.

Pathology Study of the causes, characteristics, and effects of disease.

Pathophysiology The study of disordered function.

Pauciarticular onset Affecting four or fewer joints; used in association with juvenile rheumatoid arthritis.

Pedigree Genetic lineage or family history of traits, used to trace the pattern of inheritance.

Pelvic inflammatory disease Any acute or subacute recurrent or chronic infection of the oviducts and ovaries with involvement of the adjacent reproductive organs.

Pemphigus A group of disorders including vulgaris, vegetans, foliaceus, and erythematosus. The pemphigus group disorders are characterized by bullous eruptions (blisters) thought to be caused by autoimmune reactions.

Pemphigus vulgaris Included in the pemphigus group of disorders, pemphigus vulgaris has the worst prognosis. Bullae can erupt on the skin and mucous membranes (e.g., esophagus), and toxemia and infection can cause death if proper treatment (cortisone) is not administered.

Penile urethra The longest segment of the male urethra, extending about 15 cm in length from the membranous urethra to the external meatus.

Penis Male organ of copulation and urinary excretion.

Penumbra The margin or fringe surrounding a central part. In the case of stroke, a penumbra of viable tissue surrounds the necrotic core that can survive if optimal conditions exist and if it is not subject to further insults.

Peptic ulcer disease Disorder of the upper gastrointestinal tract caused by the action of acid and pepsin. This disorder may include injury to the mucosa of the esophagus, stomach, or duodenum, and may range from a slight mucosal injury to severe ulceration.

Percutaneous Referring to a procedural approach that traverses the skin and is less traumatic than open surgical methods.

Pericardium A protective covering of the heart that is made of two layers separated by a fluid-filled space. The inner (visceral) layer is attached to the heart itself, whereas the outer (parietal) layer forms a sac around the heart.

Perimysium The connective tissue surrounding the fasciculi.

Peripheral vascular dysfunction Decreased localized blood flow resulting in coolness, often to the feet, because skin temperature depends on the amount of blood circulating through the dermis.

Peristalsis The basic propulsive movement of the gastrointestinal (GI) tract. During normal functioning, this coordinated, rhythmic, serial contraction of smooth muscle propels the contents of the GI tract in a downward direction.

Permissive hypothesis A hypothesis positing that poor dampening by serotonin of other neurotransmitter systems (e.g., norepinephrine and dopamine) allows wide variations in mood.

Permissiveness The process in which one hormone increases the number of cellular receptors for a second hormone, thus increasing the cellular response to the second hormone.

Peroxisome (microbody) Small membrane-bound organelle that uses molecular oxygen to degrade organic molecules.

Perseveration Persisting response to a previous stimulus after a new stimulus has been presented.

Personality disorder A disorder that represents immature, inflexible, and persistently maladaptive ways of dealing with the intrapersonal and interpersonal aspects of life.

Petechiae Nonblanching, pinpoint red or purple spots caused by capillary hemorrhages.

Peyronie disease Formation of palpable, fibrous plaques on the surface of the corpora cavernosa.

pH The negative logarithm of the hydrogen ion concentration; a measure of the acidity of a solution.

Phagocytosis Ingestion and destruction of pathogens by leukocytes.

Phagosome A cellular lysosome containing substances obtained by phagocytosis.

Phenotype The physical, biochemical, and biological makeup of an individual, expressed as recognizable traits.

Pheochromocytoma Tumor of the adrenal gland that secretes catecholamines, resulting in elevated blood pressure. An example of a condition that causes secondary high blood pressure.

Phimosis A condition in which the penile foreskin fits so tightly over the glans that it cannot be retracted.

Phlebitis Inflammation of a vein.

Photoreceptor A receptor found in the eye that responds to light.

Physiologic jaundice of the newborn A harmless, short-term condition caused by immature bilirubin conjugation and transport mechanisms.

Physiology The study of the specific characteristics and functions of a living organism and its parts.

Pigmentary disturbance Interruption of any organic coloring material produced in the body, such as melanin.

Pinocytosis A process of ingesting fluids and small particles that is common to most cell types. Also called "cellular drinking."

Pituitary gland A gland located at the base of the hypothalamus. It consists of anterior and posterior lobes. Also called *hypophysis.*

Pityriasis rosea A rash of unknown origin that primarily affects young adults. The characteristic lesion of a macule or papule with surrounding erythema is thought to be viral in origin, but no virus has been isolated to date.

Pivot joint A joint that allows rotation as its single axis movement. Examples include the superior radioulnar joint of the elbow and the union between the first and second vertebrae. Also called *trochoid joint.*

Placenta A highly vascularized organ through which the fetus receives nutrients and by which wastes are removed. It also is an endocrine organ, producing several hormones, most notably human chorionic gonadotropin.

Placenta previa Condition of pregnancy in which the placenta is implanted abnormally over the internal cervical os. It occurs in varying degrees of severity and may result in sudden massive hemorrhage following dilatation of the internal os.

Plasma A complex, aqueous liquid containing a number of organic and inorganic substances.

Plasma cell 1. An antibody-secreting B lymphocyte. 2. A dermal cell rarely seen in normal skin secretions, occurring in small numbers in most chronic inflammatory diseases of the skin and in larger numbers in granulomas.

Plasma membrane The membrane that surrounds a living cell.

Plasmapheresis Removal of plasma from withdrawn blood, with retransfusion of the formed elements into the donor.

Platelet A circulating cytoplasmic fragment of megakaryocytes that is essential in the formation of blood clots and in the control of bleeding.

Pleural effusion A collection of fluid in the pleural cavity resulting from a disease process.

Pleurodesis Instillation of a chemically irritating drug (e.g., tetracycline, sterile talc, bleomycin, doxycycline) into the pleural space to stimulate inflammation and adhesion.

Pneumonia An acute inflammation of lung tissue caused by an infectious agent or by aspiration of chemically irritating fluid.

Pneumothorax Accumulation of air in the pleural space.

Polyarteritis nodosa A form of systemic vasculitis that can cause inflamed arteries in visceral organs, brain, and skin.

Polyarticular onset (oligoarticular) Affecting five or more joints; used in association with juvenile rheumatoid arthritis.

Polycystic kidney disease A progressive disease characterized by multiple dilations of the collecting ducts of the kidneys, which appear as if they are fluid-filled cysts, as a result of renal pathologic processes.

Polycythemia An excess of circulating red blood cells.

Polydipsia Excessive thirst.

Polygenic Referring to a trait determined by multiple genes at different loci, all having additive effects.

Polymenorrhea An increased frequency of menstruation, which may be associated with ovulation due to endocrine or systemic factors.

Polymorphism Inherited structural differences in proteins as a result of many alleles for a particular gene locus.

Polymorphonuclear neutrophil (PMN) A cell that contains small lysosomal granules and a segmented nucleus with two to five lobes. PMNs compose 57% to 67% of leukocytes.

Polymyositis Inflammation of many muscles, usually accompanied by deformity, edema, insomnia, pain, sweating, and tension.

Polyp A general descriptive term used for any mass of protruding tissue. Polyps may be either benign or malignant, although the term usually refers to the benign form.

Polyploidy Having more than two sets of homologous chromosomes.

Polysaccharide A saccharide containing 10 to 10,000 monosaccharide units.

Polysomy Having greater than the usual number of autosomal chromosomes.

Polyunsaturated fatty acid A fatty acid with several double bonds.

Polyuria Excretion of large amounts of urine.

Portal hypertension Abnormally high blood pressure in the blood vessels draining the intraabdominal alimentary tract, pancreas, gallbladder, and spleen. It may be due to increased resistance to blood flow, as in cirrhosis, or, rarely, to abnormally increased blood flow, as in arteriovenous communications.

Portal systemic encephalopathy A neuropsychiatric syndrome caused by liver dysfunction and resulting in mental status changes ranging from mild cerebral dysfunction to deep coma (hepatic coma) and death.

Positive end-expiratory pressure A method in which a ventilator is used to maintain positive airway pressure at the end of expiration, resulting in increased functional residual capacity and decreased shunt.

Positive feedback A term used to explain homeostatic mechanisms. Positive feedback increases deviation from the set point. Although most systems of the body operate on the principle of negative feedback, sneezing and childbirth are two examples of positive feedback.

Positive nitrogen balance The condition of dietary intake of proteins exceeding output.

Positive symptoms (schizophrenia) Symptoms of schizophrenia that are thought to be due to excessive dopamine D_2 receptor activation in the brain. Disorganized thinking (inability to connect thoughts logically), disorganized speech (rambling, tangentiality), delusions (fixed system of false beliefs), and hallucinations (sensory perception when no apparent stimulus exists) are typical positive symptoms.

Positron emission tomography (PET) A technique of brain imaging. PET studies measure changes in brain utilization of glucose.

Postictal phase The phase following a seizure during which the person is sleepy and confused.

Postobstructive diuresis Increased urinary output after resolution of partial or total obstruction of the urinary tract.

Potter syndrome Congenital condition often associated with renal agenesis, but always manifesting with the following anomalies: wide-spaced eyes with epicanthal folds, low-set ears, broad and flat nose, hypoplastic lungs, and limb deformities.

Poverty of speech Speech that gives little information owing to vagueness, empty repetitions, or obscure phrases.

Preeclampsia-eclampsia Elevated blood pressure during pregnancy associated with edema and proteinuria. Blood pressure returns to normal after delivery. Eclampsia is present when preeclampsia progresses to seizures. Also known as *pregnancy-induced hypertension.*

Pregnancy-induced hypertension The rapid rise of arterial blood pressure associated with a loss of large amounts of protein in the urine occurring during pregnancy. Women at risk for pregnancy-induced hypertension include teenagers and women in their late 30s and early 40s (also known as *toxemia of pregnancy* and *preeclampsia-eclampsia*).

Preload The volume of blood in the cardiac chamber just prior to systole (end-diastolic volume).

Prepuce Also called *foreskin;* penile skin that overlies the glans and is removed with circumcision.

Presbyesophagus Presence of slow or disorganized esophageal motility in the older adult.

Pressure sores Localized areas of cellular necrosis resulting from prolonged pressure between any bony prominence and an external object such as a bed or a wheelchair. The tissues are deprived of blood supply and eventually die. Also called *decubitus ulcers.*

Priapism Painful, persistent erection.

Prickly heat A rash caused by midepidermal obstruction and rupture of the sweat glands from prolonged exposure to a warm and humid environment.

Primary biliary cirrhosis A slowly progressive disease that destroys small to medium-sized bile ducts and results in cirrhosis and liver failure.

Primary dysthymia A long-term state of chronic depression not associated with any other disorder. It is neither a prelude to major depression nor a state existing between episodes of a cyclic form of mood disorder.

Primary endocrine disorder Direct malfunction of a hormone-producing gland not induced by the pituitary.

Primary glomerulopathy Disease states resulting from alterations in the structure and function of the glomerular capillary circulation, in which the kidney is the only or primary organ involved.

Primary (essential, idiopathic) hypertension High blood pressure of unidentified cause. Accounts for 90% of cases of high blood pressure.

Primary lesion Injury that originates in the skin and has not been altered by scratching or by treatment.

Primary prevention The first level of health promotion, designed to prevent disease.

Prodromal period The period preceding the onset of a disorder. Symptoms indicate an impending seizure, migraine, or other problem.

Progesterone A hormone produced by the corpus luteum and adrenal cortex during the luteal phase of the menstrual cycle that promotes uterine changes essential for the implantation and growth of the fertilized ovum.

Prognosis A forecast about the probable outcome of a disease; the prospect of recovery from a disease indicated by the nature, signs, and/or symptoms of the case.

Progressive familial intrahepatic cholestasis A rare autosomal recessive disorder comprising severe jaundice, pruritus, and malabsorption due to a defect in bile salt excretion.

Proinsulin Precursor to insulin produced by the β cells of the pancreas.

Prokaryote A cell that does not have a membrane-bound nucleus or other membrane-bound organelles (e.g., bacteria).

Prolactin Hormone secreted by the anterior pituitary. Following birth of an infant, prolactin stimulates milk production.

Pronephros One of three distinct phases in the development of the renal system. The pronephros is the earliest state in humans, corresponding to the mature structure in primitive vertebrates.

Prostate Gland located below the bladder; its secretions help activate sperm and maintain their motility.

Prostatic urethra The widest and most distensible part of the male urethra.

Prostatitis Inflammation of the prostate.

Prostatodynia Pain in the prostate.

Protein A molecule composed of nitrogen, carbon, hydrogen, oxygen, and occasionally sulfur; when hydrolyzed, proteins yield amino acids.

Proteoglycan Any of a group of polysaccharide-protein conjugates occurring primarily in the matrix of connective tissue and cartilage, composed mainly of polysaccharide chains, particularly glycosaminoglycans, as well as minor protein components.

Proto-oncogene A normal cellular gene that is growth promoting and usually inhibited in nonproliferating cells. When erroneously activated, it becomes an oncogene and promotes cancer.

Provirus The viral DNA that is spliced into the host cell's DNA.

Pruritus Itching of the skin.

Pseudocyst A collection of fluid within or adjacent to the pancreas that often has a direct communication to the pancreatic duct. It is the most common localized complication of acute pancreatitis.

Pseudoglandular period The first stage in fetal lung development when the bronchial divisions are differentiated and the major elements of lung tissue are present except for those involved in gas exchange: the respiratory bronchioles and alveoli.

Pseudomembranous enterocolitis An acute inflammation and necrosis of the small and large intestines caused by *Clostridium difficile,* usually affecting the mucosa but sometimes extending to other layers.

Psoriasis A common chronic skin disease characterized by papules and plaques with an overlying silvery scale. Lesions can appear on any area of the body but especially the knees, elbows, lower part of the back, scalp, and nails.

Psoriatic arthritis An inflammatory arthritis associated with psoriasis occurring in approximately 0.1% population in the United States. Peak age of onset is 30 to 55 years of age, and the arthritis can occur in patients who have had psoriasis for many years.

Psychogenic Produced or caused by emotional or psychological factors rather than organic factors.

Psychosis The most serious and debilitating of mental disorders. The hallmarks of psychosis are delusions and hallucinations, thought disorders, and inappropriate emotional responses or social behavior.

Psychosomatic medicine The discipline involving the physiologic impact of psychic stress on the emergence of disease.

Pulmonic valve The cardiac valve that lies between the right ventricle and the pulmonary artery. It is open during ventricular systole and closed during ventricular diastole. Pulmonic valve closure contributes to heart sound S_2.

Pulse pressure The difference between the systolic and diastolic blood pressures.

Purpura Hemorrhagic lesions 2 to 4 mm in diameter; petechiae that occur in groups or patches, caused by a vascular or bleeding disorder.

Putamen nuclei The larger, darker, and more lateral part of the lentiform nucleus.

Pyelonephritis An infection of the kidney medulla or cortex.

Pylorus Muscular sphincter between the stomach and the duodenum that controls gastric emptying and limits the reflux of bile from the small intestine.

Pyogenic Producing or produced by fever.

Pyrosis A substernal burning sensation that may radiate to the neck or throat. It is caused by the reflux of gastric contents into the esophagus (also called *heartburn*).

R

Radical mastectomy Surgical removal of the entire breast, lymphatic drainage, and underlying pectoral muscles.

Radiolysis Lysis or splitting of water molecules into H^+ and OH^- by action of radioactive particles.

Rapidly progressing glomerulonephritis A syndrome that combines abrupt hematuria and proteinuria followed by a swift decline in renal function.

Rarefaction Decrease in density and weight of bone, but not in volume.

Raynaud phenomenon Blanching or cyanosis of fingers or hands on exposure to cold or emotional stress. The phenomenon is attributed to vasospasm and structural disease of blood vessels. Puffiness and swelling of the hands and fingers are noted clinically.

Reality testing The act of evaluating and considering the differences between internal experiences and external events.

Receptor activation Binding of a ligand to a cellular receptor, resulting in a change in intracellular cell signaling or function.

Receptor specificity The principle of allowing intracellular processes to be activated only by certain hormones. If a cell does not have the specific receptors for a hormone, it will not respond to the hormone.

Recessive Referring to a gene allele that fails to be expressed in the phenotype when a dominant allele is present. The trait carried in a recessive allele is apparent only when two identical copies are present.

Recruitment The process of calling in additional motor units in response to an increase in stimulation of motor nerves.

Rectocele Protrusion of the anterior rectal wall into the posterior vagina at a weakened part of the vaginal musculature. It usually results from an injury during either childbirth or surgery, and it may also be the result of the aging process or an inherent weakness in the vaginal wall.

Recurrent urinary tract infection Repeated infections within a short period of time following verified resolution of an earlier infection.

Red blood cell (erythrocyte) Cell responsible for transporting oxygen to the tissues, removing carbon dioxide from the tissues, and buffering blood pH.

Reed-Sternberg cell A malignant cell type found in affected lymph nodes of patients with Hodgkin disease. The presence of Reed-Sternberg cells differentiates Hodgkin disease from all other forms of malignant lymphoma.

Reentry The proposed mechanism for many dysrhythmias, including premature complexes and fibrillation. Reentry occurs when an impulse is able to activate the cardiac muscle more than once due to abnormalities in conduction through a portion of the heart.

Reflex incontinence Urine loss that occurs without sensory warning or awareness.

Reflux Retrograde flow of urine from the bladder to the kidney.

Refractory period The time during which a nerve or muscle membrane is unable to respond to a stimulus by generating an action potential.

Regurgitation (valvular) Retrograde blood flow through a cardiac valve when the valve is supposed to be closed.

Reiter syndrome Seronegative arthritis that appears 2 to 6 weeks after onset of an infection, characterized clinically by diffuse swelling of fingers and toes, swelling in the Achilles tendon or plantar fascia, and low back pain.

Relative anemia Anemia characterized by normal total red blood cell mass with disturbances in the regulation of plasma fluid volume resulting in low hematocrit.

Relative polycythemia Polycythemia characterized by normal total red blood cell mass with disturbances in the regulation of plasma volume resulting in elevated hematocrit.

Relaxation time The period between peak tension and zero tension.

Releasing hormone A hormone secreted by the hypothalamus that stimulates the anterior pituitary gland to secrete other hormones.

Remission Disappearance of clinical manifestations of disease. In leukemia, complete remission is determined by the absence of leukemic blasts in the bone marrow aspirate and peripheral blood. Malignant stem cells still may be present, and remission does not imply cure.

Renal adenoma A tumor smaller than 3 cm with a cellular makeup similar to that of renal cell carcinoma.

Renal agenesis Failure of one or both kidneys to develop.

Renal angiomyolipoma (hamartoma) Benign renal tumor composed of abdominal blood vessels, clusters of fat cells, and sheets of smooth muscle.

Renal calculus Concretion of crystals of material (e.g., uric acid, calcium phosphate, struvite) that initially form in the calices or pelvis of the kidney. Calculi may migrate down the urinary tract and cause pain, obstruction, and infection.

Renal cell carcinoma Most common malignant tumor of the kidney.

Renal or ureteral colic Intermittent flank or abdominal pain caused by spasms in the kidneys and/or ureters.

Renin An enzyme stored and released by the juxtaglomerular cells; converts angiotensinogen to angiotensin I.

Resident flora Microorganisms that usually reside in a certain environment on the host without causing disease.

Resistance In the stress response, resistance occurs when sympathetic activity declines while secretion of adrenocortical hormones is high.

Respiratory acidosis A pulmonary hypoventilation condition that tends to cause an excess of carbonic acid and that may result in acid-base imbalance.

Respiratory alkalosis A pulmonary hyperventilation condition that tends to cause a deficit of carbonic acid and that may result in acid-base imbalance.

Respiratory quotient The ratio of the volume of carbon dioxide exhaled to the volume of oxygen absorbed in the alveoli.

Respiratory syncytial virus A member of a subgroup of myxoviruses that in tissue culture cause formation of giant cells or syncytia.

Reticular formation Fibers in the brainstem that arouse the cerebrum.

Reticular layer One of two layers of the dermis; consists of a more dense reticulum (network) of fibers than the papillary layer above it. The reticular layer is made of collagen and elastin and contains skeletal (voluntary) and smooth (involuntary) muscle fibers.

Reticulocytosis Increase in the number of circulating reticulocytes (immature red blood cells).

Reticulohistiocytic group Cells of the dermis consisting of fibroblasts, histiocytes, and mast cells. Immature cells of the reticulohistiocytic group are called *reticulum cells.*

Retrodisplacement Posterior displacement, such as an alteration in the position of the uterus in which the body of the uterus is displaced from its normal location overlying the bladder to a position in the posterior pelvis.

Retroperitoneal Referring to the anatomic space in the abdomen behind the peritoneal cavity, where the kidneys reside.

Retrovirus An RNA virus capable of transcribing its own RNA into DNA, which can be integrated into the host genome through the actions of a viral polymerase, also called *reverse transcriptase.*

Reverse transcriptase An enzyme that allows certain viruses to convert RNA to DNA and incorporate their genome into the DNA of the host cell.

Reye syndrome Primarily a children's disease, it is characterized by fatty infiltration of the liver with severe hepatic dysfunction.

Rheumatoid arthritis A systemic, inflammatory, connective tissue disease of unknown cause. Enzymes are released into the joint fluid, causing inflammation, proliferation of synovium, and tissue damage. The hands, wrists, knees, and feet are most commonly involved. Joint involvement is symmetric. Other systems affected include integumentary, ocular, otolaryngologic, pulmonary, cardiac, gastrointestinal, renal, neurologic, and hematologic.

Rhinorrhea Drainage of a watery fluid from the nasal mucosa.

Rhonchus Coarse, bubbling sound usually heard on expiration, but which also can be heard on inspiration due to secretions in the airways.

Rhus dermatitis An inflammatory reaction to poison ivy, poison oak, and poison sumac. Clinically, rhus dermatitis begins within 48 hours of contact. The first symptom is pruritus, followed by erythema and vesicle formation, sometimes in linear fashion.

Rhythmicity The ability to beat regularly without external stimuli. Also called *automaticity.*

Ribonucleic acid (RNA) A nucleic acid, found in both the nucleus and cytoplasm of cells, that has several roles in the translation of the genetic code and the assembly of proteins.

Ribosome A cellular structure containing ribosomal RNA and proteins that bind to mRNA and perform the task of translating the RNA message into a protein.

Rickets A condition caused by the deficiency of vitamin D, seen primarily in infancy and childhood and characterized by abnormal bone formation.

Rigor mortis The stiffening of muscles throughout the body after death due to formation of permanent actin-myosin cross-bridges.

Risk factor Characteristic related to the probability of a certain outcome; a risk factor may be shown to cause an outcome or may be correlated with an outcome.

RNA polymerase An enzyme complex that binds to a gene segment of DNA, using it as a template for the synthesis of an RNA strand.

Rocky Mountain spotted fever An infection caused by a tick that carries *Rickettsia rickettsii.* The characteristic rash is a macular or maculopapular one that spreads to the rest of the body. Other symptoms include generalized edema, conjunctivitis, petechial lesions, photophobia, lethargy, confusion, and cranial nerve deficits.

Roseola infantum A contagious viral disease that generally affects children younger than 4 years and usually those about 1 year of age. It produces a characteristic maculopapular rash covering the trunk and spreading to the appendages.

Rostral A positional term referring to the head end.

Rough endoplasmic reticulum A portion of the endoplasmic reticulum that is studded by ribosomes. Ribosomes attached to the endoplasmic reticulum synthesize proteins that are destined for the plasma membrane or lysosomes.

Rubella Also known as *3-day measles* or *German measles.* Rubella is a childhood disease caused by the rubella virus. It is characterized by a diffuse punctate, macular rash that begins on the trunk and spreads to the arms and legs.

Rugae Folds in the lining of the body of the bladder that allow the bladder muscle to distend to accommodate urine without friction.

S

Saddle joint A joint in which the surfaces are convex in one plane and concave in the other, permitting both flexion extension and adduction-abduction movements; the surfaces of a saddle joint fit together as a saddle fits a horse. The carpometacarpal joint of the thumb is a saddle joint. Also called a *sellar joint.*

Saline deficit Extracellular fluid volume deficit.

Saline excess Extracellular fluid volume excess.

Saline imbalances Imbalances of extracellular fluid volume.

Salivary amylase Digestive enzyme (also called *ptyalin*) contained in saliva, which initiates carbohydrate digestion in the mouth.

Sarcolemma The membrane that encloses a muscle cell.

Sarcomere The unit of muscle contraction in striated muscle. A sarcomere extends from one Z disk to another and consists of overlapping actin and myosin filaments.

Sarcoplasm The cytoplasm of the muscle fiber.

Sarcoplasmic reticulum A calcium-storing structure in muscle cells analogous to the endoplasmic reticulum; it fills the space between myofibrils and forms sacs.

Saturated fatty acid Having the maximal number of hydrogen atoms present so that only single bonds exist in the carbon chain, as in saturated fatty acids.

Saturation The condition of being saturated. The degree of hydrogen saturation refers to the number of double bonds between the carbon atoms in the hydrocarbon chain.

Scabies Infestation with the mite *Sarcoptes scabiei* in humans. Scabies begins with eggs laid in the stratum corneum. These eggs hatch into larvae within 3 to 4 days and reach adulthood within 2 months.

Scarlet fever A systemic reaction to the toxins produced by group A β-hemolytic streptococci. It occurs when the person is sensitized to the toxin-producing variation of streptococci. Scarlet fever frequently occurs in association with streptococcal sore throat (strep throat), but it may also be associated with a wound, skin infection, or puerperal infection.

Schizoid Indifferent to social interaction and possessing a limited range of emotional experience and expression.

Schizophrenia A syndrome or combination of mental disorders characterized by deterioration of mental function and disturbance of psychological processes.

Scleroderma A disorder characterized by massive collagen deposition with fibrosis accompanied by inflammatory reactions and vascular changes in the capillary network.

Scoliosis A lateral deviation of the spine resulting in an S- or C-shaped spinal column. The disorder, most common in adolescent girls, can be a consequence of congenital, connective tissue, or neuromuscular disorders.

Scrotum Pouchlike sac containing the testes, epididymis, and spermatic cord.

Seasonal affective disorder A condition in which lethargy results from seasonal changes of decreased periods of daylight and longer nights.

Sebaceous gland Oil- or sebum-producing gland that anoints hair and skin.

Seborrheic keratosis Benign skin tumor common in the elderly, composed of immature epithelial cells.

Second messenger An intracellular signal that is produced in response to an extracellular signal.

Secondary dysthymia A long-term state of chronic depression that is associated with some other non-mood disorder, which may be a classic mental disorder (e.g., anorexia nervosa) or a physical illness.

Secondary endocrine disorder A malfunction of the hypothalamus/pituitary cells that control the hormone-producing gland.

Secondary glomerulopathy Alterations in the structure and function of the glomerular capillary circulation resulting from drug exposure, infections, or glomerular injury in the setting of multisystem or vascular abnormalities.

Secondary hypertension High blood pressure in which the cause can be identified.

Secondary lesion Injury modified by normal progress over time or by such external agents as scratching.

Secondary prevention The second level of health promotion, based on early detection and screening.

Second-degree burn See *superficial partial-thickness burn* and *deep partial-thickness burn.*

Secretin A digestive hormone that is produced by the S cells lining the duodenum and jejunum when protein of partially digested food enters the intestine from the stomach; it stimulates the pancreas.

Segmentation contractions A set of movements that occur in the small intestine. The primary effect of these contractions is progressive mixing of solid chyme particles with secretions of the small intestine.

Seizure A transient neurologic event of paroxysmal abnormal or excessive cortical electrical discharges that is manifested by disturbances of skeletal motor function, sensation, autonomic visceral function, behavior, or consciousness.

Self-identity disturbance In schizophrenic patients, self-identity disturbances can be profound, both in terms of the ability to differentiate one's physical self from the physical environment and the psychological discernment of self as distinct from others.

Semen Male reproductive fluid that contains spermatozoa; released with ejaculation.

Seminal vesicles Two glands that contribute rich nutrients to the seminal fluid.

Sequela, sequelae A condition or conditions caused by and following a disease.

Serotonin A major monoamine neurotransmitter that is an etiologic factor in mood disorders. See *norepinephrine.*

Sertoli cell An elongated cell that supports and provides nutrition to attached spermatids until they mature into spermatozoa.

Sex chromosome A chromosome that confers gender to the individual. In humans, females are designated as 46XX, whereas males are 46XY. The Y chromosome confers male gender.

Sexually transmitted disease One of many diseases that can be transmitted by sexual contact, regardless of whether the disease has manifestations in the genital organs (previously referred to as *venereal disease*).

Sharpey fibers Fibers that attach tendons to bones; they are continuous with the perimysium.

Shock A condition of severe hemodynamic and metabolic disturbance resulting in an imbalance between oxygen supply and oxygen demand at the cellular level. The common types of shock are cardiogenic, hypovolemic, obstructive, and distributive.

Short-bowel syndrome Severe diarrhea and significant malabsorption that develop following the surgical removal of large portions of the small intestine. The severity of the manifestations depends on the amount and location of the bowel resected.

Shunt (right-to-left) An abnormal route of blood flow through the heart or lungs that allows movement of blood into the arterial system without passing through areas of the lung.

Sickle cell A red blood cell containing abnormal hemoglobins that cause the cell to assume a sickle shape under decreased oxygen tension.

Sign Objectively identifiable aberration of the disease. Fever, reddening of the skin, and a palpable mass are *signs* of disease.

Skeletal muscle Striated muscle that is attached to bone. Constituting 40% of total body weight, skeletal muscle enables bones to move at the joint and provides strength and protection to the skeleton by distributing and absorbing shock.

Skeletal system Rigid system of bony structures designed to protect internal organs and provide bony attachments for muscles and ligaments; presents rigid levers to allow for functional movement of the body and its separate parts.

Skin A relatively flat membrane composed of an outer, thinner layer (epidermis) and an inner, thicker layer (dermis).

Skin cancer A cutaneous neoplasm caused by ionizing radiation, certain genetic defects, or chemical carcinogens, including arsenics, petroleum, tar products, and fumes from some molten metals, or by overexposure to the sun or other sources of ultraviolet light.

Sleep study Recording of electroencephalogram (EEG) motor activity and respiration during sleep to determine duration and type of sleep and number of awakenings.

Sliding filament theory This theory of muscle contraction is suggested by the anatomic configuration of the sarcomere. Muscle shortening is accomplished by increasing the amount of overlap of actin and myosin filaments. Also called *cross-bridge theory.*

Slow twitch (type I, red) A muscle fiber that develops tension more slowly than a fast-twitch fiber. This fiber is usually fatigue resistant and relies on oxidative phosphorylation for energy.

Slow-wave electrical activity One of the basic types of electrical activity in the gut. Slow waves represent an ongoing basic oscillation in membrane potential occurring in the smooth muscle of the gastrointestinal tract between 3 and 12 times per minute.

Smooth endoplasmic reticulum A portion of the endoplasmic reticulum that has no ribosomes. Smooth endoplasmic reticulum is a site of lipid synthesis.

Soft tissue injury Any trauma to soft tissue with disruption of circulatory and lymphatic systems.

Solar elastosis Wrinkled, weather-beaten appearance of skin caused by overexposure to sunlight.

Somatosensory receptors Specialized nerve endings located in the dermis of all skin areas. Receptors permit the skin to serve as a sense organ, transmitting sensations of pain, pressure, touch, and temperature.

Somatotopic Referring to the sequential arrangement of neurons related to sensory or motor function in specific anatomic regions.

Specific immune response Creation of specific antibodies by the host against a specific pathogen that leads to the destruction of the pathogen.

Spermatid An immature sperm cell.

Spermatocele A painless, cystic mass containing sperm.

Spermatogenesis Production of sperm cells.

Spermatozoon A mature sperm cell.

Spherocyte An abnormal spherical erythrocyte that is less biconvex than a normal erythrocyte.

Spike potential Sudden increase in membrane potential in the smooth muscle of the gastrointestinal tract that appears on the peaks of slow waves in response to certain conditions, including stimulation by stretching or the effects of acetylcholine or parasympathetic excitation.

Spina bifida A developmental anomaly characterized by defective closure of the bony encasement of the spinal cord (neural tube) through which the spinal cord and meninges may or may not protrude.

Spinal shock A temporary physiologic suspension of spinal cord function and reflexes below the level of cord injury.

Spiral [bacteria] Referring to any bacterium of the genus *Spirochaeta* that is motile and spiral-shaped with flexible filaments. See *spirochete.*

Spiral fracture A fracture resulting from rotational forces and causing bone to separate in the form of an S around the bone.

Spirochete Spiral-shaped bacterium.

Splinter hemorrhage A linear hemorrhage, appearing as a red or brown streak, running parallel to the finger in the nail bed; may be linked to bacterial endocarditis and trichinosis.

Spontaneous abortion Expulsion of the products of conception from the uterus before the period of fetal viability. It is usually called "miscarriage" by laypersons, and is differentiated from an elective abortion.

Squamous cell carcinoma A type of cancer that often occurs in areas of skin excessively exposed to sunlight and arising from keratinocytes.

Staging The process of determining the extent and location of cancer in an individual.

Stasis A "staying" of a substance in an anatomic location. A *stasis* of bile in the gallbladder promotes an increase in gallstone formation.

Status asthmaticus Severe asthma attack that does not respond to routine therapy.

Status epilepticus Rapid succession of seizures without intervals of consciousness. Brain damage may result.

Steatorrhea Passage of high fat content in the feces; seen in malabsorption diseases where there is lack of pancreatic enzymes.

Stenosis (valvular) Obstruction to blood flow through cardiac valves that open incompletely.

Steroid A hormone secreted by the adrenal cortex. Includes glucocorticoids, mineralocorticoids, and androgens.

Still disease Systemic-onset juvenile rheumatoid arthritis.

Stomatitis An inflammation of the oral mucosa that may extend to the buccal mucosa, lips, and palate.

Stratum Layer.

Stratum corneum Outermost layer of the epidermis, composed of flat, compact cells that have lost their nuclei.

Stratum germinativum Also known as the *basal cell layer,* the final (fifth) layer of the epidermis is a line of cuboidal cells that marks the lowest boundary of the epidermis and divides it from the dermis.

Stratum granulosum Third layer of the epidermis, comprising flatter cells that contain protein granules, called *keratohyalin granules.*

Stratum lucidum Second layer of the epidermis, appearing as a translucent line of flat cells. This layer of the skin is present only on the palms and the soles.

Stratum spinosum Fourth layer of the epidermis, composed of upwardly migrating and maturing keratinocytes. This layer forms the bulk of the epidermis over most of the body.

Strawberry hemangioma A soft vascular nevus, usually present on the face or neck, occurring at birth or shortly afterward.

Strawberry tongue Bright red papillated tongue, characteristic of scarlet fever.

Stress The sum of biological reactions produced when an organism's homeostasis is disrupted.

Stress fracture A fracture of one cortical surface of the bone, often caused by repetitive activity such as running.

Stress incontinence Loss of bladder control caused by increased intraabdominal pressure combined with pelvic muscle laxity.

Stressor An agent or condition capable of producing stress. The term denotes both physical (gravity, mechanical force, pathogen, injury) and psychological (fear, anxiety, crisis, joy) forces that an individual may experience.

Striation The typical pattern of banding apparent upon microscopic inspection of a skeletal muscle cell.

Stricture A narrowing or constriction of the lumen of a tube, duct, or hollow organ, such as the ureter or urethra.

Stroke volume The volume of blood ejected from the ventricle in one contraction (end-diastolic volume minus end-systolic volume).

Structural scoliosis A lateral curve of the spine that fails to correct itself on forced bending against the curvature and has vertebral rotation.

Subarachnoid space The space between the arachnoid and the pia mater.

Subendocardium The part of the myocardium lying in proximity to the endocardial surface.

Subluxation Displacement of a bone from its normal position (articulating surface) in a joint; less severe than dislocation.

Substantia gelatinosa Another term for areas in laminae II and III that are important in the transmission of pain signals in the spinal cord.

Substantia nigra The layer of gray matter separating the tegmentum of the midbrain from the crus cerebri; part of the basal ganglia.

Sudden cardiac death Death due to cardiac causes within 1 hour of symptom onset.

Sulcus A deep furrow or groove on the surface of a structure (e.g., cerebral cortex).

Summation The additive response to repetitive stimuli.

Superficial fascia Loose subcutaneous layer rich in fat and areolar tissue, which lies beneath the dermis. Also known as *hypodermis.*

Superficial partial-thickness burn Marked by destruction of the epidermis and dermis, a superficial partial-thickness burn is also a second-degree burn. The water vapor barrier is absent, but tactile and pain sensors are intact.

Suppurative disease A disease that produces purulent material (pus).

Surface film Thin film of emulsified material spread over the surface of skin.

Surfactant A surface tension–reducing agent produced by type II pneumocytes in the lung.

Suture joints A joint that unites bone with a thin but dense layer of fibrous tissue. Found only in the skull.

Sweat gland Most numerous of the skin glands. Sweat glands are of two types: apocrine and eccrine.

Symphysis joint A joint that connects bony segments by a fibrocartilaginous plate or disk.

Symptom Subjective feeling of discomfort that an affected individual can report to an observer. Nausea, malaise, and pain are *symptoms* of disease.

Symptomatically Defined by symptoms.

Synarthrosis A fibrous or cartilaginous (nonsynovial) joint.

Synchondrosis A joint connecting cartilage to a bony component; allows bone growth while providing stability.

Syncytium A complex of fused cells that act in concert.

Syndesmosis A fibrous joint in which opposing surfaces that are relatively far apart are connected by ligaments.

Syndrome A collection of signs and symptoms that occur together.

Syndrome of inappropriate antidiuretic hormone secretion (SIADH) Excessive antidiuretic hormone secretion either from the posterior pituitary gland or from other tissues. SIADH results in retention of water, hemodilution, and hyponatremia.

Synostosis The bony union that results from the fusion of a suture joint.

Synovial fluid A clear, pale yellow, viscous fluid similar to blood plasma but containing hyaluronic acid and a glycoprotein called lubricin. Synovial fluid reduces friction between the capsule and joint surfaces, lubricates the surface of the cartilage, resists shear forces, and provides nourishment for cartilage. Viscosity of the fluid is inversely related to joint velocity or rate of shear. High temperature decreases viscosity and low temperature increases viscosity.

Synovial joint Freely movable joint in which contiguous bony surfaces is covered by articular cartilage and connected by a fibrous connective tissue capsule lined with a synovial membrane.

Synovial sheath Also called *joint capsule.* A dense layer of connective tissue surrounding synovial joints. The capsule is solidly attached to the periosteum of the adjacent bony components. The synovial sheath provides strength to the joint and, through its neural receptors, detects motion, compression, tension, vibration, and pain.

Syphilis Sexually transmitted disease caused by the spirochete *Treponema pallidum* and characterized by distinct stages of effects over a period of years.

Systemic lupus erythematosus A chronic inflammatory disease resulting from an immunoregulatory disturbance. It is a multisystem relapsing disease that can affect skin, mucosa, lung, heart, kidneys, central and peripheral nervous systems, and blood components. Arthralgias and synovitis are common features. Skin lesions are often present as a butterfly rash. Renal failure is the leading cause of death with this disease.

Systemic vascular resistance The impedance to blood flow exerted by the arterioles; determined primarily by vascular diameter.

Systole A phase of the cardiac cycle in which the ventricles are contracting to develop force and eject blood.

Systolic blood pressure The maximal pressure in the aorta and major arteries during ventricular ejection of blood.

T

T cell Lymphocyte that provides cellular immunity, has regulatory functions, and attacks antigen in association with other cells. T cells mature in the thymus.

Tangential excision Also called *full-thickness excision.* Done to remove eschar in thin layers until viable tissue is visible.

Target cell or target organ The cell or organ that is stimulated by the effects of a hormone.

Tau protein Neuronal protein that organizes microtubules. Also known as *neural thread protein,* tau protein becomes chemically altered in Alzheimer disease and twists into abnormal bundles, known as *neurofibrillary tangles.* See *neural thread protein.*

Telangiectasia A lesion created by dilated blood vessels.

Telogen The resting phase of hair growth.

Telomerase An enzyme that permits addition of nucleotides to the tips of the chromosomes to prevent progressive shortening of the telomeres during cell division. Telomerase is produced by cancer cells, enabling them to become immortal.

Telomere The end cap of the chromosome; this section shortens with each cell division.

Tendinitis Inflammation of the tendon within the sheath.

Teratogen An agent or factor that causes damage or physical defects in a developing embryo.

Terminal hair Long, coarse, thick, visible strands of tightly fused keratinized epidermal cells.

Terminal sac period The third stage in fetal lung development when terminal sacs become thinner, preparing the lung tissue for gas exchange. Proliferation of pulmonary capillaries is also prominent during this period.

Tertiary prevention The third phase of health promotion, based on supporting independent function and preventing further disease-related deterioration.

Testis The male gonad or reproductive gland that produces spermatozoa and houses the Leydig cells.

Testosterone Male sex hormone produced by interstitial cells in the testes.

Thalamus Portion of diencephalon; mass of gray matter involved in relay of sensory information, emotion, arousal, and complex reflexes.

Thoracentesis Surgical perforation of the chest wall and pleural space with a needle to aspirate fluid for diagnostic or therapeutic purposes or to remove a specimen for biopsy.

Thoracotomy Surgical opening of the chest wall.

Threshold The lowest level at which a stimulus can produce a response.

Thrill Vibration palpated over a blood vessel reflecting turbulent blood flow.

Thrombocyte Circulating cytoplasmic fragment of a megakaryocyte that is essential in the formation of blood clots and in the control of bleeding. Also called *platelet.*

Thrombocytopenia A deficiency of platelets (thrombocytes) in the peripheral blood. Any reduction in platelet count below normal is called *thrombocytopenia,* but significant risk of bleeding does not occur until the count drops below about 20,000/μl.

Thromboembolus An embolus that originated as a thrombus, most commonly in the venous system of the lower extremities.

Thrombophlebitis Inflammation of a vein accompanied by the formation of a clot.

Thrombus Stationary blood clot formed within a vessel.

Thrush Candidiasis of the tissues of the mouth. The condition is characterized by the appearance of creamy white patches of exudates on an inflamed tongue or buccal mucosa.

Thyroid storm Extreme thyrotoxicosis. Massively elevated levels of thyroid hormones cause an increased basal metabolic rate, tachycardia, hypertension, and fever, eventually leading to cardiovascular collapse.

Thyroxine (T_4) A hormone secreted by the thyroid gland.

Tight junction Cell-to-cell junction that seals adjacent epithelial cells together and prevents the passage of most substances through the epithelial sheet.

Tinea The infection caused by fungal infections of the skin in any cutaneous area, including the hair and nails.

Tinnitus Ringing, buzzing, or roaring in the ears, commonly associated with exposure to loud noise or disorders, such as Ménière disease.

Tonic Referring to continuous stimulation or muscular contraction.

TORCH complex An acronym used to describe the usual offending infectious agents that commonly cause congenital anomalies: *t*oxoplasmosis, *o*thers, *r*ubella, *c*ytomegalovirus, *h*erpesvirus.

Torsion Act of twisting or condition of being twisted. Applies to the state of the testes when abnormally rotated.

Trabecular bone Cancellous bone cells arranged in response to mechanical stress placed on the bone. Configuration of bone cells increases strength of bone.

Tracheoesophageal fistula Congenital anomaly in which an abnormal opening between the trachea and esophagus exists. It requires immediate diagnosis and surgical correction.

Transcellular fluid Body fluid contained in special compartments, such as the synovial or cerebrospinal compartments; a component of extracellular fluid.

Transcription The process by which a segment of DNA is used as a template to produce a complementary sequence of messenger RNA.

Transient flora Microorganisms that temporarily reside in a certain environment on the host.

Transitional flow Airflow occurring in the larger airways, especially at bifurcations. Also known as *mixed pattern of airflow.*

Translation Formation of a polypeptide chain in a sequence dictated by messenger RNA.

Translocation Shifting of a segment of one chromosome into another chromosome.

Transmission of infection The process by which a pathogenic organism is transferred from one host to another.

Transmural Denoting the entire thickness of a wall (e.g., the myocardial wall). A transmural myocardial infarction extends throughout the entire cardiac muscle layer.

Transudate Fluid of low protein content that passes through membranes because of a difference in hydrostatic pressure.

Transverse fracture Occurs in a straight line at approximately a 90-degree angle to the longitudinal axis of the bone.

Traumatic alopecia Hair loss as a result of tight plaiting of hair or use of hot oil and tension on the scalp. Gradual damage to hair follicles occurs, leading to hair thinning and loss.

Triad asthma A subcategory of drug-induced asthma representing a combination of intrinsic asthma, aspirin sensitivity, and nasal polyposis.

Triaxial joint A joint that permits movement around three axes so that motion can occur in three planes. Permits gliding movement between two bones as exemplified by the carpal joints of the hand.

Tricuspid valve The cardiac valve that lies between the right atrium and right ventricle. The valve is normally closed during ventricular systole and open during ventricular diastole. Tricuspid valve closure contributes to heart sound S_1.

Triglyceride A simple fat compound consisting of three molecules of fatty acid and glycerol.

Trigone Triangular area usually referring to the bladder muscle.

Triiodothyronine (T_3) A hormone secreted by the thyroid gland.

Trisomy Having three homologous chromosomes instead of the usual pair, as in trisomy 21, also called *Down syndrome.*

Tropic/trophic hormone A hormone released by the anterior pituitary gland that stimulates the release of other hormones, which finally act on target organs.

Tropical sprue Inflammation of the mucosa of the small intestine secondary to infection.

Tropomyosin A structural protein involved in regulation of actin-myosin cross-bridge formation. Associated with the thin filament of the sarcomere in skeletal and cardiac muscle, where it blocks cross-bridge formation when intracellular calcium levels are low.

Troponin A regulatory protein involved in regulation of actin-myosin cross-bridge formation. Associated with tropomyosin and actin in the thin filament of the sarcomere. Troponin binds calcium ion in the cell and regulates the position of tropomyosin, allowing muscle contraction when intracellular calcium levels rise.

Tumor marker Biochemical substance, such as a specific enzyme, receptor, or surface protein, that helps identify the tumor cell.

Tumor suppressor gene A gene that regulates a group of growth-promoting genes and suppresses tumor formation.

Mutation and underexpression of tumor suppressor genes are associated with the development of cancer.

Tunica albuginea Fascial layer covering the testes and erectile bodies of the penis.

Turbulent flow The friction and increased resistance caused by air movement from the nasal cavity through the large bronchi.

Turnover and regeneration time Time required for a population of cells to mature and reproduce. As the surface cells of the stratum corneum are lost, replacement of keratinocytes by mitosis must occur.

Twitch The mechanical response to a single stimulus of a motor unit.

Type 1 diabetes mellitus Insulin-dependent diabetes mellitus, characterized by an absolute deficiency of insulin.

Type 2 diabetes mellitus Non-insulin-dependent diabetes mellitus, characterized by tissue insulin resistance and impaired insulin production by the pancreas.

U

Ulcerative colitis An inflammatory disease of the mucosa of the rectum and colon. Most commonly it affects the most distal portions of the colon, but eventually it may affect the entire colon. It is typically characterized by exacerbations and remissions. The clinical manifestations of ulcerative colitis are abdominal pain, diarrhea, and rectal bleeding.

Ultrafiltration Filtration through a filter capable of removing colloidal particles from a dispersion medium, as in the filtration of plasma at the capillary membrane.

Ultrasound An imaging modality that uses sound waves to assess the size, structure, and function of internal organs, tissue, or the fetus.

Uniaxial joint A joint that allows motion around a single axis.

Unipennate A muscle with a lateral tendon to which the fibers are attached obliquely, like one half of a feather.

Unipolar depression Depression without periods of mania.

Unresolved infection (UTI) A urinary tract infection (UTI) in which bacteriuria remains after initial antibiotic treatment.

Unsaturated (fatty acid) Referring to an organic compound in which one or more pairs of carbon atoms are united by double or triple bonds, as in unsaturated fatty acids.

Up-regulation An increase in the number of cell receptors for a specific hormone resulting from chronically low concentrations of the hormone. Up-regulation helps maintain the target cell response to a hormone, even when circulating hormone levels are low.

Urea Substance produced in the liver from the breakdown of protein and excreted in the urine.

Uremia A clinical syndrome related to the deleterious effects of azotemia on other body systems.

Ureter One of a pair of fibromuscular, mucosa-lined narrow tubes that connect the kidneys to the bladder.

Ureterocele Congenital cystic dilatation of the distal ureter.

Ureteropelvic junction obstruction Disruption of urinary flow from the kidney(s) into one or both ureters.

Urethral stricture A fibrotic narrowing of the urethra, usually composed of scar tissue.

Urethral valve The most common cause of urinary obstruction in male newborns and infants. Posterior in location, occurring in the distal prostatic urethra, urethral valves are mucosal folds that resemble thin membranes and cause obstruction when the child attempts to void.

Urethrorectal fistula A rare congenital anomaly almost always associated with an imperforate anus. The fistula results from failure of the urorectal septum to develop completely, leading to a persistent communication between the rectum posteriorly and the urogenital tract anteriorly.

Urge incontinence A strong and immediate urge to void brought about by involuntary detrusor overactivity.

Urinary bladder Muscular sac located in the anterior inferior pelvic cavity that holds urine until it is excreted through the urethra.

Urothelial tumor A malignant tumor of the lining of the renal pelvis, calyces, ureter, and bladder.

Urothelium Epithelial lining of the urinary tract from the renal pelvis to the bladder.

Urticaria A pruritic skin eruption characterized by transient wheals of varying shapes and sizes with well-defined erythematous margins and pale centers.

Uterine prolapse A sinking of the uterus from its normal position. It usually occurs when supporting structures, such as the uterosacral ligaments and cardinal ligaments, relax, altering the relationship of the uterus to the vaginal axis.

V

Varicose veins Incompetency of the superficial veins of the extremities, producing engorgement.

Vas deferens Thick, muscular tube that is continuous with the epididymis. It travels along the pelvic wall and joins with the seminal vesicle duct at the prostate to form the ejaculatory duct. Also called *ductus deferens*.

Vascular fluid Fluid that is in blood vessels; a component of extracellular fluid.

Vasculitis Inflammation of the lining (intima) of a blood vessel.

Vasospasm Sudden, involuntary constriction of a blood vessel, producing obstruction of flow.

Vellus Tiny hair strands that are almost unnoticeable. Vellus covers the whole body, except the palms and soles.

Ventilation The process of moving air into the lungs and distributing air within the lungs to gas exchange units (alveoli) for maintenance of oxygenation and removal of CO_2.

Ventricle A fluid-filled compartment as in brain or heart.
Ventriculoperitoneal shunt A shunt that extends all the way from the ventricular system of the brain to the peritoneal cavity of the body.
Verrucae Circumscribed elevations of the epidermis, commonly called *warts.*
Verumontanum A small elevation that is marked by a midline opening from the prostatic utricle, a remnant of the Müllerian duct system.
Vesicle A portion of the cell membrane that surrounds extracellular material and pinches off to be internalized. This is part of the process of endocytosis.
Vesicoureteral reflux Retrograde movement of urine from the bladder to the kidney as a result of a disruption in the normal valvular mechanism at the ureter-bladder junction.
Vibrissae Large hairs of the nasal cavity.
Virion A virus particle.
Virulence The capacity of a microorganism to successfully evade host defenses and cause disease.
Virulent Referring to a microorganism's ability to evade host defenses and cause disease.
Viruses Tiny genetic parasites that are totally dependent on the host cell for survival. They take over the host cell "machinery" for energy and replication.
Visual acuity The ability of the eyes to focus clearly on an image at a known distance; it is assessed with a Snellen chart and often expressed as the ability of a person to accurately discern characters of various sizes at a distance of 20 feet.
Vitamin An organic substance that is essential in the diet and is required for the body's utilization of energy-containing nutrients.
Vitiligo Patch of depigmentation; also called *leukoderma.*
Voiding dysfunction A failure in the normal process of bladder emptying that results in urinary retention and/or incontinence.
Volvulus A twisting of the bowel on itself, which results in blood vessel compression.

W

Wallerian degeneration Complete disintegration of the distal portion of an axon that has been severed from the cell body. The axon, myelin sheath, and terminal arborization all disintegrate.
Wart Also called *verruca;* caused by a virus that provokes a benign proliferation of keratinocytes.
Water imbalance Imbalance of body fluid concentration; osmolality imbalance; hypernatremia and hyponatremia.
White blood cell A cell that mediates immune function. White blood cells protect the body by phagocytosis of microorganisms and other debris. Also called *leukocyte.*
White-coat phenomenon Elevated blood pressure readings when measured in a clinic setting by a nurse or physician.
Wilson disease A rare autosomal recessive disorder in which excessive amounts of copper accumulate in the liver or other organs; also called *hepatolenticular degeneration.*
Wolffian ducts Mesonephric ducts that develop as nephric ducts but go on to form male genital ducts.
Wolff's law States that the bone is laid down where needed and resorbed where not needed.

X

Xerostomia Dryness of the mouth caused by cessation of normal salivary secretion.

Z

Z line A dark band that defines a sarcomere; Z lines are perpendicular to actin and myosin filaments. A sarcomere extends from one Z line to the next.
Zeitgeber A synchronizer of the biological clock.
Zona pellucida The thick covering of the ovum.
Zone of calcifying cartilage A very thin line of chondrocytes and the weakest segment of the epiphyseal plate.
Zone of maturing cartilage Contains the enlarged and mature cartilage cells as they migrate toward the metaphysis.
Zone of resting cartilage Maintains adherence of the plate to the epiphysis.
Zone of young proliferating cartilage Demonstrates the most active cartilage cell growth.
Zygote The developing ovum, from the time it is fertilized until it is implanted in the uterus.

INDEX

Page numbers followed by *f* indicate figures; *t*, tables; *b*, boxes.

D

E

H

U

X

Y

Z

ELSEVIER LICENSE AGREEMENT

PLEASE READ THE FOLLOWING AGREEMENT CAREFULLY BEFORE USING THIS ELECTRONIC MEDIA PRODUCT. THIS ELECTRONIC MEDIA PRODUCT IS LICENSED UNDER THE TERMS CONTAINED IN THIS ELECTRONIC MEDIA LICENSE AGREEMENT ("Agreement"). BY USING THIS ELECTRONIC MEDIA PRODUCT, YOU, AN INDIVIDUAL OR ENTITY INCLUDING EMPLOYEES, AGENTS AND REPRESENTATIVES ("You" or "Your"), ACKNOWLEDGE THAT YOU HAVE READ THIS AGREEMENT, THAT YOU UNDERSTAND IT, AND THAT YOU AGREE TO BE BOUND BY THE TERMS AND CONDITIONS OF THIS AGREEMENT. ELSEVIER. ("Elsevier") EXPRESSLY DOES NOT AGREE TO LICENSE THIS ELECTRONIC MEDIA PRODUCT TO YOU UNLESS YOU ASSENT TO THIS AGREEMENT. IF YOU DO NOT AGREE WITH ANY OF THE FOLLOWING TERMS, YOU MAY, WITHIN THIRTY (30) DAYS AFTER YOUR RECEIPT OF THIS ELECTRONIC MEDIA PRODUCT RETURN THE UNUSED ELECTRONIC MEDIA PRODUCT AND ALL ACCOMPANYING DOCUMENTATION TO ELSEVIER FOR A FULL REFUND.

DEFINITIONS

As used in this Agreement, these terms shall have the following meanings:

"Proprietary Material" means the valuable and proprietary information content of this Electronic Media Product including all indexes and graphic materials and software used to access, index, search and retrieve the information content from this Electronic Media Product developed or licensed by Elsevier and/or its affiliates, suppliers and licensors.

"Electronic Media Product" means the copy of the Proprietary Material and any other material delivered on Electronic Media and any other human-readable or machine-readable materials enclosed with this Agreement, including without limitation documentation relating to the same.

OWNERSHIP

This Electronic Media Product has been supplied by and is proprietary to Elsevier and/or its affiliates, suppliers and licensors. The copyright in the Electronic Media Product belongs to Elsevier and/or its affiliates, suppliers and licensors and is protected by the national and state copyright, trademark, trade secret and other intellectual property laws of the United States and international treaty provisions, including without limitation the Universal Copyright Convention and the Berne Copyright Convention. You have no ownership rights in this Electronic Media Product. Except as expressly set forth herein, no part of this Electronic Media Product, including without limitation the Proprietary Material, may be modified, copied or distributed in hardcopy or machine-readable form without prior written consent from Elsevier. All rights not expressly granted to You herein are expressly reserved. Any other use of this Electronic Media Product by any person or entity is strictly prohibited and a violation of this Agreement.

SCOPE OF RIGHTS LICENSED (PERMITTED USES)

Elsevier is granting to You a limited, non-exclusive, non-transferable license to use this Electronic Media Product in accordance with the terms of this Agreement. You may use or provide access to this Electronic Media Product on a single computer or terminal physically located at Your premises and in a secure network or move this Electronic Media Product to and use it on another single computer or terminal at the same location for personal use only, but under no circumstances may You use or provide access to any part or parts of this Electronic Media Product on more than one computer or terminal simultaneously.

You shall not (a) copy, download, or otherwise reproduce the Electronic Media Product in any medium, including, without limitation, online transmissions, local area networks, wide area networks, intranets, extranets and the Internet, or in any way, in whole or in part, except that You may print or download limited portions of the Proprietary Material that are the results of discrete searches; (b) alter, modify, or adapt the Electronic Media Product, including but not limited to decompiling, disassembling, reverse engineering, or creating derivative works, without the prior written approval of Elsevier; (c) sell, license or otherwise distribute to third parties the Electronic Media Product or any part or parts thereof; or (d) alter, remove, obscure or obstruct the display of any copyright, trademark or other proprietary notice on or in the Electronic Media Product or on any printout or download of portions of the Proprietary Materials.

RESTRICTIONS ON TRANSFER

This License is personal to You, and neither Your rights hereunder nor the tangible embodiments of this Electronic Media Product, including without limitation the Proprietary Material, may be sold, assigned, transferred or sublicensed to any other person, including without limitation by operation of law, without the prior written consent of Elsevier. Any purported sale, assignment, transfer or sublicense without the prior written consent of Elsevier will be void and will automatically terminate the License granted hereunder.

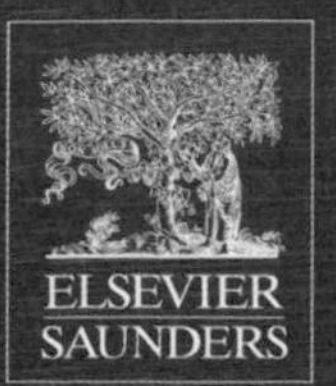

PREFIXES AND SUFFIXES COMMONLY USED IN MEDICAL TERMINOLOGY

Prefix	Meaning	Suffix	Meaning
a-	Without, not	-al, -ac	Pertaining to
af-	Toward	-algia	Pain
an-	Without, not	-aps, -apt	Fit; fasten
ante-	Before	-arche	Beginning; origin
anti-	Against; resisting	-ase	Signifies an enzyme
auto-	Self	-blast	Sprout; make
bi-	Two; double	-centesis	A piercing
circum-	Around	-cide	To kill
co-, con-	With; together	-clast	Break; destroy
contra-	Against	-crine	Release; secrete
de-	Down from, undoing	-ectomy	A cutting out
dia-	Across; through	-emesis	Vomiting
dipl-	Twofold, double	-emia	Refers to blood condition
dys-	Bad; disordered; difficult	-flux	Flow
ectop-	Displaced	-gen	Creates; forms
ef-	Away from	-genesis	Creation, production
em-, en-	In, into	-gram	Something written
endo-	Within	-graph(y)	To write, draw
epi-	Upon	-hydrate	Containing H_2O (water)
eu-	Good	-ia, -sia	Condition; process
ex-, exo-	Out of, out from	-iasis	Abnormal condition
extra-	Outside of	-ic, -ac	Pertaining to
hapl-	Single	-in	Signifies a protein
hem-, hemat-	Blood	-ism	Signifies "condition of"
hemi-	Half	-itis	Signifies "inflammation of"
hom(e)o-	Same; equal	-lemma	Rind; peel
hyper-	Over; above	-lepsy	Seizure
hypo-	Under; below	-lith	Stone; rock
infra-	Below, beneath	-logy	Study of
inter-	Between	-lunar	Moon; moonlike
intra-	Within	-malacia	Softening
iso-	Same, equal	-megaly	Enlargement
macro-	Large	-metric, -metry	Measurement, length
mega-	Large; million(th)	-oid	Like; in the shape of
mes-	Middle	-oma	Tumor
meta-	Beyond, after	-opia	Vision, vision condition
micro-	Small; millionth	-oscopy	Viewing
milli-	Thousandth	-ose	Signifies a carbohydrate (especially sugar)
mono-	One (single)	-osis	Condition, process
neo-	New	-ostomy	Formation of an opening
non-	Not	-otomy	Cut
oligo-	Few, scanty	-penia	Lack
ortho-	Straight; correct, normal	-philic	Loving
para-	By the side of; near	-phobic	Fearing
per-	Through	-phragm	Partition
peri-	Around; surrounding	-plasia	Growth, formation
poly-	Many	-plasm	Substance, matter
post-	After	-plasty	Shape; make
pre-	Before	-plegia	Paralysis
pro-	First; promoting	-pnea	Breath, breathing
quadr-	Four	-(r)rhage, -(r)rhagia	Breaking out, discharge
re-	Back again	-(r)rhaphy	Sew, suture
retro-	Behind	-(r)rhea	Flow
semi-	Half	-some	Body
sub-	Under	-tensin, -tension	Pressure
super-, supra-	Over, above, excessive	-tonic	Pressure, tension
trans-	Across; through	-tripsy	Crushing
tri-	Three; triple	-ule	Small, little
		-uria	Refers to urine condition

From Thibodeau GA, Patton KT: *Anatomy & physiology,* ed 5, St Louis, 2003, Mosby.